AHCPR Guidelines

The following list presents Clinical Practice Guidelines, Quick Reference Guides for Clinicians, and Patient Guides published by the Agency for Health Care Policy and Research (AHCPR). An agency of the U.S. Department of Health and Human Services, Public Health Service, AHCPR was established in December 1989 to enhance the quality, appropriateness, and effectiveness of health-care services as well as access to these services. AHCPR carries out its mission by conducting and supporting health research, developing clinical practice guidelines, and disseminating research findings and guidelines to health-care providers, policymakers, and the public.

Any of the following publications can be obtained by writing to the Center for Research Dissemination and Liaison, AHCPR Clearinghouse, P.O. Box 8547, Silver Spring, MD 20907, or by calling 1-800-358-9295. The Patient Guides are available in both English and Spanish.

Unstable angina: diagnosis and management. Clinical Practice Guideline. AHCPR Pub. No. 94-0602.

Diagnosing and managing unstable angina. Quick Reference Guide for Clinicians. AHCPR Pub. No. 94-0603.

Managing unstable angina. A Patient and Family Guide. AHCPR Pub. No. 94-0604.

Acute low back problems in adults: assessment and treatment. Quick Reference Guide for Clinicians. AHCPR Pub. No. 95-0643.

Management of cancer pain. Clinical Practice Guideline. AHCPR Pub. No. 94-0592.

Management of cancer pain: adults. Quick Reference Guide for Clinicians. AHCPR Pub. No. 94-0593.

Managing cancer pain. A Patient's Guide. AHCPR Pub. No. 94-0595.

Cataract in adults: management of functional impairment. Clinical Practice Guideline. AHCPR Pub. No. 93-0542.

Management of cataract in adults. Clinical Practice Guideline. Quick Reference Guide for Clinicians. AHCPR Pub. No. 93-0543.

Cataract in adults. A Patient's Guide. AHCPR Pub. No. 93-0544.

Depression in primary care, vol 1, Detection and diagnosis. Clinical Practice Guideline. AHCPR Pub. No. 93-0550.

Depression in primary care, vol 2, Treatment of major depression. Clinical Practice Guideline. AHCPR Pub. No. 93-0551.

Depression in primary care: detection, diagnosis, and treatment. Quick Reference Guide for Clinicians. AHCPR Pub. No. 93-0552.

Depression is a treatable illness. A Patient's Guide. AHCPR Pub. No. 93-0553.

Heart failure: management of patients with left-ventricular systolic dysfunction. Quick Reference Guide for Clinicians. AHCPR Pub. No. 94-0613.

Evaluation and management of early HIV infection. Clinical Practice Guideline. AHCPR Pub. No. 94-0572.

Managing early HIV infection. Quick Reference Guide for Clinicians. AHCPR Pub. No. 94-0573.

Understanding HIV. A Consumer Guide. AHCPR Pub. No. 94-0574.

HIV and your child. A Consumer Guide. AHCPR Pub. No. 94-0576.

High-quality mammography: information for referring providers. Quick Reference Guide for Clinicians. AHCPR Pub. No. 95-0633.

Managing otitis media with effusion in young children. Quick Reference Guide for Clinicians. AHCPR Pub. No. 94-0623.

Middle ear fluid in young children. Parent Guide. AHCPR Pub. No. 94-0624.

Acute pain management: operative or medical procedures and trauma. Clinical Practice Guideline. AHCPR Pub. No. 92-0032.

Acute pain management in adults: operative procedures. Quick Reference Guide for Clinicians. AHCPR Pub. No. 92-0019.

Acute pain management in infants children, and adolescents: operative and medical procedures. Quick Reference Guide for Clinicians. AHCPR Pub. No. 92-0020.

Pain control after surgery. A Patient's Guide. AHCPR Pub. No. 92-0021.

Pressure ulcers in adults: prediction and prevention. Clinical Practice Guideline. AHCPR Pub. No. 92-0047.

Pressure ulcers in adults: prediction and prevention. Quick Reference Guide for Clinicians. AHCPR Pub. No. 92-0050.

Preventing pressure ulcers. A Patient's Guide. AHCPR Pub. No. 92-0048.

Pressure ulcer treatment. Quick Reference Guide for Clinicians. AHCPR Pub. No. 95-0653.

Benign prostatic hyperplasia: diagnosis and treatment. Clinical Practice Guideline. AHCPR Pub. No. 94-0582.

Benign prostatic hyperplasia: diagnosis and treatment. Quick Reference Guide for Clinicians. AHCPR Pub. No. 94-0583.

Treating your enlarged prostate. A Patient's Guide. AHCPR Pub. No. 94-0584.

Sickle cell disease: screening, diagnosis, management, and counseling in newborns and infants. Clinical Practice Guideline. AHCPR Pub. No. 93-0562.

Sickle cell disease: comprehensive screening and management in newborns and infants. Quick Reference Guide for Clinicians. AHCPR Pub. No. 93-0563.

Sickle cell disease in newborns and infants. A Guide for Parents. AHCPR Pub. No. 93-0564.

Urinary incontinence in adults. Clinical Practice Guideline. AHCPR Pub. No. 92-0038.

Urinary incontinence in adults. Quick Reference Guide for Clinicians. AHCPR Pub. No. 92-0041.

Urinary incontinence in adults. A Patient's Guide. AHCPR Pub. No. 92-0040.

Luckmann's Core Principles and Practice of **Medical-Surgical Nursing**

ARLENE L. POLASKI, MEd, MSN, RN
Instructor
York Technical College/University of South Carolina-Lancaster Cooperative Program in Associate Degree Nursing
Rock Hill, SC

SUZANNE E. TATRO, MS, CS, RN
Instructor
York Technical College/University of South Carolina-Lancaster Cooperative Program in Associate Degree Nursing
Rock Hill, SC

W.B. SAUNDERS COMPANY
A Division of Harcourt Brace & Company
Philadelphia London Toronto Montreal Sydney Tokyo

W.B. Saunders Company
A Division of Harcourt Brace & Company

The Curtis Center
Independence Square West
Philadelphia, Pennsylvania 19106

Library of Congress Cataloging-in-Publication Data

Polaski, Arlene L.
Luckmann's core principles and practice of medical-surgical nursing / Arlene L. Polaski, Suzanne E. Tatro. — 1st ed.

p. cm.

Condensed version of: Luckmann and Sorensen's medical-surgical nursing. 4th ed. / [edited by] Joyce M. Black, Esther Matassarin-Jacobs. c1993.

ISBN 0–7216–5994–2

1. Nursing. 2. Surgical nursing. I. Tatro, Suzanne E. II. Luckmann, Joan. III. Luckmann and Sorensen's medical-surgical nursing. IV. Title.
[DNLM: 1. Nursing Care. 2. Surgical Nursing—methods. 3. Nursing Process. WY 150 P762L 1996]

RT41.P65 1996 610.73—dc20

DNLM/DLC 95–42110

Luckmann's Core Principles and Practice of Medical-Surgical Nursing ISBN 0–7216–5994–2

Cover art: Frank Lloyd Wright, *Tree of Life,* stained glass window from the D.D. Martin House, Buffalo, NY; and entry ceiling light from the W.E. Martin House, Oak Park, IL. Photographs by Thomas A. Heinz, copyright 1993 © Thomas A. Heinz.

Unless otherwise indicated, the illustrations that appear in the Anatomy and Physiology Review Sections are borrowed with permission from Applegate, E. J. (1995). *The Anatomy and Physiology Learning System Textbook.* Philadelphia: W.B. Saunders Company.

Printed in the United States of America.

Last digit is the print number: 9 8 7 6 5 4 3 2 1

To my husband, Don, who was always there
To my children, Jude, Mike, Mary, Donna, and Chuck, who always wonder what I'll do next
To my mother, Eleonore Lacey, and my siblings, who cheered me on
I cherish your love and support

AP

In loving memory of my father, Stanley Tatro,
and with deep appreciation for the love and support of my mother, Dorothy Tatro,
and many wonderful friends: Irene, Wanda, Debbie, Judith, and Jean

ST

About the Authors

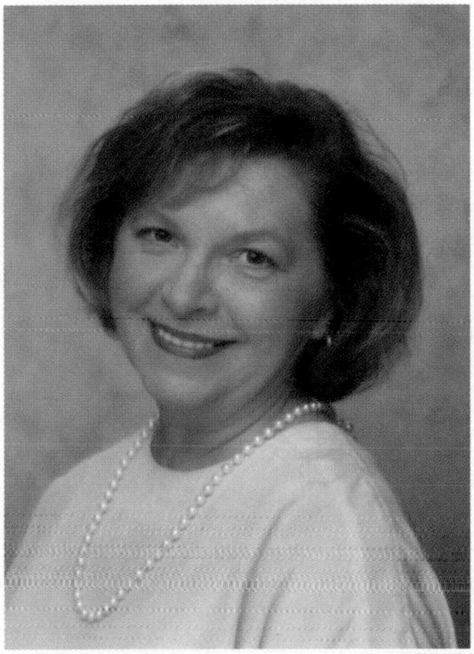

Arlene L. Polaski, MEd, MSN, RN, is an Instructor at York Technical College in the York Technical College/University of South Carolina-Lancaster Cooperative Program in Associate Degree Nursing in Rock Hill, SC. She received a Master of Education degree in Adult Education from The Pennsylvania State University at University Park, PA, and a Master of Science in Nursing from Edinboro University of Pennsylvania at Edinboro, PA. She earned a Baccalaureate of Science degree with a major in Nursing at Villa Maria College, Erie, PA, and a diploma in registered nursing from Hamot Medical Center School of Nursing, also in Erie, PA.

Arlene has taught for the past 18 years in associate degree and diploma nursing programs. Her nursing practice has included emergency, medical-surgical, and mental health nursing. She has coauthored articles published in several nursing journals. Arlene is a charter member of the Erie, PA, Eta Xi chapter of Sigma Theta Tau International and a member of the Mu Psi chapter in Charlotte, NC. She is also a member of Kappa Gamma Pi, the National League for Nursing, and the Charlotte Area Psychiatric Nurses Association.

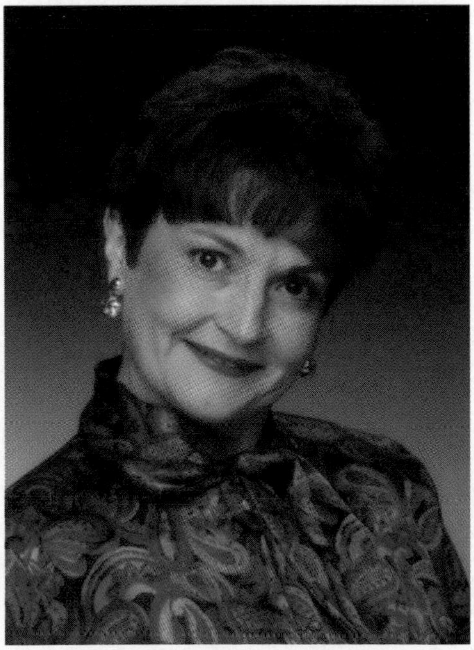

Suzanne E. Tatro, MS, CS, RN, is an Instructor at York Technical College in the York Technical College/University of South Carolina-Lancaster Cooperative Program in Associate Degree Nursing in Rock Hill, SC. She received a Master of Science degree from the University of Rochester, Rochester, NY, and a Baccalaureate of Science degree with a major in Nursing from D'Youville College at Buffalo, NY. In 1993, she became certified by the American Nurses Association as a Clinical Specialist in Gerontological Nursing.

Her career in clinical nursing includes practice in general and urological surgical nursing, as well as a Director of Health Services for a large retirement community. Suzanne has had an extensive teaching career in both baccalaureate and associate degree nursing education. While teaching at the University of Virginia, she coauthored several articles, two of which dealt with Wellness Nursing Diagnosis that were widely quoted in literature, both in the United States and Canada. Suzanne is a charter member of the Mu Psi Chapter of Sigma Theta Tau International and the American Nurses' Association.

Contributors

Edith J. Applegate, M.S.
Professor of Science and Mathematics, Kettering College of Medical Arts, Kettering, Ohio
Anatomy and Physiology Review, Units 3–15

Daryle L. Brown, M.A., M.Ed., Ed.D., R.N.
Associate Dean and Faculty Member, Department of Undergraduate Nursing, Pace University, Pleasantville, New York
Metabolic Unit

Mary Rose Chasler, B.S.N., M.S.N., R.N.
Assistant Professor, Nursing Division, Jamestown Community College, Jamestown, New York
Cardiac Unit

Carrie C. Dowdy, M.S.N., R.N., C.
Assistant Professor, Department of Nursing, Piedmont Virginia Community College, and Clinician III, University of Virginia Hospital, Charlottesville, Virginia
Gastrointestinal Unit

Catherine Eddy, M.S.N., R.N., C.C.R.N.
Assistant Professor, University of South Dakota, Rapid City, South Dakota
Respiratory Unit

Frances A. Freitas, M.S.N., R.N.C.
Assistant Professor, Kent State University, Ashtabula Campus, Ashtabula, Ohio
Immunology Unit

Renee Hyde, M.S.N., R.N.
Faculty, CMHA School of Nursing, Charlotte, North Carolina
Neurologic Unit

Susan Miller, M.B.A., M.S.N., R.N.C.
Director, Organizational Performance, Hamot Medical Center, Erie, Pennsylvania
Health-Care Delivery

Arlene L. Polaski, M.Ed., M.S.N., R.N.
Instructor, York Technical College/University of South Carolina-Lancaster, Rock Hill, South Carolina
Health-Care Delivery, Basic Concepts of Neoplastic Disorders, Treatment Modalities for Neoplastic Disorders, Sensory Unit, Hematologic Unit, Hepatic, Biliary, and Exocrine Pancreatic Unit, Integumentary Unit

Kay I. Swiger, B.S.N., M.N., R.N.C.
Nursing Faculty, York Technical College-University of South Carolina at Lancaster, and PRN Staff, L & D, Piedmont Medical Center, Rock Hill, South Carolina
Reproductive Unit

Suzanne E. Tatro, M.S., C.S., R.N.
Instructor, York Technical College University of South Carolina-Lancaster, Rock Hill, South Carolina
Acute and Chronic Illness, Fluid and Electrolyte Balance, Acid-Base Imbalances, Perioperative Nursing, Hepatic, Biliary, and Exocrine Pancreatic Unit, Multisystem Disorders Unit

Judith P. Warner, B.S.N., R.N.
Vivra Renal Care, Erie, Pennsylvania
Urinary Unit

Contributors

to Luckmann and Sorensen's Medical-Surgical Nursing, 4th edition

Steve Alderfer, M.S.N., R.N., C.C.R.N.
Clinician III, Medical Intensive Care Unit, University of Virginia Health Sciences Center, Charlottesville, Virginia
Common Respiratory Interventions

Helen A. Andrews, B.S.N.
Staff Nurse, Bergan Mercy Medical Center, Omaha, Nebraska
Common Musculoskeletal Interventions; Nursing Care of Clients with Musculoskeletal Trauma or Overuse

Bonnie Angel, Diploma, B.S.N., M.S.N.
Clinical Assistant Professor, University of North Carolina, School of Nursing, Chapel Hill, North Carolina
The Family

Minerva I. Applegate, Ed.D., R.N.
Nursing Consultant and Project Coordinator, H.C.A., L.W. Blake Hospital, Bradenton, Florida
Ethics

Ellen Barker, M.S.N., R.N., C.N.R.N.
President, Neuroscience Nursing Consultants, Newark, Delaware
Assessment of Clients with Neurologic Disorders; Nursing Care of Clients with Loss of Protective Function

Maureen B. Barrett, M.S., R.N.,C.
Assistant Professor, Loyola University of Chicago, Chicago, Illinois
Perioperative Nursing

Carol Birch, M.S., R.N., C.C.R.N.
Instructor, College of Nursing, South Dakota State University, Rapid City, South Dakota
Nursing Care of Clients with Thyroid and Parathyroid Disorders

Joyce M. Black, M.S.N., R.N.,C.
Assistant Professor, College of Nursing, University of Nebraska Medical Center, Omaha, Nebraska
Nursing Process; Theories of Health and Illness; Cross-Cultural Nursing; The Cell; Wound Healing; Assessment of Clients with Neurologic Disorders; Nursing Care of Clients with Loss of Protective Function; Nursing Care of Clients with Peripheral Vascular Disorders; Structure and Function; Assessment of Clients with Metabolic Disorders; Nursing Care of Clients with Endocrine Disorders of the Pancreas; Nursing Care of Clients with Musculoskeletal Trauma or Overuse

Barbara J. Boss, Ph.D.
Professor of Nursing, University of Mississippi Medical Center, School of Nursing, Jackson, Mississippi
Structure and Function of the Nervous System

Carol Bova, M.S., R.N.,C.
Nurse Practitioner, HIV Clinical Center, and Instructor, Graduate School of Nursing, University of Massachusetts Medical Center, Worcester, Massachusetts
Nursing Care of Clients with Altered Immune Systems

Evelyn Butera, M.S., R.N., C.N.N.
Manager, Education Services, Northwest Kidney Centers, Seattle, Washington
Nursing Care of Clients with Renal Disorders

Diane Butts-Krakoff, M.S.N., C.D.E.
Diabetes Nurse Educator, St. Vincent Hospitals, Indianapolis, Indiana
Structure and Function; Assessment of Clients with Metabolic Disorders; Nursing Care of Clients with Endocrine Disorders of the Pancreas

Lynne C. Carpenter, R.N., M.S., Ph.D.C., O.C.N.
Clinical Nurse Specialist, University of Michigan Breast Care Center, Ann Arbor, Michigan
Structure and Function of the Female and Male Reproductive Systems; Assessment of Clients with Reproductive Disorders; Nursing Care of the Client with Breast Disorders

Gretchen J. Carrougher, R.N., M.N.
Clinical Nurse Specialist, Medical-Surgical Nursing, Medical Center Hospital, and Clinical Instructor, University of Texas Health Science Center, School of Nursing, San Antonio, Texas
Nursing Care of Clients with Burn Injury

Ann J. Clark, Ph.D., R.N.
Director, Center for Nursing Research, University of Alabama at Birmingham, Birmingham, Alabama
Structure and Function of the Female and Male Reproductive Systems; Assessment of Clients with Reproductive Disorders; Nursing Care of Women with Gynecologic Disorders

Sherill Nones Cronin, Ph.D., R.N.,C.
Assistant Professor of Nursing, Bellarmine College, and Nurse Researcher, Jewish Hospital, Louisville, Kentucky
Nursing Care of Clients with Lower Airway Disorders

Pamela D. Dennison, R.N., B.S.N., M.S.N.
Assistant Professor of Nursing, University of Virginia, and Practitioner Teacher, University of Virginia Health Sciences Center, Charlottesville, Virginia
Nursing Care of Clients with Peripheral Vascular Disorders

Patricia E. Downing, M.N., R.N.
Formerly of the School of Nursing, University of California San Francisco, San Francisco, California
Nursing Care of Clients with Sexually Transmitted Diseases

Mary Elizabeth Egloff, M.S.N., R.N., C.C.R.N.
Pulmonary Clinical Nurse Specialist, Sharp Memorial Hospital, San Diego, California
Assessment of Clients with Respiratory Disorders

Darrell A. Follman, M.S., B.S., R.N., O.N.C.
Independent Consultant in Orthopedic Nursing and Quality Assurance Consultant, Health Connections, Inc., Skokie, Illinois
Structure and Function of the Musculoskeletal System; Assessment of Clients with Musculoskeletal Disorders

Mary Jane Garrett, B.S.N., M.S.N., Ph.D.
Assistant Professor, University of Nebraska at Omaha, College of Nursing, Omaha, Nebraska
Chronic Conditions

Terri Goodman, M.A.E.D., B.S.N., C.N.O.R.
Clinical Educator for Surgical Services, Shady Grove Adventist Hospital, Rockville, Maryland
Nursing Care of Clients Having Plastic Surgery

Deanna E. Grimes, Dr.P.H., R.N., M.S.N.
Associate Professor, University of Texas at Houston, Health Science Center, School of Nursing, Houston, Texas
Nursing Care of Clients with Infectious Diseases

Margie J. Hansen, Ph.D., R.N.
Assistant Professor of Pharmaceutical Science, North Dakota State University, Fargo, North Dakota
Acid-Base Imbalances

Jane H. Hawks, R.N.,C., M.S.N., D.N.Sc.,C.
Assistant Professor, Midland Lutheran College, Fremont, Nebraska
Human Sexuality

Susan Hockenberger, M.S.N., Ed.D., R.N.
Dean, Lansing School of Nursing, Bellarmine College, Louisville, Kentucky
Wound Healing

Laura Haynes Jacobson, B.S., M.S.N., C.C.R.N.
Staff Nurse IV, Coronary Care, Emory University Hospital, Atlanta, Georgia
Assessment of Clients with Cardiovascular Disorders

Linda Janusek, R.N., Ph.D.
Associate Professor, Loyola University School of Nursing, Chicago, Illinois
Structure and Function of the Immune System

Patricia F. Jassak, M.S., R.N., C.S., O.C.N.
Oncology Clinical Nurse Specialist, Loyola University Medical Center, Maywood, Illinois
Treatment Modalities for Neoplastic Disorders

Cindy Kallsen, R.N., B.S.N.
Assistant Unit Director, University of Nebraska Medical Center, Omaha, Nebraska
Nursing Care of Clients with Biliary and Exocrine Pancreatic Disorders

Joyce Kee, R.N., M.S.
Associate Professor Emerita, University of Delaware, Newark, Delaware
Fluid and Electrolyte Balance

Lynn Keegan, R.N., Ph.D.
"Consultant," University of Texas Health Science Center at San Antonio, San Antonio, TX; Director, Bodymind Systems, Temple, Texas
Spirituality; Health Promotion

Annabelle Keene, B.S.N., M.S.N., R.N.,C.
Assistant Professor, University of Nebraska at Omaha, College of Nursing, Omaha, Nebraska
Health Assessment; Physical Examination

Carol Ren Kneisl, M.S., R.N., C.S.
President and Education Director, Nursing Transitions, Inc., Williamsville, New York
Nursing Care of Clients with Substance Abuse

Mary Ann Kroi, R.N., M.S.N.
Clinical Nurse Specialist, Surgery, Loyola University Medical Center, Maywood, Illinois
Treatment Modalities for Neoplastic Disorders

Teresa Choate Loriaux, R.N., M.S.N., CDE
Managing Editor, *The Endocrinologist*, West Linn, Oregon
Nursing Care of Clients with Adrenal, Pituitary, and Gonadal Disorders

Esther Matassarin-Jacobs, R.N., Ph.D., O.C.N.
Associate Professor, Neihoff School of Nursing, Loyola University, Chicago, Illinois
Nursing Process; Pain Assessment and Intervention; Basic Concepts of Neoplastic Disorders; Nursing Care of Clients with Altered Immune Systems; Nursing Care of Clients with Connective Tissue Disorders; Structure and Function of the Urinary System; Assessment of Clients with Urinary Disòrders; Nursing Care of Clients with Disorders of the Ureters, Bladder, and Urethra; Nursing Care of Clients with Intestinal Disorders; Structure and Function of the Liver, Biliary System, and Exocrine Pancreas; Assessment of Clients with Hepatic, Biliary, and Pancreatic Disorders; Nursing Care of Clients with Hepatic Disorders; Structure and Function of the Female and Male Reproductive Systems; Assessment of Clients with Reproductive Disorders; Nursing Care of Men with Reproductive and Urinary Disorders; Nursing Care of Women with Gynecologic Disorders

Louise Nelson, M.S.N., R.N.
Assistant Professor, University of Nebraska College of Nursing, Omaha, Nebraska
Shock

Noreen Heer Nicol, M.S., R.N., E.N.C.
Dermatology Clinical Specialist/Nurse Practitioner, National Jewish Center for Immunology and Respiratory Medicine, and Clinical Senior Instructor, University of Colorado Health Sciences Center, School of Nursing, Denver, Colorado
Structure and Function; Assessment of Clients with Integumentary Disorders; Nursing Care of Clients with Integumentary Disorders

Margaret Nield, Ph.D., R.N.
Critical Researcher, Sharp Memorial Hospital, and Adjunct Professor, San Diego State University, San Diego, California
Structure and Function of the Respiratory System

Barbara Ott, R.N., Ph.D., C.C.R.N.
Assistant Professor, Wichita State University, Wichita, Kansas
Structure and Function of the Cardiovascular System; Nursing Care of Clients with Cardiac Structure Disorders

Judy Ozuna, B.S.N., M.N.
Clinical Nurse Specialist in Neurology, Veterans Affairs Medical Center, Seattle, Washington
Nursing Care of Clients with Degenerative Neurologic Disorders

Janet Pavel, R.N.
Chief Nurse, Blood Services, National Institutes of Health, Bethesda, Maryland
Basic Concepts of Hematology; Nursing Care of Clients with Hematologic Disorders

Lynn Allchin Petardi, M.S.N., R.N.
Doctoral Student, Loyola University at Chicago, Chicago, Illinois
Basic Concepts of Neoplastic Disorders

Joann Petty, M.S.N., R.N.
Nursing Staff Educator, Foster G. McGaw Hospital, Loyola University Medical Center, Maywood, Illinois
Treatment Modalities for Neoplastic Disorders

Bonita Ann Pilon, D.S.N., R.N., C.N.A.A.
Assistant Professor and Specialty Director of Nursing Administration, Graduate Program, Vanderbilt University, Nashville, Tennessee
Nursing Practice

Ann Plunkett, R.N.
Apheresis Supervisor, Blood Services, National Institutes of Health, Bethesda, Maryland
Basic Concepts of Hematology; Nursing Care of Clients with Hematologic Disorders

Nina A. Rauscher, R.N.,C., O.N.C.
Consultant, North Andover, Massachusetts
Nursing Care of Clients with Musculoskeletal Disorders

Juanita Reigle, R.N., M.S.N., C.C.R.N.
Practitioner/Teacher, University of Virginia, Charlottesville, Virginia
Nursing Care of Clients with Disorders of Cardiac Function

Marlene Reimer, R.N., M.N., C.N.N.(C).
Associate Professor, Faculty of Nursing, Val University of Calgary, Calgary, Alberta, Canada
Sleep and Sensory Disorders

Kathleen A. Ringel, D.N.S., R.N.,C.
Assistant Professor, University of Nebraska Medical Center, College of Nursing, Omaha, Nebraska
Nursing Care of Clients with Disorders of Cardiac Function

Shirley M. Ruder, B.S.N., M.S., M.S.N., Ed.D.
Coordinator of Nursing, Edison Community College, Ft. Myers, Florida
Structure and Function of the Gastrointestinal System; Assessment of Clients with Gastrointestinal Disorders; Nursing Care of Clients with Ingestive Disorders; Nursing Care of Clients with Gastric Disorders; Nursing Care of Clients with Intestinal Disorders

Sally Strong Schnell, R.N., M.S.N.
Clinical Nurse Specialist, Loyola University Medical Center, Maywood, Illinois; Clinical Instructor, Department of Medical-Surgical Nursing, Loyola University at Chicago, Chicago, Illinois
Nursing Care of Clients with Cerebral Disorders; Nursing Care of Clients with Disorders of the Spinal Cord, Cranial Nerves, and Peripheral Nerves

Linda T. Schuring, M.S.N., R.N.
Director of the Balance Disorder Clinic, Warren Otologic Group, Warren, Ohio
Structure and Function of the Ear; Assessment and Nursing Care of Clients with Ear Disorders

Barbara Sigler, R.N., M.N.Ed.
Clinical Nurse Specialist, Otolaryngology, Head and Neck Surgery Department, Eye and Ear Institute, University of Pittsburgh Medical Center, Pittsburgh, Pennsylvania
Nursing Care of Clients with Upper Airway Disorders

Bonnie Sink, R.N., B.S.N.
Clinical Nurse, Blood Services, National Institutes of Health, Bethesda, Maryland
Basic Concepts of Hematology; Nursing Care of Clients with Hematologic Disorders

Kris Strasburg, R.N., C.C.T.C.
Heart and Lung Transplant Coordinator, University of Minnesota Transplant Center, Minneapolis, Minnesota
Structure and Function of the Liver, Biliary System, and Exocrine Pancreas; Assessment of Clients with Hepatic, Biliary, and Pancreatic Disorders; Nursing Care of Clients with Hepatic Disorders

Lisa L. Strohmyer, M.S.N., R.N.
Medical-Surgical Clinical Nurse Specialist, University of Nebraska Medical Center, University Hospital, Omaha, Nebraska
Nursing Care of Clients During Medical-Surgical Emergencies

Michele J. Upvall, Ph.D., R.N.
Assistant Professor of Nursing, Northern Arizona University, Flagstaff, Arizona
Cross-Cultural Nursing

Linda A. Vader, B.S., R.N., C.R.N.O.
Head Nurse, University of Michigan, Kellogg Eye Center, Ann Arbor, Michigan
Structure and Function of the Ear; Assessment and Nursing Care of Clients with Eye Disorders

The assessment portions of chapters throughout the book were written by Annabelle Keene, B.S.N., M.S.N., R.N.,C.

All of the ETHICAL ISSUES IN NURSING features were written by Lisa Anderson-Shaw, R.N.,C., M.S.N., M.A., Clinical Nurse Specialist, Eye and Ear Infirmary, University of Illinois at Chicago.

Reviewers

Rebecca Lynn Agnew, R.N., M.S.N.
Mercy School of Nursing, Pittsburgh, Pennsylvania

Patti Altman, R.N., M.S.N.
Northwest State Community College, Archbold, Ohio

Joyce J. Esser Anderson, R.N., M.S.
Clinical Associate Professor, University of Wisconsin-Madison School of Nursing, Madison, Wisconsin

Alyce Smithson Ashcraft, M.S.N., R.N., C.S., C.C.R.N.
Blinn College, Bryan, Texas, and Doctoral Student, University of Texas, Austin, Texas

Shirley M. Bass, M.S.N., C.F.N.C./P.N.P., R.N.
Tennessee State University, Nashville, Tennessee

Linda J. Becker, B.S.N., M.S.N., R.N.,C.
Nursing Faculty, St. Clair County Community College, Port Huron, Michigan

Margaret W. Bellak, R.N., M.N.
Indiana University of Pennsylvania, Indiana, Pennsylvania

Jean Lockhart Blair, M.N.E.D., R.N.
Indiana University of Pennsylvania, Indiana, Pennsylvania

Vanessa Jones Briscoe, M.S.N., R.N., C.D.E.
Tennessee State University, Nashville, Tennessee

Sandra Brisendine, R.N., M.S.N., F.N.P.
Nursing Instructor, Seward County Community College, Liberal, Kansas

Cheryl J. Cassis, R.N., M.S.N.
Belmont Technical College, St. Clairsville, Ohio

Marcia Chorba, R.N., M.S.N.
Mercy Hospital School of Nursing, Pittsburgh, Pennsylvania

JoAnna M. Christiansen, R.N., M.S.N., F.N.S.
Laredo Community College, Laredo, Texas

Diane P. Dean, M.S.N., R.N.
Indiana University of Pennsylvania, Indiana, Pennsylvania

Shannon Ruff Dirksen, Ph.D., R.N.
Assistant Professor, College of Nursing, University of New Mexico, Albuquerque, New Mexico

Marlene A.S. Foreman, M.N., R.N.C.S., C.R.N.H.
Louisiana State University at Eunice, Division of Nursing and Allied Health, Eunice, Louisiana

Sandra Franklin, R.N., M.S.
Regis University, Denver, Colorado

Rebecca S. Frugé, R.N., M.N.
Clinical Nurse Specialist, Louisiana State University at Eunice, Eunice, Louisiana

Alma M. Harrell, R.N., M.Ed., M.S.N.
Palm Beach Community College, Lake Worth, Florida

Rebecca L. Hartman, Ed.D., R.N.
Assistant Professor of Nursing; Coordinator Health Ministries/Parish Nurse, Indiana University of Pennsylvania, Indiana, Pennsylvania

Patricia A. Hong, M.A., R.N., C.S., C.C.R.N.
School of Nursing and Health Sciences, University of Alaska Anchorage, Anchorage, Alaska

M. Regina Jennette, Ed.D., R.N.
West Virginia Northern Community College, Wheeling, West Virginia

Roseann Kaminsky, R.N., M.S.N.
Lorain County Community College, Elyria, Ohio

Veda J. King, M.N., R.N., C.S.
Seward County Community College, Liberal, Kansas

Eileen Mieras Kohlenberg, Ph.D., R.N., C.N.A.A.
Associate Professor and Chair, Adult Health Nursing Division, The University of North Carolina at Greensboro, Greensboro, North Carolina

Lauralee S. Krabill, R.N., C., C.N.O.R., M.B.A.
Instructor, School of Nursing, Providence Hospital, Inc., Sandusky, Ohio

Deborah Lewis, Ed.D., R.N-C., F.N.P., C.D.E.
West Virginia University, School of Nursing, Morgantown, West Virginia

Karen McGough Monks, R.N., M.S.N.
Arizona Western College, Yuma, Arizona

Catherine A. Myerholtz, R.N., B.S.N., M.S.N.
Providence Hospital School of Nursing, Sandusky, Ohio

Carol J. Nelson, R.N., M.S.N.
Spokane Community College, Spokane, Washington

Netha O'Meara, R.N., M.S.N.
Doctoral Student, Louisiana State University Medical Center, Graduate School of Nursing, and Associate Degree Nursing Program Director, Wharton County Junior College, Wharton, Texas

Priscilla W. Ramsey, Ph.D., R.N.C.S.
Adult Nursing Department, East Tennessee State University, Johnson City, Tennessee

Michele Dropik Rega, R.N., M.S.N.
Westmoreland County Community College, Youngwood, Pennsylvania

Donna J. Seefeldt, R.N., M.S.N., O.C.N.
D'Youville College, Buffalo, New York

Lisa K. Anderson Shaw, R.N.C., M.S.N., M.A.
Clinical Faculty, University of Illinois Medical Center, College of Nursing, Chicago, Illinois

C. Sue Snyder, Ph.D., R.N.,C.
Associate Professor, Department of Nursing, Indiana University of Pennsylvania, Indiana, Pennsylvania

Mona Newsome Wicks, Ph.D., R.N., C.C.R.N.
Assistant Professor, College of Nursing, University of Tennessee at Memphis, Memphis, Tennessee

Pamela Wilde, R.N., M.S., C.C.R.N.
School of Nursing and Health Sciences, University of Alaska Anchorage, Anchorage, Alaska

Preface

Heading toward the 21st century, health-care professionals in North America are participating in the delivery of health-care services to clients of all ages and from diverse cultures. Health promotion and disease prevention are being incorporated into what is meant to be a continuum of care offered in acute, subacute, and community settings, home care being a significant component of the last category.

Nurses need to be critical and creative thinkers to function effectively in this spectrum of settings. In clinical practice, collaboration and clinical pathways are joining—some would say displacing—the nurse-centered focus of the nursing process and care plans. Nurses, as well as other health-care professionals, are discovering innovative ways to market and deliver their services in an unstable health-care environment, while continuing their traditional commitments to promoting consumers' optimal health.

Luckmann's Core Principles and Practice of Medical-Surgical Nursing is edited from the Fourth Edition of **Luckmann and Sorensen's Medical-Surgical Nursing: A Psychophysiologic Approach**, edited by Joyce Black and Esther Matassarin-Jacobs. It has been restructured to reflect the changes taking place in the health-care system and in nursing education. The text focuses on client assessment, planning, and care of clients with the most common acute and chronic conditions, with a pronounced emphasis on client education.

Reflecting the shift toward collaborative management in health care, regardless of setting, are sample clinical pathways for selected common health conditions. Clinical pathways are being developed in all areas of the health-care delivery system. Although the nursing process remains the cornerstone for the professional nurse and is presented throughout the text, its use is evolving as the health-care delivery system is being transformed. This text continues with the nursing process format familiar to most nursing educators, using current NANDA nursing diagnoses.

Finally, this text has been carefully focused on the most essential information needed by the medical-surgical nursing student. Nursing programs have always been demanding and intensive, but the trend toward increasing numbers of second-career and second-degree nursing students seems to indicate a typical student who now more than ever needs to compress and prioritize the time available for study. To meet this need, this text emphasizes understanding of the *principles* required to address the broad spectrum of health-care problems that clients have and to build the knowledge foundation for the clinically competent and individualized nursing care that they demand.

FEATURES

Leading off each unit related to a body system is an **Anatomy and Physiology Review.** These strikingly designed presentations integrate text and illustrations to provide an overview of structure and function in a concise, highly visual format.

Critical to Remember boxes highlight key points of nursing practice, such as signs and symptoms of complications, important nursing actions, and more. Appearing throughout the text, these highlights draw the student's attention to the highest priority clinical information.

Numerous **Client Education Guides** throughout the text offer concrete recommendations for discharge planning and health promotion after discharge. These guides reflect the increasing emphasis on educating health-care consumers and encouraging them to be more active collaborators in their own care.

Pathophysiology boxes are included for many of the most common and significant disorders. These highlight key concepts in disease development, and many are illustrated to help clarify more complex physiologic processes. Similarly, **Clinical Manifestations boxes** list important signs and symptoms that alert the nurse to a disorder or a potentially dangerous complication.

Bridges to Critical Care describe the key aspects of common critical care modalities, including pulmonary pressure monitors.

Ethical Issues in Nursing, written by a nurse ethicist, are boxes describing various ethical dilemmas arising from clinical practice and raising points for reflection and discussion.

Clinical Pathways currently in use at various health-care institutions are reprinted here with their permission. These reflect the trend toward collaborative, multidisciplinary care and indicate the coordination required to achieve the continuity of care across settings that is vital to the health of each individual. In recognition of the continuing validity of the nursing process as a paradigm for clinical judgment, traditional **Nursing Care Plans** are provided for some important disorders.

Study Questions are included at the end of each chapter. These multiple choice questions at the application and analysis level of learning will help the students test their understanding of the text content. Answers to the Study Questions are provided in Appendix A.

Critical Thinking Exercises also appear at the end of each chapter. These address health promotion and disease prevention, cultural issues, and issues that cross the adult lifespan and will help sharpen the student's critical thinking skills. Response discussions for these exercises also appear in Appendix A.

TEACHING/LEARNING ANCILLARY PACKAGE

Instructor's Manual

Prepared by Carrie Dowdy, MSN, RN, this manual guides the instructor through each chapter of the textbook with a chapter outline and learning outcomes. Instructor notes suggest text features to review or discuss in the classroom. The *Critical to Remember* boxes from the text receive special emphasis. The rationale for why the material is important and suggested critical thinking questions will allow the instructor to challenge students further and deepen their understanding of essential material. Both classroom and clinical activities are suggested for each chapter, and additional recent references are provided.

Study Guide

Prepared by Charlene Morris, this guide offers students the opportunity to test their understanding of the text content using a variety of question types, including matching, true-false, and multiple choice. Knowledge-based questions require students to recall vocabulary, facts, and concepts about medical-surgical nursing. Application questions provide scenarios in which students relate knowledge to realistic situations. Evaluation questions use case studies, questionnaires, and hypothetical nursing situations to challenge students to explain, develop, and argue concepts in the text. Each chapter of the study guide specifies learning outcomes for the student.

Pocket Companion

Prepared by Mary K. Palandri, RN. BSN, and Catherine Rollman Sorrentino, RN, BSN, this companion to the text is a quick reference guide for nursing students and practicing nurses in the clinical setting. Based on content from the text, the *Pocket Companion* offers information on over 300 adult medical-surgical conditions, organized alphabetically in a format closely following the parent text. This portable guide provides reference to the page numbers of the textbook where more in-depth information can be found.

Test Bank

Edited for *Luckmann's Core Principles and Practice of Medical-Surgical Nursing* by Elaine Zimbler, RN, MA, this manual adapts the *Manual of Test Questions for Luckmann and Sorensen's Medical-Surgical Nursing,* Fourth Edition, which was written by Marie O'Toole, RN, EdD, and Diana Bubb, MSN, RN. Over 1600 questions test the student's comprehension of each chapter in the text on three cognitive levels: knowledge, application, and interpretation. The *Test Bank* is available to adopters of the text on Saunders' EXAMaster+ software to facilitate test generation for busy faculty.

Transparency Package

Two hundred transparency masters and transparencies drawn from the book (some in full color) provide exciting visual aids to assist the instructor with classroom presentations. These are available to adopters of the text.

Acknowledgments

Editing a major work is always an enormous undertaking. We extend our thanks to the many members of the team. To our family members, friends, and colleagues, thanks for always being there for us. To our Saunders family—Thomas Eoyang, Vice President and Editor-in-Chief, who encouraged our creativity and challenged us at every step of the way; Kevin Law, Senior Developmental Editor, who used humor to relieve stress and responded faithfully to our questions and comments as he guided us through the many processes required to complete such a sizeable work; Linda R. Garber, the production manager, who orchestrated the production end of the process; Annette Ferran, the copy editor, who helped us mind our grammatical p's and q's; Stacey Polk, the editorial assistant, who was always upbeat and always there; Karen O'Keefe, the designer, who faultlessly coordinated the book's complex, visually stimulating design; and the artists (especially Marjorie Domonowske and Pat Thomas), photographers, and many other individuals who lent their expertise and talents to our project—many thanks.

Our contributors deserve a special "thank you" for their efforts to present the "need to know" information to the nursing student. Their clarity and conciseness is applauded. Special thanks to Edith J. Applegate for writing the Anatomy and Physiology Review features that lead off Units 3 through 15. She has done a masterful job of condensing complex material and highlighting essential information. Thanks also to the many reviewers who offered suggestions and comments that helped us keep our focus. The individuals who created the ancillaries merit a round of applause for their efforts in supporting the concepts inherent in this textbook. We also recognize and thank Joyce M. Black and Esther Matassarin-Jacobs, who supported us, gave suggestions, and welcomed us into the world of writing for nursing students.

Contents in Brief

UNIT 8

Hematologic Disorders

UNIT 9

Urinary Disorders

UNIT 10

Gastrointestinal Disorders

UNIT 11

Hepatic, Biliary Tract, and Exocrine Pancreatic Disorders

UNIT 12

Metabolic Disorders

UNIT 13

Musculoskeletal Disorders

UNIT 14

Integumentary Disorders

UNIT 15

Reproductive Disorders

UNIT 16

Multisystem Disorders

Contents

UNIT 5

Sensory Disorders

UNIT 11

Hepatic, Biliary Tract, and Exocrine Pancreatic Disorders

Guide to Special Features

Anatomy & Physiology Reviews

Client Education Guides

Ethical Issues in Nursing

Bridge to Critical Care

Clinical Pathways

Nursing Care Plans

UNIT 1

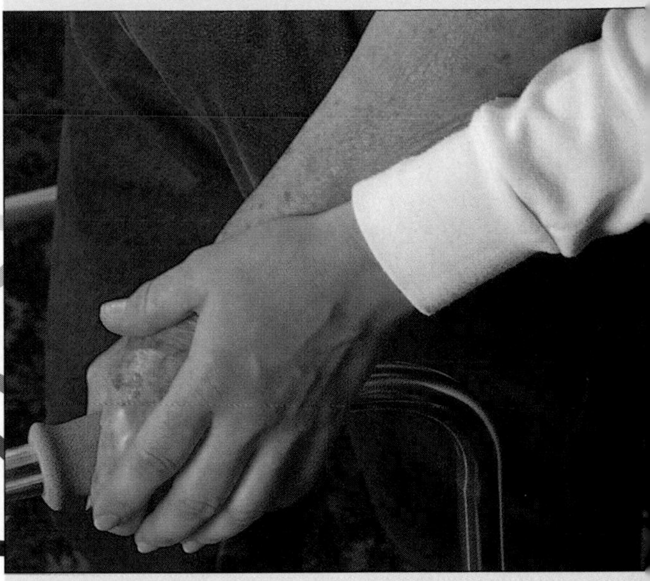

Foundations of Nursing Care

The current widespread changes in the health-care system are having a major impact on the nursing profession. The two chapters in this opening unit address important basic aspects of contemporary nursing practice. Chapter 1, Acute and Chronic Illness, explores recent developments in the traditional designations of acute care and chronic care, along with a new category—subacute care—that covers clients who do not need acute care but still are too ill to be sent home. Chapter 2, Health Care Delivery, discusses the changes that have occurred as a result of the health-care reform movement and explores how these changes are affecting health care in general and nursing in particular. It describes how health-care delivery is shifting from the traditional hospital-based system to an interconnected web of services that aims to provide a continuum of care, including subacute care, expanded outpatient and home health-care services, hospice care, and nurse-managed clinics. It also discusses case management and managed care (with an explanation of clinical pathways) and describes the changing regulatory climate and ongoing efforts to ensure quality health care for all.

Chapter 1 Acute and Chronic Illness

Learning Outcomes

After completing this chapter, the learner will be able to:

1. Assess the client with acute and chronic illnesses, using a psycho-social-cultural-physiological approach.
2. Teach the client and significant others the etiology, risk factors, and psycho-social-cultural-physiological manifestations of acute and chronic illnesses.
3. Explain the client's role in adapting to illness.
4. Develop a plan of care for the prevention and/or amelioration of illness.
5. Implement nursing interventions that optimize the quality of life for clients with acute and chronic illnesses.
6. Evaluate planned client outcomes, using outcome criteria developed in the planning phase of care.

As health-care reform makes headway, the health-care delivery system has evolved into a business-oriented system. The consumer of health care is the main player, with a new role that includes more responsibility for preventive care as well as making choices for cost-effective care. The traditional areas of acute and chronic care have expanded to include a newer service in the form of subacute care.

Changes in health care have caused a reassessment of services and new involvement with clients. The current emphasis is on prevention of illness through client education, mother and child care, and healthy living with respect to exercise, rest, healthy eating habits, and controlling stress. For clients who need health-care services, the focus on providing a seamless system of services is significant. Caregivers with multidisciplinary repertoires of skills are now found across the health-care continuum. Unlicensed personnel are being prepared for expanded roles as health-care givers. In some areas, less skilled caregivers are permitted to perform more complex tasks after education and competence are proven.

DEFINITION

Acute care is still the basis for complex care, with potential and actual serious or unpredictable outcomes, and for trauma care. The individual who is acutely ill experiences a reversible change in the structure or function of one or more body systems. An acute condition is one in which the individual can expect a return to health that may or may not be at the same level of previous functioning. Depending on the nature of the acute condition, a chronic illness can ensue. For example, a client with a fracture can expect that normal healing will occur, followed by a return to use of the body part involved. A client with an acute onset of diabetes mellitus can expect the need for life-long health care to control the disease.

An acutely ill person maybe admitted to an acute care setting for initial treatment and stabilization. In less cost-conscious days, such an individual would remain in the acute care setting until the ability to care for himself or herself returned or until the decision for 24-hour care necessitated admission to a nursing home. The advent of case management and clinical pathways has resulted in shorter but more cost-effective hospital stays.

A new option in the health-care delivery system is subacute care. A variety of medical-surgical, oncologic, rehabilitation, and other special services can be provided in alternative settings for clients who have no need for acute care but are still too ill to be sent home.[29] Some nursing homes are developing subacute units to serve this population of clients. In some areas, freestanding subacute care service is offered. The developing push for shorter stays is causing hospitals to seriously consider the shift to the provision of subacute care.

Chronic illnesses are long-term health problems caused by an irreversible disorder, an accumulation of disorders, or a latent disease state.[13] Some chronic conditions cause irreversible change in the structure or function of one or more body systems. Other illnesses are chronic because no cure has been found. Developments in the fields of bacteriology, immunology, public health, and pharmacology have led to a rapid drop in mortality from previously fatal illnesses. Decreased mortality from acute illnesses has led to lengthened lifespans and a greater risk of accidents and illness that can develop into chronic conditions. Previously fatal diseases are becoming chronic conditions. Tuberculosis is an example of a previously chronic condition for which clients were isolated in sanitariums. Today tuberculosis is treatable and is preventable with vaccines.

The terms chronic illness, long-term illness, and chronic condition are used interchangeably. The term chronic condition is preferred because it is more consistent with a definition of health that includes components of wellness and illness.

The increased prevalence of chronic conditions in our society is due to many factors. Knowledge about physiologic function continues to be generated, and advances have been made in techniques and equipment for assessing and diagnosing alterations in physical function, supporting and sustaining life, combating infection, maintaining and restoring physical function, and compensating and substituting for lost physical function. More infants survive with congenital problems. More persons of all ages survive life-threatening episodes of acute illness and trauma with different degrees of residual deficits in physical or cognitive function. Chronic conditions that were once considered rare, such as dermatophytosis and amyotropic lateral sclerosis, are becoming more common because people are living longer.

CRITICAL TO REMEMBER

Illnesses previously viewed as acute, such as myocardial infarction, cerebrovascular accidents, and congestive heart failure, are now recognized to be acute episodes of chronic conditions.

Newer illnesses such as acquired immunodeficiency syndrome (AIDS) and Lyme disease are being diagnosed. Implantable devices and transplants extend the chronic phase of chronic conditions.

Clients with chronic conditions are more visible. Beliefs about the rights of clients with chronic conditions and their role in society have changed. Having a chronic condition is no longer viewed as incompatible with maintaining social roles. Health was previously defined as the absence of illness.

CRITICAL TO REMEMBER

Health is now viewed as a continuum of wellness to death, with some degree of health being present until death.

TABLE 1–1 Comparison of Chronic Illness and Acute Illness

	CHRONIC ILLNESS	ACUTE ILLNESS
Knowledge base of health-care providers	Broad, less commonly defined than with acute illness	Focused, fairly well defined
Onset	Rapid or gradual	Rapid
Course	Ongoing process with transitions and changing demands Phases Diagnosis Chronic constant progressive remissions/exacerbations Terminal	Short, temporary
Outcome	Varying types and degrees of physical deficits Uncertain Different degrees of ongoing impact on personal, family, work, and recreational roles	Self-limiting (cure or death), no residual deficits Fairly predictable Temporary impact on personal, family, work, and recreational roles
Nursing/medical management	Long term; client/family co-managers	Short term

The revised definition of health recognizes the presence of abilities as well as deficits within illness and fits the client with a chronic condition well.

INCIDENCE

The incidence, visibility, and popular awareness of chronic conditions in our society and in acute health-care settings are greater now than at any time in history. Acute care admissions consist of those clients who experience acute trauma, abrupt onset of a life-threatening disease, or an exacerbation of an existing disease. These clients may or may not have a pre-existing chronic condition. Exact measurement of the incidence of chronic conditions is limited by variations in definitions of chronic illness found in the literature. According to the definition of chronic conditions used in the 1986 Department of Commerce census, approximately 50 per cent of the American population have one or more chronic conditions. It is estimated that more than 75 per cent of clients receiving care in acute care settings have one or more chronic conditions.

Acute as well as chronic illness can occur at any point in the lifespan. Some adults have chronic conditions that are present from birth or that are acquired during childhood or adolescence. Other clients acquire chronic conditions during adulthood.

It is important to differentiate acute conditions from chronic conditions.

CRITICAL TO REMEMBER

An acute condition is caused by a disease that produces signs and symptoms soon after exposure to the cause, typically runs a short course, and usually ends with complete recovery or abrupt termination in death.

Acute conditions may become chronic; for example, seasonal allergies may lead to lung conditions such as asthma.

A chronic condition is caused by a disease that produces signs and symptoms over a varying period of time, runs a long course, and only partially resolves. The symptoms of chronic conditions may subside with proper care. This period of time during which the client is free of symptoms is called remission. The symptoms often return, a process called exacerbation.

In the past, health-care practice, education, and research have focused on acute illnesses. The conditions were life-threatening and were the most common problems seen by health-care providers. At present, most clients are hospitalized for exacerbations of chronic conditions rather than for acute illnesses.

CRITICAL TO REMEMBER

Because most clients with chronic illness are managed by themselves or by significant others, it is common for the client and family or friends to have more factual and experiential knowledge about the condition than the average health-care provider.

A comparison of chronic and acute illnesses is listed in Table 1–1.

Many nursing leaders have advocated the inclusion of more content on chronic illness and wellness into nursing education.

THE PROCESS OF ADAPTATION

Physiologic Adaptation

Some changes in physiologic structure or function that are associated with illness are irreversible. Other physiologic changes are reversible. Treatment and life-style changes can slow the rate of some physiologic changes. Technology is available to compensate or substitute for some types of physical functioning. Adaptive tasks related to changes in physiologic structure or function are as follows:

- Changing life-style
- Controlling symptoms
- Learning about illness and treatment
- Managing the prescribed medical regimen
- Learning about techniques and devices that can substitute for lost function
- Acquiring skills in using these techniques and devices
- Monitoring body response to therapies
- Adjusting to changes in physical appearance and function during the course of the disease
- Capitalizing on physical and psychological strengths

Psychological Adaptation

Psychological adaptation to illness is an ongoing process that overlaps other biologic and psychosocial processes associated with gains, losses, and challenges throughout the remainder of a client's lifespan. Psychological adaptation to an acute illness is characterized by the demands of coping with the unexpected as well as with the progress of healing and, as with other ongoing processes, by periods of changing demands and transitions. Onset and diagnosis, hospitalizations for treatment of the condition, exacerbation of illness, failure of treatments, and loss of self-care abilities all have an impact on the course of the illness. Some clients whose illness has a terminal phase must also adapt to a shortened lifespan and the dying process.

CRITICAL TO REMEMBER

Although chronic conditions are associated with disease-specific physiologic changes and outcomes, the psychological adaptation of persons who have not experienced severe cognitive impairment has been found to be similar in clients with all conditions and is not related to the length of time since diagnosis.

The psychological health of adults with different stages of chronic illnesses has been found to be similar to that of normal adults.

CRITICAL TO REMEMBER

Clients adapt to the same diagnosis and phase of illness in very diverse ways.

During the diagnostic phase, one client may appear overwhelmed and assume a lower level of physical, psychological, or social functioning than the physical condition warrants, and another client may evidence minimal distress, maintain or regain a high level of physical, psychological, and social functioning, and continue to adapt.

THREE PHASES OF PSYCHOLOGICAL ADAPTATION

A general pattern of psychological adaptation to personal change, loss, and the threat of loss has been described by sociologists and psychologists.

Disbelief. The first phase of the pattern is commonly referred to as disbelief or resistance. Denial of the changes or the need for personal change is characteristic of this phase. This phase is similar to the stress "fight or flight" response and is believed to protect the client from being psychologically overwhelmed.

Developing Awareness. The second phase is developing awareness, which is characterized by withdrawal, preoccupation with the self, crying, depression, expression of anger toward others, or feelings of guilt, anger, being different, and being alone. In this phase, the client experiences acute awareness of and grieves for what has been lost.

Integration. The third phase is integration and is characterized by logical acceptance that change has occurred, keeping emotional distress within manageable limits, reestablishing a sense of self and meaning and purpose, revising life goals, learning to live with uncertainty, and achieving a new means to cope with one's environment.

GENERAL PSYCHOLOGICAL ADAPTIVE TASKS FOR CLIENTS WITH CHRONIC CONDITIONS

A number of general psychological adaptive tasks are related to having and living with a chronic condition. These adaptive tasks include

- coping with emotional responses of oneself and significant others to the illness experience;
- coping with the uncertainty of diagnosis and treatment;
- coming to terms with having a chronic condition;
- restructuring one's life around the chronic condition;
- restructuring schedules, priorities, and plans for the future;
- negotiating new and altered relationships with oneself, family, friends, and the health-care system;
- developing attitudes, knowledge, and skills that enable one to actively participate in regimen management;
- controlling symptoms;
- preventing and handling acute health crises;
- dealing with genetic concerns and issues in reproductive decision-making; and
- adapting to changes in physical abilities or appearance.

Personal resources that assist clients in accomplishing these adaptive tasks include life experiences, interests, memories, and the capacity to learn, change behavior, relate to others, solve problems, and express and change feelings. Literature related to psychological adaptation to chronic conditions focuses primarily on the distress component of psychological adaptation. The ways in which clients interpret physical, social, and psychological changes during the course of their illness

TABLE 1–2 Common Concerns, Fears, and Personal Changes Associated with Chronic Conditions

Concerns and Fears
Sense of self
Loss of control and predictability
Heightened sense of mortality
Loss of productivity
Loss of valued roles
Loss of relationships
Loss of opportunity or ability for sexual expression
Uncertainty about the future
Purpose and meaning in life
Fear of procedures
Fear of death
Personal Changes
Life plans and goals
Established roles and patterns of interacting within family and outside the home
Relationships with others
Daily routines
Loss of gratifying behaviors
Changes in health maintenance and management behaviors
Activity and sleep patterns
Financial resources
Appearance

and the methods that they find effective in adapting to these ongoing changes are less well understood.

Different numbers and types of physiologic, psychological, and social events are appraised as distressful by clients who have the same chronic condition for the same period of time. A number of concerns, fears, and personal change events are common to a variety of chronic conditions; these problems are identified in Table 1–2.

COPING BEHAVIORS

Clients with the same medical diagnosis and in the same phase of illness use a variety of physical, cognitive, and verbal behaviors in managing distress. The type of behaviors used and the appraised effectiveness of the same type of behaviors are highly individual. Some clients report that talking about their illness helps them cope, whereas others report that not talking about their illness helps them cope. Strategies reported as effective in managing distressful situations include avoiding, ignoring, accepting, thinking out, or changing the situation. Shopping, driving, going out to eat, and exercising are types of activities that some clients find helpful in relieving stress.

Sociologic Adaption

Health and illness roles of clients with acute, subacute, or chronic conditions overlap with social roles related to age, sex, family, work, and recreation. The degree of impact of health and illness roles on social roles ranges from minimal to severe, with health and illness roles being the dominant life roles. The degree to which clients adapt socially is influenced by changes in physical appearance, ability to communicate, ability to navigate the physical environment, and social resources (e.g., people, money, community services). Society responds differently to clients with less visible and apparent chronic conditions than to those with more visible signs of illness.

Changing social beliefs about individual rights and normalcy have influenced state and federal legislation. This legislation has contributed to a decrease in attitudinal and architectural barriers to social integration as well as the increased availability of health care, housing, employment, and transportation for persons with chronic conditions. The 1990 passage of the Americans with Disabilities Act (PL 101-336) by Congress increased social options for persons with chronic conditions. Disability is defined as "physical or mental impairment that substantially limits one or more of an individual's major life activities." (Clients with disabilities generally prefer to be known as "physically challenged" or "mentally challenged.") Passage of the act was motivated by economic as well as altruistic concerns. Equal access to society increases social independence and provides opportunities for more disabled people to be employed taxpayers rather than dependent on tax-supported services. The act addresses access to public accommodations and services, telecommunication relay services, and employment and holds the private sector accountable for the cost of compliance with the act.

COMMUNICATION PATTERNS

Communication patterns between clients and their significant others and health-care professionals have been described as changing over time and tending to move through three phases. Initially, clients and significant others have a naive trust in health-care workers. A characteristic of this phase is the belief that health-care professionals will provide a cure or do what is best for the client. This naive trust is followed by a phase of mistrust and anger.

CRITICAL TO REMEMBER

A major source of anger is lack of involvement in decision-making.

Over time, the second phase is replaced by guarded trust, with trust being placed in some health-care professionals and not in others. Health-care providers should be aware of these phases and work with the client, providing factual information without denying hope.

SOCIAL CHANGE EVENTS

The social change events commonly associated with having an illness relate to roles and interaction patterns, mobility patterns, employment, living arrangements, recreation, finances, time and place for vacations, and health insurance coverage. For the client with a chronic condition, common adjustment tasks include preventing or adjusting to social isolation, normalizing, managing symptoms and treatments in social environments, maintaining physical mobility in the environment, changing present housing or locating new housing, dealing with rejection and discrimination, developing new social skills and social networks, teaching others about the chronic condition and how it interferes with a person's abilities, and learning about community resources.

ADAPTATION OF SIGNIFICANT OTHERS

In acute and subacute illness, the client's significant others may be stressed or overwhelmed by the sudden onset of the event. Adaptive tasks include pulling together, learning to cope with the acute care environment and treatment, and establishing relationships with care givers. Response to the adaptive tasks is often telescoped into a short period of time, in which decisions may need to be made and plans for care and treatment are of immediate concern. Everyone must cope with unusual ongoing adaptive tasks related to the presence of a chronic condition. Adjustment tasks for significant others differ with different phases of the chronic condition. Adaptive tasks during the onset or diagnostic phase are the same as those related to acute illness. Additional tasks that are specific to chronic conditions include identifying the meaning of the illness, assessing potential changes in the family, moving toward integration of temporary and permanent changes while maintaining a sense of continuity between past and present, and developing an attitude of flexibility toward future personal and family goals. The client and significant others must also contend with maintaining a sense of normalcy, adjusting to changing expectations of each family member, striving to balance resources, and maintaining maximal autonomy of all family members despite the pull toward mutual dependency, care taking, or focus on the ill member. If a terminal phase is associated with the chronic illness, significant others must also manage issues related to the death of the client, achieve resolution of mourning following the death of the client, and resume normal individual and family lives.

Some families are more effective than others in accomplishing adaptive tasks. The type of physical impairments the client has, the family's resources, perception of the client's significant others, the developmental stage of family members and the family unit, behaviors of the client, and the health-care environment are interrelated factors that have an impact on adaptation. Some family units become stronger whereas others disintegrate.

ETIOLOGY

Multifactorial Etiology

Factors that converge to cause an acute condition include the suddenness of onset, the severity of the condition, the expected length of treatment, and the client's response to health care. The client may have a preexisting condition that will have an impact on the course of the illness. Age and physical condition are factors that may prolong or change the expected course of treatment. The interaction of the factors may be additive, or the factors may combine to cause increased harm. For example, asbestos workers have an increased risk of lung cancer. If the asbestos worker smokes, the risk of lung cancer increases 30 times over those coworkers who do not smoke, and the risk increases 90 times over people who neither work with asbestos nor smoke.

Impact of Aging

Young adult clients usually have short, intense, acute conditions from which they quickly recover. Elderly clients who are healthy can look forward to recovery over a somewhat longer period of time, and the degree of recovery is unpredictable. Accidental injury is common among young adults as a result of vehicular trauma and among the elderly as a result of falls. The process of aging predisposes clients to chronic conditions. It must be pointed out, however, that people in all age groups can develop a chronic illness. In elderly clients, arthritis, diabetes, hypertension, and heart disease are the most common chronic illnesses.

Technology

The use of technology has contributed to advances in acute care. Life-saving technology is used to enhance a return to wellness and to prevent complications. Technology allows a quicker and more accurate response to acute conditions such as a myocardial infarction or a cerebrovascular accident. Such medical success has contributed to the unprecedented increase in the incidence of chronic conditions. The treatment of infectious illness in children has allowed more people to live to older ages, when chronic illnesses are contracted. Likewise, the development of equipment to sustain life has changed the picture of medical care. For example, the use of dialysis for chronic renal failure has lengthened many lives, and as clients live by means of dialysis, health-care providers learn more about the ongoing process of renal failure and living while attached to a life-saving machine.

Race and Ethnic Background

Race or ethnic background predisposes clients to certain illnesses. Race-specific rates measure the association between disease occurrence and race. Data indicate that some conditions are more prevalent in certain races and, sadly, that nonwhite people (black, Native Americans, and Asians) also fail to receive necessary care for illnesses. For example, nonwhites are three times more likely to die of hypertension than whites of the same age group. In a 1985 study, six causes of death were identified that together accounted for more than 80 per cent of excess mortality in nonwhite people.[22] The diseases and degree of excess mortality listed were as follows:

- Cancer—16 per cent excess mortality among black males under age 70 and 10 per cent among black females.
- Cardiovascular disease and stroke—24 per cent excess mortality among black males and 41 per cent among black females.
- Chemical dependency, measured by deaths from cirrhosis of the liver, associated with excessive alcohol consumption—13 per cent excess mortality among Native American males and 22 per cent among Native American females.
- Diabetes—38 per cent excess deaths among Mexican-born Hispanic females.
- Homicides and accidents (unintentional injury)—60 per cent excess mortality among Hispanics under the age of 65; 44 per cent excess deaths due to unintentional injury among male Native Americans and 30 per cent among female Native Americans. Homicides and unintentional injuries account for 19 per cent excess mortality among black males under the age of 70 and 38 per cent among those under the age of 45. The figures for black females are 6 and 14 per cent, respectively. The study noted the association of these deaths with the use of drugs and alcohol.
- Infant mortality—35 per cent excess deaths in the first year of life among black females.

Cultural variations may also prevent illness. Mormons, who neither drink nor smoke, have lower cancer rates than the general population.

RISK FACTORS

Risk factors for any illness are as varied as the number of conditions. Chronic illness can develop from an acute illness that is only partially resolved or as a sequela of other illnesses, such as long-standing diabetes.

Although no one is immune from aging, the early recognition of problems can lead to early treatment in some instances. Diagnoses are made earlier in clients who have a scientific orientation to health (e.g., "I have to watch my cholesterol level"). These clients have routine check-ups to prevent illness and recognize early symptoms. Clients with a functional orientation to life ("I haven't felt well for months now") only seek medical care when they do not feel well or experience symptoms that interfere with the ability to carry out activities and demands of daily living.

In addition, some disorders have specific forms of medical management with fairly predictable outcomes. Cancer, diabetes, cardiovascular disease, and spinal cord injury have specific management regimens. These diseases can be successfully managed and leave a controllable level of residual defect. In contrast, treatment protocols are less clear for clients with multiple sclerosis, systemic lupus erythematosus, Alzheimer's disease, and severe brain injury.

PATHOPHYSIOLOGY

Illness interferes with the intake, transformation, and expenditure of physical energy for cellular metabolism, protein synthesis, and body system functioning or coordinated function of body systems. Nutrients and oxygen are primary sources of physical energy. The process by which nutrients are transformed into physical energy units may be altered by changes in the structure or function of the neurologic, musculoskeletal, circulatory, respiratory, endocrine, or digestive systems. Changes in these body systems may also interfere with the transport and use of energy. Additional energy may be required for physiologic functions and mobility. Both mechanisms can compensate for some changes in physical function; however, these mechanisms may become exhausted over time. When the physical energy demands of an illness exceed the intake and processing of nutrients over time, the body uses reserves of fat and protein as physical energy sources. Use of fat reserves is characterized by a decrease in subcutaneous tissue. Use of protein is characterized by a decrease in visceral protein and muscle mass. The client's general resistance to physiologic stressors is subsequently impaired. The client who is acutely ill or in an acute phase of a chronic condition may experience increased demands on the body for energy. Factors that contribute to increased energy demands are

- inability to ingest foods and fluids,
- infection,
- healing (as of fractures, postoperative surgical incisions, etc.), and
- anxiety and nervousness.

The client is at risk for losing weight and slowing the course of healing.

If the intake of nutrients exceeds body energy requirements for basal metabolic processes and physical activity, the excess energy is stored as muscle and fat. The client experiences an increase in body weight. Factors contributing to weight gain in clients with chronic conditions are

- polyphagia (excessive appetite) secondary to a central nervous system insult, intake of corticosteroids, pickwickian syndrome, or certain endocrine disorders;
- changes in taste;
- anxiety;
- depression; and
- decreased mobility or sedentary lifestyle.

A number of factors associated with other chronic conditions contribute to energy deficits by interfering with the intake of nutrients, metabolism, or expenditure of energy. Social, psychological, and treatment factors as well as disease-related factors may limit intake of nutrients. The following list includes several of these factors:

- Inability to procure food secondary to physical, economic, transportation, or cognitive limitations
- Lack of knowledge about adequate nutrition
- Anorexia, nausea, and vomiting secondary to the disease process, medication or treatments, depressed mood, or anxiety
- Changes in taste, smell, or vision
- Inability to feed self
- Decreased salivation
- Impaired swallowing
- Changes in the structure of the mouth or esophagus

Neuroendocrine responses to psychological distress have been associated with the development of illnesses such as cardiovascular disease, peptic ulcers, asthma, ulcerative colitis, multiple sclerosis, cancer, and accidental trauma. Neuroendocrine response to distress has also been implicated as a factor in symptoms of anorexia, pain, fatigue, shortness of breath, and decreased immune response; progression of chronic conditions; exacerbations of chronic conditions; and delayed recovery from acute episodes of illness during the course of the chronic illness. Over time, adaptive energy from neuroendocrine sources is believed to become exhausted.

CLINICAL MANIFESTATIONS

The common clinical manifestations associated with an acute illness include pain caused by the body's response to obstruction, infection, a break in the integrity of skin or bone, and trauma. There may be loss of fluid caused by hemorrhage or severe nausea and vomiting and diarrhea. Loss of consciousness may occur from a variety of assaults on the body, for example, head injury as a result of trauma or a ruptured aneurysm. Breathing may be impaired by massive infection, pneumothorax, or a crush injury.

In the case of a chronic condition, the longer the client has the condition, the greater the number of body systems involved. Some chronic conditions are characterized by an abrupt onset of symptoms, whereas others begin gradually over months or years. Anorexia, fatigue, pain, shortness of breath, sleep disturbance, and impaired mobility are common clinical manifestations.

Mobility and self-care abilities associated with the chronic phase of chronic conditions comprise a continuum ranging from complete independence, modified independence, and modified dependence to complete dependence. Many illness-related, treatment-related, and psychological factors contribute to immobility. Fatigue, pain, loss of sensation, muscle weakness, paralysis, spasticity, joint stiffness, the presence of braces or casts, and enforced chair or bed rest are common factors that contribute to immobility.

Complications

Adaptive responses to acute illness depend on the client's physical condition and pre-existing medical conditions that may interfere with healing. Multisystem trauma or illness may also predispose a client to complications.

Adaptive responses to prolonged bed rest and decreased levels of mobility occur in the neurologic, cardiovascular, respiratory, digestive, renal, metabolic, integumentary, and immune systems as well as the musculoskeletal system. These adaptive responses, which are commonly referred to collectively as disuse syndrome, increase levels of disability. Physiologic changes leading to disuse syndrome are identified in Table 1–3.

TABLE 1–3 Physiologic Changes Leading to Disuse Syndrome

BODY SYSTEM	PHYSIOLOGIC CHANGE
Neurologic	Decreased ability to concentrate Reduced stimulation of reticular activation system Brain stimulates itself with visual and auditory hallucinations Sleep disturbance
Cardiovascular	Decreased stroke volume Increased heart rate Hypovolemia Postural hypotension Increased procoagulants Shortened thromboplastin time; thromboembolism Compression of blood vessels of calves of leg
Pulmonary	Abdominal contents pushing against diaphragm Stress on inspiratory muscles Stasis of secretions Decreased lung volume Decreased intake of oxygen
Digestive	Diminished appetite Decreased metabolism Changes in insulin release pattern and effectiveness Decreased peristalsis
Integumentary	Larger surface area of skin bearing weight Evaporation of perspiration less efficient than when exposed to air Exposure to moist bed linens Pressure against bed impairs skin circulation
Renal	Stasis of urine in kidneys; urinary tract infection Increased excretion of calcium (formation of urinary calculi) Increased excretion of nitrogen
Musculoskeletal	Loss of muscle tone Loss of muscle mass Contractures Heterotrophic bone disease Osteoporosis
Immune	Decreased immunity

Diagnostic Assessment

An arsenal of diagnostic tests is available for acute and chronic conditions. In emergency situations, diagnostic studies may direct the course of immediate treatment. After the client is stabilized, further testing may be required. During an acute phase of a chronic illness, testing may determine treatment as well as follow the progression of the illness. Because there are so many types of chronic conditions, specific assessments are used for each of the conditions.

MEDICAL MANAGEMENT

Medical management varies with the condition, and surgical treatment may be required for clients with certain conditions. Health-care needs of clients with acute conditions may be addressed by delivery systems that include intensive care and step-down units, case management and the use of clinical pathways, discharge planning, and referral to subacute units when the client is in need of more recovery time under supervised care. Patterns of health-care delivery that have been expanded or implemented to address health-care needs of persons with chronic conditions include the use of rehabilitation centers, units, and programs; home health care; nurse-managed clinics; hospice care; and case management.

Rehabilitation

Traditional goals of rehabilitation have been the prevention of physical deformity, maintenance of physical function, restoration of function, education of the client and significant others, and reintegration of the client into his or her family and society. Strategies used to achieve these goals include the use of an interdisciplinary team approach, beginning discharge planning on admission, preventing deformity, maintaining skin integrity, and providing the family and the client with information and skills. Over the years, these strategies have also become integrated into acute care and are used to address the problems of chronic pain, cardiovascular disease, and chronic obstructive lung disease.

The original multidisciplinary team of physiatrist, nurses, physical therapists, occupational therapists, speech therapists, and psychologists has expanded to include dietitians, respiratory therapists, and practitioners from the newer disciplines of neuropsychology and recreational therapy. The team members apply their knowledge and skills in assisting clients in regaining functional abilities and acquiring knowledge and skills that maximize their ability to live with physical disability. Clients served are those with a severe disability secondary to neurologic or musculoskeletal trauma (accidental and surgical) or illnesses. Many clients with chronic conditions such as arthritis, cancer, amyotrophic lateral sclerosis, and multiple sclerosis would benefit from assistive devices and techniques that compensate or substitute for lost physical function.

The multidisciplinary approach and physical conditioning have been implemented in inpatient and outpatient rehabilitation programs for clients with cardiac diseases, chronic obstructive lung disease, and chronic pain. Exercise does not reverse pathophysiologic changes, but it is believed to condition muscles so that they work more efficiently and use less oxygen. Exercise also stimulates the production of endorphins, which promote feelings of well-being, increase production of high-density lipoproteins, assist in weight control, and increase exercise tolerance. Some of the strategies discussed are applicable to acute and subacute care as well.

Illness Trajectory

A trajectory is the course of something, indicating predictable direction and movement. In health care, the term trajectory is used to describe the process of any disorder. A trajectory begins with a pathophysiologic event and ends with resolution of the problem or development of another problem (e.g., a complication). By taking into account a disorder's symptoms, phases, and treatment over time, it is possible to predict potential and probable outcomes.

Illness trajectories seldom take into account the psychological aspects of a disease, because psychological adaptation is usually an individual variable in the disease. As more clients live with illness, the quality of life must become an essential aspect of any disease trajectory.

With the ongoing development and refinement of equipment and medications, the traditional disease trajectories have had to be redefined. An example of a redefined trajectory is found in the client with end-stage renal disease. In the past, clients with end-stage renal disease would have died, but today these clients live through the use of dialysis and renal transplantation. Because dialysis keeps clients with end-stage renal disease alive but does not cure them, they face an ongoing battle of dialysis versus dying and transplant versus rejection.

Compounding the issue for the client are the medical opinions. Surgeons advocate transplants, arguing that they free the client from dialysis machines. Nephrologists advocate dialysis, pointing out the number of transplant rejections. Figure 1–1 is a trajectory of the physician's view of end-stage renal disease. Figure 1–2 represents the client's view of the same illness. The difference in concerns is obvious.

A trajectory can be used to plan and intervene to shape the course of any illness. With chronic illness, these tasks may go on at home or in the hospital. Once a trajectory for a client is written out, it should be a part of the client's permanent record to provide continuity of care.

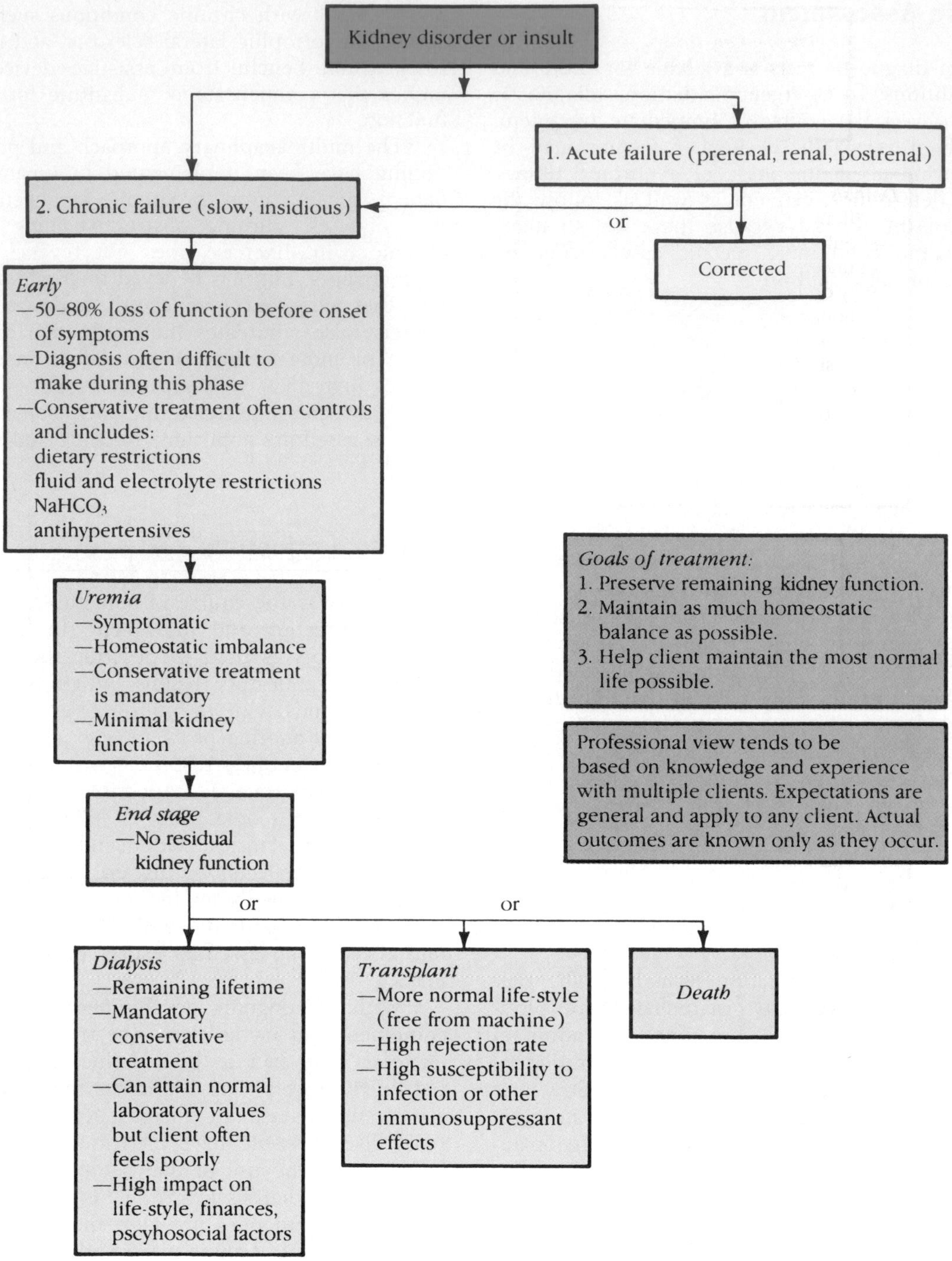

Figure 1–1
Trajectory: Professional perception of renal failure. (From Lubkin, I. [1990]. *Chronic illness:* Impact and interventions [2nd ed.]. Boston: Jones and Bartlett Publishers.)

Nursing Management

Assessment

Because illness has a tremendous impact on the client and significant others, a complete assessment should be performed in the physical, psychological, and sociologic realms of function. With acute conditions, a cure may be expected. In the event of complications or pre-existing conditions, a cure may not be realized or may be delayed.

CRITICAL TO REMEMBER

The focus of assessment for a client with a chronic condition is the client's adaptation to the condition.

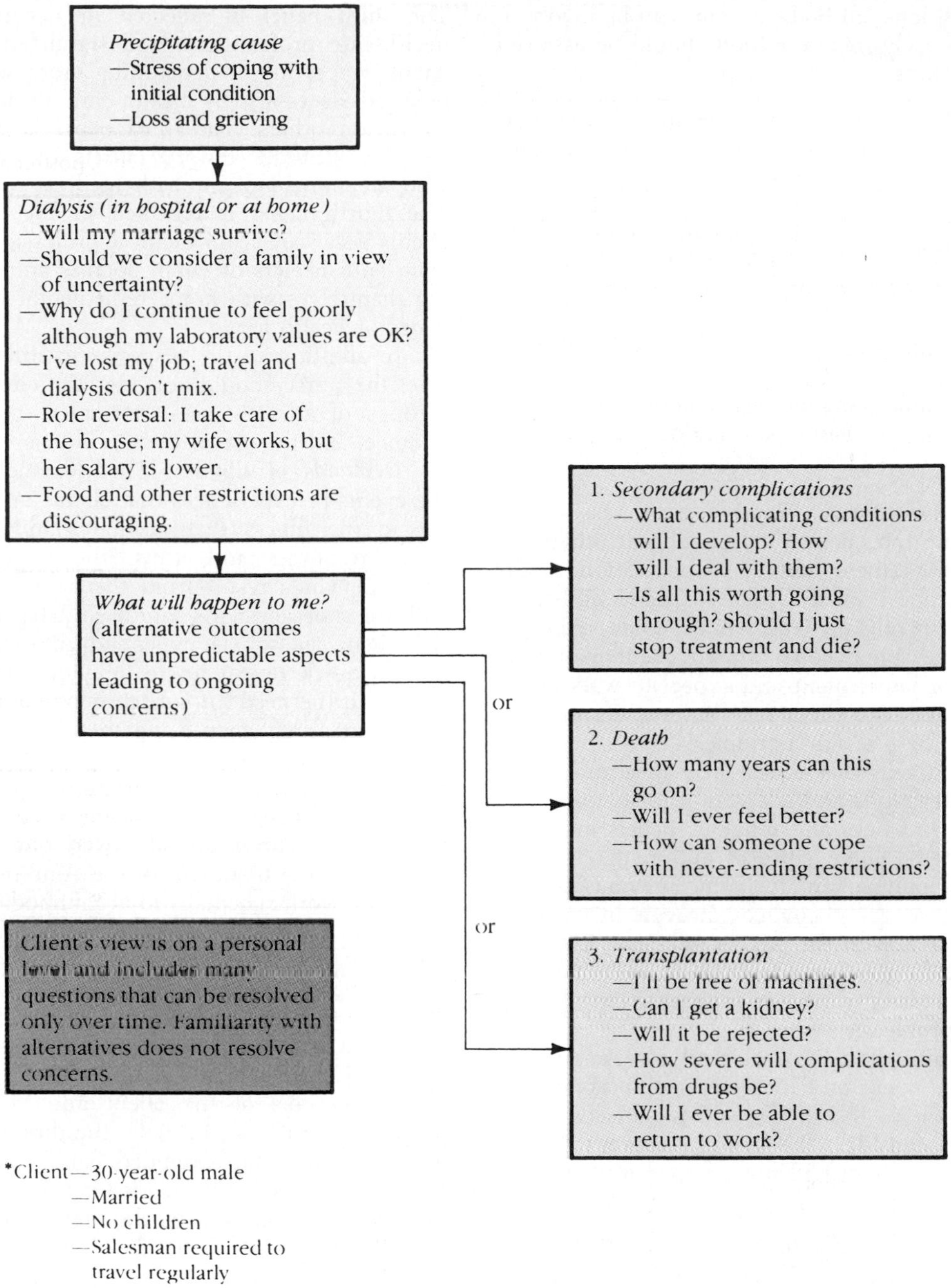
Precipitating cause
—Stress of coping with initial condition
—Loss and grieving
Dialysis (in hospital or at home)
—Will my marriage survive?
—Should we consider a family in view of uncertainty?
—Why do I continue to feel poorly although my laboratory values are OK?
—I've lost my job; travel and dialysis don't mix.
—Role reversal: I take care of the house; my wife works, but her salary is lower.
—Food and other restrictions are discouraging.
What will happen to me? (alternative outcomes have unpredictable aspects leading to ongoing concerns)
or
or
1. Secondary complications
—What complicating conditions will I develop? How will I deal with them?
—Is all this worth going through? Should I just stop treatment and die?
2. Death
—How many years can this go on?
—Will I ever feel better?
—How can someone cope with never-ending restrictions?
3. Transplantation
—I'll be free of machines.
—Can I get a kidney?
—Will it be rejected?
—How severe will complications from drugs be?
—Will I ever be able to return to work?
Client's view is on a personal level and includes many questions that can be resolved only over time. Familiarity with alternatives does not resolve concerns.
*Client—30-year-old male
—Married
—No children
—Salesman required to travel regularly

Figure 1–2
Trajectory: A client's perception of renal failure. The client is a 30-year-old man who is married and has no children. He is a salesman and is required to travel regularly. (From Lubkin, I. [1990]. *Chronic illness:* Impact and interventions [2nd ed.]. Boston: Jones and Bartlett Publishers.)

Physical Assessment: The acutely ill client should be assessed in the following spheres:

- Physical condition—a review of body systems to determine current function levels as well as the impact of the acute illness
- Psychological status—mental and emotional status and response to illness
- Pain—onset, duration, location, type (e.g., referred, constant, burning, sharp), how it is relieved, and history of previous occurrence
- Airway—patency, whether air exchange is occurring
- Breathing—rate, depth, and difficulty of breathing; lung sounds; position; and use of oxygen therapy
- Circulation—blood pressure, pulse, presence of blood and breaks in the skin, temperature and color of the skin, capillary refill, and use of anticoagulants
- Level of consciousness—pupils (equality, dilation, constriction); response to pain; alertness; orientation to person, place, and time; response to requests

Because many physical conditions can become or lead

to chronic conditions, all body systems can be involved. The client with a chronic condition should be assessed in six different areas:

- Physical condition—disorders of cardiovascular, pulmonary, gastrointestinal, skin, and endocrine systems; include usual medications used
- Mobility—structure and function of the upper and lower extremities and spine; include mobility and support devices used (e.g., wheelchair)
- Sensory limitations—speech, vision, and hearing limitations
- Renal and gastrointestinal function—bowel and bladder control
- Psychological status—mental and emotional status
- Basic functioning—ability to conduct activities of daily living

Psychological Assessment: Psychological assessment should determine the client's and significant others' attitude toward the illness, degree of adaptation to the illness, and attitude toward recovery. Clients and families may have unrealistic expectations about recovery. For example, the spinal cord–injured client may deny the extent of the impairment and expect to walk again. On the other hand, the client may become despondent, saying, "What's the use, I'm a cripple."

Cultural and religious beliefs may have an impact on the client's reactions and adaptation to the illness. A client's cultural practices and religious beliefs may be a source of strength. Some cultures and religions teach that illness is a punishment for some previous wrongdoing. In that case, the client may struggle in trying to discover which action in the past is to blame. Likewise, guilt may result from being unable to work (in cultures in which work equals worth) or from searching for the reason for the problem.

When performing a psychological assessment, the nurse must be open and nonjudgmental about the client's perception of the illness and process of recovery. If the nurse considers the client's reaction to illness wrong or silly, the client will not be open to discussing his or her true feelings.

Sociologic Assessment: Sociologic assessment considers the degree of impact the condition has on health and illness roles.

Sick Role Expectations. Medical sociologist Talcott Parsons identified four beliefs and expectations about behaviors appropriate for ill persons that have been dominant in our society and among health-care professionals. The four beliefs of "Parson's sick role model" are that the individual (1) is not responsible for his or her illness, (2) is to be released from usual role responsibilities, (3) should view illness as undesirable and try to get well, and (4) should seek medically competent help.

The first belief is reflected in professional literature that refers to clients as victims of various chronic conditions, such as cancer, stroke, Alzheimer's disease, and heart attacks. The second belief is reflected in others' assuming responsibility for personal, family, and social activities that the client is capable of doing or learning. The third belief is reflected in negative attitudes of health-care professionals and significant others toward clients' expecting or demanding more assistance than is believed necessary by health-care professionals or the significant others. The third belief is also reflected in negative attitudes toward clients or significant others who are noncompliant with medical recommendations. The fourth belief is reflected in the expectation that clients seek care from medical professionals rather than from faith healers or witch doctors and instead of treating themselves with home remedies or over-the-counter drugs or health foods.

In addition to the response to illness and the sick role, the nurse should consider the client's response to feelings of attractiveness, normalcy, productivity, self-reliance, and the use of community services.

Demands of Illness. The demands of illness are the events or experiences that clients and families attribute to the illness that tax the family's personal and social resources and, thus, the family's well-being.[9] Some demands result from the acuity of the situation and are short-term. As family and friends rally around the client, energy is expended in expectation of the client's quick return to the previous level of functioning. With the need for subacute care, a prolonged series of demands may ensue, and the client may or may not return to a previous level of functioning. As the illness progresses to a chronic condition, the roles of family and friends change as they begin to come to terms with caring for a chronically ill loved one. Some demands result from the treatment of the condition, for example, changing work schedules to accommodate treatments or the client's loss of strength due to side effects of the treatment. Likewise, the roles of the client may have to be assumed by other family members or friends. If the client is the breadwinner of the family, the tasks of earning a living will have to be assumed by another person. The demands of the illness are also affected by the perceptions of the client and family during the course of the illness. Initially, the illness may generate a lot of support from extended family members, because they can be freed from work for a few days. But as the disease process continues, the members may be difficult to call on because demands of work and family have drawn them back home. This puts all of the responsibilities on the immediate family and may create a temporary crisis until new support networks can be arranged.

Assessment Tools: Assessment tools that have been found to yield reliable data about the functional abilities of clients with chronic conditions are described in Table 1–4. The Barthel Index and the Rancho Los Amigos scale are commonly used in rehabilitation centers to quantify functional gains during the acute rehabilitation phase of recovery. The Functional Independence Measure is a more recently devised instrument that is gaining acceptance.

These assessment tools can be used to quantify physical or cognitive abilities of clients in other settings. For example, the Rancho Los Amigos scale (Table 1–5) would be useful for quantifying changes in cogni-

TABLE 1–4 Assessment Tools

Physical Function	
Barthel Index	Nine categories: feeding, transfers, grooming, toileting, bathing, walking, climbing stairs, bowel and bladder control
PULSES	Six categories: *P*resence of medical conditions, *U*pper extremity (self-care), *L*ower extremity (walking), *S*ensory, *E*limination (bowel and bladder control), *S*ocialization
Index of Activities of Daily Living (ADL)	Six categories: bed activities, transfers, hygiene, dressing, feeding, and locomotion
Functional Independence Measure (FIM)	Eighteen categories: eating, bathing, grooming, dressing–upper body, dressing–lower body, toileting, bladder management, bowel management, transfers bed, chair, wheelchair, transfers–toilet, transfers–tub or shower, locomotion–stairs, locomotion–walk/wheelchair, comprehension, expression, social interaction, problem solving, memory
Cognitive Function	
Rancho Los Amigos	Eight levels of responses: none, generalized, localized, confused-agitated, confused-inappropriate, confused-appropriate, automatic-appropriate, purposeful-appropriate
Pain	
McGill Pain Questionnaire	Comprehensive and modified versions. Modified—20 sets of sensory, affective, evaluative, and miscellaneous descriptors of pain. Includes pain intensity scale and body location of pain
Visual Analog Scales	Numbers of faces for rating intensity of pain
Coping	
Ways of Coping Scale	Fifty cognitive and behavioral strategies used in managing distress
Jaloweic Coping Scale	Forty coping behaviors used to manage distress, rated according to helpfulness

tive functioning evidenced by clients experiencing acute or chronic conditions that alter brain function. Levels of cognitive functioning on the scale are based on clinical observations of physical and cognitive behaviors evidenced by clients during recovery from severe head trauma. The scale contains indicators of changing abilities related to taking in, processing, and responding to information.

Nursing Diagnosis

Physiologic: Nursing diagnoses common to clients with acute conditions are associated with stabilizing and monitoring functions. The nursing diagnoses are related to any combination of factors such as age, extent of trauma or acute illness, pre-existing conditions, and the present health status of the individual. Common nursing diagnoses include

TABLE 1–5 Rancho Los Amigos Hospital: Scale of Cognitive Functioning

LEVEL OF RESPONSE	BEHAVIOR
I None	Unresponsive to auditory, visual, or tactile stimuli.
II Generalized	Reacts inconsistently and nonpurposefully to stimuli. Delayed and limited responses.
III Localized	Reacts specifically but inconsistently to stimuli. Responses are related to type of stimuli presented, such as visually focusing on an object or responding to sounds.
IV Confused-agitated	Extremely agitated and in a high state of confusion. Nonpurposeful and aggressive behavior. Unable to cooperate fully with treatments owing to short attention span. Requires maximal assistance with self-care.
V Confused-inappropriate, nonagitated	Alert and can respond to simple commands on a more consistent basis. Highly distractible. Needs constant cuing to attend to an activity. Memory is impaired, with confusion regarding past and present. Can perform self-care activities with assistance. May wander and needs to be watched carefully.
VI Confused-appropriate	Shows goal-directed behavior, but still needs direction. Follows simple tasks consistently, and shows carry-over for relearned tasks. More aware of own deficits and of self, family, and basic needs.
VII Automatic-appropriate	Appears oriented in home and hospital and goes through daily routine automatically. Shows carry-over for new learning, but still requires structure and supervision to ensure safety and good judgment. Able to initiate tasks in which he or she has an interest.
VIII Purposeful-appropriate	Totally alert and oriented and shows good recall of past and recent events. Independent in the home and community.

- Body Temperature, Risk for Altered
- Airway Clearance, Ineffective
- Breathing Pattern, Ineffective
- Cardiac Output, Decreased
- Confusion, Acute
- Aspiration, Risk for
- Fluid Volume Deficit or Excess
- Gas Exchange, Impaired
- Pain
- Infection, Risk for

A number of physiologic nursing diagnoses are commonly associated with a variety of chronic conditions and the medications and treatments used in managing these conditions. Owing to the great number of chronic conditions, many related factors contribute to the diagnoses. These factors include age, type and degree of irreversible change in physiologic structure or function, type of treatment, and degree of physiologic adaptation. Nursing diagnoses of a physiologic nature common to several types of chronic conditions include

- Activity Intolerance
- Disuse Syndrome, Risk for
- Fatigue
- Fluid Volume Deficit or Excess
- Health Maintenance, Altered
- Infection, Risk for
- Injury, Risk for
- Nutrition, Altered, Less than or More than Body Requirements
- Pain, Chronic
- Physical Mobility, Impaired
- Self-Care Deficit
- Thought Processes, Altered
- Urinary Elimination, Altered

Psychological: Nursing diagnoses of a psychological nature for the acutely ill individual may include

- Anxiety
- Denial, Ineffective
- Fear

Nursing diagnoses for the chronically ill client may include

- Anxiety
- Body Image Disturbance
- Diversional Activity Deficit
- Fear
- Grieving, Anticipatory and Dysfunctional
- Growth and Development, Altered
- Hopelessness
- Knowledge Deficit
- Powerlessness
- Self-Esteem Disturbance
- Spiritual Distress

Sociologic: Potential nursing diagnoses of a sociologic nature commonly associated with acute and chronic conditions include

- Communication, Impaired Verbal
- Diversional Activity Deficit
- Family Processes, Altered
- Parenting, Altered
- Powerlessness
- Role Performance, Altered
- Sexuality Patterns, Altered
- Social Interaction, Impaired
- Social Isolation

Planning: Expected Outcomes

The expected outcomes for the client are directly related to the specific diagnosis. When a cure and return to function are expected, the goals will be short-term ones. Outcomes will reflect the client's ability to return to the previous level of function. In general, when a cure is not expected, the client should be assisted to adapt to the condition. The client and family or care giver may need to be educated in order to control the condition and adapt to the change in roles. Long-term expected outcomes are usually written with months allowed for achievement.

Nursing Intervention

Interventions for the client with an acute condition require the response of a team of health-care providers until the client's condition is stabilized. Collaboration among health-care givers is important to the care planned, for example, when the client is on a clinical pathway.

Interventions for the client with a chronic illness vary depending on the disorders the client is experiencing. Many times, interventions are collaborative among all health-care providers. Regardless of the disorders the client has, there are some general tasks that the client must accomplish. Client education plans should center on these tasks. (See Client Education Guide.) In addition, the client needs to learn to adapt to the illness.

Promoting Physical Adaptation: The client's adaptation to illness can be improved by changing medications, dosages or schedules, diet, and activity patterns. Identifying environmental or behavioral factors that exacerbate symptoms or reduce sleep can also increase feelings of wellness. Early detection of clinical manifestations of complications is also part of physical adaptation.

Promoting Psychological Adaptation: Interventions to enhance psychological adaptation during the onset or diagnostic phase include encouraging the client's active involvement in the diagnostic process and treatment decisions (see Ethical Issues in Nursing), facilitating expressions of feelings, and providing or helping clients seek appropriate information. Hospitalization during a chronic condition may be perceived as a crisis episode by some clients. Other clients may view hospitalization during this phase as a reprieve from day-to-day hassles and concerns or as a period of hope. In the terminal phase of illness, one client may fear death and another client may view death as a preferred alternative to suffering and disability. Personal factors that are believed to contribute to the individual nature of psychological adaptation include hope, commitment, learned helplessness, appraisals of change, and personal and social re-

CLIENT EDUCATION GUIDE

Components of a Client Education Plan

PREVENTING AND MANAGING A MEDICAL CRISIS

Most chronic illnesses exist in a balance of control and crisis. The client needs to know the clinical indications that the disorder is becoming out of control, what to do to treat it, and when to notify the physician. For example, the diabetic client needs to recognize hyperglycemia and hypoglycemia, begin treatment, and determine when to notify the physician. The client needs to learn to plan for these crises. The diabetic client should carry a blood glucose assessment device, sugar, and insulin at all times. Likewise, the asthmatic client should carry a bronchodilator, and the client with angina should carry nitroglycerin.

MANAGING TREATMENT REGIMENS

Most chronic illnesses require some degree of daily treatment. These treatments can range from taking one pill a day, to giving injections, to running a home dialysis unit. The ability of the client and family to follow the treatment should be assessed using the following guidelines:

1. Degree of difficulty in learning to follow the regimen. Are there several steps involved? Are there potential complications that may result from not using the equipment correctly? How much manual dexterity is required?
2. Amount of time required to implement the regimen. Does the activity require several hours or just a few minutes? How many times a day does the activity have to be performed?
3. Amount of discomfort and energy associated with the regimen. If the treatment is painful, will the client comply and will the family member be persuasive enough to have the client complete the treatment?
4. Visibility of the regimen to other people, and social acceptability of the disease regimen. If the equipment must be brought with the client (e.g., oxygen), social isolation may occur. If there has been a physical alteration, such as a tracheostomy or fistula, the client may be shunned by the public.
5. Effectiveness and speed of the regimen in treating the disorder or controlling symptoms. Some clients will follow a treatment regimen if progress can be seen, and others will stop the regimen once symptoms abate.

From these data, a teaching plan can be developed. The use of visiting nurses to monitor progress and assist with financial concerns should be considered.

CONTROLLING SYMPTOMS

Clients must learn to control symptoms so that they can participate in desired activities. Some clients can plan ahead so that needed items are available, such as buying adequate supplies before leaving on a trip. In addition, the client must carry needed supplies on an airplane rather than check them with the luggage, in the event that the luggage is lost. Likewise, some clients require special equipment to perform usual activities. The client with arthritis may benefit by using Velcro closures rather than zippers or buttons.

REORDERING OF TIME

Some clients with chronic conditions have too much time or too little time. For example, clients forced into retirement because of a chronic condition may have too much time on their hands. In contrast, the client who spends hours each day conducting or undergoing the medical regimen may have very little time left to enjoy life. The client needs to be assisted to have the amount of free time desired to enjoy a high-quality life. Sometimes, a hobby or support group will help build supports and new interests. Examining the protocol used by the client in performing medical regimens may illuminate some areas in which time is wasted in the procedure, thereby freeing up time.

ADJUSTING TO CHANGES IN THE COURSE OF THE DISORDER

Some disorders have a stable course and others are very unpredictable. For example, chronic ulcerative colitis is usually quite stable, with predictable flare-ups, whereas multiple sclerosis is an erratic disorder. The client and family need to be taught the disease's trajectory and encouraged to be aware of probable changes. For example, depression is very common 4 to 6 months following stroke. The client and family need to be warned of the symptoms and taught management strategies.

PREVENTING SOCIAL ISOLATION

Because of the stigma of chronic disorders, the client and family may find it easier to withdraw from society than to face it. The nurse should prepare the client and family by easing adjustment back into society while in the hospital, especially when there is visible deformity, such as burn scars. The client should be encouraged to interact with society while in the hospital. Taking a trip to the gift shop or lobby will allow the client to experience some common reactions, such as staring. Then when the client returns, the feelings can be discussed with the nurse.

ATTEMPTING TO NORMALIZE RELATIONS WITH OTHERS

Clients should be encouraged not to become socially isolated but to normalize their lives and resume activities with others. Clients with visible deformity can often disguise the problem with scarves or makeup. Likewise, clients with dyspnea can disguise the fact that they are stopping to catch a breath while they look in a store window.

Some conditions cannot be disguised, and the client should be prepared for stares and comments by strangers. Eventually, the client becomes desensitized to these remarks and goes about his or her life.

ETHICAL ISSUES IN NURSING

Who Should Make Decisions for Clients?

Caring for clients who have chronic illnesses can be very challenging for nurses. Nurses are called on to deliver many aspects of care to these clients, including helping ease the pain of the illness, listening to clients' expressions of their feelings about their illnesses, assisting in the technological care of their disease process (e.g., dressing changes, tube feedings, intravenous infusions), and perhaps helping clients work through their decisions about treatment options. Clients who are in the chronic stages of their illness may come to rely on nurses for care that may go beyond the realm of nursing practice. When decisions become overwhelming, clients might prefer that their health-care providers make all the health-care decisions for them. On the other hand, are health-care decisions ever made for clients with chronic conditions without their input or consent simply because the client is thought to be unable to make the best choices for himself or herself?

There are three ethical principles involved here, the first being autonomy. All clients who are competent have the right to decide what medical treatments they want or do not want. Chronic illness may cause a client to become incompetent, but each client should be assessed carefully before it is decided that he or she is truly not competent. Chronic illness is not always followed by incompetence.

The second and third principles, beneficence and paternalism, are closely related. Nurses act beneficently in many ways; that is, they perform activities that benefit the client, but these actions are not seen as taking away a client's autonomy. For example, crushing a pill for a client who has dysphagia and cannot crush his or her own medications is of benefit to the client but is hardly seen as a dilemma regarding autonomy. On the other hand, paternalism in its extreme form allows health-care providers to make decisions for their clients, on their behalf, without their input.

It is sometimes the wish of a client that the nurse or doctor make decisions for him or her. Perhaps the client feels overwhelmed and simply does not know what to do, or perhaps the client feels that a nurse or doctor would make a better decision on his or her behalf. Is this any reason to act out of extreme paternalism? Clients with chronic illnesses are probably more vulnerable when it comes to making health-care decisions. Nurses should be aware of this so that they do not exercise extreme paternalism when beneficence may be more appropriate. Clients should always be allowed to make their own informed decisions. Nurses may be able to help clients gain the knowledge they need in order to do so, which is a very important act of beneficence.

sources and coping strategies. Appraisals of change are based on an individual's given set of beliefs, commitments, knowledge and skills, previous losses, and threat of loss with this crisis. The ability to manage loss, the threat of loss, or challenge also differs among individuals.

Promoting Sociologic Adaptation: Interventions that promote sociologic adaptation include referral to community resources or organizations for vocational rehabilitation and job skills training. Interventions that foster and support role changes include role playing of anticipated situations; imaginative role taking, in which the individual imagines how another person would respond to behaviors; and role modeling, in which the individual is introduced to another person who has the same condition and has positively adapted to changes presented. With the use of role modeling, the individual may gain practical tips about hunting for a job, finding accessible housing, and meeting new friends.

Role clarification is a strategy in which the individual is provided with information about behaviors necessary to accomplish a particular role. Reference group interaction is a strategy in which support groups with similar problems and concerns are found. These groups are helpful for exchanging ideas for solving problems.

Evaluation

The degree of goal attainment should be examined at regular intervals. The expected outcomes for clients with acute illness may be obtained in a short while; if the client experiences complications or the condition becomes chronic, expected outcomes may be obtained over a longer period of time. With chronic conditions, the expected outcomes are obtained over the long term, and evaluation may be used as a formal process to examine outcome achievement and movement to another level of care within a rehabilitation center. For example, the client may no longer require complete care for activities of daily living and can be moved to a less skilled area of the hospital or center. Of course, the goal may not have been met, in which case the cause should be determined, keeping in mind that the condition may have become exacerbated and the expected outcomes and interventions may require revision.

STUDY QUESTIONS

1. Which of the following areas of assessment should be included in a physical assessment of a client with a chronic condition?
   A. Basic ability to function
   B. Attitude toward condition
   C. Degree of impact of condition on health and illness role
   D. Cultural-economic status

2. Which of the following statements indicates a functional orientation to health?
   A. "I have to see my physician every 6 months for a check-up because of my high blood pressure."
   B. "I think I have hypertension, but I'm taking care of things right now. I'll go to the doctor when it gets worse."
   C. "I take several medications for my hypertension. I follow the doctor's instructions to the letter."
   D. "I believe in doing exactly what the doctor tells me. After all, we are partners in my health care."

3. Which of the following responses is an adaptive response for a client who has just learned he has diabetes?
   A. "Is it really diabetes? Couldn't it be the cola I drank before I had the blood test?"
   B. "Why me? I am a good person who never hurt anyone."
   C. "I realize that I'll have to make some changes in my life."
   D. "I can't bear to live with diabetes!"

4. An 80-year-old client has been managing declining eyesight and hearing for several years. For the last several months she has had an exacerbation of osteoarthritis. She is no longer able to bathe herself independently. The most appropriate nursing diagnosis for this client would be:
   A. Health Maintenance, Altered R/T immobility
   B. Injury, Risk for R/T immobility
   C. Self-Care Deficit: Bathing R/T inability to handle washing implements
   D. Physical Mobility, Impaired R/T osteoarthritis

5. Which of the following statements from the wife of a man who has a chronic condition indicates that her husband has successfully adjusted to his condition and thus achieved the stated outcome criteria?
   A. "Harry has decided it's best to withdraw from all his former social engagements."
   B. "Harry has begun to rejoin his buddies in many of his social activities. He says that nothing has changed. His illness is cured."
   C. "Harry has rejoined the activities that required less physical activity. He says that he'll join others as his strength improves."
   D. "Harry and I are keeping to ourselves. We need to realize nothing will remain the same. We are different people now."

CRITICAL THINKING EXERCISES

SCENARIO A

A 20-year-old Hispanic woman with severe diabetes mellitus has been able to manage her condition successfully with insulin, diet, and exercise for the past 10 years. Last month she learned she had hypertension that must be treated with medications. She tells the nurse she is not willing to "keep track" of more medications. "Insulin," she says, 'is enough to manage."

1. What behaviors would you expect her to demonstrate, given her present feelings concerning the latest regimen that has been added to her life?
2. How would her culture and age affect her acceptance of the new regimen?
3. How should the nurse proceed to help this client begin to accept her role in managing the new regimen?

SCENARIO B

An elderly man has had severe arthritis for 20 years. He tells the nurse that he will only get worse, so why should he try to continue to care for himself?

1. How would your value system influence your response?
2. Once you have examined your value system, how would you respond to his statement?

BIBLIOGRAPHY

1. Braden, B. J. (1992). Description of learned response to chronic illness: Depressed versus nondepressed self-help class participants. *Public Health Nursing, 9(2),* 103–108.
2. Bronstein, K. S., et al. (1991). *Promoting stroke recovery*. St. Louis: C.V. Mosby Co.
3. Burns, J. (1993). Subacute care feeds need to diversify. *Modern Healthcare, 23(50),* 34–36, 38.
4. Butcher, L. A. (1994). A family-focused perspective on chronic care. *Rehabilitation Nursing, 19(2),* 70–74, 126.
5. Cameron, K., & Gregor, F. (1987). Chronic illness and compliance. *Journal of Advanced Nursing,* 12, 671–676.
6. Cohen, M. H. (1993). The unknown and the unknowable: Managing sustained uncertainty. *Western Journal of Nursing Research, 15,* 77–96.
7. Douard, J. (1991). Chronic illness: A problem of passive injustice. *Journal of Clinical Ethics, 2(3),* 153–156.
8. Folkman, S., & Lazarus, R. (1988). Coping as a mediator of emotions. *Journal of Personality and Social Psychology, 54(3),* 466–471.
9. Fugate-Woods, N., et al. (1989). Supporting families during chronic illness. *IMAGE: The Journal of Nursing Scholarship, 21(1),* 46–50.
10. Gass, K. (1987). The health of conjugally bereaved older widows: The role of appraisal, coping and resources. *Research in Nursing and Health, 10(1),* 29–47.
11. Granger, C. V., et al. (1993). Performance profiles of the Functional Independence Measure. *Journal of Physical Medicine Rehabilitation, 72,* 84–89.

12. Gurkles, J., & Menks, E. (1988). Identification of stressors and use of coping methods in chronic hemodialysis patients. *Nursing Research, 37(4),* 236–239.

13. Institute of Medicine. (1990). *The second fifty years: Promoting health and preventing disability.* Washington, DC: National Academy Press.

14. Kaufman, J., Fox, R., & Swearengen, P. (1990). How a support group can help your chronically ill patient. *Nursing 90, 20(10),* 65–66.

15. Kirk, K. (1992). Confidence as a factor in chronic illness care. *Journal of Advanced Nursing, 17,* 1238–1242.

16. Lambert, C., et al. (1989). Social support, hardiness and psychological well being in women with arthritis. *Image, 21(3),* 128–131.

17. Lancaster, L. (1988). Impact of chronic illness over the life span. *American Nephrology Nurses Association Journal, 15(3),* 164–168.

18. Leidy, N., et al. (1990). Psychophysiological processes of stress in chronic physical illness: A theoretical perspective. *Journal of Advanced Nursing, 13,* 478–486.

19. Loomis, M., & Conco, D. (1991). Patients' perceptions of health, chronic illness, and nursing diagnoses. *Nursing Diagnoses, 2(4),* 162–170.

20. Miller, J. M. (1991). *Coping with chronic illness: Overcoming powerlessness,* 2nd ed., Philadelphia: F. A. Davis.

21. Miller, P., Sr., et al. (1990). Stressors and stress management one month after myocardial infarction. *Rehabilitation Nursing, 15(6),* 306–310.

22. Murray, R., & Zentner, J. (1993). *Nursing assessment and health promotion: Strategies through the life span* (5th ed.) Norwalk: Appleton & Lange.

23. Radziewicz, R. M., & Schneider, S. M. (1992). Using diversional activity to enhance coping. *Cancer Nursing, 15(4),* 293–298.

24. Raleigh, E. D. H. (1992). Sources of hope in chronic illness. *Oncology Nursing Forum, 19,* 443–448.

25. Robinson, L. A., et al. (1993). Operationalizing the Corbin & Strauss Trajectory Model for elderly clients with chronic illness. Including commentary by Corbin, J. M. *Scholarly Inquiry for Nursing Practice, 7(4),* 253–268.

26. Rolland, J. (1987). Chronic illness and the life cycle: A conceptual framework. *Family Process, 26,* 203–221.

27. Schneider, E. L. & Guralnick, J. M. (1990). The aging of America: Impact on health care costs. *JAMA, 263,* 2335–2340.

28. Schumacher, K. L., & Meleis, A. I. (1994). Transitions: A central concept in nursing. *IMAGE: Journal of Nursing Scholarship, 26(2),* 119–127.

29. Stahl, D. A. (1995). Managed care and subacute care: A partnership of choice. *Nursing Management, 26(1),* 17–19.

30. State University of New York Research Foundation. (1990). *Functional Independence Measure.* Buffalo, NY: State University of New York.

31. Sutton, T., & Murphy, S. (1989). Stressors and patterns of coping in renal transplant patients. *Nursing Research, 38(1),* 46–49.

32. Weeks, S. K., & O'Connor, P. C. (1994). Concept analysis of family + health = a new definition of family health. *Rehabilitation Nursing, 19(4),* 207–210, 258.

Chapter 2 Health-Care Delivery

Learning Outcomes

After completing this chapter, the learner will be able to:

1. Teach a client about the various modes of health-care delivery.
2. Discuss societal changes that have an impact on health care.
3. Explain aspects of health-care reform that affect health-care delivery.
4. Discuss steps that the health-care industry is taking to assure quality care.

In the United States today, we are seeing rapid change from a costly, cumbersome system of health-care delivery to a more streamlined system designed to contain and even cut costs while still providing high-quality care. Hospitals and the various other institutions that provide health-care services are carefully evaluating and refining these services in an effort to make the best use of staff, offer high-quality yet cost-effective care, provide a "seamless" system of care that extends across the health-illness continuum, and better educate clients, their families and significant others and the general public about healthy living.

The ever-present need for more cost-efficient care is spurring a shift toward a consumer-driven health-care delivery system. In this evolving system, health-care institutions and individual providers are taking a more active role in providing the health education and prevention services needed by individuals and families, while at the same time, consumers are taking a more active part in personal health care and accepting more responsibility for learning about health maintenance and illness prevention. This "partnership" should result in more efficient and economical health care.

The costs of health care have not always been controlled in a responsible manner. Today, although no definite plan for reform has yet been adopted or implemented, constraints on payment for health care are causing health-care institutions, insurers, employers, and potential consumers to rethink their responsibilities and to develop alternative approaches.

HEALTH-CARE DELIVERY MODES

Health care encompasses three primary aspects: the prevention of illness, the promotion and maintenance of health, and the restoration of health when illness occurs (Box 2–1). Traditionally, health care has been delivered primarily through acute care hospital and physician (individual or partnership) services (Box 2–2). A client who becomes acutely ill, is a victim of trauma, or experiences an exacerbation of a chronic illness needs acute care in a hospital setting. Acute care is high-cost care that relies on advanced technology and the expertise of highly trained caregivers to stabilize the client and prepare him or her for the eventual transition to a less costly health-care setting.

Driven by financial pressures and social changes, our health-care system is in the midst of evolving from a hospital-based system to an interconnecting web of facilities and services designed to care for clients in the most cost-effective manner possible. Nurses and other health-care providers are experiencing dramatic changes in their duties as the focus shifts from traditional acute care settings to new and not-so-new alternative care settings, including:

- Subacute care
- Outpatient services
- Home health care
- Hospice care
- Nurse-managed clinics
- Case management

BOX 2–1

Aspects of Health Care

Health Promotion. Assists the client to remain healthy and prevent illness while promoting a healthier life-style. Health promotion attempts to prevent the development of risk factors that may cause disease and illness. Active client participation is required.

Illness Prevention. Assists the client in reducing the consequences of risk when these are identified. Active client participation is required.

Diagnosis and Treatment. A traditional service with the purpose of detecting and treating disease once it occurs.

Rehabilitation. Restores the client to the highest level of function possible after an illness or injury. Active participation is required of the client and significant others.

BOX 2–2

Comparison of Traditional and Emerging Health-Care Services

TRADITIONAL HEALTH-CARE SERVICES	EMERGING HEALTH-CARE SERVICES
Emphasis on diagnosis and treatment of illness	Emphasis on health promotion and illness prevention
Care Settings • Acute care • Some subacute care	**Care Settings** • Subacute care • Long-term care • Rehabilitation centers • Ambulatory care • Outpatient settings (surgicenters, community clinics, etc.) • Home care
Expects passive client participation	Requires active client (and in some cases, family member) participation; client education is a hallmark

Subacute Care

As defined by the Joint Commission for Accreditation of Healthcare Organizations (JCAHO), *subacute care* is "comprehensive inpatient care designed for someone who has had an acute illness, injury, or exacerbation of a disease process. It is goal-oriented treatment rendered immediately after or instead of acute hospitalization to treat one or more specific, active complex medical conditions or to administer one or more technically complex medical treatments, in the context of a person's underlying long-term conditions and overall situation."[5]

Subacute care is generally more intensive than traditional nursing home facility care and less intensive than acute care. Like acute care, subacute care is outcome-focused and multidisciplinary and delivers complex clinical intervention through efficient and effective use of resources. Standards for subacute care delineate nursing hours per client day and average length of stay into one of four categories: transitional, general medical-surgical, chronic, or long-term transitional subacute.[5]

Skilled nursing facilities (SNFs) originally offered nursing care for chronically ill adults who could no longer care for themselves or had no family members who could provide the needed care. In recent years, SNFs have developed and implemented the subacute care model, which is now one of the fastest-growing health care services.

Subacute care services take over when the client no longer needs acute, highly technical care. Because highly trained, specialized nurses are not needed in the subacute area, the cost of care decreases. Thus, reimbursement is more easily obtained for this level of care. For this reason, many hospitals are augmenting their physical environment on a unit to meet the requirements for subacute care and are transferring clients from acute care units to this environment as soon as specific physical criteria are met.

Beds in some hospitals may serve a dual purpose. Generally, all hospital beds are occupied by acutely ill clients. The basic charge for services is essentially the same unless the client is in an intensive care unit. Certain beds are designated as "swing beds" to allow multiple uses within guidelines for levels of care. For example, a bed may be occupied by an acutely ill client for a number of days. As the client recuperates, he or she may no longer need acute care but is not yet ready to be discharged from the acute care setting. The same bed would then be designated for subacute care for that client. This "dual use" allows acute care hospitals to provide subacute care and to integrate the continuum of care philosophy into their policies and procedures.

The expected boom in subacute care will provide new employment opportunities for nurses and other health-care workers. Consumers, health-care institutions, and insurers can also benefit from this transitional, less costly health-care service.

Home Health Care

Multidisciplinary home health care is not new; rather, it developed in New York in the late 1950s in response to a hospital bed shortage. More recently, home-health-care delivery is expanding once again. Home-health-care agencies provide care to clients recovering from acute episodes of illness as well as to clients in the chronic and terminal phases of chronic illness. The home environment contains fewer microorganisms that can cause infection in a person already affected with an illness. It also promotes comfort through familiarity with people and objects in the home.

Services provided include laboratory monitoring, intravenous therapy for antibiotics and chemotherapy, pump-driven feedings, respiratory support, peritoneal dialysis, physical therapy, parenteral nutrition, and a wide range of nursing services. An important aspect of home health care includes teaching clients and family members about providing care in the home, becoming a part of the multidisciplinary health-care team, and learning to cope with the demands made by having a chronically or terminally ill person in the home.

The ability to handle special equipment and monitors with some degree of confidence contributes to an ultimately lower cost of care in many cases. For example, a client and significant others can actively learn about and control and monitor intravenous fluid administration and gastrostomy tube feedings. Some home health care agencies provide mental health services for chronically mentally ill persons in the home. When problems occur, the client and family contact the home health agency nurse for directions. Personnel from these agencies respond on a 24-hours-per-day, 7-days-per-week basis.

Ambulatory Care

The ambulatory care setting has gained a new importance as the continuum of care is increasingly emphasized. Ambulatory care includes preventive and/or maintenance care provided for clients in clinics and physicians' offices. Hospital clinics (general and specialty services), free-standing emergency services that do not require complex technological resources, and community-based walk-in services constitute this mix.

A great increase has occurred in free-standing outpatient surgery clinics. In these clinics, the client is discharged the same day as surgery (if no complications occur) and then cares for himself or herself or is cared for by a family member or friend in the home. Other emerging ambulatory care settings include medical and dental clinics established to serve the urban homeless population and clinics established in rural areas to serve that population.

Local public health departments may offer well-child care, prenatal care, adult immunizations (influenza and hepatitis B), and care for clients with sexually transmitted diseases, tuberculosis, and acquired immunodeficiency syndrome (AIDS). They may also provide teaching to the public in outreach programs, such as preventing and treating drug and alcohol abuse.

Hospice Care

The first hospice-care program in the United States, modeled after hospice programs in Great Britain, was founded in the late 1960s. Hospice-care programs address the health-care needs of clients in the terminal phase of chronic illness, particularly those expected to live less than 6 months. Some programs are based in acute-care facilities, some are based in long-term care agencies, and others are operated by community groups.

Some are accredited by an outside agency, and others are not. Some are multidisciplinary. Some hospice programs provide service for one type of client, such as programs for terminally ill cancer clients or for clients in the final stages of AIDS. Other programs may accept any client who is terminally ill.

A client accepted into a hospice-care program receives various services designed to make his or her last days comfortable in the company of loved ones and friends. These services include pain control, palliative and supportive care (including personal hygiene and nutritional needs), and supportive care and bereavement care for significant others.

Because hospice clients' illnesses will end in death, hospice staff specialize in working with clients and significant others who are facing death. An important focus is the psychological issues associated with facing one's own and a loved one's mortality. The clients and significant others are counseled about the stages leading to death and all are given support as the illness progresses. Other aspects addressed in a hospice program include care for the caregiver, assistance with financial stressors, spiritual help, and consideration for the individual's cultural diversity. Often the wish to die at home among loved ones with the intention of retaining some element of control over the illness and treatment drives a client to seek hospice care. Care is provided in the home or in a hospice facility with support staff on call to help when immediate concerns or changes in the client's status occur.

Nurse-Managed Clinics

Nurse-managed clinics represent a revival of a concept of care dating back to the early 1900s. Most of these clinics focus on health maintenance. Some address physical and psychosocial needs of clients in the chronic phase of chronic illnesses with less defined treatments, such as multiple sclerosis, myasthenia gravis, and Parkinson's disease. Some offer services on college campuses and in homeless shelters.

Nurse-managed clinics, established and operated by some nursing schools with nurse practitioner certification, provide an excellent venue for nursing students to learn about community-based health-care services. College and university faculty members have set up clinics on or near their campuses as well as in specific areas of need, such as central urban locations and rural areas, to provide services more directly to those in need. Rural nurse practitioners also offer health care services in areas of need.

Nurses who practice in these clinics obtain nursing histories and perform physical assessments for school and work physicals. They also may diagnose minor ailments such as the common cold and throat infection and monitor the progress, treatment, and client's response. The clinics may function with protocols for treatment and care or may enlist physicians for referral services. In some states, nurses with advanced practice credentials earn the privilege of writing certain prescriptions. Unfortunately, lack of consistent reimbursement for these services has limited the growth of this type of care.

Case Management

This health-care delivery mode was expanded in the late 1970s to incorporate concepts of continuity and efficiency in addressing clients' long-term physical, psychological, and social needs. The primary goals of case management are to promote self-care, enhance the quality of life, and use resources efficiently. A health care professional—usually a nurse or a social worker—assesses client needs and monitors the delivery of services. Monitoring may be intermittent or continuous. The *case manager* directly negotiates with the client, significant others, health-care providers, insurance companies, and businesses for needed health and social services.

The case manager is a consultant to clients and significant others, empowering them in planning for and obtaining needed care. This scenario offers an example: A homeless male client consented to enter a free-standing unit created for clients discharged from the acute care setting and in need of placement. The short stay enabled the client to become physically stable, provided counseling and group therapy sessions, and permitted him to see the visiting physician for medical care. The client's basic needs were met by the staff of the free-standing unit while the case manager coordinated the work of the multidisciplinary team—comprising a physician, pharmacist, therapist, registered nurse, psychologist, dietitian, activity coordinator, and social worker—assigned to the client. The client was instructed in hygiene and grooming, the need for a well-balanced diet, the importance of socializing, and how to better cope with stress. The case manager monitored length of stay; arranged for transfer to specialized housing; arranged for personal items such as clothing, a haircut, and dental care; and sought special funds to help the client with personal needs after discharge from the free-standing unit.

Multidisciplinary Care: Clinical Pathways

Health care of the future will be provided by a system known as *managed care*. Managed care encompasses all disciplines that contribute to the health and well-being of clients. The system provides for:

- coordination of health-care services
- incorporation of standards of care
- delineation of expected outcomes of care via predictable lengths of stay
- action for variances in expected outcomes of care
- inclusion of the client and significant others in the process of health care
- incorporation of teaching and health education as part of ongoing health care
- a method to monitor for quality health care

CAROLINAS HEART INSTITUTE
CAROLINAS MEDICAL CENTER
CLINICAL PATH
PTCA

Expected LOS: 2 DRG: 112

	Date: Path Day 1	Date: Path Day 2	Date: Path Day 3/Discharge
Outcomes	Patient receives post PTCA teaching and verbalizes understanding of plan of care. Chest pain absent. Peripheral pulses present. Sheath site free of redness, swelling, or bleeding. Patient hemodynamics WNL.	Chest pain absent. Sheath site free of redness, swelling or bleeding. Peripheral pulses present.	Chest pain absent. No arrhythmias. Sheath site free of redness, or sign of hematoma. Fully ambulatory.
Teaching	Orient to environment. Notify RN of chest pain. Cardiac Risk Factor Class schedule. Instruct pt./family to view "Pt. TV Channel": Cardiac Risk Factors Heart Disease & Diet Cardiac Rehab. Bedrest, leg extended, HOB < 30 degrees.	Instruct regarding bedrest following sheath removal. Instruction in meds: side effects, dose, time, food and drug interactions.	Reinforce med teaching. Groin site care. Signs of complications.
Consults	Dietary: Nurse to write order for RD to assess for post-PTCA teaching. Pt & Family Services, if needed. Pastoral Care, if needed.	Obtain order for MI Rehab Program (MIRP), if indicated. Patient and Family Services, if needed. Pastoral Care, if needed.	Patient and Family Services, if needed. Pastoral care, if needed.
Assess/Tx/Tests	12 Lead EKG post procedure. ACT protocol. Cardiac monitor. I&O Q8H. Check IV site Q1H. VS Q15MIN x 2, then Q30MIN x 4, then Q1H x 2. Sheath with transparent dressing and standard flush infusion. Monitor sheath site and pulses. HOB elevated no more than 30 degrees.	ACT protocol while sheath in. PTT QDAY if remains on Heparin after sheath removal. Cardiac monitor. I&O Q8H. Check IV site Q1H or intermittent device Q8H. Vital signs 0800-1600-2200. Pull sheath by ACT protocol or as ordered. Monitor distal pulses and cath site.	Cardiac monitor. Vital signs 0800-1600-2200. Discontinue intermittent device.
Meds	Heparin drip by ACT protocol or as ordered. IV fluids as ordered. Pain meds. Cardiac meds. ASA, prior to procedure.	Discontinue Heparin. Cardiac meds (po). ASA.	Cardiac meds (po). ASA.
Diet	Heart Disease Preventive Diet (HPDP), or as ordered. Push 1000cc po fluids over 6-8 hours.	HDPD or as ordered.	HDPD or as ordered.
Activity	Bedrest. May immobilize affected limb.	Bedrest 6-12 hours past sheath removal. Activity as tolerated.	Fully ambulatory - able to ambulate 200 ft. prior to discharge.
Spirit/Psy/So	Assess spiritual needs. Provide emotional support. Encourage patient and family to share feelings and expectations.	Assess spiritual needs. Provide emotional support. Encourage patient and family to share feelings and expectations.	Assess spiritual needs. Provide emotional support. Encourage patient and family to share feelings and expectations.
Discharge	Assess discharge needs.	Assess discharge needs. Teach discharge instructions to patient and family.	Ensure patient/family understand meds, diet, activity, food/drug interactions. Return appointment. Groin site care. Review discharge instruction sheet.
Signatures	7-3 3-11 11-7 7A-7P 7P-7A	7-3 3-11 11-7 7A-7P 7P-7A	7-3 3-11 11-7 7A-7P 7P-7A

This clinical path is a suggested guideline of care. The physician may change this plan at any time depending on the patient's individual needs.

c:\123\ptca2.wk4 11/17/94 Revised 10/10/95

Figure 2–1
Sample clinical pathway for a client after percutaneous transluminal coronary angioplasty (PTCA). (Courtesy of Carolinas Medical Center, Charlotte, NC.)

- collective responsibility for providing care
- a contribution to efficient documentation of care rendered

These characteristics are brought together in a tool known as a *clinical pathway* (also called a critical pathway, a care map, or another term specific to the institution developing the tool for its use). Developed by a team of caregivers within a health-care organization, the clinical pathway provides multidisciplinary input in an abbreviated, graphic format (Fig. 2–1). Client needs are addressed in the areas of nutrition, activity and mobility, treatment, diagnostic testing, and teaching. A column for each area shows the provision of care across disciplines and the progression during the client's hospital stay, the length of which is predetermined by the diagnosis on admission. The pathway, which becomes a standard of care protocol, is signed by the physician to cover care after admission.

The caregivers directly involved in the client's care can advance the client along the predetermined pathway without waiting for the physician to issue orders. The pathway also serves as a documentation tool, recording the basic care provided while also allowing for other, more specific documentation as it is needed. A case manager oversees the care provided under a pathway.

A copy of the pathway, with all terms readily understandable by the layperson, is shared with the client and significant others. A health-care professional explains the expectations and teaching that will occur.

If the client does not progress through the pathway as expected, a *variance* occurs. A variance is reported and documented, and the reason it occurred is investigated. A variance may be caused by the client's inability to maintain the expected progress or by a failure within the health-care system. For example, a hospitalized client may develop pneumonia from prolonged inactivity; the variance would prompt attention to the need for collaboration and cooperation to increase the client's activity levels while also treating the pneumonia.

System failure could occur when a change in a piece of equipment or a product used in care produces less than desirable results that increase the client's length of stay. Hospital administration or staff may choose a new product because it is less expensive yet works very much like the older product in use, but the newer product may cause an unexpected variance in a number of clients. This would be discovered through tracking statistics. When such a variance is found, the hospital would revert to using the known product or trying another one in an attempt to hold client length of stay to the expected minimum.

Caregiver variance may also occur, as when a health-care professional does not contribute fully to the application and evaluation of the clinical pathway for an individual client. For example, a laboratory technician may delay collection of a specimen from a client. If the delay increased the length of stay or caused a change in the client's condition, the multidisciplinary team would discuss ways to avoid future delays. When multiple variances occur, an investigation would reveal the source(s) of concern. A multidisciplinary approach is used to constantly evaluate and correct as many variances as possible.

HEALTH-CARE REFORM

Over the years, health care has become increasingly expensive, insurance premiums have climbed, businesses have been less inclined to offer health-care insurance coverage or have cut back on the breadth of coverage offered to employees, and more and more people have less health-care coverage or even no coverage at all. Citizens as well as legislators are now seeking solutions that will provide low-cost health care to all. The current health-care delivery system provides consistent services only to those who are able to pay, have health-care insurance, or qualify for health care through government programs like Medicare, Medicaid, and veterans' services.

Health-care reform is a subject of ongoing debate: who qualifies, who pays, and what care is needed. The debate will continue, but in the meantime, current market forces are causing major changes in the way health care is delivered, paid for, and evaluated.

The market approach to health-care reform—controlled primarily by insurance companies, health maintenance organizations, and other financial entities—is finance and outcome oriented. From a financial standpoint, acute-care facilities monitor client care aspects such as length of stay, readmission rates, complications, and client satisfaction. From an outcome standpoint, morbidity, mortality, clinical outcomes (e.g., functional status), access to care, human resources (e.g., retention of skilled workers and analysis of skill mix), regulatory reports (e.g., JCAHO, Department of Health, Occupational Safety and Health Administration), and customer service are examined.

Capitation is now being touted as a way to help ensure the most cost-effective care. Through capitation, a health-care institution receives a fixed dollar amount for each client, corresponding to the client's diagnosis and expected length of stay. All the care that the client receives, whether of long or short duration, is of the same quality, unless a variance occurs (e.g., the diagnosis changes or complications develop). Captitation drives health-care institutions to constantly evaluate care and to seek ways to streamline and improve care delivery.

Ultimately, services are streamlined through the use of quality assurance reviews and continuous quality improvement efforts. Services and their outcomes are constantly monitored by multidisciplinary health care teams as well as by financial entities concerned about holding down the costs of services and staffing. Streamlining is not without potential pitfalls, however: Box 2–3 lists some possible concerns related to streamlining of services.

Another service of increasing importance is education of clients and the general public. Educational services are provided by numerous organizations, including hospitals, long-term care facilities, nonprofit agencies

BOX 2-3

Special Concerns as Health Care Moves to a Capitated Environment

Access. Capacity constraints may lead providers to overbook appointments, creating long waits for service.

Client Satisfaction. Faced with crowded, capacity-constrained facilities, staff friendliness and courtesy could be compromised; under the crunch of a heavy client load, health-care providers may spend less time with each client.

such as the YMCA/YWCA and local churches, and qualified individuals who act as consultants to or owners of health education and information businesses. All of these education services are ultimately aimed at reducing health-care costs by creating better-educated health-care consumers.

Along with the market-driven changes, health-care reform is also being affected by:

- societal changes
- financial impacts
- regulatory responsibilities
- efforts to ensure quality care

Societal Changes

During the last 15 years or so, changes in our society have sparked a re-evaluation of the health-care system and the rights of the health-care consumer. Important societal changes include an aging population, widespread family life-style changes (e.g., more fragmented families, increased mobility), exposure to more stressful professional and work styles, increased speed of information flow, changes in health-care insurance regulations and coverage, increasing cultural diversity, and the appearance of new deadly communicable diseases, such as the human immunodeficiency virus (HIV).

The ever-increasing elderly population is placing more demands on the health-care delivery system as well as on family caregivers. An elderly person who becomes ill may take longer to regain health, may need more assistance while recuperating, may or may not have the means to pay for acute or alternative care (e.g., long-term care, home health care), and may not have family caregivers available to help. The children of the elderly population are themselves aging; an 85-year-old client may have a 67-year-old "child" who has her own health problems and cannot provide care for her aging parent. These factors are spurring a movement to create a healthier elderly population through education about:

- risk factors for disease and how to control them
- signs and symptoms that necessitate prompt medical-surgical intervention
- development of appropriate life-style choices, with an emphasis on a healthy diet and regular exercise
- the importance of complying with prescribed medical treatments
- a referral system of available health care and other community services

Thus, the role of the client as a health-care consumer has also evolved. Increasingly, each client is expected to:

- accept responsibility for preventive health care
- maintain health
- choose cost-effective care
- function as a partner in care

A person accepts responsibility for preventive care by maintaining a healthy life-style and participating in annual physical examinations that include recommended screening tests, such as mammograms for women and prostate examinations for men. Good health is maintained by eating a well-balanced diet, getting regular exercise, seeking health care for common illnesses, complying with treatment for chronic illness (such as hypertension), and reducing stress related to work and life-style.

Choosing cost-effective care supports the goal of lowering costs. Examples of such choices include price-comparison shopping for prescription medications, checking on physician charges for care, using outpatient facilities whenever possible, and arranging for home health care when indicated.

Functioning as a partner in care involves actively working to maintain a healthy body, complying with prescribed treatment regimens, keeping abreast of health-care trends and breakthroughs, and, when illness occurs, working with the multidisciplinary team to regain and maintain health.

Financial Impacts

Acute-care institutions have been responding to the escalating costs of health care and technology. Many of the changes that have already occurred are precursors to some of the proposed health-care reforms currently under study. These changes include:

- Increased use of multiskilled workers who are cross-trained and capable of functioning in a variety of settings; for example, a nurse who can work in an intensive care unit and an emergency department and a nursing assistant who can complete a client care assignment and also perform unit secretarial duties.
- Clinical practice guidelines, established so that all caregivers are able to respond to a client's needs in a consistent and complete manner.
- Clinical pathways, guidelines for care developed by multidisciplinary teams for clients with specific medical-surgical diagnoses.
- Case managers who coordinate, streamline, and monitor care given by the multidisciplinary teams.
- Client advocates who respond to clients' perceived needs and coordinate and negotiate so that concerns expressed by the client and/or significant others are addressed to all parties' mutual satisfaction.
- Increasingly sophisticated methods for developing and participating in information data bases, which enable

institutions to evaluate their outcomes against those of other, comparable institutions.

Each of these changes is designed to provide client-focused care that is also cost-effective care.

Hospitals continuously assess their outcomes and financial health by performing cost-benefit analyses and clinical analyses of their service lines. Cost-benefit analysis compares the cost in time, dollars, and resources to the quality of care provided, considering all components that contribute to quality care. The cost of increasingly sophisticated technology must be weighed against the benefits, in terms of outcomes of a more comfortable and extended life span.

Service lines are groupings of services, such as departments organized by service; for example, medical and surgical, or cardiac, orthopedic, and obstetric departments. Many communities with two or more hospitals collaborate and then delineate specific service lines for each institution. This is a cost- and resource-effective approach to clinical care. Expertise of staff can be maintained more easily for the acute, complex care offered in hospital settings. Acutely ill clients may have multiple diagnoses that require intensive care and treatment by experienced staff. Clinical outcomes are generally better and the work flow is more efficient when this approach is used.

To provide cost-efficient care for clients who are not acutely ill or injured, subacute care systems of delivery, as described earlier, are evolving. Subacute care may be provided in hospital-based transitional units and step-down units. Traditional nursing homes are discovering a financial advantage in providing care for clients following an acute illness or injury. One company has estimated that on a case-by-case basis, subacute care costs 30 per cent less than traditional hospital care.[1] In a subacute care setting, a highly trained professional staff with technological expertise is not required, because the clients are not as acutely ill or injured as those clients in an acute-care setting. Clients in this setting are expected to participate in as much self-care as possible (clients in the acute-care setting may not be able to assist with self-care), so that fewer numbers of highly trained personnel are required.

The home-care setting is generally considered cost-effective, with care provided by a team of caregivers often assisted by the client's significant others. The multidisciplinary team members visit the client according to need. For example, a home health-care client is visited by a nurse who completes a procedure, such as a complicated dressing change and wound evaluation, or teaches the procedure to a designated person in the home. Although the nurse would not visit daily, a nursing assistant (who also could be called a home health aide) would attend to self-care needs such as dressing, bathing, grooming, toileting, and nutrition on a daily basis.

Cooperation, rather than competition, among health-care institutions is becoming more common. Cooperative community education may be sponsored jointly by several hospitals. The shared use of high-tech, high-cost equipment reduces costs to clients. Consolidating services—one hospital, for example, providing expert care in one specialty and another hospital in a different specialty—prevents costly duplication of services. These welcome changes should lead to improved consumer satisfaction and less costly care for providers and insurers and, ultimately, the client.

On the other hand, a health-care institution's administration may compete fiercely for a certain "prize"—for example, on-site ownership of an expensive diagnostic computer—that may or may not be shared with other hospitals. Most large hospitals have developed a reputation for offering thorough and complete care for any medical or surgical need in their respective communities and thus have developed a following of loyal clients. It may be difficult to explain to clients and their significant others the reasons for changes that relate to the cost of care. Furthermore, it may be difficult for clients to accept services at another institution because of personal reasons, such as trust and loyalty.

As hospitals increasingly consolidate care, health-care professionals are also affected. Loss of employment, low morale, fear of change, more demanding job expectations (e.g., cross-training), and increased stress are all factors that can influence the health-care professional's job performance as well as personal well-being.

REGULATORY RESPONSIBILITIES

Regulatory agencies have the primary goal of enhancing the public's ability to secure adequate health care. Health-care agencies are surveyed periodically to ensure compliance with specific rules and regulations. A survey is an in-depth study of a health-care institution (e.g., a hospital or a long-term care facility) according to specific criteria set forth by the regulating agencies involved. All aspects of the institution's services are inspected. Important performance areas include client assessment, medication administration, use of restraints, client and family education, staff training, information management, and organizational performance. After the survey is completed, a report of findings is compiled, and the institution is notified of its satisfactory status. If a criterion is not met satisfactorily, the institution is notified, given time to correct the deficiency, and reevaluated at a later date.

Public disclosure of survey findings has begun. For hospital surveys completed after January 1, 1994, a status report (on 28 performance areas) will be made available to the public, including media sources, insurance companies, third-party payers, clients, and competing institutions. Other health-care delivery services function under the same disclosure rules for compliance with regulations of the inspecting agencies.

Ensuring Quality in Health Care

Amid the fast-paced changes occurring in health-care delivery, health-care professionals remain responsible for ensuring quality client care. Quality client care is the outcome of the integrated health-care team approach that involves the corporate and hospital or agency administration, medical staff, board of trustees, employees, the community, and the client. Contract services, community resources, transfer agreements, and expertise from social workers or case managers enable client transitions to alternate levels of care in a continuous, coordinated, and almost seamless fashion. Through work-redesign and skill-mix reallocation, institutions are focusing goals on achieving efficient client outcomes. Work-redesign involves studying a job over a fixed period to discover if and how a certain job function could be made more efficient. Skill-mix is determined by studying the ratio of registered nurses to licensed practical/vocational nurses and nursing assistants on a unit. The best skill-mix delivers quality care while also controlling costs.

The "one level of care" philosophy ensures that clients receive optimum care in all areas of an institution. For example, when intravenous conscious sedation is administered in the endoscopy unit, the same monitoring should be performed as is done when sedation is administered in the operating room or emergency department.

Great importance is placed on facilitating entry into the system and into the appropriate type of care (e.g., service or setting), as well as on the proper transition to various levels of care that the client later requires.

Provision of Client Care

Any plan for provision of client care involves the following aspects:

- Budgeting process, to assist the institution in studying spending and using the information to cut costs or maintain them at the present rate
- Strategic planning, to serve as a guideline for the continued and/or expanded services provided by the health care agency
- Performance improvement plan, to show the steps taken to improve performance based on monitoring and evaluation of staff performance
- Risk management input, to identify and eliminate potential safety injuries to staff and clients
- Utilization review data, to explore items such as acuity levels, outcomes, and costs, to discover what is effective care and what is not
- Client satisfaction survey results, with data gathered from clients at various stages of their stay in the agency (e.g., preprocedure, admission procedure, discharge)
- Physician input, to incorporate professional input into client care planning
- Census data, to plot current and future trends of health care in the organization
- Acuity levels (as designated by the health-care organization), to plan an appropriate skill-mix for staffing

Changes in client population, diagnoses, programs, or staffing that would necessitate changes in the type, level, or amount of care are reviewed on an ongoing basis.

Other factors contributing to quality care include the adherence to, monitoring of, and evaluation of care given according to professional standards, JCAHO and Department of Health criteria, and input from other regulatory agencies. In addition, clinical pathways, clinical practice guidelines, standards of practice and care, and competency standards serve as models for professional delivery of client care.

Clients' Rights to Quality Care

Clients have an increased awareness of the quality of care issue. They are demanding and receiving more information prior to the initiation of treatments. Increasingly, clients' requests for information about costs, risks, benefits, and alternatives to suggested therapies are being honored. No longer submissive to the suggested care, the client is becoming a participant and partner in health care, with the expectation of receiving quality care from all health-care professionals.

Client rights have reached a new level of importance for the health-care consumer. Regulating agencies, insurance carriers, third-party payers, and providers are responding to ensure that these fundamental rights are maintained and that clients receive quality services.

Staffing for Quality Care

Health-care institutions use a combination of methods to ensure a staff of caregivers who can deliver quality care to clients. Two methods include:

- daily collection of census data (a count of the number of clients occupying beds on any given day)
- determination of acuity levels (a degree of severity of illness that affects the amount and complexity of care the client requires)

Staff are assigned or reassigned to units that have the greatest need for their expertise and experience. Staffing adjustments caused by the fluctuation of census data and acuity levels are accomplished by using per diem staff and other creative measures to ensure safe client care.

Although staffing adjustment decisions in the past were typically made at higher levels of administration, now service line leaders and empowered directors and managers are instrumental in adjusting strategies based on the many shifting variables that affect client care. These individuals are closer to the actual care setting (clients and staff) and can use their expertise to make informed decisions about staffing for quality care.

Input from the employees who actually provide care is helpful in redesigning and improving the quality of care given to clients. Because caregivers are directly involved with client care, they can contribute in significant ways by reporting problems that can be addressed in a timely fashion. Such input, especially when acted on by management, contributes to staff members' feelings of being valued.

BOX 2-4

Clinical Indicators with a Focus on High-Volume, High-Risk, and Problem-Prone Issues

The community/clinic focus includes:

- Communicable diseases (TB, HIV, etc.)
- Low birth weight as a percentage of live births
- Births to mothers 10 to 17 years of age as a percentage of all live births
- Percentage of women receiving prenatal care during the first trimester
- Breast cancer rates and mammography statistics
- Immunization rates
- Return visits to the same level of care or visit within 72 hours to a higher level of care
- Accessibility, availability, and acceptability of care
- Appropriateness and relevance of care (based on diagnostic lab work, symptomology, etc.)
- Appropriateness of treatment frequency
- Intake system
- Provision for information on an emergency or after-hours basis
- Client education
- Consultation
- Documentation including transfers, advance directives, etc.
- Availability of emergency carts/equipment
- Use of leasing for expensive/alternative resources
- Client record
- Client rights, including advance directives, informed consent, special concern for abuse victims and those with cultural diversity

Unfortunately, adequate staffing is not always ensured. In the spring of 1995, nurses marched on Washington, D.C., to protest clinical staffing shortages that have already endangered and could further endanger client care.

In an attempt to make the most effective use of available nursing staff, cross-training has evolved in hospitals. Whereas earlier a nurse typically was assigned to one unit, where she or he could become familiar with the other personnel and the unit routine, today's hospital nurse may be cross-trained to work effectively in two or more units, for example, a surgical unit and a cardiac intensive care unit. The nurse is assigned to the unit where she or he is most needed that day, and may arrive for work not knowing in advance her or his work assignment for that day. This new scenario is often stress-producing for nurses and other staff members.

Performance Improvement and Measurement

Hospitals and other health-care organizations have been challenged by their goal of attaining a planned, systematic, multidisciplinary, nation-wide approach to designing, measuring, and assessing and improving performance. These institutions generally seek to enhance their measurement activities as they relate to institutional quality indicators (Boxes 2–4 and 2–5). These indicators generally include:

- Results of basic clinical indicators
- Continuous quality improvement
- Access to care issues
- Consumer satisfaction and judgment input
- JCAHO indicators
- Human resource management
- Organizational performance

Health care organizations are in the midst of a transition to performance improvement from traditional quality assurance. Relevant goals include:

- Enhancing clinical leaders' abilities to set expectations, develop plans, and manage processes to assess, improve, and maintain the quality of the organization's clinical and support activities
- Enhancing health-care outcomes and the perception of these outcomes and expectations by all consumers
- Measuring outcomes to determine priorities for improvement
- Systematically improving performance of important functions and maintaining stability of these functions
- Implementing quality improvement activities that optimally affect client outcomes and cost of services, and then measuring the ongoing effect of these changes on the services provided
- Instituting a flexible performance improvement plan so that new or changed services and clinical practices serve as triggers for new indicator development

BOX 2-5

Broad-Based Indicators

Broad-based indicators encompass both ends (pre-hospital and post-hospital) of the care spectrum. These indicators include:

- Client satisfaction in areas such as facility (cleanliness, location, comfort), the appointment process, wait time, payment (amount, clarity of billing statements, payment collection methods), staff interaction and professional service (doctor, nurse, medical assistant, receptionist/cashier), education materials, and consideration of client input into the plan of care
- Functional status and well-being (in areas such as general health perceptions and limitations in physical activities because of health problems in social activities, in usual activities [including work], general mental health, bodily pain, energy and fatigue, and depression risk)
- Access in areas such as convenience (location, hours, wait time), lead time in scheduling primary care, clinic, and outpatient diagnostic testing, cancellations (initiated by office or client)

BOX 2–6

Qualities That Enhance Performance of Services in Health-Care Settings

- Efficacy: The degree to which the care and intervention for the client have been shown to accomplish the desired or projected outcomes
- Appropriateness: The degree to which the care and intervention provided are relevant to the client's clinical needs, given the current state of knowledge
- Availability: The degree to which appropriate care and intervention are available to meet the needs of the client
- Timeliness: The degree to which the care and intervention are provided to the client at the most beneficial or necessary time
- Effectiveness: The degree to which the care and intervention are provided in the correct manner, given the current state of knowledge, in order to achieve the desired or projected outcome for the client
- Continuity: The degree to which the care and intervention for the client are coordinated among practitioners, among organizations, and over time
- Safety: The degree to which the risk of an intervention and the risk in the care environment are reduced for the client and others including health-care providers
- Efficiency: The relationship between the outcomes and the resources used to deliver client care
- Respect and caring: The degree to which the client or a designee is involved in his or her own care decisions and to which those providing services do so with sensitivity and respect for the client's needs, expectations, and individual differences[5]

- Enhancing reporting and communication mechanisms of performance improvement results so that the greatest benefit is realized
- Strengthening the client education component as a result of quality assurance and improvement information
- Supporting performance by improving existing processes
- Designing improvement activities for new processes
- Supporting client advocacy and customer response functions by responding to complaints at the closest level of client care
- Using readily available resources to produce all-inclusive information and minimize data collection by staff
- Exploring automated methods of improving the performance of clinical information systems

Qualities that enhance the important dimensions of performance are listed in Box 2–6.

Use of Performance Improvement Information

Performance improvement information is used in various ways. First and foremost, it is used to alter and enhance the delivery of client care. Other positive effects include streamlined documentation and enhanced client and staff satisfaction. Reduced lengths of stay and costs have resulted from performance improvement activities involving clinical pathways. Factors once viewed as dependent solely on medical intervention, such as morbidity and mortality, are now altered through organization-wide endeavors.

The client care performance improvement component functions as a liaison with safety, risk management, utilization review, employee performance, planning, licensure, and all clinical administrative services. It involves identifying organization-wide performance improvement endeavors, as well as promoting unit-specific and department-specific activities. Performance improvement information that reveals a need for education and/or policy and procedure development and revision is reviewed, appropriate resources are identified, and, ideally, these projects are implemented in a timely fashion.

Performance improvement can no longer be limited to hospital care. Rather, it must extend throughout the entire continuum—from pre-hospital care to post-hospital care—to ensure that both clients' and providers' needs are adequately addressed.

STUDY QUESTIONS

1. Current emphasis on health care is centered on which of the following philosophies of care?
   A. Prevention
   B. Promotion
   C. Restoration
   D. Rehabilitation
2. The health-care delivery system is focusing on which of the following components of care?
   A. Providing health care as a right
   B. Emphasizing service to others
   C. Monitoring of individual compliance
   D. Achievement of efficient client outcomes
3. Health-care reform is occurring incidentally as a result of which of the following trends?
   A. The continuous quality improvement movement
   B. Demands for services by clients and their families
   C. Changes caused by the market in health care services
   D. Legislative action by federal and state governments

CRITICAL THINKING EXERCISES

An acutely ill female client enters the hospital for care. The client states that she expects that all services will be extended to her regardless of cost.

1. What effect does health-care reform have on the individual person seeking care in the acute-care setting?
2. How does economics affect the individual as well as the health-care delivery system?
3. How has the client's role as a health-care "consumer" changed health-care delivery?

BIBLIOGRAPHY

1. Burns, J. (1993). Subacute care feeds need to diversify. *Modern Healthcare, 25(50),* 34–38.
2. Chitty, K. K. (1993). *Professional nursing: Concepts and challenges.* Philadelphia: W. B. Saunders.
3. Ellis, J. R., & Hartley, C. L. (1995). *Nursing in today's world,* 5th ed. Philadelphia: J. B. Lippincott.
4. Hydo, B. (1995). Designing an effective clinical pathway for strokes. *Nursing 95. 95(3),* 44–50.
5. The Joint Commission 1995 Accreditation Manual for Hospitals, Volume I.
6. Rasmussen, N., & Gengler, T. (1994). Clinical pathways of care: The route to better communication. *Nursing 94, 94(2),* 47–49.
7. Sowell, R. L., & Meadows, T. M. (1994). An integrated case management model: Developing standards, evaluation, and outcome criteria. *Nursing Administration Quarterly, 18(2),* 53–64.
8. Stahl, D. A. (1994). Subacute care: Creating alternatives—Subacute care: The future of health care. *Nursing Management, 25(10),* 34–38.

UNIT 2

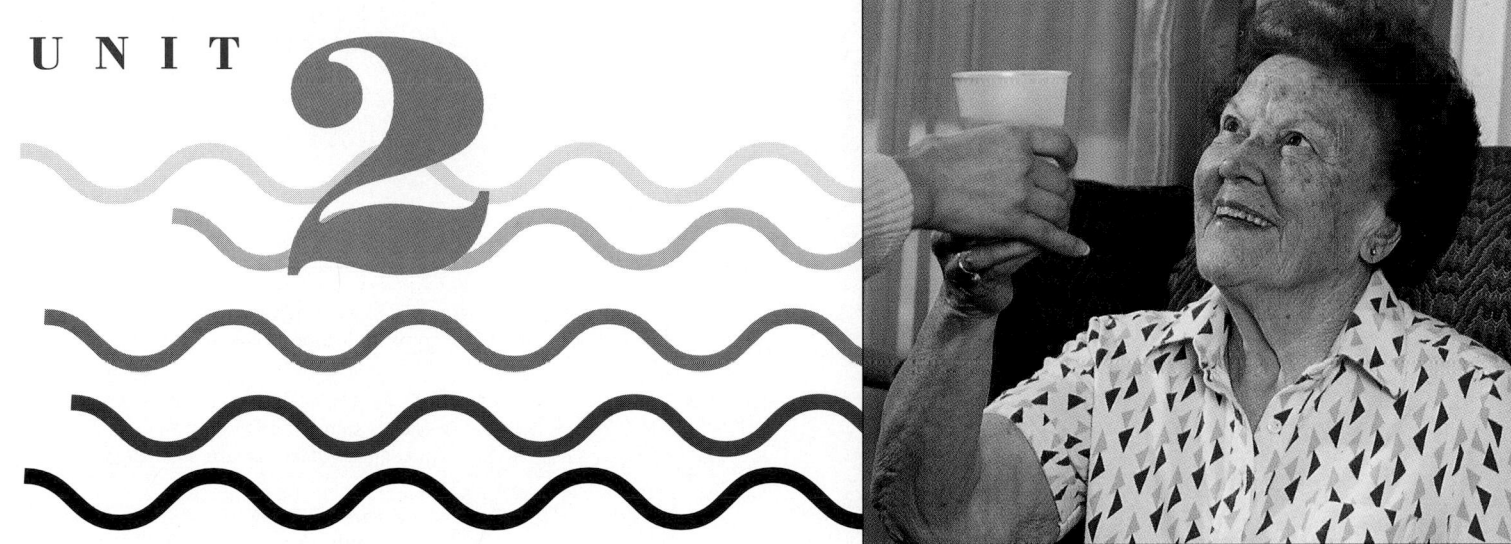

Common Health Disorders in Medical-Surgical Clients

This unit comprises five chapters addressing common health disorders and problems. These disorders commonly occur by themselves and also often occur in conjunction with many of the disorders discussed throughout the remainder of the text. The unit begins with chapters on fluid and electrolyte imbalances (Chap. 3) and acid-base imbalances (Chap. 4), disorders that reflect disturbances in cellular homeostasis. Because many clients require surgery, this unit also includes a chapter (Chap. 5) that covers the nursing aspects of the perioperative experience. The unit's final two chapters cover the basic concepts of neoplastic disorders (Chap. 6) and provide an overview of the various treatment modalities used to combat these disorders (Chap. 7). Cancers of the various body organs are discussed in more depth in specific chapters of subsequent units.

Chapter 3 Fluid and Electrolyte Balance

Learning Outcomes

After completing this chapter, the learner will be able to:

1. Assess the client for clinical manifestations of fluid and electrolyte disorders.
2. Teach the client about the etiology, risk factors, basic pathophysiology, and clinical manifestations of major fluid and electrolyte disorders.
3. Explain the client's role in the medical management of fluid and electrolyte disorders.
4. Develop plans of care for the prevention, management, and rehabilitation of clients with fluid and electrolyte disorders.
5. Implement nursing interventions that optimize the quality of life for clients with fluid and electrolyte disorders.
6. Evaluate planned client outcomes, using outcome criteria developed in the planning phase of care.

Physiologic homeostasis depends on normal fluid and electrolyte balance, and is important in both health promotion and treatment of disorders. Fluid and electrolyte imbalances commonly accompany illness. Severe imbalances may result in death. Such imbalances affect not only the acutely and chronically ill but also clients with faulty diets or those who take selected medications such as diuretics and glucocorticoid preparations. Every nurse must understand the process of fluid and electrolyte balance, identify clients at risk for imbalances, recognize early signs and symptoms of imbalances, intervene as appropriate, and evaluate the outcomes.

Fluids

Water and Fluid Balance

FLUID COMPARTMENTS

Water is the solvent responsible for the body's structure and function. Body water is located in two major fluid compartments—the intracellular fluid (ICF) compartment and the extracellular (ECF) compartment. The ECF is composed of interstitial fluid (tissues) and the intravascular fluid (plasma). Interstitial fluid lies outside the vascular fluid and cells and comprises 28 per cent of the total body water. It provides the cells with the external medium necessary for cellular metabolism. In the adult, approximately 60 per cent of body weight is water, two thirds of the water is intracellular and one third of the water is extracellular fluid.

The ICF provides the cell with the internal aqueous medium necessary for its chemical functions. The ECF transports nutrients, electrolytes, and oxygen to cells; transports waste products for excretion; regulates heat; lubricates and cushions joints and membranes; and hydrolyzes food for digestive processes. Cerebrospinal fluid, lymphatic fluid, synovial fluid, and fluids in the eye are also part of the ECF.

FLUID PRESSURES

Body fluids shift between the interstitial space and the vascular space in the capillary as a result of differences in the hydrostatic pressure and the oncotic (colloid osmotic) pressure. Hydrostatic pressure is pressure caused by water volume in the vessels. Oncotic pressure is the pressure exerted by plasma proteins. Filtration occurs at arterial ends of the capillaries because the hydrostatic pressure is greater than the oncotic pressure. Therefore, fluid is pushed out of the vessels into tissue space. At the venous end of the capillary, the oncotic pressure is greater than the hydrostatic pressure, and fluid is pulled back into the capillary from the interstitial space (Fig. 3–1).

There are some conditions in which this system does not work smoothly and fluid remains in the tissue spaces. When there is a low level of plasma/serum protein, oncotic pressure in the vascular fluid is decreased and less water is reabsorbed into the vascular space. Likewise, when the hydrostatic pressure is high because of fluid overload, the pressure gradient opposes fluid reabsorption into the venous end of the capillary. The functions of water are numerous, and without sufficient water, cells of the body deteriorate and life cannot be sustained.

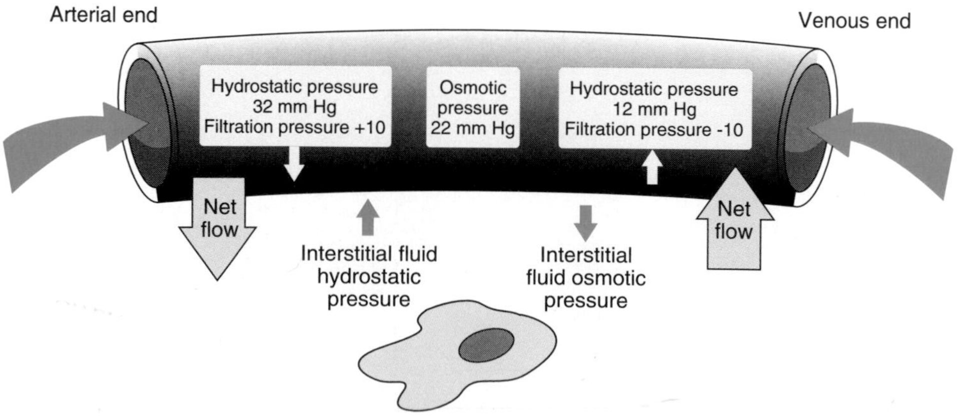

Figure 3–1
Pressure differences within the capillary are responsible for the movement of fluids. Fluid moves out of the capillary at the arterial end because hydrostatic pressure in the vessel exceeds the pressure in the tissues. Fluids return to the vessel at the venous end because the proteins (colloids) that remain in the vessel exert a pulling pressure on them. Under normal conditions, the movement of fluids is equal, and neither dehydration nor edema results. These abnormal conditions occur when too much fluid, too few proteins, or changes in the capillary wall exist.

REGULATORS OF FLUID BALANCE

Thirst, hormones, the lymphatic system, the nervous system, and the kidneys assist in the regulation of body fluids. These regulators may respond inappropriately to various stimuli and cause a fluid imbalance. Thirst is a primary factor in the maintenance of an intake of fluids. The kidneys are responsible for maintaining an adequate fluid output or retaining fluids (Fig. 3–2).

Thirst

The thirst center is located in the hypothalamus and is activated by an increase in ECF osmolality (concentration). Thirst may result from hypotension, polyuria, or fluid volume depletion.

CRITICAL TO REMEMBER

Although thirst can be reported and is an important clinical manifestation of fluid imbalances, it is not a true indicator of fluid balance in all clients.

The thirst mechanism may be depressed in the elderly and in clients with debilitating illnesses. Edematous clients, who have excess fluids, may be thirsty because the fluid is trapped in the interstitial spaces and is not contributing to cell osmolarity. (The terms *osmolarity* and *osmolality* are discussed in later paragraphs.) Comatose and confused clients may have very high osmolarity but are unable to recognize the urge to drink. Finally, the client with hypo-osmolarity of the ECF will not experience thirst even though the fluid volumes are decreased. Hypo-osmolarity inhibits the thirst mechanism.

Hormonal Influences

The antidiuretic hormone and aldosterone are the two major hormones that influence fluid balance.

Antidiuretic hormone (ADH), produced by the hypothalamus, is secreted when there is an increased plasma/serum osmolality (hyperosmolality), ECF volume depletion, pain, use of certain medications, or stress (emotional; physiologic, such as surgery, trauma, prolonged exercise). ADH promotes water reabsorption

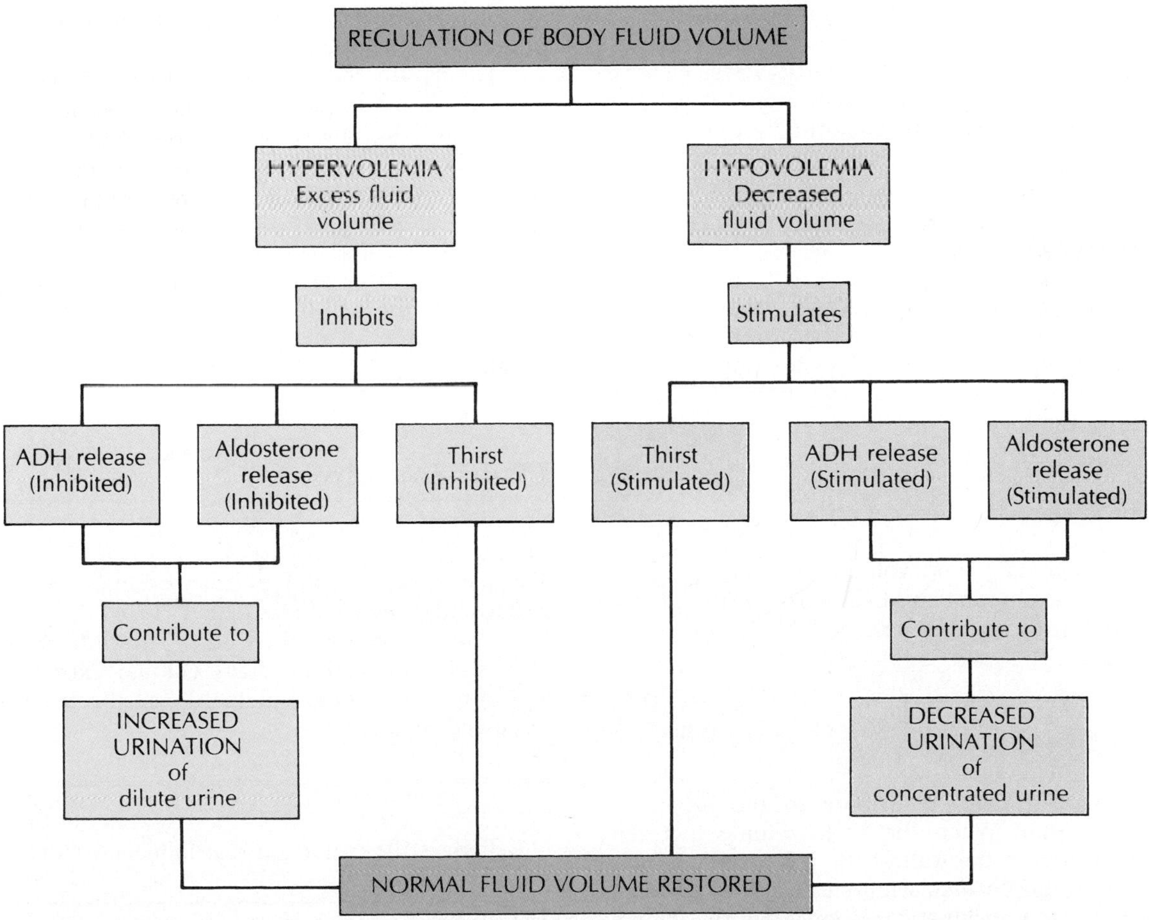

Figure 3–2
Regulation of body fluid volume depends on antidiuretic hormone (ADH), aldosterone, and thirst. (From Sorensen, K. C., & Luckmann, J. [Eds.]. [1986]. *Basic nursing: A psychophysiologic approach* [2nd ed.]. Philadelphia. W. B. Saunders.)

from the renal tubules. Stimulation of the thirst mechanism and ADH release usually occur concurrently in response to a body fluid deficit.

Factors suppressing ADH include hypo-osmolarity of the ECF, increased blood volume, exposure to cold, acute alcohol ingestion, carbon dioxide inhalation, and administration of some diuretics.

Aldosterone is secreted by the adrenal cortex and promotes sodium reabsorption and potassium excretion from the kidneys. Aldosterone secretion is stimulated primarily by the renin-angiotensin system. Renin, secreted by the kidney, converts angiotensinogen in the blood to angiotensin I. Angiotensin I is further converted to angiotensin II in the capillary beds. Aldosterone secretion can also be stimulated by an increase in potassium or a decrease in sodium concentration in interstitial fluids and by the release of adrenocorticotropic hormone from the anterior pituitary gland.

Hypovolemia is a common clinical condition in which aldosterone is secreted to maintain homeostasis. When arterial blood pressure falls, renal blood pressure falls. Hypotension decreases the stretch in vascular smooth muscle in the afferent arteriole of the kidney, which increases renin release. Renin stimulates aldosterone through multiple steps, which increases sodium retention and thereby fluid retention to raise blood pressure.

In addition to aldosterone, other circulating elements, such as cortisol or natriuretic hormone contribute to the regulation of sodium balance. These elements increase the excretion of sodium and water. Renal prostaglandins and the renal renin-kinin system also increase sodium excretion.

Lymphatic System

Plasma protein and fluid that escapes from the tissue spaces cannot be directly reabsorbed into the blood vessels. The lymphatic system plays an important role in returning excess fluid and protein from the interstitial spaces to the blood.

Kidneys

The kidneys maintain fluid volume and the concentration of urine by filtrating the ECF through the glomeruli. Reabsorption and excretion of ECF occurs in the renal tubules.

Nervous System

Neural mechanisms also contribute to the balance of water and sodium. When the ECF volume increases, mechanoreceptors in the wall of the left atrium respond to atrial distention by increasing cardiac stroke volume and triggering a sympathetic response in the kidney. Stimulation of the renal sympathetic nerves decreases renal excretion of sodium, both by increasing renin release and through a direct effect on the kidneys.

OSMOLALITY AND OSMOLARITY

Osmolarity is the concentration of all solutes or dissolved particles per liter of solution. Osmolality controls water movement and distribution between and within body fluid compartments by regulating the concentration of fluid in each compartment. The terms osmolality and osmolarity are frequently used interchangeably.

Osmolality is determined by the number of dissolved particles per kilogram of water. Electrolytes, especially sodium, contribute the largest number of particles to osmolality. Other particles that contribute to osmolality are urea and glucose.

The hypothalamus is the center of regulation of osmolarity. It manufactures ADH, which is stored in the posterior pituitary gland. The hypothalamus also contains osmoreceptors that signal the posterior pituitary gland to release ADH as needed. Increased ECF osmolarity causes the osmoreceptors to stimulate ADH release. Conversely, when ECF osmolarity decreases, the osmoreceptors inhibit ADH secretion.

Osmolality is measured by calculating the concentration of solutes per kilogram of water. Sodium is the easiest solute to measure because it is abundant and readily accessible in the plasma and serum. Elevated serum sodium (hypernatremia) indicates a state of hyperosmolality, and decreased serum sodium (hyponatremia) indicates hypo-osmolality.

The serum sodium value does not signify the total amount of sodium in the extracellular fluid, but rather it indicates the relationship of the amount of water to dissolved sodium. To illustrate this point, consider two glasses of water, one full and the other half full. One teaspoon of salt is added to each glass. The water from the half-full glass would taste saltier, even though it contains the same amount of salt as the full glass. The solution in the half-full glass is more concentrated, or, in other words, there is less water for the same amount of salt.

Fluid Imbalances

The five types of fluid imbalances that may occur are extracellular fluid volume deficit (ECFVD), extracellular fluid volume excess (ECFVE), extracellular fluid volume shift, intracellular fluid volume excess (ICFVE), and intracellular fluid volume deficit. Each imbalance is discussed separately.

CRITICAL TO REMEMBER

Sodium is the major ion that influences fluid balance and imbalance.

The relationship between sodium and water is discussed in this section; however, water imbalances and sodium imbalances are presented separately.

EXTRACELLULAR FLUID VOLUME DEFICIT

Definition and Incidence

An ECFVD is a decrease in intravascular and interstitial fluids. ECFVD is a *common* and *serious* fluid imbalance that results in vascular fluid volume loss (hypovolemia). ECFVD can lead to cellular fluid loss owing to fluid shifting from the cells to the vascular fluid to restore fluid balance.

There are two major types of extracellular fluid volume deficits: (1) *hyperosmolar fluid volume deficit,* in which the fluid loss is greater than the solute (sodium) loss; and (2) *iso-osmolar fluid volume deficit,* in which there is equal proportion of fluid and solute (sodium) loss.

Etiology and Risk Factors

CRITICAL TO REMEMBER

Extracellular fluid volume deficit commonly occurs with severe vomiting or diarrhea, traumatic injuries with excessive blood loss, third space fluid shifts, and insufficient water or fluid intake.

Clients at risk for ECFVD include those who are elderly, confused, or debilitated; in diabetic ketoacidosis; losing large volumes of blood; experiencing severe vomiting or diarrhea; having difficulty swallowing; unable to procure water because of physical restraint, or receiving an overabundance of intravenous glucose with saline or hypertonic tube feeding. The elderly are at risk because of their potential for depressed thirst mechanism. Prevention begins with adequate hydration. If fluids are being lost, fluid replacement should begin immediately with oral fluids or intravenous solutions that contain saline as well as dextrose.

Pathophysiology

The pathophysiologic changes related to ECFVD usually have to do with changes in sodium levels. Sodium has a major influence on water retention and water loss. Serum sodium concentration is increased with an ECFVD caused by insufficient water intake or massive water loss. The increased serum sodium concentration causes ECFVD by shifting water from the cells to the vascular space to decrease the hyperosmolality that occurs with water loss. This shift causes cells to shrink and cellular dehydration to occur.

The pathophysiologic changes that relate to clinical manifestations of fluid volume deficit are explained in Table 3–1.

With a severe fluid volume deficit, vascular collapse and shock may occur. The major clinical manifestations are brought about by changes in the cerebral cells. If the ECFVD develops rapidly, the manifestations are more severe. Severe brain shrinkage during water deficit may cause vascular damage and intracerebral hemorrhage. When ECFVD occurs slowly, the brain cells adapt to the increased intracellular osmolality by producing extra intracellular particles (idiogenic osmoles), which prevent large amounts of water from leaving the cell.

Clinical Manifestations

With mild ECFVD, 1 to 2 L of water and 2 per cent of the body weight is lost. Moderate ECFVD is evidenced by 3 to 5 L of water loss and a 5 per cent weight loss. In severe ECFVD, the water loss is increased to 5 to 10 L and the weight loss is increased to 8 per cent; the systolic blood pressure becomes alarmingly low, as demonstrated by a reading of less than 70 mm Hg.

CRITICAL TO REMEMBER

Immediate medical management is necessary for severe ECFVD.

Medical Management

Medical treatment of fluid volume deficit depends on the severity of the fluid deficit. If the fluid loss is mild, the fluid intake should be increased in accordance with the client's physical condition.

PHARMACOLOGIC MANAGEMENT

When a hyperosmolar fluid volume deficit is present, an intravenous solution of 5 per cent dextrose in water (D_5W) or 5 per cent dextrose in 0.2 per cent saline (D_5/0.2 per cent NaCl) may be prescribed.

CRITICAL TO REMEMBER

If a hyperosmolar fluid volume deficit has existed for more than 24 hours, it is dangerous to correct it too rapidly.

Some authorities recommend that the maximal rate at which sodium solutions should be infused is 2 mEq/L per hour. If fluid is given too rapidly, cerebral edema may result.

If hemorrhage is the cause of the ECFVD, blood replacement may be necessary when blood loss is greater than 1 L. In situations in which the blood losses are less than 1 L, normal saline and lactated Ringer's solution may be used to restore fluid volume.

The fluid needs of the client must be assessed within the context of the client's overall condition. A client with severe ECFVD and also severe heart or kidney disease cannot be given large volumes of fluid or sodium.

TABLE 3–1 Clinical Manifestations of Extracellular Fluid Volume Deficit and Their Pathophysiologic Bases

CLINICAL MANIFESTATION	PATHOPHYSIOLOGIC BASIS
Thirst	Cells shrink, stimulating "thirst" osmoreceptors in the hypothalamus; with iso-osmolar fluid loss, thirst usually does not occur
Decreased skin turgor	Decreased interstitial fluid causes skin tissue to "stick together"
Dry mucous membranes; dry, cracked lips or tongue	Cells of mucous membranes and tongue "dry out"
Eyeballs soft and sunken (severe deficit)	Water tension in eyeballs decreased
Apprehension and restlessness; coma in severe deficit	Cerebral dehydration
Elevated temperature	Less fluid available for evaporation
Tachycardia	Pulse greater than 100 bpm may be due to circulatory compensation by the heart
Postural systolic blood pressure fall >15 mm Hg and diastolic fall >10 mm Hg	With iso-osmolar fluid loss, the plasma volume is inadequate owing to hypovolemia; systolic pressure begins to fall
Narrowed pulse pressure, decreased central venous pressure and pulmonary capillary wedge pressure	Decreased venous return
Flattened neck veins in supine position	Decreased venous return
Weight loss	A lack of the water component of body weight
Oliguria (<30 mL per hour)	Due to the renal response to hypovolemia
Laboratory Findings	
Increased osmolality	Serum osmolality >295 mOsm/kg due to hypo-osmolar fluid loss (more fluid than solutes is lost)
Increased or normal serum sodium level	Hypo-osmolar fluid volume loss: serum sodium level >145 mEq/L; water is lost in greater amounts than sodium Iso-osmolar fluid volume loss: serum sodium level is within normal range
Increased blood urea nitrogen (>25 mg/dL)	Slight elevation (25–35 mg/dL) caused by hemoconcentration
Hyperglycemia (>120 mg/dL)	Sugar increases serum osmolality, thus causing diuresis and water loss; glucose levels may also be elevated owing to hemoconcentration
Elevated hematocrit (>55%)	With hypo-osmolar fluid loss, hematocrit will be increased owing to hemoconcentration; with iso-osmolar fluid loss (e.g., hemorrhage), hematocrit may be within normal range
Increased specific gravity	Increased solute-to-solvent ratio

DIETARY MANAGEMENT

Clients experiencing fluid loss from diarrhea should avoid fatty or fried foods and milk products.

Nursing Management

Assessment

The client should be assessed for the typical clinical manifestations. In addition, the nurse should assess the client's ability to participate in the treatment plan. For example, can the client swallow? At what site should the intravenous line be initiated and what size should it be?

Nursing Diagnosis, Planning, and Implementation

Nursing Diagnosis: Fluid Volume Deficit R/T insufficient fluid intake, vomiting, diarrhea, hemorrhage, or third space fluid loss (ascites, burns).

Planning: Expected Outcomes. The client's fluid balance will be restored, as evidenced by vital signs within normal range, return to baseline body weight, absence of the causative factors of ECFVD, equal intake and output, urine output of greater than 600 mL/day, skin turgor at 2 seconds or less, and moist mucous membranes.

Implementation. Vital signs should be assessed every 2 to 4 hours, depending on the severity of the fluid loss, and compared with baseline vital signs; marked differences, should be reported. Positional blood pressure should be assessed to determine the degree of orthostasis. If the standing systolic blood pressure falls 10 to 15 mm Hg or more, the results should be reported and the client protected from injury while ambulating.

Urine output should be assessed hourly if ECFVD is severe; in mild cases, the urine output per shift and per day should be compared with intake for the same time frame. Absence of a urine output in 8 to 12 hours may indicate renal insufficiency because of decreased renal perfusion.

CRITICAL TO REMEMBER

Absence of adequate renal perfusion for several hours may result in permanent renal damage.

Urine specific gravity measurements should also be

noted every shift, because these data provide very objective measurements of osmolality.

Daily weight should be monitored. A loss of approximately 1 kg is equivalent to 1 L. A 3.6 kg weight loss equals approximately 3.5 L, which is indicative of a moderate fluid volume deficit.

The nurse should apply lotion to the skin to preserve skin integrity. The client's position should be changed every 2 hours, or more often if skin assessment dictates. Oral care should be given every 2 hours with a nonalcohol-base solution. Lips should be moistened frequently.

Serum sodium, blood urea nitrogen (BUN), glucose, and hematocrit levels should be closely monitored to determine the serum osmolality.

Mild fluid volume loss can be corrected with oral fluid replacement, especially for elderly clients and debilitated clients. If the fluid loss is moderate or severe, administration of intravenous fluids is indicated. Intravenous solutions need to be closely monitored.

CRITICAL TO REMEMBER

Overhydration may occur from excessive and rapidly infused intravenous fluids or in clients with preexisting renal or cardiac disorders.

Clinical manifestations of fluid overload include dyspnea, crackles, and jugular vein engorgement.

Evaluation

The degree of expected outcome attainment should be monitored after 8 and 24 hours for determining whether the ECFVD is being corrected. Revisions of the interventions may be required.

Modification of Plan of Care for the Elderly

The elderly client must be rehydrated slowly because of the frequent problems with renal and cardiac disease in that age group. Skin breakdown is also more common, and position changes will be needed more frequently.

Client Education

Follow-up care is based on the original problem. If the client was fluid deficient because of inadequate fluid intake, the client or responsible person will need to be taught how to be certain the client gets adequate fluids. For example, if the client is dehydrated owing to the use of too highly concentrated tube feedings, the use of additional water between feedings will be needed. If the client is fluid deficient as the result of a traumatic injury, the problem will most likely be resolved before dismissal.

EXTRACELLULAR FLUID VOLUME EXCESS

ECFVE is increased fluid retention in the intravascular and interstitial spaces. When sodium and water are retained in the same proportions, the condition is referred to as iso-osmolar fluid volume excess. The serum sodium level may be within the normal range even though the actual sodium level is increased because of excess water retention.

Incidence

ECFVE frequently occurs in cases of heart disease in which there is pump failure. Excessive fluid volume and coronary insufficiency due to heart pump failure usually lead to congestive heart failure.

Etiology

ECFVE usually results from an increase in the total body sodium content. Causes of ECFVE include heart failure, renal disorders, cirrhosis of the liver, increased ingestion of foods that contain high amounts of sodium, excessive tap water enemas, and excessive amounts of intravenous fluids that contain sodium.

Risk Factors

Clients with heart, kidney, or liver disorders are prone to sodium and water retention. Likewise, clients with hyperaldosteronism or Cushing's syndrome and those using glucocorticoids are at increased risk. Other risk factors include the use of hypotonic fluids to irrigate nasogastric tubes. Men who have undergone transurethral resection of the prostate gland with sodium-free irrigation during and after surgery are also at increased risk.

Preventive measures may be simple, such as decreasing salt intake or initiating medical treatment with digoxin and diuretics.

Pathophysiology

With a fluid volume excess (fluid overload), the fluid pressure is even greater than usual at the arterial end of the capillary. Fluid is pushed into the tissue spaces with greater force because venous pressure also exceeds oncotic pressure. Peripheral and pulmonary edema may result (Fig. 3–3*A*).

When fluid overload results from renal disorders, there is a decrease in sodium and water excretion. Fluid volume rises, and the heart again must compensate for the increasing pressures; heart failure can result.

In clients with cirrhosis of the liver, the serum protein and albumin levels are decreased; therefore, the oncotic pressure is decreased in the vascular fluids, which results in less fluid reabsorption from the tissue spaces. Peripheral edema and ascites result (see Fig. 3–3*B*).

When lymphatic channels are obstructed, tissue oncotic pressure rises and leads to edema (see Fig. 3–3*C*). Edema resulting from increased capillary permeability is discussed in Chapter 49.

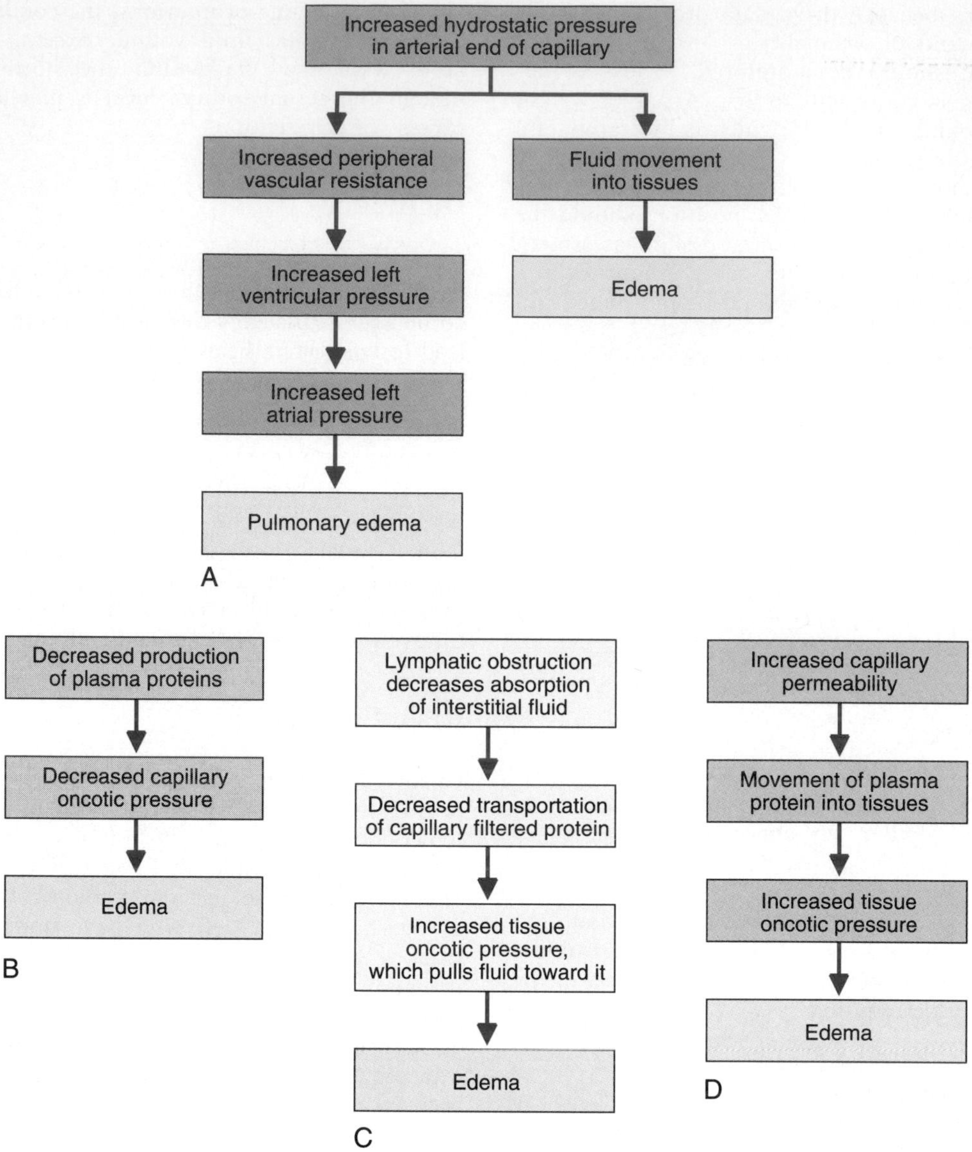

Figure 3–3
Mechanisms of edema formation. *A*, Fluid overload. *B*, Decreased serum and albumin. *C*, Lymphatic obstruction. *D*, Tissue injury.

Congestive heart failure that is not corrected leads to kidney and liver failure that may be fatal. Multiple organ failures cause body water retention in massive amounts (anasarca), which is incompatible with life.

Clinical Manifestations

Some obvious indicators of severe fluid volume excess include dyspnea, engorged neck and hand veins, a bounding pulse, moist crackles in the lungs, and edema of the extremities. Table 3–2 lists the clinical manifestations with pathophysiologic bases of fluid volume excess.

DIAGNOSTIC ASSESSMENT

With fluid volume excess or fluid overload, the concentration of solutes such as sodium is diluted. Reduced concentration of solutes lowers the serum osmolality value. Clients gain weight as a result of the excess fluid volume.

Medical Management

Diagnosis is determined by a clinical history of contributing and causative factors, history of drug use, signs and symptoms of fluid overload, and laboratory findings.

CRITICAL TO REMEMBER

The presence of pulmonary edema is a medical emergency requiring immediate interventions to prevent further respiratory distress.

TABLE 3–2 Clinical Manifestations of Extracellular Fluid Volume Excess and Their Pathophysiologic Bases

CLINICAL MANIFESTATION	PATHOPHYSIOLOGIC BASIS
Respiratory	
Constant, irritating cough	Fluid accumulation in the alveolar sacs due to hypervolemia
Dyspnea	Due to fluid congestion in lungs
Crackles in lungs	Alveoli are congested with fluid owing to increased hydrostatic pressure
Cyanosis	A late symptom of pulmonary edema that results from impaired oxygen transport due to the capillaries being filled with fluid
Cardiovascular	
Neck vein engorgement in semi-Fowler's position	Due to fluid overload and delayed right-sided heart emptying/filling
Hand vein engorgement	Due to peripheral vascular fluid overload
Bounding pulse, elevated blood pressure	Due to peripheral vascular fluid overload
S_3 gallop	Due to delayed ventricular filling and overdistention of ventricles from rapid filling during early diastole
Pitting edema of the lower extremities	Osmotic pressure in the venous end of the capillary exceeds interstitial pressure and fluid cannot return to the bloodstream
Sacral edema	Dependent edema in the supine client occurs in the sacral hollow rather than in the feet and legs, because the sacrum is the lowest place on the body
Weight gain	Due to fluid retention; for every 1 kg gained, 1 L body fluid is retained
Neurologic	
Change in level of consciousness	Malaise, confusion, headache, and lethargy are due to cerebral edema
Laboratory Findings	
Serum osmolality <275 mOsm/kg	Indicates a diluted body fluid in which there are fewer solutes in proportion to the water volume
Serum sodium <135 mEq/L to >145 mEq/L (low, normal, or high value)	Depending on the amount of sodium retention or water retention, the serum sodium level may be normal, decreased, or elevated
Decreased hematocrit	Due to hemodilution
Specific gravity below 1.010	Solvent in the urine exceeds solute

PHARMACOLOGIC MANAGEMENT

Loop and potassium-wasting diuretics and a digitalis preparation are frequently prescribed for the treatment of ECFVE. These potent diuretics cause potassium to be excreted along with the sodium and water. To preserve potassium, a combination of potassium-wasting and potassium-sparing diuretics is frequently prescribed.

Digoxin, a digitalis preparation, is ordered to increase the force of myocardial contraction or to slow the heart rate if heart failure is the cause of ECFVE.

DIETARY MANAGEMENT

A low-sodium diet is prescribed in order to reduce fluid retention. Low-sodium diets are discussed later in this chapter.

Nursing Management

Assessment

Frequent assessment of breath sounds, palpation of the lower extremities for pitting edema, observation for hand and neck vein engorgement, and observation of changes in vital signs are used to determine the presence of a fluid volume excess. When checking for neck vein engorgement, the nurse should note whether the jugular vein remains engorged when the client is in a semi-Fowler's position. Engorgement of neck veins in this position may indicate fluid overload. To check for hand vein engorgement, the nurse has the client lower the hand until the peripheral veins are engorged. The client then raises the hand above the level of the heart and the nurse observes the amount of time it takes for the veins to flatten. If the veins do not flatten within 3 to 5 seconds, fluid overload should be suspected.

Serum electrolyte values should be checked for abnormalities when the client is receiving diuretics. If the client is taking digoxin and a potassium-wasting diuretic, the client should be observed for signs and symptoms of digitalis toxicity and hypokalemia.

Nursing Diagnosis, Planning, and Implementation

Nursing Diagnosis: Fluid Volume Excess R/T compromised regulatory mechanisms or hypervolemia.

Planning: Expected Outcomes. The client's fluid balance will be within normal limits, as evidenced by the absence of dyspnea, clear chest sounds, absence of dependent edema, flat neck veins, the peripheral vein emptying in 3 to 5 seconds, decreased body weight, and the urine output exceeding intake.

Implementation. Vital signs should be monitored for bounding pulse or an elevated blood pressure every 4 to 8 hours. The nurse should auscultate breath sounds every 4 to 8 hours for crackles, noting changes and the location of adventitious sounds. The physician should be notified if there is an increase in crackles. The nurse assesses neck vein engorgement every 8 hours and monitors daily weights. Edema does not usually occur unless there are 3 L or more of excess fluids. Intake and output should be evaluated every 4 to 8 hours in cases of severe fluid excess, and once every shift in cases of moderate levels of fluid excess. The nurse assesses for changes in the client's level of consciousness and palpates the lower extremities and sacrum for pitting edema each morning.

The nurse should monitor laboratory values for changes. Pertinent values include serum osmolarity, sodium, hematocrit, and potassium levels, and specific gravity of urine.

Fluid and sodium restrictions may be necessary. The nurse should instruct the client about the fluid restriction and the rationale for it, being certain to include fluids on meal trays as part of the total fluids. The nurse should work with the dietitian in planning for fluid restrictions. Oral medications should be scheduled at the time meals are eaten (as is possible); this will decrease the chance of extra fluids being used to swallow medications. Very cold fluids rather than warm or hot liquids should be provided, because cold fluids decrease the sensation of thirst. Oral care should be offered frequently. When generalized edema is present, skin care is important for preventing pressure ulcers.

Evaluation

The client's improvement according to goal outcomes should be assessed following every shift. Revisions in the plan of care may be required.

Modification of Plan of Care for the Elderly

The elderly client commonly develops ECFVE owing to the many other diseases that are present, such as congestive heart failure. In general, the interventions are the same except that the elderly client responds more slowly to them. The potential for drug-drug interaction should be assessed before any therapy is begun.

Client Education

If the client is being discharged on a low-sodium diet, the nurse should review the foods allowed on that diet. Canned foods should be avoided; fresh and frozen foods are permissible, but should be used with caution. The client (or person who does the cooking) should be taught to read the labels on food if sodium level is not evident. The nurse should also ask if the client drinks softened water, which is high in sodium. The client may need to obtain water from another source.

EXTRACELLULAR FLUID VOLUME SHIFT: THIRD SPACE FLUID

A fluid volume shift is basically a change in the location of extracellular fluid between the intravascular and the interstitial spaces. There are two types of fluid shifts: (1) vascular fluid to interstitial space and (2) interstitial fluid to vascular fluid space. Fluid that shifts into the interstitial space and remains there is referred to as third space fluid. Third space fluid occurs in cases of tissue injury resulting from altered capillary permeability (e.g., inflammation, traumatic injury) and from increased vascular fluid volumes. Increased vascular fluid volume appears in the abdomen (ascites), pleural cavity, peritoneal cavity, and pericardial sac. Third space fluid is physiologically useless because it does *not* circulate to provide nutrients to cells.

Incidence

The incidence of third-space fluid shifts has not been recorded.

Etiology

Clinical causes of fluid shift from the vascular to the interstitial spaces may be a simple blister or sprain. Causes of massive fluid shifts from the vascular to interstitial spaces include crushing injuries, extensive burns, perforated peptic ulcer, intestinal obstruction, lymphatic obstruction, and large venous thrombosis. Pleural and pericardial fluid shifts are secondary to inflammatory responses to infectious, noninfectious, and autoimmune disorders and trauma.

Risk Factors

Clients at risk for third space fluids are those who have sustained major trauma (e.g., car accidents with major tissue injury) or had major surgery.

Pathophysiology

Tissue injury causes the release of histamine and bradykinin, which increases capillary permeability, allowing fluid, protein, and other solutes to shift into the interstitial spaces. There are two phases of fluid shift associated with tissue injury. The first phase is the fluid shift from vascular to interstitial spaces leading to a fluid volume deficit (hypovolemia) (see Fig. 3–3*D*). The second phase is the shift from the interstitial to the vascular space, leading to a fluid volume excess (hypervolemia).

Clinical Manifestations

CRITICAL TO REMEMBER

Clinical manifestations of a fluid shift from the vascular to the interstitial spaces are similar to the signs and symptoms of shock.

Typical clinical manifestations include skin pallor, cold extremities, weak and rapid pulse, hypotension, oliguria, and decreased levels of consciousness. If the fluid is obstructing an organ, nerve, or vessel, other clinical manifestations may be noted. For example, bowel sounds may change character throughout the abdomen; extremities may become pale, cool, and pulseless.

> **CRITICAL TO REMEMBER**
>
> When the fluid returns to the blood vessels, the clinical manifestations are similar to those of fluid overload.

Signs may include a bounding pulse, crackles, engorgement of peripheral and jugular veins, and an increased blood pressure.

DIAGNOSTIC ASSESSMENT

Laboratory results may indicate an elevated hematocrit measurement in relation to the hemoglobin and elevated BUN measurements. Later, after fluids return to the bloodstream, laboratory results may indicate decreased hematocrit and BUN levels. Other abnormal findings may be seen, depending on the area of the body affected.

Medical Management

Medical treatment begins with the determination of the cause of the fluid volume shift. When hypovolemia results from tissue injury such as burns or crush injury, a large volume of intravenous (iso-osmolar) fluid administration is required. The amount of fluid infusion may be three times greater than the urinary output. If replacement is overzealous, a fluid overload could occur. During the second phase, fluid administration and intake may need to be limited because of fluid influx from the tissue spaces to the vessels.

If third space fluid has occurred as a result of other processes, such as pericarditis and bowel obstruction, the fluid may have to be removed in order for the organ to retain its function (e.g., pericentesis).

Nursing Management

Shock-like symptoms are frequently present in cases of fluid volume shift, so the client's vital signs should be assessed every 1 to 8 hours (depending on the condition of the client). If fluid loss is to the peritoneum (ascites) or extremities (peripheral edema), the fluid shift is slower, and changes in the vital signs are usually subtle.

Intravenous fluid replacement should be monitored. If fluids are administered too rapidly, hypervolemia (fluid overload) may occur. Frequent checks for chest crackles, difficulty in breathing, and neck vein engorgement are essential to prevent pulmonary edema with fluid volume excess. The abdominal girth of clients with ascites should be measured every 8 hours. If the extremities are involved, the circumference of the extremity and the peripheral pulses should be measured every hour. The level of consciousness should be monitored and precautions taken for seizures. Frequent skin care to edematous areas during fluid shift is essential to prevent skin breakdown. As the fluid shifts back with the repair of tissue damage, intravenous fluid replacement is decreased.

Urine output should be monitored every hour to ensure at least 25 mL per hour. Urine output is usually reduced after tissue injury because of decreased renal circulation and the fluid shift into the injured tissue spaces. Three to 5 days after tissue injury, fluid returns to the circulation and excess fluid is excreted by the kidneys unless there is impaired renal function. The serum levels of BUN and ammonia should be monitored in clients with ascites.

A comparison of the fluids administered with the urine output and vital signs is a common practice in monitoring progress.

INTRACELLULAR FLUID VOLUME EXCESS: WATER INTOXICATION

Hypo-osmolar disorders result from either water excess or solute deficit and are mainly due to sodium loss. In the case of water excess, the number of solutes is normal, but they are diluted by excessive water. In the case of solute deficit, the amount of water is normal, but there are too few particles per liter of water. In both cases, hypo-osmolality of vascular fluids exists and cellular swelling occurs.

Although ICFVE is not as common a type of fluid imbalance as ECFVD and ECFVE, it presents a serious health problem if it is unrecognized and untreated. The most common cause of ICFVE is the administration of excessive amounts of hypo-osmolar intravenous fluids, such as 0.45 per cent saline or 5 per cent dextrose in water. ICFVE may occur in clients who receive continuous D_5W intravenous fluids; in those with brain injury or disease that causes an increased production of ADH, which increases water reabsorption from the renal tubules; or in those who are elderly and consume excessive amounts of tap water without adequate nutrient intake. Increased ADH production may also follow the stress of surgery, pain, and narcotic use. Such reactions are described as secretion of inappropriate antidiuretic hormone (SIADH). Early administration of intravenous fluids containing some sodium chloride can prevent SIADH. Saline solutions increase the osmolality of vascular fluid and prevent hypo-osmolarity.

Hypo-osmolar fluids move by osmosis to maintain fluid equilibrium, forcing fluids to move from the lesser concentration (in the vessels) to the higher concentration (in the cells). Unfortunately, too much fluid accumulates in the cells, causing cellular edema. The urine output may be normal or decreased with water intoxication. Table 3–3 lists the clinical manifestations of

TABLE 3–3 Clinical Manifestations of Intracellular Fluid Volume Excess and Their Pathophysiologic Bases

CLINICAL MANIFESTATION	PATHOPHYSIOLOGIC BASIS
Headaches, nausea, vomiting	Central nervous system changes cause increased intracranial pressure; cerebral cells absorb hypo-osmolar fluid more quickly than other cells do
Pupillary changes	Pressure on the third cranial nerve from increased cranial pressure
Behavioral changes: progressive apprehension, irritability, disorientation, confusion, drowsiness, decreased coordination	Swollen cerebral cells
Decreased muscle strength, unequal grasp, pronation drift	Cerebellar or basal ganglia swelling
Weight gain	Excess water retention
Severe central nervous system symptoms	Water excess progressively increases intracranial pressure and interferes with cell function
Vital signs: bradycardia with an increased systolic blood pressure (widened pulse pressure); increased respirations; neuroexcitability (muscle twitching); Babinski's response; flaccidity; projectile vomiting; papilledema; delirium; convulsions; coma	Vital sign changes are an ominous indicator of increased intracranial pressure and herniation of the brain stem
Laboratory Findings	
Serum sodium level <125 mEq/L	Associated with hypo-osmolality
Decreased hematocrit	Hemodilution; extracellular fluid excess often accompanies intracellular fluid excess

ICFVE and their pathophysiologic bases. The serum sodium level is decreased because of hemodilution.

Management

Treatment should begin when early signs of increased intracranial pressure are noted. ICFVE is treated by the addition of solutes to intravenous fluids. The use of D_5/0.45 per cent NaCl will help to correct ICFVE when the cause is water excess. Oral fluids such as juices or soft drinks should be given in addition to water and ice chips.

The nurse should have a high index of suspicion for clients who have received excessive amounts of D_5W or tap water or who have had a recent operation, pain, or stress, and who receive central nervous system drug depressants. The physician should be notified if the client's sensorium changes from that of the baseline assessment.

Reflexes and pupillary response should be assessed. Intravenous therapy should be monitored every hour. The nurse should offer fluids containing solutes (juices, colas, broth) every hour if permitted. He or she should monitor for changes in vital signs every 1 to 8 hours, depending on client's condition, and should monitor intake and output every 1 to 8 hours.

CRITICAL TO REMEMBER

An increase in urine output is needed to decrease ICFVE; polyuria indicates that fluid has shifted to the vascular space, from where it can be excreted.

The client's weight should be checked daily to measure fluid gain or loss.

The nurse should administer prescribed antiemetics as needed to allow food and fluids to be ingested.

Safety measures are necessary when the client displays behavioral changes (confusion, disorientation). The bed should be kept in a low position, and bedside rails should be raised. The client should be closely observed for protection from injury. An oral airway and suction equipment should be kept at the bedside in the event of seizures. (See also Chapter 14 for care of the client during a seizure.)

Electrolytes

Electrolytes are substances found in extracellular and intracellular fluid that dissociate into electrically charged particles known as ions. *Cations* are ions that carry a positive charge, and *anions* are ions that carry a negative charge. The positively charged electrolytes (cations) are sodium, potassium, calcium, and magnesium; the negatively charged electrolytes (anions) are chloride, phosphate, and bicarbonate. The electrolytes that are most plentiful in the cells are potassium, magnesium, phosphate, and proteinate. The most plentiful ions in the ECF are sodium, calcium, chloride, and bicarbonate.

CRITICAL TO REMEMBER

The principal cation in the ICF is potassium, and the principal cation in the ECF is sodium.

Electrolytes have major influences on (1) body water regulation, (2) acid-base regulation, (3) enzyme

TABLE 3–4 Concentration of Electrolytes in Body Fluids

FLUID	Na^+ (mEq/L)	K^+ (mEq/L)	Cl^- (mEq/L)	HCO_3^- (mEq/L)
Saliva	33	20	34	0
Gastric juice*	60	9	84	0
Bile	149	5	101	45
Pancreatic juice	141	5	77	92
Ileal fluid	129	11	116	29
Cecal fluid	80	21	48	22
Cerebrospinal fluid	141	3	127	23
Sweat	45	5	58	0

*The Cl^- concentration exceeds the Na^+, K^+ concentration by 15 mEq/L in gastric juice. This largely represents the secretion of H^+ by the parietal cells.
From Smith, L. H., & Thier, S. O. (1981). *Pathophysiology: The biological principles of disease.* Philadelphia: W. B. Saunders. Adapted from Narins, R. (1987). *Maxwell & Kleeman's Clinical disorders of fluid and electrolyte metabolism* (2nd ed.). New York: McGraw-Hill.

reactions, and (4) neuromuscular activity. Sodium concentration in the extracellular fluid assists in the maintenance of fluid balance.

CRITICAL TO REMEMBER

Sodium, potassium, chloride, bicarbonate, phosphate, and proteinate ions regulate acid-base balance within the body.

The cations are necessary for the transmission of nerve impulses and stimulation of muscle activity. Concentration of electrolytes in various body fluids is shown in Table 3–4.

Because intracellular levels of electrolytes cannot be measured, all values for electrolytes are expressed as serum values. Serum values for electrolytes can be expressed as mEq/L or mg/dL.

Sodium Homeostatic Mechanisms

Sodium balance is regulated by afferent and efferent mechanisms. Afferent sensing mechanisms in nerve endings recognize changes in sodium intake and extracellular fluid volume by sensing an increase or decrease in pressure. Afferent mechanisms are found in the atria, carotid sinus, liver, and kidneys. In addition, there are central nervous system receptors that respond to changes in the sodium concentration in the cerebrospinal fluid.

Efferent mechanisms include the glomerular filtration rate in the kidney. Blood enters the glomerulus and is driven by the systemic blood pressure. The pressure of the blood entering the glomeruli is high and favors filtration across the membrane. Blood proteins remaining in the vessel exert oncotic pressure to draw fluids back into the vessel. Approximately 99 per cent of the sodium that is filtered by the glomerulus is reabsorbed by the renal tubules. Considering the enormous quantities of sodium that are normally handled by the kidney, any alteration in renal function can have an impact on sodium homeostasis.

Hormonal factors also control sodium homeostasis. These mechanisms include renin-angiotensin-aldosterone, prostaglandins, kallikrein, and natriuretic hormones. Renin is a hormone excreted in response to hypotension. Renin production results in increased angiotensin; angiotensin, in turn, increases aldosterone production for the adrenal cortex. Aldosterone stimulates net sodium reabsorption across the tubule.

Prostaglandins are secreted by the kidney and stimulate the production of renin. These hormones also maintain renal blood flow during periods of reduced blood volume. Kallikreins are proteins of high molecular weight that are produced by the distal convoluted tubule and secrete kinin. Kinin is a potent renal vasodilator and increases renal excretion of sodium. The function of natriuretic hormone is not fully understood.

Sodium Imbalances

A sodium imbalance occurs when there is either a decrease in sodium or an increase in sodium concentration in the plasma. A sodium deficit is called *hyponatremia* and occurs when serum sodium levels are less than 135 mEq/L. Sodium excess is called *hypernatremia* and occurs when the serum sodium levels are greater than 145 mEq/L.

HYPONATREMIA

Hyponatremia is a serum sodium level below 135 mEq/L.

CRITICAL TO REMEMBER

Hyponatremia is said to be one of the most common electrolyte disorders, occurring in a wide variety of illnesses.

Etiology

The causes of hyponatremia are usually associated with fluid volume status. Hyponatremia may occur when the total body water is decreased.

Hyponatremia may develop from SIADH. SIADH may follow many forms of drug therapy including chemotherapy, phenothiazines, morphine, and barbiturates.

Hyponatremia may also result from the kidney's inability to excrete sufficiently diluted urine. Normally when hyponatremia and hypo-osmolality occur, diuresis (increased urine excretion) follows to promote sodium

TABLE 3–5 Causes of Hyponatremia

ETIOLOGY	CLINICAL CONDITIONS AND DISORDERS
Hypovolemic hyponatremia	Renal loss of sodium from diuretic use, diabetic glycosuria, aldosterone deficiency, intrinsic renal disease Extrarenal loss of sodium from vomiting, diarrhea, increased sweating, burns
Euvolemic hyponatremia	Sodium deficit resulting from syndrome of inappropriate secretion of antidiuretic hormone or the continuous secretion of antidiuretic hormone due to pain, emotion, medications
Hypervolemic hyponatremia	Edematous disorders resulting in sodium deficits: congestive heart failure, cirrhosis of the liver, nephrotic syndrome, acute and chronic renal failure
Redistributive hyponatremia	Pseudohyponatremia, hyperglycemia, hyperlipidemia

and water balance. Table 3–5 lists clinical conditions and disorders that may cause hyponatremia.

Risk Factors

Risk factors leading to hyponatremia are more prominent in the elderly, infants, and small children because of the variations in total body water. Clinical conditions such as vomiting and diarrhea or cardiac and renal disorders increase the risk of hyponatremia. Clients with Addison's disease are at risk. Clients who are receiving nothing by mouth (NPO), NPO and receiving intravenous solutions, or on potent diuretics without sodium replacement are also at risk. Early recognition of the high-risk status of clients may prevent a marked hyponatremic state.

Hyponatremia can also occur in healthy clients. Clients at risk include those who lose fluids through excessive perspiration and do not restore the lost sodium through fluid intake. Athletes and outdoor laborers are included in this category.

Pathophysiology

As the ECF concentration of sodium decreases, the sodium concentration gradient (difference) between the ECF and ICF also decreases. This hypo-osmolarity can lead to intracellular edema. The water in the ECF moves by osmosis into the cells. These changes also mean that there is less sodium to move across the excitable membrane, which usually results in delayed membrane depolarization. Excitable tissues vary in their response to decreased sodium; the most sensitive to changes are the central nervous system cells, leading to cerebral edema. Generally, the clinical manifestations reflect the decreased excitability or irritability of the membranes.

If the hyponatremic state and body fluid volume disorders are not corrected, potassium, calcium, chloride, and bicarbonate electrolyte imbalances may occur. Uncorrected hypovolemic hyponatremia may result in shock from continued ECF volume loss. This severe hyponatremic state leads to neurologic changes varying from confusion to convulsion and coma. A hypervolemic hyponatremic state, if not corrected, results in ECF volume excess and edema.

Clinical Manifestations

Clinical manifestations of hyponatremia vary with the cause and type of fluid volume imbalance. A sodium deficit may occur in the presence of decreased, normal, or increased total body sodium and water. An assessment of the body fluid volume is helpful in the determination of a sodium imbalance. With cardiac, renal, and liver disease, the total body sodium level is usually high, although the serum sodium level may appear normal or low. In such instances, there is generally a greater increase in total body water than the sodium indicates.

CRITICAL TO REMEMBER

A serum sodium level of less than 115 mEq/L will cause severe neurologic changes such as confusion or convulsions and may result in death due to excessive water shift to the intracellular compartment.

When the serum sodium decreases slowly or is greater than 125 mEq/L, signs and symptoms may not be apparent.

With a loss of body fluids and sodium, the heart rate increases as a compensatory mechanism to overcome fluid and sodium losses. Cellular swelling causes neurologic and behavioral changes. Clinical manifestations and their pathophysiologic bases are presented in Table 3–6.

DIAGNOSTIC ASSESSMENT

Diagnosis is based on the combination of clinical manifestations and serum laboratory values. Acute hyponatremia is a serum sodium concentration below 120 mEq/L with central nervous system manifestations.

Medical Management

Medical management begins with the attempt to determine the cause of the hyponatremia and to correct it. The goal of treatment is to correct the body water osmolarity and therefore restore cell volume by raising the ratio of sodium to water in the ECF. The increased ECF osmolarity draws water from the cells and thereby decreases cellular edema. If the client has hyponatremia

TABLE 3–6 Clinical Manifestations of Hyponatremia and Their Pathophysiologic Bases

CLINICAL MANIFESTATION	PATHOPHYSIOLOGIC BASIS
Gastrointestinal	
Nausea, vomiting, diarrhea, hyperactive bowel sounds, abdominal cramps	Sodium is abundant in the gastrointestinal tract; loss of gastrointestinal secretions causes a sodium loss
Cardiovascular	
Decrease in diastolic blood pressure, tachycardia, profound orthostatic hypotension, weak pulse	Losses of sodium and water decrease the circulating fluid volume and may result in shock-like symptoms
Elevated blood pressure; full, rapid pulse	Dilutional hyponatremia with excessive fluid volume increases circulating fluids
Pulmonary	
Changes in rate of respirations	Due to changes in central nervous system
Adventitious lung sounds	Fluid overload, congestive heart failure
Neurologic	
Headache, apprehension, lethargy, confusion, slowed problem solving, flat affect, diminished muscle tone in the extremities, decreased deep tendon reflexes, weakness and tremor	Diluted body fluids move into the brain cells, affecting both cognition and reflexes; excitable membranes are less responsive to stimuli
Integumentary	
Dry skin; pale, dry mucous membranes	Decreased interstitial fluids
Laboratory Findings	
Serum sodium <135 mEq/L	Results in hyponatremia; symptoms become apparent when the serum sodium is <125 mEq/L
Urine sodium <40 mEq/L	Body sodium losses result in a compensatory decrease in urinary excretion of sodium
Serum osmolality <275 mOsm/kg	Sodium losses result in a decreased concentration of sodium in body fluids

due to fluid volume excess, intake of fluids will be restricted to allow the sodium to regain balance. If the serum sodium level falls below 125 mEq/L, sodium replacement is needed.

Rapid elevation of serum sodium concentrations to levels greater than 125 mEq/L is hazardous. Loss of fluids in and around the brain and the shifting of electrolytes (such as potassium) are homeostatic mechanisms that prevent damage to the brain cells. The rapid correction of serum sodium levels may increase fluid volume levels and can result in damage to the central nervous system.

PHARMACOLOGIC MANAGEMENT

For a client with moderate hyponatremia, 125 mEq/L intravenous normal saline solution (0.9 per cent NaCl) or lactated Ringer's solution may be ordered. When the serum sodium level is 115 mEq/L or less, a concentrated saline solution such as 3 per cent NaCl is generally indicated. The administration of hypertonic solutions is irritating to peripheral veins. The client must be closely monitored for overhydration or hypernatremia when 3 per cent saline solution is administered. This is especially true for the client with a cardiac problem, such as congestive heart failure, or renal disease.

Many times, normal saline is administered in conjunction with the diuretic furosemide (Lasix), which increases urinary sodium loss and therefore reduces the risk of ECF volume expansion. Moreover, the urine excreted through furosemide-induced diuresis has much less sodium than does the ECF, which raises the serum sodium levels.

Drug therapy for hyponatremia from SIADH includes agents that antagonize ADH, such as demeclocycline and lithium.

DIETARY MANAGEMENT

A balanced diet is usually adequate therapy for mild hyponatremia (126 to 135 mEq/L). More severe hyponatremia may require sodium replacement. Foods high in sodium are listed in Box 3–1. If the client has hyponatremia due to excess fluids, a fluid-restricted diet may be prescribed. Fluids may be restricted to 800 to 1000 mL/day.

Nursing Management

Assessment

Nursing assessment focuses on data collection related to health problems and signs and symptoms manifested by the client with hyponatremia. The nurse should obtain a history of the cause of hyponatremia, such as vomiting, diarrhea, and decreased intake of sodium. Likewise, a history of Addison's disease, steroid use, cerebrovascular accident, and renal, cardiac, or hepatic failure should be noted. Assessment should include checking serum sodium levels and estimating the serum osmolality.

BOX 3-1

Sodium Amounts in Selected Foods

FOODS HIGH IN SODIUM (approximately 250 mg per serving)	FOODS LOW IN SODIUM (less than 50 mg per serving)
Grains	Fruits/vegetables
Cold cereal, 1 oz	Fresh or canned, ½ cup
Corn chips, 14 chips	Fresh frozen, ½ cup
Instant hot cereal, ½ cup	Grains
Potato chips, 14 chips	Unsalted pastas, ½ cup
Cheeses	Oatmeal, cooked, 1 cup
Natural cheese, 1 oz	Popcorn (unsalted), 1 oz
Processed cheese, 1 oz	Puffed rice, 1 cup
Creamed cheese, ½ cup	Shredded wheat, 1 biscuit
Meats	Meats
Sausage, 1 oz	Fresh meat, 1 oz
Luncheon meats, 1 oz	Fresh chicken, 1 oz
Frankfurters, 1 oz	Fresh fish, 1 oz
Cooked bacon, 2 slices	Beverages
Ham, 1 oz	
Convenience foods	
Pizza, 2 to 3 slices	
Pot pies, 8 oz	
Ravioli, canned, 8 oz	
Soups (canned/dehydrated), 1 cup	

Data from Laquarta, I., & Gerlach, M. (1990). *Nutrition in clinical nursing.* Albany, New York: Delmar Publishers; and Burtis, G., et al. (1988). *Applied nutrition and diet therapy.* Philadelphia: W. B. Saunders.

CRITICAL TO REMEMBER

In hyponatremic conditions such as hypervolemic hyponatremia, serum sodium levels may reveal normal to low readings.

This misleading reading occurs in response to medical conditions that cause water to be retained in greater quantities than sodium.

The usual medications and over-the-counter medications should be noted. Elderly clients are especially prone to drug-drug interactions that may alter sodium balance. Urine output as well as recent fluctuations in body weight should be assessed. A diet history should be assessed to ascertain the amount of sodium consumed.

The client and significant others should be asked about behavioral changes, headaches, and increased sleepiness.

Physical assessment should include height and weight, with a calculation of ideal body weight for body frame. Turgor and peripheral vein filling time should be noted.

Nursing Diagnosis, Planning, and Implementation

Collaborative Problem: Hyponatremia R/T vomiting, diarrhea, gastric suctioning, burns, SIADH, or surgery.

Planning: Expected Outcomes. The nurse will monitor the client for sodium levels to return to 135 mEq/L or above, the reduction of factors contributing to the hyponatremia, fluid and electrolyte losses and replacement, and symptoms of fluid and sodium imbalance.

Implementation. The nurse should have a high index of suspicion for hyponatremia in clients who have been NPO or NPO without sodium replacement in intravenous fluids; with nausea, vomiting, or abdominal cramps; and with neurologic changes or changes in mucous membranes or skin turgor.

Vital signs should be checked every 4 to 8 hours. The nurse should monitor serum sodium and osmolality levels.

CRITICAL TO REMEMBER

A serum sodium level of less than 125 mEq/L indicates the need for prompt medical care.

Estimation of the serum osmolality can be accomplished by doubling the value of the serum sodium level.

The nurse should monitor the type and amount of fluid intake. Fluid intake, whether oral or intravenous, should include sodium. If the client is receiving a 3 per cent saline solution intravenously, the nurse observes for signs and symptoms of hypervolemia such as dyspnea, chest crackles, and neck vein engorgement. The intravenous flow rate should be regulated with the aid of an intravenous pump to decrease the risk of hypervolemia.

The nurse should irrigate nasogastric tubes and wound sites with normal saline solution to prevent further sodium losses. Distilled or sterile water irrigations will increase sodium loss. The nurse should promote the intake of fluids containing sodium such as broth and juices and minimize the intake of ice chips. Ice chips can be made from saline to reduce the intake of tap water.

Intake and output should be closely monitored; hourly assessments should be performed if the client is acutely ill. Daily weights should be obtained to monitor fluid balance. The nurse should plan for fluid restriction if the hyponatremia is caused by fluid volume excess, being certain to coordinate fluid restriction with the dietitian and to schedule medications at the time of meals, as possible.

If the client is confused or agitated, the nurse needs to provide mechanisms to reorient the client as well as provide safety measures. Extraneous noise may aggravate the client's mental status and should be eliminated as much as possible. Side rails should be elevated and the bed kept in low position when the nurse is not providing direct care. As seizures may develop, the client should be protected from injury during the seizure and the airway should be maintained.

Evaluation

The client's serum sodium levels should return to normal. If the client remains hyponatremic, the interventions may require revision.

HYPERNATREMIA

Hypernatremia is a serum sodium level over 145 mEq/L. It occurs in approximately 1 per cent of hospitalized clients and carries a high mortality rate regardless of whether it has an acute or chronic onset. See Tables 3–7 and 3–8 for causes, clinical manifestations, and pathophysiology.

Medical Management

There is a high mortality rate for untreated acute and chronic hypernatremia. Neurologic manifestations and death can result from cellular dehydration. If the vascular volume decreases, the pulse rate increases, and eventually the blood pressure drops. As hypernatremia progresses, convulsions or coma or both occur.

To decrease total body sodium and replace fluid loss, either a hypo-osmolar electrolyte solution (0.2 per cent or 0.45 per cent NaCl) or D_5W is administered. These solutions will not cause a considerable dilution of body sodium; instead, the serum sodium level will be gradually decreased. D_5W, when administered continuously, is considered to be a hypo-osmolar solution because the dextrose is metabolized quickly and only water remains. When 5 per cent dextrose solutions are given, they must be given slowly to prevent osmotic diuresis, which aggravates the hypertonic state.

Sometimes normal saline is used for the volume-depleted client to provide fluid resuscitation. The saline is hypotonic in comparison with the serum and, there-

TABLE 3–7 Causes of Hypernatremia

ETIOLOGY	CLINICAL CONDITIONS AND DISORDERS
Hypovolemic hypernatremia	Renal losses: osmotic diuresis, severe hyperglycemia Extrarenal losses: profuse diaphoresis, decreased thirst, diarrhea occurring with inadequate volume replacement or fluid replacement with hyperosmolar solutions
Euvolemic hypernatremia	Excess fluid losses from the skin and lungs Hypodipsia in the elderly and infants Diabetes insipidus
Hypervolemic hypernatremia	Administration of concentrated saline solutions; hypertonic feedings, excess mineralocorticoids Accidental or intentional salt ingestions; commercially prepared soups and canned vegetables

TABLE 3–8 Clinical Manifestations of Hypernatremia and Their Pathophysiologic Bases

CLINICAL MANIFESTATION	PATHOPHYSIOLOGIC BASIS
Gastrointestinal	
Anorexia, nausea, and vomiting	Fluid retention in gastric cells
Integumentary	
Skin dry and flushed; mucous membranes dry and sticky	Decrease of interstitial fluid in tissues
Thirst; tongue dry and rough; body temperature elevated	Less interstitial fluids to cool body by evaporation
Neurologic	
Restlessness, agitation, irritability, lethargy, stupor, coma	Neurologic symptoms are the result of cerebral cellular dehydration
Muscle twitching, tremor, hyperreflexia, seizures; rigid paralysis in late stages	Neuromuscular irritability
Cardiovascular	
Tachycardia, hypotension or hypertension	Blood pressure relative to the type of hypernatremia. If hypovolemic, pressure will be decreased. If hypervolemic, pressure will be increased
Erratic heart rate and blood pressure dependent on fluid status	Myocardial depression as sodium ions compete with calcium ions in slow channels of heart
Renal	
Oliguria, dark and concentrated	Compensatory mechanism
Laboratory Findings	
Serum sodium >145 mEq/L	Hypernatremia is present when serum sodium level is >145 mEq/L
Serum osmolality >295 mOsm/kg	Sodium is the major solute of fluid concentration; hypernatremia increases serum osmolality

fore, allows the sodium level to decrease slowly. If the serum sodium level is lowered too rapidly, fluid will shift from the vascular space into the cerebral cells, causing cerebral edema. A general rule of thumb is that water replacement should be administered to reduce serum sodium levels not more than 2 mEq/L/hour for the first 48 hours.

PHARMACOLOGIC MANAGEMENT

Hypernatremia caused by sodium excess can be treated with D_5W and a diuretic such as furosemide.

DIETARY MANAGEMENT

Dietary restrictions of sodium are useful in preventing hypernatremia in high-risk clients. Dietary restriction will not bring a high sodium level down to normal, however. Clients with renal disease may need to have their sodium intake restricted to 500 to 2000 mg/day. Often fluids must also be restricted. Compliance with this degree of restriction is often difficult.

Nursing Management

Assessment

The client should be assessed for usual clinical manifestations. The nurse should have a high index of suspicion for high-risk clients (e.g., head-injured clients). A medication history should be used to assess for drugs that contain sodium, such as cough medicine and corticosteroids. Likewise, the diet history should be assessed for sodium consumption. Serum sodium levels should be checked, and the serum osmolality should be estimated.

The nurse should monitor the condition of the client's oral mucous membranes. Oral membrane assessment scores are very effective means of assessment (see Chapter 32).

Nursing Diagnosis, Planning, and Implementation

Collaborative Problem: Hypernatremia R/T decreased thirst or excessive administration of salt solutions or impaired secretion of sodium and water.

Planning: Expected Outcomes. The nurse will monitor the client for response to intravenous fluid replacement of hypo-osmolar electrolyte solutions, absence of signs and symptoms of hypernatremia, and return of normal sodium levels.

Implementation. Water and fluids should be offered frequently to the elderly and to clients with debilitating diseases in order to prevent body fluid loss and hypernatremia. However, increasing fluid intake in clients with congestive heart failure or severe renal disease is usually contraindicated. The nurse should encourage clients to drink decaffeinated fluids and to avoid alcohol. Caffeinated fluids and alcohol increase fluid loss, which can result in an increase in the serum sodium level. Overconsumption of fruit juices can also increase fluid loss.

Depending on the client's condition, vital signs should be assessed every 4 to 8 hours, and skin care given every 2 to 4 hours. Intake and output should be assessed every 8 hours, and body weight should be assessed daily.

The nurse should monitor changes in the serum sodium, serum osmolality, and symptoms of hypernatremia. Detection of the early symptoms of altered mental status (agitation, irritability, confusion) can prevent the progression of hypernatremia. Seizure precautions should be initiated.

Fluid replacement with or without sodium should be closely monitored by the nurse. The nurse should check for symptoms of osmotic diuresis when D_5W is continuously used. Signs and symptoms of cerebral edema may be apparent.

Nursing Diagnosis: Oral Mucous Membranes, Altered R/T inadequate volume of oral secretions.

Planning: Expected Outcomes. The client will have improved condition of oral mucous membranes, as evidenced by moist and intact oral mucous membranes; increased oral mucous membrane score on assessment tool; report of no oral discomfort; and ability to consume fluids without pain.

Implementation. The client should be given or offered oral care every 2 hours with a nonalcoholic mouthwash. Lemon-glycerin swabs should also be avoided because they dry the membranes and may cause pain. A soft toothbrush should be used to prevent injury to the mucosa. Lips should be moistened with a water-soluble lubricant. Cool, nonacidic fluids such as apple juice are generally tolerated best.

Evaluation

The nurse evaluates whether or not the goals of preventing and correcting fluid imbalance and hypernatremia have been met. If abnormal laboratory findings and symptoms remain, this information should be conveyed to the appropriate health professional.

The client's oral mucous membranes should be evaluated every shift to detect a lack of improvement.

Client Education

The client may require dietary education to reinforce the need for fluid and sodium restriction. The client should also be taught to avoid over-the-counter medications that are high in sodium as well as to recognize clinical manifestations of hyponatremia and hypernatremia.

Potassium Imbalances

Approximately 96 per cent of potassium is in the intracellular fluid and 4 per cent is in the intravascular fluid. Potassium is also plentiful in the gastrointestinal tract. Intracellular potassium has a value of 150 mEq. However, body potassium levels can be obtained only through the measurement of plasma. Therefore, the range of serum potassium is very narrow (3.5 to 5.0 mEq/L). It is vitally important that the potassium level be maintained within this narrow range in order to avoid potassium imbalance. Alterations in potassium level is an extremely serious problem.

CRITICAL TO REMEMBER

If the serum potassium level is less than 2.5 mEq/L or greater than 7.0 mEq/L, cardiac arrest could result.

POTASSIUM HOMEOSTATIC MECHANISMS

Potassium has many functions within the body. It assists in the regulation of intracellular osmolality. It promotes the transmission and conduction of nerve impulses and the contraction of skeletal, cardiac, and smooth muscles. It promotes enzyme action for cellular metabolism, promotes glycogen storage in the liver, and assists with the maintenance of acid-base balance.

CRITICAL TO REMEMBER

A potassium deficit is associated with alkalosis; a potassium excess is associated with acidosis.

Normal daily potassium requirements are 40 to 60 mEq/L. Potassium is poorly stored in the body, so daily potassium intake is necessary. A standard diet contains 50 to 100 mEq/day. Foods rich in potassium include vegetables, fruits, dry fruits, nuts, and meats. An increased sodium intake promotes potassium loss. Eighty to 90 per cent of potassium is excreted through the kidneys, and the remainder is excreted in feces. Renal excretion of potassium is influenced by plasma potassium concentration, blood flow into the kidney, acid-base status, and various hormones.

Acid-Base Alteration

CRITICAL TO REMEMBER

The potassium level is affected by acid-base imbalances.

Alkalosis can cause hypokalemia. In an alkalotic state, hydrogen moves out of the cells to correct the alkalosis, and potassium shifts into the cells, thus lowering the serum potassium level. In acidosis, the reverse is true, and potassium levels rise.

Hormonal Influence

CRITICAL TO REMEMBER

Insulin promotes potassium uptake by the cells. Insulin-deficient clients frequently develop hyperkalemia.

The mechanism whereby insulin promotes potassium uptake is controversial. Data suggest that insulin directly stimulates the sodium-potassium pump.

Glucagon increases plasma levels of potassium. Again, the mechanism is not fully understood; it appears that glucagon stimulates potassium release from the liver and may promote potassium movement in muscle cells.

Adrenocortical hormones such as cortisol and aldosterone promote potassium excretion and sodium retention via the kidneys. During stress, cortisol and aldosterone levels are increased; thus, potassium excretion is promoted. Catecholamines also affect potassium concentration. Beta-adrenergic agonists promote cellular uptake of potassium. Adrenergic mechanisms may also stimulate a sensor in the central nervous system for potassium homeostasis.

In contrast with beta-adrenergic stimulation, alpha-adrenergic agonists increase plasma potassium concentration. Hepatic stores of potassium are released, and muscle storage is altered.

Epinephrine, which has both alpha- and beta-adrenergic properties, causes an initial transient rise in potassium. The beta-adrenergic properties subsequently become dominant, and the major effect is a lowering of plasma potassium levels.

HYPOKALEMIA

Definition, Incidence, and Etiology

Hypokalemia is a serum potassium level of less than 3.5 mEq/L, it is a common electrolyte disorder. The many causes of hypokalemia are listed in Table 3–9.

Risk Factors

The elderly and the young are at a higher risk for the development of hypokalemia. The body does not preserve potassium; thus, potassium deficit frequently occurs in relation to an inadequate nutrient intake. Clients taking potassium-wasting diuretics or those who have a severe tissue injury are prone to develop hypokalemia.

Prevention of hypokalemia can be accomplished by the consumption of foods rich in potassium or the intake of potassium supplements. The serum potassium level should be closely monitored when a client has a renal disorder and is taking potassium supplements.

Pathophysiology

When the serum potassium levels decrease, there is an increased potassium gradient between the cell and the plasma. The increased gradient causes the resting membrane potential to increase, thus reducing excitability. Therefore, cell membranes are less responsive to stimuli.

TABLE 3–9 Causes of Hypokalemia

ETIOLOGY	CLINICAL CONDITIONS AND DISORDERS
Gastrointestinal losses	Vomiting, diarrhea, nasogastric suctioning, intestinal fistula, laxative abuse, excessive tap water enemas
Dietary changes	Malnutrition, starvation, potassium-free diet, some weight reduction diets, potassium-free intravenous solutions when there is no dietary intake
Medications	Potassium-wasting diuretics (thiazide, loop of Henle, and osmotic), steroids (cortisone preparations), large amounts of licorice (aldosterone-like effect), gentamicin, amphotericin B, digitalis preparations, and beta-adrenergics promote potassium loss
Redistribution of potassium	Insulin moves glucose and potassium back into cells; potassium loss from osmotic diuresis; in diabetic acidosis, alkalosis causes potassium to shift into cells in exchange for the hydrogen ion
Disorders	Cushing's syndrome, diuretic phase of acute renal failure, alcoholism, hyperaldosteronism

CRITICAL TO REMEMBER

The respiratory system is profoundly affected by depression of nervous and muscle synapses.

Contraction of muscle groups is slowed, and respiratory movement and ventilation are slowed. Cardiac function is also affected. The pulse is thready and often slow. Electrocardiographic changes are common. Skeletal muscle contraction is slowed. The client may experience transient irritability to profound confusion. Hypokalemia suppresses gastrointestinal function, which leads to paralytic ileus.

Clinical Manifestations

The clinical manifestations of hypokalemia include a decreased serum potassium level, abnormal electrocardiography, and signs and symptoms related to gastrointestinal, cardiac, renal, and neurologic disturbances (Table 3–10). Observable signs and symptoms may not be apparent with mild hypokalemia (3.3 to 3.4 mEq/L), especially if the decrease is gradual. In such instances, the potassium imbalance may go undetected until the serum potassium level continues to fall (Fig. 3–4). With severe hypokalemia, cardiac arrest may occur.

Medical Management

Medical management is focused on determining and correcting the cause of the imbalance. Medical care is also directed by the level of the potassium and clinical manifestations. Extreme hypokalemia requires cardiac monitoring.

PHARMACOLOGIC MANAGEMENT

Oral potassium replacement therapy is usually prescribed for mild hypokalemia (serum potassium 3.3 to 3.5 mEq/L) or for preventive purposes. Oral potassium chloride or potassium gluconate is available in liquid or tablet form. Potassium is extremely irritating to the gastric mucosa; therefore, the drug must be taken with one-half to one glass of water or juice or during meals.

Potassium chloride can be administered intravenously for moderate or severe hypokalemia.

CRITICAL TO REMEMBER

Potassium is **NOT** given intramuscularly and **NEVER** given as a bolus (intravenous push) injection. Potassium given intravenously **MUST ALWAYS BE DILUTED IN INTRAVENOUS FLUIDS.**

Administration of potassium by intravenous push may result in cardiac arrest. Potassium can be given in doses

TABLE 3–10 Clinical Manifestations of Hypokalemia and Their Pathophysiologic Bases

CLINICAL MANIFESTATION	PATHOPHYSIOLOGIC BASIS
Gastrointestinal	
Anorexia, vomiting, diarrhea, ileus, distention	Smooth muscle contraction slowed
Musculoskeletal	
Muscle weakness, paralysis, leg cramps, muscle flabbiness	Slowed smooth and skeletal muscle contraction
Cardiovascular	
Dysrhythmias, vertigo, postural hypotension, flattened T wave, prominent U wave, slow weak pulse	Increase in cell excitability; prolongation of myocardial repolarization Dysrhythmias are more pronounced when the client is taking a digitalis preparation
Respiratory	
Shallow respirations, shortness of breath	Weakness of the respiratory muscles due to a decrease in muscle contractions
Neurologic	
Fatigue, lethargy, decreased tendon reflexes, confusion, depression	Decreased transmission and conduction of nerve impulses
Renal	
Polyuria, decreased serum osmolality, nocturia	Inhibition of the kidney's ability to concentrate urine
Laboratory Findings	
Serum potassium <3.5 mEq/L	Hypokalemia is present
Serum osmolality <275 mOsm/kg	Polyuria, which leads to a loss of body potassium and other solutes

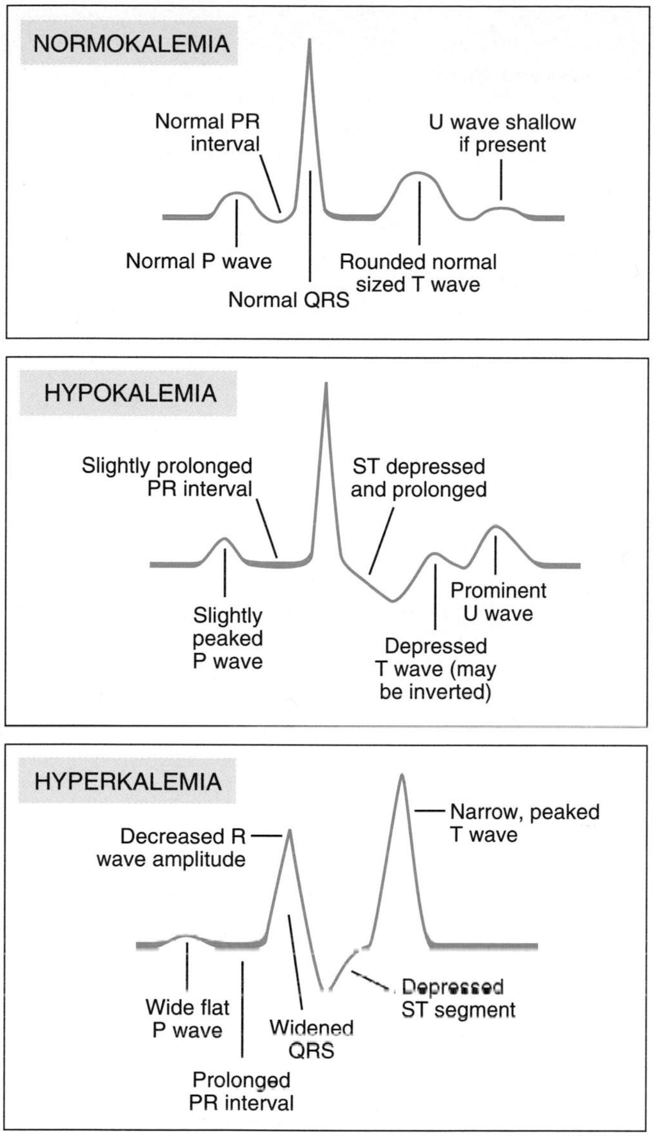

Figure 3–4
Electrocardiographic changes with potassium imbalance. (From McCance, K. L., & Huether, S. E. [1990]. *Pathophysiology: The basic biologic basis for disease in adults and children.* St. Louis: C. V. Mosby.)

of 10 to 20 mEq/hour diluted in intravenous fluids if the client is on a heart monitor.

Potassium is irritating to the blood vessels, so it has been recommended that 20 to 40 mEq of potassium be mixed in a liter of intravenous fluids for clients with mild and moderate hypokalemia. Clients with severe hypokalemia need 40 to 80 mEq in a liter of fluid. High concentrations of potassium are extremely irritating to the heart muscle. Thus, correcting a potassium deficit may take several days.

For clients who are NPO, usually after surgery or because of intestinal problems that prevent eating, a maintenance dosage of potassium is required. A common dose is 40 mEq/day in the intravenous solution.

DIETARY MANAGEMENT

The administration of foods that are high in potassium will help correct the problem as well as prevent further potassium losses. The adult recommended allowance of potassium is 1875 to 5625 mg. Common sources of foods containing potassium are listed in Box 3–2.

Nursing Management

Assessment

Nursing assessments focus on data collection related to the health problem and the clinical manifestations and laboratory findings associated with hypokalemia. The nurse should obtain a history to ascertain the cause of hypokalemia. Specific questions related to inadequate dietary intake of potassium and potassium losses due to vomiting, diarrhea, and drugs (diuretics, cortisone) are necessary. Assessment should include checking the serum potassium level and assessing for cardiac, gastrointestinal, and neuromuscular changes.

The nurse should maintain a high index of suspicion for clients who have prolonged nasogastric suctioning, are NPO without intravenous potassium supplements, or have renal disease.

Nursing Diagnosis, Planning, and Implementation

Collaborative Problem: Hypokalemia R/T vomiting, diarrhea, Cushing's disease, cortisone therapy, or decreased intake.

Planning: Expected Outcomes. The nurse will monitor the client for a return of the serum potassium level to the normal range, absence of complications related to intravenous administration of potassium chloride, and absence of signs and symptoms of cardiac and neuromuscular changes associated with hypokalemia.

Implementation. Intravenous potassium chloride is usually given for correcting potassium deficit and for maintaining potassium balance. Intravenous potassium chloride **must be diluted in intravenous fluids; it cannot be given as an intravenous push.** A large loading dose of potassium can cause cardiac arrest; thus, intravenous solution bags should always be agitated before being hung. The usual dose of intravenous potassium is 20 to 40 mEq in a liter of intravenous solution. Intravenous potassium is irritating to veins and can cause phlebitis; thus, the rate of flow must be carefully monitored. Intravenous fluids with potassium chloride are usually delivered by a controlled infusion pump to assist with maintenance of the correct intravenous flow rate.

Serum potassium levels should be closely monitored by the nurse. If the serum potassium level is less than 3.0 mEq/L, the potassium deficit will take longer to correct and requires a larger dose of potassium. Care should also be taken that continuous correction does not cause hyperkalemia. The nurse should continue to assess for signs and symptoms of potassium deficit. Neuromuscular changes are more pronounced with moderate and severe hypokalemia. Renal function should also be assessed. The nurse should monitor bowel function because constipation may be a problem. Clients on digitalis derivatives are at risk for digitalis toxicity if they are hypokalemic. The nurse should assess apical pulses for dysrhythmia.

BOX 3–2

Potassium Amounts in Selected Foods

HIGH IN POTASSIUM (average 7 mEq per serving)

Vegetables ($\frac{1}{2}$ cup cooked or 1 cup raw)
- Artichokes
- Broccoli
- Brussels sprouts
- Cabbage
- Carrots
- Celery
- Collards
- Cucumber
- Mushrooms
- Spinach
- Tomatoes

Fruits
- Apricots, fresh, 4 medium
- Apricots, canned, 4 halves
- Apricots, dried, 7 halves
- Banana, 7 inches
- Cantaloupe, $\frac{1}{4}$ small
- Guava, 1 medium
- Honeydew melon, $\frac{1}{8}$ medium
- Nectarine, $\frac{1}{2}$
- Orange, 1 small
- Prunes, 3 medium
- Strawberries, $1\frac{1}{4}$ cup
- Tangerine, 2 medium
- Watermelon, $1\frac{1}{4}$ cup

Beverages
- Brewed coffee
- Tomato juice
- Vegetable juice cocktail, unsalted

LOW IN POTASSIUM (average 3 mEq per serving)

Vegetables
- Corn, $\frac{1}{3}$ cup
- Sweet potato, yams, $\frac{1}{4}$ cup
- Lima beans, $\frac{1}{3}$ cup
- French fried potatoes, 10

Fruit
- Apple, 1 small
- Apple juice, $\frac{1}{2}$ cup
- Applesauce, $\frac{1}{2}$ cup
- Blueberries, $\frac{3}{4}$ cup
- Cranberries, $1\frac{1}{4}$ cup

Beverages
- Coffee, instant
- Cola
- Cranberry juice cocktail, $\frac{1}{3}$ cup
- Ginger ale
- Noncarbonated soft drinks
- Root beer
- Lemon-lime soda

Data from Mahan, K. L., & Arlin, M. (1992). *Krause's food, nutrition & diet therapy* (8th ed.). Philadelphia: W. B. Saunders.

Nursing Diagnosis: Injury, Risk for R/T muscle weakness and hypotension.

Planning: Expected Outcomes. The client will remain free of injury, as evidenced by no falls or near falls.

Implementation. The nurse must employ safety measures to reduce the risk of injury. The bed must be kept in low position with side rails up. Before the client ambulates, the path should be cleared of obstacles and the client should wear shoes to prevent slipping. An ambulation belt should be worn by the client and used by the nurse. Restraints should be used as needed to prevent harm.

Nursing Diagnosis: Nutrition: Less than Body Requirements, Altered R/T insufficient intake of foods rich in potassium.

Planning: Expected Outcomes. Client will increase dietary potassium intake to correct hypokalemia, as evidenced by selection of a diet consisting of potassium-rich foods such as bananas, cantaloupe, and nuts, consuming 1875 to 5625 mg of potassium each day, consumption of oral potassium supplements as prescribed to decrease or prevent potassium deficit, and an absence of signs and symptoms of hypokalemia.

Implementation. The nurse should instruct the client to choose and consume foods rich in potassium, such as fruits, fruit juices, dried fruits, vegetables including potatoes (potato skins are very rich in potassium), and nuts such as peanuts. Some fruits have more potassium than others; bananas, cantaloupe, and honeydew melons have twice as much potassium as oranges do. Meats and milk have a moderate amount of potassium. If the client is taking a liquid or tablet potassium supplement, the client should be instructed to take the potassium in or with at least one-half glass or more of water or juice.

Evaluation

The nurse evaluates whether the expected outcomes have been met: the serum potassium level is within normal range; the client is free of signs and symptoms of hypokalemia; and the client did not suffer from any preventable adverse effects of potassium therapy. A revision of the plan of care may be required if outcomes are not met.

Client Education

The client or whoever cooks in the home needs to be taught which foods are high in potassium. In addition, he or she should be taught that prolonged cooking of vegetables may result in potassium and vitamin loss. These foods should be steamed or cooked quickly.

HYPERKALEMIA

Hyperkalemia is an elevated potassium level over 5.0 mEq/L. Hyperkalemia is rare in clients with normal kidney function but may develop in clients with renal insufficiency or renal failure. Table 3–11 lists the causes of hyperkalemia.

Incidence

Because 80 to 90 per cent of potassium is excreted in the urine, clients with severe traumatic injuries—when potassium has left intracellular spaces because of direct cellular injury (e.g., burns)—develop hyperkalemia. The presence of shock in these clients compounds the problem because of low circulating vascular fluids and diminished kidney function.

Risk Factors

Clients at risk for hyperkalemia are those with insufficient renal function and decreased urinary output. Hyperkalemia may occur with excessive or rapid infusion of intravenous fluids with potassium even though there is adequate urine output.

Prevention of hyperkalemia is essential because a rapid elevation of serum potassium could cause cardiac arrest. Intravenous infusion of fluids with potassium chloride for clients with limited renal function and low urine output should be carefully monitored and given very slowly or not at all. Solutions containing potassium should be infused by intravenous pumps. Urinary output should be assessed hourly when the client is receiving a potassium supplement.

Pathophysiology and Clinical Manifestations

Hyperkalemia decreases the cell membrane's threshold, causing the cell to become more excitable (see Fig. 3–4).

Clinical manifestations are related to the serum potassium level (Table 3–12).

DIAGNOSTIC ASSESSMENT

Hyperkalemia is determined by clinical manifestations and laboratory findings as presented in Table 3–12. Low urinary output and renal function determined by BUN and serum creatinine levels are important indicators of risk of hyperkalemia because renal failure decreases potassium excretion.

Medical Management

Potassium elevation must be corrected before levels become severe. When the serum potassium level is 5.0 to 5.5 mEq/L, restriction of dietary potassium intake may be all that is needed. However, if the potassium excess is due to metabolic acidosis, correcting the acidosis with sodium bicarbonate promotes potassium uptake into the cells. Improving urine output usually decreases the elevated serum potassium level. Potassium-wasting diuretics can be used.

When hyperkalemia is severe, immediate actions are needed to avoid severe cardiac disturbances. These measures may include (1) intravenous calcium gluconate infusions to decrease the antagonistic effect of potassium excess on the myocardium and (2) infusion of insulin and glucose or sodium bicarbonate to promote potassium uptake into the cells. These methods usually provide temporary relief, and repeating them may not help.

As hyperkalemia persists or increases, a cation exchange resin such as polystyrene sulfonate (Kayexalate) may be given orally or rectally. This treatment stimulates the exchange of a potassium ion for a sodium ion in the intestinal tract; the potassium ion is then excreted in the stool. Because Kayexalate can be consti-

TABLE 3–11 Causes of Hyperkalemia

ETIOLOGY	CLINICAL CONDITIONS AND DISORDERS
Retention of potassium	Renal insufficiency, renal failure, decreased urine output after surgery, adrenal insufficiency, Addison's disease, hypoaldosteronism, potassium-sparing diuretics, blood for transfusion that is 2 weeks old or more (as blood ages, hemolysis of the red blood cell occurs, which releases the intracellular potassium into the surrounding fluids)
Excessive release of cellular potassium	Severe traumatic injuries, crushing injuries, severe burns, severe infection, metabolic acidosis; after open-heart surgery or surgery that requires a perfusion pump
Excessive intravenous infusions or oral administration of potassium	Excessive and rapid intravenous administration of potassium; excessive administration of large doses of oral potassium

TABLE 3–12 Clinical Manifestations of Hyperkalemia and Their Pathophysiologic Bases

CLINICAL MANIFESTATION	PATHOPHYSIOLOGIC BASIS
Cardiovascular	
First tachycardia and then bradycardia	Disturbances in cardiac conduction, especially through the Purkinje fibers and atrioventricular node, which may lead to ectopic beats; prolonged diastole
Electrocardiographic changes: peaked, narrow T waves; wide QRS complex; depressed ST segment; widened PR interval	
Ectopic beats	Increase in pacemaker and ectopic foci excitability
Hypotension	Cardiac arrest results with severe potassium elevation
Weaker cardiac contraction	
Gastrointestinal	
Nausea, explosive diarrhea, intestinal colic, hyperactive bowel sounds (especially over splenic flexure)	Increased smooth muscle contraction, increased peristalsis
Neuromuscular	
Paresthesia (tingling sensation), muscle weakness and later flaccid muscle paralysis, muscle cramps	Increased neuromuscular irritability of the skeletal muscles; elevated serum potassium levels cause the muscle to become weak owing to a depolarization block in the muscle
Renal	
Oliguria and later anuria	Usually due to pre-existing renal dysfunction; limits potassium excretion in the urine
Laboratory Findings	
Serum potassium >5.0 mEq/L	Hyperkalemia is present
Serum osmolality >295 mOsm/kg	Oliguria or anuria causes an accumulation of potassium and other solutes, thus increasing the osmolality of body fluids
Serum creatinine >1.5 mg/dL	Oliguria or anuria causes an elevation of creatinine and urea nitrogen in the intravascular fluids
Blood urea nitrogen >25 mg/dL	

pating, sorbitol may be combined with Kayexalate to prevent constipation and induce diarrhea. For rectal administration, it is given as a retention enema. In marked renal failure, peritoneal dialysis or hemodialysis may be needed.

Nursing Management

Assessment

Nursing assessment focuses on the clinical manifestations of and laboratory findings associated with hyperkalemia.

CRITICAL TO REMEMBER

The nurse should assess the urinary output especially when the client is to receive oral or intravenous potassium preparations. A decrease in urine output should be reported.

The serum potassium level must be closely monitored with high-risk clients and clients who are receiving potassium supplements. A serum potassium level greater than 7.0 mEq/L results in cardiac disturbances. If this is not corrected or the level rises, cardiac arrest can result. The electrocardiogram strips need to be assessed for narrowed, peaked T waves, depressed ST segment, and widening of the QRS complex and PR interval.

The flow rate of intravenous fluids with potassium should be closely monitored. A rapidly infused intravenous fluid with potassium can cause hyperkalemia. The potassium in the intravenous fluid is irritating to the vein and subcutaneous tissue. The nurse should assess for phlebitis and infiltration into the subcutaneous tissues, which can cause sloughing and tissue necrosis.

Nursing Diagnosis, Planning, and Implementation

Collaborative Problem: Hyperkalemia R/T renal dysfunction, shock from traumatic injuries, or burns.

Planning: Expected Outcomes. The nurse will monitor the client for return of serum potassium level to normal, presence of adequate (30 mL/hr) urinary output, absence of signs and symptoms of neuromuscular changes, and apical pulse rate within normal range and without dysrhythmia.

Implementation. The nurse should have a high index of suspicion for those disorders that may cause hyperkalemia. Assessment of signs and symptoms of hyperkalemia must be ongoing, and changes should be reported immediately.

CRITICAL TO REMEMBER

Numbness and tingling of the extremities are early signs of hyperkalemia.

Muscle weakness and flaccid muscle paralysis are symptoms of more severe hyperkalemia.

The urine output should be closely monitored every 1 to 8 hours, depending on the client's condition. Changes such as a urine output of less than 25 mL/hour or less than 600 mL/day should be reported immediately. Most of the body's excess potassium is excreted in urine.

CRITICAL TO REMEMBER

If the client is to receive a blood transfusion and is at risk for hyperkalemia, the nurse must notify the blood bank so that "old" blood (i.e., blood more than 2 weeks old) is not given to the client.

Methods prescribed for the correction of hyperkalemia should be closely monitored by the nurse. If the client is taking a digitalis preparation and the potassium correction is too rapid, hypokalemia may result. A hypokalemic state could enhance the action of digitalis and cause digitalis toxicity. Serum potassium levels and signs and symptoms of hyperkalemia and hypokalemia need to be continually assessed.

Collaborative Problem: Potential for dysrhythmias R/T hyperkalemia.

Planning: Expected Outcomes. The nurse will monitor for dysrhythmias, assess electrocardiographic recording every hour, and intervene according to protocols or notify the physician.

Implementation. The nurse should monitor electrocardiographic recordings and report changes that are related to hyperkalemia (see under Assessment). Cardiopulmonary resuscitation may be required but is seldom successful with severe hyperkalemia because the heart muscle will not respond. Insulin and glucose may be given to reduce potassium levels temporarily. The client should be assessed for decreased cardiac output as a result of bradycardia. The chest should be auscultated for crackles, the urine monitored for a decreased output, and the extremities assessed for peripheral edema. The nurse needs to report abnormal findings.

Evaluation

The client's status should be evaluated every hour if the client has severe hyperkalemia. Revisions in the plan of care may be required.

Client Education

The client will need to closely adhere to a diet low in potassium if the hyperkalemia is a chronic problem (e.g., renal failure). Knowledge of food preparation is important because cooking styles can affect potassium levels.

Calcium Imbalances

Calcium, an extracellular and intracellular cation, has a normal serum range of 4.5 to 5.5 mEq/L or 9 to 11 mg/dL. Approximately 99 per cent of the body's calcium is in bone and teeth. The other 1 per cent is in tissue and intravascular fluid, of which half is bound to protein, mostly albumin, and the remaining half is free, ionized calcium. The total serum calcium level does not indicate the exact amount of free, active calcium in the body.

CRITICAL TO REMEMBER

When albumin is low, it may give a false normal serum calcium level.

Instead, levels of serum ionized calcium (iCa) can be used to determine calcium deficit or excess in critically ill clients.

CALCIUM AND PHOSPHORUS HOMEOSTATIC MECHANISMS

Calcium has many functions in the body. It acts as a catalyst in the transmission and conduction of nerve impulses and stimulates the contraction of skeletal, smooth, and cardiac muscles. Calcium maintains normal cellular permeability. Increased serum calcium levels decrease cellular permeability, and decreased serum calcium levels increase cellular permeability.

CRITICAL TO REMEMBER

Calcium promotes coagulation of blood in all phases but mostly the prothrombin to thrombin phase.

It promotes absorption and utilization of vitamin B_{12}. Finally, calcium promotes strong and durable bones and teeth. Calcium is excreted in the urine and feces.

Vitamin D promotes calcium absorption from the gastrointestinal tract, whereas phosphorus (phosphate) inhibits its absorption. Therefore, calcium and phosphorus counterbalance each other.

Normal levels of serum calcium are also maintained by parathyroid hormone (PTH) in conjunction with the bones. The bones act very effectively to remove excess calcium from the blood. However, when the bones have become saturated with calcium salts, the resulting rise in calcium levels in the interstitial fluid affects the parathyroid gland. There is a decrease in PTH secretion

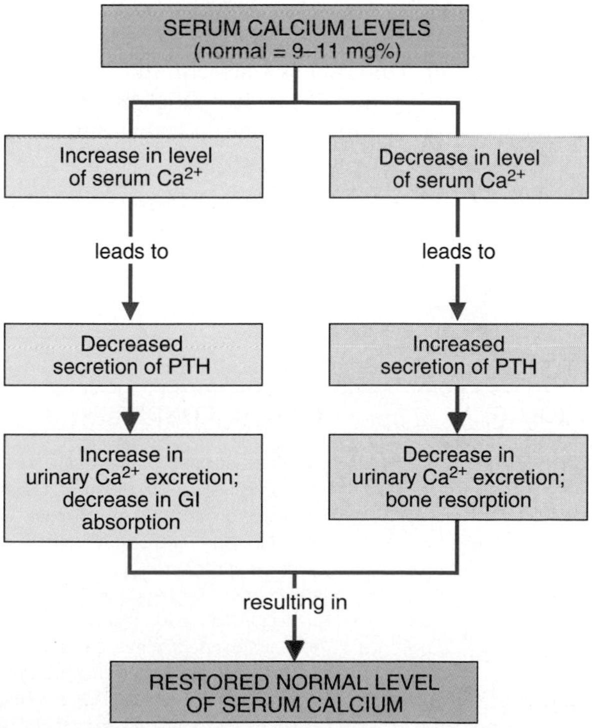

Figure 3–5
Parathyroid hormone (PTH) regulation of serum calcium level.

and an increase in urinary calcium excretion. Phosphorus and calcitonin from the thyroid gland act quickly to inhibit removal of calcium from the bone, thus decreasing the serum calcium level (Fig. 3–5).

Conversely, when the level of serum calcium falls even slightly, PTH secretion increases (see Fig. 3–5). Within minutes, calcium is reabsorbed through the kidneys; bone resorption occurs within hours, and increased absorption from the gastrointestinal tract occurs within days.

Like calcium, most phosphorus in the body resides in the skeleton. Sources of phosphorus are numerous in poultry and meat. Phosphorus is an integral part of the energy systems in the body (adenosine diphosphate and adenosine triphosphate). Deficiency is extremely rare. Phosphorus depletion can occur as a result of prolonged and excessive intake of antacids.

HYPOCALCEMIA

Definition, Incidence, and Etiology

Hypocalcemia is a serum calcium level below 4.5 mEq/L or 8.5 mg/dL. Hypocalcemia is a common and potentially serious electrolyte disorder that occurs more frequently in children and the elderly. Overcorrection of acidosis may also lead to hypocalcemia, because too much calcium is bound to protein. There are many causes of hypocalcemia (Table 3–13).

Risk Factors

Those at risk for hypocalcemia are children, the elderly, clients on reducing diets that are deficient in calcium, and clients with debilitating diseases that limit either dietary calcium intake or absorption. Primary prevention may be accomplished by teaching clients which foods are rich in calcium. Calcium supplements may be necessary for clients who have an intolerance for calcium-rich foods or clients who are on reducing diets that are calcium deficient.

Pathophysiology

A lack of PTH results in inactivity of osteoclasts and a consequent fall in serum calcium levels. Nerve fibers become more and more excitable and may discharge spontaneously, causing muscles to twitch and to go into spasms or even tetany. Spasms of the muscles of the larynx interfere with respiration and may lead to death. During hypocalcemia, the bone is stimulated to release calcium, which makes the bone osteoporotic and subject to fracture. Hypocalcemia increases capillary permeability; causes neuromuscular excitability of skeletal, smooth, and cardiac muscles; and decreases blood coagulation, which results in bleeding. Severe hypocalcemia causes neuromuscular excitability that results in tetany. If it is untreated, convulsions and death can occur. Acute hypocalcemia may cause cardiac insufficiency and cardiac dysrhythmias. Pathophysiologic changes as they relate to clinical manifestations of hypocalcemia are explained in Table 3–14.

Clinical Manifestations

Most of the clinical manifestations of hypocalcemia can be attributed to increased neuromuscular excitability. Numbness and tingling of the hands, toes, and lips, irritability, anxiety, dysrhythmias (prolonged QT interval), carpopedal spasm, seizures, laryngeal stridor, and prolonged bleeding time are common.

With prolonged hypocalcemia, cataracts may develop because of increased uptake of sodium and water by the lens. In addition, pathologic fractures and trophic changes, such as dry, sparse hair and rough skin, may be seen.

TABLE 3–13 Causes of Hypocalcemia

ETIOLOGY	CLINICAL CONDITIONS AND DISORDERS
Dietary changes	Inadequate dietary calcium intake, vitamin D deficiency, or both; excess intake of phosphorus combines with calcium, so neither electrolyte is absorbed
Gastrointestinal changes	Malabsorption of fat in the intestine
Calcium binding	Metabolic alkalosis (because there is less ionized calcium); multiple transfusion of stored blood (which is combined with citrate for storage)
Disorders	Renal failure with hyperphosphatemia, acute pancreatitis (which causes release of lipases into soft tissue spaces, so that free fatty acids that are formed bind with calcium), burns, Cushing's disease, hypoparathyroidism, liver disease, inadvertent removal of the parathyroid gland with thyroidectomy
Medications	Magnesium sulfate, colchicine, neomycin inhibit parathyroid hormone secretion; aspirin, anticonvulsants, estrogen alter vitamin D metabolism; phosphate preparations decrease serum calcium level; steroids decrease calcium mobilization; loop diuretics reduce calcium absorption from the renal tubules; antacids and laxatives decrease calcium absorption

TABLE 3–14 Clinical Manifestations of Hypocalcemia and Their Pathophysiologic Bases

CLINICAL MANIFESTATION	PATHOPHYSIOLOGIC BASIS
Neuromuscular	
Tetany symptoms: twitching around mouth, tingling and numbness of fingers, carpopedal spasms, facial spasm, laryngospasm, and later convulsions	Hypocalcemia causes increased neuromuscular excitability/irritability, producing hyperactivity of the motor and sensory nerves
Presence of Trousseau's and Chvostek's signs	
Respiratory	
Dyspnea, laryngeal spasm	Increased nerve conduction leading to tetany
Gastrointestinal	
Increased peristalsis, diarrhea	Calcium absorption from the intestine is decreased; decreased calcium increases smooth muscle contraction
Cardiovascular	
Dysrhythmias, palpitations	Increase in cell excitability
Musculoskeletal	
Pathologic fractures	Calcium loss from bone due to osteoporosis causes bone to be brittle
Hematologic	
Prolonged bleeding time	Intrinsic pathway for blood coagulation is inhibited
Laboratory Findings	
Serum calcium < 4.5 mEq/L (< 9 mg/dL) Serum ionized calcium < 2.2 mEq/L (< 4.4 mg/dL)	Hypocalcemia is present

BOX 3–3

Calcium Content of Selected Foods

FOODS HIGH IN CALCIUM (more than 100 mg per serving)

Dairy Products
- Cheese, all types
- Ice cream, 1 cup
- Milk, 1 cup
- Yogurt, low-fat with fruit, 1 cup

Other Foods
- Oatmeal, instant, $\frac{3}{4}$ cup
- Rhubarb, cooked, 1 cup
- Spinach, frozen, $\frac{1}{2}$ cup
- Tofu, regular, $\frac{1}{2}$ cup

FOODS LOW IN CALCIUM (less than 25 mg per serving)

- Apple, 1 medium
- Banana, 1 medium
- Chicken breast, baked, 3 oz
- Ground beef, lean, 3 oz
- Oatmeal, cooked, 1 cup
- Pasta, cooked, 1 cup
- Vegetable juices

Data from Laquarta, I., & Gerlach, M. (1990). *Nutrition in clinical nursing*. Albany, New York: Delmar Publishers; and Burtis, G., et al. (1988). *Applied nutrition and diet therapy*. Philadelphia: W. B. Saunders.

Medical Management

Medical management is focused on determining and correcting the cause of the hypocalcemia. Other medical management is dictated by the level of the serum calcium.

PHARMACOLOGIC MANAGEMENT

Asymptomatic hypocalcemia is usually corrected with oral calcium gluconate, calcium lactate, or calcium chloride. It is best to administer the calcium supplement 30 minutes before meals for better absorption and with a glass of milk because vitamin D is necessary for the absorption of calcium from the intestine.

CRITICAL TO REMEMBER

Acute hypocalcemia with tetany needs immediate correction.

Intravenous calcium chloride or calcium gluconate (10 per cent) is given slowly to avoid hypotension, bradycardia, and other arrhythmias. Usually intravenous calcium is diluted in a liter of D_5W. Saline solutions are not used because sodium tends to promote calcium loss.

DIETARY MANAGEMENT

Chronic or mild hypocalcemia can be treated in part by having the client consume a diet high in calcium. Foods high in calcium are listed in Box 3–3. If hypocalcemia is secondary to parathyroid deficiency, the client must avoid high-phosphate foods (e.g., milk products, carbonated beverages). Maintenance needs are met through calcium and vitamin D supplements.

Nursing Management

Assessment

The nurse should have a high index of suspicion for those clients at risk for hypocalcemia who present with clinical manifestations. If neuromuscular and cardiac symptoms are present, the hypocalcemic state is usually severe. Assessing the medications and diet the client is taking is important.

CRITICAL TO REMEMBER

If the client is taking a digitalis preparation, administration of calcium will enhance the action of digitalis and may cause digitalis toxicity.

Clinical manifestations of digitalis toxicity include bradycardia (pulse rate <60), nausea, vomiting, and blurred vision. The client's diet may also give clues to hypocalcemia due to malnutrition or lack of calcium intake.

The nurse needs to assess the client's cardiac status by noting changes in the electrocardiogram and the heart rate. Changes would include a weak pulse, and the electrocardiographic recording may show a prolonged QT interval.

Two tests used to check for increased neuromuscular excitability and tetany are the Trousseau's and Chvostek's signs. The Trousseau's sign is carpopedal spasm (contraction of the fingers and hand). It is best elicited by inflating a blood pressure cuff on the upper arm for 1 to 5 minutes, constricting circulation. A positive test result is carpopedal spasm. The Chvostek's sign is spasm of the muscles innervated by the facial nerve. It is best determined by tapping the client's face lightly (over the facial nerve) below the temple. Spasm of the face, lip, or nose would indicate a positive finding for tetany (Fig. 3–6).

Nursing Diagnosis, Planning, and Implementation

Collaborative Problem: Hypocalcemia R/T diarrhea, pancreatitis, renal failure, or decreased intake.

Planning: Expected Outcomes. The nurse will monitor the client for resolution of hypocalcemia: increased serum calcium level, no dysrhythmias, absence of tetany symptoms, and adequate peripheral perfusion.

Implementation. The nurse monitors peripheral pulses and vital signs, especially the heart rate and electrocardiographic recordings, every 1 to 4 hours depending on the client's condition. The nurse should check the arterial blood gases for the presence of acid-base imbalances. As the acidotic state is being corrected, the nurse needs to monitor for tetany.

If the client is receiving intravenous calcium, the nurse needs to monitor the intravenous site for infiltration or phlebitis every hour.

CRITICAL TO REMEMBER

Calcium chloride is extremely irritating to the subcutaneous tissue; if infiltration occurs, sloughing of the tissue can result.

Symptomatic hypocalcemia should be assessed by testing of the Chvostek's and Trousseau's signs. The serum calcium level should be closely monitored and changes reported.

Nursing Diagnosis: Injury, Risk for R/T increased neuromuscular irritability resulting from hypocalcemia.

Planning: Expected Outcomes. The client will be free of injury associated with calcium deficit, as evidenced by no falls or near falls and no pathologic fractures.

Implementation. The nurse should use caution in turning or moving the client to prevent inadvertent pathologic fractures. He or she should walk the client with an ambulation belt and use precautions (e.g., extra personnel) in lifting or moving the client into and out of bed.

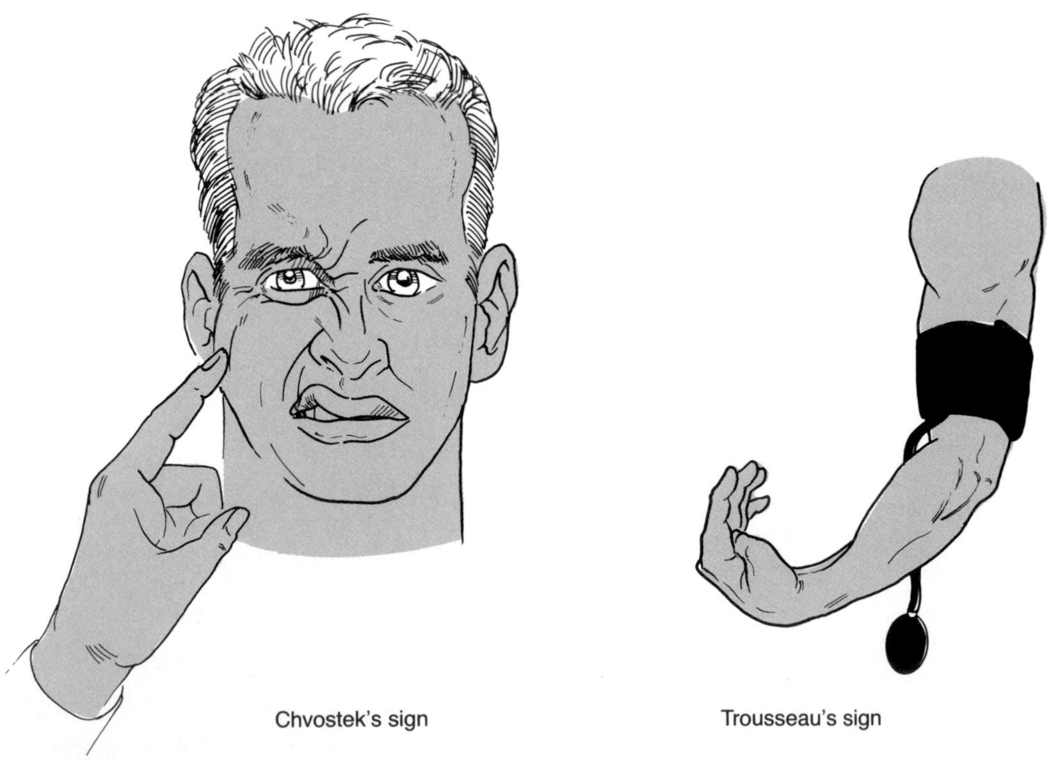

Figure 3–6
Chvostek's and Trousseau's signs.

Nursing Diagnosis: Health Maintenance, Altered R/T knowledge deficit regarding foods high in calcium.

Planning: Expected Outcomes. The client will have an improved knowledge base regarding dietary correction of hypocalcemia, as evidenced by selecting a diet to replace calcium loss and using oral calcium supplements or providing intravenous calcium replacement.

Implementation. The client should be instructed about foods that are rich in calcium, such as milk, cheese, yogurt, and vegetables. Oral calcium supplements should be taken before meals and with milk that contains vitamin D for better absorption. The nurse should instruct the client who is on a reducing diet to check with the physician for diet approval and to use caution if hypocalcemia is due to hypoparathyroidism. For these clients, phosphorus intake should be decreased by omitting milk and milk products. Instead, calcium and vitamin D supplements should be used.

Evaluation

The degree of attainment of expected outcomes should be reviewed and modifications made in the plan of care as needed.

Modification of Plan of Care for the Elderly

Elderly clients may have difficulty incorporating large amounts of food and fluids containing calcium into the diet. Part of the difficulty is in adjusting long-established eating habits. Many elderly clients drink very little milk because milk used to be a high-priced food item that adults gave up in favor of children drinking it. Also, many older adults are lactose intolerant, making selection of foods rich in calcium even more difficult. The nurse can help the client find other sources of milk that are palatable and obtainable. For example, yogurt is well-tolerated and is an excellent source of calcium.

HYPERCALCEMIA

Hypercalcemia is a serum level over 5.5 mEq/L or 11 mg/dL.

Incidence

Hypercalcemia can occur in any age group. It is a common electrolyte disorder that can create serious physical complications.

Etiology

The three most common causes of hypercalcemia are metastatic malignancy, hyperparathyroidism, and thiazide diuretic therapy. Severely high levels of calcium are usually the result of a malignancy. The most common of malignancies that may cause hypercalcemia include lung, breast, ovarian, prostatic, bladder, multiple myeloma, leukemia, lymphoma, kidney, and head and neck cancers. These cancers can cause bone destruction from metastasis or increase secretion of ectopic PTH.

Other causes of hypercalcemia include prolonged immobilization, excessive intake of calcium supplements and vitamin D, calcium-containing antacids, and hypophosphatemia. With hypophosphatemia, the serum calcium level is increased and the kidneys are unable to excrete the excess calcium. Metabolic acidosis can also decrease calcium elimination, thus increasing the serum calcium levels. Severe hypercalcemia may result in hypercalcemic crisis, which carries a 30 to 50 per cent mortality rate.

Risk Factors

Calcium loss from the bone, which increases the serum calcium level, can occur with many malignancies. Severe hypercalcemia may be fatal; thus, serum calcium levels must be monitored. Early treatment may prevent a hypercalcemic crisis. Mobilization is an important factor in the prevention of calcium loss from the bone. Bones maintain calcium because of the pressure exerted on them by carrying body weight; therefore, during a period of bed rest, the bone can lose calcium.

Pathophysiology

Because calcium levels are increased, there is a lesser gradient between the cell and the serum. There is also an increased amount of calcium in the cell. Therefore, the threshold becomes more difficult to achieve, and the cell membrane becomes refractory to depolarization. As a result, cardiac and smooth muscle activity is decreased. Calcium in the bloodstream impairs renal function, and it precipitates as a salt, forming renal stones. Some cancer tumors destroy the bone, whereas others, such as lung and breast cancers, cause ectopic PTH production. Hypophosphatemia is a complication of excessive PTH production that promotes calcium retention. A shortened QT segment and depressed T waves may be seen on the electrocardiogram. Pathophysiologic changes as they relate to clinical manifestations of hypercalcemia are explained in Table 3–15.

Hypercalcemic Crisis

A hypercalcemic crisis occurs when calcium levels reach 15 mg/dL. This level of serum calcium can cause cardiac dysrhythmias (widened T wave and shortened QT interval). Hypokalemia may occur as the body wastes potassium rather than calcium. Usual treatment includes hydration with 6 to 10 L normal saline in 24 hours and etidronate disodium (Didronel) therapy. These actions are designed to lower the calcium level in 36 to 48 hours.

TABLE 3–15 Clinical Manifestations of Hypercalcemia and Their Pathophysiologic Bases

CLINICAL MANIFESTATION	PATHOPHYSIOLOGIC BASIS
Gastrointestinal	
Anorexia, nausea, vomiting, constipation, decreased peristalsis, distention	Slowed gastrointestinal transit time Increased calcium enhances hydrochloric acid, gastrin, and pancreatic enzyme release
Neuromuscular	
Mild to moderate hypercalcemic state: weakness, fatigue, depression, difficulty in concentrating Severe hypercalcemic state: extreme lethargy, depressed sensorium, confusion, and coma	Neurologic depression
Cardiovascular	
Dysrhythmias, heart block Electrocardiographic changes: shortened ST segment and lengthened QT interval Digitalis toxicity Critical: cardiac arrest	Delayed transmission due to prolonged repolarization
Renal	
Polyuria, kidney stones, renal failure	Decreases the glomerular filtration rate; causes osmotic diuresis and volume depletion; reduces the kidney's ability to concentrate urine and results in polyuria
Musculoskeletal	
Bone pain, fracture	Metastatic cancer to the bone causes bone pain, which can be severe; decalcification of bones may cause osteoporosis and spontaneous fractures
Laboratory Findings	
Serum calcium >5.5 mEq/L (>11.5 mg/dL)	Hypercalcemia is present
Arterial blood gases pH <7.45 HCO_3^- >26 mEq/L	Acidotic state inhibits calcium excretion from the kidneys

Clinical Manifestations

The clinical manifestations of hypercalcemia are determined by the serum calcium level but in general are nonspecific. Mild hypercalcemia (near 11.5 mg/dL or 5.5 mEq/L) is usually asymptomatic. In mild cases, the serum calcium level may increase momentarily when the client consumes calcium-containing antacids or a large dose of an oral calcium supplement and the kidneys are initially unable to eliminate the excess. In moderate hypercalcemia (serum calcium level of 13 mg/dL or 6.2 mEq/L), symptoms usually include anorexia, nausea, vomiting, polyuria, fatigue, lethargy, and dehydration. As the hypercalcemic state progresses to severe levels, the client becomes more lethargic and confused, and coma may result. In some instances, clients may complain of deep bone pain.

DIAGNOSTIC ASSESSMENT

Hypercalcemia is determined by clinical manifestations and laboratory findings (see Table 3–15).

Medical Management

Treatment consists of correcting the underlying cause. In addition, the clinical manifestations may require some additional forms of treatment.

PHARMACOLOGIC MANAGEMENT

Immediate correction of moderate and severe hypercalcemia is essential. Intravenous normal saline (0.9 per cent NaCl), given rapidly with furosemide to prevent fluid overload, promotes urinary calcium excretion. Antitumor antibiotics such as plicamycin (mithramycin) inhibit the action of PTH on osteoclasts in bone tissue and result in a reduction of decalcification and a decrease in the serum calcium level. Calcitonin decreases the serum calcium level by inhibiting the effects of PTH on the osteoclasts and increasing urinary calcium excretion. Corticosteroid drugs decrease calcium levels by competing with vitamin D, thus resulting in decreased intestinal absorption of calcium. Intravenous phosphate decreases the serum calcium level; however, it should be used cautiously because it may result in severe calcification of various tissues. Sometimes thiazide diuretics are changed to furosemide or some other diuretic that does not retain calcium. If the cause is excessive use of calcium or vitamin D supplements or calcium-containing antacids, these agents should be either avoided or used in a reduced dosage. A newer form of therapy is the use of etidronate disodium. This drug reduces serum calcium by reducing normal and abnormal bone reabsorption of calcium and secondarily by reducing bone formation. The client needs to be hydrated with normal saline before administration and given loop diuretics to enhance urine output and calcium excretion following administration of the drug.

DIETARY MANAGEMENT

Forcing fluids will assist in adequately hydrating the client and flushing excess calcium through the kidney.

Surgical Management

Surgery may be used to remove an ectopic PTH-secreting tumor.

Nursing Management

Assessment

The nurse should have a high index of suspicion for those clients at risk for hypercalcemia or with early symptoms of this disorder. When the nurse notes an elevated serum calcium level, he or she should assess the client for signs and symptoms of neuromuscular and cardiac changes associated with hypercalcemia. An accurate nursing history may identify factors such as excessive use of calcium supplements or calcium-containing antacids that could cause mild to moderate hypercalcemia. A drug history is important for determining whether the medications the client is taking could be affected by the hypercalcemic state.

CRITICAL TO REMEMBER

An increased calcium level enhances the action of digoxin; thus, digitalis toxicity may result.

The client's hydration status should be assessed for fluid volume depletion caused by hypercalcemia. Electrocardiographic changes and the state of the client's sensorium should be reported.

Nursing Diagnosis, Planning, and Implementation

Collaborative Problem: Hypercalcemia R/T metastatic lesions, hyperparathyroidism, thiazide therapy, or increased intake of calcium.

Planning: Expected Outcomes. The nurse will monitor the client for resolution of hypercalcemia: serum calcium levels returning to normal, adequate urine output, no cardiac dysrhythmias, no neurologic changes, no pathologic fractures, and no severe weakness.

Implementation. Vital signs, including electrocardiographic readings, should be assessed every 4 to 8 hours. The presence of dysrhythmias or changes in sensorium should be reported. Bowel sounds should be assessed every 8 hours. Calcium levels should be closely monitored. Fluid intake should be increased, unless contraindicated (e.g., in cases of congestive heart failure), to dilute the calcium level. Acid-ash foods and fluids that contain acid should be encouraged, such as cranberry and prune juices. Urine should be strained to capture renal calculi (stones). Caution should be used with mobilization to reduce the risk of fractures.

Nursing Diagnosis: Health Maintenance, Altered R/T excessive ingestion of calcium supplements and/or calcium-containing antacids.

Planning: Expected Outcomes. The client's knowledge of the complications of calcium-containing drugs will be improved, as evidenced by decrease in or elimination of supplemental dosage of calcium, substitution of calcium-free antacids or decrease in the use of calcium-containing antacids, and return of serum calcium level to normal range.

Implementation. The nurse should instruct the client to avoid the use of calcium supplements. Sodium intake is increased, unless contraindicated (sodium promotes calcium loss through the kidney). High-fiber foods may be suggested to prevent constipation associated with hypercalcemia.

Nursing Diagnosis: Injury, Risk for R/T potential pathologic fractures, mental confusion, and immobility.

Planning: Expected Outcomes. The client will sustain no injury as evidenced by no falls or near falls and no reports of bone pain or extremity swelling, loss of motion, or ecchymosis.

Implementation. Safety precautions are necessary when the client is displaying symptoms of confusion or is extremely lethargic or comatose. The client should be turned and moved with extreme caution, and adequate assistance should be given for prevention of injury. Back braces, tripod canes, and walkers can be used to facilitate safer ambulation. The bed should be in low position with side rails elevated. Clinical manifestations of fractures (bone pain, ecchymosis) should be reported immediately.

Evaluation

The nurse evaluates whether the expected outcomes have been achieved and the client's serum calcium level is normal. Revisions in the plan of care may be required.

Client Education

The client and significant others should be taught to continue an acid-ash diet, force fluids, and avoid calcium-containing medications. The client should also be taught to report clinical manifestations of renal calculi (flank pain, hematuria) or cardiac dysrhythmias (irregular pulse, palpitations).

Magnesium Imbalances

Magnesium is the second most abundant intracellular cation. Magnesium's actions in the body and the clinical manifestations of its imbalances are similar to those of potassium. Magnesium is absorbed from the small intestine and excreted in the urine. Fifty per cent of the body's magnesium is stored in bone, 49 per cent is in intracellular fluid, and 1 per cent is in the extracellular fluid. Magnesium is absorbed from the small intestine in the same site where calcium is absorbed; therefore, malabsorption problems will affect both electrolytes. Magnesium is excreted in the urine and in small amounts in feces.

The functions of magnesium include the transmission and conduction of nerve impulses and the contraction of skeletal, smooth, and cardiac muscles. It is responsible for the transportation of sodium and potassium across the cell membrane, through the sodium-potassium pump. It influences utilization of potassium, sodium, and protein and activates enzymes that are necessary for the metabolism of carbohydrates and protein. Finally, magnesium promotes vasodilation of peripheral arteries and arterioles.

An increased calcium or phosphorus intake can decrease magnesium absorption from the intestines. Conversely, a low calcium level increases magnesium absorption from the intestines. Magnesium inhibits PTH, which results in a decrease in the amount of calcium released from the bone, thus promoting a calcium deficit.

Magnesium has been used for the treatment of acute myocardial infarction. It acts to decrease dysrhythmias, especially the digoxin-induced ventricular dysrhythmias. It is frequently selected when other treatment modalities have failed, especially when the client has hypokalemia.

HYPOMAGNESEMIA

Hypomagnesemia is a serum magnesium level below 1.5 mEq/L or below 1.8 mg/dL. Magnesium deficits are rare among healthy individuals because magnesium is abundant in foods and water. Magnesium deficits are seen in critically ill clients and alcoholic clients. Administering magnesium-free parenteral fluid solutions may increase the hypomagnesemic state.

Hypomagnesemia may be present but overlooked because tests for serum magnesium levels are not routinely ordered until there is a severe deficit. Magnesium deficits often accompany a potassium or calcium deficit. Cellular magnesium deficits can occur in the presence of normal serum values.

Clients who are prone to an inadequate intake of magnesium include those with severe or chronic malnutrition, alcoholism, and prolonged intravenous or hyperalimentation therapy without magnesium replacement.

Hypomagnesemia can lead to increased transmission of action potentials owing to an increased release of acetylcholine. Therefore, magnesium deficiencies can cause cardiac dysrhythmias as a result of myocardial irritability and neuromuscular changes such as tetany. The client can also develop psychological disorders such as depression, psychosis, and confusion. Gastrointestinal changes include decreased contractility leading to anorexia, nausea, and abdominal distention.

Alcoholism, when accompanied by liver disease, decreases intestinal absorption as the enzymes necessary for absorption are decreased. In addition, excessive amounts of phosphorus in the intestine (usually from antacids) will inhibit the uptake of magnesium from the intestinal villi. Clients with prolonged losses of fluids from the gastrointestinal tract (diarrhea, draining intestinal fistulas, laxative abuse), hyperparathyroidism, prolonged diuretic therapy, and in the diuresis phase of acute renal failure are prone to excessive loss of magnesium. There are also medications that interfere with renal handling of magnesium as either a primary action or side effect. The primary drugs are diuretics and antibiotics. Furosemide, osmotic and thiazide diuretics, aminoglycoside antibiotics (gentamicin, tobramycin), amphotericin B, corticosteroids, and digitalis are the usual offenders.

Severe hypomagnesemia causes neuromuscular symptoms such as the presence of Chvostek's and Trousseau's signs, tetany, and convulsions. Cardiac dysrhythmias include premature ventricular contractions and atrial or ventricular fibrillation. Clients who have a magnesium deficit and are taking digoxin could experience toxic effects from digitalis.

A magnesium deficit affects the potassium-sodium pump, causing hypokalemia. Hypomagnesemia also inhibits PTH, so the serum calcium levels may also be low.

Management

Treatment of hypomagnesemia includes oral magnesium replacement in the form of magnesium-containing antacids or parenteral magnesium sulfate. Increasing dietary intake of magnesium will also help prevent further loss.

Nursing diagnoses for magnesium imbalances are similar to the diagnoses for other electrolyte imbalances: injury, high risk for; nutrition, altered; decreased cardiac output. The majority of nursing intervention falls within the collaborative problem of hypomagnesemia.

Vital signs and electrocardiographic recordings should be monitored every 4 to 8 hours depending on the client's condition. Tachycardia and cardiac dysrhythmias may indicate hypomagnesemia. Serum magnesium, potassium, and calcium levels should be monitored. Clients who are extremely confused will need protection from harm with restraints or constant monitoring.

The administration of magnesium replacements needs to be closely monitored. The nurse should slowly administer magnesium diluted in intravenous solution. Rapid infusion of magnesium sulfate can cause a hot or flushed feeling.

Clients should be taught which foods are rich in magnesium to prevent magnesium deficiency or to correct a mild deficit. These foods are listed in Box 3–4.

BOX 3–4

Magnesium Content of Selected Foods

FOODS HIGH IN MAGNESIUM (more than 75 mg per serving)

Cashews, roasted, 1 cup
Chili, with beans, 1 cup
Halibut, baked, 3 oz
Swiss chard, cooked, $\frac{1}{2}$ cup
Tofu, $\frac{1}{2}$ cup
Wheat germ, toasted, $\frac{1}{4}$ cup

FOODS LOW IN MAGNESIUM (less than 25 mg per serving)

Chicken breast, 3 oz
Fruits
Egg, 1
Green peas, frozen, $\frac{1}{2}$ cup
Ground beef, 3 oz
White bread, 1 slice

Data from Mahan, K. L., & Arlin, M. (1992). *Krause's food, nutrition & diet therapy* (8th ed.). Philadelphia: W. B. Saunders.

STUDY QUESTIONS

1. The best clinical indication of ECFVD in an elderly client is
   A. A pulse between 70 and 90 beats per minute.
   B. Thirst.
   C. Urinary output of below 30 mL per hour.
   D. Decreased skin turgor.
2. A nurse is teaching a woman about risk factors of ECFVE. Which of the following nursing actions would enable the woman to identify clinical manifestations of ECFVE?
   A. Teaching about the importance of checking her finger tips and lips for cyanosis
   B. Recommending the inclusion of instant hot cereals and vegetable juice in her diet
   C. Demonstrating the techniques for checking for hand vein engorgement
   D. Teaching her about the importance of not driving when she feels dizzy or lightheaded
3. The nurse tells a client his serum potassium level is 3.0 mEq/L. The nurse explains that the client should
   A. Eat more vegetables, especially lima beans and sweet potatoes.
   B. Stay in bed with the side rails elevated at all times.
   C. Expect some discomfort from intramuscular injections of potassium.
   D. Report any burning or tingling after the nurse starts the intravenous infusion of potassium.
4. A nurse reviews lab values. The lab values reveal a low albumin level, a low folic acid level, and an above normal level of phosphorus. Considering these lab values, which of the following would be an appropriate nursing diagnosis?
   A. Injury, Risk for R/T increased neuromuscular irritability resulting from hypocalcemia
   B. Fluid Volume Excess R/T hypovolemia
   C. Hyponatremia R/T diarrhea
   D. Hyperkalemia R/T burns
5. A nurse designs nursing interventions for a client who has insulin-dependent diabetes. Of the following interventions, which intervention would help to prevent an electrolyte imbalance?
   A. Teaching the client about foods high in potassium
   B. Teaching the client about foods high in calcium
   C. Teaching the client about foods high in magnesium
   D. Teaching the client about foods high in phosphorus

CRITICAL THINKING EXERCISES

SCENARIO A

An elderly client is admitted to a surgical unit in preparation for major abdominal surgery. The nurse manager asks you to develop a one-page assessment tool that will enable the nursing staff to monitor this man and all other elderly clients for major fluid and electrolyte imbalances. The nurse manager asks you to include:

ECFVD
ECFVE
Hyponatremia and hypernatremia
Hypokalemia and hyperkalemia

1. Can you think of any other deficit or excess that would be appropriate to assess in this client considering his age and impending surgery?
2. How will you proceed to design the tool?
3. What instructions would you give to every R.N. before he or she uses this tool?

SCENARIO B

Consider how culture may affect dietary counseling for electrolyte imbalances. If you had to advise a client regarding a high potassium diet, how would you proceed if the client were Greek? How would you change your teaching plan for a Jewish client?

BIBLIOGRAPHY

1. Bryce, J. (1994). S.I.A.D.H. *Nursing 94, 24(4),* 33.
2. Bullock, B., & Rosendahl, P. (1992). *Pathophysiology: Adaptations and alterations in function* (3rd ed.). Philadelphia: J. B. Lippincott Co.
3. Cannon, P. (1989). Sodium retention in heart failure. *Cardiology Clinics, 7(1),* 49–59.
4. Carroll, H., & Oh, M. (1989). *Water, electrolyte and acid-base metabolism* (2nd ed.). Philadelphia: J. B. Lippincott Co.
5. Chernow, B., et al. (1989). Hypomagnesemia in patients in postoperative care. *Chest, 95(2),* 391–396.
6. Davis, K., & Attie, M. (1991). Management of severe hypercalcemia. *Critical Care Clinics, 7(1),* 175–189.
7. DeAngelis, R., & Lessig, M. L. (1991). Hypokalemia. *Critical Care Nurse, 11(7),* 71–75.
8. Gershan, J., et al. (1990). Fluid volume deficit: Validating the indicators. *Heart and Lung, 19(2),* 152–156.
9. Giesecke, A., Grande, C., & Whitten, C. (1990). Fluid therapy and the resuscitation of traumatic shock. *Critical Care Clinics, 6(1),* 61–71.
10. Hawthorne, J., Schneidner, S., & Workman, M. L. (1992). Common electrolyte imbalances associated with malignancy. *AACN Clinical Issues in Critical Care Nursing, 3(3),* 714–723.
11. Heitkemper, M., & Bond, E. (1988). Fluid and electrolytes:

Assessment and interventions. *Journal of Enterostomal Therapy, 15(1),* 18.

12. Kamel, K. S., et al. (1990). Urine electrolytes and osmolality: When and how to use them. *American Journal of Nephrology, 10(2),* 89–102.
13. Karb, V. (1989). Electrolyte abnormalities and drugs which commonly cause them. *Journal of Neuroscience Nursing, 21(2),* 125–128.
14. Kee, J. (1991). *Laboratory and diagnostic tests with nursing implications* (3rd ed.). Norwalk, CT: Appleton & Lange.
15. Kokko, J., & Tannen, R. (1996). *Fluids and electrolytes* (3rd ed.). Philadelphia: W. B. Saunders.
16. Kositzke, J. (1990). A question of balance: Dehydration in the elderly. *Gerontological Nursing, 16(5),* 4–11.
17. Laquarta, I., & Gerlach, M. (1990). *Nutrition in clinical nursing.* Albany, New York: Delmar Publishers.
18. Mahan, K. L., & Arlin, M. (1992). *Krause's food, nutrition & diet therapy* (8th ed.). Philadelphia: W. B. Saunders.
19. McCance, K., & Huether, S. (1994). *Pathophysiology: The basic biologic basis for disease in adults and children* (2nd ed.). St. Louis: C. V. Mosby.
20. Mendyka, B. (1992). Fluid and electrolyte disorders caused by diuretic therapy. *AACN Clinical Issues in Critical Care Nursing, 3(3),* 672–680.
21. Metheny, N. (1992). *Fluid and electrolyte balance: Nursing considerations* (2nd ed.). Philadelphia: J. B. Lippincott Co.
22. Olinger, M. (1989). Disorders of calcium and magnesium metabolism. *Emergency Medical Clinics of North America, 7(4),* 795–819.
23. Salem, M., et al. (1991). Hypomagnesemia in critical illness. *Critical Care Clinics, 7(1),* 225–247.
24. Stein, J. H. (1988). Hypokalemia, common and uncommon causes. *Hospital Practice, 23(3A),* 55–70.
25. Sterns, R. (1991). The management of hyponatremic emergencies. *Critical Care Clinics, 7(1),* 127–141.
26. Van Hook, J. (1991). Hypermagnesemia. *Critical Care Clinics, 7(1),* 215–223.
27. Votey, S., et al. (1989). Disorders of water metabolism: Hyponatremia and hypernatremia. *Emergency Medical Clinics of North America, 7(4),* 749–765.
28. Williams, M. (1991). Hyperkalemia. *Critical Care Clinics, 7(1),* 155–173.
29. Williams, S. (1994). *Essentials of nutrition and diet therapy* (6th ed.). St. Louis: C. V. Mosby.
30. Zaloga, G. (1991). Hypocalcemic crisis. *Critical Care Clinics, 7(1),* 191–199.
31. Zull, D. (1989). Disorders of potassium metabolism. *Emergency Medical Clinics of North America, 7(4),* 771–793.

Chapter 4 Acid-Base Imbalances

Learning Outcomes

After completing this chapter, the learner will be able to:

1. Assess the client for clinical manifestations of acid-base imbalances.
2. Teach the client about the etiology, risk factors, basic pathophysiology, and clinical manifestations of major acid-base imbalances.
3. Explain the client's role in the medical management of acid-base imbalances.
4. Develop plans of care for the prevention, management, and rehabilitation of clients with acid-base imbalances.
5. Implement nursing interventions that optimize the quality of life for clients with acid-base imbalances.
6. Evaluate planned client outcomes, using outcome criteria developed in the planning phase of care.

The normal function of body cells depends on the regulation of hydrogen ion (H^+) concentration within very narrow limits. Acid-base imbalances occur when these limits are exceeded and are recognized clinically as abnormalities of serum pH. Because acid-base imbalances can result from disease of virtually any body system, their incidence in clinical settings is very high. The nurse is responsible, along with other health professionals, for the prevention and detection of and the intervention in acid-base disorders.

REGULATION OF ACID-BASE BALANCE

The symbol pH stands for the negative log (logarithm) of the hydrogen ion concentration. It is used to express the degree of acidity or alkalinity of a solution. A solution with a pH of 7.0 is neutral, having equal parts of acids and bases. An acidic solution has a pH below 7.0; an alkaline solution has a pH above 7.0. Because pH is the *negative* log, a rise in pH reflects a fall in H^+ concentration and vice versa.

Normal serum pH is 7.35 to 7.45. Cell function is seriously impaired when pH falls to 7.2 or lower or rises to 7.55 or higher. Rapid *rates* of change in pH are especially detrimental. Serum pH below 6.8 or above 7.8 may be incompatible with life.

Three physiologic systems act interdependently to maintain normal serum pH: excretion of acid by the *lungs,* excretion of acid or reclamation of base by the *kidneys,* and buffering of excess acid or base by the *blood buffer systems.*

Regulation of Volatile Acid by the Lungs

The lungs are the major organs of acid elimination. The lungs excrete carbonic acid (H_2CO_3) in its gaseous form, carbon dioxide (CO_2).

Produced by body cells as an end product of aerobic carbohydrate metabolism, CO_2 diffuses into the blood, where it reacts with water to form carbonic acid. Carbonic acid may then dissociate, releasing free H^+ into the blood to decrease pH. As CO_2 rises, acid rises (pH falls), and as CO_2 falls, acid falls (pH rises). As carbonic acid reaches the lungs via venous blood, CO_2 is exhaled. The lungs are able to respond relatively quickly to pH changes, acting within a matter of hours to restore normal or near-normal acid-base proportions. The rate of CO_2 excretion by the lungs depends on the rate of alveolar ventilation. As ventilation increases (i.e., as tidal volume or respiratory rate increases), CO_2 excretion increases, and pH rises. Conversely, when ventilation is decreased, less acid is excreted, and pH falls.

Some of the CO_2 entering the blood ultimately forms the base bicarbonate (HCO_3^-). A small amount of HCO_3^- is formed in the plasma, but most is formed in erythrocytes. CO_2 diffuses into erythrocytes, in which the hydrolysis reaction occurs rapidly owing to the presence of *carbonic anhydrase,* a catalytic enzyme. The bicarbonate anion then diffuses out of the erythrocyte into the plasma while the chloride anion moves in. This *chloride shift* is necessary to maintain electroneutrality inside the red blood cell.

Regulation of Fixed Acids and Bicarbonate by the Kidneys

Acids that cannot be converted to a gaseous form must be eliminated in the urine. These include sulfuric and phosphoric acid produced by protein metabolism, ketoacids produced by incomplete lipid metabolism (as in diabetic ketoacidosis), and lactic acid produced by anaerobic carbohydrate metabolism (as in shock or hypoxemia). Regulation of acid-base balance by the kidneys is slower than that of the lungs; it takes several days for significant changes in urine pH to be clinically apparent.

Renal tubular cells are able to secrete H^+ into the urine until the pH of the urine falls to about 4.5. Presence of *urinary buffer systems* allows the tubular fluid to accept large quantities of H^+ while the degree to which urinary pH falls is limited.

BUFFER SYSTEMS

Buffer systems consist of a weak acid (one that does not readily release free H^+) and a salt of its conjugate base. The pH of buffered solutions tends to be fairly stable in spite of the addition of strong acid or base because the buffer system combines with the added acid or base to convert it to a weaker form. Buffer systems do *not* eliminate acid or base from the body; rather, they minimize pH changes by forming acids or bases that do not readily dissociate into free ions. Because only the free H^+ contributes to pH, changes in pH are minimized.

The three principal buffers in renal tubular fluid are bicarbonate, ammonia, and phosphate. All three systems start within the renal tubular cell.

In the *bicarbonate* system, the conjugate pair consists of carbonic acid and sodium bicarbonate ($NaHCO_3$). H^+ ions from the hydrolysis reaction are secreted into the urinary filtrate in exchange for sodium from the dissociated salt. The sodium is then actively transported to the extracellular fluid, accompanied by HCO_3^-, which was also formed in the tubular cell from the hydrolysis reaction. It is important to note that for each H^+ secreted, a bicarbonated ion is returned to the blood. Meanwhile, in the tubule, the H^+ ions combine with HCO_3^- from the dissociated salt, forming carbonic acid, which in turn forms CO_2 and H_2O in a reversal of hydrolysis. CO_2 is reabsorbed into the blood for excretion by the lungs; the H_2O is eliminated in the urine.

Ammonia (NH_3) is generated in renal tubular cells from amino acids such as glutamine. NH_3 gas diffuses into the tubular fluid, in which it can combine with H^+ to form ammonium (NH_4^+), which cannot be reabsorbed into the tubular cell. NH_4^+, "trapped" in the tubule, combines with Cl^- (from NaCl) and is excreted in the urine. Na^+ is reabsorbed along with HCO_3^- from the tubular cell.

The phosphate buffer operates in a similar fashion. $Na_2^{2+}HPO_2^{2-}$, present in the filtrate, exchanges hydrogen for sodium. $H_2PO_4^-$ is then excreted in the urine; Na^+ and HCO_3^- enter the blood.

THE ROLE OF OTHER ELECTROLYTES

The role of the kidneys in regulating serum bicarbonate and hydrogen ion concentrations is greatly influenced by the concentrations of other electrolytes. When potassium (K^+) is present in excessive amounts in tubular cells (hyperkalemia), K^+ is secreted in place of H^+. In hypokalemia, increased amounts of H^+ are secreted. When H^+ is low, selective K^+ loss occurs. In acidosis at the tissue level, extracellular H^+ tends to shift intracellularly while K^+ moves into the blood. Early in acidosis, K^+ excess occurs in the extracellular fluid because of this exchange. True hyperkalemia develops more gradually, as the kidney secretes H^+ instead of K^+. This concept has clinical implications in that if acidosis is corrected too rapidly (as with rapid infusion of sodium bicarbonate), an undetected hypokalemia may result as K^+ moves back into cells.

Bicarbonate reabsorption is also influenced by sodium regulation, which is in turn dependent on blood volume. As a consequence of hypovolemia, the renin-angiotensin-aldosterone system is activated, and the adrenocortical hormone aldosterone stimulates sodium bicarbonate ($NaHCO_3$) reabsorption in the distal tubule of the nephron.

Because of the chloride shift in the red blood cells, chloride levels in the blood vary inversely with bicarbonate. When a chloride deficit exists (as is often the case with hyponatremia), bicarbonate is reabsorbed in increased amounts by the kidney. Chloride levels may, therefore, be elevated in acidosis caused by loss of bicarbonate in the urine, as in renal tubular acidosis, or by intestinal losses through enteric drainage or diarrhea.

Serum calcium (Ca^{2+}) exists in both ionized and nonionized forms in the plasma; however, only the ionized form is electrochemically active. The proportion of ionized calcium increases in an acid environment, because more hydrogen ions are present to occupy binding sites on blood proteins. Conversely, in alkalosis, binding sites are more abundant. Calcium binds to these sites, reducing the proportion of unbound (ionized) calcium. Because of this competition for binding sites, acidosis thus promotes hypercalcemia, whereas alkalosis may result in hypocalcemia.

Modulation of Serum pH by Blood Buffer Systems

Several buffer systems are present in the blood, both within red blood cells (e.g., hemoglobin, phosphate, bicarbonate) and in the plasma (e.g., bicarbonate, plasma proteins, phosphate). These systems act instantaneously to minimize the impact of the addition of strong acid or base to the blood by converting these to weaker forms.

CRITICAL TO REMEMBER

Blood buffers constitute the body's first line of defense against acid-base imbalance.

Whereas hemoglobin is present in the greatest concentration, *plasma bicarbonate* is the most effective buffer because it is an *open* buffer system. That is, the end products of acid buffering reactions can be continuously eliminated from the body by the lungs and kidneys, allowing the reaction to continue unimpeded. When bases must be buffered, the CO_2 consumed by carbonic acid formation is readily replenished by normal metabolism.

Interaction of Acid-Base Regulatory Systems

Clinical evaluation of total acid-base homeostasis is aided by an understanding of the Henderson-Hasselbalch equation, which describes the relationship of pH, acid (H_2CO_3), and base (HCO_3^-).

$$pH = pKc + \log(HCO_3^-/H_2CO_3)$$

The clinical importance of this equation becomes evident when the normal value for pH (7.4) is substituted. Because pKc is a constant (6.1), the equation reveals that a ratio of 20 parts base to 1 part acid must be present to yield a normal pH. An increase in the numerator (base) tends to increase blood pH; a decrease tends to decrease pH. An increase in the denominator (acid) lowers pH; a decrease causes a rise in pH.

ACID-BASE COMPENSATION

In terms of commonly reported laboratory tests, normal acid-base translates the 20:1 ratio to 24:40 (24 mEq/L HCO_3^- to 40 mm Hg $PaCO_2$). $PaCO_2$ is the partial pressure of carbon dioxide in arterial blood. When primary disease processes alter either the acid or base component of the ratio, the lungs or the kidneys (whichever is unaffected by pathologic change) act to restore the 20:1 ratio and normalize pH. This process is known as acid-base compensation. When kidney disease impairs excretion of fixed acids, for example, the respiratory system can increase ventilation to "blow off" excess acid as CO_2. The kidneys can compensate for retention of acid (CO_2) in respiratory failure by retaining more HCO_3^-.

The blood buffers act to modulate pH changes but do not eliminate acid or base from the body. The lungs or kidneys alter actual amounts of acid and base, but regulation by these systems is not instantaneous. The lungs respond within minutes, but maximal compensation takes up to 24 hours. The kidneys may require up to 72 hours to achieve optimal compensation. Compen-

TABLE 4–1 Overview of Acid-Base Imbalances

MECHANISM	ETIOLOGY	CLINICAL MANIFESTATIONS	TREATMENT
Respiratory Acidosis			
Hypoventilation	COPD Neuromuscular disease Guillain-Barré syndrome Myasthenia gravis Respiratory center depression Drugs Barbiturates Sedatives Narcotics Anesthetics Central nervous system lesions Tumor Stroke Iatrogenic disorders Inadequate mechanical ventilation CO_2 narcosis	Dyspnea Disorientation or coma Dysrhythmias pH below 7.35 $PaCO_2$ above 45 mm Hg Hyperkalemia Hypoxemia	Treat underlying cause Support ventilation Correct electrolyte imbalance Intravenous $NaHCO_3$*
Excess CO_2 production	Hypermetabolism Sepsis Burns Excess carbohydrate intake Total parenteral nutrition Enteral feeding		
Respiratory Alkalosis			
Hyperventilation	Hypoxemia Emphysema Pneumonia ARDS Impaired lung expansion Pulmonary fibrosis Ascites Scoliosis Pregnancy† Thickened alveolar-capillary membrane Congestive heart failure ARDS Pneumonia Pulmonary embolism Chemical stimulation of respiratory center	Tachypnea Hyperpnea‡ Giddiness, dizziness, syncope, convulsions, or coma Weakness, paresthesias, tetany pH above 7.45 $PaCO_2$ below 35 mm Hg Hypokalemia Hypocalcemia	Treat underlying cause Increase CO_2 retention Mechanical hypoventilation CO_2 rebreathing§ Sedation

sation does not usually result in complete return of pH to the normal range. More typically, compensation brings pH to within 50 to 75 per cent of normal.

ACID-BASE CORRECTION

Although compensatory responses for primary acid-base disorders may nearly restore the 20:1 ratio of base to acid, the actual amounts of acid and base remain abnormal. Thus, compensation must be differentiated from *correction,* in which not only is the ratio restored, but absolute quantities of $PaCO_2$ and HCO_3^- are returned to the normal range. Correction occurs only with resolution of the underlying disorder.

DISORDERS OF ACID-BASE BALANCE

The four general classes of acid-base imbalance are respiratory acidosis, respiratory alkalosis, metabolic acidosis, and metabolic alkalosis. *Acidosis* refers to any pathologic process causing a relative excess of acid in the body. *Acidemia* is excess acid in the blood. The presence of acidemia does not necessarily confirm an underlying pathologic process; technically, it is merely a laboratory finding. The same distinction may be made between the terms *alkalosis* and *alkalemia.* Alkalosis in-

TABLE 4–1 Overview of Acid-Base Imbalances *Continued*

MECHANISM	ETIOLOGY	CLINICAL MANIFESTATIONS	TREATMENT
	Bacterial toxins (sepsis) Ammonia (hepatic failure) Salicylates (aspirin overdose) Traumatic stimulation of respiratory center Central nervous system trauma Central nervous system tumor Increased intracranial pressure Excessive exercise Extreme stress Severe pain		
Metabolic Acidosis			
Fixed acid excess	Renal failure Diabetic ketoacidosis Lactic acidosis Injested toxins Aspirin Antifreeze	Hyperventilation (compensatory) Drowsiness, confusion, or coma Headache pH below 7.35 HCO_3^- less than 22 mm Hg Anion gap greater than 16 if excess acid Hyperchloremia if base deficit $PaCO_2$ normal or slightly decreased	Treat underlying cause Correct electrolyte imbalance Intravenous $NaHCO_3$*
Base deficit	Renal tubular acidosis Carbonic anhydrase inhibitors Acetazolamide (Diamox) Mafenide acetate (Sulfamylon Acetate Cream)		
Metabolic Alkalosis			
Fixed acid loss (with resultant base excess)	Hypokalemia Diuresis Steroids Gastric fluid loss Vomiting Nasogastric aspiration	Hypoventilation (compensatory) Dysrhythmias pH above 7.45 Hypokalemia Hypocalcemia $PaCO_2$ normal or slightly increased	Treat underlying cause Administer HCl Intravenous acidifying salts* (e.g., NH_4Cl) in extreme cases
Excessive HCO_3^- intake	Milk-alkali syndrome Overcorrection of acidosis with $NaHCO_3$ Massive transfusion of whole blood		
Excessive HCO_3^- reabsorption	Hyperaldosteronism		

* Use of therapeutic compensation, e.g., intravenous acid or base administration, is controversial. (See text.)
† In the third trimester of pregnancy, the hormone progesterone also stimulates respiration.
‡ Restrictive lung disorders may preclude increased tidal volume.
§ Specific measures include breathing into a paper bag or increasing tubing dead space with mechanical ventilation.

dicates a primary condition resulting in excess base in the body. Although efforts have been made to standardize acid-base terminology, the terms are often used interchangeably in clinical practice.

Incidence

The incidence of acid-base imbalances in clinical settings is high. A recent study of 110 consecutive admissions to a general hospital revealed an overall incidence of acid-base imbalances of 56 per cent. The most common disorder was respiratory alkalosis, followed in order by respiratory acidosis, metabolic alkalosis, and metabolic acidosis. Eleven persons had more than one acid-base imbalance concurrently.[11]

Overview of Acid-Base Disorders

Table 4–1 summarizes pathophysiologic mechanisms, common etiologic factors, clinical manifestations, and medical management of the four imbalances.

RESPIRATORY ACIDOSIS AND ALKALOSIS

Respiratory acidosis is nearly always caused by hypoventilation. Chronic respiratory acidosis is most commonly caused by chronic obstructive pulmonary disease (COPD). In end-stage disease, pathologic changes lead to airway collapse, air trapping, and disturbance of ventilation-perfusion relationships. Acute respiratory acidosis also occurs in clients with end-stage disease when superimposed respiratory infection or concurrent cardiac disease increases the work of breathing. Hypoventilation with resultant respiratory acidosis is also seen in diseases of the neuromuscular junction in which diaphragmatic movement is impaired (such as Guillain-Barré syndrome) and in depression of the medullary respiratory center by drugs or lesions of the central nervous system.

Respiratory acidosis may be caused iatrogenically by inadequate mechanical ventilation or by excessive oxygen administration to clients with COPD. In the latter case, CO_2 narcosis results when blunting of the central respiratory drive occurs. It was formerly thought that hypoventilation in CO_2 narcosis was caused by desensitization of chemoreceptors to CO_2 (normally the primary respiratory stimulus), leaving only hypoxemia as a stimulus for ventilation. Current theory holds, however, that worsening of ventilation-perfusion relationships is the responsible mechanism. The second, much less common mechanism of respiratory acidosis is excessive CO_2 production because of excessive metabolic rate or excessive metabolism of carbohydrate.

Respiratory alkalosis is caused by alveolar hyperventilation, in which excess CO_2 is eliminated. The most common cause of respiratory alkalosis is hypoxemia. Low levels of oxygen (PaO_2) in the blood are sensed by the peripheral chemoreceptors in the carotid bodies and aortic arch. These receptors then increase their rate of firing to the respiratory center in the medulla, and rate and depth of ventilation increase. The peripheral chemoreceptors are also stimulated in states of low blood flow, such as shock.

Conditions that physically impede expansion of the lungs (such as pulmonary fibrosis) stimulate activation of the respiratory center via stretch reflex. The J receptors, located in the alveolar-capillary membrane, are thought to stimulate increased ventilation in disorders such as adult respiratory distress syndrome, which causes thickening of the alveolar-capillary membrane.

The central chemoreceptors and respiratory center may be stimulated excessively by chemicals or toxins. In the case of salicylate (aspirin) overdose, it is interesting that adults usually exhibit respiratory alkalosis. The reason for this is unknown. Other conditions that may overstimulate the respiratory center include central nervous system lesions or trauma, fever, exercise, extreme emotional stress, or severe pain.

METABOLIC ACIDOSIS AND ALKALOSIS

Metabolic acidosis can be caused by two different mechanisms: accumulation of fixed acid or loss of base. These mechanisms may be differentiated clinically by the presence or absence of a high *anion gap* (A^-). When acidosis is the result of addition of fixed acid (as in lactic acidosis), bicarbonate is consumed in buffering, and the anion gap increases. When acidosis is the result of loss of bicarbonate, however, chloride levels increase to maintain electroneutrality, and the anion gap does not change.

Common causes of high anion gap acidosis include azotemic renal failure, in which end products of protein metabolism cannot be effectively excreted because of impaired glomerular filtration; diabetic ketoacidosis, in which ketoacids accumulate owing to accelerated lipid metabolism in the absence of insulin; and lactic acidosis, a consequence of anaerobic carbohydrate metabolism. Less commonly, ingestion of toxins with acid metabolites is the cause.

Normal anion gap acidosis, due to loss of base, is also called *hyperchloremic metabolic acidosis*. Chloride is retained by the kidney when excess bicarbonate is lost in order to maintain electroneutrality. Excess bicarbonate may be lost through either the kidneys or the intestinal tract. In renal tubular acidosis, the renal tubular cells are unable to reabsorb bicarbonate; thus, it is lost in the urine. (Because glomerular filtration is normal in renal tubular acidosis, accumulation of fixed acids, or azotemia, does not occur.)

Intestinal secretions, high in bicarbonate, may be lost through enteric drainage tubes (e.g., ileostomy) or with diarrhea. Drugs such as acetazolamide (Diamox), which inhibit carbonic anhydrase, interfere with bicarbonate reclamation during urinary buffering.

Metabolic alkalosis may be caused by either abnormal loss of fixed acid or excess accumulation of bicarbonate. In actuality, these mechanisms are interdependent, because H^+ excretion is accompanied by HCO_3^- reclamation in the kidney and in gastric cells.

The most common cause of metabolic alkalosis is hypokalemia, frequently seen in hospitalized clients secondary to diuretic or steroid therapy. When potassium is deficient, the kidneys secrete H^+ into the urine in exchange for sodium. This process, in turn, stimulates bicarbonate reabsorption.

Loss of gastric fluid via nasogastric suction or vomiting causes metabolic alkalosis due to loss of hydrochloric acid (HCl). When HCl is lost, new HCl must be produced by gastric cells via the hydrolysis reaction. H^+ is secreted into the stomach with Cl^-; the HCO_3^- produced in the reaction is reabsorbed into the blood in exchange for chloride.

Hyperaldosteronism leads to metabolic alkalosis via increased renal tubular reabsorption of sodium and subsequent loss of potassium. Overcorrection of acidosis with $NaHCO_3$ administration may cause alkalosis, as can massive transfusion of whole blood. The citrate anticoagulant used for storage of blood is metabolized to bicarbonate. Packed red blood cells contain much less citrate; thus, their use in multiple transfusion is preferred.

MIXED ACID-BASE DISORDERS

Mixed acid-base disorders, in which two primary acid-base imbalances coexist, are frequently seen in clinical situations. In cardiac arrest, for example, lactic acid quickly accumulates as a result of anaerobic metabolism; carbonic acid is elevated because of respiratory arrest. In COPD, underlying respiratory acidosis may be complicated by metabolic alkalosis secondary to diuretic or steroid therapy.

Prevention

The nurse must maintain a high index of suspicion for clients at risk for acid-base imbalance. These include (1) clients with known disease of the pulmonary, cardiovascular, or renal systems; (2) clients who manifest hypermetabolic states, as in fever, sepsis, or burns; (3) clients receiving total parenteral nutrition or enteral tube feedings high in carbohydrate; (4) mechanically ventilated clients; (5) insulin-dependent diabetics; (6) clients with vomiting, diarrhea, or enteric drainage; and (7) the elderly, whose age-related decreases in respiratory and renal function may limit their ability to compensate for acid-base disturbances.

The normal aging process results in decreased ventilatory capacity as well as loss of alveolar surface area for gas exchange; thus, the elderly are prone to respiratory acidosis due to hypoventilation and to respiratory alkalosis due to hypoxemia. Elderly persons are frequently taking multiple medications for hypertension or cardiovascular disease; these drugs may contribute to hypokalemia and metabolic alkalosis. Respiratory compensation in this condition is compromised owing to the structural and functional changes mentioned. Decreased cardiac output in the aging person diminishes renal perfusion and glomerular filtration. Aldosterone is less effective in the elderly, as is ammonia buffering. These changes limit renal compensation for respiratory imbalances and place the individual at higher risk for metabolic imbalance.

Clinical Manifestations

Ventilatory disturbance is present in all imbalances, either as a contributing cause in respiratory imbalances or as a compensatory response in metabolic imbalances.

CRITICAL TO REMEMBER

Acidosis depresses the central nervous system; alkalosis stimulates it.

Ultimately, severe untreated acidosis and alkalosis both lead to coma.

DIAGNOSTIC ASSESSMENT

Electrolyte imbalance nearly always coexists with acid-base imbalance owing to the mechanisms previously discussed. Symptoms resulting from abnormal levels of specific ions are seen. Abnormalities of serum pH, $PaCO_2$, or HCO_3^- typical of the specific disturbance are seen on arterial blood gas (ABG) reports. (See later discussion of ABG analysis.)

Medical Management

Treatment of acid-base imbalances is directed toward removing the underlying cause, if possible. Respiratory infections contributing to ventilatory failure are managed with appropriate antibiotic therapy. Use of pharmaceutic agents that depress the respiratory control center is curtailed. Enteral feedings that supply more than 50 per cent of calories in the form of carbohydrate are replaced if metabolic CO_2 production is excessive. Dialysis may be indicated in the case of renal failure or overdose of toxins. Support of ventilation may be required in the form of pharmacologic intervention, hydration, pulmonary hygiene, oxygen therapy, and possibly continuous mechanical ventilation. Correction of any coexisting electrolyte imbalance is also indicated.

Therapeutic compensation for severe pH derangement is controversial. In acidosis, for example, intravenous administration of sodium bicarbonate may have an immediate beneficial effect on pH. Eventually, however, blood levels of CO_2 rise because HCO_3^- fuels the hydrolysis reaction in reverse. In severe alkalosis, intravenous administration of HCl or an acidifying salt such as ammonium chloride or arginine hydrochloride might be employed. These agents are highly toxic to the liver and kidneys, however, and cause red blood cell hemolysis if they are administered too rapidly.

Nursing Management

Assessment

Findings of comprehensive physical assessment of ventilatory status, cardiovascular function, and fluid balance must be documented with careful analysis of trends. Laboratory values that should be noted include electrolytes, blood urea nitrogen, creatinine, serum lactate, and ABGs.

The nurse's knowledgeable interpretation of ABGs is critical for timely, appropriate intervention in acid-base disturbances. Often, ABG results are first reported to the nurse, who is the communication link between respiratory therapists and physicians regarding potential changes in client status or treatment. ABG interpretation is essential to diagnosis and treatment of acid-base imbalance.

CRITICAL TO REMEMBER

ABG findings are of value only when they are considered in the context of the total clinical picture.

The recommended procedure for evaluation of ABGs is detailed in Box 4–1.

Nursing Diagnosis, Planning, and Implementation

Nursing Diagnosis: Several nursing diagnoses may apply to the management of underlying causes and clinical manifestations of acid-base disturbances. Examples of these diagnoses, along with priority nursing interventions, are shown in the Care Plan for the Client

BOX 4–1

Analysis of Arterial Blood Gases

STEP 1: CLASSIFY THE pH

Normal: 7.35–7.45
Acidemia: below 7.35
Alkalemia: above 7.45

STEP 2: ASSESS $PaCO_2$

Normal: 35–45 mm Hg
Respiratory acidosis: above 45 mm Hg
Respiratory alkalosis: below 35 mm Hg

STEP 3: ASSESS HCO_3^-*

Normal: 22–26 mEq/L
Metabolic acidosis: below 22 mEq/L
Metabolic alkalosis: above 26 mEq/L

STEP 4: DETERMINE PRESENCE OF COMPENSATION

Compensation present: $PaCO_2$ *and* HCO_3^- are abnormal (or nearly so) in *opposite* directions, e.g., one is acidotic and the other alkalotic.†
Compensation absent: One component ($PaCO_2$ or HCO_3^-) is abnormal, the other normal.

STEP 5: IDENTIFY PRIMARY DISORDER, IF POSSIBLE

If pH is clearly abnormal: Acid-base component with value most consistent with pH deviation is primary.
If pH is normal or near-normal: The more deviant component is probably primary.‡ To verify, note whether pH is on acidotic or alkalotic side of 7.4. The more deviant value should be consistent with this pH.

STEP 6: CLASSIFY DEGREE OF COMPENSATION, IF PRESENT

Partial compensation: Evidence of compensation, but pH is still abnormal.
Complete compensation: Evidence of compensation, pH is normal.

* Base excess (BE) is also reported with arterial blood gases and is a second index of metabolic status. Normal BE is −2 to +2. Because fluctuation in BE exactly parallels that of bicarbonate, it is not necessary to classify both.
† It is possible, but less likely, that two opposing primary imbalances (e.g., a mixed disorder) are present, which results in the *appearance* of compensation. The detection of mixed disorders is facilitated by the use of acid-base maps or nomograms, but a mixed disorder cannot always be differentiated from compensation.
‡ It is unlikely that the more deviant value represents compensation, because the body does not overcompensate for imbalance. When pH approaches the normal range, compensatory mechanisms are no longer triggered.

with Acid-Base Imbalance. Acid-base imbalances per se are perhaps best conceptualized as collaborative problems, however, in that the interventions of several health-care professionals, including nurses, respiratory therapists, and physicians, are required for effective treatment.

Planning: Expected Outcomes: Expected outcomes for nursing diagnoses are shown in the Care Plan for the Client with Acid-Base Imbalance. When the collaborative approach is used, the nurse monitors for clinical manifestations of the imbalances during and following treatment.

Implementation. Protection of the client from injury during diagnostic procedures is a priority nursing responsibility. Before radial puncture for obtaining an arterial specimen for ABGs, the Allen test should be performed to ascertain adequate ulnar circulation. The Allen test is done by first having the client tightly close the hand into a fist. The nurse then occludes both the radial and ulnar arteries by applying pressure over the pulse points. The client's hand is then opened; it will have a blanched appearance because of lack of blood. The nurse then releases the ulnar pressure. If ulnar circulation is adequate, color will return to the hand within 10 to 15 seconds. The test should then be repeated with release of the radial artery.

CRITICAL TO REMEMBER

Failure on the nurse's part to assess collateral circulation could result in severe ischemic injury to the client's hand if damage to the radial artery occurs with arterial puncture.

Critically ill clients commonly have femoral or radial arterial catheter systems from which blood specimens are drawn. Frequent sampling can result in significant blood loss if an open system is used. Nursing research has demonstrated that a minimum discard specimen of 2 mL is sufficient to clear the arterial line of heparinized solution before aspiration of blood for ABG testing. Recently introduced closed systems allow reinstillation of initially aspirated heparinized solution and blood. Nursing responsibilities for clients with arterial lines are discussed in Chapter 25.

The nurse is also responsible for minimizing errors in ABG analysis due to faulty specimen collection and handling. Potential sampling errors and their consequences and nursing implications are summarized in Table 4–2.

Despite quality control procedures, erroneous blood gas data are sometimes reported. The nurse should suspect sampling error or transcription error when the reported values lack internal consistency or external congruity. Internal consistency means that the values make sense when considered as a whole. An alkalotic pH, for example, is inconsistent with excess $PaCO_2$ and a deficit of HCO_3^-. External congruity means that the ABG findings are consistent with other laboratory data as well as with clinical assessment findings. For example, the client with a pH of 7.10 should appear profoundly ill.

Supportive Care

Supportive care involves preserving an *acceptable* (not necessarily normal) pH and preventing life-threatening deviations in pH. The nurse optimizes respiratory and renal function through positioning, pulmonary hygiene, and hydration. The nurse intervenes in helping clients cope with the anxiety that often accompanies—and may contribute to—acid-base imbalance. The nurse

CARE PLAN: The Client with Acid-Base Imbalance

Nursing Diagnosis/ Collaborative Problem	Planning: Expected Outcomes	Implementation: Nursing Interventions	Rationales
Breathing Pattern, ineffective; Gas Exchange, impaired	Client will have improved breathing patterns and gas exchange as evidenced by • respiratory rate within normal limits • no dyspnea • clear breath sounds • ABGs within normal limits • SAO_2 above 95%	Monitor respiratory status: rate, volume, patterns, breath sounds, ABGs, SAO_2	There are clinical manifestations of respiratory impairments.
		Position for optimal ventilation; reposition frequently	Ventilatory problems exist in all acid-base disorders. Repositioning allows ventilation of all lung fields.
		Offer fluids if allowed	Fluids help thin secretions, facilitating expectoration.
		Intervene if pain, fever, or anxiety is present	Pain, fever, and anxiety increase respiratory rate.
		Teach and encourage coughing and deep-breathing; suction as necessary	Coughing, deep breathing, and suctioning help maintain airway patency and ventilation.
Sensory/Perceptual Alterations	Client will have decreased sensory/perceptual alterations as evidenced by orientation in all spheres	Observe and attend as necessary to ensure safety	
		Assess level of consciousness and orientation	Decreasing levels of consciousness and disorientation may indicate cerebral hypoxia.
		Reorient as necessary	Reorientation assists the client to understand and participate in care.
Tissue Perfusion, Altered: cardiopulmonary	Client will have adequate peripheral tissue perfusion as evidenced by • full pulses in extremities • immediate capillary refill • warm and dry skin	Assess skin color, temperature, peripheral pulses, capillary refill	Decreased peripheral tissue perfusion causes pallor, cool skin, decreased pulse quality, and slowed capillary refill.
		Maintain comfortable room temperature and provide warm blankets if needed	External warmth will improve peripheral tissue perfusion.
		Assess pressure points for skin breakdown	Decreased perfusion to the skin increases risk of pressure ulcers.
Anxiety	Client will have decreased anxiety as evidenced by • fewer statements about anxiety • fewer nonverbal signs (eyes darting, fidgeting)	Assess verbal and nonverbal behavior for cues to anxiety	Anxiety is seen in conditions leading to cerebral hypoxia. Clients often report anxiety prior to other objective symptoms.
		Assess client and family coping	Ineffective coping increases anxiety, and anxiety is contagious.
		Reduce environmental stress if possible	Stressors in the environment may increase anxiety and oxygen consumption.
		Establish therapeutic relationship: acknowledge client's anxiety, listen to client's concerns, provide factual information, reinforce positive coping	The nurse's calm manner and therapeutic communication can decrease anxiety.

Care Plan continued on following page

CARE PLAN: The Client with Acid-Base Imbalance *Continued*

Nursing Diagnosis/ Collaborative Problem	Planning: Expected Outcomes	Implementation: Nursing Interventions	Rationales
Injury, Risk for	Client will remain free of injury as evidenced by: • maintenance of adequate (or previous) quality of pulses and perfusion of extremities • no development of clinical manifestations of complications from mechanical ventilation or oxygen therapy	Perform Allen test prior to arterial puncture	Determines patency of ulnar and radial arteries.
		Monitor infusion rates of fluids, $NaHCO_3$, or HCl if ordered; observe carefully for response	These drugs are tissue irritants.
		Use quality control measures to maximize ABG accuracy	Prevents unnecessary redrawing for ABGs.
		Monitor mechanical ventilation parameters carefully; assess for deteriorating status	Impairment of lung tissue may result from mechanical ventilation which would further impair oxygen.
		Monitor response to oxygen therapy; assess for possible CO_2 narcosis if indicated	The client's response to oxygen should be monitored before oxygen levels are increased.
		Monitor electrolyte levels; assess for symptoms specific to imbalance associated with identified acid-base abnormality	Early detection of abnormalities improves treatment.
Fatigue	Client will have improved energy level as evidenced by • being able to perform more of own ADLs • fewer statements of fatigue • ambulating to chair or walking with less assistance • remaining up for longer periods of time	Assess client's energy level	Ongoing assessments provide data to monitor fatigue.
		Assist client with ADLs as indicated	Client should be encouraged to perform ADLs within energy limits to prevent further muscle wasting.
		Provide a quiet environment	Decreases oxygen consumption.
		Organize nursing care to provide periods of uninterrupted rest	Stress and illness increase need for rest.
		Promote optimal nutrition	Fatigue may be due to inadequate nutrition.
Fluid Volume Deficit and Decreased Cardiac Output	Client will have adequate fluid volume and cardiac output as evidenced by • blood pressure within normal limits • urine output >30 mL per hour • skin turgor responsive <2 seconds • immediate capillary refill • no abnormal heart sounds (S_3 and S_4) • stable body weight intake = output	Monitor for signs related to contributing cause, e.g., shock, dehydration, diabetic ketoacidosis	There are multiple etiologies of acid-base imbalances.
		Monitor for signs of azotemia	Elevation of blood urea nitrogen and creatinine may increase risk of metabolic acidosis.
		Assess vital signs, skin turgor, capillary refill, heart sounds	Signs of dehydration and cardiac disorders which may increase risk of acid-base imbalance.
		Promote rest to decrease metabolic demand	Decreases oxygen demand.
		Monitor weight and fluid balance	Weight change is the most accurate measure of fluid balance. Fluid imbalance may lead to acid-base imbalance.

ABGs, arterial blood gases; ADLs, activities of daily living; SAO_2, arterial oxygen percent saturation.

TABLE 4–2 Sources of Error in Sampling of Arterial Blood Gases

SAMPLING ERROR	EFFECT	NURSING IMPLICATIONS
Air bubbles in syringe	↑ PaO_2 ↓ $PaCO_2$ ↑ pH	Expel all air bubbles immediately Do not agitate syringe Do not use any sample that appears frothy
Inadvertent venous sample or venous contamination of arterial sample	↓ PaO_2 ↑ $PaCO_2$ ↓ pH	Avoid use of femoral artery Use short-beveled needle Do not overshoot artery and then withdraw to "catch" it Watch for autofilling of syringe with arterial puncture Verify questionable results with new sample
Anticoagulant effects: alteration of pH	↓ pH	Use lithium heparin, if possible Use 1:1000 units/mL concentration Use minimum 2 mL discard sample with arterial line aspiration
Anticoagulant effects: dilution of sample	↑ pH ↓ in all other values	Use syringe with minimal dead space Use dried heparin if available
Effects of metabolism of white blood cells in sample	↓ PaO_2 ↑ $PaCO_2$ ↓ pH	Place sample in ice water immediately Have sample analyzed within 20 minutes Have sample analyzed immediately if client has leukocytosis

Data from Malley, W. J. (1990). *Clinical blood gases: Application and noninvasive alternatives.* Philadelphia: W. B. Saunders.

collaborates in the administration of drug therapy, oxygen therapy, and mechanical ventilation when indicated. In extreme circumstances in which therapeutic compensation (intravenous administration of acid or base) is required, the nurse is knowledgeable about potential risks of this therapy and carefully monitors administration rates and therapeutic response.

Corrective interventions address the underlying causes of primary acid-base imbalances and are the mainstay of treatment in such disorders. Compensatory imbalances are not treated but instead resolve spontaneously as the primary disorder is reversed. Chapters on the specific diseases responsible for acid-base imbalances should be consulted for detailed discussion of appropriate nursing intervention.

Evaluation

The client's status should be evaluated frequently, because many acid-base imbalances are life threatening. Revisions in the plan of care may be required.

STUDY QUESTIONS

1. A nurse is performing a physical assessment of a client with Adult Respiratory Distress Syndrome. Which of the following laboratory findings indicates the acid-base and electrolyte imbalances that occur with this syndrome?
   A. pH below 7.35, $PaCO_2$ above 45 mm Hg, and hyperkalemia
   B. pH above 7.45, $PaCO_2$ below 35 mm Hg, and hypokalemia
   C. pH below 7.35, normal $PaCO_2$, and hyperchloremia
   D. pH above 7.45, normal $PaCO_2$, and hypocalcemia

2. A client has experienced several episodes of respiratory acidosis. He asks the nurse what he can do to decrease these episodes. Which of the following responses by the client provides the best indication that he understands the etiology of respiratory acidosis?
   A. "I'll breathe into a paper bag every time I experience rapid breathing so I can rebreathe my own carbon dioxide."
   B. "I'll need to stop eating so many carbohydrates."
   C. "I'll take my prescribed sedatives as often as possible in order to decrease my anxiety."
   D. "I'll cut down on my excessive aspirin intake."

3. An 80-year-old client with chronic kidney disease presents with a normal $PaCO_2$, a pH of 7.31, and an HCO_3^- concentration of 22 mm Hg. Of the following collaborative nursing diagnoses, which would take priority, considering the data?
   A. Sensory/Perceptual Alteration R/T respiratory acidosis
   B. Anxiety, Moderate R/T respiratory alkalosis
   C. Fatigue R/T metabolic alkalosis
   D. Injury, Risk for R/T metabolic acidosis

4. A client presents with subjective and objective data that indicate metabolic alkalosis. The nurse should monitor for which of the following signs or symptoms?
   A. Headache
   B. Hyperventilation
   C. Dysrhythmia
   D. Coma

CRITICAL THINKING EXERCISES

SCENARIO A

A 70-year-old woman who has remained essentially healthy for her entire adult life falls while lifting a heavy object. She does not have any broken bones but does have muscle spasms and some bruising. To relieve her "aches and pains" she takes 10 grains of aspirin every 4 hours for a week. Consider the client's age, present condition, and medication usage.

1. What could happen to this client physiologically?
2. How would a nurse proceed to decrease or eliminate further health problems for this client?
3. What are the signs and symptoms of an acid-base imbalance that might occur in this client?
4. How would the nurse proceed if the imbalance occurred?

SCENARIO B

Using your knowledge of acid-base imbalances, interpret the following laboratory results:

1. pH 7.32
   $PaCO_2$ 47 mm Hg
   HCO_3^- 22 mEq/L
2. pH 7.36
   $PaCO_2$ 35 mm Hg
   HCO_3^- 22 mEq/L
3. pH 7.30
   $PaCO_2$ 35 mm Hg
   HCO_3^- 20 mEq/L
   Which are uncompensated and which are compensated?

BIBLIOGRAPHY

1. Anderson, S. (1990). ABGs: Six easy steps to interpreting blood gases. *American Journal of Nursing, 90(8)*, 42–45.
2. Brenner, M., & Welliver, J. (1990). Pulmonary and acid-base assessment. *Nursing Clinics of North America, 25(4)*, 761–770.
3. Bullock, B., & Rosendahl, P. (1992). *Pathophysiology: Adaptations and alterations in function* (3rd ed.). Philadelphia: J. B. Lippincott Co.
4. Carpenito, L. (1991). *Nursing care plans and documentation: Nursing diagnoses and collaborative problems*. Philadelphia: J. B. Lippincott Co.
5. Feeney-Stewart, F. (1990). The sodium bicarbonate controversy. *Dimensions of Critical Care Nursing, 9(1)*, 22–28.
6. Holloway, N. (1993). *Nursing the critically ill adult* (4th ed.). Menlo Park, CA: Addison-Wesley Publishing Co.
7. Malley, W. (1990). *Clinical blood gases: Application and noninvasive alternatives*. Philadelphia: W. B. Saunders Co.
8. Maxwell, M., et al. (1987). *Clinical disorders of fluid and electrolyte metabolism* (4th ed.). New York: McGraw-Hill Book Co.
9. Mendyka, B. (1992). Fluid and electrolyte disorders caused by diuretic therapy. *AACW Clinical Issues in Critical Care, 3(3)*, 672–680.
10. Metheny, N. (1992). *Fluid and electrolyte balance: Nursing considerations* (2nd ed.). Philadelphia: J. B. Lippincott Co.
11. Mountain, R., et al. (1990). Acid-base disturbances in acute asthma. *Chest, 98(3)*, 651–655.
12. Palange, P., et al. (1990). Incidence of acid-base and electrolyte disturbances in a general hospital: a study of 100 consecutive admissions. *Recenti Progressi in Medicina (Roma), 81(12)*, 788–791.
13. Preusser, B., et al. (1989). Quantifying the minimum discard sample required for accurate blood gases. *Nursing Research, 38(5)*, 276–279.
14. Russell, J. (1991). Successful method for arterial blood gas interpretation. *Critical Care Nurse, 11(5)*, 14–19.
15. Shapiro, B., et al. (1994). *Clinical application of blood gases* (5th ed.). St. Louis: Mosby–Year Book, Inc.
16. Stringfield, Y. (1993). Back to basics: Acidosis, alkalosis, and ABGs. *American Journal of Nursing, 93(11)*, 43–44.
17. Taylor, L., & Stephens, D. (1990). Arterial blood gases: clinical application. *Journal of Post-Anesthesia Nursing, 5(4)*, 264–272.

Chapter 5 Perioperative Nursing

Learning Outcomes

After completing this chapter, the learner will be able to:

1. Assess the client for clinical manifestations of preoperative, intraoperative, and postoperative complications.
2. Teach the client about the etiology, risk factors, basic pathophysiology, and clinical manifestations of postoperative complications.
3. Explain the client's role in preoperative, intraoperative, and postoperative stages.
4. Develop plans of care for the prevention of postoperative complications.
5. Implement nursing interventions that optimize the quality of life for clients in the preoperative, intraoperative, and postoperative stages.
6. Evaluate planned client outcomes, using outcome criteria developed in the planning phase of care.

Caring for perioperative clients is a challenging and gratifying specialty. A major change in the past decade is the emergence of outpatient surgery centers and ambulatory surgery. For many types of surgery, the client is admitted, surgery is performed, and the client is discharged the same day. To decrease the cost of care and client recovery, and to decrease the infection rate, many types of surgery are performed in ambulatory care settings (also known as surgicenters, same-day surgery centers, or outpatient surgery centers). This development will change the focus of nursing care because of the brief time the client spends in the hospital or clinic. Knowledge of nursing processes, technical skills, and responsibility for all phases of the client's perioperative experience become essential to the nursing care of the surgical client.

Perioperative nursing requires some special skills. The perioperative nurse prepares clients and their significant others physically and emotionally for surgery. Surgery is traumatic. Any surgical procedure, however minor, carries some degree of risk. The nurse also helps prepare clients and significant others cognitively, emotionally, and spiritually following psychosocial assessment.

CRITICAL TO REMEMBER

The client being prepared for surgery is awaiting the unknown and is often in a state of anxiety.

Experienced perioperative nurses are alert to the emotional turmoil many clients and their significant others experience preoperatively. These nurses recognize that surgery inevitably involves expense, discomfort, emotional and physiologic stress, and disruption of the client's life. Nursing assessment and interventions are planned accordingly.

The scope of perioperative nursing practice consists of three phases: preoperative, intraoperative, and postoperative.

Preoperative Phase. The scope of perioperative practice commences with the preoperative phase. This phase begins when the decision for surgical intervention is made and ends with transfer of the client to the operating room bed. Nursing activities range from a baseline assessment of the client during the preoperative interview at the clinic or at home, to an assessment in the preoperative area or surgical suite on the day of surgery.

Intraoperative Phase. The scope of perioperative nursing practice continues into the intraoperative phase of the surgical experience. This phase begins when the client is transferred to the operating room bed and ends when the client is admitted to the postanesthesia care unit (PACU). In this phase, nursing interventions range from recognizing improper positioning and the potential for injury, to implementing corrective measures and evaluating cardiopulmonary assessment data.

Postoperative Phase. The scope of perioperative nursing practice ends with the postoperative phase of the surgical experience. The client's postoperative period begins with admission to the PACU and ends with the resolution of the surgical sequelae. Nursing activities range from communicating pertinent information about the client's surgery to post-anesthesia nursing staff, to a postoperative evaluation in the clinic or the client's home.

The nursing process is applied throughout the entire perioperative period to ensure that the client's physical and emotional needs are met. Meeting these needs enhances the client's ability to withstand the trauma of surgery and return quickly to preoperative condition.

BASIC CONCEPTS

Definitions and Surgical Procedures

Common prefixes and suffixes can explain the type of procedure the client will undergo. Surgical procedures are categorized by purpose, extent, and urgency of the procedure. Knowledge of these categories may aid nurses in planning care for all phases of the client's surgery. Table 5–1 outlines the main categories of surgical procedures.

TABLE 5–1 Categories of Surgical Procedures

PROCEDURE	DEFINITION
Purpose	
Diagnostic	Confirms a diagnosis
Exploratory	Estimates the extent of disease and/or confirms a diagnosis
Curative	Removes or repairs damaged or diseased tissue or organs
Ablative	Involves removal of diseased organ
Reconstructive	Partial or complete restoration of a damaged organ or tissue to its original appearance and function
Constructive	Repair of a congenitally defective organ by improving its function or appearance
Palliative	Relieves symptoms but does not cure underlying disease
Urgency	
Emergency	Must be performed immediately to (1) maintain life; (2) maintain organ or limb function; (3) remove a damaged organ; or (4) stop hemorrhage
Imperative	Requires surgical intervention within 24–48 hours
Planned or required	Surgical intervention is important, but it can be scheduled several weeks or months in advance
Elective	Performed for the person's well-being but is not absolutely necessary
Optional	Surgery performed simply for individual's preference. It is not needed

Stress and the Perioperative Client

Stress must be considered in the care of the perioperative client. Surgery increases stress on all body systems. Stressors in the perioperative client include pain, tissue damage, blood loss, anesthesia, fever, and immobilization.

In response to the stress of surgery, the body mobilizes its defenses to maintain homeostasis. The systemic responses to surgical stress are outlined in Table 5–2. The success of the stress response in maintaining homeostatic balance is determined by a person's age, physical condition, and the duration of stress.

CRITICAL TO REMEMBER

The ability to withstand the stress of surgery and anesthesia is decreased significantly in aged or debilitated clients.

In the perioperative period, the nurse must be able to assess stress in the client and intervene to prevent and reduce complications.

The Practice of Perioperative Nursing

Technologic advances and a change in the surgical setting have contributed to the expanded practice of perioperative nursing. The safety and welfare of the client is the primary goal during all phases of the perioperative experience.

Nurses have different roles and have varied responsibilities for the care of the surgical client. All contribute to the safe recovery of the operative client. The *staff nurse* is responsible for the care of the client in the preoperative and postoperative period. This nurse's role includes teaching, physical preparation, assessment, and discharge of the client. The *operating room nurse* is responsible for the safe care of the client during surgery. The operating room nurse's role may include visiting clients preoperatively to assess their needs and prepare them for surgery. *Nurse anesthetists* are responsible for the safe delivery of anesthesia during surgery. *Postanesthesia care unit nurses* care for clients in the immediate postanesthesia and postoperative period. After a client is stable and ready to be transferred, the client is cared for by a *staff nurse* on a general surgery floor or in an intensive care or specialized unit, or he or she may go home. Because so many types of surgery are now performed on an outpatient basis, some staff nurses in ambulatory care units or outpatient centers care for clients throughout the entire perioperative period.

The Association of Operating Room Nurses (AORN) has developed standards of nursing care and provides a basic model by which the quality of nursing practice can be measured for the operative client. Other nursing organizations have developed standards of practice for nurses associated with care of the perioperative client. In the following units, the nurse's role in each phase of the operative experience is discussed.

TABLE 5–2 Responses to Surgical Stress

RESPONSE	ADAPTIVE	MALADAPTIVE
Vasoconstriction peripherally with increased coagulability	Blood increased to vital organs, away from periphery; increased clotting to decrease blood loss	Decrease in renal perfusion possible; clotting and thrombus formation increase
Tachycardia with increased cardiac output, blood pressure, and coronary artery dilation	Increased perfusion of myocardium; increased oxygen perfusion to vital organs	Increased demand on heart possibly leading to heart failure; hypertension
Sodium and water retention secondary to increased antidiuretic hormone and aldosterone secretion	Increased volume to prevent hypovolemia, maintenance of blood pressure and cardiac output	Hypervolemia, circulatory overload, hypertension, and heart failure
Increased gastric acidity and decreased peristalsis	Blood shifted from large intestine to more vital areas	Paralytic ileus and stress ulcers
Bronchial dilation	Increased oxygen exchange, improved ventilation	No maladaptive change
Protein catabolism	Increased amino acids for wound healing	Negative nitrogen balance, eventual lack of tissue repair unless reversed
Proliferation of granulation and connective tissue	Increased wound healing	Development of excessive scar tissue and adhesions
Increased blood sugar and mobilization of fat stores	Increased energy available	Increased blood sugar detrimental to diabetic clients
Increased cortisol with increased anti-inflammatory response	Increased blood sugar	Possible infection if anti-inflammatory effect is prolonged
Increased metabolic rate	Increased energy available for adaptation	Increased heat loss may lead to hypothermia and shivering, with increasing oxygen demand

PREOPERATIVE NURSING

Careful preparation during the preoperative period of clients undergoing surgery decreases operative risk and promotes postoperative recovery. In the case of emergency surgery, time may not permit complete preoperative assessment, care planning, and teaching. Nevertheless, essential preparation must be thorough.

Generally, preoperative preparation can take place in any of four times and places: (1) in the physician's office before admission to the health-care facility, (2) on admission and during the days before the operation, (3) the night before surgery if the client is in the hospital, and (4) the morning of surgery on admission.

General Preoperative Preparation

PHYSIOLOGIC NURSING ASSESSMENT OF THE CLIENT UNDERGOING SURGERY

Physiologic nursing assessment before surgery includes information about age, presence of pain, nutritional status, fluid and electrolyte balance, presence of infection, cardiovascular function, pulmonary function, renal function, gastrointestinal function, liver function, endocrine function, neurologic function, hematologic function, medication history, presence of trauma, health habits, and social history.

Age. Older adults have the lowest tolerance to the stressful effects of surgery. Consequently, their perioperative needs differ from those of younger or even middle-aged adults.

Older Adults. Like extreme youth, old age produces physiologic changes that increase surgical risk. Physiologic changes and presence of disease in the older adult's cardiovascular, pulmonary, musculoskeletal, gastrointestinal, hepatic, and renal systems may affect surgical outcomes. Chronic conditions also increase risk for older adults undergoing surgery.

Some of the conditions that increase the risk include malnutrition, anemia, dehydration, atherosclerosis, chronic obstructive pulmonary disease (COPD), diabetes mellitus, and many others. These problems should be corrected or controlled before surgery, if possible. A nutritious diet and adequate fluids help to counteract these problems, thus reducing the client's operative risk (Table 5–3).

Presence of Pain. Pain is an important physiologic indicator that must be carefully monitored. During the preoperative nursing assessment, the client should be asked to describe the pain and how it began. The nurse should learn if the pain developed rapidly, gradually, or in one explosive burst and determine the regularity of the pain—whether it is constant or intermittent—and if anything has helped relieve it.

Judging the client's reaction to pain is as important as assessing the nature of the pain. Reactions vary from panic to apparent indifference, making it difficult to observe exactly what an individual is experiencing.

TABLE 5–3 Interventions for Physical Changes in Older Adults Undergoing Surgery

PHYSICAL CHANGE	NURSING INTERVENTIONS
Cardiovascular	
Decreased cardiac output Moderate increase in blood pressure Decreased peripheral circulation Arrhythmias	Know what anesthesia is used Monitor vital signs carefully Encourage early ambulation and leg exercises Assess for hypotension or hypertension or hypothermia Note any changes to baseline electrocardiogram
Respiratory	
Decreased vital capacity Reduced oxygenation of blood Decreased cough reflex	Assess for pulmonary aspiration Monitor respirations carefully Vigorous pulmonary hygiene Postoperative: auscultate lung sounds Oxygen saturation monitor
Renal	
Decreased renal blood flow and glomerular filtration rate Decreased ability to excrete waste products	Monitor urine output every 1 to 2 hours during immediate postoperative period Evaluate intake and output Monitor fluid and electrolyte status
Musculoskeletal	
Decrease in lean body mass Increase in spinal compression Increased incidence of osteoporosis and arthritis	Assess level of mobility Position on operating table with padding to reduce trauma to bones and joints Spine, limbs, and pressure points may be padded to prevent fractures Early ambulation or exercises to individual's ability Provide adequate nutrition Provide effective pain management
Sensorimotor	
Decreased reaction time Decreased visual acuity Decreased auditory acuity	Orient client to environment Plan individual teaching, allow time to reinforce teaching Provide a safe environment

Nutritional Status

CRITICAL TO REMEMBER

A client's nutritional status directly correlates with intraoperative success and postoperative recovery.

The client who is well nourished preoperatively is better prepared to handle surgical stress and to return to optimal health after surgery.

Two major problems are nutritional deficiencies and excess. Nutritional deficiencies primarily affect clients with chronic illnesses, cancer, gastrointestinal conditions (e.g., ulcerative colitis, pyloric stenosis, bulimia), and advanced age. Nursing intervention for clients who are malnourished preoperatively includes encouraging a high intake of carbohydrates (for energy), protein (for wound healing), and vitamins (for healing), especially vitamin K (for proper blood coagulation). Total parenteral or enteral nutrition may be administered for several days to a week before surgery.

Total parenteral nutrition plus lipids involves total nutritional replacement with vitamin and mineral supplements. Enteral nutrition involves feeding directly through a tube placed into the stomach or small intestine. Enteral nutrition is also called tube feeding. Both methods help improve a client's nutritional status before surgery and are often continued postoperatively until satisfactory gastrointestinal function returns.

If possible, obesity should be corrected before elective surgery. A severely obese client faces a greater surgical risk than a client of normal weight because of the following problems:

- Obese clients frequently suffer from hypertension, congestive heart failure, and metabolic problems such as diabetes mellitus. These complicate the operative and postoperative course.
- Adipose tissue increases the technical difficulty of surgery. Incisions are usually larger than normal, and the tissue is weaker. This increases the risk of postoperative infection, incisional hernias, and wound dehiscence and evisceration.
- An obese client is more susceptible to postoperative pulmonary complications. Obesity decreases the efficiency of coughing and deep breathing. The pressure of the abdominal contents on the diaphragm and lungs decreases expansion, leading to hypotension.

Treating obesity before surgery requires a reducing diet; mild exercise, if possible; and assessing and controlling conditions such as hypertension and diabetes mellitus, often with medications.

Fluid and Electrolyte Balance. Dehydration and hypovolemia (fluid volume deficit) predispose a client to complications during and after surgery. Dehydration results from prolonged vomiting, diarrhea, and bleeding, coupled with inadequate fluid intake. To correct dehydration, fluids are usually administered intravenously during the preoperative period.

Electrolyte imbalances also increase operative risk. Assessment and management of fluid and electrolyte imbalances is discussed in detail in Chapter 3.

Presence of Infection. Any infection, even a minor cold, can adversely affect surgical outcome. When the surgical site is near the lymphatic glands draining an infection, the likelihood of postoperative wound infection increases. During preoperative assessment, the nurse should document such symptoms as sneezing, coughing, sore throat, elevated temperature, and the presence of skin lesions, boils, or rashes. He or she should also note an elevated or low white blood count and communicate these findings to the surgeon or anesthesiologist, because all these factors increase surgical risk. It may be necessary to reschedule surgery.

Cardiovascular Function. Cardiac conditions that increase operative risk include angina pectoris, a myocardial infarction within the last 6 months, uncontrolled hypertension, congestive heart failure, and peripheral vascular disease. All cardiac conditions could lead to decreased tissue perfusion, and peripheral vascular disease could impair wound healing in an extremity.

All clients should be assessed for elevated blood pressure; slow, rapid, or irregular pulse; edema; cold, cyanotic extremities; weakness; and shortness of breath. Laboratory and diagnostic studies, which are often ordered before surgery to determine cardiovascular function, include electrocardiogram and hemoglobin, hematocrit, and serum electrolyte measurements.

Preoperative treatment of clients with cardiovascular disease includes rest, a low-sodium or low-cholesterol diet, heart medications, and the judicious administration of fluids. An attempt is made to get the client's cardiovascular system in the best condition possible before surgery.

Pulmonary Function. Pulmonary conditions such as COPD, emphysema, asthma, and bronchitis increase operative risk because they impair CO_2 and O_2 diffusion in the alveolus and predispose the client to pulmonary infection.

To evaluate pulmonary conditions, the nurse should assess the client for shortness of breath, wheezing, clubbed fingers, chest pain, and coughing with expectoration of copious or purulent mucus. The client should be questioned carefully about smoking habits, and a history obtained of any respiratory allergies and infections. A chest x-ray study is ordered for diagnostic purposes on all clients.

Often a baseline arterial blood gas study is obtained to evaluate pulmonary function in a client with known respiratory disease, as are pulmonary function studies (see Chaps. 19 and 20). Clients with severe respiratory disease are usually treated preoperatively with aerosol therapy, postural drainage, and antibiotics. Clients who still smoke are strongly encouraged to stop before surgery. To help prevent postoperative respiratory complications, these clients need careful preoperative instruction and practice in deep breathing and coughing exercises.

Renal Function. The surgical client needs adequate renal function to eliminate protein wastes, maintain fluid and electrolyte balance, and clear anesthetic agents. Conditions that increase operative risk include advanced renal insufficiency, acute nephritis, and benign prostatic hypertrophy. In older men, benign prostatic hypertrophy may obstruct the normal flow of urine and make voiding difficult.

To assess renal status, the nurse should assess for symptoms of frequency, dysuria, and anuria and observe the appearance of the urine. Urine that is cloudy or bloody rather than a clear amber color should be documented and reported.

The most commonly ordered preoperative tests to assess renal function are urinalysis, blood urea nitrogen, and creatinine.

Gastrointestinal Function. The client should be questioned about normal bowel functioning, so postoperative expectations for return of function are appropriate. Clients with a long history of constipation may have more difficulty postoperatively than those with regular bowel function.

Liver Function. Liver disease, such as cirrhosis, increases risk because an impaired liver is unable to detoxify medications and anesthetic agents or to metabolize carbohydrates, fats, and amino acids. In addition, inadequate liver function is associated with poor wound healing and a higher rate of infection. Clients with a history of alcoholism or ascites should be assessed for jaundice or ascites. If either condition is found, it should be reported to the surgeon before surgery. Because these clients are usually malnourished and debilitated, the surgeon generally orders a high-calorie diet, intravenous solutions, and vitamins during the preoperative period.

Endocrine Function. Endocrine function, particularly that of the thyroid, must be monitored carefully preoperatively to minimize operative risk. Hyperthyroidism can lead to thyroid storm or thyroid crisis, with symptoms of hypertension, tachycardia, and hyperthermia and, therefore, should be treated medically preoperatively (see Chap. 41). Likewise, hypothyroidism increases the risk of hypotension and cardiac arrest during the administration of anesthesia, and it should be recognized and treated before surgery.

Diabetes mellitus predisposes a client to infection and to poor tissue healing and swings of blood sugar levels that are more profound than usual. Cardiovascular and renal complications also increase surgical risk for a client with diabetes. The client with well-controlled diabetes is more likely to respond well to surgery. Chapter 40 discusses in detail the care of clients with diabetes mellitus.

Neurologic Function. The nurse should conduct a thorough neurologic physical assessment before surgery to determine the client's baseline function. Testing generally includes assessing cranial nerves, reflex response of the upper and lower extremities, sensory reflexes, and cerebellar response (see Chap. 12).

Serious neurologic conditions, such as uncontrolled epilepsy or severe Parkinson's disease, increase surgical risk. Important neurologic preoperative findings include severe headache, frequent dizziness, lightheadedness, ringing in the ears, unsteady gait, unequal pupils, and a history of convulsions.

Hematologic Function. Clients with blood coagulation disorders are at risk for hemorrhage and hypovolemic shock during and following surgery. Five factors pointing to abnormal hematologic factors are

- a history of bleeding tendencies
- symptoms such as easy bruising, excessive bleeding following dental extractions and shaving, and severe nosebleeds
- the presence of hepatic or renal disease
- use of anticoagulants
- abnormal bleeding time, prothrombin time, or platelet counts (see Chaps. 27 and 28)

Blood tranfusions are used less frequently than in past years because of the fear of AIDS and hepatitis B transmission. If possible, clients are encouraged to donate their own blood before surgery (autologous blood transfusion) for use during or after. Blood transfusions are discussed in Chapter 28.

Use of Medications

CRITICAL TO REMEMBER

Many clients take prescribed and nonprescribed medications that may increase operative risk by increasing coagulation time or interacting unfavorably with the anesthetic.

Some of the medications that may result in complications include

- anticoagulants including aspirin, which cause clotting abnormalities
- antibiotics, which combine with some muscle relaxants to increase postoperative respiratory depression
- tranquilizers, which decrease blood pressure and thus increase the risk of shock; they also potentiate the effects of narcotics and barbiturates
- thiazide diuretics, which can create potassium depletion
- steroids, which cause hypofunction of the adrenal cortex and, thus, impair physiologic response to the stress of anesthesia and surgery; their anti-inflammatory effects also delay wound healing and increase the risk of infection
- monoamine (MAO) inhibitors, which can cause hypertensive crisis when combined with anesthetic agents
- antiparkinsonian drugs, which cause hypotension or hypertension when combined with anesthetics
- street drugs and alcohol abuse, which increase the tolerance to narcotics
- hypoglycemics, which require dosage alteration and close monitoring of the blood sugar

CRITICAL TO REMEMBER

Steroid replacement also must be increased before, during, and after surgery.

When performing a nursing preoperative assessment, document whether the client has any drug allergies or reactions or is currently taking any prescribed or over-the-counter medications. Surgical risk is increased if the client is allergic to the anesthetic or if the medications the client is taking interact adversely with the anesthesia. Clients often forget to list some medications they are taking. They also sometimes fail to recognize that nonprescription medications may pose a threat and, consequently, do not mention them. Therefore, the nurse should question clients very carefully and obtain as complete a list of medications as possible. The physician's decision to discontinue, reduce, or continue preoperative medications is based on the client's surgical risk.

Presence of Trauma. When surgery must be performed following a traumatic incident (e.g., gunshot wound, stab wound, serious accident, severe fall), the details of the event should be documented as precisely as possible. Questioning the client and significant others may help determine whether there is an underlying, undetected condition that may increase surgical risk (e.g., epilepsy, coronary artery disease, uncontrolled diabetes mellitus, and elder abuse).

Health Habits. The client undergoing surgery who smokes or abuses drugs has an increased surgical risk. The client who smokes has reduced hemoglobin levels and, therefore, less oxygen available for tissue repair. Smokers are more susceptible to thrombus formation because of the hypercoagulability of their blood and their increased rate of arteriosclerosis. Smokers are also more likely to have damage to their lung tissue, including COPD and chronic bronchitis. Smokers should stop smoking at least 1 week before elective surgery.

Clients undergoing surgery who use alcohol or drugs may experience withdrawal symptoms during hospitalization. Their surgical course may be complicated by poor nutrition, as well as unpredictable reactions to the anesthetic agents. Remember, even two drinks a day can lead to withdrawal symptoms and the need for increased analgesia and anesthesia.

Clients who lead a sedentary life-style may have a complicated postoperative course because of poor muscle tone, limited cardiac and respiratory reserve, and decreased stress response to the physical demands of surgery.

Clients who are HIV-positive have several areas of increased surgical risk. If their immune systems are affected, they are at a much higher risk for developing a postoperative infection and for being unable to fight that infection. If they have developed *Pneumocystis carinii* pneumonia, they are at increased risk of anesthetic and postoperative pulmonary complications.

Social History. The client's marital status, significant others, and support systems should be thoroughly explored. The client's occupation should also be identified because it may be a source of difficulty after surgery if the client is unable to return to work. It is also important to determine whether the client has insurance or whether this surgery will cause severe financial hardship.

Because all of these factors could increase the client's stress and interfere with healing, the nurse should be aware of these potential risks that may jeopardize a successful surgical intervention.

Psychosocial Aspects of Preoperative Preparation

Effectively handling clients' fears can smooth the preoperative experience. Studies show that clients who are calm and emotionally prepared for surgery withstand anesthesia better and experience fewer postoperative complications.

Fear of the unknown is one of the most important causes of preoperative anxiety. During the preoperative phase, clients also may fear postoperative pain, the discovery of cancer, the loss of an organ or limb, anesthesia, vulnerability while unconscious, threat of loss of job or financial security, loss of social and familial roles, disruption of life-style, separation from significant others, and even death.

CRITICAL TO REMEMBER

Clients respond differently to fear. Some respond by becoming silent and withdrawn, childish, belligerent, evasive, tearful, or clinging.

Most clients feel helpless when admitted to a health-care facility. Nurses need to remember that although surgery may become commonplace to the health-care professional, it is a frightening experience to the client.

Based on the nursing assessment, a number of interventions may be appropriate for the preoperative client. First, the nurse should provide explanations and printed information about the health-care facility routines, visiting hours, mealtimes, the location of the chapel and waiting room, and so forth. The nurse should explain the procedures involved in the planned surgery to allay the client's anxiety; the client should have a complete idea of what the preoperative, intraoperative, and postoperative course entails. The nurse should consult with the physician before speaking to the client about specific or technical details. He or she should explain all nursing care and any possible discomfort that may result as a consequence of nursing interventions and tell the client what the nurse will do to minimize any discomfort. If the client is scheduled to go to the intensive care unit after surgery, the nurse should ask what the client already knows or has heard about intensive care. At this point, time should be taken to clarify any misconceptions or incorrect information.

The client should be allowed to take the lead in asking questions concerning surgery and the postoperative period. The nurse provides the client with essential information, such as nothing-by-mouth (NPO) status and preoperative procedures, but then only as much additional information as the client wishes to know. If the client is very withdrawn, depressed, or apprehensive, the nurse's communication skills should be used to encourage expression of fears and concerns. For example, he or she can tell the client that preoperative fear is normal and that it is not unusual to experience anxiety and invite the client to share concerns. The nurse can find out if the client knows someone who had similar surgery and what the outcome was. Often a client's fears may be rooted in the stories of unpleasant experiences that happened to others.

Whenever possible, the nurse should introduce the client or significant others to other people who have successfully undergone similar surgery. If this is not possible preoperatively, it may be done after surgery. Support groups such as the local laryngectomy or colostomy organization, for instance, can be contacted and asked for a volunteer to visit the client.

Discharge needs of the client based on planned surgical procedures and current health status should be identified. Referrals for assistance could include

- Local visiting nurse or home health-care services
- Local chapters of the Cancer Society, Heart Association, and Diabetes Association
- Local mastectomy, laryngectomy, colostomy support groups
- Medic Alert Foundation
- Malignant hyperthermia hotline
- Local senior citizens' assistance program
- Substance abuse treatment programs or groups
- Emergency social services
- Local sexual assault center (United States law requires that suspected sexual abuse of minors be reported)
- Child protection services
- Emergency legal assistance

The nurse should find out the client's religious preference and arrange for a visit from clergy, if the client so desires. Finally, the client's significant others should be included in preoperative discussions whenever possible and provided with information they can use to assist in reducing the client's preoperative anxiety.

Preoperative Assessment

HISTORY

CRITICAL TO REMEMBER

Data gathered during a purposeful history taking help detect problems that may arise preoperatively or postoperatively. The manner in which the history is conducted plays a large part in determining the degree of preoperative and postoperative anxiety the client experiences.

The history allows clients to explain their understanding of impending surgery. This information can be used to determine clients' learning needs. The preoperative history also allows the nurse to

- Establish rapport with the client and significant others.
- Begin a psychosocial assessment of the client. A client who is apprehensive preoperatively may need more frequent or repetitive instruction and more reinforcement than a less anxious client.
- Reassure the client and significant others and answer general questions about the surgery, the health-care facility, and so forth.

Specific information to obtain during the preoperative history concerns

- previous surgery and experience with anesthesia;
- responses of significant others to previous surgery and anesthesia;
- whether the client has had any serious illnesses;
- previous and current medications (prescription or over-the-counter);
- allergies and reactions and dietary restrictions;
- alcohol, nicotine, or recreational drug use;
- current symptoms or discomforts;
- occupation;
- religious affiliation;
- significant others (Is the client single or married? How many dependents does the client have?);
- whether the client has any questions about the surgery; and
- chronic illnesses, such as arthritis, migraines, back pain.

In addition to helping the nurse establish valuable preoperative baseline data, this information uncovers the need for supportive services. If a client will need assistance after returning home, the nurse can initiate discharge plans.

PHYSICAL EXAMINATION

A physical examination is performed on all clients undergoing surgery to determine baseline data and identify conditions that may interfere with the administration of anesthesia or produce problems postoperatively.

A complete physical examination should be performed, with special attention paid to cardiac and respiratory systems. Baseline vital signs are obtained as one determination of the client's risk for postoperative complications. Any abnormal vital sign is significant and may cause a postponement of surgery until the problem is treated. Abnormal breath sounds may indicate the need for respiratory therapy both before and after surgery, or the need for bronchodilators. Clients with abnormal cardiac findings will need further evaluation to determine whether they can withstand the stress of surgery and anesthesia. Physical examination also should reveal any problems with joint mobility or deformities that may interfere with operative positioning as well as their postoperative course. Special consideration of the elderly should include cardiac, respiratory, renal, and musculoskeletal assessment.

PREOPERATIVE DIAGNOSTIC TESTS

Routine diagnostic tests are ordered less often than in past years. Currently, clients have specific tests ordered based on their health status to identify potential problems that would interfere with the surgery. Table 5–4 identifies commonly requested preoperative laboratory tests.

INFORMED CONSENT

Anyone undergoing any invasive procedure must sign a permit. This legal document signifies that the client is giving informed consent for the procedure. The permit guards the client against unwanted invasive procedures. It also protects the health-care facility and health-care professionals.

A signed consent is necessary for each invasive procedure. The client must receive a full explanation of the operation before signing the permit. The surgeon

TABLE 5–4 Preoperative Diagnostic Tests

TEST	NORMAL RANGES*	PURPOSE
Serum potassium	3.5 to 5.0 mEq/L	To identify hyperkalemia or hypokalemia
Serum sodium	136 to 145 mEq/L	To identify hypernatremia, hyponatremia, dehydration, or overhydration
Serum chloride	96 to 106 mEq/L	To identify hyperchloremia, hypochloremia, or metabolic alkalosis
Glucose	60 to 100 mg/dL	To identify hypoglycemia or hyperglycemia
Creatinine	0.7 to 1.4 mg/dL	To identify acute or chronic renal disease
Blood urea nitrogen	10 to 20 mg/dL	To identify impaired liver or kidney function or excessive protein or tissue catabolism
Hemoglobin	Female: 12.0 to 15.0 g/dL Male: 13.0 to 17.0 g/dL	To identify the presence and extent of anemia
Hematocrit	Female: 36 to 45 per cent Male: 39 to 51 per cent	To identify the presence and extent of anemia
Prothrombin time	11 to 18 seconds	To identify dysfunction of blood clotting (prothrombin level)
Partial thromboplastin time	35 to 45 seconds	To identify deficiencies of coagulation factors
Chest x-ray study	No abnormal heart or lung lesions	To determine size and contour of heart, lungs, and major vessels
Electrocardiogram	Baseline rate and rhythm	To determine the electrical activity of the heart

* May vary with different laboratories.

should explain the procedure in terms the client readily understands. The client must be told about potential risks, complications and disfigurement that may result from the surgery; about anesthesia; who will perform the surgery; and whether or not organs or body parts may be removed. The client should be informed about alternative treatments.

The procedure for obtaining a signed consent varies from state to state and according to the policy of the health-care facility. Generally, the surgeon explains the surgical procedure, possible risks and complications, and alternatives.

Adults sign their own operative permit unless they are unconscious or mentally incompetent. In such cases, a relative or guardian is responsible for consent. If the relative or guardian is out of state, the physician can secure consent over the telephone in the presence of one or two witnesses on the same line. If no relative or guardian can be found, the court can appoint one.

Once the operative permit is signed, it becomes a permanent part of the client's record. The nurse needs to make sure it accompanies the record to the operating room.

The client may choose to obtain a second opinion regarding the need for surgery. Most insurance carriers, Medicare, and Medicaid encourage second opinions and will pay for them.

SPECIAL CONSIDERATIONS

Medications. In preparing clients for surgery, it is important to assess what routine medications they are taking so care can be planned safely. Clients must be interviewed carefully about what medications they are taking, and nurses need to assess the individual's medication history. Nurses, in consultation with the physician, must intervene to stop medications, reduce dosage, or anticipate possible medication side effects.

The Older Adult. Another consideration in the care of the operative client is the care of the older surgical client. Normal physiologic changes place the older client at increased risk when surgical intervention is needed. Table 5–3 outlines major physiologic changes that occur as a result of surgery and appropriate nursing interventions.

Preoperative Teaching

Preoperative teaching is an important component in the client's operative experience.

CRITICAL TO REMEMBER

> Numerous research studies have supported the value of preoperative instruction in both decreasing the incidence of postoperative complications and decreasing the length of hospital stay.

Client's teaching needs must be assessed individually.

In many cases, clients are admitted the same day of the surgery. Hopefully, they will have received written or verbal instructions prior to this time and the nurse will be able to reinforce instructions and answer questions. A phone interview is conducted in many ambulatory surgery units.

Preoperative teaching decreases anxiety and encourages clients to participate actively in their own care. The basic areas that must be covered in preoperative teaching are

- deep breathing and coughing exercises
- turning and extremity exercises
- pain control methods that will be offered
- postoperative equipment

DEEP BREATHING EXERCISES

Breathing and coughing exercises help expand collapsed lungs and prevent postoperative pneumonia and atelectasis. The nurse demonstrates correct deep breathing by inhaling slowly through the nose, distending the abdomen, and exhaling slowly through pursed lips. After the demonstration, the client should be asked to perform the exercise (Fig. 5–1).

The nurse should instruct the client to use this breathing method as often as possible, preferably five to ten times every hour during the postoperative, immobilized period.

COUGHING EXERCISES

For this exercise, the client may be in a sitting or lying position. The nurse shows the client how to splint an incision. Splinting minimizes pressure and helps to control pain when the person is coughing. The nurse instructs the client to lace the fingers and hold them tightly across the incision before coughing. A small pillow or folded towel held over the incision also facilitates splinting. The client takes a deep breath, exhaling through the mouth, before coughing from deep in the lungs.

CRITICAL TO REMEMBER

The nurse should encourage the client to perform deep breathing exercises *before* coughing, to stimulate the cough reflex.

Incentive spirometers are used to promote lung expansion. They promote alveolar inflation and strengthen respiratory muscles. Their use also helps prevent atelectasis in the postoperative client. They should be used at least four times a day.

TURNING EXERCISES

The client also needs to practice turning from side to side, using the side rails to assist movements. Turning prevents venous stasis and respiratory problems. The nurse should teach the client to turn every 1 to 2 hours while awake until the client is out of bed and ambulatory.

EXTREMITY EXERCISES

Finally, the client should practice extremity exercises. The client flexes and extends each joint, particularly the hip, knee, and ankle joints, keeping the lower back flat as the leg is lowered and straightened, and moves each foot in a circular motion. These exercises help prevent circulatory problems, such as thrombophlebitis, by facilitating venous return to the heart.

Antiembolism stockings are used on the lower extremities preoperatively, intraoperatively, and postoperatively combined with turning and leg exercises to help to prevent thrombophlebitis or thromboemboli formation. Sequential compression stockings to massage legs rhythmically are now being used for even more effective prevention of clots.

Ambulation after the surgery should be encouraged when appropriate.

CRITICAL TO REMEMBER

Ambulation helps prevent postoperative complications.

The nurse should include a projected schedule for postoperative ambulation in the preoperative teaching program.

PAIN CONTROL

A common concern among preoperative clients is the pain they will experience in the postoperative period. It is important to assure clients they will be kept as comfortable as possible while regaining their strength and mobility.

During the immediate postoperative period, clients will receive medication by intravenous, intramuscular, or epidural routes. If the pain medication is given intravenously or epidurally, it may be given by an infusion pump. Patient-controlled analgesia (PCA) allows clients to administer their own pain medication. If it is anticipated the client will use PCA postoperatively, the nurse should explain the operating instructions and allow the client time to practice operating it.

POSTOPERATIVE EQUIPMENT

Clients should be instructed about equipment they may anticipate postoperatively. Depending on the surgery, various tubes, drains, and intravenous lines will be used. Discussion should focus on the purpose of specific equipment and how it relates to the client's specific surgery.

Tubes. The most common type of tube is an indwelling catheter for the purpose of bladder drainage. Another common tube is the nasogastric tube. The purpose is to decompress the stomach and upper bowel and to drain stomach contents.

Drains. Drains are usually inserted during surgery to promote evacuation of fluid from the operative site. They act by either wick action, such as with a Penrose drain, or with a mild amount of suction, such as with a Hemovac or Davol drain.

Intravenous Infusion Devices. Intravenous infusions are usually started prior to surgery. The purpose of the infusion is to administer medications and fluids before, during, and after surgery.

Physical Preparation

PREPARING THE SKIN

Usually the operative area is cleansed the night prior to surgery with an antiseptic such as povidone-iodine (Betadine or Hibiclens) to decrease the number of microorganisms on the skin.

Opinions differ as to preoperative skin preparation. Research studies show that not removing hair at all, clipping hair, or using an electric razor is associated with a lower rate of infection than traditional shav-

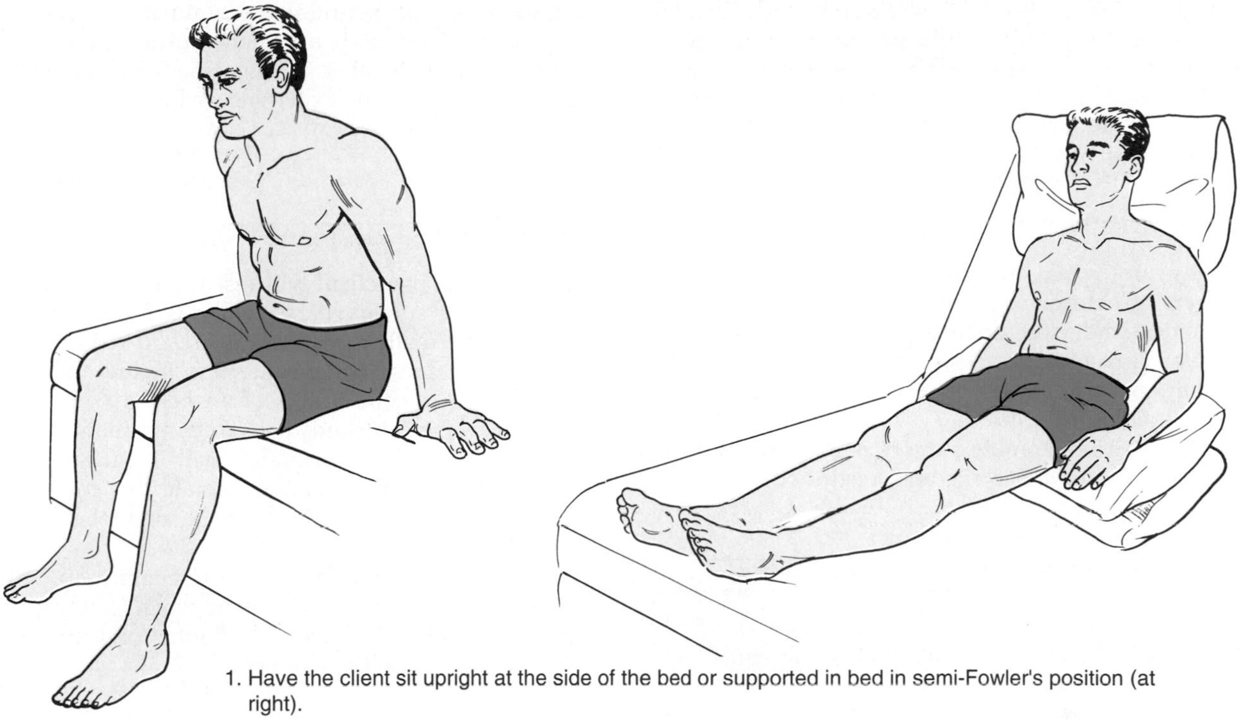

A

1. Have the client sit upright at the side of the bed or supported in bed in semi-Fowler's position (at right).

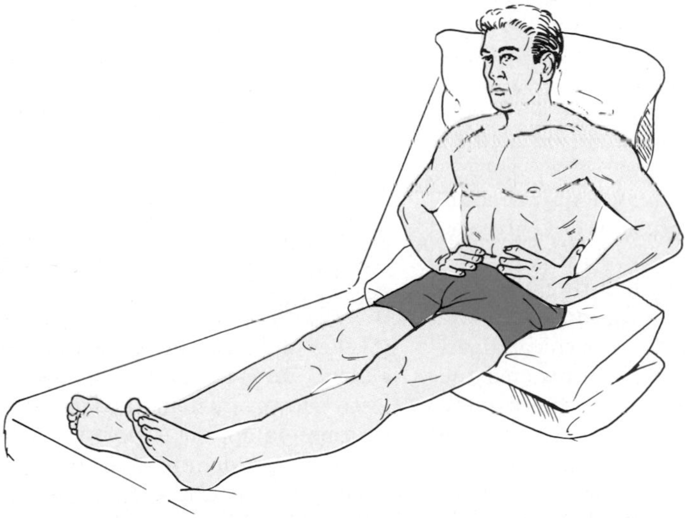

2. Instruct the client to place his or her hands on the abdomen to feel whether the chest rises to indicate that the lungs are expanding.
3. Have the client inhale through the nose until the abdomen distends.
4. Instruct the client to exhale through pursed lips while contracting the abdominal muscles.
5. Have the client repeat this exercise every hour during the first postoperative day.

B

Figure 5–1

Deep (diaphragmatic) breathing after surgery.

ing.[19] The Centers for Disease Control and Prevention recommends that if shaving is necessary, it can be performed in the operating room prior to surgery. The nurse responsible for skin preparation should conduct a preoperative assessment for any skin abrasions, lacerations, or signs of infection at the operative area.

PREPARING THE GASTROINTESTINAL TRACT

The gastrointestinal tract needs special preparation on the evening before surgery to (1) reduce the possibility of vomiting and aspiration during anesthesia, (2) reduce the possibility of a bowel obstruction, and (3) prevent contamination from fecal material during intestinal tract or bowel surgery.

If a client undergoing surgery is to receive a general anesthetic, foods and fluids are restricted for 8 to 10 hours before the operation.

CRITICAL TO REMEMBER

This restriction significantly reduces the possibility of aspiration of gastric contents, which can cause aspiration pneumonia.

Because solid food must be withheld 8 to 10 hours before surgery, most clients have an NPO status after midnight. When surgery is not scheduled until late afternoon, the client may eat a light breakfast in the morning if the surgeon permits. The nurse should teach the client and family the importance of maintaining NPO status.

If the client who is NPO consumes food or fluids, the surgeon and the anesthesiologist should be notified because the surgery may be cancelled.

Clients who are extremely debilitated or malnourished may receive intravenous infusions of glucose, amino acids, or plasma prior to surgery.

Enemas are not routinely ordered during the preoperative period except for surgical procedures involving the gastrointestinal tract, perianal or perineal areas, and pelvic cavity. Enemas are usually administered the evening before surgery. Clients who are admitted the same day as the surgery may be instructed to take one or more enemas at home the night before surgery. This will require excellent teaching to ensure the client knows how to administer the enemas correctly and what results to expect. Some clients may require further bowel cleansing on the morning of surgery after admission to the facility.

Gastrointestinal tubes are usually inserted during surgery, if they are to be used at all. This procedure is usually performed for clients undergoing major abdominal or intestinal tract surgery.

Some types of surgery require special bowel preparations. The specific protocol for each surgical procedure is ordered to meet the client's need.

PREPARING FOR ANESTHESIA

The anesthesiologist or nurse anesthetist visits the client before surgery to perform a complete respiratory, cardiovascular, and neurologic examination. Generally, the topics discussed with the client during the examination include the type of anesthesia planned and the sensations the client will experience when undergoing anesthesia. The client's fears concerning anesthesia also are addressed.

PROMOTING REST AND SLEEP

The preoperative client will rest more completely on the night before surgery if he or she is physically comfortable and mentally at ease. Measures to reduce preoperative sleeplessness and restlessness include a well-ventilated room, a comfortable clean bed, a backrub, and a warm beverage (if fluids are not contraindicated). These measures will work equally well in the hospital or home. Apprehensive clients should be encouraged to take ordered sleep medication the night before surgery to help them to sleep.

The nurse should always remember to talk in a positive manner with the client when giving preoperative care and to listen to any doubts or fears the client may have concerning surgery.

Preparing the Client on the Day of Surgery

EARLY MORNING CARE

Immediate preoperative preparation begins at least 1 to 2 hours before surgery for clients in the hospital and as soon as same-day-admission clients come into the hospital. At this time, the nurse asks whether the client has any questions or concerns and continues to assess for signs of anxiety. The nurse should communicate any surgical delays to the client and significant others.

The following preoperative interventions on the part of the nurse help promote safety during surgery:

- Take and record the vital signs. Some increase in blood pressure or pulse is common because of anxiety. However, if marked differences from baseline information appear, report them to the surgeon.
- Check the identification band to make sure it is legible, accurate, and securely fastened to the client.
- If a skin preparation has been ordered, check that it has been completed accurately and thoroughly.
- Check for and carry out any special orders such as administering enemas or starting an intravenous line.
- Verify that the client has not eaten for the last 8 hours. Check that fluids have been restricted, although sometimes the physician will order clients to take their usual oral medications with a small sip of water.
- Ask the client to void; record the time and amount of urine voided.
- Assist the client with oral hygiene, if necessary.
- Remove dentures or bridgework that could obstruct the airway if left in place. Store these and other valuable items according to health-care facility policy or give them to family members.

- Have the client remove jewelry. Many facilities allow the client to keep wedding bands on as long as they are taped securely. If jewelry is removed, store it according to policy or give it to the family. Assist the client with the removal of hairpins, wigs, or prostheses.
- If the client is wearing a hearing aid, notify the operating room nurse. Leave it in place so operating room personnel know it is there and can communicate with the client.
- Assist the client in donning a hospital gown, protective head cap, Ace wraps, or antiembolic hose, if these items have been ordered.
- Remove colored nail polish from at least one nail for the pulse oximeter (although the device can accurately read oxygen saturation levels through light-colored polish). Remove make-up so skin color can be observed.

To prevent omissions in preoperative nursing interventions, most facilities supply nurses with a preoperative checklist. As each intervention on the list is completed, the nurse initials it.

PREOPERATIVE MEDICATIONS

Prior to administering preoperative medications, the nurse should check to be sure that the operative permit and transfusion permit (if required) are correctly signed and attached to the client record.

CRITICAL TO REMEMBER

Permits must be signed and witnessed before the client receives any medication that will alter his or her consciousness (such as a narcotic or tranquilizer).

The purposes of various preoperative medications are to allay anxiety, decrease pharyngeal secretions, reduce side effects of anesthetic agents, and create amnesia.

Table 5–5 presents an overview of common preoperative medications. Specific drug choices are based on the individual client variables, the goals for sedation, and the potential for undesirable side effects. Preoperative medications may be given in the preoperative area or on the nursing unit prior to the client's leaving for

TABLE 5–5 Commonly Used Preoperative Medications

GENERIC NAME	TRADE NAME	DESIRED EFFECTS	UNDESIRED EFFECTS
Tranquilizers			
Diazepam	Valium	Decreases anxiety	May cause dizziness, clumsiness, or confusion
Droperidol	Inapsine	Decreases anxiety Produces an antiemetic effect	Anxiety Hypotension during and after surgery
Sedatives			
Midazolam hydrochloride	Versed	Induces desired sleepiness and reduces anxiety	Hypotension, undesired respiratory depression
Promethazine	Phenergan	Same as for droperidol	Hypotension during and after surgery
Secobarbital sodium	Seconal sodium	Decreases anxiety Promotes sedation	Disorientation, especially in elderly patients
Pentobarbital sodium	Nembutal sodium	Same as for secobarbital sodium	Same as for secobarbital sodium
Analgesics			
Morphine sulfate	—	Relieves pain Decreases anxiety Sedation	Respiratory depression Hypotension Circulatory depression Decreased gastric motility causing potential for vomiting
Meperidine hydrochloride	Demerol	Same as for morphine sulfate	Same as for morphine sulfate
Anticholinergics			
Atropine sulfate	—	Controls secretions	Excessive dryness of mouth, tachycardia
Glycopyrrolate	Robinul	Same as for atropine sulfate	Same as for atropine sulfate
Histamine H_2-Receptor Antagonists			
Cimetidine	Tagamet	Inhibits gastric acid production	Some mild dizziness, diarrhea, somnolence, and rash

surgery. If the preoperative medication is given on the unit, the nurse is responsible for raising the bed's side rails, lowering the window shades, and turning off bright lights.

CRITICAL TO REMEMBER

The nurse should instruct the client not to get up without assistance, because medications may cause drowsiness or dizziness.

Once the client is calm and drowsy, he or she should be disturbed only when necessary and then briefly and quietly. The nurse observes the client for side effects from medication such as hypotension or respiratory depression.

TRANSPORTING THE CLIENT TO SURGERY

When surgical personnel call for the client, the client is gently transferred to a stretcher (the nurse needs to make sure he or she has enough help to transfer the client safely). The client is covered with blankets for protection from drafts and then secured with a restraining belt. The nurse should make sure the client record accompanies the client to the operating room.

Caring for Significant Others

During surgery, the significant others usually wait in a designated surgical lounge. If they must leave the facility for any reason, the nurse should ask them for a phone number where they can be reached and provide the phone number of the client's unit.

When discussing surgery with significant others, the nurse should be aware of information previously given by the surgeon regarding the immediate surgical outcome and eventual prognosis. The nurse can then answer questions with confidence that the information given agrees with previous statements.

The client's significant others should be prepared for the sight of nasogastric tubes, chest tubes, suction equipment, respiratory equipment, intravenous infusions, dressing, or monitoring equipment. They should be informed when the surgery is completed (this can be done by waiting room personnel). The nurse should make certain the surgeon knows who is waiting for information on the client.

The nurse should reassure significant others that the length of time the client is gone may not reflect the actual length of surgery. There are often unpredictable delays that might cause the client to wait before surgery. Significant others should be reassured if this has happened to the client so they will not worry.

INTRAOPERATIVE NURSING

The intraoperative phase of the perioperative experience begins as the client is placed on the surgical bed and ends with admission to the PACU.

CRITICAL TO REMEMBER

Nursing care during the intraoperative phase focuses on the client's emotional well-being as well as physical factors such as safety, positioning, maintaining asepsis, and controlling the surgical environment.

Clients are highly dependent on the nurse for their needs during this phase.

In the preoperative area, the nurse is responsible for reviewing the record for completeness, ensuring proper identification of the client, client safety, and providing emotional support. It is important to deal with the fears and concerns of a frightened or agitated client. A relaxed client undergoes anesthetic induction more easily than one who is anxious. If the client still seems anxious despite sedation and reassurance, the surgeon or anesthesia personnel should be notified.

Procedures vary among institutions, but after admission to the operating room, the client is moved to the operating room bed. At this time, the client is identified by the surgeon, anesthetized, positioned, has the skin prepared, and is draped for surgery.

Anesthesia in Surgery

Anesthesia means the absence of pain ('an' meaning without, and 'esthesia' meaning awareness or feeling). Anesthesia is an artificially induced state of partial or total loss of sensation, occurring with or without loss of consciousness. The purpose of anesthesia is to produce muscle relaxation, block transmission of nerve impulses, suppress reflexes, and cause loss of consciousness.

Clients are generally anxious about receiving anesthesia. Reviewing the preoperative nursing assessment reveals some of the client's fears and concerns and allows the surgical nursing staff to offer continued support.

The decision as to the type of anesthesia to be used is made largely by the anesthesiologist in consultation with the surgeon and client. The anesthetic agents chosen for a client's surgical procedure depend on many variables. These include (1) age and physical condition of the client; (2) type, location, and duration of the surgery; (3) degree of technical intricacy of the surgery; (4) previous anesthetic history; and (5) personal preference, expertise, and judgment of the anesthesiologist or nurse anesthetist. Also, the client undergoing surgery may prefer one type of anesthesia over another (e.g., spinal anesthesia rather than general anesthesia). A client's preference should be considered as part of the total profile when the type of anesthesia is selected.

There are two major classifications of anesthesia: general and regional. General anesthetics block pain stimulus at the cerebral cortex. General anesthesia is a drug-induced depression of the central nervous system that is reversed either by metabolic elimination in the body or by pharmacologic means. General anesthetic agents produce analgesia, amnesia, and unconsciousness, characterized by the loss of reflexes and muscle tone.

TABLE 5–6 Types of Anesthesia

TYPE	GOAL	ADMINISTRATION	ASSESSMENT
General	Total loss of consciousness and sensation; produces amnesia by blocking awareness centers in brain	Intravenous Inhalation Rectal	Loss of reflexes and muscle tone
Regional	Reduces all painful sensations in one region of the body without inducing unconsciousness:		
	• Blocks transmission of nerve impulses at their origin	Topical Local infiltration	Produces analgesia over specific tissue area
	• Blocks transmission of nerve impulses along afferent neurons	Field block Nerve block Intravenous regional	Produces analgesia over specific area of body
	• Blocks transmission of nerve impulses along spinal cord	Spinal Epidural block	Produces analgesia over specific region of body

Regional anesthetics block the pain stimulus at its origin, along afferent neurons, or along the spinal cord. Unlike general anesthesia, regional anesthesia produces a loss of painful sensation in only one region of the body and does not result in unconsciousness. The client also may receive sedative agents that produce drowsiness. The client might receive epidural narcotics, which have a systemic effect and produce some drowsiness. Table 5–6 illustrates the purpose, method of administration, and assessment of these two major types of anesthesia.

GENERAL ANESTHESIA

Effects of General Anesthesia. The body systems affected by general anesthetics are the neurologic, respiratory, and cardiovascular systems. General anesthesia is best suited for surgery of the head, neck, and upper torso; prolonged surgical procedures; or for clients who are unable to lie quietly for a prolonged period of time. General anesthetic agents affect all tissues in the body to some degree.

The anesthesiologist or nurse anesthetist continually monitors body systems and tissues during induction of anesthesia, maintenance of the anesthetized state, and emergence of the client from anesthesia. The depth of anesthesia is monitored by observing changes in respirations, oxygen saturation and tidal CO_2, heart rate, urine output, and blood pressure.

Stages of General Anesthesia. The four stages of anesthesia are described in Table 5–7. Although not apparent with all anesthetics, all stages may be seen if

TABLE 5–7 The Four Stages of Anesthesia

STAGE	FROM	TO	ASSESSMENT OF CLIENT	NURSING INTERVENTIONS
I: Onset	Anesthetic administration	Loss of consciousness	May be drowsy or dizzy May experience auditory or visual hallucinations	Close operating room doors. Keep room quiet. Stand by client to assist, if necessary
II: Excitement	Loss of consciousness	Loss of eyelid reflexes	Increase in autonomic activity Irregular breathing May struggle	Remain quietly at client's side. Assist anesthetist, if needed
III: Surgical anesthesia	Loss of eyelid reflexes	Loss of most reflexes Depression of vital functions	Is unconscious Muscles are relaxed No blink or gag reflex	Begin preparation (if indicated) only when anesthetist indicates stage III has been reached and client is under good control
IV: Danger (death)	Vital functions too depressed	Respiratory and circulatory failure	Not breathing May or may not have a heartbeat	If arrest occurs, respond immediately to assist in establishing airway. Provide cardiac arrest tray, drugs, syringes, long needles. Assist surgeon with closed or open cardiac massage

TABLE 5–8 General Anesthetic Agents

DRUG	ACTION	SIDE EFFECTS	NURSING IMPLICATIONS
Inhalation Agents			
Nitrous oxide	Gas with very low anesthetic potency, so it must be used with other agents. Highest analgesic effect of all agents; little or no effect on BP or pulse, no muscle relaxant properties	Minimal side effects; little or no hypotension or respiratory depression. Low incidence of malignant hypothermia	Monitor vital signs, especially BP and pulse; monitor effects of central nervous system depressants for 24 hours after administration
Halothane (Fluothane)	Volatile liquid with high anesthetic potency, so it could be used alone. Has weak analgesic effect; causes a moderate decrease in BP and a large decrease in respirations, and is only a mild muscle relaxant	Hypotension, depression of myocardium with decreased cardiac output, bradycardia, respiratory depression, sensitizes heart to catecholamines, malignant hyperthermia, hepatitis, postoperative mild nausea and vomiting, and decreased urine output	Monitor all vital signs closely; monitor temperature for signs of malignant hyperthermia; keep client warm during recovery, and watch for severe shivering; avoid use of catecholamines (epinephrine or norepinephrine); monitor liver function after surgery; monitor urine output closely
Enflurane (Ethrane)	Volatile liquid with fairly high anesthetic potential. Has weak analgesic effect, causes moderate decrease in BP, a large decrease in respirations, and is moderate muscle relaxant	Hypotension, respiratory depression, blocks labor, minimal sensitization of heart to catecholamines, and seizures with high doses	Do not give to clients with history of seizures; monitor vital signs, especially BP, pulse, and respirations; not for use during labor
Isoflurane (Forane)	Volatile liquid with high anesthetic potential. Has weak analgesic effect, causes moderate decrease in BP, a large decrease in respirations, and is a moderate muscle relaxant. Produces profound vasodilation	Hypotension related to vasodilatory effect; respiratory depression; and suppresses uterine contractions	Does not sensitize heart to catecholamines, so it can be used with epinephrine and norepinephrine; monitor vital signs; avoid rapid position changes, which may lead to hypotension due to vasodilation

the drug is given slowly. Clients emerge through the first three stages after the anesthetic agents are discontinued.

Administration of General Anesthesia. General anesthesia can be administered by inhalation, intravenous, rectal, or oral routes. Inhalation and intravenous methods are the most common routes of administration. Table 5–8 describes the most common general anesthetic agents in use and their implications for nursing.

Balanced Anesthesia. Balanced anesthesia is the practice of selecting drug combinations based on the individual client's need with consideration of the type of surgery. Balanced anesthesia is typically achieved with a combination of inhalation agent, narcotic, and muscle relaxants.

TYPES OF GENERAL ANESTHESIA

Intravenous Anesthesia. When general anesthesia is administered intravenously, the client experiences an extremely rapid induction. Unconsciousness generally occurs about 30 seconds after the initial intravenous administration. Intravenous anesthesia is most commonly used as an induction agent before inhalation anesthetics are given. However, intravenous anesthesia is sufficiently potent to be used alone in such minor procedures as dental extractions or pelvic examinations. Examples of intravenous anesthetics include thiopental sodium and ketamine.

Inhalation Anesthesia. Inhalation anesthesia is a mixture of volatile liquids or gas and oxygen. The mixture is given through a mask or through an endotracheal tube inserted directly into the trachea (Fig. 5–2). These anesthetics are advantageous because of their ease of administration and elimination through the respiratory system.

When inhalation anesthesia is administered by mask, the gases generally flow into the mask via a finely calibrated vaporizer controlled by a machine. When an endotracheal tube is used to give anesthetic,

TABLE 5–8 General Anesthetic Agents *Continued*

DRUG	ACTION	SIDE EFFECTS	NURSING IMPLICATIONS
Intravenous Drugs			
Thiopental sodium (Pentothal)	Short-acting barbiturate that produces rapid unconsciousness. It is a weak analgesic and muscle relaxant	Respiratory depression with momentary apnea after injection, retrograde amnesia, myocardial depression, hypotension, headache, and shivering	Monitor for allergic reactions; monitor respiratory function closely, especially during induction; monitor vital signs; can not be mixed with solutions containing atropine, diturbocurare, or succinylcholine; and avoid extravasation
Fentanyl citrate with droperidol (Innovar)	A potent opioid (fentanyl) combined with a neuroleptic (droperidol). Produces indifference to surroundings and insensitivity to pain. Central nervous system depressant, which produces calming, analgesia, and reduced motor activity	Emergence delirium with hallucinations, hypotension, vasodilation, nausea and vomiting, laryngospasms, respiratory depression, shivering, and apnea	Use with caution in elderly clients and clients with head injuries, increased intracranial pressure, COPD, hepatic or renal dysfunction, or bradyarrhythmias; monitor vital signs; maintain patent airway; decrease narcotic doses to $\frac{1}{4}$ or $\frac{1}{3}$ for the first 24 hours postoperatively; when Innovar is used for induction, fentanyl (Sublimaze) alone is used for maintenance of anesthesia
Ketamine hydrochloride (Ketamine)	Produces state of dissociative anesthesia. Causes sedation, immobility, analgesia, amnesia, and unresponsiveness to pain	Delirium, hallucinations, disturbing dreams, tonic and clonic movements, respiratory depression, hypotension or hypertension, decreased or increased pulse, nystagmus, increased salivation, laryngospasms, and mild nausea and vomiting	Contraindicated in clients with history of cerebrovascular accident and severe hypertension; use with caution in clients with alcoholism, or elevated cerebrospinal fluid; maintain airway; do not give in same syringe as barbiturates; keep all stimulation to a minimum as client emerges from anesthesia; use diazepam if hallucinations occur or delusions are severe; excellent for anesthesia in young and elderly

BP, blood pressure; COPD, chronic obstructive pulmonary disease.

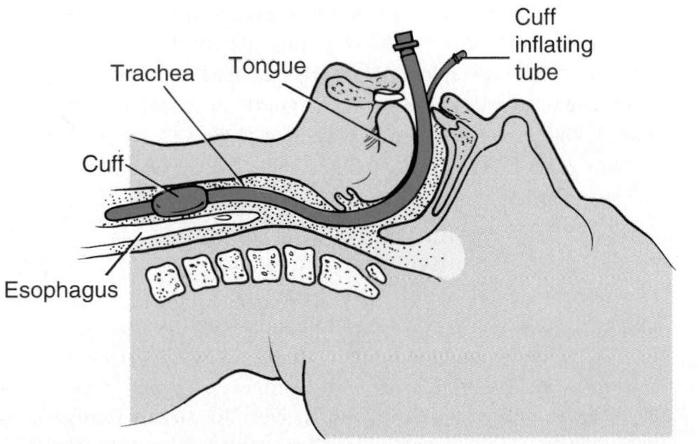

Figure 5–2
Correct placement of the endotracheal tube for the administration of anesthesia.

the gases flow directly into the client's tracheobronchial tree.

Many different liquids and gases are used in inhalation anesthesia. Two commonly employed volatile liquid anesthetics are halothane and isoflurane. A commonly used gas anesthetic is nitrous oxide.

As mentioned earlier, an intravenous anesthetic is often administered before the use of inhalation anesthetic. This process promotes a rapid transition from the conscious stage to the surgical anesthesia stage (from stage 1 to stage 3). In this case, the early stages of anesthesia typically are not seen.

Ether produces a deep and prolonged anesthesia that rarely results in cardiovascular complications, the leading medical cause of perioperative mortality in adults. Consequently, although ether is sometimes used for high-risk individuals, its highly explosive properties make it a dangerous and less desirable choice.

MUSCLE RELAXANTS

Muscle relaxants are administered intravenously and are given mainly to facilitate intubation, relax the muscles within the surgical field, ease laryngospasms, and relax muscles for controlled ventilation. When given with muscle relaxants, potent general anesthetics can be administered in smaller, and thus safer, doses.

Muscle relaxants are classified as depolarizing and nondepolarizing agents that block the transmission of nervous impulses to the muscle fibers (Table 5–9). This block produces temporary paralysis of voluntary muscles, including the muscles that control respiration. Hence, respiration must be supported mechanically when muscle relaxants are employed. Respirations in clients who have received muscle relaxants must be closely monitored for at least 1 hour after the relaxants appear to have worn off because paralysis may recur.

Examples of the common muscle relaxant agents include succinylcholine (Anectine), D-tubocurarine (DTC), pancuronium (Pavulon), and vecuronium (Norcuron).

LOCAL ANESTHESIA

Local anesthetics are useful in many clinical situations. They can be used for local effects and also can be administered to function as central, peripheral, intravenous, regional, retrobulbar, or transbronchial nerve blocks. These anesthetic agents block the conduction of impulses in nerve fibers without depolarizing the cell membrane (Table 5–10).

Sometimes epinephrine is added to the local anesthetic agent to provide a more prolonged effect. Epinephrine causes local blood vessels to constrict, thus delaying absorption of the anesthetic agent. Epinephrine should be used with caution in elderly clients with cardiovascular or liver disease.

Types of Local Anesthesia

Several anesthetic techniques are applied to local anesthesia: topical, local infiltration, field block, peripheral nerve block, spinal, epidural, caudal, and intravenous regional block.

Topical Anesthesia. Topical anesthesia may be directly applied to an area to be desensitized. The anesthetic may be a solution, ointment, gel, cream, or powder. This short-acting form of anesthesia can block peripheral nerve endings in the mucous membranes of the vagina, rectum, nasopharynx, and mouth. Topical anesthesia is used in minor procedures such as a rectal examination when painful hemorrhoids are present, or before a bronchoscopic examination to desensitize the bronchi.

One drug commonly used for topical anesthesia is cocaine, in a 4 to 10 per cent solution. This agent is for *topical use only,* and it is primarily used to anesthetize the eye and the mucous membranes of the nose, mouth, and urethra. Cocaine is highly toxic. If accidentally injected, it may cause severe excitement and seizures, followed by shock, respiratory failure, and cardiac arrest. Emergency resuscitation equipment must be available.

TABLE 5–9 Muscle Relaxants

DRUG	ACTION	SIDE EFFECTS	NURSING IMPLICATIONS
Pancuronium bromide (Pavulon)	Nondepolarizing agent; prevents acetylcholine from binding to receptors on muscle end plate, blocking depolarization	Tachycardia, hypertension, prolonged dose-related apnea, allergic reaction, and excessive sweating and salivation	Use carefully in older or debilitated clients or in clients with renal, hepatic, or pulmonary disease, myasthenia gravis, or thyroid disease; measure intake and output carefully; have resuscitation equipment available; do not mix in syringe or solution with barbiturates; neostigmine reverses effect
Vecuronium bromide (Norcuron)	Nondepolarizing agent; prevents acetylcholine from binding to receptors on muscle end plate, blocking depolarization	Transient tachycardia; prolonged dose-related apnea, redness, itching, and induration	Has no effect on cardiovascular system. Use with caution in clients with hepatic disease, obesity, or neuromuscular disease; tolerated well in renal disease; reversed with anticholinesterase and neostigmine. Have emergency resuscitation equipment available
Succinylcholine chloride (Anectine)	Depolarizing agent that prolongs depolarization of muscle end plate	Increased or decreased pulse rate and blood pressure, dysrhythmias, increased intraocular pressure, prolonged respiratory depression, malignant hyperthermia, postoperative muscle pain, excessive salivation, and hypersensitivity	Monitor vital signs; maintain patent airway; postoperative stiffness is normal; drug of choice for short procedures; keep emergency resuscitation equipment on hand; repeat infusions can prolong apnea; is reversible with neostigmine

TABLE 5–10 Local and Topical Anesthetic Agents

DRUG	ACTION	SIDE EFFECTS	NURSING IMPLICATIONS
Local Agents			
Bupivacaine (Marcaine)	Amide type local anesthetic that blocks depolarization, preventing generation and conduction of nerve impulses. When combined with epinephrine, it has prolonged action	Edema, anaphylaxis. Rarely: anxiety, convulsions, respiratory arrest, cardiac arrest, blurred vision, and shivering	Contraindicated for children under 12, for spinal or paracervical block or topical anesthesia; use with caution in older clients, or clients with hepatic disease or allergies; onset 4 to 15 minutes, duration 3 to 6 hours; keep resuscitative equipment available
Chloroprocaine hydrochloride (Nesacaine)	Ester type local anesthetic that blocks depolarization, preventing generation and conduction of nerve impulses	Anaphylaxis, edema. Rarely: anxiety, convulsions, respiratory arrest, cardiac arrest, blurred vision, and shivering	Contraindicated for clients with allergies to "caines," central nervous system disease; use cautiously with older adults; check solution for particles or discoloration; keep resuscitative equipment available; do not use solution with preservative for caudal or epidural blocks
Lidocaine hydrochloride (Xylocaine)	Amide type local anesthetic that blocks depolarization, preventing generation and conduction of nerve impulses. When combined with epinephrine, it has prolonged action	Edema, anaphylaxis, arrhythmias. Rarely: anxiety, respiratory arrest, cardiac arrest, and tinnitus	Contraindicated in clients with hypersensitivity, severe hypertension, septicemia, spinal deformities, or neurologic disorders; use cautiously with older clients and clients with heart block, general drug allergies, or in severe shock; use solutions with epinephrine only in body areas with good blood supply; use preservative-free solution for spinal, epidural, and caudal blocks
Topical Agents			
Benzocaine (Americaine)	Blocks conduction of impulses at sensory nerve endings	Sensitization rash, possible tolerance	Contraindicated in clients with history of hypersensitivity to "caines"; discontinue if rash develops; avoid contact with eyes; avoid inhalation when using spray; has short duration of action; do not use over infected area; if used rectally, clean area well first
Ethyl chloride (spray)	Produces local anesthesia by producing sensation of cold	Frostbite, tissue necrosis from prolonged use, muscle spasms, and increased pain	Do not apply over broken skin; protect adjacent skin; avoid contact with eyes; avoid inhalation; highly flammable, do not use near open flame; very short duration
Tetracaine hydrochloride (Pontocaine)	Blocks conduction of impulses at sensory nerve endings	Local sensitization and rash	Do not use in hypersensitive clients; cleanse rectal area well before applying; do not use if rash develops
Cocaine	Ester type topical anesthetic, blocks uptake of norepinephrine by adrenergic neurons	Central nervous system stimulation, euphoria, decreased fatigue, tachycardia, vasoconstriction, and hypertension	For topical use only; produces psychological dependence with prolonged or repeated use, schedule II narcotic; use cautiously with clients with history of severe hypertension or heart disease; when combined with epinephrine, it can lead to cardiovascular toxicity; monitor vital signs closely

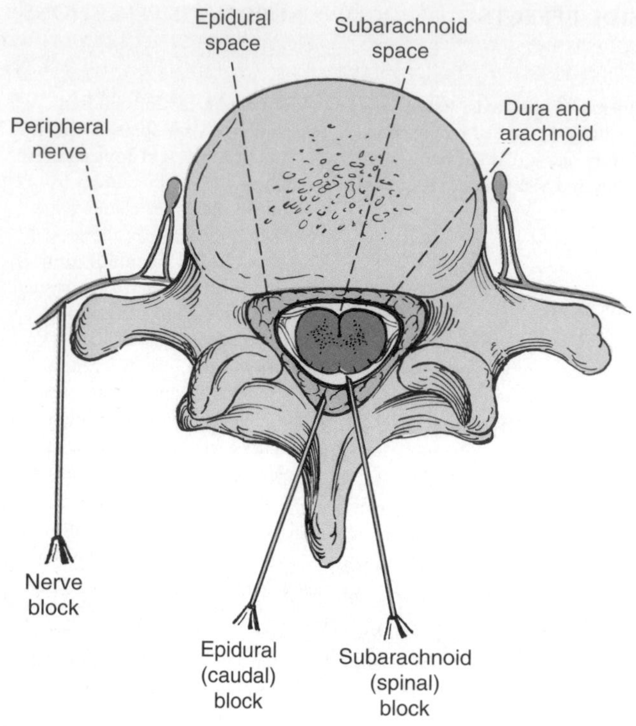

Figure 5–3
Cross section of the spinal cord, showing injection sites for anesthesia.

Other agents used for topical anesthesia include tetracaine, procaine, mepivacaine, bupivacaine, and lidocaine (see Table 5–10).

CRITICAL TO REMEMBER

To avoid an anaphylactic reaction from previous sensitization to anesthetic agents, check the client's drug allergies before topical anesthesia is applied.

Infiltration Anesthesia. Local anesthesia involves the injection of an anesthetic agent, such as lidocaine (Xylocaine), into the skin and subcutaneous tissue of the area to be incised. Local anesthesia blocks only the peripheral nerves around the area of the incision.

When a local anesthetic is administered, the physician must not allow the needle to slip into one of the veins. If a local anesthetic agent is given intravenously by accident, cardiovascular collapse or convulsions may result. For this reason, the physician must always aspirate before injection to ensure the needle is not in a vein.

Field Block Anesthesia. In a field block, the area proximal to the incision is injected and infiltrated with local anesthetics, thereby forming a barrier between the incision and the nervous system. This procedure contrasts with that of local anesthesia, in which only the area of the incision is injected.

Peripheral Nerve Block Anesthesia. A nerve block anesthetizes individual nerves or nerve plexuses rather than all the local nerves anesthetized by a field block. Nerve blocks may be used to anesthetize, for example, a finger (digital nerve block), the entire upper arm (brachial plexus nerve block), or the chest or abdominal wall (intercostal nerve block). Nerves most commonly blocked are those within the brachial plexus and the intercostal, sciatic, and femoral nerves. Drugs commonly used as nerve blocks are lidocaine, bupivacaine, and mepivacaine. The anesthetist attempts to inject the anesthetic along the nerve rather than into the nerve, to decrease the risk of nerve damage. Once the drug has been injected, it takes several minutes for the area to become anesthetized.

Nerve blocks, like local infiltration blocks, can produce severe systemic responses if the drug is accidentally injected into a blood vessel. Because epinephrine causes vasoconstriction, particularly of the extremities, surgery performed below the wrist or ankle typically uses anesthetics that do not contain epinephrine.

Spinal Anesthesia. Spinal anesthesia is achieved by injecting certain local anesthetics into the subarachnoid space (Fig. 5–3). Autonomic nerve fibers are the first to be affected by spinal anesthesia and the last to recover. Following autonomic blockage, spinal anesthesia blocks the following fibers in this order: touch, pain, motor, pressure, and proprioceptive fibers. Recovery is in reverse order.

Spinal anesthesia can be used for almost any type of major procedure performed below the level of the diaphragm, such as hysterectomy and appendectomy. Figure 5–4 illustrates the proper positioning for spinal anesthesia.

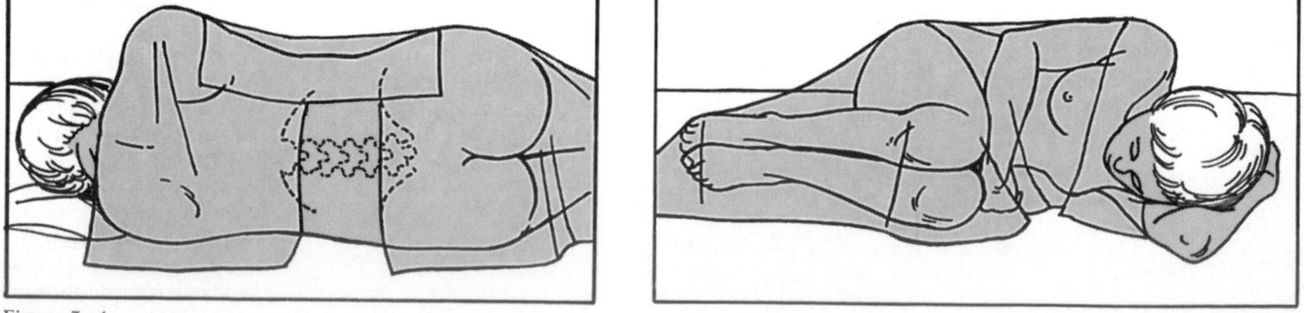

Figure 5–4
Proper positioning for administration of spinal anesthesia.

Within minutes after induction of spinal anesthesia, the client experiences a loss of sensation and paralysis of first the toes, then the feet and legs, and finally, the abdomen.

Spinal anesthesia offers many advantages for clients undergoing surgical procedures involving the lower half of the body. Major benefits are that it

- is a relatively safe method of anesthesia
- provides excellent muscle relaxation
- does not cloud the client's consciousness or alertness (anxious clients, however, can be given a small dose of barbiturates to enable them to rest or even sleep throughout the operation)
- can be used for clients with a full stomach, because they will be awake to maintain their airway if they vomit

Complications of spinal anesthesia are listed in Table 5–11, with their causes, prevention, and intervention. The nurse should remember that a client who has undergone spinal anesthesia is a candidate for serious neurologic, respiratory, or cardiovascular problems.

As the anesthetic agent wears off, the nurse should monitor the client carefully. Return of motion to the extremities is checked by asking clients to move their toes. However, clients who can wiggle their toes have not necessarily recovered completely from the spinal anesthetic. An ability to move the toes simply means that the motor blockade is wearing off, although autonomic blockade may still be present..

CRITICAL TO REMEMBER

Clients who are still experiencing autonomic blockade are prone to hypotension despite having the ability to move toes and extremities.

The nurse should continue to monitor vital signs and for return of sensation.

Epidural Anesthesia. Epidural block is achieved by the introduction of an anesthetic agent into the epidural space (see Fig. 5–3). The epidural space is generally entered by a needle at the thoracic, lumbar, sacral, or caudal interspaces. The needle is carefully positioned in the epidural space, without penetrating the dura and entering the subarachnoid space. When the needle is properly positioned, the cerebrospinal fluid cannot be aspirated.

TABLE 5–11 Complications and Discomforts of Spinal Anesthesia

COMPLICATIONS AND DISCOMFORTS	CAUSES	INTERVENTION	PREVENTION
Hypotension	Paralysis of vasomotor nerves; usually occurs shortly after induction of anesthesia	Administer oxygen by inhalation Vasoactive drugs Trendelenburg position if level of anesthesia is fixed, 10 to 20 minutes after induction	In people who are not prone to congestive heart failure, 500 to 800 mL of intravenous fluids, administered rapidly prior to block
Nausea and vomiting	Occur mainly during abdominal surgery, owing to traction placed on various structures within abdomen or hypotension	Ephedrine Antiemetics Oxygen fluids Mouth care	
Headache (can be extremely painful and may last a week)	Cerebrospinal fluid (which cushions the brain) is lost through dural hole; leakage of fluid and loss of cushioning effect increased by • use of a large spinal needle • poor hydration	Apply tight abdominal binder Fluids Analgesics In severe cases, inject 10 mL of person's blood to plug hole	Use of very small spinal needle reduces incidence of spinal headache to 0.9 per cent Administer intravenous and oral fluids (especially those with caffeine) before and after induction of spinal anesthesia Keep person flat and quiet as much as possible postoperatively
Respiratory paralysis	Occurs if drug reaches upper thoracic and cervical cord in large amounts or in heavy concentrations	Artificial respiration	Avoid extreme Trendelenburg position before level of spinal anesthesia set, i.e., 10 to 20 minutes following induction
Neurologic complications (e.g., paraplegia, severe muscle weakness in legs)	Paralysis postoperatively may be due to pre-existing diseases of central nervous system (e.g., multiple sclerosis and spinal cord tumors), which cause paralysis, rather than spinal anesthesia itself		Strict sterile technique Heat-sterilized medications and instruments Careful preoperative neurologic examination to ascertain presence of neurologic disease

CRITICAL TO REMEMBER

Epidural block, like spinal anesthesia, produces autonomic blockade. Hypotension can result. Respiratory depression or paralysis also may occur if the level of the block is too high and affects respiratory muscles.

Caudal Anesthesia. This type of anesthesia is produced by injecting the local anesthetic into the caudal or sacral canal. Caudal anesthesia is a variation of epidural anesthesia.

Intravenous Regional (Extremity) Block Anesthesia (Bier Block). Regional anesthesia of a limb can be achieved through an agent such as lidocaine, which is injected into a vein of the limb to be anesthetized. A pneumatic tourniquet applied to the anesthetized area prevents the lidocaine from circulating beyond the area undergoing the procedure. This type of anesthesia is used most commonly for short procedures on the extremities.

OTHER TYPES OF ANESTHESIA

Acupuncture. Acupuncture is an age-old Chinese pain-killing technique that is performed by the insertion of long, thin needles into specific points located along channels called *meridians* that run throughout the body.

Some advantages of acupuncture as an anesthetic include (1) no anesthesia-related side effects during or after surgery, (2) less blood loss during surgery, and (3) reduced need for postoperative analgesia, because acupuncture's pain-killing effects persist for several hours.

Hypnoanesthesia. Hypnosis is an altered state of consciousness in which the person experiences a heightened state of concentration. As an anesthetic, hypnosis alleviates pain through relaxation, suggestion, and intense concentration on a particular object or sound to the exclusion of other distractions, including pain. Exactly how hypnosis relieves pain is unknown.

Hypnoanesthesia has been used successfully in obstetrics and in certain dental procedures, but not every person is susceptible to hypnotic suggestion. Moreover, it must be carried out by a carefully and specially trained practitioner. There are better alternatives to anesthesia, especially for major surgery.

Nursing Care During Surgery

PROVIDING EMOTIONAL CARE

The client's emotional well-being is paramount during the operative phase. Before anesthesia, the nurse is responsible for ensuring that the client feels secure and that anxieties have been addressed.

If the client is awake during the procedure, the nurse should explain the procedure and support and reassure the client. When the client is recovering from the anesthesia, explanations and reinforcement of teaching should be given.

ASSISTING WITH CLIENT POSITIONING

The operating room nurse understands the various operative positions as well as the physiologic changes that occur when a client is placed in a specific position. Essential factors to consider when positioning a client on the operating room bed include (1) site of operation, (2) age and size of client, (3) type of anesthetic used, and (4) pain normally experienced by the client on movement, such as from arthritis. The position must not hinder respiration or circulation, apply excessive pressure to the skin surfaces, or limit surgical exposure. The following surgical positions are shown in Figure 5–5:

- The *dorsal recumbent* position is commonly used for hernia repair, mastectomy, or bowel resection.
- The *Trendelenburg* position permits displacement of the intestines into the upper abdomen and is often used during surgery of the lower abdomen or pelvis.
- The *lithotomy* position exposes the perineal and rectal areas, and is ideal for vaginal repairs, dilatation and curettage, and most rectal surgeries.
- The *laminectomy* position is used during surgical procedures involving the spine.
- The *lateral* position is used for clients undergoing kidney, chest, or hip surgery.

Whatever the client's position on the operating room bed, the nurse should observe certain general considerations and rules of safety:

- Explain to the client in simple, understandable terms, why the positions and restraints are necessary.
- Preserve the client's dignity and avoid undue exposure.
- Secure the client to the table with well-padded straps, usually placed above the knees. Nerves, muscles, and bony prominences are padded to prevent nerve and tissue damage.
- Maintain adequate respiratory excursion and vascular circulation. Avoid pressure on the chest and on body parts, because pressure can impair or slow circulation, predisposing a client to thrombus formation.
- Do not allow the client's extremities to dangle over the sides of the table, because this may impair circulation or cause nerve and muscle damage.
- Avoid excessive strain on the client's muscles.
- Be certain the client's body does not rest on hands or fingers; circulation may be occluded.
- Always move both lower extremities at the same time when putting them up in the stirrups and when lowering them so the hips are not dislocated or muscles strained.

Remember that the client may remain in one position for hours. Even with careful positioning, most clients feel stiff and sore after long operations. Therefore, observe the client throughout surgery, protect any bony prominences or pressure points, and readjust the client's position as needed.

MAINTAINING SURGICAL ASEPSIS

The nurse is responsible for maintaining surgical asepsis during the operative procedure. The circulating nurse is

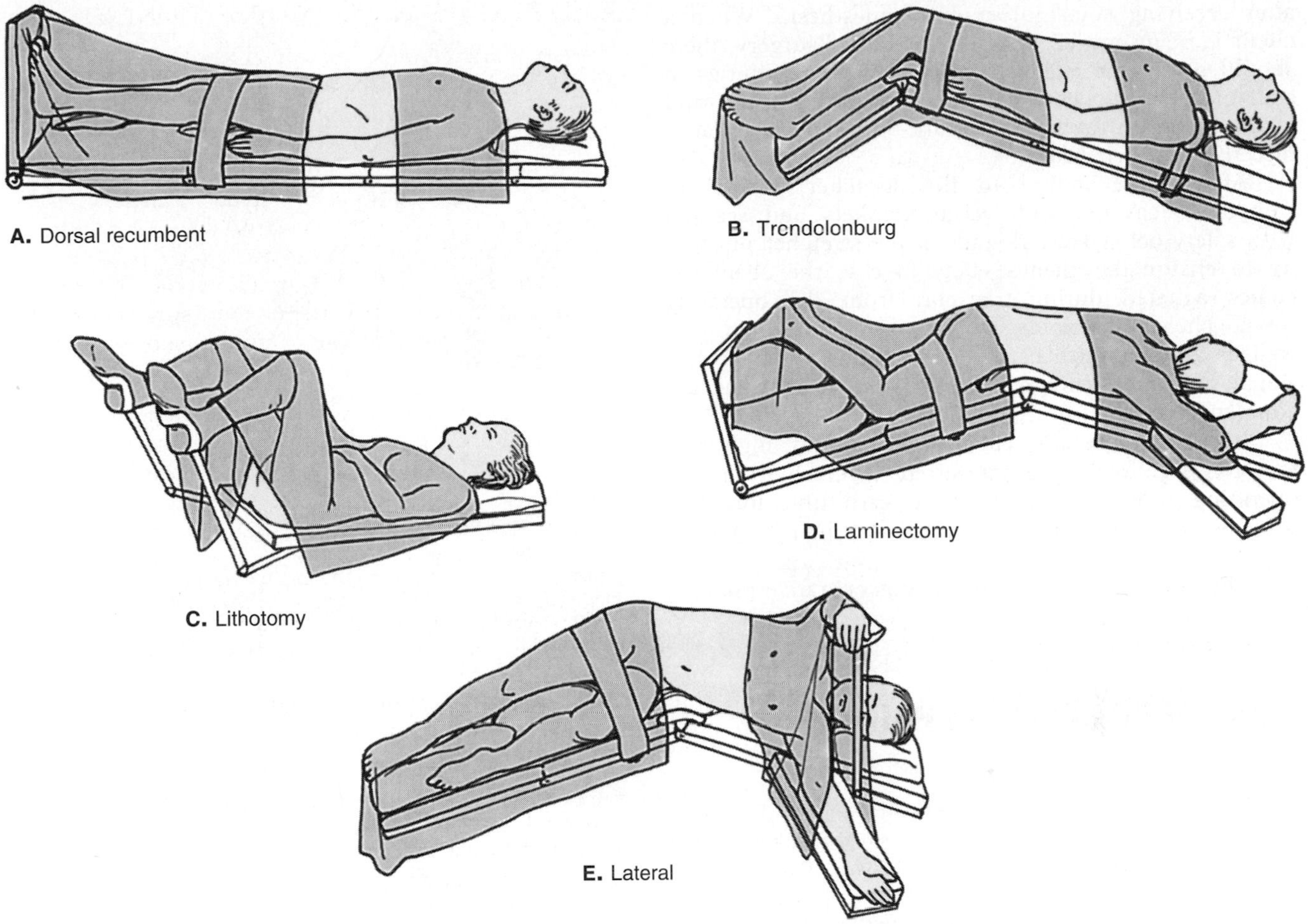

Figure 5–5
Five surgical positions.

responsible for ensuring the sterility of supplies and equipment and is also responsible for ensuring that all members of the health-care team use sterile technique. If a suspected or actual break in the sterile field occurs, the contaminated instruments or clothing are replaced with sterile ones immediately.

PREVENTING CLIENT HEAT LOSS

The temperature in the operating room is maintained at a standard cool level, and humidity is regulated to inhibit bacterial growth. The client usually feels cold in the operating room if he or she is not well covered. The client loses heat from the skin and from the area open for surgery. When tissues that are not covered with skin are exposed to the air, the heat loss is greater. The client should be kept as warm as possible to minimize the loss without causing vasodilation that could result in more bleeding.

ASSESSING DRAINAGE

A drain may be placed in a stab wound to drain blood, serum, and debris from the operative site. If they are allowed to collect, these contents may delay wound healing and promote infection. There are several types of surgical drains. A specific type of drain is chosen based on the size of the wound and type of drainage expected. Drains may be free-draining, attached to suction, or self-contained drainage with suction.

The nurse is responsible for assessing that the drainage is flowing freely through the system. Drains are usually removed when the drainage is reduced to an insignificant amount.

TRANSPORTING THE CLIENT TO THE POSTANESTHESIA OR INTENSIVE CARE UNIT

Following the operation, a member of the surgical team generally dresses the client in a clean gown, then assists with the transfer of the client to a stretcher. During this transfer, the operating room personnel avoid exposure, which may be embarrassing and predisposes the client to heat loss, respiratory infections, and shock. Also, rough handling is to be avoided, as it may strain the client's sutures and conveys lack of concern for the client's comfort and feelings. Finally, hurried movements and rapid changes in position that predispose the client to hypotension should be avoided. In particular, the client must be moved gradually from the lithotomy to the horizontal position and from the prone to the supine position, and he or she must be moved carefully after receiving spinal or epidural anesthesia. When a client is being moved or transferred after surgery, there should always be adequate help to prevent injuries to staff or the postoperative client. Very large clients and clients going to the intensive care unit are often placed directly into their beds.

After being moved to the stretcher, the client should be covered with warm blankets and secured with safety belts. The side rails of the stretcher must be up to ensure the client's safety in case the client becomes agitated during transport from the operating room. The anesthesiologist or the nurse anesthetist, as well as another member of the operating room professional staff and sometimes the surgeon or assistant, accompany the client to the PACU.

In some hospitals, clients who are at high risk for complications are transferred directly from the operating room to the intensive care unit for continued specialized care and constant nursing supervision.

The client has just begun the postoperative phase.

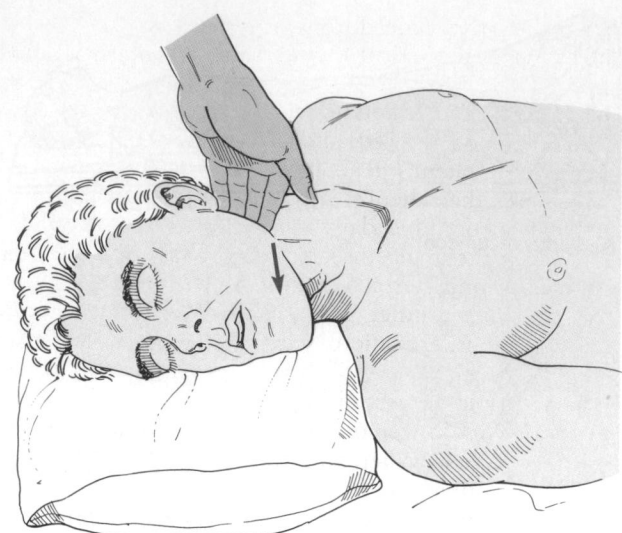

Figure 5–6
Proper positioning of the hand to move the jaw forward after anesthesia. Fingers are placed behind the angle of the jaw. As the jaw is moved, the tongue comes forward, opening the airway.

POSTOPERATIVE NURSING

The postoperative phase of surgery is the third and final phase of the surgical experience. Nursing plays a critical role in returning the client to an optimal level of functioning. The postoperative period can be divided into two phases. The first phase, the immediate postanesthesia and postoperative period, is the first few hours after surgery when the client is recovering from the effects of anesthesia. The second phase, or later postoperative phase, is a time for healing and preventing complications. This period may last for weeks or months after surgery. There is certainly an overlap of these two phases, but for purposes of discussion, they will be dealt with separately.

Postoperative Nursing in the Postanesthesia Care Unit

The immediate postanesthesia period is a critical time for the client. Close observation is important. The client's vital physiologic functions must be supported until the effects of the anesthesia abate. Until then, the client is dependent, drowsy, and may be unable to call for assistance. In the PACU, nurses assess the client during recovery from the immediate effects of surgery and intervene as appropriate.

ADMISSION TO THE POSTANESTHESIA CARE UNIT

The PACU nurse has special education in the care of clients recovering from surgery. Before the arrival of each client from the operating room, the nurse checks that all equipment is functioning and ready for use.

The client is left on the stretcher while in the PACU. Proper positioning of an unconscious or semiconscious client ensures airway patency. The adult client's head should be kept to the side and the chin extended forward; the nurse may need to extend the neck and thrust the jaw forward (Fig. 5–6). The lateral Sims position allows the client's tongue to fall forward and mucus or vomitus to drain out. There may be specific surgical or anatomic reasons to keep a client lying flat on the back while in the PACU. If this is the case, the nurse should carefully monitor the client's respiratory status and have suction equipment ready to suction vomitus or oral secretions.

IMMEDIATE BASELINE ASSESSMENT

On the client's admission, the PACU nurse

- assesses airway patency and support as needed; assesses for the presence of hoarseness, croup, stridor, wheezes, or decreased breath sounds
- applies humidified oxygen via nasal cannula or face mask
- records baseline data including blood pressure; heart rate, strength, and regularity; respiratory rate and depth; oxygen saturation; skin color; and temperature
- assesses the client's level of consciousness, muscle strength, and ability to follow commands
- observes the client's intravenous infusions, dressings, drains, and special equipment
- remains at the client's bedside, continuing close observation of the client's condition

After the client has been positioned safely and the return to baseline of vital signs has been ascertained, the nurse receives a verbal report from the members of the operating room team and a detailed report of events from the anesthesia personnel.

The following questions should be answered during the report:

- What operative procedure was performed?
- What were the client's vital signs in the operating room?
- What were the amounts of the client's blood loss, fluids or blood infused, and urine output?
- What is the client's general condition?
- What are the client's medical diagnosis, pertinent medical history, and daily medications?
- What anesthetic agents, narcotics, muscle relaxants, antibiotics, and steroids has the client received?
- Did the client suffer any complications during surgery? What interventions were instituted? What were the outcomes?
- What pathologic disorders were encountered during surgery? Was cancer or some other unexpected problem discovered? When will the client be told that the cancer (or other problems) is present?
- Are there any specific symptoms or complications to observe? What symptoms should be reported immediately?
- Are there physician orders to be carried out immediately?

With the anesthesiologist present, the PACU nurse then reviews the client's record, noting specifically (1) the anesthesia record for intravenous medications and blood received during surgery, and (2) the length of time the client was in surgery. Ideally, a preoperative nursing assessment and nursing history are available in the record for comparison with the postoperative assessment.

Following the baseline nursing assessments, review of the client's record, and postoperative verbal report, the PACU nurse assesses and documents routine observations. Observations to document include

- Time of admission of the client to the PACU.
- The absence of reflexes, such as the pharyngeal reflex. Clients admitted to the PACU without pharyngeal reflex are positioned on their side.

CRITICAL TO REMEMBER

The nurse stays at the bedside until the client's gag reflex returns.

- Level of consciousness. What is the response to stimuli such as light or touch? Does saying the client's name or giving simple commands bring a response? Is the client moving voluntarily or making audible or intelligible sounds?
- Temperature and vital signs. Monitor the vital signs every 15 minutes until they are stable, or more often as necessary. In some hospitals this assessment continues until the client leaves the PACU. Monitor the temperature on admission and at intervals until the client is discharged as established by PACU policy. Usually, clients must achieve a minimum temperature of greater than 36° C (96.8° F) before they are discharged from the PACU.
- Skin color and dryness. Dusky, pale, cold, wet skin is one important sign of shock and should be considered with blood pressure. Also, observe the lips and nail beds for pallor and cyanosis. Consider this information in relationship to oxygen saturation and hemoglobin.
- Condition of the dressing (whether it is dry or soiled, or intact). If soiled, note the color, type, and amount of drainage.
- Drainage tubes, such as T-tube, gastric tube, urinary catheter, or wound drains. Is the T-tube unclamped and attached to a gravity drainage system? Are gastric, chest, and intestinal tubes attached to suction as ordered? Ensure that tubes drain freely, that there are no kinks in the tubes, and that the client is not lying on them. Note the volume of drainage and color. Note any abnormalities in the appearance of the urine.
- Intravenous infusion. Note the type of intravenous solutions that are running. Also, check the amount of intravenous solution left in the bag and the rate of infusion. Redness, soreness, and swelling at the insertion site may indicate that the solution has infiltrated. Note medications added to the intravenous solution or orders.
- Infusion of blood products or colloid infusion, or if one is ordered. Check the rate of drip, and watch carefully for signs of a reaction.
- Maintenance of the client's comfort and safety. Side rails always must be up. Maintain proper body alignment, and turn the client from side to side if he or she is still unconscious. Offer psychological support.
- Pain. Observe and interview client about pain. Initiate analgesia in consultation with anesthesia personnel or PACU policy.

After completing the assessment, the nurse performs an assessment that relates to the specific surgical procedure. In most health-care facilities, the nurse and other PACU staff record their observations on a postanesthesia recovery assessment form. Finally, the nurse carefully reviews the physician's order sheet for further instructions and medication orders.

ASSESSMENT AND INTERVENTIONS FOR IMMEDIATE POSTOPERATIVE COMPLICATIONS

Nursing intervention during the immediate postoperative period centers on performing interventions to prevent or treat complications. The most common immediate postoperative complications that occur are those related to spinal anesthesia and those affecting respiratory, cardiovascular, and renal systems and those affecting fluid and electrolyte balance.

Complications of Spinal Anesthesia. An important nursing intervention for the client who has received spinal anesthesia is to check the blood pressure, heart rate, and depth of breathing every 10 to 15 minutes during the recovery period.

CRITICAL TO REMEMBER

If the blood pressure begins to fall rapidly or if breathing becomes labored, the nurse should notify the surgeon or anesthesiologist at once so interventions can be started promptly.

Transient hypotension may occur as blood pools in the lower extremities. Elevating the client's feet can quickly reverse this problem. Clients who have undergone spinal anesthesia and who are discharged from the PACU still require monitoring. The nurse should watch them for sudden drops in blood pressure and other signs of shock.

Respiratory Complications. Respiratory complications that occur in the PACU are usually caused by airway obstruction or hypoventilation. Airway obstruction is caused by mucus or vomitus collecting in the back of the throat, the tongue relaxing to obstruct the airway passage, aspiration, or pre-existing problems such as COPD or pulmonary edema.

The primary intervention to prevent respiratory complications is ensuring that the airway is patent. All clients receive oxygen while recovering from anesthesia. In the immediate postoperative period, the minimally responsive client's head may be turned to the side and the chin extended forward to prevent respiratory obstruction. An oral or nasal airway may be placed to help maintain airway patency and tongue control. This artificial airway is a hollow rubber or plastic tube, through the nose or mouth, that passes over the base of the tongue and keeps the tongue from falling back and obstructing the anatomic airway (Fig. 5–7). Airways should not be taped in place. As the client awakens and the gag reflex returns, he or she may spit it out. When the gag reflex has returned, the PACU nurse may remove the airway for the responsive client who is unable to remove it himself or herself. Its continued presence could irritate or stimulate vomiting or laryngospasm. The client who is unable to clear mucus or vomitus from the throat requires suctioning immediately.

Some clients are intubated and ventilated. They require close monitoring and suctioning as needed.

CRITICAL TO REMEMBER

When the client is extubated, the nurse should observe for the development of laryngospasms.

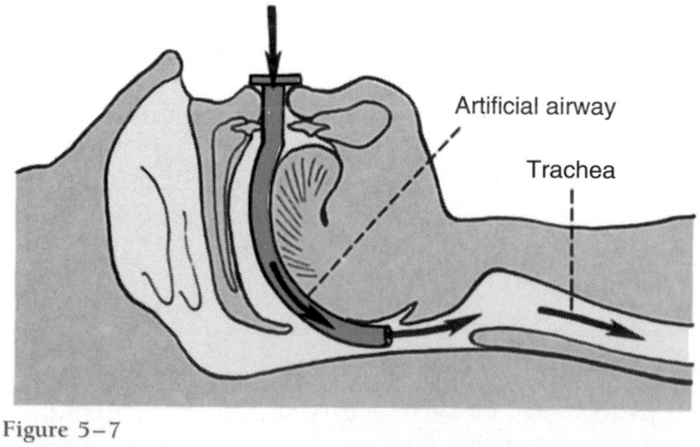

Figure 5–7
Artificial airway. The flattened, hollow tube prevents the tongue from falling back and occluding the natural airway.

If the client develops crowing respirations after extubation and is not moving air, he or she is probably experiencing a laryngospasm. If this problem develops, the client could progress to respiratory arrest. The nurse should immediately attempt to ventilate the client using an Ambu bag. If the spasm cannot be broken, the client may require a tracheostomy.

Other major respiratory problems include respiratory distress or depression and aspiration. Interventions may include the continued administration of oxygen, positive pressure airway support, or narcotic antagonists. Reversal agents such as naloxone hydrochloride (Narcan) are administered to reverse the narcotic effect or neostigmine with glycopyrrolate (Robinul) to reverse muscle relaxants.

Cardiovascular Complications. Common cardiovascular complications include cardiac arrhythmias, hypertension, and hypotension resulting in shock. When assessing a client for postoperative cardiovascular complications, remember that a slight increase in a client's heart rate after surgery may be normal. However, a significant increase or decrease in the preoperative heart rate or the development of new dysrhythmias requires observation. Clients in the PACU are usually connected to a cardiac monitor. In this way, diagnosis and treatment can be started immediately.

Causes of postoperative cardiac dysrhythmias include hypovolemia, pain, electrolyte imbalances, hypoxemia, and acidosis. When dysrhythmias develop, the PACU nurse monitors the client's blood pressure, oxygen saturation, and ventilation. When ventilatory status is inadequate, the nurse institutes airway management. The nurse also consults with the surgeon and anesthesiologist, and intervenes with prescribed medications.

Postoperative hypotension can have numerous causes, including inadequate ventilation, effects of anesthetic agents or preoperative medications, rapid position change, pain, fluid or blood loss, and peripheral pooling of blood after regional anesthesia. A drop in blood pressure slightly below a client's preoperative baseline range is common after surgery. However, a significant drop in blood pressure, accompanied by an increase or decrease in heart rate, may indicate hemorrhage, circulatory failure, or fluid shifts. In addition to hypotension, symptoms of shock include a weakened, thready pulse; cold, moist, pale, or cyanotic skin; and increased restlessness and apprehension.

When a client appears to be going into shock, the PACU nurse (1) applies oxygen or increases the rate of delivery; (2) elevates the client's feet, keeping his or her head flat or elevated to a 30-degree angle, if the position is not contraindicated by the surgical procedure, or raises the client's legs above the level of the heart; (3) increases the rate of the intravenous fluids; (4) notifies the anesthesiologist and surgeon; (5) administers medication or additional fluid volume as ordered; and (6) continues assessment on a one-to-one basis.

Clients in the PACU also may develop hypertension. Older clients with a history of hypertension may exhibit hypertensive episodes after the stress of surgery. If the blood pressure rises above the baseline, the PACU nurse should consult with the anesthesiologist or surgeon and administer antihypertensive medications as ordered.

Complications Involving Renal Function and Fluid and Electrolyte Balance. Changes in renal function and fluid and electrolyte balances also may develop soon after surgery. Surgery and anesthesia stimulate the secretion of antidiuretic hormone (ADH) and aldosterone, which cause fluid retention. Urine volume decreases regardless of the fluid intake. Fluid and electrolyte maintenance following surgery requires astute nursing assessment and intervention to avoid fluid overload while maintaining blood pressure, cardiac output, and adequate urinary output. Nursing interventions must include assessment of intake and output, blood pressure, pulse, and serum electrolytes. Any significant changes should be reported to the anesthesiologist or surgeon.

Temperature Alterations. Hypothermia is a potential problem in the PACU. The heat loss from the operating room can continue in the PACU if the client is not warmed sufficiently. Warming is a delicate procedure involving maintaining the client's temperature without overwarming and causing excessive vasodilation (which could cause fluid shifts and a decrease in blood pressure). Warm blankets are applied to maintain the client's body temperature.

Pain. Clients must be assessed carefully in the PACU for postoperative pain. If clients become restless and state that they are in pain, they should be medicated. The nurse consults with the anesthesiologist to determine the appropriate medication and dosage for such a client. After clients receive a pain medication, many PACUs have a policy requiring them to be closely monitored for another hour or until stable.

Other Complications. Diabetic clients require extra monitoring and care in the PACU. The stress of surgery can cause fluctuations in the client's blood sugar. Blood glucose monitoring is conducted in the PACU and, based on the results, intravenous regular insulin or subcutaneous insulin, based on blood glucose may be ordered.

Clients who are on steroids also require special care in the PACU. If the blood pressure drops, the pulse increases, and the client is in shock, a low level of cortisol may be the problem. Intervention is immediate replacement with intravenous hydrocortisone.

DISCHARGE FROM THE PACU

Common criteria to evaluate the client's readiness for discharge from the PACU are as follows:

- The client has recovered (a criterion score of 10 on the PACU assessment form) from the effects of anesthesia. This requires a stay of about 1 to 2 hours in the PACU.
- The vital signs are stable at the preoperative level.
- There is only moderate or light drainage from any site.
- The physiologic effects of narcotic medication have stabilized. This requires about ½ hour from the time of administration.
- The client has regained a satisfactory level of consciousness and can maintain a patent airway.
- Essential postoperative care has been completed by the PACU personnel.
- Urine output is adequate, at least 30 mL/hour for an adult. The amount must be monitored and recorded.
- Staff on the clinical unit to which the client is to be transferred have been alerted, a report has been given on the client's condition, and the unit is prepared to receive the client.
- Thorough documentation of the client's progress in the PACU is included in the client's permanent medical record.

A client who has undergone ambulatory surgery, in an inpatient or outpatient facility, requires the same level of monitoring and support whether general or regional anesthesia was used. After surgery, the client remains in the PACU until fully awake, possibly until he or she voids and tolerates oral fluids. Then the client may be transported to a special area to prepare for discharge.

To prepare for discharge following ambulatory surgery, the client (1) receives complete postoperative written and verbal instructions, (2) knows when and how to seek help for any problems that may arise, and (3) has transportation home with assistance by a competent individual. The next day there will be a follow-up phone call by the staff.

TRANSFER TO THE CLINICAL UNIT

After meeting the PACU discharge criteria, the client can be returned to the appropriate clinical unit to complete recovery. Clients who have experienced complications in the PACU generally may be transferred to the intensive care unit for continued close observation.

Postoperative Nursing on the Clinical Unit

To carry out postoperative care, certain preparations need to be made on the clinical unit. These preparations include the following:

- A clear passageway to the client's bed to ensure easy transfer.
- Clean bed linen, with pads if excessive drainage is anticipated. Keep additional blankets available.
- Necessary equipment that is contingent on the type of surgery, such as an emesis basin, intravenous pole, tissues, suction apparatus, and oxygen administration equipment.

The PACU nurse calls the clinical unit to notify the staff that the client is ready for transfer. The client is transferred to the unit, accompanied by a PACU nurse. The nursing staff helps move the client into bed, ensuring that the client's body is in correct alignment and a comfortable position. All tubes and equipment are identified and adjusted appropriately. The PACU nurse gives a verbal report that includes the client's history and condition, the operative and PACU course, and any special orders that were initiated or need to be initiated.

The client's significant others should be notified of the client's status. The surgeon usually discusses the surgical procedure and outcome with the client and significant others. Thus, the nurse needs to be aware of the client's condition and of the information given to the client and significant others by the surgeon.

ASSESSMENT ON THE CLINICAL UNIT

The nurse on the unit makes an initial assessment of the client after the transfer. The assessment should include the status of respiratory, cardiovascular, and neurologic systems, and assessment of the surgical wound, intravenous lines, tubes, client position, and level of pain.

Respiratory Status. The nurse should assess for a patent airway; listen for breath sounds and assess their character; check the quality, depth, and rate of respirations; and remember that skin color and temperature also indicate the degree of oxygen exchange. Pale or dusky skin may signal poor oxygen exchange and the possible recurrence of narcotic effects.

CRITICAL TO REMEMBER

Cyanosis is a very late sign of hypoxia.

Cardiovascular Status. The nurse should assess vital signs, skin color, temperature, and degree of moistness and assess for any abnormal pulse rate or rhythm.

Neurologic Status. The nurse should assess the client's level of consciousness or ability to move extremities and assess the lingering effects of regional anesthesia.

Surgical Wound. The nurse should assess the dressing and any drainage present. The nurse should measure and record the area of drainage to compare later assessments for changes.

Intravenous Lines. The nurse should assess the intravenous line for patency, type of fluid infusing, and rate.

Tubes. The nurse should assess any drainage tubes (e.g., catheters, nasogastric tubes, hemovacs, Jackson-Pratt drains, etc.) as to whether to attach the tube to suction or to use gravity drainage. He or she should note and record the amount of drainage.

Position. The nurse should assess the client for proper positioning to promote ventilation and decrease pain.

Pain. The nurse should assess the client for pain and initiate comfort measures. The need for pain control through the use of narcotic analgesics is assessed. It is vital that pain be managed if the client is to comply with instructions for coughing, deep breathing, and ambulation.

ESTABLISHMENT OF POSTOPERATIVE GOALS

The client has now entered the next phase of the postoperative course. At this point, a postoperative care plan is developed based on a thorough assessment. Nursing diagnoses are used to specify and define postoperative problems and guide the plan of nursing care.

Goal 1: Restore Optimal Functioning and Prevent Complications. One of the nurse's primary goals in caring for the postoperative client is to prevent complications after surgery. No matter how seemingly minor the surgery, the danger of postoperative complications is present. Complications have caused death following relatively simple surgeries such as tonsillectomies and hernia repairs.

Postoperative complications can develop (1) directly in the wound, (2) in organs bordering on the operative site or far removed from it, (3) in body cavities, or (4) as a result of the client's medical condition. Complications may arise immediately after surgery or may develop later.

Complications are particularly common after a devastating illness or difficult surgery. These include disorders such as stress ulcer, renal failure, and hepatic failure. Most cardiovascular complications (e.g., cerebrovascular accident, myocardial infarction, pulmonary embolism) and virtually all life-threatening infections (e.g., peritonitis) follow some critical event such as postoperative shock or hemorrhage, or preoperative rupture of an organ.

Preventing postoperative complications promotes rapid convalescence and saves time, expense, worry, pain, and even life itself. The nurse must know the symptoms of postoperative complications and be able to recognize them quickly. Once postoperative problems develop, they are difficult to treat.

CRITICAL TO REMEMBER

One of the most common complications following surgery is postoperative shock.

Causes include bleeding and hemorrhage (hypovolemic shock), sepsis (septic shock), cardiac arrest and myocardial infarction (cardiogenic shock), drug sensitivity (anaphylactic shock), transfusion reactions, pulmonary embolism, and adrenal failure.

Table 5–12 discusses, in brief, each type of shock, its causes, assessments, and interventions. See Chapter 56 for further information on shock.

Goal 2: Maintain and Promote Adequate Airway and Respiratory Function. Respiratory complications are among the more common complications that may occur in the postoperative period. Early assessment of respiratory problems can lead to immediate treatment.

Symptoms of pulmonary complications include increased temperature, restlessness, dyspnea, tachycardia, hemoptysis, pulmonary edema, altered breath sounds, and thick viscous sputum (with chest pain, if the client has pneumonia).

Pulmonary problems typically develop in the first 48 hours after surgery. Postoperative respiratory complications may be caused by one or several of the following risk factors:

TABLE 5–12 Types of Shock

CAUSE	ASSESSMENT	INTERVENTION
Bleeding (hypovolemic shock)	Check wounds, drain sites, open wounds; central venous pressure low; bleeding usually in peritoneal or pleural cavities or retroperitoneal areas	Blood administration and immediate ligation of bleeding vessel by surgeon; measure arterial blood gases
Sepsis (septic shock)	Culture of blood or suspicion of gram-negative bacterial source of septicemia; tachycardia, hypotension, oliguria, fluid retention, respiratory failure	Massive intravenous antibiotics, fluids, corticosteroids may be ordered
Cardiac arrest, myocardial infarction or arrhythmias (cardiogenic shock)	Check for pulse irregularities, electrocardiogram; absence of pulse and cyanosis suggest cardiac arrest; angiotensin sensitivity test aids diagnosis of infarction; central venous pressure is high	Dependent on specific cause; general measures: oxygen, sedation, and cardiopulmonary resuscitation, if needed
Drug sensitivity (anaphylactic shock)	Obscure clinical picture; history of drug sensitivities is vitally important; urticaria and edema may aid diagnosis	Epinephrine, antihistamines, corticosteroids may be ordered; maintain airway, O_2 by mask or prongs, intravenous line, cardiac monitor, reassurance, arrange for intensive care unit bed
Transfusion reaction (contaminated or incompatible blood)	Smears of blood show gram-negative organisms; shock rapidly follows blood administration	Discontinue blood; corticosteroids, massive doses of antibiotics intravenously may be ordered
Pulmonary embolism	No specific signs; chest pain, hemoptysis suggest diagnosis; angiography can make diagnosis; obesity, previous cardiac difficulties, cancer, pelvic operations, immobility, and increased age are associated factors	Embolectomy, fibrinolytic agents to dissolve clots are promising and may be ordered. O_2 by mask or prongs, arterial blood gases, electrocardiogram, cardiac monitor, pain relief, chest film
Adrenal failure	Must be diagnosed by suspicion or history of steroid therapy, lack of other causes	Intravenous corticosteroids (hydrocortisone) may be ordered

Adapted by permission from Liechty, R. D. (1985). Postoperative care. In R. D. Liechty & R. T. Soper (Eds.), *Synopsis of surgery* (5th ed.). St. Louis: C. V. Mosby Co.

- Pre-existing respiratory infections (colds, flu, and sore throats) that were not resolved during the preoperative period
- Respiratory infection following surgery
- Use of anesthetics, endotracheal tubes, and oxygen, all of which irritate the tracheobronchial tree and cause increased mucous secretions
- Aspiration of vomitus
- Prolonged immobility of the client on the operating table during lengthy surgery
- A history of smoking
- Respiratory disease prior to surgery (e.g., asthma, chronic bronchitis, COPD)
- Depressive effects of many narcotics (especially codeine) on the cough reflex
- Collapse of the lung during surgery or inadequate re-expansion of lung tissue following surgery
- Severe postoperative pain, which makes the client reluctant or unable to turn, cough, or breathe deeply
- Surgery with a high abdominal or chest incision, which causes the client to neglect deep breathing exercises because of pain
- Extreme debilitation and old age, which lower the client's resistance to pulmonary infections
- Prolonged postoperative immobility, which leads to decreased chest expansion, pooling of mucus in the bronchi, and hypostatic pneumonia

CRITICAL TO REMEMBER

Older adults are especially prone to pulmonary complications because of their decreased cough reflex.

The most common postoperative respiratory problems are atelectasis, pneumonia, and pulmonary emboli (Box 5–1).

Although the etiology of each respiratory complication is different, some basic nursing interventions may prevent these and other pulmonary complications. Rigorous attention to these interventions is essential to prevent respiratory complications.

- Perform respiratory assessment and chest auscultation as part of routine postoperative care.
- Provide preoperative instruction regarding moving, coughing, and deep breathing exercises.
- Coach the client during the performance of postoperative exercises.
- Encourage the client to breathe deeply every 1 to 2 hours in the manner described earlier.
- Encourage the client to cough every 1 to 2 hours.
- Splint the client's incision so coughing will be less painful and less likely to cause the incision to rupture.
- Check the color and consistency of mucus expecto-

BOX 5–1

ATELECTASIS

Defined as collapse of the alveoli in sections of a lung.
Assess for increased pulse, increased temperature, and decreased breath sounds on auscultation.

PNEUMONIA

An acute infection causing inflammation of lung tissue.
Assess for elevated temperature, tachycardia, tachypnea, productive cough, dyspnea, crackles, and a dullness over the area of consolidation.

PULMONARY EMBOLI

Occurs with the passage of thrombi into the pulmonary vasculature.
May be a blood clot or a fat embolism.
Assess for severe dyspnea, intense pleural pain, apprehension, fever, and hemoptysis.

rated following coughing. (If a respiratory infection is present, the mucus may be thick, colored, and emit an odor.)

- Adequately hydrate the client. (Fluids thin mucous secretions.)
- If the client is receiving intravenous infusions, make certain the infusions drip properly and are administered on time.
- If the client can tolerate oral fluids, encourage fluid intake.
- Assist the client to ambulate as early as possible.
- Assess the client for respiratory depression and suppression of cough, especially if the client is receiving narcotics (e.g., morphine) for pain.
- If respirations are depressed, notify the surgeon so a different narcotic can be prescribed.
- Assess and report symptoms of respiratory infection. Nasotracheal suctioning may be necessary to stimulate a cough if pneumonia develops.
- Encourage the client to stop smoking prior to surgery and postoperatively.
- Encourage the use of an incentive spirometer every 1 to 2 hours after surgery (Fig. 5–8).

Goal 3: Maintain Adequate Cardiac Function and Promote Tissue Perfusion. Any surgical client is at risk for developing cardiac or perfusion problems, but clients at most risk are the elderly and clients with a history of cardiac or peripheral vascular disease. Two common problems that may occur in the postoperative client are thrombophlebitis (and possibly embolism) and myocardial infarction.

Thrombophlebitis usually involves a thrombus of the peripheral veins, usually the calf veins. It develops because of direct pressure on the walls of veins during surgery or from venous stasis.

Postoperative thrombophlebitis generally occurs 7 to 14 days after surgery. Dehydration and inadequate circulation resulting from hemorrhage can result in circulatory stasis and increased blood coagulability, both of which can cause thrombophlebitis. The great danger of thrombophlebitis is that a clot will break loose from the vein wall and travel as an embolus to the client's lungs, heart, or brain.

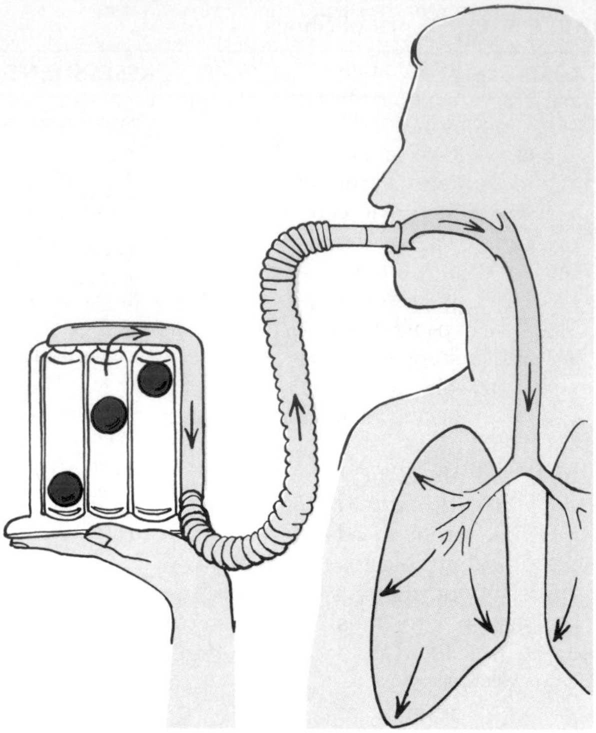

Figure 5–8
Use of an incentive deep-breathing exerciser to promote alveolar inflation, restore and maintain lung capacity, and strengthen respiratory muscles.

Symptoms of phlebitis include redness, swelling, and tenderness of the extremity and the presence of a Homans' sign. Preventive measures for thrombophlebitis include postoperative leg exercises, early ambulation, antiembolic support stockings and/or sequestral compression device, adequate hydration, and low-dose heparin.

Myocardial infarction occurs during the first 72 hours after surgery. The nurse must assess high-risk clients—those with a history of dysrhythmias or heart disease and those over 70 years of age. Because anesthesia might mask chest pain, the nurse should observe the client for dyspnea, tachycardia, cyanosis, or dysrhythmias. Interventions and nursing care for the client with a myocardial infarct are discussed in depth in Chapter 24.

Another postoperative condition that can occur related to tissue perfusion is blood loss. In the postoperative client, this can be the result of a pre-existing condition, blood loss during the surgery, or a postoperative complication.

Clients who are at a high risk for experiencing blood loss postoperatively are those with pre-existing medical conditions, a history of aspirin use, a history of anemia or clotting disorders, and the elderly.

Signs and symptoms of blood loss in the postoperative client include postural hypotension, tachycardia, tachypnea, decreased urine output, cool clammy skin, and decreased level of consciousness. Laboratory data should include hemoglobin, hematocrit, and clotting studies (prothrombin time, partial prothrombin time, and platelet count).

Treatment of blood loss is accomplished with plasma expanders, albumin, large volumes of fluid, salvage of blood with the cell saver, and possibly, transfusion therapy. Packed red blood cells are administered; however, whole blood may be used. Fresh frozen plasma or coagulation factors are used if the client has a coagulation problem. Blood transfusions are covered in detail in Chapter 28. The importance of intelligent nursing care for the client needing transfusion therapy is critical to success in maintaining adequate tissue perfusion.

Goal 4: Maintain Adequate Fluid and Electrolyte Balance and Adequate Renal Function. After surgery, it is crucial to promote adequate fluid and electrolyte intake and output. Postoperative imbalances can lead to retention of metabolic wastes, neurologic and cardiac problems, and problems of overhydration or underhydration. See Chapter 3 for indepth discussion of fluids and electrolytes.

To help promote and maintain renal function following surgery, the nurse should encourage fluids when the client is able to tolerate them. Before administering oral or parenteral fluids, the fluid limits set by the physician should be checked. The nurse must remember to administer fluids cautiously during the early postoperative period while ADH is being released.

The nurse should record intake and output for at least 48 hours after surgery. A client with a fluid restriction, or anyone whose intake is being monitored, may need close observation for a week or more. The nurse should check the physician's order, consult with the physician and nursing staff, and use his or her own judgment to decide when documentation of fluid intake and output can be discontinued.

The well-hydrated client generally is able to void 6 to 8 hours after surgery. An inability to void after surgery may be caused by anesthesia (especially spinal or epidural), postoperative medications (e.g., morphine), pain, fear, unfamiliar surroundings, or the client's position.

Signs of bladder distention are fullness above the symphysis pubis that can be palpated (usually indicating more than 240 mL in the bladder) and voiding 30 to 60 mL of urine every 20 to 30 minutes (indicating retention with overflow).

Possible nursing interventions include

- running tap water so the client hears it
- pouring warm water over the female perineum
- assisting the male to sit or stand at the bedside (if not contraindicated)
- administering prescribed pain medication
- inserting a straight or indwelling catheter, as ordered

Symptoms of urinary tract infection generally occur between the third to fifth day after catheterization and include dysuria, frequency of urination, and fever.

CRITICAL TO REMEMBER

Catheterization is the most common cause of postoperative urinary tract infection and therefore should be used only if necessary.

Intervention for urinary tract infections involves first sending a specimen of the urine to the laboratory for culture and sensitivity testing. The culture results reveal the organism causing the infection. The results of the sensitivity test indicate which antibiotic will be most effective in treating the infection. Appropriate antibiotics are prescribed on the basis of the laboratory results. To prevent bladder infections, catheterization should be avoided if possible.

Goal 5: Promote Comfort and Rest. Being comfortable and free from pain enables a client to progress more quickly and more easily through the postoperative period.

Nursing assessment of pain, especially prior to the administration of narcotics involves carefully checking for

- Hypotension or hypertension, although pain can cause either an increase or a decrease in blood pressure
- Pressure points beneath a case or splint; relieving pressure by splitting the cast or cutting a window (usually done by a physician) may decrease pain
- Distended bladder; obtain an order for catheterization if the client is unable to void
- Abdominal distention and flatulence; Flatus is a common postoperative problem that is often alleviated by ambulation

Nursing measures that help alleviate pain include

- Comfort measures, such as changing the client's position, straightening bed linen, giving a back rub with lotion, and applying a cool cloth to the hands and face
- Administration of narcotics, such as morphine, meperidine, and codeine; narcotics are used primarily during the first 24 to 72 hours after surgery to relieve pain

A newer option is the use of PCA, which allows the client to self-administer postoperative analgesia (often morphine, meperidine, or fentanyl). Note in Figure 5–9 that the PCA system is basically a pump that can be programmed to deliver a precise dose of analgesic when the client pushes the control button.

CRITICAL TO REMEMBER

Assessing intravenous catheter patency during PCA is the nurse's responsibility. He or she ensures that the intravenous line remains patent (so the analgesic is not deposited subcutaneously) and that the intravenous tubing is not occluded.

Narcotics should be given routinely during the first 24 hours after surgery and as needed for up to 72 hours. There is little danger of overmedication as long as careful assessment is performed. The client will re-

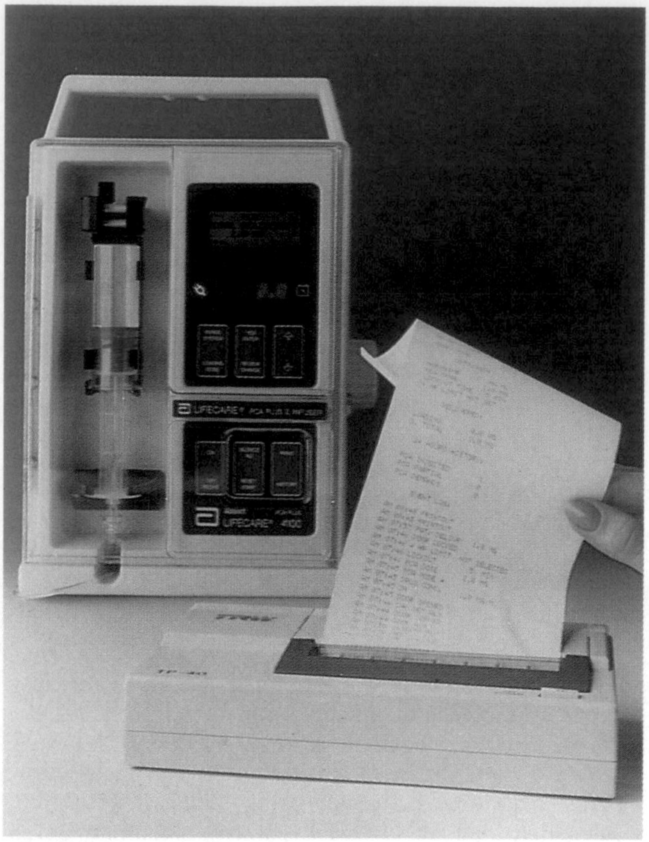

Figure 5–9
A Patient-controlled analgesic device allows individuals to control their own pain relief postoperatively. (Courtesy of Abbott Laboratories, Hospital Products Division, North Chicago, IL.)

cover faster if he or she is comfortable and able to comply with postoperative breathing exercises and ambulation.

As convalescence progresses, pain medications are administered in decreasing doses and strengths. Comforting and reassuring can help to relieve any anxiety that might cause tension and increase the pain. Most clients require less medication as the pain associated with the surgical procedure decreases. Drug dependence or tolerance is not a common problem for most surgical clients, and medication should never be withheld from a client who is in pain.

If the client is having difficulty resting during the postoperative period or if restlessness is severe, a thorough assessment should be made of possible causes. Restlessness may be caused by pain, bladder or abdominal distention, fear, anxiety, hypoxia, wet or tight dressings, or hemorrhage.

Nursing interventions to promote rest include

- Changing the client's position when necessary
- Keeping the bed linen clean, dry, and free of wrinkles
- Giving a back rub with lotion
- Administering pain medication as ordered and as needed
- Specific interventions for other potential causes of restlessness (e.g., administering oxygen, loosening the dressings, assisting with voiding, assisting ambulation to decrease abdominal distention)

Goal 6: Promote Adequate Nutrition and Elimination. It is beneficial for the client to resume a normal diet as soon as possible after surgery. A normal diet promotes an early return of gastrointestinal function, aids in wound healing, and is psychologically healthy for the client.

Nursing assessments to be made prior to feeding a client postoperatively are the presence of positive bowel sounds, that the abdomen is soft and palpable, and that the client is passing flatus.

Certain surgical procedures (e.g., abdominal exploration and cholecystectomy) may require that the client abstain from oral fluids and food until the bowel sounds return, usually within about 24 to 48 hours after surgery. Clients who are unable to eat for longer periods (after gastric or bowel resection) may have a nasogastric tube in place, which, because of its decompressive properties, removes flatus and stomach secretions. Clients who are NPO for a prolonged period after surgery usually receive nutritional support with hyperalimentation.

For the first 24 to 36 hours following surgery, many clients are nauseated and have episodes of vomiting. Antiemetics may be ordered for the nausea. If nausea persists, the surgeon should be notified. The initial postoperative diet is usually clear liquids. These liquids may include broth, tea with lemon and sugar, fruit juices, jello, and soups. Early solid foods may include toast, light cornstarch puddings, and easily digested meats and vegetables. As the client regains his or her appetite and begins to eat well, a full diet is ordered to promote vitamin and mineral balance and proper nitrogen balance. Muscle substance and strength return, and the client may regain weight slightly.

Normal peristalsis returns during the first 48 to 72 hours after surgery. It is important for the nurse to record any bowel movements in the postoperative period. Bowel function can be impaired by immobility, anesthesia, manipulation of abdominal organs, and the use of pain medications.

A common postoperative discomfort related to a decrease in peristalsis is abdominal distention. This causes the client a feeling of fullness and discomfort. Nursing measures to prevent and treat abdominal discomfort are early ambulation, adequate fluid intake, and an increase in dietary fiber. A rectal tube may be inserted if none of these interventions work.

Paralytic ileus is a postoperative complication that may occur when a portion of the bowel stops normal peristalsis. Nursing assessment includes diminished or absent bowel sounds, abdominal distention, and feelings of fullness. X-ray studies often reveal a distended bowel. A nasogastric tube may be inserted to prevent distention and vomiting until bowel function resumes.

Goal 7: Promote Wound Healing. Factors affecting wound healing are location of the incision, type of surgical closure, nutritional status, presence of disease, presence of infection, and the presence of drains and dressings.

Nursing assessments include

- Assessing the wound for signs of infection, such as redness, drainage, odor, pain, and induration
- Observing the wound for edema, bleeding, and color
- Observing the wound for approximation of the suture line
- Monitoring drains and assessing the color, consistency, and amount of drainage

Wound infections are often evident within 36 to 48 hours postoperatively, although most symptoms appear about 5 to 7 days after surgery. Important factors that predispose a client to develop wound infections are

- *Obesity.* Adipose tissue is difficult for the surgeon to approximate and suture, and it does not heal readily.
- *Debilitation.* Clients debilitated by cancer, malnutrition, or ulcerative colitis have a lowered resistance to infections.
- *Advanced age.* Elderly clients, particularly those with arteriosclerosis and poor circulation, have lowered defenses against infection.
- *Lengthy, complicated operations.* Complex operations are stressful and lower resistance. The longer the client is in surgery, the longer the tissues are exposed, making them more susceptible to infection.
- *Therapy with steroids, irradiation, and anticancer medications.* Certain medications and treatments affect the immune system and reduce the body's leukocyte counts dramatically.
- *The presence of other diseases.* Hypogammaglobulinemia, diabetes mellitus, obstructive jaundice, ulcerative colitis, uremia, leukemia, aplastic anemia, and malignant neoplasms, in particular, lower resistance to wound infection.
- *Failure to maintain asepsis* in the operating room or during wound dressing changes.
- *Preoperative organ rupture or sepsis,* such as occurs with a ruptured appendix, perforated ulcer, or abscess drainage. When the organ is also infected prior to surgery, the wound is usually considered contaminated and infected.

The organism most commonly responsible for wound infections is methicillin-resistant *Staphylococcus aureus* (MRSA), a gram-positive, nonmotile organism. Staphylococci produce a golden-yellow pus. These organisms can be transmitted to the surgical wound from contaminated wound-dressing equipment or from staff who harbor the organism in their noses and throats as resident flora.

Clients with infected surgical wounds must be isolated from clients with clean wounds in order to stem the transmission of infections. Other organisms frequently responsible for wound infections are *Escherichia coli, Proteus vulgaris, Aerobacter aerogenes,* and *Pseudomonas aeruginosa.* Infectious diseases are covered in more detail in Chapter 10.

Wound dehiscence and evisceration are possible complications of improper wound healing. Wound dehiscence is an opening of the wound edges. Wound evisceration is the protrusion of internal organs (such as loops of bowel) through the incision (Fig. 5–10).

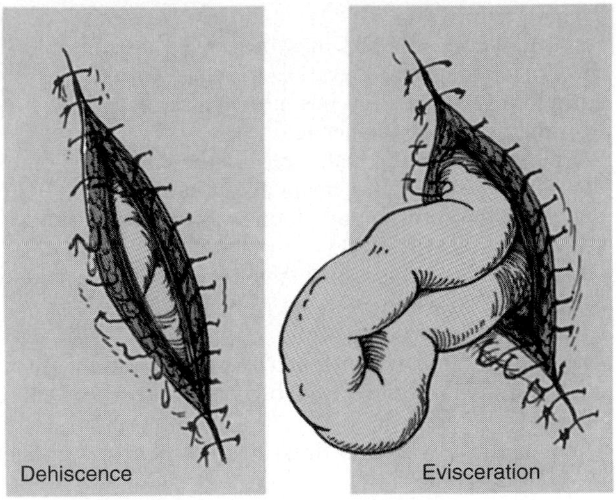

Figure 5–10
Wound dehiscence and evisceration require immediate attention. The attending nurse should have someone notify the surgeon. Using sterile technique, the nurse should cover the wound site with gauze or a sterile towel moistened in sterile saline and take measures to prevent shock (see text). The nurse should not leave the client's side.

Malnourished, chronically ill, or obese clients are most prone to wound dehiscence and evisceration. Related causal factors are wound infection, faulty closure of the wound in surgery, and severe stretching of the abdominal wall as a result of coughing and vomiting.

Although wound dehiscence and evisceration can occur at any time, they generally develop on the sixth to seventh day after surgery. At this time, the client's incision is weakest because the sutures may have been removed, wound infection is likely to be present, and pulmonary complications may cause excessive pressure when the client coughs. Preventing wound dehiscence and evisceration includes splinting the wound during vigorous coughing or movement, preventing wound infection, and providing adequate nutrition and hydration. Obese or debilitated clients can wear a binder to increase the support to the suture line. Any wound can rupture; however, midline abdominal incisions are the most prone to dehiscence and evisceration.

When an abdominal wound ruptures suddenly, evisceration may occur because coils of intestine protrude from the incision. When the wound edges part slowly, a gush of pinkish serous drainage is usually the major sign of dehiscence. The client feels something give way.

CRITICAL TO REMEMBER

In any postoperative client, sudden, profuse, pink, serous drainage from the wound is an ominous sign and must be investigated immediately.

Intervention for wound dehiscence and evisceration involves immediate closure of the wound under general or local anesthesia. The nurse's role in the event of wound dehiscence and evisceration includes the following:

- Remain calm.
- Place the client in bed in semi-Fowler's position with the knees slightly elevated. If the wound has not completely opened or has not eviscerated, this position may prevent further tear.
- Ring the emergency bell, pull on the call light, or use the phone to tell the hospital operator to notify the nurse's station on your floor to send help immediately.
- Have another nurse notify the surgeon while you remain with the client.
- Cover any protruding coils of intestine with sterile dressings moistened with sterile normal saline; if sterile supplies are not available, use clean towels or dressings.
- Moisten the towels and dressings frequently with sterile normal saline.
- Monitor the client's vital signs because shock may ensue.
- Reassure the client that the physician is on the way.
- Do not medicate the client with narcotics until after the client has signed an operative permit to reclose the wound.
- Set up intravenous equipment, and prepare the client for surgery.
- Notify surgery that the client will be returning to the operating room.

Goal 8: Promote and Maintain Activity and Mobility. After surgery, complications from immobility may be prevented by encouraging the client to (1) move around in bed, (2) cough and deep breathe, and (3) flex the ankles and legs. Allow the client to assume personal care as soon as possible to promote early movement. Encourage and assist with ambulation, if it is not contraindicated by the physician. Remember that clients vary. Some clients are ready to move or walk about more quickly than others.

CRITICAL TO REMEMBER

Allowing the client to return to physical activity as soon as possible after surgery can hasten recovery, shorten his or her hospital stay, and decrease expenses.

Goal 9: Provide Adequate Emotional Support and Foster Positive Body Image. Surgery has different means and implications for each client. Recognize these differences and individualize your psychological approach to each client and significant others as they progress through the surgical experience. The degree of psychological support the client needs depends on the client's social support as well as the type of surgery performed. A client whose postoperative course is complicated needs much more psychological support than the client who recovers quickly.

Assessment may reveal passivity, depression, reduced involvement in self-care, sleep disturbances, increased pain and use of analgesics, and hyperactivity. The client also may experience the onset of stress-related symptoms, such as gastrointestinal dysfunction and cardiovascular problems.

Nursing intervention primarily involves providing psychological support. The nurse should draw the client and significant others into discussions of anticipated changes and about how they feel these postoperative changes will affect their lives. He or she should encourage the expression of feelings, provide empathetic listening, reassure these clients that the grieving process they are going through is normal and that it will pass with time, and arrange support groups and community referrals for the client and significant others.

Goal 10: Plan for Discharge. The type of planning and instruction required varies with each individual and type of surgery. Discharge teaching instructions need to be clear, and they must reinforce the material the client learned during the preoperative period and recovery. Teaching plans and the client's understanding need to be included in the care plan and documented in the chart.

Because of the anxiety associated with discharge, written instructions should be given to the client and family or significant others for reference. (See the Client Education Guide.)

Finally, the nurse should know the quality of the client's support systems, because community resources for follow-up care may need to become involved. Contacting community resources such as mental-health facilities and home health agencies helps to ensure continuity of care.

CLIENT EDUCATION GUIDE

Postoperative Client

Discharge planning and teaching should begin at the time of the client's admission to the hospital. Most clients are discharged within 5 to 7 days after major surgery and sometimes even sooner. Early discharge planning is a necessity.

Specific instructions that the client needs to receive prior to discharge should include

Wound care (signs of infection)
Activity restrictions
Dietary instructions
Postoperative medication instruction
Personal hygiene
Follow-up appointment with surgeon or clinic

STUDY QUESTIONS

1. Obese individuals are at risk for postoperative complications because they have
   A. Hypertension
   B. Sodium and potassium deficiencies
   C. Decreased cough strength and depth
   D. An increased tendency to bleed
2. When teaching clients about the prevention of postoperative pulmonary complications, the nurse should instruct the client to
   A. Exhale through the mouth, while keeping the mouth wide open.
   B. Use deep breathing and coughing exercises every 4 hours after surgery.
   C. Use deep breathing exercises before trying to cough.
   D. Use the incentive spirometer rather than deep breathing exercises.
3. The nurse is explaining spinal anesthesia to a client. Which of the following statements by the client indicates the client understands spinal anesthesia?
   A. "Spinal anesthesia may make me unaware of my surroundings."
   B. "Spinal anesthesia will numb my belly first, then my toes."
   C. "Spinal anesthesia may lower my blood pressure."
   D. "Spinal anesthesia has no side effects."
4. A nurse is monitoring an elderly client in the recovery room. The nurse observes cyanosis of the client's lips and nail beds. The nurse should
   A. Call the doctor immediately
   B. Assess the client's skin temperature and moisture content
   C. Assess blood pressure and pulse and oxygen saturation
   D. Both B and C
5. A nurse is preparing care plans to prevent postoperative respiratory complications. Which of the following interventions should be included in the plan?
   A. Tape oral airways in place to ensure airway patency.
   B. Turn the client's head to the side and extend his or her chin forward.
   C. Hyperextend the client's head and stabilize with sandbags.
   D. Maintain the oral/nasal airway even after the gag reflex returns.

CRITICAL THINKING EXERCISES

SCENARIO A

A nurse is asked to orient a group of new graduates to the PACU. The nurse must design a teaching plan that includes assessment and interventions for postoperative complications that occur most frequently in adult clients. How should the nurse proceed? (Suggestion: Consider assessing the learners' age, education, readiness to learn, etc.)

SCENARIO B

A middle-aged man has been transferred to a surgical unit from the PACU after major abdominal surgery. He has a large, bulky abdominal dressing and has received several doses of morphine for his pain.

1. What is the client's greatest postoperative risk?
2. What other factors might influence the severity of this risk?
3. How should the nurse intervene?

BIBLIOGRAPHY

1. Alexander, J. W. (1983). The influence of hair-removal methods on wound infection. *Archives of Surgery, 118,* 347–352.
2. American Society of Postanesthesia Nurses (1995). *Standards of perianesthesia nursing practice.* Thorofare, NJ: Author.
3. Association of Operating Room Nurses (1993). *Standards and recommended practices.* Denver: Author.
4. Atkinson, L. J., & Kohn, M. L. (1986). *Berry and Kohn's introduction to operating room techniques* (6th ed.). New York: McGraw-Hill Book Co.
5. Bailes, B. K. (1989). Perioperative nursing research, part IV: Intraoperative phase. *AORN Journal, 49,* 1397–1409.
6. Birdsall, C., et al. (1988). How is autotransfusion done? *American Journal of Nursing, 88,* 108–111.
7. Cuzzell, J. Z. (1988). The new RYB color code. *American Journal of Nursing, 88,* 1342–1346.
8. Davis, N. B. (1992). Suturing techniques and material. In Rothrock, J. C. (Ed.). *The RN first assistant* (2nd ed.). Philadelphia: J. B. Lippincott Co.
9. Drain, C. B. (1995). *The post anesthesia care unit: A critical care approach to post anesthesia nursing* (3rd ed.). Philadelphia: W. B. Saunders Co.
10. Dripps, R. D., et al. (1988). *Introduction to anesthesia* (7th ed.). Philadelphia: W. B. Saunders Co.
11. Erbostoesser, M. (1989). Care of the patient with malignant hyperthermia. *Journal of Post Anesthesia Nursing, 3,* 71–74.
12. Fairchild, S. S. (1993). *Perioperative nursing: Principles and practice.* Boston: Jones & Bartlett Publishers.
13. Feldman, M. E. (1988). Inadvertent hypothermia: A threat to homeostasis in the postanesthetic patient. *Journal of Post Anesthesia Nursing, 3,* 82–87.
14. Felver, L., & Pendarvis, J. H. (1989). Electrolyte imbal-

ances: Intraoperative risk factors. *AORN Journal, 49,* 992–1008.

15. Fraulini, K. E., & Borchardt, A. C. (1988). Guide to solving postanesthesia problems. *Nursing '88, 18(5),* 66–86.
16. Fromm, C. G., & Metzler, D. J. (1993). Preparing your older patient for surgery. *RN, 56(1),* 38–43.
17. Girard, N. J., et al. (1988). Autologous salvage of blood: Perioperative nursing considerations. *AORN Journal, 47,* 492–502.
18. Groah, L. K. (1990). *Operating room nursing: Perioperative practice* (2nd ed.). Norwalk, CT: Appleton & Lange.
19. Hallstrom, R., & Beck, S. L. (1993). Implementation of the AORN skin shaving standard: Evaluation of a planned change. *AORN Journal, 58(3),* 498–506.
20. Hardy, E. B., et al. (1988). Rewarming patients in the PACU: Can we make a difference? *Journal of Post Anesthesia Nursing, 3,* 313–316.
21. Hardy, J. D. (1988). *Hardy's textbook of surgery* (2nd ed.). Philadelphia: J. B. Lippincott Co.
22. Hill, G. J. (1988). *Outpatient surgery* (3rd ed.). Philadelphia: W. B. Saunders Co.
23. Iscenheur, M. L. (1988). Quality of interpersonal care: A study of an ambulatory surgery patient's perspective. *AORN Journal, 47,* 1414–1419.
24. Jackson, M. F. (1989). High risk surgical patients. *Journal of Gerontological Nursing, 14,* 8–15.
25. Jacox, A., et al. (1992). A guideline for the national management of acute pain. *American Journal of Nursing, 92(5),* 49–55.
26. Kneedler, J. A., & Dodge, G. H. (1993). *Perioperative patient care* (3rd ed.). Boston: Jones & Bartlett Publishers.
27. Kneedler, J. A., & Purcell, S. K. (1989). Perioperative nursing research, part II: Intraoperative chemical and physical hazards to personnel. *AORN Journal, 49,* 829–854.
28. Kneedler, J. A., & Purcell, S. K. (1989). Perioperative nursing research, part III: Potential intraoperative biological hazards to personnel. *AORN Journal, 49,* 1066–1079.
29. Kuhn, M. (1994). *Pharmacotherapeutics: A nursing process approach* (2nd ed.). Philadelphia: F. A. Davis.
30. Lawler, M. (1991). Managing other complications beyond the respiratory system. *Nursing '91, 21(11),* 40–48.
31. Lindeman, C. A. (1988). Patient education. *Annual Review of Nursing Research, 6,* 29–60.
32. Litwak, K., & Parnass, S. (1988). Practical points in the management of postoperative nausea and vomiting. *Journal of Post Anesthesia Nursing, 3,* 275–277.
33. Marshall, M. (1993). Postoperative confusion: Helping your patient emerge from the shadows. *Nursing '93, 23(1),* 44–47.
34. Matassarin-Jacobs, E. (Ed.). (1994). *Saunders review for NCLEX-RN* (2nd ed.). Philadelphia: W. B. Saunders Co.
35. Matteson, M., & McConnell, E. A. (1988). *Gerontologic nursing: Concepts and practice.* Philadelphia: W. B. Saunders Co.
36. McConnell, E. A. (1991). Minimizing respiratory problems. *Nursing '91, 21(11),* 34–39.
37. Meeker, M. H., & Rothrock, J. C. (1991). *Alexander's care of the patient in surgery.* St. Louis: C. V. Mosby Co.
38. Metzler, D. J., & Fromm, C. G. (1993). Laying out a care plan for the elderly postoperative patient. *Nursing '93, 23(4),* 67–74.
39. Nyamathi, A., & Kashiwabara, A. (1988). Preoperative anxiety: Its effects on cognitive thinking. *AORN Journal, 47,* 164–170.
40. Pierce, S. F., & Campbell, M. (1988). Return of bladder function: A research study. *AORN Journal, 47,* 702–703, 706–712.
41. Rothrock, J. C. (1989). Perioperative nursing research. Part I. Preoperative psychoeducational interventions. *AORN Journal, 49,* 597–614.
42. Rowland, M. (1990). Myths and facts about postop discomfort. *American Journal of Nursing, 90(5),* 60–64.
43. Sabiston, D. C., Jr. (1991). *Textbook of surgery: The biological basis of modern surgical practice* (14th ed.). Philadelphia: W. B. Saunders Co.
44. Schwartz, S. I., et al. (Eds.) (1994). *Principles of surgery* (6th ed.). New York: McGraw-Hill Book Co.
45. Shapira, J., et al. (1993). Managing delirious patients. *Nursing '93, 23(5),* 78–83.
46. Silo, H. M. S. (1989). Perioperative nursing research, part V: Intraoperative recommended practices. *AORN Journal, 49,* 1627–1635.
47. Spearing, C., & Cornell, D. J. (1988). Incentive spirometry: Inspiring your patients to breathe deeply. *Nursing '88, 17(9),* 50–51.
48. Taylor, D. L. (1988). The healing process: From the inside out. *Nursing '88, 18(6),* 36–67.
49. Taylor, T. H., & Major, E. (Eds.). (1993). *Hazards and complications of anaesthesia* (2nd ed.). New York: Churchill-Livingstone.
50. Williams, B., & Baer, C. (1994). *Essentials of clinical pharmacology* (2nd ed.). Springhouse, PA: Springhouse Corp.
51. Wolcott, M. W. (1988). *Ambulatory surgery and the basics of surgical care* (2nd ed.). Philadelphia: J. B. Lippincott Co.
52. Woodlin, L. M. (1993). Cutting postop pain. *RN, 56(8),* 26–34.
53. Young, M. E. (1988). Malnutrition and wound healing. *Heart and Lung, 17(1),* 60–65.

Chapter 6 Basic Concepts of Neoplastic Disorders

Learning Outcomes

After completing this chapter, the learner will be able to:

1. Teach the client about the pathogenesis, etiology, and predisposing factors for the occurrence of cancer.
2. Discuss with the client the physical, psychosocial, and financial impact of cancer on the client and significant others.
3. Explain to the client the differences between normal and malignant cells.
4. Explain to the client the differences between benign and malignant neoplasms.
5. Describe screening tests that are used for early detection of cancer.
6. Conduct a nursing history and physical assessment of the client with actual or potential neoplasm.
7. Teach the client about diagnostic studies used to detect a neoplasm.

BASIC PRINCIPLES

Caring for clients with cancer is one of the most difficult tasks facing health care professionals today. Currently, cancer is the second leading cause of death in the United States, exceeded only by cardiovascular disease. Cancer will strike at least one in four people in this country and about one in three will survive the encounter. Within the United States and throughout the world, cancer has a tremendous economic and sociologic impact. It influences people in every realm of their lives: physical, emotional, spiritual, cognitive, social, and economic.

Nurses in all areas of practice are likely to care for people who are ill with cancer and, therefore, must be familiar with its diagnosis and treatment. More important, the nurse is often the professional in closest contact with clients and is in a unique position to teach prevention and early detection.

The first task in understanding the complex disease of cancer is being able to define some commonly used terms associated with the disease. It is vital that both the client and the health-care provider have a mutual understanding of the terms associated with cancer so the disease and its treatment can be discussed without confusion.

The word cancer, abbreviated Ca, is a term that frightens most people. Cancer is synonymous with the term malignant neoplasm. Other terms that suggest malignant neoplasm include tumor, malignancy, carcinoma, and aberrant cell growth. Strictly speaking, these words are not interchangeable.

The term cancer is a collective term describing a large group of diseases characterized by uncontrolled growth and spread of abnormal cells. This group of diseases (1) arises from different tissues and organs, (2) differs greatly from one another in appearance and growth, (3) may follow very different courses of development in their hosts, and (4) responds differently to the variety of therapies applied to them.

The word neoplasm is derived from the Greek words neos, which means new, and plasia, which means growth of new tissue. Therefore, a neoplasm is defined as an abnormal new growth of tissue that serves no useful purpose and may harm the host organism.

A neoplasm can be either benign or malignant. Benign is defined as a usually harmless growth that does not spread or invade other tissue. Malignant is defined as a harmful tumor, capable of spread and invasion of other tissues far removed from the site of origin. Other important terms can be found in Table 6–1.

Cancer is a disease of the cell in which the normal mechanisms of control of growth and proliferation are disturbed.

TABLE 6–1 Cancer Terminology

TERMS	DEFINITIONS
Anaplastic	Tumor cells that are completely undifferentiated and bear no resemblance to cells of tissues of their origin
Hyperplasia	An increase in the number of normal cells in a normal arrangement in a tissue or organ; usually leads to an increase in the size or part and an increase in functional activity
Metaplasia	The replacement of one type of fully differentiated cell by another fully differentiated cell in another part of the body where the second cell type does not normally occur
Dysplasia	An alteration in the size, shape, and organization of differentiated cells; cells lose their regularity and show variability in size and shape, usually in response to an irritant; they revert to normal when the irritant is removed but may transform to a neoplasia
Metastasis	The ability of neoplastic cells to spread from the original site of the tumor to distant organs, spreading as the same cell type as the original neoplastic tissue
Carcinoma	A form of cancer that is composed of epithelial cells that tend to infiltrate surrounding tissues and may eventually spread to distant sites
Oncogene	Cancer genes that are altered versions of normal genes
Proto-oncogenes	Repressed oncogenes existing in normal cells, which can be activated by many different factors and cause the host cell to become malignant
Tumor	Usually synonymous with neoplasm

The Challenge of Cancer Nursing

Nurses are involved in all phases of the cancer experience: prevention, detection, diagnosis, treatment, rehabilitation, survivorship, and palliative and terminal care. Cancer nursing skills are vital in all health-care settings because clients are seen in the home, office, clinic, acute care setting, rehabilitation setting, and hospice.

CRITICAL TO REMEMBER

Perhaps the greatest role any nurse can play is by assisting individuals in the prevention and early detection of cancer.

Nurses meet a variety of people daily (family, friends, coworkers), and there is always an opportunity to teach and encourage good health habits. Nurses can and must take advantage of time spent with the general public to engage in health promotion teaching and encourage individuals to follow cancer prevention guidelines.

Cancer occurs in all strata of our society. It strikes people of all ages, all socioeconomic and cultural backgrounds, and both sexes. It is the second leading cause of death in the United States, affecting one in three to four persons.

Epidemiology

Epidemiology is the study of the distribution and determinants of diseases and health problems in human populations. The goal of an epidemiologic study is the control or prevention of the health problem. An epidemiologic approach to cancer evaluates patterns of the disease, identifies possible causes, and infers relationships between patterns of disease and determining factors. Although the etiologic factors (causes) of many cancers remain unknown, some epidemiologic studies have helped to identify those factors that underlie theories of causation. The knowledge gained from epidemiologic findings gives the nurse greater insight into the magnitude of cancer risk or complications.

Incidence

The incidence rate for cancer reflects the number of new cases occurring in a given population at risk during a specified time. The incidence gives a perspective on the current magnitude of the problem and provides a source for establishing future priorities in cancer control programs (Fig. 6–1). Factors that influence cancer incidence and deaths include sex, age, geographic location, socioeconomic status, ethnic background, personal habits (including diet), occupation, and personal and family histories of cancer or precancerous conditions.

The incidence of reported cases of cancer has been increasing steadily since 1900. The apparent rise in the incidence of cancer is somewhat misleading. It may simply reflect more precise diagnostic and statistical methods combined with the trend toward a longer lifespan.

Mortality

The mortality rate is the number of deaths that occur in the population at risk in a specific period. Although there is a chance some of the information is inaccurate or incomplete, it is a solid beginning in helping describe and determine the number of deaths attributed to cancer.

Survival

Generally, clinicians consider the client who is alive and without evidence of the disease for at least 5 years after diagnosis of cancer as cured. Although the 5-year determination is arbitrary, in many cancers, this waiting period decreases the probability that the condition will recur or spread.

Analysis of survival data is used to evaluate the effectiveness of cancer therapies, determine whether or not the interval between disease onset and treatment

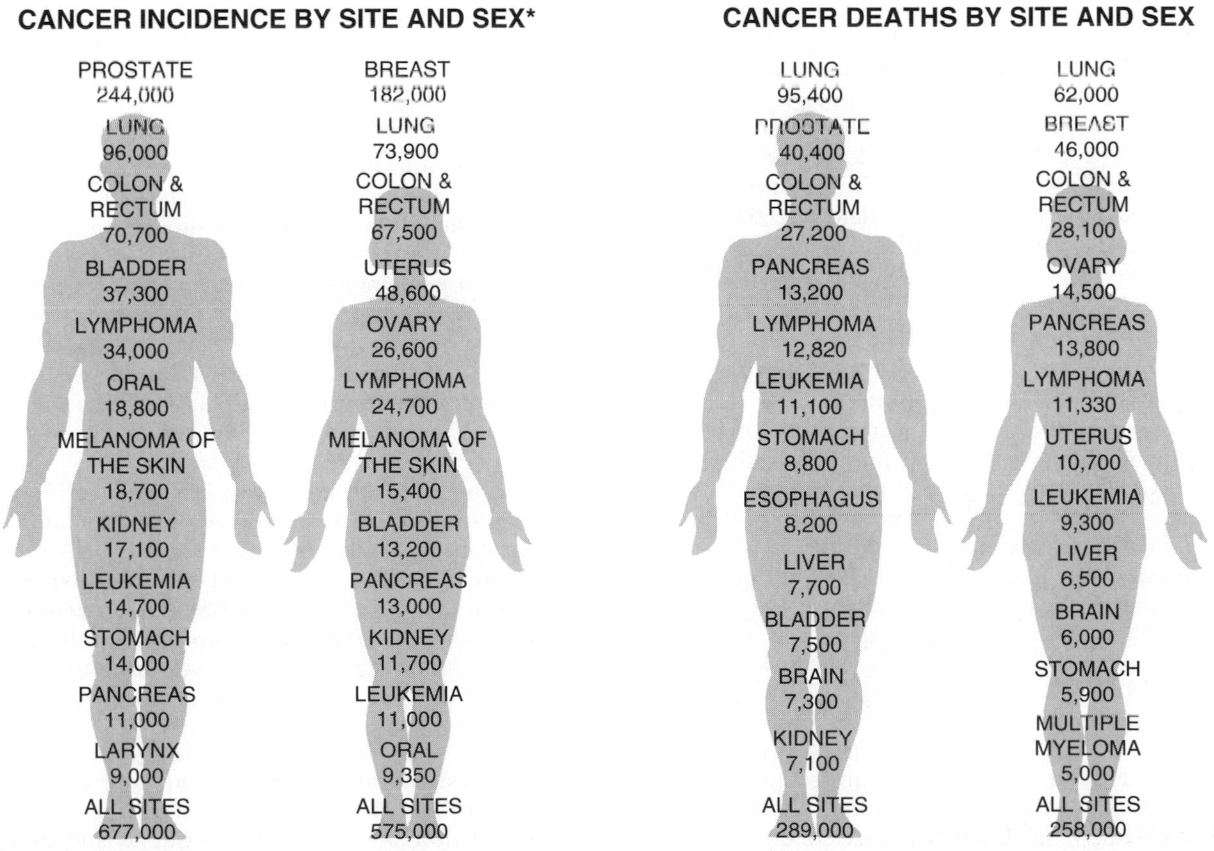

*Excluding basal and squamous cell skin cancer and carcinoma in situ.

Figure 6–1
Cancer incidence and deaths by site and sex, 1992 estimates. (From American Cancer Society [1995]. *Cancer facts and figures—1995.* Atlanta, GA: American Cancer Society.)

initiation could be modified to reduce cancer morbidity or mortality, and develop hypotheses regarding cancer risk factors.

Trends

Despite significant advances in detection, diagnosis, and treatment, cancer continues to be a significant health problem. It is believed that many cancers could be prevented if primary prevention (such as stopping smoking) was initiated against known causative factors by the government, industry, and the public. Prevention and early detection of cancer must be a high priority to further decrease cancer morbidity and mortality rates.

Pathogenesis

The exact causes and methods of the development of cancer are unknown. The following two theories are common explanations for the development of cancer.

CELLULAR TRANSFORMATION AND DERANGEMENT

Although scientists have learned a great deal about the etiologic agents responsible for cancer, the exact mechanism by which these agents transform healthy cells into neoplastic cells remains obscure. One accepted premise is that cancer develops as a result of genetic alteration caused by one or more etiologic agents, resulting in uncontrolled cellular reproduction and growth. When a defective cell divides, the new cells contain the defective genetic code within the deoxyribonucleic acid (DNA). Over time, defective cells divide and multiply, and the malignancy grows.

IMMUNE RESPONSE FAILURE

According to the immune theory of cancer control, cancer cells continually form within the body. The immune system perceives these cancer cells as foreign and destroys them. However, certain conditions either cause a breakdown or overwhelm the immune system. Thus, the malignant cells reproduce more rapidly than the immune system can destroy them.

Supporting this theory are the data from postoperative heart and kidney transplant clients. These clients are intentionally immunosuppressed to prevent the rejection of their transplanted organs. The risk of cancer is at least 80 times greater among clients who have undergone transplantation surgery than among the population as a whole. Further support for this theory comes from data on clients with acquired immunodeficiency syndrome (AIDS). These clients have a much higher incidence of a number of cancers such as non-Hodgkin's lymphoma and Kaposi's sarcoma. The immunodeficiency of AIDS makes these clients more susceptible to cancers.

Etiology

Approximately 150 types of cancers are found in humans, and there are probably at least 500 different cancer-causing agents. Researchers suspect that cancer results from multiple agents working together.

VIRUSES

The study of viruses as carcinogens is one of the most rapidly advancing areas in cancer research today. Researchers now have proof that viruses cause cancer in animals.

The study of viruses in tumors has led researchers to discover oncogenes. Oncogenes are small segments of genetic DNA that have the ability to transform normal cells into malignant cells, independently or incorporated with a virus.

Viruses probably do not, as single agents, cause cancer. However, viruses may be one of multiple agents acting to initiate carcinogenesis.

CHEMICAL AGENTS

Some of the most common chemical carcinogens include tar, soot, asphalt, aniline dyes, hydrocarbons, crude paraffin oil, fuel oils, nickel, and arsenicals. Most of these agents cause cancer only after close and prolonged contact, and persons affected are usually workers in industries in which these chemicals are used or occur as by-products, such as tanning, die making, refineries, and battery-making factories.

PHYSICAL AGENTS

Physical carcinogens cause cellular damage just as chemical carcinogens do, except their action is physical in nature. Radiation and asbestos are both physical carcinogens.

Two forms of radiation can lead to cancer: ultraviolet radiation and ionizing radiation. Ultraviolet radiation from the sun can cause changes in DNA structure that can lead to malignant transformation if it is not repaired. Both basal and squamous cell carcinomas of the skin as well as melanoma are linked to ultraviolet exposure.

Ionizing radiation can cause permanent DNA mutation when exposure is excessive. This mutation may transform into a malignant growth if the DNA repair is incomplete. The vast majority of radiation exposure is from natural sources (radon, cosmic, terrestrial, and internal radiation). Preventive measures are usually focused on minimizing exposure to manufactured sources of radiation such as x-rays and isotopes, which are used in medical diagnosis and treatment.

In the United States, asbestos, a carcinogenic fiber, contributes significantly to the occurrence of bronchogenic cancer and mesothelioma. There is a strong synergistic relation between tobacco smoke and asbestos. The mechanism of action of asbestos is unknown, but it is thought to be a promoter rather than an initiator of the cancer.

DRUGS AND HORMONES

Scientists have demonstrated that a relationship exists between hormonal secretion and action, tumor development, and growth. Exactly what the relationship is remains obscure.

One of the most controversial topics in carcinogenesis is the role of estrogen. Animal studies have shown that estrogen is involved in the development of breast cancer. Human studies indicate that estrogen is related to human breast cancer but in a poorly defined manner.

Cancer chemotherapeutic agents are carcinogenic, and cancer clients are at risk for future development of leukemia and other cancers (see Chap. 7 for further discussion of this topic).

Predisposing Factors

In addition to the carcinogens described, there are also predisposing factors that influence the host's susceptibility to various etiologic agents.

AGE

Cancer affects people of all ages. However, cancer develops more readily in older people than in younger individuals. Many cancers, such as prostate, colon, and some chronic leukemias, have increased incidence in older clients. Older people may be more susceptible to cancer simply because they have been exposed to carcinogens longer than younger people. Also, as individuals age, their immune system ages and becomes less active. The immune response failure theory suggests that this problem alone could make clients more susceptible to cancers.

Also, there are cancers that occur within very narrow age ranges. Testicular cancer is found in men from about 20 to 40 years of age. Ovarian cancer is more common in women older than 55 years. A number of cancers occur mainly in childhood, such as Ewing's sarcoma, certain acute leukemias, Wilms' tumor, and retinoblastoma.

SEX

Women are more susceptible to certain types of cancer than men are, and vice versa. Since 1949, more men than women have died from all types of cancer.

GEOGRAPHIC LOCATION

The incidence of different types of cancer varies on a geographic basis. For example, the incidence of stomach cancer is higher in Japan than in the United States. On the other hand, breast cancer is rare in Japan but has a high incidence in the United States, Europe, and Israel. These differences may reflect the influence of environmental factors (diet, customs, pollutants in the environment) rather than genetic differences between races and nationalities. This explanation seems likely because the rate of breast cancer among Japanese women living in the United States is the same as that of other women in the United States.

Differences exist among parts of this country also. In highly urbanized areas, colon cancer is more prevalent than in rural areas. The industrialized areas have higher amounts of polluted air, so rates of lung cancer are higher. In rural areas, particularly among farmers, skin cancer is more common. Colon cancer is more common in the industrialized Northeast and Great Lakes region. The greater susceptibility in certain geographic areas is probably related to exposure to different carcinogens, especially environmental ones.

OCCUPATION

People with particular occupations are more susceptible to certain cancers because of their greater contact with specific carcinogens. For example, workers in asbestos factories have a higher incidence of lung cancer as a result of their chronic exposure to asbestos. People who work near hydrocarbons, especially benzene, have a higher rate of bladder cancer. Radium miners and those who paint the iridescent dials on watches have a higher incidence of leukemia from the exposure to radioactivity. Radiologists also have a high rate of leukemia.

HEREDITY

A number of cancers provide evidence of a heritable predisposition to cancer. Fanconi anemia, ataxia-telangiectasia, and xeroderma pigmentosum are examples of autosomal recessive conditions that predispose persons to a variety of malignancies. Familial polyposis coli, retinoblastoma, Wilms' tumor, and neurofibromatosis are examples of autosomal dominant disorders that follow classic mendelian patterns of inheritance.[33] Breast, ovarian, and colon cancers also show a familial pattern.

DIET

The role of diet in the causation of cancer, for the most part, is unclear. What is known is that intake of cured, pickled, smoked, salted, preserved, and unrefrigerated food has been linked to stomach cancer. The high amount of fat in the average diet of people in the United States and the incidence of breast and colon cancer show a striking correlation. There is a similar correlation between excessive meat consumption in this country and colon cancer.[42]

STRESS

Recent research suggests a strong link between stress and cancer. In brief, stress may increase the risk of cancer. Chronic physical or emotional stress preys on the hypothalamus, the portion of the pituitary gland that regulates hormone and immune systems. Increased stress causes hormonal or immunologic changes, or both, which, in turn, spur the growth and proliferation of cancer cells.

PRECANCEROUS LESIONS

Precancerous lesions and some benign tumors may undergo transformation later into cancerous lesions and tumors. Common precancerous lesions include pigmented moles, burn scars, senile keratosis, leukoplakia, and benign adenomas or polyps of the colon or stomach. All of these lesions need to be periodically assessed for malignant changes.

Impact of Cancer

PHYSICAL

Physical changes can occur in the client throughout the cancer experience. The malignant tumor itself may cause obvious disfigurement or internal organ changes even before diagnosis. For example, some skin cancers are potentially disfiguring and colon cancer can cause a great deal of internal change, including obstruction, before diagnosis.

Treatment for a malignant tumor also may cause the client to experience physical changes. Surgery may cause mutilation, as in the amputation of a breast or an arm. Radiation therapy may cause changes in body functions and skin integrity. Chemotherapy may lead to hair loss, weight gain or loss, and skin pigmentation changes.

It is important for the health care provider to recognize the fact that even though the body has been changed by treatment to increase survival, it has still been changed. Clients, along with their significant others, need to adjust to the changes that treatment may produce.

PSYCHOSOCIAL

CRITICAL TO REMEMBER

It is important for the nurse to remember that clients will experience both physical and psychosocial reactions to cancer.

Anxiety, along with depression, has been described as the most common psychosocial reaction among clients with cancer.[13] It is vital to realize that each client diagnosed with cancer reacts to the diagnosis differently and has unique concerns and problems regarding the diagnosis and treatment. Each client copes with the cancer experience in his or her own way.

Health professionals can guide and facilitate open communication among the client, significant others, and health-care provider to reduce anxiety and depression and increase feelings of hopefulness. There are many support groups (such as I Can Cope, Make Today Count, New Voice Club) available for these clients to help them establish effective support systems.

FINANCIAL

Impact on Client and Significant Others. The diagnosis and treatment of cancer are expensive. Medical intervention is technical and lengthy. Not surprisingly, the financial consequences of the illness are a major concern to the cancer client. Sometimes, even if the client has health insurance, the amount the client is required to pay can be astronomic. The client without private insurance may be unable to afford needed care. Primary and secondary prevention methods also can help lower the cost either by preventing the cancer or by treating it sooner.

Depending on the type and stage of cancer, a client may find it necessary to work fewer hours, to find a different line of work, or, in extreme cases, to stop working altogether. If the client is the main source of income and insurance benefits, a change, decrease, or loss of work may have catastrophic consequences. It has been reported that a majority of clients with cancer return to work after diagnosis and treatment of cancer.

Because a social stigma is still associated with the diagnosis of cancer, clients may be denied their former jobs or job benefits (insurance included) when their cancer becomes known to those in the work place. It is, however, illegal to terminate employment on the basis of the diagnosis of cancer. The Federal Rehabilitation Act of 1973 prohibits discrimination against an employee on the basis of a real or perceived handicap. Many states also protect cancer clients against job discrimination.

To help the client and significant others deal with the overall cancer experience, it is necessary to discuss personal financial obligations and responsibilities and the changes diagnosis and treatment may bring.

Impact on the Economy. Cost may be direct or indirect. Direct costs involve cancer prevention, diagnosis, and treatment. Indirect costs include loss of national productivity as a result of the absence of clients with cancer from the work force.

Cancer care cost an estimated $104 billion in 1990. As technology advances and medical costs increase, the cost of cancer care will become even greater in the future. It is unlikely that this nation can afford the ever-increasing cost of health care.

Research

Both physicians and nurses contribute to cancer research. Medical research focuses on the natural history of the disease, new treatment approaches, and singular versus multimodal approaches to medical treatment. Nursing research focuses on the client with cancer and the client's significant others rather than on the cancer and may include biologic, psychological, and social aspects.[24]

CLINICAL TRIALS

The National Cancer Institute (NCI) has developed a method of testing new cancer treatments, especially chemotherapy. There are several stages to this method, commonly known as phase I, II, III, and IV clinical trials. Information is available on these trials from the Physician's Data Query, a computer program accessible by modem, through a medical library, or by calling

1-800-4-CANCER. If an agent successfully meets the criteria of the clinical trials, U.S. Food and Drug Association approval is granted, and the agent is approved to treat specific cancers.

ETHICAL ISSUES

Ethical issues related to cancer research include informed consent, which encompasses client competence; disclosure and understanding of information; voluntariness; and confidentiality. Although in any given institution it may be the physician's responsibility to obtain informed consent before the client's inclusion in a research protocol, it is always the nurse's responsibility to ascertain a client's competence, understanding of the given information, and voluntariness before the initiation of any treatment or therapy.

CHARACTERISTICS OF NORMAL CELLS

Specific characteristics of normal cells that help us understand changes that occur in neoplastic cells are (1) the cell cycle, (2) differentiation, and (3) contact inhibition.

The Cell Cycle. The concept of the cell cycle has increased researchers' understanding of how both normal and neoplastic cells replicate. The cell's replication cycle is divided into the following intervals, or steps, with the letter G standing for "gap"—the interval separating mitosis (M) and synthesis (S).

Step 1a: G_0. This is the interval in which the cell is at rest (until a trigger in the immediate environment signals the beginning of the G_1 interval). Some cells do not replicate, or they replicate so infrequently that they are always said to be in G_0 state.

Step 1b: G_1. The interval in which ribonucleic acid (RNA) and protein are synthesized. The acquisition of the ability to begin DNA synthesis marks the termination of G_1.

Step 2: S. Synthesis of both the DNA and proteins of new chromosomes occurs.

Step 3: G_2. Biochemical processes, including synthesis of some RNA, occur in preparation for mitosis.

Step 4: M. Actual division of the cell—mitosis—occurs, producing two daughter cells.

In the normal mature organ, cell cycling is carefully controlled so that the organ maintains its function. Cells that die are replaced, but no extra cells are produced. Researchers are investigating the mechanisms of this control, which is not fully understood at this time.

Differentiation. In the embryo, genetically identical cells assume various structures and functions. One muscle cell looks like all the other muscle cells but not much like a kidney or liver cell. This process is called differentiation.

Contact Inhibition. When normal cells are grown outside the body on culture plates, they exhibit an interesting characteristic called contact inhibition. Normal cells spread freely about the culture medium until they contact another cell. Then they adhere to each other and align themselves in parallel fashion. The cells grow until they reach the edges of the container, covering the surface in a single layer. At this point active growth stops.

PREVENTION AND ASSESSMENT

Cancer Cell Growth

Tumor growth is related to increased numbers of cells. Cells may increase in number by the following:

- Shortening the length of the cell cycle
- Increasing the fraction of cells going through the cell cycle
- Decreasing cell loss

The current belief is that the fraction of proliferating cells in a tumor is higher, thus accounting for the tumor mass. There is also a decrease in cell death, with the ratio of cell death to cell birth being altered.

The concept of doubling time is central to the study of tumor growth. Theoretically, cancer could start as a single abnormal cell that divides to form two cells, then four cells, and so on. Provided that the amount of time for the cell cycle remains constant, the tumor mass would double each time the cell cycle went from mitosis to mitosis (Fig. 6–2).

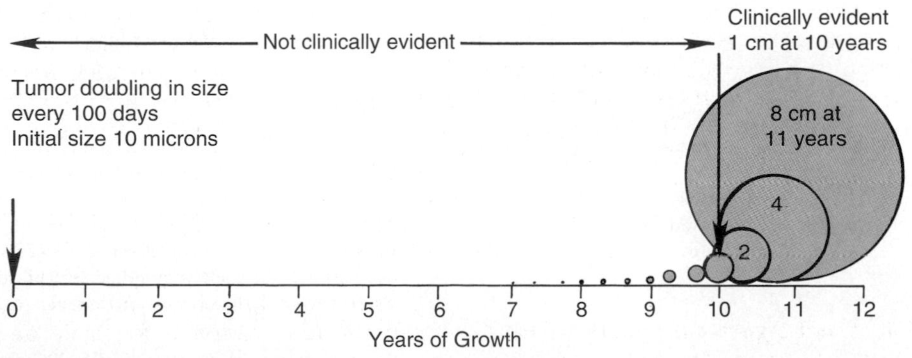

Figure 6–2
Tumor growth: doubling time related to tumor size.

Clearly, the cell cycle of a tumor is of great clinical significance. First, the slower the cell cycle of the tumor, the longer it is before the tumor can be identified. Second, Figure 6–2 shows that the preclinical period of growth is approximately two thirds of the total growth period. This fact helps us to understand how metastasis or spread of a tumor occurs, even when the original tumor is small. It also explains why the physician requires a long period of time after removal of the tumor before being assured that the client is cancer free.

Neoplastic Cell Division and Differentiation

Neoplastic cells differ from normal cells in appearance, pattern of growth, and physiologic function. Neoplastic tissue that differs radically from the host tissue is referred to as anaplastic cells. These anaplastic cells lack the differentiated cell characteristics, specific functions, and organization of normal cells (Table 6–2). Differentiated cells are functionally and structurally specialized and are often nondividing.

Growth of Neoplastic Tumors

Neoplastic cells mass together to form neoplastic tissue growths or tumors. What accounts for the growth and spread of these tumors?

Some neoplastic cells have the ability to spread through the circulation from the original site of the tumor to distant organs of the body. This characteristic is called metastasis. The word is derived from the Greek words meta, meaning beyond, and stasis, meaning

TABLE 6–2 Normal Cells Versus Malignant Cells

CHARACTERISTIC	NORMAL CELLS	MALIGNANT CELLS
Mitotic cell division	Mitotic division leads to two daughter cells	Mitosis leads to multiple daughter cells that may or may not resemble the parent; multiple miotic spindles
Appearance	1. Cells of same type homogeneous in size, shape, and growth 2. Cells cohesive, form regular pattern of expansion 3. Uniform size to nucleus 4. Have characteristic pattern of organization 5. Mixture of stem cells (precursors) and well-differentiated cells	1. Cells larger and grow more rapidly than normal; pleomorphic (i.e., heterogeneous in size and shape) 2. Cells not as cohesive; irregular patterns of expansion 3. Larger, more prominent nucleus 4. Lack characteristic pattern of organization of host cell 5. Anaplastic, lack of differentiated cell characteristics, specific functions
Growth pattern	1. Do not invade adjacent tissue 2. Proliferate in response to specific stimuli 3. Grow in ideal conditions (e.g., nutrients, oxygen, space, correct biochemical environment) 4. Exhibit contact inhibition 5. Cell birth equals or is less than cell death 6. Stable cell membrane 7. Constant or predictable growth rate 8. Cannot grow outside specific environment (e.g., breast cells grow only in breast)	1. Invade adjacent tissue 2. Proliferate in response to abnormal stimuli 3. Grow in adverse conditions such as lack of nutrients 4. Do not exhibit contact inhibition 5. Cell birth exceeds cell death 6. Loss of cell control a result of cell membrane changes 7. Growth rate erratic 8. Able to break off cells that migrate through blood stream or lymphatics, or seed to distant sites and grow in other sites
Function	1. Have specific, designated purpose 2. Contribute to the overall well-being of the host 3. Cells function in specific predetermined manners, such as cells in the thyroid secrete thyroid hormone	1. Serve no useful purpose 2. Do not contribute to the well-being of the host, parasitic, actually feed off host without contributing anything 3. If cells function at all, they do not function normally, or they may actually function to cause damage, such as malignant lung cancer cells that secrete ACTH and cause excessive stimulation of the adrenal cortex
Other	1. Develop specific antigens, characteristic of the particular cell formed 2. Chromosomes remain constant throughout cell division 3. Complex metabolic and enzyme pattern 4. Cannot invade, erode, or spread 5. Cannot grow in presence of necrosis or inflammation	1. Develop antigens completely different from a normal cell 2. Chromosomal aberrations occur as cell matures 3. Have more primitive and simplified metabolic and enzyme pattern 4. Invade, erode, and spread 5. Grow in presence of necrosis and inflammatory cells such as lymphocytes and macrophages 6. Exhibit periods of latency that vary from tumor to tumor 7. Have own blood supply and supporting stroma

ACTH, adrenocorticotropic hormone.

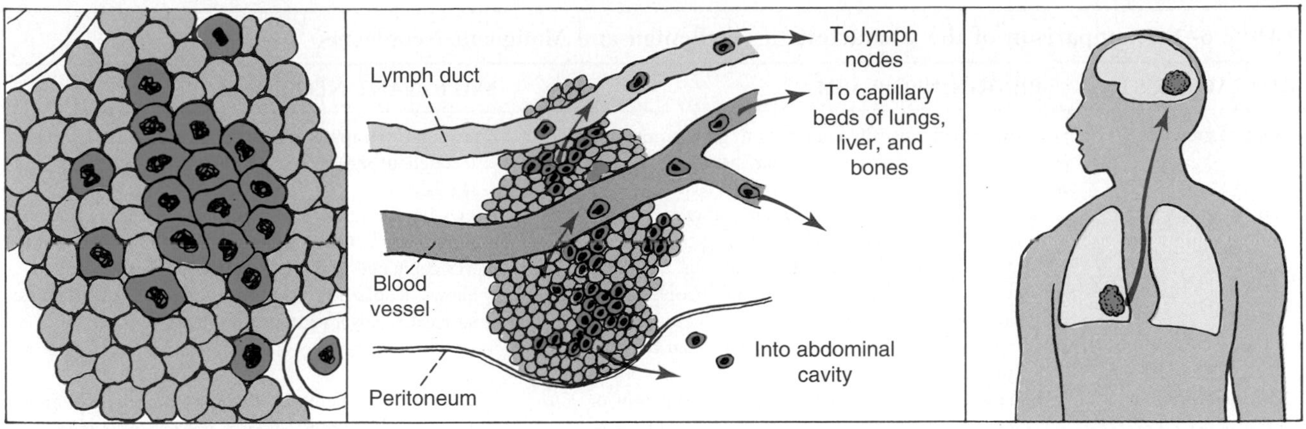

STAGE 1. Invasion of cancer cells into adjacent tissue
STAGE 2. Spread of cancer cells
STAGE 3. Establishment and growth at secondary site

Figure 6–3
Three stages of the metastatic process.

standing. The capacity of a neoplastic tumor to metastasize to other sites is a major characteristic of malignancy, and it distinguishes malignant from benign growths.

For the purposes of study, the metastatic process may be divided into three stages (Fig. 6–3).

Stage 1 involves invasion of neoplastic cells from the primary tumor into surrounding tissue and penetration of blood and lymph vessels. Tumor invasion may be caused by any of the following:

- Increasing tumor size, leading to tissue pressure and mechanical expansion
- Loss of tumor cell cohesiveness, with increasing motility
- Destruction of the host stroma (the supporting tissues of an organ)
- Factors in the host response to tumor cell invasion

Stage 2 involves spread of tumor cells via the lymph or blood circulation or by direct expansion. The lymphatic system provides the most common pathway for initial spread of cancer cells. Lymph node involvement is seen in about one half of all fatal cancers. The blood vessels (including both veins and arteries) carry cancer cells from the primary tumor to the capillary beds of the lungs, liver, and bones. Metastatic spread to distant organs and tissues is almost always the result of cells moving through the bloodstream. Direct expansion of tumors in body cavities occurs as cells travel throughout the cavity to develop new growth on other serosal surfaces. Cancers of the ovary are often said to seed the entire peritoneal cavity.

Stage 3 involves establishment and growth of tumor cells at the secondary site. The tumor develops its own vascularization in the new site and has the ability to infiltrate adjacent tissue.

The growth of metastatic tumors puts severe stress on the person both physiologically and psychologically. As the tumor burden (the amount of tumor in the body) increases, fewer metabolic resources are available for normal cells.

Common Metastatic Sites. The metastatic sites of many tumors are fairly predictable. The predilection of certain tumors for particular sites may be due either to the ability of the tumor to live within only certain tissues or to some other unknown factor. The five most common sites of metastasis are the lymph nodes, liver, lung, bone, and brain.

Factors Influencing Metastasis. The spread of cancer, although not fully understood, appears to be dependent on a variety of factors. These include the host factors such as the immune system, age, and hormonal environment. Many other factors such as pregnancy, stress, and trauma to the malignant tumor seem to increase spread. Other factors such as steroids, aspirin, the immune system, and radiation and chemotherapy appear to both increase and decrease the spread, but these factors are not predictable. Anticoagulants, conversely, seem to decrease the spread of malignant cells.

Classification of Neoplasms

BENIGN VERSUS MALIGNANT

Neoplastic tumors are classified as either benign or malignant. Deciding whether a tumor is benign or malignant is probably the most important decision a physician must make when treating a person with a neoplastic growth.

The word benign comes from the Latin bene, meaning good, and genus, which means sort. Thus, a benign tumor is a "good sort of tumor," a tumor of limited growth. A benign tumor, however, does occupy space. Consequently, if it is located near a vital tube or organ, it could be fatal. As a rule, though, the person with a benign tumor has a good prognosis.

Malignant tumors, on the other hand, represent a serious threat to the life and well-being of the host. Table 6–3 compares the characteristics of these two major types of neoplasms.

TABLE 6–3 Comparison of the Characteristics of Benign and Malignant Neoplasms

CHARACTERISTIC	BENIGN NEOPLASM	MALIGNANT NEOPLASM
Speed of growth	Grows slowly, usually continues to grow throughout life unless surgically removed; may have periods of remission	Usually grows rapidly, tends to grow relentlessly throughout life; rarely, neoplasm may regress spontaneously
Mode of growth	Grows by enlarging and expanding; always remains localized; never infiltrates surrounding tissues	Grows by infiltrating surrounding tissues; may remain localized (in situ) but usually infiltrates other tissues
Capsule	Almost always contained within a fibrous capsule; capsule does not prevent expansion of neoplasm but does prevent growth by infiltration; capsule advantageous because encapsulated tumor can be removed surgically	Never contained within a capsule; absence of capsule allows neoplastic cells to invade surrounding tissues; surgical removal of tumor difficult
Cell characteristics	Usually well differentiated; mitotic figures absent or scanty; mature cells; anaplastic cells absent; cells function poorly in comparison with normal cells from which they arise; if neoplasm arises in glandular tissue, cells may secrete hormones	Usually poorly differentiated; large numbers of normal and abnormal mitotic figures present; cells tend to be anaplastic (i.e., young, embryonic type); cells too abnormal to perform any physiologic functions; occasionally a malignant tumor arising in glandular tissue secretes hormones
Recurrence	Recurrence extremely unusual when surgically removed	Recurrence common after surgery because tumor cells spread into surrounding tissues
Metastasis	Metastases never occur	Metastases very common
Effect of neoplasm	Not harmful to host unless located in area where it causes compression of tissues or obstruction of vital organs; does not produce cachexia (weight loss, debilitation, anemia, weakness, wasting)	Always harmful to host; results in death unless removed surgically or destroyed by radiation or chemotherapy; causes disfigurement, disrupted organ function, and nutritional imbalances; may result in ulcerations, sepsis, perforations, hemorrhage, and tissue slough; almost always produces cachexia, which leaves person prone to pneumonia, anemia, and so forth
Prognosis	Very good; tumor generally removed surgically	Depends on cell type and speed of diagnosis; poor prognosis indicated if cells are poorly differentiated and evidence exists of metastatic spread; good prognosis indicated if cells still resemble normal and there is no evidence of metastasis

TISSUE OF ORIGIN

Neoplasms are classified not only as benign or malignant but also according to the tissue from which they arise. Almost all names for tumors end in the suffix oma, meaning tumor. This suffix is usually attached to a term for the parent tissue of the tumor. Thus, adenoma comes from the Greek aden, or gland, plus oma. When more than one parent tissue enters into the formation of a neoplasm, the names of the tumors are even more descriptive. For example, an adenomyoma is a benign neoplasm that contains both glandular and muscle cells.

Three common benign tumors are the fibroma, lipoma, and leiomyoma.

Let us now consider the classification of malignant tumors. A malignant tumor that arises from epithelial tissue is called a carcinoma, whereas a malignant neoplasm that arises from mesenchymal origins (i.e., blood vessels, lymphatics, nerve tissue) is called a sarcoma (Greek sarc means flesh).

Three representative examples of malignant neoplasms are carcinoma in situ, fibrosarcoma, and bronchogenic carcinoma.

Prevention

RISK ANALYSIS AND MODIFICATION

Although cancer is the second most common cause of death in this country, many forms of cancer have identifiable risk factors and are preventable (Table 6–4). Some cancers can be prevented through primary prevention. However, some cancers cannot be prevented. For these cancers, there is secondary prevention, or early detection. Dietary modifications are among the important ways to reduce the occurrence of cancer in general (Fig. 6–4).

The nurse needs to know the risk factors for each client and the common factors for each type of cancer. Table 6–5 identifies specifics of primary prevention with which the nurse should be familiar.

SCREENING

Primary prevention is the ideal method of cancer control. Not all cancers can be prevented, however, so early detection is also a major tool in the fight against cancer. Nurses must emphasize to the public the importance of

TABLE 6–4 Risk Factors and Prevention Levels for Common Cancers

TYPE OF CANCER	RISK FACTORS AND LEVEL OF PREVENTION
Lung	Smoking, all types (P); high levels of indoor radon (P); occupational and environmental industrial pollutants (P); air pollution (P); family history of lung cancer (S); secondary cigarette smoke (P)
Breast	Family history of breast cancer, especially on maternal side and occurring before menopause (S); history of breast or other gynecologic cancer (S); Jewish (S); single (P,S); nulliparity (P,S); early menarche, late menopause (S); birth of first child after 30 (P,S); ? history of benign breast disease (S); diet high in fat (S); high alcohol intake (S); higher socioeconomic groups (S); increasing age (S); whites (S)
Colorectal	Low-fiber, high-fat diet (P); history of ulcerative colitis, colon cancer, breast or female genital cancer, or bladder cancer (S); increasing age (S); obesity (P); sedentary life-style (P); family predisposition (S); history of colorectal adenomas (S)
Bladder	Smoking (P); men (S); whites (S); high alcohol consumption (P); aniline dye, print, coal, tar, and pitch workers (S); apparel, textile, and leather industries (S); painters (S); ? saccharin use (P); schistosomiasis (S); treatment with cyclophosphamide (S); exposure to asbestos (P,S)
Cervical	Black women (S); early, frequent intercourse with multiple sex partners (P,S); multiparity (S); intercourse with uncircumcised males (P,S); chronic cervicitis (S); history of genital herpes or HPV (P,S)
Skin	Exposure to ultraviolet light (P); history of excessive sunbathing or sunburn before age 20 years (P); fair skinned, fair hair (S); increasing age (S); history of dysplastic nevi, burns, topical ulcers, scars from squamous or basal cell carcinoma (S); family history of melanoma (S); PUVA treatment for psoriasis (S); outdoor workers (P,S); organ transplant recipients (S)
Prostate	Increasing age (S); black men (S); industrial exposure to cadmium (P,S); ? diet high in fats and sugar (P); ? history of venereal disease (P,S); ? sexual activity (P,S)
Ovarian	History of breast cancer (S); nulliparity or first pregnancy after age 30 years (S); white, upper income groups (S); history of pelvic radiation (S)
Uterine-endometrial	Obesity (P); history of hypertension, diabetes mellitus, or menstrual disorders (P,S); higher socioeconomic groups (S); nulliparity (P,S); infertility related to anovulation (S); long-term use of conjugated estrogens (P,S); Stein-Leventhal syndrome (S)
Testicular	Whites (S); cryptorchidism (S); age, 20 to 40 years (S); family history (S); DES exposure in utero (S); atrophic testicles (S)
Oral	Smoking (P); smokeless tobacco or snuff (P); heavy alcohol use (P); vitamin B complex and iron deficiencies (P); poor oral hygiene, poor dental care, or ill-fitting dentures (P); pipe smoking or long-term exposure to sun (lip) (P,S)
Gastric	Family history (S); blood group A (S); atrophic gastric mucosa (S); gastric ulcers (P,S); pernicious anemia (S); history of gastric resection (S); stomach polyps (S); lower socioeconomic groups (S), intake of nitrates and nitrosamines (P); nonwhites (S); eating smoked foods, especially fish and mutton (P); eating pickled foods (P); eating rice treated with talc (P)
Leukemia	Age, childhood for acute and old age for chronic (S); exposure to benzene (P,S); poultry farmers (S); exposure to radiation (P,S); explosive and rubber cement workers, radiologists, distillers, dye users and painters, radium miners and chemists, and radium dial painters (P,S); Down's or Klinefelter's syndrome (S); men (S); an identical twin with leukemia (S); viruses (S); immunologic factors (S); genetic factors (S); intake of drugs such as melphalan, cyclophosphamide (Cytoxan), or chloramphenicol (P,S)

DES, diethylstilbestrol; HPV, human papillomavirus; P, primary prevention; PUVA, ultraviolet light; S, secondary prevention; ?, possible risk factor, not yet proved.
Data from Groenwald, S., et al. (1990). *Cancer nursing: Principles and practice* (2nd ed.). Boston: Jones & Bartlett Publishers.

finding the cancer and eradicating it early, before the cancer begins to metastasize from the primary site. The public needs to realize that manifestations of a malignant disease can mimic those of other less serious disease processes. Currently, two of three people diagnosed with cancer die from it. Early detection could raise the survival rate to 50 per cent.

The individual's age, personal health history, and family history may indicate risk factors and are vital to the early detection of cancer. Nurses can help in this educational process by emphasizing the need for an annual physical examination, by stressing the importance of a yearly Papanicolaou (Pap) test for women, and by teaching women the technique for breast self-examination and teaching men the technique for testicular self-examination. Chapter 51 describes these examinations in detail.

Increasing public awareness of cancer's warning signals is the role of every nurse (Box 6–1). Table 6–6 summarizes the American Cancer Society's (ACS) most recent guidelines for screening asymptomatic populations.

BOX 6–1

Cancer's Seven Warning Signals (Caution)

Change in bowel or bladder habits
A sore that does not heal
Unusual bleeding or discharge
Thickening or lump in breast or elsewhere
Indigestion or difficulty in swallowing
Obvious change in wart or mole
Nagging cough or hoarseness
If you have a warning signal, see your physician!

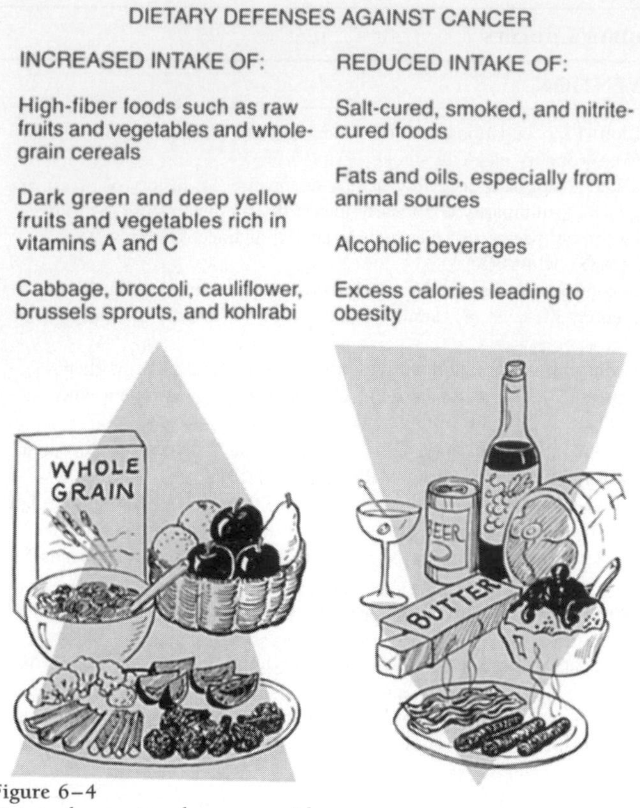
DIETARY DEFENSES AGAINST CANCER
INCREASED INTAKE OF:
High-fiber foods such as raw fruits and vegetables and whole-grain cereals
Dark green and deep yellow fruits and vegetables rich in vitamins A and C
Cabbage, broccoli, cauliflower, brussels sprouts, and kohlrabi
REDUCED INTAKE OF:
Salt-cured, smoked, and nitrite-cured foods
Fats and oils, especially from animal sources
Alcoholic beverages
Excess calories leading to obesity
WHOLE GRAIN
BEER
BUTTER

Figure 6–4
Dietary changes to reduce cancer risks.

The nurse should remember that it is a normal human response to procrastinate in scheduling an examination when cancer is suspected. People are frightened by the thought of cancer. They do not always realize that cancer is curable when found early. Early detection always improves survival. Part of the process of screening clients is educating them as well.

The ACS strongly supports public education programs for cancer prevention and early detection. The nurse needs to support these measures to help reduce the risk of cancer.

Diagnosis

What specifically is involved in cancer detection? The primary health-care provider uses both general and special techniques in a complete cancer diagnostic examination. General techniques include obtaining the client's history, including familial and environmental histories, performing a thorough physical examination, and ordering and evaluating laboratory examinations of the client's blood, tissue, sputum, urine, and other specimens.

PSYCHOSOCIAL ISSUES DURING DIAGNOSIS

When people undergo the diagnostic process associated with suspicious lumps or other cancer symptoms, they are usually somewhat afraid and anxious. They are experiencing unfamiliar and possibly painful tests.

TABLE 6–5 Factors to Be Avoided That Might Lead to the Development of Cancer (Primary Prevention)

FACTOR	DISCUSSION
Smoking	Cigarette smoking is responsible for 90 per cent of lung cancer cases among men and 79 per cent among women—about 87 per cent overall. Smoking accounts for about 30 per cent of all cancer deaths. Those who smoke two or more packs of cigarettes a day have lung cancer mortality rates 15 to 25 times greater than nonsmokers.
Sunlight	Almost all of the more than 800,000 cases of basal and squamous cell skin cancer diagnosed each year in the United States are considered to be sun related. Epidemiologic evidence shows that sun exposure is a major factor in the development of melanoma and that the incidence increases for those living near the equator.
Ionizing radiation	Excessive exposure to ionizing radiation can increase cancer risk. Most medical and dental radiographs are adjusted to deliver the lowest dose possible without sacrificing image quality. Excessive radon exposure in homes may increase risk of lung cancer, especially in cigarette smokers. If levels are found to be too high, remedial actions should be taken.
Nutrition and diet	Risk for colon, breast, and uterine cancers increases in obese people. High-fat diets may contribute to the development of cancers of the breast, colon, and prostate. High-fiber foods might help reduce risk of colon cancer. A varied diet containing plenty of vegetables and fruits rich in vitamins A and C may reduce risk for a wide range of cancers. Salt-cured, smoked, and nitrite-cured foods have been linked to esophagus and stomach cancer.
Alcohol	Oral cancer and cancers of the larynx, throat, esophagus, and liver occur more frequently among heavy drinkers of alcohol especially when accompanied by cigarette smoking or chewing tobacco.
Smokeless tobacco	Use of chewing tobacco or snuff increases risk of cancer of the mouth, larynx, throat, and esophagus and is a highly addictive habit.
Estrogen	Estrogen treatment to control menopausal symptoms can increase risk of endometrial cancer. However, including progesterone in estrogen replacement therapy helps to minimize the risk. Consultation with a physician will help each woman to assess personal risks and benefits.
Occupational hazards	Exposure to several different industrial agents (nickel, chromate, asbestos, vinyl chloride, etc.) increases risk of various cancers. Risk from asbestos is greatly increased when combined with cigarette smoking.

Adapted from American Cancer Society. (1995). *Cancer facts and figures—1995.* New York: American Cancer Society. By permission.

TABLE 6–6 American Cancer Society Guidelines (1995) for Early Detection of Cancer in Asymptomatic Populations

TEST	AGE (YR)	SEX	FREQUENCY
Chest x-ray study			No longer recommended for smokers to screen for lung cancer
Sputum cytology			No longer recommended for smokers to screen for lung cancer
Physical examination	40+	M,F	Yearly for all people older than 40 years, including examination of skin, lymph nodes, mouth, thyroid, breast, testes, rectum, and prostate
Health teaching	20	M,F	Teach proper diet, exercise, health habits, breast and testicular self-examination, avoidance of sunlight, and stop smoking
Breast self-examination	20+	F	Every month after menses before menopause; after menopause, monthly, on any specified day such as the first or last of the month
Mammography	35–40	F	Baseline mammogram between 35 and 40 years; between 40 and 49 years a mammogram should be done every 1 to 2 years and yearly after 50 years; high-risk women should check with their physician
Pap smear	18+	F	Sexually active women should have Pap smears regardless of age; should be performed yearly until there are three negative examinations in a row; at this point, they can be performed yearly or as physician advises
Pelvic examination	20–40, 40+	F	Every 3 years, earlier if sexually active; yearly after 40 years
Endometrial tissue sample	At menopause	F	High-risk women (obese, abnormal uterine bleeding, estrogen therapy, history of infertility, diabetes, hypertension, and failure to ovulate) should have this test performed at menopause
Testicular self-examination	20–40	M	Monthly, on a set date such as the first of the month, after a shower
Digital rectal examination	40+	M,F	Annually for rectal cancer in men and women and prostate in men
Fecal occult blood	20–40,	M,F	Done per physician's recommendation, women at higher risk
	40–49, 50+		Done per physician's recommendation, yearly
Proctoscopy, flexible sigmoidoscopy	50+	M,F	Examination annually for 2 years and, if negative, then every 3–5 years
Oral examination	20+	M,F	Annually
Breast physical examination	20–40,	F	Every three years
	40+		Annually

Pap, Papanicolaou.
Adapted from American Cancer Society. (1995). *Cancer facts and figures—1995.* New York: American Cancer Society by permission.

When working with clients undergoing diagnosis, the nurse should consider the following points. First, it usually is helpful to give clients the information over time. If they know the alternatives that are being ruled out during the diagnostic process, the confirmation of one alternative, even if unpleasant, will not be as much of a shock. Having time to prepare for an event is part of successful coping. Second, the nurse should gear explanations to the clients' level of understanding. Listen to the clients and the terms they are choosing. Sometimes they avoid the word cancer and use tumor or growth instead. If the diagnosis of cancer is made, make sure that clients understand the terms the physician is using. Third, clients will need to hear information several times and often from several people they trust. Often, clients repeat the same questions several times. Sometimes, clients are reluctant to take up the time of the busy nurse or physician with their repeated questions. Clients need to feel that the nurse is willing to take the time to talk with them. The nurse should communicate clients' needs to other members of the health-care team as well. Finally, at the time the diagnosis is confirmed, clients need to know what alternatives are available. There should be time for clients to assimilate the information before being asked to make choices about interventions. The nurse needs to be informed about the diagnosis and plan of care, about the disease and interventions in general, and about what the clients actually know.

The goal of care during this time is to help clients cope with the diagnosis, recommended treatment, and prognosis. People cope in different ways during a crisis situation. They may react with fear, denial, withdrawal, anger, and other coping behaviors. Nevertheless, the nurse can help clients explore new and more effective coping strategies. The foundation for successful coping is receiving accurate information about the situation and possible solutions.

It is also important for clients to be both physiologically and psychologically capable of understanding and using the information. They should not be in pain and they should have a sense of control over the situation. The nurse must be especially aware of clients' feelings. Hospitalization makes most people feel helpless and out of control, all of which interferes with coping.

If the nurse can help clients cope successfully during the period of diagnosis and beginning of treatment, they may cope better during the entire course of the disease. People with cancer and their significant others often demonstrate great strength as they learn to deal with their fears and with the difficulties of being treated for cancer.

HISTORY AND PHYSICAL ASSESSMENT

The first step in the diagnostic process is obtaining a complete history and physical examination of the client.

Nurses must learn about the health of the client's family members, the work history of the client, and the environment in which the client lives.

When a malignant tumor is in its early stages, there are often few symptoms. Clinical manifestations usually appear once the tumor has grown to a sufficiently large size to cause one or more of the following problems:

- Pressure on surrounding organs or nerves
- Distortion of surrounding tissues
- Obstruction of lumina of tubes
- Interference with the blood supply of surrounding tissues
- Interference with organ function
- Disturbance of body metabolism
- Parasitic use of the body's nutritional supplies
- Mobilization of the body's defensive responses, resulting in inflammatory changes

Common clinical manifestations that may arise secondary to cancer include weight loss, weakness or fatigue, central nervous system (CNS) alterations, pain, and hematologic and metabolic alterations. Close assessment of such symptoms may reveal that they are directly or indirectly related to the tumor growth.

Anorexia, weight loss, weakness, and fatigue are related to the body's inability to consume and use nutrients appropriately. Mechanical interference by tumors, malabsorption, paraneoplastic endocrine secretions (such as excessive secretion of thyroid hormones), and tumor use of nutrients may all contribute to a cycle that must be interrupted to prevent general physical debilitation.

The client who has difficulty with vision, speech, coordination, or memory may be experiencing primary or metastatic CNS disease. Increased intracranial pressure caused by tumor growth may result in headache, lethargy, nausea, or vomiting.

Although pain is not a common early symptom of cancer, it may occur as a result of obstruction or destruction of a vital organ, pressure on sensitive tissues or bone, or involvement of nerves. If it occurs and is not adequately treated, it may become constant and progressively severe. Bone cancer is particularly painful because the rigidity of bone allows for little or no expansion as the tumor cells proliferate. It also becomes more painful because pathologic fractures produce instability and muscle spasms.

Unexplained anemia often indicates a malignancy. Hematologic changes also include leukopenia, leukocytosis, and bleeding disorders, which, in some diseases, may occur before local symptoms. Metabolic manifestations such as Cushing's syndrome, hypercalcemia, inappropriate antidiuretic hormone secretion, and carcinoid syndrome also signify the possibility of malignant disease.

A localized tumor usually produces symptoms related to increased pressure or obstruction in a single region. Metastatic disease and extensive tumors of major organs may display a variety of local and systemic symptoms.

CANCER-SPECIFIC DIAGNOSTIC EXAMINATIONS

The ideal diagnostic test would find cancer at the beginning, when it is composed of only a few cells. It would be specific for one type of cancer, and a positive test would provide a definitive diagnosis. It would also be inexpensive, easy to perform, and noninvasive. Unfortunately, no such test exists.

RADIOGRAPHIC PROCEDURES

Basic X-Ray Studies. X-ray studies are particularly useful in diagnosing obstructive tumors of the gastrointestinal, respiratory, and renal tracts. They are also valuable in identifying bone malignancies and, aided by computers, help pinpoint the location of brain tumors and the degree to which the tumors are compressing surrounding tissues.

Radioisotope Studies (Scans). Isotopes are capable of entering into the same chemical reactions and the same metabolic processes in the body as stable elements. Thyroid, bone, brain, liver, lung, and spleen are areas of the body most frequently scanned for diagnostic purposes.

When utilized diagnostically, radioisotopes are used as tracers. A tracer is a material that can be administered to the client either orally or by injection. The isotope is then identified, located, and traced by a radiosensitive apparatus as the radioactive material circulates through the body and concentrates in particular organs and tissues.

The scintillation scanner is a device for locating and pinpointing malignant growths by measuring the uptake of a radioisotope. This scanner is passed back and forth over the area of the body that is being studied.

Radioisotopes can be

- Administered in very small doses so there is no destruction of body cells
- Used to study the functions of specific organs and tissues
- Used to measure blood volume, blood circulation rate, red cell turnover, cardiac output, and lung blood flow
- Used to locate tumors and lesions within the brain, kidneys, liver, lungs, pericardium, and bones

An organ scan is a simple and completely painless procedure. There are three steps involved.

1. Administration of the radioisotope. The client receives a tracer dose of the appropriate radioisotope either orally or by injection.
2. Waiting period. Before the scanning procedure can be performed, the radioisotope must be assimilated by the organ under study. The length of time required for assimilation varies. A brain scan should be performed $1\frac{1}{2}$ hours after an injection of radioactive mercury and 18 to 48 hours after an injection of radioiodinated human serum albumin.

3. The scanning procedure. The client is asked to lie still and breathe normally while the scintillation scanner measures the radioactive atoms concentrated in the organ under study and records its findings. Sedation before this procedure may help the restless, agitated, or anxious client.

Computed Tomography Scan. The computed tomogram is an x-ray technique that produces sequential cross-sectional body images at progressive depths. Computed tomographic (CT) scans can help differentiate malignant and nonmalignant masses and accurately identify their size and location. Occasionally, an oral or intravenous contrast agent is administered to increase the sensitivity of the CT scan. Always check for an allergy to the dye.

Depending on the area to be scanned, clients may be placed on a restricted diet. Clients should be taught that they will lie on a table and the x-ray machine will move around them. This is a painless test unless an intravenous contrast dye, which may cause a burning sensation on injection, is given. The dye also may cause nausea, vomiting, flushing, itching, and a bitter taste. The x-ray machine is very noisy and could frighten clients if they are not warned.

Mammogram. A mammogram is a radiologic examination using a minimal and safe amount of radiation to allow visualization of breast masses, differentiating tumors from fibrocysts. The breast is compressed between two plates. The use of compression decreases the amount of radiation that must be used to visualize the tumors. Some women, particularly those with multiple fibrocysts in the breast, will find the compression uncomfortable; otherwise, the examination is painless. Two views are taken of the breast: a craniocaudal view and a lateral view.

Angiogram. Angiography is used infrequently to check the resectability of tumors. This examination involves the injection of a radiopaque dye that circulates to the tumor; a radiographic study is then performed. This procedure clearly outlines the blood supply of the tumor and surrounding structures.

Depending on the site of the angiography, the client may be placed on a restricted diet. Clients may be sedated before the examination to help them relax and lie still during the test. The skin over the injection site is cleaned, shaved if necessary, and anesthetized. The radiopaque dye injected may cause some feelings of nausea, vomiting, flushing, itching, or a bitter or salty taste. Before it is administered, the nurse should check whether or not the client has an allergy to the dye.

After the test, a pressure bandage is applied to the site of the cannulization. This site is then immobilized for up to 24 hours. If a cutdown (an incision to locate the vein) is used, then the site is sutured and wound care should be done.

Lymphangiogram. The lymphangiogram is a very useful diagnostic test because it examines the lymphatic system, the primary site of metastasis for tumors with good lymphatic drainage. Although the test cannot rule out metastasis, it is an excellent marker when there is known disease because it can show tumor growth or remission.

The lymphangiogram cannot be performed for 48 hours after another contrast study. There is no preparation before this examination except client teaching. The nurse should explain to the client that the test is fairly long and uncomfortable. The test is performed by injecting blue dye into the interdigital webs of the feet. This dye is picked up by the lymphatic system so it can be cannulized. The skin on each foot over the lymphatics is anesthetized and cutdown performed so cannulas can be inserted to infuse the dye. The dye may take several hours to infuse into the lymphatics of the abdomen. X-ray studies are then obtained.

After the test, the client should drink plenty of fluids. The dye may continue to discolor the urine for several days. The feet also will remain tinted blue for a long time after the test. The client must return the following day for follow-up x-ray studies.

BLOOD STUDIES

A variety of blood tests can be performed to help diagnose cancer (Table 6–7). Some of the more routine tests, such as the complete blood count and differential, do not test for specific types of cancer but indicate the presence of any number of problems. Other blood tests, such as tumor markers produced by the specific tumor cells and biochemical tests, including the acid phosphatase, identify the extent of a particular type of cancer. These specific tests, however, are not used to make the diagnosis of cancer but only to check its progression.

CYTOLOGIC EXAMINATION

Papanicolaou Test (Pap Smear). This valuable diagnostic test was developed by George N. Papanicolaou in 1943. Its original purpose was to discover cancer of the cervix during the early, noninvasive, asymptomatic stage. Today, the test is also used to detect early cancers of the digestive, respiratory, and renal tracts and, occasionally, those of the breast. The Pap smear is used to evaluate responses to chemotherapy and radiation therapy as well as to detect malignant disease when it recurs postoperatively.

Materials that can be examined by Pap smears include (1) cervical scrapings, (2) bronchial secretions and washings obtained by bronchoscopy, (3) urine sediment, (4) coughed-up sputum, (5) aspirated gastric secretions, and (6) mammary gland discharge fluid.

The method for obtaining a Pap smear is fairly simple. First, the examiner either scrapes cells from a tissue (e.g., the cervix) or obtains cells by aspirating fluid or sediment from an organ (e.g., the stomach or bronchi). Next, the examiner fixes the smear by immersing it in a chemical solution of equal parts of ether and 95 per cent ethyl alcohol. Finally, the fixed slide is allowed to dry. It is then stained and evaluated.

The laboratory technique used to analyze the Pap smear is called exfoliative cytology, which means the examination of desquamated or sloughed-off cells.

TABLE 6–7 Laboratory Blood Tests for Cancer

TEST	REFERENCE VALUES	CONDITIONS IN WHICH LEVELS ARE ALTERED
Hematologic Tests (CBC)		
Hemoglobin	M: 14–18 g/dL F: 12–16 g/dL	↓ in anemia, nonspecific, may indicate malignancy
Hematocrit	M: 40–54 mL/dL F: 37–47 mL/dL	↓ in anemia, nonspecific, may indicate malignancy
Leukocytes (white cell count)	4500–11,000 mm^3	↑ in leukemia and lymphomas ↓ in leukemia and metastatic disease to bone marrow
Per cent neutrophils	54–62 per cent	↑ in AML, CML, and lymphoma ↓ in leukemia, carcinoma, myeloma, sarcoma, and bone marrow depression
Per cent lymphocytes	25–33 per cent	↑ in ALL and CLL, multiple myeloma, lymphoma, and carcinoma ↓ in Hodgkin's disease, nonlymphocytic leukemias, lymphosarcoma, and bone marrow depression
Per cent monocytes	3–7 per cent	↑ in Hodgkin's disease, lymphoma, monocytic leukemia, CML, and multiple myeloma ↓ in hairy cell leukemia
Per cent eosinophils	1–3 per cent	↑ in CML ↓ in Hodgkin's disease and bone marrow depression
Per cent basophils	0–1 per cent	↑ in CML and Hodgkin's disease
Platelets	150,000–300,000 mm^3	↑ in myeloproliferative disorders, CML, and Hodgkin's disease ↓ in ALL, AML, multiple myeloma, and bone marrow depression
Blood/Serum Tests		
Acid phosphatase	0.11–0.60 mU/mL	↑ in metastatic prostate cancer
ACTH	10–80 pg/mL (in AM)	↑ in lung cancer
Alkaline phosphatase	20–90 mU/mL	↑ in cancer of bone or bone metastasis, liver cancer, lymphoma, and leukemia
Calcitonin	Undetectable	↑ in medullary thyroid cancer > 100 pg/mL
Calcium	9.0–11.0 mg/dL	↑ in bone metastasis, breast cancer, leukemia, lymphoma, multiple myeloma, lung, kidney, bladder, liver, and parathyroid cancers
Gastrin	< 200 pg/mL	↑ in gastric and pancreatic cancer
IgG	500–1900 mg/dL	↑ in IgG myeloma
IgA	60–333 mg/dL	↑ in IgA myeloma
IgM	45–145 mg/dL	↑ in IgM Waldenstrom's macroglobulinemia
IgD	0.5–3.0 mg/dL	↑ in IgD myeloma
IgE	500 ng/mL	↑ in IgE myeloma
LDH	100–190 mU/dL	↑ in liver cancer and liver metastasis, lymphoma, acute leukemia
Lysozyme	4–13 mg/L	↑ in AML and CML
Parathyroid hormone	430–1860 ng/L	↑ in squamous cell lung, kidney, pancreatic, and ovarian cancers
Serotonin	50–200 ng/mL	↑ in carcinoid syndrome
SGPT	5–35 mU/mL	↑ in metastatic liver cancer
SGOT	7–40 mU/mL	↑ in metastatic liver cancer
Testosterone	M: 275–875 ng/dL F: 23–75 ng/dL	↑ in adrenal and ovarian cancers
Uric acid	M: 2.5–8.0 mg/dL F: 1.4–7.0 mg/dL	↑ in leukemia and multiple myeloma ↓ in Hodgkin's disease, multiple myeloma, and lung cancer
Tests for Tumor Markers		
AFP	< 10 ng/mL	↑ in lung, nonseminomatous testicular, pancreatic, colon, and stomach cancers, and choriocarcinoma
CA-125	< 35 U	↑ in ovarian cancer
Calcitonin	< 100 pg/mL	↑ in medullary thyroid, small cell lung, and breast cancers and carcinoid
CEA	Nonsmokers: 0–2.5 ng/mL Smokers: < 3.0 ng/mL	↑ in colorectal, breast, lung, stomach, pancreatic, and prostate cancers
Estrogen receptors	Positive > 10 fmol/mg	↑ in breast cancer
HCG	0–5 IU/L	↑ in choriocarcinoma, germ cell testicular, lung, liver, stomach, pancreatic, endometrial, and liver cancers
Progesterone receptor assay	Positive > 10 fmol/mg	↑ in breast cancer
Prostatic acid phosphatase	0.26–0.83 U/L	↑ in metastatic prostate cancer
PSA	0–4 ng/mL	↑ in prostate cancer
CA-19-9		↑ in pancreatic and colon cancer
CA-15-3		↑ in breast cancer

ACTH, adrenocorticotropic hormone; AFP, alpha-fetoprotein; ALL, acute lymphocytic leukemia; AML, acute myelogenous leukemia; CBC, complete blood count; CEA, carcinoembryonic antigen; CLL, chronic lymphocytic leukemia; CML, chronic myelogenous leukemia; F, females; HCG, human chorionic gonadotropin; Ig, immunoglobulin; LDH, lactate dehydrogenase; M, males; PSA, prostate-specific antigen; SGOT, serum aspartate aminotransferase; SPGT, serum alanine aminotransferase.

Under the microscope, the cells may have either a normal or an anaplastic appearance. Cells are graded on the following five-point scale:

Class I: normal
Class II: inflammation
Class III: mild to moderate dysplasia
Class IV: possibly malignant
Class V: probably malignant

If the Pap smear indicates a class II finding, the smear is simply repeated in 3 months. If the test reveals a class III finding, the Pap smear will be repeated in 6 weeks to 3 months, and if it is still class III, a biopsy is performed. If the Pap smear is class IV or V, a biopsy is performed immediately.

BIOPSY

A biopsy is the surgical excision of a small piece of tissue for microscopic examination. Physicians most commonly use this method to either rule out or confirm a diagnosis of malignancy.

The client is usually scheduled for minor surgery. If the site for biopsy is easily accessible (e.g., cervix, breast), the nurse drapes the person appropriately and assists with the administration of a local anesthetic. Then, the surgeon removes a piece of the suspicious tissue. Additional procedures (e.g., bronchoscopy, cystoscopy, and sigmoidoscopy) are necessary for an internal tumor.

There are two types of biopsy procedures. The type used depends on the size of the tumor and the purpose of the biopsy. If the suspicious tumor is small, the entire tumor is excised for examination. This is called a total or excisional type of biopsy. If the tumor is large, only a part of the neoplasm is excised. This procedure is termed a subtotal or incisional type of biopsy. There is some question as to the safety of the subtotal biopsy. Some surgeons believe that this procedure opens vascular channels and releases tumor cells, which may then metastasize to other sites during the time when the excised tissue is being examined. However, there are no studies to date that definitely confirm this fear.

After the excision, the pathologist prepares a frozen section or a permanent paraffin section to examine the specimen. To prepare a frozen (or rapid) section, the tissue is immediately frozen. Then the pathologist cuts the tissue into thin sections and examines the tissue slices under the microscope. The main advantage of the frozen section is the speed with which the section can be prepared and the diagnosis made. Only minutes are required. In contrast, the slower, more classic method of embedding the tissue in paraffin takes about 24 hours. However, the paraffin section provides the pathologist with clearer detail than does the frozen section.

Needle or aspiration biopsy is used mainly to obtain tissue samples for identification from the liver, kidney, spleen, lung, or breast. The physician aspirates a core of tissue from a suspicious nodule or mass rather than excising it.

ULTRASOUND PROCEDURES

The ultrasonogram uses high-frequency sound waves to visualize the interfaces around organs and within pathologic masses. Special equipment is used to detect and map echoes of varying densities from various organs and tumors. This technique is used to detect lesions in the female pelvis, abdominal lymph nodes, prostate through a transrectal approach, and other areas of the body. One advantage of this procedure is that it noninvasively demonstrates and follows the growth of neoplasms without radiation exposure.

Preparation for the test includes cleansing the bowel with enemas if the abdominal area is to be tested and having the client drink six to eight glasses of water without voiding before the test. The water distends the bladder, used as a landmark for a pelvic ultrasonogram, and the client is not allowed to void until after the test. The test is painless, with only a slight pressure being felt. A lubricant gel is applied but is easily wiped off after the test. The client is allowed to void after the test is completed.

DIRECT VISUALIZATION

An endoscopy involves direct visualization of the gastrointestinal tract, bronchoscopy of the lungs, laryngoscopy of the larynx, colposcopy of the cervix and vagina, cystoscopy of the bladder, laparoscopy of the pelvic or abdominal cavities, and so on. These tests use a rigid or flexible scope, which allows the physician to view the internal anatomy directly without major surgery. During these tests, suspicious areas can be examined, tissue samples and aspirates taken for biopsies, the extent of the disease staged, and pathologic processes excised. These tests are discussed in detail in later chapters.

MAGNETIC RESONANCE IMAGING

Magnetic resonance imaging (MRI) identifies abnormalities by creating sectional images of the body without the use of contrast dyes or radiation. MRI provides clear images of internal structures in response to the magnetic field created by harmless, low-energy radio waves. MRI can be used to detect, localize, and stage malignancies of the CNS, spine, head and neck, and musculoskeletal system.

All materials that might be affected by a magnet should be removed before the test. This test cannot be performed if any material affected by a magnet cannot be removed such as a pacemaker or surgical clips. The test is painless, although some clients may feel somewhat claustrophobic because of the narrow tunnel in the machine where they must lie. The nurse must inform clients that the machine makes a loud, hammering sound during the test, so they will not be frightened. If an intravenous contrast dye is used to enhance the image, clients may experience some nausea, vomiting, and itching. There is no specific nursing care required after the test. As with all diagnostic tests, clients must be provided with emotional support while awaiting the results.

TABLE 6–8 TNM Staging System

STAGE	DESCRIPTION
Tumor	
T0	No evidence of primary tumor
TiS	Carcinoma in situ
T1, T2, T3, T4	Progressive increase in tumor size and involvement
TX	Tumor cannot be assessed
Nodes	
N0	Regional lymph nodes not demonstrably abnormal
N1, N2, N3	Increasing degrees of demonstrable abnormality of regional lymph nodes (for many primary sites, the letter a, e.g., N1a, may be used to indicate that metastasis to the node is not suspected; and the letter b, e.g., N1b, may be used to indicate that metastasis to the node is suspected or proved)
NX	Regional lymph nodes cannot be assessed clinically
Metastasis	
M0	No evidence of distant metastasis
M1, M2, M3	Ascending degrees of distant metastasis, including metastasis to distant lymph nodes

ANTIGEN SKIN TESTING

The immune system apparently plays a vital role in preventing tumor growth and in destroying those tumors that do develop. The immune response can be suppressed by (1) immunosuppressive medications, (2) physical or emotional stress (which stimulates the release of plasma cortisol), (3) smoking, (4) alcohol, and (5) blocking agents released by the tumor. A suppressed immune response usually indicates a poor prognosis. The dinitrochlorobenzene (DNCB) skin test is one method currently used to assess whether or not the person has a properly functioning immune system. Approximately 90 to 95 per cent of healthy clients can be sensitized to the chemical DNCB when it is placed on a small area of the skin. In the healthy individual a positive response (redness, itching, perhaps blistering) develops within 24 to 48 hours. When given a second (challenge) dose of DNCB 14 days later, a delayed cutaneous hypersensitivity response (a raised red site) develops on the skin.

The DNCB skin test is useful in several ways. First, it acts as a diagnostic aid. For example, clients who have a negative reaction or who cannot be sensitized to DNCB are said to be anergic (i.e., have diminished ability to react to specific antigens). This signals inadequacy of the immune response. Second, DNCB can assess the client's immunocompetence before and during radiotherapy and chemotherapy. Remember that both of these modalities can suppress the immune system. Candidates for immunotherapy (see Chap. 7) are tested before therapy to determine their immune function. Clients in immunotherapy programs are monitored throughout their therapeutic regimen to determine their response to therapy.

Staging and Grading

When a neoplastic growth is definitely diagnosed, it must be further defined in terms of its extent. This diagnostic process, called staging, involves a systematic search for (1) the characteristics of the primary tumor (using clinical examination and pathologic examination), (2) involvement of the lymph nodes (using clini-

TABLE 6–9 Karnofsky Performance Status Scale

CONDITION	PERCENTAGE	COMMENTS
Able to carry on normal activity and to work; no special care is needed	100	Normal; no complaints; no evidence of disease
	90	Able to carry on normal activity; minor signs or symptoms of disease
	80	Normal activity with effort; some signs or symptoms of disease
Unable to work; able to live at home, care for most of personal needs; a varying degree of assistance is needed	70	Cares for self; unable to carry on normal activity or to do active work
	60	Requires occasional assistance but is able to care for most needs
	50	Requires considerable assistance and frequent medical care
Unable to care for self; requires equivalent of institutional or hospital care; disease may be progressing rapidly	40	Disabled; requires special care and assistance
	30	Severely disabled; hospitalization is indicated, although death is not imminent
	20	Hospitalization is necessary; very sick; active supportive treatment necessary
	10	Moribund; fatal processes progressing rapidly
	1	Unconscious
	0	Dead

Adapted from Baird, S. B., et al. (1991). *Cancer nursing: A comprehensive textbook.* Philadelphia: W. B. Saunders Co.

cal examination, lymphangiography, and perhaps needle biopsy), and (3) evidence of metastasis, based on knowledge of the natural history of the disease.

The TNM system is the accepted system for staging today. In this system, T stands for tumor, and T1 to T4 defines the increasing tumor size. N refers to the regional lymph nodes, and N1 to N3 indicates advancing nodal disease. M refers to metastasis, with M0 meaning no evidence of metastasis and M1 referring to the presence of metastasis. Table 6–8 summarizes the TNM staging system.

Several types of tumors are still staged using older systems, such as Clark's classification for malignant melanomas and Duke's classification for colorectal cancer. Clark's classification considers the level of invasion of melanomas, and Duke's system refers to the depth of invasion of colorectal cancer. Hodgkin's disease uses the Ann Arbor classification, which refers to both the distribution of the tumor and the associated symptoms.

The tumor grade is an evaluation of the extent to which tumor cells differ from their normal precursors. Low numeric grades, grade I or II, mean the cells are well differentiated and deviate minimally from the normal cells. High grades, grade III or IV, refer to cells that are poorly differentiated and the most aberrant compared with the normal cells.

The histologic grade is determined by a pathologist. Tumor grading involves a histologic and anatomic description of the malignant neoplasm. Staging and grading information guides the physician in the choice of intervention and in estimating the client's prognosis.

Assessment of Clients' Physical Performance

There are scales that help assess the client's ability to continue activity. A common scale is the Karnofsky Performance Status Scale (Table 6–9). This scale can help the nurse assess the effect of the cancer on clients' physical activity and guide interventions to assist with deficits.

STUDY QUESTIONS

1. Which one of the following physical agents is a carcinogen?
   A. Asphalt
   B. Fuel oils
   C. Asbestos
   D. Hydrocarbons
2. Which one of the following statements regarding the impact of cancer on the client is true?
   A. The client is referred to a support group as a last resort.
   B. The cost of treatment of cancer is entirely covered by medical insurance.
   C. Anxiety and depression are common reactions to the diagnosis of cancer.
   D. Physical changes occur in the client after the diagnosis has been confirmed.
3. A client states to the nurse, "Cancer is just a lot more cells than usual." The nurse should respond by teaching that malignant cells
   A. Do not invade adjacent tissue.
   B. Can grow in the presence of necrosis.
   C. Have a specific, designated purpose in the body.
   D. Cannot invade, erode, or spread to surrounding tissue.
4. A middle-aged woman states she has a benign tumor. She is sure that she has cancer but is willing to listen to an explanation about the kind of tumor she has. The nurse should explain that
   A. Metastases never occur with a benign tumor.
   B. The prognosis with a benign tumor is very poor.
   C. The tumor may recur or spread after surgery.
   D. Cancer cells grow rapidly and spread into surrounding tissue.
5. Which one of the following diagnostic tests can be used to detect early cancer of the cervix, respiratory, digestive, and renal tracts?
   A. Acid phosphatase
   B. Aspiration biopsy
   C. Papanicolaou test (Pap smear)
   D. Computed tomography (CT) scan
6. During a physical assessment, a client states, "I can't have cancer because I never had any pain until this week." The nurse should respond by saying:
   A. "Are you sure you didn't have abdominal pain for the past few months?"
   B. "Pain can occur if a tumor interferes with the way an organ is functioning."
   C. "If you're worried about having pain, we have some good medications that will help you."
   D. "It's pretty early in the disease process for you. The tumor won't cause any pain until it metastasizes."
7. A client with a suspected neoplasm is scheduled for a radioisotope study. He emphasizes to the nurse and his spouse that he will be radioactive. Which one of the following statements by the client will help the nurse evaluate the success of teaching about radioisotopes and their use in diagnostic testing?
   A. "I'll be radioactive for about a month, so I need to stay away from my grandchildren."
   B. "Radioisotopes are used only in extreme cases and I know that you have protected me from extra exposure."
   C. "I'll be able to resume my usual daily activities after the test because the dose is so small it won't cause any harm."
   D. "I'll remember to take my prescription faithfully so that the radioactivity clears from my body as soon as possible."

CRITICAL THINKING EXERCISES

SCENARIO A

A client who is newly diagnosed with cancer is very inquisitive about his disease. How should the nurse answer the following questions?

1. "What is the difference between the terms malignant and benign?"
2. "What term should I use? The word cancer makes me afraid and I wonder how my friends and family will react when I tell them I am ill."
3. If the client's type of cancer originated from his life-style, what information will help the nurse plan care?
4. What kind of teaching should be done when the client asks whether a virus caused his cancer?

SCENARIO B

A client is being prepared for a series of diagnostic studies relative to a suspected carcinoma. The client is asking why there is not one test that can tell whether cancer is present in her body. She is very frightened of the diagnosis and the upcoming tests. She is anticipating pain and discomfort associated with diagnostic testing. How should the nurse caring for her react to the following questions?

1. "Why do I have to have so many kinds of tests?"
2. "Will the tests hurt? Will they give me something to help with the pain?"
3. "Why is a biopsy so important? Can it be done during my surgery?"

BIBLIOGRAPHY

1. American Cancer Society. (1994). *Cancer facts and figures.* New York: American Cancer Society.
2. American Cancer Society. (1992). *Cancer facts and figures.* New York: American Cancer Society.
3. American Nurses' Association & Oncology Nursing Society. (1987). *Standards of oncology nursing practice.* Kansas City, MO: American Nurses' Association.
4. Applebaum, J. (1992). The role of the immune system in the pathogenesis of cancer. *Seminars in Oncology Nursing, 8(1),* 51–62.
5. Baird, S. B., et al. (1991). *Cancer nursing: A comprehensive textbook.* Philadelphia: W. B. Saunders Co.
6. Barrere, C. C. P. (1994). Hospital employee cholesterol screening: Modification of dietary behavior. *AAOHN Journal, 42(6),* 261–269.
7. Bast, R., Fenoglio-Preiser, C. M., Ozer, H., & Sidransky, D. (1993). Clinical applications of tumor markers. *Patient Care, 27(6),* 61–64, 67–68, 71–72.
8. Beahrs, O. H., et al. (1992). *Manual for staging of cancer* (4th ed.). Philadelphia: J. B. Lippincott Co.
9. Benner, P., & Wrubel, J. (1989). *The primacy of caring.* Menlo Park, CA: Addison-Wesley Publishing Co.
10. Breslow, L., & Cumberland, W. G. (1988). Progress and objectives in cancer control. *Journal of the American Medical Association, 259,* 1690–1694.
11. Cannon-Albright, L. A., et al. (1988). Common inheritance of susceptibility to colonic adenomatous polyps and associated colorectal cancers. *New England Journal of Medicine, 319,* 533–537.
12. Cartmel, B., Loescher, L., & Villar-Werstler, P. (1992). Professional and consumer concerns about the environment, lifestyle, and cancer. *Seminars in Oncology Nursing, 8(1),* 20–29.
13. Clark, J. (1990). Psychosocial dimensions: The patient. In S. L. Groenwald, et al. (Eds.), *Cancer nursing: Principles and practice* (2nd ed., pp. 346–364). Boston: Jones & Bartlett Publishers.
14. Consolidated Omnibus Budget Reconciliation Act (COBRA). (1986). 42 U.S.C. 300 bb et seq.
15. Cooper, G. (1990). *Oncogenes.* Boston: Jones & Bartlett Publishers.
16. Cooper, G. (1992). *Elements of human cancer.* Boston: Jones & Bartlett Publishers.
17. Feldstein, M. A., & Rait, D. (1992). Family assessment in an oncology setting. *Cancer Nursing, 15(3),* 161–172.
18. Frank-Stromborg, M. (1986). The role of the nurse in early detection of cancer: Population 66 years of age and older. *Oncology Nursing Forum, 13,* 107–115.
19. Frank-Stromborg, M. (1988). Nursing's role in cancer prevention and detection. Vital contributions to attainment of the Year 2000 Goal. *Cancer, 62(8, Suppl),* 1833–1838.
20. Frank-Stromborg, M. (1989). Reaction to the diagnosis of cancer questionnaire (RDCQ): Development and psychometric evaluation. *Nursing Research, 38,* 364–369.
21. Frank-Stromborg, M., & Rohan, K. (1992). Nursing's involvement in the primary and secondary prevention of cancer: Nationally and internationally. *Cancer Nursing, 15(2),* 79–108.
22. Frost, P., & Fidler, I. J. (1986). Biology of metastasis. *Cancer, 58,* 550–553.
23. Fucile, J. (1992). Functional rehabilitation in cancer care. *Seminars in Oncology Nursing, 8(3),* 186–189.
24. Grant, M. M., & Padilla, G. V. (1990). Cancer nursing research. In S. L. Groenwald, et al. (Eds.), *Cancer nursing: Principles and practice* (2nd ed., pp. 1270–1279). Boston: Jones & Bartlett Publishers.
25. Greenwald, P., & Sondik, E. (Eds.). (1986). Cancer control objectives for the nation. *National Cancer Institute Monograph, 1985–2000* (NIH Publication No. 86–2880). Washington, DC: United States Government Printing Office.
26. Griffith, H. M., & DiGuiseppi, C. (1994). Guidelines for clinical preventive services: Essentials for nurse practitioners in practice, education, and research. *Nurse Practitioner: American Journal of Primary Health Care, 19(9),* 25, 27–28.
27. Groenwald, S., et al. (1990). *Cancer nursing: Principles and practice.* Boston: Jones & Bartlett Publishers.
28. Halstead, M. T., & Fernsler, J. I. (1994). Coping strate-

gies of long-term cancer survivors. *Cancer Nursing, 17(2),* 94–100.

29. Jenkins, J. (1992). Biology of cancer: Current issues and future prospects. *Seminars in Oncology Nursing, 8(1),* 63–69.
30. Kaye, J. M., & Gracely, E. J. (1993). Psychological distress in cancer patients and their spouses. *Journal of Cancer Education, 8(1),* 47–52.
31. Lamkin, L. Outpatient oncology settings: A variety of services. *Seminars in Oncology Nursing, 10(4),* 229–236.
32. Lassauniere, J., & Vinant, P. (1992). Prognostic factors, survival, and advanced cancer. *Journal of Palliative Care, 8(4),* 52–54.
33. Levine, E. G., et al. (1989). The role of heredity in cancer. *Journal of Clinical Oncology, 7,* 527–540.
34. McMillan, S. (1992). Carcinogenesis. *Seminars in Oncology Nursing, 8(1),* 63–69.
35. Muzzin, L. J., Anderson, N. J., Figueredo, A. T., & Gudelis, S. O. (1994). The experience of cancer. *Social Science Nursing, 38(9),* 1201–1208.
36. Nicolson, G. L. (1993). Growth mechanisms and cancer progression. *Hospital Practice, 28(2),* 43–53.
37. Palos, G. (1994). Cultural heritage: Cancer screening and early detection. *Seminars in Oncology Nursing, 10(2),* 104–113.
38. Redler, N. (1994). A triumphant survival, but at what cost? Meeting the long-term needs of cancer survivors. *Professional Nurse, 10(3),* 166–170.
39. Scharlach, A. E., Mor-Barak, M. E., & Birba, L. (1994). Evaluation of a corporate-sponsored health care program for retired employees. *Health and Social Work, 19(3),* 192–198.
40. Srivastava, S., & Kramer, B. S. (1992). Oncogenes in cancer detection. *Contemporary Oncology, 2(3),* 63–65, 69–72.
41. Weisburger, J. H., & Wynder, E. L. (1991). Dietary fat intake and cancer. *Hematology Oncology Clinics of North America, 5(1),* 7–23.
42. Willet, W. (1989). The search for the causes of breast and colon cancer. *Nature, 338,* 389–394.
43. Yarbro, J. (1992). Oncogenes and cancer suppressor genes. *Seminars in Oncology Nursing, 8(1),* 30–39.

Chapter 7 Treatment Modalities for Neoplastic Disorders

Learning Outcomes

After completing this chapter, the learner will be able to:

1. Conduct a psychosocial assessment of the client and significant others during the cancer experience.
2. Teach the client and significant others to cope with the diagnosis of cancer.
3. Teach the client about surgery, radiation therapy, chemotherapy, bone marrow transplantation, and biologic response modifiers as modalities in the treatment of cancer.
4. Consider safety precautions when administering radiation and chemotherapy.
5. Assess the client for side effects and toxic effects of radiation and chemotherapy.

PSYCHOSOCIAL ASPECTS OF CANCER

Cancer is a feared and dreaded disease for several reasons. It may present in an advanced stage with no symptoms. Compliance with vigorous and sometimes disfiguring treatment does not guarantee a cure. In addition, cancer may recur after many years of remission. A healthy life-style does not ensure that a person will escape the disease.[39]

Cancer can affect the client at all levels of functioning. Intellectual function can be clouded by physical distress or medication. The client's self-concept is affected by the physical changes and changes in role or function. The client who was the caretaker of the family may become dependent on others and the consumer of family savings and resources. The young adult, striving for independence, may need to revert to an earlier level of dependency. Changes in body image occur in most clients. Weight loss, alopecia, and skin changes can result from treatment. Radical surgical procedures can produce changes that may be humiliating and overwhelming to the client.

The diagnosis of cancer has an impact on the entire family. The daily life of the family is changed. If the client is the caretaker, other family members will need to assume this role. If the family functions poorly before the illness, then the additional stress may increase the dysfunction.

All clients undergo a period of diagnosis and initial treatment. If the cancer is considered curable and the client completes definitive treatment for the cancer, a period of survivorship ensues. This is characterized by watchful waiting for disease recurrence. Those clients who have metastatic disease at the time of treatment or who have a cancer recurrence must deal with the chronicity of the disease.

Specific psychosocial problems, assessment, and intervention strategies are addressed for each of the distinct phases of the cancer continuum: (1) diagnosis and treatment, (2) survivorship, (3) recurrent disease and palliation, and (4) terminal illness.

DIAGNOSIS AND TREATMENT

Cancer clients reach the point of diagnosis in many ways. Clients may have had vague symptoms, that is, weight loss and fatigue, that have been ignored or the cause of some anxiety for weeks or months. They may have symptoms such as pain or abdominal bloating that evaded diagnosis. Many times, cancer is found inadvertently during routine examinations. Often, the client suspects cancer, but many clients are shocked when the diagnosis is made. The diagnostic period may be lengthy and extremely distressful. This period is filled with anxiety over each test result, especially when staging procedures are done. Many clients consider the time of diagnosis and treatment as the most distressful in the cancer experience.

During diagnosis, the magnitude of the problems becomes apparent. Is the disease curable or not? Will the disabilities be temporary or permanent? What types of physical impairment will occur? What will be the side effects of treatment? Will the symptoms be relieved? Will the client be able to return to work? What adjustments have to be made in family life or work? Will finances be adequate? What plans need to be abandoned? Which changes in life-style will be temporary and which permanent?

Clients must not only deal with specific problems but also the emotional distress experienced throughout this time. They may feel angry and frustrated because their lives have been changed; they may feel isolated or may worry about being abandoned by family and friends. They may be shocked and disbelieving that they are the ones with cancer.

It must be stressed that there is great variability in clients' reactions. Some have minimal distress, whereas others may be overwhelmed and devastated. The magnitude and intensity of emotions and problems depend on the clients' psychological make-up, social support, resources, and the disease itself.

Coping is the dynamic process by which a client responds to a problem to bring about relief or equilibrium. The nurse must assess clients for coping strategies that have helped them in the past.[30]

Families also should be assessed for their coping ability. Families who use excessive denial, exhibit strong anger and guilt, or are particularly demanding may be at increased risk of dysfunction. When the client is the pivotal family person or when the family has had a previous experience of cancer, family needs may be increased.[38]

Coping strategies of the clients must be identified. Once defined, interventions to help clients deal with their emotions and solve specific problems can be used.

Expressing emotions may be difficult for many clients. Nurses can help clients by listening actively to them and maintaining a noncritical relationship that allows expression of negative feelings. Referrals to counseling or more formal methods of emotional expression such as music or art therapy may be appropriate, if available. Providing social support and improving clients' sense of control helps reduce anxiety. Stress reduction or relaxation techniques can be taught. Many clients are encouraged by speaking with former clients. Programs such as Reach to Recovery and Cansurmount (American Cancer Society) provide this opportunity.

CRITICAL TO REMEMBER

The nurse should assess clients' readiness to learn during the diagnostic and treatment periods.

Informational needs predominate during the diagnostic and treatment periods. Tests, procedures, and treatments, which are often very technical and complicated, need to be taught to clients. During this time of anxiety and stress, the simplest explanation is usually the most appropriate and all that clients can assimilate. Misconceptions need to be identified and corrected.

The diagnostic period is one of great distress. Clients are vulnerable and fragile. They need compassion and caring, sensitivity, and understanding. A relationship of trust and confidence helps carry clients through this time of uncertainty and threat.

SURVIVORSHIP

Clients who have completed curative treatment enter an indeterminate period of survivorship. As increasing numbers of clients are being cured of cancer, more attention is being focused on the physiologic and psychological needs of this group (see Client Education Guide: Post-Treatment Care at Home). Clients have organized into advocate groups to provide mutual support and to lobby for legislation to address some of their specific needs in employment and insurance coverage.

Employment discrimination has been a problem for cancer survivors. Although clients with a cancer history have proved themselves to be dependable and productive, studies show that as many as 84 per cent of blue collar workers and 38 per cent of white collar workers experience some type of discrimination in employment.[49] Over the years, these issues have been rectified by state laws protecting the rights of the disabled.

Like employment, obtaining insurance coverage for clients with a cancer history has been difficult, exorbitantly expensive, and sometimes impossible. Legislative efforts over the past decade have rectified some of these problems. Insurance discrimination can be legally appealed. Federal programs such as COBRA (Consolidated Omnibus Budget Reconciliation Act) protect the insurance coverage of an employee for 18 months after employment termination. Many states have passed comprehensive health insurance plans to provide coverage for clients who are unable to obtain commercial insurance. Clients who have difficulty with insurance coverage should be directed to the American Cancer Society, their state department of human rights, or insurance department. The booklet *Facing Forward* from the National Institutes of Health provides detailed informational resources.

CLIENT EDUCATION GUIDE

Post-Treatment Care at Home

The home health-care nurse functions as a vital link that ensures continuity of care as the cancer client goes home after surgery, chemotherapy, or radiation therapy. Still stunned by the reality of the disease, the cancer client requires considerable emotional support to aid in the management of symptoms. It is hoped that symptom management will result in a renewed sense of well-being and determination to continue to participate in life despite the illness. Emotional support means simply showing you care through touch and active listening. When all else is forgotten, that touch and that kind word will provide comfort.

Teaching quickly becomes the focus of the home health nurse's visit as the cancer client begins to relax again in his or her own home and really hears other information that will help him or her feel better. Be familiar with the rationale for your suggestions and present them when appropriate. Start with simple basic information about nutrition and fluid intake. Teaching should include information such as eating a sizeable breakfast because the appetite wanes with the day, eating small, frequent meals, eating foods at room temperature, avoiding fatty or fried foods, avoiding spicy foods, using a supplement such as a powdered instant breakfast between meals to boost caloric intake and give energy, and taking nausea medication regularly so eating is possible. Drink lots of water to support blood pressure, flush the bladder, and replace fluids that might be lost through vomiting and diarrhea. Pay attention to mouth care, watch for the development of mouth sores and report them immediately, use a soft toothbrush, keep lips moist, and rinse the mouth before and after meals. Elimination is always a major concern of clients. If diarrhea is the problem, increase fluids; use nutmeg, apples, or bananas to slow peristalsis; use vitamins A and D ointment on the rectum after washing; and use prescribed medication. If constipation is the problem, increase fluids, fiber, and activity. A concoction of prune juice, milk of magnesia, and sodium biphosphate (Phospho-Soda) is just one remedy.

Fatigue remains a troublesome and universal symptom. Clients must be reminded that it is okay to take the time needed for recovery and that a longer recovery period is likely with each succeeding treatment. Clients in treatment are likely to be affected by low blood counts. Stress the necessity of avoiding sick people, have the client take his or her temperature twice a day, teach good hand washing, suggest avoiding bumping or cutting the skin, and have the client use an electric shaver. Pain, actual or potential, frightens all cancer clients. Two simple suggestions go a long way to promote comfort. They are (1) take medication on a scheduled rather than an as-needed basis, and (2) reorder medication 1 week before the supply is depleted.

RECURRENT DISEASE AND PALLIATION

The recurrence of cancer provides the basis for a chronic phase of the cancer experience. Most clients with cancer live with the threat or reality of recurrent disease. Recurrence, at the very least, signifies that the disease is in control and that the individual is not.

With recurrent disease, therapy may once again be used to eradicate or stabilize the disease process. Yet, although subsequent recurrent disease may occur, it is usually the first recurrence that involves surprise, shock, and disbelief. Thus, it is important for the nurse to assess the client's coping skills and provide assistance in helping to mobilize resources and support.

Physical impairment may be increased and quality of life may be limited owing to disease or treatment. Clients who previously verbalized an optimistic outlook may now express a more guarded attitude. It is vital for the nurse to maintain open communication and to be sensitive to the informational and support needs of clients with cancer and their significant others.

Palliative care and palliative treatment are two distinct options for clients with cancer. Palliative treatment (surgery, radiation therapy [RT], or chemotherapy) may be used to alleviate complications caused by persistent tumor growth. For example, surgery may be used to manage a malignant obstruction or RT to reduce or prevent paralysis from spinal cord compression.

Palliative care is the provision of symptom management and psychosocial support provided by a multidisciplinary health-care team. It is important that the nurse communicate that symptoms can be managed successfully and that resources are available to assist in providing supplies and support.

THE TERMINALLY ILL

More than 50 per cent of clients with cancer die from their disease. The time from diagnosis to death ranges from weeks to years. Not all clients with cancer become terminally ill. Some clients die during the initial treatment, whereas others die from treatment complications. Many clients, however, reach an endpoint at which their cancer no longer responds to treatment and disease progression cannot be controlled. Now the goals of treatment are directed toward supportive care of clients and significant others until death occurs.

During the past 25 years, hospice care has become the standard of care for terminally ill cancer clients in the United States. This philosophy of care emphasizes symptom control and pain management, providing comfort and dignity for the client during the dying process.

The hospice can be connected with a hospital, community, home care agency, or skilled nursing facility. The basic characteristics of a hospice program include:

- Control of client symptoms and pain relief
- Treatment of client and family as a unit
- Provision of care by a physician-directed interdisciplinary team
- 24-hour, 7-day coverage
- An autonomous hospice administration providing coordinated home care with back-up inpatient services
- Use of trained volunteers to augment staff services
- Structured systems of staff support
- Bereavement follow-up
- Services given based on need and not ability to pay

To qualify for hospice services, clients must have a life expectancy of fewer than 6 months and be on only supportive treatment.

When cancer clients reach the point at which treatment is no longer effective, they are considered terminally ill (see Ethical Issues in Nursing). Some clients can accept or resign themselves to the approaching end of their life; others cannot and will continue to seek treatment beyond reasonable limits.

Cancer clients approach death in as many ways as they approach life. Some try to remain active despite tremendous physical limitations. Others may withdraw into depression. This period is a time of suffering for both clients and significant others as the physical loss of function and the psychological pain of anticipated and real losses in relationships and roles are intensified.

Nursing care of the terminally ill addresses pain and symptom management while maintaining the dignity of clients and promoting the maximum quality of life. As significant others become caretakers, they must be taught simple nursing skills and pain management. Family members and significant others need constant reassurance that they are providing good care. Although it is often a new and unfamiliar experience, most are able to focus their energies and strengthen their family bonds through the experience of caring for a dying family member. When death occurs, families are usually physically exhausted but psychologically strengthened.

Clients without families or friends to function as primary caretakers have few options for their care. A few free-standing hospices exist to provide them with care. Many nursing homes have hospice programs. Clients without insurance or financial means are less fortunate.

Nurses are encouraged to plan, implement, and evaluate the care of the client during each phase of the cancer experience.

ETHICAL ISSUES IN NURSING

Who Should Decide the Continuation or Cessation of Cancer Treatment?

Are there times when a client should accept from the health-care provider that nothing more can be done, that treatment options are futile? Are physicians obligated to treat clients with therapies that are hopeless even if the client might want such therapies? On the other hand, are there times when clients can say they wish no more treatment—no more chemotherapy, radiation therapy, or even surgery—even if there is a chance that such treatments might be helpful? Perhaps they believe the end stages of their life would be better lived without the side effects of such treatments.

Nursing care for clients with cancer presents many challenges. The nurse must be sensitive to the emotional aspect of their client's illness, be skilled with the technical aspects of care (such as in chemotherapy), be available to teach clients and significant others about the disease process and treatments, and be a health-care advocate for the clients. If clients decide that they no longer want treatment, the nurse must put all of his or her skills to work to help meet clients' current and anticipated needs. If treatment is no longer an option for clients, the nurse is there to provide care for them and perhaps their significant others.

MEDICAL AND SURGICAL TREATMENT AND NURSING CARE FOR CLIENTS WITH CANCER

Goals of Intervention

The major goal of cancer therapy is to treat clients effectively with the appropriate therapy for a sufficient duration so a cure results with minimal functional and structural impairment.[6] If a cure is not possible, important alternate goals are to prevent further metastasis, relieve symptoms, and maintain a high quality of life for as long as possible. Decisions made at the time of first diagnosis are crucial because early aggressive intervention usually offers the best hope of cure.

Methods for treating clients with cancer include chemotherapy, surgery, RT, biotherapy, and bone marrow transplantation. The choice of method depends on the tumor type, extent of disease, and clients' physical status. Often, clients are treated with a combination of methods rather than a single therapy. This approach is called combined modality therapy.

Surgery

Surgery plays a major role in the diagnosis, staging, and treatment of cancer. It is also an integral part of rehabilitation and palliation of clients with cancer. It is used with less frequency as a method of cancer prevention.

DIAGNOSTIC SURGERY

The diagnosis of cancer is established by microscopic identification of malignant cells from tumor tissue. There are a variety of methods used to obtain tissue for diagnostic purposes. The biology of the tumor, size, location, and proposed method of treatment determine which method of biopsy should be used.

Cytology Specimens. Cytology specimens can be obtained from tumors that tend to shed cells from their surface. Tumor cells can often be obtained from cytologic examination of fluids aspirated from effusions, ascitic fluid, or endoscopic brushings.

Needle Biopsy. Needle biopsy is a simple method of obtaining tissue samples. In a fine-needle aspiration, tumor cells are withdrawn from the tumor by a needle and syringe. A core-needle biopsy is essentially the same procedure; however, the needle is larger and a core of tissue is obtained. Needle biopsies are useful in obtaining samples from tumors in subcutaneous tissue, muscle, breast, pancreas, liver, and lung.

Care must be taken to obtain needle biopsies from areas that will be surgically removed if the tumor is malignant, because malignant cells can be deposited in the needle tract. A negative biopsy does not prove the absence of cancer but rather may be an indication of inadequate or misplaced tissue sampling. Negative biopsies must be pursued with additional biopsies.

Incisional Biopsy. An incisional biopsy surgically removes a small sample of tissue for examination. It is performed during endoscopic examinations of the bronchus, stomach, bladder, and colon and in removal of samples of large tumor masses in which a diagnosis must be made before definitive surgical treatment. Surgical techniques are used to prevent seeding of tumor cells in the biopsy site. As with the needle biopsy, cancer can be proved with a positive result but not ruled out with a negative one. When negative results are obtained, additional biopsies may be attempted.

Excisional Biopsy. An excisional biopsy removes all of the tumor mass and provides the pathologist with an entire sample. It is used for small tumors (2–3 cm in size) in which the biopsy also may serve as the treatment if the tissue margins contain no tumor cells. If tumor cells remain, a wider excision is required. Excisional biopsies are useful in skin cancers, melanomas, and breast cancer.

STAGING

Cancer staging is the process of determining the extent of disease as the basis for treatment decisions. Clinical staging, such as x-ray studies or scans, is sufficient for most types of cancer. Staging information is also obtained during surgery for cancer treatment. For example, the true stage of colon cancer is usually determined after surgery, when the regional lymph nodes are examined for the presence of tumor cells.

CURATIVE SURGERY

Primary Lesions. Surgery is performed in the treatment of 55 per cent of clients with cancer. Forty per cent of clients are treated with surgery alone. Cancers that are localized to the organ of origin and the regional lymph nodes are potentially curable by surgery.

Current concepts in tumor growth hold that tumors probably begin shedding cells into the systemic circulation throughout their growth; therefore, combinations of local therapies, surgery, and radiation must be combined with systemic therapies, chemotherapy, and biotherapy to improve survival.

When surgery is performed with curative intent, the extent of the excision is determined by the type of tumor. For slow-growing tumors, such as those of the skin, a wide local excision may be sufficient. Tumors of the colon and breast that spread to the regional lymph nodes are removed with an en bloc excision of the tumor and the regional lymph nodes. Large tumors, such as sarcomas, which tend to spread locally without metastasizing, are removed with radical excisions, such as amputations. In all surgical procedures, various operative techniques, such as glove changing, instrument cleaning, and wound irrigation with cytotoxic agents, are used to prevent dissemination of tumor cells into the operative field.

Recurrent Lesions. Cancer that recurs locally can be resected, resulting in occasional cure, remission, or both. Local recurrences of sarcomas, colon, breast, and skin cancers have been successfully excised, resulting in cures.

Metastatic Lesions. Excision of metastatic lesions is considered if no other evidence of disease exists and the metastatic lesion appeared after a relatively long, disease-free interval. The metastatic lesion must exhibit some degree of stability and be refractory to chemotherapy and radiotherapy. Metastatic renal cell carcinomas, sarcomas, melanomas, and colon carcinomas have been removed in selected clients, resulting in cures or prolonged survival times.

PALLIATIVE SURGERY

Because surgical procedures carry an inherent potential for morbidity, use of surgery in palliative care is carefully considered and used only if the benefits outweigh the risks. Examples of palliative surgery that can benefit clients with cancer and improve quality of life include procedures that (1) reduce pain, (2) relieve airway obstructions, (3) relieve obstructions in the gastrointestinal and urinary tracts, (4) relieve pressure on the brain or spinal cord, (5) prevent hemorrhage, (6) remove infected and ulcerating tumors, and (7) drain abscesses.

RECONSTRUCTIVE SURGERY

Advances in reconstructive surgery offer a different perspective of rehabilitation to clients who have experienced curative surgery. Restoration of form and function is possible in varying degrees, depending on the site and extent of surgery. Reconstructive surgery may be performed concurrently with the radical procedure or delayed for optimal outcome. The major goal of reconstructive surgery is to improve clients' quality of life by restoring maximal function and appearance.

PREVENTIVE SURGERY

The client at unusually high risk for cancer may elect to have preventive surgical intervention. Certain conditions or diseases increase the risk of cancer occurrence so significantly that removal of the target organ is justified to prevent cancer development. Clients with familial polyposis are at a 50 per cent risk for colon cancer by the age of 40 years. Clients with ulcerative colitis also have an increased risk for colon cancer. Prophylactic subtotal colectomies are indicated for this group of clients.[53]

Nursing Management

Although many aspects of surgical care for clients with cancer are similar to those of all surgical clients (see Chap. 5 and those chapters that address surgery of a specific body system), some differences exist.

Preoperatively, clients with cancer may be nutritionally compromised and require hospitalization before surgery. Those who have had adjuvant or palliative chemotherapy or radiotherapy may have low blood counts, which need correction before surgery.

CRITICAL TO REMEMBER

Clients undergoing a palliative surgical procedure must have their pain assessed from the perspective of normal postoperative pain in addition to pain secondary to tumor invasion.

Unfortunately, the current insurance-driven practices of shortened hospital stays leave little time for preoperative assessment of clients' psychological equilibrium. It is critical, however, that nurses preoperatively evaluate clients' understanding of the proposed surgery and the changes it involves.

Radiation Therapy

One half of all clients with cancer receive RT at some point during their disease course. RT may be used as a primary, adjuvant, or palliative treatment modality. As a primary treatment modality, RT is the only treatment used and provides local cure of the cancer (e.g., early-stage Hodgkin's disease). In the adjuvant setting, RT can be used either preoperatively or postoperatively to aid in the destruction of cancer cells. In addition, it can be used in conjunction with chemotherapy to treat disease in sites not readily accessible to systemic chemotherapy, such as the brain. Chemotherapy also can be combined with RT and is administered before the RT dose in an attempt to potentiate the effects of RT. RT also can be used as a palliative treatment modality to relieve pain caused by obstruction, pathologic fractures, spinal cord compression, and metastasis.

HOW RADIATION THERAPY WORKS (RADIOBIOLOGY)

RT is the use of high-energy ionizing rays that destroy the cell's ability to reproduce by damaging the cell's deoxyribonucleic acid (DNA). Rapidly dividing cells, such as some cancer cells, are more vulnerable to radiation than are slower dividing cells. Furthermore, normal cells have a greater ability than cancer cells to repair the DNA damage from radiation.

TYPES OF RADIATION THERAPY

RT can be administered from a variety of sources. Sources can be divided into those used outside the body (external RT) and those used inside the body (internal RT).

External Radiation Therapy. External RT is usually administered by high-energy x-ray machines (e.g., the betatron and linear accelerator) or machines containing a radioisotope (cobalt 60).

The major advantage of the high-energy x-ray machines is their skin-sparing effect. This means that the maximum effect of radiation occurs within the tumor deep in the body and not on the skin surface.

Neutron beam therapy delivered from a cyclotron particle accelerator is currently used to treat many types of cancers, including salivary gland tumors, sarcomas, and tumors of the prostate and lung.

Internal Radiation Therapy. Internal RT involves the placement of specially prepared radioisotopes directly into or near the tumor itself or into the systemic circulation. The two major types of internal RT are the sealed source, in which the radioactive material is enclosed in a sealed container, and the unsealed source, in which the radioactive material is administered systemically, such as by injection or orally. Sealed-source RT includes intracavity and interstitial therapy. Unsealed sources are used in systemic therapy.

FACTORS THAT DETERMINE SIDE EFFECTS OF RADIATION THERAPY

Several factors determine the side effects of RT, including the following:

- Size of the treatment field (A higher dose is tolerated if the treated area is small.)
- Area of the body exposed (Areas are affected differently by radiation.)
- Total dose administered.

In general, skin toxicities, fatigue, and anorexia may occur with RT to any site, whereas other side effects occur only when specific areas are involved in the treatment field (Box 7–1).

The goal of RT is to destroy the malignant tumor without harming the surrounding tissues. Several factors help achieve this goal. Fractionation refers to dividing the total radiation dose into small, frequent doses. A common dosage schedule for external radiation therapy is 150 to 200 cGy, 5 days per week for a total of 4 to 5 weeks. Fractionation increases the probability that tumor cells will be in a vulnerable phase of the cell cycle when treated. Fractionation also allows normal cells time to repair themselves.

Another way in which normal cells are spared is to alternate the sites of entry (ports) of radiation. For example, radiation for cervical cancer can be directed at the cervix through the front, back, and sides of the body. The maximum effect of the radiation beam is on the cervix, with the normal tissues receiving only a portion of the total dose. Additionally, customized shielding "blocks" may be created to protect normal tissues from ionizing rays.

BOX 7–1

Side Effects of Radiation

AREA OF THE BODY	EFFECT
Head and neck	Irritation of the mucous membranes, stomatitis Oral pain and infection Loss of taste Increased intracranial pressure
Skin	Change in color or texture, alopecia (usually temporary)
Chest	Inflammation, infection, tissue destruction
Abdomen	Anorexia, nausea, vomiting, diarrhea
Pelvis	Cystitis, urethral and rectal stenosis, diarrhea, sexual dysfunction
Blood	Bone marrow depression, anemia, leukopenia, compromised immune function, thrombocytopenia
General	Fatigue

ROLE OF RADIATION IN CANCER RESEARCH

Radiation is a vital area in medical research. Radioactive isotopes are being attached to monoclonal and polyclonal antibodies to treat certain tumors on an investigational basis.[4, 11] Intraoperative radiation is being used in several centers in the United States in an attempt to deliver a high dose of radiation directly to the tumor, with little damage to normal structures in the beam pathway.[10]

Another area of research involves the use of hyperthermia with RT.

Hyperthermia can be provided locally, regionally, or to the entire body. Local hyperthermia is usually generated with electromagnetic coupling or ultrasonography. Regional hyperthermia may involve perfusion with heated solutions. Whole-body hyperthermia can be accomplished by placing clients in a heated enclosure, such as a heated water tank or a water-heated space suit. Studies involving hyperthermia continue and may prove to potentiate the efficacy of radiation therapy significantly.[62]

In addition, the use of radiosensitizers and radioprotectors is being explored. Radiosensitizers and radioprotectors are chemical compounds that may be used to change the effect of radiation on cells and tissues.[63]

RADIATION SAFETY

Three key principles to follow to protect nurses and others from excessive radiation exposure are distance, time, and shielding.

Distance. The greater the distance maintained from the radiation source, the less is the exposure to ionizing rays. Distance and radiation exposure are inversely related. Thus, as the square of the distance from the source increases, the intensity of radiation decreases. For example, if a person stands 4 feet away from a source of radiation, the person is exposed to approximately one fourth the amount of radiation the person would receive at 2 feet (Fig. 7–1).

Time. The less time spent close to the radiation source, the less is the amount of radiation exposure. Minimal exposure time should be promoted, although client care needs must still be met. A nurse's exposure time is generally limited to 30 minutes of direct care per 8-hour shift.[24]

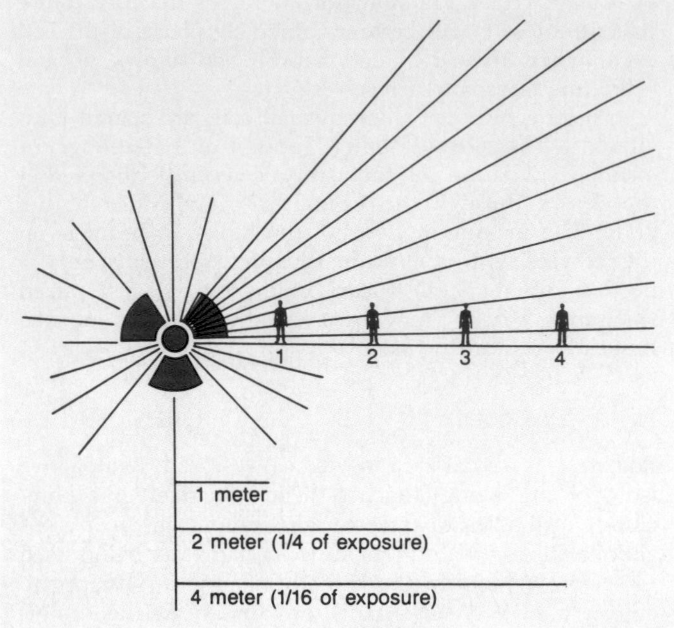

Figure 7–1
Radiation safety. (From Sedhom, L. N., & Yann, M. I. Y. [1985]. Radiation therapy and nurses' fears of radiation exposure. *Cancer Nursing, 8,* 129–134.)

Shielding. The choice of whether or not to use shielding devices to decrease exposure depends on the source of radiation. X-rays and gamma rays are blocked as the thickness of the lead shield increases. Individuals routinely working with x-rays or gamma rays wear lead gloves or aprons in situations that present the risk of exposure.

Radiation Safety Standards. The U.S. Nuclear Regulatory Commission requires that radiation exposure be kept as low as reasonably achievable.[61] All institutions using radioactive materials must have written policies concerning radiation protection. In addition, a radiation safety officer who is licensed by the U.S. Atomic Energy Commission to work with radioactive materials must be available at all institutions using radioactive materials.

Monitoring devices such as a film badge are required by law and provide a record of an individual's exposure.[25] Film badges should not be shared. The film badge provides a measure of whole-body exposure.

Nursing Management

The general precautions listed earlier apply to all forms of internal RT, both sealed and unsealed sources. However, because sealed and unsealed sources differ from each other in certain respects, each type requires additional precautionary measures for safe use.

Sealed Sources. Sealed sources of internal radiation differ from unsealed sources in that the radioisotope is completely enclosed by nonradioactive material.

CRITICAL TO REMEMBER

The radioisotope cannot circulate through the client's body, nor can it contaminate urine, sweat, blood, or vomitus.

Consequently, excretions are not radioactive. However, radiation exposure can result from direct contact with the sealed radioisotope, such as touching the container with bare hands or from lengthy exposure. Afterloading devices have been developed in which an empty applicator (the product that holds the radiation source) is placed during the operative procedure, and the radioactive source is not loaded until clients return to the hospital room. The radioactive source can then be automatically removed each time entry by health-care personnel is necessary. Thus, the use of afterloading devices has helped to decrease exposure. Clients with radioactive implants require a private room and bath. Client rooms at the ends of halls or stairwells may be designated for use because their location provides a decreased chance of exposure to others. Institutions with a high volume of radiation implants may have specially designed rooms with lead-shielded walls.

A lead container and a pair of long-handled forceps should always be present in a client's room. If the source becomes dislodged from the client, forceps should be used to pick up the source, which should then be placed immediately in the lead container. Generally, the radiation therapist and the radiation safety officer are notified immediately of the situation.[5]

Unsealed Sources. Unsealed sources used for internal radiation therapy are colloid suspensions and come into direct contact with body tissues. Unsealed sources are given intravenously, orally, or by instillation directly into a body cavity. Because the source is not encased in a protective container, a potential contamination hazard exists. The isotope may be excreted in any body fluid. Clients are instructed to flush the toilet several times after each use for several days, depending on the radiation source used.[10]

Table 7–1 summarizes radiation safety precautions. Nurses use these guidelines for their own protection as well as for the protection of other staff and visitors. Clients receiving internal radiation therapy should be taught about the precautions that must be followed and why they are necessary.

Alterations in skin integrity are a common side effect of radiation therapy. The nurse should teach the client to keep the skin dry and avoid the use of topical skin products (lotions, creams, deodorants, astringents, etc.). The client should maintain an intact skin surface by avoiding damage to skin surfaces caused by razors, tight fitting garments, and inadvertent contact with sharp or blunt objects. The client may be taught to use corn starch to help maintain dryness and decrease friction and to apply a thin coating of A & D ointment. The client should avoid exposure to direct sunlight by wearing protective clothing. If the skin is marked for the course of radiation, the client should be taught not to remove the markings. Radiation therapy and chemo-

TABLE 7–1 Safety Precautions and Rationales for the Care of the Client Receiving Radiation

SAFETY PRECAUTION	RATIONALE
Place the client in a private room.	This prevents undue exposure to other clients and to nurses caring for these clients.
Plan care well so minimal time is spent in direct contact with client with implant.	The nurse should not spend more than ½ hour per shift with the client to limit amount of radiation exposure. Plan care well in advance, change linens less frequently, prepare meal trays outside the room, and work as quickly as possible. If client can get up, have him or her sit as far as possible from bed while the nurse changes the linen. The nurse can spend more time with the client at a distance of 20 feet, where exposure will be minimal.
Provide care for client standing at client's shoulder (for cervical implants) or at foot of bed (for head and neck implants), avoiding any close contact with unshielded areas.	The client's body will provide increased shielding for the nurse.
If contact or care of unshielded area is prolonged, use lead aprons or lead shield.	Lead will decrease radiation exposure to the nurse.
Never care for more than one client with a radiation implant at the same time.	Caring for more than one client with an implant could expose the nurse to unnecessarily high amounts of radiation.
All health-care personnel should wear appropriate monitoring devices.	Records must be kept to monitor the exact amount of radiation exposure for each person in contact with the client. If any one employee is receiving too high an amount, this person should not be assigned to care for radiation clients for a while.
The room should be marked with appropriate signs stating the presence of radiation. The care plan should also be appropriately marked, and a sign should be posted in the room.	All personnel (and visitors) should be adequately warned of the presence of radiation so that undue exposure does not occur.
Carefully check all linens or other materials removed from the bed for the presence of foreign bodies.	If the client has excessive drainage requiring frequent linen changes, the linen may be examined with a Geiger counter to be certain no portion of the implant is lost. Careless discarding of the linens could lead to unnecessary exposure of personnel to radiation.
Keep long-handle forceps and a lead-lined container available on the nursing unit or in the client's room while the implant is in place.	In case of accidental dislodgement of implant, use long-handled forceps to pick up implant and place it in the lead-lined container. Notify radiation therapy department immediately.

therapy have many side effects in common: fatigue, nausea and vomiting, anorexia and altered taste sensation, alterations in oral mucosa, alterations in skin integrity, alopecia, diarrhea, and bone marrow depression. Some side effects correlate with the specific organ being irradiated. See the discussion following Chemotherapy.

Chemotherapy

DRUG DEVELOPMENT AND CLINICAL TRIALS

The National Cancer Institute methodically screens 50,000 compounds each year, of which only a few become commercially available. First, pharmacologic studies are carried out in the laboratory. If these experiments demonstrate antitumor activity and the absence of prohibitive toxicity, the drug advances to supervised clinical trials in humans.

Nursing responsibilities associated with caring for a client participating in a clinical trial include documentation of treatment benefits and side effects, anticipation of adverse reactions and early recognition of toxicity, management of side effects, preparation for diagnostic procedures, and client education. Important questions clients should ask when considering participation in a clinical trial are described in the client education pamphlet prepared by the National Cancer Institute.[43]

OBJECTIVES OF CHEMOTHERAPY

The objective of cancer chemotherapy is to destroy all malignant tumor cells without excessive destruction of normal cells. Chemotherapy is a systemic intervention and is appropriate when disease is widespread or when the risk of undetectable disease is high.

Chemotherapy leads to a cure for many clients with cancer. Guidelines for treating curable cancers stress early aggressive therapy. Another important use of chemotherapy is to control tumor growth when a cure is not possible. Chemotherapy may also be given for palliation (alleviation of symptoms such as pain or obstructions) without curing the underlying disease. Many clients with cancer have benefited from an extended lifespan and an improved quality of life as a result of chemotherapy.

In recent years, chemotherapeutic agents have come into use as adjuvant therapy. This means that, after initial treatment with either surgery or radiotherapy, medications are used to eliminate any remaining cancer cells.

BOX 7–2

Chemoresponsiveness of Selected Tumors

CURES IN ADVANCED CANCERS

- Gestational trophoblastic tumors
- Acute lymphoblastic leukemia (children)
- Acute lymphoblastic leukemia (adults)
- Acute myeloblastic leukemia
- Non-Hodgkin's lymphoma (children)
- Diffuse large cell lymphoma
- Hodgkin's disease
- Burkitt's lymphoma
- Testicular tumors

CURES WITH ADJUVANT CHEMOTHERAPY

- Wilms' tumor
- Osteogenic sarcoma
- Rhabdomyosarcoma

MINOR RESPONSES WITH CHEMOTHERAPY/ADJUVANT CHEMOTHERAPY, NO DEMONSTRABLE PROLONGATION OF LIFE

- Non-small cell lung cancer
- Head and neck cancer
- Large bowel cancer
- Cancer of the adrenal cortex
- Soft tissue sarcoma
- Stomach cancer
- Pancreatic cancer
- Liver cancer
- Cervical cancer
- Melanoma

COMPLETE AND PARTIAL REMISSIONS WITH UNCERTAIN PROLONGATION OF SURVIVAL WITH CHEMOTHERAPY/ADJUVANT CHEMOTHERAPY

- Multiple myeloma
- Ovarian cancer
- Endometrial cancer
- Neuroblastoma

COMPLETE REMISSIONS WITH INCREASED SURVIVAL WITH CHEMOTHERAPY/ADJUVANT CHEMOTHERAPY

- Small cell carcinoma of the lung
- Acute myeloblastic leukemia
- Non-Hodgkin's lymphoma, indolent
- Chronic granulocytic leukemia
- Breast cancer
- Prostate cancer
- Hairy cell leukemia

From Krakoff, I. H. (1991). Cancer chemotherapeutic and biologic agents. *Ca: A Journal for Clinicians, 41,* 265–266. Reprinted with permission.

Significant advances in the field of chemotherapy have been made in the last 30 years. Twelve types of cancer are now considered curable with chemotherapy, even in advanced stages.[34] Unfortunately, these 12 tumors account for only about 10 per cent of all cancers. The chemosensitivity of specific neoplasms is summarized in Box 7–2. See Table 7–2 for a discussion of antineoplastics.

BASIS OF ACTION OF CHEMOTHERAPY

The phases of mitosis are common to all cells. Normally, cells respond to the body's need for growth, repair, or regeneration in an orderly manner and cease production by entering a resting phase or slowing growth when the need is met. At any given time, normal cells may be found in all phases of growth. Cancer cells reproduce in the same manner as normal cells. However, growth occurs in an uncontrolled manner. In general, cells that are actively dividing are the most sensitive to chemotherapy.

Only a percentage of cancer cells will be killed with each course of chemotherapy. Repeated doses of chemotherapy, therefore, must be used.

The use of medications in combination, known as combination chemotherapy, has been consistently far superior to single-agent therapy.[34, 35] When combined, medications destroy malignant cells more effectively and produce fewer side effects. Combination chemotherapy is now the standard, and the regimens are complex and cyclic. An example of a chemotherapy regimen for Hodgkin's disease is shown in Table 7–3.

CLASSIFICATION OF CHEMOTHERAPY

Chemotherapeutic agents generally are classified according to their pharmacologic action and effect on the cell generation cycle. However, the method by which cancer cells are inhibited or destroyed is not always known. Common chemotherapeutic drugs are classified in Box 7–3.

ADMINISTRATION OF CHEMOTHERAPY

Depending on the clinical setting, chemotherapy may be administered by the physician, staff nurse, or specialized team member, such as the oncology clinical nurse specialist or intravenous therapist. Only adequately prepared registered professional nurses who are skilled in administering chemotherapy should assume responsibility for its administration to ensure quality of client care and maintain the highest standards of client and personnel safety.[46]

Safe Preparation, Handling, and Disposal. The safe administration and disposal of chemotherapeutic agents are controversial. Although evidence suggests that these agents may be carcinogenic, no valid and reliable studies have verified the risks of exposure to the health-care provider.

TABLE 7–2 Antineoplastics

CLASS	EXAMPLE	ACTION	USE	COMMON SIDE EFFECTS	NURSING IMPLICATIONS
Alkylating agents	Cyclophosphamide (Cytoxan)	Wide variety of drugs that act to destroy rapidly dividing cells; classified as cell-cycle specific (those that attack cells at a specific point in the process of cell division) or cell-cycle nonspecific (those that act at any time during cell division)	To treat a wide variety of cancers including leukemia, lymphoma, multiple myeloma, breast, lung, ovarian	Bone marrow depression in 7–14 days, nausea and vomiting, anorexia, alopecia, hemorrhagic cystitis, amenorrhea, sterility	Monitor blood counts closely; teach client safety precautions about low blood counts; use antiemetics preventively; increase fluid intake; administer IV slowly
	Cisplatin (Platinol)		To treat testicular, lung, ovarian, head and neck cancer	Severe nausea and vomiting, anorexia, nephrotoxicity, peripheral neuropathy, ototoxicity, moderate bone marrow depression at 14–21 days with high-dose therapy, potassium and magnesium wasting, hypersensitivity	Hydrate well with IV fluids and mannitol before therapy; monitor hearing; assess motor and sensory function; check weight daily; use antiemetics preventively; monitor for allergic reactions; monitor renal function, potassium, magnesium, and CBC
Antimetabolites	Methotrexate (Mexate)		To treat leukemia, lymphoma, ovarian, breast	Gastrointestinal ulceration, severe stomatitis, bone marrow depression in 10–14 days, nephrotoxicity, diarrhea, hepatotoxicity, pulmonary toxicity, neurological symptoms with intrathecal use, photosensitivity	With high-dose therapy, give leucovorin to prevent toxicity, hydrate well, and maintain alkaline urine; monitor CBC and renal function closely; oral hygiene and comfort measures; avoid sun exposure, use sunblock
Antibiotics	Doxorubicin (Adriamycin)		To treat breast, lung, head and neck, pancreas, soft-tissue sarcoma, ovarian	Bone marrow depression in 10–14 days, severe tissue necrosis with extravasation, nausea and vomiting, anorexia, cardiotoxicity, alopecia, stomatitis, diarrhea, red discoloration of urine	Avoid extravasation; monitor cardiovascular function; warn about red urine; provide antiemetic therapy; warn about alopecia; monitor CBC; treat stomatitis
Plant alkaloids	Vincristine (Oncovin)		To treat testicular, neuroblastoma, leukemia, lymphoma, breast, lung, multiple myeloma	Neurotoxicity, constipation, peripheral neuropathies, abdominal pain, rare and mild bone marrow depression, alopecia, tissue necrosis with extravasation	Monitor for sensory or motor changes; administer stool softeners; avoid extravasation; observe for neurotoxicity; administer IV slowly

Table continued on following page

TABLE 7–2 Antineoplastics (*Continued*)

CLASS	EXAMPLE	ACTION	USE	COMMON SIDE EFFECTS	NURSING IMPLICATIONS
Hormones: Androgens	Testosterone propionate	Growth of certain tumors (breast, thyroid, prostate, uterine) depends on specific hormonal environment; altering this environment impairs/arrests tumor growth	Replacement therapy for males; to treat dysmenorrhea and menopause in women; to treat inoperable breast cancer in women	Males: impotence, gynecomastia, epididymitis, bladder irritation; females; hirsutism, amenorrhea, masculinization; both: nausea and vomiting, fluid retention, hypercalcemia with bone metastases	Warn about possible changes in sexual characteristics; use with caution in patients on oral anticoagulants; monitor input and output; check for edema; monitor calcium levels
Antiandrogens	Flutamide (Eulexin)	Antagonizes androgen effects at cellular level; decreases growth in androgen-sensitive tumor	To treat metastatic prostate cancer; used with leuprolide	Diarrhea, nausea, vomiting, loss of libido, impotence, gynecomastia, hot flashes, edema, hypertension	Monitor for gastrointestinal effects, warn about side effects concerning sexuality; encourage compliance
Estrogens	Diethylstilbestrol (DES)		Postmenopausal syndrome, amenorrhea due to ovarian failure, suppression of lactation; prostatic cancer; breast cancer	Nausea and vomiting, anorexia, abdominal distension and bloating, spotting, menstrual changes, fluid retention, depression, hypercalcemia, migraines, breast tenderness and enlargement, reduced glucose tolerance, possible uterine cancer, thromboemboli, increased incidence of cardiovascular-associated deaths; males: similar but also development of female secondary sexual characteristics, impotence, loss of libido	Contraindicated in pregnancy, some breast cancers, thrombophlebitis, thyroid and liver disease; use cautiously in clients with hypertension, migraines, diabetes, and asthma; monitor for edema and congestive heart failure; watch for depression; monitor serum calcium; counsel about sexual dysfunction
Anti-estrogens	Tamoxifen (Nolvadex)		To treat estrogen receptor positive breast cancer	Rare transient bone marrow depression, nausea, menstrual irregularity, hot flashes, "flare" reaction (bone and tumor pain), hypercalcemia in women with bone metastases, induces ovulation in premenopausal women	Monitor menstrual function; advise premenopausal women to use birth control; monitor serum calcium level; reassure that flare reaction will subside (not an indication of disease progression; rather of drug effectiveness)
Synthetic luteinizing hormone	Leuprolide (Lupron)	Lowers testosterone level with continuous use	To treat advanced prostate cancer; used with flutamide; used in clients who cannot tolerate an orchiectomy or estrogen therapy	Dizziness, headache, decreased libido, impotence, anorexia, increased bone pain, hot flashes, paresthesias	Monitor for increase in bone pain; with vertebral metastasis, watch for loss of function; monitor acid phosphatase for response to therapy; teach client about side effects

TABLE 7–2 Antineoplastics *(Continued)*

CLASS	EXAMPLE	ACTION	USE	COMMON SIDE EFFECTS	NURSING IMPLICATIONS
Miscellaneous antineoplastic	Paclitaxel (Taxol)	Inhibits microtubular function, causing cell death	To treat metastatic breast and ovarian cancer	Bone marrow depression at 11 days, hypersensitivity reactions, peripheral neuropathy, nausea and vomiting	Monitor blood counts closely; teach clients about low blood counts; monitor for hypersensitivity reactions (dyspnea, urticaria); severe reactions may occur in the first hour of treatment; use antiemetics preventively

CBC, complete blood count; IV, intravenous dose.
Modified from Matasserin-Jacobs, E. (1994). Saunders Review for NCLEX-RN (2nd ed.). Philadelphia: W. B. Saunders Co.

Undue exposure to antineoplastic drugs can occur from three major routes: (1) inhalation of aerosols, (2) absorption through the skin, and (3) ingestion of contaminated materials.[21] Several organizations including the U.S. Occupational Safety and Health Administration, the National Study Commission on Cytotoxic Exposure, and the Oncology Nursing Society have prepared guidelines for the safe preparation, handling, and disposal of antineoplastics.[44–46] The use of gloves and gowns during preparation and administration and the use of a Biologic Safety Cabinet for drug preparation are included in these guidelines.

Antineoplastic agents and their metabolites are found in the excreta and body fluids of clients undergoing chemotherapy. For this reason, it is recommended that gloves and disposable gowns be worn when handling body secretions such as blood, vomitus, or excreta from clients who have received chemotherapy within the previous 48 hours.[46]

CHEMOTHERAPY ADMINISTRATION ROUTES

Appropriate routes of medication administration are determined by the properties of the medication and the purpose of the therapy. Some agents may be safely administered by a variety of routes. Therapy may be systemic or local.

TABLE 7–3 MOPP Regimen

DRUG	REGIMEN
M = Nitrogen mustard	6.0 mg/m² IV, days 1 and 8
O = Oncovin	1.4 mg/m² IV, days 1 and 8
P = Procarbazine	100.0 mg/m² PO, days 1–14
P = Prednisone	40.0 mg/m² PO, days 1–14

Repeat cycle every 28 days for a minimum of 6 cycles.
IV, intravenously; PO, orally.

Intravenous Routes

Peripheral Access. Large veins in the forearm are the preferred peripheral access sites. Avoid areas of impaired lymphatic drainage, phlebitis, invading neoplasm, hematoma, inflamed or sclerosing areas, areas of impaired venous circulation, the lower extremities, and sites distal to a recent venipuncture site.

Vascular Access. Vascular access devices (VADs) are placed in clients with poor venous access. Because chemotherapy regimens are complex and supportive care is extensive, they are used during the initial treatment of clients with leukemia and in those requiring continuous chemotherapy, total parenteral nutrition, multiple access, parenteral fluids and antibiotics, and frequent blood draws.

These catheters are usually inserted into one of the major veins of the upper chest. The brachial or cephalic vein in the forearm is used for nontunneled peripheral access devices. The distal catheter tip is advanced to the level of the superior vena cava at or above the junction of the right atrium. Proper catheter tip placement is confirmed by fluoroscopy or radiography.

The most frequently reported complications are infection and catheter occlusion. The prevention of VAD infections centers on catheter care, daily assessment for signs and symptoms of infection, and client education. Intraluminal occlusion may occur secondary to a blood clot or precipitate. Prevention strategies include proper flushing, vigilance for drug incompatibilities, and adherence to proper drug dilutions. Procedures for the care and maintenance of VADs vary with each clinical setting. Nursing management strategies for VADs are extensively described elsewhere.[47, 69]

Extravasation Management. Careful assessment of the intravenous site is required during and after the infusion of antineoplastic agents because some agents have the potential to cause tissue damage if extravasated (infiltrated). Criteria to determine whether or not an extravasation is present include pain, erythema, swelling, and lack of a blood return.

BOX 7-3

Classification of Chemotherapy

ALKYLATING AGENTS

- Busulfan (Myleran)
- Chlorambucil (Leukeran)
- Cyclophosphamide (Cytoxan)
- Cisplatin (Platinol)
- Carboplatin (Paraplatin)
- Ifosfamide (Ifex)
- Mechlorethamine (Mustargen)
- Melphalan (L-PAM, Alkeran)
- Thiotepa

ANTIMETABOLITES

- Cytarabine (Ara-C, Cytosar)
- Methotrexate
- 5-Azacytidine
- 5-Fluorouracil (5-FU)
- Floxuridine (FUDR)
- 6-Mercaptopurine (6-MP)
- 6-Thioguanine (6-TG)
- Hydroxyurea (Hydrea)

ANTITUMOR ANTIBIOTICS

- Bleomycin (Blenoxane)
- Dactinomycin (actinomycin-D)
- Daunorubicin (Daunomycin)
- Doxorubicin (Adriamycin)
- Mitomycin C (Mutamycin)
- Mitoxantrone (Novantrone)
- Plicamycin (mithramycin)

NITROSUREAS

- Carmustine (BCNU)
- Lomustine (CCNU)
- Semustine (methyl-CCNU)
- Streptozocin (Zanosar)

VINCA (PLANT) ALKALOIDS

- Vinblastine (Velban)
- Vincristine (Oncovin)
- VP-16 (etoposide, VePesid)
- VM-26 (teniposide)
- Vindesine (Eldisine)

STEROIDS AND HORMONES

Androgen

- Testosterone propionate
- Fluoxymesterone (Halotestin)
- Testolactone (Teslac)
- Methyltestosterone

Estrogen

- Diethylstibestrol (DES)
- Ethinyl estradiol (Estinyl)

Antiestrogens

- Tamoxifen (Nolvadex)
- Leuprolide (Lupron)

Progestins

- Delalutin
- Megestrol (Megace)
- Medrocyprogesterone (Depo-Provera, Provera)

Adrenal Cortical Compounds

- Cortisone acetate
- Prednisone
- Dexamethasone (Decadron)
- Methylprednisolone sodium succinate (Solu-Medrol)
- Hydrocortisone sodium succinate (Solu-Cortef)

Antiadrenal

- Aminoglutethimide

MISCELLANEOUS AGENTS

- DTIC (dacarbazine)
- *m*AMSA
- Hexamethylmelamine (HXM)
- L-Asparaginase (Elspar)
- Procarbazine hydrochloride (Matulane)
- Paclitaxel (Taxol)

Data from Chabner, B. A., & Myers, C. E. (1989). Clinical pharmacology of cancer chemotherapy. In V. T. DeVita, S. Hellman, & S. A. Rosenberg (Eds.), *Cancer: Principles and practice of oncology* (3rd ed.). Philadelphia: J. B. Lippincott; Krakoff, I. H. (1991). Cancer chemotherapeutic and biologic agents. *Ca: A Journal for Clinicians, 41,* 270–276.

Procedures for management of extravasation are controversial and unique to each clinical setting. Institutionally approved guidelines for the management of extravasation should be readily available.

Less Common Administration Routes. Regional chemotherapy allows high concentrations of chemotherapy to be directed to localized tumors. Methods of regional administration include topical, intrathecal, intracavitary, and intra-arterial chemotherapy.

Most medications given systemically are not effective against central nervous system (CNS) tumors because they cannot cross the blood-brain barrier. The physician may instill chemotherapeutic agents into the CNS through a reservoir placed in the ventricle (Fig. 7–2) or via a lumbar puncture.

HYPERSENSITIVITY REACTIONS TO CHEMOTHERAPY

Hypersensitivity reactions to chemotherapy, although rare, can be serious and life threatening. The antineoplastic agents commonly implicated in the development of immediate hypersensitivity reactions are L-asparaginase, cisplatin, and bleomycin.

The signs and symptoms of an immediate hypersensitivity reaction include dyspnea, chest tightness or

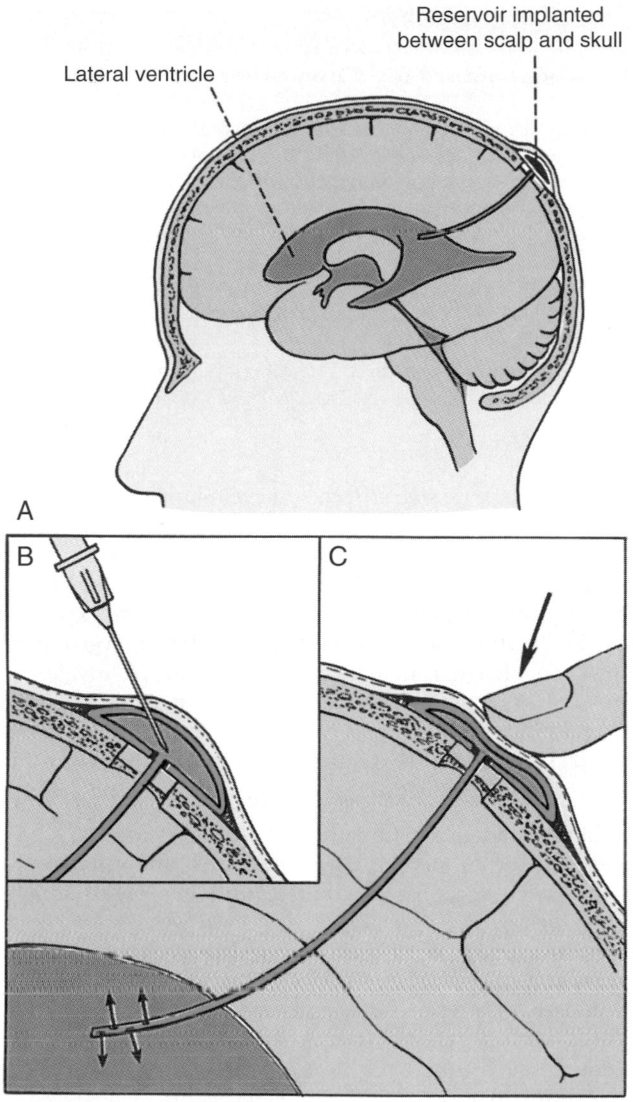

Figure 7–2
Omaya reservoir. *A,* Placement of Omaya reservoir in the ventricle. *B,* Injection of chemotherapeutic agent into the reservoir. *C,* Delivery of chemotherapeutic agent into the ventricle and into the cerebrospinal fluid. (Adapted from Ratcheson, R. A., & Omaya, A. [1968]. Experience with the subcutaneous cerebrospinal fluid reservoir. *New England Journal of Medicine, 279,* 1026. Reprinted by permission of The New England Journal of Medicine.)

pain, pruritus, urticaria, tachycardia, dizziness, anxiety, agitation, inability to speak, abdominal pain, nausea, hypotension, decreased sensorium, flushed appearance, and cyanosis.

CRITICAL TO REMEMBER

If an anaphylactic reaction is suspected, the nurse should immediately stop drug administration, maintain intravenous access with 0.9 per cent saline, and notify the physician.

Maintain the airway, and place the client in a supine position with the feet elevated unless contraindicated. Monitor the client's vital signs every 2 minutes until he or she is stable. Administer epinephrine, aminophylline, diphenhydramine, and corticosteroids on the basis of the physician's orders.

OUTPATIENT CHEMOTHERAPY ADMINISTRATION

Aggressive, complex, and sophisticated cancer therapies are currently delivered in ambulatory, office, and home care settings. This shift in the provision of services from the traditional hospital setting is a result of cost-containment efforts, consumerism, advanced technology, competition, and nursing competence.[73]

Different nursing challenges exist in outpatient settings. First, a high level of commitment is required from clients and care givers. Both require education regarding complex treatment regimens; identification, prevention, and treatment of symptoms experienced at home; the operation of medical equipment; and the care of a variety of VADs. Second, a mechanism for immediate access to health-care personnel is required. Finally, when chemotherapy is administered in the home setting, provisions must be made for the safe handling and disposal of cytotoxics to minimize client, family, and nurse exposure.

When the chemotherapeutic medication is obtained from the health-care facility, it should be labeled as cytotoxic, carefully capped and securely sealed, and packed in an impervious material for transportation.

When preparing the medication in the home for administration, the nurse should be sure to work in an area away from food and anywhere the family, particularly children, congregate. The area should be cleaned and covered with a plastic-backed pad. The nurse can then assemble all needed materials for the chemotherapy administration on this absorbent surface. The nurse should use the same precautions for administering the chemotherapy used in the hospital setting.

The waste materials can be disposed of in biohazard containers obtained from medical supply companies, or empty coffee cans with reinforced lids can be used for sharp instruments. All empty containers and tubing should be placed in sealable plastic bags with appropriate labels and disposed of properly.

If a spill occurs in the home, the nurse should wear a protective gown, gloves, and goggles to clean it up. The area should be wiped completely with disposable absorbent towels and then washed three times with detergent and rinsed. All materials used should be placed in sealable plastic bags and disposed of as hazardous waste.

The client may excrete the chemotherapeutic agents for 48 hours after administration. Blood, emesis, and excreta may be considered contaminated during this time. The client should not share a bathroom with children or pregnant women during this time. Any contaminated linens or clothing should be washed separately and then can be washed a second time with the rest of the laundry. All contaminated disposable items should be sealed in plastic bags and disposed of as hazardous waste.

TOXIC EFFECTS OF CHEMOTHERAPY

Antineoplastic medications are capable of damaging and destroying not only malignant cells but also certain normal cells. Normal cells most vulnerable to antineoplastic medications are those that divide and proliferate rapidly, specifically cells of the bone marrow, hair, and mucosa. Damage to these cells can result in myelosuppression, alopecia, oral mucositis, and diarrhea. In addition to these effects on proliferative cells, drugs may exert organ-specific toxicities resulting in cardiac, renal, pulmonary, hepatic, reproductive, and neurologic dysfunction. A summary of the many potential side effects and toxicities of antineoplastic agents is found in Box 7–4.

Side effects are evaluated or graded according to the degree of severity. Mild to moderate side effects generally do not warrant discontinuing the drug or decreasing the dose. More severe or unexpected toxicities require careful evaluation and dose reduction. Risk factors for the development of toxicities are listed in Box 7–5.

The onset of side effects of chemotherapy may be acute or delayed. Acute toxicities tend to occur in tissues composed of rapidly dividing cells, are frequently intermittent in nature, and generally resolve with complete recovery; in contrast, late effects tend to occur in different tissues and may produce life-long problems.[62] Clients and all health-care providers must be aware of, monitor for, and report side effects. A discussion of the more common acute side effects of chemotherapy follows.

BOX 7–4

Systemic Chemotherapeutic Effects

Gastrointestinal: nausea and vomiting, constipation, anorexia, stomatitis, esophagitis, taste alterations, diarrhea, weight loss, pharyngitis
Integumentary: dermatitis, alopecia, perianal ulcers, vulvular ulcers, hyperpigmentation, photosensitivity, nail changes
Hematopoietic: anemia, thrombocytopenia, neutropenia
Genitourinary: nephrotoxicity, urine color change, hemorrhagic cystitis, hyperuricemic nephropathy
Hepatic: hepatotoxicity, cirrhosis, hepatic fibrosis, portal hypotension
Reproductive: amenorrhea, sterility, loss of libido, impotence, azoospermia, gonadal dysfunction, menopausal symptoms, irregular menses, gynecomastia, oligospermia
Cardiac: electrocardiographic changes, arrhythmias, cardiomyopathy, chronic heart failure, tachycardia
Pulmonary: pneumonitis, pulmonary fibrosis
Metabolic: tumor lysis syndrome
Neurologic: ototoxicity, subacute meningeal irritation, peripheral neuropathy, cranial nerve neuropathy, autonomic neuropathy, cerebellar toxicity

Data from Hydzik, C. A. (1990). Late effects of chemotherapy: Implications for patient management and rehabilitation. *Nursing Clinics of North America, 25,* 423; and Ruccione, K., & Weinberg, K. (1989). Late effects in multiple body systems. *Seminars in Oncology Nursing, 5,* 4.

BOX 7–5

Risk Factors for Chemotherapy Toxicity

- Drug dose, route, method of administration
- Extent of cancer and overall physical condition
- Prior chemotherapy or radiation therapy or both
- Concomitant organ dysfunction or illness
- Age
- Nutritional status
- Self-care behavior
- Combination versus single-agent therapy

Adapted from Goodman, M. S. (1989). Managing the side effects of chemotherapy. *Seminars in Oncology Nursing, 5(2)(Suppl. 1),* 29.

Myelosuppressive Effects. Myelosuppression is one of the most common side effects of chemotherapeutic drugs. It is also one of the most lethal. Infection and bleeding as a result of diminished white cell and platelet production are two common causes of death in cancer clients. For this reason, complete blood counts must be checked before administration of myelosuppressive drugs and must be monitored periodically after drug administration.

It is essential that clients are taught measures to protect against infection:

- Maintain adequate nutrition and fluid intake.
- Avoid crowds, people with infections, and clients who have been recently vaccinated with live or attenuated vaccines.
- Avoid contact with animal excrement, such as bird, cat, and dog feces.
- Immediately report any signs and symptoms of infection, such as temperature greater than 38° C (100° F), cough, sore throat, chills or sweating, or frequent or painful urination.
- Maintain personal hygiene, especially hand washing.
- Get adequate rest and exercise.
- Avoid indiscriminate use of antipyretics because they can mask fever.

Because infections are associated with increased morbidity and mortality, infection must be treated promptly and aggressively in neutropenic clients. The development of fever in neutropenic clients should be treated as a medical emergency and mandates prompt assessment, diagnosis, and initiation of antibiotic therapy. Management includes culturing all suspected infection sites, use of protective isolation, and the administration of broad-spectrum antibiotics.

Thrombocytopenia increases the client's risk for bleeding. A high risk of hemorrhage exists when the platelet count is less than 20,000/mm^3. Fatal CNS hemorrhage or massive gastrointestinal hemorrhage can occur when the platelet count is less than 10,000/mm^3. Clients should be instructed to report

- Bleeding gums
- Increased bruising, petechiae, or purpura, especially on lower extremities
- Hypermenorrhea

- Tarry colored stools, blood in urine, coffee-ground emesis
- Hemoptysis
- Epistaxis

Clients should be taught to avoid the use of razors, aspirin and ibuprofen, and enemas and suppositories.

Controversy exists as to whether or not clients should receive prophylactic transfusions when platelet counts reach a certain level or emergent transfusions when bleeding is noted.[18] Platelet products include multiple or random donor, single donor, and human leukocyte antigen (HLA) matched.

Anemia may cause fatigue, headache, dizziness, fainting, pallor, dyspnea, palpitations, and tachycardia. Packed red cell transfusions may be required to relieve symptomatic anemia.

Gastrointestinal Effects. Gastrointestinal effects of chemotherapy include nausea and vomiting, anorexia, taste alteration, weight loss, oral mucositis, diarrhea, and constipation.

Nausea and vomiting are two of the most dreaded side effects of chemotherapy. Adequate control is an essential aspect of client compliance with chemotherapy. Uncontrolled nausea and vomiting can result in anorexia, malnutrition, dehydration, metabolic imbalances, psychological depression, and treatment noncompliance.[41]

Management of nausea and vomiting has greatly improved during the last decade because of heightened interest and research.

Three common patterns of nausea and vomiting have been described. Anticipatory nausea and vomiting occur before the administration of therapy. Acute, post-therapy nausea and vomiting occur within the first 24 hours after therapy. Delayed nausea and vomiting refer to symptoms that persist or develop 24 hours after chemotherapy.

Antiemetics are usually prescribed 6 to 12 hours before the administration of chemotherapy and are continued every 4 to 6 hours for at least 12 to 24 hours, or as long as the symptoms persist.[72] Specific drug combinations, doses, and schedules are described elsewhere.[26, 41] Ongoing evaluation is essential to find the most effective dose, schedule, and combination of drugs for each client.

Nonpharmacologic interventions include adjusting oral and fluid intake, relaxation, exercise, hypnosis, biofeedback, guided imagery, and systemic desensitization.[26]

Anorexia and weight loss occur as a result of the disease process as well as the treatment. The client with cancer is at risk for protein-calorie malnutrition. Many variables may alter the client's ability to ingest food via the oral route. Common problems that may interfere with oral intake include anorexia, nausea and vomiting, early satiety, taste alterations, dry mouth, stomatitis, esophagitis, viscous saliva, lactose intolerance, pain, diarrhea, and constipation.

When medically appropriate, the nurse should enhance oral nutrition by relaxing any dietary restrictions and emphasizing the need for a high-protein, high-calorie diet with fortification from either natural food sources or commercial supplements. The nurse should also monitor the client's nutritional status by daily calorie counts and assessment. If the nutritional requirements cannot be met orally, another method must be considered. Enteral feedings and total parenteral nutrition are two possibilities (see Chaps. 34 and 35 for a discussion of these alternate methods).

Stomatitis and oral mucositis are terms used to describe inflammation and ulceration of the mucosal lining of the mouth. Consequences of stomatitis include pain, decreased nutritional and fluid intake, and oral infections.

An oral hygiene program should start before therapy and continue throughout treatment. Dietary modifications during periods of stomatitis include avoiding extremely hot or cold foods, spices, and citrus juices; eating soft foods; and taking nutritional supplements.

Diarrhea is most often the result of antimetabolite drugs. A low-residue or liquid diet is usually advised. Electrolytes and intake and output should be carefully monitored. Scrupulous perineal hygiene is encouraged, especially in the neutropenic client. Antidiarrheals may be prescribed.

Constipation is frequently the result of Vinca alkaloid effects on bowel peristalsis. Other causes of constipation include narcotics, immobility, decreased fluid and bulk intake, tumor invasion of the gastrointestinal tract, and depression. Preventive measures include increasing fluid and bulk intake, administering stool softeners prophylactically, increasing activity, and administering laxatives when necessary.

Cutaneous Effects. Alopecia is a common side effect of many antineoplastic agents. The degree of hair loss depends on the specific drug, dosage, and method of administration. Alopecia is temporary, with regrowth often occurring before chemotherapy ends, although the hair color and texture may change.

A variety of skin reactions may occur in the client receiving chemotherapy, such as the following:

- Red patches (erythema) or hives (urticaria) at the drug injection site or on other body parts. These reactions generally disappear within several hours.
- Darkening of the skin (hyperpigmentation) in the nail beds and mouth, on the gums or teeth, or along the veins used for chemotherapy, or the condition may be generalized. Hyperpigmentation usually occurs 2 to 3 weeks after the administration of chemotherapy and continues for 10 to 12 weeks after therapy completion.
- Sensitivity to sunlight (photosensitivity). This may result in an acute sunburn after just a short exposure to the sun. The sensitivity disappears once treatment stops.
- Radiation recall. This skin reaction may occur in clients who received radiation therapy before the administration of chemotherapy. When chemotherapy is given several weeks or months later, a recall reaction occurs in the previously irradiated skin area. Skin effects range from redness, shedding, or peeling to blisters and oozing. After the skin heals, it is permanently darkened.[73]

Reproductive Effects. The effects of chemotherapy on gonadal function and reproductive capacity may be temporary or permanent. Azoospermia, oligospermia, and sterility have been documented in males. Amenorrhea, menopausal symptoms, and sterility have been noted in females.

However, not all clients experience these effects to the same degree. Preliminary studies suggest that the effects of chemotherapy on gonadal function vary with respect to the client's age at time of therapy, drugs administered, and total drug dosage.[2]

Although successful pregnancy outcomes have been reported, many physicians advise the use of birth control during cancer treatment and for up to 2 years after completion of treatment.

Pregnancies occurring after cytotoxic chemotherapy have about the same chance for successful outcomes as do normal pregnancies.[2] However, the genetic effects of chemotherapy may not be evident for several generations of offspring. Therefore, the unpredictability of the occurrence, degree, and duration of genetic damage should be discussed with the client and spouse or significant other.

Pretreatment sperm banking offers the possibility of retaining reproductive capacity for some clients.

Nursing Management

Assessment. A thorough client evaluation is necessary before cytotoxic drugs can be administered. By reviewing the client's medical history, the nurse can identify potential risk factors for chemotherapy toxicity, such as a history of impaired cardiac, pulmonary, or renal function. The severity and duration of side effects experienced since the previous course of therapy must be carefully assessed as well.

Abnormal laboratory values may indicate the development of organ-specific toxicities. Drug doses may be modified or delayed on the basis of these results.

The client's chart should have either a copy of the formal drug protocol or a written summary of the planned chemotherapy regimen. Chemotherapy doses are usually based on body surface area (square meters), which is determined by the client's height and weight. Clear and complete chemotherapy prescriptions include the name of the drug, dosage per square meter and total dose, administration route, administration rate for intravenous infusions, and frequency of administration. Plans for antiemetic coverage, hydration, diuresis, and electrolyte supplementation are frequently included as well.

CLIENT EDUCATION GUIDE

Side Effects of Chemotherapy

The nurse should

- Teach the client and significant others about common side effects for drugs the client is receiving. The client needs information to maintain comfort and safety, since many of the medications disrupt bodily functions and are potentially harmful.
- Explain the importance of diagnostic studies that monitor for side effects (which studies are needed, how often, and precautions to take).
- Teach about rapidly dividing (tumor) cells in the body and how antineoplastic agents affect them, causing side effects.

Common Side Effects	Implications for the Client
Signs of infection (increased temperature, sore throat, malaise). Infections may occur when white cell counts drop.	Avoid crowds and people with infections. Avoid any situation that increases exposure to infection. Clients with catheters and ports should be monitored closely.
Fatigue, lightheadedness, shortness of breath, and headache may be associated with anemia, a result of a low red cell count.	Pace activities to tolerance. Rest as frequently as needed. Follow through on prescribed therapy for replacement of red cells in the blood.
Bleeding problems because of a low platelet count.	Avoid the use of razors for shaving. Do not use aspirin or ibuprofen. Avoid the use of enemas and suppositories.
Alopecia (hair loss) occurs because of damage at the cellular level.	Suggest that women wear scarfs or hats; men, caps. Hair resumes growth when treatment is completed. Hair that grows back may be different in color and texture.
Alterations in oral mucosa are common. They may also occur during radiation therapy.	Frequent oral hygiene is needed. Maintain fluid intake for hydration of tissue. Suck on hard candy or ice chips. Changes in taste and solid food intake may occur. Avoid hot, spicy foods.
Nausea and vomiting, usually occur early in therapy and are most feared of expected side effects.	Use antiemetics preventively. They may be used alone or in combination with another medication. Use relaxation techniques and distraction (television, music, reading, etc.).
Anorexia may occur as a side effect of medication or the cancer itself.	Eat six small meals from all food groups. Use prescribed medications (e.g., corticosteroids) that stimulate appetite.
Diarrhea, a more common side effect than constipation.	Maintain hydration. Use antidiarrheals as prescribed.

- Explain that any body system may be affected by chemotherapy, and that the client should report all signs and symptoms of changes in body function to the physician.

Before administering antineoplastic agents, consult with the pharmacist and review chemotherapy drug handbooks and investigational drug protocols for detailed information regarding drug actions, dosages, administration guidelines, and potential side effects.

Client and Family Education. Client and family education about chemotherapy and the identification, prevention, and management of side effects are primarily nursing functions. (See Client Education Guide: Side Effects of Chemotherapy.)

Bone Marrow Transplantation

Bone marrow transplantation (BMT) is a unique treatment modality with the singular goal of cure. It is a complex therapy with a high potential for complications.

BMT allows the client to receive lethal and potentially more effective doses of chemotherapy and radiation therapy without regard to hematopoietic toxicity. The damaged bone marrow is replaced by healthy donor marrow.

There are three types of donor bone marrow: allogeneic, syngeneic, and autologous. An autologous BMT is the most common type of transplantation performed and is often referred to as a rescue. The marrow donor is also the recipient. The bone marrow is generally harvested during disease remission, may or may not be chemically treated, and is stored (frozen) to be reinfused later.

In an allogeneic BMT, the marrow donor is usually a sibling or parent with a similar HLA tissue type. In rare instances, an unrelated donor, found through the National Bone Marrow Registry or through a local tissue-typing drive, may be the donor.[65] A syngeneic BMT uses bone marrow from an identical twin.

Another type of BMT is the peripheral blood stem cell (PBSC) harvest. In a PBSC transplant, the client's peripheral blood stem cells are harvested by leukopheresis, processed, and stored. The client then receives lethal doses of chemotherapy, RT, or both and then the PBSCs are reinfused.

The transplant process consists of several phases: conditioning, harvest, marrow infusion, pre-engraftment, and engraftment. The time of the bone marrow harvest depends on the type of transplantation being performed. Conditioning refers to the immunosuppression treatment regimen (chemotherapy, RT, or both) used to eradicate all malignant cells, provide a state of immunosuppression, and create space in the bone marrow for the engraftment of the new marrow.

Marrow is usually infused 48 to 72 hours after the last dose of chemotherapy or RT. Potential side effects include fluid overload, development of micropulmonary emboli, and hypersensitivity reactions to the white cells present in the marrow.[66]

Once the marrow has been infused, the client starts an arduous upward battle. Potential complications include infection; bleeding; renal insufficiency; gastrointestinal effects; veno-occlusive disease (VOD), a condition in which the small veins of the liver become obstructed; and graft-versus-host disease. Management of these transplantation complications is beyond the scope of this chapter.[15]

Biologic Response Modifiers

The search to understand and manipulate the human immune system has fascinated scientists for decades. Evidence exists that, under the proper circumstances, malignant tumors are susceptible to immune surveillance and subsequent destruction. Thus, the quest to isolate and identify effective biologic agents continues.

Biologic response modifiers are defined as those agents that are capable of modifying the relationship between the tumor and the host by strengthening the host's immune function.

Those currently in use in the clinical setting include a variety of interleukins (ILs), including IL-1, IL-2, IL-3, and IL-4; interferon-α (IFN); monoclonal antibodies (MoAbs); tumor necrosis factor; and colony-stimulating factors (CSF), granulocyte-macrophage (GM-CSF), granulocyte (G-CSF), and erythropoietin (EPO). Several of these agents, such as G-CSF, GM-CSF, and EPO, have received U.S. Food and Drug Administration approval and are available on the market.

Interleukins are substances produced by lymphocytes that function to promote normal hematopoiesis. IL-2 is responsible for the growth of T cells, augments various other T-cell activities, and enhances natural killer cell function. Major toxicities reported with IL-2 therapy include an increased capillary permeability that may produce hypotension, ascites, pulmonary edema, and generalized weight gain.[33] Additionally, integumentary changes occur and may include generalized redness, rash, pruritus, and, occasionally, skin desquamation. Toxicities with IL-2 vary greatly with the dose of drug administered. Higher doses produce greater toxicities and require astute clinical management.

The IFNs are small proteins that have cellular activity in three areas: antiviral, immunomodulatory, and antiproliferative. Toxicities appear to be dose related, with lower doses of IFN exhibiting few side effects, whereas high doses may require therapy to be interrupted or stopped.[23] A flulike syndrome is a common side effect of IFN therapy. Premedication with acetaminophen and diphenhydramine assists in providing client comfort.

The MoAbs have the potential of providing the specificity now lacking in other types of treatment modalities. They can be used either diagnostically or therapeutically. Diagnostic use may include the early detection of cancer. Therapeutically, MoAbs may be used to deliver immunotoxins, such as ricin, chemotherapeutic agents, and radioactive isotopes directly to the tumor site.[11] To date, MoAbs have demonstrated limited success as a therapeutic option, and clinical trials continue for a variety of cancers.

Colony-stimulating factors are naturally occurring growth factors that mediate hematopoiesis.[22] G-CSF is administered by subcutaneous injection, intravenous short infusion, or intravenous continuous infusion daily, starting at least 24 hours after chemotherapy is completed. It is important to note that G-CSF (Neupogen) is not compatible with saline.

The most commonly reported side effect with G-CSF is bone pain, and the problem appears to occur more frequently in high doses administered intravenously. It is hypothesized that the bone pain is the result of the marrow expansion that occurs from the rapid increase in the neutrophil pool. Clients report pain in bone areas that have large marrow reserves, such as the pelvis, sternum, and long bones.

The agent GM-CSF can be administered by continuous intravenous infusion (over 2 hours) or by subcutaneous injection daily. GM-CSF (Leukine and Prokine) is not compatible with dextrose. It should be discontinued if the absolute neutrophil count exceeds 20,000 cells/mm^3. For clients receiving either G-CSF or GM-CSF, monitoring of the complete blood count with a differential is recommended twice weekly during therapy to avoid potential complications of excessive leukocytosis. Currently, the use of erythropoietin in clients with cancer is under clinical investigation.

Because most biologic agents are still investigational, it is important for the nurse to understand the potential side effects of the agent to be administered and to be prepared for and continually assess and document the client's response to therapy. Client and family teaching is of the utmost importance because many clients will seek investigational therapy when standard therapy fails to achieve a tumor response.

SECOND MALIGNANCIES

The term second malignancy refers to the occurrence of new, unrelated neoplasms after initial cancer therapy.

An increased risk of leukemia and solid tumors has been noted after treatment of childhood malignancies, Hodgkin's disease, multiple myeloma, non-Hodgkin's lymphomas, gastrointestinal cancers, lung cancer, and ovarian cancer.[16] Acute nonlymphocytic leukemia after treatment with alkylating agents and solid tumors after RT account for the majority of second cancers.

Most treatment-related leukemias occur within the first 10 years after treatment. Acute nonlymphocytic leukemia that occurs after cancer therapy is exceedingly refractory to therapy and almost uniformly fatal within 6 months of diagnosis.

In contrast to leukemia, most radiation-related cancers appear after 10 years. The majority of these cancers occur either within the direct field of radiation or in the organs surrounding it. The relationship of chemotherapy alone to subsequent solid tumor development is not as clear.

When instructing clients and significant others about treatment-related risks, it is important to remember that the risk of second malignancy is small and must be balanced against the benefits of therapy for a life-threatening disease. Once therapy is completed, the nurse should emphasize the importance of life-long surveillance.

CANCER RESOURCES

Many resources (patient or professional emphasis or both) are available on request. The following list identifies a few key resources for the nurse caring for the client with cancer and significant others to contact for further information.

Oncology Nursing Society (ONS)
501 Holiday Drive
Pittsburgh, PA 15229-2749
(412) 921-7373

American Cancer Society (ACS)
1599 Clifton Road NE
Atlanta, GA 30329
(404) 320-3333

Office of Cancer Communications
National Cancer Institute
Building 31, Room 10A24
Bethesda, MD 20892
1-800-4-CANCER

National Coalition for Cancer Survivorship
323 Eighth Street SW
Albuquerque, NM 87102
(505) 764-9956

STUDY QUESTIONS

1. Before the nurse can intervene to help the client and significant others, which one of the following must be completed first?
   A. The coping strategies must be identified.
   B. The client must have a verified diagnosis of cancer.
   C. The client and significant others must verbalize an understanding of the diagnosis.
   D. The nurse should seek a mental health consultation to assist the client and significant others to accept the diagnosis.
2. The nurse has completed discharge teaching for a client diagnosed with cancer. Which one of the following statements by the client will help the nurse evaluate that learning has occurred?
   A. "I believe that when the time comes, we'll look into having hospice care."
   B. "I've learned not to worry so much now that my palliative treatment has cured my cancer."
   C. "Whenever I face a tough situation, I work harder and things seem to sort themselves out."
   D. "I've always reacted quickly and angrily to situations I can't control; that should work very well for me now."
3. A client is concerned about his scheduled surgery because he has heard that "having surgery causes the cancer to spread." The best response by the nurse is:
   A. "I've heard many people say that, but I don't think it is true."
   B. "It depends on what stage the cancer is in when the original surgery is performed."

C. "Tumors probably begin shedding cells into the body throughout the period of their growth."
D. "Tumors are cells that are growing in a capsule and remain contained in one area of the body unless they metastasize."

4. When radiation therapy is used as the primary treatment modality, it is the:
A. Only treatment used
B. Preferred treatment followed by surgery
C. Preferred treatment followed by chemotherapy
D. Treatment preceding surgery and chemotherapy

5. The nurse is assisting a client after she has received a chemotherapy treatment. The client is nauseated and has vomited twice since the medication finished infusing. The nurse should:
A. Position the client in the mid-Fowler's position
B. Place a cool washcloth on the client's forehead
C. Don a pair of clean gloves when giving care to the client
D. Seek an order to delay the next scheduled course of chemotherapy

6. The nurse caring for the client who is receiving radiation therapy via intravenous infusion should:
A. Wear a radiation monitoring device
B. Realize that body excretions are contaminated
C. Care for all the radiation implant clients on the unit
D. Keep long-handle forceps and a lead container in the room

7. Diminished white cell and platelet production during chemotherapy can cause:
A. Nausea
B. Alopecia
C. Anorexia
D. Infection

CRITICAL THINKING EXERCISES

SCENARIO A

A client who is experiencing cancer is a first-grade school teacher. As a result of chemotherapy, she is experiencing myelosuppression.

1. What might be a psychosocial loss facing the client?
2. How would the myelosuppressive effects influence the client's functioning?
3. When would the client be ready for teaching about the myelosuppressive effects of the chemotherapy?

SCENARIO B

A male client is receiving the third of a series of treatments for cancer. There is a 75% hair loss with daily evidence of continued loss.

1. How do men react to hair loss as a side effect of treatment compared with women?
2. How does society, in general, view a person who has complete loss of hair?
3. How can individuals show acceptance of the person who is displaying side effects of cancer treatment?

BIBLIOGRAPHY

1. American Nurses' Association & Oncology Nursing Society. (1987). *Standards of oncology nursing practice.* Kansas City, MO: American Nurses' Association.
2. Averette, H. D., et al. (1990). Effects of cancer chemotherapy on gonadal and reproductive capacity. *Ca: A Cancer Journal for Clinicians, 40,* 199–209.
3. Baird, S. B., McCorkle, R., & Grant, M. (1991). *Cancer nursing: A comprehensive textbook.* Philadelphia: W. B. Saunders Co.
4. Boyle, N., Bertin-Matson, K., & Bratschi, A. (1994). A patient's guide to Taxol. *Oncology Nursing Forum, 21(9),* 1569–1572.
5. Bucholtz, J. (1992). Implications of radiation therapy for nursing. In J. Clark & R. McGee (Eds.), *Core curriculum for oncology nursing* (2nd ed., pp. 319–328). Philadelphia: W. B. Saunders.
6. Bucholtz, J. (1987). Radiolabeled antibody therapy. *Seminars in Oncology Nursing, 3(1),* 67–83.
7. Carbone, P. P. (1990). Progress in the systemic treatment of cancer: Concepts, trials, drugs, and biologics. *Cancer, 65,* 625–633.
8. Chabner, B. A., & Myers, C. E. (1989). Clinical pharmacology of cancer chemotherapy. In V. T. DeVita, S. Hellman, & S. A. Rosenberg (Eds.), *Cancer: Principles & practice of oncology* (3rd ed., pp. 349–395). Philadelphia: J. B. Lippincott.
9. Chisholm, L. G., et al. (1993). Programmed instruction: Cancer chemotherapy: Alternative administration routes. *Cancer Nursing, 16(3),* 237–246.
10. Clark, R. A., et al. (1989). Antiemetic therapy: Management of chemotherapy-induced nausea and vomiting. *Seminars in Oncology Nursing, 5(2, Suppl. 1),* 53–57.
11. DeLaPena, L. B., & Pyron, S. (1993). Taxol: A case study. *Cancer nursing, 16(6),* 423–430.
12. DeVita, V. T., Hellman, S., & Rosenberg, S. (1993). *Cancer: Principles and practice of oncology* (4th ed.). Philadelphia: J. B. Lippincott.
13. Dillman, J. B. (1988). Toxicity of monoclonal antibodies in the treatment of cancer. *Seminars in Oncology Nursing, 4,* 107–116.
14. Dow, K. H., & Hilderley, L. J. (1992). *Nursing care in radiation oncology.* Philadelphia: W. B. Saunders Co.
15. Dreifke, L., & DeMeyer, E. (1992). Total body irradiation for bone marrow transplant patients. *Cancer Nursing, 15(1),* 206–212.

16. Dudjak, L., & Fleck, A. (1991). New drug therapy comes of age. *RN, 54(10),* 41–48.

17. Ford, R., & Ballard, B. (1988). Acute complications after bone marrow transplantation. *Seminars in Oncology Nursing, 4(1),* 15–24.

18. Fraser, M. C., & Tucker, M. A. (1989). Second malignancies following cancer therapy. *Seminars in Oncology Nursing, 5(1),* 43–55.

19. Freedman, S. E. (1988). An overview of bone marrow transplantation. *Seminars in Oncology Nursing, 4(1),* 3–8.

20. Fuller, A. K. (1990). Platelet transfusion therapy for thrombocytopenia. *Seminars in Oncology Nursing, 6(2),* 123–128.

21. Goodman, M. (1989). Managing the side effects of chemotherapy. *Seminars in Oncology Nursing, 5(2, Suppl. 1),* 29–52.

22. Groenwald, S. L., et al. (1993). *Cancer nursing: Principles and practice* (3rd ed.). Boston: Jones & Bartlett.

23. Gullo, S. M. (1988). Safe handling of antineoplastic drugs: Translating the recommendations into practice. *Oncology Nursing Forum, 15,* 595–601.

24. Haeuber, D., & DiJulio, J. E. (1989). Hemopoietic colony stimulating factors: An overview. *Oncology Nursing Forum, 16(2),* 247–255.

25. Hahn, M. B., & Jassak, P. F. (1988). Nursing management of patients receiving interferon. *Seminars in Oncology Nursing, 4(2),* 95–101.

26. Hassey, K. (1987). Principles of radiation safety and protection. *Seminars in Oncology Nursing, 3(1),* 23–29.

27. Hilderley, L. J., & Hassey Dow, K. (1991). Radiation oncology. In S. B. Baird, R. McCorkle, & M. Grant (Eds.), *Cancer nursing: A comprehensive textbook* (pp. 246–265). Philadelphia: W. B. Saunders.

28. Hogan, C. M. (1990). Advances in the management of nausea and vomiting. *Nursing Clinics of North America, 25,* 475–497.

29. Holcombe, A. (1987). Bone marrow harvest. *Oncology Nursing Forum, 14(2),* 63–65.

30. Hood, L. A., & Abernathy, E. (1991). Biologic response modifiers. In S. Baird, R. McCorkle, & M. Grant (Eds.), *Cancer nursing: A comprehensive textbook* (pp. 321–343). Philadelphia: W. B. Saunders.

31. Hydzik, C. A. (1990). Late effects of chemotherapy: Implications for patient management and rehabilitation. *Nursing Clinics of North America, 25,* 423–446.

32. Jalowiec, A., & Dudas, S. (1991). Alterations in patient coping. In S. Baird, R. McCorkle, & M. Grant (Eds.), *Cancer nursing: A comprehensive textbook* (pp. 806–820). Philadelphia: W. B. Saunders.

33. Jassak, P. F. (1990). Biotherapy. In S. L. Groenwald, M. Frogge, M. Goodman, & C. Yarbro (Eds.), *Cancer nursing: Principles and practice* (2nd ed., pp. 284–306). Boston: Jones & Bartlett.

34. Jassak, P. F., & Porter, N. A. (1990). Bone marrow transplantation. In K. M. Sigardson-Poor & L. M. Haggerty (Eds.), *Nursing care of the transplant recipient* (pp. 280–306). Philadelphia: W. B. Saunders.

35. Jassak, P. F., & Sticklin, L. A. (1986). Interleukin-2: An overview. *Oncology Nursing Forum, 13(6),* 17–22.

36. Krakoff, I. H. (1987). Cancer chemotherapeutic agents. *Ca: A Cancer Journal for Clinicians, 37,* 93–105.

37. Krakoff, I. H. (1991). Cancer chemotherapeutic and biologic agents. *Ca: A Cancer Journal for Clinicians, 41,* 264–277.

38. Levy, W., et al. (1993). Programmed instruction: Chemotherapy agents: Part I. *Cancer Nursing, 16(4),* 321–336.

39. Loescher, L. J., et al. (1989). Surviving adult cancers, part I: Physiologic effects. *Annals of Internal Medicine, 111(5),* 411–432.

40. McCaffery, D. (1989). Family issues in cancer care: Current dilemmas and future directions. *Journal of Psychosocial Oncology, 6(1/2),* 199–211.

41. McGee, R. F. (1990). Overview of psychosocial dimensions. In S. L. Groenwald, M. Frogge, M. Goodman, & C. Yarbro (Eds.), *Cancer nursing: Principles and practice* (2nd ed., pp. 342–345). Boston: Jones & Bartlett.

42. McGuire, D. B., & Braine, H. G. (Guest Eds.). (1990). Blood component therapy. *Seminars in Oncology Nursing, 6(2),* 89–177.

43. Morrow, G. R. (1989). Chemotherapy-related nausea and vomiting: Etiology and management. *Ca: A Cancer Journal for Clinicians, 39,* 89–104.

44. Morton, D. L., et al. (1989). Principles of surgery. In S. I. Schwartz (Ed.). *Principles of surgery* (pp. 331–381). New York: McGraw-Hill.

45. National Cancer Institute. (1986). *What are clinical trials all about?* (NIH Publication No. 86-2706). Washington, DC: U.S. Government Printing Office.

46. National Study Commission on Cytotoxic Exposure. (1984). *Recommendations for handling cytotoxic agents.* Providence, RI: Rhode Island Hospital.

47. Occupational Safety and Health Administration. (Jan. 29, 1986). *Work practice guidelines for personnel dealing with cytotoxic (antineoplastic) drugs* (OSHA Instruction Publication No. 8-11). Washington, DC: Office of Occupational Medicine.

48. Oncology Nursing Society. (1988). *Cancer chemotherapy guidelines: Module I, II, III, IV, V.* Pittsburgh, PA: Author.

49. Oncology Nursing Society. (1989). *Access device guidelines: Recommendations for nursing education and practice: Module I, II, III.* Pittsburgh, PA: Author.

50. Oniboni, A. C. (1990). Infection in the neutropenic patient. *Seminars in Oncology Nursing, 6(1),* 50–60.

51. Quigley, K. M. (1989). The adult cancer survivor: Psychosocial consequences of cure. *Seminars in Oncology Nursing, 5(1),* 63–69.

52. Quint-Kasner, S., et al. (1993). Programmed instruction: Cancer chemotherapy—Basic principles. *Cancer Nursing, 16(1),* 63–78.

53. Quint-Kasner, S., et al. (1993). Programmed instruction: Chemotherapy agents: Part II. *Cancer Nursing, 16(5),* 398–418.

54. Relman, D. A., et al. (1992). Identification of the uncultured bacillus of Whipple's disease. *New England Journal of Medicine, 327(5),* 293–301.

55. Rosenberg, S. A. (1989). Principles of surgical oncology. In J. T. DeVita, S. Hellman, & S. A. Rosenberg (Eds.), *Cancer: Principles and practice of oncology* (3rd ed., pp. 236–246). Philadelphia: J. B. Lippincott.

56. Ruccione, K., & Weinberg, K. (1989). Late effects in multiple body systems. *Seminars in Oncology Nursing, 5(1),* 4–13.

57. Scheid, L., et al. (1994). Will you recognize these oncological crises? *RN, 57(9),* 22–28.

58. Schryber, S., et al. (1987). Autologous bone marrow transplantation. *Oncology Nursing Forum, 14(4),* 74–80.

59. Skidmore-Roth, L. (1995). *Mosby's nursing drug reference.* St. Louis: Mosby-Year Book.

60. Somerville, E. T. (1991). Knowledge deficit related to chemotherapy. In J. C. McNally, et al. (Eds.), *Guidelines for oncology nursing practice* (2nd ed., pp. 57–61). Philadelphia: W. B. Saunders.

61. Strohl, R. (1988). The nursing role in radiation oncology: Symptom management of acute and chronic reactions. *Oncology Nursing Forum, 15(4),* 429–434.

62. Tenenbaum, L. (1994). *Cancer chemotherapy and biotherapy: A reference guide.* Philadelphia: W. B. Saunders.

63. Theisen, A. (1991). The irreplaceable gift. *Journal of the American Medical Association, 266(9),* 1283.

64. U.S. Department of Health and Human Services. (1990). *Facing forward: A guide for cancer survivors* (NIH Publication No. 90-2424). Washington, DC: National Cancer Institute.

65. U.S. Nuclear Regulatory Commission. (1981). *Instruction concerning risks from occupational radiation exposure.* Regulatory Guide 8:29. Washington, DC: Office of Nuclear Regulatory Research.

66. Valdagni, R., et al. (1988). Important prognostic factors influencing outcome of combined radiation and hyperthermia. *International Journal of Radiation Oncology, Biology, Physics, 15,* 959–972.

67. Wasserman, T. H., & Kligerman, M. (1987). Chemical modifiers of radiation effect. In C. A. Perez & L. W. Brady (Eds.), *Principles and practice of radiation oncology* (pp. 360–376). Philadelphia: J. B. Lippincott.

68. Weber, M. S. (1995). Chemotherapy-induced nausea and vomiting. *American Journal of Nursing, 95(4),* 34.

69. Weinberg, P. A. (1991). The human leukocyte antigen (HLA) system, the search for a matching donor, national marrow donor program development, and marrow donor issues. In M. Whedon (Ed.), *Bone marrow transplantation: Principles, practice, and nursing insights* (pp. 3–19). Boston: Jones & Bartlett.

70. Whedon, M. (1991). Autologous bone marrow transplantation: Clinical indications, transplant process and outcomes. In M. Whedon (Ed.), *Bone marrow transplantation: Principles, practice, and nursing insights* (pp. 49–69). Boston: Jones & Bartlett.

71. Whedon, M. (Ed.). (1991). *Bone marrow transplantation: Principles, practice, and nursing insights.* Boston: Jones & Bartlett.

72. Wickham, R. (1988). Techniques for long-term venous access. In *Nursing management of the patient receiving chemotherapy* (pp. 9–20) (ACS No. 3480.03-PE). New York: American Cancer Society.

73. Wickham, R. S. (1990). Advances in venous access devices and nursing management strategies. In C. Liaskowski (Ed.), *Nursing Clinics of North America, 25,* 345–364.

74. Wingard, J. R. (1991). Historical perspective and future directions. In M. Whedon (Ed.), *Bone marrow transplantation: Principles, practice, and nursing insights* (pp. 3–19). Boston: Jones & Bartlett.

75. Workman, M., Ellerhorst-Ryan, J., & Koertge, V. (1993). *Nursing care of the immunocompromised patient.* Philadelphia: W. B. Saunders.

76. Yasko, J. M., & Greene, P. (1987). Coping with problems related to cancer and cancer treatment. *Ca: A Cancer Journal for Clinicians, 37(2),* 106–125.

77. Yasko, J. M., & Rust, D. (1989). Trends in chemotherapy administration. *Seminars in Oncology Nursing, 5(2, Suppl. 1),* 3–7.

78. Youngblood, M., et al. (1994). A comparison of two methods of assessing cancer therapy-related symptoms. *Cancer Nursing, 17(1),* 37–44.

UNIT 3

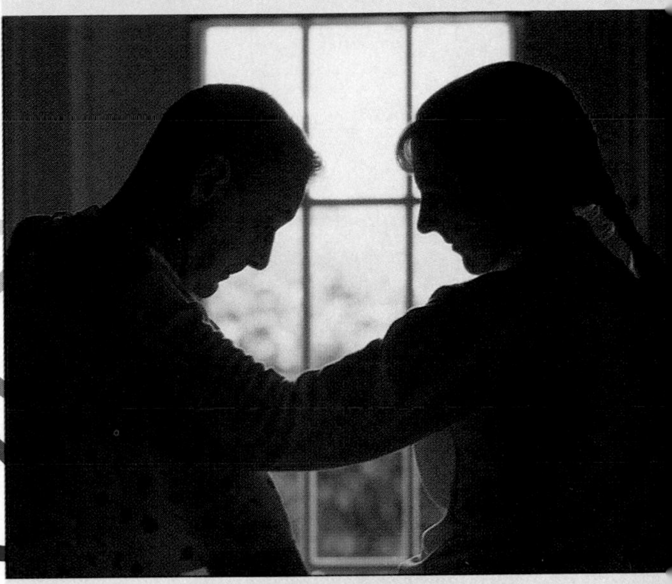

Immunologic Disorders

Bacteria and viruses have always plagued humans and animals. These tiny, unseen enemies cause damage by entering and attacking the internal milieu of the body, creating homeostatic disturbances. Living creatures have been forced to develop some means of defense against these minute and dangerous organisms to survive and reproduce. This unit discusses the body's nonspecific defenses, such as the inflammatory process, and specific defenses, such as immunity. Although the discussion separates nonspecific and specific responses, all of the body's defenses function together to afford maximum protection and maintain homeostasis.

After a concise review of immune system structure and function, Chapter 8 focuses on assessment and diagnosis of immune disorders. Chapter 9 examines specific immune protective responses and the implications of these responses for transplantation, and Chapter 10 covers the processes of infection and their implications. Finally, Chapter 11 concludes the unit with a discussion of connective tissue disorders.

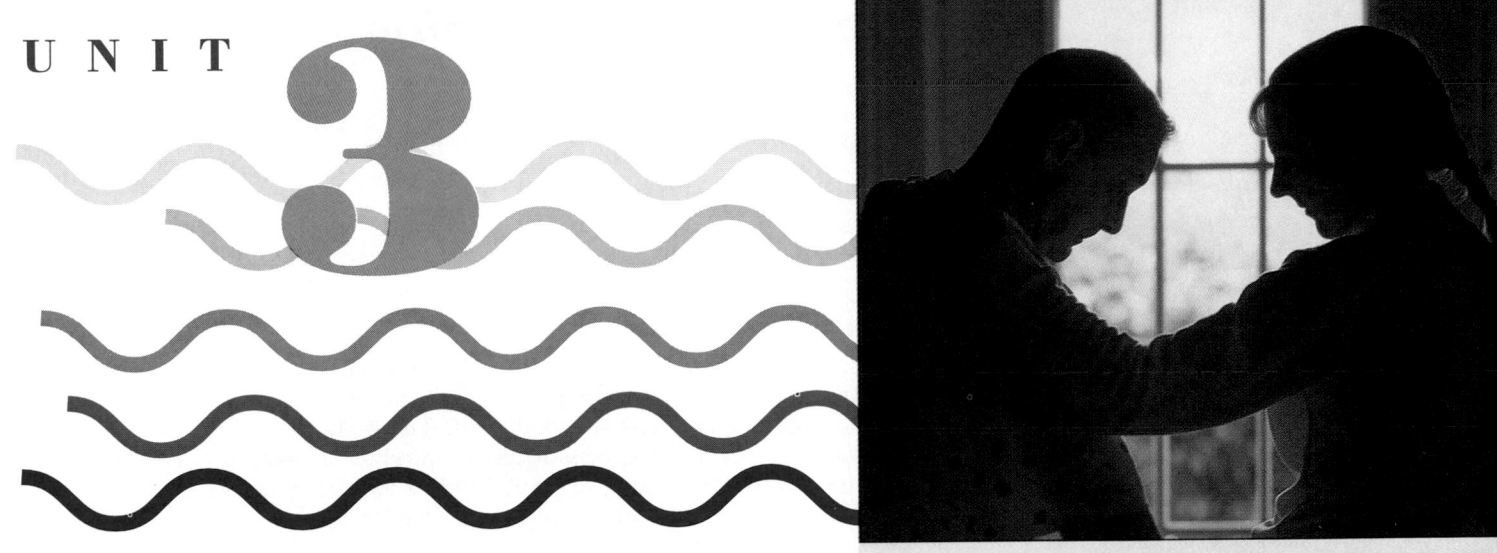

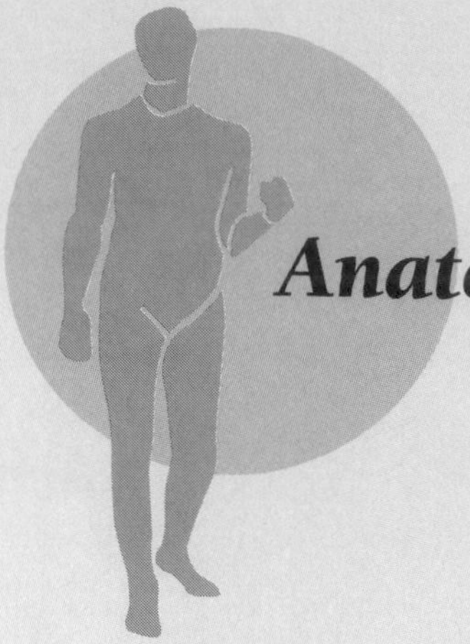

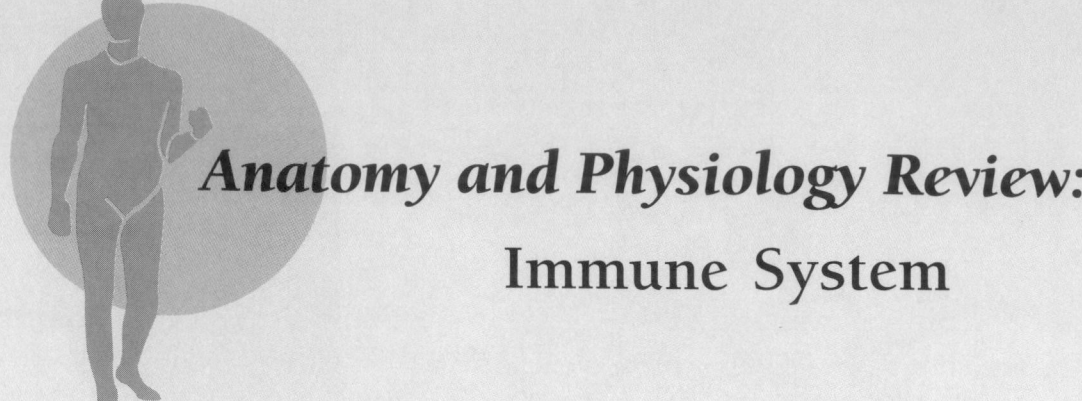

Anatomy and Physiology Review: Immune System

The human body has an intricate system of specialized cells, tissues, and organs that work together to protect it against invasion by bacteria, viruses, fungi, and parasites. This protection is called the immune system. In addition to defending the body against invasion from the outside, the immune system seeks out and destroys malignantly transformed cells internally. Without an effective immune system, an individual is likely to develop overwhelming infection, malignant disease, or both. Excessive or inappropriate activity of the immune system can result in autoimmune disease or hypersensitivity conditions. The body's ability to counteract the effects of disease-producing organisms is called resistance. Susceptibility is a lack of resistance.

Because the lymph nodes and other lymphatic organs have a vital role in the effectiveness of the immune system, the lymphatic system is presented first, followed by descriptions of body defense mechanisms.

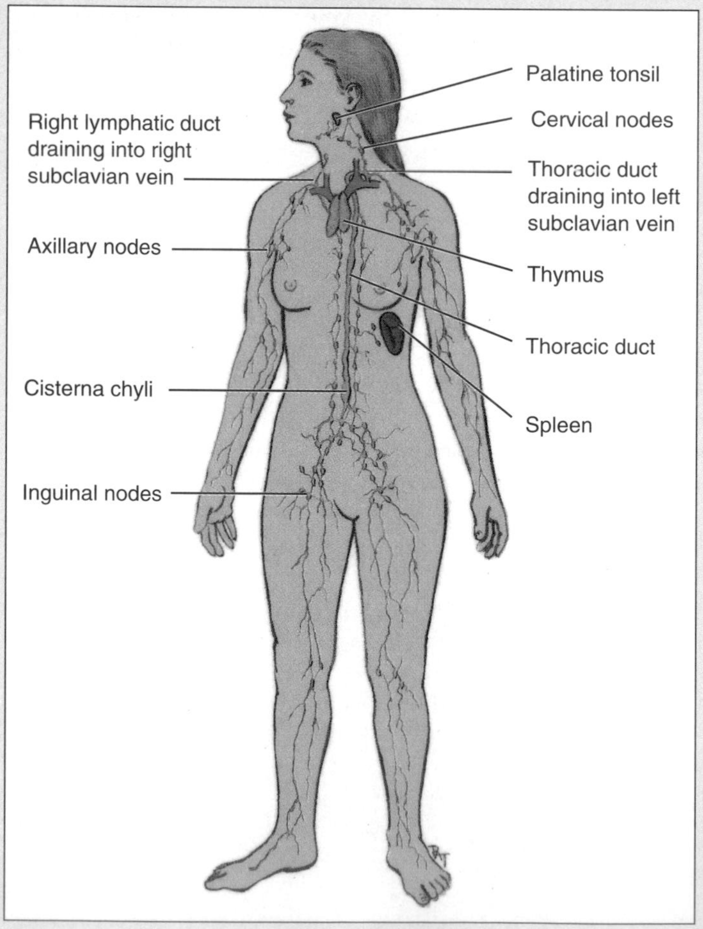

Organs of the lymphatic system.

Functions of Lymphoid Organs

LYMPHOID ORGAN	FUNCTION
Primary lymphoid organs	Proliferation and maturation of cells
Bone marrow	Proliferation and maturation of immune system cells
Thymus	Proliferation and maturation of certain lymphocytes; produces immunoregulatory hormones
Secondary lymphoid organs	Create appropriate environment for immune reactions
Lymph nodes	Filter and cleanse lymph before it enters the blood
Tonsils	Provide protection against pathogens that may enter through the nose and mouth
Spleen	Filters blood; reservoir for blood
Mucosal lymphoid tissue of gastrointestinal, respiratory, and urogenital tracts	Defends against pathogens that enter through mucus-lined passages that open to the exterior

LYMPHATIC SYSTEM

The lymphatic system has three primary functions:

- Returning excess interstitial fluid to the blood
- Absorbing and transporting fats and fat-soluble vitamins
- Defending against invading microorganisms and disease

The organs of the lymphatic system are widely distributed and located near points of entry for microorganisms. The primary lymphoid organs generally provide for the proliferation and maturation of the immune system cells. The mobility of the cells allows them to move into and out of tissues and circulate throughout the body to provide surveillance against potentially harmful entities. Lymphatic vessels collect fluid from the interstitial spaces of tissues and transport it to the lymph nodes. As the fluid moves through the nodes, infectious agents, damaged cells, cancerous cells, and cellular debris become trapped and are destroyed. Secondary lymphoid organs create an appropriate environment for the immune reactions.

THE NATURE OF BODY DEFENSE MECHANISMS

For the immune system to function properly, the cells must be able to distinguish self from nonself. All cells of the body have specific markers, usually proteins, that identify them as belonging to self. If the markers are not present or the immune system does not recognize them, the cells are identified as nonself, and reactions are elicited to destroy them. Any substance in the body that is interpreted as nonself and triggers an immune reaction is called an antigen.

The leukocytes, or white blood cells, provide the immune system with an army that protects the body

Types of Leukocytes (White Blood Cells)

COMPONENT	DESCRIPTION	FUNCTION	PER CENT OF TOTAL LEUKOCYTES
Granulocytes			
Neutrophils Bands (immature cells with horseshoe-shaped nuclei) Segmented (mature cells with lobed nuclei)	Light-staining granules in the cytoplasm; multilobed nucleus	Phagocytosis and destruction of bacteria and cellular debris	40–75; number increases during infections, resulting in more immature cells in the blood
Eosinophils	Granules in the cytoplasm that stain red with eosin dyes	Phagocytosis; suppress inflammation and granulocyte migration	2–5; increases in response to allergies
Basophils	Granules in the cytoplasm that stain blue with basic dyes; granules contain heparin; similar to mast cells	Release chemicals that stimulate inflammation, especially in response to allergens	0.2–0.5
Agranulocytes			
Monocytes	Large cells without granules in cytoplasm; mature into macrophages in the tissues	Phagocytosis; process antigens; secrete chemicals that assist in immune responses	2–6
Lymphocytes	Small cells without granules in cytoplasm; large nucleus that nearly fills the cell	Specific, or adaptive, immunity; cell-mediated immunity and antibody-mediated immunity	30–25

against foreign invasion. The total number of leukocytes is 4000 to 10,000 cells per cubic millimeter of blood. This number does not include the cells that have entered the tissue spaces or lymph vessels. Infections stimulate hematopoietic tissue to increase production, which leads to leukocytosis. Bone marrow suppression or increased destruction of leukocytes leads to a decrease in the number of circulating leukocytes, called leukopenia. There are five types of leukocytes, each with a specific function in the immune response. A differential count measures the relative number of each type and provides important diagnostic information about disease processes.

NONSPECIFIC DEFENSE MECHANISMS

Nonspecific defense mechanisms are directed against all pathogens and foreign substances, regardless of their nature. They present the initial barriers against invading organisms. The first line of defense is the barrier against invasion provided by:

- Intact skin and mucous membranes
- Flow of fluids such as tears, saliva, and urine
- Chemicals that are present in tears and other fluids

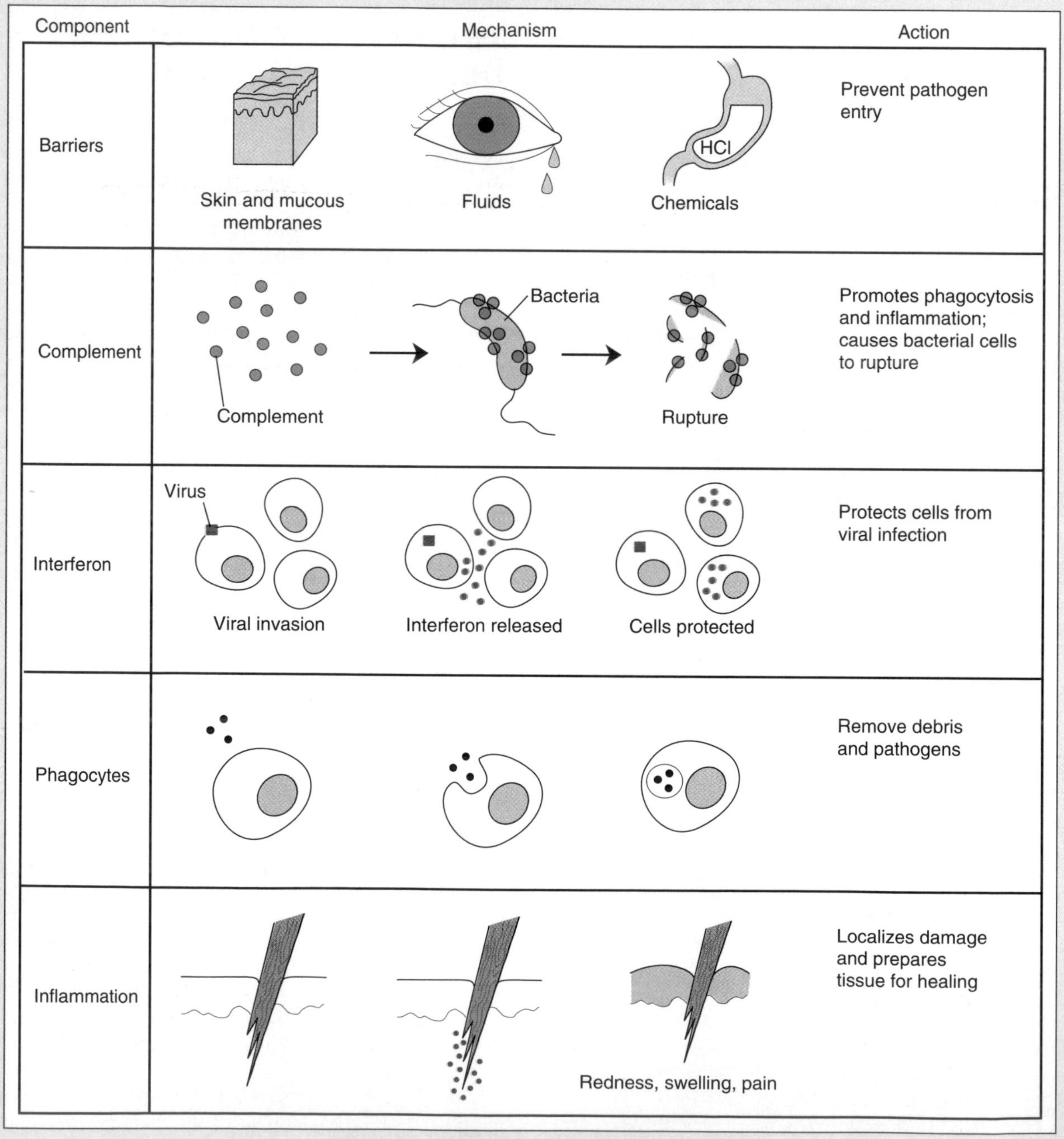

Component
Mechanism
Action
Barriers
Skin and mucous membranes
Fluids
HCl
Chemicals
Prevent pathogen entry
Complement
Complement
Bacteria
Rupture
Promotes phagocytosis and inflammation; causes bacterial cells to rupture
Interferon
Virus
Viral invasion
Interferon released
Cells protected
Protects cells from viral infection
Phagocytes
Remove debris and pathogens
Inflammation
Redness, swelling, pain
Localizes damage and prepares tissue for healing

Components of nonspecific defense mechanisms.

Overview of defense mechanisms.

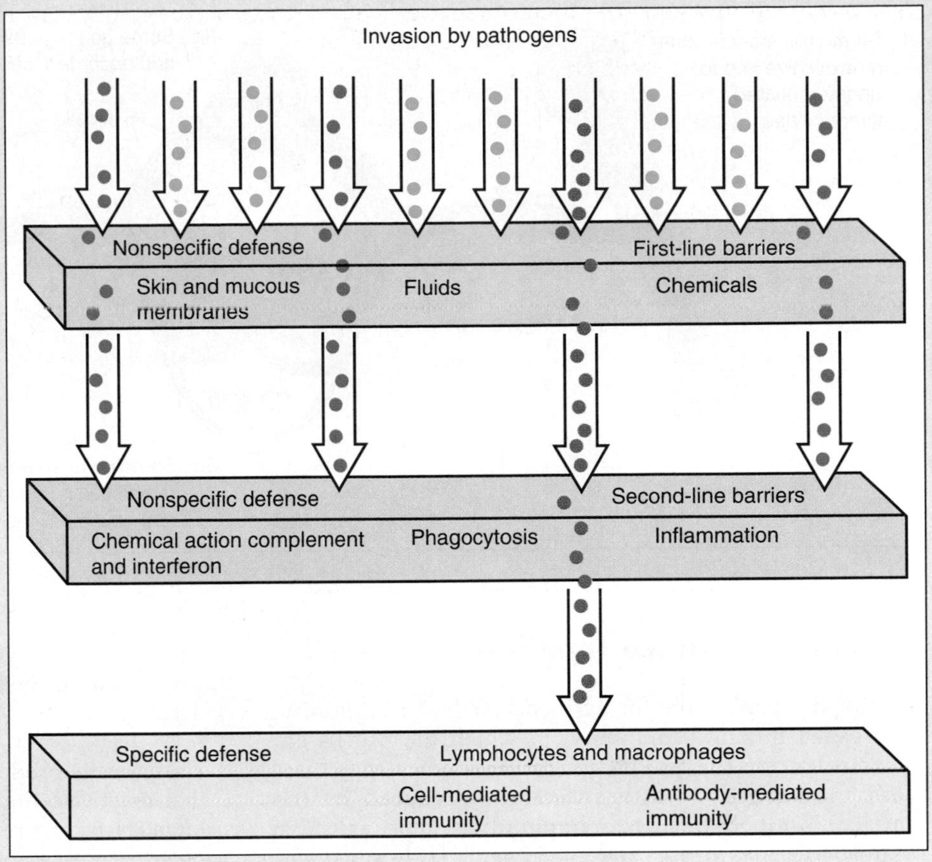

If a foreign agent penetrates the first-line barriers, it meets a second line of defense that includes:

- Chemical action of complement
- Chemical action of interferon
- Phagocytosis
- Inflammation

SPECIFIC DEFENSE MECHANISMS

Specific defense mechanisms, or immune responses, provide the third line of defense against microbial invasion. The primary cells involved in immune responses are lymphocytes and macrophages. Two characteristics of these responses are:

- Specificity: defending agents are programmed to be selective.
- Memory: once exposed, defending agents "remember" for a quicker response with a second exposure.

Development of Lymphocytes

Like all other blood cells, lymphocytes develop from stem cells in the bone marrow. Some of the lymphocytes go to the thymus and differentiate into T lymphocytes, or T cells. Others go elsewhere, probably the fetal liver, and differentiate into B lymphocytes, or B cells. Both T cells and B cells are distributed to lymphoid tissue.

Cell-Mediated Immunity

T cells are responsible for cell-mediated immunity, in which T cells directly attack and destroy foreign antigens. Cell-mediated immunity is most effective against virus-infected cells, cancer cells, foreign tissue cells (transplant rejection), fungi, and protozoan parasites. Macrophages phagocytize and process antigens and present them to T cells with receptor sites for that specific antigen. This activates the T cells to reproduce and produce large clones, which are divided into four subgroups:

- Killer T cells directly destroy the offending antigens.
- Helper T cells secrete substances that stimulate B cells and promote the immune response. Interleukin-2 is one of the substances secreted by helper T cells, and researchers are using interleukin-2 produced by genetic engineering to stimulate the immune system. Cyclosporine, a drug that inhibits the production of interleukin-2, is used to prevent transplant rejection.
- Suppressor T cells are regulatory cells that control the response. Normally in a correctly operating immune system, there are twice as many helper cells as suppressor cells.
- Memory T cells "remember" the specific antigen and stimulate a faster and more intense response if the same antigen is introduced another time.

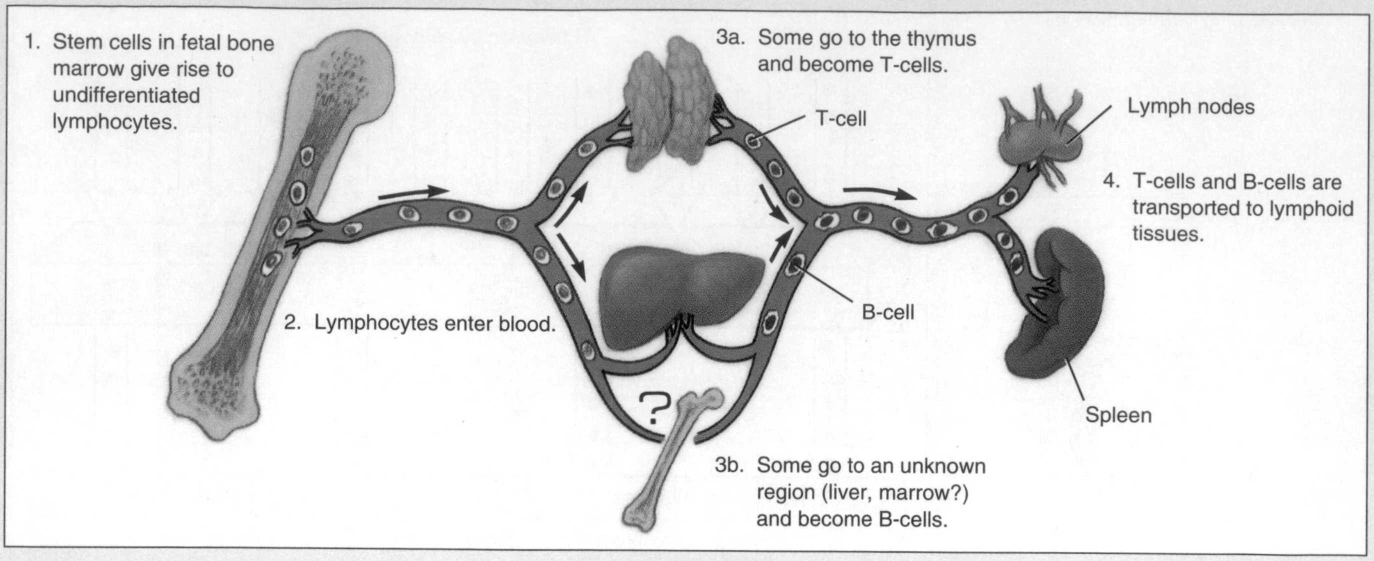

1. Stem cells in fetal bone marrow give rise to undifferentiated lymphocytes.
2. Lymphocytes enter blood.
3a. Some go to the thymus and become T-cells.
T-cell
B-cell
3b. Some go to an unknown region (liver, marrow?) and become B-cells.
Lymph nodes
4. T-cells and B-cells are transported to lymphoid tissues.
Spleen

Development of lymphocytes.

Antibody-Mediated Immunity

B cells are responsible for antibody-mediated immunity, also called humoral immunity, in which the B cells are responsible for the production of antibodies that react with the antigen or with substances produced by the antigen. Antibody-mediated immunity is most effective against bacteria, viruses that are outside body cells, and toxins produced by antigens. It is also involved in allergic reactions.

When antigens enter the body, macrophages engulf and process them, then present them to B cells and helper T cells. The activated helper T cells secrete substances that stimulate the activated B cells to divide and form a clone of cells consisting of memory B cells and plasma cells.

- Plasma cells produce large quantities of antibodies that inactivate the invading antigens.
- Memory B cells remember the antigen, and subsequent exposure to the same antigen changes memory B cells to plasma cells for a rapid production of antibodies.
- All antibodies have a similar structure, but one portion of the molecule differs so that each antibody is capable of reacting with only a specific antigen.

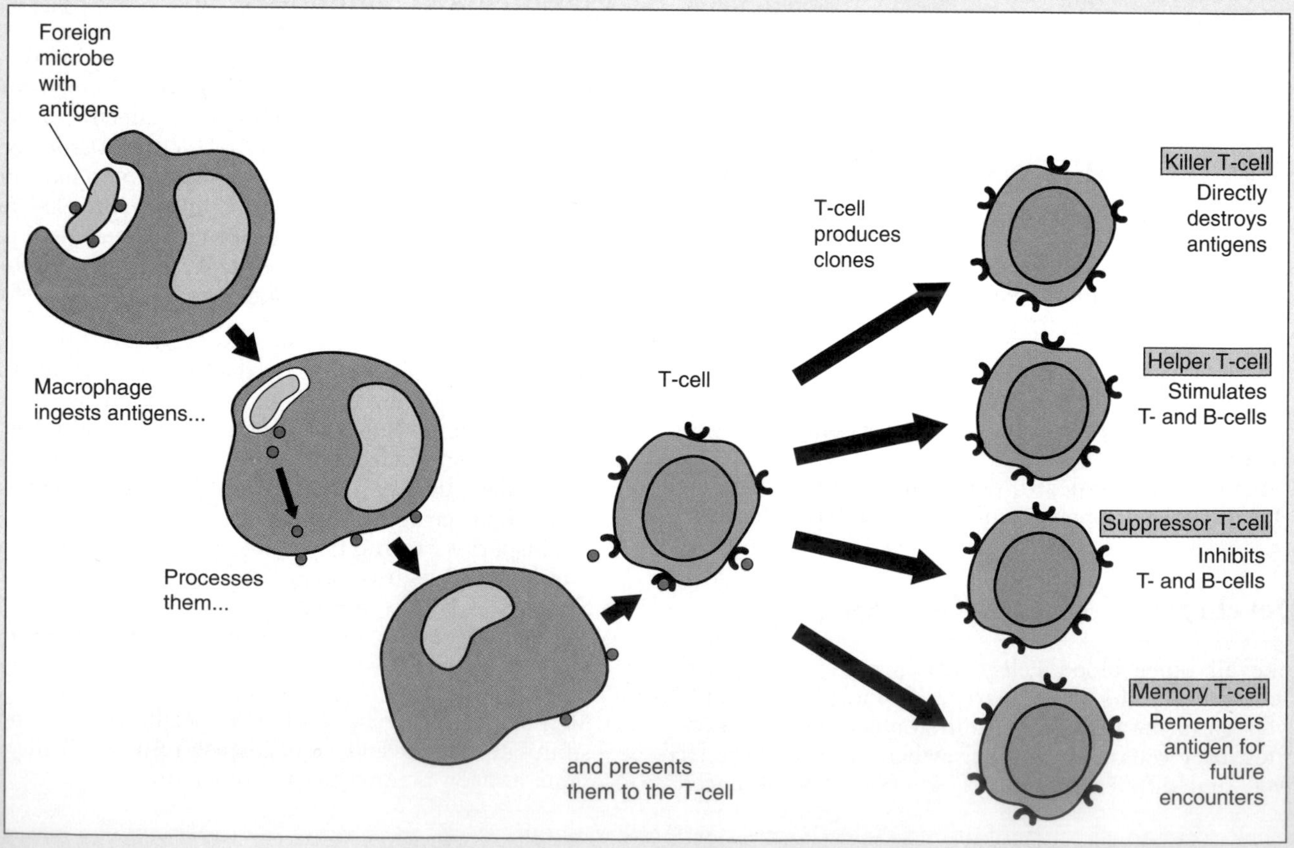

Foreign microbe with antigens
Macrophage ingests antigens...
Processes them...
and presents them to the T-cell
T-cell
T-cell produces clones
Killer T-cell
Directly destroys antigens
Helper T-cell
Stimulates T- and B-cells
Suppressor T-cell
Inhibits T- and B-cells
Memory T-cell
Remembers antigen for future encounters

Cell-mediated immunity.

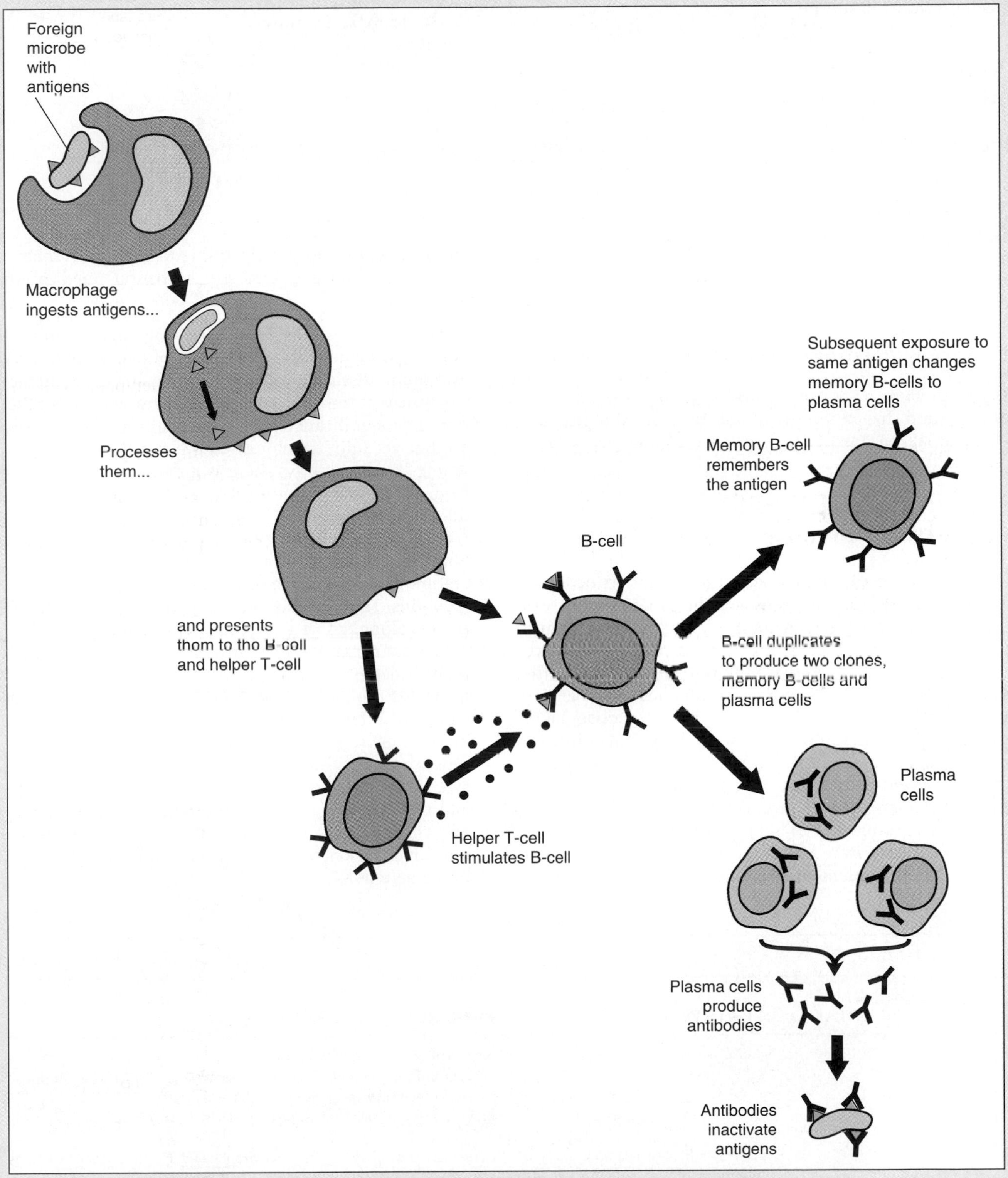
Foreign microbe with antigens
Macrophage ingests antigens...
Processes them...
and presents them to the B-cell and helper T-cell
B-cell
Helper T-cell stimulates B-cell
B-cell duplicates to produce two clones, memory B-cells and plasma cells
Subsequent exposure to same antigen changes memory B-cells to plasma cells
Memory B-cell remembers the antigen
Plasma cells
Plasma cells produce antibodies
Antibodies inactivate antigens

Antibody mediated immunity.

Immunoglobulins

Antibodies belong to a class of proteins called globulins, which, because they are involved in immune reactions, are also called immunoglobulins. There are five main classes of antibodies, or immunoglobulins, each with a specific role in immunity.

Primary and Secondary Immune Responses

After the initial exposure to an antigen, there is a latent period, or delay, in which little or no antibody can be measured in the serum. During this time, the B cells recognize the antigen and differentiate into plasma cells and memory cells, and the plasma cells start producing antibodies. After 4 to 10 days, serum antibody levels (titer) increase; however, the peak levels decrease rapidly. This is the primary immune response. Memory cells continue to circulate for several years and, on re-exposure to the same antigen, antibodies are produced within 1 to 2 days. This is a secondary immune response. This response occurs more quickly, is more intense, and has a longer duration than the primary response, all because of the presence of memory cells.

Classification of Specific (Adaptive) Immunity

The recognition of antigens and the formation of memory cells against the antigens are the hallmark features of specific, or adaptive, immunity. This specific immunity, mediated by T cells and B cells, can be acquired actively or passively. Active immunity occurs when the individual's own body produces antibodies and memory cells in response to an antigen. This response takes several days to develop but lasts a long time because memory cells are produced. Passive immunity results when the immune agents develop in another person (or animal) and are transferred to an individual who was not previously immune. This type of treatment provides immediate protection but is effective for only a short time because no memory cells are produced. The terms natural and artificial refer to how the immunity is obtained. Natural immunity is acquired through normal activities. Artificial immunity requires some deliberate action. Combining the terms gives the four types of specific immunity.

- Active natural immunity
- Active artificial immunity
- Passive natural immunity
- Passive artificial immunity

FACTORS AFFECTING BODY DEFENSE MECHANISMS

Immune function is greatly influenced by a number of factors, including genetics, age, nutrition, medications, and stress.

- Genetics provides the foundation for one's immune system, influences the expression of allergy and autoimmune disease, and may account for the tendency for certain forms of cancer to develop within families.
- Age is of significance because the immune responses are not yet fully developed in the newborn and very young. In the elderly, there is a decrease in hormones from the thymus, diminished T-cell activity, and reduced antibody titer.
- Nutrition is of vital importance to the immune system. Appropriate proteins are necessary for the proliferation of leukocytes and the synthesis of immunoglobulins. High-calorie diets appear to be involved in the development of autoimmune disease.
- Medications can depress the immune system. Some may be taken for that specific purpose, but others, taken for unrelated conditions, have side effects that suppress immunity. Many drugs also produce bone marrow depression as a side effect.
- Stress has been linked to suppression of the immune system for decades. Physical stressors, such as trauma and burns, and emotional stress, such as grief, are known to depress immune cell function. A number of hormones associated with stress also decrease immune activity.

Classes of Antibodies

CLASS	PER CENT OF TOTAL	LOCATION	FUNCTION
IgG	75–85	Blood plasma	Major antibody in primary and secondary immune responses; inactivates antigen; neutralizes toxins; crosses placenta to provide immunity for newborn; responsible for Rh reactions
IgA	5–15	Saliva, mucus, tears, breast milk	Protects mucous membranes on body surfaces; provides immunity for newborn
IgM	5–10	Attached to B cells; released into plasma during immune response	Causes antigens to clump together; responsible for transfusion reactions in the ABO blood typing system
IgD	0.2	Attached to B cells	Receptor sites for antigens on B cells; binding with antigen results in B cell activation
IgE	0.5	Produced by plasma cells in mucous membranes and tonsils	Binds to mast cells and basophils, causing release of histamine; responsible for allergic reactions

Ig, immunoglobulin.
Modified from Applegate, E. J. (1995). *The Anatomy and Physiology Learning System Textbook*. Philadelphia: W. B. Saunders.

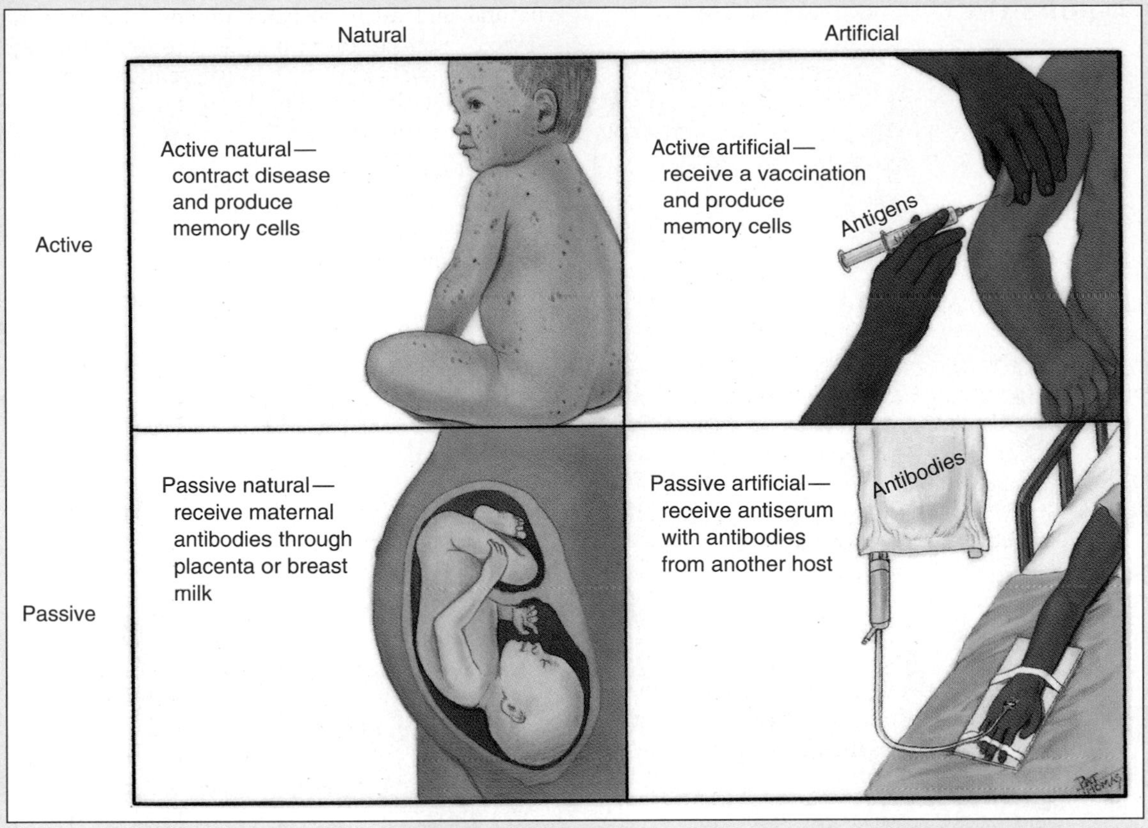
Natural
Artificial
Active
Passive
Active natural—
contract disease
and produce
memory cells
Active artificial—
receive a vaccination
and produce
memory cells
Antigens
Passive natural—
receive maternal
antibodies through
placenta or breast
milk
Passive artificial—
receive antiserum
with antibodies
from another host
Antibodies

Classification of specific immunity.

AGE-RELATED CHANGES

Most lymphoid tissues, such as the spleen, thymus, tonsils, bone marrow, and lymph nodes, undergo structural changes with age. They reach their maximum development at the time of puberty, then slowly regress after that period. Structural changes in the thymus are accompanied by a decrease in production of the hormone thymosin. This affects the differentiation and functional activity of T lymphocytes, which leads to an increase in immature T cells and a decrease in the number or activity, or both, of mature T cells. The number of B lymphocytes does not appear to decline with age; however, their responsiveness to antigens and their ability to form plasma-cell clones to produce antibodies do appear to decline. This may be because helper T cells are less active and do not stimulate the B cells as they normally do.

In general, but not always, aging is accompanied by a decrease in immune sensitivity and an increase in autoimmune reactions in which the body fails to recognize its own cells. The declining immune system also accounts, in part, for the increased incidence of cancer in the elderly.

Chapter 8 Assessment of Clients with Immune Disorders

Learning Outcomes

After completing this chapter, the learner will be able to:

1. Teach the client about the normal structure and function of the immune system.
2. Explain to the client the abnormalities of structure and function of the immune system.
3. Conduct a nursing history and physical assessment of the client with actual or potential disorders of the immune system.
4. Teach the client about diagnostic studies common to the immune system.

The immune system is extremely complex. Understanding its structure, function, and assessment helps the nurse provide more consistent and appropriate care for clients with inflammations, infections, and immune disorders.

Assessment of the Immune System

Allergies always follow sensitization to an allergen, so one of the primary diagnostic tools is a complete history to determine possible allergies, including food, medication, insect, or pollen sensitivities. The history is followed by a complete physical examination.

HISTORY

The health history focuses on the chief complaint and present allergies, the medical history for allergies, family history, psychosocial history, including life-style and stress management, and review of systems (ROS). The client ideally is the source for the history, although significant others such as parents or spouse or other family members may be valuable sources of information.

Chief Complaint

The client may report a variety of symptoms associated with an allergy. Symptoms vary depending on the nature of the allergen and the client's individual sensitivity pattern. The nurse completes a symptom analysis for each reported symptom to assist in the identification of the allergen. The major types of allergens include inhalants (e.g., pollens, molds, spores, dust, mites, and animal dander); contact agents (e.g., dyes in clothing, fibers, cosmetics, metals in jewelry, plant oils and secretions, topical drugs, and numerous chemicals); ingested agents (e.g., foods, food additives, drugs); and injectable agents (e.g., drugs, vaccines, and insect venom).

Medical History

The nurse asks the client about past episodes of allergic reactions. The client is asked to relate whether or not there is a seasonal pattern associated with these episodes, the symptoms that developed, and the treatment for these allergies and their effectiveness. Specifically, inquire about drug allergies and food allergies or sensitivities. Has the client ever suffered an anaphylactic reaction? Has the client ever been hospitalized for an allergic reaction? Has the client had previous series of treatment for desensitization with allergy shots? If so, were the treatments effective?

Family History

The client is asked to identify allergies and sensitivities in family members, particularly atopic reactions. The nurse attempts to determine the specific problem, the accompanying symptoms, and course of treatment.

Psychosocial History and Life-Style

Information about the client's physical environment and psychosocial patterns is important in obtaining a complete allergy history. The nurse asks about both the home and work (or school) environments as well as suspicious stressors such as food, plants, and heating and cooling systems. The nurse also asks how the client reacts to outbreaks of allergic symptoms. For example, some clients break out in hives when they are under psychological or emotional stress. Their appearance triggers more emotional stress, which, in turn, leads to further outbreaks of hives. A cycle develops that is difficult to interrupt.

Review of Systems

Before the physical examination, the nurse asks the client about the following problems associated with allergies.

- General: fatigue, malaise, unusual reactions to insect bites or medications, including over-the-counter drugs
- Integumentary: rashes, urticaria, itching, scratching, dryness, scaling
- Eyes: dark circles around the eyes, excessive tearing, rubbing or blinking, conjunctivitis, sties
- Ears: altered hearing acuity, feeling of fullness in the ears, ruptured tympanic membranes
- Nose: sneezing, sniffling, rhinitis, nasal polyps, nasal voice quality, nose twitching or rubbing, nasal stuffiness, recurrent epistaxis, postnasal drip
- Throat: swollen lips or tongue, frequent clearing of the throat, sore throat, itching of the throat or neck, hoarseness
- Respiratory: wheezing, dyspnea, frequent cough, ineffective cough
- Gastrointestinal: diarrhea, vomiting, cramping, food intolerances

PHYSICAL EXAMINATION

The client with allergies should receive a head-to-toe physical examination. The nurse focuses on the area that is the target for the allergen for in-depth assessment.

Assessment of the Lymphatic System

Disorders of the lymphatic system may result from inflammation (lymphangitis), an increased amount of lymph (lymphedema), or enlargement of the lymph nodes (lymphadenopathy). A complete history and physical examination help determine the cause of the problem and direct the eventual treatment. Included in the assessment of the lymphatic system are the peripheral lymph nodes, liver, and spleen. Assessment of the liver and spleen is discussed in Chapter 36.

HISTORY

The history for the lymphatic system focuses on the client's chief complaint, history of present illness, medical history, psychosocial history and life-style, and ROS.

Chief Complaint

The client may report localized swelling over an underlying lymph node (or nodes) or generalized swelling and edema of an extremity. Other symptoms include pruritus, increased redness or streaks (indicating cellulitis), pain, tenderness, fever, malaise, anorexia, headache, and irritability. The nurse conducts a symptom analysis to determine the location, onset, and duration of the problem and accompanying symptoms such as drainage and increased warmth over the area.

History of Present Illness

The nurse asks the client about infections, both systemic and local. Lymphedema can result from congenital deformity of the lymph vessels or altered structure and function. Therefore, the nurse asks the client about surgery or trauma to extremities, radiation therapy, and presence of a malignancy or neoplasm, which may have interrupted lymphatic flow and drainage from an area. The nurse also asks whether elevation relieves swelling of an affected extremity and whether or not a dependent position leads to increased swelling.

Medical History

The nurse inquires about previous problems with swelling, injury, or trauma to extremities, including surgery. Has the client had a systemic infection, immunologic reaction, or neoplastic disorder? If so, the nurse should ask the client to describe the specific disorder and its treatment. For example, a client who has had axillary node dissection accompanying a mastectomy often has upper extremity edema of the ipsilateral side. The nurse also asks about disorders affecting the vascular system, such as congestive heart failure, renal disease, and peripheral vascular problems, because these disorders are often accompanied by edema of the extremities. Specifically, the nurse asks about allergies to iodine or seafoods such as shellfish. Diagnostic studies of the lymphatic system use an iodine-based contrast medium.

Psychosocial History and Life-Style

The nurse inquires about the effect the problem has had on the client's emotional status and coping abilities. Disorders involving the lymphatic system may result in a variety of psychological and emotional reactions ranging from disregard to obvious distress. The client may be disturbed by an altered body image, particularly if the deformity is evident. If symptoms are related to a neoplastic disorder, the client may express fear or anxiety, especially if it is a recurrent problem. The nurse remains sensitive to the client's expressed and unexpressed emotions during the history and physical examination.

Review of Systems

The client is asked to describe problems in the following areas:

- General: malaise, fatigue, fever, lassitude, chills, sweating, pruritus
- Head and neck: localized swelling, pain or tenderness; swollen nodes; headache; irritability
- Cardiovascular: hypertension; congestive heart failure; peripheral vascular disorders such as varicose veins; edema of the hands, feet, or legs
- Gastrointestinal: anorexia; hepatomegaly, splenomegaly
- Renal: kidney disease including renal failure
- Immunologic: recent infections such as influenza, measles, mononucleosis, viral infections; neoplasms including lymphoma; injury or trauma resulting in break in the skin barrier; date of last tetanus toxoid injection.

PHYSICAL EXAMINATION

The portions of the lymphatic system accessible to physical examination are the superficial lymph nodes, liver, and spleen. Examination of the liver and spleen is discussed in Chapter 36. The techniques used to examine superficial lymph nodes are inspection and palpation. The nurse uses a methodical approach when examining lymph nodes in order not to overlook single nodes or chains of nodes. The nodes of the head and neck, supraclavicular areas, axilla, and epitrochlear areas are most easily palpated while the client is sitting.

TABLE 8–1 Sequence and Palpation Technique for Lymph Nodes in the Head and Neck

NODES	LOCATION	PALPATION TECHNIQUE
Occipital	Posterior at base of skull and lateral to cervical spine	Flex client's neck forward slightly to relax trapezius. Palpate right and left node centers simultaneously.
Posterior auricular (mastoid)	Behind auricle of ear, over outer surface of mastoid process	Palpate over both mastoid processes simultaneously.
Posterior cervical chain	Along anterior edge of trapezius, in the posterior triangle	Flex client's neck to relax trapezius muscles. Palpate slowly against the trapezius muscles, progressing from the mastoid processes toward the clavicles.
Supraclavicular (scalene)	Above the clavicle, in the angle formed by the clavicle and the sternocleidomastoid	Flex client's neck sharply with one hand and encourage the client to relax the shoulders so that clavicles drop. Palpate one side at a time with fingers over client's right clavicle lateral to sternocleidomastoid. Ask the client to inhale deeply while pressing in and behind clavicle. Repeat using right hand to palpate client's left node centers.
Superficial (anterior) cervical chain	Along and over (anterior to) the sternocleidomastoid, in the anterior triangle	Flex client's neck forward to relax sternocleidomastoid. Palpate one side at a time. Palpate slowly against the sternocleidomastoid, progressing from the clavicle toward the jaw.
Deep cervical chain	Under the sternocleidomastoid	Flex client's neck laterally toward the side being examined to relax muscles and soft tissue. Palpate one side at a time. Hook thumb (on one side) and fingers (on the other side) around the sternocleidomastoid muscle to feel deep to the muscle. Progress from the jaw toward the sternum.
	Along anterior edge of sternocleidomastoid, in the anterior triangle	With client's neck still flexed laterally, palpate along anterior edge of sternocleidomastoid from the sternum to the jaw angle. Repeat on opposite side of neck.
Tonsillar	Near angle of jaw at the jaw margin	Flex client's neck slightly in midline. Palpate behind both jaw angles simultaneously.
Submandibular (submaxillary)	Along medial border of mandible, between the angle of the jaw and the chin	Palpate along medial borders of mandible from angle of jaw toward the chin. Palpate right and left node centers simultaneously.
Submental	At the midline, posterior to the tip of the mandible under the chin	Palpate with one hand under client's chin just behind tip of mandible. Steady client's head with free hand if necessary.
Anterior auricular	In front of tragus of ear	Palpate right and left sides simultaneously, anterior to tragus and posterior to the temporomandibular joint.

Inguinal and popliteal nodes are more accessible when the client is lying down.

Inspection

The nurse inspects the surface overlying nodes for masses or scars, looking for bilateral symmetry. If masses are seen, the nurse palpates the area and compares it with the contralateral side.

Palpation

Palpation is used to assess lymph nodes for size, shape, consistency, discreteness, mobility, and tenderness. The nurse uses the finger pads of the middle three fingers in a gentle, circular motion to palpate over the nodes. The finger tips stay in contact with the skin and slide the skin's surface over the underlying nodes. Excessive pressure is avoided because it obliterates small, palpable nodes. Lymph nodes are not normally palpable, yet it is common to find small (1 cm or less diameter), round, soft, single, mobile, nontender nodes, particularly in the cervical and inguinal areas. Nodes that are large (greater than 1 cm diameter) or hard, feel matted together, are fixed to underlying structures, or are tender are abnormal findings, and their characteristics are described thoroughly. The sequence and palpation technique for lymph nodes in the head and neck are given in Table 8–1.

If an extremity appears edematous, the nurse measures its circumference and compares it with that of the contralateral extremity. Differences of less than 1 cm (about $\frac{1}{2}$ inch) are considered within normal limits.

DIAGNOSTIC TESTS

Human Immunodeficiency Virus Testing

ENZYME-LINKED IMMUNOSORBENT ASSAY

This test is the first one performed when human immunodeficiency virus (HIV) infection is suspected in the client who has unexplained generalized enlarged lymph nodes. Although this is a relatively inexpensive, quick, and easy test, there tends to be a high rate of false-positive results; in other words, the enzyme-linked immunosorbent assay (ELISA) is a highly sensitive test but not necessarily very specific for HIV. The ELISA detects antibodies produced in response to the HIV antigen.

WESTERN BLOT

The Western blot is a more specific test for the presence of the HIV antibody. It is also more expensive and labor intensive compared with the ELISA.

The usual course of events when a client requests testing for HIV includes the following steps: (1) Pretest counseling is provided, and the informed consent is signed; (2) serum is drawn and tested by ELISA for the presence of the HIV antibody, and if this test is negative, the tests stop here; (3) if the test is positive twice by ELISA, then a Western blot is performed, and if this is also positive, the client is considered HIV positive and, therefore, infected with HIV; (4) if the Western blot is negative, a confirmatory test is often run, and if this is still negative, the client is considered HIV negative. Most laboratories will confirm positive results by running the Western blot a second time.

CD4 CELL COUNT

The CD4 cell count is a pivotal test in the evaluation of any client with HIV infection to stage the disease for diagnostic purposes, to provide a guideline for differential diagnosis, and to make therapeutic decisions. The CD4 count represents the product of three variables: the white cell count × the percentage of lymphocytes × the percentage of lymphocytes that are CD4 cells. A change in any one of the three variables will alter the result. The majority of clients who have a diagnosis defining acquired immunodeficiency syndrome (AIDS) have a CD4 count of less than 200 mm^3.[2]

Allergic Skin Testing

In addition to blood tests, skin testing confirms sensitivity to a specific allergen. These tests involve placing a known antigen on or directly below the skin (intradermal) to check for the presence of antibodies. The antigen can be applied in one of three methods: (1) scratch test, (2) patch test, or (3) intradermal test. In the first test (also known as a tine or prick test), the allergen is applied to a superficial scratch that cuts the outer layer of skin. For a patch test, the antigen is applied directly to the skin and then covered with a gauze dressing. Intradermal testing involves injecting a small amount of the antigen into the intradermal layer of the skin. Intradermal testing is the most accurate method but carries a higher risk of severe allergic reactions.

Often, nurses administer skin tests and interpret test results. To interpret results, the nurse must observe for several reactions. An immediate reaction (i.e., appearing within 10–20 minutes after the injection) marked by erythema and wheal formation denotes a positive reaction. Positive reactions indicate an antibody response to previous exposure to this antigen and suggest that the client is allergic to the particular substance causing the reaction. Negative reactions may be inconclusive, indicating the need for further assessment. Negative results may indicate that (1) antibodies have not formed to this antigen, (2) the antigen was deposited too deeply into the skin (e.g., subcutaneously), or (3) the client is immunosuppressed as a result of disease or therapies (e.g., chemotherapy, steroids, and radiation therapy).

Problems arising from skin testing range from minor itching to anaphylaxis. Itching and discomfort at the injection site, for example, are common and can be relieved by the application of cool compresses and topical steroids. Ulceration of the injection site is best treated by keeping the area clean and dry. Anaphylactic shock is a rare but potentially lethal complication of skin testing. A client with a history of an anaphylactic reaction to a substance should never be skin tested for an allergy to that substance.

Food Allergy Testing

Food allergies can be tested by skin testing or by either food challenges or an elimination diet. In the challenge test, suspected foods are given to the client in progressively larger doses until a reaction is evoked. Symptoms of a reaction range from the typical erythema, itching, and rash to vomiting or diarrhea. Symptoms such as fatigue, depression, or restlessness are not conclusive of an allergy.

In the elimination diet, foods are eliminated from the diet one by one until the symptoms are relieved. This may indicate allergies to food additives or foods themselves.

Radioallergosorbent Test

The radioallergosorbent test (RAST) identifies the immunoglobulin E antibodies that are a response to antigens such as dust and pollen. A sample of blood is needed for this expensive test.

Bone Marrow Assessment

Chapter 27 discusses bone marrow aspiration.

Lymphatic Assessment

Diagnostic assessment of the lymphatic system can be found in Chapters 27, 28, 36, and 55.

Lymphangiogram

A lymphangiogram is a test that allows visualization of the lymphatic system to assess the presence of malignancy (lymphoma) or metastatic disease (testicular cancer) in tumors involving the lymphatic system or with typical lymphatic spread. The test involves the injection of an oil-based dye into the lymphatic system. First, local anesthesia is applied to the tops of the feet and a blue dye is injected into the top of the feet, which is picked up by the lymphatics. A cutdown is performed with a catheter inserted into the lymphatic channel and an oil-based dye is injected. The feet are elevated to aid in distribution of the dye throughout the lymphatic system. X-ray studies are taken to visualize the lymphatic system.

The test takes several hours on the first day, and follow-up x-ray studies are performed the next day. The dye itself is excreted very slowly, taking months to more than a year for it to be completely excreted. The dye is excreted through both the urine and respiratory system.

Possible adverse reactions associated with the test include fever, allergic reaction to the dye, infection at the incision site, and possible pulmonary oil embolism. The client should monitor the site of the incision closely for infection. The client should be told that the urine will have a bluish discoloration for a while after the test and the tops of the feet may remain blue for months. The client also should be told to report any fever, signs of redness or swelling at the incision, or respiratory distress to the physician.

Other Diagnostic Studies

A complete blood count (CBC) with differential and immunoglobulin studies may also be completed.

STUDY QUESTIONS

1. Which of the following organs produces immunologic defense for a client?
   A. Liver
   B. Lung
   C. Heart
   D. Bone marrow
2. Immunoglobulin G is found in:
   A. Tears
   B. Mucus
   C. Blood plasma
   D. Breast milk
3. The client most susceptible to disease resulting from a compromised immune system is:
   A. A newborn with combined immunodeficiency
   B. An adult who was exposed to the human immunodeficiency virus
   C. A teenager who is taking glucocorticoids for asthma
   D. An elderly client whose spouse died and who has asthma
4. Prevention of immunocompromise in clients consists of which of the following behaviors?
   A. Sexual activity with multiple partners
   B. Balanced nutritional intake
   C. Increasing emotional and physical stress
   D. Use of recreational drugs
5. The laboratory study that best indicates immunocompromise is:
   A. Electrolytes
   B. Blood urea nitrogen
   C. Complete blood count with differential
   D. Erythrocyte sedimentation rate

CRITICAL THINKING EXERCISES

SCENARIO A

A client has a suspected disease that suppresses the immune system.

1. Which diseases suppress the immune system?
2. Which drugs suppress the immune system?
3. How are alterations in the immune system diagnosed?
4. Assuming the client has an appropriately functioning immune system, which diseases stimulate an immune response?

SCENARIO B

A young woman has reactive airway disease and has acquired a respiratory infection. She was treated with oxygen per nasal cannula, dexamethasone (Decadron) intravenously (IV), aminophylline IV, erythromycin IV, and acetaminophen (Tylenol) orally. Her diet is clear liquids.

1. What components of this client study put the woman at risk for compromise of the immune system?
2. What part of the immune system is specifically involved in reactive airway disease?
3. What must occur in the immune system for an infection to require external intervention for a cure?
4. How can people enhance their immune system without the use of medications?

BIBLIOGRAPHY

1. Baigis-Smith, J., Coombs, U. J., & Larson, E. (1994). HIV infection, exercise, and immune function. *IMAGE: Journal of Nursing Scholarship, 26*(4), 277–281.
2. Bartlett, J. G. (1992). Recommendations for the medical care of persons with HIV infection. In *A guide to HIV care from the AIDS Care Program of the Johns Hopkins Medical Institutions* (pp. 23–25). Baltimore, MD: Johns Hopkins University.
3. Calianno, C., & Pino, T. (1995). Getting a reaction to anergy panel testing. *Nursing '95, 25*(1), 58–61.
4. Campbell, N. A., Mitchell, L. G., & Reece, J. B. (1994). *Biology: Concepts and connections*. Redwood City, CA.: Benjamin/Cummings.
5. Golde, D. W. (1991). The stem cell. *Scientific American, 261,* 86–93.
6. Grady, C. (1988). Host defense mechanisms: An overview. *Seminars in Oncology Nursing, 4,* 86–94.
7. Hokyt, N. J. (1989). Host defense mechanisms and compromises in the trauma patient. *Critical Care Clinics of North America, 1,* 753–765.
8. Klein, D. M., & Witek-Janusek, L. (1992). Advances in immunotherapy for sepsis. *Dimensions in Critical Care Nursing, 11,* 75–89.
9. Klein, J. (1990). *Immunology*. Boston: Blackwell Scientific.
10. Mackey, R. B. (1995). Discover the healing power of therapeutic touch. *American Journal of Nursing, 95*(4), 26–33.
11. Paul, W. E. (1989). *Fundamental immunology* (2nd ed.). New York: Raven Press.
12. Reckling, J. (1987). Understanding immune system dysfunction. *Nursing '87, 87,* 34–42.
13. Rennie, J. (1990). The body against itself. *Scientific American, 260,* 106–115.
14. Roit, I. M., Brostoff, J., & Male, D. K. (1989). *Immunology*. Philadelphia: J. B. Lippincott.
15. Rosenthal, C. H. (1989). Immunosuppression in pediatric critical care patients. *Critical Care Nursing Clinics of North America, 1,* 775–785.
16. Sande, M. A., & Volberding (1995). *The medical management of AIDS* (4th ed.). Philadelphia: W. B. Saunders.
17. Schwab, R. (1989). Host defense mechanisms and aging. *Seminars in Oncology, 16,* 20–27.
18. Sheehan, C. (1990). *Clinical immunology*. Philadelphia: J. B. Lippincott.
19. Stites, D. P., & Terr, A. I. (Eds.). (1991). *Basic and clinical immunology* (7th ed.). Norwalk, CT: Appleton & Lange.
20. Tribett, D. (1989). Immune system function: Implications for critical care nursing practice. *Critical Care Nursing Clinics of America, 1,* 725–740.
21. Virella, G., Goust, J. M., & Fudenberg, H. H. (Eds.). (1990). *Medical immunology*. New York: Marcel Dekker.
22. Weigle, W. (1989). Effects of aging on the immune system. *Hospital Practice, 24,* 112–119.
23. Young, J. D., & Cohn, Z. A. (1988). How killer cells kill. *Scientific American, 258,* 38–44.

Chapter 9 Nursing Care of Clients with Altered Immune Systems

Learning Outcomes

After completing this chapter, the learner will be able to:

1. Conduct a nursing history and physical assessment of the client with an altered immune system.
2. Identify nursing diagnoses pertinent to the client with an altered immune system.
3. Identify goals for the client with an altered immune system.
4. Implement appropriate nursing interventions for the client with an altered immune system.
5. Evaluate nursing care for the client with an altered immune system.

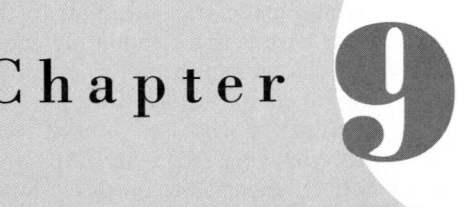

The immune system controls the body's response to invading foreign substances. A functioning immune system can help protect the body from a wide variety of pathogens. On the other hand, an immune system that is malfunctioning predisposes the client to the development of a wide variety of disorders ranging from severe infection to autoimmune disease. Chapter 8 describes the normally functioning immune system; this chapter looks at alterations in the immune system and how these changes affect the client.

HUMAN IMMUNODEFICIENCY VIRUS

In 1981, astute observation by several physicians in San Francisco and New York witnessed the onset of a new spectrum of diseases known as acquired immunodeficiency syndrome (AIDS). Because of the prevalence of AIDS in the homosexual community, it was suspected that the causative agent was sexually transmitted, similar to that of hepatitis B. By 1982, AIDS was identified in other populations, including injection drug users, recipients of blood or blood products, heterosexual partners of clients with AIDS, and children. The causative agent, human immunodeficiency virus (HIV), was isolated from clients with AIDS in 1983. Shortly after this discovery, screening tests for the detection of HIV antibody were developed. Since March 1985, all blood products have been routinely screened for the presence of HIV antibody. Anonymous testing sites have been established to facilitate voluntary screening of those who participate in high-risk behaviors.

The development of AIDS represents an advanced stage of disease along a continuum that ranges from asymptomatic HIV infection to the development of this most serious and debilitating condition.

The nomenclature of HIV infection and HIV disease has taken on several forms over the past decade. The Centers for Disease Control (CDC) revised the case definition for AIDS and AIDS-related complex (ARC) until it reached the proposed form in 1991 (Box 9–1).

BOX 9–1

1993 Revised Human Immunodeficiency Virus Classification System for Adolescents and Adults

The revised Centers for Disease Control classification system for human immunodeficiency virus–(HIV) infected adolescents and adults emphasizes the importance of CD4+ lymphocyte testing in the clinical management of HIV-infected clients. The classification system is divided into laboratory and clinical categories as follows.

LABORATORY CATEGORIES

Category 1: greater than or equal to 500 CD4+ cells
Category 2: 200 to 499 CD4+ cells
Category 3: less than 200 CD4+ cells

CLINICAL CATEGORIES

Category A: One or more of the following conditions occurring in an adolescent or adult with documented HIV infection. Conditions listed in categories B and C must not have occurred.

- Asymptomatic HIV infection
- Persistent generalized lymphadenopathy
- Acute (primary) HIV infection with accompanying illness or history of acute HIV infection

Category B: Symptomatic conditions occurring in an HIV-infected adolescent or adult that are not included among conditions listed in clinical category C and that meet at least one of the following criteria:

The conditions are attributed to HIV infection or are indicative of a defect in cell-mediated immunity.
The conditions are considered by physicians to have a clinical course or management that is complicated by HIV infection.

Examples of conditions in clinical category B include but are not limited to

- Bacterial endocarditis, meningitis, pneumonia, or sepsis
- Candidiasis, vulvovaginal; persistent for more than 1 month, or poorly responsive to therapy
- Candidiasis, oropharyngeal (thrush)
- Cervical dysplasia, severe; or carcinoma
- Constitutional symptoms, such as fever (>38.5° C) or diarrhea lasting more than 1 month
- Hairy leukoplakia, oral
- Herpes zoster (shingles), involving at least two distinct episodes or more than one dermatome
- Idiopathic thrombocytopenic purpura
- Listeriosis
- *Mycobacterium tuberculosis* infection, pulmonary
- Nocardiosis
- Pelvic inflammatory disease
- Peripheral neuropathy

Category C: Any condition listed in the 1987* surveillance case definition for AIDS and affecting an adolescent or an adult. For classification purposes, once a Category C condition has occurred, the person will remain in category C.

- The conditions in clinical category C are strongly associated with severe immunodeficiency, occur frequently in HIV-infected clients, and cause serious morbidity or mortality.
- According to the proposed classification system, HIV-infected clients would be classified on the basis of both.

The lowest accurate (not necessarily the most recent) CD4+ lymphocyte determination
The most severe clinical condition diagnosed regardless of the client's current clinical condition

* As of January 1, 1993, three clinical conditions (pulmonary tuberculosis, recurrent pneumonia, and invasive cervical cancer) were added to the 1987 surveillance case definition for AIDS.

Adapted from the CDC. (1992). Revised classification system for HIV infection and expanded surveillance case definition for AIDS among adolescents and adults. *Morbidity and Mortality Weekly Report, 41*(51), 961–962.

Incidence

HIV disease represents one of the most devastating conditions to appear in modern times. Current research suggests that HIV is probably a new disease that has occurred as a result of mutation of a closely related virus, called the simian immunodeficiency virus. Retrospective studies have shown that HIV was present in Africa, Europe, and the United States over the past 30 years. The disease has grown to epidemic proportions since 1981. Because only AIDS is reportable to the CDC, statistical information is somewhat limited concerning those with the earlier form of infection or disease. It is estimated that worldwide more than 10 million people are HIV positive.

Etiology

The CDC first used the name AIDS in the fall of 1982. In 1986, the virus was renamed HIV. This term is now commonly accepted throughout the world.

Besides the logarithmic increase in incidence, AIDS has an extremely high mortality rate; more than 90 per cent of clients who experience the most severe form of the disease will die within 4 years of an AIDS diagnosis.

In the United States, the incidence of HIV disease is not evenly distributed. Cases of HIV infection tend to occur in areas with high concentrations of participants in high-risk behaviors. According to the CDC, states with the highest occurrence are New York, California, Florida, Texas, and New Jersey.

Since 1989, there has been a decrease in the incidence of AIDS among white gay men but an increase among intravenous drug users. Black and Hispanic communities are disproportionately represented in the number of AIDS cases in the United States. The incidence of infection is especially increasing in women. Minority women are even more dramatically affected by AIDS.

Risk Factors

Transmission of HIV occurs through horizontal transmission (from either sexual contact or parenteral exposure to blood and blood products) or through vertical transmission (from HIV-infected mother to infant). Several cases of HIV transmission through breast milk have been reported. No other routes of transmission have been shown to exist.

CRITICAL TO REMEMBER

HIV is not transmitted by casual contact. Transmission always involves exposure to some body fluid from an infected client.

The greatest concentrations of virus have been found in blood, semen, cerebrospinal fluid, and cervical-vaginal secretions. HIV has been found in low concentrations in tears, saliva, and urine, but no cases have been transmitted by these routes. It is believed that the amount or concentration of the virus, the length of exposure, and the route of transmission all play important roles in transmission of the virus.

CRITICAL TO REMEMBER

Sexual activity remains the number one route of transmission of HIV in the United States.

Sexual activity between men and women can result in transmission of HIV. The incidence of heterosexual transmission is on the rise. Some factors that increase the risk of sexual transmission include multiple sexual partners, receptive anal intercourse, the presence of open lesions in the genital area, and sexual exposure without some form of barrier such as a condom.

Parenteral transmission occurs when there is direct blood-to-blood contact with a client infected with HIV. This can occur through sharing of contaminated needles and drug paraphernalia (works), through transfusion of blood or blood products, by accidental needle-stick injury to a health-care worker, or from blood exposure to nonintact skin or to mucous membranes. The rate of transmission to a health-care worker from a needle stick involving a known HIV-positive client is 0.47 per cent.

There is recent evidence that the use of crack cocaine (which is smoked, not injected) results in an alarmingly high rate of HIV infection. Some investigators have speculated that this may occur because of the frequent practice of exchanging this drug for sexual favors, which, therefore, increases the number of sexual partners. The fact that crack costs significantly less than other drugs has led to its use in younger populations; therefore, there is concern that this will lead to an increased incidence of HIV in adolescents.

There is consensus that the spread of HIV, similar to any communicable disease, is preventable through education that focuses on knowledge about transmission and risk-reduction strategies. Interventions aimed at reducing a client's risk of acquiring HIV infection need to be based on a thorough assessment of the client's sexual practices and past or present use of drugs. Clients need to be counseled on safer sexual practices, avoidance of sharing needles, and methods of cleaning drug paraphernalia. Assisting the injection drug user to gain access to drug-treatment facilities is an essential aspect of nursing care aimed at reducing the risk of HIV transmission both for the individual and the client's family.

Women considering pregnancy who participate in high-risk behaviors, or have sexual partners who do, should be offered HIV testing and counseling. The risk to the infant and the mother as well as methods of reducing risks during pregnancy need to be discussed.

Health-care workers need to use universal precautions (Box 9–2) when handling all body fluids and when they engage in procedures that may possibly place them at risk (i.e., phlebotomy, handling of specimens).

Pathophysiology

HIV-1 is a member of the lentivirus subfamily of human retroviruses. Diseases caused by lentiviruses are

BOX 9–2

Universal Precautions

Universal precautions are intended to prevent parenteral, mucous membrane, and nonintact skin exposures of health-care workers to blood-borne pathogens. Universal precautions apply to blood and to other body fluids containing visible blood, semen, vaginal secretions, cerebrospinal fluid, synovial fluid, pleural fluid, peritoneal fluid, pericardial fluid, and amniotic fluid. Universal precautions do not apply to feces, nasal secretions, sputum, sweat, tears, urine, and vomitus unless they contain visible blood.

BARRIER GUIDELINES

1. Disposable gloves (vinyl, latex) should be worn when in contact or when there is potential for contact with blood, body fluids, or other fluids that may contain human immunodeficiency virus (HIV). Gloves should be removed after each client contact. Rubber gloves can be used for equipment cleaning.
2. Hands should be washed between clients, after any exposure, and after removal of gloves.
3. Protective eyewear, face shields, or masks or a combination should be worn during procedures that may aerosolize blood.
4. Impervious gowns should be worn when there is potential for exposure to large quantities of blood, such as in the labor and delivery area or emergency room.

NEEDLE PRECAUTIONS

1. Needles should never be recapped after use; keep in mind that most needle sticks are the result of missed needle recapping.
2. Do not cut, break, or bend needles after use; this may release aerosolized blood from the needle shaft.
3. Do not leave used needles lying around.
4. Do not dispose of needles in ordinary receptacles; instead, use appropriately labeled, impermeable needle containers.

Adapted from the Centers for Disease Control (1988). Update: Universal precautions for prevention of transmission of human immunodeficiency virus, hepatitis B virus, and other bloodborne pathogens in health-care setting. *Morbidity and Mortality Weekly Report, 37(3),* 377–388.

characterized by an insidious onset with progressive involvement of the central nervous system and may result in disorders of the immune system. A retrovirus belongs to the family *Retroviridae* and is characterized by the presence of a viral enzyme called reverse transcriptase. This enzyme converts the virus' RNA into DNA, which becomes incorporated into the host cell nucleus. HIV infects helper T cells (T4 lymphocytes), macrophages, B cells, and certain cells in the brain and central nervous system. Helper T cells are infected more readily than are other cells, and their subsequent depletion is responsible for the devastating symptoms and opportunistic infections associated with HIV disease.

Once the initial HIV infection takes place, the virus may remain latent inside the cell for an undetermined length of time. Some form of activation must occur for viral replication to begin. The exact mechanism that causes activation is still being investigated.

HIV-2 is distinctly different from HIV-1 but has many similarities. HIV-2 was first described in West Africa in 1986. The majority of clients with HIV-2 infection in Africa experience a syndrome similar to AIDS; others have AIDS-related complex (ARC)–type symptoms, whereas others remain asymptomatic. HIV-2 is most commonly spread through sexual intercourse. To date, cases of HIV-2 are rare in the United States, but the CDC and the U.S. Food and Drug Administration initiated a surveillance program for HIV-2 in 1987, anticipating that occasional cases of infection with this virus will occur.

The main target of HIV infection is the T4 or CD4+ cell. The normal number of T4 cells for clients with an intact immune system is between 700 and 1300 T4 cells/mm^3. Once these cells are infected, either they are changed and rendered nonfunctional or their actual number is depleted.

CRITICAL TO REMEMBER

Opportunistic infections most commonly occur when the T4 cell count drops below 200.

HIV-related malignancies and neurologic disease can occur at higher T4 cell counts. Remaining T4 cells may become dysfunctional.

Infection by HIV can also result in leukopenia, which frequently results in a white cell count less than 3500 cells/mm^3. Immune thrombocytopenia is also seen along the entire spectrum of HIV infection. Platelet counts may drop to a level that requires frequent intervention to prevent hemorrhage. Zidovudine, intravenous immune globulin, and steroids have been shown to be effective in treating HIV-related thrombocytopenia. In rare cases, splenectomy may be indicated when thrombocytopenia is unresponsive to conventional therapy.

The CDC also developed a classification system in 1987 in an attempt to outline the stages of illness (Table 9–1). This system viewed HIV disease in stages rather than as a continuum of disease states.

Clinical Manifestations

The first stage is often one of acute infection (CDC category A) or the process of being exposed to HIV and becoming antibody positive (also known as seroconversion). Some clients experience a mononucleosis-like ill-

TABLE 9–1 Centers for Disease Control (CDC) Classification System for Human Immunodeficiency Virus Infection

GROUP	DESCRIPTION
I	Acute Infection
II	Asymptomatic infection
III	Persistent generalized lymphadenopathy with nodes 1 cm or more at two or more extrainguinal sites for more than 3 months
IV	Other disease
Subgroup A	Constitutional symptoms
Subgroup B	Neurologic disease
Subgroup C	Secondary infectious diseases
Category C-1	Specified secondary infectious diseases listed in the CDC surveillance definitions for acquired immunodeficiency syndrome
Category C-2	Other specified secondary infectious diseases
Subgroup D	Secondary cancers
Subgroup E	Other conditions

Adapted from the Centers for Disease Control. (1986). Classification system for human T-lymphotropic virus III/lymphadenopathy-associated virus infection. *Morbidity and Mortality Weekly Report, 35,* 334–339.

ness consisting of fever, malaise, lymphadenopathy, rash, and, at times, aseptic meningitis; others remain asymptomatic throughout the seroconversion phase.

Once a client is HIV positive, the continuum begins with a period of remaining asymptomatic. Although the length of the asymptomatic state varies for each client, it commonly ranges from 7 to 10 years. These clients usually feel well and are able to carry on their usual activities. They are faced, however, with risks of transmission and anxiety over planning for the future. Persistent generalized lymphadenopathy (PGL), defined as lymph node enlargement persisting for longer than 3 months, with greater than 1-cm enlargement at more than one extrainguinal site and with no other explanation for the lymphadenopathy, is frequently found in the earlier phase of HIV infection. Early HIV infection is classified by the CDC as category A (see Box 9–1).

HIV disease begins to develop as the immune system becomes depleted or ineffective as a result of the virus's effect on the helper T cell. During this phase, symptoms develop, either alone or in combination, that reflect the damage done to the body's defenses. Some of these symptoms include skin rashes, fevers, fatigue, drenching night sweats, persistent diarrhea, weight loss, PGL, oral thrush, oral hairy leukoplakia, and vaginal yeast infections. The CDC classification system describes these clients as belonging to clinical category B.

The most severe form of HIV disease (CDC category C) involves the development of clinical disease indicative of severe immunosuppression. Although clients with constitutional signs may have debilitating symptoms (i.e., severe diarrhea and weight loss), clients with clinical category C disease, in general, have more severe immune suppression. The AIDS-associated malignancies and neurologic disease may occur at higher helper T cell counts, whereas opportunistic infections more commonly occur when the helper T cell count drops below 200.

These clients are usually very ill and frequently require hospitalization during their acute infection. It is not unusual, however, for these clients (especially when first diagnosed) to return to a high level of functioning once the infection is treated and maintenance therapy is begun.

Another phase of HIV disease is advanced or terminal AIDS. Within this phase, clients often have experienced multiple opportunistic infections or malignancies, have some form of neurologic disease, experienced toxic reactions such as bone marrow suppression or intolerance to known therapies, and have little in the way of energy or nutritional stores to combat the persistent devastation of HIV infection on an already depleted immune system. In addition to the more common constitutional symptoms, clients with advanced AIDS often experience some form of pain. Pain may be related to physical symptoms such as peripheral neuropathies, myalgias, or malignancies; but psychogenic pain may be experienced by these clients as well.

DIAGNOSTIC ASSESSMENT

Many clients infected with HIV will develop the antibody in about 6 to 12 weeks. Testing for the presence of the antibody is done in two stages: first with the enzyme-linked immunosorbent assay (ELISA) and then for confirmation with the Western blot.

CRITICAL TO REMEMBER

It is important that clients receive post-test counseling, whether they test positive or negative.

HIV-positive clients will have many questions and concerns about insurance, medical care, and access to support services. Clients who test HIV negative need to be counseled about any high-risk behaviors as well as the need for retesting if it has been 12 weeks or less since a possible exposure. Several other HIV detection tests are available, but are expensive and still investigational.

OPPORTUNISTIC INFECTIONS

Because nurses frequently care for clients with opportunistic infections, it is important that these unusual infections be demystified by acquiring an understanding of the type of infection, the target organs, and the methods of treatment and prevention.

***Pneumocystis Carinii* Pneumonia.** *Pneumocystis carinii* pneumonia (PCP) is the primary killer of clients with AIDS. PCP is caused by the protozoal pneumocyst. The target organ is the lung, although extrapulmonary pneumocystosis has occurred in clients with AIDS. Those clients who experience PCP almost always have clear evidence of immunosuppression, such as a low helper T cell count (often less than 200). PCP commonly has an insidious onset. Clients with the HIV infection often have nonspecific symptoms such as fever, fatigue, and weight loss for weeks to months before the onset of respiratory symptoms.

CRITICAL TO REMEMBER

Nonproductive cough and dyspnea are the most common presenting symptoms of PCP.

Clients may be mildly or very symptomatic.

Definitive diagnosis requires seeing *Pneumocystis* organisms in bronchial secretions or in lung tissue. This can be accomplished by bronchoscopy, transbronchial lung biopsy, or sputum induction. Treatment options include a 3-week course of trimethoprim-sulfamethoxazole (Bactrim or Septra), parenteral pentamidine, or dapsone-trimethoprim. It is important to note that, in clients with AIDS, there is a high frequency of adverse reactions (especially rash and fever) to trimethoprim-sulfamethoxazole. Because PCP ultimately occurs in 80 to 90 per cent of clients with AIDS, it is important to prevent either the first episode or recurrences of this opportunistic infection.

Cytomegalovirus. Infection with cytomegalovirus (CMV), a member of the herpesvirus family, is extremely common in clients with AIDS. Depending on the socioeconomic conditions of the population, anywhere from 40 to 100 per cent of adults have been infected with CMV and have formed an antibody to it; yet, in immunocompetent hosts, it remains latent and does not cause clinical disease. In clients with AIDS, infection with CMV can cause various clinical illnesses, including chorioretinitis, pneumonitis, esophagitis, colitis, encephalitis, adrenalitis, and hepatitis.

Diagnosis of CMV disease is made by biopsy. Autopsy reports and clinical studies have indicated that almost 90 per cent of AIDS clients experience invasive CMV during the course of their illness.

Herpes Simplex. Herpes simplex virus (HSV) can cause disease in both normal and immunocompromised hosts.

CRITICAL TO REMEMBER

Ulcerative HSV infection that lasts longer than 1 month in a client with the HIV infection is diagnostic of AIDS.

Reactivation of HSV is common in clients with AIDS and includes extensive disease of the mouth, esophagus, and genital and perirectal areas. In severe cases, HSV may result in encephalitis. Tingling and burning at the site of the vesicle and later blister formation are the first symptoms. Severe pain at the location of the lesions is not unusual. In the case of esophageal HSV, pain and difficulty swallowing are the presenting symptoms. Diagnosis is made by clinical evidence, viral culture, or biopsy. Acyclovir is the agent of choice for all HSV infections. Acyclovir is available in oral, topical, and intravenous preparations; the best route of administration is based on the location and severity of the infection. Foscarnet has also been used to treat severe HSV infections when acyclovir resistance was suspected.

Toxoplasmosis. Toxoplasmosis, or infection with *Toxoplasma gondii,* a protozoan, causes focal neurologic symptoms in clients with AIDS and is recognized as the major opportunistic infection of the central nervous system. Infection with *T. gondii* is the result of reactivation of a latent infection that causes headache, seizures, hemiparesis, lethargy, and focal encephalitis. Some clients may experience a subtle change in personality or cognitive ability. A computed tomographic scan of the head with contrast will usually show multiple ring-enhancing mass lesions. Brain biopsy is the only definitive diagnostic method but is rarely used because of the risks associated with this procedure. Standard medical management includes the combination of pyrimethamine and sulfadiazine.

Cryptosporidium. *Cryptosporidium* is also a protozoan parasite that results in intestinal infection manifested by watery diarrhea, malaise, nausea, and abdominal cramps. Diarrhea and abdominal pain usually occur after food ingestion. Clients with AIDS have been known to lose 10 to 15 L of stool per day, which results in severe dehydration. The diagnosis of cryptosporidiosis is made by stool culture. Clinical trials are under way using various medications to control the symptoms. Management focuses on alleviation of symptoms associated with dehydration, fluid and electrolyte imbalance, and weight loss.

Mycobacterium Avium Complex. *Mycobacterium avium* complex is an environmental bacterium, present in soil and water, that causes gastrointestinal, respiratory, or disseminated disease in immunocompromised hosts. In clients with AIDS, it is usually found when severe immunosuppression is present and after multiple opportunistic infections have occurred. Symptoms of infection include fever, weight loss, anemia, and neutropenia; it may cause chronic diarrhea, malabsorption, and extrabiliary obstruction. Multiple drug regimens, including amikacin, ethambutol, clofazimine, ciprofloxacin, and rifampin, produce profound side effects and their use is controversial.

The incidence of *Mycobacterium tuberculosis* (MTB) infection is increasing in clients with HIV infection. Tuberculosis is a more rapidly progressing disease in these clients and may occur at any time throughout the spectrum of HIV infection. Fever, weight loss, night sweats, fatigue, and lymphadenitis are the most common presenting symptoms. HIV-associated MTB infection is often extrapulmonary and disseminated to other organs, particularly the kidneys, liver, spleen, lymph nodes, blood, skin, gastrointestinal tract, and bone marrow. Diagnosis is made by culture or by chest radiography if the lungs are involved. A tuberculin skin test should be done with use of a control such as *Candida;* because anergy is frequently found in clients with HIV infection, false negatives may result. Two- or three-drug regimens are used to treat MTB infection; most commonly, ethambutol, isoniazid, rifampin, and pyrazinamide are among the choices. All clients with HIV infection should be screened for tuberculosis by having a Mantoux skin test with a control done every 6 months. Clients with advancing HIV disease may need periodic chest radiographs because they are likely to be anergic.

Other Fungal Infections. Fungal infections that can occur in clients with HIV infection include *Candida albicans, Cryptococcus neoformans,* histoplasmosis, and coccidioidomycosis. Candidiasis appears as a thick, cottage cheese–like exudate on the affected oral, esophageal, and vaginal mucosa. *C. neoformans* presents with headache and subtle mental status changes, which may progress to fever, focal neurologic signs, seizures, and coma. With histoplasmosis, symptoms may include persistent fever and weight loss. Coccidioidomycosis presents with nonspecific symptoms such as malaise, fever, weight loss, cough, and fatigue. Topical or systemic antifungal therapies, or both, are used as indicated.

MALIGNANCIES ASSOCIATED WITH HUMAN IMMUNODEFICIENCY VIRUS

Malignancies associated with HIV include Kaposi's sarcoma (KS) and AIDS-associated lymphoma. KS, a neoplasm of the vascular endothelium, is the most common neoplasm affecting clients with AIDS. AIDS-associated KS is often aggressive and disfiguring. KS is more common among homosexual and bisexual men compared with other high-risk groups. It typically presents as a purplish-red lesion that is not painful or pruritic. The lesion can be flat or indurated and will frequently progress to a nodule over time. Lesions may appear anywhere on the skin and may include the lymph nodes, mucous membranes, and viscera. Treatment for KS centers on balancing the risk of treatment with the risk of opportunistic infection. Radiation therapy, chemotherapy, and interferon α are all used, depending on the location and extent of involvement. Symptomatic therapy is also used for palliation of disfigurement, lymphedema, skin breakdown, and pain.

Non-Hodgkin's lymphoma, Burkitt's-like lymphomas, and malignant lymphomas of the central nervous system can be classified as AIDS-associated malignancies. Prognosis tends to be poor because of an inadequate response to chemotherapy and lack of adequate bone marrow reserve for completion of needed therapy. Although these neoplasms occur less often than KS does, survival is significantly shorter when they are present.

HUMAN IMMUNODEFICIENCY VIRUS NEUROLOGIC DISEASE

Neurologic disease in HIV can involve the central and peripheral nervous systems. AIDS dementia complex is characterized by cognitive, motor, and behavioral dysfunction.

Neuropsychiatric testing may be performed at various intervals to monitor symptoms. Cerebral atrophy on neurodiagnostic imaging is a nearly universal finding in AIDS dementia complex. The use of zidovudine (Retrovir, ZDV, and formerly known as AZT) has been used successfully in treating AIDS dementia. Symptomatic therapy is aimed at treating the depression or mania; ensuring safety is essential. Prognosis is poor, and end-stage dementia leaves the client lying in bed with a vacant stare, unable to ambulate and often incontinent.

Peripheral nerve disease, although not an AIDS-defining condition, is a common complication of the HIV infection. The most common of these neuropathies presents as a burning or tingling sensation of the feet, legs, or hands. Neuropathies may be further complicated by the addition of certain antiviral medications (dideoxyinosine, or ddI, dideoxycytidine, or ddC) that are discussed later. Treatment involves symptomatic therapy. Amitriptyline has been reported to have some benefit in treating these neuropathies.

Medical Management

PHARMACOLOGIC MANAGEMENT

The medical management of HIV infection is aimed at controlling the replication of the virus and thereby delaying further destruction of the immune system. Zidovudine (also known as Retrovir, ZDV, and formerly AZT) is an antiretroviral agent that has been shown to prolong survival and reduce mortality in clients with HIV infection. The use of zidovudine is indicated for anyone with HIV infection with a helper T4 cell count less than 500. The most worrisome side effects associated with zidovudine include anemia and neutropenia. Complete blood counts are monitored at frequent intervals throughout the course of therapy. Serious side effects are easily managed by blood transfusion, temporary withholding of the medication, or dosage reduction. Some additional adverse experiences that have been reported include nausea, headaches, muscle pain and weakness, and fatigue. The dose of zidovudine has been modified to include the current standard of 100 mg every 4 hours five times per day. Various doses and schedules are being investigated, including 300 mg/day and a schedule of 200 mg every 8 hours.

Dideoxyinosine (ddI) is approved for use in clients with HIV infection who have demonstrated intolerance to zidovudine or who have had significant disease progression despite treatment with this drug. Dideoxycytidine (ddC) is still under investigation. Both ddI and ddC are antiretroviral agents that inhibit replication of the virus. The main side effects include peripheral neuropathy, diarrhea, and pancreatitis (Table 9–2).

A host of other medications are administered for a variety of associated conditions. These include

- Antifungals (for candidiasis, histoplasmosis)
- Antitubercular agents (for mycobacterium tuberculosis, mycobacterium avium complex infection)
- Antineoplastics (for Kaposi's sarcoma, non-Hodgkin's lymphoma)
- Antiinfectives (for Kaposi's sarcoma, *Pneumocystis carinii* pneumonia, mycobacterium avium complex infection, toxoplasmosis)
- Antivirals (for herpes simplex, herpes zoster, cytomegalovirus infection)
- Hormones (for immunomodulation, muscle wasting)
- Colony stimulating factors (for neutropenia)

TABLE 9–2 Antiretroviral Agents*

GENERIC NAME (TRADE NAME)	SIDE EFFECTS	NURSING IMPLICATIONS
Zidovudine (Retrovir, AZT)	Anemia, granulocytopenia, headache, malaise, nausea, abdominal pain, diarrhea, rash	Monitor complete blood counts, (anemia in 2–4 weeks; granulocytopenia in 6–8 weeks), teach client to take medication around the clock and to report signs of infection.
Didanosine (ddI, Videx)	Pancreatitis, peripheral neuropathy, diarrhea, abdominal pain, liver function abnormalities, headache, granulocytopenia, possibly seizure and liver failure	Monitor for and teach client to monitor for and report signs and symptoms of pancreatitis, infection, and peripheral neuropathy. Monitor appropriate laboratory test results.
Zalcitabine (ddC, Hivid)	Peripheral neuropathy, pancreatitis, esophageal and oral ulcers, rash	Monitor for and teach client to monitor for and report signs and symptoms of pancreatitis and peripheral neuropathy. Monitor appropriate laboratory test results.
Stavudine† (Zerit)	Peripheral neuropathy, hepatitis, anemia, headache	Monitor appropriate laboratory test results. Follow protocols established for this investigational medication. Client should be informed that the drug is in clinical trials and written consent is required for participation.

* In combination therapy, these drugs can be combined for an enhanced effect.
† Not approved by the Food and Drug Administration.

Vaccines both to prevent HIV transmission and to treat those already infected are being developed. Scientists predict that the availability of such vaccines will take another 5 to 10 years before general distribution is possible.

DIETARY MANAGEMENT

The immune system needs protein, carbohydrates, fat, vitamins, and minerals in sufficient quantity to maintain optimal functioning. Therefore, nutrition is an essential component of the management of clients with the HIV infection. Eating well not only enhances the immune system but can serve to maintain a normal life-style and appearance.

A complete nutritional assessment is key to any educational strategy aimed at improving general nutrition. Weight loss may be caused by symptoms associated with gastrointestinal reactions to the infectious process or side effects of the drug regimen. Many of these symptoms are amenable to medical and nursing management. Routine dental care is essential for clients with HIV infection. Progressive disease to the gingivae and teeth can occur as a result of HIV infection and thereby affect the desire (taste changes) and ability to eat a well-balanced diet.

HIV wasting syndrome or the profound involuntary weight loss that occurs in some clients with advanced HIV disease is characterized by a weight loss of greater than 10 per cent of baseline body weight, either chronic diarrhea for more than 30 days, or chronic weakness and fever that is present constantly without any other explanation. This syndrome places extraordinary demands on available nutrients. Oral and enteral nutritional supplements are frequently used to combat the rapid weight loss and debilitation.

A well-balanced diet is generally recommended for all clients with the HIV infection. Dietary guidelines need to include foods that take into account the cultural and economic background of the client. Many experts also suggest that the addition of a multiple vitamin with B complex is desirable for ensuring adequate intake of essential vitamins and minerals.

Because of the increased energy requirements during times of infection, the body often demands more than is able to be consumed. For these clients, nutritional supplements are used. These supplements provide vitamins and minerals besides extra protein and calories. Products such as Ensure Plus, Sustacal HC, and Carnation Instant Breakfast are frequently added two to three times per day to the daily diet.

HOLISTIC THERAPIES

Many clients with HIV turn to holistic or complementary therapies in addition to traditional Western health-care practices. Some of these therapies include acupuncture, meditation, guided imagery, massage, and spiritual healing. The goal of such interventions is to empower clients to take an active part in the healing process.

Surgical Management

The surgical management of clients with HIV is limited to the placement of a venous access device, surgical intervention for treatment of malignancies, or biopsy. Venous access devices, such as a Groshung catheter, are used to facilitate frequent blood drawing, administration of intravenous medications (ganciclovir), hyperalimentation, and transfusions.

Nursing Management

Assessment

Understanding the real risk of HIV transmission is the first step in providing comprehensive nursing care. HIV is a fragile virus that demands a set of conditions in order to cause infection.

CRITICAL TO REMEMBER

For health-care workers, there must be mucous membrane contact or a break in the skin in contact with infected blood in order for the virus to invade the bloodstream.

HIV infection is the most difficult to contract in the health-care setting, but its potential devastation warrants careful adherence to universal precautions (see Box 9–2).

Most of the infections that afflict clients with HIV infection cannot be transmitted. Opportunistic infections, such as with *P. carinii, T. gondii, Mycobacterium avium-intracellulare,* and *Candida,* are not transmissible. Viruses such as herpes and bacteria such as *M. tuberculosis* can be transmitted to the immunocompetent host. Careful adherence to good hygiene and universal precautions is essential. Hepatitis B infection tends to be very common in clients with the HIV infection; therefore, immunization is recommended for health-care workers who have regular contact with these clients.

The skin is the body's first line of defense and is frequently affected by HIV infection. Cutaneous hypersensitivity reactions to medications and environmental antigens is seen often, and skin breakdown resulting from various viruses (HSV, varicella zoster) and fungi (tinea) can lead to further invasion and systemic disease. Open wounds may take slightly longer to heal and frequently cause scarring. Clients with a history of psoriasis or eczema may have severe exacerbations of these conditions. Nail changes are frequent and occur as a result of fungal infection or medications. Zidovudine has been shown to cause hyperpigmented changes in nails, especially in black and Hispanic clients. Hair changes are also seen; thinning of the hair is the most common. The nursing assessment includes a complete history of any skin conditions and allergies. Examining for rashes, ulcerations, vesicles, lesions, pruritus, dryness, scaling, bruising, color changes, and violaceous lesions is essential. Intervention is aimed at defining the cause and eliminating it, if possible (medication or environmental allergen), or treating the infection or dermatologic condition.

CRITICAL TO REMEMBER

The oral, vaginal, and rectal mucosa are particularly susceptible to the effects of HIV.

The history should include information about history of oral, vaginal, or rectal lesions (i.e., HSV); oral hygiene and dental practices; history of vaginal infections; and the presence of pain or bleeding in any of these locations. Assessment includes examination for oral ulcerations or lesions (violaceous lesions in the mouth may be suggestive of KS); thick, white, curdlike exudate suggestive of oral thrush; linear white striations on the lateral aspect of the tongue, or white plaques, suggestive of oral hairy leukoplakia; bleeding or hypertrophy of the gums; and the condition of existing teeth or dentures. The presence of a white, thick vaginal discharge is suggestive of vaginal candidiasis. The presence of vesicular lesions, ulcerations, and condylomata (warts) in the vaginal and rectal areas needs to be ascertained. The nasal mucosa is susceptible to herpetic lesions and may contain perforations when clients use inhaled cocaine. Intervention is based on defining the cause and initiating appropriate treatment.

Appetite and weight changes are frequent occurrences associated with HIV infection and disease. Whether these changes lead to obesity or cachexia, both can adversely affect immune system functioning. Profound weight loss is readily associated with HIV infection; however, some clients, especially early in the course of disease, actually have a weight gain. Sometimes this is a result of appetite changes caused by medication, stress, or drug detoxification. Nursing care needs to focus on identification of the underlying cause, monitoring weight and dietary intake, and evaluating the effect that the weight change has on the client's self-image.

Substance abuse, whether of alcohol or drugs such as heroin or cocaine, has potential deleterious effects on the immune system. Nursing care focuses on assessment of the potential or actual substance abuse and includes defining the substance of choice, the frequency of use, financial considerations, and how these affect family, job, and interpersonal relationships as well as omission of prescribed medications, poor dietary intake, inadequate rest, and missed follow-up appointments. Nurses need to evaluate the client's desire to change this behavior and to refer the client to appropriate services. It is important to call attention to the substance abuse and offer assistance even if it is refused. Many experts in the field of substance abuse agree that most clients are approached numerous times before they finally obtain help.

Many studies have proposed a connection between stress and coping and the immune system. Nurses need to assess the current stressor and coping patterns. If substance abuse has been a past coping mechanism, it is important to identify this by discussing the potential for relapse with the client. Using stress-reduction techniques and referral to counseling or support groups may also be helpful.

Besides supporting immunocompetence, nurses play an important role in evaluating the client's level of functioning. Because intervention strategies need to be tailored to the client's ability to carry out such an intervention, it is essential to obtain an adequate data base. This data base should include assessment of the client's energy level, sleep patterns, comfort level, mobility, spirituality, sexual functioning, and relationships.

Because many clients with HIV disease experience multiple losses, it is important for nurses to assist these clients in maintaining a realistic sense of hope in the face of multiple changes.

The nurse should maintain universal precautions for all clients as well as needle disposal protocols to prevent infection with HIV. When infection is suspected, the caregiver should follow institutional policy for care. A person who is a victim of rape, has experienced exposure to used (shared) needles or bodily secretions, or has not practiced safe sex can seek help at a public health department or a private physician.

A report of the possible infection is completed and pretest counseling is begun. Pretest counseling should include an information component during which a review of testing protocols, meaning of test results, confidentiality, and information on HIV and AIDS occur. A consent form for testing is signed. The pretest counselor should attend to the person's psychosocial needs, as the person may feel "infected" and fearful of infecting loved ones, experience guilt when a break in procedure occurs, and harbor thoughts of helplessness, denial, and anger.

During post-test counseling, results of the testing and their meaning are explained. A retest is completed after 3 months, especially if safe sex practices are not followed. Information on safe sex is taught (single partner, protection via condoms). If test results are seropositive, a repeat test is ordered. Information regarding transmission of the disease and symptoms are reviewed. The appropriate referrals are made for psychosocial support (e.g., support groups, psychologist or psychiatrist). The affected person should develop a plan for a healthy life-style; medical care and continuing follow-up should be established.

Nursing Diagnosis, Planning, and Implementation

There are many nursing diagnoses appropriate for the client with AIDS (Box 9–3). The five highest priority diagnoses are discussed in detail. Nursing care for clients with symptomatic AIDS centers on management of the symptoms, support of immunocompetence, and psychosocial support and counseling.

Nursing care for clients with AIDS focuses on the response to the opportunistic infections or malignancy, issues of death and dying, support for the family or significant others, and restoration to an optimal level of functioning.

Nursing Diagnosis: Breathing Pattern, Ineffective R/T congestion and weakness secondary to PCP, CMV, pulmonary KS, MAC, tuberculosis, pneumonitis, pneumothorax, and anxiety.

Planning: Expected Outcomes. The client will breathe with minimal difficulty, as evidenced by a decrease in dyspnea and less effort with breathing.

Implementation. Nurses need to assess the client's respiratory status for rate, rhythm, regularity of respirations, use of accessory muscles, presence of adventitious breath sounds, cough, skin color, general appearance, and level of consciousness. A patent airway must be maintained at all times. Administer medications and

BOX 9–3

Common Nursing Diagnoses for Clients with Human Immunodeficiency Virus Infection Diseases

- Infection (any body organ), Risk for R/T cellular immunodeficiency
- Breathing Pattern, Ineffective R/T PCP, CMV infection, pulmonary KS, MAC infection, tuberculosis, pneumonitis, pneumothorax
- Nutrition, Altered: Less than Body Requirements R/T persistent diarrhea, malabsorption, increased metabolic rate, anorexia, stomatitis, infection
- Skin Integrity, Impaired R/T malnutrition, KS, immobility, infection (HSV, histoplasmosis, CMV, varicella zoster, candidiasis)
- Social Isolation R/T stigma, fear, cultural and religious mores, risk for HIV transmission
- Diarrhea R/T infection, diet, medications
- Sleep Pattern Disturbance R/T anxiety, depression, withdrawal from drugs (heroin, cocaine, methadone), pain, night sweats, side effect of medications
- Pain R/T side effects of medications, infections, immobility, lymphadenopathy, lymphedema secondary to KS, lymphoma, headaches caused by central nervous system infection, peripheral neuropathy, severe myalgias, psychogenic pain related to anxiety and fear of death
- Activity Intolerance R/T fatigue, weakness, arthralgia, myalgia, side effects of medications, dyspnea, fever, malnutrition
- Thought Processes, Altered R/T central nervous system disease (toxoplasmosis, cryptococcosis), CMV infection, KS, lymphoma, HIV infection
- Body Image Disturbance R/T diagnosis, KS lesions, alopecia from chemotherapy or HIV infection, weight loss, depression, social stigma, change in sexuality
- Grieving, Anticipatory R/T multiple losses, including health, independence, friends, social activities, job, housing, life, and loss of control
- Anxiety R/T HIV diagnosis, fear of death, fear of disclosure
- Knowledge Deficit R/T disease progression, treatment options, transmission, and methods of preventing transmission
- Sexual Patterns, Altered R/T safer sex practices, abstinence, fear of transmission, impotency secondary to medications
- Injury, Risk for R/T weakness, HIV encephalopathy and cognitive changes, neuromuscular changes
- Sensory/Perceptual Alterations: Auditory/Visual R/T hearing loss secondary to medications and visual loss related to infection (CMV)
- Role Performance, Altered R/T parenting, childbearing, supporting
- Individual Coping, Ineffective R/T the diagnosis of HIV disease

PCP, *Pneumocystis carinii;* CMV, cytomegalovirus; KS, Kaposi's sarcoma; MAC, *Mycobacterium avium* complex; HSV, herpes simplex virus; HIV, human immunodeficiency virus.

oxygen as ordered and monitor for side effects. The head of the bed should be elevated and the client monitored frequently to lessen anxiety during times of dyspnea. The results of arterial blood gas analyses, pulmonary function tests, and other pertinent laboratory studies must be monitored. In addition, the nurse should provide teaching before any procedures, including bronchoscopy, lung biopsy, or radiographic imaging. One must encourage the client to report any changes such as increased dyspnea or cough, help the client with activities of daily living (ADLs), and provide emotional support for the client and significant others.

Nursing Diagnosis: Activity Intolerance R/T fatigue, weakness, anemia, arthralgia, myalgia, dyspnea, fever, malnutrition, or motor dysfunction secondary to neurologic disease.

Planning: Expected Outcomes. The client will maintain a level of activity compatible with the stage of disease, avoiding immobility as long as possible, as evidenced by a balance of rest and activity and absence of complications associated with immobility.

Implementation. A change in activity tolerance becomes a common finding as AIDS progresses. Nurses need to assess the pre-illness activity tolerance to establish the client's usual energy level.

The current degree of activity needs to be determined. The nurse must assess the client's need for sleep and rest and assist the client with ADLs. The client should be encouraged to engage in regular exercise and rest as tolerated. He or she must be taught energy conservation measures, and the nurse should evaluate response to instructions. One must establish a time with the client and family or significant others for rest while the client is hospitalized and educate other staff about this protected time. The client should be encouraged to eat and maintain an adequate dietary intake during periods of activity intolerance. Ordered treatment for underlying infections, pain, anxiety, sleeplessness, or malnutrition should be administered.

Nursing Diagnosis: Pain R/T lymphadenopathy, peripheral neuropathy, lymphedema secondary to KS, lymphoma, severe myalgia, headache secondary to central nervous system infection, and psychogenic pain related to fear and anxiety over death.

Planning: Expected Outcomes. The client will have pain controlled or relieved, as evidenced by client's statements and increased activity for the client.

Implementation. The pain experienced by clients with AIDS needs to be carefully assessed. Nurses and clients alike expect to have pain with cancer, whereas clients with AIDS are expected to waste away without significant painful experiences. Nurses need to perform a thorough pain assessment. In collaboration with the physician, appropriate pain relief in the form of anti-inflammatory, antianxiety, or analgesic agents may be used.

Clients with a history of injectable drug abuse are particularly concerned about the potential of being inadequately medicated because of either past illicit drug use or a high tolerance for narcotics. The use of established schedules or client-controlled analgesia works well in these situations. Provide alternative measures for pain relief such as massage, visualization, and touch. Assess the effectiveness of any therapy that is administered and monitor for side effects. Support is essential at this phase because clients with AIDS frequently associate the need for chronic pain medication with death and dying and, therefore, delay requesting pain relief.

Nursing Diagnosis: Knowledge Deficit R/T transmission of the disease and the need for proper nutrition, adequate rest and exercise, and good health practices.

Planning: Expected Outcomes. The client will understand disease transmission and the need for proper nutrition, adequate rest and exercise, and good health practices, as evidenced by client's statements and absence of transmission to others, maintenance of body weight, adequate activity level, and good health practices.

Implementation. Nursing care of asymptomatic AIDS clients includes education strategies aimed at reducing the risk of transmission. This includes safe sex counseling, avoidance of sharing of needles or instructions on cleaning the works (paraphernalia used in the injection of drugs) or both, care of household items, and proper disposal of items soiled with body fluids (see Client Education Guide).

Health maintenance also is important at this stage. This includes instruction on maintaining adequate nutrition, weight management, exercise, smoking cessation, and stress reduction. Early disease-detection methods need to be included in care planning, including screening mammography, Pap smears, breast self-examination, testicular self-examination, and Mantoux testing. Counseling and support around the issue of social stigma, potential losses to body image and childbearing potential, changes in sexuality, and premature loss of life need to be included in the nursing care planning.

Nursing Diagnosis: Spiritual Distress, Risk for R/T terminal illness.

Planning: Expected Outcomes. The client will come to terms with terminal nature of disease, as evidenced by client's statements and acceptance of approaching death.

Implementation. Nursing care in the late stages focuses on palliative care, symptom management, and emotional support for the client, family, and significant others. The ethical dilemmas of advanced life support, ability to care for surviving children, and use of experimental treatments are major concerns.

Evaluation

The nurse must evaluate client outcomes on the basis of the established plan of care. If these goals have not been achieved, the plan and interventions must be revised to meet the client's needs.

Modification of Plan of Care for the Elderly

To date, there is little information regarding HIV infections in the elderly because this tends to be a disease

CLIENT EDUCATION GUIDE

Guidelines for Caregivers and Clients with Human Immunodeficiency Virus

Maintain personal hygiene; wash hands frequently. Caregivers should wear gloves for actual or potential contact with body fluids or if the caregiver's hands are chapped or have open sores. Kitchen and bathroom facilities may be shared provided normal sanitary practices are observed.

- Wash dishes and silverware in hot, soapy water, or use dishwasher.
- Clean kitchen counters with sponges and scouring pads to remove food particles. Do not use the same sponge to clean bathroom spills.
- Clean refrigerator frequently to control molds.
- Clean up spills of body fluids or waste immediately with a solution of 1 part bleach to 10 parts water. A bleach solution should be used to disinfect kitchen and bathroom floors, showers, sinks, and toilet bowls.
- Towels and washcloths should not be shared without laundering.
- Toothbrushes, razors, enema equipment, and sexual objects should not be shared.
- Clothes and linens can be washed in the usual manner unless soiled with body fluids; bleach should then be used.
- Sanitary napkins, tampons, and any bloody dressings should be wrapped in a plastic bag and then placed in a plastic-lined trash collector.
- Needles or sharp instruments should be handled carefully. Needles should not be recapped; they should be disposed of in an impenetrable sealed container, for example, a coffee can with a plastic lid or a plastic milk jug.

Clients with acquired immunodeficiency syndrome do not have to remove pets from the household if certain precautions are taken:

- Do not allow outdoor cats to use an indoor litter box. Have someone else change litter boxes and birdcages, when possible; if this is not feasible, use gloves.
- Do not handle animals with diarrhea or those that appear ill.
- Wash hands after handling animals.

Teach specific information about each of the following to the client and caregiver in the home:

- Discuss the methods of transmission of AIDS.
- Teach about the immunocompromised status of the client and how to prevent exposure to infection from contact with people or items in the environment.
- Teach about the dosage and actions of medications. The client should be informed about the expected side effects. Provide information about experimental drugs.
- Demonstrate how to care for any central or peripheral catheters when appropriate.
- Provide information about support groups and hospice services available in the client's community.

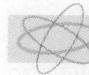

that affects a younger population (ages 20–49 years). Limited experience has suggested that clients with HIV who are older (more than 45 years of age) may have a more rapid rate of disease progression than do their younger counterparts.

HYPERSENSITIVITY DISORDERS

Although the immune system protects the body from harmful invaders, an overactive or overzealous response is detrimental. Over-reaction to a substance, or hypersensitivity, is often referred to as an allergic response. Although "allergy" is widely used, the word "hypersensitivity" is more appropriate; this term designates an increased immune response to the presence of an antigen (in this case referred to as an allergen) that results in tissue destruction.

Predisposing Factors

The occurrence and intensity of hypersensitivity responses depend on several factors: host defenses, the nature of the allergen, the concentration of the allergen, the route of allergen entrance into the body, and the exposure to the allergen. Some clients are more prone to allergies than others are for reasons that are unclear. About one in four Americans have serious allergies. Higher concentrations usually result in hypersensitivity responses of greater intensity. Routes include inhalation, injection, ingestion, or direct contact. Most allergens are inhaled.

Hypersensitivity responses occur after initial exposure. The first contact with the substance causes a primary immune response, slower and less severe than the secondary immune response, which occurs with subsequent exposure to the allergen. Also, if much time elapses between each contact with the allergen (e.g., several years), the immune response diminishes.

Types of Hypersensitivity Reactions

There are two general categories of hypersensitivity reaction: immediate and delayed. These designations are based on the rapidity of the immune response. Recent research, however, suggests there is a biochemical and a cellular component in both types of reaction. Immune globulins mediate immediate reactions, whereas T cells

TABLE 9–3 Types of Hypersensitivity Reactions

	TYPE	CAUSATIVE COMPONENT	PATHOLOGIC PROCESS	REACTION
I	Immediate-anaphylactic	IgE	Mast cell degranulation ↓ Histamine and leukotriene release	Anaphylaxis Atopic diseases Skin reactions
II	Cytolytic-cytotoxic	IgG IgM Complement	Complement fixation ↓ Cell lysis	ABO incompatibility Drug-induced hemolytic anemia
III	Immune complex	Antigen-antibody complexes	Deposition in vessels and tissue walls ↓ Inflammation	Arthus reaction Serum sickness Systemic lupus erythematosus Acute glomerulonephritis
IV	Cell-mediated delayed	Sensitized T cells	Lymphokine release	Tuberculosis Contact dermatitis Transplant rejection

Ig, immunoglobulin.

govern delayed hypersensitivity responses. Humoral responses occur more rapidly than cell-mediated responses do.

In addition to the delayed and immediate categories, hypersensitivity reactions are divided into four main types (Table 9–3): (1) immediate-anaphylactic, (2) cytolytic-cytotoxic, (3) immune complex, and (4) cell-mediated delayed.

TYPE I ANAPHYLACTIC HYPERSENSITIVITY

Anaphylactic shock represents the most severe form of type I hypersensitivity. Initial manifestations of anaphylaxis may include localized itching, edema, and sneezing. These seemingly innocuous problems are followed in minutes by wheezing, dyspnea, cyanosis, and circulatory shock.

Anaphylaxis requires immediate emergency treatment. Common causes of anaphylaxis are listed in Table 9–4. See Chapter 56 for a discussion of emergency care of clients with anaphylaxis.

CRITICAL TO REMEMBER

Prevention is the key in anaphylaxis.

A careful nursing history reveals individual susceptibility to such reactions. Always mark known allergies clearly on the permanent health record, and nursing care plans.

Special identification bracelets worn by the client at all times or signs placed on the client's bed also help. If the physician suspects a client might be allergic to a certain medication or substance, the physician will order an intradermal skin test. A localized reaction to such a test may be an indication that a more severe reaction will occur if the full dose is given.

Atopic allergies are less severe forms of type I response. These reactions commonly occur; 15 to 25 per cent of people in developed countries suffer from atopic allergies. Atopic allergies include hay fever (allergic rhinitis), some types of bronchial asthma, atopic der-

TABLE 9–4 Common Agents Causing Anaphylaxis

Drugs	
Penicillins (most common)	Vancomycin
Cephalosporins	Amphotericin B
Tetracyclines	Polymyxin
Streptomycin	Bacitracin
Kanamycin	Aspirin, other anti-inflammatory agents
Neomycin	Colchicine
Heparin	Tranquilizers
Protamine	
Foods	
Seafoods	Citrus fruits
Eggs	Strawberries
Nuts	Legumes
Insect Venoms	
Hymenoptera (honeybees, wasps, yellow jacket, hornets, fire ants)	
Biologic Agents	
Heterologous antisera (especially equine)	
Enzymes	
Hormones	
Vaccines (especially egg-cultured types)	
Blood Products	
Plasma	
Cryoprecipitate	
Whole blood	
Gamma globulin	
Allergen Extracts	
Skin-testing agents	
Desensitization	
Diagnostic Agents	
Bromsulphalein dye	
Iodinated contrast media	

TABLE 9–5 Clinical Manifestations of Allergic Reactions to Selected Medications

DRUG	SYSTEMIC MANIFESTATIONS	CUTANEOUS MANIFESTATIONS
Penicillin	Anaphylaxis Serum sickness syndrome Pulmonary alterations (e.g., bronchial asthma) Vasculitis	Contact dermatitis Urticaria Rash Pruritus
Sulfonamides	Hepatic alterations Vasculitis Polyarteritis Renal disturbances Hematologic alterations	Rash Pruritus Exfoliative dermatitis Erythema multiforme Purpuric eruptions Photosensitivity
Salicylates	Bronchial asthma	Angioneurotic edema Urticaria Pruritus
Para-aminosalicylic acid	Fever Löffler's syndrome (pulmonary infiltrate with eosinophilia) Hepatic alterations Hematologic alterations	—
Phenytoin sodium (Dilantin)	Eosinophilia Lymphadenopathy Hepatic alterations	Erythema multiforme
Barbiturates	—	Rash Exfoliative dermatitis Fixed eruptions

matitis, some food and drug allergies, and urticaria. Urticaria is an area of localized edema and itching resulting from exposure to an allergen, most commonly a food or drug. Table 9–5 lists some clinical manifestations of allergic reactions to selected medications.

TYPE II CYTOLYTIC OR CYTOTOXIC HYPERSENSITIVITY

These reactions are complement dependent and thus involve immunoglobulin (Ig) G or IgM antibodies. The antigen-antibody complex and complement attach to a cell, usually a circulating blood cell, with resultant cell lysis. During blood transfusion, blood group incompatibility causes cell lysis, which results in a transfusion reaction. The antigen responsible for initiating the reaction is a part of the donor red cell membrane.

Manifestations of a transfusion reaction result from intravascular hemolysis of red cells. They include

- Headache and back pain (flank)
- Chest pain similar to angina
- Nausea and vomiting
- Tachycardia and hypotension
- Hematuria
- Urticaria

Transfusions of more than 100 mL of incompatible blood can result in severe, permanent renal damage, circulatory shock, and death.

Other Type II hypersensitivity reactions include autoimmune TTP, Graves' disease, and autoimmune or allergic hemolytic anemia.

TYPE III IMMUNE COMPLEX HYPERSENSITIVITY

Immune complex disease results from the formation or deposition of antigen-antibody complexes in tissues. The molecular size of the antigen-antibody complexes is an important feature in eliciting immune complex disease. Larger complexes are rapidly cleared by phagocytic cells. The smaller complexes formed in antigen excess persist longer in the circulation because they are not as easily captured by phagocytic cells in the spleen and liver. Inflammation results and leads to acute or chronic disease of the organ system in which the immune complexes were deposited.

The antigen may be tissue fixed or released locally, as in Goodpasture's disease, in which circulating antibodies react with autologous antigens in the glomerular basement membranes of the kidneys and result in inflammation of the glomerulus. Alternatively, antigen-antibody complexes may form in the joint space, with resultant synovitis, as in rheumatoid arthritis. The antigen may also be circulating, as in serum sickness. Antigen-antibody complexes are formed in the bloodstream and get trapped in capillaries or deposited in vessel walls, causing urticaria, arthritis, arteritis, or glomerulonephritis. The Arthus reaction is a localized area of tissue necrosis that results from immune complex hypersensitivity.

Serum sickness is another type III hypersensitivity response. The serum sickness–like reaction may occur after administration of such medications as penicillin, sulfonamides, streptomycin, thiouracils, and hydantoin compounds. Manifestations include fever, arthralgias, lymphadenopathy, and urticaria. This illness is usually benign and self-limiting. It resolves after the offending medication is discontinued.

TYPE IV CELL-MEDIATED OR DELAYED HYPERSENSITIVITY

In cell-mediated hypersensitivity, sensitized T cells respond to antigens by releasing lymphokines, which direct phagocytic cell activity. This reaction occurs 24 to 72 hours after exposure to an allergen. Delayed hypersensitivity is induced by chronic infection (e.g., tuberculosis) or by contact sensitivities, as in contact dermatitis.

Type IV reactions occur after the intradermal injection of tuberculosis antigen or purified protein derivative. If the client has been sensitized to tuberculosis, sensitized T cells react with the antigen at the injection site. The reaction leads to edema and fibrin deposits, which result in the induration characteristic of a positive tuberculosis reaction.

Graft-versus-host disease (GVHD) and transplant rejection are also type IV reactions. In GVHD, immunocompetent donor bone marrow cells (the graft) react against various antigens in the bone marrow recipient (the host), which results in a variety of clinical manifestations, including skin, gastrointestinal, and hepatic lesions. Further details of transplant rejection and GVHD are discussed later.

Contact dermatitis is another type IV reaction that occurs after sensitization to an allergen, commonly a cosmetic, adhesive, topical medication, drug additive (such as lanolin added to lotions), or plant toxin (such as poison ivy). With the first exposure, no reaction occurs; however, antigens are formed. On subsequent exposures, hypersensitivity reactions are triggered, which leads to itching, erythema, and vesicular lesions.

Diagnostic Assessment

Laboratory tests also provide valuable data, especially when they are evaluated with consideration of a history of allergic responses. Common tests include assays of IgE levels: radioallergosorbent test, radioimmunosorbent test, and paper radioimmunosorbent test. These tests reveal elevated levels of IgE, but a normal or even decreased level may occur in IgE-mediated sensitivities. The last two tests are more sensitive. Elevated serum eosinophil levels also suggest hypersensitivities.

In addition to blood tests, skin testing confirms sensitivity to a specific allergen. These tests involve placing a known antigen on or directly below the skin (intradermal) to check for the presence of antibodies. The antigen can be applied in one of three methods: scratch test, patch test, or intradermal test. In the first (also known as a tine or prick test), the allergen is applied to a superficial scratch that cuts the outer layer of skin. For a patch test, the antigen is directly applied to the skin and then covered with a gauze dressing. Intradermal testing involves injecting a small amount of the antigen into the intradermal layer of the skin. Intradermal testing is the most accurate method but carries a higher risk of severe allergic reactions.

Problems arising from skin testing range from minor itching to anaphylaxis. Itching and discomfort at the injection site, for example, are common and can be relieved by the application of cool compresses and topical steroids. Ulceration of the injection site is best treated by keeping the area clean and dry.

Anaphylactic shock is a rare but potentially lethal complication of skin testing. A client with a history of an anaphylactic reaction to a substance should never be skin tested for an allergy to that substance.

Food allergies can be tested by skin testing or by either food challenges or an elimination diet. In the challenge test, suspected foods are given to the client in progressively larger doses until a reaction is evoked. Symptoms of a reaction range from the typical erythema, itching, and rash to vomiting or diarrhea. Symptoms such as fatigue, depression, or restlessness are not conclusive of an allergy.

In the elimination diet, foods are eliminated from the diet one by one until the symptoms are relieved. This may indicate allergies to food additives or foods themselves.

Medical Management

Allergies are chronic problems that require prolonged and often multiple treatments. The client often requires a combination of treatments ranging from avoidance of known allergens to environmental control and immunotherapy.

Avoidance of the allergen is often the easiest, cheapest, and safest way of dealing with allergies. However, identification of the specific allergen is sometimes difficult, especially if the client refuses or cannot afford or locate allergen-testing services. Sometimes, even if the allergen can be identified, complete avoidance may not be possible, such as with pollens, dust, and some food additives.

Environmental control sometimes helps eliminate airborne allergens. Figure 9–1 illustrates ways to desensitize a room. These environmental controls, combined with air filters that remove small particles from the air, can help eliminate many allergens for the client.

PHARMACOLOGIC MANAGEMENT

Clients with atopic allergies can have their symptoms alleviated or controlled by many prescription and over-the-counter medications. Usually, clients will self-administer these agents, although in some settings the nurse or family members administer them. Instructing clients about these medications, however, is always an important nursing responsibility.

Antihistamines are the major group of prescription and over-the-counter drugs used to alleviate symptoms. These medications decrease sneezing, rhinorrhea, itching, and other symptoms of allergic rhinitis. Newer

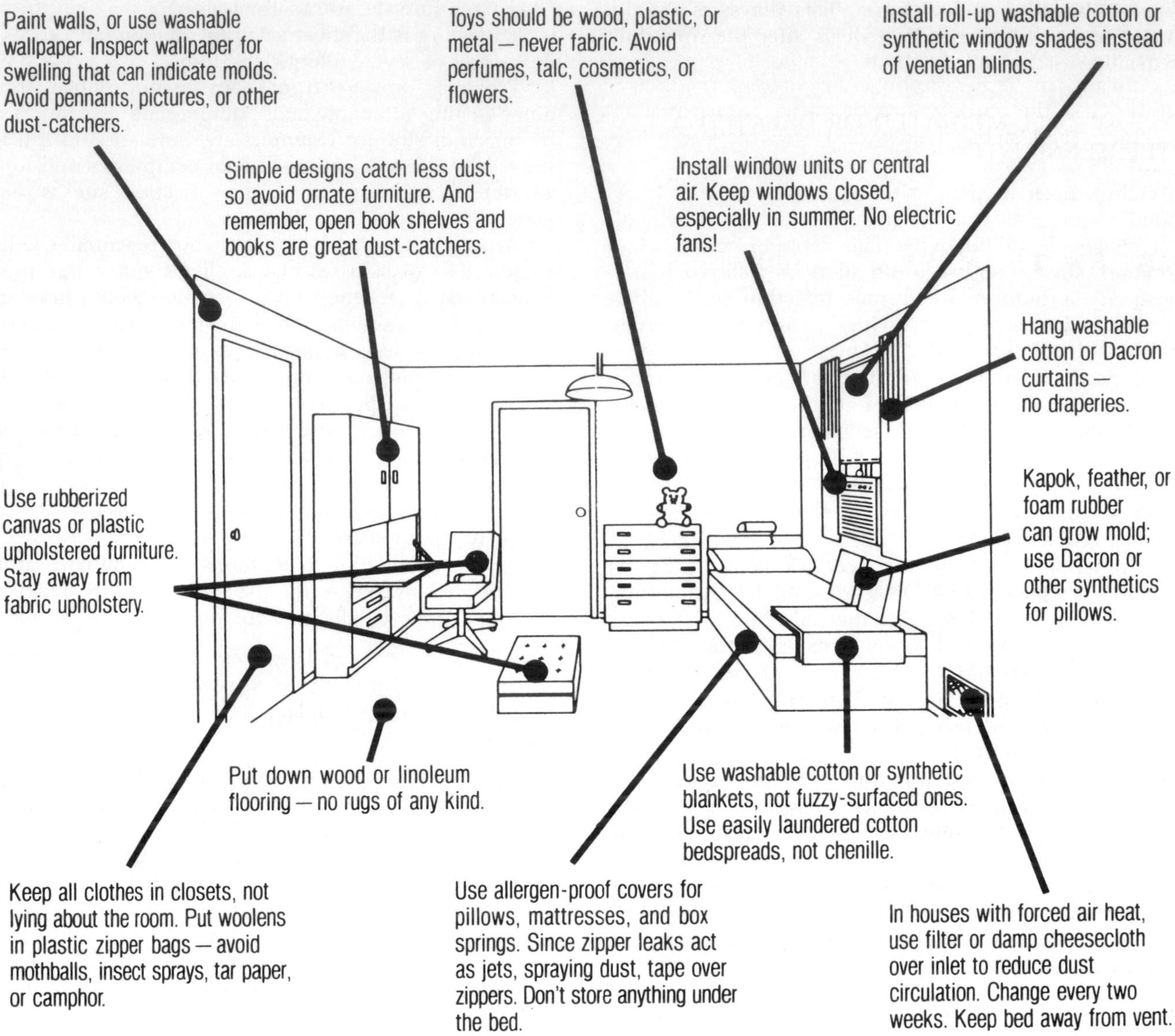

Paint walls, or use washable wallpaper. Inspect wallpaper for swelling that can indicate molds. Avoid pennants, pictures, or other dust-catchers.
Toys should be wood, plastic, or metal — never fabric. Avoid perfumes, talc, cosmetics, or flowers.
Install roll-up washable cotton or synthetic window shades instead of venetian blinds.
Simple designs catch less dust, so avoid ornate furniture. And remember, open book shelves and books are great dust-catchers.
Install window units or central air. Keep windows closed, especially in summer. No electric fans!
Hang washable cotton or Dacron curtains — no draperies.
Kapok, feather, or foam rubber can grow mold; use Dacron or other synthetics for pillows.
Use rubberized canvas or plastic upholstered furniture. Stay away from fabric upholstery.
Put down wood or linoleum flooring — no rugs of any kind.
Use washable cotton or synthetic blankets, not fuzzy-surfaced ones. Use easily laundered cotton bedspreads, not chenille.
Keep all clothes in closets, not lying about the room. Put woolens in plastic zipper bags — avoid mothballs, insect sprays, tar paper, or camphor.
Use allergen-proof covers for pillows, mattresses, and box springs. Since zipper leaks act as jets, spraying dust, tape over zippers. Don't store anything under the bed.
In houses with forced air heat, use filter or damp cheesecloth over inlet to reduce dust circulation. Change every two weeks. Keep bed away from vent.

Figure 9–1
Controlling the environment of a room. (Courtesy of A. H. Robins Company, Richmond, VA.)

agents (such as terfenadine [Seldane]) do not cause the drowsiness that limited the use of older medications.

Decongestants (oral sympathomimetics) help relieve the nasal congestion. These drugs can be combined with antihistamines to treat multiple symptoms of the allergy. The nasal sprays of these agents can be used for several days to treat the nasal congestion; however, overuse of these agents can lead to rebound congestion and exacerbation of the nasal symptoms secondary to chemical rhinitis.

Corticosteroids, anti-inflammatory agents, and immunosuppressant agents can be used to treat a variety of symptoms associated with allergies. Topical steroids can be used to treat dermatitis and other skin manifestations. Beclomethasone dipropionate (Beconase) is a steroidal aerosol useful in treating allergic rhinitis. It has fewer side effects than dexamethasone does. This drug is also available via inhalation for asthma.

Cromolyn sodium is another topical or aerosol medication used to treat allergic rhinitis and asthma. It helps prevent the release of chemical mediators, such as histamine and leukotrienes from mast cells.

Immunotherapy (sometimes called desensitization therapy) is designed for type I, IgE-mediated hypersensitivity reactions. Precise doses of allergens are injected at intervals over a prolonged period. The doses are increased gradually over time. Immunotherapy increases IgG antibody levels and may increase suppressor T-cell function. It also decreases IgE binding to allergens. Although there is some controversy regarding the efficacy of this treatment, it is widely used. The greatest success has been achieved with allergic rhinitis (hay fever) and Hymenoptera sensitivity (bee, yellow jacket, wasp, and hornet stings).

Nurses often administer these injections and assess and treat side effects. Clients are asked to wait at least

20 minutes after receiving the injections so immediate reactions can be treated. Side effects are similar to those seen in skin testing. Sometimes, clients are taught to administer the desensitization injections to themselves. In this case, the nurse will teach clients proper injection technique and signs of any untoward reactions to the medication.

ORGAN TRANSPLANTATION

Histocompatibility

With recent advances in technology and immunology, organ and tissue transplantation is becoming commonplace. Thus, nurses need to (1) gain a clear understanding of the immunology on which this intervention is based and (2) learn how to assess and provide intervention for clients with their transplants. See the specific chapters (such as Chap. 31 for renal transplants) for specific information on each type of transplant.

There are several different types of transplant. Syngeneic transplants are between genetically identical members of the same species (identical twins); they are also called isograft. Allogeneic transplants are between individuals of the same species (e.g., human to human). Autologous transplants are grafts within the same species (e.g., skin graft from leg to hand, on the same client). Xenogeneic transplants are between individuals of different species.

In all cases of graft rejection, the cause is incompatibility of cell-surface antigens. As expected, there is a better chance of graft acceptance with autologous or syngeneic transplants because the cell-surface antigens are identical.

A major role of the immune system is to distinguish between self and nonself. This fact is the major problem facing the candidate for transplantation: the immunologic response of the client to the donor's tissues. This ability to distinguish between self and nonself is central to proper immune function.

The closer the match between the donor's and recipient's antigens, the less chance rejection will occur. Although many hundreds of antigens may differ between donor and recipient, certain antigens are critical for a successful transplant. These are (1) ABO and Rh antigens present on red cells and (2) histocompatibility antigens. Most important in this latter group is the human leukocyte antigen, also known as MHC in humans.

The process of finding compatible donors and recipients is called tissue typing. After tissue typing of the donor and recipient, the laboratory performs a matching procedure called the mixed lymphocyte culture. Various lymphocyte antibodies form after blood transfusions, pregnancy, (prior) exposure to foreign bodies, or infections. In the mixed lymphocyte culture, lymphocytes from the donor are mixed with serum from the recipient and then observed for immune responses. This test can determine whether antibodies incompatible with the donor have been formed by the recipient (a positive crossmatch). If the crossmatch is positive, the transplant will fail; therefore, a negative test is necessary for a successful transplant.

Graft Rejection

Rejection is actually the body's normal immune response to the invasion of foreign tissue (the transplanted tissue or organ). Although this response is normal, it is not the desired response after a transplant. The physiologic mechanisms in rejection (the normal immune response) involve B lymphocytes forming antibodies and T lymphocytes producing cell-mediated immunity. Acute rejection is caused by the T-lymphocyte activity and chronic rejection by that of B lymphocytes.

There are three basic kinds of rejection: hyperacute, acute, and chronic.

HYPERACUTE REJECTION

Allografts transplanted into presensitized recipients may be rejected very quickly. This rejection may occur from the time of the transplant up to 48 hours after the transplant.

The symptoms of hyperacute rejection include general malaise and fever. In renal transplants, the kidney becomes infiltrated with leukocytes, which results in thrombosis of arterioles and glomerular capillaries. In cardiac transplants, the heart becomes hard and a mottled purple.

Hyperacute rejection is not treatable; removal of the rejected tissue or organ is the only way to stop the reaction. The client must then be maintained until another transplant can be arranged.

ACUTE REJECTION

This occurs usually within 3 months but may occur as late as 2 years after the transplant. The graft becomes vascularized in 2 to 3 days. In acute rejection, the response is primarily a cell-mediated one. The reaction begins when the recipient becomes sensitized to the donor antigens. Memory cells are formed that can trigger rapid rejection of a subsequent transplant of the same histocompatibility type.

In 6 to 10 days, the first signs of rejection may be observed. Sensitized lymphocytes and macrophages appear at the graft site. Later, the vascular bed itself begins to deteriorate, and the graft becomes necrotic.

Acute rejection is treatable with immunosuppressant medications including corticosteroids, azathioprine, cyclophosphamide, antithymocyte globulin, cyclosporin A, and OKT_3 (Table 9–6). Intravenous methylprednisolone sodium succinate (Solu-Medrol) is usually given first with good response (i.e., rejection reversed). Repeated episodes of acute rejection can lead to permanent damage of the organ.

TABLE 9–6 Medications Used in Transplantation

MEDICATION	ACTION	SIDE EFFECTS	NURSING IMPLICATIONS
Azathioprine (Imuran)	Inhibits DNA and RNA, blocks antibody production	Leukopenia, bone marrow depression, pancreatitis, liver dysfunction, immunosuppression	Monitor for signs of liver dysfunction; monitor CBC; warn client to avoid people with known infections; teach client signs of even mild infection to report; avoid intramuscular injections if client is thrombocytopenic
Cyclosporine (Sandimmune)	Inhibits action of T lymphocytes and cell-mediated immunity	Hypertension, tremor, infection, gum hyperplasia, hirsutism, nephrotoxicity, hepatotoxicity, flushing	Monitor BUN and creatinine, liver function studies; always given in conjunction with corticosteroids; monitor levels of drug because oral absorption is erratic; give dose daily, at same time of day; give with meal to decrease nausea; comes suspended in olive oil, so administer in juice or milk, in glass so container does not absorb drug; stress to client importance of never varying or stopping medication without physician's approval
Antithymocyte globulin (ATG)	Either alters T-cell function or eliminates antigen-reactive T cells to inhibit cell-mediated immunity	Leukopenia, hemolysis, hypotension, chest pain, dyspnea, laryngospasms, nausea, vomiting, serum sickness (horse serum), anaphylaxis	Client should be skin tested before first dose; do not use in clients allergic to horse serum; solution very heat sensitive, keep refrigerated; monitor client for signs of infection; use filter when administering drug
Muromonab-CD3 (OKT_3)	IgG antibody, reacts in T-lymphocyte membrane to block T-cell function and proliferation; may reverse rejection, but carcinogenic and used with caution	Chest pain, fever, nausea, vomiting, severe pulmonary edema, dyspnea, increased incidence of malignant lymphomas	Used only in cases of acute rejection not responding to other agents; monitor cardiopulmonary system closely during administration; assess for signs of fluid overload; administer antipyretic before drug to decrease chills and fever
Methylprednisolone sodium succinate (Solu-Medrol)	Anti-inflammatory, prevents leukocyte infiltration during rejection, decreases antibody production and inhibits antigen-antibody reaction	Infection, delayed wound healing, peptic ulcers, hypertension, congestive heart failure, hypokalemia, weight gain, hyperglycemia; withdrawal symptoms if stopped suddenly	Monitor client for infection; teach client to prevent infection; tell client not to decrease or stop dose suddenly because of possibly life-threatening reaction; treat side effects symptomatically; give with food or antacids to prevent ulcers
Cyclophosphamide (Cytoxan)	Action similar to azathioprine, used mainly when cyclosporine or azathioprine not tolerated	Bone marrow depression, leukopenia, nausea, vomiting, hemorrhagic cystitis, alopecia	Monitor for infection; teach client to avoid infections and notify physician at first sign of infection; increase fluid intake and encourage client to void every 2 hours; monitor CBC regularly

BUN, blood urea nitrogen; CBC, complete blood count; DNA, deoxyribonucleic acid; RNA, ribonucleic acid; Ig, immunoglobulin.

CHRONIC REJECTION

Months or even years after the transplant, function of the transplanted tissue or organ may deteriorate gradually. The problem is a recurring, continuing one. Antibodies and complement play a role in this type of rejection, causing arteriolar narrowing as a result of deposition of fibrin, platelets, and complement along vessel walls. The body tries to repair the endothelial damage that leads to intimal proliferation, necrosis, and collagen deposits, which further blocks circulation.

Clients with chronic rejection may be asymptomatic. Others will demonstrate symptoms directly related to failure of the transplanted organ.

Treatment is not usually successful for chronic rejection. It is a gradual, progressive deterioration. Antirejection medications may slow the process, so it is years before the organ fails completely and retransplantation is required.

Graft-Versus-Host Disease (GVHD)

A different type of rejection occurs when the transplanted material is an allogeneic bone marrow transplant. GVHD is a variation of the traditional graft rejection but involves the same immunologic principles. GVHD occurs with bone marrow transplantation in which immunocompetent donor cells are infused into an immunosuppressed recipient. Thus, if rejection occurs, it is the immunocompetent T lymphocytes from the graft (i.e., the donated marrow) rather than the host cells that cause the problem.

GVHD has acute and chronic forms. Acute GVHD manifests itself as early as 1 to 100 days after transplant, with a peak time of onset in 30 to 50 days. Chronic GVHD usually occurs or persists later than 100 days. The major organs affected by GVHD are the skin, liver, and gastrointestinal tract.

Prevention of GVHD is similar to that of transplant rejection and involves immunosuppression of the recipient. For further information on bone marrow transplants, see Chapters 7 and 28.

Criteria for Transplantation

The basic criteria for transplantation include the following:

- The presence of end-stage disease in a transplantable organ
- Failure of conventional therapy to treat the condition successfully
- Progression of problems associated with the organ failure that in themselves may be fatal
- The absence of untreatable malignancy or irreversible infection
- The absence of disease that would attack the transplanted tissue
- The client is able to survive the surgical procedure

The first, fourth, fifth, and sixth criteria apply to all transplants, whereas the second is mainly for liver and heart and the third for pancreas and kidney. Different institutions apply other criteria, such as age limits and the absence of drug or alcohol abuse.

Candidates for transplantation of the heart, lung, kidney, or liver usually have an end-stage disease associated with that organ. The client should not have severe complications that might have a negative impact on the transplanted organs.

Corneal transplantations are performed on clients with corneal opacity or ulceration. Skin transplantations are typically done on clients with severe burns, which make autografts impossible. Bone marrow transplantations are done for clients with leukemia, aplastic anemia, or genetic hematopoietic disorder or experimentally on others with late-stage malignant disease (however, these are usually autologous transplants). Criteria for selection of bone marrow transplant candidates are mainly based on the stage of disease and the potential for improvement.

Donor Procurement and Preparation

Organ procurement is a subject that makes many health-care professionals uncomfortable. They hesitate to approach a family of a potential donor when the family is suffering the potential loss of their loved one. There is, however, a federal requirement that request protocols for donation exist in the hospital, or the hospital risks losing Medicare and Medicaid reimbursement. Most states now have laws requiring that families be given the opportunity for organ donation.

Families often have been very receptive to possible donation as a living memorial to their loved one. The approach must be sensitive, sincere, and stated in the most positive way possible. Many institutions have set up organ-procurement teams that handle this process. The request for organ donation occurs only after the family has been completely informed about the hopelessness of the situation. The discussion can be initiated by asking the family whether their loved one ever thought about organ donation and how they feel about this option.

Organ donors typically have been either living relatives or cadavers. More recently, however, living unrelated donors have been used for bone marrow transplants (see Chaps. 7 and 28). The most ideal living donor is an identical twin, who will have the same genetic make-up. Close relatives with similar genetic make-up are the most common living donors.

Bone marrow is transplanted only from living donors. For autologous transplants, the marrow is donated by the client, frozen, and then returned to the client after treatment.

All living donors must be in good health without severe disease. Kidney donors must have normally functioning kidneys. Kidney disease is often genetic, so with living donors, assessment must be made for the presence of the same genetic disorder. The donor's ability to withstand the transplant must be a prime consideration.

Living donors and the families of cadaver donors must be given a great deal of psychological support. The living donor often seems to be forgotten in the joy of a successful transplant. This client has undergone major surgery and requires expert physical and psychosocial nursing care. The families of cadaver donors often find the usefulness of their loved one's organs of help in their grief. These families should not be forgotten in the rush to transplant the organs successfully.

The organ to be transplanted is removed under sterile conditions for both living and cadaver donors. With living donors, the organ is transplanted immediately. With cadaver donors, once the organs are removed, they must be transplanted immediately or preserved at 4° C in a special electrolyte solution. The organs are then transported to the recipient's hospital as soon as possible for transplantation. The kidney can last about 48 hours with hypothermic preservation, the liver 18 to 24 hours, the pancreas about 18 hours, and the heart-lung about 4 hours. Corneas and skin can be preserved for longer periods.

Nursing Management

Pretransplantation

Before the transplant, the priority nursing intervention is to maintain the health of the recipient. The client's disease as well as any other problems that develop during the pretransplant period must continue to be vigorously treated. Clients should have careful dental screening and receive any needed treatment before the transplant. Also, any chronic condition, such as ulcers or gastritis, should be adequately treated before the stress of a transplant.

Immunosuppressants may begin before the transplantation in some cases. In the case of clients undergoing bone marrow transplantation, the recipient's marrow must be destroyed before the transplantation (see Chaps. 7 and 28 for further information).

The psychosocial care of the transplant recipient is very important for the nurse. Many transplant programs include psychological evaluation and follow-up, but expert nursing care is of vital importance. All concerns are usually addressed in multidisciplinary conferences. The family or significant others should also be assessed for their coping abilities and strategies.

Once the decision is made to undergo transplantation, the client is placed on a transplant list with others awaiting the availability of the same organ. This wait can be unbearable for the client and significant others. The client, however, must continue treatment of the underlying disease and maintain a high level of wellness.

One issue that is often discussed before the transplantation is the client's ability to comply with post-transplantation therapy. Often, it is the client's failure to comply with therapy that has led to the organ failure and the need for a transplant. Clients are screened, and the reasons for past noncompliance are explored. If there is strong evidence that clients will not be able to comply with the complex posttransplant regimen, they will probably not be placed on the transplant list.

Nutrition is important before transplantation. Many clients may be malnourished and need extra vitamins and protein before the procedure. Liver transplant clients need to have the ascites reduced and may need total parenteral nutrition to reach a better physical condition for the transplant.

A great deal of teaching must be done before the transplantation. The client must be instructed in pulmonary exercises for preventing postoperative respiratory problems. Teaching about the post-transplantation medication and treatment regimen is also begun preoperatively. The client should also be thoroughly taught about what to expect throughout the transplantation, from the uncertainty of the waiting period to the intensive care required postoperatively. Some of the appropriate nursing diagnoses for transplant clients are listed in Box 9–4. Specific care for each type of transplant can be found in the appropriate chapter.

The financial impact of the transplant on the family and on society must also be considered. The transplant surgery is extremely expensive. Many clients are not employed at the time of the transplant, having left their jobs as their diseases progressed. Post-transplant medications alone may cost between $5000 and $10,000 a year. Many of these clients have only Medicare, and perhaps Medicaid, to provide insurance coverage. Those with coverage often find they have reached their policy limit.

BOX 9–4

Common Nursing Diagnoses and Collaborative Problems for the Client Undergoing a Transplantation

- Knowledge Deficit R/T transplant procedure, postoperative course, post-transplantation self-care requirements, and medication regimen
- Anxiety R/T end-stage organ disease and pending transplant
- Breathing Pattern, Ineffective, Risk for R/T surgical procedure and need for ventilator
- Fluid Volume Excess, Risk for R/T postoperative fluid management
- Pain R/T surgical procedure
- Infection, Risk for R/T immunosuppressant medications
- Individual and Family Coping, Ineffective, Risk for R/T possible rejection phenomena
- Tissue Perfusion, Altered, Risk for R/T leakage or thrombosis at graft anastomosis sites
- Injury, Risk for R/T side effects of immunosuppressant medications
- Activity Intolerance R/T post-transplantation weakness and fatigue
- Home Maintenance Management, Impaired Risk for R/T post-transplantation activity intolerance

Post-Transplantation Period

In many ways, care after transplantation is the same as the care after any major abdominal or cardiothoracic surgery (see Chap. 5).

CRITICAL TO REMEMBER

Infection control is extremely important for these clients because of the immunosuppression required by the transplant.

Nosocomial (hospital-associated) infections can be fatal in these clients, so the nurse must be meticulous about preventing them. Strict aseptic technique must be used

TABLE 9–7 Potential Post-Transplantation Complications

ORGAN	POTENTIAL COMPLICATIONS
Kidney	Rejection, fluid and electrolyte imbalances, acute tubular necrosis, post-transplantation diabetes, problems related to immunosuppression (e.g., infections), renal artery thrombosis or leakage at anastomosis sites, decreased renal function, hypertension, renal abscess
Liver	Rejection, fluid and electrolyte imbalance, clotting disorders, post-transplant diabetes, problems related to immunosuppression (e.g., infections), hepatic artery or vein thrombosis or leakage at anastomosis sites, liver failure, subphrenic abscess, atelectasis and pneumonia secondary to ascites, peritonitis.
Heart (lung)	Rejection, post-transplantation diabetes, problems related to immunosuppression (e.g., infections), thrombosis or leakage at anstomosis sites, heart (lung) failure, pulmonary hypertension, mental status changes, effusion
Pancreas	Rejection, problems related to immunosuppresion (e.g., infections), thrombosis or leakage at anastomosis sites for total replacement, decreased pancreatic function, peritonitis, pancreatic abscess
Bone marrow	Graft-versus-host disease, clotting disorders, problems related to immunosuppression (e.g., infections), agranulocytosis, failure of engraftment

in working with these clients, especially with indwelling urinary catheters and intravenous catheters.

A variety of complications, other than organ rejection, are possible after transplantation (Table 9–7). These must be anticipated and, if possible, prevented. Postoperative nursing care of clients receiving specific transplants is discussed in the appropriate chapters.

Client teaching about these potential problems is an important nursing function. The educational program for a transplant client is complex and often must be taught and mastered in a short time under less than ideal conditions. The nurse must do everything possible to facilitate client learning.

The focus of nursing care after transplantation, in addition to the prevention of infection, is on the prevention of rejection. Early recognition of rejection leads to early treatment, which improves the chances that rejection can be reversed. The pathophysiology of rejection has been covered earlier in this chapter. The actual symptoms of rejection vary with the affected organ (see appropriate chapters for each specific organ).

All clients receive immunosuppressant therapy, but when rejection actually occurs, the doses of the immunosuppressants must be increased. The nurse must then watch the client closely for the side effects and potentially toxic effects of these medications.

Each medication administered has its own particular side effects (see Table 9–6). These drugs produce immunosuppression and, therefore, possible infection. Clients and significant others must understand their medications, the side effects, and adverse effects. Often clients with transplants are also taught to keep track of their own laboratory values as well as to understand them.

Psychosocial care is also extremely important at this point. The client often plummets from the joy of survival to the dark depression of possible rejection. The client needs a great deal of emotional support at this point and needs to focus on the reality of the situation.

Long-Term Follow-Up Care

The post-transplantation client requires follow-up care for a prolonged period. The client will continue immunosuppressant therapy, which can usually be gradually decreased over time.

Infection is one of the most serious prolonged problems after transplant. The client must be continually vigilant to avoid obvious potential sources of infection. This includes precautions such as avoiding crowds, wearing a mask when out in public, and immediately seeking treatment for even a minor infection. Prevention of infection, however, remains the priority.

CRITICAL TO REMEMBER

Immunosuppressant medications have major side effects, and much of the post-transplantation client's long-term care needs revolve around controlling these side effects.

Clients must learn what to do to control these problems. The common side effects are given in Table 9–6. It is important to help the client understand that, although the side effects from these medications can be severe and even fatal, these medications are necessary to maintain the viability of the transplant.

Future Considerations

The future for organ transplantation continues to grow. The use of living donors who share their liver, kidney, pancreas, or bone marrow with the recipient exemplifies this. As improvements in antirejection medications continue, transplants are increasingly successful with prolonged survival.

The nurse has a major role to play in the future of transplantation. Nurses are becoming increasingly involved in procurement. Nurses also provide care to the potential donors in intensive care units. The nurse must provide increasingly complex care to keep the organs viable and then provide the complex care required by the recipient.

Organ transplantation will continue to grow in this country, and the nurse's involvement should grow with it. The role of the nurse in helping this client learn self-care is vital.

STUDY QUESTIONS

1. To gather subjective data from a client with HIV, which one of these questions should the nurse ask?
   A. "How have you been feeling lately?"
   B. "Is your urine bloody?"
   C. "What color is your stool?"
   D. "How is your vision?"
2. The mode of transmission for HIV is contact with an infected person's:
   A. Skin or clothing
   B. Nasal secretions
   C. Body fluids
   D. Tears or sweat
3. A client demonstrating a transfusion reaction from intravascular hemolysis of red cells would present with:
   A. Bradycardia and hypertension
   B. Thirst and diarrhea
   C. Joint pain and rash
   D. Tachycardia and hypotension
4. Which of the following persons would be most appropriate to donate organs?
   A. An elderly client who has died from cancer
   B. A middle-aged client with head trauma who was promptly resuscitated and died
   C. A young adult who had juvenile-onset diabetes and died from burns in a fire
   D. An infant who has died from AIDS.
5. Which activity would be safest for the immunocompromised client?
   A. Work at a day-care center with children.
   B. Volunteer to serve meals at a homeless shelter.
   C. Work at a computer center.
   D. Go door to door to register voters.
6. The nursing diagnosis most appropriate for a client with HIV wasting syndrome is:
   A. Infection (any body organ), Risk for R/T cellular immunodeficiency
   B. Diarrhea R/T infection, diet, medications
   C. Nutrition: Less than Body Requirements, Altered R/T persistent diarrhea, malabsorption, increased metabolic rate, anorexia, stomatitis, infection
   D. Body Image Disturbance R/T diagnosis, KS lesions, alopecia from chemotherapy or HIV infection, weight loss, depression, social stigma, change in sexuality

CRITICAL THINKING EXERCISES

SCENARIO A

A 30-year-old client is diagnosed as having acquired immunodeficiency syndrome (AIDS). His CD4+ cells are less than 200. He has candidiasis of the esophagus and trachea and *Pneumocystis carinii* pneumonia (PCP).

1. Teach the client how a differential diagnosis of PCP is made.
2. What is the treatment for PCP?
3. Which clients are treated prophylactically for PCP?
4. What is the treatment for systemic candidiasis?

SCENARIO B

A young man who is positive for human immunodeficiency virus (HIV) has an acute case of *Candida albicans* of the mouth and a CD4+ level of 250.

1. According to the Centers for Disease Control, what group from the control classification system for HIV infection is this client in?
   A. What laboratory category?
   B. What clinical category?
2. According to the case definition for AIDS, does this client have AIDS?
3. What supportive measures should the nurse perform to enhance the client's response to treatment?
4. What precautions should the client take to prevent the spread of the HIV disease?

BIBLIOGRAPHY

1. Anastasi, J. K., & Lee, V. S. (1994). HIV wasting: How to stop the cycle. *American Journal of Nursing, 94(6),* 18–24.
2. Anderson, J. A., & Adkinson, N. F., Jr. (1987). Allergic reaction to drugs and biologic agents. *Journal of the American Medical Association, 258,* 2834–2840.
3. Bartlett, J. G. (1992). Recommendations for the medical care of persons with HIV infection. *A guide to HIV care from the AIDS Care Program of the Johns Hopkins Medical Institutions,* 23–25.
4. Bernard, E. M., et al. (1992). Pneumocystosis. *Medical Clinics of North America, 76(1),* 107–119.
5. Brostoff, J., et al. (1991). *Clinical immunology.* New York: Gower Medical.
6. Centers for Disease Control. (1987). Recommendation for prevention of HIV transmission in health care settings. *Morbidity and Mortality Weekly Report, 36(Suppl. 2),* 1–3.
7. Centers for Disease Control. (1987). Revision of the CDC surveillance case definition for acquired immunodeficiency

syndrome. *Morbidity and Mortality Weekly Report, 36(Suppl. 1),* 3–15.

8. Centers for Disease Control. (1988). Update: AIDS worldwide. *Morbidity and Mortality Weekly Report, 37,* 286–295.
9. Centers for Disease Control. (1991). Women and AIDS: The growing crisis. *HIV/AIDS Prevention Newsletter, 2(1),* 1–19.
10. Centers for Disease Control. (1992). 1993 Revised classification system for HIV infection and expanded surveillance case definition for AIDS among adolescents and adults. *Morbidity and Mortality Weekly Report, 41(51),* 961–962.
11. Centers for Disease Control. (1993). Update: Barrier protection against HIV infection and other sexually transmitted diseases. *Morbidity and Mortality Weekly Report, 42(30),* 589–591.
12. Dault, L. A., et al. (1989). Reversing cardiac transplant rejection with orthoclone OKT_3. *American Journal of Nursing, 89,* 953–955.
13. Deglin, J. H., & Vallerand, A. H. (1993). *Davis's drug guide for nurses* (3rd ed.). Philadelphia: F. A. Davis.
14. Flaskerud, J. H., & Ungvarski, P. J. (1995). *HIV/AIDS: A guide to nursing care* (3rd ed.). Philadelphia: W. B. Saunders Co.
15. Flye, M. W. (1989). *Principles of organ transplantation.* Philadelphia: W. B. Saunders.
16. Gallo, R. C. (1988). HIV—the cause of AIDS: An overview on its biology, mechanisms of disease induction, and our attempts to control it. *Journal of AIDS, 1,* 521–535.
17. Gawlikowski, J. (1992). White cells at war. *American Journal of Nursing, 92(3),* 44–51.
18. Gee, G., & Moran, T. (1988). *AIDS: Concepts in nursing practice.* Baltimore: Williams & Wilkins.
19. Grady, C. (1988). Host defense mechanisms: An overview. *Seminars in Oncology Nursing, 4(2),* 86–94.
20. Graziano, F. M., & Lemanske, R., Jr. (1989). *Clinical immunology.* Baltimore: Williams & Wilkins.
21. Greene, W. C. (1993). AIDS and the immune system. *Scientific American, 269(3),* 99–105.
22. Griffin, J. (1986). *Hematology and immunology: Concepts for nursing.* Norwalk, CT: Appleton-Century-Crofts.
23. Gurka, A. M. (1990). The immune system: Implications for critical care nursing. *Critical Care Nurse, 9(7),* 24–35.
24. Hollander, H., & Katz, M. H. (1994). HIV infection. In L. M. Tierney, S. J. McPhee, & M. A. Papadakis, eds. (1994). *Current medical diagnosis & treatment* (34th ed.). Norwalk, Connecticut: Appleton & Lange.
25. Hoth, D. F., & Myers, M. W. (1991). Current status of HIV therapy: Antiretroviral agents. *Hospital Practice, 1,* 94–117.
26. Kaplan, A. P. (1992). Anaphylaxis. In J. B. Wyngaarden, L. H. Smith, Jr., & J. C. Bennett (Eds.), *Cecil textbook of medicine* (19th ed., pp. 1462–1465). Philadelphia: W. B. Saunders.
27. Kelly, P. J., & Holman, S. (1993). The new face of AIDS. *American Journal of Nursing, 93(3),* 26–32.
28. Kirton, C. A. (1994). AIDS: When your patient refuses HIV testing. *American Journal of Nursing, 94(12),* 49–54.
29. Macalinao, M., & Kirton, C. A. (1994). The AIDS patient with respiratory failure. *American Journal of Nursing, 94(12),* 5–10.
30. Maddeux, M. S. (1989). The pharmacology and complications of immunosuppressive therapy. *Problems of General Surgery, 6(2),* 85–96.
31. Meisenhelder, J. B., & La Charite, C. L. (1989). *Comfort in caring: Nursing the person with HIV infection.* Philadelphia: J. B. Lippincott.
32. Montagnier, L. (1988). Origin and evolution of HIV's and their role in AIDS pathogenesis. *Journal of AIDS, 1,* 517–520.
33. Ruggiero, M. (1988). The donor in bone marrow transplantation. *Seminars in Oncology, 4(1),* 9–14.
34. Sande, M. A., & Volberding, R. A. (1995). *The medical management of AIDS* (4th ed.). Philadelphia: W. B. Saunders.
35. Santangelo, J., & Schnack, J. (1991). Primary care intervention and management for adults with early HIV infection. *Nurse Practitioner, 16(6),* 9–15.
36. Selwyn, P. A. (1989). Issues in the clinical management of intravenous drug users with HIV. *AIDS, 3(Suppl. 1),* 201–206.
37. Shannon, M. T., Wilson, B. A., & Stang, C. L. (1995). *Govoni & Hayes drugs and nursing implications* (8th ed.). Norwalk, Connecticut: Appleton & Lange.
38. Sinclair, B. P. (1991). Epidemiology and transmission of infection by human immunodeficiency virus. *NAACOG's Clinical Issues in Perinatal Women's Health Nursing, 1(1),* 1–9.
39. Sipes, C. (1995). Guidelines for assessing HIV in women. *MCN, 20(1),* 29–33.
40. Smith, S. (Ed.). (1990). *Tissue and organ transplantation: Implications for nursing practice.* St. Louis: C. V. Mosby.
41. Stites, D. P., & Terr, A. I. (1991). *Basic and clinical immunology* (7th ed.). Norwalk, CT: Appleton & Lange.
42. Williams, A. B. (1991). Women at risk: An AIDS educational needs assessment. *IMAGE: Journal of Nursing Scholarship, 23(4),* 208–213.
43. Widman, F. K. (1989). *An introduction to clinical immunology.* Philadelphia: F. A. Davis.
44. Williams, B. A. H., et al. (1991). *Organ transplantation: A manual for nurses.* New York: Springer.
45. Workman, M. (1993). The immune system: Your defensive partner and offensive foe. *AACN Clinical Issues in Critical Care, 4(3),* 568–593.
46. Workman, M., Ellerhost-Ryan, J., & Koertge, V. (1993). *Nursing care of the immunocompromised patient.* Philadelphia: W. B. Saunders.
47. Wyngaarden, J. B., L H. Smith, Jr., & Bennett, J. C. (Eds.). (1992). *Cecil textbook of medicine* (19th ed.). Philadelphia: W. B. Saunders.

Chapter 10 Nursing Care of Clients with Infectious Diseases

Learning Outcomes

After completing this chapter, the learner will be able to:

1. Assess the client for clinical manifestations of infectious disorders.
2. Teach the client and significant others about the etiology, risk factors, basic pathophysiology, and clinical manifestations of major infectious disorders.
3. Explain the client's role in the management of infectious disorders.
4. Develop plans of care for the prevention of illness and for the management and rehabilitation of clients with infectious disorders.
5. Implement nursing interventions that optimize the quality of life for clients with infectious disorders.
6. Using outcome criteria developed in the planning phase of care, evaluate planned client outcomes.

For one brief moment in human history (circa 1950–1980), management of infectious disease did not dominate health-care practice. During those years, morbidity and death from infectious diseases had plummeted as a result of multifaceted efforts in social, public health, and medical control. This brief moment in history did not last. The 1980s brought new infectious agents, such as *Legionella* and the human immunodeficiency virus (HIV), further reminders of human vulnerability to infectious disease. Hepatitis, tuberculosis, sexually transmitted diseases, and the vaccine-preventable diseases persist, spread, and continue to kill. Antibiotic-resistant organisms flourish, particularly in the hospital; and organisms that are normally nonpathogenic create devastating disease in the immunocompromised. In addition, many of the major killers of the past, such as cholera and yellow fever, continue to cause death and destruction in many parts of the world, thus reminding us of the need for vigilance everywhere.

All persons, particularly health-care professionals, must maintain a vigilant attitude (see Ethical Issues in Nursing). Such an attitude centers on preventing infectious disease rather than relying on treating it. Prevention requires understanding of the infection process, the transmission chain, and the control measures that break the chain. This chapter describes the process of infection, the chain of transmission, and selected aspects of control. The tables summarize major information highlighted in this chapter for each disease. The reader is referred to other chapters for information on nursing care of clients with specific infectious diseases.

THE PROCESS OF INFECTION

Infection is a process by which an organism establishes a parasitic relationship with its host. The process begins with transmission of an infectious organism (sometimes called an agent, pathogen, or pathogenic agent). The agent, host, and environment interaction is a prerequisite to infectious disease occurrence, and all infectious diseases must be viewed in their unique multicausal context.

Even after successful transmission of a pathogen, the host may experience more than one possible outcome. The pathogen may merely contaminate the body surface. The process ends there if the host's first-line defenses, such as intact skin or mucous membranes, block the pathogen from further invasion. Disease symptoms herald the end of the incubation period. By definition, infectious disease is the pathophysiologic response of a host to the destructive action of the pathogen, to its toxic products, or to the host's immune responses to fight the pathogen. This pathophysiologic response is generally symptomatic. An asymptomatic pathologic response is called subclinical infection.

CRITICAL TO REMEMBER

An asymptomatic host may transmit a pathogen.

The host may harbor a pathogen in sufficient quantities to be shed at any time after latency and toward the end

ETHICAL ISSUES IN NURSING

Do Health Care Workers Have the Right to Refuse Care to Clients with Human Immunodeficiency Virus?

The ethical question that must be addressed is whether health-care workers have a right not to provide care to human immunodeficiency virus (HIV)–infected clients. This question is important for several reasons. One is the severity of the disease. Clients infected with HIV become very ill and are in great need of health care. Another reason is the fatal nature of the virus. In caring for an infected client, there may be a chance that this fatal disease could be transmitted to the heath-care worker. A third consideration is the availability of care—do all clients, no matter what the circumstances, have a right to health care? Also, do health-care workers have a blind obligation to care for all clients, even if it places their own health at risk? On the other hand, do clients have the right to know the HIV status of their health-care workers? Should HIV-infected health-care workers be allowed to work, even if their work involves little or no risk of transmission of the disease to their clients?

The Centers for Disease Control have set up guidelines for the care of all clients regarding precautions for the transmission of disease. These universal precautions should be used on all clients regardless of their disease status. If such precautions are used, the transmission of any disease by blood or body fluids is extremely limited. Nurses care for clients from all walks of life. Some clients may have the HIV virus and not know it. Some might have other diseases, such as hepatitis, which are similarly transmitted. It is of the utmost importance that nurses and all other health-care providers exercise universal precautions with all clients.

Nurses do need to examine their own feelings about caring for clients who may have infectious diseases. There are no easy answers to the dilemmas that have surrounded HIV. Nurses and other health-care workers do have an obligation to keep up with research regarding infectious diseases and should be responsible for taking appropriate precautions in caring for all clients. Such precautions are in the best interest of both the health-care workers and the clients.

of the incubation period. This time period when an organism can be shed is called the period of communicability. It usually precedes symptoms and coincides with part or all of clinical disease, sometimes extending to convalescence. The communicable period, like the incubation period, varies with different pathogens and different diseases. The chain of transmission tables, which are presented later in this chapter, describe specifics on these time periods for each disease.

THE CHAIN OF TRANSMISSION

Infection begins with transmission of a pathogen to a new host. The sequence of events that result in infection is called the chain of transmission. Each of the links in the chain is described.

CRITICAL TO REMEMBER

Determinants of successful transmission include a

- Pathogenic agent
- Reservoir
- Portal of exit from the reservoir
- Mode (mechanism) of transmission through the environment
- Portal of entry into a new host
- Susceptible host

Pathogen

Humans coexist with many micro-organisms in complex, mutually beneficial relationships. The ability of pathogens to elicit disease in the host explains why they are sometimes called etiologic agents of infectious disease. One must remember, however, that pathogens can produce disease only when the host is susceptible. Nonpathogens, that is, normal flora organisms, can also produce disease when the host is immunocompromised and defenseless. So, the cause of infectious disease is always multicausal even though the term "etiologic agent" may be used to describe a pathogen. See the chain of transmission tables for the etiologic agents for each of the diseases summarized.

All micro-organisms can be distinguished by certain intrinsic properties. The property of viability is important because it determines the pathogen's ability to survive in a free state outside its host. Viability is a function of how well an organism can withstand environmental conditions such as drying, sunlight, or heat. It is important in considering ways of interfering with the mechanisms of indirect transmission.

Pathogens also vary in how they interact with their human host. Means of interaction encompass the pathogen's mode of action, infectivity, pathogenicity, virulence, toxigenicity, and antigenicity. The mode of action of a pathogen refers to how the organism produces a pathologic process. The deadly HIV virus causes immune suppression by destroying helper T lymphocytes. Infectivity refers to the pathogen's ability to invade and replicate in the host. Pathogenicity is the ability of the organism to always induce disease. Virulence refers to the potency of the pathogen in producing severe disease and is measured by case-fatality rate (the proportion of cases that result in death). Toxigenicity, the amount and destructive potential of released toxin, is closely related to virulence. Some bacteria secrete water-soluble antigenic exotoxins that are quickly disseminated in the blood, causing potentially severe systemic and neurologic manifestations. Antigenicity, the ability of a pathogen to stimulate an immune response in the host, varies greatly between organisms and with the site of their invasion and dissemination in the body. Generally, organisms that invade and localize in tissue initially stimulate a cellular (T-cell) response. Organisms that disseminate quickly stimulate a humoral or antibody response. Some organisms, such as the influenza virus, have the potential to alter their antigenic characteristics.

One additional characteristic of pathogens and their interaction with their host is worth noting. Many parasites have the ability to adapt to new hosts over time. An example is the plague bacillus, *Pasteurella pestis*. Before 1900, this organism resided in domestic rats and fleas. With environmental control of domestic rats, the bacillus has taken up residence in wild rodents and their parasites, thus maintaining its viability in nature.

Reservoir

A reservoir is an environment in which an organism can live and multiply. Both human and animal reservoirs may be diseased and, therefore, also be hosts. If diseased, the host may be a symptomatic or asymptomatic case or be a carrier of the pathogen. A carrier maintains an environment that promotes growth, multiplication, and shedding of the parasite without exhibiting signs of disease.

Portal of Exit

The portal of exit is the place from which the parasite escapes the reservoir. Generally, this is the site of growth of the organism and corresponds to the system of entry into the next host. For example, the portal of exit for gastrointestinal parasites is generally the feces, and the portal of entry into a new host is the mouth. Some organisms, such as HIV, have more than one portal of exit. Knowledge of the portal of exit is essential for preventing transmission of a pathogen.

Mode of Transmission

Organisms can have one or more than one route of transmission from the reservoir to a new host. Two main routes are direct and indirect transmission. Direct refers to immediate transfer from one person to another as in sexual contact, biting, touching, kissing, or direct projection of respiratory mucous droplets. Indirect transmission implies a vehicle of transmission: a living vector, a common vehicle, or a fomite (inanimate object). Living vectors can carry the pathogen internally as a biologic vector or externally by mechanical means. Common vehicles include water, soil, food, milk, biologic products, and air. Airborne transmission requires that the pathogen survive in dried form in the air until it is inhaled. Fomites include inanimate objects like needles, eating utensils, and urinary catheters.

Portal of Entry

A pathogen may enter a new host by ingestion, by inhalation, through contact with mucous membranes, percutaneously, or transplacentally. There is variation with each infectious disease as to the number of organisms and the duration of the exposure required to start the infectious process in a new host.

Susceptible Host

When it comes to infectious diseases, not all humans are created equal; some are more susceptible than others. Biologic and personal characteristics such as age, gender, ethnicity, and heredity influence this probability. General health and nutritional status, hormonal balance, and the presence of concurrent disease also play a role. Likewise, living conditions and personal behaviors such as drug use, eating, hygiene, and sexual practices all influence the risk of exposure to pathogens and resistance once exposed. Susceptibility is also influenced by the presence of anatomic and physiologic defenses, sometimes called lines of defense.

The first-line defenses are external and act to bar invasion of pathogens. Physical barriers include intact skin and mucous membranes; oil and perspiration on skin; cilia in respiratory passages; gag and cough reflexes; peristalsis in the gastrointestinal tract; and the flushing action of tears, saliva, and mucus. All act to remove organisms before they have an opportunity to invade. The chemical composition of body secretions such as tears and sweat together with the pH of saliva, vaginal secretions, urine, and digestive juices further prevents or inhibits growth of organisms. Compromise in any of these natural defenses increases host susceptibility to pathogen invasion.

Another important first-line defense is the normal flora of micro-organisms that inhabit the skin and mucous membranes in the oral cavity, gastrointestinal tract, and vagina. These parasites are indigenous to specific tissue. They generally coexist with their host in a mutually beneficial relationship as long as they do not wander from the specific tissue. Through a mechanism called microbial antagonism, they control the replication of potential pathogens. The importance of this mechanism is evident when it is disturbed. An example of disturbance is the overgrowth of *Candida albicans* (thrush), which results from extensive antibiotic therapy that destroys normal flora in the oral or vaginal cavity. Some normal flora can become pathogenic under specific conditions, such as immunosuppression or displacement of the pathogen to another area of the body.

The second line of defense, the inflammatory process, and the third line, the immune response, share several physiologic components. These include the lymphatic system, leukocytes, and a multitude of chemicals, proteins, and enzymes that facilitate the internal defenses. For discussion of inflammation and wound healing, refer to Chapter 5. See Chapter 8 for a description of the structure and function of the immune system.

CONTROL OF TRANSMISSION

Transmission of infectious disease can be controlled by breaking the transmission chain at only one link. In general, the aim is to break the chain at the most cost-effective point or points. That is the point at which the greatest number of people can be protected with available technology with use of the least amount of resources.

Some pathogens can be controlled by interventions directed at inactivating them through disinfection, sterilization, or use of anti-infective drugs. Other pathogens can be controlled best by eradicating their nonhuman reservoirs. This is accomplished through environmental sanitation, particularly water treatment; food and milk safety programs; and control of animals, vectors, rodents, sewage, and solid wastes.

Transmission from the portal of exit can often be prevented by detecting and treating clients shedding a pathogen, such as gonococcus. Other prevention methods include proper handling and disposal of secretions, excretions, and exudates; isolation of infected clients; and quarantine of contacts. Specific isolation precautions, based on knowledge of the transmission chain for individual infections, have been recommended by the Centers for Disease Control (CDC). The precautions were designed to prevent transmission of pathogens among hospitalized patients, health-care personnel, and visitors (see Box 10–1). The category-specific recommendations from the CDC (1983) together with the 1991 recommended universal precautions are given in Box 10–2 and Chapter 9. Chains of transmission for specific diseases are also highlighted in Tables 10–1 and 10–2.

CRITICAL TO REMEMBER

Transmission to a new portal of entry can be prevented by environmental disinfection:

- Use of barrier precautions (gloves, masks, condoms)
- Proper handling of food, milk, and water
- Protection from vectors
- Personal hygiene
- Avoidance of high-risk behaviors (unsafe sexual practices, intravenous drug use, recapping needles)
- Effective hand washing

Text continued on page 212

BOX 10–1

Methicillin-Resistant *Staphylococcus aureus*

Methicillin-resistant *Staphylococcus aureus* (MRSA) is a strain of staphylococci that is resistant (cannot be killed) to antibiotics, including the aminoglycosides, penicillins, cephalosporins, and others. Over the past 10 years, MRSA and other resistant strains of *S. aureus* have become the most common causes of hospital- and community-acquired infections. MRSA is virulent and because of its resistance to antibiotics is a feared organism. MRSA usually develops when multiple antibiotics are used in the treatment of infection and in clients who are elderly, debilitated, having surgery or multiple invasive procedures, or being treated in critical care units. Unfortunately, inanimate objects can also serve as reservoirs for the bacterium. Items such as the telephone, sphygmomanometer, side rails, and tray tables have been infected.

Not only are clients at risk, but also health-care providers can become "colonized" by the bacterium. The term "colonized" means that a healthy person carries the organism and potentially can infect others with it, although she or he does not feel ill.

MRSA is difficult to eradicate once it has been introduced into a hospital or nursing home by a client. A client infected with it is usually treated with intravenous vancomycin. Colonized carriers can be treated with a variety of medications, including topical antibiotics for colonized nasal passages and shampoos with disinfectants for skin and hair colonization. Some health-care providers have lost their jobs because of chronic colonization with MRSA.

It is perhaps more important to prevent MRSA infection because it is not easily treated. Some suggested precautions include thorough hand washing with a mild iodine-containing soap and establishing community-wide infection control policies on the placement of clients who are infected with MRSA. Sometimes potentially infected clients are isolated when they are transferred to other agencies until all culture reports are returned. Honest reporting of infected clients would reduce unnecessary costs.

BOX 10–2

Category-Specific Isolation Precautions

STRICT ISOLATION

Strict isolation is an isolation category designed to prevent transmission of highly contagious or virulent infections that may be spread by both air and contact.

Specifications for Strict Isolation

- Private room is indicated; door should be kept closed. In general, clients infected with the same organism may share a room.
- Masks are indicated for everyone entering the room.
- Gowns are indicated for everyone entering the room.
- Gloves are indicated for everyone entering the room.
- Hands must be washed after touching the client or potentially contaminated articles and before taking care of another client.
- Articles contaminated with infective material should be discarded or bagged and labeled before being sent for decontamination and reprocessing.

Diseases Requiring Strict Isolation

Diphtheria, pharyngeal
Lassa fever and other viral hemorrhagic fevers, such as Marburg virus disease*
Plague, pneumonia
Smallpox*
Varicella (chickenpox)
Zoster, localized in immunocompromised client or disseminated

CONTACT ISOLATION

Contact isolation is designed to prevent transmission of highly transmissible or epidemiologically important infections (or colonization) that do not warrant strict isolation.

Specifications for Contact Isolation

- Private room is indicated. In general, clients infected with the same organism may share a room. During outbreaks, infants and young children with the same respiratory clinical syndrome may share a room.
- Masks are indicated for those who come close to the client.
- Gowns are indicated if soiling is likely.
- Gloves are indicated for touching infective material.
- Hands must be washed after touching the client or potentially contaminated articles and before taking care of another client.
- Articles contaminated with infective material should be discarded or bagged and labeled before being sent for decontamination and reprocessing.

Disease or Conditions Requiring Contact Isolation

Acute respiratory infections in infants and young children, including croup, colds, bronchitis, and bronchiolitis caused by respiratory syncytial virus, adenovirus, coronavirus, influenza viruses, parainfluenza viruses, and rhinovirus
Conjunctivitis, gonococcal in newborns
Diphtheria, cutaneous
Endometritis, group A streptococcus
Furunculosis, staphylococcal in newborns
Herpes simplex, disseminated, severe primary or neonatal
Impetigo
Influenza, in infants and young children
Multiple resistant bacteria, infection, or colonization (any site) with any of the following:

* A private room with special ventilation is indicated.

Box continued on following page

BOX 10-2

Category-Specific Isolation Precautions *Continued*

- Gram-negative bacilli resistant to all aminoglycosides that are tested (in general, such organisms should be resistant to gentamicin, tobramycin, and amikacin for these special precautions to be indicated.)
- *Staphylococcus aureus* resistant to methicillin (or nafcillin or oxacillin if they are used instead of methicillin for testing)
- *Pneumococcus* resistant to penicillin
- *Haemophilus influenzae* resistant to ampicillin (beta-lactamase–positive) and chloramphenicol
- Other resistant bacteria may be included if they are judged by the infection control team to be of special clinical and epidemiologic significance

Pediculosis
Pharyngitis, infectious, in infants and young children
Pneumonia, viral, in infants and young children
Pneumonia, *Staphylococcus aureus* or group A streptococcus
Rabies
Rubella, congenital and other
Scabies
Scalded skin syndrome, staphylococcal (Ritter's disease)
Skin wound or burn infection, major (draining and not covered by dressing or dressing does not adequately contain the purulent material) including those infected with *Staphylococcus aureus* or group A streptococcus
Vaccinia (generalized and progressive eczema vaccinatum)

RESPIRATORY ISOLATION

Respiratory isolation is designed to prevent transmission of infectious diseases primarily over short distances through the air (droplet transmission).

Specifications for Respiratory Isolation

- Private room is indicated. In general, clients infected with the same organism may share a room.
- Masks are indicated for those who come close to the client.
- Gowns are not indicated.
- Gloves are not indicated.
- Hands must be washed after touching the client or potentially contaminated articles and before taking care of another client.
- Articles contaminated with infective material should be discarded or bagged and labeled before being sent for decontamination and reprocessing.

Diseases Requiring Respiratory Isolation

Epiglottitis, *Haemophilus influenzae*
Erythema infectiosum
Measles
Meningitis
  Haemophilus influenzae, known or suspected
  Meningococcal, known or suspected
Meningococcal pneumonia
Meningococcemia
Mumps
Pertussis (whooping cough)
Pneumonia, *Haemophilus influenzae,* in children (any age)

TUBERCULOSIS ISOLATION (AFB ISOLATION)

Tuberculosis isolation (AFB isolation) is an isolation category for clients with pulmonary tuberculosis who have a positive sputum smear or a chest film that strongly suggests current (active) tuberculosis. Laryngeal tuberculosis is also included in this isolation category.

Specifications for Tuberculosis Isolation (AFB Isolation)

- Private room with special ventilation is indicated; door should be kept closed. In general, clients infected with the same organism may share a room.
- Masks are indicated only if the client is coughing and does not reliably cover mouth.
- Gowns are indicated only if needed to prevent gross contamination of clothing.
- Gloves are not indicated.
- Hands must be washed after touching the client or potentially contaminated articles and before taking care of another client.
- Articles are rarely involved in transmission of tuberculosis. However, articles should be thoroughly cleaned and disinfected or discarded.

ENTERIC PRECAUTIONS

Enteric precautions are designed to prevent infections that are transmitted by direct or indirect contact with feces.

Specifications for Enteric Precautions

- Private room is indicated if client's hygiene is poor. A client with poor hygiene does not wash hands after touching infective material, contaminates the environment with infective material, or shares contaminated articles with other clients. In general, clients infected with the same organism may share a room.
- Masks are not indicated.
- Gowns are indicated if soiling is likely.
- Gloves are indicated for touching infective material.
- Hands must be washed after touching the client or potentially contaminated articles and before taking care of another client.
- Articles contaminated with infective material should be discarded or bagged and labeled before being sent for decontamination or reprocessing.

Diseases Requiring Enteric Precautions

Amebic dysentery
Cholera
Coxsackievirus disease
Diarrhea, acute illness with suspected infectious cause
Echovirus disease
Encephalitis (unless known not to be caused by enteroviruses)
Enterocolitis caused by *Clostridium difficile* or *Staphylococcus aureus*
Enteroviral infection
Gastroenteritis caused by
  Campylobacter species
  Cryptosporidium species
  Dientamoeba fragilis
  Escherichia coli (enterotoxic, enteropathogenic, or enteroinvasive)
  Giardia lamblia
  Salmonella species

BOX 10-2

Category-Specific Isolation Precautions *Continued*

Shigella species
Vibrio parahaemolyticus
Viruses—including Norwalk agent and rotavirus
Yersinia enterocolitica
Unknown cause but presumed to be an infectious agent

Hand, foot, mouth disease
Hepatitis, viral, type A
Herpangina
Meningitis, viral (unless known not to be caused by enteroviruses)
Necrotizing enterocolitis
Pleurodynia
Poliomyelitis
Typhoid fever (*Salmonella typhi*)
Viral pericarditis, myocarditis, or meningitis (unless known not to be caused by enteroviruses)

DRAINAGE-SECRETION PRECAUTIONS

Drainage-secretion precautions are designed to prevent infections that are transmitted by direct or indirect contact with purulent material or drainage from an infected body site.

Specifications for Drainage-Secretion Precautions

- Private room is not indicated.
- Masks are not indicated.
- Gowns are indicated if soiling is likely.
- Gloves are indicated for touching infective material.
- Hands must be washed after touching the client or potentially contaminated articles and before taking care of another client.
- Articles contaminated with infective material should be discarded or bagged and labeled before being sent for decontamination and reprocessing.

Diseases Requiring Drainage-Secretion Precautions

The following infections are examples of those included in this category provided they are not (1) caused by multiple resistant microorganisms; (2) major draining (and not covered by a dressing or dressing does not adequately contain the drainage) skin, wound, or burn infections, including those caused by *Staphylococcus aureus* or group A streptococcus; or (3) gonococcal eye infections in newborns. See contact isolation if the infection is one of these three.

Abscess, minor limited
Burn infection, minor limited
Conjunctivitis
Decubitus ulcer, infected, minor or limited
Skin infection, minor or limited
Wound infection, minor or limited

AFB, acid-fast bacilli.
Centers for Disease Control. (1983). *CDC guidelines for isolation precautions in hospitals.* HHS publication number CDC 83-8314. Atlanta: Centers for Disease Control.

TABLE 10–1 Chain of Transmission for Meningitis and Encephalitis

VARIABLE	MENINGOCOCCAL MENINGITIS	PNEUMOCOCCAL MENINGITIS	*HAEMOPHILUS* MENINGITIS	VIRAL MENINGITIS (ASEPTIC)	VIRAL ENCEPHALITIS
Pathogen	*Neisseria meningitidis,* with many subgroups	*Streptococcus pneumoniae,* many serotypes	*Haemophilus influenzae,* six serotypes; type B responsible for 90% of *Haemophilus* meningitis	Most viruses (e.g., mumps, herpes, and polio) produce the syndrome	A variety of viruses, commonly the *herpes virus*
Reservoir	Humans	Humans; many carriers	Humans	Humans	Humans
Transmission	Direct contact with droplets from respiratory passages of infected clients and carriers	Direct and indirect contact with discharges from respiratory passages	Direct contact with droplets from respiratory passages	Not transmitted at this stage	Direct contact with droplets from respiratory passages or other excretions harboring the virus
Host susceptibility	Children younger than 5 years and clients in crowded living conditions; susceptibility to clinical disease is low; many carriers; group-specific immunity of unknown duration follows infection	Infants and elderly most susceptible; follows pneumococcal pneumonia; immunity for specific type persists for years	Children 2 months to 3 years of age most susceptible; otitis media may be a precursor; immunity of unknown duration follows infection	Children, elderly, and immunocompromised clients and those unimmunized against vaccine-preventable viral diseases	Depends on viral disease

Table continued on following page

TABLE 10–1 Chain of Transmission for Meningitis and Encephalitis *Continued*

VARIABLE	MENINGOCOCCAL MENINGITIS	PNEUMOCOCCAL MENINGITIS	*HAEMOPHILUS* MENINGITIS	VIRAL MENINGITIS (ASEPTIC)	VIRAL ENCEPHALITIS
Incubation period	2–10 days; usually 3–4 days	1–3 days for pneumonia	2–4 days	Depends on virus and associated viral disease	Depends on viral disease
Period of communicability	Until organism is not present in discharges; within 24 hours of treatment with sulfonamides	Until organism is not present in respiratory discharges: 24–48 hours after antibiotic treatment	Prolonged; until organism is not present in nasal discharge		Depends on viral disease
Isolation precautions	Respiratory isolation for 24 hours after initiation of antibiotic therapy	Respiratory isolation for 24 hours after initiation of antibiotic therapy	Respiratory isolation for 24 hours after initiation of antibiotic therapy	Respiratory isolation for duration of hospitalization	Respiratory isolation for duration of hospitalization

Adapted from Grimes, D. (1991). *Infectious diseases.* St. Louis: Mosby-Year Book.

Host susceptibility can be decreased through active and passive immunization, positive health practices, avoiding risky behaviors, and maintaining the first-line defenses. The last is an important consideration for the nurse caring for clients whose health status has already been compromised by disease or diagnostic and treatment procedures. Specifically, the nurse can strengthen defenses of clients by providing preprocedure instruction and postprocedure assistance to encourage deep breathing, coughing, ambulation, bladder emptying, and asepsis of invasive sites. Turning and providing skin care to an immobilized client also protect the defenses. Maintaining hydration and electrolyte balance and ensuring adequate fluid and nutrition intake strengthen resistance. Administering anti-infectives as ordered and instructing clients and care givers on the proper use of anti-infectives are important not only in treatment but also in preventing drug resistance. In addition, using asepsis with all invasive procedures and avoiding all unnecessary invasive procedures are essential for preventing transmission of infection (see the Client Education Guide).

TABLE 10–2 Chain of Transmission for Streptococcal Throat, Scarlet Fever, and Rheumatic Fever

VARIABLE	STREPTOCOCCAL THROAT	SCARLET FEVER	RHEUMATIC FEVER
Pathogen	*Streptococcus pyogenes* (group A streptococcus of approximately 70 serologically distinct types)		
		Three erythrogenic toxins	Group A beta-hemolytic streptococcus
Reservoir	Humans	Humans	Humans
Transmission	Direct or intimate contact with person or carrier; may follow ingestion of contaminated food	Contact with respiratory secretions containing *Streptococcus*	Contact with respiratory secretions containing *Streptococcus*
Host susceptibility	Children age 3–15 years most susceptible	Permanent acquired immunity from active disease with type of toxin; second attacks caused by different toxin	Persons who have suffered one attack are predisposed to a recurrent episode after group A streptococcal upper respiratory tract infections
Incubation period	1–3 days	2–4 days (range, 1–7 days)	3–35 days after clinical strep throat (average, 19 days)
Period of communicability	Untreated uncomplicated cases: 10–21 days; complicated: weeks to months; antibiotic-treated: 24–48 hours	Not communicable	Not communicable
Isolation precautions	Respiratory isolation for 24 hours after onset of antibiotic therapy	None	None

Adapted from Grimes, D. (1991). *Infectious diseases.* St. Louis: Mosby-Year Book.

CLIENT EDUCATION GUIDE

Infection Control at Home

How the disease is transmitted from person to person is the basis for client, family, and caregiver education. For example, a feces-borne illness such as hepatitis A requires a good sewer system, easy access to toileting, and means to wash the hands. One must teach the client and all care givers about the chain of infection so that transmission of infection will be avoided.

- Hand washing is the best protection against transmission of infectious diseases, and it is essential after the caregiver provides direct care and when gloves are removed. The nurse must teach that gloves should be worn for all contact with body fluids.
- Caregivers should leave all extraneous clothing and equipment outside the client's room and take in only items that are needed for care. Equipment needed on a regular basis such as the blood pressure cuff and stethoscope should stay in the client's room.
- Supplies at the entrance to the room should include gloves, masks, gowns to cover clothing and arms or disposable plastic aprons as indicated, and plastic bags for disposal of used items. The nurse must demonstrate to the caregivers how to handle soiled linens and trash and teach them to wash their hands afterward.
- Paper towels can be used to create a clean work surface and to wipe the hands.
- Isolation or precautions can have a negative effect on the client and family. One must help the care givers feel comfortable with the techniques needed for isolation and encourage family and caregivers to visit with the client and not just be with him or her during care.
- If the client has hepatitis A or salmonellosis, the client should be instructed not to handle raw food, such as lettuce or tomatoes, until the physician believes the client is past the infectious stage.
- If the client is recovering from a disease that is spread by stool, the client should be instructed not to prepare food until the physician believes the client is past the infectious stage.
- If the client is severely immunocompromised, the client should be instructed not to handle feces from pet animals or birds until the physician believes the infectious stage is past.
- In helping client with blood-borne illness, caregivers should be taught what to do if the client accidentally cuts himself or herself; for example, to clean the blood off the bathroom counter with a solution of one part household bleach to 10 parts water. Sharing razors, toothbrushes, or other personal items should be discouraged.

Health professionals should be concerned about improving their own resistance and decreasing their own susceptibility to infectious diseases. One important approach is to maintain one's immunization status. This means being adequately immunized for hepatitis B, measles, mumps, rubella, polio, tetanus, and diphtheria. The 1991 CDC recommendations for immunization of health-care workers are given in Table 10–3.

According to government regulations, certain diseases must be reported to the local health authority. Some states require that additional diseases endemic to their area be reported. State laws vary regarding who is responsible for reporting. In general, the responsibility falls to physicians, laboratories, and others who are aware that a reportable disease has not been reported (nurses!).

TABLE 10–3 1991 Centers for Disease Control Recommendations for Immunization of Health-Care Workers

DISEASE	RECOMMENDATION
Hepatitis B	Three-dose series of hepatitis B vaccine for pre-exposure protection
Polio	Primary series of oral poliovirus vaccine in childhood is sufficient
Tetanus-diphtheria	Booster dose of tetanus-diphtheria every 10 years after primary series of diphtheria and tetanus toxoids; tetanus toxoid may be repeated in 5 years if a dirty wound is sustained
Measles	College entrants and health-care workers who do not have evidence of immunity to measles (physician-diagnosed measles or laboratory evidence of immunity) should have documentation of two doses of measles vaccine received on or after their first birthday; vaccine can be given as MMR*
Mumps	A single dose of live mumps vaccine received on or after the first birthday is sufficient; vaccine can be given as MMR*
Rubella	A single dose of live attenuated rubella vaccine received on or after the first birthday is sufficient; vaccine can be given as MMR*

* There is no evidence suggesting an increased risk from live MMR vaccination to persons already immune to these diseases as a result of previous vaccination or natural disease.
MMR, measles, mumps, rubella.
From Centers for Disease Control. (1991). Update on adult immunization: Recommendations of the Immunization Practices Advisory Committee (ACIP). *Morbidity and Mortality Weekly Report, 40* (RR–12):1–19.

STUDY QUESTIONS

1. The use of which of the following is indicated for family or staff caring for clients with meningitis?
   A. Gloves
   B. Gowns
   C. Masks
   D. Semiprivate room

2. In teaching about infection control, the client and family should know that the first line of bodily defense is the:
   A. Skin
   B. Environment
   C. Inflammatory process
   D. Immune response

3. The nurse teaches the client that his or her disease *cannot* be transmitted during which phase of the disease process?
   A. The asymptomatic phase
   B. The latent period
   C. The incubation period
   D. The symptomatic phase

4. The client with the greatest risk of transmission of disease to others is the one with:
   A. Pertussis who wears a mask and washes his or her hands.
   B. Cholera who washes his or her hands and keeps personal items separate from others.
   C. Conjunctivitis who washes his or her hands and separates infected materials for discard.
   D. Smallpox who washes his or her hands and wears a mask.

5. Which of the following is the *best* way to determine how to treat a suspected infectious disease?
   A. Send samples of bodily substances to the laboratory for analysis and report
   B. Current history and physical examination
   C. Perform a culture of all known sources of infection to which the client has been exposed
   D. Observe client behaviors for indications of transmission and reservoir sources

6. Successful treatment and prevention of transmission are identified when the client has:
   A. No further symptoms
   B. Changed his or her hand-washing behavior
   C. Completed his or her therapeutic regimen
   D. Identified how to prevent further reinfection

CRITICAL THINKING EXERCISES

A client is admitted to the hospital with nausea, vomiting, diarrhea, and diagnosed dehydration. Serum electrolytes, complete blood count, urinalysis, and gastric and stool samples for culture and sensitivity as well as ova and parasites are sent to the laboratory. The client is ordered to have nothing by mouth, and intravenous feeding is begun. The client is noted to have poor hygiene, and compliance with hand washing is questionable.

1. What type of isolation would be most appropriate for this client until culture results are available?
2. What specific precautions would you take in managing this client's care?
3. The physician orders diphenoxylate/atropine (Lomotil), which is an antidiarrheal medication. Would you question this order? If so, why?
4. On admission, in what type of a room would you put this client?

BIBLIOGRAPHY

1. Benenson, A. (Ed.). (1990). *Control of communicable diseases in man* (15th ed.). Washington, DC: The American Public Health Association.
2. Brown, K. K. (1994). Critical interventions in septic shock. *American Journal of Nursing, 94(10),* 21–26.
3. Bryant, J., & Lewicki, L. J. (1992). Infection control. In G. M. Bulacheck, & J. C. McCloskey (Eds.), *Nursing interventions: Essential nursing treatments.* (2nd ed., pp. 247–253). Philadelphia: W. B. Saunders.
4. Centers for Disease Control. (1983). *CDC guidelines for isolation precautions in hospitals.* HHS publication number CDC 83-8314. Atlanta: Centers for Disease Control.
5. Centers for Disease Control. (1987). Recommendations for prevention of HIV transmission in health-care settings. *Morbidity and Mortality Weekly Report, 36(2S),* 3–17.
6. Centers for Disease Control. (1991). Update on adult immunization: Recommendations of the Immunization Practices Advisory Committee (ACIP). *Morbidity and Mortality Weekly Report, 40(RR-12),* 1–19.
7. Centers for Disease Control. (1993). 1993 sexually transmitted disease treatment guidelines. *Morbidity and Mortality Weekly Report, 42(RR-14),* 1–102.
8. Ealer, R., et al. (1994). Patient-centered pneumonia care: A case management success story. *American Journal of Nursing, 94(11),* 34–38.
9. Fecht-Grasley, M. E. (1994). Recognizing compartment syndrome. *American Journal of Nursing, 94(10),* 41.
10. Grawlikowski, J. (1992). White cells at war. *American Journal of Nursing, 92(3),* 44–51.
11. Grimes, D. (1993). Potential for infection. In J. Thompson, et al. (Eds.), *Mosby's clinical nursing* (3rd ed.). St. Louis: Mosby-Year Book.
12. Grimes, D. (1991). *Infectious diseases.* St. Louis: Mosby-Year Book.

13. Kolodner, D. E. (1993). The new federal bloodborne pathogens standard: Significance to the health care worker. *MEDSURG Nursing, 1(1)*, 29–32.
14. Much, J. K., & Cotteta, T. A. (1993). Stress of occupational exposure to blood or body fluids: Managing the response. *MEDSURG Nursing, 2(1)*, 49–56.
15. Shovein, J., & Young, M. S. (1992). MRSA: Pandora's box for hospitals. *American Journal of Nursing, 92(2)*, 49–52.
16. Stites, D. P., & Terr, A. I. (1991). *Basic and clinical immunology*. Los Altos, California: Appleton & Lange.
17. Valenta, A. L. (1994). Using the vaccuum dressing alternative for difficult wounds. *American Journal of Nursing, 94(4)*, 44–45.

Chapter 11

Nursing Care of Clients with Connective Tissue Disorders

Learning Outcomes

After completing this chapter, the learner will be able to:

1. Assess the client for clinical manifestations of connective tissue disorders.
2. Teach the client and significant others about the etiology, risk factors, basic pathophysiology, and clinical manifestations of major connective tissue disorders.
3. Explain the client's role in management of connective tissue disorders.
4. Develop plans of care for the management and rehabilitation of clients with connective tissue disorders.
5. Implement nursing interventions that optimize the quality of life for clients with connective tissue disorders.
6. Using outcome criteria developed in the planning phase of care, evaluate planned client outcomes.

OVERVIEW

Connective tissue disorders (collagen diseases) include diseases such as rheumatoid arthritis, systemic lupus erythematosus (SLE), polyarteritis nodosa, polymyositis, dermatomyositis, and scleroderma. Genetic factors appear to be significant in the development of these conditions. They are also classified as autoimmune disorders.

Collagen diseases produce widespread changes in collagenous connective tissue, cause problems involving almost every organ, may be autoimmune in nature, are difficult to diagnose, have no cure, and are not preventable. Treatment for autoimmune conditions (mainly to control the symptoms) includes corticosteroids, ionizing radiation, and salicylates. Common features include myocarditis, endocarditis, pericarditis, pleuritis, peritonitis, vasculitis, myositis, and sometimes, nephritis.

Laboratory tests may reveal Coombs-positive hemolytic anemia, thrombocytopenia, leukopenia, immunoglobulin excesses or deficiencies, antinuclear antibodies, antibodies to deoxyribonucleic acid (DNA) and ribonucleic acid, rheumatoid factors, false-positive serologic tests for syphilis, elevated muscle enzymes, and changes in acute phase–reactive proteins. Some of these laboratory findings also may occur in asymptomatic clients, suggesting the possibility of the presence or future development of a connective tissue disease.

Often anatomic, immunologic, and histologic findings overlap from one disease to another. Although serologic tests may help establish a differential diagnosis, they are not specific. The various conditions do tend to differ in their prognosis, clinical patterns, and response to treatment.

The term *autoimmune disease* implies that autoantibodies are important in the cause or pathogenesis of the disorder. These diseases have been classified as systemic or organ specific. Rheumatoid arthritis (RA), for example, is classified as system specific, whereas Graves' disease is organ specific.

Etiology

The cause of autoimmunity remains obscure, but five factors are thought to contribute to this state: altered antigens, cross-reactive antibodies, viral factors, hormonal factors, and genetic factors (Box 11-1). None of these elements are a complete explanation for autoimmune disease, but they do offer clues to the direction of future research in this area.

Pathophysiology

There are three ways in which the autoimmune response causes disease:

- Action of autoantibodies on cell surfaces
- Circulation and deposition of small immune complexes
- Activation of sensitized T lymphocytes.

BOX 11-1

Possible Contributing Causes of Autoimmunity

ALTERED ANTIGENS

Tissues may break down naturally, or in response to some stimulus, so autoantibody production may occur. Tissue injury may cause cells that do not normally circulate to be released into the bloodstream and to be recognized as foreign. For example, testicular cells may be released after a vasectomy. They may elicit an autoantibody response because the immune cells do not recognize them as self, a normally circulating cell.

CROSS-REACTIVE ANTIBODIES

The body may elicit an immune response to a foreign antigen that is structurally very similar to a self-antigen. For example, the streptococcal antigen that causes rheumatic fever is very similar to heart tissue antigen. The antibodies produced to the streptococcal antigen may cross-react with heart tissue and damage the heart.

VIRAL FACTORS

Viruses may damage cells, allowing the release of antigens that do not normally circulate (i.e., causing altered antigens). Viruses also may damage the regulatory T cells, promoting faulty regulation of the immune response. The occurrence of multiple autoimmune disorders in the same client suggests a breakdown in suppressor T-cell activity.

HORMONAL FACTORS

Autoimmune diseases have a much higher incidence in women than in men. In SLE, for example, the female-to-male ratio is 10:1. This suggests hormonal influence on the immune response.

GENETIC FACTORS

Identical twins have a higher incidence of the same autoimmune disease than do nonidentical twins. Thus, it may not be simply environmental factors that lead to autoimmunity. Autoimmune disease increases with age, which may indicate that genetic errors accumulate in cells as one ages. It is known that regulatory T-cell function decreases with age, so there may be a link between the loss of this suppressor regulation and the development of autoimmunity.

ACTION OF AUTOANTIBODIES ON CELL SURFACES

Destruction of cells or tissues occurs by direct antibody-mediated cellular cytotoxicity (e.g., autoimmune hemolytic anemia and thrombocytopenia), interference with receptors (e.g., myasthenia gravis and Graves' disease), or complement activation (e.g., basement membrane disease).

CIRCULATION AND DEPOSITION OF SMALL IMMUNE COMPLEXES

Soluble antigen-antibody complexes (made up of one antibody and one or more antigens) are small enough to invade and deposit in the capillaries (butterfly rash of SLE), the synovium of joints (rheumatoid arthritis), and the basement membrane of cells (as occurs with renal damage in SLE and Goodpasture's syndrome). These complexes cause tissue damage via activation of the complement system.

THE ACTIVATION OF SENSITIZED T LYMPHOCYTES

Sensitized T cells cause tissue destruction by the release of lymphokines (e.g., polymyositis).

RHEUMATOID ARTHRITIS

Arthritis is defined as joint inflammation. Rheumatoid arthritis (RA) is a chronic, systemic, progressive, inflammatory connective tissue disorder affecting mainly the small, peripheral joints in a pattern of symmetric distribution (Fig. 11–1).

Incidence

Women are affected with rheumatoid arthritis two to three times more often than are men; however, women who are taking or have taken oral contraceptives are less likely to experience RA. Although it may occur at any age, RA is most common in people between the ages of 20 and 40 years. The incidence of RA is about 1 to 3 per 100. It is characterized by unexplained periods of exacerbation and remission.

Etiology

The cause of RA is unknown, although there are many and varied theories about its cause. A genetic basis may exist, and RA may be caused by a combination of factors.

The immunologic theory is currently the most prevalent. Rheumatoid factor, unusual antibodies of the immunoglobulin (Ig)M or IgG type or both, develops against the IgG antigens. These complexes lodge in the synovium and other connective tissues. The result is local and systemic inflammation.

Risk Factors

There are no specific risk factors for the development of RA. There are risk factors, however, for exacerbation of the disease, including the presence of physical and emotional stress. Controlling stress can help the client keep the disease in remission.

Pathophysiology

The pathologic processes involved in RA are type III (immune complex) and type IV (cell-mediated) reactions. If unarrested, pathologic changes in RA pass through four stages:

- Synovitis
- Pannus formation
- Fibrous ankylosis
- Bony ankylosis

(See the Pathophysiology Box.)

Although joint involvement is the most obvious manifestation of RA, other body tissues also are affected by this inflammatory process. RA is a systemic disease, attacking all connective tissue. Nonarticular connective tissue may be diffusely involved, such as the collagen in lungs, heart, muscles, blood vessels, pleura, or tendons. Collagen is a scleroprotein present in connective tissue. Vasculitis may occur in the eyes, nervous system, and skin, producing thrombosis and ischemia.

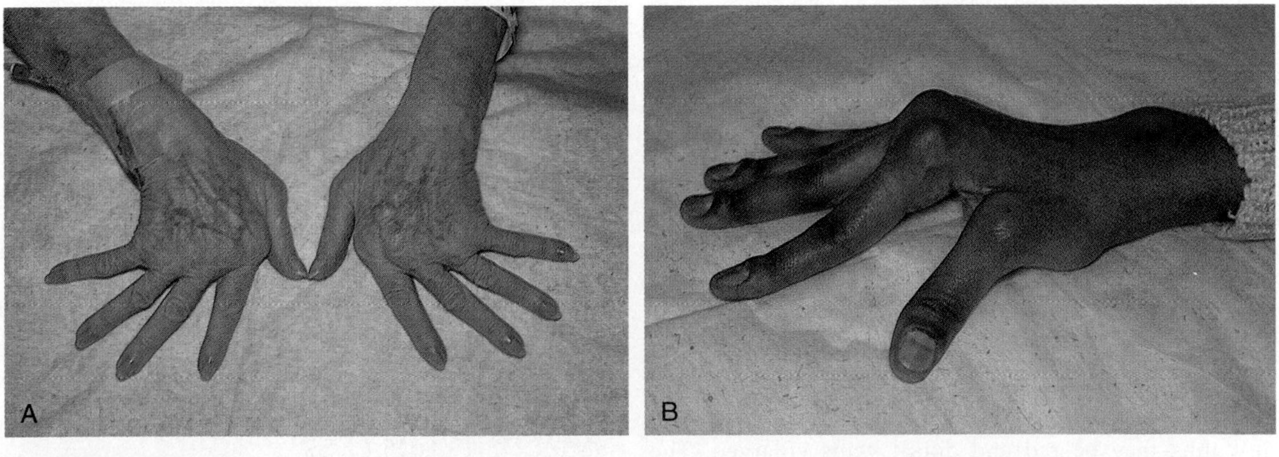

Figure 11–1
Hand deformities characteristic of chronic rheumatoid arthritis. *A*, Subluxation of metacarpophalangeal joints with ulnar deviation (ulnar drift) of digits. *B*, Hyperextension ("swan neck") deformities of proximal interphalangeal joints. (From Swartz, M. H. [1994]. Textbook of physical diagnosis: History and examination [2nd ed.]. Philadelphia: W. B. Saunders Co.)

PATHOPHYSIOLOGY

Four Stages of Rheumatoid Arthritis

In **stage 1,** involved joints become inflamed with a proliferative type of inflammation, initially localized in the joint capsule, primarily in the synovial membrane (synovitis). Tissue thickens with edema and congestion (Illustration A).

In **stage 2,** pannus gradually develops. This layer of inflammatory granulation tissue is derived from synovial membrane extending over the articular surface into the joint interior. It appears reddish and rough and adheres tightly to the underlying cartilage by invasion and lysis, interfering with cartilage nutrition (Illustration B).

In **stage 3,** fibrous ankylosis, with subluxation and distortion of the affected joint, occurs as granulation tissue becomes invaded with tough fibrous tissue and is converted to scar tissue that inhibits or prevents joint movement (Illustration C).

In **stage 4,** bony ankylosis (firm bony union) may then develop as the fibrous tissue calcifies and changes into osseous tissue (Illustration D).

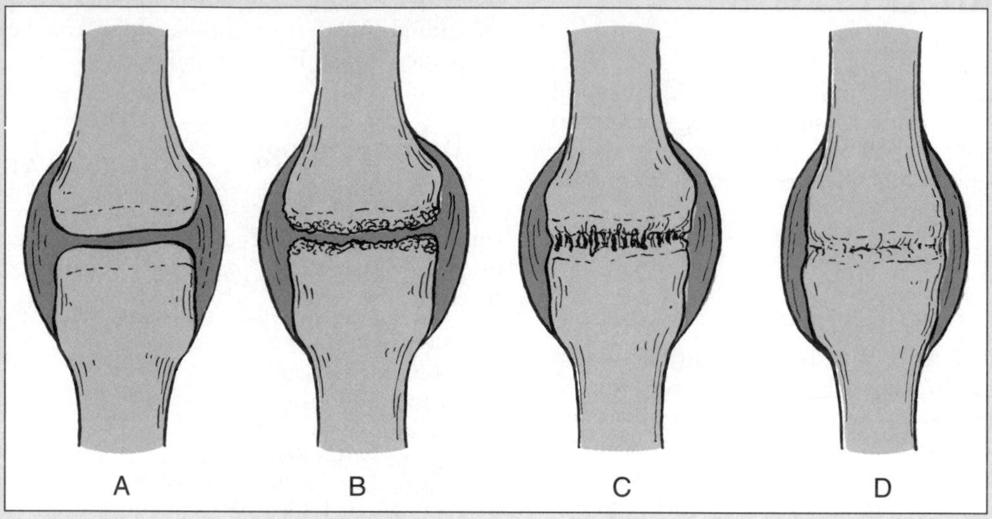

As the disease destroys the joints, the client experiences pain, stiffness, and swelling. If the disease can be diagnosed early and treated successfully, permanent joint deterioration may not occur. About 25 per cent of clients with RA have a remission possibly lasting up to 25 years. Some clients experience spontaneous remissions without any treatment. Some clients, however, seem to progress rapidly to deformity and limitation of joint movement in spite of aggressive therapy.

Clinical Manifestations

Even in well-established, chronic arthritis, the client typically has periods of increased and severe symptoms and times of relative comfort and remission. Remissions occur most often, however, early in the disease. Each exacerbation seems more difficult to treat than the previous one, with more residual damage occurring. Although permanent remission can occur rarely, RA is usually progressive and deformity producing. (See Clinical Manifestations: Rheumatoid Arthritis.)

During an exacerbation of the disease, the joints are red, warm, swollen, stiff, and tender when examined. The palms may be red and dorsal veins enlarged. The client may be slightly febrile. The client exhibits guarded movement and limited range of motion and strength. Prodromal signs and symptoms include vague articular pain and stiffness, malaise, weight loss, and vasomotor changes such as paresthesias (numbness of the hands and feet). Symptoms are usually worse in the morning and subside during the day with moderate activity.

The onset of RA, or exacerbations of the disease, often coincides with stress (anxiety, exposure to temperature extremes, overwork, and acute infections), which depletes the client's physical and emotional reserves.

RA commonly begins insidiously, although it may begin abruptly. When RA develops insidiously, the client usually experiences pain (on use) and stiffness in one or several joints, followed by swelling. Muscle aching may occur anywhere in the body. The client's temperature may be normal or slightly elevated. Although almost any joint may be affected initially, within several weeks, the smaller joints of the hands and feet are typically involved. In acute-onset RA, numerous joints suddenly become painful and swollen. The client experiences chills, prostration, and fever.

DIAGNOSTIC ASSESSMENT

Laboratory findings help establish a diagnosis of RA. Serum protein abnormalities are often present, such as

CLINICAL MANIFESTATIONS

Rheumatoid Arthritis

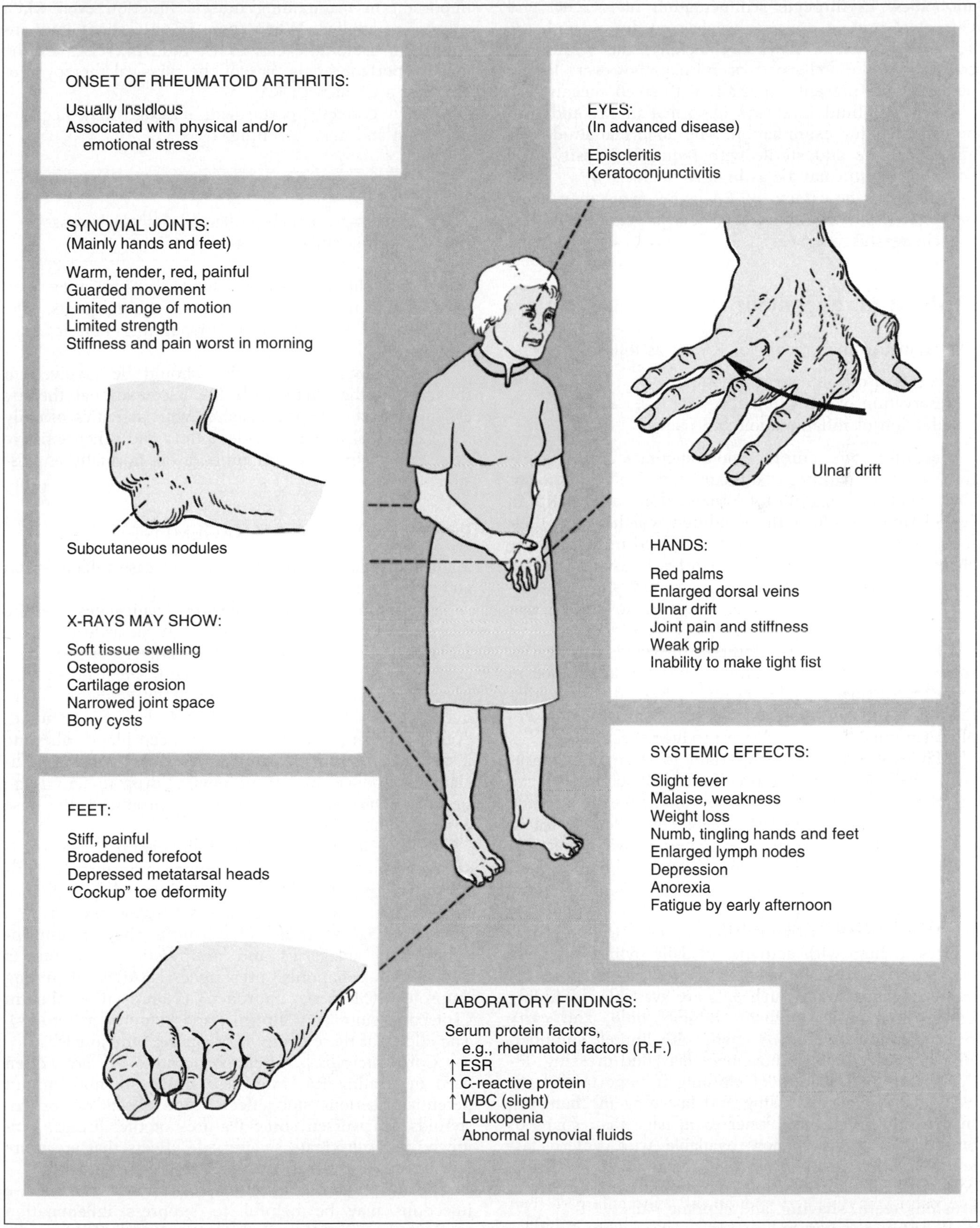
ONSET OF RHEUMATOID ARTHRITIS:
Usually insidious
Associated with physical and/or emotional stress
EYES:
(In advanced disease)
Episcleritis
Keratoconjunctivitis
SYNOVIAL JOINTS:
(Mainly hands and feet)
Warm, tender, red, painful
Guarded movement
Limited range of motion
Limited strength
Stiffness and pain worst in morning
Subcutaneous nodules
Ulnar drift
HANDS:
Red palms
Enlarged dorsal veins
Ulnar drift
Joint pain and stiffness
Weak grip
Inability to make tight fist
X-RAYS MAY SHOW:
Soft tissue swelling
Osteoporosis
Cartilage erosion
Narrowed joint space
Bony cysts
SYSTEMIC EFFECTS:
Slight fever
Malaise, weakness
Weight loss
Numb, tingling hands and feet
Enlarged lymph nodes
Depression
Anorexia
Fatigue by early afternoon
FEET:
Stiff, painful
Broadened forefoot
Depressed metatarsal heads
"Cockup" toe deformity
LABORATORY FINDINGS:
Serum protein factors, e.g., rheumatoid factors (R.F.)
↑ ESR
↑ C-reactive protein
↑ WBC (slight)
Leukopenia
Abnormal synovial fluids

rheumatoid factors (RFs) (large protein molecules). Antinuclear antibodies (ANAs) are found in a speckled pattern with anti-DNA antibodies and many other autoantibodies. Erythrocyte sedimentation rate (ESR) and C-reactive protein are usually elevated during both the acute and chronic phases. Generally, the white cell count is slightly elevated or normal; however, leukopenia may be present, especially with splenomegaly.

Synovial fluid is always abnormal in RA and may be aspirated for examination. The abnormal fluid usually is opaque and sterile with reduced viscosity. The white cell count may be as high as 50,000/mm^3.

Early in the course of RA, x-ray films may show only soft tissue swelling. After several years, degenerative changes may appear.

Medical Management

The main treatment goals for RA are as follows:

- Prevention of joint deformity
- Preservation of joint function
- Reduction of inflammation and pain

Because of its chronic and sometimes crippling nature, arthritis requires a difficult period of adjustment. The client and significant others often need help in considering the effect the condition will have on their lives. Several disciplines may be involved in helping the client and significant others. Arthritis is usually treated conservatively, with salicylates, rest, and physical therapy, unless activities of daily living are so limited that surgery (e.g., joint replacement) is necessary.

Local pain control of joints is managed with heat in some clients and cold in others. Heat can be applied in a variety of forms, including moist heat, dry heat, diathermy, ultrasound, and whirlpools. Cold is usually applied via crushed ice packs to produce anesthesia.

Physical therapy is important to strengthen weakened muscles and to improve function. Deformities can be minimized and corrected by an active positioning and exercise program. Pain can be controlled by teaching clients how to regulate activities in ways that will not increase pain. Clients can be taught isometric exercises and progressive resistance methods of isotonic strengthening exercises.

Most clients with arthritis do not need assistive devices to help with activities of daily living, but these may be used occasionally if severe loss of range of motion occurs. Many such aids are available, including devices that assist a client to grab, hold, and carry objects or to cut food. A client with limited shoulder, elbow, wrist, or hand movement may find dressing difficult. Careful selection of clothing is important, especially the choice of closing and fastening mechanisms. In general, zippers are easier to manage than snaps or buttons. Clothing is now available with Velcro fasteners, which are ideal for clients with arthritis. Grooming aids are available to help with combing hair, brushing teeth, shaving, and clipping nails.

Continuous immobility can increase pain. Exercise of all joints can actually relieve pain (Fig. 11–2). It may be helpful to take aspirin 1/2 hour before exercising, providing the client does not overexercise, because aspirin raises the pain threshold. Isometric exercises are important in maintaining muscle function even when splints are applied. When there is only slight joint involvement, isotonic exercises are best. Exercises are the most important single part of the physical therapy program for a client with RA.

When correctly performed, massage may help relieve pain and muscle aching.

CRITICAL TO REMEMBER

Never massage acutely inflamed joints, because it may aggravate inflammation.

The nurse should instruct clients because they may have a tendency to rub inflamed, aching joints. The client should massage over surrounding muscles, not over joints.

Occupational therapy also should be involved in the care of the client with RA. Occupational therapy can provide the client assistance with activities of daily living. They also can provide splints and other assistive devices to help the client function as normally as possible.

PHARMACOLOGIC MANAGEMENT

Medication may be prescribed to decrease inflammation and reduce pain.

Aspirin or Sodium Salicylate. Salicylates are the mainstay of pharmacologic treatment for arthritis. They are analgesic, anti-inflammatory, relatively safe, and inexpensive. Analgesia is achieved with small doses, and large doses are needed to reduce inflammation. Frequent doses (three to four times a day) are required, even when pain is not present, to keep blood salicylate levels high. Aspirin is usually prescribed in doses sufficient to produce mild symptoms of drug toxicity (e.g., tinnitus). Once such symptoms are produced, the dose is reduced slightly.

Other Nonsteroidal Anti-Inflammatory Drugs. If aspirin is ineffective or not tolerated, nonsteroidal anti-inflammatory drugs (NSAIDs) may be used. Compliance may be better with these agents because they have a simpler dosage schedule. Like aspirin, they are anti-inflammatory, analgesic, and antipyretic. There are a number of commonly prescribed NSAIDs, including ibuprofen (Motrin), naproxen (Naprosyn), tolmetin (Tolectin), sulindac (Clinoril), and ketoprofen (Orudis). The effects of these drugs vary among individuals.

Corticosteroids. Adrenocorticosteroids are often used in treating RA, but these drugs are not without potentially serious side effects. Side effects of corticosteroids can worsen some features of the disease. Prolonged use can create severe side effects that are more serious and difficult to treat than the arthritis itself.

Intra-Articular Injections of Corticosteroids. These injections may be helpful to suppress inflammation temporarily in specific joints and are most effective with acute inflammation in smaller joints. Fluid is removed

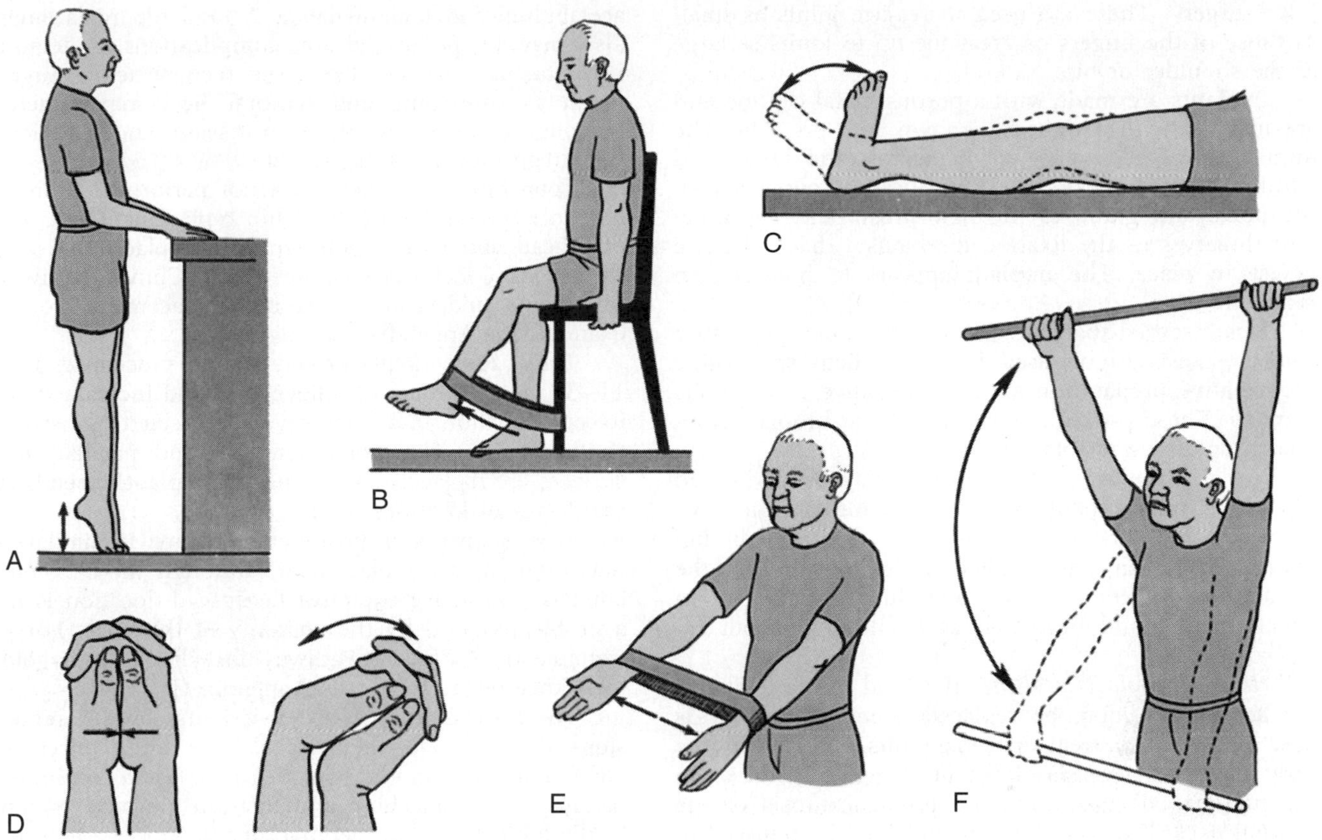

Figure 11–2
Exercises helpful for arthritic people to increase flexibility, improve circulation and muscle tone, and prevent further movement restriction. *A*, Stand alternately on tiptoes and flat of foot. *B*, Knee scissor. Loop a cloth ring (e.g., bandage) around chair leg. Move leg from normal position to extend cloth ring. *C*, Quadriceps setting. *D*, Palm presses. Press palms together. Bend wrists as shown. *E*, Side pull. Loop cloth ring over wrists. Pull arms against resistance of cloth ring. *F*, Wand exercise. Holding a short pole, move arms from thigh level to above head.

from the joint before injecting the medication. If there is any possibility of infection, corticosteroids are *never* injected.

Antimalarials, Gold Salts, and D-Penicillamine. These are remissive agents used to treat RA, sometimes with NSAIDs or steroids, if these medications alone are not sufficient to control the disease. Although they are not immunosuppressants, these drugs seem to halt progression of RA. The onset of action is slow (1–8 weeks) so prolonged administration is necessary. Gold salts and D-penicillamine may lead to leukopenia, thrombocytopenia, proteinuria, and skin rashes.

Immunosuppressive (Cytotoxic) Agents. The most common cytotoxic agent used to treat RA is methotrexate. This drug acts as an immunosuppressant, blocking the inflammatory process of RA. The dosage used to treat RA is much lower than the dose used to treat cancer. The side effects are also fewer than those associated with doses to treat cancer.

DIETARY MANAGEMENT

There is no particular dietary modification required in the management of RA. The client is encouraged to eat a nutritious diet. If clients are overweight, they are taught to lose weight to relieve stress on the affected joints.

Surgical Management

Surgical procedures may be helpful for clients with arthritis. Surgery may be used to relieve symptoms such as pain, improve function, and correct deformities. Preventive surgery (to prevent deformities) is now used during early phases of the disease. Surgery may be performed when there is active arthritis.

Among the numerous types of surgical procedures used in the treatment of RA are tendon transfers and osteotomy. Tendon transfers can prevent progressive deformity caused by muscle spasm. Osteotomy (excising or cutting through bone) may improve the function of deformed joints or limbs.

Synovectomy (removal of synovia), such as of the elbows, wrists, fingers, or knees, may be used in treating RA to help maintain joint function. Early synovectomy helps prevent recurrent inflammation.

Implants composed of Vitallium, stainless steel, and polyethylene (for cups, such as those used to replace the acetabulum) have been developed for reconstructive joint surgery. These are used to replace joints as small as those of the fingers or great toe up to joints as large as the shoulder or hip.

Implants are made with a porous metal coating and are inserted with a tight fit, known as a press fit. The implant is placed very snugly against the bone, and within about 6 weeks, new bone tissue grows between the pores and grafts to the new prosthesis. The bony growth serves as the fixation mechanism that holds the device in place. The implant appears to hold for an indefinite time.

It is essential that nurses know the exact procedure and prosthesis to be used for each client so specific preoperative preparation and postoperative care can be planned. These procedures include the arthroplasty, hemiarthroplasty, and total hip replacement.

Hip Arthroplasty. Arthroplasty may be performed for RA to relieve pain and restore joint motion. Two types of hip arthroplasty may be performed: hemiarthroplasty, in which either the femoral head or the acetabulum is replaced, and total hip replacement, in which the femoral head and acetabulum are both replaced.

Hemiarthroplasty. Either the head of the femur or the acetabulum may be replaced. Hemiarthroplasty is used not only to treat arthritic joints but also in the early stages of necrosis of the head of the femur or in the presence of post-traumatic pseudoarthrosis of the femoral neck. The acetabulum would not be replaced in the latter two examples.

Total Hip Replacement. Total hip replacement (Fig. 11–3*A*) is performed if arthritis involves both acetabulum and femoral head. A total hip replacement also may be performed for complications of femoral neck fractures, failure of previous reconstructive surgery (such as osteotomy and femoral head replacement), complications of congenital hip disease, and pathologic fractures from metastatic cancer.

Total hip replacements are not performed if an infection is present. With total hip replacement, the femoral head and acetabulum are both replaced by prostheses. Some facilities have developed Clinical Pathways for clients undergoing total hip replacement. For an example, see Appendix C.

Total Knee Replacement. This procedure (Fig. 11–3*B*) is performed to relieve pain and increase stability and function in a knee severely affected by osteoarthritis or RA. The tibial, femoral, and patellar joint surfaces are replaced. The choice of implant depends on the degree of joint destruction.

Preoperative and postoperative care is similar to that for total hip replacement, although there is more emphasis on active exercises because dislocation is not a problem caused by the anatomy of the knee. For an example of a Clinical Pathway for clients undergoing total knee replacement, see Appendix C.

The knee is kept in extension first by a compressions dressing and then by a knee immobilizer for about 1 month. Another practice is to use a continuous passive motion machine and institute physical therapy in the immediate postoperative phase.

Exercise progresses from isometric quadriceps setting to straight leg raising to increase muscle strength and range of motion in the operated knee.

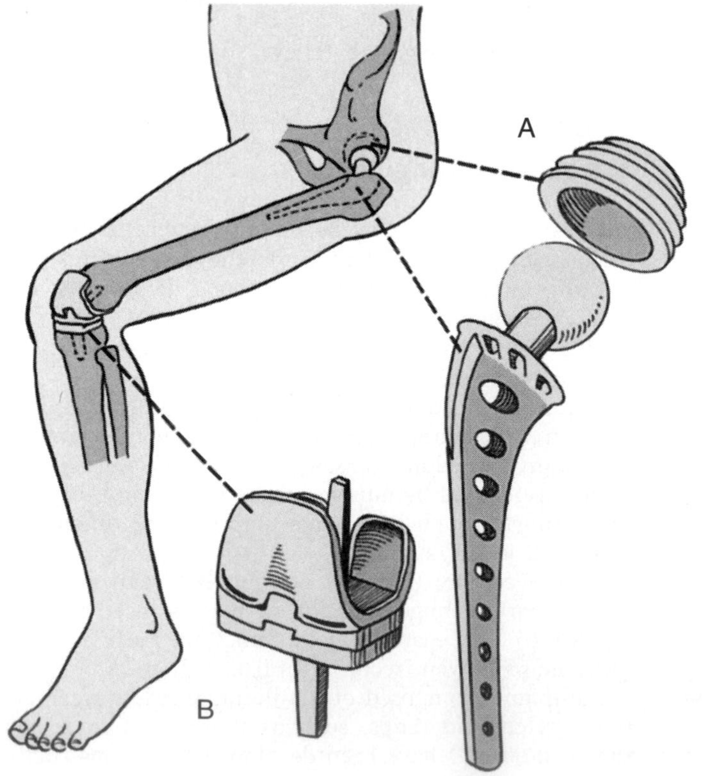

Figure 11–3

A, Total hip joint replacement. A cementless prosthesis allows porous ingrowth of bone. *B*, Total knee joint replacement using a tibial metal retainer and a femoral component. The femoral component is chosen individually for each person according to the amount of healthy bone present.

Once the client has 90-degree knee flexion and good voluntary quadriceps muscle control (can actively raise a straight leg and initiate active knee extension against gravity), ambulation should start. Partial weightbearing usually begins about 1 week after surgery or sooner. At about 2 weeks or less, weightbearing is permitted to the point of pain.

The client is discharged with detailed instructions for a home exercise program. Stationary bicycle exercise can be helpful for at least 1 year after surgery.

Flexion contractures can develop after total knee replacement. To prevent this complication, the operated knee must remain extended whenever the client is in bed. A trochanter roll can be used beside the affected leg in bed to prevent external rotation.

Swelling also can be a problem. The nurse must keep the leg elevated with a pillow under the leg (including the ankle). This position also promotes full extension with the aid of gravity. Whirlpool baths may help the person obtain knee flexion and full extension.

Other Total Joint Replacements. Replacement surgery is possible for elbow, shoulder, finger, and ankle joints, although they are not as common as hip and knee replacements.

Infection and dislocation are the two most common postoperative complications following any joint replacement. Methods of preventing these problems are discussed later.

Nursing Management

Assessment

The assessment of the client with RA varies slightly depending on whether this is a new condition or an ongoing one.

Physical assessment includes inspecting all joints for signs of inflammation, deformity, or limitation of normal movement. Assessment of the whole client is required, not just the joints, because arthritis is a systemic disease. Organs possibly affected include the heart, blood vessels, eyes, and peripheral nerves.

All clients with rheumatoid disease require a thorough psychosocial assessment. The disease affects the client's whole life. The impact of the disease and how the client is coping with it are vital areas for the nurse to assess. Chronic disease such as RA requires the client to cope and adapt to an entire new lifestyle.

Nursing Diagnosis, Planning, and Implementation

For the client with RA, the following plan of care would be appropriate.

Nursing Diagnosis: Chronic Pain R/T inflammation, joint deformity, and joint destruction.

Planning: Expected Outcomes. The client will have chronic pain controlled, as evidenced by client's report and ability to perform activities of daily living.

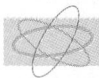

Implementation. Control of the chronic pain is vital in the care of the client with RA. Pain limits mobility, leading to further deformity and loss of function. Pain control can be achieved through medication (aspirin and other anti-inflammatory agents), the use of heat, cold, and massage, controlled exercise, and splinting. See the Client Education Guide: Techniques to Protect Joints.

Nursing Diagnosis: Physical Mobility, Impaired R/T pain, stiffness, impaired joint function, and systemic inflammation.

Planning: Expected Outcomes. The client will maintain physical mobility to the maximal level, as evidenced by ability to perform activities of daily living.

Implementation. Impaired physical mobility is an-

CLIENT EDUCATION GUIDE

Techniques to Protect Joints

The following techniques reduce stress to joints, tendons, ligaments, and capsules.

- Respond to pain. If pain lasts more than an hour or two after activity, stop doing that particular activity for a while.
- Use your largest muscles. For example, women should carry a shoulder bag rather than a handbag; push doors open with your arms rather than with your hands or fingers.
- Alternate between light and heavy tasks. Do not do all your heavy tasks at once. Take frequent breaks and rest between tasks.
- Minimize joint stress that may lead to deformity; for example, use a large, wide pen rather than a thin one; use lightweight equipment and devices; maintain a good, comfortable posture; change position frequently.
- Plan for rest, for example, take a walk where you can sit down if you need to.
- Conserve energy. Make activities that are really important to you a priority. Eliminate unnecessary tasks.
- Assess your joints. If they are warm or swollen, use them as little as possible. Put them through range-of-motion exercises only once a day.
- Assess the tasks you must do, such as your work. What is the least painful way to accomplish these tasks? Be sure you do the tasks in this way.
- What are your horizontal and vertical reaching areas? Move items into these ranges.
- Avoid prolonged or unnecessary bending, stretching, reaching, stair climbing, or prolonged grip.
- Use simultaneous motion with smooth, continuous movements, such as dusting or putting dishes away with both hands.
- Sit to work as much as possible because standing places more stress on hip and knee joints and uses more energy. Do remember to get up and move around at intervals.

other serious problem facing the client with RA. Prescribed activity helps a client with arthritis attain and maintain optimal function and independence. Activity also helps the client feel more mentally focused. Occupational therapy often encourages purposeful movements and makes exercising seem less burdensome. Encouraging self-care is an important part of therapy.

During exercise, a client may experience pain for a short time. If pain lasts for several hours after exercise, the program may be excessive and need modification.

The amount of systemic rest needed varies, depending on the severity of the disease at any given time. With extensive systemic and articular involvement, complete bedrest is indicated for a limited time for its anti-inflammatory effect.

For bedrest to be effective, the bed must be firm and the client positioned to prevent deformities (footdrop, fixation of the joints in extension, flexion contractures).

Resting joints involved with RA helps reduce articular inflammation. Weightbearing joints may be rested by complete bedrest. Splints may be used to rest inflamed joints. Splints are removed periodically and the joints exercised to prevent fibrous ankylosis. Intervention is needed to prevent complications of immobility during periods of limited activity, such as during bedrest or while in a wheelchair (see Chaps. 43 and 44).

During periods when the client is not on bedrest, the client must learn to balance rest and activity. Rest periods should be planned between all activities causing fatigue. The client needs to learn to do the most important activities first while his or her energy is at the highest. Activities that can be eliminated should be in order to save the client's strength.

Nursing Diagnosis: Self-Care Deficit, Risk for Possibly Total, R/T joint deformity, pain, fatigue, and immobility.

Planning: Expected Outcomes. The client will be able to perform self-care activities with minimal pain, as evidenced by client's maintaining activities of daily living.

Implementation. Proper posture and body alignment are important for clients with RA. The nurse must teach clients to look at their posture in a mirror and consciously attempt to sit and stand erect.

When hips, knees or both are involved, it may be most comfortable for the client to sit on a straight-backed armchair elevated 3 to 4 inches higher than ordinary chairs. The added height prevents excessive hip and knee flexion and makes it easier for the client to get in and out of the chair. Similarly, elevation of toilet seats also helps. Grab bars on or beside the toilet are helpful. It also may help to have the client's bed raised between 10 and 30 degrees.

Often, the knees of a client with arthritis become stiff after sitting for a while. The nurse must teach the client to flex and extend the knees several times before standing up. Limbering up helps the client stand up more easily and feel steadier. Similarly, periodic flexion and extension of the knees while seated may make sitting more comfortable.

Self-care is important for the client. Occupational therapy is often involved in this intervention. The occupational therapist can help with assistive devices to make self-care possible, even with joints that have become deformed. They also can provide splints for the client so further joint deformity can be limited.

Nursing Diagnosis: Health Maintenance, Altered R/T knowledge deficit regarding the disease, physical therapy, medication, and alterations in life-style.

Planning: Expected Outcomes. The client will understand the disease, physical therapy, medication, and alterations in life-style, as evidenced by client's statements and compliance with treatment regimen.

Implementation. When providing the client with medications to control the symptoms of RA, the nurse should use this opportunity to teach the client about them. The client should be taught to take aspirin with food to reduce gastric irritation. It also may help to take aspirin with antacids. There is increasing concern, however, about the aluminum content of antacids. One must advise the client to watch for signs of bleeding, such as dark stools, bruising.

When the client is taking NSAIDs, advise the client to take the medication with food to minimize possible gastric irritating effects. Some clients also may be given histamine receptor antagonists such as ranitidine (Zantac) to prevent any gastrointestinal irritation or ulcer formation. In older clients, piroxicam (Feldene) appears to increase the risk of peptic ulcer disease, so it should be used with caution in this age group. Also, warn the client that the effects of these medications may not be apparent for several weeks.

Clients who take corticosteroids should always carry identification stating they are receiving steroid therapy. Such identification advises health professionals of the client's condition if emergency treatment is required.

For the client who has a total joint replacement, an appropriate plan of care would include the following items.

Nursing Diagnosis: Knowledge Deficit R/T surgery, postoperative restrictions, and rehabilitation.

Planning: Expected Outcomes. The client will understand the proposed surgery, postoperative restrictions, and rehabilitation, as evidenced by client's statements and compliance with postoperative regimen.

Implementation. The care of the client who will have joint replacement is another focus of the plan of care. Preoperative preparation is similar to that for any client undergoing major surgery (see Chap. 5). Besides the usual preparation, the client requires specialized teaching about the postoperative course.

One must teach the client and significant others about the procedure and what the client can expect after surgery. One must also discuss the procedure and goals of treatment with the client and significant others. The nurse should assess ambulation and identify areas in which the client may need extra help postoperatively. The client should be taught how to use crutches, a walker, or both and encouraged to practice using them.

The client should be assisted to practice moving from bed to a chair or a wheelchair without flexing the hip more than 90 degrees to prevent dislocation of the prosthesis.

With nursing assistance, physical therapists assess the client preoperatively and teach postoperative exercise. If the exercises are not understood preoperatively, the client may not be able to do them effectively after surgery, when pain and anxiety may be present. Exercises include quadriceps setting, gluteal setting, isometric hip extension and abduction exercises, as well as upper extremity strengthening exercises to prepare for crutch walking or use of a walker. The nurse must encourage the client to practice the exercises regularly.

Nursing Diagnosis: Injury, Risk for R/T postoperative complications such as dislocation of the prosthesis, thrombophlebitis.

Planning: Expected Outcomes. The client will not suffer injury related to postoperative complications and will heal normally, as evidenced by absence of dislocation of the prosthesis and no thrombophlebitis.

Implementation. General postoperative nursing interventions are discussed in Chapter 5. Postoperative interventions for clients following hip surgery are discussed in Chapter 45. Here, it is necessary to emphasize only those points that are particularly relevant for clients after total hip replacement.

Postoperatively, the affected leg must be maintained in an abducted position and in straight alignment while the client is recumbent. The surgeon may order support hose or sequential compression pumps to prevent deep vein thrombosis. An abduction splint or four pillows are used postoperatively. Most splints can be adjusted for the desired amount of abduction.

The nurse must encourage and supervise prescribed exercises such as quadriceps setting. Muscle strengthening of the gluteal muscles helps prevent dislocation, because muscular control replaces the function of the hip capsule. Dislocation of the prosthesis and infection are possible early postoperative complications. One must document and report indications of complications immediately. Following hip replacement, hip flexion greater than 90 degrees and leg adduction must be prevented. Both can cause dislocation.

The client is usually mobilized at the bedside on the first or second postoperative day. This may mean standing at the bedside briefly or being assisted to a chair.

CRITICAL TO REMEMBER

Care must be taken *not* to flex the hip joint greater than 90 degrees, and maintain abduction of the legs to prevent dislocation.

While the client is supine, the client should be turned to the unaffected side and given back care every 2 hours. The client is turned with the splint in place so abduction is maintained. The client should be medicated well before this procedure to prevent any pain caused by the turning. The client's position must be changed frequently to help prevent complications of immobility.

Nerve function and circulation must be assessed in the affected leg every 1 or 2 hours (or as directed by the physician) for the first day or so and then as often as the client's condition warrants. This includes assessment of bilateral pulses and quality, skin color and temperature, capillary refill in the toes, and movement of joints distal to the surgery.

Pink-tinged sputum may appear postoperatively and is believed to result from some of the cement leaking into circulation and being excreted through pulmonary alveoli. It is important, therefore, to know the type of replacement procedure that has been performed. This complication is not dangerous, but it should be documented and must be distinguished from pulmonary emboli.

Physical therapy may be started as early as the fourth or fifth postoperative day. In addition to helping the client ambulate, physical therapy may include gentle, active assisted range-of-motion exercises in sling suspension (within the pain-free range). Until discharge, the client continues exercises that increase range of motion and strengthen hip muscles.

On the third to fifth postoperative day, the physician may allow the client to lie prone twice a day for 20 to 30 minutes to prevent hip flexion contractures. The client may be required to continue this practice at home after discharge.

The client is also at risk for thrombophlebitis after total hip replacement. The surgery itself, positioning during surgery, and impaired mobility all contribute to the development of thrombophlebitis. To prevent the development of phlebitis, support stockings are applied to the client preoperatively and are maintained postoperatively. Another preventive measure used by some physicians is low-dose heparin. Heparin can be given subcutaneously in doses of 5000 U every 12 hours. This helps to prevent thrombophlebitis without significantly increasing the risk of hemorrhage. Exercising the unaffected leg also helps prevent clot formation.

The usual period of hospitalization for total hip replacement varies from 5 to 10 days. If clients still require extensive rehabilitation, they are sent to rehabilitation centers or extended-care facilities until they are able to function independently or with limited assistance. Total hip replacement often produces dramatic results. Clients often find their pain relieved and movement increased markedly and rapidly.

Before discharge, the client and significant others should be given a list of written instructions for home health care. The most important instruction is that the client not flex the hip greater than 90 degrees to prevent the hip from dislocating and to avoid extremes of internal rotation, adduction, and flexion of the hip. Exercises to be performed also should be included in the instructions (Fig. 11–4). These restrictions continue for 6 months to 1 year after surgery.

Nursing Diagnosis: Infection, Risk for R/T implanted prosthesis and possible immunosuppression related to drug therapy.

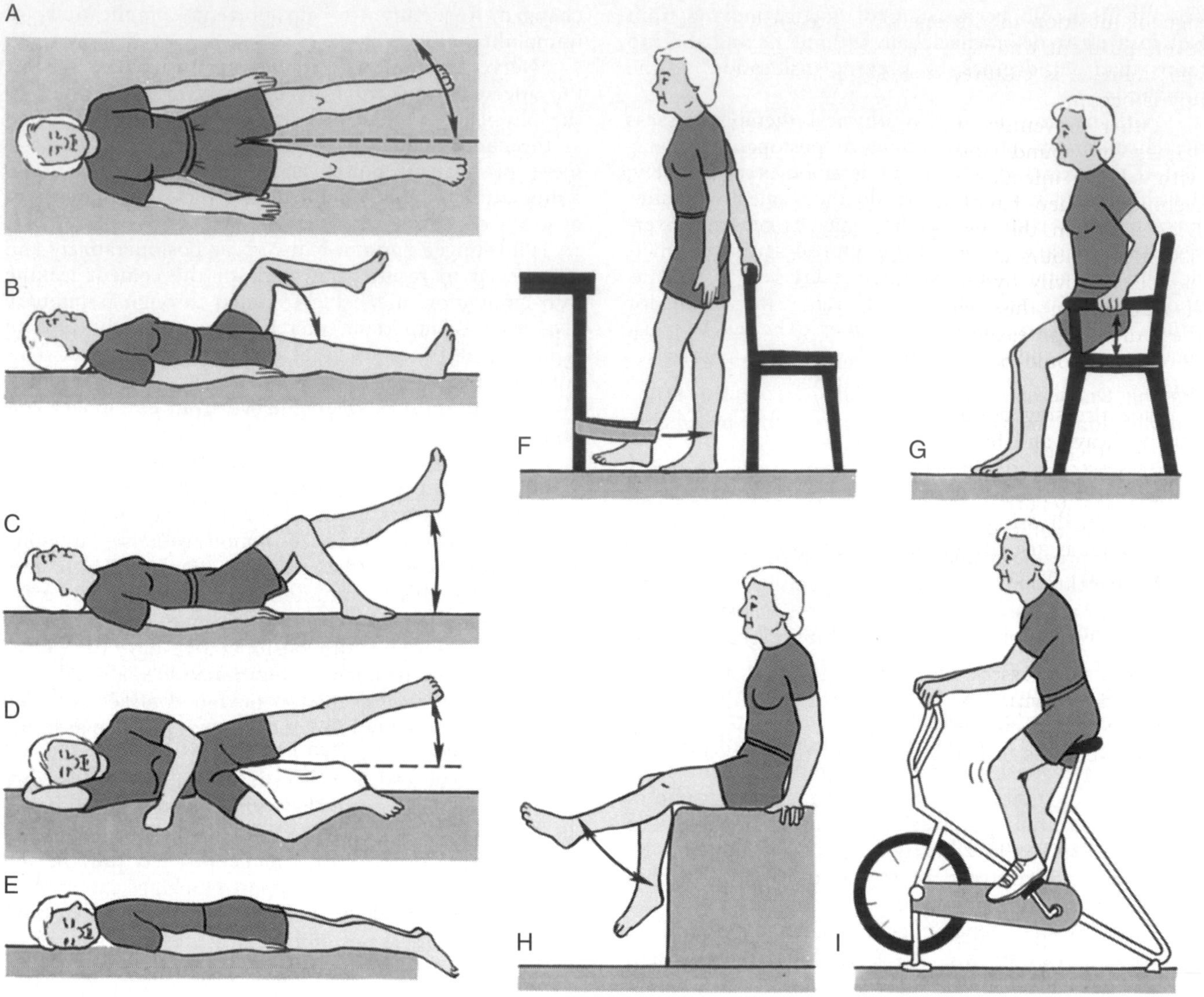

Figure 11–4
Rehabilitative exercises after total hip replacement. *A,* Lie on back and gently swing leg away from body and return to midline. *B,* While supine, raise hip and knee as shown to increase range of motion and strengthen hip flexors. *C,* While supine, raise the leg straight to strengthen quadriceps muscle. *D,* Lie on unoperated side and raise operated leg straight up toward ceiling to strengthen hip abductors and adductors. *E,* Lying prone stretches flexor muscles of the hip and prevents flexion contractures. *F,* Put a ring of resistive material (such as rubber tubing) on ankle and secure to sturdy object. Try to pull operated leg back to midline to increase power of quadriceps. *G,* Raise self gently out of a chair to increase strength of upper extremities. Good preparation for crutch walking. *H,* Raise leg from a sitting position to increase range of motion and strengthen quadriceps tone. *I,* Stationary bicycling is one of the last exercises to be added to a post-total hip replacement exercise program. This increases range of motion, provides warm-up before and after exercises, and increases cardiovascular capacity.

Planning: Expected Outcomes. The client will not experience an infection in implanted prosthesis, as evidenced by a normal white cell count, temperature, absence of purulent drainage, and no sign of inflammation.

Implementation. Prevention of infection is another priority in the client after hip replacement. These clients are at high risk for infection for several reasons. First, a foreign body has been implanted in the client. Although the material used produces little inflammation, it is a potential source of infection because of the trauma of surgery. The client also may have been receiving anti-inflammatory agents, especially steroids or cytotoxics, which increase the risk of infection. This places the total joint replacement client at a greater risk of infection.

Usually the client is started on prophylactic broad-spectrum antibiotics during surgery, and this therapy is continued for several days after surgery, even if there is no sign of infection. If the client begins to exhibit any sign of infection in the operative site such as redness, fever, purulent drainage, or increasing incisional pain, any drainage is cultured and aggressive antibiotic therapy is begun.

Other preventive measures range from the use of staples for wound closure because they are associated with a lower infection rate and the use of strict aseptic technique when handling dressings or wound drains. Drainage from the wound drains is usually less than 600 mL/24 hours or 200 mL/8 hours unless the client has been heavily hydrated with plasma expanders such as dextran. In this case, the amount of output from these drains can easily triple. Therefore, intake and output totals should be carefully calculated to assess fluid balance.

The dressing applied immediately after surgery is usually heavy and bulky and is left in place (but carefully assessed) until the surgeon removes it 2 to 3 days postoperatively. The wound is either then recovered with a light dressing or sometimes left open to the air. The wound is usually cleansed each shift according to the surgeon's orders.

Evaluation

The nurse must assess whether the goals have been met for the client with RA who has had surgery. If these goals have not been met, the nurse must revise the plan and interventions to better meet the client's needs.

Modification of Plan of Care for the Elderly

Although the age of onset for RA is between 20 and 40 years of age, the client who is treated for the disease is often an older adult. The care is essentially the same; however, immobility, deformity, and joint destruction can be more severe in this age group. Elderly clients are more susceptible to the side effects their decreased mobility may cause, including more rapid loss of function.

Older clients may have adapted to the RA very well but often find any further deterioration more difficult to handle. Elderly clients also may have more trouble recovering after an acute exacerbation of the disease. They also may be slower in their recovery from total joint replacement. They may require prolonged hospitalization in an extended-care facility until they regain adequate mobility to function independently or with some assistance and safely.

Posthospital Care

DISCHARGE TEACHING

The discharge instructions that the client and significant others must receive are given in the Client Education Guide: Discharge Instructions for the Client After a Total Hip Replacement and Figure 11–4. It is important for the client to know which activities are allowed and which may cause problems. Clients should be reminded that this surgery does not cure their arthritis and that they will need to continue therapy for their disease.

Some alterations need to be made to the home for the client with severe arthritis and for the client after total hip surgery. These alterations include devices such as ramps, good lighting, and modifications in floor plans that help the client maintain independence longer.

The client who has a total hip replacement needs assistive devices added to the home such as a riser on the toilet seat, a good chair for sitting, and grab bars in

CLIENT EDUCATION GUIDE

Discharge Instructions for the Client After a Total Hip Replacement

- Do not cross one leg over the other—keep the knees apart.
- Do not flex the hip when putting on shoes and stockings. Use assistive devices such as long-handled shoe horns and extenders with clothespins, or have someone help you put them on.
- Do not sit continuously for longer than 1 hour. Stand, stretch, and take a few steps periodically to prevent hip flexion contractures.
- Do not sit in low, reclining, or rocking chairs. Low, soft seats require more than 90 degrees of hip flexion to stand up. Sit in a firm, high chair with arms. Use a raised toilet seat. Place a very secure bar beside the toilet to help you stand up. Use of tub baths are not allowed.
- Do lie prone twice a day for 30 minutes.
- Do place a pillow between the knees when lying down to prevent hip adduction and maintain abduction.
- Follow detailed exercise prescriptions, including quadriceps setting, range-of-motion exercises, and activity limitations. The most important exercises to rebuild hip muscles are abduction exercises (spreading legs apart) and extension exercises (pushing the knee backward into the bed). Stationary bicycle exercises may help when an adequate range of hip flexion is achieved (see Fig. 11–4).
- Avoid actions that place a strain on the hip joint, such as excessive bending, heavy lifting, jogging, and jumping.
- Use crutches or a walker for as long as prescribed by the physician. (Full weightbearing without crutches may be allowed as early as 4 weeks after surgery or later if the physician requires.) Then use a cane in the hand opposite the operated leg. See Chapter 44 for proper use of assistive devices.
- Climb stairs carefully after discharge from the health-care facility.
- Wear support stockings on the unaffected leg and an elastic wrap on the affected leg until there is no swelling in the legs or feet and full activities are resumed.
- Do not drive a car for 6 weeks after surgery unless authorized by the physician.
- Take prophylactic antibiotics if undergoing procedures that may cause bacteremia, such as tooth extraction.

the bathroom. These devices should be installed before the client returns from the hospital.

OSTEOARTHRITIS

Osteoarthritis (OA) is a noninflammatory joint disease characterized by a degeneration and loss of articular cartilage in synovial joints. OA was previously called degenerative joint disease (DJD), but the term DJD is generally considered inaccurate because there is no biochemical or metabolic degeneration.

Osteoarthritis is classified as primary or secondary, based upon its etiology. Primary (or idiopathic) OA is associated with aging, but recently a genetic basis for the disorder has been described. An autosomal recessive trait has been implicated as one cause, through which the genes encoded for articular cartilage structure are altered. Primary OA is the most common type, existing in about 60 million people in the United States. It occurs in about 50 per cent of all people by the age of 16 years. Weight-bearing joints are the most commonly affected.

Secondary OA is caused by conditions that lead to damage to joint surfaces, sometimes from "wear and tear" of the joints. Other etiologies of OA are joint injury such as repetitive strain and sprains, joint dislocation, fractures, disorders that lead to abnormal movements (e.g., neurologic disease), and medications that stimulate the activity of collagen-digesting enzymes in the synovial membrane (e.g., steroids, colchicine).

Primary prevention of OA can occur with the reduction of injury, as in sports with the use of protective gear and warm-ups. Also, the reduction of repetitive motions, such as those in assembly-line work, decreases wear and tear on joints.

The pathophysiology of OA is the loss of articular cartilage due to enzymatic destruction. Destruction begins in the matrix, leading to damage to proteoglycans and collagen. Layers of the cartilage loosen, and eventually the subchondral bone becomes unprotected, then dense. In addition, cysts and fissures often develop in the bone. If the fluid content inside the cyst breaks open into the synovial space through the cartilage, further destruction of the joint occurs. When the cartilage is ruptured, osteophytes, or small pieces of bone that coat its surface, may form abnormal bony growths in the joint space and surrounding bone. Osteophytes of new bone may break off and lodge in the synovial space, possibly leading to inflammation of the joint capsule.

It is important to differentiate OA from rheumatoid arthritis (RA). Clients with OA tend to be older. There are no specific laboratory tests to confirm OA. X-rays of OA show reduced joint space, and osteophytes may be visible. Laboratory studies for rheumatoid factor are normal in clients with OA. Sometimes, the sedimentation rate is elevated if the client has synovitis.

Clinical manifestations of OA are aching pain, crepitation, and stiffness in involved large weight-bearing joints. The client may also have enlarged joints, contractures, and muscle spasms. New bone growth in joints may lead to swelling, called Heberden's nodes. When osteophytes lodge in the joint, swelling, called joint effusion, occurs.

Management

Medical management of the client with OA includes pain management, reduction of inflammation, and improvement of range-of-motion and strength. Nonsteroidal anti-inflammatory drugs are used to reduce inflammation and pain. Narcotics are not used because of the chronic nature of OA. In addition, local injections of steroids such as cortisone may be used for acute pain in a single joint. When joints become inflamed or acutely painful, they may be rested in splints that limit motion in the joint. Splints are not used for prolonged periods, because the joint tends to stiffen when immobilized, and the client may find difficulty in regaining range of motion. Skin traction or cervical collars may be used for OA of the vertebrae. Heat treatments can also be used to control pain and decrease inflammation. Other methods for pain control should also be used. There is no specific diet for OA, nor is there a diet that will "cure" OA. Obese clients are encouraged to lose weight and increase activity as allowed by their pain levels. Decrease in activity is not advised for any client with OA; the client should be taught to exercise daily despite mild discomfort. Improved muscle tone and strength can decrease the chronic pain of OA. Low levels of exercise are as beneficial as high-intensity exercise.

Surgical management of OA includes osteotomy and joint replacement. Osteotomy is the removal of a section of bone to realign a joint and decrease joint strain. It is commonly performed for valgus (bowleg) and varus (knock-knee) deformities. After surgery, the leg is wrapped from toes to groin and elevated. Ambulation is allowed with toe-touch weight-bearing.

Total hip and total knee replacements are the most common types of joint reconstruction. Both surfaces of the joint are replaced to eliminate bone-on-bone articulation.

Nursing management for the client with OA includes encouragement of activity. Walking and swimming or water aerobics are some of the best activities. Ambulatory aids may be helpful by reducing the weight on involved joints. Weight reduction should be encouraged, if needed, because being closer to ideal body weight lessens strain on joints.

Pain should be managed with nonsteroidal anti-inflammatory agents. Ice or heat may be applied to the joints. Positions of comfort should be used only for short times. Clients should be discouraged from propping a joint in flexion without stretching the joint. The continual use of flexion encourages contracture.

Self-care should be promoted. There are several devices that can be purchased to facilitate self-care. Rubber grips can be used to open jars. Velcro closures can be placed on clothing rather than zippers or buttons. Front-closing garments and slip-on shoes should be worn.

GOUT/GOUTY ARTHRITIS

Gout is a metabolic disorder in which purine (protein) metabolism is altered and the by-product, uric acid, accumulates. In the body, uric acid is made by the enzymatic breakdown of tissue and dietary purines. Hyperuricemia develops because of undersecretion or overproduction of uric acid. In addition to accumulating in the blood, uric acid accumulates in the synovial fluid, myocardium, kidneys, and ears. When uric acid levels reach a certain level, they crystalize and the crystals, called tophi, are deposited in connective tissue. Because the crystals are deposited in connective tissue, gout is classified as a form of arthritis.

Gout is classified as primary or secondary. Primary gout is caused by an inherited defect of purine metabolism leading to increased or decreased renal excretion. Primary gout accounts for 80 per cent of all cases, of which 95 per cent are males. The initial attack of gout occurs in the fourth or fifth decade of life.

Secondary gout is an acquired condition, following hematopoietic or renal disorders. Multiple myeloma, polycythemia vera, and leukemia are disorders of blood cell formation. In these disorders there is an increase in cell turnover and increased uric acid production. In addition, gout may develop from the rapid induction of chemotherapy or radiation therapy when there is massive destruction of cells. Renal disorders that decrease the excretion of uric acid may lead to gout. Hyperuricemia may also result from the use of aspirin, thiazide, and mercurial diuretics, and some antituberculosis medications.

Alcohol intoxication and starvation increase serum urate levels by inhibiting renal excretion due to lactic acidosis and ketosis, respectively. In addition, alcohol ingestion increases urate production by stimulating purine breakdown.

Clinical manifestations of gout develop in stages:

Stage I: asymptomatic hyperuricemia

Stage II: acute attack with redness, swelling, and exquisite tenderness in one joint (toes, fingers, wrists, ankles, knees, or other joints). The great toe is the most common site. This first attack develops quickly, often overnight. Fever, tachycardia, malaise, and anorexia may be noted. The acute episode usually subsides within a week. As the edema subsides, pruritus and local desquamation (tissue loss) may be noted. Following the initial attack, the affected joint returns to normal and the client may be asymptomatic for years. Eventually, other attacks occur.

Stage III: permanent changes in multiple joints with restrictions in movement. Tophi may be detected on the ears, hands, elbows, feet, and knees. Renal and cardiac disorders may also develop. The client may have uric acid renal stones, renal colic, and hypertension. Atherosclerosis occurs in about half of all clients.

Gout is diagnosed by the presence of persistent hyperuricemia (>7.0 mg/dL) in addition to the clinical manifestations. The presence of uric acid in an aspirated sample of synovial fluid confirms the diagnosis.

Management

The management of the client with gout has two components: (1) management of the acute attack and (2) long-term management of hyperuricemia.

Management of the acute attack includes the use of colchicine and nonsteroidal anti-inflammatory agents to reduce pain and inflammation. Colchicine reduces the migration of leukocytes to the synovial fluids. The initial dose of colchicine is 0.6 to 1.2 mg followed by 0.6 mg per hour until pain is relieved or signs of toxicity develop. The therapeutic dose is close to the toxic dose. Signs of toxicity include nausea, vomiting, and diarrhea. Other nonsteroidal anti-inflammatory agents can be used, such as indomethacin. In resistant cases of gout, adrenocorticotropic hormone or steroids may be required. Ice over the inflamed joints may also relieve pain.

Medications to lower uric acid include allopurinol, which blocks formation of uric acid, and probenecid, which promotes resorption of uric acid deposits and excretion of uric acid. Long-term medication use is advised in clients who have more than two attacks of gout a year, secondary forms of gout, or persistent hyperuricemia.

CRITICAL TO REMEMBER

Salicylates (aspirin) antagonize the action of uricosuric agents and must not be used concurrently.

Dietary management of gout includes avoiding foods high in purine. Food containing high amounts (150–1000 mg) of purine include liver, kidneys, sweetbreads, brains, heart, mussels, anchovies, sardines, herring, and consomme. Moderate levels (50–150 mg) of purine are found in other meats, poultry, beans, peas, lentils, asparagus, cauliflower, mushrooms, and spinach.

Ample fluids should be given and encouraged to promote excretion of uric acid. A moderate intake of distilled forms of alcohol does not seem to precipitate gouty attacks. Beer, ale, and wine may precipitate them. Excessive alcohol of any form should be avoided.

Gradual weight loss should be encouraged after the initial attack. Weight loss alone may reduce the incidence of attacks and uric acid levels. A sudden loss of weight may precipitate an attack due to the destruction of cells.

Clients who can recognize early symptoms of gout can avert the attack in many cases by prompt use of colchicine or indomethacin. Long-term side effects (alopecia, bone marrow suppression, hepatic damage) from these agents, although rare, should be explained to the client.

Nursing management of the client with gout includes pain management. The client is usually placed at bedrest until pain subsides. Once ambulating, the client's need for crutches or a walker should be considered until gait is stable. The client is taught dietary restrictions, fluid requirements, and long-term self-management. Clients should be instructed to expect close monitoring of the blood in long-term drug therapy. Long-term drug therapy for gout has serious side effects (e.g., hepatotoxicity).

SYSTEMIC LUPUS ERYTHEMATOSUS

SLE is a chronic, inflammatory, autoimmune disease. Lupus comes from the Latin word for wolf, referring to a belief in the 1800s that the rash of this disease was caused by a wolf bite. The characteristic rash of lupus is red, leading to the term erythematosus.

Incidence

SLE occurs most commonly in younger women between the ages of 15 and 40 years. It is almost 10 times more common in women than in men. It is more common in black women, with a rate of about 1 per 250, with the rate for white women about 1 per 700.[27] SLE has a familial tendency, and when one twin has the disease, the other twin has a 60 to 70 per cent chance of acquiring it.

SLE may be drug induced. Four features separate this condition from spontaneous SLE. In the drug-induced syndrome, (1) men and women are affected equally, (2) nephritis and central nervous system features do not usually occur, (3) depressed serum complement and antibodies to DNA are present, and (4) symptoms revert to normal when the offending drug is withdrawn, although serologic abnormalities may persist for months or years.

Etiology

SLE is an autoimmune disease involving diffuse inflammatory changes of the vascular and connective tissue. There is some evidence of a genetic predisposition to the disease because of the incidence in families and twins. There is a theory that the genetic predisposition for the disease is present in some clients and a virus or some other agent triggers it and the disease occurs. This theory is as yet unsupported.

Although the exact cause of SLE is unknown, causes of disease exacerbation have been identified. These include sunlight and other forms of ultraviolet light, physical and emotional stress, and pregnancy.

There is a form of drug-induced SLE associated with adverse reactions to some drugs, including procainamide (Pronestyl) and hydralazine (Apresoline). Some drugs, phenytoin (Dilantin) and phenobarbital, are known to produce an SLE-like syndrome. The drug-induced problems resolve when the drugs are discontinued. Sometimes, a short course of steroids are needed to completely eradicate the symptoms.

Risk Factors

This is not a preventable disease; however, the exacerbations might be prevented. Control of stress, avoidance of sunlight and ultraviolet light, and prevention of pregnancy can help delay exacerbations of SLE.

Pathophysiology

SLE is a chronic, progressive, systemic, inflammatory connective tissue disease. It produces inflammatory, biochemical, and structural changes in the vascular and connective tissue as well as in the viscera, joints, fascia, tendons, and bursae. SLE is characterized by remissions and exacerbations and often has an insidious onset.

Several abnormal serum protein factors and ANA may be found with SLE that suggest an autoimmune mechanism is occurring. These ANA mainly affect the DNA within the cell nuclei, leading to the formation of immune complexes in serum and organ tissues. The complexes can cause vasculitis, or inflammation of the vessels, leading to a decrease of oxygen in the organs and tissues. They may also directly invade the organs, causing inflammation and damage.

Characteristic histologic findings are lupus erythematosus (LE) cells and extracellular masses called hematoxylin bodies. However, LE cells may be found in many diseases and may or may not be demonstrated with SLE. Most clients with SLE have a mild to moderate, normochromic anemia. The ESR is usually elevated, a mild leukopenia is often present, and serum globulins may be increased.

The leading cause of death in clients with SLE is renal failure from the kidney involvement. There is some degree of kidney involvement causing progressive changes within the glomeruli in most clients with SLE. With progression of SLE nephritis, the glomeruli become increasingly abnormal and accumulate immune complex deposits. Once 50 per cent of the glomeruli have been affected, the client will show signs of renal failure.

In general, the clinical pattern and prognosis of SLE are variable. The illness may develop rapidly and have an acute fulminant course. More commonly, it develops insidiously and becomes chronic with remissions and exacerbations.

Clinical Manifestations

Clients with SLE often present with nonspecific symptoms, such as weight loss, fever, malaise, and lethargy. In some clients, the symptoms are very insidious and resemble other conditions such as arthritis because of the joint involvement. Many of the clinical hallmarks of SLE are due to the deposition of immune complexes in the tissues (see Clinical Manifestations: Chronic Systemic Lupus Erythmatosus).

Assessment findings in acute disease may include fever, musculoskeletal aches and pains, butterfly rash on the face, pleural effusion, basilar pneumonia, gener-

CLINICAL MANIFESTATIONS

Chronic Systemic Lupus Erythematosus

Assessment findings in chronic systemic lupus erythematosus vary with specific organ involvement but may include the following:

- Fever
- Malaise
- Anorexia and weight loss
- Cutaneous discoid lupus erythematosus lesions
- Erythema of exposed skin
- Generalized lymphadenopathy
- Severe hemolytic anemia
- Thrombocytopenic purpura
- Hypersplenism
- Pericarditis
- Tachycardia
- Gallop rhythm
- Peripheral vascular syndromes (e.g., Raynaud's phenomenon, gangrene)
- Ulcerative mucous membrane lesions
- Abdominal pain
- Nausea and vomiting
- Bloody stools
- Hepatic dysfunction, hepatomegaly
- Focal glomerulitis progressing to glomerulonephritis
- Myalgia, arthralgia, and neuritis
- Hemiplegia
- Psychosis
- Convulsions
- Coma

alized lymphadenopathy, pericarditis, tachycardia, gallop rhythm, hepatosplenomegaly, nephritis prostration, delirium, convulsions, psychosis, and coma.

DIAGNOSTIC ASSESSMENT

In addition to the physical findings of SLE, laboratory tests reveal

- Presence of LE cells (autoantibodies); the severity of SLE usually correlates with the degree of LE cell formation
- Decreased complement levels
- Presence of immune complexes in the serum
- Presence of immune antibodies to DNA and antinuclear antibodies
- Decreased levels of red cells, white cells, and platelets
- Increased gamma globulin fraction as a result of increased antibody production
- An elevated ESR

Medical Management

Treatment of SLE is based on the organ systems involved in the disease. The treatments are essentially pharmacologic in nature. Dialysis may be used to treat the renal failure if it develops.

PHARMACOLOGIC MANAGEMENT

Treatment of SLE is similar to that of RA and other autoimmune, connective tissue disorders. These treatments include the following:

- Nonsteroidal anti-inflammatory agents such as aspirin and ibuprofen
- Antimalarial drugs, although the action of these medications in SLE is unclear; these agents are helpful, especially in clients with predominantly cutaneous and joint involvement
- Corticosteroids, agents that ameliorate the systemic inflammatory manifestations of the disease
- Cytotoxic agents, the use of which is controversial because of the serious side effects; however, they are used in severe, refractory cases of SLE, including alkylating agents (cyclophosphamide) and antifolates (methotrexate)
- Plasmapheresis, which is used to remove circulating autoantibodies and immune complexes from the blood before organ and tissue damage occurs; the efficacy and safety of this therapy is also controversial.

Note the order of these therapies. The agents associated with the least serious side effects are tried first. Success of pharmacologic intervention is often difficult to evaluate because spontaneous remissions may occur.

DIETARY MANAGEMENT

Dietary factors are thought to influence the development of autoimmune diseases. Therefore, some clinicians recommend dietary alterations. Restriction of L-canavanine (a nonprotein amino acid found in alfalfa sprouts) is sometimes suggested because this substance is thought to be an inducer of autoimmune diseases. Other studies suggest that diets high in calories may enhance autoimmunity. If this is true, a reduction in calories may decrease the formation of antibodies to DNA. However, dietary modifications are still in the experimental stages.

Nursing Management

The goals of care for the client with SLE focus on:

- Maintenance of skin integrity
- Promotion of a healthy life-style and reduction of stress
- Maintenance of proper nutrition
- Relief of discomfort

- An increase in the client's independence
- Maintenance of emotional well-being

Intervention for clients with SLE depends on how they respond to the condition and on the severity and specific types of clinical manifestations. In a newly diagnosed client, the nurse can expect knowledge deficits with respect to the diagnosis itself, prescribed drug therapies, and the prognosis. One must provide the client and significant others with teaching to help relieve anxiety and avoid misunderstandings. This is particularly important in terms of the prescribed medications. The client and significant others should be advised of the actions, side effects, and potential interactions of prescribed medications.

During exacerbations, one must provide physiologic support to prevent skin breakdown, maintain nutritional and metabolic status, and minimize the risk of opportunistic infection. Also, the nurse should provide emotional support to the client facing a chronic, potentially fatal disease.

PROGRESSIVE SYSTEMIC SCLEROSIS (SCLERODERMA)

Progressive systemic sclerosis (PSS), commonly known as scleroderma, is a connective tissue disease characterized by fibrosis and degenerative changes of the skin, synovium, digital arteries, and parenchymal and small arteries of the internal organs.

PSS is less common than SLE but has a higher mortality rate. It is two to three times more common in women as men, occurs between the ages of 30 to 50 years, and is not more common in any race.

The cause of PSS is unknown, although abnormal serologic features suggest an altered immune status.

There are two forms of PSS:

- CREST syndrome
- progressively fatal PSS.

CREST syndrome is a group of symptoms involving *c*alcinosis (calcium deposits), *R*aynaud's phenomenon (vasospasms of small peripheral arteries or arterioles), *e*sophageal dysfunction (impaired motility), *s*clerodactyly (scleroderma of the digits), and *t*elangiectasia (spider-like hemangiomas). This condition can progress rapidly but is still characterized by periods of exacerbation and spontaneous remission.

Progressively fatal PSS is associated with a generalized skin thickening and invasion into internal organs.

Common clinical manifestations include subcutaneous edema, fever, and malaise. The skin becomes thickened and hidelike and loses normal skinfolds. Ulcerations around the finger tips and subcutaneous calcification occur. Polyarthritis and polyarthralgias are also present. Dysphagia caused by esophageal dysfunction, from abnormalities in motility and later from fibrosis, occurs in about 90 per cent of clients. Fibrosis and atrophy of the gastrointestinal tract cause hypermotility and malabsorption.

Diffuse pulmonary fibrosis and pulmonary vascular disease are reflected by low oxygen-diffusing capacity and decreased lung compliance. Hypertensive uremic syndrome, resulting from obstruction in small renal vessels, is serious.

Mild anemia is often present. An elevated ESR and hypergammaglobulinemia are also common. RF may be present in a small number of clients.

PSS typically progresses slowly. When death occurs, it is usually from infection, or renal or cardiac failure. Treatment for the disease is supportive and symptomatic. The primary goal of medical treatment is to trigger a remission of the disease. Steroids and immunosuppressants are used to treat the disease, often in high doses.

Nursing interventions are directed at control of symptoms. One of the major areas of concern is skin care to prevent breakdown and ulceration. The skin should be carefully inspected daily so any injury or breakdown is noted and treatment begun immediately. The client should be taught to use gentle soaps and nonalcohol astringent lotions to maintain skin integrity.

Helping the client control acute pain, which is sometimes associated with Raynaud's phenomenon, polyarthralgia, and polyarthritis, is another important nursing function. The client must learn to avoid activities that might trigger pain. This includes actions such as joint protective behaviors, avoiding extreme cold, wearing gloves when hands are exposed to cold (even when removing food from the freezer), eliminating smoking, and resting the painful part when pain is acute.

If the client is experiencing esophageal dysfunction, modification of the diet may be necessary. Clients usually tolerate small, frequent, bland feedings better than three regular meals a day. The client also should learn to sit up for at least 1 hour after meals to help the food move into the stomach. Histamine receptor antagonists and antacids may be prescribed to help the acidity some clients feel.

The client will need continued follow-up care and monitoring. As with SLE, the client also will need psychosocial support to cope with this chronic debilitating disease. Encourage the client to continue to receive psychological support as needed after hospitalization.

POLYMYOSITIS AND DERMATOMYOSITIS

Polymyositis is an acute or chronic inflammatory disorder of the striated muscles causing symmetric weakness. When there is a rash associated with polymyositis, it is referred to as dermatomyositis. As with other connective tissue diseases, they are characterized by periods of remission and exacerbation and are chronically progressive.

These disorders are treated with high-dose corticosteroids and immunosuppressants. Nursing care is mainly supportive. The client's ability to swallow should be monitored closely so that aspiration does not occur.

VASCULITIS

This is actually a group of disorders including polyarteritis nodosa, systemic necrotizing vasculitis, and allergic granulomatous angiitis, all of which result in necrotizing inflammation of the blood vessels. With these disorders, the circulating immune complexes are deposited in the blood vessels.

With these disorders, there is inflammation and damage to large and small vessels, resulting in end-stage organ damage. The specific symptoms vary depending on the organs affected. Steroids are the treatment of choice for these disorders.

SPONDYLOARTHROPATHY

This group of diseases includes ankylosing spondylitis (also known as Marie-Strümpell disease, or rheumatoid spondylitis), Reiter's syndrome, and psoriatic arthritis. The first two disorders are more common in men, and the latter disorder is more common in women. The disease is associated with the HLA-B27 antigen. RF is absent in the serum.

The major characteristics of these disorders are progressive joint fibrosis (especially of the vertebral column with ankylosing spondylitis), synovitis, and inflammation of skin, of mucous membranes, and at the site of ligament insertion into the bone.

All the disorders are treated with steroid therapy and aggressive physical therapy. Nonsteroidal anti-inflammatory agents may be used to treat the joint pain.

POLYMYALGIA RHEUMATICA AND CRANIAL (GIANT CELL) ARTERITIS

Polymyalgia rheumatica is a clinical syndrome occurring more commonly in women than in men. It is a disease of aging, rarely occurring before the age of 60 years. It is characterized by pain and stiffness in the neck, shoulder, back, and pelvic girdle, especially in the morning. Headaches or painful areas on the head may be present. The client also may have a low-grade fever or temporal arteritis.

Laboratory findings include an elevated ESR, mild anemia, and possible elevation of immune globulins. Steroids usually produce symptomatic relief within days.

The onset of this disorder is usually sudden, with severe pain often appearing in the temporal area. The pain also may be felt in the occipital area, face, jaw, or side of the neck. It is usually associated with hyperesthesia, which makes any touch exquisitely painful. The client may experience visual changes including sudden onset of blindness in one or both eyes.

It is very important to diagnose and treat this disorder before blindness occurs. Because older women are often affected, their complaints of decreased vision and headaches are sometimes ignored as normal aging. Treatment is with corticosteroids, which are highly effective in controlling this disorder.

OTHER DISEASES

Other conditions that may produce arthritis include Crohn's disease, Lyme disease, ulcerative colitis, tuberculosis, hyperthyroidism, hyperparathyroidism, sickle cell anemia crisis, and psoriasis. Treatment for the primary condition usually leads to a decrease in the severity of the arthritis.

STUDY QUESTIONS

1. A client receiving corticosteroids for rheumatoid arthritis would demonstrate the best response by having:
   A. Increased weight
   B. Decreased joint pain
   C. Increased susceptibility to infection
   D. Decreased bone density
2. Which client is most at risk for acquiring systemic lupus erythematosus?
   A. A 15-year-old white girl taking estrogen and progesterone as an oral contraceptive
   B. A 25-year-old white man taking furosemide (Lasix)
   C. A 35-year-old black woman taking hydralazine (Apresoline)
   D. A 45-year-old black man taking aspirin
3. Which of the following will assist clients in preventing exacerbations of systemic lupus erythematosus?
   A. Exposure to sunlight
   B. Pregnancy
   C. Anticonvulsant medications
   D. Control of stress
4. Fluid balance is an important nursing intervention for clients with SLE, because the major cause of death for these clients is from involvement of which system?
   A. Renal
   B. Cardiac
   C. Pulmonary
   D. Cerebrovascular

5. Which of the following medications is usually given during surgery to prevent infection?
   A. Antibiotics
   B. Anti-inflammatories
   C. Antipyretics
   D. Antifungals

6. Which of the following behaviors demonstrates the most successful treatment for a client with joint pain from rheumatoid arthritis?
   A. Joint mobility
   B. Decreased discomfort
   C. Decreased redness and swelling
   D. Improved laboratory and diagnostic studies

CRITICAL THINKING EXERCISES

SCENARIO A

A client is diagnosed as having an acute exacerbation of rheumatoid arthritis. An assessment identifies that her joints are red, warm, swollen, stiff, and tender. Rheumatoid factors, erythrocyte sedimentation rate, and C-reactive protein are elevated.

1. The treatment for local pain control in an acute exacerbation of rheumatoid arthritis is:
   A. Continuous range-of-motion exercises
   B. Massaging the involved joints
   C. Administration of aspirin
   D. Surgical joint replacement
2. In teaching clients to protect their joints, the nurse should teach them to:
   A. Do all heavy tasks at once
   B. Move articles to the outer limits of reach to improve stretching
   C. Plan for rest
   D. Use warm or swollen joints as much as possible
3. When taking nonsteroidal anti-inflammatory drugs (NSAIDS), the client needs to know that:
   A. They are ineffective for arthritis
   B. They should be taken with food
   C. Piroxicam (Feldene) should be used routinely in the elderly.
   D. Histamine receptor antagonists should not be given with NSAIDS.
4. Care of the postoperative client who had joint replacement of the hip consists of:
   A. Adduction of the affected hip and leg
   B. Affected hip flexion of greater than 90 degrees
   C. Neurovascular assessment of the affected leg
   D. External rotation of the affected leg and hip

SCENARIO B

At the nursing home at which you are employed, two clients are being admitted to your floor. The first is a 90-year-old woman who has rheumatoid arthritis and has had a total hip replacement. Ambulation for this client is still slow and difficult because only 4 days have elapsed since surgery. This client is taking naproxyn (Naprosyn) and rantidine (Zantac). The second client is a 65-year-old female with systemic lupus erythematosus who is taking ibuprofen (Motrin) and has congestive heart failure. The renal system is also involved, and the client has recently been prescribed corticosteroids to decrease the acute systemic involvement.

1. Which of the following clients would be best as a roommate for the client with rheumatoid arthritis?
   A. An 80-year-old man with cataracts and hypertension
   B. A 70-year-old woman with renal failure on hemodialysis
   C. A 60-year-old woman with congestive heart failure on diuretics
   D. An 85-year-old woman with diabetes mellitus who is an amputee and is legally blind.
2. Which of the following clients would be inappropriate to place as a roommate for either client? A female client with:
   A. Pneumonia
   B. A stroke
   C. Polyarthralgia and polyarthritis
   D. Pulmonary fibrosis
3. Would the two clients mentioned in the scenario be appropriate roommates for each other? If yes, why? If no, why not?
4. Which client is most at risk for acquiring an infectious process? Why?

BIBLIOGRAPHY

1. Bailey, J. M., & Nielson, B. I. (1993). Uncertainty and appraisal in women with rheumatoid arthritis. *Orthopaedic Nursing, 12(2)*, 63–67.
2. Balow, J. E. (1988). Lupus as a renal disease. *Hospital Practice, 23*, 129–135, 139–140, 142–144.
3. Benson, C. H. (1988). Arthritis and sexuality. *Journal of Urological Nursing, 7*, 370–372.
4. Blake, S. A. (1985). Non-cemented femoral prostheses: Intraoperative focus. *Orthopaedic Nursing, 4(1)*, 42–44.
5. Brassel, M. P. (1988). Pharmacologic management of rheumatic diseases. *Orthopaedic Nursing, 7(2)*, 43–51.
6. Burlinghame, M. B., & Delafuente, J. C. (1988). Treatment of systemic lupus erythematosus. *Drug Intelligence and Clinical Pharmacology, 22*, 283–288.

7. Clough, D. H. (1991). The effects of cognitive distortion and depression on disability in rheumatoid arthritis. *Research in Nursing and Health, 14,* 439–446.
8. Crosby, L. (1991). Factors which contribute to fatigue associated with rheumatoid arthritis. *Journal of Advanced Nursing, 16,* 974–981.
9. Dunajcik, L. M. (1989). The hip: When the joint must be replaced. *RN, April:* 62–71.
10. Fessel, W. J. (1988). Epidemiology of systemic lupus erythematosus. *Rheumatic Disease Clinics of North America, 14,* 15–23.
11. Hahn, B. H. (1990). Lupus nephritis: Therapeutic decisions. *Hospital Practice, 25(3A),* 89–93, 96–97, 103–104.
12. Hynes, D. (1992). Oral NSAIDs: The best choice in practice. *Practitioner, 236,* 328–330.
13. Joseph, N. (1989). Arthritis medications from A to Z. *Caring, 8(1),* 14–16.
14. Klipple, J. H. (1990). Systemic lupus erythematosus. Treatment-related complications superimposed on chronic disease. *JAMA, 263(13),* 1812–1815.
15. Kuper, B. C., & Failla, S. (1994). Shedding new light on lupus. *American Journal of Nursing, 11,* 26–32.
16. Lambert, V. A. (1991). Arthritis. *Annual Review of Nursing Research, 9,* 3–18.
17. Lambert, V. A. (1987). Coping with rheumatoid arthritis. *Nursing Clinics of North America, 22,* 551–558.
18. Lorish, C., et al. (1989). Missed medication doses in rheumatic arthritis patients: Intentional and unintentional reasons. *Arthritis Care Research, 2(1),* 3–9.
19. Magee, D. (1992). *Orthopedic physical assessment* (2nd ed.). Philadelphia: W. B. Saunders Co.
20. McCaffery, M., & Beebe, A. (1989). *Pain: A clinical manual for nursing practice.* St. Louis: C. V. Mosby.
21. McCarthy, D. J. (Ed.). (1989). *Arthritis and allied conditions: A textbook of rheumatology* (11th ed.). Philadelphia: Lea & Febiger.
22. Mirabelli, L. (1990). Caring for patients with rheumatoid arthritis. *Nursing '90, 20(9),* 67–68, 70, 72.
23. Morrey, B. F., & Kavanagh, B. F. (1987). Cementless joint replacement: Current status and future. *Bulletin on the Rheumatic Diseases, 37(4),* 1–7.
24. Mourad, L., & Droste, M. (1988). *The nursing process in the care of adults with orthopedic conditions* (3rd ed.). Albany: Delmar.
25. Nordin, M., & Frankel, V. (1989). *Basic biomechanics of the musculoskeletal system* (2nd ed.). Philadelphia: Lea & Febiger.
26. Pellino, T. A. (1994). How to manage hip fractures. *American Journal of Nursing, 94(4),* 46–50.
27. Relman, D. A., et al. (1992). Identification of the uncultured bacillus of Whipple's disease. *New England Journal of Medicine, 327(5),* 293–301.
28. Richardson, J. K., & Iglarsh, Z. A. (1993). *Clinical orthopedic physical therapy.* Philadelphia: W. B. Saunders.
29. Rothfield, N. F. (1989). The diagnostic pictures of systemic lupus erythematosus. *Hospital Practice, 24,* 37–46.
30. Schlegel, S. I., & Paulus, H. E. (1986). Update on NSAID use in rheumatic diseases. *Bulletin on the Rheumatic Diseases, 36(6),* 1–8.
31. Schumacher, H. R., Jr., et al. (Eds.). (1993). *Primer of rheumatic disease* (10th ed.). Atlanta: The Arthritis Foundation.
32. Smeltzer, K. J. (1987). Fibromyalgia: The frustration of diagnosis and treatment. *Orthopaedic Nursing, 6(3),* 28–31.
33. Steinberg, A. D., & Klinman, D. M. (1988). Pathogenesis of systemic lupus erythematosus. *Rheumatic Disease Clinics of North America, 14,* 25–41.
34. Whitney, R. (1989). Unlock the mystery of lupus. *Today's OR Nurse, 11(3),* 10–12, 30–32.

UNIT 4

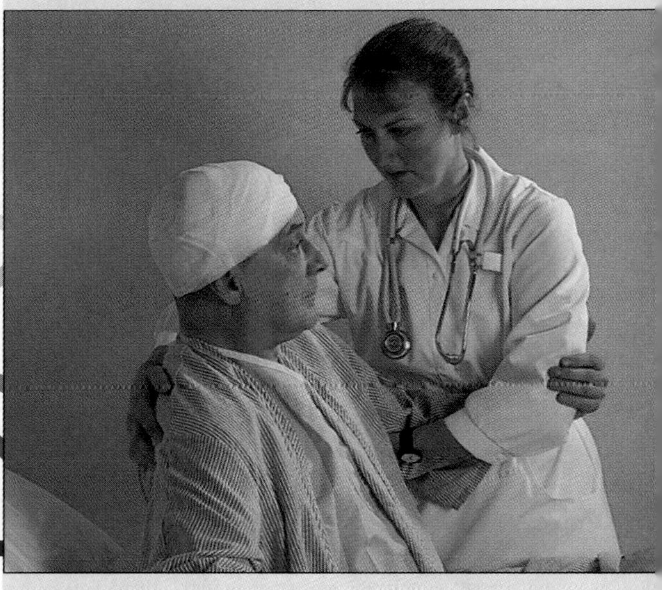

Neurologic Disorders

The body's most organized and complex system, the nervous system, profoundly affects both psychological and physiologic function. The onset of neurologic disorders may be sudden (e.g., spinal cord trauma or ruptured aneurysm) or insidious (e.g., Parkinson's disease or multiple sclerosis). These disorders can be frightening, even devastating, to clients and their significant others—especially if the process is irreversible. Providing nursing care for clients with neurologic disorders is challenging and demands extensive knowledge of neurologic structure and function and neurologic disease processes.

This unit provides the information necessary to plan appropriate nursing care for clients who experience neurologic problems in both acute and rehabilitative stages. Chapter 12 describes the overall assessment of clients with neurologic problems. The next four chapters discuss the care of clients with specific neurologic disorders: Chapter 13, loss of protective function; Chapter 14, cerebral disorders; Chapter 15, degenerative neurologic disorders; and Chapter 16, disorders of the spinal cord, cranial nerves, and peripheral nerves.

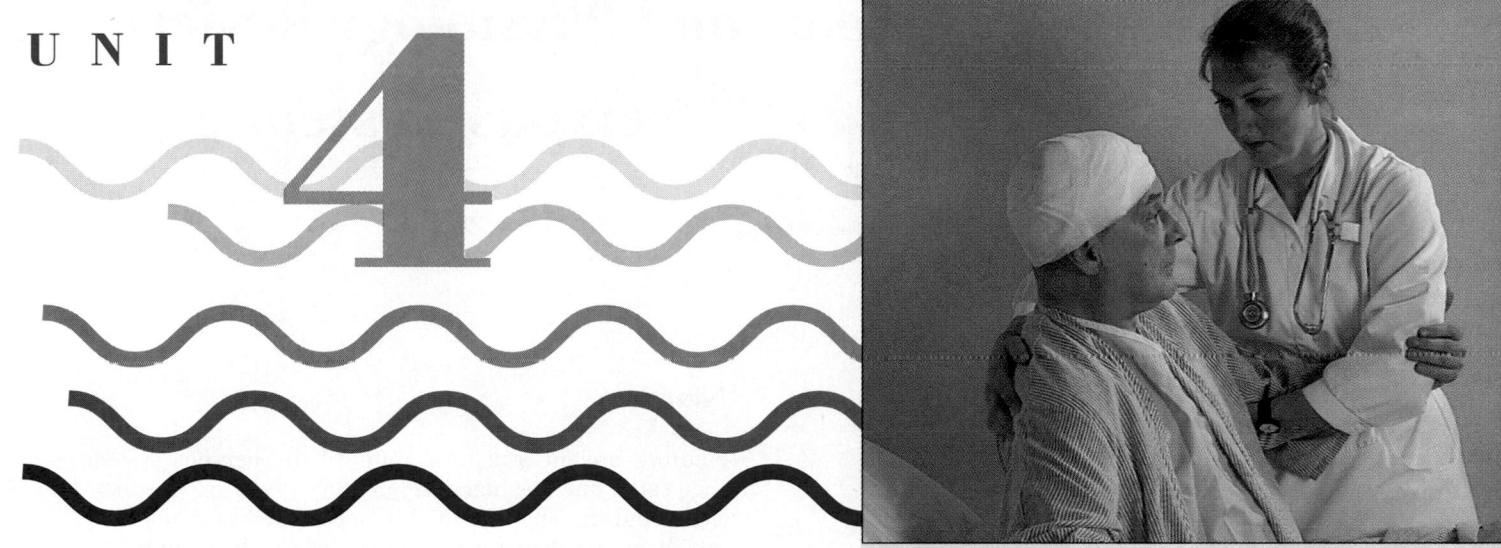

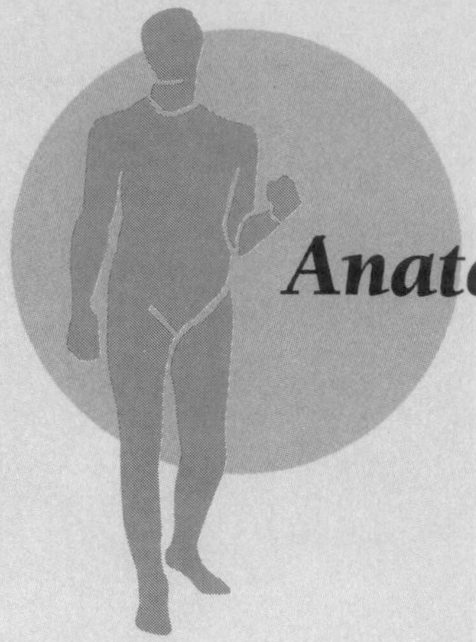

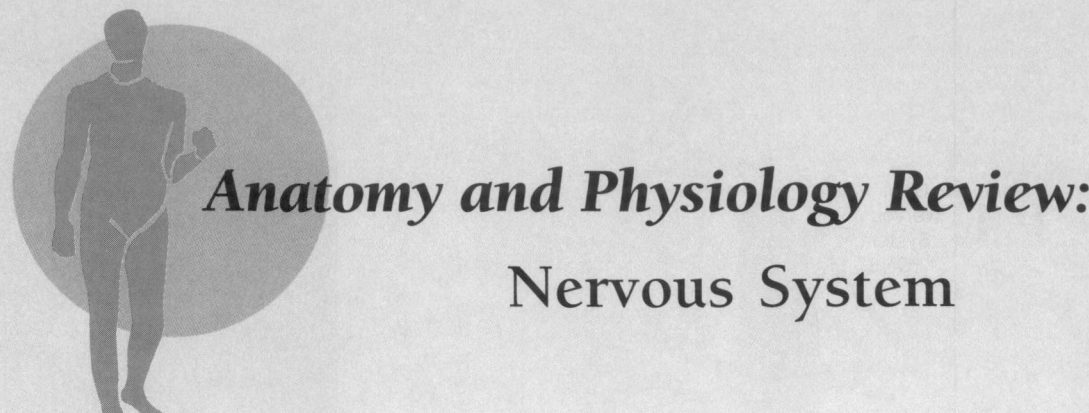

Anatomy and Physiology Review: Nervous System

FUNCTIONS OF THE NERVOUS SYSTEM

The various activities of the nervous system can be grouped as three general, overlapping functions that work together to maintain homeostasis:

- *Sensory functions* detect changes that occur inside and outside the body. They monitor such things as temperature, light, sound, internal and external pressures, pH, and carbon dioxide concentrations.
- *Integrative functions* create sensations, produce thoughts, add to memory, and make decisions based on sensory input.
- *Motor functions* cause an effect such as muscle contraction or glandular secretion in response to sensory input and integration in the nervous system.

ORGANIZATION OF THE NERVOUS SYSTEM

The nervous system is divided into two subsystems: the central nervous system, which includes the brain and spinal cord, and the peripheral nervous system, which includes the nerves and ganglia. The peripheral nervous system is further divided into sensory and motor systems, and each of these has a portion that supplies the viscera and a portion that innervates the somatic tissues.

NERVE TISSUE

Although the nervous system is very complex, there are only two main types of cells in nerve tissue: nerve cells, called *neurons,* and supporting cells, called *neuroglial cells* or, as a structure, the *neuroglia.*

Neurons

Neurons are the structural units of the nervous system that carry out the functions of the system by conducting impulses. They are highly specialized and amitotic, which means that if a neuron is destroyed it cannot be replaced. Functionally, neurons are classified as afferent, efferent, or association neurons, according to the direction in which they transmit impulses relative to the central nervous system. Each neuron has three basic parts:

- Cell body, which is similar to other types of cells
- One or more dendrites, which transmit impulses to the cell body
- A single axon, which transmits impulses away from the cell body

Dendrites and axons are cytoplasmic extensions, or processes, that project from the cell body. They are sometimes referred to as nerve fibers. Axons are often long and surrounded by a fatty substance called myelin that increases the rate of impulse conduction.

Neuroglia

The neuroglia does not conduct nerve impulses; instead, it supports, nourishes, and protects the neurons. Neuroglial cells are far more numerous than neurons. Because neuroglial cells are capable of mitosis, primary tumors of the brain are formed from them. There are six types of neuroglial cells, each with its own specific function.

NERVE IMPULSE GENERATION AND CONDUCTION

All the functions associated with the nervous system are based on two fundamental characteristics of neurons: excitability and conductivity. Excitability is the ability

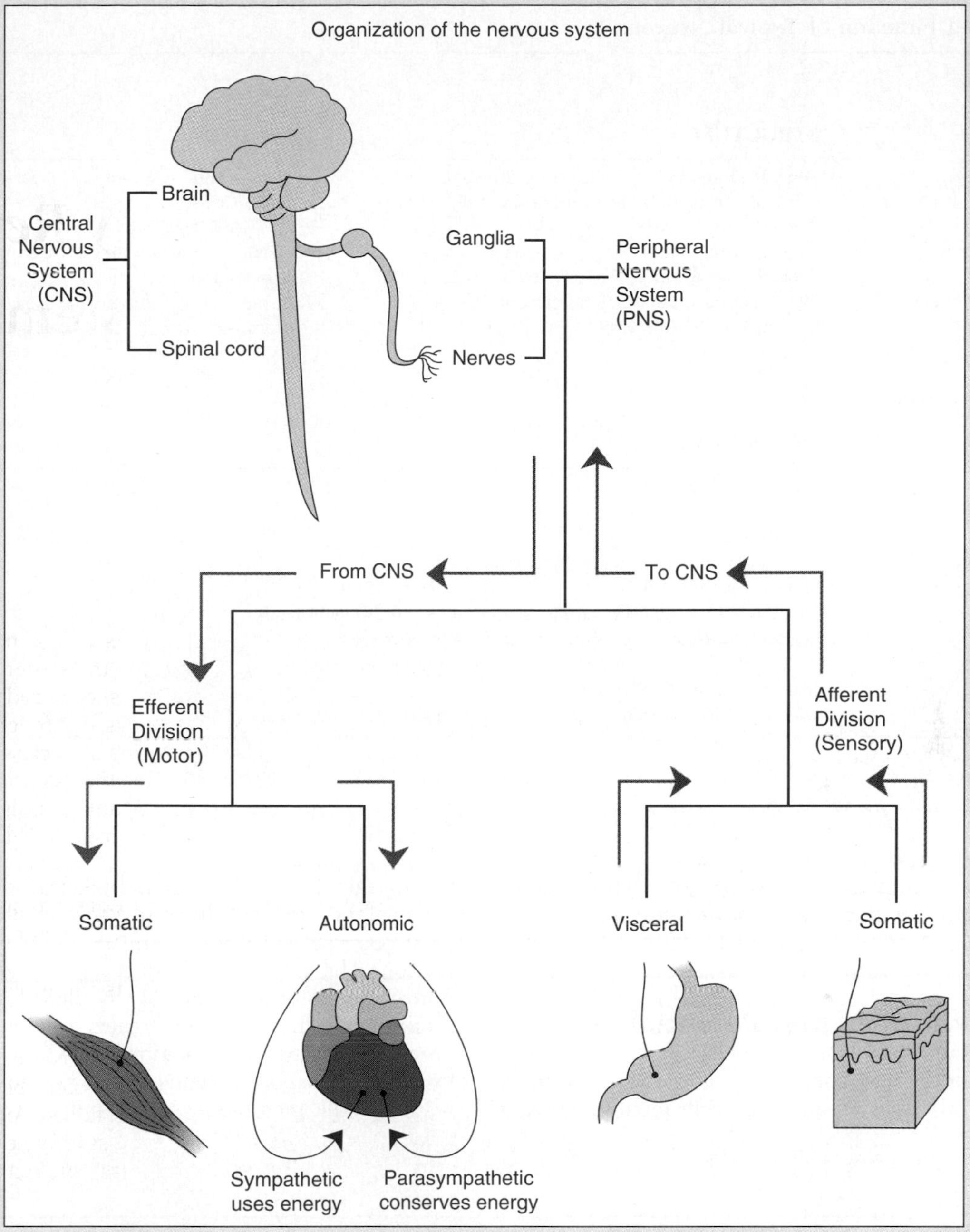

Organization of the nervous system.

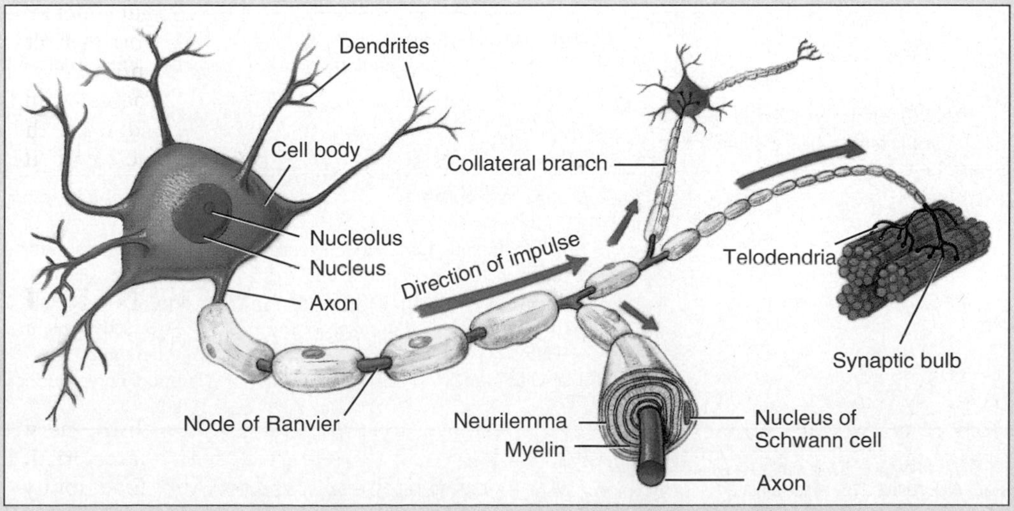

Structure of a typical neuron.

Structure and Function of Typical Neurons

Types

NAME	STRUCTURE	FUNCTION
Afferent (Sensory)	Long dendrites and a short axon; cell body located in ganglia in the PNS; dendrites in the PNS; axon extends into the CNS	Transmits impulses from peripheral sense receptors to the CNS
Efferent (Motor)	Short dendrites and a long axon; dendrites and cell body located within the CNS; axons extend to PNS	Transmits impulses from the CNS to effectors such as muscles and glands in the periphery
Association (Interneurons)	Short dendrites; axon may be short or long; located entirely within the CNS	Transmits impulses from afferent neurons to efferent neurons

Structural Elements

NAME	DESCRIPTION
Axon collateral	Branches of the axon
Synaptic bulb	Slight enlargement at the end of telodendria
Node of Ranvier	Gap between myelin segments
Unmyelinated axon	Axon without myelin; makes up gray matter of CNS
Oligodendrocytes	Make myelin in the CNS
Telodendria	Numerous short branches at the ends of axons and axon collaterals
Myelin	Segmented, white, fatty substance around some axons
Myelinated axon	Axon with myelin around it; makes up white matter of CNS
Schwann cells	Make myelin in the PNS
Neurilemma	Schwann cells that form a tight covering around myelin and axons in PNS; function in nerve regeneration

CNS, central nervous system; PNS, peripheral nervous system.
Data on types of neurons from Applegate, E. J. (1995). *The Anatomy and Physiology Learning System Textbook.* Philadelphia: W. B. Saunders Co.

to respond to a stimulus and generate an action potential; conductivity is the ability to transmit an impulse (action potential) from one point to another.

Development of Action Potential

A neuron that is not conducting a nerve impulse is called a resting neuron, and its cell membrane is a resting membrane. The interstitial fluid outside the cell has a higher concentration of sodium ions and is more positively charged than the intracellular fluid inside the neuron. The intracellular fluid has a higher concentration of potassium and negatively charged ions than the fluid outside the cell. This creates a potential difference, or charge, across the membrane, which is maintained by active transport systems (biologic pumps). A stimulus alters the membrane permeability, which allows the

Neuroglial Cell Types

CELL TYPE	LOCATION	DESCRIPTION	SPECIAL FUNCTION
Astrocytes	CNS	Star-shaped; numerous radiating processes with bulbous ends for attachment	Bind blood vessels to nerves; regulate the composition of fluid around neurons
Ependymal cells	CNS (line the ventricles of the brain and central canal of spinal cord)	Columnar cells with cilia	Active role in formation and circulation of cerebrospinal fluid
Microglia	CNS	Small cells with long processes; modified macrophages	Protection; become mobile and phagocytic in response to inflammation
Oligodendrocytes	CNS	Small cells with few, but long, processes that wrap around axons	Form myelin sheaths around axons in the CNS
Schwann cells*	PNS	Flat cells with a long, flat process that wraps around an axon in the PNS	Form myelin sheaths around axons in PNS; active role in nerve fiber regeneration
Satellite cells*	PNS	Flat cells, similar to Schwann cells	Support nerve cell bodies within ganglia

* Some authorities do not consider these to be neuroglia because they are in the PNS.
CNS, central nervous system; PNS, peripheral nervous system.
Modified from Applegate, E. J. (1995). *The Anatomy and Physiology Learning System Textbook.* Philadelphia: W. B. Saunders Co.

Components of a synapse.

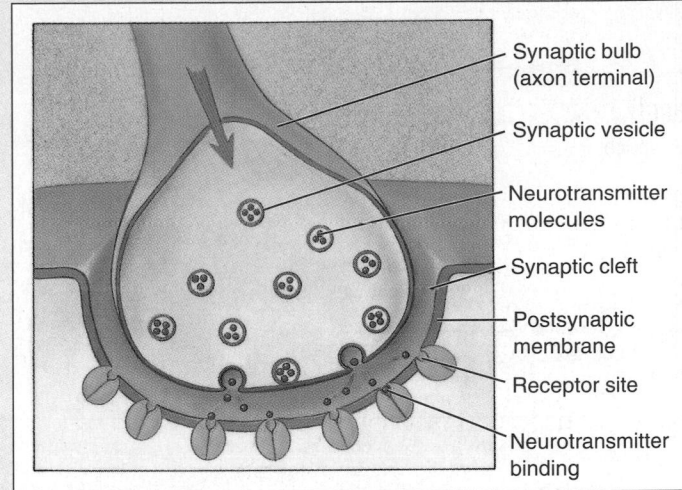

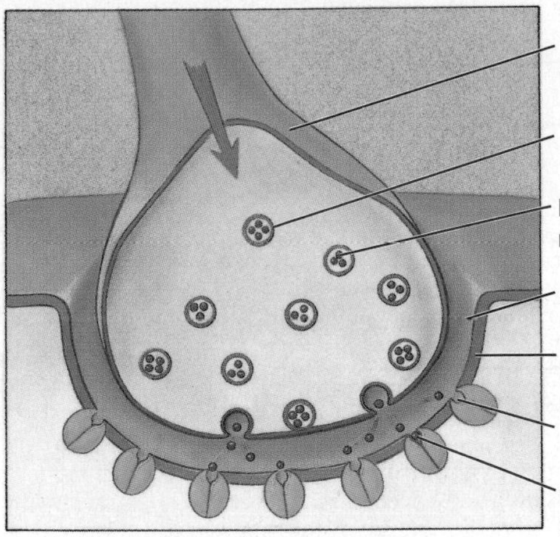

ions to move across the membrane and generate an action potential, or nerve impulse.

Calcium plays a role in membrane excitability. When the calcium level is low, sodium leaks across the membrane and makes it more excitable. When the calcium level is high, sodium is less able to enter the neuron, making it less excitable. During the time that the membrane is permeable to sodium ions, it cannot respond to a second stimulus, no matter how strong that impulse is. This is the absolute refractory period. For a brief period after the absolute refractory period, roughly comparable to the time of altered permeability to potassium, it takes a stronger than normal stimulus to reach threshold. This is the relative refractory period.

Conduction Along a Neuron

The minimum stimulus necessary to initiate an action potential is called a threshold, or liminal, stimulus. If the threshold is reached, the axon responds with an all-or-none response. A strong stimulus will produce the same action potential as a weaker one if they are both above the threshold. A threshold stimulus causes a localized action potential, which then acts as a stimulus for an adjacent point, and the action potential is propagated along the fiber. In an unmyelinated fiber, there is a smooth progressive movement of the action potential along the entire length of the fiber. In a myelinated fiber, the action potential "jumps" from one node of Ranvier to the next. This is called saltatory conduction and results in a faster rate of impulse conduction. In diseases like multiple sclerosis, the myelin is damaged and nerve impulse conduction is impaired.

Synapse

A nerve impulse travels along a nerve fiber until it reaches the end of the axon; then it must be transmitted to the next neuron. The region of communication between two neurons is called a synapse and acts as a one-way valve, allowing transmission in only one direction. A synapse consists of three parts: a synaptic knob (bulb) on the presynaptic neuron, a synaptic cleft between the two neurons, and the postsynaptic membrane. Neurotransmitters from the presynaptic neuron bind with specific receptors on the postsynaptic membrane and alter its permeability. Some neurotransmitters have an excitatory effect at the synapse and result in depolarization. Others have an inhibitory effect by hyperpolarizing the membrane, which makes it more difficult to transmit an impulse.

CENTRAL NERVOUS SYSTEM

The central nervous system consists of the brain and spinal cord. These are vital to each person's well being and have protective features that help preserve their integrity against the physical stresses of everyday life.

Protective Features

The brain and spinal cord are protected by:

- Bone: Eight bones of the cranium surround the brain, and the vertebral column encases the spinal cord.
- Meninges: Three layers of connective tissue coverings, called meninges, surround the brain.
- Cerebrospinal fluid: Cerebrospinal fluid, similar to blood plasma, is produced by specialized capillary networks, called choroid plexus, within the ventricles of the brain. It flows through the ventricles and subarachnoid space, then returns to the vascular system through arachnoid granulations. The flow is caused by the pressure difference between the vascular system and the subarachnoid space. The fluid serves as a shock-absorbing medium, provides an optimal chemical environment for production of action potentials, and is a medium for exchange of nutrients and waste products between the blood and nervous tissue.
- Blood-brain barrier: Brain barriers are either physical barriers or physiologic processes that slow movement of certain substances. An intact blood-brain barrier prevents these substances from crossing into the

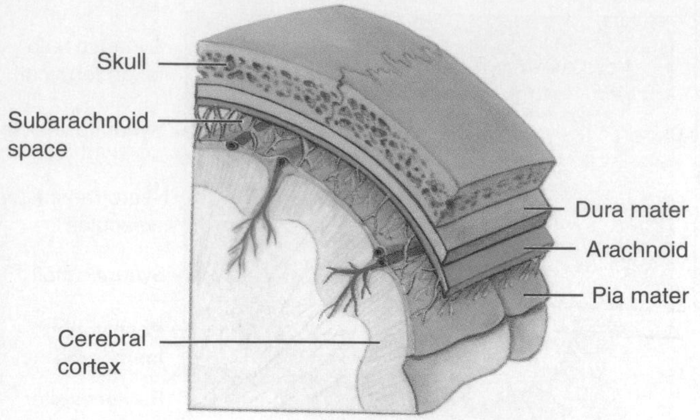

Pia mater: thin, delicate, vascular layer that is so closely adherent to the brain and spinal cord that it follows every contour and cannot be dissected from the surface.
Arachnoid: middle, thin layer of meninges with numerous threadlike strands that attach it to the innermost pia mater; does not extend into the sulci, but follows along the top of the gyri; together, the arachnoid and pia mater are referred to as the leptomeninges.
Dura mater: outer, tough, white fibrous connective tissue layer that forms an envelope around the brain and spinal cord.
Subarachnoid space: space between the arachnoid and pia mater; contains cerebrospinal fluid.

Meninges of the central nervous system.

brain. This barrier must be taken into consideration when medications are prescribed for nervous system disorders.

Brain

The brain is divided into the cerebrum, diencephalon, brain stem, and cerebellum.

- Cerebrum—the largest and most obvious portion of the brain. It is divided by a deep longitudinal fissure into two cerebral hemispheres, which are connected by a band of white fibers called the corpus callosum. The surface of the cerebrum is marked by convolutions, or gyri, separated by grooves, or sulci. Most of the cerebrum is white matter consisting of myelinated nerve fibers. The white matter is covered by the cerebral cortex, which is gray matter. Regions of gray

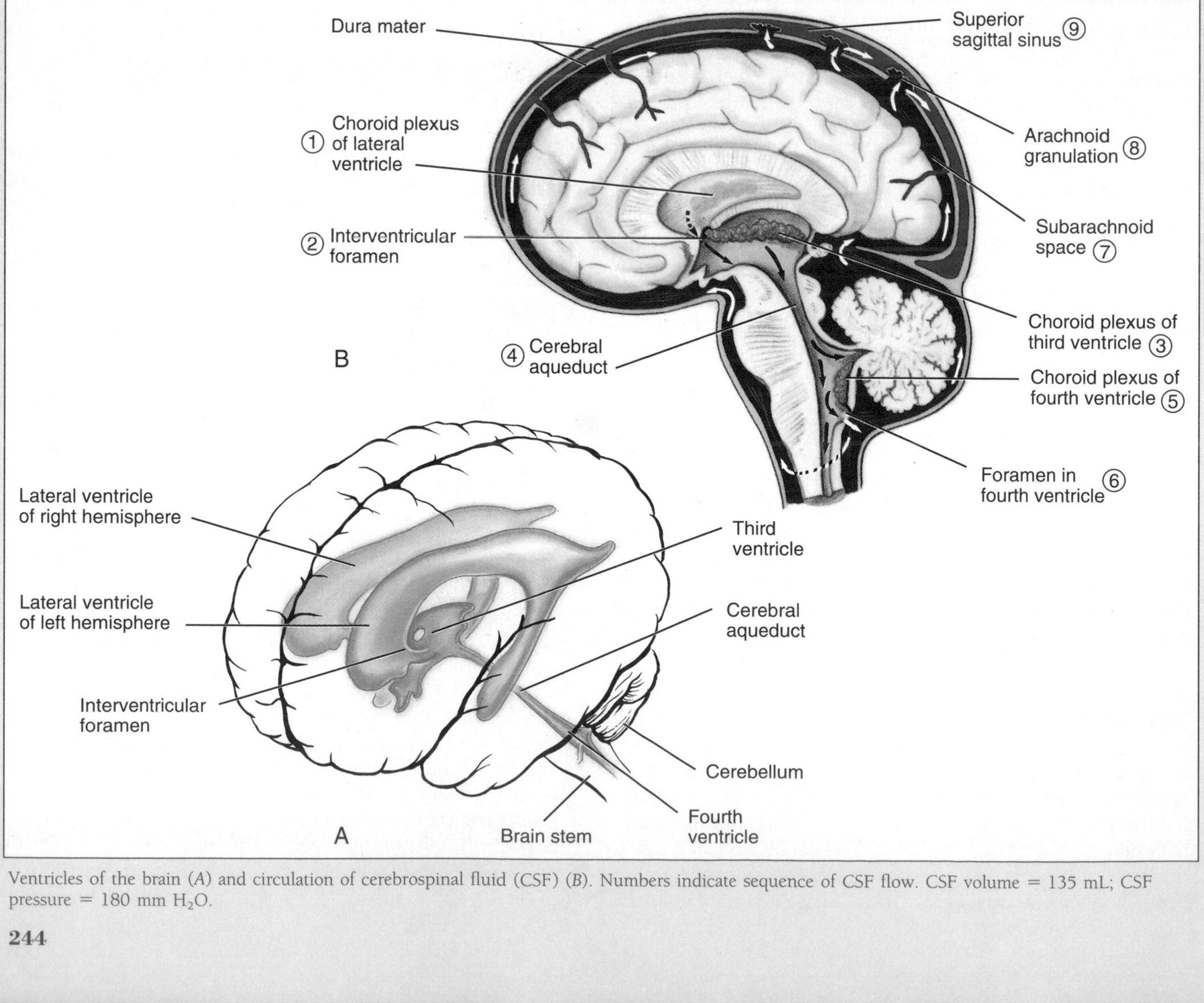

Ventricles of the brain (*A*) and circulation of cerebrospinal fluid (CSF) (*B*). Numbers indicate sequence of CSF flow. CSF volume = 135 mL; CSF pressure = 180 mm H_2O.

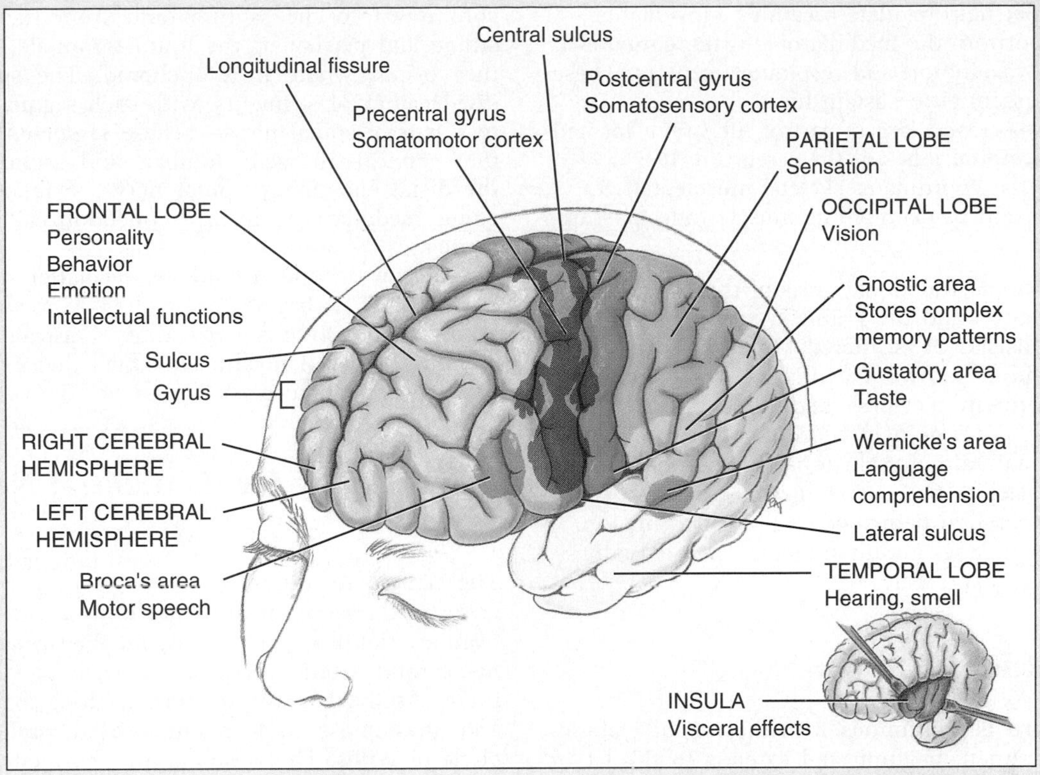

Lobes and functional areas of the cerebrum.

matter, called basal ganglia, are scattered throughout the white matter. These regions are integrating or processing areas where synapses occur, and their major effect relates to muscle tone and production of dopamine. Each cerebral hemisphere is divided into five lobes, each with designated functions.

- Diencephalon—centrally located and nearly surrounded by the cerebral hemispheres. About 80 per cent of the diencephalon is the thalamus, which serves as a relay station for sensory impulses going to the cerebral cortex. The hypothalamus plays a key role in homeostasis by regulating endocrine activity and the autonomic nervous system. The epithalamus is involved with the rhythmic cycles in the body.
- Brain stem—between the diencephalon and the spinal cord. The upper portion, the midbrain, is primarily bundles of nerve fibers going to and from the cerebrum. The middle portion, the pons, contains respira-

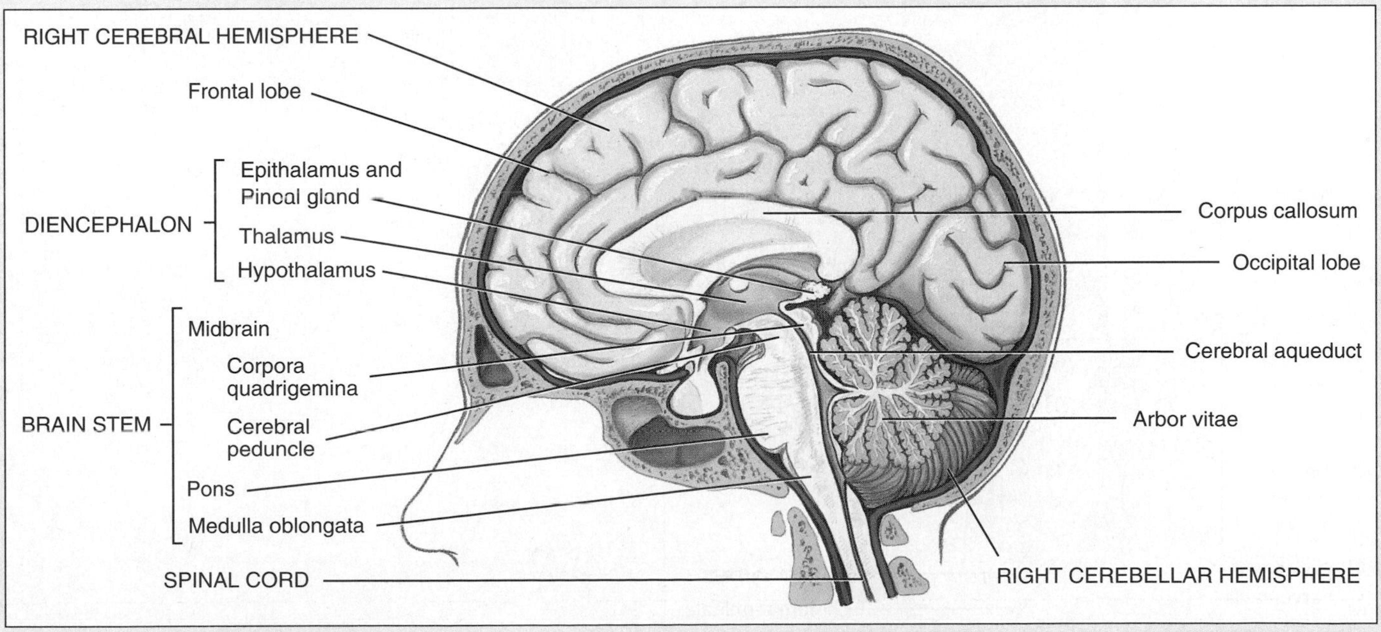

Midsagittal section of the brain showing the major portions of the diencephalon, brain stem, and cerebellum.

tory areas that help regulate breathing movements. The lower portion, the medulla oblongata, contains the cardiac, vasomotor, and respiratory centers. These centers are essential to sustain life.

- Cerebellum—second largest part of the brain, located below the occipital lobes of the cerebrum. It is a motor area that coordinates skeletal muscle activity and is important in maintaining muscle tone, posture, and balance.

Two additional functional areas of the brain are the reticular formation and the limbic system. The reticular formation consists of scattered, but interconnected, neurons and fiber pathways in the midbrain and brain stem that maintain alertness and filter out repetitive stimuli. Motor portions help coordinate skeletal muscle activity and maintain muscle tone. The limbic system consists of scattered, but interconnected, regions of gray matter in the cerebral hemispheres and diencephalon. It is involved in memory and in emotions such as sadness, happiness, anger, and fear.

Spinal Cord

The spinal cord is continuous with the medulla oblongata at the foramen magnum and extends to the L1 or L2 vertebral level, where it terminates in the conus medullaris. The meninges extend beyond the end of the cord down to the sacrum, and from there, a fibrous strand and pia mater, the filum terminale, continues to the coccyx, where it is anchored. The spinal cord is divided into 31 segments, with each segment giving rise to a pair of spinal nerves. These segments are grouped into cervical, thoracic, lumbar, and sacral regions. At the distal end, many spinal nerves extend beyond the conus medullaris to form a collection called the cauda equina.

Within the spinal cord, white matter surrounds the butterfly- or H-shaped gray matter. The white matter is arranged in columns consisting of ascending and descending tracts of myelinated fibers that extend up and down the spinal cord.

Blood Supply for the Central Nervous System

The central nervous system does not store glucose and oxygen; therefore, it must receive a constant supply from arterial blood. The vertebral arteries and the internal carotid arteries provide the arterial supply to the brain. At the base of the brain, these arteries branch and anastomose to form an arterial circle, called the circle of Willis. The vertebral artery system supplies the brain stem, cerebellum, lower portion of the diencephalon, occipital lobe, and portions of the temporal lobe.

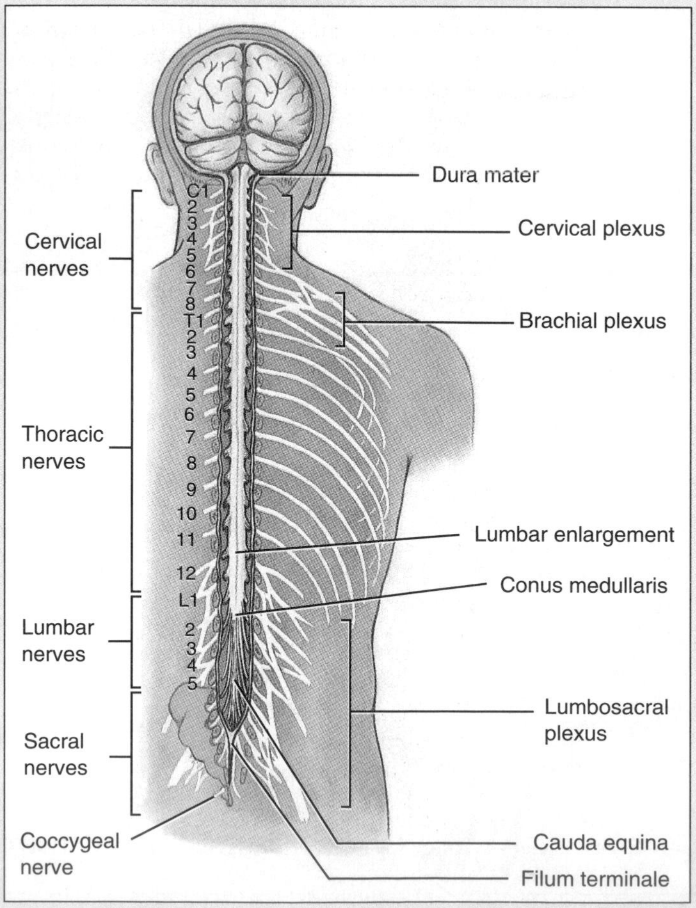

Surface anatomy of the spinal cord.

Cross section of the spinal cord showing gray matter and white matter.

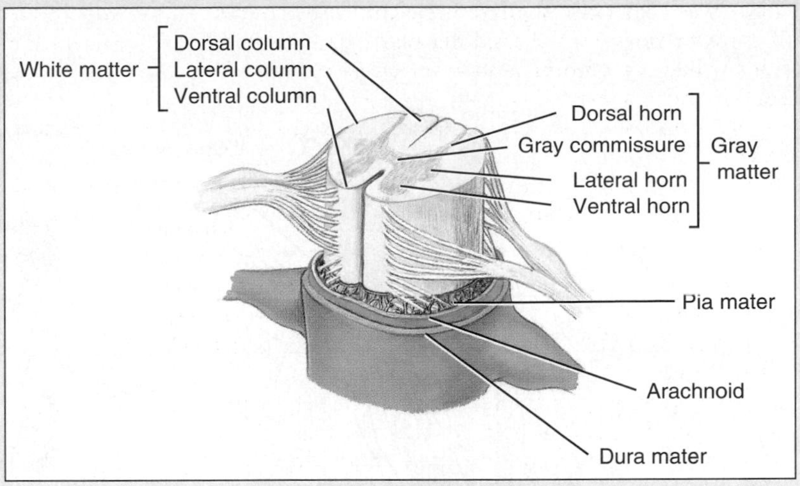

The internal carotid artery system supplies the remainder of the brain. Obstruction of blood flow in any of the arteries supplying parts of the brain may result in a cerebrovascular accident (stroke). Venous blood is drained through cerebral veins into the venous sinuses, and then into the internal jugular veins.

The spinal cord receives its arterial supply from small spinal arteries that branch from larger arteries, including the vertebral, cervical, intercostal, lumbar, and sacral arteries. These vessels form two posterior spinal arteries and a single anterior spinal artery that extend the length of the cord. The distribution of veins is similar to the distribution of arteries.

PERIPHERAL NERVOUS SYSTEM

The peripheral nervous system consists of the nerves that branch out from the brain and spinal cord to form the communication network between the central nervous system and body parts. A nerve contains bundles of nerve fibers, either axons or dendrites, surrounded by connective tissue. Most nerves are mixed nerves because they contain both afferent (sensory) and efferent (motor) fibers. A few contain only afferent fibers and are called sensory nerves, while some others contain only efferent fibers and are called motor nerves.

Ascending and Descending Tracts Within the Spinal Cord

Ascending Tracts: Sensory pathways that terminate in the cerebral or cerebellar cortex

TRACT	COLUMN	FUNCTION
Fasciculus cuneatus and fasciculus gracilis	Dorsal (posterior)	Touch, pressure, and sense of position of body limbs
Lateral spinothalamic	Lateral	Pain and temperature
Anterior spinothalamic	Ventral (anterior)	Crude (nonlocalized) touch and pressure
Spinocerebellar	Lateral	Subconscious proprioception from muscles and tendons; necessary for coordinated muscle contractions

Descending Tracts: Motor pathways that originate in the cerebrum

Pyramidal		Precise, voluntary movements
Lateral corticospinal	Lateral	Voluntary muscle movement on opposite side of the body
Anterior corticospinal	Ventral	Voluntary muscle movement on same side of the body
Extrapyramidal		Automatic movements
Tectospinal	Ventral	Movement in response to visual and auditory stimuli
Vestibulospinal	Ventral	Muscle tone and posture
Rubrospinal	Lateral	Muscle tone and posture
Reticulospinal	Ventral and lateral	Muscle tone and sweat gland activity

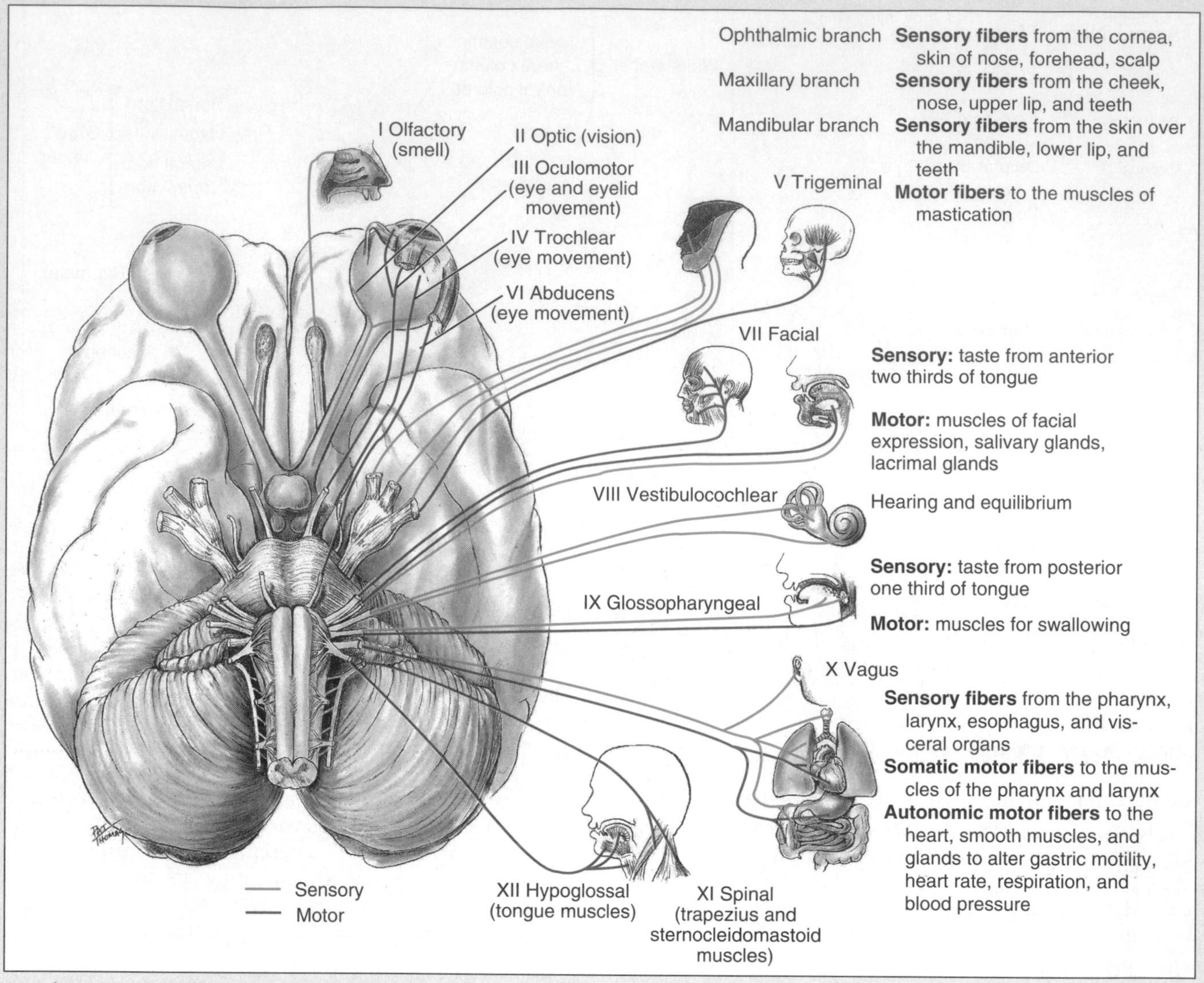

Cranial nerves and their functions.

Cranial Nerves

Twelve pairs of cranial nerves emerge from the inferior surface of the brain. All of these nerves, except the vagus nerve, pass through the foramina of the skull to innervate structures in the head, neck, and facial region. The vagus nerve has numerous branches that supply the viscera in the body.

Spinal Nerves

Thirty-one pairs of spinal nerves emerge from the spinal cord and are attached to it by dorsal and ventral roots. All spinal nerves are mixed nerves because they contain both afferent and efferent fibers. Each pair of nerves corresponds to a segment of the cord. Immediately after they leave the vertebral column, the spinal nerves divide into several branches. The dorsal and ventral branches provide the nerve supply to the muscles and skin of the body wall. The area of skin surface supplied by a single spinal nerve is called a dermatome.

In the thoracic region, the main portion of a spinal nerve becomes an intercostal nerve. In all other regions, the main portions of the nerves form complex networks called plexuses. The three main ones are the cervical plexus, the brachial plexus, and the lumbosacral plexus.

Autonomic Nervous System

The autonomic nervous system sends motor impulses to the visceral organs to regulate and coordinate visceral activities. Its primary function is to help maintain a stable internal environment. The system has two divisions, the sympathetic and the parasympathetic nervous systems. The sympathetic division is concerned primarily with preparing the body for stressful or emergency situations. It stimulates the responses that are needed to meet the emergency and inhibits those visceral activities that can be delayed momentarily. It is an energy-expending system with widespread and long-lasting effects. The parasympathetic nervous system is associated with conservation and restoration of energy and is most active under ordinary relaxed conditions. It has localized, discrete, and brief effects.

Most organs, but not all, have both sympathetic and parasympathetic innervation. Many drugs used to

Spinal Nerve Plexuses

PLEXUS	LOCATION	SPINAL NERVES INVOLVED	REGION SUPPLIED	MAJOR NERVES LEAVING PLEXUS
Cervical	Deep in the neck, under the sternocleidomastoid muscle	C1–C4	Skin and muscles of neck and shoulder; diaphragm	Phrenic
Brachial	Deep to the clavicle, between the neck and axilla	C5–C8, T1	Skin and muscles of upper extremity	Musculocutaneous Ulnar Median Radial Axillary
Lumbosacral	Lumbar region of the back	T12, L1–L5, S1–S4	Skin and muscles of lower abdominal wall, lower extremity, buttocks, external genitalia	Obturator Femoral Sciatic Pudendal

From Applegate, E. J. (1995). *The Anatomy and Physiology Learning System Textbook*. Philadelphia: W. B. Saunders Co.

treat various health problems affect one of these systems. Side effects occur because all the innervated organs are affected, not just the one organ needing treatment.

AGE-RELATED CHANGES

Aging of the nervous system is of major importance because changes in this system affect organs in other systems, cause disturbances of many body functions, and alter patterns of daily living. Like other cells, neurons undergo an aging process with intracellular, cellular, and biochemical changes. Lipofuscin accumulates, tangles and senile plaques develop, and neurons decrease in number. Because neurons are amitotic, those that are lost or damaged are not replaced. Fortunately, the brain has a large reserve supply of neurons, so the decrease in neuron number alone is not devastating. Loss of the specialized neurons in the cerebellum, however, may affect balance and cause difficulty in coordinating fine movements. Another change associated with aging is a decrease in the rate of impulse conduction along an axon and across a synapse. A reduction in the amount of myelin around the axon probably accounts for the diminished conduction along the axon. Decreases in the quantity of neurotransmitters and in the number of receptor sites cause slower conduction across the synapses. These factors contribute to the slower reflexes and longer response time sometimes seen in elderly people.

Comparison of Sympathetic and Parasympathetic Actions on Selected Visceral Effectors

VISCERAL EFFECTORS	SYMPATHETIC ACTION	PARASYMPATHETIC ACTION
Pupil of the eye	Dilates	Constricts
Lens of the eye	Lens flattens for distance vision	Lens bulges for near vision
Sweat glands	Stimulates	No innervation
Arrector pili muscles of hair	Stimulates contraction; goosebumps	No innervation
Heart	Increases heart rate	Decreases heart rate
Bronchi	Dilates	Constricts
Digestive glands	Decreases secretion of digestive enzymes	Increases secretion of digestive enzymes
Digestive tract	Decreases peristalsis	Increases peristalsis
Digestive tract sphincters	Stimulates—closes sphincters	Inhibits—opens sphincters
Blood vessels to digestive organs	Constricts	No innervation
Blood vessels to skeletal muscles	Dilates	No innervation
Blood vessels to skin	Constricts	No innervation
Adrenal medulla	Stimulates secretion of epinephrine	No innervation
Liver	Increases release of glucose	No innervation
Urinary bladder	Relaxes bladder and closes sphincter	Contracts bladder and opens sphincter

From Applegate, E. J. (1995). *The Anatomy and Physiology Learning System Textbook*. Philadelphia: W. B. Saunders Co.

Chapter 12

Assessment of Clients with Neurologic Disorders

Learning Outcomes

After completing this chapter, the learner will be able to:

1. Assess the client for clinical manifestations of common nervous system disorders.
2. Teach the client about the basic pathophysiology of major nervous system disorders.
3. Explain the client's role in diagnostic tests and procedures used in the diagnosis of neurologic disorders.
4. Evaluate subjective and objective data of a basic assessment of the nervous system in relation to nursing diagnoses.

The assessment of a client experiencing a neurologic disorder is a nursing challenge. Neurologic disorders can range from simple to complex, with widespread involvement of the central nervous system. Some neurologic disorders have profound consequences on activities of daily living and even on survival. There are three main components to a neurologic assessment: (1) a comprehensive history, which includes symptom analysis; (2) a neurologic physical examination; and (3) general and specific neurodiagnostic studies.

The focus of the nurse's assessment is both anatomic and functional. The nurse makes continuous observations of the client and compares them with baseline data. Astute observations are essential because most neurologic changes occur subtly. Nurses also collect data on the ability of the client to function physically (e.g., self-care deficit) and mentally (e.g., confusion and altered problem solving). Finally, because many neurologic disorders are very serious, the nurse provides skillful, crisis-oriented support for the client and significant others.

HISTORY

The purpose of the history is to determine past and present health status and to obtain a description of the onset of the current illness. It includes biographic data, the chief complaint and history of present illness, past medical history, family history, psychosocial history, and review of systems.

Biographic Data

Biographic data include demographic, administrative, and financial data. Often included is (1) personal profile, or brief description of the client, (2) source of the history (e.g., client or significant other), and (3) the client's mental status (indicating the reliability of the data). Neurologic problems often affect mental status, sometimes making it difficult to get an accurate history directly from the client.

Chief Complaint

The nurse obtains a detailed description of the events leading the client to seek care. The sequence of signs and symptoms development is explored, including onset, precipitating factors, and duration. The nurse avoids suggesting symptoms to the client and uses open-ended questions. For example, the nurse should ask the client to describe what a headache feels like rather than asking whether it feels throbbing or dull.

It is important to determine the onset of symptoms and their progress. Neurologic disease processes should be described with great accuracy, to facilitate the diagnostic process.

The health history guides the nurse in performing the physical examination. For example, a complaint of dizziness cues the nurse to focus on examination of the eyes, ears (vestibular), and cerebellar function instead of motor and sensory functions. A detailed neurologic examination by a physician is indicated in situations in which the client reports behavioral changes, altered level of consciousness, growth and development problems, pain, changes in motor or sensory function, infection, or trauma. The nurse is alert to assess for neurologic problems that may be related to other problems such as alcohol and recreational drug use, metabolic imbalances, or metastatic lesions.

Past Medical History

The past medical history encompasses previous illnesses, hospitalizations, childhood and infectious diseases, medications, perinatal period, growth and development, family history, and psychosocial history and lifestyle. Neurologic illnesses often subtly affect a client's ability to function in an integrated fashion. The nurse asks about changes in consciousness, vision, speech, motor or sensory functions, headaches, seizures, dizziness, vertigo, and gait and body posture (motor assessment parameters).

CHILDHOOD AND INFECTIOUS DISEASES

Data are collected regarding common childhood diseases and immunizations. Diseases associated with neurologic sequelae include rubeola (measles), influenza, and meningitis. The nurse should ask whether or not the client has been immunized for polio, tetanus, and measles.

MAJOR ILLNESSES AND HOSPITALIZATIONS

A number of major illnesses are associated with neurologic changes, for example, diabetes mellitus, pernicious anemia, cancer, infections, and hypertension. Advanced liver disease and renal disease result in metabolic disturbances such as fluid and electroyte imbalances and acid-base changes that affect mental function. The nurse should inquire about hospitalization, injury, or surgery for problems related to the neurologic system such as head trauma, seizures, stroke, or crushing tissue injury. He or she should ascertain whether the client has had any neurologic diagnostic studies performed, such as an electroencephalographic (EEG), electromyographic (EMG), or computed tomographic (CT) scan. Results of such diagnostic studies provide valuable data for future comparison.

MEDICATIONS

The medication history includes all medications that the client is taking or has taken, both prescription and over-the-counter medications. The nurse should ask specifically about aspirin, anticonvulsants, central nervous system stimulants and depressants, sedatives, anticoagulants, narcotics, tranquilizers, and antihypertensive medications. Many preparations for allergies and colds contain ingredients that cause drowsiness. The nurse should inquire about the past or current use of recreational drugs, type of drug, and duration of use.

FAMILY HISTORY

The nurse asks the client about the family history of neurologic disorders to determine whether genetic risk factors are present. He or she should inquire about the familial occurrence of epilepsy, Huntington's disease, amyotrophic lateral sclerosis, muscular dystrophy, hypertension, stroke, mental retardation, and psychiatric disorders.

PSYCHOSOCIAL HISTORY AND LIFESTYLE

The nurse should question the client concerning personal psychosocial factors, such as educational background, level of performance, and personality changes; this enhances accurate assessment. The nurse specifically inquires about changes that have occurred in the client's daily routines. He or she should ask about changes in sleep patterns, exercise routines, hobbies and recreation, occupation, perceived stressors, and sexual interest and performance. Is the client at risk from exposure to neurotoxic fumes or chemicals, such as pesticides, paints, or glue, or is he or she in an inadequately ventilated living or work space?

The client with a neurologic problem may be unaware of its presence. The nurse attempts to supplement and verify the client's history and review of systems with a family member or significant other who knows the client well. The nurse should ask specifically about mental or physical changes that have been noticed.

PHYSICAL EXAMINATION

The neurologic physical examination is intended to detect abnormalities in neurologic functioning. Variations in the client's age, physical condition, and level of consciousness determine how detailed the examination can be. The components of a comprehensive neurologic examination are described here. Adaptations to the examination in response to various situations are presented.

The comprehensive neurologic examination consists of mental status, language and communication, cranial nerve assessment, motor response, sensory response, reflexes, and vital signs. A suggested sequence of physical examination is as follows:

1. Mental status, including language and communication
2. Cranial nerves
3. Head, neck, and back
4. Motor system
5. Sensory function
6. Reflex activity
7. Vital signs

Mental Status

The nurse documents general data about the client's mental status (e.g., level of consciousness, orientation, memory, mood and affect, intellectual performance, judgement and insight, speech, and thought content).

CRITICAL TO REMEMBER

The *level of consciousness* (LOC) is the most sensitive indicator of changes in the neurologic status of a client.

Consciousness is maintained by function of the cerebral hemispheres and the reticular activating system. LOC is tested with the use of stimuli to determine arousability. Stimuli include verbal, visual, tactile, and noxious agents or painful pressure.

When the nurse is assessing LOC, stimuli are provided and observations are made regarding the response. He or she should start with visual cues, such as walking in front of the client, and note the response. If a response is not elicited, stimulation should be provided by use of the voice. Touch and painful (noxious) stimuli are used only if the client does not respond to the milder forms of stimulation. If the nurse must use painful stimuli to elicit a response, nailbed pressure or pinching the trapezius muscle is recommended.

The Glasgow Coma Scale is an assessment tool designed to note trends in a client's response to stimuli (see Chap. 13). The LOC should be documented with a description of the client's behavior in response to stimulation.

The nurse should establish orientation to time, place, person, and event (or situation). (What is your name? What day is this? What kind of place is this? Where are you? What brought you to the hospital today?) Identify gross deficits in long-term and short-term memory by using simple tests. For example, long-term memory is tested during history taking when the client is asked to give a past medical history. There must be another source to validate such data. Short-term memory is tested by the nurse's giving the client three unrelated words to remember and asking the client to repeat the words immediately and again in a few minutes.

The nurse assesses mood and affect both by the way the client appears (e.g., euphoric, depressed) and the reports of significant others. Is the client's affect appropriate to the situation?

Intellectual performance includes fund of knowledge and calculation ability. The nurse should ask the client to identify commonly known people, places, and events. However, the nurse should ensure that these and other questions are consistent with the client's cultural and educational background. He or she assesses calculation ability by asking the client to subtract 7 from 100, then 7 from the remainder, and so on. Judgment and insight include reasoning, abstract thinking, and problem solving, as well as the client's perception of the situation and should be assessed for indications of major thought content problems. The nurse should listen to the way the client answers questions. Are the answers logical? Do they relate to the question? Clients can be asked to explain a proverb such as "a rolling stone gathers no moss," or to give a solution to a problem situation. The nurse must be careful to ask such questions in a way that does not appear to judge the client's intelligence. Insight can be assessed by asking the client to give an opinion of what may be the cause of the chief complaint.

Language and communication are used to assess the client's speech as well as thought processes, comprehension, and intellectual abilities. Speech should be assessed for articulation problems (usually motor disorders) or problems in language understanding or expression (aphasic disorders). The nurse should assess the client's ability to communicate and understand verbally, in writing, mathematically, and nonverbally. During the initial interview, the nurse notes the client's speech characteristics (e.g., fluency, words used, composition of sentences, questions asked). Does the client spontaneously initiate speech? Does the client repeat the examiner's words? Are the words appropriate? (Note the client's nonverbal behavior.) Does the client understand the questions that are asked? Can the client follow commands? (Ask the client to identify the right and left thumbs.) This tests the client's ability to comprehend the spoken word. The nurse should ask the client to read from a newspaper or magazine and give the meaning of the words. Reading comprehension should be tested, not the ability to read. The client can copy several words or sentences on a piece of paper while the nurse notes the client's ability to form letters as well as to copy. The client should be asked to perform simple addition, subtraction, multiplication, and division without aid of pencil and paper. The client should be asked to verbally identify several common objects, such as a pen, a key, and a coin.

If the client is expressively aphasic, mental status can still be assessed. The nurse should ask questions that can be answered with a yes or no response, or a head nod. Asking the same question using different phrasing will help identify whether or not the client is actually oriented.

Cranial Nerves

The cranial nerves (CN) are referred to by specific name or number. Cranial nerve examination is important for three reasons.

First, half of all the cranial nerves innervate eye function. Therefore, careful examination of eye function provides considerable information about the cranial nerves.

Second, cranial nerves III through XII arise in the brain stem. Thus, testing their functions gives information about the brain stem.

Finally, normal cranial nerve function requires an appropriately received input stimulus that produces an appropriate response (output). The pairs of cranial nerves are tested separately and then compared for normal function (Fig. 12–1 and Table 12–1).

OLFACTORY (CRANIAL NERVE I): SMELL

The nurse asks the client to smell and then identify an aromatic, nonirritating odor (e.g., coffee, toothpaste) with each nostril with the eyes closed. Several different odors should be tested. If the client can perceive any one smell, the nerve is considered functional. Although inability to smell (called anosmia) may develop in elderly people, it may indicate problems such as basal skull fracture or olfactory groove tumor. Other possible causes of anosmia include cribriform plate fracture and an olfactory bulb or tract tumor.

OPTIC (CRANIAL NERVE II): VISION

Assessing the optic nerve involves (1) inspecting the globe for foreign bodies, cataracts, inflammation, or other obvious abnormalities; (2) testing visual acuity; (3) testing visual fields; and (4) examining eye fundus with an ophthalmoscope. (Details of eye assessment are in Chap. 17.) The nurse tests visual acuity generally by having the client read from a newspaper, a sign (from a distance), or a Snellen chart. The client should be tested with glasses if they are worn for far or near vision. The nurse should test visual fields to determine whether vision is absent in one or more directions or a portion of the visual field, such as half of the visual fields, the middle portion, or both sides. Such losses may indicate various problems and may correlate with the area of the brain involved. Gross inspection of the eyes and examination of the fundus can provide information about neurologic disease. Possible causes of abnormal findings include trauma to orbit or eyeball; fracture of optic foramen; diabetic retinopathy; laceration or blood clot in the brain's temporal, parietal, or occipital lobes; and increased intracranial pressure (e.g., papilledema).

OCULOMOTOR (CRANIAL NERVE III), TROCHLEAR (CRANIAL NERVE IV), AND ABDUCENS (CRANIAL NERVE VI): EYES AND EYE MOVEMENT

Cranial nerve III controls pupil constriction and elevation of the upper lid. Pupils should be equal in size and round. The nurse should note pupil size prior to shining a light into the client's eyes and document each pupil's size and shape. The nurse then approaches the pupil from the temporal side while the client looks straight ahead and tests each pupil for both direct and consensual responses (pupillary constriction) to a light. A direct response occurs in the eye being tested. A consensual response occurs in the other eye at a slightly slower rate. The nurse tests accommodation (eyes able to focus on both near and far objects) by having the

Text continued on page 259

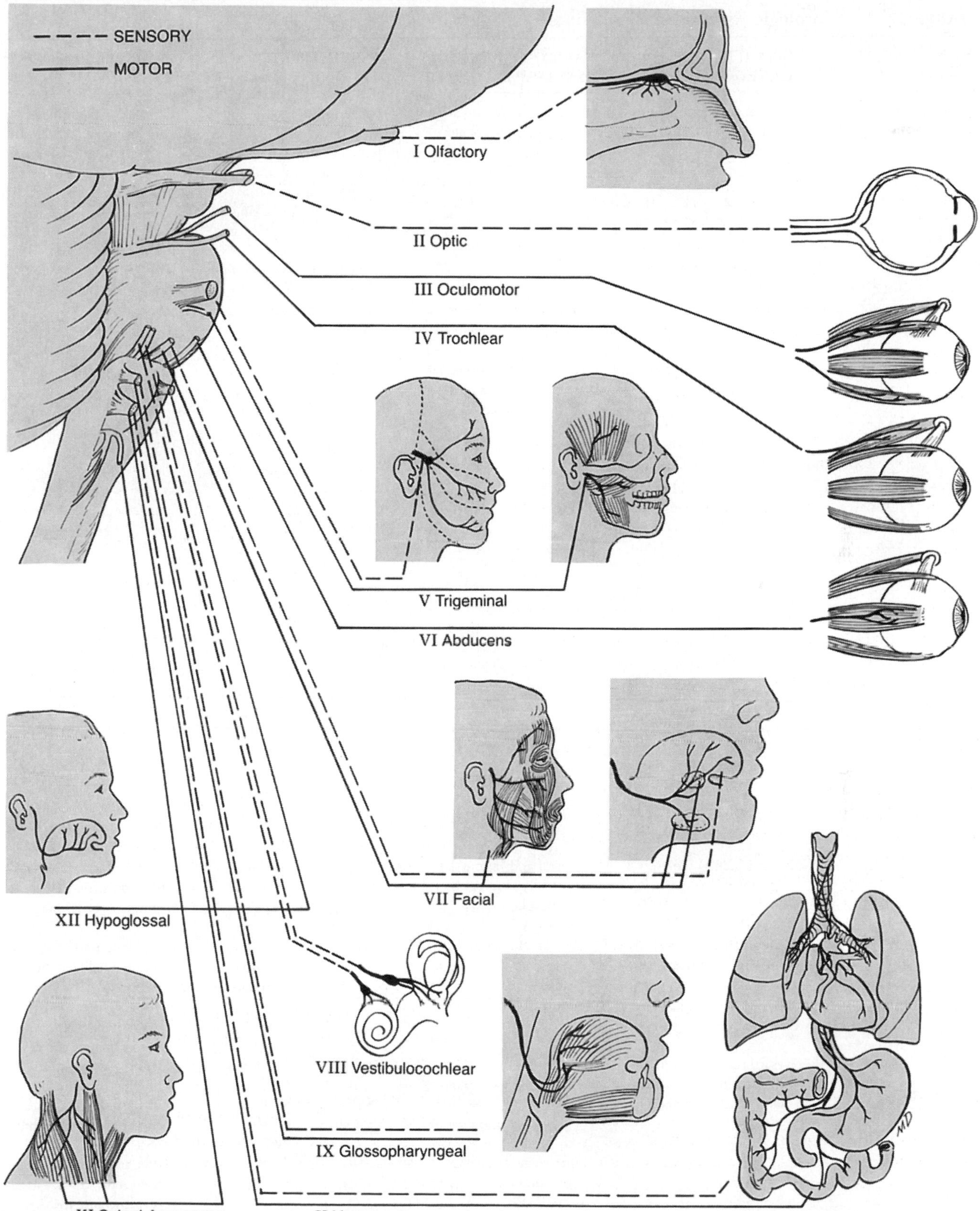

Figure 12–1
Distribution of cranial nerves.

TABLE 12–1 Neurologic Assessment Guidelines

FUNCTIONAL CATEGORY	SPECIFIC CATEGORY	AREA OF NERVOUS SYSTEM INVOLVED	ASSESSMENT TECHNIQUE	EXAMPLES OF DYSFUNCTION
1. Consciousness (awareness of self and environment)	Arousal response to verbal, tactile, and visual stimuli	Reticular activating system (mesencephalon, diencephalon); both hemispheres	Is client alert, what is attention span? Is there normal response to visual and auditory stimuli? Reaction to loud noises, shaking, deep pressure over eye orbits or sternum? Are vital signs, pupils, and reflexes normal?	Elevation: Insomnia, agitation, mania, delirium Depression: Somnolence, lethargy, semicoma, coma
2. Mentation	Thinking	Cerebral hemispheres plus specific regional functions	Is client oriented (time, place, person)?	Disorientation
	Insight, judgment, planning	Frontal lobe, with association fibers to other areas of cerebrum	Does client recognize implications of illness? Are goals congruent with abilities? How would client respond to given situation (e.g., house on fire)?	Lack of judgment, inattention to grooming, appearance, and personal habits
	Fund of information	Basic biologic intellect (frontal lobe) integrated into other areas	Calculation ability, knowledge of current events consistent with educational level. Who is U.S. President?	Impairment-functioning not congruent with level of education
	Memory	Temporal lobe and association to most other areas of cortex		
	Recent:		What was eaten for breakfast? What happened one day ago?	Organic brain disease
	Past:		Recall past events during taking of history	Lapses of memory for past events may coincide with past central nervous system problems (i.e., trauma, infection, psychic trauma)
	Feeling (affect) (congruence of response to stimulus)	General and bifrontal (usually involves both hemispheres)	Compare observed with expected reactions. Are emotions labile? Appropriate?	Blunted affect. Hysteria, schizophrenia, bilateral frontal lobe lesions
	Perceptual distortions (illusions, hallucinations)	General and specific cortical areas in hallucinations	Observations for behavior indicating perceptual problems; ask client	Irritative lesions of cortex may → hallucinations. (Occipital cortex → visual, postcentral gyrus → somatic sensation uncus → smell)
3. Language and speech	Dysarthria (defects in articulation, enunciation, and rhythm in speech)	Impairment of muscles of tongue, palate, pharynx, or lips (may be due to ↓ impulses or incoordination) Brain stem, cerebellum, or extraneural causes; CN V, VII, IX, X, XII	Have client repeat a difficult phrase (e.g., "Susie sells seashells by the seashore")	Slurring, slowness, indistinctness, nasality, break in normal speech rhythm (e.g., speech of a drunk, amyotrophic lateral sclerosis, pseudobulbar palsy, myasthenia gravis)
	Dysphonia (abnormal production of sounds from larynx)	Many extraneural causes; recurrent laryngeal nerve problems (part of vagus); CN X	Is client hoarse? Is whispered voice intact? Use indirect laryngoscopy findings	Compression of recurrent laryngeal nerve by bronchogenic CA of left main stem bronchus; left atrial hypertrophy

TABLE 12–1 Neurologic Assessment Guidelines *Continued*

FUNCTIONAL CATEGORY	SPECIFIC CATEGORY	AREA OF NERVOUS SYSTEM INVOLVED	ASSESSMENT TECHNIQUE	EXAMPLES OF DYSFUNCTION
		Medulla (area of nucleus of vagus nerve)		Brain stem tumors, occlusion of posterior inferior cerebellar or vertebral artery
	Aphasia (inability to use and understand written and spoken words)	Fluent (receptive) left temporal and parietal lobes Nonfluent (expressive) Broca's area (lateral) inferior portion of frontal lobe of dominant side Global (combined)	Observe vocal expression, written expression, comprehension of spoken and written language, and gesture communication	Cerebrovascular disease of middle cerebral artery Trauma, tumor, abscess, etc., in left temporal and parietal lobe areas
	Agnosia (inability to recognize objects or symbols by means of senses)	Primarily in parietal temporal and occipital areas	Sense organs intact? Can the client recognize objects by sight, touch, hearing, etc?	Cerebrovascular disease
4. Motor function	Expression (facial)	CN VII	Symmetry of smile, frown, raising eyebrows	Central facial weakness (upper motor neuron dysfunction); weakness of lower half of face Causes: Cerebral vascular accident, corticobulbar tract Peripheral facial weakness (lower motor dysfunction); weakness of entire half of face Causes: Bell's palsy, brain stem tumor, fracture of temporal bone
	Eating (chewing, swallowing)	CN V, VII, IX, X, XII	Strength of masticator muscles, gag reflexes, ability to swallow	Tetanus, peripheral spasm of muscle. Amyotrophic lateral sclerosis, medullary tumor. Pseudobulbar palsy may be associated with dysarthria
	Eye movements	CN III, IV, VI	Extraocular movement, pupil size, reactivity, pupils equally react to accommodation, diplopia, nystagmus	Cerebral peduncle pressure → CN III dysfunction, cavernous sinus thrombus → CN III, IV, VI problems Muscular problems (e.g., myasthenia gravis, hyperthyroid), Horner's syndrome (ptosis, constricted pupil), anisocoria
	Moving	Motor precentral gyrus (pyramidal) and cerebellar systems, basal ganglia, CN XI, spinal cord, upper motor neuron, (brain → anterior horn cell via corticospinal tract)	Gait, heel-to-toe walking, presence or absence of involuntary movements, coordination, muscle tone, mass, strength, Romberg reflex, ability to shrug shoulders and to rise from chair	*Upper motor neuron:* Brain and cord-sparing anterior horn cell Tone ↑ ↑ (spastic) Bulk ↓ due to atrophy of disuse Reflexes ↑ ↑ due to loss of central inhibition

Table continued on following page

TABLE 12–1 Neurologic Assessment Guidelines *Continued*

FUNCTIONAL CATEGORY	SPECIFIC CATEGORY	AREA OF NERVOUS SYSTEM INVOLVED	ASSESSMENT TECHNIQUE	EXAMPLES OF DYSFUNCTION
		Lower motor neuron (motor cells of cranial nerves and anterior horn cells → peripheral muscles)		No fasciculations Frequent clonus
		Involves brain, midbrain, cerebellum, and spinal cord		*Lower motor neuron:* Segment anterior horn cell peripheral nerve Tone ↓ ↓ (flaccid) Bulk ↓ due to tone loss Reflexes ↓ or absent due to loss of anterior horn cell Fasciculations No clonus *Cerebellar problem:* Loss of coordination and balance
5. Sensory function	Seeing	CN II Optic, occipital lobe	Acuity, visual fields, fundoscopy	Field test: loss in retina or optic nerve → loss in eye involved, optic chiasm → bitemporal hemianopia. Optic tract → homonymous hemianopia, parietal lobe → quadrant problems (inferior), temporal lobe → superior quadrant problems ↑ intracranial pressure → papilledema (raised disc → hemorrhage)
	Smelling	CN I Temporal lobe (uncus)	Ability to detect familiar odors	Usually ↓ smell due to extraneural causes (i.e., upper respiratory infection, allergy, smoking), olfactory groove Meningioma, olfactory hallucinations
	Hearing	CN VIII Cochlear division, temporal lobe	Acuity of hearing, presence or absence of unusual sounds, Weber and Rinne tests	May have conductive (nerve ok) or neural hearing loss. Meniere's syndrome (tinnitus, hearing loss, vertigo, and nystagmus), basilar skull fracture → otorrhea Brain stem vascular dysfunction or tumors → ↓ hearing
	Taste	CN VII, IX	Ability to differentiate sweet, salt, sour, and bitter	Brain stem lesions → ↓ taste Extraneural causes, smoking, poor oral hygiene

TABLE 12–1 Neurologic Assessment Guidelines *Continued*

FUNCTIONAL CATEGORY	SPECIFIC CATEGORY	AREA OF NERVOUS SYSTEM INVOLVED	ASSESSMENT TECHNIQUE	EXAMPLES OF DYSFUNCTION
	Feeling (sensory)	Peripheral nerves → Dermatomes → Spinal cord → Tracts (leading to) Pain-temperature tactile, anterolateral system, proprioception, stereognosis, dorsal roots thalamus (leading to) somasthetic area (postcentral gyrus) (parietal lobe)	Pain: pinprick Touch: cotton touched to skin Proprioception: check where digit is in space Vibration: place vibrating tuning fork on bony prominence Temperature: test tubes of cold and warm water laid against skin; client identifies whether hot or cold	Polyneuropathy, (i.e., diabetes, anemia) Spinal cord lesions → dermatome alterations Upper pons → thalamus, contralateral loss Thalamus → contralateral loss + paresthesia Thalamus → cortex → cortical sensory loss
6. Bowel and bladder function	Bowel function	Afferent Spinal nerve S3-S5 External sphincter (voluntary control)	Check for fecal impaction or incontinence Check muscle tone	Fecal incontinence with lesions of S3, S4, S5 Anal anesthesia–conus medularis and tabes dorsalis
		Internal sphincter Spinal nerve S3-S5 Autonomic nervous system		May be extraneural causes
	Bladder function	Autonomic nervous system Afferent Spinal nerve T9-L2 and S2-S4 Pudendal nerve	Feel when bladder is full, complete emptying. Does client have urgency, frequency?	Urinary incontinence Flaccid bladder
		Efferent Spinal nerve T11-L2 External sphincter (voluntary) Spinal nerve S2-S4		Spastic bladder May be extraneural causes

CN, cranial nerve; ↑, increased; ↓, decreased; →, lead(s) to.

client look across the room (away from the light source) and then look at the examiner's fingers, held about 6 inches from the client's nose. Normally, the lens shape changes and the pupils constrict. The notation "PERRLA" indicates that these functions are normal (i.e., *p*upils *e*qual, *r*ound, *r*eactive to *l*ight, and *a*ccommodation). Approximately 20 per cent of the population has unequal pupils (anisocoria). Destruction of part of CN III can cause ptosis (drooping) of the eyelid. Disorders or pressure on a specific side of CN III can cause the ipsilateral pupil to dilate, the eyelid to droop, and the eye to deviate outward.

Assessment of direct and consensual pupillary reactions provides information about the functioning of CN III and intracranial pressure. As intracranial pressure increases, the oculomotor nerve is compressed. Depending on the cause, the compression may be unilateral, as in a right-sided subdural hematoma, or bilateral, as seen with generalized edema secondary to head injury. If the pressure is not relieved, the pupils become larger in size and less reactive until they are fixed and dilated (blown pupil). A fixed and dilated pupil indicates increased intracranial pressure of such severity that the oculomotor nerve is unable to function. This is a poor prognostic sign, because herniation of the brain and death may be imminent. The nurse should inform the physician as the pupil becomes larger and less responsive to light so that medical interventions can be instituted to relieve the increased intracranial pressure.

Cranial nerves III, IV, and VI coordinate to control eye movements in all six cardinal directions of gaze (see Chap. 17). The function of these nerves is tested in various ways. The nurse asks the client to move the eyes in the six directions. Alternatively, he or she moves an object in the six cardinal directions and asks the client to follow it with the eyes.

CRITICAL TO REMEMBER

A fixed and dilated pupil in a client who has had previously reactive pupils is a neurologic emergency. The physician should be notified immediately.

If a client has diplopia (double vision), but no muscle weakness can be demonstrated, the nurse can shine a light so that it reflects on both eyes. The area of reflection is normally symmetric, meaning that the client has a conjugate gaze. With dysconjugate gaze, the light's reflection is asymmetric (i.e., not the same in both eyes). If extraocular movements are intact, the nurse documents as "EOMs intact." The nurse should observe for nystagmus, the rapid back-and-forth movement of the eyes. The movement may be horizontal or vertical. Although some individuals are born with nystagmus, the condition usually indicates brain stem dysfunction, dilantin toxicity, or a side effect of medication. Possible causes of abnormal findings include pressure on oculomotor, trochlear, or abducens nerves at the brain stem due to fractured orbit, increased intracranial pressure, or tumor at or trauma to the base of the brain. An inability to look down or to walk down steps because of a visual disturbance could be related to CN IV dysfunction. Failure of an eye to move laterally in an outward direction is associated with compression of or damage to CN VI.

TRIGEMINAL (CRANIAL NERVE V)

Cranial nerve V has a motor and a sensory division. The motor division innervates the muscles of mastication. The nurse tests CN V function by asking the client to clamp the jaws, open the mouth against resistance, open the mouth widely, move the jaws from side to side, and make chewing movements. A normal CN V allows all these activities. The nurse should document any asymmetry in the temporal muscles. The sensory division mediates all sensations for the entire face, scalp, cornea, and nasal and oral cavities. With the client's eyes closed, the nurse tests sensations such as pain (e.g., pinprick), touch (e.g., wisp of cotton), and temperatures (e.g., hot and cold test tubes of water) on both sides of the face from the top of the head (vertex) to the chin. The nurse tests the corneal reflexes by gently touching the cornea with a sterile wisp of cotton or gently stroke the eyelash. The normal response is brisk eyelid blinking. The corneal reflex involves CN V and CN VII. CN V is the afferent (sensory) arc while CN VII controls closure of the eye (motor). Possible causes of abnormal findings include tumor at or trauma to the base of the brain, fractured orbit, and trigeminal neuralgia.

FACIAL (CRANIAL NERVE VII)

Cranial nerve VII has a motor and sensory division. The motor division innervates muscles controlling facial expression. The nurse should observe the face for symmetry and the ability to use facial muscles. He or she asks the client to smile, frown, raise the forehead and eyebrows, tightly close the eyes and resist attempts to open them, whistle, show the teeth, and puff out the cheeks. The nurse tests the anterior part of tongue for taste by asking the client to close the eyes and protrude the tongue, and then place a taste substance on one side of the anterior tongue. The client should keep the tongue protruded while identifying the taste. The client should rinse the mouth or drink a small amount of water before the other side is tested. Taste should be tested on each side with sweet, salty, acidic or sour (e.g., vinegar or lemon), and bitter (e.g., coffee). Common abnormalities noted include loss of the nasolabial fold, inability to close the eye and blink reflexively, facial asymmetry, drooling, difficulty swallowing secretions, loss of tearing, and loss of taste on the anterior two thirds of the tongue. Possible causes of abnormal findings include Bell's palsy, temporal bone fracture, and peripheral laceration or contusion to the parotid region.

VESTIBULOCOCHLEAR OR ACOUSTIC (CRANIAL NERVE VIII)

Cranial nerve VIII is a sensory nerve with two divisions, cochlear and vestibular. The cochlear nerve permits hearing. The nurse tests auditory acuity by having the client listen to and report on a whispered voice, rustling fingers, or a tuning fork at various distances from the ear. Bone and air conduction are tested with a tuning fork. Audiometry may be used for a precise assessment. The vestibular nerve helps maintain equilibrium by coordinating the muscles of the eye, neck, trunk, and extremities. Equilibrium tests include the Romberg and caloric tests (oculovestibular reflex) and electronystagmography. (For details on hearing and equilibrium assessment, see Chap. 18.) Possible causes of abnormal findings include Meniere's syndrome and acoustic neuroma.

GLOSSOPHARYNGEAL (CRANIAL NERVE IX) AND VAGUS (CRANIAL NERVE X)

Because of the overlapping innervation of the pharynx, CNs IX and X should be assessed together. The nurse asks the client to open the mouth widely and say "Ah" and then observes the position and movement of the uvula and palate. Do they rise midline? The nurse tests the gag reflex by gently touching the pharynx on each side with a tongue depressor. This normally elicits a brisk gag response.

CRITICAL TO REMEMBER

Clients with decreased or absent gag responses are at risk for aspiration.

The client's ability to swallow is assessed with a small amount of water. The nurse tests the posterior third of the tongue for taste, as with the seventh cranial nerve (may be performed when testing CN VII). Dysfunction of CN IX includes loss of taste and sensation of glossopharyngeal pain. The nurse should ask the client to cough and to speak to test CN X. Damage to CN X causes an ineffectual cough and a weak, hoarse voice. To differentiate areas of weakness, the client can be asked to vocalize different sounds: "kuh kuh" (soft palate), "mi mi" (lips), "la la" (tongue). Possible causes of abnormal findings include brain stem trauma, neck trauma, brain stem tumors, and stroke.

SPINAL ACCESSORY (CRANIAL NERVE XI)

Cranial nerve XI innervates the sternocleidomastoid muscle and the upper portion of the trapezius muscle. To test, the nurse asks the client to (1) elevate the shoulders (with and without resistance), (2) turn (not tilt) the head to one side (and then the other), (3) resist attempts to pull the chin back toward midline, and (4) push the head forward against resistance. Disorders may produce drooping of a shoulder, muscle atrophy, weak shoulder shrug, or turn of the head. Possible causes of abnormal findings include neck trauma, radical neck surgery, and torticollis.

HYPOGLOSSAL (CRANIAL NERVE XII)

Cranial nerve XII innervates the tongue. The nurse should ask the client to open the mouth widely, stick out the tongue, and rapidly move the tongue from side to side and in and out. The nurse documents any deviation of the tongue to the side or any fasciculation of the tongue. He or she assesses tongue strength by having the client push the tongue strongly against the inside of the cheek while pressure is applied to the area externally. Possible causes of abnormal findings include neck trauma associated with major blood vessel damage.

Head, Neck, and Back

The head, neck, and spine are examined by inspection, palpation, auscultation, and percussion. The head is inspected for size, shape, contour, and symmetry. The nurse notes any ecchymosis or bruising around the eyes or behind the ears. "Raccoon eyes" are indicative of an anterior basilar skull fracture and appear as bruising around the eyelids. The nurse also notes any drainage from the nares, bruising behind the ears over the mastoid (Battle's sign), and presence or absence of drainage from the ears.

CRITICAL TO REMEMBER

If drainage is present in a client with a neurologic disorder, it should be tested for glucose. If the drainage is glucose positive, the physician should be informed of a possible cerebrospinal fluid leak.

The skull is palpated lightly for nodules or masses and to supplement abnormal inspection findings. If there are open or draining areas, the nurse wears gloves. The skull normally feels smooth and firm. Areas of bogginess or depressions are abnormal. Palpation of neck muscles may identify masses or areas of tenderness.

The nurse inspects and palpates the spine for alignment, noting any deviation from the normal curvatures. Gentle percussion over the spinous processes may produce pain or tenderness. The paravertebral muscles are palpated for masses, tenderness, and spasm. Auscultation of major neck vessels and other vessels may reveal bruits or other abnormal sounds indicative of pathology. Tumors, vascular disorders, traumatic disorders, and problems involving the vertebrae and surrounding muscles may be detected through examination.

Motor System

Thorough assessment of the motor system involves numerous procedures. The following discussion focuses on the screening examinations and common abnormalities.

Included in the motor examination are muscle size, muscle strength, tone, coordination, gait, station, and movement disorders.

MUSCLE SIZE

The nurse inspects major muscle groups bilaterally for symmetry. He or she should inspect the trunk, and intercostal and abdominal muscles.

MUSCLE STRENGTH

The nurse should assess muscle power in the following way: Ask the client first to walk on the heels, then on the toes. Ask the client to stand and hold the arms straight out in front with palms up, and then to maintain this posture with eyes closed. A "drift" is said to be present if one arm moves upward or if one hand begins to pronate and fall lower than the other arm. The nurse should also assess major muscle groups against resistance (see Chap. 43). Muscle strength is assessed and rated on a five-point scale in all four extremities, comparing one side to the other as follows:

- 5/5 = Normal full strength. Muscle is able to move actively through full range of motion against the effects of gravity and applied resistance
- 4/5 = Muscle is able to move actively through full range of motion against the effect of gravity with weakness to applied resistance
- 3/5 = Muscle is able to move actively against the effect of gravity alone
- 2/5 = Muscle is able to move with support against the effect of gravity
- 1/5 = Muscle contraction is palpable and visible; trace or flicker movement occurs
- 0/5 = Muscle contraction or movement is undetectable

Assessment of specific muscle groups can be completed to assess deficits in certain areas, such as spinal cord disorders. Disorders of muscle strength may be exhibited by weakness on one side of the body, in both lower extremities, or in both upper and lower extremities.

If an asymmetry is detected, the client and significant others are asked if this is a long-standing or new finding.

CRITICAL TO REMEMBER

The age and physical condition of the client should be considered when interpreting the results of muscle strength testing. One would not expect the same strength from a physically fit young client as from an elderly or debilitated client.

If abnormalities are found in muscle power, more detailed assessment may be conducted with procedures such as EMG, discussed later in this chapter.

MUSCLE TONE

Muscle tone is assessed while the client is moving each extremity through passive range of motion. When tone is decreased (hypotonic), the muscles are soft, flabby, or flaccid. Increased muscle tone exists if the muscles are resistant to movement, rigid, or spastic. The nurse should note the presence of fibulation or tremor.

MUSCLE COORDINATION

Muscle coordination assessment includes testing rapid alternating movements, point-to-point maneuvers, and maintenance of truncal balance and head position. To test rapid alternating movements, the nurse asks the client to touch (approximate) each finger to the thumb quickly in succession. Alternatively, ask the client to pat the thighs first with the palms, then with the back of the hands. In point-to-point testing, the examiner holds up an index finger approximately 18 inches away from the client. The client is asked to touch first his or her nose with a finger, then the examiner's index finger. This is repeated several times while the examiner moves the index finger to different points. The test is performed bilaterally for the client's right and left hands. Lower extremity coordination is tested by asking the client to place the heel of the foot below the opposite knee and then to slide the heel down the shin toward the great toe. Repeat for the opposite leg.

GAIT AND STATION

The nurse assesses gait and station by having the client stand still, walk, and walk in tandem (i.e., one foot in front of the other in a straight line). Walking involves the functions of motor power, sensation, and coordination. The ability to stand quietly with feet together requires coordination and intact proprioception. If the client has difficulty standing, further assessment is needed to determine whether the client is weak or unsteady. If the client is weak, the nurse needs to protect the client from falling.

The nurse should examine the muscles for fine and gross abnormal movements. Examples of fine movements are fasciculations (involuntary ripples or twitches occurring while the client is relaxed), which may indicate lower motor neuron disease.

The client should move all joints through a full range of passive motions. Abnormal findings include pain, contractures, and muscle resistance.

The nurse tests for apraxia (inability to carry out a learned movement on command in the absence of weakness or paralysis) by asking the client to perform common activities, such as tying shoes or combing hair. True apraxia is present only if a client can do the activity spontaneously but cannot do it on request.

Sensory Function

Sensory assessment involves testing for touch, pain, vibration, position (proprioception), and discrimination. Assessing hearing, vision, smell, and taste is also sensory assessment. Sensory assessment may identify dermatomes (skin area innervated by various nerves) that have absent, reduced, exaggerated, or delayed sensation.

An unresponsive patient can only be tested for response to painful stimuli (e.g., reflex withdrawal of limbs, wincing, grimacing). A complete sensory examination is only possible on a conscious client because it requires cooperation. Sensation should always be tested with the client's eyes closed. The nurse should help the client become as relaxed as possible.

The nurse conducts the sensory assessment systematically by testing a particular area of the body and then testing the corresponding area on the opposite side. This system should be followed until all dermatomes are tested. The extremities should be tested first, then the trunk. The nurse documents any asymmetric findings, that is, those varying from one side to the other. If the client has a sensory loss, the nurse should document the area of loss and where normal sensation begins. Sensation assessment may be documented on a body chart of dermatomes.

SUPERFICIAL SENSATION

Superficial sensations are tested by stimulating the skin in symmetric areas on each side of the body according to the dermatome distribution. Superficial pain is tested by alternating the sharp and dull ends of a sterile safety pin. After testing, the safety pin should be disposed of properly in a sharps container.

Touch and Pain. The nurse asks the client to close the eyes and says that there will be a sharp and a dull stimulus. The nurse should then proceed as follows: Demonstrate how sharp and dull feel. Touch the client with the dull end of the safety pin, then apply a painful stimulus by using the pin's sharp end. Moving from the fingers to the shoulders, alternate the two stimuli inconsistently (so the client cannot predict which is being used) and ask the client to distinguish between which is sharp and which is dull. Then test the toes to the thigh. Finally, test the anterior and posterior trunk and buttock. The nurse must keep in mind the dermatomal pattern while testing. Where there is a loss of the sense of pain, he or she should test for temperature awareness. Otherwise, it is not necessary to test for temperature, because pain and temperature travel on related pathways.

In an unconscious client, deep pain is used to elicit a sensory response when superficial pain does not produce such a response. The minimal amount of stimulus is used. The nurse should take special precautions not to bruise the client or repeat noxious stimuli in the absence of significant change in client status. Means of producing noxious stimuli include nailbed pressure, sternal rubs, and pinching the trapezius muscle. The client's response to noxious stimuli is noted. The following responses are those most commonly seen when painful stimuli are applied:

Localization–the client pushes the stimulus away
Flexion withdrawal–the client pulls away from the stimulus

Decorticate posturing (abnormal flexion)–the client pulls the fists up toward the chest and extends the legs; this indicates damage to the cortex of the brain

Decerebrate posturing (abnormal extension)–the client extends and outwardly rotates the arms and extends the legs; this indicates damage to the brainstem

No response–there is no visible movement on painful stimulus.

Other Modalities. Other modalities for testing superficial sensation in the conscious client include using a cotton wisp to assess light touch. The nurse should follow the same guidelines as for testing superficial pain sensation, stimulating symmetric areas of the dermatomes.

MECHANICAL SENSATION

Mechanical sensations are assessed by vibration and proprioception.

Vibration. A tuning fork is used to test for vibration. The nurse places the end of a vibrating tuning fork on a distal bony prominence such as a finger or great toe joint. The nurse should ask the client to indicate when and where vibration (not touch) is felt. If vibration is not felt, the tuning fork is moved proximally to the wrist or elbow or foot or ankle.

Proprioception. The nurse tests sense of body position by holding the side of the client's great toes, between the thumb and index finger. As the toes are gently flexed and extended, the client should be asked to state when movement is felt and in what direction. If impairment is detected, more proximal joints are tested.

DISCRIMINATION

Cortical discrimination depends on the ability to discriminate superficial and deep sensations. Included are tests for stereognosis, graphesthesia, extinction phenomenon, and two-point stimulation.

To test stereognosis (i.e., discernment of the form and configuration of objects felt, or three-dimensional discrimination), three small, familiar objects are placed one at a time in the client's hands, such as coins, keys, or a paper clip, and the client is asked to identify each.

To test graphesthesia (recognition of the form and configuration of written symbols), the nurse traces different separate letters and numbers on the client's palm with the blunt end of a pen, asking the client to identify each.

To test for the extinction phenomenon (simultaneous stimulation), the nurse pricks the client's skin simultaneously at the same place on both sides of the body and asks the client to say whether one or two pricks are felt.

To perform two-point stimulation, the nurse pricks the client's skin simultaneously with two pins at varying distances apart to identify the smallest distance in which the client can perceive two pricks.

Figure 12–2 summarizes patterns of sensory loss. Sensory changes are part of the normal aging process. Careful assessment of such changes is the basis of nursing intervention for elderly clients. Table 12–2 is an assessment guide.

Reflex Activity

Muscles normally contract and relax promptly. This response can be elicited by striking a muscle with a reflex hammer. Reflex activity assessment provides information about the nature, location, and progression of neurologic disorders.

NORMAL REFLEXES

Two types of reflexes are normally present: (1) superficial, or cutaneous, reflexes and (2) deep tendon, or muscle-stretch, reflexes.

Superficial (Cutaneous) Reflexes. Superficial reflexes are elicited by cutaneous or mucous membrane stimulation. The stimulus is produced by stroking a sensory zone with an object that will not cause damage. Examples of superficial reflexes are the abdominal reflex, plantar reflex, corneal reflex, pharyngeal ("gag") reflex, and anal reflex.

Abdominal Reflex. Scratching the skin on an abdominal quadrant normally causes the abdominal muscle to contract in that quadrant, and the umbilicus moves toward the stimulated side.

Plantar Reflex. Scratching the foot's outer aspect of the plantar surface (outer sole) from the heel toward the toes normally causes the toes and sometimes the foot to contract or flex.

Corneal Reflex. Gently touching the cornea with a wisp of sterile cotton causes reflex blinking. (For example, to test the left eye, the nurse has the client look up and to the right and brings the cotton wisp in from the side so the client cannot see the hand. The nurse then very gently touches the outer edge of the cornea.)

CRITICAL TO REMEMBER

In an unconscious client, the corneal reflex can be tested by holding the eyelids open and placing a drop of sterile saline on the cornea.

This technique prevents inadvertent corneal abrasions.

Pharyngeal ("Gag") Reflex. Gentle stimulation with a tongue blade at the back of the throat and pharynx normally produces gagging. The corneal and pharyngeal reflexes are usually assessed with the cranial nerves, discussed later in this chapter.

Anal Reflex. The nurse stimulates the perianal skin or gently inserts a gloved finger into the rectum. Normal response is contraction of the rectal sphincter ("anal wink").

Deep Tendon (Muscle-Stretch) Reflexes. Deep tendon reflexes are also called muscle-stretch reflexes because reflex muscle contraction normally results from rapid stretching of the muscle. This is produced by striking a muscle's tendon of insertion sharply with a

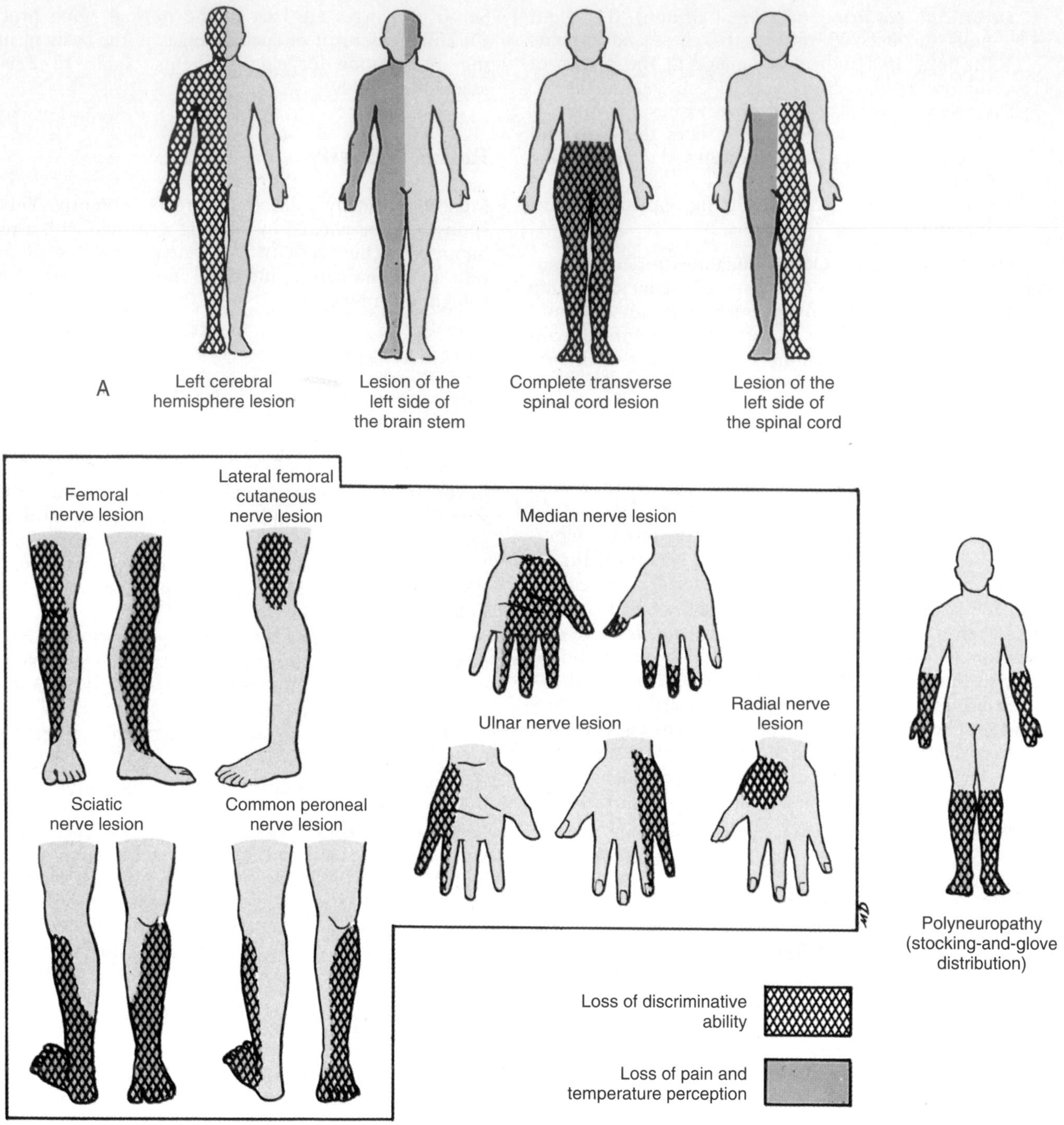

Figure 12–2
Patterns of sensory loss with brain and spinal cord disorders *(A)* and peripheral nerve lesions *(B)*.

sudden, brief blow using a reflex hammer (Fig. 12–3 and Box 12–1).

Reflex sites commonly assessed include the Achilles tendon, patella, biceps, and triceps.

- An *ankle jerk* (plantar flexion of the foot) is produced by tapping the Achilles tendon.
- A *knee jerk, quadriceps jerk,* or *patellar reflex* (leg extension) is produced by tapping the quadriceps femoris tendon just below the patella.
- A *biceps jerk* (forearm flexion) is produced by tapping the biceps brachii tendon.
- A *triceps jerk* (forearm extension) is produced by tapping the triceps brachii tendon at the elbow.

ABNORMAL REFLEXES

Pathologic (abnormal) reflexes are reflexes that do not normally occur. Their presence indicates neurologic

TABLE 12–2 Assessment of Neurologic Sensory Changes in the Elderly

SENSORY FUNCTION	ASSESSMENT TECHNIQUE	OBSERVATION
Hearing	Ask client questions using normal voice tone and volume. Vary position in relationship to client, such as face-to-face or facing away from client	Note client's response to direct questions when asked by examiner from the varying positions. Does client respond or not respond when face to face with examiner? When examiner's back is toward client?
	Rub thumb and index finger together lightly next to client's ear. Test each ear separately	Note client's ability to hear the sound in each ear, as well as discern the distance between examiner's fingers and client's ear
Vision (instruct client to wear corrective lenses, if usually worn)	*Acuity* Ask client to read from a newspaper, first with one eye then the other eye (instruct client to cover one eye then the other eye with hand), and second with both eyes together	Note client's ability to see regular size print versus the headlines and fine print. Note distance at which client holds printed material from eyes
	Color Ask client to identify colors from a color wheel containing red, orange, yellow, green, blue, and purple	Note client's ability to identify primary colors (red, yellow, blue) as well as inability to identify any color
	Peripheral Vision Instruct client to look straight ahead while examiner holds one finger on each side of client's head at eye level, just outside client's shoulder line	Note whether client can see both fingers. If one or no fingers is seen, visual deficit is present
	Depth Perception Ask client to identify which one of two objects is nearer (select two objects in the room)	Note client's ability to identify which object is nearer. Also note whether client is able to estimate the distance between the two objects accurately within 1 inch
Position sense (instruct client to keep eyes closed)	Instruct client to identify when various body parts are flexed or extended passively by the examiner. Test each arm (at shoulder), thumbs and index fingers (grasp at the sides), and legs (at hip). Ask client to identify whether body part is being flexed or extended	Note client's ability to identify whether a body part is being moved or not. Also note whether client can identify whether joint is being flexed or extended
Vibration (instruct client to keep eyes closed)	Ask client to identify when vibration is felt. Use a tuning fork, set it into vibration, and place on bony prominences. Begin at distal carpal and phalangeal joints and progress proximally to wrists and ankles, elbows and knees, and iliac crests and acromion processes. Alternate vibration with nonvibrating tuning fork	Note client's ability to identify vibration versus lack of vibration, as well as whether sensation is diminished or absent at distal joints. If vibration is felt at distal joints, more proximal joints are usually not tested
Temperature (instruct client to keep eyes closed)	Ask client to identify whether an object feels hot or cold when placed against the skin. Use two test tubes, one filled with hot water, the other with cold water. Place tubes in an alternating pattern against the hands then arms, as well as the feet then legs	Note client's ability to discriminate hot from cold. Also note whether client is able to identify both hot and cold distally as well as proximally, that is, below the elbow and knee versus above elbow and knee
Smell (instruct client to keep eyes closed)	Ask client to identify various aromas. Test each nare separately by instructing client to occlude one nare at a time with index finger. Use familiar smells such as instant coffee or chocolate	Note client's ability to identify various aromas accurately
Taste (instruct client to keep eyes closed)	Ask client to differentiate between two flavors of familiar foods with similar textures, such as two flavors of hard candy or a cracker and a firm cookie	Note client's ability to discriminate between two flavors as well as ability to identify the different flavors
Light touch (instruct client to keep eyes closed)	Brush client's skin lightly with cotton wisp over scattered areas including face, hands, arms, trunk, feet, and legs	Note client's ability to discriminate sensation of being touched, comparing one side to the other. Does client feel cotton on both sides, one side, or not at all?
Deep pressure	Gently squeeze client's Achilles tendons, calf muscles, and forearm muscles	Note whether client verbalizes discomfort and/or withdraws extremity

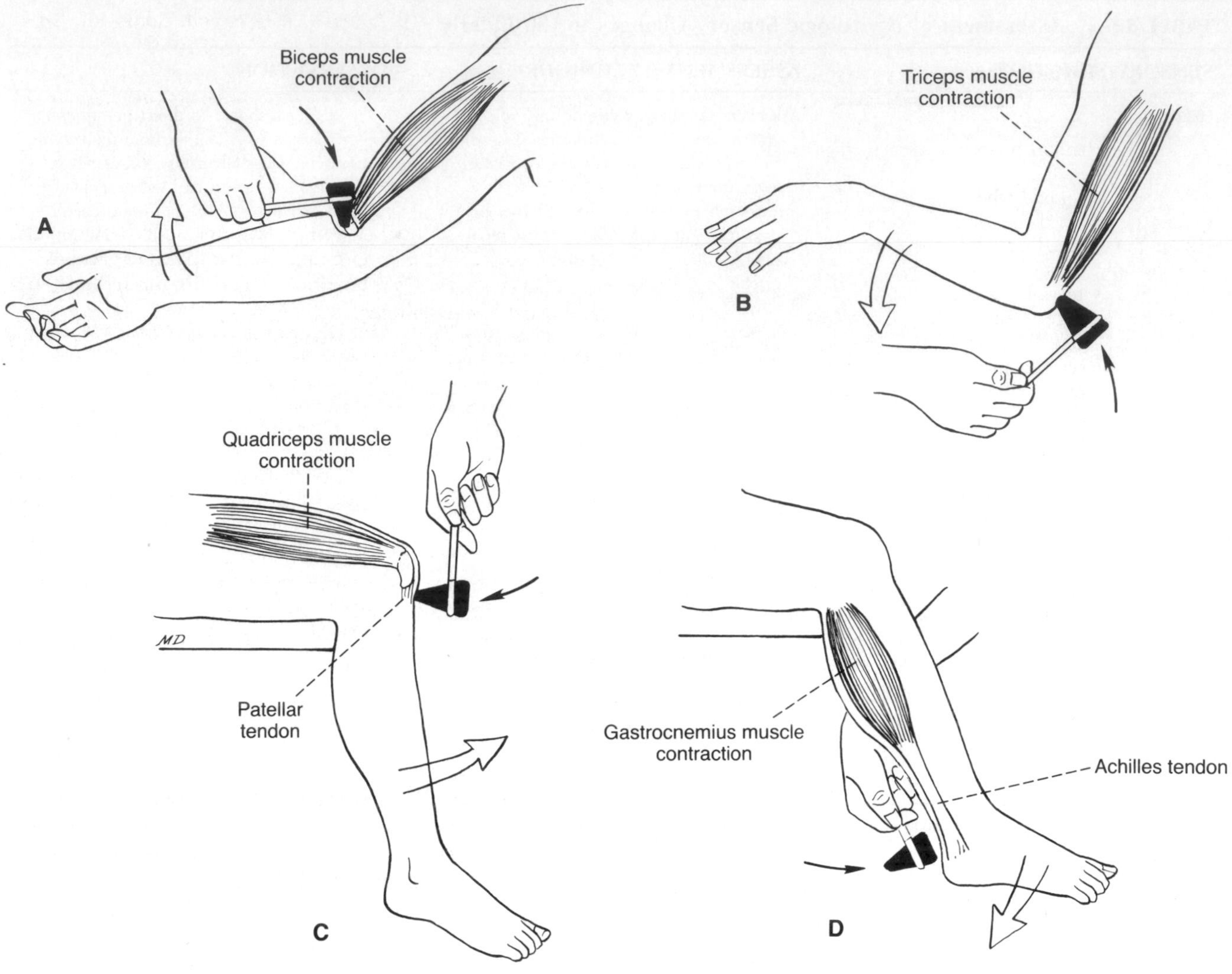

Figure 12–3
Deep tendon (muscle stretch) reflexes. *A,* Biceps jerk (C5–C6); *B,* triceps jerk (C7–C8); *C,* patellar reflexes (C5–C6); *D,* ankle jerk (L3–L4).

disorders, often related to the spinal cord or higher centers.

These responses include Babinski's, jaw, palm-chin (palmomental), clonus, snout, rooting, sucking, glabella, grasp, and chewing reflexes.

Babinski's Reflex. Babinski's reflex is tested by gently scraping the sole of the foot with a blunt point. To elicit Babinski's reflex, the stimulus should start at the midpoint of the heel and be carried upward and lateral along the outer border of the sole to the ball of the foot. The stimulus is then directed across the ball of the foot (without touching the toes) toward the medial side and off the foot. Alternatively, the stimulus is started at the midlateral sole and carried down toward the heel. A normal response (absent Babinski's reflex) is plantar flexion of the toes. An abnormal response (present Babinski's reflex) is dorsiflexion of the great toes and often fanning of the other toes (Fig. 12–4). In extreme circumstances, a present Babinski reflex may be accompanied by dorsiflexion of the foot at the ankle and flexion at the knee and hip.

When exaggerated deep reflexes are present, superficial reflexes are usually diminished or absent, and pathologic reflexes (e.g., Babinski's reflex) also exist.

Jaw Reflex. Jaw reflex, in which the jaw contracts and closes the mouth as a result of downward tapping on the lower jaw when the mouth is relaxed and passively hanging partially open, occurs rarely in healthy individuals but is noticeably present in some disorders, e.g., sclerosis of the lateral columns of the spinal cord. Jaw reflex is also called mandibular reflex or jaw jerk.

Palm-Chin (Palmomental) Reflex. Vigorous, rapid irritation on the mound of the palm at the thumb's base with a blunt instrument causes the chin muscles to pull up on the same side.

BOX 12-1

Guidelines for Assessment of Deep Tendon Reflexes

- Test deep tendon reflexes with the client either sitting or supine.
- Support the joint where the tendon is being tested so that the attached muscle is relaxed.
- Use the pointed end of a triangular reflex hammer to strike over small areas, such as the thumb placed over the biceps tendon. Use the flat end of the hammer to strike over larger areas, such as the Achilles tendon.
- Hold the reflex hammer loosely between the thumb and fingers so it can swing in an arc.
- Swing the reflex hammer using only wrist motion, not the arm or elbow.
- Tap the tendon briskly.
- Note the speed, force, and amplitude of reflex responses.
- Compare reflex responses bilaterally.
- Ask the client to perform isometric contraction of other muscles, which may increase the generalized reflex response.
- For the upper extremities, have the client either clench the teeth together or contract the quadriceps muscles (i.e., push the thighs against the table).
- For the lower extremities, have the client lock fingers together and try to pull them apart at the same time the tendon is tested.

Clonus. Clonus is rapidly alternating joint flexions and extensions, resulting from continuous rhythmic contractions of a stretched muscle. This is not like a normal stretch reflex, which typically produces one reflex action. With clonus, the action continues.

Snout Reflex. A brisk midline tap above or below the mouth results in pursing of the lips.

Rooting Reflex. Stroking the side of the face causes the mouth to open and the head to turn to the stimulated side.

Sucking Reflex. Touching the lips with a blunt object results in movement of the tongue, lips, and jaws.

Glabella Reflex. Tapping the forehead between the eyebrows results in sustained closure of the eyelids.

Grasp Reflex. Placing an object in the palm of the hand causes the fingers to curl around the object.

Chewing Reflex. A tongue blade placed between the teeth results in the jaws closing tightly.

GRADING REFLEX ACTIVITY

Superficial reflexes are graded 0 (absent), ± (slightly present), and + (normally active). Deep reflexes are graded from 0 through 4+; 2+ is normal. Although 1+ or 3+ responses are not considered normal, they may not be significant findings (Fig. 12–5). Asymmetric responses are much more significant. Abnormal reflexes may be present in both neurologic and metabolic disorders. Table 12–3 summarizes important reflexes.

Vital Signs

Neurologic disorders can cause life-threatening changes in a client's vital signs. An example is the classic triad of hypotension, bradycardia, and hypothermia seen in spinal cord injuries. Inadequate perfusion of vital organs may result from hypotension if the blood pressure is not supported.

Another example of a neurologically mediated change in vital signs is the rise in pulse pressure that accompanies a rise in intracranial pressure. The body

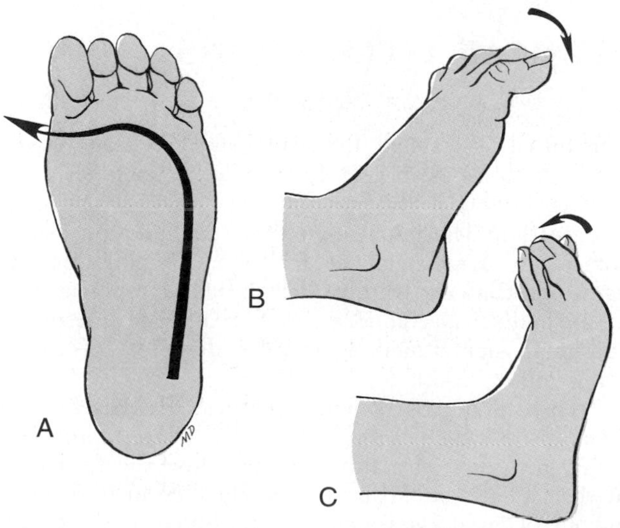

Figure 12–4
Babinski's response. *A,* Test maneuver: Scratch the sole of the foot as shown, using a blunt point. *B,* Normal response (absent Babinski's response) is plantar flexion of the toes. *C,* Abnormal response (present Babinski's response) is dorsiflexion of the big toe and often fanning of the other toes.

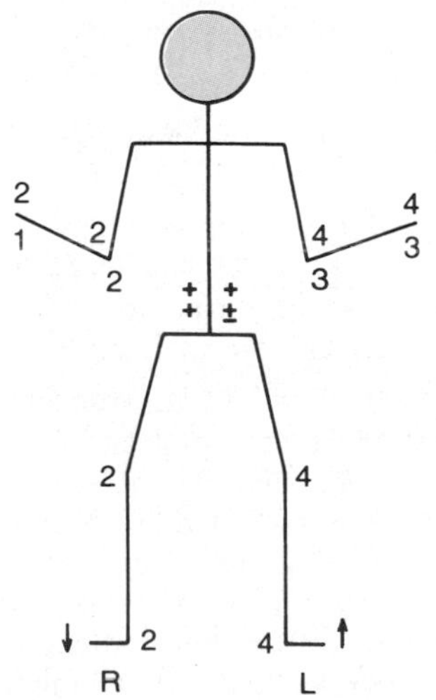

Figure 12–5
Documentation of muscle stretch and superficial reflexes in left hemiparesis. Muscle stretch reflex grades: grade 0, absent; grade 1, diminished; grade 2, normal; grade 3, brisker than normal; grade 4, hyperactive (clonus). Superficial reflex grades: grade 0, absent; grade ±, equivocal or barely present; grade +, normally active.

TABLE 12–3 Important Reflexes

REFLEX	METHOD	EFFECT	LOCALIZATION
Tendon Reflexes			
Biceps reflex	A blow on the examiner's thumb placed over the biceps tendon	Flexion of elbow	C5 and C6
Brachioradialis reflex (supinator)	Styloid process of radius is tapped while forearm is in semiflexion and semipronation	Flexion of elbow, fingers, and hand with supination of forearm	C5 and C6
Triceps reflex	Strike on triceps tendon just above the olecranon	Extension of elbow	C6 to C8 (C7 primarily)
Patellar reflex (knee jerk)	Tap on patellar tendon	Leg extends	L2 to L4
Achilles reflex (ankle jerk)	Tap on Achilles tendon	Plantar flexion of foot	S1 and S2
Superficial Reflexes			
Corneal reflex	Light touch at the corneoscleral junction	Closure of eyelids	CN V and CN VII
Palatal and pharyngeal reflexes	Light touch to soft palate and pharynx	Elevation of palate; gagging	CN IX and CN X
Abdominal reflexes	Stroke skin of upper, middle, and lower abdomen toward umbilicus	Contraction of abdominal wall toward stimulus	Upper—T7 to T9 Middle—T9 to T11 Lower—T11 to T12
Cremasteric reflex	Stroke medial surface of upper thigh	Elevation of scrotum and testicle	T12 to L2
Anal reflex	Stroke perianal region	Contraction of external anal sphincter	S3 to S5
Plantar reflex (normal)	Stroke sole of foot	Flexion of toes	L4 to S2
Plantar reflex (pathologic; Babinski's sign)	Stroke sole of foot	Dorsiflexion of great toe and fanning of other toes	L4 to S2

Adapted from Mitchell, P. A., et al. (1988). *AANN's neuroscience nursing: Phenomena and practice.* Norwalk, CT: Appleton & Lange.

attempts to provide adequate supplies of oxygen and glucose to the brain by increasing the blood flow to the brain to compensate for increased intracranial pressure. Changes in vital signs can indicate neurologic changes in clients in whom the neurologic examination has limited usefulness, such as in unresponsive clients or those who are pharmacologically paralyzed.

See Table 12–1 for an overall neurologic assessment guide.

FUNCTIONAL ASSESSMENT

A client with a neurologic disorder is usually experiencing problems that disrupt basic function either permanently or temporarily. The client's ability to cope effectively with activities of daily living (ability to meet basic needs) is often altered. For example, a client may have problems seeing, hearing, breathing, walking, talking, or eating. Remember that a client with a neurologic disorder may be frustrated just trying to do the things most people take for granted.

There are many tools for functional neurologic nursing assessment. They are based on the principle that the main purpose of nursing is to help clients cope effectively with changes (actual or potential) in daily living and self-care. The tools provide a systematic method of using daily observations that may become the basis for nursing intervention.

CLINICAL APPLICATIONS

The initial assessment for diagnosis and triage of the clients with a possible neurologic deficit includes a history, a brief physical examination, and a neurologic examination. The initial neurologic examination usually consists of assessment of the level of consciousness using the Glasgow coma scale, pupillary response, focal motor and sensory abnormalities in all four extremities, and brain stem function via assessment of corneal response (Box 12–2).

The initial assessment provides the baseline for comparison when serial assessments are completed. When recorded on a time-oriented flow sheet, changes in the client's status can be quickly identified. The frequency of serial assessment is determined by the client's diagnosis and may be as frequent as every 15 minutes. The nurse has an important responsibility to monitor the client's progress and report any unexpected deviations.

Thorough assessment and reporting of changes in a

BOX 12-2

The Initial Neurologic Examination

The sequence in which the neurologic examination is performed and the amount of time devoted to each section is dictated by the client's situation. For example, assessment of the head-injured client in the emergency room requires evaluation of vital signs, pupil reactivity, level of consciousness, and motor response. These clients may not be stable or cooperative enough for the nurse to complete the cranial nerve and sensory response assessment. Spinal cord–injured clients, however, are usually coherent and able to participate in the sensory examination. This information is essential for documenting changes in the status of spinal cord–injured clients.

As clients become more stable and cooperative, the examination can be performed in more depth and with less frequency. It should be remembered that neurologically impaired clients frequently experience fluctuations in status. This requires the nurse to alter the assessment schedule and technique to detect and report these fluctuations.

The following are suggested modifications in the screening neurologic examination based on the client's initial presentation.

- Initial examination for diagnosis and triage:
  - Client history based on chief complaint
  - Physical examination including vital signs
  - Level of consciousness
  - Pupil response
  - Brain stem function (corneal reflex)
  - Motor and sensory function in all four extremities
- If the client is conscious and stable:
  - Complete baseline neurologic examination
  - Focused examination at prescribed intervals
- If the client is conscious and unstable:
  - Quick baseline physical assessment
  - Frequent focused examinations until stable
  - Vital signs
  - Level of consciousness
  - Pupil response
  - Brain stem function
  - Motor and sensory function in extremities
  - Spinal cord function
- If the client is unconscious yet stable:
  - Vital signs
  - Level of consciousness and arousal
  - Cranial nerve function
  - Motor and sensory function
  - Pathologic reflexes
- If the client is unconscious and unstable:
  - Vital signs
  - Level of consciousness
  - Cranial nerve function
  - Motor and sensory function relative to the ability to test for these
  - Pathologic reflexes
  - Frequent focused examination on ongoing basis (hourly or more often)
- If the client is suspected to have spinal cord involvement:
  - Motor function in detail with testing of specific muscle groups
  - Sensory function
  - Reflexes
  - Bowel and bladder function
  - Vital signs

client serve a major role in determining the plan of care. Often, the client's current condition, for example, a decreased level of responsiveness and a change in pupillary reaction, is compared with initial data.

Because nurses are with clients continuously, it becomes the nurse's responsibility to develop sound assessment skills and recognize trends in the client's condition that warrant further care. In no other area of practice are subtle changes as important to detect and act on than in the care of the client with neurologic disorders.

DIAGNOSTIC TESTS

The complexity of the central nervous system combined with the relative inaccessibility of the brain requires indirect techniques to study it. Early techniques such as lumbar puncture, plain x-ray study, pneumoencephalography, and EEG have provided the foundation for new techniques that allow direct visualization of the brain structure, blood supply, and metabolism. Air contrast studies, such as pneumoencephalogram and ventriculogram, were performed for client assessment prior to the development of CT and magnetic resonance imaging (MRI). The nurse may find the results of these tests recorded in the history of a client who has had neurologic disorders for many years. These tests use air to provide contrast so that various portions of the brain can be viewed by x-ray study. The tests were painful and had potentially serious side effects. Today's neurodiagnostic studies are much safer for the client. The tests begin with the least invasive and move to the most invasive forms.

The focus of nursing care for the client undergoing a diagnostic assessment is centered on physical and psychological preparation for the study. The nurse also plans for the specific assessments that will need to be made after the study is completed, such as continued neurologic assessment. Prior to the study, the nurse should provide education to the client and family about the purpose of the study, the preparation needed, and the client's role during the test. The nurse may also have to assist the client to reduce anxiety about the test, and can usually reduce anxiety by providing information and answering questions.

After the diagnostic procedures have been performed, the nurse assesses the client for possible side effects and neurologic changes and assists the client to understand the results of the studies as needed.

Noninvasive Tests

SKULL AND SPINAL X-RAY STUDIES

Skull x-ray studies reveal the size and shape of the skull bones, suture separation in infants, fractures or bony defects, erosion, calcification, sella turcica erosion, and pineal gland shift (after age 12). Spinal x-ray studies show fractures, dislocation, compressions, curvature, erosion, narrowed spinal cord, and degenerative processes.

Nursing Intervention: Some clients with neurologic disorders require nursing support throughout an x-ray study, especially clients who are confused, combative, or dependent on a ventilator. If the client has a suspected spinal fracture, the neck is immobilized prior to moving the client to make the x-ray films. A lateral view of the cervical spine is taken first because the x-ray study can usually be taken with minimal movement to determine whether fractures have occurred. Metal items should be removed from the body parts that are undergoing the x-ray procedure, for example, barrettes. Nurses should document thick or heavy hair, because hair may affect interpretation of the x-ray film.

COMPUTED TOMOGRAPHY AND MAGNETIC RESONANCE IMAGING

Computed Tomography. The primary purpose of CT scans is to detect intracranial bleeding, space-occupying lesions, cerebral edema, and shifts of brain structures. Infarctions, hydrocephalus, and cerebral atrophy can also be identified. Aneurysms and arteriovenous malformations (AVMs) are best detected by angiogram. CT scans are completed by having x-ray beams pass through the brain in many slices to provide cross-sectional pictures (Fig. 12–6). The computer amplifies tissue density differences to visualize structures, such as bone, blood vessels, and tissues. CT scans can be performed with or without contrast.

The CT scan can be performed quickly—within about 20 minutes—not including data analysis. The radiation exposure from CT scans has been reduced to a level similar to that of a chest x-ray study. The results of the CT scan are usually recorded on x-ray film for a permanent record.

Nursing Intervention: Providing information about the CT scan is the major focus of nursing intervention. Prior to the test, the nurse should ascertain that informed consent has been obtained and answer any questions the client and family have about the CT scan.

Unless a contrast medium will be used, there are usually no dietary restrictions prior to the procedure. However, some physicians may restrict intake to liquids.

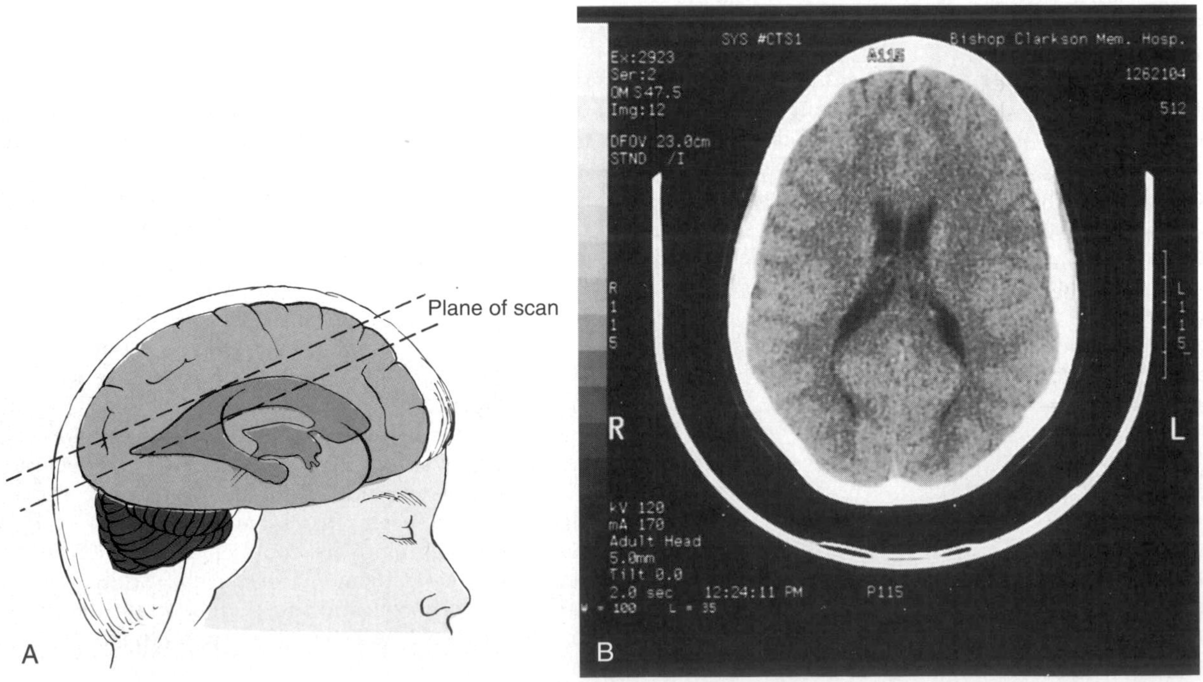

Figure 12–6
Computed tomographic scans are taken at various cross sections of the brain. *A*, Cross section used for the scan shown in part *B*.

The nurse should explain that a contrast agent is often given. Because the agent (also called dye) is iodine-based, ask whether the client has known allergies to iodine, contrast dyes, or shellfish. (See the section on the use of contrast.)

The nurse removes all objects from the head before the examination, including wigs, barrettes, earrings, and hair pins. The client's hair should be combed smoothly.

The client's role in the scan should be explained. The client will be positioned supine and the head placed into the donut-shaped ring of the scanner. The table is moved by the technologist from a control room during the scan to direct the study toward different levels of the head. The client should expect to hear mechanical noises coming from the scanner as it scans. Some clients will feel claustrophobic during the test but should be assured that it is possible to communicate with the technologist during the scan. Finally, the client will be asked to remain still during the scan. If the client is unable to comply, sedation, or even general anesthesia, may be required.

Following the test, the client should be assessed for reactions to contrast media as well as other specific assessments, such as presence of hematoma at the injection site and the quality of pulses in the extremity used to inject the dye. The client can resume normal activities, unless other diagnostic tests are planned. Diuresis from the dye should be expected.

Use of Contrast Agents. Certain pathologic conditions are better visualized with the use of a contrast agent. For example, tumors are better visualized with contrast, whereas bleeding and edema can be seen better without it. The use of the contrast agents is potentially dangerous. They may irritate blood vessels. Clients who are sensitive to contrast agents may have allergic reactions, and if untreated, these clients may develop anaphylactic shock.

The nurse should instruct the client that it is common to feel a hot, flushed sensation and a metallic taste in the mouth when the dye is injected. The client should report any difficulty breathing or pruritus (itching) to the personnel in the radiology department. After the procedure has been completed, the client can usually resume normal activities. Diuresis will occur shortly after the use of contrast agents. Replacement fluids may be needed, and the client should be assessed for fluid balance.

CRITICAL TO REMEMBER

The fluid balance in clients with renal or cardiac disease should be assessed carefully after a series of tests requiring intravenous contrast agents.

Complications rarely occur but may include local and systemic allergic reactions, spasm or occlusion of the vessels by a clot, and bleeding at the injection site. The nurse should assess the affected extremity for color, warmth, pulses distal to the injection site, bleeding or hematoma formation, and ability to move the site.

In addition, the nurse should assess the client for clinical manifestations of an allergic reaction, which include restlessness, tachypnea, respiratory distress, facial flushing, urticaria, nausea, and vomiting. The client should be assessed for these reactions after the dye is injected, because clients have had respiratory and cardiac arrests while undergoing x-ray study. Emergency equipment always should be available.

Magnetic Resonance Imaging. This procedure is a diagnostic tool similar to CT. The advantages are that MRI provides much more anatomically detailed pictures than are provided by a CT scan, and it does not have the associated radiation exposure. In fact, the MRI images look strikingly like anatomic slices of the brain. An MRI uses powerful magnetic fields and radio frequency pulses to produce an image; therefore, the client is not exposed to ionizing radiation. The magnet in the scanner is 30,000 times more powerful than the earth's magnetic field. A contrast agent is often used to augment the images (Fig. 12–7).

Nursing Intervention: The client and family should be taught about the purpose of the test, the sensations that the client will hear and feel during the examination, and the client's role during the test.

Prior to the test, the client should remove all metal-containing objects, such as the bra, jewelry, and watches. Such objects may be drawn into the magnetic field by the powerful magnet and become harmful projectiles. Any internal metal objects should be noted for the physician, such as prostheses and pacemakers. Intravenous fluid pumps need to be removed from the client during the test. Special precautions are needed for clients with pulse oximeters. The cord from the sensor to the finger cannot be coiled around the body or any body part because it may cause a burn.

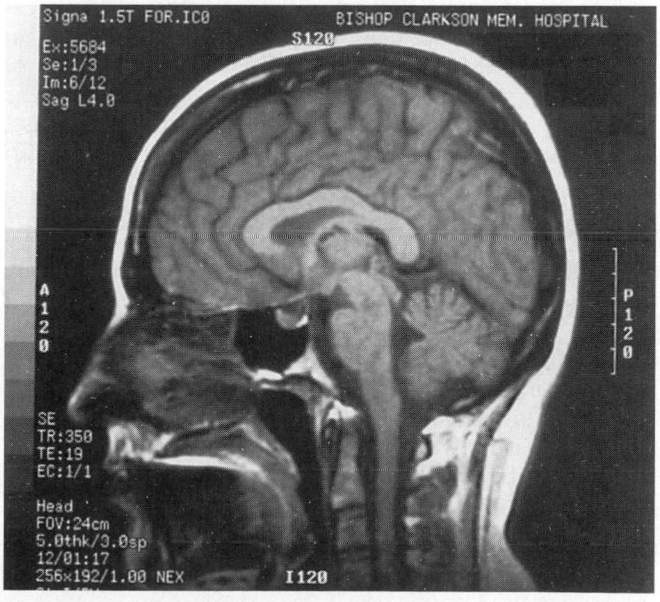

Figure 12–7
Normal magnetic resonance image. Sagittal section showing cerebrum, ventricles, cerebellum, and medulla of the brain.

Normally, the client can eat and take any prescribed medication prior to the examination. If the use of a contrast agent is planned, the nurse should ask whether the client tends to become nauseated easily and should adjust the intake of food and fluids accordingly. For example, some clients prefer a light breakfast to reduce nausea and others prefer to have an empty stomach.

The client lies supine on a padded table and moves through the imager. The client is asked to lie still while the test is in progress. There are tapping noises from the scanner while the images are being taken. Some clients feel claustrophobic during the test but should be assured that it is possible to communicate with the technologist during the scan. The examination takes about an hour. Following the test, the client can resume previous activities. Diuresis can be expected if a contrast agent was used.

Clinical Aspects of Computed Tomography and Magnetic Resonance Imaging. The ability to clearly visualize the brain with the use of the CT scan and MRI has been a significant step in the care of the client with neurologic disorders. The specific location of tumors and areas of bleeding has allowed neurosurgeons greater precision with surgical procedures. Other disorders such as multiple sclerosis can be diagnosed with the aid of the CT and MRI scans.

POSITRON-EMISSION TOMOGRAPHY

Positron-emission tomography (PET) allows the visualization of physiologic function in body areas. Often, the function of diseased tissue is different from that of normal tissues. The client is given doses of strong radioactive tracers, and the high concentration of tracers creates signals that are picked up by a scanner. The tracers, although potent, have a very short half-life, which makes their use safe. PET can be used to measure cerebral blood flow, cerebral glucose metabolism, and oxygen extraction. It is used in the diagnosis of stroke, brain tumors, and epilepsy, and to chart the progress of Alzheimer's disease, Parkinson's disease, head injury, schizophrenia, and manic-depressive illness.

One major disadvantage is that PET is expensive. It requires its own positron to manufacture high-energy radioactive tracers; a system can cost 5 million dollars initially. As a result of the cost of PET, a modification of the test has been developed. It is called a single photon emission computed tomography. This test uses less precise but more stable and more readily available isotopes to measure cerebral blood flow rather than metabolic activity, as is measured with PET. The test appears to be an effective diagnostic tool.

Nursing Intervention: The client and family should be informed about the purpose of the test, the sensations that the client will hear and feel during the examination, and the client's role during the test. In contrast to CT and MRI, the PET scanner is absolutely quiet. Clients need to fast for 4 hours prior to the scan. If the client is diabetic, it is preferred that the blood sugar be below 150 g/dL. Clients who are agitated may require sedation prior to the scan.

ELECTROENCEPHALOGRAM

An EEG is a measurement of the electrical activity of the superficial layers of the cerebral cortex. It demonstrates the electrical potentials from neuron activity within the brain in the form of wave patterns.

Electrodes are attached to the client's scalp (Fig. 12–8). The waveforms are amplified and recorded on a moving paper strip, similar to an electrocardiogram. EEGs are interpreted according to brain wave characteristics, frequency, and amplitude.

Brain activity as recorded on an EEG correlates with the cerebral blood flow. A constant supply of oxygen, blood, and glucose is needed to meet the metabolic demands of the brain. Decreased cerebral blood flow causes cerebral hypoxia and causes changes in mentation and decreased electrical activity on the EEG. EEG can detect hypoxia in the brain prior to permanent damage to cerebral tissues.

If the client is comatose or unable to be moved, EEG can be performed at the bedside. For routine diagnostic examination, the client is taken to an EEG laboratory for a more controlled environment. The client's scalp is cleaned, and electrodes are applied to the scalp and earlobe (for reference) with collodion. Leads can also be placed in the nasopharynx to assess disorders in the temporal lobe. The first portion of the test is performed with the client as relaxed as possible to obtain a baseline recording. Further readings are taken while the client is hyperventilating, sleeping, or viewing flickering lights. Hyperventilation alters acid-base balance (respiratory alkalosis) and decreases cerebral blood flow. Flickering lights may trigger seizures. Sleep may evoke abnormal EEG patterns not present while the client is awake. The client may be kept awake the night preceding the test or sedated to induce sleep.

An EEG is useful in assessing clients with any type of seizure disorder. An EEG is diffusely abnormal in various metabolic disturbances, toxic conditions (e.g., drug overdose), coma, organic brain syndrome, and in-

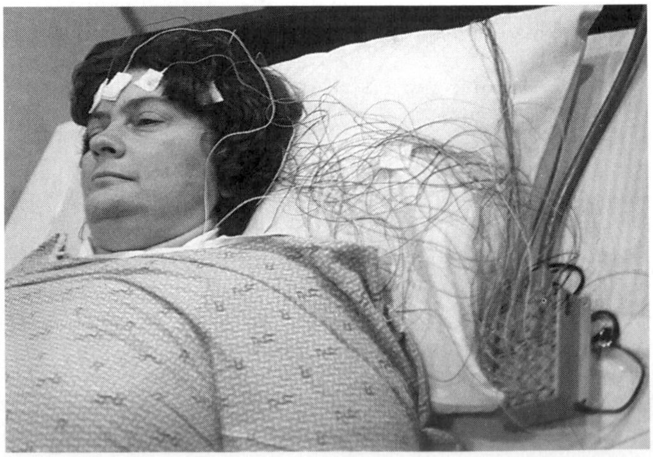

Figure 12–8
Client undergoing electroencephalography.

fections such as meningitis and encephalitis. The EEG may be used in the operating room to monitor cerebral activity during surgery on the blood vessels in the head or neck. Sleep patterns in depressed clients may also be assessed with EEGs. Some clients are assessed for temporal lobe epilepsy with the use of a 24-hour EEG recording.

Absence of EEG waves (flat lines) on EEG is one of the criteria for defining brain death. Studies on comatose patients show that findings of the EEG have a high correlation with the survival or death of the client in a coma.

Nursing Intervention: The purpose of the test and the procedure should be explained to the client and significant others, who may need to be reassured that electricity does not enter the brain (shock is not given) and the machine is not able to read the mind. Before the EEG is performed, the client's hair must be shampooed. Stimulants, (e.g., coffee, alcohol, tea, cola, and cigarettes), antidepressants, tranquilizers, and anticonvulsants should be avoided for 24 to 48 hours prior to the test. Normal meals should be consumed because a lowered serum glucose will alter the test results. If the client will be asked to sleep for a portion of the test, sleep should be minimized the night before the test. The client will be asked to relax during the test, because anxiety can block alpha rhythms and produce artifacts from increased muscle tone in the head and neck. The nurse should be sure to send adequate supplies (i.e., intravenous fluids or oxygen) to the laboratory.

If the EEG is being performed to evaluate the possibility of brain death, it is important to keep artifacts to a minimum. Artifacts can be caused by the manipulation of electrodes, electrical interference, cycling of respirators, and even walking in the room. Institutional guidelines should be followed for the avoidance of artifacts when EEG is performed at the client's bedside.

Following the EEG, the client can resume previous activity, medications, and diet. If seizure activity is possible, seizure precautions need to be followed. The hair can be washed and acetone may be required to remove the collodion from the scalp and hair.

EVOKED POTENTIAL STUDIES

Evoked potential (EP) studies are a form of EEG in which the client's brain waves are monitored as the client is given various stimuli. The test is used to assess the function of the cerebral hemispheres and the brain stem. A variety of types of stimuli are used, such as auditory, somatosensory, and visual. Typical stimuli include flashing lights, buzzing tones, and peripheral nerve stimulation. EP can be used to assess blindness, deafness, and brain stem injury. EP studies are carried out in the same fashion as EEGs. EP studies can detect abnormalities even if the client is sedated or paralyzed with neuromuscular blocking agents. Some clinicians believe that EP studies are more reliable than clinical assessments in predicting neurologic recovery in comatose head-injured clients.

Nursing interventions are the same as for the client undergoing an EEG, except in the explanation of the variations between the tests.

Invasive Tests

LUMBAR PUNCTURE

A lumbar puncture (LP, or spinal tap) is the insertion of a needle into the subarachnoid space in the lumbar region of the spine below the level of the spinal cord. Cerebral spinal fluid can be withdrawn or substances can be injected into this space.

LP is performed for assessment and therapeutic purposes. LP enables assessment of cerebrospinal fluid (CSF) pressure and collection of CSF for evaluation. When meningitis or subarachnoid hemorrhage is suspected, the CSF is examined for white blood cells and blood.

Therapeutically, LP is used to administer spinal medications and anesthetics.

Even though LP is generally a safe procedure, it does have some potential hazards. The procedure can be uncomfortable for the client. The client will feel pressure in the lower back and may experience pain if a nerve root is touched with the needle during insertion. The potential complications of LP are CSF leakage (see spinal headache), infection, intervertebral disc damage, and herniation of the brain due to increased intracranial pressure. A space-occupying lesion within the cranium, such as a tumor or bleeding, increases intracranial pressure. Therefore, LP is not performed in clients with papilledema (a sign of increased intracranial pressure), suspected intracranial lesions, or increased intracranial pressure or infection of the skin at the puncture site. CT scans are used in these clients to rule out masses before a LP is performed. If an LP were performed in clients with increased intracranial pressure, there would be a rapid decrease in pressure within the CSF around the spinal cord. This change in pressure might allow the structures within the brain to drop (herniate) into the spinal canal. The process of herniation creates pressure on the vital centers in the medulla (cardiac and respiratory centers) and could cause sudden death.

Nursing Intervention:

Prior to Procedure. The client and the significant others need to be taught about the purpose of lumbar puncture, the sensations that the client will feel during the examination, and the client's role during the examination. An informed consent form must be signed by the client prior to the test. The bladder and bowels should be emptied, if possible. It is important for the client to lie still during the test.

The necessary equipment should be assembled in the client's room. Spinal tap trays are available, which contain all needed equipment. In addition, the nurse should have laboratory request forms and a marking pencil to label the bottles of spinal fluid.

During the Procedure. The nurse assists in positioning the client as follows: (LP to remove a sample of

CSF is described here. The same general principles apply to any LP procedure, however.)

Position the client on the side (lateral recumbent) with the back close to the edge of the bed. Place a pillow under the flank so that the spinous processes are horizontal. Use additional pillows between the client's knees and under the head to keep the spine horizontal. Ask the client to draw the knees up to the abdomen and chin onto the chest (Fig. 12–9). Help the client maintain this curved position to separate and increase spaces between the vertebrae so that the needle can be inserted more easily. Stand in front of the client and place one hand behind the client's knees and the other around the neck. Keep the client's upper shoulder from falling forward, thus preventing rotation of the spine. (An alternative position is with the person sitting up with head and chest bent toward the knees.)

After a local anesthetic is given, a needle will be placed into the space between the vertebrae in the lower back. The needle is inserted well below the end of the spinal cord, so there is no danger of paralysis. A little local pain may occur as the needle passes the dura mater. The client should be asked to mention additional discomfort because it may indicate misplacement of the needle.

When the needle has entered the subarachnoid space, the physician removes the stylus and attaches a stopcock and manometer. A manometer measures CSF pressure.

Specimens of CSF are collected in a series of small sterile test tubes, numbered in sequence of collection (e.g., No. 1, No. 2). Two to three mL of CSF are collected in each tube; 8 to 10 mL may be removed. The needle is withdrawn, and a dry sterile dressing is placed over the puncture site.

In adults, CSF is assessed for cells, chloride, glucose, protein, pressure, and lactate dehydrogenase. Table 12–4 lists common abnormalities of CSF. The first vial of CSF obtained is not assessed for blood because it may contain blood from the puncture.

Following the Procedure. Vital signs should be recorded after an LP. The client can eat and drink, as was done prior to the test. Forcing fluids will help restore CSF volume. If the CSF measurement indicated a high intracranial pressure, the client should be assessed for decreasing levels of consciousness, which indicates increasing intracranial pressure.

Postlumbar puncture headache (spinal puncture headache, spinal headache) is typically throbbing, bifrontal, and suboccipital, developing a few hours to

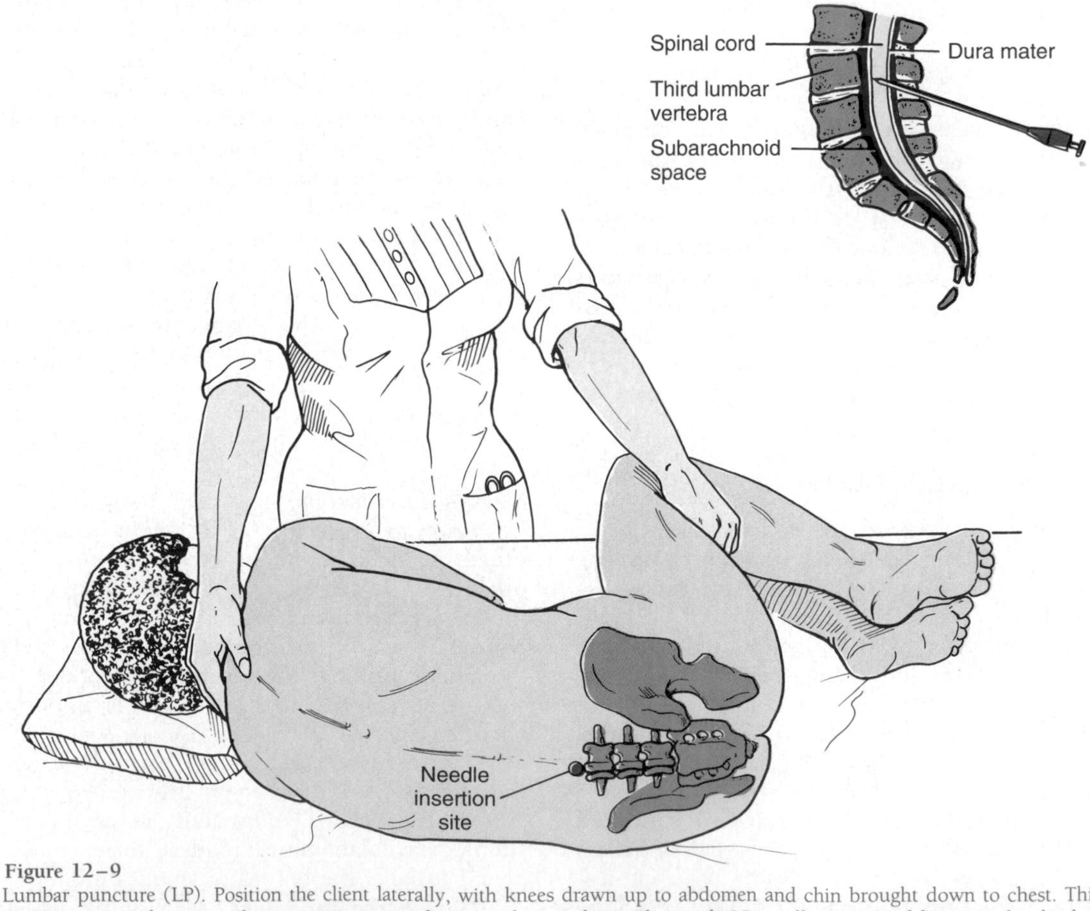

Figure 12–9
Lumbar puncture (LP). Position the client laterally, with knees drawn up to abdomen and chin brought down to chest. This position curves the spine, thus increasing space between the vertebrae. The sterile LP needle is inserted between the third and fourth (or fourth and fifth) vertebrae and enters the subarachnoid space.

TABLE 12–4 Normal Cerebrospinal Fluid Values and Significance of Abnormal Values

SUBSTANCE	NORMAL VALUE (CONVENTIONAL UNITS)	SIGNIFICANCE OF ABNORMAL VALUES
Blood	None; CSF should be clear	Gross blood is seen in central nervous system hemorrhage. Rarely, there are some blood cells in the first tube of CSF collected, because of trauma during the tap. The collection of specimens in sequence should be marked, so that it is possible to determine whether the blood in the first tube is more than the last tube. If the CSF is grossly bloody, other tests may not be able to be performed
Cells	0 to 5 mononuclear	Increased neutrophils may be seen in bacterial infections such as bacterial meningitis. Lymphocytes may be increased in tuberculosis and some viral disorders
Enzymes (lactate dehydrogenase)	10% of serum level	Elevated with inflammations and bacterial meningitis
Glucose	50 to 75 mg/DL, should be 20 mg less than serum glucose level	Glucose level is lowered in bacterial infections because bacteria use sugar. Some types of tumors also lower CSF glucose. Be certain to compare CSF glucose with serum glucose. Ideally, a serum specimen should be drawn 30 minutes before a lumbar puncture, because it takes glucose about 30 to 60 minutes to diffuse into the CSF
Protein Albumin	15 to 45 mg/dL 29.5 mg/dL (80%)	Increased proteins may be seen in degenerative disorders and brain tumors. Lesions that interrupt the blood-brain barrier also increase proteins because there is an increased diffusion from the blood into the brain tissues
Immunoglobulin G Oligoclonal bands	<14% of total protein Absent	Immunoglobulin G and oligoclonal bands (an abnormal type of protein band seen on immunoelectrophoresis) are often present in multiple sclerosis and neurosyphilis
Pressure	70 to 180 mm H_2O	Elevated in bacterial meningitis, cerebral bleeding, and tumors. Decreased in conditions that obstruct CSF flow, such as tumors of the spinal canal

CSF, cerebrospinal fluid

several days after an LP. The headache is probably caused by continuing CSF leakage through the opening in the dura made by the needle. The headache is usually relieved when the client lies down and is made worse by sitting up or a sudden jolt of the head. Such headaches usually disappear within 24 hours but may last for several days.

To reduce the risk of postlumbar puncture headache, the client should remain in bed following the examination. Although physician's orders may differ on the length of time, an average time in bed is 3 hours. Fluids should be encouraged to replace the CSF withdrawn during the test. Once a headache begins, treatments may include bed rest in a dark, quiet room, and the administration of analgesics and fluids. If the headache continues, an epidural blood patch may be required. Blood is withdrawn from the client and injected into the epidural space, usually at the LP site. The blood acts as a fibrin patch to seal the hole in the dura and prevent further CSF leakage. Blood patches cannot be performed when the client has bleeding tendencies or infection at the puncture site.

MYELOGRAPHY

Myelography is an x-ray examination of the spinal cord and vertebral canal following introduction of a contrast medium into the spinal subarachnoid space (Fig. 12–10). It is used to study the spinal canal and subarachnoid space. This study is a particularly valuable assessment tool when the spinal cord is thought to be compressed by a herniated intervertebral disc or a tumor encroaching on the spinal subarachnoid space. Myelography is also useful in diagnosing such spinal cord pathology as intramedullary tumors, syringomyelia, and AVMs.

Preparation for a myelogram includes hydration for at least 12 hours before the procedure. In the radiology department, a lumbar puncture is performed, a small amount of CSF is withdrawn, and the contrast material is injected. With the needle in place, the client is turned on the abdomen and secured to the table by foot and shoulder supports. While the radiologist follows carefully with fluoroscopy, the table is slowly tilted. This procedure causes the column of dye to move up or down within the subarachnoid space, permitting visualization of the desired areas. Standard films are taken of these areas. If metrizamide (a water-soluble medium) is used, it mixes with the CSF and cannot be removed. However, if iophendylate (an oil-based medium) is used, the solution is withdrawn after the films are obtained.

Nursing Intervention: Following the myelogram, the client may have to remain flat in bed or with the head

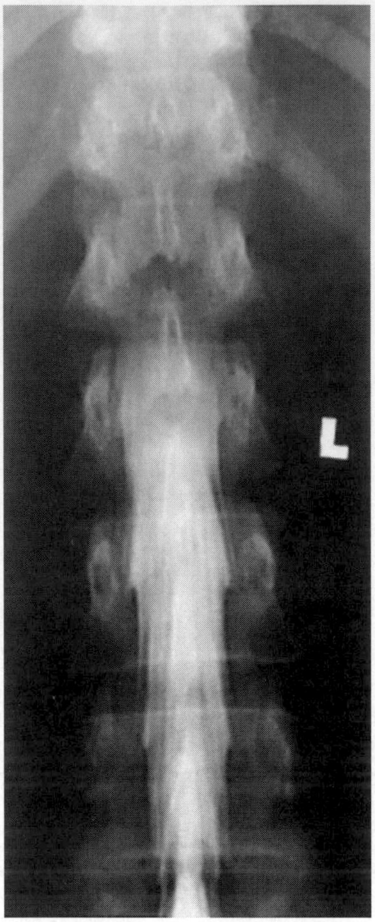

Figure 12–10
Myelogram of lumbar spine shows contrast material flowing throughout subarachnoid space without obstruction.

of the bed elevated 15 to 30 degrees, depending on the type of dye used. Usually, the client remains in bed 6 to 8 hours and then resumes normal activity. The nurse should encourage the person to take extra fluids and should assess neurologic status frequently. Back pain (ranging from mild discomfort to severe pain) in the area of the needle insertion may develop and may last a few days. Also, the client may experience a stiff neck and headache for a few days, particularly if the contrast medium was allowed to rise to high cervical levels. This discomfort is usually relieved by the client's lying flat and taking fluids and analgesics. (See also nursing intervention for LP.)

CISTERNAL PUNCTURE

When access to the CSF cannot be made by LP, cisternal puncture may be used. Cisternal puncture is puncture of the cisterna magna (a small reservoir of CSF between the cerebellum and medulla). Cisternal puncture is performed either to drain CSF or to obtain a CSF specimen when there is a block in the spinal subarachnoid space or if LP is contraindicated. If the client has a lesion on the spinal cord, the top edge of the lesion can be determined by means of contrast, with the agent injected via the cisternal puncture.

The nurse positions the client at the edge of a treatment table or bed, lying on the side with a sandbag under the head to keep the cervical spine and head straight with the thoracic spine. The client's head is flexed forward and held firmly in position. Following skin preparation, local anesthetic may or may not be injected. A cisternal needle with stylet in place is inserted to a depth of about 5 cm.

Subsequent assessments and interventions are essentially the same as with LP.

CEREBRAL ANGIOGRAPHY

A cerebral angiogram is the injection of a contrast medium into an artery to visualize intracranial circulation (Fig. 12–11). Angiography is the procedure used most often to visualize aneurysms, AVMs, major vessel displacement, vascular occlusion, and thrombi. Not only is cerebral angiography an invasive procedure, but it is a test in which small errors can result in permanent disability or death. Meticulous attention must be given to the client before, during, and following angiography.

The procedure is performed by inserting a catheter (a soft needle) into the femoral artery and then guiding the catheter through the use of a fluoroscope into the carotid-vertebral arteries. Once the vessels are reached, the contrast agent is injected and a series of x-ray studies are taken. Sequential views of the vessels show the movement of the dye in the vessels. After the catheter is removed, a sterile dressing is placed over the puncture site and firm pressure is applied to the site for 10 minutes to prevent hematoma formation. Sandbags and a pressure dressing may be used to provide firm pressure. Ice bags may also be used to provide pressure and relieve tenderness. The injection site may be tender.

Interventional Angiography. Interventional angiography is a recent advance in client care. This technique uses a polymer glue or Gelfoam (a material that stops bleeding) to occlude feeding vessels in tumors or AVMs.

Digital Venous Angiography. Computerized digital video subtraction systems allow visualization of vascular structures. Much less contrast material is required than for cerebral angiography. A central venous line is necessary to inject the contrast medium. The nurse instructs the client to be well hydrated and take no solid food for 2 hours before the procedure. Three to four venous injections are usually required for a complete diagnostic craniocerebral study. The only potential complication is a reaction to the contrast material.

Pancerebral Angiography. Pancerebral angiography is a technique used to assess cerebral blood flow through the four major blood vessels. This test may be given to patients who have received high doses of barbiturates as part of their treatment and in whom it is difficult to determine cerebral perfusion. The lack of intracranial blood flow through the four major vessels is an absolute indication of brain death.

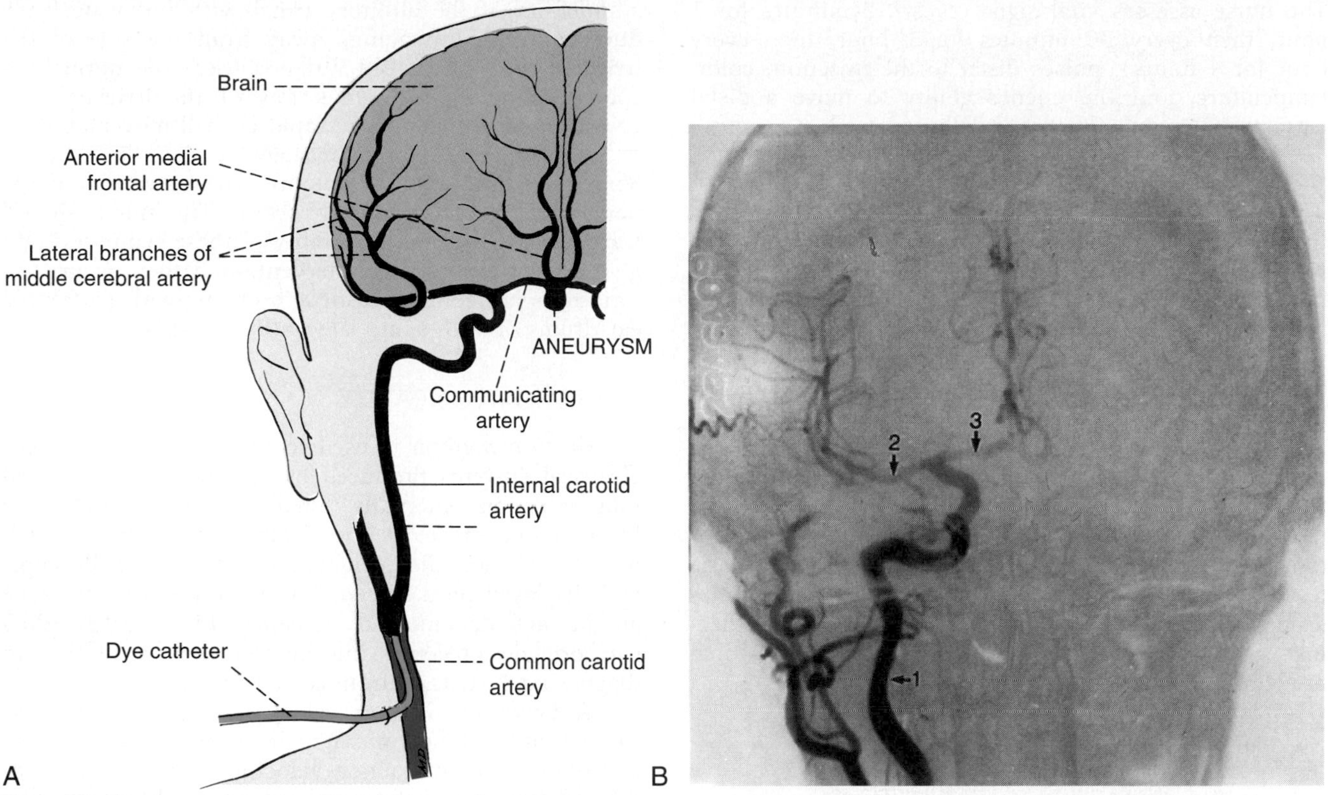

Figure 12–11
Cerebral angiography allows x-ray visualization of the brain's vascular system when a contrast dye is injected arterially. *A*, Insertion of dye through a catheter in the common carotid artery. The dye subsequently outlines vessels of the brain. *B*, Angiogram using subtraction technique. *1*, Internal carotid, *2*, middle cerebral, and *3*, middle meningeal arteries.

Nursing Intervention: The client and significant others should be informed about the purpose of the test, the sensations that the client will experience during the test, and the client's role during the procedure. Prior to the test, the client may not take anything by mouth for 4 to 6 hours but should be well hydrated prior to that time. Intravenous fluids may be prescribed. The nurse should document the neurologic status of the client to serve as a baseline after the examination. The client should remove metal items from the hair, such as barrettes, and earrings. Allergies to iodine should be reported. During the test, the client will be given an injection of local anesthetic prior to the placement of the catheter. There will also be a warm flushed feeling when the dye is injected. (See also the section entitled "The Use of Contrast Dye.") While the angiogram is being conducted, the client is continually assessed for neurologic deterioration.

Following the test, the nurse must assess the client closely for complications. Complications are rare but include (1) local and systemic allergic reactions to the contrast dye, (2) spasm or occlusion of the vessel by a clot, (3) hemorrhage, and (4) obstructive clot formation above a femoral injection site. The nurse assesses for reactions to the contrast dye. Spasm or occlusion of the target vessels causes symptoms similar to those of a stroke. (Stroke, or cerebral vascular accident, is discussed in Chap. 14.) Clot formation at the injection site also causes ischemic reactions in the affected area. These adverse reactions are usually reversible, and rarely cause permanent damage.

Potential complications vary, depending on their cause. For example, indications of centrally located reactions may include changes in LOC, aphasia, hemiplegia, hemiparesis, convulsive seizures, or increased focal symptoms. A hematoma in the neck may cause difficulty in breathing or swallowing. If it is large, it may compress the trachea and esophagus, requiring emergency tracheostomy. Nausea, vomiting, extremity numbness or weakness, speech disturbances, profuse sweating, and alterations in LOC may indicate a delayed reaction to the contrast material.

Following angiography, the client should be positioned safely and comfortably and maintain bed rest for as long as prescribed (often about 12 hours).

CRITICAL TO REMEMBER

The nurse should check the injection site frequently for bleeding and hematoma formation. The affected extremity (arm or leg) or neck must be kept straight to prevent kinking the vessel and clot formation.

The nurse assesses vital signs (every 15 minutes for 1 hour, then every 30 minutes for 1 hour, then every hour for 4 hours), pulses distal to the injection, color, temperature, and the client's ability to move a distal extremity. A regular diet is usually resumed.

CEREBRAL PERFUSION STUDIES

Cerebral perfusion can be assessed when brain death is suspected. The patient is injected with technetium, a radioactive substance. The ability of the substance to perfuse from blood vessels into brain tissue is assessed with a scanner. In patients who are clinically brain dead, there is no uptake of the substance by the cerebrum or cerebellum. This test allows appropriate medical care to continue when brain death cannot be determined, and conversely, medical care can stop for those patients who are brain dead. The nurse's role in this test is supporting the client's significant others after they have been informed about the significance of the test and its findings. Once the patient is declared brain dead, it is the end of meaningful life. Significant others may need help accepting the results of this very final test.

CALORIC TESTING

The oculovestibular reflex, or caloric test, is a diagnostic examination providing information about the function of the vestibular portion of the eighth cranial nerve. It aids in the differential diagnosis of cerebellum and brain stem lesions (see also Chap. 13).

The test is performed by introducing either cold or hot water into the external auditory canal. A current then flows through the endolymphatic fluid. Typically, when the vestibular eighth cranial nerve is normal, stimulation of the auditory canal with hot water produces a rotary nystagmus away from the side of the irrigated ear. When cold water is used, the normal response is rotary nystagmus toward the irrigated ear. (Nystagmus is involuntary, rapid eyeball movement.)

If pathology exists, nystagmus does not occur. Sometimes unpleasant symptoms, such as vertigo, dizziness, nausea, and vomiting occur. The nurse should warn the client of the possibility of these symptoms and give supportive nursing intervention if they occur. Caloric tests are contraindicated in clients with perforated ear drums or with acute labyrinthine disease.

ELECTROMYOGRAPHY

An electromyograph is used to measure and document electrical currents produced by skeletal muscles, called muscle action potentials. Small needle electrodes are inserted into muscles. The electrical potentials of each muscle are amplified, transmitted to an oscilloscope, and displayed on a screen. The recording can be made audible and documented on paper (Fig. 12–12). EMG can provide objective information that is helpful in diagnosing various neuromuscular diseases.

A nerve conduction velocity study is often performed in conjunction with EMG, which studies the excitability and conduction velocities of motor and sensory nerves. It is helpful in diagnosing diseases of peripheral nerves. A stimulating electrode and a recording electrode are placed to test specific nerves (usually on a limb). The time required for the passage of a nerve impulse from the point of stimulation to the point of recording is measured precisely. Conduction velocity is calculated. Both motor and sensory modalities are altered in peripheral nervous system disorders (e.g., carpal tunnel syndrome), whereas only motor fibers are

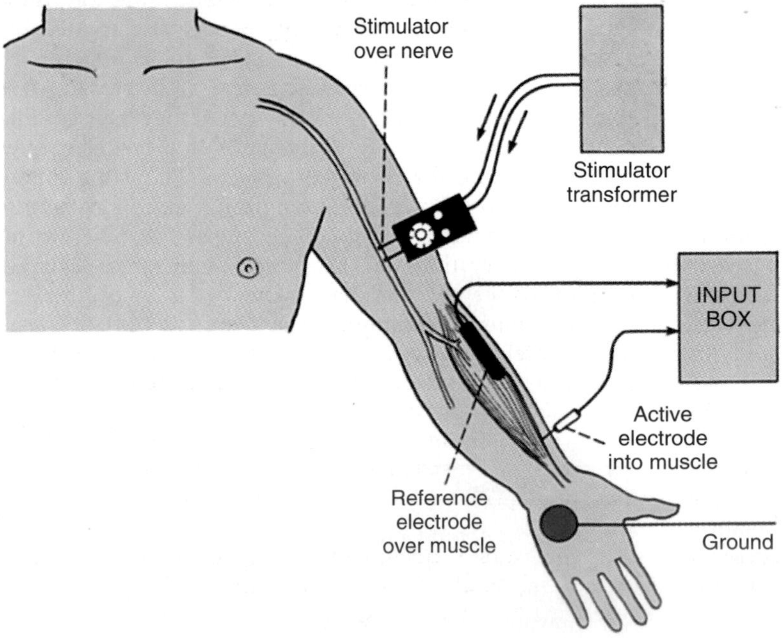

Figure 12–12
Electromyography measures and documents electrical currents produced by skeletal muscles. A stimulator is placed over the peripheral nerve being tested. A small pin is inserted into the muscle being assessed for innervation, and a ground is placed on the client's skin.

affected in chronic diseases of the anterior horn cell or motor nerve roots.

Nursing Intervention: The nurse explains the procedure to the client and significant others. They are often concerned about the outcome of the test and may be very anxious and stressed. The client should avoid all stimulants, depressants, or sedatives for 24 hours before the test. There may be discomfort when the electrodes are inserted. If many muscles are tested, there may be some residual discomfort. The client may experience a mild electrical shock during the procedure. The client lies flat and may be asked to move various muscles at specific times during the test.

CELLULAR ASSESSMENT

Chromosome analysis is used to (1) assist diagnosis of some abnormal neurologic conditions and (2) provide the basis for genetic counseling in families with evidence of congenital neurologic malformations. Chromosomes can be prepared for microscopic examination from tissue culture of cells obtained from peripheral blood, bone marrow, or skin.

Mental retardation and convulsive seizures may result from neurologic dysfunction associated with inborn errors of metabolism. Diagnosis of disorders of carbohydrate and lipid metabolism may require measurements of specific enzyme concentration in blood cells or tissue biopsied from brain, muscle, liver, or peripheral nerve. Usually, protein metabolism disorders are indicated by increased amounts of particular amino acids in the urine or blood.

NEUROPSYCHOLOGICAL TESTING

Neuropsychological testing involves a series of tests to evaluate the presence of cortical function and impairment by localizing the area and degree of impairment, and determining the rate of progression or recovery. The tests are sensitive to brain function and gauge many types of abilities (e.g., motor, perceptual, language, visual-spatial, cognitive).

With careful interpretation, inferences can be made about the extent of brain function impairment and the effect it may have on the client's ability to function. Results from the neuropsychological evaluations, clinical manifestations, neurologic examinations, and neurodiagnostic studies are correlated and used to predict the client's potential functioning in 6 months, 12 months, and so on.

Results of neuropsychological testing assist in the diagnosis of specific cognitive dysfunction and the development of an individualized rehabilitation program. Serial testing is valuable in monitoring rehabilitative progress and recovery in clients with problems such as head injury and epilepsy.

There is poor correlation between the degree of brain damage as revealed, for example, by CT scan and neuropsychological testing. A small lesion can create a large functional deficit, and in contrast, a large lesion may only cause small changes. There are even instances in which testing clearly demonstrates brain dysfunction in the absence of a demonstrable lesion on CT scan.

A client may be referred for neuropsychological assessment in the acute phase or months after an injury. For example, after a head injury in which the physical neuro-assessment is normal and the EEG reveals only mild generalized abnormalities, the client may complain of being unable to work because of persistent headaches. Recommendations from testing may be made about treatment, including educational and vocational rehabilitation.

Neuropsychological tests measure deficits in coping skills by assessing the skills directly. They may be helpful when deficits in adaptive abilities are suspected. An individual test may be performed in the case of a disorder with only one specific symptom, or a complete series of tests with extended evaluation may require several hours or days of testing. The client's level of performance is compared with scores that represent normal levels of performance. General measures of intelligence (e.g., Wechsler Adult Intelligence Scale) as well as tests for emotional and personal adjustment, such as the Minnesota Multiphasic Personality Inventory, are used.

Testing may be nonspecific in implicating the presence of brain damage or very narrow in scope, with sensitivity to certain areas of the brain. Results may indicate that something is wrong but not be able to identify the problem specifically.

Memory loss is common following head injury and in neurologic disorders. Skills such as reading, which have been stored in the brain over the years, may be retained in contrast to new learning or short-term memory, which may be impaired. The client's impaired memory may interfere with the nurse's ability to teach and the client's ability to learn. Knowing that a brain-injured client has damage to the limbic system or areas of the temporal and prefrontal lobe is a good indicator for neuropsychological testing to determine memory loss.

Testing will identify problems in cognitive, psychomotor, and affective domains. Left hemisphere lesions impair factual information functions like problem solving, decision making, and judgment. Teaching of the client and significant others must be modified to address these deficits.

Both the right and left hemispheres are involved with psychomotor learning, with the right hemisphere controlling visual and spatial abilities, and the left verbal instructions and sequencing of activities. Repetition and time are needed for the individual to perform activities automatically.

Memory loss diagnosed from damage to the right or left hemisphere causing affective learning deficits can be improved with role modeling, one-to-one, and group therapy.

The nurse's documentation of client behavior and functional abilities assists the neuropsychologist in following the individual's progress and recovery.

STUDY QUESTIONS

1. Damage to the prefrontal cortex of the frontal lobe may result in:
   A. Loss of movement on the contralateral side of the body
   B. Loss of auditory function
   C. Inability to interpret sensory information
   D. Difficulty with problem solving
2. In assessing pupillary reflex, the nurse should:
   A. Instruct the client to hold his or her breath
   B. Shine the light in both eyes simultaneously
   C. Approach the pupil from the temporal side while the client looks straight ahead
   D. Have the client focus on an object across the room and then look at the nurse's fingers
3. The nurse is assessing a client with a decreased level of consciousness. It would be most important for the nurse to document:
   A. The behavior exhibited by the client in response to a specific stimulus
   B. The presence of corneal reflexes
   C. The presence of pathologic reflexes
   D. By using descriptive terms such as stupor, obtunded, etc.
4. Which of the following positions should the nurse help the client to assume in preparation for a lumbar puncture?
   A. Lying on the stomach with the head turned to the right
   B. Lying on the side with the legs extended
   C. Lying on the side with the knees bent up and head bent forward
   D. Lying flat in the Trendelenburg position
5. A client with a seizure disorder is scheduled to undergo an electroencephalogram. Which of the following nursing actions is appropriate prior to the procedure?
   A. Assure the client that only a small amount of hair will be shaved
   B. Ask the client to avoid coffee, cigarettes, and alcohol
   C. Ask the client to empty his or her bladder
   D. Administer a mild sedative

CRITICAL THINKING EXERCISES

SCENARIO A

A 68-year-old client has experienced a stroke that involves both the parietal and temporal lobes on the left. As the nurse performs the initial neurologic assessment he or she anticipates neurologic dysfunction.

1. What dysfunctions are anticipated with damage to the parietal lobe?
2. What dysfunctions are anticipated with damage to the temporal lobe?
3. In general, how does the function of the left side of the brain differ from that of the right?

SCENARIO B

A 42-year-old client is scheduled for a magnetic resonance imaging (MRI) scan.

1. Describe the procedure as you would explain it to a client.
2. List the advantages and disadvantages of MRI.
3. Describe any client preparation required prior to the procedure.

BIBLIOGRAPHY

1. Barker, E., & Moore, K. (1992). Neurological assessment. *RN, 55(4),* 28–35.
2. Carnevali, D., & Patrick, M. (1993). *Nursing management of the elderly* (3rd ed.). Philadelphia: J. B. Lippincott.
3. Chipps, E., et al. (1992). *Neurological Disorders: C. V. Mosby's Clinical Nursing Series.* St. Louis, Mosby–Year Book.
4. el Mallakh, R. (1987). CSF evaluation in neurologic disease. *American Family Physician, 35(6),* 112–118.
5. Fuller, J., & Schaller-Ayers, J. (1994). *Health assessment: A nursing approach* (2nd ed.). Philadelphia: J. B. Lippincott.
6. Henneman, E. (1989). Clinical assessment and neurodiagnostics. *Critical Care Nursing Clinics of North America, 1(1),* 131–142.
7. Hickey, J. V. (1992). *The clinical practice of neurological and neurosurgical nursing* (3rd ed.). Philadelphia: J. B. Lippincott.
8. Jarvis, C. (1992). *Physical examination and health assessment.* Philadelphia: W. B. Saunders.
9. Lauren, N., et al. (1989). Cerebral perfusion imaging with technetium-99m HM-PAO in brain death and severe central nervous system injury. *Journal of Nuclear Medicine, 30(10),* 1627–1635.

10. Lower, J. (1992). Rapid neuroassessment. *American Journal of Nursing, 92(6),* 38–48.

11. Lundgren, J. (1990). Computerized EEG: Applications and interventions. *Journal of Neuroscience Nursing, 22(2),* 108–112.

12. Malasanos, L., et al. (1990). *Health assessment* (4th ed.). St. Louis: Mosby–Year Book.

13. Marshall, S., et al. (1990). *Neuroscience critical care.* Philadelphia: W. B. Saunders.

14. McDonagh, A. (1991). Getting your patient ready for a nuclear medicine scan. *Nursing 91, 21(2),* 53–57.

15. Morton, P. (1993). *Health assessment in nursing* (2nd ed). Philadelphia: F. A. Davis.

16. Norris, M., et al. (1989). Needle bevel direction and headache after inadvertent dural puncture. *Anesthesiology, 70(5),* 729–731.

17. Potter, P. & Perry, A. (1993). *Fundamentals of nursing. Concepts, process, and practice* (3rd ed.). St. Louis: Mosby–Year Book.

18. Reid, R., et al. (1989). Clinical use of technetium-99m HM-PAO for determination of brain death. *Journal of Nuclear Medicine, 30(10),* 1621–1626.

19. Rogers, A., & Dykstra, C. (1989). EEGs: A closer look at a familiar diagnostic test. *Journal of Neuroscience Nursing, 21(4),* 227–233.

20. Sand, T. (1989). Which factors affect reported headache incidence after lumbar myelography? A statistical analysis of publications in the literature. *Neuroradiology, 31(1),* 55–59.

21. Solomon, E. P., et al. (1990). *Human anatomy & physiology* (2nd ed.). Philadelphia: W. B. Saunders.

22. Swartz, M. H. (1994). *Textbook of physical diagnosis: History and examination* (2nd ed.). Philadelphia: W. B. Saunders.

23. Thomas, C. L. (Ed.) (1993). *Taber's cyclopedic medical dictionary* (17th ed.). Philadelphia: F. A. Davis.

Chapter 13

Nursing Care of Clients with a Loss of Protective Function

Learning Outcomes

After completing this chapter, the learner will be able to:

1. Assess the client for information and physical examination data essential to the assessment of the unconscious client.
2. Develop nursing diagnoses, related expected outcomes, and nursing care interventions associated with the care of the unconscious client.
3. Implement a plan of care for clients with confusional states.
4. Implement the medical plan of care and nursing interventions used in the care of clients with increased intracranial pressure.

The brain serves many functions in the body. Other body systems monitor and regulate a group of functions; the nervous system monitors and regulates all other body systems. Some functions of the brain are self-protective and include the ability to think, be awake, respond appropriately to the environment, and move about. Other functions are automatic and include the regulation of body temperature and protective reflex responses. When these protective functions are lost, the symptoms reflect the complexity of the nervous system. Clients with a loss of protective function may have mild symptoms, such as the inability to blink; or more serious symptoms, such as the inability to move; or life-threatening symptoms, such as irreversible coma.

The term "patient" is used in this chapter to describe the client who is comatose. It is assumed that such a client cannot be an active participant in care, and the family serves as the client in these circumstances.

DISORDERS OF CONSCIOUSNESS

Consciousness is a state of being that has two important aspects: wakefulness and awareness of self, others, and time. Awareness of time includes the past, present, and future events. Therefore, a client can be awake but confused about the time of day or year. The nurse should never assume that a client who is awake and looking about is aware of self, others, surroundings, and time without fully assessing the client.

Unconsciousness can be sustained, lasting for a few hours or longer, or brief, lasting for a few seconds to an hour or so. To produce unconsciousness, a disorder must (1) disrupt the ascending reticular activating system that is found in the center of the brain stem and thalamus; (2) significantly disrupt the function of both cerebral hemispheres; or (3) metabolically depress the cerebrum or reticular activating system, as in the case of drug overdose. Coma is a state of sustained unconsciousness in which the patient does not respond to verbal stimuli, may have varying responses to painful stimuli, may not move voluntarily, may have altered respiratory patterns, may have altered pupil responses to light, and does not blink. In general, the longer the state of unconsciousness lasts, the more likely that it is caused by a permanent disorder in the structure of the brain (and irreversible) rather than a temporary alteration in the function (and reversible).

Etiology

Three kinds of disorders produce sustained unconsciousness. They are: (1) structural lesions in the brain that place pressure on the brain stem or in the posterior fossa, which destroy the reticular formation; (2) metabolic disorders, which impair the cerebrum and the arousal functions by decreasing the supply of oxygen or allowing waste products to accumulate; and (3) psychogenic causes, in which the patient looks comatose but self-awareness is usually intact, such as is seen in catatonia. The reader should refer to a psychiatric nursing text for discussion of psychogenic coma.

Structural causes of unconsciousness include brain tumors, concussion and head trauma, and cerebral hemorrhage. Automobile and motorcycle accidents, assault with guns and knives, and falls are common etiologic factors for head injury. Trauma physically damages the brain, and the brain is further damaged as a result of the edema and hemorrhage that follow.

There are many metabolic causes of coma. The term "metabolic" is used to describe problems that did not begin in the brain but began in another system and eventually caused a disorder in the nervous system. Hypoxia is a common cause of metabolic brain disorders. Blood loss, high altitudes, or carbon monoxide poisoning may deprive the brain of oxygen. Ischemia, the loss of blood to the brain, may occur with cardiac disorders in which the cardiac output is decreased, such as cardiac arrest or even fainting. Disorders of the liver, lungs, and kidney may produce coma because of the accumulation of metabolic waste products. Finally, there are many agents that have impact on the metabolism of neurons: poisons; hypoglycemia; fever; infection, such as encephalitis; and fluid, electrolyte, or acid-base imbalance.

Pathophysiology

Decreased levels of consciousness are most often due to disorders in the reticular activating system of the brain stem and thalamus. Conditions such as confusion and decreased attention span can be due to disorders of one of the cerebral hemispheres, such as stroke. Coma itself is caused by extensive damage to both cerebral hemispheres or the reticular activating system.

Masses within the brain alter the functioning of the brain in many ways; a common symptom is a decreasing level of consciousness. Masses or lesions, whether they are growing tumors, edema, or bleeding, place pressure on the brain. Because the brain is encased in the cranium, there is no space within the skull for the expanding brain. The pressure is exerted down toward the spinal canal. This pressure slows blood and cerebrospinal fluid (CSF) flow in and out of the brain and reduces cerebral function. The level of consciousness and ability to move purposefully are affected. When pressure reaches the midbrain or diencephalon, vital functions such as heart rhythm and respiration are affected. The client's outcome is based on the location of the mass, the size and rate of enlargement, and the amount of edema and necrosis in brain tissues (see also the section on Increased Intracranial Pressure).

A blow to the head is a common cause of decreased consciousness and coma. At the time of impact, the brain can be lacerated, bruised, or contused as it is jarred within the cranium. In addition, the brain can suffer diffuse injury as tissues are torn and sheared. A common problem after head injury is the accumulation of blood between the skull and dura (epidural hematoma) or beneath the dura (subdural hematoma). Epidural hematomas are common when an unprotected head is injured, such as in assault victims, bicyclists and motorcyclists without helmets, and baseball players. Subdural hematoma is common in the elderly who fall and hit their heads as well as in clients with alcohol abuse problems because of decreased platelet aggregation. In addition to the direct injury to the brain tissue and the pressure caused by accumulating blood, clients with head injury may also have injury to their chests or airways, which increases the risk of hypoxia.

Metabolic disorders that produce coma do so through various mechanisms. Infection of the brain, such as encephalitis, causes inflammation of the meninges and brain tissues. Hyperglycemia and hypoglycemia starve the cells of needed glucose for metabolism. Overdoses of sedative drugs suppress the central nervous system, especially the centers for breathing. Failure of the liver, kidney, and lungs allows metabolic waste to accumulate, which poisons the neurons.

There is a marked increase in the metabolic needs of the patient in a coma. When these nutritional needs are not met, malnutrition increases the patient's morbidity and mortality. Malnutrition and negative nitrogen balance also retard healing. Immunodeficiency, which follows protein malnutrition, increases the risk of infection and sepsis. Malnutrition can also lead to pressure ulcers, stress ulcers, weight loss, skeletal muscle wasting, and lung tissue catabolism.

Some patients in coma slowly awaken and begin to respond normally. They often require physical and speech therapy for restoration of previous levels of function. Irreversible coma, also called cerebral death, is caused by damage to the cerebral hemispheres so that the patient is unable to respond to the environment. The brain stem and cerebellum remain intact and functional so that vital functions, such as heart, lung, and gastrointestinal, continue. Patients can remain in irreversible coma for years. It is these patients, and the maintenance of their feeding and fluids, that have inspired great ethical and legal debates.

Brain death is irreversible damage to cerebrum, cerebellum, and brain stem. The damage is so severe that there is no hope for recovery and the patient's life must be maintained with a respirator and vasoactive drugs. General agreement is that brain death has occurred when there is no discernible evidence of cerebral activity or brain stem activity (see Box 13–1).

Clinical Manifestations

If a client has a mass in the temporal lobe, early symptoms may include headaches or focal seizures (those located in one area, such as the hand). As the mass expands, symptoms change. The mass places pressure on nearby areas as well as the diencephalon. The client may develop a unilateral sensorimotor deficit (cannot raise the right leg or has numbness in the right leg), aphasia, and a deficit in the visual field (blind in the left visual field). These clients usually have intact pupillary reflexes and oculovestibular reflexes. If the mass is not detected or cannot be treated and progresses, the client will eventually develop coma.

BOX 13–1

Clinical Criteria for Brain Death

- Completion of all appropriate and therapeutic procedures
- Unresponsive coma with absence of motor and reflex response
- No spontaneous respiration (apnea)
- No oculocephalic response or oculovestibular response with fixed and dilated pupils
- Isoelectric (flat) electroencephalogram
- Persistence of the above signs for 30 minutes to 1 hour and for 6 hours after the onset of coma and apnea
- Confirming tests indicating the absence of cerebral circulation (optional)[15]

Infratentorial lesions produce different symptoms. Infarct or bleeding in the midbrain or pons produces coma from the start. Clients with these lesions may have a history of brain stem dysfunction or a sudden onset of coma. Oculovestibular abnormalities are present. Abnormal respiratory patterns also develop as the cranial nerves are trapped by the mass or edema (Fig. 13–1).

CRITICAL TO REMEMBER

An important difference in coma caused by a metabolic disorder is the presence of bilateral or symmetric symptoms, because the disorder affects the entire brain rather than just one section.

The client usually develops confusion and stupor before any physical signs are noticed. Physical signs include tremor, asterixis (flapping tremors of the hands), myoclonus (a single, sudden jerking movement), and seizures. Pupillary response is normal. Depending on the underlying cause, acid-base imbalances may be noted. For example, metabolic acidosis would be present in a patient in a diabetic coma.

Clients with unresponsiveness from a psychiatric disorder, rather than a true coma, do not have the same manifestations. These clients have intact eyelid muscles and their eyelids close tightly; the pupils are small but react normally; oculocephalic responses are unpredictable; and oculovestibular stimulation produces the normal nystagmus. Motor tone is inconsistent, no pathophysiologic reflexes are present, and the electroencephalogram (EEG) is normal.

LEVEL OF CONSCIOUSNESS

The level of consciousness is the most critical clinical piece of data assessed in the comatose patient and clients with decreasing levels of consciousness. There are many components of level of consciousness assessments, such as degree of orientation, level of alertness, and ability to solve problems or follow directions. A

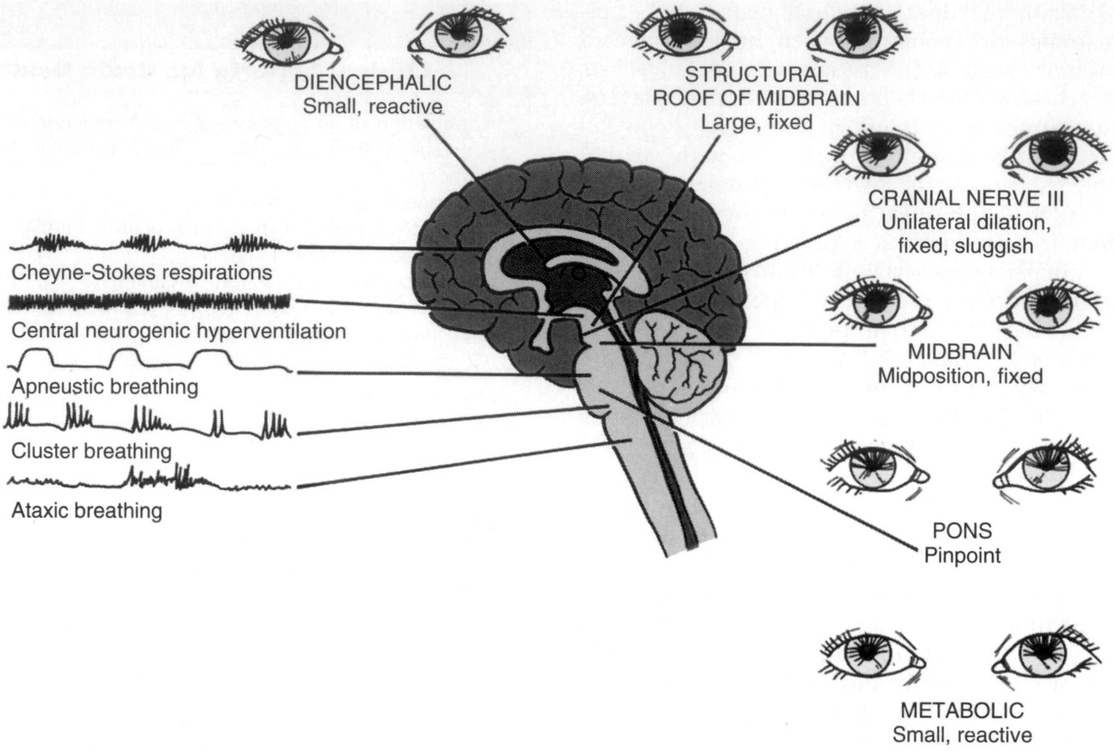

Figure 13–1
Respiratory patterns and pupil appearances associated with lesions of various neurologic structures.

client who is awake, alert, and fully oriented to self, others, place, and time is considered to be fully conscious. As changes in the level of consciousness occur, the client can be improving or deteriorating. From the normal alert state, consciousness deteriorates in stages, each having its own definition.

- *Confusion:* the loss of the ability to think rapidly and clearly; an impairment in judgement and decision making.
- *Disorientation:* beginning loss of consciousness. Disorientation to time is followed by disorientation to place and the inability to recognize others. The last step of disorientation is the inability to know self.
- *Lethargy:* a lack of spontaneous movement or speech. The client is easily aroused with speech or touch but is not oriented to person, place, or time.
- *Obtundation:* reduced ability to be aroused and limited response to the environment. The client sleeps unless stimulated with speech or touch. Verbal response to questions is minimal, perhaps a grunt or nod.
- *Stupor:* a condition of deep sleep or unresponsiveness from which a patient may be aroused only with vigorous, sometimes painful, stimulation. Patients respond by withdrawing from or grabbing at the source of pain.
- *Coma:* no motor or verbal response to the environment or any stimuli, even deep pain or suctioning.[10]

In the clinical setting, these terms can be confusing and their true meaning is debatable. As previously stated, the nurse should document the level of consciousness by stating a description of the client's behavior in response to stimulation.

PATTERN OF BREATHING

Respiration is a complex process controlled by the cerebrum, pons, and brain stem. Disorders that cause coma and decreased levels of consciousness also commonly cause respiratory abnormalities. Changes in respiratory rate and rhythm occur from many different processes. Compression of the medulla causes respiratory failure, and rapidly expanding lesions in the cerebellum may lead to respiratory arrest. Common abnormal respiratory patterns are shown in Figure 13–1.

Airway obstruction and aspiration are common complications in unconscious patients. An obstructed airway leads to inadequate gas exchange, which in turn causes (1) carbon dioxide retention, contributing to vasodilation, and cerebral edema, increasing intracranial pressure; or (2) decreased arterial oxygen levels, resulting in decreased oxygen delivery to the brain. Respiratory failure will occur if a patient has insufficient lung ventilation and inadequate gas exchange. Respiratory failure may be prevented by oxygen administration and assisted ventilation.

EYE MOVEMENT

The cranial nerves exit through the brain stem; when the cranial nerves are compressed, eye movement is impaired. Eye movements in the comatose patient are uncoordinated, and pupillary response is abnormal. The eyes of an awake and alert client at rest normally gaze straight ahead. Eyes normally track together to look at something. When the eyes move in such a way, gaze is said to be conjugate. Dysconjugate gaze or *conjugate* deviation of the eyes at rest indicates a disorder of one or more of the ocular muscles or damage to the cranial nerves supplying the eye muscles (CN III, IV, and VI). Several types of abnormal involuntary eye movements may occur: ocular bobbing, in which the eyes appear to be slowly jumping up and down; or roving eye movements, in which the eyes slowly wander or move around. Doll's eyes (oculoreflexic response) are said to be present if, when the head is rotated, the eyes move in the direction opposite to the head. Doll's eyes are absent if the eyes remain fixed straight ahead regardless of head position (Fig. 13–2).

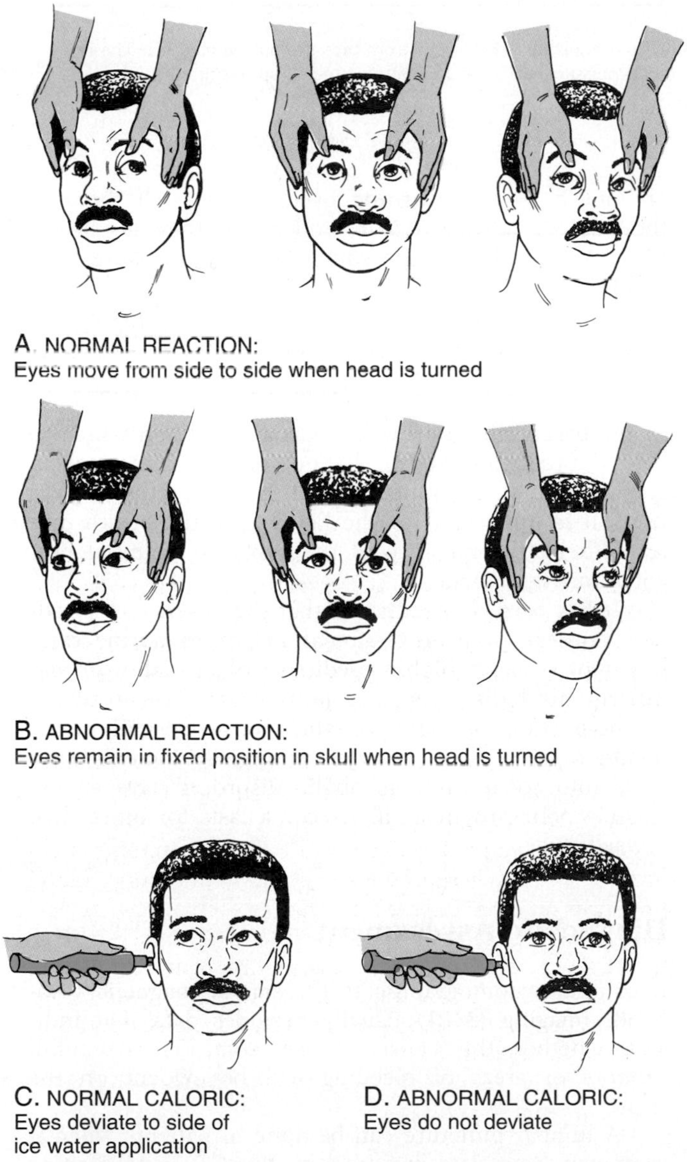
A. NORMAL REACTION:
Eyes move from side to side when head is turned
B. ABNORMAL REACTION:
Eyes remain in fixed position in skull when head is turned
C. NORMAL CALORIC:
Eyes deviate to side of ice water application
D. ABNORMAL CALORIC:
Eyes do not deviate

Figure 13–2
A and B, Normal and abnormal doll's eye test (oculocephalic response). *C and D,* Normal and abnormal caloric test (oculovestibular response).

PUPILLARY CHANGES

The reticular activating system within the brain stem is adjacent to the area that controls the pupil's size and reaction to light. Therefore, pupillary changes are used in the assessment of brain stem function. Severe cerebral hypoxia and ischemia cause pupils to become fixed and dilated. Hypothermia may also fix the pupils. There are also several medications that affect pupil size and reaction to light. These medications include large doses of atropine and scopolamine, which fix and fully dilate the pupil; miotics, which constrict the pupil; midriatics, which dilate the pupil; narcotics (especially morphine), which cause the pupils to become pinpoint in size; and barbiturates, which produce fixed pupils (see Fig. 13–1).

MOTOR RESPONSE

Motor response is the most powerful predictor of outcome in patients with severe neurologic impairment.[14] The client may respond to commands such as "raise your right arm" within a reasonable time. Other clients may not respond to verbal requests but are noted to have purposeful movement, that is, to withdraw from a painful stimulus. For example, the patient may push away a suction catheter. As consciousness decreases further, the patient may only draw up the knees and arms without directing any response toward the stimuli.

Decorticate posturing is abnormal flexion of the arms, wrists, and fingers with the arms abducted. The legs are fully extended and internally rotated, with the feet in plantar flexion. Decerebrate posturing is abnormal extension of the legs in a position similar to decorticate posture. The arms are stiffly extended and abducted and the hands hyperpronated. Decorticate and decerebrate postures are shown in Figure 13–3.

Other motor signs in a patient with cerebral hemisphere damage may include

- primitive sucking or snout reflexes
- strong reflexic hand grasp

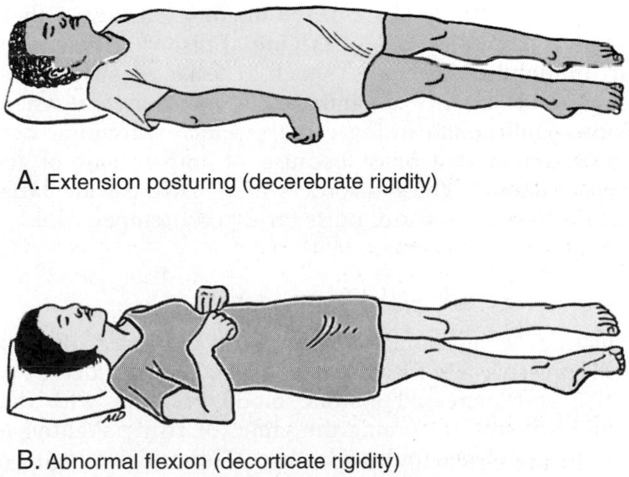
A. Extension posturing (decerebrate rigidity)
B. Abnormal flexion (decorticate rigidity)

Figure 13–3
A and B, Pathologic posturing in clients with severe brain injury.

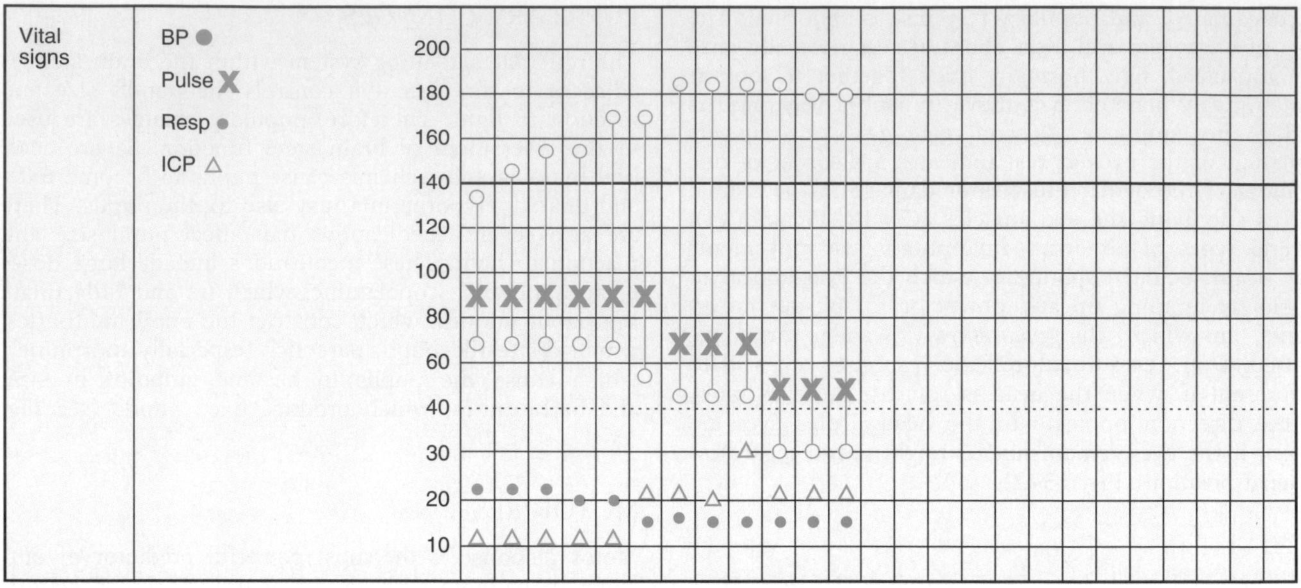

Figure 13–4
Cushing's response (Cushing's triad) includes bradycardia, systolic hypertension, and bradypnea that occur from pressure on the medulla. These signs often occur with intracranial hypertension or herniation syndrome. BP, blood pressure; ICP, intracranial pressure; Resp, respiration.

- restlessness
- resistance to passive movement
- hemiplegia
- hemiparesis
- seizures

The most severe impairment of motor function is bilateral flaccidity. True flaccidity, the absence of any movement or tone in response to deep painful stimuli, is one of the criteria for measuring brain death. Therefore, great caution is used in determining whether flaccidity is present. Disorders such as stroke and spinal cord injury also may produce flaccidity.

VITAL SIGNS

Wide variations in vital signs may occur in patients with various levels of consciousness. Some changes relate directly to the cause of the unconsciousness. Others relate to complications of the initial disorder, treatment, or immobility, such as shock, cardiac dysrhythmias, fluid and electrolyte imbalances, and hypertension. Some conditions causing coma produce autonomic nervous system instability because of impairment of the hypothalamus. These disorders may cause a wide variation in blood pressure, pulse, and body temperature.

CUSHING'S CHANGES

Cushing's changes may develop with increased intracranial pressure (ICP). These changes include decreased pulse and increased systolic blood pressure with diastolic pressure remaining the same (or rising slightly) to create a widened pulse pressure. These physiologic responses are an attempt to restore adequate blood flow through compressed cerebral vessels. Cushing's changes are not a reliable warning of increasing ICP because they do not always occur, and when they do occur, they are often late in the course of rising pressure (Fig. 13–4).

Prognosis

In the past, little information was available on which to base a prediction about the outcome of a patient in coma. Most of the time, a "wait and see attitude" was used. It is important for the family and the health care team to have some idea of the probable eventual outcome for the patient.

It has been demonstrated that the absence of pupillary, corneal, or oculovestibular responses during early stages of coma is highly predictive of mortality or significant morbidity (e.g., vegetative state). The recovery of these responses and a return to purposeful movement correlate with a better prognosis. Patients who lapse into coma from metabolic disorders have an extremely poor prognosis if the coma lasts for more than 1 week.

Diagnostic Assessment

A computed tomographic (CT) scan or magnetic resonance imaging (MRI) usually provides data that indicate whether the cause of the coma is structural. Tumors or areas of bleeding will be evident on the scan.

A lumbar puncture can be done in patients when it is known from data provided by the CT or MRI scans that there is no expanding intracranial mass. Lumbar puncture can assist with the diagnosis of infection or bleeding as a cause of coma. CSF may be cloudy or bloody when the client has an infection or bleeding into the ventricles or the subarachnoid space.

An EEG can be used to determine whether the patient is comatose because of continuous seizures. EEG results are abnormal in many patients in metabolic coma and do not serve as a clear diagnostic tool.

In some comatose clients, doll's eyes can be noted without specially testing for the response. Doll's eyes can also be tested, and this is a rapid method for detecting potential abnormalities of the brain stem. This test can be done only on unconscious patients because the response does not occur in awake clients. The doll's eye test should not be performed on comatose patients with suspected or known cervical spine injury. The head movement could produce permanent spinal cord damage.

Patients in metabolic coma, except barbiturate and phenytoin (Dilantin) poisoning, retain ocular reflexes. The presence of brisk doll's eyes movement indicates a decrease in the level of consciousness with an intact brain stem. The absence of doll's eyes movement in a comatose patient does not always mean that the brain stem is not functioning. Other agents and disorders can block the eye's response. Neuromuscular drugs, such as succinylcholine, and Meniere's disease, which destroys the labyrinth in the ear, cause absent oculocephalic response.

If oculocephalic responses are absent, oculovestibular (caloric) tests can be performed to test the third, sixth, and eighth cranial nerves (see Chap. 12). A normal response occurs when the eyes have conjugate movement and nystagmus. Nystagmus is the involuntary oscillation of the eyeballs and may be horizontal, vertical, oblique, rotary, or mixed, with various rates of movement. The occurrence of roving eye movements and the failure to produce nystagmus with the instillation of warm or cold water into the ear canal indicates a decrease in consciousness with an intact brain stem. Absent cold caloric responses do not always indicate brain stem disorder. The use of ototoxic drugs, barbiturates, sedatives, phenytoin, or tricyclic antidepressants or the presence of Meniere's disease may produce a false caloric test. The nurse should use caution when assessing the oculovestibular response in clients with head trauma because they may have sustained a ruptured tympanum (eardrum).

Medical Management

The goal of medical management of the patient in coma is to remove or correct the cause. Frequently, time is required to perform all the tests to find the specific cause. In the interim, the patient's brain must be protected from further injury.

The patient's airway and circulation must be maintained. A nasal or oral airway may be inserted for a short time. If the patient is completely unresponsive, an endotracheal tube is carefully inserted, avoiding injury to the cervical spine. The head-injured patient may be hyperventilated while on a ventilator for reducing $PaCO_2$ to between 27 and 30 mm Hg. Hyperventilation is an effective way to reduce cerebral blood flow when coma is due to bleeding. Caution is used, however, to avoid decreasing blood supply to areas of the brain where blood flow is already reduced because of effects of the injury. Circulation is maintained by monitoring blood pressure and using vasoactive agents to keep mean systolic blood pressure above 80 mm Hg. If the patient is breathing without assistance, the airway and respirations need to be closely monitored because the airway may become obstructed and aspiration may occur as consciousness decreases.

If the patient is having repetitive seizures, coma and brain damage can follow; the patient is given intravenous diazepam to stop the seizures. If the patient is not intubated, the airway needs to be closely monitored because of the effects of the diazepam.

Many metabolic causes of coma lead to acid-base and fluid imbalances. The patient's acid-base balance should be restored quickly. Fluid imbalances should be restored slowly for preventing rebound fluid shifts into the brain. Fluids may be given if the patient is dehydrated or withheld if the patient is fluid overloaded. Normal saline and hypertonic saline are the fluids of choice because these fluids will not passively move into the brain and increase edema.

At one time, barbiturates were the most common cause of overdose, but there are many more choices of drugs today. Most emergency deparments have lists of antidotes to reverse specific agents. Many times, however, the specific drug ingested is not known. Narcotic overdose is common and reversed with naloxone (Narcan). The nurse needs to be aware that the duration of action of naloxone is 2 to 3 hours shorter than that of most narcotics, and the dose may need to be repeated. Cocaine overdose can be treated with diazepam. Patients with cocaine overdose often have cardiac arrhythmias and irregular respirations also. Gastric lavage may be used to remove ingested agents.

Once the emergency care is given, medical management centers on trying to diagnose and treat the cause of the coma. Body functions are maintained, and complications that may slow recovery or cause residual problems are prevented. If the coma is prolonged, the patient is begun on nasogastric tube feeding for promotion of nutrition and prevention of muscle wasting. The complications from immobility, such as pneumonia and pressure ulcers, are continually assessed and treated.

Nursing Management

Assessment

Frequent, systematic, and objective nursing assessment including neurologic status and mental status is essential. Serial observations are important for comparison. Even if assessment findings seem insignificant for long periods, documentation provides an objective pattern and an important baseline for future observations.

The nurse should take "neuro checks" as often as every 15 minutes during the first few hours of unconsciousness. They are often continued hourly for several days.

The nurse periodically assesses the entire body, observing for lacerations, bruises, ulcerations, fractures, dislocations, and contractures. He or she also notes skin color, texture, and temperature and inspects dressings frequently for purulent or bloody drainage and head dressings for CSF leakage.

The following questions may guide nursing assessment of an unconscious patient.

- What is the patient's level of consciousness?
- Is the airway patent? Is the patient hemodynamically stable? Are circulation and respiration adequate? Is skin, nail bed, and mucous membrane color appropriate?
- Is heart rate slowing and diastolic and systolic blood pressure widening? If so, these indicate increased ICP. Document and report immediately.
- Are pupil responses normal, that is, equal size and reactive to light? Are corneal responses present? Are eye movements abnormal?
- Are any normal reflexes absent (e.g., corneal, blink, gag reflexes)? Are any abnormal reflexes present (e.g., Babinski's reflex)? Absence of the corneal reflex usually indicates problems in the first division of the fifth cranial nerve (see Chap. 12).
- In what position are the head, limbs, and trunk? Does the patient change these positions? Is the neck rigid or stiff? Are there other indications of meningeal irritation? Are there changes in muscle tone? Is paralysis evident? Is the patient making any voluntary movements?
- Are any focal or generalized seizures occurring? Carefully document their onset and progression.
- Is the patient incontinent? Is the abdomen distended?
- Are there any indications of fluid-electrolyte imbalances?
- If the patient has sustained head injuries or had cranial surgery, is there any periorbital or facial edema?
- Does the patient respond to painful stimuli? Is the patient resistive to care? Is spontaneous behavior occurring?

Glasgow Coma Scale: The most commonly used neurologic assessment tool in clinical care is the Glasgow Coma Scale (GCS). This scale provides objective measurement of three essential components of the neurologic examination. Eye opening, best motor response, and best verbal response are scored. Vital signs are also recorded. The total of the three scores can range from 3 to 15. The patient who is unresponsive to painful stimuli, does not open the eyes, and is flaccid has a score of 3. The client who is oriented, opens the eyes spontaneously, and follows commands scores 15. Because the scoring of the GCS is based on the client's ability to respond and communicate, the nurse should always note whether the client (1) is intubated and cannot speak; (2) has eyes that are swollen closed; (3) is unable to communicate in English; (4) has a hearing loss; or (5) is blind.

The first GCS score recorded on the patient becomes the baseline coma score. Subsequent scores allow assessment of trends or changes in neurologic status. The scale can also be used to recognize disorders as well as predict outcomes. It is imperative that the nurse use consistent criteria for patient assessment. Specific behaviors indicating a given score should be used. If there are variations in scoring criteria, the value of the scale is lost and serious changes in the client's condition can be overlooked or treated unnecessarily (Fig. 13–5).

Eye Opening. The nurse should observe the eye opening without speaking to the client. Does the client open the eyes and look around? If the eyes are closed, the nurse calls the client's name. If there is no response, he or she raises the voice or shouts. If there is still no response, a painful stimulus should be used to see if a response can be elicited. Supraorbital pressure should be avoided if the face is traumatized. Nail bed compression can be used in an older client with thin skin.

Verbal Response. Verbal responses assess orientation of the client to self, environment, and time. The nurse should ask appropriate questions, such as, What is your name? Where are you? What is the date today? and so on. The conversation should include information that can be verified by family, such as address or employer. Many times slight degrees of confusion will not be noticeable until the nurse spends some time with a client. The nurse may find the apparently oriented client asking the same question a few hours after it was originally answered. Likewise, the client may have "learned" the answers to common questions such as "What is your name?" and "What hospital are you in?" Therefore, it is helpful to reassess a client after a few hours to check memory, or challenge the client with varying questions.

Motor Response. Motor responses are assessed by asking the client to follow specific commands, such as "raise your right arm" or "wiggle your toes." The client should not be asked to squeeze the nurse's hand because grasp is a reflexic response that occurs in clients with head injury. If agency protocol lists grasp as a neurologic assessment, the nurse can ask the client to "let go" after grasping, to measure the cognitive ability to control movement. Clients who are unable to follow commands are given a painful stimulus, and their response is assessed. The patient may respond by localizing (trying to remove the stimulus), withdrawing, or posturing; or no response may be elicited, with the patient remaining motionless and flaccid. The nurse compares the right and left sides and upper and lower extremities and records the best reponse while noting any abnormality as all four limbs are scored.

These three components are scored on the GCS. In addition to documentation on the GCS with a number, at times the nurse will document the neurologic status on the chart. Phrases such as "disoriented times 3" or "stuporous" should be avoided. Instead, the specific data are recorded, such as "states it is 1968 and that Taft is president." In addition, the nurse should describe the most obvious findings, such as aphasia and inability to move a specific limb. If the GCS score decreases, the nurse should perform a detailed neurologic assessment and notify the physician immediately. A significant change in the level of consciousness, including a decrease of one point of the GCS, indicates cerebral dysfunction.

Pupillary Response. A pupil check includes assessing pupil appearance and physiologic response. The nurse should remember that the affected pupil is usually on the same side (ipsilateral) as the brain lesion, whereas the motor and sensory deficits are usually on the opposite side (contralateral).

CRITICAL TO REMEMBER

The nurse must be sure to determine whether the patient has an artificial eye before doing a pupil assessment.

This mistake has occurred, and the pupil in the prosthetic eye has been reported as "fixed."

Pupil Equality. The nurse documents pupil equality with a labeled drawing of the relative size of each pupil, for example, R • L ●.

Pupil Size. The nurse estimates the size of each pupil in millimeters.

Pupil Position. The nurse notes, for example, whether the pupil is at midline or deviated from midline.

Pupil Reaction to Light. To assess pupil reaction, the nurse brings the light toward the eye from the side of the patient's head and shines it directly into the pupil. Constriction of the pupil should occur. The nurse assesses whether the other pupil responds to the light (consensual response) and determines how quickly the pupils react (e.g., briskly, sluggishly). This examination tests the fact that the light stimulus, once it travels along the optic nerve, stimulates the brain stem bilaterally.

Pupil Shape. If the shape is not round, the nurse describes the shape (e.g., oval) and documents it with a drawing. The nurse should assess whether each pupil has regular borders. Irregular borders may mean midbrain damage.

Pupil Accommodation. Normally, the size of the pupil adjusts to accommodate varying focal lengths. This is usually tested by having the client focus on a distant object and then quickly focus on something close. Pupils should change size depending on focal length.

Eye Movement. The nurse documents eye movement changes. He or she observes the position of the eyes when checking pupils and involuntary movements.

Motor Activity. Motor activity assessment is the measure of strength on voluntary movement of the arms and legs.

If a client cannot cooperate with testing, paralysis may be difficult to detect. The nurse should observe the client carefully. If a client is restless, paralysis may become obvious because the paralyzed part will not move as other body parts move. Additional information may be obtained by (1) comparing the tone of one side of the body with the other, (2) lifting the arms or legs on both sides and watching them return to the bed, and (3) observing the position of the limbs at rest.

If a client can cooperate, assessing "drift" may show subtle tone alterations. To do this, the nurse should have the client hold both arms up in front of the body with palms upward and eyes closed. Muscles are weak if one arm "drifts" (i.e., moves downward) or the hand pronates.

Vital Signs. Vital signs should be assessed every 15 minutes until the client's condition becomes stable. Body temperature should be monitored every 2 hours. If hypothermia or hyperthermia occurs, a rectal probe should be used. Trends in vital signs and respiratory patterns should be analyzed. Vital signs change in a Cushing's response when ICP increases, but vital signs change much later than do other neurologic signs.

Nursing Intervention for Comatose Patients

Unconscious patients are completely dependent on others because their protective reflexes are impaired. Nursing intervention provides the safety normally afforded by protective reflexes. The nurse should recall what the normal protective mechanisms are and identify critical areas of nursing intervention required for unconscious clients. For example, because

- spontaneous movement is lost, the patient needs protection from skin breakdown due to prolonged pressure, pooling of secretions in the lungs, and joint contractures.
- ability to swallow or cough is lost, the patient needs protection from choking and alternative ways of maintaining nutrition and fluid-electrolyte balance.
- blink reflex is lost, the eyes need protection (especially if they are open).
- ability to respond to the environment is lost, the patient needs protection from environmental hazards.
- ability to alter body position is lost, the patient needs protection from injury by being positioned in correct alignment.

Nursing Diagnosis, Planning, and Implementation

This section discusses intervention appropriate for all unconscious patients regardless of the cause of the coma. Intervention specific to particular etiologic factors is discussed in other sections of the book. Unconsciousness is often life-threatening and requires aggressive medical intervention.

Collaborative Problem: Airway Obstruction, Risk for R/T loss of swallowing, gag, and coughing reflexes.

Planning: Expected Outcomes. The nurse will monitor the patient for signs of airway obstruction, as evidenced by abnormal lung sounds, unequal lung expansion, stridor, cyanosis or pallor, abnormal arterial blood gas values, and increasing ICP.

MISSION HOSPITAL
REGIONAL MEDICAL CENTER

ADULT NEURO FLOW SHEET

				TIME
GLASGOW COMA SCALE			Eyes Open	
			Best Motor	
			Best Verbal	
			TOTAL	
VOLUNTARY MOTOR	Right		upper extremity	
			lower extremity	
	Left		upper extremity	
			lower extremity	
CRANIAL NERVES	PUPILS	Right	Size	
			Reaction	
		Left	Size	
			Reaction	
	EOMS		Conjugate	
			Dysconjugate	
		Tracking	Right	
			Left	
	Blink Reflex			
	Gag Reflex			
	Facial Symmetry			
			Date	
				TIME

KEY

MOTOR
5+ Normal Power
4+ Weakness
3+ Anti-gravity
2+ Not anti-gravity
1+ Trace
0 No movement

Pupil Size
B = Brisk
S = Sluggish
A = Absent

2mm 3mm 4mm 5mm

6mm 7mm 8mm

✓ = Present
O = Absent
S = Symmetrical
A = Asymmetrical

Speech Patterns: ______

Comments: ______

GLASGOW COMA SCALE		
Eyes Open	4	Spontaneously
	3	To verbal command
	2	To Pain
	1	No Response
Best Motor Response	6	Obeys Commands
	5	Localize Pain
	4	Flexion to pain withdraw
	3	Flexion Decorticate
	2	Extension to pain (decerebrate)
	1	No Response to pain
Best Verbal Response	5	Oriented
	4	Confused
	3	Inappropriate words
	2	Incomprehensible sounds
	1	No Response

Unit ______

R.N. Signature ______ Shift: ______

R.N. Signature ______ Shift: ______

R.N. Signature ______ Shift: ______

ADDRESSOGRAPH

#408 10/89

Adult Neuro Flow Sheet

Figure 13–5
Neurologic observation chart. (Courtesy of Mission Hospital Regional Medical Center, Mission Viejo, CA.)

NEUROLOGIC FLOW SHEET

1. Glasgow Coma Scale (GCS). Three areas are assessed: Best eye opeing, Best motor response, and Best verbal response. Assign the appropriate numerical score for each category (1st box—best eye, 2nd box--best motor, and 3rd box—best verbal). Place the total score in the fourth box (total score 3-15).

2. Voluntary Motor is evaluated by assessing each extremity on both the right and left side. Note **symmetry vs. asymmetry.** In the cooperative patient, voluntary motor strength is assessed by asking the patient to close their eyes and hold their arms straight ahead with palms up for about 30 seconds. The leg strength is evaluated by asking the patient to push downward against the examiner's hands.

Scoring: Normal power (5+) is the score given if the patient's arms stay in the same position and/or if the legs have equal strong power.

Weakness (4+) is the score given if one of the pt.'s arm drifts downward (hands may pronate) or if the leg strength is diminished. Some resistance to force is noted.

Anti-gravity (3+) is the score given if the patient is able to move an extremity above the plane of gravity (ie flexing & extending a hand up/down against gravity).

Not anti-gravity (2+) is the score given to a patient who can move the extremity back and forth on the bed but not against the forces of gravity.

Trace movement (1+) is the score given to a patient who can move an extremity slightly.

No movement (0) is the score given if a patient cannot move the extremity.

3. **Cranial Nerve Exam:**

Pupillary response: Each pupil is assessed individually. Note the size of the pupil prior to shining the light into the eye. Place your hand at the bridge of the nose to block light to the opposite eye. Using the penlight, shine the light from outside the right eye to midpoint across the eye to assess the direct light reflex. Note the pupillary constriction (Brisk, sluggish, or non-reactive) in the right eye. Also, observe for constriction in the left pupil (consensual light reflex). Repeat the above steps for the left eye observing the direct light reflex in the left eye and the consensual reflex in the right eye. Document the pupil size (prior to light in the eye) and the reaction on the flow sheet.

Extra-ocular movements (EOMS's) are tested on patients who are awake enough to follow instructions. Ask the patient to follow your fingers with his eyes without moving the head. Move your fingers in a figure H and observe both eyes as they move across/up/down. **Conjugate eye movements** occur when both eyes move in parallel motion. **Dysconjugate eye movements** occur when the eyes do not move in a lateral direction together (one eye may move laterally while the other is fixed or moves in another direction). **Tracking** occurs when the patient is consciously following someone's or something's movement around the room. Place a check for present or a 0 for absent.

The Blink reflex is elicited by lightly stroking the patient's eyelashes. When the eyelids are closed, the eyelids will flutter slightly if the reflex is present. In the conscious alert patient, observe for blinking. Place a check for present or a 0 for absent.

The Gag reflex is evaluated by asking the alert, cooperative patient to cough or swallow. If the patient is unable to do so or is unconscious, take a long cotton tipped swab and stroke the back of the patient's throat. Note if the reflex is present (place a check) or absent (place a 0).

Muscles of the face: Note the muscle symmetry of the facial muscles. Note the ability of the eyelids to open spontaneously and equally. Ask the patient to close their eyes as tightly as possible. Note asymmetry. Ask the patient to smile—note the corners of the mouth to identify symmetrical patterns. Ask the patient to frown/wrinkle his forehead—note the symmetry of the muscles. Place a S for symmetrical and an A for asymmetrical.

Speech patterns: Note if speech is clear, slurred, rambling, or aphasic.

Comments: Utilize this section to elaborate on any abnormal findings or document other pertinent data.

Sign your name and document shift worked. Complete the date/unit and addressograph. The Neurological flow sheet is for a 24 hour period. Each day at 7 am, obtain a new flow sheet. Document your findings in the appropriate time box.

Figure 13–5 *Continued*

CRITICAL TO REMEMBER

Airway obstruction is the most common source of harm to patients with decreased consciousness.

Implementation. Initial care of an unconscious patient includes clearing the airway immediately and loosening all tight clothing, especially around the neck. A recently injured or unconscious patient should never be moved without the use of a cervical collar to protect the neck if there is any possibility of spinal injury. The nurse can maintain a patent airway by the jaw-thrust method (i.e., place fingers at the angle of the jaws and pull the jaw forward). He or she should remove and store any dentures or bridge work. These could cause airway obstruction or could be swallowed and broken.

Noisy respirations or obvious efforts to breathe indicate partial airway obstruction. When possible, the cause of obstruction should be removed. The nurse places the patient in a lateral position to facilitate drainage of pulmonary secretions and to prevent the tongue from falling into the posterior pharynx and occluding the airway. The patient should not be positioned on the back, unless intubated, because this position can compromise respirations. In addition to the tongue's occluding the airway, secretions may pool in the pharynx and be aspirated.

For initial airway management, an oral airway can be inserted in an unconscious patient. Endotracheal intubation may be required to maintain airway patency or improve ventilation with the use of a ventilator. For extended airway management, a tracheostomy may be required.

Nursing Diagnosis: Aspiration, Risk for R/T ineffective airway clearance and absent gag reflex.

Planning: Expected Outcomes. The patient will exhibit no signs of aspiration, as evidenced by clear lung sounds, no stridor, afebrile, minimal amounts of clear mucus upon suctioning, and PaO_2, $PaCO_2$, and pH within normal limits.

Implementation. Aspiration is a common cause of death in unconscious patients. Suctioning equipment must be kept available. The nurse assesses breath sounds every hour or two in acutely ill patients. He or she monitors the results of arterial blood gas analysis and pulse oximetry to determine the degree of oxygenation provided by ventilators or oxygen and performs tracheobronchial suctioning only when necessary to prevent or decrease the accumulation of secretions from immobility, the lack of a cough and sigh reflex, or pneumonia. Even though suctioning increases ICP, the damage from hypoxia and hypercapnia requires that the removal of secretions be ongoing. While suctioning, the nurse should monitor the EEG for dysrhythmias (e.g., premature ventricular contractions), arterial pressure, and SpO_2 (PaO_2).

A comatose patient may lack pharyngeal reflexes and is therefore unable to swallow. A comatose patient should never be given fluids to swallow. Secretions accumulate in the posterior pharynx and may be aspirated. The nurse should turn the patient from side to side every 2 hours to facilitate drainage of secretions and prevent pneumonia. He or she should suction the posterior pharynx and upper trachea frequently.

While performing mouth care, the nurse should place a comatose patient well over onto the side to prevent aspiration. If facial paralysis is present, the affected side should be kept uppermost. At times, a second nurse assisting will facilitate oral care by holding the mouth open and suctioning. The nurse must pay close attention to the roof of the mouth in patients who mouthbreathe for long periods. Crusts may form, break off, and be aspirated.

CRITICAL TO REMEMBER

The nurse should never suction the nasal passages in patients who have had brain surgery or head injuries.

The suction catheter can cause further trauma and increase the risk of CSF leak.

Nursing Diagnosis: Tissue Perfusion, Altered Cerebral, Risk for R/T increased ICP.

Planning: Expected Outcomes. The patient will maintain normal cerebral perfusion, as evidenced by maintaining or improving level of consciousness; maintaining or improving GCS score; ICP is less than or equal to 15 mm Hg, having no restlessness, irritability, or headache; and having no pupillary changes, no seizures, no widening pulse pressure, no respiratory irregularity, and no hypertension or bradycardia.

Implementation. The nurse places the patient supine with the head of the bed elevated 30 degrees. The patient's head should be maintained in a neutral position to facilitate venous drainage from the brain.

CRITICAL TO REMEMBER

Extreme rotation and flexion of the neck are avoided because these positions compress the jugular veins and increase ICP. Extreme hip flexion is also avoided because this position increases intra-abdominal and intrathoracic pressure, which increases ICP.

As coma lightens, the patient may become disoriented and combative, making it challenging to keep him or her positioned in an ideal position. The nurse will have to assess each patient to determine whether the use of restraints is necessary or if their use will cause further agitation. Agitation will further increase ICP. The patient will probably be treated with osmotic or loop diuretics or corticosteroids to reduce cerebral edema. The nurse needs to monitor the response to these medications. Because the signs of increasing ICP may develop slowly, the continued assessment of the patient is critical. Cerebral edema usually peaks within 72 hours after trauma and gradually subsides over the next few weeks. Additional interventions for clients with increased ICP are discussed later in this chapter. Some patients have ICP monitors inserted for close monitoring of increasing pressure. The monitors are described in the Bridge to Critical Care.

BRIDGE TO CRITICAL CARE

Intracranial Pressure Monitoring

GUIDELINES FOR MANAGEMENT OF ICP

Unstable: ICP >20 for 5 minutes or pupillary changes (dilating pupil)
↓
Drain cerebrospinal fluid → ICP <20 → Monitor/assess
↓
Hyperventilate → ICP <20 → Monitor/assess
$PaCO_2$ 25–30
PaO_2 >90
↓
Medicate/sedate → ICP <20 → Monitor/assess
Morphine sulfate/midazolam (Versed)
↓
Mannitol 25 g IV
15 minutes later give furosemide 20 mg IV
↓
STAT CT of brain
↓
If ICP remains above 20 mm Hg, consider pentobarbitol sodium coma

Stable: ICP <20
↓
Monitor/assess
↓
Maintain airway
Maintain $PaCO_2$ 25–30
Maintain PaO_2 >90
Head of bed elevated 30 degrees
Maintain alignment
Maintain fluid volume status

- Monitor serum osmality (up to 315)
- Monitor serum sodium levels
- Monitor cardiac output, pulmonary artery wedge pressure, and central venous pressure

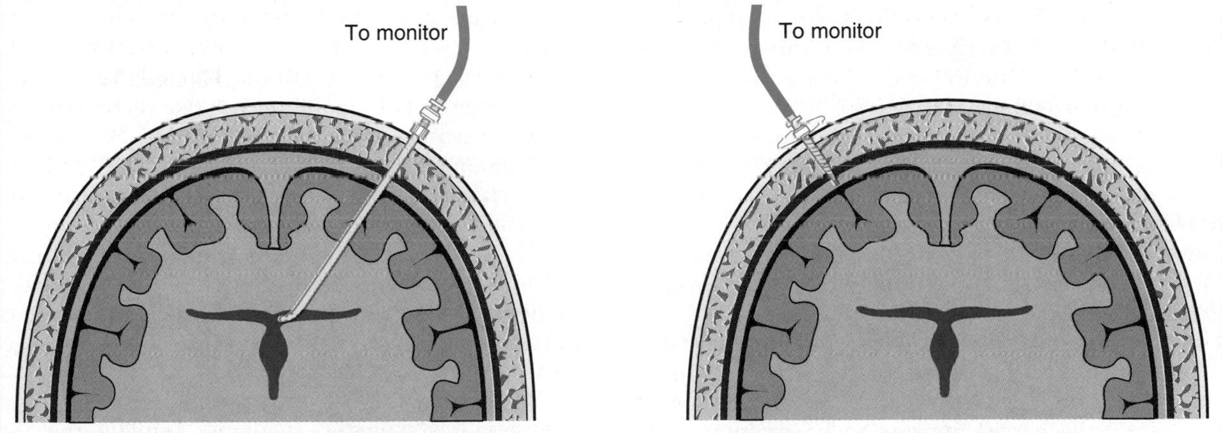

Ventricular Catheter (Ventriculostomy)
Subarachnoid Screw (bolt)

GENERAL INTERVENTIONS FOR INTRACRANIAL PRESSURE MONITORING

- Ensure that the tubing is long enough to allow the client to be moved in bed but not longer than 14 feet. Tubing longer than 14 feet may cause inaccurate readings.
- Be careful to prevent kinks in the tubing.
- Place the transducer and screw (or catheter) at the preset level of the transducer to take a reading.
- Use sterile technique when working with the device.
- Monitor for signs of infection.
- Flush the catheter if the readings dampen.
- Check for the following if inaccurate readings occur:
  - Leaks in the system
  - Differences in the height of the transducer and the device
  - Kinks in the tubing
  - Client performing the Valsalva maneuver
  - Obstruction in the system

CT, computed tomography; ICP, intracranial pressure; IV, intravenously

Nursing Diagnosis: Oral and Nasal Mucous Membranes, Altered, Risk for R/T NPO status (nothing by mouth), inability to swallow, mouth breathing, and unconsciousness.

Planning: Expected Outcomes. The patient will maintain intact oral and nasal mucous membranes, as evidenced by having oral and nasal mucous membranes pink, moist, and without lesions, crusts, or bloody drainage.

Implementation. The nurse should inspect the patient's mouth daily, using a flashlight and tongue depressor. The nurse should keep the lips coated with a water-soluble lubricant to prevent encrustation, drying, and cracking. He or she should carefully inspect a paralyzed cheek for crusts or other conditions requiring care.

The nurse provides oral hygiene to prevent excessive drying of oral mucous membranes and complications such as parotitis, aspiration, and respiratory tract infections. He or she should perform the following:

Brush the patient's teeth with a small toothbrush at least twice a day. Clean the oral mucous membranes (especially the roof of the mouth), tongue, and gums with toothettes. Agents containing lemon or alcohol should be avoided (or diluted) because they dry the membranes. Then, rinse the mouth. Gauze wrapped around a tongue depressor or toothbrush may help with aspects of oral care.

While performing mouth care for an unconscious patient, the nurse should suction excess secretions to prevent aspiration. It is easier if two nurses perform mouth care together. One nurse does the cleaning while the other suctions as necessary.

Nasal passages may become occluded because an unconscious patient is unable to sniff, blow, sneeze, or clear the nose. To clear the nasal passages of mucus and crust formations, gently swab the nose with an applicator moistened with water or normal saline and then apply a thin coat of water-soluble lubricant with a cotton-tipped applicator.

The nurse should *not* clean the nasal passages or ears of patients who have had brain surgery or head injuries. If bleeding occurs from the ears or nose, or if CSF (a watery discharge) appears to be draining from these areas, the nurse must notify the physician.

Nursing Diagnosis: Skin Integrity, Impaired, High Risk for R/T immobility and loss of protective reflexes.

Planning: Expected Outcomes. The patient will have intact skin, as evidenced by no reddened areas over bone prominences, no areas or signs of skin irritation or dryness, and no signs of corneal irritation.

Implementation. The nurse should provide intervention for all "self-care" needs, including bathing, hair care, and skin and nail care. Patients often scratch themselves as the depth of unconsciousness lessens; therefore, nails should be kept trimmed. It may be helpful to apply superfatted solutions (e.g., castile, baby oil, or cold cream) instead of a bath every fourth or fifth day to prevent loss of cutaneous oils and skin irritation and dryness. Unconscious women need perineal care, especially during menstruation.

The nurse should keep the cornea moist by instilling methyl cellulose (0.5 to 1 per cent) solution. Protective eye shields can be applied or the eyelids closed with adhesive strips if the corneal reflex is absent, if the eyes are open, or if the eyes appear irritated. These measures prevent corneal abrasion and irritation.

When the patient cannot respond to local tissue hypoxia from being in one position for an extended period of time, the risk of pressure ulcers increases. Patients in a coma should be placed on special mattresses or beds (Fig. 13–6). However, the use of these special beds does not eliminate the need to assess the skin and rub the skin every 4 hours. In addition, the nutritional needs of the patient must be met in order to reduce the risk of pressure ulcers.

Collaborative Problem: Risk for contractures, R/T immobility.

Planning: Expected Outcomes. The patient will have no signs of contractures, as evidenced by full range of motion in all joints; no evidence of flexion contractures in wrists, elbows, and knees; and no signs of footdrop.

Implementation. The nurse should maintain the client's extremities in functional positions by providing proper support. An occupational or physical therapist should be consulted for appropriate supportive devices. Remove support devices every 4 hours for skin care and passive exercises.

Nursing Diagnosis: Nutrition, Altered: Less than Body Requirements R/T inability to eat secondary to unconsciousness.

Planning: Expected Outcomes. The patient will demonstrate signs of adequate nutrition, as evidenced by weight remaining stable; consuming adequate calories for age, height, and weight; intake equaling output; incisions or wounds healing within 12 to 14 days; hemoglobin, blood urea nitrogen, total lymphocyte count, and albumin levels within normal limits for age and sex.

Implementation. Intravenous fluids are begun on admission for comatose patients. Initially the intravenous site provides access to the circulatory system for the administration of medications. Because fluid intake is restricted and glucose is avoided to control cerebral edema, an intravenous infusion cannot be considered nutritional support.

Just because a client is comatose, the nurse should never assume that hunger is not present and calorie requirements are decreased. In fact, the opposite is true; caloric needs are increased in patients with head injury. Nutritional and fluid needs of comatose patients are usually met through nasogastric feedings. If the patient does not have paralytic ileus or delayed gastric emptying, and if bowel sounds are audible and gastric residual volumes are less than 100 mL/hr, nasogastric feedings are started. An unconscious patient cannot swallow fluids normally. To prevent aspiration, food and liquids should not be given by mouth.

Nursing responsibilities in tube feeding uncon-

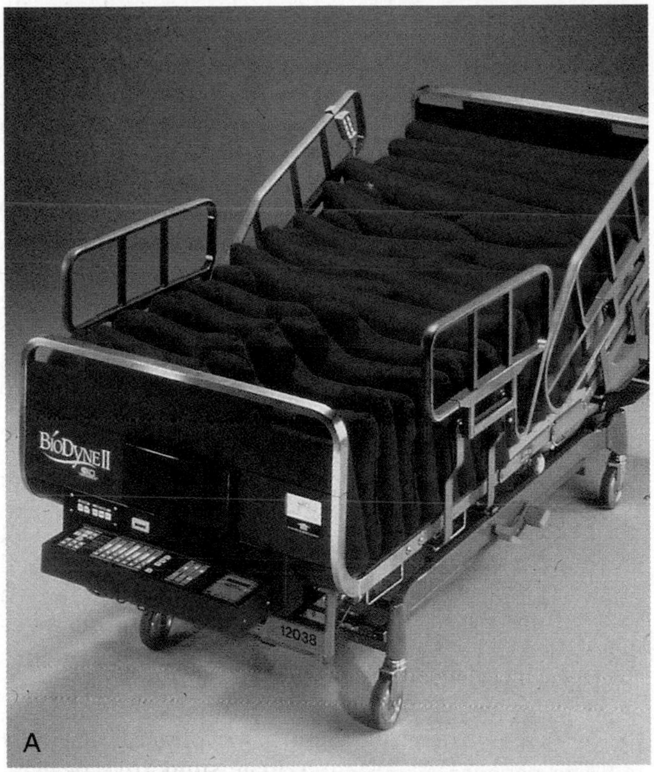

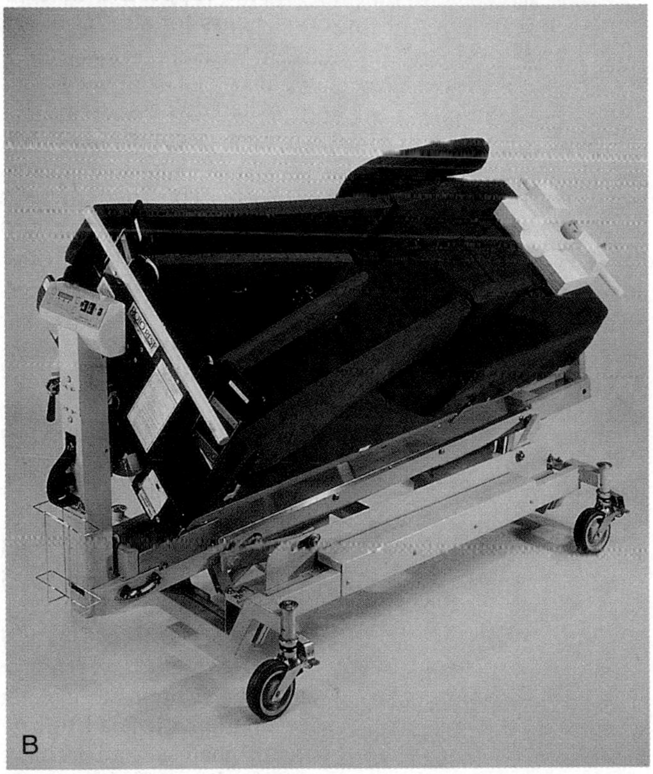

Figure 13–6
A, BIODYNE, an oscillating air support surface. *B*, ROTO REST, an oscillating bed. Both devices are used to treat hypoxemia and to reduce the incidence of nosocomial pneumonia. ROTO REST is also used for clients with spinal cord injury and skeletal traction. (Courtesy of Kinetic Concepts, Inc., San Antonio, TX.)

scious patients are critical because these patients cannot communicate and may have lost protective cough and gag reflexes. The reader should consult a fundamentals text or procedure manual for complications from nasogastric tube feedings.

As consciousness returns and the client begins to respond to verbal stimuli and has a gag reflex, the nurse tests the client's ability to suck and swallow liquid. Before the test, the nurse positions the client sitting up, with suction equipment nearby in case it is needed. A thick juice, nectar, or ice chips should be used rather than water, as thick consistency is easiest to swallow. The nurse places about 1 teaspoonful of liquid into the back of the client's mouth and observes for swallowing. Suction should be used as needed to prevent aspiration. If a client cannot suck through a straw or drink from a glass owing to facial paralysis, fluids can be placed into the unaffected side of the mouth with an Asepto syringe. The nurse should watch for difficulty in swallowing and suction as needed.

Swallowing can be stimulated by having the client lean the head forward and, after taking fluid, quickly tipping the head backward. Stroking the anterior neck may also promote swallowing.

Once a client can safely swallow, small oral liquid feedings can be started, progressing to a soft diet. Tube feedings should be discontinued only when the client can take adequate nutrition orally. Many clients are fed orally during the daytime and tube fed at night to maintain adequate nutrition. When a client begins to eat independently, the nurse should be reassuring and encouraging. He or she should remind the client to eat slowly and to swallow and should position the client sitting up as tolerated.

Nursing Diagnosis: Fluid Volume Deficit, Risk for R/T inability to drink fluids and respond to normal thirst mechanisms.

Planning: Expected Outcomes. The patient will demonstrate signs of fluid balance, as evidenced by equal intake and output for 24, 48, and 72 hours; stable body weight; no signs of excessive perspiration, diarrhea, or vomiting; serum glucose, blood urea nitrogen, creatinine, sodium, potassium, and chloride levels within normal limits.

Implementation. Important aspects in maintaining fluid-electrolyte balance in unconscious patients are (1) accurate intake and output documentation; (2) daily weighing; and (3) assessing and documenting symptoms that may increase fluid volume deficit (e.g., excessive sweating, polyuria, diarrhea, or vomiting).

Before fluid and electrolyte intervention is planned for a comatose patient, the nurse should carefully assess the fluid-electrolyte status. The coma itself may be caused by fluid-electrolyte imbalances. Blood tests such as blood sugar, blood urea nitrogen or creatinine, serum sodium, potassium, chloride, and carbon dioxide help determine fluid-electrolyte status (see Chaps. 3 and 4). Dehydration and water intoxication (true hyponatremia) are common causes of electrolyte imbalance associated with coma.

CRITICAL TO REMEMBER

Overhydration and intravenous fluids with glucose are always avoided in comatose patients because cerebral edema may follow.

Diuretics may be prescribed to correct fluid overload and reduce edema. The nurse should monitor the response to these medications. For evaluating the response to any diuretic, the indwelling catheter should be emptied before the diuretic is administered. When evaluating the response, the nurse should consider the diuretic given, the dose, and renal status.

Nursing Diagnosis: Injury, Risk for R/T unconsciousness and immobility.

Planning: Expected Outcomes. The patient will sustain no injury, as evidenced by no abrasions or bruises and no falls from bed.

Implementation. The side rails must be kept up on the bed and the bed kept in lowest position whenever the patient is not receiving direct care or is unattended. Seizure precautions should be observed for anyone with a history of seizure and for patients who could have a seizure for the first time.

The nurse should give adequate support to limbs and head when moving or turning an unconscious patient. Limbs without tone may dislocate if they are allowed to fall unsupported. An unconscious patient should always be turned toward the nurse or someone else, to stop the patient's rolling off the bed. The nurse should protect an unconscious patient from external sources of heat (e.g., heating pads, radiators).

The nurse should protect the patient from injury during seizures or periods of agitation (e.g., use padded side rails, keep the patient's nails short and clean). Medication may be prescribed to control seizures or hyperexcitability.

Oversedation should be avoided because it impedes assessment of level of consciousness and impairs respiration. The nurse should not restrain the patient unless it is absolutely necessary because restraint is likely to increase confused and combative behavior. Unstable patients should not be unattended.

Nursing Diagnosis: Incontinence, Bowel, Risk for R/T unconsciousness.

Planning: Expected Outcomes. The patient will have reduced risk of bowel incontinence, as evidenced by a bowel movement every 2 to 3 days and no signs of fecal impaction.

Implementation. The nurse plans an intervention to (1) control bowel movements, (2) maintain the patient's normal schedule, and (3) prevent fecal impaction or constipation. As soon as the patient is able, the nurse begins a program of bowel retraining. He or she should maintain a regular schedule of stool softeners, suppositories, and digital removal at approximately the same time each day. The abdomen should be examined frequently for distention, as constipation and fecal impaction may occur.

Nursing Diagnosis: Family Processes, Altered, R/T family member in a coma.

Planning: Expected Outcomes. The family members will exhibit positive coping behaviors, as evidenced by showing an ability to solve problems, not neglecting needs of other family members, and asking questions about the patient that indicate that previous teaching has been understood.

Implementation. The significant others of a comatose patient are often very stressed. It is difficult for the family not to be able to communicate with the patient and at times not know whether the patient will recover. The nurse should include them in the patient's care as much as they can and wish to be involved. It is important that the significant others see the patient receiving quality, professional, caring nursing care. A very caring behavior for the comatose patient and significant others is for the nurse to talk to the patient as if he or she could understand. Initially, this behavior will seem awkward for the nurse, but in time it will feel appropriate. The nurse can tell the patient that he or she will be turned to the side, bathed, and so on. Because the sense of hearing is the first sense to return as consciousness returns, the patient may hear the nurse speaking. Comatose patients have awakened and reported that they remember hearing specific voices.

The patient's significant others are often in a state of shock, needing someone to recognize their need and help them through this difficult situation. They may experience various conflicting, perhaps irrational emotions, for example, guilt and anger. The nurse should reinforce information provided by the physician to the significant others, for example, what happened to the patient and the treatment being planned or given. The explanation may not be understood initially and will need to be repeated. Be sure to explain the function of all the "tubes" that can be seen, as people can be overwhelmed by the presence of many tubes (i.e., intravenous line, catheter, ventilator) and perceive the patient to be in critical condition, when this may not be the case. When the patient is not expected to survive, the significant others should be told of the prognosis and be given the opportunity to be as involved as possible with the decisions about care.

The significant others should be allowed to stay with the patient, when and where this is possible. At times, some significant others may become vigilant in attending and stay at the patient's bedside continuously. The nurse should encourage them to care for themselves also by encouraging adequate meals and sleep. The nurse should have them consider using external support systems (e.g., neighbors and church groups), tell them that they will be called if any significant changes occur, and ask them to leave a phone number where they can be reached. Significant others should be encouraged to call the nurses if they have questions or concerns.

Evaluation

The patient may remain comatose for a few hours or even months. Therefore, some expected outcomes have brief time frames (e.g., airway obstruction) and others are prolonged, requiring frequent re-evaluation (e.g., family coping).

Modification of Plan of Care for the Elderly

The aged patient in a coma requires no different care than the young patient, except that the nurse should be vigilant in assessing for the complications of immobility. The aged patient is at higher risk of all complications of immobility, especially pressure ulcers and pneumonia. For male patients, urinary retention is common because of prostatic enlargement. Finally, the patient should be fully assessed for the common disorders of aging that might be the cause of the coma (e.g., diabetes).

Posthospital Care

The site for discharge from an acute care setting is totally dependent on the condition of the patient and the cause of the coma. If the patient is still in a coma and recovery is expected, placement in a rehabilitation center may be planned. If the patient is in a coma and is not expected to awaken but may live for a time with nutritional support, placement in a skilled nursing center is common. Some comatose patients awaken and make a complete recovery while in the hospital. If it is determined that the comatose patient is brain dead, the family may be approached for organ donation. Funeral arrangements can begin from the hospital for these patients.

DISCHARGE TEACHING

The nurse's role in discharge of the comatose patient centers on communication with the receiving nurses and the client's significant others. If the patient is ventilator-dependent or combative, special consideration will be required for transport to the new facility. A complete plan of care should be provided also.

CONFUSIONAL STATES

Confusion is a mental state marked by alterations in thought and attention deficit, followed by problems in comprehension. Confusion is accompanied by a loss of short-term memory and often irritability alternating with drowsiness.

Etiology

Common causes of acute confusion are alcohol withdrawal and drug ingestion. Confusion can also follow fever, heart failure, head injury, or anesthetics. Other causes of confusion are hypoxia, hypoglycemia, severe fluid and electrolyte disorders, sepsis, liver and renal failure, poisons, and drug overdose. Dementia is a chronic form of severe confusion that affects memory, judgement, and abstract thought, resulting in the loss of personal and social independence in a previously competent individual. Alzheimer's disease is the most common cause of dementia. The remaining cases of dementia are caused by stroke, other neurologic diseases, and other treatable disorders. This section discusses the care of clients who have varying degrees of cognitive changes. The specific care required by the client with Alzheimer's disease and other disorders is discussed in Chapter 15.

Risk Factors

Risk factors leading to confusion vary with the specific etiologic factors. In general, the proper management of various diseases, such as diabetes mellitus, would reduce the incidence of confusion. Disorders such as Alzheimer's disease have no known prevention at this time.

Pathophysiology

Three mechanisms account for the development of acute confusion:

- Damage to the brain with swelling or loss of oxygen, blood, or both (functional disorder)
- Impairment of the action of the nervous system by chemicals or other substances (metabolic disorder)
- The rebound overactivity of a previously depressed center in the brain. Injury to the brain results in increased ICP (see later).

Chemicals that cross the blood-brain barrier, such as alcohol, impair the metabolism of the neuronal cells. When the drug action wears off or the client is withdrawn from the drug, the lower centers in the brain are overactive. This overactivity accounts for the development of acute confusion, combativeness, and other abnormal behaviors.

Chronic confusional states are the result of disorders that cause brain tissue destruction, biochemical imbalances, or compression of the brain. For example, clients with Alzheimer's disease have a lack of acetylcholine, a neurotransmitter that is necessary for short-term memory. Other disorders may be inherited, be caused by viruses (e.g., Creutzfeldt-Jakob disease), or follow diseases (e.g., encephalitis).

Clinical Manifestations

The earliest sign of a metabolic brain disorder is a disorder of attention. The client may report the loss of concentration or appear preoccupied. At the same time, restlessness, emotional lability, insomnia or drowsiness, and vivid nightmares may begin. Clients may appear anxious and fear that they are "going crazy." As the disorder progresses, stupor and coma develop. Symptoms seen in the client are reflective not of personality but of the cause of the disorder. For example, barbiturate or alcohol abuse and withdrawal and liver disorders cause agitated delirium. In contrast, anoxia and kidney and lung disorders cause a more quiet response. Disorders that develop rapidly are more likely to cause an agitated response than are those that develop slowly.

Fluctuations in cognition (the ability to think and reason) are common in clients with metabolic brain disorders. Clients may be totally out of context one moment and lucid the next. Some of the fluctuations are due to the environment, and delirious clients become more disoriented at night, in unfamiliar surroundings, and in situations in which restraints are used, unfamiliar noises are heard, or unfamiliar people are seen. The lack of a window in the room has caused many clients to become disoriented.

The client will commonly have difficulty with immediate recall and ability to abstract. Loss of memory for recent events is a hallmark of metabolic brain disorders. Clients who are delirious quickly lose orientation to time. Normal subjects can readily recall six or seven digits forward and five or six backward and identify the commonalities between an orange and an apple or a tree and a bush. Delirious clients cannot do this. However, the client's general intelligence level can have an impact on the data seen. If possible, the client's level of education and cultural background should be known before assessment.

Perceptual errors (e.g., mistaking the nurse for a daughter) as well as hallucinations, illusions, and delusions are common accompaniments of delirium.

Hallucinations are sensations that occur in the absence of external stimuli. A client may hear, see, feel, smell, or taste something that is not present. The client may or may not realize that the experience is "unreal."

Illusions differ from hallucinations in that illusions are the misinterpretation of something in the environment. For example, if a client sees a shadow on the drape and mistakes it for a real person, the client is experiencing an illusion.

Delusions are thoughts or beliefs that have no basis in fact. For example, a client may think that he or she has been robbed or poisoned, when there is no basis for this thought.

DIAGNOSTIC ASSESSMENT

There are no specific diagnostic tests for confusion. The client would undergo a CT or MRI scan for determining whether there is a structural cause of the confusion, such as a tumor. In addition, a series of laboratory studies would be performed to determine whether there is a metabolic cause. Common studies include a complete blood count, electrolyte determinations, vitamin B_{12} and folate levels, thyroid and liver function studies, drug toxicity screening tests, and an electroencephalogram. A lumbar puncture may be performed for the analysis of CSF.

Medical Management

The medical management of the confused client begins with determining the cause of the confusion and correcting it if possible. When no specific cause is found, the medical management focuses on controlling symptoms.

Surgical Management

There are no operations for the correction of confusion, unless the confusion is the result of a structural disorder such as a tumor or hematoma. For those clients, craniotomy may be performed to remove the growth or accumulation of blood.

Nursing Management

Assessment

The confused client needs a thorough history, which should include the onset of the confusion, past medical illness, work and occupational history, and past injuries. Past medical illness, such as diabetes or liver failure, may be out of control and the cause of the confusion. The client may have been exposed to heavy metals or toxic waste during employment. Past injuries, especially head injury, are important to record. Depending on the level of confusion, the client may not be able to answer each question, and the nurse may need to rely on the family or others who have been with the client. Specific questions to determine how well the client was able to handle routine financial transactions or home safety in situations such as cooking, dressing, and driving will help determine whether the client can return home or needs placement in a nursing home at discharge. At times the family or significant others may report a change in personality, such as apathy, social isolation, disinterest in current events, and irritability. These data should be recorded because they may be symptoms of Alzheimer's disease.

The confused client needs ongoing assessment with use of the Glasgow Coma Scale (see Fig. 13–5) or the mini–mental state form. The nurse should analyze the data collected to determine whether the confusion is improving, worsening, or remaining the same.

The confused client is often combative and argumentative. The nurse should assess whether the client is able to refrain from self-injury or injury to others.

Nursing Diagnosis, Planning, and Implementation

Nursing Diagnosis: Thought Processes, Altered R/T memory loss and lack of self-protective behavior.

Planning: Expected Outcomes. The client will have improved thought processes, as evidenced by improving score on mini–mental state form and reported fewer hallucinations, illusions, and delusions.

Implementation. The confused client will benefit from consistency in the environment and routine. Objects should be kept in the same place, such as the tray table and bedside chair. If possible, the same staff should care for the client. When the routine is changed, the client should be given short explanations as the events occur.

The nurse should reorient the client as often as necessary. The nurse should speak quietly and slowly and repeat as necessary.

CRITICAL TO REMEMBER

Clients with chronic untreatable confusion do not benefit from reorientation and may become more agitated when the nurse attempts to reorient them.

For these select clients, the nurse can avoid reorienting and "go along" with the confusion. Of course, when the client has a risk of injury, safety precautions must be foremost. Clocks and calendars in the room will also help with reorientation. The use of familiar objects is helpful because remote memory is intact. For example, the use of a quilt from home on the bed may help the confused client recognize the bed as his or her own.

Unfamiliar noise should be reduced because it adds to the confusion. The client's room should be quiet and softly lit without producing shadows.

Nursing Diagnosis: Injury, Risk for R/T unpredictable behavior.

Planning: Expected Outcomes. The client will be harmless to self and others.

Implementation. The client must be protected from self-injury. The client should be in a room near the nursing station so that frequent assessments can be performed. In addition, the bed should be in low position and the side rails should be up at all times when the client is not attended. The use of side rails and the low bed position do not guarantee that the client will not fall, but they do remind the client of the location and slow the client down as he or she attempts to get out of bed. Therefore, the nurse must continue frequent assessments. Physical restraints should be used *cautiously*. Some clients become more agitated as they resist the restraint. When restraints are used, the nurse must be certain to remove the restraint every 2 hours to assess the skin beneath it and allow or provide range-of-motion exercises. Chemical restraint (e.g., tranquilizers) should also be used cautiously, and the nurse should assess for the side effects of the drugs, including increased confusion and tremors (extrapyramidal symptoms). The nurse must remember that the client is not in control of his or her behavior. It is unpredictable, irrational, and impulsive. The client may be frightened and suspicious. Comments made by the client should not be taken as personal insults by the nurse. The client should never be "punished" for inappropriate behavior or comments.

Nursing Diagnosis: Sleep Pattern Disturbance R/T daytime napping and nighttime hallucinations.

Planning: Expected Outcomes. The client will have improved sleep patterns, as evidenced by sleeping 4 to 6 hours continuously at night and not sleeping as often during the day hours.

Implementation. Nighttime interventions should be planned to allow 4 to 6 hours of uninterrupted sleep. When the nurse enters the room at night, the client should be assessed for rapid eye movement (REM). When REM is present, the client should be allowed to complete the REM portion of the sleep cycle and the nurse should return later to care for the client. (Recall that a sleep cycle requires 2 to 3 hours and the loss of REM sleep can increase confusion.)

The client should be kept active during the day hours so that there is some fatigue by nighttime. Daytime sleeping is a difficult pattern to break, and the client may have to be "kept awake" in order for the pattern to be reversed. For the elderly client, the normal changes in sleep with aging need to be considered, such as the increased use of short naps and less sleep during the night. Sleeping medications are seldom given to confused clients because they often alter sleep cycles and deplete the client of REM sleep.

Nursing Diagnosis: Family Coping, Ineffective R/T unfamiliar behavior of the client or stress of providing continual care for the client at home.

Planning: Expected Outcomes. The client's significant others will demonstrate improved coping strategies, as evidenced by improved use of support systems and appropriate analysis of the client's condition.

Implementation. When confusion is a new problem for the client, significant others will be distressed by the behavior. The nurse should explain to the family that the client is not able to control behavior or speech at this time. This nurse should assess whether the client becomes calm or agitated when the family or significant others are present and advise visitation accordingly. If possible, the need for and use of restraints should be explained to the family *before* they see the client.

If the client's confusion is the result of a chronic disease, such as Alzheimer's disease, the family may need to find support systems to provide continual supervision of the client in the home. The nurse should be prepared to direct significant others to appropriate resources for determining the client's competency and determine the need for guardianship or durable power of attorney.

Evaluation

The degree of goal attainment should be assessed at regular intervals.

Modification of Plan of Care for the Elderly

The confused aged client is a common problem; therefore, most interventions discussed in the preceding paragraphs are directed at that population.

CRITICAL TO REMEMBER

It is common, but incorrect, to think that elderly clients always have a marked deterioration in mental function.

In general, most elderly clients have difficulty recalling new information, but the remote memory is intact. In addition, depression occurs in 20 to 30 per cent of the elderly. Depression may follow the loss of friends, spouse, health, and independence and may lead to symptoms such as memory loss and confusion.

Posthospital Care

The discharge of a confused client from the hospital varies with the cause of confusion. If the confusion is acute and full recovery is expected, the client can sometimes go home under the care of family members or significant others. If the confusion is chronic, the client will need either care or supervision at home or placement in a nursing home. See also discussion of the care of the client with Alzheimer's disease at home in Chapter 15.

INCREASED INTRACRANIAL PRESSURE

Intracranial pressure is the pressure exerted in the cranium by its contents: the brain, blood, and CSF. The pressure is measured via the CSF. The normal pressure of CSF is 5 to 15 mm Hg or 60 to 180 mm H_2O. Pressures over 250 mm H_2O are called increased ICP and are a symptom of a serious underlying disorder. The pressure of CSF at the lumbar area, such as that recorded during a lumbar puncture, may not reflect the ICP. If the CSF flow is obstructed between the brain and the spinal cord, the lumbar pressure could be normal and the ICP very high.

Incidence and Etiology

Increased ICP occurs commonly in clients with brain tumors, head injury, meningitis, encephalitis, subarachnoid hemorrhage, and disorders that alter the flow of CSF, such as stenosis of the aqueducts and hydrocephalus.

Increased ICP is most often associated with a rapidly expanding lesion (e.g., bleeding), an obstruction to the outflow of CSF (e.g., tumor), or increased CSF formation (e.g., cerebral edema).

Risk Factors

Clients at the highest risk of developing increased ICP are those who have expanding masses in the brain, such as those caused by an injury to the head, surgery on the brain, hydrocephalus, brain tumors, and bleeding (e.g., subarachnoid hemorrhage).

Increased ICP can be reduced by proper positioning of the high-risk client, use of diuretics, and intracranial monitoring for early detection of rising pressures. The use of seat belts in motor vehicles decreases the incidence of serious head injury and therefore would reduce problems from increased ICP.

Pathophysiology

The skull is a hard bony container filled with the brain tissue, blood, and CSF. The pressure within the cranium is maintained by the amount of brain tissue and the pressure of the blood and CSF. A theory for understanding ICP states that since the bony skull cannot expand, when one of the three compartments expands, the other two must compensate by decreasing in volume in order for the total brain volume and pressure to remain constant.

As a mass enlarges, initial compensation in the skull is through displacement of CSF into the spinal canal or back into venous blood through the arachnoid mater. The ability of the brain to adapt to increasing pressure without increasing ICP is called compliance. The movement of CSF is the first and the major compensatory mechanism, but it can offset increasing intracranial volume only to a point. When the ability of the brain to be compliant is exceeded, the ICP rises, the client develops symptoms, and other compensation efforts to reduce pressure begin.

The second form of compensation is by reducing blood volume in the brain. When blood flow is reduced by 40 per cent, cerebral tissue becomes acidotic. When 60 per cent of blood flow is lost, the EEG begins to change. This stage of compensation alters cerebral metabolism and eventually produces brain tissue hypoxia and areas of brain tissue necrosis.

The last stage of compensation and the most lethal is displacement of brain tissue across the tentorium, under the falx cerebri or through the foramen magnum into the spinal canal. This process is called herniation and often results in death.

HERNIATION SYNDROMES

There are four types of herniation syndrome. These conditions occur late in the course of increased ICP and represent the body's last attempt to restore normal brain volume and pressures (Fig. 13–7).

Central Transtentorial Herniation. Central transtentorial herniation is the end result of downward displacement of one or both of the cerebral hemispheres. As the cerebrum is compressed, it displaces the diencephalon and midbrain through the tentorial notch. An early indication of central transtentorial herniation is a change in the level of consciousness. The client may have headache and other symptoms such as nausea and vomiting. If tissue displacement continues, the level of consciousness deteriorates until coma occurs. As the

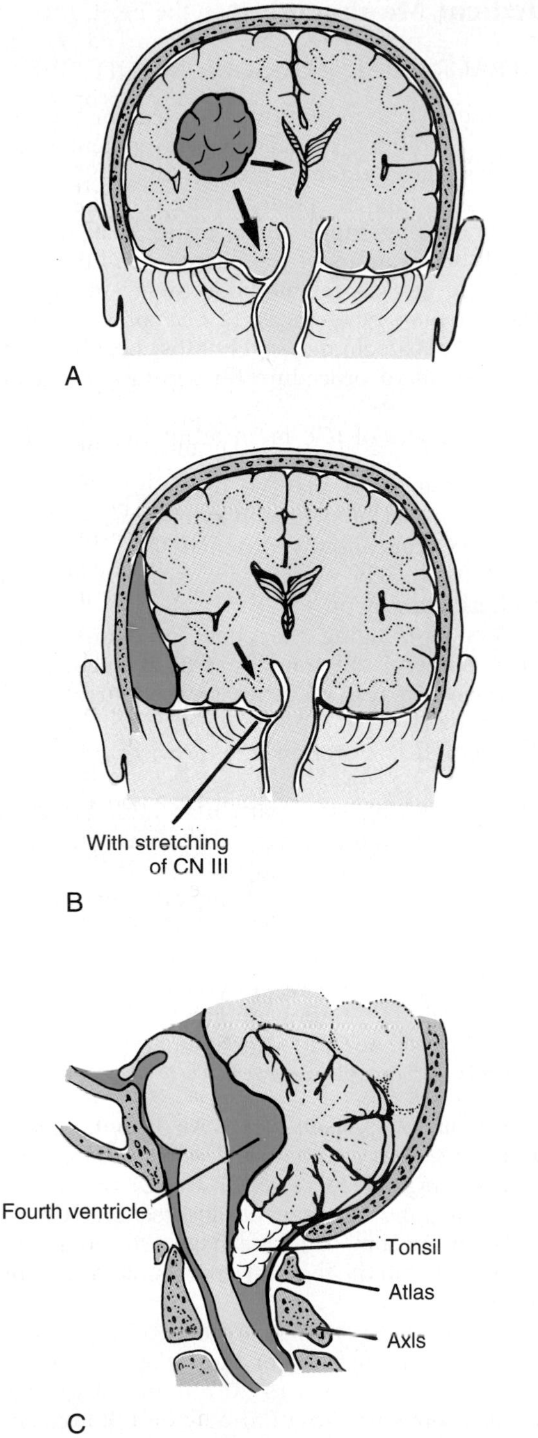

Figure 13–7
Types of herniation syndromes. *A,* Central transtentorial herniation syndrome. A lesion centrally placed or superior in the cranium may compress central and midbrain structures. Assessment findings include confusion and loss of consciousness. This may be followed by a dilated pupil and other signs of herniation. *B,* Lateral or uncal herniation syndrome. Lateral lesion within the cranium causes pressure on the midbrain. Assessment findings include headache, some confusion, and often a dilated pupil on same side of lesion. Client may lapse into coma. *C,* Tonsillar herniation syndrome occurs when the cerebellar tonsils are driven between the posterior arch of the atlas and the medulla and compressed.

midbrain and the upper pons are compressed, Cheyne-Stokes respirations change to central neurogenic hyperventilation, and the pupils dilate and fix at midposition. As herniation continues, the medulla becomes compressed. Breathing stops, the pupils dilate widely, and death occurs.

Lateral Transtentorial Herniation. Lateral transtentorial herniation occurs from masses in or along the temporal lobe. As the temporal lobe is compressed, the uncus and hippocampal gyrus will herniate through the incisura, compressing the third cranial nerve, the midbrain, and the posterior cerebral artery. Symptoms include loss of oculomotor and pupil function from third cranial nerve compression, dilation of the ipsilateral pupil, and decerebrate posturing. At times, a respiratory dysfunction called central neurogenic hyperventilation will be noted also.

Tonsillar Herniation. Herniation of the cerebellar tonsils through the foramen magnum, compressing the medulla and the upper portion of the spinal cord, is called tonsillar herniation. Symptoms include quadriparesis and erratic changes in blood pressure, pulse rate, and breathing. The pupils become small, and there are disturbances in conjugate gaze. This syndrome occurs most often in clients with cerebellar bleeding and occurs rapidly over just a few minutes.

Cingulate Herniation. When the frontal lobes of the cerebrum are compressed, the cingulate gyrus is pressed under the falx cerebri; this process is called cingulate herniation. Symptoms include signs of severe increased ICP as the ipsilateral anterior cerebral artery is compressed, causing ischemia, congestion, and edema.

BRAIN SWELLING AND BRAIN EDEMA

The terms "cerebral edema," "brain swelling," and "increased ICP" are sometimes used interchangeably, but they are not the same. Cerebral edema and brain swelling are causes of increased ICP. An increase in brain bulk due to an increase in cerebral blood volume is called brain swelling.

CRITICAL TO REMEMBER

Brain edema, in contrast to brain swelling, is an increase in the water content surrounding the tissues of brain, such as the extracellular spaces or the white matter, or within the cells themselves.

The distinction between these two conditions is important because the interventions differ.

After head injury, edema develops as a result of a disruption of the blood-brain barrier. This type of edema is similar to other forms of edema, such as that seen in a sprained ankle. The fluid contains electrolytes, proteins, and even blood. Edema reaches its maximum within 48 to 72 hours after brain surgery or injury. The fluid returns to the systemic circulation via the CSF or the venous systems. This form of edema is treated with corticosteroids to stabilize the cell walls and reduce fluid shifts.

Brain swelling occurs when blood vessels within the brain dilate. Brain swelling appears to be the major mechanism responsible for increasing ICP and decreasing the size of the ventricles when compensation occurs. This form of swelling is usually treated with hyperventilation, which causes the cerebral vessels to constrict.

Clinical Manifestations

Symptoms of increased ICP are due to the pull on the cerebral blood vessels by swelling tissues and pressure on the pain-sensitive dura mater and various structures within the brain and back of the eye. Increased ICP is actually several entities occurring at the same time, rather than one process. No single set of clinical manifestations occurs in all clients. Indications of increased ICP relate to the location and the cause of the raised pressure and the speed and extent of its development.

The symptoms of increased ICP are subtle, and the nurse must be diligent in observing for changes in the client's condition. Symptoms include any alteration in level of consciousness, restlessness, irritability, confusion, and a decrease in the GCS score. In addition, the client may have changes in speech, pupillary reactions, motor or sensory changes, or cardiac rate and rhythm changes. Headache, nausea, vomiting, or blurred or double vision (diplopia) may be reported. The optic nerve is an extension of the brain, and increased tension within the skull is transmitted to the optic nerve, where it can be directly observed.

CRITICAL TO REMEMBER

Papilledema has no symptoms, and often the client is surprised to hear about the seriousness of the disorder on the basis of an eye examination.

Cushing's triad of increased systolic pressure, widened pulse pressure, and irregular respirations is a late response to increased ICP and often indicates that herniation is occurring.

The variety of symptoms and the vagueness of those indicating increased ICP have led to the development of more reliable forms of determining ICP, such as ICP monitors. Early detection and treatment of increased ICP can greatly improve client outcome because increased ICP precedes clinical signs and symptoms.

DIAGNOSTIC ASSESSMENT

Clients with symptoms of increased ICP have various studies performed to locate the lesion or other cause. Common diagnostic studies include the CT and MRI scans. Usually a lumbar puncture is not performed because of the risk of herniation of the brain stem when the pressure of CSF in the cord is lower than in the cranium. Continuous ICP monitoring is commonly used in clients with increased ICP.

Medical Management

INTRACRANIAL PRESSURE MONITORING

Continuing ICP monitoring is used for clients experiencing conditions associated with potentially elevated ICP (e.g., head trauma, preoperative and postoperative aneurysms, tumors, posterior fossa lesions). However, ICP monitoring supplements rather than replaces serial clinical observations of the client's condition.

There are several methods of ICP monitoring. The most common types measure CSF pressure in the ventricles or subarachnoid space. Most health care facilities have a standard procedure for setting up and maintaining the monitors.

Advantages of ICP monitoring are the following.

- Pressure increase may be recognized and treated before the onset of signs and symptoms.
- Some systems allow ventricular fluid drainage above a set pressure. The system becomes part of treatment as well as assessment.
- Delays in bringing the client to definitive treatment (e.g., surgery) can sometimes be avoided.
- The effectiveness of other types of treatment can be monitored.
- Level of ICP elevation can provide prognostic information.
- ICP monitoring is of particular value for clients who require paralyzing drugs (e.g., curare for mechanical ventilation) or are being treated with barbiturate-induced coma or induced hypothermia, because key changes in the "neuro signs" of these clients are not easily assessed.
- The effect of nursing intervention on ICP can be monitored. The timing of procedures known to raise ICP (e.g., suctioning) can be altered to coincide with periods of "lower" pressure.

Nursing Responsibilities. An ICP monitor requires continuous observation. Nursing responsibilities include (1) observing for increased ICP, (2) intervening when this occurs, and (3) preventing infection. ICP should be less than 15 mm Hg, mean arterial pressure above 70 mm Hg, and cerebral perfusion pressure above 50 mm Hg.

Increased ICP may be recognized by observing the number on the monitor or by noting elevated (plateau) waves continuing for 5 to 20 minutes. These periods of sustained pressure elevation may be followed or accompanied by signs and symptoms such as extension posturing or disorientation.

Nursing intervention should be planned so that activities known to increase ICP are not performed when elevations are present (e.g., suctioning, excessive hip flexion, turning the client). Administration of endotracheal lidocaine has been helpful in limiting the effect of suctioning on ICP. The nurse should space out interventions so that a stair-step rise in ICP does not occur. Other problems that may contribute to increased ICP are (1) excess water in the respirator tubing, (2) excess secretion production causing a rise in PCO_2, (3) an endotracheal tube taped tightly over the jugular veins, retarding venous circulation from the head, and (4) discussing the client's condition at the bedside.

The nurse can avoid ICP catheter infections by (1) keeping the area around the catheter site clean and dry, (2) documenting and reporting leakage from the catheter, and (3) maintaining a closed system from the catheter to the monitor. If CSF drainage is required, most systems have a stopcock where the tubing and a drainage bag are attached. To drain fluid from the ventricles, the stopcock is turned to the drainage tubing. The system is therefore opened only to change the drainage bag.

PHARMACOLOGIC MANAGEMENT

Osmotic Diuretics. The most commonly used diuretic is mannitol, which removes fluid from the normal brain tissue and not from edematous tissue. Side effects of large doses of mannitol include (1) production of hyperosmolar states, (2) decreased effectiveness with repeated use, and (3) aggravation of edema in some clients.

Loop Diuretics. Treatment with a nonosmotic diuretic like furosemide (Lasix) inhibits reabsorption of sodium and chloride at the proximal portion of the ascending loop of Henle. This drug is often given in varying doses ranging from 10 to 40 mg, alone or in combination with hyperosmolar agents to control cerebral edema. For older clients at risk for congestive heart failure, furosemide may improve the cardiovascular status. The nurse should watch for electrolyte disturbances, ototoxic effects, nausea, and vomiting and monitor vital signs carefully.

Steroids. Steroids, such as dexamethasone (Decadron), may be used. The exact mechanism by which steroids work is unknown, but some physicians believe they are useful in controlling edema, especially brain tumor edema. Their use is controversial. Antacids or H_2-blockers may also be prescribed to control gastrointestinal irritation and hemorrhage.

Antihypertensives. Sustained arterial hypertension over 160 mm Hg is treated. Caution is used to avoid agents that cause peripheral vasodilation along with cerebral vasodilation. Beta blockers have been used in conjunction with other antihypertensives to block effects on cerebral vessels.

Anticonvulsants. Treatment of seizures after head injury requires anticonvulsants. Seizures increase metabolic requirements, cerebral blood flow, cerebral blood volume, and ICP even in paralyzed patients. Phenytoin (Dilantin) and phenobarbital are the usual agents. Seizures are discussed in Chapter 14.

Barbiturate Therapy for Uncontrolled ICP. Some clients require large doses of barbiturates for treatment of uncontrolled ICP. The use of this treatment requires sophisticated monitoring capacity and trained personnel, but its use has shown an increased rate of survival.

The client must be placed on a ventilator and have a Swan-Ganz catheter inserted. Pentobarbital is the drug of choice. While the drug is slowly infused, the client's mean arterial blood pressure is closely monitored because pentobarbital is a cardiac depressant. If the loading dose is sufficient to reduce ICP, a maintenance dose is administered until pressure is under control. Pentobarbital is tapered slowly. It is important to monitor the serum level of the drug daily; the dose should be reduced if the serum levels exceed 5 mg/100 mL.

Assessment of the pupils should continue while the client is being treated. Even though the client is in a deep coma, the pupils will dilate if the brain stem becomes compressed. If pupils become dilated, the physician should be notified. Arterial pressure must be monitored closely, and systemic arterial pressure should not be allowed to fall below 70 mm Hg.

CRITICAL TO REMEMBER

The client's body temperature should also be monitored because barbiturates reduce metabolism and have a concurrent cooling effect on the body.

If temperature falls below 91.4° F (33° C), the patient should be warmed.

MECHANICAL VENTILATION

Hyperventilation, induced by a ventilator or by manual ventilation, is an important adjunct to management. It induces hypocapnia, which reduces cerebral blood volume and ICP. This intervention may be lifesaving while a client is being prepared for other treatments. Manual hyperventilation is sometimes performed during ICP elevations or when sudden clinical signs of deterioration appear.

Surgical Management

Various surgical techniques are used to treat clients with increased ICP. Optimally, the cause is located and removed. Other techniques include (1) surgical placement of a shunt to allow drainage if CSF is blocked and (2) decompressive surgery. The latter is done by removing some brain tissue (e.g., part of the temporal lobe) to give the remaining structures room to expand. If compliance is low at surgery, the bone flap removed to gain access to the brain is not replaced or the dura may not be closed. Subsequent surgery is then required to repair the defect.

Nursing Management

Whether or not hyperventilation is used, the nurse should pay meticulous attention to maintaining respiratory function and assess an intubated client often. Frequent arterial blood gas samples are drawn. Acid-base imbalances are corrected to ensure adequate oxygenation.

The nurse maintains a patent airway by judicious suctioning to prevent buildup of carbon dioxide and elevation of ICP. Intubated clients should be adequately intubated before each passage of a suction catheter.

CRITICAL TO REMEMBER

Because hyperinflation as well as the addition of positive end-expiratory pressure raises ICP, the nurse should keep the passage of a suction catheter as brief as possible. Never exceed 15 seconds.

The use of lidocaine via the endotracheal tube may reduce elevations in ICP. Suction should not be done via the nose because drainage may indicate CSF leak and it is important to be able to observe it.

It is also important to prevent venous obstruction. The head of the bed should be raised 30 degrees. The nurse should avoid turning the client's head sharply to either side and keep the head in alignment with the rest of the body. A regular bowel program should be maintained because excessive strain can cause a Valsalva maneuver, which can result in venous back-up and increased ICP.

Fluid administration for clients with increased ICP is controversial. The nurse should administer fluid exactly as prescribed. Currently the tendency is to use a slightly hypertonic solution (e.g., 5 per cent dextrose in half-normal saline). Such fluid remains in the vascular space and therefore contributes less to cerebral edema. Balanced salt solutions are generally used, but other solutions may be required if complications occur that render the client hemodynamically unstable.

It is important to avoid the use of fluid (e.g., dextrose 5 per cent in water) that moves rapidly into the brain to cause edema. The nurse must remember to document the fluid administered with medications and in keeping monitoring devices open (e.g., indwelling arterial catheter lines). A large amount of fluid can be administered by these routes. The types and amounts of such fluids must be taken into account.

The actual amount of fluid infused per hour is determined by various factors. The nurse should never infuse more than the prescribed amount.

CRITICAL TO REMEMBER

If fluid therapy falls behind, the physician must be consulted.

This is especially important for a client with low intracranial compliance. Mechanical ventilation causes a client to retain fluid.

Increased temperature in clients with increased ICP raises the metabolic rate and aggravates ICP further. Therefore, hyperthermia requires vigorous treatment with cooling measures and prescribed medication.

ALTERATIONS IN BODY TEMPERATURE

For maintenance of a normal body temperature, heat gain must equal heat loss. Heat is produced by metabolism or acquired from the environment. The regulation of body temperature is primarily through blood flow to the skin. Cutaneous blood flow is regulated by the hypothalamus. When the blood flow to the skin increases, the skin becomes red and warm. Heat is lost through the skin by conduction, radiation, or convection. When these mechanisms are not effective in reducing temperature, sweating begins, and evaporation is used to lose heat. If the body is too cold, cutaneous vessels control temperature by vasoconstriction. The skin becomes pale and cool as blood is shunted toward warm internal organs. If it is necessary to increase temperature, metabolic heat production increases, and shivering occurs.

There is a small range of normal temperature in the body. There is no one "normal" temperature. Norms vary according to the client's age and physiology. Central nervous system function is impaired when the body temperature varies 4 degrees from the client's norm. Seizures commonly occur when the temperature exceeds 106° F (41° C). Irreversible changes in the brain occur with a temperature of 111° to 113° F (44° to 45° C).

The term *hyperthermia* is often used to describe a client who has an elevation in body temperature. There are many etiologic agents of hyperthermia, including malfunction of the thermoregulatory center in the hypothalamus, prolonged exposure to heat, loss of water, infection, cocaine toxicity, alcohol withdrawal, and salicylate overdose.

Disorders in the Hypothalamic Centers

The body's thermoregulatory centers in the hypothalamus may malfunction as a result of cerebral edema, after a cerebrovascular accident (stroke), after head injury, as a result of brain tumors, or in association with herniation syndrome. Hyperthermia exceeding 106° F (41.4° C) is most common in clients with central nervous system hemorrhage.

Fever is best understood from the hypothalamus level, and the best example is the thermostat used to regulate the home. The anterior hypothalamus regulates body temperature by balancing the heat gain and loss. During fever, the "thermostat" in the hypothalamus increases, and the common symptoms of fever occur. Heat is produced from shivering muscles and heat conservation (feeling cold) until the blood reaching the hypothalamus matches the thermostat setting. When the temperature of the blood exceeds the hypothalamic thermostat, sweating and vasodilation occur until the body cools to the thermostat setting. In clients with injury to the brain, the action of the hypothalamus can be impaired, and the client can develop hyperthermia. Hyperthermia also increases the demand for oxygen, cardiac output, and pulse rate. These changes can increase ICP and decrease cerebral perfusion. When untreated, hyperthermia can lead to acidosis, hypovolemia, cardiac dysrhythmias, and electrolyte imbalance.

Comatose patients may develop central nervous system hyperthermia (hyperpyrexia) because of damage to the hypothalamus. These fevers are difficult to control. Symptoms of hyperthermia include prolonged temperatures over 106° F (41.4° C), warm skin over the trunk, and cool extremities. The fever is not preceded by chilling. The client does not perspire, and cutaneous blood vessels do not dilate, so body temperature continues to rise. Hyperventilation and seizures may occur. Before hyperthermia from central nervous system disorders is diagnosed, other causes of fever, such as infection, must be considered.

Interventions for hyperthermia are aimed at reduction of body temperature. When body temperature is 101° F (38.4° C), the nurse should keep the room temperature at 70° F (21° C) and remove excess blankets and clothing. He or she should keep the client from being improperly exposed. Cooling blankets can be used if temperature continues to rise. When the cooling blanket is used, the nurse should be certain to provide frequent skin care. He or she inspects the skin every hour or two and covers the cooling blanket with a sheet or bath blanket. The client's temperature should be monitored continuously with a rectal probe. Rapid cooling may induce serious dysrhythmias and hypothermia. These physical methods of reducing temperature are combined with the use of antipyretics for improved therapeutic effects.

Antipyretics are administered as prescribed. These drugs inhibit prostaglandin synthesis and reduce the set point (thermostat) in the hypothalamus. If physical methods to reduce temperature are used when the thermostat in the hypothalamus is set higher, shivering and vasoconstriction will occur in an effort to raise core temperature to match the thermostat. The ideal treatment of fever is the combination of antipyretics and physical methods to promote heat dissipation.

Heatstroke

Heatstroke is an emergency and requires immediate treatment for survival. There are two forms of heatstroke: classic heatstroke and exertional heatstroke.

Classic heatstroke is seen most commonly in the poor, the elderly, the chronically ill, clients with heart disease, the obese, and alcoholics. Hot humid weather lasting 3 days or more increases the risk of heatstroke in these clients. The stress of the heat increases the demand on the heart. In addition, certain medications increase the risk of heatstroke. Some medications decrease the ability to sweat: antihistamines, betablockers, anticholinergics, and phenothiazines. Other medications increase heat production: amphetamines and neuroleptics.

Exertional heatstroke is more common in laborers, farmers, military recruits, athletes (especially football players and long-distance runners), and clients who work in boiler rooms or foundries. Symptoms of this form of heatstroke are similar to classic heatstroke except that these clients sweat. They tend to develop lactic acidosis and have more severe bleeding problems.

Heat Exhaustion

Heat exhaustion is a common disorder that occurs after sustained exposure to heat for more than 3 days. It is caused by a lack of water or salt or both.

Heat exhaustion from loss of water occurs most often in the elderly, the infirm, or unconscious patients because they are unable to verbalize their thirst. It is also seen in clients who supplement their diet with salt tablets but inadequate water. Heat exhaustion from a loss of water is dangerous because it increases the risk of heatstroke. Symptoms of heat exhaustion include intense thirst with dehydration, fatigue, muscle incoordination, agitation, and impaired judgement.

Symptoms of central nervous system disorders are present with heat exhaustion and may include coma and bizarre behavior. In addition, the body temperature exceeds 104° F (40.6° C); the skin is hot, dry, and flushed; and the client is hypotensive as a result of shunting of blood into the peripheral circulation for cooling. Once cooling begins, the client may develop seizures, muscle rigidity, and tremors. Other symptoms may include respiratory alkalosis, hemorrhage, liver and renal problems, and dysrhythmias.

Heat exhaustion from lack of salt occurs mainly in clients who have moved to hot climates and not yet acclimated to the weather. These clients fail to replace the fluid and salt lost through perspiration with lightly salted fluids. The symptoms include weakness, fatigue, severe headache, and muscle cramps. Dehydration, thirst, and weight loss do not commonly occur.

MANAGEMENT

Prevention is key to treatment of heat exhaustion. The rooms of elderly clients in nursing homes should be well supplied with fresh water during hot summer months. Ample water should be included in tube feedings when there is risk that water is being lost through evaporation, perspiration, or respiration. Further treatment includes replacement of water and salt, rest, and removal of the client from the source of the heat. If the client requires rehydration by intravenous therapy, hypertonic fluids are usually given at 2 mEq of sodium per hour. Acclimatization, the process of cardiovascular, endocrine, and exocrine adaptation to warm environments, requires about 2 weeks. During this time, the client should increase oral intake of fluids even though thirst is not felt.

Hypothermia

Hypothermia can occur accidentally through exposure to environmental cold or as a response to illness, or can be induced as a form of treatment. Hypothermia can also occur with central nervous system disorders, congestive heart failure, uremia, diabetes mellitus, drug overdose, and acute respiratory failure.

Hypothermia is induced during some surgical procedures to reduce blood flow to the area and blood loss.

Some near-drowning victims and clients being treated for Reye's syndrome have been treated with hypothermia. Hypothermia decreases tissue metabolism by reducing demands for oxygen and glucose. It also reduces blood pressure, pulse, and cerebral function. Cerebral blood flow is reduced about 6 per cent for every centigrade degree the body temperature is reduced below normal.

Hypotension and somnolence often accompany hypothermia. When body core temperature drops to 86° F (30° C), ventricular dysrhythmias occur. At temperatures below 80° F (26.7° C), unconsciousness develops, and below 75° F (24° C), apnea and asystole occur. Rewarming of the client (in induced hypothermia) occurs slowly by either turning off the cooling blanket or warming the client through the blanket. The client may develop acidosis from the return of acidotic blood and waste from the peripheral tissues that were not completely perfused during the hypothermic state.

The use of cooling blankets is a common technique for induction of hypothermia. The client may be placed in barbiturate coma before hypothermia to control physiologic response to the rapid cooling, such as shivering.

Interventions for the client during hypothermia include continuous assessment. Hemodynamic lines are placed to monitor cardiac and pulmonary function. Internal temperature probes are required to monitor temperature. The remainder of the care is the same as for any patient in coma.

STUDY QUESTIONS

1. With the unconscious client, which of the following positions would *not* be appropriate for airway maintenance?
   A. Sitting up in a chair
   B. Lying flat on the back
   C. Lying on the side
   D. Semi-Fowler
2. A comatose client is receiving tube feedings via a gastrostomy tube. Which of the following actions by the nurse is important to prevent complications?
   A. Check residual volume before feedings.
   B. Feed the client in the supine position.
   C. Feed the client large amounts three times a day.
   D. Stimulate the gag reflex prior to feedings.
3. A 62-year-old client is admitted to the hospital with symptoms of increasing forgetfulness, irritability, and decreasing concentration. In preparing the nursing plan of care, which of the following interventions should the nurse include?
   A. Restrain the client at all times.
   B. Remind the client of her forgetfulness every 2 hours.
   C. Answer questions using short, simple sentences.
   D. Keep the blinds drawn and the lights on at all times.
4. Which of the following nursing measures is appropriate to decrease intracranial pressure?
   A. Encourage vigorous coughing and deep breathing.
   B. Elevate the head of the bed 30 to 45 degrees.
   C. Group nursing activities to provide for long rest periods.
   D. Apply wrist restraints to an agitated client to prevent movement.
5. The nurse is caring for a client with increased intracranial pressure. Which of the following would indicate to the nurse that the client's condition is deteriorating?
   A. Pupillary response to light changes from sluggish to brisk.
   B. The client coughs when the endotracheal tube is suctioned.
   C. The client now responds only to painful stimuli.
   D. The client's EKG shows sinus tachycardia.

CRITICAL THINKING EXERCISES

SCENARIO A

A 76-year-old client has been admitted to the hospital for evaluation of confusion. Her family tells the nurse that the client often appears preoccupied, has difficulty concentrating, and often cries for "no reason." On physical examination, the nurse finds that the client has difficulty with immediate recall and the ability to abstract and appears agitated, often picking at the bed linen.

1. What information should be included in the nursing history of a confused client?
2. A nursing diagnosis of Thought Processes, Altered R/T memory loss is established for the client. Discuss the nursing interventions that are associated with this diagnosis.

SCENARIO B

A 32-year-old woman was involved in a single-car motor vehicle accident. On arrival at the hospital the client was unresponsive, had an irregular respiratory pattern, and was exhibiting decorticate posturing. CT scan revealed a head injury with diffuse cerebral swelling and edema. The client was intubated with an endotracheal tube and had an ICP monitor placed for continuous monitoring.

1. The nurse notices that when the client is suctioned, her ICP rises and remains elevated. What measures may help to prevent this rise in ICP?
2. What are some of the advantages of ICP monitoring?
3. Would 5 per cent dextrose in water be an acceptable intravenous fluid for the client?

BIBLIOGRAPHY

1. Cammermeyer, M., & Appledorn, C. (1990). *Core curriculum for neuroscience nursing* (3rd ed.). Chicago: American Association of Neuroscience Nurses.
2. Crosby, L. J., & Parsons, L. C. (1992). Cerebrovascular response of closed head injured patients to a standardized endotracheal tube suctioning and manual hyperventilation procedure. *Journal of Neuroscience Nursing, 24*, 40–49.
3. Crutchfield, J., et al. (1990). Evaluation of a fiberoptic intracranial pressure monitor. *Journal of Neurosurgery, 72(3)*, 482–487.
4. Cutchins, C. (1991). Blueprint for restraint free care. *American Journal of Nursing, 91(7)*, 36–44.
5. DiIorio, C., & Price, M. E. (1990). Swallowing: An assessment guide. *American Journal of Nursing 90(7)*, 38–41.
6. Folstein, M., et al. (1985). The meaning of cognitive impairment in the elderly. *Journal of the American Geriatric Society, 33(4)*, 228–235.
7. Foreman, M. (1990). Complexities of acute confusion. *Geriatric Nursing, 11(3)*, 136–139.
8. German, K. (1988). Interpretation of ICP pulse waves to determine intracerebral compliance. *Journal of Neuroscience Nursing, 20(6)*, 344–348.
9. Glass, C., & Grap, M. (1995). Ten tips for safer suctioning. *American Journal of Nursing, 95(5)*, 51–53.
10. Hickey, J. V. (1992). *The clinical practice of neurological and neurosurgical nursing.* Philadelphia: J. B. Lippincott.
11. House, M. (1990). Cocaine. *American Journal of Nursing, 90(4)*, 40–45.
12. Laurin, N., et al. (1989). Cerebral perfusion imaging with technetium 99m HM-PAO in brain death and severe central nervous system injury. *Journal of Nuclear Medicine, 30(10)*, 1627–1635.
13. McCance, K., & Huether, S. (1994). *Pathophysiology* (2nd ed.). St. Louis: Mosby–Year Book.
14. Marshall, S., et al. (1990). *Neuroscience critical care.* Philadelphia: W. B. Saunders Co.
15. Newbern, V. (1991). Is it really Alzheimer's? *American Journal of Nursing, 91(2)*, 50–54.
16. Sherman, D. (1990). Managing acute head injury. *Nursing 91, 20(4)*, 46–51.
17. Youmans, J. (1995). *Neurological surgery* (4th ed.). Philadelphia: W. B. Saunders Co.
18. Zegeer, L. (1989). Oculocephalic and vestibulo-ocular responses: significance for nursing care. *Journal of Neuroscience Nursing, 21(1)*, 46–55.

Chapter 14

Nursing Care of Clients with Cerebral Disorders

Learning Outcomes

After completing this chapter, the learner will be able to:

1. Assess the client for clinical manifestations of cerebral disorders, including cerebrovascular disorders, tumors, head trauma, and infections.
2. Teach the client and significant others about the etiology, risk factors, and basic pathophysiology of cerebral disorders.
3. Develop plans of care for the prevention, management, prevention of complications, and rehabilitation of clients with cerebral disorders.
4. Explain the role of the client and significant others in medical and surgical management of cerebral disorders.
5. Implement nursing interventions that optimize the quality of life for clients with cerebral disorders.
6. Evaluate planned client outcomes based on criteria established in the nursing plan of care.

Cerebrovascular Disorders

Cerebrovascular disorders are those problems that result from inadequate blood supply to the brain. Although stroke is the most common problem, cerebrovascular disorders encompass other disorders of blood supply to the brain. This section addresses vascular lesions of the brain including aneurysms and arteriovenous malformations (AVMs).

CEREBROVASCULAR ACCIDENT

A cerebrovascular accident (CVA) or stroke is infarction (death) of a specific portion of the brain due to insufficient blood supply. Stroke can occur from an occlusion (blockage) of one of the major vessels feeding the brain, a partial or complete obstruction of a major intracranial vessel, or hemorrhage within the brain.

CRITICAL TO REMEMBER

The blood vessel affected determines the area and extent of infarction.

Incidence

Cerebrovascular disorders are the third most common cause of death in the United States (preceded by heart disease and cancer). Fortunately, the incidence of stroke has been declining for the past 30 years, in part as a result of the improved control of hypertension, increased diet consciousness, and a reduction in smoking in some segments of the population.

Several other important facts about stroke are noteworthy. There is a higher incidence and death rate for stroke among black people than among white in the United States. Stroke is found equally in men and women, with a greatly increased incidence after age 75.[20]

Etiology

The most common causes of CVA are thrombi and emboli, which result in narrowing or complete closure of one of the vessels supplying the brain, and hemorrhage. Stroke from vascular compression or arterial spasm is less common (Fig. 14–1).

Risk Factors

Box 14–1 lists risk factors related to stroke. Primary prevention focuses on education of the public. Mainte-

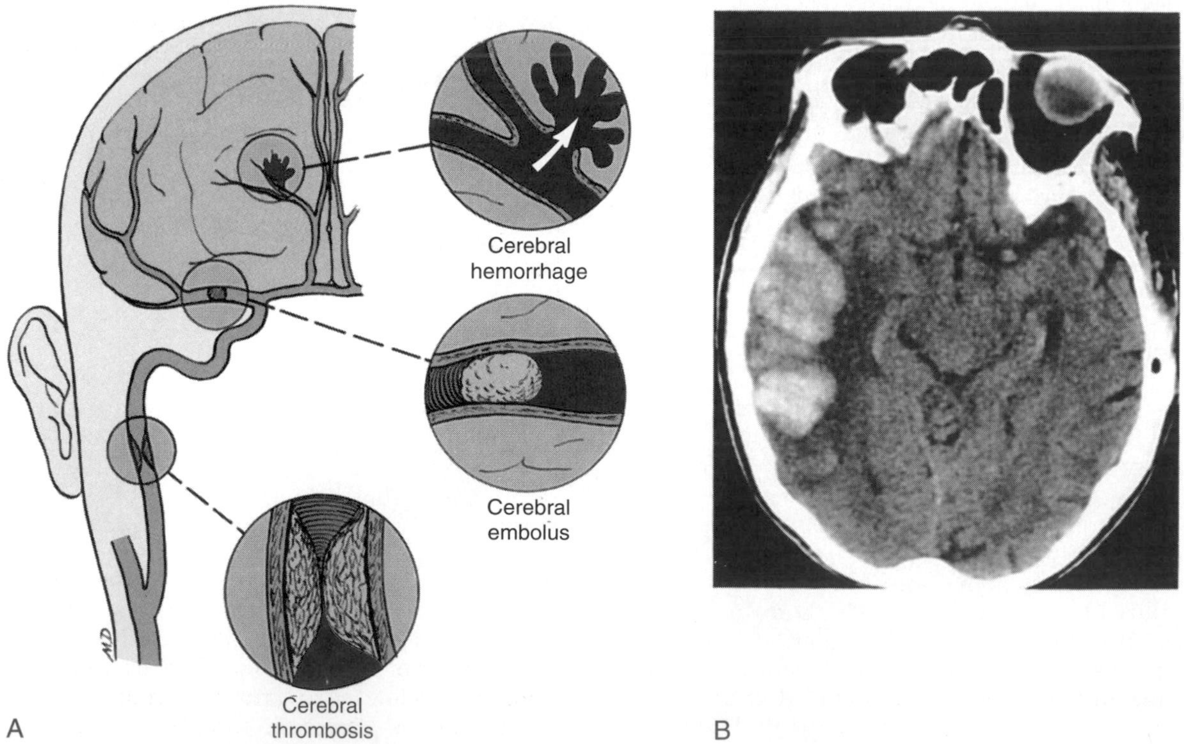

Figure 14–1
A, Events causing stroke. *B*, A magnetic resonance image showing hemorrhagic stroke in the left cerebrum.

BOX 14-1

Risk Factors Related to Stroke

Prior ischemic episodes
Cardiac disease: myocardial infarctions (emboli of the heart, especially with arrhythmias), coronary artery disease, left ventricular hypertrophy, congestive heart failure
Diabetes mellitus
Atherosclerotic disease of intracranial and extracranial vessels
Hypertension
Polycythemia
Hypercholesterolemia
Smoking
Oral contraceptive use
Emotional stress
Obesity
Family history of stroke
Age (incidence increases with age)
Note: With some of these risk factors, the client has a choice (e.g., whether to smoke, overeat, or use oral contraceptives). Also, some strokes may be prevented or minimized by activities such as stress reduction and by a proper balance of diet, rest, and exercise.

nance of appropriate body weight and of cholesterol levels within normal limits lessens the likelihood of stroke, as does avoidance of smoking and oral contraceptives.

Medical management and control of diabetes, hypertension, and cardiac disease decrease the stroke risk factors these diseases present. Clients need education regarding the interaction of various disease processes and how these diseases can increase the severity of one other.

Tertiary prevention addresses those individuals who have already experienced CVA. In such a situation, the goal is to prevent complications related to the present stroke and future infarctions. Immobility carries significant complication risks. Injury related to paralysis and aspiration are other potential complications. Prevention of future CVAs involves minimizing all identifiable risk factors.

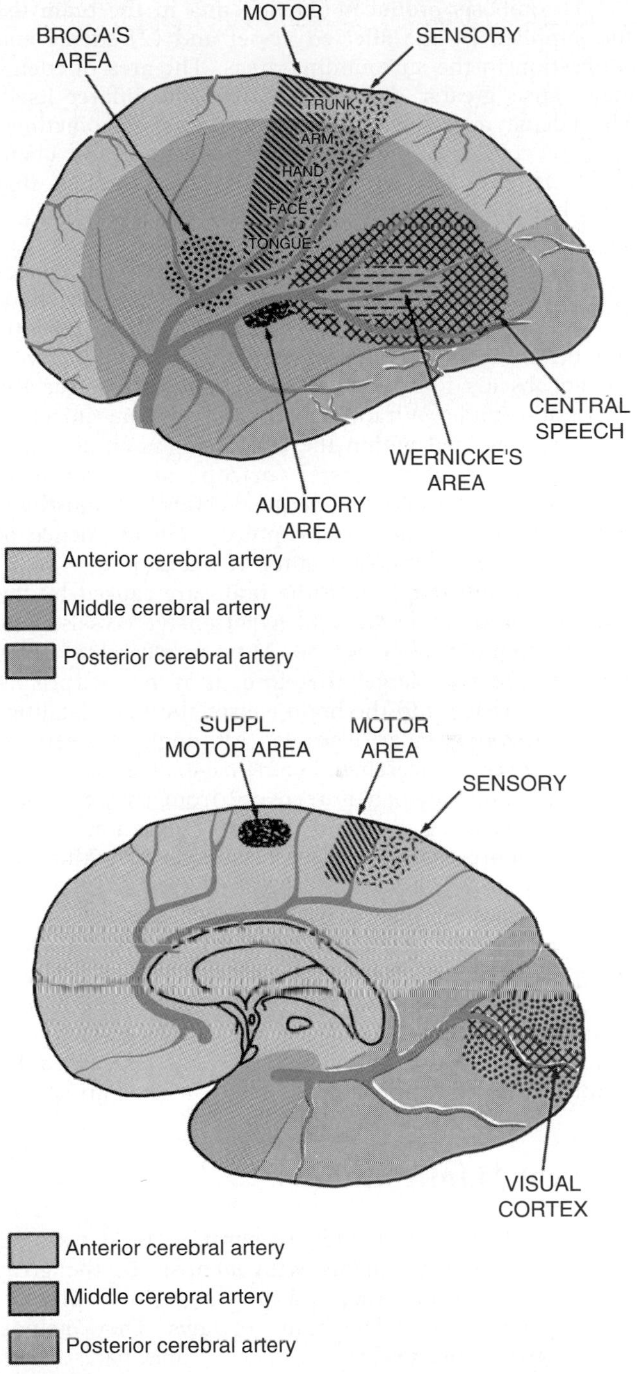

Figure 14–2
Areas of the brain supplied with blood from the branches of the cerebral artery. (From Wyngaarden, J. & Smith, L. [1988]. *Cecil textbook of medicine.* [18th ed.]. Philadelphia: W. B. Saunders.)

Pathophysiology

To understand the pathophysiology of cerebrovascular diseases, it is important to review (1) how the brain receives its blood supply, (2) what areas of the brain are supplied by various major vessels (Fig. 14–2), and (3) the physiology of cerebral circulation (see Chap. 12).

Cerebral infarction is deprivation of blood supply to a localized area of the brain. The extent of infarction depends on factors such as the location and size of an occluded vessel and the adequacy of collateral circulation to the area supplied by the occluded vessel.

Blood supply to the brain may be altered (slowly or rapidly) by local disorders (e.g., thrombi, emboli, hemorrhage, or vascular spasms) or by generalized disorders (e.g., hypoxia from lung and heart disorders). Atherosclerotic disease often affects arteries leading to the brain but affects vessels within the brain much less often. Thrombi may form on atherosclerotic plaques, or blood may clot in an area of stenosis in which the bloodstream is slowed or turbulence occurs. Thrombi that break loose from a blood vessel wall become emboli carried in the bloodstream.

Thrombosis produces (1) ischemia in the brain tissue supplied by the affected vessel and (2) edema and congestion in the surrounding areas. The area of edema may cause greater dysfunction than the infarct itself. The edema may subside in a few hours or sometimes after several days. As the edema subsides, the client begins to improve and may regain some functions that were impaired by the edema. CVA from thrombosis is usually not fatal, unless the infarct is massive.[9]

Occlusion of cerebral vessels by an embolus causes necrosis and edema similar to that following thrombosis, unless the embolus contains bacteria. If it is septic and the infection extends beyond the walls of the vessel, an abscess forms or encephalitis develops (see the discussion under Viral Encephalitis). If the infection remains contained within the occluded vessel, an aneurysmal dilation of the vessel (mycotic aneurysm) may develop. This is dangerous because cerebral hemorrhage may occur if the aneurysm ruptures. The incidence of cerebral embolism increases after 40 years of age.

Most hemorrhages into the brain are caused by the rupture of arteriosclerotic and hypertensive vessels. This is most common after age 50. Most intracerebral hemorrhages are very large; therefore, it is not surprising that hemorrhage into the brain causes the most fatalities of all cerebrovascular diseases. Although recovery is possible after intracerebral hemorrhage, it is less likely and less complete than is recovery from stroke caused by thrombosis or embolus. Brain herniation causes death in more than 50 per cent of clients within the first 3 days after intracerebral hemorrhage.

If cerebral circulation is interrupted extensively, cerebral anoxia develops, that is, lack of oxygen to the brain. In an adult, the changes caused by cerebral anoxia may be reversible for up to 4 to 6 minutes. Changes are irreversible if cerebral anoxia lasts longer than 10 minutes. Cerebral anoxia may be caused by various disorders, the main one being cardiac arrest.

TABLE 14–1 Clinical Manifestations of the Various Causes of Cerebrovascular Accident

CAUSE	CLINICAL MANIFESTATIONS
Thrombosis	Tends to develop during sleep or within 1 hour of arising Ischemia is produced gradually; therefore, the clinical manifestations develop more slowly than those caused by hemorrhage or emboli Relative preservation of consciousness Hypertension
Embolism	No discernible time pattern, unrelated to activity Clinical manifestations occur rapidly, within 10–30 seconds and often without warning; no headache May have rapid improvement Relative preservation of consciousness Normotension
Hemorrhage	Typically occurs during active, waking hours Severe headache occurs (if client is able to report symptoms) Rapid onset of complete hemiplegia, occurs over minutes to 1 hour; most likely form to be fatal Usually results in extensive, permanent loss of function with slower, less complete recovery Rapid progression into coma Nuchal rigidity

Clinical Manifestations

Although they are not often recognized, focal warning signs may occur in clients with stenosis of the great vessels in the neck. Such warning signs may precede severe paralysis by a few hours or days. They include hemiplegia, transient loss of speech, and paresthesias involving half of the body. These manifestations are called transient ischemic attacks (TIAs) and should not be ignored (see later discussion).

Five events that may precede cerebral hemorrhage in hypertensive clients are

- severe occipital (back of head) or nuchal (nape of neck) headaches
- vertigo (dizziness) or syncope (fainting)
- motor or sensory disturbances (e.g., tingling, paresthesias, transient paralysis)
- nosebleeds (epistaxis)
- retinal hemorrhages

Other findings associated with strokes include headache, vomiting, seizures, coma, nuchal rigidity, fever, hypertension, electrocardiographic abnormalities (e.g., prolonged ST segment), sclerosis of peripheral and retinal vessels, confusion, disorientation, memory impairment, and other mental changes. Depending on the hemorrhage or infarct site, focal neurologic findings may be present (e.g., weakness or paralysis, sensory loss, language disorder, and reflex changes).

Table 14–1 correlates clinical manifestations of CVA with the cause. See Clinical Manifestations: Cerebrovascular Accidents Affecting Various Areas of the Brain for manifestations correlated with the area of brain affected.

SPECIFIC DEFICITS AFTER CEREBROVASCULAR ACCIDENT

Many deficits can occur with CVA, depending on the area of the brain damaged as well as the side of the brain (e.g., dominant). The client may have more than one of the following deficits or have very little impairment after CVA.

Hemiplegia. Hemiplegia is paralysis of one side of the body. Hemiplegia results from damage to the motor area of the cortex or the pyramidal tract fibers. Hemorrhage or clot in the brain's right side causes left-sided hemiplegia, and vice versa. This is because nerve fibers cross over in the pyramidal tract as they pass from the brain to the spinal cord. Other cortical areas may be affected, producing localized symptoms (e.g., hemianesthesia, hemianopia, apraxia, agnosia, aphasia).

Muscles of the thorax and abdomen are usually not paralyzed because they are innervated from both cerebral hemispheres. Sudden hemiplegia usually results from cerebral thrombosis.

CLINICAL MANIFESTATIONS

Cerebrovascular Accidents Affecting Various Areas of the Brain

	Location						
	Middle Cerebral Artery	*Anterior Cerebral Artery*	*Posterior Cerebral Artery*	*Internal Carotid Artery*	*Vertebral-Basilar System*	*Anteroinferior Cerebellar (Lateral Pontine)*	*Posteroinferior Cerebellar*
Motor changes	Contralateral hemiparesis or hemiplegia	Contralateral hemiparesis, foot and leg deficits greater than arm, footdrop, gait disturbances	Mild contralateral hemiparesis (with thalamic or subthalamic involvement) Intention tremor	Contralateral hemiparesis with facial asymmetry	Alternating motor weaknesses Ataxic gait, dysmetria (uncoordinated actions)	Ipsilateral ataxia Facial paralysis	Ataxia Paralysis of larynx and soft palate
Sensory changes	Contralateral hemisensory alterations Neglect of involved extremities	Contralateral hemisensory alterations	Diffuse sensory loss (thalamic)	Contralateral sensory alterations	Numbness of the tongue	Ipsilateral loss of sensation in face, sensation changes on trunk and limbs	Ipsilateral loss of sensation on face, contralateral on body
Visual or ocular changes	Homonymous hemianopia Inability to turn eyes toward affected side	Deviation of eyes toward affected side	Pupillary dysfunction (brain stem) Loss of conjugate gaze, nystagmus Loss of depth perception Cortical blindness Homonymous hemianopia	Hemianopia Ipsilateral periods of blindness (amaurosis fugax)	Double vision Homonymous hemianopia Nystagmus, conjugate gaze paralysis	Nystagmus	Nystagmus
Speech changes	Dyslexia, dysgraphia, aphasia	Expressive aphasia	Perseveration Dyslexia	Dysphagia	Dysarthria, dysphagia		Dysarthria, dysphagia, dysphonia
Mental changes		Confusion, amnesia Flat affect, apathy Shortened attention span Loss of mental acuity	Memory deficits		Memory loss Disorientation		
Other changes	Vomiting may occur	Apraxia (inability to carry out purposeful movements in nonaffected areas)	Visual hallucinations	Mild Horner's syndrome Carotid bruits	Drop attacks Tinnitus, hearing loss	Horner's syndrome Tinnitus, hearing loss	Horner's syndrome Hiccoughs and coughing

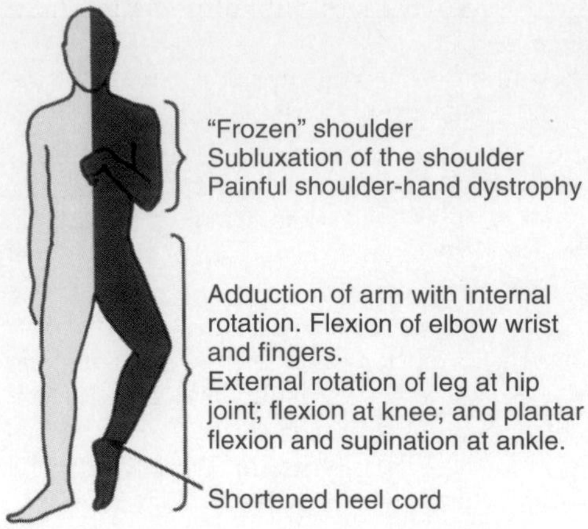

Figure 14–3
Hemiplegic deformities to be prevented. Note that the elbow is bent, the wrist is flexed, and the fingers are curled into palmar flexion; the knee is bent and the heel cord shortened. (Illustration by K. C. Sorensen.)

When voluntary muscle control is destroyed, strong flexor muscles overbalance the extensors. This can cause serious deformities (Fig. 14–3).

Aphasia. Aphasia, a defect in using and interpreting the symbols of language, is caused by a cerebral cortex disorder. Aphasia may involve any or all aspects of language use, such as speaking, reading, writing, and the understanding of spoken language. Aphasia may be (1) sensory (receptive or fluent aphasia), affecting speech comprehension, or (2) motor (expressive or nonfluent aphasia), affecting speech production.

Sensory aphasias involve loss of the ability to comprehend written, printed, or spoken words. For example, with auditory or acoustic aphasia clients have difficulty understanding what is being said. They hear sound but cannot make sense out of it because they cannot understand the symbolic communication associated with the sound. Visual aphasia is similar. Affected clients cannot read words but can see them. They cannot understand the symbolic content of printed or written symbols.

Motor aphasias include aphasias in which the ability to write, make signs, or speak is lost. For example, with motor aphasia, words may be recalled, but the client cannot combine speech sounds into words and syllables. Most aphasias are mixed (expressive-receptive), affecting both expressive and receptive elements.

Most aphasias are partial rather than complete. The severity of aphasia varies with the area and the extent of cerebral damage. Severe damage may deprive the client of any meaningful relationship with the environment. Global aphasia (total aphasia) is so extensive that neither expressive nor receptive language abilities are retained.

TABLE 14–2 Types of Aphasia

TYPE OF APHASIA	CLINICAL MANIFESTATIONS	AFFECTED BRAIN AREA
Global aphasia	Spontaneous speech absent or limited to a few stereotyped words Comprehension reduced to client's name or few words	Posterior and anterior cortical areas
Nonfluent aphasia	Telegraphic speech, conjunctions and pronouns not used Repetition and reading aloud impaired Naming may show paraphasias Auditory and reading comprehension intact Frustration, agitation, depression	Anterior speech area Right-sided hemiplegia
Fluent aphasia	Severe disturbance in auditory comprehension Speech is well articulated but lacks meaningful content, is unrelated to questions, has paraphasias Client seems unaware he or she does not make sense; reading and writing are impaired	Posterior language area
Conduction aphasia	Fluent, halting speech; word finding pauses; paraphasias Comprehension good, naming disturbed, reading unimpaired; writing shows errors in spelling, word choice, syntax	Supramarginal gyrus and arcuate fasciculus between anterior and posterior areas
Anomic aphasia	Word finding difficulty, inability to name objects on confrontation Repetition good May have alexia (inability to read) and/or agraphia (inability to write)	Can be caused by lesions in many parts of dominant hemisphere
Articulation disturbances (dysarthrias)	Buccofacial apraxia (inability to control muscles needed for speech) Dysfluency (stuttering or stammering)	Lesions between supramarginal gyrus and frontal lobe Etiology not known

From Chenitz, W., et al. (1991). *Clinical gerontological nursing.* Philadelphia: W. B. Saunders; adapted from Strub, R., & Black, F. W. (Eds.) (1985). *The mental status examination in neurology.* Philadelphia: F. A. Davis.

Aphasia is caused by pathologic lesions affecting specific locations in the cortex (Table 14–2). The most common cause of aphasia is vascular disease of the brain, especially involving the middle cerebral artery. Aphasia may occur if blood supply to the speech center is cut off. Aphasia is associated with hemiplegia involving the dominant hemisphere. The speech center for a right-handed client is located in the left cerebral hemisphere. The speech center for a left-handed client may be in the brain's right side. Thus, a right-handed client with a right-sided hemiplegia may have aphasia, because the speech center is in the damaged left hemisphere.

Apraxia. Apraxia is a condition in which a client can move the affected part but cannot use it for specific purposeful actions (e.g., walking, speaking, or dressing). The part is not paralyzed or uncoordinated. An apraxic client can conceive or conceptualize the content of messages to send to muscles (e.g., "stand"). However, it is impossible to reconstruct the motor patterns or schema necessary to convey the impulse message. Thus, accurate "instructions" do not reach the limb from the brain, and the desired action or movement does not happen.

Apraxia ranges from relatively simple to highly complex disorders. It may occur in any or all modalities and may vary from one modality to another; for example, a client may have less difficulty writing than speaking, or vice versa.

In hemiplegic clients, apraxic and agnosic states generally occur along with other symptoms. Such clients are at great risk of injury and have a poor prognosis for functional recovery.

Visual Changes. Lesions in the parietal and temporal lobes may interrupt visual fibers of the optic tract (en route to the occipital cortex) and produce visual defects. A lesion on one side of the brain produces a defect in the opposite half of the visual field. Such defects occur in the same visual field of each eye.

Visual deficiency problems are often associated with hemiplegia and may prevent the client from seeing recognizable cues. Visual disorders may interfere with a client's ability to relearn motor skills and increase the risk of accidents.

Homonymous Hemianopia. Homonymous hemianopia (Fig. 14–4) is defective vision or visual loss in the same half of the visual field of each eye, so the client sees only one half of normal vision. Clients with homonymous hemianopia cannot see past the midline toward the side opposite the lesion without turning the head toward that side.

Depth perception and visual perception of horizontal and vertical planes may also be impaired. In clients with hemiplegia, this causes motor performance prob-

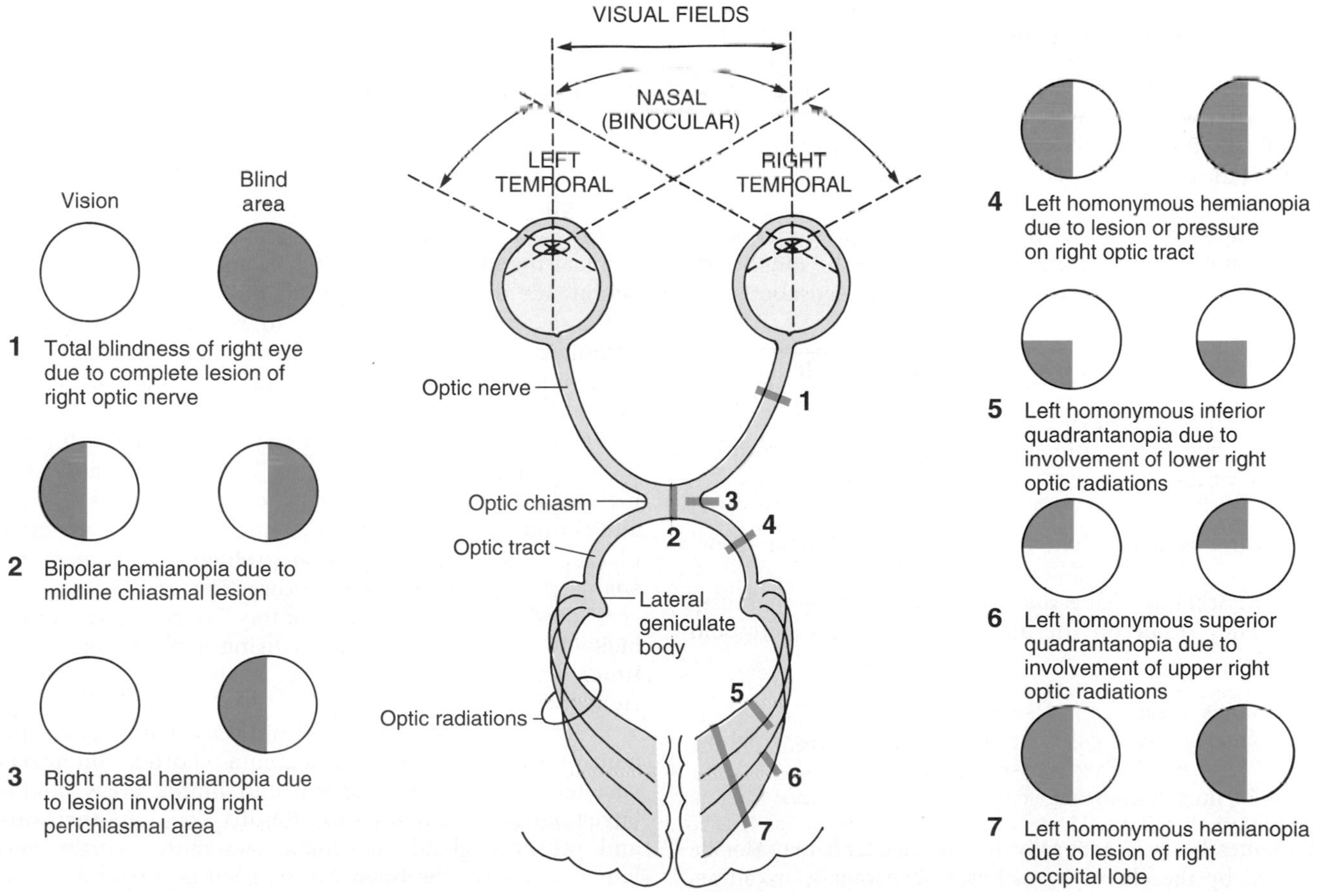

Figure 14–4
Visual field defects associated with optic nerve lesions.

lems in gait and posture. Clients may or may not be aware of a perceptual difficulty, but it may cause them to be accident prone and their behavior to appear bizarre.

Agnosia. Agnosia is a disturbance in interpreting visual, tactile, or other sensory information. The client is unable to recognize objects. Agnosia may be visual, auditory, or tactile but is not the same as blindness, deafness, or loss of touch. Loss of muscle-joint sensation may be accompanied by inaccurate beliefs about the position of a limb in space or its existence or ownership. For example, a man with agnosia may not feel his arm is part of his body, may be unaware of his arm's position, or may deny that a limb is paralyzed when it is.

A client with visual agnosia sees objects but is unable to recognize or attach meaning to them. Disorientation occurs because of inability to recognize environmental cues, familiar faces, or symbols. Such a client may examine objects curiously but be unable to know their function. This can cause considerable self-care deficit when common, necessary objects such as silverware, clothing, or toilet articles are unfamiliar.

Visual agnosia greatly increases risk of injury because the client cannot recognize danger or symbols warning of danger. Extensive visual agnosia can produce such extreme behavioral effects that the client may be inaccurately diagnosed as having diffuse dementia.

Dysarthria. Dysarthria is imperfect articulation that causes difficulty in speaking. It is important to differentiate between dysarthric and aphasic speech. With dysarthria, the client understands language but has difficulty pronouncing words and may slur them, enunciating poorly. There is no disturbance in grammar or in phrase or sentence construction. A dysarthric client can understand verbal speech and can read and write (unless the dominant hand is paralyzed, absent, or injured).

Dysarthria is caused by cranial nerve dysfunction. It may result from weakness or paralysis of the muscles of lips, tongue, and larynx or from a loss of sensation.

CRITICAL TO REMEMBER

In addition to speaking problems, clients with dysarthria often have difficulty chewing and swallowing food because of poor muscle control.

Dysarthria is a problem for clients with bulbar disorders.

Kinesthesia. Kinesthesias are alterations in sensation. They occur on the affected side of the body and include

- hemianesthesia (loss of sensation)
- paresthesia (feelings of heaviness, numbness, tingling, prickling, heightened sensitivity)
- loss of muscle-joint sense

Hemianesthesia is generally incomplete and may not be noticed by the client. Paresthesia occasionally manifests in a hemiplegic client as persistent, boring pain. Proprioception and postural sense disturbance may occur with loss of muscle-joint sense. This may interfere seriously with the ability to ambulate because of lack of balance control and inappropriate movements. The risk of falling is high because of the tendency to misplace the feet when walking.

Incontinence. Bowel and bladder incontinence do not result from all types of stroke. There is no physiologic reason for a client with a unilateral hemisphere lesion to be incontinent. Incontinence in hemiplegic clients occurs because of

- inattention
- memory lapses
- emotional factors
- inability to communicate

Shoulder Pain. Many clients have severe pain in the affected shoulder after CVA. This pain can be so severe that it restricts mobility and self-care because of the lack of balance and loss of range of motion (ROM). The problem can be aggravated by overstretching from turns and transfers. Some clients have experienced subluxation (partial dislocation) of the shoulder both from having the shoulder pulled on and from the weight of the arm pulling it. Chronic subluxation results in shoulder-hand syndrome (characterized by a painful or frozen shoulder and hand edema).

Horner's Syndrome. Horner's syndrome is the paralysis of sympathetic nerves to the eye, causing sinking of the eyeball, ptosis of the upper eyelid, slight elevation of the lower lid, constriction of the pupil, and lack of tearing in the eye.

Unilateral Neglect. Unilateral neglect is described as a deficit of looking, listening, touching, and searching as opposed to a deficit of seeing, hearing, feeling, or moving. Clients with neglect often have intact vision but will not look at or search for specific areas of the environment. Because of the dominance of the right hemisphere in directing attention, neglect is most commonly seen in clients with right hemisphere damage. Clinical manifestations of neglect appear on the contralateral side to the lesion and include failure to attend to one side of the body, failure to report or respond to stimuli on one side of the body, failure to use one extremity, and failure to orient the head and eyes to the one side.[11]

Other Deficits. The client may also have difficulty in localizing objects within the environment and estimating their size or distance. The client may have difficulty finding routes or following directions to new places. This is due in part to problems with memory, spatial perception, and loss of direction.

Some clients lose their ability to recognize numbers; this prohibits them from using a phone or telling time. The client may also be unable to discriminate right from left.

Various portions of the brain assist with behavioral control and coping. The cerebral cortex interprets various stimuli. The temporal and limbic areas modulate emotional responses to stimuli. The hypothalamus and pituitary gland coordinate the motor cortex and language areas. The brain can be seen as an inhibitor of emotions, and when the brain is not fully functional, emotional reactions and responses lack this inhibition.

After CVA, clients are often emotionally labile, confused, forgetful, and frustrated. They tend to burst into tears or (less commonly) laughter without provocation. Clients may also use profanity, which is often termed automatic language. Also, they may appear highly distressed but not feel distress.

Other emotional or behavioral reactions may occur, including

- severe mood swings
- social withdrawal (especially in aphasic and dysphasic clients)
- inappropriate sexual behavior
- outbursts of frustration and anger
- regression to earlier behavior, perhaps childlike

Complications

Complications of stroke depend primarily on the location of the lesion or infarcted tissue. If the brain stem is affected, blood pressure fluctuations, altered respiratory patterns, and cardiac dysrhythmias are all possible. Aspiration, immobility, and injury related to the client's not realizing his or her physical limitations are other potential complications.

Coma can follow stroke from various causes. The blood supply to the brain stem or reticular activating system may have been directly occluded. Likewise, the deep structures of the thalamus that relay information to the cerebral cortex may be involved. Vascular occlusion of the internal carotid artery or one of its major branches may also decrease the level of consciousness. Sometimes, the cerebral edema that follows stroke may produce midline shifts, resulting in coma.

Strokes resulting from occlusal disease (thrombus, embolus) rarely cause sudden death. When sudden death does occur, it is usually due to heart failure. However, if an intracerebral hemorrhage ruptures into the ventricles, symptoms of increased intracranial pressure (ICP) develop, and the outcome is fatal. When stroke is fatal, death may occur within 3 to 12 hours but is more usual between 1 and 14 days after the original episode. Typically, with any type of fatal stroke, a rise in temperature, heart rate, and respiratory rate occurs along with deepening coma several hours or days before death. This is because of damage to the vasomotor and heat-regulating centers.

There are two primary causes of death with stroke: (1) respiratory infection and (2) brain stem failure. Impaired consciousness, altered attention, and feeding and swallowing problems all predispose to respiratory infections, which can lead to death from progressive hypoxia. Increasing ICP, central herniation, and brain stem hemorrhage lead to death from depression of the vital centers in the medulla, that is, brain stem failure.

DIAGNOSTIC ASSESSMENT

The tests used to diagnose CVA are summarized in Table 14–3.

Medical Management

Medical management of the client after CVA is directed toward

- preserving life
- minimizing residual deformity
- reducing ICP
- preventing extension or recurrence

Specific treatment goals and interventions are used in the treatment of the various causes of CVA. Some facilities have developed clinical pathways for clients who have sustained a CVA; see Appendix C for an example.

The client is placed at bed rest with the head elevated to 30 degrees to reduce ICP and facilitate venous drainage. Sometimes, external ventriculostomy drainage is used for a few days to reduce pressure from cerebrospinal fluid (CSF) accumulation. Blood pressure and level of consciousness (LOC) are closely monitored. The goal is to maintain blood pressure enough to prevent another stroke or hemorrhage but not to the point at which cerebral perfusion is decreased. Because many clients with hemorrhagic stroke have a history of hypertension, it is common to maintain their systolic blood pressure at 150 to 160 mm Hg. Fluids are administered carefully for avoidance of fluid volume excess and further cerebral ischemia. The client may require continuous mechanical ventilation and may develop coma.

CRITICAL TO REMEMBER

Rehabilitation begins during this acute period after the CVA.

Interventions directed at preserving ROM and muscle tone are beneficial. In addition, the family and significant others are taught about the condition and what they can do to promote the client's independence.

OCCLUSIVE STROKE

The sudden occlusion of a major artery or blood supply to a large portion of the brain is usually poorly tolerated, especially in the elderly. If the dominant hemisphere is involved, aggressive medical management may not be considered if there is slim potential for rehabilitation. The choices of whether to pursue aggressive treatment focus on a number of factors. At present, the treatment for most clients with large infarctions is supportive care. Hopefully, future research can improve the treatment outcomes for these clients.

EMBOLIC STROKE

The usual cause of embolism is cardiac disorders. Atrial fibrillation, cardiac valve disorders, valve prostheses, and bacterial endocarditis are common disorders that result in thrombus formation. The thrombi break loose from the left side of the heart (embolize) and travel to the brain. Treatment is directed at resolution of the underlying problem for preventing further emboli.

TABLE 14–3 Diagnostic Assessment Findings in Cerebrovascular Disorders

	INTRACEREBRAL HEMORRHAGE	CEREBRAL THROMBOSIS	CEREBRAL EMBOLISM	SUBARACHNOID HEMORRHAGE	VASCULAR MALFORMATION AND INTRACRANIAL BLEEDING
History and related disorders	Suspect diagnosis, especially if other hemorrhagic manifestations are present, and in acute leukemia, aplastic anemia, thrombocytopenic purpura, and cirrhosis of the liver	Evidence of arteriosclerosis, especially coronary, peripheral vessels, aorta; associated disorders: diabetes mellitus, xanthomatosis	Evidence of recent emboli: (1) other organs (spleen, kidneys, lungs), extremities, intestines; (2) several regions of brain in different cerebrovascular areas	History of recurrent stiff neck, headaches, subarachnoid bleeding	History of repeated subarachnoid hemorrhages, epilepsy
Special findings	Hypertensive retinopathy, cardiac hypertrophy, and other evidence of hypertensive cerebrovascular disease may be present	Evidence of arteriosclerotic cardiovascular disease frequently present	Cardiac dysrhythmias or infarction (source of emboli usually in the heart)	Subhyaloid (preretinal) hemorrhages Focal neurologic signs frequently absent; nuchal rigidity, positive finding of Kernig's and Brudzinski's signs	Subhyaloid (preretinal) hemorrhages and retinal angioma Focal neurologic signs; cranial bruit
Cerebrospinal fluid	Grossly bloody	Clear	Clear	Grossly bloody	Grossly bloody
Skull radiography	Shift of pineal to opposite side	Calcification of internal carotid artery siphon visible; shift of pineal to opposite side may occur	Pineal apt to show little if any displacement	Partial calcification of walls of aneurysm sometimes noted	Characteristic calcifications in skull films may be present
Cerebral angiography	Hemorrhagic area seen as vascular zone surrounded by stretched and displaced arteries and veins	Arterial obstruction or narrowing of circle of Willis (internal carotid, etc.)	Arterial obstruction of circle of Willis branches (internal carotid, etc.)	Typical aneurysmal pattern in circle of Willis arteries (internal carotid, middle cerebral, anterior cerebral, etc.)	Characteristic pattern showing cerebral arteriovenous malformation
Brain scan	May show increased uptake in affected cerebral area; most marked in 2–3 weeks, with diminution or clearing thereafter			Apt to be normal	Increased uptake may be seen in area of arteriovenous malformation
Echoencephalography	May show shift of midline toward opposite side in clients with a cerebral lesion acting as a mass				
Computed tomography and magnetic resonance imaging	May show area of hematoma, infarct, or the like with distortion or shift of ventricles				

From Chusid, J. G. (1985). *Correlative neuroanatomy and functional neurology* (19th ed.). Los Altos, CA: Lange Medical Publications.

HEMORRHAGIC STROKE

Treatment of hemorrhagic stroke depends in part on the condition of the client when first seen. A client who is seen with a severe headache but who is fully conscious will probably survive no matter what the therapy. The client who is in a coma is likely to do poorly despite intensive medical or surgical intervention.[15]

Hypoxia often occurs in clients with hemorrhagic stroke because of inadequate ventilatory effort. Intubation and continuous mechanical ventilation may be required to prevent injury to the brain from hypoxia.

Often intracranial hemorrhage is accompanied by

hyperthermia. This condition increases oxygen use by the brain at a time when the oxygen supply is compromised. Antipyretics may be prescribed. In addition, a hypothermia blanket or ice packs may be required to reduce body temperature. Causing the client to shiver should be avoided, however, because shivering increases oxygen consumption and ICP.

STROKE IN EVOLUTION

In clients in whom the cerebral infarction is still evolving, the eventual area of defect is controllable. Treatment centers on improving cerebral blood flow by avoiding fluid volume deficits and hypotension. In addition, hypoxia is also controlled by administration of oxygen and maintenance of a patent airway.

Pharmacologic Management

Steroids or osmotic diuretics may be used to reduce ICP. Hypertension is commonly controlled with antihypertensives and diuretics.

Anticoagulants are commonly used initially through intravenous routes and then orally. Monitoring of clotting times is important for preventing over-anticoagulation, which increases the risk of bleeding.

Headache and neck stiffness can usually be treated with mild analgesics, such as codeine and acetaminophen. Stronger narcotics are usually avoided; these agents sedate the client and can make neurologic assessment inaccurate.

If the client develops seizures, phenytoin (Dilantin) or phenobarbital may be used. Barbiturates and other sedative agents are avoided. If the client develops fever, antipyretics may be prescribed.

Dietary Management

CRITICAL TO REMEMBER

Because of the high risk for aspiration, choking, excessive coughing, and vomiting, oral food and fluids are generally withheld for 24 to 48 hours in clients with CVA.

If the client cannot eat or drink after 48 hours, alternative feeding routes are used, such as tube feeding or hyperalimentation. When the swallowing mechanism has returned, the client can be fed orally.

Surgical Management

Several criteria are used to determine candidates for rapid evacuation of the hematoma in clients with hemorrhagic stroke or bleeding on the dominant side. Clients who usually survive surgery are those who are under the age of 70, or who open their eyes and follow commands on the unaffected side. Another guide commonly used in determining the need for surgery is ICP. Pressures below 20 mm Hg are usually managed without surgery; pressures above 30 mm Hg often require surgery. Clients with relatively large areas of superficial cerebral bleeding or shifts may also require surgery. Likewise, clients who suddenly deteriorate from lethargy to unconsciousness may benefit from surgery. Surgery is usually not performed on clients with bleeding in the basal ganglia or thalamus.

Surgery is also performed on some intracranial aneurysms and on the carotid arteries (carotid endarterectomy) to reduce the risk of CVA. These operations are discussed later in this chapter.

Nursing Management

Assessment

The initial assessment of the client with CVA is very important, providing baseline for ongoing assessments. The client who is awake and alert should be taught about the pathologic process and instructed to inform the nurse about any changes in sensation, movement, or function regardless of how minor they may seem. Increasing neurologic deficit indicates either progression of the infarct or ischemia of the area from cerebral edema or bleeding. Changes in neurologic assessments must be reported promptly to the physician.

A complete history of the presenting problem as well as past medical and social history will provide data about the problem source of the CVA.

Ongoing assessments of the neurologic status and vital signs are imperative. These assessments may be required as often as hourly or even more frequently for unstable clients. Assessment data must be analyzed, and if the client is deteriorating (decreasing LOC, changes in motor or sensory function, pupillary changes, respiratory difficulty, development of visual or perceptual defects or aphasia), the physician should be notified. Assessment of hemiplegia includes the repeated assessment of motor function (spontaneous movement), sensation, and reflex activity.

Nursing Diagnosis, Planning, and Implementation

Nursing Diagnosis: Tissue Perfusion, Altered Cerebral, Risk for R/T increased ICP.

Planning: Expected Outcomes. The client will maintain cerebral tissue perfusion as evidenced by no reports of headache, no decreases in LOC, and stable or improving Glasgow Coma Scale score.

Implementation. The client's ICP should be monitored hourly. The client should be positioned with his or her head elevated and neck straight. The physician should be notified of sustained rises in pressure. Ongoing neurologic assessments must be performed frequently and comparisons made with previous data.

Delirium and restlessness should be controlled, with sedatives if necessary. The nurse should be certain, however, that preventable causes of restlessness, such as a full bladder, bowel impaction, or pain, are not the cause. Restraints should be avoided, because they often increase agitation.

Straining with defecation or excessive coughing, vomiting, lifting, or the use of the arms to change position should be avoided as should suctioning, noise, and light. Mild laxatives and stool softeners are often prescribed.

Nursing Diagnosis: Physical Mobility, Impaired R/T paralysis.

Planning: Expected Outcomes. The client will have maximal physical mobility, as evidenced by absence of tendon contractures, joint ankylosis, and muscle shortening and by effective use of adaptive devices.

Implementation. Proper positioning, turning, and exercising of a hemiplegic client can prevent many deformities and complications.

Positioning. The nurse should change a hemiplegic client's position every 2 hours. The client should be positioned mainly on the unaffected side, with brief periods on the affected side or supine to relieve pressure. When positioning on the affected side, the nurse should make sure that body weight does not harm paralyzed limbs. The client should be allowed to sit upright for short periods only, because this position can contribute to hip flexion deformity. The nurse should not place a pillow under the affected knee when the client is supine. This encourages flexion deformity and impedes circulation. If there is a tendency to develop hyperextension of the knee, however, the nurse can place a folded towel under the knee for short periods while the client is lying supine. When the client is on one side, the upper thigh should not be flexed acutely (also to avoid hip flexion deformity). The nurse should position the client prone for 15 to 30 minutes several times a day, with a small pillow under the pelvis (from the umbilicus to the upper third of the thigh) to hyperextend the hip joints.

The nurse can prevent footdrop by avoiding pressure, performing frequent passive ROM exercises, and having the client sit in a chair as soon as possible with the feet flat on the floor.

A trochanter roll, extending from the crest of the ilium to midthigh, prevents external hip rotation by wedging under the projection of the greater trochanter and stopping the femur from rolling.

The nurse should support the affected leg when turning and positioning a hemiplegic client. Complete hip dislocation can occur if the flaccid leg falls forward and downward when the client is turned onto the unaffected side. The nurse can place a pillow between the client's legs to provide support. At night, a padded posterior splint can be applied to the affected leg to maintain correct positioning and prevent leg flexion.

When the client is in bed, the nurse should prevent adduction of the affected shoulder by placing a pillow in the axilla, between the upper arm and chest wall, to keep the arm abducted about 60 degrees. The arm should be slightly flexed in a neutral position. The nurse can place the client's forearm on another pillow in a modified "Statue of Liberty" position, with the elbow above the shoulder and the wrist above the elbow. This position stretches the shoulder's internal rotators. Elevating the arm also helps prevent edema and resultant fibrosis.

The nurse should place the client's affected hand in a position of function, that is, slight supination with fingers slightly flexed and thumb in opposition. A hand roll or splint can be used to prevent finger flexion and thumb adduction. Frequent passive ROM exercises are important. If the wrist and fingers are spastic, a splint can be used to prevent flexion contracture (Fig. 14–5).

Exercises in Bed. Encouraging clients with hemiplegia to exercise while they are still in bed not only prepares for later activities but also offers hope and a sense of optimism about recovery. A hemiplegic client can learn to move the paralyzed leg by sliding the unaffected leg under it to lift and move it. Hourly gluteal muscle setting and quadriceps muscle setting exercises during the day help prepare for later ambulation.

Range-of-Motion Exercises. The nurse should perform passive ROM exercises four times daily after the first 24 hours following a stroke unless otherwise prescribed. Motor impulses usually begin to return between 2 and 14 days afterward. The affected part (initially flaccid) becomes spastic as the spinal cord motor systems establish their autonomy. Potential for contractures increases.

CRITICAL TO REMEMBER

Passive exercises are more difficult to perform once affected muscles begin to tighten.

The nurse must not force extremities beyond the point of initiating pain or continuous spasm.

Once some voluntary movement returns, the nurse should encourage the client with assisted movements. Paralyzed arms during such movements can be sup-

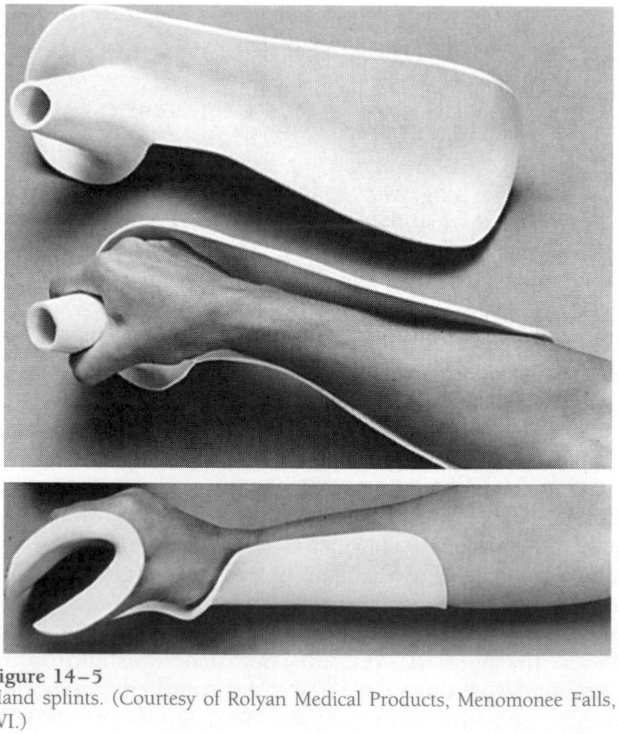

Figure 14–5
Hand splints. (Courtesy of Rolyan Medical Products, Menomonee Falls, WI.)

ported with sling suspensions. As movement strength increases, resisted movements may strengthen weakened muscles and help restore muscle bulk.

The weight of an immobile arm may cause (1) pain and movement limitation ("frozen shoulder") due to shoulder joint fibrositis or (2) subluxation (incomplete dislocation of the shoulder joint). The nurse can prevent these by supporting a completely flaccid arm in a sling when the client is walking and on a pillow when the client is in bed or seated in a chair. He or she can teach the client to use the unaffected hand to lift the paralyzed arm from the sling periodically and put it through ROM exercises. Each finger should be exercised separately. The nurse can also teach the client, while in bed, to (1) exercise the affected arm by grasping it at the wrist with the unaffected hand and raising it above the head and (2) stretch and rub the fingers of the affected hand several times each day.

Sitting Up. The nurse should help the client out of bed as soon as it is medically permitted, remembering however, that hemiplegia severely affects the client's balance. Assistance is needed to provide security and safety. The client's head should be raised slowly in bed to reduce the risk of injury from orthostatic hypotension.

When the client first sits up, the nurse supports the paralyzed side, especially the back and head. Gradually the client learns to sit alone with the head of the bed elevated, and then to sit on the edge of the bed, with feet on a firm surface. The nurse helps the client maintain balance by extending the affected arm and placing its palm flat on the bed. The nurse should be patient and encouraging as the client regains balance.

Eventually the client learns to raise the paralyzed leg with the unaffected leg and swing both legs laterally over the side of the bed onto the floor.

CRITICAL TO REMEMBER

It is safest to have the client pivot on the unaffected leg. Therefore, the chair should be positioned at a right angle to the unaffected side.

Wheelchair. A hemiplegic client needs to learn safe transfers from bed to chair, commode, or wheelchair. One method is shown in the Client Education Guide: Transfer to Wheelchair. The client with unilateral paralysis can propel a wheelchair with the unaffected arm and leg; also, one-arm-drive wheelchairs are available. Once in a wheelchair, a client's level of independence increases greatly.

Using a wheelchair is helpful, but walking is best. A tilt table may be used to assume a standing position if there is difficulty with balance. Standing practice should begin as soon as the quadriceps muscles on the unaffected side have normal strength. The nurse should have the client seated on the edge of the bed. He or she encourages the client to rise, using the muscle power of the unaffected leg. The client may tend to swing around toward the affected side. Gradually, the client learns to take increasing amounts of weight onto the weaker side. In spite of weakness in the affected limb, a hemiplegic client often develops an extensor reflex (reflex patterns of extension), which facilitates standing.

Most hemiplegic clients can be taught to walk. The nurse can remind them to keep body weight forward over the feet. Practice is important for learning to walk correctly. The nurse should supervise clients carefully until they can safely walk alone without fear of falling. When walking, the client should not show circumduction, toe scraping, or any other characteristics of hemiplegic gait. Heel-toe walking with a reciprocal gait pattern is the goal of ambulation.

Bracing. Hemiplegic clients often do not need leg braces. However, if needed, the most commonly used short leg brace for hemiplegic clients is a double-bar 90-degree ankle stop with a posterior metal calf band. An orthopedic-type oxford shoe, properly fitted, is the support for the brace. The nurse should teach the client and significant others how to

- apply and remove the brace
- observe skin for breakdown and give proper skin care
- care for the brace itself.

Nursing Diagnosis: Self-Care Deficit R/T paralysis.

Planning: Expected Outcomes. The client will perform as many activities of daily living (ADLs) as possible, as evidenced by use of adaptive devices and techniques and recognition of limitations.

Implementation. At first, a client experiencing a stroke may need considerable help with all self-care activities (e.g., washing, eating, grooming).

It is important for hemiplegic clients to do as much for themselves as possible. Because this is often difficult, a lot of encouragement is needed. The nurse should help them use the paralyzed arm as much as possible and avoid a tendency to do everything with the unaffected limb. As soon as hemiplegic clients can sit up in bed, the nurse should encourage them to do all the self-care activities they can using the unaffected hand (e.g., brushing teeth, eating, combing hair, shaving, bathing). This helps preserve independent self-care and prevents immobility complications. The nurse should assist clients as necessary but not "rush in."

To protect the eye if the eyelid is paralyzed, the nurse can irrigate it with physiologic saline and instill artificial tears as prescribed and cover it with an eye patch as necessary. An eye patch over one eye in clients with diplopia removes the second image and ensures better vision. The nurse should provide mouth care at least three or four times a day, giving special attention to the paralyzed side of the tongue and mouth. Rehabilitation plans should focus extensively on self-care deficits and ADLs.

Nursing Diagnosis: Injury, Risk for R/T paralysis.

Planning: Expected Outcomes. The client will be without signs and symptoms of injury, as evidenced by no abrasions, burns, or falls.

Implementation. Bedside rails should be kept raised for clients with recent hemiplegia to protect them from rolling out of bed. As recovery proceeds, the client may pull against side rails when sitting up or turning. Once the client can get out of bed unassisted, half side

CLIENT EDUCATION GUIDE

Transfer to Wheelchair

Instructions to a hemiplegic client to transfer from bed to wheelchair. (Shading on right side of client indicates the affected side.)

1. Lock the wheelchair for safety and keep it placed beside the bed on your nonaffected side.
2. Use your nonaffected arm and leg (*A* and *B*) to move your affected arm and leg.
3. As your legs drop over the edge of the bed, swing your torso up to a sitting position (*C*).
4. Push yourself up to a standing position (*D*) by using your nonaffected arm and leg.
5. Reach across the wheelchair (*E*) to grasp the far arm of the chair, and turn to seat yourself.

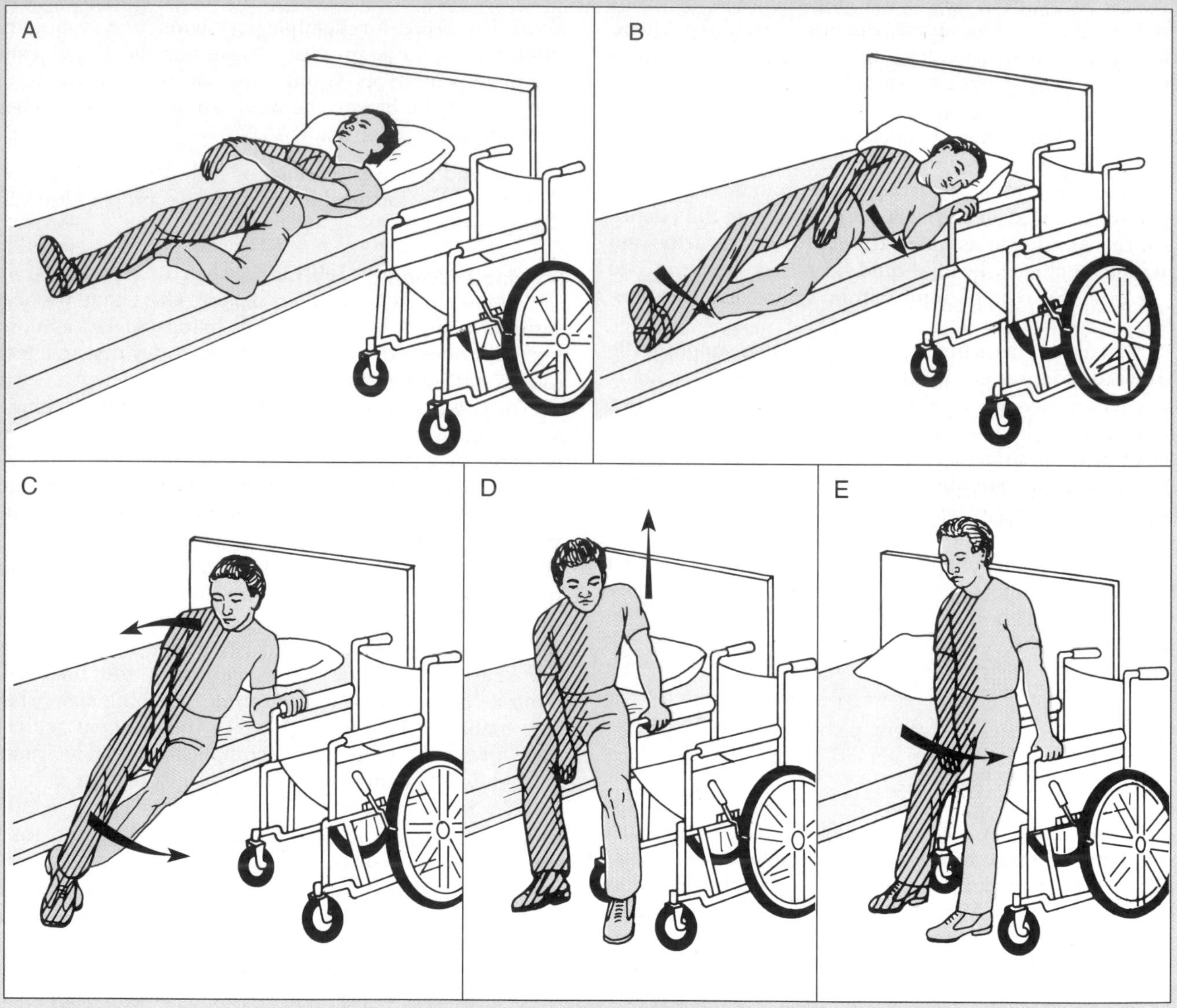

rails may be more useful. Full side rails hinder ambulation.

A client with impaired sensation is especially prone to injury. Frequent skin inspections for signs of injury are essential. Visual disturbances may also increase a hemiplegic client's potential for injury (see earlier discussion of agnosia). Paralysis on one side makes clients prone to falls. The nurse should remind them to walk slowly, rest adequately between intervals of walking, use effective lighting, and look where they are going.

Nursing Diagnosis: Aspiration, Risk for R/T loss of swallowing reflex.

Planning: Expected Outcomes. The client will develop no clinical manifestations of aspiration, as evidenced by no choking while eating, no coughing while eating, no fever, and no rales or rhonchi.

Implementation. The nurse assesses the client for clinical manifestations of aspiration, such as fever, dyspnea, crackles and rhonchi, confusion, and decreased PaO_2 in arterial blood gases. He or she should use caution in feeding the client, either orally or by tube (see later discussion).

Nursing Diagnosis: Nutrition, Altered: Less than Body Requirements R/T inability to swallow secondary to paralysis.

Planning: Expected Outcomes. The client will demonstrate signs of adequate nutrition, as evidenced by weight remaining stable; consuming adequate calories for age, height, and weight; intake equaling output; incisions or wounds healing within 12 to 14 days (as applicable); hemoglobin level within normal limits for age and sex; and lymphocyte level within normal limits.

Implementation. The nurse should carefully assess the client's diet to ensure adequate nutrition. Total intake should also be assessed.

Feeding clients with partial paralysis of the tongue, mouth, and throat requires patience and care for prevention of choking and aspiration. Clients often fear choking and are embarrassed and frustrated by eating difficulties. Consequently, they may avoid eating and not get sufficient nutrition. The nurse should give supplemental meals as necessary. If the client is not able to swallow at all, tube feeding may be used. With help and encouragement, hemiplegic clients can usually learn to feed themselves. Many helpful devices are available. The nurse can make mealtimes pleasant and unhurried. Food should be served attractively and at an appropriate temperature.

Feeding can be very frustrating for a dysphagic client, especially if the nurse is not familiar with the client's specific disabilities (Box 14–2).

Nursing Diagnosis: Communication, Impaired Verbal R/T aphasia secondary to CVA.

Planning: Expected Outcomes. The client will be able to communicate effectively, as evidenced by the client's needs being understood and met, and the client indicating understanding of the communication of others.

Implementation. Communication involves the dual processes of sending and receiving language. Although either can be affected, after initial recovery, the expressive defect is usually greater than the receptive, clients may understand more than they can respond to.

Most aphasic clients regain some speech through speech therapy or spontaneously recover. Because this does not always occur, speech therapy should be started early. If speech therapy was not initiated early, clients may be helped by speech therapy 2 years or more after the time of origin of the speech disorder.

Nurses often continue and reinforce lessons a speech therapist has initiated. The client may have a short attention span, so the nurse should use every encounter to encourage and support communication, being careful not to cause fatigue. Box 14–3 gives guidelines that may help in communicating with aphasic clients.

The nurse should always try to put aphasic clients at ease and to reduce the feelings of panic that may occur when they first realize that they cannot communicate as before.

Assessment of dysarthria usually includes examination of the peripheral speech mechanism, tests for specific speech skills, otolaryngologic consultation, and as-

BOX 14–2

Guidelines for Feeding a Client With Dysphagia

To facilitate feeding, the nurse should assess the following and intervene as necessary:

- Head control. If the client has limited or no voluntary head control, placing a hand on his or her forehead may help. Have the client face forward rather than to the side. Remind the client not to throw the head back to propel food, because this can cause aspiration.
- Position. Have the client in an upright position either in bed or in a chair. Support the head to counteract hyperextension.
- Mouth opening. If the client cannot open his or her mouth, lightly touch both lips with the tip of the spoon. If this does not work, apply light pressure with a finger to the chin just below the lower lip. Ask the client to open the mouth at the same time. Stroking the muscle under the chin (digastric muscle), without crossing the midline, also stimulates mouth opening.
- Mouth closing. If the client cannot close his or her lips, swallowing is more difficult. Stimulate lip closure by stroking the lips with a finger or ice or applying gentle pressure just above the upper lip with your thumb or forefinger.
- Sucking. If the client cannot remove food from a spoon, the sucking reflex needs strengthening. Place a small disc at the end of a short straw and have the client drink through it. Gradually lengthen the straw and use thicker liquids as sucking ability improves.
- Tongue movement. Tongue movement can be improved by (1) lightly touching various parts of the cheek with a tongue blade to encourage the tongue to move to that place, (2) icing weak tongue muscles, (3) applying pressure to soft tissue under the mandible to correct tongue protrusion, and (4) walking a tongue blade from the tip of the tongue to the back (this inhibits tongue thrust and stifles the gag reflex).
- Saliva secretion. Ice (plain or a popsicle) stimulates saliva secretion.
- Swallowing. A dysphagic client must concentrate on swallowing. A quiet environment, free from distractions, is helpful. Feed the client slowly and offer small amounts. Alternate liquids with solids whenever possible to prevent food from being left in the mouth. Place food in the unaffected side of the client's mouth. After the client has swallowed, teach him or her to check for food on the paralyzed side by turning the head to the unaffected side and checking with the tongue.

BOX 14-3

Communicating With Aphasic Clients

The nurse can use many techniques to improve communication with aphasic clients:

1. When a client cannot understand spoken words (receptive or fluent aphasia), repeat simple directions until they are understood (e.g., "Drink this juice"). Do not shout; the client can hear. Speak slowly and clearly. Talk without pressing for a response. Also use nonverbal methods of communication.
2. When talking to a client with receptive difficulty, stand within 6 feet and face the client directly. Shift topics of conversation gradually and say when you are going to change the topic before you do so.
3. When a client cannot identify objects by name (naming aphasia), give practice in receiving and recalling word images. For example, point to frequently used objects and clearly state their names (e.g., "hand," "glass").
4. When a client has difficulty with verbal expression (motor or nonfluent aphasia), give practice in repeating words after you. Begin with simple words and then progress (e.g., "Yes," "No," "Here is breakfast").
5. When working with any aphasic client, practice expanded speech (a slower rate) and self-pacing (give the client time to respond).
6. Help the client's significant others communicate with hm or her. Act as a model for such communication. Be calm, patient, and gentle. Explain how damaging it can be to the client's self-image if others appear embarrassed or amused by his or her attempts to communicate. Likewise, remind significant others not to do all the speaking for the client.
7. Listen and watch carefully when the client attempts to communicate. Try hard to understand. This can help reduce the client's frustration.
8. Anticipate the client's needs to reduce feelings of communication helplessness.

sessment of the client's functional ability based on the clarity of speech in conversation. Speech therapy is beneficial for many dysarthric clients.

Nursing Diagnosis: Thought Processes, Altered R/T impaired cerebral blood flow, altered sensations, and faulty interpretation of environmental stimuli.

Planning: Expected Outcomes. The client will have reduced confusion, as evidenced by recall of information, improved Glasgow Coma Scale scores, decreased agitation, and cooperation with interventions.

Implementation. Reorient the client as consciousness returns. Continually reorient a confused and aphasic client. Position a calender and a clock where the client can see them. Cerebrovascular diseases contribute to many behavioral deviations including confusion, memory loss, language disorders, and lability. Additional changes in behavior may be due to alterations such as in body image, sensation, vision, mobility, and perception.

Nursing Diagnosis: Sensory/Perceptual Alterations: Visual R/T physiologic changes associated with CVA.

Planning: Expected Outcomes. The client will successfully compensate for altered sensory perceptions, as evidenced by safely performing ADLs and safely moving through the environment.

Implementation. The nurse should approach the client from the side that is not visually impaired and position the call light and phone on that side. If possible, the bed should be positioned so that the side of the client that is not visually impaired is toward the center of the room. The nurse can teach clients to position the head to increase the visual field and warn hemiplegic clients to be very careful when crossing streets because they may not see traffic approaching from the affected side.

A client with perceptual defects benefits from simplicity. A busy or noisy environment is difficult to interpret and may increase confusion.

The nurse should reduce decision-making and complexity for the client by, for example, (1) obtaining clothing that is simply designed and easy to put on; (2) giving brief, simple directions; and (3) preparing food trays with a minimum number of utensils, dishes, and foods.

Nursing Diagnosis: Unilateral Neglect R/T damage to portions of the right hemisphere.

Planning: Expected Outcomes. The client will be free of unilateral neglect, as evidenced by being free from injury, demonstrating an awareness of the neglected body side, and developing an ability to compensate for neglect.

Implementation. Initially, the nurse adapts the environment to the deficit by focusing on the client's unaffected side. He or she assists client from affected side and has the client groom the affected side first. The nurse should cue the client to scan the entire environment.[11]

Nursing Diagnosis: Individual Coping, Ineffective R/T physiologic changes and frustration associated with CVA.

Planning: Expected Outcomes. The client will develop effective coping strategies, as evidenced by appropriate life-style modifications, utilization of the assistance of others, and appropriate social interactions.

Implementation. The term "coping" refers to the use of all forms of coping strategies: emotional, cognitive, support systems, and risk appraisal. After CVA, the client may experience grief over lost motion, inability to speak, alterations in sensation and vision, and loss of roles within society (see Ethical Issues in Nursing).

ETHICAL ISSUES IN NURSING

Who Should Judge Quality of Life?

The quality of life is important to most clients, in sickness or in health. "Quality" is a relative term and is best described by each client at a given stage of his or her life. What clients consider quality in health might be significantly altered when illness strikes or any time there is a change in life-style (e.g., employment, financial situation, family, and the like). Clients assess and reassess the quality of their lives day by day. We may not always consciously state what the quality of life is today, but nevertheless, how we feel about our life at a given moment is an important part of who we are. The best judge of the quality of life is each individual client, not someone else. However, health-care workers are constantly being placed in positions of judging the quality of their clients' lives.

Cerebrovascular disorders can significantly change a client's life. Clients who have had a stroke may experience such life changes, which in turn alter the way they view the quality of life. Perhaps they can no longer speak clearly or perform many of the tasks that they used to. Perhaps their stroke was so severe they can no longer care for themselves. In severe cases, perhaps the stroke has left them dependent on machines and unaware of their existence.

When possible, nurses should be aware of how their clients feel their illness has affected the quality of their lives. This may help health-care providers better understand how illness has emotionally affected their clients. In cases in which clients are unable to make their quality-of-life judgements known, it is easy for health-care providers to make judgements for them. It is not uncommon to hear a nurse say, "I don't understand why we are continuing to treat Mr. X. I would not want to live that way." This statement may be true for the nurse, but it may not be true for the client being described.

Quality-of-life judgements are best made by each client about himself or herself, with the situation of life at the present time taken into account. Nurses who care for clients who can no longer judge their own quality of life must be sensitive and not judge the client's quality of life from their own personal perspectives.

These reactions can be understood when the extent of the change and dysfunction in a client's life is appreciated. The nurse should be understanding and kind. Supportive statements are often helpful.

Care for clients with hemiplegia should be given so that their dependency is minimized. The nurse should praise all successes, however small. When necessary, he or she should point out disruptive or inappropriate behavior kindly and ask them to stop. The nurse can arrange the environment and anticipate needs to reduce frustration. Significant others often need help to understand these behaviors.

Psychosocial Nursing Diagnoses: Various psychosocial nursing diagnoses may be appropriate for clients experiencing stroke, depending on the client and the circumstances. These include Family Processes, Altered; Diversional Activity Deficit; Anxiety; Fear; Powerlessness; Self-Esteem Disturbance; and Social Isolation. Significant others should be included in the plan of care and allowed to help care for the client if they want to. The nurse should provide them with the information they need to understand the client's condition. Many clients with strokes are in intensive care units (ICUs) during their acute phase. The complexity of equipment and activity within an ICU may be frightening to the client and significant others. The nurse should provide opportunities for questions and discussion, explain carefully what is happening, and give frequent reassurance and support.

Intervention After the Acute Phase of Stroke

During the convalescent stage, residual defects from a stroke are treated, and intervention is directed toward helping the client function at the maximum capacity. Clients with stroke and their significant others face difficult adjustments as the acute stages pass and residual disabilities become obvious. A multidisciplinary rehabilitative team may help to assist and support clients during this time. Assessing the functional abilities of the client and setting realistic goals are part of this approach. Tasks the client and significant others face include

- learning to use intact strengths and abilities to compensate for impaired functions;
- learning to become independent in ADLs, such as bathing, dressing, and eating;
- developing behavior patterns that are likely to prevent symptom recurrence. Medications should be taken as prescribed. Diet may require modification. The nurse should advise the client to stop smoking and to engage in stress-reducing activities. The client should be encouraged to follow a prescribed exercise program to promote better physical health and mental well-being.

Evaluation

The degree of outcome attainment should be evaluated on an ongoing basis. After CVA, some outcomes are achieved early (e.g., cerebral perfusion); others may require rehabilitation (e.g., self-care deficit). It is important for the nurse to monitor progress toward outcomes, working with both the client and the family.

TRANSIENT ISCHEMIC ATTACKS

Transient ischemic attacks (TIAs) are brief, reversible episodes of neurologic dysfunction caused by temporary, focal cerebral ischemia. A TIA is analogous to angina pectoris. TIAs are also called intermittent cerebrovascular insufficiency or "mini stroke."

Incidence

Because of the variable presentation and duration, it is difficult to determine the incidence of TIAs. It is estimated that 25 to 50 per cent of all clients who experience CVA had a previous TIA.

Etiology

During a TIA, a transient decrease occurs in blood supply to a focal area of the cerebrum or brain stem. Many factors can cause this ischemia. Occlusive disease of the extracranial cerebral vessels is the most common cause of TIAs. Emboli can also cause TIAs. Common sources of emboli include the heart valves and breakdown of plaque.

Risk Factors

The risk factors and preventive measures of TIAs are essentially the same as those of CVAs. The pathophysiology is also similar; the major differences are the duration and permanency of symptoms.

Clinical Manifestations

Clinical manifestations vary, depending on which area of brain is affected. Transient symptoms may include

- visual, auditory, or vestibular disturbances
- motor and sensory disturbances
- headache
- slowed mental processes
- seizures

Generally, TIAs last only minutes (often 2 to 15 minutes) to an hour. Sometimes they last only a few seconds; other times, for as long as 24 hours. Although TIAs are often recurrent, some clients have only one or two episodes. TIAs may occur for as long as 2 years before cerebral infarction, or clusters of TIAs may first appear only a few hours or days before a cerebral infarction. Between episodes, neurologic assessment findings are usually normal.

Clients experiencing TIAs are often afraid that they are having a CVA. They need emotional support and education during this stressful time. The diagnostic work-up as well as the symptoms themselves can produce anxiety. Thorough, simple explanations of upcoming events can help.

DIAGNOSTIC ASSESSMENT

Diagnosis of a TIA is made by the client's reported symptoms. The causes of the TIA and potential risk of CVA are diagnosed by

- auscultation and palpation of a carotid bruit
- Doppler studies of the carotid artery
- computed tomography (CT) to rule out CVA
- echocardiogram to rule out mural thrombosis

Doppler studies revealing 70 per cent narrowing of the carotid are considered significant for cerebrovascular disease. Angiograms are used to illuminate niches in the carotid plaque, which may have broken free.

Medical Management

Preventing the progression of a TIA to a CVA is the goal of medical management. Antihypertensives, antiplatelet drugs, or aspirin may be prescribed. In some instances, warfarin (Coumadin) may be administered to prevent clot development. Every effort is made to determine the cause of the TIAs.

Surgical Management

If vascular insufficiency is detected in the distribution of the middle cerebral artery, an extracranial-intracranial bypass may be performed. This procedure connects the superficial temporal artery to the middle cerebral artery, thereby increasing blood flow to the brain.

A more frequently performed procedure is carotid endarterectomy. Surgery is usually performed only on stenotic arteries, not those that are totally occluded. A client may require bilateral extracranial-intracranial bypass and endarterectomy. Duration between surgeries is determined by the client's tolerance of the procedure and the likelihood of symptom progression from the remaining stenotic vessel. The client is at increased risk of decreased cerebral perfusion during the operation. For some clients, a temporary blood supply is created by shunting blood through other vessels to the brain. Clients treated with shunts include those with contralateral stenosis of the carotids, neurologic deficits, known decreases in cerebral blood flow, a history of CVA, and a stroke in evolution. Once the plaque is resected, the incision is closed with a drain in place. A pressure dressing is applied to reduce the risk of hematoma formation (Fig. 14–6).

Serious neurologic complications include

- embolization during surgery, causing cerebral occlusion and ischemia
- clotting (thrombosis) of the artery at the endarterectomy site, causing cerebral ischemia
- increased ICP due to intracranial hemorrhage
- inadequate cerebral perfusion from intolerance of the temporary artery clamping during surgery

Nursing Management

The care of clients undergoing an extracranial-intracranial bypass is the same as that of clients undergoing other types of cranial surgery. In addition, the surgical anastomosis creates a pulse just below the curve of the incision that should be palpated during assessment of

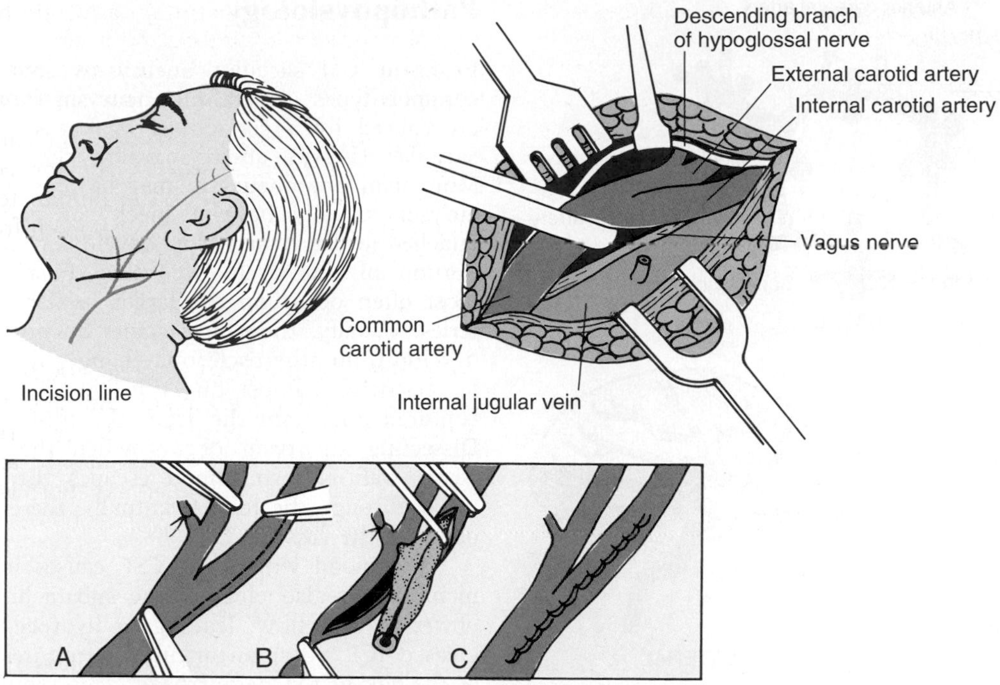

Figure 14–6
Carotid endarterectomy. An incision is made along the carotid bifurcation, and plaque is removed. Sometimes portions of the artery are removed also and reconstructed with vein grafts or Dacron.

vital signs. If the pulse changes in character, the surgeon should be notified immediately.

Postoperative care after carotid endarterectomy is most important during the first 24 hours. The client's head should be kept in a straight position to help maintain airway patency and to minimize stress on the operative site. The nurse should elevate the head of the bed when vital signs are stable and should frequently assess breathing pattern, pulse, and blood pressure. Blood pressure must be maintained between 120 and 170 systolic to ensure cerebral perfusion. Labile blood pressure is a common problem after surgery. Baroreceptors located in the lining of the carotid sinus are one of the primary mechanisms of maintaining normotension. Manipulation of the baroreceptors during surgery causes a short-term disruption in regulation. The nurse should observe the operative site; airway obstruction can occur from excessive swelling of the neck or hematoma formation. The nurse also should assess the client's pupillary reactions, LOC, and motor and sensory function and promptly report indications of deterioration of neurologic impairment.

The nurse assesses the function of the following cranial nerves: facial (VII), vagus (X), spinal accessory (XI), and hypoglossal (XII) (see Chap. 12). Cranial nerve damage is usually temporary but may last for months. The most common cranial nerve damage causes vocal cord paralysis or difficulty managing saliva and tongue deviation. Horner's syndrome may result from damaged sympathetic nerve fibers. This is usually temporary.

Some facilities have developed clinical pathways to guide care of clients who have sustained a TIA. See Appendix C for an example of such a pathway.

INTRACRANIAL ANEURYSM AND SUBARACHNOID HEMORRHAGE

Intracranial aneurysms are congenital, traumatic, arteriosclerotic, or septic weakenings or outpouchings in vessel walls. Ninety per cent of aneurysms are congenital. Cerebral aneurysms most often occur on the circle of Willis (Fig. 14–7).[29] Sometimes these aneurysms weaken, leak, or rupture and cause bleeding into the subarachnoid space. This is called subarachnoid hemorrhage (SAH).

Incidence

Subarachnoid hemorrhage from ruptured intracranial aneurysms occurs in about 18,000 people annually in the United States. Females are more commonly affected. Ruptures occur most frequently between the ages of 30 and 60 years; the peak incidence is in the fifth decade.[15]

Etiology

The most common cause of spontaneous SAH is leaking or rupture of an intracranial aneurysm. This is the cause of death in over half of all fatal cerebrovascular lesions in clients under the age of 45 years. It is not clear why some aneurysms bleed (rupture), but it is probably related to degenerative changes in the vessel wall at the site of the aneurysm, hypertension, and constant stress caused by the force of blood flow, par-

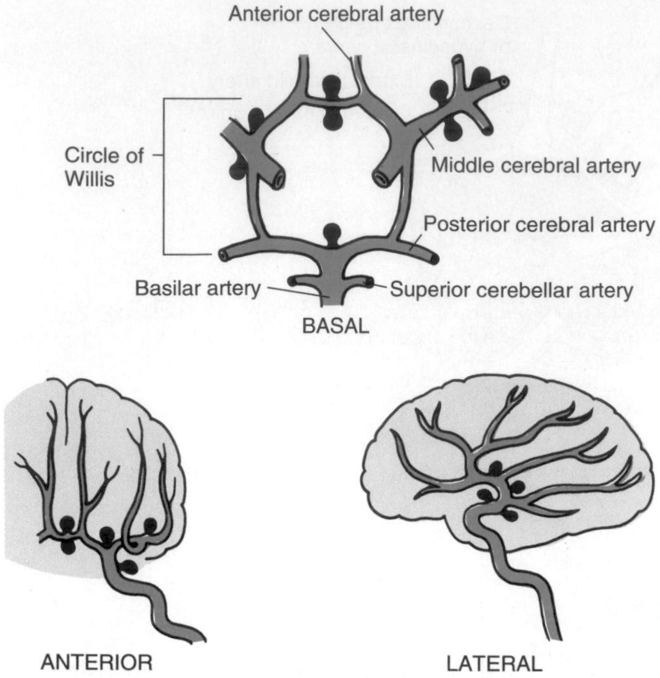

Figure 14-7
Common aneurysm sites.

ticularly at a bifurcation. Meningeal vessel rupture from head trauma is another cause of subarachnoid bleeding. Spontaneous hemorrhage that is not associated with trauma may be caused by blood dyscrasias, primary or metastatic intracranial tumors, vascular anomalies (e.g., angiomas or AVMs), central nervous system infections, or intracerebral hemorrhages spreading to the subarachnoid space.

Risk Factors

Risk factors for SAH include head trauma, hypertension, and cocaine use. Primary prevention focuses on education. Nurses often participate in campaigns to prevent driving after alcohol consumption and to promote the use of bicycle and motorcycle helmets. Similarly, information regarding the ability of cocaine to elevate blood pressure and possibly trigger rupture of a blood vessel needs to be made available and reinforced.

Secondary prevention involves treating hypertension appropriately. High blood pressure can increase the flow of blood against a weakened blood vessel wall and possibly increase the chance of aneurysm rupture.

Tertiary prevention focuses on those clients who have already experienced SAH. The goal in this case is to prevent rebleeding and complications of the initial hemorrhage. Rebleeding is prevented by early clipping of the aneurysm if the client's condition allows. In the case of traumatic or cocaine-induced SAH, hypertension is controlled as closely as possible. The nurse can minimize or prevent the complications associated with immobility, aspiration, or injury related to paralysis.

Pathophysiology

Fusiform and saccular aneurysms are the two most common types of cerebral aneurysm (Fig. 14-8). Both are caused by a congenital weakness in artery walls. Saccular (berry) aneurysms are the most common. More than one aneurysm may be present. Saccular aneurysms usually have a "neck" or narrowed portion attached to the vessel. Most develop around the anterior portion of the circle of Willis. Fusiform aneurysms most often occur on the larger basilar and carotid arteries. Usually, these aneurysms do not rupture. They develop from atherosclerotic changes that impair vascular elasticity. Almost one third of clients who have a ruptured aneurysm die from the initial hemorrhage.[10] Dissecting aneurysm occurs when the intima of the vessel wall is torn. Blood escapes the lumen of the vessel through the tear. Eventually, the expanding mass occludes the vessel.

The blood within the CSF causes irritation of the meninges. It also clots in the subarachnoid space and obstructs CSF flow, leading to hydrocephalus and increased ICP. After an aneurysm ruptures, a clot forms at the site of the hemorrhage. This reduces the risk of rebleeding for a few days. As the clot begins to dissolve, the possibility of rebleeding increases. The greatest risk is about 1 week after the initial hemorrhage.

Complications of SAH that may affect intervention include rebleeding, vasospasm, and hydrocephalus.

REBLEEDING

Rebleeding is a major complication that may occur at any time in an untreated SAH. Rebleeding commonly occurs within the first few days after hemorrhage, but may occur anytime over the first few months. Mortality is high following rebleeding. Definitive management of rebleeding is clipping of the aneurysm. Antifibrinolytic agents may be used in situations in which surgery is not an option. These agents prevent dissolving of the clot. A disadvantage is that the agents cause vasospasm.[14]

VASOSPASM

Vasospasm is a narrowing of a vessel lumen. Vasospasm is a major concern because of its location. Aneurysms

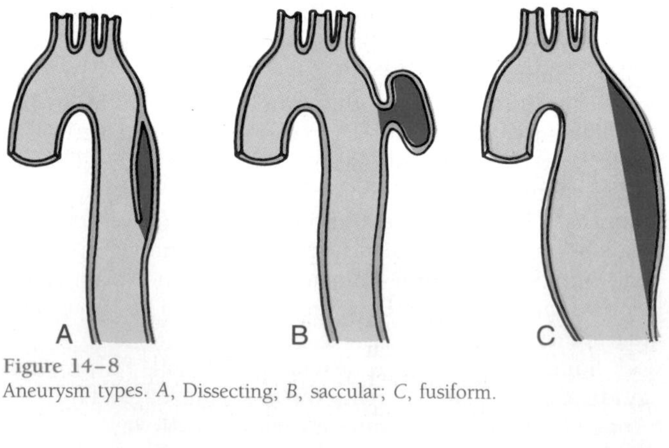

Figure 14-8
Aneurysm types. *A*, Dissecting; *B*, saccular; *C*, fusiform.

commonly occur in the circle of Willis; therefore, when vasospasm occurs in the major vessels, the major cerebral vessels are affected. Spasm usually occurs in the vessel adjacent to a ruptured aneurysm and may spread throughout all the major vessels at the base of the brain. Vasospasm produces symptoms of ischemia and, if extensive and prolonged, results in infarction and permanent neurologic deficit.

HYDROCEPHALUS

Hydrocephalus is caused by blood in the subarachnoid space that prevents adequate CSF circulation. It often occurs in the acute stage that follows SAH and contributes to increased ICP. Hydrocephalus often resolves spontaneously but may be treated by short-term external ventriculostomy to help decrease ICP. Hydrocephalus may develop again after several weeks, this time more slowly, producing dementia and ataxia. Chronic hydrocephalus is usually treated with a ventriculoperitoneal or a ventriculoatrial shunt.

Clinical Manifestations

An aneurysm is usually asymptomatic until it ruptures. Occasionally, there are mild premonitory indications such as mild headache, confusion, fainting, or vertigo. However, the onset of the hemorrhage is usually sudden.

CRITICAL TO REMEMBER

The client experiences a sudden, severe headache, typically in the occipital area and often accompanied by vomiting. Often the client says, "This is the worst headache I have ever had."

The client may lose consciousness immediately, may become confused and lethargic and gradually comatose within hours, or may remain conscious and coherent. Generalized seizures may occur. There are often signs of meningeal irritation (e.g., stiff neck and leg and back pain) due to blood in the subarachnoid space. Focal neurologic deficits include cranial nerve involvement (usually the third and sixth cranial nerves) and motor weakness (usually monoparesis or hemiparesis).

Clinical manifestations of SAH have been divided into five grades for classification of severity of the neurologic deficits (see Box 14–4). Clients over age 50 are classified one grade higher than their signs indicate. Prognosis varies from good to grave as the client progresses from grade I to grade V.

BOX 14–4

Grading the Severity of Subarachnoid Bleeding

Grade I	Minimal bleeding, alert, no neurologic deficit, no symptoms, slight nuchal rigidity
Grade II	Mild bleeding, alert, headache, minimal neurologic deficit (e.g., third nerve palsy, stiff neck)
Grade III	Moderate bleeding, drowsy or confused, headache, stiff neck, with or without neurologic deficit
Grade IV	Moderate to severe bleeding, semicoma, moderate to severe hemiparesis, early decerebrate posturing
Grade V	Severe bleeding, coma, decerebrate or decorticate posturing, moribund appearance

DIAGNOSTIC ASSESSMENT

Diagnosis of SAH is usually based on history and physical examination. CT scan (without contrast) may identify blood in the subarachnoid space, intracerebral clots, and large clots surrounding an aneurysm. Lumbar puncture usually confirms the presence of blood in the CSF. Variations occur in the pressure, color, and cell content of CSF, depending on the timing of the lumbar puncture in relation to the hemorrhage. Angiography is the definitive diagnostic test.

Medical Management

Medical intervention focuses on management of the systemic effects of SAH and vasospasm. Systemic effects include neurogenic pulmonary edema, cardiac arrhythmias, and stress ulcers. Although no definitive prevention or cure exists for cerebral vasospasm, there are treatment modalities. Hypertensive, hypervolemic hemodilution can minimize the impact of vasospasm. Systolic blood pressure is maintained between 100 and 150 mm Hg. The increase in volume and pressure forces blood through spastic vessels. Untreated vasospasm leads to ischemic stroke. This is usually accomplished by infusion of serum albumin. This colloid helps maintain the high intravascular volume by osmosis. Albumin also results in hemodilution. Low hematocrit reflects decreased blood viscosity. The less viscous the blood is, the more easily it flows through narrowed vessels. If the hypervolemia does not adequately elevate blood pressure, the vasopressors may be instituted.

Another theory of etiology for vasospasm is the influx of calcium into the muscular layer of the blood vessel wall. Nimodipine, which is a calcium channel blocker, has been administered in an effort to inhibit this influx. Research is ongoing in the use of this and other drugs in the treatment of vasospasm.

Nonsurgical measures to decrease ICP often include

- administering dexamethasone (Decadron) and osmotic agents
- elevating the head of the bed 20 to 30 degrees
- maintaining a patent airway to prevent increased PCO_2

Surgical Management

Surgical obliteration of the aneurysm with a metal clip or suture eliminates the risk of rebleeding. Clipping is performed through a craniotomy to expose the aneurysm. The aneurysm is isolated, and a clip is placed over the neck of the aneurysm. Many neurosurgeons advocate surgery as soon as possible after rupture. Early surgery is not recommended for all clients, however. Clients with grades IV and V SAH are not operated on because early surgery may contribute to morbidity or mortality. Also, if vasospasm is present, most surgeons will delay surgery. Operating while vessels are in spasm has been shown to increase the morbidity and mortality. Unfortunately, medical instability, delay in transfer from one hospital to another, or client or family reluctance to consent to surgery may delay prompt surgery. Studies have shown that clients who enter the hospital in relatively good condition after the rupture of an aneurysm have only a 50 per cent chance of leaving the hospital in good condition when surgery is delayed.[22]

Nursing Management

Nursing care of the client with SAH is a complex task taking place in an ICU. The condition of the client may range from alert and oriented to comatose and ventilator-dependent.

Assessment

Assessing arterial blood pressure is especially important after SAH. Elevated arterial pressure may contribute to further bleeding from the ruptured aneurysm. At the same time, pressure sufficient to maintain cerebral perfusion pressure must be maintained. The nurse administers vasoactive agents as prescribed and evaluates the effects carefully. He or she should ask the physician for an ideal blood pressure range. If the blood pressure goes above or below that range, the nurse should contact the physician. Vital signs should be assessed and documented frequently, especially blood pressure. The nurse should observe carefully for changes in the client's status, particularly a decrease in LOC, progression of motor weakness, or pupil changes, and notify the physician of significant changes.

Nursing Intervention

The nurse should attempt to provide a quiet, calm environment for clients with SAH. This may be difficult to do in a busy ICU. He or she can evaluate the client's response to visitors and adjust visiting schedules as needed. Keeping a restless client quiet and in bed for an extended period of time is difficult, especially if visual problems or attention deficits preclude reading or watching television as diversion. Sedation should be avoided whenever possible.

Individualized aneurysm precautions are followed during the acute stages of SAH in an attempt to prevent rupture of the vascular abnormality. They may also be used after surgery and in clients with AVMs. The nurse can take the following typical aneurysm precautions.

Elevation of the Head: Elevate the head of the bed 15 to 30 degrees, as prescribed. Advise the client to avoid straining. Place necessary items such as the call bell within easy reach. Assist with position changes and turning. During these activities, encourage the client to relax and not to tighten muscles. Advise the client to minimize turning the head and not to rotate or flex the neck. Isometric or active exercises are not permitted. Passive ROM exercises are acceptable.

Avoidance of Valsalva's Maneuvers: Avoid creating a vagal effect and limit the duration and frequency of Valsalva's maneuvers. Valsalva's maneuvers occur with activities such as passing urine, sneezing, coughing, straining at stool, bending, and vomiting and during suctioning. Avoid rectal stimulation or straining at stool. Enemas are contraindicated, because a vagal effect may result from distention of the lower colon. Do not use rectal thermometers; they may precipitate Valsalva's maneuver. Manage bowel elimination with prescribed stool softeners and mild laxatives. A client whose condition allows (grades I and II) may be permitted by the physician to use a commode. Constipation, bedpan use, and the effort of expelling even a soft stool with weakened abdominal muscles increase Valsalva's effort. Taking a deep breath when it is necessary to perform Valsalva's maneuver reduces the strain. Teach this activity to the conscious client.

Administration of Analgesics and Sedatives: Administer prescribed medications such as analgesics for comfort and sedatives to promote rest. Avoid oversedation, because the client must be easily aroused as necessary for neurologic assessment. Phenobarbital may be prescribed for sedation and because it also helps prevent seizures.

Careful monitoring of neurologic status, hemodynamic parameters, and systemic functioning is required. See care of the client after craniotomy later in this chapter. Prompt identification of changes, notification of the physician, and intervention are the keys to improving client outcome.

ARTERIOVENOUS MALFORMATION

These congenital malformations consist of tangles of thin-walled blood vessels without intervening capillaries. Arterial and venous blood shunt together; hence, perfusion of brain tissue cannot occur through them. The vessels may "leak" small amounts of blood or they may rupture, causing hemorrhage into the subarachnoid space or brain, depending on the location of the bleeding AVM. Whereas some AVMs are huge, others are microscopic. Most commonly, they occur in the posterior portions of the cerebral hemispheres. Over time, they may change in size, and large AVMs may decrease somewhat, whereas small ones may enlarge. Bleeding into brain tissues usually produces focal neurologic clinical manifestations; however, cerebral infarction or ischemia may occur without rupture. A ruptured AVM produces clinical manifestations and laboratory results similar to those of SAH. The smaller AVMs are most prone to rupture.

Aneurysm precautions (see the discussion of SAH) may be prescribed. About half of AVMs can be completely removed surgically. Laser intervention may be used preoperatively to decrease the size of the AVM, or neuroradiologic procedures may be performed to reduce the AVM's blood supply. (These procedures may also be used on inoperable AVMs.) Other techniques that may be used to reduce the size of AVMs include (1) use of radiation energy from a proton beam, (2) detachable balloon procedures, (3) artificially embolizing (clotting) the AVM, or (4) ligating the AVM's feeding arteries. These interventions are not without such hazards as initiating hemorrhage or infarction or enlarging the area of ischemia.

Tumors

INTRACRANIAL TUMORS

Intracranial tumors can be defined in several different ways. Primary tumors develop from central nervous system tissue. Secondary tumors have metastasized from other locations in the body. Intra-axial tumors originate from glial cells within the cerebrum, cerebellum, or brain stem. These tumors infiltrate and invade brain tissue. Extra-axial tumors have their origin in the skull, meninges, cranial nerves, or pituitary gland. These tumors have a compressive effect on the brain.

Incidence

Intracranial tumors are second only to cerebrovascular disease as the most common endogenous neurologic problem; 14,000 new cases of primary brain tumor develop yearly in the United States. Tumors of this type occur equally in males and females of all age groups. Heredity is not a significant risk factor in brain tumors, except for tumors of neurofibromatosis and tuberous sclerosis (Table 14–4). Metastatic brain tumors are even more frequent than primary tumors.[17]

Etiology

The etiology of secondary tumors can be traced to the primary site from which they metastasized. This site is often the lung or breast. No clear etiologic factor has

TABLE 14–4 Types of Intracranial Tumors in Adults

TYPE OF TUMOR	FREQUENCY OF OCCURRENCE	CHARACTERISTICS
Glioma (malignant)	50% of all intracranial tumors	Rapid growth and infiltration
Astrocytoma	38% of all gliomas 6–10% start as benign but may become malignant	Can infiltrate large areas of brain, making complete excision impossible
Glioblastoma multiforme	50% of all primary brain tumors	Very invasive, vascular tumor Often causes cerebral edema Originates from various cell types
Oligodendroglioma	Less than 5% of all gliomas	Client may present with a long history of seizures
Metastases	20% of all intracranial tumors	It may be the increased ICP that causes death rather than the primary tumor
Pituitary adenomas (benign)	7–10% of all intracranial tumors	May cause visual disturbances, Cushing's syndrome, hypertension, acromegaly, and dysfunction of the reproductive system
Acoustic neuroma (benign)	5% of all intracranial tumors	Arises from Schwann's cells in the vestibular portion of CN VII Slow-growing, encapsulated tumor Often symptoms of unilateral nerve compression are seen
Granuloma (benign)	Unknown	Composed of granulation tissue May develop after sarcoidosis, fungal infection, tuberculosis, syphilis infection, or intestinal parasite infections
Cholesteatoma (benign)	Unknown	Slow-growing epidermal tumor Extensive spread may make complete excision impossible
Chordoma (malignant)	Unknown	Locally invasive, slow-growing Usually originates at the base of the cranium Complete removal is often impossible
Meningioma (benign)	Unknown	Frequently recur if partial excision is done
Primary brain lymphoma	Increasing in frequency in AIDS and non-AIDS populations	Involves the brain diffusely, producing infiltrating, multicentric tumors that lie deep within the brain, unresectable; responds temporarily to radiation

AIDS, acquired immunodeficiency syndrome; CN, cranial nerve, ICP, intracranial pressure.

been established for any of the primary intracranial tumors. Although the type of cell that gave rise to the tumor can often be identified, the mechanism causing the cells to act abnormally remains unknown. Primary intracranial tumors do not metastasize to other sites in the body.

Risk Factors

Because the etiologic mechanism of primary intracranial tumors is uncertain, no specific risk factors or primary and secondary preventive measures have been identified. Aggressive treatment of the primary site may prevent the development of metastatic tumors. Unfortunately, such treatment is not always successful, and not all clients can tolerate aggressive treatment. These clients may develop metastatic tumors.

Tertiary prevention addresses those clients who have an intracranial tumor. Depending on the location of the lesion and type and extensiveness of medical intervention, the client may exhibit various neurologic deficits. Tertiary prevention focuses on preventing complications associated with these deficits.

Pathophysiology

CRITICAL TO REMEMBER

Both benign and malignant intracranial tumors are potentially fatal. The outcome depends on the tumor location, size, and type.

Benign tumors (e.g., neurinomas, meningiomas) may be cured with early diagnosis and surgery. However, gliomas and metastatic intracranial tumors are often fatal.

Intracranial tumors cause death by infiltration and compression of brain tissue. Not only are the tumors space-occupying lesions, but they often produce considerable cerebral edema. The skull is rigid and has little room for expansion of the contents. Brain tumors progressively increase ICP, which causes brain stem herniation and death.

Cranial nerves may be compressed or invaded by benign or malignant tumors, or they may be the primary site of tumors. Papilledema (edema and hyperemia of the optic disc) occurs from optic nerve head swelling and retinal vein enlargement and eventually hemorrhages into the nerve and adjacent retina.

Clinical Manifestations

As with other cranial disorders, the symptoms associated with an intracranial tumor correlate with the area of the brain involved (see Clinical Manifestations: Intracranial Tumor).

DIAGNOSTIC ASSESSMENT

A complete history from the client or family, followed by a thorough physical examination, is especially important. If intracranial tumor is suspected, the following diagnostic studies may be performed: (1) CT scan or magnetic resonance imaging (MRI) scan; (2) plain skull and chest radiographs (to rule out metastatic carcinoma); and (3) electroencephalogram and radionuclide scans. An angiogram is used when an intracranial tumor is strongly suspected but a CT scan does not provide sufficient information. Angiograms are very helpful in making a differential diagnosis of masses and for planning surgery. A lumbar puncture is performed provided increased ICP does not exist.

Medical Management

Intervention depends on the type and location of the intracranial tumor and the client's condition. Sometimes chemotherapy is used (e.g., methotrexate, CCNU, and BiCNU). Intrathecal (placed within the CSF) methotrexate is currently used. Nitrosourea (carmustine, BiCNU), and lomustine (CCNU), are lipid-soluble compounds that easily cross the blood-brain barrier. Carmustine can be administered directly into the tumor with biodegradable, timed-release wafers.

Surgical Management

STEREOTACTIC RADIATION THERAPY

A stereotactic needle biopsy may confirm the diagnosis of a brain tumor and help in planning chemotherapy and radiation therapy. Radiation therapy is often used to slow tumor growth and improve the quality of life. Radiation may be administered in the conventional manner or via several innovative systems. The Gamma Knife uses multiple lower-dosage radiation sources. These sources are arranged around the client's head in a helmet device to focus on the tumor. In radiosurgery, a linear accelerator is used to deliver the radiation. The single radiation source is moved in arcs around the client's head, again focusing on the tumor. The benefit of these systems is that the area being irradiated can be clearly identified. This minimizes the effect on healthy brain tissue. These techniques can also be used on tumors or AVMs that are surgically inaccessible. In brachytherapy, radioactive seeds are inserted, through catheters, into the tumor. These seeds are left in place for approximately 2 days and then removed to minimize radiation to healthy brain tissue. This technique can be used after traditional radiation treatments.

CRANIOTOMY

A craniotomy is a surgical opening into the skull made in various ways:

- Osteoplastic bone flap: The bone flap remains attached and hinged to muscles and other structures.
- Free-form flap: A section of cranium is cut away from its attachments and temporarily removed.
- Enlarging burr hole: Bone is gradually removed by a rongeur until enough brain is exposed for the procedure.

CLINICAL MANIFESTATIONS

Intracranial Tumor

Localized signs and symptoms are caused by destruction, irritation, or compression of the part of the brain in or near the tumor. Blood supply to the affected area is also impaired. Localized manifestations include:

- focal weaknesses (e.g., hemiparesis)
- sensory disturbances (e.g., anesthesia or paresthesia)
- language disturbances
- coordination disturbances (e.g., staggering gait)
- visual disturbances (e.g., diplopia [double vision], visual field deficit [hemianopia])

As an intracranial tumor enlarges, it shifts intracranial structures and may produce brain stem herniation.

General signs and symptoms are caused by generalized cerebral function disturbance resulting from edema and increased intracranial pressure. They include the following:

HEADACHES

Headaches (localized or generalized) are often most severe in the frontal or occipital region. They are usually intermittent, are of increasing duration, and may be intensified by a change in posture or straining. Recurrent, severe headaches in a client previously free of them or recurrent headaches in the morning, increasing in frequency and severity, suggest intracranial tumor and need assessment.

NAUSEA AND VOMITING

Nausea and vomiting may occur late in tumor progression. Vomiting may not be related to meals. Nausea may be marked.

PAPILLEDEMA

Papilledema ("choked disc") is common in clients with intracranial tumors and may be the first sign. Early papilledema does not cause visual acuity changes. Prolonged papilledema causes optic atrophy and severely diminished visual acuity.

SEIZURES

Seizures, focal or generalized, are common in clients with intracranial tumors, especially cerebral hemisphere tumors. Seizures are often the first indication of intracranial tumors, especially in clients without an obvious seizure cause (e.g., head injury).

DIZZINESS AND VERTIGO

Dizziness and vertigo may develop from intracranial circulatory impairment.

MENTAL STATUS CHANGES

Mental status changes may accompany intracranial tumor (e.g., lethargy and drowsiness, confusion, disorientation, and personality changes).

The clinical course of a client with an intracranial tumor varies with the specific type of tumor present. For example, a client with a low-grade glioma who has undergone partial surgical excision of the tumor followed by radiation may survive 5 to 15 years. In contrast, a glioblastoma multiforme grows rapidly and may cause death within 6 months to a year, even with radiation.

A craniectomy (in which a portion of cranium is permanently removed) is sometimes performed for decompression, that is, to relieve pressure on brain structures by providing space for expansion. After some craniectomies (e.g., if large), a protective prosthesis made of methyl methacrylate is later surgically inserted.

Intraoperative Care. Local or general anesthetics can be used for intracranial surgery. Local anesthesia is used when the client's response to manipulation of the brain must be assessed during surgery. Potential problems associated with local anesthesia include discomfort, inability to control the airway, nausea, vomiting, straining, and coughing. Some of these activities may detrimentally increase ICP. All general anesthetics alter cerebral dynamics. However, they facilitate control of the client's vital functions.

Positioning. The client must be carefully positioned during intracranial surgery for prevention of postoperative positioning complications. Pressure sores may form because intracranial surgery may be prolonged (e.g., 12 hours; typical length is 4 to 12 hours), and position changes (to prevent pressure damage to nerves and tissues) may be impossible. The client's head is supported in a special frame. The frame may cause pressure sores on the client's head, edema of the face, and muscle soreness, especially in the neck. Improper positioning of the client during surgery may also injure peripheral nerves (e.g., peroneal, brachial plexus) and the eyes and eyelids.

Complications of Intracranial Surgery

General postoperative complications after intracranial surgery may include atelectasis, pneumonia, cardiac irregularities, fluid and electrolyte imbalances, and renal and gastrointestinal disorders.

Potential complications with any major surgery may be very serious, possibly fatal. Complications from intracranial surgery may be fatal or psychosocially and physically devastating because of the significant functions performed by the structures involved. Some postoperative complications gradually improve; others are permanent. Potential complications with intracranial surgery may vary, depending on the area of surgery and the procedure being performed.

Increased ICP (due to cerebral edema or bleeding) is the major complication of intracranial surgery. Assessment findings may include decreased LOC with associated headaches, visual and speech disturbances, muscle weakness or paralysis, pupil changes, seizures, vomiting, and respiratory changes (see Chap. 13).

Conventional management of increased ICP includes osmotic diuretic therapy, intubation with hyperventilation to reduce ICP and prevent hypoxia, steroid administration, and elevation of the client's head (see Chap. 13). Further surgical intervention may be necessary, depending on the suspected cause of the increased ICP. The surgeon may place a catheter in the brain to drain excess fluid or blood from a ventricle or another fluid-filled space. A Jackson-Pratt suction drain (Fig. 14–9) may be surgically inserted if a large cavity remains after removal of a tumor or large hematoma. During brain surgery, the brain may become quite edematous and expand so that the surgeon cannot close the dura. Sometimes a craniectomy is performed to permit expansion of such an edematous brain.

Leak of CSF may be apparent postoperatively by saturation of the surgical head dressing or drainage from the ear (otorrhea) or nose (rhinorrhea) of clear, thin fluid that dries in concentric circles. CSF leaks are managed with antibiotics. If they do not spontaneously close, a dural patch may be used to repair the site.

Management. Nursing intervention includes observing the client carefully for serous (or blood) drainage from the ears or nose. CSF drainage from the nose

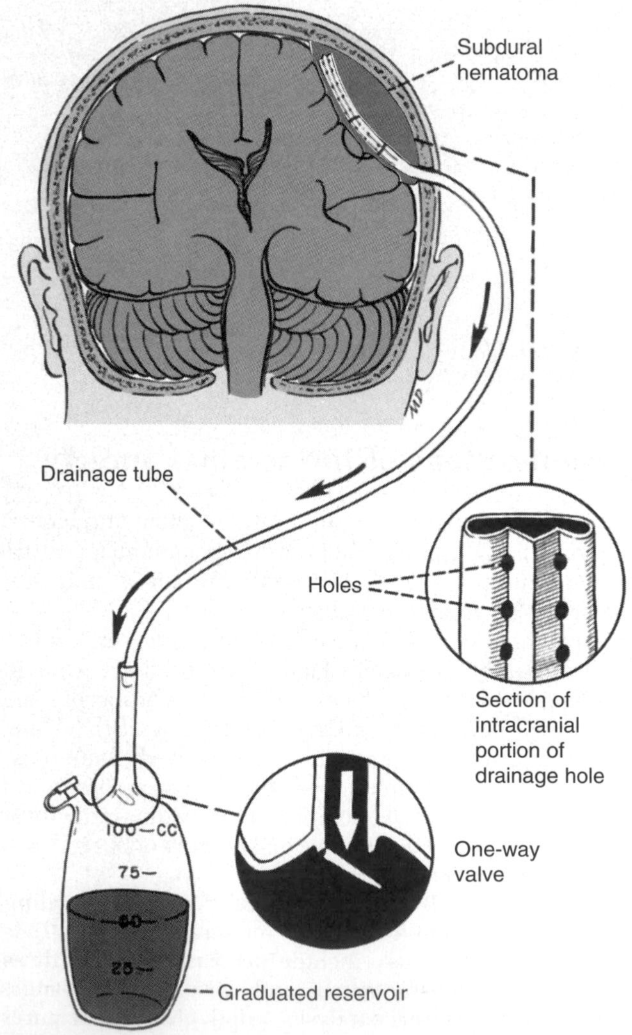

Figure 14–9
Jackson-Pratt suction drain. (See text for discussion.)

(CSF rhinorrhea) is usually preceded by bleeding from the nose and may not be recognized until bleeding stops.

Drainage from the nose or ears may be clear, serosanguineous, or frankly bloody. The nurse must distinguish between blood that is draining from local trauma (fractured nose) and blood containing CSF from a meningeal tear. A clear wet "halo" or watery pale ring encircles a bloody spot on sterile gauze when CSF is in the drainage. Clear fluid draining from the nose may be either CSF or normal watery mucus. Keto-Diastix helps distinguish these fluids (i.e., a positive sugar reaction is often present with CSF; a negative sugar reaction may occur with mucus).

The nurse gently places a sterile pad near the outer opening of the client's ear or nose for absorbency or places a loosely slung external bandage (e.g., sterile pad) over the external ear to absorb the discharge. These dressings should be replaced as soon as they become moist. The nurse should not pack cotton or gauze in the nose or ear. This obstructs the free flow of fluid and acts as a reservoir for infection.

The nurse assesses and documents color, consistency, and approximate amount of drainage. The client should be positioned as prescribed so that free drainage of the CSF is possible. A position with the client's head elevated about 20 degrees is often prescribed. The nurse should not allow the client to remain for long in a position that allows stasis of the CSF drainage. He or she should teach the client to observe the drainage and to be aware of signs of infection.

The nurse must never attempt to clean or suction the ears or nose of any head-injured client until the physician allows. These activities can introduce infection into the central nervous system. A head-injured client must be taught not to cough, sneeze, or blow the nose. These activities increase the likelihood of meningitis and may allow air to enter the cranial cavity.

Body temperature regulation may be erratic after intracranial surgery. Hypothermia can result from excessive body dehydration due to the client's condition before surgery. Hyperthermia may be secondary to blood in the cranium or underlying infection. Postoperative respiratory complications are the most common cause of hyperthermia. When the hypothalamus has been operated on or manipulated, wide variations in temperature regulation may occur if nerves governing temperature regulation have been disturbed.

Seizures may occur in clients with intracranial surgical lesions (see Seizure Disorders later in this chapter). There may be only one seizure or many, possibly progressing to status epilepticus. Because seizures increase metabolic activity, which increases ICP, they are suppressed by anticonvulsants (usually phenytoin). These are often prescribed prophylactically, preoperatively or during surgery, if the surgeon manipulates the cerebral cortex. Typically, seizure activity greatly increases the brain's metabolic needs and may cause further brain damage.

Meningitis (see later in chapter), when it develops, typically appears 2 to 3 days after surgery. Usually it is caused by irritation of the meninges due to infection or blood in the subarachnoid space. Meningitis may also develop with prolonged use of intracranial monitoring devices. Assessment findings indicating meningitis may include chills, fever, nuchal rigidity, headache, irritability, decreased LOC, and increased sensitivity to light. It is essential for all care providers to practice infection prevention measures.

Ecchymosis and periorbital edema are commonly present after intracranial surgery but are usually transient. Nursing intervention to promote comfort may include use of cool moist packs of normal saline over the eyes and insertion of prescribed lubrication (artificial tears or ointment) into the eyes.

Stress ulcer is a frequent complication if the acute postoperative course is prolonged and requires complex management in an ICU setting. Hyperacidity of gastric secretions and decreased production of gastric mucus can cause gastritis with ulceration and frank hemorrhage. The development of stress ulcer is probably secondary to insult to one or several major organ systems. Steroid administration and mechanical ventilation are also predisposing factors. Intervention includes administering prescribed antacids or histamine-blocking agents and monitoring gastric contents to keep the pH above 4.5.

Clients who have had surgery in the posterior fossa have the risk of additional postoperative complications because the surgical site is close to vital brain stem structures. Cardiac arrhythmias and air embolism may relate to the positioning of the client during surgery. Other complications relate to eighth, ninth, tenth, eleventh, and twelfth cranial nerve dysfunction (e.g., hearing loss, inability to swallow, aspiration, and impaired airway protection).

Nursing Management

Preoperative Assessment

The nurse should assess and document the following about the client:

- Vital signs; LOC; orientation to person, place, time; ability to follow instructions; pupil size, equality, and reaction to light (Glasgow Coma Scale score); skin color and palpable skin temperature (cool, warm).
- Limb movements; limited or exaggerated movements; strength in extremities (grip); any paresis or paralysis; sensory abnormalities; edema; indications of skin pressure, burns, irritations, abrasions, bruises, or hematomas.
- Manifestations of increasing ICP or pulmonary congestion. Report these findings immediately.
- Any other abnormal findings (e.g., indications of dehydration, seizures, aphasia, visual or auditory problems).

These assessment findings provide preoperative baseline data for comparison with postoperative assessment findings. It is thus possible to determine if a client's condition is improved, is worsened, or remains unchanged in the various assessed parameters as a result of the neurosurgery.

Clients with suspected or known brain tumors are frightened and apprehensive. The nurse should answer questions as appropriate.

Preoperative Intervention

Psychosocial Preparation: Having one's skull opened and brain structures operated on is major surgery and obviously a frightening experience. This is true both for the client undergoing the surgery and for the significant others. All these individuals require sensitive, skilled psychosocial support. The nurse should provide this for the conscious client before, during, and after surgery.

Medications. Preoperative orders are naturally individualized. Parenteral corticosteroids may be prescribed to reduce cerebral edema preoperatively and also in the early postoperative phase.

Atropine and scopolamine are common preoperative medications. They reduce tracheobronchial secretions and vagal influences on the heart (bradycardia) caused by intubation, anesthesia, or the surgical procedure. Vagal effects may occur with posterior fossa surgery and with manipulation of the carotid artery.

A client requiring neurosurgery often has an altered ability to tolerate other conventional premedications. Thus, for example, if narcotics are prescribed, the nurse should be sure to reconfirm these orders with the neurosurgeon before administering the narcotics. Hypoventilation and circulatory depression may cause major problems, particularly for comatose clients or those with increased ICP.

Scalp Preparation: The client's surgical site is shaved immediately before surgery. Then, if the scalp is accidentally cut, the wound does not become infected. If scalp preparation is done in the nursing care unit, the nurse places a clean neuro-cap (made of tubular stockinette) on the head immediately after the preparation to retain body warmth. A lot of body heat is lost through a shaved head. The cut hair is typically saved for the client. The nurse prepares the scalp according to the situation and the preoperative instructions. A shampoo may be ordered before the head is shaved. If so, during the shampoo, the nurse should examine the scalp closely for unusual conditions (e.g., lesions, dermatitis, infection).

Antiembolism stockings and sequential compression devices are typically applied before the client goes to the operating room.

Postoperative Assessment

The frequent and thorough neurologic assessment of the client after neurologic surgery is essential. These clients can deteriorate quickly. Vital signs and neurologic signs are usually assessed every hour until the client is stable and then every 2 hours. LOC, ability to move extremities, and speech are assessed. The dressing is inspected for drainage. Intake and output must be carefully documented each hour. The nurse must monitor laboratory values, especially serum glucose, sodium potassium, osmolarity, and hematocrit, and take appropriate measures to keep these values within normal range while avoiding extremes of hydration. The response of the client and significant others to the surgery should be evaluated. This is a very stressful experience, particularly if the tumor was malignant or the client experiences neurologic deficits after surgery.

The nurse should observe the client carefully for focal or generalized seizure activity. Such activity requires prompt, aggressive nursing and medical intervention. The client must be protected from harm and seizures stopped as quickly as possible, because continuous seizures damage the brain. The nurse should immediately report a seizure to the physician. The client's movement should not be restricted during the seizure, but provide physical protection. Medication should be administered promptly, if ordered.

The nurse should frequently assess the condition of the head dressing, inspecting it and the underlying sheet for evidence of bleeding or CSF leak. He or she should immediately report and document such evidence (see discussion under Head Trauma). The nurse should assess (character, estimated amount) and document prolonged oozing bleeding or oozing wound drainage. Sometimes a small amount of bloody drainage occurs on the dressing if a catheter or drain is in place. This should be brought immediately to the attention of the neurosurgeon, who may elect to place a stitch at the insertion site to stop this localized bleeding and to anchor the catheter or drain.

The nurse assesses whether the dressing is comfortable. It should not be constrictive around the client's head or ears or over the eyes. Sometimes the dressing fits tightly and is down over the eyes; it should remain above the eyes. Does the dressing appear to be too tight? Neurosurgeons usually prefer to perform the first head dressing change personally after intracranial surgery. The nurse may reinforce the initial dressing if it becomes contaminated before the first dressing change (e.g., from serosanguineous drainage). Nurses usually perform subsequent dressing changes.

Postoperative Intervention

Nursing Diagnosis: Tissue Perfusion, Altered Cerebral, R/T increased ICP.

Planning: Expected Outcomes. The client will maintain normopressure cerebral perfusion, as evidenced by maintaining or improving level of consciousness; maintaining or improving Glasgow Coma Scale score; no restlessness, irritability, or headache; no pupillary changes; no seizures; and no widening pulse pressure, respiratory irregularity, hypertension, or bradycardia.

Implementation. The nurse continuously monitors the client's neurologic status, comparing postoperative findings to preoperative status. The parameters within the Glasgow Coma Scale are common indicators.

During the acute phase of care after intracranial surgery, correct postoperative positioning of the client is extremely important to prevent pressure on the brain's operative site, prevent or minimize ICP increases, facilitate tissue perfusion (circulation), and prevent pressure sores or promote their healing.

Positions allowed vary with the type of surgery performed and specific postoperative orders. If in doubt, the nurse should always double-check orders before placing the client in a questionable position. Incorrect positioning of a client after intracranial surgery may have serious, possibly fatal consequences. The nurse should make certain to know whether the client's head is to be elevated or kept flat. The client may not be positioned on the operative side if there is no bone flap. To help ensure proper positioning, a sign should be posted that clearly states safe and unsafe positions for the client. Some guidelines for typical positions after intracranial surgery are presented.

Supratentorial Surgery. After surgery above the brain's tentorium, the client's head is usually elevated 30 degrees to promote venous outflow through the jugular veins. If central lines are present for hemodynamic monitoring purposes, the nurse monitors and documents pulmonary artery or central venous pressure readings at least every 4 hours. If the client is to remain in this head-elevated position, the nurse must be certain to take these readings consistently while the client is in this position and document the position.

CRITICAL TO REMEMBER

The nurse must not lower the client's head (or the head of the bed) in the acute phase of care after supratentorial surgery for any procedure without a written order from the neurosurgeon.

The neurosurgeon may order the client's head to remain flat after supratentorial surgery to remove a chronic subdural hematoma. Clients with this problem are usually older and their brains are less expandable. When the hematoma is removed, a large space may remain between the dura and brain. To allow the brain to re-expand, the client lies flat. There may also be a Jackson-Pratt drain to remove fluid buildup in the space. Increased ICP rarely occurs with chronic subdural hematomas.

Infratentorial Surgery. After surgery below the brain's tentorium, the client may be kept flat, without head elevation, to prevent pressure on brain stem structures. The client is turned every 2 hours but never onto the back. This would cause very serious, possibly life-threatening pressure on vital brain stem structures.

CRITICAL TO REMEMBER

The nurse must not elevate the client's head (or the head of the bed) in the acute phase of care after infratentorial surgery for any procedure without written permission from the neurosurgeon.

Posterior Fossa Surgery. The client is typically positioned on the side, with a pillow under the head for support, and not on the back. This protects the operative site from pressure and minimizes tension on the suture line (very important if wound closure was difficult).

If a bone flap was surgically removed for decompression (to allow further expansion of an already edematous brain), the client should be placed only on the unoperated side or back. This facilitates brain expansion. The client should be turned from the back to the unoperated side, but not to the operated side if a bone flap is not present.

Other interventions to reduce ICP are discussed in Chapter 13 and include diuretics and CSF drainage techniques.

Also, if a client is neurologically unstable (loses consciousness, is sleepy, or is weak) and the ICP elevation is within a critical range (more than 20 mm Hg), the nurse should avoid procedures that require a flat position (e.g., daily weight-taking). Such a position dangerously elevates ICP.

When a client who must remain head-elevated is positioned on the side (for a position change), the head must be supported. For example, the nurse can prop the head on a small pillow or folded blanket or apply a soft cervical collar to prevent the head from turning and thus decreasing venous outflow (reduced venous outflow from the head elevates ICP). When the client is in the side-lying position, the nurse places a pillow between the legs to maintain good body alignment, to make the client comfortable, and to protect the knees from pressure sores. Sharp hip flexion, which increases ICP, should be avoided. Increased intra-abdominal pressure in turn increases intrathoracic pressure, and this decreases venous outflow.

Nursing Diagnosis, Planning, and Implementation

Body Temperature, Risk for Altered R/T loss of primary defenses (incision).

Planning: Expected Outcomes. The client will exhibit no signs or symptoms of infection, as evidenced by no fever, timely wound healing, no induration or abnormal drainage amounts or color from wound, and no clinical manifestations of meningitis.

Implementation. For preventing wound infection and possible meningitis, the nurse should use sterile technique during dressing changes and should follow these procedures: Place a Telfa dressing over the incision site or around a drain or catheter insertion site to keep this area clean, dry, and free from abrasion by the overlying bulky dressings. During dressing changes, inspect the operative site and sites around drains or catheters for edema and signs of infection. Document and report these assessment findings.

As postoperative edema subsides and the client's wound heals and improves, bulky dressings can be replaced with modified dressings to suit individual needs. For example, sutures are usually kept covered with Telfa pads, and a stockinette cap is placed over the client's head. To remove dried flaky skin and residue, the nurse can soften the scalp with baby oil or glycerin and then gently wash the head with soap and water, taking care not to cause any tension on the suture line. While giving wound care, the nurse should assess the suture line and wound healing and document and report any sutures inadvertently left in place, openings in the suture line, or other complications of wound healing.

Nursing Diagnosis: Nutrition, Altered: Less than Body Requirements R/T inability to eat secondary to unconsciousness.

Planning: Expected Outcomes. The client will demonstrate signs of adequate nutition, as evidenced by weight remaining stable; consuming adequate calories for age, height, and weight; intake equaling output; incisions or wounds healing within 12 to 14 days; hemoglobin level within normal limits for age and sex; and lymphocyte level within normal limits.

Implementation. A client with an uncomplicated postoperative course after intracranial surgery usually requires minimal intravenous maintenance and electrolyte therapy. As the level of wakefulness improves and the swallowing and gag reflexes return, the client usually begins a clear liquid diet and progresses to diet as tolerated. Total food and fluid intake may be curtailed to minimize overhydration and cerebral edema.

If complications delay recovery and nutritional needs are not being met, or if the client's nutritional status is impaired by ill health, enteral feedings may be prescribed once the swallowing reflex and peristalsis are present.

Collaborative Problem: Airway Clearance, Ineffective R/T cerebral edema, decreased level of consciousness, or neck edema.

Planning: Expected Outcomes. The client will show no signs of airway obstruction, as evidenced by clear lung sounds; full, equal lung expansion; and quiet respirations.

Implementation. The nurse assesses respiratory parameters frequently to avoid hypercapnia and to ensure maximal oxygenation of the brain (cerebral oxygenation). Arterial lines or pulse oximetry may be used, airway patency must be maintained. However, the nurse should not suction through the nose. CSF is protected by the nasal membrane. If the nasal membrane is torn during suctioning, CSF will leak and infection may result. If ICP is markedly increased, suction should not be performed longer than 15 seconds at one time. Prolonged suctioning increases thoracic pressure. This, in turn, increases ICP because of decreased venous return.

The nurse monitors arterial blood gases after intracranial surgery to ensure adequate oxygenation. If cerebral edema is a problem, the client may require hyperventilation for prevention of hypercapnia.

Nursing Diagnosis: Communication, Impaired Verbal R/T aphasia or dysarthia.

Planning: Expected Outcomes. The client will be able to effectively communicate, as evidenced by the client's needs being understood and met, and the client indicating understanding of the communication of others.

Implementation. After intracranial surgery, speech disorders may occur as a result of decreased circulation to the brain during surgery or surgical trauma to the areas of the brain governing speech. Interventions for aphasia are discussed earlier.

Nursing Diagnosis: Physical Mobility, Impaired R/T bed rest.

Planning: Expected Outcomes. The client will have no signs of contractures, as evidenced by full ROM in all joints; no evidence of flexion contractures in wrists, elbows, and knees; and no signs of footdrop.

Implementation. After intracranial surgery, the client remains on bed rest for at least 24 hours. Nursing care to prevent complications of immobility is imperative. After 24 hours, passive ROM exercises are usually begun. Increased ICP or physiologic instability may delay these activities beyond 24 hours.

Frequent position changes (to other safe positions) are important. The nurse should prepare the client (and other nurses) for the move and explain what each nurse should or should not do during the move. The client's head and any weak extremities must be protected and supported to prevent injury and to maintain a safe position.

When the client's condition is stabilized, movement to the bedside chair is ordered. Once the client is secured in the chair, the head of the chair is slowly elevated. This is done in gradual increments until the full upright position is tolerated. If a chair is not available, the nurse helps the client to dangle his or her legs over the side of the bed. The nurse should remain present for safety and support in both situations and closely assess for dizziness or faintness. Before and after the transfer, the nurse auscultates and documents the blood pressure to assess for postural hypotension. As improvement continues, self-care and other activities are gradually resumed.

Nursing Diagnosis: Self-Care Deficit, Risk for R/T weakness, cognitive impairments.

Planning: Expected Outcomes. The client will perform as many ADLs as possible, as evidenced by the use of adaptive devices and techniques and recognition of limitations.

Implementation. Extensive self-care deficits may be present after intracranial surgery. They may be due to factors such as neuromuscular impairment, perceptual or cognitive impairment, pain, severe anxiety, or weakness. Self-care deficits may include those related to bathing and hygiene, feeding, toileting, or dressing and grooming. Careful nursing assessment is required to meet the client's needs in these areas and to promote a return to maximal possible self-care. The client should be encouraged to perform ADLs as he or she is able.

Nursing Diagnosis: Self-Esteem Disturbance R/T operative or postoperative complications.

Planning: Expected Outcomes. The client will develop effective coping strategies, as evidenced by appropriate life-style modifications, use of the assistance of others, and appropriate social interactions.

Implementation. Postoperative complications of devasting proportions may occur after intracranial surgery. They can profoundly disturb the client's self-esteem, role performance, and personal identity. Also, there may be body image changes that are difficult for the client to accept. Nurses can assist the client and significant others to deal with these threatening issues.

If a defect remains in the skull after surgery, it may be helpful for the surgeon to discuss possible cranioplasty before the client sees the defect. Cranioplasty is the surgical repair of the defect with a custom-made implant.

Nursing Diagnosis: Thought Processes, Altered R/T surgical resection, cerebral edema, sleep deprivation.

Planning: Expected Outcomes. The client will recognize limitations and attempt to minimize them, as evidenced by participation in prescribed therapies, consideration of physical capabilities during activities, and verbalization of limitations and adaptations.

Implementation. Alteration in thought processes may be temporary (e.g., due to sleep deprivation, cerebral swelling) or permanent (e.g., due to surgical trauma) after intracranial surgery. If thought process disturbances continue to persist, the nurse may make suggestions for living with this problem. For any brain function change (verbal thought, memory), neuropsychological testing helps establish parameters of dysfunction.

Nursing Diagnosis: Pain R/T scalp incision.

Planning: Expected Outcomes. The client will experience adequate pain relief, as evidenced by verbalization of improvement in comfort level without excessive drowsiness or lethargy, the ability to rest without interruption by pain, and the ability to participate in therapies without hindrance by pain.

Implementation. The nurse must be careful not to jar the client's bed or otherwise cause sudden movements that worsen the pain. The environment should be kept quiet, calm, and dimly lit. The nurse administers prescribed medications as indicated for pain relief. Acetaminophen or codeine may be prescribed for pain relief. The nurse evaluates the effectiveness of pain-relieving medications and checks for allergies to medications. If the client vomits from the inability to tolerate medication, ICP may be seriously elevated.

Nursing Diagnosis: Family Processes, Altered R/T irreversible changes in client after surgery.

Planning: Expected Outcomes. The client's significant others will exhibit positive behaviors, as evidenced by the ability to solve problems; care for all members of the family as needed; and ask questions about showing concern toward the client as appropriate, showing that they have understood previous conversations.

Implementation. Significant others are also affected by the client's postoperative changes. Some are able and willing to help the client and themselves grow and meet postoperative challenges. Others are unable to adapt effectively in this way, finding it difficult to accept changes in the client.

Facilitating the expression of concerns, providing support and understanding, careful listening, and an unhurried empathetic manner may all help the client and significant others if postoperative problems occur (e.g., paralysis, infection, speech disorders, skull defects) or if the surgery seems unsuccessful. The client and significant others may also experience spiritual distress, powerlessness, or anticipatory grieving if the surgery was not successful and the client is unimproved, has postoperative complications, or is dying.

Evaluation

The degree of expected outcome attainment should be evaluated on a regular basis. Some expected outcomes, such as ICP and cerebral perfusion, will need to be met before discharge from the ICU. Other expected outcomes, such as improved cognition and speech, may require months to obtain. Setting appropriate and achievable outcomes with the client and family is important.

Posthospital Care

Many clients can be discharged home and return to a gratifying life after brain surgery. Others require short-term or ongoing rehabilitation to achieve complete recovery. Still others never regain complete competence because of the amount of brain tissue damaged from the disorder and surgery. For these clients, the greater burden rests on the family and significant others to provide ongoing care either at home or in a nursing home.

Family support groups are available through many hospitals to families with brain-damaged members. These groups help the significant others to know they are not alone. Clinical nurse specialists in neuroscience are often the facilitators for these groups. Participation by both client and significant others should be encouraged. Care should be taken to include everyone who is important to the client, not just those who are legal relatives.

PITUITARY TUMORS

Pituitary tumors cause the client to develop visual field defects, irregular or absent menstrual cycles, infertility, decreased libido, impotence, decreased body hair, and decreased production of other stimulating hormones. Most of these tumors occur in the anterior lobe and are benign, small, and encapsulated. They can usually be removed successfully with surgery. The procedure is called transsphenoidal hypophysectomy. The operation is performed through the nose to avoid entering the cranium (Fig. 14–10).

After surgery, the client is positioned with the head elevated. The nose is packed to control bleeding. Postoperative care is similar to that of other clients after craniotomy.

A fairly common effect from pituitary edema is the development of transient diabetes insipidus due to a lack of secretion of antidiuretic hormone. Clients with diabetes insipidus have large volumes (2 to 15 L/day) of dilute urine. Aside from the inconvenience of polyuria, the client often suffers no serious side effects from diabetes insipidus, unless the client is deprived of water. When this happens, circulatory collapse (hypovolemic shock) and hypertonic encephalopathy will occur as a result of fluid shifts in the brain.

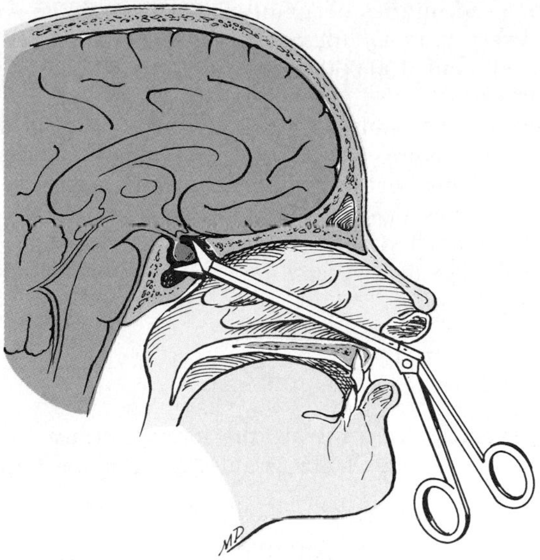

Figure 14–10
Transsphenoidal hypophysectomy for the excision of pituitary tumors.

Usual treatment is with intravenous or inhalation vasopressin (Pitressin) or desmopressin (DDAVP). Long-acting forms of these agents can be used for chronic diabetes insipidus. After pituitary surgery, the client will also require hormones for replacement of those lost with tissue resection.

Nursing intervention for diabetes insipidus or syndrome of inappropriate antidiuretic hormone involves

- accurate intake and output documentation
- assessing urine specific gravity every 2 hours
- assessing for indications of fluid and electrolyte imbalances
- documenting and reporting changes in the client's status or therapy
- explaining the condition to the client and significant others, emphasizing the need for fluid balance (i.e., avoiding overhydration or dehydration)
- explaining the reasons for medication, when and how to take it, and any side effects to the client and significant others

Head Trauma

INJURIES TO THE SCALP, SKULL, OR BRAIN

Incidence

In the United States, a head injury is experienced approximately every 16 seconds. Head injury is often classified as minor or mild, moderate, and severe.

Minor head injuries occur in over half a million Americans every year. Of these, more than 290,000 are hospitalized, and 150,000 experience disability lasting 1 month or more.

Moderate injuries, resulting in disability for 3 months or more, occur to approximately 60,000 to 75,000 clients per year. Fatal head injuries occur over 140,000 times per year. Head trauma results in more deaths than all other causes combined for Americans under the age of 34 years.

Etiology

Motor vehicle accidents are the foremost cause of head injuries. Other causes are assaults, falls, and accidents.

MECHANISMS OF INJURY

Head injuries are caused by a sudden force to the head (Fig. 14–11). The results are complex. Three mechanisms contribute to head trauma: (1) acceleration, (2) deceleration, and (3) deformation. An acceleration injury occurs when the immobile head is struck by a moving object. If the head is moving and hits an immobile object, a deceleration injury occurs. This can be seen in an auto accident when the head hits the steering wheel. In an acceleration/deceleration injury, a moving object hits the immobile head, and then the head hits an immobile object. Deformation refers to injuries in which the force results in deformation and disruption of the integrity of the impacted body part (e.g., skull fracture).

Head trauma is also categorized by describing the injury (e.g., blunt or penetrating trauma or a coup or contrecoup injury). Acceleration/deceleration injuries often result in blunt trauma. These are complex injuries involving several cranial structures, including brain parenchyma and vessels. Because the brain is able to move within the skull, movement of the brain can result in injuries at different locations.

Penetrating injuries include those made by foreign bodies (e.g., knives or bullets) or those made by bone fragments from a skull fracture. The damage caused by a penetrating injury often relates to the velocity with which a penetrating object pierces the skull and brain. Bone fragments from a skull fracture may cause local brain injury by lacerating brain tissue and damaging other structures (e.g., nerves and blood vessels). If a major blood vessel is severed or ruptured, a large clot (hematoma) may form, with damage to adjacent or even remote structures (e.g., brain compression from one of the herniation syndromes). Thus, a secondary event, a hematoma, can also cause extensive brain tissue damage.

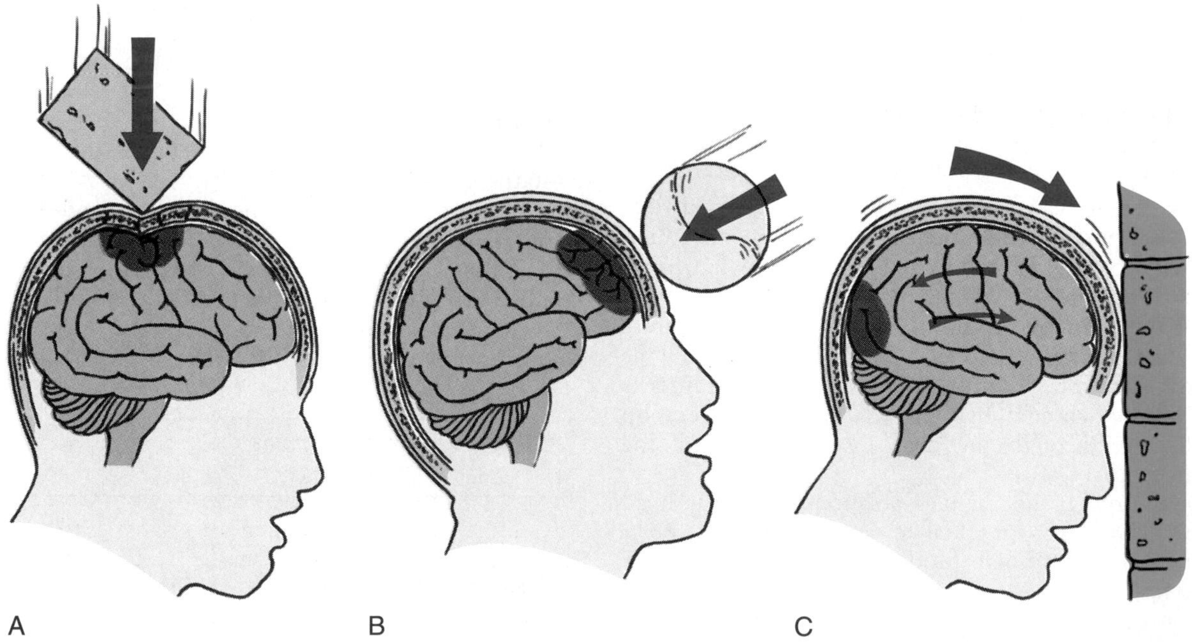

Figure 14–11
Some mechanisms of head injury. Head injury results from penetration or impact. *A*, A direct injury (blow to skull) may fracture the skull. Contusion and laceration of the brain may result from fractures. Depressed portions of the skull may compress or penetrate brain tissue. *B*, In the absence of skull fracture, a blow to the skull may cause the brain to move enough to tear some of the veins going from the cortical surface to the dura. Subsequently, subdural hematoma may develop. Note the areas of cerebral contusion *(shaded)*. *C*, Rebound of the cranial contents may result in an area of injury opposite the point of impact. Such an injury is called a contrecoup injury. In addition to the three injuries depicted, secondary phenomena may result from the injury and cause additional brain dysfunction or damage. For example, ischemia, especially cerebral edema, may occur, elevating intracranial pressure.

Frequently, low- and high-velocity penetrating wounds create an open communication between the external environment and the cranial cavity. Thus, infection is a possible complication. These penetrating wounds are commonly treated surgically with débridement and wound closure.

A coup injury occurs immediately at the point of impact. Because of movement within the skull, the same blow may cause injury on the opposite side of the brain, that is, a contrecoup injury. (Contrecoup is derived from a French word meaning reverse-blow.) In addition there are often multiple areas of injury along the line of the blow's force. Tissues around major injured areas often swell, which increases damage to the brain.

Injuries may also be classified according to the structure damaged (e.g., brain stem) and whether they are primary or secondary. Primary head injury refers to impact damage, the severity of which is estimated by initial signs and symptoms. Secondary or delayed events that follow head injury include edema, hemorrhage, or infection. These processes can significantly impede recovery or even cause death from what initially appeared to be a mild injury.

Risk Factors

The major factor contributing to the occurrence of head injury is alcohol consumption. Alcohol slows reflexes and alters cognitive processes and perception. These physiologic changes increase the chances of a person's being involved in an accident or altercation.

Primary prevention centers on the education of clients of all ages. Children should be taught the importance of safety restraints in cars and of bicycle helmets. The use of motorcycle helmets and the dangers of driving after drug or alcohol ingestion are necessary information for older children and adults.

Tertiary prevention focuses on preventing or minimizing the complications of head trauma. At-the-scene care by trained professionals, stabilization, and transportation to tertiary care centers improve outcomes. At the time of an accident, many clients suffer primary, irreversible brain injury, which ultimately causes death. The most common causes of such deaths are brain stem hemorrhage and diffuse axonal injury throughout the brain as a result of the impact.

Pathophysiology

Primary head injuries include injuries to the scalp, skull, or brain or all of these. The injuries result from the original impact.

SCALP INJURIES

Scalp injuries can cause lacerations, hematomas, and contusions or abrasions to the skin. These injuries may be unsightly and bleed profusely. Clients with minor scalp injuries not accompanied by damage to other areas do not require hospitalization.

SKULL INJURIES

Skull fractures are often caused by a force sufficient to cause both fracture and brain injury. The fractures in themselves do not mean brain injury is also present. However, skull fractures often cause serious brain damage. Depressed skull fractures injure the brain by bruising it (abrasion) or by driving bone fragments into it (lacerations). The site of a fracture and the extent of brain injury may not correlate.

There are three types of skull fracture: linear, depressed, and basilar.

Linear Skull Fractures. These fractures appear as thin lines radiographically and do not require treatment. They are important only if there is significant underlying brain damage.

Depressed Skull Fractures. These fractures may be palpated and are seen radiographically. Surgery may be required within the first 24 hours after injury if the depression is as deep as the skull thickness. Depressed fractures may be associated with bone fragments penetrating into brain tissue. When this occurs, the area is usually surgically explored and débrided.

Basilar Skull Fractures. These fractures occur in bones over the base of the frontal and temporal lobes. They are rarely seen radiographically.

Basilar skull fractures, depressed fractures, and other open (compound) fractures all allow communication between the exterior environment and the brain. Infection is therefore a possible complication. (See later discussion of brain abscess and meningitis.)

BRAIN INJURIES

There is a wide variety of brain injuries (see discussion under Mechanisms of Injury). A single classification of brain injuries does not exist. However, the terms open, closed, contusion, and concussion are often applied to brain injuries. Open head injuries are those that penetrate the skull. Closed injuries are from blunt trauma.

Concussions. A concussion is head trauma that may result in loss of consciousness for 5 minutes or less and retrograde amnesia. There is no break in the skull or dura, and no visible damage on the CT or MRI is seen. The client usually presents with headache and dizziness and may complain of nausea and vomiting. The duration of amnesia may directly correlate with severity of the concussion.

Contusions. Contusions cause more extensive damage than do concussions. Contusions damage the brain substance itself, causing multiple areas of petechial and punctate hemorrhage and bruised areas. Abnormalities may be mainly in one area of the brain, but other areas may also be injured. This is particularly true of brain stem contusions, which are a very serious type of lesion.

Clinical Manifestations

SKULL FRACTURES

Other than a history of head injury, clients with skull fractures may not have clear symptoms of their injury. They may develop other clinical signs including

- CSF or other drainage from the ear or nose
- various cranial nerve injuries
- blood behind the eardrum
- periorbital ecchymosis (bruise around the eyes)
- a delayed bruise over the mastoid (Battle's sign)

Indications of cranial nerve damage may occur at the time of the initial injury or may develop later. They include

- vision loss (e.g., blindness, blurred vision) from optic nerve damage
- hearing loss with postural vertigo and nystagmus from auditory nerve damage
- loss of the sense of smell (bilaterally or unilaterally) from olfactory nerve damage
- squint or fixed dilated pupil and loss of some of the eye movements from oculomotor nerve damage
- facial paresis or paralysis (unilateral) from facial nerve damage

CONTUSIONS

There are various clinical manifestations in clients with contusions. This is partly because of the numerous areas of damage. Contusions are often associated with other serious injuries, including cervical fractures. Secondary effects (e.g., brain swelling and edema) accompany serious contusions. Increased ICP and herniation syndromes may result.

Contusions can be divided into cerebral contusions and brain stem contusions.

Cerebral Contusions. These contusions can be diagnosed only if the client is alert, although they may be present in comatose patients. Assessment findings vary, depending on which areas of the cerebral hemispheres are damaged. The nurse must remember that although findings correlate with cerebral contusion, they do not rule out other abnormalities such as a developing mass or lesion. Adverse changes in the client's condition require immediate medical attention. They may indicate treatable complications.

Brain Stem Contusions. Brain stem contusions render a client immediately unresponsive or partially comatose because of significant brain stem disruption. Typically, an altered LOC continues for at least several hours and usually days or weeks. The client may regain partial consciousness within hours or remain in a coma.

Damage to the reticular activating system may render the client permanently comatose. Other neurologic abnormalities are present and are usually symmetric (i.e., on both sides of the body). Some may be lateralized (asymmetric, on one side of the body only), indicating development of a secondary event such as a hematoma.

In addition to the altered LOC that is always present with brain stem contusion, respiratory, pupillary, eye movement, and motor abnormalities may occur.

- Respirations may be normal, ataxic, periodic, or very rapid.
- Pupils are usually small, equal, and reactive. Damage to the upper brain stem (third cranial nerve) may cause pupillary abnormalities.
- Loss of normal eye movements may occur because pathways controlling eye movements traverse the midbrain and pons.
- The client may respond to light or noxious stimuli by purposeful movements, pushing the stimulus away. Or the client may have no response to stimuli, that is, may be flaccid. In the presence of profound LOC alterations, flexion and extension posturing may be elicited with or without noxious stimuli (see Chap. 12).

Brain stem contusions do not usually injure the brain stem alone. Swelling or direct injury to the hypothalamus may produce autonomic nervous system effects. The client has a high temperature, has rapid pulse and respiration, and perspires profusely. These effects may wax and wane but, if sustained, can lead to serious complications.

These clinical manifestations often vary from one observation to another (whereas findings indicating a developing hematoma are more consistent). Careful documentation of assessment findings is important to identify patterns or trends in the client's condition.

DIAGNOSTIC ASSESSMENT

CRITICAL TO REMEMBER

There is a high association of cervical fracture with head injury; therefore, lateral cervical spine radiographs are obtained before the client's head is moved.

CT scans and radiographs are also obtained to assess for fractures and areas of bleeding or brain shift. Lumbar puncture can also be used to assess for bleeding within the subarachnoid space.

Medical Management

A complete history is taken of the mechanism of injury. These data allow the physician to determine the probable extent of injury. Diagnostic findings are reviewed.

Open head wounds should be covered and pressure applied to control bleeding unless there appears to be underlying depressed or compound skull fracture.

CRITICAL TO REMEMBER

The nurse should not attempt to remove foreign objects or any penetrating objects from the wound.

Uncomplicated scalp wounds (that do not lie over depressed or compound skull fractures) are anesthetized locally, cleansed, and sutured.

Simple skull depressions are electively treated by surgically elevating the depressed bone fragment and repairing the dura if it is lacerated. All bone fragments are removed. Compound depressed skull fractures are immediately treated surgically. The scalp, skull, and devitalized brain are débrided, and the wound is cleansed thoroughly. Unless all foreign material is removed, a brain abscess develops. Débridement of a penetrating wound or depressed skull fracture frequently leaves a cranial defect that is cosmetically unsightly. The defect is surgically corrected by cranioplasty.

SEVERE HEAD INJURY

Major goals in the care of severely head-injured clients are (1) the prompt recognition and treatment of hypoxia and acid-base disturbances that can contribute to cerebral edema, increasing ICP resulting from factors such as cerebral edema, or expanding hematoma and (2) stabilization of other conditions.

Few clients die instantly from head injury. However, many head-injured clients die within the first few minutes after injury from shock or impaired respiration. Early death may also result from brain stem damage. Rigorous intervention is started immediately because severe brain trauma is associated with high morbidity and mortality rates.

Some clients survive initial head trauma only to develop intracranial mass lesions such as expanding hematomas (e.g., epidural and subdural hemorrhages), which may be fatal unless promptly diagnosed and treated. Severe cerebral swelling often follows brain injury. It is probably the most common cause of death in clients who survive the initial injury and who do not develop intracranial mass lesions.

Clients with traumatic head injuries often have other major injuries. These include facial fractures, lung and heart injuries, cervical fractures, abdominal injuries, and musculoskeletal injuries. Facial fractures and lung injuries may contribute to respiratory insufficiency. Airway obstruction and decreased ability to breathe (e.g., from pulmonary contusion, flail chest, pneumothorax) contribute to respiratory insufficiency and poor oxygenation of the brain and other tissues. Brain death may result.

CRITICAL TO REMEMBER

Hemorrhagic shock in clients with multiple trauma is rarely caused by head injury alone.

Frequently it relates to ruptured abdominal organs or musculoskeletal injuries (e.g., fractured femur and pelvis). Circulation may be further compromised by cardiac contusion and associated arrhythmias. Head injuries can also cause arrhythmias and further complicate the client's recovery.

The medical management of severely head-injured clients focuses on supporting all organ systems while recovery from the injuries takes place. This involves ventilatory support, management of nutrition and gastrointestinal function, and management of fluid balance and elimination. Head trauma has impact on all systems of the body, and managing these effects requires a holistic perspective. Clinical manifestations must be evaluated as stemming from the head injury or arising from a complicating process.

Fluids are usually managed carefully for avoidance of either over- or underadministration. Parameters such as central venous pressure and urinary output are used to guide fluid intake. Because severely head-injured clients are given nothing by mouth, potassium is commonly given through the intravenous line.

PHARMACOLOGIC MANAGEMENT

Antiseizure medications, such as phenytoin, are begun on admission. Even though seizures early in the course of head injury are uncommon, if they occur, brain injury can intensify because of alterations in oxygenation from impaired ventilation and increased ICP. Histamine antagonists are given to reduce the risk of stress ulcers. Mild analgesics may be prescribed, such as acetaminophen or codeine. Antibiotics may also be prescribed. Osmotic diuretics may be required to reduce ICP.

DIETARY MANAGEMENT

Initially the client is given nothing by mouth until peristalsis returns, commonly after 5 days. Enteral tube feedings are utilized because metabolic needs increase after head injury. The risk of aspiration with enteral tube feeding must be prevented by feeding the client with the head elevated and monitoring pulmonary changes. Hyperalimentation can also be used, but some clients develop hyperglycemia from the solution. Hyperglycemia can further cerebral anoxia, and blood glucose levels should be monitored carefully.

Nursing Management

Assessment

A history of how a client was injured is helpful in understanding the nature of a head injury. When accident witnesses accompany a newly head-injured client to the care facility, the nurse should obtain as much information as possible about the accident and the client's neurologic responses at the scene of the accident. The nurse should try to find out if the client lost consciousness.

As soon as possible after head injury, the nurse assesses and documents the client's vital signs and neurologic status. This initial assessment establishes a baseline for later observations. The nurse should carefully document all assessment findings.

In the health-care facility, the frequency of assessing vital signs and neurologic status varies according to the client's condition. However, it is usually every 15 minutes until the client is stable and within limits for age and previous conditions. It may be necessary to awaken a head-injured client hourly for assessment during the first 24 to 48 hours after injury. Parameters assessed include

- LOC and responsiveness
- pupillary diameters and responses to light
- vital signs
- motor strength
- speech
- vision
- reaction to auditory and painful stimuli
- response to command
- spontaneous activity
- general responsiveness to stimulation.

The Glasgow Coma Scale is commonly used.

The nurse should promptly report to the physician any findings that indicate the possible development of complications. It is particularly difficult to assess the condition of a head-injured client who has ingested large amounts of alcohol or other drugs before injury because these substances may obscure significant clinical assessment findings.

Nursing Intervention

Nursing of the head-injured client is found in the Care Plan for the head-injured client.

Evaluation

The degree of attainment of expected outcomes should be assessed often in the early phases of care. Later in

Text continued on page 41

CARE PLAN: The Head-Injured Client

Nursing Diagnosis/ Collaborative Problem	Planning: Expected Outcomes	Implementation: Nursing Interventions	Rationales
Paralysis, Risk for R/T undiagnosed cervical fractures	The nurse will monitor for development of progressive motor/sensory deficit; increased neck pain, stiffness, bruising; bilateral paralysis	Immobilize head and neck until cervical injury ruled out by examination/x-ray study (cervical collar, sandbags, spine board)	The cervical spine needs to be immobilized until it is certain no fracture exists
		Avoid flexion, hyperextension, rotation of neck	
		If respiratory resuscitation needed, use jaw thrust maneuver	Hyperextension of the neck increases risk of injury
		Assess/document leg, hand, arm, and shoulder movement and strength hourly and as necessary	Cervical fracture may cause weakness or paresthesias in the extremities
		Assess sensory deficits	
		Assess for neck pain, stiffness, bruising	Bleeding in the subarachnoid space causes tissue irritation
Airway Clearance, Ineffective R/T coma or bleeding into airway	Client will have effective airway clearance, as evidenced by: • Upper airway free of secretions • Regular respiratory rate (16–22), rhythm, amplitude • Breath sounds present both lung bases • Symmetric chest movement • Trachea midline • Absence of dyspnea, agitation, confusion, yawning • Absence of aspiration • ABGs normal with PaO_2 greater than 90 mm Hg and PCO_2 between 30 and 35 mm Hg • Chest film clear	Maintain a patent airway	The airway may be occluded from blood, vomitus, or secretions
		Clear mouth/oropharynx of foreign bodies (e.g., teeth)	
		Suction oropharynx and trachea every 1–2 hr and as necessary (suction nasopharynx after basilar fracture is ruled out)	
		Assess respiratory rate, rhythm, amplitude every 1–2 hr or as necessary	Respiratory rate may be altered if brain stem is injured
		Check breath sounds and chest excursions every 1–2 hr	Breath sounds indicate air movement
		Monitor ABGs (initially, daily, and as necessary)	Indicate arterial oxygen, carbon dioxide, and pH
		Position semiprone, lateral position	Facilitates drainage of secretions and prevents aspiration *after* cervical spine is stabilized
		Administer humidified oxygen as indicated	Oxygen is used to prevent cerebral hypoxia
		Assist or maintain endotracheal intubation, tracheostomy, and mechanical ventilation as needed	Mechanical ventilation may be required to supplement ventilatory efforts

CARE PLAN: The Head-Injured Client *Continued*

Nursing Diagnosis/ Collaborative Problem	Planning: Expected Outcomes	Implementation: Nursing Interventions	Rationales
Tissue Perfusion, Altered Cerebral R/T hypotension, intracranial hemorrhage, hematoma, or other injuries	Client will have adequate cerebral tissue perfusion, as evidenced by	Assess LOC/responsiveness hourly or as necessary, including alertness, orientation	Alterations in LOC are first indications of increasing ICP
	• Stable, improving LOC • Glasgow Coma Scale score of 9 or above • Temperature less than 38.5° C • Equal and reactive pupils • Intact consensual light reflex	Assess pupillary size, position, response to direct and consensual responses every 1–4 hr	Pupillary changes commonly accompany head injury
	• Intact extraocular movements	Assess extraocular eye movements every 1–4 hr	Increasing ICP often traps third cranial nerve, affecting eye movement
	• Stable or improving motor response (hand, arm, and leg movements) • Stable or improving response to painful stimulation • ICP remains less than 15 mm Hg • Mean arterial pressure at about 100 mm Hg	Cognitive function may be impaired by edema and inadequate blood flow Note verbalization and response to verbal command by checking hand grip and release, leg movement, dorsiflexion, and plantar flexion every 1–4 hr	Voluntary movement requires functional brain areas (cerebrum, cerebellum, and parietal lobes)
	• Systolic pressure greater than 90 mm Hg	In unconscious client, note spontaneous movement, withdrawal to pain every 1–4 hr	Denotes level of coma
	Stable vital signs Normal sinus rhythm Urine output of at least 30 mL/hr Absence of hemorrhage Hgb and Hct within normal limits Central venous pressure within normal limits	Report, record, and assess more frequently if any deterioration is evident	Early recognition of neurologic changes is imperative
		Monitor temperature every 2 hr; report temperature greater than 38.5° C and maintain normothermia with antipyretic agents or hypothermia blanket	Hyperthermia commonly accompanies head injury; blood is an irritant to the meninges; temperature is reduced as it increases cerebral metabolism
		Monitor cardiovascular and pulmonary status	Maximizes oxygenation and perfusion of brain tissue
		Vital signs every 1–4 hr	Changes may indicate increasing ICP
		Maintain head of bed elevation at least 30 degrees or as prescribed; keep head in neutral position (use sandbags)	Facilitates venous and CSF drainage
		Monitor input and output every 1–4 hr	Fluid overload and dehydration can impair cerebral circulation
		Avoid extreme hip flexion	Increases intrathoracic pressure and thereby intracranial pressure
		Monitor electrocardiographic pattern continuously	Dysrhythmias reduce cardiac output
		Massage every 2–4 hr; avoid bony prominences if red	Massage stimulates blood supply, rubbing bony prominences may increase tissue shear
		Turn every 2 hr	Permits tissue perfusion

Care Plan continued on following page

CARE PLAN: The Head-Injured Client *Continued*

Nursing Diagnosis/ Collaborative Problem	Planning: Expected Outcomes	Implementation: Nursing Interventions	Rationales
Tissue Integrity, Impaired R/T lack of reflexic movement	Client will have intact tissues, as evidenced by • Eyes free of irritation, inflammation • Mucous membranes moist, absence of infection	Check corneal reflex, eye care every 4 hr: apply artificial tears and tape eye(s) closed prn	Blinking or use of artificial tears resupplies the cornea with fluid
		Mouth care every 4 hr; check for infection (thrush)	Stomatitis can occur in clients who are NPO; thrush may also develop, a side effect from antibiotics
Nutrition, Altered: Less than Body Requirements	Client will maintain usual weight, as evidenced by • Caloric intake range of 2000–3000 (NG) daily • Protein intake 50–60 g daily (adults) not to exceed 1 g/kg body weight • Minimal residual NG feeding	Monitor daily weights Assess input and output every 8 hr Monitor daily caloric and protein intake (note: for every gram protein, 50 mL of water is required for excretion) Monitor NG residuals Hold next feeding per orders	Weight is an accurate indicator of nutrition Intake should equal output to avoid fluid overload or dehydration A catabolic state will delay wound healing Residuals indicate delayed gastric emptying
Fluid Volume Deficit, Risk for R/T tube feeding and lack of ability to respond to thirst	Client will have fluid balance, as evidenced by • Input and output nearly equal every 24 hr • Urine specific gravity within normal limits • Skin turgor at 3 seconds • Tongue moist and pink • Normal serum electrolyte, blood urea nitrogen, creatinine, and Hct	Assess for signs of dehydration, electrolyte imbalance, and uremia by monitoring skin turgor, electrolytes, blood urea nitrogen, creatinine, Hct, urine specific gravity, input and output	Skin turgor will increase with dehydration because of loss of interstitial fluids Electrolytes and specific gravity will rise with dehydration
		Give additional free water with tube feeding to meet daily requirements	Free water will replace water lost to perspiration and respiration that is not replaced by drinking
Injury, Risk for R/T restlessness and confusion	Client will remain free of injury, as evidenced by • Oriented to time, place, person • Absence of neurologic changes • Absence of pain or other sources of discomfort • ABGs within normal limits	Orientate as necessary Assess client for pain or other sources of discomfort	Assists client in understanding what has happened Pain and pain response increase ICP
		Decrease stressors: noxious stimuli, visceral discomfort (pain, chills, fever) Provide appropriate sedation as ordered, e.g., Haldol, Sublimaze Restrain if only alternative Give emotional support	Noxious stimuli increase ICP Facilitates management and ventilation Restraints may increase agitation May decrease anxiety
Sleep Pattern Disturbance R/T frequent assessments and loss of REM sleep	Client will obtain sleep, as evidenced by two 90-minute periods of uninterrupted sleep	Allow visiting only to the extent client can tolerate it Keep environmental stimuli to a minimum	Visitors may stimulate client and prohibit sleep Promotes a quiet environment for rest

CARE PLAN: The Head-Injured Client *Continued*

Nursing Diagnosis/ Collaborative Problem	Planning: Expected Outcomes	Implementation: Nursing Interventions	Rationales
Urinary Elimination, Altered R/T lack of awareness of bladder distention, unconsciousness	Client will have adequate urinary elimination, as evidenced by • Urine output 30–50 mL/hr • Absence of bladder distention • Absence of urinary infection	Assess input and output every 8 hr (when stable)	Data to assess urine output
		Assess client for urinary retention, overflow, incontinence	Symptoms of urinary disorders
		Intermittent catheterization preferred to indwelling urinary catheter	Decreases risk of infection
		Bladder training program as soon as possible	Promotes self-care
		Monitor daily for signs of urinary tract infection	Catheterization increases risk of urinary tract infection
Constipation, R/T loss of muscle tone, reflexes, and inactivity	Client will regain usual bowel habits, as evidenced by • Normal bowel sounds • Absence of paralytic ileus, distention, impaction • Regular bowel evacuation	Auscultate for bowel sounds every shift	Bowel sounds indicate peristalsis
		Check for impaction daily	Unconscious patients will not have an urge to move their bowels
		Administer stool softeners, laxatives, suppositories, or enemas as needed	Treatments for constipation cause bowel evacuation
		Add water to diet	Replaces water loss with colonic reabsorption
		Use tube feedings	
		Increase the bulk in stool with fiber	
Thought Processes, Altered R/T memory deficit, impaired reasoning ability, altered LOC, confusion, speech impairment, sensory deprivation	Client will have intact thought processes, as evidenced by • Minimal or absent memory impairment • Appropriate verbalizations • Appropriate behavior patterns • Establishes method of communication • Participates in retraining and rehabilitation activities	Orientate to person, time, and place daily and prn	Assists clients' memory
		Explain all nursing activities before initiating	Decreases agitation
		Avoid sensory overload	Decreases agitation
		Devise alternative methods of communication as needed	Provides a mechanism to communicate with client
		Side rails up, bed low	Decreases risk of injury
		Consult with rehabilitation therapists	Develops continuity of plans
		Involve client and significant others in care planning and goal setting	Family members and client need to have mutual goals
Seizures, Risk for R/T brain injury, hypoxia, electrolyte imbalance, hyperthermia, fluid volume alterations	The nurse will monitor for seizure development, protect from injury, and maintain airway during seizure	Prevent/protect from injury	Client is unable to protect self
	Patent airway	Check adequate airway; do not force a tongue blade into mouth	Clients do not "swallow their tongues" during seizures
		Observe onset, progression, duration of seizures	Assists with diagnosis of location of epileptogenic focus
		Position client on side postictally; suction prn; monitor vital signs, duration postictal phase, onset status epilepticus	Maintains patent airway
		Administer antiepileptic drugs as prescribed	Head injury increases risk of seizure

Care Plan continued on following page

CARE PLAN: The Head-Injured Client *Continued*

Nursing Diagnosis/ Collaborative Problem	Planning: Expected Outcomes	Implementation: Nursing Interventions	Rationales
Altered Health Maintenance R/T knowledge deficit on seizure management	Client will be able to manage seizure risk, as evidenced by verbalizing of understanding of seizures, medications, precipitating factors, community resources, safety measures by client and significant others	Initiate client education opportunities to include medication instruction, precipitating factors, safety measures, community resources	Epilepsy is a chronic disorder, education is a critical aspect of nursing management
At Risk for CSF leak, meningitis, and diabetes insipidus	The nurse will monitor for complications of head injury: CSF leak, meningitis, diabetes insipidus	Observe for otorrhea or rhinorrhea	CSF may leak through nose or ears
		Test clear watery fluid for glucose	CSF rhinorrhea is clear
		Observe blood-tinged fluid for "halo sign"	CSF contains glucose and dries in concentric rings
		Apply a drip pad, change when wet	Wet dressings facilitate movement of organisms
		Do not suction nasally if anterior fossa fracture is present or if basilar fractures have not been ruled out	Suction catheter may pierce dura
		Instruct not to blow nose or cough or inhibit sneeze; sneeze through open mouth	Withholding a sneeze forces bacteria backward
		Aseptic technique when working with Richmond screws, incisions, drains	Prevents central nervous system infection
		Give antibiotics as prescribed	Reduces risk of infection
		Monitor input and output every 1–8 hr	Diabetes insipidus causes polyuria
		Assess skin turgor daily Daily weights if indicated Report urine output over 200 mL/hr for 2 consecutive hr	Clients can become dehydrated if fluid not replaced
		Monitor electrolytes and serum/urine osmolality and urine specific gravity	Sodium and osmolality can become altered because of fluid imbalance
		Monitor Hgb and Hct	Continued loss of blood decreases cerebral perfusion
		Assess for signs of bleeding: abdomen, chest, pelvis, long bones, extremities	Other injuries may be undetected
		Check for hematuria	Indication of renal or urinary trauma
		Control active bleeding from scalp by compression	Compression is effective in reducing blood loss
		Administer blood and blood products	Restore blood volume
Physical Mobility, Impaired R/T motor, sensory, or proprioceptive deficits, depressed consciousness level	Client will maintain physical mobility, as evidenced by not developing contractures and maintaining baseline ROM in all uninvolved joints	Early ROM exercises	Maintains joint mobility and muscle tone
		Prevent contractures: splints to maintain functional position of hands, arms, legs, and feet	Maintains functional strength and alignment of extremities
		Physical therapy as needed	
Skin Integrity, Risk for Impaired R/T immobility and lack of awareness to turn	Client will have intact skin, as evidenced by Absence of skin redness, abrasions, breakdown	Check signs of skin redness, especially over ears, shoulders, elbows, sacrum, hips, heels, and toes every 4–8 hr	Bone prominences are the first body areas to develop skin impairment

ABGs, arterial blood gases; CSF, cerebrospinal fluid; Hct, hematocrit; Hgb, hemoglobin; ICP, intracranial pressure; LOC, level of consciousness; NG, nasogastric; NPO, nothing by mouth; REM, rapid eye movement; ROM, range of motion.

rehabilitation, expected outcomes may require weeks for full attainment. Because the care of the head-injured client goes on in many areas of a health-care setting (i.e., ICU, a general nursing unit, a rehabilitation unit), complete communication about the client, significant others, and goals should always be a part of any care plan.

Modification of Plan of Care for the Elderly

Although most head injuries do not occur in the elderly population, these clients experience more complications. An elderly client may be less able to tolerate respiratory problems or cardiac dysrhythmias. The presence of chronic obstructive pulmonary disease or congestive heart failure can make managing ventilation and fluid balance more difficult. If any type of mental impairment was present before the injury, recovery to full independence is less likely. Rehabilitation may be impeded by poor stamina and medical complications.

Posthospital Care

DISCHARGE TEACHING

Clients with possible head injury or mild head injury are usually hospitalized for observation for a minimum of 6 hours (ideally for 48 hours) because of the risk of extradural hemorrhage (see later discussion). This observation period is essential for clients who lose consciousness after the head injury, even if the period of unconsciousness lasts only minutes or seconds. If the client is sent home, clear instructions are required to assess for complications (see Client Education Guide: Assessment for Complications After Head Injury).

REHABILITATION

Almost any client who is hospitalized for more than 48 hours because of a head injury will require some rehabilitation. This treatment may take place in an inpatient or outpatient setting, depending on the client's condition. Rehabilitation, which can include physical, occupational, speech, and cognitive therapy, is essential in returning the client to maximal function. Nurses play a major role in the rehabilitation of a head-injured client and significant others. Even if physical disabilities are not present, cognitive rehabilitation can greatly improve the likelihood of the client's leading a productive life. The rehabilitation of clients with brain injuries is challenging. Often, community reintegration is unsuccessful. Some problems have found improved success with interdisciplinary techniques that include development of cognitive skills, comprehensive techniques, social skills, emotional adjustment, leisure skills, physical fitness, and health maintenance. Most clients require 6 months in such a program.[24]

CLIENT EDUCATION GUIDE

Assessment for Complications After Head Injury

Any client who has sustained a head injury should be observed for 24 hours. The client should be taken to the hospital immediately if any of the following occurs:

- Increased drowsiness or confusion
- Inability to be awakened
- Vomiting
- Convulsions
- Bleeding or drainage from the nose or ears
- Weakness in either arm or either leg
- Blurring of vision
- Slurred speech
- Enlargement or shrinkage of one pupil

COMPLICATIONS AFTER HEAD TRAUMA

Secondary events after head injury (problems occurring soon after the primary injury) often cause rapid deterioration in the injured client's condition. Among these secondary events are

- hemorrhage, with hematoma formation (epidural, subdural, and intracerebral)
- infections, including meningitis and brain abscess
- secondary brain swelling and edema
- carotid artery occlusion

All may turn a relatively "benign" head injury into a disastrous event (Fig. 14–12).

EARLY COMPLICATIONS

Epidural Hematoma (Extradural Hematoma). An epidural hematoma forms between the skull and the dura (i.e., outer meninges). It occurs in about 1 to 2 per cent of all head injuries and is usually associated with skull fracture. An epidural hematoma occurs from injury to the extracerebral blood vessels, most often the middle meningeal artery and vein.

Assessment findings usually reveal acute clinical manifestations because the bleeding is often arterial. Bleeding is almost always continuous, and a large clot forms, separating the dura from the skull. Bleeding ceases only with medical interventions or death. Occasionally, an epidural clot develops slowly, and the client remains asymptomatic for a week or even a month before neurologic changes become evident.

With a "classic" epidural hematoma, the client (1) is unconscious immediately after head trauma, (2) then awakens and is quite lucid, and (3) later lapses into coma. Focal signs usually appear first (e.g., rapid deterioration in LOC, pupil dilation and eye movement paralysis on the same side as the hematoma). Hemiparesis on the opposite side or seizures may also occur. The client may deteriorate rapidly, showing signs of increas-

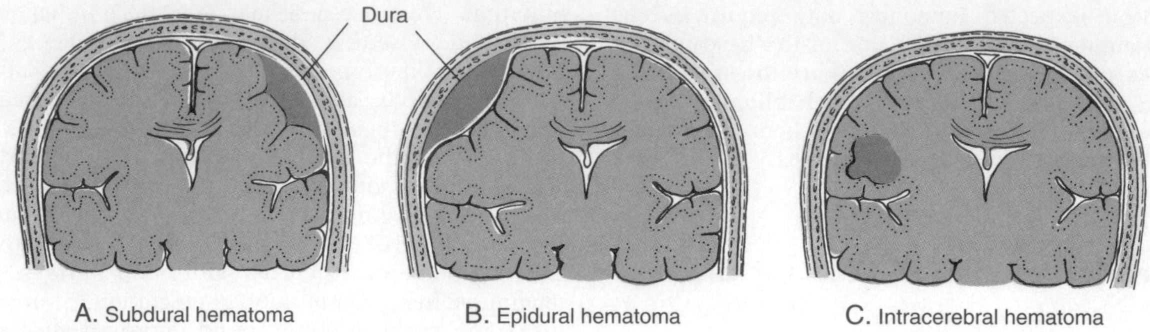

Figure 14–12
The formation of hematoma after head injury.

ing ICP and tentorial herniation until death occurs from respiratory arrest.

There may be no indications of extradural hemorrhage immediately after the initial trauma. Within several hours, the hematoma may grow to a critical level, and the client deteriorates rapidly and may die. For this reason, head-injured clients are usually hospitalized for observation even after apparently minor injuries.

Skull radiography, CT scan, and arteriography may confirm the diagnosis. Rapid diagnosis and prompt intervention are essential with epidural hematoma. Careful, ongoing assessment of neurologic status is also necessary. The nurse should notify the physician immediately of significant changes.

Management. Intervention includes lowering the ICP with hyperventilation by mechanical ventilation or by manually ventilating the client with an Ambu bag. An epidural clot may be surgically evacuated through burr holes (Fig. 14–13), twist drills, or a craniotomy.

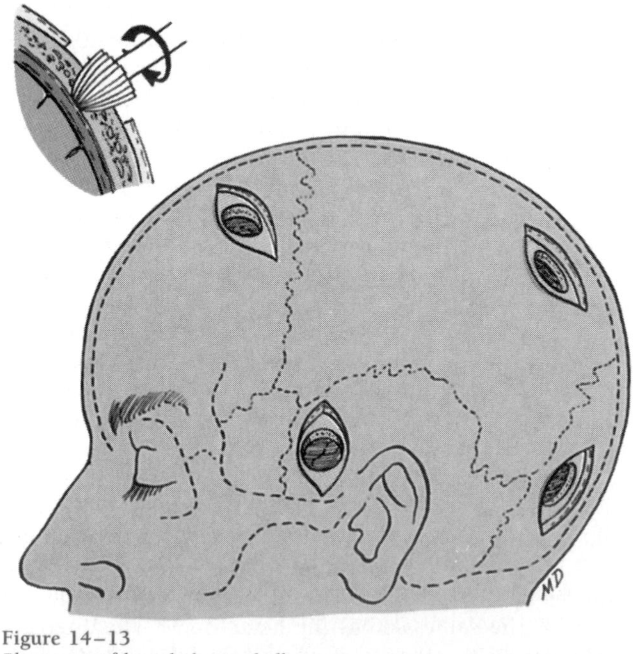

Figure 14–13
Placement of burr holes in skull.

Reasons for surgery include removing the hematoma and draining and ligating bleeding vessels.

Subdural Hematoma. Subdural hematoma (SDH) is a collection of blood in the subdural space (i.e., between the dura [outer meninges] and arachnoid [middle meninges]). Blood escaping into the subdural space is not absorbed but becomes organized or encapsulated by the dura. As a blood clot forms, blood cells within the clot's membrane lyse, forming a fluid of high osmotic character. This draws water from the surrounding subarachnoid space into the clot, which produces a gradually increasing intracranial mass. Large clots may produce such high ICP that cerebral herniation occurs, and death may result.

SDH may be classified as acute, subacute, or chronic, depending on how rapidly signs and symptoms develop. Another classification recognizes only acute and chronic, combining the acute and subacute categories.

- Acute SDH is symptomatic within 24 hours of injury.
- Subacute SDH is symptomatic several weeks after injury.

Acute and Subacute SDH. Acute SDH usually results from brain laceration. In addition to brain damage, severe brain swelling is usually present. Occasionally, acute SDH results from a ruptured saccular aneurysm or an intracerebral hemorrhage if tearing of the arachnoid over the source of the hemorrhage occurs. Acute SDH is seen in approximately 24 per cent of clients with severe head injuries.

Acute subdural hematomas are a serious complication requiring prompt treatment because they compress and distort an already damaged, edematous brain.

The assessment findings with an acute SDH are similar to those with acute epidural hematoma. The onset and development of the clinical manifestations may be somewhat slower because the bleeding is more often venous (rather than arterial, as in most epidural hematomas). Symptom recognition may be difficult because SDH is often associated with moderate or severe brain injury. Subtle changes in LOC and development of lateralizing (on one side) changes (e.g., hemiparesis, pupillary dilation, extraocular eye movement paralysis) are important findings.

A client developing an acute SDH may remain unconscious after injury or may have a variable LOC (depending on the extent of injury). A conscious client usually has a headache. The client may become irritable and confused and lapse into coma or show fluctuating LOC. Symptoms of increasing ICP occur.

Chronic SDH. Chronic SDH often develops weeks or months after the initial head injury. Gradually the blood clot causes pressure on the brain. There is an interval during which the client appears to be recovering or seems completely recovered; then later, progressive neurologic signs and symptoms develop. The initial injury may have been relatively minor, and the client may not associate current symptoms with the past injury. Chronic SDH is most common in the elderly and in alcoholic clients. These clients experience atrophy of the brain, which results in stretching of the bridging veins. These stretched veins are easily ruptured in a fall, even if it does not result in other injuries. Elderly or alcoholic clients may not even recall the mechanism of injury.

The client may become drowsy, inattentive, and incoherent and display personality changes. Headaches are another prominent symptom. These indications of chronic SDH may be overlooked until focal or lateralizing signs appear (e.g., hemiparesis, pupil signs). Changes in LOC continue and may fluctuate widely. An injured client and significant others need to be aware of indications of this possible complication so that they can seek medical help early if necessary.

Clinical assessment of subdural hematomas is similar to that for epidural hematomas. CT scan is definitive, but if it is unavailable, arteriography may be used. Surgical intervention usually consists of placing several burr holes or performing craniotomy to remove the hematoma. Treatment results depend on the client's condition before surgery.

A client who has had evacuation of a chronic SDH usually has a drain placed in the cavity to prevent reaccumulation of the fluid and blood. These clients are typically kept flat during the immediate postoperative period. This allows the brain to re-expand and fill the cavity, without the effects of gravity hindering the reexpansion.

Intracerebral Hematoma. Intracerebral hematomas occur less often than epidural or subdural hematomas do and are caused by bleeding directly into brain tissue. They may occur at the area of injury or some distance away. These hematomas are often hypertensive in nature and may occur deep within the brain. Assessment findings are similar to those occurring with epidural or subdural hematomas, although hemiplegia is more common than hemiparesis.

Brain Swelling and Edema. Serious head injuries are almost always associated with brain swelling and edema. The skull is a closed box with little room to accommodate these changes. A "mass effect" occurs once the space is filled and ICP increases. Clinical manifestations of compromised brain function develop.

Infections. Meningitis and brain abscess may occur after head injury. They are most common after "open" head injuries.

Acute Hydrocephalus. Acute hydrocephalus develops when increased CSF accumulates in the ventricles. This results from the defective reabsorption of CSF or blockage of the CSF flow. Traumatic or infectious blockage of CSF flow can occur with head injuries. As the CSF pressure rises, signs of increased ICP develop. Intervention includes surgical shunting or the placement of a ventriculostomy.

Adult Respiratory Distress Syndrome. Some clients with head injuries and other trauma develop adult respiratory distress syndrome that may not respond well to conventional therapy. In the head-injured client, perhaps damage to the hypothalamus leads to massive sympathetic outflow. (See also Chap. 22.)

Traumatic Delirium, Automatic Behavior. On regaining consciousness after several days of unconsciousness that follow head injury, a client's behavior may be noisy, generally disturbed, and confused. Such a client is usually experiencing traumatic delirium resulting from cerebral irritation. It is important to remember that a client experiencing traumatic delirium is not deliberately being difficult. During this temporary phase, the client needs protection, reassurance, and care such as during other delirious states. This partially confused state may remain even after the client can speak clearly and is able to cooperate in some activities. The family and significant others need complete explanations and reassurance. They are often upset with the client's behavior.

After this phase comes a time in which the client appears to have fully regained mental faculties. The client may be up and about, may recognize others, and may cooperate, yet memory of these events is impaired. This is a state of automatic behavior during which the client has no memory of day-to-day events and yet is able to carry on activities in a seemingly normal manner.

Post-traumatic Syndrome (Postconcussional Syndrome). This is a set of complications emerging in the recovery phase after head injury that may continue for months or years. Posttraumatic syndrome generally occurs in clients who have sustained a "minor" head injury. Assessment findings include headache, poor concentration (especially in reading), dizziness, unsteadiness related to sudden head movements, irritability, sensitivity to noise, insomnia, restlessness, hyperhidrosis, depression, personality changes, nervousness, impaired memory, anxiety, alcohol intolerance, and easy fatigability. Although as many as half of head-injured clients may experience these symptoms in mild form for a short time, the symptoms are not appropriately referred to as post-traumatic unless they persist for weeks or even years and impair the client's employability.

Post-traumatic syndrome is seen in clients whose condition progressively worsens, whose extent of injury does not correlate with the severity of the syndrome, and who tend to have complex overlapping neurologic and psychogenic symptoms. Whether the symptoms arise from brain damage or are psychogenic in origin is not known and is the subject of much controversy.

Management. Intervention for post-traumatic syndrome is usually supportive. The client and significant others may be relieved to know that this syndrome does sometimes occur after head injury. The nurse should explain that the problems usually diminish and eventually clear. Professional counseling may be helpful. Cognitive rehabilitation may be useful to help the client compensate for memory impairment and attention deficits.

LATE COMPLICATIONS

Unfortunately, a head-injured client is prone to various complications and sequelae. These include not only problems related to the head injury itself but also the complications of any serious illness that requires immobilization for a period of time. See the discussion of Complications of Intracranial Surgery earlier in the chapter for a complete discussion.

Seizure Disorders

EPILEPSY

Epilepsy, derived from the Greek word *epilepsia,* means to take hold of or to seize. Today, it is known that epilepsies are paroxysmal neurologic disorders causing recurrent episodes of (1) loss of consciousness, (2) convulsive movements or other motor activity, (3) sensory phenomena, or (4) behavioral abnormalities.

Epilepsy is always recurrent. An isolated, single seizure does not mean a client has epilepsy. Epilepsy is not a single disorder. There are many types of recurrent seizures. Acute cerebral disturbance, producing seizures, can usually be demonstrated on an electroencephalogram. Box 14–5 presents some important definitions.

Occasionally, simulated convulsive episodes occur in clients with psychiatric disorders. Clients experiencing this type of seizure seldom have epilepsy. These may be termed pseudoepileptic seizures.

Incidence

Approximately 0.5 to 1.0 per cent of people in the United States experience epileptic seizures.[1]

Etiology

The etiology of seizures varies remarkably in adults, brain tumors being the most common. When a seizure disorder begins after the age of 20 years in the absence of head trauma, the client has a 10 per cent chance of having a brain tumor. Seizures are often the first symptom of an intracranial mass. Head trauma is another common cause of seizures in young adults. With severe closed head injuries, seizures occur in a small percentage of clients. However, with open head injuries in which skull and dura are penetrated, the incidence of seizures rises markedly. Post-traumatic seizures most often occur within the first year after head injury. Hence, many neurosurgeons prescribe prophylactic anticonvulsants for clients with head injuries for a year after injury.

Risk Factors

Arteriosclerotic cerebrovascular disease is the most common cause of seizures in clients over age 50 years. These episodes usually accompany a stroke due to infarct or intracerebral hemorrhage. In other vascular lesions (e.g., AVMs), seizures may be the first symptom.

Central nervous system infections frequently produce seizures, either in their acute phase or chronically thereafter. Viral infections, which cause brain destruction, and postinfectious encephalitis can cause persistent seizures.

Toxic substances that interfere with brain metabolism or with the supply of oxygen or glucose to the brain can cause seizures. Alcohol is one of the most frequently ingested toxins and can cause seizures either during ingestion or during withdrawal. Chronic sub-

BOX 14–5

Terms Used to Describe Epilepsy

- Seizure: a paroxysmal, uncontrolled, abnormal discharge of electrical activity in the brain's gray matter; causes events that interfere with normal function; a symptom rather than a disease.
- Prodromal phase: precedes some seizures and may last minutes or hours; a vague change occurs in emotional reactivity or affective responses (e.g., depression or anxiety).
- Aura: generally, a brief sensory experience (e.g., a feeling of weakness, dizziness, strange sensations in an arm or leg, numbness, an odor) that occurs at the onset of some seizures. An aura may localize the area of the brain from which the seizure originates. For instance, a seizure arising from a focus in the motor strip could produce twitching in the client's thumb. A focus in the temporal lobe could cause a client to experience an unpleasant odor. Usually, an aura precedes other manifestations of the seizure by only a few seconds. Occasionally, an aura gives the client enough time to lie down before seizure activity occurs or may not be followed by a complete seizure.
- "Epileptic cry": a cry, occurring in some seizures, caused by a thoracic and abdominal spasm, which expels air through the narrowed spastic glottis.
- Ictus, postictal: ictus is synonymous with seizure; postictal refers to that time immediately after a seizure during which the client usually experiences some change in consciousness, behavior, or activity.

stance abuse, especially of barbiturates, can lead to seizures when the drug is withdrawn.

The causes of symptomatic epilepsy (due to organic or other known factors) are multiple, including hyperpyrexia, central nervous system infections, cerebral hypoxia, toxic agents or poisons, metabolic intoxications and disturbances, convulsive agents, cerebral trauma, brain defects, electrical stimulation, expanding brain lesions, anaphylaxis, and degenerative brain disorders. Seizures resulting from these factors may be transient symptoms and may not recur after treatment of the primary disorder. However, if a permanent lesion or scar remains in the central nervous system, seizures may persist.

Genetic factors are associated with epilepsy beginning in childhood but decrease in importance with age. A tendency to cerebral dysrhythmia is inherited, not the actual seizure disorder itself. These seizures are usually labeled idiopathic epilepsy, because no specific causes can be found.

The causes of seizures relate somewhat to the age of onset. Idiopathic epilepsy most often begins before age 20 years and rarely after age 30 years. After age 20 years, generalized seizures usually have an identifiable cause.

Pathophysiology

Seizures occur from a malfunction of hypersensitive neurons in the cerebral cortex and the limbic centers in the hippocampus. The membrane of the cell is more permeable, which makes the cell more likely to become activated by hyperthermia, hypoxia, hypoglycemia, hyponatremia, sensory overload, and certain phases of sleep. These cells begin by firing in increasing frequency and amplitude. When the intensity of the discharges reaches a threshold, it spreads to adjacent normal neurons and spreads over the entire cerebral cortex, the basal ganglia, thalamus, and brain stem. Discharges in the brain stem cause muscle contraction and loss of consciousness. The excitation of the cells can further spread to the spinal cord.

Eventually, inhibitory neurons in the cortex, anterior thalamus, and basal ganglia slow the neuronal firing. This inhibition interrupts the seizure and produces an intermittent contraction-relaxation phase. As the epileptogenic neurons are exhausted and inhibitory processes build, the seizure stops. These later events depress central nervous system action and impair consciousness. This period of impaired consciousness after a seizure can be seen as sleep, confusion, or fatigue. It is called a postictal state.

Seizure activity increases the need for adenosine triphosphate and cerebral oxygen consumption. To meet these demands, the cerebral blood flow increases by 250 per cent during a seizure, but supplies of oxygen and glucose are readily consumed. If the seizure is ongoing (such as in status epilepticus), severe hypoxia and lactic acidosis may occur. These conditions may result in brain tissue destruction.

Clinical Manifestations

There are various types and classifications of seizures. Table 14–5 presents one classification. Seizures can be divided into two major groups:

- generalized seizures, which begin bilaterally without local onset and show diffuse electroencephalographic abnormalities
- partial seizures (focal epilepsy), which begin in one localized area of the brain's cortex and produce abnormalities in one area of the electroencephalograms

GENERALIZED SEIZURES

About one third of seizures are generalized. The most common types of generalized seizures are

- grand mal (generalized tonic-clonic)
- petit mal (absence)
- "minor motor" seizures (e.g., akinetic, myoclonic, and atonic.)

Generalized (Tonic-Clonic) Seizures. Although these are the type of seizures most associated with epilepsy, they actually make up only about 10 per cent of all seizures. A grand mal seizure typically proceeds as follows.

- Sudden loss of consciousness.
- Tonic phase, in which the entire body stiffens in rigid tonic contraction (Fig. 14–14*A*). If standing or sitting, the client falls stiffly to the floor. A cry may be uttered. Respirations are interrupted temporarily, and the client may become cyanotic. Jaws are fixed and the hands clenched. Eyes may be opened widely; the pupils are dilated and fixed. This tonic phase lasts 30 to 60 seconds.
- Clonic phase begins next with rhythmic, jerky contraction and relaxation of all body muscles, especially the extremities (Fig. 14–14*B*). The client is usually incontinent of urine or feces and may bite the lips, tongue, and inside of the mouth. Excessive saliva is blown from the mouth, which creates a froth at the lips.

An entire grand mal seizure may last from 2 to 5 minutes, after which the client relaxes and remains to-

TABLE 14–5 Classification of Seizures

Generalized
Tonic-clonic seizures (grand mal)
Absence (petit mal)
Minor motor seizures (akinetic, myoclonic, atonic)
Partial (focal)
Partial seizures with motor components
Partial seizures with sensory components
Partial seizures with complex symptoms
Partial seizures that secondarily generalize

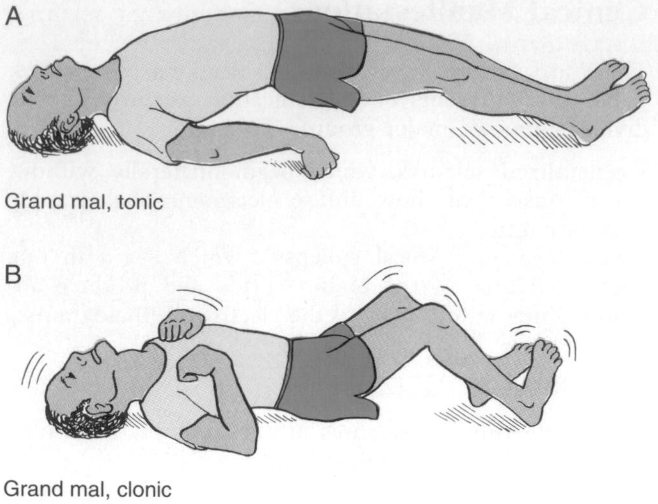

Figure 14–14
Tonic (*A*) and clonic (*B*) phases of grand mal seizures.

tally unresponsive for a time. The client may rouse briefly and then go into a postictal sleep lasting 30 minutes to several hours. This may be followed by general fatigue, depression, confusion, or headache, all of which gradually clear. The client has complete amnesia for the seizure episode and may feel nauseated, stiff, and sore. Falling during the seizure may cause injury. Grand mal seizures may vary in frequency from many times daily to once or twice a year.

Petit Mal (Absence) Seizures. These "little," or minor, seizures usually begin during childhood and are primarily limited to childhood and early adolescence. Petit mal seizures consist of brief periods of altered consciousness (periods of "absence") lasting 5 to 30 seconds. They may diminish or disappear after puberty. Grand mal or partial seizures may develop at any time in clients who have had petit mal seizures.

Minor Motor Seizures. Three other types of generalized seizures, referred to as minor motor seizures, are myoclonic, akinetic, and atonic. Minor motor seizures are often difficult to treat. Myoclonic seizures are characterized by involuntary jerking contractions of major muscles. The contractures are often so intense that the client is thrown to the floor. Akinetic seizures are characterized by momentary loss of muscle movement. Atonic seizures cause a total loss of muscle tone, and the client falls to the floor. Occasionally, a client may have atonic along with myoclonic seizures. Often, the client needs to stay in bed with side rails up or must wear a protective helmet to prevent head injuries from frequent violent falls.

PARTIAL (FOCAL) SEIZURES

Partial seizures are the most common type of epilepsy. Various symptoms occur, depending on the part of the cerebral cortex involved; partial motor seizures, partial sensory seizures, and partial seizures with complex symptoms (partial complex seizures, psychomotor seizures) are discussed.

Partial Motor Seizures. Partial seizures with motor symptoms arise from a focus in the region of the brain's motor cortex (posterior frontal lobe). The resulting motor activity (seizure) occurs in that part of the body innervated by motor neurons originating in the affected region of the cortex. Because the hand and fingers have the largest cortical representation, most focal motor seizures begin with convulsive twitching in an upper extremity. Involuntary movements may spread centrally and involve the entire limb, and even that side of the face and the lower extremity. This progression or "spread" is known as the jacksonian march.

Partial Sensory Seizures. Partial seizures with sensory symptoms may be transient. If such a seizure arises from a focus in the parietal area, the client experiences sensory phenomena such as numbness and tingling in the affected area. If the focus is in the occipital region, the client may experience bright, flashing lights in the field of vision opposite the side of the focus. Involvement in the posterior temporal area of the dominant hemisphere (usually the left) causes difficulty with speaking or total speech arrest.

Partial Seizures with Complex Symptoms. These seizures usually arise in the anterior temporal lobe. They are also called psychomotor seizures and partial complex seizures. These seizures frequently begin with an aura, or recognizable sensation, that helps localize the focus. Often the aura consists of a sense of "rising" or "welling up" in the epigastric region or the experiencing of an unpleasant odor. Visual distortions and feelings such as "déjà vu" are common.

The most characteristic parts of a psychomotor seizure are the automatisms during the seizure (i.e., purposeless, repetitive activities such as lip-smacking, chewing, patting a part of the body, or picking at clothes) while the client is in a dreamy state. Inappropriate or asocial behavior may also automatically occur during the seizure. This unusual behavior may cause the client to be viewed as psychotic or otherwise mentally disturbed. However, some abnormalities are very subtle and may not be detected by an untrained observer.

Temporal lobe seizures usually last 2 to 3 minutes but may last up to 15 minutes. The client is usually unaware of any activity during the seizure and may be confused or drowsy postictally. Attempts to restrain the client during a seizure may cause combative and uncooperative behavior.

Partial Seizures that Secondarily Generalize. Such a seizure starts from a particular focus, and then the electrical discharges spread throughout the brain. Clinically, the client first shows focal signs; one side of the face moves, and then the whole body becomes involved. Consciousness is lost if the discharges spread through the brain.

Complications

STATUS EPILEPTICUS

Status epilepticus is a state in which a client has continuous seizures or seizures in rapid succession lasting at least 30 minutes. A client experiencing status epilepticus may remain comatose and have repetitive seizures for hours. This state is exhausting and dangerous to the client. There are many kinds of status epilepticus.

CRITICAL TO REMEMBER

Status epilepticus may be precipitated by the sudden withdrawal of anticonvulsant medication.

Status epilepticus is a medical emergency. During a seizure, the brain's metabolic needs increase dramatically. If these heightened requirements continue without opportunity for the body to recover, the supply of glucose and oxygen to the brain becomes inadequate, and permanent brain damage may occur.

Treatment of status epilepticus is best carried out in a setting with emergency equipment and skilled personnel (see Box 14–6).

If status epilepticus is not controlled by medication, general anesthesia may be used. If the client is placed on general anesthesia or neuromuscular blockade agents such as vecuronium bromide (Norcuron), there must be continuous electroencephalographic monitoring. Absence of signs of seizure does not mean the seizure has stopped.

Clients in status epilepticus are especially difficult for significant others to watch. They need ongoing support. The nurse should always explain to them the treatment that is being used. After the seizures have been controlled, maintenance anticonvulsants are prescribed.

DIAGNOSTIC ASSESSMENT

Assessment of a client experiencing seizures includes

- history: prenatal, birth, and developmental history; family history; age of seizure onset; history of all illness and trauma; complete description of seizures including precipitating factors and postictal symptoms
- psychosocial assessment including mental status examination
- complete physical examination, including a detailed neurologic examination
- skull radiographs
- electroencephalogram, which helps to (1) locate the focus of abnormal electrical discharges if present, (2) establish a diagnosis of epilepsy, and (3) identify specific types of seizures. However, a normal electroencephalogram does not always exclude a diagnosis of epilepsy, and electroencephalographic abnormalities do not always confirm the diagnosis. During a seizure, electroencephalographic abnormalities involve all portions of the cortex. Between seizures, clients with epilepsy may show abnormalities not characteristic of seizure disorders.
- CT scan to detect congenital abnormalities or any masses (e.g., tumors)

Medical Management

Intervention for epilepsy includes (1) eliminating factors that may cause or precipitate seizures, (2) improving the client's physical and mental health, (3) specific medical treatment, and (4) possible surgical treatment. The main focus in intervention for epilepsy is preventing seizures from occurring.

PHARMACOLOGIC MANAGEMENT

The most effective method of controlling seizures that have no treatable cause (tumors, infections, metabolic disturbances) or no identifiable cause is the use of anticonvulsant drugs, also called antiepileptic drugs. Large doses of a single anticonvulsant are often more helpful

BOX 14–6

Interventions for Status Epilepticus

Nursing intervention for status epilepticus includes

- maintaining a clear airway. Prevent aspiration by positioning and suctioning, and provide adequate oxygenation. Pulmonary edema may occur. Intubation may be necessary.
- assessing the client constantly. Even when seizures are controlled, the client may be unconscious for a while. If a client does not awaken within 2 hours, careful reassessment is needed. Document and report recurrent seizures immediately.
- protecting the person from injury (e.g., padded side rails).
- administering prescribed emergency anticonvulsant therapy to terminate seizures and prevent exhaustion. Intravenous infusion is begun immediately and maintained during treatment. The medication of choice is intravenous lorazepam (Ativan) given slowly until the seizures stop. Other possible medications include diazepam (Valium), phenobarbital, or phenytoin (Dilantin). Because all of these medications may depress respirations, emergency ventilation equipment should be readily available. Phenobarbital may depress consciousness for a prolonged period. Intravenous phenytoin may cause cardiac arrhythmias, so it is given slowly while the heart rate is monitored.

If status epilepticus is not controlled by medication, general anesthesia may be used. If the client is placed on general anesthesia or neuromuscular blockade agents such as vecuronium bromide (Norcuron), there must be continuous electroencephalographic monitoring. Absence of signs of seizure does not mean the seizure has stopped.

Clients in status epilepticus are especially difficult for significant others to watch. The significant others need ongoing support. Always explain to them the treatment that is being used. After the seizures have been controlled, maintenance anticonvulsants are prescribed.

TABLE 14–6 Antiepileptic Agents

CLASSIFICATION OF SEIZURE	MEDICATION	SIDE EFFECTS
Focal and generalized	Primary	
	Phenytoin (Dilantin)	Mental dullness, ataxia, diplopia, hypertrophy of gums
	Carbamazepine (Tegretol)	Nystagmus, ataxia, rash, blood dyscrasias
	Phenobarbital	Mental changes, withdrawal seizures if drug is stopped abruptly
	Primidone (Mysoline)	Emotional and mental changes including depression, irritability, impotence; withdrawal seizures if drug is not discontinued slowly
	Valproate (Depakene)	Transient nausea, potential bleeding problems, liver damage
	Secondary	
	Succinimides	
	Phensuximide (Milontin)	Drowsiness, headache
	Methsuximide (Celontin)	Drowsiness, headache
	Benzodiazepines	
	Diazepam (Valium)	Respiratory depression, lethargy, ataxia
	Clonazepam (Klonopin)	Drowsiness, exacerbation of childhood hyperactivity, withdrawal seizures, and status epilepticus if drug is removed too quickly
	Ancillary	
	Acetazolamide (Diamox)	Anorexia, numbness of extremities
Petit mal seizures	Primary	
	Ethosuximide (Zarontin)	Gastric distress, nausea, dizziness, drowsiness
	Valproate (Depakene)	See above
	Clonazepam (Klonopin)	See above
	Secondary	
	Trimethadione (Tridione)	Hemeralopia ("glare effect"), blood immune disorders
Other minor motor seizures		
Akinetic-atonic seizures	Same drugs as for focal and major generalized seizures	See above
Myoclonic seizures	Phenytoin (Dilantin)	See above
	Valproate (Depakene)	See above
	Clonazepam (Klonopin)	See above

than are smaller doses of several drugs. Ideally, initial treatment begins with a single drug (primary anticonvulsant) until either seizure control is attained or unacceptable side effects appear. If side effects become intolerable before seizures are controlled, other drugs are used. Combining medications does not appear to be effective because drug-drug interactions decrease effectiveness.[1] Promising new medications are being investigated, including lamotrigine and vigabatrin. Current antiepileptic agents are listed in Table 14–6.

Medical intervention focuses on prescribing anticonvulsants that will arrest or prevent a client's seizures. Developing such a program requires weeks of medication trial and error and adjustment. During this time, the client and significant others must closely observe the effects of the medication and carefully document any seizure activity. The client must take the medication regularly as prescribed to maintain a blood level of the medication. Antiepileptic agents require time to take effect. Taking this medication after a seizure or when a seizure feels imminent is not effective. A certain antiepileptic level in the blood must be continually maintained. If a client feels a need to change the medication regimen, medical consultation is essential before acting.

Surgical Intervention

For approximately 75 per cent of people with seizures, medical management with antiepileptic agents and follow-up suffice. The remaining people continue to have seizures. For about 5 per cent of people with epilepsy, surgery is a last resort to control the disease. The safest and most effective surgical treatment is cortical resection of the anterior temporal lobe for complex partial seizures.[7, 9] Criteria for resection include (1) failure of the medical approach and (2) localization and identification of a focus of abnormal discharge that is easily accessible surgically and is located in dispensable cortex. Cortical resection is a lengthy surgery. The client must be awake during most of it. It is important that the client be highly motivated and psychologically well prepared.

Thorough assessment is necessary before cortical resection, including (1) several electroencephalograms and/or positron emission tomographic studies to locate the epileptogenic site, (2) neuropsychological testing, (3) CT scan, and (4) cerebral angiogram with Wada's procedure to determine hemisphere dominance and location of the speech center. The functional supremacy of one cerebral hemisphere is critical to language function. Wada's test is a method of determining which side of the brain is dominant.

Other surgical interventions may be considered. Epileptic foci are not identified by standard scalp electroencephalograms in some clients. Electrodes may then be surgically implanted into the brain's deeper structures to help localize the focus. Some neurosurgeons advocate stereotactic procedures in an effort to (1) destroy foci, (2) interrupt pathways of electrical activity, or (3) alter the activity of cortical neurons. These procedures have not been very successful. Occasionally, more drastic surgical procedures, such as division of the corpus callosum and anterior commissure or hemispherectomy, are used.

Nursing Management

Epilepsy is not usually treated by hospitalization. However, a client may initially be hospitalized for assessment, diagnosis, and education and again later if seizures become uncontrolled or if status epilepticus develops.

Nurses have a role in supporting and educating clients with epilepsy and their significant others. They should provide information about (1) how anticonvulsants prevent seizures, (2) the importance of taking prescribed medication regularly, and (3) care during seizures. The nurse can plan with the client ways to make taking medication part of daily activities (e.g., keeping medication by the toothbrush). The nurse can also help the client identify factors that precipitate seizures and ways of avoiding these factors. Such factors include increased stress, lack of sleep, emotional upset, and alcohol use.

It is important for a client with epilepsy to live as normal a life as possible. The client and significant others must learn to accept the condition and not exaggerate it or overprotect the client. Whereas certain dangerous activities should be avoided or performed with special safeguards (e.g., swimming or horseback riding), a wide range of activities can still be enjoyed. Driving motor vehicles depends on local laws and the client's medical control of seizures.

A regular pattern of adequate diet, fluid intake, sleep, and moderate recreation and exercise is helpful. Alcoholic beverages are contraindicated.

Clients with epilepsy should always wear or carry identification stating that they have epilepsy and providing the name of their physician.

Clients with epilepsy often have a poor self-image, feelings of inferiority, self-consciousness, guilt, anger, depression, and other emotional problems. These can be overcome by education and the support and understanding of significant others and care providers.

The client may be frightened and anxious about future seizures (e.g., Where will I be when it happens? What will I be doing? Who will be with me?). Some adults with epilepsy have difficulty finding or keeping employment and may benefit from vocational rehabilitation or counseling.

Various organizations are working at public education, introduction of appropriate legislation, and assisting people with epilepsy. In the United States, these include the Epilepsy Foundation of America, at 4351 Garden City Drive, 5th Floor, Landover, MD 20785, (301–459–3700).

Nursing Management During a Seizure

The client who is experiencing a seizure usually requires only protection from the environment. For example, objects should be moved out of the way and the client placed in bed so he or she does not strike the floor. Some clients will require airway management, and this usually can be done by turning the client over onto one side.

Observers' comments about a client's seizures can be very helpful in making a diagnosis, especially if they can describe minute detail, including the sequence in which phenomena occurred.

Assessment during the seizure involves:

- Duration of the seizure
- Where the seizure began
- Did eyes deviate?
- Were the respirations labored or frothy?
- Was client incontinent?

When seizure continues in a client without periods of rest or no seizure activity, the client is in *status epilepticus*. This is an emergency condition and, if not treated swiftly, will result in irreversible brain damage or death (see previous discussion).

Posthospital Care

DISCHARGE TEACHING

The client and significant others should be taught that epilepsy is a chronic disorder and requires long-term management. Even though the client does not actively experience seizure, it is important to take medication daily. Phenytoin, a common antiepileptic medication, leads to excessive gum tissue (gingival) growth. Brushing 2 to 3 times daily helps retard its growth. Some clients have excess gingival tissues excised every 6 to 12 months. Medications may also cause diplopia and ataxia.

If the client is able to recognize that certain activities trigger the seizure, the activities can be avoided or the client can be desensitized in some cases. For example, flickering lights can trigger seizures. Fluorescent lights and flickering shadows from trees on the road while driving during the late afternoon are common culprits. If the client has an aura, precautions should be taken immediately to prevent self-injury from the impending seizure; for example, lying down on the ground.

For some clients, the psychosocial impact of epilepsy is overwhelming. Because most seizures occur without warning, many clients spend their lives anticipating inappropriate behavior, embarrassment, and self-injury. In many states, clients with epilepsy may be prohibited from driving a car until they are seizure-free for 1 year. Some epileptics cannot find work if they admit to having seizures. These factors contribute to a higher incidence of depression among clients with epilepsy.

When discussing the long-term impact of epilepsy with the client, the nurse needs to be empathetic as well as realistic. It is hoped the client can accept the limitations of the disorder on life-style and not be overwhelmed by it.

Family Education. The client's family needs to know what to do for the client in the event of a seizure. The client should be protected from self-injury. Clothing should be loosened, the client's head protected from impact, and sharp objects in the environment removed. The client should not be forcibly restrained during a seizure but protected from self-injury. Hard objects or fingers should not be inserted into the mouth; epileptic clients do not swallow their tongues. When the seizure is over, the client should be positioned on the side to allow oral secretions to drain from the airway. Someone should stay with the client until full consciousness has returned.

CRITICAL TO REMEMBER

An ambulance should be called if the client's seizure lasts for over 10 minutes; another seizure occurs before consciousness returns; or there is respiratory difficulty, there is evidence of injury, or the client is pregnant.

Infections

NEUROLOGIC INFECTIONS

Almost any pathogenic micro-organism can invade the nervous system and related structures (e.g., neurologic parenchyma, coverings, and blood vessels). Neurologic infectious syndromes may be categorized according to the main area of involvement (e.g., meningeal subdural and epidural infections) or by causative mechanism. This section discusses (1) bacterial or pyogenic infections, (2) viral infections, (3) fungal infections, and (4) parasitic infections.

Bacterial or Pyogenic Neurologic Infections

In bacterial infections, the invading organisms reach the central nervous system by (1) the vascular system after systemic or bloodstream infection or (2) direct extension from adjacent cranial structures (e.g., infection entering through cranial fracture or fracture through mastoid or nasal sinuses). Infection may also be accidentally introduced into the central nervous system during invasive procedures.

BACTERIAL MENINGITIS

Overview. Bacterial meningitis is an inflammation of the arachnoid, pia, and intervening CSF. The infection spreads throughout the subarachnoid space about the brain and spinal cord and usually involves the ventricles. Approximately 20,000 to 25,000 cases of meningitis occur yearly in the United States.[26] Factors predisposing to bacterial meningitis include

- head trauma
- systemic infection
- postsurgical infection
- meningeal infection
- anatomic defects
- other systemic illness

When pathogenic organisms enter the subarachnoid space, an inflammatory reaction occurs, with resultant CSF clouding, exudate formation, changes in subarachnoid arteries (e.g., engorgement with blood, rupture, thrombosis), and congestion of adjacent tissues. The pia-arachnoid becomes thickened, and adhesions form, especially in the area of the basal cisterns. Little change occurs in brain structure in the early stages of meningitis.

Almost any bacteria entering the body can cause meningitis. The most common are meningococcus (*Neisseria meningitidis*), pneumococcus (*Streptococcus pneumoniae*), and *Haemophilus influenzae*. These organisms are often present in the nasopharynx. It is not known how they enter the bloodstream and the subarachnoid space. *S. pneumoniae* and *N. meningitidis* occur most often in adults.

Clinical manifestations initially include headache, prostration, chills, fever, nausea, vomiting, back pain, stiff neck, and generalized seizures. The client may be irritable at first, but as the infection progresses, the sensorium often becomes clouded, and coma may develop. Clients experiencing meningitis appear acutely ill and confused, stuporous, or semicomatose. A petechial or hemorrhagic rash may develop. Temperature is moderately elevated, and pulse and respiratory rate are increased. Blood pressure is usually normal. Signs of meningeal irritation include

- nuchal rigidity (rigidity of the neck)
- positive finding of Brudzinski's sign
- positive finding of Kernig's sign

Eliciting Brudzinski's and Kernig's signs is described in Clinical Manifestations: Eliciting Brudzinski's and Kernig's Signs.

Medical diagnosis is made by assessment of signs and symptoms and is confirmed by isolating the causative organism from CSF. Gram's stain is performed on the CSF and reveals the organisms in 70 to 80 per cent of cases.[27] In cases in which the organism cannot be identified, bacterial antigens can be determined. Cases of *H. influenzae* are frequently diagnosed with this technique. Clients with bacterial pneumomeningitis show

- moderately elevated CSF pressures
- elevated CSF protein (over 100 mg/dL)
- decreased CSF glucose (40 mg/dL)

CLINICAL MANIFESTATIONS

Eliciting Brudzinski's and Kernig's Signs

Brudzinski's sign. With the client supine, the nurse lifts his or her head up from the bed rapidly. If meningeal irritation is present, forward neck flexion produces flexion of both thighs at the hips and flexure movements of the ankles and knees. (Illustration A.)

Kernig's sign. Beginning with the client recumbent and his or her thigh flexed at a right angle to the abdomen, with the knee flexed at a 90-degree angle to the thigh, the nurse then extends the client's lower leg. In meningeal irritation, extending the leg upward causes pain, spasm of the ham string muscles, and resistance to further leg extension at the knee. (Illustration B.)

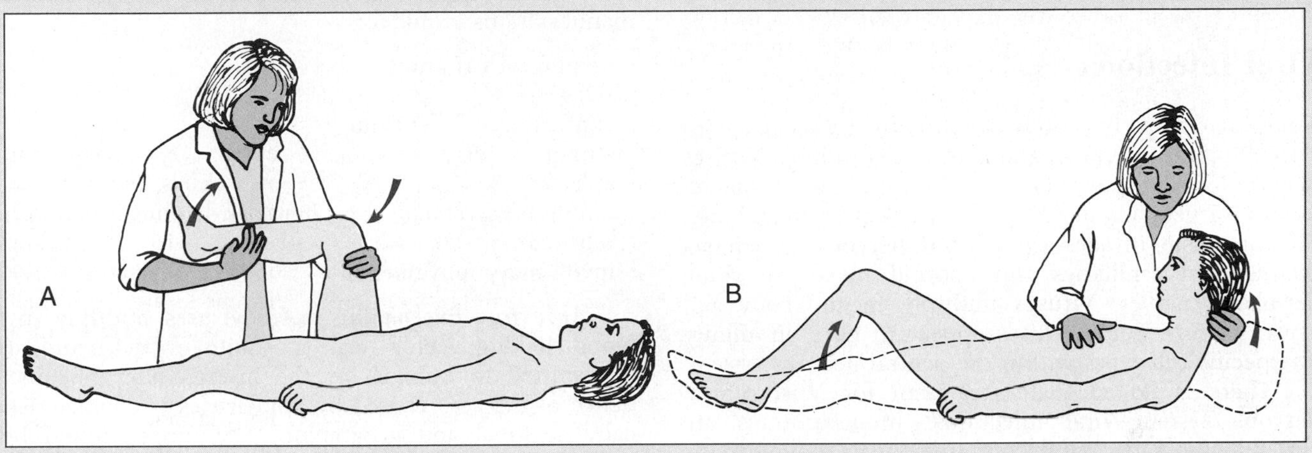

- usually increased cell count (100–10,000/cm) with predominantly polymorphonuclear leukocytes

CRITICAL TO REMEMBER

Bacterial meningitis is a medical emergency.

Management. If untreated, it can be fatal within hours to days. Intervention for bacterial meningitis depends on the causative microorganism and the source of the infection. Large doses of the appropriate antibiotic are usually prescribed four to six times daily for 10 days. With the exception of chloramphenicol, the common antibiotics do not readily penetrate the normal blood-brain barrier. Fortunately, meningeal inflammation improves passage. High doses of penicillins and third-generation cephalosporins are preferred agents. Antibiotics are given intravenously; their dosage is not reduced as the client improves because the blood-brain barrier recovers as inflammation subsides and high doses are required in order to reach the CSF. Adequate fluid and electrolyte balance are maintained. The nurse should assess neurologic status frequently (possibly as often as hourly) to detect early signs of increasing ICP and seizures. Anticonvulsants may be prescribed for seizures. If the primary focus of infection is located (e.g., in parasinuses or mastoid, cranial osteomyelitis), surgery may be indicated when the acute phases of meningitis have subsided.

The use of antibiotics has reduced the mortality rate of all types of bacterial meningitis. Prognosis varies according to the causative organism. Mortality is less than 5 per cent.[26] Deaths most often occur in newborn infants and elderly clients, and complications are rare.

DISORDERS DUE TO BACTERIAL TOXINS

Toxins produced by several pathogenic bacteria have a special affinity for the nervous system, causing, for example, tetanus, diphtheria, and botulism.

Tetanus. Tetanus is caused by the anaerobic spore-forming rod *Clostridium tetani.* The spores produce a toxin when introduced into a wound. The toxin suppresses spinal and brain stem inhibitory neurons and may act directly on skeletal muscle at the point of entry.

Clinical manifestations may be limited to painful muscular spasms and contractions in the affected extremity. However, generalized tetanus is more common, with production of spasms beginning with trismus of the jaw muscles and progressing to spasms of muscles of the neck, trunk, limbs, and the respiratory and pharyngeal muscles. Seizures and impaired respiration may occur. The affected muscles become constantly rigid, with painful paroxysms of tonic contractions in response to slight external stimuli. This is followed by a full course of immunization.

Intervention includes

- surgery to débride any associated wounds
- single dose of antitoxin (hyperimmune serum [Hyper-Tet])
- 10-day course of penicillin G (Tetracycline, erythromycin, and chloramphenicol are alternate agents.)

- respiratory support, including possible mechanical ventilation
- Chlorpromazine, meprobamate, or diazepam to control muscle spasms
- nasogastric feeding if client has dysphagia
- prophylactic anticoagulation to prevent thrombus

The overall mortality rate for tetanus is 25 to 50 per cent, even in modern facilities with extensive resources. Tetanus is best prevented by immunization and regular booster doses of toxoid.

Viral Infections

Neurologic viral infections are usually associated with systemic viral infections and can be devastating. Viruses may enter the body (1) via the respiratory system, mouth, or genitalia or (2) from an insect or animal bite. The organism invades the central nervous system via the cerebral capillaries and choroid plexus or along peripheral nerves. Viruses multiply in the body and cause viremia. Some viruses appear to have an affinity for specific cell types within the central nervous system.

There is no adequate treatment for most central nervous system viral infections. Immunizations are available for a few viral conditions (e.g., poliomyelitis and rabies). They are not available for most viral encephalitides, however. Currently, mass immunization is practical only for acute anterior poliomyelitis. The best control of other viral disorders is probably to identify and eliminate vectors responsible for their transmission.

VIRAL MENINGITIS

Acute viral meningitis ("aseptic" meningitis) is most often due to mumps virus or one of the picornaviruses. Aseptic meningitis infecting the subarachnoid space usually resolves within 2 weeks.

Clinical manifestations include mild symptoms. The client may be drowsy and photophobic, may have a headache and pain when moving the eyes, and may experience neck and spine stiffness on flexion. Other generalized symptoms include weakness, rash, and painful extremities. Fever and signs of meningeal irritation may be present. Physical examination reveals presence of Brudzinski's and Kernig's signs. Acute and convalescent serologic testing and appropriate viral cultures may identify the specific virus involved.

Intervention for clients with aseptic meningitis is symptomatic. The nurse should keep the client at bed rest during the acute phase and plan intervention to relieve headache, control fever, and increase comfort. If seizures occur, anticonvulsants are prescribed.

VIRAL ENCEPHALITIS

Encephalitis is inflammation of the brain parenchyma. Many viruses can cause encephalitis. The two most common are arthropod-borne (arbo)virus encephalitis and herpes simplex type I virus encephalitis. Also, the viruses that cause viral meningitis (see preceding discussion) may cause severe viral encephalitis. They become very destructive when they invade brain parenchyma. The course of the illness is unpredictable. Death occurs in about 10 per cent of affected clients. Herpes simplex encephalitis has a much higher mortality rate (10 to 40 per cent). Of the clients who recover, about 20 per cent have some disability (e.g., mental deterioration, personality changes, hemiparesis). (Residual disability is even higher in eastern equine encephalitis.)

Viral encephalitis is an acute febrile illness. Clinical manifestations include

- meningeal irritation
- seizures
- confusion and delirium
- stupor or coma
- aphasia
- motor involvement (e.g., hemiparesis and asymmetric reflexes)
- involuntary movements

Arbovirus Encephalitis. Arboviruses multiply in a blood-sucking vector (e.g., mosquito or tick) and are transmitted to humans by the insect's bite. The incidence of diseases caused by arboviruses is characteristically seasonal and geographic. The nurse should become familiar with those in his or her location. In the United States, they occur in late summer and early fall. The most common types are St. Louis and eastern and western equine encephalitis.

The infection sites are usually microscopic and scattered throughout the cerebral gray and white matter, except for eastern equine encephalitis, which may destroy major parts of a lobe or hemisphere. Two thirds of clients who develop eastern equine encephalitis either die or develop severe residual disabilities (e.g., mental retardation, seizures, blindness, deafness, speech disorders, hemiplegia).

Clinical manifestations with all arbovirus encephalitides are similar. The onset is gradual in adults and older children, with headache, nausea, vomiting, listlessness, and fever. After a few days, seizures, stiff neck, stupor, and coma develop. Photophobia, hemiparesis, and asymmetric reflexes may be present. Fever and neurologic signs subside within 2 weeks if the client does not develop irreversible central nervous system changes or die.

Herpes Simplex Virus Encephalitis. This form of encephalitis occurs any time of year and throughout the world, particularly in middle-aged adults. The gradually evolving initial clinical manifestations are similar to those with other acute encephalitides. However, because this virus has an affinity for the inferomedial portions of the frontal and temporal lobes, the client soon becomes acutely ill with headache, fever, vomiting, and, often, seizures. Signs of a localized lesion develop, including visual field deficits. If not aggressively treated, temporal lobe swelling leads to transtentorial herniation, coma, and brain death.

The prognosis is grave but not hopeless. The mortality rate is above 30 per cent, and the client may die within 2 weeks. Of those who survive, many are left with severe neurologic and mental disabilities (e.g., global dementia, seizures, aphasia).

Intervention for herpes simplex encephalitis is a 10-day course of intravenous acyclovir, an antiviral agent. To be effective, it must be given early in the course of the disease. A biopsy may be done in an attempt to identify the herpes virus. Although biopsy is definitive for the disease, there are risks. MRI has been shown to be an effective diagnostic tool. Despite treatment, the course of the disease may continue.

Nursing intervention is a challenge. An acutely ill client is often restless and combative and exhibits bizarre behavior. Such clients need careful protection from injury, and the family requires sensitive support. If residual behavior changes and mental deterioration develop, the nurse must help the family and significant others adjust to changes in the client.

ACUTE ANTERIOR POLIOMYELITIS

Since the 1950s, mass immunization programs have significantly reduced the incidence of acute anterior poliomyelitis worldwide. The best time for this immunization is in infancy. Trivalent oral poliomyelitis vaccine has almost completely replaced both the inactivated (Salk) and monovalent (Sabin) vaccines because it is so easy to administer and supervise. A few infections secondary to other enteroviruses in unvaccinated clients occasionally occur.

Acute anterior poliomyelitis ("polio," infantile paralysis) is characterized by (1) destruction of motor cells (particularly anterior horn cells in the spinal cord and brain stem, especially the medulla) and (2) flaccid paralysis of muscles innervated by affected neurons. Poliomyelitis is caused by one of three types of poliovirus and spreads from the gastrointestinal tract to the nervous system.

Associated paralysis may or may not occur. If present, paralysis may be spinal or bulbar. Spinal paralysis, restricted to spinal segments, is flaccid, asymmetric, and scattered in distribution. It tends to be more severe in one extremity (most often a leg). Involvement of the diaphragm and intercostal muscles or damage to the respiratory center in the medulla oblongata may produce respiratory paralysis. Occasionally, transient bladder paralysis occurs. Bulbar paralysis involves the muscles supplied by the cranial nerves because bulbar nuclei are affected. These muscles may be paralyzed alone or in combination with spinal musculature. Bulbar paralysis is often unilateral. Respiratory paralysis results from reticular formation lesions. Protein levels in the CSF are elevated. It is difficult to distinguish polio from Guillain-Barré syndrome (see Chapter 15). However, for practical purposes, no other acute disorder produces headaches, stiff neck, fever, and asymmetric flaccid paralysis without sensory loss coupled with an increase in white blood cells in the CSF.

Clients with respiratory muscle paralysis need intensive care. Mechanical ventilation at the first sign of respiratory embarrassment greatly increases the client's chances of recovery.

Post-polio Syndrome. Post-polio syndrome is a recently recognized disorder affecting survivors of polio. This syndrome is characterized by new onset of progressive muscle weakness, fatigue, decreased endurance, pain in the joints and muscles, and respiratory problems beginning 30 or more years after the original attack. Clients may experience any or all of these symptoms. The etiology and pathophysiology of this syndrome are not well understood, particularly because the interval between the original illness and the post-polio syndrome is so long.

Post-polio syndrome can be very discouraging to clients who have successfully adapted to a certain level of disability. Further restriction of physical capabilities is difficult for the client and significant others to accept. Emotional support is as vital as teaching the client to balance rest and activity and to utilize new adaptive techniques. Development of respiratory difficulty may be particularly frightening to those clients who required ventilatory support with an iron lung (a respirator that encompassed all of the body except the head) during their initial illness.

Bulbar Disorders, Syncope, and Head Pain

BULBAR DISORDERS

Some neurologic disorders involve the lower brain stem and alter bulbar function (e.g., difficulties in respiration, talking, swallowing, and coughing). Such conditions include tetanus, myasthenia gravis, and bulbar poliomyelitis.

Bulbar involvement is evidenced by hoarseness, dysarthria, pooling of food and saliva in the pharynx, increased oropharynx secretions, inability or difficulty swallowing (dysphagia), hypoxia, and laryngeal stridor. Airway obstruction, pulmonary aspiration, and asphyxia may occur. Mortality is high with bulbar disorders.

When caring for clients with bulbar dysfunction, the nurse should watch for early indications of hypoxia (e.g., anxiety, restlessness, apprehension, sleeplessness, increasing respiratory effort, increasing pulse rate). Early indications of hypoxia may be very subtle (e.g., apparently insignificant requests by the client).

The nurse should quickly assess for possible causes of airway obstruction if hypoxia is possible. A tracheostomy and possibly mechanical ventilation may be needed. Many clients with bulbar problems are conscious but immobile and have difficulty speaking. Their progressive loss of respiratory function is terrifying. Thorough, ongoing assessment and supportive communication help reduce distress. Technical skills also reassure the client that respiration will be maintained.

Nursing intervention for clients with bulbar involvement is similar to that described for clients with altered states of consciousness. This is especially true for assessing vital signs, preventing deformities, and maintaining patent airway and fluid balance.

To test clients' ability to swallow, the nurse has them sit up with head slightly flexed. The head should not be tilted backward because this opens the airway. The nurse offers a small amount of nectar (e.g., thick, fruity juice such as apricot nectar) or firm gelatin. (The consistency of these foods is easier to swallow than water.) He or she watches to see if the clients are able to swallow. If aspiration occurs, the fluid should be quickly suctioned from the back of the mouth and throat.

Before feeding, the nurse should give mouth care to keep the mouth clean and induce salivation. Soft foods are easiest for dysphagic clients to swallow. Milk products should be avoided. Liquids should be offered in a small glass or cup, as the client may not be able to suck or swallow when using a straw. Clients with progressive dysphagia may need tube feeding or gastrostomy to maintain adequate nutrition. The nurse should make sure that clients obtain enough calories.

The extent of bulbar paralysis and return of muscle function varies. A client with persisting partial bulbar paralysis is particularly disabled and may need a permanent tracheostomy tube. When suction equipment is needed in the client's home, someone must be taught to use it efficiently. Eating, drinking, and common colds are all potentially hazardous for clients with bulbar problems.

HEADACHES

Headache is a symptom of an underlying disorder, rather than a disease itself. The cause of headache must be identified so that appropriate treatment can be given.

Clients often self-treat headaches with over-the-counter medications available without prescription. Most headaches do not indicate serious disease. However, the nurse should encourage clients with persistent or recurrent headaches to seek neurologic assessment. Serious disorders that typically produce headache include intracranial tumors and infections; bacterial or viral meningitis; acute systemic infections; head injuries; cerebral hypoxia; severe hypertension; and acute or chronic diseases of the eye, ear, nose, or throat.

The most common types of headaches are

- migraine
- cluster
- tension (muscle contraction headaches)
- pain related to the eyes, ears, teeth, and paranasal structures (Fig. 14–15).

Some clients experience several types of headaches (e.g., migraine and tension headaches are often associated).

Assessment of client with headache includes detailed history, psychosocial assessment, and physical examination. Neurologic assessment is particularly important. Possible neurologic diagnostic tests include skull radiographs, CT scan, electroencephalogram, and lumbar puncture with CSF examination.

History includes asking about

- pain localization, intensity, and paths of radiation
- character of the headache (sharp, dull, throbbing)
- mode of headache onset, duration, and frequency
- way in which headaches stop
- presence of localized tenderness
- associated phenomena or precipitating factors
- familial incidence

Migraine Headaches

Migraine headaches are paroxysmal disorders characterized by recurrent throbbing headaches. Headache episodes begin during puberty or ages 20 to 40 years.

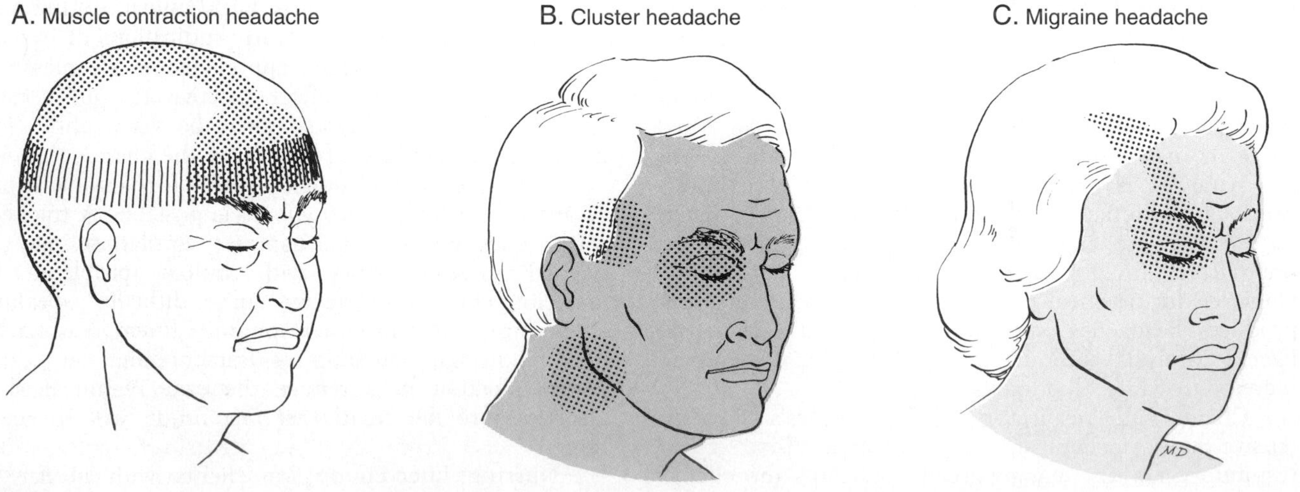

Figure 14–15
Types of headache. *Shaded areas* show regions of greatest pain.

Generally, they decrease in frequency and severity with advancing years. Migraines affect about 5 to 10 per cent of the population. Women are more susceptible than men are. Migraine headaches usually occur at irregular intervals. Their frequency varies from several times a week to only several times a year.

The pathophysiology of migraine is complex. The vascular theory is currently accepted, which states that early neurologic symptoms are due to constriction of intracranial vessels. The later intense, throbbing headache is due to dilation of extracranial and intracranial branches of the external carotid artery. The underlying mechanism causing this periodic spasm and dilation of vessels is not known.

Psychosocial factors also influence migraine headaches. They tend to occur in clients who have "perfectionist" tendencies. Migraine episodes may be precipitated by various, often repetitive conditions such as fatigue, excess sleep, hunger, refractive errors, bright light, surprises, mental and emotional excitement, excessive smoking, high altitudes, or drinking alcoholic beverages. Certain foods seem to precipitate migraine episodes (see Client Education Guide: Preventing Migraine Headaches). There appears to be a familial character to these headaches. Oral contraceptives may exacerbate migraines or induce their onset in women previously free from significant headaches. Headaches often occur during menstruation and are rare during pregnancy.

There are numerous variants of the migraine syndrome and many variations among clients.

CLIENT EDUCATION GUIDE

Preventing Migraine Headaches

Many things can trigger a migraine headache. It is important for the client to find out what triggers the headache and avoid the trigger, if possible; If avoidance of the trigger is not possible, the dose of medication can be adjusted.

Adjusting Medications During Menstrual Cycles. Menstruation and ovulation may trigger migraines. If medications are taken for migraines, a larger dose may be required during these times.

Recognizing Dietary Triggers. Alcohol increases the size of blood vessels (vasodilation) and may increase headache. Some foods contain beta-phenylethylamine and should be considered possible triggers. These items include chocolate, cheese, citrus fruits, coffee, pork products, and dairy products. The lack of eating may lower blood sugar and also lead to headache. In this case, small frequent meals may avert headaches.

Identifying the Role of Stress. Stress may trigger migraines. If stressors cannot be reduced, then medications may need to be increased. Heat intolerance (such as vacationing in warm climates) may increase headaches. Other factors related to stress that may trigger headaches include fatigue, excess sleep, and bright sunlight causing a glare from water, roads, or car hoods.

Classic or Typical Migraine. The headache may be preceded by an aura or prodromal phase in which the client may feel depressed, irritable, restless, and perhaps anorexic. The client may also experience transient neurologic disturbances, including visual phenomena (flashes of lights, bright spots, distorted vision, diplopia, transitory impaired vision), vertigo, nausea, diarrhea, abdominal pain, paresthesias (numbness or tingling of lips, face, or extremities), or transient hemiparesis. Prodromal symptoms may last a few minutes or several hours.

A migraine headache has a "crescendo" quality. It gradually increases in severity until the pain becomes intense and all-encompassing. Pain varies in intensity from mild discomfort to a prostrating, throbbing pain that forces the client to seek seclusion and lie in bed in a darkened room. The pain may be described as vise-like, dull and boring, pressing, throbbing, or hammering. Initially throbbing in nature, the pain may later become a steady ache. The pain is usually unilateral and may be localized to the front, back, or side of the head. It may begin at any part of the head, often the temple and the eye areas. Prodromal symptoms and head pain rarely occur in the same location in every episode.

During an acute migraine episode (often 4 to 6 hours), the client is acutely ill and may be extremely irritable. Various somatic signs and symptoms accompany severe episodes (e.g., photophobia, nausea, vomiting, vertigo, tremor, diarrhea, and excessive sweating or chilliness). The common symptoms of nausea and vomiting explain why many clients call migraine headaches "sick headaches." There is usually a general hypersensitivity of all the sensory organs, and the client withdraws from light and sound. Arteries of the head may become prominent, and the amplitude of their pulsations increases. The client's scalp may be very tender. Swelling, redness, and excessive tearing of the eyes and swelling of the nasal mucosa (sometimes accompanied by epistaxis) may occur.

Atypical or Common Migraine. This headache begins suddenly, with or without prodromal symptoms; may be generalized or unilateral; and may or may not be accompanied by nausea and vomiting.

MANAGEMENT

Treatment of migraine headaches involves prevention of episodes and treating the two phases of migraine, that is, vasoconstriction and vasodilation. Treatment of an acute migraine episode varies with symptom intensity. The transient neurologic symptoms are not treated. Analgesics such as acetaminophen or acetylsalicylic acid may relieve a mild headache. More severe headaches respond to ergot preparations, but only if they are taken 30 to 60 minutes after headache onset. Ergot must be taken before the vessels become rigid from edema in their walls. Ergot may be prescribed orally, intravenously, or rectally. Once a migraine headache becomes intense, ergot is of little value, and a stronger analgesic such as codeine sulfate, diphenhydramine hydrochloride (Benadryl), or meperidine may be more effective.

Some sources recommend reducing the pain of migraine by applying pressure on the common carotid artery and the affected superficial artery. Lying in a dark, quiet room with ice on the back of the neck is often helpful during an acute episode.

Between migraine attacks, the client is usually in a normal state of health. If migraine episodes occur as often as once a week or more, preventive treatment may be possible. Beta-adrenergic blockers (propranolol [Inderal]), the medication most often used, may reduce the frequency of episodes or abolish them completely. Some clients with migraine benefit from relaxation techniques, biofeedback, or counseling directed at preventing episodes by helping the client understand tensions and resolve major life conflicts. Another prophylactic measure is following a restrictive diet directed at trying to avoid food and beverages that contain tyramine and have vasoactive qualities that seem to predispose to migraine headaches.

Cluster Headaches (Histamine Headaches)

Cluster headaches are sometimes classified as a form of migraine. Most clients experiencing cluster headaches do not have a history of migraine headaches. Cluster headaches are excruciatingly painful, are unilateral, and tend to occur in clusters. There is usually no aura. Numerous episodes may occur within a few days, weeks, or occasionally months, followed by a remission with no symptoms for months or years. Then the headaches again recur in clusters. Men are affected five times more often than are women. Episodes usually begin in middle life and are often worsened by alcohol consumption. Recurrent episodes are dreaded by the client because of the intense suffering they cause.

A cluster of episodes subsides as suddenly and inexplicably as it began. Cluster headache may recur at irregular intervals for many years, often related to times of stress, anxiety, or emotional upset. The mechanism underlying cluster headaches is not well understood but is believed to be vascular in origin. These headaches were formerly believed to be caused by sensitivity to histamine.

Individual cluster headaches begin suddenly and may last only a few minutes or as long as 2 to 3 hours. Often they begin at night at approximately the same time. During an episode, the client experiences excruciating, throbbing, or steady pain arising high in the nostril and spreading to one side of the forehead, around and behind the eye on the affected side. The nose and affected eye water, and the skin reddens on the affected side. Nasal congestion and conjunctival infection are common.

Intervention for cluster headaches is ineffective because of the shortness of episodes. The client is acutely ill during the attack and desires to be alone and quiet. Applying cold relieves some clients. Indomethacin (Indocin) is the medication of choice. Tricyclic antidepressants can also be used in treatment. Supportive care is important, because clients with cluster headaches often become depressed over their condition and fearful of recurrent episodes. Some feel they cannot survive another episode.

Tension Headaches (Muscle Contraction Headaches)

Tension headaches result from the long-sustained contraction of skeletal muscles around the scalp, face, neck, and upper back. The muscles become tender, and as a result, the client then tenses more. This prolonged muscle contraction is the primary source of many headaches associated with excessive emotional tension, anxiety, and depression. Vasodilation of associated cranial arteries may also contribute to muscle irritability and head pain.

Tension headaches begin in adolescence but occur most often in middle age. They may increase significantly with menopause. Premenstrual headaches are usually of this type.

Sustained muscle contraction may also cause headaches secondary to painful stimuli from other cranial structures (e.g., brain tumor; distended arteries; eye, ear, nose, paranasal, or tooth inflammation).

Assessment of tension headaches typically reveals a steady, nonpulsatile ache (unilateral or bilateral) in any region of the head. Pain often occurs in the occipital and upper cervical regions and extends diffusely over the top of the head. The pain is frequently described as feelings of tightness, fullness, drawing sensations, or pressure. The pain of tension headache may be localized, or frequent changes may occur in location and intensity. Sometimes these headaches are fleeting but recurrent.

The onset of tension headaches is more gradual than with migraine headache. Nausea and vomiting may accompany tension headache but occur as a late reaction to pain. Also, the headache may be accompanied by dizziness, tinnitus, or lacrimation, or these symptoms may be elicited by pressing on the tender muscles. Palpation may demonstrate contracted muscles with localized painful areas or nodules. Pain may be precipitated or aggravated by combing the hair, by wearing a hat, or by exposure to cold. Tension headaches may be unrelieved for weeks, months, or years.

Tension headaches are treated when possible by removing the primary source of stimulation (e.g., treating diseased teeth). Clients with prolonged or recurrent muscle tension headaches of psychological origin may be helped by psychotherapy. Symptomatic treatment for the headaches themselves includes massaging affected muscles, applying local heat, rest, and various relaxation techniques. Sometimes, local injections of procaine are helpful. Tension headaches respond best to a medication that combines a non-narcotic analgesic with an anxiety-relieving drug. Occasionally, a stronger analgesic is needed (e.g., codeine sulfate).

Head Pain Related to Other Structures

Headaches may result from errors of refraction, glaucoma (with increased intraocular pressure), inflammation, and ocular muscle equilibrium disturbances (see Chap. 17).

Pain associated with sinus infection is usually due to irritation and inflammation of sinus openings. (Sinus walls are less sensitive.) The pain of a sinus headache may be relieved or eliminated by decongestants and analgesics. Sometimes antibiotics are needed. Surgery to drain the sinuses may also be required (see Chap. 21).

STUDY QUESTIONS

1. The nurse recognizes that which of the following clients is at greatest risk of stroke?
   A. A caucasian client, age 43
   B. A 60-year-old client with uncontrolled diabetes
   C. A client who maintains a low-fat diet
   D. A 55-year-old client who stopped smoking 5 years ago
2. The client tells the nurse, "The doctor said that my brain tumor is benign. Now I don't have to worry about it." In assessing the need for further teaching, the nurse bases her evaluation on the fact that benign brain tumors:
   A. Do not require surgery, chemotherapy, or radiation therapy.
   B. Are easily treated regardless of location.
   C. Can cause increased intracranial pressure and herniation.
   D. Rarely produce life-threatening symptoms.
3. A 24-year-old client is being discharged from the emergency department after sustaining a head injury with a 1 minute loss of consciousness. Which of the following statements by the family indicates understanding of the nurse's discharge teaching?
   A. "I won't be worried if vomiting occurs as this often is common after a bump on the head."
   B. "I will check his pulse and blood pressure every hour tonight."
   C. "I will bring him back to the emergency department if he gets irritable and does not easily awaken."
   D. "I will make an appointment with our doctor if he complains of a severe headache."
4. A client has been experiencing seizures in rapid succession. The physician orders intravenous lorazepam (Ativan) given slowly until the seizures stop. After the administration of IV lorazepam, the nurse should assess for:
   A. Tachycardia
   B. Hypertension
   C. Respiratory depression
   D. Tissue hypoxia
5. Of the following clinical manifestations, which would *not* be expected in clients with a diagnosis of meningitis?
   A. Chills and fever
   B. Nausea and vomiting
   C. Bradycardia and hypotension
   D. Confusion and seizures

CRITICAL THINKING EXERCISES

SCENARIO A

A 43-year-old client was singing at choir practice when she experienced a severe headache and an episode of syncope. She was taken to the local emergency department, where she described the headache as "the worst headache that I have ever had." After CT scan, she was diagnosed as having a subarachnoid hemorrhage (SAH).

1. What findings are commonly seen in clients with SAH?
2. Describe the characteristics and classifications of cerebral aneurysms.
3. What are the common nursing interventions for clients with SAH?

SCENARIO B

A 24-year-old college student is being admitted to the hospital with a diagnosis of complex partial seizures. She is being evaluated for a possible temporal lobectomy.

1. Describe the various clinical manifestations of complex partial seizures.
2. What are the criteria for being a candidate for temporal lobectomy?

BIBLIOGRAPHY

1. Adams, B. A., Clancey, J. K., & Eddy, M. S. (1991). Malignant glioma: Current treatment and perspectives. *Journal of Neuroscience Nursing, 23(1),* 15–20.
2. Andrus, C. (1991). Intracranial pressure: Dynamics and nursing management. *Journal of Neuroscience Nursing, 23(2),* 85–91.
3. Chipps, E., Clanin, N., & Campbell, V. (1992). *Neurological Disorders,* St. Louis: Mosby-Year Book.
4. Dean, E. (1991). Clinical decision making in the management of the late sequelae of poliomyelitis. *Physical Therapy, 71(10),* 752–761.
5. Dring, R. (1989). The informal caregiver responsible for home care of the individual with cognitive dysfunction following brain injury. *Journal of Neuroscience Nursing, 21(1),* 42.
6. Fontaine, D. K. (1989). Measurement of nocturnal sleep patterns in trauma patients. *Heart and Lung, 18(4),* 402.
7. Gilman, S. (1992). Advances in neurology. Part 2. *New England Journal of Medicine, 326(25),* 1671–1676.
8. Godbole, K. B., et al. (1991). A head injured patient: Caloric needs, clinical progress and nursing care priorities. *Journal of Neuroscience Nursing, 23(5),* 290.
9. Hauser, W. A., & Hesdorffer, D. C. (Eds.) (1990). *Epilepsy: Frequency, causes and consequences.* New York: Demos Press.
10. Hodges, K., & Root, L. M. (1991). Surgical management of intractable seizure disorders. *Journal of Neuroscience Nursing, 23(2),* 93–98.
11. Kalbach, L. R. (1991). Unilateral neglect: Mechanisms and nursing care. *Journal of Neuroscience Nursing, 23(2),* 125–129.
12. Keller, C., et al. (1989). Psychological responses in aphasia: Theoretical considerations and nursing implications. *Journal of Neuroscience Nursing, 21(5),* 290–294.
13. Krause, E. A., et al. (1991). Radiosurgery: A nursing perspective. *Journal of Neuroscience Nursing, 23(1),* 24–28.
14. MacDonald, E. (1989). Aneurysmal subarachnoid hemorrhage. *Journal of Neuroscience Nursing, 21(5),* 313–321.
15. Marshall, S. B., et al. (1990). *Neuroscience critical care: Pathophysiology and patient management.* Philadelphia: W. B. Saunders Co.
16. Mattson, A. J., & Levin, H. S. (1990). Frontal lobe dysfunction following closed head injury. *The Journal of Nervous and Mental Disease, 178(5),* 282.
17. McCance, K. L., & Huether, S. E. (1994). *Pathophysiology: The biological basis for disease in adults and children.* (2nd ed.). St. Louis: Mosby-Year Book.
18. Mitchell, M. (1989). *Neuroscience nursing: A nursing diagnosis approach.* Baltimore: Williams & Wilkins.
19. Origitano, T. C., et al. (1990). Sustained increased cerebral blood flow with prophylactic hypertensive hypovolemic hemodilution ("triple-H" therapy) after subarachnoid hemorrhage. *Neurosurgery, 27(5),* 729.
20. Plylar, P. A. (1989). Management of the agitated and aggressive head injury patient in an acute hospital setting. *Journal of Neuroscience Nursing, 21(6),* 353.
21. Pulsinelli, W. & Levy, D. (1992). Cerebrovascular diseases—principles. In J. Wyngaarden, L. Smith, & J. Bennett. (Eds.), *Cecil textbook of medicine* (19th ed.). Philadelphia: W.B. Saunders.
22. Rivara, F. P., et al. (1988). The public cost of motorcycle trauma. *Journal of the American Medical Association, 260(2),* 221.
23. Sabiston, D. (1991). *Textbook of surgery* (14th ed.). Philadelphia: W.B. Saunders.
24. Simon, R. (1992). Parameningeal infections. In J. Wyngaarden, L. Smith, & J. Bennett (Eds.), *Cecil textbook of medicine* (19th ed.). Philadelphia, W.B. Saunders.
25. Smigielski, J., et al. (1992). Mayo Medical Center brain injury outpatient program: Treatment procedures and early outcome data. *Mayo Clinic Proceedings, 67(8),* 767–774.
26. Stewart-Amidei, C. (1989). Hypervolemic hemodilution: A new approach to subarachnoid hemorrhage. *Heart and Lung, 18(6),* 590.
27. Swartz, M. N. (1992). Bacterial meningitis. In J. Wyngaarden, L. Smith, & J. Bennett (Eds.), *Cecil textbook of medicine* (19th ed.). Philadelphia, W.B. Saunders.
28. Thelan, L. A., et al. (1994). *Textbook of critical care nursing: Diagnosis and management* (2nd ed.). St. Louis: Mosby–Year Book.
29. Tosch, P. (1988). Patients' recollections of their posttraumatic coma. *Journal of Neuroscience Nursing, 20(4),* 223–228.
30. Vick, N. A. (1992). Intracranial tumors: General considerations. In J. Wyngaarden, L. Smith, & J. Bennett, (Eds.), *Cecil textbook of medicine* (19th ed.). Philadelphia: W.B. Saunders.
31. Willis, D. (1991). Intracranial astrocytoma: Pathology. Diagnosis and clinical presentation. *Journal of Neuroscience Nursing, 23(1),* 7.
32. Willis, D., & Harbit, M. D. (1989). A fatal attraction: Cocaine related subarachnoid hemorrhage. *Journal of Neuroscience Nursing, 21(3),* 171.
33. Wyngaarden, J., Smith, L., & Bennett, J. (Eds.). (1992). *Cecil textbook of medicine* (19th ed.). Philadelphia: W.B. Saunders.
34. Youmans, J. R. (Ed.) (1995). *Neurological surgery: A comprehensive reference guide to the diagnosis and management of neurosurgical problems* (4th ed.). Philadelphia: W.B. Saunders.

Chapter 15

Nursing Care of Clients with Degenerative Neurologic Disorders

Learning Outcomes

After completing this chapter, the learner will be able to:

1. Assess the client for clinical manifestations of degenerative neurologic disorders.
2. Develop plans of care for the prevention of complications, nursing management, and rehabilitation of clients with degenerative neurologic disorders.
3. Implement nursing interventions that optimize the quality of life for clients with degenerative neurologic disorders.
4. Evaluate the needs of the client and family for information, emotional support, and planning for home care.

ALZHEIMER'S DISEASE

Alzheimer's disease is a form of dementia. Dementia involves progressive decline in two or more areas of cognition, usually memory and one or more of the following: language, calculation, visuospatial perception, constructional praxis, judgment, abstraction, and personality change. Dementia of the Alzheimer's type (DAT) comprises at least half of all dementias (see Chap. 13 for a general discussion of dementia).

Incidence

Recent studies have shown that the prevalence of DAT is higher than previously expected.[7,23] DAT occurs in 10 to 15 per cent of people older than age 65, 19 per cent of people older than age 75, and 47 per cent of people older than age 85. The incidence of DAT increases greatly with increasing age.

Etiology and Risk Factors

The cause of DAT has not been found, although several risk factors have been identified. As can be seen by the statistics listed earlier, increasing age is a risk factor. DAT can be a genetic disorder. A defect associated with chromosome 21 has been found in some families with early-onset DAT, and a defect associated with chromosome 19 has been found in some families with late-onset DAT. However, the lack of 100 per cent concordance in studies of identical twins implies that environmental, metabolic, and other factors also may play a role. Head trauma, lack of education, and myocardial infarction have been shown to be risk factors,[15] although the reasons for their being risk factors are not fully understood. Some have postulated that aluminum intoxication, disordered immune function, and viral infection are causes of DAT; however these factors have not yet been proved.[4]

Pathophysiology

Alois Alzheimer first described presenile dementia in 1907. He used a new staining technique of human brain tissue to demonstrate the disease. The changes he noted are now termed *neurofibrillary tangles* and *neuritic plaques.* These are abnormal proteins that accumulate in the brain. The neuritic plaque is a cluster of degenerating nerve terminals, both dendritic and axonal, that contains amyloid protein. The precursor of this protein, amyloid precursor protein, is coded by a gene on chromosome 21 and an adjacent "housekeeping" gene that regulates the daily functioning of cells. Neurofibrillary tangles are abnormal neurons in which the cytoplasm is filled with bundles of abnormal protein called *paired helical filaments.* Neuritic plaques and neurofibrillary tangles are located in areas of cell loss in the brain of the person with DAT. These areas are the association areas of the neocortex and the hippocampus, which account for the cognitive decline. The term "association" is used to describe all the intellectual activities of the cerebral cortex. These functions include learning and reasoning, memory storage and recall, language abilities, and even consciousness.

In addition to structural changes, there are neurotransmitter changes in the brains of clients with DAT. A decline in cholinergic neurons in the basal nucleus leads to loss of choline acetyltransferase in the neocortex and hippocampus.

Clinical Manifestations

Clinically, Alzheimer's disease is characterized by a relentless impairment of decision making that generally begins insidiously and can progress for a decade or so. The onset of DAT typically occurs in late middle age (age 65 and older), although some familial cases occur in the fifth and sixth decades. The clinical progression of symptoms is usually divided into three stages (Table 15–1). The sequence of loss of higher cognitive func-

TABLE 15–1 Common Clinical Manifestations in Each Stage of Dementia of the Alzheimer's Type

STAGE I (DURATION OF DISEASE 1 TO 3 YEARS)
Memory—new learning defective, remote recall mildly impaired
Visuospatial skills—topographic disorientation, poor complex constructions
Language—poor word list generation, anomia
Personality—indifference, occasional irritability
Psychiatric features—sadness or delusions in some
Motor system—normal
EEG—normal
CT/MRI—normal
PET/SPECT—bilateral posterior parietal hypometabolism/hyperfusion
STAGE II (DURATION OF DISEASE 2 TO 10 YEARS)
Memory—recent and remote recall more severely impaired
Visuospatial skills—poor constructions, spatial disorientation
Language—fluent aphasia
Calculation—acalculia
Praxis—ideomotor apraxia
Personality—indifference or irritability
Psychiatric features—delusions in some
Motor system—restlessness, pacing
EEG—slowing of background rhythm
CT/MRI—normal or ventricular dilatation and sulcal enlargement
PET/SPECT—bilateral parietal and frontal hypometabolism/hypoperfusion
STAGE III (DURATION OF DISEASE 8 TO 12 YEARS)
Intellectual functions—severely deteriorated
Motor—limb rigidity and flexion posture
Sphincter control—urinary and fecal incontinence
EEG—diffusely slow
CT/MRI—ventricular dilatation and sulcal enlargement
PET/SPECT—bilateral parietal and frontal hypometabolism/hypoperfusion

EEG, electroencephalogram; CT, computed tomography; MRI, magnetic resonance imaging; PET, positron emission tomography; SPECT, single photon emission computed tomography.

From Cummings, J. L., & Benson, D. F. (1992). *Dementia: A clinical approach.* Boston: Butterworth-Heinemann. Reprinted by permission.

tions is a helpful clue for establishing the clinical diagnosis. Memory disturbance is usually the first feature of the disease. Family members or coworkers often notice the memory loss before the individual does. The individual may demonstrate poor judgment and problem-solving skills and become careless in work habits and household chores. He or she may do well in familiar surroundings and be able to follow well-established routines but lack the ability to adapt to new challenges. The person may become irritable, suspicious, or indifferent.

In the second stage of illness, the client may demonstrate language disturbance, characterized by impaired word finding and circumlocution (talking around a subject rather than directly about it). Later, spontaneous speech becomes increasingly empty and paraphasias (words used in the wrong context) are used. The person may repeat words and phrases used by him- or herself (palilalia) or others (echolalia). Motor disturbance (apraxia) is characterized by difficulty in using everyday objects like a toothbrush, comb, razor, and utensils. Apraxia combined with forgetfulness can create serious safety problems. The individual may leave a burner on in the kitchen or forget to extinguish a cigarette. Indifference worsens and restlessness with frequent pacing appears. Hyperorality (the desire to take everything into the mouth to suck, chew, or taste) may develop. Swallowing may become difficult. Depression and irritability may worsen, and delusions and psychosis may appear. The person fears personal harm, theft of property, or infidelity of the spouse. He or she may see bugs crawling in the bed or throughout the house. Wandering at night is common. Occasional incontinence may occur.

In the final stage, virtually all mental abilities are lost, including speech. Voluntary movement is minimal, and the limbs become rigid with flexor posturing. Urinary and fecal incontinence is frequent. The person has lost all ability for self-care.

DIAGNOSTIC ASSESSMENT

Because there is no definitive test for DAT, the diagnosis is made by exclusion of known causes of dementia (e.g., toxic-metabolic alterations, drug side effects, cerebrovascular disease, neoplasm, and infection). Diagnosis of DAT requires the presence of dementia involving two or more areas of cognition, insidious onset, steady progression, and normal alertness.[27] When these criteria are applied, 9 of 10 individuals given this diagnosis have DAT confirmed at autopsy. Postmortem examination of the brain is the only way DAT can be definitively diagnosed. The brain is viewed under the microscope for the presence of neuritic plaques and neurofibrillary tangles.

Diagnostic assessments such as the electroencephalogram (EEG), computerized tomography (CT), and magnetic resonance imaging (MRI) are sometimes used in the diagnosis of DAT. In general, these studies rule out other causes of dementia, such as seizures and cerebral bleeding, but do not diagnose DAT. Changes on EEG, CT, and MRI do not appear until the later stages of DAT. Finally, laboratory studies are currently being performed to assist in the diagnosis of DAT looking at beta-amyloid protein.

Medical Management

There is no cure for DAT. Results of studies in which acetylcholine precursors (choline, lecithin, and deanol) and anticholinesterase agents (physostigmine and tetrahydroaminoacridine) are used to enhance memory and cognitive function have been disappointing. Pharmacologic therapy is primarily aimed at treating behavior problems, although behavioral and environmental manipulations are often more effective (see later). Low-dose antipsychotic agents, like haloperidol, can be effective for agitation and confusion. The lowest effective dose should be used and should be given just before bedtime. Sometimes, twice-a-day dosing is required. Adverse side effects such as akathisia (motor restlessness), parkinsonian symptoms, tardive dyskinesias, orthostatic hypotension, anticholinergic symptoms (urinary retention and confusion), and sedation should be monitored. Antidepressants (e.g., nortriptyline and desipramine) that have few anticholinergic side effects, fluoxetine, and trazodone are helpful for depression.[15] Table 15–2 lists drugs that can be used to treat behavioral problems in DAT.

Nursing Management

Assessment

When DAT is suspected, a complete history should be taken to assess for other causes of dementia. Data should be obtained from the client, family, and coworkers (if possible). Secondary sources are used because the client is often unaware of a problem with thought processing and minimizes it. The nurse should ask specific questions about difficulties with activities of daily living (ADLs), increasing forgetfulness, and changes in personality. Medical history should be assessed for head injury or surgery, recent falls, headache, and family history of DAT. A mini mental state examination may provide objective data for ongoing evaluation of the client (see Chap. 13).

DAT has a profound impact on psychosocial behaviors. The nurse should ask about the client's reactions to changes in routine or in the environment. It is not uncommon for a client with DAT to become very agitated over small changes. Likewise, apathy, social isolation, and irritability may be noted. As the brain continues to atrophy and the limbic system becomes dysfunctional, the client displays paranoia, uses abusive language, and becomes suspicious of others.

DAT also has a profound impact on the family. The nurse needs to assess the family for strengths and weaknesses, the ability to provide care for the client, and financial concerns. In large centers, the assessment of the client and family is performed through a team approach.

TABLE 15–2 Pharmacologic Treatment of Behavioral Problems in Dementia of the Alzheimer's Type

PROBLEM	TREATMENT
Suspiciousness, paranoia, sundowning:	1. Behavioral 2. Environmental 3. Correct sensory impairment 4. Low-dose antipsychotics a) Haloperidol 0.25–1 mg/day b) High-potency phenothiazine 1–4 mg/day c) Watch for akathisias, parkinsonism, sedation, falls
Anxiety:	1. Treat underlying physical problems (pain, dyspnea, urinary urgency, sensory impairment) 2. Acute, short-lived—reassurance 3. Related to confusion—antipsychotics 4. Diffuse, chronic—long-acting benzodiazepine (low dose)* 5. Avoid: non-benzodiazepine sedative-hypnotics, esp. barbiturates 6. Role of buspirone unclear
Acute catastrophic reactions:	1. Haloperidol 2–5 mg IM 2. Lorazepam 1 mg IM
Insomnia:	1. Environmental/behavioral 2. If associated confusion, low-dose antipsychotic 3. If associated depression, antidepressant a) Nortriptyline b) Trazodone 4. Intermediate-acting benzodiazepine (e.g., temazepam, lorazepam, oxazepam)* 5. Antihistamine (diphenhydramine) a) Particularly useful if restlessness with antipsychotic rx (?treating akathisia or parkinsonian symptoms) 6. Chloral hydrate
Angry or violent outbursts:	1. Very difficult to control 2. Behavior log key 3. ?Relationship to pain or other physiologic stimuli a) Arthritis b) GU problems c) Constipation 4. Low-dose antipsychotic 5. Trazodone 6. Carbamazepine 7. Propanolol (?) 8. Lithium (dubious)

* May cause disinhibition or increased confusion. Rebound anxiety at the end of a dosing interval may be a problem with chronic use.
IM, intramuscularly; GU, genitourinary.
Reprinted with permission of the American Geriatrics Society, Alzheimer disease: Basic and Clinical Advances, by Katzman, R., & Jackson, J., *Journal of the American Geriatrics Society, 39,* 517–525, 1991.

Nursing Diagnosis, Planning, and Implementation

Nursing Diagnosis: Communication, Impaired Verbal R/T neuronal degeneration.

Planning: Expected Outcomes. The client's needs will be communicated effectively, as evidenced by making his or her needs known and interacting meaningfully with others.

Implementation. In the initial stage of DAT, the client's receptive and expressive language skills are relatively intact. The nurse must be prepared to adapt to the communication level of the client. If the client speaks only single words or short phrases, the nurse should do likewise. It is best to speak slowly and simply, with firm volume and low pitch. The tone of voice should always be calm and reassuring and project control of the situation. However, when language becomes impaired in the second stage of the illness, the nurse must be prepared to apply new techniques for communicating with the client.

Bartol[2] wrote in 1979 a very useful guide for nurses that is still appropriate today. Nonverbal behavior can provide the nurse with clues. Clients with DAT often avert their eyes, look down, back away, and increase hand gesturing when they do not understand. If they are frustrated, angry, or hostile, they may increase motor activity by pacing, rattling doorknobs, waving their arms or shaking their fists, frowning, raising their voice volume and pitch, and tightening their face muscles. These behaviors should signal staff to increase their alertness, search for the cause of the distress, and prepare to intervene. Interventions can include:

- Decreasing environmental stimuli
- Approaching the client calmly and with assurance
- Taking care not to place any more demands on the client
- Distracting the client
- Making sure that all verbal and nonverbal communication cues are concordant
- Using multiple sensory modalities (visual, auditory, and tactile) to send the message.

The client's memory loss can be an advantage in distracting him or her from the stressful situation. If removed from the situation and provided a calm, nonthreatening environment, the client may forget why he was upset. Bartol suggested that nurses can elicit listening behavior from DAT clients by reaching out and touching, holding a hand, putting an arm around the waist, or in some way maintaining physical contact with the client. Dementia sufferers can perceive nonverbal behavior from others and can become agitated or upset if they sense negative nonverbal behavior from others.

The identification of pain or discomfort in clients with advanced DAT is also difficult. Hurley and colleagues[13] developed a tool to facilitate assessment. Behavioral indicators of discomfort include noisy breathing, negative vocalization (constant muttering, making noise with a negative quality), sad or frightened facial expression, frown, tense body language, and fidgeting.

Nursing Diagnosis: Thought Processes, Altered R/T neuronal degeneration.

Planning: Expected Outcomes. The client will have improved thought processing, as evidenced by exhibiting retention of information to maximal capacity, maintaining orientation to maximal capacity, and sharing meaningful life experiences.

Implementation. Because memory deficit occurs in all stages of DAT, the nurse must continually apply interventions to enhance memory. The nurse should reorient the client as necessary by placing a calendar and clock in obvious places. Because DAT clients' long-term memory is retained longer than their short-term memory, the nurse should allow clients to reminisce. The nurse should be aware of a client's past so experiences can be shared meaningfully. Repetition is useful for ensuring maximal retention of information by the client.

Nursing Diagnosis: Injury, Risk for R/T impaired judgment and forgetfulness.

Planning: Expected Outcomes. The client's physical and environmental safety will be maintained, as evidenced by the absence of physical injury and the existence of a safe living environment.

Implementation. Impaired judgment, forgetfulness, and motor impairment can make any environment unsafe for the client with DAT. In the home, electrical devices, toxic substances, loose rugs, hot tap water, inadequate lighting, and unlocked doors can be sources of injury. Family members should be educated on how to eliminate these safety hazards. In the inpatient setting, nurses should ensure that clients cannot leave the premises without being noticed, that they wear an identification badge in case they become lost, and that doors and windows be secured. Dangerous objects should be kept out of reach, and potentially dangerous activities, like cooking, should be supervised.

Nursing Diagnosis: Self-Care Deficit R/T loss of memory and motor praxis.

Expected Outcomes. The client will have ADLs completed, as evidenced by completing the tasks he or she is capable of performing and receiving assistance with ADLs he or she is incapable of performing.

Implementation. The client with DAT should be encouraged to do as much as possible as long as it is safe and appropriate. The nurse must carefully balance helping the client with maintaining his or her autonomy. This will boost the client's confidence and self-respect, which can be very fragile during the early and middle stages of the disease. The client should be given plenty of time to complete a task. Constant encouragement, urging, and reminding the client in a step-by-step approach is necessary.

Nursing Diagnosis: Incontinence, Urge R/T neuronal degeneration and forgetfulness.

Planning: Expected Outcomes. The client will have optimal continence of bladder and bowel, as evidenced by having clean, dry clothing and bedding as much as possible; having intact skin; and voiding appropriately in the bathroom.

Implementation. DAT clients experience urge incontinence as cortical neurons degenerate and no longer provide inhibition of the micturition and defecation responses. Anticipation of elimination needs and scheduled voiding and defecation times can help in the initial stages. The client may show nonverbal signs of needing to void or defecate, like restlessness, grasping the genital area, or picking at clothing. Sometimes, the client may forget where the bathroom is located. Having clear, bright signs indicating where the bathroom is and frequently taking the client there may help control incontinence. Fluid intake after the dinner meal can be restricted to help maintain continence during the night. A bowel program can be arranged to coincide with the client's usual pattern. In the later stages of DAT, clients may need to wear incontinence pads during the day and external urinary drainage devices at night. Indwelling catheters should be avoided because of the risk of infection and injury.

Nursing Diagnosis: Care Giver Role Strain R/T grieving the loss of a family member to DAT, change in social role, and intense demands for time commitment and provision of care.

Planning: Expected Outcomes. The family will demonstrate decreased role strain, as evidenced by voicing their emotional concerns, seeking appropriate assistance, and providing adequate care for the client.

Implementation. Family members and especially care givers (usually a spouse or adult child) of clients with DAT face a great deal of emotional and physical burden. Family members grieve the loss of the person they used to know. Each decline in cognitive function becomes another source of grief. Jones and Martinson[14] described two stages of grief in the family. The process of grief begins during the care-giving stage and continues after the client's death. Normal family routines are lost, and the relationship between the family member and the dementia sufferer changes. The Alzheimer's Disease and Related Disorders Association has local chapters that offer support groups in many major cities in the United States. The toll free number is 1-800-272-3900 for information on nearby local chapters.

A variety of options are available to care givers. Chore service workers can help with household chores and relieve the care giver of these duties. Other paid help can provide in-home respite care by observing the dementia sufferer while the care giver tends to business outside the home, seeks social interaction, or meets recreational needs. Adult day care provides time away from home for the dementia sufferer. Day care usually offers a lunchtime meal as well as several hours of scheduled activities that are tailored to the client's abilities. These activities may include games, crafts, music, and exercise. Respite care involves admission to an extended-care facility for a few days to a few weeks to allow the care giver time to recover from the demands of providing 24-hour care. Nursing home care is usually the final, and most difficult and trying, option for a care giver. This decision creates guilt, self-doubt, and anxiety. However, it is often the only option when the care giver suffers burnout and becomes unable to provide adequate care. Table 15–3 lists helpful nursing guidelines for meeting family needs.

When the person with DAT reaches the terminal stage of illness, questions about end-of-life treatments arise. Should a feeding tube be used to provide nour-

TABLE 15–3 Nursing Guidelines for Meeting the Needs of the Family of the Client with Dementia of the Alzheimer's Type

GOALS	SELECTED INTERVENTIONS
Physical	
Monitor chronic health problems or physical limitations of family care giver.	Obtain health history of family care giver to identify past and new health problems.
	Support family in following through with routine health examinations.
Identify development of new health problems.	Refer family member(s) to physician when health problems are observed.
	Assess family's understanding of medical management of own health problems.
	Teach family members to preserve own health in order to continue caring for patient with AD.
Identify cues for stress.	Emphasize family's need for adequate nutrition, hydration, exercise, and rest.
Examine somatic health problems.	Help family members to be alert to signs of care giver stress.
Psychosocial	
Assist family to cope positively with stress.	Instruct family to get respite regularly for rest and relaxation.
	Teach stress-management techniques (i.e., relaxation, supportive relationships, goal setting, time management, diversion).
Identify destructive methods of coping (i.e., alcohol, drugs, tobacco, over- or undereating, physical abuse of patient).	Refer family to physician, therapist when stress remains unmanageable even with social or psychological resources.
	Refer signs of physical abuse to adult protective services.
Assess family dynamics.	Recognize the family's role, discuss capacity to provide care, and give reinforcement for care provided.
Assist family members to deal with role change and conflict.	Counsel family in dealing with role conflicts, unmet expectations, or interpersonal conflicts.
	Teach family the need to maintain roles and social activities outside care-giving experience.
	Administer burden interview.
	Reinforce family's attempt to cope.
	Acknowledge family fears of being unable to continue with care giving.
If need for support identified, direct family members to sources.	Refer family to a support group to share with others in similar situations.
	Refer family to nearest office on aging or Alzheimer's Disease and Related Disorders Association, Inc. (ADRDA) to identify benefits in community available to AD patients.
Identify family's mixed emotions (i.e., depression, anger, resentment, pity, embarrassment, guilt).	Listen to family and facilitate sharing of emotions and feelings in supportive, empathetic environment.
Identify alternative plans for care if family members or social support systems become unable to provide care or are ineffective.	Counsel and support family if patient placed in care of other (i.e., day care, respite service, home care, nursing home); allay feelings of guilt.
	Facilitate family meeting to identify time for socialization.
Identify financial limitations.	Encourage family to be specific about financial limitations.
	Offer family referrals (legal, financial, or social service) for information on eligibility for private, county, state, or federal financial support for home services, and advice and counsel regarding power of attorney or guardianship, trust or estate planning.
Assess family's ability to make funeral plans.	Help family anticipate and cope with grief process.
	Assist family in making prefuneral arrangements.
	Address family's fear regarding the possible role of heredity in development of AD and assist in making decision regarding autopsy.
Environmental	
Identify compatibility of environment with family and patient.	Conduct a family meeting to discuss relationship of family, patient, and environment.
Assess learning needs regarding patient care tasks.	Teach management of concurrent physical health problems of the AD patient.
	Include family in development of patient care plan.
	Teach family to encourage AD patient to continue daily habits to extent possible.
	Complete behavior problems checklist.
	Anticipate likely problems and teach how to manage them.
	Teach environmental modification (consistent, simple, calm routines) to maximize family endurance and enhance safety.
	Teach family to relate to patient with creative connectiveness (touch, humor, flexibility, reminiscence, music, planned activities).
Assess family need and desire for information about AD and how it affects patient's behavior.	Assist family to understand symptoms related to memory loss, nature of the illness, symptoms, stages of disease progression, and behavior manifestations.
	Provide written material to reinforce education and understanding (i.e., *The 36 Hour Day, Coping and Caring: Living with Alzheimer's Disease;* literature from local, state, or national ADRDA chapters).
	Supply ADRDA 24-hour hotline number: 1-800-621-0379.

AD, Alzheimer's disease.
Adapted from Stevenson, J. P. (1990). Family stress to home care of Alzheimer's disease patients and implications for support. *Journal of Neuroscience Nursing, 22*(3), 185.

ishment? Should antibiotics be used to treat pneumonias or other infections? Should cardiopulmonary resuscitation be used? Ideally, decisions about these questions are raised and discussed with the client before he or she loses decisional capacity, and with family members.

Evaluation

The nurse continually evaluates the degree of expected outcome attainment. In the case of the client with DAT, this includes evaluation of outcomes focused on improving verbal communication; facilitating memory; preventing injury; enhancing self-care; maintaining continence; and, perhaps most important, bolstering care giver and family coping strategies. Most of the nursing care of persons with DAT is provided in an outpatient setting or in a nursing home.

Posthospital Care

Family members should be interviewed to determine their understanding of the diagnosis and prognosis of DAT and to allow them to discuss their concerns about caring for the client. Do they know about community resources? Do they have someone to call when they can no longer cope with care giving? The home environment should be evaluated before the client is sent home from the hospital to ascertain safety issues (see Client Education Guide). Is the home on a busy street? Can doors be secured so that the client cannot get out without supervision? Are potentially dangerous appliances out of reach?

MULTIPLE SCLEROSIS

Multiple sclerosis (MS) is a progressive degenerative disease that affects the myelin sheath of neurons in the central nervous system (CNS). The myelin sheath is essential for normal conduction of nerve impulses to and from the brain and spinal cord. Patches of myelin deteriorate at irregular intervals along the nerve axon, causing slowing of nerve conduction.

Incidence

The onset of MS usually occurs between ages 20 and 40 years, and it affects women twice as often as men. Whites are affected more often than Hispanics, blacks, or Asians. The disease is most prevalent in the colder climates of North America and Europe. If someone is born in an area of high risk for MS and moves to an area of low risk after age 15 years, he or she carries the risk of the country of origin.

Etiology

The exact cause of MS is unknown. Most theories suggest that MS is an immunogenetic-viral disease: that is, an immune-mediated demyelination triggered by viral infection. A genetic susceptibility apparently alters the body's immune response to viral infection. MS is 15 to 20 times more common in first-degree relatives of affected persons.[24]

Risk Factors

A variety of precipitating factors can precede the onset or an exacerbation of MS. They include infection, physical injury, emotional stress, pregnancy, and fatigue.

Pathophysiology

Myelin is a highly conductive fatty material that surrounds the axon and speeds conduction of nerve impulses along the axon. In MS, plaques form along the myelin sheath, causing inflammation, edema, and

CLIENT EDUCATION GUIDE

Safety for a Client with Alzheimer's Disease

Ensuring safe home health care for a client with Alzheimer's disease requires creativity and good communication with the client's physician and care givers as well as with the client. Following is a description of some topics to discuss.

Nocturnal wandering, a common problem, presents significant safety problems and a constant challenge to care givers. The use of sedatives and restraints has been found to be counterproductive, leading to confusion, injuries, and increased physical care needs such as toileting and positioning. Safe home care necessitates a thorough assessment of the client's sleeping habits, activity during the day, number of and reasons for arousals during the night, amount of daytime sleeping, sleep aids used, and side effects of medication.

White noise from a fan, air conditioner, or sound generator may prove effective in promoting sleep. Using a Wanderguard, which sounds an alarm if the client leaves the house or enters a potentially dangerous room, such as the kitchen, may allow care givers to rest at night.

Other important safety measures to discuss include removing knobs from stoves and other potentially hazardous appliances, keeping living areas free of clutter and throw rugs, and keeping rooms well lighted. A quiet, well-structured environment also helps minimize the client's confusion and enhances safety.

eventually scarring and destruction. Plaques are characterized by primary demyelination and death of oligodendrocytes in the center of the lesion. Initially, perivascular inflammatory cells invade the myelin-covered axons in the CNS. This is followed by extensive gliosis or scarring by astrocytes and aberrant attempts at remyelination, with oligodendrocytes proliferating at the edges of the plaque. When edema and inflammation subside, some remyelination occurs but is often incomplete. Although plaques may occur anywhere in the white matter of the CNS, the areas most commonly involved are the optic nerves, cerebrum, and cervical spinal cord.

MS has two major courses: exacerbating remitting and chronic progressive. In the former case, the client has episodes of neurologic dysfunction (exacerbations) from which he or she recovers and is able to function normally (remission). In some cases, the recovery from each exacerbation is not complete, causing a stepwise decline in function with each exacerbation. In the second major course of MS, the client experiences a steady decline in neurologic function that can occur over several years. In acute, fulminant cases, the decline may occur rapidly within a year or two. Life expectancy is about 85 per cent of the general population. The usual cause of death is bacterial infection of the lungs, bladder, or pressure ulcers.

Clinical Manifestations

The random distribution of MS plaques leads to a variety of clinical manifestations, including:

- Weakness or tingling sensations (paresthesias) of one or more extremities as a result of involvement of the cerebrum or spinal cord
- Vision loss from optic neuritis
- Incoordination caused by cerebellar involvement
- Bowel and bladder dysfunction as a result of spinal cord involvement.

Seizures may develop in some clients.

Bladder dysfunction can have several forms, depending on which neural pathways are affected. Dysfunction may involve hesitancy, frequency, loss of sensation, incontinence, and retention. Proper diagnosis of the type of bladder dysfunction requires a good history, laboratory assessment of kidney function, and a search for and identification of infection. If bladder emptying is defective, further investigation using urography, cystoscopy, and urodynamic studies should be performed.

Stool incontinence and constipation are common. Dysfunction can result from one or more of the following factors: spinal cord lesion, immobility, dehydration, medications, and nutritional deficiencies.

Fatigue is a common symptom in MS. It usually worsens as the day progresses. Spasticity can reduce energy; inhibit motor control; and interfere with self-care, sexuality, vocational responsibilities, and recreation.

Because MS strikes young adults during their years of establishing a family and an occupation, the impact of the disease can be devastating. Cognitive and psychosocial problems may be caused by frontal or parietal lobe involvement. Emotional lability and euphoria may result from loss of connections between the cortex and the basal ganglia. Depression often occurs in MS clients, but it is not clear whether depression is a reaction to disability or a function of the disease itself.[1]

DIAGNOSTIC ASSESSMENT

Because there is no definitive test for MS, clinicians rely on a detailed history, clinical findings, and a variety of diagnostic tests. The history should reveal at least two episodes of neurologic dysfunction, separated in time and in different locations in the CNS. Diagnostic tests include spinal fluid evaluation for the presence of oligoclonal banding, evoked potentials of the optic pathways and auditory system to assess presence of slowed nerve conduction, and MRI of the brain and spinal cord to determine the presence of MS plaques.

Medical Management

Several treatments for MS have been tested, but because many clients experience spontaneous remission within days to weeks, the effects of treatment are difficult to evaluate. Corticosteroids, which have both anti-inflammatory and immunosuppressive properties, are often used to enhance recovery from an exacerbation. These include adrenocorticotropic hormone and prednisone. Despite the popularity of these therapies, clear evidence of their efficacy does not exist.[8] Likewise, there is no convincing evidence that either cyclophosphamide (Cytoxan), an alkylating agent with broad immunosuppressive properties, or plasma exchange is an effective treatment for chronic progressive MS.[8]

Interferon-β_{1b} (Betaseron) may be of benefit for clients with exacerbating remitting MS. A recently completed multicenter study of the effectiveness of Betaseron has demonstrated that alternative-day subcutaneous injection is effective in reducing the rate and severity of exacerbations in clients and in decreasing the size of MS plaques in the CNS. The effect of Betaseron on progressive MS is currently being studied. The mechanism of action is unknown. Unfortunately, the limited supply of medication and the expense have limited the number of clients who can be treated with Betaseron.[16]

Several strategies are available for the variety of complications that occur with MS.[6] Interventions for bladder and bowel dysfunction, fatigue, weakness, spasticity, and ataxia are described later under the nursing diagnoses. Areas of numbness should be inspected regularly to prevent injury and development of pressure ulcers. Skin should be kept dry and free of urine and feces. A pressure-distributing seat cushion should be used for wheelchair-bound clients with insensate buttock skin. Some clients may experience painful dysesthesias or pain syndromes like trigeminal neuralgia. Drugs like carbamazepine (Tegretol), phenytoin (Dilantin), and amitriptyline (Elavil) are often helpful. Transcutaneous electrical stimulation is also helpful. Blindness or severely impaired vision may occur and will require referral to services for the blind for rehabilitation. Cognitive and perceptual impairment necessitates psychometric and functional testing for accurate assessment and rehabilitation services.

Nursing Management

Assessment

If the client is being assessed for possible MS, the nurse should assess the client for clinical manifestations of the disorder. Ocular symptoms are very common. Likewise, as a result of the fluctuations of clinical manifestations, the client may report a history of similar findings that went away.

If the client is being hospitalized for an exacerbation of MS, the nurse should focus on the client's ability to perform ADLs as well as other areas that require fine motor movements. Gross motor activities such as walking may also be impaired and lead to problems with bowel and bladder continence.

Nursing Diagnosis, Planning, and Implementation

Nursing Diagnosis: Urinary Elimination, Altered R/T bladder dysfunction.

Planning: Expected Outcomes. The client will maintain urinary continence and normal bladder filling, as evidenced by residual volumes of less than 100 mL, application of appropriate bladder-elimination procedures, and verbalization of personal satisfaction with urinary elimination status.

Implementation. The following interventions are for neurogenic bladder, the most common type of bladder dysfunction in MS. Fluid intake should be maintained at 2000 mL/24 hr (ideally, 400 to 500 mL with each meal and 200 mL at midmorning, midafternoon, and late afternoon). Avoidance of fluid intake after the evening meal reduces the need for bladder emptying during the night. Voiding should be attempted every 3 hours during waking hours. If voiding is not successful, a catheter should be inserted into the bladder and then removed once emptying is complete. This is called *intermittent catheterization.* If the volume of catheterized urine exceeds 500 mL, the catheterization schedule may need to be more frequent. The client should be instructed on how to perform self-catheterization if he or she is capable. A clean red rubber catheter can be reused for up to 1 week as long as it is washed thoroughly with soap and water and placed in a clean, tightly sealed plastic bag after every catheterization. Sterile equipment is not required for ongoing self-catheterization.

Nursing Diagnosis: Constipation R/T immobility and demyelination.

Planning: Expected Outcomes. The client will have bowel movements of normal consistency and frequency.

Implementation. A high-fiber diet, bulk formers, and stool softeners are useful for maintaining stool consistency. Adequate fluid intake also assists bowel elimination; 2000 mL should be taken. Laxatives and enemas should be avoided. A bowel program should be performed every other day, approximately 45 minutes after the largest meal, to take advantage of the gastrocolic reflex. Rectal evacuation may be augmented by the use of glycerin or bisacodyl (Dulcolax) suppositories or digital stimulation.

Nursing Diagnosis: Activity Intolerance R/T fatigue.

Planning: Expected Outcomes. The client will demonstrate improved activity tolerance, as evidenced by maintaining a balance among work, rest, and exercise and recreation; performing ADLs without excessive fatigue; using energy-saving devices and techniques; avoiding elevations in environmental and body temperatures; and consuming a diet adequate in calories and protein for body size, frame, and age.

Implementation. Because fatigue can be precipitated by warm temperatures, the environment should be kept cool. If air conditioning is unavailable, cool baths and ice packs may help lower body temperature.

The nurse should assist the client to plan activities at his or her peak energy level, which is usually in the morning. This schedule promotes optimal synchrony between circadian rhythms and the client's physical demands. The client should plan for periods of rest throughout the day. Collaboration with the physical and occupational therapists can reveal methods to reduce energy consumption with repeated tasks and apply adaptive devices for ambulation and toileting. The drug amantadine (Symmetrel) may alleviate fatigue in some clients.

Nursing Diagnosis: Physical Mobility, Impaired R/T spasticity, ataxia, weakness, and contractures.

Planning: Expected Outcomes. The client will achieve optimal physical mobility, as evidenced by improved or maintained range of motion in all joints, optimal control of spasticity, and effective use of adaptive aids.

Implementation. Although some clients are bothered by painful muscle spasms, others may rely on spasticity to stabilize weak limbs during transfers and ambulation. Spastic muscles must be stretched at least twice daily through their full range of motion. The drug baclofen (Lioresal) provides synaptic inhibition of spinal reflexes, which can reduce spasticity, although it can increase weakness and fatigue in some clients. Diazepam (Valium) and dantrolene (Dantrium) are other antispasmotic drugs. Surgical intervention or nerve blocks may be necessary if contractures develop.

Strengthening exercises for muscle weakness (paresis) must be done with caution because they can aggravate paresis by causing muscle fatigue. However, selective strengthening of nonaffected or less affected muscles can enhance physical function and well-being. Range-of-motion exercises should be performed at least twice daily. Active movement is preferable to passive movement. Correct body alignment should be maintained to reduce the risk of contractures. Splints may help maintain position and provide support for weak hands and ankles. Ataxia and tremor of the extremities can be lessened by the use of small weights applied to the distal extremities or the use of weighted utensils. Weakness and fatigue can aggravate ataxia. Ambulation aids such as a cane or a walker may be necessary.

Nursing Diagnosis: Self-Esteem Disturbance R/T loss of independence and fear of disability.

Planning: Expected Outcomes. The client will achieve improved self-concept, as evidenced by verbalizing awareness that personal goals and body image will need to be adjusted, willingness to maintain appropriate independence, and positive self-thoughts and statements about self.

Implementation. Regardless of the cause of disturbance in self-concept, the nurse should carefully assess the individual and family history for presence and type of depressive episodes and the clinical manifestations. Previous treatment for depression should be identified, including psychotherapy and drug therapy. By assessing the client's problem-solving strategies, the nurse can identify coping behavior strengths and defense mechanisms such as denial, avoidance, or intellectualization that the client may use to mask depression. The client's social support system should also be evaluated because this contributes to his or her sense of well-being. Grieving the loss of function in MS can lead to a reactive depression and require provision of support group therapy for both the client and family. Some clients may not benefit from this kind of therapy, however, because they may see people whose condition is much worse than their own and may fear experiencing that level of disability.

EVALUATION

The degree of expected outcome attainment should be evaluated on an ongoing basis. Most outcomes are long term and may require weeks to months to attain.

Posthospital Care

The client with MS needs to have a clear understanding about the unpredictableness of this disorder. The client may be symptom free for many weeks to months, even years, and then experience further symptoms. If the client can identify stressors that exacerbate the symptoms, sometimes these stressors can then be avoided.

HOME HEALTH CARE

Clients experiencing a decline in self-care abilities may require aids to perform ADLs and ambulate, such as wheelchairs or canes. The performance of ADLs may be enhanced if the counters and table tops are adjusted to a comfortable working height. The nurse works in combination with the physical therapist, occupational therapist, social worker, and home health nurse to identify, purchase, and teach the client how to use ADL aids.

PARKINSON'S DISEASE

Parkinson's disease (PD) is an idiopathic syndrome characterized by disability from tremor and rigidity. PD involves degeneration of dopamine-producing cells in the substantia nigra, which leads to degeneration of neurons in the basal ganglia. Once cell loss in the substantia nigra reaches 80 per cent, symptoms appear. The cause of nigral cell degeneration is not known.

PD most often develops in people in their 60s. It occurs worldwide. About 1 per cent of people older than 50 years have PD. PD has three cardinal features: tremor, rigidity, and bradykinesia. Early in the disease, the client may notice a slight slowing in the ability to perform ADLs. This is called *bradykinesia.* A general feeling of stiffness (rigidity) may be noticed, along with mild diffuse muscular pain. Tremor is a common early sign that usually occurs in one of the upper limbs. It occurs at rest and involves a coarse "pill-rolling" movement of the thumb against the fingers, which can vary in intensity and distribution. Voluntary movement stops or reduces the tremor in some people; however, others have tremor during voluntary movement (intention tremor).

Bradykinesia makes voluntary movements difficult to execute. When symptoms are severe, total lack of movement (akinesia) may occur and the client is literally frozen in one spot. Bradykinesia also affects the gait. Initially there may be a slight stiffness of one leg while walking, and the corresponding arm may be held flexed at the elbow and abducted at the shoulder. The person may catch or drag one foot. Later, when both sides of the body are involved, the typical shuffling gait with short steps may develop. There is lack of associated swinging of the arms while walking. In advanced PD, the client stands with head, shoulders, and spine flexed forward, giving the appearance of a stooped posture.

The face of someone with advanced PD appears stiff, masklike, and without expression. The speech is low in volume, monotonous in tone, and slow. Words are poorly articulated (dysarthria). Saliva may flow involuntarily from the mouth because of the lack of spontaneous swallowing. Various autonomic effects may accompany PD, including decreased lacrimation (tearing) and sexual capacity, constipation, incontinence, excessive perspiration, and heat intolerance. PD does not usually affect intellectual ability; however, 15 to 20 per cent of PD sufferers do experience a dementia similar to Alzheimer's disease. Mood disturbance can occur, and emotional stress may intensify signs and symptoms.

Management

PHARMACOLOGIC MANAGEMENT

The symptoms of PD can be relieved by various medications, particularly levodopa and anticholinergic drugs. The purpose of these medications is to provide dopamine to the basal ganglia. The most common drug for this purpose is carbidopa-levodopa (Sinemet). Levodopa is a synthetic metabolic precursor of dopamine. Dopamine itself cannot be used because it cannot cross the blood-brain barrier. Carbidopa must be given with levodopa because it prevents peripheral metabolism of levodopa, allowing levodopa to reach the brain. Initiation of carbidopa-levodopa therapy is usually delayed until symptoms affect ADLs because the benefit of the drug seems to decline with prolonged use. The therapy is more effective in treating bradykinesia and rigidity than tremor. The dosage of levodopa is gradually increased until the optimal therapeutic response is achieved. This process may take several months. When the daily dose of levodopa approaches the desired level, the client often has involuntary dyskinesias (jerky, writhing movements), especially of the face, mouth, and tongue. Some clients prefer this state to being severely bradykinetic, because at least they can be mobile and perform voluntary movements more easily. Table 15–4 lists the drugs used in PD.

Occasionally, clients with PD experience parkinsonian crisis as a result of emotional trauma or sudden or inadvertent withdrawal of antiparkinson medication. Severe exacerbation of tremor, rigidity, and bradykinesia, accompanied by acute anxiety, sweating, tachycardia, and hyperpnea, occurs. Intervention for parkinsonian crisis includes respiratory and cardiac support. The person should be placed in a quiet room with subdued lighting. Barbiturates may be prescribed, as well as antiparkinson medication.

An "on-off response" (rapid fluctuation of symptoms) may occur in clients with PD. A person may be mobile and active ("on") one moment and akinetic and rigid ("off") the next. This transition may happen quickly, within 1 to 2 minutes. Initially, the "off" periods tend to occur 3 to 4 hours after a dose of antiparkinson medication. Later, the transition may happen at any time and be unrelated to medication ingestion. Apparently "off" periods are due to dopamine deficit, but this factor is not clear. A person experiencing on–off response may be temporarily helped by shortening the interval between medication doses or by gradually increasing the total dosage.

SURGICAL MANAGEMENT

Surgical intervention is not often used for PD. However, intractable tremor may be improved by thalamotomy. Autologous transplantation of adrenal medullary tissue into the brains of PD clients, in the hope that these cells will produce dopamine, has yielded disappointing results. Fetal tissue transplantation conducted in the United States is very controversial for ethical reasons. Federal funding for this procedure has been put on hold, although some medical centers are doing this procedure with private funds.

Nursing Management

Nursing care for the PD client includes health assessment, medication instruction and monitoring, liaison with other members of the health-care team, and client and family education.[32]

The client should be advised to maintain fluid intake of 2000 mL/24 hr and increase intake of dietary fiber. Stool softeners and mild laxatives can be used. A regular time for bowel movements should be established, usually a half hour after the morning or evening meal.

The client should be taught various techniques to enhance voluntary movement. Clients often need to try different things on their own to find what helps most. Some clients grasp coins in the pocket to reduce embarrassing hand tremor. Others grip the arms of a chair. Mental thoughts, such as walking over imaginary lines, can aid ambulation. Daily range-of-motion exercises should be encouraged to avoid rigidity and contractures. The client should be reminded to maintain good posture and to avoid flexion of the neck and shoulders. The client should sleep on a firm mattress. When resting, the client should avoid using a pillow to prevent flexion of the spine. Periodically lying prone also helps.

Because self-care activities are performed more slowly by the client with PD, extra time should be allowed for completion of tasks like dressing, bathing, and eating. Warming trays can keep food hot. Rest periods should be encouraged during meals to avoid aspiration.

As PD progresses, clients become rigid and unresponsive to verbal stimuli. During these stages, nurses continue to treat the client with dignity, speaking to the client rather than ignoring him or her.

The client should be taught about home safety. Loose carpeting should be removed. Grab bars should be placed in the bathroom. An elevated toilet seat should be installed. Clients with severe tremor should avoid carrying hot liquids. Walking aids such as a cane or walker can provide added stability.

The client and family need emotional support. Support groups are available in most major cities. The client and family can be referred to the Parkinson's Disease Foundation, William Black Medical Research Building, Columbia University Medical Center, 650 West 168th Street, New York, NY 10032, (212) 923-4700.

MYASTHENIA GRAVIS

Myasthenia gravis (MG) is an autoimmune disease that presents as muscular weakness and fatigue that worsens with exercise and improves with rest. It is caused by loss of acetylcholine (ACh) receptors in the postsynaptic neurons of the neuromuscular junction. The cause of MG is unknown, but 80 per cent of people with the generalized form of the disease have elevated titers of antibodies to the ACh receptor in their serum. MG may appear at any age, although there are two peaks of onset. In early-onset MG, at age 20 to 30 years, women

TABLE 15–4 Pharmacologic Management of Parkinson's Disease

DRUG CLASSIFICATION AND EXAMPLE	ACTION	INDICATIONS	COMMON SIDE EFFECTS	NURSING IMPLICATIONS
Anticholinergics				
Trihexyphenidyl (Artane) Benztropine (Cogentin) Procyclidine (Kemadrin) Ethopropazine (Parsidol)	Inhibit action of endogenous acetylcholine and muscarine agonists to block the excitatory effect of the cholinergic system	Tremor, rigidity, drooling	Dry mouth, constipation, blurred vision, confusion, hallucination	Usually contraindicated in clients with acute-angle glaucoma and tachycardia; monitor pulse and blood pressure during periods of dosage adjustment; administer with meals; do not withdraw medication suddenly
Antihistamines				
Diphenhydramine (Benadryl)	Mild anticholinergic	Tremor, rigidity, insomnia	Dry mouth, lethargy, confusion	Use with caution in clients with seizures, hypertension, hyperthyroidism, heart and renal disease, and diabetes; administer with meals or antacids
Dopaminergics				
Amantadine (Symmetrel)	Cause the release of dopamine in the central nervous system	Rigidity, bradykinesia	Dizziness, ataxia insomnia, leg edema	Monitor client for postural hypotension; do not administer at bedtime
Carbidopa/levodopa (Sinemet)		Tremor, rigidity, bradykinesia	Orthostatic hypotension, nausea, hallucinations, dystonia, dyskinesias	Monitor blood pressure; use elastic stockings to increase venous return; monitor client for urinary retention
Dopamine Agonists				
Bromocriptine (Parlodel)	Activate dopamine receptors in the central nervous system	Fluctuation of symptoms, dyskinesia, dystonia	Hallucinations, mental fogginess, orthostatic hypotension, confusion	Monitor blood pressure and mental status
Pergolide (Permax)			Orthostatic hypotension, nausea, insomnia	Monitor blood pressure; do not administer at bedtime
Monoamine Oxidase Inhibitors				
Selegiline (Deprenyl)	Inhibit monamine oxidase B, an enzyme that converts chemical by-products in the brain into neurotoxins that prevent substantia nigra cell death	Adjuvant treatment	Being researched; look up side effects	Being researched; look up recent information on use

are more often affected than men. In late-onset MG, after age 50, men are more often affected.

The primary feature of MG is increasing weakness with sustained muscle contraction. For instance, if the person is asked to hold the arms up, the power of muscle contraction diminishes and the arms gradually drift downward. After a period of rest, the muscles regain their strength. Muscle weakness is greatest after exertion or at the end of the day. Ocular symptoms are most common, with ptosis (drooping of the upper eyelid) or diplopia (double vision) occurring in the majority of clients. Other symptoms are weakness of the orbicularis oculi muscles (which help close the eye), the facial muscles, the muscles of chewing and swallowing, and the limbs. Weakness of the facial and levator palpebrae muscles produces an expressionless face, with droopy eyelids, smoothed features, and a tendency for the mouth to hang open. An attempt to smile often turns into a snarl because of the weakness. A client may hold a hand under the jaw to keep it closed. Dysphagia and a nasal quality to speech occur when the muscles of chewing and swallowing are involved. In severe cases, respiratory muscle weakness may occur, which may necessitate intubation and mechanical ventilation (see discussion of myasthenic crisis in complications).

The course of MG varies, and there may be remissions and exacerbations. Clinical manifestations may progress quickly or slowly and may fluctuate from day to day. The severity of the disease varies greatly from person to person.

The diagnosis of MG is based on the clinical presentation. It can be confirmed by testing the client's response to anticholinesterase drugs. These drugs inhibit cholinesterase, an enzyme that breaks down ACh in the neuromuscular junction, thereby allowing more ACh to bind to the remaining ACh receptors. Edrophonium (Tensilon) is a short-acting drug that is given intravenously. A test dose of 2 mg (for adults) is injected first. If no untoward reaction occurs (such as increased weakness, change in heart rate or rhythm, nausea, or abdominal cramps), the remaining 8 mg is injected. The client is then observed for objective signs of improvement in muscle strength. The effect is transitory, wearing off after 3 to 5 minutes. Another drug, neostigmine methylsulfate (Prostigmin), may be used because the longer duration of effect on muscle strength (1–2 hours) allows better analysis of its effect. When either drug is used, atropine sulfate should be available to inject intravenously. This medication counteracts any severe cholinergic reactions (cardiac arrhythmias or abdominal cramping). Electromyography (EMG) helps confirm the diagnosis. Repetitive stimulation of the nerve with recording from the involved muscle shows a characteristic decrementing response of the muscle action potential.

Medical Management

There is no cure for MG. Pharmacologic intervention consists of two groups of medications: (1) short-acting anticholinesterase compounds and (2) corticosteroids. The most effective anticholinesterase drugs are pyridostigmine (Mestinon) and neostigmine (Prostigmin). Dosages are highly individualized, based on physiologic response to the medication. The goal is to achieve the maximum benefit (muscle strength and endurance) with the least side effects (excessive salivation, sweating, nausea, diarrhea, abdominal cramps, or tachycardia). Corticosteroids (usually prednisone) are directed toward reducing the levels of serum ACh receptor antibodies. However, clinical improvement can occur when there has been no significant decrease in antibodies, so this cannot be the sole mode of steroid action.[23] Corticosteroids may temporarily worsen symptoms; however, this is followed by gradual improvement in muscle strength. After a peak of improvement is reached and maintained for several weeks, the dosage of both prednisone and anticholinesterase medication may be gradually decreased. A low maintenance dose of alternate-day prednisone may be effective for many months or years. The precautions of any steroid therapy are important, including potassium supplements if indicated and liberal use of antacids. Potential complications of steroid use are cataracts, hypertension, diabetes, fluid retention, delayed wound healing, insomnia, and osteoporosis.

Complications

Two major complications of MG may occur. In *myasthenic crisis,* clients with moderate or severe generalized MG, especially those who have difficulty swallowing or breathing, may experience a sudden worsening of their condition. This is usually precipitated by an intercurrent infection, but it may occur spontaneously. If an increase in the dosage of the anticholinesterase drug does not improve the weakness, endotracheal intubation and mechanical ventilation may be required. In many instances, drug responsiveness returns in 24 to 48 hours, and weaning from the respirator can proceed.[3]

The other major complication of MG, *cholinergic crisis,* results from overmedication. The muscarinic effect of a toxic level of anticholinesterase medication causes abdominal cramps, diarrhea, and excessive pulmonary secretions. The nicotinic effect paradoxically worsens weakness and can cause bronchial spasm. If respiratory status is compromised, the client may need intubation and mechanical ventilation, and treatment is similar to that of the client in myasthenic crisis. Table 15–5 outlines the features and interventions of cholinergic and myasthenic crises.

Plasmapheresis is an adjunctive therapy for clients with refractory MG. It is a process by which plasma is separated from formed elements of blood. The plasma is discarded and the packed red cells are joined with albumin, normal saline, and electrolytes and returned to the client. The purpose is to remove plasma proteins containing antibodies that are believed to cause MG. Plasmapheresis produces transient improvement in clients who have actual or pending respiratory failure. Usually three to five treatments are required.[3] Potential complications include myasthenic or cholinergic crisis and, rarely, hypovolemia. Muscle strength should be assessed before and after the procedure, with particular attention paid to vital capacity, swallowing ability, diplopia, and ptosis to evaluate the effectiveness of the treatment.

Another intervention for MG is thymectomy. The thymus gland, located in the superior mediastinum, is important during fetal development for development of the immune system. It is usually atrophied and nonfunctioning in adulthood. The effect of thymectomy is not fully understood. It may alter some immunologic control mechanism that affects the production of antibodies to the ACh receptor, or it may eliminate a trigger to antibody production.[22]

TABLE 15–5 Myasthenic and Cholinergic Crises in Clients Experiencing Myasthenia Gravis

Myasthenic Crisis Is Caused by Undermedication
Clinical Manifestations
Sudden marked rise in blood pressure caused by hypoxia
Increased heart rate
Severe respiratory distress and cyanosis
Absent cough and swallow reflex
Increased secretions, increased diaphoresis, increased lacrimation
Restlessness, dysarthria
Bowel and bladder incontinence
Intervention
Increased doses of cholinergic drugs as long as the person responds positively to Tensilon treatment
Possible mechanical ventilation if respiratory muscle paralysis is acute
Cholinergic Crisis Is Caused by Depolarization Block Resulting from Excessive Medications
Clinical Manifestations
Weakness with difficulty swallowing, chewing, speaking, and breathing
Apprehension, nausea, and vomiting
Abdominal cramps, diarrhea
Increased secretions and saliva
Sweating, lacrimation, fasciculations, blurred vision
Intervention
Discontinue all cholinergic drugs until cholinergic effects decrease
Provide adequate ventilatory support
1 mg IV of atropine may be necessary to counteract severe cholinergic reactions

IV, Intravenous.

Nursing Management

Clients with MG are usually managed in an outpatient setting. When they are hospitalized for diagnosis or during a crisis, the following nursing management procedure may be pertinent.

Because MG may involve the muscles of respiration, the client may experience dyspnea and ineffective cough and swallow mechanisms. This may lead to aspiration and pneumonia. Deep breathing and coughing should be encouraged. Suction equipment should be available at the bedside, and the client should be instructed on how to use it. When eating, the client should be instructed to sit upright, swallow only when the chin is tipped downward toward the chest, and never speak while food is in the mouth. Oxygen and, in severe cases, mechanical ventilation may be required for some clients.

In MG, weakness is usually greatest after exertion and at the end of the day. Activities should be carefully planned to include rest periods so that energy is conserved and the muscles have a chance to regain their strength. Rearrangement of the home environment may help prevent unnecessary energy expenditure. Vocational retraining may be indicated for those who can no longer meet the physical demands of their jobs. Clients with severe disease or an acute exacerbation will be totally dependent on nursing care for ADLs. This level of care requires that complications of immobility be avoided.

The client and family should be provided with information about MG and its treatment. They should be aware of adverse reactions of both anticholinesterase drugs and steroids and should be taught that timing of anticholinesterase medication is critical. It is important to instruct the client to administer the medication on time to maintain a chemical balance at the neuromuscular junction. If the medication is not given on time, the client may be too weak to swallow. They also should know how to recognize myasthenic and cholinergic crises and have a plan to seek medical intervention, if necessary. The Myasthenia Gravis Foundation, 53 West Jackson Boulevard, Suite 660, Chicago, IL 60604, publishes educational materials that can be helpful to the client and family. The number is (202) 546-0807.

AMYOTROPHIC LATERAL SCLEROSIS

Amyotrophic lateral sclerosis (ALS) is the most common of the motor neuron diseases. The onset of ALS usually occurs in middle age. Men are affected more often than women. ALS involves degeneration of both the anterior horn cells and the corticospinal tracts. Consequently, both upper and lower motor neuron clinical manifestations are seen. Lower motor neuron clinical manifestations include weakness, atrophy, cramps, and fasciculations (irregular twitchings of muscle fibers or bundles). Upper motor neuron signs include spasticity and hyperreflexia. Involvement of the corticobulbar tracts causes dysphagia (difficulty swallowing) and dysarthria (slurred speech). The sensory system is not involved.

The course of the disease is relentlessly progressive. Death usually results from pneumonia caused by respiratory compromise within 2 to 5 years. Weakness typically begins in the upper extremities and progressively involves the upper arms and shoulders and then the muscles of the neck and throat. The trunk and lower extremities are usually not affected until late in the disease. When the intercostal muscles and diaphragm become involved, respirations become shallow and coughing is ineffective. Cognition as well as bowel and bladder sphincters remain intact, even when the client is totally debilitated. In some cases, weakness begins in the brain stem, causing problems with speech and swallowing. This is called *bulbar ALS*.

Diagnosis of ALS is made by the clinical presentation and EMG. EMG criteria for the diagnosis of ALS include the presence of widespread anterior horn cell dysfunction with fibrillations, positive waves, fasciculations, and chronic neurogenic motor unit potential changes in multiple nerve root distribution in at least three limbs and the paraspinal muscles in the presence of normal sensory responses.[20]

Management

Supportive therapy is the only intervention for ALS. Results of therapeutic trials have been depressingly negative.[20] Clients with ALS are usually admitted to health-care facilities only twice in their illness, first for diagnosis and later in the final stage of debilitation.

Supportive nursing care is an important aspect of managing the ALS client. In the outpatient arena, the nurse can provide ongoing assessment of daily living needs and make suggestions for modifications in activity level, clothing, and diet. Often, just allowing the client or family to talk about problems reduces anxiety and helps them find solutions to problems. Interventions should be aimed at conserving energy. Activities should be spaced during the day. Muscle stress, strenuous activity, and extremes of hot and cold should be avoided. Leg braces, canes, and walkers can prolong independence in ambulation. Hand braces, special utensils, and adaptive devices such as button hooks can enhance dressing and self-feeding. Pressure ulcers are not usually a problem because the sensory system remains intact and the client can feel when pressure on a body part is too great.

In the acute care setting, the nurse should gather information from the client and family about communication needs and what positions are best for respiration, handling secretions, eating, and turning routines.[31]

Fluid intake should be encouraged regularly, when the client is not fatigued. Proper positioning is imperative. Providing a cup with a spout may prevent liquid from running out of the corners of the mouth. Liquids may be given by using a large syringe with short tubing on the tip. The tube is placed at the back of the tongue, and gentle force is used to deliver small amounts of liquid.

Small, frequent, high-nutrient feedings should be encouraged. The client should be told to sit upright, with the head slightly flexed forward while eating. Papase tablets placed under the tongue 10 minutes before meals can make thick saliva less sticky. Plenty of time should be allowed for eating, and the client should not attempt to speak while food is in the mouth. Suction equipment should be available during meals to reduce the risk of aspiration of food and secretions that become lodged in the mouth and pharynx. The head may need to be stabilized by placing a soft cervical collar on the neck. The dietitian should be consulted for special diet recommendations.

Although speech remains intelligible, the client can be trained to slow the rate of speech and exaggerate articulation. As symptoms progress, the client may need to repeat words or have an interpreter (usually the spouse). At this stage, it is important to eliminate extraneous noise, face the client when he or she is talking, and maintain eye contact. When speech contains only one-word phrases or is no longer possible, writing can be an effective means of communicating and should be encouraged. When writing is no longer possible, a speech pathologist can provide communication devices such as alphabet boards and portable memo writers.[10]

If the client is a smoker, he or she should be encouraged to stop. Exposure to people with respiratory infections should be avoided. The client should be reminded to use good posture. Pulmonary function tests should be performed regularly to assess ventilatory status. Clients generally experience respiratory fatigue when vital capacity is less than 1.5 L. Some clients can be taught to use abdominal muscles to enhance respirations when the intercostal muscles and diaphragm become weak. A sign of pending respiratory insufficiency is shortness of breath while eating.

The client and family should be encouraged to talk about the losses they are experiencing and the feelings associated with them. Family members should be encouraged to take time for rest and activities away from the client. The client and family can be referred to an ALS support group.

Eventually, clients face the difficult choice of deciding whether or not they will accept artificial ventilation. They should be encouraged to discuss this with family and friends and to seek input from ALS support groups. Information about these groups can be obtained from the Amyotrophic Lateral Sclerosis Association, 21021 Ventura Boulevard, Suite 321, Woodland Hills, CA 91364, (818) 990-2151, or the Muscular Dystrophy Association, 810 Seventh Avenue, New York, NY 10019, (212) 586-0808.

Clients should be encouraged to complete advance directives to indicate whether they desire life-sustaining treatments such as cardiopulmonary resuscitation, but this should be reassessed at regular intervals. Clients may change their minds on the basis of their experience with their illness, changes in their subjective appreciation of their quality of life, or changes in their evaluation of the benefits and burdens of life-sustaining measures as they realize the imminence of death.[27]

HUNTINGTON'S DISEASE

Huntington's disease (HD), also known as Huntington's chorea, is a genetically transmitted degenerative neurologic disease. It is characterized by abnormal movements (chorea), intellectual decline, and emotional disturbance. Clinical manifestations usually begin in the fourth and fifth decades, although occasionally they begin in young adulthood or even in children. Women and men are equally affected. The disease is relentlessly progressive, leading to disability and death within 15 to 20 years. Death usually results from respiratory complications caused by aspiration.

The disease is autosomal dominant, meaning that offspring of an affected person have a 50 per cent chance of inheriting the disease. Because HD does not skip generations, offspring who have not inherited the disease will not pass it on to their offspring. New developments in molecular biology and linkage analysis of inherited diseases have identified that the abnormal gene for HD lies on the short arm of chromosome 4.[9]

The pathology of HD involves degeneration of the striatum (caudate and putamen) in the basal ganglia.

ETHICAL ISSUES IN NURSING

In Revealing Information About Huntington's Disease, Which Should Take Precedence: Client Confidentiality or Beneficence?

Huntington's disease is a degenerative neurologic disorder that is autosomal dominant and afflicts 50 per cent of an affected parent's offspring. The disease usually appears in the 30- to 40-year age range, bringing on irreversible dementia that leads to death within approximately 10 years after onset. The disease, at present, is incurable. Often a parent has had children before he or she knows he or she has the disease. Currently, there are diagnostic tests that detect the disease long before symptoms are present. Because offspring of a parent with Huntington's disease have a 50 per cent chance of acquiring it, early testing may assist them in their own decision to procreate. One dilemma that could surface from this would be whether or not the results of testing were positive, the person has a duty to disclose the results to his or her spouse, children, fiancé, or significant other.

Several ethical principles must be considered in this case. First, there is confidentiality. A person has the right not to have medical information disclosed to anyone unless he or she consents to do so. Is this right absolute even if it means that others may be harmed by such confidentiality? The American Nurses' Association code states that there is a duty of veracity (i.e., to tell the truth and not to deceive others). If a family member asks the nurse if another family member has a positive test for Huntington's chorea, what should the nurse do? Is there any duty of beneficence toward family members in disclosing information that could ultimately affect their own lives?

The profession of nursing is one that assists others in maintaining or improving their health status. Information gathered from diagnostic tests can greatly influence the treatment decisions of health-care providers. Information regarding a positive test for Huntington's disease may assist in the counseling of those family members at risk for acquiring the disease. However, if information is withheld from those family members, counseling may not be given. Nurses must be sensitive to their client's desire for confidentiality, but should also use this opportunity to teach their client about the effect the disease may have on other family members.

Other subtle changes occur in the cortex and cerebellum, namely, loss of neurons and an increased number of glial cells (gliosis). The degeneration of the caudate nucleus leads to a reduction in several neurotransmitters, including gamma-aminobutyric acid, ACh, substance P, and met-enkephalin, and their synthetic enzymes. This leaves relatively higher concentrations of the other neurotransmitters, dopamine and norepinephrine.

The abnormal movements in HD are subtle at first. The person may appear restless or fidgety. The person may be aware of these movements and try to mask them by making them seem to be parts of intentional movements, such as head scratching or leg crossing. As the disease progresses, the rapid, jerky choreiform movements become more pronounced and involve all muscles. The person is constantly in motion. Stress, emotional situations, and attempts to perform voluntary movement can aggravate the abnormal movements. During sleep, the movements diminish or disappear.

Emotional disturbances and mental deterioration may precede the abnormal movements. The person may become negative, suspicious, and irritable. This condition may progress to depression and psychosis. Temper outbursts and sexual promiscuity may also occur. Severe mood swings are common. Cognitive decline progresses, and eventually, the person becomes demented, unkempt, incontinent, and completely helpless.

The diagnosis of HD is made on the basis of clinical signs and symptoms and family history, because there is no specific diagnostic test for the disease itself. CT or MRI imaging of the brain may show atrophy of the head of the caudate, but this factor alone is not diagnostic of HD.

Management

There is no known treatment to cure or alter the course of HD. Haloperidol (Haldol), a dopamine blocker, can control the abnormal movements and some behavioral manifestations. Diazepam (Valium) can be used to lower anxiety, aiding in control of movements. Antidepressants can help depression.

One of the most common and dangerous middle- to late-stage problems is dysphagia. Several interventions should be tried.[11] Medications need to be evaluated for their anticholinergic and sedative effects, which may impair swallowing. Mealtime should be free of stress and clutter and have an unhurried atmosphere. Use of adaptive eating utensils can encourage and extend independence in eating. The diet should include foods that are easy to swallow, those that form a bolus in the mouth (e.g., canned peaches, chopped meat in gravy and mashed potatoes, custards). Because many clients with HD require high caloric intake because of excessive movements, they should try eating frequent, small meals containing high-calorie foods. Clients should sit upright while eating. While swallowing they should keep the chin down toward the chest. They can be trained to hold their breath before swallowing and cough after each mouthful is swallowed to clear the throat of any residual food.

If the client continues to have difficulty eating and loses weight despite dietary and environmental modifications, a feeding tube may become necessary. However, artificial feeding methods can often frighten families and represent ethical dilemmas about prolonging life. Nurses can help clients and their families make these difficult decisions by clarifying the issues and providing information on the types, risks, benefits, and long-term effects of artificial feeding methods.[11]

Poor control of oral and respiratory muscles can make communication difficult. The nurse can assist the family to develop signals such as raising a hand or keeping the eyes open or closed for yes-no responses. If physical signals are not an option, cards with printed words may be helpful. Keep communication simple and unstrained. Repeat words that are understood to let the client know that communication has been successful.

Excessive movements and falls may cause physical injury and can decrease independence. Pads on wheelchairs and beds, shin guards, and walking belts can prevent injury. Aids for ambulation (e.g., walking behind a wheelchair) can extend independence. Clothing should be light and simple to get on and off.

HD has a major impact on the family, not only because of the burden of care giving but also because of the risk to offspring of inheriting the disease (see Ethical Issues in Nursing). The discovery of linked polymorphic DNA markers for HD has led to the development of predictive testing programs. These programs can modify the risk of having inherited the gene, from 50 per cent to as high as 95 or as low as 5 per cent. However, the marker test requires blood samples from multiple family members and is costly.[12]

GUILLAIN-BARRÉ SYNDROME

Guillain-Barré syndrome (GBS) is an inflammatory disease of unknown cause that involves degeneration of the myelin sheath of peripheral nerves. GBS is seen worldwide and affects people of all ages and races. Since the virtual elimination of poliomyelitis, GBS has become the most common cause of acute generalized paralysis, with an annual incidence of 0.75 to 2 cases per 100,000 population. In one half to two thirds of cases, an upper respiratory or gastrointestinal infection precedes the onset of the syndrome by 1 to 4 weeks. Cytomegalovirus and Epstein-Barr virus have been implicated in these antecedent illnesses, as have *Mycoplasma pneumoniae, Salmonella typhosa,* and *Campylobacter jejuni.* An association between human immunodeficiency virus (HIV) and GBS has also been reported, so clients with GBS should be tested for HIV.

The characteristic feature of GBS is ascending weakness, usually beginning in the lower extremities and spreading, sometimes rapidly, to the trunk, upper extremities, and even the face. The weakness evolves over days to weeks, with maximal deficit by 4 weeks in 90 per cent of cases. Deep tendon reflexes are lost. Paresthesia (tingling sensation) in the limbs may occur early in the course of the illness. Deep, aching muscle pain in the shoulder girdle and thighs is common. The two most dangerous features of the disease are respiratory muscle weakness and autonomic neuropathy involving both the sympathetic and parasympathetic systems. The latter feature can involve orthostatic hypotension, hypertension, pupillary disturbances, sweating dysfunction, cardiac dysrhythmias, paralytic ileus, and urinary retention. Improvement and recovery occur with remyelination. However, if nerve axons are damaged, some residual deficits may remain. Recovery is usually maximal at 6 months, although severe cases may take up to 2 years for maximal recovery. Fortunately, 85 to 90 per cent of clients with GBS recover completely.

Diagnosis of GBS is based on history and physical examination, cerebrospinal fluid (CSF) examination, and electrophysiologic studies. The CSF contains increased protein, with few or no white cells. Nerve conduction velocity is slowed, although it may be normal in the early stage of the illness. "Conduction block," a diminution in amplitude or an absence of elicited muscle action potentials from stimulation of a peripheral nerve, also occurs.

Management

The focus of therapy is supportive care. Respiratory or cardiovascular status must be monitored carefully. This includes vital signs, serial measurement of vital capacity, peripheral oxygen saturation, and electrocardiography. When vital capacity falls to 15 mL/kg of body weight, intubation and artificial ventilation are usually necessary. Plasmapheresis accelerates recovery, although the exact mechanism for this effect is not known (hypotheses include the removal of circulating antibodies or other humoral myelinotoxic or immunopathogenic factors[5]). Gamma-globulin infusion may prove to be the treatment of choice because of its ease and rapidity of administration and its relative safety, even in unstable patients.[26] However, further research must be performed.

Interventions to control infection and prevent complications of immobility are important. Proper body alignment should be maintained to prevent deformities and injury to paralyzed limbs. Once the client's condition has stabilized, rehabilitative interventions can be implemented.

The nurse also assists the client to cope with the progressive nature of GBS. During the early stages, clients are frightened because each day their paralysis has climbed upward. They are often admitted to an acute care agency with progressive weakness and within days are completely paralyzed. Clients fear they will never recover. Nurses assist clients in verbalizing their fears and offer support and encouragement that although the disorder is progressive, most clients gain full recovery. Encouragement is not hollow, however. The client is not taught to expect immediate resolution but is assisted to realize the usual time frames for recovery.

STUDY QUESTIONS

1. A 76-year-old client with stage I dementia of the Alzheimer's type frequently talks about playing with his brothers during his childhood. Which of the following actions by the nurse is most appropriate?
   A. Frequently reorient the client to time and place.
   B. Listen to his stories, allowing the client to reminisce.
   C. Distract the client by asking him what he ate for breakfast.
   D. Place the client in a less stimulating environment.
2. The nurse knows that clients with multiple sclerosis (MS) experience a variety of symptoms. Which of the following is atypical of MS?
   A. Double vision
   B. Sudden bursts of energy
   C. Weakness in the extremities
   D. Urinary retention
3. Which of the following neurologic findings would the nurse find when assessing the client with Parkinson's disease?
   A. Masklike expression and drooling
   B. Hyperreflexia and jerking movements of the arms
   C. Decreased mental capacity and confusion
   D. Flaccid extremities and decreased range of motion
4. In planning the care for a client with myasthenia gravis, which of the following nursing interventions is most appropriate?
   A. Arrange activities to include rest periods so that energy is conserved.
   B. Schedule physical therapy just before mealtime.
   C. Allow the client to delay anticholinesterase medications if sleeping.
   D. Perform active and passive range-of-motion exercises to the point of fatigue.
5. Which of the following clinical manifestations would the nurse expect to find in a client diagnosed with Guillain-Barré syndrome?
   A. Disorientation to time and place
   B. Ascending weakness, beginning in the lower extremities
   C. Hyperreflexia
   D. Loss of sensation

CRITICAL THINKING EXERCISES

SCENARIO A

A 72-year-old client has lived with her daughter and son-in-law since being diagnosed with Alzheimer's disease 1 year ago. Lately, she has become increasingly confused at night, often getting lost trying to find the bathroom. She often becomes hostile and angry when unable to find misplaced objects, often accusing her son-in-law of taking them.

1. What safety precautions should be taken to prevent injury?
2. What interventions can be used to decrease wandering at night to find the bathroom?
3. What interventions can be used when the client is hostile or angry?

SCENARIO B

A 32-year-old client has been recently diagnosed with multiple sclerosis (MS). The client complains of weakness and tingling in the lower extremities, fatigue, and urinary difficulty.

1. What is the usual course of MS?
2. What interventions can be used to combat fatigue?
3. What interventions promote self-esteem in clients with MS?

BIBLIOGRAPHY

1. Acorn, S., & Andersen, S. (1990). Depression in multiple sclerosis: Critique of the research literature. *Journal of Neuroscience Nursing, 22(4),* 209–214.
2. Bartol, M. (1979). Nonverbal communication in patients with Alzheimer's disease. *Journal of Gerontological Nursing, 5(4),* 21–31.
3. Chipps, E. (1991). Myasthenia Gravis: The patient in crisis. *Critical Care Nurse, 7,* 18–26.
4. Cummings, J. L., & Benson, D. F. (1992). *Dementia, a clinical approach.* Boston: Butterworth-Heinemann.
5. England, J. D. (1990). Guillain-Barré syndrome. *Annual Review of Medicine, 41,* 1–6.
6. Erickson, R. P., Lie, M. R., & Wineinger, M. A. (1989). Rehabilitation in multiple sclerosis. *Mayo Clinic Proceedings, 64(7),* 818–828.
7. Evans, D. A., et al. (1989). Prevalence of Alzheimer's disease in a community population of older persons. *Journal of the American Medical Association, 262(18),* 2552–2556.
8. Goodin, D. S. (1991). The use of immunosuppressive agents in the treatment of multiple sclerosis: A critical review. *Neurology, 41(7),* 980–985.
9. Gusella, J. F., et al. (1983). A polymorphic marker genetically linked to Huntington's disease. *Nature, 306(5940),* 234–238.

10. Hillel, A. D., & Miller, R. (1989). Bulbar amyotrophic lateral sclerosis: Patterns of progression and clinical management. *Head and Neck, 11(1),* 51–59.

11. Hunt, V. P., & Walker, F. O. (1989). Dysphagia in Huntington's disease. *Journal of Neuroscience Nursing, 21(2),* 92–95.

12. Hunt, V. P., & Walker, F. O. (1991). Learning to live at risk for Huntington's disease. *Journal of Neuroscience Nursing, 23(3),* 179 182.

13. Hurley, A. C., et al. (1992). Assessment of discomfort in advanced Alzheimer patients. *Research in Nursing & Health, 15(5),* 369–378.

14. Jones, P. S., & Martinson, I. M. (1992). The experience of bereavement in care givers of family members with Alzheimer's disease. *Image: Journal of Nursing Scholarship, 24(3),* 172–176.

15. Katzman, R., & Jackson, J. E. (1991). Alzheimer disease: Basic and clinical advances. *Journal of the American Geriatrics Society, 39(5),* 517–525.

16. Kelly, C. L., & Smeltzer, S. C. (1994). Betaseron: The new MS treatment. *Journal of Neuroscience Nursing, 26(1),* 52–56.

17. Kim, T. (1989). Hope as a mode of coping in amyotrophic lateral sclerosis. *Journal of Neuroscience Nursing, 21(6),* 342–347.

18. Lanska, D. J. (1990). Indications for thymectomy in myasthenia gravis. *Neurology, 40(12),* 1828–1829.

19. Miller, C. M., & Hens, M. (1993). Multiple sclerosis: A literature review. *Journal of Neuroscience Nursing, 25(3),* 174–179.

20. Mitsumoto, H., Hanson, M. R., & Chad, D. A. (1988). Amyotrophic lateral sclerosis: Recent advances in pathogenesis and therapeutic trials. *Archives of Neurology, 45(2),* 189 202.

21. Morris, R. G., Morris, L. W., & Britton, P. G. (1988). Factors affecting the emotional wellbeing of the caregivers of dementia sufferers. *British Journal of Psychiatry, 153,* 147–156.

22. Pearlman, A. L. (1990). Neuromuscular junction. In A. L. Pearlman & R. C. Collins (Eds.), *Neurobiology of disease* (pp. 44–61). New York: Oxford University Press.

23. Pfeffer, R. I., Afifi, A. A., & Chance, J. M. (1987). Prevalence of Alzheimer's disease in a retirement community. *American Journal of Epidemiology, 125(3),* 420–424.

24. Ransonott, R. M. (1991). Understanding multiple sclerosis: New immunological insights and prospects for specific therapy. *Comprehensive Therapy, 11,* 3–6.

25. Rodriguez, M. (1989). Multiple sclerosis: Basic concepts and hypothesis. *Mayo Clinic Proceedings, 64(5),* 570–576.

26. Ropper, A. H. (1992). The Guillain-Barré syndrome. *New England Journal of Medicine, 326(17),* 1130–1136.

27. Shapira, J. (1994). Research trends in Alzheimer's disease. *Journal of Gerontological Nursing, 20(4),* 4–10.

28. Silverstein, M. D., et al. (1991). Amyotrophic lateral sclerosis and life-sustaining therapy: Patients' desires for information, participation in decision making, and life-sustaining therapy. *Mayo Clinic Proceedings, 66(9),* 906–913.

29. Stolley, J. (1994). When your patient has Alzheimer's disease. *American Journal of Nursing, 94(8),* 34–40.

30. Stone, N. (1987). Amyotrophic lateral sclerosis: A challenge for constant adaptation. *Journal of Neuroscience Nursing, 19(3),* 166–173.

31. Tidwell, J. (1993). Pulmonary management of the ALS patient. *Journal of Neuroscience Nursing, 25(6),* 337–341.

32. Vernon, G. M. (1989). Parkinson's disease. *Journal of Neuroscience Nursing, 21(5),* 273–282.

Chapter 16

Nursing Care of Clients with Spinal Cord and Peripheral and Cranial Nerve Disorders

Learning Outcomes

After completing this chapter, the learner will be able to:

1. Assess the client for clinical manifestations of spinal cord injury and intervertebral disc disease.
2. Develop plans of care for the prevention of complications, management, and rehabilitation for clients with spinal cord injury.
3. Teach the client about the etiology, basic pathophysiology, and clinical manifestations of common peripheral nerve and cranial nerve disorders.
4. Implement nursing interventions that optimize the quality of life for clients with a spinal cord disorder related to trauma, tumor, or intervertebral disc disease.
5. Evaluate planned client outcomes based on criteria established in the nursing plan of care.

Disorders of the Spinal Cord

SPINAL CORD INJURY

Injury to the spinal cord can range in severity from mild flexion-extension "whiplash" injuries to complete transection of the cord with quadriplegia. Trauma to the cord can occur at any level but most commonly occurs in the cervical and lower thoracic-upper lumbar vertebrae.

Although this discussion focuses on nursing management of acute spinal cord injury, it should be remembered that there are approximately 200,000 spinal cord–injured people living in America. Those nurses who do not routinely care for neurologically impaired individuals may find themselves caring for a client who has a spinal cord injury in addition to his or her presenting symptoms.

Incidence

Each year approximately 10,000 individuals sustain a spinal cord injury. Most of these individuals are males younger than 40 years.

Etiology

Trauma is the most common cause of spinal cord injury. Traumatic spinal injury may be due to automobile or motorcycle accidents, gunshot or knife wounds, falls, or sporting mishaps. Disorders that may result in spinal cord injury include the following:

- Cervical spondylosis with myelopathy, producing spinal canal narrowing and causing progressive injury to the cord and roots
- Myelitis (infective or noninfective inflammatory processes)
- Osteoporosis causing compression fractures of the vertebrae
- Syringomyelia (central cavitation of the cord)
- Tumors, both infiltrative and compressive
- Vascular diseases, usually infarction or hemorrhage (hematomyelia)

Whatever the cause, spinal cord injuries produce distinctive and debilitating syndromes. Nowhere else in the body can local insult produce such devastation in proportion to the extent of tissue involved.

Risk Factors

The feeling of immortality often held by adolescents and young adults contributes strongly to their risk for spinal cord injury. Young people may believe they can engage in dangerous behavior without being injured. The use of alcohol and illicit drugs can add to this belief.

Pathophysiology

Spinal cord injuries most often occur as a result of injury to the vertebrae. The cord is injured as a result of acceleration, deceleration, or deformity that occurs from various forces (e.g., impact) applied to the spine. The forces injure the spinal cord by compressing, pulling, or tearing the tissues. The most common sites of injury are at the 1st to 2nd cervical, 4th to 6th cervical, and 11th thoracic to 2nd lumbar vertebrae. These segments of the spine are the most mobile and thus injured more easily.

MECHANISM OF INJURY

Flexion-Rotation, Dislocation, or Fracture Dislocation. This type of injury most often occurs in the cervical spine, usually at C5 to C6. When it occurs in the thoracic-lumbar spine, it is commonly seen at T12 to L1. This form of injury ruptures supporting ligaments, fractures the vertebrae, damages blood vessels, and leads to ischemia of the spinal cord (Fig. 16–1*A*).

Hyperextension. This type of injury is commonly seen in elderly clients who have degenerative vertebral changes, young people who have been in an automobile accident in which they hit the windshield or steering wheel, and young people who sustained neck injuries while diving. This type of injury stretches the spinal cord against the ligamenta flava and can lead to dorsal column contusion and posterior dislocation of the vertebrae. Complete transection of the cord can follow a hyperextension injury. Complete lesions of the cord result in loss of all voluntary movement below the lesion and loss of reflex function in isolated segments of the cord (Fig. 16–1*B*).

Compression. Compression injuries are often caused by falls or jumps in which the individual lands on the feet or buttocks. The force of impact fractures the vertebrae and they compress the cord. Disc and bone fragments may be propelled backward into the spinal cord on impact. The lumbar and lower thoracic vertebrae are most commonly injured; about 50 per cent of these injuries result in incomplete lesions. Incomplete lesions occur when some of the spinal tracts are intact (Fig. 16–1*C*).

Edema and microscopic bleeding occur after injury. The site of injury has the most edema and bleeding, but there is some edema and bleeding for at least two cord segments to either side of the injury. Edema of the cord leads to temporary loss of sensation and function. Therefore, initially after injury it is not easy to determine the degree of permanent impairment. After the edema and bleeding, there is massive necrosis and, finally, parenchymal and vessel destruction. The axon sheath begins to disintegrate within hours after injury.

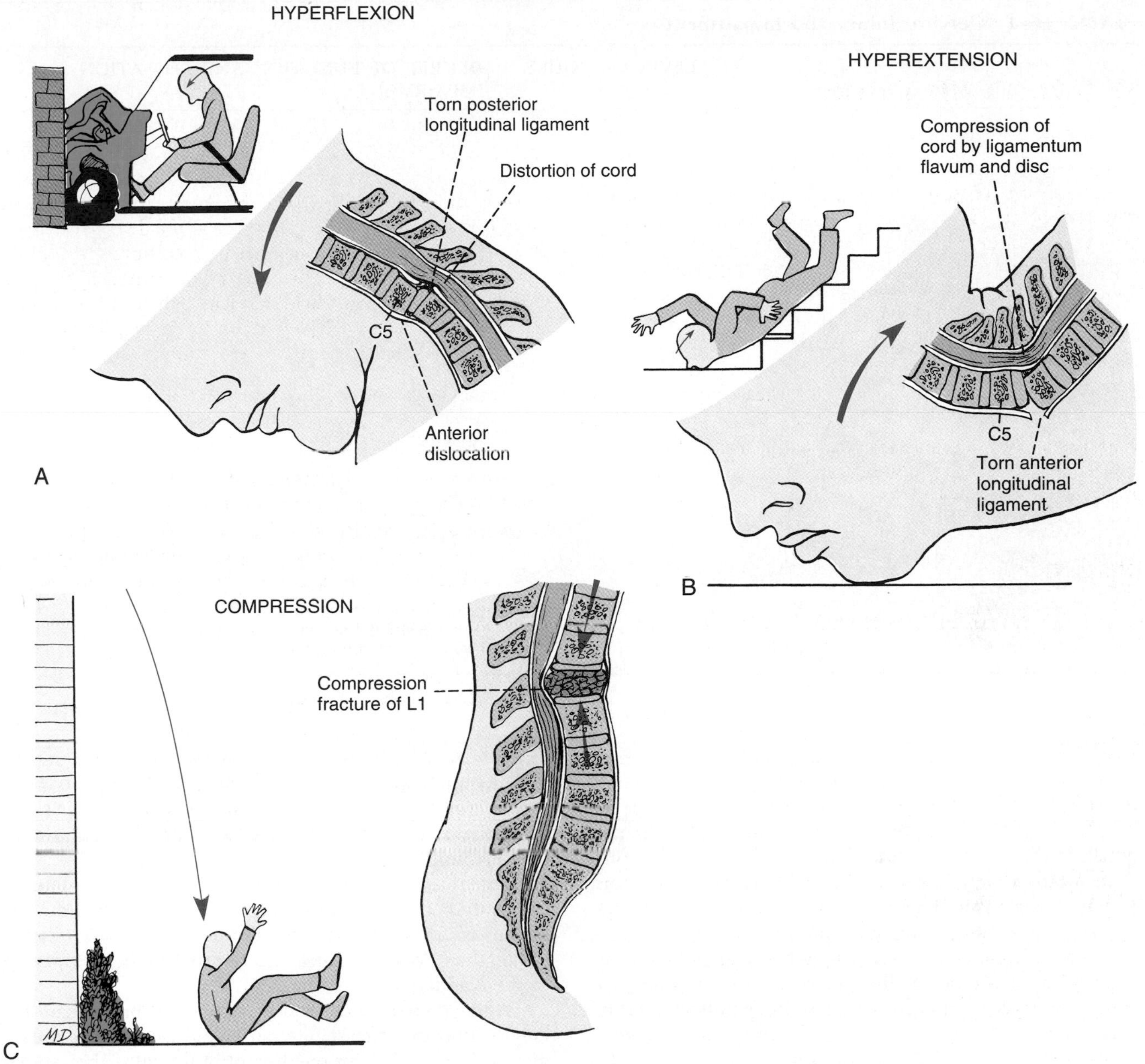

Figure 16–1
Mechanisms of spinal cord injury. Many situations can produce these consequences. This figure shows examples only.

LEVEL OF INJURY

Injury to the cervical spine and cord produces quadriplegia. Injuries above the fourth cervical vertebra (C4) may be fatal because of the loss of innervation to the diaphragm and intercostal muscles. Without immediate rescue breathing after the accident, the individual will die of respiratory failure. Today, because of the general public's knowledge of cardiopulmonary resuscitation, many people live after injuries to the cervical spine. Injuries to the remainder of the cervical spine create very specific patterns of motor loss (Table 16–1).

Injuries to the thoracic or lumbar spine produce paraplegia. Clients with such injuries have function of their upper extremities and can be mobile in a wheelchair or with crutches and braces.

SYNDROMES CAUSING PARTIAL PARALYSIS

There are three spinal cord syndromes, each characterized by distinctive neurologic findings: central cord syndrome, anterior cord syndrome, and Brown-Séquard syndrome.

Central Cord Syndrome. Central cord syndrome (most common with hyperextension-hyperflexion injuries) produces more weakness in the upper extremities than in the lower. The weakness is caused by edema

TABLE 16–1 Cervical Injury and Impairment

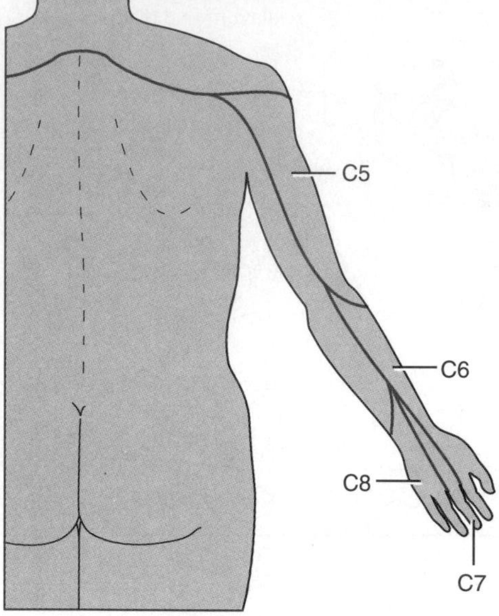

LEVEL OF INJURY	DEGREE OF FUNCTION AND SENSATION IMPAIRMENT
C5	Able to lift shoulder, elbow (partial) No sensation below clavicle
C6	Able to lift shoulder, elbow and wrist (partial) Sensation as C5, except more in arms and thumb
C7	Able to lift shoulder, elbow, wrist, and hand (partial) Loss of sensation below midchest
C8	Arm function normal, hands weak Loss of sensation below midchest

and hemorrhage in the central area of the cord, which is predominantly occupied by nerve tracts to the hands and arms.

Anterior Cord Syndrome. A lesion to the anterior spinal cord causes anterior cord syndrome, with complete motor function loss and decreased pain sensation. Touch, position, and vibration sensation remain intact. Cervical cord concussion may produce varying degrees of motor and sensory deficit, which completely resolve within hours. Occasionally, cervical cord trauma produces only root injuries, which may paralyze isolated muscles or muscle groups in the arms and shoulders. These deficits are usually permanent.

Brown-Sêquard Syndrome. Brown-Séquard syndrome is caused by lateral hemisection of the cord (i.e., when a lesion cuts or affects half the cord) such as a bullet wound or knife wound. This results in ipsilateral motor paralysis, loss of vibratory and position sense, and contralateral loss of pain and temperature sensation.

COMPLETE TRANSECTION

Total transection of the spinal cord results in immediate loss of all sensation and voluntary movement in areas below the transection. Initially, all reflex activity is also lost, but it does recover; and sometimes reflexes may become hyperactive.

Spinal Shock. The immediate response to cord transection is called spinal shock or post-traumatic areflexia. There is complete loss of skeletal muscle function, bowel and bladder tone, sexual function, and autonomic reflexes. There is also a loss of venous return and hypotension. The hypothalamus cannot control temperature by vasoconstriction and increased metabolism; therefore, the client assumes the temperature of the surrounding air.

Spinal shock may last for 7 days to 3 months. Indications that spinal shock is resolving include the return of reflexes, the development of hyperreflexia rather than flaccidity, and the return of reflex emptying of the bladder.

After spinal cord transection, the brain can no longer influence the segmental spinal cord reflex movements (i.e., reflex movements built into the spinal cord). The lower part of the cord eventually works automatically. Spinal automatisms are spinal reflex activities that occur automatically after spinal cord severance, such as flexor withdrawal reflex and reflex emptying of the bladder and bowel. These primitive, spinal mechanisms, normally kept inactive by higher centers, are "released" when the normal inhibitions of the higher centers are destroyed.

Clinical Manifestations

The initial clinical manifestations of acute spinal cord injury depend on the level and extent of injury to the cord. Below the level of injury or lesion, there is loss of:

- Voluntary movement
- Sensation of pain, temperature, pressure, and proprioception

- Bowel and bladder function
- Spinal and autonomic reflexes

After a traumatic complete transverse spinal cord lesion and cessation of spinal shock, painful, intense muscular spasms of the lower extremities occur. The nurse should explain to the client and family that these muscle spasms are involuntary and do not mean that voluntary movement is returning.

Muscle spasms vary from mild muscular twitchings to vigorous mass reflex states, depending on the posture. Violent, involuntary muscle spasms can actually throw a client off a bed. Bed side rails should be kept up and restraining straps kept comfortably secured over the client when lying on a stretcher. Muscle spasms are often aggravated by cold weather, prolonged periods of sitting, or emotionally upsetting events. Reflex spasms may become intolerable. They may be triggered by extrinsic or visceral stimuli, such as a distended bladder.

When the spinal cord is severed, blood pressure and temperature in the body part supplied by the isolated spinal cord fall markedly and respond poorly to reflex stimuli. Other functions may occur reflexively (e.g., control of the urinary bladder), but they lack integration with other visceral activities. Visceral activities may be initiated by atypical stimuli (e.g., scratching the skin may cause vasodilatation, sweating, and urination).

Nervous system lesions may produce defective urinary bladder functions known as cord bladder. For example, stimulation of the skin of the lower abdomen or thighs may cause reflex urination. This form of cord bladder is called an automatic bladder. Such stimulation may also cause reflex ejaculation and priapism (i.e., persistent abnormal penile erection without sexual desire in paralyzed men).

AUTONOMIC DYSREFLEXIA

Autonomic dysreflexia is a cluster of clinical manifestations that results when multiple spinal cord autonomic responses discharge simultaneously (Fig. 16–2). This life-threatening syndrome occurs in clients with injury above T7 and can occur for up to 6 years after injury. The manifestations of autonomic dysreflexia result from an exaggerated sympathetic response to a noxious stimulus. Stimuli commonly are bladder and bowel distention but can be pressure ulcers, spasms, pain, pressure on the penis, or uterine contractions. Exaggerated sympathetic responses cause the blood vessels below the level of injury to constrict. As a result, the client experiences hypertension (possibly as high as 300 mm Hg), pounding headache, flushing, diaphoresis, blurred vision, bradycardia (30–40 beats per minute), restlessness, and nausea. Immediate intervention is required to prevent cerebral bleeding or seizures. The head of the bed is elevated, tight clothing is loosened, and the noxious stimulus is found and removed. Sometimes nitrates, nifedipine, or hydralazine ganglionic blocking agents are given. Most commonly, a distended bladder is the problem. The client may need catheterization, straightening of a kinked catheter tube, or emptying of a collection bag. Impacted feces should be removed with the use of anesthetic ointments to decrease the risk of aggravating the dysreflexia.

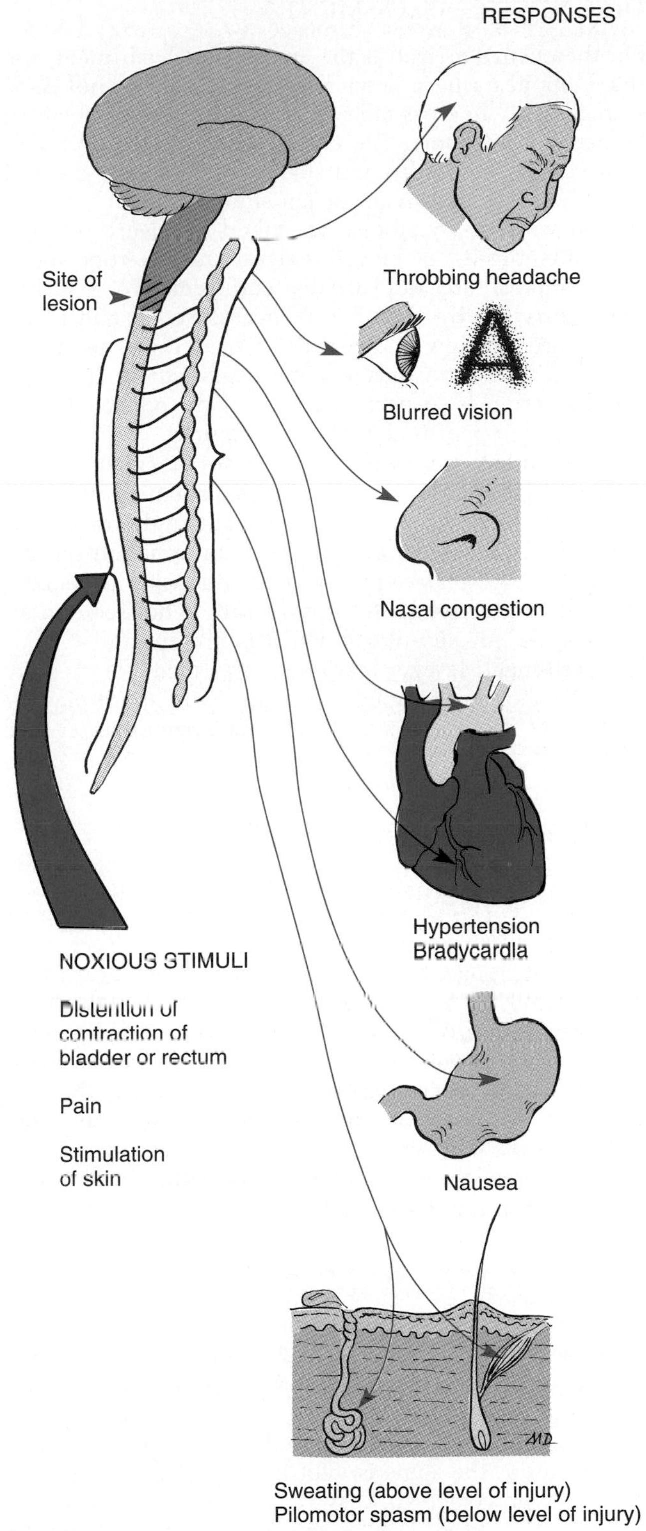

Figure 16–2
Causes of hyperreflexia and assessment findings.

DIAGNOSTIC ASSESSMENT

On the client's arrival in the emergency department, the nurse applies a hard cervical collar if this was not done at the scene. A cross-table lateral x-ray film is obtained before any transport. The client is transported on a flat, firm stretcher, usually with halter traction if a cervical injury is suspected. A physician should remain with the person while x-ray studies are taken to ensure that the cervical spine is not moved. Lateral and anteroposterior x-ray studies are not usually sufficient. To visualize lower cervical fractures, it is necessary to either use downward traction to the arms or have the arms in the swimmer's position during x-ray examination. If a high cervical lesion is suspected, a view of the odontoid bone through the open mouth may be required.

Computed tomographic (CT) or magnetic resonance imaging (MRI) scans may be obtained after the client has achieved hemodynamic and pulmonary stability. These tests can provide more information regarding the nature of fractures and the status of the spinal cord. They are also useful if a fracture is not seen on an x-ray study but neurologic deficit is present.

Peritoneal lavage may be performed for acutely quadriplegic or paraplegic clients with multiple injuries, to rule out intra-abdominal hemorrhage (see Chap. 57).

Medical Management

IMMEDIATE CARE

Both the initial (especially during the first hour after injury) and long-term intervention provided for a client experiencing spinal cord injury significantly influences the extent of the injury and associated deficits, how well the person survives the acute phase of injury, and the success of recovery and rehabilitation. People with spinal cord injury can lead productive and, in some cases, independent lives.

Spinal trauma is often associated with other injuries such as head and abdominal injuries.

CRITICAL TO REMEMBER

Anyone who has sustained multiple trauma should be handled as if there are spinal injuries until assessment procedures prove otherwise.

For handling a client suspected of having a cervical spinal injury, the spine is kept in neutral alignment and flexion is prevented. If turning is required, a log-rolling maneuver is used. The client is placed in a supine position on a firm surface. The head is supported in alignment with the body and is immobilized by placing sandbags on either side of it or by taping it to the board, and a firm, padded cervical collar is applied. Some physicians use halter traction immediately to keep the cervical spine aligned and prevent movement. Clothing is cut off rather than removed.

Cervical injury may produce respiratory distress. In this case, immediate action is taken to maintain a patent airway and provide adequate oxygenation. Damage at the C3 to C5 levels can involve the phrenic nerve, causing diaphragmatic paralysis and respiratory failure. It is important that the client's neck is not hyperextended during intubation; therefore, the jaw thrust technique is used. Suction is performed as necessary to maintain a patent airway. Mechanically assisted respiration may be required when definite loss or impairment of respiratory muscle function occurs.

Careful monitoring of hemodynamic parameters is essential. Heart rate, blood pressure, temperature, respirations, and fluid balance should be monitored continuously. Hypotension associated with spinal shock is initially treated with intravenous fluid. It is important to remember that hypotension with cervical injury is due to vasodilation and the inability to vasoconstrict, not volume depletion. Therefore, fluid resuscitation should be carefully monitored to avoid fluid overload, which can lead to pulmonary edema. Vasopressor agents are often used in the acute phase of spinal cord injury to maintain adequate blood pressure.

A brief but thorough neurologic examination is made to assess the extent of injury and establish a baseline of function and involvement for later comparison.

If the client is conscious, the nurse asks where any pain is occurring. Sensation is tested by determining whether or not the person can feel touch or a pinprick in the feet, legs, trunk, hands, and arms. Levels of sensation are documented according to dermatomes. To assess motor function, the nurse asks the client to wiggle toes, move ankles, flex knees, and move hands and arms. The location, symmetry, and strength of muscle movement are documented (Table 16–2). The major reflexes (i.e., the ankle, knee, biceps, and triceps) are briefly tested. The nurse looks for areas of sensory

TABLE 16–2 Motor Assessment After Spinal Cord Injury

SPINAL NERVE	ASSESSMENT TECHNIQUE
C4–C5	Shoulders are shrugged against downward pressure of examiner's hands.
C5–C6	Arm is pulled up from resting position against resistance.
C7	From the flexed position, arm is straightened out against resistance.
C7	Index finger is held firmly to thumb against resistance to pull apart.
C8	Hand grasp strength is evaluated.
L2–L4	Leg is lifted from bed against resistance.
L5–S1	Knee is flexed against resistance.
	From flexed position, knee is extended against resistance.
L5	Foot is pulled up toward nose against resistance.
S1	Foot is pushed down (stepping on the gas) against resistance.

Modified from Marshall, S. B., et al. (1990). *Neuroscience critical care: Pathophysiology and patient management* (p. 327). Philadelphia: W. B. Saunders.

sparing, such as sacral sparing, in which the perineum retains sensation.

If the client is unresponsive, assessment is more limited. The nurse observes for spontaneous movement and assesses respiratory status and thorax expansion. Sensation and movement of extremities are assessed by watching the client for a few moments or by applying a painful stimulus (pinprick) and observing for withdrawal. The nurse obtains details of the injury and the client's condition immediately after the injury from anyone who observed the incident.

A person who has sustained a severe cervical injury should be placed immediately in skeletal traction to immobilize the cervical spine and reduce the fracture and dislocation. Various types of tongs may be used for this: Crutchfield, Barton, or Gardner-Wells. Tongs are inserted through the skull's outer table. Traction is applied to the tongs via rope, pulleys, and weights. Weights begin with 10 to 20 lb (4.5–9.1 kg) and gradually increase to accomplish bony reduction. When proper alignment is obtained and verified by x-ray examination, the amount of traction may be reduced to that which is sufficient to maintain the position. Traction is not used to stabilize and immobilize thoracic or lumbar spinal fractures or fracture-dislocations because there is no effective way to provide it.

PHARMACOLOGIC MANAGEMENT

Vasoactive agents are commonly used to support blood pressure immediately after injury. High doses of methylprednisolone (15 mg/kg) started within 8 hours of injury have resulted in both improved motor and sensory function.

Long-term pharmacologic management may include urinary anti-infectives, anticoagulants, laxatives, and antispasmotics.

DIETARY MANAGEMENT

Nutritional intake may be compromised by respiratory impairment, position, emotional status, and gastrointestinal function. Intubation eliminates the possibility of oral intake, whereas a tracheostomy does not. Clients with a tracheostomy require time to adjust to swallowing with the tube in place and must be carefully monitored to prevent aspiration.

Aspiration is also a risk for clients who must remain flat while in tongs and traction. Although these clients may be capable of swallowing, it is unlikely that they will be able to consume safely enough food to meet their metabolic needs. Clients in halo jackets often experience difficulty eating because their head is immobile. They should be encouraged to take small bites, eat slowly, and concentrate on swallowing.

Depression is a common reaction to spinal cord injury and may have an inhibitive effect on the appetite. Also, choosing when and what to eat may be one of the few areas of control left to an individual with spinal cord injury. As much free choice of dietary intake as is feasible should be encouraged.

Paralytic ileus is a common sequela of spinal cord injury. By frequently assessing bowel sounds and documenting the passage of stool, the nurse can determine when the peristalsis has returned and the client is capable of digesting food.

Any of these conditions can severely limit a spinal cord–injured client's oral intake at a time when a high-calorie, high-protein diet is needed. Enteral feeding or total parenteral hyperalimentation, or both, is often prescribed until oral intake is sufficient to meet body needs.

Surgical Management

Surgical intervention during the initial treatment of cervical spine injuries is controversial. Some neurosurgeons and orthopedic surgeons recommend decompressive laminectomy for complete spinal cord injuries. Others believe that laminectomy should not be used routinely to treat spinal cord injury. Similarly, some surgeons recommend stabilization by surgical fusion within the first few days after trauma, whereas others do not.

Cervical fractures can also be allowed to heal with bony stability by immobilization in a brace or halo jacket. The halo jacket has a ring that is fixed to the skull with pins. This ring is then attached to the jacket by rods. This system provides the traction required to maintain cervical alignment. A halo jacket allows early mobilization and rehabilitation. The wrench that comes with the brace should always be taped to the front of the jacket. This allows quick removal in case of emergency.

CRITICAL TO REMEMBER

The nurse should never grasp the rods to help turn the client.

If the client has some mobility remaining, the nurse always assists during the client's first attempt at any activity. The halo jacket changes the client's center of gravity and makes it easy for him or her to fall.

Burst fractures of the thoracic and lumbar spine can be treated with body casts, Harrington rods, or other forms of spine stabilization. Spine stabilization devices are commonly inserted through an anterior incision. After the operation, the client has the usual postoperative assessments, including assessment of neurovascular status of the legs. Chest tubes and nasogastric tubes are inserted during surgery. The client is logrolled to faciliate respiration and skin perfusion. Pain is managed with continuous or injected narcotics. The client usually ambulates on the fourth day and is fitted for a body brace.

Complications of surgery include infection and poor wound healing as well as the complications of anesthesia. Both infection and impaired wound healing are more likely to occur in a malnourished client.

Long-Term Management

ESTABLISHING FUNCTIONAL GOALS

Prediction of functional ability after spinal cord injury can generally be guided by the degree of residual muscle function (Table 16–3). Clients with all levels of injury and of all ages will benefit from rehabilitation. The client and family are involved in all phases. The client is taught skills that he or she cannot perform so that he or she can teach those who will provide this skill at home. Likewise, skills learned in a rehabilitation setting must be generalizable to a home environment and community setting before discharge. This process can be accomplished by the use of therapeutic weekend passes and participation in community activities as a part of the rehabilitation process.

CRITICAL TO REMEMBER

In all phases of rehabilitation, it is imperative that a motivated client be given the opportunity to perform any skill, even if it can be accomplished more quickly by the nurse or physician.

Allowing the client to attempt a complex skill demonstrates support of the client's self-care abilities (see Table 16–3).

Promoting Mobility. Wheelchairs provide mobility, and having the proper wheelchair is critical. The wheelchair design must provide the client the ability to propel the chair and prevent the development of spinal deformities and pressure ulcers. A high back and head support are needed for clients without arm function.

TABLE 16–3 Functional Goals in Spinal Cord Injury

SPINAL CORD LEVEL	MUSCLE FUNCTION	FUNCTIONAL GOALS
C1–C2	Has no phrenic nerve function	Respirations managed with phrenic pacemaker
C3–C4	Neck control Scapular elevators Diaphragm function may be weak or absent	Manipulate electric wheelchair with breath control, chin control, or voice activation Limited self-feeding with ball-bearing feeders Operate environmental control units
C5	Fair-to-good shoulder control Functional deltoids and biceps Elbow flexion	Dress upper trunk Turn self in bed with or without arm slings Propel wheelchair with or without friction-surface hand rims Self-feeding with hand splints or after tenodesis Assist getting to and from bed May learn to write or type
C6	Good shoulder control Wrist extension Supinators	Dress upper trunk, sometimes dress lower trunk Turn self in bed with arm slings Propel wheelchair with hand-rim projections Self-feeding with hand splints Transfer from wheelchair to bed with or without minimal assistance (e.g., sliding board) Assist getting to and from commode chair Self-catheterization
C7	May have weak shoulder depression Weak elbow extension Some hand function Triceps	Independent in transfer to bed, car, and toilet Total dressing independence Wheelchair without hand-rim projections Self-feeding with no assistive devices
T1–T4	Good-to-normal upper extremity muscle function Intrinsic muscles of the hand No trunk control	Independent in transfer to bed, car, and toilet Total dressing independence Wheelchair with standard hand rims Self-feeding with no assistive devices Transfer from wheelchair to floor and return Wheelchair up and down curb Transfer from wheelchair to tub and return
T5–L2	Partial-to-good trunk stability	Total wheelchair independence Limited ambulation with bilateral long leg braces and crutches (injury at T12 or below)
L3–L4	All trunk-pelvic stabilizers intact Hip flexors Adductors Quadriceps	Ambulation with short leg braces with or without crutches, depending on level
L5–S3	Hip extensors Abductors, knee flexors, ankle control	No equipment needed if plantar flexion is strong enough for push off at end of stance

Modified from Rancho Los Amigos Hospital, Physical Therapy Department, Downey, CA.

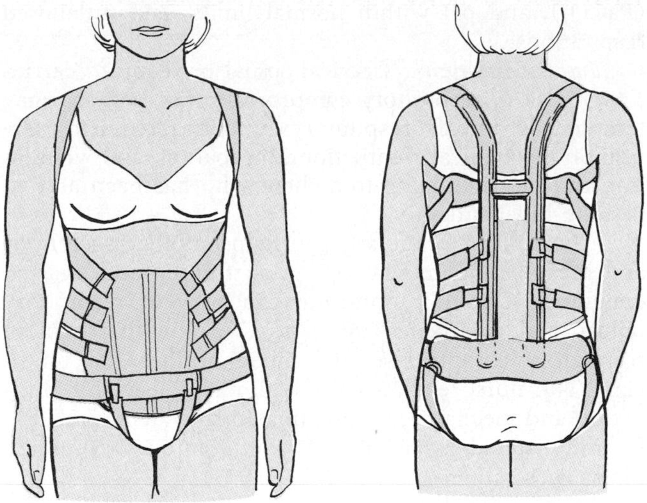

Figure 16–3
Taylor splint.

Clients who can use their arms should have the back of the wheelchair at the level of the scapula. Cushions help decrease pressure and the risk of pressure ulcers. However, cushions do not prevent pressure ulcers, and the client still needs to shift weight every 10 to 15 minutes while in the chair.

Current emphasis is on strengthening muscles rather than using braces. However, back braces may be prescribed after lumbar spinal injury or intervertebral disc problems. A Taylor back brace (Fig. 16–3), splint, or heavy muslin corset with stays may be initially worn while the client is in bed. More frequently, a thoracic lumbar sacral orthosis (TLSO) is used. This is a custom-made plastic brace with front and back pieces that fasten together with Velcro straps. This brace provides stability for the healing spine.

LONG-TERM COMPLICATIONS

Long-Term Pain. Long-term pain occurs in almost all spinal cord–injured clients. Dysesthetic pain, which is distal to the site of injury, is extremely disabling. It is similar to phantom pain seen after amputation. It is described as cutting, burning, piercing, radiating, or tightening. Usual treatment is with non-narcotic analgesics and transcutaneous nerve simulators.

Spasticity. Spasticity is an increase in tonic stretch reflexes and often interferes with positioning and functional activities. Spasticity does maintain muscle bulk and venous return and serves as an aid for transfers. Treatment includes range-of-motion (ROM) exercises and pharmacologic agents such as baclofen, dantrolene sodium, and clonidine. Medications for the treatment of spasms are given only when the spasms cause discomfort or safety concerns.

Neurogenic Bladder. A neurogenic bladder occurs with both upper and lower motor neuron disorders. Upper motor neuron disorders produce a spastic or reflex bladder. Lower motor neuron disorders produce a flaccid bladder. There are many ways to manage the bladder, and treatment options must be tailored to fit the client's preferences and life-style as well as functional abilities.

Most clients with arm function are taught to empty their bladder using the Credé method to tap over the bladder and relax the sphincter (discussed later in the chapter). To ensure complete emptying, this method is often combined with other techniques such as catheterization and external catheters. Intermittent catheterization decreases the risk of infection and bladder stone formation caused by indwelling catheters. Clients with C6 and lower injuries can perform self-catheterization, although the technique requires adequate hand function and the ability to manage lower extremity clothing. External catheters are used for men who can void between catheterizations. Suprapubic catheters can also be inserted and seem to offer the advantages of decreased infection and urethral injury over indwelling catheters. A neurogenic bladder may also be treated with medications such as bethanechol (Urecholine) to stimulate bladder contraction. Urine-acidifying agents may also be prescribed to reduce the risk of infection.

Neurogenic Bowel. A neurogenic bowel is similar to a neurogenic bladder because the client cannot defecate. The goal is to develop a bowel elimination method that is convenient, effective, and least expensive for the client. Sufficient fluid and fiber intake is essential. When fiber is added to or increased in the diet, it must be done slowly to avoid cramping and diarrhea. Stool softeners and bulk laxatives may also be used.

The bowel movements of clients with upper motor neuron damage are generally regulated with suppositories or digital stimulation every day or every other day. A lower motor neuron neurogenic bowel is more difficult to regulate, and often the client requires manual disimpaction.

Respiratory Dysfunction. Respiratory dysfunction is a significant cause of morbidity and mortality after spinal cord injury. The diaphragm is often the only functional muscle because the intercostal and abdominal muscles are paralyzed. Vital capacity and inspiratory reserve volume are markedly diminished. The client should be taught to use incentive spirometry and diaphragmatic breathing to enhance vital capacity. Glossopharyngeal breathing uses the muscles of the mouth, pharynx, and larynx to swallow air into the lungs. This technique enhances vital capacity and promotes chest expansion.

Sexual Dysfunction. Sexual dysfunction in spinal cord–injured males depends on the location of the lesion. Erection is possible in clients with upper motor neuron lesions. Reflex erections occur in lower motor neuron lesions. Ejaculation is possible with lower motor neuron lesions and if the lesion is more caudal. Unfortunately, fertility is about 5 per cent, but it is hoped that this rate will improve as technological developments progress.

Female clients retain fertility after spinal cord injury. Problems with sexual function generally relate to positioning and the lack of vaginal lubrication. These problems can usually be addressed through client education.

Psychological Counseling. Psychological counseling is ongoing. Commonly, spinal cord–injured clients participate in peer group sessions to share experiences, help newly injured clients gain insight, and cope better with their situation. Vocational rehabilitation may help clients reach their maximum rehabilitation potential.

Nursing Management

Assessment

Rehabilitation begins on the client's admission to the health-care facility. During the acute stage, nursing and medical attention appropriately focuses on immediate needs. However, it is also imperative to remember that the client probably has severe residual disabilities and must make major life-style changes. Care provided in the acute period can significantly affect the client's later life. Prevention of complications such as infection, pressure sores, and contractures facilitates rehabilitation and reduces suffering, disability, and expense. See Appendix C for a sample clinical pathway for clients with spinal cord injury.

A holistic assessment is essential when caring for clients with spinal cord injury. Every system of the body is affected in spinal cord injury. A complete baseline assessment is obtained initially. The results of subsequent serial assessments are then compared with the baseline. The most important questions for spinal cord–injured clients are the following:

- Is the client hemodynamically stable? Are vasopressor agents required to maintain adequate blood pressure? Is circulation adequate, as evidenced by palpable peripheral pulses and appropriate skin, nail bed, and mucous membrane color?
- Is respiration adequate? Are accessory muscles being used for respiration? Is the client exhibiting diaphragmatic breathing or nostril flaring? Does the client complain of shortness of breath? If pulse oximetry is available, are oxygen saturation levels adequate?

Other questions that may guide nursing assessment are: Are pupil responses, corneal responses, and eye movements normal? At what spinal cord level is sensation diminished or lost? At what level is motor function diminished or lost? Do the levels differ in different areas of the body? Is there any voluntary movement? Are normal reflexes (e.g., deep tendon, bulbocavernosus, and anal reflexes) absent? Is the client incontinent? Are there bowel sounds? Is the abdomen distended? Is the client edematous? Is the skin intact? What is the emotional condition of the client and family?

Nursing Diagnosis, Planning, and Implementation

Collaborative Problem: Ventilatory Insufficiency or Atelectasis, Risk for.

Planning: Expected Outcomes. The client will show no signs of respiratory compromise, as evidenced by clear lung sounds, partial pressure of arterial oxygen (PaO_2), partial pressure of arterial carbon dioxide ($PaCO_2$), and pH within normal limits, and unlabored respirations.

Implementation. Cervical spinal cord injury carries a high risk of respiratory compromise. Cord edema may temporarily impair respiratory function, requiring the use of mechanical ventilation. Intubation and ventilation can be frightening to a client who has been able to breathe independently.

Chest physical therapy can help mobilize secretions and prevent pneumonia, as can suctioning and assisted coughing. Careful monitoring can prevent respiratory failure and emergency intubation. At the first sign of respiratory compromise, the nurse notifies the physician. The nurse explains the equipment used for intubation and mechanical ventilation to the client. Sedation is administered as needed after intubation, within the physician's orders.

For extended airway management, a tracheostomy may be required to allow for long-term controlled ventilation, facilitate the removal of tracheobronchial secretions, and seal off the esophagus from the trachea to prevent aspiration.

Nursing Diagnosis: Aspiration, Risk for R/T ineffective airway clearance and absent gag reflex.

Planning: Expected Outcomes. Client will exhibit no signs of aspiration, as evidenced by clear lung sounds; absence of stridor and fever; minimal amounts of clear mucus on suctioning; and PaO_2, $PaCO_2$, and pH within normal limits.

Implementation. Aspiration is a common cause of morbidity in spinal cord–injured clients. Suctioning equipment should be kept available, and breath sounds assessed every 1 or 2 hours in acutely ill clients. The results of arterial blood gases and pulse oximetry are monitored to determine the degree of oxygenation provided by ventilators or oxygen. Tracheobronchial suctioning is performed frequently to prevent or decrease the accumulation of secretions from immobility, the lack of a cough and sigh reflex, or pneumonia. The nurse should monitor the electrocardiogram for dysrhythmias (e.g., premature ventricular contractions [PVCs]) while suctioning as a result of hypoxia.

Nursing Diagnosis: Skin Integrity, Impaired, Risk for R/T immobility and loss of protective reflexes.

Planning: Expected Outcomes. Client will have intact skin, as evidenced by no reddened areas over bony prominences, no areas or signs of skin irritation or dryness, and no signs of corneal irritation.

Implementation. When the client cannot respond to local tissue hypoxia resulting from being in one position for an extended period of time, the risk of pressure ulcers increases. Spinal cord–injured clients should be placed on pressure-reducing beds or mattresses. However, the use of these special beds does not eliminate the need to assess the skin every 2 to 4 hours. In addition, the client's nutritional needs must be met to reduce the risk of pressure ulcers.

A Roto-Rest bed is currently popular for clients with spinal cord injuries or other disorders requiring prolonged immobilization (see Chapter 13, Fig. 13–8). It is equipped with supportive packs and straps that keep the body in alignment while it continuously oscillates from side to side. The continuous motion helps (1) prevent skin breakdown, (2) reduce urinary stasis, and (3) promote lung aeration. Unfortunately, the constant movement may also stimulate peristalsis, resulting in severe diarrhea. Some clients also experience disorientation from the constant movement. These clients also express fear of falling. Staff members should remain with the client during the initial rotations to provide emotional support and reassurance.

Once the client is able to be responsible for some activities of daily living (ADLs), the nurse teaches the client about the risk of pressure ulcers and techniques to reduce risk. The client should shift body weight every 10 to 15 minutes while sitting in a wheelchair. Shifting weight promotes reactive hyperemia and vasodilation to bring blood into hypoxic tissues. Finally, the client should use a mirror to inspect for signs of pressure ulcers each evening before bedtime.

Nursing Diagnosis: Oral and Nasal Mucous Membranes, Altered, Risk for R/T nothing by mouth (NPO) status, inability to swallow, and mouth breathing.

Planning: Expected Outcomes. The patient will maintain intact oral and nasal mucous membranes, as evidenced by having oral and nasal mucous membranes pink, moist, and without lesions or bloody drainage.

Implementation. The client's teeth are brushed with a small toothbrush at least twice a day. The oral mucous membranes (especially the roof of the mouth), tongue, and gums are cleaned with toothettes. Agents containing lemon or alcohol should not be used for any length of time, because they dry the membranes. The mouth is then rinsed. Gauze wrapped around a tongue depressor or toothbrush and saturated with dilute mouthwash may help with aspects of oral care.

Nursing Diagnosis: Nutrition, Altered: Less Than Body Requirements, Risk for R/T inability to eat and increased metabolic needs.

Planning: Expected Outcomes. Client will demonstrate signs of adequate nutrition, as evidenced by stabilization of weight; consumption of adequate calories for age, height, and weight; equal intake and output; healing of incisions and wounds within 12 to 14 days; and hemoglobin, blood urea nitrogen, lymphocyte, and albumin levels within normal limits for age and sex.

Implementation. Intravenous fluids are begun on admission for newly injured clients. Initially, the intravenous site provides access to the circulatory system for the administration of medications, but an intravenous infusion cannot be considered nutritional support.

The nutritional and fluid needs of comatose patients are usually met through nasogastric feedings. If the client does not have paralytic ileus or delayed gastric emptying and if bowel sounds are audible and gastric residual volumes are less than 100 mL/hr, nasogastric feedings are started.

Collaborative Problem. Autonomic Dysreflexia, Risk for R/T spinal cord injury.

Planning: Expected Outcomes. The nurse will assess for, prevent, and respond to complications, as evidenced by assessing for clinical manifestations and intervening quickly to reduce dysreflexia.

Implementation. The nurse assesses the client for sudden indications of severe hypertension, severe throbbing headache, profuse diaphoresis, flushing of the skin above the level of the lesion, nasal stuffiness, pilomotor spasm, blurred vision, nausea, and bradycardia. If autonomic dysreflexia occurs, the nurse follows interventions mentioned previously in this chapter.

Once symptoms have subsided, the client is observed closely for 3 to 4 hours. If medication has been given, the client may become hypotensive after the stimulus is removed. Autonomic dysreflexia may recur if the stimulus is not completely removed. If the identified source of irritation is bowel distention, the nurse must be very careful when disimpacting the client. An anesthetic lubricant is used, and another nurse must monitor the client's blood pressure every few minutes. The stimulation of trying to remove the impaction can increase the severity of the autonomic response.

Nursing Diagnosis: Injury, High Risk for R/T uncompensated sensory deficit.

Planning: Expected Outcomes. Client will be free of injury, as evidenced by no abrasions, reddened areas, ulcerations, or burns.

Implementation. Sensory loss poses serious problems for paralyzed clients because they cannot feel the pain or pressure that normally warns of tissue damage. These clients should not wear tight, restrictive clothing or ill-fitting shoes or braces. They need to develop the habit of preventive thinking to avoid potential danger. Dangerous situations include getting too close to heaters, radiators, and fireplaces and using heating pads or hot water bottles. Burns can be a serious problem because impaired circulation delays healing. External heat should not be applied if there is a loss of sensation, and the bath water should not be too warm.

Regular foot and nail care is required to prevent nails rubbing or cutting the skin and to prevent ingrown nails. Foot infections may be prevented by instructing the person not to cut corns or calluses.

CRITICAL TO REMEMBER

Injections should be given above the level of the cord lesion whenever possible. Adequate absorption is not likely to occur in denervated areas of the body with impaired capillary and precapillary circulation.

Clients can also be injured from involuntary spasms. The nurse must avoid unnecessary stimulation of areas that elicit reflex spinal automatisms. When such reactions do occur, an unembarrassed, accepting response helps relieve the client's anxiety and embarrassment. The release of spinal automatisms makes people respond to stimuli in ways that may be puzzling to them and others unless the origin of such responses is explained. For example, stimulation of the limbs (perhaps toe flexion while the person's foot is being dried) may cause mass flexion of the upper and lower extremities. Mass flexion reactions may be accompanied by massive contractions of the abdominal wall; evacuation of the urinary bladder and bowel; and automatic response such as sweating, flushing, and pilomotor reactions below the level of the lesion.

Nursing Diagnosis: Incontinence, Total, R/T atonic bladder.

Planning: Expected Outcomes. The client will have improved bladder control, as evidenced by no infection and emptying of the bladder every 4 to 6 hours.

Implementation. Nursing intervention is planned to (1) prevent urinary tract infection, (2) preserve existing bladder capacity and muscle tone, and (3) establish and maintain a routine pattern of elimination requiring minimal artificial assistance.

The nurse observes the client carefully for indications of faulty bladder control and infection, including incontinence, retention, urgency, dribbling, frequency, enuresis, and precipitate micturition. The nurse documents such observations and informs the physician.

Urinary bladder atony (absence of tone) may last several weeks or months after spinal cord injury. In clients with upper motor neuron lesions, when spinal shock subsides and the reflex arc returns, as evidenced by increase in rectal tone, the bladder empties reflexively. During the period of atony, a retention catheter may be inserted to prevent bladder distention and keep the client dry and comfortable. Bladder overdistention causes stretching and fissure formation and a predisposition to infection and may result in bladder rupture. When sensory pathways are damaged, the client does not feel the discomfort of bladder distention. However, prolonged catheter use also predisposes to infection.

Urinary complications may be avoided by

- Periodically examining the client for bladder distention
- Accurately documenting fluid intake and output
- Using aseptic technique when handling urinary catheters
- Observing for signs of bladder infection

The client should also be encouraged to drink cranberry juice to keep the urine acidic and decrease the possibility of infection. Urine acidifiers may be prescribed. Urinary complications occur because of incomplete emptying of the bladder, necessitating catheterization. Catheterization may predispose the client to infection and vesicoureteral reflux, which may lead to kidney complications. Renal calculi, pyelonephritis, and hydronephrosis are major causes of death and considerable disability in paralyzed clients.

To prevent development of renal calculi, the nurse encourages the client to drink about 3000 mL of fluid/day, unless contraindicated by other medical conditions. This is sufficient to maintain a minimal urinary output of 2000 mL/day. Drinking this much fluid may increase incontinence but is necessary to prevent renal calculi.

When the initial indwelling catheter is removed, a program of intermittent catheterization is commonly prescribed to empty the bladder regularly every 4 to 6 hours for several weeks. During this time, the client is taught methods of emptying the bladder without catheterization. Such methods promote urination by increasing intra-abdominal pressure on the bladder. Urinary flow may be initiated by Credé's maneuver, Valsalva's maneuver, and the rectal stretch (Box 16–1).

Nursing Diagnosis: Bowel Incontinence or Constipation, Risk for R/T paralysis.

Planning: Expected Outcomes. The client will have reduced risk of bowel incontinence or constipation, as evidenced by a bowel movement every 1 to 2 days, no signs of fecal impactions, and no incontinence.

Implementation. Nursing intervention is planned to:

- Prevent constipation, distention, and impaction
- Detect and treat these conditions if they occur
- Re-establish habitual, controlled bowel movements by conditioned reflex activity

BOX 16–1

Techniques to Initiate Urine Flow

CREDÉ'S MANEUVER

The client makes a fist and presses it directly over the bladder and down toward the pubic bone with a kneading motion. Continue until the bladder is empty.

VALSALVA'S MANEUVER

The client inhales deeply, holds the breath and bears down as hard as possible, as if for a bowel movement.

RECTAL STRETCH

The client inserts a finger into the rectum. When the anal sphincter is relaxed, the client maintains the relaxation by gently pulling on the sphincter. This relaxes the perineal floor. A Valsalva maneuver is performed at the same time.

Urination may also be stimulated by reflex stimulation. The following stimuli may be successful: tapping the suprapubic area; stroking the glans penis, thigh, or vulva; tugging pubic hairs; or flexing the toes. The stimulation may be applied by the client or care giver. As training continues, less stimulation is needed to initiate urination.

Catheterization may be required at home. Teach the client and care giver clean, rather than sterile, technique. This technique has the same infection rate as sterile insertion methods for home catheterization. Suprapubic catheters may be inserted for long-term bladder management. Occasionally, a surgical procedure such as sphincterotomy may be necessary. The bladder then empties continuously. An external, condom-type catheter connected to a straight closed drainage bag may be used to collect drainage in men. External appliances for females do not work as well.

The client is observed carefully for indications of constipation, diarrhea, or tenesmus (ineffective, painful straining at stool). If a client becomes impacted, a cleansing enema is usually prescribed to initially empty the lower bowel. However, enemas should be avoided for long-term bowel management. A paraplegic or quadriplegic client cannot retain enema solution; nor can the degree of intestinal distention be felt. Therefore, enemas must be administered carefully without overdistending the intestine with excessive fluid.

The client's intake of fluid and food and elimination pattern are documented. The routine daily pattern of bowel elimination is established, with the client using suppositories and other means of stimulating evacuation until reflex evacuation occurs.

A daily fluid intake of 3000 to 4000 mL/day is important for proper bowel function as well as bladder function. Also, the diet must be high in bulk and roughage such as bran, whole grains, fresh and dried fruits, and leafy green and raw vegetables. A stool softener such as docusate sodium (Colace) may be taken daily, but laxatives should be avoided. Metamucil is very effective for spinal cord–injured clients if they drink enough fluid.

Bowel retraining is possible for most paraplegic and quadriplegic clients. It involves developing controlled bowel movements by conditioned reflex activity. The nurse must begin bowel retraining as soon as possible. The nurse should also ensure privacy during the daily bowel routine and, if possible, have the client sit upright. When possible, appropriate family members should be included in the bowel-retraining program because they may be involved in this aspect of long-term management. One must always assess the family members' willingness to participate in such care. If the sexual partner is also responsible for hygiene and personal care, problems in role separation and intimacy may result. These issues should be openly discussed between partners.

With an effective bowel program, a client has a bowel movement once a day or every other day and is not incontinent at other times. Attaining continence may influence a paralyzed client's vocational future and positively affect his or her ability to have satisfying social relationships. It can also give the client the self-esteem to withstand other problems.

Nursing Diagnosis: Pain R/T spinal cord injury.

Planning: Expected Outcomes. The client will experience adequate pain relief, as evidenced by verbalization of improvement in comfort level, ability to rest without interruption by pain, and ability to participate in therapies without hindrance by pain.

Implementation. Clients with spinal injuries may experience pain at the level of the injury and radiating along spinal nerves originating in the area. Phantom pain may also be experienced. Pain usually occurs later than muscular spasms. Some paraplegic and quadriplegic clients experience both pain and spasm. Pain most often occurs in the lower extremities. Analgesics such as acetylsalicylic acid and nonsteroidal anti-inflammatory agents may be prescribed. Narcotics are seldom used after the initial injury and are contraindicated in clients with high cervical injuries because of the risk of respiratory depression.

Clients with thoracic injuries often tend to breathe shallowly to avoid pain. This can lead to respiratory complications. The nurse gives prescribed pain medication and encourages deep breathing and coughing to aerate the lungs and remove secretions from the respiratory tract.

Antispasmotics, nonsteroidal anti-inflammatory agents, and non-narcotic analgesics are prescribed for pain associated with spasticity. Surgery (e.g., neurectomy or chordotomy) is sometimes required for pain relief.

Collaborative Problem. Thrombophlebitis, Risk for R/T loss of muscle contraction in lower extremities and loss of venous return.

Planning: Expected Outcomes. The nurse will monitor for thrombophlebitis as evidenced by unilateral leg edema, erythema, and warmth.

Implementation. Muscular activity is a major factor in venous circulation. A paralyzed client experiences slowed venous return and pooling of blood in dependent limbs. These phenomena increase the risk of intravascular clotting. In the acute phase of spinal cord injury, antiembolic stockings, sequential compression devices, and subcutaneous heparin may be used prophylactically.

Education is vital to preventing vascular complications and minimizing their impact. Each time the nurse applies stockings and performs ROM exercises, the client is taught the importance of these activities. During assessment of the legs for signs of clot formation (i.e., redness and unilateral swelling and warmth), the nurse explains what is being done and why the client needs to incorporate this activity into daily routines. Clients are also taught not to cross their legs while sitting in a wheelchair.

Nursing Diagnosis: Impaired Physical Mobility R/T paralysis.

Planning: Expected Outcomes. Client will have maximum physical mobility, as evidenced by absence of tendon contractures, joint ankylosis, and muscle shortening, and effective use of adaptive devices.

Implementation. Spinal cord injury causing permanent mobility impairment produces problems with ambulation and potential complications arising from immobility.

Throughout the acute and rehabilitative phases of nursing care, every effort should be made to maximize the client's functional abilities and independence by encouraging the client to perform independently any ADLs for which capability remains.

Tendon Contractures, Joint Ankylosis, and Muscle Shortening. These problems are caused by improper positioning of a client in the bed or chair and lack of joint movements (e.g., because of spasticity or immobility). Interventions to prevent such problems include:

- Frequent position changes
- Proper positioning of joints
- Use of splints and removable casts
- Intermittent turning to a prone position

- Positioning of upper extremities away from the body
- Draping of bedding over frames to keep pressure off feet
- Keeping knee joints flexed 15 degrees when supine
- Use of active and passive conditioning exercises

Passive exercises prevent contractures and painful reflex dystrophies of the hand and shoulder. Such exercises may be prescribed as soon as 48 to 72 hours after the injury. Active exercises, massage, and electrical stimulation may also be prescribed. One must begin shoulder and arm exercises early. Strength in these areas and in the chest and back is essential for effective self-transfers and ambulation when the lower spine is stable enough to permit mobilization.

Muscle Weakness and Fatigue. Wristdrop and footdrop will develop in paralyzed extremities unless prevented. Footdrop may be prevented by keeping the client's feet firmly supported in dorsiflexion at right angles to the hips to counteract the force of gravity on weakened muscles. The nurse must support a paralyzed arm in a sling when the client is out of bed and a cock-up splint while in bed. Usually, the hand end of the splint is elevated 2 inches to support the wrist, and the fingers are maintained in a position of function. Posterior molded casts may be used instead of splints to support a paralyzed wrist while the patient is in bed.

Rehabilitative programs often require strength and endurance. To prepare a client for ambulation, the unaffected parts of the body must be strengthened and suitable exercises started early. Tolerance for activity gradually increases. The nurse must take care not to fatigue the client. Periods of planned rest and recreation are important.

Physical therapy is essential for all clients with spinal cord injuries. Paraplegic clients need to learn various transfers to become self-sufficient. Learning to sit up precedes learning to transfer. Many paralyzed clients become mobile by using a wheelchair. Many types of wheelchairs are available, and selection needs to be made carefully, according to individual needs. Prolonged, unrelieved periods of immobility can create renal calculi and pressure ulcers. When sitting up, a paralyzed client needs to shift body weight every 10 to 15 minutes and lift the body by pushing with the arms and hands against the chair arms or seat. This relieves pressure on the buttocks and prevents skin breakdown. By using a wheelchair, clients may become completely independent in all ADLs. Many clients drive and hold outside jobs.

The nurse must apply the brace or corset before helping the client out of bed. After fracture of a cervical vertebra, cervical disc rupture, or whiplash injury, the person may wear a neck brace (fitted so the chin rests on a cup and the neck is kept hyperextended), a hard collar (which extends up under the chin and prevents flexion of the neck), or a soft collar. Neck braces tend to limit vision, because people wearing them cannot look down at their feet. Safety awareness is important to prevent falls.

A thin, knitted undershirt is worn under the brace or corset to protect the skin and keep the appliance clean. To apply the brace or corset, the nurse turns the client to one side, places the appliance against the back, and then rolls the client back into it. The brace or corset is secured while the client lies supine. As recovery and rehabilitation progress, many clients learn to apply their own braces and corsets while in bed. Others continue to need help. The degree of the client's arm and hand function determines the ability to apply a brace.

Weightbearing begins as early as possible after spinal cord injury. This stimulates osteoblastic activity and thus decreases the demineralization of bone (osteoporosis) that develops with prolonged immobilization. Standing boards or tilt tables assist the person gradually to a standing position. Having the person assume a standing position periodically each day also helps prevent contractures (e.g., hip contractures from long periods of sitting). Care must be taken when helping clients to stand or sit in a chair for the first time. Because of the loss of muscular activity on the peripheral venous system, these clients are very prone to orthostatic hypotension. Blood pressure should always be checked before and after transfers.

Clients easily lose their balance when wearing braces, particularly the halo brace, and must be very careful not to fall. A brace feels surprisingly heavy at first, especially if the client is weak. Some braces are now made from plastic and are considerably lighter. For safety, shoes, rather than slippers or just stockings, should be worn during ambulation. Shoes should tie or have Velcro straps for firm support and have a low heel. High-top athletic shoes give added support. Slick soles, high or narrow heels, or stockinged feet are hazardous. Wearing shoes also helps prevent footdrop when the client lies down.

The fit, comfort, and appearance of braces, corsets, and shoes are important to the client. Try to assist clients who want to be as stylish as possible as well as benefit from therapeutic garments. Disabled clients are helped by being encouraged to express their feelings concerning self-image and having their feelings taken into consideration when fitting therapeutic garments. Some garments can be painful when first worn. The pain worsens if the garments do not fit properly. The client's skin should be inspected frequently, especially at first, because pressure sores can develop very quickly.

Nursing Diagnosis: Self-Care Deficit R/T loss of function secondary to spinal cord injury.

Planning: Expected Outcomes. The client will independently perform as many ADLs as possible. If the client is unable to independently perform an activity, he or she will be able to direct a care giver's performance. These goals will be evaluated by successful performance of an ADL by the client or at client's direction.

Implementation. Spinal cord injury is often accompanied by a feeling of powerlessness. Assisting the client to maximize independence can lessen this feeling. The client is assisted with muscle-strengthening exercises and use of adaptive devices. Clients with high cervical injuries are able to perform very few activities independently. The nurse must allow them adequate time to accomplish whatever tasks they can do. If the client is dependent in ADLs, nursing care should be adapted to the client's routine.

Nursing Diagnosis: Sexual dysfunction R/T spinal cord injury.

Planning: Expected Outcomes. The client will develop personally satisfying and socially acceptable means of expressing sexuality, as evidenced by interacting appropriately in social situations, verbalizing the effects of the injury on sexual function, discussing sexual issues with a team member, verbalizing methods of sexual expression, and verbalizing understanding of contraceptive implications.

Implementation. Spinal cord–injured clients are often concerned about sexuality and their ability to achieve sexual fulfillment. They often worry about such concerns long before they express them to others. Nurses are often asked about sexuality issues before other professionals are approached, perhaps because nurses provide intimate care activities. Such care can promote a high degree of trust between those involved.

Some clients discuss their own sexual potential directly. Others refer to it obliquely or appear crude in the way they introduce the topic (e.g., by making inappropriate sexual comments or gestures). Such behaviors are attempts to acknowledge sexuality. Nurses try to look beyond the behavior to the underlying emotional concerns. They acknowledge the client's concerns and offer discussion, by saying, for example, "You seem concerned about your sexuality, Janet. I understand that and I would like to talk with you about it if you want."

To be helpful, nurses need to be able to talk about sexuality without embarrassment. They also need accurate information about "normal" sexuality and how physiologic changes that occur because of injury affect sexual function.

The client can be referred to another person or an agency if appropriate. Referral should not be done too hastily, though. If someone talks with a nurse about this personal subject, it is probably because at that time that person feels most comfortable speaking with that nurse about it. The nurse should allow the client to lead the conversation, which may be difficult. Professionals often think they know what someone needs and wants without listening to the person.

To some extent, sexual function can be predicted by the level of spinal cord lesion (Table 16–4). However, although physical limitations certainly occur,

TABLE 16–4 Sexual Function in Clients with Spinal Cord Injury

SEXUALITY	REPRODUCTIVE FUNCTIONING	SPECIAL CONSIDERATIONS FOR CONTRACEPTIVE METHODS
Females Lesions at C1–C3: Reflex lubrication is probable. Erogenous areas may develop above injury. Libido is intact. Lesions at C4–C6: Psychogenic lubrication is unlikely. Nongenital orgasm may be experienced. Lesions at C7: Able to use hands for holding and caressing. Lesions at T12–L5: Psychogenic stimulation of the clitoris, lubrication, labial swelling, and skin flush are possible but unlikely.	Menstruation and fertility are unaffected. Pregnancy is not affected. Incidence of bladder infection during pregnancy increases. Risk of autonomic hyperreflexia during delivery and labor increases.	Birth control pills are contraindicated when circulatory problems present; thrombophlebitis could go undetected owing to lack of sensation in extremities. Intrauterine device may be contraindicated because pelvic inflammatory disease and other problems could remain undetected owing to lack of sensation. Client must be able to assess for vaginal bleeding.
Males Lesions at C1–C3: Reflex erection is caused by genital stimulation. Psychogenic erection is not possible. Erogenous areas above injury site may develop. Libido is intact. Lesions at C4–C6: Reflex erection is possible. Nongenital orgasm may be experienced.; no ejaculation. Oral sex is possible. Libido is intact. Lesions at C7: Holding and caressing with hands are possible. Lesions at T12–L6: Psychogenic stimulation and erection are possible; no reflex erection. Lesions at S2–S4: Reflex erection is possible. Ejaculation is possible but may retrograde.	Semen can be obtained from the bladder of those clients who have retrograde ejaculation. For clients who cannot ejaculate, semen can be obtained through glandular vibratory stimulation. In general, semen quality is impaired, with poor motility the most common abnormality. Some clients are candidates for penile prosthesis.	Client or partner may apply condom.

every individual is different. Many men do have erections after spinal cord injury. Many disabled people enjoy paraorgasm (phantom orgasm) by developing alternative erogenous zones. The genitals are not the only body areas that can be sexually excited, and intercourse is not the only means of sexual expression.

Some individuals find it disappointing, perhaps devastating, if they can no longer function sexually as they did before an injury. However, they can be helped to learn new ways of giving and receiving sexual pleasure. Sex and relationship counseling is sometimes helpful. The nurse's role is to facilitate expression of feelings and convey hope that new and real sexual enjoyment can be experienced. Some form of sexual expression is possible for anyone, regardless of disability. Before making specific suggestions of alternative expressions of sexuality, the nurse should interview the client regarding past sexual behavior and cultural taboos. Some clients may find specific methods of giving and receiving sexual pleasure unacceptable.

Society as a whole is becoming progressively more open about sexuality. Increasingly, the parenting potential of disabled people is receiving serious attention. Physical assessment is needed to determine a client's ability to reproduce. Male infertility is a frequent complication of spinal cord injury because of testicular atrophy, decreased sperm formation, and ejaculation infrequency. Most men are unable to ejaculate after spinal cord injury. Women usually remain fertile and can conceive and deliver a child. Adoption is a viable option, and conception by artificial insemination is possible.

Disabled people may have contraception concerns. Little is known about the effects of various kinds of contraceptives on disabled people. Oral contraceptives may be contraindicated. Paralyzed women often have slowed circulation, increasing the potential circulatory complications of oral contraceptives. To use an intrauterine device, a woman must have feeling in her pelvis. Then she can recognize early symptoms of pelvic inflammatory disease. Many paralyzed women do not have such feeling. Barrier devices (e.g., a diaphragm, a condom, or foam) may be used if at least one partner has enough manual dexterity to insert the diaphragm or foam or put on the condom.

Nursing Diagnosis: Anticipatory Grieving R/T sudden change in body image, loss of independence, and feelings of inadequacy.

Planning: Expected Outcomes. The client will progress through the grieving process and develop adaptive coping strategies, as evidenced by verbalizing feelings about the degree of injury and the future, participating in community activities, and expressing positive thoughts about the future.

Implementation. Adjusting to paralysis is difficult physically and psychosocially for the client and family. The family may experience the same reactions and need the same kind of help as the disabled client. Sudden paralysis in a previously healthy, active individual can be devastating. Typically, the sudden life-style changes brought about by serious spinal cord injury cause a grief reaction. This may involve initial shock and denial, leading to depression and anger. Crying and talking about the injury repeatedly may be helpful.

It takes time to accept disability and develop ways of coping. Psychological adjustment occurs when the client can accept and deal with reality.

A client may use psychological defense mechanisms in adjusting to paralysis. When caring for such a client, the nurse assesses the possible reasons for the behavior. Hostility, depression, anger, or withdrawal may be upsetting to the staff and family. These behaviors are coping mechanisms and should not be taken personally. Paralysis may cause complex changes in self-concept and body image. In the acute phase, immobilization can contribute to sensory deprivation (e.g., hallucinations). This may be minimized by providing visual, auditory, and tactile stimulation as desired by the client.

Paralyzed clients are often helped initially by being with others who are experiencing similar problems. Clients should be allowed to wear their own clothing as soon as possible and encouraged to be out of bed and out of their rooms. Planned social activities may reduce feelings of social isolation and help clients regain self-confidence. Peer counseling may be helpful (e.g., newly disabled clients talking with others who have adjusted to similar disabilities).

A sense of security is particularly important for a newly paralyzed client adjusting to enforced dependency. A paralyzed client should always have a means of summoning available help, yet needs to learn that it is safe to be alone at times. Gradually, trust develops in the client's abilities and resources, and some reliance on others is relinquished. These feelings and attitudes develop slowly as people experience truly trustworthy relationships.

To avoid unnecessary frustrations, the nurse should try to keep each person's environment comfortable, with necessary items conveniently placed. It is difficult and depressing for the client to have to ask for help repeatedly. Although recent advances have been made in the rehabilitation prognosis of paraplegic and quadriplegic people, it is important to be realistic as well as optimistic. The nurse needs to understand the tremendous life-style changes disabled clients must make. Some can be rehabilitated to a level of near independence, walking (maybe with braces or other appliances), driving a car, and coping with full-time employment outside their home. Quadriplegic individuals usually rely on a wheelchair and other devices and appliances.

Most paralyzed clients can become productive. Even if some are unable to be "productive," all disabled clients have a right to satisfying lives. Although many paralyzed clients achieve complete rehabilitation, others lead lives that are difficult, frustrating, and psychophysiologically complex. At times, severe mental depression may develop. Depression is assessed and professional counseling offered as indicated. Suicide frequently occurs.

Nursing Diagnosis: Family Coping, Ineffective R/T spinal cord injury, loss of independence, perceived or actual change in future plans.

Planning: Expected Outcomes. The client and family identify areas of significant or potential loss and changes in family roles, work together to overcome obstacles, seek appropriate support services, and are able to restore a supportive family structure.

Implementation. Spinal cord injury has a devastating impact on the lives of the injured client and everyone connected with him or her. The injury affects not only physical functioning but also the psychological, vocational, educational, and social aspects of life. An organized team approach is vital to helping the injured client and family cope with life-style changes. Nurses are often the first professionals to assess client and family coping. An open, empathetic manner can allow these individuals to express their grief and uncertainty and ask questions. The nurse teaches the family about the normal grief response. The nurse also carefully probes about persistent denial of grief or lack of progression through grieving. Encouraging as much optimism as possible while remaining truthful and realistic may help spinal cord injury survivors to face the future.

The nurse assesses the previous roles of the client and other family members and how they handle stressful situations or losses. Sources of strength for the family are identified. The nurse assesses patterns of interaction between family members and the family's spiritual, social, and economic status and usual life-style and cultural or ethnic influences. These variables often have an impact on grief responses.

Nursing Diagnosis: Health Maintenance, Altered R/T spinal cord injury.

Planning: Expected Outcomes. The client and family members will be able to successfully meet the client's needs, as evidenced by intact skin, bowel and bladder continence, ability to transfer in and out of wheelchair, absence of infection, maintenance of appropriate weight, and satisfying personal relationships.

Implementation. The learning needs of spinal cord–injured clients and their family members are complex and ongoing. In the acute phase, information regarding spinal anatomy and physiology is needed. When the reality of the injury and the permanency of deficit are understood, coping skills may need to be taught. New means of performing activities and managing bodily functions must be learned. This teaching begins in the acute phase of hospitalization and should be incorporated into all aspects of care. Successful learning in this stage affects the client's entire life.

Teaching should be conducted in short sessions, using easily understood terms. Complex tasks should be taught in steps with return demonstrations.

Evaluation

Spinal cord–injured clients are hospitalized for a long time. Therefore, some expected outcomes need to be evaluated frequently, such as respiratory and cardiac functions. Other expected outcomes will not be met for months, such as independence in ADLs. The plan of care for each client needs to reflect these individual problems. (See the Client Education Guide: Rehabilitation After Spinal Cord Injury.)

CLIENT EDUCATION GUIDE

Rehabilitation After Spinal Cord Injury

- Prevention of skin breakdown in the desensitized and paralyzed areas of the body must be a top priority with clients and care givers. Pressure sores develop mainly over bony prominences that are exposed to unrelieved pressure in the lying or sitting position. Clients can use a mirror to examine areas they cannot view directly. Clients unable to inspect their own skin must take responsibility and ask for assistance from their care givers.
- Frequent relief of skin pressure is necessary to prevent breakdown. Regular turning in bed not only relieves pressure but also aids renal function by preventing stagnation in the urinary tract. Using a special mattress such as a water bed or an alternating pressure pad can lengthen the time required between turning. Skin should be kept clean and dry. It is important that all wrinkles and debris are removed from bed linen. Removing pockets from clothing and selecting clothing with few seams also decrease skin pressure. Use pillows, foam rubber, blankets, or any other form of soft padding to protect vulnerable bony prominences.
- Wheelchair cushions need to be inspected regularly for wear and replaced when necessary. Encourage clients who are able to lift up from the wheelchair seat to do so every 15 minutes. Clients unable to lift themselves will require a special cushion such as a Bye Bye Decubiti or ROHO Dry Flotation Cushion.
- Passive movements of the paralyzed limbs are essential to stimulate circulation, maintain full mobility of joints and soft tissue, and prevent contractures. The client should have a daily range-of-motion program for the paralyzed limbs and a strengthening program for the uninvolved extremities.
- Spasticity is a common complication that could prevent a client from performing some self-care activities. If a spasm occurs during a movement, hold the limb firmly and wait for the spasm to relax before completing the motion. Slow, steady movement works better than trying to hurry. Forced passive movement against spasticity may cause injury or even fracture a limb.
- Clients with spasticity commonly have adductor spasticity. To prevent development of pressure sores, use a wedge large enough to keep thighs abducted. The core of the wedge can be made of an old blanket or other firm material covered with thick foam rubber and encased in stockinette. The wedge can be used in bed and in the wheelchair.
- Provide clients with information about available community resources. Possibilities include transportation, care giver assistance, home adaptations, health services, financial assistance, and recreation.

Modification of Plan of Care for the Elderly

For elderly clients, the most important modification of the nursing care plan is increased vigilance. Elderly people are more prone to the complications of immobility. A person with congestive heart failure may have difficulty breathing when lying flat. Elderly people are also more susceptible to sensory deprivation. The nurse must make sure the individual has his or her eyeglasses and hearing aid. If the person is not able to see a window or clock, he or she should be reoriented as needed. Discharge plans for elderly clients may be complicated if the care giver is also elderly. The spouse of an elderly spinal cord–injured person may not have the physical strength to provide the needed care. Learning to provide the care may also be problematic.

HERNIATED INTERVERTEBRAL DISC

Displacement of intervertebral disc material may be referred to as prolapse, herniation, rupture, or extrusion of the disc. These interchangeable terms indicate loss of integrity of the disc between two vertebrae. Ruptured intervertebral discs may occur at any level of the spine. As in spinal cord injury, thoracic involvement is the least common. Lumbar discs are more likely to rupture than cervical discs because of the forces of gravity.

Incidence

Approximately 80 per cent of all individuals experience low back pain at some point in their lives. One third of these individuals also experience sciatica. This is inflammation of the sciatic nerve, usually caused by compression. The pain follows the course of the sciatic nerve down the leg. It is estimated that 10 per cent of individuals who seek medical attention for back pain have herniated discs.

Etiology

More than one half of the people with symptoms of a herniated disc give a history of a back injury. Flexing the back without bending the knees and making rotating movements create significant stress on the intervertebral disc. Repeated stress progressively weakens the disc, resulting in bulging and herniation. It is postulated that the pain is caused by stretching of the posterior annulus and the posterior longitudinal ligament.

Risk Factors

Heavy physical labor, strenuous exercise, and weak abdominal and back muscles all increase the risk of herniated disc. Use of proper body mechanics is the foundation of primary prevention of back injuries. Strengthening of the back and abdominal muscles provides a strong support for the spine. Bending the legs and keeping the back straight minimize the stress of lifting. Shifting of positions is important for individuals with sedentary employment, such as truck drivers and office workers. Exercise should be encouraged and carried out in a planned and controlled fashion.

Secondary prevention addresses the individual who already has sustained a back injury and wishes to prevent recurrence. Slow, gentle exercise to strengthen muscles is helpful; this may be best supervised by a physical therapist. Weight reduction, if appropriate, reduces stress on the disc. A change in employment may be suggested if occupation is contributing to back pain.

Tertiary prevention focuses on minimizing the complications of a herniated disc. This involves careful monitoring of neurologic signs to detect further deterioration. Muscle strength and deep tendon reflexes are sequentially assessed. Spinal cord or nerve root compression is usually treated surgically.

Pathophysiology

The intervertebral disc is composed of three parts. The cartilaginous plates act as the superior and inferior limits of the disc. These are composed of hyaline cartilage and cover the top and bottom of the vertebrae. The annulus fibrosus is the ring of tissue that gives size and shape to the disc and holds the nucleus pulposus in place. This semigelatinous material forms the center of the disc and provides the cushioning effect.

The annulus fibrosus is weaker in the back than in the front, which explains why most discs herniate in a retrograde fashion. In the case of a disc bulge, the annulus remains intact. With herniation, the annulus is usually torn, allowing extrusion of nucleus pulposus (Fig. 16–4).

Compression of spinal nerve roots may result from herniation of the disc. If compression remains untreated, weakness or paralysis of the innervated muscle group may result.

Clinical Manifestations

Assessment findings with a ruptured lumbar intervertebral disc include:

- Lower back pain that radiates down the posterior thigh
- Muscle spasm
- Aggravation of pain by straining (coughing, defecation, bending, lifting, and straight-leg raising)
- Depression of deep tendon reflexes
- Hyperesthesia in the area of distribution of affected nerve roots

Rupture of a small, laterally placed cervical disc typically causes stiff neck, shoulder pain that radiates down the arm into the hand, and paresthesias and sensory disturbances in the hand. Electromyography or

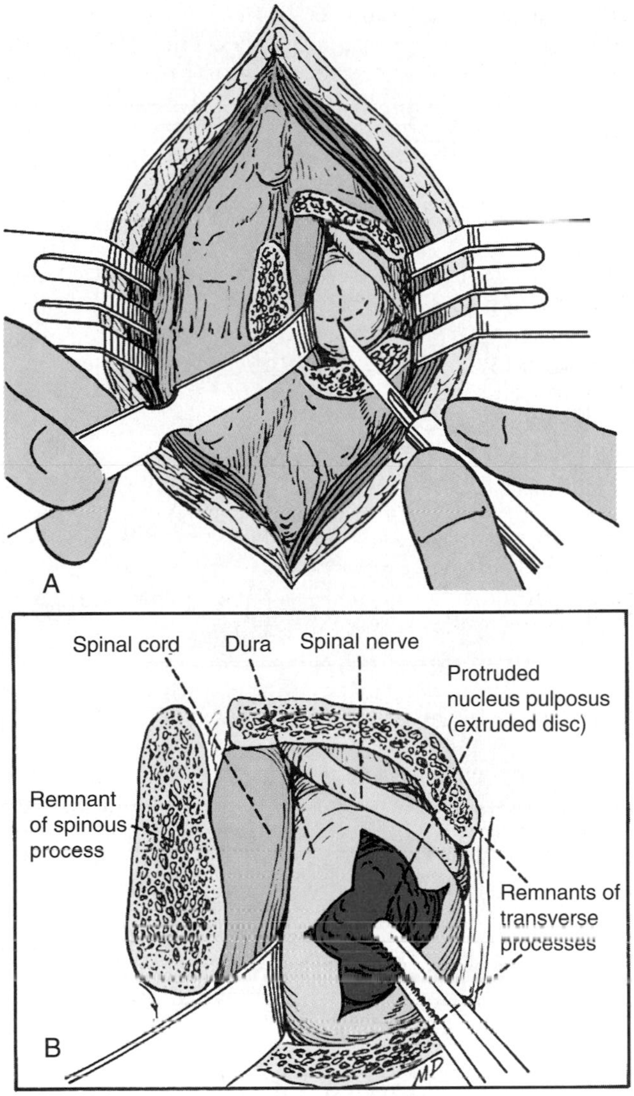

Figure 16–4
Laminectomy for the interlaminal removal of a herniated disc.

electrical testing of the peripheral nerves may localize the ruptured disc site.

DIAGNOSTIC ASSESSMENT

Plain x-ray studies may show spinal degenerative changes (at any level) that may indicate disc problems but usually do not show a ruptured disc. Osteophytes and narrowed disc interspaces are degenerative changes visible on plain x-ray films. Also, other spinal disorders (e.g., spinal tumors, vertebral fracture, rheumatoid arthritis, osteoarthritis) that are useful in establishing an accurate diagnosis may be demonstrated.

MRI may demonstrate spinal stenosis (narrowing of the spinal canal), extrusion of disc material into the spinal canal, or impingement of a spinal nerve root.

Myelography may show narrowing of the disc space or impingement of a spinal nerve root. Myelography identifies the level of herniation and may rule out other spinal diseases. It is typically performed if the MRI is not conclusive. A CT scan is usually done following a myelogram. This sequence allows better imaging with only one administration of contrast material. CT scanning may demonstrate spinal stenosis or other changes associated with degenerative disc disease. CT scans are more useful at the thoracic or lumbar level than the cervical level.

Medical Management

Most cases of intervertebral disc herniation are initially treated conservatively unless there is progressive neurologic dysfunction. Then surgery is indicated.

Conservative intervention for disc problems at any spinal level includes prescribed medications such as anti-inflammatory agents, muscle relaxants, and analgesics. Muscle spasm (which often triggers a cycle of pain and increased muscle spasm) can be severe. Narcotics may be prescribed. Sufficient medication must be administered to achieve pain relief or adequate pain reduction. Deep ultrasonic heat treatment and moist local heat applications may also help. However, one must avoid prolonged heat because it increases congestion. Recently, the use of ice has been found to reduce pain and spasm.

Activities should be reduced during episodes of back or neck pain. Thus, conservative intervention also includes bedrest. Bedrest relieves back pain by relieving the back muscles and vertebrae of the stresses. The forces of gravity (e.g., weight of the head with cervical problems) and motion can increase back pain during activity. Lying in a prone position and sleeping with thick pillows under the head should always be avoided. For clients on bedrest, antiembolic stockings and periodic flexion and extension of the feet are important to prevent thrombophlebitis. Bedside items (e.g., call light) should be placed conveniently to prevent the client from twisting the back to reach them.

Provide psychosocial support to the client and family. Disc problems often create fears and concerns related to pain, treatments, sexual activity, possible length of illness, and possible life-style changes. Socioeconomic considerations about employment and finances should be referred to a social worker.

Client education is an important aspect of back care. See the Client Education Guide: Back Care.

For severe lumbar disc problems, conservative intervention involves bedrest on a firm mattress. Use of traction for lumbar disc problems is controversial. The client should be encouraged to systematically change positions (unless in traction) while on bedrest. If the client requires assistance to turn, or when turning to place a bedpan, the nurse turns the client in a logrolling manner. Use of a fracture bedpan or a child's bedpan instead of a higher, regular-sized bedpan reduces back strain.

Sometimes, with severe lumbar disc pain, a semisitting position is prescribed to promote forward lumbar spine flexion and thus reduce back strain. A client with lumbar pain may be most comfortable when supine, with the bed's backrest elevated 10 to 30 degrees and

CLIENT EDUCATION GUIDE

Back Care

The following points should be included in client teaching about back care:

- Get out of bed by rolling onto one side near the edge of the mattress. Push up to a straight position by pushing off the bed with the arms while keeping the spine straight and swing the legs over the edge. Avoid twisting while getting up.
- Do not sleep while partially reclined or sitting in chair. Sleep on a bed with a firm (not hard) mattress. Avoid riding in or driving a car for a long distance or time. Sit erect without slouching. Avoid low couches and chairs, and use leg muscles when rising from a chair; a recliner chair is usually comfortable.
- When required to stand for a long time, bend one knee to reduce stress on the low back.
- Maintain a body weight that is close to ideal. Exercise and walk or swim to strengthen back muscles. Wear low-heeled shoes.
- Eat a diet high in fiber and fluids to soften bowel movements and reduce strain. (When adding fiber to the diet, add it slowly over days.)
- Use proper body mechanics when lifting. Get adequate help if the object is heavy. Use the muscles of the legs, not the back, by bending at the knees to get close to the object being lifted. Never turn and lift at the same time.

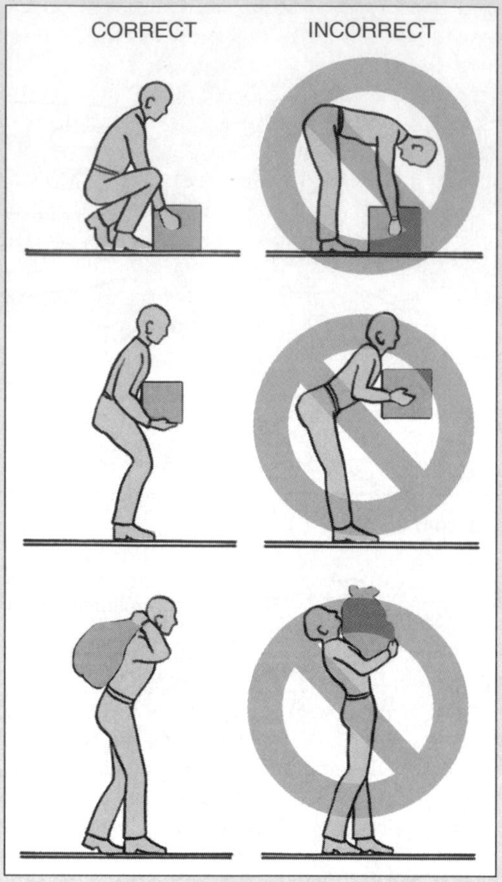

the knees slightly flexed. Other positions of comfort include the supine position with pillows under the legs or the lateral position, in which the client lies on the unaffected side with a thin pillow between the knees and the painful leg flexed to reduce tension on the sciatic nerve. Use of an over-bed trapeze is contraindicated.

A back brace or corset is often prescribed for a client with a ruptured lumbar disc. However, back supports are usually not recommended once symptoms are relieved, because restricted back motion progressively weakens musculature and causes further degeneration of spinal structures. Once the acute pain episode passes, progressive muscle strengthening exercises (usually William's flexion exercises or simple isometric exercises) may be prescribed. Strengthening the back and abdominal muscles helps prevent further problems if the exercises are done daily throughout life. See also the discussion of sciatic nerve injury.

Opinions differ concerning the advisability of performing head and neck ROM exercises in the presence of significant cervical disease. Teach the client to avoid activities that increase cervical disc pain. To prevent neck extension when in bed, only one flat pillow (to prevent neck flexion) is recommended in the presence of cervical disc problems. A soft cervical collar may be prescribed for mild-to-moderate cervical disc problems to keep the head slightly flexed. The neck should not be hyperextended. Intermittent traction may be applied for cervical disc herniation (5–8 lb weight) to relieve pain. The head of the bed may be slightly elevated with cervical traction. Otherwise, it is best kept flat when cervical pain is present.

Conservative intervention often produces satisfactory results in treating herniated discs unless there are obvious neurologic symptoms. Ruptured discs often recede into intervertebral spaces but protrude again upon exertion or change of position.

Surgical Management of Back and Neck Disorders

Spinal surgery is performed to correct spinal deformity (e.g., scoliosis); remove tumors, herniated spinal discs, and hematomas; correct spinal arteriovenous malformations; and fuse unstable vertebrae.

Laminectomy and spinal fusion are the most common spinal surgeries. Laminectomy is the surgical removal of the posterior arch of a vertebra, exposing the spinal cord. This gives access to the spinal canal for (1) removing a spinal cord tumor, (2) removing a portion of nucleus pulposus that is ruptured or protruding from a herniated intervertebral disc, or (3) decompressing (relieving pressure on) the spinal cord.

A bone graft (bone chips) may be placed in the disc interspace during spinal surgery. This is called a spinal fusion, because the new bone that grows fuses the two vertebrae together and immobilizes them. Not all spinal surgeries include spinal fusion, but it is sometimes indicated to strengthen the spine. The bone graft may be obtained from a bone bank or the anterior, superior region of the person's iliac crest. (This graft site is often quite painful postoperatively.) Bone chips may be placed between vertebral bodies where a disc was removed to provide stabilization. Usually no more than five vertebrae are fused; fusing more than five causes loss of movement in the spine. During healing the graft gradually grows onto the vertebrae and fuses them permanently together in a firm, bony union. This causes permanent stiffness in the area. After a while, the stiffness is hardly noticed in the lumbar area but is more noticeable in the cervical area. Metal rods may also be used to straighten and fuse the spine in disorders such as scoliosis.

An anterior or posterior surgical approach may be taken to perform spinal fusions. The anterior approach is usually used only to perform cervical spine fusions. However, when unusual circumstances make a posterior approach impossible, the anterior approach may also be used for thoracic and lumbar fusions.

INDICATIONS

Surgery is indicated with spinal disc problems when conservative intervention is ineffective, neurologic deficits are increasing, and repeated attacks of pain occur despite optimal treatment. Some surgeons use other criteria. A surgical approach is selected that gives the best exposure with the least risk.

Microsurgical techniques in disc removal cause less trauma to the surgical site than standard surgery and preserve more tissue integrity. Advantages of microsurgery include minimal nerve root retraction, preservation of an intact joint capsule (no bone is removed), improved hemostasis, and minimal stripping of the muscle and fascia from the spine. Sometimes foraminotomy is performed to enlarge the intervertebral foramen if it is narrowed and osteophytic processes (overgrowths of bone) entrap the nerve root and impinge on neural structures.

COMPLICATIONS

General potential complications following spinal disc surgery at any level include infection and inflammation; injury to nerve roots, the dural sac, the spinal cord, or other nearby structures; mechanical instability of the spine; inadequate disc removal; spinal cord compression; and hemorrhage.

Specific complications after posterior cervical surgery may include soft tissue hematoma, air embolism, and subcutaneous wound dehiscence. Specific complications following anterior cervical surgeries may include laryngeal nerve damage and injury to neck structures such as the carotid arteries, trachea, esophagus, and soft tissue. Following lumbar discectomy, chronic adhesive arachnoiditis, delayed epidural hematoma, or muscle spasms may occur. Also, severe pain may be experienced owing to improved sensation after nerve root decompression.

CRITICAL TO REMEMBER

The postoperative development of a spinal epidural hematoma is a surgical emergency because it may compress the spinal cord and cause irreversible damage.

Nursing Management

Preoperative Management

The client and significant others are included in preoperative education. The nurse explains to the client that frequent turning follows surgery and that correct turning protects the back and helps the recovery process. The logrolling method of turning is explained.

A baseline neurologic assessment is obtained for comparison after surgery. Assessment should include motor and sensory function of extremities, and psychological readiness for surgery.

The nurse explains that deep breathing, coughing, and turning after surgery help prevent pulmonary complications and that limitations of activity (flexion, extension, or twisting) are necessary to prevent damage to the surgical site and to eliminate straining. The client is also taught to roll onto the side and push the torso from the bed with his or her arms to rise from bed. This technique has often been used by clients with long-standing back pain and may be familiar to the client. In this case, the nurse reviews the client's technique for rising from bed. Clients with a recent injury may not be permitted to ambulate before surgery. For these clients, the nurse explains and demonstrates. The client is advised to ask for help rather than stretching to reach for objects. Stool softeners are given daily while the client is in the hospital to minimize straining at bowel movement.

The nurse encourages the client and family to express their concerns and fears about the spinal surgery. Many people fear postoperative problems such as paralysis and chronic pain. Concerns and fears should be allayed whenever possible.

When the client is being transferred to bed postoperatively, at least four people should assist. Transfer devices such as a sliding board may be used with adequate help. The client should be transferred gently and smoothly, with the spine supported and properly aligned at all times.

Postoperative Management

After spinal surgery, assessment is similar to that of other surgical clients. In addition, neurologic function is assessed by asking the client to move all four extremities and comparing the results with those of the baseline evaluation. The client is questioned about the presence of numbness and tingling and changes in sensation or pain compared with preoperatively. Although there will be incisional pain, often the pain in an extremity associated with a herniated disc will be significantly decreased after surgery. In addition, many surgeons inject long-acting local anesthetics into disc spaces during surgery. This gives the client immediate relief from pain and promotes a positive attitude toward the outcome of surgery. Often the pain recurs on the second postoperative day. This is due to both the increase in swelling and the fact that the local anesthetic is wearing off. The nurse observes the client's movements in bed and reinforces preoperative teaching as needed.

Immediately after a posterior cervical discectomy, a soft cervical collar is worn. The client's head is kept flat except for a folded small blanket or folded sheet beneath the head to maintain spinal alignment while the client lies supine or on the side. Laryngeal nerve damage during surgery may cause permanent vocal impairment, such as a hoarse voice. Difficulty swallowing and throat discomfort are usually present for several days. A drain may be present and is usually removed by the surgeon on the first postoperative day. A hard cervical collar may or may not be prescribed following such a fusion. However, a postoperative x-ray study is typically taken before the client is permitted to assume an upright position, and follow-up x-ray studies are taken to assess healing. During recovery, jiggling movements such as from riding in a car should be avoided (except to go home initially). The graft could be displaced.

Positioning and Turning the Client. Postoperatively, immediately following lumbar discectomy, the person typically is not turned for an hour or so but remains flat to aid hemostasis. Side-to-side logrolling then begins and is done every 2 hours. If a dural tear was repaired, the surgeon may order the person to remain flat longer to minimize the risk of cerebrospinal fluid leak or a tear in the dural sutures. Sometimes, around the third postoperative day, a temporary increase in pain occurs owing to muscle spasm or improved nerve root sensation.

Postoperative care, turning, and positioning after spinal fusion depend on whether the surgical approach was anterior or posterior and the surgeon's preference. The goal of nursing intervention is to prevent strain or flexion at the surgical site.

After lumbar fusion, the bed is generally kept flat. Sometimes the head of the entire bed is elevated on 6-inch blocks, but the bed itself is not flexed, in order not to flex the client's spine. The mattress is firm and a bedboard may be placed under it. A client who will be in bed for a long time may be switched to an alternating air mattress bed or a bed that rocks from side to side. These beds aid turning and promote cardiopulmonary function and circulation. Use of special beds facilitates turning after spinal surgery.

After microdiscectomy, in which the herniated fragment of disc is removed under microscopic visualization, the client may have the head of the bed elevated to whatever position is comfortable. Following cervical spine surgery, the surgeon often permits the head of the bed to be elevated slightly for comfort and to reduce edema.

If a client is lying supine after spinal surgery (e.g., after removal of infection with an open incision remaining), the lower back muscles may be relaxed somewhat if pillows are placed under the entire length of the legs. This may also prevent possible thrombophlebitis in the femoral vessels. The nurse must not flex the client's knees by placing anything under the popliteal space; this is hazardous because it increases the risk of deep vein thrombosis.

When positioning a client in a side-lying position after spinal surgery, strain on the back may be prevented by keeping the spine straight, pulling the hips slightly back so the person is balanced, flexing the upper leg and placing a pillow between the legs, and placing a pillow to support the upper arm and prevent the upper shoulder from sagging. A client who has had cervical surgery is positioned in essentially the same manner. The nurse makes sure the spine is in line at the cervical area and places a small pillow under the head to keep the spine straight.

When turning a client to the side, the nurse uses a logrolling maneuver. Twisting the client's spine or twisting at the hips must be avoided. Safety needs to be ensured during turning to prevent straining of the spine or rolling off the bed. It is beneficial to have extra help in turning a client the first few times after spinal surgery, and adequate help is advisable even after the client is able to participate in the turning process. Spinal bone grafts are delicate and heal slowly. Eventually, turning is permitted without help, while keeping the spine rigid.

The call light is placed so the client can touch it without straining, and all calls are answered promptly so the client does not strain in trying to move. Once a client is allowed to reach for things, the objects needed should be conveniently placed.

Circulation in the client's back, head, and neck after spinal surgery is stimulated by giving frequent gentle back rubs, avoiding the area of surgery.

A sign is placed on the bed stating the prescribed position for the bed, which is discussed with the client. The nurse also instructs the client clearly about contraindicated activities and positions.

Progressive Activity. When helping the client up, the nurse uses the technique specified by the surgeon and has ample help to prevent a fall or other injury to the spine. Blood pressure is assessed before the move is begun. Postural hypotension may occur. If collapse occurs, proper spinal alignment is maintained, and the client is carefully returned to bed.

To prevent falls and enhance proper posture, the

client should wear stockings and firm walking shoes when ambulating, rather than slippers or just stockings.

People with lumbar laminectomies or microdiscectomies are typically out of bed by the first or second postoperative day. Those with cervical fusions are usually out of bed by the first day postoperatively, normally wearing a cervical collar. A spinal fusion usually requires longer bedrest for healing. The surgeon should be consulted about permitted active or passive exercises. Some are contraindicated because they strain the back (e.g., toe touching and straight-leg raises).

Complications. The nurse continues to assess for clinical manifestations of complications and notifies the physician if they occur. The client's neurologic status is assessed and documented frequently, and the development or worsening of a neurologic deficit promptly reported to the surgeon. During the first 24 hours after an anterior cervical discectomy, the nurse assesses the client's ability to breathe, the operative site for excessive swelling, and the client's voice. A soft diet, throat lozenges, viscous lidocaine (Xylocaine), humidified air, minimal talking, and other comfort measures are appreciated. If a spinal fusion was performed with the anterior cervical discectomy, the surgeon is notified if radicular pain suddenly recurs. This could mean that the bone graft has moved out of place and surgery needs to be repeated.

After surgery on the cervical spine, the nurse watches for indications of respiratory paralysis resulting from cord edema. Emergency tracheostomy equipment is kept readily available. Postoperatively, flexion of the neck is prevented.

Skin incisions for laminectomies and posterior spinal fusions are made directly over the spinous processes. The person is logrolled for position changes to maintain skin integrity. The wound or dressing is observed for indications of hemorrhage or cerebrospinal fluid leakage. If present, the nurse notifies the surgeon. The dressing is reinforced as necessary with sterile compresses. The dressing must be changed if contaminated (e.g., with urine). Surgeons usually perform the first dressing change.

Every 2 to 4 hours during the first 48 postoperative hours, client's motor abilities and sensation in the extremities are assessed (see Chap. 12). After lumbar surgery, the person focuses on moving the legs; if cervical, the shoulders and legs. The nurse checks pinprick and light touch with an alcohol wipe on the extremities. Progressive worsening of motor and sensory functions may indicate spinal cord edema or hemorrhage compressing the spinal cord. Assessment findings indicating cord damage or cord compression should be promptly documented and reported. If motor or sensory losses are present, injury from, for example, falls or heat must be prevented.

The client is assessed for indications of postoperative improvement (e.g., "The tingling I had in my leg before surgery is gone now"). These findings are documented.

Pain Management. Compression of various structures caused by edema may cause pain for some time after spinal surgery. Muscle spasms may occur in the back and thigh as a result of irritation of nerves during surgery. Antispasmodics may be prescribed for muscle spasms. The area from which the bone was taken for a spinal fusion may also be painful for several days. Pain relief is provided as indicated. Pain medication is given readily. Narcotics are administered, commonly through epidural sites and patient-controlled analgesia devices. Then acetaminophen (Tylenol) with codeine (or an equivalent) is used. Eventually plain Tylenol is all that is required. The nurse should not wait until the client is in great pain. Appropriate nursing actions are taken to prevent or minimize pain. Keeping the operative leg and the spine correctly and comfortably positioned helps reduce pain and muscle spasms. Massage (not directly over the operated area) may also be relaxing and prevent or reduce pain. The client must always be kept in proper alignment.

Urinary Management. After spinal surgery, urinary retention may occur. Most commonly, it occurs when the cauda equina is affected. Cervical surgery may affect the parasympathetic chain, causing urinary retention. If present, assessment typically reveals a urinary bladder that may feel distended and painful or an inability to urinate. An indwelling catheter may be used for the first few days. Intermittent catheterization may also be used rather than indwelling catheters. When the client is able to void spontaneously, the use of a fracture pan allows the client to remain fairly flat. After 24 to 48 hours, bladder function usually resumes. It helps if the client is permitted to sit up when trying to urinate. After the client voids, the nurse checks residuals. If the bladder is full or cannot be emptied completely, the physician may order straight catheterization to check for residual urine. If the client cannot void voluntarily and the bladder is full, the excess urine will overflow. It may appear that the client is urinating, but actually the bladder remains full. Intermittent catheterization is required.

Men are accustomed to urinating standing up. Lying flat while using a urinal is an unnatural position. Their inability to pass urine does not necessarily indicate bladder dysfunction. Catheterization may be required for a full bladder until standing to void is permitted.

Bowel Management. The most common bowel problem after laminectomy and spinal fusion is paralytic ileus. This loss of bowel sounds and abdominal distention is due to lack of peristalsis from a sudden loss of parasympathetic function innervating the bowels. Assessment findings with paralytic ileus include nausea, vomiting, a hard abdomen, and absence of bowel sounds. Intervention typically includes insertion of a nasogastric tube on low suction and nothing by mouth. When bowel sounds return or the client passes gas or has a bowel movement, a clear fluid diet usually begins, progressing to a regular diet.

The client is assessed every 4 hours postoperatively for bowel distention. Bowel dysfunction may occur for several days postoperatively. Inactivity often causes problems with bowel elimination. Bowel movements are documented. Fluids are forced as ordered; a regular time for bowel movements and bowel care is encouraged; roughage is provided in the diet (when allowed); and medications and enemas as ordered (e.g., stool softeners, mild bulk laxative, or suppository) are administered. The client is instructed not to strain at bowel movement because this increases pain and cerebrospinal fluid.

Often clients find it difficult or impossible to defecate when lying flat. A bowel movement may not occur until sitting up is possible.

Braces, Corsets, and Casts. After spinal surgery, a brace or corset may be temporarily required to support the spine. Persons who have lumbar or thoracic spinal fusions wear a fiberglass brace. Initially, back braces or corsets may be worn all the time, whether the client is in or out of bed. As the client's muscles strengthen, decreased use of braces or corsets is usually recommended. Casts may be used for a while after any thoracic spinal surgery for clients with unstable thoracic spines (e.g., thoracic spinal cord trauma). This is not the only external method of stability for this region of the spinal cord.

Posthospital Care

Clients need clear instructions on ability to walk, lift, drive, and return to work. Most clients can resume activity 6 weeks after surgery. Specific physician instructions need to be followed.

Contraindicated activities vary. The person is instructed to ask the surgeon when it will be safe to perform activities that could damage the back (e.g., climbing stairs, lifting any weight greater than 5 lb, prolonged travel, sexual activity, sports, exercises, driving a car). See also Client Education Guide: Back Care.

SPINAL TUMORS

Spinal tumors are similar in nature and origin to intracranial tumors but occur much less often. They are most common in young or middle-aged adults and most often involve the thoracic region. Spinal tumors may occur outside of the spinal cord (extramedullary) or within the substance of the spinal cord (intramedullary). Extramedullary tumors may be intradural, extradural, or extravertebral. Neurofibromas and meningiomas are the most common spinal cord tumors. Both are benign and operable and may not produce permanent damage if removed early enough.

Clinical manifestations of spinal tumors vary according to their location. Spinal cord compression is the common pathologic feature of all tumors within the spinal canal because it has little room for expansion. Compression of the spinal cord interrupts the function of nerve fibers in the cord's peripheral portions.

Extramedullary tumors cause signs and symptoms by compressing the spinal cord or some of its nerve roots or by occluding blood vessels supplying the cord. Early characteristics of spinal cord compression include pain, sensory loss, muscle weakness, and wasting. Progressive cord compression is manifested by spastic weakness below the level of the lesion, decreased sensation, and increased reflexes. Severe cord compression destroys the cord and produces paraplegia or quadriplegia.

Intramedullary tumors produce more variable signs and symptoms. High cervical cord involvement causes spastic quadriplegia and sensory changes. Tumors in descending areas of the spinal cord produce motor and sensory changes appropriate to functions of that level.

Medical diagnosis is made after a complete general neurologic examination. The diagnostic tests that are used are x-ray study, CT scan, MRI, and myelogram.

Management

Intervention for spinal tumors is usually surgery, radiation therapy, or both. Immediate surgery is indicated if compression of the cord or nerve roots is evident. Often, marked improvement or even complete restoration of function results, especially if the tumor is encapsulated (e.g., meningioma or lipoma). However, surgery often does not have good results if cord necrosis is present (e.g., from compression or interrupted blood supply). Complete surgical removal of an intramedullary tumor is rare, but partial resection followed by radiation may clinically improve the client's condition. The course of the condition is usually gradually progressive.

Injuries to the Peripheral Nerves

Peripheral nerves can be injured in many ways—from bone fractures, stretching of the nerves, constriction by fascial bands, pressure, trauma associated with perforating wounds, or injection of drugs. The peripheral nerves most commonly subjected to external pressure are the radial, common peroneal, ulnar, and long thoracic nerves. The median nerve is most often affected by constriction by fascial bands. The axillary nerve may be affected from an allergic reaction to serum injections. The sciatic nerve may be injured directly during medication injections. Any peripheral nerve can be injured by bone fractures or perforating wounds.

If a peripheral nerve is traumatically severed, the ends should be surgically anastomosed to enable healing. The nearer the site of injury is to the central nervous system, the poorer is the chance of regeneration. When nerves are only slightly damaged, mild edema occurs at the injury site. This may cause temporary symptoms that recede in a few days or possibly weeks.

MEDIAN NERVE COMPRESSION AT THE WRIST

Carpal Tunnel Syndrome

Carpal tunnel syndrome is an entrapment neuropathy that occurs when the median nerve is compressed as it passes through the carpal tunnel in the wrist. This compression causes sensory and motor changes. Carpal tunnel syndrome typically produces increased pain and paresthesia at night, which may awaken the client. The syndrome may develop spontaneously without a known cause or may result from disease or injury. A common cause is trauma to the wrist involving the distal end of the radius and the carpal bones. Another common cause is repetitive movements of the hands and wrists, such as during typing or factory work (Fig. 16–5).

When the symptoms of carpal tunnel syndrome are mild and of short duration, or if the client does not want surgery, the wrist may be splinted in a neutral position with the hand resting to prevent mechanical irritation of the nerve. Temporary relief may be obtained by injection of a steroid suspension into the flexor tendons in the carpal tunnel. Pain relief may occur immediately but is usually transitory. Surgery is indicated with severe symptoms of long duration, muscle atrophy, or progressive sensory loss in the fingers and hand. Usually, surgery for carpal tunnel syndrome involves decompression of the medial nerve by transecting the transverse carpal ligament.

Tarsal Tunnel Syndrome

Tarsal tunnel syndrome is the counterpart of the carpal tunnel syndrome in the lower extremity. In this syndrome, the posterior tibial nerve is trapped beneath the flexor retinaculum and deep fascia along the foot's medial border.

ULNAR NERVE COMPRESSION AT THE ELBOW

Lying within a bony groove at the elbow, the ulnar nerve is susceptible to compression from direct trauma to the elbow (hitting the funny bone) or from changes within the groove that gradually squeeze the nerve. Repeated mild trauma (e.g., habitual leaning on the elbows on a hard surface) can injure the ulnar nerve. Sensory changes occur in the ulnar aspect of the hand

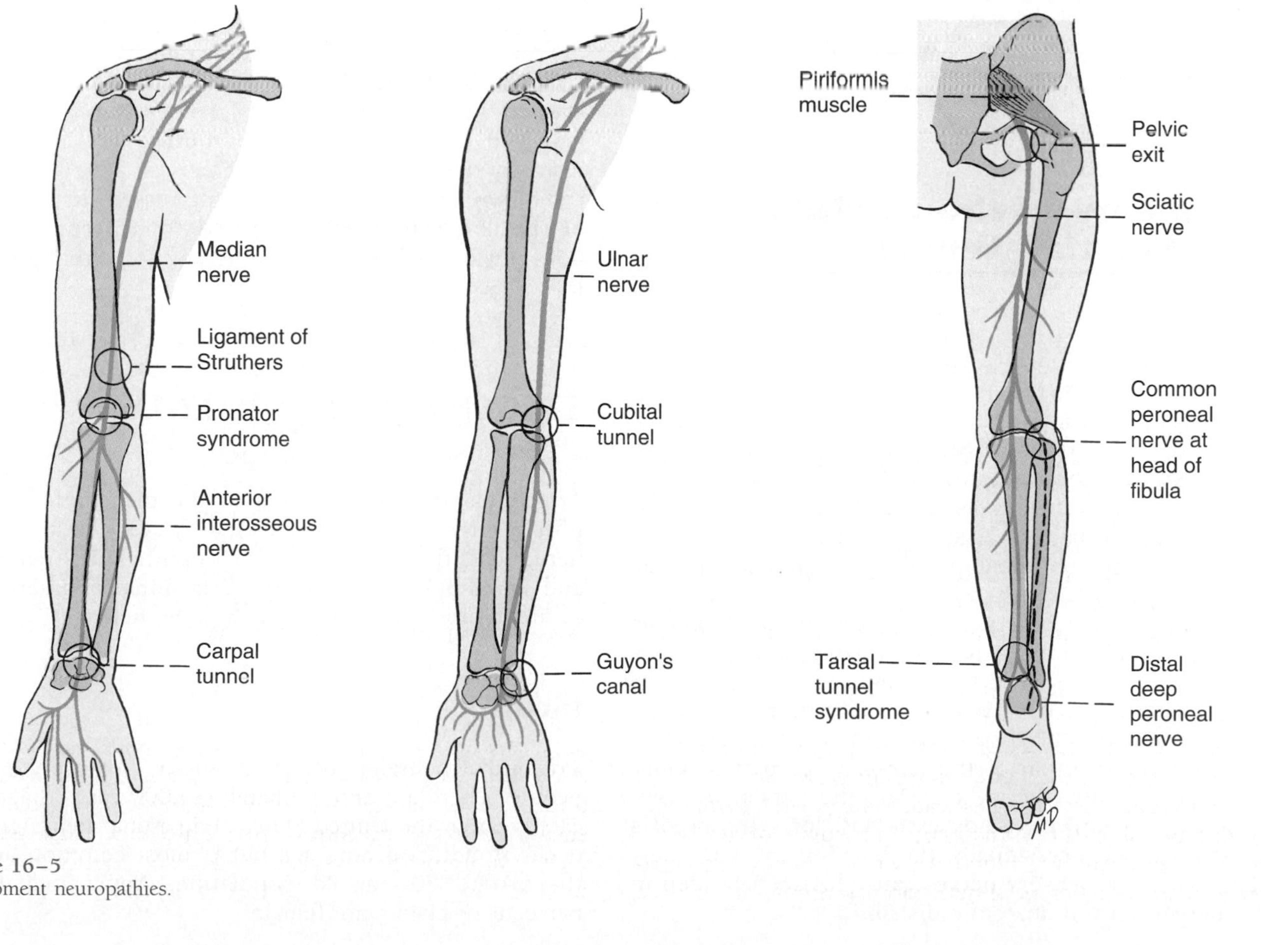

Figure 16–5
Entrapment neuropathies.

and wrist. The usual treatment for ulnar nerve compression at the elbow is surgical transplantation of the ulnar nerve.

SCIATIC NERVE INJURY

The sciatic nerve is the longest nerve in the body. The common peroneal nerve (a terminal branch of the sciatic) is injured more frequently than any other nerve. Because of its particular course and distribution, the sciatic nerve is exposed to internal and external trauma and inflammation more than any other nerve.

Sciatica is severe, usually constant pain in a lower extremity that occurs along the course of the sciatic nerve and its branches. There are many causes of sciatica. However, in about 90 per cent of people, the causes are ruptured intervertebral disc or osteoarthritis of the lumbosacral spine, producing mechanical pressure on the nerve or its spinal roots. Sciatic nerve injury can also result from incorrect medication injection technique.

Typically, the pain of sciatica begins in the buttocks and extends down the back of the thigh and leg to the ankle. Any movement of the lower extremities that stretches the nerve causes pain and involuntary resistance. Straight-leg raising on the affected side is limited. Complete extension of the leg is not possible when the thigh is flexed on the abdomen (Lasègue's sign). Treatment of sciatica is based on treating the underlying cause when possible. Laminectomy may be necessary.

Disorders of the Peripheral and Cranial Nerves

Cranial and peripheral nerves may be damaged by tumors, infections, trauma, vascular and metabolic disturbances, and toxic agents. Neuritis is nerve damage from any cause. Mononeuritis is injury to a single nerve as a result of localized injury. Polyneuritis is diffuse damage to many nerves as a result of toxic agents or metabolic disturbances. Assessment findings with nerve damage depend on the type of nerve injured and the extent of damage.

Damaged motor nerves cause clinical manifestations such as flaccid paralysis, muscle wasting, and reflex loss in the muscle innervated by the injured nerve.

Damaged mixed nerves or sensory nerves cause vasomotor and trophic disturbances after either partial or complete interruption of the nerve. After partial injury or incomplete division of a nerve, the person may experience stabbing pains, dysesthesias (pins-and-needles sensation), and occasionally the burning pains of causalgia. Damaged sensory nerves cause loss of sensation in the nerves' area of anatomic distribution.

PERIPHERAL NERVE TUMORS

Although solitary tumors (generally neurofibromas) may develop on any peripheral nerve, multiple tumors most often occur and are part of a syndrome known as neurofibromatosis (von Recklinghausen's disease). This hereditary disorder is characterized by multiple tumors of spinal and cranial nerves along with the involvement of many other systems. The disease is usually not life threatening, and lesions are excised only when they interfere with normal activity. Intracranial and intraspinal tumors are usually removed.

Management

Surgery for peripheral nerve entrapment is often done on an outpatient basis. In the recovery room, the dressings are checked for drainage and circulation, motion, and sensation to the extremity are assessed. Clients are encouraged to perform ROM exercises. Clients and family members are taught the signs of circulatory compromise and infection, medication management, and care of the dressing and incision.

CRANIAL NERVE DISORDERS

Cranial nerves can be affected in many ways by various nervous system disorders. For example, they may be secondarily affected by compression resulting from increased intracranial pressure, or they may be directly damaged as a result of head injuries. In this section, diseases specific to the cranial nerves, not those associated with other disorders, are discussed. Regeneration of the first (olfactory) or second (optic) cranial nerve does not occur because these nerves are actually part of the CNS.

TRIGEMINAL NEURALGIA

Trigeminal neuralgia is pain in the distribution of the fifth cranial nerve, the trigeminal nerve. The trigeminal nerve has three branches: the ophthalmic, maxillary, and mandibular (Fig. 16–6). Trigeminal neuralgia may occur in any one or more of these branches.

Incidence

Trigeminal neuralgia occurs in about 1 of every 25,000 people. There are approximately 15,000 cases diagnosed each year in the United States. Trigeminal neuralgia can occur in adults of any age but is most common among the 50- to 70-year-old population. Approximately 60 per cent of clients are female.

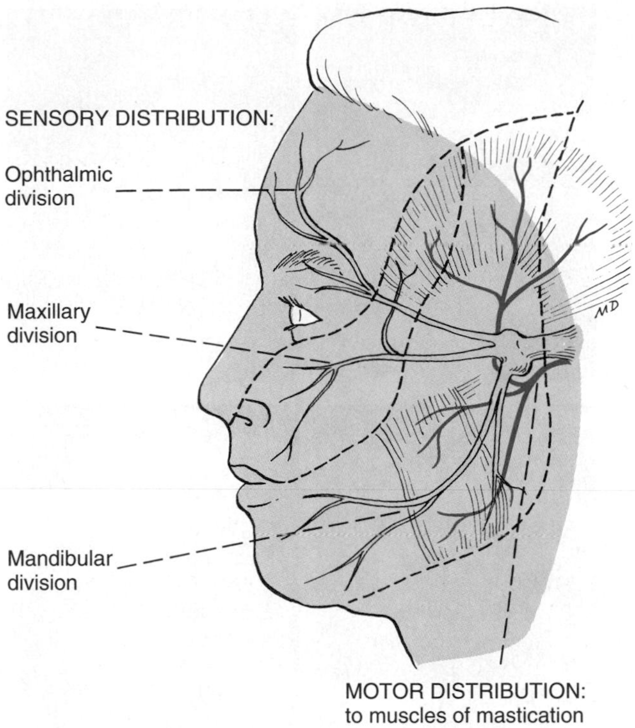

Figure 16–6
Distribution of the trigeminal nerve.

Etiology

The causative mechanisms for trigeminal neuralgia can be divided into intrinsic and extrinsic lesions. Intrinsic lesions are those that occur within the nerve itself. These include gross abnormalities of the axon or myelin and multiple sclerosis.

Extrinsic lesions are outside the trigeminal root and cause distortion, stretching, or compression of the nerve. Mechanical compression is the most common extrinsic cause. This compression may arise from a tumor or from vascular anomalies. Compression of the nerve by a blood vessel is a very common cause. Dental abscesses may also result in irritation of the trigeminal nerve.

Risk Factors

There are no identified risk factors for trigeminal neuralgia. Consequently, there are no primary or secondary preventive measures. Tertiary prevention centers on minimizing the complications that can accompany any cranial pathology.

Pathophysiology

The current theory is that chronic irritation of the trigeminal nerve sets up a cascade of responses. The first response is that segmental inhibition within the trigeminal nucleus fails. This leads to hyperactivity of the primary afferent fibers because action potentials arise from ectopic foci. Tactile stimulation leads to paroxysmal neuronal discharges, triggering of nociceptive neurons, and a trigeminal neuralgia episode.

Clinical Manifestations

Trigeminal neuralgia is characterized by intermittent episodes of intense pain with sudden onset. This pain is not relieved by analgesics. Tactile stimulation, such as touch and facial hygiene and even talking, may trigger an attack. Trigeminal neuralgia is more prevalent in the maxillary and mandibular distributions and on the right side of the face. Bilateral trigeminal neuralgia is rare.

DIAGNOSTIC ASSESSMENT

The actual diagnosis is made on the basis of an in-depth history, with attention paid to triggering stimuli and the nature and site of the pain.

Medical Management

The anticonvulsants carbamazepine (Tegretol) and phenytoin (Dilantin) are often prescribed as initial treatment for trigeminal neuralgia. The rationale for using these drugs is that they may dampen the reactivity of the neurons within the trigeminal nerve. For some clients, these medications are all the treatment that is ever needed. Liver impairment may result from administration of both Tegretol and Dilantin. Liver enzymes must be monitored before and during therapy. These medications should be used cautiously in clients with a history of alcohol abuse. Baclofen (Lioresal) is an antispasmodic that may be used alone or in conjunction with the anticonvulsants. Narcotics are not particularly effective in relieving trigeminal neuralgia pain.

Surgical Management

Surgical procedures can be categorized according to invasiveness. Less invasive procedures are nerve blocks using alcohol and glycerol, peripheral neurectomy, and percutaneous radiofrequency lesions. The relief obtained with these procedures is not always permanent. Complications include development of facial paresthesias and muscular weakness. These procedures, being less invasive, are often better tolerated by elderly or debilitated clients.

The more invasive techniques involve major surgical procedures. Microvascular decompression involves removing the vessel from the posterior trigeminal root. Rhizotomy is actual resection of the root of the nerve. These procedures require a craniotomy to allow access to the nerve. Complications include those of any surgical procedure as well as facial weakness and paresthesias.

Nursing Management

A careful history is obtained from the client regarding stimuli that trigger an attack. This information is used to plan care so as to minimize triggering events. The client's dental hygiene and nutritional intake are evaluated. These clients often do not eat enough to meet their daily nutritional needs and neglect their teeth because of the pain.

The nurse helps clients use and improve any pain control strategies they have developed. Individuals with trigeminal neuralgia need emotional support to help them deal with pain that has often been present for a long time.

Clients should be taught to use a water jet device instead of a toothbrush for dental hygiene, and a visit to the dentist as soon as possible after surgery should be recommended. If facial anesthesia is present following surgery, clients must learn to test the temperature of food before putting it into their mouth. They should chew on the unaffected side and inspect mucous membranes for irritation. The nurse assesses for aspiration and advances the diet slowly.

If the corneal reflex has been impaired, the client will need to be taught eye care. During the acute postoperative period, the nurse needs to apply eye drops and a protective shield. The client assumes these tasks with supervision and then independently.

BELL'S PALSY: SEVENTH CRANIAL (FACIAL) NERVE

This discussion concerns motor aspects of the facial nerve, the main motor nerve of the facial muscles. The facial nerve becomes paralyzed more often than any other. Facial paralysis may be central or peripheral in origin. Central facial palsy is an upper motor neuron paralysis or paresis. Sometimes it produces dissociation of motor function. In this situation, the client cannot voluntarily show the teeth on the paralyzed side, but can show them with emotional stimulation such as that causing smiles or laughter. This phenomenon is called voluntary emotional dissociation.

Bell's palsy is the most common type of peripheral facial paralysis. Bell's palsy is a unilateral paralysis of the facial muscles of expression with no evidence of a pathologic cause. Assessment findings on the affected side include:

- Upward movement of the eyeball on closing the eye (Bell's phenomenon)
- Drooping of the mouth
- Flattening of the nasolabial fold
- Widening of the palpebral fissure
- A slight lag in closing the eye

Eating may be difficult. Bell's palsy affects both women and men in all age groups. However, it is most common between ages 20 and 40 years (Fig. 16–7).

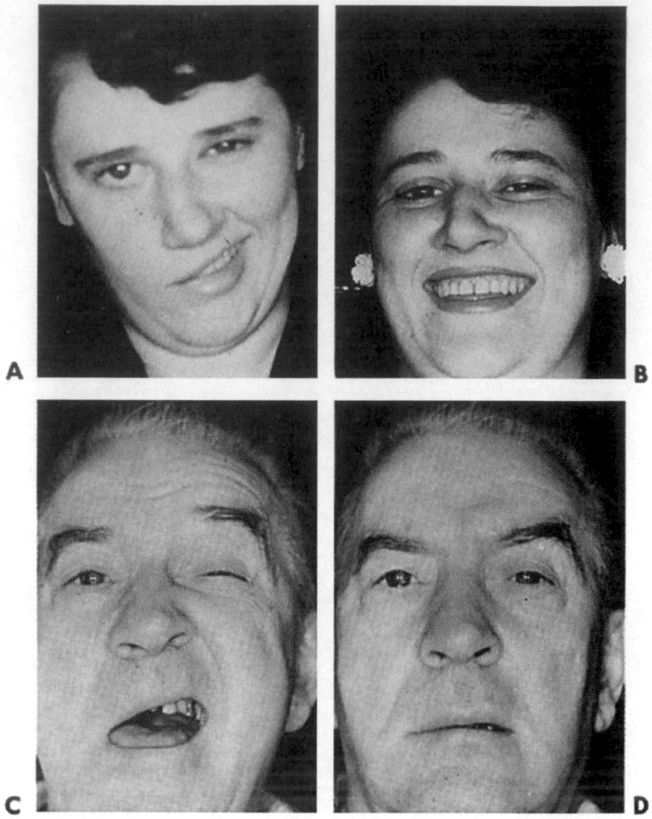

Figure 16–7
A, Bell's palsy of 1 week's duration. *B,* After treatment, the paralysis of the seventh nerve disappeared. *C,* Bell's palsy following exposure to cold. Note the right-sided paralysis and inability to close the right eye. *D,* Drooping of the right lip. (From Archer, W. H. [1975]. *Oral and maxillofacial surgery* [5th ed.] [pp. 1669, 1672]. Philadelphia: W. B. Saunders Co.)

Management

There is no known cure for Bell's palsy. Palliative measures include the following:

- Analgesics if discomfort occurs from herpetic involvement
- Corticosteroids to decrease nerve tissue edema
- Physiotherapy, moist heat, gentle massage, stimulation of facial nerve with faradic current
- Corneal protection with artificial tear solution, sunglasses, eye patch at night, and periodic gentle closure of the eye

Clients experiencing Bell's palsy often think they have had a stroke. One must reassure the client that this is not true. Most clients recover from Bell's palsy within a few weeks without residual symptoms. If permanent complete facial paralysis occurs, surgery may be necessary. Anastomosis of the peripheral end of the facial nerve with the spinal accessory or the hypoglossal nerve allows closure of the eye during sleep and restores tone to the facial musculature.

STUDY QUESTIONS

1. While the nurse is caring for a client who is a C5 quadriplegic, the client complains of severe headache, nausea, and nasal congestion. On assessment the client has a pulse of 40 and a blood pressure of 190/110. Which of the following nursing actions is most appropriate at this time?
   A. Place the client flat in bed.
   B. Assess for bladder distension.
   C. Administer oxygen.
   D. Administer medication for pain.
2. In assessing the client with an incomplete spinal cord lesion, the nurse would anticipate:
   A. Loss of all voluntary movements and sensation below the level of the lesion
   B. No loss of motor or sensory function
   C. Varying degrees of motor and sensory loss below the level of the lesion
   D. Only loss of reflex function below the level of the lesion
3. Which of the following practices places the client at greatest risk for the development of back pain?
   A. Heavy physical labor
   B. Strenuous exercise
   C. Weak abdominal and back muscles
   D. All of the above
4. After a lumbar laminectomy, the client complains of increasing back pain on the second postoperative day. The nurse knows that the increased amount of pain:
   A. Is a sign of the development of a complication
   B. Is normal as a result of swelling and local anesthetic wearing off
   C. Often signals a chronic back pain problem
   D. Occurs before sensory impairment
5. In assessing the client with trigeminal neuralgia, the nurse would expect to find:
   A. Ptosis of the eyelid
   B. Intermittent episodes of intense pain
   C. Flattening of the nasolabial fold
   D. Upward movement of the eyeball on closing the mouth

CRITICAL THINKING EXERCISES

SCENARIO A

A 23-year-old construction worker is admitted to the emergency department after a fall from a scaffold. He momentarily lost consciousness after the accident but is now fully alert and oriented. Cervical spine x-ray films show a compression fracture with damage to the cord at C4. He is to be fitted with a halo brace.

1. What assessment data should the nurse gather during the emergency care of this client?
2. What are the priority nursing diagnoses for this client?
3. Describe the nursing care for the client with a halo brace.

SCENARIO B

A 43-year-old client has been experiencing back and leg pain. Magnetic resonance imaging showed an L4-L5 herniated intervertebral disc. She is admitted to the hospital to undergo a lumbar laminectomy.

1. In planning preoperative teaching for this client, what should the nurse include?
2. The client asks about her activity level after surgery. What should the nurse tell her?
3. What teaching should be included in the discharge planning?

BIBLIOGRAPHY

1. Aisen, M. (1993). Differential diagnosis of spinal cord disease. In L. Barclay (Ed.), *Clinical geriatric neurology*. Philadelphia: Lea & Febiger.
2. Beretta, G., et al. (1989). Reproductive aspects in spinal cord injured males. *Paraplegia, 27*(2), 113–118.
3. Dunnum, L. (1990). Life satisfaction and spinal cord injury: The patient perspective. *Journal of Neuroscience Nursing, 22*, 43–47.
4. Frank, R. G., & Elliott, T. R. (1989). Spinal cord injury and health locus of control beliefs. *Paraplegia, 27*(4), 250–256.
5. Gaehle, K. E., et al. (1992). Thoracolumbar burst fractures. *AORN Journal, 55*(3), 721–731.
6. Huang, C., et al. (1990). Anemia in acute phase of spinal cord injury. *Archives of Physical Medicine and Rehabilitation, 71*.
7. Hickey, J. V. (1992). *The clinical practice of neurological and neurosurgical nursing*. Philadelphia: J. B. Lippincott.
8. Maeda, C. J., et al. (1990). The effect of halovest and body position on pulmonary function in quadriplegia. *Journal of Spinal Disorders, 3*(1), 47–51.
9. Marshall, S. B., et al. (1990). *Neuroscience critical care: Pathophysiology and patient management*. Philadelphia: W. B. Saunders.
10. Mitchell, M. (1989). *Neuroscience nursing: A nursing diagnosis approach*. Baltimore: Williams & Wilkins.
11. Nieves, C. C., Charter, R. A., & Aspinall, M. J. (1991). Relationship between effective coping and perceived quality of life in spinal cord injured patients. *Rehabilitation Nursing, 16*, 129–133.
12. Preksto, D. (1992). The Kaneda device: A new anterior spine stabilization system. *AORN Journal, 55*(3), 734–746.
13. Youmans, J. R. (Ed.) (1995). *Neurological surgery* (4th ed.). Philadelphia: W. B. Saunders.

UNIT 5

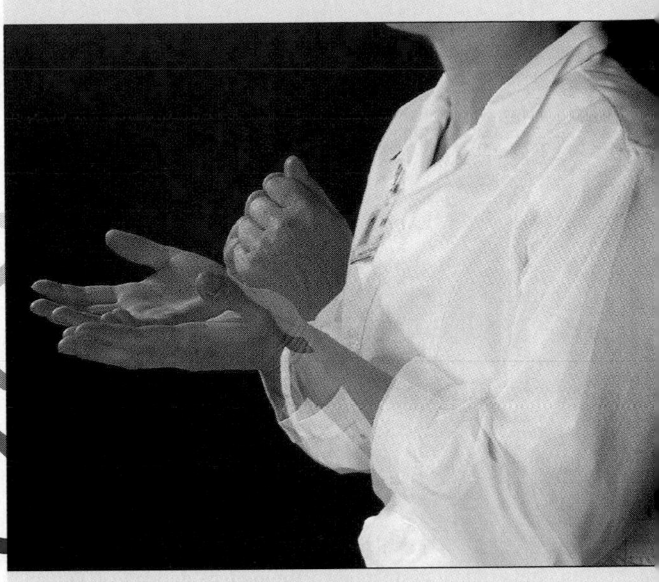

Sensory Disorders

Communicating is a basic human need. Essential to this interaction is the adequate functioning of the senses. A person unable to receive sensory input (e.g., through sight, sound, smell, taste, and touch) has a communication disability. For example, children born deaf or in whom hearing loss develops before they learn to speak have difficulty not only hearing sounds but also learning to talk effectively. Likewise, persons with impaired vision are limited in the amount of visual stimuli they can take in, interpret, and respond to.

Our senses are also a source of pleasure. Consider the joys of looking at the face of a loved one, hearing a bird sing, smelling the fragrance of a flower, tasting a favorite food, and stroking a companion animal. Clients experiencing sensory disorders live with the reality and hardships of sensory deprivation.

This unit's chapters cover the problems experienced by clients with sensory disorders and other problems of the eyes and ears. Chapter 17 focuses on problems with the eyes and vision. Discussion includes assessment and diagnostic tests, general care and protection of the eyes and vision, and nursing care related to eye disorders and their management. Chapter 18 discusses problems with the ears and hearing, covering assessment and diagnosis, general care and protection, and nursing care for clients with ear and hearing problems.

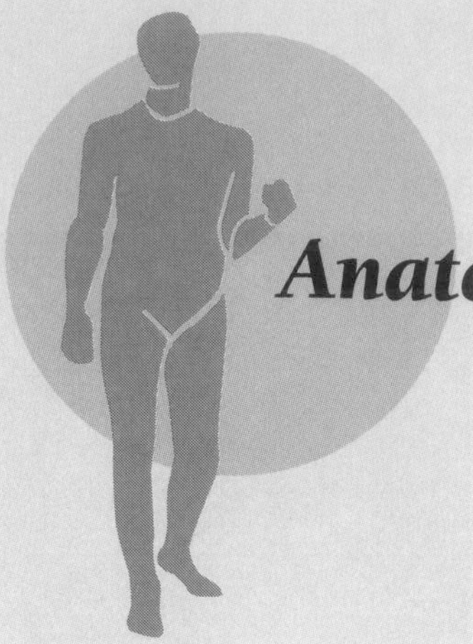

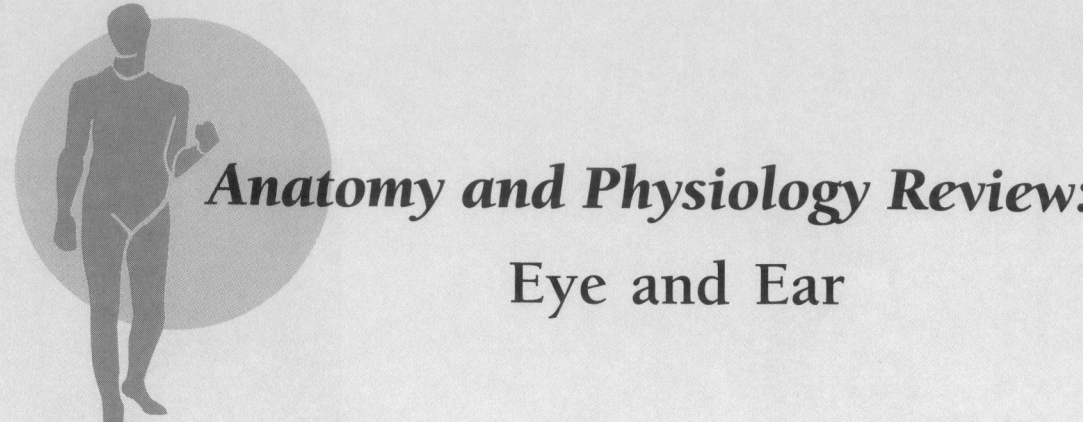

Anatomy and Physiology Review: Eye and Ear

EYE

The visual system is a complex group of structures that includes the eyeballs, muscles, nerves, fat, and bones. The eyes contain the photoreceptors and are the external portion of the visual pathway. Electrical impulses travel along the visual pathway from the photoreceptors to the brain, where the impulses are interpreted as vision. Accessory structures protect and move the eye.

Ocular Adnexa

The ocular adnexa are the accessory structures of the eye that support and protect it. These structures include the bony orbit, fat, eyelids, lacrimal apparatus, and the ocular muscles.

Bony Orbit. The bony orbit, or eye socket, surrounds and protects most of the eye so that only a small portion is visible from the exterior. It is formed from portions of the frontal, lacrimal, ethmoid, maxilla, zygomatic, sphenoid, and palatine bones. In addition to the eyeball, the orbit contains fat, various connective tissues, blood vessels, and nerves.

Eyelids. The upper and lower eyelids are folds of skin that close the eye to keep foreign objects from entering. Movement of the eyelids helps distribute a film of tears across the surface of the eye. Eyelashes along the margin of the eyelids help trap foreign particles. Conjunctiva, a thin transparent layer of mucous membrane, lines the eyelids.

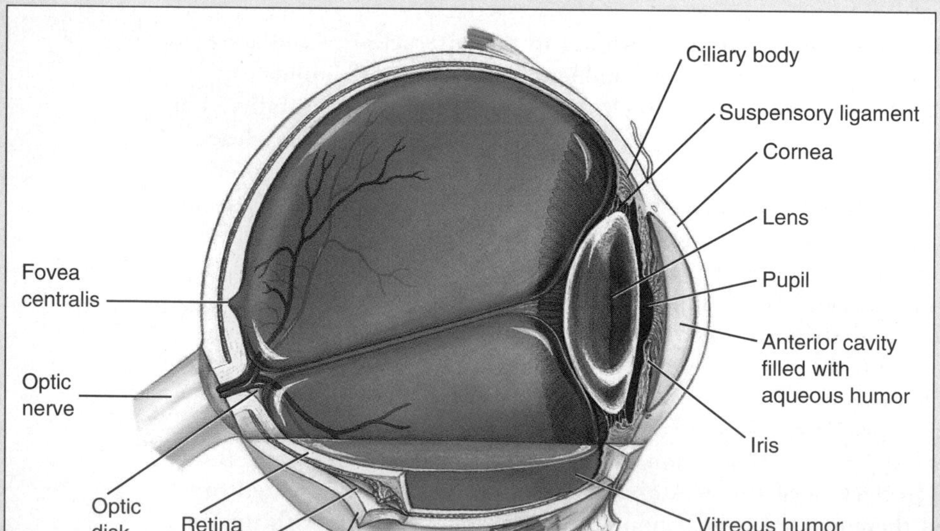

Anatomy of the eye.

The lacrimal apparatus. (From Jarvis, C. [1992]. *Physical Examination and Health Assessment.* Philadelphia: W. B. Saunders Co.)

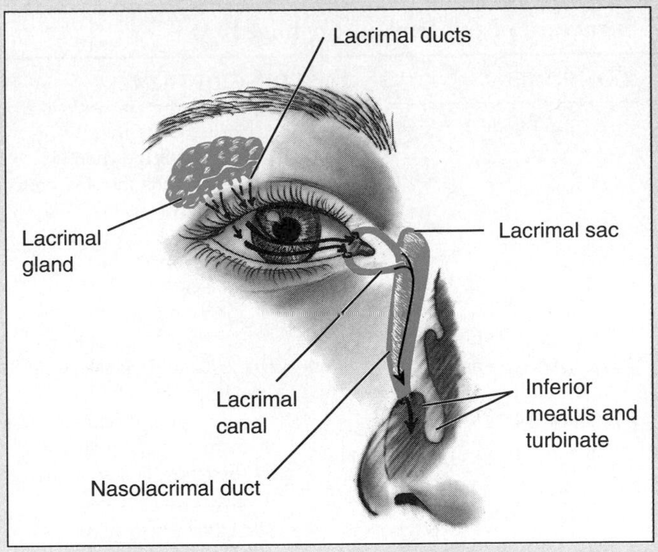

Lacrimal Apparatus. The lacrimal apparatus consists of a lacrimal gland in the superior and lateral margin of the orbit, and a duct system for drainage. The gland produces tears that reach the ocular surface through secretory ducts. The tears moisten and clean the ocular surface. The nasolacrimal duct drains the tears into the nasal cavity.

Ocular Muscles. Six extrinsic ocular muscles are attached to the surface of the eyeball and are responsible for its movements.

Eyeball (Bulbus Oculi)

In the normal adult, the eyeball, or bulbus oculi, measures approximately 24 mm in diameter and is protected by orbital fat within the bony orbit. The conjunctiva that lines the eyelids is continuous with the bulbar conjunctiva that covers the anterior surface of the eyeball. The elasticity of the conjunctiva permits the eye to move freely within the orbit. The components of the eyeball include the wall, lens, humors, and angle structures.

Structure of the Eyeball

COMPONENT	DESCRIPTION	FUNCTION	COMMENTS
Wall			
Outer fibrous tunic			
Sclera	White, opaque, fibrous layer that covers the posterior five sixths of the eyeball; continuous with the cornea	Support and protection	Extraocular muscles attached to sclera; may become yellowish due to degenerative changes
Cornea	Transparent, avascular, convex covering of the anterior one sixth of the eyeball; continuous with the sclera; about 0.5 mm thick with numerous nerve fibers	"Window" of the eye where light rays enter; refracts (bends) light rays	Derives its oxygen from the atmosphere; sensitive to pain
Middle vascular tunic (uvea)			
Iris	Thin, pigmented, doughnut-shaped diaphragm with a central aperture called the pupil	Regulates the amount of light that enters the eye by changing the size of the pupil	Colored portion of the eye
Choroid	Highly vascular, dark pigmented layer between the sclera and retina and firmly attached to the retina; attached anteriorly to the ciliary body and posteriorly to the optic nerve	Dark pigment absorbs excess light rays; blood vessels nourish interior of eye	Only loosely connected to the sclera, can be stripped away easily

Table continued on following page

Structure of the Eyeball *Continued*

COMPONENT	DESCRIPTION	FUNCTION	COMMENTS
Ciliary body	Circular structure that is continuous with the choroid and surrounds the lens; contains ciliary processes and ciliary muscle; suspensory ligaments attach ciliary body to the lens	Ciliary processes produce and secrete aqueous humor; ciliary muscles regulate the shape of the lens by increasing or decreasing tension in the suspensory ligaments; suspensory ligaments also support the lens	The area anterior to the ciliary body and lens, but posterior to the cornea, is called the anterior cavity, which is divided into anterior and posterior chambers by the iris
Inner nervous tunic (retina)			
Pigmented epithelium	Single layer of dark cells firmly attached to the choroid	Absorbs excess light	Region where a retina "detaches"
Photoreceptor cells	Rods and cones; rods are more numerous in the periphery of the retina; cones are more localized near the center of the retina	Rods function in black and white vision and for vision in dim light; cones are for color vision and acuity	Damage to rods results in night blindness; very active metabolically, adequate oxygen supply from capillaries in the choroid is critical to normal vision
Bipolar neurons and ganglion cells	Numerous layers of neural tissue between the photoreceptor cells and the interior of the eye	Transmit impulses created by the rods and cones	Axons of the ganglion cells converge to form the optic nerve
Optic disc	Region in the posterior part of the retina where the optic nerve emerges from the eye	Optic nerve transmits visual impulses from the retina to the brain	Optic disc represents a blind spot in the eye because it contains no rods or cones; can be seen with an ophthalmoscope
Macula lutea	Yellowish region, about 5 mm in diameter, in center of retina; central depression of macula is the fovea	Fovea contains only cones, so it is area of sharpest vision	Damage to macula can severely reduce vision
Lens	Biconvex, avascular, colorless, and transparent; supported by suspensory ligaments attached to the ciliary body; posterior to the iris; surrounded by transparent capsule	Refracts light rays to focus them on the retina	Change of focus from distant objects to near objects (accommodation) achieved by interaction between the elasticity of the lens and tension in the suspensory ligaments
Humors			
Aqueous humor	Fluid similar to plasma in the anterior cavity; secreted by ciliary processes, flows through the pupil and drains through the canal of Schlemm into the blood	Maintains a constant intraocular pressure; helps nourish lens and cornea; transmits light rays	Aqueous humor normally replaced about every 90 minutes; glaucoma is increased intraocular pressure due to imbalance between production and drainage of aqueous humor
Vitreous humor	Clear, avascular, viscous, jelly-like substance in posterior chamber; also called vitreous body	Helps maintain shape of eye; pressure from vitreous helps keep retina attached to choroid; transmits light rays	Not continually replaced; formed during embryonic life and lasts a lifetime
Angle structures	Trabecular meshwork and venous canal (of Schlemm) where the cornea and iris meet	Aqueous humor filtered through the trabecular meshwork into the venous canal and then into the blood	Normally there is a balance between the production of aqueous humor and drainage into the venous canal to maintain normal intraocular pressure

Optic Nerve and Visual Pathway

The visual pathway begins with the rods and cones in the retina where the visual impulses are generated. From there the impulses travel along the optic nerves, optic chiasma, optic tracts, thalamus and midbrain, and optic radiations and are finally interpreted in the visual cortex of the occipital lobe.

Age-Related Changes

Several age-related changes occur in the eye and surrounding tissue. The eyebrows and eyelashes turn gray, skin around the eyes may become wrinkled, and lacrimal gland secretion may decrease, resulting in dry eyes.

The most significant changes occur in the lens. It tends to become thicker and less elastic, which makes it less able to change shape to accommodate for near vision. This condition, called presbyopia, or farsightedness of aging, is probably the most common age-related dysfunction of the eye. The lens also tends to become cloudy or opaque, developing cataracts. About 90 per cent of people over age 70 have some degree of cataract formation; however, it is not always significant enough to affect vision seriously. The cornea tends to become more translucent and less spherical, which contributes to an increase in astigmatism in older people.

Older people require more light to see well because atrophy of the muscles in the iris reduces the ability of the pupil to dilate and decreases the amount of light that reaches the retina. The chemical processes that rebuild the visual pigment, rhodopsin, are slower in older people, so dark adaptation takes longer and is not as complete as in young people. This puts older people at greater risk for falls and injuries, particularly when there is a sudden change in light intensity.

Glare from the cornea and lens is a particular problem at night. This and a decrease in peripheral vision are often reasons older people stop driving at night. The vitreous humor begins to liquefy and collapse, resulting in pieces of debris that are annoying even if they do not obstruct vision. Additionally, the retina may degenerate because of local ischemia.

EAR

Structure of the Ear

The ears are a pair of complex sensory organs that function both in hearing and in balance. Pathology in the ear may reduce a person's ability to communicate, limit social activities and the use of leisure time, and compromise career opportunities and financial security. The visible portion of the ears on the sides of the head

Visual pathway from the retina, where impulses are generated, to the occipital lobe, where they are interpreted.

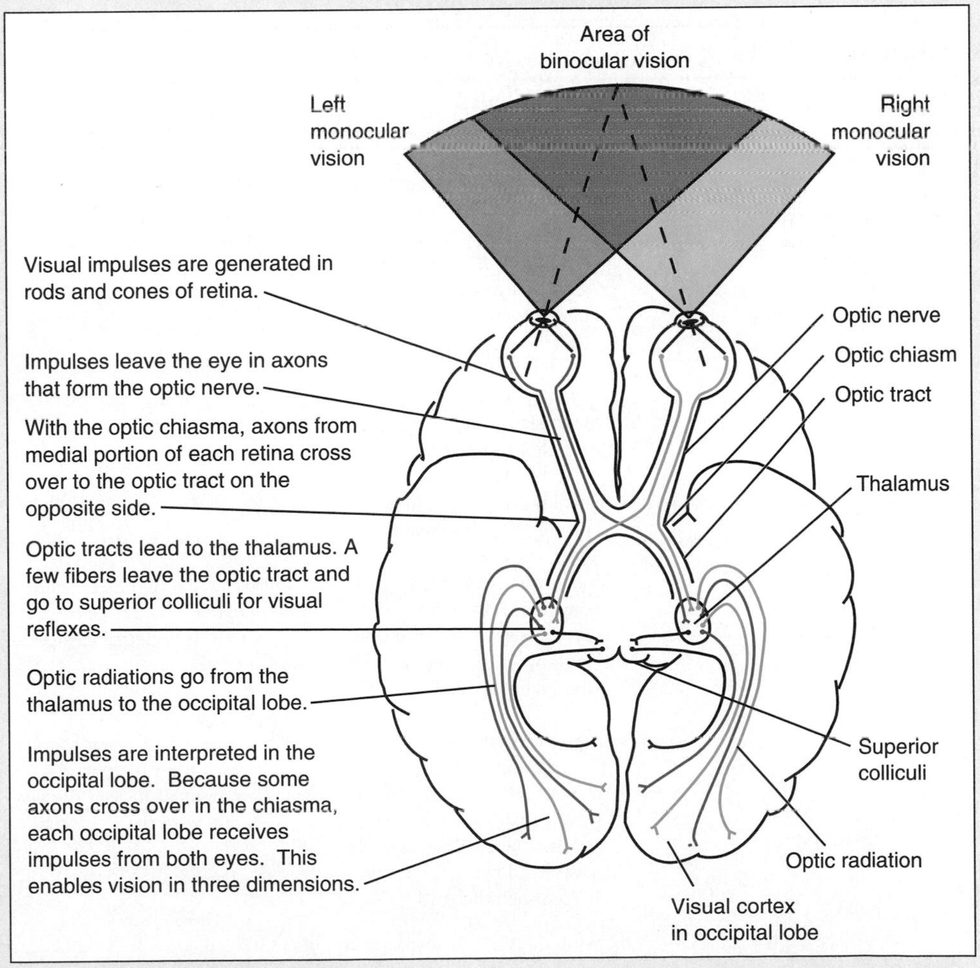

Area of binocular vision
Left monocular vision
Right monocular vision
Visual impulses are generated in rods and cones of retina.
Impulses leave the eye in axons that form the optic nerve.
With the optic chiasma, axons from medial portion of each retina cross over to the optic tract on the opposite side.
Optic tracts lead to the thalamus. A few fibers leave the optic tract and go to superior colliculi for visual reflexes.
Optic radiations go from the thalamus to the occipital lobe.
Impulses are interpreted in the occipital lobe. Because some axons cross over in the chiasma, each occipital lobe receives impulses from both eyes. This enables vision in three dimensions.
Optic nerve
Optic chiasm
Optic tract
Thalamus
Superior colliculi
Optic radiation
Visual cortex in occipital lobe

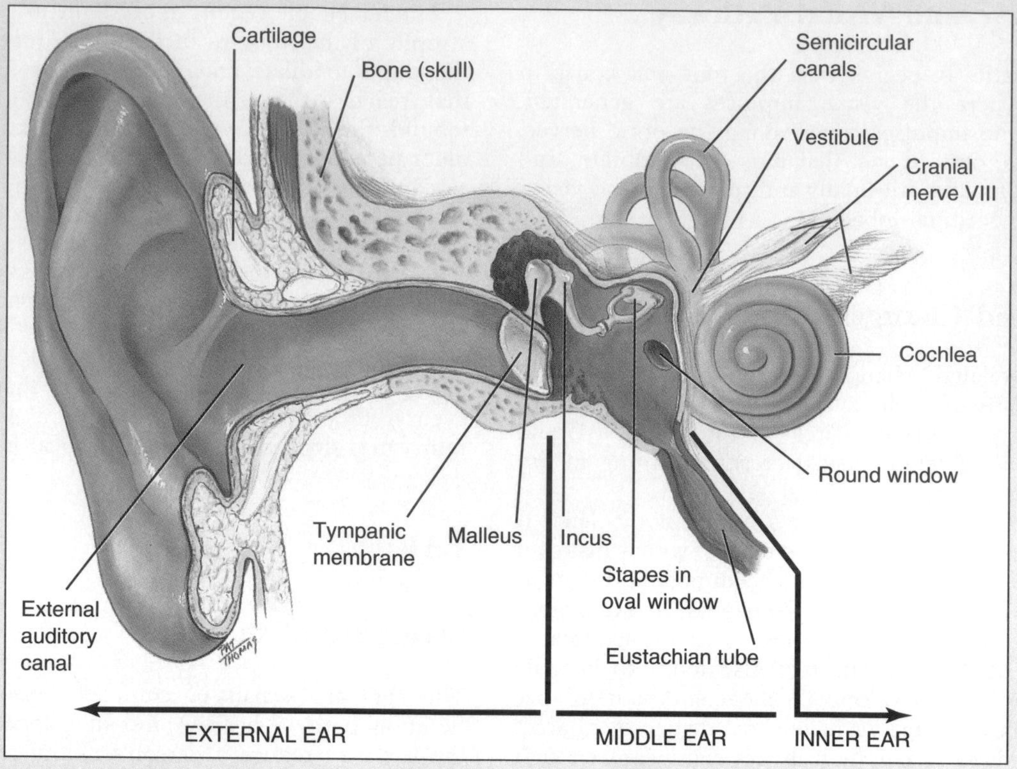

Anatomy of the ear. (From Jarvis, C. [1992]. *Physical examination and health assessment.* Philadelphia: W. B. Saunders.)

Structure of the Ear

COMPONENT	DESCRIPTION	FUNCTION	COMMENTS
External ear			
Auricle or pinna	Visible portion of the ears on the sides of the head; formed primarily of cartilage covered with skin; sebaceous glands and rudimentary hairs cover most of the surface	Collects sound waves and directs them toward the auditory meatus	The temporomandibular joint (TMJ) is immediately anterior to the external opening of the ear; TMJ problems frequently produce referred pain to the ear
External auditory meatus (external auditory canal)	S-shaped cartilaginous tube, about 2.5 cm long, lined with skin, extends from the auricle to the tympanic membrane; skin contains sebaceous and ceruminous glands that, together, produce cerumen (ear wax)	Canal directs sound waves to the tympanic membrane; hairs and cerumen help cleanse the canal of foreign matter	Retention of wax may become a problem in elderly people; impacted cerumen can cause hearing loss at any age, sometimes must be mechanically removed
Tympanic membrane (eardrum)	Thin, translucent, pearly gray membrane, oval disc approximately 1 cm in diameter; covers the inner end of the auditory canal	Protects the middle ear and conducts sound vibrations from the external ear to the ossicles	May be ruptured or perforated by shock waves from an explosion, scuba diving, trauma, or acute middle ear infections
Middle ear (tympanic cavity)			
Ossicles	Three tiny bones within the middle ear; malleus, the largest, is firmly attached to the tympanic membrane; stapes, the smallest, is in the oval window; incus lies between the other two	Mechanically transmit sound waves from the tympanic membrane through the oval window to the inner ear	Smallest bones in the body

Structure of the Ear *Continued*

COMPONENT	DESCRIPTION	FUNCTION	COMMENTS
Windows			
Oval	Opening between middle ear and inner ear filled with the stapes foot plate, where sound waves enter the inner ear	Transmits sound vibrations from the stapes to the fluids in the inner ear	
Round	Membrane-covered opening where sound vibrations exit the inner ear	Relieves pressure as vibrations exit the inner ear	
Eustachian tube (auditory tube)	Narrow channel approximately 35 mm long and 1 mm wide, connects the middle ear to the nasopharynx; normally closed to both the middle ear and the nasopharynx	Provides an air passage from the nasopharynx to the middle ear; during yawning, sneezing, and swallowing, the tensor veli palatini muscle opens the tube to equalize pressure on both sides of the tympanic membrane	Throat infections may spread to the middle ear through the eustachian tube
Mastoid	Portion of the temporal bone posterior to the pinna; contains an interconnected arrangement of air-filled spaces	Air-filled spaces aid the middle ear in adjusting to changes in pressure	Mastoid cavity is close to the dura mater of the brain, the sigmoid sinus, and internal carotid artery; infections from middle ear may pass through mastoid to these structures
Inner ear			
Bony labyrinth	Series of interconnecting chambers in the temporal bone; contains a fluid called perilymph	Surrounds and protects the delicate membranous labyrinth	
Vestibule	Central portion	Contains the utricle and saccule, which function in the sense of balance	Vestibular branch of cranial nerve VIII emerges from this region
Cochlea	Coiled portion	Contains the cochlear duct, which contains the auditory receptors; the portion above the cochlear duct is the scala vestibuli and the portion below is the scala tympani	Cochlear branch of cranial nerve VIII emerges from this region
Semicircular canals	Portion that consists of three semicircles and extends from the vestibule opposite the cochlea	Contains the semicircular canals of the membranous labyrinth, which function in the sense of balance	Nerve fibers from this region enter the vestibular branch of cranial nerve VIII
Membranous labyrinth	Series of membranous tubes within the bony labyrinth; contains a fluid called endolymph, is surrounded by perilymph	Contains the receptor cells for hearing and balance	
Utricle and saccule	Two saclike portions of the membranous labyrinth located within the vestibule of the bony labyrinth; each contains a small structure called a macula	The macula, within the utricle and saccule, is the organ of static equilibrium	Static equilibrium (balance) is involved in evaluating the position of the head relative to gravity
Cochlear duct	Membranous tube within the bony cochlea; contains the organ of Corti	Organ of Corti, within the cochlear duct, contains the receptors for sound	Cochlear duct, like all other regions of the membranous labyrinth, contains endolymph
Semicircular canals	Three membranous tubes within the bony semicircular canals; canals are positioned in three different planes, at right angles to each other; each canal has an enlargement, or ampulla, at its base	Each ampulla contains a crista ampullaris, which has hair cells that function in dynamic equilibrium	Dynamic equilibrium (balance) is involved in detecting rotational or angular movement

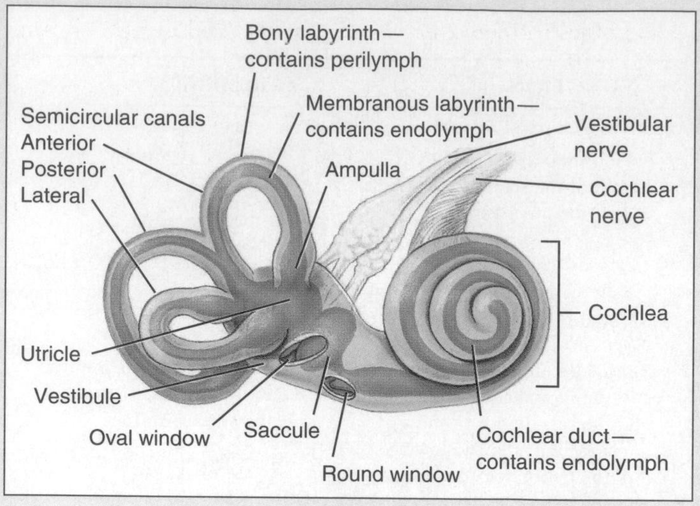

Labyrinths of the inner ear.

is only a small part of the actual organ. The most important part, the receptor organs and nerves, lies hidden from view within the temporal bones, which form a portion of the base and lateral walls of the skull. Anatomically, the ear is divided into the external ear, the middle ear, and the inner ear.

Physiology of Hearing

Hair cells are specialized sensory cells in the organ of Corti, which is located within the cochlear duct of the membranous labyrinth. A gelatinous layer, called the tectorial membrane, extends over the hair cells. It is easier to follow the pathway of the pressure waves created by sound in an uncoiled or straightened cochlea than in the normal coiled structure. The list following summarizes the sequence of events in the initiation of auditory impulses.

- Tympanic membrane vibrates in response to sound waves.
- Malleus, incus, and stapes transfer vibrations to the oval window.
- Movement in the oval window starts oscillations in the perilymph.
- Perilymph oscillations cause vibrations in the vestibular and basilar membranes.
- When the basilar membrane moves, hair cells in the organ of Corti rub against the tectorial membrane and bend.
- Bending of the hair cells initiates the formation of nerve impulses.

Auditory impulses are transmitted along the cochlear branch of cranial nerve VIII to the medulla oblongata where some fibers cross to the opposite side. From the medulla oblongata, the impulses go to the midbrain for auditory reflexes, then to the thalamus, and finally to the auditory cortex on the temporal lobe.

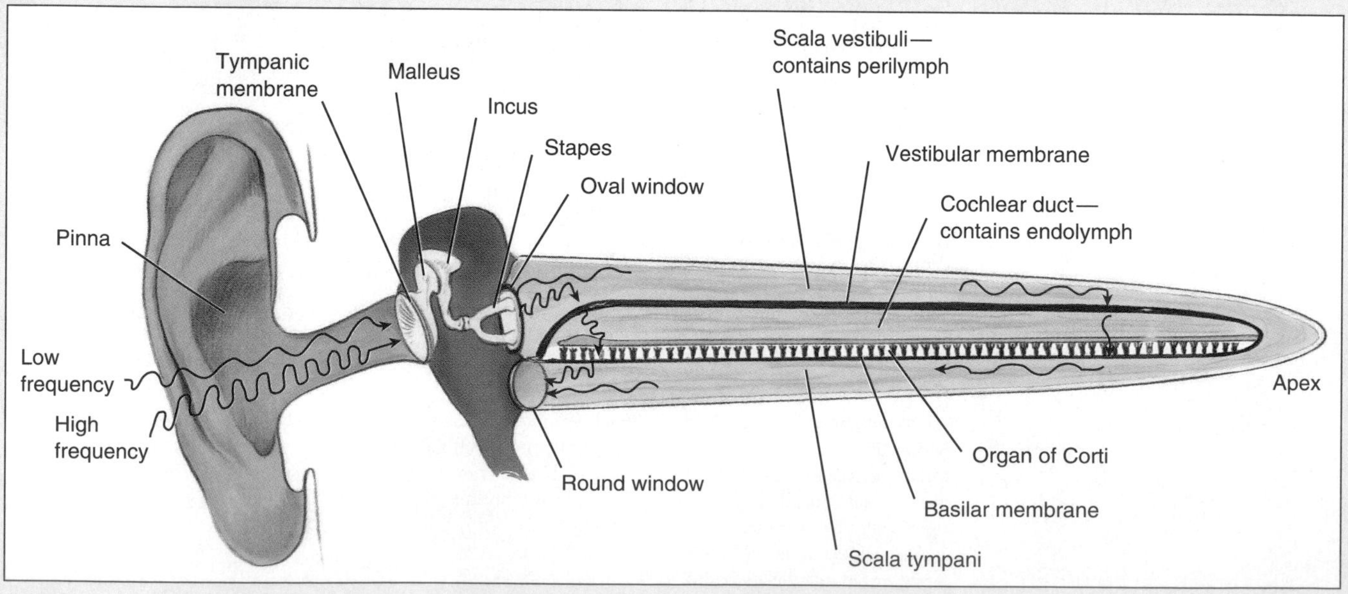

The uncoiled cochlea, showing the pathway of pressure waves.

Pitch is determined by the portion of the basilar membrane that vibrates and stimulates hair cells. Different regions of the membrane are sensitive to different pitches. The portion near the middle ear vibrates in response to high frequencies (high pitch), and the region near the apex is more sensitive to low frequencies (low pitch). Loudness is determined by the intensity of the sound waves. Louder sounds cause more vibration in the basilar membrane, more hair cells are stimulated, and more impulses travel to the auditory cortex.

Physiology of Balance

Balance is a combination of static equilibrium and dynamic equilibrium. The sense receptors for static equilibrium are hair cells in the macula, which is found in both the utricle and saccule of the vestibule. When the head is in an upright position, the hair cells are straight. When the head bends forward or tilts, calcium carbonate crystals called otoliths and the gelatinous mass over the hair cells move. This bends some of the hair cells and initiates an impulse, which is transmitted on the vestibular branch of cranial nerve VIII to the central nervous system.

Rotational or angular movements, called dynamic equilibrium, are detected by hair cells of the crista ampullaris located in the ampulla at the base of each of the three semicircular canals. Each crista ampullaris has hair cells embedded in a gelatinous mass called the cupula. When the head turns, endolymph pushes against the cupula and it tilts. This bends the hair cells and initiates an impulse. The canals are positioned in three different planes so their cristae are stimulated differently by the same motion. This creates a mosaic of impulses that are transmitted to the central nervous system on the vestibular branch of cranial nerve VIII. The central nervous system interprets the information and initiates appropriate responses to maintain balance.

Age-Related Changes

Most age-related changes in the external ear and middle ear have little effect on hearing. Cerumen, or earwax, may accumulate in the external ear and contribute to hearing loss, especially in the low frequency range. This is corrected by removal of the impacted cerumen. The joints between the ossicles may become less movable and interfere with transmission of sound waves. Most of the gradual loss of hearing due to aging, called presbycussis, is caused by degeneration of the receptor cells in the organ of Corti. Another factor is a reduction in the number of nerve fibers in the vestibulocochlear nerve, cranial nerve VIII. A decrease in the cochlear branch contributes to hearing loss, and reduction in the vestibular branch interferes with balance and equilibrium. Bacterial and viral infections in the temporal bone may also cause a sensorineural hearing loss.

Chapter 17 Assessment and Nursing Care of Clients with Eye Disorders

Learning Outcomes

After completing this chapter, the learner will be able to:

1. Teach the client about the normal structure of the eye.
2. Explain to the client abnormalities of ocular structure and function.
3. Conduct a nursing history and physical assessment of the client with actual or potential disorders of the eye and vision.
4. Teach the client about diagnostic studies common to functions of the eye.
5. Assess the client for clinical manifestations of ocular disorders.
6. Teach the client about the etiology, risk factors, basic pathophysiology, and clinical manifestations of major ocular disorders.
7. Explain the client's role in the medical and surgical management of ocular disorders.
8. Develop plans of care for the prevention of illness, management, and rehabilitation of the client with an ocular disorder.
9. Implement nursing interventions that optimize the quality of life for the client with an ocular disorder.
10. Evaluate planned client outcomes, using outcome criteria developed in the planning phase of care.

The eye is a complex organ that involves intricate microscopic structures capable of bringing the entire world into the mind. The visual pathway is a multidimensional system that transcends anatomic description. Although there have been great technologic advances in understanding ocular physiology, there remains an element of mystery regarding the science of vision.

The use of sight is an integral part of early life experiences. Most individuals are not consciously aware of the degree to which they depend on it for daily functioning. Once vision becomes significantly limited, the degree to which sight influences the activities of daily living (ADLs) becomes acutely apparent. Even simple tasks become difficult to perform. Seeing what food is being served at the table, selecting clothes for color and design, avoiding objects while walking, and reading books, magazines, or personal mail are no longer possible. The visually impaired person must adapt to this loss to maintain independence and control.

It is essential for nurses to understand the complexity of ocular structures and the physiology of vision to provide comprehensive nursing care to their clients. The specialty practice of ophthalmic registered nursing is devoted to caring for clients with eye disorders. Ophthalmic registered nurses perform the roles of care giver, advocate, educator, counselor, technician, coordinator, and researcher. Not only is ophthalmic nursing care directed at those biologic systems that are affected by an actual or potential deficit, but it is an integration of how actual or potential visual deficits affect the individual as an entire being.

Assessment of Clients with Eye Disorders

One of the most important considerations in an ocular assessment is that many ophthalmic disorders are asymptomatic. The four most common preventable causes of permanent vision loss in developed nations are

- Amblyopia (reduced visual acuity that is uncorrectable with glasses in the absence of anatomic defects in the eye or visual pathways)
- Diabetic retinopathy
- Age-related maculopathy
- Glaucoma

It is for these reasons that routine eye examinations are imperative.

The eye is a unique organ of the body in that the external anatomy of the eye may be easily assessed. Even the internal eye is visible through the cornea where blood vessels and central nervous system (CNS) tissue (the retina and the optic nerve) may be visualized without the use of x-ray films or invasive procedures. The effects of many systemic disorders, such as infections, neoplasms, vascular disorders, and autoimmune disorders, are detectable with an internal eye examination.

HISTORY

An ophthalmic history includes demographic data, the chief complaint, medical history, family history, psychosocial history, and review of systems.

Demographic Data

Demographic data relevant to ocular assessment include age and sex. The incidence of cataracts, dry eye, retinal detachment, glaucoma, entropion (eyelid inversion), and ectropion (eyelid eversion) increases with age. Males have hereditary color vision deficits. Women do not have as many hereditary visual problems.

Chief Complaint

The most common chief complaint is often a change or loss of vision but may also be less specific, such as headache or eyestrain. It is common that the client is unable to verbalize a specific complaint. The chief complaint may be as vague as "Something is wrong with my eyes." Whenever possible, symptoms are characterized according to the rapidity of onset, the location, duration, and characteristics (such as frequency and severity). The associated circumstances surrounding onset are important as is the client's response to treatment. Current eye medications being used and all other current and past ocular disorders are recorded.

Ocular symptoms may be divided into three basic categories of abnormalities: vision, appearance, and ocular sensation—pain and discomfort.

ABNORMAL VISION

Visual changes or loss of vision may be due to abnormalities in the eye or anywhere along the visual pathway. Considerations in this category include a refractive (focusing) error, lid ptosis (drooping of the eyelid), clouding or interference in the cornea, lens, aqueous or vitreous space, malfunction of the retina, optic nerve, and intracranial visual pathway.

Glare or halos may result from uncorrected refractive error, scratches on glasses, dilated pupils, corneal edema, and cataract. Flashing or flickering lights may indicate retinal traction or migraine. Floating spots may represent normal vitreous strands or the pathologic presence of blood, pigment, or inflammatory cells in the vitreous. Diplopia (double vision) may occur in one eye or both and may be due to refractive correction, muscle imbalance, or neuromuscular disorders.

ABNORMAL APPEARANCE

The most common abnormal appearance is the red eye. Causes of red eye include minor irritation, vascular congestion, subconjunctival hemorrhage, inflammatory disorders, infection, allergy, and trauma. Other external changes in appearance include growths or lesions, edema, redness, or abnormal position.

ABNORMAL SENSATION

Eye pain is often poorly localized. Nonspecific complaints may be eyestrain, pulling, pressure, fullness, or generalized headache. The pain may be periocular, ocular, or retrobulbar (behind the globe). Foreign body sensation produces a sharp superficial pain relieved by topical anesthesia. Deeper internal aching may indicate glaucoma, inflammation, muscle spasm, or infection. Reflex spasm of the ciliary muscle and iris sphincter that occurs with inflammation may produce brow ache and *photophobia* (sensitivity to light) or a constricted pupil (miosis). Itching is usually a sign of an allergic response. Dryness, burning, grittiness, and mild foreign body sensation can occur with dry eyes or mild corneal irritation. Tearing may be due to irritation or an abnormality of the lacrimal system. Increased ocular secretions usually indicate viral or bacterial infections and may also be present in allergic and noninfectious irritations.

Medical History

The medical history focuses on the client's general state of health. Specifically, the nurse should ask about systemic disorders commonly associated with ocular manifestations, such as diabetes mellitus, arthritis, hypertension, thyroid disease, and myasthenia gravis. If glasses or contact lenses are worn currently, the client should be questioned as to when the last eye examination was and when the prescription was last changed. The nurse should inquire whether the client has been hospitalized or has had surgery related to the eyes or brain. Is there a history of head trauma or eye trauma related to motor vehicle accidents or sports injury? Has the client had surgery on the eyes such as laser treatment?

CHILDHOOD AND INFECTIOUS DISEASES

Diseases occurring in childhood with possible ocular sequelae include diabetes mellitus, retinoblastoma, thyroid disorders, rheumatoid arthritis, exposure to sexually transmitted diseases such as syphilis and acquired immunodeficiency disease (AIDS), and muscular dystrophy. Inquire about immunizations, particularly for measles (rubella).

MEDICATIONS

Many medications affect the eyes. Prescription drugs include insulin, corticosteroids, oral hypoglycemics, and thyroid replacement hormones. The nurse should ask whether or not the client uses eye drops and note the name, dose, and frequency taken. Specifically, one must determine whether or not the client uses over-the-counter eye drops, such as natural tears. Over-the-counter preparations that may dry the eyes include antihistamines and decongestants.

ALLERGIES

Note allergies to medications and other substances. Has the client ever had an allergic reaction to eye drops or other medications that have affected the eyes? Allergic symptoms include eye redness, tearing, and itching. One should determine past allergic reactions not only to medications but also to inhalants (dust, chemicals, or pollens) and contactants (cosmetics or woolens).

Family History

Because there are many ocular disorders with familial tendencies, it is important to ask questions specifically about strabismus, glaucoma, myopia (nearsightedness), and hyperopia (farsightedness). Other common familial disorders include migraine, retinoblastoma, macular degeneration, retinitis pigmentosa, sickle cell anemia, keratoconus, and diabetes mellitus. Lack of a family history does not necessarily rule out the possibility of a genetic disorder. Some clients do not know the ocular history of family members, and some may be embarrassed or hesitant to share the information.

Psychosocial History and Life-Style

Psychosocial history and life-style factors that influence ocular health include occupational hazards and leisure activities and hobbies. Is the client exposed to irritating fumes, smoke, or airborne particles? Are safety goggles worn in situations in which eye injury may occur from fragments of metal or sand? Is there a problem with insufficient lighting, leading to eyestrain, or harsh, glaring lighting? Participation in active outdoor activities such as gardening, hiking, cross-country skiing, baseball, and contact sports increases risk of foreign body injury, abrasion, or penetrating injury. Does the client wear sunglasses or other protective eye gear when outdoors?

Health-management behaviors related to the eyes are explored. If the client has a systemic disease that affects the eyes, are self-care measures practiced? For example, does the diabetic client aggressively manage the disease by attempting to regulate blood glucose levels with diet and ordered medication? If the client wears contact lenses, are the lenses cleaned and stored as recommended? Is the client capable of safely taking care of the lenses?

Review of Systems

The review of systems relevant to the eyes includes asking about symptoms such as headaches and problems with sinusitis. Specifically, one should ask whether symptoms occur in association with pain or discomfort, visual changes, swelling, redness, or drainage from the eye.

PHYSICAL EXAMINATION

The role and scope of practice of the nurse in ophthalmic assessment and examination varies according to state nurse practice acts, institutions, and employer guidelines. Regardless of the level of responsibility in any practice situation, the nurse must be knowledgeable about ophthalmic clinical manifestations and diagnoses as they relate to the holistic approach in client care.

Examination of the eyes includes assessment of external structures, using inspection and palpation, extraocular movements, visual acuity, and visual fields (peripheral vision). Nurses may perform tonometry and examine the internal eye structures with an ophthalmoscope. When documenting observations, the abbreviations OD (right eye), OS (left eye), and OU (both eyes) should be used.

The client's body structure and features are observed for obvious deformities and apparent age. For example, the hand deformities or abnormal gait of an arthritic may be a clue to the diagnosis of an associated eye disorder of keratoconjunctivitis sicca (dry eye syndrome) in a client who complains of itching and burning eyes.

External Eye Examination

External eye structures include the eyebrows, eyelashes, eyelids, lacrimal apparatus, anterior portion of the eyeballs, conjunctivae, sclerae, corneas, anterior chambers, pupils, and irises. Inspect and palpate these structures while the client sits at eye level to the examiner.

EYE POSITION

Assess eye position for symmetry and alignment. Sunken or protruding eyes are abnormal findings, as is protrusion of one eye or both eyes, as in exophthalmos.

EYEBROWS

Inspect the eyebrows for symmetry, hair distribution, skin condition, and movement. Hair loss of the lateral aspects occurs with aging. The skin may be dry and flaking (i.e., dandruff), which is abnormal.

EYELIDS AND EYELASHES

Examine the eyelids and eyelashes for placement and symmetry. When open, the upper lids rest at the top of the irises and the lower lids at the bottom so that the sclerae are not visible above or below the irises. Sagging of the upper lids that covers part of the pupil is abnormal and called ptosis. Ptosis may occur with aging but also results from edema, third cranial nerve disorders, and neuromuscular disorders. Check for effective closure by asking the client to close the eyes. Eyelids that turn inward (entropion) or outward (ectropion) can result in corneal irritation.

BLINK RESPONSE

Blinking is an involuntary reflex that occurs bilaterally up to 20 times a minute. Rapid, infrequent, or asymmetric blinking is abnormal.

EYEBALLS

The eyeballs are palpated for symmetry and firmness. Instruct the client to close the eyes and look down. Place the tip of the index fingers on the upper eyelids, over the sclerae, and palpate gently. Normally, the eyeballs feel firm and symmetric, not asymmetric, hard, or soft. Nurses may perform tonometry to measure ocular pressure. See the section on internal eye examination for discussion of tonometry.

LACRIMAL APPARATUS

The lacrimal apparatus is examined by retracting the upper lid and having the client look down so that part of the lacrimal gland may be visualized. Observe this area for swelling or tenderness. The eye surface should be moist, without excess tearing. Inspect the area between the lower lid and the nose, which should be free of edema. The area over the lower orbit rim near the inner canthus (over the lacrimal sac) is palpated gently. There should be no regurgitation of fluid from the sac or puncta.

CONJUNCTIVAE AND SCLERAE

The conjunctivae and sclerae are inspected for color changes, texture, vascularity, lesions, thickness, secretions, and foreign bodies. Small blood vessels may be visible. In white individuals, the sclerae are white, whereas they may appear light yellow in clients with dark skin tones. To inspect the palpebral conjunctivae, the nurse is advised to wear gloves. Regardless of whether gloves are worn, meticulous hand washing is advised both before and after the conjunctivae are examined. The lower eyelids are retracted to expose the conjunctivae without applying pressure to the eyeballs. The nurse (or the client) gently pushes the lower lids down against the bony orbit while the client looks up. Healthy conjunctivae are pink to light red; paleness or bright red color are abnormal. If the lower palpebral conjunctivae are normal, the upper palpebral conjunctivae usually are not inspected.

CORNEA

Inspect the cornea from an oblique angle while shining a penlight on the corneal surface. The irises are easily visible. In the elderly, a thin, white ring around the corneas' edges may be seen (arcus senilis). Abnormalities include surface irregularity and cloudiness or opacity.

CORNEAL REFLEX

The corneal reflex test is performed to assess the function of the fifth (trigeminal) cranial nerves. The client is instructed to keep the eyes open and look straight ahead. A sterile cotton wisp is brought from behind the client and lightly touched to the cornea. The client should blink and tear, indicating that the nerves are intact. A separate wisp is used for each eye. Clients who wear contact lenses may not respond to the same degree as clients who do not wear them because they become somewhat insensitive to the stimulus.

ANTERIOR CHAMBER

The anterior chamber is inspected with the cornea using the same oblique angle and penlight. The chambers should appear clear and transparent with no cloudiness or shadows cast upon the irises.

IRIS AND PUPIL

The iris and pupil are inspected. The irises should light up with the oblique lighting from the penlight and have a consistent color. Bulging or uneven coloring are abnormal. When light shines into the eyes, the irises constrict as the optic nerves are stimulated, making the pupils smaller. Dim lighting causes the pupils to dilate. The nurse inspects the pupils for size, shape, equality, and ability to react to light and accommodation. Box 17–1 presents the steps in assessing pupil reactions to light and accommodation. Results of the pupil assessment that are normal are recorded as PERRLA (pupils equal, round, and reactive to light and accommodation). Abnormal results include light intolerance (photophobia), irregular or unequal pupils, or pupils that do not react to light or accommodation. Abnormalities of the pupil may be due to neurologic disease, intraocular inflammation, iris adhesions, the effect of systemic or ocular medications, or surgical alteration, or they may be benign variations of normal findings.

BOX 17–1

Testing Pupil Reactions to Light and Accommodation

- Dim the lights and instruct the client to look straight ahead.
- To test **direct response to light,** bring the penlight in from the side to shine directly over the center of the pupil. The illuminated pupil should constrict briskly and evenly.
- Repeat this maneuver on the other eye. Both eyes should react to the same degree.
- Test **consensual response** by observing one pupil while shining the penlight on the opposite pupil. Both pupils should constrict to the same degree, although the consensual response will be slightly slower.
- Test **accommodation** by holding the penlight 4 to 6 inches (10–15 cm) away from the client's nose. Instruct the client to look first at the penlight, then at the distant wall straight ahead, and then again at the penlight.
- While the client gazes from near to far and back again, observe the pupils' response to changes in distance. They should dilate when looking at the far point and constrict when looking at the near object.
- Then move the penlight toward the bridge of the client's nose and observe for the pupils to converge and constrict.

Examination of Ocular Motility

Evaluation of ocular motility provides information about the extraocular muscles; the orbit; cranial nerves III, IV, and VI; their brain stem connections; and the cerebral cortex. The client is asked to track a target with both eyes as it is moved in each of the six cardinal directions of gaze (Fig. 17–1). The examiner notes the speed, smoothness, range, and symmetry of movements and observes for unsteadiness of fixation (nystagmus).

Extraocular Muscle Tests

The eyes normally move in parallel to each other, smoothly and in unison. To test the function of the oculomotor, trochlear, and abducens, the nurse asks the client to look straight ahead while standing directly in front, holding a penlight approximately 12 inches (30 cm) from the eyes. The nurse instructs the client to keep the head still and to follow the penlight's movements with the eyes only. The penlight is moved slowly and smoothly through the six cardinal positions of gaze; care is taken not to go beyond the client's field of vision. The penlight is moved in an orderly manner from the center outward along each of the six directions; one must pause briefly to observe for nystagmus and then return to the center. Nystagmus is an involuntary rapid, oscillating movement of the eyeball and is considered an abnormal finding except for slight nystagmus in the extreme lateral gazes (i.e., endpoint nystagmus). If the eyes do not move in parallel motion or if the upper eyelid covers more than a tiny portion of the iris, the conditions are noted as abnormal findings.

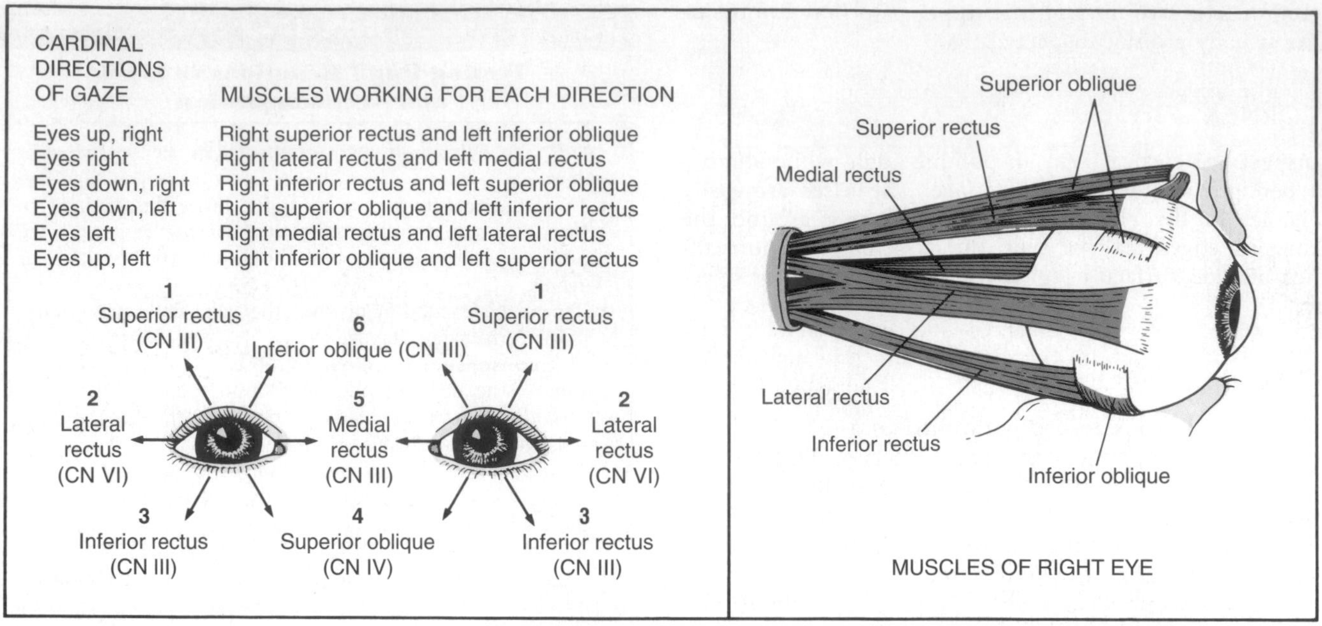

Figure 17–1
The six cardinal directions of gaze and the muscles responsible for each.

Assessment of Vision

VISUAL ACUITY

Testing visual acuity is the standard and routine method used to determine the clarity of the ocular media (cornea, lens, and vitreous) and the function of the visual pathway from the retina to the brain. It is important to remember that while an abnormal acuity implies an uncorrected refractive error or pathologic process, normal acuity does not exclude disease of the visual system. Visual acuity is assessed in one eye at a time, then in both eyes together, with the client comfortably seated. Begin with the right eye while the left eye is covered by an occluder or an opaque card. Test visual acuity with and without corrective lenses. Visual acuity is traditionally measured with the Snellen chart (the letter chart used in schools and physicians' offices) at a distance of 20 feet; at this distance, rays of light from an object are practically parallel and little effort of accommodation is required. There must be adequate lighting for the client to see.

Begin by asking the client to read the smallest line of symbols or letters that are seen. The client is credited for the smallest line of print that is read with more than 50 per cent accuracy. Record the results according to the standardized numbers printed by the lines on the Snellen chart. The sizes of the symbols are identified according to the distances at which they are normally visible. For example, the largest symbols can be read 200 feet away by people with unimpaired vision. The results of visual acuity testing are expressed in a fraction. Vision that is 20/20 is normal, that is, the client is able to read from 20 feet what a person with normal vision can read from 20 feet. A client with a visual acuity of 20/60 sees at a distance of 20 feet to read what a client with normal vision can read at 60 feet. The client with myopia (i.e., nearsightedness) will have results of 20/30 or greater, signifying that the client can only read at 20 feet what a person with normal vision can read at 30 feet (or greater). Hyperopia (i.e., farsightedness) results are 20/15 or less, meaning the client can read at 20 feet what a person with normal vision can read at 15 feet (or less). It is not uncommon for a client to have a test result of 20/15, which indicates better than average visual acuity. Legal blindness is defined as 20/200 or less with corrected vision (glasses or contact lenses) or less than 20 degrees of visual field (see later) in the better eye.

When a client is unable to distinguish the largest letter on the chart, vision may be assessed by asking the client to read the number of fingers held up in front of him or her at a distance of 3 feet (CF = count fingers). If the client is unable to distinguish fingers, one should ask whether the client perceives hand movements (HM = hand motion). Finally, determine whether the client can perceive light (LP = light perception). NLP indicates no light perception.

Near vision is tested with a handheld card or newsprint 12 to 14 inches (30–36 cm) from the client's eyes. Corrective lenses are worn if needed. The client with normal vision is able to read the material at that distance. Complaints of blurring or attempts by the client to move the card either closer or farther away signal abnormal near vision.

VISUAL FIELDS

Visual field testing evaluates peripheral vision. It may be accomplished by the confrontational method or with the use of a computerized instrument. The confrontational method assumes that the examiner has normal peripheral vision.

The client sits facing the nurse approximately 2 feet (60 cm) away. The eyes of the client and the nurse should be at the same level. Both the nurse and the client cover the eye directly opposite to one another with an opaque cover (e.g., the nurse's right eye and the client's left eye) and stare at each other's uncovered eye. The nurse holds a small object such as a penlight in the free hand and holds it equidistant between herself and the client, just out of view at the periphery of the visual field. Starting with the superior field, the nurse slowly brings the penlight down between the client and herself until the client states that he or she can see it (the nurse should be able to see the penlight at the same time). This maneuver is repeated at 45-degree angles, progressing through the superior, temporal, inferior, and nasal fields until all are tested. The test is repeated for the other eye.

A variety of manual and computerized visual field testing equipment may be used to permit more accurate, reproducible detection and quantification of scotomas (areas of decreased visual function). Visual fields can be altered by CNS disorders, such as a brain lesion or syphilis, and ocular disorders, such as glaucoma or retinal detachment.

Internal Eye Examination

Internal eye structures are visible only with illumination such as that provided by an ophthalmoscope. The ophthalmoscope is used to inspect the structures posterior to the iris, including the lens and fundus (which includes the retina, retinal vessels, choroid, optic disc, macula, and fovea). The ophthalmoscope requires considerable skill and practice.

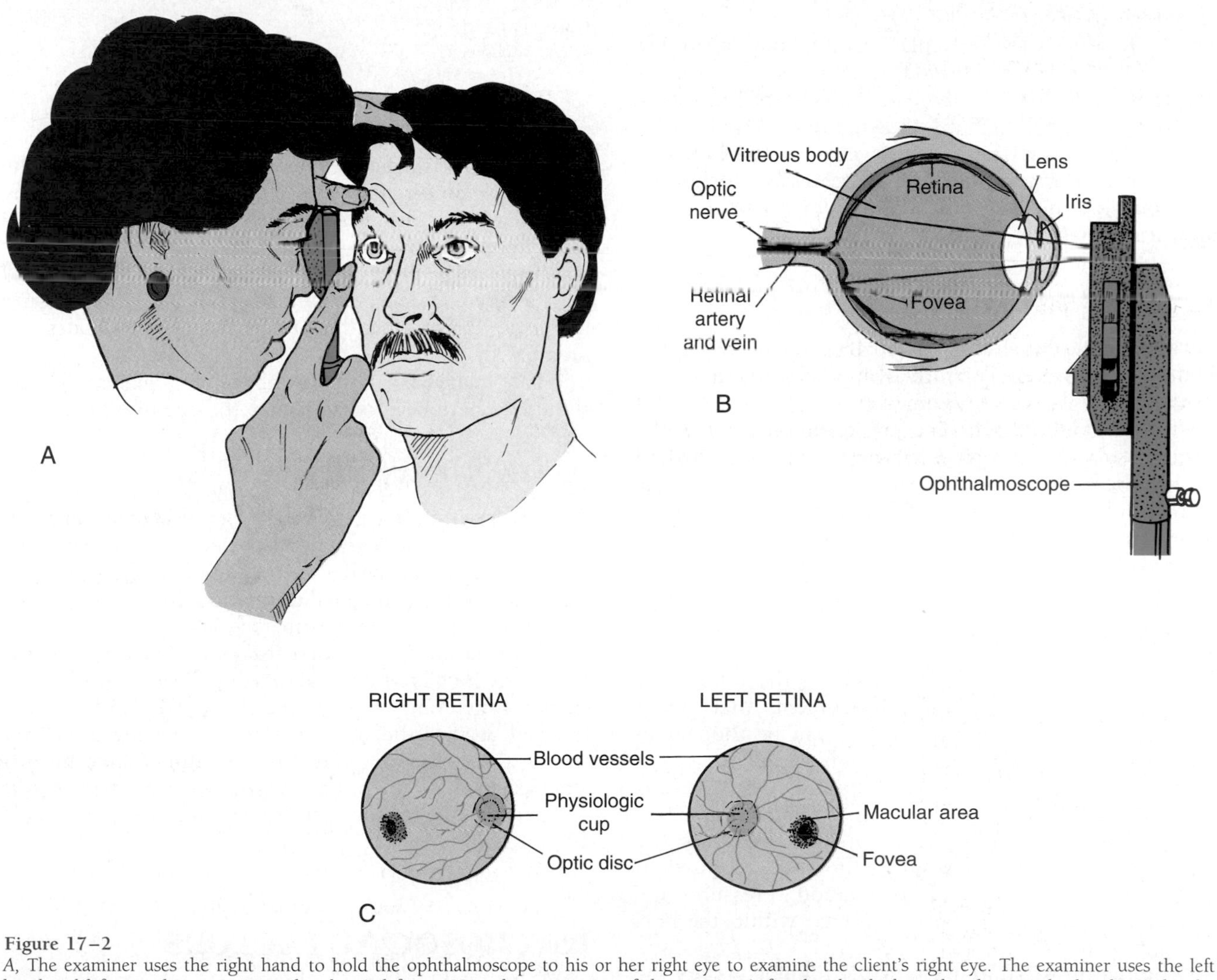

Figure 17–2
A, The examiner uses the right hand to hold the ophthalmoscope to his or her right eye to examine the client's right eye. The examiner uses the left hand and left eye when examining the client's left eye. Note the positioning of the examiner's free hand, which is placed to steady the client's head and to slightly retract the eyebrow. *B,* The examiner sees what appears in the angle of light through the viewing aperture. *C,* The actual area of retina visualized depends on the pupil dilation. Note the structures that may be examined.

DIRECT OPHTHALMOSCOPY

The handheld direct ophthalmoscope provides a detailed view of the disc and retinal vasculature and is a part of a general physical examination as well as an ophthalmologic examination (Fig. 17–2). Dilating the eye enhances the examiner's view, although a darkened room may cause adequate dilation. The examiner's view may be impaired by a cloudy cornea or the presence of a cataract.

The red reflex is a bright red-orange glow seen through the pupil. The optic disc normally appears round, with well-defined margins (except in the nasal margin), and a creamy pink color. The physiologic cup should be no larger than half the diameter of the optic disc. Retinal veins are darker than arteries and radiate from the disc. Veins are slightly thicker than arteries and should be free of pulsation. Tortuous vessels or straightened arteries are abnormal, as is nicking (i.e., the appearance that a vessel disappears where an artery and vein cross each other so that one vessel looks discontinuous). The retinal background is pink in white people and dark and heavily pigmented in clients with a dark complexion. Choroidal vessels may appear as linear orange streaks.

The fundus is the only place in the body where the vascular bed may be observed directly. Thus, examination yields information about many systemic diseases. Abnormal findings include altered arteriovenous (AV) ratio, narrowed arteries, widened veins, pinched-off vessels, abnormal arterial light reflex, excessive tortuosity, numerous AV nickings, exudates, white patches, and focal hemorrhage.

INDIRECT OPHTHALMOSCOPY

The indirect ophthalmoscope enables the examiner to obtain a stereoscopic picture over a large area of the retina. The light source comes from a head-mounted light. The examiner holds a convex lens in front of the client's eye and, through a viewing device attached to the headband, sees an inverted reversed image. The indirect ophthalmoscope has the advantage of binocular vision with depth perception for the examiner and permits a wider field of view.

TONOMETRY

Tonometry is the method of measuring the intraocular fluid pressure using calibrated instruments that indent or flatten the corneal apex. The eye can be thought of as an enclosed compartment through which there is a constant circulation of aqueous humor. The aqueous maintains the shape of the eye with a relatively uniform pressure within the globe. As the pressure increases, the eye becomes firmer and a greater force is required to cause the same amount of indentation. Pressures between 8 and 21 mm Hg are considered within the normal range.

The two most common types of tonometers are the Schiøtz and applanation. The Schiøtz tonometer (Fig. 17–3) is a portable handheld instrument that may be used in an office, clinic, emergency room, operating room, or at the bedside. The applanation tonometer is attached to a slit-lamp microscope and measures the amount of force required to flatten the corneal apex by a standard amount. Anesthetic eye drops are used before either examination method.

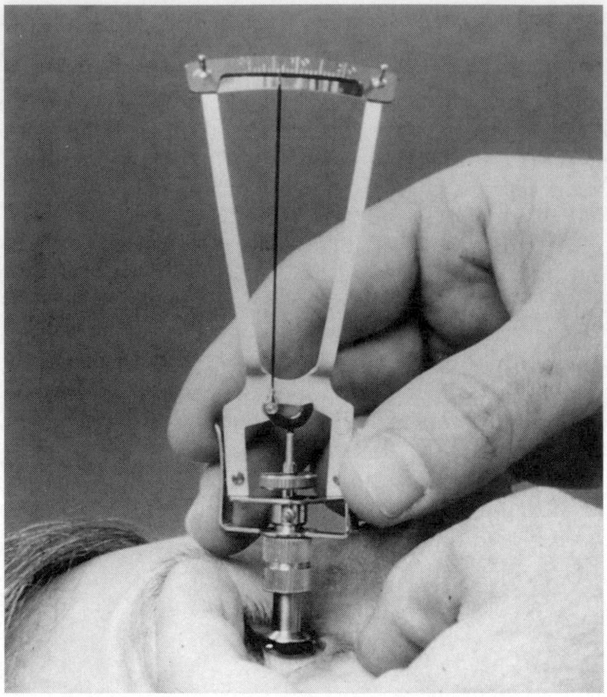

Figure 17–3
Schiøtz's tonometer.

Intraocular pressure is noted in the client record with a large T. The top number indicates the pressure in the right eye, and the bottom number indicates the pressure in the left eye.

Tonometry is used to check for glaucoma and should be performed yearly after the age of 40.

SLIT-LAMP EXAMINATION

The slit-lamp microscope is used to illuminate and examine the anterior segment of the eye under magnification. A linear slit beam of incandescent light is projected onto the globe, illuminating an optical cross section of the anterior chamber.

Fluorescein dye is often used in a slit-lamp examination to highlight corneal irregularities. Sterile paper strips containing fluorescein dye are wetted and touched against the inner surface of the lower lid, instilling the yellow dye into the tear film. A blue filter is attached to the light beam, causing the dye to fluoresce.

Specific diagnostic studies are discussed in Table 17–1.

PSYCHOSOCIAL FACTORS

The social stigma of blindness underlies the anxiety that clients experience with actual or potential vision loss.

TABLE 17–1 Diagnostic Tests for Ocular Problems

DIAGNOSTIC TEST	USE	ABNORMALITY
Fundus photography	Documents fine details of the fundus	Optic nerve changes
Exophthalmometry	Measures forward protrusion of the eye	Thyroid disease and tumors of the orbit
Ophthalmic radiology	Evaluates orbital and intracranial conditions	Neoplasms, inflammatory masses, fractures, extraocular muscle enlargement, foreign body
Magnetic resonance imaging	Provides multidimensional views	Edema, areas of demyelination, vascular lesions
Ultrasonography	Evaluates tissue characteristics and size and growth of tumors	Growth of tumor
Ophthalmodynamometry	Gives an approximate measurement of pressures within the central retinal arteries; indirectly assesses carotid arterial flow	Changes in carotid blood flow
Electroretinography	Measures change in electrical potential of the eye	Retinitis pigmentosa (progressive degeneration of photoreceptor cells), massive ischemia, disseminated infection, or toxic effects from chemicals or drugs
Visual evoked response	Same as electroretinography	Retinal or optic nerve disease
Fluorescein angiography	Enhances fundus photography	Optic nerve changes

Total loss of vision isolates an individual within a different reality. Although most clients are successfully rehabilitated, some losses are permanent. There are also individuals who, for a variety of reasons, remain socially isolated. The image of a blind person who is pitied and must accept the charity of others is disturbing.

Not all jobs and work environments are adaptable for a person who can no longer see. Clients with actual or potential vision loss may be faced with barriers in their vocations that force an unwanted change. Age may be a major factor in the client's ability to meet this challenge.

Self-esteem is closely related to the roles of the client in his or her particular life-style. Loss of control in personal, family, and work situations can be devastating. The issue of dependence versus independence for an individual may also be a factor in the client's ability to cope with the stressors of vision loss.

Nursing Care of Clients with Eye Disorders

GLAUCOMA

Glaucoma includes a group of ocular disorders characterized by increased intraocular pressure, optic nerve atrophy, and visual field loss. The degree of increased pressure that causes ocular damage is not the same in every eye, and some individuals may tolerate a pressure for long periods of time that would rapidly blind another.

Incidence

It is estimated that more than 50,000 persons in the United States are blind as a result of glaucoma. The incidence of glaucoma is about 1.5 per cent, and in blacks, between the ages of 45 and 65 years, the prevalence is at least five times that of whites in the same age group. In most cases, blindness can be prevented if treatment is begun early.

Pathophysiology

Intraocular pressure is determined by the rate of aqueous production in the ciliary body and the resistance to outflow of aqueous from the eye. Increased intraocular pressure (usually greater than 23 mm Hg) indicates the need for further evaluation. Normal variations do not usually exceed 2 to 3 mm Hg.

CRITICAL TO REMEMBER

Increased intraocular pressure may result from hyperproduction of aqueous or obstruction of the outflow.

As aqueous fluid builds up in the eye, the increased pressure inhibits blood supply to the optic nerve and the retina. These delicate tissues become ischemic and gradually lose function.

Etiology and Risk Factors

Many terms are used to describe the various types of glaucoma. The terms primary and secondary refer to whether the cause is the disease alone or is due to another condition. Acute and chronic refer to the onset or duration of the disorder. The terms open (wide) and closed (narrow) describe the width of the angle between the cornea and the iris. Anatomically narrow anterior chamber angles predispose clients to an acute onset of angle-closure glaucoma.

PRIMARY OPEN-ANGLE GLAUCOMA

Approximately 90 per cent of primary glaucoma cases occur in clients with open angles. It is a multifactional disorder that is often genetically determined, bilateral, insidious in onset, and slow to progress. Symptoms appear late when vision is impaired by damage to the optic nerve. Because there are no early warning symptoms, it is imperative that regular ophthalmic examinations include tonometry and assessment of the optic nerve head (disc). The most common cause of chronic open-angle glaucoma is degenerative change in the trabecular meshwork, resulting in the decreased outflow of aqueous humor.

ANGLE-CLOSURE GLAUCOMA

An acute attack of angle-closure glaucoma can develop only in an eye in which the anterior chamber angle is anatomically narrow. The attack occurs as a result of a sudden blockage of the anterior angle by the base of the iris. When the aqueous flow is obstructed, intraocular pressure becomes markedly elevated, causing severe pain and blurred vision or vision loss. Some clients will see rainbow halos around lights, and some will experience nausea and vomiting.

SECONDARY GLAUCOMA

Increased intraocular pressure may occur as a postoperative complication. Edematous tissue may inhibit the outflow of aqueous through the trabecular meshwork. Delayed healing of corneal wound edges may result in epithelial cell growth into the anterior chamber.

Glaucoma may occur as a result of trauma. Lens displacement, hemorrhage into the anterior chamber, lacerations, and contusions can disrupt the flow pattern of aqueous humor.

Inflammation of filtering structures in uveitis may cause increased intraocular pressure. Encroachment by a rapidly growing tumor and chronic use of topical corticosteroids may also produce the symptoms of open-angle glaucoma.

Clinical Manifestations

Clinical manifestations of glaucoma include the following:

- Increased intraocular pressure
- Cupping or indentation of the optic nerve head (disc)
- Visual field defects

DIAGNOSTIC ASSESSMENT

An ophthalmoscopic examination shows atrophy (pale color) and cupping (indentation) of the optic nerve head. The visual field examination is used to determine the extent of peripheral vision loss (see the section on visual fields). In chronic open-angle glaucoma, a small crescent-shaped scotoma (blind spot) appears early in the disease. In acute angle-closure glaucoma, the fields demonstrate larger areas of significant vision loss.

Slit-lamp examination may reveal significant changes associated with glaucoma. Intraocular pressure is measured at the slit lamp with the applanation tonometer. Gonioscopy is performed to determine the depth of the anterior chamber angle and to examine the entire circumference of the angle for any abnormal changes in the filtering meshwork.

Medical Management

The goal of medical management is to facilitate the outflow of aqueous through remaining channels. This is achieved through the daily use of

- Topical miotics (e.g., pilocarpine), which constrict the pupil and increase outflow
- Topical epinephrine (e.g., Epifrin), which also increases the outflow
- Topical beta-blockers (e.g., timolol [Timoptic]), which suppress the secretion of aqueous humor
- Oral carbonic anhydrase inhibitors (e.g., acetazolamide [Diamox]), which also reduce the production of aqueous humor

When medical management is no longer effective, surgical intervention may be indicated.

Surgical Management

When maximum medical therapy has failed to halt the progression of visual field loss and optic nerve damage, surgical intervention is recommended. Many procedures are used to correct the aqueous outflow; however, there is no operation that is uniformly successful.

LASER TRABECULOPLASTY

The use of the laser to create an opening in the trabecular meshwork is often indicated before filtration surgery is considered. The laser produces scars in the trabecular meshwork, causing tightening of meshwork fibers. The tightened fibers allow increased outflow of aqueous. Intraocular pressure is reduced through improved outflow in about 80 per cent of cases. The effect of the laser treatment decreases with time, and the procedure may need to be repeated. Treatment with medications is usually continued.

FILTERING PROCEDURES

Operative procedures such as trephination, thermal sclerostomy, or sclerectomy create an outflow channel from the anterior chamber into the subconjunctival space. These are called filtering procedures. Aqueous is absorbed through the conjunctival vessels. In about 25 per cent of cases, the opening closes as a result of scar tissue formation, and reoperation is necessary.

A more common filtering procedure called trabeculectomy reduces some of the complications of surgery but achieves a somewhat lesser reduction in pressure. Filtering procedures are less successful in young and black clients because of their increased ability to produce thicker fibroblastic healing tissue. Topical corticosteroids are used postoperatively because their anti-inflammatory action inhibits the proliferation of fibroblasts at the surgical site.

5-Fluorouracil and other antimetabolites are sometimes injected subconjunctivally because they also inhibit fibroblast proliferation and, thereby, reduce postoperative scarring.

Ocular implantation devices such as the Molteno implant are sometimes used to control the flow of aqueous in patients with complicated types of glaucoma.

CILIODESTRUCTIVE PROCEDURES

When other surgical procedures have failed, cyclocryotherapy (the application of a freezing tip) or cyclophotocoagulation may be used to damage the ciliary body and decrease the production of aqueous.

Nursing Management

Assessment

The nursing assessment of the client includes establishing demographic data of age and race because open-angle glaucoma occurs most often in clients older than 40 years and in blacks. It is also important to determine whether there is a family history of glaucoma or other eye problems or whether the client has had ocular surgery, infections, or trauma. An accurate list of current medications is imperative because over-the-counter medications such as antihistamines may dilate the pupil, putting the client at risk for angle-closure glaucoma. A history of allergic reactions, particularly to medications or dye studies, should always be noted.

The nurse should ask the client to describe any changes in vision. Although the symptoms of primary open-angle glaucoma are insidious, the client may describe blind spots in the periphery or an overall decreased visual acuity with loss of contrast sensitivity.

CRITICAL TO REMEMBER

Decreased uncorrectable visual acuity usually occurs when there has been irreversible damage to the optic nerve.

The nurse assesses the client's perception of glaucoma and the effect it has on the client's life. The nurse assists the client in identifying effective coping skills the client may have used in the past.

Nursing Diagnosis, Planning, and Implementation

Nursing Diagnosis: Visual Sensory/Perception Alterations R/T increased intraocular pressure.

Planning: Expected Outcomes. The client will maintain as much functional vision as possible, as evidenced by reporting no further loss of vision and adapting to any visual loss, demonstrate an ability to perform ADLs, instill his or her own eye medications, and recognize clinical manifestations of complications.

Implementation. The nurse must first determine the client's current level of knowledge and then provide necessary information about glaucoma and its treatment in understandable terms using diagrams. Because treatment for glaucoma is often complex, involving both oral and topical ophthalmic medications, a written plan of care in large print should be reviewed with the client and family. To maximize compliance, the plan of care must fit into the client's life-style. The nurse should reinforce that, although some vision has been lost and cannot be restored, further loss may be prevented by adhering to the treatment plan.

The administration of eye drops is a critical component of self-care for the client with glaucoma. After instructing the client and family on instillation technique, the nurse should validate the client or significant others' ability to instill eye drops properly by asking for a return demonstration. The discussion of side effects of medications is also very important (Table 17–2).

In emergent situations in which intraocular pressure must be brought under control, an oral osmotic agent may be administered in the form of glycerin (Osmoglyn). The diuretic action of glycerin lowers intraocular pressure. Because the high sugar content affects some diabetic clients, a synthetic glycerin such as isosorbide (Ismotic) may be used. The average dose for an adult is 4 oz, which may be repeated several times until the intraocular pressure is reduced to a tolerable level. Intravenous mannitol, a potent intravenous osmotic diuretic, may be used to arrest extremely high intraocular pressure. It should be used only for the management of a glaucoma crisis under close nursing and medical supervision.

Preoperative nursing care includes preparing the client for a surgical procedure that may be performed in either an outpatient or an inpatient setting.

Outpatient Treatment. Laser therapy is most often performed in a clinic or office using topical anesthetic. It is important for the nurse to explain not only the expected outcome of the procedure but also the popping sounds and flashing lights that the client will experience. The client should be informed that there will be a waiting period (usually 1–2 hours) after the procedure to evaluate a possible rise in intraocular pressure. Because of the instability of the intraocular pressure, the client should arrange to have a friend or family accompany him or her to provide transportation.

Inpatient Treatment. Preoperatively, the nurse should evaluate the level of the client's anxiety and knowledge about the procedure. Mild preoperative sedation is usually prescribed.

TABLE 17–2 Teaching the Client About Eye Drops for Glaucoma

MEDICATION	USUAL FREQUENCY	TEACHING ASPECTS
Pilocarpine hydrochloride	3–4 times/day	A miotic, causes pupillary constriction to open the canal of Schlemm Space out the administration, beginning on waking and ending at bedtime May cause blurred vision after instillation Brow ache has been reported Consider the use of thin gel strips (a timed-release form) to improve compliance
Timolol maleate and other beta-blockers such as levobunolol	Every 12 hours	Decreases production of aqueous humor Space out the administration Contraindicated in clients with asthma and COPD Assess for bradycardia before administration
Carbonic anhydrase inhibitors (acetazolamide [Diamox])		Inhibits the production of aqueous humor Available as tablets and in sustained-release capsules Side effects include anorexia and tingling in the hands and feet

COPD, chronic obstructive pulmonary disease.

Postoperative nursing care may need to be accomplished in a matter of hours or days, depending on the expected length of stay. When the client returns from the operating room, the eye is covered with a patch and a metal or plastic shield for protection. The nurse should instruct the client not to lie on the operative side to avoid pressure on the operative site. When the effects of the perioperative sedation have diminished, the client may ambulate and eat as desired.

The plan for discharge must include client education and evaluation of the home environment and available care. (See Client Education Guide: Care After Glaucoma Surgery.)

CLIENT EDUCATION GUIDE

Care After Glaucoma Surgery

Client and family education for postoperative eye care includes a review of the following:

- Signs and symptoms of infection (redness, swelling, drainage, blurred vision, pain)
- Signs and symptoms of increased intraocular pressure (unrelieved pain, nausea, decrease in vision)
- The need to report any of the above signs and symptoms to the physician
- The rationale for eye protection (shield or glasses at all times, although not all physicians order eye protection)
- Medications and eye drop instillation technique
- How to cleanse the area carefully around the eye with warm tap water and a clean wash cloth, avoiding direct contact with the eye
- The need to avoid rubbing or applying pressure over the closed eye, which could damage healing tissue
- Return visit date and time

The nurse uses information supplied by the client, family, or significant others to assess how much support may be needed. Referrals may need to be made to visiting nurses for home health care or social services for assistance with rehabilitation or finances. The nurse assists the client and significant others to plan for housekeeping and meal preparation, safety in the home environment with decreased vision, transportation, and assistance with eye care.

Evaluation

The nurse determines the degree of expected outcome attainment. Generally, the care of these clients is very short in the hospital setting. If long-term expected outcomes are important, other modes of quality assurance will be needed.

CATARACTS

A cataract is an opacity of the lens.

Incidence

Although cataract formation is usually associated with aging, cataracts may be due to a variety of other causes. A person with a normal lifespan is more likely to undergo a cataract operation than any other major surgical procedure.

Etiology and Risk Factors

AGE-RELATED CATARACTS

The most common cataract is age-related or senile cataract. Worldwide, it is the primary cause of reduced vision and blindness. Senile cataracts usually begin around the age of 50 years and consist of cortical, nuclear, or posterior subcapsular opacities. These three forms may coexist in various combinations.

In cortical cataracts, spokelike opacifications are found in the periphery of the lens. They progress slowly, infrequently involve the visual axis, and often do not result in severe vision loss.

Nuclear sclerotic cataracts are a result of a progressive yellowing and hardening of the central lens (nucleus). Most individuals older than 70 years have some degree of nuclear sclerosis.

Posterior subcapsular opacities occur centrally on the posterior lens capsule. They cause visual loss early in their development because they lie directly in the visual axis.

OTHER FORMS OF CATARACTS

Cataracts may develop as a result of many other ocular, systemic, and congenital disorders. Systemic disorders include diabetes and Down syndrome. Intraocular disorders that may be associated with cataract are iridocyclitis, retinitis, retinal detachment, and onchocerciasis. Trauma, radiation, exposure to infrared light, and chronic use of corticosteroids may also result in cataracts. Infections (German measles, mumps, hepatitis, poliomyelitis, chickenpox, infectious mononucleosis) during the first trimester of pregnancy may cause congenital cataracts.

Pathophysiology

Cataract formation is characterized chemically by a reduction in oxygen uptake and an initial increase in water content followed by dehydration. The protein in the lens undergoes numerous age-related changes, including yellowing, which is from the formation of fluorescent compounds and molecular changes. These changes, along with the photoabsorption of ultraviolet radiation throughout life, suggest that cataracts may be due to a photochemical process. (See Pathophysiology: Stages of Cataract Development.)

Clinical Manifestations

Clients experience blurred vision, sometimes monocular diplopia, photophobia, and glare. Clients usually see better in low-lit conditions when the pupil is dilated, which allows for vision around a central opacity. There is no complaint of pain. A cloudy lens can be observed (Fig. 17–4).

DIAGNOSTIC ASSESSMENT

A cataract should be suspected when the red reflex seen with the direct ophthalmoscope is distorted or absent.

PATHOPHYSIOLOGY

Stages of Cataract Development

Cataracts progress through the following clinical stages of development:

- *Immature* cataracts, which are not completely opaque and transmit some light, allowing useful vision
- *Mature* (formerly known as "ripe") cataracts, which are completely opaque, significantly reducing vision
- *Intumescent* cataracts, in which the lens takes on water and increases in size, and *hypermature* cataracts, in which lens proteins leak out through the lens capsule. Either of these stages may result in glaucoma.

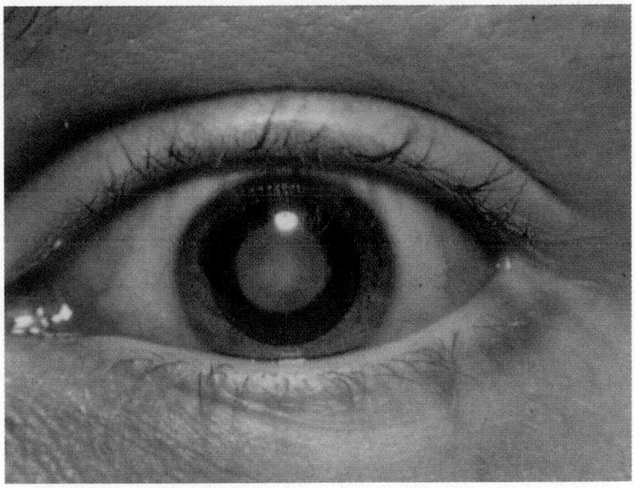

Figure 17–4
Cloudy appearance of the lens affected by cataract. (Courtesy of Ophthalmic Photography at the University of Michigan W. K. Kellogg Eye Center.)

Although cataracts can usually be diagnosed easily with the direct ophthalmoscope, an accurate determination of the type and extent of the lens change requires a slit-lamp examination.

Medical Management

There is no known medical treatment that either prevents or reduces cataract formation.

Surgical Management

The objective of cataract surgery is to remove the opacified lens. The lens is surgically removed by an intracapsular or extracapsular procedure (Fig. 17–5).

Intracapsular cataract extraction consists of removing the lens including the lens capsule. Extracapsular cataract extraction consists of removing the lens and the anterior portion of the lens capsule. The posterior lens capsule is left intact. The primary reason for performing extracapsular surgery is to allow the insertion of a posterior chamber intraocular lens inside the remaining capsule, which results in fewer postoperative complications.

Phacoemulsification is an extracapsular technique that uses ultrasound vibrations to break up the lens material. Pieces of the anterior lens capsule and the lens are removed by suction through the phacoemulsifier tip.

Cataract surgery is usually performed under local anesthesia with sedation. The client is given an intravenous injection of methohexital sodium (Brevital) or thiopental (Pentothal) to induce a few minutes of light anesthesia while the retrobulbar injection of local anesthetic is given.

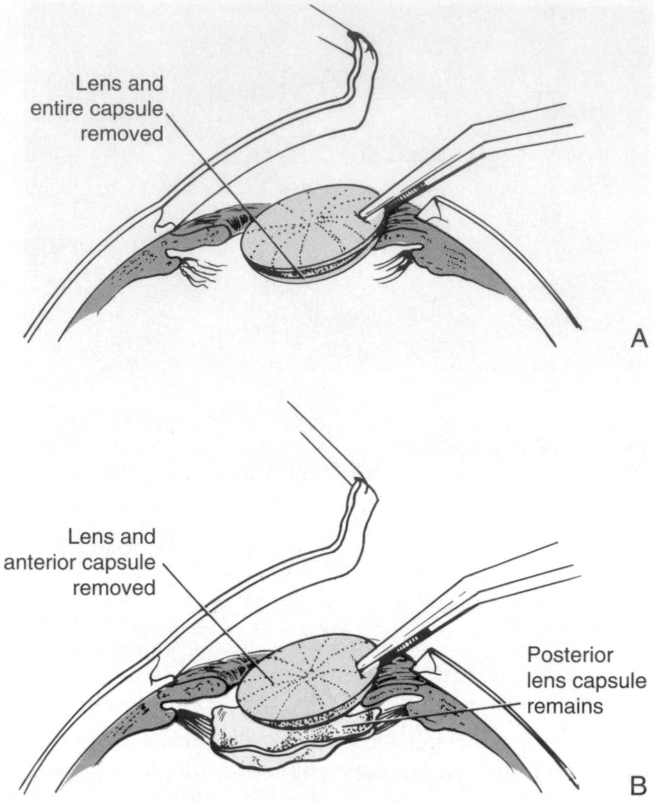

Figure 17–5
Surgical approaches to lens removal for cataracts. *A*, Intracapsular cataract extraction. *B*, Extracapsular cataract extraction.

INTRAOCULAR LENS IMPLANTATION

After the extraction of the cataract, a new lens is inserted in the posterior chamber, or the client is left without a lens. Although there are many styles of lenses, they all consist of two basic parts: a clear spherical optic usually made of polymethylmethacrylate (Plexiglas) and footplates or haptics to hold the lens in place. Foldable lenses made of silicone or hydrogel material have been developed, but data on long-term use are not available yet.

APHAKIA

Aphakia (absence of the lens) is corrected by the use of eyeglasses, contact lenses, or intraocular lenses. Without the lens, the eye has no accommodative power and has lost a great deal of its refractive power. Depth perception is greatly altered. The safest and least expensive method of correcting aphakia is with eyeglasses (with very thick lenses). Contact lenses are also available and are able to achieve visual correction with much less distortion. The client, however, must have the manual dexterity necessary to handle the lenses. Intraocular lens implants offer the best visual correction with immediate return of binocular vision. The main disadvantage is a somewhat higher incidence of postoperative complications.

COMPLICATIONS

Secondary glaucoma is one of the major complications that may occur after cataract extraction. As a result of postoperative edema in the ocular tissues, a certain rise in intraocular pressure is anticipated and expected. It most often resolves within 24 to 72 hours. If prolonged intraocular pressure persists, medical therapy may be necessary. Postoperative infection, bleeding, macular edema, and wound leaks are also a possibility. The incidence of retinal detachment is higher in the first 12 months after cataract surgery.

After extracapsular cataract extraction, the posterior capsule may become opacified and it is called an after cataract or secondary membrane. Subcapsular lens epithelial cells may regenerate lens fibers, which can obstruct vision. This postoperative complication occurs fairly frequently and, in the past, required a second operation to remove the opacified tissue. More recently, the neodymium-yttrium-aluminum-garnet laser is being used to create an opening in the capsule through pulses of laser energy that cause tiny "explosions" in the target tissue. Complications of this technique include a transient rise in intraocular pressure and possible damage to the intraocular lens.

Nursing Management

Assessment

During the history and physical examination, the nurse directs questions to the client about any predisposing factors (trauma, systemic diseases, medications such as corticosteroids, and other ocular problems). Visual acuity (both distant and near) in each eye is documented. It is important for the nurse to ask the client to describe visual disturbances. It is possible for the client's visual acuity to be relatively close to normal ranges, and yet the client experiences difficulty in performing ADLs, for example. The client's individual perception of the quality of vision is an important factor in determining the need for surgery.

Nursing Diagnosis, Planning, and Implementation

Nursing Diagnosis: Visual Sensory/Perceptual Alterations R/T cataract formation.

Planning: Expected Outcomes. The client will gain improved vision and will adapt to changes in visual correction, as evidenced by verbalization of ability to see with the prescribed correction.

Implementation. Adaptation is the key issue in caring for the client having cataract surgery. Nursing interventions are based on assisting the client to gain or maintain as much independence as possible.

Unless there are other ocular complications or health factors, cataract surgery is performed on an outpatient basis. At the time of admission to the hospital or surgical facility, the nurse determines the client's current level of knowledge and understanding about the perioperative events. Preoperative sedation may include an oral sedative or medication to reduce intraocular pressure in the eye (a lower than normal intraocular pressure facilitates the surgical procedure). Preoperative eye drops may include a dilating agent such as the mydriatic tropicamide (Mydriacyl) to dilate the pupil, facilitating the surgery. A cycloplegic, cyclopentolate (Cyclogyl), may also be administered to paralyze the ciliary muscles.

Postoperative care includes observation of the ocular dressing, if present, and assessment of the client's ability to perform ADLs at the preoperative level. The eye patch is usually removed the next morning but may be removed after a few hours if the client has limited vision in the other eye. The client is instructed to wear a metal or plastic shield to protect the eye from accidental injury or rubbing of the eye. Glasses may be worn during the day.

Discharge teaching includes education for the client and significant others regarding postoperative activities, eye care, medications, home care, and adaptation to visual correction. Eye care after cataract surgery is the same as that after glaucoma surgery (see Client Education Guide: Care After Glaucoma Surgery).

Evaluation

The degree of expected outcome attainment should be assessed. Adaptation to restored normal vision is usually rapid. Adaptation to limited vision will require more time based on individual variations.

Retinal Disorders

RETINAL DETACHMENT

Retinal detachment is the separation of the retina from the choroid layer, which is its blood supply. It may take the form of small holes or tears or the actual peeling of the retina from the choroid.

Incidence

Retinal detachment occurs mainly in the adult eye. The overall incidence is 1 in 10,000 people per year, but the risk of detachment increases after the fourth decade and most often occurs between the ages of 50 and 70 years.

Etiology and Risk Factors

Predisposing factors to retinal detachment include cataract extraction, degeneration of the retina, trauma, and high myopia. Retinal holes and tears usually occur from spontaneous vitreous traction, but there may be abnormal adhesions between the retina and vitreous secondary to diabetic retinopathy, injury, or other ocular disorders. Atrophy of the vitreous may also result in a retinal tear.

Pathophysiology

When the retina is separated from its choroidal blood supply, it will die. Without intervention, the detachment continues to spread and the detached retina will lose the ability to function. It may become increasingly detached over a period of hours to years. The retinal tissues are at a high risk for avascular necrosis because they are delicate structures and have a high metabolic rate.

Clinical Manifestations

Characteristic symptoms of retinal detachment are described by clients as a shadow or curtain falling across the field of vision (Fig. 17–6). There is no pain associated with detachment of the retina. The onset is usually sudden and may be accompanied by a burst of black spots or floaters, indicating that bleeding has occurred as a result of the detachment. Clients may also see flashes of light caused by separation of the retina.

Medical Management

Surgery is required to repair a detached retina because spontaneous reattachment of the retina is an uncommon occurrence. The indirect ophthalmoscope with a handheld magnifying lens is used to evaluate the extent and source of the detachment. Areas of detachment appear bluish gray as opposed to the normal red-pink color (Fig. 17–7). Tears are most often horseshoe shaped but may be round.

Surgical Management

Surgical repair is required for retinal detachment. The goal is to place the retina back in contact with the choroid and to seal the accompanying holes and breaks. Often cryopexy (the use of a freezing probe) or laser photocoagulation is used to seal the hole if it has not progressed to detachment. Both methods create inflammation around the area, which scars and seals the hole.

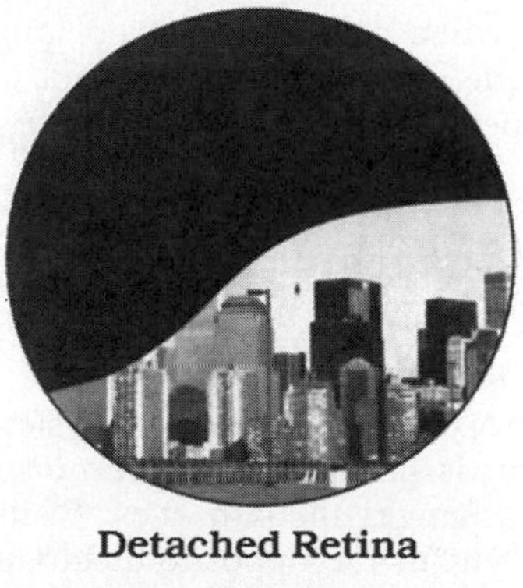

Figure 17–6
Vision of a client with retinal detachment. (Courtesy of National Industries for the Blind, Wayne, NJ.)

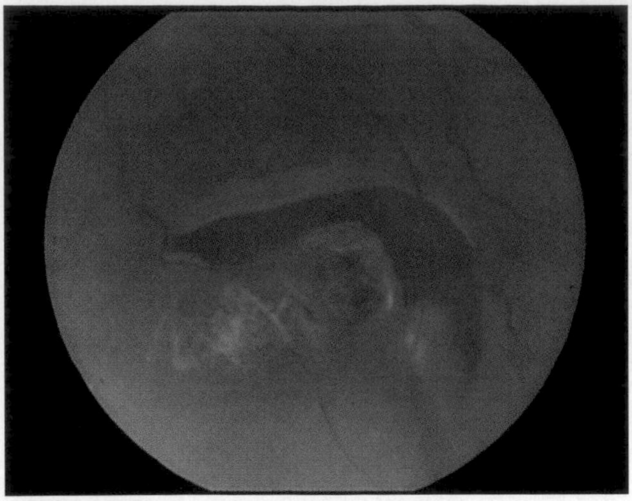

Figure 17–7
Bluish gray appearance of areas of retinal detachment. (Courtesy of Ophthalmic Photography at the University of Michigan W. K. Kellogg Eye Center.)

The surgical procedure to place the retina back in contact with the choroid is called scleral buckling (Fig. 17–8). The sclera is actually depressed from the outside by Silastic sponges or silicone bands that are sutured in place permanently. Prior to the buckling procedure, an intraocular injection of air or sulfahexafluoride gas bubble, or both, may be used to apply pressure on the retina from the inside of the eye. This bubble holds the retina in place by gravitational force during the healing phase. Postoperative positioning of the client maximizes the tamponade effect of the air-gas bubble. The air-gas bubble is slowly absorbed. If the condition is not corrected, scleral buckling is performed.

COMPLICATIONS

Postoperative swelling of tissues and cells in the anterior chamber caused by the inflammatory process or compromise of the venous drainage system may result in increased intraocular pressure. Because of the fragility of the tissues involved in the repair, redetachment of the retina may occur at any time. At times, the retina has been separated from its blood supply long enough so that, even when reattached, it no longer has useful function and the client's vision does not improve significantly. Postoperative infection is also a risk.

Nursing Management

Assessment

When the history is obtained and physical examination is performed, it is important for the nurse to assess the client's visual changes in both eyes. Visual field loss is seen by the client in the opposite quadrant of the actual detachment. For example, a tear in the temporal region, which is affected more frequently, creates a visual defect in the nasal area.

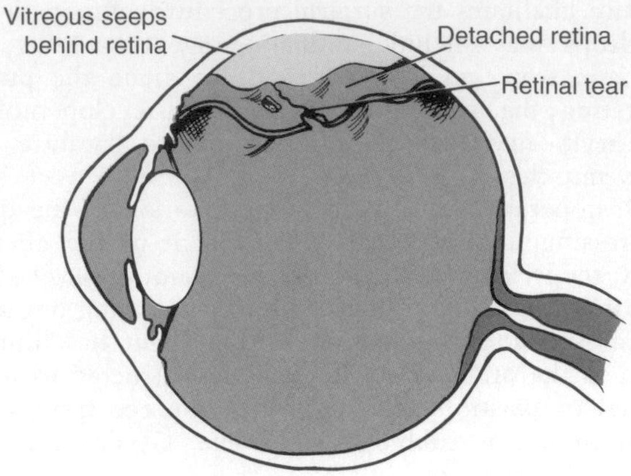

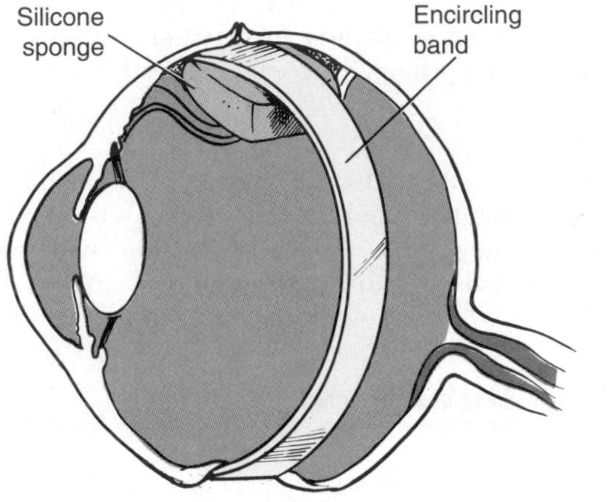

Figure 17–8
Scleral buckling to repair a detached retina. A silicone sponge implant is placed over the tear and held in place with an encircling band. When the buckle is tightened, the implant indents the sclera, holding the choroid and retina together.

The pupil must be widely dilated for a retinal examination. The nurse explains that the client will see an extremely bright light and be asked to change gaze frequently to facilitate the examination.

Nursing Diagnosis, Planning, and Implementation

Nursing Diagnosis: Visual Sensory/Perceptual Alterations R/T compromised retinal function.

Planning: Expected Outcomes. The client will maintain as much functional vision as possible, as evidenced by reporting no further loss of vision and adapting to any visual loss, demonstrate an ability to perform ADLs, instill his or her own eye medications, and recognize clinical manifestations of complications.

Implementation. The focus of the care plan is assisting the client to cope with the fears and reality of vision loss and to adapt to changes in vision. The client must be aware of the clinical manifestations of further vision loss.

Surgery may require a 1- to 3-day hospital stay or may be performed on an outpatient basis. The client may be placed on activity restrictions before surgery based on the size and location of the detachment. If the macula is threatened, the risk of further detachment is greater and the potential for vision loss is also greater. Most often, bathroom privileges are allowed.

The nurse should assess the client's current level of knowledge and understanding about the implications of retinal detachment and the expectations from the surgical procedure. Because retinal detachment repair may take several hours in the operating room, general anesthesia is used in many cases. The pupil must be widely dilated before the operation, and the client may be given a sedative.

Postoperatively, the nurse observes the eye patch for any drainage. Blood loss in retinal detachment surgery is minimal, and only serous drainage is expected on the postoperative dressing. Activity restrictions may be necessary if an air-gas bubble has been injected. The client will need to be positioned so that the bubble can apply maximal pressure on the retina by the force of gravity. The position is usually maintained for several days. The nurse provides comfort and support to assist the client with positioning and monitors the client during sleep.

Narcotics may be needed during the first 24 hours after surgery, particularly for scleral buckling procedures (resulting from manipulation during surgery). Nausea and vomiting may also require management. Intravenous acetazolamide (Diamox) may be used to reduce increased intraocular pressure. The intraocular pressure is monitored closely during the first 24 hours. The client should be encouraged to resume a regular diet and fluids as tolerated.

The eye patch and shield are removed the next morning. Redness and swelling of the lids and conjunctiva should be expected from the surgical manipulation. After several days, the swelling and ecchymosis of the lids subside, but the conjunctiva may remain red or pink for a few weeks.

Postoperative eye medications generally include an antibiotic-steroid combination drop to prevent infection and reduce inflammation. Cycloplegic agents are prescribed to dilate the pupil and relax the cilliary muscles, which decreases discomfort and helps prevent the formation of iris adhesions to the corneal endothelium (synechiae). The client should not expect immediate return of vision. Postoperative inflammation and the dilating drops interfere with vision. As healing takes place over weeks and months, vision may improve on a gradual basis. Either warm or cold compresses may be applied for comfort several times a day.

Evaluation

The nurse evaluates the expected outcomes for the client. Revisions in the plan of care may be required.

Posthospital Care

The client is instructed to clean the eye with warm tap water using a clean wash cloth. Warm compresses may be continued at home. Either an eye shield or glasses should be worn during the day, and the shield should be worn during naps and at night. The client is usually instructed to avoid vigorous activities and heavy lifting during the immediate postoperative period. If an air-gas bubble has been injected, it may take several weeks to totally absorb. Clients are advised to avoid air travel during this time because the gas and air expand at high altitudes.

Although the eye patch is usually removed early in the postoperative period, the client likely has decreased functional vision in the operative eye. A discussion of safety in the home environment should be completed as part of discharge teaching.

DIABETIC RETINOPATHY

Diabetic retinopathy is a progressive disorder of the retina characterized by microscopic damage to the retinal vessels, resulting in occlusion of the vessels. As a result of inadequate blood supply, sections of the retina deteriorate and vision is permanently lost.

Diabetic retinopathy is one of the leading causes of blindness in the United States and the world. All diabetics are prone to experience retinopathy; approximately 30 to 40 per cent of the diabetic population has some degree of retinopathy.

There are two types of retinopathy: background, or nonproliferative diabetic retinopathy and proliferative diabetic retinopathy. In background retinopathy, early pathologic changes include development of tiny dotlike outpouchings called microaneurysms, and the retinal veins become dilated and tortuous (Fig. 17–9*A*). Multiple hemorrhages occur from these defective vessels. Retinal edema is caused by leaking capillaries. Hemorrhages, exudates, and ischemia contribute to impaired vision, particularly if these occur on or around the macula.

Progressive retinal ischemia stimulates the growth of blood vessels into the vitreous. These vessels leak, hemorrhage, and undergo fibrous changes that may form bands that pull on the retina, causing detachment. This process is called proliferative retinopathy (see Fig. 17–9*B*).

Clients experience a wide range of visual disturbances and fluctuations. Retinal vessel hemorrhage into the vitreous space obstructs vision with black spots or floaters or may result in complete loss of vision. Areas of retinal ischemia become blind spots. Macular edema causes decreased central vision.

Management

To reduce the occurrence of hemorrhage and retinal detachment in progressive retinopathy, the argon laser is used to photocoagulate the blood vessels. Hundreds and even thousands of microscopic photocoagulation applications (burns) are systemically placed around the peripheral retina, avoiding the central area that includes the macula and the optic disc.

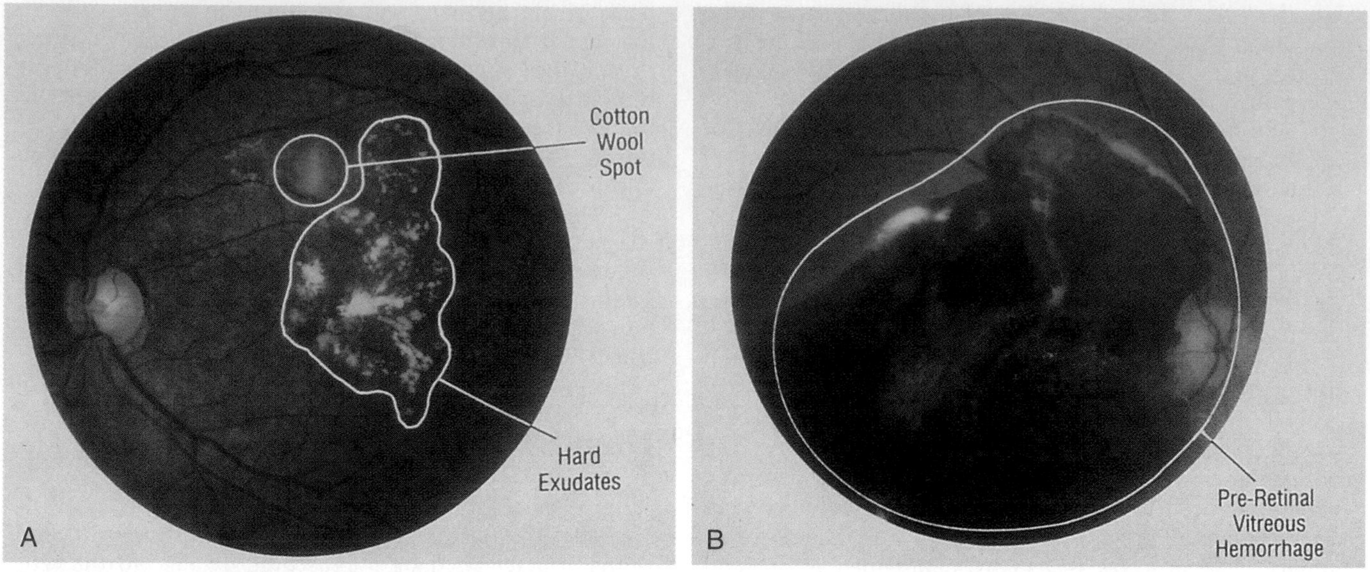

Figure 17–9
Diabetic retinopathy. (From Ignatavicius, D. D., & Bayne, M. V. [Eds.]. *Medical-surgical nursing: A nursing process approach [2nd ed.]*. Slide Set. Philadelphia: W. B. Saunders Co.)

When a hemorrhage does not clear spontaneously, over time, a vitrectomy (removal of a portion of the vitreous) may be performed. A vitrectomy may also need to be performed to release the traction of membranes on the retina.

Nursing interventions for the client with diabetic retinopathy are focused on assessment and management of diabetes (see Chap. 40).

AGE-RELATED MACULAR DEGENERATION

Previously known as senile macular degeneration, age-related macular degeneration is an atrophic degenerative process that affects the macula and surrounding tissues, resulting in central visual deficits.

Age-related macular degeneration can be found to some degree in most adults older than 65 years. It is one of the most common causes of visual loss in the elderly. The exact cause is unknown, but the incidence increases with each decade over 50. It may also be hereditary.

Age-related macular degeneration falls into two groups: nonexudative and exudative. Both are usually bilateral and progressive.

The client may notice a blurred scotoma, decreased central visual acuity (Fig. 17–10), or a blurred, wavy distortion of vision. Fundus photography and angiography may be performed on a regular basis to document and evaluate changes.

Management

There is no known means of medical treatment or prevention for age-related macular degeneration. Further damage from exudative macular degeneration sometimes may be arrested by the use of argon photocoagulation, even though laser damage to the retina in this area results in a blind spot. When the fovea is involved, central vision is lost and the only helpful measures are low-vision aids.

The client with age-related macular degeneration is threatened with the loss of central vision. To evaluate changes in vision, the client is taught to use an Amsler grid at home. The nurse may be able to assist the client to maximize remaining vision with low-vision aids and community referral to a low-vision specialist and low-vision support groups.

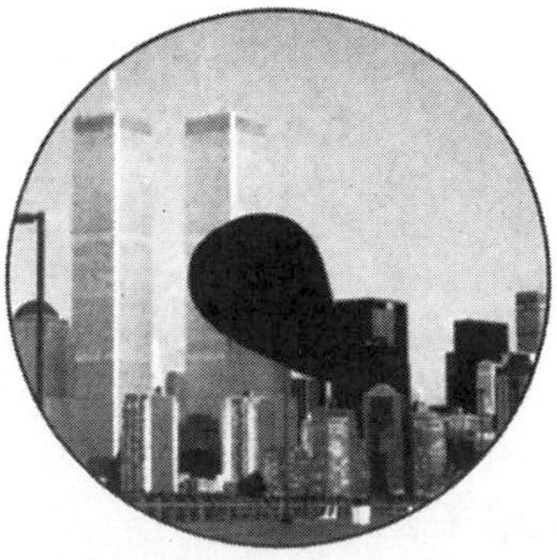

Figure 17–10
Vision of a client with macular degeneration. (Courtesy of National Industries for the Blind, Wayne, NJ.)

Corneal Disorders

CORNEAL DYSTROPHIES

Corneal dystrophies are a group of hereditary and acquired disorders of unknown cause characterized by deposits in the layers of the cornea and alteration of the corneal structure.

Specific corneal dystrophies characteristically appear at different ages. They may be stationary or slowly progressive throughout life. The most common, Fuchs' dystrophy, usually begins in the third or fourth decade, affects more women than men, and is slowly progressive.

Corneal dystrophies are associated with all five layers of the cornea. Although the disease usually originates in the inner layers, the degeneration, erosion, and deposits affect all layers.

Fuchs' dystrophy is characterized by deposits that look like warts. Because the integrity of the cornea is compromised, it becomes edematous and cloudy. Vision is compromised not only by the corneal deposits but by the altered structure of the cornea secondary to the edema.

Medical Management

The cornea is evaluated by slit-lamp examination. Fluorescein staining is used to enhance visualization of surface corneal defects. Corneal scrapings may be taken with a sterile spatula for further staining and microscopic evaluation. Specular micrography (see the section on diagnostic tests) may be used to evaluate the corneal endothelium.

Surgical Management

Corneal transplantation, or keratoplasty, may be indicated for a number of serious corneal conditions including corneal dystrophy. Penetrating keratoplasty denotes full-thickness corneal replacement; lamellar keratoplasty denotes a partial-thickness procedure.

Donor eyes are obtained from cadavers and must be enucleated soon after death because of rapid endothelial cell death, and the eyes must be stored in a preserving solution.

Corneal transplantation surgery is usually performed under local anesthesia (Fig. 17–11).

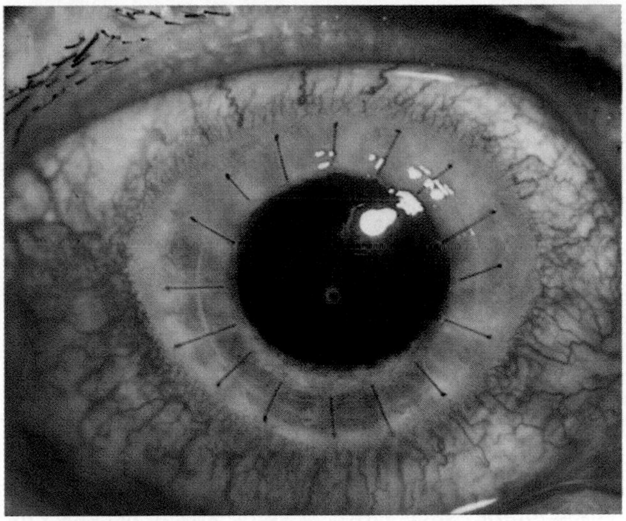

Figure 17–11
Keratoplasty. (Courtesy of Ophthalmic Photography at the University of Michigan W. K. Kellogg Eye Center.)

COMPLICATIONS

Graft rejection or failure may occur at any time after the transplantation. It can result from unsuitable storage of donor tissue, dystrophy of the donor's endothelium, surgical trauma, or immunologic rejection. Because the cornea is an avascular structure, blood typing, which is necessary for other types of grafts, is not necessary.

At the first sign of graft rejection, when the cornea becomes cloudy and edematous and when there is an anterior chamber reaction (presence of white cells or protein) (Fig. 17–12), topical steroids are prescribed in frequent doses to control the inflammatory response and reverse the rejection reaction. In severe cases, a repeat transplantation may be necessary.

Wound leakage, bleeding into the anterior chamber,

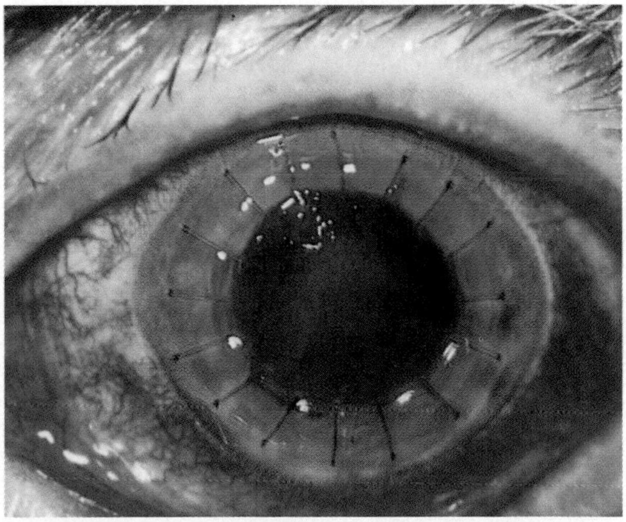

Figure 17–12
Acute graft rejection. (Courtesy of Ophthalmic Photography at the University of Michigan W. K. Kellogg Eye Center.)

glaucoma, cataract, and infection are also complications that may occur.

Nursing Management

Assessment

It is important for the nurse to assist the client in describing symptoms. Because the cornea is extremely sensitive, pain is a common occurrence.

Nursing Diagnosis, Planning, and Implementation

Nursing Diagnosis: Visual Sensory/Perceptual Alterations R/T decreased corneal function.

Planning: Expected Outcomes. The client will have improved visual sensation and perception, as evidenced by functioning safely with current visual deficits and maintaining improved vision with corneal transplantation, recognizing clinical manifestations of graft failure, instilling eye drops correctly, and performing a daily check of vision.

Implementation. The focus of nursing care is to help the client adapt to the limitations in vision and to prepare the client to undergo surgery.

Because some corneal dystrophies and other disorders may progress slowly, the nurse assists the client in adaptation to vision loss (see nursing care for the client with cataracts). Corneal transplantation surgery is usually performed on an outpatient basis or may involve an overnight stay in the hospital.

The client is usually notified the day before the surgery that donor tissue has become available. Receiving a call with short notice for the surgery usually produces a relatively high level of anxiety for the client and significant others. The nurse assists the client in coping with the rush of preoperative activities by using a calm and assured manner and providing education about perioperative events.

Postoperatively, the client returns from the operating room with an eye patch and protective shield in place. The nurse observes the patch for signs of drainage. There is no blood loss associated with this procedure. The client should experience only mild to moderate discomfort, which should be relieved by acetaminophen. Unrelieved pain may indicate a rise in intraocular pressure and is reported to the surgeon. The eye patch will be in place until the following morning when the eye is examined with the slit lamp. Depending on the extent of preoperative visual limitations, most clients experience improved vision immediately. Clients are instructed, however, not to place their expectations too high. Vision continues to improve gradually because the healing process may take up to a year or more. Glasses or contact lenses are usually needed to obtain the best visual result.

Postoperative eye drops usually include an antibiotic and a corticosteroid. Topical corticosteroid therapy may be needed indefinitely. Discharge instructions include the rationale for the medications and proper instillation technique. (See Client Education Guide: Care After Corneal Transplantation.)

CLIENT EDUCATION GUIDE

Care After Corneal Transplantation

Teach the client and significant others about the prescribed medications and proper instillation technique. It is important for the client to wear eye protection in the form of regular glasses, sunglasses, or a protective shield to prevent any injury to the eye. The client is advised never to rub the eye. The area around the eye may be cleaned with warm tap water using a clean wash cloth.

Teaching the client and significant others to recognize the signs and symptoms of graft rejection is a critical component of discharge education. The following teaching tool may be useful in teaching the client to remember the signs of graft rejection. It involves the use of the letters RSVP, which are familiar to most people:

R = Redness
S = Swelling
V = Decreased Vision
P = Pain

The client is advised to evaluate the vision in the operative eye each day. A picture on the wall or some object in a well-lighted room should be selected to use as a point of reference. If a change in vision from the day before is noted, the client should re-evaluate his or her vision in a few hours. If no improvement is noted or if vision is worse, the client should notify the physician. Because graft rejection may occur at any time (even years) after the surgery, the client is advised to make the vision check a routine part of his or her activities of daily living for the rest of his or her life.

The nurse also teaches the client and significant others to recognize the signs of increased intraocular pressure and infection.

Evaluation

The expected outcomes are evaluated. Because many months may be required for visual restoration, revisions in the plan of care may be needed.

KERATITIS

The corneal epithelium is normally an effective barrier against microorganisms. Once it is compromised from disease or trauma, the underlying stromal layer becomes an excellent culture media for a variety of organisms.

Dry eyes or ineffective eyelid closure predispose the eye to keratitis. Clients who have a systemic collagen disorder such as rheumatoid arthritis are particularly susceptible to corneal infections and ulceration.

Tearing and photophobia are common, and blurred vision results from the inability of the cornea to provide the proper refractive surface. The client with a corneal defect from an infection will experience a great deal of discomfort, which is worsened by eyelid movement. The eye appears infected and indurated. Fluorescein staining of the cornea outlines the affected area, which can be viewed through the slit lamp or with a handheld flashlight.

CORNEAL ULCERS

Corneal infections may develop into ulcerations (Fig. 17–13) that severely compromise the integrity of the eye. Sources of infection include bacteria (e.g., *Staphylococcus aureus, Pseudomonas aeruginosa,* and *Streptococcus pneumoniae*), fungi *(Candida, Aspergillus)*, viruses (adenovirus, herpes simplex, herpes zoster), and protozoa *(Acanthamoeba)*. Clinical findings under slit-lamp examination are specific to particular organisms. Hypopyon (a layer of white cells in the anterior chamber) may accompany corneal ulceration.

MANAGEMENT

Topical antibiotic, antifungal, and antiviral therapy is prescribed, with the frequency of instillation based on the severity of the infection to prevent the progression to perforation and to promote healing. Maximal therapy includes the instillation of two broad-spectrum eye drops every 15 minutes around the clock and may require hospitalization. As the infection begins to respond to the medication, frequency is gradually decreased. Systemic intravenous medication may be prescribed as well.

To aid the healing process, surgical intervention may be necessary. Tarsorrhaphy (suturing the eyelid shut) promotes healing by decreasing eyelid blinking and by decreasing evaporation of the corneal tear film. Tissue adhesive, a kind of super glue, may also be used to seal the perforation. A soft contact lens may be used as a bandage to maintain the seal. Large perforations may require either lamellar (partial-thickness) or penetrating (full-thickness) keratoplasty.

Eye drops are given alternately every 15 minutes around the clock.

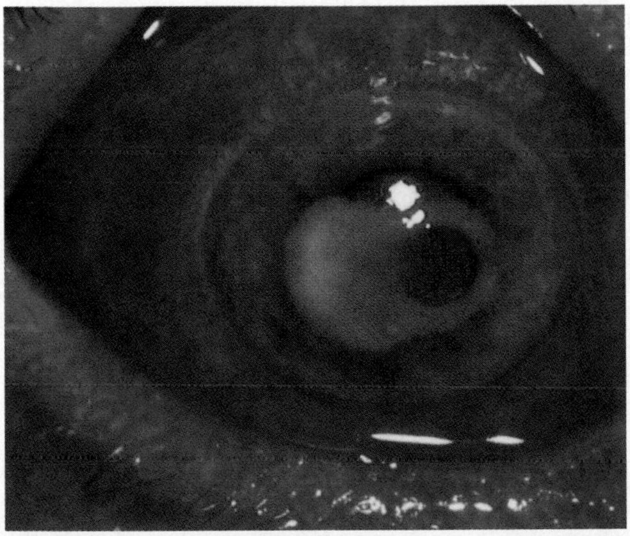

Figure 17–13
Corneal ulcer. (Courtesy of Ophthalmic Photography at the University of Michigan W. K. Kellogg Eye Center.)

CRITICAL TO REMEMBER

Hand washing is particularly important in this situation and is carried out even if gloves are worn to instill the drops.

The threat of losing eyesight compels many clients to watch the clock for fear that the nurse will forget to administer an eye drop. The nurse can build the client's trust and reduce anxiety by maintaining the time schedule for the eye drops.

Effective sleep and rest are nearly impossible with interruptions every 15 minutes. The client rarely reaches the deeper stages of sleep, and most experience restless light sleep in stage one and two. In addition to the eye pain the client may already be experiencing, some of the eye drops, such as fortified bacitracin, may cause stinging that lasts several minutes.

Oral analgesics are given at regular intervals, and mild sleeping medications may be helpful at bedtime.

The client's eye may need to be cleansed frequently because the medications and excessive tearing will become dried and the lids will stick together. Warm tap water applied with soft gauze pads is used. The combination of tearing, medications, and cleaning may cause the skin of an elderly client to become excoriated. Antibiotic ophthalmic ointment may be applied to the lower lid margin and cheek to reduce irritation.

Clients usually become adapted to this regimen of interruptions after the first 48 hours. As the cornea begins to show signs of improvement, the eye drops may be reduced in frequency to every 30 minutes and then every hour.

At discharge, the client should be able to demonstrate how to instill eye drops properly. The client will also understand the importance of complying with the medication regimen. The nurse should instruct the client and significant others about the signs and symptoms of increasing infection. The eye may continue to be cleansed with warm tap water at home. The nurse also assesses the home environment if the client's vision is greatly reduced. Referrals for rehabilitation may be necessary as well.

KERATOCONUS

Keratoconus is a degenerative disease of the cornea characterized by a thinning and protrusion of the cornea in a cone shape (Fig. 17–14). Blurred vision is the result of the change in the shape of the cornea, which may be corrected by contact lenses. Keratoconus is often slowly progressive between the ages of 20 and 60 years.

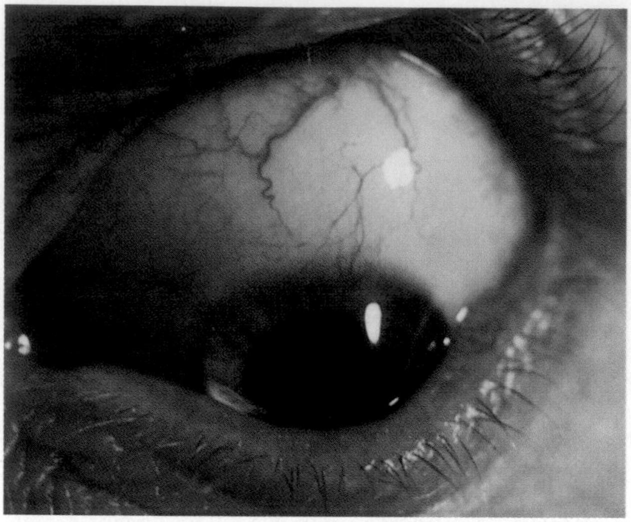

Figure 17–14
Keratoconus. (Courtesy of Ophthalmic Photography at the University of Michigan W. K. Kellogg Eye Center.)

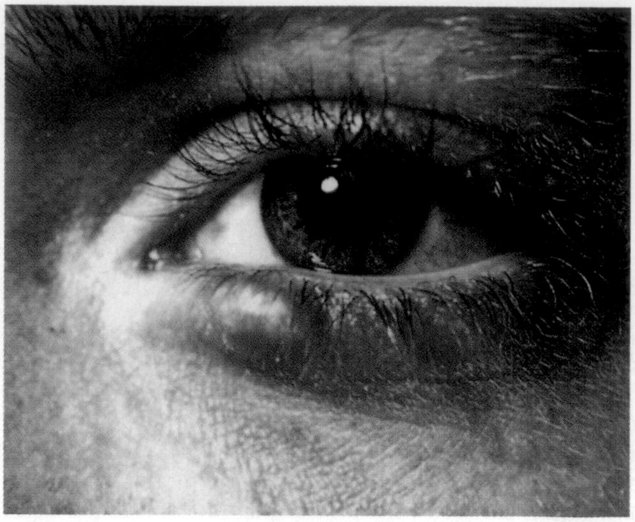

Figure 17–15
Chalazion. (Courtesy of Ophthalmic Photography at the University of Michigan W. K. Kellogg Eye Center.)

At some point, the conical shape of the cornea may no longer allow for contact lenses to correct vision. Corneal transplantation for keratoconus is highly successful.

Uveal Tract Disorders

UVEITIS

Uveitis is an inflammation of the uveal tract that can affect one or more parts (iris, ciliary body, and choroid). Uveitis commonly occurs from a hypersensitivity reaction in its acute form or after microbial infection in its chronic form. Clients with this condition complain of pain, blurred vision, and photophobia. There is marked redness of the eye, and the pupil is usually constricted.

A cycloplegic medication such as atropine effectively relieves spasm of the ciliary body muscle, and the dilation of the pupil prevents the inflamed iris from adhering to the lens and the corneal endothelium from forming synechiae. Topical steroid drops are prescribed to reduce the inflammation.

Photophobia (sensitivity to light) and eye discomfort are the chief complaints. The nurse should advise the client to wear dark glasses and to avoid bright light. Reduced lighting at home may be hazardous because the client's pupil is dilated, causing blurred vision. Oral analgesics usually relieve the ocular discomfort.

The nurse should be sure that the client and significant others understand the rationale for the prescribed medications. The client should also be able to recognize signs and symptoms of increased intraocular pressure.

Eyelid, Lacrimal, and Conjunctival Disorders

Infection and inflammation cause most common diseases of the eyelid, lacrimal, and conjunctival areas. Hordeolum (stye) is an infection of the glands of the eyelids that is treated with warm compresses and antibiotics. Incision and drainage of purulent material may be indicated. Chalazion is a sterile, chronic, granulomatous inflammation of a meibomian gland (Fig. 17–15). If it is large enough to distort vision or to be a cosmetic blemish, it may be surgically excised. Blepharitis is a common chronic bilateral inflammation of the eyelid margins that is treated by keeping the scalp clean, removing scales with baby shampoo and cotton-tipped applicators. Antibiotic ophthalmic ointment is used for treatment if infection occurs. Conjunctivitis is an inflammation of the conjunctiva; it is treated with antibiotic eye drops or systemic medications.

Benign tumors of the lids are very common and often increase in frequency with age. They may be removed for cosmetic reasons. Basal cell and squamous cell carcinomas of the lids are the most common malignant tumors of the eyelids. Malignant tumors may be treated by a variety of methods such as electrodesiccation, cryotherapy, or surgical removal.

Refractive Disorders

Light is bent (refracted) as it passes through the cornea and lens of the eye. Refractive errors exist when light rays are not focused appropriately on the retina of the eye.

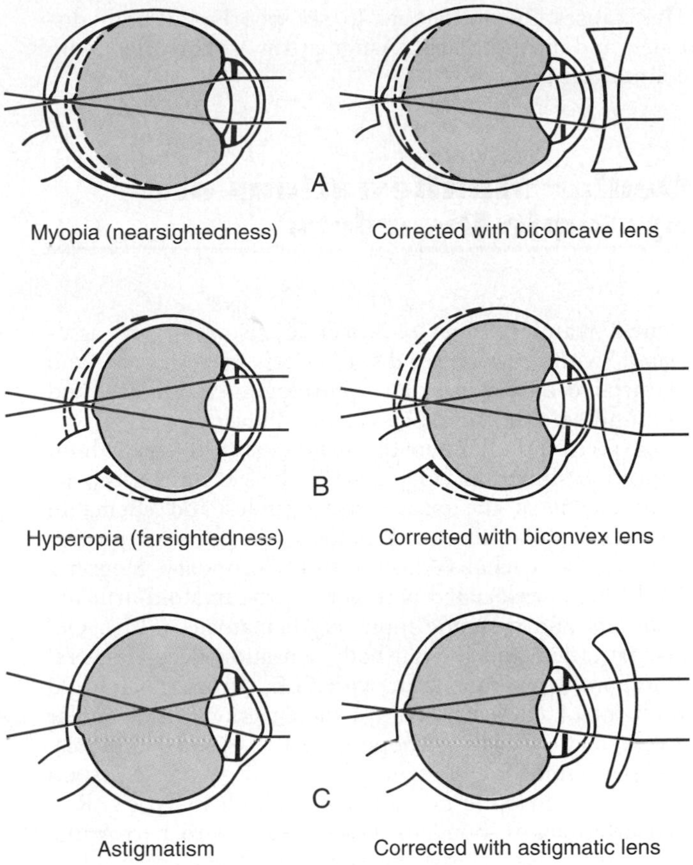

Figure 17–16
Common refractive disorders and their correction. *Dashed lines* in parts *A* and *B* indicate normal eye contour.

Three basic abnormalities of refraction occur in the eye: myopia, hyperopia, and astigmatism. Optical correction is important to distinguish between visual loss caused by disease and visual loss caused by refractive error.

MYOPIA

Myopia, or nearsightedness, is a condition in which the light rays come into focus in front of the retina (Fig. 17–16*A*). In this case, the refractive power of the eye is too strong and a concave, or minus, lens is used to focus light rays on the eye. In the great majority of cases, myopia is caused by an eyeball that is longer than normal, which may be a familial trait.

In some cases of myopia, surgical intervention (radial keratotomy) may be performed on the cornea to reduce or eliminate the need for myopic refractive correction. In one type of procedure, eight partial-thickness incisions are made in the cornea with a diamond blade to flatten the curvature of the cornea. Radial keratotomy is an elective procedure, and although it has been somewhat controversial over the past few years, it has been successful. Risks associated with this procedure include unsatisfactory correction, corneal glare, and postoperative infection. The excimer laser is used in this type of corneal surgery to evaporate tissue cleanly, with almost no damage to adjacent cells. The excimer laser is able to make extremely precise incisions in the cornea and may be useful in refractive surgery as well as keratoplasty.

HYPEROPIA

The hyperopic, or farsighted, eye is deficient in its ability to focus light rays. The focal point falls behind the eye (see Fig. 17–16*B*) and, consequently, the image that falls on the retina is blurred. Vision may be brought into focus by placing a convex, or plus, lens in front of the eye. The lens supplies the magnifying power that the eye is lacking. Hyperopia may be caused by an eyeball that is shorter than normal or a cornea that has less curvature than normal.

ASTIGMATISM

Astigmatism is a refractive condition in which rays of light are not bent equally by the cornea in all directions, so that a point of focus is not attained (see Fig. 17–16*C*). In most instances, astigmatism occurs because the curvature of the cornea is not perfectly spherical.

This causes the individual to see poorly for both distance and near objects. Astigmatism is corrected with cylindric lenses.

Ocular Manifestations of Systemic Disorders

Ocular manifestations of systemic disorders are associated with endocrine disturbances; rheumatoid and connective tissue disorders; neurologic, circulatory, and immunologic disorders; and Lyme disease.

Graves' ophthalmopathy may exist with or without thyroid dysfunction (Fig. 17–17). It is characterized by enlargement of the extraocular muscles and edema in the extracellular tissues. Proptosis (the forward protrusion of the eyeballs) may result. Secondary Sjögren's syndrome is associated with certain rheumatoid-arthritic disorders and systemic lupus erythematosus (SLE). Ocular irritation and foreign body sensation occur. Several other problems can occur with SLE. Approximately 90 per cent of clients with myasthenia gravis have ocular involvement. Ptosis (drooping of the eyelid), diplopia, and nystagmus are present. There is also a close association between optic neuritis and multiple sclerosis. Retinal arterioles respond to hypertension with narrowing; the client is also at risk for retinal vein occlusion. Ocular complications affect approximately 75 per cent of all clients with AIDS. The conjunctiva and eyelids may be the first sites of Kaposi's sarcoma. Opportunistic infections may also involve the eyes of the AIDS client. If untreated, blindness can result. Lyme disease, caused by a tick bite, may cause uveitis, optic neuropathy, keratitis, choroiditis, and exudative retinal detachments.

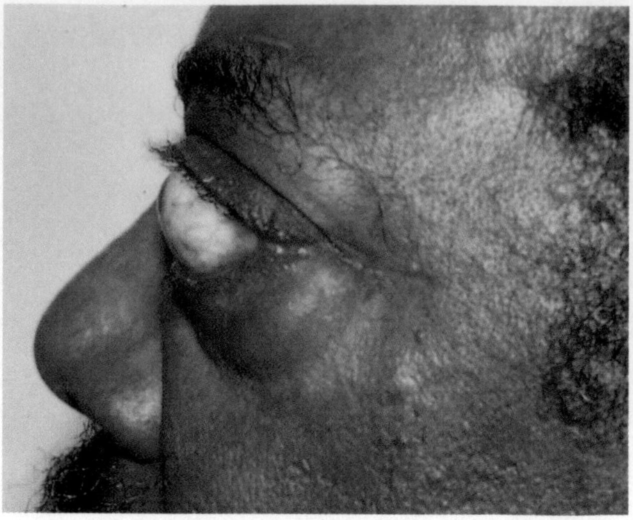

Figure 17–17
Graves' exophthalmos. (Courtesy of Ophthalmic Photography at the University of Michigan W. K. Kellogg Eye Center.)

STUDY QUESTIONS

1. Normal intraocular pressure is maintained as long as there is a balance between the:
   A. Daily production and outflow of tears.
   B. Aqueous production and the aqueous outflow.
   C. Internal and external atmospheric pressure affecting the conjunctiva.
   D. Smooth and elastic functioning of the accessory structures of the eye.

2. Which is the most important question the nurse should ask an elderly client who is being treated for an ocular problem?
   A. "Do you use eye drops every day?"
   B. "When was your last eye examination?"
   C. "Can you read without wearing your eyeglasses?"
   D. "How long have you been wearing contact lenses?"

3. A client with a foreign body in her eye is frightened and asks the nurse, "What kind of test will they have to do on my eye?" Which one of the following should the nurse teach the client?
   A. "The most common test for a foreign body in the eye is fundus photography."
   B. "The physician will use a noninvasive instrument called the exophthalmometer."
   C. "The physician will use a slit-lamp microscope to look directly into the eye to locate the foreign body."
   D. "A visual evoked response is performed to ascertain that the electrical potential of the eye is functioning correctly."

4. Which of the following would be assessed in the client with angle-closure glaucoma?
   A. Tearing and photophobia
   B. Ocular pain on waking
   C. Rainbow halos around lights
   D. A shadow falling across the field of vision

5. A man who has a "mature" cataract needs to know that:
   A. He should not drive a car.
   B. He must have his eyes examined more frequently.
   C. Special lenses will enable him to see more clearly.
   D. Special eye drops must be inserted into the conjunctival sac daily.

6. A client states, "I'm worried that I'll have a retinal detachment just like my cousin." She needs to be taught that:
   A. Retinal detachment can be prevented by having yearly ophthalmic examinations.
   B. She should prevent trauma to the eye because trauma can cause retinal detachment.
   C. Chances are very high that she will experience a retinal detachment when she is older.
   D. If she feels pain behind the eyeball and is dizzy and nauseated, she should seek medical assistance immediately.

7. A client has a nursing diagnosis of Visual Sensory/Perceptual Alterations R/T increased intraocular pressure secondary to glaucoma. Which of the following is an appropriate intervention?

A. Instruction about the instillation of eye drops
B. Preparing the client for a lens implant in the affected eye
C. Demonstrating how to apply eye shields to wear during sleep
D. Showing the client how vision is restored with proper treatment

8. The client with a cataract will exhibit:
A. Photophobia and glare.
B. Blurred vision and headache.
C. The need for more light in order to see.
D. Nausea and will see rainbow halos around lights.

9. Instructions for the client who is discharged after cataract surgery should include which one of the following statements?
A. "There are no restrictions on lifting."
B. "Avoid sleeping on the operative side."
C. "Take aspirin for any discomfort you experience."
D. "There are no eye drops to use after cataract surgery."

10. The plan of care for the client who has surgery for a retinal detachment should include instruction about medications. Which medication might be used to reduce intraocular pressure?
A. Miotic ointment
B. Cycloplegic agents
C. Intravenous acetazolamide (Diamox)
D. Combination antibiotic-steroid eye drops

11. Which one of the following is an expectation of the client who has an ocular disorder requiring daily treatment? Most important, the client should have the ability to:
A. Apply the eye shields for use during the day.
B. Perform required ocular exercises on a daily basis.
C. Understand the actions of the medications that are ordered.
D. Instill medication in the eye the required number of times each day.

CRITICAL THINKING EXERCISES

SCENARIO A

An elderly man is a client at the clinic. He is being treated for glaucoma. During his visit, he states that he is not using his eye drops every day because he can see without any problems. He has had glaucoma for about 3 years.

1. What might occur as a result of untreated glaucoma?
2. What assessment should the nurse complete during the examination?
3. What information should be included in discharge teaching for this client?

SCENARIO B

Clients who have ocular surgery are usually given instructions for postoperative care at home.

1. What instructions are given for the client after cataract surgery?
2. What instructions are given for the client after surgery for a retinal detachment?
3. What modifications might be necessary for an elderly client?

BIBLIOGRAPHY

1. Anderson, W., et al. (1991). *Atlas of ophthalmic surgery* (Vol. 1). St. Louis: Mosby-Year Book.
2. Bienkowski, J. (1994). An overview of the progression of diabetic retinopathy with treatment recommendations. *Nurse Practitioner: American Journal of Primary Health Care, 19(7),* 50–58.
3. Boyd-Monk, H., & Steinmetz, C. (1987). *Nursing care of the eye.* Norwalk, CT: Appleton & Lange.
4. Burlew, J. (1991). Preventing eye injuries—the nurse's role. *Journal of the American Society of Ophthalmic Registered Nurses, 16(6),* 24–28.
5. Capino, D., & Leibowitz, H. (1990). Glaucoma: Screening, diagnosis, and therapy. *Hospital Practice. 25(5A),* 73–74, 77–80, 85–88.
6. Carpenito, L. (1993). *Nursing diagnosis: Application to clinical practice* (5th ed.). Philadelphia: J. B. Lippincott.
7. Char, D. (1989). *Clinical ocular oncology.* New York: Churchill Livingstone.
8. Charlton, J. F. (1995). *Ophthalmic surgery complications: Prevention and management.* Philadelphia: J. B. Lippincott Co.
9. Chingnell, A. (1989). *Retinal detachment surgery.* New York: Springer-Verlag.
10. Clanton, C., & Means, M. (1988). Retinal reattachment—Quality and appropriateness of care. *Journal of Ophthalmic Nursing and Technology, 7(4),* 130–133.
11. Copstead, L. C. (1995). *Perspectives on pathophysiology.* Philadelphia: W. B. Saunders Co.
12. deSmet, M., & Nussenbatt, R. (1991). Ocular manifestations of AIDS. *JAMA, 266(21),* 3019–3022.
13. Duane, T., & Jaeger, E. (1990). *Clinical ophthalmology* (Vol. 1). Philadelphia: J. B. Lippincott.

14. Duane, T., & Jaeger, E. (1990). *Clinical ophthalmology* (Vol. 2). Philadelphia: J. B. Lippincott.
15. Duane, T., & Jaeger, E. (1990). *Clinical ophthalmology* (Vol. 3). Philadelphia: J. B. Lippincott.
16. Duane, T., & Jaeger, E. (1990). *Clinical ophthalmology* (Vol. 4). Philadelphia: J. B. Lippincott.
17. Duane, T., & Jaeger, E. (1990). *Clinical ophthalmology* (Vol. 5). Philadelphia: J. B. Lippincott.
18. Friedlaender, M. (Ed.). (1988). *Prevention of eye disease.* New York: Liebert.
19. Gallagher, C. (1991). The young adult with recent vision loss: A pilot case study. *Journal of The American Society of Ophthalmic Registered Nurses, 16(6),* 8–14.
20. Garber, N. (1991). Basic ocular motility assessment. *Journal of Ophthalmic Nursing and Technology, 10(5),* 215–219.
21. Gills, J., & Sanders, D. (1990). *Small incision cataract surgery.* Thorofare, NJ: Slack.
22. Goodman, D. F., et al. (1989). Complications of cataract extraction with intraocular lens implantation. *Ophthalmic Surgery, 20(2),* 132–140.
23. Hosein, A. (1989). Exenteration—The nursing approach. *Journal of Ophthalmic Nursing and Technology, 8(3),* 91–96.
24. Kaufman, H. (1989). Refractive surgery through the looking glass. *Acta Ophthalmologica, 192(Suppl. 67)*; 30–37.
25. Kaye, G., et al. (1990). IOL implant patients need your help. *Journal of Ophthalmic Nursing and Technology, 4(4),* 18–23.
26. Larson, P. M. (1992). Double vision. *Journal of Ophthalmic Nursing and Technology, 11(2),* 79–83.
27. Latham, B., Higgins, L., & Ambrose, P. (1992). Cataract patients' postop eye care: Development and evaluation of a teaching program. *Australian Journal of Advanced Nursing, 10(1),* 4–9.
28. Legro, M. (1991). Quality of life and cataracts: A review of patient-centered studies of cataract surgery outcomes. *Ophthalmic Surgery, 22,* 431–443.
29. Matteson, M. A., Linton, A., & Byers, V. (1993). Vision and hearing screening in cognitively impaired older adults. *Geriatric Nursing: American Journal of Care for the Aging, 14(6),* 294–297.
30. McGrory, A., & Assmann, S. (1994). A study investigating primary nursing, discharge teaching, and patient satisfaction of ambulatory cataract patients. *Insight, 19(2),* 8–13, 29.
31. Meissner, J. E. (1995). Caring for patients with glaucoma. *Nursing '95. 25(1)*, 56–57.
32. Mills, K. (Ed.). (1989). *Glaucoma.* Proceedings of the 4th International Symposium of the Northern Eye Institute, Manchester, UK, July 14–16, 1988. Oxford: Pergamon Press.
33. Morgan, C., et al. (1988). Ocular complications associated with retrobulbar injections. *Ophthalmology, 95(5),* 660–665.
34. Newell, F. (1992). *Ophthalmology: Principles and concepts* (7th ed.). St. Louis: C. V. Mosby.
35. Obstbaum, S. (1991). *Glaucoma surgery atlas.* Norwalk, CT: Appleton & Lange.
36. Perkins, R., & Olson, R. (1991). A new look at postoperative instructions following cataract extraction. *Ophthalmic Surgery 22(2),* 66–68.
37. Perry, A. (1990). Integrated orbital implants. *Advances in Ophthalmic Plastic and Reconstructive Surgery, 8,* 75–81.
38. Phillips, W. B. II. (1994). Ocular manifestations of diabetes mellitus. *Journal of Ophthalmic Nursing and Technology, 13(6),* 255–261, 276–277.
39. Portnoy, S., et al. (1989). Surgical management of corneal ulceration and perforation. *Survey of Ophthalmology, 34(1),* 47–58.
40. Rozakis, G. (1990). *Cataract surgery.* Thorofare, NJ: Slack, Inc.
41. Ruehl, C. A., & Schremp, P. S. (1992). Nursing care of the cataract patient: Today's outpatient approach. *Nursing Clinics of North America, 27(3),* 727–743.
42. Sardegna, J., & Paul, T. (1991). *The encyclopedia of blindness and vision impairment.* New York: Facts on File Publishing.
43. Servodidio, C. (1991). Teaching aids to patients diagnosed with choroidal melanoma. *Journal of American Society of Ophthalmic Registered Nurses, 16(6),* 21–23.
44. Singerman, L., & Jampol, L. (1991). *Retinal & choroidal manifestations of systemic disease.* Baltimore: Williams & Wilkins.
45. Smith, R. S. (1989). Refractive surgery. In R. D. Reincke (Ed.), *Ophthalmology annual* (pp. 361–362). New York: Raven Press.
46. Vade, L. (1992). Vision and vision loss. *Nursing Clinics of North America, 27(3),* 705–714.
47. Vine, A. K., et al. (1989). A new inexpensive customized plaque for choroidal melanoma iodine-125 plaque therapy. *Ophthalmology, 96(4),* 543–546.
48. Weingeist, T. A. (1992). *Laser surgery in ophthalmology: Practical applications.* Philadelphia: F. A. Davis.
49. Werner, E. (1991). *Manual of visual fields.* New York: Churchill Livingstone.
50. Wilson, S., & Kaufman, H. (1990). Graft failure after penetrating keratoplasty. *Survey of Ophthalmology, 34(5),* 325–356.
51. Woods, S. (1992). Macular degeneration. *Nursing Clinics of North America, 27(3),* 761–775.
52. Young, R. (1991). *Age related cataract.* New York: Oxford University Press.

Chapter 18

Assessment and Nursing Care of Clients with Ear Disorders

Learning Outcomes

After completing this chapter, the learner will be able to:

1. Teach the client about the normal structure of the ear.
2. Explain to the client structural and functional abnormalities of the ear.
3. Conduct a nursing history and physical assessment of the client with actual or potential disorders of the ear.
4. Teach the client about common diagnostic studies common to functions of the ear.
5. Assess the client for clinical manifestations of ear disorders.
6. Teach the client about the etiology, risk factors, basic pathophysiology, and clinical manifestations of major ear disorders.
7. Explain the client's role in the medical and surgical management of ear disorders.
8. Develop plans of care for the prevention of illness, management, and rehabilitation of the client with an ear disorder.
9. Implement nursing interventions that optimize the quality of life for the client with an ear disorder.
10. Evaluate planned client outcomes, using outcome criteria developed in the planning phase of care.

Hearing and balance problems can reduce the ability to communicate, limit social activities, and hinder the constructive use of leisure time. Career options, job opportunities, and financial security can also be compromised. Ear problems can interfere with the client's ability to remain independent, which can lead to isolation. Also, the aesthetic enjoyment of life and the ability to share human experiences can be temporarily or permanently diminished. All these situations can result in feelings of anger, anxiety, frustration, uncertainty, and loneliness, which ultimately may affect the quality of life.

Assessment of the Ear

HISTORY

The otologic history can be the most important assessment tool and should be obtained before audiometric testing.

An otologic history includes demographic data, the chief complaint, past medical history, family history, psychosocial history, and review of systems. Ear problems often result from childhood illnesses or problems associated with adjacent structures. The history interview is essential for determining current problems related to the ear.

Demographic data relevant to otologic assessment include the client's age. Hearing loss occurs as a consequence of the aging process (presbycusis). It is caused by changes in the delicate labyrinthine structures over time or a slow decrease in the blood supply or infection. The majority of clients will eventually experience presbycusis during the aging process. Presbycusis cannot be treated medically or surgically.

Chief Complaint

The most common chief complaints include hearing loss, pain, tinnitus, ear drainage, loss of balance, vertigo, and dizziness. The client may also complain of associated nausea or vomiting. The nurse completes a symptom analysis to determine onset, duration, frequency, and precipitating and relieving factors for the presenting symptom. The client's past medical history is explored carefully in order to determine the chronicity of the problem and to determine the cause.

Hearing loss can occur suddenly or gradually and can vary according to whether loss is conductive, sensorineural, or related to a central nervous system disorder. The client may report inability to hear certain words or sounds or that sounds are muffled. Pain may be perceived by the client as a feeling of fullness in the ear. It may be intensified by movement and relieved by holding the head still or by application of heat. Ear pain may occur as a result of related problems of the nose, sinuses, oral cavity, or pharynx. Ear drainage can be bloody (sanguineous), clear (serous), mixed (serosanguineous), or pus (purulent). Drainage may also be accompanied by an odor. Tinnitus (ringing in the ears) may be reported as high- or low-pitched, roaring, humming, hissing, or loud and persistent. Tinnitus may occur more commonly at certain times of the day. Loss of balance may be accompanied by vertigo or dizziness.

Past Medical History

CHILDHOOD AND INFECTIOUS DISEASES

Childhood diseases that commonly occur include acute middle ear infections (otitis media), eardrum perforations resulting from otitis media, complications of ear infections such as chronic otitis media, frequent upper respiratory tract infection, and acute and chronic sinus infections. Infectious diseases with ear problem sequelae include mumps, measles, and meningitis. Specifically inquire whether the client has been immunized for mumps and measles and against *Haemophilus influenzae* type B. In utero exposure to maternal influenza or rubella may result in congenital hearing loss in the child. Premature birth is also associated with hearing problems.

MAJOR ILLNESSES AND HOSPITALIZATIONS

Inquire about a history of tonsillitis. Has the client had a tonsillectomy or adenoidectomy? Is there a history of ear surgery? Has the client had trauma to the head or ear, such as a severe blow or sustained loud noise exposure or concussion from sudden changes in air pressure (such as may occur in an explosion)? Is there a history of a chronic eardrum perforation?

MEDICATIONS

Certain medications can damage the vestibulocochlear nerve (eighth cranial nerve), with resultant hearing loss, tinnitus, or disturbances in equilibrium. Aspirin is a common cause of tinnitus. Other drugs include aminoglycosides, analgesics, salicylates, and antiprotozoal agents. (Box 18–1 lists drugs that have ototoxic effects.) The nurse should inquire whether the client has taken or is currently taking medications and for how long. Signs of ototoxicity include dizziness, nausea, vomiting with motion, vision impairment, tinnitus, ear pain, and nystagmus.

ALLERGIES

In addition to asking about allergies to medications and other substances, the nurse should inquire about allergies resulting in nasal stuffiness and congestion. Close proximity of the eustachian tubes may also result in edema, which obstructs the flow of air between the middle ear and nose so that air pressure cannot be equalized.

Family History

The nurse asks about family members and whether there is a history of hearing loss. Age of onset for presbycusis is determined.

BOX 18-1

Selected Ototoxic Drugs*

AMINOGLYCOSIDE ANTIBIOTICS	OTHER DRUGS
Streptomycin	Chemotherapeutic agents
Neomycin	Cisplatin
Gentamicin	Nitrogen mustard
Tobramycin	Salicylates
Amikacin	Quinine drugs
Kanamycin	Bleomycin
Netilmicin	Quinidine
OTHER ANTIBIOTICS	CHEMICALS
Vancomycin	Metals
Viomycin	Lead
Polymyxin B (Aerosporin)	Mercury
Polymyxin E (colistin; Coly-Mycin)	Gold
Erythromycin	Arsenic
Minocycline	Alcohol
Capreomycin	DIURETICS
	Furosemide (Lasix)
	Ethacrynic acid (Edecrin)
	Acetazolamide (Diamox)

*Substances toxic to the ear.

Psychosocial History and Life-Style

Psychosocial and life-style factors that influence the occurrence of ear problems include occupational hazards, environmental exposure, and leisure activities and hobbies. The nurse asks about exposure to loud noises, their type, frequency, and duration. Is protective ear gear worn? Does the client swim, especially in water that may be contaminated? Has the client had problems with "swimmer's ear"? Does the client use ear plugs to prevent water from entering the ear canal?

The nurse should explore health management behaviors the client practices regarding ear hygiene. Does the client have a habit of putting objects into the ear, such as pencils, bobby pins, or cotton-tipped applicators?

Review of Systems

The review of systems related to the ear includes asking about problems with the nose, sinuses, mouth, pharynx, and throat. The nurse should ask whether the client has experienced head trauma, loss of balance, dizziness, or vertigo.

PHYSICAL EXAMINATION

Physical examination of the ear includes assessment of hearing acuity, balance, and equilibrium. Because the external ear is completely visible, it is easy to identify anatomic landmarks and assess any abnormalities. The eardrum reveals significant information regarding the middle ear. However, much of the middle ear and inner ear is inaccessible to direct examinations, and inferences must be made by testing auditory and vestibular function.

Inspection and Palpation

EXTERNAL EAR

Gross examination of both ears should precede individual examination of either ear. Inspection and palpation are used for assessment of the external ear. The external ear should be inspected for size, configuration, and angle of attachment to the head. The skin of the ear should be smooth and without breaks or inflammation, especially in the crevice behind the ear. Lumps, skin lesions, and cysts should be noted and their approximate size and location recorded.

Palpation and manipulation of the pinna produce information regarding tenderness, nodules, or tophi (small, hard nodules). In palpation, the nurse should move the pinna, feel the mastoid area, and press on the tragus. He or she should note whether any of the manipulations produces pain or discomfort, which could indicate inflammation or infection.

EAR CANAL

Direct Observation. Inspection of the ear canal is carried out by direct observation, otoscopy, or microscopic examination. For direct observation, the adult is asked to tip the head slightly to the opposite side while the nurse pulls the pinna up, back, and out. A penlight is then used to inspect the ear canal for any abnormalities such as extreme narrowing of the ear canal, excessive wax, redness, scaliness, swelling, drainage, cysts, or foreign objects. Normally, none of these signs are present. Visualization of the eardrum with this method would be unlikely.

Otoscopy. The eardrum is located at the end of the only skin-lined canal in the body. Therefore, visualization is difficult and requires illumination and magnification for accurate assessment. An otoscope is portable, and otoscopic examination is the most common method used. An otoscope is a device consisting of a handle, a light source, a magnifying lens, and an attachment for visualizing the ear canal and eardrum. An otoscope with a pneumatic device for injecting air may be used if fluid is suspected behind the ear drum.

Specula for the otoscope come in a variety of sizes. The diameter of the meatus and the length of the ear canal vary; thus, the speculum with the largest diameter that fits comfortably into the ear canal should be selected. The light source must be checked for brightness. If the light appears yellowish or dim (like a flashlight with weak batteries), the batteries must be recharged or replaced.

The otoscope is held with the dominant hand, with the hand resting against the client's head. In this manner, should the client move suddenly, the otoscope will also move, so that the examination will be less likely to damage the external canal. With the nondominant hand, the pinna is pulled up, back, and out (in the adult); thus, the ear canal is straightened. While this is done, the client's head is gently tilted away from the nurse, and the speculum is inserted slowly and carefully into the ear canal. The nurse's eye is brought close to the magnifying lens in order to visualize the ear canal and eardrum (tympanic membrane).

The ear canal of the unaffected ear is observed first while the speculum is entering and leaving. The otoscope is moved in a circular fashion to visualize the entire ear canal; abnormalities such as extreme narrowing of the ear canal, nodules, redness, scaliness, swelling, drainage, cysts, foreign objects, or excessive wax are noted. Visualization of the eardrum will be impaired by most of these abnormalities. Sometimes the ear canal must be cleaned of wax, dead skin, and other debris. Wax and debris can be removed with a cerumen spoon (wax curet), suction aspirator, or irrigation. Cerumen that is impacted in the ear canal is a cause of hearing loss. Therefore, assessment of the amount of cerumen is important.

CRITICAL TO REMEMBER

The normal eardrum is slightly conical, quite shiny and smooth, and pearly gray in color.

In the presence of disease, not only does the color of the eardrum change, but also other abnormalities such as retraction of the eardrum, bulging of the eardrum, perforation of the eardrum, or a white plaque (tympanosclerosis) in the eardrum can exist.

The nurse should carefully inspect the entire eardrum, again rotating the otoscope in a circular fashion.

Indirect Testing for Auditory Acuity

Assessment of the middle and inner ear for hearing is accomplished by sophisticated methods of indirect testing. However, a gross assessment of hearing can be made simply through conversation, by evaluating the logical sequence of replies and the appropriateness of the responses.

The client is asked whether hearing is better in one ear than in the other ear. If the auditory acuity is different, the ear that hears better should be tested first. Each ear must be tested separately to estimate the hearing. The nurse begins by occluding one of the client's ears with a finger. Then while standing 1 to 2 feet away, the nurse whispers two-syllable numbers softly toward the unoccluded ear, and the client is asked to repeat the numbers. The intensity of the nurse's voice can be increased from a soft, medium, or loud whisper to a soft, medium, or loud voice. If the nurse suspects that the client is lip reading, the client's face should be turned away.

The tuning fork also provides a general estimate of hearing loss. The three major tuning fork tests date from the 19th century and are named after their originators: Weber, Rinne, and Schwabach.

WEBER TEST

The tuning fork is set into vibration by striking the tines on the examiner's hand or knee. The rounded tip of the handle is placed on the center of the client's forehead or nasal bone (Fig. 18–1). Placement on the teeth (even if the client has false teeth) is a reliable option. Normally the sound is heard equally in both ears by bone conduction. If the client has a sensorineural hearing loss in one ear, the sound is heard in the other ear. If the client has a conductive hearing loss in one ear, the sound is heard in that ear.

RINNE TEST

The vibrating tuning fork is shifted between two positions: against the mastoid bone (bone conduction) and 2 inches from the opening of the ear canal (air conduction) (see Fig. 18–1). As the position is changed, the client is asked to indicate which tone is louder (in front of the ear or behind the ear) or when one of the tones is no longer heard. The Rinne test is useful for differentiating between conductive and sensorineural hearing losses.

Normally sound is heard twice as long or loud by air conduction than it is by bone conduction. Therefore, a normal response is one in which air conduction is greater than bone conduction, or a positive Rinne test finding. With a conductive hearing loss, a client hears bone conduction louder or longer than air conduction, or a negative Rinne test finding. With a sensorineural hearing loss, the client hears better by air conduction, or a positive Rinne test finding.

SCHWABACH TEST

This test is also used to detect a hearing loss. The Schwabach test compares the hearing of the examiner (who must have normal hearing) with the client's. When the client no longer hears the tuning fork, the examiner listens. Results of the test are determined by who can hear the tuning fork longer, the client or the examiner.

Vestibular Acuity

ROMBERG TEST

To assess the inner ear for balance, the nurse performs a Romberg test. The client stands with feet together, arms out in front, and eyes open. The nurse notes the ability to maintain an upright posture. The same test is then performed with the client's eyes closed. Normally, only a minimal amount of swaying exists. If the client loses balance, this may indicate a vestibular ear problem

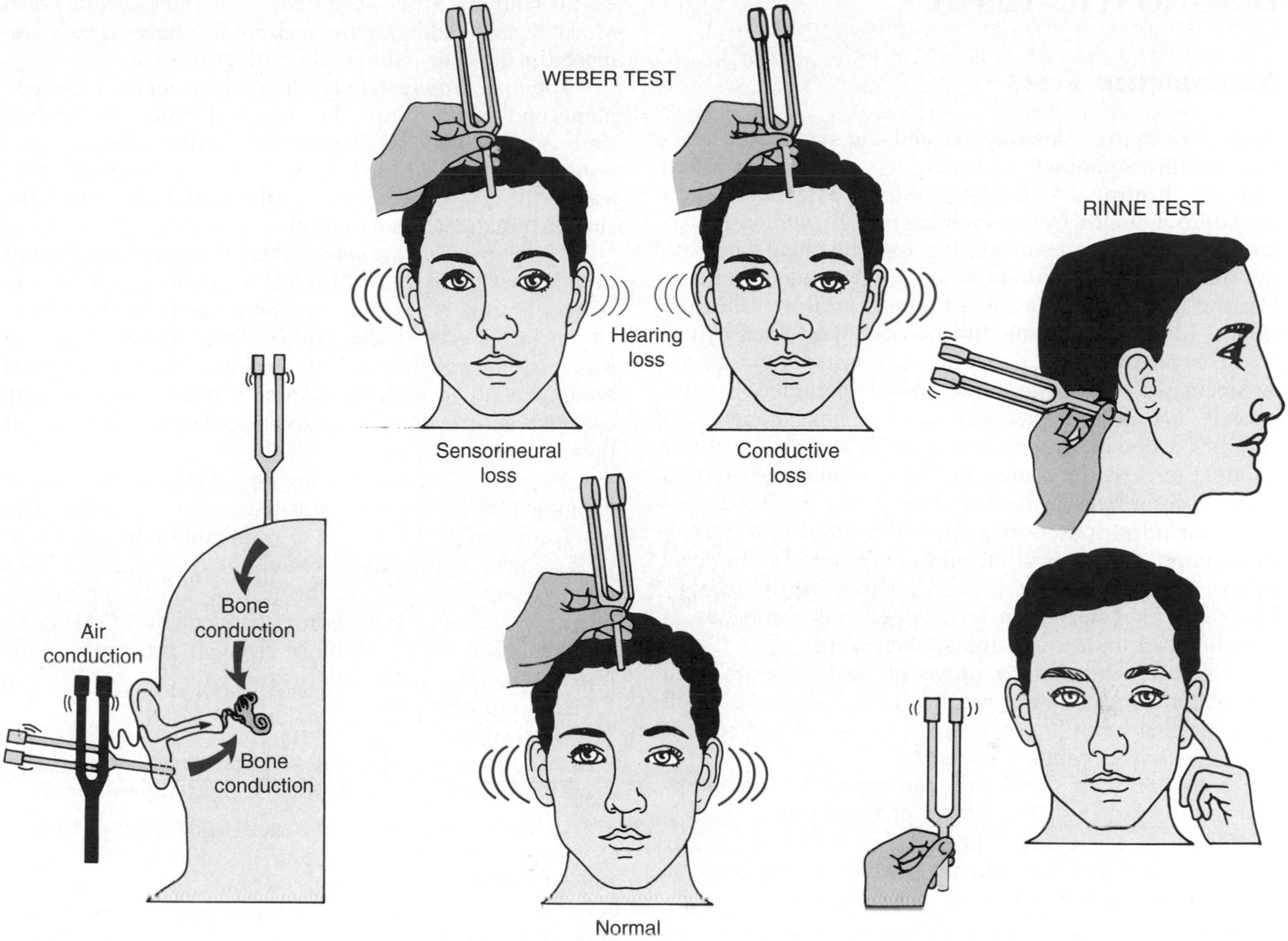

Figure 18–1
The Weber and Rinne tests for hearing loss. The Weber test is used to detect lateralization of hearing damage; the Rinne test distinguishes between conductive hearing loss and sensorineural hearing loss. The two tests should be performed consecutively. The Weber test uses a vibrating tuning fork placed on the client's head or nose to produce a centrally located stimulus. The client should hear the sound equally in both ears. The tone is louder in an ear with unilateral conductive loss and quieter in an ear with unilateral sensorineural loss. The Rinne test then characterizes the unilateral hearing loss as conductive or sensorineural. The Rinne test is performed by holding a vibrating tuning fork about 2 inches from the external ear. When the client cannot hear the sound, the tuning fork is placed on the mastoid bone. When the tone is louder through air than through bone, the client has a positive Rinne finding, which indicates normal hearing or sensorineural hearing loss. A negative Rinne finding (louder bone conduction than air conduction) indicates a conductive loss.

or cerebellar ataxia. A dysfunction is called a positive Romberg test finding.

A tandem Romberg should also be assessed. The nurse instructs the client to walk forward and backward, heel to toe. A peripheral vestibular lesion may cause marked swaying or falling. A client without pathologic change is usually able to maintain balance, depending on age.

TEST FOR NYSTAGMUS

Nystagmus is the involuntary, rhythmic oscillation of the eyes, associated with vestibular dysfunction. Nystagmus occurs normally when a client watches a rapidly moving object or looks beyond 30 degrees laterally (end-point nystagmus). To check a client for gaze nystagmus, the nurse's finger is placed directly in front of the client at eye level. The client is asked to follow the finger without moving the head. The nurse's finger is moved slowly from the midline toward the right ear and left ear, but not more than 30 degrees. The eyes are observed for any jerking movements. For example, if the eyes jerk quickly to the left, and drift slowly back to the right, the client has left spontaneous (horizontal) nystagmus. Nystagmus can be horizontal, vertical, or rotary.

DIAGNOSTIC TESTS

Audiometric Tests

Audiology may be broadly termed the science of hearing. Specific audiometric hearing tests are performed to measure hearing. A hearing test is performed in a soundproof booth by an audiologist. An audiometer is an electronic instrument used to test the client's hearing by producing sounds of varying tones and loudness. Hearing is assessed by a special unit of measure called the decibel (dB), a logarithmic function of sound intensity.

The components of hearing are tested through assessment of air conduction, bone conduction, and speech. A difference between air and bone conduction signifies a conductive hearing loss. When air and bone conduction are the same, either normal hearing or a nerve (sensorineural) hearing loss exists. Speech evaluation includes speech reception threshold and speech discrimination. Speech reception threshold is the level of speech hearing and serves as a check on the reliability of the air conduction test. Speech discrimination is the ability to understand the spoken word.

Normal hearing is a range of hearing established nationally by testing the hearing levels of people of all ages. A client with "normal hearing" has 80 per cent or more hearing, depending on age.

Some of these tests are performed by computer-assisted instruments. The object of these special tests is to differentiate whether a problem or lesion within the hearing system is located in the cochlea, in the acoustic nerve, or in the brain stem.

Vestibular Tests

The vestibular system also can be tested by electrophysiologic means. Although the physical assessment of balance is important, the most common objective measurement of balance is accomplished by electronystagmography (ENG). The ENG instrument was developed to measure nystagmus (involuntary, rapid eye movement) in response to stimulation of the vestibular system.

Platform posturography, which is performed while the client is standing, is one of the newest computerized balance tests. This test can help isolate the etiologic basis as vestibular, visual, or proprioceptive. This platform test helps to identify, quantify, and localize the source of balance disorders.

Rotary chair or harmonic acceleration can also be used. Rotation of the client in a chair in darkness provides information about vestibular dysfunction and level of central compensation.

Other Otologic Tests

IMAGING TESTS

The temporal bone and its structures are easily examined by x-ray study. The oldest but not necessarily most useful study is x-ray examination of the mastoid bone. More recent radiographic techniques have largely replaced plane film radiography.

Polytomography. Polytomography focuses on one plane and "opened up" the temporal bone for the first time, so that very small structures within the temporal bone could be identified. In addition, the surgeon could assess the problems before surgery and anticipate the surgical treatment more closely.

Computed Tomography. The computer in a computed tomographic (CT) scan mathematically reconstructs a cross section of the temporal bone from measurement of the radiographic film transmission. In order to show better soft-tissue detail in the temporal bone, a contrast agent is generally used. CT scan with contrast is the most commonly ordered CT scan for the ear.

Magnetic Resonance Imaging. Magnetic resonance imaging (MRI) enhances soft-tissue details rather than bony structures. Therefore, the membranous organs as well as nerves and blood vessels of the temporal bone can be examined. MRI is the test of choice for tumors of the temporal bone. For enhancement of MRI, an intravenous contrast agent is given at the time of the test. For certain diagnostic assessments, both MRI and CT scan are obtained.

Arteriography. Arteriography and venography are contrast blood vessel studies. These tests are specially used for vascular abnormalities in the temporal bone.

Laboratory Tests

BLOOD TESTS

Blood tests that are diagnostic for systemic abnormalities are only secondarily significant for ear disease. For example, an elevated white blood cell count points to an infection but is not diagnostic of ear disease. However, in the presence of ear infection, and in the absence of other infection, blood tests are necessary for assessing acute ear infection. Other blood tests are useful for diagnosis of autoimmune diseases and other systemic illnesses that can affect hearing and balance.

EAR DRAINAGE CULTURES

Drainage from the ear canal or a surgical incision is usually cultured to identify the organism. This is especially necessary in acute infections in order to choose the appropriate antibiotic. When a long-term drainage is present, such as in chronic otitis media, cultures are less helpful because gram-negative bacillus growth covers up the original pathogen. In these cases, many physicians do not culture the drainage but begin broad-spectrum antibiotics.

TESTING FOR PRESENCE OF CEREBROSPINAL FLUID

When clear drainage is found in the ear, a dilemma is presented. Is this fluid cerebrospinal fluid or serous drainage? A fistula from the inner ear to the middle ear can drain cerebrospinal fluid. This pathway can also lead to meningitis by retrograde contamination. Therefore, an analysis of clear fluid drainage from the ear or nose is often helpful in diagnosing the problem.

Disorders of the External Ear

OVERVIEW

Infections

The most common problems found in the external ear are infections, primarily bacterial or fungal. The most frequent infection, called external otitis, involves the external ear canal. The most common form of external otitis is also called swimmer's ear, because it is prevalent when water remains in the ear canal. In addition, opportunistic fungal infections are common. When a debilitating systemic disease such as diabetes is present, the external otitis can spread wildly through cartilage and bone and is then called malignant external otitis.

Another form of infection is seen as an ear canal furuncle or abscess.

Masses

Benign masses of the external ear canal are usually cysts arising from a sebaceous gland and more rarely from the cerumen glands. Cysts can also be congenital in nature. Infectious polyps found in the ear canal arise from either the tympanic membrane or, more commonly, the middle ear through a hole in the tympanic membrane. Malignant tumors are also found in the external ear. The cutaneous carcinomas are most often basal cell carcinoma on the pinna and squamous cell carcinoma in the ear canal.

Trauma

Trauma, either sharp or blunt, is becoming a more common finding. A residual finding of repeated blunt trauma is a hypertrophic scar formation known as cauliflower ears, an occupational hazard for boxers. Acute trauma should be treated quickly to decrease the incidence of perichondritis. With prompt treatment, traumatic injuries seldom leave residual deformity.

Obstructions

On inspection of the external canal, the most frequent problem is impacted cerumen. Although the ear canal is self-cleaning, cerumen may become impacted from a disorder or improper cleaning. Removal of cerumen must be done carefully and may be necessary for examination of the tympanic membrane.

Surprisingly, a wide array of foreign bodies fit into the ear canal. The most common foreign body found in the adult ear is either a piece of cotton or, most annoying, an insect. The least traumatic method of removing a foreign body is with the aid of an operating microscope. For removal of a live insect, the ear canal is filled with mineral oil, not water, to kill the insect. Water will cause the insect to swell, and it will become more difficult to remove.

Pain in the external ear is the most common symptom of infection. Pain is more intense when the ear canal is swollen. A clue to early external otitis is tenderness when the pinna is gently pulled. A forerunner of pain in external otitis is itching in the ear canal. Inflammation (redness) is easily identified with an otoscope. At different stages of infection, drainage will be found from the ear canal. In early infectious disorders, the drainage may be clear and not discolored by pus.

A common complaint of clients with occlusion of the ear canal is loss of hearing. Both infection and cerumen can cause a sudden hearing loss.

MANAGEMENT

Medical Management

The most common external ear problems are infections, which are treated with both local and systemic antibiotics. However, the first rule of treating infection is meticulous cleaning of the site in order for the local antibiotic to reach the infected area. Thus, external otitis must be treated by microscopic cleaning before antibiotic drops or ointments are applied. If the infection is generalized or severe, systemic antibiotics are used. If debris accumulates in the ear canal, irrigations (with an ear syringe) can be used. Because external otitis is one of the most painful disorders of the ear, appropriate analgesics are required.

The surgical treatment of infections involves incision and drainage in the acute phase for abscesses and, at times, for perichondritis. The most common surgical treatment is excision of cysts and cutaneous carcinomas. For conditions that occlude the ear canal, more extensive surgery involving skin grafting, known as a canalplasty, is performed.

Nursing Management

The most frequent conditions of the external ear that are seen by the nurse are inflammation and infection. Pain is the most common subjective symptom, followed by decreased hearing, sense of fullness, throbbing sensation, and itching. The information to be collected includes the onset, duration, frequency, and intensity of symptoms, as previously described.

The nurse should observe the external ear for signs of redness, swelling, lumps, scaling, crusting, or drainage, either serous or purulent.

Clients with inflammations or infections of the external ear are usually diagnosed and treated on an ambulatory basis. These problems are not life-threatening or life-shortening and are easily treated with topical antibiotic solutions. During the infection, the client should avoid getting water in the ear while bathing or showering by using either earplugs or cotton coated with petroleum jelly.

Analgesics are often helpful. After the physician has prescribed the analgesic, the nurse clarifies for the client the amount, frequency, and duration of action. Ear pain usually results from the buildup of matter in the small ear canal, which leads to pressure and pain. Once the swelling and drainage are reduced by treatment, the pain subsides.

Instillation of Medications

Eardrops: Antibiotics and anti-inflammatory agents are usually administered locally rather than systemically in problems involving the external ear. The procedure and directions for administration of eardrops and ointment can be found in a fundamentals textbook.

Softening and Removal of Cerumen

Eardrops: Wax visible in the ear canal can be removed with a cotton-tipped applicator. One should not put more than the cotton portion in the ear. Impacted accumulations of earwax can be softened and loosened for removal by alternate instillation of glycerin and hydrogen peroxide eardrops. The eardrops are warmed to body temperature and used daily as directed for 1 to 2 weeks. The ear is then irrigated gently with warm water for removal of the softened wax or cleaned under magnification with a cerumen spoon. Wax that is on the tympanic membrane should be removed by a physician or a clinical nurse specialist in otology.

Ear Irrigation: The ear is commonly irrigated to cleanse the external auditory canal or to remove impacted wax, debris, or foreign bodies. Irrigations are not used in clients with a history of or who are suspected of having a perforated eardrum. The irrigating solution (usually water) is warmed to body temperature and placed in the irrigating syringe. The client's clothes are protected with a plastic drape, and a kidney-shaped basin is placed below the ear to catch the irrigating solution. The client sits with the ear to be irrigated toward the nurse, with the head tilted toward the opposite ear. The external ear is pulled upward and backward in adults, and the tip of the syringe is directed along the upper wall of the ear canal. The canal should not be completely obstructed by the syringe to allow the backflow of solution. When charting the ear irrigation, the nurse should include the nature of returned solution regarding amount, texture, color of cerumen, or type of debris. The nurse instructs the client to report pain, vertigo, or nausea during the procedure.

Disorders of the Tympanic Membrane, Middle Ear, and Mastoid

Tympanic Membrane

OVERVIEW

Infections

Infections of the external ear canal can involve the surface of the tympanic membrane, and the tympanic membrane will be a "window" for infection of the middle ear. Infection can cause hard deposits in the tympanic membrane known as tympanosclerosis (see later discussion). Holes or perforations of the tympanic membrane can be caused by infection and can be accompanied by drainage.

Tumors

Both benign and malignant tumors can involve the tympanic membrane but seldom arise from it. However, an infectious glandular polyp can be isolated to the tympanic membrane. Tumors in the middle ear can be seen through or protrude through the tympanic membrane.

Trauma

The tympanic membrane is the most common ear structure damaged by trauma. Increased pressure from a hand slap or falling in water can rupture the thin membrane. Sports injuries, cleaning the ear with a sharp instrument, or industrial accidents involving welding sparks can also cause a perforation. When the tympanic membrane is perforated, infection is likely.

Because the tympanic membrane is a semitransparent membrane, it can reflect what lies underneath it as well as discoloration and displacement of the membrane. Therefore, both fluid in the middle ear and infection can be seen. The tympanic membrane may be dull or red instead of the normal pearly gray.

The tympanic membrane can be altered by either positive or negative pressure. The membrane may be bulging as a result of positive pressure in the middle ear that results from infection. This pressure is strong enough in some cases to "burst" the eardrum and cause drainage. A ruptured eardrum is more common in children than in adults and usually heals spontaneously. Disorders involving the tympanic membrane are painful, perhaps the most painful of all middle ear disorders. A negative pressure in the ear causes a retraction of the tympanic membrane, outlining the ossicles. In these cases, fluid is usually found.

The major finding in tympanic membrane disorders is a perforation. A perforation may be either acute, as seen in trauma and acute infection, or chronic, as seen in repeated infection. A perforation causes hearing loss, depending on its size and location. The largest hearing loss found with a perforation is approximately 35 dB (one third of the hearing). If a perforation is present, damage to the ossicles should be suspected, which will cause a greater hearing loss.

MEDICAL AND SURGICAL MANAGEMENT

The medical management of tympanic membrane disorders involves both systemic and local antibiotics. Local antibiotics are used in the form of eardrops.

Surgery can be performed on the tympanic membrane with use of an operating microscope to magnify the area. The major surgical procedure performed is closure of a perforation. This procedure is called a myringoplasty if only the perforation is addressed, or a tympanoplasty if the middle ear is also involved. Tympanoplasty is a common surgical procedure with a high rate of success.

Other surgical treatments of the tympanic membrane include incision and drainage of vesicles, excision of polyps, and office patching of perforations. Myringotomy is discussed later.

Middle Ear

OVERVIEW

Infections

OTITIS MEDIA

The most prevalent disorder of the middle ear is infection known as otitis media. Otitis media is caused by various types of bacteria, depending on the age of the client and type of infection. When the infection is sudden in onset and short in duration, the diagnosis is acute otitis media. When the infection is repeated, usually causing drainage and perforation, the problem is called chronic otitis media. In between bouts of otitis media, fluid may form in the middle ear, known as serous otitis media. At times, serous otitis media is found in conjunction with upper respiratory infections or allergies. If the fluid remains over a period of years, it causes tympanic membrane retraction, or adhesive otitis media. Because of the extraordinary anatomy of the temporal bone, middle ear infection can also lead to brain abscesses that are life-threatening if not treated properly. Cholesteatoma is a complication from otitis media but is also a problem of the mastoid and is discussed later.

TYMPANOSCLEROSIS

Tympanosclerosis is a result of repeated infection and deserves special emphasis. Tympanosclerosis is a deposit of collagen and calcium within the middle ear that can harden around the ossicles, causing a conductive hearing loss.

Otosclerosis

Otosclerosis or "hardening of the ear," which involves the stapes, is an important middle ear disorder. This bony disease of the otic capsule causes excess bone to form, which impedes normal movement of the stapes. The progressive conductive hearing loss that results is one of the most common correctable middle ear disorders, second only to an infection of the ear. Tinnitus is an early symptom. This disease begins in the late teens and early 20s and affects twice as many women as men.

Tumors

The most common benign growth in the middle ear is an infectious polyp. Next in frequency is a cholesteatoma, which is not a true tumor but acts like one. Malignant tumors involving the middle ear can be primary or secondary in nature.

Trauma

Trauma to the tympanic membrane from a blast or blunt injury can involve the middle ear, causing a fracture or dislocation of the ossicles and tearing of the tympanic membrane. Also, the facial nerve is vulnerable to trauma. A basal skull fracture involves the temporal bone and, depending on the fracture site, causes ossicular damage as well as facial nerve paralysis and usually sensorineural hearing loss.

Eustachian Tube Disorders

The eustachian tube is part of the middle ear but has separate problems. Because the eustachian tube connects the middle ear to the nasopharynx, pharyngeal disorders will also cause eustachian tube dysfunction and, thus, secondary middle ear problems. The most common blockage in adults is swelling of the mucosa in the eustachian tube during an upper respiratory infection that can lead to serous otitis media. Acute blockage from barotrauma (altitude changes) caused by flying or underwater diving will also cause middle ear problems. The incidence of barotrauma is increased when an upper respiratory infection is present. Any long-term blockage of the eustachian tube leads to serous otitis media and a hearing loss.

Because the middle ear is the transformer for hearing (transmitting sound vibrations from the tympanic membrane to the inner ear), a hearing loss is the most frequent symptom of middle ear disorders. Pain is also quite common because of pressure from infection or fluid behind the tympanic membrane. If the tympanic membrane perforates, pus, blood, and other material may drain from the ear. In chronic middle ear and mastoid problems, a thick yellow discharge is common. With acute otitis media, all three findings (hearing loss, pain, and discharge) can be present.

MEDICAL AND SURGICAL MANAGEMENT

With any form of otitis media, appropriate antibiotic therapy may be necessary. If drainage is present, culture and sensitivity study should be performed. However, most episodes of acute otitis media do not produce drainage, and the most probable bacterial cause need not be identified. In chronic ear discharge, the normal contaminants of the ear abound and unfortunately do not respond to the common antibiotics. Thus, local treatment involving ear irrigations, antibiotic drops, and antibiotic powders is used.

Blood coming from the ear canal usually points to a minor problem such as a scratch and not a major disease. Persistent hemorrhage must be checked by an otologist.

Because the eustachian tube is an integral part of middle ear disorders, decongestants and antihistamines are used to decrease the swelling and open the eustachian tube. Pain medication may be needed.

An incision into the tympanic membrane through which fluid is removed by suction is called myringotomy. To keep the incision open and prevent a recurrence of fluid, various types of transtympanic tubes can be inserted into the incision. These tubes extrude in 3 to 12 months by themselves and rarely have to be removed.

Other middle ear lesions are often excised in combination with recognized middle ear procedures. For example, tympanosclerosis is routinely removed during tympanoplasty or ossiculoplasty. Reconstruction of the necrotic ossicles is not yet an exact science. Various synthetic prostheses have been used to reconnect the ossicles to carry sound. In an attempt to prevent extrusion of the prostheses, tissue is combined with the prostheses in order to rebuild the ossicles. This semibiologic method is used in different forms by the majority of otologic surgeons. The surgical procedure of ossicular reconstruction is called ossiculoplasty.

Stapedectomy, removal and replacement of the stapes, was once a common middle ear procedure. However, the pool of clients with otosclerosis is dwindling, and today stapedectomy is performed less and less.

Mastoid

OVERVIEW

Infections

Before the discovery of antibiotics, a mastoid infection was a life-threatening event. Now, acute mastoiditis is rare, although chronic mastoiditis still occurs. With repeated middle ear infections, the mastoid cavity becomes a significant part of the problem, which increases the amount of drainage. A chronic infection also leads to the development of cholesteatoma. Although a benign growth, the cholesteatoma causes erosion of the surrounding structures. A cholesteatoma is a skin-lined sac that sheds debris into the center, thus enlarging in size. Often infection is present in the mass of the cholesteatoma.

Tumors

The same tumors that arise in the middle ear can be found in the mastoid cavity. Because the mastoid cavity is connected to other air cells throughout the temporal bone and is close to the brain, malignant tumors in the mastoid carry a poor prognosis.

MANAGEMENT

Medical and Surgical Management

Antibiotics are the most common medical therapy in use today. Because infection starts in the middle ear, the problems in the mastoid cavity are avoided by early use of antibiotics. Various irrigations of the mastoid and middle ear are used in chronic infections along with antibiotic eardrops or powders.

Radical mastoidectomy removes the mastoid bone for control of infection and cholesteatoma. However, because the radical mastoidectomy sacrificed hearing, a modified radical mastoidectomy was developed that saved the remaining middle ear structures.

Nursing Management

Nursing assessment of the client with problems of the tympanic membrane, the middle ear, or the mastoid cavity is the same, regardless of the need for surgery. A thorough history should precede the ear examination.

Hearing loss is the most frequent symptom of blockage of the tympanic membrane or the ossicles. Pain may also be present because of pressure from infection or fluid behind the tympanic membrane. Data are collected about the onset, duration, and severity of these symptoms.

The tympanic membrane is the only structure that can be visualized directly; the middle ear and mastoid cavity must be evaluated by indirect means. The eardrum may be normal, perforated, infected, retracted, or bulging according to the disease process involved. Pain is not usually elicited on palpation of the external ear; this phenomenon usually provides a differential diagnosis between problems of the external ear and middle ear structures. Serous, purulent, or bloody drainage may be present.

Surgical intervention normally follows unsuccessful attempts to treat the client medically. Eardrops and ear ointment may be necessary for the client with problems of the tympanic membrane, middle ear, or mastoid cavity. In addition, oral antibiotics and analgesics may be needed. The client is instructed in the amount, frequency, and duration of medications. In addition to other treatment, the client may be asked to use a medicinal ear irrigation. A family member or significant other performs the irrigation for the client. Usually, the ear irrigation is followed by the use of eardrops. Hospitalization is rarely necessary for the client with ear disorders that do not require surgery. For those clients undergoing surgery, the hospital stay usually does not exceed 2 to 3 days.

The Perioperative Client

The client undergoing ear surgery should be told what to expect during surgery because frequently the client is given only local anesthesia. The client is awake but sedated during surgery. Instructions should be given about the length of the procedure, the estimated length of hospital stay, and immediate postoperative instructions. Very often, fear of the unknown can be decreased by understanding of events that will occur.

Immediate postoperative instructions may include the following:

- Specified positions, such as lying with operated ear up for several hours after surgery.
- If necessary, blow nose gently one side at a time.
- Sneeze or cough with mouth open.
- Normal occurrences in the initial period may include decreased hearing in operated ear from the packing (possibly, the sound of talking in a barrel); noises in the ear such as cracking or popping; minor earache and discomfort in cheek and jaw; and swelling of ear.

Pain is not usually a major problem. Vertigo or light-headedness may occur when the client ambulates for the first time; clients should be supervised when ambulating on the day of surgery to protect them from falling. Nausea may also be a problem.

The ear rarely bleeds after surgery. A small amount of serosanguineous drainage on a cotton ball is expected. Most ear surgeries require only a cotton ball in the ear postoperatively, although a dressing over the ear may be necessary after tympanomastoidectomy. Postoperative client teaching is listed in the Client Education Guide: Discharge Teaching After Ear Surgery.

CLIENT EDUCATION GUIDE

Discharge Teaching After Ear Surgery

The nurse should give the following instructions to the client:

- Continue to blow nose gently one side at a time and to sneeze or cough with mouth open for 1 week after surgery.
- Avoid physical activity for 1 week and exercises or sports for 3 weeks after surgery.
- Return to work as recommended, usually 3 to 7 days after surgery (3 weeks if work is strenuous).
- Avoid heavy lifting, especially after stapedectomy.
- Change cotton ball in ear daily as prescribed.
- Keep ear dry for 4 to 6 weeks after surgery.
- Do not shampoo for 1 week after surgery.
- Protect ear when necessary with two pieces of cotton (outer piece saturated with petroleum jelly).
- Avoid airplane flights for first week after surgery. For sensation of ear pressure, hold nose, close mouth, and swallow to equalize pressure.
- Wear noise defenders for loud noise environment.
- Report any drainage other than a slight amount of bleeding to the physician.

Disorders of the Inner Ear

HEARING IMPAIRMENT

Hearing impairment ranges from difficulty in understanding words or hearing certain sounds to total deafness. Up to 80 per cent of all hearing impairments are due to hearing nerve disorders, for which presently there is no cure.

Incidence

Hearing impairment is the nation's number one disability; 1 of every 15 Americans is affected. Of the 10 million people in the United States with a hearing loss who are 65 years of age or older, over 90 per cent have a sensorineural hearing loss. Because of fear, misinformation, lack of information, and vanity, many clients do not admit that they have a hearing problem.

Etiology

Factors that influence the type and amount of hearing loss include hereditary disease, toxic substances, trauma, age, and noise exposure. Infectious diseases (measles, mumps, and meningitis), arteriosclerosis, ototoxic drugs, neuromas of the eighth cranial nerve, otospongiosis, trauma to the head or ear, or degeneration of the organ of Corti are also etiologies of hearing loss and occur most commonly from age (presbycusis).

Conductive hearing loss may be caused by anything that blocks the external ear, such as wax, infection, or a foreign body; a thickening, retraction, scarring, or perforation of the tympanic membrane; or any pathophysiologic changes in the middle ear affecting or fixing one or more of the ossicles.

Noise-induced hearing loss can be traumatic, for example, a sudden loud noise such as a blast injury. More commonly, this hearing loss occurs over time from repeated injury from loud noise. The major cause is industrial noise, use of firearms, and listening to loud music.

Infection can also lead to hearing loss. An infection of the inner ear called labyrinthitis can be either viral or bacterial in origin. Viral labyrinthitis is usually isolated to the inner ear, whereas the rarer bacterial labyrinthitis is from infection in the middle ear and mastoid.

Both benign and malignant tumors of the temporal bone can involve the inner ear and lead to hearing loss. Malignant tumors invade the entire inner ear, spreading from the middle ear and mastoid.

Pathophysiology

SENSORINEURAL HEARING LOSS

Sensorineural hearing loss is the most common inner ear disorder. It results from disease or trauma to the sensorineural structures or nerve pathways of the inner ear leading to the brain stem. The hearing loss may at times fluctuate, but usually a progressive hearing loss results. Sensorineural hearing losses are usually permanent and not correctable by medical or surgical treatment.

CONDUCTIVE HEARING LOSS

Any interference with the conduction of sound impulses through the external auditory canal, the eardrum, or the middle ear results in a conductive hearing loss. The inner ear is usually not involved in a conductive loss, and sound amplification can reach the inner ear. Most conductive hearing losses are correctable by medical or surgical treatment.

NOISE-INDUCED HEARING LOSS

Noise-induced hearing loss is characterized by a greater loss in the higher frequencies. The only treatment for noise-induced hearing loss is to prevent further injury by avoiding noise or by wearing ear protection.

SUDDEN OR FLUCTUATING HEARING LOSS

Sudden or fluctuating hearing loss is recognized as a separate hearing disorder because of the isolated finding and dramatic outcome. Because it is thought to be vascular in nature, attempted treatments are made to alter the vascular system in some way. Occasionally, the hearing may return to normal without the reason being understood. Unfortunately, most clients do not regain normal hearing. If a fistula is suspected, it is surgically closed by a tissue graft.

CENTRAL DEAFNESS

Central deafness is also known as central auditory dysfunction. With this phenomenon, the central nervous system cannot interpret normal auditory signals. Therefore, the hearing test findings are normal, although the client is "deaf."

OTHER TYPES OF HEARING LOSS

Different types of hearing loss are listed in Box 18–2. A client has a mixed hearing loss when both a conductive and sensorineural hearing loss are present simultaneously. A functional loss is a hearing loss for which no

BOX 18–2

The Types of Hearing Loss

Air conduction hearing loss: loss of hearing through the external and middle ears.

Bone conduction hearing loss: loss of hearing through the inner ear.

Central hearing loss: loss of hearing from damage to the brain's auditory pathways or auditory center.

Conductive hearing loss: loss of hearing in which air conduction is worse than bone conduction and involves the external and middle ear.

Fluctuating hearing loss: a sensorineural hearing loss that varies with time.

Functional hearing loss: loss of hearing for which no organic lesion can be found.

Mixed hearing loss: sensorineural and conductive hearing loss occurring together.

Neural hearing loss: a sensorineural hearing loss originating in the eighth nerve or brain stem.

Sensorineural hearing loss: loss of hearing involving the cochlea and hearing nerve; bone and air conduction equal but diminished.

Sensory hearing loss: a sensorineural hearing loss in the cochlea and involving the hair cells and nerve endings.

Sudden hearing loss: a sensorineural hearing loss with a sudden onset.

Conductive hearing loss results from interference with conduction in the external and middle ear; sensorineural hearing loss, in the inner ear; and mixed hearing loss, in all three areas.

organic lesion can be found and special testing suggests normal hearing. A hearing loss may also be congenital or acquired. The majority of clients with ear problems have some degree of hearing loss.

Prevention

A major nursing responsibility is the identification of hearing impairment in clients in both hospital and community settings. Detection and referral of an ear problem are the first steps in limiting the client's disability. For maintaining normal ear function, adequate protection of the ears is important and involves several activities:

- Early, adequate treatment of disease
- Prevention of trauma to the ear
- Early detection of hearing loss
- Monitoring for side effects of ototoxic drugs
- Monitoring for noise pollution
- Periodic ear examination

EARLY, ADEQUATE TREATMENT OF DISEASE

The nurse must teach clients to see a physician for any condition that causes prolonged symptoms of the ear, such as pain, swelling, drainage, "plugged" feeling, or decreased hearing.

During upper respiratory infections (colds), the nose should be blown with at least one nostril open. Excessive pressure can force infected secretions up the eustachian tube into the middle ear.

PREVENTION OF TRAUMA TO THE EAR

Clients should be taught to avoid inserting any objects into the ear canal, obstructing the ear canal with objects, inserting unclean articles or solutions into the ear, or swimming in water identified as being polluted. These activities can lead to damage of the tympanic membrane or to ear infections.

EARLY DETECTION OF HEARING LOSS

The hearing nerve does not usually regain function; thus, early detection of hearing loss is important so the cause of the loss can be diagnosed and, it is hoped, the problem treated. However, the signs of a small loss of hearing are elusive.

A hearing loss in both ears may first be detected by a family member rather than by the client. The earliest sign is not hearing what was once heard. Another common sign is asking for a repetition of what was said. Usually the request is in the form of a question, such as "What did you say?" Sometimes the hard-of-hearing client may repeat the information, even incorrectly, to provoke a response and thus a repetition of the information.

A hearing loss in one ear is also difficult to detect. The client can notice the loss when using a telephone or by having difficulty with the direction of sounds.

MONITORING SIDE EFFECTS OF OTOTOXIC DRUGS

Some medicines can affect the cochlea, the vestibular labyrinth, or the eighth cranial nerve (see Box 18–1). Clients taking ototoxic drugs need to know the signs and symptoms of side effects of these medicines so that the development of loss of hearing or balance can be prevented. If these symptoms (discussed previously) occur, the next dose of the drug should be omitted and the physician consulted. Audiometric and vestibular testing may be necessary.

MONITORING NOISE POLLUTION

Industrial and occupational noise is a primary cause of hearing loss in our society. The most common type of occupational hearing loss is caused by continuous loud noises. In the United States, the Occupational Safety and Health Administration has established acceptable levels of noise in work environments. The nurse must participate in teaching the proper use of protective ear devices or earplugs. Courses are available to educate nurses about industrial hearing conservation requirements.

A client firing guns who notices tinnitus (ringing in the ear), a sensation of fullness in the ear, or a temporary hearing loss should stop firing the guns or wear suitable ear protection. Sound in front of rock band speakers can be very high, and hearing losses have been measured in some members of rock bands.

CRITICAL TO REMEMBER

If proximity to the high noise level cannot be avoided, earplugs should be worn during exposure.

Earplugs are inserted into the external auditory canal and are capable of reducing the noise by 10 to 30 dB. Usually standardized plugs are effective, but custom-made plugs molded to the client's ear canal can also be purchased and are better tolerated. For noise levels reaching 120 dB and above, clients must wear both earmuffs and earplugs.

PERIODIC EAR EXAMINATIONS

Periodic ear examinations for evaluation of hearing are important in the adult because aging frequently causes degenerative changes in the ear as well as in other body tissues.

Clinical Manifestations

A sensorineural hearing loss is found with almost any inner ear disorder. The hearing loss is usually incomplete but can be progressive in some illnesses. A characteristic of a severe hearing loss is the loss of discrimination (understanding of words). To some clients, a hearing loss feels like a blockage in the ear.

Tinnitus accompanies most sensorineural hearing losses and is very annoying. Clients with a hearing loss can also experience distorted or abnormal sounds that can cause discomfort.

Medical Management

AURAL REHABILITATION

If hearing loss is irreversible or not amenable to surgical intervention or if the client elects not to have surgery, aural rehabilitation may improve communication. The purpose of aural rehabilitation is to maximize the hearing-impaired client's communication skills by teaching the client more effective use of the senses of vision, touch, and vibration plus maximizing the use of any remaining hearing ability. Rehabilitation is affected by all demographic variables and the severity of impairment. As with other forms of rehabilitation, success depends partly on the degree of motivation.

Hearing Aids. Because most hearing losses are permanent, the use of a hearing aid should always be considered. A client should undergo a trial period before purchasing the aid. Bilateral (binaural) aids are desirable.

The evolution in hearing aid development has led to smaller and more effective aids. Today, small hearing aids are available that fit into the ear canal. The latest advancement in hearing aids is the ability to produce digital hearing aids, some with remote control.

Hearing aids are instruments made of miniature parts working together as a system to amplify sound in a controlled manner. They are used by both hearing-impaired clients (slight or moderate hearing loss) and deaf clients (severe or profound hearing loss). Hearing aids make sound louder but may not improve the ability to hear. Therefore, clients with decreased discrimination (the ability to understand what is spoken) benefit less from a hearing aid. The hearing aid amplifies all background noises, such as hospital machinery, footsteps, and department store noises, as well as speech. These noises may mask conversation or confuse the hearing-impaired client, especially the elderly.

There are several types of hearing aids, which vary according to the size to be worn and location. Hearing aids can be worn

- In the ear
- In the canal
- Behind the ear (postauricular)
- In the temple of eyeglasses (eyeglasses aid)
- In the middle of the chest (body-worn aid)

Regardless of the type of aid, the hearing aid consists of the following parts:

- Microphone to receive sound waves from the air and change sounds into electrical signals
- Amplifier to increase the strength of electrical signals
- Receiver (loudspeaker) to change the electrical signals back into sound waves
- Battery to provide the electrical energy needed to operate the hearing aid

On all types of hearing aids but the body-worn type, all four components are housed in one small case. The louder sounds are then directed into the ear through a custom-fitted earmold.

The hearing aid user should know how to care for the aid and what to do if the aid does not work. The nurse must also have a basic knowledge of the hearing aid to assist the client who is ill. The client is encouraged to use the hearing aid and to provide safe storage when it is not in use.

Implantable Hearing Devices. Three types of implantable hearing devices are either available for use or in the investigation stage. They are cochlear implants, bone hearing devices, and semi-implantable hearing devices.

Cochlear implants for those clients with no hearing at all are now available (Fig. 18–2). This device has a small computer that changes the spoken word to electrical impulses. The impulses are transmitted across the skin to an implanted coil that carries the impulse to the hearing nerve endings in the cochlea by an electrode introduced through the round window. The success of a cochlear implant varies widely and ranges from minimal improvement in auditory awareness to understanding of speech on the telephone.

In some cases of hearing loss, sound can be transmitted through the skull to the inner ear. For clients with a conductive hearing loss, a device is available in which the receiver is implanted under the skin into the skull. The external device transmits the sound through the skin. This device is worn above the ear and not in the ear canal. Because some conductive hearing losses cannot be repaired, this device may provide an alternative rehabilitative method to conventional hearing aid potential.

The implantable device with the greatest potential usage will be for those clients now using a hearing aid. It eliminates several bothersome problems of hearing aids, such as feedback and hearing-in noise. This method of hearing aid technology is still in the research stage.

Assistive Listening Devices. In addition to hearing aids, many practical devices are on the market that use hearing aid technology. These devices help the hard-of-hearing client hear the television or radio as well as use the telephone. For the client who cannot use a hearing aid, other assistive devices are available.

Hearing Education. Clients with a hearing loss need to have special education. Auditory training is an approach to enhance listening skills. The primary purpose of auditory training exercises is to help the client concentrate on the speaker. For some clients, only gross differences between sounds may be recognized.

Speech reading is the current term used for lip reading and is an important means of communication. Speech reading is the process of understanding vocal communication by the integration of lip movements with facial expressions, gestures, environmental clues, and conversation contexts. Speech reading is difficult without auditory cues. A high percentage of the words have to be guessed by the hearing-impaired client. Knowledge of this fact alone will help the nurse to be more understanding of the client using this approach.

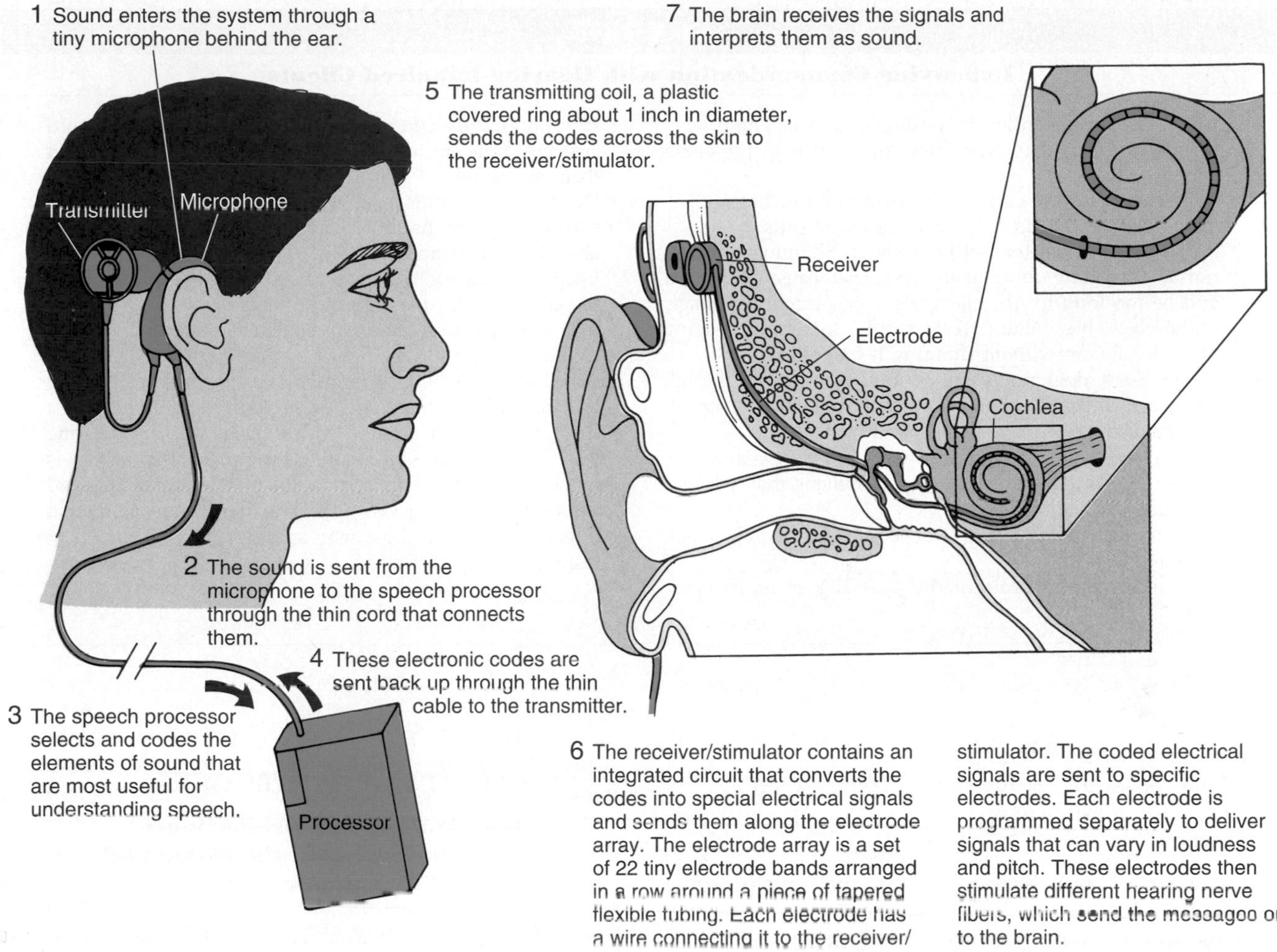
1 Sound enters the system through a tiny microphone behind the ear.
7 The brain receives the signals and interprets them as sound.
5 The transmitting coil, a plastic covered ring about 1 inch in diameter, sends the codes across the skin to the receiver/stimulator.
Transmitter
Microphone
Receiver
Electrode
Cochlea
2 The sound is sent from the microphone to the speech processor through the thin cord that connects them.
4 These electronic codes are sent back up through the thin cable to the transmitter.
3 The speech processor selects and codes the elements of sound that are most useful for understanding speech.
Processor
6 The receiver/stimulator contains an integrated circuit that converts the codes into special electrical signals and sends them along the electrode array. The electrode array is a set of 22 tiny electrode bands arranged in a row around a piece of tapered flexible tubing. Each electrode has a wire connecting it to the receiver/stimulator. The coded electrical signals are sent to specific electrodes. Each electrode is programmed separately to deliver signals that can vary in loudness and pitch. These electrodes then stimulate different hearing nerve fibers, which send the messages on to the brain.

Figure 18–2
Cochlear implant to restore hearing.

Because of reduced auditory feedback (the inability of hearing-impaired clients to monitor their own speech), the clearness, pitch quality, or rate of the client's speech may deteriorate. These changes may alter the efficiency of communication and reduce the intelligibility of speech. The goal of speech training is to conserve, develop, or prevent deterioration of speech skills.

Last, but still important today, is sign language. Sign language allows communication by hand signals. Various hand signals represent different letters of the alphabet, words, or phrases.

Other than antibiotics for infections, the medical treatment of hearing loss is dismal. General modalities include steroids and vasodilators, but specific treatment is still lacking. The purpose of medication is to attempt to lessen the progressive hearing loss or, it is hoped, to reverse a sudden loss.

Surgical Management

When a sensorineural hearing loss occurs, surgery is usually not warranted. However, because mixed hearing loss exists (both conductive and sensorineural hearing loss), surgery may be performed to alleviate the conductive hearing loss component. Also, some surgery is performed today to try to stop progressive hearing loss. However, surgery for sensorineural hearing loss does not yet have a successful history.

Nursing Management

Assessment

The history is often the most important part of the clinical assessment. All nurses should be able to inspect the outer ear and grossly assess the client's auditory acuity. The nurse can identify clients with impaired hearing and encourage them to seek professional diagnosis and treatment. Indications of a hearing loss may include the following:

- Failure to respond to oral communication
- Inappropriate response to oral communication
- Excessively loud speech
- Abnormal awareness of sounds
- Strained facial expressions

BOX 18–3

Improving Communication with Hearing-Impaired Clients

- Get the client's attention by raising an arm or hand.
- Stand with a light on your face; this will help the client speech read.
- Talk directly to the client while facing him or her.
- Speak clearly, but do not overaccentuate words.
- Speak in a normal tone; do not shout. Shouting overuses normal speaking movements and may cause distortion and be too loud for the client with sensorineural damage. If the client has conductive loss only, sometimes making the voice louder without shouting is helpful.
- If the client does not seem to understand what is said, express it differently. Some words are difficult to "see" in speech reading, such as "white" and "red."
- Move closer to the client and toward the better ear.
- Write out proper names or any statement that you are not sure was understood.
- Do not smile, chew gum, or cover the mouth when talking.
- Inattention may indicate tiredness or lack of understanding.
- Use phrases to convey meaning rather than one-word answers. State the major topic of the discussion first and then give details.
- Do not show annoyance by careless facial expression. Clients who are hard-of-hearing depend more on visual clues for understanding.
- Encourage the use of a hearing aid if it is available; allow the client to adjust it before speaking.
- In a group, repeat important statements and avoid asides to others in the group.
- Avoid the use of the intercommunication system, because this may distort sound and cause poor communication.
- Do not avoid conversation with a client who has hearing loss. It has been said that to live in a silent world is much more devastating than to live in darkness, and clients with hearing loss appear to have more emotional difficulties than do those who are blind.

- Tilted head when listening
- Constant need for clarification of conversation
- Faulty speech articulation
- Behavioral clues

The impact of not hearing others may make some clients withdraw from social situations and become anxious and insecure. Clients with hearing losses can experience fears of inadequacy, feelings of inferiority, depression, and varying degrees of stress and isolation. Important nursing assessments include the extent and duration of the hearing loss, how the client has coped with stress previously, and what support systems are available.

Nursing Diagnosis, Planning, and Implementation

Nursing Diagnosis: Social Isolation, Risk for R/T perceived inability to interact with others secondary to hearing loss.

Planning: Expected Outcomes. The client will exhibit a willingness to be involved in social situations, as evidenced by attempting to become a part of social events, conversing with others, indicating fewer feelings of inadequacy, and responding appropriately to questions asked (not fabricating answers to cover hearing loss).

Implementation. Common nursing interventions to facilitate communication for clients with hearing loss are listed in Box 18–3. They can apply to all clients, regardless of the type or severity of hearing loss. (See the Client Education Guide: The Hearing-Impaired Client: Communication in the Home and Social Environment.)

Evaluation

The degree of outcome attainment should be evaluated at predetermined intervals. A client with a new hearing

CLIENT EDUCATION GUIDE

The Hearing-Impaired Client: Communication in the Home and Social Environment

The client and significant others should be instructed about adaptations that can be made in the home and social environment so that the client will be able to respond appropriately and not feel isolated:

- Services for hearing tests and hearing aids are available in the home. The yellow pages can be checked for information. Services are offered by audiology clinics sponsored by universities, hospitals, community or state programs, the Veterans Administration, and national organizations.
- If hearing loss is severe, writing may be the only form of communication available to the client.
- During conversation, create a quiet, nondistracting environment (turn off the television and radio).
- A TDD (telephone device for the deaf) transmits typed words over the phone line. The community section of the phone book can be checked for this service. One TDD is needed to call another one.
- To enable the client to answer the door, the doorbell can be connected to an electrical device that will cause the light of a room lamp to flicker on and off. Such a device can be purchased in an electronics store.
- To enable the client to respond to an alarm, special devices are light-activated rather than sound-activated.
- To allow the client to enjoy television programming, a device to provide closed-caption services is available.
- The client and significant others can be referred to sign language classes provided by community agencies as a service.
- The client should be taught to avoid environments that are noisy or crowded, such as restaurants. When a hearing aid is used, it often amplifies all sounds; therefore, background noise is amplified also.

loss disorder will need frequent evaluation for determination of the degree of hearing regained as well as the coping strategies used. Because many forms of hearing loss are permanent or progressive, long-term evaluation should also be performed to be certain the client is adapting positively.

TINNITUS (HEAD NOISES)

Tinnitus literally means "ringing." Not all ear noises are ringing sounds, but they fall under the broad classification of tinnitus. Tinnitus is not a disease but a very distressing symptom and often a warning of hearing loss or other more serious problems. Ear noise may or may not be heard by an observer.

The major nursing responsibility should be to perform a thorough history and assessment about the onset, frequency, constancy, and level of intensity of the tinnitus. Unilateral tinnitus merits a complete neuro-otologic evaluation with the goal of ruling out the potential of a tumor, most likely an acoustic neuroma.

Many approaches have been tried to alleviate this distressing symptom, such as biofeedback, electrostimulation, hypnosis, medication, hearing aids, and tinnitus maskers. Tinnitus maskers are quite similar to hearing aids except that they generate noise. However, every approach for the relief from tinnitus is only moderately successful, at best. Nurses need to educate clients to avoid unproven treatments for tinnitus.

BALANCE DISORDERS

Disorders of balance and coordination result from problems of the vestibular system and righting reflexes. Very few symptoms are more private than those involving one's sense of balance. Balance problems may be debilitating and also cause embarrassing gait problems, which can jeopardize safety.

Incidence

More than 90 million Americans, 17 years of age or older, have experienced vertigo or a balance problem.

Etiology

In considering the etiology of "vertigo," there are two major categories: disequilibrium, or lightheadedness, and vertigo. Vertigo is further subdivided to determine whether the disease is central or peripheral. Central disorders involve the central nervous system, whereas peripheral disorders are lesions of the eighth cranial nerve or inner ear. Although the cause of vertigo can be either central or peripheral, at least 70 per cent of all cases are due to labyrinthine/inner ear disorders.

VIRAL INFECTIONS

The most common balance disorder is a viral neuronitis, a self-limiting disorder characterized by a sudden onset of vertigo without a hearing loss. The first episode is usually the worst one, with subsequent episodes manifesting less and less vertigo.

Another disorder is viral labyrinthitis, which affects both hearing and balance. These clients have extreme vertigo for longer periods plus varying degrees of hearing loss. Although most clients recover their balance, the hearing loss is usually permanent. In this same category of labyrinthitis are bacterial labyrinthitis and toxic labyrinthitis. Whereas bacterial labyrinthitis is self-explanatory, toxic labyrinthitis is caused by many different agents. The best understood cause is certain antibiotics. Other medicines can also cause this permanent disorder, which, unfortunately, is usually in both inner ears.

PRESBYASTASIS

A disorder that is recognized more and more today is presbyastasis, or balance disorder of aging. Because of the generalized degenerative changes that occur in aging, balance and stability are also affected. Whereas the labyrinth has been focused on primarily, balance also depends on several other systems, namely, the visual system and the proprioceptive changes in the muscles. Because all three systems are involved in aging, the elderly have difficulty with stability, which causes falls and subsequent trauma.

MENIERE'S DISEASE

One of the best known balance disorders is Meniere's disease. This disorder is characterized by a triad of symptoms: vertigo, hearing loss, and tinnitus. The cause is unknown but is thought to be from an abnormality of either the formation or absorption of endolymph. Recurring episodic incapacitating bouts of vertigo and hearing loss characterize this disorder. Because of the violent nature of Meniere's disease, the diagnosis is usually dreaded. Initially, the associated hearing loss fluctuates, but it worsens in time.

Pathophysiology

The ability to maintain balance depends on four systems being intact: the vestibular system (the labyrinth or inner ear); the visual system (the eyes); the proprioceptive system (the somatosensors of joints and muscles); and the cerebellar system (the coordinator). The sensations transmitted from the ears, the eyes, and the somatosensors are integrated in the brain stem and cerebellum and perceived in the cerebral cortex. Balance problems are most likely to occur when one or more systems are impaired or when the sensory information is contradictory.

Risk Factors

There is little that can be done to reduce the risk of balance disorders. Clients should be treated early for symptoms of ear problems. Clients at high risk of falling as a result of vertigo should rise slowly to prevent injury. Finally, situations that lead to vertigo should be avoided. Motion sickness occurs normally if the provocative stimulus is present. Special environmental situations such as deep-sea diving, high-speed flying, and space travel are situations for which humans have not been evolutionarily adapted.

Clinical Manifestations

Vertigo is the most common clinical manifestation in a client with a balance problem. The symptoms of balance disorders vary widely depending on the cause, the location (one or both ears), the client's age at onset, the extent of the loss, and the rapidity with which damage occurs. Clinical manifestations include, but are not limited to, spinning vertigo, sensation of falling, imbalance, staggering, giddiness, lightheadedness, disorientation, visual blurring, veering in one direction while walking, unsteadiness, reeling, faintness, wooziness, shakiness, instability, wobbly feeling, bewilderment, confusion, dazed feeling, clumsiness, floaty feeling, falling, weakness, or a vague feeling of uncertainty. In most instances, vertigo is present without a hearing loss.

Because the balance system can compensate, and certain disorders recur, vertigo is usually not present constantly but is episodic in nature. Vertigo, like pain, is subject to psychological influences. Vertigo is second only to chronic pain as the most common symptom found in America today.

Diagnostic Assessment

For the client with vertigo, the differential diagnosis may be accomplished by a thorough medical assessment, including audiometry, vestibular tests, imaging evaluation, and laboratory studies. The nurse may be involved in any or all of these procedures, according to the setting, and must be able to explain the procedure to the client to promote understanding and to gain trust. Clients may have a positive Romberg finding; a positive platform posturography examination is usually graded 1 to 6, with 6 being complete loss of balance. Nystagmus may also be evoked with electronystagmography.

Medical Management

The treatment of acute vertigo involves several medicines, which are called antivertiginous medicines. These medicines tend to suppress the balance system or the central nervous system. In chronic vertigo, vasodilators are used.

Vestibular rehabilitation is now a recognized form of control for vertigo. Because the balance system can compensate for a partial or complete absence, head and total body exercises are performed by the client to hasten compensation. Usually, physical therapists are involved in structuring this treatment. Vestibular rehabilitation uses all three organ systems that provide balance.

Control of Meniere's episodes is usually possible, although a cure is not yet available. Clients are treated with low-sodium diets, diuretics, and balance exercises.

Surgical Management

The delicate inner ear does not lend itself to surgical treatment, except for procedures that destroy the balance system on purpose. The intent of these procedures is to lessen the fluid pressure within the labyrinth and control the vertigo of Meniere's disease. A destructive procedure to remove the membranous labyrinth, either subtotally through the oval window or totally through the mastoid bone, is called labyrinthectomy. Of course, any remaining hearing is sacrificed. Also, vestibular nerve resection can be performed to alleviate vertigo. Vestibular nerve resection can be performed through the labyrinth (sacrificing hearing) or around the labyrinth (saving hearing). The retrolabyrinthine surgical choice is the most common form of surgical control for vertigo today. Alleviation of the client's vertigo is usually immediate. Because of the compensation by all of the other structures related to maintaining balance, a client can function with only one labyrinth.

The necessity of removing tumors of the inner ear and internal auditory canal has also led to various approaches through and around the temporal bone.

Nursing Management

Because vertigo is only a symptom, the diagnosis and treatment of the underlying disease are frustrating to both the client and health care providers. The nurse's role becomes even more important because psychological factors complicate the illness. The nurse's ability to understand and assess the client with vertigo aids in providing care that will contribute to the client's recovery. Most clients with vertigo are managed as outpatients.

Assessment

Nursing assessment of the client with a balance problem should include the following:

- A client interview to obtain a health history and specific information about the onset and characteristics of the balance problem and associated hearing problems.
- An interview with a family member or significant other to identify the effect of the client's balance problem on others.
- Physical examination with specific emphasis on eyes, ears, thyroid, heart, and lungs, including a specific neurologic examination.
- Review of laboratory tests.

The importance of the history and interview cannot be overemphasized. All clients bring some degree of anxiety regarding this illness to the examination. Balance problems can have devastating effects on the client's behavior. The disruption of the client's routine, the severity of the "attacks," and the fear of the unknown can make the client agitated, anxious, or depressed. The nurse must be aware of these feelings and demonstrate self-confidence, patience, courtesy, and gentleness.

A gross assessment of the client's balance can be made by watching the client's gait. Evidence of instability may be noted if the client touches the wall or walks with a wide-based gait.

The same inspection, palpation, and otoscopic examination should be performed for the client with a balance problem as was performed for the client with a hearing loss (see earlier). The client should be assessed for the loss of hearing and tinnitus, symptoms that can accompany a balance problem.

Nursing Diagnosis, Planning, and Implementation

Nursing Diagnosis: Injury, Risk for R/T tendency to fall and lose balance.

Planning: Expected Outcomes. The client will reduce the risk of injury, as evidenced by moving slowly, remaining immobile when dizzy, and using aids for ambulation if gait and balance are unstable.

Implementation. Responsibilities of the nurse caring for a client with vertigo include the promotion of comfort and safety. Clients who are experiencing vertigo are sometimes reluctant to move because movement aggravates the symptoms. Specific nursing care activities include the following:

- Encourage the client to move slowly.
- Encourage and facilitate eating by providing the client with desired foods and fluids (vertigo may cause nausea and vomiting).
- Assist the client with hygiene as needed while encouraging independence.
- Keep side rails up when the client is in bed.
- Assist the client as needed in ambulation.
- Encourage the client to verbalize specific problems created by the vertigo.

Client teaching should include:

- Nature of the disorder
- Diagnostic tests and planned medical or surgical therapy for the vertigo
- Ways to protect self from injury when dizzy, such as remaining immobile or using an aid for walking
- Information about prescribed medications
- Symptoms requiring medical attention

Approximately 5 per cent of all clients with vertigo undergo surgical intervention at present. However, an increasing number of clients will undergo surgical procedures in the future because of new surgical developments and advanced technology. The care of the client experiencing surgery of the inner ear was described earlier.

Evaluation

The degree of goal attainment should be assessed every day. If vertigo is increasing, the client may need to remain at bed rest to reduce the risk of falls.

STUDY QUESTIONS

1. A client, diagnosed with labyrinthitis, asks for an explanation. The best response by the nurse is:
   A. "The labyrinth, part of the inner ear, is infected."
   B. "You have an infection of the small bones of the ear."
   C. "A part of the eustachian tube, called the labyrinth, is infected."
   D. "Labyrinthitis is often associated with infections of the middle ear."

2. Which of the following are common observations associated with disorders of the ear?
   A. Pain, tinnitus, loss of balance
   B. Discomfort, itching of the ear, headache
   C. Tinnitus, headache, impaired visual acuity
   D. Impaired visual acuity, loss of balance, discomfort

3. To teach a client about the Romberg test, the nurse should:
   A. Explain that the test is used to assess the inner ear for balance.
   B. Explain that a prone position is needed for best conduction of sound.
   C. Demonstrate to the client how the tuning fork conducts sound waves.
   D. Show how to position earphones for best sound conduction during the test.

4. To assess the tympanic membrane, the nurse should use an otoscope to visualize:
   A. A normal pinkish-red color of the membrane.
   B. The oval window at the center of the membrane.
   C. The presence or absence of perforations of the membrane.
   D. The presence or absence of pressure within the eustachian tube.

5. Removal of an insect from the external ear canal is accomplished by using which of the following methods?
   A. Instilling alcohol
   B. Irrigating with sterile water
   C. Filling the ear canal with mineral oil
   D. Allowing the insect time to leave the ear canal on its own

6. Ototoxic drugs may cause hearing loss, tinnitus, or disturbances in equilibrium by:
   A. Damaging the eighth cranial nerve.
   B. Decreasing the fluid in the semicircular canals.
   C. Thickening the tympanic membrane of the ear.
   D. Weakening the function of the ossicles of the inner ear.

7. Discharge teaching for the client after ear surgery should include which one of the following?
   A. Avoid inserting cotton balls in the ear.
   B. Hearing may not return for 6 months or more.
   C. Keep ear dry for 4 to 6 weeks after the surgery.
   D. Sneeze or cough with mouth closed for 1 week after surgery.

CRITICAL THINKING EXERCISES

SCENARIO A

An elderly client has a history of ear infections. She is experiencing sensorineural hearing loss associated with presbycusis that affects many elderly people. She has come to the clinic for a follow-up appointment and tells the nurse that her right ear is painful and keeping her awake at night. She states that she has been using her eardrops as directed but has stopped taking her antibiotic because she felt better 2 days ago. She asks if medicine or surgery will help her hearing loss.

1. What observations should be made during the appointment interview with this client?
2. How should the nurse respond to questions of treatment for the hearing loss the client has experienced?
3. Can hearing loss also occur as a result of recurrent ear infections?
4. Since there have been recurrent infections with a variety of treatments, what are the possibilities for problems due to ototoxic drugs? What signs and symptoms should be made to evaluate the effect of ototoxic drugs?
5. What teaching should the nurse complete regarding the prescribed treatment for the present ear infection?

SCENARIO B

A 40-year-old client has worked as a telephone lineman for about 10 years. He enjoys working out-of-doors. Lately, he has been feeling dizzy while on the pole. Today he fell about 15 feet to the ground and struck his head on a stabilizing wire on the way down. He has come to the Trauma Center because his head hurts him over the left ear. He tells the nurse that sometimes when he is falling asleep, he feels like he is at the center of a spinning plate.

1. What focused assessment should be completed by the nurse?
2. The client states he is feeling fine and wishes to return to his work station. A diagnosis of head injury is ruled out. What teaching should the nurse complete before discharge?
3. How might the client react to a diagnosis of vertigo? What defense mechanisms would most likely be used? What implications might this have?

BIBLIOGRAPHY

1. Acute otitis media in adults. (1994). *Emergency Medicine, 26*(6), 44.
2. Adams, G. L., Boies, L. R., & Hilger, P. A. (1989). *Boies Fundamentals of otolaryngology: A textbook of ear, nose, and throat diseases* (6th ed.). Philadelphia: W. B. Saunders.
3. Ballenger, J. (1991). *Diseases of the nose, throat, ear, head, and neck.* Philadelphia: Lea & Febiger.
4. Bates, B. (1991). *A guide to physical examination* (4th ed.). Philadelphia: J. B. Lippincott.
5. Brackman, D. F. (1994). *Otologic surgery.* Philadelphia: W. B. Saunders.
6. Brinkman, K. (1991). Why can't your patient hear you? *RN, 54*(1), 46–48.
7. Britton, B. H. (Ed.) (1991). *Common problems in otology.* St. Louis: Mosby-Year Book.
8. Bulechek, G. M., & McCloskey, J. C. (1992). *Nursing interventions, treatments for nursing diagnosis* (2nd ed.). Philadelphia: W. B. Saunders.
9. Chen, H. (1994). Hearing in the elderly: Relation of hearing loss, loneliness, and self-esteem. *Journal of Gerontological Nursing, 20*(6), 22–28.
10. Cleveland, P., & Morris, J. (1990). Meniere's disease. *RN, 53*(8), 28–32.
11. Cohen, H. (1994). Vestibular rehabilitation improves daily life function. *American Journal of Occupational Therapy, 48*(10), 919–925.

12. Copstead, L. C. (1995). *Perspectives on pathophysiology*. Philadelphia: W. B. Saunders.

13. DeWeese, D. D., & Saunders, W. H. (1988). *Textbook of otolaryngology* (7th ed.). St. Louis: Mosby-Year Book.

14. Erber, N. P. (1994). Communicating with elders: Effects of amplification. *Journal of Gerontological Nursing, 20(10)*, 6–10.

15. Goldenberg, R. A., Brown, M., & Cunningham, S. (1992). Laser stapedotomy: A new method of correcting deafness. *AORN Journal, 55(3)*, 759, 761–762, 764.

16. Goldstein, J. C., et al. (1989). *Geriatric otolaryngology*. Philadelphia: B. C. Decker.

17. Hahn, A. B., et al. (1982). *Pharmacology in nursing* (15th ed.). St. Louis: C. V. Mosby.

18. Haybach, P. J. (1993). Tuning in to ototoxicity: The inside story. *Nursing 93, 23(6)*, 34–40.

19. Hughes, G. B. (1985). *Textbook of clinical otology*. New York: Thieme-Stratton.

20. Jahn, A. F., & Santos-Sacchi, J. (1988). *Physiology of the ear*. New York: Raven Press.

21. Lauder, W. (1993). Preventive measures to maintain control: Management and treatment of vertigo. *Professional Nurse, 8(8)*, 508–509.

22. Martin, R. L. (1994). How to care for the external ear. *Hearing Journal, 47(2)*, 43–44.

23. Matteson, M. A., Linton, A., & Byers, V. (1993). Vision and hearing screening in cognitively impaired older adults. *Geriatric Nursing: American Journal of Care for the Aging, 14(6)*, 294–297.

24. Reiner, A. (1988). *Manual of patient care standards*. Rockville, MD: Aspen Publishers.

25. *Report of the task force on the National Strategic Research Plan of the National Institute on Deafness and Other Communication Disorders* (1989). Bethesda, MD: Institute of Health.

26. Riley, M. A. K. (1987). *Nursing care of the client with ear, nose and throat disorders*. New York: Springer.

27. Schuring, L. T. (1995). Assessment of the ear. In Phipps, et al. (Eds.), *Medical-surgical nursing: Concepts and clinical practice* (5th ed., pp. 2113–2126). St. Louis: Mosby-Year Book.

28. Schuring, L. T. (1995). Management of persons with problems of the ear. In Phipps, et al. (Eds.), *Medical-surgical nursing: Concepts and clinical practice* (5th ed., pp. 2127–2154). St. Louis: Mosby-Year Book.

29. Sigler, B. A., & Schuring, L. T. (1994). *Ear, nose, and throat disorders*. St. Louis: C. V. Mosby.

30. Smelzer, C. D. (1993). Primary care screening and evaluation of hearing loss. *Nurse Practitioner: American Journal of Primary Health Care, 18(8)*, 50–55.

UNIT 6

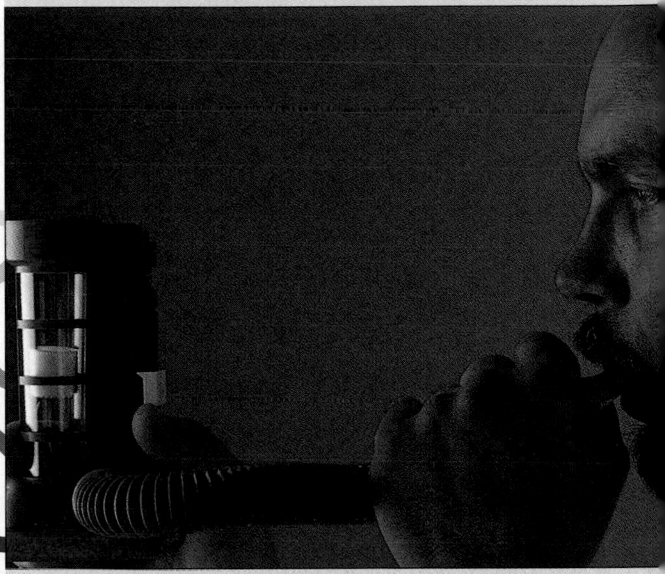

Respiratory Disorders

Breathing is a physiologic function that is almost synonymous with being alive. We experience difficulty in breathing as a threat to life itself. Persons with respiratory disorders are often very anxious, fearing that they may die. Whether death is a real possibility often has nothing to do with the fear.

Respiratory problems are widespread and may be acute or chronic. Acute disorders range from minor inconveniences such as colds or flu to more life-threatening problems such as asthma, some types of pneumonia, and chest trauma. Chronic respiratory problems, such as chronic obstructive pulmonary disease (now called chronic airflow limitation) and certain restrictive lung diseases, can cause significant disability.

The many causes of respiratory problems include allergies, occupational exposures, genetic factors, smoking, infection, neuromuscular disorders, chest abnormalities, trauma, pleural conditions, and pulmonary vascular abnormalities. The most significant factor in chronic respiratory illness and lung cancer is cigarette smoking.

Nurses are involved both in providing care for clients with respiratory conditions and in preventing such problems, through encouraging clients to take care of their lungs and especially to stop smoking. In acute care settings, nursing intervention focuses on relieving existing respiratory problems and preventing possible respiratory complications.

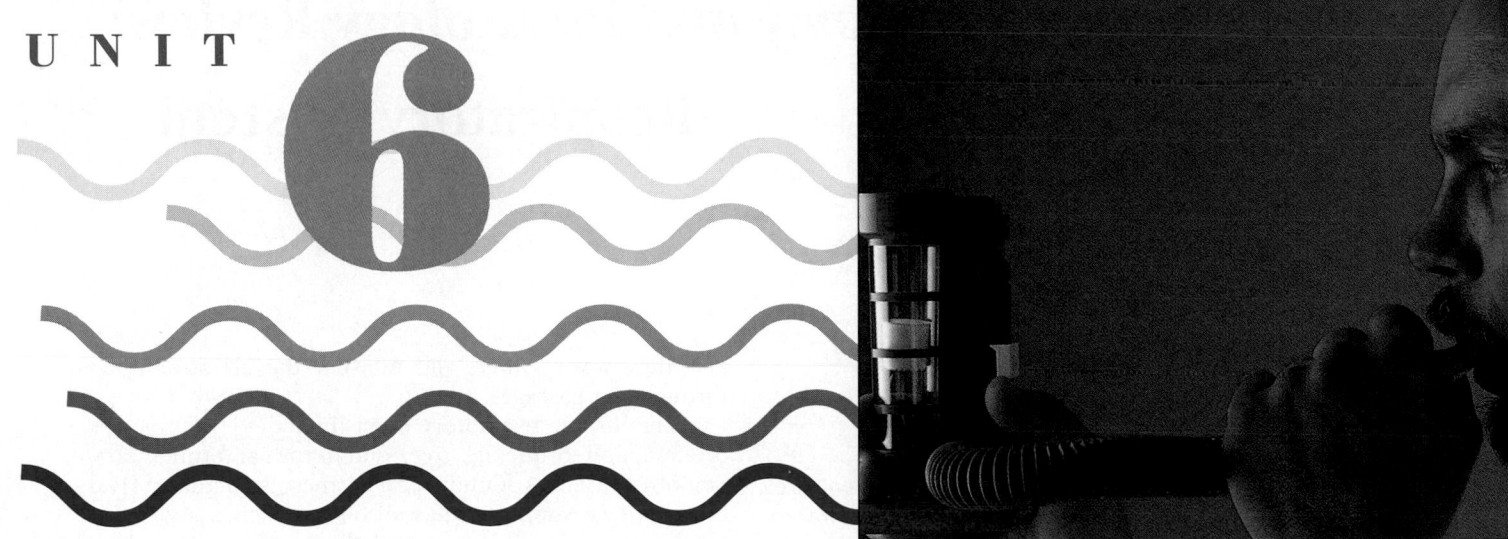

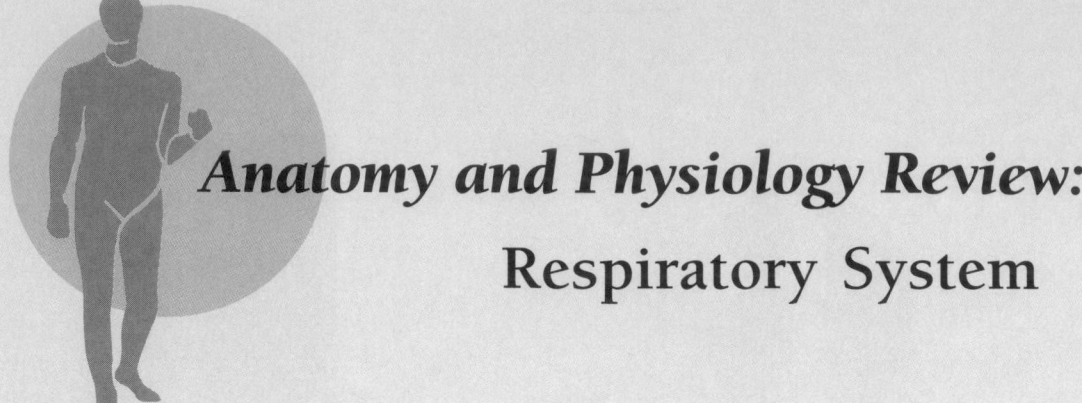

Anatomy and Physiology Review: Respiratory System

CONDUCTING PASSAGES OF THE RESPIRATORY SYSTEM

The conducting passages of the respiratory system are divided into the upper respiratory tract and the lower respiratory tract. The upper respiratory tract (airway) includes the nose with associated structures, pharynx, and larynx. The trachea, bronchial tree, and lungs are regions of the lower respiratory tract. Upper regions of the tract protect the lower airway from foreign matter and they warm, filter, and moisten the air as it flows through the passages.

The lower respiratory tract includes the trachea, bronchi and bronchial tree, and terminal bronchioles. Smooth muscle is found in all of these structures. Hyaline cartilage supports the wall of the trachea and bronchial tree so that it does not collapse. The point where the trachea divides into the right and left bronchi is reinforced with cartilage and is called the carina. The terminal bronchioles, the final portion of the lower airway, lead into the respiratory zone, which consists of

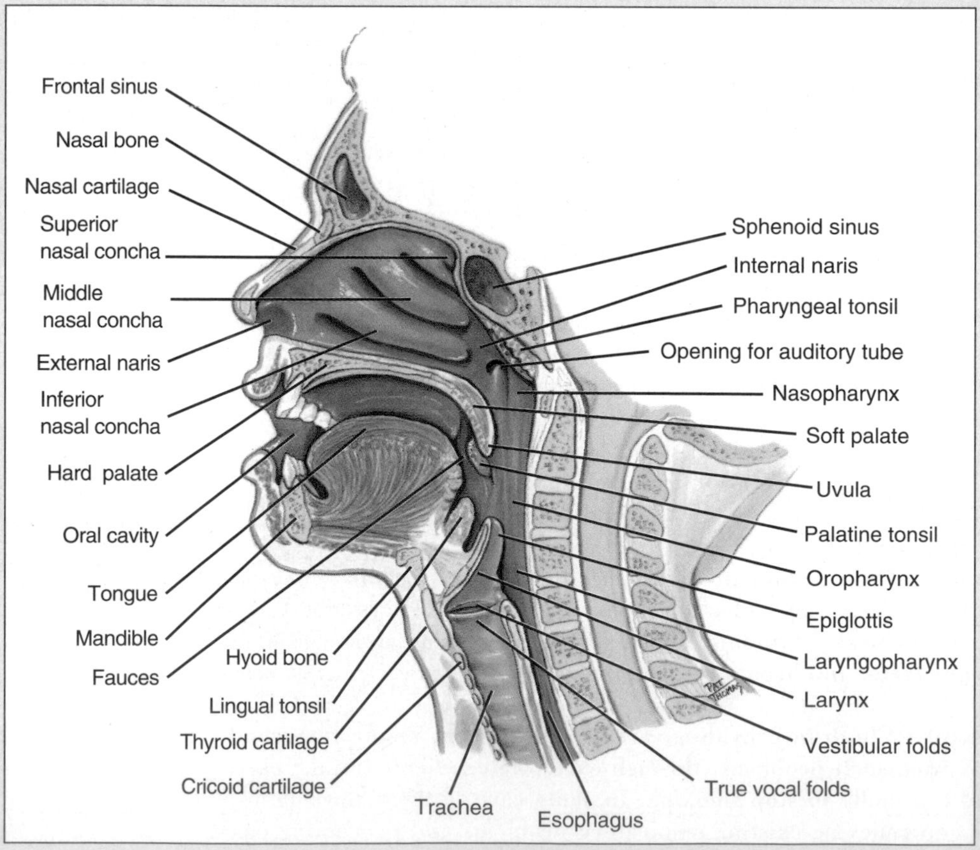

The upper respiratory tract.

Regions of the Upper Respiratory Tract

REGION	DESCRIPTION/COMMENTS
Nose	Formed from bone, cartilage, and connective tissue; internal cavity divided into two parts by the nasal septum
External nares	Openings of the nose on the face; also called nostrils
Vestibule	Cavity on either side of nasal septum; each nostril opens into a vestibule
Turbinates	Projections on the lateral wall of each vestibule; covered by a mucous membrane with a rich blood supply to warm and moisten the air
Internal nares	Openings from the vestibule into the pharynx
Paranasal sinuses	Cavities within the maxillae, frontal, ethmoid, and sphenoid bones; lined with mucous membrane; drain into the nose; lighten the weight of the skull and act as resonating chambers for sound
Mouth	Not actually part of the respiratory tract, but can deliver air to the lungs, especially when nose is obstructed; does not perform nasal functions efficiently
Pharynx	Funnel-shaped tube that extends from base of the skull to the larynx; divided into three regions
Nasopharynx	Located behind the nose and above the soft palate; posterior wall has masses of lymphoid tissue, called pharyngeal tonsils, that help protect against bacterial infection; adenoids are infected pharyngeal tonsils
Oropharynx	Located behind the mouth, between the soft palate and hyoid bone; receives air from nasopharynx and food from oral cavity; associated with palatine tonsils and lingual tonsils
Laryngopharynx	Most inferior portion of pharynx; also called hypopharynx; serves both respiration and digestion
Larynx	Commonly called the voice box; located between the pharynx and trachea, anterior to cervical vertebrae IV through VI
Endolarynx	Inner portion of larynx formed by two pairs of tissue folds; upper folds are the false vocal cords, lower folds are the true vocal cords; slit between vocal cords forms the glottis
Cartilages	Three pairs of small cartilages (cuneiform, corniculate, arytenoid) and three large cartilages (thyroid, cricoid, epiglottis) form the framework of the larynx; thyroid forms the Adam's apple; cricoid is the most inferior and is the anatomic site for a tracheostomy; epiglottis is leaf-shaped and closes over larynx during swallowing to prevent food from entering the lower airway

the respiratory bronchioles, the alveolar ducts, and the alveolar sacs.

The two lungs contain all the components of the respiratory zone and the bronchial tree beyond the primary bronchi. The lungs occupy most of the space in the thoracic cavity and are separated from each other by the mediastinum, which contains the heart. Elastic and collagen fibers contribute to the alveolar walls, which makes the lungs capable of stretching if a pulling force is exerted on them from outside or if they are inflated from within. The elastic recoil helps return the lungs to their resting volume. Each lung is enclosed by a double-layered serous membrane called the pleura. The visceral pleura is firmly attached to the surface of the lung. At the hilum, the visceral pleura is continuous with the parietal pleura that lines the wall of the

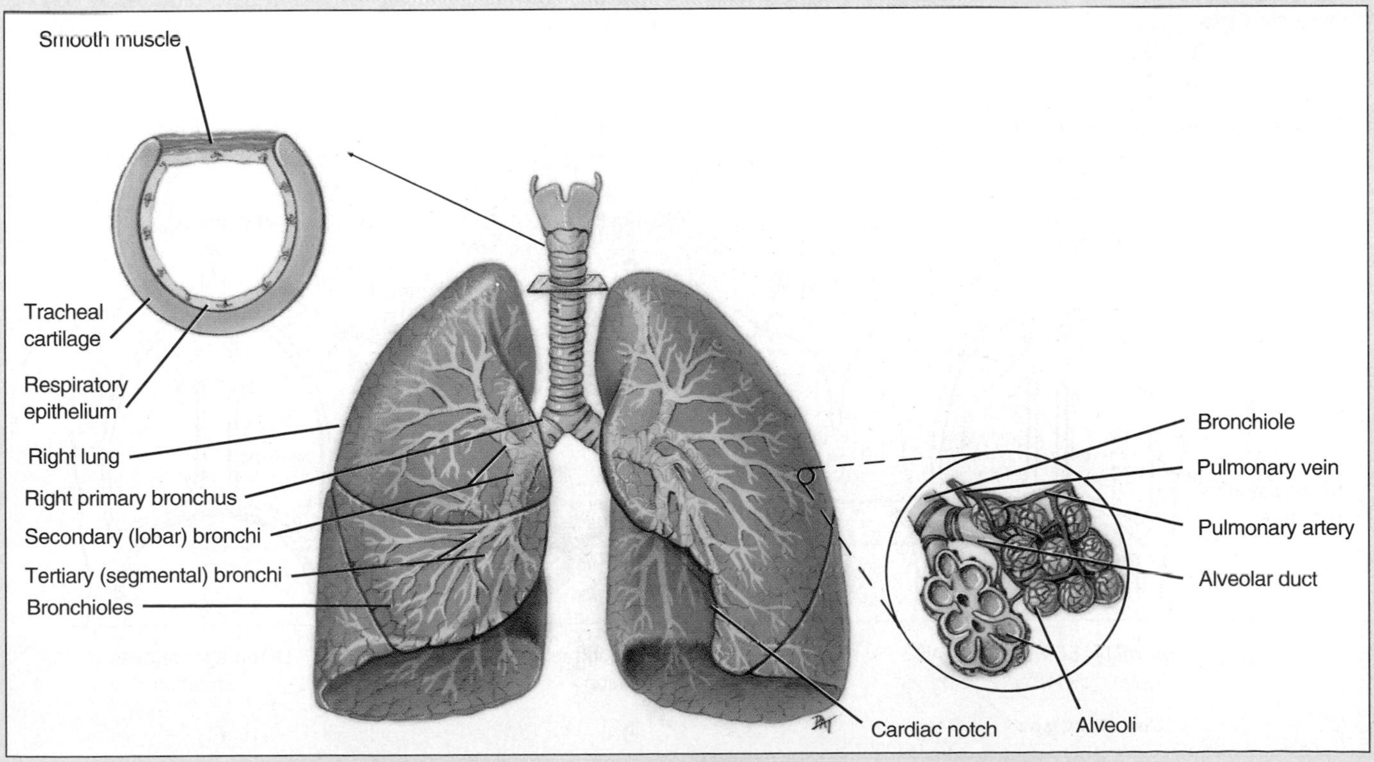

The lower respiratory tract.

thorax. Normally, there is no space between the pleurae, but there is a potential space called the pleural space. A thin film of serous fluid acts as a lubricant in this potential space. The fluid causes the pleural membranes to adhere, creating a pulling force that helps expand the lungs. If air or fluid accumulates in the space, the lungs are compressed and respiratory difficulties follow.

FUNCTIONS OF THE RESPIRATORY SYSTEM

The primary function of the respiratory system is the exchange of oxygen and carbon dioxide between the air and the tissues. For this to occur, there must be (1) ventilation, or air flow into and out of the lungs through the conducting passages; (2) respiration, which is the exchange of oxygen and carbon dioxide between the blood and alveoli in the lungs, and between the blood and tissues; and (3) transport, or movement of oxygen and carbon dioxide between the lungs and tissues via the blood.

Ventilation

Pulmonary ventilation is commonly referred to as breathing. It is the process of air flowing into the lungs during inspiration (inhalation) and out of the lungs during expiration (exhalation). Air, like other gases, flows from a region with higher pressure to a region with lower pressure. Muscular contraction and recoil of elastic tissues create the pressure gradients that result in ventilation. Pulmonary ventilation involves three different pressures:

- Atmospheric pressure: pressure of the air outside the body
- Intra-alveolar (intrapulmonary) pressure: pressure inside the alveoli of the lungs
- Intrapleural pressure: pressure within the pleural space, between the two layers of pleura

Inspiration is an active process that begins with the contraction of the respiratory muscles. The primary muscle is the diaphragm, but the external intercostal, scalene, and sternocleidomastoid muscles may also be involved. Contraction of these muscles increases the size of the thoracic cavity. Surface tension causes the two layers of pleura to adhere to each other so that when the thoracic cavity enlarges, the lungs expand or increase in volume. This decreases the intra-alveolar pressure to below the atmospheric pressure, and air flows into the lungs.

Expiration is a passive process involving the relaxation of respiratory muscles and the elastic recoil of the alveoli. This decreases the volume of the thoracic cavity and the lungs, which increases the intra-alveolar pressure to above the atmospheric pressure, and air flows out of the lungs.

Compliance is a measure of the force required to distend the lungs. Diseases that cause fibrosis of the lungs result in stiff lungs (low compliance) that require greater force (pressure) to expand or increase in volume so that air flows into the alveoli. Changes in the surface tension of the liquid film lining the alveoli also affect compliance. The surface tension restricts alveolar expansion. Surfactant, produced by certain alveolar cells, reduces the surface tension and increases compliance. This aids ventilation by reducing the force required to expand the lungs.

The respiratory center in the medulla oblongata establishes the basic rhythm and depth of breathing by sending impulses along the phrenic and intercostal nerves to the diaphragm and intercostal muscles to

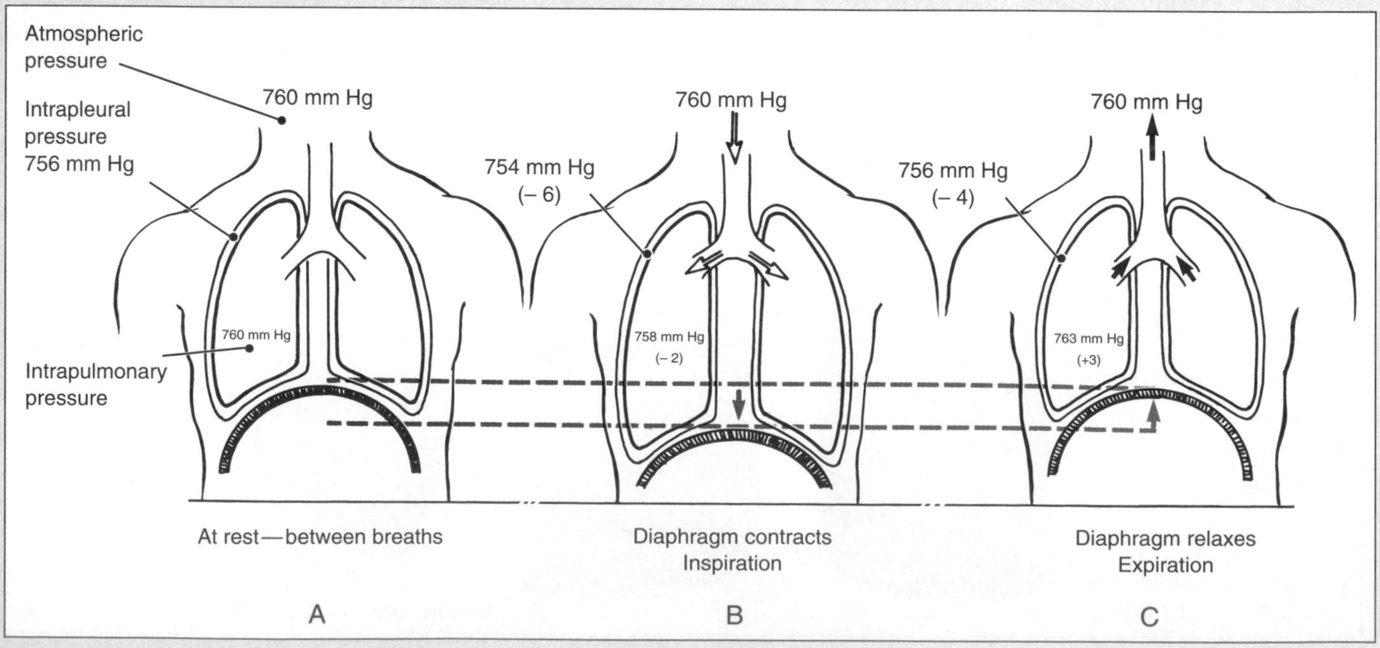

Pressures in pulmonary ventilation.

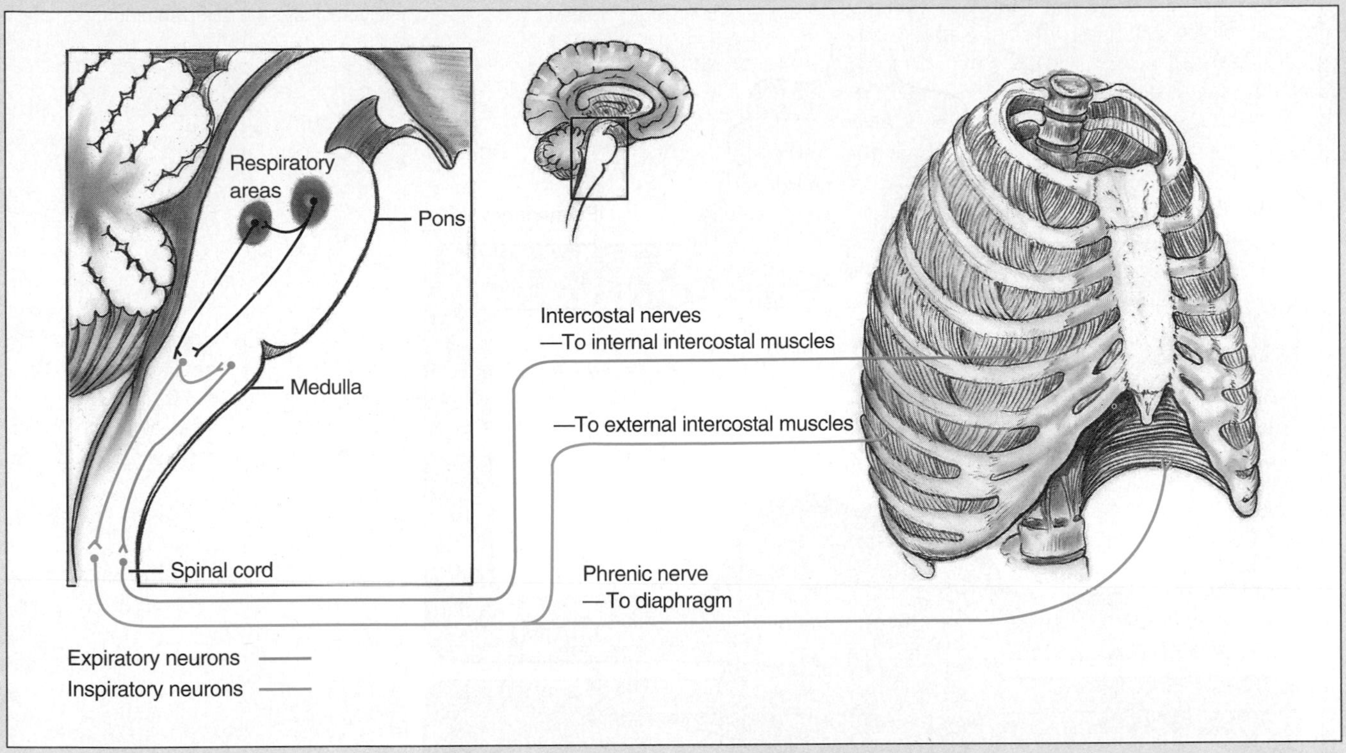

Respiratory centers in the brain stem.

stimulate muscle contraction. Pneumotaxic and apneustic respiratory centers in the pons modify ventilation in response to external and internal stimuli by sending impulses to the medulla. Central chemoreceptors in the medulla are sensitive to changes in carbon dioxide and hydrogen levels.

Gas Exchange

External respiration is the exchange of oxygen and carbon dioxide between the air in the lungs and the blood in the surrounding capillaries. Oxygen diffuses from the alveoli of the lungs, where the partial pressure of oxygen is high, into the blood, where the partial pressure of oxygen is low. Carbon dioxide diffuses from the blood into the air in the alveoli. The diffusion rate across the respiratory membrane in the lungs depends on

- The surface area of the membrane
- The thickness of the membrane
- The solubility of the gas
- The difference in partial pressure of the gas on the two sides of the membrane

Internal respiration is the exchange of gases between the tissue cells and the blood in the tissue capillaries. The concentration gradients that exist drive the diffusion of oxygen from the capillaries into the tissue cells and the carbon dioxide from the tissue cells into the capillaries.

The relationship between ventilation (air flow) and perfusion (blood flow) in the lungs determines the efficiency of gas exchange. Both low and high ventilation-to-perfusion ratios result in lower oxygen levels in the blood. Gravity also affects ventilation and perfusion. Blood flows to the more dependent lung segments, and air flows more easily to the upper lung segments.

Transport of Gases

The blood transports oxygen and carbon dioxide between the lungs and tissue cells. Erythrocytes have the major role in transporting both gases. The plasma has a lesser but still significant function.

After oxygen diffuses across the respiratory membrane into the capillary, it dissolves in the plasma. About 3 per cent of the oxygen remains in the plasma, dissolved, and is transported this way. The remaining 97 per cent quickly diffuses from the plasma into the erythrocytes, where it combines with hemoglobin to form oxyhemoglobin and is transported in this form. The bonds between oxygen and hemoglobin are relatively unstable and reversible. When the blood reaches the tissue capillaries, where the partial pressure of oxygen is low, the bonds break and oxygen is released to the tissues. Dissolved oxygen is also released when the partial pressure of oxygen is low.

Carbon dioxide, which is a by-product of cellular metabolism, diffuses from the tissue cells into the blood in the capillaries. The blood transports the carbon dioxide to the lungs by three mechanisms:

- Dissolved in plasma (about 7%)
- Combined with hemoglobin to form carbaminohemoglobin (about 23%)
- As part of bicarbonate ions in the plasma (about 70%)

In the lungs, where the partial pressure of carbon dioxide is relatively low and that of oxygen is high, the reactions reverse. The carbon dioxide diffuses into the alveoli and is exhaled.

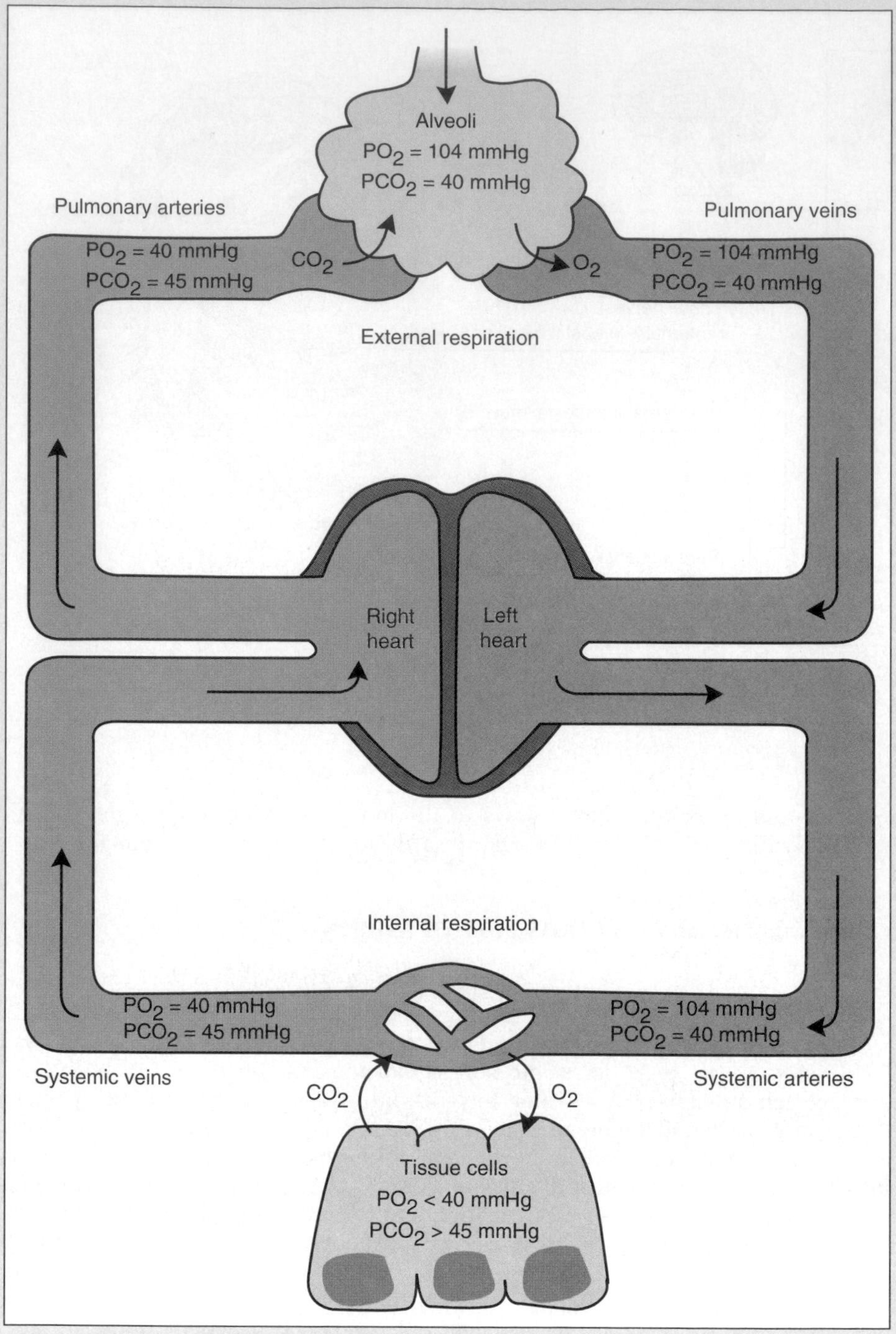

External and internal respiration.

AGE-RELATED CHANGES

Various harmful substances, including cigarette smoke, air pollution, and pathogens, continually bombard the respiratory system and take their toll. Some, like cigarette smoke, can be decreased, but others are inescapable. Because of the continual contact between the respiratory system and the environment, it is difficult to distinguish between the changes that are related solely to aging and those that are the result of external factors. Long-term exposure to irritants results in deterioration of the cilial lining of the respiratory tract and hinders the cleansing action of the cilia. Diminishing effectiveness of the immune system makes elderly people more susceptible to microbial diseases.

One type of structural change that is the result of aging is the loss of elasticity in the tissues of the respiratory tract. The cartilage in the walls of the trachea and bronchi undergoes progressive calcification. Smooth muscle fibers are replaced by fibrous tissue, making them less able to stretch and contract, and the alveoli lose some of their elastic recoil capabilities. Another type of structural change is a deterioration of the walls between adjacent alveoli. This increases the size of each individual alveolus but reduces the total surface area for diffusion of gases. These two types of structural changes affect ventilation-to-perfusion ratios and result in a decreased ability to acquire and deliver oxygen to the arterial blood.

Chapter 19 Assessment of Clients with Respiratory Disorders

Learning Outcomes

After completing this chapter, the learner will be able to:

1. Assess clients for clinical manifestations of disorders or trauma of the respiratory system.
2. Compare the assessment findings to the underlying anatomic structures and normal physiologic processes.
3. Utilize knowledge of diagnostic tests when interpreting the client's role in diagnostic tests.
4. Evaluate diagnostic outcomes in light of nursing assessment.
5. Perform a physical assessment appropriate to the respiratory system.

General Respiratory Assessment

Nurses who care for clients experiencing respiratory disorders perform and interpret a variety of assessment procedures. The data obtained during the respiratory assessment are used to plan client care.

HISTORY

A respiratory history gathers information about a client's present condition and previous respiratory problems. The nurse interviews the client or significant others and focuses on the clinical manifestations of the chief complaint, events leading up to the current condition, past medical history, family history, and psychosocial history.

The detail and time taken for a respiratory history depend on the client's condition (e.g., acute, chronic, or emergency). The nurse should state questions simply, using short, easy-to-understand sentences and ask questions in the context of the client's daily activities (e.g., "Are you able to carry the groceries in from the car?" or "Are you able to make your bed, vacuum, bathe, or dress yourself without stopping to rest and catch your breath?").

The history begins with obtaining biographic data from the client. Included are the client's name, age, sex, and living situation. The living situation, whether it is alone or with children or disabled significant others, will be important in planning for discharge.

Chief Complaint

The chief complaint is determined to establish priorities for intervention and to assess the client's level of understanding of the current condition.

- What are the client's current respiratory symptoms?
- When did each symptom start?
- What is the perceived cause of the symptom (after exercise, a respiratory infection)?
- When do the symptoms affect the client?
- What helps to relieve the symptoms?

In emergency or acute situations, these questions are all that may be asked until the client is stabilized and comfortable. Whenever possible, the nurse should seek further details from significant others.

Symptom Analysis

DYSPNEA

Dyspnea is one of the most common symptoms experienced by clients with pulmonary and cardiac disorders. Dyspnea is difficulty breathing. It is a subjective symptom and a reflection of the client's assessment of his or her degree of work of breathing for a given task and/or effort. According to Gift and Nield,[5] the most supported objective sign of dyspnea is accessory muscle use.

COUGH

The nurse asks the client when the cough started, how long the cough has been present, and whether it is painful. The nurse also asks whether the client is having any sputum production.

SPUTUM PRODUCTION

Sputum is the substance expelled by coughing or clearing the throat. The tracheobronchial tree normally produces about 3 ounces of mucus a day as part of the normal cleansing mechanism. However, sputum production with coughing is *not normal.* The nurse questions the client about the color (clear, yellow, green, rust, bloody), odor, quality (watery, stringy, frothy, thick), and quantity (teaspoon, tablespoon, or cup).

CRITICAL TO REMEMBER

Changes in color, odor, quality, or quantity are important to document in the client's medical record.

HEMOPTYSIS

Hemoptysis is blood expectorated from the mouth in the form of gross blood, frankly bloody sputum, or blood-tinged sputum. The nurse attempts to identify the source of the blood—lungs, nosebleed, stomach. Most hemoptysis is associated with frothy bright red blood. The nurse asks the client if the hemoptysis was produced as a result of forceful coughing. Also, an estimate of the amount of blood expectorated is obtained.

WHEEZING

Wheezing sounds are produced when air passes through partially obstructed or narrowed airways on expiration. Clients with advanced disorders may also have inspiratory wheezing. Wheezing may be audible or heard only via a stethoscope.

CRITICAL TO REMEMBER

The client may not complain of wheezing but may complain of chest tightness or chest discomfort instead.

The client is asked to identify when the wheezing occurs and if the wheezing relieves itself or if medication is required for relief.

STRIDOR

Stridor sounds are produced when air passes through partially obstructed or narrowed upper airways on inspiration. The nurse inquires about changes in voice character, hoarseness, difficulty swallowing, sleep-related disorders such as insomnia, degree of snoring (has sleep partner moved to another room?), hypersomnolence in the morning, early morning headaches, weight gain, fluid retention, apnea, and restlessness. Aspiration of a foreign body into the upper airway may lead to stridor.

CHEST PAIN

Chest pain may be associated with pulmonary and cardiac problems, and differentiation between the two is important. Coughing and pleuritic infections can cause chest pain. Retrosternal pain (behind the sternum) is usually burning, constant, and aching in nature. Pleuritic chest pain is commonly a sharp, stabbing pain that increases with movement or deep breathing. Pain can also originate in the bony and cartilaginous parts of the thorax. The location of the chest pain is important to obtain from the client.

CRITICAL TO REMEMBER

The nurse must differentiate pleuritic pain from cardiac pain or angina.

(See Chap. 23 for comparison of selected causes of chest pain.) The nurse should ask whether there are other symptoms, problems, or situations related to the chest pain (e.g., occurs only with deep breathing or with certain body movements).

Past Medical History

The past medical history examines the health history of the client and family members for data related to the upper and lower respiratory systems.

Nursing assessment of upper respiratory history includes questions about past problems with frequent colds, sinus infections, or nasal trauma. Episodes of epistaxis are explored for cause (such as hypertension), frequency, and treatment. Questions related to the lower respiratory system history focus on changes in their chronic respiratory symptoms (e.g., sputum production and characteristics, cough, and dyspnea).

Initial assessment of a hospitalized client should include the following areas.

CHILDHOOD AND INFECTIOUS DISEASES

Data about the usual childhood diseases and immunizations are obtained. Special attention should be focused on any past episodes of tuberculosis, bronchitis, influenza, asthma, pneumonia, and any upper respiratory infection followed by a lower respiratory infection.

RESPIRATORY IMMUNIZATIONS

The nurse should review with the client the dates for last administration pneumovax and flu shots. Pneumovax was once believed to provide life-ling immunity against pneumococcal pneumonia. Currently, revaccination is recommended at periodic intervals.

MAJOR ILLNESSES AND HOSPITALIZATIONS

The client is asked about previous hospitalizations or treatment of respiratory problems. Questions should include:

- Dates of the problem and any related hospitalizations
- Description of the specific problem
- Medical treatment (surgery, use of ventilator, and oxygen therapy and/or inhalation therapy)
- Diagnostic tests (chest x-ray, arterial blood gases, etc.)
- Current status of the problem

MEDICATIONS

Detailed information is obtained about both prescribed and over-the-counter medications. Questions should include not only the current medications, but any that relate to past respiratory problems.

ALLERGIES

Precipitating factors such as foods, medications, pollens, smoke, fumes, dust, and animal dander are explored. Many respiratory problems have an initial relationship with allergies. The client is asked to describe his or her allergic reaction to any of the usual allergens.

Family History

The nurse questions the client about the family history of respiratory diseases. Asthma, emphysema, chronic obstructive pulmonary disease, lung cancer, respiratory infections, tuberculosis, and allergies are identified for any blood relatives or other family members.

Psychosocial History and Life-Style

Respiratory status is affected by numerous factors that may lead to acute problems or will impact on chronic problems.

OCCUPATIONAL OR ENVIRONMENTAL EXPOSURE AND GEOGRAPHIC LOCATION

The nurse should ask specifically about home, hobbies and work environment, focusing on exposure to dust, asbestos, beryllium, silica, or other toxins or pollutants. Crowded living quarters increases exposure to upper respiratory infections and communicable disease such as tuberculosis. Farmers are exposed to airborne particles such as grain dust, fertilizers, and animal danders. Other workers are exposed to welding gases, toxic fumes, cotton fibers, and rock dust. The client should be questioned about travel to areas where certain respiratory diseases are prevalent, such as Asia (tuberculosis), the Ohio River valley (histoplasmosis), or the San Joaquin valley (coccidioidomycosis). Whether the client lives in a major metropolitan area with pollution must also be evaluated.

PERSONAL HABITS

The use of tobacco and nontobacco products needs to be evaluated. The client is asked about the use of cigarettes, cigars, pipes, smokeless tobacco (snuff, chewing tobacco), and marijuana or clove cigarettes.

CRITICAL TO REMEMBER

In addition to asking if the client smokes now, the nurse must be sure to ask if the client *ever* smoked. Calculation of pack years is made to estimate exposure using the following formula: years of smoking × packs per day = pack years.

Alcohol use slows ciliary action and decreases mucus clearance from the lungs. Ingestion of large amounts of alcohol depresses the gag reflex; and therefore, increases the risk of aspiration. The use and abuse of recreational drugs increase the risk of drug overdose and respiratory failure. Intravenous drug use and sharing of needles puts the client at risk for acquired immunodeficiency syndrome and *Pneumocystis carinii*. Exercise intolerance (dyspnea on exertion) is an important indicator of the status of chronic respiratory condition. The nurse needs to determine if exercise tolerance has remained stable or decreased. He or she can have the client describe the impact of dyspnea on activities of daily living.

Weight loss can be a significant problem for clients with chronic respiratory problems. A combination of factors influence the client's nutritional status. Large meals are not tolerated because of the decreased lung capacity and greater workload of the lungs and cardiovascular system. Anorexia and nausea are common side effects of respiratory medications.

Fatigue can be caused by protein depletion and interferes with the client's ability to consume adequate nutrition. The client often has to choose between breathing and eating.

PHYSICAL EXAMINATION

Physical examination follows the health history. The techniques of inspection, palpation, percussion, and auscultation are used. Successful examination requires that the nurse be familiar with the anatomic landmarks of the posterior, lateral, and anterior thorax (Fig. 19–1). These landmarks are used by the nurse to locate and visualize the underlying structures, particularly the lobes of the lungs, the heart, and major vessels.

CRITICAL TO REMEMBER

It is essential to compare the findings on one side of the thorax with the other side. Palpation, percussion, and auscultation proceed in a back-and-forth or side-to-side manner so that the nurse is continually evaluating findings by using the opposite side of the client as the standard for comparison.

Inspection

The physical examination actually begins during the history taking as the nurse observes the client and his or her response to questions. Signs and symptoms of respiratory distress are noted at this time: tachypnea, gasping, grunting, central cyanosis, open mouth, flared nostrils, dyspnea, color of facial skin and lips, and use of accessory muscles. The nurse notes the inspiratory to expiratory ratio; the normal ratio is 1:2. The client's speech pattern is observed. How many words or sentences can be said before another breath is taken? Clients who are short of breath may be able to say only three or four words before taking another breath. During the physical examination, the client should be undressed to the waist while privacy and warmth are maintained. Inspection and palpation are often performed together but are discussed separately here.

HEAD AND NECK

The key to any assessment technique is to develop a systematic approach. Logically, it is easiest to start with the head and work down. Inspection begins with observation of the head and neck area for any gross abnormalities that would interfere with respiration. The examiner also notes the odor of the breath and whether any sputum is present.

CHEST WALL CONFIGURATION

Inspection continues as the nurse observes the chest wall configuration. Chest size and contour are observed while the anteroposterior (AP) diameter is noted. The AP-transverse diameter refers to the ratio of the side view compared with the front view. The transverse diameter is generally twice the size of the AP diameter. Increased AP diameter, or barrel chest, is a characteristic finding in clients with chronic obstructive pulmonary disease.

CHEST MOVEMENT

Chest movement is observed during respiration. Normal respiratory rate is 12 to 22 breaths per minute. Rate is observed for amplitude, or depth of expansion, and rhythm. Abdominal breathing is more apparent in men, whereas women are more often thoracic breathers. Use of accessory muscles, retractions, symmetry, and any paradoxical movements are noted.

FINGERS AND TOES

Examination of the fingers and toes may reveal clubbing, which may be present in clients with pulmonary

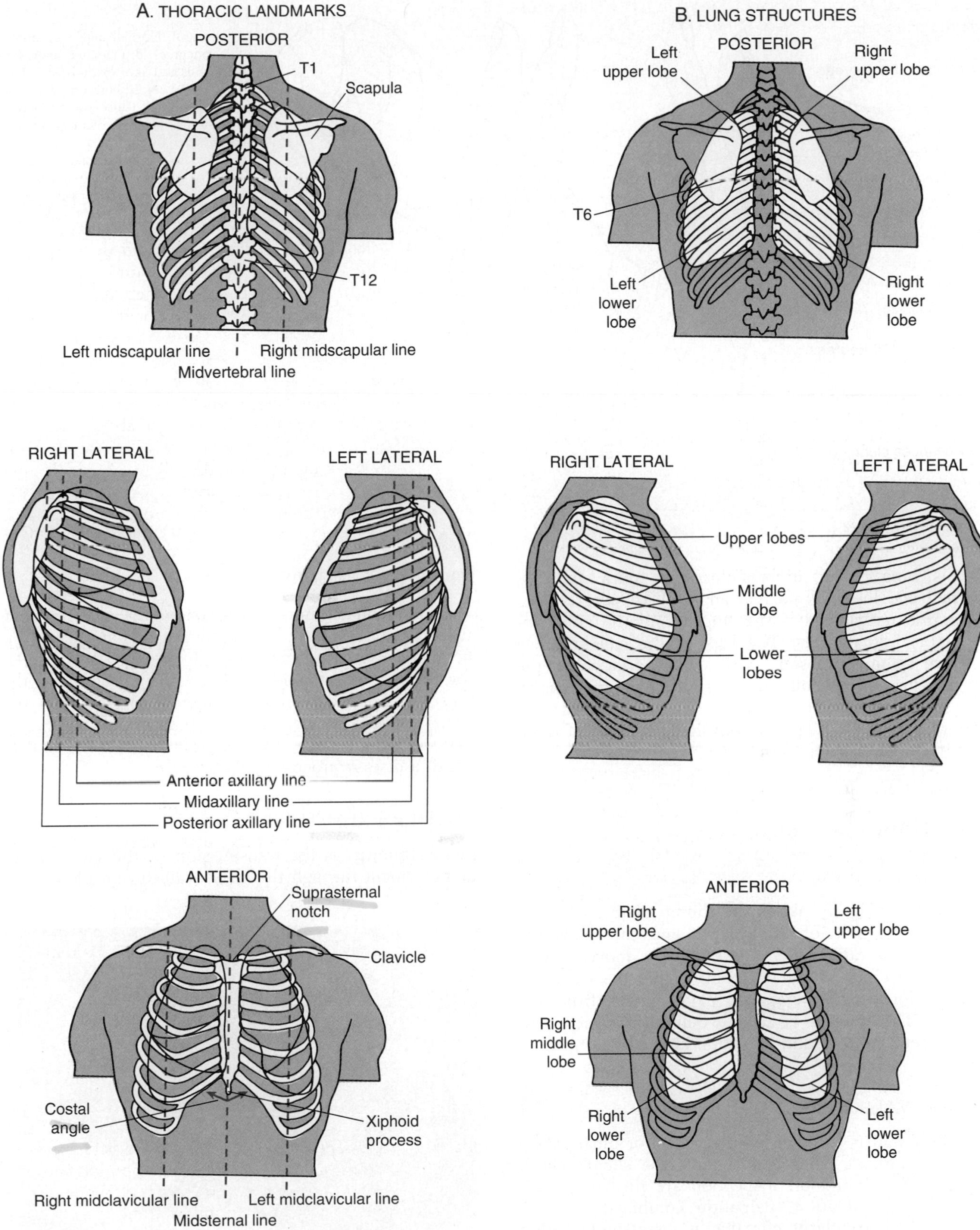

Figure 19–1
Respiratory examination. *A,* Thoracic landmarks; *B,* underlying lung structures. During chest examination, it is important to document the location of unusual or abnormal findings in a universally understood manner. Use the thoracic landmark and lung structure terminology shown.

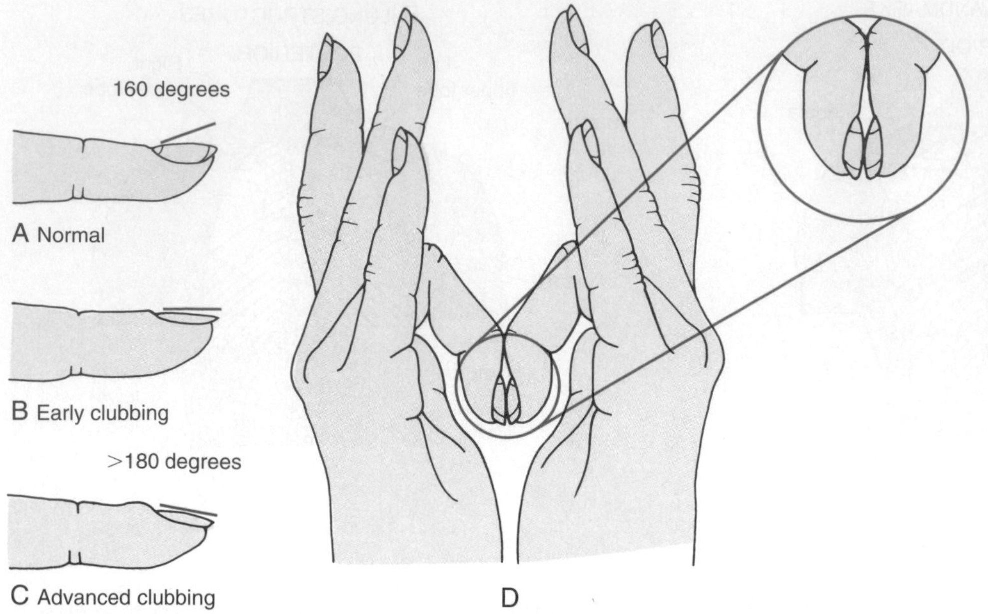

Figure 19–2
Clubbing. *A,* Normal digit with angle of 160 degrees. *B,* Flattened angle between nail and skin exceeds 180 degrees. *C,* Advanced clubbing with rounded nail. *D,* Clubbing is assessed with the use of the Schamroth technique, whereby the nurse instructs the client to place the nails of the fourth (ring) fingers together while extending the other fingers and to hold the hands up. A diamond-shaped space between the nails is a normal finding, that is, clubbing is absent.

fibrosis, lung cancer, or bronchiectasis. With clubbing, the nail bed loses its normal angle of 160 degrees between the nailplate and the finger, and the angle increases to 180 degrees. The base of the nail bed may also feel spongy and soft. With advanced clubbing, the finger takes on a bulbous or spoon-like appearance. Early clubbing may be assessed by use of the Schamroth technique (Fig. 19–2). The physiologic cause of clubbing has not yet been identified.

Palpation

TRACHEA

The examiner gently places the thumb of the palpating hand on one side of the trachea and the remaining fingers on the other side. The trachea is moved gently from side to side along its length while the examiner palpates for masses, crepitus, or deviation from the midline. The trachea is usually slightly movable and quickly returns to midline position after displacement.

CHEST WALL

The chest wall is palpated with the heel or ulnar aspect of the examiner's hand held against the client's chest. Abnormalities found on inspection are further investigated during palpation. Palpation combined with inspection is particularly effective in assessing whether the movements, or thoracic excursion of the chest during inspiration and expiration, are symmetric and equal in amplitude. During palpation, the nurse assesses for any crepitus, tenderness of the chest wall, muscle tone, swelling, and tactile fremitus.

THORACIC EXCURSION

For evaluation of thoracic excursion, the client is in a sitting position, and the examiner's hands are placed on the client's posterior chest wall (Figs. 19–3 and 19–4). The thumbs meet midline over the spine, and the fingers face upward and out like a butterfly. As the client inhales, the examiner's hands should move up and out symmetrically. Any asymmetry may be indicative of a disease process in that region.

TACTILE FREMITUS

Tactile fremitus is the transmission of the vibration of air movement through the chest wall during phonation.

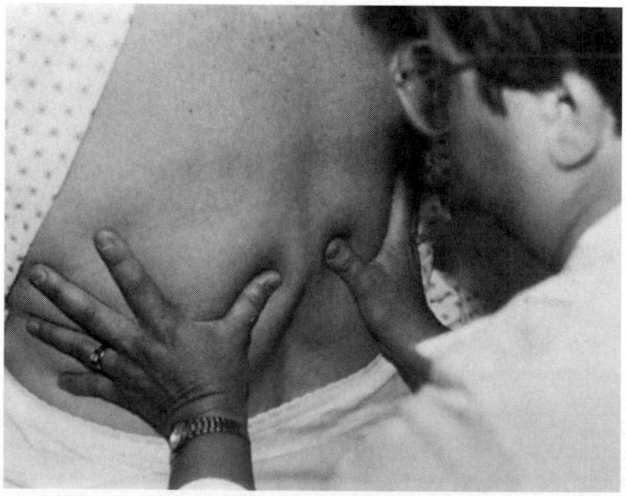

Figure 19–3
Thoracic excursion assesses the degree and symmetry of chest movement.

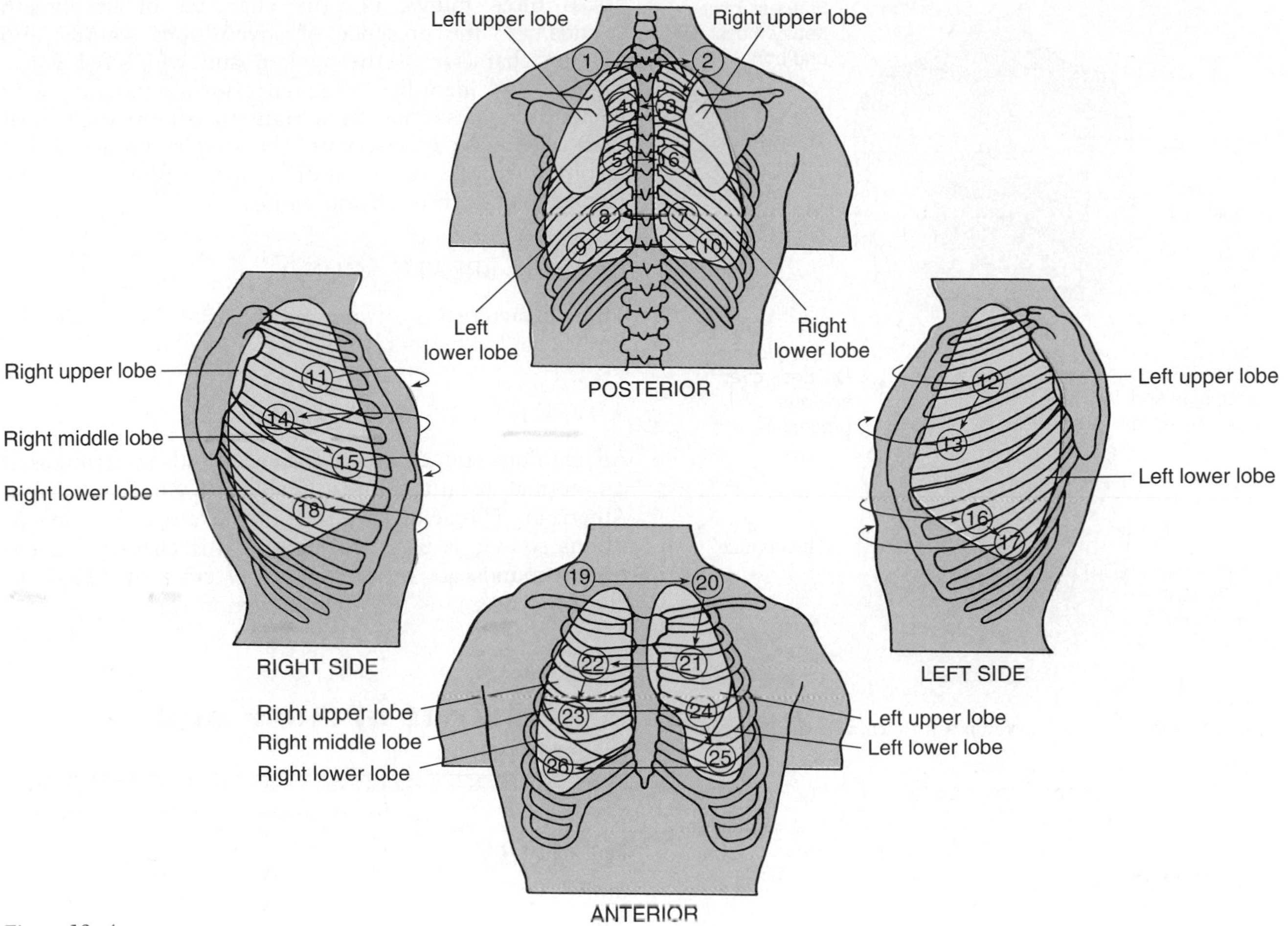

Figure 19–4
Lung assessment. Sequence for palpation, percussion, and auscultation of the thorax (posterior, lateral, and anterior)

The nurse palpates the posterior chest wall while the client says phrases that produce relatively intense vibrations (e.g., "99"). The vibrations are transmitted from the larynx via the airways and can be palpated on the chest wall (see Fig. 19–4). The intensity of vibrations on both sides is compared. Stronger vibrations are felt over areas where there is consolidation of the underlying lung (e.g., pneumonia). Decreased tactile fremitus is usually associated with abnormalities that move the lung farther from the chest wall, such as pleural effusion and pneumothorax.

Percussion

Percussion is an assessment technique of producing sounds by tapping on the chest wall with the hand. Tapping on the chest wall between the ribs produces various sounds that are described in regard to their acoustic properties—resonant, hyper-resonant, dull, flat, or tympanic (Fig. 19–5).

Percussion begins at the apices and proceeds to the bases, moving from the posterior areas to the lateral areas and then to the anterior areas (see Fig. 19–4). The posterior chest is best percussed with the client in an upright position and with arms crossed to separate the scapulae. Percussion sounds of the chest are described in Fig. 19–5.

DIAPHRAGMATIC EXCURSION

Percussion is also used to assess diaphragmatic excursion. The client is asked to take a deep breath and hold it as the examiner percusses down the posterior lung field and listens for the percussion note to change from resonant to dull; this area is marked. The process is repeated after the client exhales, and again the area is marked. Both right and left sides are assessed. The distance between the two marks should be 3 to 6 cm; smaller spans are found in females, and larger spans in males. The marks on the right will be slightly higher because of the presence of the liver. A client with an elevated diaphragm related to a pathologic process will have a decreased diaphragmatic excursion. If the client has lung disease in the lower lobes (e.g., consolidation or pleural fluid), the same dull percussion note will be heard. When abnormalities are found, it is recommended that other diagnostic tests be scheduled.

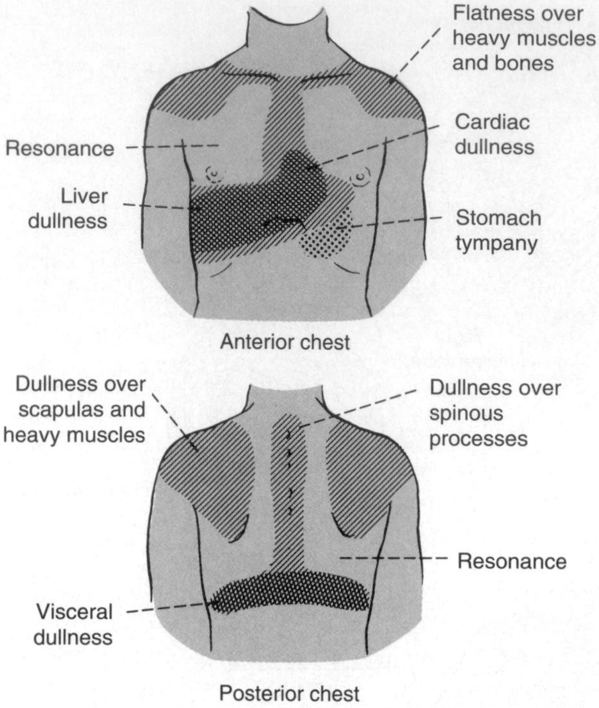

Figure 19–5
The location of thoracic percussion tones and their associated structures.

Auscultation

Auscultation is listening to the sounds of the chest with a stethoscope. By listening to the lungs while the client breathes with the mouth open, the examiner is able to assess three things: (1) the character of the breath sounds, (2) the presence of adventitious sounds, and (3) the character of the spoken and whispered voice. Figure 19–4 identifies a sequence for auscultation with comparison of sounds from right to left. At each position, the nurse listens with the diaphragm for a full respiratory cycle of inspiration and expiration as the client breathes through the mouth.

NORMAL BREATH SOUNDS

The characteristics of normal breath sounds are described in Table 19–1.

ADVENTITIOUS BREATH SOUNDS

Adventitious sounds are abnormal sounds superimposed on normal breath sounds (Table 19–2). The current American Thoracic Society nomenclature for adventitious sounds is used throughout this chapter. Adventitious sounds are described as (1) crackles, (2) rhonchi, (3) wheeze, or (4) pleural friction rub.

Assessment of Nose and Sinuses

HISTORY

Upper respiratory problems can occur alone or progress to lower respiratory complications, such as in viral infections.

TABLE 19–1 Characteristics of Normal Breath Sounds

	PITCH	AMPLITUDE	DURATION	QUALITY	NORMAL LOCATION
Bronchial (tracheal) 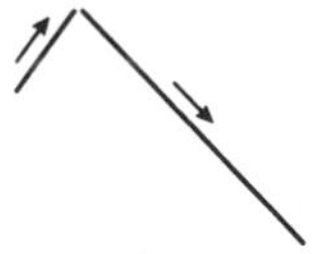	High	Loud	Inspiration < expiration	Harsh, hollow, tubular	Trachea and larynx
Bronchovesicular 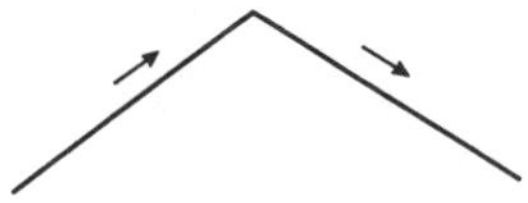	Moderate	Moderate	Inspiration = expiration	Mixed	Over major bronchi where fewer alveoli are located: posterior, between scapulae especially on right; anterior, around upper sternum in first and second intercostal spaces
Vesicular 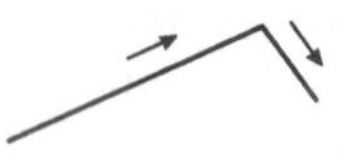	Low	Soft	Inspiration > expiration	Rustling, like the sound of the wind in the trees	Over peripheral lung fields where air flows through smaller bronchioles and alveoli

From Jarvis, C. (1992). *Physical examination and health assessment.* Philadelphia: W. B. Saunders.

TABLE 19–2 Adventitious Sounds

SOUND*	DESCRIPTION	MECHANISM	CLINICAL EXAMPLE
Discontinuous Sounds			
Crackles—fine (rales, crepitations) 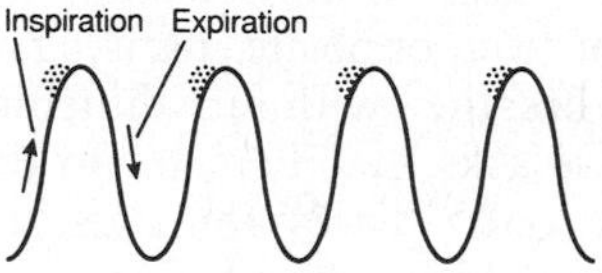	Discontinuous, high-pitched, short crackling, popping sounds heard during inspiration that are not cleared by coughing; this sound can be simulated by rolling a strand of hair between the fingers near the ear, or by moistening thumb and index finger and separating them near the ear	Inhaled air collides with previously deflated airways; airways suddenly pop open, creating crackling sound as gas pressures between the two compartments equalize	*Late inspiratory crackles* occur with restrictive disease: pneumonia, congestive heart failure, and interstitial fibrosis *Early inspiratory crackles* occur with obstructive disease: chronic bronchitis, asthma, and emphysema
Crackles—coarse (coarse rales) 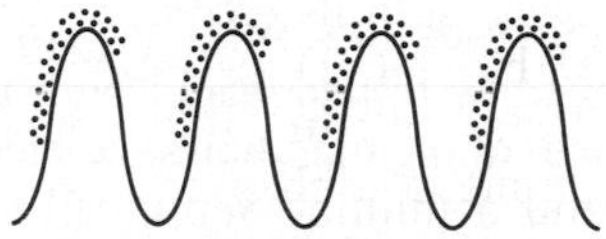	Loud, low-pitched, bubbling and gurgling sounds that start in early inspiration and may be present in expiration; may decrease somewhat by suctioning or coughing but will reappear shortly; sound like opening a Velcro fastener	Inhaled air collides with secretions in the trachea and large bronchi	Pulmonary edema, pneumonia, pulmonary fibrosis, and in the terminally ill who have a depressed cough reflex
Atelectatic crackles (atelectatic rales) 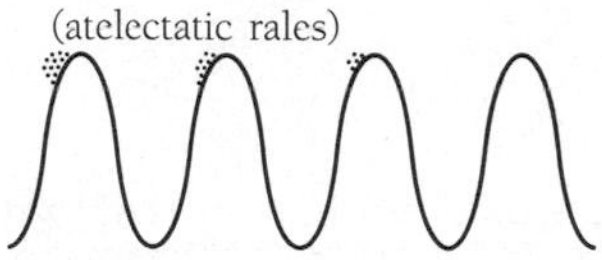	Sound like fine crackles, but do not last and are not pathologic; disappear after the first few breaths; heard in axillae and bases (usually dependent) of lungs	When sections of alveoli are not fully aerated, they deflate and accumulate secretions; crackles are heard when these sections re-expand with a few deep breaths	In aging adults, bed-ridden persons, or in persons just aroused from sleep
Pleural friction rub 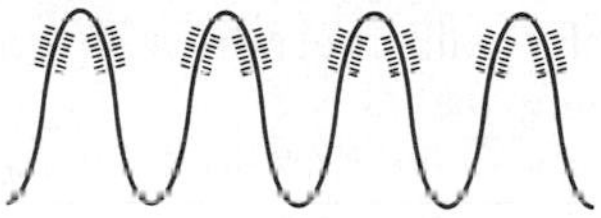	A very superficial sound that is coarse and low-pitched; it has a grating quality as if two pieces of leather are being rubbed together; sounds just like crackles, but close to the ear; sounds louder if the stethoscope is pushed harder onto the chest wall; sound is inspiratory and expiratory	Caused when pleurae become inflamed and lose their normal lubricating fluid; their opposing roughened pleural surfaces rub together during respiration; heard best in anterolateral wall where there is greatest lung mobility	Pleuritis, accompanied by pain with breathing (rub disappears afrter a few days if pleural fluid accumulates and separates pleurae)
Continuous Sounds			
Wheeze—high-pitched (sibilant rhonchi) 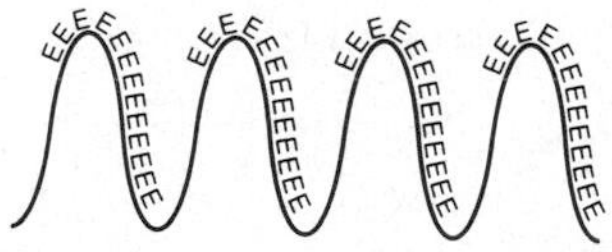	High-pitched, musical squeaking sounds that predominate in expiration but may occur in both expiration and inspiration	Air squeezed or compressed through passageways narrowed almost to closure by collapsing, swelling, secretions, or tumors; the passageway walls oscillate in apposition between the closed and barely open positions; the resulting sound is similar to a vibrating reed	Obstructive lung disease such as asthma and emphysema
Wheeze—low-pitched (sonorous rhonchi) 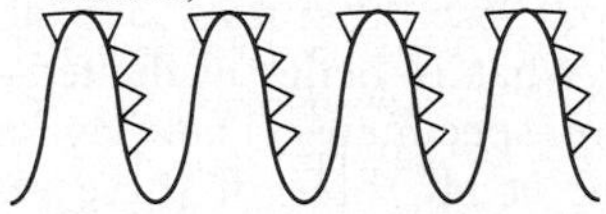	Low-pitched, musical snoring, moaning sounds; they are heard throughout the cycle, although they are more prominent on expiration; may clear somewhat by coughing	Airflow obstruction as described by the vibrating reed mechanism above; the pitch of the wheeze cannot be correlated to the size of the passageway that generates it	Bronchitis

* Although nothing in clinical practice seems to differ more than the nomenclature of adventitious sounds, most authorities concur on two categories: (1) discontinuous, discrete crackling sounds and (2) continuous, coarse, or musical sounds.

From Jarvis, C. (1992). *Physical examination and health assessment.* Philadelphia: W. B. Saunders.

Chief Complaint

The client may present with a current complaint of nosebleeds (epistaxis), sinus infection, hayfever, postnasal drip, rhinitis, sneezing, or nasal, facial, or referred ear pain. Obstruction from engorged mucous membranes or nasal polyps may occlude the upper airway. A loss or decreased sense of smell may accompany symptoms of the common cold and allergies or may signal a more serious neurologic problem. The nurse inquires whether the client has experienced these symptoms previously and, if so, when and how often. The client is asked to describe self-treatment measures such as nasal sprays, decongestants, antihistamines, and other over-the-counter cold and allergy medications. A complete symptom analysis is performed to determine the nature of the problem including onset, duration, and severity. The nurse asks the client to relate factors that alleviate or aggravate the symptoms such as increased humidity, sitting upright, lying supine, weather and season changes, or allergies.

Nasal and sinus problems may be allergy-related and provoked by pollen, fumes, smoke, animal dander, or dust particles. Epistaxis episodes may increase during the winter months if insufficient humidity dries mucous membranes. A foul taste in the mouth, unpleasant breath odor (halitosis), nasal obstruction, and facial pain (particularly over the frontal and maxillary sinuses) accompany sinusitis. Chronic sinusitis may be accompanied by headache or facial pain present on awakening and diminishing during the day.

Past Medical History

The nurse asks about past problems with frequent colds, sinus infections, nasal stuffiness, or trauma (fracture). Episodes of epistaxis are explored for cause (such as hypertension), frequency, and treatment (such as cauterization or nasal packing).

PHYSICAL EXAMINATION

The nurse uses inspection and palpation to examine the nose and sinuses.

Nose

EXTERNAL NOSE

The external nose is inspected and palpated for deviations from normal alignment, symmetry, color, discharge, nasal flaring, lesions, and tenderness. Normal findings are listed:

- The skin color over the nose is the same as that of the facial skin.
- Alignment is straight and symmetric without deviation from midline.
- Discharge from the nares is absent, and the nares do not flare (spread) with respirations.
- The client is able to breathe quietly through the nose rather than mouthbreathe.
- Masses, lesions, and tenderness are absent.

The nurse checks the nasal canals for patency by asking the client to occlude one naris with a finger and to breathe through the open naris while closing the mouth. This is repeated for the opposite naris. The client should be able to breathe without difficulty through both nares. The nurse asks the client to tip the head back and inspects the outer nares for crusting, bleeding, or dryness, which should be absent.

INTERNAL NOSE

The nurse next inspects the vestibules with use of a penlight while the client's head is tipped back. Normal findings include the presence of coarse hairs, a clear passage without discharge, and a midline septum. Further examination of the internal nose requires use of a nasal speculum; this is not done unless it is indicated.

Nasopharynx

The nasopharynx is best examined with a mirror with the tongue depressed with a tongue blade or gauze. The nurse can prevent the mirror's fogging by warming it before putting it into a mouth. Hold the mirror to one side of the uvula and focus light on it.

Paranasal Sinuses

The nurse assesses the paranasal sinuses by inspecting and palpating the soft overlying tissues and observing any nasal secretions (it is possible to determine which sinus is infected according to where purulent discharge appears).

DIAGNOSTIC TESTS

Diagnostic procedures augment the assessment of clients experiencing respiratory disorders. In order to help the new nurse remember which diagnostic test is used when and for what purpose, the tests are discussed in the framework of what is being evaluated—functional status, anatomy, or specimens. The diagnostic test may be used for one or all three of these reasons. This listing is by no means all-inclusive but identifies the most commonly used diagnostic tests.

Diagnostic Tests for Function

The diagnostic tests that evaluate the functional status of the pulmonary system include (1) arterial blood gas analysis, (2) pulmonary function tests, (3) pulse oximetry, and (4) ventilation/perfusion studies.

ARTERIAL BLOOD GAS ANALYSIS

Arterial blood gas (ABG) analysis directly measures the partial pressures of oxygen (PaO_2), carbon dioxide ($PaCO_2$), and pH. Other data are calculated such as oxygen saturation and HCO_3. PaO_2 reflects the efficiency of gas exchange (ventilation/perfusion), whereas $PaCO_2$ reflects the effectiveness of ventilation. The acid-base status of the body (see Chap. 4) is indicated by the pH of arterial blood.

Arterial blood gases are essential for the assessment of clients who are acutely ill with pulmonary and nonpulmonary disorders, require artificial airways, are dependent on mechanical ventilation, and are experiencing chronic respiratory diseases.

A sample of arterial blood is obtained by arterial puncture. This procedure is done by inserting a sterile needle (connected to a heparinized syringe) into the radial, brachial, or femoral artery. The radial artery is most commonly used because it is readily accessible, is easily palpated, and is not associated with as severe complications as the other two sites are. Low complication rates are related to ease of access and presence of collateral circulation via the ulnar artery. For serial ABG analyses or ongoing respiratory monitoring, multiple punctures may be avoided by using an arterial line (i.e., a sterile cannula inserted into one of the arteries) (Fig. 19–6).

Interpretation. A systematic approach to ABG interpretation, in conjunction with the client's overall

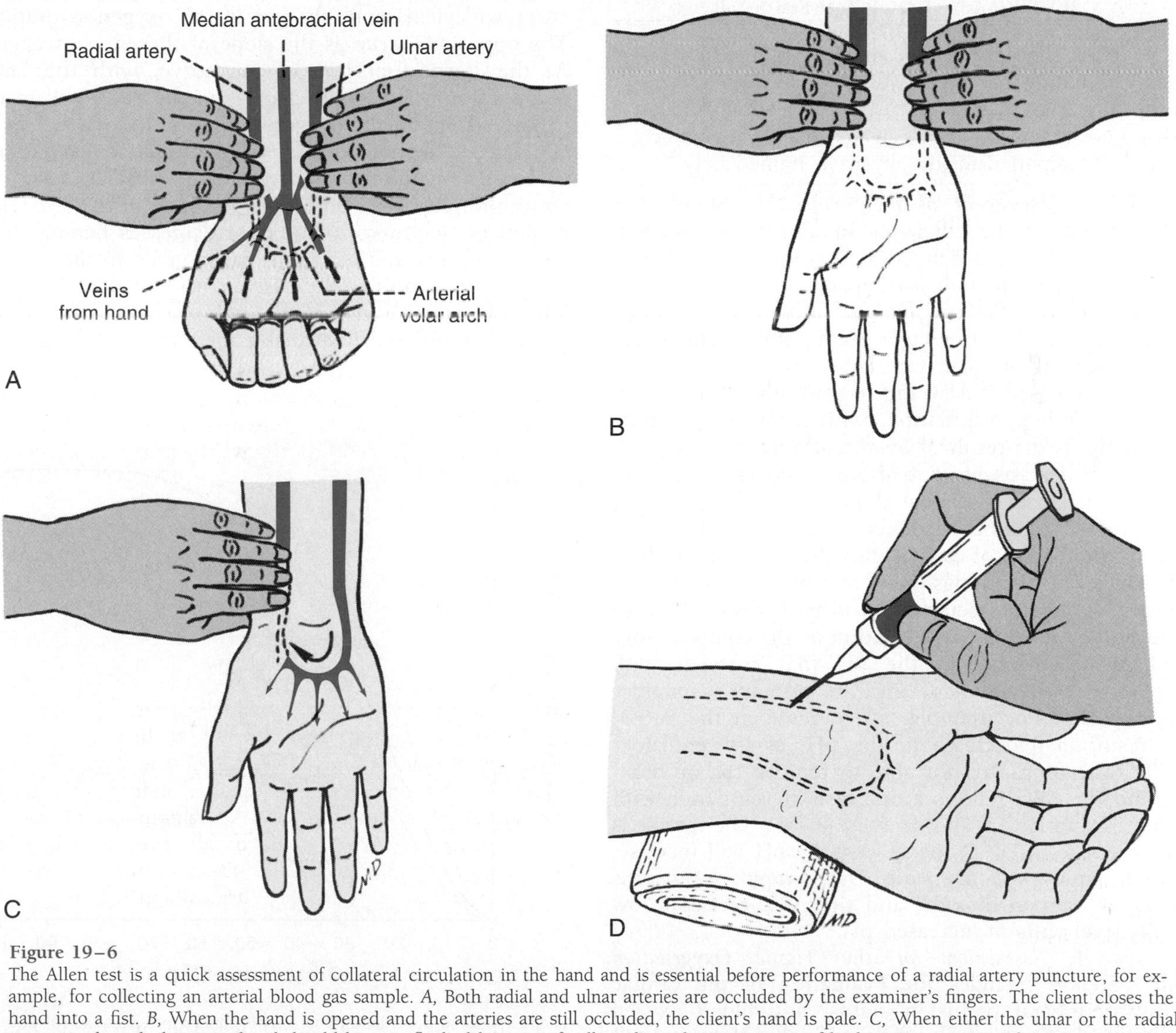

Figure 19–6
The Allen test is a quick assessment of collateral circulation in the hand and is essential before performance of a radial artery puncture, for example, for collecting an arterial blood gas sample. *A,* Both radial and ulnar arteries are occluded by the examiner's fingers. The client closes the hand into a fist. *B,* When the hand is opened and the arteries are still occluded, the client's hand is pale. *C,* When either the ulnar or the radial artery is released, the entire hand should become flushed because of collateral circulation. Patency of both arteries is assessed one at a time. *D,* An arterial blood gas sample is drawn from the radial artery with a heparinized needle and syringe.

status, can lead to the identification of potentially life-threatening abnormalities.

Four steps can be used for interpretation:

- Assessment of the hypoxemic state
- Assessment of the ventilatory state
- Assessment of acid-base balance
- Assessment of the tissue oxygenation state

Step 1: Assessment of the Hypoxemic State. The PaO_2 is evaluated first because of the seriousness of hypoxemia. Hypoxemia is a reflection of the tension of oxygen in the arterial blood but does not reflect the status of tissue oxygenation. Mild hypoxemia is a PaO_2 less than 80 mm Hg on breathing room air. Moderate hypoxemia is a PaO_2 less than 60 mm Hg; severe hypoxemia is a PaO_2 less than 40 mm Hg. Baseline normal values decrease with age at a rate of 1 mm Hg per year of age over 60. Nonetheless, the same values are used to label levels of hypoxemia. Hypoxemia is treated with oxygen.

CRITICAL TO REMEMBER

The nurse should carefully monitor prescribed oxygen concentrations and length of time of administration. Blood gas analysis during oxygen administration that indicates PaO_2 levels greater than 100 mm Hg should be reported to the physician immediately.

Step 2: Assessment of the Ventilatory State. The $PaCO_2$ evaluates the efficiency of alveolar ventilation. Alveolar ventilation is defined as that inspired air which reaches the alveoli and participates in gas exchange. Alveolar hypoventilation or ventilatory failure is diagnosed when a $PaCO_2$ greater than 50 mm Hg is observed. Normal alveolar ventilation is evident with a $PaCO_2$ between 30 and 50 mm Hg, ideally 35 to 45 mm Hg. Alveolar hyperventilation, with a $PaCO_2$ less than 30 mm Hg, is the result of overbreathing.

Step 3: Assessment of Acid-Base Balance. The pH–acid-base balance is evaluated next. The lungs play a major role in acid-base balance. Changes in the retention or elimination of carbon dioxide will directly affect pH. However, the lungs may act in a compensatory manner to correct metabolic acid-base disorders with hypoventilation or hyperventilation as the compensatory mechanism. Changes in the pH that correlate with changes in carbon dioxide indicate primary respiratory abnormalities. For example, an increase in the $PaCO_2$ will result in a decrease in the pH, as in ventilatory failure. The lungs are not able to remove carbon dioxide, and the ABG reflects a decrease in ventilation with an increase in $PaCO_2$ and decrease in pH. The reverse is also true; as the $PaCO_2$ decreases, the pH will increase, as in a hyperventilatory state. Deep, rapid respirations "blow off" carbon dioxide, and the ABG reveals a low $PaCO_2$ level with an increased pH.

Step 4: Assessment of the Tissue Oxygenation State. Step 4 includes the evaluation of the cardiac status, peripheral perfusion status, and blood oxygen transport. Cardiac status and peripheral perfusion status are evaluated together and include blood pressure, cardiac output, heart rate, skin color, capillary refill, mental status, electrolyte balance, and urine output. The blood oxygen transport mechanisms include the arterial oxygen tension, blood oxygen content, and hemoglobin-oxygen affinity. Disorders of myocardial pumping, red blood cell count, and blood volume have a potential impact on tissue oxygenation.

Oxygenation can be understood with the help of the oxyhemoglobin dissociation curve. The oxyhemoglobin dissociation curve represents the relationship between the partial pressure of oxygen in the blood and the saturation of hemoglobin. This relationship is represented in Figure 19–7 as an S-shaped curve. A PaO_2 of 60 mm Hg or greater provides an oxygen satuation of 90 per cent or greater. At higher PO_2 tensions (above 90 mm Hg), the curve flattens, and the percentage of oxygen saturation does not rise as steeply. The flat portion of the curve is advantageous to the lung because despite significant decreases in the alveolar PO_2, the hemoglobin circulating through the pulmonary capillaries is nearly saturated to full capacity with oxygen. Changes in the PaO_2 at the flat, top portion of the curve will yield small changes in the oxygen saturation. The opposite is true as the slope of the curve steepens. At the steepest portion of the curve, with the PaO_2 below 60 mm Hg, small changes in the PaO_2 will result in large drops in the oxygen saturation.

The oxyhemoglobin curve is affected by a number of factors, including temperature, pH, $PaCO_2$, and the concentration of 2,3-diphosphoglycerate in the red cells. A shift of the curve to the right decreases hemoglobin-oxygen affinity and oxygen is easily given to the tissues. Thus, with a similar decrease in PaO_2 to low levels (a left shift), increased amounts of oxygen will be bound to hemoglobin and unavailable for tissues. During a left

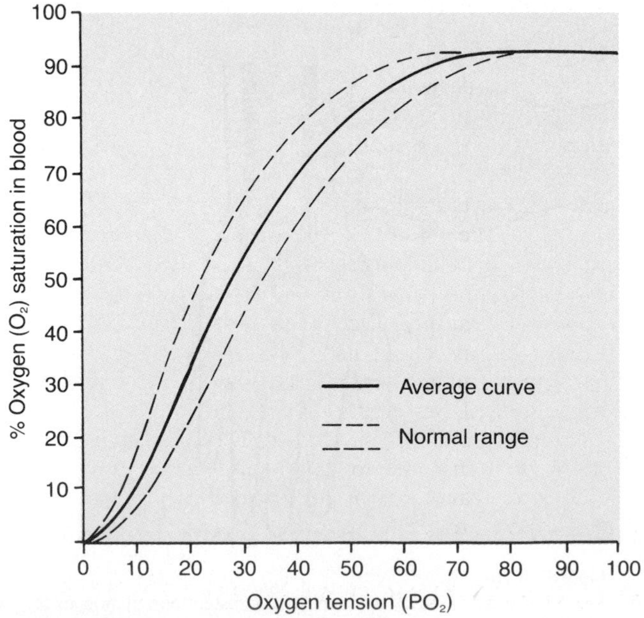

Figure 19–7
Oxyhemoglobin dissociation curve. This curve represents the relationship between the partial pressure of oxygen (PO_2) in the blood and the saturation of hemoglobin with oxygen (O_2).

shift, hemoglobin has a high affinity for oxygen, so less oxygen is available for tissues. The body's tissues benefit from the steep portion of the curve. As even a small decrease in the oxygen tension occurs, oxygen is rapidly released to the tissues by the hemoglobin. This is illustrated by the way the curve quickly drops off as the saturation curve reflects the lower saturation of hemoglobin. The oxyhemoglobin saturation curve shifts upward to the left when conditions occur that cause oxygen and hemoglobin to bind more tightly, so that less oxygen is actually released to the tissues. The curve shifts down and to the right when conditions occur that cause hemoglobin to be released more readily to the tissues.

Nursing Management

The physician or other clinician skilled in arterial puncture must collect the blood sample. In most hospitals, physicians are the only personnel allowed to draw from the femoral artery, whereas nurses with special training can draw radial or brachial samples.

Before the sample is drawn, the site must be treated with a disinfectant and allowed to dry. The client should be told the stick will be painful for a moment. If the client is quite anxious about the test or other problems and is hyperventilating, the results of the test may be altered. If the client is not likely to cooperate, the nurse may need to hold the client's arm still during the stick in order to avoid inadvertent injury to nerves, vessels, and tendons. The amount of blood needed for the sample varies with each laboratory but may be as small as 0.5 mL or as large as 10 mL.

CRITICAL TO REMEMBER

After the sample is drawn, continuous pressure should be applied to the site for 5 minutes for radial and brachial sites and 10 minutes for femoral sites. Pressure bandages are commonly used. If the client has a tendency to bleed, pressure will be needed for a longer period of time.

It is important to note whether the client is receiving oxygen; the amount and source of oxygen should be recorded on the laboratory request form. The results will be examined in light of the degree of oxygen needed. For example, if a client's PaO_2 is 85 on 50 per cent oxygen, this client has a more significant problem with oxygen transport than does the client who is at 85 on room air (21 per cent oxygen).

Complications from arterial sampling include bleeding or hematoma formation at the site and injury to the artery and surrounding structures. The nurse should report any of these signs to the physician.

PULMONARY FUNCTION TESTS

Pulmonary function tests (PFTs) help the practitioner further evaluate the lungs. PFTs can provide information related to lung volumes, lung mechanics, and diffusion capabilities of the lung. The obtained data allow the practitioner to determine the

- Presence of pulmonary disease or abnormality of lung function
- Extent of abnormalities
- Severity of impairment
- Progression of the disorder
- Appropriate treatment

Preparation for PFTs includes education about the purpose of the test, how the tests are done, and what to expect during the tests. Explicit instructions will be given during the testing, and complete patient cooperation is important. The nurse should instruct the clients that they may feel short of breath after the test. Clients should also be instructed not to smoke or use a bronchodilator 6 hours before undergoing a PFT.

Pulmonary function tests performed in a pulmonary function laboratory cover the entire range of respiratory volumes. On the other hand, PFTs done outside of a laboratory are modified to ventilation tests of forced expiratory volume, vital capacity, and maximal voluntary ventilation measures. Table 19–3 defines common lung volumes. Lung capacities are figures calculated from two or more lung volumes. They include the inspiratory capacity, functional residual capacity, and vital capacity.

Clients with obstructive and restrictive diseases will have disease-specific changes in lung volumes and capacities. Table 19–4 categorizes the diseases and outlines the differences in the PFTs. Clients with obstructive lung diseases have air trapping and associated symptoms. The total lung capacity will be increased, with severe disease along with lung hyperinflation as seen on the chest radiograph. Restrictive disorders are characterized by decreased total lung capacity, a decreased residual volume, and, usually, difficulty taking a deep breath.

Lung Mechanics. Lung mechanics evaluate the flow of gas in and out of the lung. These measurements evaluate the respiratory muscles, lung and chest wall compliance, and airway resistance, which is sometimes called the lung's bellow function. The flow rates are measured during the exhalation phase of the respiratory cycle. Depending on the test, the client may be asked to exhale forcefully or to the maximal expiratory level. See Table 19–4 for definitions of maneuvers that test lung mechanics. Lung mechanics are measured with a spirometer. The client exhales or inhales into a mouthpiece, causing displacement of air or water. Flow volume loops can be created as visual patterns.

Clients with obstructive diseases will have decreased FEV_t (forced expiratory volume; subscript *t* is number of seconds). The client can still exhale, but because of the nature of the disease, exhalation takes much longer, compared with exhalation of air from a normal lung. Restrictive diseases cause a decreased FEV, because lung volumes are decreased.

Lung mechanics are a reflection of the efficacy of the lung's bellow function. Typically with obstructive lung disorders, chest bellow function is impaired and

TABLE 19–3 Pulmonary Function Test Components

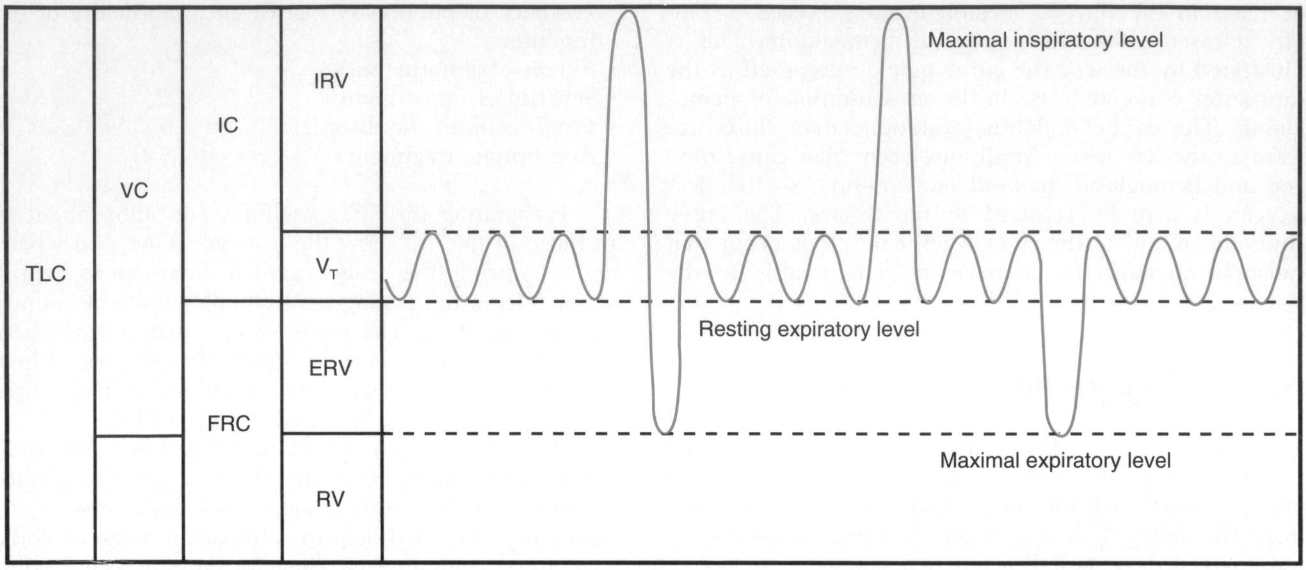

ABBREVIATION	COMPONENT	DESCRIPTION
Lung Volumes and Capacities		
VC	Vital capacity	Volume of air that is measured during a slow, maximal expiration after a maximal inspiration; normal range varies with age, sex, and body size
IC	Inspiratory capacity	Largest volume of air that can be inhaled from resting expiratory volume
ERV	Expiratory reserve volume	Largest volume of air exhaled from resting end-expiratory level
FRC	Functional residual capacity	Volume of air remaining in lungs at resting end-expiratory level
RV	Residual volume	Volume of air remaining in the lungs at the end of maximal expiration
TLC	Total lung capacity	Volume of air contained in the lungs after maximal inspiration
V_T	Tidal volume	Volume of air inhaled or exhaled during each respiratory cycle; normal range is 400 to 700 mL
f	Respiratory rate	Frequency of breathing is the number of breaths per minute; normal range is 12 to 22
Lung Mechanics		
FVC	Forced vital capacity	Maximal volume of air that can be forcefully expired after a maximal inspiration to total lung capacity
FEV_t	Forced expiratory volume	Volume of air expired during a given time interval (t in seconds) from the beginning of an FVC maneuver
$FEF_{25\%-75\%}$	Forced expiratory $flow_{25\%-75\%}$	Average of flow during the middle half of an FVC maneuver
PEFR	Peak expiratory flow rate	Maximal flow rate attained during an FVC maneuver
MVV	Maximal voluntary ventilation	Largest volume that can be breathed during a 10- to 15-second interval with voluntary effort
MIP	Maximal inspiratory pressure	Greatest negative or subatmospheric pressure that can be generated during inspiration against an occluded airway
MEP	Maximal expiratory pressure	Highest positive pressure that can be generated during a forceful expiratory effort against an occluded airway

the client is dyspneic. Home testing of peak flow is commonly performed by clients with asthma.

Lung mechanics are measured before and after administration of beta-adrenergic agents. Reversible lung disease is said to be present if a 15 per cent change in the FVC, FEV_t, and $FEF_{25\%-75\%}$ (forced expiratory flow) is noted.

PULSE OXIMETRY

Pulse oximetry combines the principles of plethysmography and spectrophotometry to measure arterial oxygen saturation noninvasively. The pulse oximeter (Fig. 19–8) passes a beam of light through the tissue, and a sensor measures the amount of light absorbed by the

TABLE 19–4 Categorization of Obstructive and Restrictive Pulmonary Disorders and PFT Findings

	OBSTRUCTIVE	RESTRICTIVE
	Disorders or diseases affecting the patency or elasticity of the airways, leading to an increase in airway resistance; expiration primarily affected	Disorders or diseases causing interference or change in chest wall or lung parenchyma; inspiration primarily affected
	Emphysema Chronic bronchitis Asthma Bronchiectasis Airway inflammation in response to irritants, infections, or allergies	Kyphoscoliosis Abdominal distention/obesity Pulmonary fibrosis Neuromuscular diseases and disorders Chest wall trauma Congenital chest wall changes Inflammatory changes of the lung tissue or pleura Tumors Pulmonary edema
PFTs and Findings		
VC (vital capacity)	Decreased	Normal or decreased
FEV_t (forced expiratory volume)	Decreased	Decreased, but not as severe as in obstructive disease
FEV_t/VC ratio	Decreased	Normal to increased
RV (residual volume)	Increased	Decreased
FRC (functional residual capacity)	Increased	Decreased
TLC (total lung capacity)	Increased	Decreased

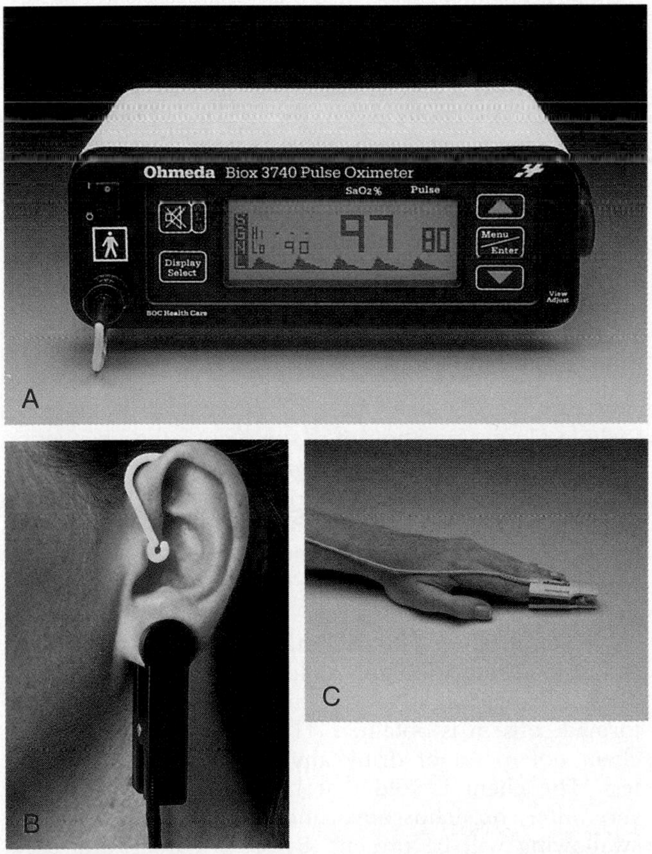

Figure 19–8
Oximetry. Noninvasive monitoring of oxygen saturation is done with a pulse oximeter. This unit (*A*) has an ear probe and a finger probe. The ear probe (*B*) is used for measurements of oxygen saturation during exercise. The finger probe (*C*) is most frequently used for stationary measurements. (Courtesy of Ohmeda, Boulder, CO.)

oxygen-saturated hemoglobin. Arterial saturations have a close correlation with the saturations obtained from the pulse oximeter if the arterial saturation is above 70 per cent. The following provides a quick guide for comparison of oxygen saturation and PaO_2:

Oxygen saturation	*PaO_2*
50%	25 mm Hg
75%	40 mm Hg
90%	55 mm Hg

Limitations with pulse oximetry are still present despite the advancement of the technology. Hypotension, hypothermia, and vasoconstriction reduce arterial blood flow, and movement of the finger interferes with the interpretation of the oxygen saturation.

VENTILATION/PERFUSION SCANNING (LUNG SCAN)

Ventilation/perfusion scanning is used to assess lung ventilation and lung perfusion. This scan is often called a V/Q scan. V/Q scans are valuable in diagnosing pulmonary embolism, pulmonary infarction, emphysema, fibrosis, or bronchiectasis. Quantitative perfusion scans may be helpful in preoperative assessment of clients for surgical resection of thoracic malignancy. The test has two parts (done together or separately): (1) assessing the pulmonary vasculature (perfusion scan) and (2) assessing the distribution of ventilation (ventilation scan).

- *Perfusion scan.* Radioactive dye is injected intravenously and carried into the pulmonary vasculature. Decreased blood flow to any part of the lung is revealed as a decrease in the amount of radioactivity shown on either x-ray film with use of a rectilinear

scanner or on Polaroid film with use of a gamma or scintillation camera. Scanning is done in both the anterior and posterior views.
- *Ventilation scan.* Radioactive gas is inhaled, which produces an image of the areas where ventilation is occurring. Assessment of the pattern of deposition of radioactive gas in the alveoli is also possible.

Ventilation images are compared with the pictures taken during the perfusion scan. There should be an equal amount of radioactivity discernible on both ventilation and perfusion pictures. If there are areas in which there is ventilation but little or no perfusion, a pulmonary embolus is suspected. Further assessment may be needed. If there is doubt as to the cause of impaired perfusion, pulmonary angiography may be needed.

There is no specific preparation for a lung scan. With the exception of local discomfort from the injection of radioactive dye, the procedure is painless.

Diagnostic Tests to Evaluate the Anatomy

The following diagnostic procedures are used to assess the anatomy:

- Chest radiography
- Computed tomography
- Bronchoscopy
- Magnetic resonance imaging
- Pulmonary angiogram

CHEST X-RAY STUDIES

Chest x-ray studies provide information about the chest that may not be available through other assessment means. Also, they often graphically illustrate the cause of respiratory dysfunction. Chest films may reveal abnormalities when there are no physical signs or symptoms of pulmonary disease.

Chest films show the bony structures (e.g., ribs, sternum, clavicles, scapulae, and upper portion of the humerus). The vertebral column is visible vertically through the middle of the thorax. The two hemidiaphragms normally appear rounded, smooth, and sharply defined, with the right hemidiaphragm slightly elevated above the left. The junction of the rib cage and the diaphragm, called the costophrenic angle, is normally clearly visible and angled. Heart tissue is dense and appears white but less intensely white than bony structures. The heart shadow is normally clearly outlined and extends primarily onto the left side of the thorax and occupies no more than one third of the chest width. Close observation shows the trachea in the upper middle chest almost superimposed over the cervical and thoracic vertebrae. The trachea bifurcates at the level of the fourth thoracic vertebra into the right and left mainstem bronchi. The pulmonary blood vessels, bronchi, and lymph nodes are located in the hilum on both the right and left sides of the midthorax. Lung tissue appears black on x-ray film. Vascular lung structures are visible as white, thin, wispy strings fanning out from the hilum (Fig. 19–9).

Chest x-ray studies may be taken (1) as part of routine screening procedures, (2) when pulmonary disease is suspected, (3) to monitor the status of respiratory disorders and abnormalities (e.g., pleural effusion, atelectasis, and tuberculous cavitary lesions), (4) to confirm endotracheal or tracheostomy tube placement, (5) after traumatic chest injury, or (6) in any other situation in which radiographic information helps the management of a respiratory problem.

COMPUTED TOMOGRAPHY

Computed tomography, also called CAT scan, provides more sophisticated tomography than is possible with conventional x-ray equipment. By using a computer to regulate the layers or "slices" of tissue examined, the camera rotates in a circular pattern, and three-dimensional assessment of the thorax (or other body area) is possible. Still photographs are taken at each level. Computed tomography is able to visualize most abnormalities, but small early lesions may be missed.

Often computed tomographic studies are done before and after the intravenous administration of a contrast medium containing a radioactively tagged iodine isotope. If a contrast medium is used, it is extremely important to find out whether the client is allergic to iodine or shellfish.

Computed tomography is particularly helpful in diagnosing peripheral (e.g., pleural) or mediastinal disorders. Special techniques can be used to view pulmonary nodules. "Thin cuts" of the computed tomographic scan are used in diagnosing interstitial lung disorders such as pulmonary fibrosis and bronchiectasis.

BRONCHOSCOPY

Bronchoscopy is the passage of a lighted bronchoscope into the bronchial tree (Fig. 19–10). Bronchoscopy may be performed with rigid steel or flexible fiberoptic instruments. Bronchoscopy may be performed for diagnostic or therapeutic purposes. The diagnostic purposes include (1) examination of tissue, (2) further evaluation of a tumor for potential surgical resection, (3) collection of tissue specimens for diagnosis, and (4) evaluation of bleeding sites. Therapeutic bronchoscopy is used to (1) remove foreign bodies, (2) remove thick, viscous secretions, (3) treat postoperative atelectasis, and (4) destroy and remove lesions.

Nursing interventions include client preparation, assisting during the study, and observation. The procedure is explained to the client and family and an informed consent is obtained. The nurse also instructs the client not to eat or drink anything 6 hours before the test. The client is told that his or her throat may be sore after bronchoscopy, and some initial difficulty swallowing will be present. Before preprocedural sedation, dentures, contact lenses, and other prostheses are removed. Sedation is given to suppress the cough, sedate the patient, and relieve anxiety. A topical anesthetic is also sprayed into the back of the throat.

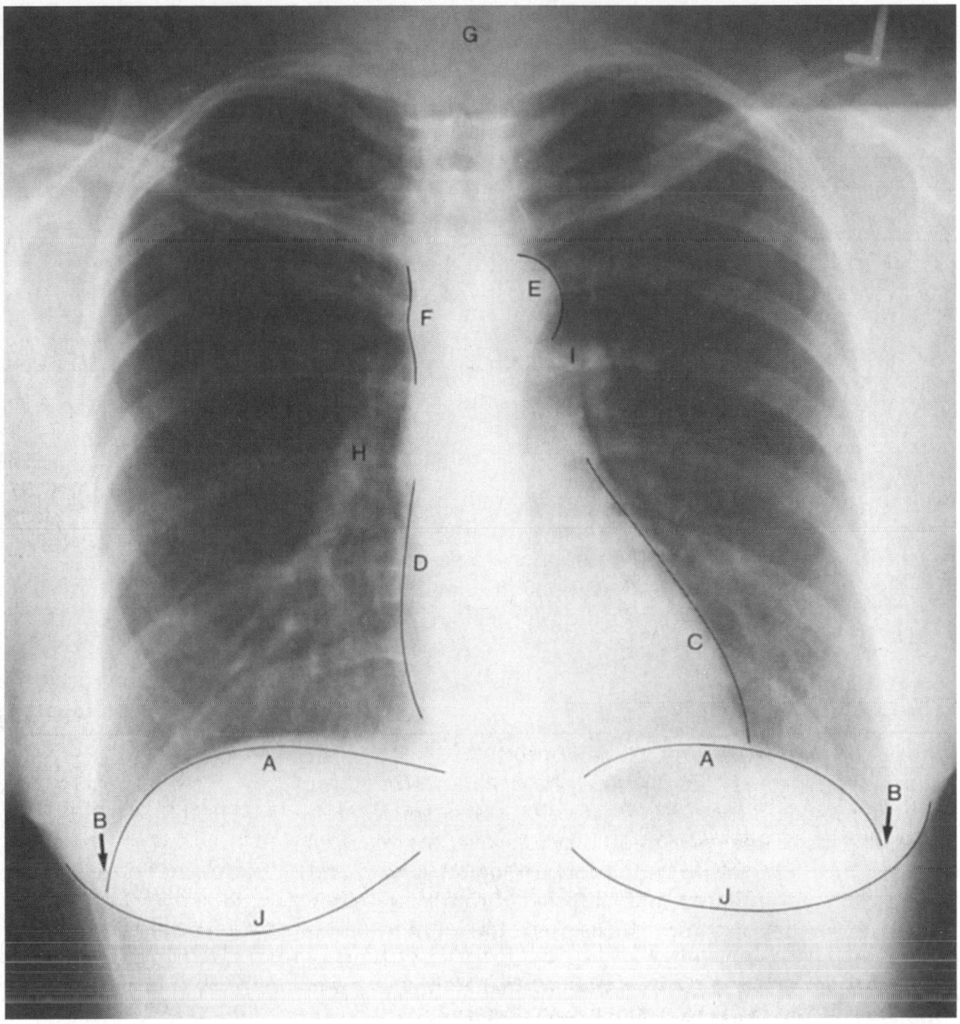

Figure 19–9
Normal chest x-ray study taken from a posteroanterior view. The backward L in the upper right corner is placed on the film to indicate the client's left side of the chest. Some anatomic structures can be seen on the x-ray study. *A*, diaphragm; *B*, costophrenic angle; *C*, left ventricle; *D*, right atrium; *E*, aortic arch; *F*, superior vena cava; *G*, trachea; *H*, right bronchus; *I*, left bronchus; and *J*, breast shadows.

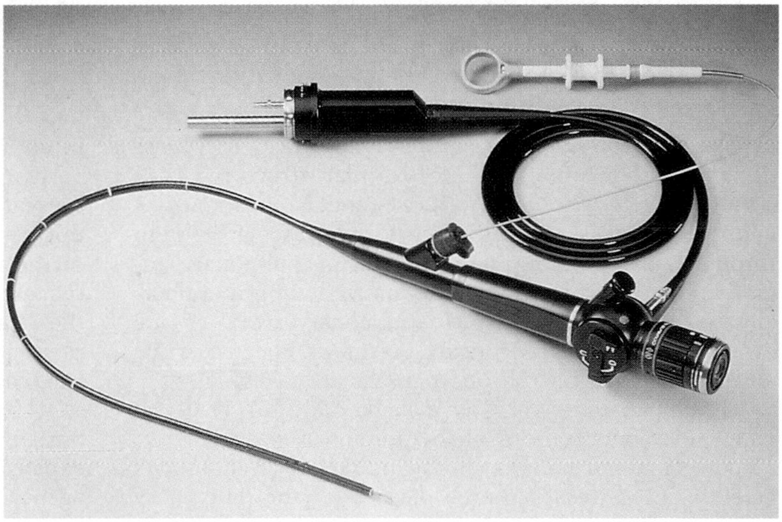

Figure 19–10
A flexible fiberoptic bronchoscope. (Courtesy of The Olympus Corporation, New Hyde Park, NY.)

During the procedure, the client lies supine with head hyperextended. The nurse monitors vital signs, talks to and reassures the client, and assists the physician as necessary.

CRITICAL TO REMEMBER

After bronchoscopy, vital signs are monitored per hospital protocol. The client is observed for signs of respiratory distress including dyspnea, changes in respiratory rate, use of accessory muscles, and changes in or absent lung sounds. Expectorated secretions are inspected for evidence of any hemoptysis. Nothing is given by mouth until the cough and swallow reflexes have returned.

Cough and swallow reflexes usually return in 1 to 2 hours. Once the client can swallow, feeding may begin with ice chips and small sips of water. Lung sounds are monitored for 24 hours. Development of adventitious sounds should be reported to the physician.

THORASCOPY

Thorascopy is a new diagnostic procedure that is an alternative to open lung biopsy and thoracotomy for pleural surface disorders. Typically, three small incisions are made into the middle chest wall. A camera is inserted through the first incision to inspect tissue, and tissues are manipulated and biopsied through the other incisions. A chest tube is inserted to promote lung re-expansion.

Advantages of the procedure include reduced anesthesia time, less pain, and shortened hospital stay. In addition, biopsies may be obtained from the lower lobes, which are not routinely biopsied during open lung biopsy procedures.

PULMONARY ANGIOGRAPHY

Sometimes the vascular structure of the thorax may need to be assessed. Angiography and other procedures designed to examine specific vascular structures (i.e., aortography for the aorta) all use similar techniques. A contrast agent is injected into the vascular system through an indwelling catheter. During pulmonary angiography, the catheter may be inserted either peripherally or directly into the main pulmonary artery or one of its branches. The contrast agent is injected while cinefluorographs or still photographs are taken.

Pulmonary angiography may be done to (1) detect congenital abnormalities of the pulmonary vascular tree, (2) detect abnormalities of the pulmonary venous circulation, (3) assess acquired diseases of the pulmonary arterial and venous circulation (e.g., primary pulmonary arterial hypertension), (4) assess the destructive effects of emphysema, (5) investigate the potential benefit of resection for bronchogenic carcinoma, (6) assess peripheral pulmonary lesions, and (7) assess the extent of thromboembolism in the lungs.

CRITICAL TO REMEMBER

As with any procedure in which a catheter is inserted into the peripheral or central vasculature, it is important after the procedure to observe the site of catheter entry for infection, hematoma formation, or local reaction to contrast media. The nurse should continue to observe for signs of adverse reaction to contrast media (e.g., increasing respiratory distress, hypotension, stridor, and other indications of anaphylaxis).

MAGNETIC RESONANCE IMAGING

Magnetic resonance imaging is the use of magnetic fields rather than radiation to create images of body structures. Magnetic resonance imaging has limited usefulness in pulmonary assessment. It may be used to diagnose chest wall invasion by peripheral lung cancer.

Specimens

The following procedures are used for the recovery and analysis of pulmonary specimens: (1) thoracentesis, (2) biopsy, and (3) sputum collection.

THORACENTESIS

Thoracentesis is the drainage of fluid or air found in the pleural space. Therapeutic thoracentesis will remove an accumulation of pleural fluid or air that has caused lung compression and respiratory distress. When the main goal is to determine the cause of an infection or empyema, diagnostic thoracentesis is performed. The fluid collected is sent to the laboratory and assessed for specific gravity, glucose, protein, pH, culture, sensitivity study, and cytology. The color and consistency of the pleural fluid are also documented.

Before thoracentesis, the client is prepared and positioned. The client is instructed about the importance of holding still during the procedure. Sudden movement may force the needle through the pleural space and injure the visceral pleura or lung parenchyma.

Figure 19–11 is an example of appropriate positioning during thoracentesis. With the client in the upright position, pleural fluid accumulates in the base of the thorax. An alternative is to place the client in a recumbent position with his or her arm resting under the head. During the procedure, the nurse assists the physician, monitors vital signs, and observes for dyspnea, complaints of difficulty breathing, nausea, or pain.

After the procedure, the client is usually turned onto the unaffected side for 1 hour to facilitate lung expansion. Vital signs should be assessed according to agency policy. The respiratory rate and character and breath sounds should be assessed carefully. Tachypnea, dyspnea, cyanosis, retractions, or diminished breath sounds, which may indicate pneumothorax, should be reported to the physician.

The amount of fluid withdrawn should be recorded as fluid output. A chest x-ray study may be performed

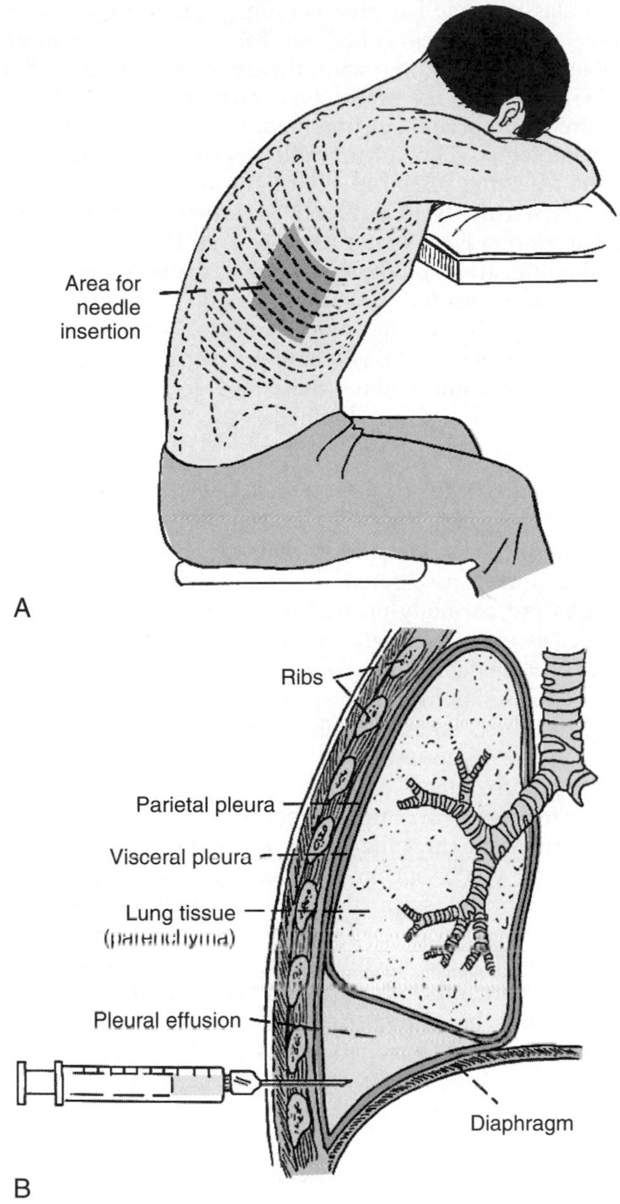

Figure 19–11
A, Thoracentesis position. Arms are raised and crossed. Head rests on folded arms. This position allows the chest wall to be pulled outward in an expanded position. If an overbed table is not available, the arms may be left down but positioned forward of the hips or crossed in front of the chest. *B,* The usual site for the insertion of a thoracentesis needle for a right-sided effusion. The actual site varies with each client, depending on the location and volume of the effusion. The physician tries to keep the needle as far away from the diaphragm as possible while at the same time inserting the needle close to the base of the effusion so that gravity can help with drainage.

to evaluate the degree of lung re-expansion and pneumothorax.

Subcutaneous emphysema may follow this procedure, because air in the pleural cavity leaks into subcutaneous tissues. The tissues feel like lumpy paper and crackle when palpated (crepitus). Usually subcutaneous emphysema causes no problem unless it is increasing and constricting vital organs (e.g., trachea). The client often needs reassurance about this disorder.

If the client has pleural effusion due to a malignancy, cytotoxic medications may be inserted into the pleural space after thoracentesis. Some of these agents burn, and others require the client to roll about in order to have the medication coat the entire pleural space. The nurse will need to review the interventions used with the various medications.

BIOPSY

Biopsy specimens may be taken from various respiratory tissues for assessment. As previously mentioned, biopsy of tracheobronchial structures may be performed during bronchoscopy. Biopsies of scalene and mediastinal nodes may be done (with local anesthesia) to obtain tissue for pathogenic analysis by culture or cytologic assessment.

Pleural biopsies may be performed surgically through a small thoracotomy incision or during thoracentesis, with use of a Cope needle. Needle biopsy is a relatively safe, simple diagnostic procedure useful in determining the cause of pleural effusions. The needle removes a small fragment of parietal pleura, which is used for microscopic cellular examination and culture. If bacteriologic studies are needed, the biopsy specimen should be obtained before chemotherapy is begun.

The preparation and positioning of a client for pleural biopsy is similar to that for thoracentesis. Rare complications include temporary pain from intercostal nerve injury, pneumothorax, and hemothorax. After the biopsy procedure, the nurse observes for indications of complications (e.g., dyspnea, pallor, diaphoresis, excessive pain). There is a possibility of the development of pneumothorax associated with needle biopsy. Chest tubes and chest drainage equipment must be available. Follow-up chest x-ray studies are usually taken after the procedure. The development of hemothorax is indicated by a substantial increase in fluid in the pleural space and requires immediate thoracentesis.

As with pleural biopsy, lung biopsy may be done by surgical exposure of the lung (open lung biopsy) or by use of a needle designed to remove a core of lung tissue. Tissue is then examined for abnormal cellular structure and bacteria. Lung biopsies are most often done to identify pulmonary tumors or parenchymal changes (e.g., sarcoidosis).

Needle puncture (aspiration) biopsy of chest lesions is done under fluoroscopy. After a lesion is found on a chest x-ray study and localized under fluoroscopy, topical anesthesia is administered, and the needle is inserted through the chest wall into the lung tissue and lesion. A small sample of cells is aspirated for microscopic study, and the needle is withdrawn. Aspiration biopsy may enable definitive diagnosis of malignant neoplasms, granulomas, or other nonmalignant growths. Possible complications of needle aspiration lung biopsy are hemoptysis, hemothorax, and pneumothorax. After the procedure, the nurse should examine any sputum closely for evidence of blood, observe for respiratory distress (which may indicate pneumothorax), and monitor vital signs, breath sounds, skin color, and temperature.

SPUTUM COLLECTION

Normally, the goblet cells produce 100 mL of mucus a day, but an infectious process can lead to excessive mucus production, commonly called sputum. Assessment of sputum for bacteria, fungus, or cellular elements assists the practitioner in treating the underlying infection. The sputum is initially inspected for color, quantity, quality, presence of blood, food particles, or other unusual contents. If possible, sputum should be collected before antimicrobial treatment is begun. Acid-fast smear and culture specimens are collected in the morning, when it is more plentiful and concentrated from pooling through the night. Sputum can be collected by the direct method or the indirect method, or by gastric lavage.

To obtain a specimen by the direct method, the client first brushes the teeth to reduce contamination, then he or she coughs into a sputum specimen container. The client should be encouraged to cough and not spit so as to obtain sputum. Sputum can be thinned by inhaling nebulized saline or water.

Indirect techniques to obtain sputum use a sterile suction catheter with a sputum trap attached to the catheter. Sputum can be obtained by transtracheal aspiration also. A puncture is made with a needle through the cricothyroid membrane into the trachea, and sputum is aspirated.

Gastric lavage is not a common technique to obtain sputum but can be used in uncooperative or extremely ill clients. Lavage is based on the assumption that sputum is swallowed while sleeping and sometimes after coughing. A nasogastric tube is inserted using appropriate techniques. Gastric juice is aspirated with a syringe and sent to the laboratory. The tube is then removed.

Once collected, the sputum is sent to the laboratory for Gram stain, culture, and sensitivity study. The Gram stain classifies the bacteria as gram-positive or gram-negative and provides guidelines for appropriate antimicrobial therapy, along with the sputum culture. After the Gram stain, the sputum is incubated for 24 hours on the appropriate culture medium and studied by a microbiologist. The culture allows further identification of the infecting organism. Once the organism is identified, its sensitivity to antibiotic treatment will be tested and appropriate antibiotic therapy prescribed.

Identification of organisms that cause tuberculosis and similar diseases (acid-fast bacilli) requires tests other than the Gram stain, culture, and sensitivity study. Regardless of the technique used to obtain the specimen, the nurse notes the color, consistency, odor, and amount of sputum obtained.

NOSE AND THROAT CULTURES

Bacteria in the nose and throat can be identified by culture during assessment of the upper airway. Some bacteria are normally present (e.g., streptococci, staphylococci, pneumococci, *Haemophilus influenzae,* and *Klebsiella pneumoniae*). Other organisms are abnormal (e.g., those causing diphtheria or tuberculosis).

The nurse takes a swab from the nose and throat using a sterile cotton swab and places the swab in a sterile culture tube. Some laboratories require the swab to be suspended in a tube containing 2 mL of fluid (to keep the air in the tube moist and prevent evaporation and drying of the specimen). The fluid is not a culture medium, so the swab should *not* touch the fluid. If Loeffler's medium is used in the tube (i.e., if diphtheria is suspected), the medium should touch the swab. When culture tubes without fluid are used, the specimen should be taken to the laboratory immediately, where the swab is streaked across a culture plate.

STUDY QUESTIONS

1. A client with a total laryngectomy will no longer have which of the following:
   A. The ability to communicate verbally
   B. The ability to filter or humidify air
   C. The ability to produce an effective cough
   D. All of the above
2. While the nurse is assessing the characteristics of a client's respiration, the client is hyperventilating. Hyperventilation would affect the central chemoreceptors because of:
   A. Changes in the PaO_2 in the blood
   B. Changes in pH of the blood
   C. Changes in pH in the cerebrospinal fluid
   D. Changes in PaO_2 in the cerebrospinal fluid
3. Client teaching prior to obtaining a sputum specimen should include all of the following instructions *except:*
   A. Brush the teeth to reduce oral bacteria
   B. Spit whatever is in the mouth into the container
   C. Take a few deep breaths prior to coughing
   D. Spit into a container upon first rising
4. Adventitious breath sounds that can be simulated by rolling a strand of hair between the fingers near the ear are called:
   A. Crackles–coarse
   B. Wheezes
   C. Crackles–fine
   D. Atelectatic crackles
5. The nurse reads the results of the client's ventilation-perfusion scan and notes that there is an obstruction of pulmonary blood flow. This result could occur because:
   A. Perfusion exceeds ventilation
   B. There is an absence of perfusion and ventilation
   C. Ventilation exceeds perfusion
   D. Ventilation and perfusion are equal

CRITICAL THINKING EXERCISES

SCENARIO A

A 74-year-old man is admitted for diagnostic workup of a potential carcinoma. He is scheduled for a bronchoscopy.

1. What anatomical structures are being evaluated by this procedure?
2. Which nursing interventions are appropriate prior to the bronchoscopy?
3. Shortly after the bronchoscopy, the client's wife asks the nurse if her husband can have something to eat. How would you respond?
4. You monitor the client for potential complications of a bronchoscopy. What parameters do you monitor?

SCENARIO B

A client is admitted with excess air on the left lung. She is to have a thoracentesis to remove this excess air.

1. What are the nursing responsibilities prior to the procedure?
2. Which positions would be most comfortable for the client during the thoracentesis?
3. The doctor asks you to expose the left chest. Which anatomic landmarks must you use?
4. After the thoracentesis, what do you need to monitor?

BIBLIOGRAPHY

1. Bates, B. (1991). *A guide to physical assessment and history taking* (5th ed.). Philadelphia: J. B. Lippincott.
2. Bolgiano, C. S., Bunting, K., & Shoenberger, M. M. (1990). Administrating oxygen therapy: What you need to know. *Nursing 90, 20(6).* 47–51.
3. Cherniack, R. M., & Cherniack, L. (1983). *Respiration in health and disease* (3rd ed.). Philadelphia: W. B. Saunders.
4. Comroe, J. H. (1974). *Physiology of respiration* (2nd ed.). Chicago: Year Book.
5. Gift, A. G., & Nield, M. D. (1991). Dyspnea: A case for nursing diagnosis status. *Nursing Diagnosis, 2(2),* 66–71.
6. Guyton, A. C. (1991). *Textbook of medical physiology* (8th ed.). Philadelphia: W. B. Saunders.
7. Holden, T. (1992). What keeps oxygenation on track? *American Journal of Nursing, 92(12),* 32–40.
8. Jarvis, C. (1992). *Physical examination and health assessment.* Philadelphia: W. B. Saunders.
9. Kersten, L. D. (1989). *Comprehensive respiratory nursing.* Philadelphia: W. B. Saunders.
10. McCord, M., & Cronin-Stubbs, D. (1992). Operationalizing dypsnea: Focus on measurement. *Heart & Lung, 21(2),* 167.
11. Murray, J. F. (1986). *The normal lung* (2nd ed.). Philadelphia: W. B. Saunders.
12. Murray, J. F., & Nadel, J. A. (1994). *The textbook of respiratory medicine* (2nd ed.). Philadelphia: W. B. Saunders.
13. Ruppel, G. (1994). *Manual of pulmonary function testing* (6th ed.). St. Louis: Mosby-Year Book.
14. Rutherford, K. A. (1989). Principles and application of oximetry. *Critical Care Nursing Clinics of North America, 1(4),* 649–657.
15. Shapiro, B. A., et al. (1991). *Clinical application of respiratory care* (4th ed.). St. Louis: Mosby-Year Book.
16. Shapiro, B. A., et al. (1994). *Clinical application of blood gases* (5th ed.). St. Louis: Mosby-Year Book.
17. Stiesmeyer, J. (1993). A four-step approach to pulmonary assessment. *American Journal of Nursing, 93(8),* 22–28.
18. University of Washington, School of Medicine (1989). *The respiratory system.* Seattle Health Sciences Academic Services.
19. Von Rueden, K. T. (1990). Noninvasive assessment of gas exchange in the critically ill. *AACN Clinical Issues in Critical Care Nursing, 1(2),* 239–247.
20. West, J. B. (1990). *Respiratory physiology* (4th ed.). Baltimore: Williams & Wilkins.

Chapter 20 Common Respiratory Interventions

Learning Outcomes

After completing this chapter, the learner will be able to:

1. Formulate a plan of care based on nursing assessment of the respiratory system.
2. Differentiate between interventions that can be performed by specifically trained specialists and nursing personnel.
3. Develop a teaching plan for the client with chronic obstructive pulmonary disease.
4. Perform invasive respiratory interventions such as suctioning.

It is important for nurses to understand the interventions administered by other health-care professionals as well as the interventions that are specifically nursing procedures. The most appropriate intervention is chosen for each client after consideration of both physical and psychosocial factors.

This chapter discusses in sequence the least invasive respiratory interventions (e.g., positioning, hydration) to the most invasive interventions (e.g., endotracheal intubation, mechanical ventilation).

General Interventions

POSITIONING AND POSTURE

Clients with respiratory problems can usually breathe more comfortably if they are positioned so that the head and chest are elevated. Elevating the chest and head promotes expansion of the lungs and increases the efficiency of the respiratory muscles. The client's rotating the shoulders backward will enable unrestricted movement of the diaphragm, thus facilitating diaphragmatic breathing. A semi-Fowler's position may be suitable for those clients with moderate respiratory distress. A client who is weak or severely dyspneic is often most comfortable sitting upright leaning on a padded overbed table. By resting the arms on the table, the client will increase the effectiveness of the secondary inspiratory muscles. While standing, clients with chronic respiratory disorders can often breathe most effectively by maintaining a straight posture leaning slightly forward.

ENVIRONMENTAL CONTROL

The single most important cause of respiratory irritation is cigarette smoke. Chronic pulmonary diseases (e.g., chronic bronchitis, pulmonary emphysema) and lung cancer are major health problems that are adversely affected by air pollution and cigarette smoking.

ACTIVITY AND REST

Some respiratory problems force clients to alter their normal activities of daily living. Certain acute disorders (e.g., influenza) require bed rest for several days before normal activity is resumed. Clients who experience chronic respiratory disorders may need to permanently modify their activities of daily living, change to sedentary work, or even retire. Remaining active for as long as possible is physically as well as psychosocially helpful for clients who suffer from chronic respiratory disorders. The nurse should encourage and facilitate activity and ambulation within the limits of the client's abilities and the physician's recommendations.

ORAL HYGIENE

Most clients with breathing difficulty breathe through the mouth. Mouth breathing dries the oral mucosa, and dry mucosa increases the risk of stomatitis. Coughing is common in this population of clients, and sputum may dry to the oral mucosa. For these reasons, thorough oral hygiene is important for clients with respiratory problems. It may improve appetite and promote a general feeling of well being.

CRITICAL TO REMEMBER

Oral hygiene is essential after the administration of aerosolized mucolytics, steroids, antibiotics, and enzymes because these medications may interfere with the balance of normal flora that prevents infection.

Gas-forming foods (e.g., beans, cabbage) are undesirable because they produce abdominal distention, which may lead to decreased ventilation.

HYDRATION

Optimal hydration (1) helps liquefy bronchopulmonary secretions for easier removal (thick, tenacious secretions are difficult to cough up and expectorate) and (2) prevents constipation and fluid imbalances. The nurse should encourage a client with tenacious secretions to take 3000 to 4000 mL of fluid a day.

CRITICAL TO REMEMBER

Before encouraging a client to drink this much water, the nurse should be certain the client has no pre-existing cardiac or renal disorders that might impair fluid excretion.

A client confined to bed needs fresh fluids that are within easy reach. The nurse should document fluid intake and output.

INFECTION PREVENTION AND CONTROL

Opportunistic infections are of increasing importance. They may be drug-induced or nosocomial. To control infection or prevent its development, the nurse must employ prophylactic measures (Box 20–1).

BOX 20-1

Infection Control Prophylaxis

To control infection or prevent its development, the nurse should use prophylactic measures such as

- proper handwashing with a bacteriostatic soap
- observing universal precautions to prevent cross-contamination
- turning and repositioning clients confined to bed
- encouraging activity, coughing, and deep breathing to mobilize secretions
- maintaining a clear airway
- changing respiratory therapy equipment daily (e.g., aerosol tubes, humidifiers)
- restricting contact with clients who have respiratory or other infections
- isolating clients with infectious disorders to reduce spread
- maintaining resistance to disease in clients with respiratory problems by adequate rest, nutrition, and hydration
- teaching how to prevent the spread of airborne infections; e.g., cover nose and mouth with disposable tissues when sneezing or coughing, dispose of tissues carefully, wash hands frequently
- assessing for indications of infection in clients receiving chemotherapeutic agents or corticosteroids and for development of superinfections in clients receiving antibiotics
- administering antibiotics as prescribed. Specific antibiotic prescriptions are based on bacteriologic culture and sensitivity reports. Sometimes broad-spectrum antibiotics are prescribed before culture sensitivity reports are available.

Clients with chronic respiratory problems can try to avoid repeated respiratory infections by

- wearing warm, dry, protective clothing while outside in cold or damp weather
- avoiding excessive exertion in very cold or humid environments
- balancing work, rest, and recreation
- avoiding crowded places when respiratory infections are prevalent
- avoiding smoke-filled environments and not smoking
- taking influenza shots and antibiotics as prescribed
- observing sputum for signs of infection (e.g., increased amounts, change in color)
- consulting a physician if a new infection seems to be developing. Even infections that appear "minor" need vigorous treatment to prevent progressive, serious superinfections
- receiving pneumococcal vaccine

PSYCHOSOCIAL SUPPORT

Reducing anxiety is very important because anxiety worsens symptoms such as dyspnea and bronchospasm. Some respiratory conditions produce frightening feelings such as suffocation or choking, causing the client to panic and fight for air. Some symptoms may be disturbing for the client, significant others, and nurses. The nurse should teach the client to dispose of tissues properly and to cover the mouth and nose when coughing.

Many respiratory conditions are difficult to accept and live with (e.g., lung cancer, emphysema). The nurse can support the client and significant others in making realistic future plans.

Chronic respiratory disease necessitates many changes and adaptations. The goals of care are to preserve and make the most of existing lung function and to prevent further deterioration. These limitations are often hard for clients to accept. The acceptance process is an individual one. Denial of respiratory symptoms is not unusual until the severity of symptoms eventually forces recognition of the illness by the client and significant others. Even when professional help is sought, some clients resist recommended treatment. Such clients may need extra education to obtain information and planning sessions to experience some control in decision making.

Self-care is essential with respiratory disorders and should start with relieving specific self-care problems in daily living. For example, clients may need to learn more effective ways to control breathing before they can learn about postural drainage and exercises. Self-care activities may include (1) performing postural drainage and breathing exercises, (2) increasing daily fluid intake, (3) taking prescribed medication, and (4) performing specific respiratory therapies. The nurse should praise clients who faithfully follow their recommended regimens and encourage those who are unable to do so and who feel discouraged.

CRITICAL TO REMEMBER

The nurse should allow clients to develop their own daily routine. Dyspneic clients often need frequent rest periods and usually know when they can be most comfortably active during the day.

Clients producing sputum usually know when postural drainage is most effective (e.g., before getting out of bed). Some clients develop ritualistic and apparently compulsive patterns around their daily routines. The nurse should not interfere with these patterns, as the client perceives them as useful and necessary.

Whenever possible, significant others should be in teaching and planning sessions on long-term respiratory intervention. The nurse must remember that family members are experiencing stress also and may become tired, despondent, and frustrated. They too may need professional support.

Respiratory Pharmacologic Agents

Various pharmacologic agents are used to treat clients with respiratory disorders. Some of the more common classifications are presented in Table 20–1. Medications are discussed further throughout the unit in relation to specific respiratory conditions.

Respiratory Therapy

ADMINISTERING OXYGEN

Oxygen (O_2) is administered to treat the harmful and possibly lethal effects of hypoxemia (lowered blood oxygen). The need for oxygen is assessed by arterial blood gases (ABGs), oxygen saturation measuring devices (oximeters), and monitoring for indications of hypoxemia. Oxygen, used for both acute and chronic conditions, does not cure a disease. Examples of pulmonary and nonpulmonary disorders that may cause hypoxemia and the need for supplemental oxygen include airway obstruction, pulmonary edema, acute respiratory failure, chronic respiratory insufficiency, cardiac disorders, metabolic disorders, and shock.

CRITICAL TO REMEMBER

Oxygen should never be withheld from a hypoxic client. However, like any drug, oxygen is prescribed in dosages safe for the client.

Indications

Oxygen administration is required whenever hypoxemia occurs or is expected to occur. With the relief of hypoxemia, hypoxia (reduced oxygen in tissues) can be prevented.

There are three major indications for oxygen administration: reduced arterial blood oxygen, increased work of breathing, and need for decreased myocardial workload (Box 20–2).

Complications

OXYGEN-INDUCED HYPOVENTILATION

A normal respiratory drive occurs when blood carbon dioxide rises slightly and stimulates the primary respiratory centers in the medulla and pons. Secondary respiratory centers in the carotid bodies and the arch of the aorta are activated by decreases in blood oxygen tension (e.g., lower than 60 mm Hg). Clients with chronic respiratory dysfunction may retain carbon dioxide. When carbon dioxide is retained over a long period of time, the medullary center in the brain is no longer stimulated by the increased level of carbon dioxide in

Text continued on page 512

BOX 20–2

Indications for Oxygen Administration

REDUCED ARTERIAL BLOOD OXYGEN

Tissue hypoxia is impossible to measure accurately because levels vary greatly in different body parts. Hypoxemia, however, may be assessed by measuring the amount of oxygen in a sample of arterial blood (ABG analysis). Normal arterial blood oxygen levels range from 80 to 100 mm Hg. If the arterial blood oxygen level (PaO_2) falls below normal, supplemental oxygen usually corrects the hypoxemia if the hypoxemia is caused by hypoventilation or small ventilation or perfusion defects. If the hypoxemia is caused by ventilation or perfusion mismatch that is greater than 25 per cent, such as in adult respiratory distress syndrome (ARDS) or pneumonia, other methods of oxygen administration may be needed.

INCREASED WORK OF BREATHING

The body responds to hypoxemia by increasing the rate and depth of respirations in an effort to bring more oxygen into the blood. Consequently, a hypoxemic client shows signs of respiratory distress (e.g., use of accessory muscles, diaphoresis, cyanosis). A vicious cycle develops as respiratory effort increases, the body requires more and more oxygen to support the effort, and oxygen consumption increases accordingly. The result is fatigue and possibly respiratory arrest or cardiac complications. Hypoxemia can be relieved when supplemental oxygen is administered to a client with signs of increased work of breathing. As hypoxemia is relieved, the client no longer requires additional respiratory effort and resumes a normal breathing pattern.

NEED FOR DECREASED MYOCARDIAL WORKLOAD

When the body becomes hypoxemic, the heart attempts to compensate for the lack of oxygen by increasing the cardiac output. Although the heart's increased output circulates the available oxygen to the tissues more quickly and efficiently, the myocardial workload increases. Administering supplemental oxygen increases the amount of oxygen available to the tissues, thus decreasing hypoxemia and myocardial workload. Because hypoxemia stresses the myocardium, oxygen is prescribed for clients experiencing myocardial infarction, congestive heart failure, coronary artery disease, or other cardiac problems.

TABLE 20–1 Pharmacologic Management of Respiratory Disorders

CLASS	EXAMPLE	ACTION	USE	COMMON SIDE EFFECTS	NURSING IMPLICATIONS
Antimicrobials					
Penicillins	Penicillin G sodium Penicillin G procaine (Wycillin) Penicillin V potassium (Pen-Vee K) Nafcillin (Unipen) Ampicillin Amoxicillin Carbenicillin Ticarcillin		Bactericidal against a wide variety of gram-positive and some gram-negative organisms Most effective in the treatment of bacterial pneumonia	Allergic reactions (skin rashes, anaphylaxis) Gastrointestinal disturbances (nausea and vomiting, epigastric distress) Central nervous system toxicity manifested by hallucinations, hyperreflexia, seizures when administered in very large doses to patients with neurologic reactions (thrombocytopenia, agranulocytosis, anemia) Impaired renal function	Check for history of penicillin allergy before administration of drug Observe for allergic manifestations and other side effects Evaluate effects of drug especially when given concurrently with drugs that may increase or decrease its action, e.g., gentamicin is synergistic to penicillin; probenecid decreases its renal excretion; tetracycline and erythromycin both inhibit bactericidal activity of penicillin Monitor for development of resistant organisms; susceptibility testing should be done before and during the course of therapy
Cephalosporins	Cephalexin (Keflex) Cefamandole (Mandol) Cefazolin (Ancef, Kefzol) Cephalothin (Keflin) Cefoxitin (Mefoxin) Cephapirin (Cefadyl)		Effective against numerous infections but used primarily for *Klebsiella pneumoniae* along with aminoglycoside	Gastrointestinal disturbances Nephrotoxicity (decreased urine output and creatinine clearance, hematuria, proteinuria) Phlebitis with intravenous administration	Assess for allergic reactions to cephalosporins and penicillins; it is controversial whether cephalosporins can be given without causing allergic reactions when there is a known hypersensitivity to penicillin Monitor for toxic side effects Assess effectiveness when administered with bacteriostatic antibiotics, e.g., tetracyclines and erythromycins, which may decrease or destroy their effects

Table continued on following page

TABLE 20–1 Pharmacologic Management of Respiratory Disorders *Continued*

CLASS	EXAMPLE	ACTION	USE	COMMON SIDE EFFECTS	NURSING IMPLICATIONS
Aminoglycosides	Kanamycin (Kantrex) Neomycin Amikacin sulfate Gentamicin (Garamycin) Tobramycin Streptomycin		Bactericidal against a wide range of gram-positive and gram-negative bacteria and mycobacteria; however, they differ in clinical uses Streptomycin: used in the treatment of tuberculosis in combination with other tuberculostatic drugs Neomycin: used for reducing intestinal flora and thereby decreasing blood ammonia levels Gentamicin: used to treat bacteremia caused by *Proteus, Pseudomonas, Escherichia coli,* and *Klebsiella* Amikacin and tobramycin: used to treat gentamicin-resistant infection	Ototoxicity Nephrotoxocity Neuromuscular blockage Peripheral neuritis Resistant infection	Assess client for beginning auditory and vestibular damage, e.g., vertigo, ataxia, roaring in the ears, hearing loss Monitor renal function, especially when administered to elderly clients or to those with renal insufficiency Monitor peak and trough levels and drug dosages Assess neuromuscular effects, especially when administered with muscle relaxants and sedatives
Tetracyclines	Chlortetracycline HCl (Aureomycin) Demeclocycline HCl (Declomycin) Doxycycline hyclate (Vibramycin)		Bacteriostatic for many gram-negative and gram-positive organisms, including mycobacteria, rickettsiae, mycoplasma, and agents of psittacosis	Gastrointestinal disturbances Allergic reactions Hepatotoxicity Enamel hypoplasia Permanent staining of teeth when used during tooth development	Avoid use in children, during pregnancy, and when there is impaired hepatic or renal function Do not administer with food, milk, milk products, antacids because they inhibit tetracycline absorption Monitor client for a developing superinfection Monitor liver function in long-term therapy Instruct client to avoid direct sunlight because sunburn reaction or erythema is likely to occur

TABLE 20–1 Pharmacologic Management of Respiratory Disorders *Continued*

CLASS	EXAMPLE	ACTION	USE	COMMON SIDE EFFECTS	NURSING IMPLICATIONS
Bronchodilators					
Beta-adrenergics	Albuterol (Ventolin) Isoproterenol (Isuprel) Terbutaline (Brethine)	Relaxation of constricted airways by stimulating beta-adrenergic receptors	Symptomatic relief of asthma and bronchial spasms	Gastrointestinal upset Nausea Nervousness, anxiety Frequency Diarrhea Insomnia Tachycardia Palpitations Esophageal reflux Tremors	Use with caution in clients with hypertension, tachycardia, hypoxemia, glaucoma, hyperthyroidism, benign prostatic hypertrophy, diabetes Monitor for central nervous system symptoms Give with food or antacids; avoid smoking
Theophylline	Theophylline (Theo-Dur)	Bronchial relaxation by inhibition of the breakdown of cyclic adenosine monophosphate			
Adrenal glucocorticoids	Prednisone Beclomethasone (Vanceril)	Reduce inflammation and inflammatory response in bronchial walls	Symptomatic relief and preventive care of asthma	With systemic agents—gastrointestinal upset, gastric irritation and ulceration, euphoria, hunger, insomnia, adrenal shutdown	Administer in morning if dosage is four times daily; give with food Plan to supplement clients with cortisone agents during periods of stress
Antitussives	Narcotics: any product with codeine Non-narcotics: dextromethorphan	Suppress cough reflex Act centrally on the cough center or peripherally within the tracheobronchial tree to decrease sensitivity to irritant receptors	To treat dry, nonproductive coughs that interfere with sleep or other activities	Dizziness Sedation Sweating Nausea Dry mouth Constipation Urinary retention Palpitations	Caution client about possible sedation Administer with caution to patients with asthma, COPD, cardiac disease, convulsions, renal or hepatic disease, central nervous system depression, benign prostatic hypertrophy, alcoholism, or hypothyroidism
Mucolytics	Water Acetylcysteine (Mucomyst)	Thin mucus	Chronic pulmonary conditions that lead to thick, dry sputum	Bronchospasm with Mucomyst	Administer Mucomyst by aerosolized bronchodilator
Antiallergenics	Cromolyn sodium (Intal)	Stabilizes mast cell	Asthma, especially due to exercise or allergen exposure	Headache Rash Cough Worsening of asthma	Require 3 weeks of continuous therapy before they are effective Use in decreased dosages for clients with liver or renal disorders

Table continued on following page

TABLE 20–1 Pharmacologic Management of Respiratory Disorders *Continued*

CLASS	EXAMPLE	ACTION	USE	COMMON SIDE EFFECTS	NURSING IMPLICATIONS
Antihistamines	Diphenhydramine HCl (Benadryl)	Block action of histamine at H_1-receptor sites, smooth muscles of the blood vessels, bronchioles, and gastrointestinal tract	Relieve symptoms of allergies Adjunct in treatment of anaphylaxis	Sedation Epigastric distress Hypotension Palpitations Tachycardia Thickening of bronchial secretions Vertigo Urinary frequency	Warn about sedation Use carefully in clients with convulsions, hyperthyroidism, cardiovascular and renal disease, hypertension, diabetes Avoid use with alcohol Monitor for dry mucous membranes Give with meals or antacids
	Terfenadine (Seldane)	Specific, selective histamine H_1-receptor antagonist		Dryness of nose, mouth Dysrhythmias when used to toxic levels	Do not use in conjunction with ketoconazole or levamisole (Ergamisole). Use cautiously with erythromycin
Cough preparations Expectorants	Guaifenesin (Robitussin)	Facilitate removal of thick mucus from lungs and act as soothing demulcent by stimulating secretion of a lubricant	Facilitate productive cough	Nausea and vomiting Gastrointestinal irritation Drowsiness	Instruct client not to use more than 1 week without seeing physician Use high fluid intake and humidity to loosen secretions Do not follow with water, except potassium iodide
Decongestants	Ephedrine sulfate (Efedron)	Dry mucous membranes and reduced mucus production	Reduce allergy and cold symptoms	Rebound inflammation of mucous membranes	Instruct client not to use for more than 1 week without seeing physician

COPD, Chronic obstructive pulmonary disease.
Adapted from Matassarin-Jacobs, E. (1990). *Saunders review for NCLEX-RN*. Philadelphia: W. B. Saunders.

the blood. In these clients, respiration is stimulated by low levels of oxygen in the blood (arterial oxygen tension [PaO_2]). Administration of unspecified and unmonitored doses of oxygen may depress ventilation (hypoventilation) or even cause apnea. Serial ABGs alert the nurse to increasing arterial carbon dioxide tension ($PaCO_2$) levels. However, the risk of oxygen-induced hypoventilation in clients with suspected chronic pulmonary disease should not prevent the administration of oxygen in life-threatening situations. Chronic carbon dioxide retention is diagnosed by a baseline $PaCO_2$ above 45 mm Hg with a compensated pH (pH in the normal range or slightly acidotic).

OXYGEN TOXICITY

Oxygen toxicity is a medically induced, potentially fatal, progressive condition in which ventilatory failure occurs in clients who inspire a high concentration of oxygen for a prolonged period of time. The development of oxygen toxicity is related to both time and dose. Pathophysiologic changes begin within the lungs after 24 to 48 hours of exposure to high oxygen concentrations.

Early indications of oxygen toxicity may include a mild tracheobronchitis that begins as a substernal soreness, nasal congestion, pain on inspiration, and increased coughing. As the condition worsens, the cough becomes more severe, substernal soreness increases, and dyspnea develops. Prolonged exposure to oxygen in high concentrations may cause structural damage to the lung tissue (e.g., interstitial edema, thickening of the alveolar capillary membranes, intra-alveolar hemorrhage, and atelectasis). These changes impair the transport of oxygen. Clients at risk for oxygen toxicity are those on bleomycin or steroids and those with hyperthermia, hyperthyroidism, protein deficiency, vitamin E deficiency, and adrenergic stimulation.

Assessment findings at the end stage of oxygen toxicity include progressive atelectasis, consolidation, and fibrosis of the lung. Chest films show progressive opacification of the lungs. Oxygenation is greatly impaired and breathing is difficult owing to decreasing compliance. Auscultation may reveal diminished breath sounds and audible crackles.

Analysis of ABGs is monitored to prevent oxygen toxicity. If a client develops oxygen toxicity, ABG values show a decreasing PaO_2 with an increased fractional inspired oxygen (FIO_2) requirement. At the same time, an increase in the pressure required to deliver a mechanical ventilator breath is noted. This increased pressure may indicate a decrease in lung compliance or the ability of the lung to stretch or distend.

Intervention for oxygen toxicity is aimed at maintaining adequate oxygenation at the lowest FIO_2 possible and treating the underlying, precipitating disease. The best intervention is to prevent oxygen toxicity from occurring.

Even when a client demonstrates oxygen toxicity, oxygenation must be supported. Unfortunately, a dangerous cycle occurs because the "stiff" or noncompliant lungs require high levels of oxygen for hypoxemia to be prevented, and yet the oxygen itself is the cause of the problem.

Nursing assessment and intervention for clients with oxygen toxicity include

- emotional support for the client and family
- assessment of fluid and electrolyte status
- monitoring and documenting ABG response to changes in treatment (ABGs are usually taken every 3 to 4 hours or as needed)
- assessing and documenting inspired oxygen concentration after any change in FIO_2
- aseptic airway care (lung damage increases the risk of infection)
- prevention of any further damage or complications by using positive end-expiratory pressure to reduce FIO_2

Atelectasis. As a result of increased oxygen concentrations in the inspired air, alveoli may collapse. The mechanism for this oxygen-induced side effect is the elimination of nitrogen from the lungs. Most nitrogen remains in the alveoli, adding volume to the alveoli, which in turn helps to prevent alveolar collapse. When the level of inspired oxygen rises, the oxygen molecules replace the nitrogen molecules. However, oxygen molecules are readily absorbed into the bloodstream, leaving the alveoli empty and thus predisposing them to collapse. In addition to the loss of intra-alveolar volume, hyperoxia retards the production of surfactant. Loss of surfactant also allows the forces of surface tension to collapse the affected alveolar units. These collapsed alveoli continue to be perfused with blood, which leads to hypoxemia. Hypoxemia results from unoxygenated blood passing these closed alveolar units without receiving oxygen, a condition known as intrapulmonary shunting.

The nurse should carefully assess clients receiving high concentrations of oxygen for indications of atelectasis, including vague discomfort, anxiety, tachypnea, fever, cough, tachycardia, shortness of breath, and substernal retractions. Assessment findings vary, depending on the extent of atelectasis. The physician should be made aware of ABG and x-ray results. Auscultation demonstrates diminished or absent breath sounds in the affected areas. Serial parameter checks of vital capacity, inspiratory force, and tidal volume indicate the degree of impairment.

Nursing interventions appropriate for clients with atelectasis may include early ambulation, coughing, deep breathing, incentive spirometry, hydration, and frequent position changes. The nurse should watch for changes in oxygenation with position changes. Gravitational effects on the blood flow can result in hypoxemia owing to the intrapulmonary shunting. ABG analysis with supplemental oxygen administration may be necessary if hypoxemia occurs.

Atelectasis may occur in other situations, including hypoventilation, impingement of a portion of the lung by space-occupying lesions, mucous plugs, effects of anesthesia, immobility, pleural effusion, and pneumothorax.

OCULAR DAMAGE

Retinal injury can occur in adults exposed to 100 per cent oxygen. Arterial oxygen tensions of 150 mm Hg for a period of greater than 4 hours can cause retrolental fibroplasia. Clients with previous retinal disease (e.g., retinal detachment) are especially vulnerable. Tearing, edema, and visual impairment result from the toxic effects of high concentrations of oxygen on the cornea and lens of adults.

Nursing Management

The nurse must become familiar with the various methods of oxygen administration and be knowledgeable about oxygen therapy so that he or she can administer as well as detect equipment malfunction. The percentages of oxygen delivered by most equipment are approximate.

A nurse responsible for oxygen therapy must know about the hazards of oxygen therapy and the clinical indications of hypoxia, respiratory acidosis, carbon dioxide narcosis, respiratory alkalosis, and oxygen toxicity. (Respiratory acidosis and alkalosis are discussed in Chap. 4.)

Nursing intervention during oxygen administration includes

- correctly administering the prescribed amount of oxygen
- maintaining a patent airway by correct positioning, suctioning, and productive coughing
- giving mouth and nose care every 3 to 4 hours
- changing the client's position periodically and providing skin care
- changing equipment as necessary (e.g., changing tanks before they become empty)
- providing appropriate education
- offering psychosocial support to the client and family

When oxygen is administered for the first time, the nurse should explain the process to the client, demonstrate the equipment, and explain the expected outcomes of the oxygen therapy. A dyspneic person may initially remove an oxygen administration device if the equipment increases the feeling of suffocation. An oxygen nasal cannula is usually more comfortable than a mask. Careful assessment of clients on oxygen systems is important, especially during the first 30 to 60 minutes when oxygen-induced hypoventilation can develop.

Some clients become dependent on oxygen and are afraid to have it discontinued even when it is no longer necessary. The oxygen should be withdrawn gradually. Sometimes it helps to keep oxygen available for 2 to 3 days to be used only for respiratory distress. When clients realize that most activities are possible without oxygen, the dependency on it diminishes.

Oxygen Delivery Systems

Oxygen is supplied for administration from either a portable tank (cylinder) or a wall outlet (which leads via pipes to large stores of oxygen). Oxygen can be administered by masks, nasal cannula, face tent, ventilator, or nebulizer. The equipment used to administer oxygen is divided into two categories: low-flow and high-flow systems. The terms refer to the rates of oxygen delivered by the equipment. Low-flow systems deliver oxygen at flow rates that supplement the oxygen contained in ambient (room) air. High-flow systems meet or exceed the client's inspiratory flow rate, allowing an accurate delivery of inspired oxygen (Table 20–2).

HUMIDITY AND AEROSOL THERAPY

Humidity is water vapor in the air. An aerosol is a suspension of solid or liquid particles in a flow of gas. Because oxygen and other compressed gases are dry (contain no water vapor), humidity may be added to them before they are inhaled. If an inhaled mist is needed to prevent mucosal drying and secretion retention, an aerosol is indicated.

Humidification. Humidifiers are devices that add water vapor (humidity) to inspired gas. Humidity is needed to decrease the drying effects of the gases and increase comfort. Moist air (1) prevents drying and irritation of respiratory mucous membranes, (2) prevents drying and thickening of respiratory tract secretions, and (3) loosens secretions, making them more easily removed. Dry, thick secretions form plugs and crusts within the tracheobronchial tree. Mucous plugging may result in inadequate ventilation and obstruction.

Nebulization (Aerosolization). Nebulizers are used (1) for airway hydration, (2) for administration of aerosolized medication, and (3) as an adjunct therapy for the mobilization of retained secretions. Water, isotonic saline, and 0.25 to 0.45 per cent saline may be nebulized to hydrate the airways and liquefy inspissated secretions that occlude the airway. However, bronchospasm can be induced by aerosolization of any substance. Clients who develop bronchospasm from nebulized saline are probably better treated with bronchodilator therapy.

Nebulizers used for hydration, large-volume nebulizers, are most often used for continuous aerosol therapy. Small-volume nebulizers (e.g., bronchodilators, mucolytics) are used to administer medication to the respiratory system.

Mist therapy is sometimes ordered before or during intermittent positive-pressure breathing treatments or postural drainage. The nurse should prepare clients carefully for mist treatments and stay with them

TABLE 20–2 Oxygen Concentration in Various Delivery Systems

TYPE OF FACE MASK	FLOW SYSTEM	L/MIN	O_2, %*
Nasal cannula	Low flow	1 to 6 L/min	24 to 44
Simple face mask	Low flow	5 to 8 L/min	40 to 60
Partial rebreather mask	Low flow	6 to 10 L/min	60 to 80
Non-rebreather mask†	Low flow	6 to 15 L/min	95 to 100
Venturi mask‡	High flow	4 to 15 L/min	24 to 40 or 50
Face tent	Low flow	4 to 8 L/min	30 to 55

* All oxygen masks must fit securely to provide the highest percentage of oxygen.

† The non-rebreather mask gives the highest oxygen concentration possible other than intubation or mechanical ventilation.

‡ The Venturi mask delivers oxygen concentrations precise to within 1%. This mask can deliver a very controlled amount of oxygen, e.g., 4 L/min blue adapter = 24%; 8 L/min green adapter = 35%. When the O_2 is jetted into the tube, air is pulled from the room and oxygen is mixed, providing a precise mixture within 1% accuracy. When using the Venturi mask, prevent occlusion of air entrainment ports by bed linen, clothing, or other objects. Obtain an order from physician for O_2 per nasal cannula while client is eating. If the client is on Venturi O_2 concentration of 24%, he or she should receive O_2 by nasal cannula at 1 L flow (20% atmospheric oxygen + 4% O_2 = 24%), 28% Venturi = 2 L flow. The Venturi mask is replaced when client is finished eating.

throughout the treatment to ensure that they are familiar with the procedure and benefit from it. The nurse should teach them to cough effectively during and after the mist treatment and document tolerance of the procedure (emotionally and physically) and the effectiveness of the treatment (e.g., amount of sputum produced).

Nebulization may be prescribed as a continuous or intermittent procedure. Nebulized medication is specifically prescribed, including amount and frequency. If metered dose inhalers are used, a specific number of inhalations is prescribed. If other types of aerosol generators are used, treatment may take 10 to 20 minutes.

The nurse should assess the client carefully, documenting the effectiveness of treatment and any adverse reactions. For example, if bronchospasm was evident before therapy, did a nebulized bronchodilator improve the quality of breath sounds?

Nebulized air is also used in clients with tracheostomy. Tracheostomy creates an artificial air passage that bypasses the upper airway (see Chap. 21). Thus, the "new airway" is exposed to air that is not warmed, moistened, or filtered by upper respiratory mucosa. Nebulization or a cool mist is therefore used immediately after tracheostomy is established. A relative humidity of 100 per cent is desirable. The temperature of the nebulized mist may need to be monitored to prevent possible hyperthermia.

CRITICAL TO REMEMBER

For preventing infection, it is important to use sterile nebulized solution and to change and sterilize the tubings, nebulizer, and connections at least every 24 hours.

After aerosol treatments, postural drainage, chest percussion, and expulsive coughing may be carried out. Nasal and oral hygiene should be performed to remove the secretions from the mucous membranes.

FACILITATING EFFECTIVE COUGHING

Effective coughing is of utmost importance. An effective cough augments the body's own ciliary clearance mechanisms, thus helping to maintain patent airways. Ineffective (forced) coughing may cause adverse effects in clients with severe chronic lung disease. It may (1) collapse airways, producing air trapping; (2) rupture thin-walled alveoli (blebs); or (3) cause pneumothorax. Ineffective coughing is especially dangerous for clients with unstable cardiac and cerebral function. An effective cough is one in which the client uses (1) the diaphragm; (2) posture; (3) slow, deep, stacked breaths; and (4) short expulsive blasts of air to mobilize and expectorate secretions.

Five steps that the client can take to create an effective cough while ensuring that muscular energy is not wasted are to

- assume a position that will facilitate effective use of the abdominal muscles. Assume a sitting position with the knees slightly flexed. If sitting in a chair or on the side of the bed is not possible, sit with the head of the bed raised and flex the knees with the feet planted firmly on the mattress.
- take slow, deep inspirations, using diaphragmatic breathing
- bear down against the glottis to produce a Valsalva-type maneuver. When the pressure inside the thorax peaks, a cough will be produced.
- exhale through pursed lips. Prolonged exhalation will move secretions to one of the tracheobronchial cough reflex centers.
- learn coughing technique before it is needed. Preoperative teaching about proper coughing techniques has been shown to be very effective. Coughing and pain medication administration should be maximized. Splinting of the operative site may help to alleviate some of the discomfort as well.

Box 20–3 lists some nursing interventions that can facilitate effective coughing. Modifications of the coughing technique are needed in those clients with chronic obstructive pulmonary disease (COPD) and early airway collapse. Effective coughing can be produced if smaller amounts of air are inspired before coughing. This technique creates less change in the intrathoracic pressure, which may help to prevent early airway collapse.

Incentive Spirometry

When performed properly, deep breathing plays a key role in preventing and treating atelectasis. A deep

BOX 20-3

Nursing Interventions to Facilitate Effective Coughing

- Position change. Roll the client from side to side to cause secretions to drain into large airways.
- Increased level of activity. Have the client sit in a chair or walk around. Encourage deep, diaphragmatic breathing with slow exhalation during ambulation.
- Vibrations/end-expiratory assist. Place your hands around the client's lower ribs. As the client exhales or coughs, apply firm, upward vibrating pressure. This often supports the thorax enough to achieve an expulsive cough.
- Sips of water. A few sips of water or a cup of hot tea or coffee may stimulate coughing.
- Manually stimulated cough. Use a manual, self-inflating resuscitation bag to give a deep inflation to a client who has a tracheostomy or endotracheal tube. This often loosens secretions and promotes a cough in a client with an artificial airway.
- Splinting with a pillow over the client's abdomen.
- As a last resort, consider alternatives to coughing, such as suctioning.

breath is a very potent bronchodilator and is essential for effective coughing.

Incentive spirometry is used to encourage maximal deep breathing; it is a form of goal-directed therapy. The incentive to perform is provided by visualizing the amount of volume that is being achieved with each inspiration. The goal or volume to be achieved with each inspiration is set by the practitioner. The goals are individualized for each client. The goals set should be obtainable but only after some reasonable effort. Incentive breathing devices affect the inspiratory capacity and work on the principle of sustained, voluntary, maximal inflation.

Incentive spirometry is most effective if taught to the client before it is needed (e.g., preoperatively) rather than when a client is sedated or in pain. It is often used to encourage deep breathing after surgery. People with pneumonia and neuromuscular weakness, and those on prolonged bed rest are also helped by incentive spirometry. The nurse should teach the client to perform a minimum of 8 to 10 sustained, voluntary, maximal inflation maneuvers an hour. He or she should leave the device near the client and supervise the client and increase the goals frequently (see the Client Education Guide: Incentive Spirometry).

Other types of respiratory therapy that may be used with incentive spirometry to optimize bronchopulmonary hygiene include (1) hydration; (2) aerosolized medications; (3) mobilization maneuvers such as turning, position changes, and ambulation; (4) chest physiotherapy; (5) breathing retraining; (6) assistance with and encouragement in effective coughing techniques; and (7) postural drainage.

BREATHING RETRAINING

Acute or chronic respiratory dysfunction often predisposes to ineffective breathing habits. Breathing retraining involves various methods to improve breathing patterns and ensure maximal use of the available respiratory function. It allows clients to "get the most out of what they have" and teaches them how to control breathing.

To be effective, breathing retraining must be correctly learned and performed constantly as a part of the client's way of life.

Breathing retraining must be adapted to a client's needs and not cause undue stress or increase dyspnea. The nurse should teach the client to do the following before beginning breathing exercises:

- Clear the respiratory tract of secretions by coughing. Suctioning may be necessary.
- Use an aerosolized bronchodilator to open the air passages and loosen tenacious mucus, then cough.
- Perform postural drainage to help remove secretions.
- Clear nasal passages. If blowing the nose does not bring relief, decongestant medications may be prescribed.

DIAPHRAGMATIC BREATHING (ABDOMINAL BREATHING)

Clients with COPD (e.g., emphysema) have lost much of the elastic tissue in the lung. These clients use accessory muscles to breathe, such as the shoulder muscles, which are much less effective. This change results in pulmonary distention, gas trapping, and inefficient use of the respiratory muscles. By learning diaphragmatic breathing, the diaphragm is used more effectively, thereby decreasing the use of accessory muscles and the work of breathing.

CRITICAL TO REMEMBER

Expected benefits of diaphragmatic breathing include an increased tidal volume, a decreased respiratory rate, an increased exercise tolerance, and an increase in alveolar ventilation.

When performed properly, diaphragmatic breathing causes the abdomen to rise visibly during deep inhalation and contract during exhalation. Tightening the abdominal muscles during exhalation helps the diaphragm squeeze air out of the lungs. By placing one hand on the abdomen and the other on the chest, the client can feel if breathing is correct while sitting up or reclining (see the Client Education Guide: Diaphragmatic Breathing).

Diaphragmatic breathing requires practice to become part of one's normal breathing. Gradually the client adjusts this controlled breathing pattern to the rhythm of body movements (e.g., walking) and develops rhythm in which exhalation takes at least twice as long as inhalation. A metronome may help establish this rhythm.

Some breathing exercises emphasize forced exhalation to force "trapped" air out of the lungs while using a diaphragmatic breathing pattern. One method is to push on the chest with the flattened palms of the hands while exhaling. Another exercise is to pull a band of material snugly around the chest while exhaling and

CLIENT EDUCATION GUIDE

Incentive Spirometry

The nurse should set attainable goals for the client and give the following instructions:

1. Exhale slowly to a point of comfort.
2. Place the mouthpiece between the teeth and place the lips around the mouthpiece.
3. Inhaling through the mouth only (a noseclip may be necessary), take in a slow, deep breath (using the diaphragm, not the accessory muscles), until the preset goal is attained.
4. Hold the breath for 3 to 5 seconds.
5. Exhale normally.
6. Rest between attempts.
7. Repeat steps 2, 4, 5, and 6.

CLIENT EDUCATION GUIDE

Diaphragmatic Breathing

1. Help the client get comfortable, both physically and mentally.
2. Help the client assume a comfortable semi-Fowler's position with shoulders rotated slightly inward and with the knees bent.
3. Place your thumbs in the client's epigastric notch, i.e., just below the xiphoid process. Comfortably spread your fingers around the lower ribs. Maintain this position.
4. Ask the client to inhale through the nose while relaxing the abdomen and pushing your thumbs "out" with the abdominal wall. The practitioner should provide gradual abdominal pressure during inspiration.
5. Instruct the client to pause naturally and briefly at the end of inspiration. This creates a smooth ventilation pattern and an even distribution of air in and out of the lungs.
6. Ask the client to exhale gently as you press inward and upward on the epigastric notch with your thumbs. Have the client contract the abdominal muscles and purse the lips during exhalation.
7. Ideally, the length of exhalation should be two to three times that of inhalation. This is especially important for clients who have difficulty breathing out effectively, e.g., those with chronic lung disease. However, do not overemphasize the length of exhalation time. If the client places undue effort on counting, anxiety and dyspnea may occur, defeating the purpose of breathing retraining.
8. When diaphragmatic breathing has been mastered in a semi-Fowler's position, the client should practice it in other positions (lying, standing, and sitting) and then during exercise. A hand or a weighted object, e.g., 5-lb sandbag or a book, placed on the upper abdomen may remind the client to use the diaphragm.

relax the band when inhaling. Using a piece of tightly woven fabric at least 3 inches wide (e.g., drapery pleating tape) and maintaining even tension are important during this exercise.

INSPIRATORY RESISTIVE BREATHING

Inspiratory resistive breathing involves simply imposing additional work on the inspiratory muscles during diaphragmatic breathing. With use of this method, over time, inspiratory muscle strength as well as endurance will be improved. Exercise tolerance will be enhanced with stronger, more efficient inspiratory muscles.

To strengthen inspiratory muscles, a flow resistor with a one-way valve is used. When the client inhales, the valve closes, forcing air to be drawn through the resistive openings. On exhalation, the valve opens, allowing passive exhalation against minimal resistance.

On the client's beginning to use the flow resistive device, the resistive setting should be set on the least resistive setting. The client should be instructed to inhale and exhale slowly through the device. Respirations should not exceed 15 breaths per minute. The nurse should encourage the client to exercise with the device for 15 minutes at a time using good diaphragmatic breathing technique. As the client's endurance improves, the exercise time and inspiratory resistance can be gradually increased.

PURSED-LIP BREATHING

Pursed-lip breathing during exhalation is a useful technique for preventing early airway collapse. It can be practiced during any activity. The nurse teaches the client as follows:

- Encourage the client to relax and breathe in through the nose.
- Next, instruct the client to exhale slowly and completely through pursed lips for a comfortable length of time.

With chronic lung disorders, airways lose their elasticity and may collapse during exhalation (especially during forced or labored exhalation). This traps air beyond (distal to) the point of collapse. The client is unable to exhale efficiently and becomes short of breath, anxious, and increasingly dyspneic. Pursing the lips slows or retards the flow rate of exhaled air. This (1) creates a back pressure in the airways, which keeps the "flabby" airways open and prevents airway collapse, and (2) helps empty the lungs more completely.

COACHING BREATHING RETRAINING

Breathing retraining helps a client with respiratory dysfunction develop a sense of normality without creating undue respiratory distress. Coaching is a very important component of any breathing retraining technique. It improves instruction, demonstration, discussion, and practice. During teaching sessions, the nurse should discuss the ways the technique will help the client (e.g., increased activity without shortness of breath). The technique is demonstrated, and the client practices it while the nurse observes and offers support.

CRITICAL TO REMEMBER

It is important that the client develop a habit of using the breathing techniques all the time rather than just "practicing" them periodically. Pursed-lip and diaphragmatic breathing can be used during all activities of daily living.

RELAXATION

To develop maximal breathing control, the client must learn to relax. When helping a client learn to relax, the nurse must assume an unhurried and calm manner. The client should wear loose clothing. The nurse teaches the client the dyspnea positions which facilitate diaphragmatic breathing without increasing the work of other muscle groups. He or she instructs the client to use diaphragmatic breathing and slow, relaxed, pursed-lip exhalation. Various relaxation exercises can be used. Many self-relaxation tapes and books are available. Meditation is also a powerful means of relaxation. In addition, the following exercises may promote relaxation.

- Slow head rolling to the left and right in a circular pattern coordinated with breathing. The client inhales as the head goes from left to right and exhales as the head swings from right to left.
- Shoulder rolling (backward and forward) coordinated with breathing. The client inhales while rolling the shoulders backward and exhales while bringing them forward.
- Arm swinging (backward and forward) coordinated with breathing. The client inhales while the arms swing upward and forward and exhales on the downward and backward swing.
- Tightening all muscle groups from head to toe while inhaling and relaxing all muscle groups while exhaling.

During these exercises, the client should inhale through the nose and exhale through pursed lips. The nurse can teach the client to make a conscious effort to exhale slowly and as completely as possible. The ventilation pattern must be relaxed, unhurried, and comfortable.

Chest Physiotherapy

Chest physiotherapy (CPT) is a combination of percussion over the chest wall, vibration, coughing, and deep breathing. CPT combined with postural drainage is an effective method of mobilizing secretions.

The goals of CPT may include mobilization and clearance of sputum, an increase in exercise tolerance, improving ventilation, and restoring effective breathing patterns.

PERCUSSION AND VIBRATION

Percussion (Fig. 20–1*A*) is performed by clapping on the chest wall with a cupped hand over an affected area of the lung. A cupped hand "captures" a pocket of air as it strikes the chest. The nurse should not slap the chest wall. He or she places a towel on the chest of the client over the area in which the percussion is being performed. A hollow, deep sound is produced when percussion is done correctly.

Vibration is applied to the chest; energy waves from the hand are used to move secretions from affected lung areas during the expiration phase of respiration, as shown in Figure 20–1*B*. The nurse must not attempt to perform percussion or vibration on a client without first receiving adequate practice and direct supervision.

CRITICAL TO REMEMBER

CPT should be performed at least 2 hours after a meal to reduce the risk of vomiting and aspiration. This is especially true in confused or tube-fed clients. The nurse should never percuss or vibrate over soft tissue, over the spine, in areas of increased pain, or below the rib cage.

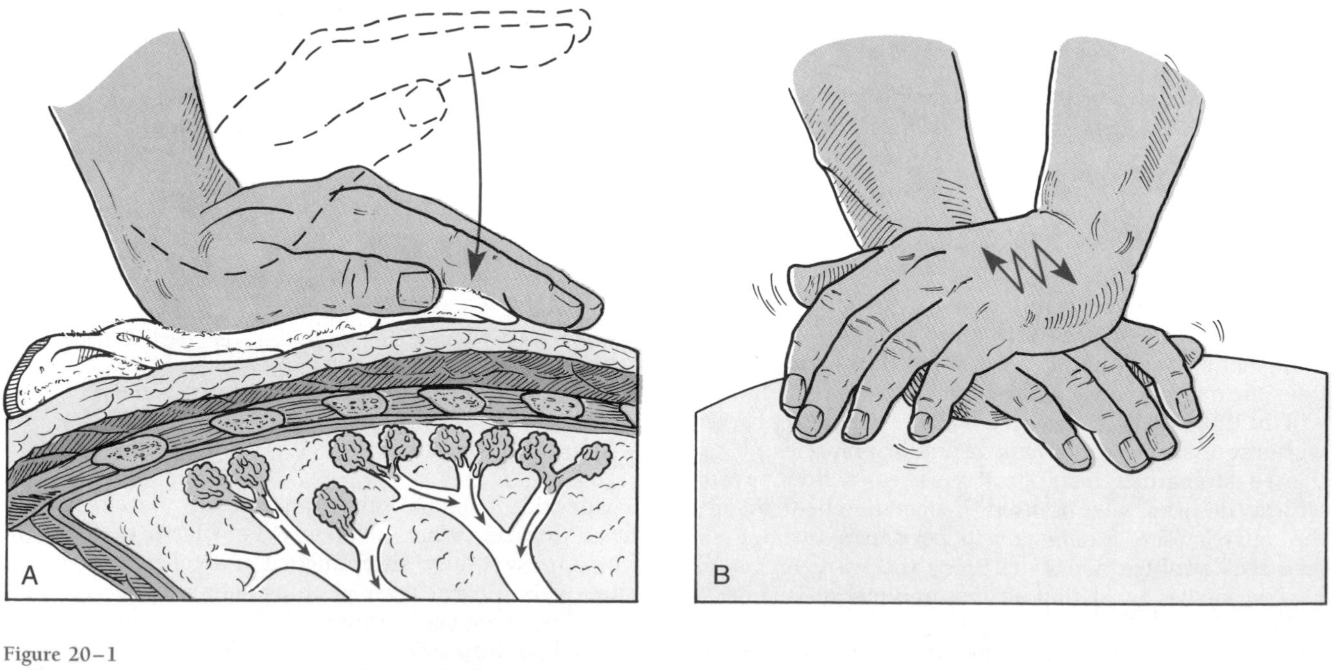

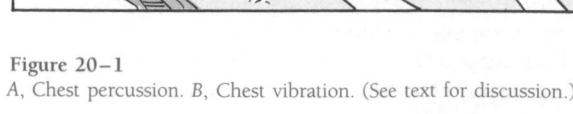

Figure 20–1
A, Chest percussion. *B*, Chest vibration. (See text for discussion.)

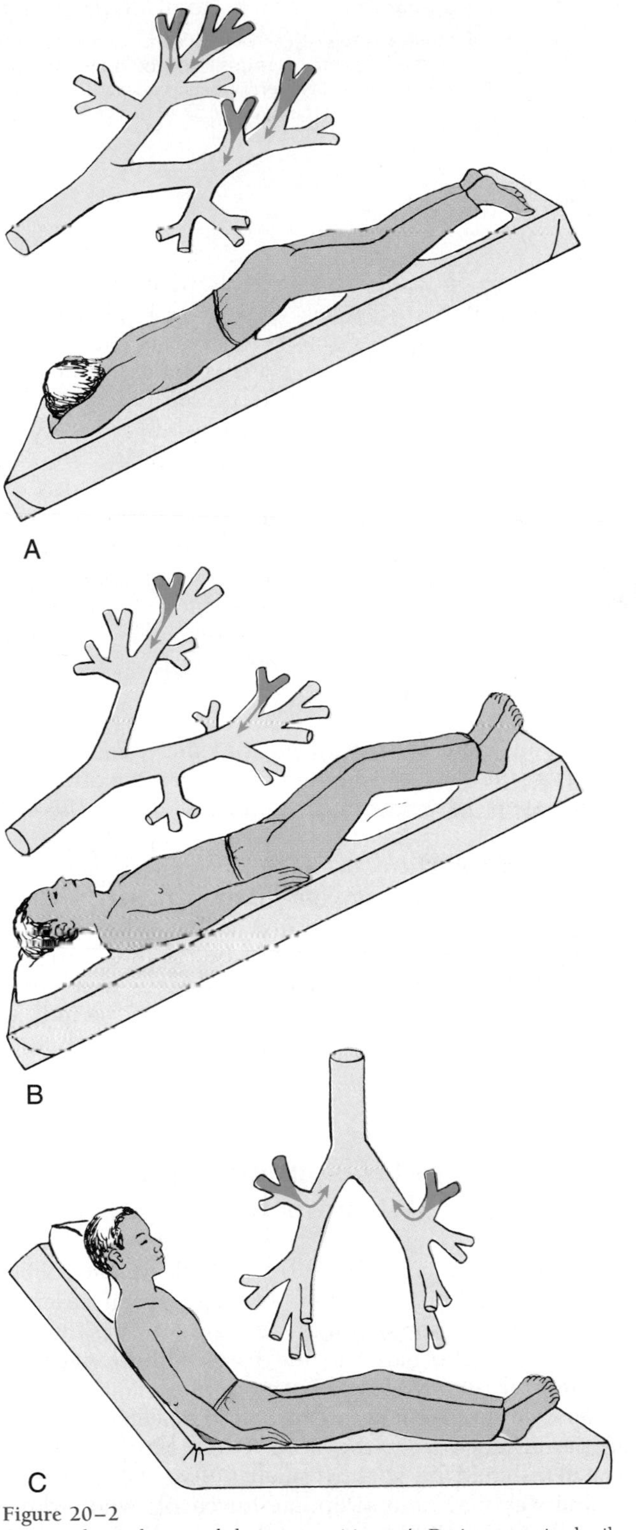

Figure 20–2
Commonly used postural drainage positions. *A*, Drains posterior basilar segments; *B*, drains middle lobes; and *C*, drains upper lobes.

If several areas require drainage, the nurse can plan apical section drainage positions (sitting position) in the middle of the series to allow the client to rest.

POSTURAL DRAINAGE

Postural drainage is accomplished by positioning a client so that gravity is used to drain specific lung segments of retained secretions. The segment of lung to be drained is placed vertical to the force of gravity. The positions used for postural drainage differ, depending on which lung segments need draining. Also, positions may be modified according to the client's condition and tolerance (Figs. 20–2 and 20–3).

The nurse properly positions the client, using pillows or towels to support the joints. Each position is maintained for 5 to 10 minutes.

CRITICAL TO REMEMBER

However, drainage should be stopped or the position changed (1) if the client can no longer tolerate it as evidenced by cyanosis, dyspnea, or significant changes in vital signs, or (2) when no more secretions are heard, felt, or drained or the cough is no longer productive.

During postural drainage, proper breathing and effective coughing should be encouraged.

Indications for postural drainage, percussion, and vibration include the management of clients with

- excessive secretions (e.g., due to chronic bronchitis, smoking) prior to surgery
- excessive secretions due to an ineffective cough (e.g., from pain, sedation) after surgery
- any chronic disease process producing abnormal sputum that increases the risk of recurrent infection (e.g., cystic fibrosis, bronchiectasis, chronic bronchitis); also, for bronchial or lobar pneumonia that is productive of secretions and lung abscess (if abscess does not involve the vascular system)
- bronchospasm or extreme sputum tenacity that makes it difficult or exhausting to raise secretions (e.g., asthma, bronchiectasis)
- musculoskeletal abnormalities that interfere with effective coughing (e.g., scoliosis, quadriplegia, "barrel chest")

Contraindications for postural drainage include the presence of

- increased cyanosis or exhaustion after its use
- secretions that, once mobilized, could obstruct the airway, especially when suction equipment is not available
- unstable vital signs, including increased intracranial pressure
- any pre-emergent medical or surgical situation

Contraindications for percussion and vibration include the presence of

- known or suspected carcinoma or metastatic disease in the area to be treated
- bronchospasm that increases by their use
- pain during the treatment
- possible hemorrhage or seizure activity
- a predisposition to pathologic rib fractures

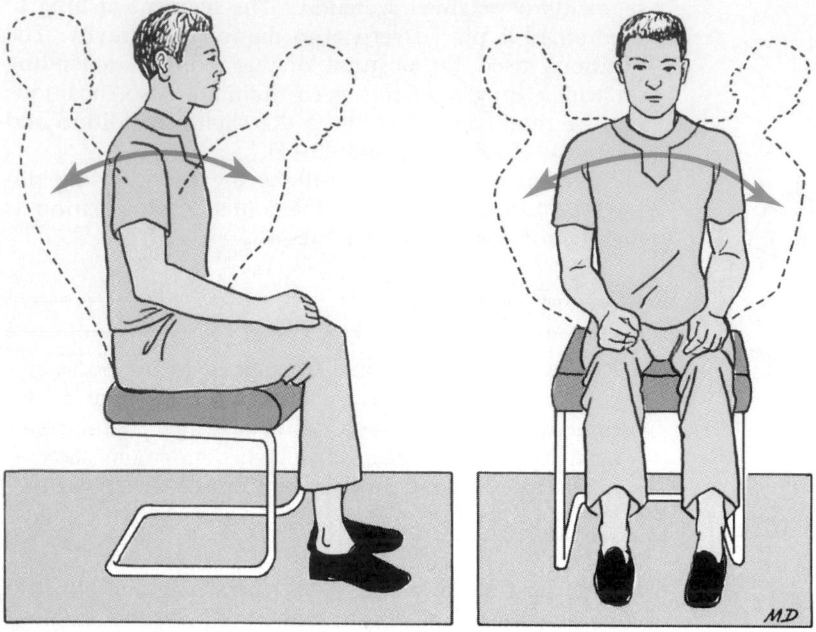

Figure 20–3
Postural drainage exercises to drain the upper lobes of the lungs. Have the person sit upright in a chair and rock the upper torso forward and backward several times, then sway the upper torso from side to side.

CLIENT TEACHING

It is important to teach clients who have respiratory problems (and their significant others) these techniques so that they can participate in their care. In large health-care facilities, CPT is usually performed by respiratory therapists. In smaller settings, it is often a nursing responsibility.

The treatment is used in various respiratory disorders (e.g., bronchiectasis, COPD) and after chest surgery and chest injury. It often takes several weeks of treatment for a client with a chronic respiratory problem to experience any benefit. The nurse should help clients understand the length of time needed so they do not become discouraged.

ARTIFICIAL AIRWAYS

Comatose or obtunded clients often require an artificial airway to maintain airway patency. There are various kinds of artificial airways: oral airway, nasal airway, endotracheal tube, tracheostomy tube. It is often necessary to quickly select an appropriate airway that will only minimally traumatize the client.

Oral (Oropharyngeal) Airways

Oral airways come in varied sizes (Fig. 20–4). The length of an airway should match the distance between the lips and the angle of the jaw. An oral airway that is too long causes gagging or coughing. One that is too short may push the tongue back into the throat and increase airway obstruction. Contraindications for the use of oral airways may include consciousness, facial fractures, or a foreign body in the oral cavity.

A conscious client or someone with an intact gag reflex cannot tolerate an oral airway. Hence, a client who can expel an airway probably does not need one. If gagging occurs, the airway should be removed. An oral airway is a temporary, short-term device. If a client requires an artificial airway for an extended period, an endotracheal tube is more appropriate.

Nasal Airways (Nasopharyngeal Airways, Nasal Trumpets)

The nasal airway (Fig. 20–4*B*) is a hollow, soft rubber tube that fits into the nasal passage. When inserted correctly, the nasopharyngeal airway provides a passageway from the nares to the base of the tongue. In selecting the airway, length is more important than diameter. The proper length can be estimated by measuring the distance from the nose to the earlobe. Airway diameter should be slightly smaller than the nostril. A nasal airway may be appropriate for clients who require an artificial airway but cannot tolerate an oral airway. A nasal airway is ideal for clients who require frequent nasotracheal suctioning. The suction catheter can be passed through the nasal tube; thus, trauma to the nasal mucosa is avoided. When a nasal airway is required for long periods, it should be rotated from one side to the other every 8 hours. If frequent nasotracheal suctioning is required for longer than a week, a nasal airway is replaced by an endotracheal or tracheostomy tube.

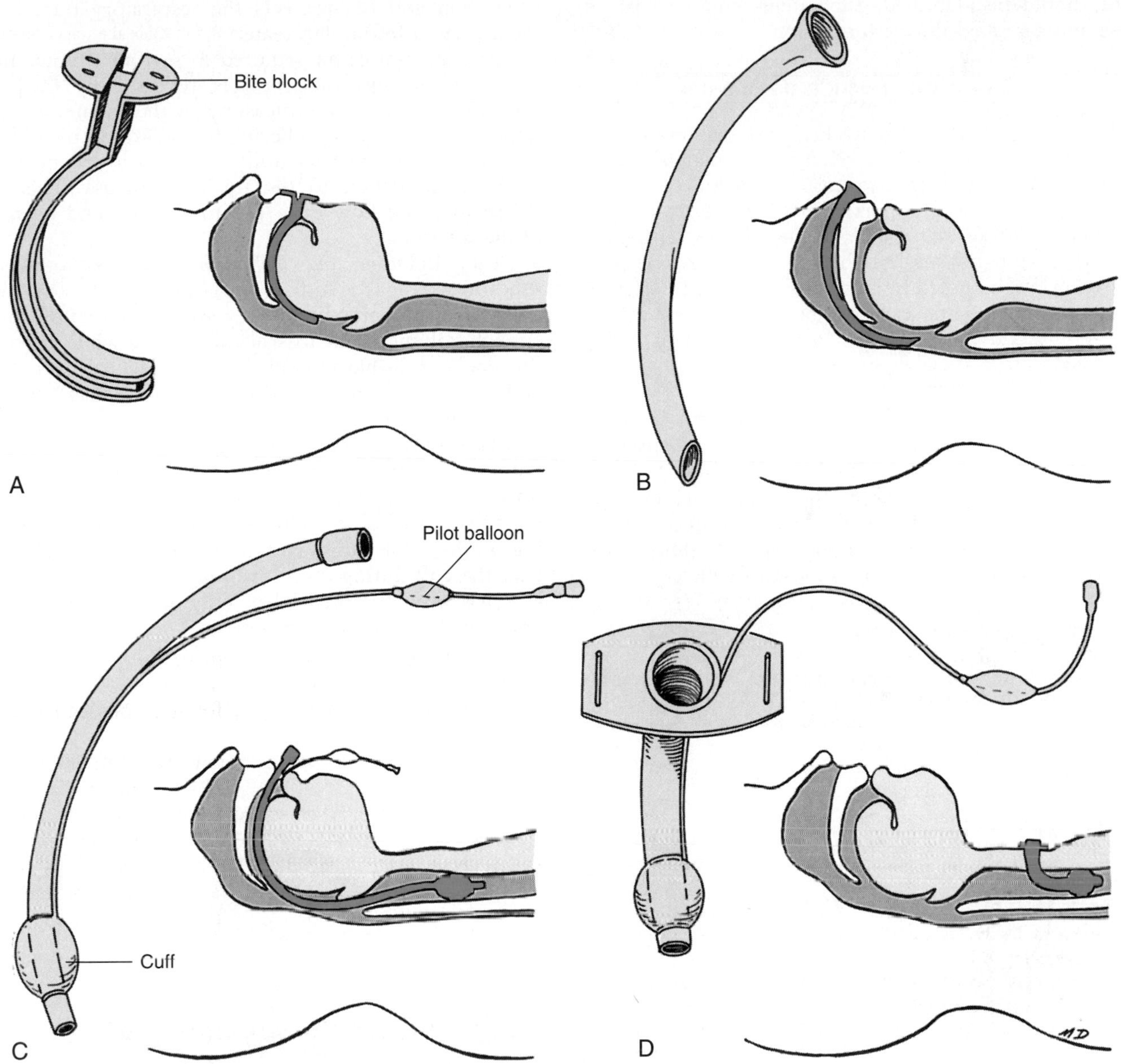

Figure 20–4
Artificial airways. *A*, Oral airway; *B*, nasal airway; *C*, endotracheal tube; *D*, tracheostomy tube. Endotracheal tubes have several parts: 15-mm adapter on the proximal end, pilot balloon, radiopaque pilot line, and cuff. All respiratory therapy and anesthesiology equipment is designed to connect with a 15-mm adapter. Consequently, a client can easily be manually ventilated, mechanically ventilated, or anesthetized via the same endotracheal tube.

Endotracheal Tubes

An endotracheal tube is a long, slender, hollow tube (Fig. 20–4*C*), usually made of polyvinylchloride, inserted into the trachea via the mouth or nose. It passes through the vocal cords, and the distal tip is positioned just above the bifurcation of the main stem of the bronchus (carina). Oral intubation is usually used for short-term airway management. Nasal intubation is generally more secure and is believed to be more comfortable because it does not move as much in the airway. However, many institutions are not using nasal intubation because of the risk of sinusitis. If a client requires prolonged intubation, a tracheostomy may be performed (Fig. 20–4*D*).

Indications for endotracheal intubation include

- relief of airway obstruction
- prevention of aspiration
- facilitation of tracheal suctioning
- facilitation of artificial ventilation

Inserting the Tube. The client is positioned supine with all dental bridgework and plates removed. Loose teeth should be identified. Such items could be jarred loose and aspirated during intubation.

CRITICAL TO REMEMBER

Immediately after an endotracheal tube has been inserted, tube placement is verified by auscultation and chest x-ray examination to ensure aeration of both sides of the chest. The nurse should record in his or her notes and on the respiratory flow sheet the point at which the tube meets the lips or nostrils. This position can be noted by using the numbers listed on the side of the endotracheal tube. Then, if the tube slips, its correct position can be re-established quickly.

The endotracheal tube should be secured immediately after intubation with adhesive tape or specially designed endotracheal tube holders (Fig. 20–5). A nasotracheal tube is secured in the same way, but the second of the small strips is placed across the bridge of the nose instead of on the upper lip. Retaping is required only if the tape becomes loose or soiled.

MONITORING THE CUFF

The cuff of an endotracheal tube (1) seals the tube against the tracheal wall to facilitate positive-pressure ventilation and (2) protects the respiratory tract from the aspiration of foreign material.

The amount of air required to seal an endotracheal (or tracheostomy) tube cuff is reflected by the cuff pressure. Cuff pressure, measured with a manometer, is important because it reflects the pressure the cuff is exerting on the tracheal wall. Too high a cuff pressure impedes circulation to the tracheal mucosa. This decrease in blood flow may lead to stenosis and necrosis of the trachea.

Cuff Inflation and Deflation. Most endotracheal tubes are designed with soft plastic cuffs to use high volumes at low pressures. They are inflated with a high enough volume of air to seal the trachea while exerting the lowest possible pressure on the tracheal wall. Low cuff pressure is necessary to prevent damage to the tracheal mucosa.

The most common method of cuff inflation is the minimal leak technique. The aim of this technique is to provide an adequate seal in the trachea at the lowest possible cuff pressure. This is attained by slowly injecting air into the cuff while auscultating the neck area over the cuff during a positive-pressure breath. Minimal leak has been achieved when only a very small leak is noted at the peak inflation pressure.

Generally, endotracheal cuffs should remain inflated at all times. Tracheostomy cuffs are occasionally deflated when the client is no longer on mechanical ven-

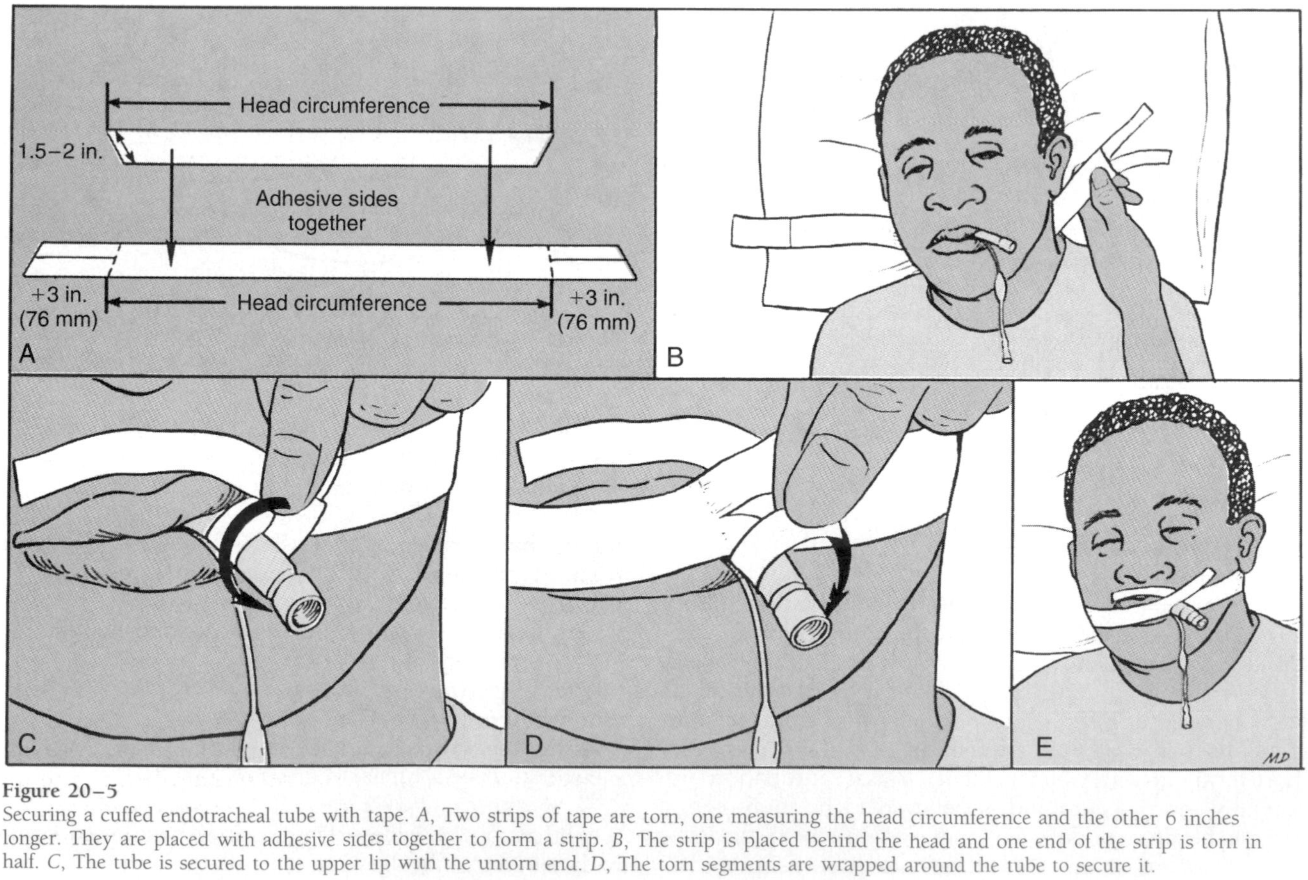

Figure 20–5
Securing a cuffed endotracheal tube with tape. *A*, Two strips of tape are torn, one measuring the head circumference and the other 6 inches longer. They are placed with adhesive sides together to form a strip. *B*, The strip is placed behind the head and one end of the strip is torn in half. *C*, The tube is secured to the upper lip with the untorn end. *D*, The torn segments are wrapped around the tube to secure it.

tilation and has begun to eat. Swallowing effectiveness is improved with the cuff down in some clients. Also, fenestrated tracheostomy tube cuffs are always deflated when the inner cannula is removed and the outer opening is closed or "plugged." This decreases the amount of airway resistance by allowing air to move around the tracheostomy tube as well as providing for adequate sputum clearance.

Cuff Leaks. Cuff leaks are a major problem. They may be caused by a rupture or tear in the cuff or pilot system and by the endotracheal tube's changing positions in the trachea.

CRITICAL TO REMEMBER

Signs of a leak in or around the endotracheal tube cuff include (1) the pilot balloon's not filling when air is injected, (2) the client's ability to talk when the cuff is inflated, (3) air heard leaking during positive-pressure breathing, and (4) food suctioned up through the tube.

Because the system is not functional, the endotracheal tube is replaced. Before replacement, increasing tidal volume may help maintain ventilation by compensating for the escaping gas.

CRITICAL TO REMEMBER

The client is at high risk for aspiration while the cuff is leaking.

REMOVING THE TUBE (EXTUBATION)

Extubation is the removal of the endotracheal tube. The client's respiratory function is monitored throughout the time of intubation (heart rate, ABGs, lung sounds, and lung expansion). When the client demonstrates adequate arterial oxygen levels, tidal volume, vital capacity, and negative inspiratory force as well as a level of consciousness to sustain spontaneous respiration, the endotracheal tube may be removed. Endotracheal tubes are removed with physician's orders and only by health-care team members qualified to reintubate if necessary. The occurrence of laryngospasm and tracheal edema after extubation may occlude the airway and require reintubation. If the client has been on mechanical ventilation, weaning from the ventilator is accomplished before extubation; this process is discussed later (see discussion under Mechanical Ventilators).

CRITICAL TO REMEMBER

Immediately after extubation, the client is usually placed on oxygen. The client is also assessed for signs of respiratory distress and hypoxia as evidenced by restlessness, irritability, tachycardia, tachypnea, and decreased PaO_2 or increased $PaCO_2$. If these signs are noted, the physician should be notified, and the nurse should prepare for reintubation.

Some clients are restless and extubate themselves. Because the cuff is not deflated, there can be damage to the tracheal wall and bleeding. In most cases, the client requires reintubation, and this is done swiftly to prevent hypoxia and to avoid having to insert the endotracheal tube through swollen tissues.

Complications. Fig. 20–6 illustrates the complications of endotracheal intubation.

Noninvasive Positive-Pressure Ventilation

Noninvasive positive-pressure ventilation (NIPPV) is being used to treat individuals who have acute or chronic respiratory failure resulting from a variety of respiratory conditions. It is also used to assist in the weaning of respirator-dependent individuals, treating postextubation respiratory decompensation, and in the reversal of acute respiratory failure associated with the exacerbation of COPD.

The NIPPV apparatus connects to a standard ventilator and then is affixed to an individual's head. It delivers air by nasal mask, nasal pillow, oral mask, or mouthpiece. The choice of the delivery device depends on individual comfort and the provision of an airtight seal. Adverse effects of NIPPV include skin breakdown, gastric distention, and nasal congestion and irritation.

Nursing Management

Suctioning

Suctioning secretions is a common nursing intervention used to (1) remove secretions from the nose, mouth, and tracheobronchial tree and (2) stimulate productive coughing. Suctioning the nose and mouth is a relatively simple, safe procedure.

CRITICAL TO REMEMBER

Oral and nasal tracheal suctioning should not be the first-line therapy for removal of secretions.

The nurse should try other techniques to stimulate productive coughing before using tracheal suctioning for this purpose. Tracheal suctioning is needed only for clients (1) with tenacious secretions that require suction removal, (2) with impaired pulmonary function that interferes with the cough reflex, or (3) with debilitation and weakness who cannot bring up secretions even after vigorous coughing.

Many complications can be avoided by hyperinflating a client's lungs and providing oxygen before, during, and after tracheal suctioning. Possible complications from tracheal suctioning include infection, hypoxemia, mechanical trauma to the mucosa, alveolar collapse (atelectasis), bradycardia, tachycardia, rupture of a bronchial suture line, and cardiac arrhythmias. Complications and nursing precautions are presented in Table 20–3 and Figure 20–6.

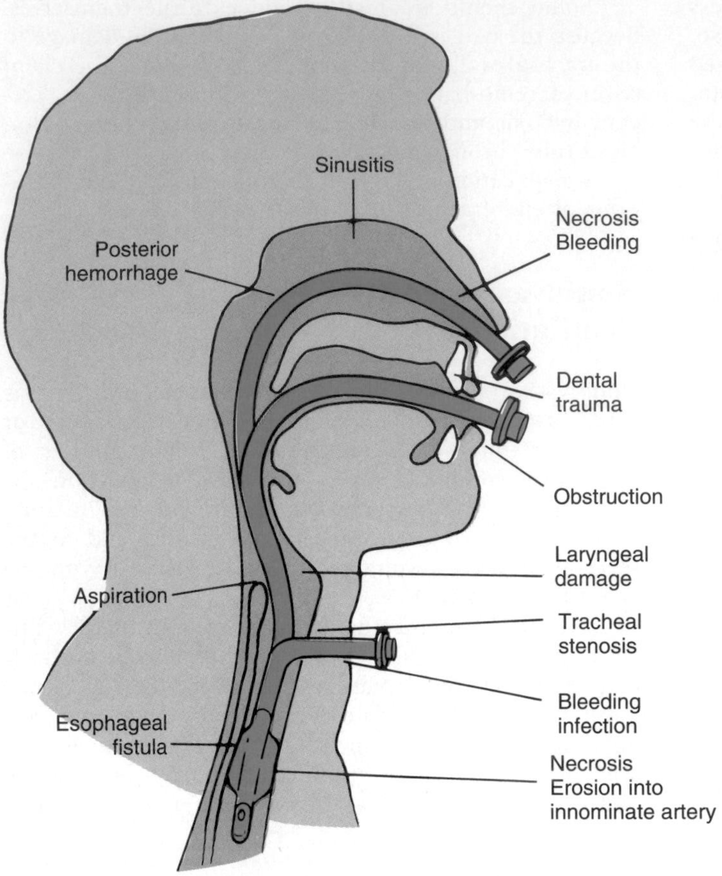

Figure 20–6
Complications of endotracheal intubation and tracheostomy. (From Marino, P. [1991]. *The ICU book*. Philadelphia: Lea & Febiger.)

Nursing Precautions

Assessment: The nurse assesses for clinical manifestations of airway obstructions requiring suctioning. These include noisy, wet respirations; restlessness; increased pulse and respirations; visible mucus bubbling into an artificial airway; rhonchi identified by auscultation; an increase in peak airway pressure visible on a manometer if the client is on continuous mechanical ventilation.

CRITICAL TO REMEMBER

Cyanosis is a late sign of upper airway obstruction.

A conscious client is usually aware of airway obstruction and can ask for help. Obtunded clients need careful and constant assessment with prompt suctioning when indicated.

Thinning Secretions. Clients with excessive tracheobronchial secretions are often helped by humidification of their inspired air to loosen secretions. Tracheobronchial hydration may be done by parenteral or oral methods or aerosolization of liquid.

Providing Oxygenation. Before suctioning, the nurse should oxygenate the client with use of a manual resuscitation bag. He or she hyperinflates the lungs with 100 per cent oxygen for five or six breaths to increase the PaO_2 before suctioning. Tracheal suctioning removes oxygen and therefore lowers the PaO_2, which may trigger cardiac dysrhythmias. When possible, the nurse should assess pulse and heart rhythm before and during suctioning. Tachycardia is a result of agitation and hypoxemia. If tachycardia occurs during tracheal suctioning, the nurse should assess its severity and proceed only if it is mild. Bradycardia results from vagal stimulation of the larynx and carina.

CRITICAL TO REMEMBER

If bradycardia develops, discontinue suctioning immediately and ventilate the client with 100 per cent oxygen.

The nurse reports and documents untoward effects of suctioning immediately.

Performing Psychosocial Interventions: Tracheal suctioning can be an uncomfortable, often frightening procedure. Once the catheter passes between the vocal cords, the client cannot talk because the cords cannot approximate. Naturally, the client may become very anxious and restless. The nurse should explain the procedure and gently tell the client what to do throughout the procedure, e.g., not to swallow while the catheter is being inserted, and not to cough or talk. He or she should reassure the client that the procedure will be very quick, 15 seconds at most. The nurse's skill and competence will be the most reassuring of all.

Loss of a sense of personal dignity may accompany tracheal intubation or tracheostomy. The whole experi-

TABLE 20–3 Complications of Tracheal Suctioning

COMPLICATION	PATHOPHYSIOLOGIC BASIS	NURSING PRECAUTIONS
Hypoxemia	Suctioning removes the oxygen from the airways	Preoxygenate the client with manual ventilation or ventilator sighing, to 1½ the usual tidal volume and with a high FIO_2 (0.6–1.0)
Dysrhythmias (premature ventricular contractions, tachycardia, bradycardia, asystole)	Hypoxemia can be caused by prolonged suctioning, stimulating pacemaker cells within the heart; a vasovagal response may also occur, causing bradycardia	Limit suctioning to 10 seconds, preoxygenate Monitor the electrocardiogram during suctioning Use extra caution in clients (1) with PaO_2 below 70 mm Hg (suctioning further reduces PaO_2), (2) with a large alveolar-arterial gradient (indicating very low cardiopulmonary reserve), and (3) in generally poor condition, e.g., with inadequate oxygenation, hypotension, arrhythmias, acid-base imbalances
Bronchospasm	Respiratory reflex caused by irritation of the tracheal membranes, improper ventilation, and coughing	Be certain to time the inflation stage of mechanical ventilation with the client's own inspiratory effort Do not forcibly inflate the bag against the client's exhalation May require bronchodilators
Airway trauma	Direct trauma to the airway or excessive pressures used to suction	Keep the suction level below 120 mm Hg Suction only as the client needs it, usually no more often than every hour
Infection	Introduction of pathogens into the sterile airway	Use sterile technique for suctioning procedures Change reservoirs of water for humidification daily Assess the color and quantity of sputum
Atelectasis/lobar collapse	Use of excessive wall suction pressure and a suction catheter that is too large for the airway causes a vacuum, collapsing the lung units distal to the tip of the catheter	Use suction catheter that does not exceed one third to one half of the diameter of the airway being suctioned Use smaller catheters if the endotracheal tube size is less than a 7-French Suction pressure is kept at less than 120 mm Hg

ence is very frightening. The client cannot speak or breathe normally, and the presence of the tube may limit physical mobility. The nurse should spend time with the client (and encourage significant others to do the same) and communicate concern and understanding, both verbally and nonverbally.

Helping Clients Cope with Inability to Speak. An endotracheal tube passes through the vocal cords. A tracheostomy bypasses them altogether. Therefore, a client with either cannot cough effectively or speak, requiring the nurse to create other means of communication.

Providing Oral Hygiene. Careful oral hygiene is essential every few hours for a client requiring suctioning or with an endotracheal tube. Secretions pool in the oropharynx because of the inflated tracheal cuff. Frequent oral suctioning above the cuff is highly recommended.

CRITICAL TO REMEMBER

The client's teeth should be brushed and oral mucosa moistened with solutions without alcohol or lemon because these solutions dry mucous membranes.

Tracheostomy

A tracheotomy is a surgical opening made into the trachea for airway management (see Fig. 20–4*D*). A tracheostomy is the surgical creation of a stoma from the trachea to the overlying skin. Even though the terms indicate different procedures, they are often used interchangeably. For the benefit of simplicity, the term tracheostomy is used in the text.

Indications for tracheostomy are

- Need for long-term artificial airway
- Upper airway obstruction
- Upper airway bleeding
- Altered level of consciousness, such as increasing lethargy or obtundation, producing inability to protect the lower airway
- Inability to clear lower airway secretions
- Need for continuous mechanical ventilation
- Prolonged endotracheal tube insertion, causing erosion or pain
- Sleep apnea
- Laryngeal or tracheal fracture
- Airway burns

Tracheostomy is by far the most satisfactory artificial airway. It totally bypasses the upper airway and glottis, avoiding complications in those areas. It is easier to stabilize, suction, and attach respiratory equipment. The client can eat and, with some adjustments, can talk.

TYPES OF TRACHEOSTOMY TUBES

Tracheostomy tubes vary in their composition, number of separate parts, shape, and size. The type to be used is determined before the tracheostomy procedure is begun. Incorrectly fitting tubes can precipitate permanent or life-threatening damage.

The length and curve of a tracheostomy tube are important. Short to moderately short tubes with an angle of about 60 degrees are most often used. A tube must be long enough to avoid dislodgement into paratracheal tissue when the person coughs or turns the head. The lower end of a tracheostomy tube should be located above the carina. The tube's curve must allow the tip to be in a straight line with the trachea rather than to press on the anterior or posterior tracheal wall.

Tracheostomy tubes may be cuffed or uncuffed. Inflated cuffs permit mechanical ventilation and protect the lower airway by creating a seal between the upper and lower airways.

CRITICAL TO REMEMBER

Tracheostomy cuffs do not hold the tube in place.

Rather, when inflated, they seal the area between the outer cannula and the tracheal wall. A pilot balloon reflects the presence or absence of air in the cuff. However, it cannot be considered an absolute indicator of cuff inflation.

Most tracheostomy tube cuffs are designed to exert a low pressure against the tracheal wall through use of an easily distensible cuff that accepts a high volume of air without generating excessive force (i.e., high volume–low pressure cuffs). See Table 20–4 for cuff inflation and deflation technique. Low cuff pressure is necessary to prevent tracheal mucosa damage. The volume of air in the cuff determines the pressure exerted on the tracheal mucosa. Cuff pressures should not exceed 20 cm H_2O.

Tracheostomy tubes are made of various substances (e.g., nonreactive plastic, stainless steel, sterling silver). Plastic tubes are used for only one person. Metal tubes can be reused for different people following sterilization. The most common "trach" tube is a universal, or standard, tracheostomy tube with three parts, outer and inner cannulas and an obdurator.

TABLE 20–4 Inflation and Deflation of Tracheostomy Tube Cuff*

Inflation (Minimal Leak Technique)

Objective

Inflate the cuff with the minimum volume of air required to adequately seal the trachea during positive-pressure ventilation and to prevent aspiration of foreign material while exerting the lowest possible cuff-to-tracheal wall pressure.

Intervention

1. Withdraw all residual air from the cuff
2. Place 6 mL air in a syringe
3. Place the diaphragm of a stethoscope over the client's neck in the area of the tracheostomy tube cuff
4. On inhalation, slowly inject air through the one-way valve into the pilot line in 1 mL increments
5. Auscultate the neck area over the cuff
6. Apply positive pressure to the tracheostomy tube with a manual self-inflating bag. An audible air leak will be heard via the stethoscope unless the cuff is inflated
7. Continue slowly injecting air until the air leak is no longer present during inhalation
8. When a leak is no longer auscultated, withdraw a small amount of air from the cuff until a very small leak is heard. This is called a minimal leak
9. Note the amount of air necessary to achieve the minimal leak. This is the minimal occluding volume (MOV)
10. Once minimal leak is attained, measure the cuff pressure with a manometer
11. Routinely measure and document cuff pressures

Deflation

Objective

Allow air to flow around tracheostomy tube to (a) permit phonation and (b) provide opportunity to blow secretions above the cuff into the oropharynx where they may be removed by suctioning

Intervention

Routinely deflating the cuff is not necessary, provided safe cuff inflation and cuff pressure measurements are performed

1. Remove ventilator assembly (if present), and attach a self-inflating bag to the 15 mm adapter on the inner cannula
2. Hyperoxygenate, hyperinflate, and suction trachea to remove secretions below the cuff. Remove secretions above the cuff by gently applying suction deep into the oropharynx
3. Insert an empty syringe into the one-way valve, and pull back on the plunger to remove the air in the cuff. At the same time, apply positive pressure with the manual self-inflating bag. This will blow secretions lying directly above the cuff into the mouth, which will prevent secretions accumulated above the cuff from draining into trachea and lower airway
4. Suction oropharynx again
5. If the client is ventilator-dependent, remember that with the cuff "down" or deflated, a portion of ventilation volume will not reach the lungs. Air will escape through the upper airway and may compromise the client's ventilatory status. This volume loss will create an audible leak. Phonation is possible during the exhalation phase of the ventilator

* The same procedure is used for inflation and deflation of endotracheal tube cuffs.

Single-Cannula Tracheostomy Tube. This tube is slightly longer than a double-cannula tube. Because it does not have an inner cannula, it requires less tube care. However, it is not appropriate for clients who are producing secretions, because maintaining airway patency is difficult. This tube requires optimal airway humidification.

Fenestrated Tracheostomy Tube. This tube differs from a universal tracheostomy tube in that it has an opening (fenestration) on the curvature of the posterior wall of the outer cannula. This tube may be used while a client is being weaned from a tracheostomy and for a client needing long-term tracheostomy. When the inner cannula is in place, the tube functions as a universal tracheostomy tube. When the inner cannula is removed, however, the fenestration permits air to flow through both the upper airway and the tracheostomy opening. This permits speech, more effective coughing, and other uses of the upper airway. When the inner cannula is replaced with a short decannulation stopper (tracheostomy plug), all airflow passes through the upper airway. When the tube is plugged, the person can speak, cough normally, breathe deeply, and breathe through the upper airway. If oxygen is required through the tracheostomy, the nurse can administer nasal oxygen when a tracheostomy tube is plugged with a decannulation stopper. Fenestrated tracheostomy tubes may be cuffed or cuffless.

CRITICAL TO REMEMBER

If a fenestrated tube has a cuff, it is imperative to deflate it before plugging the tracheostomy. If the cuff is left inflated, sufficient air cannot pass in or out of the lungs and asphyxiation results.

Talking Tracheostomy. This is a one-way valve in a plastic T-piece attached to the 15 mm end of the inner cannula of a universal tracheostomy tube. It permits talking without the need to plug the tracheostomy tube. The one-way valve allows air (and supplemental humidification and oxygen) to flow into the arm of the T-piece during inspiration. Then on exhalation, the one-way valve closes, directing air from the lungs up through the vocal cords and upper airway. Phonation and effective coughing are facilitated by this normal passage of air.

A talking tracheostomy is *never* used unless there is enough room around the tracheostomy tube to permit sufficient airflow for breathing.

CRITICAL TO REMEMBER

The nurse should always deflate a cuffed tracheostomy tube before using a talking tracheostomy adapter. Cuff inflation prevents exhalation, causing suffocation.

Communitrach. This tube allows speech but requires coordination. It functions similarly to a universal tracheostomy tube, with some modifications. An airflow tube (which looks like a second pilot tube) runs outside the Communitrach and opens just above the cuff. There is a port at the distal end of the airflow tube. When occluded, compressed air or oxygen flow is directed through the airflow tube, generating an airflow up through the vocal cords. This airflow enables speech, although it does not sound "normal."

A Communitrach may be successful for a person who can coordinate occluding the airflow with speech. Before inserting the tube, it is important for the person to realize that speech with a Communitrach will not sound normal.

Tracheostomy Button. This button is sometimes used during weaning as an intermediate device between using a standard tracheostomy tube and complete extubation. A button is a short, straight tracheostomy tube that fits into the stoma of a tracheostomy but is not deep enough to enter the tracheal lumen. It has a removable cap with a one-way flap inside that permits inhalation but not exhalation. When the cap is on the tube, the person can talk. The cap is removed for suctioning.

A button cannot be used with a ventilator. It replaces (once the tracheostomy tract is well established) a standard tracheostomy tube, for people with retained secretions who do not require ventilatory assistance. A button creates less airway resistance than a plugged standard tracheostomy tube. Hence, breathing is easier. Artificial humidification of inspired air is necessary with a button (as with any tracheostomy tube), since the natural airway is bypassed.

Permanent Tracheostomies. Many people with permanent tracheostomies lead a full life (see Chap. 21). Uncuffed tracheostomy tubes are most often recommended for these individuals. To minimize the tracheostomy's appearance, many persons prefer a low-profile inner cannula. This does not have a 15-mm adapter incorporated. Instead, it fits into the outer cannula and lies flush with the neck. "Breathable" (i.e., not plastic or rubber) clothing may be arranged to conceal the tracheostomy. Sometimes, the margins of the entire tracheal opening are sutured to the skin, creating a permanent stoma. This is often performed when a permanent opening, such as after laryngectomy, is necessary. However, a permanent stoma is not satisfactory for people with chronic pulmonary disorders. They need a tracheostomy tube so that secretions can be removed.

Metal Tracheostomy Tube. These tubes are made of sterling silver or stainless steel. Metal tubes are most often used following a permanent tracheostomy or laryngectomy. The inner cannula locks together with the outer cannula. Because metal tubes do not have a standard 15-mm adapter, rapid adaptation to respiratory or anesthesia equipment is impossible unless a specific adapter is available.

POTENTIAL PROBLEMS ASSOCIATED WITH TRACHEOSTOMY TUBES AND CUFFS

Problems develop from prolonged contact between tube cuffs at high pressure and the tracheal wall. These include obstruction, cuff inflation problems, tracheoesophageal fistula, and malposition of the tube.

Factors contributing to tracheal wall breakdown include long-term ventilation requiring a cuffed tracheostomy tube, infection, misalignment of the tracheostomy tube such that the tube's tip lies directly against the tracheal wall, incorrect tracheostomy tube size (e.g., too small a tube not only compromises airway patency but also necessitates high cuff pressures to obtain an adequate seal), and the client's general poor condition. Shock, hypoxemia, general debilitation, impaired defense mechanisms, use of immunosuppressive agents or radiation or both, anemia, and malnutrition all affect tissue well-being.

When long-term tracheostomy is required, uncuffed tracheostomy tubes are usually used. Even people who require long-term mechanical ventilation tolerate uncuffed tracheostomy tubes. Tidal volumes and respiratory rates are adjusted on the ventilator to produce satisfactory ventilation and ABGs while eliminating the risks associated with tracheostomy tube cuffs.

Other possible complications associated with tracheostomy tubes include tube displacement, accidental extubation, airway obstruction, and infection.

Accidental Extubation (Tube Removal). A tracheostomy tube that is not properly secured may be accidentally dislodged from the stoma. This may occur while the nurse is changing the tube-securing ties. Manipulation of a tracheostomy tube often produces vigorous coughing. Coughing can expel the tube from the stoma unless it is held firmly. The nurse must hold the tube with two fingers placed on the flange or neck plate on either side of the adapter. With accidental extubation, if the stoma is less than 4 days old, it may close because a tract is not yet formed. If this occurs, the nurse should call for help immediately while maintaining ventilation and oxygenation by bag and mask.

CRITICAL TO REMEMBER

If the tracheostomy tube cannot be reinserted in 1 minute, the nurse must call a code for respiratory arrest. Unless the client is breathing adequately, an emergency cricothyroidotomy will be necessary (see Chap. 57).

Airway Obstruction. The flow of air through a tracheostomy tube may become occluded for several reasons. The tracheostomy tube may be misaligned so its opening lies against the tracheal wall, preventing airflow. Cuff overinflation causes the cuff to herniate over the tip of the tube, obstructing airflow. Without adequate airway care, the inner cannula can occlude with dried secretions or excessive bronchial secretions.

Infection. Tracheostomies increase the risk of bronchopulmonary infection because (1) they bypass upper airway protective mechanisms (i.e., filtering, warming, and humidifying) and (2) cuffs decrease mucociliary transport and coughing, thus increasing retained secretions. Stoma site infection may also occur. Nosocomial infection is also a potential problem. The lower airway (below the larynx) is normally sterile. Therefore, all solutions, devices, and so forth entering the trachea must be sterile. Organisms (e.g., *Pseudomonas aeruginosa* and other gram-negative bacteria) grow readily in respiratory equipment and contaminate the lower airway. Some bacteria may colonize a tracheostomy without causing infection.

Nursing Management

Following tracheostomy, frequent assessment is required, including (1) monitoring vital signs; (2) assessing mucous membrane color; and (3) observing for indications of shock, hemorrhage, respiratory insufficiency, or complications from the client's general condition or the surgical intervention.

Nursing Diagnosis: Airway Clearance, Ineffective R/T secretion accumulation.

A client with a tracheostomy is unable to perform the Valsalva maneuver and therefore has a limited ability to cough and deep breathe. Thus, the client's ability to maintain a clear airway is compromised. Intervention to promote airway clearance and pulmonary aeration includes (1) changing the client's position frequently, (2) providing humidification and hydration, (3) eliminating factors that impair airway clearance (e.g., reduce fever, use sedatives cautiously), and (4) performing frequent manual ventilation, hyperinflation, and suctioning to promote lung expansion and reduce the risks of atelectasis, pulmonary infection, and ineffective gas exchange. Hyperinflation creates an "artificial sigh," improving lung aeration and facilitating removal of tracheobronchial secretions by enhancing the cough effort. When the client's condition is stabilized sufficiently, coughing may be enhanced by having the client place a finger over the tracheostomy tube opening while attempting to cough.

CRITICAL TO REMEMBER

It is important that the client's hands be washed before he or she places a finger over the tracheostomy tube opening.

The client should cough into paper tissues and carefully dispose of them.

When a cuffed tracheostomy tube is used, secretions collect above the cuff. It is difficult to reach such secretions by oropharyngeal suctioning. However, the secretions can be "blown" into the mouth by simultaneously deflating the cuff and giving a deep manual inflation. If secretions above the cuff are not "blown up," they will fall into the lower airway when the cuff is deflated. Infection from oral contaminants or impaired gas exchange, or both, can result.

The nurse should suction the airway as needed. Careful technique reduces mucosal trauma, which can lead to tracheal infection. Mucosal trauma is indicated by (1) tracheal irritation and tracheitis, and (2) bloody tracheal secretions.

If tracheal secretions are thick and not easily removed, a small amount of sterile normal saline can be directly instilled (if agency policy permits) into the trachea to try to reduce the viscosity of the secretions. The saline can be instilled directly into the tracheostomy tube during inhalation. The lungs are immediately manually inflated with a self-inflating bag. If the inner cannula is encrusted, the nurse can soak it in hydrogen peroxide (H_2O_2) and rinse it with sterile distilled water or normal saline to remove the crusts. This increases airway patency (Table 20–5).

The nurse should provide adequate hydration. The normal hydrating mechanisms of the upper airway are bypassed by a tracheostomy. Hydration can be ensured

TABLE 20–5 Tracheostomy Care

Preprocedure

- Auscultate chest to assess need for suctioning
- Assemble equipment: tracheostomy care kit* or individual supplies (i.e., hydrogen peroxide [H_2O_2], scissors, fresh tracheostomy tape or other type of tracheostomy-securing device, sterile normal saline, two sterile basins, plastic or paper bag for disposal of used items)

Prepare Client

- Tell the client what you are going to do
- If teaching self-care, describe the items you have assembled and the purpose of each
- Loosen the caps on the hydrogen peroxide and normal saline
- Open tracheostomy kit on a firm surface
- Pour H_2O_2 into one basin and normal saline into the other
- Close the caps on the H_2O_2 and normal saline
- Remove used tracheostomy dressing and discard
- Wash hands and clean under fingernails

Tracheostomy Care

- Put on sterile gloves
- Dip cotton-tipped applicator into H_2O_2 and clean skin around stoma. Repeat as many times as needed to remove mucus from the skin. Clean area behind the neck plate. Observe the condition of the skin
- Dip another applicator into normal saline. Rinse H_2O_2 and mucus from skin
- Use a dry 4 × 4 gauze sponge to wipe area if necessary
- Hold neck plate steady with the fingers of one hand and remove inner cannula with the other. Tracheostomy tube motion may stimulate a cough or produce an uncomfortable sensation similar to strangling or choking
- Place inner cannula in H_2O_2. Use small brush or pipe cleaners to scrub mucus from the inside of the inner cannula. If the mucus is very thick, let the inner cannula soak at least 3 minutes. Repeat process until the inner cannula is clean
- Carefully reinsert inner cannula and lock it in place
- If a tracheostomy dressing is needed, use a pre-cut one from the care kit, use a pre-cut drain dressing, or fold a 4 × 4 dressing into a V. *Do not cut standard 4 × 4's unless they are tightly woven and do not fray or leave gauze filaments when cut.*

Changing Tracheostomy Ties

- Changing tracheostomy ties always requires two people. At least one person must be experienced in this procedure and capable of handling accidental extubation. The tube is easily dislodged by coughing when the tracheostomy tube is manipulated
- One person holds the tracheostomy tube in place by placing two fingers directly on the neck plate. Apply firm pressure. Never remove fingers until the new ties are tied and secured
- $\frac{3}{4}$-inch twill tape is most comfortable for ties
- Always tie the twill with a square knot
- Never position knots directly over the carotid artery or the spinal cord
- Tie knots with tension that allows two fingers to slip between the skin and the tapes
- Change tracheostomy ties when soiled and at least every 8 hours, initially. People with permanent tracheostomies usually need them changed once a day

Postprocedure

- Discard soiled disposable supplies, solutions, and equipment. Send nondisposable items for decontamination
- Note the size and type of the tracheostomy tube. Make sure there is an identical tube placed at the head of the bed
- Make sure the obturator is taped in an easily visible place
- Replace equipment used
- Document procedure. Note quality and quantity of any blood or mucus, and the skin integrity. Document any unusual observations and notify physician
- If the client or significant others are being taught the procedure, document their progress
- Ensure that emergency situations may be handled appropriately, e.g., a tracheal dilator or tracheal hook kept in the room to assist in emergency tracheostomy tube replacement. (This is not usually needed when the stoma has become well established)

* Prepackaged tracheostomy care kits are expensive for prolonged or permanent use. People discharged from the hospital with a tracheostomy often find it more cost-effective to assemble individual items. Most United States third-party payers do not provide an unlimited supply of packaged tracheostomy care kits.

by oral, parenteral, or inhalation routes. Inhalation may be provided by (1) increasing the humidity of room air (room humidifier) or of dry gases (e.g., oxygen) or (2) administering aerosols.

If humidification is insufficient, the body tries to make up the deficit by taking fluid from body water. The result is thick mucus, which compromises airway patency and increases the risk of secretion pooling and subsequent infection. Many factors can impair the mucociliary mechanisms of the lungs, e.g., dehydration, fever, anesthesia, anticholinergic drugs, sedatives, and immobility. All of these factors may be experienced by a person with a tracheostomy. Dried mucus occludes air passages and leads to atelectasis, pneumonia, and potentially severe gas exchange abnormalities. Nursing intervention for insufficient hydration includes careful monitoring of fluid intake and output and administering prescribed additional parenteral hydration.

Nursing Diagnosis: Gas Exchange, Impaired. Following tracheostomy, impaired gas exchange may occur because of various factors.

- Factors affecting oxygen delivery include (1) aspiration of blood, oral secretions, or gastric contents; (2) restricted lung expansion from immobility; (3) excessive tracheobronchial secretions; (4) inability to cough and deep breathe; and (5) pre-existing medical conditions (e.g., obesity, fever, inadequate hydration, pneumonia, tracheal injury such as from burns).
- Factors affecting the removal of carbon dioxide include (1) sedatives or anesthesia, (2) deteriorating level of consciousness, and (3) any other condition potentially affecting ventilation efficiency and leading to hypoventilation and retention of carbon dioxide.

CRITICAL TO REMEMBER

Assessment of gas exchange by ABG analysis is important immediately following tracheostomy and whenever there is a change in the person's condition or a change in treatment.

Noninvasive monitoring is appropriate once baseline values are established by ABG.

Nursing Diagnosis: Infection, Body Temperature, Altered Risk for R/T tracheostomy's bypassing normal upper airway protective mechanisms and R/T surgical incision.

Nursing intervention is required to prevent respiratory infection as well as oral and skin infection following tracheostomy. The nurse should use aseptic technique for all intervention directly involving the tracheostomy. Careful handwashing, appropriate use of gloves, use of sterile supplies and solutions, and changing and decontaminating respiratory equipment every 24 hours are essential. The nurse cleans and inspects the skin around the stoma and the stoma itself and observes for indications of irritation, inflammation, skin breakdown, and purulent drainage. If skin or stomal infection does occur, a topical antibacterial ointment may be prescribed.

Tracheostomy dressings (Fig. 20–7) are often used, especially in the early postoperative stage. Damp blood-and-mucus-soaked dressings are a perfect medium for the growth of micro-organisms. They also promote tissue irritation and breakdown. The nurse should change dressings whenever they are damp. Using H_2O_2 and cotton-tipped applicators, the nurse should carefully clean the skin each time the dressing is changed, rinse with normal saline, and dry the area. Plastic-backed or water-proofed dressings should not be used. Moisture, secretions, and blood may seep behind them, and these dressings hold warmth and moisture in. Skin then becomes irritated and macerated.

Nursing Diagnosis: Fluid Volume Deficit and Nutrition, Altered: Less Than Body Requirements, Risk for. Intravenous fluids are usually given during the first 24 hours following tracheostomy. Then, if the person is alert and swallowing and if gag mechanisms are intact, oral fluid intake and food intake may be attempted.

If a cuffed endotracheal tube was used before the tracheostomy, the nurse assesses for tracheoesophageal fistula before permitting oral feedings.

CRITICAL TO REMEMBER

The risk of a tracheoesophageal fistula increases if both a cuffed endotracheal tube and a nasogastric feeding tube were used. To assess for the presence of such a fistula, the client is given a "test swallow" of water (room temperature and colored blue with vegetable dye) before receiving fluid or food.

Severe coughing or blue fluid suctioned from the tracheostomy tube indicates a fistula. The nurse should withhold oral food and fluid and continue feeding by nasogastric tube or other methods.

If the client's swallowing mechanism is impaired following tracheostomy, intravenous fluid may be prescribed for a short time. A client with a long-term or permanently impaired swallowing mechanism (e.g., following a cerebrovascular accident) requires a permanent feeding tube or gastrostomy feedings (G-tube) (Chap. 33). G-tube feedings may cause reflux and be aspirated into the trachea.

CRITICAL TO REMEMBER

Before administering G-tube feedings, the nurse should inflate the tracheostomy tube's cuff. It should be left inflated for at least 1 hour after feeding. The nurse suctions above the cuff before deflating it to remove any tube-feeding material.

When feeding a client with a tracheostomy, the nurse should have him or her sit upright. Often, food and fluids with texture (e.g., pudding) are easier to swallow than water. Tipping the chin toward the chest narrows the airway and helps food enter the esophagus.

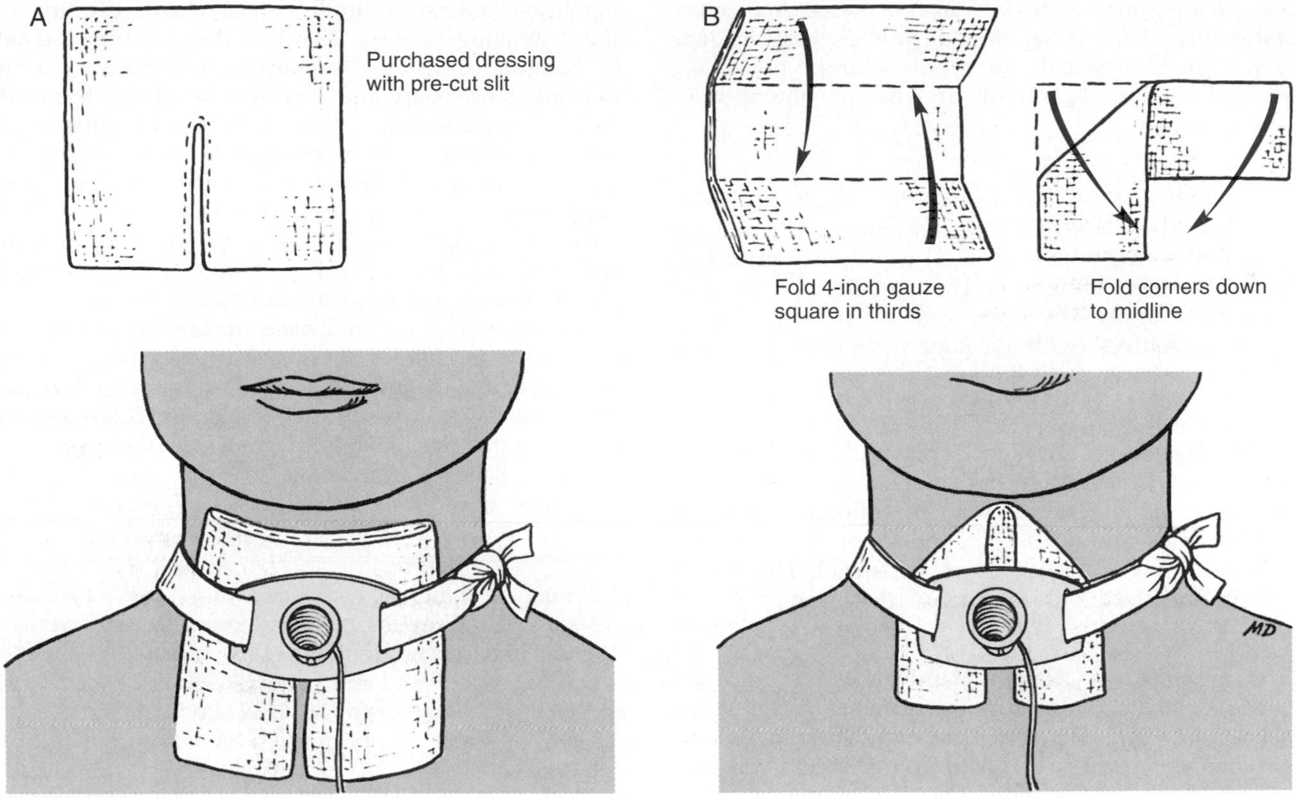
A
Purchased dressing
with pre-cut slit
B
Fold 4-inch gauze
square in thirds
Fold corners down
to midline
MD

Figure 20–7
Tracheostomy dressings. If there is significant bleeding or tracheal secretions, cleaning the skin and changing the dressing frequently may prevent infection and skin breakdown. *A,* A manufactured dressing with a precut slit has no fine threads that could unravel and enter the stoma. Place dressing around the tracheostomy tube with the slit downward (as shown) or upward. *B,* A 4 × 4 gauze pad folded and placed under the tracheostomy tube. There should be no cut edges on the pad that could unravel.

Overinflation of a tracheostomy tube's cuff causes swallowing difficulty. If oral fluid intake is limited, intravenous fluids should be continued to make up the deficit.

Nursing Diagnosis: Communication, Impaired Verbal R/T bypassing of vocal cords by tracheostomy. The nurse should make sure the client can always reach an emergency call system to summon help. An intercom system should not be used because the client cannot talk. The nurse must be sure all personnel know this. The nurse can make a written list of common needs, words, and phrases so the client can point on the list to communicate needs (e.g., "I want to pass urine"; "I need a drink"; "I have pain"). A paper and pencil can be used to facilitate communication.

Nursing Diagnosis: Injury, Risk for. The nurse must secure a tracheostomy tube properly. If tracheostomy tube–securing tapes require knotting, a square knot should always be used. The nurse should avoid placing the knot over the person's carotid artery or spine and make sure the tapes are not too tight (i.e., allow room for two fingers to slide comfortably under the tape). The nurse should inspect the skin under the securing tape for skin irritation. Clients requiring a long-term tracheostomy may use more comfortable securing devices (e.g., padded straps with Velcro fasteners). The nurse should secure the tube in midline tracheal alignment and create a "loop" in aerosol or ventilator tubing assembly; i.e., let the tube loop down to catch condensate. Water and condensate in the tubing should be drained away from the tracheostomy. The ventilator and aerosol tubing should be supported to prevent pulling on the tracheostomy tube. The nurse must be careful not to disconnect tubing when turning the client.

The nurse must not allow smoking in the room of a person who has a tracheostomy and must not use aerosol spray cans (e.g., room deodorizers) near the person. The nurse should not shake bedding or create dust clouds and should be careful when shaving or tending the person's hair that whiskers or hairs do not fall into the trachea. The tracheostomy should be covered with a thin cloth towel during shaving.

Nursing Diagnosis: Oral Mucous Membrane, Altered. Oral hygiene is important to prevent oral infection and lower airway infection from oral bacteria passing downward. Oral hygiene performed on a regularly scheduled basis (at least once each shift) also makes a client more comfortable. The nurse should provide oral hygiene every 2 hours, especially for people who are not taking any food or fluid by mouth or who are obtunded or unconscious.

Nursing Diagnosis: Constipation R/T absence of Valsalva maneuver. When the glottis and vocal cords are bypassed (as with tracheostomy), a person cannot perform a Valsalva maneuver. This impairs the person's ability to defecate. The nurse can use prescribed stool softeners, laxatives (with adequate hydration), and even enemas as necessary.

Nursing Diagnosis: Anxiety. This problem is due to various factors affecting individuals with tracheostomies, e.g., inability to talk, fear of suffocating, anxiety about diagnosis, fear that the tracheostomy tube will come out. Frequent observation is essential. The nurse's presence and skillful care are most reassuring.

Nursing Diagnosis: Health Maintenance, Altered R/T knowledge deficit regarding permanent or long-term tracheostomy care. When a client's tracheostomy is long term or permanent, the nurse should begin teaching during routine care as appropriate. He or she can use a mirror to allow the client to observe procedures. Family members and significant others should be included. Before discharge from the health-care facility, the client and significant others need to be confident about performing tracheostomy care, suctioning, preoxygenating, safety measures, aerosol therapy, and other aspects of the individual's airway maintenance. The nurse should arrange home follow-up by a home health agency that has expertise in caring for people with complex airway needs. A pulmonary nurse specialist can be involved in the teaching opportunities when available. If the client requires mechanical ventilation, an audible disconnect alarm must be incorporated into the ventilator system.

WEANING FROM THE TRACHEOSTOMY TUBE

For clients who do not require continuous mechanical ventilation, weaning begins by plugging the tracheostomy tube's opening. At first, the tube is plugged for short periods of time, e.g., 5 to 20 minutes. The time is gradually lengthened according to the client's respiratory status, condition, and confidence. Eventually, the tracheostomy tube can be removed. The weaning process takes a varying length of time (typically 7 to 14 days), depending on a person's ability to ventilate through the upper airway. If the client still requires some intervention via the tracheal opening, an uncuffed tube, a fenestrated tube, or a tracheal button can be used at different times during the weaning process.

Ideally, tracheostomy plugging is attempted only when an uncuffed or fenestrated tracheostomy tube is in place.

The nurse explains the process to the client and significant others. Naturally, most clients are anxious about weaning because they fear they may not be able to breathe. Constant, supportive observation during weaning is necessary and reassures the client. The nurse should encourage the client to begin to think about breathing through the nose again. This breathing is a strange sensation for people who have used a tracheostomy tube for a long time. The nurse can explain to them ways to facilitate optimal respiration and to maintain control of breathing (e.g., inhale slowly and completely through the nose; avoid holding the breath).

Analysis of ABGs and measurement of spontaneous respiratory mechanics (respiratory rate, tidal volume, vital capacity, inspiratory effort, expiratory effort) are important assessments during weaning. Oximetry and other noninvasive assessment may also be used once baseline ABGs are established.

CRITICAL TO REMEMBER

During weaning from tracheostomy, the nurse assesses for indications of respiratory distress or ventilation impairment. Findings may include (1) abnormal respiratory rate and pattern, (2) use of accessory muscles to assist breathing, (3) abnormal pulse and blood pressure, (4) abnormal skin and mucous membrane color, and (5) abnormal ABGs. The nurse should remove the tracheostomy plug immediately if any indication of respiratory distress or ventilation impairment appears.

He or she also assesses the client's quality of phonation and ability to deep breathe and cough effectively. If oxygen has been administered via the tracheostomy, it should be administered at the prescribed liter flow with nasal prongs.

REMOVAL OF TRACHEOSTOMY TUBE (EXTUBATION)

A tracheostomy tube is removed after successful tracheostomy plugging and when the client's respiratory status and function are stable. Successful tracheostomy plugging is indicated by (1) a client's ability to breathe comfortably with the tracheostomy plugged, (2) normal ABG analysis, and (3) a client's ability to cough and raise secretions. The nurse gradually increases the length of plugging sessions until the client is comfortable and confident.

After a tracheostomy tube is removed, the nurse places a dry sterile dressing over the stoma. Initially, every 8 hours, he or she cleans the skin around the stomas, removes mucus with hydrogen peroxide, rinses the area with normal saline, and applies a fresh dry dressing over the healing stoma.

CRITICAL TO REMEMBER

The nurse should document the condition of the stoma and surrounding skin and notify the physician if they appear irritated or infected.

Topical antibiotic ointment may be prescribed. A tracheostomy stoma closes gradually (over a period of 2 weeks or longer). As long as the stoma is open, an air leak is present. To correct this the client may need to place clean fingers firmly over the dressing to facilitate normal speech and coughing.

Following extubation, ongoing respiratory function assessment is necessary. Some complications of tracheostomy do not appear for months following tracheostomy tube removal, e.g., tracheal stenosis.

PERMANENT TRACHEOSTOMY

Most clients with a permanent tracheostomy use a universal, or fenestrated, cuffless, tracheostomy tube or an Olympic trach button. However, some do not need a tracheostomy tube (e.g., a "laryngectomee" with a permanently constructed stoma). Care of a client who has had a laryngectomy is discussed in Chapter 21. The same principles apply to a client with a permanent tracheostomy.

Learning self-care is important for individuals with permanent tracheostomies. It provides a sense of self-control and reduces dependency on others. However, significant others must also be able to provide tracheostomy care and other aspects of airway management. The client and significant others are often anxious about home management. Careful preparation before discharge reduces this anxiety. Close follow-up is essential. Home health services are necessary. Home health care equipment should be ordered from medical suppliers who employ respiratory therapists or nurses. Ideally, the equipment should be initially delivered to the hospital, so the client and significant others can learn its use with the supervision of professionals.

TRACHEOSTOMY TUBE CHANGES

Recommendations for changing tracheostomy tubes vary. Most physicians and health-care facilities have established protocols. Although some facilities change tracheostomy tubes as often as every month, others wait longer. Ideally, the tube should be changed every 6 to 8 weeks, or more frequently if the person is at risk of recurrent tracheobronchial infections. Each person has a unique set of circumstances that may dictate the frequency of tracheostomy tube changes.

EMERGENCY RESUSCITATION

Emergency mouth-to-neck (mouth-to-tracheostomy or mouth-to-stoma) resuscitation may be necessary if a person with a tracheostomy or laryngectomy experiences respiratory depression or respiratory arrest. The nurse should consult the agency procedure manual for appropriate interventions.

MECHANICAL VENTILATORS

Some clients are not able to ventilate their lungs adequately because of various disorders resulting in respiratory insufficiency or failure. These clients require immediate intervention, including the establishment of an artificial airway (e.g., by endotracheal intubation or tracheostomy) and mechanical lung ventilation with a positive-pressure ventilator.

Indications

The decision to use mechanical ventilation is a separate issue from the decision to intubate. In emergency situations, however, mechanical ventilation nearly always follows intubation, at least until a more complete assessment of the client can be performed.

The two main indications for mechanical ventilation are inadequate ventilation and hypoxemia. Clients who have indications other than these are those clients with COPD (emphysema). Mechanical ventilation is delayed for as long as possible in these cases, as such clients can tolerate higher $PaCO_2$ levels, and acute respiratory failure is likely to reverse with bronchodilator therapy, respiratory therapy, and other supportive measures.

Common clinical indications and disorders that frequently require mechanical ventilation are presented in Table 20–6 and the Bridge to Critical Care.

Positive-pressure ventilators may be broadly categorized as those for short-term use (intermittent positive-pressure breathing) and those for continuous supportive use (continuous mechanical ventilation), which provide for all aspects of ventilation and oxygen administration.

Intermittent Positive-Pressure Breathing

Intermittent positive-pressure breathing (IPPB) uses a pressure-cycled ventilator to deliver pressurized breaths to a spontaneously breathing client in 10 to 20 minute treatments.

Currently IPPB is infrequently prescribed, as it is uncomfortable, and its benefits have not been substantially proved. IPPB can be an effective therapy if the candidates are carefully screened and goals and outcomes are clearly understood.

Continuous Mechanical Ventilation

The use of continuous mechanical ventilation (CMV) is now an ordinary level of care for clients managed in critical care and on general care units. The client on CMV is a challenge to the nurse providing care. The nurse must be familiar with the equipment, complications of CMV, and nursing management. The goals of CMV are to (1) maintain adequate ventilation, (2) deliver precise concentrations of FIO_2, (3) deliver adequate tidal volumes in order to obtain an adequate minute ventilation and oxygenation, and (4) decrease the work of breathing in those clients who cannot sustain adequate ventilation on their own. Continuous mechanical ventilators can be either pressure-cycled or volume-cycled.

TABLE 20–6 Common Clinical Indications and Disorders Requiring Mechanical Ventilation

DISORDERS	CLINICAL INDICATIONS
Lung or airway disorders or trauma (pneumonia, adult respiratory distress syndrome, rib fractures, asthma, pulmonary edema)	PaO_2 below 60 mm Hg with $FIO_2 > 0.4$ $PaCO_2$ above 45 mm Hg pH below 7.3 Hemodynamic instability
Circulatory disorders (myocardial infarction, cardiogenic shock)	Same as for lung and airway disorders
Acute exacerbations of chronic obstructive pulmonary disease	PaO_2 below 35 to 45 on oxygen pH below 7.2 to 7.25 Respiratory rate above 30 to 40/min
Neuromuscular disorders and trauma (Guillain-Barré syndrome, myasthenia gravis, head injury)	Maximum inspiratory pressure per 25 cm H_2O Vital capacity less than 10 to 15 mL/kg body weight Respiratory rate above 30 to 40/min
Airway obstruction (facial trauma, aspiration)	Presence of inspiratory stridor
Prophylactic management following surgery	Major cardiac, pulmonary or gastrointestinal surgery. Hemodynamic instability during surgery.

BRIDGE TO CRITICAL CARE

The Ventilator-Dependent Client

PARAMETERS FOR WEANING

Inspiratory force (IF)	> − 20 cm Hg
Tidal volume (V_T)	10–15 mL/kg
Vital capacity (VC)	> 10–15 mL/kg
Expiratory force (EF)	> + 60 cm H_2O
Resting minute ventilation (VE)	> 10 L/min
$PaCO_2$	Within normal range
PaO_2	Minimally 70–80 mm Hg on 0.5 FIO_2
Dead space to tidal volume (V_D/V_T)	0.55–0.60
PaO_2 on 100% O_2	> 300 mm Hg
Shunt fraction	< 15%

PARAMETERS INDICATING AN UNSUCCESSFUL WEANING ATTEMPT

Change in blood pressure: a rise or fall of 20 mm Hg systolic and/or 10 mm Hg diastolic
Pulse rate: increase of 20 beats/min or pulse > 110
Respiratory rate: an increase of 10/min or a rate of more than 30 to 35/min
Tidal volume: less than 250 to 300 mL (adult)
Significant electrocardiographic changes

PaO_2	60 mm Hg	Acceptable values in clients with COPD may be lower PaO_2 and pH and higher $PaCO_2$
$PaCO_2$	55 mm Hg	
pH	7.35	

TROUBLESHOOTING MECHANICAL VENTILATOR ALARMS

High-Pressure Alarms

1. Check to see whether the client is biting on the endotracheal tube.
2. Check to see whether the ventilator tubing is kinked.
3. Listen to lung sounds. Is there bronchospasm or pulmonary embolus?
4. Question the possibility of mucus plugging. Suction vigorously.
5. Is the client coughing?
6. Check for water in the tubing.
7. Is the client out of rhythm with the ventilator? The client may be breathing against an incoming mechanical breath.

Low-Pressure/Low Exhaled Tidal Volume Alarms

1. Check for disconnected tubing.
2. Listen for a cuff leak.
3. Is the client on an IMV mode of ventilation? If so, he or she may need small spontaneous breath tidal volumes.

Minute Ventilation Alarms

1. Assess the client's respiratory rate. If it is rapid, this may produce a larger minute ventilation than normal, especially if he or she is on an assist/control mode of ventilation.
2. The alarms may not have been reset after a rate or volume change on the ventilator.

Oxygen Alarms

1. Check the oxygen to ensure that it is set on the proper amount.
2. Check to make sure that the alarms were changed after a change in FIO_2 on the ventilator.

NOTE: If at any time an alarm is sounding and the nurse cannot quickly ascertain the problem, the client should be disconnected from the ventilator and a manual resuscitation bag should be used to support him or her until the problem can be corrected.

Physiologic Effects

Decreased cardiac output is the most common physiologic effect of positive pressure, with either intermittent or continuous mechanical ventilation. Normal, unassisted respiration begins with subatmospheric pressure. Negative pressure increases during inhalation and decreases during exhalation. Positive pressure applied to the airway has the opposite effect. As positive pressure inflates the lungs, pressure in the thorax builds, decreasing the flow of blood to the vena cava, and reducing blood flow to the right atrium of the heart. Exhalation is passive, and pressures return to their normal, resting, subatmospheric level. Positive pressure also briefly affects the left side of the heart by increasing filling and output. This increase is caused by the displacement of blood from the pulmonary system into the left ventricle. However, this effect is noted only immediately after the institution of positive-pressure ventilation.

CRITICAL TO REMEMBER

If positive-pressure ventilation is continued for more than a few minutes, the blood flow to and from the right ventricle is decreased. This in turn decreases the filling of the left ventricle, leading to a lowered cardiac output. The lowered cardiac output will be reflected in the hypotension that clients commonly exhibit immediately after being placed on mechanical ventilation. It is imperative that nurses monitor blood pressure closely.

Other body systems are also affected by positive pressure. As the diaphragm descends into the abdomen during the inspiratory phase, blood flow to the splanchnic area decreases. This decrease in splanchnic blood flow may lead to ischemia of the gastric mucosa. Ischemia of the gastric mucosa may be one of the reasons that clients who receive positive-pressure ventilation for an extended period of time have a high incidence of gastrointestinal bleeding and stress ulcerations. Decreasing blood flow to the splanchnic region also results in a decreased blood flow to the kidneys. This decrease in blood flow signals the posterior pituitary gland to increase secretion of vasopressin or antidiuretic hormone. Elevated vasopressin levels lead to reabsorption of free water in the renal tubular cells, thereby increasing water retention. Lymphatic flow also decreases as a result of positive pressure.

Positive pressure can cause neurophysiologic changes. When ABG values improve in acute, uncompensated respiratory failure, improved cerebral oxygenation results. A client with compensated respiratory acidosis (chronic carbon dioxide retention) may be adversely affected by positive-pressure breathing owing to "blowing off" of carbon dioxide. Acute alkalosis may occur, producing faintness, dizziness, lightheadedness, and anxiety. If severe alkalosis persists, convulsions, cardiac arrhythmias, and cerebral edema may occur. Cerebral edema may contribute to intensive care unit psychosis.

Assisted and Controlled Ventilation

Ventilators cycle as a result of either inspiration effort, i.e., assisted (person-cycled) ventilation, or an automatic, preset number of breaths, i.e., controlled (machine-cycled) ventilation.

With assisted (person-cycled) ventilation, the client's own inspiratory effort turns on ("trips") the ventilator, thus initiating the mechanical inspiratory phase. Some clients are able to make only weak inspiratory efforts. However, because the ventilator can be adjusted to respond to the respiratory abilities of each client, even a slight inspiratory effort may activate the positive-pressure phase, inflating the lungs at a preset flow rate. When the flow of gas stops, the client passively exhales without assistance from the machine. Assist/control ventilation allows the clients to take as many breaths as they desire. Every breath that they receive will be delivered by the machine at the same preset tidal volume and FIO_2. Assisted ventilation is indicated for clients who can control their own respiratory rate and pattern.

Controlled (machine-cycled) ventilation governs a client's rate of ventilation by automatically cycling the ventilator at a predetermined number of cycles per minute; the ventilator does all of the work of breathing, and the client does none. The respiratory cycle allows an expiratory time conducive to the return of blood flow to the right side of the heart. This mode is independent of the client's efforts or pattern of breathing. This mode of ventilation is the only mode that allows consistent physiologic results, but only if the client is chemically paralyzed with neuromuscular blocking agents, such as vecuronium bromide (Norcuron) or pancuronium bromide (Pavulon).

Clients who are on controlled mechanical ventilation and have spontaneous respirations may "fight" or "buck" the ventilator because they cannot synchronize their respirations with the machine's cycle. If the client continues to fight the ventilator, exhaustion and ineffective alveolar ventilation will result. If the nurse is unable to help such a client relax and breathe in cycle with the machine, the physician should be notified. With an artificial airway in place, the client who is fighting the ventilator may be safely sedated to reduce ventilatory efforts, and thus ventilatory control can be maintained. Medications that can be prescribed for this include morphine and diazepam (Valium). If additional control is required, the use of neuromuscular blocking agents may be indicated. These agents include pancuronium bromide (Pavulon), curare, vecuronium bromide (Norcuron), and atracurium besylate (Tracrium). These drugs block the transmission of nerve impulses, resulting in muscle paralysis. Because these agents do not affect sensorium, or perception of pain, they should *always* be used in conjunction with sedation or analgesics. Clients with these problems are not comatose or deaf, and the nurse should talk to them and explain what is happening. These clients are in great need of reassurance and support because of their helplessness.

Muscle-paralyzing agents may be administered in continuous intravenous drip, with the rate of infusion titrated to control the prolonged paralytic effects. Reversal of these effects is accomplished by drugs that inhibit acetylcholinesterase and allow an excess of acetylcholine to accumulate at the myoneural junction, e.g., neostigmine (Prostigmin) and edrophonium (Tensilon). Serial doses may be needed because recurrence of paralysis is possible. Careful assessment is important.

Controlled respiration and muscle paralysis are often used if a client (1) has muscle spasms, (2) is confused or tachypneic, or (3) is making respiratory efforts out-of-phase with the mechanical ventilator. Paralyzing agents may also be used to ensure effective mechanical ventilation for clients who have sustained head injury, flail chest, seizure disorders, or tetanus.

Positive End-Expiratory Pressure and Continuous Positive Airway Pressure

Positive end-expiratory pressure (PEEP) and continuous positive airway pressure (CPAP) are ventilator techniques applied during expiration whereby intrathoracic pressures are not allowed to return to ambient pressure. This increased pressure helps to keep the alveoli open, increase functional residual capacity, and enhance oxygenation as a result of the enlarged surface area that is available for diffusion. With the implementation of PEEP or CPAP, oxygenation is improved, thus allowing the use of lower levels of FIO_2. In this way, the body's metabolic oxygen requirements are met without the toxic effects of higher concentrations of oxygen.

PHYSIOLOGIC EFFECTS

Functional residual capacity is the volume of air remaining in the lung after normal expiration. If end-expiratory alveolar volumes remain above their critical closing point, the alveoli remain open and functioning. However, if they fall below the closing point, the alveoli have a tendency to collapse. If alveolar collapse occurs, the volume of functional residual capacity also decreases. When alveoli collapse, hypoxemia results, and the lungs become "stiffer" or less compliant.

When alveoli collapse, pulmonary blood flow continues. Although perfusion (blood flow) continues, oxygenation of blood flow to that alveolus does not occur (Fig. 20–8). As alveoli collapse, the residual volume is decreased. A decreased residual volume also causes reduced functional residual capacity. This results in a true intrapulmonary shunt (perfusion without oxygenation). Lung compliance is also affected. Once alveolar collapse occurs, reinflation requires very high opening pressures, the generation of which significantly increases the work of breathing. The hypoxemia resulting from alveolar collapse and the increased oxygen consumption caused by the increased work of breathing may severely compromise the client.

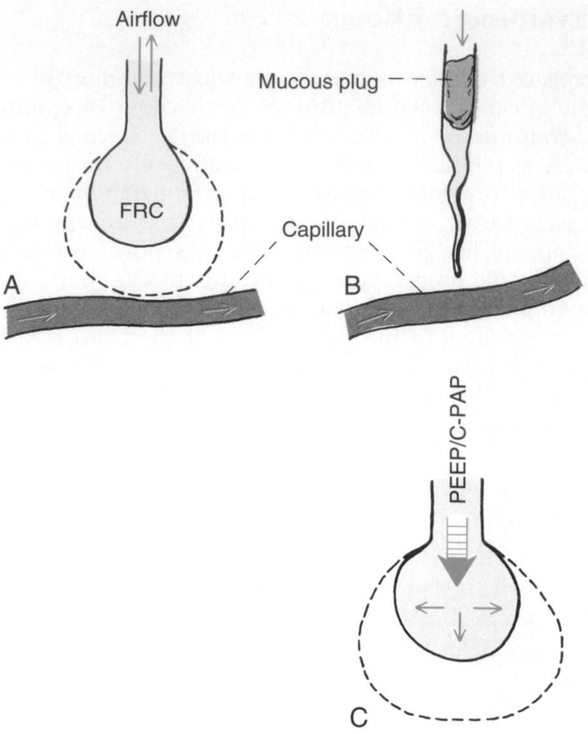

Figure 20–8
Effects of positive airway pressure on alveolus. *A*, Normal alveolus. Dotted line represents expansion during inspiration. *B*, Collapsed alveolus. Perfusion continued. *C*, Alveolus opened by positive pressure. *Dotted line* indicates alveolus during inspiration and *solid line* indicates end-expiratory alveolar volume.

Hazards

The physiologic effects of positive airway pressure on inspiration and expiration are basically the same as those effects discussed for IPPB and CMV. There are a few added risks, such as (1) rupture of the lung from increased intrathoracic and intra-airway pressures (barotrauma), (2) pneumothorax, (3) subcutaneous emphysema, (4) pneumomediastinum, and (5) cardiovascular embarrassment. Cardiovascular embarrassment results from the increased intrathoracic pressure caused by the PEEP, which leads to a decrease in cardiac output. If cardiac output cannot be improved with vasopressor or increased blood volume, hepatic and renal function become compromised.

CRITICAL TO REMEMBER

CPAP and PEEP also increase intracranial pressure. In neurologically injured clients, this is an added risk.

Assessment of clients on CPAP and PEEP includes

- blood pressure and heart rate
- breath sounds
- urinary output
- signs of increased heart failure

- chest films (before and after institution of CPAP and PEEP)
- observing for subcutaneous emphysema (palpate both the posterior and anterior subcutaneous tissue)
- ABGs

Intermittent Mandatory Ventilation

Intermittent mandatory ventilation (IMV) is a popular method of weaning a client from mechanical ventilation in which the ventilator is set to deliver a specific respiratory rate. If a client breathes at a rate higher than the machine rate, the breaths will not be positive-pressure ventilations.

Nearly all mechanical volume ventilators are equipped with an intermittent mandatory ventilation mode. Rather than being put on assisted or controlled ventilation, an intubated client may be immediately placed on intermittent mandatory ventilation. This may facilitate a more rapid progression through the weaning process. Disconnecting the ventilator can then be considered. Extubation is done when all the initial criteria for intubation and mechanical ventilation are reversed.

Pressure Support Ventilation

Pressure support is a recent ventilation method that has been adapted to most modern volume ventilators. Pressure support ventilation is a form of ventilation that augments spontaneous inspiratory effort with a preset level of positive airway pressure. When the client on pressure support ventilation initiates a breath, the machine is triggered and delivers a flow of gas at the preset pressure. The flow rate remains constant until the inspiratory flow rate drops to one fourth the original rate. Pressure support ventilation cannot be used with assist and control ventilation because every time the machine senses a spontaneous breath it delivers a machine breath at the preset tidal volume.

Pressure support ventilation allows the client to set his or her own tidal volume, respiratory rate, and rhythm.

High-Frequency Ventilation

High-frequency ventilation is another mode of mechanical ventilation used for clients who cannot be adequately ventilated with conventional techniques. High-frequency ventilation is often useful for clients with severe noncompliant lungs. The overall advantage of high-frequency ventilation over conventional forms of ventilation is that there is a reduction in peak and mean airway pressure, resulting in better ventilation of noncompliant lungs, for example, in the case of adult respiratory distress syndrome.

Unilateral Lung Ventilation

Unilateral lung ventilation requires tracheal intubation with a special tube that permits the separate ventilation of each lung. In this way, one lung can be ventilated at a different volume and rate from the other lung. A client with a bronchopulmonary fistula who requires mechanical ventilation can benefit from unilateral lung ventilation.

Nursing Management

Because clients with respiratory difficulties are usually tense and apprehensive, the transition to mechanical ventilation needs to be done in as smooth and calm a fashion as possible. A common fear that clients have is that the machine will fail and they will be unable to breathe or summon help in time. Careful preparation of clients receiving ventilator therapy may help to relieve these fears and also contribute to successful treatment. (A client receiving CMV who is inadequately prepared may panic and offset the positive effects of mechanical ventilation.) Explain the basic mechanics of the ventilator, how the machine will help breathing, what it will feel like, and how to cooperate. Never leave clients on CMV unattended. Around-the-clock nursing care by nurses experienced in the care of clients on CMV is essential.

Assessment

Assessment is essential to maintain effective breathing patterns with CMV. The nurse should

- Monitor the respiratory status by ABG analysis, chest films, auscultation, and tracheal aspirate cultures.
- Ensure that ordered arterial blood samples are taken for regular ABG analysis. Document and inform the physician of ABG results.
- Assess and document vital signs for cardiovascular depression, inspiratory pressures, breath sounds, arterial oxygen tension, and ventilatory parameters hourly. Report trends or abnormal findings to the physician.

Continuous mechanical ventilation is almost entirely automatic, but there are some nursing problems: maintaining prescribed inspired oxygen concentrations and the patency of endotracheal and tracheostomy tubes; supplying adequate humidification; and preventing trauma, infection, and mechanical problems such as loose connections and kinks in tubing.

Nursing care for clients with inadequate ventilation requires skill in assessing for indications of respiratory distress, i.e., restlessness, apprehension, irritability, wakefulness, use of the accessory muscles of respiration, pallor, increasing pulse rate, and labored respirations.

Nursing Intervention: When surrounded by machines, health-care providers may sometimes overlook the client and focus on the machines exclusively. Clients on

ETHICAL ISSUES IN NURSING

How Should the Decision to End Continuous Mechanical Ventilation Be Made?

Continuous mechanical ventilation (CMV) is used for many different reasons. Ventilator support may be needed for short-term care, as in certain cases of severe pneumonia, or for more long-term care, as for some stroke patients. In some emergency cases, ventilator support is required to stabilize a client's condition. No matter why CMV is initiated, there are degrees of benefit it offers to the patient. A positive benefit is that CMV allows the lungs to rest in order that healing may take place (such as in severe pneumonia). However, CMV may produce an unwanted effect such as artificially prolonging death and causing suffering, as with severe stroke patients or patients in terminal states.

The decision to place a person on CMV is made by the client, or his or her surrogate, and the medical team. This decision may be a very difficult one, e.g., when a client is in a persistent vegetative state, and the wishes of the client regarding CMV are not known. However, it is even more difficult for persons to decide for another whether to discontinue CMV. To many persons, this decision is viewed as somehow causing the client's death and this is very uncomfortable for them.

The best alternative to this dilemma is for all persons, while in a state of health, to decide what they would want done should a situation arise requiring resuscitative measures, including CMV. Advance directives such as a living will or a health-care power of attorney can help people guide their own treatment should certain health-care situations arise. In fact, as of December 1991, all health-care facilities who take Medicare and Medicaid reimbursement must include, on admission, an advance directive assessment of all their clients.

Nurses have a great deal of influence over the health-care teaching of their clients. Information about advance directives may be shared with clients, community members, family members, and friends. The more the public is made aware of such directives, the easier it is for health-care professionals to guide their care. In many cases, people have strong feelings about the initiation of certain treatments, such as CMV. Advance directives allow all persons to decide, in advance of crisis situations, what they wish to have done in such situations. By allowing all persons to exercise advance directives, health-care providers may avoid many legal and ethical dilemmas that occur in the initiation, continuation, or discontinuation of certain treatments.

ventilators are highly dependent and need comprehensive, holistic care with meticulous attention to detail. They need health-care providers who are not only skillful in managing the machines but also understanding and supportive during stressful experiences.

The nurse should check the machine frequently to ensure proper functioning and the adequate operation of all alarm systems, check the electrical cords frequently to avoid disconnection, and safely place them so that they cannot be pulled loose or cause falls.

A self-inflating resuscitation bag should always be readily available. Manual ventilation may be used during tracheobronchial suctioning, temporary disconnection of the ventilator for tests or treatments, when an apparatus on the machine is being changed, or to ventilate the client if the ventilator fails.

When clients are initially placed on a ventilator, they must be closely observed so that the effectiveness of the therapy can be evaluated and complications can be prevented from occurring. Serious complications that may arise during initial mechanical ventilation include rapid electrolyte changes, severe alkalosis (frequently with convulsions), and hypotension due to decreases in cardiac output.

The Care Plan for the client on mechanical ventilation discusses other interventions.

ETHICAL IMPLICATIONS

Placing a client on CMV involves ethical considerations. CMV does not necessarily "save life," but it may prolong life. For some, it allows the body time to heal. For others (those with terminal illness), it may prolong suffering (see Ethical Issues in Nursing).

WEANING

The physician decides when to begin weaning a client from CMV. The decision is often based on assessments made by nurses and respiratory therapists. Weaning may cause psychological and physiologic changes. The length of time required for successful weaning generally relates to the underlying disease process and to the client's state of health before a ventilator is used.

Careful assessment of ventilatory status before and during weaning is necessary, including spontaneous tidal volume; vital capacity; maximal voluntary ventilation; inspiratory effort; breath sounds; cardiovascular, renal, and cerebral status; and ABGs.

Respiratory Home Care

Clients with chronic respiratory diseases often require frequent hospitalization because of the recurrent nature of their diseases (e.g., COPD). However, whenever possible, it is desirable to help clients manage at home rather than in an acute-care facility.

Respiratory home care can require a range of interventions from simple oxygen therapy to CMV. The principles for intervention are the same at home or in a

CARE PLAN: The Mechanically Ventilated Client

Nursing Diagnosis/ Collaborative Problem	Planning: Expected Outcomes	Implementation: Nursing Interventions	Rationales
Altered Respiratory Function (Airway Clearance, Ineffective; Gas Exchange, Impaired; Breathing Pattern, Ineffective) R/T pathologic processes in the lung, trauma, anesthesia, surgery on the chest or abdomen, neuromuscular disorders	Client will have improved respiratory function as evidenced by • less crackles and rhonchi • ventilation in both lungs • no signs of hypoxia • ABGs returning to preintubation level or normal parameters	Auscultate lung sounds every hour and as needed	Indicates the amount of fluid and secretion in the lungs; validates that endotracheal tube is placed correctly so that both lungs can be ventilated
		Suction as needed, provide pre- and post-hyperinflation and hyperoxygenation	Suctioning removes airway secretions, facilitating ventilation; oxygen and inflation reduce hypoxia during suctioning
		Provide adequate humidity via the ventilator or nebulizer	Replaces the function of the upper airway to warm and humidify the inspired air; thins secretions to facilitate their removal
		Turn and reposition every 2 hours	Allows both lungs to be fully ventilated, mobilizes secretions
		Position with affected lung upper most	Facilitates drainage into large airways
		Secure endotracheal tube properly	Prevents accidental dislodgement
		Use a bite block or oral airway	Prevents compression of endotracheal tube If the client is biting it; bite block is more comfortable for the conscious client
		Assist in changing endotracheal tube as necessary	Assures adequate ventilation
		Monitor ABG values and arterial oxymetry	Indicates the degree of oxygenation; lack of improvement in ABGs may require a change in interventions
		Perform range-of-motion exercises; ambulate to chair when feasible	Immobility leads to decreased respiration muscle strength
Individual Coping, Ineffective R/T dependency while on CMV	Client will exhibit positive coping strategies as evidenced by • reduction in the level of stress or anxiety • decreased feelings of powerlessness	Develop a means of communication	Allows client to have needs met
		Place nurse call device within reach	Allows client to contact nurse
		Be available and visible	Reduces anxiety in client
		Provide distractions (e.g., TV, radio)	Reduces anxiety because client does not focus on ventilator and noises
		Explain all procedures	Allows client to feel respected
		Monitor for behavior and physiologic signs and symptoms that indicate increased levels of anxiety	Antianxiety medications and narcotics may be needed, but use with caution in clients being weaned because these drugs suppress respiratory drive
		Provide privacy	Demonstrates client respect
		Respect client's rights and opinions	Demonstrates client respect and maintains dignity
		Provide a calm environment	Anxiety is contagious, and if the client becomes anxious, ventilation will be more difficult and oxygen needs will increase

Care Plan continued on following page

CARE PLAN: The Mechanically Ventilated Client *Continued*

Nursing Diagnosis/ Collaborative Problem	Planning: Expected Outcomes	Implementation: Nursing Interventions	Rationales
		Explain to client and family that vocal cords have been bypassed, which prevents talking; encourage them to use other modes of communication	Clients can hear and respond even though they cannot talk
Collaborative Problem, Risk for complications of continuous mechanical ventilation positive-pressure ventilation	The nurse will monitor the client for pulmonary barotrauma, cardiovascular depression, inadvertent extubation, and malposition of endotracheal tube	Assess for acute, increasing, or severe dyspnea, agitation, panic, decreased or absent breath sounds, localized hyperresonance, increased breathing effort, tracheal deviation away from the side with abnormal findings, subcutaneous emphysema, and decreasing PaO_2 levels	Barotrauma is damage to the lungs from extrapulmonary air changing intrapleural pressures during positive-pressure ventilation
		Have a high index of suspicion for clients' pre-existing lung lesions, high positive end-expiratory pressure, and invasive thoracic procedures; contact the physician if symptoms occur	Barotrauma can lead to pneumothorax or tension pneumothorax
		Assess for acute or gradual fall in blood pressure, tachycardia (early sign), bradycardia (late sign), dysrhythmias, weak peripheral pulses, acute or gradual increase in pulmonary capillary wedge pressure, and respiratory "swing" (depression) in arterial or pulmonary artery waveforms during inspiration	Cardiovascular depression can occur after an increase in tidal volume, PEEP, CPAP, or with hyperinflation; the positive pressure decreases venous return and afterload due to an increase in intrathoracic pressure
		Monitor for signs of inadvertant extubation: vocalization, low-pressure alarm, bilateral decrease in upper lobe airway sounds, gastric distention, clinical manifestations of inadequate ventilation; if inadvertent extubation occurs, notify physician because reintubation is necessary; manage ventilation and oxygenation with a self-inflating resuscitation bag	Inadvertent extubation can be obvious, such as when the tube is found in the client's hand; it can also be obscure, such as when the tube slips into the hypopharynx or esophagus
Infection, Risk for R/T impaired primary defenses in respiratory tract	Client will remain free of infection as evidenced by: • clear sputum • no fever • lung sounds clearing • no increased difficulty with ventilation • white blood cell count within normal limits	Wash hands thoroughly	Proper handwashing will decrease the spread of infection
		Use sterile technique for: • suctioning • changing dressings	The respiratory tract is considered sterile
		Monitor for increased breathing effort, localized changes in auscultation, and changes in PaO_2	Infected lung segments transmit sound differently (more solid) and do not permit O_2/CO_2 exchange
		Provide oral care every 2 hours	The client's mouth becomes dry, and stomatitis may develop from the lack of oral secretions

CARE PLAN: The Mechanically Ventilated Client *Continued*

Nursing Diagnosis/ Collaborative Problem	Planning: Expected Outcomes	Implementation: Nursing Interventions	Rationales
		Drain water from ventilator tubing; do not drain water back into the humidifier	Water may become a source of contamination, especially with *Pseudomonas*
		Monitor laboratory values, white blood cell count	White blood cell increases may indicate pulmonary infection
		Monitor sputum for changes in color, consistency, amount, and odor	Infection may cause sputum to increase, darken, thicken, and become malodorous
Nutrition, Altered: Less than Body Requirements R/T lack of ability to eat while on ventilator	Client will exhibit adequate nutrional intake as evidenced by: • stable weight, or weight appropriate to height • intake of 1200 kcal/day per nasogastric tube • no signs of catabolism • wounds healing • no infection	Provide adequate nutrition	Intake of 1200 kcal (approx.) is adequate to maintain weight; inadequate nutrition decreases diaphragmatic muscle mass, decreases pulmonary function performance, and increases mechanical ventilation requirements
		Begin tube feeding as soon as it is evident that client will remain on CMV for a length of time	The client should not be allowed to develop a catabolic state
		Avoid excessive carbohydrate loads	Carbohydrate loads may increase carbon dioxide production to the point of producing hypercapnia
		Weigh daily	Changes in body weight are a reliable indicator of nutritional balance
		Monitor intake and output	Fluids are still required, and output should match intake
		Assess for complications of tube feeding. • aspiration • diarrhea • constipation	Feed client sitting upright, with cuff inflated Check for residual tube feeding every shift or before beginning another feeding Diarrhea is most often due to osmotic changes from a too-high concentration of tube feeding or the use of sorbitol based elixirs; consider decreasing the concentration or changing to crushed pills Constipation is due to a lack of free water within the feeding; add 100 mL of water every 4–6 hours if allowable
		Monitor laboratory values (calcium, magnesium, phosphorus, total protein, and albumin)	These trace elements and proteins may not be adequately supplied by a tube feeding
		Monitor bowel sounds	Bowel obstruction and ileus present as changes in bowel sounds
		Before tube feeding or between bolus feedings, test pH and guaiac every shift	Changes in pH may indicate an increased risk of gastric stress ulcers; positive guaiac tests indicate bleeding

ABGs, arterial blood gases; CMV, continuous mechanical ventilation; CPAP, continuous positive airway pressure; PEEP, positive end-expiratory pressure.

health-care facility. Some modifications are necessary, however, for a home environment.

MULTIDISCIPLINARY APPROACH

Before a client with respiratory disease is discharged from a health-care facility, it is important to assess the type of care needed at home. A team of allied health professionals meets to assess specific needs. A typical team consists of nurse, physician, respiratory therapist, physical therapist, occupational therapist, dietitian, discharge coordinator, home health nurse, social worker, and pastoral services person. Consultants from other health-care services may also be present (see the Client Education Guide: The Ventilator-Dependent Client).

Many criteria must be met before instituting "home care" to ensure safety and optimize the client's quality of life (Box 20–4). Much depends on the client's attitude and motivation and the attitude and resources of significant others.

Many respiratory devices require electricity, and electrical outlets must be readily available. The supplier of the equipment usually helps to arrange for all necessary equipment and home adaptations. Duplicate equipment and circuits must be available so that when one piece of equipment is being cleaned and dried the other can be used.

An important aspect of home respiratory care is cleaning and disinfecting equipment. Contaminated respiratory care equipment is a serious potential source of infection.

Providing education and ongoing support for the client and significant others is probably the most essential component of respiratory home care. Motivation is key to the success of the plan. Goals include developing skills and habits to ensure overall safety and a self-determined, quality life-style in the home.

The nurse should plan education according to the established attainable short- and long-term goals. For success, the client and significant others must be involved in goal setting because they are often most aware of what they need. The amount and type of training required depend on the client's condition and capabilities, the intervention needed, and the capabilities of the significant others.

All education must be individually designed for each unique home situation. When mechanical skills are involved, it is important to explain a procedure, then demonstrate it, and have clients perform the procedure under supervision.

CRITICAL TO REMEMBER

The client and significant others must practice all necessary skills with professional support (probably in the health-care facility) before they are expected to perform them without supervision at home. The nurse should be sure they know how to get professional help if needed.

CLIENT EDUCATION GUIDE

The Ventilator-Dependent Client

Good communication between the ventilator-dependent client, family members and/or caregivers, and the home health nurse, the physician, and specific community resources is essential. As soon as the nurse obtains physician's orders and establishes a plan of care, the nurse calls the durable medical equipment supplier. All the equipment and supplies that will be required in the home are reviewed. The nurse may want to plan a shared home visit with the equipment supplier. Next, the nurse needs to check with the local electric company to make sure the community has a list of persons who, in case of an electrical failure, receive priority in getting their service turned back on immediately. It is very important to have a portable, battery-operated ventilator in the home in case of a power failure.

The nurse should plan to spend several hours with the family and caregivers on initial visits. They need to be taught about the equipment, ventilator alarms, suctioning, dressing changes, and other care requirements. The nurse should be certain that they give satisfactory return demonstrations. Often, the equipment is very intimidating to the family and significant others. The nurse should write as much information down as possible, such as phone numbers of the home health nurse, the equipment suppliers, and the physician and instructions about the use of the equipment. Writing this information on a large piece of paper in large print is helpful. The paper should be kept close to the client. This will prevent the family or caregivers from shuffling through various papers or pamphlets to obtain pertinent information. It is not unusual for caregivers to forget everything the nurse has said once she or he leaves. The nurse should remember that the client is probably happy to be home in his or her own environment, but that the family and significant others may be very anxious and frightened. The nurse also addresses the use of help to provide periods of rest for the family.

Equipment noise may be quite a nuisance for clients and caregivers. The nurse should suggest a radio, TV, or cassette player with earphones. If clients can communicate through writing, the nurse should make sure they have a small chalkboard or dry erase board in which to communicate messages or needs to others. The family or client may want to hire a tutor to teach sign language, but most persons learn to read lips. The room should be kept light and open; a bed by a window provides extrasensory stimuli. The nurse must be sure to caution the family to avoid irritants or pollutants such as smoke, animal fur or dander, bird feathers, and/or heavy dust in the environment.

BOX 20-4

Criteria for Respiratory Home Care

The following areas are among those assessed for determining the feasibility of providing home care:

- availability of a strong, positive support system
- motivation and trainability of family or other care providers
- financial resources
- physical resources of the home, e.g., access to electrical outlets, accessibility of bathroom and bedroom, absence of long flights of stairs
- client's physiologic needs and status, e.g., dyspnea and exercise tolerance, and psychosocial status and needs
- client's maximal capabilities
- specific professional support needed, e.g., personnel, equipment, services

Respiratory intervention that may be required at home by clients experiencing chronic respiratory conditions includes oxygen therapy, aerosolization and humidification, chest physiotherapy, IPPB, and mechanical ventilation.

Oxygen Therapy. Home oxygen administration uses the same delivery systems as in health-care facilities (e.g., cannulas, masks). The oxygen source is different, however. Clients who require continuous oxygen may purchase or rent an oxygen concentrator to extract oxygen from room air. This may be more cost effective than large oxygen cylinders. Cylinder oxygen is also used in the home, and lightweight liquid oxygen systems are available for clients requiring oxygen while ambulatory.

Mechanical Ventilation. Continuous mechanical ventilation is being increasingly used outside of health-care facilities. Small, portable, electrically powered ventilators are available for home use. Some models can be adapted to a 12-volt care battery and attached to a wheelchair. Supplemental oxygen must be bled into the inspiratory side of the circuit to provide an FIO_2 greater than 0.21. Family members need to learn daily maintenance checks and how to manage machine problems. The nurse should develop emergency plans with the client and family in case machines fail. A second ventilator must always be readily available.

Aerosolization and Humidification. Humidification can be provided at home by steam from boiling water or a hot shower, and mist therapy can be provided by vaporizers or room humidifiers. The latter are usually available over-the-counter at pharmacies and are often useful for upper airway disorders. They are not so helpful for lower airway disorders, however. Humidifiers produce an aerosol output that is typically restricted to particles of a larger size that are unable to penetrate deep within the lungs. Small-volume medication nebulizers and metered dose inhalers are easily used at home. Small air compressors can be rented or purchased to power small-volume nebulizers.

Chest Physiotherapy. The client's family can learn the techniques of chest physiotherapy, percussion, vibration, and diaphragmatic breathing. If the client has an adjustable "hospital" bed at home, the various positions required are easier to assume. If not, pillows can be used for positioning.

Intermittent Positive-Pressure Breathing. This intervention is seldom used, but if necessary, portable, electrically powered IPPB units are available. Disposable incentive spirometers can be used at home but are rarely necessary.

STUDY QUESTIONS

1. When performing postural drainage, the nurse should include which of the following nursing actions?
   A. Encouraging the client to cough after the procedure
   B. Auscultating the lungs before and after the procedure
   C. Encouraging the client to exhale through pursed lips
   D. All of the above
2. A client has been receiving 100% oxygen therapy by way of a nonrebreather mask for several days. The nurse notes that he is extremely restless and states that he is short of breath and has pain beneath his breastbone. The nurse should suspect:
   A. Oxygen-induced hypoventilation
   B. Oxygen toxicity
   C. Oxygen-induced atelectasis
   D. All of the above
3. When suctioning a tracheostomy tube, the nurse needs to remember that each aspiration should not exceed:
   A. 15 seconds
   B. 30 seconds
   C. 45 seconds
   D. 60 seconds
4. A client is being medicated with a bronchodilator to reduce airway obstruction. Nursing actions include teaching the client to observe for the side effect(s) of:
   A. Dyrhythmias
   B. Central nervous system excitement
   C. Tachycardia
   D. All of the above
5. Diaphragmatic breathing is taught to the client because it does all of the following except:
   A. Decrease respiratory rate
   B. Decrease tidal volume
   C. Increase alveolar ventilation
   D. Reduce functional residual capacity

CRITICAL THINKING EXERCISES

SCENARIO A

A Hispanic client has had emphysema for the last 5 years. He was just admitted to the hospital with his third episode of pneumonia in 2 years. The nurse is to prepare him for discharge on 2 liters of oxygen.

1. Who should be involved in teaching about the client's oxygen therapy?
2. What information should be taught about the oxygen therapy?
3. What preventive measures need to be taught regarding exposure to respiratory infections?

SCENARIO B

An 18-year-old trauma victim suffered from multiple rib fractures. He is to be weaned from his ventilator today.

1. What are the indications for the use of mechanical ventilation?
2. What weaning criteria need to be performed prior to this procedure?
3. What nursing interventions will assist the client in a successful rapid weaning attempt?

BIBLIOGRAPHY

1. Barnes, T. A. (Ed.) (1994). *Core textbook of respiratory care practice* (2nd ed.). St. Louis: Mosby-Year Book.
2. Brown, L. H. (1990). Pulmonary oxygen toxicity. *Focus on Critical Care, 17(1),* 68–75.
3. Bolgiano, C. S., et al. (1990). Administering oxygen therapy: What you need to know. *Nursing 90, 20(6),* 47–51.
4. Bolton, P., & Line, K. (1994). Understanding modes of mechanical ventilation. *American Journal of Nursing, 94(6),* 36–42.
5. Burton, G., et al. (Eds.) (1991). *Respiratory care: A guide to clinical practice* (3rd ed.). Philadelphia: J. B. Lippincott.
6. Cherniack, N. S. (Ed.) (1991). *Chronic obstructive pulmonary disease.* Philadelphia: W. B. Saunders Co.
7. Clark, A. P., et al. (1990). Effects of endotracheal suctioning on mixed venous oxygen saturation and heart rate in critically ill adults. *Heart and Lung, 19(5) (Suppl),* 552–557.
8. Dabbs, A., & Olslund, L. (1994). The new alternatives to intubation. *American Journal of Nursing, 94(8),* 42–45.
9. DeLetter, M. C. (1991). Nutritional implications for chronic airflow limitation patients. *Journal of Gerontological Nursing, 17(5),* 21–26.
10. Deshpande, V., et al. (1988). *A comprehensive review in respiratory care.* Norwalk: Appleton & Lange.
11. Dettenmeier, P. A. (1990). Planning for successful home mechanical ventilation. *AACN Clinical Issues in Critical Care Nursing, 1(2),* 267–279.
12. Dolan, J. T. (1991). *Critical care nursing: Clinical management through the nursing process.* Philadelphia: F. A. Davis.
13. Fedorovich, C., & Littleton, M. T. (1990). Chest physiotherapy: Evaluating the effectiveness. *Dimensions of Critical Care Nursing, 9(2),* 68–74.
14. Ferland, P. (1991). Are you ready for ventilator patients? *Nursing 91, 21(1),* 42–47.
15. Freichels, T. (1993). Orchestrating the care of mechanically ventilated patients. *American Journal of Nursing, 93(10),* 26–34.
16. Glass, C., & Grap, M. J. (1995). Ten tips for safer suctioning. *American Journal of Nursing, 95(5),* 51–53.
17. Gray, J. E., et al. (1990). The effects of bolus normal saline instillation in conjunction with endotracheal suctioning. *Respiratory Care, 35(8),* 785–790.
18. Gregg, B. L. (1989). Inspiratory muscle training with a weighted incentive spirometer in subjects with chronic airway obstruction. *Respiratory Care, 34(10),* 860–867.
19. Hee, M. K., et al. (1992). Intubation of critically ill patients. *Mayo Clinic Proceedings, 67(6),* 569–576.
20. Hudak, C. M., & Gallo, B. M. (Eds.) (1994). *Critical care nursing: A holistic approach* (6th ed.). Philadelphia: J. B. Lippincott.
21. Jeffrey, A. A., et al. (1989). Accuracy of inpatient oxygen administration. *Thorax, 44(12),* 1036–1037.
22. Kersten, L. (1989). *Comprehensive respiratory nursing.* Philadelphia: W. B. Saunders.
23. Kirby, M. J., et al. (Eds.) (1990). *Clinical applications of ventilatory support.* New York: Churchill Livingstone.
24. MacIntyre, N. R. (1989). Pressure support in perspective. *Respiratory Care, 34(2),* 134–135.
25. Marino, P. (1991). *The ICU book.* Baltimore: Williams & Wilkins.
26. Mathews, P. J., et al. (1992). Airway monitoring and ventilation. *Nursing 92, 22(2),* 48–51.
27. McPherson, S. P., & Spearman, C. B. (Eds.) (1994). *Respiratory therapy equipment* (5th ed.). St. Louis: Mosby-Year Book.
28. Nelson, D. M. (1992). Interventions related to respiratory care. *Nursing Clinics of North America. 27(2),* 301–323.
29. *Physicians' desk reference* (48th ed.). (1994). Oradell, NJ: Medical Economics Data.
30. Scanlan, C. L., et al. (Eds.) (1994). *Egan's fundamentals of respiratory care* (6th ed.). St. Louis: Mosby-Year Book.
31. Shapiro, B., et al. (1991). *Clinical applications of respiratory care* (4th ed.). St. Louis: Mosby-Year Book.
32. Sonnesso, G. (1991). Are you ready to use pulse oximetry? *Nursing 91, 21(8),* 60–64.
33. Stiesmeyer, J. K. (1991). What triggers a ventilator alarm? *AJN, 91(10),* 60–65.

34. Stone, K. S., & Turner, B. (1989). Endotracheal suctioning. *Annual Review of Nursing Research, 7(1),* 27–49.

35. Weilitz, P. B. (1991). *Pocket guide to respiratory care.* St. Louis: Mosby-Year Book.

36. Weilitz, P., & Dettenmeier, P. (1994). Test your knowledge of tracheostomy tubes. *American Journal of Nursing, 94(2),* 46–50.

37. Wilson, S. F., & Thompson, J. M. (1990). *Respiratory Disorders.* St. Louis: Mosby-Year Book.

38. Wyngaarden, J. B., et al. (Eds.) (1992). *Cecil textbook of medicine* (19th ed.). Philadelphia: W. B. Saunders.

39. Yeaw, E. M. J. (1992). Good lung down? *American Journal of Nursing, 92(3),* 27–32.

Chapter 21

Nursing Care of Clients with Upper Airway Disorders

Learning Outcomes

After completing this chapter, the learner will be able to:

1. Assess the client for clinical manifestations resulting from upper airway disorders.
2. Teach the client about the risk factors, basic pathophysiology, and clinical manifestations of upper airway disorders.
3. Explain the client's and significant others' role in the prevention and treatment of upper airway disorders.
4. Develop plans of care for the prevention, management, and treatment of clients with upper airway disorders.
5. Implement nursing interventions that optimize the quality of life for clients with upper airway disorders.
6. Evaluate planned outcomes using outcomes developed in the planning phase of care.

TUMORS

CANCER OF THE LARYNX

Cancers of the larynx account for only 2 to 3 per cent of all malignancies. However, clients with these tumors present a unique challenge to the nurse because of the cosmetic and functional deformities commonly seen with this disorder and its treatment.

Cancer of the larynx, or voice box, is classified and treated by its anatomic site. Supraglottic tumors occur on the posterior surface of the epiglottis to the vocal cords, including the false vocal cords. Glottic tumors are tumors of the true vocal cords. Subglottic tumors occur on the undersurface of the true vocal cords.

Incidence

There will be an estimated 12,500 cases of laryngeal cancer each year. Eighty per cent of those cases will involve men. Over the past 30 years, the incidence of cancer of the larynx has remained steady in men; it is up 150 per cent in women.[2] If untreated, cancer of the larynx is inevitably fatal; 90 per cent of untreated clients die within 3 years. Like other cancers, however, it is potentially curable if discovered early enough.

Etiology and Risk Factors

Considerable data indicate that the etiologic agent of laryngeal cancer is cigarette smoking. Three of four clients in whom laryngeal cancer develops have smoked or currently smoke. Other contributing agents include noxious fumes, polluted air, chronic laryngitis, and voice and alcohol abuse.

BOX 21–1

Clinical Warning Signs of Laryngeal Cancer

- Change in voice quality
- A lump anywhere in the neck or body
- Persistent cough, sore throat, or earache
- Hemoptysis
- Sores within the throat do not heal
- Difficulty swallowing or breathing

In this regard, laryngeal cancer is one of the most preventable cancers. Primary prevention is to decrease the number of people who smoke and drink to excess. Secondary prevention is through the early detection of signs of laryngeal cancer, as shown in Box 21–1. Tertiary prevention, the reduction of morbidity, is discussed throughout this section.

Pathophysiology

Cancer of the larynx is most often squamous cell carcinoma. It begins as a small, hard patch, and in time it ulcerates and abscesses. Cancer of the glottis grows slowly owing to limited lymphatic supply. Cancer elsewhere in the larynx spreads more quickly because there are abundant lymphatic vessels. Metastatic disease often may be palpated as neck masses. Distant metastasis occurs in the lungs. Patterns of spread of laryngeal cancer are shown in Figure 21–1.

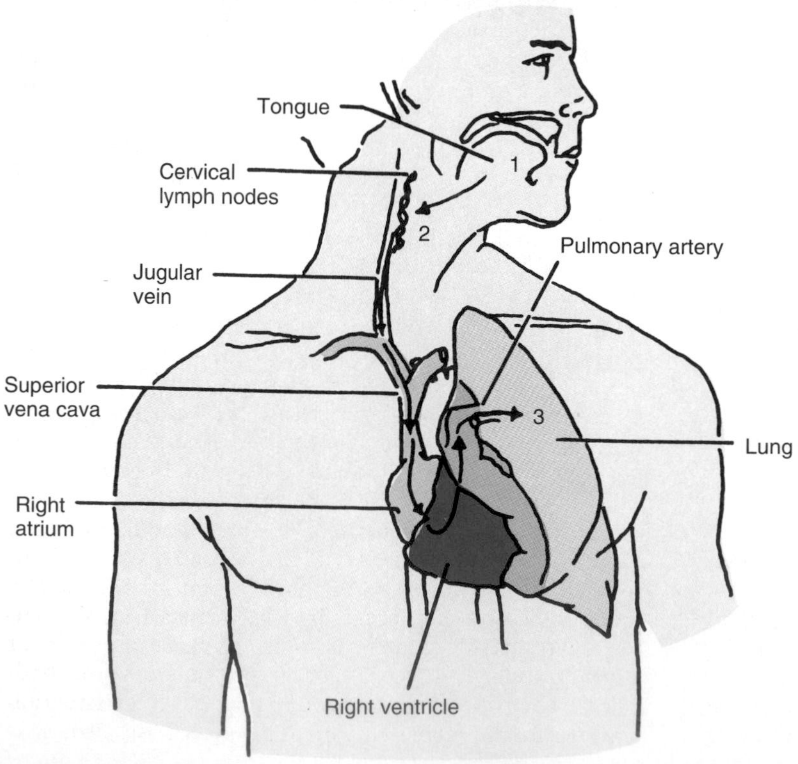

Figure 21–1

The pattern of spread of head and neck cancer. (From Black, J. [1991]. Reconstructive surgery in the elderly. *Plastic Surgical Nursing, 11[4],* 157.)

CLINICAL MANIFESTATIONS

Laryngeal Cancer

AREA	SIGNS AND SYMPTOMS
Glottic tumor	Early: voice change, hoarseness, hemoptysis Late: Dyspnea, respiratory obstruction, dysphagia, weight loss, pain Metastasis: Through regional lymph nodes (rare except in superior or inferior tumors)
Supraglottic tumor	Early: Aspiration on swallowing (especially liquids), persistent unilateral sore throat, foreign body sensation, dysphagia, weight loss, neck mass, hemoptysis Late: Dyspnea, pain in the throat or referred to the ear
Subglottic tumor	Early: None Late: Dyspnea, airway obstruction, dysphagia, weight loss, hemoptysis

Clinical Manifestations

The earliest symptoms of laryngeal cancer are dependent on the location of the tumor (see Clinical Manifestations). In general, hoarseness that lasts longer than 2 weeks should be evaluated. Unfortunately, most clients wait before seeking a diagnosis for chronic hoarseness.

DIAGNOSTIC ASSESSMENT

The diagnosis of laryngeal cancer is made from visual examination of the larynx with direct or indirect laryngoscopy (Fig. 21–2*A*). The nasopharynx and posterior soft palate are inspected indirectly with a small mirror or an instrument resembling a telescope. While the mirror is inserted, slight pressure is applied to the tongue, and the client is instructed to say "uh-hah," which elevates the soft palate. The instrument should not touch the tongue or the client will gag. The nasopharynx is then inspected for drainage, bleeding, ulceration, or masses.

Direct visualization of the larynx may be accomplished with use of several different instruments; most are lighted scopes. The client is instructed to protrude the tongue, and the examiner *gently* pulls the tongue forward with a gauze sponge. A laryngeal mirror or telescopic rod is inserted into the oropharynx; again, contact with the oral cavity is avoided. The client is instructed to breathe in and out rapidly through the mouth or to "pant like a puppy." Panting decreases the gagging sensation caused by the examination. During quiet respiration, the base of the tongue, epiglottis, and vocal cords are examined for signs of infection or tumor (Fig. 21–2*B*). The client is instructed to say a high-pitched "*e*" to close the vocal cords. The examiner observes the movement of the cords, the color of the mucous membrane, and the presence of any lesions. If the client is unable to cooperate with this examination, it may be performed with a fiberoptic endoscope inserted through the nose.

Before any definitive treatment for tumor is initiated, a panendoscopy and biopsy should be performed to determine exact location, size, and extent of the primary tumor. Sometimes computed tomography (CT) or magnetic resonance imaging is used to assist with this process. Laboratory analysis includes a complete blood count, electrolytes, serum calcium levels, and kidney and liver function tests. These data help determine the physiologic state of the client for surgery. Because the airway will be altered after surgery, the client requires a thorough pulmonary assessment with arterial blood gas determinations for identification of any pre-existing pulmonary disorders that would interfere with breathing. Clients who will have a partial laryngectomy must have an adequate pulmonary reserve to produce an effective cough.

CRITICAL TO REMEMBER

The surgery places clients at increased risk of aspiration, and they must be able to cough to rid the airway of aspirated secretions.

Finally, for ascertaining possible tumor spread or other primary tumors, a chest radiograph and barium swallow or esophagogram are performed.

Medical Management

Once the tumor has been located and a biopsy performed, the tumor can be staged. Staging has important implications for treatment choice and outcome. It is essential to determine the extent of the primary tumor to select the most appropriate intervention. Staging is accomplished by measuring the size of the primary tumor, determining the presence of enlarged lymphatic nodes, and determining the presence of distant metastasis. The TNM classification system for laryngeal cancers is shown in Box 21–2. See also Chapter 6 for more information on staging.

Treatment of glottic cancer depends on the degree of tumor involvement. If the tumor is limited to the true vocal cord, without causing a limitation of the cord's movement, radiation therapy is usually the best treatment, with cure rates of 85 to 95 per cent. The dosage of radiation therapy depends on the size and location of the tumor over 5 to 7 weeks. During radiation therapy, the client needs to be assessed for signs of destruction of normal tissue, ability to eat, and other side effects.

Supraglottic tumors may be treated with radiation therapy or a partial laryngectomy with or without lymph node dissection. Subglottic tumors are usually more advanced carcinomas in which metastasis is common. Treatment requires a total laryngectomy with or without radical neck dissection on the same or both sides. The operative site may require reconstruction with pectoralis myocutaneous flaps (see Chap. 50).

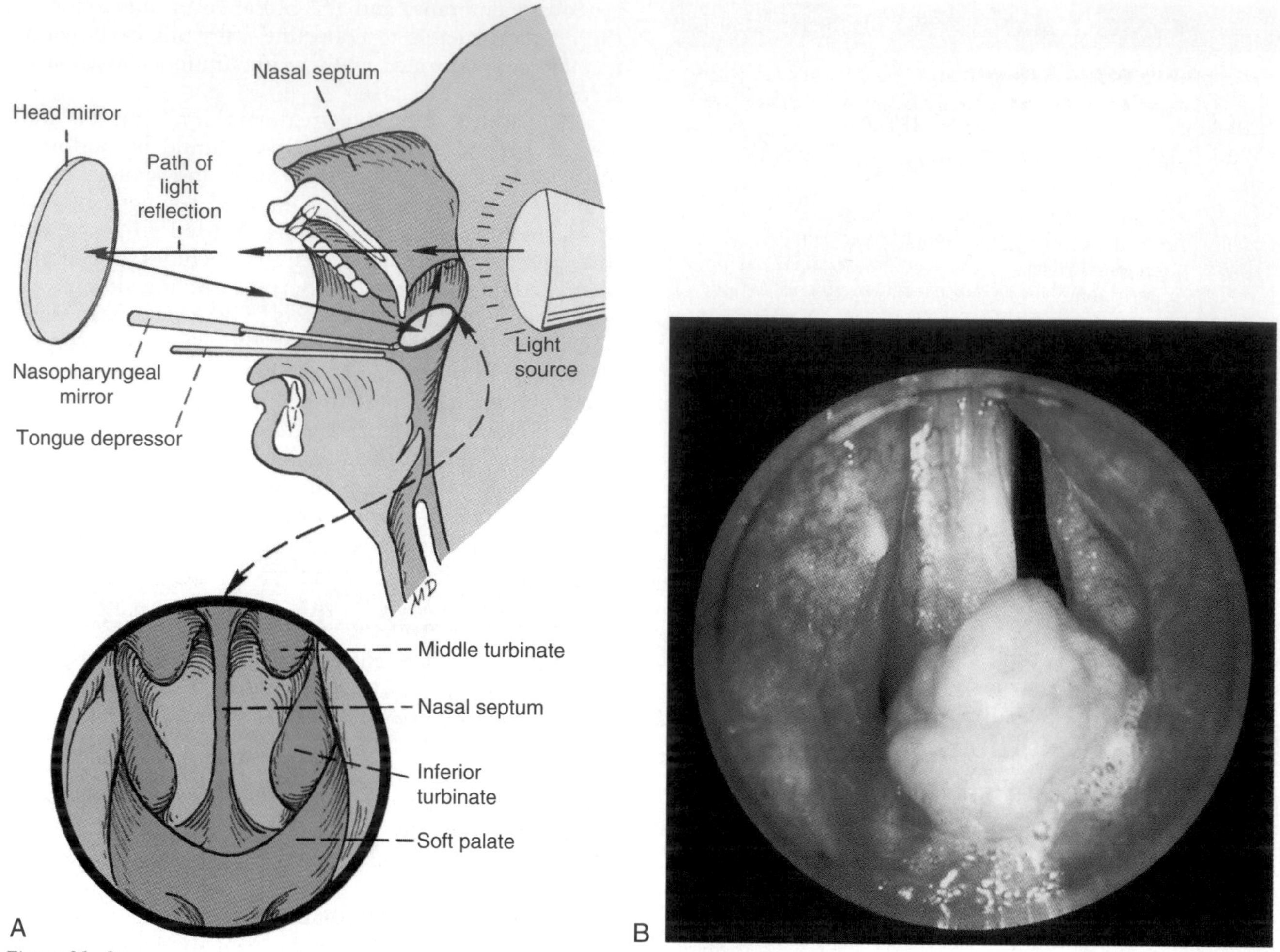

Figure 21–2

A, Indirect laryngoscopy enables assessment of the pharynx and buccal cavity and some visualization of the larynx. (Laryngeal structure and function are best assessed by direct visualization, such as flexible or rigid laryngoscope or flexible fiberoptic bronchoscopy.) Indirect laryngoscopy is performed using a head mirror, tongue depressor, light source, and small examining mirror. The mirror is positioned behind the soft palate after the tongue is depressed. To visualize the larynx, the tongue is gently grasped with a gauze sponge and pulled forward. A mirror is placed against the soft palate in front of the uvula and moved gently until the cords are visualized. The sound "eee" will cause the larynx to move. The larynx is assessed for symmetric cord motion. *B,* Large granular cell tumor of the true vocal cord as seen during laryngoscopy. (From Wenig, B. M. [1993]. *Atlas of head and neck pathology.* Philadelphia: W. B. Saunders Co.)

PHARMACOLOGIC MANAGEMENT

Chemotherapy is generally not effective in advanced laryngeal cancer, but it may have the ability to control the development of new primary tumors through a process called chemoprevention.

DIETARY MANAGEMENT

Most clients with advanced laryngeal cancer also have malnutrition from not being able to eat as well as from the effects of the cancer. Before surgery, the client should receive enteral feedings.

Surgical Management

The goals for surgical intervention for laryngeal cancer are to

- Remove the cancer
- Maintain adequate physiologic function of the airway
- Achieve a personally acceptable physical appearance

Laser surgery for small vocal cord tumors can preserve much of the normal glottis and leave the client with a usable voice. Sometimes laser is combined with radiation therapy. Nursing considerations for the use of laser are in Chapter 5.

BOX 21-2

Criteria for Staging Head and Neck Cancer (American Joint Committee on Cancer)

PRIMARY TUMOR (T)

TX	Minimal requirements to assess the primary tumor cannot be met
T0	No evidence of primary tumor
Tis	Carcinoma in situ
T1	Greatest diameter of primary tumor 2 cm or less
T2	Greatest diameter of primary tumor less than 4 cm
T3	Greatest diameter of primary tumor more than 4 cm
T4	Massive tumor more than 4 cm in diameter with deep invasion to involve antrum, pterygoid muscles, base of tongue, skin of neck

NODAL INVOLVEMENT (N)

NX	Minimal requirements to assess the regional nodes cannot be met
N0	No clinically positive node
N1	Single clinically positive homolateral node 3 cm or less in diameter
N2	Single clinically positive homolateral node more than 3 cm but less than 6 cm in diameter of multiple clinically positive homolateral nodes, none more than 6 cm in diameter
N2a	Single clinically positive homolateral node more than 3 cm but less than 6 cm in diameter
N2b	Multiple clinically positive homolateral nodes, none more than 6 cm in diameter
N3a	Clinically positive homolateral node or nodes, one more than 6 cm in diameter
N3b	Bilateral clinically positive nodes (in this situation, each side of the neck should be staged separately, i.e., N3b: right, N2a: left, N1)
N3c	Contralateral clinically positive nodes only

TUMOR METASTASIS (M)

M0	No metastases present
M1	Metastases clinically demonstrable

STAGE GROUPING

Stage I	T1, N0, M0
Stage II	T2, N0, M0
Stage III	T3, N0, M0
	T1, T2, T3; N1, M0
Stage IV	T4, N0 or N1, M0
	Any T, N2 or N3, M0
	Any T, any N, M1

PARTIAL LARYNGECTOMY

For cancer of one true vocal cord or one true vocal cord and a portion of the other, a partial laryngectomy is feasible. This operation is also called a vertical partial laryngectomy and is the removal of half or more of the larynx (Fig. 21–3). A horizontal neck incision is made, and the diseased portion of one vocal cord is removed. Sometimes up to one third of the contralateral cord is also removed. This operation is generally well tolerated,

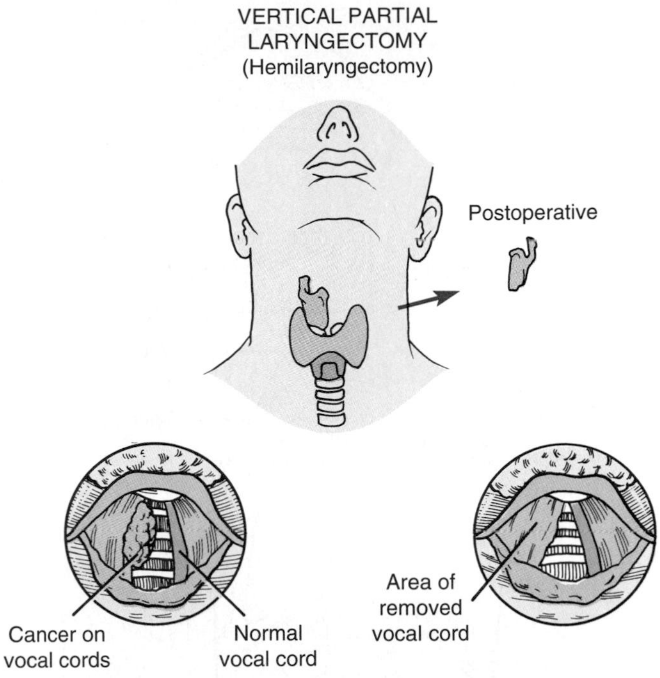

Figure 21–3
The technique of partial laryngectomy.

and the client has only mild difficulty swallowing and an altered, but adequate, voice.

Another form of partial laryngectomy is the supraglottic laryngectomy. This surgery is performed for cancer of the supraglottis. The operation removes the superior portion of the larynx from the false vocal cords to the epiglottis and may extend upward to remove a portion of the base of the tongue. Lymph node dissection also may be performed. Because the true vocal cords are preserved, the voice quality is excellent. The major postoperative problem is risk of aspiration because the epiglottis, which closes over the larynx, has been removed. Airway is managed with a tracheostomy after surgery; when the edema subsides in surrounding tissues, it can usually be removed. The client will need to be taught how to swallow to avoid aspiration.

Possible complications after laryngeal surgery are airway obstruction, hemorrhage, carotid artery rupture, fistula formation, and tracheostomy stenosis.

Airway obstruction is due to edema in the surgical site, bleeding into the airway, or loss of airway from a plugged tracheostomy tube. These problems constitute an emergency and require immediate intervention for restoration of the airway. See care of the obstructed airway.

Hemorrhage is usually the result of inadequate hemostasis during surgery. Some blood-tinged sputum is expected in the tracheal secretions for the first 48 hours, but frank bleeding from the tracheotomy site or tube is a sign of hemorrhage and must be reported to the physician immediately. The nurse should also assess the client for other signs of bleeding such as evident hematoma or unilateral swelling, tachycardia, hypotension, and changes in respiratory patterns.

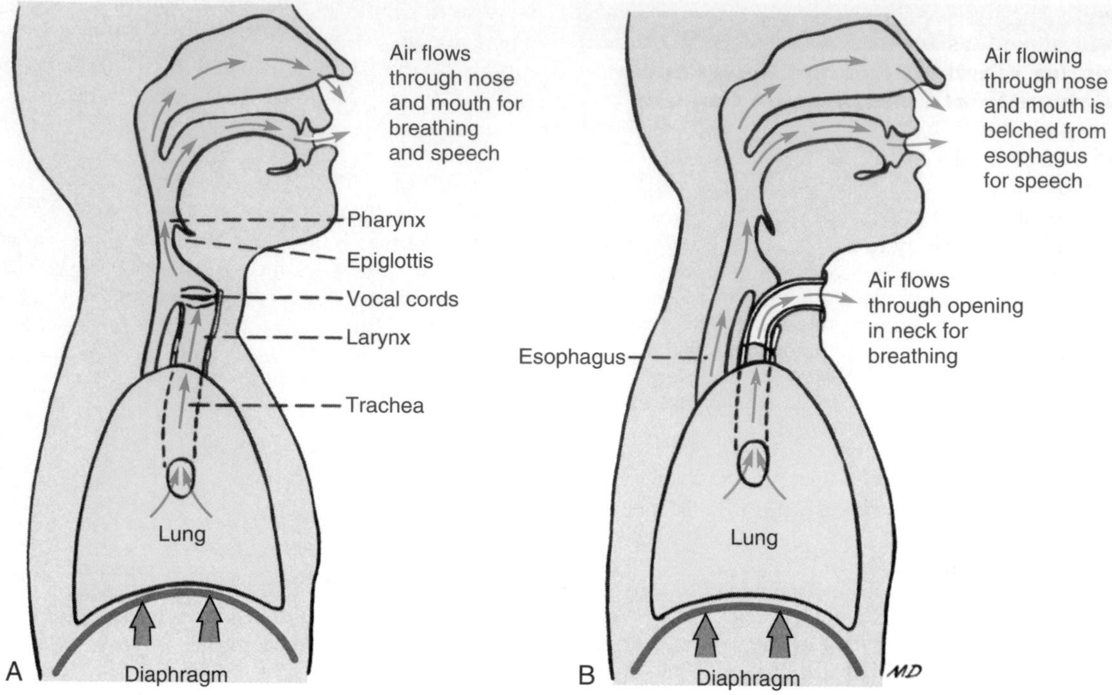
Air flows
through nose
and mouth for
breathing
and speech
Pharynx
Epiglottis
Vocal cords
Larynx
Trachea
Lung
A
Diaphragm
Air flowing
through nose
and mouth is
belched from
esophagus
for speech
Air flows
through opening
in neck for
breathing
Esophagus
Lung
B
Diaphragm
MD

Figure 21–4
Prior to laryngectomy, air flow is through the nose and mouth. Surgical removal of the larynx requires that a new opening be made for air passage. The trachea and esophagus are separated.

Carotid artery rupture is usually a late complication resulting from poor neck tissue integrity. It may be the result of prior radiation therapy to the area, bronchocutaneous fistula, recurrent tumor, or infection. Again, this is a life-threatening emergency and carries an extremely high mortality rate.

CRITICAL TO REMEMBER

Mild bleeding from the oral cavity, neck, or trachea may precede an impending rupture by 24 to 48 hours.

A pulsating tracheostomy tube may indicate that the tip of the tube is resting on the innominate artery and may cause injury to the artery.

A fistula is an abnormal opening between two body cavities. Fistulas between the hypopharynx and the skin are the most common. Many fistulas heal on their own, but surgery may be required, depending on the location and size.

Tracheostomy stenosis is the scarring and narrowing of the ostomy site in the neck. It usually occurs weeks or months after surgery. In some clients, it may lead to a narrowed airway and difficult breathing. The stenotic stoma may be stretched open by use of increasingly larger tracheostomy tubes.

TOTAL LARYNGECTOMY

For large glottic tumors with fixation of the vocal cords, a total laryngectomy is required. When the larynx is removed, a permanent opening is made into the trachea for breathing and the voice is lost. The esophagus remains attached to the pharynx (Fig. 21–4). Because no air can enter the nose, the client loses the sense of smell. The greatest problem for the client after laryngectomy is loss of voice. The client should be made aware that without surgery, the voice quality will worsen as the tumor spreads, but in any case the loss of voice is a serious psychological problem. Because the trachea and pharynx are permanently separated by surgery, there is no risk of aspiration unless a fistula forms from the trachea to the esophagus. Besides this, the potential complications of the total laryngectomy are the same as for the partial laryngectomy (see earlier).

NECK DISSECTION

Metastasis to the cervical lymph nodes is common with tumors of the upper aerodigestive tract. Surgical management of laryngeal tumors often includes neck dissection. Radical neck dissection (also called en bloc) is the removal of lymphatic drainage channels and nodes, sternocleidomastoid muscle, spinal accessory nerve, jugular vein, and submandibular area. A modified radical neck dissection leaves various structures in the neck to minimize deformity.

Nursing Management for the Client Undergoing Partial Laryngectomy

Assessment

Before Surgery: In addition to usual preoperative assessments, the nurse should assess the client's nutritional status. The nurse should assess current body weight to ideal and usual body weight, usual caloric intake, lymphocyte levels, and hemoglobin and hematocrit. The client's state of dentition and oral care should also be assessed. Because many of these clients have abused tobacco and alcohol, their dentition and oral cavity are frequently in poor repair. In addition, if the client is still an active alcoholic, plans should consider support through the period of alcohol withdrawal. The ideal plan would allow some nutritional support and oral care before surgery.

The client's work history and financial concerns should also be investigated during this initial assessment. A lack of medical insurance or money may account for the client's lack of personal and medical care.

The client's usual coping strategies and family support should also be noted. There will be some degree of disfigurement after surgery and a period of time during which the client is unable to speak. Preoperative plans should consider alternative methods of communication and family support networks.

Because of the multiple problems common in these clients, a team approach to their care is used. Members of the team usually include physician-surgeon, nurses, social worker, dietitian, speech-swallowing therapist, physical therapist, and home health-care coordinator. If extensive surgery is required, a plastic surgeon and maxillofacial prosthodontist may also care for the client during reconstruction.

After Surgery: In addition to the routine assessments of any postoperative client, after a partial laryngectomy the client needs to have careful assessment of the airway, lung sounds, position of the tracheostomy tube, and potential complications of the surgery (see earlier).

Nursing Diagnosis, Planning, and Implementation

Nursing Diagnosis: Aspiration, Risk for R/T loss of normal reflexes and excessive secretions secondary to surgery.

Planning: Expected Outcomes. The client will be free from aspiration, as evidenced by clear breath sounds throughout the chest, normal (for age) respiratory rate and rhythm, chest secretions that are clear or only slightly blood tinged, and ability to cough.

Implementation. In the immediate postoperative period, priority is given to the management of the upper airway. The client should be positioned in semi-Fowler's to high-Fowler's position to decrease edema of the airway, facilitate breathing, and improve comfort.

A cuffed tracheostomy tube is generally inserted during surgery and is maintained for the first several days after surgery to minimize aspiration of secretions and for assisted or controlled ventilation. Secretions collect above the cuff and need removal. For removal of the secretions, the cuff should be deflated during exhalation. The client should be instructed to cough during deflation of the cuff. If the client cannot cough, suctioning should be used to prevent secretions from being aspirated. The cuff should be reinflated during inspiration.

When the edema has subsided, the tracheostomy tube may be removed. The decannulation process is slow and begins by observing the client for aspiration. The cuff of the tube is deflated, and the client is observed for the ability to swallow saliva and other secretions without coughing or requiring additional suctioning. If there are increased secretions through and around the tracheostomy tube, aspiration is occurring and the cuff should be reinflated. If no aspiration is occurring, the tracheostomy tube can be replaced with a smaller uncuffed tube. If this is tolerated without aspiration, the tube is capped to determine the client's ability to breathe through the upper airway. If the client can breathe through the upper airway for 24 hours, the tracheostomy tube is removed, and the stoma is taped closed and covered with an occlusive dressing.

Nursing Diagnosis: Airway Clearance, Ineffective R/T physical alteration in airway and presence of tracheostomy tube.

Planning: Expected Outcomes. The client will have improved airway clearance, as evidenced by effortless, quiet respirations at baseline rate and clear breath sounds.

Implementation. The client may have copious secretions because of the presence of the tracheostomy tube, history of chronic obstructive lung disease, and aspiration. There may also be oral secretions that cannot be swallowed. In the alert and conscious client, coughing and deep breathing will mobilize and eliminate many of these secretions. However, in the client having head and neck surgery and just emerging from anesthesia, this may not be possible. Suctioning of the trachea will be needed for the first 24 to 48 hours after surgery. The frequency of suctioning depends on the client's needs, but suctioning every hour is common for the first 24 hours. Sterile technique must be used to avoid introducing micro-organisms into the tracheobronchial tree in a client with impaired immune defenses resulting from malignancy and surgery. (Suctioning techniques can be found in a fundamentals of nursing textbook.)

A tracheostomy tube with an inner cannula is commonly used in these clients. Mucus collects in the inner cannula, which can be removed and cleaned without removing the entire tube. The inner cannula should be cleaned as often as necessary to provide a clear airway for the client. In the immediate postoperative phase, the inner cannula is cleaned after suctioning. Once the client is ambulatory and handles secretions safely, it can be cleaned as necessary but at least three times a day.

Chest physiotherapy, ultrasonic nebulization, or aerosol administration of medications in addition to ambulation, coughing, and deep breathing is recommended to prevent pulmonary complications. These treatments are performed every 4 hours for the first few days after surgery and then usually decreased to four times a day once the client can ambulate.

Collaborative Problem: Risk for Acute Airway Distress R/T accidental decannulation.

Planning: Expected Outcomes. The nurse will monitor for a patent airway, as evidenced by clear breath sounds; quiet, effortless respirations; and a patent, intact cannula.

Implementation. Tracheostomy tube displacement or accidental decannulation may result in acute airway distress. To prevent this emergency, many surgeons are attaching long sutures (called stay sutures) from the tracheal wall to the client's chest. If the tube is accidentally removed, the sutures can be loosened on the chest and pulled upward and outward to open the stoma for tube reinsertion. If stay sutures are not used and the tracheostomy tube is displaced or removed, a tracheal dilator and an emergency tracheostomy tray must be available for reinsertion of the tube. After approximately 72 hours, a tract will form between the skin and trachea, and the tube can be reinserted with little difficulty.

Collaborative Problem: Risk for Tracheal Necrosis and Stenosis.

Planning: Expected Outcomes. The risk of tracheal necrosis or stenosis will be reduced, as evidenced by use of a high-volume, low-pressure tracheostomy cuff, routine deflation of the cuff, and avoidance of the minimal leak technique to reinflate the cuff.

Implementation. A high-volume, low-pressure cuff should be used to prevent excess pressure on the tracheal mucosa. Excessive pressure can result in tracheal ischemia with eventual necrosis and stenosis. Although low-pressure cuffs are used, cuffs should be deflated every shift to improve circulation to the cuff site and remove accumulated secretions. Only a minimal amount of air should be used to reinflate the cuff to prevent overinflation and excess pressure. The minimal occlusion volume technique should be used to seal the space between the tracheal wall and the cuff. The minimal leak technique should not be used; it is not effective in clients who have had head and neck surgery because of edema of the airway. (These techniques are discussed in Chapter 20.) To assist with the minimal occlusion technique, the nurse should ascertain and document on the medical record the amount of air used to inflate the cuff during surgery as a point of reference.

Nursing Diagnosis: Infection, Risk for (Respiratory) R/T loss of normal filtration systems in the mouth and nose with use of an artificial airway.

Planning: Expected Outcomes. The client will not experience clinical manifestations of a respiratory infection, as evidenced by afebrile state, clear or slightly blood-tinged secretions, white cell count remaining within normal limits, and clear lung sounds.

Implementation. Once a tracheostomy is performed, the nose and upper airway are no longer able to provide filtration, warming, and moistening of inspired air. Supplemental humidification and airway protection will be required. Commonly, 40 per cent oxygen with high humidity is delivered at 4 to 6 L/minute. Oxygenation is assessed through arterial blood gases, and fraction of inspired oxygen (FIO_2) may be adjusted. If the client has pre-existent chronic lung disease, oxygen may have to be delivered at lower percentages or not at all. Compressed air with high humidity may be substituted for these clients. Humidified oxygen or compressed air is administered through a tracheostomy mask or universal adaptor to a cuffed tracheostomy tube. The supplemental humidification is usually given for the first 48 hours and then on a supplemental basis.

Nursing Diagnosis: Nutrition, Altered: Less than Body Requirements R/T malignancy and swallowing difficulties.

Planning: Expected Outcomes. The client will have an improved nutritional status, as evidenced by maintaining baseline body weight or losing less than 5 pounds; consuming adequate fluid, protein, fat, and carbohydrate each 24 hours; swallowing without aspirating or choking; hemoglobin, hematocrit, and lymphocyte count remaining within normal limits.

Implementation. Immediately after surgery, it is likely the client will have a nasogastric tube for removal of gastric secretions until postoperative ileus subsides. The nurse should assess for bowel sounds, passing of flatus, and hunger as signs of returning gastrointestinal function. Some clients will be tube fed with commercial supplements. The nurse must continually ascertain the correct placement of the tube before each feeding. (Techniques to check tube placement can be found in a fundamentals of nursing textbook.) The tube feeding can be administered by pump, slow drip, or bolus feeding depending on the client's tolerance. Aspiration remains a high risk with partial laryngectomy, and precautions to guard the client from it are critical.

Because the epiglottis has been removed, when to begin oral feeding after a partial laryngectomy is controversial. One approach is to begin oral feedings with the tracheostomy tube in place, when edema has subsided and the client is able to swallow secretions. The advantage of this technique is that aspirated liquid can be suctioned. A second technique is to delay oral feeding until the client has been decannulated and the stoma has healed. The advantage of this technique is that, with a closed stoma, the client will be able to increase intrathoracic pressure and remove any aspirated material through an effective cough.

Whenever the client eats, eating should begin with a nonpourable pureed diet; liquids are reserved until swallowing has been relearned (see the Client Education Guide: Swallowing Technique After a Partial Laryngectomy). Once swallowing can be accomplished without aspiration, carbonated beverages may be added. Thin liquids should be withheld until the risk of aspiration is minimal.

Nursing Diagnosis: Infection (Wound), Risk for R/T loss of primary defenses (incision) and malignancy.

Planning: Expected Outcomes. The client will experience no clinical manifestations of wound infection, as evidenced by incisional edges remaining approximated; amounts of wound drainage decreasing; absence of redness, swelling, tenderness, or warmth beyond the suture lines; remaining afebrile; and white cell count remaining within normal limits.

Implementation. During surgery, a wound drain is placed into the surrounding tissues of the neck and attached to constant suction. A common mechanism for collecting the drainage is a Hemovac container, which is attached to the client's gown to prevent accidental dislodgement. Using universal precautions, the amount

CLIENT EDUCATION GUIDE

Swallowing Technique After a Partial Laryngectomy

The nurse should:

1. Have the client begin with soft or semisolid foods.
2. Stay with the client during meals until the technique of swallowing is mastered without choking.
3. Offer encouragement; learning to reswallow is frustrating.
4. Guide the client in the following steps:
   - Take a deep breath.
   - Bear down to close the vocal cords.
   - Place food into mouth.
   - Swallow.
   - Cough to rid the closed cord of accumulated food particles.
   - Swallow.
   - Cough.
   - Breathe.

and color of the drainage should be assessed by the nurse every 4 hours for the first 24 hours. The wound should be assessed for signs of hematoma or seroma formation by noting whether the amount of drainage is increasing or whether there is change in the color or consistency of the drainage. The color of the incision lines should also be assessed. If the drainage is subsiding, the drain may be removed by the physician. Dressings are placed over the drain puncture sites on the skin. Small to moderate amounts of serosanguineous drainage should be expected for another 48 to 72 hours.

The suture lines should be cleansed at least twice daily with hydrogen peroxide followed by water or saline rinse. A thin film of antibiotic ointment may be applied to the suture line to prevent crusting of secretions and promote healing.

Evaluation

The degree of goal attainment is evaluated, and revisions are made in the interventions as needed to meet the revised goals. Depending on the client's preoperative condition (e.g., malnourished), additional time may be required to meet the various goals.

Nursing Management for the Client Undergoing Total Laryngectomy

The nursing management of the client after a total laryngectomy is the same as the care given a client with a partial laryngectomy except for feeding and teaching about the permanent stoma care. Clients who have a total laryngectomy will have a permanent tracheostomy and need to learn how to speak using alternative methods.

Immediately after surgery, the client's nutrition is supplemented with nasogastric feedings. When the client exhibits signs of swallowing his or her own secretions, the edema has subsided and feeding can begin. The diet usually begins with soft or semisoft foods and progresses as healing occurs.

Communication: For the first few days after surgery, the client should communicate by writing. If the client is very fatigued, common client requests such as "I need something for pain" may be written on a pad of paper, and the client can just point to the statement.

CRITICAL TO REMEMBER

Even though the client cannot speak, conversation should still include the client's input through nodding and pointing and not be directed only to others such as the family. Avoiding conversation with the client because of the difficulty in communication is demeaning and leads to client frustration.

An artificial larynx may be used as early as 3 to 4 days after surgery. These electronic devices are held alongside the neck, or a plastic tube is inserted in the mouth; vibration produces mechanical speech (Fig. 21–5). The air inside the mouth is vibrated, and the client articulates as usual. The speech quality is monotone and artificial, but it is better than no speech at all.

Esophageal speech is a technique that requires the client to swallow and hold air in the upper esophagus. By controlling the flow of air, the client can pronounce as many as 6 to 10 words before stopping to reswallow air. The voice is deep, but it is loud and entirely effective once the technique is mastered.

Tracheoesophageal puncture (Fig. 21–6) is a surgical technique that may also restore speech. A small puncture is made into the upper tracheostoma to the cervical esophagus for creation of a fistula. Once the fistula is healed, a small one-way valve is inserted, called a voice button or trapdoor prosthesis. By occlusion of the valve, air can be shunted into the esophagus, producing speech. These devices require maintenance; therefore, only clients who are highly motivated, are able to perform self-care, and have good manual dexterity are eligible for this procedure.

The techniques to restore speech require much time for mastery; the client is seen by a speech therapist after discharge from the hospital. Community support groups exist for clients after laryngectomy, called the Lost Cord Club and International Association of Laryngectomees, that may offer needed reassurance.

Much patience is required by the client and significant others while the client is relearning to speak. The process is time consuming and frustrating and requires more time to speak. Significant others should be encouraged to give the client enough time to formulate the words and not speak for the client.

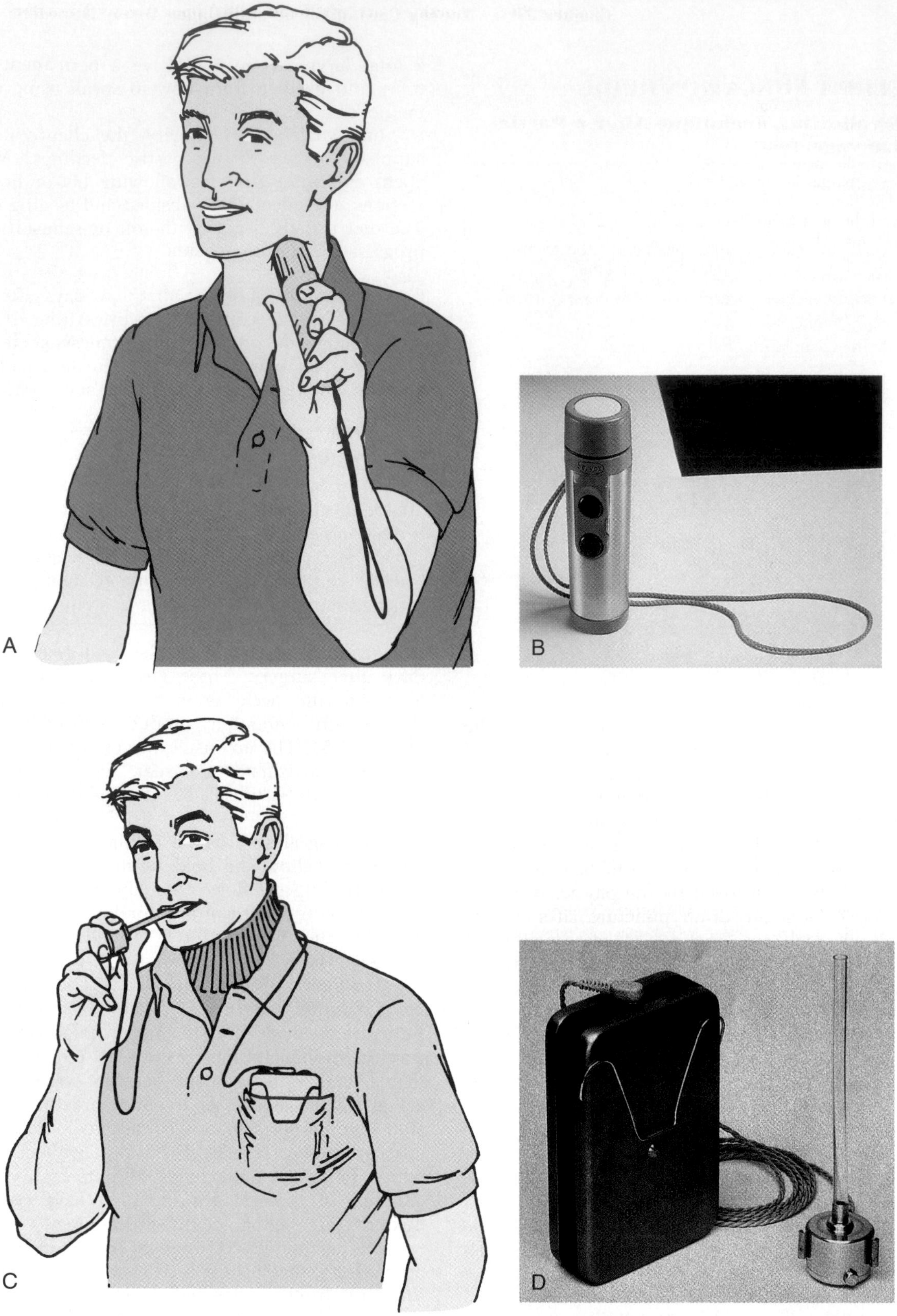

Figure 21–5
A and *B,* Artificial larynx (electrolarynx). This handheld, battery-powered speech aid is placed against the neck. *A,* When activated, it creates a vibration that is transmitted to the neck and into the mouth. Words silently formed by the mouth become sounds from the vibrations emitted by the device. Any type of artificial larynx requires muscle and tongue control and hand strength. It normally is not used until immediate postoperative neck tenderness has subsided. (Part *B,* Courtesy of Servox Electrolarynx Mfg. by Siemans Hearing Instruments, Inc., Union, NJ.) *C* and *D,* Electronic speech aid (Cooper Rand). This instrument allows the person to adjust tone, pitch, and volume. An oral connector permits speech without the necessity for placing the device against the neck. This is an advantage immediately after surgery, when the neck is too sensitive for a neck-vibrating device. (Part *D,* Courtesy of Luminaud, Inc., Mentor, OH.)

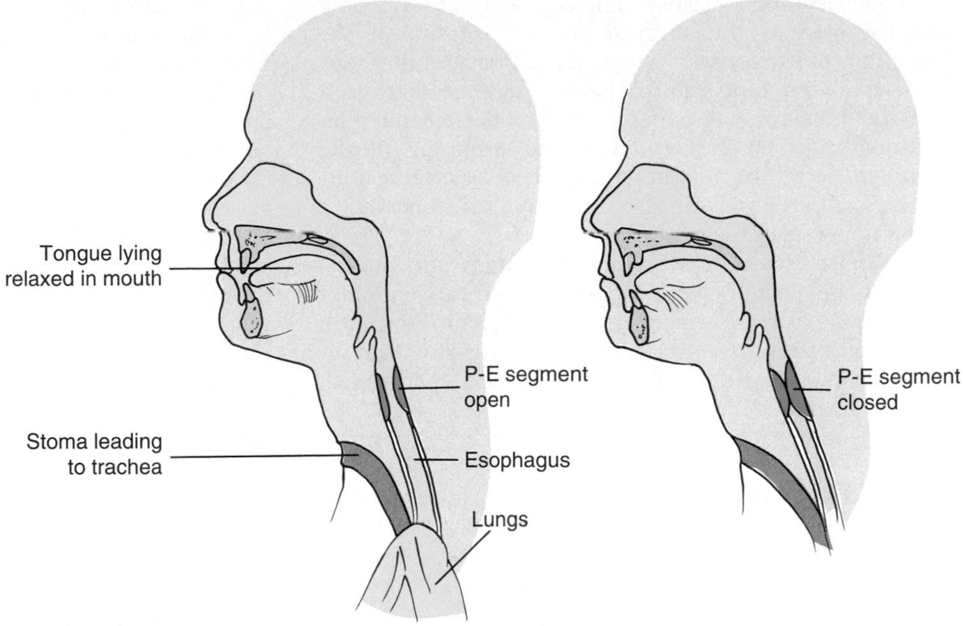

Figure 21–6
Tracheoesophageal puncture for voice rehabilitation after laryngectomy. A prosthesis is inserted into a created fistula in the neck. The prosthesis has a one-way valve that permits air to pass into the esophagus but prevents accidental aspiration. To speak, the client occludes the prosthesis with a finger or attachment. Exhaled air is then shunted through the prosthesis, where it vibrates, and exits the mouth as spoken word.

Nursing Management for the Client Undergoing Neck Dissection

Assessment

Before surgery, the client's understanding of the plans for surgery should be assessed. The nurse should determine what the surgeon has told the client and how much information has been retained or lost because of anxiety. In addition, the fears the client has about the diagnosis of cancer and fears of deformity after surgery should be addressed. The nurse can explain to the client and significant others what to expect after surgery (e.g., placement in the intensive care unit, tracheostomy, drainage tubes) and review postoperative care (e.g., communication technique if a tracheostomy will be placed).

The client's support systems and degree of coping should be assessed. If the client is an alcoholic, the use of alcohol may be the usual coping tool. Because alcohol will not be available, the nurse should assess the other coping mechanisms available to the client and encourage the client to motivate them. Sources include friends, family, and insurance and other finances. If new support systems are needed, these should be identified as soon as possible, such as other clients who have had the same surgery or diagnosis.

After surgery, the usual postoperative assessments are performed, with special attention given to the airway. Airway patency can be lost as a result of edema of the neck or bleeding within the area. If the surgical defect was repaired with musculocutaneous flaps, the flap should be assessed for arterial inflow and venous outflow. The temperature, color, and blanching should be noted every hour for the first 24 hours and every 4 hours after that time.

Nursing Diagnosis, Planning, and Implementation

Collaborative Problem: Airway Obstruction, Risk for R/T to edema or bleeding.

Planning: Expected Outcomes. The client will have no airway distress, as evidenced by normal breathing patterns, no cyanosis or pallor, no stridor, and no hematoma formation.

Implementation. The nurse must assess the client for signs of airway edema or bleeding and auscultate lung sounds every 2 hours for the first 24 hours. Signs of airway obstruction should be reported immediately.

The client should be placed in a semi-Fowler's position to minimize postoperative edema. Neck drainage catheters, inserted into the surgical wound, are monitored for amount of drainage. The drains should be aspirated under strict aseptic technique at least every 4 hours to maintain patency of the drains and allow drainage of blood or serum from the wound. Sanguineous or serosanguineous drainage is expected for the first 72 hours after surgery. Once drainage has stopped, the catheters are removed.

Pressure dressings may be used in the immediate postoperative period, depending on physician preference. If a dressing is used, it should be reinforced as needed and observed for any drainage. If musculocutaneous flaps are needed for coverage, pressure dressings will not be used, and special flap care will be required. (See Chap. 50 for specific care of flaps.)

Nursing Diagnosis: Physical Mobility, Impaired R/T shoulder dysfunction.

Planning: Expected Outcomes. The client will retain usual shoulder function, as evidenced by full (or previously normal) range of motion in shoulder and maintenance of shoulder strength.

Implementation. Most clients will report only minimal pain in the surgical site as a result of the disruption of the sensory nerve fibers from the incisions used. If an en bloc radical neck dissection has been performed, clients will experience shoulder dysfunction, resulting in a forward rotation and dropping of the shoulder. Sectioning of the spinal accessory nerve during neck dissection will also interrupt the innervation to the upper trapezius muscle.

Exercises to increase range of motion and muscle strength are encouraged to prevent a frozen shoulder and restore full movement (see the Client Education Guide: Exercises After Radical Neck Surgery). If a selective or modified neck dissection has been performed, minimal change will occur.

Client Education Guidelines

THE CLIENT UNDERGOING PARTIAL LARYNGECTOMY

After discharge from the hospital, therapy may be needed for swallowing and sometimes for speech (see the Client Education Guide: Esophageal Speech). If the client needs to continue wound care until full healing occurs, instructions should be given in writing. Ongoing assessment for potential malignancy will be required.

THE CLIENT UNDERGOING TOTAL LARYNGECTOMY

Client Education. Clients should be discharged with an extra tracheostomy tube to allow daily changes at home. To provide humidified air, normal saline may be instilled into the stoma several times each day to stimulate coughing, moisten the mucosa, and loosen dried secretions and crusts. A bedside humidifier or vaporizer will also aid in humidifying the inspired air. So that foreign bodies are prevented from entering the stoma, a stoma bib or covering should be worn. These coverings can be purchased, or the client may improvise by using a scarf, necktie, or turtleneck shirt.

The client should be encouraged to continue speech therapy as begun in the hospital.

Once the incision has completely healed, the tracheostomy tube will not be required. This process varies but usually takes about 6 to 8 weeks. Occasionally, the tube will be required at night, if the stoma is small or the client does not get adequate air exchange during sleep. Once the tracheostomy has been removed, the client will be able to disguise the stoma with clothing and begin to regain a sense of normalcy.

Tub baths or showers are permitted, but the client must use caution to prevent introduction of water into the stoma. Commercial stoma shower covers are available, and the water spray should be aimed at midchest. Water sports are prohibited. If the client fishes, a life preserver will need to be worn at all times on the boat.

The client should wear a Medic Alert bracelet to identify the fact that resuscitation cannot be performed through the mouth. The client will need mouth-to-stoma rescue breathing.

The client may require a nutritional plan for the first few weeks at home. The dietitian should work with the client and significant others to determine the consistency of food easiest to swallow as well as the kinds of foods required to obtain needed protein and calories.

It is essential that the client not smoke so that lung function is preserved and the formation of other aerodigestive tract tumors is prevented. For some clients after laryngectomy, the process of smoking cessation seems pointless. Some clients continue to smoke by inhaling the cigarette smoke through the stoma. The attitude is one of "Why quit now? What else could happen to me?" The nurse should use extra support and encouragement with the client, remembering to be an advocate of the client's choice as well as providing assurance that the quality of life after smoking cessation improves.

Follow-Up Care. Follow-up care is important to assess the healing process, evaluate coping mechanisms, and examine the client for possible metastasis or new tumors. The client should be taught to report any of these signs or symptoms to the physician:

- A lump anywhere in the neck or body
- Persistent cough, sore throat, or earache
- Hemoptysis
- Sores around the stoma or within the trachea that do not heal
- Difficulty swallowing or breathing

THE CLIENT UNDERGOING NECK DISSECTION

Clients should be cautioned about potential injury to the neck tissue because of lack of sensation. The use of a heating pad or exposure to temperature extremes may result in tissue injury (burns, frostbite) in a client who cannot feel these temperatures. Clients with tracheostomy will need specific instructions for its management. Ongoing malignancy care should be explained.

CLIENT EDUCATION GUIDE

Esophageal Speech

When learning esophageal speech, the client may experience indigestion from excessive air intake. The nurse can help with the following:

- Inform the client that decreased appetite may result from air in the digestive tract.
- Encourage the client to speak slowly and practice the correct technique.
- Remind the client of the inability to speak and eat at the same time.
- Follow the communication techniques learned to converse with any client with impaired communication ability.
- Teach the client that mucus buildup in the tracheostomy and stoma site will decrease the ability to maintain adequate air intake.

CLIENT EDUCATION GUIDE

Exercises after Radical Neck Surgery

Step 1: Begin by gently moving your head from side to side, tipping your ear toward your shoulder on the same side and moving your chin toward your chest.

Step 2: To exercise your shoulders using the hand on your unoperated side, lean or hold onto a low table or chair. Bend your body slightly at the waist and:

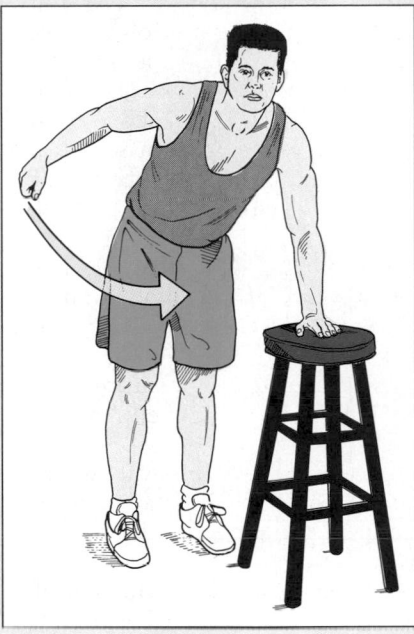

a. Swing shoulder and arm from left to right.

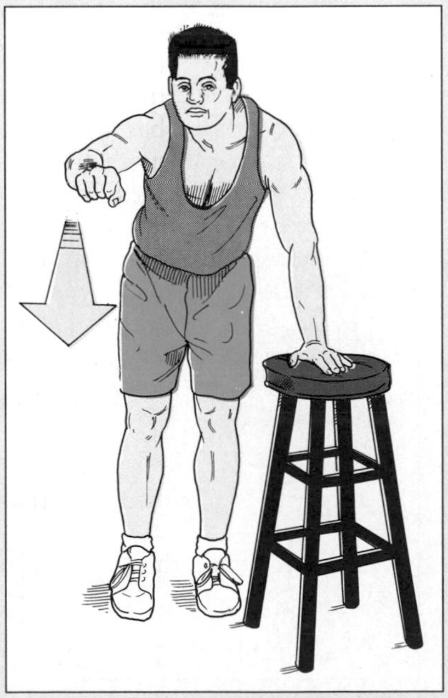

b. Swing shoulder and arm from front to back.

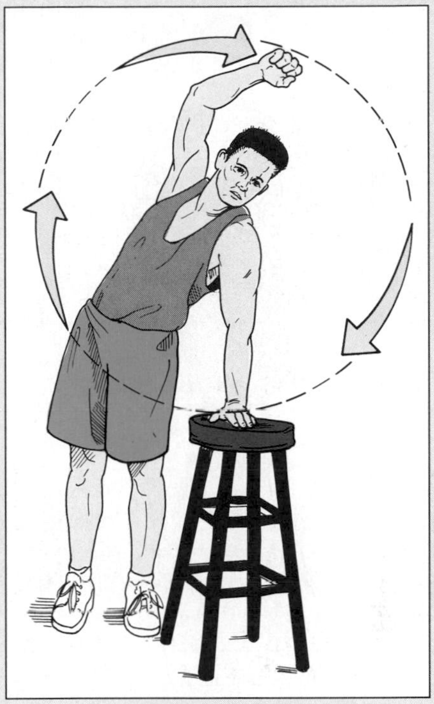

c. Swing shoulder and arm in a wide circle, gradually bringing your arm all the way over your head.

Step 3: It would be helpful to do this exercise before a mirror. Sit straight and:

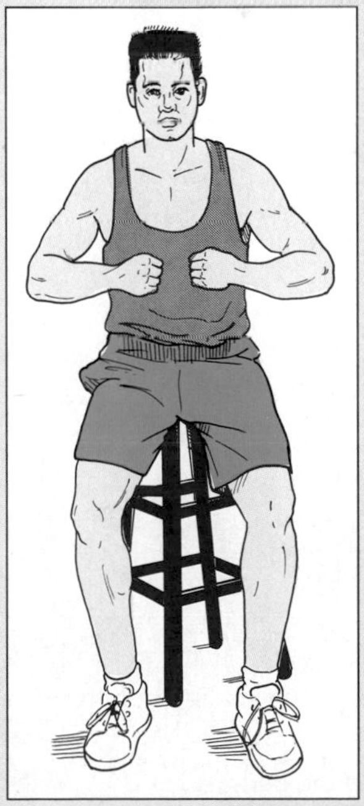

a. Place hands in front of you with your elbows at right angles, sticking out from your body.

Client Education Guide continued on following page

CLIENT EDUCATION GUIDE

Exercises after Radical Neck Surgery Continued

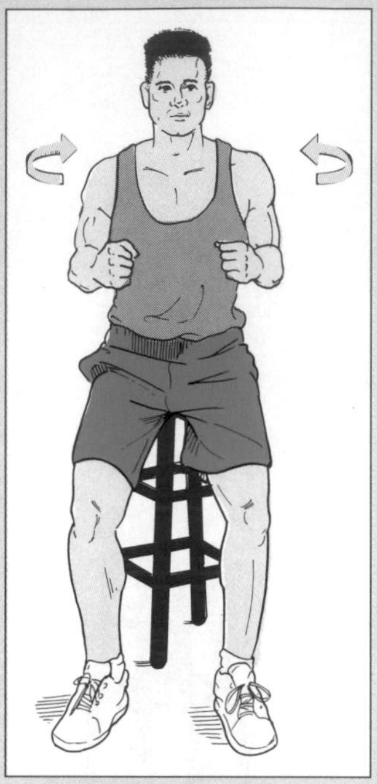

b. Rotate your shoulders back, bringing elbows to your side.

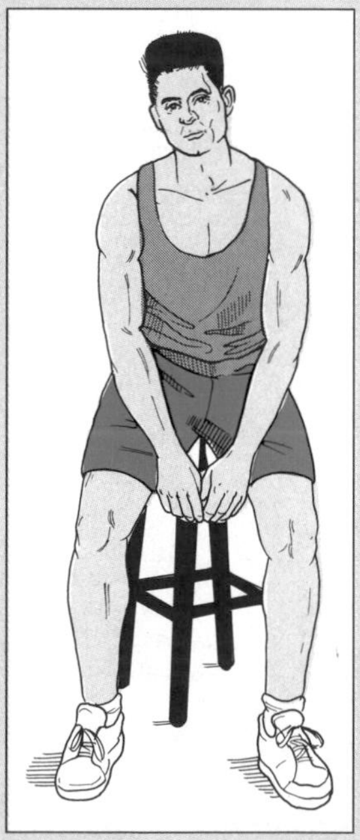

c. Relax your whole body.

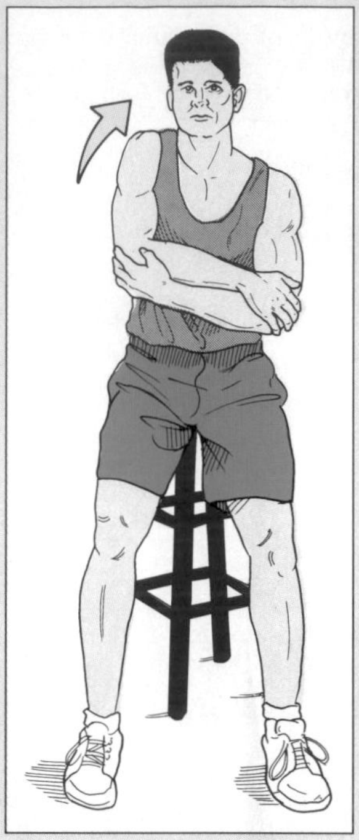

d. With arms crossed in front of you, support the elbow on the operated side with our opposite hand, and help lift the arm and shoulder while shrugging.

Step 4: Stand sideways at arm's length from the wall.

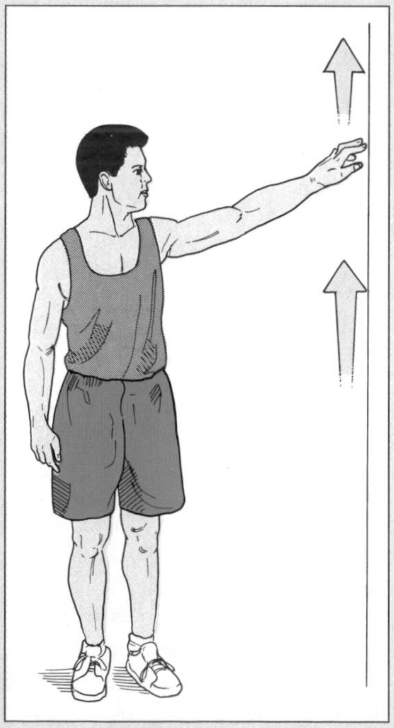

a. Walk your fingers slowly up the wall.

b. As your fingers climb up, begin to move your body closer to the wall.

c. Continue until your arm is high above your head and shoulder.

CLIENT EDUCATION GUIDE

Exercises after Radical Neck Surgery Continued

Step 5: Attach a hook to a wall or door. Hang a short rope knotted at each end over the hook. Under the hook, place a straight-back chair or stool.

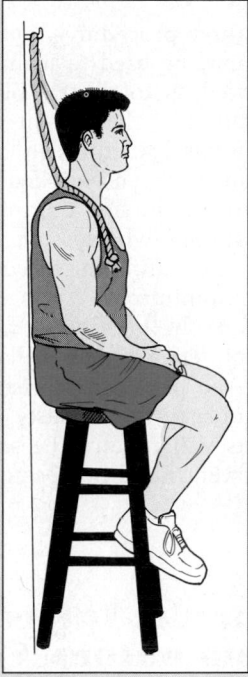

a. Sit straight, with your back against the wall.

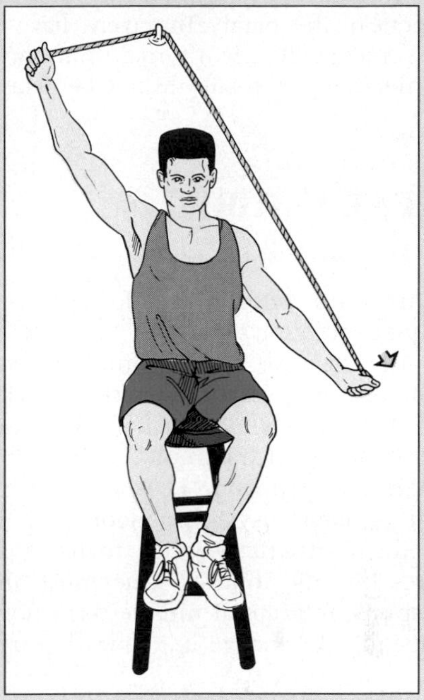

b. Pull one arm and shoulder up with the rope by bringing the other arm and shoulder down. Repeat with the other arm. It is important in this exercise not to bend your body. Keep the motion in the shoulder.

Obstructions of Upper Airway

Acute Airway Obstruction

ACUTE LARYNGEAL EDEMA

This may be associated with inflammation, injury, or anaphylaxis. It is manifested by hoarseness and dramatic shortness of breath. Dyspnea progresses rapidly, and unless a patent airway is established, respiratory arrest occurs. Endotracheal intubation may be very difficult because the larynx is edematous and is likely to bleed. Emergency tracheostomy may be required. If anaphylaxis is the precipitating cause, subcutaneous epinephrine, 1:1000, is given. Intravenous corticosteroids are also used.

LARYNGOSPASM

Spasm of laryngeal muscles may occur

- After administration of some general anesthetic agents
- After repeated and traumatic attempts at endotracheal intubation
- As a response to some inhaled agents and foreign material, such as industrial fumes and dusts, and chemicals
- From hypocalcemia

CRITICAL TO REMEMBER

Management is directed at re-establishing the airway as quickly and efficiently as possible. Administer 100 per cent oxygen until the airway is fully re-established and the larynx relaxes and stops spasming.

Titrate FIO_2 according to pulse oximetry values. If the laryngospasm persists, paralysis with neuromuscular blocking agents, such as succinylcholine, may be required to allow intubation until the spasm breaks. Manual or mechanical ventilation is then necessary until the effects of the paralyzing agent have worn off. Occasionally, emergency cricothyroidotomy or tracheotomy may be necessary and should not be delayed.

LARYNGEAL INJURY

Laryngeal injury most often results form trauma during a motor vehicle accident, such as when the driver's neck strikes the steering wheel. Other causes include the inhalation of hot gases or aspiration of caustic liquids. If complete airway obstruction does not occur, carefully assess for post-traumatic edema, which may lead to complete obstruction. Few outward signs may be present. It is often easy to overlook potential problems in the neck structures while focusing on other, possibly more dramatic injuries. One must observe for increased dyspnea, intercostal muscle retraction, stridor, inability to speak, and change in respiration patterns.

Chronic Airway Obstruction

DEVIATED NASAL SEPTUM AND NASAL FRACTURE

The nasal septum, the dividing structure of the nose, is usually straight and divides the nose into two equal chambers. After trauma, the septum may become deviated creating asymmetric breathing passages. For some clients, the deviation may cause an obstruction to nasal breathing, dryness of the nasal mucosa causing bleeding, and occasionally a cosmetic deformity.

If a nasal fracture occurs, immediate medical management is advised. Within several hours of nasal injury, severe edema may occur, which causes difficulty in reducing the fracture. Immediately after the injury, ice should be applied. A simple nasal fracture may be reduced in an emergency facility with use of local anesthesia. If immediate reduction of the nasal fracture is not possible, it is advisable to wait several days until edema subsides but before healing begins.

Surgical management of a client for correction of a deviated nasal septum, reconstruction of a cosmetic deformity of the nose, or reduction of a nasal fracture is similar. All three procedures are usually performed under local anesthesia with use of mild sedation in conjunction with the anesthesia. Because of the vasoconstrictor properties of local anesthetics, they appear to decrease the bleeding during and immediately after surgery. Surgery to correct a deviated nasal septum is known as a nasal septoplasty and consists of making an incision on either side of the septum, elevating the mucous membrane, and straightening or removing the offending portion of the cartilage. If a cosmetic deformity is also of concern or if the deformity interferes with septal reconstruction, a rhinoplasty (reconstruction of the external nose) may be done in conjunction with the nasal septoplasty or as a separate procedure. (See also Chap. 50.)

After these three procedures, intranasal packing and internal splints may be used to maintain the position of the septum as well as to control bleeding and prevent hematoma formation. If the patient has had rhinoplasty or reduction of a nasal fracture, an external splint and a small dressing may also be applied. Some clients may return directly to the nursing unit after surgery because of the local anesthesia, whereas others may be observed in the recovery area until the effects of intraoperative medications are minimized. Areas of concern for the nurse regardless of the location of recovery include airway management, edema, hemorrhage, and pain control. Because of the presence of bilateral nasal packing, after nasal septoplasty, rhinoplasty, and nasal fracture reduction, clients will require the same care as the patient who underwent nasal polypectomy.

Hemorrhagic, Infectious, and Inflammatory Conditions

EPISTAXIS

Epistaxis (nosebleed) may result from irritation, trauma, infection, or tumors. In addition, epistaxis may also be the result of systemic disease (such as atherosclerosis, hypertension, blood dyscrasias) or systemic treatment (such as chemotherapy or anticoagulants).

The initial treatment of epistaxis is application of pressure by pinching the anterior portion of the nose for a minimum of 5 to 10 minutes. This is often successful because most common epistaxis occurs in the anterior part of the septum. In addition, the application of ice compresses to produce vasoconstriction may also decrease bleeding. If these initial measures do not stop bleeding, nasal packing may be necessary. Once the location of the bleeding vessel is located, cauterization of the bleeding vessel with silver nitrate is attempted, and nasal packing may be inserted. For a client with anterior nasal bleeding, anterior nasal packing may be all that is required. Antibacterial ointment such as bacitracin or Neosporin is applied to half-inch gauze and gently, but firmly, inserted into the anterior nasal cavities to apply pressure to the bleeding vessels. Petrolatum gauze packing should be avoided because it has no antimicrobial properties, and a malodorous discharge may develop within 1 to 2 days with its use. Nasal packing should remain in place for a minimum of 48 to 72 hours.[14]

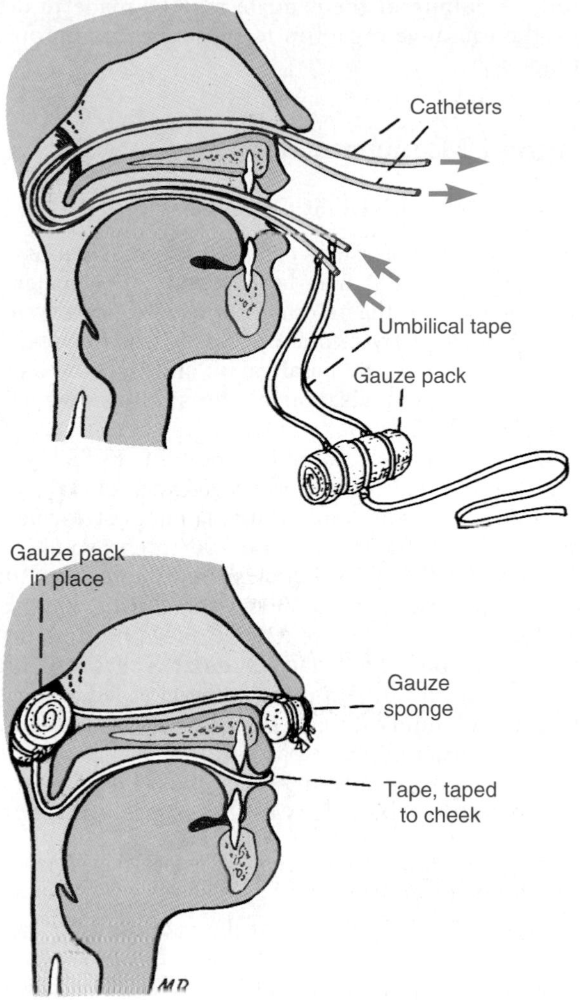

Figure 21–7
Instillation of posterior nasal pack (plug, typically used in emergency). (See text.)

Posterior Plugs. For those clients with posterior epistaxis, a posterior plug may be necessary in addition to the anterior nasal packing (Fig. 21–7). Insertion of a posterior plug is very uncomfortable for clients, and a mild analgesic may be required to reduce anxiety and discomfort. A small, red rubber catheter is passed through the nose into the oropharynx and mouth. A gauze pack is tied to the catheter, and the catheter is withdrawn; this moves the pack into proper placement in the nasopharynx and posterior nose to apply pressure. The nasal cavity is packed with half-inch gauze, and the strings from the posterior pack are tied around a rolled gauze or bolus for maintaining its position. The ties from the oral cavity are taped to the client's face to prevent loosening or dislodgement of the plug. Clients with posterior plug and anterior nasal packing are admitted to the hospital. Clients with nasal packing and posterior plugs are monitored closely for hypoxia. General comfort measures, such as humidification, the use of a drip pad to collect bloody drainage and mucus, and the use of water-soluble ointment around the nares to provide lubrication will alleviate some discomfort. The client should be monitored closely for any signs of bleeding from the anterior or posterior nares. The nurse must inspect the oral cavity for the presence of blood and proper placement of the posterior plug. If the posterior plug is visible, the nurse should notify the physician for readjustment of the packing. Posterior nasal packs remain in place for 5 days.[14] Prophylatic antibiotics are used to prevent toxic shock syndrome and sinusitis.

Arterial Ligation. If medical measures are not sufficient to eliminate epistaxis, surgical interventions may be necessary. Internal maxillary or ethmoid artery ligations may be required to control nasal bleeding. An incision is made in the gum line above the incisor on the affected side, and the maxillary sinus is entered. The artery that supplies the area of bleeding is identified, and a metal clip or suture is used to ligate the artery. Clients will have nasal packing inserted for a minimum of 24 hours, during which time they must be observed for additional bleeding, hyper- or hypotension, and infection. On discharge, the client is instructed to minimize activity for approximately 10 days. This is most frequently accomplished by avoiding strenuous exercise; not blowing the nose; sneezing with the mouth open; and no lifting, stooping, or straining. The use of water-soluble ointment at the entrance of the nose and around the nares may provide comfort, and mouth rinses of half-strength hydrogen peroxide mixed with water or saline should be provided for oral hygiene. The use of a humidifier or vaporizer will add supplemental moisture to prevent dryness and crusting of secretions.

SINUSITIS

Definition and Incidence

Sinusitis is an infection of one of the paranasal sinuses. Pansinusitis is infection of more than one sinus. It is a common medical condition that affects an estimated 35 million people a year.[24]

Pathophysiology

The sinuses are protected against infection by mucociliary action. The normal mucus produced by the sinuses is removed through small openings into the nose called ostia. When the ciliary action is impaired or the ostia are obstructed, mucus can accumulate in the sinus and become infected.

Clinical Manifestations

Sinusitis is considered by evaluation of the client's symptoms and confirmed by x-ray study. Generalized symptoms of fever and chills with local symptoms of pain in the sinuses exacerbated with bending, pain or numbness in the upper teeth, and a purulent or discolored nasal discharge may be present.

DIAGNOSTIC ASSESSMENT

Sinus radiographs or CT may show opacification of the sinus, thickened mucous membranes, and an air-fluid level, all indicative of sinusitis.

Medical Management

The medical management of sinusitis includes use of the appropriate antibiotic to manage the bacterial infection; decongestants to reduce edema; steroid nasal sprays to reduce mucosal inflammation; and humidification by way of normal saline solution irrigations or a vaporizer-humidifier to prevent nasal crusting and to moisten secretions.

Antral Irrigation. Antral irrigation or sinus lavage may be performed in clients who are not responding to treatment or who have increased purulent exudate in the maxillary sinus. Antral irrigation is performed with the use of a local anesthetic. A trocar is inserted through the ostium in the lateral wall of the nose into the sinus. The client should be prepared for the procedure with thorough explanations of the anesthetic, the sensation of the trocar passing through the ostium, and feelings of pressure. Normal saline solution is then injected through the cannula to rinse the sinus of purulent exudate. The client is placed in a sitting position, leaning slightly forward with the mouth open to allow drainage of the irrigating solution through the nose and mouth. A culture of the exudate may be made to determine the causative organism to prescribe an appropriate antibiotic.

Surgical Management

FUNCTIONAL ENDOSCOPIC SINUS SURGERY

If nonoperative measures fail, functional endoscopic sinus surgery (FESS) may be necessary. The major objective of FESS is the re-establishment of sinus ventilation and mucociliary clearance.[6] Small sinus endoscopes are passed through the nasal cavity and into the sinuses to allow direct visualization of the sinuses in order to remove diseased tissue and enlarge sinus ostia (Fig. 21–8). The possible complications of FESS include nasal bleeding, pain, scar formation, and, on rare occasion, blindness from intraorbital hematoma formation, direct injury to the optic nerve, or cerebrospinal fluid leak. Complications are minimized by meticulous surgical technique. Hemostasis is achieved during the procedure for minimizing postoperative bleeding and hematoma formation. Anatomic landmarks are identified frequently during the procedure, thereby decreasing the possibility of injury to the optic nerve or intracranial structures.[6] After FESS, nasal packing may be inserted. Nasal packing is used to minimize nasal bleeding and is removed within a few hours of the surgical procedure.

CALDWELL-LUC PROCEDURE

Caldwell-Luc is another surgical procedure for maxillary sinusitis. An incision is made into the gingival buccal sulcus above the lateral incisor teeth under gen-

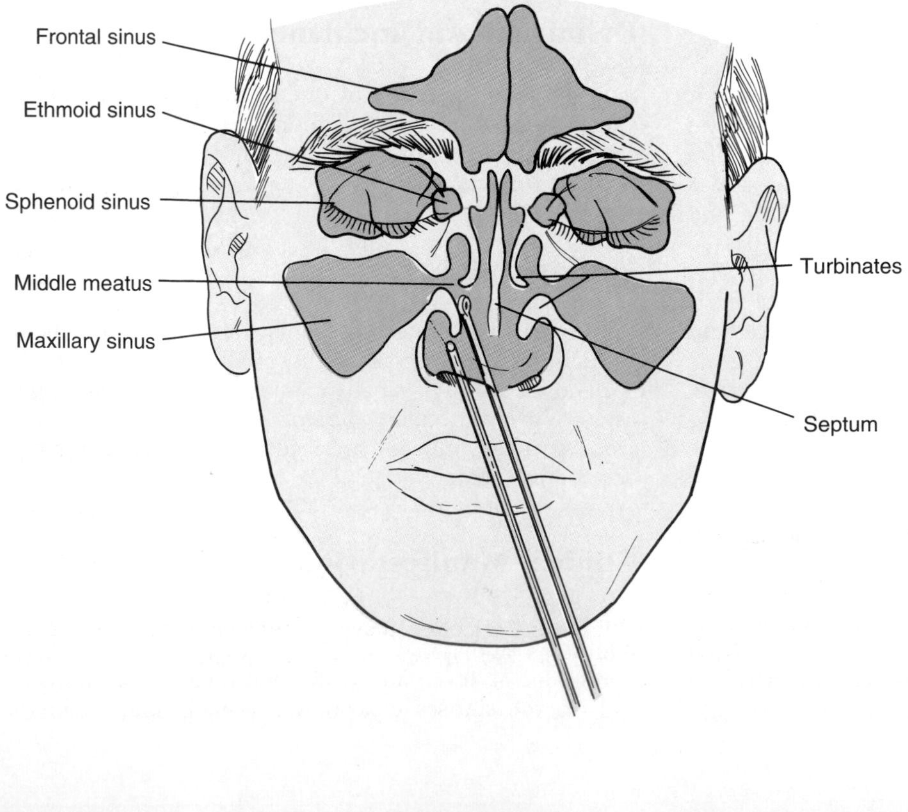

Figure 21–8
Functional endoscopic sinus surgery. The middle meatus is the site where most of the sinuses drain and, if plugged, obstructs drainage. With an endoscope the sinuses can be seen, and the obstructions removed.

eral or local anesthesia. Through this opening, the diseased mucous membrane is removed. In addition, an opening between the maxillary sinus and lateral nasal wall (nasal antral window) may be created to increase aeration of the sinus and to permit drainage into the nasal cavity. After a Caldwell-Luc procedure, the maxillary sinus and anterior nasal cavity are packed with half-inch gauze. Because of the packing, nasal breathing is obstructed. The oral cavity is frequently evaluated for the presence of blood or packing that may have become dislodged, obstructing the pharynx. If packing is present in the pharynx, the visible portion may be held with a hemostat and cut with scissors. One must be certain the hemostat is holding the trimmed gauze; otherwise, it could be aspirated.

EXTERNAL SPHENOETHMOIDECTOMY

External sphenoethmoidectomy is a surgical procedure to remove diseased mucosa from the sphenoid or ethmoid sinuses. A small incision is made over the ethmoid sinus on the lateral nasal bridge, and the diseased mucosa is removed. The client will have nasal and ethmoid packing inserted. In addition to the instructions given after a Caldwell-Luc operation (see later), an eye pressure patch is usually applied to decrease periorbital edema.

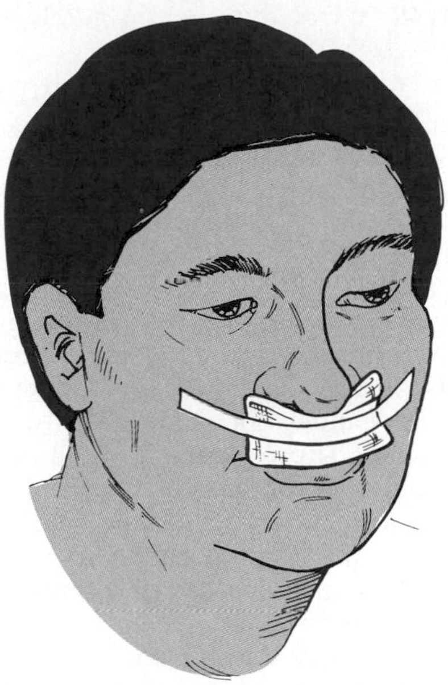

Figure 21–9
A nasal drip pad is taped beneath the nares to absorb drainage after nasal or sinus surgery. The usual technique is to fold 3 × 3 dressings into thirds and tape in place. These dressings can be changed at the nurse's discretion.

Nursing Management

After sinus surgery, the client is observed for an increase in bleeding, respiratory distress, and edema for the first 24 hours after surgery. Ice compresses are applied to the nose and cheek to minimize edema and control bleeding. The client is placed in a semi- to high-Fowler's position for 24 to 48 hours after surgery to minimize postoperative edema. The nasal packing is generally removed the morning after surgery; however, antral packing remains in place for 36 to 72 hours. Mild analgesics should be given to the patient to minimize discomfort after surgery and before removal of the packing.

After a Caldwell-Luc procedure, the client receives the same instructions as after FESS. Postoperative sequelae include numbness of the upper teeth as a result of interruption of sensory nerves from the mucosal incision. This sensation may remain for several weeks.

DISCHARGE TEACHING

Clients are instructed to increase fluids to moisten secretions. Although there may be some pain, a mild analgesic is all that is required. Minimal nasal bleeding is expected for 24 to 48 hours after surgery. A "drip pad" under the nose may eliminate the need to be constantly wiping the nose (Fig. 21–9). Clients are instructed to avoid blowing the nose for 7 to 10 days after surgery; clients are told to sniff backward or spit, not blow. Nasal saline sprays may be started 3 to 5 days after surgery to moisten the nasal mucosa. Clients are requested to have minimal physical exercise and avoid strenuous activity, lifting, and straining for approximately 2 weeks. After FESS, clients will be required to return to the physician's office for removal of crusts and debris and examination of the nose.

PHARYNGITIS

Pharyngitis is inflammation of the pharynx and may be viral or bacterial in origin. A culture of the pharyngeal mucosa is sometimes indicated before treatment. Clients may complain of a sore throat, difficulty swallowing, fever, malaise, and cough and have an elevated white cell count. Treatment of pharyngitis depends on the causative agent. Both viral and bacterial types of pharyngitis are contagious by droplet spread. Good handwashing technique is essential, and the use of a mask may prevent spread. Antibiotics are used to treat the bacterial pharyngitis; comfort measures are required for viral types. Bed rest, fluids, warm saline irrigations or gargles, analgesics, and antipyretics are recommended until the symptoms are alleviated.

Chronic pharyngitis (chronic pharyngeal inflammation) is most common in people who habitually use tobacco and alcohol, have a chronic cough, are employed or live in dusty environments, or use their voices excessively. Clinical manifestations vary according to the degree of irritation and inflammation.

RHINITIS

Rhinitis is inflammation of the nasal mucosa. Symptoms of rhinitis include increased nasal drainage. Normally, this drainage is clear mucus. If the infection spreads to the sinuses, however, drainage may become yellow or green. Rhinitis may be classified as acute, allergic, or vasomotor. Acute rhinitis is also known as the common cold or coryza. Acute rhinitis may be bacterial or viral in origin; it is treated symptomatically. Acute rhinitis usually lasts 5 to 7 days with or without treatment. Common interventions for acute rhinitis are symptomatic and include supplemental humidification, decongestants to reduce the edema of the nasal mucosa, increased fluids to prevent dehydration, and analgesics to relieve the generalized myalgia. Sometimes antibiotics are given not to treat the virus but to prevent a secondary infection by bacteria.

Allergic rhinitis is most often seen as a seasonal disorder. In addition to obstruction to nasal breathing, the client with allergic rhinitis may also experience irritation of other mucous membranes (i.e., the conjunctiva, causing tearing and edema of the eyelids). Treatment of allergic rhinitis is also symptomatic. A complete allergy evaluation may be required to determine the offending allergen. Most clients are placed on a desensitization program, told to avoid the antigen, and treated symptomatically with antihistamines, steroids, or mast cell–stabilizing sprays.

Vasomotor rhinitis causes the same symptoms as do acute rhinitis and allergic rhinitis but has no known specific cause. Clients complaining of vasomotor rhinitis who have a negative culture and negative allergy evaluation are treated symptomatically. If medications have been prescribed for clients with rhinitis (especially nasal sprays), they must be taught about the use of the medications, including side effects and possible interactions with other medications.

LARYNGITIS

Laryngitis is inflammation of the larynx, or hoarseness. Hoarseness is a common symptom that may be due to inflammation of the vocal cords, abnormal movements of the vocal cords, or a benign or malignant tumor of the vocal cords. All of these interfere with normal mobility of the vocal cords, which produces an abnormal sound.

Laryngitis, inflammation of the vocal cords, may be due to an inflammatory process or vocal abuse. The laryngeal membrane is continuous with the lining of the upper respiratory tract, and infections in other areas of the nose and throat may include the larynx. Edema of the vocal cords caused by the chronic irritation of an upper respiratory tract infection inhibits the normal mobility of the vocal cords, which causes an abnormal sound.

Laryngitis may also be the result of gastroesophageal reflux disorder (GERD). In this syndrome, the sphincter between the stomach and esophagus relaxes, and gastric acid is allowed to enter the esophagus. Reflux of gastric secretions, especially during sleep, may result in the aspiration of gastric secretions into the larynx, causing a chemical irritation or burning of the mucous membrane lining the larynx.[13] Clients with gastroesophageal reflux may complain of hoarseness from the chemical irritation of the gastric acid on the vocal cords, increased mucus production from the body's natural tendency to protect the irritated membrane, foreign body sensation, or sore throat. Chronic cough and asthma may also be associated symptoms of GERD.

Abnormal voice may also be the result of vocal abuse. Screaming, shouting, and loud speaking over a period of time may produce edema of the vocal cords and the formation of nodules or polyps, outpouchings of inflamed mucous membranes.

The initial treatment of laryngitis is to treat the causative factors. If inflammatory laryngitis is suspected, the inflammation should be treated. Antibiotics may be used if a bacterial infection is suspected. In severe cases, systemic steroids (such as methylprednisolone [Medrol Dosepak]) may be prescribed to reduce inflammation and edema. Supplemental humidification may add increased moisture to liquefy secretions, and mucolytic agents may be prescribed to thin and mobilize mucus. Clients with laryngitis may also be placed on voice rest to allow the edema of the vocal cords to subside without added strain. The client should be cautioned to avoid whispering, which will also cause excessive vocal cord strain.

Gastroesophageal reflux is initially treated symptomatically. The client is instructed to elevate the head of the bed to minimize reflux; to avoid eating or drinking for 2 to 3 hours before going to sleep; to avoid caffeine, alcohol, and tobacco, which are known to increase gastric secretions; and to use antacids and hydrogen inhibitors (famotidine [Pepcid], ranitidine [Zantac]) to neutralize and decrease acid production.[13]

Chronic laryngitis may stem from repeated infections, allergy, chronic irritant exposure, long-term voice abuse, and reflux esophagitis of acidic gastric contents.

Chronic laryngitis is manifested by a tickling sensation in the throat, voice huskiness, and painful or difficult phonation. Management involves correction or removal of the irritation in addition to the measures to increase comfort (see acute laryngitis). Long-term voice retraining may be necessary if improper use or overuse of the voice is the main cause of chronic laryngitis. This retraining includes learning to use the voice without straining and forming and projecting words to use the diaphragm without shouting.

STUDY QUESTIONS

1. A client reports a 40 pack per year history of cigarette smoking and moderate alcohol intake. The nurse assesses the client for which of the following findings on the basis of the understanding of early symptoms of cancer of the larynx.
   A. Foul breath
   B. Hoarseness
   C. Dyspnea
   D. Throat pain
2. The nurse is providing the preoperative teaching for the client who will be undergoing a total laryngectomy. It is most important for the nurse to develop a plan relating to:
   A. Aspiration
   B. Wound infection
   C. Dyspnea
   D. Communication
3. The most comfortable postoperative position for the laryngectomy client is:
   A. Sims'
   B. Fowler's
   C. Trendelenburg's
   D. Recumbent
4. A client has had a total laryngectomy. The nurse is suctioning blood-tinged secretions from his tracheostomy on the first postoperative day. What is the most appropriate nursing intervention at this time?
   A. Page the attending physician immediately.
   B. Reduce the frequency of suctioning.
   C. Instill normal saline into the lumen of the tracheostomy.
   D. Reassure the client that this is normal.
5. After his laryngectomy, the client becomes withdrawn. Which of the following interventions will be most successful in decreasing his sense of isolation?
   A. Allow his family to stay with him ad libitum.
   B. Encourage him to look at himself in a mirror.
   C. Tell him to sit in the visitor's lounge.
   D. Arrange for a visit from another laryngectomee.
6. A client has been involved in a motor vehicle accident. He reports that his neck struck the steering wheel. Trauma to the face and neck:
   A. Frequently results in a fatality
   B. Can result in airway obstruction
   C. Seldom results in significant blood loss
   D. Almost never occurs with head injury
7. A client needs to be monitored for signs of laryngeal edema. Which of the following symptoms should be reported as an early sign of edema?
   A. Rales
   B. Rhonchi
   C. Stridor
   D. Wheezes
8. While you are visiting with a friend, she tells you that she frequently experiences epistaxis. What initial treatment should you teach her that is best to help control the bleeding?
   A. Assume Fowler's position with her head back.
   B. Apply ice to the back of her neck for 5 to 10 minutes.
   C. Pinch her anterior nose for 5 to 10 minutes.
   D. Assume Fowler's position with her head forward.

CRITICAL THINKING EXERCISES

SCENARIO A

A 65-year-old rancher is admitted for a diagnostic work-up and potential total laryngectomy. He is a widower and is accompanied by his daughter and her 16-year-old son. The client reports to the nurse a 50 pack per year history of smoking "hand-rolled" cigarettes and "boozing on Saturday nights." The daughter tells you that her son is "just like Grandpa" except he does not drink yet.

1. Identify the client's risk factors related to laryngeal cancer.
2. Teach the grandson the warning signs of laryngeal cancer.
3. If the client is scheduled for the total laryngectomy, what does the preoperative teaching need to include?
4. The client wants to know how soon before he'll be able to eat his daughter's biscuits and gravy after the surgery. What nutritional teaching does the client need?

SCENARIO B

A college student is sent to the school nurse for epistaxis.

1. What initial measures should the school nurse carry out?
2. The bleeding is not controlled by these early measures, and the student must go to the hospital emergency room. What is the next step in the care of epistaxis?
3. The student's bleeding is from both an anterior epistaxis and a posterior epistaxis and both require nasal packing. What additional precautions are necessary?

BIBLIOGRAPHY

1. Albarren, J. W. (1991). A review of communication with intubated patients and those with tracheostomies within an intensive care environment. *Invensive Care Nursing, 7(3),* 179–186.
2. American Cancer Society. (1995). *Cancer facts and figures.* Atlanta: Author.
3. Applegate, E. J. (1994). *Anatomy & physiology learning system.* Philadelphia: W. B. Saunders Co.
4. Baker, C. A. (1992). Factors associated with rehabilitation in head and neck cancer. *Cancer Nursing, 15(6),* 395–400.
5. Hillel, A., et al. (1989). Radical neck dissection: A subjective and objective evaluation of postoperative disability. *Journal of Otolaryngology, 18(1),* 53–61.
6. Kennedy, D. W., & Zinreich, S. J. (1989). Functional endoscopic surgery. In E. N. Myers et al. (Eds.), *Advances in otolaryngology—Head and neck surgery* (Vol. 3, pp. 1–27). Chicago: Year Book Medical Publishers.
7. Krakoff, I. (1991). Cancer chemotherapeutic and biologic agents. *CA: A Cancer Journal for Clinicians, 41(5),* 264–278.
8. Lavertu, P., et al. (1989). Secondary tracheoesophageal puncture for voice rehabilitation after laryngectomy. *Archives of Otolaryngology—Head and Neck Surgery, 115(3),* 350.
9. Litwack, K. (1991). Managing postanesthetic emergencies. *Nursing 91, 21(9),* 49–51.
10. Lockhart, J., Troff, J., & Artim, L. (1992). Total laryngectomy and radical neck dissection. *AORN Journal, 55(2),* 458–479.
11. Logemann, J. A. (1983). *Evaluation and treatment of swallowing disorders.* Austin, TX: PRO-ED.
12. Maas, A. (1991). A model for quality of life after laryngectomy. *Social Science and Medicare, 33(12),* 1373–1377.
13. Olson, N. R. (1986). The problem of gastroesophageal reflux. *Otolaryngologic Clinics of North America, 19(1),* 119–113.
14. Petruzzelli, G. J., & Johnson, J. T. (1989). How to stop a nosebleed. *Postgraduate Medicine, 86(4),* 44–56.
15. Sabiston, D. (1991). *Textbook of surgery* (14th ed.). Philadelphia: W. B. Saunders Co.
16. Sigler, B. A. (1987). Nursing care for head and neck tumor patients. In S. E. Thawley & W. R. Panje (Eds.), *Comprehensive management of head and neck tumors* (pp. 79–100). Philadelphia: W. B. Saunders Co.
17. Sigler, B. A. (1989). Nursing care of patients with laryngeal carcinoma. *Seminars in Oncology Nursing, 5(3),* 160–165.
18. Sigler, B. A., & Hooper, J. A. (1989). Nursing care of the head and neck cancer patient. In E. N. Myers & J. Y. Suen (Eds.), *Cancer of the head and neck* (pp. 1045–1071). New York: Churchill Livingstone.
19. Singer, M. I., & Blom, E. D. (1990). Medical techniques for voice restoration after total laryngectomy. *CA: A Cancer Journal for Clinicians, 40(3),* 166–173.
20. Slavin, R. G. (1991). Recalcitrant asthma: Could sinusitis be the culprit? *The Journal of Respiratory Diseases, 12(2),* 182–194.
21. Weber, M., & Reiner, M. (1993). Laryngectomy: Grieving, disfigurement and dysfunction. *The Canadian Nurse, 89(3),* 31–34.
22. Weimert, T. A. (1992). Common ENT emergencies: The acute nose and throat, part 2. *Emergency Medicine, 24(6),* 26–28, 31–32, 34–36.
23. Wyngaarden J., et al. (Eds.) (1992). *Cecil textbook of medicine* (19th ed.). Philadelphia: W. B. Saunders Co.
24. Yoshida, G. Y., et al. (1989). Primary voice restoration at laryngectomy: 1989 update. *Laryngoscope, 99,* 1093–1095.

Chapter 22 Nursing Care of Clients with Lower Airway Disorders

Learning Outcomes

After completing this chapter, the learner will be able to:

1. Assess the client for clinical manifestations resulting from lower airway disorders.
2. Teach the client about the risk factors, basic pathophysiology, and clinical manifestations of lower airway disorders.
3. Explain the role of the client and significant others in the prevention and treatment of lower airway disorders.
4. Develop plans of care for the prevention, management, and treatment of clients with lower airway disorders.
5. Implement nursing interventions that optimize the quality of life for clients with lower airway disorders.
6. Evaluate planned client outcomes, using outcomes developed in the planning phase of care.

Airway Disorders

ASTHMA

Asthma is a complex disorder of the bronchial airways characterized by periods of bronchospasm (spasms of prolonged contraction of the airway).

Incidence and Etiology

Asthma affects about 2 to 3 per cent of the United States population, and its incidence is rising. It is the most common chronic disease in children and adults. Asthma occurs in families, which indicates that it is an inherited disorder. Apparently environmental factors (e.g., viral infection) interact with inherited factors to produce disease.

Risk Factors and Prevention

Methods of primary prevention include reduction of air pollution and cigarette smoking. Secondary smoke inhalation is known to increase the incidence of respiratory disorders. Secondary prevention through early detection in known asthmatics is through the daily monitoring of peak airflow volumes. In many clients, peak airflow volume decreases about 24 hours before asthma symptoms begin. Tertiary prevention in clients who are known asthmatics mainly consists of avoiding known allergens. Clients who develop asthma along with respiratory infections can begin early treatment when clinical manifestations of upper respiratory infection begin.

Pathophysiology

Asthma can be divided into two main categories: extrinsic (allergic) and intrinsic (nonallergic). Extrinsic asthma is caused by agents such as dust, lint, pollen, insects, mold spores, smoke, medications, and foods. This form of asthma usually begins in childhood. In contrast, intrinsic asthma does not have easily identifiable allergens and is triggered by many internal disorders, such as the common cold or upper respiratory infection, or even exercise. This form of asthma usually begins in adults over the age of 35 years. Both forms of asthma can be triggered by changes in environmental temperature, strong odors (perfumed soaps and cosmetics), stress, emotion, exercise, and exposure to specific allergens (mold spores, pollen). Clients with intrinsic asthma may also have nasal polyps and aspirin allergy (called triad disease).

In both forms of asthma, the airway is hyperreactive. Extrinsic asthma is an example of type I hypersensitivity reaction (see Chap. 9). Mast cells and basophils release chemical mediators (i.e., histamine, bradykinin, prostaglandins, and slow-releasing substance of anaphylaxis, also called leukotrienes). These chemical mediators cause bronchial smooth muscle to contract and close the airways. These substances also increase vascular permeability, which leads to airway edema.

Intrinsic asthma begins with both a parasympathetic and a sympathetic response. The parasympathetic nervous system causes a release of acetylcholine, which leads to bronchoconstriction. The sympathetic nervous system stimulates the mast cells (see preceding).

Both alpha- and beta-adrenergic receptors of the sympathetic nervous system are found in the bronchi. Stimulation of the alpha-adrenergic receptors causes bronchoconstriction; conversely, stimulation of the beta-adrenergic receptors causes bronchodilation. Cyclic adenosine monophosphate balances the two receptors. Some theories on the cause of asthma suggest that the client lacks beta-adrenergic stimulation.

Once the airway is in spasm, mucus plugs the airway, trapping distal air. Ventilation/perfusion (V/Q) mismatch, hypoxemia, and increased workload of breathing follow. Hyperventilation eventually occurs as the lung attempts to respond to the increased volume and pressure.

Asthma symptoms commonly worsen at night. The mechanisms of nighttime asthma are not fully understood, but more is involved than simply being exposed to bedding or bedroom allergens. Some possible mechanisms include decreased levels of epinephrine, cyclic adenosine monophosphate, and cortisol. Clinical manifestations may also be caused by increased levels of histamine, increased inflammatory cells in the airway, airway cooling, and airway secretions.

Complications

Status asthmaticus is a severe, life-threatening complication of asthma. It is an acute episode of bronchospasm that tends to intensify. With severe bronchospasm, the workload of breathing increases 5 to 10 times, which can lead to acute cor pulmonale. Pneumothorax commonly develops. If status asthmaticus continues, hypoxemia worsens, and acidosis begins. If the condition is untreated or not reversed, respiratory or cardiac arrest will ensue.

Clinical Manifestations

The signs and symptoms of bronchial asthma are summarized in Clinical Manifestations: Bronchial Asthma.

The severity of asthma can be classified as mild, moderate, or severe, depending on the symptoms. A scoring system is depicted in Table 22–1.

DIAGNOSTIC ASSESSMENT

Spirometry reveals decreased peak expiratory flow rate, forced expiratory volume (FEV_1), and forced vital capacity (FVC). Functional residual capacity, total lung capacity (TLC), and residual volume are increased.

CLINICAL MANIFESTATIONS

Bronchial Asthma

GENERAL APPEARANCE

Anxious: as asthma becomes more severe, $PaCO_2$ rises, and central nervous system depression occurs

AGE RANGE

All ages; is a component of CAL

ASSESSMENT FINDINGS

- Nasal flaring as respiratory distress increases
- Lips pursed in an effort to exhale
- Use of accessory muscles as work of breathing increases
- Paradoxic pulse increases as bronchospasm worsens
- Wheezing, cough, or dyspnea; if no breath sounds, status asthmaticus (life-threatening), intubation, and mechanical ventilation are urgent
- Cyanosis is late development

CARDIAC INVOLVEMENT

- Tachycardia
- Electrocardiogram may show right-sided heart strain

SMOKING HISTORY

Uncommon; smoke is often an allergen that triggers bronchospasm

DIAGNOSTIC FINDINGS

Pulmonary Function

Increased FRC; FEV_1 decreased; peak flow decreased

Arterial Blood Gases

- If untreated, asthma progresses in severity; $PaCO_2$ goes from below normal to normal and finally elevates
- A normal $PaCO_2$ indicates tiring; elevated $PaCO_2$ indicates significant tiring leading to respiratory arrest
- As $PaCO_2$ rises, PaO_2 falls, effects of hypercapnia and hypoxia are noticeable
- If $PaCO_2$ rises and remains uncorrected, pH falls, causing respiratory acidosis

Chest Film

Hyperinflation

OVERVIEW

- Swollen mucous membranes of bronchioles and surrounding tissue
- Muscles of bronchioles become spastic, causing narrowing
- Thick mucus fills bronchioles and alveoli; breathing becomes labored; expiration difficult

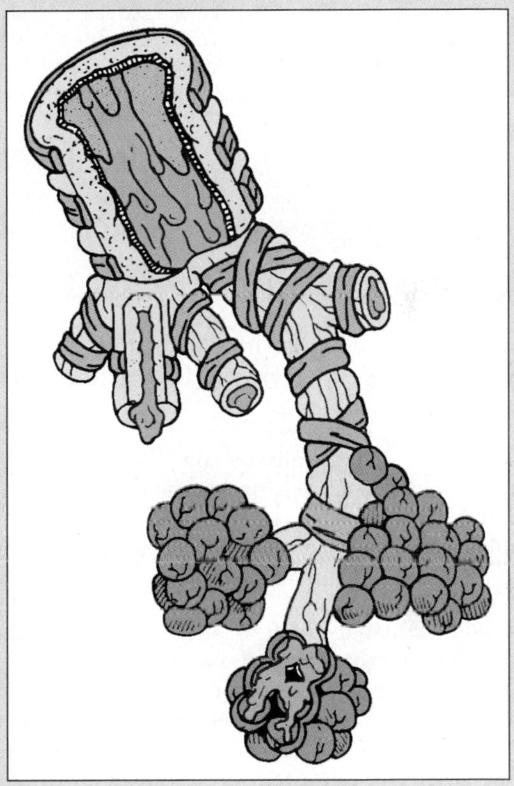

Blood gas analysis reveals hypoxemia and respiratory alkalosis. Chest radiography may reveal hyperinflation.

Baseline assessment of pulmonary status will include arterial blood gas (ABG) analysis (Table 22–2 for typical ABG changes during an asthma attack) and essential pulmonary function studies (i.e., peak flow rate and forced expiratory volume, measured with spirometry or peak flowmeter). A 20 per cent improvement in FVC, FEV, and peak expiratory flow rate following inhaled administration of a beta-agonist bronchodilator implies a reversible airflow obstruction, i.e., asthma.

Auscultation of breath sounds will usually reveal wheezing, especially during expiration.

CRITICAL TO REMEMBER

The inability to auscultate wheezing in an asthmatic client with acute respiratory distress may be an ominous sign. It may indicate that the small airways are too constricted to allow any airflow. This client may require immediate, aggressive medical intervention.

A problem with the use of diagnostic tests for asthma is that when the client is not having an acute attack, blood gases, pulmonary function tests, and chest film are often normal.

TABLE 22–1 Assessing the Severity of Asthma

CLINICAL MANIFESTATIONS	SCORE 0	SCORE 1
Loss of exercise tolerance, capable of work?	Yes	No
Using accessory muscles, tracheal tug and intercostal retraction present?	Absent	Present
Wheezing?	Absent	Present
Respiratory rate per minute	Under 25	Over 25
Pulse rate per minute	Under 120	Over 120
Palpable pulsus paradoxus	Absent	Present
Peak expiratory flow rate (L/min)	Over 100	Under 100

Score the client in each area. A score of 4 or more suggests severe asthma, and the client will require careful observation to determine whether there is a response to therapy or hospitalization is necessary.

From Cochrane, G., & Rees, P. (1989). *A colour atlas of asthma.* London: Wolfe Medical Publications.

Medical Management

An acute asthma episode may constitute a medical emergency. Medical intervention for such episodes is primarily aimed at

- maintaining a patent airway by relieving bronchospasm and clearing excess or retained secretions
- maintaining effective gas exchange
- preventing complications such as acute respiratory failure and status asthmaticus.

Emergency management of the client includes inhaled beta-adrenergics and intravenous theophylline. If the asthma does not abate, that is, FEV_1 remains less than 40 per cent of predicted, intravenous steroids are given. If these treatments do not reverse the symptoms, the client is usually admitted to the hospital for further treatment.

Status asthmaticus is treated with aggressive use of intravenous corticosteroids and frequent administration of inhaled beta-adrenergics to avoid intubation and mechanical ventilation.

Supplemental oxygen is indicated if the alveolar oxygen tension (PaO_2) levels fall below 60 mm Hg. The client should be monitored closely for signs of increasing anxiety, increased work of breathing, and indications of tiring. Endotracheal intubation and mechanical ventilation may be necessary. Medically induced paralysis may be necessary in rare cases.

After the acute asthma attack is over, the client is assessed for determination of the precipitating event or factors and is instructed in self-care activities.

PHARMACOLOGIC MANAGEMENT

Beta-adrenergic agents are the mainstay of bronchodilator therapy. Beta-adrenergic agents with varying degrees of beta-2 selectivity are used by nebulizer or metered-dose inhaler. Some beta-adrenergic agents can be administered parenterally also. The use of parenteral agents in adults is not common because inhaled agents have equal effect and do not have systemic side effects that accompany parenteral agents. Common agents include albuterol (Proventil) and isoetharine (Bronkosol).

Clients with very mild asthma (fewer than three to four attacks per year) can use the inhalers on an as-needed basis. Clients with moderate asthma (six to eight attacks annually) should use inhalers on a regular, daily basis. Clients with severe asthma combine the use of inhalers with other agents.

CRITICAL TO REMEMBER

Treatment with metered-dose inhalers consists of two puffs about 3 to 5 minutes apart. The first dose dilates the narrowed airways, allowing the second breath to extend further. The client begins by exhaling fully and then inhaling with a slow sustained breath, attempting to reach TLC.

Aerosol "spacers," extensions that collect the medication in a chamber from which the client inhales, are available for clients who have difficulty coordinating inhalation with the spray.

In addition to beta-adrenergic agents, theophylline and aminophylline are moderately potent bronchodilators used to manage asthma. The use of theophylline is limited by its toxicity and by the wide variations in the rate of metabolism. Theophylline levels are monitored to evaluate the effectiveness of the drug.

Antihistamines had been ineffective in the treatment of asthma until recently. In the past decade, more potent H_1-receptor agonists, such as terfenadine (Seldane), have emerged, with fewer central nervous system side effects. Early clinical trials indicate that they produce bronchodilation and alleviate asthmatic symptoms. It is likely that H_1-receptor agonists will become part of the treatment of asthma.

TABLE 22–2 Alterations in Arterial Blood Gases Associated with Asthma

	MILD	MODERATE	SEVERE	STATUS ASTHMATICUS
PaO_2	Slightly elevated	Normal to mild hypoxemia	Hypoxemia	Severe hypoxemia
$PaCO_2$	Decreased	Decreased to normal	Elevated	Significantly elevated
pH	Alkalosis	Alkalosis	Alkalosis	Acidosis

Anticholinergics, corticosteroids, and mast cell stabilizers have also been used in treating asthma. Medications used in management of respiratory disorders are discussed in Chapter 20.

Nursing Management

Assessment

Initially, the client should be assessed for signs or symptoms of airway distress. If the client is having acute airway distress, this emergency must be managed before a detailed history of the disease is performed. Known medication allergies should be determined so that these medications are avoided in treatment.

> **CRITICAL TO REMEMBER**
>
> Ascertaining whether the client has a history of cardiac disease is important initially, because the medication used to treat the asthma may worsen a diseased heart.

Once the asthma is controlled, the history of the client's asthma should be explored. The nurse should assist the client to determine if there is a pattern to the symptoms. These data may help identify a trigger to the asthmatic symptoms. If an extrinsic trigger can be identified, then many times it can be reduced or eliminated. For example, if the client is allergic to mold, common sources of mold can be avoided. The nurse should also ask about current medications, especially those used to treat other illnesses. Some clients are inadvertently placed on medications that may induce bronchospasms. For example, if a noncardioselective beta-blocker, such as propranolol (Inderal), is prescribed for hypertension, it may cause bronchospasm.

Within the psychosocial domain, the nurse can ask about the client's ability to manage the asthma and general adaptation to the illness. Denial of the illness can lead to a lack of treatment of early symptoms. It is important to determine whether the client feels control over the illness and feels capable of managing it. Clients who have this feeling of control, called an internal locus of control, may demonstrate improved compliance with treatments.

Another area of assessment lies in determining whether the client is experiencing an increased number of stressors. Stressful lifestyles may increase the number of asthmatic symptoms.

The attitude of the client's family and significant others should also be assessed. The family can be a great source of support and assist the client to recognize early symptoms. In contrast, an unsupportive family may contribute to denial or be an additional source of stress to the client.

The client with a new diagnosis of asthma may be asked to assess the home and work environment for likely triggers to the symptoms. The presence of pets that shed hair or dander, cigarette smoke, or occupational exposure may require some lifestyle changes. Elimination of irritants is generally performed in a reasonable fashion. Improvements in a client's symptoms that may result from a major lifestyle change, such as job change or loss of a pet, may be quickly offset by the stress felt from such a move.

Nursing Diagnosis, Planning, and Implementation

Nursing Diagnosis: Breathing Pattern, Ineffective R/T impaired exhalation and anxiety.

Planning: Expected Outcomes. The client will have improved breathing patterns, as evidenced by a decreasing respiratory rate to within normal limits; decreased signs of dyspnea, nasal flaring, and use of accessory muscles; decreased signs of anxiety; ABG levels returning to normal limits; and vital capacity measurements within normal limits or greater than 40 per cent of predicted, including FEV_1, TLC, and residual volume.

Implementation. The nurse should assess the client frequently, observing the respiratory rate and depth and the breathing pattern for shortness of breath, pursed-lip breathing, nasal flaring, sternal and intercostal retractions, and a prolonged expiratory phase. In acute asthma, these assessments may be needed continually or every hour.

Arterial blood gases should be monitored to determine the effectiveness of treatments. Pulmonary function test results should be compared with normal levels. The degree of dysfunction will assist the nurse to plan for activity.

The client should be placed in Fowler's position and given oxygen as ordered. Bronchodilators and steroids are commonly prescribed. Tachycardia and tremors are common side effects of bronchodilator therapy. The nurse should monitor for therapeutic levels of theophylline (8 to 20 μg/mL).

Nursing Diagnosis: Airway Clearance, Ineffective R/T increased production of secretions and bronchospasm.

Planning: Expected Outcomes. The client will have an effective airway clearance, as evidenced by decreased inspiratory and expiratory wheezing; decreased sonorous wheezing; PaO_2 over 60 mm Hg, alveolar carbon dioxide tension ($PaCO_2$) equal to or less than 40 mm Hg, and pH greater than 7.35; and decreasing dry, nonproductive cough.

Implementation. Lung sounds should be assessed every hour during acute episodes for determining the adequacy of air movement. If the airway is compromised, the client may require suctioning. Some clients develop asthma as a result of pulmonary infection. The nurse should monitor the color and consistency of the sputum and assist the client to cough effectively. Fluids should be encouraged to thin the secretions and replace fluids lost through rapid respirations. The humidity in the room may be increased slightly. If chest secretions are thick and difficult to expectorate, the client may benefit from chest physiotherapy (postural drainage, percussion, and vibration) and frequent position changes. The client should be given frequent oral care, every 2 to 4 hours, to remove the taste of the secretions.

Refer to the care plan for the client with chronic obstructive pulmonary disease (COPD) when working

CLIENT EDUCATION GUIDE

Asthma Management

The nurse should teach the client with asthma:

1. How to identify early symptoms of an asthma attack and how to treat them at home.
2. When to seek help during an asthma attack.
3. To avoid known allergens.
4. To monitor pollen indexes, pollen counts, and air quality reports and to avoid outdoor activity during periods of increased risk.
5. The purpose and common side effects of prescribed medications:
   - Although bronchodilators may interfere with sleep, they should be taken when the client is tired and close to bedtime to counteract the increased symptoms of asthma at nighttime.
   - Oral steroids can cause gastric irritation and should be taken with meals or food.
   - After the use of inhaled steroids, the client should perform mouth care to prevent the onset of fungal infections.
6. How to use and care for equipment:
   - How to use a metered dose inhaler.
   - How to clean the metered dose inhaler after use.
   - How to perform pulmonary function testing.

with clients with diagnoses of Activity Intolerance; Anxiety; Nutrition, Altered; or Sleep Pattern Disturbance.

Evaluation

The degree of expected outcome attainment should be evaluated. Revisions in the plan of care may be necessary. Generally, asthma can be reversed quickly, if there is no underlying problem such as infection (see the Client Education Guide: Asthma Management).

CHRONIC AIRFLOW LIMITATIONS

Chronic obstructive pulmonary disease, also called chronic obstructive lung disease, refers to a number of disorders that affect movement of air in and out of the lungs. The most important of these disorders are obstructive bronchitis, emphysema, and asthma.

Whereas bronchitis, emphysema, and asthma may occur in a "pure form," they most commonly coexist, and assessment findings overlap. Although the term COPD is commonly used, to specialists in pulmonary medicine it is not completely accurate, and the nurse may see the term "chronic airflow limitation" (CAL) in its place.

Chronic airflow limitation can occur either as a result of increased airway resistance secondary to luminal narrowing as a result of bronchial mucosal edema or smooth muscle contraction, or as a result of decreased elastic recoil (seen in emphysema). Decreased elastic recoil results in a decreased driving force to empty the lung.

Incidence

Chronic airflow limitation is a widespread disorder; it affects 1 of 14 people over the age of 45 years.[24] The disorder usually begins in the fifth or sixth decade of life and is predominant in the elderly. CAL is more common in men, although the incidence in women is increasing. It is more frequent in clients living in urban environments and among the socioeconomically disadvantaged. Morbidity and mortality rates for CAL are increasing as the effects of chronic irritation and pollution increase.

Etiology

The specific causes of CAL are not clearly understood. However, the effects of numerous irritants found in cigarette smoke make smoking the leading risk factor for the development of the disorder.

Chronic respiratory infections, including sinusitis, contribute to the development of CAL, as does the aging process. In addition, heredity and genetic predisposition seem to have a role.

Risk Factors

The primary prevention for COPD is smoking cessation or never starting in the first place. In addition, the control of air pollution will reduce the incidence of COPD. Secondary prevention consists of early treatment and diagnosis of diseases that cause COPD, such as pneumonia. Early COPD detection in high-risk clients through lung function studies is beginning to be used.

Pathophysiology

Two major components are involved in COPD: chronic obstructive bronchitis and emphysema.

Chronic Obstructive Bronchitis. Chronic obstructive bronchitis is inflammation of the bronchi, which causes increased mucus production and chronic cough. In order for a diagnosis of chronic bronchitis to be made as opposed to acute bronchitis, the symptoms must continue for 3 months of the year and for 2 consecutive years. Additionally, if the client has a decreased FEV_1/FVC ratio less than 75 per cent and chronic bronchitis, then the client is said to have chronic obstructive bronchitis. This term implies that the client has obstructive lung disease combined with chronic cough.

This disorder is caused by exposure to irritants, especially cigarette smoke. Clients with chronic bronchitis have (1) an increase in the size and number of submucous glands in the large bronchi, which increases mucus production; (2) thicker, more tenacious mucus; and (3) impaired ciliary function, which reduces mucus clearance. Therefore, the lungs' mucociliary defenses are impaired, and there is increased susceptibility to infection. When infection occurs, the mucus production is even greater, and the bronchial walls inflame and thicken. Chronic bronchitis initially affects only the larger bronchi, but eventually all airways are involved. The thick mucus and enlarged bronchi obstruct airways, especially during expiration. The airways collapse, and air is trapped in the distal portion of the lung. This obstruction leads to reduced alveolar ventilation, hypoxia, and acidosis. The client has poor tissue oxygenation; an abnormal V/Q ratio develops, with a corresponding fall in PaO_2. Impaired ventilation may also result in increased levels of $PaCO_2$. The client appears cyanotic. As compensation for the hypoxemia, polycythemia (an overproduction of erythrocytes) occurs. Cyanosis and peripheral edema have led to the slang term "blue bloater" for the client with chronic bronchitis.

As the disease progresses, copious amounts of sputum are produced; pulmonary infection is common. During infections, the client has marked reduction in FEV_1 with increased residual volume and FRC. If these problems are not reversed, hypoxemia will lead to cor pulmonale (see Chap. 25) and congestive heart failure (see Chap. 24).

Emphysema. Emphysema is a disorder in which the alveolar walls are destroyed, which leads to permanent overdistention of the air spaces. Air passages are obstructed as a result of these changes, rather than from mucus production as in chronic bronchitis. Difficult expiration in emphysema is due to the destruction of the walls (septa) between the alveoli, partial airway collapse, and loss of elastic recoil. As the alveoli and septa collapse, pockets of air form between the alveolar spaces (called blebs) and within the lung parenchyma (called bullae). This process leads to increased ventilatory "dead space," or areas that do not participate in gas or blood exchange. The work of breathing is increased because there is less functional lung tissue to exchange oxygen and carbon dioxide. Emphysema also causes destruction of the pulmonary capillaries, further decreasing the oxygen perfusion and ventilation. Some degree of emphysema is considered normal with aging, but if it occurs earlier in life, it is usually due to chronic bronchitis and cigarette smoking.

There are three types of emphysema. Centrilobular emphysema, the most common type, produces destruction in the bronchioles, usually in the upper lung regions. Inflammation develops in the bronchioles, but usually the alveolar sac remains intact. Panlobular emphysema destroys the air spaces of the entire acinus and most commonly involves the lower lung. These forms of emphysema, collectively called centriacinar emphysema, occur most often in smokers. Paraseptal (or panacinar) emphysema destroys the alveoli in the lower lobes of the lungs, resulting in isolated blebs along the lung periphery. Paraseptal emphysema is believed to be the likely cause of spontaneous pneumothorax. A small number of clients with CAL have an inherited deficiency of alpha$_1$-antitrypsin, a nonspecific proteolytic enzyme inhibitor. Normally, alpha$_1$-antitrypsin inhibits the action of enzymes that break down proteins. Clients without alpha$_1$-antitrypsin have increased risk of CAL because the walls of the lung are at higher risk of destruction. Panacinar emphysema occurs in the elderly and in clients with AAT deficiency (Fig. 22–1).

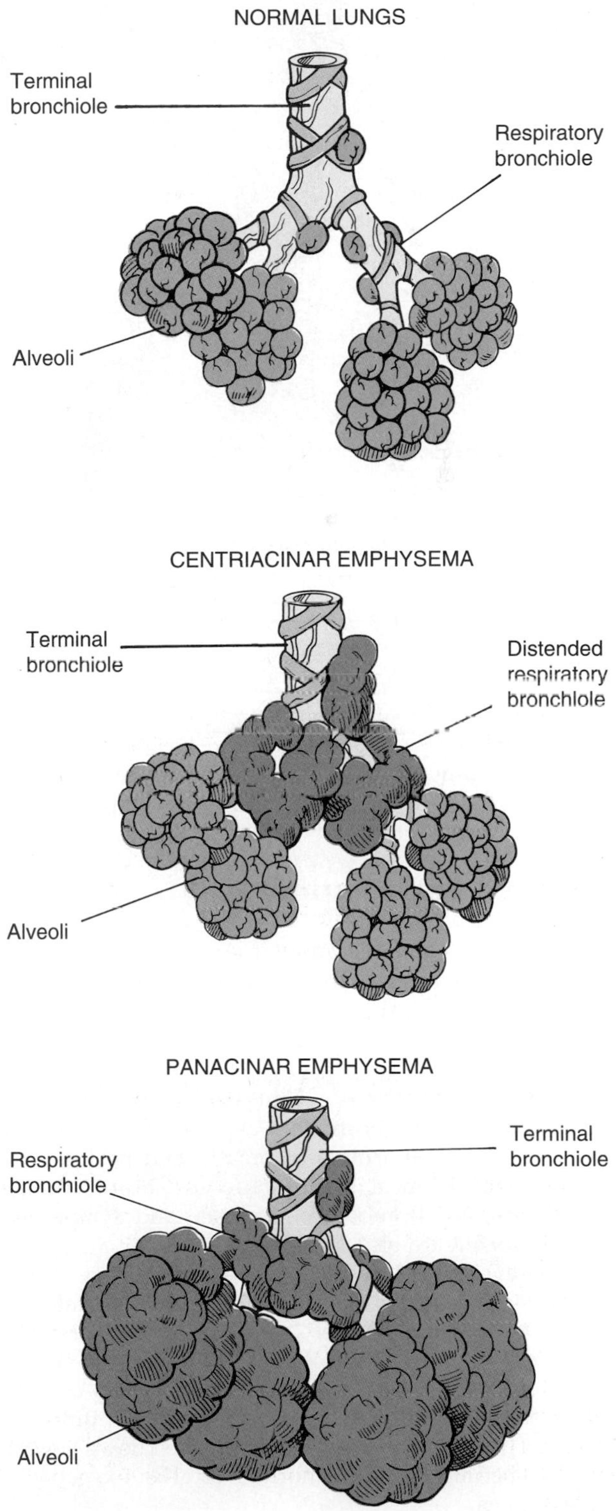

Figure 22–1
Types of emphysema.

CLINICAL MANIFESTATIONS

Chronic Airflow Limitation

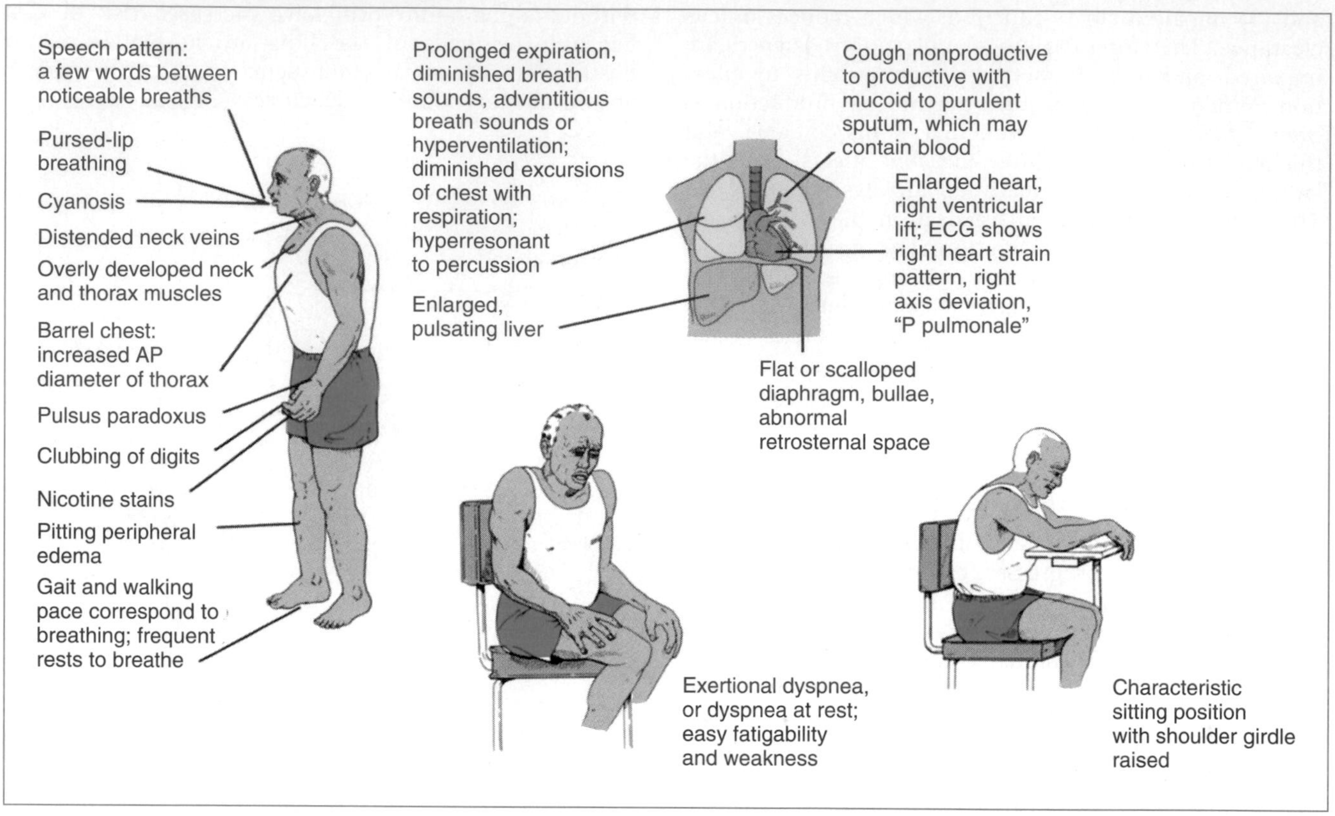

As the disease progresses, there is increasing dyspnea and pulmonary infection. Eventually cor pulmonale (right-sided congestive heart failure) develops.

Clinical Manifestations

Recall that all three disorders, asthma, chronic bronchitis, and emphysema, are present to some degree in the client with CAL. Clinical Manifestations: Chronic Airflow Limitation illustrates the common physical findings in the client with CAL.

Chronic Bronchitis. Clients whose major disease is chronic obstructive bronchitis experience decreased exercise tolerance, shortness of breath, and prolonged expiration (see Clinical Manifestations: Chronic Bronchitis). A history of smoking, cyanosis, and symptoms of cor pulmonale are also common.

Emphysema. Clients who have primary emphysema have marked dyspnea on exertion that later progresses to dyspnea at rest (see Clinical Manifestations: Emphysema). The client often leans forward with arms braced on the knees to support the shoulders and chest for breathing. ABGs are usually normal until later stages. These clients have come to be known as "pink puffers" because of their normal arterial oxygen levels and dyspnea.

Asthma. Asthma is one component of the triad of CAL. Asthma is a reactive airway disorder because allergens cause the airways to react in bronchospasm. Reactive airways increase mucus production (bronchitis). The two disorders of bronchospasm and increased mucus are called asthmatic bronchitis. Many clients with CAL have some degree of asthma in that they have wheezing and bronchospasm. Asthma can also occur alone.

Complications

Respiratory infections commonly develop in clients with CAL as a result of alterations in the normal respiratory defense mechanisms and decreased immune resistance. Because respiratory status is already compromised, infection frequently leads to acute respiratory failure and is a common reason for hospitalization.

The client often develops cor pulmonale (chronic enlargement of the heart's right ventricle) owing to increased cardiac workload. As CAL progresses, hypoxemia leads to pulmonary vasoconstriction. To pump blood through the narrowed vessels, the right side of the heart must generate high pressures; over time, the right ventricle enlarges and thickens. Additionally, hypoxemia stimulates erythropoiesis (production of red

CLINICAL MANIFESTATIONS

Chronic Bronchitis

GENERAL APPEARANCE

Tendency to overweight; cyanotic secondary to polycythemia; dependent edema secondary to right-sided heart failure; barrel chest

AGE RANGE

45–65 years

ASSESSMENT FINDINGS

Persistent cough, copious sputum production; variable levels of dyspnea; variable wheezing on expiration; frequent respiratory infections

Symptoms usually occur over a long period of time

DIAGNOSTIC FINDINGS

Pulmonary Function

Small airways affected early (reduced $FEF_{25-75\%}$); FEV_1 reduced later as airway damage progresses; normal to variable diffusion capacity

Arterial Blood Gases

Increased $PaCO_2$ common; hypoxemia usually present and increasing in severity as disease progresses

Chest Film

Chest film shows normal or "dirty" chest with increased bronchovascular markings

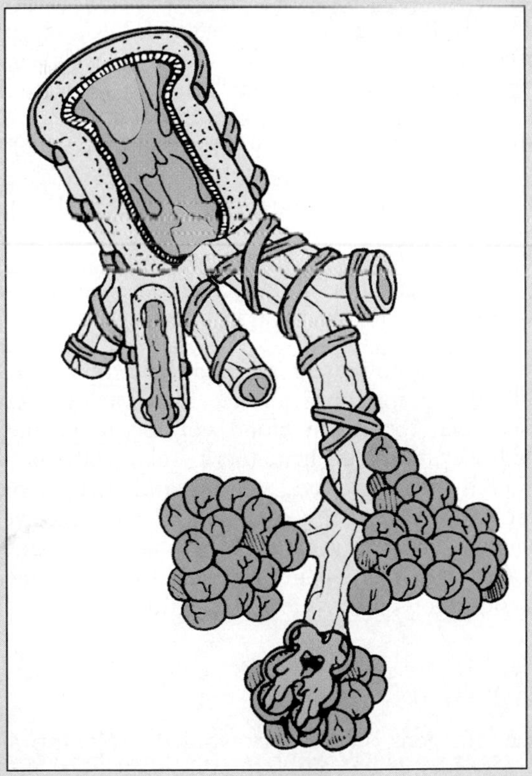

CARDIAC INVOLVEMENT

Enlarged heart; cor pulmonale; hematocrit > 60%

SMOKING HISTORY

Invariably, a long history of smoking

OVERVIEW

Bronchioles narrowed as a result of thickened mucous membrane; surrounding tissue inflamed

Mucus and pus impede action of respiratory cilia

CLINICAL MANIFESTATIONS

Emphysema

GENERAL APPEARANCE

Thin; pink skin color; flattened hemidiaphragms

No signs of right-sided heart failure with dependent edema until end stage

AGE RANGE

65–75 years

ASSESSMENT FINDINGS

Persistent shortness of breath with gradual progressive exertional dyspnea

Infrequent respiratory infections

On auscultation, diminished breath sounds even with deep breathing

DIAGNOSTIC FINDINGS

Pulmonary Function

Reduced $FEF_{25-75\%}$ and FEV_1; reduced diffusion capacity due to destruction of alveoli

Arterial Blood Gases

$PaCO_2$ usually low or normal until end stage; mild to moderate hypoxemia

Chest Film

Chest film shows overinflation, flattened diaphragms, increased retrosternal air space, and increased lucency of lower lung fields

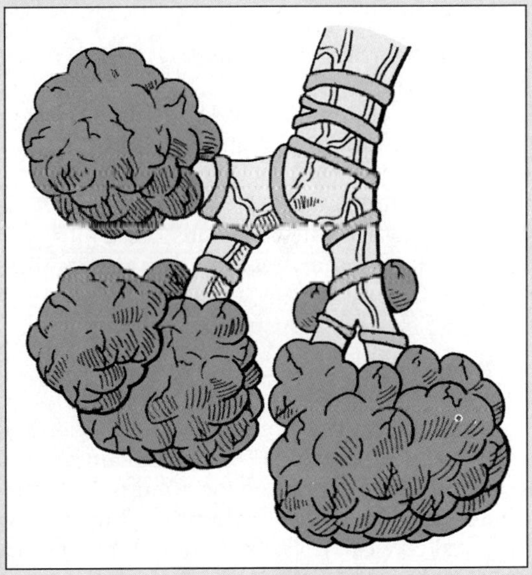

Expiratory wheezing not a prominent finding

Rare sputum production and cough

CARDIAC INVOLVEMENT

No cardiac enlargement; cor pulmonale late; hematocrit < 60%

SMOKING HISTORY

Usually, but not always, a smoking history

OVERVIEW

Walls of individual air sacs torn; repair not possible

Small bronchioles collapse, trapping air; exhalation difficult

Lung tissue becomes inelastic; lungs enlarged

blood cells), which leads to polycythemia. The overworked, hypertrophied right side of the heart must work even harder to circulate the blood, which is now viscous from the increased number of red blood cells.

Heart failure may or may not accompany cor pulmonale. If it does, assessment findings are similar to those of congestive heart failure (see Chap. 24).

Spontaneous pneumothorax may develop from rupture of an emphysematous bleb. This results in a closed pneumothorax.

Like asthma, chronic obstructive bronchitis and emphysema worsen at night. Clients often report sleep onset insomnia and frequent or early morning awakenings. During sleep, there is a decrease in the muscle tone and activity of the respiratory muscles. This leads to hypoventilation, an increase in the resistance of the airways, and V/Q mismatch. Eventually the client becomes hypoxemic. There appears to be an increased risk of pulmonary hypertension and nocturnal hypoxemia.

Medical Management

The main goals for the client with CAL are to improve oxygenation and decrease carbon dioxide retention. These are accomplished by

- relieving the portion of the airway obstruction that is reversible (asthma)
- facilitating the elimination of bronchial secretions
- preventing and treating respiratory infection
- increasing exercise tolerance
- controlling complications
- avoiding airway irritants/allergens
- relieving anxiety and treating depression that often accompany CAL

PHARMACOLOGIC MANAGEMENT

Common classifications of medications used in the treatment of CAL include bronchodilators, antihistamines, steroids, antibiotics, expectorants, and mast cell membrane stabilizers. In addition, the flu vaccine should be taken yearly. Clients should also be urged to take the Pneumovax vaccine. The medications are listed in Table 20–1.

CRITICAL TO REMEMBER

Narcotics, tranquilizers, and sedatives are used with caution in treatment of CAL because they depress the respiratory center.

Some ongoing studies are examining the effect of AAT replacement therapy. The future looks promising for the treatment of early emphysema with the replacement of this protective enzyme inhibitor.

Oxygen is used when the client has severe exertional or at rest hypoxemia (PaO_2 below 40 mm Hg). One to 3 L oxygen by nasal cannula is required to raise PaO_2 to 60 to 80 mm Hg. Oxygen is used cautiously in clients with emphysema; the normal respiratory drive is obliterated because of the long-standing hypercapnia, and carbon dioxide retention can occur. Cautions for use of oxygen are discussed in Chapter 20.

PULMONARY HYGIENE

Pulmonary hygiene is used to rid the lungs of secretions and thereby improve ciliary action and reduce the risk of infection. In the hospital, the client may be treated with nebulized bronchodilators and the use of positive-pressure airflow or positive end-expiratory pressure devices to increase the caliber of the airways. In addition, postural drainage and chest physiotherapy may be prescribed to move the secretions from the small to the large airways, from which they can be expelled.

EXERCISE

Exercise does not improve lung function. Instead, it is used to enhance cardiovascular fitness and train skeletal muscles to function more effectively. Progressively increased walking is the most common form of exercise. Before a walking program is begun, ABGs should be assessed and compared with resting levels. Supplemental oxygen should be used during exercise if the client becomes severely hypoxemic.

Breathing exercises may also be prescribed. Diaphragmatic breathing should be encouraged, and the client should be discouraged from rapid, shallow "panic" breathing.

CONTROLLING COMPLICATIONS

Edema and cor pulmonale are treated with diuretics and digitalis for improving cardiac function. Phlebotomy may be used to reduce blood volume in clients with marked elevations in hematocrit (over 60 per cent). Phlebotomy reduces blood volume and thereby reduces cardiac workload. At times, the client must receive continuous mechanical ventilation for adequate oxygenation, although it is usually difficult to wean the client from continuous mechanical ventilation.

AVOIDING IRRITANTS

Known allergens should be avoided. Smoking should cease. All clients with CAL should avoid high altitudes, and supplemental oxygen may be required for air travel. No specific climate has been shown to alter the course of the disorder.

PSYCHOLOGICAL SUPPORT

Clients with CAL often continue to deteriorate despite the medical care given. It is difficult to cope with failing health that limits activity and employment. As much as possible, the client should be encouraged to live an active life with daily exercise.

DIETARY MANAGEMENT

Clients with CAL often have difficulty eating because of dyspnea. The client should be offered frequent small meals, rather than large meals. Oxygen delivery devices should be adjusted so that the mouth is not obstructed but oxygen is delivered through the nose during eating.

Nursing Management

Assessment

Nursing History: The nursing history can assist the nurse in determining many aspects about the client. The nurse can ascertain whether the client's symptoms are those of chronic bronchitis, emphysema, or asthma. In addition, the nurse can determine the ability of the client to recognize the signs and symptoms that require further care. For example, if a client says, "I knew I was developing an infection and went to the doctor," the statement indicates an understanding of the disorder. In contrast, if another client does not fully understand the reasons for hospitalization, the nurse will need to teach the client about CAL. A review of past medical history will help determine whether the client has other disorders that have impact on treatment (such as heart disease) and the current medications.

A thorough history may need to be delayed until the client is able to breathe comfortably, or it may be taken over short periods of time or obtained through the family.

Physical Assessment: The nurse should collect data with an emphasis on the respiratory and cardiac system. The degree of dyspnea, amount of activity, and signs of congestive heart failure should be noted. ABGs should be analyzed to determine the adequacy of oxygenation and possible need for oxygen in the activities of daily living.

Psychosocial Assessment: When assessing the client with CAL, the nurse should consider the possible effects of decreased oxygenation on the central nervous system. Hypoxemia may result in impaired cognition.

The nurse should consider the impact of stressors that may have led to exacerbations of CAL. Possible factors may include the progressive illness itself, marital problems, or financial concerns. Another portion of the psychosocial assessment is reviewing coping strategies that the client normally uses. It is important to determine whether these strategies are working now and if not, why not. Support systems, such as friends and family, are also important components of psychosocial stability. The reliability of the client's support system should be determined.

Nursing Intervention

There are several nursing diagnoses that can occur in the client with CAL. They are listed in the Care Plan for the client with CAL.

Modification of Plan of Care for the Elderly

The elderly client frequently has other problems that influence the treatment of CAL. For example, the client may have decreased exercise tolerance, impaired nutrition, or a long-standing habit of smoking that retards rehabilitation. The nurse should also consider the possibility of drug-drug interactions.

Posthospital Care

Home oxygen therapy may be required by the client with COPD. Clients and their significant others should be instructed in the proper use of this therapy, including potential hazards and complications (see Client Education Guide: Oxygen Conservation, and the discussion in Chap. 20).

CLIENT EDUCATION GUIDE

Oxygen Conservation

At home, the client with chronic airflow limitation needs to think of himself or herself as an active person. At the same time, he or she must choose activities that will conserve oxygen, improve breathing, and prevent infection. The nurse should teach the client and significant others:

1. To alternate periods of rest and activity.
2. To use pursed-lip breathing during activity.
3. To eat smaller, more frequent, well-balanced meals to decrease shortness of breath when eating.
4. To identify irritants around the house (e.g., hair spray, cigarette smoke, pet dander) and remove or avoid them.
5. In cold weather, to wear a scarf or face mask when outside or until the air in the vehicle has warmed.
6. To gradually increase exercise to build strength and endurance. Walking is ideal.
7. To use infection control techniques:
   - Drink eight 10-ounce glasses of water a day to thin mucus and make expectoration easier.
   - Avoid crowds and people with upper respiratory infections.
   - Avoid smoke-filled environments.
   - Receive an annual flu vaccine.
   - Ask the family physician about the Pneumovax vaccine.
8. To monitor for signs of infection:
   - changes in the color or amount of sputum produced.
   - increased confusion or drowsiness.
   - peripheral edema and/or weight gain of more than 2 pounds a week.
9. Include the same teaching that is contained in the Client Education Guide: Asthma Management.
10. Encourage membership in any local support groups, such as Better Breathers or Huffers and Puffers.
11. Encourage the client and significant others to view the client as an active person.

Text continued on page 584

CARE PLAN: The Client with Chronic Airflow Limitation

Nursing Diagnosis/ Collaborative Problem	Planning: Expected Outcomes	Implementation: Nursing Interventions	Rationales
Gas Exchange, Impaired R/T decreased ventilation and mucus plugs	The client will maintain adequate gas exchange, as evidenced by blood gas values (i.e., PaO_2 of at least 60 mm Hg, pH within normal limits, and $PaCO_2$ at baseline).	1. Regularly monitor respiratory rate and pattern, ABG results, and signs of hypoxia/hypercapnia. Report significant changes promptly.	1. Prompt recognition of deteriorating respiratory function can reduce potentially lethal outcomes.
		2. Administer low-flow oxygen therapy (1–3 L/min 24–31% FIO_2) as needed via nasal prongs or high-flow venturi mask (24 to 31 per cent FIO_2).	2. Oxygen corrects existing hypoxemia. Excessive increases in oxygen (55 to 70 per cent FIO_2) may diminish respiratory drive and further increase carbon dioxide retention.
		3. Assist client into high-Fowler's position.	3. The upright position allows full lung excursion and enhances air exchange.
		4. Administer bronchodilators if ordered. Monitor for side effects.	4. Bronchodilators relax bronchial smooth muscle, facilitating airflow. Common side effects include tremor, tachycardia, and other cardiac dysrhythmias.
		5. Use caution when administering narcotics, sedatives, and tranquilizers.	5. These medications are respiratory depressants and can further impair ventilation.
Airway clearance, Ineffective R/T excessive secretions and ineffective coughing	The client will have improved airway clearance, as evidenced by effective coughing techniques and maintaining patent airways.	1. Teach client to maintain adequate hydration by a. drinking at least 8–10 glasses of fluid/day (if not contraindicated). b. increasing humidity of environmental air.	1. Hydration helps to thin secretions.
		2. Teach and supervise effective coughing techniques (Chap. 20).	2. Proper coughing techniques conserve energy, reduce airway collapse, and lessen client frustration.
		3. Perform chest physical therapy, if needed, and instruct client/significant others in these techniques (Chap. 20).	3. Chest physical therapy techniques utilize forces of gravity and motion to facilitate secretion removal.
		4. Assess breath sounds before and after coughing episodes.	4. This assessment will help in the evaluation of coughing effectiveness.

CARE PLAN: The Client with Chronic Airflow Limitation *Continued*

Nursing Diagnosis/ Collaborative Problem	Planning: Expected Outcomes	Implementation: Nursing Interventions	Rationales
Activity Intolerance R/T inadequate oxygenation and dyspnea	The client will have improved activity tolerance, as evidenced by maintaining a realistic activity level and demonstrating use of energy conservation techniques.	1. Advise client to avoid conditions that increase oxygen demand, such as smoking, temperature extremes, excess weight, and stress.	1. These factors increase peripheral vascular resistance, which increases cardiac workload and oxygen requirements.
		2. Instruct client in energy conservation techniques such as pacing activities throughout the day, interspersed with adequate rest periods, and alternating high- and low-energy tasks.	2. Conservation techniques allow the client to accomplish more tasks, with a limited energy supply.
		3. Assist client to schedule a gradual increase in daily activities and exercise.	3. Gradual increases in physical activity improve respiratory and cardiac conditioning, thus improving activity tolerance.
		4. Teach the client to use pursed-lip and diaphragmatic breathing techniques during activities (Chap. 20).	4. Breathing retraining ensures maximal use of available respiratory function. Pursed-lip breathing leaves positive end-diastolic pressure in the lungs and helps keep airways open.
		5. Schedule active exercise after respiratory therapy or medication (e.g., bronchodilator in metered dose inhaler).	5. Lung function is maximized during peak periods of treatment/drug effect.
		6. Maintain supplemental oxygen therapy, as needed.	6. Supplemental oxygen helps alleviate exercise-induced hypoxemia, thus improving activity tolerance.
		7. Assess client for signs of a negative response to activity (e.g., significant change in respiratory rate, failure of pulse to return to near resting rate within 3 minutes of activity, changes in mental status).	7. Significant changes in respiratory, cardiac, or circulatory status signal activity intolerance.
Anxiety R/T acute breathing difficulties and fear of suffocation	The client will express an increase in psychological comfort and demonstrate use of effective coping mechanisms.	1. Remain with client during acute episodes of breathing difficulty and provide care in a calm, reassuring manner.	1. Reassure the client that competent help is available, if needed. Anxiety can be contagious. The nurse must remain calm.
		2. Provide a quiet, calm environment.	2. Reduction of external stimuli helps promote relaxation.
		3. During acute episodes, open doors and curtains and limit number of people and unnecessary equipment in client's room.	3. Environmental changes may lessen the client's perceptions of suffocation.
		4. Encourage the use of breathing retraining and relaxation techniques (Chap. 20).	4. A feeling of self-control and success in facilitating breathing will help reduce anxiety.
		5. Use sedatives and tranquilizers with extreme caution. Nonpharmaceutical methods of anxiety reduction are more useful.	5. Oversedation may cause respiratory depression.

Care Plan continued on following page

CARE PLAN: The Client with Chronic Airflow Limitation *Continued*

Nursing Diagnosis/ Collaborative Problem	Planning: Expected Outcomes	Implementation: Nursing Interventions	Rationales
Nutrition, Altered: Less than Body Requirements R/T reduced appetite, decreased energy level, and dyspnea	The client will maintain body weight within normal limits for sex and body build and hemoglobin and albumin levels within normal range	1. Promote mouth care before meals and as needed.	1. Coughing and sputum production may impair appetite. Mouthbreathing dries mucous membranes.
		2. Advise client to eat small, frequent meals (e.g., six meals a day).	2. Large meals may create an excessive feeling of fullness that may make breathing uncomfortable and difficult.
		3. Advise client to avoid gas-producing foods, such as beans and cabbage.	3. Gas-forming foods may cause abdominal bloating and distention and thus impair ventilation.
		4. Instruct client in the use of high-calorie liquid supplements, if indicated.	4. Increased calorie intake is needed to provide energy for increased work of breathing. Liquid supplements provide high-calorie concentrations in a relatively small volume.
		5. Advise hypoxemic clients to use oxygen via nasal cannula during meals.	5. Adequate oxygenation increases energy available for eating.
		6. Suggest methods to make meal preparation more convenient (e.g., Meals on Wheels program).	6. Reducing energy expenditure on preparation will maximize energy availability for eating.
		7. Monitor food intake, weight, and serum hemoglobin and albumin levels.	7. Changes in body weight reflect the degree of nutrition or malnutrition. Hemoglobin and albumin levels reflect protein intake.
Sleep Pattern Disturbance R/T dyspnea and external stimuli	The client will report feeling adequately rested	1. Promote relaxation by providing a darkened, quiet environment; ensuring adequate room ventilation; and following bedtime routines, as possible.	1. The hospital environment can interfere with relaxation and sleep. Using established bedtime rituals increases relaxation.
		2. Schedule care activities to allow periods of uninterrupted sleep.	2. For most people, completing four to five complete sleep cycles (60–90 minutes) per night promotes a feeling of being rested.
		3. Instruct client in measures to promote sleep:	3.
		a. Plan physical exercise during the day and passive, nonstimulating activities in the evening.	a. Activity increases the need for sleep and contributes to a feeling of "tiredness."
		b. Avoid stimulants, such as caffeine.	b. Stimulants increase metabolism and inhibit relaxation.
		c. Maintain a consistent bedtime and a regular bedtime routine.	c. Consistency promotes relaxation and prevents disruptions of the biologic clock.
		d. Eat a high-protein snack before bedtime.	d. Protein digestion produces tryptophan, an amino acid that has a sedative effect.
		e. Use relaxation techniques (e.g., meditation, massage, warm bath, warm beverage).	e. Sleep is difficult unless the client is relaxed.

CARE PLAN: The Client with Chronic Airflow Limitation *Continued*

Nursing Diagnosis/ Collaborative Problem	Planning: Expected Outcomes	Implementation: Nursing Interventions	Rationales
		4. If the client awakens during the night, suggest the use of a quiet, diverting activity, such as reading, in another room.	4. Frustration over being awake will further deter sleep efforts. The bedroom should be mentally associated with sleep to enhance future sleep promotion.
		5. If dyspnea is severe, a recliner chair or hospital bed may be more comfortable than a regular bed.	5. The upright position facilitates ventilation.
Family Processes, Altered R/T chronic illness of a family member	The family will verbalize their feelings, participate in the care of the ill family member, and seek external resources as needed	1. Plan intervention considering the client and significant others as the unit of care. Encourage participation in the planning process.	1. CAL affects not only the client experiencing the condition but also the client's significant others.
		2. Assess family communication patterns and intervene if ineffective. Family counseling may be needed.	2. Effective communication helps each member to understand his or her own and others' feelings. Counseling may facilitate healthy interaction.
		3. Encourage as wide a social support system as feasible.	3. The use of various support people prevents a few family members from being overloaded with responsibility.
		4. Encourage the client and family to seek support from other sources (e.g., self-help groups and support groups such as Better Breathers Clubs sponsored by the American Lung Association).	4. Clients may benefit from opportunities to share common experiences and learn from others in similar situations.
		5. Provide the family with anticipatory guidance as client's CAL progresses.	5. Knowing what to expect facilitates family adjustment.
Sexual Dysfunction R/T dyspnea, reduced energy, and changes in relationships	The client will report increased satisfaction with sexual function	1. Provide opportunity for client to discuss concerns.	1. Many people are embarrassed or reluctant to talk about their sexual concerns.
		2. Suggest measures that may facilitate sexual activity (e.g., alternative positions, use of bronchodilator therapy before beginning sexual activity).	2. Such measures can reduce physical exertion and maximize available oxygen levels.
		3. Encourage client and partner to consider other forms of sexual expression (e.g., hugging, cuddling, stroking, kissing).	3. Alternative methods require less energy expenditure than does intercourse.
		4. Refer to a professional skilled in sexuality, if appropriate.	4. Talking with a skilled professional may further assist client with constructive problem solving.

ABG, arterial blood gas; CAL, chronic airflow limitation.

FOLLOW-UP

Ongoing respiratory assessment is essential. Annual ABG analysis, pulmonary function tests, and noninvasive monitoring (see Chapter 20) are often required.

BRONCHIECTASIS

Bronchiectasis is a form of obstructive lung disease. It is an extreme form of bronchitis. This disorder causes permanent, abnormal dilation and distortion of bronchi and bronchioles. It develops when bronchial walls are weakened by chronic inflammatory changes in the bronchial mucosa.

Bronchiectasis most often develops after recurrent inflammatory conditions, following infection or obstruction. However, any condition producing a narrowing of the lumen of the bronchioles may create bronchiectasis, including tuberculosis, adenoviral infections, and pneumonia. Bronchiectasis is usually localized to a lung lobe or segment rather than generalized throughout the lungs. At times, however, persistent, nonresolving infection may cause the disorder to spread to other parts of the same lung. Diagnosis may be confirmed through chest x-ray study, bronchogram, or chest computed tomographic scan.

Clinical manifestations vary according to the etiologic agent. The main manifestations are cough and purulent sputum production in voluminous quantities. Fever, hemoptysis, nasal stuffiness, and drainage from sinusitis are also common. The client may complain of fatigue and weakness, and clubbing may be found on physical assessment.

Medical and nursing management of bronchiectasis are the same as for CAL. Severe cases may be treated by surgical resection if the pathologic process is well localized in one lobe or two adjacent lobes and when no contraindications to surgery exist.

Parenchymal Disorders

ATELECTASIS

Atelectasis denotes the collapse of lung tissue at any structural level (e.g., segmental, basilar, lobar, microscopic). It develops when there is interference with the natural forces that promote lung expansion. Examples of the causes are given in Box 22–1. It is particularly common in postoperative clients, especially those undergoing high abdominal or thoracic surgeries.

Atelectasis may be diagnosed by physical examination, although it is usually detected first by chest x-ray examination. Some clients are asymptomatic. If significant hypoxemia is present, dyspnea, tachypnea, tachycardia, and cyanosis may occur. Chest auscultation may reveal diminished breath sounds or crackles over the involved area. In severe forms, physical assessment findings may include (1) tracheal shift toward the side of the atelectasis, (2) decreased tactile fremitus over the affected lung area, (3) decreased percussion note over the atelectatic region, and (4) a decrease in size of the chest and decreased movement on the involved side. However, none of these signs is specific for atelectasis, and the entire clinical picture must be considered.

BOX 22–1

Causes of Atelectasis

- Decreased lung distention forces
  - Pleural space encroachment (e.g., pneumothorax, pleural effusion, pleural tumor)
  - Chest wall disorders (e.g., kyphoscoliosis, flail chest)
  - Impaired diaphragmatic movement (e.g., ascites, obesity)
  - Central nervous system dysfunction (e.g., coma, neuromuscular disorders, oversedation)
- Localized airway obstruction
  - Mucus plugging
  - Foreign body aspiration
  - Bronchiectasis
- Insufficient pulmonary surfactant
  - Respiratory distress syndrome
  - Inhalation anesthesia
  - High concentrations of oxygen (oxygen toxicity)
  - Lung contusion
  - Aspiration of gastric contents
  - Smoke inhalation
- Increased elastic recoil
  - Interstitial fibrosis (e.g., silicosis, radiation pneumonitis)

Management

CRITICAL TO REMEMBER

One of the primary goals of nursing intervention is to prevent atelectasis in the high-risk client.

Frequent position changes and early ambulation help promote drainage of all lung segments. Deep breathing and effective coughing enhance lung expansion and prevent airway obstruction. Hyperinflation therapy with the use of an incentive spirometer (see Chap. 20) may also be helpful.

If atelectasis develops, treatment is directed toward the underlying cause. If the client becomes hypoxic, oxygen should be administered as prescribed. More aggressive measures to maintain airway patency, such as postural drainage, chest physiotherapy, or tracheal suctioning, may also be ordered. If an airway obstruction is causing atelectasis, bronchoscopy may be used to remove the material.

PNEUMONIA

Pneumonia (pneumonitis) is an inflammatory process of lung parenchyma usually associated with a marked increase in interstitial and alveolar fluid.

Incidence and Etiology

Pneumonia remains a major cause of morbidity and mortality, especially among the elderly. It accounts for more than 10 per cent of hospital admissions and occurs in about 5 per cent of clients who are admitted with other diagnoses.

There are many causes, including bacteria, viruses, mycoplasmas, fungal agents, and protozoa. Pneumonia may also result from (1) aspiration of food, fluids, or vomitus or (2) inhalation of toxic or caustic chemicals, smoke, dusts, or gases. Pneumonia may complicate immobility and chronic illnesses. It often follows influenza.

Risk Factors

Pneumonia is most likely to occur when normal defense mechanisms are weakened or overcome by the virulence, quality, or number of organisms. Box 22–2 lists risk factors that predispose a client to pneumonia. Young or otherwise healthy clients may develop pneumonia as a consequence of upper respiratory or viral infections. Group living or working conditions may facilitate wide transmission.

General measures to reduce the incidence of pneumonia involve decreasing the proliferation and spread of pneumonia-causing organisms. Adequate nutrition and fluid intake and proper hygiene measures help maintain normal defenses. Resistance is also enhanced by avoiding cigarette smoke, which decreases the ciliary clearance of secretions. Clients at risk for the development of pneumonia, especially those with chronic diseases, should avoid exposure to infected clients.

In the hospital, rigorous handwashing by medical personnel is essential for reducing the transmission of infectious agents. Proper infection control measures of respiratory equipment are vital. Effective airway clearance and mobilization (e.g., coughing, turning, early ambulation) should be promoted, particularly in clients at risk.

BOX 22–2

Risk Factors Predisposing a Client to Pneumonia

- Smoking
- Air pollution
- Upper respiratory infection
- Altered consciousness: alcoholism, head injury, seizure disorder; drug overdose; general anesthesia
- Tracheal intubation (bypassing the upper airway)
- Prolonged immobility
- Immunosuppressive therapy: corticosteroids; cancer chemotherapy
- Nonfunctional immune system: AIDS
- Severe periodontal disease
- Prolonged exposure to especially virulent organisms
- Malnutrition
- Dehydration
- Chronic diseases: diabetes mellitus; heart disease; chronic lung disease; renal disease; cancer
- Prolonged debilitating disease
- Inhalation of noxious substances
- Aspiration of oral or gastric material
- Aspiration of foreign material (e.g., petroleum products)
- Chronically ill, elderly clients who generally have poor immune systems, often residing in group-living situations where there is an increased probability of disease transmission, especially through the respiratory system

Pathophysiology

The common feature of all types of pneumonia is an inflammatory pulmonary response to the offending organism or agent. Infectious agents are usually introduced by inhalation. The defense mechanisms of the lungs lose effectiveness and allow organisms to penetrate the lower airways, in which inflammation develops. Organisms may also be introduced into the pulmonary system via the bloodstream. Circulating organisms that are too large to flow through the pulmonary capillary bed become lodged in the lungs, leading to a potential source of infection.

BACTERIA ASSOCIATED WITH PNEUMONIA

Gram-Positive Bacteria

Streptococcus Pneumoniae (Pneumococcal Pneumonia). This is the most common cause of community-acquired pneumonia. Pneumococcal pneumonia often follows influenza and is frequently seen in clients with chronic diseases, immunosuppression, and alcohol abuse.

Staphylococcus Aureus. This organism usually reaches the lungs through the blood or by aspiration. Incidence is highest among hospitalized adult clients, but it is also common in diabetes, drug abusers, and clients on hemodialysis. The organism can be quite virulent, causing considerable morbidity and mortality despite appropriate antibiotic therapy. Toxins associated with the staphylococcus organism can cause extensive parenchymal tissue necrosis.

Gram-Negative Bacteria

Haemophilus Influenzae. This organism is a common cause of infection in children and in clients with chronic debilitating diseases, chronic airway limitations, or immune defects. *H. influenzae* may affect multiple lobes of the lungs and has a high mortality rate, especially among the elderly. It may also cause infections at other sites (e.g., epiglottitis, endocarditis, meningitis).

Pseudomonas Aeruginosa. This is the most common cause of hospital-acquired gram-negative pneumonia. This organism thrives in warm, moist environments such as respiratory therapy equipment and liquid soap dispensers. It is common in the respiratory tract of hospital employees and in clients with cystic fibrosis. In addition to the lungs, *Pseudomonas* may infect wounds, burns, tracheostomies, and the urinary tract.

Klebsiella Pneumoniae (Friedländer's Bacillus). This is the most common gram-negative organism encountered outside the hospital setting. The incidence of *Klebsiella* pneumonia is increased among the elderly and those with chronic debilitating disease. It is also common in hospitalized clients with complicated or prolonged illnesses. The organism reaches the lung most frequently through aspiration of oropharyngeal secretions. Necrosis, abscess formation, hemoptysis, and permanent fibrotic lung changes may occur, leading to a high mortality rate.

Anaerobic Bacteria. Anaerobic bacterial pneumonias are commonly caused by anaerobic streptococcus, *Fusobacteria,* and *Bacteroides* species. Infection usually develops after aspiration of oropharyngeal secretions. Altered consciousness (from alcohol, coma, or seizures), impaired swallowing mechanisms, or poor dentition are often the precipitating causes. The chest film typically reveals lung abscess, empyema, and necrotizing pneumonia, with primary involvement in dependent lung zones (especially the right lung, in which aspirated secretions tend to settle). Accurate culture identification may require the use of a sheathed brush to obtain a specimen during fiberoptic bronchoscopy. This device allows the maintenance of an environment that is as anaerobic as possible and reduces cross-contamination with other upper airway flora.

Atypical Bacteria

Legionella Pneumophila (Legionnaires' Disease). This organism was first identified in 1976 after a major outbreak of pneumonia at an American Legion convention in Philadelphia that resulted in 29 deaths. The organism was traced to a contaminated air conditioning system but has also been isolated from soil; construction workers and those living near soil excavations are at risk. Legionnaires' disease is most commonly seen in older adults, smokers, or others with impaired lung defenses. Diagnosis may be made through serologic testing.

Mycoplasma Pneumoniae. This organism has characteristics of both bacteria and viruses. It is transmitted by droplet infection and spreads rapidly in settings where people live or work closely together (e.g., dormitories, military units). *M. pneumoniae* accounts for about 20 to 40 per cent of the pneumonias affecting ambulatory clients. Onset is often insidious, with slowly rising fever, headache, malaise, and nonproductive cough.

VIRUSES ASSOCIATED WITH PNEUMONIA

Many different viruses are responsible for pneumonias in adults, including influenza, parainfluenza, and adenovirus. Most are community acquired; the resulting infection follows an insidious course, which is similar to the one seen in atypical pneumonias. Viral pneumonias are usually self-limiting and are treated symptomatically. However, they will frequently lower the client's resistance, which increases the risk of a secondary bacterial pneumonia.

FUNGI AND PROTOZOA ASSOCIATED WITH PNEUMONIA

Fungi and protozoa are opportunistic organisms; they become pathogenic only when the client's physiologic state is altered and normal bacterial flora are suppressed. Opportunistic pneumonias are commonly seen after extended antibiotic use and in clients who are immunosuppressed (e.g., those taking corticosteroids or antineoplastics, those with acquired immunodeficiency syndrome [AIDS]) or severely debilitated. These forms of pneumonia are not spread by person-to-person contact. Common fungal infections include candidiasis, histoplasmosis, aspergillosis, coccidioidomycosis, and cryptococcosis. Protozoan infection is most common with *Pneumocystis carinii* pneumonia, typically seen in the client with AIDS.

Clinical Manifestations

The onset of all pneumonias is generally marked by any or all of the following: fever, chills, sweats, pleuritic chest pain, cough, sputum production, hemoptysis, dyspnea, headache, and fatigue.

CRITICAL TO REMEMBER

The elderly client, however, may present not with fever or respiratory symptoms but with altered mental status and volume depletion.

Chest auscultation reveals bronchial breath sounds over areas of consolidation (i.e., dense areas on the chest film). Consolidated lung tissue transmits bronchial sound waves to outer lung fields. Crackling sounds (from fluid to interstitial and alveolar areas) and whispered pectoriloquy may be heard over affected areas. Tactile fremitus is usually increased over areas of pneumonia. Percussion is dulled over affected areas. Unequal chest wall expansion may occur during inspiration if a large area of lung tissue is involved. This is due to decreased distensibility in the affected area.

Assessment findings with specific types of pneumonia are shown in Table 22–3.

DIAGNOSTIC ASSESSMENT

Definitive diagnosis is usually determined through sputum culture and sensitivity or serologic testing. At times, fiberoptic bronchoscopy or transcutaneous needle aspiration or biopsy may be necessary for confirmation. Additional diagnostic testing may include (1) skin tests, if tuberculosis or coccidioidomycosis is suspected; (2) blood and urine cultures to assess systemic spread; and

TABLE 22–3 Assessment and Treatment of Pneumonias

COMMON NAME	CLINICAL MANIFESTATIONS	MANAGEMENT
Pneumococcal pneumonia (caused by *Streptococcus pneumoniae*)	Sudden onset with a single shaking chill, high fever, stabbing, pleuritic chest pain, malaise, weakness, occasional vomiting, tachypnea, dyspnea, and elevated white blood cell count; single or multiple lobar consolidation on the chest film; cough productive of rusty brown or blood-streaked purulent sputum that turns yellow and mucoid	Primary: penicillin G intravenously or penicillin V orally Alternative: cephalosporins or erythromycin Prevention: vaccine available
Staphylococcal pneumonia (caused by *Staphylococcus aureus*)	Sudden onset with fever, multiple chills, pleuritic pain, dyspnea, rales, decreased breath sounds, elevated white blood cell count, and exaggerated cough productive of purulent golden-yellow or blood-streaked sputum; chest film may show patchy infiltrates, empyema, abscesses, and pneumothorax; disease may start with headache, cough, and myalgia	Primary: nafcillin or oxacillin Alternative: cephalosporins or vancomycin if client is sensitive to penicillin
H. flu pneumonia (caused by *Haemophilus influenzae*)	Similar to pneumococcal pneumonia; cough productive of apple- or lime-green purulent sputum, which may be blood-tinged	Primary: ampicillin or third-generation cephalosporins such as cefotaxime and moxalactam Alternative: chloramphenicol
Gram-negative bacterial pneumonia (most commonly caused by *Klebsiella pneumoniae*)	Sudden onset with high fever, multiple chills, pleuritic pain, dyspnea, cyanosis, and elevated white blood cell count; lobar consolidation and cavitation on the chest film; cough productive of red sputum resembling currant jelly—mucoid, sticky, and difficult to expectorate	Cephalosporins such as cefotaxime and aminoglycosides such as tobramycin
Anaerobic bacterial pneumonia, hypostatic pneumonia (caused by normal oral flora)	Insidious onset with low-grade fever, dyspnea, rales, cyanosis, hypertension, tachycardia, and elevated white blood cell count; patchy infiltrates in dependent lung segments on the chest film; cough productive of purulent greenish-yellow foul-smelling sputum	Primary: third-generation cephalosporins (such as cefotaxime) or penicillin G Alternative: cefoxitin, clindamycin, or chloramphenicol
Legionnaires' disease (caused by *Legionella pneumophila*)	Prodrome of 24–48 hours with fever, headaches, and malaise followed by high fever with pulse-temperature dissociation, dyspnea, hypoxia, pleuritic pain, nausea, vomiting, diarrhea, confusion, and elevated white blood cell count; single or multilobar consolidation and small pleural effusions on the chest film; dry cough productive of scant mucoid or blood-tinged sputum	Primary: erythromycin Alternative: tetracycline or rifampin
Mycoplasma pneumonia (caused by *Mycoplasma* microorganisms)	Insidious onset with slowly rising fever, headache, myalgia, malaise, and normal white blood cell count; pulmonary infiltrate—sometimes extensive—on the chest film; cough productive of scant mucoid sputum; client may show only minimal signs and symptoms	Primary: erythromycin in severe cases Alternative: tetracycline
Viral pneumonia (caused by influenza A virus)	Prodrome with headache and myalgia followed by high fever, dyspnea, normal breath sounds with occasional wheezing and rales, and normal or slightly elevated white blood cell count; diffuse, patchy infiltrates on the chest film; dry cough with initial mucoid sputum that later turns purulent; cough may be unproductive	None indicated

From Coleman, D. A. (1986). Pneumonia: where nursing care really counts. *RN, 49,* 23.

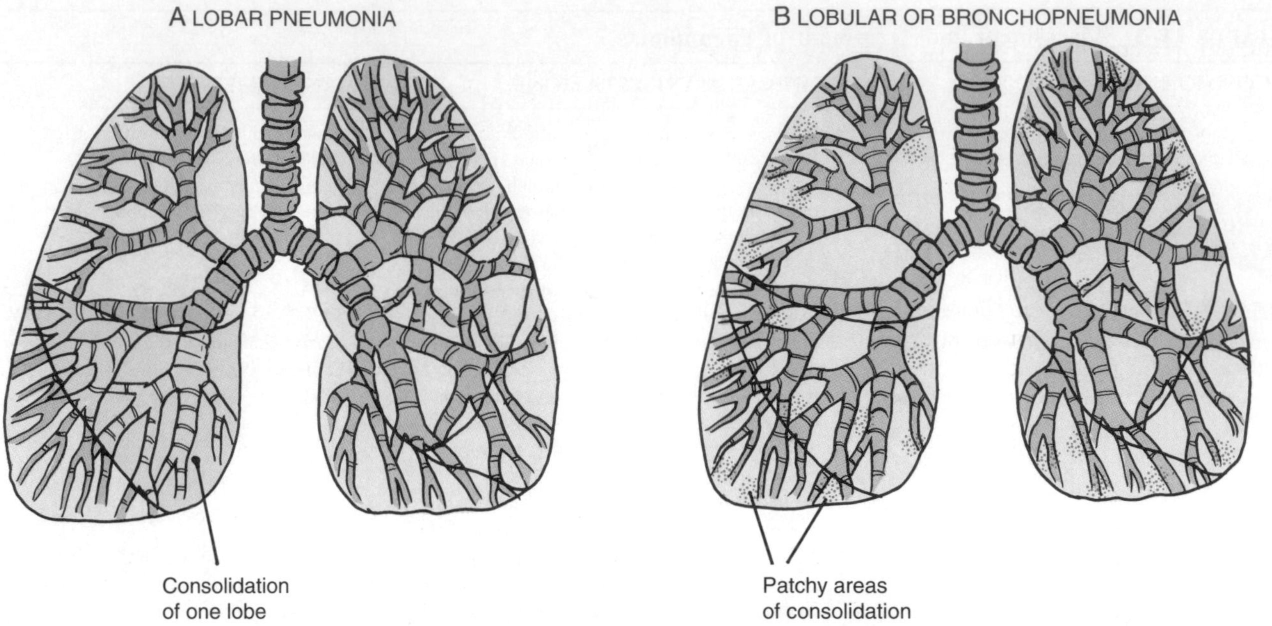

Figure 22–2
Two types of pneumonia. *A*, Lobar pneumonia with consolidation in one lobe of one lung. *B*, Lobular, or bronchopneumonia, with patchy consolidation throughout both lungs.

(3) ABG analysis to assess the need for supplemental oxygen.

Chest x-ray examination provides information about the location and extent of pneumonia. Pneumonia may involve one or more lobe segments of the lungs (segmental pneumonia), one or more entire lobes (lobar pneumonia) (Fig. 22–2*A*), or entire lobes or segments of lobes in both lungs (bilateral pneumonia). On the basis of location and radiologic appearance, pneumonias may be classified as bronchopneumonia, interstitial pneumonia, alveolar pneumonia, or necrotizing pneumonia.

Bronchopneumonia (bronchial pneumonia) (Fig. 22–2*B*) involves the terminal bronchioles and alveoli. Interstitial (reticular) pneumonia involves inflammatory responses within lung tissue surrounding the air spaces or vascular structures, rather than the air passages themselves. In alveolar (acinar) pneumonia, fluffy shadows are caused by fluid accumulation in a lung's distal air spaces. Necrotizing pneumonia causes the death of a portion of lung tissue, surrounded by viable tissue. Necrotic lung tissue, which does not heal, constitutes a permanent loss of functioning parenchyma.

Medical Management

The primary treatment for most forms of pneumonia is antibiotic therapy. Table 22–3 lists the drugs of choice for each form.

Hospitalization is not always necessary for clients with pneumonia. If the client has intact defense mechanisms and good general health, recuperation can often take place at home with rest and supportive treatment. The term "walking pneumonia" is sometimes used to describe this situation.

Clients who are ambulatory but have an ongoing health problem that predisposes them to pneumonia may require hospitalization. Similarly, clients who are already hospitalized for other reasons are at risk for developing nosocomial (hospital-acquired) pneumonias because of their decreased ability to combat infection and their potential exposure to resistant strains of organisms.

Nursing Management

Assessment

The following should be determined through the nursing history:

- contact with other clients experiencing similar symptoms (suggesting viral or mycoplasma pneumonia)
- factors suggesting the presence of noninfectious diseases that produce symptoms similar to those of pneumonia (e.g., pulmonary embolism, allergic or hypersensitivity reaction to drugs or other substances, neoplasm)
- presence of tuberculosis or contact with others who have active tuberculosis
- exposure to animals or birds (suggests certain diseases such as histoplasmosis or cryptococcosis)
- travel to areas where certain pulmonary diseases are common (e.g., Asia, Africa, South America)

Assess and monitor the client for possible hypersensitivity reactions, superinfections, altered renal function, and blood dyscrasias.

Nursing Diagnosis, Planning, and Implementation

Nursing Diagnosis: Airway Clearance, Ineffective R/T inflammation and increased secretions.

Planning: Expected Outcomes. The client will maintain effective airway clearance, as evidenced by maintaining patent airway and effectively clearing secretions.

Implementation. Measures should be taken to promote airway patency. These may include increasing fluid intake, effective coughing and deep-breathing techniques, and frequent turning. Clients with an altered level of consciousness should be turned at least every 2 hours and should be positioned in side-lying positions, unless contraindicated, for prevention of aspiration. The nurse should administer bronchodilating medications as prescribed. If indicated, more aggressive measures to maintain airway patency may be required (e.g., chest physiotherapy, suctioning, artificial airway). These procedures are fully discussed in Chapter 20.

Nursing Diagnosis: Breathing Pattern, Ineffective R/T tachypnea secondary to chest pain, hypoxia, and increased body temperature.

Planning: Expected Outcomes. The client will have improved breathing patterns, as evidenced by respiratory rate within normal limits, adequate chest expansion, clear breath sounds, and decreased dyspnea.

Implementation. The client should be positioned for comfort and to facilitate breathing (e.g., at 45 degrees). The nurse teaches the client how to splint the chest wall with a pillow for comfort during coughing and administers prescribed cough expectorants and analgesics. The nurse should be cautious, however, because such medications may depress respirations. He or she should routinely auscultate the chest and document findings. The nurse monitors ABGs and observes for signs of hypoxia or hypercapnia.

Nursing Diagnosis: Activity intolerance R/T depleted energy reserves and impaired oxygen/carbon dioxide transport.

Planning: Expected Outcomes. The client will have improved activity tolerance, as evidenced by ability to perform activities of daily living and demonstrating progressively increasing physical activities.

Implementation. The nurse assesses the client's baseline of activity and response to activity.

CRITICAL TO REMEMBER

Note whether client tolerates any activity by assessing for changes in respiratory and pulse rate, marked dyspnea, pallor or cyanosis, and dysrhythmias.

Activity should be scheduled after treatments or medications and oxygen used as needed. Activity can be gradually increased on the basis of tolerance.

The nurse teaches the client to avoid conditions that increase oxygen demand such as smoking, temperature extremes, weight gain, and stress. Pursed-lip and diaphragmatic breathing as well as techniques to decrease energy use should be reinforced. High-energy activities should be interspersed with rest.

The nurse should provide psychosocial support and a quiet environment to reduce anxiety and promote rest. Nursing care and visitors should be paced, as warranted by the client's condition.

EVALUATION

The degree of expected outcome attainment is monitored every 2 to 3 days. Elderly clients may require additional time to fully recover.

Modification of Plan of Care for the Elderly

Because many cases of pneumonia go undiagnosed in the elderly, the nurse must maintain a high index of suspicion for the common clinical manifestations (see earlier discussion).

CRITICAL TO REMEMBER

In addition, the nurse assesses the aged client for changes in cognition (confusion and lethargy), anorexia, tachypnea, and deterioration of pre-existing disorders (heart failure and CAL).

The most common bacterial source of pneumonia is bacteria from the gastrointestinal tract. Elderly clients who are immobile or debilitated are at highest risk.

Another common situation increasing risk of pneumonia is aspiration from tube feeding, or following the administration of medications or anesthesia.

The elderly are managed as previously discussed, with caution exercised in the use of fluids for hydration so as to not aggravate pre-existing renal or cardiac disorders. Likewise, oxygen is used as needed in clients with CAL to maintain blood oxygen levels without impairing the drive to breathe.

Posthospital Care

The client and significant others are taught techniques of deep breathing and coughing. Chest physical therapy may be prescribed until the chest clears. The client is taught the importance of completing prescribed antibiotics. Plans for rest and gradual resumption of activity should be discussed. A list of complications that require physician notification (return of fever, chest pain, hemoptysis, chills) should be provided.

The client is followed in a clinic setting until the chest clears according to x-ray study, and clinical manifestations abate. The client is encouraged to plan for immunization the next winter. People who live with the client are also monitored for the onset of pneumonia.

LUNG ABSCESS

A lung abscess is a collection of pus within lung tissue. In its early stages, it resembles a localized pneumonia. If lung abscess is undiagnosed and untreated, tissue necrosis may occur.

Single lung abscesses occur most often behind a bronchial obstruction. They nearly always create putrid (foul) material. The bronchial obstruction may be caused by

- aspirated foreign material (e.g., vomitus, teeth, blood, or food or tissue during upper airways surgery)
- benign or malignant tumors
- inspissated (thickened through evaporation or absorption) mucus in bronchial tree
- accumulated mucus due to impaired airway clearance during unconsciousness (e.g., during oversedation, alcohol-induced unconsciousness, or epileptic seizure)

Multiple lung abscesses follow pneumonia caused by necrotizing bacteria (i.e., bacteria that create necrotic lung tissue). These organisms spread through the bloodstream. Bacteria may also arise from septic emboli from infected foci such as septic phlebitis (especially with chronic, debilitating conditions such as congestive heart failure, cirrhosis, malnutrition, or alcoholism). Lung abscesses frequently occur in immunosuppressed clients (e.g., after organ transplantation). Multiple abscesses are usually not putrid.

Early assessment findings in a client with a lung abscess are the same as with bronchopneumonia (i.e., chills, fever, pleuritic pain, cough). The body attempts to wall off the abscess with fibrous tissue. If the attempt is unsuccessful, the abscess ruptures into a bronchus, causing a cough producing copious amounts of sputum. With a single abscess, the sputum is purulent, foul smelling, and foul tasting. After bronchial rupture, hemoptysis often occurs.

Chest auscultation reveals decreased breath sounds and dullness to percussion over the affected area. Crackles may be present when the abscess drains.

Management

Antibiotics are used to treat lung abscesses, most commonly penicillin. If performed early, bronchoscopy may be helpful in removing foreign matter and promoting the drainage of abscess contents. In severe cases, surgical removal of a portion of the lung, or of the entire lung, may be indicated.

Caring for a client with a lung abscess is similar to caring for a client with pneumonia. Lung abscesses produce copious volumes of sputum. Nursing intervention focuses on removing sputum from the lungs through drainage, expectoration, and antibiotic therapy. The nurse notes the color, quantity, quality, and odor of the expectorated material, including the presence of blood. Expectorated material is sent for microbiologic assessment. Universal precautions are followed when handling sputum.

The sputum may have a foul taste. The nurse should provide the client frequent opportunities to use mouthwashes and to perform tooth brushing and flossing. Because long-term antibiotic administration is usually necessary, the nurse should observe oral mucous membranes for indications of *Candida albicans* overgrowth (i.e., white, cheesy patches) and encourage long-term dental care.

CRITICAL TO REMEMBER

Antibiotic therapy for lung abscess may be necessary for up to 6 weeks. Clients with lung abscesses must understand the importance of compliance with the medication schedule. The entire course of antibiotics must be taken.

Teaching regarding medications includes (1) reasons for taking them; (2) specific directions such as time of day, frequency, and when to take in relation to food; (3) potential side effects; and (4) what to do if side effects occur. Reassessment after antibiotics are completed (e.g., reculture of sputum, chest films) is essential to evaluate the effectiveness of the treatment.

PULMONARY TUBERCULOSIS

Tuberculosis (TB) is a chronic, infectious disease that is characterized by the formation of tubercles, or granulomas, in the lungs.

Incidence

Despite improved methods of detection and treatment, TB remains a worldwide health problem with an estimated 3 million new cases diagnosed each year.[38]

Before the development of anti-TB drugs in the late 1940s, TB was the leading cause of death in the United States. Drug therapy, along with improvements in public health and general living standards, resulted in a marked decline in incidence. However, recent influxes of immigrants from developing third world nations, along with the emergence of the human immunodeficiency virus (HIV) epidemic, led to an increase in reported cases in 1986, reversing a 40-year period of decline.

Etiology

Tuberculosis is a reportable communicable disease caused by *Mycobacterium tuberculosis*. This aerobic organism is an acid-fast bacillus that produces niacin. The tubercle bacillus is airborne, transmitted by aerosolization. Droplet nuclei (1 to 5 μm in size) are emitted during coughing, laughing, sneezing, or singing. Infected droplet nuclei may then be inhaled by a susceptible client (host). Before pulmonary infection can occur, the inhaled organisms must resist the lung's defense mechanisms and actually penetrate lung tissue.

Brief exposure to TB does not usually cause infection. Clients most commonly infected are those who have repeated close contact with an infected individual who is not yet diagnosed. When a client is diagnosed as having TB, public health officials (often nurses) talk with the client and develop a contact list. Everyone with whom the client has had contact is then assessed with a tuberculin skin test and chest radiograph to determine whether they have been infected with TB.

Risk Factors

Although TB may affect anyone, certain segments of the population have an increased risk of contracting the disease. These high-risk groups include

- the elderly, who constitute nearly half of the newly diagnosed cases of TB in the United States
- racial and ethnic groups such as Native Americans, Eskimos, and African Americans, especially the economically disadvantaged or homeless; also, immigrants from Southeast Asia, Ethiopia, Mexico, and Latin America
- clients dependent on alcohol or other chemicals, because of malnutrition, debilitation, and generally poor health; older alcoholics who are of minority races are at even greater risk
- infants and children under the age of 5 years
- clients with reduced immunity, including those with HIV infection, with malnutrition, on cancer chemotherapy, or on steroid therapy

Pathophysiology

PRIMARY (FIRST) INFECTION

The first time a client is infected with TB, it is said to be a "primary infection." Only a small proportion of clients infected with TB (about 5 per cent of North Americans) actually develop active, clinical disease. Primary TB infections are usually located in the apices of the lungs or near the pleurae of the lower lobes. Although a primary infection may be only microscopic in size (and hence never even appear on x-ray film), the following sequence of events typically occurs.

A small area of bronchopneumonia develops in the lung tissue. Many of the infecting tubercle bacilli are phagocytized by wandering macrophages. However, before the development of hypersensitivity and immunity, many of the bacilli may survive within these blood cells and be carried into regional bronchopulmonary (hilar) lymph nodes via the lymphatic system. The bacilli may even spread throughout the body. Thus, the infection, although small, rapidly spreads.

The primary infection site may or may not undergo a process of necrotic degeneration (caseation), which produces cavities filled with a cheeselike mass of tubercle bacilli, dead white blood cells, and necrotic lung tissue. In time, this material liquefies and may drain into the tracheobronchial tree and be coughed up as sputum. The air-filled cavities remain and may be detected radiologically.

Most primary tubercles heal over a period of months through the formation of fibrous scars and, ultimately, calcified lesions. These lesions may contain living bacilli that can reactivate (even after many years) and can cause reinfection or secondary TB (see later discussion).

Primary TB infections cause the body to develop a state of sensitivity (allergic reaction to tubercle bacilli or their proteins). This cell-mediated immune response appears in the form of sensitized T cells and is detectable by a positive reaction to a tuberculin skin test. The development of this tuberculin sensitivity occurs in all body cells 2 to 6 weeks after the primary infection. It is maintained as long as living bacilli remain in the body (perhaps for life). This acquired immunity usually inhibits the further growth of the bacilli and the development of active infection (discussed later).

The term "tuberculin converter" refers to a client who does not show radiologic or bacteriologic evidence of pulmonary TB but whose tuberculin skin test converts from a known negative reaction to a known positive reaction (i.e., from less that 5 mm of induration with a Mantoux skin test to 10 mm or more with the same test).

CRITICAL TO REMEMBER

It is important to know that the absence of a positive (reactive) tuberculin test does not always mean that TB is absent.

Primary TB infections are often not recognized because usually they are relatively asymptomatic. Calcified lesions and a positive skin test are frequently the only reminders that a primary TB infection has occurred. Most clients harbor tubercle bacilli for life and never develop actual disease. Usually, their body defenses are adequate to arrest primary infection, and they heal by fibrosis and calcification. However, a primary TB infection is occasionally not controlled, and progressive primary disease develops. In this situation, the primary complex sites progress and worsen, possibly causing cavitation and the spread of active infection, and the client becomes clinically ill.

The reason active TB disease develops in some clients (instead of being controlled by the acquired immune response) is poorly understood. However, factors that seem to play a role in the progression from TB infection to active disease include

- advancing age
- immunosuppression
- hormonal changes
- malnutrition
- alcoholism
- presence of other disease states (e.g., poorly controlled diabetes mellitus, chronic renal failure, or silicosis)
- gastrectomy

REINFECTION

In addition to progressive primary disease, reinfection (or secondary disease) may also lead to a clinical form of active TB. Primary sites of infection containing TB bacilli may remain latent for years and then reactivate if the client's resistance is lowered. Because reinfection is possible (infection does not provide total immunity) and because dormant lesions may reactivate, it is extremely important for clients who have had a TB infection to be reassessed periodically for evidence of active disease.

Clinical Manifestations

Typical findings with pulmonary TB include fatigue; anorexia; weight loss; persistent, long-term, low-grade fever; chills and sweats (often at night); nonresolving bronchopneumonia; dyspnea; hemoptysis; persistent, progressive, and often productive cough; chest pain that may be pleuritic or dull in nature; and chest tightness.

The detection and diagnosis of TB is achieved by objective tests and subjective assessment findings. The diagnosis can be difficult because TB mimics many other diseases. Also, TB may occur concurrently with other diseases. Often, a diagnosis of TB is not considered or obtained until a client with pulmonary symptoms fails to improve after treatment for other pulmonary disorders such as pneumonia.

History includes assessing the probability of recent or past exposure to TB as well as the client's occupation, other usual activities, and travel or residence in countries with a high incidence of TB. A history of exposure to TB is certainly significant, but most clients are not aware of exposure. Also, during assessment for TB, it is advisable to determine whether the client has been previously tested for TB and to obtain the results of that testing.

DIAGNOSTIC ASSESSMENT

Culture of *M. tuberculosis* from sputum or other body secretions or tissue is the only method of confirming the diagnosis. If TB is disseminated throughout the body or is suspected in another organ system, an acid-fast smear and culture is performed on appropriate tissue or fluid (e.g., urine for suspected TB of kidney).

Tuberculin test results, of which a Mantoux test is most reliable, are also used in diagnosis.

Chest x-ray examination is valuable for detecting old lesions or new ones once they are large enough to be seen. Cavities may be present with far-advanced disease. Inflammation that accompanies a new infection may also be apparent.

Medical Management

Figure 22–3 summarizes detection, diagnosis, and medical intervention related to TB.

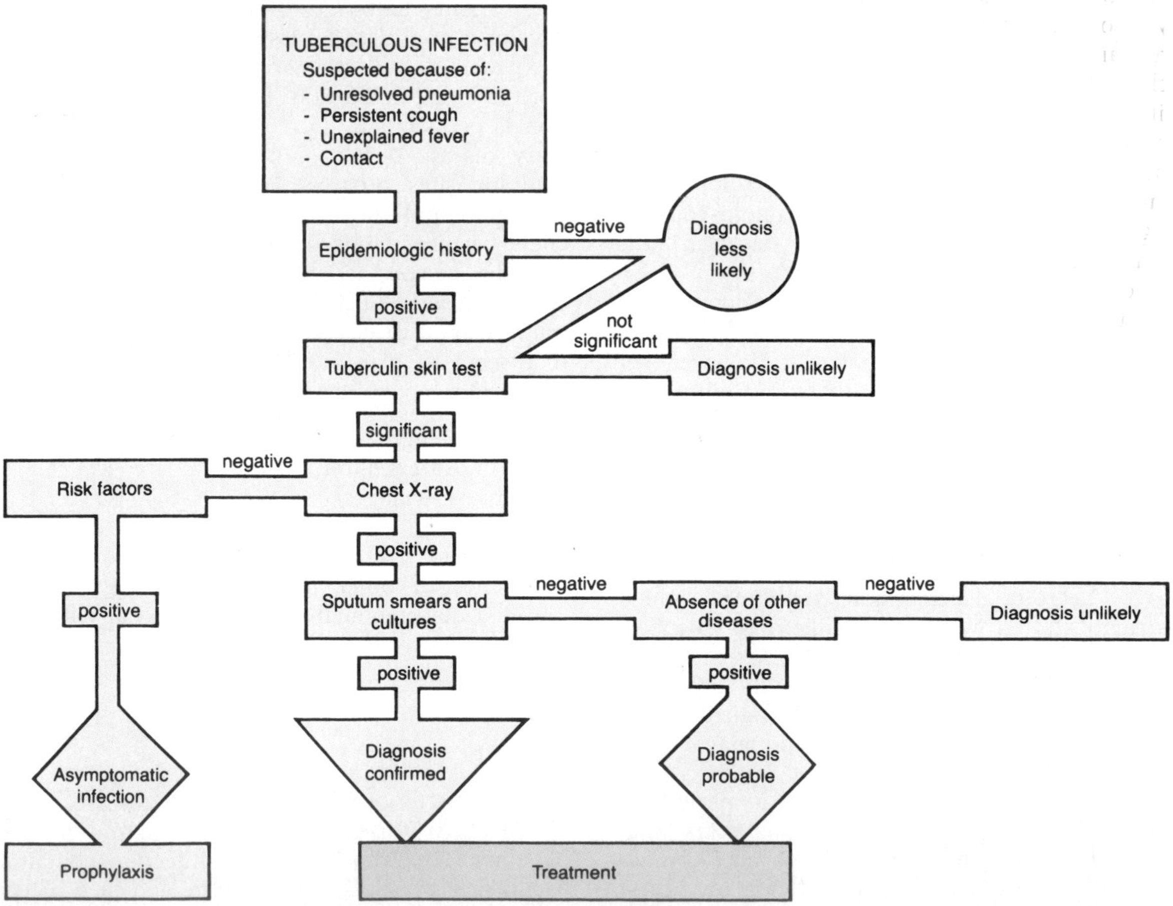

Figure 22–3
Algorithm for diagnosis and management of tuberculosis: a logical progression. (From the American Lung Association, The Christmas Seal People ©.)

Clients with active TB must be identified and properly treated not only for their own welfare but also to prevent the transmission of TB to others. Screening programs can effectively detect the presence of TB infection. However, they are cost-effective only for groups at high risk of developing or having TB. In addition to the groups previously discussed, these may include (1) health care providers at risk of exposure to TB, (2) children entering schools in areas where TB is prevalent, (3) food handlers (not because TB is food-borne, but because immigrants from countries with prevalent TB often work in food-related occupations where they have numerous contacts), and (4) clients living or working in institutions, if there is an increased risk or a high prevalence of TB in the population, environmental factors that facilitate TB transmission, or the potential for infecting young children or immunosuppressed clients.

PHARMACOLOGIC MANAGEMENT

Preventive Measures. Prevention of active TB with isoniazid preventive therapy consists of taking 300 mg of isoniazid daily for 9 to 12 months. Isoniazid preventive therapy stops the growth of the bacilli, thus preventing active pulmonary or extrapulmonary TB. Isoniazid preventive therapy is recommended for clients who (1) are newly infected (have converted tuberculin skin tests but no other indication of active disease), (2) live or closely associate with others who have active TB, (3) have significant tuberculin skin test reactions and abnormal chest films compatible with inactive TB, (4) have positive tuberculin skin tests and conditions (e.g., steroid therapy, diabetes mellitus, AIDS) placing them at increased risk for TB, and (5) are less than 35 years old and have significant tuberculin skin test reactions, even though they may have a normal chest film and no other risk factors (because of the cumulative risk, over time, of reactivation).

Therapeutic Measures. Clients with diagnosed active TB are usually started on three or more medications to be certain the resistant organisms are eliminated. The dose of some drugs may initially be large because the bacilli are difficult to kill. Treatment continues long enough to eliminate or substantially reduce the number of dormant or semidormant bacilli. Long-term, uninterrupted chemotherapy is important.

Medications used for TB may be divided into first- and second-line drugs. Table 22–4 lists and discusses medications in these categories. First-line drugs are almost always initially prescribed until culture and sensitivity laboratory reports are available. Clients with a previous history of incomplete TB chemotherapy may have developed resistant organisms.

The duration of treatment varies. Some programs have a two-phase approach: (1) an intensive phase using two or three drugs, aimed at destroying large numbers of rapidly multiplying organisms, and (2) a maintenance phase, usually with two drugs, directed at eliminating most remaining bacilli. The length of each phase depends on the success of treatment and the client's compliance. Some courses are as short as 6 months; others last 24 months. The average is 9 to 12 months. Some TB protocols call for medication two or three times a week rather than daily. These programs are often used for noncompliant clients, and the drugs are administered in a clinic or physician's office to ensure that they are received.

If the medication regimen does not seem effective (e.g., worsening symptoms, continued acid-fast bacilli in sputum, increasing infiltrates, or cavity formation), the program needs re-evaluation, and the client's compliance should be assessed. At least two medications (never just one) are added to a failing TB chemotherapy program.

Because medications used to treat TB have potentially serious side effects (see Table 22–4), baseline studies (depending on the specific drugs prescribed) are performed. Drug toxicity can limit the treatment of TB. Drug tolerance, drug effect, and drug toxicity depend on factors such as age, medication dosage, time since last dosage, the medication's chemical formula, renal and intestinal function, and compliance with chemotherapy program.

HOSPITALIZATION

If pulmonary TB is diagnosed in the hospitalized client, the client is often kept in the hospital for 1 to 2 weeks until therapeutic drug levels are established. The newly diagnosed client should be cared for in a private room that has fresh, circulating air and is irradiated with ultraviolet light, if possible. Further hospitalization is not usually necessary.

Some clients with active TB may be hospitalized if (1) they are acutely ill, (2) their living situation is considered a high risk, (3) they are suspected of noncompliance, (4) there is a history of previous TB and noncompliance and the disease has reactivated, (5) concomitant diseases are present and acute, (6) improvement does not occur after chemotherapy, or (7) their organisms are highly resistant to usual treatment, requiring second- or third-line drugs. In this last situation, brief hospitalization is necessary to monitor the effects and side effects of the drugs.

Clients whose TB is not improving or who are unable to tolerate medication may require assessment and treatment at medical facilities specializing in the treatment of complicated pulmonary TB and other forms of mycobacterial disease.

Nursing Management

Nursing management of the client with TB may include many of the interventions discussed earlier in this chapter and in Chapter 20, depending on the specific nursing diagnoses identified. Possible nursing diagnoses for the client with TB include Anxiety; Airway Clearance, Ineffective; Gas Exchange, Impaired; Pain; Individual Coping, Ineffective; Family Coping, Ineffective; Altered Health Maintenance; Noncompliance; and Sleep Pattern Disturbance.

TABLE 22–4 Tuberculosis Medication

	DOSAGE*				
	DAILY	TWICE WEEKLY	MOST COMMON SIDE EFFECTS*	TESTS FOR SIDE EFFECTS*	COMMENTS/ INTERVENTION
First-Line Drugs					
Isoniazid	5–10 mg/kg up to 300 mg PO or IM	15 mg/kg PO or IM	Peripheral neuritis, nausea, hepatitis, hypersensitivity	AST/ALT (not as a routine)	Bactericidal; pyridoxine 10 mg/day as prophylaxis for neuritis; 50–100 mg as treatment; take at bedtime if nausea occurs
Ethambutol	15–25 mg/kg up to 2.5 g PO	50 mg/kg PO	Optic neuritis (reversible with discontinuation of drug; very rare at 15 mg/kg), skin rash	Red/green color discrimination and visual acuity†	Use with caution with renal disease or when eye testing is not feasible; check red/green discrimination with each follow-up visit
Rifampin	10–15 mg/kg up to 600 mg PO	600 mg PO	Hepatitis, febrile reaction, purpura (rare)	AST/ALT (not as a routine)	Bactericidal; orange urine color; affects action of other drugs (e.g., inactivates birth control pills)
Streptomycin	15 mg/kg up to 1 g IM	25–30 mg/kg IM	Eighth nerve damage, nephrotoxicity	Vestibular function, audiograms†; blood urea nitrogen and creatinine	Use with caution in older clients or those with renal disease
Pyrazinamide	25 mg/kg up to 2 g PO	50 mg/kg, up to 3.5 g PO	Hyperuricemia, hepatotoxicity	Uric acid, AST/ALT	Rapidly bacteriostatic and slowly bacteriocidal, thus kills bacilli not attacked by other anti-TB drugs
Second-Line Drugs					
Capreomycin, kanamycin	12–15 mg/kg up to 1 g IM		Auditory toxicity, nephrotoxicity, vestibular toxicity (rare)	Vestibular function, audiograms†; blood urea nitrogen and creatinine	Use with caution in older clients; rarely used with renal disease
Ethionamide	15 mg/kg up to 1 g PO		Gastrointestinal disturbance, hepatotoxicity, hypersensitivity	AST/ALT	Divided dose may help reduce gastrointestinal side effects; antinausea drugs may be prescribed
Para-aminosalicylic acid (aminosalicylic acid)	200–300 mg/kg up to 12 g PO		Gastrointestinal disturbance, hypersensitivity, hepatotoxicity, sodium load	AST/ALT	Gastrointestinal side effects very frequent, making compliance difficult
Cycloserine	15 mg/kg up to 1 g PO		Psychosis, personality changes, convulsions, rash	Psychological testing	Very difficult drug to use; side effects may be blocked by pyridoxine, ataractic agents, or anticonvulsant drugs; monitor closely

AST/ALT, aspartate aminotransferase/alanine aminotransferase; IM, intramuscularly; PO, orally.
* Check product labeling for detailed information on dose, contraindications, drug interaction, adverse reactions, and monitoring.
† Initial levels should be determined on start of treatment.
Modified from Pérez-Stable, E. J., & Hopewell, P. C. (1989). Current tuberculosis treatment regimens: choosing the right one for your patient. *Clinics in Chest Medicine, 10*:323–337.

Posthospital Care

Treatment of TB is a long process. Nurses in clinics and public health facilities are often responsible for follow-up assessment and monitoring. Determining medication compliance, understanding the pharmacologic actions of medications, monitoring unwanted side effects, collecting sputum specimens for acid-fast smear and culture, obtaining serial chest films, and observing for reversal or worsening of initial assessment findings are all part of the ongoing follow-up of clients with TB. It is essential that clients experiencing TB, and their significant

CLIENT EDUCATION GUIDE

Pulmonary Tuberculosis

The nurse should teach the client as follows:

- TB is infectious, but it may be cured or arrested if you take your medication as prescribed.
- TB is transmitted by droplet infection and is not carried on articles such as clothing, books, or eating utensils. You do not need to dispose of any possessions.
- Cover your nose and mouth when coughing, laughing, or sneezing.
- Wash your hands very carefully after any contact with body substances, masks, or soiled tissues. Sputum is highly contaminated. Cough into paper tissues and dispose of them properly.
- Wear masks in appropriate situations when advised. Make sure they are tight-fitting, and change them frequently.
- People with TB are usually not restricted in their activities for more than 2 to 4 weeks after medication is begun, and they are not isolated from others, as long as compliance is maintained. TB is no longer treated by isolation in sanatoriums.
- Treatment may be necessary for a long time. Take your medication exactly as prescribed and report all side effects to your doctor. Do not stop the medication for any reason without the doctor's supervision. Keep an adequate supply of medication available at all times to avoid running out. Compliance with treatment is essential.

The nurse should provide information regarding side effects of prescribed medications, as indicated in Table 22–4.

others, receive the information in the Client Education Guide: Pulmonary Tuberculosis.

Suspicion of noncompliance is dealt with in various ways. In the United States, public health departments have regulations that may be enforced regarding noncompliance with TB treatment. In some cities, a noncompliant client can be arrested, taken to court, and even jailed as a public health hazard. Less drastic means usually ensure compliance. Providing complete information, as outlined in the Client Education Guide, and ongoing support helps. The more information clients have, and the more personal control they perceive, the more likely they are to comply with treatment. Each client should be treated as an individual.

FUNGAL PULMONARY DISEASES

Most fungi that are pathogenic to humans limit their activities to the skin. However, the spores of some fungi become airborne and can be inhaled into the respiratory tract, causing pulmonary diseases that, in their chronic forms, produce granulomatous conditions similar to TB. The most common of these are coccidioidomycosis and histoplasmosis. Each has a specific geographic distribution and occurs in people living or traveling in the regions where these fungi are found. Person-to-person transmission is virtually unknown.

Coccidioidomycosis is found in the Western Hemisphere, primarily in California (the San Joaquin Valley), New Mexico, Arizona, western Texas, and northern Mexico. The disease is most likely to develop in those engaging in desert recreational activities or working in construction or other occupations that involve digging (e.g., archaeology). The disease is mild and self-limiting in 60 per cent of those affected. Such clients are either symptomatic or have only mild upper respiratory assessment findings. The remaining 40 per cent develop a syndrome similar to influenza with cough, fever, pleuritic chest pain, myalgias, and arthralgias. Erythema multiforme (a flat, red rash that erupts with dark red papules) occurs in a few people.

The causative organism of histoplasmosis, the fungus *Histoplasma capsulatum,* is endemic to the central and eastern portions of North America, most notably in the Ohio, Missouri, and Mississippi River valleys. It is also found in South and Central America, India, and Cyprus. This fungus lives in moist soil of appropriate chemical composition, in mushroom cellars, on the floors of chicken houses and bat caves, and in bird droppings (especially from starlings and blackbirds). As with coccidioidomycosis, histoplasmosis infections are usually asymptomatic or mild.

The diagnosis of fungal pulmonary diseases is usually based on history and clinical assessment findings. Skin testing is also used for coccidioidomycosis. Chest films may show hilar adenopathy, small areas of infiltrates, or signs of pneumonia. Sometimes, cavities and calcified nodules may form, usually remaining in the lungs as permanent indicators of previous infection.

A few clients may develop disseminated or chronic forms of pulmonary fungal diseases. When disseminated disease occurs, central nervous system, liver, spleen, gastrointestinal tract, or musculoskeletal involvement may be present. Chronic disease may result in progressive cavitary changes similar to those seen with TB. Emphysema-like pulmonary structural changes may also occur.

Management

Mild, primary forms of fungal pulmonary disease usually do not require treatment. Progressive, disseminated, or chronic forms are treated with intravenous amphotericin B. This fungicidal antibiotic is quite toxic, and acute reactions (e.g., seizures, anaphylaxis, headache, or decreased renal function) may occur during infusion. Antiemetics, antihistamines, antipyretics, or hydrocortisone may be prescribed as premedications. In order to reduce the incidence of thrombophlebitis at the intravenous site (a common problem), a small amount of heparin may be added to the infusion. Ketoconazole, a less toxic oral medication, may also be used. However, the long-term effectiveness of this medication has not yet been determined. If the disorder is not responsive to drug therapy, surgical removal of affected areas (e.g., lung cavities) may be necessary.

Nursing management includes providing (1) preventive education to minimize exposure of clients to infectious fungi (i.e., teach to avoid high-risk situations and to recognize early indications of infection) and (2) appropriate support and education for infected clients and their significant others, along with symptomatic management of the disease. Education involves teaching about not only the disease and intervention measures but also reportable indications of complications.

OTHER FUNGAL AND FUNGUS-LIKE INFECTIONS

In addition to the pathogenic fungi, other common fungi spores may cause serious, potentially fatal pulmonary disease in immunocompromised clients (e.g., clients with AIDS, clients receiving cancer chemotherapy). These fungi include *Aspergillus, Blastomyces dermatitidis, Candida,* and *Cryptococcus neoformans.* Treatment of these infections is also with amphotericin B.

Pulmonary infections caused by actinomycetes (gram-positive organisms), once classified as fungi, may also be seen. Nocardiosis is caused by the *Nocardia* species and is treated with sulfadiazine. Surgical drainage may be required. Actinomycosis (caused by *Actinomyces israelii*) develops from dental, facial, or neck infections. Pulmonary disease may result if the organism is aspirated; treatment with penicillin is required.

BOX 22–3

Common Causes of Noncardiogenic Pulmonary Edema

- Aspiration of gastric contents, especially if significant amount of hydrochloric acid is present
- Drug-induced (e.g., after administration of narcotics)
- Fluid overload from intravenous fluids
- Hypoalbuminemia (e.g., nephrotic syndrome, hepatic disease, malnutrition)
- Smoke inhalation (e.g., in people or firefighters trapped in a burning building)
- Inhalation of toxic chemicals (e.g., sulfur dioxide, paraquat, phosgene, chlorine, nitrogen oxides)
- High altitudes (i.e., greater than 8000 ft)
- Neurogenic stimulus (e.g, conditions causing increased intracranial pressure, epileptic seizures, head trauma, profound infection)
- Near-drowning syndrome (i.e., inhalation of large quantities of fresh or sea water)
- Mechanical ventilation, oxygen toxicity, acute (adult) respiratory distress syndrome
- Malignancies blocking outflow of lymph within the lungs
- Unilaterally, after re-expansion of collapsed lung (pneumothorax)

NONCARDIOGENIC PULMONARY EDEMA

Noncardiogenic pulmonary edema is an abnormal accumulation of fluid in the interstitial and alveolar spaces of lung tissue. It results from an imbalance between hydrostatic and colloidal osmotic pressures within the respiratory circulation. It may result from a variety of conditions (Box 22–3) but is not related to left-sided heart failure (see Chap. 24). Sometimes the precipitating event has occurred 12 to 24 hours earlier (e.g., smoke inhalation). At other times, noncardiogenic pulmonary edema develops rapidly, as with neurogenic causes.

Pulmonary manifestations of pulmonary edema are the same, regardless of the cause. In the noncardiogenic form, however, no signs of cardiac involvement (i.e., cardiac enlargement, presence of S_3 heart sound, jugular vein distention, and elevated pulmonary wedge pressures) will be seen.

ACUTE RESPIRATORY FAILURE

Respiratory failure is a broad, nonspecific clinical diagnosis used to indicate that the respiratory system is unable to supply the oxygen necessary to maintain metabolism or cannot eliminate sufficient carbon dioxide. Acute respiratory failure is defined as a PaO_2 of 50 mm Hg or less or a $PaCO_2$ of 50 mm Hg or more. In clients with chronic hypercapnia, $PaCO_2$ elevations of 5 mm Hg or more from their previously stable levels indicate acute respiratory failure superimposed on chronic respiratory failure. Various factors may precipitate respiratory failure. If these factors are not recognized and corrected, other organ systems are affected. Box 22–4 lists some causes of acute respiratory failure.

Classically, a client in acute respiratory failure has an elevated arterial carbon dioxide level. Elevated $PaCO_2$ directly relates to alveolar hypoventilation from either (1) decreased minute ventilation with normal dead space ventilation or (2) normal or increased minute ventilation with increased dead space ventilation. In the first category are clients with normal lungs whose respiratory status is impaired by drugs or diseases affecting respiration (e.g., neuromuscular disorders). In the second category are clients with intrinsic lung diseases such as COPD or severe pneumonias. Lung damage in these clients increases the amount of dead space (wasted ventilation). Thus, even with normal or increased minute ventilation, they cannot blow off a sufficient amount of carbon dioxide.

Diagnosis of respiratory failure is sometimes difficult. Assessment findings indicating hypoxemia and hypercapnia often occur subtly. By the time abnormalities are recognized, an emergency may exist. If respiratory failure is suspected, confirmation with ABG analysis is essential. Diagnosis is made by clinical observation and blood gas analysis.

BOX 22–4

Causes of Acute Respiratory Failure

FACTORS DECREASING VENTILATORY DRIVE

- Depression of respiratory drive with drugs (e.g., barbiturates, sedatives, narcotics, tranquilizers)
- Brain disorders (e.g., stroke, brain tumor, brain trauma)
- Obstructive sleep apnea syndrome
- Obesity

CHEST WALL DYSFUNCTION AND NEUROMUSCULAR FACTORS

- Anesthetic blocking agents
- Cervical spinal cord injury
- Neuromuscular disorders (e.g., muscular dystrophy, Guillain-Barré syndrome, amyotrophic lateral sclerosis, polio, and post-polio effects)
- Neuromuscular blocking agents (e.g., curare)
- Kyphoscoliosis

FACTORS IN LUNG PARENCHYMA

- Near-drowning
- Pneumonia
- Interstitial lung diseases
- Pulmonary edema
- Chronic airflow limitation
- Acute (adult) respiratory distress syndrome
- Inhalation of toxic chemicals, gases, or smoke
- Pulmonary contusion

OTHER FACTORS

- Carbon monoxide inhalation
- Upper airway obstruction (e.g., foreign body, tumor, micrognathia)
- Abdominal distention due to intestinal obstruction
- Ascites

Management

Intervention for acute respiratory failure is directed toward (1) treating the underlying cause of the respiratory failure and (2) restoring gas exchange to maintain physiologic function. Nursing intervention focuses on

- promoting effective airway clearance and effective gas exchange
- preventing complications of immobility
- monitoring and documenting indications of altered tissue perfusion
- monitoring and promoting effective breathing patterns
- reducing anxiety and fear
- promoting comfort

If endotracheal intubation and mechanical ventilation are required, the client must communicate nonverbally. When acute respiratory failure is superimposed on chronic respiratory disease or chronic respiratory failure, nursing intervention is directed to promoting self-care and performing teaching activities to prevent complications and to increase treatment compliance. Discussions earlier in this chapter and in Chapter 20 outline interventions appropriate for clients with acute respiratory failure A sample clinical pathway for clients with acute respiratory failure is presented in Appendix C.

ADULT RESPIRATORY DISTRESS SYNDROME

Adult Respiratory Distress Syndrome (ARDS) is the most common form of noncardiogenic pulmonary edema seen in hospitals today. The syndrome was first described in 1967 and has been referred to by a variety of terms, including shock lung, wet lung, Da Nang lung (in reference to the high number of cases observed during the Vietnam era), post-traumatic lung, congestive atelectasis, capillary leak syndrome, and adult hyaline membrane disease. ARDS can affect children as well as adults, and therefore a name change has been recommended by the American-European Consensus Conference on ARDS. They suggest changing from "adult" to "acute" respiratory distress syndrome.[25]

Incidence

An estimated 150,000 cases of ARDS occur each year in the United States.[20] Despite major advances in intensive pulmonary care, mortality remains high, approximately 30 per cent to 60 per cent. Furthermore, 90 per cent of deaths from ARDS occur within 2 weeks of disease onset.[32] Most clients die from complications of multiple organ dysfunction syndrome.[25]

Etiology and Risk Factors

The syndrome develops as a result of an insult, condition, or noxious event that traumatizes the lung tissue. The insult may be directly to lung tissue or indirect, occurring in other body areas.

Conditions at high risk of leading to ARDS are listed in Box 22–5. A comparison of the causes of noncardiogenic pulmonary edema (Box 22–3) and ARDS (Box 22–5) will demonstrate many similarities between predisposing clinical states.

Pathophysiology

The initial insult is followed by a period of apparently normal lung function that may last from 1 to 96 hours. ARDS may follow one of several possible courses (see Pathophysiology: Acute [Adult] Respiratory Distress Syndrome):

- full healing and recovery
- mild pulmonary fibrosis followed by healing and recovery
- healing initially, followed by severe fibrosis and death
- rapid progression to fibrosis and death.

BOX 22–5

Clinical States that May Lead to Acute (Adult) Respiratory Distress Syndrome

DIRECT PULMONARY TRAUMA

- Viral, bacterial, or fungal pneumonias
- Lung contusion
- Fat embolus
- Aspiration (e.g., foreign material, drowning, vomitus)
- Massive smoke inhalation
- Inhaled toxins
- Prolonged exposure to high concentrations of oxygen

INDIRECT PULMONARY TRAUMA

- Sepsis
- Shock
- Multisystem trauma
- Disseminated intravascular coagulation
- Pancreatitis
- Uremia
- Drug overdose
- Anaphylaxis
- Idiopathic
- Prolonged cardiobypass surgery
- Massive blood transfusions
- Pregnancy-induced hypertension
- Increased intracranial pressure
- Radiation therapy

In addition to lung fibrosis, a number of other complications may arise during supportive management of the client with ARDS. These include cardiac dysrhythmias due to hypoxemia, oxygen toxicity, renal failure, thrombocytopenia, gastrointestinal bleeding secondary to stress ulcers, sepsis from invasive lines, and disseminated intravascular coagulation (see Chap. 28).

Clinical Manifestations

The earliest clinical sign of ARDS is usually an increased respiratory rate. Breathing becomes increasingly labored; the client may exhibit air hunger, retractions, and cyanosis. Chest auscultation may or may not reveal the presence of adventitious sounds. Table 22–5 summarizes the four phases of ARDS relating the pathophysiology to the diagnostic assessment and the clinical manifestations. The chest x-ray usually demonstrates diffuse, bilateral, and rapidly progressing interstitial or alveolar infiltrates.

DIAGNOSTIC ASSESSMENT

Blood gas analysis reveals increasing hypoxemia (PaO_2 $<$70 mm Hg when fractional inspired oxygen [FIO_2] $>$0.4) that does not respond to increased FIO_2 levels and compensatory hypocapnia. In the early stages, respiratory alkalosis is present because of hyperventilation. Later metabolic acidosis develops from increased work of breathing and hypoxemia. The chest film usually demonstrates diffuse, bilateral, and rapidly progressing interstitial or alveolar infiltrates.

Medical Management

The key to the successful management of ARDS is early detection and initiation of treatment. The goals of therapy are respiratory support, treatment of the underlying cause when possible, and prevention of complications.

Endotracheal intubation, mechanical ventilation, and positive end-expiratory pressure are usually required to maintain adequate blood oxygen levels. Sedation may be necessary to reduce anxiety and restlessness during ventilator management. If tachypnea, restlessness, or respirations out of phase with the ventilator ("bucking") cannot be managed by sedation, pharmacologic paralysis (e.g., pancuronium bromide, curare) may be induced (see Chap. 20).

The use of pharmacologic agents in the treatment of ARDS will vary according to the client's underlying disease process. Inotropic agents (e.g., dopamine) may be indicated to improve cardiac output and increase systemic blood pressure. Antibiotics are administered if suspected or confirmed infection is present. Although it remains controversial, the use of large doses of corticosteroids is also common. The rationale for steroid ad-

PATHOPHYSIOLOGY

Acute (Adult) Respiratory Distress Syndrome

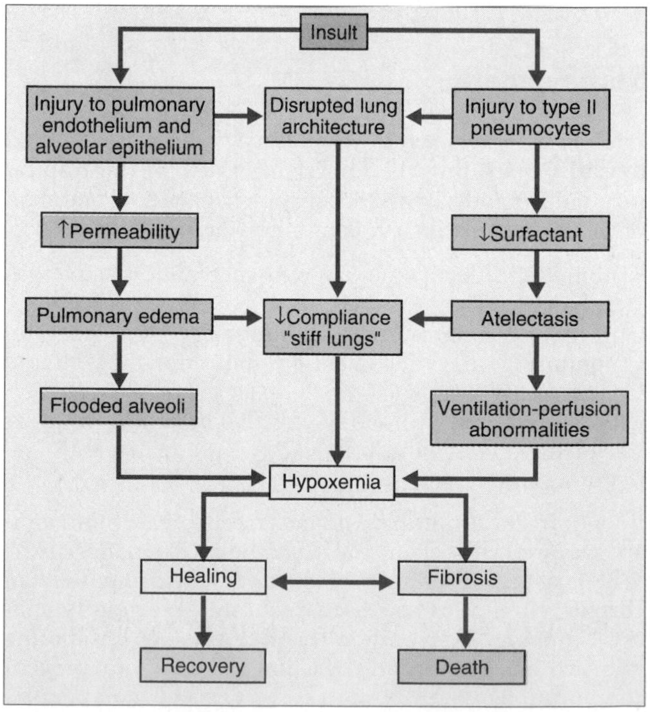

From Bradley, R. B. (1987). Adult respiratory distress syndrome. *Focus on Critical Care, 14,* 48.

TABLE 22–5 Four Phases of Acute (Adult) Respiratory Distress Syndrome

PHASE	PROCESS	OUTCOME	SIGNS AND SYMPTOMS
I	• Direct or indirect injury to the lung. • Systemic release of mediators. • Mediators activate or stimulate other cells to release toxic by-products. • Toxic by-products cause pansystemic microvascular injury. • Fluid leaks into the interstitial space.	Disruption of capillary endothelium • Onset of interstitial edema • ↓ CL • ↑ V/Q mismatch • ↓ PaO_2	• Mild hypoxemia • Tachypnea • Lungs clear on auscultation • Pulmonary capillary wedge pressure < 18 mm Hg
II	• As leakage of fluid continues, the lung becomes increasingly stiff and lung compliance decreases. • As compliance decreases, alveoli are underventilated and hypoxemia increases	Interstitial edema increases and causes: • ↓ ↓ CL • ↑ ↑ V/Q mismatch • ↓ ↓ PaO_2	• Restlessness • Tachypnea • Tachycardia • Dyspnea • Fine crackles
III	• Leakage of fluid into the alveoli. • Flooding of alveoli increases shunt (perfusion without ventilation). The greater the alveolar filling the greater the shunt and the lower the PaO_2. • Fluid in alveoli damages surfactant	Disruption of alveolar membrane • ↑ alveolar edema • ↓ ↓ ↓ CL • ↑ ↑ ↑ V/Q mismatch • ↓ ↓ ↓ PaO_2	• Worsening hypoxemia • Coarse crackles
IV	• Alveoli lack surfactant and collapse. • Shunt increases, causing severe hypoxemia. • Inflammation leads to fibrosis (stiff lungs) with increased gas exchange impairment. • $PaCO_2$ increases.	Alveolar collapse/massive atelectasis • ↓ ↓ total lung volume • ↓ ↓ ↓ functional residual capacity • ↓ ↓ ↓ ↓ CL • ↓ ↓ ↓ ↓ PaO_2	• Severe hypoxemia despite ↑ FIO_2 • ↑ $PaCO_2$ • Pulmonary hypertension

CL, lung compliance; V/Q ventilation/perfusion.
From Jones, M. A., Hoffman, L. A., & Delgado, F. (1994). ARDS revisited. *Nursing 94, 24*(12), 34–45, with permission from Springhouse Corp.

ministration is to reduce inflammatory response and promote pulmonary membrane stability. However, controlled clinical trials of corticosteroid use have failed to demonstrate their effectiveness in ARDS.[33]

Nursing Management

The principles of nursing management of clients with pneumonia, pulmonary edema, and other pulmonary disorders that affect gas exchange are also appropriate in the care of the client with ARDS. In addition, nursing interventions associated with CMV will also be used. Evaluation of the client's response to treatment, as well as careful monitoring for potential complications, is essential.

Emotional support for the client's family or significant others is also important. The disease can progress very rapidly, leaving family members unprepared for the severity of the client's condition. Clear communications and frequent condition updates are essential for keeping the family adequately informed.

RESTRICTIVE LUNG DISORDERS

Restrictive lung disorders are a major category of pulmonary problems. The category includes any disorder that limits lung expansion and produces a pattern of abnormal function on pulmonary function tests characterized by a decrease in lung volume (TLC).

There are many causes of restrictive lung diseases. They may result from conditions affecting interstitial lung tissues (there are over 100 identified interstitial lung diseases) or from extrapulmonary causes. Extrapulmonary causes include neurologic and neuromuscular disorders and disorders affecting the thoracic cage, pleura, and diaphragm movement. Obesity may also lead to restrictive lung disorders. Peripheral (obstructive) sleep disorders may also be categorized as restrictive lung diseases. Box 22–6 is a representative list of restrictive lung disorders.

Clinical manifestations vary according to the cause of the restrictive disorder. For example, kyphosis, scoliosis, and kyphoscoliosis result in changes in the thoracic cage. Generally, clients with restrictive lung disease exhibit a rapid, shallow respiratory pattern. Chronic hyperventilation occurs in an effort to overcome the effects of reduced lung volume and compliance. Shortness of breath is experienced, at first only with exertion but later at rest also. ABGs reveal alveolar hyperventilation (i.e., reduced $PaCO_2$) during the initial and intermediate phases of the disease process. As the disease progresses, respiratory muscle fatigue may occur, leading to inadequate alveolar ventilation and carbon dioxide retention. Hypoxemia is a common finding, especially in the later stages of restrictive lung disease.

Pulmonary function tests demonstrate impairment

BOX 22-6

Restrictive Lung Diseases

INTRAPULMONARY

- Pulmonary fibrosis
- Sarcoidosis and other interstitial lung diseases
- Pneumonia
- Atelectasis
- Pneumoconioses
- Surgical lung resection
- Neoplastic disease

EXTRAPULMONARY

- Head or spinal cord injury
- Amyotrophic lateral sclerosis
- Myasthenia gravis
- Muscular dystrophy
- Congenital chest wall deformity
- Acquired chest wall changes (e.g., kyphosis or scoliosis)
- Abdominal distention restricting the diaphragm and respiration
- Sleep disorders
- Poliomyelitis
- Pleural effusion
- Pleurisy
- Excessive obesity

These are representative of the many disorders affecting lung volumes and compliance of either chest wall or lung tissue (i.e., restrictive lung diseases).

of the lungs' bellows action. Commonly, the FEV_1/FVC ratio will be normal or increased (i.e., 75 per cent or more of expected values). The FEV_1/FVC ratio by itself is not an absolute indicator of restrictive lung disorders. The TLC is the primary indicator of the disease. TLC is less than 80 per cent of expected values in these clients. Some clients have a mixture of restrictive and obstructive lung disorders.

Often, a specific diagnosis of restrictive lung disease is made only after extensive testing, including biopsy, immunologic testing (e.g., blood studies to determine increased globins and autoantibodies), and tests to differentiate neurologic dysfunction such as electromyography or spinal fluid analysis.

Interstitial lung diseases cause characteristic chest x-ray findings. Chest films may also show extrapulmonary disorders (e.g., large abdominal tumor restricting diaphragm movement).

Management

The management of the client is based on the degree of impairment and the ability to reverse the condition. Clients with spinal deformities may be helped with spinal surgery. Likewise, obese clients will breathe better after weight loss. Clients with restrictive lung disorders due to interstitial disease are discussed later. Selected clients may benefit from the use of transtracheal oxygen administration or nocturnal mechanical ventilation with a mask or both, especially those clients with postpoliomyelitis syndrome.

The primary goals for nursing management of the client with restrictive lung disease are (1) promotion of adequate oxygenation, (2) maintenance of a patent airway, and (3) achievement of the highest possible functional level. Interventions to attain these goals are similar to those used in the treatment of COPD (see earlier). ABG analysis is important for monitoring oxygen needs and assessing the effects of physical activity. $PaCO_2$ levels should be monitored because rising carbon dioxide levels are an indicator of impending respiratory failure.

Most restrictive lung disorders are not reversible. End-stage disease is characterized by the development of pulmonary hypertension, cor pulmonale, severe oxygenation problems, and eventual ventilatory failure. Efforts should be made to maintain the client's functional status and quality of life at as high a level as possible.

LUNG TRANSPLANTATION

Some clients with end-stage disease may be candidates for single-lung transplantation. This procedure involves replacement of one of the diseased lungs with a lung from a cadaver donor. Although the procedure is still relatively uncommon, the success of lung transplantation is increasing with advanced surgical techniques and antirejection medications (immunosuppressives).

Following surgery, the client is observed for excessive bleeding. The nurse monitors vital signs, hemodynamic pressures, electrocardiogram, and chest tube drainage. Pulmonary edema may develop in the denervated transplanted lung. Therefore, the client is placed on continuous mechanical ventilation with positive end-expiratory pressure for 24 to 48 hours. Fluids are restricted, lung sounds are auscultated, and the degree of peripheral edema is monitored. Following extubation, the client is assisted to cough and deep breathe and use incentive spirometry to expand the lung.

The client is at high risk of infection and transplant rejection. Protective isolation is used to decrease inadvertent exposure to pathogens. The client is also monitored for clinical manifestations of infection such as changes in vital signs, local infections at intravenous access sites and incision lines, and changes in respiratory status (excessive secretions, tachypnea, dyspnea, fatigue). Rejection of the lung may present as dyspnea, changes in chest x-ray (the development of white-out on the film), a need for ventilatory support, and fatigue.

Following the intial surgery, the client may develop alterations in self-concept related to changes in appearance from the side effects of medications such as steroids and immunosuppressants, a change in lifestyle, or a change in work ability and role performance. The nurse is sensitive to these issues and encourages the client and significant others to discuss their feelings and explore options.

Prior to discharge, the client is taught about the medication regimen and the nurse stresses the need for daily medication despite a lack of symptoms. The client should report fever, dyspnea, excessive weight gain, and fatigue to the physician. In addition, the client begins a physical rehabilitation program.

During follow-up visits the client is monitored for signs of rejection and compliance with immunosuppressive therapy.

Lung transplantation offers some hope for extended life to clients with previously fatal conditions. However, it is a very frightening and stressful surgery. Clients undergoing lung transplants are always critically ill before coming to surgery. In addition, they must undergo a radical, major surgery; endure prolonged intensive care and isolation procedures; tolerate a certain degree of public, and sometimes media, attention; and adapt to an altered self-concept. The client and significant others need constant and ongoing emotional support for achievement of a successful outcome.

INTERSTITIAL LUNG DISEASE

Interstitial lung diseases (ILDs) are a group of diffuse, inflammatory lower respiratory tract disorders. The term interstitial is used to describe the fact that the interstitium of the alveolar walls is thickened and usually fibrotic. The alveolar walls thicken as a result of the accumulation of inflammatory cells. The thick alveolus becomes nonfunctional.

The etiology of ILD is not clearly defined. It most commonly develops from idiopathic pulmonary fibrosis, sarcoidosis, and collagen vascular disorders. ILD can also result from the inhalation of inorganic dust, such as crystalline silica, asbestos and coal dust, and organic dust from organisms encountered in farming, air conditioner use, and animal husbandry.

Clinical manifestations are insidious and nonspecific, such as dyspnea and nonproductive cough. Because the symptoms are nonspecific, ILD may go undiagnosed for years.

The diagnosis of ILD can be complex, because many other disorders can produce similar clinical manifestations. The client history plays a major part in diagnosis, because it is important to determine to what agents the client has been exposed. Clients report progressive dyspnea and often have dyspnea at rest. Chest expansion is normally reduced, reflecting a decreased TLC. Inspiratory and expiratory crackles are frequently heard. The crackles have a characteristic sound, like the sound of Velcro being pulled apart. Clubbing of the finger tips may be evident. Diagnostic assessment may include gallium ventilation perfusion scans. Bronchoscopy and biopsy may also be used to confirm ILD.

Management

The management of a client with ILD is based on the degree of impairment. The inflammation is controlled with corticosteroids. The client is taught that corticosteroids reduce further impairment, but previously damaged alveolar-capillary units are lost forever. Many clients have subjective improvement on steroids and can eventually be tapered off of the drugs. If the offending agent is known, the initial treatment is to remove the client from exposure to the agent. As the disorder progresses, clients are usually treated with bronchodilators to help mobilize secretions and oxygen during periods of exercise.

Nursing management is the same as for clients with restrictive lung disorders.

SARCOIDOSIS

Sarcoidosis is an inflammatory condition that affects many body systems. The disease is characterized by the formation of widespread granulomatous lesions. In addition to lung involvement, which occurs in over 90 per cent of cases, clients may present with clinical manifestations involving the peripheral lymphatic system, skin, liver, eyes, spleen, bones, salivary glands, joints, and heart. The onset of sarcoidosis is generally between the ages of 20 and 40 years. The incidence in the United States ranges from 11 to 40 per 100,000 people. The disorder is approximately 14 times more common in blacks than in whites, and although the male to female ratio is about even in the nonblack population, black females develop sarcoidosis twice as frequently as do black males.[23]

The exact cause of sarcoidosis remains unknown. However, the disease itself is becoming more fully understood. There is now evidence that a triggering agent, which may be genetic, infectious, immunologic, or toxic, stimulates enhanced cell-mediated immune processes at the site of involvement.[23] A series of interactions between T lymphocytes and monocytes/macrophages leads to the formation of noncaseating granulomas (i.e., those that do not undergo necrotic degeneration), which are characteristic of the disease. Granuloma formation may regress with therapy or as a result of the disorder's natural course but may also progress to fibrosis and restrictive lung disease.

About a third of the clients with sarcoidosis are asymptomatic; diagnosis is made by chest x-ray study findings of hilar adenopathy and pulmonary fibrosis. Clients with pulmonary manifestations usually present with a dry cough and shortness of breath. Chest pain, hemoptysis, or pneumothorax may also be present. Systemic symptoms may include fatigue, weakness, malaise, weight loss, and fever. A definitive diagnosis of sarcoidosis is made by tissue biopsy. When lung involvement is suspected, bronchoscopy, bronchoalveolar lavage, mediastinoscopy, or open lung biopsy may be performed.

Medical management is primarily determined by the degree to which the client's life is disturbed by the symptoms experienced. If the client with sarcoidosis is asymptomatic, management involves ongoing assessment for further disease progression. Repeat chest films at 6-month intervals are often indicated. When symptoms are present, medical treatment usually consists of systemic corticosteroids. When corticosteroids are administered, dramatic improvement may occur.

Nursing intervention for clients with sarcoidosis is the same as that for other restrictive lung diseases and hypoxemia. The nurse should assess for drug side effects, especially adverse responses to corticosteroids. The nurse should also assess for signs of improvement, such as (1) increased exercise tolerance, (2) disappearance of initial assessment findings, (3) improved pulmonary function studies, (4) side effects of steroids (weight gain, change in mood, development of diabetes mellitus), and (5) improved oxygenation. If assessment findings worsen, the nurse should document them and notify the physician.

OCCUPATIONAL LUNG DISEASES

Lung diseases are among the most common occupational health problems. They are caused by the inhalation of various chemicals, dusts, and other particulate matter that are present in certain work settings. Not all clients exposed to occupational inhalants will develop lung disease. Harmful effects depend on the (1) nature of the exposure; (2) duration and intensity of the exposure; (3) particle size and water-solubility of the inhalant (the larger the particle, the lower the probability of its reaching the lower respiratory tract; highly water-soluble inhalants tend to dissolve and react in the upper respiratory tract, whereas poorly soluble substances may travel as far as the alveoli); (4) smoking history; and (5) presence of underlying pulmonary disease.

The most commonly encountered occupational lung diseases are described in Table 22–6. Acute respiratory irritation results from the inhalation of chemicals such as ammonia, chlorine, and nitrogen oxides in the form of gases, aerosols, or particulate matter.

Occupational asthma is defined as variable airflow obstruction caused by a specific agent in the workplace. By far the greatest number of occupational agents causing asthma are those with known or suspected allergic properties, such as plant and animal proteins (e.g., wheat flour, cotton, flax, and grain mites).

Hypersensitivity pneumonitis, or allergic alveolitis, is most commonly due to the inhalation of organic

TABLE 22–6 Characteristics of Occupational Lung Diseases

	ONSET OF SYMPTOMS	DIAGNOSIS	TREATMENT	CLINICAL COURSE
Acute respiratory irritation	Usually within minutes of exposure to irritant, but pulmonary edema may be delayed several hours	Consistent history; physical findings of respiratory tract irritation and damage	Prevention of exposure; respiratory support as needed	Upper respiratory tract signs resolve in hours to days; pulmonary edema resolves in days to weeks; residual damage rare
Occupational asthma	Usually within minutes of exposure to precipitant but possibly delayed 4 to 6 hours or more	Pulmonary function tests showing obstructive pattern during exacerbations; chest film usually normal; skin tests, IgE measurement, and history of atopy helpful only if the disorder is IgE-mediated	Prevention of exposure; asthma medications	Usually resolves within hours; airways may remain persistently hyperreactive
Hypersensitivity pneumonitis	Usually 4 to 8 hours after exposure to antigen; possible subacute or chronic presentation	Specific IgG antibodies; radiographic findings ranging from normal to pulmonary edema to interstitial fibrosis; pulmonary function tests giving restrictive or restrictive/obstructive pattern	Prevention of exposure; respiratory support as needed; steroids helpful in some cases	Symptoms usually resolve in several days; radiographic and pulmonary function findings normalize in a few weeks; however, there may be permanent lung damage
Pneumoconioses	Requires long-term exposure; first symptom often cough progressing to dyspnea	Restrictive pattern on pulmonary function tests; on chest film, asbestosis is associated with interstitial markings in lower lobes and silicosis with opacities in upper lobes	Prevention of exposure; cessation of smoking	Gradual worsening

From Mardel, J. H., & Baker B. A. (1989). Recognizing occupational lung disease. *Hospital Practice,* 24:21.

antigens of fungal, bacterial, or animal origin. The nature of the exposure and the client's immunologic reactivity will determine the pulmonary response. Nonatopic people (i.e., those with no history of allergies) develop a pulmonary response to organic dusts more often than do atopic individuals, although they too may exhibit pulmonary reactions.

Pneumoconioses, or the "dust diseases," result from inhalation of minerals, notably silica, coal dust, or asbestos. These diseases are most commonly seen in miners, construction workers, sandblasters, potters, and foundry and quarry workers. Early symptoms may include cough and dyspnea on exertion. Chest pain, productive cough, and dyspnea at rest develop as the condition progresses.

Early detection is one way to prevent progression of the disease process. When the nurse takes a respiratory history, it should include a complete occupational history and questions about (1) the actual job performed rather than title or job description, (2) past as well as current occupations, and (3) exposure to organic and inorganic substances in each job. Assess dyspnea, cough, chest tightness, or other symptoms indicating potential lung disease. Some employers support ongoing assessment programs (e.g., routine pulmonary function studies or chest films) for workers at risk for occupational disorders.

Exposure precautions are essential for avoiding permanent pulmonary disability. Safety measures include adequate ventilation, wearing masks, and using care when handling garments worn in dusty environments.

Nursing intervention for clients experiencing occupational lung diseases is similar to that for clients with other restrictive lung disorders (see the discussion under Restrictive Lung Disorders). Supportive measures can help these clients to adjust their lifestyles to their condition.

If occupational lung disease is significant, the client may qualify for disability allowances. Nurses can refer clients to community resources, such as federal or state departments of labor, if they have questions concerning eligibility. Because of legal problems that may surround compensation claims, the nurse may have to deal with much hostility and resentment on the part of the client aimed toward the employer and the legal system. These clients may also experience much anxiety and uncertainty about their future health status. A calm, positive approach is often needed.

MALIGNANT LUNG TUMORS

Lung cancer is malignancy in the epithelium of the respiratory tract. At least a dozen different cell types of tumors are included under the classification of lung cancer. Clinically, lung cancers are grouped into two divisions—small cell lung cancer, and non–small cell lung cancer. The term lung cancer excludes other disorders such as sarcomas, lymphomas, blastomas, and mesotheliomas.

Incidence

The incidence of lung cancer is rising at a faster rate than that of any other cancer type. In 1986, lung cancer exceeded breast cancer as the leading cause of death from cancer in American women. It continues to be the number one cause of cancer deaths in men, as it has been for the past 30 years. Mortality rates are similar for white and nonwhite women but greater in nonwhite versus white men. The incidence of specific types of cancer is discussed later.

Etiology

The most common cause of lung cancer is cigarette smoking. Cigarette smoke contains several organ-specific carcinogens. Genetic predisposition to the development of lung cancer also plays a role in the etiology. Other carcinogens include inhaled toxins, such as asbestos, and pollutants.

Risk Factors

Cigarette smoking is the leading risk factor for the development of lung cancer; as many as 80 to 90 per cent of lung malignancies occur in clients who smoke. Heavy smokers (i.e., those who smoke more than 25 cigarettes a day) have 20 times the risk of developing lung cancer than do nonsmokers. Whereas smoking cessation lowers the risk, the decrease is gradual and the risk does not approach that of a nonsmoker until 15 to 20 years later. Recent studies have also suggested that passive smoke (i.e., smoke inhaled from the environment surrounding an active smoker) may be responsible for up to 5 per cent of all lung cancers.[41]

The risk of lung cancer is increased even further in the smoker who is also exposed to other carcinogenic agents, such as radioactive isotopes, polycyclic hydrocarbons, vinyl chloride, metallurgical ores, and mustard gas. Whether these occupational factors increase the risk of cancer development in the nonsmoker is still unclear. The inhalation of asbestos fibers, however, is associated with higher cancer risks for both smokers and nonsmokers.

Air pollution has also been implicated in increasing the risk of lung cancer, although its exact role is not known. The rate of lung cancer in clients who live in urban areas is 2.3 times greater than in those living in rural areas.

Pathophysiology

Lung cancers are divided into two major categories: small cell lung cancers (SCLC) and non–small cell lung cancers (NSCLC), which include epidermoid or squamous cell, adenocarcinoma, and large cell. The characteristics of each of these types are described in Table 22–7. In general, survival rates are best for NSCLC, especially with treatment in its early stages. Despite

TABLE 22–7 Overview of Malignant Pulmonary Neoplasms

CELL TYPE	APPROXIMATE INCIDENCE	SPECIFIC CHARACTERISTICS	GROWTH RATE
Epidermoid (squamous cell)	30–35% of lung cancer	Arises from bronchial epithelium; as growth occurs, cavitation may develop in lung distal to tumor. Pancoast's tumors arise in apex and upper lung zones Abundant keratin formation noted microscopically Secondary infections distal to obstructive tumor in bronchioles frequently occur	Slow growth, metastasis not common If tumor metastasizes, usually to lymph, adrenals, and liver (in that order)
Adenocarcinoma	25–30% of lung cancer	May arise proximally but more often peripherally (60–70%); arises from bronchial mucus gland Often subpleural; often difficult to distinguish from other tumors in the body; rarely cavitates; often arises in previously scarred lung tissue Incidence strongly linked to cigarette smoking Increasing incidence in women Bronchiolo-alveolar cell carcinomas are a subtype	Slow growth May metastasize throughout lung or to other organs of the body
Large cell	10–20% of lung cancer	More often peripheral mass, either single or multiple masses Cavitation common May be located centrally, midlung, or peripherally Rare hilar involvement Often grows to large tumor mass before diagnosis	Slow; metastasis may occur to kidney, liver, and adrenals, in that order
Small cell (oat cell)	20–25% of lung cancer	65–75% present with hilar or central mass May narrow bronchi through compression Involvement of diaphragm through paralysis of phrenic nerve and hoarseness through paralysis of recurrent laryngeal nerve Pleural, pericardial effusions and tamponade Does not form cavities	Rapid growth Metastasis to mediastinum, thoracic and extrathoracic structures occurs early

increasing knowledge and technology, however, overall survival from lung cancer remains low, especially for clients with small cell carcinomas.

Metastatic spread of pulmonary tumors is usually to the long bones, vertebral column (especially the thoracic vertebrae), liver, and adrenal glands. Brain metastasis is also common, occurring in as many as 50 per cent of cases.

Paraneoplastic syndromes (i.e., remote effects of a malignancy) occur in 10 to 20 per cent of lung cancer clients. These usually result from the secretion of substances (e.g., hormones) by the tumor itself. These substances then act on target organs, producing a variety of symptoms, such as hypercalcemia, mental changes, gynecomastia, and Cushing's syndrome. Occasionally, symptoms of paraneoplastic syndrome may occur before detection of the primary lung tumor.

Clinical Manifestations

The warning signals of lung cancer are presented in Box 22–7. In many instances, lung cancer may mimic other pulmonary conditions. Lung cancer may also be manifested by extrapulmonary symptoms that occur before pulmonary symptoms appear. Specific clinical assessment findings vary according to tumor type, location, and extent as well as pre-existing pulmonary health.

Centrally located pulmonary tumors usually obstruct airflow, producing symptoms such as coughing, wheezing, stridor, and dyspnea. As obstruction in-

BOX 22–7

Warning Signals of Lung Cancer

- Any change in respiratory patterns
- Persistent cough
- Sputum streaked with blood
- Frank hemoptysis
- Rust-colored or purulent sputum
- Chest, shoulder, or arm pain
- Recurring episodes of pleural effusion, pneumonia, or bronchitis
- Dyspnea, unexplained or out of proportion

creases, bronchopulmonary infection often occurs distal to the obstruction. Chest, shoulder, and back pain may develop as the tumor invades the perivascular nerves. Squamous and small cell tumors often cause hemoptysis. Small cell tumors may also extend into the pericardium, causing pericardial effusion and, possibly, tamponade. Cardiac rhythm disturbances are also likely. Centrally located pulmonary tumors are easiest to locate and identify with fiberoptic bronchoscopy and sputum cytologic study. Positive tissue diagnosis is possible 90 per cent of the time.

Peripheral pulmonary tumors often do not produce assessment findings initially. In time, pleural pain develops that increases on inspiration, is sharp and severe, and is usually localized. Pleural effusion also develops and, along with the pain, limits lung expansion. Only 30 per cent of peripheral lung tumors are successfully categorized by bronchoscopic and cytologic examination.

Pancoast's tumors occur in the apices of the lungs in both squamous cell and adenocarcinomatous cancers. Assessment findings do not occur until the tumor growth extends into surrounding structures. Pancoast's tumors often involve the first thoracic and eighth cervical nerves within the brachial plexus. This causes arm and shoulder pain on the affected side and atrophy of the arm and hand muscles on that side. With continuing tumor growth, the ribs over the tumor (usually the first and second ribs) may be invaded. Bone pain and later involvement of the sympathetic nerve ganglia lead to Horner's syndrome. This syndrome consists of miosis (pupil contraction), partial eyelid ptosis, and anhidrosis (absence of sweating) on the affected side of the face.

The primary assessment finding with pleural tumors (malignant mesotheliomas) is chest pain. Dyspnea, cough, weight loss, and fever may also be present. Thoracotomy is usually required for a definitive diagnosis.

Metastasis. Tumor spread, by either direct extension or metastasis, may produce further clinical symptoms. Direct extension to the recurrent laryngeal nerve produces hoarseness. Compression of the esophagus may produce dysphagia. Invasion or compression of the superior vena cava produces superior vena cava syndrome, a potentially life-threatening emergency. Obstruction of venous blood flow leads to clinical manifestations that may include shortness of breath; facial, arm, and trunk swelling; distention of the thoracic veins; chest pain; and venous stasis. Immediate, palliative surgical treatment may be necessary.

Regional lymph node involvement may produce symptoms that result from impaired lymph drainage. Involvement of the mediastinal lymph nodes may result in vocal cord paralysis, dysphagia, diaphragm paralysis on the affected side (due to phrenic nerve compression), vena cava compression, and malignant pleural effusion. When mediastinal lymph nodes are involved, surgical excision of the pulmonary tumor is usually no longer possible.

DIAGNOSTIC ASSESSMENT

Numerous diagnostic tests may be used to determine the presence and extent of the disease. Sputum cytology and chest radiography are most commonly used. Tomograms and computed tomographic scans may be used when visualization on standard chest radiographs is unclear or suggests a pulmonary lesion. Bronchoscopy may be performed with centrally located lesions; bronchial washing and brushing is done to obtain tumor cells for cytologic and pathologic assessment. In addition, percutaneous needle biopsy, mediastinoscopy, or direct surgical biopsy may be required to confirm the diagnosis. Radionuclide scans may be used to detect metastasis to the bone, liver, or brain (see Chap. 6).

Staging is performed to provide a guideline for the selection of appropriate therapies and the estimation of prognosis. Staging information is valuable for helping clients and their families to make treatment decisions and to set appropriate short- and long-term goals.

The TNM classification scheme is used for lung cancer staging (Box 22–8). The definitions and stage groupings were recently revised to provide more descriptive information for classifying limited versus extensive disease for SCLC as well as for NSCLC. This revised system appears to provide a better basis for predicting 5-year survival rates than did previously used systems.[32]

Medical Management

The key to increasing the survival rate of clients with lung cancer is early detection. When premalignant changes begin, dysplastic cells are identifiable with fiberoptic bronchoscopy and sputum cytologic studies. At this stage, lesions are potentially curable. However, a tumor must be at least 1 cm in diameter before it is detectable on chest film. Unfortunately, invasion and metastasis have usually already occurred.

Management of the client with lung cancer depends on tumor type and stage as well as the client's underlying health status. Primary treatment modalities include radiation therapy, chemotherapy, and surgery.

RADIATION THERAPY

Radiotherapy may be used as a potentially curative treatment in clients with locally advanced disease who are poor surgical risks, who have technically inoperable tumors, or who refuse thoracotomy. Radiation therapy may also be used in combination with surgery or chemotherapy to improve treatment outcomes. Radiotherapy is administered over a period of 5 to 6 weeks, either consecutively or in split courses. Doses are limited by other structures in the treatment area and by normal tissue tolerance. Irreversible fibrotic changes and other pulmonary side effects may occur. To delineate the area to be irradiated precisely, computed tomographic scanning is often performed before treatment begins. This method also minimizes tissue damage to surrounding areas.

Radiotherapy may also be used for palliation of symptoms such as hemoptysis and obstruction or compression of bronchi, blood vessels, or esophagus. Irradiation of metastases to the brain and bone may reduce

BOX 22–8

Classification of Pulmonary Malignancies

PRIMARY TUMOR (T)

- T_x Tumor proven by presence of malignant cells in bronchopulmonary secretions but not visualized roentgenographically or bronchoscopically, or any tumor that cannot be assessed, as in a retreatment staging
- T_0 No evidence of primary tumor
- T_{is} Carcinoma in situ
- T_1 A tumor that is 3 cm or less in greatest dimension, surrounded by lung or visceral pleura and without evidence of invasion proximal to a lobar bronchus at bronchoscopy
- T_2 Tumor more than 3 cm in greatest dimension or a tumor of any size that either invades the visceral pleura or has associated atelectasis or obstructive pneumonitis extending to the hilar region; at bronchoscopy, the proximal extent of demonstrable tumor must be within a lobar bronchus or at least 2 cm distal to the carina; any associated atelectasis or obstructive pneumonitis must involve less than an entire lung
- T_3 A tumor of any size with direct extension into the chest wall (including superior sulcus tumors), the diaphragm, or the mediastinal pleura or pericardium without involving the heart, great vessels, trachea, esophagus, or vertebral body; or a tumor in the main bronchus within 2 cm of the carina without involving the carina
- T_4 A tumor of any size with invasion of the mediastinum or involving the heart, great vessels, trachea, esophagus, vertebral body, or carina in the presence of malignant pleural effusion

NODES (N)

- N_0 No demonstrable metastases to regional lymph nodes
- N_1 Metastasis to lymph nodes in the peribronchial or the ipsilateral hilar region or both, including direct extension
- N_2 Metastases to ipsilateral mediastinal lymph nodes and subcarinal lymph nodes
- N_3 Metastasis to contralateral mediastinal, contralateral hilar, ipsilateral or contralateral scalene, or supraclavicular lymph nodes

DISTANT METASTASIS (M)

- M_0 No (known) distant metastasis
- M_1 Distant metastasis present, specify site(s)

From Mountain, C. F. (1986). A new international staging system for lung cancer. *Chest 89,* 225S–233S.

the distressing symptoms associated with these sequelae as well.

CHEMOTHERAPY

The response of lung cancer to chemotherapy depends on the tumor's cell type. SCLC responds well to chemotherapeutic agents because of its rapid growth rate. However, this rapid growth pattern also causes metastasis to occur readily. As a result, long-term survival rate for SCLC is still low.

Chemotherapy's effectiveness in the treatment of NSCLC remains controversial. It is commonly used in clients treated with surgery or radiation who experience recurrent disease or distant metastasis. However, large-scale studies have failed to demonstrate a significantly improved overall survival rate for these clients.[11] As a result, the decision to use chemotherapy is usually made on an individual basis, depending on the client's previous history, current condition, and acceptance of the risks and side effects involved.

Surgical Management

Surgical intervention is the treatment of choice in early stage NSCLC. Cure is possible if the disease is still localized to the thoracic cavity and no distant metastases are present. However, only 20 to 25 per cent of clients with NSCLC meet these criteria at time of diagnosis. Surgical survival rates (over a 5-year period) drop from 50 per cent survival for stage I to 15 per cent survival for stage III cancers.

The role of surgical resection in the treatment of SCLC remains under investigation. Surgery may be effective for clients in the early stages of SCLC, after chemotherapy. For clients with more advanced disease, surgery causes unnecessary risk and stress, with no valid benefits.

The primary aim of surgical resection is to remove the tumor completely while as little of the surrounding lung tissue as possible is removed. The extent of the surgery will depend on the location and size of the pulmonary tumor and the degree of the underlying pulmonary pathologic process. Clients with pre-existing pulmonary disease may not be able to tolerate extensive lung tissue removal.

Pulmonary Resection. Common pulmonary resection procedures are shown in Figure 22–4.

Wedge Resection. This procedure involves the removal of a small, localized area of diseased tissue near the surface of the lung. Because the resected area is small, pulmonary structure and function are relatively unchanged after healing.

Segmental Resection. This procedure involves the removal of one or more lung segments (a bronchiole and its alveoli). The remaining lung tissue overexpands to fill the space previously occupied by the removed segment.

Lobectomy. Lobectomy refers to removal of an entire lobe of the lung. After lobectomy, some compensatory nonpathologic emphysema occurs as the remaining lung tissue overexpands to fill in that portion of the thoracic space previously occupied by the resected tissue.

Pneumonectomy. This procedure involves removal of an entire lung. Once the lung is removed, the involved side of the thoracic cavity is an empty space. In order to reduce the size of this cavity, the phrenic nerve is severed on the affected side to paralyze the diaphragm in an elevated position. A thoracoplasty may

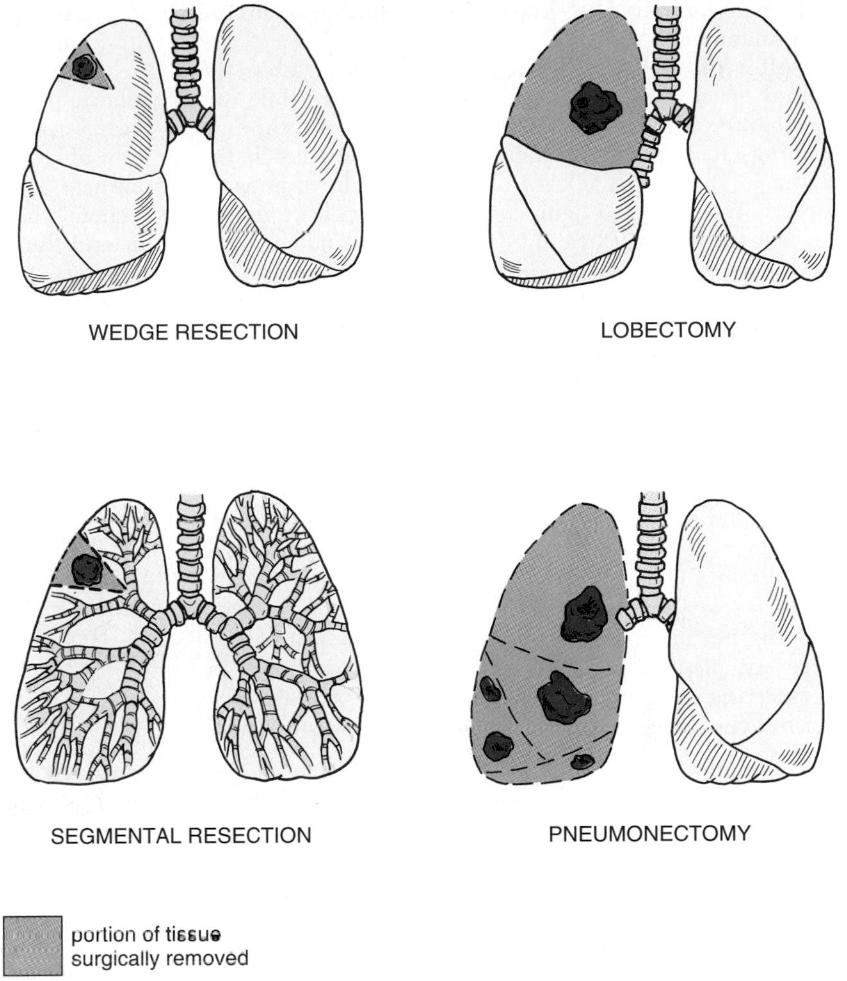

Figure 22–4
Pulmonary resections.

also be performed, which is removal of several ribs or portions of ribs to further reduce the thoracic space.

Closed chest drainage is usually not used after pneumonectomy. The serous fluid that accumulates in the empty thoracic cavity, and eventually consolidates, prevents extensive mediastinal shift of the heart and remaining lung.

LASER THERAPY

Another surgical treatment modality is laser therapy. Currently, laser use is palliative for the relief of endobronchial obstructions caused by nonresectable lung tumors. Lasers do not produce systemic or cumulative toxic effects and are well tolerated. Laser therapy may be done in the outpatient setting. However, in order to use the laser, the tumor mass must be accessible by bronchoscope. Therefore, tumors pressing on bronchial tissue from outside the bronchial lumen are not amenable to laser therapy. The use of laser as an operative modality is discussed in Chapter 5.

CLOSED CHEST DRAINAGE

Closed chest drainage is commonly used after chest surgery. It is also used to treat empyema or pneumothorax (spontaneous or following injuries). This section discusses the principles and purpose of chest drainage, the specific apparatus used, guidelines for assessing the functioning of closed chest drainage systems, precautions, and indications of complications.

Closed chest drainage means that the chest drainage system is closed to atmospheric pressure. Various equipment may be used. Historically, closed chest drainage was performed using a glass bottle water-seal apparatus (one or two bottle set-ups) with or without controlled mechanical suction. Most health care facilities have replaced glass bottle water-seal drainage systems with disposable single units (e.g., Pleur-Evac). However, an understanding of the principles of bottle chest drainage is basic to understanding any type of closed chest drainage. A clear understanding of normal ventilation mechanisms (structure and function) is also essential to understand the principles of closed chest drainage (see Chap. 19).

Purposes of Closed Chest Drainage. Chest surgery actually causes a pneumothorax on the operated side. During thoracotomy, the parietal pleura is incised and the pleural space is entered. Atmospheric air then rushes into the pleural space. This changes the normally negative pressure in that pleural space to a positive pressure. As a result, the lung recoils to its unexpanded size and remains collapsed. Cohesion of the parietal and visceral pleurae is disrupted. Chest trauma, such as fractured ribs, leads to pneumothorax in the same manner.

After the chest wall is closed, pressure within the pleural space is initially atmospheric. For a while, air may continue to escape into the pleural space through openings in the visceral pleural incision. Although the pleura is sutured, it takes time to heal. The trauma of surgery causes serosanguineous fluid to collect in the thoracic cavity until healing occurs. Unfortunately, such fluid is a good culture medium and predisposes the client to infection. Also, the fluid may cause pleural thickening, reducing pulmonary compliance and the lung's ventilatory and diffusion capacities by stiffening the lung.

Because of the above-mentioned factors, it is often necessary to use closed chest drainage following thoracotomy to

- foster and permit the drainage of air and/or serosanguineous fluid from the pleural space and to prevent their reflux (back-, or return, flow)
- help re-expand the remaining lung tissue by re-establishing normal negative pressure in the pleural space
- prevent mediastinal shift and lung tissue collapse by equalizing pressures on both sides of the thoracic cavity (operated and nonoperated sides)

Principles Used in Closed Chest Drainage Systems. Three principles are used in all closed drainage systems: gravity, water seal, and suction.

Gravity. Air and fluid flow from a higher level (pressure) to a lower level (pressure). Therefore, the chest drainage apparatus should always be kept below the level of the client's chest.

Water Seal. A water seal provides a barrier between atmospheric pressure (pressing on the outside of the body) and subatmospheric (negative) intrapleural pressure (normal, 754 to 758 mm Hg).

On expiration, air and fluid in the pleural space travel through the drainage tubing into the first compartment. The air bubbles up through the bottle and enters atmospheric air.

On inspiration, the water seal prevents atmospheric air from being sucked back into the pleural space (which would collapse the lung). The fluid in the water-seal compartment is not drawn into the chest cavity, because the fluid is heavier than air.

As air and fluid drainage commences, the pressure in the pleural space becomes more negative. The greater this negative pressure is, the more the lung expands. Lung expansion, in turn, forces more fluid and air out of the pleural space. This cycle continues until the lung is fully expanded and intrathoracic negative pressure returns to its normal (subatmospheric) level.

A water-seal drainage system must be airtight between the pleural space and the water seal. Any air leak is an entry for atmospheric air into the pleural space, creating a positive pressure that collapses the lung. However, a water-seal chamber *must* have an air vent to provide an escape route for air passing through the water seal from the pleural space.

If there is no air vent, air from the pleural space builds up in the water-seal chamber, creating a buildup of positive pressure in the pleural space and collapsing the lung.

Suction. Suction is a pull force of less than atmospheric pressure (760 mm Hg). A suction of 20 cm H_2O creates a subatmospheric pressure of 746 mm Hg. Suction of 10 to 20 cm H_2O can be applied to a chest drainage system if gravity drainage is not adequate or if a client's cough and respirations are too weak to force air and fluid out of the pleural space through the chest catheters. Additionally, suction may be applied to closed chest drainage (1) if air is leaking into the pleural space faster than it can be removed by a water-seal apparatus or (2) to speed up the removal of air from the pleural space.

CRITICAL TO REMEMBER

Suction must never be applied to the same chamber as the drainage and/or water-seal chambers. A separate suction chamber is needed.

Suction can be applied to a two- or three-bottle water-seal system. A suction chamber contains a long tube with its top end open to atmospheric air and its lower end immersed in water. Suction is regulated by pulling atmospheric air through the long tube that is immersed in 10 to 20 cm of water. The immersed tube provides a barrier between the atmospheric air and the water.

CRITICAL TO REMEMBER

The deeper the tube is immersed in water, the more suction (subatmospheric pressure) is created.

With suction, air travels from the client's pleural cavity via the water seal, through the air vent, into the suction chamber, and then to the suction source.

If the long tube in the suction bottle were not immersed in water, atmospheric air would go straight from the air vent into the suction source as fast as the suction was applied. Passing through water slows the air, and the suction force is controlled. Increasing the source of suction only causes more air to travel through the air vent. The suction applied to the client remains stable.

CRITICAL TO REMEMBER

An occluded atmospheric air vent is dangerous because it would cause the suction to be directly applied to the pleural cavity.

Suction force greater than 50 cm H_2O can cause lung damage.

Insertion of Chest Catheters. Chest catheters are usually inserted in an operating room during chest surgery. However, in some emergencies or to treat problems such as empyema, a chest catheter may be inserted in a treatment room or at the bedside.

Two catheters are usually placed in the chest following resectional surgery (except pneumonectomy).

One of these (the upper, or anterior, tube) is placed anteriorly through the second intercostal space to permit the escape of air rising in the pleural space. The other catheter (the lower, or posterior, tube) is placed posteriorly through the eighth or ninth intercostal space in the midaxillary line to drain off serosanguineous fluid accumulating in the lower portion of the pleural space. The lower tube may have a larger diameter than the upper tube, to enhance fluid drainage.

Chest catheters are brought out of the chest wall through stab wounds or through the incisional line. The catheters are secured to the client's skin with sutures. The tubes should be taped to the outside of the dressing for extra security against tube displacement.

The two chest catheters are attached to separate drainage systems. This makes it possible to monitor air and fluid drainage from each tube and later to remove a nondraining tube without disrupting the rest of the system. Flexible drainage tubing connects the chest catheter to the drainage apparatus. Usually, chest catheters are connected to a closed chest drainage apparatus before the client leaves surgery.

Three-Bottle Water-Seal Apparatus. The first bottle collects drainage from the pleural cavity, the second bottle acts as the water seal, and the third bottle is the suction control. The three-bottle system allows for separate drainage collection and measurement, a stable water-seal system, and controlled suction. A Pleur-Evac is a common commercially made three-bottle system that is less cumbersome than the three separate bottle system.

Nursing Management

Assessing Chest Drainage

CRITICAL TO REMEMBER

It is important to measure *and* document the amount of drainage coming from the pleural space.

This record helps determine the amount of blood loss and the flow rate of drainage from the pleural space. Pleur-Evac systems are manufactured with a marked strip to record the amount of drainage. This is important in planning blood replacement therapy and assessing the client's status. Usually as much as 500 to 1000 mL of drainage occurs in the first 24 hours after chest surgery. Between 100 and 300 mL of drainage may accumulate during the first 2 hours. After this, the drainage should lessen. Excessive drainage may require further surgery to determine its cause.

Chest drainage is normally grossly bloody immediately following surgery. However, it should not continue to be so for more than several hours. The nurse should assess blood loss by monitoring the rising fluid level in the collection bottle. Hemorrhage is suspected if the blood pressure drops and the pulse is rapid. The nurse should check fluid in the drainage collection bottles. If the fluid level has not risen, the nurse checks the tubes for patency.

CRITICAL TO REMEMBER

The nurse should notify the surgeon if the drainage remains frankly bloody for longer than the first few postoperative hours, if bleeding recurs after it has stopped, or of any other signs of hemorrhage.

The client may be bleeding rapidly within the chest.

Assessment of Water-Seal Functioning

Observe the Water Seal: Fluid in the water-seal compartment rises with inspiration and falls with expiration, a process sometimes referred to as tidaling. When tidaling occurs, the drainage tubes are patent, and the apparatus is functioning properly. Tidaling stops when the lung has re-expanded or if the chest drainage tubes are kinked or obstructed. If tidaling does not occur, the nurse should (1) check to be sure the tube is not kinked or compressed, (2) try milking (or stripping if necessary) the tube to remove any obstructions (this procedure may not be permitted in some facilities), (3) change the client's position, and (4) have the client deep breathe and cough. If these measures do not restore tidaling, the nurse should notify the surgeon. (*Note:* Tidaling may not occur or may be minimal in systems using suction.)

Observe for Bubbling in the Water-Seal Compartment: Bubbling in the water-seal compartment is caused by air passing out of the pleural space into the fluid in the bottle. Intermittent bubbling is normal. It indicates that the system is accomplishing one of its purposes, that is, removing air from the pleural space. Intermittent bubbling may occur with the normal expiration, because expiration increases intrapleural pressure and forces air through the tube.

CRITICAL TO REMEMBER

Continuous bubbling during both inspiration and expiration indicates that air is leaking into the drainage system or pleural cavity. This situation must be corrected, because air entering the system also enters the pleural space.

The nurse must locate the source of the air leak, and repair it if possible. He or she begins by inspecting the chest wall where the catheters are inserted. If a chest catheter is loose, the nurse gently squeezes the skin up around the catheter or applies sterile petrolatum gauze around the insertion. He or she then determines whether this stops the continuous bubbling in the bottle. If this does not stop it, the tubing should be checked, inch by inch, and all the connections. A break in the tubing or a loose connection may be found that can be sealed with tape. If the leak still cannot be located, it may be necessary to replace the water-seal bottle.

CRITICAL TO REMEMBER

Rapid bubbling in the absence of an air leak indicates considerable loss of air, such as from an incision or tear in the pulmonary pleura. The physician must be notified *immediately* so that appropriate intervention is taken to prevent collapse of the lung or mediastinal shift.

Suction may be needed, or the amount of suction may need to be increased, or thoracotomy may be necessary.

When caring for a person on water-seal drainage, the nurse should find out whether this particular person's water-seal bottle should be "bubbling." Knowing this facilitates accurate assessment of the drainage pattern (e.g., if intermittent bubbling changes to constant bubbling or if the apparatus that has not been "bubbling" begins to bubble).

Assessment of Suction Apparatus Function

Because most suction motors can create potentially damaging amounts of suction, the degree of suction in the system (and thus in the pleural space) must be controlled. To control the amount of pressure exerted by a wall suction outlet, a suction valve or meter is inserted between the wall outlet and the water-seal bottle. A suction control compartment sometimes is not used so that higher suction pressures can be obtained via a wall suction outlet. In these circumstances, it is essential to maintain the exact pressure prescribed. When portable suction machines are used, a suction control bottle is used to govern the amount of negative pressure permitted to build up within the system.

Proper functioning of a suction control compartment is indicated by continuous bubbling. Vigorous bubbling does not increase the amount of suction, it just causes the water in the bottle to evaporate more rapidly.

Absence of bubbling in a suction control bottle means that the system is not functioning properly and that the correct level of suction is not being maintained. Possible reasons for malfunction of a mechanical suction apparatus include (1) large amounts of air leaking into the pleural space or into the drainage apparatus and (2) mechanical problems in the pump or suction power source. The most serious problem is air leaking into the pleural space.

If bubbling in the suction control bottle stops, the nurse should check for air leaks by briefly clamping the chest drainage tube and observing the suction control bottle. If bubbling begins in the suction control bottle, there is nothing wrong with either the drainage apparatus or the pump. The problem is therefore an air leak into the pleural space around the chest tubes. If the air leak cannot be sealed off (e.g., with petrolatum gauze), the nurse should notify the surgeon immediately. If bubbling does not begin in the suction control bottle when the chest catheter is clamped, the problem is in the drainage connections or the pump. The nurse should check the system carefully, looking for loose connections, air leaks around bottle tops, or air leaks in the tubing (e.g., split tubing). He or she should also make sure that the tubing is not kinked, is correctly positioned, and has no dependent loops. If the suction power source appears to be causing the problem (i.e., bubbling in the suction control bottle does not recommence after all the tubing and all connections are checked), another pump or power source should be obtained immediately.

Because the chest catheter remains clamped during this inspection, the nurse must observe the client closely for indications of tension pneumothorax. As soon as the problem is corrected, the fluid in the suction control bottle will begin to bubble. The nurse then immediately removes the clamps on the chest catheter.

Promoting Chest Drainage. Apparatus for closed chest drainage must always be placed lower than the client's chest (unless for some reason the catheters are clamped). Drainage by gravity is thus maintained, and air and fluid are not forced back into the pleural space. Chest drainage systems must be placed in a box or rack (secured to the bed or on wheels at the bedside) or taped securely to the floor so they will not be knocked over. The preferred arrangement is a rack secured to the bed. This reduces the danger of breaking, elevating, or upsetting the device.

If the drainage apparatus is on the floor, the nurse must be careful not to lower a high-low bed or side rails onto it. The drainage apparatus should be kept about 2 to 3 feet below the client's chest. If a client with closed chest drainage is to be moved, care must be taken to always keep the chest drainage system below the level of the person's chest.

If the apparatus is placed above the level of the client's chest, even for a moment, fluid from the drainage bottle is siphoned back into the pleural cavity. If absolutely necessary, chest tubes may be double-clamped very briefly during momentary movement of the apparatus above the level of the person's chest (e.g., when moving drainage apparatus from one side of the bed to the other if the tubing is not long enough to allow movement around an end of the bed).

The nurse must follow positioning orders carefully. If an individual can be positioned on the side that has chest catheters, the nurse should be sure that the client is not lying on (compressing or kinking) the catheters or tubing. This could (1) impair drainage and cause retrograde pressure (forcing drainage back into the pleural cavity) and (2) increase the client's discomfort. When the client is in a lateral position, small sandbags or folded towels can be placed on either side of the tubing to prevent the client's body weight from compressing the tubing.

Drainage tubing (connecting the chest catheters to the drainage apparatus) should be neither too short nor too long. Excessive tubing length causes tangling and kinking. The drainage tubing should be attached to the edge of the client's mattress so it falls straight to the drainage apparatus, with no dependent loops. Dependent loops of tubing that contain fluid obstruct fluid flow and create back-pressure, thus impairing air or fluid drainage. Drainage tubing may be secured to bedding in various ways:

- Place a rubber band or strip of adhesive tape around the drainage tubing, then pin the other end of the band or tape to the mattress.

- Coil the tubing near the client's side on the bed.

The nurse should make sure the tubing is long enough to allow the client to turn and sit up without pulling on the chest catheters. Each time the client is turned or moved, chest catheters must be checked to be sure they are not being pulled or displaced, and drainage tubing to be certain it is properly positioned.

The nurse should check the patency of drainage tubing and chest catheters frequently and observe the fluid collecting in the drainage bottles. He or she must be sure the client is not lying on the tubing and that it is not kinked or compressed and ensure that the tube is not internally plugged, such as with blood clots. The flow of drainage fluids can be observed easily through clear plastic tubing. If the tubing is not patent, drainage of air and fluid from the pleural space is impossible.

Routine milking or stripping chest tubes is not performed because it creates excessive negative pressure.

CRITICAL TO REMEMBER

Accumulations of blood, fluid, or air in the pleural space may eventually compress the lung, precipitating tension pneumothorax or mediastinal shift. Therefore, if the drainage apparatus malfunctions, the nurse must correct the problem immediately and observe the person closely for indications of complications.

Early detection of tension pneumothorax, for example, can prevent mediastinal shift if appropriate treatment is given promptly.

The nurse should notify the surgeon immediately if complications are suspected. While waiting for the surgeon, the nurse can try to locate and correct the cause of any problems within the drainage system. A relatively simple action may correct a malfunctioning system, such as straightening a kinked tube or setting upright a water-seal bottle that has been knocked over.

Preventing Infection. When properly used, closed chest drainage helps prevent infection in the pleural space by removing serosanguineous fluids. However, unless careful aseptic technique is used when caring for chest catheters, the drainage system, and the insertion site, infection may be introduced into the pleural space. The nurse must observe strict asepsis whenever he or she is changing a chest drainage apparatus or any of its connections. The open tube ends must always be protected with sterile dressings and the nurse must always wash the hands thoroughly before and after caring for chest tubes. Because infection can occur along the tube tract, chest catheters are usually not used for longer than 5 to 7 days.

Activity with Chest Drainage. The nurse should encourage a client on closed chest drainage to cough and deep breathe frequently. In addition to clearing the bronchi of secretions, these activities promote lung expansion and the expulsion of air or fluid or both from the pleural space (by increasing intrapulmonic and intrapleural pressure).

A client with a chest drainage system can sit up in bed, get in and out of bed, and ambulate without clamping the chest catheters as long as the apparatus stays upright. Traction (pulling) should not be exerted on the tubing. Various arrangements are used to hold a client's chest water-seal bottles during ambulation. Most commonly the device is placed in a wheelchair in front of the client. If suction is to be maintained, the client can walk only those few steps permitted by the length of tubing.

Clamping Chest Drainage Tubing. Rubber-shod clamps should always be kept at the bedside of a client on closed chest drainage. The clamps are 6- to 8-inch, strong forceps with protective rubber on the tips. Two clamps should be available for each chest catheter so that each can be double-clamped (for extra safety) if clamping is required. When not in use, the clamps should be kept in a visible, readily available place, for example, at the head of the bed. The clamps should not be taped to the bed, or they will be too difficult to release for emergency use. They should not be left lying on the bedside stand or in a drawer, as they are likely not to be there when the nurse needs them, or they may be hidden by other articles.

Except for those emergencies in which clamping is clearly indicated, the nurse should *never* clamp chest drainage tubes without an order to do so.

If clamps must be used, the best time to apply them to a chest catheter is following an expiration. They should be removed as soon as possible.

Potential Emergencies

Intervention if Water-Seal Bottle Is Accidentally Elevated Above the Level of the Client's Chest. The nurse should immediately lower the bottle and contact the surgeon. This serious accident causes fluid in the bottle to be siphoned or to flow by gravity into the pleural space, precipitating collapse of the lung or mediastinal shift or both.

Intervention if Apparatus Is Broken. If the chest drainage device is broken, atmospheric air enters the pleural space through the drainage tubing. Intervention depends on whether the client has been "bubbling" or not.

In such an emergency, rapid assessment is necessary to determine (1) the extent to which exposing the pleural space to atmospheric air would disrupt the treatment and (2) the pros and cons of shutting off air flow into and out of the chest cavity with clamps. Such decisions must be made quickly. Knowing whether the person was "bubbling" or not before the accident is important, because there is no way to observe this after a device has broken. If the person has not been "bubbling," the nurse should immediately clamp the chest catheter, wipe the exposed ends of the catheter with an antiseptic solution, reconnect it to another chest drainage apparatus, and unclamp. If clamps have been applied to a chest tube and it is noticed that the client is beginning to experience respiratory distress before being reconnected to another apparatus, tension pneumothorax (and possibly mediastinal shift) is probably occurring. (Indications of respiratory distress include rapid, shallow breathing, apprehension, chest pain, and cyanosis.) The nurse should immediately release the clamps on the chest catheter and call for the surgeon. It is best to open the clamps and create an open pneumothorax. Then at least air can move both in and out of the pleural space and is not trapped there, building up pressure.

Intervention if the Chest Tube Is Accidentally Removed. Cover the insertion site with sterile petroleum gauze and notify the surgeon. Observe the client for respiratory distress.

Alternative Chest Drainage Equipment

Flutter Valve. A flutter valve can be used instead of water-seal drainage bottles in closed chest drainage setups. The B-P Heimlich Chest Drainage Valve (Fig. 22–5) is presterilized, disposable, and about 7 inches long. When inserted between a chest catheter and a drainage collecting apparatus, the valve permits the unidirectional flow of air and fluid from the pleural space into a collection apparatus and prevents the reflux of air or fluid back into the chest.

A flutter valve is a single piece of wide, thin rubber tubing. It is open at the end that attaches to a chest catheter and is compressed at the other end so that its flattened sides (valve leaflets) remain in contact with each other. Air and fluid draining from the intrapleural space enter the "open" end and pass out through the valve's flattened ends. The air and fluid cannot re-enter the flattened sides of the tubing because these two sides remain in contact with each other. A flutter valve offers minimal resistance to air or fluid leaving the intrapleural space. The valve is enclosed in a clear plastic case that (1) protects the tubing from being kinked and (2) facilitates assessment of the passage of fluid and blood through the valve. Expansion and contraction of the valve leaflets (caused by changes in intrapleural pressure associated with ventilatory chest movements) can also be observed.

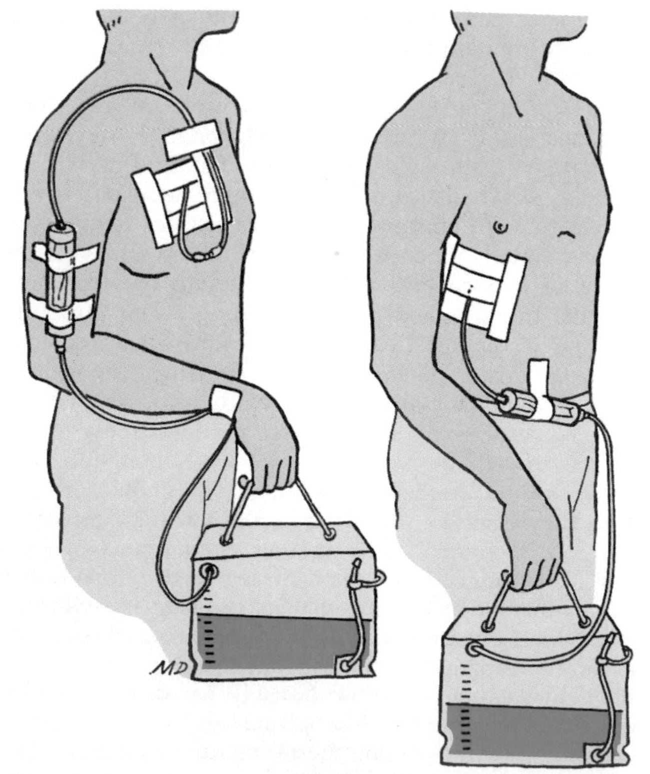

Figure 22–5
Heimlich flutter valve: an alternative to water-seal drainage. A valve allows chest drainage while preventing reflux of air and fluid back into the chest. It allows ambulation and greater mobility than other systems. The valve may be attached to the arm or body, and the drainage bag may be carried at any level, because reflux is prevented.

A flutter valve functions in any position, allowing the client to assume any position desired. It allows greater freedom of movement than a water-seal system. The client can be comfortably ambulatory if the drainage tube is connected to a vented portable plastic bag or even a rubber glove. Because a flutter valve functions in the same way as a water-seal bottle, it can be attached to controlled chest suction if necessary.

McSwain's Dart System. This system can replace water-seal drainage bottles for clients with a pneumothorax. A McSwain dart system is a presterilized, disposable small-bore catheter with built-in polyvinyl chloride tubing and a molded, one-way injection valve. It operates on the same principle as a flutter valve (see earlier discussion). Air from the intrapleural space can escape through the catheter, but the one-way valve prevents air from being sucked back into the chest. Controlled suction may be applied to the end of the tubing for rapid evacuation of air from the pleural space. As with the flutter valve, the McSwain dart system functions in any position and allows the client to move freely.

Removal of Chest Catheters. A physician determines when to remove water-seal chest drainage. As mentioned earlier, one indication that the evacuation of intrapleural air and fluid is completed and that the lung has re-expanded is the cessation of fluctuation in the long tube of the water-seal bottle (if suction is not applied). The re-expanded lung blocks the catheters' openings into the pleural space. Thus, fluctuations of intrapleural pressure during inspiration and expiration are no longer transmitted to the water-seal apparatus. When the lung is completely re-expanded, no air or fluid passes through the chest catheters.

Usually, a lung is fully re-expanded after 2 to 3 postoperative days of chest drainage. Generally, chest catheters are left in place connected to drainage bottles for 24 hours after all air drainage and significant fluid drainage have stopped. Sometimes, the catheters are temporarily clamped to see how the client will tolerate their removal. Chest catheters may not be removed if the chest is draining more than 50 to 70 mL of fluid daily. The sooner the chest catheters can be removed, the better. Their presence often contributes to postoperative pain and inactivity. Also, the longer the catheters are in place, the greater the risk of infection. When treating empyema, chest catheters may be used longer than when following chest surgery.

Chest auscultation, chest percussion, and chest x-ray study confirm lung re-expansion. The surgeon removes the chest catheter when convinced it is safe to do so. Although both chest catheters can be removed at the same time, it is more common for the upper one to be left in place longer than the lower.

CRITICAL TO REMEMBER

Removal of chest catheters can be moderately painful. The prescribed premedication for pain relief should be administered about one half hour before the procedure.

The nurse assembles equipment as necessary, such as sterile scissors, knife or suture set to cut sutures securing the catheter(s), sterile petrolatum gauze, 4 × 4 gauze to cover the wound, and three strips of tape 2 inches wide and about 6 inches long.

Diagnostic Phase

The client who is undergoing diagnostic tests for lung cancer faces an uncertain future. If the diagnosis is confirmed, the client can anticipate a variety of physical difficulties, potentially extensive medical treatment, and many emotional changes. The nursing assessment plays a critical role in developing a plan of care that will provide needed support.

The nursing history should include an exploration of the client's chief complaints, particularly cough (productive or nonproductive), dyspnea, pain, or recurrent infection. The client should be asked about the presence of risk factors, including a smoking history, exposure to occupational respiratory carcinogens, or a family history of the disease. Socioeconomic situation and available social support should also be assessed because these factors will affect subsequent management options.

Nursing management during the diagnostic phase will focus on emotional support and client education, along with required physical care. The nurse can help clients maintain a sense of control by keeping them informed about all scheduled tests. Once a diagnosis of lung cancer is confirmed, nursing care must incorporate aspects of assisting the client to cope with anxiety and fear, family responses, financial considerations, absence from work and social activities, and possible changes in life goals.

Treatment Phase

Preoperative Assessment: Preoperative preparation is the same as for any surgical client but with greater emphasis on assessment and preparation of the respiratory system (see Chap. 5 for discussion of preoperative nursing care). Extensive pulmonary function testing may be ordered before chest surgery for determining the client's ability to tolerate the proposed surgical intervention. Clients with impaired pulmonary function may be treated with antibiotics, bronchodilating medications, intermittent positive-pressure breathing procedures, and supervised breathing exercises to improve respiratory efficiency. Clients are encouraged to refrain from smoking during the preoperative period, because smoking will increase pulmonary secretions and decrease blood oxygen saturation.

Preoperative Nursing Intervention. Nursing interventions during the preoperative period are primarily aimed at reducing the client's anxiety level. Anxiety results from fear of cancer and its prognosis, as well as from fear of the surgical procedure and insufficient knowledge of surgical routines and postoperative self-care activities. The client and significant others are taught about

- the anticipated surgical procedure. The nurse should assess the client's (and significant others') understanding and give further information as needed.
- the early postoperative period. The nurse should talk specifically about what will be happening to the client and how he or she can participate in recovery activities. Specific explanations should be given about the presence of chest tubes (except with pneumonectomy) and drainage tubes, intubation and mechanical ventilation, oxygen therapy, and available pain relief measures.
- postoperative exercises (Figs. 22–6 and 22–7). These include (1) respiratory exercises to maintain effective pulmonary function; (2) leg exercises to prevent thrombophlebitis; and (3) arm and shoulder exercises to maintain normal range of motion and correct posture. These exercises should be demonstrated, and opportunity should be given for practice and return demonstration.

Postoperative Assessment: During the immediate postoperative period, thorough assessment is essential. The nurse should make observations as often as the client's condition warrants. This will be determined by factors such as (1) amount of anesthesia received and the client's reaction to it, (2) amount of intraoperative blood loss, (3) preoperative client condition (e.g., presence of pre-existing medical conditions such as diabetes, heart disorders), (4) client's response to pain, and (5) facility protocols. In general, the nurse should make assessments every 15 minutes until the client is stable, then every 30 minutes for several hours. Hourly assessment is usually indicated throughout the first postoperative night. More frequent assessments may be required if the client's condition changes.

Postoperative Nursing Intervention. Nursing interventions are based on careful assessment and appropriate nursing diagnoses. General postoperative nursing measures will be applicable (see Chap. 5). Nursing management specific to thoracic surgery is discussed in the Care Plan. Chest tubes are placed to facilitate drainage and lung re-expansion in all clients undergoing chest surgery, except following pneumonectomy.

Terminal Phase

During the end stage of lung cancer, the emphasis of nursing care is on physical and emotional support of the client and significant others. Effective physical care and comfort for the terminally ill client can greatly contribute to a peaceful death. Extensive measures may be required to control the client's pain, including epidural or intrathecal analgesia. Measures should be taken to enhance the therapeutic effects of pain-relieving medications as well as to minimize potential side effects.

Clients in the terminal phase of the disease can be expected to experience some degree of anger or depression. These emotions may be expressed through abusive or aggressive behavior toward family and care givers, thus adding to stress and anxiety levels. The nurse should find ways to help the client to ventilate thoughts and feelings as well as to assist significant others in understanding and coping with the situation.

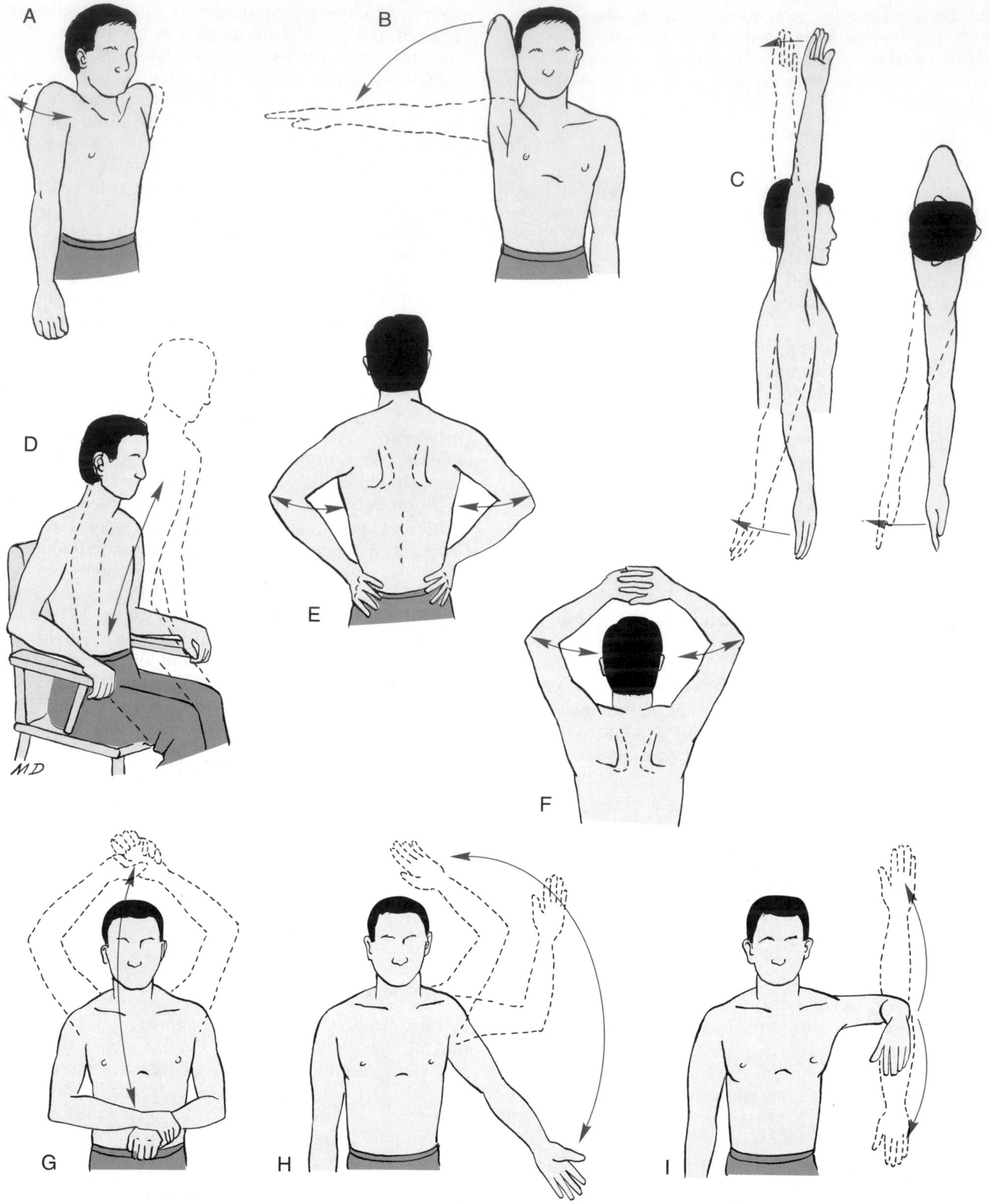

Figure 22–6
Arm and shoulder exercises often prescribed after chest surgery.

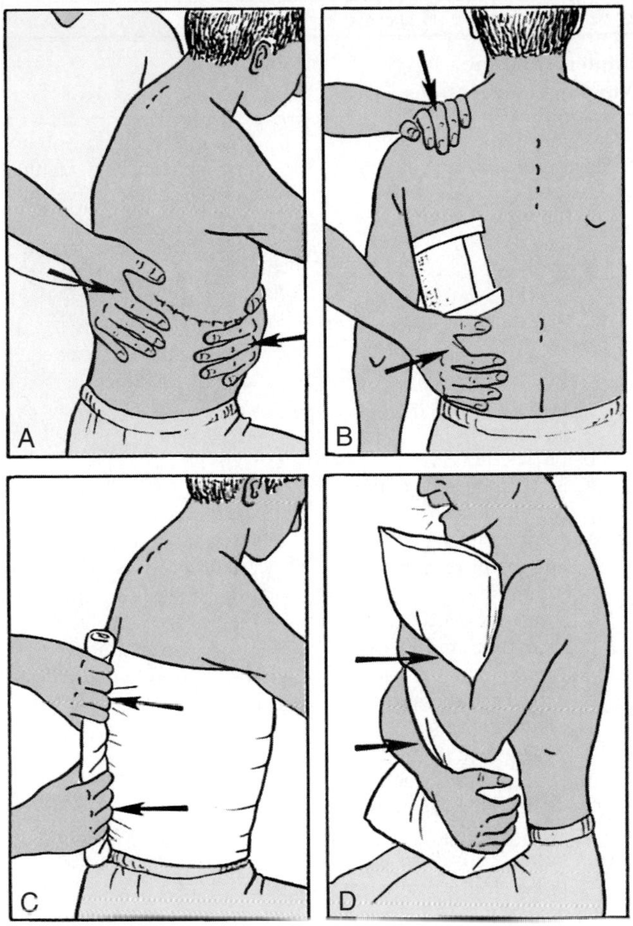

Figure 22–7
Splinting techniques to promote effective coughing and deep breathing. Apply firm, even pressure after the person has taken a deep breath and during forced expiratory cough. Do not squeeze the chest or interfere with chest inspiratory expansion. *A*, Place one hand around the person's back and the other around the incisional area. *B*, Support the area below the incision with one hand while exerting downward pressure on the shoulder on the affected side with the other. *C*, Place a towel or draw sheet snugly (but not tightly) around the chest. *D*, Have the person hug a pillow during forced expiratory cough.

BENIGN LUNG TUMORS

Benign pulmonary neoplasms account for less than 10 per cent of all primary pulmonary tumors. The term "benign" may be misleading, because although they are not directly harmful to the body, some of these tumors may still have serious physiologic effects. Mechanical interference with lung function (e.g., obstruction of a major bronchus) may occur, depending on the tumor's location. In addition, some of these tumors may become malignant over time.

The most common benign lung tumor is the hamartoma, which usually arises in peripheral lung parenchyma. This tumor is more common in older men. Other benign tumor types include the fibroma, hemangioma, lipoma, and papilloma.

Benign tumors may also arise from pleural (mesothelial) tissue. Benign mesotheliomas occur in both sexes, usually between the ages of 40 and 60 years. They may be a postinflammatory response (i.e., subsequent to pulmonary infections), although their specific cause is unknown.

Benign lung tumors are often difficult to diagnose because clients may be asymptomatic. Unless there is pre-existing lung disease or major airway obstruction, pulmonary function studies and ABGs are usually within normal limits. The tumor may be first detected through chest radiography. Confirmatory diagnosis usually requires bronchoscopy or, more commonly, thoracotomy.

Until the diagnosis is confirmed, most clients will be quite anxious and fearful of the possibility of cancer. Emotional support is an important adjunct to the physical preparation required for diagnostic procedures.

Surgical intervention is the treatment of choice for all benign neoplasms. Tumor removal promptly alleviates any respiratory symptoms that may be present. Postoperative management is the same as that used with the surgical treatment of malignant lung disease.

Disorders of the Pulmonary Vasculature

PULMONARY EMBOLISM

Pulmonary embolism (PE) is an occlusion of a portion of the pulmonary blood vessels by an embolus. An embolus is defined as a detached intravascular solid, liquid, or gaseous mass that is carried by the bloodstream from its point of origin to a distant site. A PE is an acute and potentially lethal disorder.

Incidence

Pulmonary embolism is one of the four most common causes of sudden death in the United States. Over 600,000 people develop pulmonary emboli each year and half of these individuals die within 2 hours after embolization.[31] Several autopsy studies indicate that major pulmonary emboli occur in as many as 25 per cent of hospitalized patients. The diagnosis of pulmonary embolism is often difficult to make because of the vagueness of the clients' clinical symptoms. The importance of making the diagnosis is confirmed by studies revealing that the mortality rate for untreated PE is between 20 per cent and 35 per cent; the mortality rate is 8 per cent when the condition is recognized and appropriately managed.[48]

Text continued on page 621

CARE PLAN: The Client Undergoing Thoracic Surgery

Nursing Diagnosis/ Collaborative Problem	Planning: Expected Outcomes	Implementation: Nursing Interventions	Rationales
Potential complications of thoracic surgery: • Respiratory insufficiency • Tension pneumothorax and mediastinal shift • Subcutaneous emphysema • Pulmonary embolus • Pulmonary edema • Cardiac dysrhythmias • Hemorrhage, hemothorax, hypovolemic shock • Thrombophlebitis	The nurse will monitor for respiratory, cardiac, and vascular complications.	1. Monitor for signs and symptoms of respiratory failure: a. increased respiratory rate b. dyspnea c. use of accessory muscles and/or retractions d. cyanosis e. decreased PaO_2 levels and increased $PaCO_2$ levels f. restlessness g. increase in adventitious breath sounds	1. Postoperatively, respiratory insufficiency may result from an altered level of consciousness due to anesthesia and pain medications, incomplete lung reinflation, decreased respiratory effort due to chest pain, and inadequate airway clearance.
		2. Monitor for signs and symptoms of tension pneumothorax: a. severe dyspnea b. tachypnea and tachycardia c. extreme restlessness and agitation d. progressive cyanosis e. laryngeal and tracheal deviation to unaffected side f. Point of maximal impulse shift laterally or medially	2. Postoperative tension pneumothorax can result from air leaking through pleural incision lines if closed chest drainage fails to function properly.
		3. Observe for subcutaneous emphysema around incision and in the chest and neck. a. Assess progression by periodically marking the chest with a skin-marking pencil at outer periphery of emphysematous tissue. b. If neck involvement occurs, measure neck circumference at least every 2–4 hours.	3. Subcutaneous emphysema may result from air leakage at pulmonary incision site. a. Rapid progression (i.e., an increase of more than a hand's width in 1 hour) may indicate leakage through bronchial stump. b. Severe subcutaneous emphysema in the neck may compress the trachea and may require tracheostomy.
		4. Monitor for signs and symptoms of pulmonary embolus: a. chest pain b. dyspnea and tachypnea c. fever d. hemoptysis e. indications of right-sided heart failure	4. Pulmonary embolism is a serious potential complication after chest surgery and a significant cause of postoperative hypoxemia.

CARE PLAN: The Client Undergoing Thoracic Surgery *Continued*

Nursing Diagnosis/ Collaborative Problem	Planning: Expected Outcomes	Implementation: Nursing Interventions	Rationales
		5. Monitor for signs of acute pulmonary edema: a. dyspnea b. rales c. persistent cough d. frothy sputum e. cyanosis	5. Circulatory overload may result from the reduced size of the pulmonary vascular bed due to surgical removal of pulmonary tissue and delayed re-expansion of the operated lung. Additionally, hypoxia increases capillary permeability, causing fluid to enter pulmonary tissue.
		6. Monitor intravenous flow rates. Consult physician if fluid amounts (maintenance plus intermittent medications [e.g., antibiotics]) exceed 125 mL/hr.	6. After chest surgery, intravenous fluids should not exceed 125 mL/hr because of possible circulatory overload.
		7. Assess cardiac monitor for the development of cardiac dysrhythmias, particularly atrial fibrillation, atrial flutter, and paroxysmal atrial tachycardia.	7. Cardiac dysrhythmias are fairly common after chest surgery. Rhythm disturbances result from a combination of factors, including increased vagal tone, hypoxia, mediastinal shift, and abnormal blood pH.
		8. Assess dressing/incisional area every 4 hours for evidence of bleeding (increase to every 1–2 hours if bleeding develops). 9. Assess drainage in closed chest drainage system for signs of bleeding.	8 & 9. Blood loss may be great with major thoracic surgery because a. blood vessels in the thorax are of large caliber b. the incision is often large and produces considerable capillary oozing c. adhesion and tissue planes within the thorax are generally quite extensive and vascular
		10. Monitor for signs of hypovolemic shock: a. increased pulse b. decreased blood pressure c. restlessness and decreased level of consciousness d. decreased urine output (< 30 mL/hr) e. cool, pale, clammy skin f. increased respirations	10. The body compensates for lost blood volume by increasing blood flow (through increased heart rate) to vital organs and decreasing peripheral circulation.
		11. Monitor for thrombophlebitis: a. unilateral leg edema b. calf tenderness, redness, unusual warmth	11. Anesthesia and immobility reduce vasomotor tone, leading to decreased venous return and peripheral pooling of blood.
		12. Encourage client to perform leg exercises. Discourage placing pillows under knees, crossing the legs, or prolonged sitting.	12. These measures prevent venous stasis, thus reducing the risk of thrombophlebitis.

Care Plan continued on following page

CARE PLAN: The Client Undergoing Thoracic Surgery *Continued*

Nursing Diagnosis/ Collaborative Problem	Planning: Expected Outcomes	Implementation: Nursing Interventions	Rationales
Airway Clearance, Ineffective R/T increased secretions and decreased coughing effectiveness due to pain	The client will demonstrate effective airway clearance, as evidenced by clear breath sounds, effective coughing, and adequate air exchange in the lungs	1. Once the vital signs are stable, place client in semi-Fowler's position.	1. The upright position enhances lung expansion and facilitates ventilation with minimal effort.
		2. Assist client to cough and deep breathe at least every 1 or 2 hours during the first 24 to 48 postoperative hours.	2. Coughing helps to move tracheobronchial secretions out of the lung. Deep breathing dilates the airways, stimulates surfactant production, and expands lung tissue.
		3. When possible, schedule coughing and deep breathing sessions at times when pain medication is maximally effective (i.e., 15–20 minutes after intravenous administration and 30–45 minutes after intramuscular or subcutaneous administration). (If client-controlled analgesia is used, timing is not as crucial because analgesia level is more consistent.)	3. The less postoperative pain a client experiences, the more effective are coughing and deep breathing.
		4. Assess breath sounds before and after coughing.	4. This will help in evaluation of coughing effectiveness.
		5. Provide support and reassurance:	5.
		a. Explain that breathing exercises will not damage lungs or suture line.	a. Fear of "splitting open" the incision may hamper coughing efforts.
		b. Manually splint the incision area during coughing and deep breathing	b. Physical support of the incision is both comforting and reassuring.
		c. Offer sips of warm water.	c. Warm water can aid relaxation and produce more effective coughing.
		6. Maintain adequate level of hydration and adequate humidity of inspired air.	6. Fluids and moisture help to thin secretions, making them easier to expectorate.
		7. Monitor results of chest x-ray examination.	7. Frequent chest films help detect atelectasis and infection.
		8. Evaluate need for suctioning.	8. If coughing is ineffective, suctioning may be required to remove pulmonary secretions. Suctioning should be performed cautiously so that disruption of pulmonary suture lines is avoided.
Pain R/T surgical procedure	The client will have improved comfort, as evidenced by verbalizing that discomfort is reduced, using fewer narcotics, moving in bed with less pain.	1. Administer pain medication as ordered.	1. After chest surgery, the client's chest will be quite painful because of the trauma of surgery and the presence of chest tubes. The severance of intercostal nerves during surgery may also produce sensations of pain, numbness, or heaviness in the operative area.

CARE PLAN: The Client Undergoing Thoracic Surgery *Continued*

Nursing Diagnosis/ Collaborative Problem	Planning: Expected Outcomes	Implementation: Nursing Interventions	Rationales
		2. Offer pain medication before pain becomes severe.	2. A preventive approach to pain control provides a more consistent level of relief and reduces client anxiety.
		3. Assess medication effectiveness and avoid overmedication.	3. A delicate balance with pain management is essential. Adequate pain relief must be obtained. However, overmedication can depress respirations and the cough reflex.
		4. Use nonpharmacologic pain relief measures concurrently.	4. Proper positioning, relaxation techniques, and the like can augment effects of medications.
Physical Mobility, Impaired R/T pain and muscle dissection and restricted positioning	The client will maintain physical mobility in arm and shoulder, as evidenced by regaining preoperative arm and shoulder function	1. Position client as indicated by phase of recovery and surgical procedure.	
		a. Nonoperative side-lying position may be used until consciousness is regained.	a. This position promotes hemodynamic stability in the immediate postoperative period and prevents aspiration.
		b. Semi-Fowler's position (head of bed elevated 30 to 45 degrees) is recommended once vital signs are stable.	b. The upright position enhances lung expansion and facilitates chest tube drainage.
		c. Avoid positioning client on operative side if a wedge resection or segmentectomy has been performed.	c. Lying on the operative side hinders expansion of remaining lung tissue.
		d. Avoid complete lateral positioning after pneumonectomy.	d. Because the mediastinum is no longer held in place on both sides by lung tissue, extreme turning may cause mediastinal shift and compression of the remaining lung.
		2. Gently turn the client every 1 to 2 hours, unless contraindicated.	2. Frequent turning promotes mobilization and drainage of air and fluid from the pleural space. Turning also improves circulation, promotes lung aeration, and enhances comfort.
		3. Avoid traction on chest tubes while changing client position. Check for kinking or compression of tubing.	3. Traction may dislodge the chest tubes. Kinking or compression inhibits drainage and re-establishment of negative intrapleural pressure.
		4. Encourage regular ambulation, once client's condition is stable. Maintain supplemental oxygen, if ordered.	4. Early ambulation improves ventilation, circulation, and morale. Oxygen therapy should be maintained during activity to avoid hypoxia.

Care Plan continued on following page

CARE PLAN: The Client Undergoing Thoracic Surgery *Continued*

Nursing Diagnosis/ Collaborative Problem	Planning: Expected Outcomes	Implementation: Nursing Interventions	Rationales
		5. Begin passive ROM exercises of the arm and shoulder on the affected side 4 hours after recovery from anesthesia. Exercises should be performed two times every 4 to 6 hours through the first 24 postoperative hours, with progression to 10 to 20 times every 2 hours.	5. ROM exercises help prevent adhesion formation in the operative area, which can lead to dysfunction syndrome (i.e., "frozen" shoulder).
		6. Active ROM exercises are begun once the client's condition permits (see Fig. 22–8).	6. Active ROM exercises prevent adhesions of the incised muscle layers.
		7. Encourage client to use arm on affected side in daily activities (e.g., eating, reaching, grooming). Keep bedside stand on operative side to encourage reaching.Teach importance of continued use after discharge.	7. Regular use of the affected arm and shoulder reduces the possibility of contractures.
		8. Carefully assess client's response to activity and exercise. Observe for signs of dyspnea, shortness of breath, and fatigue.	8. It may take time for client's activity tolerance to increase, because the body must adjust to reduced respiratory capacity after resectional surgery.
		9. Allow adequate rest periods between activities.	9. Adequate rest will allow the client to cooperate more fully with activities.
Individual Coping, Ineffective, Risk for R/T temporary dependence and loss of full respiratory function	The client will use adaptive coping mechanisms, as evidenced by verbalizing feelings related to emotional state and taking appropriate actions to regain self-care capabilities.	1. Provide opportunity for client to ventilate feelings.	1. Loss of normal body function and self-care capabilities can lead to feelings of powerlessness, anger, and grief. Open expression of these feelings can help client to begin the coping process.
		2. Encourage use of positive coping strategies that have been successful in the past.	2. The use of effective coping actions can decrease feelings of hopelessness and helplessness.
		3. Allow client to have as much control over daily activities and decision making as is possible.	3. Active involvement in the plan of care gives the client a sense of control and promotes return to independence.
		4. Support and praise all independent activities that promote recovery.	4. Emotional support and encouragement helps motivate client to continue progress toward independence.
Altered Health Maintenance R/T self-care after discharge	Client will be able to maintain health, as evidenced by stating or demonstrating discharge plans.	1. Provide thorough instruction and preparation for hospital discharge:	1. Thorough understanding promotes compliance and enhances self-care capabilities.
		a. proper wound care	a. Wound care will vary according to condition of incision and client.

CARE PLAN: The Client Undergoing Thoracic Surgery *Continued*

Nursing Diagnosis/ Collaborative Problem	Planning: Expected Outcomes	Implementation: Nursing Interventions	Rationales
		b. continuation of exercise program	b. Continued exercise increases activity tolerance and prevents complications.
		c. precautions regarding activity and environmental irritants	c. Heavy lifting should be avoided. Return to work will depend on client's condition and type of job. However, it is usually possible within 4 to 6 weeks. Environmental irritants can cause severe coughing episodes.
		d. Clinical manifestations to be reported to health care professional	d. Evidence of infection, deteriorating respiratory status, or other complications should be reported promptly.
		e. importance of regular follow-up care	e. The client should be followed closely for signs of surgical complications, recurrence of malignancy, and metastasis.
		f. community agencies that can provide resources, as needed	f. Community resources can facilitate home management.

ROM, range of motion.

Etiology

Virtually 99 per cent of all emboli develop from thrombi (clots).[14] Other sources of emboli include tumors, air, fat, bone marrow, amniotic fluid, septic thrombi, and vegetations on heart valves that develop with endocarditis. The most common source of pulmonary emboli is venous thrombosis in the thigh and pelvis.

Risk Factors

Clients at the highest risk of developing pulmonary embolism are those who have had surgery on the pelvis or legs, have had trauma to the pelvis or lower legs, are immobile for other reasons, are obese, require estrogen therapy, or have clotting abnormalities.

Measures to reduce the risk of PE include early ambulation of all clients, leg exercises in bedridden clients, and avoidance of smoking. Prophylactic heparin is often administered.

Clients with deep vein thrombosis must be carefully assessed for early clinical manifestations of PE (see later discussion). Clients with a past history of deep vein thrombosis or a previous occurrence of PE also have an increased risk. These clients should avoid restrictive clothing on the legs and prolonged sitting or standing.

Pathophysiology

Emboli travel to the lungs and lodge in the pulmonary vasculature. The size and number of emboli determine the location. Blood flow is obstructed, leading to decreased perfusion of the section of lung supplied by the vessel. The client continues to ventilate the lung portion but because the tissue is not perfused, a V/Q mismatch occurs, and hypoxemia develops.

If the embolus lodges in a large pulmonary vessel, it increases proximal pulmonary vascular resistance, causes atelectasis, and eventually decreases cardiac output. If the embolus is in the smaller vessels, less dramatic clinical manifestations follow but perfusion is still altered.

The arterioles constrict due to platelet degranulation, accompanied by a release of histamine, serotonin, catecholamines, and prostaglandins. The chemical agents result in bronchial and pulmonary artery constriction. This vasoconstriction probably plays a major role in the hemodynamic instability that follows PE.

Clinical Manifestations

Chest pain is the most common symptom of PE, but it is not diagnostic of the condition. The pain most often associated with PE is pleuritic. Pleuritic pain is caused by an inflammatory reaction of the lung parenchyma or by pulmonary infarction or ischemia caused by obstruction of small pulmonary arterial branches. Typical pleuritic chest pain is sudden in onset and aggravated by breathing. The client is also dyspneic, especially if the embolus has occluded major arteries or major portions of lung tissue. Apprehension, cough, diaphoresis, syncope, and hemoptysis may occur. The presence of hemoptysis indicates that the infarction or areas of atelectasis have produced alveolar damage.

Respirations typically increase; the client also develops crackles, an increased physiologic split of the second heart sound, tachycardia, and fever. Less common findings include heart gallops, edema, heart murmur, and cyanosis.

DIAGNOSTIC ASSESSMENT

The diagnosis of pulmonary embolism is suggested by chest pain, especially pleuritic in nature; hemoptysis; dyspnea; a low arterial PO_2; and a wedge-shaped density on chest x-ray study.

Ventilation-perfusion lung scan (V/Q scan) is one of the most important studies to determine PE. A negative perfusion scan rules out PE.

Arterial blood gas analyses indicate arterial hypoxemia (low PO_2) and hypocapnia (low PCO_2) in massive pulmonary embolism. There may be a severe respiratory alkalosis.

A radioisotope lung scan is performed by intravenously injecting particles of human serum albumin that have been labeled with radioactive iodine (^{131}I) or technetium (^{99m}Tc). These macroaggregated particles are trapped in the pulmonary microvasculature and are distributed according to pulmonary flow. Both lungs are scanned with a scintillation counter, and the amount of radioactivity counted gives an indication of obstruction to flow.

Pulmonary angiograms provide the most effective means of diagnosing pulmonary emboli. This procedure is performed by injecting a radiopaque contrast agent into the right atrium and pulmonary artery via a catheter threaded through a peripheral vein.

Medical Management

Successful management of PE depends on the prompt recognition of the condition and immediate treatment. Medical management focuses on anticoagulation to reduce the size of future thrombi, slow the development of emboli from thrombi, and maintain cardiopulmonary stability.

Anticoagulation is begun with intravenous heparin sodium. The client is administered anticoagulants until the partial thromboplastin time is 2 to 2.5 times the normal value. Administration of sodium warfarin (Coumadin) is begun about 3 days before heparin is stopped to provide a transition, because the half-life of heparin is very short. Clients are maintained on warfarin for 3 to 6 months.

Cardiopulmonary support varies with the client's symptoms. Sometimes hypoxemia can be reversed with low-flow oxygen by nasal cannula. Other clients require endotracheal intubation to maintain PaO_2 over 60 mm Hg.

Hypotension is treated with fluids. If fluids do not raise the preload (right ventricular end-diastolic pressure) enough to raise blood pressure, inotropic agents may be required.

Chest pain and apprehension are usually treated with intravenous analgesics (e.g., morphine sulfate). Because the usual cause of PE is thrombus from the lower legs, the legs are usually elevated with caution to avoid severe flexure of the hips. Such flexure will again slow blood flow and increase the risk of new thrombi.

The use of fibrinolytic therapy in the management of massive PE is not clear. Some clinicians have found that although the treatment dissolves the clot, it does not improve the mortality rate.

Surgical Intervention

There are three surgical interventions for pulmonary embolus: (1) vein ligation to prevent the embolus from traveling to the heart; (2) vena cava plication, or insertion of an umbrella filter to allow blood flow while trapping emboli (Figure 22–8); and (3) embolectomy.

An embolectomy involves surgical removal of emboli from the pulmonary arteries. Before the advent of the cardiopulmonary bypass, the procedure had an extremely high mortality rate. Even now, embolectomy during anticoagulant therapy carries a high risk, partly

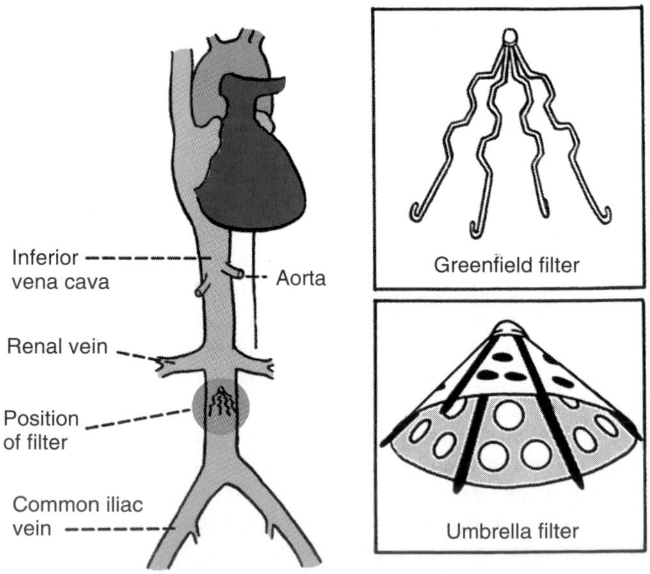

Figure 22–8
Inferior vena cava filters, such as Greenfield and umbrella filters, prevent emboli from traveling to the lung.

because of possible misdiagnosis and partly because operating on clients in profound shock is dangerous.

Nursing Management

The client is closely monitored for hypoxemia and respiratory compromise. Vital signs are assessed every 15 minutes until they are stable. Lung sounds are auscultated every 2 to 4 hours. Blood gas values are monitored. To facilitate breathing, the client is placed in semi-Fowler's position, and oxygen is applied per doctor's orders.

The client is also monitored for clinical manifestations of right-sided heart failure. Heart sounds are ascultated every 4 hours, assessing for murmurs or extra heart sounds. The nurse monitors for right-sided heart failure (e.g., peripheral edema, distended neck veins, liver engorgement).

The nurse assesses for effectiveness by monitoring the partial thromboplastin time. The usual goal is 2 to 2.5 times the control (normal) value. The nurse also monitors for manifestations of excess anticoagulation, bleeding (evidenced by blood in the urine, stool, and along the gums or teeth), subcutaneous bruising, or flank pain. When invasive studies are necessary, such as arterial blood gases, pressure is applied for 30 minutes to the puncture site.

The client typically experiences fear associated with the sudden onset of severe chest pain and inability to breathe. The person becomes anxious, restless, and apprehensive. Many times, the client will not reveal his or her innermost fears. The nurse's firm emotional support can be a stabilizing factor at this time. This support can effectively be shown by staying with the client. In addition, the nurse should give intensive care efficiently but should not display fear.

Analgesics are given as needed to reduce pain and anxiety. Anxiety and pain increase oxygen demand and dyspnea. Oral care is given while oxygen is in use, especially if the client breathes through the mouth.

PULMONARY HYPERTENSION

Pulmonary hypertension is defined as a prolonged elevation of the mean pulmonary artery pressure (PAP) above 18 mm Hg (norm, 10 to 20 mm Hg) and systolic PAP above 30 mm Hg (norm, 20 to 30 mm Hg) at rest or during exercise. Normally, the pulmonary circulation is a low-pressure, low-resistance system. Increased cardiac output in the healthy person, as with exercise, causes minimal elevations in PAP because of the large pulmonary vascular reserve. When pulmonary vasoconstriction is present, however, pressure elevation occurs because the pulmonary vasculature cannot accommodate increased blood flow.

Mild forms of pulmonary hypertension are generally caused by pulmonary vasoconstriction due to chronic hypoxia, acidosis, or both. The administration of oxygen, correction of acid-base imbalance, and use of vasodilating medications in select cases will generally return PAP to normal, either completely or partially.

Severe forms of pulmonary hypertension are classified as either secondary or unexplained (previously known as primary). Secondary pulmonary hypertension is usually associated with underlying heart or lung disease (e.g., pulmonary emboli, venocclusive disease, COPD). The cause of the unexplained form remains unclear. However, it occurs most often in young adults between the ages of 20 and 40 years; females are affected more often than are males. The condition is progressive, leading to right-sided heart failure and severe dyspnea.

Clients with mild pulmonary hypertension may be relatively asymptomatic. In moderate to severe forms, the main (and occasionally only) symptom is dyspnea. Fatigue, syncope, angina-like chest pain, palpitations, and muscular weakness may also occur. Chest x-ray examination reveals right ventricular hypertrophy, enlarged pulmonary arteries, prominent hilar vessels, and normal or reduced intrapulmonary vascular markings. Cardiac catheterization provides the most valuable diagnostic measurements. Typical findings include elevated PAP and increased arteriovenous oxygen differences accompanied by normal systemic blood pressure and normal to low cardiac output. Pulmonary wedge pressures remain normal because left ventricular function is typically unchanged.

The overall prognosis in severe pulmonary hypertension is poor. There is no known cure for the disorder, although treatment of the underlying cause of secondary forms may slow its progression. Vasodilator therapy may also be employed with some success. Additionally, supportive intervention will be used to reduce hypoxemia. A few clients with severe, unexplained pulmonary hypertension have undergone heart-lung transplantation, but data regarding long-term effectiveness are not yet available.[27] Interventions appropriate for underlying diseases and preparation for diagnostic procedures are incorporated into nursing care.

Disorders of the Pleura and Pleural Space

PLEURAL PAIN

Pleural pain is a common pulmonary symptom associated with a variety of disorders. It arises from the parietal pleura, which is richly supplied with sensory nerve endings. Pleuritic pain indicates the presence of pleural inflammation (pleurisy) due to pneumonia, pulmonary infarction, or other cause; pleural effusion; or pneumothorax. It is often accompanied by a pleural friction rub that is discovered during chest auscultation.

Pleuritic chest pain often develops abruptly and is usually severe enough that the client seeks medical attention. It frequently occurs only on one side of the chest, usually in the lower lateral portions of the chest wall, and is aggravated by deep breathing or coughing. Most of the time, the client can point directly to the exact location of the pain. However, pleural pain may also be referred to the neck, shoulder, or abdomen. Because other types of chest pain (e.g., cardiac pain, chest wall pain) may be misinterpreted as pleuritic pain, careful assessment is necessary.

Pleuritic chest pain may restrict normal respiratory efforts, leading to problems with gas exchange and airway clearance. If pain-relieving measures, including administration of prescribed analgesics, do not relieve the pain, the physician may perform an intercostal nerve block.

PLEURAL EFFUSION

A pleural effusion is an accumulation of fluid in the pleural space. Pleural fluid normally seeps continually into the pleural space from the capillaries lining the parietal pleura and is reabsorbed by the visceral pleural capillaries and lymphatics. Any condition that interferes with either the secretion or drainage of this fluid will lead to pleural effusion.

Causes of pleural effusion can be grouped into four major categories:

- conditions that increase subpleural capillary pressure (e.g., congestive heart failure)
- conditions that decrease capillary oncotic pressure (e.g., liver or renal failure)
- conditions that cause inflammation of the pleura, pleural spaces, or underlying structures (e.g., infections or tumors)
- conditions that impair lymphatic function (e.g., lymphatic obstruction)

Clinical manifestations of pleural effusion will depend on the amount of fluid present and the degree of lung compression. If the effusion is small (i.e., < 250 mL), its presence may be discovered only by chest x-ray examination. With large effusions, lung expansion may be restricted and the client may experience dyspnea, primarily on exertion. Tactile fremitus may be decreased or absent, and percussion notes may be dull or flat.

Management

PRIMARY PLEURAL EFFUSION

Thoracentesis (see Chap. 19) is used to remove excess pleural fluid. The fluid is then analyzed to determine if it is transudate or exudate. Transudates are substances that have passed through a membrane or tissue surface. They occur primarily in conditions in which there is protein loss and low protein content (e.g., left ventricular failure, cirrhosis, nephrosis). Transudative effusions are sometimes referred to as hydrothorax. Exudates are substances that have escaped from blood vessels. They contain an accumulation of cells, have a high specific gravity and a high lactate dehydrogenase level, and occur in response to malignancies, infections, or inflammatory processes. Exudates occur when there is an increase in capillary permeability. Differentiating between transudates and exudates helps establish a specific diagnosis. Diagnosis may also require analysis of the fluid for (1) white and red blood cells, (2) malignant cells, (3) bacteria, (4) glucose content, (5) pH, and (6) lactate dehydrogenase.

Pleural fluid may be (1) hemorrhagic, or bloody (e.g., if tumor is present, after trauma, or after pulmonary embolus with infarction), (2) chylous, or thick and white-colored (e.g., after lymphatic obstruction or trauma to the thoracic duct), or (3) rich in cholesterol (e.g., chronic, recurrent effusions due to tuberculous rheumatoid arthritis).

If there is a high white blood cell count and the pleural fluid is purulent, the effusion is called an empyema. An empyema of any amount requires drainage and treatment for the infection. If the pus is not drained, it may become thick and almost solidified or loculated (containing cavities). This is called fibrothorax. Fibrothorax may significantly restrict lung expansion and may require surgical intervention. The procedure, known as decortication, involves the removal of the restrictive mass of fibrin and inflammatory cells. Decortication is usually not performed until the fibrothorax is relatively solid, so it can be easily removed. After the procedure, closed chest drainage with suction (see Chap. 20) is used to re-expand the lung rapidly and fill the pleural space. If the fibrous material has restricted the lung for some time, the lung may not re-expand effectively, and further intervention (usually thoracoplasty), may be needed.

RECURRENT PLEURAL EFFUSION

In some cases, pleural effusions may recur despite repeated thoracenteses (e.g., malignancy-induced effusions), with resultant compromise of lung function or persistent pleural pain. Treatment of recurrent effusions is accomplished through obliteration of the pleural space. Methods of obliterating the pleural space include

- pleurectomy (pleural stripping). This procedure consists of surgically stripping the parietal pleura away from the visceral pleura. This produces an intense inflammatory reaction that promotes adhesion formation between the two layers during healing.
- pleurodesis. This involves the instillation of a sclerosing substance (e.g., unbuffered tetracycline, nitrogen mustard, talc) into the pleural space via a thoracotomy tube. This creates an inflammatory response that scleroses tissues together.

Because pleural space obliteration creates permanent changes, the client's existing and predicted postprocedure respiratory status must be carefully determined. If a large area is involved, significant alterations in ventilatory mechanics (e.g., deep breathing, coughing) may occur, leading to compromised respiratory function.

After the procedure, the nurse should closely monitor lung function, including respiratory rate and ventilation pattern. He or she documents alleviation or persistence of pleural pain and watches for indications of a return of the pleural effusion. Pulmonary function studies (see Chap. 19) and ABGs should also be evaluated.

BRONCHOPLEURAL FISTULA

A bronchopleural fistula is a connection between the pleural space and a bronchus. It may occur when an undrained empyema erodes into a bronchus or the pleural space does not heal spontaneously after chest tube removal (see Chap. 20). A bronchopleural fistula increases the risk of pleural infection. It may also compromise ventilation and oxygenation.

The management of a client with a bronchopleural fistula is often complex, requiring a critical care setting. Bronchopleural fistulas may be slow to heal. The client may be discharged home with a chest tube connected to a collection system. It is important that the client and family understand how to care for the chest tube and collection system, signs and symptoms of irritation at the chest puncture site, and changes in chest drainage that require the physician to be notified (e.g., blood).

METASTATIC PLEURAL TUMORS

Primary tumors in the lungs and other organs often metastasize to the pleura. The primary tumor is usually in a lung but may occur in the breast, ovaries, liver, kidneys, uterus, testicles, or larynx, or it may result from leukemia or lymphoma. Metastatic pleural disease causes about half of all pleural effusions.

Assessment findings with malignant pleural effusion are the same as for pleural effusion from other causes. Diagnosis of pleural effusion is by chest x-ray examination. The source of the effusion is determined by cytologic examination of pleural fluid obtained by thoracentesis. Intervention is the same as for pleural effusion and the primary malignancy (see previous discussion).

STUDY QUESTIONS

1. A client is admitted with the diagnosis of rule-out lung cancer. The nurse knows that lung cancer survival rates are poor because:
   A. Radiation therapy is ineffective because of the shielding effect of the ribs and sternum.
   B. Medical oncology therapeutic agents do not cross the alveolar-capillary membrane.
   C. Lung cancer often metastasizes before it creates noticeable symptoms in a client.
   D. Surgical intervention can never completely resect the tumor.

2. The nurse is caring for the client with chronic airflow limitation. Which of the following indicates that the client's respiratory status is deteriorating?
   A. Cough productive of thick, tenacious sputum
   B. Dyspnea and confusion
   C. Prolonged expiration and pursed-lip breathing
   D. Wheezes on auscultation

3. The nurse is caring for the client with the following nursing diagnosis: Gas Exchange, Impaired R/T decreased functional lung tissue, and hypoventilation secondary to pneumonectomy for lung cancer. Which nursing intervention is *not* appropriate for this client?
   A. Monitor closely for signs of mediastinal shift.
   B. Place the client in the high-Fowler's position.
   C. Turn the client side to side every 2 hours.
   D. Teach the client to splint the incision during coughing and deep breathing.

4. A client is admitted with the diagnosis of pneumonia, and the nurse assesses the following: increased respiratory rate, fever, dry mucous membranes, and a cough productive of thick, tenacious sputum. These assessment data support which of the following nursing diagnoses?
   A. Activity Intolerance R/T hypoxemia.
   B. Ineffective Breathing Pattern R/T pleuritic chest pain.
   C. Gas Exchange Impaired R/T ventilation-perfusion mismatch
   D. Fluid Volume Deficit, Risk for R/T insensible fluid loss

5. Diagnostic workup for tuberculosis involves multiple tests. However, the only method of confirming the diagnosis is:
   A. Chest x-ray
   B. Mantoux test
   C. Sputum culture
   D. Bronchoscopy

6. Which of the following clients is most at risk for developing acute respiratory distress syndrome?
   A. An 18-year-old with a fractured femur
   B. A 74-year-old who aspirates tube feeding
   C. A 45-year-old who is near drowning
   D. A 24-year-old with pregnancy-induced hypertension

7. Cigarette smoking is the most common cause of lung cancer. All of the following are also risk factors, *except:*
   A. Air pollution
   B. Radon gas exposure
   C. Chewing tobacco
   D. Chronic airflow limitation

8. The intensive care unit nurse is counseling family members of a client newly diagnosed with acute respiratory distress syndrome. The nurse should base his or her comments on the understanding that:
   A. The mortality rate is over 75 per cent.
   B. Multiple invasive therapies may be required.
   C. Intubation and mechanical ventilation are rarely utilized.
   D. Most deaths from ARDS occur in the first 24 hours.

CRITICAL THINKING EXERCISES

SCENARIO A

A 76-year-old resident of a nursing home aspirated a portion of her dinner on Tuesday and has been receiving appropriate treatment. Thursday, she was no longer responding to treatment and now is being admitted to your unit with a diagnosis of acute respiratory distress syndrome (ARDS).

1. As the nurse doing the admission to the Medical Intensive Care Unit, which respiratory assessment data do you anticipate?
2. Symptoms of cerebral hypoxia were responsible for the client's diagnosis of ARDS. Which symptoms would you anticipate in the elderly?
3. You apply supplemental oxygen at 6 L/minute via nasal cannula. What is the expected FIO_2 for this oxygen delivery device?
4. If this does not provide enough oxygen support for the client, she will have to be intubated and placed on mechanical ventilation. What criteria will be used to determine when to intubate?
5. Frequently with the ARDS client, positive end expiratory pressure needs to be added to the therapeutic regimen to maintain adequate tissue oxygenation at the lowest possible FIO_2. What is the therapeutic value of positive end expiratory pressure?

SCENARIO B

A 33-year-old divorced mother with two sons is a sales clerk at a busy retail store and has recently been diagnosed with bacterial pneumonia.

1. Sputum for culture and sensitivity are obtained and an antibiotic is prescribed based on the most common strain of bacterial pneumonia. What is this most common infecting agent?
2. The client describes the symptoms that brought her to the emergency room. What are the clinical manifestations of bacterial pneumonia?
3. What antibiotic do you think was prescribed for the client? How long will it take before the client starts to respond to antibiotic therapy? How long should she continue to take her antibiotics?

BIBLIOGRAPHY

1. Borkgren, M, & Gronkiewiez, C. (1995). Update your asthma care from hospital to home. *American Journal of Nursing, 95(1),* 26–34.
2. Boutotte, J. (1993). TB the second time around, *Nursing 93, 23(5),* 2–50.
3. Burrows, B. (1990). Airways obstructive diseases: Pathological mechanisms and natural histories of the disorders. *Medical Clinics of North America, 74(3),* 547–560.
4. Carpenito, L. J. (1992). *Nursing diagnosis: Application to clinical practice* (4th ed.). Philadelphia: J. B. Lippincott.
5. Carpenito, L. J. (1991). *Nursing care plans and documentation.* Philadelphia: J. B. Lippincott.
6. Caruthers, D. D. (1990). Infectious pneumonia in the elderly. *American Journal of Nursing, 90(2),* 56.
7. Coleman, D. A. (1986). Pneumonia: Where nursing care really counts. *RN, 49(2),* 23.
8. Davidson, P. T. (1989). The diagnosis and management of disease caused by M. avium complex, M. kansasii, and other mycobacteria. *Clinics in Chest Medicine, 10(9),* 431.
9. DeVito, A., & Kleven, M. (1987). Dyspnea. *RN, 50(6),* 38–46.
10. Eggland, E. T. (1987). Teaching the ABC's of COPD. *Nursing 87, 17(1),* 60.
11. Elpern, E. H. (1992). Lung cancer. In S. L. Groenwald, et. al. (Eds). *Cancer nursing principles and practices.* (2nd ed., pp. 952–973). Boston: Jones & Bartlett Publishers.
12. Epps, M. E. (1992). Diagnostic testing for patients with lung cancer. *Nursing Clinics of North America, 27(3),* 615–630.
13. Faber, L. P. (1991). Lung cancer. In A. Holleb, et. al. (Eds.) *American Cancer Society textbook of clinical oncology.* (pp. 194–211). Atlanta: American Cancer Society.
14. Fahey, V. A. (1994). *Vascular nursing* (2nd ed.). Philadelphia: W. B. Saunders.
15. Feinsilver, S. H. (1988). Respiratory failure in asthma and COPD. *Emergency Medicine, 21(4),* 90.
16. Goft, A. (1989). Clinical measurement of dyspnea. *Dimensions of Critical Care Nursing, 8(4),* 210–216.
17. Gross, N. (1990). Chronic obstructive pulmonary disease: Current concepts and therapeutic approaches. *Chest, 97(2),* 195–235.
18. Haas, F., & Axen, K. (1991). *Pulmonary therapy and rehabilitation: Principles and practice.* (2nd ed.). Baltimore: Williams & Wilkins.
19. Hahn, K. (1989). Sexuality and COPD. *Rehabilitation Nursing, 14(7),* 191.
20. Hunter, F. C., & Mitchell, S. (1993). Managing ARDS. *RN, 56(7),* 52–58.
21. Jess, L. W. (1992). Chronic bronchitis and emphysema: Airing the difference. *Nursing 92, 22(3),* 34–41.
22. Jess, L. W. (1992). When your patient has asthma. *Nursing 92, 22(4),* 48–51.
23. Johns, C. J., Scott, P. P., & Schonfeld, S. A. (1989). Sarcoidosis. *Annual Review of Medicine, 40,* 353.
24. Johnson, A. P. (1988). The elderly and COPD. *Journal of Gerontological Nursing, 14(12),* 20–24, 35–36.
25. Jones, M. A., Hoffman, L. A., & Delgado, E. (1994). A.R.D.S. revisited. *Nursing 94, 24(12),* 34–45.
26. Kersten, L. D. (1989). *Comprehensive respiratory nursing: A decision making approach.* Philadelphia: W. B. Saunders.

27. Lareau, S., & Larson, J. (1987). Ineffective breathing pattern related to airflow limitation. *Nursing Clinics of North America, 22(1),* 179.
28. Mandel, J. H., & Baker, B. A. (1989). Recognizing occupational lung disease. *Hospital Practice, 24(1),* 21.
29. Martin, R. (1990). The sleep-related worsening of lower airways obstruction: Understanding and intervention. *Medical Clinics of North America, 74(3),* 701–714.
30. Masden, L. A. (1990). Tuberculosis today. *RN, 53(3),* 44–50.
31. McCance, K., & Huether, S. (1994). *Pathophysiology.* (2nd ed.) St. Louis: Mosby-Year Book.
32. Meredith, J. W. (1988). Emergency management of chest injury, including complications and immediate life-threatening injury. *Topics in Emergency Medicine, 10(7),* 60.
33. Mitchell, R. S., Petty, T. L., & Schwarz, M. I. (1989). *Synopsis of clinical pulmonary disease* (4th ed.). St. Louis: Mosby-Year Book.
34. Naccarato, M., & Kresevic, D. (1989). Caring for adults who have cystic fibrosis. *American Journal of Nursing, 89(11),* 1462.
35. Nelson, D. M. (1992). Interventions related to respiratory care. *Nursing Clinics of North America. 27(2),* 301–323.
36. Noll, M. L. (Ed.). (1990). Respiratory care in adults. *AACN Clinical Issues in Critical Care Nursing, 1(2),* 237–326.
37. O'Brien, R. J. (1989). The epidemiology of nontuberculous mycobacterial disease. *Clinics in Chest Medicine, 10(9),* 407.
38. Perez-Stable, E. J., & Hopewell, P. C. (1989). Current tuberculosis treatment regimens: Choosing the right one for your patient. *Clinics in Chest Medicine, 10(3),* 323.
39. Raffin, T. A. (1986). Pancoast syndrome. *Hospital Medicine, 22(5),* 218.
40. Rostad, M. (1990). Advances in nursing management of patients with lung cancer. *Nursing Clinics of North America, 25(2),* 393.
41. Sexton, D. L. (1990). *Nursing care of the respiratory patient.* Norwalk, CT: Appleton and Lange.
42. Sheehy, S. B. (1992). *Emergency nursing: Principles and practice* (3rd ed.). St. Louis: Mosby-Year Book.
43. Shuey, K. M. (1989). Case studies in thoracic surgery. *Dimensions in Oncology Nursing, 3(4),* 14.
44. Vork, K. L., & Olson, D. K. (1990). Asbestos review and update. *American Association of Occupational Health Nurses, 38(4),* 160–164.
45. Votava, K. M., & Bartock, B. S. (1990). Home rehab for cardiopulmonary patients. *RN, 53(10),* 79.
46. Webster, J. R., & Kadak, H. (1991). Unique aspects of respiratory diseases in the aged. *Geriatrics, 46(7),* 31–43.
47. Wilson, S. F., & Thompson, J. M. (1990). *Respiratory disorders.* St. Louis: Mosby-Year Book.
48. Wyngaarden, J. B., Smith, L. H., & Bennett, J. C. (1992). *Cecil textbook of medicine* (19th ed.). Philadelphia: W. B. Saunders.
49. Young, J. R., Olin, J. W., & Bartholomew, J. R. (1991). *Peripheral vascular diseases.* St. Louis: Mosby-Year Book.

UNIT 7

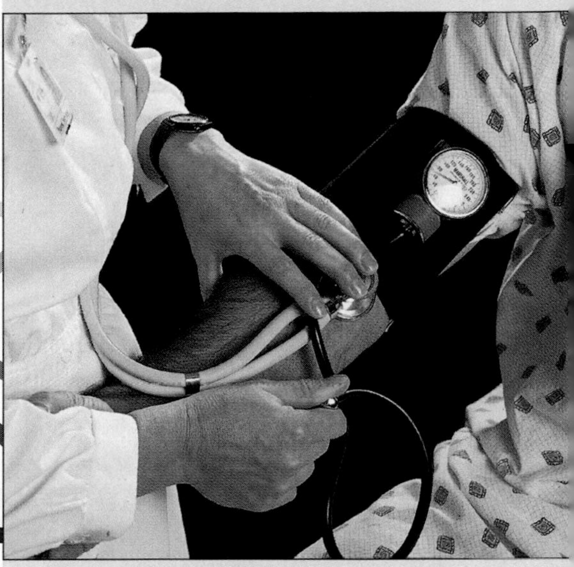

Cardiovascular Disorders

The heart is one of the few truly vital organs. Disorders related to the heart are currently the leading cause of death throughout the Western world. In the United States alone, nearly 1 million people die every year from cardiovascular ailments.

Fortunately, heart disease as a cause of death has been gradually declining since the early 1970s. With continued advances in research and clinical practice, the coming decades may see additional breakthroughs in the prevention and treatment of cardiovascular disorders.

Through research, the understanding of cardiovascular disease continues to expand. As a result, the care of clients with these disorders is currently one of the most progressive areas in nursing. This care is not confined to the critical care unit but extends throughout the scope of nursing practice, on medical-surgical units, in pediatric wards, on obstetric units, in surgery, and in the community.

Nurses caring for clients with cardiovascular disorders must understand cardiac structure and function. They must be able to identify life-threatening dysrhythmias on an electrocardiogram swiftly and be ready to initiate emergency intervention when appropriate. Because cardiovascular disorders are long-term, another important component of nursing care is client education about self-management of the disorder.

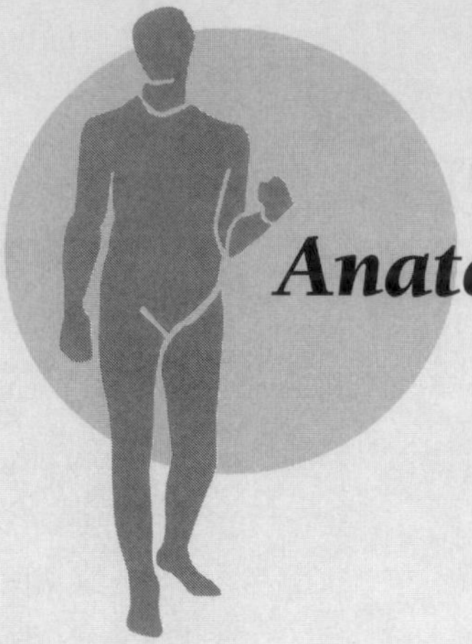

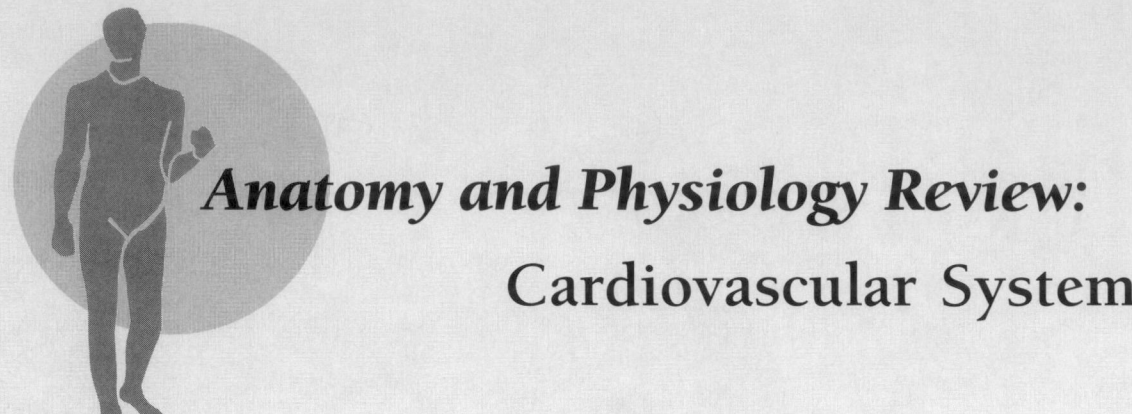

Anatomy and Physiology Review: Cardiovascular System

STRUCTURE OF THE HEART

Pericardium

The heart, located in the mediastinum between the two lungs, is enclosed by a loose-fitting sac called the pericardium, which protects it from trauma and infection. The sac is of tough fibrous connective tissue lined with a parietal layer of serous membrane. A visceral layer of serous membrane forms the outermost layer of the heart wall. A potential space known as the pericardial space (cavity) contains a thin layer of fluid that lubricates the tissue surfaces as they move against each other when the heart beats.

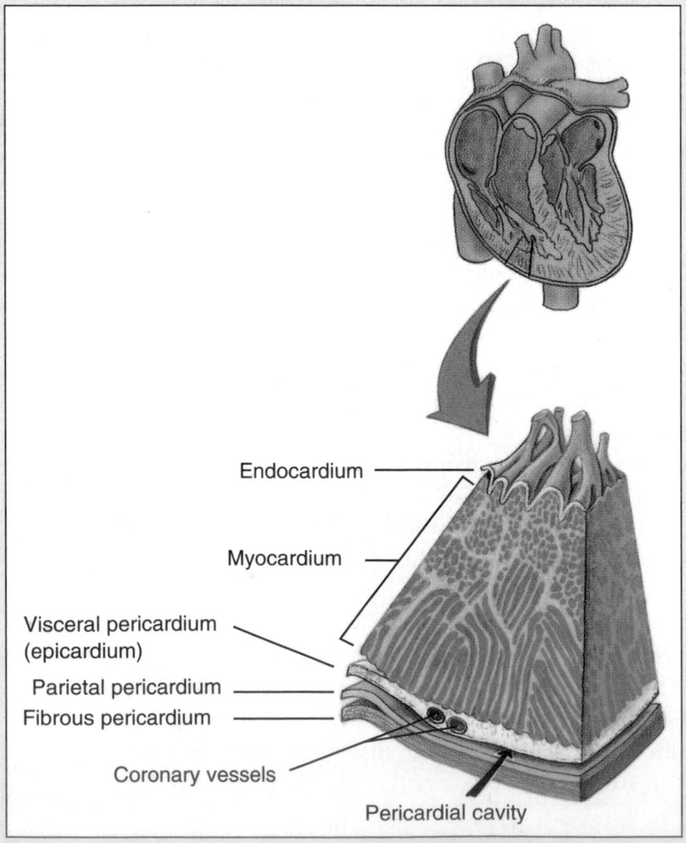

Layers of the heart wall.

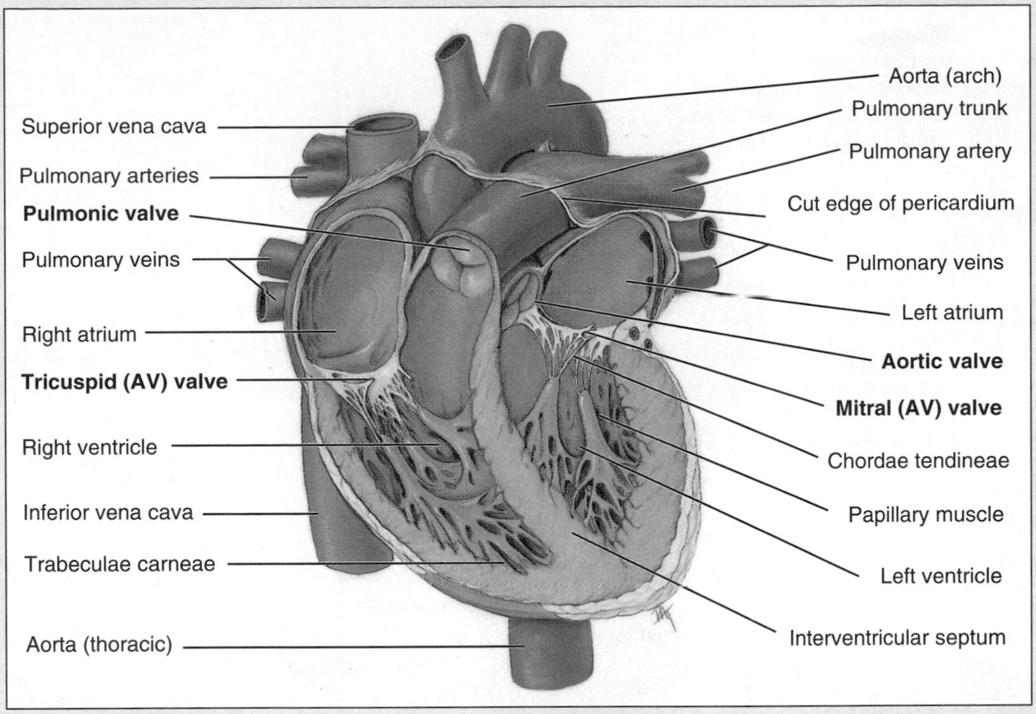

Chambers of the heart. (From Jarvis, C. [1992]. *Physical Examination and Health Assessment.* Philadelphia: W. B. Saunders Co.)

Layers of the Heart Wall

The heart wall consists of three distinct layers. The epicardium forms the outer surface and is the same as the visceral pericardium. The thick middle layer, the myocardium, is cardiac muscle. The thin innermost layer, the endocardium, is endothelium, which also covers the valves of the heart and is continuous with the lining of the blood vessels.

Heart Chambers

Each side of the heart consists of two chambers, a thin-walled collecting chamber (atrium) and a thick-walled pumping chamber (ventricle). A muscular septum separates the chambers on the right side of the heart from those on the left. Oxygen-poor blood enters the right atrium from the superior and inferior venae cavae and flows into the right ventricle, which pumps the blood to the lungs through the pulmonary arteries. Oxygen-rich blood from the lungs returns to the left atrium through four pulmonary veins. From the left atrium, the blood flows into the left ventricle, which pumps the blood through the aorta into systemic circulation.

Heart Valves

The heart has two types of valves that keep blood flowing in the correct direction. The valves between the atria and ventricles are called atrioventricular valves, and those between the ventricles and the large vessels that exit the heart are semilunar valves. Both types consist of fibrous connective tissue covered with endothelium.

Blood Supply to the Heart Wall

The myocardium of the heart wall is working muscle that needs a continuous supply of oxygen and nutrients to function with efficiency. Two main coronary arteries branch from the ascending aorta just above the aortic semilunar valve and encircle the heart; their branches penetrate the myocardium. The right coronary artery extends to the right and continues in the right atrioventricular sulcus to the posterior surface of the heart. The left coronary artery extends to the left for about 2 cm, then divides into two major branches: the left anterior descending and circumflex arteries. Unlike in other arteries, 75 per cent of the coronary artery blood flow occurs during diastole, when the heart is relaxed. Cardiac veins, which usually run parallel to the arteries, return blood from the myocardium to the right atrium.

PHYSIOLOGY OF THE HEART

The work of the heart, to pump blood, is accomplished by systematic contraction and relaxation of the cardiac muscle in the myocardium. Effective contractions depend on the electrophysiologic properties of the muscle and are coordinated by the conduction system of the heart.

Electrophysiologic Properties of the Heart

The electrophysiologic properties of cardiac muscle (excitability, automaticity, conductivity, refractoriness) regulate the heart rate and rhythm.

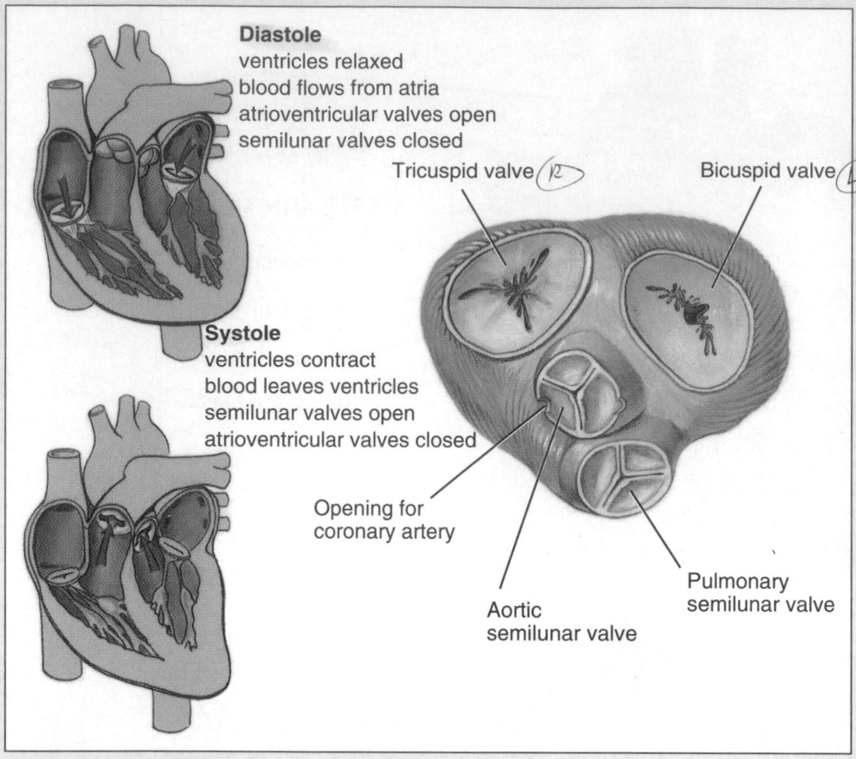

Valves of the heart as viewed from above.

- *Excitability* is the ability of cardiac muscle cells to depolarize in response to a stimulus. The unique nature of cardiac muscle cells enables them to function collectively as a unit, rather than as individual cells, so that once stimulated the whole heart muscle contracts. Excitability is influenced by hormones, electrolytes, nutrition, oxygen supply, medications, infection, and nerve characteristics.
- *Automaticity*, or rhythmicity, is the ability of cardiac cells to initiate an impulse spontaneously and repetitively, without external neurohormonal control. In contrast to other muscle tissue, which must be stimulated by a nerve in order to depolarize and contract, heart muscle can depolarize spontaneously and stimulate its own contraction. Cells with the highest rate of automaticity assume the role of pacemaker. Under

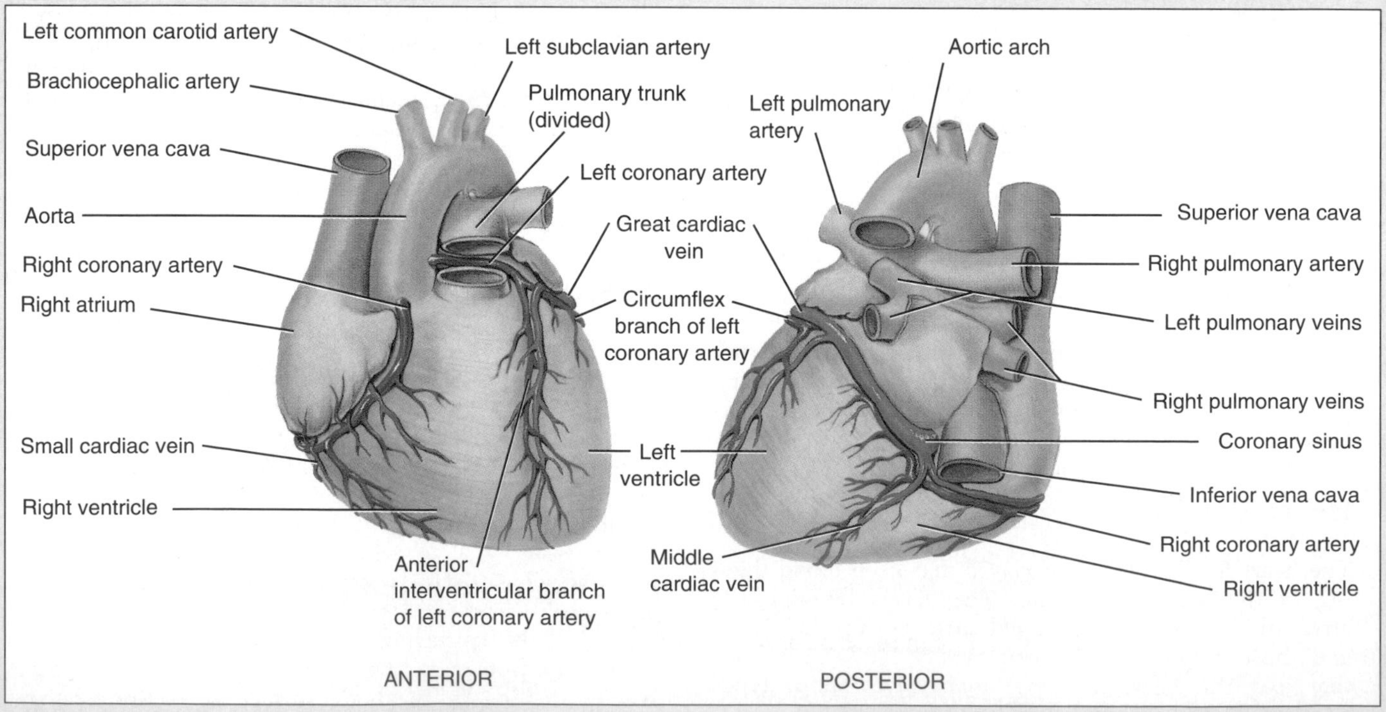

Blood supply to the myocardium.

Cardiac conduction system.

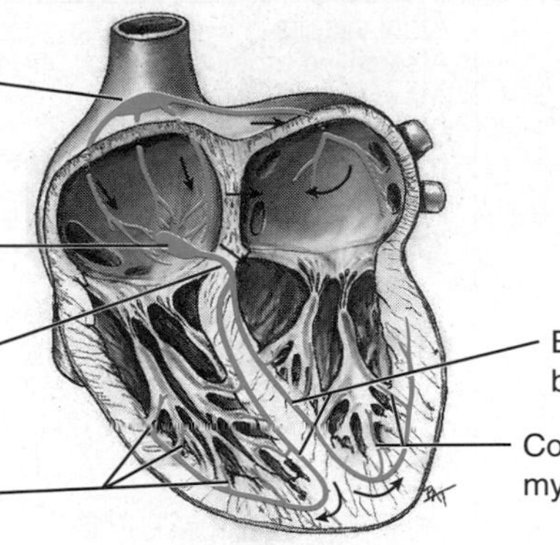

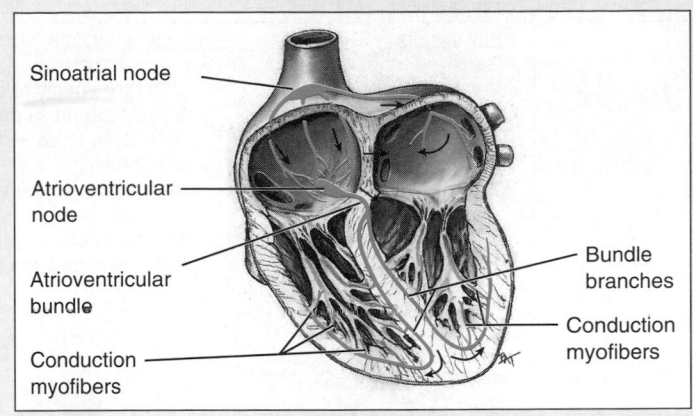

normal circumstances, this is the sinoatrial node.

- *Conductivity* is the ability of heart muscle fibers to propagate action potentials along and across cell membranes. Intercalated discs permit impulses to travel rapidly between adjacent cells so that the entire muscle mass acts together as a single unit.
- *Refractoriness* is the heart's inability to respond to a new stimulus while still in a state of contraction from an earlier stimulus. During the absolute refractory period, cardiac cells do not respond to any stimulus, however strong. During the relative refractory period, a stronger-than-normal stimulus can cause contraction. Myocardial refractoriness normally prevents uncontrolled rapid cardiac contractions and helps to preserve heart rhythm.

Cardiac Conduction System

The conduction system of the heart consists of modified cardiac muscle cells. Instead of contracting, these cells act somewhat like neural tissue by initiating impulses and rapidly conducting them throughout the myocardium to coordinate the contraction of the atria and ventricles. The conduction system has the following major components:

- *Sinoatrial (SA) node*—in the right atrium near the superior vena cava. Under normal circumstances the SA node has the fastest rate of spontaneous depolarization and initiates each heartbeat. For this reason, it is referred to as the pacemaker. Any myocardial tissue has the capability of taking over the role of pacemaker if that tissue generates impulses at a higher rate than the SA node. The sympathetic and parasympathetic nervous systems control the SA node. Impulses from the SA node stimulate atrial contraction.
- *Atrioventricular (AV) node*—in the lower portion of the interatrial septum. The AV node receives impulses from the SA node and delays the impulses about 0.07 second while the atria contract. This delay enables atrial contraction (atrial kick) to complete before the ventricles contract.
- *Atrioventricular bundle*—also called the bundle of His. The AV bundle is a short segment attached to the AV node. It divides into the right and left bundle branches.
- *Bundle branches*—course down either side of the interventricular septum. The right and left bundle branches terminate in conduction myofibers.
- *Conduction myofibers*—also called Purkinje fibers. These represent a diffuse network of conducting fibers that rapidly spread the wave of depolarization throughout the ventricular myocardium.

Cardiac Cycle

The cardiac cycle is the alternating contraction and relaxation of the heart chambers during one heartbeat. The two atria contract at the same time, and then they relax while the two ventricles simultaneously contract. The contraction phase of the chambers is called systole, and the relaxation phase is called diastole. Blood is returned to the atria from circulation during atrial diastole. Ventricular systole pumps blood from the ventricles into the circulatory pathways. When the terms systole and diastole are used alone, they refer to action of the ventricles. With a heart rate of 72 beats/minute, one cardiac cycle lasts 0.8 second.

Cardiac Output

Cardiac output is the volume of blood pumped by each ventricle in 1 minute. Because the primary function of the heart is to pump blood, this is a measure of its effectiveness. Cardiac output is calculated by multiplying the volume pumped out in one cardiac cycle (stroke volume) by the number of cycles or heartbeats in 1 minute (heart rate). Cardiac output ranges widely, averaging in adults between 4 and 8 L per minute. Adjustments in either stroke volume or heart rate can compensate for fluctuations in the other, or both can rise or fall at the same time. Cardiac index is another measure of heart function. It gives a better indication of how well the tissues are being perfused than does the cardiac output alone. The cardiac index is the cardiac output divided by the body surface area. Normal cardiac index range is from 2.5 to 4.0 L/min/m^2.

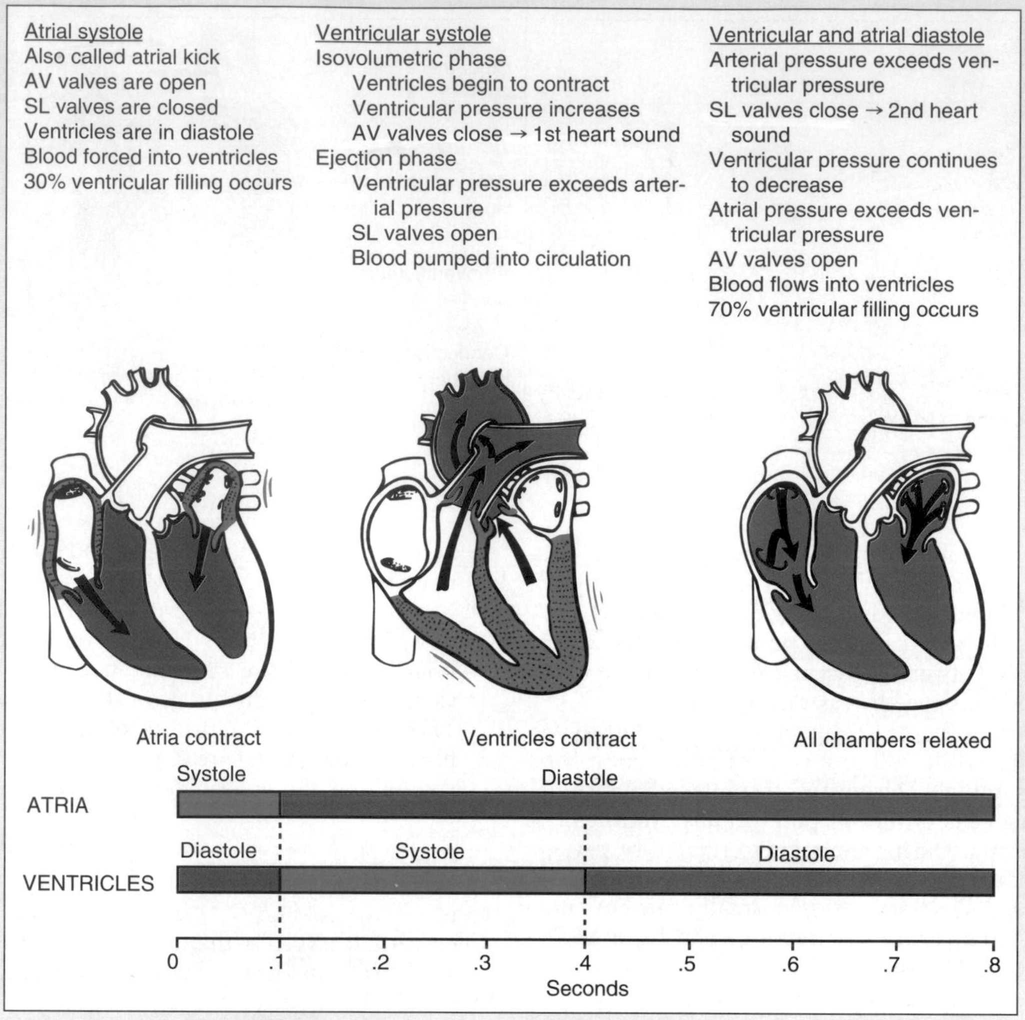
Atrial systole
Also called atrial kick
AV valves are open
SL valves are closed
Ventricles are in diastole
Blood forced into ventricles
30% ventricular filling occurs
Ventricular systole
Isovolumetric phase
Ventricles begin to contract
Ventricular pressure increases
AV valves close → 1st heart sound
Ejection phase
Ventricular pressure exceeds arterial pressure
SL valves open
Blood pumped into circulation
Ventricular and atrial diastole
Arterial pressure exceeds ventricular pressure
SL valves close → 2nd heart sound
Ventricular pressure continues to decrease
Atrial pressure exceeds ventricular pressure
AV valves open
Blood flows into ventricles
70% ventricular filling occurs
Atria contract
Ventricles contract
All chambers relaxed
Systole
Diastole
ATRIA
Diastole
Systole
Diastole
VENTRICLES
0
.1
.2
.3
.4
.5
.6
.7
.8
Seconds

Cardiac cycle.

Factors Relating to Cardiac Output

FACTOR	DESCRIPTION	RELATIONSHIP
Afterload	Resistance against which heart must work, i.e., arterial blood pressure	Increased afterload decreases stroke volume
End diastolic volume (EDV)	Amount of blood in ventricle when it is ready to contract; depends on venous return; sometimes called preload	Increased EDV increases stroke volume
Ejection fraction	Portion of EDV that is pumped from the ventricle during systole	Normally equals about $\frac{2}{3}$ EDV
Contraction strength	Force generated by myocardium during systole; increased by sympathetic stimulation and by increased EDV; decreased by hypoxia and metabolic acidosis	Increased contraction strength increases stroke volume
Starling's law	The greater the length of muscle fibers (stretch), the greater will be the contraction strength	Directly relates EDV to contraction strength
Heart rate	Number of cardiac cycles per minute; sinus tachycardia > 100 beats/min; sinus bradycardia < 60 beats/min; parasympathetic impulses decrease rate; sympathetic impulses increase rate; other variations caused by exercise, body size, age, gender, hormones, temperature, blood pressure, anxiety, stress, pain	Within limits and with similar stroke volumes, increased heart rate increases cardiac output

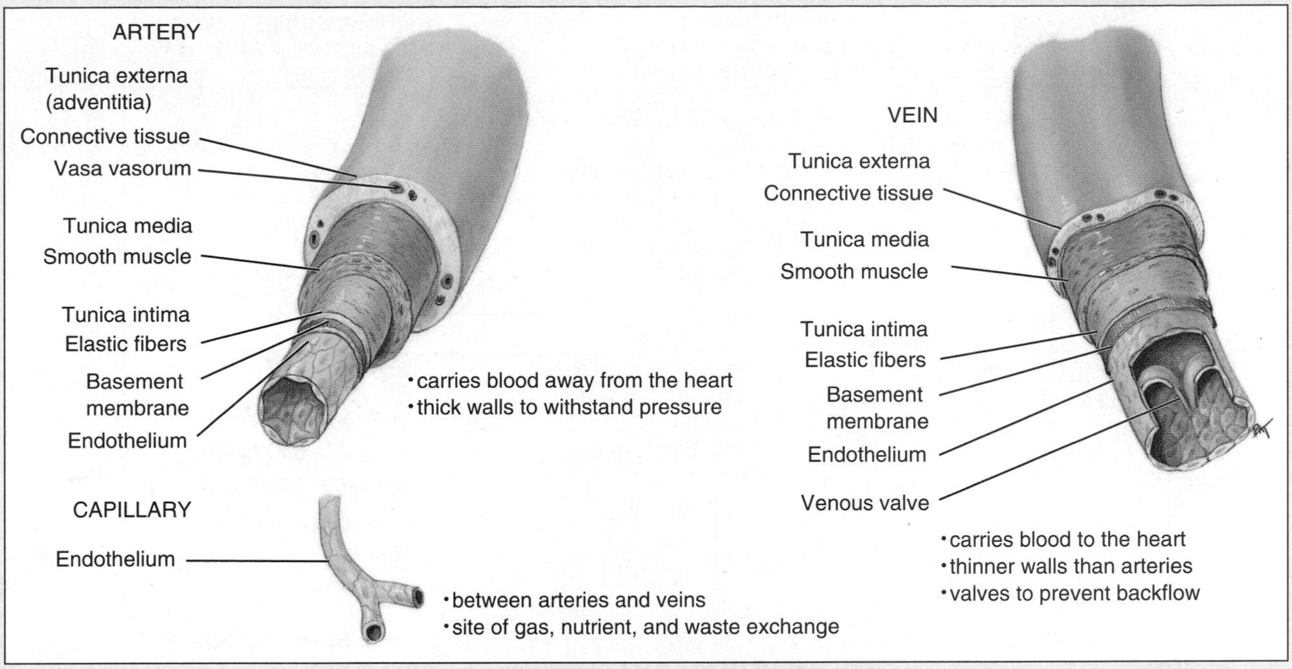

Structure of blood vessels.

BLOOD VESSELS

Blood vessels are the channels through which blood is distributed to body tissues. The vessels make up two closed systems of tubes that begin and end at the heart. One system, the pulmonary vessels, transports blood from the right ventricle to the lungs and back to the left atrium. The other system, the systemic vessels, carries blood from the left ventricle to the tissues in all parts of the body and then returns the blood to the right atrium. Based on their structure and function, blood vessels are classified as either arteries, capillaries, or veins.

Structure of Blood Vessels

The wall of an artery or vein consists of three layers, the tunica intima, tunica media, and tunica externa. The thickness of the wall and the amount of connective tissue and smooth muscle depends on the pressure the vessel must endure. Large arteries near the heart have elastic fibers in the tunica externa to allow expansion to accommodate the surge of blood ejected from the heart with each cardiac cycle. Smooth muscle in the tunica media changes vessel diameter to regulate blood flow and blood pressure.

Role of Capillaries

Capillaries have a vital role in the exchange of gases, nutrients, and metabolic waste products between the blood and tissue cells. Their distribution varies with the metabolic activity of the tissues. Metabolically active tissues have extensive capillary networks, while other tissues have a less abundant supply. Blood flow from the arterioles into the capillaries is regulated by smooth muscle cells, called precapillary sphincters, in the small arterioles. When the sphincters are open, blood flows through the capillary bed. When they are closed, blood passes directly from small arterioles into small venules. This allows blood to be diverted from one capillary bed to another for distribution to the regions that need it most at any given time.

Distribution of Systemic Blood Vessels

The systemic circulation provides the functional blood supply to all body tissues. The arteries carry oxygen-rich blood from the left ventricle to the capillaries in the tissues of the body. From the tissue capillaries, the veins carry oxygen-poor blood to the right atrium.

Blood Pressure

Blood pressure is the pressure of blood against vessel walls. Specifically, there is arterial pressure, venous pressure, and capillary pressure, to correspond to the three types of vessels. Both cardiac output and peripheral vascular resistance have a direct relationship to arterial blood pressure. Since stroke volume and heart rate affect cardiac output, they also influence arterial pressure. Blood volume and venous return also affect arterial pressure. Anything that narrows the opening in

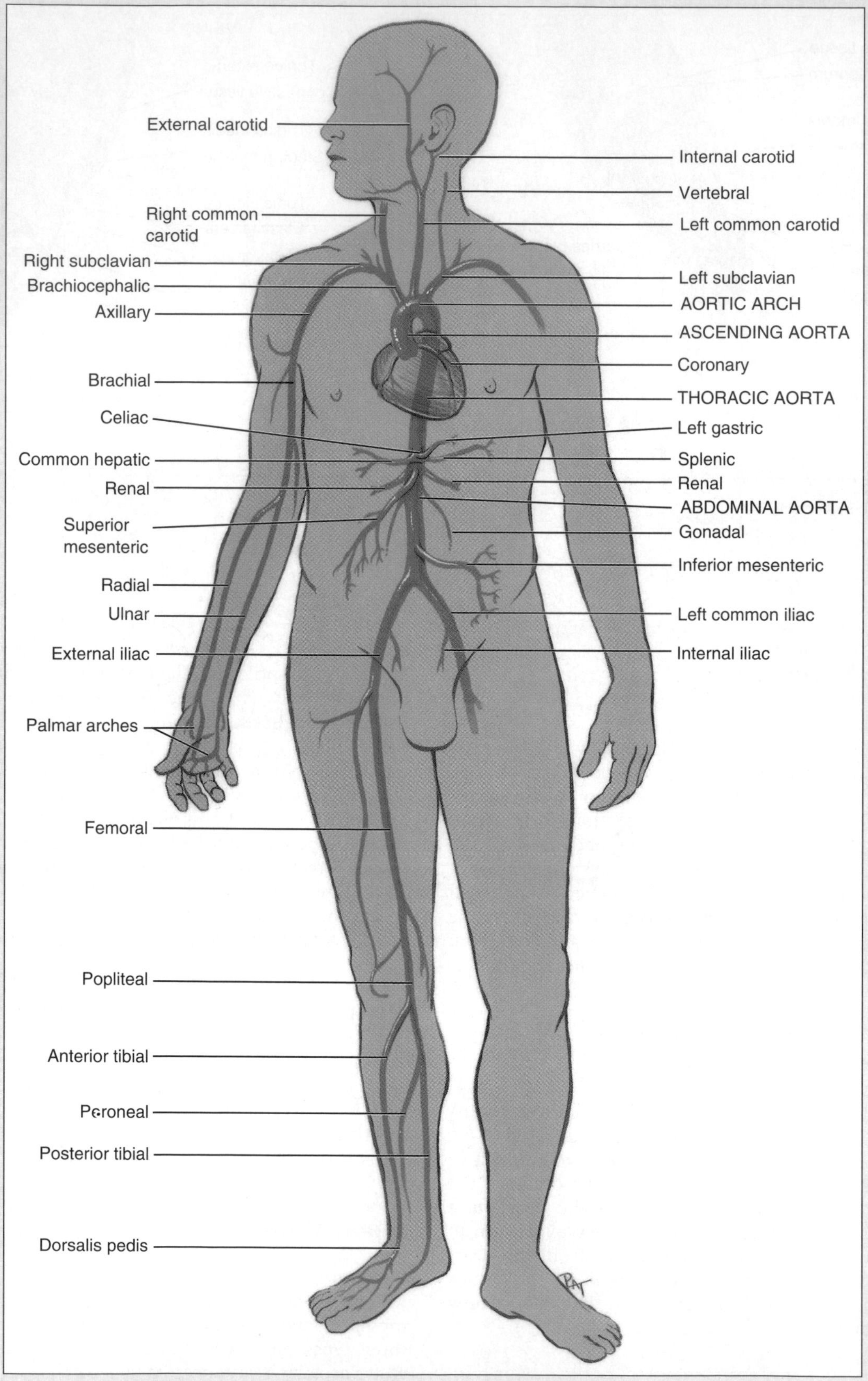
External carotid
Internal carotid
Vertebral
Right common carotid
Left common carotid
Right subclavian
Brachiocephalic
Left subclavian
Axillary
AORTIC ARCH
ASCENDING AORTA
Coronary
Brachial
THORACIC AORTA
Celiac
Left gastric
Common hepatic
Splenic
Renal
Renal
ABDOMINAL AORTA
Superior mesenteric
Gonadal
Inferior mesenteric
Radial
Ulnar
Left common iliac
External iliac
Internal iliac
Palmar arches
Femoral
Popliteal
Anterior tibial
Peroneal
Posterior tibial
Dorsalis pedis

Major systemic arteries.

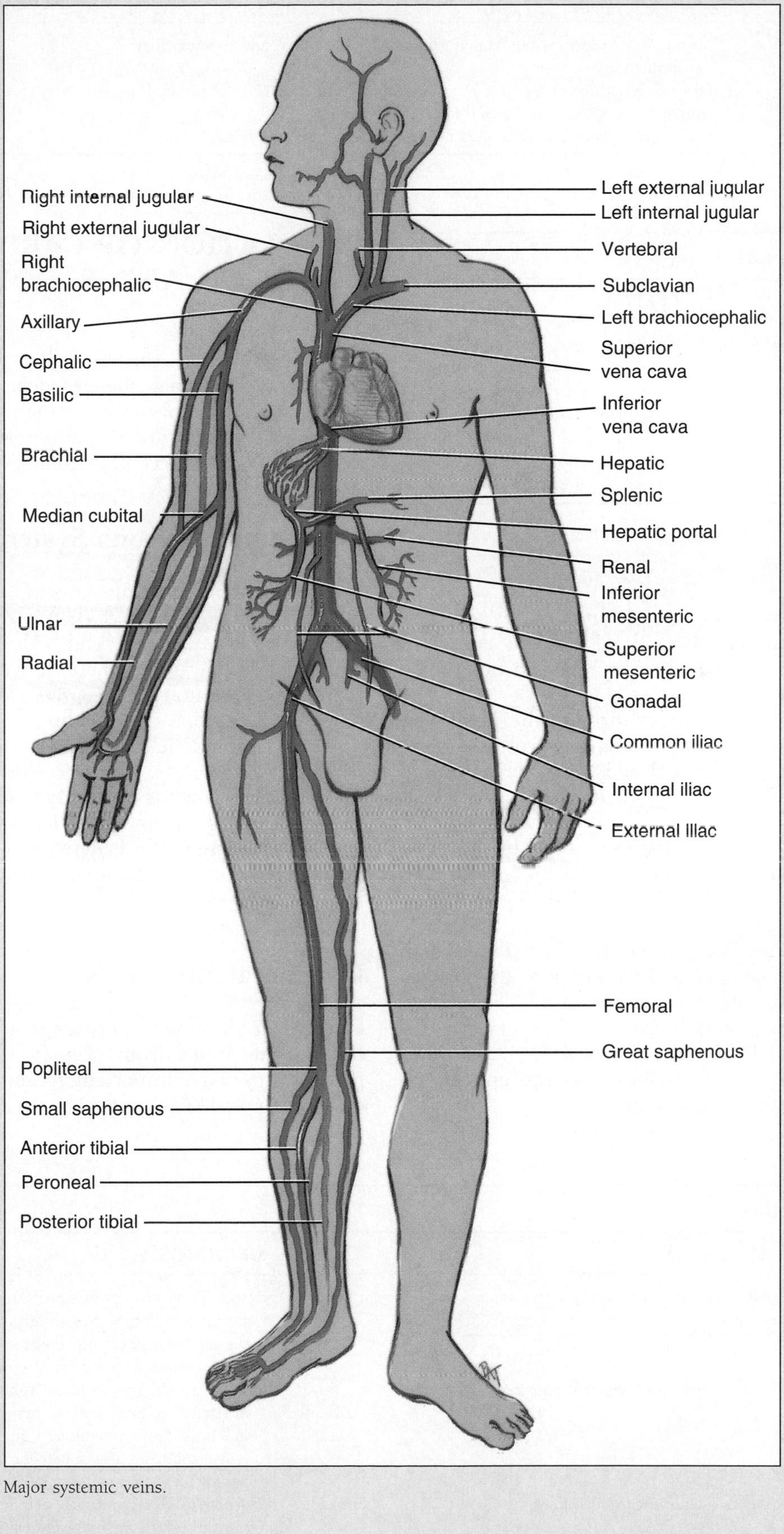
Right internal jugular
Right external jugular
Right
brachiocephalic
Axillary
Cephalic
Basilic
Brachial
Median cubital
Ulnar
Radial
Popliteal
Small saphenous
Anterior tibial
Peroneal
Posterior tibial
Left external jugular
Left internal jugular
Vertebral
Subclavian
Left brachiocephalic
Superior
vena cava
Inferior
vena cava
Hepatic
Splenic
Hepatic portal
Renal
Inferior
mesenteric
Superior
mesenteric
Gonadal
Common iliac
Internal iliac
External iliac
Femoral
Great saphenous

Major systemic veins.

Types of Arterial Pressure

PRESSURE	DESCRIPTION	NORMAL VALUE, mm Hg
Systolic pressure	Maximum pressure blood exerted on arterial walls as a result of ventricular contraction	100–140
Diastolic pressure	Force of blood exerted on arterial walls during relaxation (filling) phase	60–90
Pulse pressure	Difference between systolic and diastolic pressures	40–60
Mean arterial pressure	Equivalent to $\frac{1}{3}$ of the pulse pressure plus the diastolic pressure	70–105

Adrenergic Receptors

TYPE	LOCATION	EFFECT
$Alpha_1$	Arteries and veins	Peripheral vasoconstriction
$Alpha_2$	Arteries and veins	Peripheral vasoconstriction
$Beta_1$	Heart wall	Increases heart rate and myocardial contraction, which may increase cardiac output and blood pressure
$Beta_2$	Arterial walls	Arterial vasodilation

a vessel increases peripheral resistance, so it also increases arterial blood pressure. Blood viscosity and elasticity of the arterial walls also have a role in peripheral resistance.

By the time the blood passes through the capillaries and enters the veins, the force remaining from the contraction of the heart is minimal and there are no pulsations. Venous pressure is about 12 to 15 mm Hg. Pressure gradients to assist venous return to the heart against the force of gravity develop from (1) the contraction of surrounding skeletal muscles; (2) smooth muscle tone in the vessel walls; and (3) negative thoracic pressure during inspiration.

Capillary pressure is 25 to 30 mm Hg at the arterial end of the capillary and 12 to 15 mm Hg at the venous end. A high capillary pressure causes capillary filtration to increase and fluid to shift from the vascular system into the interstitial fluid (edema). Low capillary pressure moves fluid from the tissues into the circulatory system and increases blood volume.

REGULATION OF CARDIAC FUNCTION AND BLOOD PRESSURE

The ability of the cardiovascular system to adapt to internal and external changes depends on the integration of several factors. Among the most important regulatory mechanisms are the autonomic nervous system, various peripheral receptors, and several hormones.

Autonomic Nervous System

The sympathetic nervous system, through the neurotransmitter norepinephrine, increases (1) heart rate, (2) myocardial contractility, and (3) peripheral vasoconstriction. The parasympathetic nervous system, through the neurotransmitter acetylcholine, decreases both heart rate and myocardial contractility.

The sympathetic division also stimulates the adrenal gland to secrete norepinephrine and epinephrine. The response depends on the type and location of adrenergic receptors within the cell membranes of the heart and blood vessels. In general, epinephrine influences $alpha_2$ and $beta_2$ receptors, whereas norepinephrine predominantly affects $alpha_1$ and $beta_1$ receptors.

Peripheral Receptors

Changes in autonomic nervous system activity occur in response to input from sensory receptors in various parts of the body. Important receptors involved in cardiovascular reflexes include the baroreceptors, the

Peripheral Receptors

TYPE	LOCATION	MECHANISM
Baroreceptors	Walls of aortic arch and carotid sinus	Detect changes in arterial pressure; increases in pressure stimulate baroreceptors to send additional signals to the medulla, parasympathetic system responds; sympathetic system responds to low pressure
Stretch receptors	Right atrium and terminal regions of venae cavae	Respond to changes in blood volume reflected by amount of stretch in atrial wall; in hypovolemia, stretch receptors send fewer impulses to medulla, sympathetic system responds; parasympathetic system responds to hypervolemia
Chemoreceptors	Aortic arch and carotid bodies	Sensitive to changes in O_2, pH, and CO_2; information is transmitted to medulla, sympathetic or parasympathetic system responds as appropriate

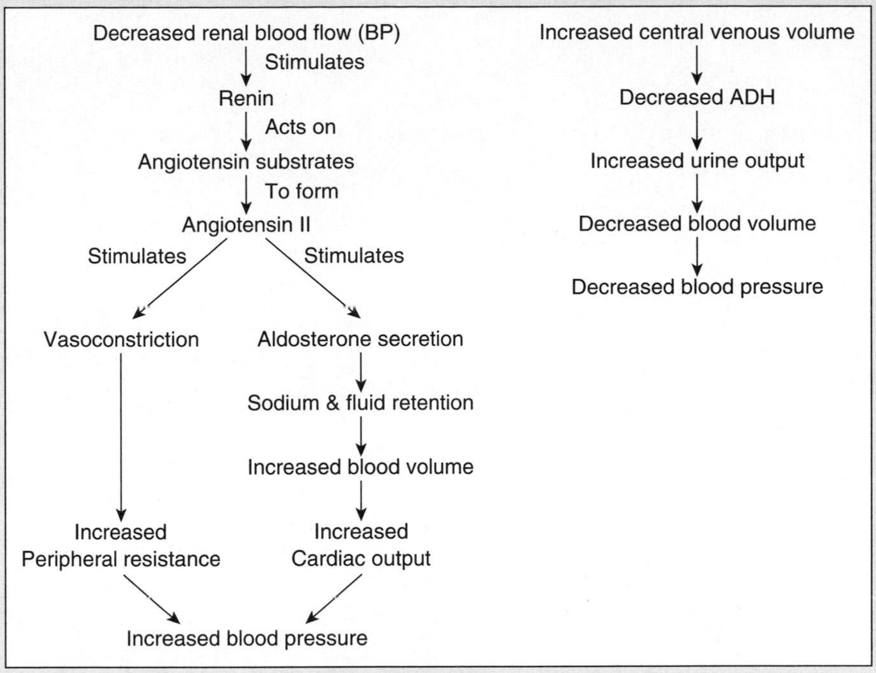

Hormonal mechanisms for increasing and decreasing blood pressure.

stretch receptors, and the chemoreceptors. These receptors send impulses to the medulla oblongata, which responds by altering sympathetic and parasympathetic activity.

Hormones

In addition to epinephrine and norepinephrine, the most important hormones regulating cardiovascular activity are antidiuretic hormone (ADH) and the renin angiotensin-aldosterone mechanism. ADH influences blood pressure indirectly by regulating vascular volume.

Renin is an enzyme that is synthesized, stored, and released from the kidney in response to a decrease in renal blood flow. Renin influences the production of angiotensin II, leading to vasoconstriction and release of aldosterone, which result in increased blood pressure and increased renal flow.

AGE-RELATED CHANGES

It is difficult to isolate the aging process of the cardiovascular system because it is so closely related to diet, exercise, and disease processes, but even when these factors are excluded, a clinical pattern of age-related changes emerges:

- Decreased myocardial contractility. This appears to have little effect on resting stroke volume but reduces cardiac reserve.
- General thickening of endocardium and valves. The valves tend to become more rigid and incompetent. Heart murmurs develop.
- Conducting fibers are replaced by fibrous tissue. This reduces the effectiveness of pacemaker cells, decreases conductivity, and leads to arrhythmias.
- Coronary arteries become rigid and thickened. This reduces the ability to respond to additional demands and increases the likelihood of coronary artery disease.
- Decrease in elastic fibers in vessel walls and increase in collagen. This makes the vessels less elastic and results in systolic hypertension and increased pulse pressure.
- Decrease in internal diameter of vessels. Generally this is due to an accumulation of lipids in the vessel walls. The decreased diameter leads to increased peripheral vascular resistance.

Chapter 23

Assessment of Clients with Cardio-vascular Disorders

Learning Outcomes

After completing this chapter, the learner will be able to:

1. Teach the client about the normal structure and function of the heart and blood vessels.
2. Explain to the client abnormalities of structure and function of the heart and blood vessels.
3. Conduct a nursing history and physical assessment of the client with actual or potential heart and blood vessel disorders.
4. Teach the client about diagnostic studies common to heart and blood vessel function.

Cardiovascular disease remains the most common cause of death in the United States. Because of the high incidence of heart disease and the seriousness of its complications, nurses must know how to assess the cardiovascular system. Assessment of the cardiovascular system incorporates data obtained from history taking, physical examination, and diagnostic studies. From these data, nursing and medical diagnoses are derived and the approach to client management is formulated.

Assessment of the Heart

HISTORY

Assessment is a dynamic process beginning with a health history, which includes information about the client's chief complaint, current health status, and medical history including family history.

Chief Complaint

The nurse inquires about the client's chief complaints to establish priorities for intervention and also to evaluate how well the client understands the presenting condition.

Common clinical manifestations of cardiovascular disorders include chest pain or discomfort, shortness of breath, palpitations, fainting, fatigue, and peripheral skin changes, such as edema. A client may have more than one major symptom. When this occurs, the nurse prioritizes them. Symptoms should be documented in chronologic order and any changes in their frequency or quality noted.

CHEST PAIN

Pain in the chest is a common symptom, occurring in various cardiac, pulmonary, musculoskeletal, gastrointestinal, neurologic, and anxiety-related disorders (Table 23–1). Common cardiac causes include myocardial ischemia, myocardial infarction, and pericarditis. Because chest pain is caused by a number of different conditions, it is highly variable in nature. To evaluate chest pain and its cause and to set care priorities, the nurse obtains and documents sufficient descriptive data about the pain in the following areas.

CRITICAL TO REMEMBER

A client experiencing chest pain who has a history of coronary artery disease should be treated as having cardiac ischemia until medical evaluation and laboratory studies are completed.

Characteristics. Chest pain may be described as a "strange feeling;" indigestion; dull, heavy pressure; burning; crushing; constricting; aching; stabbing; or tightness.

Location. Chest pain occurs in the substernal or precordial areas. It may be diffuse or localized. The pain may also radiate to the jaw, teeth, neck, one or both shoulders, arms, elbows, or the back. If the pain radiates down the arm, it may cause a sensation of numbness or tingling. Sometimes the client feels only the radiated pain and no precordial (in the chest) pain.

Duration. The nurse notes the time pain begins and ends to determine the duration of discomfort. Several intermittent, small episodes of chest pain are not considered as one long period of pain. Generally, the pain of myocardial infarction lasts longer than one-half hour or until intervention is instituted. Conversely, anginal pain typically lasts fewer than 20 to 30 minutes.

Severity. To assist the client in better quantifying the chest pain, the nurse may use a scale of 1 (least severe) to 10 (most severe). This recorded scale can then be used to compare future episodes of chest pain.

Precipitating or Aggravating Factors. The pain may sometimes be associated with certain factors or conditions. Such factors as emotional excitement, temperature extremes, exertion, deep sleep, position changes, deep breathing, straining during bowel movements, and eating may trigger the onset of chest pain.

Associated Symptoms. The nurse asks the client whether other symptoms accompany the onset of chest pain (i.e., anxiousness, shortness of breath, nausea, diaphoresis, vertigo, or palpitations).

Alleviating Factors. Anginal pain may be relieved by resting, sublingual nitroglycerin, and oxygen. Pain that is not relieved with these interventions and lasts 20 minutes or longer is highly suggestive of myocardial infarction.

SHORTNESS OF BREATH

Labored breathing, or shortness of breath, is termed *dyspnea*. Like chest pain, this common symptom affects clients with cardiac and pulmonary disorders.

CRITICAL TO REMEMBER

In about 25 per cent of clients with myocardial ischemia, dyspnea, not angina, is the chief complaint. This group includes the elderly as well as clients with diabetes mellitus.

Dyspnea also may occur in clients experiencing anxiety, depression, and various psychosomatic conditions.

Dyspnea occurs in several forms: exertional dyspnea, orthopnea, and paroxysmal nocturnal dyspnea.

Exertional Dyspnea. The most common form of cardiac-related dyspnea, exertional dyspnea, occurs during mild to moderate exercise or activity and disappears with rest. If severe, exertional dyspnea can greatly limit activity tolerance. The nurse asks the client to describe the degree of activity that typically precipitates the onset of dyspnea (e.g., walking up one flight of stairs or walking to the mailbox). The nurse also asks whether there was a sudden or gradual change in activity tolerance.

Orthopnea. This form of dyspnea occurs when the client is resting flat in bed and is relieved when the client assumes an upright or semivertical position. The nurse records the degree of head elevation that the client needs to breathe easily. Orthopnea usually indicates a more serious compromise of the cardiovascular system than does exertional dyspnea.

Paroxysmal Nocturnal Dyspnea. This form of dyspnea occurs in terrifying "attacks" during the night, waking the individual from sleep, and is associated with left ventricular failure.

FATIGUE

Easy fatigability on mild exertion is a frequent problem for clients experiencing cardiac disease. Progressive deterioration in activity tolerance results from the heart's inability to pump an effective volume of blood to meet the varying metabolic demands of the body.

PALPITATIONS

This common symptom of heart disease is a sensation of rapid, skipping, irregular, thumping, or pounding heartbeat, often accompanied by anxiousness. Tachycardia (rapid heart rate), increased force of myocardial contraction (as can occur with ingestion of caffeine or with emotional or physical stress), or premature ventricular beats may cause palpitations. The onset and termination of palpitations are often abrupt.

SYNCOPE

Syncope, or fainting, is a momentary loss of consciousness resulting from a reduction in cerebral blood flow. Certain cardiac and valvular disorders may cause an adverse change in circulatory hemodynamics and cause syncope or vertigo. Clients who are prone to syncopal episodes (e.g., those with Stokes-Adams syndrome) should wear Medic Alert bracelets to inform emergency health-care providers.

WEIGHT GAIN

As a result of fluid accumulation, an expanded blood volume may result when the heart fails. An increase in body weight of 3 pounds or more within 24 hours results from fluid rather than body mass changes. The nurse asks the client about trends in weight changes. Body weight is a sensitive indicator of water and sodium retention and will increase even before edema occurs.

Medical History

The medical history explores the health history of both the client and family members in an attempt to identify nonmodifiable and modifiable risk factors that may have contributed to the development of cardiovascular symptoms. The client is asked about several areas, discussed next.

CHILDHOOD AND INFECTIOUS DISEASES

Besides obtaining the usual data regarding common childhood diseases and immunizations, the nurse also asks about the client's experiences with rheumatic fever and severe streptococcal infections. These two conditions are associated with structural heart disease. The presence of known congenital anomalies is also ascertained.

MAJOR ILLNESSES AND HOSPITALIZATIONS

The history or presence of any major illness is determined. Particular attention is paid to those conditions that have the greatest influence on the client's current cardiovascular performance (i.e., diabetes mellitus, chronic obstructive lung disease, kidney disease, anemia, hypertension, stroke, gout, thrombophlebitis, collagen diseases, and bleeding disorders). The nurse inquires about previously performed cardiovascular diagnostic studies, such as an electrocardiogram (ECG) or an exercise stress test. Results of such studies provide baseline data for comparative analysis when later studies are performed.

MEDICATIONS

Prescription, over-the-counter, and recreational drug use is evaluated and documented. Whenever possible, brand names or simple descriptors should be used instead of generic names. For example, the nurse asks whether the client is currently taking "water pills," "heart pills," or "blood pressure" medications. Numerous medications can affect the overall performance of the cardiovascular system. The nurse asks specifically about the use of the following agents: antihypertensives, diuretics, vasodilators (nitroglycerin), cardiotonic drugs (digoxin), anticoagulants, bronchodilators, contraceptives, and steroids. Certain noncardiac medications can also have profound secondary effects on cardiovascular performance. For example, tricyclic antidepressants and other psychotropic medications can potentiate dysrhythmias; oral contraceptives increase the incidence of thrombophlebitis; steroid use may cause hypertension and increases fluid retention; and various antineoplastic agents may be cardiotoxic, causing dysrhythmias and cardiomyopathy.

Cocaine toxicity is a major threat to the cardiovascular system. Its systemic sympathomimetic effects result in a "fight or flight" response, which increases heart rate, contractility, blood glucose levels, and peripheral vasoconstriction. Cocaine also potentiates the effects of the circulating catecholamines (epinephrine and norepinephrine).

PSYCHOSOCIAL HISTORY AND LIFE-STYLE

Information in this area provides abundant data about risk factors, such as tobacco use, for the development of

TABLE 23–1 Assessment of Chest Pain

CONDITION	LOCATION	QUALITY	SEVERITY	COURSE	AGGRAVATING OR RELIEVING FACTORS	SYMPTOMS OR SIGNS
Angina	Retrosternal region; radiates to neck, jaw, epigastrium, shoulders, arms—left common	Pressure, burning, squeezing, heaviness, indigestion	Moderate to severe	< 10 minutes	Aggravated by exercise, cold weather, emotional stress, or after meals; relieved by rest or nitroglycerin; atypical (Prinzmetal's) angina may be unrelated to activity and caused by coronary artery disease	S_4, paradoxical split S_2 during pain
Intermediate syndrome or coronary insufficiency	Same as angina	Same as angina	Increasingly severe	> 10 minutes	Same as angina, with gradually decreasing tolerance for exertion	Same as angina
Myocardial infarction	Substernal; may radiate like angina	Heaviness, pressure, burning, constriction	Severe, sometimes mild (in 25% of patients)	Sudden onset; lasting longer than 15 minutes	Unrelieved	Shortness of breath, sweating, weakness, nausea, vomiting, severe anxiety
Pericarditis	Usually begins over sternum and may radiate to neck and down left upper extremity	Sharp, stabbing knifelike	Moderate to severe	Lasts many hours to days	Aggravated by deep breathing, rotating chest or supine position; relieved by sitting up and leaning forward	Pericardial friction rub, syncope, cardiac tamponade, pulsus paradoxus (Kussmaul's sign)
Dissecting aortic aneurysm	Anterior chest; radiates to thoracic area of back; may be abdominal; pain shifts in chest	Tearing	Excruciating, tearing, knifelike	Sudden onset, lasts for hours	Unrelated to anything	Lower blood pressure in one arm, absent pulses, paralysis, murmur of aortic insufficiency, pulsus paradoxus, stridor; myocardial infarction can occur
Mitral valve prolapse syndrome	Substernal; sometimes radiates to the left arm, back, jaw	Stabbing, sharp	Variable; generally mild but can become severe	Episodes are paroxysmal, may be prolonged	Not related to exertion, not relieved by nitroglycerin or rest	Variable palpitations, dizziness, syncope, dyspnea

Pulmonary embolism (most pulmonary emboli do not produce chest pain)	Substernal "anginal"	Not pleuritic unless infarction exists	Can be severe	Sudden onset; lasts minutes to < hour	May be aggravated by breathing	Fever, tachypnea, tachycardia, hypotension, elevated jugular venous pressure, right ventricular lift, accentuated P_2, occasional murmur of tricuspid insufficiency and right ventricular S_4; with infarction usually in the presence of congestive heart failure, rales, pleural rub, hemoptysis, clinical phlebitis present in minority of cases
Pulmonary hypertension	Substernal	Pressure; oppressive	Variable		Aggravated by effort	Pain usually associated with dyspnea; right ventricular lift, accentuated P_2
Spontaneous pneumothorax	Unilateral	Sharp, well localized		Sudden onset; lasts many hours	Painful breathing	Dyspnea, hyperresonance, and decreased breath and voice sounds over involved lung
Pneumonia with pleurisy	Localized over area of consolidation	Pleuritic, well localized	Moderate		Painful breathing	Dyspnea, cough, fever, dull to flat percussion, bronchial breathing, rales, occasional pleural rub
Gastrointestinal disorders	Lower substernal area, epigastric, right or left upper quadrant	Burning, colic-like aching			Precipitated by recumbency or meals	Nausea, regurgitation, food intolerance, melena, hematemesis, jaundice
Musculoskeletal disorders	Variable	Aching		Short or long duration	Aggravated by movement, history of muscle exertion	Tender to pressure or movement
Neurologic disorders (herpes zoster)	Dermatomal in distribution, usually localized to a point	Sharp burning; commonly, location of pain moves from place to place		Prolonged period of time	Unassociated with external events	Rash appears in area of discomfort with herpes
Anxiety states			Mild to moderate	Varies; usually very brief	Situational anger	Sighing respirations, often chest wall tenderness

P_2, pulmonic second sound.
From Andreoli, K., et al. (1987). *Comprehensive cardiac care* (6th ed., pp. 54–55). St. Louis: C. V. Mosby.

cardiovascular disease. From this background information, the nurse formulates a plan to assist the client in making necessary life-style adaptations to promote health and lessen disease. Chapter 24 covers such risk factors in more detail.

Review of Systems

The nurse asks the client about past problems involving the cardiovascular system, including chest pain, palpitations, shortness of breath (including exertional dyspnea, orthopnea, and paroxysmal nocturnal dyspnea), fatigue, edema, wheezing, fainting (syncope), weight gain, heart murmurs, hypertension, and history of rheumatic fever.

Because cardiovascular problems also affect the pulmonary, renal, and neurologic systems, the nurse asks about productive cough, decreased urination, dark or concentrated urine, edema of the legs, dizzy spells, and memory loss.

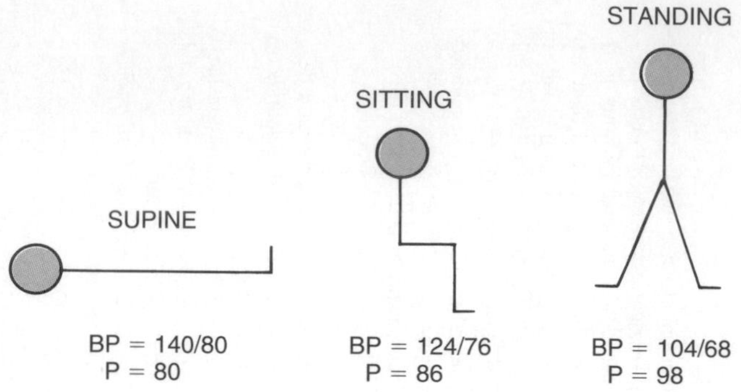

Figure 23–1
Recording postural blood pressure (BP). After measuring the client's BP and pulse in the supine position, leave the BP cuff in place and assist the client to sit. Then measure the BP within 15 to 30 seconds. Assist the client to stand, and measure again. A drop of more than 10 to 15 mm Hg systolic and more than 10 mm Hg diastolic pressure indicates postural hypotension. Postural hypotension is typically accompanied by a 10 to 20 per cent increase in heart rate (pulse). Sample measurements given earlier indicate postural hypotension.

PHYSICAL EXAMINATION

Every nurse should be able to perform a basic cardiovascular examination. Assessment of the client's cardiovascular status must be ongoing because the underlying condition can change dramatically within minutes. A physical examination involves obtaining objective data via observation, palpation, and auscultation. Percussion is rarely performed to assess cardiovascular status.

Blood Pressure

The nurse measures blood pressure (BP) in both arms to rule out dissecting aortic aneurysm, coarctation of the aorta, vascular obstruction, vascular outlet syndromes, and errors in measurement. If the client's arms are inaccessible, pressures are obtained using the thighs and popliteal artery or the calves and posterior tibial artery. If pressures are difficult to auscultate, systolic pressures can be determined through palpation or by using a Doppler ultrasound flowmeter.

POSTURAL BLOOD PRESSURE

A postural BP reading is taken when an extracellular volume depletion or decreased vascular tone is suspected. Blood pressure is recorded in relation to the client's position (Fig. 23–1).

PARADOXICAL BLOOD PRESSURE (PULSUS PARADOXUS)

An abnormal drop in systolic BP of greater than 10 mm Hg during inspiration, paradoxical BP is common in pericardial tamponade, constrictive pericarditis, and pulmonary hypertension. To check for paradoxical BP, the nurse places a sphygmomanometer on the client's arm and a stethoscope over the brachial artery and instructs the client to breathe normally. The nurse inflates the cuff 20 mm Hg above the systolic BP, then slowly deflates (1–2 mm Hg/sec) the cuff, and listens for Korotkoff's sounds to appear only during expiration. (Sounds are first heard during expiration and then during inspiration.) The nurse continues deflating the cuff until Korotkoff's sounds are heard equally well during inspiration and expiration. The degree of paradoxical BP is the difference between the BP when sounds were first heard during expiration and the BP when sounds were heard on both expiration and inspiration. Normally, this difference is less than 10 mm Hg. If the client has normal breathing and a systolic difference greater than 10 mm Hg, possible cardiac compression, including a cardiac tamponade, is considered.

Pulse

Pulses can have varying characteristics (Box 23–1). If the pulse is irregular, the nurse assesses for a pulse deficit by taking apical and radial pulses simultaneously, noting differences in rate. Peripheral pulse assessment is discussed in Chapter 26.

Respirations

In assessing breathing pattern, the nurse notes the rate, rhythm, depth, and quality. Variations in respiratory rate and character could indicate heart failure or pulmonary edema. The nurse auscultates the lungs for crackles, rhonchi, or other abnormal breath sounds. Severe left ventricular failure may produce pulmonary congestion and resulting frothy sputum with deep respiratory effort.

BOX 23–1

Abnormal Pulse Variations

Water-hammer pulse is a large, bounding pulse with a rapid rise and fall. It is associated with an increased stroke volume and widened pulse pressure, such as occurs with emotional excitement. It may be seen in aortic regurgitation and patent ductus arteriosus.

Pulsus tardus is a weak and feeble pulse, with a slow upstroke and prolonged peak. It is associated with a decrease in stroke volume and diminished pulse pressure, as seen in hypovolemic shock.

Pulsus alternans has a regular rhythm along with alterations in pulse amplitude. Strong beats alternate with weak ones. This type of pulse may be seen in myocardial infarction and congestive heart failure when the left ventricle function is depressed.

Bigeminal pulse results primarily from an underlying rhythm disturbance, which is most commonly associated with premature ectopic beats. A strong beat alternates with a premature (early), weak beat. The irregularity of the pulse differentiates this type of pulse from pulsus alternans.

Pulsus bisferiens is characterized by a rapid upstroke and has two systolic peaks. This pulse may be present in aortic regurgitation (with or without stenosis) and large left-to-right shunts, and idiopathic hypertrophic subaortic stenosis (hypertrophic obstructive cardiomyopathy). This pulse is best felt in the carotid artery.

Head and Neck

In examining the head, the nurse pays particular attention to the lips, ear lobes, and buccal mucosa. A bluish tinge or duskiness indicates central cyanosis, implying serious heart or lung disease in which the hemoglobin is not able to saturate fully with oxygen. Peripheral cyanosis usually accompanies this condition.

EXAMINATION OF NECK VEINS

The nurse examines the neck veins to estimate central venous pressure (CVP). The distensibility of the neck veins reflects the pressure and volume changes within the right atrium. The internal jugular veins, although harder to detect than the external jugular veins, are more reliable indicators of CVP (Figs. 23–2 and 23–3). The external jugular vein can be easily engorged with only slight provocation (i.e., breath holding, neck twisting, and constrictive clothing). Exceptions may be found in weight lifters, football players, and professional speakers and singers, who often have overdeveloped neck muscle tendons. The vessels are prominent and visible but soft and compressible.

To assess jugular vein distention, one must follow the steps listed in Box 23–2.

The timing and amplitude of the jugular vein pulsations may also be assessed to evaluate right-sided heart function, tricuspid valve performance, and the presence of certain dysrhythmias.

EXAMINATION OF CAROTID ARTERIES

Examining the carotid arteries provides evidence regarding the adequacy of stroke volume and the patency of the arteries.

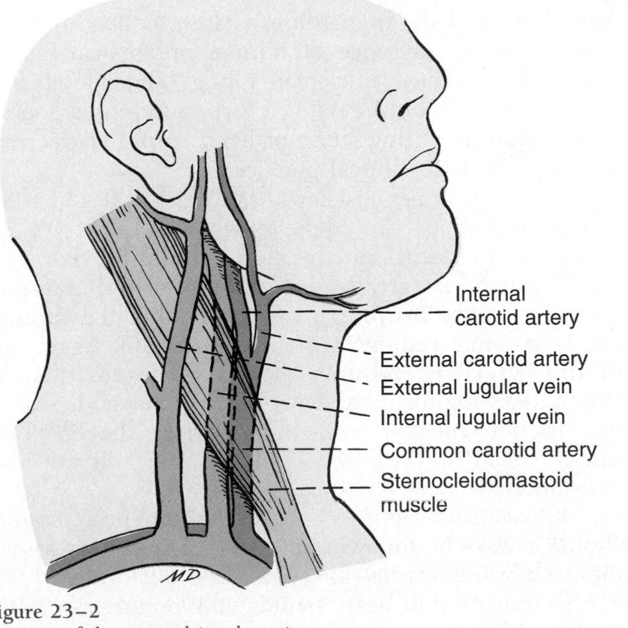

Figure 23–2
Location of the internal jugular vein.

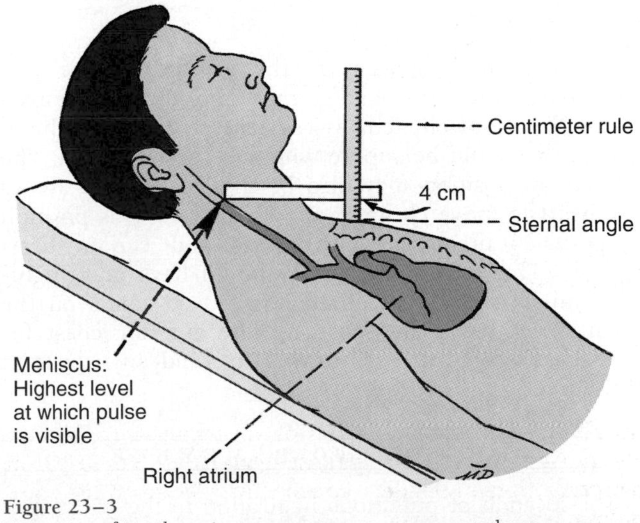

Figure 23–3
Estimation of jugular vein measurement to assess central venous pressure.

BOX 23–2

Assessing Jugular Vein Distention

- The client should assume a relaxed supine position with the head of the bed at an angle of comfort. Ideally, the head of the bed should be inclined between 15 and 30 degrees to maximize jugular vein prominence. In clients with greatly increased right atrial pressure, head elevations from 45 to 90 degrees may be required.
- A small pillow should be used to support the client's head, avoiding sharp neck flexion. The head should be turned slightly away from the examiner. Any clothing that compresses the neck or upper thorax must be removed.
- Tangential (oblique) lighting should be used so that small shadows are cast on the neck, making the veins more apparent. Observe both sides of the neck. The internal jugular vein lies deep to the sternocleidomastoid muscle and runs in the same direction along its length to the jaw and ear lobe (see Fig. 23–2). The pulsations of the internal jugular should be identified. The external jugular may be used if the internal jugular is not visible.
- The highest point at which the internal jugular pulses can be seen (the meniscus) should be noted. The sternal angle (manubrial joint) should be used as a reference point to measure the height of venous pulsation. This point is approximately 4 to 5 cm above the center of the right atrium. Using a centimeter ruler, one measures the vertical distance between the sternal angle and the point of highest venous pulsations. Figure 23–3 demonstrates the method of jugular vein measurement.
- Normally, the value is less than 3 or 4 cm above the sternal angle with the head of the bed elevated at 30 to 40 degrees. Higher values indicate increased right atrial or right ventricular pressure as seen in right ventricular failure, tricuspid regurgitation, or pericardial tamponade. Flat jugular veins noted with the client lying supine may suggest extracellular volume depletion. Unilateral distention may indicate vessel obstruction on that side.

CRITICAL TO REMEMBER

With the finger tips, the nurse gently palpates the carotid arteries one side at a time, checking and comparing pulse rate, rhythm, and amplitude.

A bruit (a blowing sound) may be heard by listening to the carotid arteries with the diaphragm of a stethoscope while the client holds his or her breath. Tracheal breath sounds are heard if respiration is ongoing. A bruit generally indicates that the carotid artery has narrowed. Bruits typically result from atherosclerosis or radiation of sounds from an aortic valve murmur.

Chest

INSPECTION AND PALPATION OF THE PRECORDIUM

Inspection and palpation of the precordium are performed together to detect normal and abnormal pulsations. For more efficient assessment of the precordium, the client should be supine with the chest exposed. The left lateral position may also be used because it allows the heart to move closer to the chest wall. This position accentuates precordial movements and certain heart sounds. The examination area should have good lighting and be warm and quiet. The nurse stands on the client's right side and observes the anterior chest for size, shape, symmetry of movement, and any apparent pulsations.

CRITICAL TO REMEMBER

The location of pulsations in relation to the intercostal space and the midclavicular line is recorded.

Palpation is used to confirm the observed phenomenon. When palpating, the fingers and palmar aspect of the hand are used.

Normally, the point of maximum intensity (PMI) or apical impulse is seen at the apex. The PMI is palpated as a single, faint, instantaneous tap and is no more than 2 cm in diameter beneath the examiner's fingers. Turning the client to the left side may assist in locating the PMI, but this maneuver will displace its location. With left ventricular enlargement and aneurysm, the PMI is more diffuse, sustained, and displaced downward and to the left of the midclavicular line.

AUSCULTATION OF HEART SOUNDS

Auscultation of the precordium yields valuable information about the presence of normal or abnormal heart rate and rhythm, ventricular filling, and blood flow across heart valves. Assessing heart sounds is a sophisticated skill, requiring study of heart sound characteristics and extensive clinical practice.

The environment is key to successful auscultation. The surroundings should be warm and quiet. An exposed chest is ideal, but the nurse should prevent shivering, which can greatly distort heart sound transmission. The nurse instructs the client to breathe through the nose while resting in a supine position. Again, use of the left lateral position may facilitate auscultation. When assessing for early diastolic murmers and pericardial friction rubs, it is helpful to have the client sit upright, lean forward, and hold his or her breath after exhalation.

A systematic approach to evaluating heart sounds should always be followed to ensure a thorough assessment each time cardiac auscultation is performed.

Examination of heart sounds may progress from the base (right second intercostal space) of the heart to the apex or from the apex to the base. Whichever approach is used, special attention must be paid to each of the precordial locations shown in Figure 23–4. The nurse listens carefully, noting the quality (crisp or muffled), intensity (loud or soft), rhythm (irregular or regular), and presence of extra sounds (murmurs, gallops, rubs, or clicks). Then this process is repeated using the bell over each of the precordial areas.

Normal Heart Sounds. The first heart sound (S_1) marks the onset of systole (ventricular contraction). It occurs just after or in concert with the carotid pulse. It is heard best with the diaphragm at the apex (the mitral valve area) and at the left lower sternal border at the fourth intercostal space (the tricuspid valve area). S_1 results from abrupt closure of the atrioventricular (AV) valves, which causes some blood turbulence and vibration of structures within the ventricles. This vibration is transmitted across the chest wall as a heart sound. Phonetically, if both heart sounds are appreciated as "lub-dup," S_1 is "lub." The intensity of S_1 may vary in certain pathologic conditions.

The second heart sound (S_2) relates to closure of the pulmonic and aortic (semilunar) valves and is heard best with the diaphragm at the base of the heart. Phonetically, it is the "dup" of the heart sound. It signifies the end of systole and the onset of diastole (ventricular filling). Physiologic (normal) splitting of S_2 occurs during inspiration. Normal splitting results from delayed closure of the pulmonic valve. At the base of the heart, normal S_2 is always louder than S_1, whereas both sounds usually are of nearly equal intensity at the left sternal border over Erb's point. Usually S_1 is the louder of the two sounds at the apex.

Figure 23–5 illustrates the relationship of heart sounds to events in the cardiac cycle.

Abnormal Heart Sounds. Certain abnormal heart sounds indicate a serious heart disorder or change in cardiac function. The nurse may not be able to label each abnormality but, with a thorough understanding of the normal sounds, should be able to recognize the abnormal sound, identify where it is best heard on the chest wall, and refer the problem to the physician.

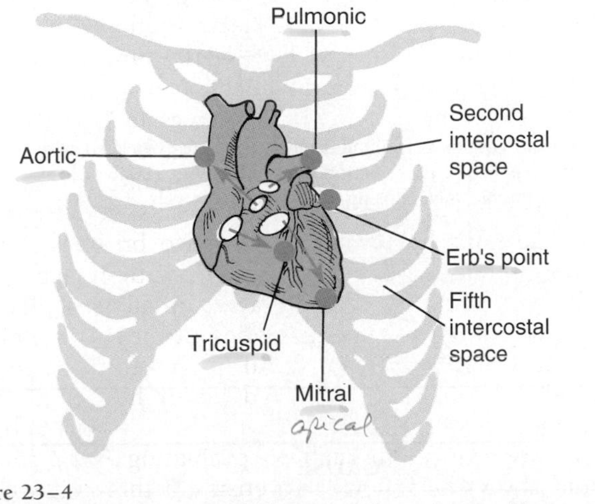

Figure 23–4
Precordial locations for cardiac palpation and auscultation of heart sounds. Closure of the mitral and tricuspid valves produces the S_1 heart sound; closure of the pulmonic and aortic (semilunar) valves produces the S_2 heart sound.

Pathologic Splitting of S_2. Forms of pathologic splitting of S_2 include a wide splitting, heard during both inspiration and expiration, with an increase during inspiration; fixed splitting, which is continuous and does not vary with respirations; and paradoxical splitting, heard during expiration but not during inspiration (Table 23–2).

Gallops. Diastolic filling sounds, or gallops (S_3 and S_4), occur during the two phases of ventricular filling. Sudden changes of inflow volume cause vibrations of the valves and ventricular supporting structures, producing low-pitched sounds that occur either early (S_3) or late (S_4) in diastole. Such sounds can originate from either side of the heart. These extra heart sounds create a triplet rhythm, acoustically mimicking a horse's gallop. For that reason the term *gallop* is often used to denote these heart sounds.

A gallop sound that occurs in early diastole, during passive, rapid filling of the ventricles, is known as the third heart sound (S_3). It is heard best with the bell at the apex and with the client in the left lateral decubitus position. An S_3 immediately follows the S_2 and is a dull, low-pitched sound. An S_3 gallop is considered a normal finding in children and young adults. In adults older than 30 years, an S_3 is considered characteristic of left ventricular dysfunction.

Clinical conditions associated with an S_3 gallop are those precipitating congestive heart failure (e.g., myocardial infarction and valvular incompetence). Third heart sounds arising in the left ventricle are best heard at the apex, with the person on the left side. Right ventricular gallops are best detected along the left sternal border, with the person assuming a supine position.

A fourth heart sound, or S_4 gallop, occurs in the later stage of diastole, during atrial contraction and active filling of the ventricles. This soft, low-pitched sound is heard immediately before the S_1 and is also referred to as an atrial gallop. An atrial gallop is found most commonly in disorders in which there is an increased stiffness of the ventricle, such as ventricular hypertrophy, ischemia, and fibrosis. These conditions are often associated with elevated diastolic ventricular pressures and a vigorous atrial contraction. The ventricles become resistant to filling, and the structures within the ventricles vibrate in response to the added blood input during the "atrial kick." The presence of an S_4 may result from myocardial infarction (transient S_4), hypertension, hypertrophy, fibrosis, cardiomyopathy, cor pulmonale, aortic stenosis, or pulmonic stenosis. An S_4 is never heard in the absence of atrial contraction (i.e., atrial fibrillation). An S_4 is heard best with the bell of the stethoscope at the apex and with the client in the supine, left lateral position.

Quadruple Rhythm. At times, a quadruple rhythm is noted when both S_3 and S_4 become audible. Clients manifesting this unusual heart sound often have tachycardia, which causes the diastolic filling sounds to fuse, forming a summation gallop that may be louder than the first or second heart sounds. It can be heard best

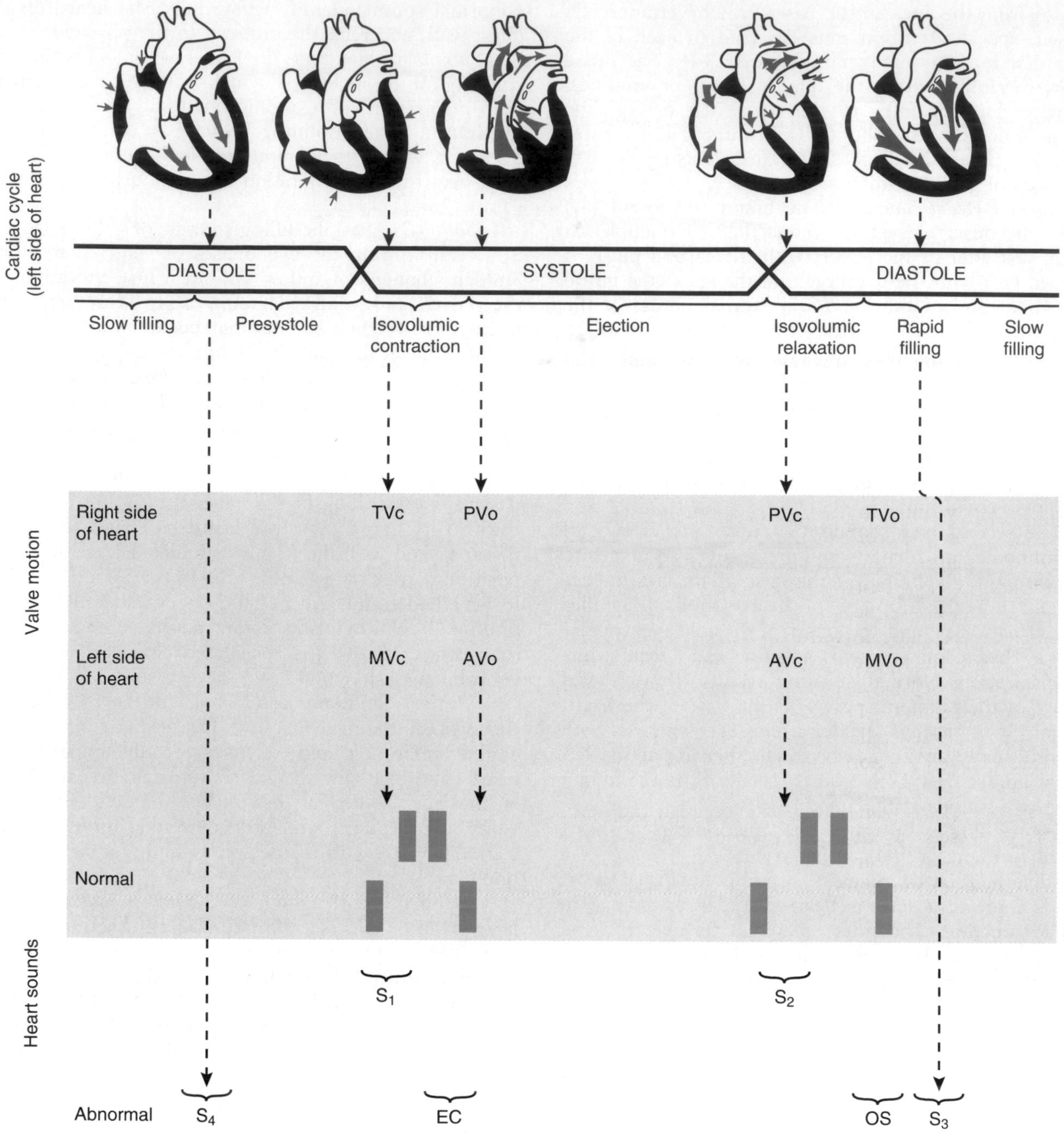

Figure 23–5
Relationship of heart sounds to events during the cardiac cycle. An understanding of heart sounds is facilitated when they are correlated with cardiac cycle events and valvular movements. AVc, aortic valve closing; AVo, aortic valve opening; EC, ejection click; MVc, mitral valve closing; TVc, tricuspid valve closing; MVo, mitral valve opening; OS, opening snap; PVc, pulmonic valve closing; PVo, pulmonic valve opening; TVo, tricuspid valve opening.

TABLE 23–2 Pathologic Splitting or S_2

PATHOLOGIC SPLIT S_2	TIMING	CAUSE
Wide splitting	Heard throughout respiratory cycle, increased on inspiration	Right bundle branch block; delayed closure pulmonic valve; early closure aortic valve
Fixed splitting	Continuous, does not vary with respiration	Atrial septal defect
Paradoxical splitting	Heard with expiration; disappears on inspiration	Left bundle branch block, aortic stenosis

TABLE 23–3 Opening Sounds

SOUND	PITCH	TIMING	CAUSE	BEST HEARD
Opening snap	High pitch, brief	Diastole	Opening stenotic aortic valve or tricuspid valve	Apex Diaphragm stethoscope
Ejection click	High pitch	Systole	Opening semilunar valve; prolapsed mitral valve; calcified aortic valve, mitrial insufficiency	Apex Diaphragm stethoscope

with the bell at the apex and resembles the sound of a galloping horse.

Opening Sounds. Valve opening normally occurs silently. Opening snaps or ejection clicks are always associated with valve disease (Table 23–3).

Pericardial Friction Rub. A pericardial friction rub is produced by inflammation of the pericardial sac (pericarditis) as the roughened parietal and visceral layers of the pericardium rub against each other during cardiac motion. It is best detected with the diaphragm at the apex and along the left sternal border. It may be accentuated by leaning forward or lying prone and exhaling. Friction rubs produce a sound that is described as "to-and-fro," scratchy, grating, rasping, and much like "squeaky leather." Friction rubs may be present during the first week following a myocardial infarction. Newly auscultated friction rubs should be reported to the physician.

Murmurs. Turbulent blood flow through the heart and large vessels produces vibrations within these structures that are heard as blowing or swooshing sounds. Causes of murmurs include the following:

- Increased rate or velocity of blood flow
- Abnormal forward or backward flow across stenosed or incompetent valves
- Flow into a dilated chamber
- Flow through an abnormal passage between heart chambers

Bruits are due to turbulence in vessels. Box 23–3 lists characteristics of murmurs. Box 23–4 presents a grading system used to characterize murmurs. Table 23–4 provides a discussion of types of heart murmurs.

EXAMINATION OF THE LUNGS

Because of the intimate relationship between the cardiovascular and respiratory systems, assessment of the cardiovascular system must include evaluation of the respiratory system. A more thorough discussion of respiratory assessment is found in Chapter 19. Some common respiratory findings related to cardiovascular disease are discussed next.

Tachypnea. Tachypnea, or rapid respirations, is often associated with the pain and anxiety that may accompany myocardial ischemic pain. Tachypnea also commonly occurs as a compensatory mechanism in congestive heart failure and pulmonary edema.

Crackles. Rales or crackles are a frequent sign of left ventricular failure and usually occur just after the onset of an S_3 gallop. Crackles may also result from atelectasis caused by limited chest wall excursion from prolonged bedrest, chest splinting from pain, and the effects of sedatives and narcotics.

Blood-Tinged Sputum. A pink, frothy sputum may indicate acute pulmonary edema. This symptom accompanies diffuse pulmonary crackles and denotes very se-

BOX 23–3

Characteristics of Cardiac Murmurs

Timing. When does the murmur occur during the cardiac cycle? Is it in the systolic phase or the diastolic phase? It is imperative to identify S_1 and S_2 to determine the phase. The murmur is then described as either systolic (between S_1 and S_2) or diastolic (between S_2 and S_1).

Quality. What is the quality or sound of the murmur? Is it blowing, harsh, rumbling, or musical?

Pitch. What is the frequency (pitch) of the murmur? Is it high and heard best with the diaphragm or low and heard best with the bell?

Location. Where is the murmur loudest? Murmurs, like all sounds, are loudest at their point of origin.

Radiation. The sound of the murmur is transmitted in the direction of blood flow. Therefore, the sound may be transmitted to the axilla, neck, back, and other locations on the chest.

Configuration. Note the shape of the sound. Does the sound begin soft and become louder (crescendo)? Does it do just the opposite (decrescendo)? Does it seem to have a "diamond shape" (crescendo-decrescendo)? The sound may be fairly constant (plateau).

Intensity. The degree of intensity (loudness) is typically measured using a rating system that does not necessarily reflect the seriousness of disease. Six grades (I to VI) of intensity are noted. A grade II murmur would be recorded as II/VI.

BOX 23-4

Grading Heart Murmurs

Grade I:	Faint; heard after listener has "tuned in"
Grade II:	Faint murmur heard immediately
Grade III:	Moderately loud, without accompanying thrill
Grade IV:	Loud, may be associated with a thrill
Grade V:	Very loud
Grade VI:	Very loud; heard with the stethoscope off the chest wall

rious left ventricular failure. Frank hemoptysis may be associated with pulmonary embolus. A cough frequently occurs in association with hemoptysis.

Cheyne-Stokes Respirations. These abnormal respirations are characterized by abnormal periods of deep breathing alternating with periods of apnea. This is a common finding in heart failure, anemia, and brain damage (from anoxic encephalopathy).

Abdomen

Examination of the abdomen provides data regarding cardiac competency. It is, however, of less value than other assessment parameters discussed in this section. Abdominal assessment is discussed in Chapter 32.

INSPECTION AND PALPATION

On inspection, the nurse may note abdominal distention. Palpation may confirm the presence of ascites (fluid accumulation within the peritoneal cavity) and an enlarged liver. Both of these findings indicate liver dysfunction, which can be a sequela of chronic right ventricular failure.

AUSCULTATION

Auscultation can yield the following clues about cardiovascular function:

- Decreased bowel tones can accompany potassium (K^+) depletion. Potassium depletion can complicate chronic diuretic use without sufficient K^+ replacement.
- Increased bowel tones, indicative of hypermotility, may result from laxative use or may be a side effect of certain antiarrhythmics (such as quinidine).
- Loud bruits, heard with the bell just over or above the umbilicus, may herald the presence of an aortic obstruction or aortic aneurysm (the latter can be detected by a palpable abdominal pulsation). Bruits heard over the upper midline or toward the back typically arise from renal arterial stenosis.

DIAGNOSTIC TESTS

The four most common types of diagnostic procedures used to diagnose cardiovascular disease are graphic procedures, laboratory tests, x-ray studies, and hemodynamic studies. Nursing responsibilities in diagnostic testing include the following:

- Explaining the purpose and procedure and answering any questions
- Scheduling the test
- Performing any necessary preliminary care (e.g., adjustments in medications and special diets)
- Promoting maximum emotional and physical comfort

Laboratory Tests

Data obtained from laboratory tests are used to diagnose a variety of cardiovascular ailments (e.g., myocardial infarction), screen individuals considered at risk for cardiovascular disease, determine baseline values, identify the presence of concurrent conditions (e.g., diabetes mellitus, electrolyte imbalance) that may affect the course of intervention, and evaluate the effectiveness of intervention. We consider here only those tests that are more commonly used to determine cardiovascular function and disease.

COMPLETE BLOOD CELL COUNT

The erythrocyte red cell count usually decreases in rheumatic fever and infective endocarditis. It usually increases in heart diseases characterized by inadequate oxygenation of tissues (e.g., right-to-left congenital shunts and heart conditions accompanied by obstructive lung disease).

An elevated hematocrit can result from obstructive lung disease and conditions of vascular volume depletion with hemoconcentration (e.g., hypovolemic shock and excessive diuresis). Decreases in hematocrit and hemoglobin indicate anemia, which is commonly caused by hemorrhage, hemolysis (from prosthetic valves), and chronic disease states. Clients with anemia have a significant reduction in red cell mass and a decrease in the oxygen-carrying capacity. Anemia can manifest as angina or aggravate congestive heart failure and produce heart murmurs.

The leukocyte (white cell) count is elevated in infectious and inflammatory diseases of the heart (e.g., infective endocarditis and pericarditis). It is also elevated after myocardial infarction because large numbers of white cells are necessary to dispose of the necrotic tissue resulting from the infarction.

CARDIAC ENZYMES

Enzymes are special proteins that catalyze chemical reactions in living cells. Cardiac enzymes are organ-specific enzymes that are present in high concentrations in

TABLE 23–4 Heart Murmurs

TYPE OF HEART SOUND	ORIGIN	PREFERRED METHOD OF AUSCULTATION
Systolic murmurs Ejection type 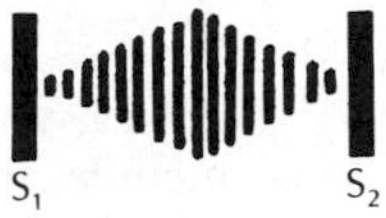	Systolic ejection murmurs are associated with forward blood flow during ventricular contraction across stenotic aortic or pulmonic valves.	Use of the stethoscope diaphragm is indicated. Ejection murmurs are typically of medium pitch and harsh quality and may be associated with an early ejection click. Aortic ejection murmurs are best heard over the aortic valve with radiation into the neck, down the left sternal border, and occasionally to the apex. They may be accompanied by a decreased S_2. Pulmonic ejection murmurs are heard best over the pulmonic valve, with radiation toward the left shoulder and left neck vessels. These murmurs may be accompanied by a wide-split S_2.
Pansystolic regurgitant murmurs 	Pansystolic murmurs occur when blood regurgitates through incompetent mitral and tricuspid valves (AV valves) or a ventricular septal defect as pressures rise during systole and blood seeks chambers of lower pressure. Damage to valve leaflets, papillary muscles, and chordae tendineae results in mitral valve insufficiency (blood regurgitates from left ventricle to left atrium) and tricuspid valve insufficiency (blood regurgitates from the right ventricle to right atrium). A ventricular septal defect results in blood regurgitation from the left ventricle to the right ventricle.	All regurgitant murmurs are high pitched, and those of AV valve incompetence have a blowing quality. Mitral regurgitant murmurs are heard at the apex with radiation into the left axilla and may be accompanied by an ejection click and signs of left ventricular failure. Tricuspid regurgitant murmurs are heard loudest over the tricuspid area, with radiation into the sternum. Ventricular septal defects are usually loud, harsh, and heard best over the left sternal border in the fourth, fifth, and sixth intercostal spaces with radiation over the precordium but not the axilla.
Early systolic murmurs 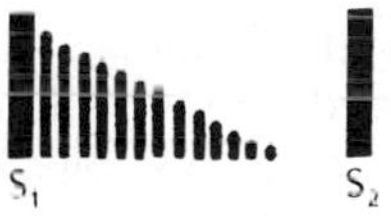	Early systolic murmurs (innocent murmurs) are associated with high cardiac outputs because there is increased blood flow velocity across normal semilunar valves. Causes include anemia, tachycardia, thyrotoxicosis, and fever. The murmur disappears with correction of the underlying condition. These are a normal variant in children.	These murmurs are best heard with the bell over the base of the heart or along the lower left sternal border. They are usually no greater than a grade II, are of medium pitch, and have a blowing quality. Intensity may increase during inspiration with the patient in a left recumbent position or with increased heart rates.
Late systolic murmurs 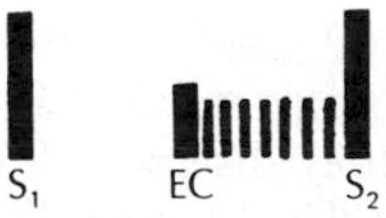	Late systolic murmurs imply mild mitral regurgitation as the mitral valve balloons into the left atrium late in ventricular systole.	These are best heard with the diaphragm of the stethoscope over the apex and are often preceded by a mid or late systolic ejection click.
Diastolic murmurs Early diastolic murmur 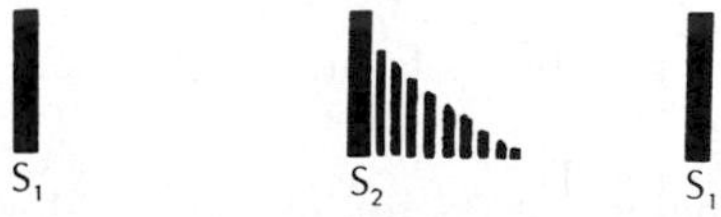	Early diastolic murmurs (decrescendo murmurs) are usually caused by semilunar valve insufficiency, with regurgitation resulting from valvular deformity or dilation of the valvular ring. They are heard immediately after the second heart sound and then diminish in intensity as the pressure in the aorta or pulmonary artery falls and the ventricles fill.	These murmurs are heard best with the diaphragm at the base of the heart with the patient leaning forward in deep expiration. They are high-pitched and blowing and radiate down the left sternal border, perhaps to the apex or down the right sternal border. Accompanying signs of heart failure may be present.
Diastolic filling rumbling 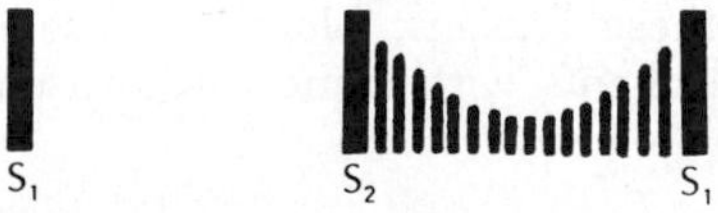	Diastolic filling rumbles are caused as blood flows across stenotic AV valves (more often mitral). They may also occur during augmented blood flow across normal AV valves. The murmur has two phases, becoming louder as the blood flow from the atrium to the ventricle increases with passive ventricular filling just after AV valve opening and again during atrial contraction (presystole).	With the bell, this murmur is heard over only a small area at and just medial to the apex. Exercise and a left lateral position of the patient increase the intensity of the sound. It is a low-pitched, rumbling sound often accompanied by an augmented S_1 and an opening snap.

AV, atrioventricular.
From Huang, S. L., et al. (1989). *Coronary care nursing* (2nd ed., p. 19). Philadelphia: W. B. Saunders.

myocardial tissue. Tissue damage causes a release of enzymes from their intracellular storage areas. For example, myocardial infarction causes cellular anoxia, which alters membrane permeability and causes spillage of enzymes into the surrounding tissue. This leakage of enzymes can be detected by rising plasma levels.

The enzymes most commonly used to detect myocardial infarction are creatine kinase (CK) and lactic acid dehydrogenase (LDH). Serum elevations of these two enzymes after myocardial insult occur in sequence. Because these enzymes are also found in other organs and tissues (e.g., skeletal muscle and liver), cardiac specificity must be determined by measuring isoenzyme activity. Isoenzymes are the various forms of CK and LDH, identified only by a process known as electrophoresis. There are three isoenzymes of CK: CK-MM (skeletal muscle), CK-MB (myocardial muscle), and CK-BB (brain). An elevated CK-MB, then, indicates myocardial damage. Elevation of CK-MB may occur within 4 to 6 hours and peaks 18 to 24 hours after the acute ischemic event. Of particular importance is the fact that up to a threefold elevation of CK may follow an intramuscular injection. Intramuscular injections should be avoided when treating a client with a suspected myocardial infarction.

There are five isoenzymes for LDH, of which only LDH_1 and LDH_2 are cardiac specific. If the serum concentration of LDH_1 is higher than the concentration of LDH_2, the pattern is said to have flipped, signifying myocardial necrosis. Eighty per cent of individuals demonstrate elevations in LDH within 48 hours after myocardial infarction.

As well as indicating the presence of myocardial damage, these elevations in serum cardiac enzymes can reveal the timing of the acute cardiac event. This is discussed in further detail in Chapter 24.

BLOOD COAGULATION TESTS

Blood coagulation tests are used to examine the ability of the blood to clot. It is important to evaluate coagulation tests such as prothrombin time and partial thromboplastin time in individuals with a greater tendency to form thrombi (e.g., those with atrial fibrillation, infective endocarditis, or prosthetic valves). They are also used to monitor anticoagulation therapy for clients receiving heparin or warfarin (Coumadin). Research has shown an increase in coagulation factors during and after a myocardial infarction. Therefore, the client is at greater risk of thrombophlebitis and extension of clots in the coronary artery. Chapter 27 discusses coagulation tests in detail.

SERUM LIPIDS

Serum lipids play a major role in the development of atherosclerosis. Serum lipids are composed of fatty substances that are insoluble in water. They are derived from dietary intake of fats or synthesized in the liver. The lipid profile measures serum cholesterol, triglycerides, and lipoprotein levels and is used to assess a client's degree of risk for coronary artery disease.

SERUM ELECTROLYTES

Cardiovascular disorders may impact on fluid and electrolyte regulation. In addition, certain medications alter electrolyte balance.

Potassium. The serum potassium level decreases as a result of diuretic therapy, vomiting, diarrhea, and alkalosis. Cardiac effects of hypokalemia include increased electrical instability, ventricular dysrhythmias, and increased risk of digitalis toxicity. Characteristic changes on the ECG include flattening and inversion of the T wave, the appearance of a U wave, and sagging of the ST segment.

A high serum potassium level is usually associated with kidney and endocrine disorders. The cardiac effects of hyperkalemia include asystole and ventricular dysrhythmias.

Sodium. The serum sodium level reflects water balance and may decrease (indicating water excess) in congestive heart failure, stress, excessive intravenous infusion of hypotonic fluids, and vomiting. Extensive use of diuretics and severely restricted sodium intake also lower serum sodium.

Calcium. The serum calcium level lowers as a result of multiple transfusions of citrated blood, renal failure, alkalosis, and laxative and antacid abuse (phosphate excess). Cardiac manifestations of hypocalcemia include serious ventricular dysrhythmias, prolonged QT interval, and cardiac arrest. Hypercalcemia occurs in thiazide diuretic use, acidosis, adrenal insufficiency, immobility, and vitamin D excess. A high serum calcium level shortens the QT interval and causes AV block, tachycardia, bradycardia, digitalis hypersensitivity, and cardiac arrest.

BLOOD UREA NITROGEN

Blood urea nitrogen (BUN) is a test of renal function: specifically, the ability of the kidney to excrete urea and protein. The BUN level elevates in kidney diseases, during water and saline depletion, and in heart disorders that adversely affect renal circulation (e.g., congestive heart failure and cardiogenic shock).

BLOOD GLUCOSE

Diabetes mellitus is a major risk factor in the development of atherosclerosis. In addition, the stress of an acute cardiac event can greatly elevate blood glucose, causing unstable hyperglycemia in clients with latent diabetes mellitus. For these reasons, blood glucose is routinely assessed in all clients with acute cardiovascular disorders.

Electrocardiogram

Each heartbeat is the result of an electrical impulse. This impulse, which begins in the sinoatrial node of the right atrium, is conducted through a network of fibers (the conduction system) within the heart and causes the heart to contract. This same electrical impulse spreads outward from the heart to the skin, where it can be detected by electrodes attached to the skin. The ECG is a display of the electrical activity of the heart. There are several types of ECG: continuous monitoring, 12-lead, and signal-averaged ECG. Through analysis of the ECG waveforms, any disorder of cardiac rate, rhythm, or conduction can be identified.

ECG is a common test. It is performed preoperatively on clients older than 40 years to assess for unknown heart disease, and it is a frequent noninvasive diagnostic test in almost all clients with known or suspected heart disease.

CONTINUOUS ELECTROCARDIOGRAM MONITORING

Four steps are required for ECG monitoring (Box 23–5):

- Attaching the electrodes to the client's skin
- Connecting the electrodes to the monitor by way of a cable
- Adjusting the monitor to obtain a readable ECG
- Setting the alarms for desired high and low rates

The client should be reassured that the ECG does not cause electrical shock and does not hurt.

CRITICAL TO REMEMBER

At times, false alarms may occur as a result of poor electrode contact. The nurse may be tempted to set the alarm limits widely apart (e.g., 40–180 BPM) or, worse, to turn the alarm off completely. This practice defeats the purpose of the alarm system and should never be adopted.

ELECTROCARDIOGRAM TRACINGS

Once the client is attached to continuous ECG monitoring, the heart rhythm is assessed regularly. Routine rhythm strips and strips of any dysrhythmias are logged into the medical record. Dysrhythmias are discussed in Chapter 24.

The impulse waves, recorded by the ECG machine onto graph paper, are arbitrarily designated by the letters P, Q, R, S, and T. The QRS letters are generally referred to as the QRS complex. Figure 23–7 depicts the typical ECG pattern formed by these waves.

The components of the ECG are defined as follows:

- The P wave represents depolarization of the atria.
- The PR interval represents the time it takes for the impulse to spread from the atria to the ventricles.
- QRS represents depolarization of the ventricles.
- The T wave represents repolarization of the ventricles.
- The ST segment indicates that ventricular depolarization is complete and that repolarization is about to begin.

BOX 23–5

Electrocardiographic Monitoring

Attaching the Electrodes. Electrodes pick up the electrical impulses from the heart on the skin. It is apparent that unless the signal is detected accurately, the remaining phases of electrocardiographic (ECG) monitoring have little value. The most common form of electrodes are disc-type or floating electrodes, which are deliberately separated from direct contact with the skin by a spacer filled with conductive gel. The gel is used to improve the signal by reducing local electrical interference on the skin. The gel is surrounded by a ring of adhesive. By peeling a paper backing off the pad, the electrode can be immediately applied to the skin. Three electrodes are required for continuous ECG monitoring. Two of these serve to detect the heart's activity; the third is an electrical ground.

The electrodes should be attached to the lead wires before they are applied to the chest wall. This process avoids applying pressure to the electrode, which could hurt the client and squeeze the gel outward, reducing contact and avoiding artifacts.

Some clients require special preliminary steps before the electrodes are attached. If the client has a lot of hair on the chest, it should be shaved to provide contact. If the client is wet or has been sweating, the sites should be dried off before the electrodes are applied.

In positioning the electrodes on the chest wall, locations are selected that will provide the clearest ECG waveforms. The two most common positions are the conventional position and the modified chest lead position (Fig. 23–6). Electrodes should be changed if the tracing is not clear or if they become dry or lose skin contact.

Connecting the Monitor. The electrodes are connected to the monitor by lead wires. These wires are 12 to 18 inches in length. One end snaps on to the electrodes, and the other end is attached to a cable that is connected to the monitor. At the cable is a cable receptacle for the attachment of each wire. The receptable and lead wires are color coded to facilitate connection.

Adjusting the Monitor. If the electrodes were applied properly and the wires are secure, the ECG pattern should be clear and distinct. If the pattern is not clear, the first steps should be checked. If the client's chest is large, the pattern may appear small and the gain (degree of magnification) should be adjusted until the pattern is clear.

Setting the Alarms. If the client's heart rate is between 60 and 100 beats per minute (BPM), it is customary to set the low alarm at 50 BPM and the high alarm at 140 BPM.

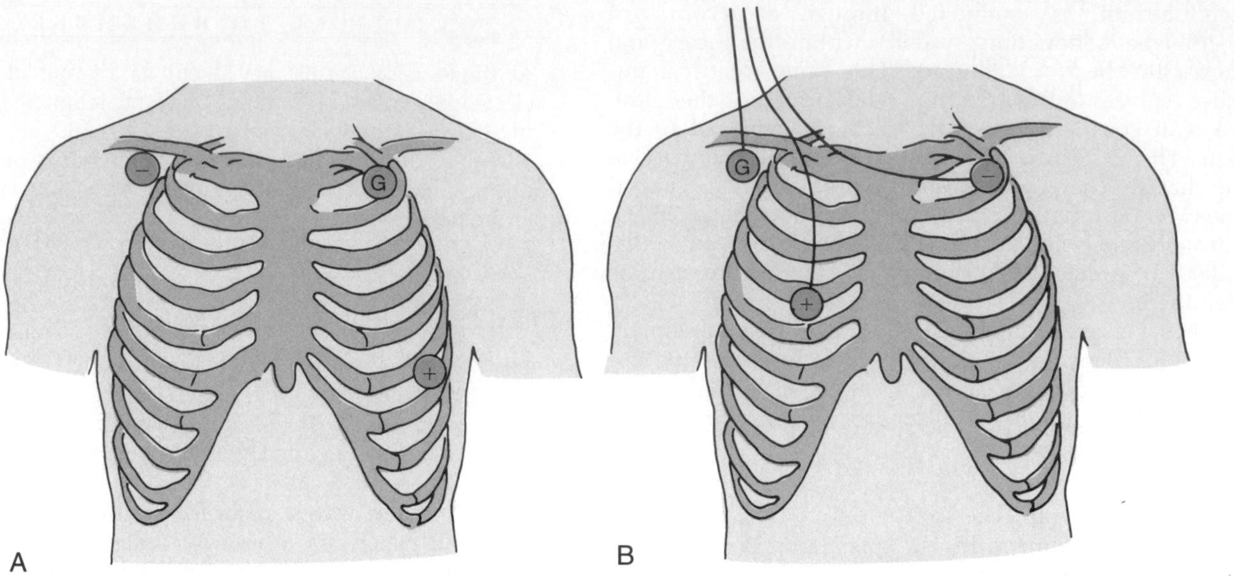

Figure 23–6
Common positions for continuous monitoring lead placement. Use lead II *(A)* or lead V_1 *(B)*. (From Phillips, R. E. & Feeney, M. K. [1990]. The cardiac rhythms: A systematic approach to interpretation [3rd ed.]. Philadelphia: W. B. Saunders.)

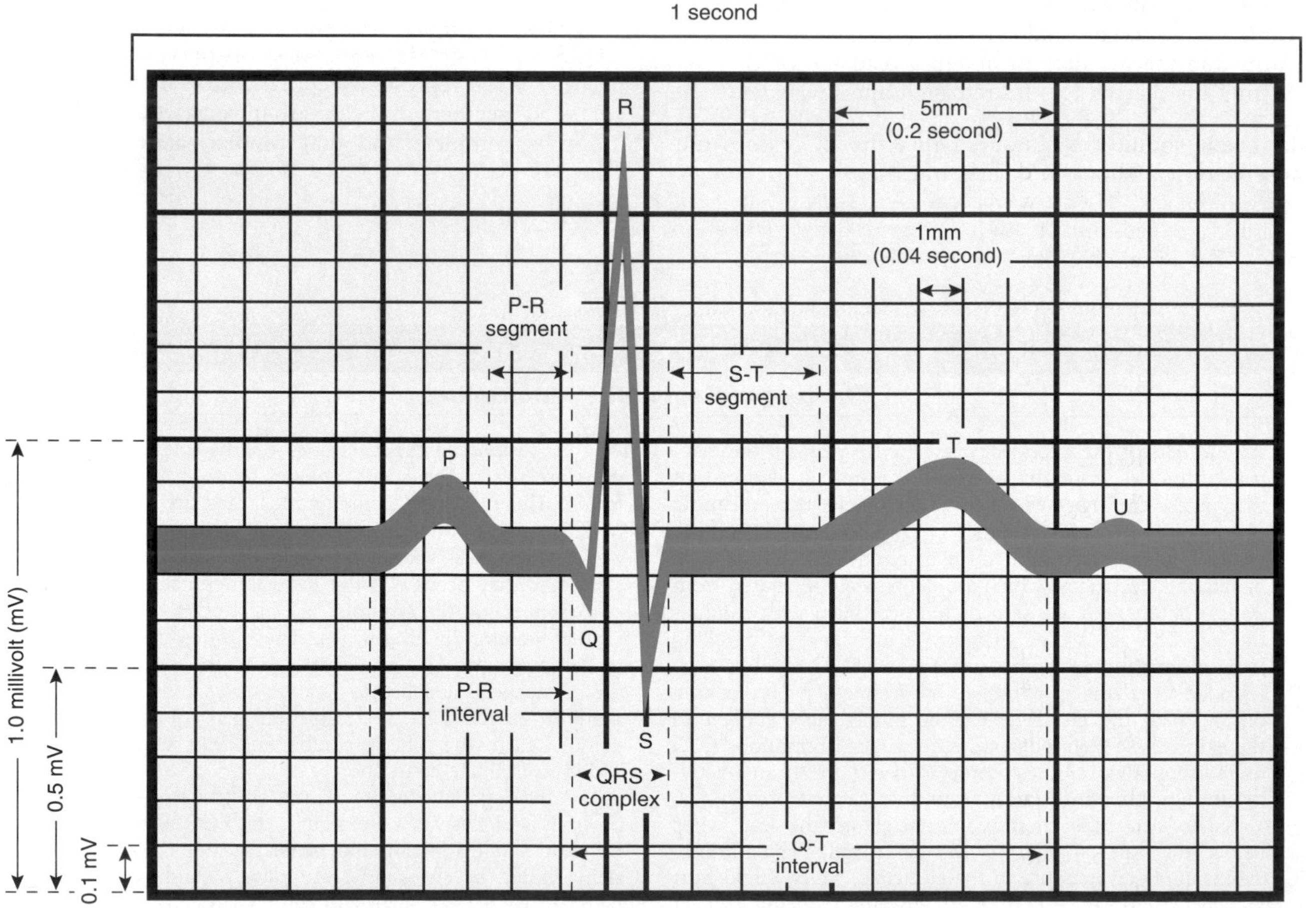

Figure 23–7
Normal electrocardiograph (ECG) pattern. The P wave represents depolarization of the atria to the ventricles. The QRS complex represents depolarization of the ventricles, and the T wave represents repolarization of the ventricles. The small U wave is sometimes seen following the T wave. Time and voltage lines of ECG paper: vertically, 1 mm = 0.1 millivolt (mV), 5 mm = 0.5 mV, and 10 mm = 1.0 mV. Horizontally, 1 small box = 0.04 second; 5 small boxes = 0.20 second, and 25 small boxes = 1 second.

- The QT interval represents electrical systole and varies with age, sex, and heart rate.
- The U wave is a small wave that sometimes follows the T wave. It may indicate hypokalemia.

An ECG tracing also shows the voltage of the waves and the time duration of both the waves and the intervals. Note that ECG graph paper is divided into horizontal lines and vertical lines and large squares and small squares. Voltage is represented on the vertical axis of the ECG paper. Each small square is 1 mm in height. Five small squares are equivalent to 5 mm, which, in turn, is equivalent to 0.5 mV. Voltage yields information regarding the presence and degree of atrial or ventricular hypertrophy. Time duration is measured on the horizontal axis. Each small square signifies the passage of 0.04 second. Each large square indicates the passage of 0.20 second. By studying the duration of the waves and intervals, the examiner can diagnose abnormal impulse formation and conduction (Fig. 23–8). Normal time durations for waves and intervals are as follows:

- P wave: less than 0.11 second
- PR interval: 0.12 to 0.20 second (average, 0.16 sec)
- QRS complex: 0.4 to 0.11 second
- QT interval: in women, up to 0.43 second; in men, up to 0.42 second (normal duration is inversely related to heart rate).

Because of its normal variation in configuration, a little more must be said about the QRS complex. The Q wave is always the first downward (negative) deflection of the complex. The R wave is always the first upward (positive) deflection. If there is a negative deflection (below the baseline) after an R wave, it is labeled an S wave. In most instances, a Q wave is not obvious on the ECG of the normal heart. The QRS complex may appear as a mostly positive or mostly negative deflection, depending on the recording electrode used.

ELECTROCARDIOGRAM VARIATIONS

12-Lead Electrogram. Indications for a 12-lead ECG are listed in Box 23–6.

The standard ECG has a 12-lead system, offering 12 points of reference for recording electrical activity of the heart. This can be conceptualized as 12 different views of the heart, looking in both horizontal and vertical planes. The standard 12-lead ECG has 6 limb leads, used to view the heart in a frontal or vertical plane, and 6 precordial leads, used to view the heart in a horizontal plane (Figs. 23–9 and 23–10).

Together, the 12 leads permit multidirectional examination of the electrical events going on in the heart. The location of pathologic change within the heart, which alters electrical activity, can be pinpointed with the use of the ECG. Views from the different leads are oriented to various surfaces of the myocardium:

- Leads I, aVL, V_5, and V_6 record electrical events occurring on the lateral surface of the left ventricle.
- Leads II, III, and aVF record electrical events occurring on the inferior surface of the left ventricle.

BOX 23–6

Indications for a 12-Lead Electrocardiogram

- Dysrhythmias
- Chest pain
- Myocardial infarction
- Heart rate determination
- Chamber dilation or hypertrophy
- Preoperative assessment
- Pericarditis
- Effect of medications (especially cardiac)
- Effects of systemic diseases on the heart (i.e., renal or pulmonary disease)
- Effects of electrolyte disturbances (especially potassium)

- Leads V_1 and V_2 record electrical events occurring on the surface of the right ventricle and anterior surface on the left ventricle.
- Leads V_3 and V_4 record electrical events occurring within the septal region of the left ventricle.

The placement of 12-lead electrodes is shown in Figure 23–9.

It is important that good contact be made between the skin and the electrodes. To facilitate this, the electrodes are placed firmly on the flat surface just above the wrists and ankles. There are many varieties of electrodes: adhesive back, foam, cloth, plastic, and suction cups. In clients with an amputation, the electrodes are applied to the residual limb of the affected extremity. The leg and arm electrodes must remain attached to obtain the precordial leads. Some ECG machines are able to record only one lead at a time, whereas others can record 3, 6, or all 12 leads simultaneously.

The nurse notes any unusual chest deformities, respiratory distress, or tremors that may account for alterations in the recording and whether the client experiences angina pectoris or chest discomfort at the time of the ECG.

Signal-Averaged Electrocardiogram. A signal-averaged ECG is used to identify the presence of electrical impulses called *late potentials.* These impulses occur during diastole late into the QRS and ST segment. This noninvasive test may be done at the bedside and is used to predict those clients who may be prone to ventricular tachycardia resulting in sudden death. The presence of late potentials in patients with normal sinus rhythm identifies the risk for ventricular tachycardia and sudden cardiac death.[20]

Holter Monitoring. When the client wears a portable Holter monitor, an ECG tracing may be recorded continuously over a period of a day or longer on an outpatient basis. Whereas a standard ECG is obtained over a relatively short period with the client at rest, Holter monitoring continues for an extended period with the client active. Thus, Holter monitoring is done to determine which dysrhythmias may be causing clinical manifestations that may not occur during a routine ECG but do occur when the client is ambulating at home or work. Holter monitoring also helps clinicians

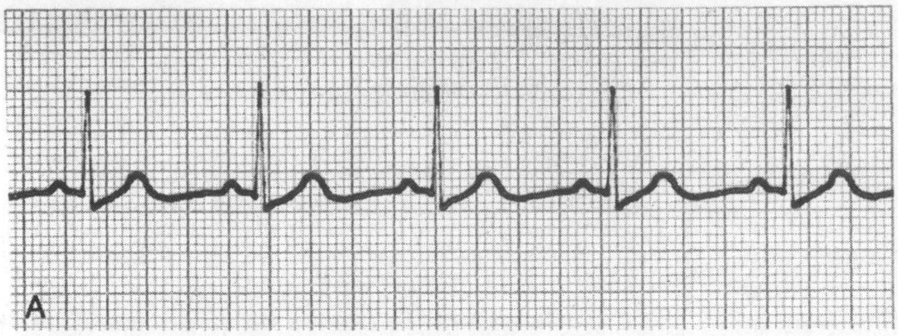

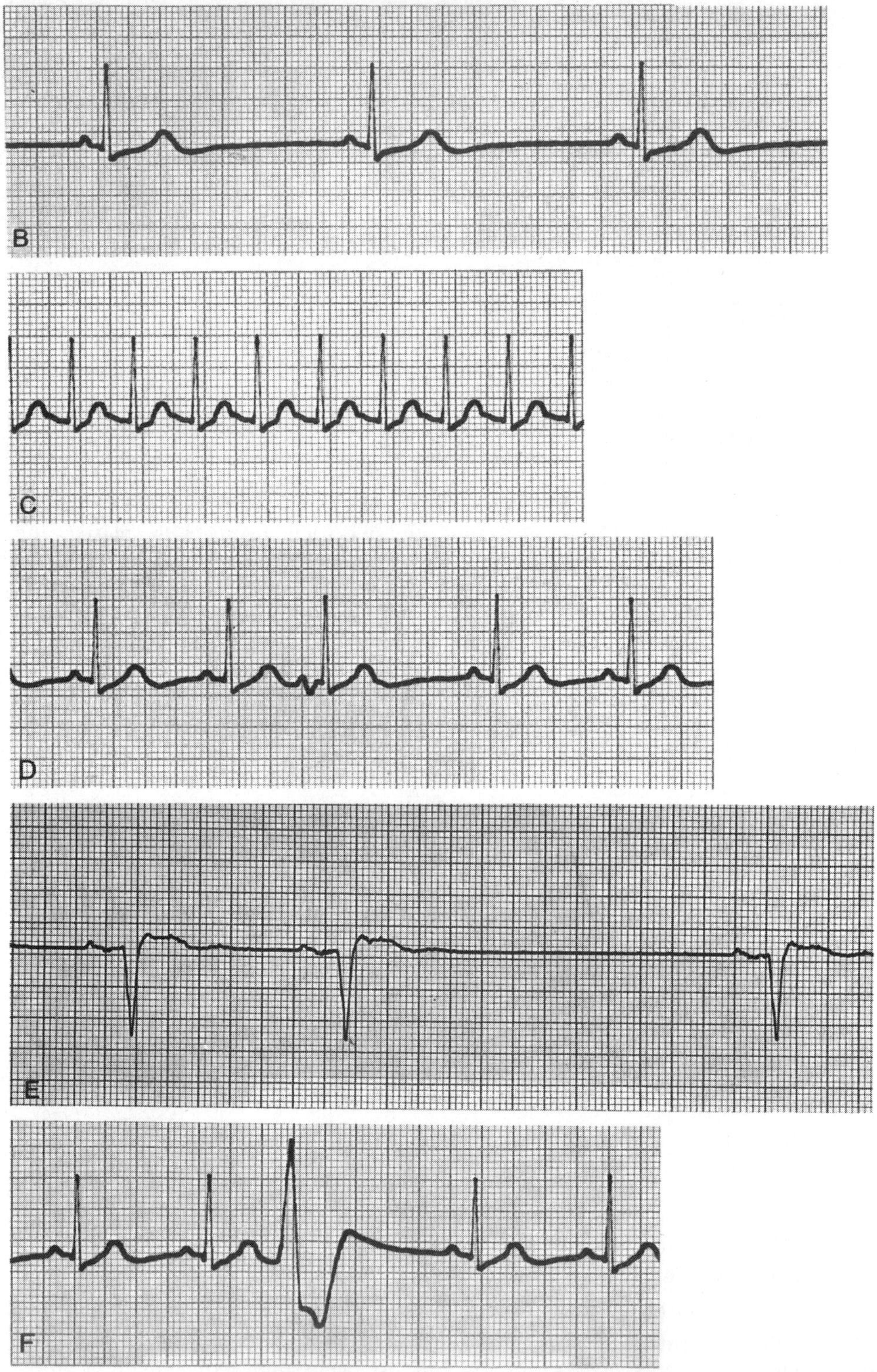

Figure 23–8
Electrocardiogram. *A*, Normal sinus rhythm; *B*, sinus bradycardia; *C*, sinus tachycardia; *D*, normal sinus rhythm with a premature atrial contraction; *E*, sinus rhythm with sinus arrest; and *F*, sinus rhythm with a premature ventricular contraction.

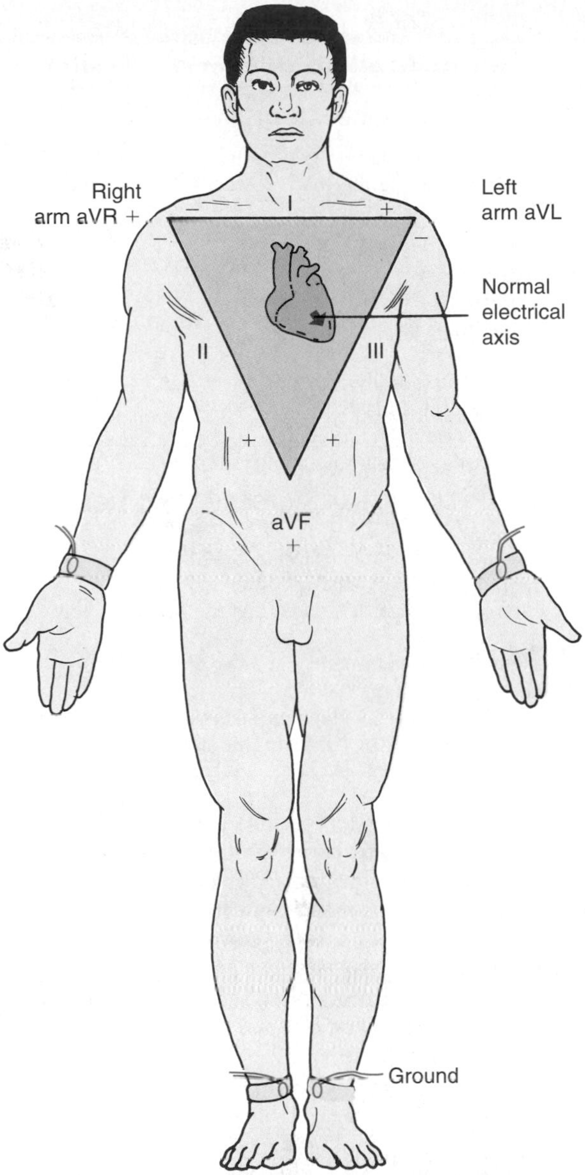

Figure 23–9
Standard positions for electrocardiographic leads. Bipolar limb leads are I, II, and III (Einthoven's triangle). Augmented unipolar limb leads are aVR (right arm), aVL (left arm), and aVF (left leg).

evaluate the effectiveness of pacemaker and pharmacologic antiarrhythmic therapy. See Client Education Guide: Holter Monitoring, for more information.

Exercise Electrocardiogram (Stress Testing). Exercise ECGs, referred to as stress testing, are valuable tools in detecting and evaluating coronary artery disease. Stress testing involves using controlled and carefully supervised exercise to increase myocardial oxygen demands and evaluating the coronary arteries' ability to meet the increased demands successfully. Its greatest advantage is that it provides information about the cardiovascular system in a dynamic state. The two major modes of exercise used for stress testing in the United States are bicycle ergometry and treadmill.

Exercise testing may have single or multiple stages.

CLIENT EDUCATION GUIDE

Holter Monitoring

The nurse should give the client the following explanations and instructions:

- In this procedure, which detects cardiac dysrhythmias occurring during normal daily activity, two or three electrodes are placed on your chest and connected to a portable monitoring system, called a *telemetry unit,* that you wear around your waist or over your shoulder. For 24 to 48 hours, the telemetry unit records your heart rhythm at preset intervals or when it senses an abnormal rhythm.
- Do not remove the electrodes and telemetry unit or get them wet.
- Record any unusual symptoms, such as chest pain, dizziness, or palpitations, in the diary that you have been given.
- Return to the hospital or clinic at the scheduled time for removal of the electrodes and telemetry unit.

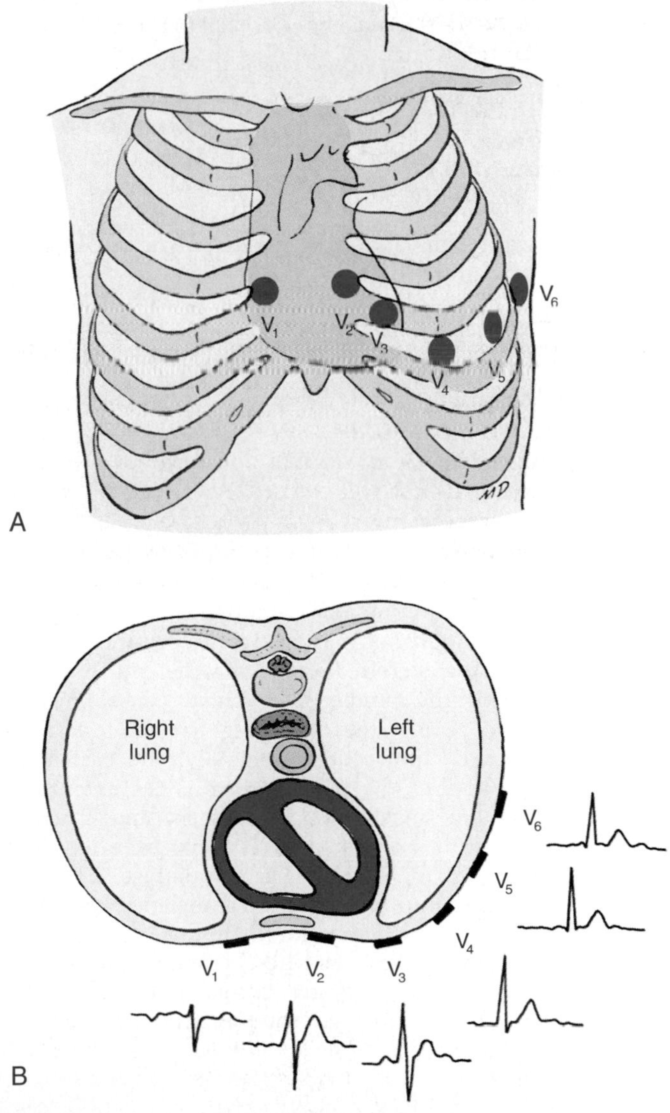

Figure 23–10
Placement of chest (V) leads. *A,* Precordial (chest) lead placement. *B,* Normal electrocardiographic findings with corresponding chest leads to cross section at fourth rib level.

A single-stage test is one in which exercise workload is constant throughout. Multiple-stage testing involves increasing the exercise workload in increments until a desired point is reached. These incremental increases in workload may occur every 1 to 5 minutes. The duration of testing varies with the type of test being used and the client's tolerance for testing.

Before stress testing, the nurse informs the client of the purposes and risks of exercise testing and obtains a signed consent for testing. The client must have a detailed physical examination before testing. In addition, the examiner must take a baseline, resting ECG immediately before testing begins. During the exercise test, the client's BP (using an automatically inflating cuff) and ECG are closely monitored by a physician or an appropriately trained individual.

A multilead monitoring system is most often used to provide maximal views of the heart wall. The examiner makes frequent observations throughout testing for any untoward manifestation related to impaired cardiovascular performance. The nurse should be alert for signs of client fatigue or claudication (leg pain due to vascular disease). Reasons for terminating the test include the following:

- Chest pain or fatigue
- Greatly increased heart rate (age related): 20 to 29 years, 170 beats per minute (BPM); 30 to 39 years, 160 BPM; 40 to 49 years, 150 BPM; 50 to 59 years, 140 BPM; and 60 to 69 years, 130 BPM
- Untoward signs and symptoms of myocardial ischemia or heart failure
- Failure of systolic BP to rise or a drop in BP (below resting levels)
- Sudden development of bradycardia
- Serious cardiac dysrhythmia
- Severe hypertension
- Severe dyspnea
- ST segment depression (greater than 2–4 mm)
- A sudden loss of coordination (cerebral ischemia)

Because these symptoms occur with some frequency, an emergency cart containing cardiac drugs and resuscitation equipment is kept close at hand at all times. Clients rarely die from this procedure.

A positive exercise test is one that must be terminated before the predicted maximal (or submaximal) limits have been achieved owing to manifestations of cardiovascular intolerance. Generally, the earlier these symptoms appear, the more serious is the extent of the disease. Alterations in the ST segment and T wave on the ECG during exercise and recovery are often considered diagnostic of coronary artery disease. This is because these alterations reflect an imbalance between the myocardial oxygen demand and supply.

Although the exercise test is very helpful as an adjunct diagnostic study for coronary artery disease, it can produce false-positive findings in some cases, especially in women. In some individuals, alterations in ST segments may occur during exercise, even though no coronary artery disease exists. Hyperventilation, certain drugs, and electrolyte imbalances can produce false-positive readings. For this reason, diagnosis cannot be made on the basis of exercise findings alone.

False-negative findings can also occur, although with less frequency. Medications such as beta-blocking agents and nitrates are capable of producing false-negative results. Another limitation of exercise stress testing study is that it is absolutely contraindicated in various cardiovascular and noncardiac conditions. See Box 23–7 for contraindications to exercise testing. When exercise stress testing is contraindicated, the client may undergo a dipyridamole (Persantine) stress test in conjunction with thallium scintigraphy (see Thallium-201 Scintigraphy).

BOX 23–7

Contraindications to Exercise Testing

ACUTE CARDIOVASCULAR DISEASE

Acute myocardial infarction (usually avoided in those individuals for whom fewer than 2 weeks have elapsed since infarction)

- Unstable angina pectoris
- Heart failure
- Pericarditis
- Myocarditis
- Endocarditis
- Life-threatening dysrhythmias
- Thrombophlebitis
- Recent systemic embolus
- Dissecting or enlarging aneurysm

OTHER SEVERE DISEASES RESTRICTING MOBILITY

Renal failure

- Severe pulmonary disruptions
- Orthopedic disorders affecting the spine or lower extremities
- Neurologic impairment (e.g., stroke or paralysis)
- Systemic infection
- Left ventricular outflow obstruction (aortic stenosis, hypertension, or hypertrophic cardiomyopathy)

CLIENT EDUCATION GUIDE

Stress Testing

The nurse should give the client the following instructions:

- Obtain sufficient rest the night before the test.
- Avoid eating a heavy meal just before the test, although it is advisable to eat a light meal 1 to 2 hours before the test.
- Avoid smoking and consuming alcohol and caffeine-containing beverages the day of testing.
- Wear nonconstrictive, comfortable clothing and rubber-soled, supportive shoes during testing. Only a loose-fitting, front-buttoning shirt (or blouse) should be worn. (Women should wear a bra.)
- Continue all usual medications unless specified otherwise by the physician. (An inquiry about this should be made to the physician.)
- After the test, rest and keep the physician informed of any lingering symptoms of cardiovascular distress (i.e., chest pain, shortness of breath, or dizziness).
- Avoid taking a hot shower for 1 to 2 hours after the test because this may potentiate hypotension, resulting in a fainting episode. If bathing is desired, use only tepid water.

Nurses need to be familiar with the stress-testing procedure to provide clear teaching guidelines to clients scheduled to undergo exercise testing. Many clients harbor misconceptions and unnecessary fears about the procedure. Although the procedure is not painful, it can produce a great deal of fatigue. The nurse warns the client that this test may trigger chest pain and dyspnea. Along with this warning, the nurse points out that the procedure is performed in a controlled environment with prompt nursing and medical attention close at hand. It is very important that the client arrive for the exercise testing appointment relaxed and well rested. Teaching guidelines for stress testing are given in the Client Education Guide.

Electrophysiologic Studies

The electrophysiologic study is an invasive method of recording intracardiac electrical activity. It is used to shed light on the mechanisms of dysrhythmias, to differentiate between supraventricular and ventricular dysrhythmias, to evaluate sinoatrial or AV node dysfunction, to determine the need for a pacemaker, and to evaluate the effect of antiarrhythmic agents used to prevent tachycardias.

Under fluoroscopy, an electrophysiologic catheter is threaded into the heart via the femoral, basilic, or subclavian vein. The catheter site selected depends on the purpose of the examination.

The procedure is designed to reproduce any dysrhythmia so that its origin may be isolated. Ventricular tachycardia is induced by using programmed stimulation to fire an impulse at different times during the cardiac electrical cycle. If the dysrhythmia is induced, the person's BP and hemodynamic responses are observed. It is possible for arterial pressure, surface ECGs, and ECGs from intracavitary catheters to be recorded simultaneously.

Antiarrhythmic drugs may be administered during the study to evaluate their effect. After the initial antiarrhythmic has been given, induction of ventricular tachycardia is attempted. If ventricular tachycardia is induced, the dosage may be increased or other drugs administered, and the electrophysiologic studies are repeated in several days to determine the effectiveness of the antiarrhythmic drug therapy.

Frequently, when the irritable focus has been identified (e.g., accessory pathway or bundle of His), an ablation may be performed. Ablation of the irritable focus may be accomplished by the use of radiofrequency, direct current, ethyl alcohol, or cryosurgery. Radiofrequency ablation is the most popular method because its effect may be localized, with less damage to surrounding tissue.

Chest X-Ray Studies

The physician routinely orders posteroanterior, lateral, and oblique chest x-ray films to determine the size, silhouette, and position of the heart. In the acutely ill client, an anteroposterior x-ray film is taken at the bedside. Specific pathologic changes of the heart are difficult to determine on x-ray examination, but anatomic changes in the heart and pulmonary sequelae of various cardiac conditions can be seen. Valvular and pericardial calcifications; pulmonary congestion (from heart failure); pericardial effusion; and placement of central catheters, endotracheal tubes, hemodynamic monitoring devices, and intra-aortic balloon catheters are all assessed on x-ray film.

CLIENT EDUCATION GUIDE

Magnetic Resonance Imaging

The nurse should give the client the following explanations and instructions:

- MRI shows images of tissue that cannot be seen with other radiologic techniques.
- You may be asked to sign a consent for the procedure.
- This procedure takes approximately 45 to 60 minutes.
- If you are prone to feelings of claustrophobia, alert the nurse or technician before the procedure begins. The physician may need to prescribe a sedative to help you relax.
- If you feel the need for additional support, ask the technician if a family member or friend may accompany you in the magnetic resonance imaging (MRI) room during the procedure.
- You can talk to and hear the staff via microphones placed in the scanner.
- Before the procedure, remove all metal items, including watch, eyeglasses, and jewelry. You may be allowed to wear special mirrored glasses that allow you to see outside of the scanner.
- Be aware that the MRI unit normally makes a loud, knocking noise as it scans your body.
- The only discomfort is caused by lying still on a hard, flat surface.
- An open MRI is a newer unit with open areas that enable you to see outside the machine.

Magnetic Resonance Imaging

Although magnetic resonance imaging (MRI) is the most expensive noninvasive diagnostic option, a variety of information may be obtained in a single image. Magnetic resonance imaging provides the best information on chamber size, wall motion, valvular function, and great vessel blood flow.[30] Magnetic resonance imaging is commonly used for examination of the aorta, detection of tumors or masses, cardiomyopathies, and pericardial disease. In MRI, a strong magnetic field and radiowaves are used to detect and define the differences between healthy and diseased tissue. MRI can image over three spatial dimensions and over time. It can actually show the heart beating and the blood flowing in any direction.

Information obtained from MRI includes the following:

- Normal morphology and structural disease
- Wall thickness, chamber volumes, valve areas, vessel cross-sections, and extent, location, and size of lesions
- Global and regional biventricular function, including ejection fraction, stroke volume, and cardiac output
- Blood flow quantifications within vessels over the cardiac cycle
- Tissue characterization of paracardiac and intracardiac masses, pericardial effusion, and myocardial infarction

Clients with pacemakers, prosthetic valves, or recently implanted clips or wires are not eligible for MRI scans. See Client Education Guide: Magnetic Resonance Imaging.

Positron Emission Tomography

The positron emission tomographic (PET) scanner is a diagnostic imaging tool that allows visualization of regional physiologic function and images the biochemistry that often separates normal from diseased myocardium. Cellular metabolic information is obtained by mapping regional myocardial glucose metabolism. Combining information from the perfusion and the metabolism images provides a thorough assessment of regional cardiac viability.

Compounds found normally in the body are radiolabeled. After infusion, the radiopharmaceuticals travel through the client's blood stream, serving as tracers of normal physiologic activity. These tracer isotopes have a very short half-life and deliver only a very low radiation dose. The circular array of scanning around the body detects these paired gamma rays, which are associated with positron decay events. A computer then reconstructs images of the radionuclide distribution within the body.

The scanner looks like a standard computed tomographic unit and is silent. The scanning procedure takes about 2 to 3 hours. An intravenous radiopharmaceutical, (N)-ammonia, is administered and a 20-minute blood flow image is begun. Next, an intravenous injection of fluorene 18 fluorodeoxyglucose follows. It takes this about 40 minutes to localize in the myocardium. Final uptake of this tracer is proportional to the glucose metabolic activity of myocardial cells and provides an excellent indication of regional tissue viability.

Clinical indications for PET scanner use include the following:

- Detection of coronary artery disease
- Assessment of myocardial viability
- Assessment of progression of coronary artery stenosis
- Documentation of collateral coronary circulation
- Differentiation of ischemia and dilated cardiomyopathy

The terms *match* and *mismatch* describe the relationship between the perfusion and the metabolism study. A perfusion study that shows similarities between a perfusion study with poor blood flow and a metabolic study showing decreased glucose uptake of necrotic tissue is described as a "match." A perfusion study that shows poor blood flow and a metabolic study that shows only stunned viable myocardium that has survived the initial insult is described as a "mismatch."

Echocardiography

The echocardiogram, a noninvasive diagnostic procedure based on the principles of ultrasound, is used to evaluate structural and functional changes in a wide variety of heart ailments. It is one of the mainstays of diagnostic cardiology because it is totally noninvasive, can be used at the bedside, and provides accurate information at no risk to the client.

An echocardiogram is performed by placing a transducer on several areas of the chest wall. This transducer emits short pulses of high-frequency sound through the chest wall and heart. Wave pulses bounce off tissues of varying densities and are reflected back to the transducer as a series of echoes, thus creating an image via an oscilloscope graph. The bursts of ultrasound are directed at the part of the heart under investigation. The echocardiogram records the structure and motion of that area in relation to its distance from the anterior chest wall. An electrocardiogram is recorded simultaneously on the graph. Two-dimensional echocardiography generates a continuous picture of the beating heart. These images are recorded on videotape for analysis.

Echocardiograms are used to help assess and diagnose pericardial effusion, cardiomyopathy, valvular disorders (including prosthetic valves), cardiac shunts, myocardial ischemia, chamber size, left ventricular function, ventricular aneurysms, and cardiac tumors (atrial myxoma). In addition, they are very useful during heart biopsies because the physician can view the heart on a monitor while taking tissue samples.

Nursing intervention for clients undergoing echocardiography involves explaining the procedure and reassuring the client that the study is noninvasive, painless, and without complication. An echocardiogram can be performed at the bedside, although it is preferable to send the client to the echocardiography laboratory.

Transesophageal Echocardiography

Transesophageal echocardiography (TEE) is an invasive test that gives a higher quality picture of the heart than does a regular echocardiogram. It is especially useful in clients who have thickened lung tissue or thick chest walls or who are obese. The procedure may also be used intraoperatively, in which conventional echocardiography is ineffective. The client needs to be in bed or on a table with ECG leads attached. ECG and BP are monitored. The throat is anesthetized and sedation is given. An esophageal scope is inserted through the mouth and passed into the esophagus by the physician. Because the probe is placed behind the heart, it allows the left atrium to be viewed. TEE allows clearer visibility of the heart and its structures and is most useful in diagnosis of cardiac masses, prosthetic valve function, and aneurysm.

CRITICAL TO REMEMBER

The nurse should instruct the client to avoid eating and drinking for 8 to 10 hours before the procedure. After the procedure, the nurse assesses the client for the return of the gag reflex before allowing the client to eat or drink anything

CLIENT EDUCATION GUIDE

Myocardial Scintigraphy

The nurse should give the client the following explanations and instructions:

- In this procedure, electrodes will be placed on your chest and an intravenous catheter inserted for the administration of a radioisotope. Generally, total exposure to radiation during these scans is less than or equal to that of one chest x-ray study.
- Notify the physician if you are pregnant or suspect that you may be pregnant because these studies involve some (although minimal) radiation exposure.
- Wear comfortable clothing and walking shoes if you will be exercising on the treadmill or bicycle.
- Follow the prescribed preprocedure dietary instructions. A light meal is preferred over a heavy meal if the scan will be taken during exercise. This prevents nausea and stomach cramping during exercise and allows for better uptake of the radioisotope.
- If ordered by the physician, avoid taking your usual prescribed dosage of beta-blockers, calcium channel blockers, and xanthines before the procedure.
- Notify the nurse or technologist of any chest pain during or after the procedure.

Phonocardiography

Recordings of audible vibrations coming from the heart and great vessels, phonograms assist in diagnosing the timing of cardiac sounds and murmurs. Microphones are placed under elastic straps, usually at the base and apex of the heart. No client preparation is required for this assessment.

Myocardial Scintigraphy

Myocardial function, motion, and perfusion may be studied by a method called *scintigraphy,* which involves the intravenous injection of a radioactive isotope. As the isotope is absorbed by the blood cells of the heart muscle, photons are emitted. These photons are detected by an external gamma camera, which produces a radionuclide image. Because these nuclear imaging techniques are relatively noninvasive, they are frequently used diagnostic tests. See Client Education Guide: Myocardial Scintigraphy, for client teaching information related to these tests.

Thallium-201 Scintigraphy. Thallium-201 is the most widely used isotope for myocardial perfusion because of its short (73 hours) half-life and low total body radiation dose. Thallium-201 is a radioactive analogue of potassium, which is easily extracted by smooth skeletal and cardiac muscle fibers. The amount of thallium-201 found in the myocardium after an intravenous injection depends on the regional myocardial perfusion via the coronary arteries and on the efficiency of cellular extraction.

A high concentration of thallium-201 is present in well-perfused cells, and a lower concentration remains in the blood, setting up a concentration gradient for the diffusion of thallium-201. Areas of the myocardium receiving less blood flow (resulting from coronary atherosclerosis) receive less thallium-201. Infarcted or scarred areas of myocardium do not extract any thallium-201 and show up as "cold spots." If the defective area is ischemic, then the cold spots fill in or become "warm" on the delayed images. Infarcts continue to appear cold with little or no perfusion of thallium-201 either during a stress test or with delayed images.

The perfusion scanning is performed with a special camera that records the source of the radioactivity emitted. A computer refines and enhances the images and then provides quantitative information about the myocardial walls.

Thallium-201 imaging can be performed before or after an exercise ECG study or as a resting study only. Ischemic myocardium may show up on a resting thallium-201 study. The thallium-201 stress test begins with a graded exercise protocol on a treadmill. The client has a slow infusion of intravenous normal saline. The ECG is monitored continuously. About 1 minute before the peak of the stress test, thallium-201 is injected intravenously. The client exercises for the last minute to ensure thallium-201 distribution to the heart during 85 per cent maximum stress. The client then cools down and reclines on an examination table for the perfusion scan. Continuous imaging in a 180-degree arc over the chest is obtained. The client then waits for 3 hours and returns for repeat films. Before the delayed images are obtained, the client receives additional thallium-201 by intravenous injection. The two sets of images are then carefully compared.

Dipyridamole–Thallium-201 Test. This test may be used as an alternative to standard treadmill exercise when the client is not able to achieve a vigorous level of exercise. Dipyridamole (Persantine) serves as a pharmacologic stress agent. It is given intravenously to dilate the coronary arteries, which would normally dilate during the stress of exercise. Arteries that are narrowed as a result of coronary artery disease do not expand as much as normal arteries. Infusion of dipyridamole for 5 minutes is followed by an injection of thallium-201. Thallium-201 travels easily through normal arteries that have dilated and travels less freely through narrowed arteries. At 7 minutes, images are taken.

Any form of caffeine as well as medications for asthma, such as theophylline or aminophylline, should be omitted before this test. Aminophylline is the antagonist to dipyridamole and may be given slowly intravenously to reverse any adverse side effects.

Technetium 99m Ventriculography (Gated Blood Pool Imaging or Multiple Gated Acquisition). This test studies the motion of the left ventricle wall and measures the ventricle's ability to eject blood (ejection fraction). If a coronary artery is narrowed, causing ischemia, the segment of the myocardium it serves exhibits diminished wall motion or contractility. In addition, hemodynamic changes may be measured by observing the actual filling and emptying of the cardiac chambers. Changes in cardiac output as well as ejection fraction may be obtained. Gated blood pool images represent the blood pool within the ventricular and atrial chambers.

Intravenous stannous pyrophosphate is given to allow the red cells to tag onto the technetium 99m. Approximately 20 minutes after the PYP is injected, the technetium 99m is injected. The client is then placed on a heart monitor and images are begun.

Gated blood pool scans use counts from any one of a number of consecutive beats. Multiple serial images are obtained using a gamma camera.

In a stress gated blood pool study, the client is put on a bicycle ergometer with a gamma camera positioned to project the right and left blood pools. The ECG is monitored continuously. Images are obtained at rest and during each stage of exercise.

First-Pass Cardiac Study. During a first-pass study, a single intravenous injection of technetium 99m is administered intravenously and traced as it passes through the heart. Only the initial pass of the technetium 99m is recorded as it passes through the cardiac chambers. Ejection fraction and information about ventricular wall motion are obtained. A first-pass study may be performed during exercise or rest.

Cardiac Catheterization

This complex procedure involves the insertion of a catheter into the heart and surrounding vessels to obtain detailed information about the structure and performance of the heart, valves, and circulatory system. Specifically, cardiac catheterization is performed to:

- Confirm a diagnosis of heart disease and determine the extent to which the disease has affected the structure and function of the heart
- Determine congenital abnormalities
- Obtain a clear picture of cardiac anatomy before heart surgery
- Obtain pressures within the heart chambers and the great vessels (aorta and pulmonary artery)
- Measure blood oxygen concentration, tension, and saturation within the heart chambers
- Determine cardiac output
- Perform angiography for better coronary artery visualization
- Obtain endocardial biopsies
- Allow infusion of fibrinolytic agents directly into an occluded coronary artery in the hope that coronary blood flow may be restored

Cardiac catheterization is usually performed in the controlled environment of a cardiac catheterization laboratory. Typically, only one side of the heart is catheterized, although it is sometimes necessary to insert the catheter into both sides of the heart. A clinician continuously monitors the ECG during the procedure.

COMPLICATIONS

Although cardiac catheterization has become a safer and more useful diagnostic tool in recent years, it is far from innocuous and has inherent complications. Most complications are related to the puncture site. Clot formation during catheterization is prevented by administering moderate amounts of anticoagulant (usually 4000 to 5000 units of heparin), which increases the risk of bleeding at the insertion site or into the retroperitoneal area. In addition, trauma from arterial cannulation may potentiate vasospasm or clot formation, causing temporary or permanent arterial occlusion to the affected extremity. Dysrhythmias frequently develop during catheterization owing to direct catheter stimulation of the atrium and ventricle. In addition, the client may experience anginal pain. Pain occurs when contrast dye replaces the blood flowing through the coronary arteries under study. Lack of blood flow causes a painful regional cardiac hypoxia. Occasionally, clients may have an allergic reaction to the iodine-based contrast media. Allergic symptoms include flushing, nausea, and vomiting, tingling and numbness, weakness, and urticaria. Fortunately, anaphylactic shock is rare. Osmotic diuresis after injection of the hypertonic radiographic contrast agents can produce significant dehydration. Finally, myocardial and aortic perforations are rare but potentially fatal complications of cardiac catheterization.

NURSING ASSESSMENT AND INTERVENTION

Before cardiac catheterization, the client must be physically and emotionally prepared. Major steps in preparing the client are as follows:

CLIENT EDUCATION GUIDE

Cardiac Catheterization

The nurse should give the client the following description of the procedure:

- In this procedure, you will lie on an x-ray table in the special cardiac catheterization room. Electrocardiographic leads will be attached to your arms.
- After you receive an injection of local anesthesia in your groin area, the physician will make a small incision and insert a small, flexible catheter into a blood vessel. You should feel little or no discomfort during this procedure.
- The physician then will carefully thread the catheter through the vessel to your heart. You may feel a fluttering sensation as the catheter enters the heart chamber.
- Once the catheter is in place in your heart, contrast dye will be injected through the catheter. The dye will flow through the heart's chambers and into the circulatory system. You may feel flushed or experience a "hot flash" as the dye is injected and may feel some heart palpitations, but you should not feel any pain.
- Once the dye is injected, a series of x-rays will be taken of your heart. The room lights will be dimmed as the x-rays are taken.
- After the procedure is completed, you will lie flat for 4 to 6 hours, during which time you will be monitored closely by a nurse.

- The nurse should explain the procedure, its purpose, and its hazards. (See Client Education Guide: Cardiac Catheterization.)
- The client must sign a consent for the procedure after he or she has been carefully informed and questions have been answered satisfactorily.
- The nurse determines whether there is any history of allergies, particularly to iodine-containing substances or shellfish. The physician may order a skin test with an iodine-containing solution the day before the procedure.
- Solid food must be withheld for 6 to 8 hours and liquids for at least 4 hours (or according to institutional protocol) before the procedure to prevent vomiting and aspiration.
- The client's height and weight must be recorded in the chart. This is needed for calculating the amount of dye that will be administered.
- The peripheral pulses must be marked distal to the probable cannulation sites with a felt-tipped pen and the quality of the pulses recorded in the chart. This will aid in locating the pulses after the procedure. Extremities are checked at this time for postprocedure comparisons and to detect possible occlusion of the vessel that will be undergoing cannulation.
- The prescribed medications (often a sedative and, sometimes, an antibiotic) must be administered. The insertion site may be prepared by shaving and cleansing it with an antiseptic solution.
- An intravenous catheter must be inserted.

After cardiac catheterization, assessment, prevention, and early detection of complications are the primary goals. Postcatheterization care varies, depending on the institution, but the following are basic points:

- Vital signs must be assessed every 15 minutes for 1 hour, every 30 minutes for 2 hours, and then less frequently, as specified by institutional policy.
- The extremity in which the catheter was inserted must be kept straight for 4 to 6 hours after the procedure. If the antecubital vessel was used, the arm must be immobilized on an arm board. If the femoral artery was used, strict bedrest must be enforced for 6 to 12 hours after the procedure. The client must be allowed to turn from side to side. However, to keep the leg straight at the groin and to prevent arterial occlusion, the head of the bed must not be elevated more than 15 degrees.
- The pressure dressing over the puncture site must be checked for intactness and for evidence of bleeding. Occasionally, a sandbag is applied to the insertion site for 4 to 6 hours. The site must be monitored for hematoma formation and the client questioned about the presence of increasing pain or tenderness.
- The pulses, color, warmth, and sensation of the extremity distal to the insertion site must be checked and documented every 30 minutes during the first hour and then as specified by institutional policy. Cardiac rhythm must be monitored for dysrhythmias.

CRITICAL TO REMEMBER

The nurse must notify the physician at once if:

- The client complains of numbness or tingling in the extremity
- The extremity becomes cool, pale, or cyanotic
- The distal pulse is not palpable or has changed
- Cardiac dysrhythmias occur
- The client complains of chest pain

- Fluid intake should be encouraged (if the underlying condition allows) for adequate fluid replacement and renal elimination of the contrast medium.
- The nurse must observe for nausea, vomiting, rash, and other signs of hypersensitivity to the contrast medium.
- Because the procedure is lengthy as well as a psychological drain on the client, supportive measures to promote comfort must be instituted. Whatever the findings of the procedure, the client needs clear explanation of their significance and consequences.
- Sometimes cardiac catheterization is an emergency procedure and not elective. In such instances, the client gets caught in a whirlwind of activity that ends not on completion of the catheterization but on completion of either balloon angioplasty or cardiac surgery. The nurse must provide emotional support to the client and significant others.

Angiography

This procedure involves intravenous injection of contrast medium into the heart during cardiac catheterization. Immediately after the injection, a series of x-ray films are taken that reveal the course of the contrast medium as it circulates through the heart, lungs, and great vessels. Angiography is an invaluable tool in cardiac diagnosis and aids in understanding heart and vessel disease.

Coronary angiography involves injecting contrast medium directly into the coronary arteries (via the coronary ostia) during cardiac catheterization. Cineangiography involves taking moving pictures during cardiac catheterization. This is particularly valuable because the examiners can view the film at both rapid and slow speeds, permitting detailed and unlimited review of the study.

Hemodynamic Studies

Four important parameters are used to assess early hemodynamic status: CVP, pulmonary artery (PA) pressure, cardiac output, and intra-arterial pressure. All of these parameters require invasive procedures. Critical care nurses perform all of these routinely at the bedside.

Hemodynamic pressure monitoring provides information about blood volume, fluid balance, and how well the heart is pumping. Current technology allows us to measure right atrial pressure (CVP), PA pressures during systole and diastole (reflecting right and left ventricular pressures), and pulmonary capillary wedge pressure (PCWP), a direct indicator of left ventricular pressure.

The Pulmonary Artery Catheter. Development of the balloon-tipped, flow-directed catheter has enabled continuous direct monitoring of PA pressure.

The most commonly used PA flow-directed catheter, the Swan-Ganz catheter, has four lumens (see the Bridge to Critical Care). The proximal lumen terminates in the right atrium, allowing CVP measurement, fluid infusion, and venous access for blood samples. The distal lumen terminates in the PA and measures PA systolic pressure, PA diastolic pressure, PA mean pressure, and PAWP. There is a small lumen that is used for inflation and deflation of the balloon. The fourth lumen is the thermistor port, which permits the measurement of cardiac output. In addition, some catheters have an additional port for the infusion of fluids and capabilities for cardiac pacing and measuring of the oxygen saturation of the blood. Five-lumen catheters also exist.

Inserting the Catheter. Insertion of a Swan-Ganz catheter is not risk free for the client. The potential complications of the catheter are PA infarction, pulmonary embolism, injury to the heart valves, injury to the myocardium, and infection. In addition, while the catheter is in place, the heart valves have less ability to close completely.

PA monitoring must be carried out in a critical care unit under careful scrutiny of an experienced nursing staff. Before insertion of the catheter, the nurse should explain to the client that the procedure may be uncomfortable but not painful and a local anesthetic will be given at the catheter insertion site. The nurse's support of the critically ill client at this time helps promote cooperation and lessens the client's anxiety.

Maintaining the Catheter. To maintain patency of the system, a small amount of heparinized solution is delivered under pressure at a constant flow rate. The nurse should ensure that the connections between the catheter and attachments are secure to prevent air embolism. The nurse applies an occlusive dressing at the insertion site and changes it regularly according to institutional protocol. Potential complications to watch for include pneumothorax, dysrhythmias, sepsis, and microelectric shock.

Obtaining Measurements. The nurse takes PA and PCWP measurements at routine intervals with the client in a supine position and the head of the bed at an angle of no more than 25 degrees.[11] For accurate PA and PCWP measurements, the baseline transducer position must be established. The zero point of the transducer must be level with the right atrium at the midaxillary line at the fourth intercostal space. This landmark is marked on the client's chest wall with a felt-tipped pen for future reference. The transducer must be releveled each time the client's head is raised or lowered. Also, measurements should be taken on end-expiration, especially if the client is on a mechanical ventilator.

Measurements of the PA systolic and diastolic pressures are taken with the balloon deflated. PA systolic pressure indicates the peak pressure generated by the right ventricle. PA diastolic pressure indicates the lowest pressure in the pulmonary artery. Mean PA pressure is an average of the systolic and diastolic pressures. The normal adult PA systolic and diastolic pressure is 20 to 30/10 mm Hg.

The balloon is inflated to measure PCWP. Pulmonary capillary wedge pressure reflects the pressure in the distal branches of the PA, thus estimating pressures within the left atrium or the end-diastolic pressure in the left ventricle. The normal PCWP is 8 to 13 mm Hg.

CRITICAL TO REMEMBER

The only time the balloon should be inflated after it is in place is to obtain further PCWP readings. Leaving the catheter in a wedged position can lead to infarction of the lung tissue being supplied by that vessel. If a fixed-wedge waveform occurs, the nurse should

- Check to see whether the balloon is inflated
- Change the client's position
- Instruct the client to cough
- Perform chest percussion
- Notify the physician for catheter repositioning.

From the PCWP, the function of the left ventricle is known. The client can be given fluids, inotropic agents, or other treatments to support and improve peripheral circulation.

BRIDGE TO CRITICAL CARE

Swan-Ganz Monitoring

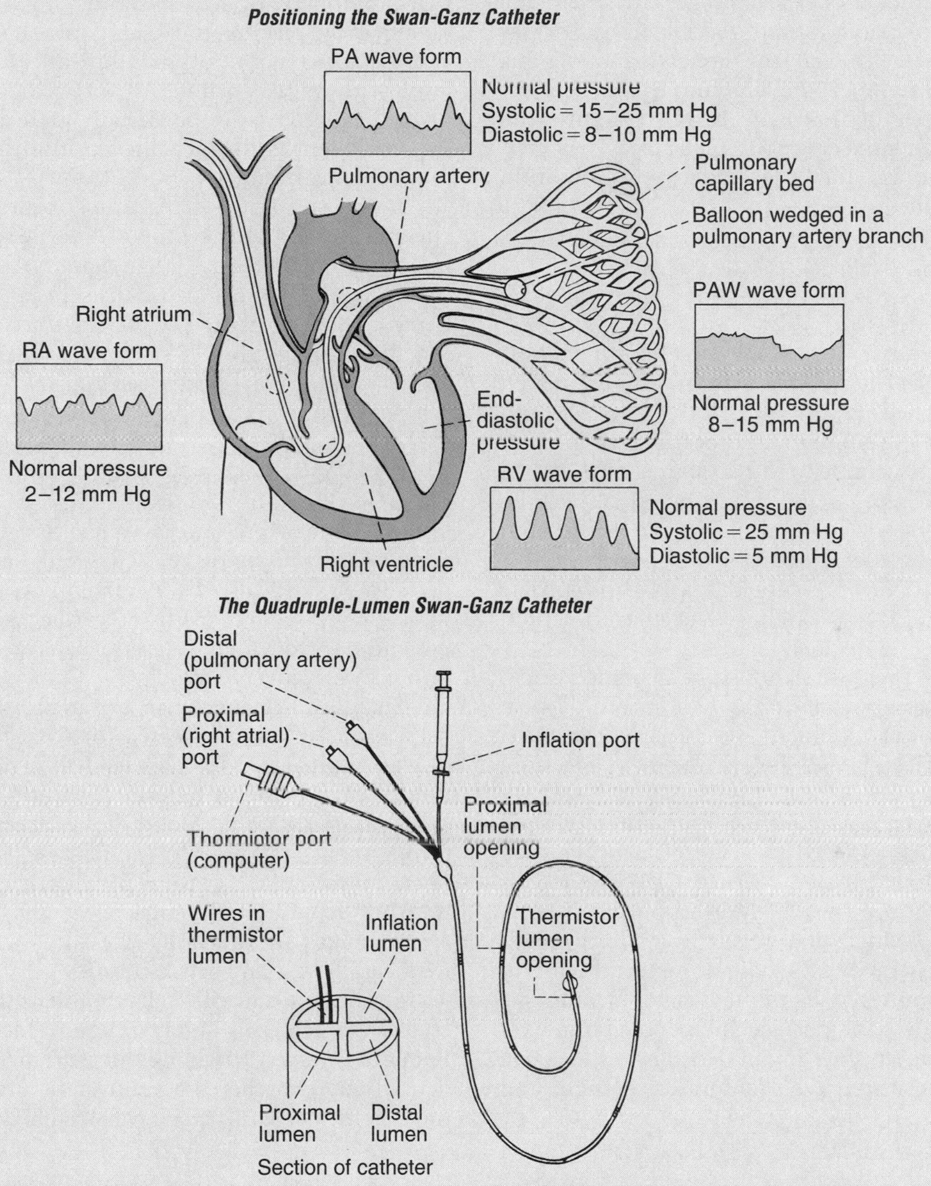

Conditions with Expected Pressure Changes

Condition	RA	RV	PAP	PAWP
	Pressure Changes			
Heart failure (volume overload)	↑	↑	↑	↑
Hypovolemia	↓	↓	↓	↓
Cardiogenic shock*	— or ↑	— or ↑	— or ↑	— or ↑ (Diastolic)
Pulmonary hypertension	↑	↑	↑	— or ↑
Cardiac tamponade	↑	↑	↑	↑ (Diastolic)
Pulmonary emboli	↑	↑	↑	↑ (Systolic)
Mitral valve stenosis-insufficiency†	↑	↑	↑	↑

RA, right atrial pressure; RV, right ventricular pressure; PAP, pulmonary artery pressure; PAWP, pulmonary artery wedge pressure.
* Pressure readings depend on the heart's ability to handle circulating volume. Chronic lung disease elevates all readings.
† Mitral valve disease produces unreliable pressure readings.

Obtaining Blood Samples. The PA catheter also provides a means of readily obtaining samples of mixed venous blood from the PA. Mixed venous blood refers to blood from both the inferior and superior vena cava and the coronary veins. The normal oxygen saturation of mixed venous blood is 75 per cent, whereas the normal oxygen saturation for arterial blood is 95 per cent. The difference between the arterial and venous oxygen saturation signifies the amount of oxygen extracted by the tissues of the body. In heart failure, the oxygen saturation of mixed venous blood may fall considerably, even though the arterial oxygen saturation may remain the same.

CENTRAL VENOUS PRESSURE

Central venous pressure is the pressure within the superior vena cava, reflecting the pressure under which the blood is returned to the superior vena cava and right atrium. Central venous pressure is determined by vascular tone, blood volume, and the ability of the right side of the heart to receive and pump blood. When the tricuspid valve is open at the end of diastole, the atrium and ventricle are, in effect, one chamber. At this time, the CVP is equal to the pressure in the right ventricle and is a good indicator of right ventricular function. (See Table 23–5.)

Central venous pressure can also be seen as a measurement of preload on the right side of the heart. Preload is the amount of blood presented to the heart or when the ventricle is full before the next ejection. Preload is the right ventricular end-diastolic pressure.

Central venous pressure can be measured with a central venous catheter placed in the superior vena cava or a balloon flotation catheter. Normal CVP pressure is 2 to 12 mm Hg. A drop in CVP indicates a decrease in circulating volume, which may result from fluid imbalance, hemorrhage, or severe vasodilation and pooling of blood in the extremities with limited venous return. A rise in CVP indicates an increase in blood volume resulting from a sudden shift in fluid balance, excessive intravenous fluid infusion, renal failure, or sodium and water retention.

For an accurate CVP measurement, a baseline must be established for the transducer position. The zero point on the transducer needs to be at the level of the right atrium. (See Obtaining PCWP Measurements.)

If the client has orthopnea or another condition that prohibits lying flat or supine, a CVP reading can be obtained by placing the client in a 45-degree position and the zero point of the transducer adjusted to the level of the right atrium. To obtain a comparison of the data, the nurse must be certain with any CVP reading that the client is in the same position he or she was for previous measurements.

In measuring CVP, the nurse makes certain that the client is relaxed at the time of the measurement. Straining, coughing, or any other activity that increases the intrathoracic pressure causes falsely high measurements. If the CVP is measured while the client is on a ventilator, the readings should always be taken at the point of end expiration for greatest accuracy.

PULMONARY ARTERY PRESSURE

Central venous pressure is not a satisfactory means of determining the status of left-sided heart function, especially in critically ill persons (e.g., those who are immediately recovering from cardiac surgery, have experienced myocardial infarction, have cardiomyopathy, or are in cardiogenic shock).

Significant changes can occur in the left side of the heart without being reflected for some time in the right side of the heart. This can lead to a delay in intervention or even inappropriate intervention.

During diastole, blood flows freely from the PA through the pulmonary capillaries, left atrium, and open mitral valve to the left ventricle. Therefore, the pressure in the left ventricle at the end of diastole approximates the diastolic pressure in the PA, pulmonary capillaries, and left atrium.

Starling's principle tells us that the heart muscle contracts most effectively when under slight stretch. Pulmonary artery pressure measurements can assist in determining whether the ventricle is understretched and the client needs fluids, overstretched and the client

TABLE 23–5 Indications for Central Venous Pressure (CVP) and How They May Affect the Readings

TO ASSESS	↑ CVP (>11 CM H_2O)	↓ CVP (<3 CM H_2O)
Right-sided heart hemodynamics	Right-sided heart failure (including chronic CHF, LVF) Constrictive pericarditis Cardiac tamponade Valvular stenosis Pulmonary hypertension	Early LVF
Blood volume	↑ Circulating volume	↓ Circulating volume
Vascular tone	Vasoconstriction Hypertension	Vasodilation-peripheral pooling Septic shock

CHF, congestive heart failure; LVF, left ventricular failure.
From Huang, S. H., et al. (1989). *Coronary care nursing* (2nd ed., p. 101). Philadelphia: W. B. Saunders.

TABLE 23–6 Conditions That Cause a Change in Cardiac Output

CONDITIONS THAT DECREASE CARDIAC OUTPUT	CONDITIONS THAT INCREASE CARDIAC OUTPUT
Acute congestive heart failure	Hypoxia
Pericarditis with effusion	Hyperthyroidism
Old age	Excitement
Arterial hemorrhage	Exercise
Standing motionless, which decreases the venous return to the heart	Food intake
Myxedema	Oral and intravenous fluid intake
Shock	Early stage of septic shock
Valvular heart disease	Pregnancy
Myocardial ischemia	Sepsis
Dysrhythmias	
Paroxysmal atrial tachycardia	
Atrial fibrillation	
Heart block	
Ventricular tachycardia	
Heat stroke	

needs diuretics, or appropriately stretched and at maximum function.

CARDIAC OUTPUT MEASUREMENT

Cardiac output is the amount of blood pumped out of the left ventricle into the arterial system every minute (i.e., cardiac output is equal to the stroke volume [volume of blood pumped out with each beat] multiplied by the heart rate). Table 23–6 lists the conditions that change cardiac output.

Currently, the most common method for determining cardiac output is thermodilution. This method requires a cardiac output computer and a quadruple-lumen PA catheter and can be obtained by the nurse at bedside.

Normal cardiac output in adults ranges widely from 4 to 8 L/min. However, these values do not take into account individual needs, which vary according to body size.

NONINVASIVE HEMODYNAMIC MONITORING

Thoracic electrical bioimpedance (TEB) is a noninvasive hemodynamic monitoring system first developed by NASA in the 1960s. This technique is currently being perfected for use in clients who are not good candidates for invasive monitoring (e.g., clients receiving thrombolytic therapy). This computerized system uses electrodes placed on the client's chest that emit low-level electrical signals. Although the signals are conducted by body fluids, they are not felt by the client. Thoracic electrical bioimpedance can measure cardiac output, stroke volume, preload and afterload, contractility, and ejection fraction and can help detect pleural effusion, pneumonia, and pulmonary edema.[26]

INTRA-ARTERIAL PRESSURE MONITORING

Systemic intra arterial monitoring has become a common method for obtaining BP measurements in acutely ill clients. This method provides continuous detection of arterial BP via an indwelling catheter. It is of greatest benefit in the client with low cardiac output, fluctuating hemodynamic status, and excessive peripheral vasoconstriction and in whom cuff BP measurements are undetectable or unreliable. (Note that intra-arterial pressure readings are at least 10 mm Hg higher than cuff BP readings.) The intra arterial catheter offers one other advantage: It simplifies obtaining blood samples for arterial blood gas and blood studies, minimizing the need for arterial or venous punctures.

The major complications of intra-arterial monitoring include hemorrhage caused by loose connections of the monitoring system, hematoma at the insertion site, infection (local or systemic), and embolization of the artery that supplies the distal portion of the cannulated extremity.

Besides accurate monitoring and recording of arterial pressure, nursing responsibilities focus on preventing complications of arterial cannulation. The nurse should:

- Check all connections frequently to ensure that they remain tight and secure. Accidental blood loss from a disconnected catheter can be as much as 200 mL in 4 to 5 minutes.
- Evaluate the cannulated extremity for neurovascular function every 2 hours. Assess and document color, temperature, capillary filling, and sensation distal to the site of cannulation.
- Check the insertion site for redness or signs of infection daily and change dressing per institutional policy.
- Maintain the potency of the system with a small amount of heparinized fluid delivered under pressure at a constant flow rate.

STUDY QUESTIONS

1. When assessing a client with the chief complaint of chest pain, the nurse should inquire about:
   A. The onset and duration
   B. The location and quality
   C. The aggravating and alleviating factors
   D. All of the above
2. When listening to heart sounds, the nurse is aware that simultaneous palpation of the carotid pulse helps identify:
   A. S_1
   B. S_2
   C. S_3
   D. S_4
3. Depolarization of the ventricles is represented by what on the electrocardiogram?
   A. PR interval
   B. T wave
   C. QRS
   D. ST segment
4. The client complains of substernal chest pain that is aggravated by exercise and alleviated by rest. This pain is most likely associated with:
   A. Pericarditis
   B. Myocardial infarction
   C. Myocardial ischemia
   D. Musculoskeletal deformity
5. After cardiac catherization using the femoral artery, the client complains of numbness and tingling in the extremity. The nurse assesses that the foot is cool and cyanotic. These manifestations represent:
   A. Infection at the insertion site
   B. Impaired circulation to the extremity
   C. A normal postprocedure finding
   D. Evidence of arterial spasm

CRITICAL THINKING EXERCISES

SCENARIO A

A client enters the emergency room complaining of shortness of breath that is worse with exertion. On assessment the nurse notes that the client is diaphoretic, tachycardic, and hypertensive. The history is significant for diabetes mellitus and coronary heart disease. The nurse initiates the myocardial infarction protocol for the client.

1. What data alerted the nurse to the possible diagnosis of myocardial infarction?
2. Why would the nurse immediately initiate the myocardial infarction protocol for the client?

SCENARIO B

A client says to you, "My father died of a heart attack when he was 50 years old. My grandfather also died of a heart attack. Why should I bother to stop smoking. I know that I am going to die young too."

How should the nurse respond?

BIBLIOGRAPHY

1. Adler, L., Brundage, B., & Shapiro, B. (1991). Tomorrow's cardiac imaging—Today. *Patient Care, 25(11),* 143–161.
2. Ahrens, T., & Taylor, L. (1992). *Hemodynamic waveform analysis.* Philadelphia: W. B. Saunders.
3. American Heart Association. (1991). *Heart and stroke facts.* Dallas: Author.
4. Apple, S., & Thurkauf, G. (1994). Preparing your client for and understanding transesophageal echocardiography. *Critical Care Nurse, 12(6),* 29–34.
5. Bates, B. (1991). *A guide to physical exam and history taking* (5th ed.). Philadelphia: J. B. Lippincott.
6. Braunwald, E., et al. (Ed.). (1990). *Harrison's principles of internal medicine* (12th ed.). New York. McGraw-Hill.
7. Burke, M., & Walsh, M. (1992). *Gerontology nursing: Care of the frail elderly.* Chicago: Mosby-Year Book.
8. Canobbio, M. (1990). *Cardiovascular disorders.* St. Louis: Mosby-Year Book.
9. Copstead, L. C. (1995). *Perspectives on pathophysiology.* Philadelphia: W. B. Saunders.
10. Dennison, R. (1990). Understanding the four determinants of cardiac output. *Nursing 90, 20(7),* 35–42.
11. Ehman, R. L., & Julsrud, P. R. (1989). Magnetic resonance imaging of the heart: Current status. *Mayo Clinic Proceedings, 64(9),* 1134–1146.
12. Emerson, R. J., & Banasik, J. L. (1994). Effect of position on selected hemodynamic parameters in postoperative cardiac surgery patients. *American Journal of Critical Care, 3(4),* 289–299.
13. Fahey, V. (1994). *Vascular nursing.* (2nd ed.) Philadelphia: W. B. Saunders.
14. Guyton, A. C. (1991). *Medical physiology* (8th ed.). Philadelphia: W. B. Saunders.
15. Huang, S., et al. (1989). *Coronary care nursing* (2nd ed.). Philadelphia: W. B. Saunders.

16. Hudak, C., Gallo, B., & Betz, T. (1994). *Critical care nursing: A holistic approach* (6th ed.). Philadelphia: J. B. Lippincott.
17. Izor-Povenmire, K., & House, M. A. (1989). Acute crack cocaine intoxication: A case study. *Focus on Critical Care, 16(2),* 112–119.
18. Jarvis, C. (1992). *Physical examination and health assessment.* Philadelphia: W. B. Saunders.
19. Kinney, M., et al. (1991). *Comprehensive cardiac care* (7th ed.). St. Louis: Mosby-Yearbook.
20. Loveys, B., & Woods, S. (1986). Current recommendations for thermodilution cardiac output measurements. *Progress in Cardiovascular Nursing, 1(4),* 242–247.
21. Messerli, F. H. (Ed.). (1993). *Cardiovascular disease of the elderly* (3rd ed.). Boston: Kluwer Academic.
22. Nelson, S. (1989). Clinical utility of signal averaged electrocardiography. *Practical Cardiology, 15(3),* 59–72.
23. Purcell, J. (1990). Advances in treatment of dilated cardiomyopathy. *AACN Clinical Issues in Critical Care Nursing, 1(1),* 31–45.
24. Schelbert, H. (1989). Myocardial ischemia and clinical applications of positron emission tomography. *American Journal of Cardiology, 64,* 46–52.
25. Smith, M. (1994). Noninvasive hemodynamic monitoring with thoracic electrical bioimpedance. *Critical Care Nurse, 14(5),* 56–59.
26. Stein, E. (1991). *Electrocardiographic interpretation: A self-study approach to clinical electrocardiography.* Baltimore: Williams & Wilkins.
27. Thelan, L. A., et al. (1994). *Critical care nursing* (2nd ed.). St. Louis: Mosby-Yearbook.
28. Underhill, S., et al. (1989). *Cardiac nursing* (2nd ed.). Philadelphia: J. B. Lippincott.
29. Vitello-Cicciu, J. M., & O'Sullivan, C. K. (1993). Introduction to hemodynamics. In J. Hartshorn, et al. (Eds.), *Introduction to critical care nursing.* Philadelphia: W. B. Saunders, 71–104.
30. Weeks, L. (Ed.). (1986). *Advanced cardiovascular nursing.* Boston: Blackwell Scientific.
31. Wolf, G. (1989). Magnetic resonance imaging and the future of cardiac imaging. *American Journal of Cardiology, 64,* 60–63.

Chapter 24

Nursing Care of Clients with Disorders of Cardiac Function

Learning Outcomes

After completing this chapter, the learner will be able to:

1. Teach the client about the pathophysiology associated with disorders of cardiac function.
2. Assess the client for risk factors associated with disorders of cardiac function.
3. Assess the client for changes in body function associated with cardiac disorders.
4. Develop plans of care for the prevention, management, and rehabilitation of clients with cardiac disorders.
5. Teach the client with cardiac disorders about prevention, management, and rehabilitation factors that optimize health.
6. Monitor the client for changes in cardiac function that may be life-threatening.

Coronary Artery Disease

The heart muscle must have an adequate blood supply to contract properly. The coronary arteries carry oxygen and blood to the myocardium. When a coronary artery is narrowed or blocked, the area of the heart muscle supplied by that artery becomes ischemic and injured, and infarction may result. The major disorders that result from insufficient blood supply to the myocardium are angina pectoris, congestive heart failure (CHF), and myocardial infarction (MI). These disorders are collectively known as coronary artery disease (CAD), also called coronary heart disease or ischemic heart disease.

Incidence

Coronary artery disease is the leading cause of death in Americans today. Nearly 1 million Americans died in 1991 from cardiovascular disease.[4] As high as this figure may seem, mortality from cardiovascular disease, including coronary heart disease and stroke, has actually declined over the last 40 years. Contributing to this decline are such factors as improved technologies and therapies for treatment of cardiovascular disease, use of thrombolytic drugs in acute MI, improved surgical techniques, and successful modification of risk factors in populations at risk.

Etiology

Although CAD claims more lives each year than any other disease, its causes are poorly understood. CAD results from the development of obliterative atherosclerotic lesions within the coronary arteries that narrow or obstruct these vessels. Atherosclerosis, a disorder of lipid metabolism, is characterized by deposits of fat-containing substances along the intima of blood vessels and smooth muscle cell proliferation. It underlies most causes of cardiovascular disease and death.

Risk Factors

The concept of risk factors helps categorize the causes of CAD and prevent them. Risk factors that precipitate CAD can be classified as

- nonmodifiable risk factors
- modifiable risk factors
- contributing factors

NONMODIFIABLE RISK FACTORS

Heredity. Genetic factors contribute to four traits that increase the incidence of atherosclerosis: hypertension, dyslipidemia, diabetes, and obesity.

Age. Symptomatic CAD appears predominantly in clients over 40 years of age. However, clients in their 30s, and even their 20s, sometimes suffer anginal attacks or MI.

Gender. Women of childbearing age display one fourth the risk of developing CAD, compared with men of the same age. This obvious difference in susceptibility diminishes after menopause; however, even after age 65 years, women continue to be less likely than are men to develop CAD.[69] Women who take oral contraceptives are more likely to develop CAD. This risk is particularly significant in women who smoke. Once oral contraceptives are discontinued, the increased risk of CAD does not continue.[69] Women with an early menopause face three times the risk of CAD as women with a normal or late menopause.

Two life-style changes during the past decade may increase the incidence of CAD among women. More women (many with the full responsibility of the household and children) have entered the work force. Also, more women begin smoking at an earlier age.

Race. Black men die more frequently from CAD than white men.[4] The mortality rate of black women is lower than that of white men but higher than that of white women.[4]

MODIFIABLE RISK FACTORS

Environment, smoking, hypertension, elevated serum cholesterol levels, and diabetes constitute other major risk factors.

Environment. CAD is seven times more prevalent in North America, Australia, Europe, and New Zealand than in Japan, Switzerland, and Italy. Also, urban populations have a higher incidence of CAD than do rural populations. In developing countries, CAD is most prevalent among the affluent; in Great Britain and the United States, the opposite is true.[69]

Cigarette Smoking. One of the three major risk factors in CAD is cigarette smoking. How smoking causes CAD remains unknown. Male adult smokers have a 70 per cent higher mortality rate than do male nonsmokers, and all smokers have more than twice the risk of heart attack than do nonsmokers. Clients who smoke have two to four times the risk of sudden cardiac death. Clients who quit smoking lose their increased risk within 24 months.[72]

Hypertension. High blood pressure afflicts nearly 60 million American adults and children. Men over 45 years of age with blood pressure exceeding 140/90 and all adult women with pressures above 160/95 have a 50 per cent higher chance of mortality. As blood pressure increases, the risk for cardiovascular events also escalates. When hypertension is controlled, the risk of CAD decreases. Therefore, hypertension should be treated to lower the risk of CAD and premature death.

Elevated Serum Cholesterol. An elevated serum cholesterol level definitely increases the risk of developing CAD. A client with a serum cholesterol level greater than 259 mg/dL is three times more likely to develop CAD than is one with a serum level of 200 mg/dL.

The body produces endogenous cholesterol, primarily in the liver. Additional cholesterol is ingested through dietary intake, primarily from dairy products and meats. Cholesterol circulates in the blood in combination with triglycerides and protein-bound phospholipids. This complex is called a lipoprotein. There are four basic groups of lipoproteins, all produced in the intestinal wall. Elevation of lipoproteins is called hyperlipoproteinemia. Elevation of lipids, a component of lipoproteins, is called hyperlipidemia.

Lipoproteins and their functions are as follows:

- Chylomicrons primarily transport dietary triglycerides and cholesterol.
- Very-low-density lipoprotein mainly transports the triglycerides synthesized by the liver.
- Low-density lipoprotein (LDL) has the highest concentration of cholesterol and transports endogenous cholesterol to body cells.
- High-density lipoprotein (HDL) has the lowest concentration of cholesterol and transports endogenous cholesterol to body cells.

Recent investigations have documented how the presence of lipoproteins may predispose the body to development of CAD. The ratio of total cholesterol to HDL or of LDL to HDL is the best test for predicting the risk of CAD.[69] High concentrations of HDL seem to have a protective effect against the development of CAD. Exercise and low-fat, low-cholesterol diets increase the amount of HDL in the blood.

Diabetes. Diabetes frequently appears in middle-aged, overweight clients. Diabetes leads to early atherosclerosis. For women in particular, diabetes is a contributing factor to the development of CAD.[72]

CONTRIBUTING FACTORS

Obesity, lack of exercise, and response to stress also increase the risk of CAD. Obesity places an extra burden on the heart, requiring the muscle to work harder to pump enough blood to support added tissue mass. In addition, obesity is often associated with a sedentary life-style, elevated serum cholesterol, and high blood pressure.

Several studies suggest that effective, routine aerobic exercise may decrease the likelihood of a coronary event. Research confirms that a sedentary life-style potentiates the lethality of a myocardial infarction, and it is considered a significant risk factor in the development of CAD. The Framingham Study demonstrated an inverse relationship between exercise and the risk of CAD. Exercise may reduce the risk of CAD by decreasing weight, reducing blood pressure, and elevating the protective HDL.[72] The prevailing thought is that exercise, along with general body conditioning, makes the heart use oxygen more efficiently. To be effective, aerobic exercise should raise the heart rate from 50 to 100 per cent of baseline (depending on age and physical condition) for at least 20 to 30 minutes. Such exercise must be performed at least three times a week to be beneficial.

Stress appears to be associated with elevated blood pressures. Although moderate stress plays a role in modern life, excessive response to stress can be a health hazard. Significant stressors include major changes in residence, occupation, or status.

It has recently been reported that the electrocardiographic (ECG) abnormality seen with left ventricular hypertrophy is independently associated with CAD. The mechanism that accounts for this fact is unknown.[72]

The role that some of the modifiable risk factors have in precipitating heart disease is controversial. Hypertension, hyperlipidemia, and cigarette smoking have been objectively identified as predictive of CAD.[4]

Pathophysiology

The broad term arteriosclerosis, or hardening of the arteries, encompasses the following conditions: atherosclerosis, Mönckeberg's sclerosis, and arteriolar sclerosis.

Atherosclerosis is an occlusive arterial disease most commonly involving the aorta and the femoral, coronary, and cerebral arteries. The process of atherosclerosis includes the accumulation and deposit of cholesterol and lipids in the arterial wall (Fig. 24–1). Electron microscopic studies also document that structural changes occur in the layers of the arterial wall.

Mönckeberg's sclerosis involves calcium accumulations in the medial layer of the arteries. Arteriolar sclerosis is thickening of the small artery walls.

ALTERATIONS IN THE ARTERIAL WALL DUE TO ATHEROSCLEROSIS

There are three layers in the arterial wall separated by elastic laminae: the intima, the media, and the adventitia (Fig. 24–1*A*). Atherosclerosis primarily affects the intima of the arterial wall. The lesions affecting this layer and commonly seen in atherosclerosis are the fatty streak, the fibrous plaque, and the complicated lesion.

The fatty streak appears as a smooth, yellowish, slightly raised streak on the inner surface of the artery (Fig. 24–1*B*). It is characterized by the presence of lipoprotein deposits (mostly cholesterol). These deposits are located in the intima of the artery, inside smooth muscle cells and macrophages.

The raised fibrous plaque appears as a yellowish-gray bump on the surface of the artery. The plaque is made up of three types of material: (1) smooth muscle cells from the medial layer, (2) collagen, and (3) accumulated lipid within the intimal layer.

A complicated lesion (Fig. 24–1*C*) contains the fibrous plaque, calcium deposits, and a thrombus caused by hemorrhage into the plaque.

THEORIES OF PATHOGENESIS

The cause of arteriosclerosis is unknown. One theory suggests that certain changes occur in response to a nonspecific injury to the inner surface of the arterial wall. These changes then produce a classic lesion (see

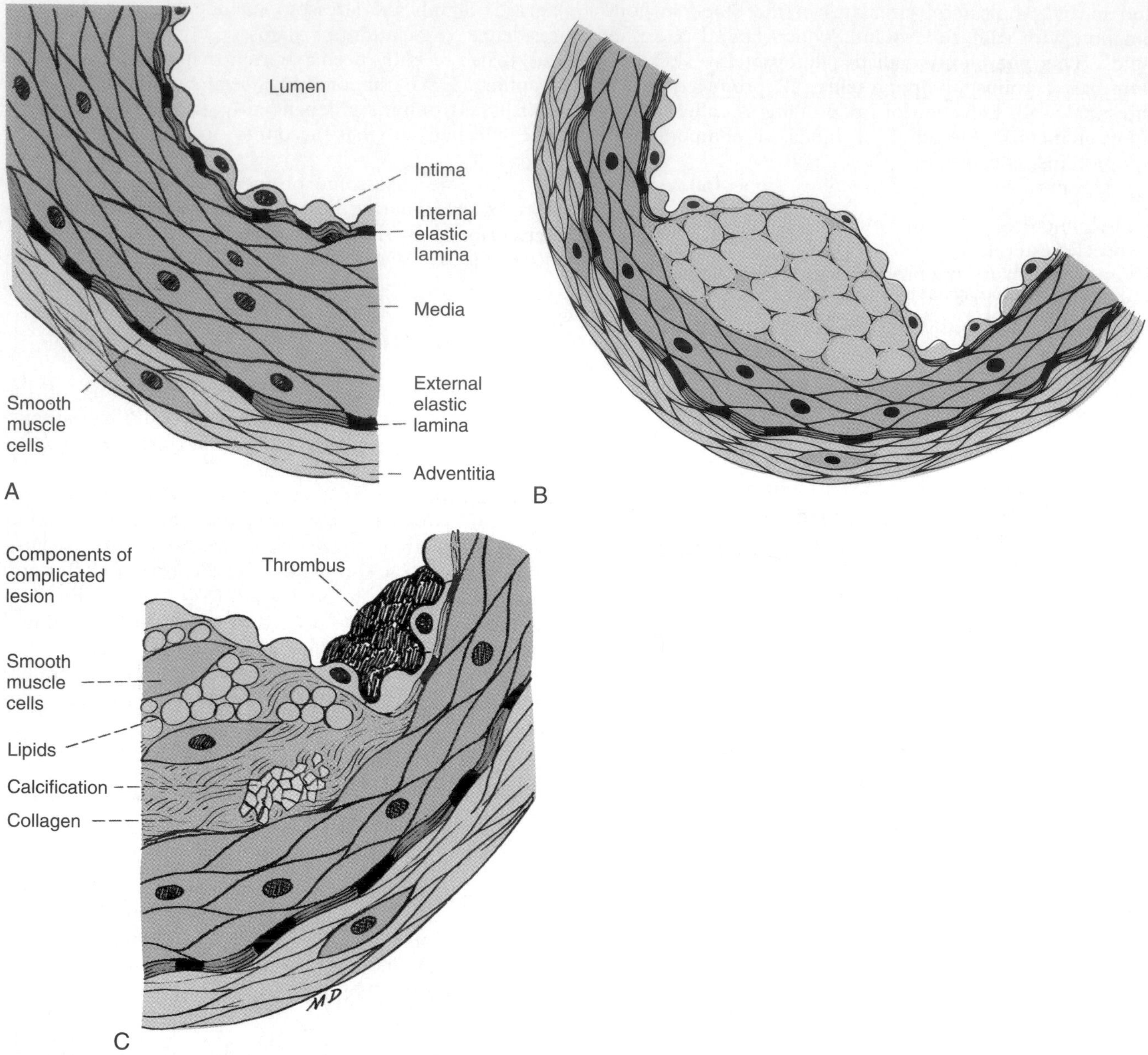

Figure 24–1
Cross section of artery. *A*, Normal; *B*, with fatty lesion; *C*, with complicated lesion.

Pathophysiology: The Response to Injury Theory of Atherogenesis). Nonspecific injury (mechanical, chemical, hormonal, or immunologic) may arise from such diverse causes as hypertension, hydrocarbons from smoking, cholesterol, catecholamines, angiotensin, or hormones. In turn, nonspecific injury results in the shedding or desquamation of the superficial layer of the artery. Continued exposure to the source of intimal injury results in continued lipid deposit and proliferation of smooth muscle cells.

Other theories for explaining the development of CAD include the monoclonal hypothesis, the senescence hypothesis, the thrombogenic hypothesis, the lipid-irritation hypothesis, and the hemodynamic hypothesis.

In general, most theories include the following major events in the development of atherosclerotic plaque:[72]

- endothelial injury
- platelet/fibrin interaction
- smooth muscle cell proliferation
- lipid entry and accumulation
- fibrosis
- thrombus formation
- ulceration and calcification

SEQUELAE OF CORONARY ARTERY DISEASE

It is important to recognize that CAD is a progressive disorder; if not prevented or treated in early stages, it

PATHOPHYSIOLOGY

The Response to Injury Theory of Atherogenesis

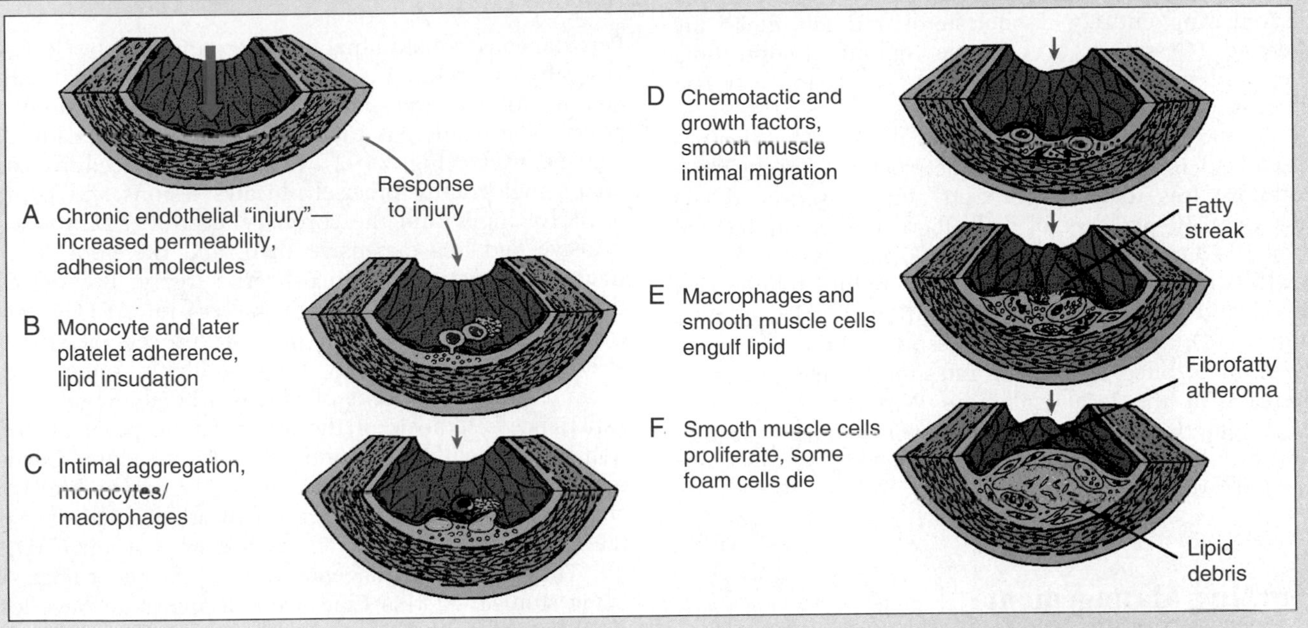

A, The process begins with focal areas of endothelial injury, usually very subtle, that result in increased endothelial permeability.
B, Lipids and platelets assimilate into the area. The lipoproteins commonly include low density lipoproteins (LDLs) and very low density lipoproteins (VLDLs).
C, Oxidized LDL attracts monocytes and macrophages to the site.
D, Plaques begin to form from cells, which imbed in the endothelium.
E, Lipids are engulfed by the cells, and smooth muscle cell develops leading to a fatty atheroma *(F).*

From Kumar, V., et al. [1992]. *Basic pathology* [p. 281]. Philadelphia: W. B. Saunders.

will progress to more severe forms of cardiac disorders. Common sequelae of CAD include sudden cardiac death, angina pectoris, and MI. In addition, clients may develop heart failure, chronic arrhythmias, conduction disturbances, and unstable angina. Sudden cardiac death is presented here; the other sequelae are the focus of the rest of this chapter.

Sudden cardiac death is not a clinical diagnosis but rather a descriptive term to identify clients who die from cardiac causes within 24 hours of the onset of symptoms. Each year, 250,000 Americans experience sudden cardiac death. In 20 per cent of these cases, sudden cardiac death is the first sign of cardiac disease. CAD accounts for 75 per cent of all causes of sudden cardiac death. Other risk factors include hypertrophic and dilated cardiomyopathies, Wolff-Parkinson-White syndrome, long QT syndrome, valvular abnormalities, and electrolyte abnormalities (hypomagnesemia and hypokalemia).

CRITICAL TO REMEMBER

Primary ventricular fibrillation is the major cause of sudden cardiac death. Dyspnea and fatigue are the most commonly reported symptoms experienced immediately preceding sudden cardiac death. Angina is a primary symptom in fewer than 35 per cent of cases.[21]

Clinical Manifestations

Atherosclerosis by itself does not necessarily produce symptoms. For manifestations to develop, there must be a critical deficit in blood supply to the heart in proportion to the demands of the myocardium for oxygen and nutrients. In other words, there must be a supply and demand imbalance. When atherosclerosis progresses slowly, the collateral circulation that develops generally can meet the heart's demands. Thus, whether symptoms of CAD develop depends on the total blood supply to the myocardium (by way of coronary arteries and collateral circulation) and not solely on the condition of the coronary arteries (see the discussion of angina, which appears later in this chapter). Often, symptoms of CAD do not appear until the lumen of the coronary artery narrows by 75 per cent.

DIAGNOSTIC ASSESSMENT

Techniques to determine the extent of CAD and identify the affected vessels include electrocardiogram, nuclear scanning, and angiography. (See Chap. 23 for a complete discussion.)

Medical Management

Prevention, rather than treatment, is the goal for clients with CAD. Fatty streaks are capable of regressing and disappearing entirely if cholesterol and fat intake are reduced. Cessation of cigarette smoking, controlling diet, and managing diabetes and hypertension can also decrease the risk of CAD.

Dietary modification is an initial step. The client is instructed to alter his or her diet so that saturated fats compose less than 10 per cent and nonsaturated fats less than 30 per cent of daily food intake. Cholesterol intake is also reduced to 250 to 300 mg/day.

Medications can be given to reduce cholesterol levels and reduce the risk of clotting. Cholestyramine (Questran) and colestipol (Colestid) inhibit the reabsorption of bile acids in the intestine, which causes an increase in the fecal excretion. With the increase in fecal excretion of bile acids, the liver increases production of bile acids from cholesterol; thereby, serum levels are lowered.

Nursing Management

Nurses need to have a high index of suspicion for clients at increased risk for CAD. These clients should be encouraged to reduce their risk by decreasing dietary intake of fats and cholesterol, increasing exercise, controlling diabetes and hypertension, keeping body weight at near-ideal levels, and ceasing smoking. The risk and incidence of CAD are so pervasive that many clients are engaged in these activities on an ongoing basis. The nurse should reinforce these healthy behaviors.

The client's level of motivation to reduce cardiovascular risk factors is the primary predictor of success. Nursing researchers are studying methods to improve motivation.

Surgical Management

PERCUTANEOUS TRANSLUMINAL CORONARY ANGIOPLASTY

Percutaneous transluminal coronary angioplasty (PTCA) is a surgical technique in which a balloon-tipped catheter is inserted and "floated" into a blocked coronary artery. The balloon is then inflated to mechanically dilate the artery (Fig. 24–2). Prior to the procedure, coronary angiography precisely locates lesions and points of narrowing within the coronary arteries. PTCA is less invasive and less expensive than, and therefore an attractive alternative to, open-heart surgery. But despite these advantages and its high success rate, PTCA only eases symptoms; it cannot halt the process of atherosclerosis, although it may prolong life in some cases. From 25 to 50 per cent of clients who undergo PTCA experience restenosis of the artery at the point of dilation, usually within 6 months of the procedure. Clients must be taught about and encouraged to make life-style changes to slow the progression of atherosclerosis (see the Client Education Guide: Decreasing Risk for CAD).

The surgical management of CAD in women is being studied. At this time, women appear to have less short-term benefit from surgery (i.e., suffer more immediate complications) but have similar, if not better, long-term results than men.[23]

The guidelines for selection of clients for PTCA are rapidly changing. Clients with no symptoms or mild symptoms to clients with unstable angina may be suitable candidates. PTCA may also be successful in single-vessel or multiple-vessel disease.[24]

Along with PTCA, new therapeutic devices for coronary application continue to evolve as alternatives to bypass surgery. Atherectomy is a procedure that uses a device consisting of a balloon and motorized cutter. The cutter is positioned against the blockage and mechanically débrides the plaque.

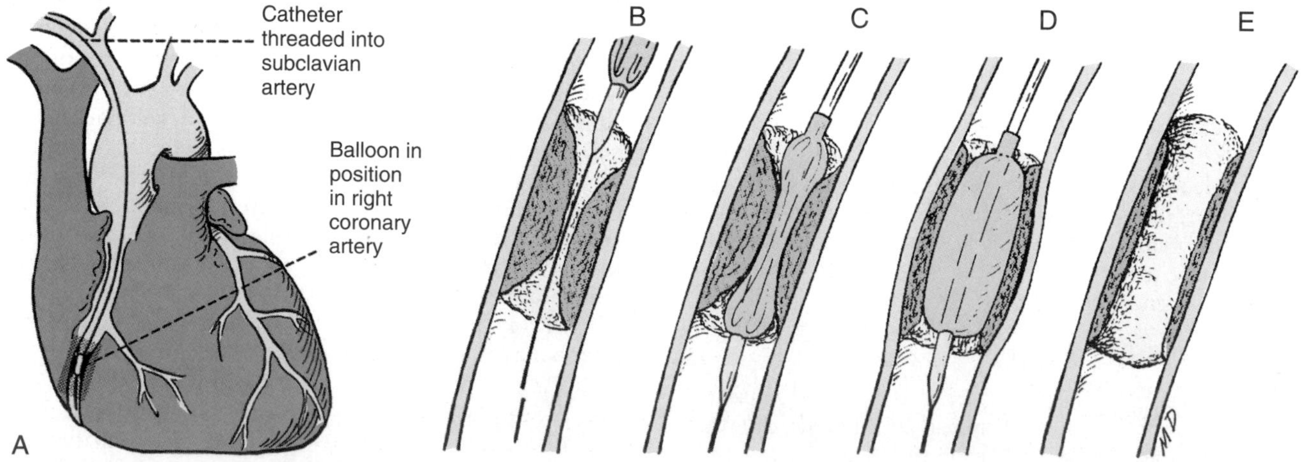

Figure 24–2
Percutaneous transluminal coronary angioplasty. *A*, Balloon-tipped catheter positioned in blocked artery. *B*, Balloon is centered. *C*, Balloon expands to *(D)* compress blockage. *E*, Artery diameter opened.

CLIENT EDUCATION GUIDE

Decreasing Risk for Coronary Artery Disease

The nurse should include the following information in client teaching sessions:

- Daily management of hypertension: Take medication as prescribed. Do not stop.
- Stop smoking immediately. Smoking reduces oxygen available to the heart and can precipitate angina. Smoking increases heart rate and blood pressure. Seek help from smoking cessation clinics or other resources in your community.
- Avoid passive smoke. Two hours of passive smoke decreases oxygen to the heart, decreases exercise time, and increases heart rate and blood pressure.
- Plan a regular exercise program under medical supervision.
- If overweight, lose weight. Seek help from professionals.
- Follow a healthy heart diet. Reduce cholesterol and increase fiber.
- Reduce stress. Seek help from professionals.
- Allow adequate time for rest and relaxation.
- These are life-long life-style changes.

An intravascular stent is a coil-spring tube, placed in the coronary artery, that acts as a mechanical scaffold to reopen the blocked artery. Early research results indicate that clients with stents have a decreased incidence of restenosis but an increased risk of bleeding and vascular complications. The client is at increased risk of bleeding at the time of the procedure because of the use of anticoagulation to prevent clot formation at the site of the stent. Clients with intravascular stents typically receive anticoagulation therapy for approximately 3 months.[60]

Lasers are currently being used with balloon angioplasty to vaporize atherosclerotic plaque. After the initial balloon angioplasty, a brief burst of laser radiation is administered, and additional remaining plaque is removed.[37]

Nursing Management

Before PTCA, the client is usually given an anticoagulant, most commonly aspirin, to help reduce the risk of arterial occlusion. During the procedure, the client is given heparin or calcium agonists, or both, or nitrates to reduce coronary artery spasm.

The client is also typed and crossmatched for blood in the event that emergency coronary artery bypass grafting becomes necessary. A consent is signed for angioplasty and surgery if required for spasm, perforation of the artery, or occlusion.

Following PTCA, the client is monitored for changes in vital signs and ECG readings and for angina. Additional postprocedural nursing care guidelines are the same as those following cardiac catheterization. Complications to watch for include acute myocardial infarction resulting from perforation of an artery, refractory arterial spasm, or occlusion.

CORONARY ARTERY BYPASS GRAFT

Coronary artery bypass graft (CABG) surgery involves the bypass of a blockage in one or more of the coronary arteries using the saphenous or mammary veins as replacement vessels.

Advances such as the development of calcium channel blockers and nonsurgical techniques such as PTCA have reduced the number of CABG surgeries performed. Nevertheless, because CABG can reduce angina in 80 to 90 per cent of patients refractory to medical management, it continues to be an important intervention in the management of CAD.

In CABG surgery, the surgeon harvests a length of saphenous vein from the client's thigh or lower leg. The heart is accessed through a median sternotomy. While the client is on cardiopulmonary bypass and the heart is not beating, the surgeon sews the distal end of the vein to the aorta and the proximal end to the coronary vessel distal to the blockage (Fig. 24–3). The veins are reversed so that their valves do not interfere with blood flow. In some cases, the internal mammary artery can be grafted to a coronary artery.

More than one half of all CABGs are performed on people over age 65, and approximately 73 per cent of them on men.[4] Elderly clients have a postoperative recovery similar to that of younger clients, but at a slower pace. Elderly clients are hospitalized for 4 more days on the average. They also have a higher mortality rate.[30] Postoperative complications that are more prevalent in the elderly include dysrhythmias related to aged sinoatrial node cells, drug toxicity related to impaired hepatic and renal perfusion, multiple drug-drug interactions, and decreased physical stamina.

During the first and second weeks after discharge, depression, fatigue, incisional chest discomfort, dyspnea, and anorexia are common. By the fourth to fifth weeks, clients typically report improved mood, comfort, and appetite. At 1 year, almost all clients are pleased with the outcome and improved quality of life.[30]

Nursing management of clients undergoing heart surgery is discussed in Chapter 25. A sample clinical pathway for clients undergoing CABG surgery is presented in Appendix C.

ANGINA PECTORIS

As vessels become lined with atherosclerotic plaques, symptoms of inadequate blood supply develop in the tissues supplied by these vessels. Problems such as cerebrovascular accident (or stroke), claudication, and angina develop. This section discusses angina; a discussion of cerebrovascular accident can be found in Chapter 14, and claudication in Chapter 26.

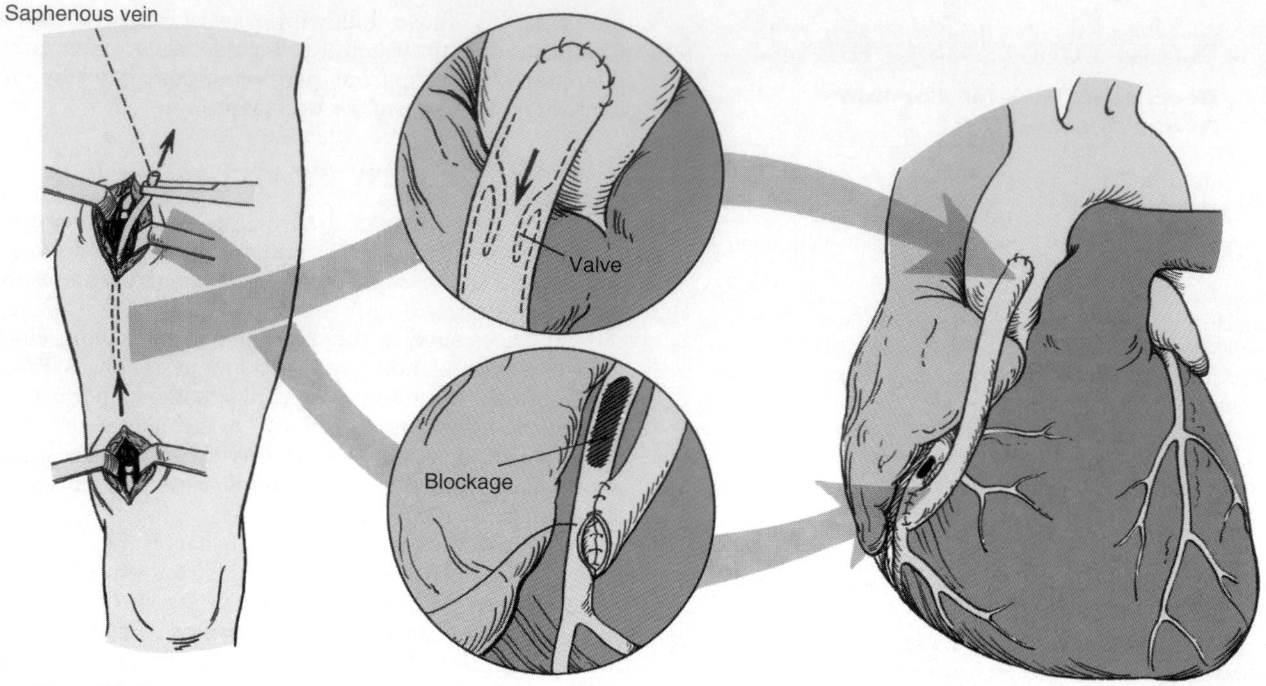

Figure 24–3
Coronary artery bypass graft. A section of saphenous vein is harvested from the leg and anastomosed to coronary artery to bypass the obstruction.

Definition, Incidence, and Etiology

Angina pectoris is a term used to describe chest pain resulting from myocardial ischemia (lack of blood supply). Angina pectoris is common, although its exact incidence is not recorded. The cause of angina pectoris is CAD or any cardiac disease impeding blood flow.

Risk Factors

Risk factors for angina are similar to those for CAD. Primary prevention is achieved through a life-long commitment to decreasing these risk factors. Secondary prevention focuses on the recognition and early treatment of anginal attacks. Tertiary prevention involves the resolution of angina before myocardial damage occurs.

Pathophysiology

The coronary arteries normally supply the myocardium with blood to meet its metabolic needs during varying workloads. When the heart needs more blood, the vessels dilate. As the vessels become occluded, they cannot dilate sufficiently to supply the myocardium with blood for normal workloads. A growing mass of plaque in the vessel collects platelets, fibrin, and cellular debris. Platelet aggregations are known to release prostaglandins, which can cause vessel spasm. This in turn promotes platelet aggregation, and a vicious cycle begins.

Myocardial ischemia develops if the blood supply through the coronary vessels or oxygen content of the blood is not adequate to meet the metabolic demands. Disorders of the coronary vessels (i.e., atherosclerosis, arterial spasm, and coronary arteritis), the circulation (i.e., hypotension and aortic stenosis or insufficiency), or the blood (i.e., anemia, hypoxemia, and polycythemia) may lead to decreases in blood or oxygen supply.

Conditions that increase demands on the myocardium include conditions that increase cardiac output (e.g., exercise, emotion, digestion of a large meal, anemia, and hyperthyroidism) and conditions that increase myocardial need for oxygen (e.g., damage to the myocardium, hypertrophy of the myocardium, aortic stenosis, aortic insufficiency, diastolic hypertension, thyrotoxicosis, strong emotion, exposure to cold, and heavy exertion). Damaged myocardium is unable to utilize oxygen properly. Hypertrophied myocardium has "outgrown" its normal blood supply and requires added supplies of oxygen. Aortic stenosis or insufficiency and diastolic hypertension cause the heart to work harder. Thyrotoxicosis increases oxygen consumption. Finally, strong emotions, cold exposure, and heavy exertion increase the heart's and the body's need for oxygen.

Myocardial ischemia occurs when either supply or demand is altered. In some clients, the coronary arteries can supply adequate blood when the client is at rest; but when the client attempts activity or becomes taxed in some other manner, angina develops. Myocardial cells become ischemic within 10 seconds of coronary artery occlusion. After several minutes of ischemia, the heart pumping function is reduced. The reduction of pumping deprives the ischemic cells of much needed oxygen and glucose. The cells convert to an anaerobic metabolism, which leaves lactic acid as a waste product.

As lactic acid accumulates, pain develops. Angina pectoris is transient, lasting for only 3 to 5 minutes. If blood flow is restored, no permanent myocardial damage occurs.

Clinical Manifestations

Characteristics. Angina pectoris produces transient paroxysmal attacks of substernal or precordial pain that may radiate to the left shoulder and down the inner side of the left arm. Less frequently, pain may be referred to the right shoulder and arm, epigastrium, jaw, neck, or left scapular region (see Clinical Manifestations: Characteristics of Anginal Pain).

Patterns. Classic angina pectoris may be subdivided into the following basic patterns.

Stable Angina. Stable angina is paroxysmal chest pain or discomfort triggered by a predictable degree of exertion or emotion. Stable angina characteristically has a stable pattern of onset, duration, and intensity of symptoms.

Unstable Angina. Unstable angina (preinfarction angina, crescendo angina, or intermittent coronary syndrome) is paroxysmal chest pain triggered by an unpredictable degree of exertion or emotion, which may occur at night. Unstable angina attacks characteristically increase in number, duration, and intensity over time.

Variant Angina. Variant angina (Prinzmetal's angina) is chest discomfort that is similar to classic angina but is of longer duration and may occur while at rest. These attacks tend to happen in the early hours of the day. Variant angina may result from coronary artery spasm and may be associated with elevation of the ST segment on the ECG.

Nocturnal Angina. Nocturnal angina occurs only during the night and is possibly associated with the rapid-eye-movement, or REM, sleep that accompanies dreaming.

Angina Decubitus. Angina decubitus is paroxysmal chest pain that occurs when the client reclines and lessens when the client sits or stands up.

Intractable Angina. Intractable angina is chronic incapacitating angina unresponsive to intervention.

Postinfarction Angina. Postinfarction angina occurs after MI, when residual ischemia may cause episodes of angina.

CLINICAL MANIFESTATIONS

Characteristics of Anginal Pain

SENSATION

The sensation of anginal pain is described as squeezing, burning, pressing, choking, aching, or bursting. The client often says the pain feels like "gas," "heartburn," "indigestion," or "a heavy weight on the chest." Clients do not describe anginal pain as sharp or knifelike.

SEVERITY

The pain of angina is usually mild or moderate in severity. Rarely is the pain described as severe.

LOCATION

Eighty to 90 per cent of clients experience the pain as retrosternal or slightly to the left of the sternum.

RADIATION

The pain usually radiates to the left shoulder and upper arm. It may then travel down the inner aspect of the left arm to the elbow, wrist, and fourth and fifth fingers. The pain may also radiate to the right shoulder, neck, jaw, or epigastric region. On occasion, the pain may be felt only in the area of radiation and not in the chest. The client rarely experiences the pain localized to any one single small area over the precordium.

DURATION

Anginal attacks usually last a short time, typically less than 5 minutes. However, attacks precipitated by a heavy meal or extreme anger may last 15 to 20 minutes.

RELIEF

Most anginal attacks quickly subside with the administration of nitroglycerin and with rest.

The typical "exertion-pain-rest-relief" symptom pattern is the major clue to the diagnosis of angina pectoris. Other symptoms accompanying the pain include dyspnea, pallor, sweating, faintness, palpitations, dizziness, and digestive disturbances.

DIAGNOSTIC ASSESSMENT

Electrocardiogram. The ECG tracings remain normal in 25 to 30 per cent of clients with angina pectoris. An ECG taken in the presence of pain may document transient ischemic attacks with ST segment elevation. An ECG taken during an episode of pain may also suggest the coronary artery involved and the amount of cardiac muscle affected by the ischemic event.

Exercise Electrocardiogram ("Stress Test"). An ECG may also be taken while the client exercises on a treadmill or stationary bicycle. The client increases exercise performance according to a defined program until reaching 85 per cent of maximal heart rate. ECG or vital sign changes may indicate ischemia.

Radioisotope Imaging. Various nuclear imaging techniques are used as diagnostic tools to evaluate the myocardial muscle. Regions of poor perfusion or ischemia appear as areas of diminished or absent activity ("cold" spots).[36]

Coronary Angiography. Angiography provides the most accurate information about the patency of the coronary arteries. This diagnostic assessment allows visualization of the artery and any partial or complete blockages.

These diagnostic assessments are fully described in Chapter 23.

Medical Management

Medical management of clients with angina pectoris focuses on two goals: relieving the acute attack and preventing further attacks to reduce the risk of MI.

Angina pectoris is diagnosed by history and various diagnostic assessments. Risk factors for CAD are investigated. A complete history of the pain and its pattern is taken. Clients are encouraged to describe the pain in their own words, to provide a baseline that can be used in ongoing care.

Most physical findings are transient. The client exhibits pallor or has cold and clammy skin. Tachycardia and hypertension may be recorded. Pulsus alternans may be present at the onset of ischemic attacks. On auscultation, an S_3 or S_4 gallop or a paradoxical split of S_2 may be noted. If the client has a mitral regurgitation

TABLE 24–1 Antianginal Agents

CLASS	EXAMPLE	ACTION	COMMON SIDE EFFECTS	NURSING IMPLICATIONS
Opiate analgesic	Morphine sulfate	Opiate analgesic used to relieve severe pain and anxiety associated with acute MI Also reduces venous return: thereby, myocardial workload is decreased	Sedation, confusion, hypotension, nausea and vomiting, constipation, dry eyes, and respiratory depression	When administering IV, administer slowly over 3 to 5 minutes; monitor closely for hypotension and respiratory depression
Vasodilators	Nitrates/nitrites: nitroglycerin SL and nitroglycerin IV, translingual spray Long-acting: isosorbide dinitrate (Isordil, Sorbitrate, and other manufacturers) Nitroglycerin topical (Nitro-Bid, Transderm-Nitro, and other manufacturers)	Relax smooth muscle of coronary and peripheral blood vesels, causing an increase in their diameter: thereby, blood flow is improved and resistance is decreased As peripheral resistance decreases, workload on heart is reduced, and oxygen demand to supply ratio improves May enhance collateral circulation	Flushing, headache, dizziness, hypotension, tachycardia	Assess baseline cardiac function, heart rate, and blood pressure Postural hypotension may occur; caution clients to change position slowly, to sit or lie down, especially when taking nitroglycerin tablets SL Can take up to 3 nitroglycerin tablets SL at 5-minute intervals if necessary; if pain is not relieved after 15 minutes, physician should be contacted immediately or client should report to hospital Tablets are inactivated by light, heat, air, and moisture; store at room temperature, in tight-fitting amber glass container A potent nitroglyerin tablet should produce a burning sensation under tongue when taken SL: check expiration date
Calcium channel blockers	Diltiazem (Cardizem) Nifedipine (Procardia)	Reduce vascular smooth muscle tone by interfering with the ability of free calcium ions to initiate muscular contraction Act on coronary and peripheral arteries, causing vasodilation, increased myocardial oxygen supply, and decreased peripheral resistance	Dizziness, hypotension, bradycardia with diltiazem, diarrhea, abdominal cramps, nausea, vomiting, rash, dermatitis	Assess baseline cardiac function, electrocardiogram, heart rate, and blood pressure Monitor hepatic and renal function Food delays absorption and decreases plasma levels Decrease dosage gradually Administer slowly by IV
Beta-blocking agents	Propranolol (Inderal), metoprolol, atenolol	Block beta receptors, slow heart rate, increase exercise tolerance, reduce workload of heart	Nausea, vomiting, mental depression, fatigue, mild diarrhea, impotence	Propranolol should not be given to clients with a history of asthma. Administer with food. Give with extreme caution in clients with (and assess for) heart failure. Assess for bradycardia. Do not stop abruptly.

IV, intravenously; SL, sublingually; MI, myocardial infarction.

from ischemia of the papillary muscle, a murmur will be heard.

PHARMACOLOGIC MANAGEMENT

The primary goal of pharmacologic treatment of angina is to reduce myocardial oxygen consumption by altering the various components of the process. The components of myocardial oxygen consumption that can be pharmacologically treated are blood pressure, heart rate, contractility, and left ventricular volume.

The three major types of medications used in angina pectoris are vasodilators, calcium channel blockers, and beta-adrenergic blocking agents (e.g., propranolol). Specific drugs, along with their actions, common side effects, and nursing implications, are listed in Table 24–1.

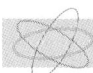

Vasodilators. Nitroglycerin, a short-acting nitrate, has been the medication of choice against anginal attacks since 1867. Today, nitroglycerin remains the major weapon against acute attacks. Administered sublingually, nitroglycerin acts to relieve the pain of angina within 1 to 2 minutes (see Client Education Guide: Sublingual Nitroglycerin). Nitroglycerin may also be administered orally, transdermally, and intravenously.

Long-acting nitrates act to maintain coronary artery vasodilation, thereby promoting a greater flow of blood and oxygen to the heart. This may be achieved with the use of isosorbide dinitrate (Isordil). Nitroglycerin decreases the oxygen requirements of the myocardium by causing systemic vasodilation and decreasing preload. Decreased preload and decreased left ventricular filling eases cardiac workload. Vasodilation also decreases afterload, further decreasing myocardial oxygen demand.

Long-acting nitrates produce the same general side effects as nitroglycerin (i.e., severe headache, flushing of the skin, nausea and vomiting, hypotension, vertigo, and syncope).

Approximately two thirds of clients taking long-acting nitrates develop a tolerance to the medication. Therefore, it is generally suggested that a 12-hour drug-free interval be maintained to preserve responsiveness to the nitrate. For most clients, this drug-free time is at night.[15]

Calcium Channel Blockers. Calcium plays a major role in the electrical excitation of cardiac cells and in the contraction of vascular and cardiac muscle cells. The resultant vascular smooth muscle relaxation decreases afterload and leads to decreased myocardial oxygen demand. The Food and Drug Administration has accepted three calcium channel blockers for use in the United States: nifedipine, verapamil, and diltiazem. The clinical use of each medication varies with the way each agent affects the heart. Physicians usually order nifedipine (Procardia) to treat angina. Nifedipine appears to complement the antianginal action of the vasodilators and beta blockers. Common side effects include flushing, dizziness, headache, and pedal edema. Verapamil (Calan, Isoptin) primarily acts as an antiarrhythmic. Because of verapamil's effect of decreasing heart rate and blood pressure, give it with caution when it is combined with beta blockers that have a similar effect. Diltiazem (Cardizem) has become popular because it has effects similar to verapamil and nifedipine with a lower incidence of side effects.

Beta-Blocking Agents. Administration of a beta-adrenergic blocking agent (e.g., propranolol, metoprolol, atenolol) will reduce the workload of the heart and may decrease the number of anginal attacks. Beta-blocking agents reduce myocardial oxygen requirement by blocking beta receptors and slowing heart rate. This in turn raises the exercise tolerance of clients with reduced coronary blood flow. Because beta-blocking agents reduce myocardial contractility and decrease the heart rate, extreme caution must be used when administering these drugs to clients with any degree of heart failure. Side effects of beta-blocking agents include nausea, vomiting, mental depression, mild diarrhea, fatigue, and impotence. Beta-blocking agents given in combination with nitrates on an around-the-clock schedule appear to be superior to either type of medication given alone. Propranolol should not be administered to clients with a history of bronchial asthma, significant mitral or aortic valvular disease, allergic rhinitis during the pollen season, or brittle diabetes. Propranolol should never be given in conjunction with monoamine oxidase inhibitors.

Because of the adverse effects of propranolol on the bronchial tree, pharmaceutical companies have developed other beta blockers that act more specifically on the heart (cardioselective). Examples of beta-blocking agents that are cardioselective are metoprolol (Lopressor) and atenolol (Tenormin). In small doses, these medications can induce full cardiac beta blockage without causing wheezing in clients with pulmonary disease. At larger doses, cardioselective beta blockers may become nonselective and block both the heart and bronchial beta receptors. Beta blockers should not be discontinued suddenly, which can increase the risk of myocardial infarction.

CLIENT EDUCATION GUIDE

Sublingual Nitroglycerin

The nurse should provide the client with the following instructions:

- Carry nitroglycerin at all times. Avoid carrying it close to the body's warmth.
- Keep the drug in its original container.
- Replace unused nitroglycerin every 6 months.
- Sublingual nitroglycerin tablets should cause a "tingling" sensation in the mouth.
- Place tablets under the tongue to dissolve.
- Dizziness may develop; sit, lie down, or change positions slowly.
- For angina, take one tablet every 5–10 minutes for three doses.
- **If you feel no relief, call the physician or go to the hospital. Do not drive yourself.**
- You may take a tablet prior to an activity that is known to precipitate chest pain.

DIETARY MANAGEMENT

In the average American diet, approximately 45 per cent of the total calories come from fat—a level in excess of the prudent diet recommended by the American Heart Association. Dietary fat comes in many forms and disguises. A high intake of cholesterol and saturated fats is associated with the development of coronary heart disease, whereas a proportional intake of polyunsaturated and monounsaturated fats is linked with lower risk. The prudent diet should include no more than 30 per cent of calories from fat, 55 per cent from carbohydrate (at least half of these should be complex carbohydrates), and 15 per cent from protein. When fat intake does not exceed 30 per cent of total calories, the expected rise in triglycerides from a high carbohydrate diet is minimal. Saturated fats should account for no more than 10 per cent of the caloric intake.

Overweight clients should be urged to lose excess weight. They should be encouraged to eat small meals, avoid high-calorie and high-cholesterol diets, abstain from gas-forming foods, and rest for short periods after meals. They also should increase their dietary fiber intake, which may not only prevent constipation and other intestinal tract ailments but also decrease the number and severity of anginal attacks. A high-fiber diet may also lower serum cholesterol and triglyceride levels. CAD is less common among clients with high intake of dietary fiber than in those with low intake. A high-fiber diet has also been shown to decrease hypertension.

Nursing Management

Besides documenting the clinical manifestations of angina, the nurse should attempt to determine how long the client has had angina, risk factors of CAD, and emotional reaction to the chest pain. Cardiac monitoring should be started, a 12-lead ECG obtained, and ongoing angina controlled. If the client reports angina, the nurse should assess the pain and ask the client whether it is the same pain experienced in the past. New characteristics or increased pain should be noted. Sublingual nitroglycerin should be given as prescribed. Because nitroglycerin causes vasodilation and hypotension, blood pressure should be monitored. If the pain is not relieved after three nitroglycerin tablets 5 to 10 minutes apart or by morphine, the physician should be notified. In addition, an environment that provides rest and security as well as decreases fear and anxiety will help reduce pain.

CRITICAL TO REMEMBER

Until the angina is controlled and coronary blood flow re-established, the client is at risk of myocardial damage from myocardial ischemia.

Client Teaching

The client must be knowledgeable in the care of episodes of angina and how to reduce the risk factors that exacerbate the process. See Client Education Guide: Managing Angina Pectoris and Client Education Guide: Decreasing Risk for CAD.

CLIENT EDUCATION GUIDE

Managing Angina Pectoris

The nurse should provide the client with the following instructions:

- Avoid known activities that precipitate angina (e.g., eating large meals, smoking, strenuous exercise, extremes in weather, increased humidity, excess stress).
- If angina occurs, stop the activity, sit down and rest, and take nitroglycerin if prescribed (three tablets taken 5–10 minutes apart).
- If the pain does not subside, worsens, or radiates, **Notify the physician or go to the emergency room. Do not drive yourself.**

ACUTE MYOCARDIAL INFARCTION

Acute MI, also known as a heart attack, coronary occlusion, or just "a coronary," is a life-threatening condition characterized by the formation of localized necrotic areas within the myocardium. MI usually follows the sudden occlusion of a coronary artery and the abrupt cessation of blood and oxygen flow to the heart muscle.

Because the heart muscle must function continuously, blockage of blood to the muscle and the development of necrotic areas within the myocardium represent a serious event, which may claim the client's life. Indeed, even if the client survives the initial attack, complications may arise, and the likelihood of suffering a subsequent fatal heart attack increases.

Incidence, Etiology, and Risk Factors

Every year approximately 1,500,000 Americans fall victim to heart attacks. MI is the leading cause of death in America, causing an estimated 500,000 deaths each year.[4] Approximately 300,000 persons die each year before they reach the hospital. Most deaths occur within the first 2 hours after the onset of symptoms, yet studies indicate that, unfortunately, half of all heart attack victims wait more than 2 hours before getting help because they are in denial. Public education to increase awareness of MI symptoms and thus decrease delays in treatment continues to be a challenge for health professionals. On the basis of data from the Framingham Study, approximately 45 per cent of all heart attack clients are under the age of 65 years, and 5 per cent are under the age of 40 years.

The risk factors that predispose a client to heart attack are the same as for all forms of CAD.

The most common cause of MI is complete or nearly complete occlusion of a coronary artery due to ongoing atherosclerosis. The vessel lumen slowly occludes and is often blocked with a thrombus. When blood flow ceases abruptly, the myocardial tissue supplied by that artery becomes ischemic, and infarction follows. Other causes of acute occlusion include coronary artery spasm and hemorrhage into a plaque.

Pathophysiology

Myocardial infarction can be considered the endpoint of CAD. Unlike the temporary ischemia that occurs with angina, prolonged unrelieved ischemia causes irreversible damage to the myocardium. Cardiac cells can withstand ischemia for about 20 minutes before cellular death occurs. Because the myocardium is very metabolically active, signs of ischemia can be seen within 8 to 10 seconds of decreased blood flow. Acidosis leads to conduction system disorders, and dysrhythmias develop. Contractility is also reduced, decreasing the heart's ability to pump. As the myocardial cells necrose, certain intracellular enzymes are introduced into the bloodstream, where they can be detected by laboratory tests.

The infarcted site is called the zone of infarction and necrosis. Around it is a zone of hypoxic injury. This zone is able to return to normal but may also necrose if blood flow is not restored. The outermost zone is called the zone of ischemia; damage to this area is reversible.

The most common site for myocardial infarction is the anterior wall of the left ventricle near the apex. Infarction of the anterior left ventricle results from thrombosis of the descending branch of the left coronary artery (see Pathophysiology: Areas of Myocardium Affected by Arterial Insufficiency of Specific Cardiac Arteries).

PATHOPHYSIOLOGY

Areas of the Myocardium Affected by Arterial Insufficiency of Specific Cardiac Arteries

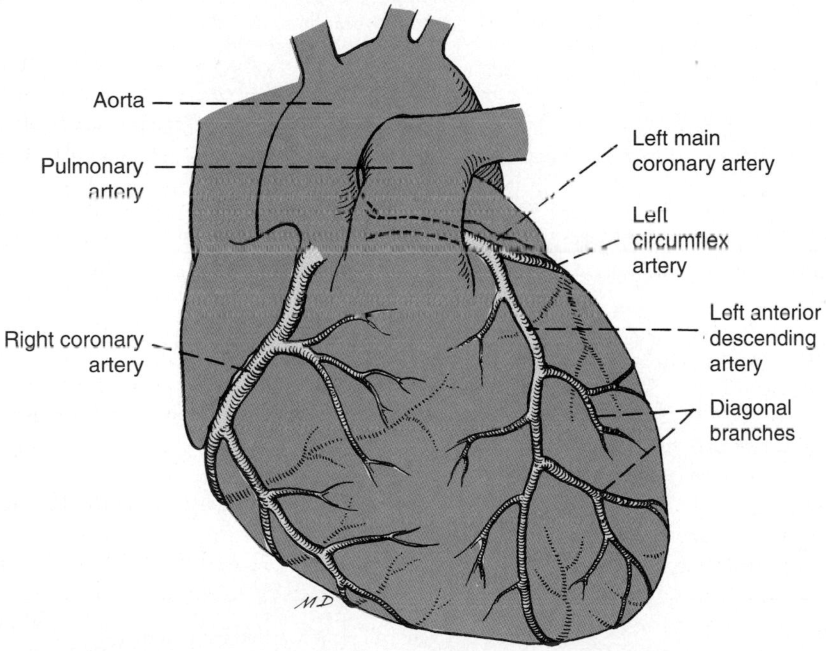

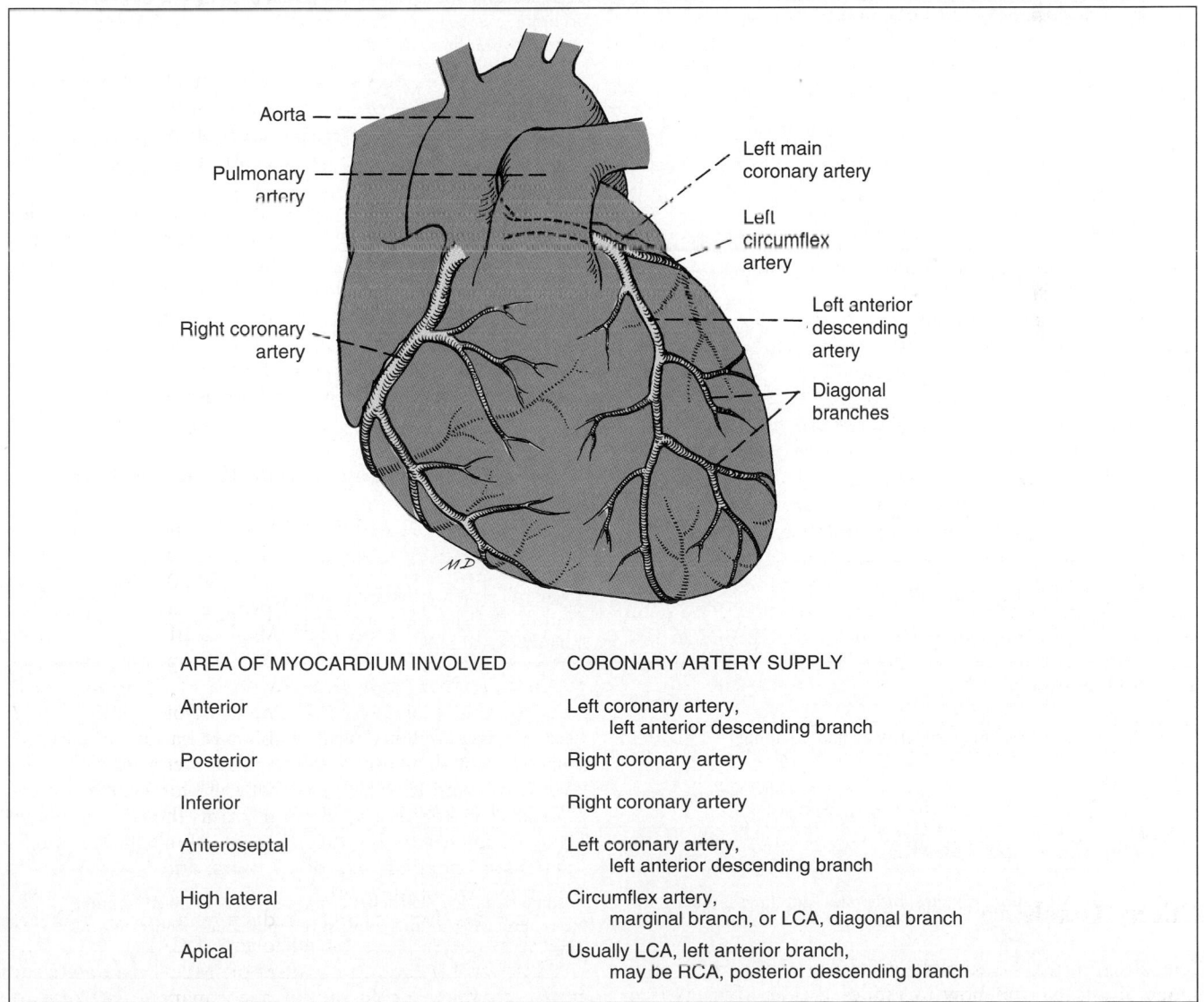

AREA OF MYOCARDIUM INVOLVED	CORONARY ARTERY SUPPLY
Anterior	Left coronary artery, left anterior descending branch
Posterior	Right coronary artery
Inferior	Right coronary artery
Anteroseptal	Left coronary artery, left anterior descending branch
High lateral	Circumflex artery, marginal branch, or LCA, diagonal branch
Apical	Usually LCA, left anterior branch, may be RCA, posterior descending branch

Clinical Manifestations

The cardinal symptom of MI is chest pain, similar to angina pectoris but more severe in character and duration and unrelieved by nitroglycerin. The pain may radiate to the neck, jaw, shoulder, back, or left arm (Fig. 24–4). Also, the pain may present near the epigastrium, simulating that of indigestion. See Clinical Manifestations: Myocardial Infarction for the signs and symptoms of MI along with their pathophysiologic bases.

DIAGNOSTIC ASSESSMENT

ECG Changes. Ischemia and myocardial infarction typically cause the ECG changes shown in Figure 24–5. Through the course of an MI, changes occur first in the ST segment, then in the T wave, and finally in the Q wave. As the myocardium heals, the ST segment and T waves return to normal, but the Q wave changes remain evident. Daily (serial) ECGs are routinely done for 3 days to diagnose MI.

Laboratory Studies. Laboratory findings include elevated serum creatine phosphokinase (CK-MB), elevated lactate dehydrogenase isoenzyme (LDH_1), leukocytosis, and elevated erythrocyte sedimentation rate.

Serum levels of CK-MB (an isoenzyme of CPK found only in cardiac muscle) increase 4 to 6 hours after the onset of chest pain, reach a peak in 12 to 18 hours, and return to normal levels in 3 to 4 days.

The LDH_1 is plentiful in the heart muscle and is

CLINICAL MANIFESTATIONS

Myocardial Infarction: Clinical Manifestations and Pathophysiologic Bases

Clinical Manifestations	Pathophysiologic Bases
Pain	
Crushing, severe, prolonged, unrelieved by rest or nitroglycerin; often radiating to one or both arms, the neck, and back	Cessation of blood supply to myocardium caused by thrombotic occlusion causes accumulation of metabolites within ischemic part of myocardium; this affects nerve endings
Shock	
Systolic blood pressure below 80 mm Hg, gray facial color, lethargy, cold diaphoresis, peripheral cyanosis, tachycardia or bradycardia, weak pulse	In some cases, shock caused primarily by severe pain; in others, by severe reduction in cardiac output and by inadequate tissue perfusion resulting in tissue hypoxia
Oliguria	
Urine flow of less than 30 mL/hr	Indicates renal hypoxia due to inadequate tissue perfusion resulting from hypotension. Cardiogenic shock is seen with damage to more than 40 per cent of left ventricle
Fever	
Temperature rises within 24 hours and lasts 3 to 7 days; usually 37.5° to 39.5° C (100° to 103° F), accompanied by leukocytosis and elevated sedimentation rate	Fever and elevated white blood cell counts result from destruction of myocardial tissue and ensuing inflammatory process; fever drops when fibroblasts begin to replace leukocytes and scar tissue starts to form
Apprehension	
Feeling of "doom," restlessness	Severe pain of a heart attack is terrifying; also, most clients are aware of the significance of a heart attack; restlessness results from shock and pain
"Indigestion"	
"Gas pains around the heart," nausea and vomiting	Client may prefer to believe that pain is caused by "gas" or "indigestion" rather than by heart disease; nausea and vomiting may result from severe pain or from vagovagal reflexes conducted from area of damaged myocardium to gastrointestinal tract
Acute Pulmonary Edema	
Sense of suffocation, dyspnea, orthopnea, gurgling; bubbling respirations	In some cases, left ventricle becomes severely crippled in pumping action owing to infarction; severe pulmonary congestion results

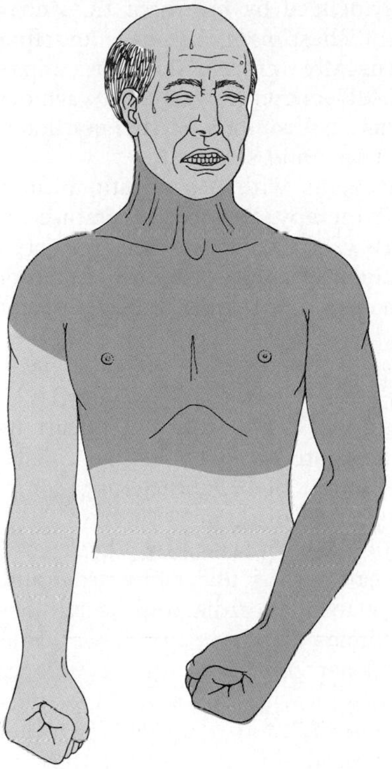

Figure 24–4
Possible extent of pain from myocardial infarction.

released into the serum when myocardial damage occurs. LDH_1 elevates 12 hours after onset of myocardial damage, peaks within 24 to 48 hours, and slowly returns to normal over the next 10 days.

Leukocytosis of 10,000 to 20,000 cells/mm^3 appears on the second day after MI and disappears in 1 week.

As discussed in Chapter 23, multiple tests are used to evaluate myocardial viability, ischemia, and wall motion. These include

- radionuclide imaging
- positron emission tomography
- magnetic resonance imaging
- echocardiography
- transesophageal echocardiography

As a rule, these studies are not used in the acute phase to diagnose MI.

Prognosis

Since the advent of coronary care units and devices that aid in promptly recognizing and treating life-threatening arrhythmias, 70 to 80 per cent of those suffering from an acute MI survive the initial attack. The following factors greatly diminish the chance of survival:

- advanced age (persons age 80 years or older have a 60 per cent mortality rate)
- evidence of other cardiovascular disease, respiratory diseases, or uncontrolled diabetes mellitus (presence of angina or previous MI is associated with a mortality rate exceeding 30 per cent)
- anterior location of MI (clients with an anterior MI have a 30 per cent mortality rate)
- hypotension (systolic blood pressure of less than 55 mm Hg on admission is associated with a 60 per cent mortality rate)

Deaths generally result from severe dysrhythmias, cardiogenic shock, congestive heart failure, rupture of the heart, and recurrent MI. Recent research shows a

Figure 24–5
Areas of change and the electrocardiographic patterns that accompany these changes during myocardial infarction.

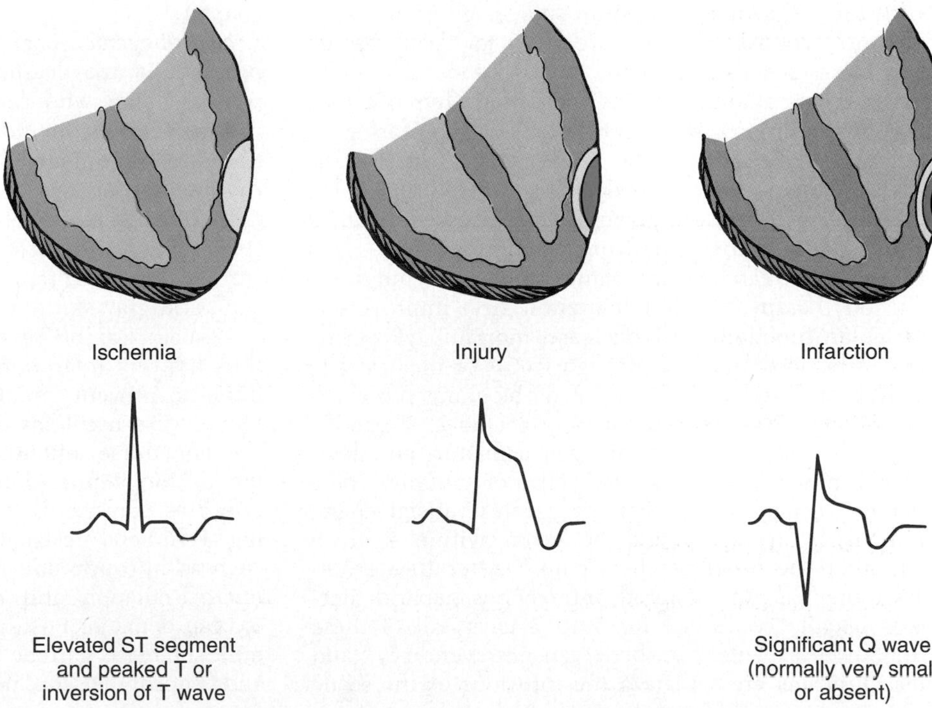

correlation between post-MI mortality and hypomagnesemia, although the etiology is not yet understood.[36]

Clients fortunate enough to avoid developing complications after MI still require a period of 6 to 12 weeks for complete recovery. Unfortunately, however, 50 per cent of those who completely recover from their first coronary will die within 5 years; 75 per cent will die within 10 years from massive infarction.[68]

Medical Management

Major goals of care for clients with acute MI are

- successful treatment of the acute attack and prompt alleviation of manifestations
- prevention of complications and further attacks
- rehabilitation and education of the client and significant others

MANAGEMENT OF THE ACUTE ATTACK

The client who suffers an acute MI needs immediate admission to a hospital with a coronary care unit, if possible. Invasive monitoring (arterial and pulmonary artery pressure lines) are commonly used. (See Chap. 23 for information on intra-arterial pressure monitoring and pulmonary artery pressure lines.)

The first goal of treatment is to decrease the heart's workload and increase oxygen supply to the myocardium, to limit the area of infarction. Workload is decreased through rest, decreasing preload, and eliminating tachycardia. The first 6 hours after the onset of pain is the crucial time frame for the salvage of the myocardium. Pain control is a priority. Continued pain is a symptom of continuing myocardial ischemia. Pain also stimulates the autonomic nervous system and increases preload, increasing myocardial demands. The drug of choice for MI pain is morphine sulfate, given in small doses intravenously. Nitrates are given for their vasodilating effect (see Table 24–1).

Oxygen is administered to treat tissue hypoxia. Because dysrhythmias are common, ECG monitoring is essential. Administration of antiarrythmics is begun. Anticoagulants are given to decrease the risk of embolism. Stool softeners are given to decrease constipation and the risk of bradycardia from straining.

Standard treatment for acute MI also includes reperfusion therapy, to limit infarction size, improve left ventricular function, and decrease mortality. Reperfusion can be accomplished through PTCA or medications that lyse or dissolve the clot that is blocking the coronary artery. Thrombolytic therapy includes streptokinase, urokinase, tissue-plasminogen activator, and acylated plasminogen streptokinase activator complex. It is generally recommended that for greatest effectiveness, thrombolytic agents should be given within 3 to 6 hours after the onset of chest pain.[32] After the thrombolytic agent is administered, intravenous heparin therapy is usually continued for 5 to 7 days. All of these thrombolytic agents can be given intravenously, and some clinicians are initiating the infusions at the scene of the infarction. Successful reperfusion of the coronary arteries is evidenced by return of ECG changes to normal, relief of chest pain, presence of reperfusion dysrhythmias (usually ventricular), and a rapid, early peak of the CK-MB enzymes (called "washout"). Possible complications of thrombolytic therapy include bleeding, allergic reactions, and stroke.[32]

Not all clients with MI are suitable candidates for thrombolytic therapy. Possible contraindications include age above 76 years; recent trauma, surgery, or cerebrovascular accident; history of bleeding disorder or gastric ulcer; pregnancy; and pericarditis or endocarditis.

PREVENTION OF COMPLICATIONS

The possibility of death from complications always accompanies an acute MI. Thus, prime collaborative goals include prevention of life-threatening complications, or at least recognition of them.

Dysrhythmias. Specifically, these are ventricular premature beats, ventricular tachycardia and fibrillation, supraventricular tachycardia, and heart block.

Dysrhythmias are the major cause of death after an MI; 40 to 50 per cent of deaths occur because of dysrhythmias. Ectopic rhythms arise in or near borders of intensely ischemic and damaged myocardial tissues. Damaged myocardium may also interfere with the conduction system, causing bradycardia or heart block. Supraventricular tachycardia sometimes occurs as a result of heart failure. Spontaneous or pharmacologic reperfusion of a previously ischemic area may also precipitate ventricular arrhythmias.

The nurse should provide continuous cardiac monitoring and frequent counts of premature ventricular contractions (PVCs) (many monitoring systems count continuously) and notify the physician if more than three PVCs occur per minute. The nurse provides prompt intervention for dysrhythmias per protocol or orders. Dysrhythmias are discussed later in this chapter.

Cardiogenic Shock. Cardiogenic shock results in 9 per cent of the deaths from MI. An estimated 80 per cent of clients who develop shock die from the complications. Causes include decreased myocardial contraction and diminished cardiac output, undetected dysrhythmias, and sepsis.

Clinical manifestations include systolic blood pressure significantly below a client's normal blood pressure, diaphoresis, rapid pulse, restlessness, cold clammy skin, and gray skin color.

Shock can be prevented with rapid relief of pain, thus limiting infarction size, and sufficient intravenous fluids to prevent circulatory collapse. It is also vital to identify dysrhythmias rapidly.

The nurse administers vasopressors such as levarterenol, dopamine, dobutamine, and metaraminol (Aramine) as prescribed to raise blood pressure by increasing peripheral resistance. In other cases, vasodilators such as nitroprusside promote better blood flow in the microcirculation and reduce preload, thus decreasing oxygen demand. Positive inotropic agents such as dopamine increase cardiac contractility and cardiac output and improve tissue perfusion. The nurse administers oxygen therapy and antiarrhythmic agents as prescribed and continuously monitors interarterial and pulmonary artery pressures. Chapter 56 discusses shock in detail.

Heart Failure and Pulmonary Edema. The most common cause of in-hospital death for clients with cardiac disorders is CHF, which is responsible for one third of deaths after an MI.[61]

Heart failure may develop at the onset of the infarction, or it may occur weeks later. Clinical manifestations include dyspnea, orthopnea, weight gain, edema, enlarged tender liver, distended neck veins, and crackles. CHF is managed by correcting the underlying etiology, relieving symptoms, and enhancing cardiac pump performance. CHF is discussed later in this chapter.

Pulmonary Embolism. Pulmonary embolism may develop secondary to phlebitis of the leg or pelvic veins (venous thrombosis). Pulmonary embolism occurs in 10 to 20 per cent of clients at some point either during the acute attack or in the convalescent period.

Prevention is the best treatment for pulmonary embolism. The client should be encouraged to move legs and feet frequently. The nurse should avoid placing pressure under the knees with pillows or by gatching the bed and should apply Ace bandages or elastic stockings to legs. Sufficient fluids must be administered to prevent dehydration and increased blood viscosity; anticoagulant therapy should be used. Anticoagulant therapy as a general preventive measure against thrombus formation and embolization after MI is considered standard practice. Intravenous administration of heparin is initiated on the client's admission to the hospital and may be continued for 3 to 7 days. See Chapter 22 for information on the diagnosis and treatment of pulmonary embolism.

Recurrent Myocardial Infarction. Recurrent MI occurs in about 5 per cent of clients during the period of recovery from the first acute attack.[61] Possible causes include overexertion, embolization, or further thrombotic occlusion of a coronary artery by an atheroma. The clinical manifestation is the return of angina. Management is the same as for the acute MI.

Complications Due to Necrosis of the Myocardium. Complications due to necrosis of the myocardium include ventricular aneurysm, rupture of the heart, ventricular septal defect, and ruptured papillary muscle. These problems are infrequent but serious complications that usually occur 7 to 10 days after an MI. Weak, friable necrotic myocardial tissue increases vulnerability to these complications.

Manifestations of CHF develop with ventricular aneurysm, rupture of the ventricular septum, and rupture of the papillary muscle. Symptoms of severe mitral insufficiency often develop when the papillary muscle of the left ventricle ruptures.

CRITICAL TO REMEMBER

The presence of a new mitral murmur should be reported to the physician immediately.

Ventricular dysrhythmias (e.g., frequent PVCs and ventricular tachycardia) often occur in the presence of a ventricular aneurysm (the necrotic tissue is very irritable). Signs of cardiac tamponade may develop with rupture of the heart.

The goal of medical therapy is to increase oxygen supply and decrease oxygen demand to minimize the necrotic area.

Surgery is performed in 4 to 6 weeks to (1) excise the ventricular aneurysm, (2) replace the mitral valve if the papillary muscle is ruptured, or (3) repair the ventricular septal defect. Pericardiocentesis and immediate surgery help relieve cardiac tamponade that occurs after rupture of the heart. Also, the surgeon repairs the rupture.

Pericarditis. Up to 28 per cent of clients suffering an acute transmural MI will develop early pericarditis (within 2 to 4 days). The inflamed area of the infarction rubs against the pericardial surface and causes it to lose its lubricating fluid. A pericardial friction rub can be auscultated across the precordium. The client complains of chest pain that is aggravated with movement, deep inspiration, and cough. The pain of pericarditis is relieved when the client sits up and leans forward.

Frequent assessment may lead to early identification and intervention. Pain is relieved with analgesics, such as acetaminophen, or other anti-inflammatory agents such as aspirin or indocin. The nurse can reduce the client's anxiety by differentiating the pain of pericarditis from the pain of MI.[77] Dressler's syndrome is a form of pericarditis that occurs 6 weeks to months after an MI.

REHABILITATION

A successful rehabilitation program begins the moment a client with a "coronary" enters the coronary care unit for emergency care, and it continues for months and even years after the client is discharged home from the health-care facility (see Client Education Guide: Discharge After Myocardial Infarction).

CLIENT EDUCATION GUIDE

Discharge After Myocardial Infarction

The nurse should teach the client and significant others about:

- Medications, including action, side effects, dosage, and method of administration
- How to take a pulse and why
- Progressive exercise based on the discharge MET level
- The need to avoid extremes of weather and increased humidity
- Walking in environmentally controlled areas, such as shopping malls
- When to stop exercise
- When to resume sexual activity
- Symptoms of congestive heart failure and myocardial infarction

See also Client Education Guides for Decreasing Risk for Coronary Artery Disease and Managing Angina Pectoris.

Goals of Rehabilitation. The overall goal of rehabilitation is twofold: to help the client (1) live as full, vital, and productive a life as possible and (2) remain within the limits of the heart's ability to respond to increases in activity and stress.

Six important subgoals of the rehabilitation process are

- To develop a program of progressive physical activity.
- To teach the client and significant others about the cause, prevention, and treatment of CAD.
- To help the client accept the limitations imposed by illness.
- To aid the client in adjusting to changes in occupational goals.
- To lessen avoidable risk factors.
- To change the psychosocial factors that adversely affect recovery from CAD.

Program of Physical Activity. Clients who have suffered a heart attack usually remain on bed rest for only 24 hours unless complications such as CHF or dysrhythmias develop. The nurse must remember that protracted bed rest produces numerous complications.

The client must increase activities gradually to avoid overtaxing the heart as it pumps oxygenated blood to the muscles. The metabolic equivalents (METs) system provides one way of measuring the amount of oxygen needed to perform an activity: 1 MET equals 3.5 mL of oxygen per kilogram of body weight per minute. One MET is approximately equivalent to the oxygen uptake a client requires when resting. Early mobilization activities after an acute MI should not exceed 1 to 2 METs (e.g., shaving, washing, and self-feeding). Later activities can increase up to 10 or 11 METs (e.g., cycling, running).

With each increase in activity level, the nurse should monitor heart rate, blood pressure, and fatigue and adjust the client's activity level accordingly. During early activities, the heart rate should not rise more than 25 per cent above resting level. Resting tachycardia is a contraindication to activity. Blood pressure must not rise more than 25 mm Hg above normal.

CRITICAL TO REMEMBER

- Monitor and record baseline vital signs
- Monitor and record activity vital signs
- Monitor and record vital signs 3 minutes after activity or until return to baseline

The typical program of activity for clients recuperating from an acute MI is designated by phases.

Phase I (In-Hospital). Phase I begins with admission to the coronary care unit. Complete bed rest is provided for the first day or so with use of a bedside commode for bowel movements. A liquid diet is provided for the first 24 hours.

Clinicians may allow the client to shave and feed himself or herself, move around in bed, and brush his or her teeth once blood pressure and vital signs stabilize. A coronary care nurse or physiotherapist should start passive exercises.

As strength is regained, the nurse should have the client sit for brief periods on the side of the bed and dangle the feet. The client can be allowed to ambulate to a bedside chair for 15 to 20 minutes if permissible after the first day.

When the client is transferred from the coronary care unit to an intermediate or regular unit, bathroom privileges and self-care activities are encouraged. Telemetry heart monitoring may continue. Brief walks in the hall are allowed with supervision. The length and duration of these walks progressively increase according to the client's endurance.

The nurse can help the client avoid fatigue by pacing activity. Dyspnea, chest pain, tachycardia, and a sense of exhaustion warn that the client is attempting to do too much. The nurse should instruct the client regarding these warning signs of overexertion.

Client education during phase I should include anatomy and physiology of the heart and CAD, risk factors and management of CAD, behavioral counseling, and home activities.

Phase II (Intermediate). In 7 to 10 days, the client will be discharged. Clients may be monitored by a home health nurse or referred for outpatient cardiac rehabilitation.

After an acute MI, many clients will be instructed to take one aspirin daily. Aspirin decreases platelet aggregation and may be useful in preventing MIs. Side effects include epigastric distress, gastrointestinal bleeding, and nausea.

Clinicians need to correct pre-existing health problems that might have contributed to the development of CAD (e.g., hypertension, anemia, hyperthyroidism, aortic valve disease). In addition, the client is encouraged to make life-style changes that enhance health. This includes eliminating modifiable risk factors for CAD (see the Client Education Guide: Decreasing Risk for CAD).

Clients should be discharged on a progressive ambulation program that includes specific guidelines (MET) for aerobic exercise. The walking program aims at a goal of 2 miles in less than 60 minutes. A monitored outpatient cardiac rehabilitation program is encouraged when available. The goal of cardiac rehabilitation is overall conditioning, thus decreasing the oxygen need of the body. This can decrease the cardiac workload. Collateral circulation may be enhanced by exercise. The client benefits from the physical conditioning and an extensive education program about the disease process and treatment. In either case, it is the nurse's responsibility to educate the client concerning

- Pacing activities of daily living
- Progressive exercise
- Signs and symptoms of inability to tolerate exercise
- Medication (dose, action, route, side effects, schedule)
- When to call the doctor
- Risk factor reduction
- Follow-up appointments

Between the sixth and the tenth weeks, the client requires a complete physical examination, including ECG, exercise stress test, lipid analysis, and chest radiography. About 80 per cent of clients with uncomplicated MI return to work after 8 or 9 weeks. Some

Text continues on page 695

CARE PLAN: The Client with a Myocardial Infarction

Nursing Diagnosis/ Collaborative Problem	Planning: Expected Outcomes	Implementation: Nursing Interventions	Rationales
Pain, Acute (Chest) R/T myocardial ischemia resulting from coronary artery occlusion with loss/restriction of blood flow to an area of the myocardium and necrosis of the myocardium • typically substernal pain, tightness, pressure, or heaviness • pain radiating to arms, especially on the left side • complaints of neck, shoulder, back, and arm pain • nausea and vomiting • diaphoresis • weakness • anxiety • shortness of breath • dysrhythmias • palpitations • feeling of "doom"	Client will have improved comfort in chest, as evidenced by the following: • states a decrease in the rating of the chest pain • is able to rest, displays reduced tension, sleeps comfortably • requires decreased analgesia or nitroglycerin	Assess characteristics of chest pain, including location, duration, quality, intensity, presence of radiation, precipitating and alleviating factors, and associated symptoms; have client rate pain on a scale of 1 to 10 and document findings in nurses' notes	Pain is an indication of myocardial ischemia. Assisting the client in quantifying pain may differentiate preexisting and current pain patterns as well as identify complications Duration of pain has an impact on thrombolytic therapy
		Assess respirations, blood pressure, and heart rate with each episode of chest pain	Respirations may be increased as a result of pain and associated anxiety; release of stress-induced catecholamines will increase heart rate and blood pressure
		Obtain a 12-lead ECG on admission, then each time chest pain recurs for evidence of further infarction	Serial ECG and stat ECGs record changes that can give evidence of further cardiac damage and location of myocardial ischemia
		Monitor response to drug therapy. Notify physician if pain does not abate	Pain control is a priority, as it indicates ischemia
		Provide care in a calm, efficient manner that will reassure the client and minimize anxiety; stay with client until discomfort is relieved	Decreases external stimuli, which may aggravate anxiety and cardiac strain and limit coping abilities
		Limit visitors	Prevent overstimulation, promote rest, and decrease cardiac workload
Dysrhythmias R/T electrical instability or irritability secondary to ischemia or infarcted tissue • increase or decrease in heart rate • change in rhythm • dysrhythmias	Client will have no dysrhythmias, as evidenced by • normal sinus rhythm • normotension	Teach client and significant others about need for continuous monitoring; keep alarms on and limits set at all times	Continued monitoring keeps staff aware of myocardial changes. Family anxiety decreased
		Assess apical heart rate; auscultate for change in heart sounds (murmurs, rub, S_3 and S_4)	Indicative of early cardiac decompensation and potential loss of cardiac output
		Document rhythm strip every shift and as necessary if dysrhythmias occur; measure pulse rate and QRS segments with each strip; note and report any deviations from the client's baseline	Dysrhythmias are the most common complication after an MI
		Report three or more multifocal PVCs per minute to physician	Indicate ventricular irritability, which decreases cardiac output and may lead to life-threatening dysrhythmias
		Administer antidysrhythmics as ordered	Antidysrhythmics reduce myocardial irritability
		Monitor effects of antidysrhythmic agents	Desired result is increased diastolic threshold potential and decreased action potential duration
		Monitor serum potassium levels	Altered potassium levels can affect cardiac rhythms

Care plan continued on following page

CARE PLAN: The Client with a Myocardial Infarction *Continued*

Nursing Diagnosis/ Collaborative Problem	Planning: Expected Outcomes	Implementation: Nursing Interventions	Rationales
		Maintain a patent intravenous line or heparin lock at all times	Administration of intravenous cardiac medications in emergency
Decreased Cardiac Output R/T negative inotropic changes in the heart secondary to myocardial ischemia, injury, or infarction • change in level of consciousness • weakness/dizziness • loss of peripheral pulses • abnormal heart sounds • hemodynamic compromise • cardiopulmonary arrest	Client will have improved cardiac output, as evidenced by • cardiac rate, rhythm, and hemodynamic parameters within normal limits • dysrhythmias controlled or absent • absence of angina • respiratory parameters within normal limits	Assess for and document the following as evidence of myocardial dysfunction with decreasing cardiac output 1. Mental status—be alert to restlessness and decreased responsiveness 2. Lung sounds—monitor for crackles and rhonchi 3. Heart sounds—note the presence of gallop, murmur, and increased heart rate 4. Urinary output—be alert to output less than 30 mL/hr 5. Peripheral perfusion—monitor for pallor, mottling, cyanosis, coolness, diaphoresis, and peripheral pulses 6. Vital signs—note any abnormalities in client's vital signs 7. Presence of jugular neck vein distention 8. Dependent edema (sacral) 9. Weakness, fatigue 10. Decreased activity level 11. Shortness of breath with activity 12. Monitor arterial blood gases	Cerebral perfusion is directly related to cardiac output and aortic perfusion pressure and is influenced by hypoxia and electrolyte and acid-base variations; crackles may develop, reflecting pulmonary congestion related to alterations in myocardial function; hypotension related to hypoperfusion, vagal stimulation, or ventricular dysfunction may occur; S_3 is an early sign of heart failure; hypertension may be related to pain, anxiety, catecholamine release, or preexisting vascular problems; urinary output less than 30 mL/hr may reflect reduced renal perfusion and glomerular filtration as a result of reduced cardiac output
		If client has pulmonary artery catheter, record hemodynamic parameters every 2 to 4 hours and as necessary, be alert to pulmonary capillary wedge pressure greater than 18 mm Hg, cardiac output less than 4 L/min, and cardiac index less than 2.5 L/min	Hemodynamic pressures reflect intravascular responses and ventricular function; use to assess drug therapy and for prevention or early detection of complications of myocardial infarction (i.e., extension, heart failure, cardiogenic shock)
		Maintain hemodynamic stability by monitoring the effects of beta-blockers and inotropic agents	Assess effect of drug therapy on myocardial contractility and function

CARE PLAN: The Client with a Myocardial Infarction

Nursing Diagnosis/ Collaborative Problem	Planning: Expected Outcomes	Implementation: Nursing Interventions	Rationales
Gas Exchange, Impaired R/T decreased cardiac output • increased or decreased heart rate • decreased blood pressure • decreased temperature • dusky color • impaired capillary refill • reduced arterial PaO_2 • dyspnea	Client will have improved gas exchange, as evidenced by • vital signs within normal limits for client • absence of cyanosis • absence of dyspnea • arterial blood gases within normal limits	Administer oxygen as ordered; continuous oximetry	Increases amount of oxygen available for myocardial uptake; oximetry measures peripheral oxygenation
		Monitor arterial blood gases as ordered	Presence of hypoxia indicates need for supplemental oxygen
		Continue to assess client's skin, capillary refill, level of consciousness, and vital signs every 2 to 4 hours and as necessary	Provides data on adequacy of tissue perfusion and oxygenation
		Prepare for intubation and mechanical ventilation if hypoxia increases	With increasing hypoxia, mechanical ventilation may be necessary to oxygenate the client adequately
Powerlessness R/T hospital environment and anticipated life-style changes • withdrawn • verbalizes "feelings of doom" • crying • anger	Client will have an improved feeling of control, as evidenced by • verbalizing feelings of powerlessness • verbalizing a sense of control over present situation and future outcomes	Provide opportunities for the client to express feelings about self and illness	Creates supportive climate, sends message that care givers are willing to help
		Explore reality perceptions and clarify if necessary	Listening to the feelings as well as to the words of the client can help client see a more hopeful outlook
		Eliminate unpredictability of events by allowing adequate preparation for tests/procedures	Information can help client or significant others feel more hopeful about situation and more willing to participate in care
		Reinforce the client's right to ask questions	Keep a supportive climate to let client feel free to ask questions or have information repeated
		Allow choices when possible	Allows client to feel independent
		Provide positive reinforcement for increased involvement in self-care	When clients participate in planning for care, they are more apt to feel a sense of control and to follow through with actions
		Help client identify strengths and areas of control	Self-confidence and security come with a sense of control; allow full client participation
Anxiety/Fear R/T hospital admission and fear of death • client/significant others appear restless, hostile, or withdrawn • client/family verbalize fatalism or act extremely emotional as if in grieving process	Client will have reduced feelings of anxiety/fear, as evidenced by the following: • demonstrates appropriate range of feelings and initial signs of effective coping, such as participation in treatment regimen • ability to rest • client and significant others ask fewer questions	Limit nursing personnel; provide continuity of care	Continuity of care promotes security and development of rapport with and trust of health-care providers
		Allow and encourage client/significant others to ask questions; do not avoid questions. Bring up common concerns	Accurate information about the situation reduces fear, strengthens client-nurse relationship, assists client and family to deal realistically with situation
		Allow client and significant others to verbalize fears	Sharing information elicits support and comfort and can relieve tension and unexpressed worries
		Stress that frequent assessments are routine and do not necessarily imply a deteriorating condition	Client may feel reassured to know that frequent assessments may prevent development of more serious complications

Care plan continued on following page

CARE PLAN: The Client with a Myocardial Infarction *Continued*

Nursing Diagnosis/ Collaborative Problem	Planning: Expected Outcomes	Implementation: Nursing Interventions	Rationales
		Repeat information as necessary because of reduced attention span of client and significant others	Attention span is short, and time perception may be altered. Anxiety decreases learning and attention
		Provide a comfortable, quiet environment for client and family	Enhances coping mechanisms as well as reduces myocardial workload and oxygen consumption
Constipation, Risk for R/T bedrest, pain medications, and NPO/soft diet • subjective feeling of fullness • abdominal cramping • painful defecation • palpable impaction	Client will have improved bowel elimination, as evidenced by eliminating a stool without straining or having a vasovagal response	Ensure adequate bulk in diet and adequate fluid intake	Bulk and fluid within the colon prevent straining
		Monitor effectiveness of softeners or laxatives; instruct on prevention of straining and avoiding Valsalva's (vasovagal) maneuver	Stool softeners decrease myocardial workload of straining; Valsalva's maneuver causes bradycardia, decreasing cardiac output
		Use bedside commode rather than bedpan	Bedpan use requires more straining and increases vasovagal response
Health Maintenance, Altered R/T myocardial infarction and implications for life-style changes	Client and significant others will have improved knowledge of medical regimen and life-style changes, as evidenced by verbalizing an understanding of a heart attack and the necessary life-style changes regarding diet; medications; stress reduction; quitting smoking; and cholesterol, weight, and blood pressure reduction	Discuss the following with clients and family, providing both oral instructions and written materials: • anatomy and functions of the heart muscle • coronary arteries and the atherosclerotic process • definition of "heart attack" • healing process of the heart and the role of collateral circulation	Use of multiple learning methods enhances retention of material; information helps client understand the underlying problems or overall heart functions
		Assist client with identifying his or her own risk factors	Risk factor identification is the first step before changes can be implemented
		Assist client in devising a plan for risk factor modification (e.g., diet; smoking cessation; cholesterol, stress, and blood pressure reduction)	Information helpful in providing opportunity for client to identify risk factors, assume control, and participate in a treatment regimen
		Provide guidelines for a diet low in cholesterol and saturated fat; arrange for dietary consultation before client is discharged from hospital	Consultation with other health professionals enhances client learning from others; guidelines developed with the client and family before discharge will help once they are home
		Discuss post–myocardial infarction activity progression; arrange for cardiac rehabilitation consultation	Continued follow-up will let client know how he or she is doing; outpatient cardiac rehabilitation will support and assist client in the life-style changes necessary for a healthy recovery and life
		Teach client and significant others about medications that will be taken after hospital discharge, including name, purpose, dosage, schedule, precautions, and potential side effects	The more the client understands the medical regimen and potential side effects, the more adept he or she will be in monitoring for them

CARE PLAN: The Client with a Myocardial Infarction

Nursing Diagnosis/ Collaborative Problem	Planning: Expected Outcomes	Implementation: Nursing Interventions	Rationales
Activity Intolerance, Risk for R/T imbalance between oxygen supply and demand • weakness, fatigue • change in vital signs • dysrhythmias • dyspnea • pallor • diaphoresis	Client will have improved activity tolerance, as evidenced by • participating in desired activities • meeting own activities of daily living • reduced fatigue and weakness • vital signs within normal limits during activity • absence of cyanosis, diaphoresis, and pain	Monitor vital signs before, immediately after activity, and 3 minutes later	Trends determine client's response to increase in activity. Vital signs should return to baseline in 3 minutes. Pulse rate over established limits and development of chest pain or dyspnea may indicate need for alterations in exercise regimen or medication changes
		Monitor for tachycardia, dysrhythmias, dyspnea, diaphoresis, or pallor after activity	Indicators of myocardial oxygen deprivation that may require decrease in activity, changes in medications, or use of supplemental oxygen
		Encourage verbalization of feelings or concerns regarding fatigue or limitations	Knowing limitations prevents exertion and increasing myocardial workload
		Provide assistance with self-care activities and provide frequent rest periods, especially after meals	Large meals may increase myocardial workload and cause vagal stimulation, with resultant bradycardia or ectopic beats; caffeine, a direct cardiac stimulant, increases heart rate
		Increase activity per cardiac rehabilitation nurse and physician orders	Gradual increase in activity increases strength and prevents overexertion, enhances collateral circulation, and restores normal life-style as much as possible

ECG, electrocardiogram, MI, myocardial infarction; PVCs, premature ventricular contractions

clients need to return to work on a part-time basis or to a less strenuous or stressful job.

Resuming sexual activity may be one of the most difficult phases of returning to normal life after an MI. The physician may allow sexual intercourse 4 to 8 weeks after an MI. Research shows that the cardiac workload (METs) associated with sexual intercourse with a known partner is equal to climbing one flight of stairs. The nurse should caution clients not to eat or drink alcoholic beverages immediately before intercourse. Taking nitroglycerin before intercourse may help prevent exertional angina.

Phase III (Long-Term). Clinicians trained in cardiac rehabilitation may provide detailed, written instructions for a life-long exercise program. Various methods are used to determine the appropriate exercise routines, including stress testing. Periodic evaluation is necessary to assess the client's endurance and tolerance to the prescribed exercise program.

Nursing Management

Initial nursing care includes a focused history, rapid assessment, and implementing MI protocols. The focus of the plan of care for the MI client includes

- Recognizing and treating potentially life-threatening dysrhythmias
- Monitoring for complications from decreased cardiac output
- Maintaining a therapeutic critical care environment
- Identifying the psychosocial impact of the MI on the client and family
- Educating the client in life-style changes and rehabilitation after the MI

Nursing diagnoses or collaborative problems that may apply to the client after an acute MI are discussed in the Care Plan.

CONGESTIVE HEART FAILURE

Heart failure can be defined as a physiologic state in which the heart is unable to pump enough blood to meet the metabolic needs of the body (determined as oxygen consumption) at rest or during exercise, even though filling pressures are adequate. The heart fails because of damage (disease or structural defects) or because of an increased workload (strenuous exercise). Heart failure is not a disease itself; instead, the term denotes a group of manifestations related to inadequate pump performance. Whatever the cause, pump failure results in hypoperfused tissue followed by pulmonary and systemic venous congestion. Because heart failure causes vascular congestion, it is often called congestive heart failure. Other terms used to denote heart failure include cardiac decompensation, cardiac insufficiency, and ventricular failure.

Incidence

Estimates from the American Heart Association[4] indicate that between 2.3 and 3 million Americans have CHF and are alive. The incidence of those developing the condition is around 400,000. Annually, 37,371 clients die from CHF.

Etiology

The performance of the heart depends on two essential components: fiber length (Frank-Starling mechanism) and the inherent contractility (inotropic state) of the muscle. The normal heart automatically responds to maintain the cardiac output. In health and disease, a complicated interplay automatically adjusts the stroke volume and the cardiac output. Five interrelated factors are involved: preload, afterload, contractility, the coordinated pattern of contraction, and heart rate (Table 24–2). Adverse changes in these determinants of myocardial performance ultimately cause the heart to fail. If the heart is damaged (MI), these automatic physiologic responses may be a detriment, not a benefit, further stressing the client.

Pathophysiology

The myocardium of the left ventricle may either (1) be diseased and unable to meet normal circulatory demands or (2) be intrinsically normal but unable to meet increased circulatory needs. When failure first begins, the left ventricle fails to eject a sufficient amount of blood. At this point, the compensatory mechanisms of sympathetic nervous system activation (tachycardia, dilation, and hypertrophy) come into play. When these mechanisms fail, the amount of blood remaining in the left ventricle at the end of diastole increases. This increase in residual blood in turn decreases the ventricle's capacity to receive blood from the left atrium. The left atrium, having to work harder to eject blood, dilates and hypertrophies. It is unable to receive the full amount of incoming blood from the pulmonary veins, and left atrial pressure increases. This leads to subsequent pulmonary congestion, pulmonary edema, and respiratory symptoms.

TABLE 24–2 Terms Used to Describe Cardiac Function

TERM	FUNCTION
Afterload	Force that the ventricle must develop during systole in order to eject the stroke volume
Cardiac output	Stroke volume × heart rate
Diastole	The normal period in the heart cycle during which the muscle fibers lengthen, the heart dilates, and cavities fill with blood
Inotropic state	A measure of contractility
Preload	Stretch of myocardial fibers at end diastole
Stroke volume	The amount of blood ejected from the ventricle with each contraction
Systole	That part of the heart cycle in which the heart is in contraction; the myocardial fibers are tightening and shortening

The right ventricle, because of the increased pressure in the pulmonary vascular system, must now dilate and hypertrophy in order to meet its increased workload. It too eventually fails. Engorgement of the venous system then extends backward to produce congestion in the gastrointestinal tract, liver, viscera, kidneys, legs, and sacrum, with edema as the main manifestation. Right ventricular failure thus results.

Right ventricular failure usually follows left ventricular failure. Occasionally, right ventricular failure develops independently of left ventricular failure. Causes include

- pulmonary diseases (e.g., pulmonary hypertension, recurrent pulmonary embolism, chronic obstructive pulmonary disease, and cor pulmonale), which force the right ventricle to pump against increased pressure within the lungs
- constrictive pericarditis, which obstructs the inflow of blood to the heart from the venous system
- tricuspid and pulmonic valvular disorders, which produce greater demands on the right ventricular myocardium
- right ventricle infarction (rare)

The healthy heart can meet the demands of life through the use of cardiac reserve. Cardiac reserve is the heart's ability to increase output in response to stress. The normal heart has the ability to increase its output up to five times the resting level. However, the failing heart, even at rest, is pumping near its capacity and thus has lost much of its reserve. The compromised heart has a limited ability to respond to the body's needs for increased output in situations of stress.

The heart in failure has recourse to three main compensatory mechanisms to meet the body's demands: (1) ventricular dilation, (2) ventricular hypertrophy, and (3) increased sympathetic nervous system stimulation (tachycardia). Tachycardia is an adaptive mechanism available only to the chronically failing heart (see Pathophysiology: Compensatory Mechanisms in Congestive Heart Failure). Cardiac compensation exists when these three mechanisms—ventricular dilation, ventricular hypertrophy, and sympathetic nervous system stimulation—succeed in maintaining an adequate

PATHOPHYSIOLOGY

Compensatory Mechanisms in Congestive Heart Failure

VENTRICULAR DILATION

Ventricular dilation causes an increase in preload and thus cardiac output, because a stretched muscle contracts more forcefully (Starling's law). However, dilation has limits as a compensatory mechanism. Muscle fibers, if stretched beyond a certain point, cease to increase the ventricular contractility. Second, a dilated heart requires more oxygen. Thus, the dilated heart with a normal coronary blood flow can suffer from a lack of oxygen. Hypoxia of the heart further decreases the muscle's ability to contract. A dilated heart with coronary artery disease is at even greater risk of hypoxia.

VENTRICULAR HYPERTROPHY

In ventricular hypertrophy, the walls of the heart chamber thicken, and the weight of the heart increases. Hypertrophy generally follows persistent dilation, further increasing the contractile power of the muscle fibers. Like dilation, hypertrophy has limits as a compensatory mechanism. A hypertrophied heart does far greater work than does a normal-sized heart and, as a consequence, has a greater demand for oxygen. Unfortunately, as the heart's muscle mass increases, the number of capillaries supplying the muscle fibers remains the same. Thus, the hypertrophied heart may simply outgrow its coronary blood supply and become hypoxic. As the myocardium becomes hypoxic, the contractile force of the heart decreases. Ventricular hypertrophy may also impede ventricular emptying if the enlarged muscle blocks the valve areas.

INCREASED SYMPATHETIC NERVOUS SYSTEM STIMULATION

Increased sympathetic nervous system stimulation is the least effective compensatory mechanism and often proves to be more of a burden than a blessing. Sympathetic activity produces venous and arteriolar constriction, thus increasing peripheral vascular resistance (afterload) and myocardial workload. In addition, sympathetic stimulation reduces renal blood flow, and the kidneys respond by activating the renin-angiotensin system and retaining water and sodium. The expanded blood volume increases the load on an already compromised heart.

cardiac output and blood flow to the tissues in the presence of pathologic changes. Cardiac decompensation occurs when the heart, despite these mechanisms, fails to cope with the demands put on it and must expend most of its reserve. At this point, symptoms of congestive heart failure develop because the heart cannot maintain adequate circulation.

Risk Factors

Some clients have pre-existing mild to moderate heart disease with no evidence of CHF. In these clients, adequate cardiac output depends on functional compensatory mechanisms. When the heart undergoes undue stress, these compensatory mechanisms may prove inadequate, and the heart fails. Careful assessment helps identify precipitating causes for the great increase in cardiac workload. Recognition of these factors allows prompt treatment and long-term prevention. Precipitating factors include those listed in Box 24–1.

Clinical Manifestations

Heart failure may be categorized as left versus right ventricular, backward versus forward, high versus low output, and systolic versus diastolic.[48]

LEFT VERSUS RIGHT VENTRICULAR FAILURE

The heart is composed of two pumps; a right and a left. Each pump bears its own stressors and has its own role in maintaining the circulation. For this reason, one pump or ventricle can fail independently of the other.

The theory of left-sided versus right-sided failure is based on the fact that fluid accumulates behind the chamber that first fails. However, because the circulatory system is a closed circuit, impairments of the one ventricle will frequently progress to failure of the other. This is referred to as ventricular interdependence.

Left Ventricular Failure. Left ventricular failure causes either pulmonary congestion or a disturbance in the respiratory control mechanisms. These problems in turn precipitate respiratory distress. The degree of distress varies with the client's position, activity, and level of stress.

Dyspnea is a subjective problem, and it does not always correlate with the extent of heart failure. An apprehensive client with only moderate ventricular failure may be more aware of dyspnea than a client with advanced disease. To some degree, exertional dyspnea occurs in all clients. Therefore, it is important for the nurse to elicit from the client a description of the degree of exertion that results in the sensation of breathlessness.

Cheyne-Stokes respirations sometimes occur in clients with severe forms of heart failure.

Cough is a common symptom of left ventricular heart failure. The cough, often hacking, may produce large amounts of frothy, blood-tinged sputum. The client coughs because a large amount of fluid is trapped in the pulmonary tree, irritating the lung mucosa. On auscultation, bilateral crackles may be heard.

Orthopnea is a more advanced stage of dyspnea. Orthopnea develops because the supine position increases the amount of blood returning from the lower extremities to the heart and lungs (preload). This gravitational redistribution of blood increases pulmonary congestion and dyspnea.

Paroxysmal nocturnal dyspnea resembles the frightening sensation of suffocation. The client suddenly awakens with the feeling of severe suffocation and seeks

BOX 24-1

Conditions that Precipitate or Exacerbate Heart Failure

PHYSICAL OR EMOTIONAL STRESS

Strenuous physical exercise and strong emotions (fear, excitement, anxiety) increase myocardial work by increasing heart rate, myocardial contractility, and blood pressure.

DYSRHYTHMIAS

Cardiac dysrhythmias, most notably tachycardia (rapid heart rate), are the most common factors precipitating heart failure. A rapid heart beat shortens the time for ventricular filling (diastole), which in turn reduces cardiac output. In addition, the workload and oxygen requirements of the myocardium increase.

INFECTION

Any systemic infection increases the oxygen demands of the body tissues. Fever and hypoxemia, which occurs in some pulmonary infections, further tax the ailing heart and may precipitate failure.

ANEMIA

Reduction in the oxygen-carrying capacity of the blood, as in anemia, necessitates increased cardiac output to meet the body's need for oxygen. Wheras a normal heart may adjust to the increased workload, a compromised heart cannot, and failure ensues.

THYROID DISORDERS

Thyrotoxicosis, associated with hyperthyroidism, augments the metabolic needs of the body, accelerating heart rate and the workload of the heart. If thyrotoxicosis is untreated, heart failure may occur. In hypothyroidism, the thyroid produces an inadequate amount of thyroxine (thyroid hormone). This can indirectly lead to heart failure by predisposing the client to coronary atherosclerosis.

PREGNANCY

Heart failure ranks high among causes of death during pregnancy. Like anemia and hyperthyroidism, pregnancy increases the metabolic needs of the body, thereby increasing the workload of the heart. Pregnant women with rheumatic valvular disease are particularly prone to heart failure.

PAGET'S DISEASE

In some cases, Paget's disease also increases myocardial workload. This disease causes vascular proliferation in the bones. When the disease involves over one third of the skeleton, a high cardiac output state exists and may tax the compromised heart (see Chap. 45).

NUTRITIONAL DEFICIENCY

Thiamine deficiency interferes with cardiac function by reducing myocardial contractility and causing tachycardia and ventricular dilation. Thiamine deficiency, which causes beriberi, is associated with alcoholism (especially Wernicke's syndrome).

PULMONARY DISEASE

Increased pressure in the pulmonary system due to chronic obstructive lung disease, severe pulmonary embolization, or primary pulmonary artery hypertension can produce sizable resistance to right ventricular emptying. Such resistance may lead to right ventricular hypertrophy and failure.

HYPERVOLEMIA

An excess in circulating blood volume can result from poor renal function, cardiac disease, medications (such as steroids), or excessive intake of sodium (promoting water retention). Iatrogenic causes include overadministration of intravenous fluids. Expanded circulatory volume augments venous return, increasing preload. A diseased heart may not be able to pump the increased load, and cardiac decompensation occurs.

MYOCARDIAL INFARCTION (MI)

After MI, some of the heart muscle is replaced by noncontracting scar tissue, and the ventricles pump less efficiently. Some degree of heart failure, either chronic or transient, appears in over one half of clients after MI.

RESTRICTIVE PERICARDITIS AND CARDIAC TAMPONADE

Disorders that greatly restrict cardiac chamber filling and myocardial fiber stretch include: constrictive pericarditis, which is an inflammatory and fibrotic process of the pericardial sac, and cardiac tamponade, which involves the accumulation of fluid or blood within the sac. Because the pericardium encases all four chambers, compression of the heart will (1) decrease diastolic relaxation, (2) elevate diastolic pressure, and (3) hamper forward flow through the heart.

relief by sitting upright or opening a window for a breath of "fresh air." Respirations may be labored and wheezing (cardiac asthma). Paroxysmal nocturnal dyspnea stems from (1) a combination of increased venous return to the lungs due to recumbency and (2) suppression of the respiratory center to sensory input from the lungs during sleep. Once the client is in the upright position, relief from the attack of paroxysmal nocturnal dyspnea may not occur for 30 minutes or longer.

Pulmonary edema may develop. Clinical manifestations of it include extreme breathlessness, anxiety, frothy sputum, nasal flaring, use of accessory breathing muscles, tachypnea, noisy and wet breathing, diaphoresis, vasoconstriction, and hypoxia in arterial blood gas findings.

Cardiovascular signs also denote left ventricular failure. Inspecting and palpating the precordium may reveal an enlarged or left laterally displaced apical impulse. This occurs because the left ventricle dilates in an effort to augment ventricular contraction and emptying. Also, heart gallop (S_3) sounds may be an early finding in heart failure as the left ventricle becomes less compliant and its walls vibrate in response to filling during diastole. The appearance of pulsus alternans (alternating strong and weak heart beats) may also herald the onset of left ventricular failure.

Cerebral hypoxia may occur as a result of a decrease in cardiac output causing inadequate brain perfusion. On assessment, the client may appear anxious, restless, confused, or irritable.

Fatigue and muscular weakness are often associated with left ventricular failure. Inadequate cardiac output leads to hypoxic tissue and slowed removal of metabolic wastes, which in turn causes the client to tire easily. Disturbances in sleep and rest patterns may aggravate fatigue.

Renal changes can occur in both right- and left-sided heart failure but are more striking in the latter. Nocturia occurs early in heart failure. During the day, the client is upright, blood flow is away from the kidneys, and the formation of urine is reduced. At night, urine formation increases as blood flow to the kidneys improves. Nocturia may interfere with effective sleep patterns, which may contribute to fatigue. As cardiac output falls, decreased renal blood flow may result in oliguria, a late sign of heart failure.

In addition, if renal artery pressure falls, lowered glomerular filtration increases retention of sodium and water. In response to a continued reduction in renal blood flow, the renin-angiotensin-aldosterone mechanism activates. Aldosterone, released from the adrenal cortex, promotes further retention of sodium and water by the renal tubule. This results in an expansion in blood volume of up to 30 per cent and edema. As the sodium concentration in the extracellular fluid increases, so does the osmotic pressure of the plasma. The hypothalamus responds to the higher osmotic pressure by releasing antidiuretic hormone from the posterior pituitary. This, in turn, promotes renal tubular reabsorption of water. However, aldosterone is more important than is antidiuretic hormone in the production of edema. Reabsorption of water increases the preload and oxygen needs of the heart.

Right Ventricular Failure. When the right ventricle fails, peripheral edema and venous congestion of the organs develop. Liver enlargement (hepatomegaly) and abdominal pain occur as the liver becomes congested with venous blood. If this occurs rapidly, stretching of the capsule surrounding the liver causes severe discomfort. The client may notice either a constant aching or a sharp pain in the right upper quadrant. In chronic heart failure, abdominal tenderness generally disappears.

In severe CHF, lobules of the liver may become so congested with venous blood that they become anoxic. Anoxia leads to necrosis of the lobules. In long-standing CHF, these necrotic areas may become fibrotic and then sclerotic. As a result, a condition called cardiac cirrhosis develops, manifested by ascites and jaundice, which are symptoms of liver damage.

In chronic heart failure, the increased workload of the heart and the extreme work of breathing increase the metabolic demands of the body. Anorexia, nausea, and bloating develop secondary to venous congestion of the gastrointestinal tract. The combination of increased metabolic needs and decreased caloric intake results in a marked wasting of tissue mass and cardiac cachexia.[44] Anorexia and nausea may also result from digitalis toxicity. This is a common problem because digitalis is usually prescribed for CHF.

Dependent edema is one of the early signs of right ventricular failure. The pitting edema is usually symmetric and occurs in the dependent parts of the body where venous pressure is the highest. In ambulatory clients, edema begins in the feet and ankles and ascends the lower legs. It is most noticeable at the end of a day and often decreases after a night's rest. In the recumbent client, pitting edema may develop in the presacral area and, as it worsens, progress to the genital region and medial thighs. Concurrent jugular vein distention differentiates the edema of CHF from that of lymphatic obstruction, cirrhosis, and hypoproteinemia. Anasarca, a late sign in heart failure, is substantial and generalized edema. It can involve the upper extremities, genital area, and thoracic and abdominal walls. Cyanosis of the nail beds appears as venous congestion reduces peripheral blood flow.

Clients with CHF often feel anxious, frightened, and depressed. Almost all clients realize that the heart is a vital organ and that when the heart begins to fail, health also fails. As the course of the disease progresses and symptoms worsen, the client may develop an overwhelming fear of permanent disability and death. Clients express their fears in varying ways: experiencing frightening nightmares, insomnia, acute anxiety states, depression, or withdrawal from reality.

BACKWARD VERSUS FORWARD FAILURE

The clinical presentation of heart failure arises from inadequate cardiac output or the pooling of blood behind the failing chamber, or both. Backward failure is the term used to refer to the venous congestion arising from the damming of blood behind the failing chamber. Forward failure refers to the problems of inadequate perfusion. It results when reduced contractility produces a decrease in stroke volume and cardiac output. As cardiac output falls, blood flow to vital organs and peripheral tissue diminishes. This causes mental confusion, muscular weakness, and renal retention of sodium and water. Extracellular fluid retention increases circulating blood volume, further taxing the ailing heart.

Backward failure may develop concurrently with forward failure. As the ventricles fail to expel their contents, blood accumulates and pressure rises in the ventricles and in the atria and venous systems that empty into them. A rise in blood volume within the venous systems causes hydrostatic pressure to exceed capillary oncotic pressure; thereby, fluid is forced out of the vascular beds and into the interstitium. The fluid shift results in pulmonary edema, peripheral (dependent) edema, and serous effusion.

HIGH VERSUS LOW OUTPUT FAILURE

High output failure occurs when the heart, despite normal to high cardiac output levels, is simply not able to meet the accelerated needs of the body. Causes of high output failure include sepsis, Paget's disease, beriberi, anemia, thyrotoxicosis, arteriovenous fistula, and pregnancy.

Low output failure occurs in most forms of heart disease, including congenital, valvular, rheumatic, coronary, and cardiomyopathic heart diseases. Because the heart is unable to pump an adequate supply of blood to the body, low output failure results in hypoperfused tissue cells.

SYSTOLIC VERSUS DIASTOLIC FAILURE

Heart failure may be caused by the inability of a ventricle to eject an adequate volume of blood (systolic failure) or the inability of the ventricle to accept sufficient blood (diastolic failure).[44]

Systolic heart failure refers to a decrease in the ability of the ventricle to contract forcefully and maintain an adequate forward cardiac output. Situations in which the inotropic state is impaired include MI, coronary atherosclerosis, dilated cardiomyopathy, and massive pulmonary embolus.

Diastolic heart failure occurs when ventricular relaxation is incomplete and the chamber is unable to accept sufficient blood. Examples of heart diseases in which diastolic dysfunction may occur include coronary atherosclerosis, amyloidosis, restrictive cardiomyopathy, or subendocardial fibrosis.

CLINICAL MANIFESTATIONS

Right and Left Ventricular Failure

Left Ventricular Failure	Right Ventricular Failure
Weakness	Weight gain
Fatigue	Jugular vein distention
Mental confusion	Neck vein pulsations
Isomnia	Increased central venous pressure
Anorexia	Parasternal life (heave)
Anxiety	Subcostal pain
Diaphoresis	Abdominal distention
Breathlessness	Anorexia, nausea, gastric distress
Cough	Ascites
Pulmonary crackles	Hepatomegaly
Orthopnea or paroxysmal nocturnal dyspnea	Pitting edema (in dependent areas; sacral, ankle, pretibial)
Tachycardia, premature atrial contractions	Ankle or pretibial swelling and pigmentation
Gallop heart sounds (S_3, S_4)	
Diminished S_3	
Pulsus alternans	
Elevated pulmonary artery wedge pressure	
Enlarged point of maximal impulse	

Adapted from Michaelson, C. (1983). *Congestive heart failure.* St. Louis: C. V. Mosby.

Complications

The symptoms of heart failure depend on the specific ventricle involved, the precipitating causes of failure, the degree of impairment, the rate of progression, the duration of the failure, and the client's underlying condition. Symptoms of pulmonary congestion and edema dominate the clinical picture of left ventricular failure. Right ventricular failure is associated with signs of abdominal organ and peripheral edema (see Clinical Manifestations: Right and Left Ventricular Failure).

ACUTE PULMONARY EDEMA

Acute pulmonary edema, a medical emergency, usually results from left ventricular failure. In clients with severe cardiac decompensation, the capillary pressure within the lungs becomes so elevated that fluid is pushed from the circulating blood into the interstitium, then into the alveoli, bronchioles, and bronchi. Clients with pulmonary edema literally drown in their own fluids.

CRITICAL TO REMEMBER

Pulmonary edema, if untreated, can cause death from suffocation.

The dramatic symptoms of acute pulmonary edema terrify the client and significant others. Typical manifestations include severe dyspnea; orthopnea; expectoration of large amounts of frothy, blood-tinged sputum; wheezing; sweating; bubbling respirations; tachycardia; pallor; cyanosis; and fear.

REFRACTORY HEART FAILURE

Heart failure is termed refractory or intractable when recommended diet, medications, and interventions fail to alleviate symptoms and restore partial cardiac reserve. To treat refractory heart disease, the physician usually (1) reviews the client's entire course of treatment, (2) reassesses the medical intervention, and (3) prescribes the following interventions:

- a prolonged period of complete bed rest in a health-care facility
- severe sodium restriction (e.g., 250 mg sodium diet)
- fluids restricted to less than 500 mL/day
- diuretic therapy using several different types of diuretics

Prognosis

The prognosis for the client with CHF depends on (1) the degree of cardiac hypertrophy, (2) the amount of cardiac reserve, and (3) the presence of other heart or associated disorders. The prognosis can generally be predicted by the client's response to therapeutic measures. A very slow or inadequate response to prescribed medications, special diets, activity limitations, and so forth signals a poor prognosis. Nevertheless, thorough ongoing assessment, early intervention, therapeutic compliance, and prevention of complications can control this disorder.

Diagnostic Assessment

The diagnosis of CHF rests primarily on presenting manifestations and pertinent data from the client's health history. Diagnostic studies assist in determining the underlying cause and the degree of heart failure. Such studies include a chest radiography, ECG, and echocardiogram.

Arterial blood gases are drawn. Early CHF with pulmonary edema may lead to respiratory alkalosis because of hyperventilation. However, as the disorder progresses and oxygenation becomes more impaired, acidosis will develop.

Liver enzymes document the degree of liver failure. Elevated blood urea nitrogen and creatinine levels reflect decreased renal perfusion.

Abnormalities in the ECG arise from the underlying cardiac disorder and from therapeutic agents. For instance, cardiac dysrhythmias may occur because of myocardial ischemia or electrolyte imbalance induced by diuretics or digitalis excess. Therefore, the ECG plays an important role in the management of heart failure.

Echocardiography, a noninvasive diagnostic technique, uses ultrasonography to assess cardiac function. This procedure provides information about cardiac chamber size and ventricular wall motion and aids in assessing myocardial, valvular, congenital, and pericardial heart diseases.

Medical Management

Clients with acute CHF are usually admitted to an intensive care unit where they receive continuous assessment and intervention. Those with chronic CHF require continuing assessment, emotional support, and assistance.

The goals in the management of CHF are to improve ventricular pump performance and reduce myocardial workload.

Positioning. The client is placed in a high Fowler's position or chair to reduce pulmonary venous congestion and ease dyspnea. The legs are maintained in a dependent position as much as possible.

Oxygen Administration. Oxygen is administered in high concentrations by mask or cannula to (1) relieve hypoxia and dyspnea and (2) lessen pulmonary capillary permeability. For hypoxemia, the physician may order a partial-rebreather mask with a flow rate of 8 to 10 L/min to deliver oxygen concentrations of 40 to 70 per cent or a non-rebreather mask to achieve higher oxygen concentrations. If these methods fail to raise the arterial oxygen tension above 60 mm Hg, the client may need intubation and ventilatory management.

PHARMACOLOGIC MANAGEMENT

Improving Ventricular "Pump" Performance

Digitalis. Digitalis exerts a direct and beneficial effect on myocardial contraction in the failing heart. Digitalis acts to

- increase ventricular contractility (inotropic effect)
- increase ventricular emptying and the capacity of the heart for work
- slow conduction of impulses through the atrioventricular (AV) node and Purkinje fibers
- increase the AV nodal refractory period
- augment stroke volume
- increase cardiac output

Improved cardiac output enhances kidney perfusion, which may create a mild diuresis of sodium and water.

A number of different digitalis preparations are available, and all have approximately the same effect on the heart. However, digitalis medications differ significantly in their potency, speed of action, elimination from the body, and gastrointestinal irritation. Table 24–3 lists digitalis preparations and their distinguishing characteristics.

The effectiveness of digitalis in heart failure depends on the severity and underlying cause of the condition. Digitalis is contraindicated in heart failure caused by constrictive pericarditis or cardiac tamponade. Digitalis should be used with caution in acute MI because it increases myocardial oxygen demand.

When administering digitalis, the nurse should assess for signs of digitalis toxicity. Clients most prone to the toxic effects of digitalis include the elderly and those with advanced heart disease, severe arrhythmias, or acute MI. Also, clients with cor pulmonale, hypothyroidism, hepatic disease, renal disease, metabolic alkalosis, or hypokalemia (lowered serum potassium) more readily develop toxic effects. Digitalis toxicity occurs in approximately one of every five clients. It may present with systemic or cardiac manifestations.

The major signs and symptoms of digitalis toxicity are outlined in Table 24–4. Any of these manifestations

TABLE 24–3 Pharmacologic Properties of Selected Cardiac Glycosides

AGENT	ABSORPTION	EXCRETION	ONSET OF ACTION	PEAK EFFECT	HALF-LIFE	THERAPEUTIC PLASMA LEVEL	TOXIC PLASMA LEVELS
Digoxin	55–75% gastrointestinal	Principally renal; some hepatic	5–30 min	1–5 hr (IV)	30–40 hr	0.5–2.0 ng/mL	2.4 ng/mL
Digitoxin	90–100% gastrointestinal	Principally hepatic; some renal excretion	30 min–2 hr	4–12 hr	5–7 days	14–26 ng/mL	35 ng/mL

IV, intravenous.
Based on data in Kuhn, M. (1991). *Pharmacotherapeutics.* Philadelphia: F. A. Davis.

TABLE 24–4 Signs and Symptoms of Digitalis Toxicity

Gastrointestinal tract	Anorexia, nausea, vomiting, diarrhea, abdominal cramps (these symptoms are common in 50 per cent of clients with digitalis toxicity and are often the first indication of toxicity)
Central nervous system	Headache, fatigue, lethargy, depression, restlessness, irritability, drowsiness; profound symptoms may include convulsions, neuralgia, delusions, hallucinations, aphasia, memory loss
Cardiovascular system	Bradycardia, ventricular bigeminy or trigeminy, ventricular tachycardia, atrioventricular conduction block, and atrial tachycardia with block
Eyes	Flickering flashes of light; "colored vision" usually yellow or blue, halo vision, photophobia, blurring; diplopia, scotomata (blind spots in visual field)

should be reported to the physician, digitalis should be withheld, and interventions to abate the undesirable symptoms should be initiated.

Digitalis toxicity may be a life-threatening condition. The guidelines in Box 24–2 should be carefully followed and are critical to remember.

Dopamine and Dobutamine. Other inotropic agents (e.g., dopamine, dobutamine, and amrinone) may be ordered for clients with severe low output heart failure. These medications facilitate myocardial contractility and enhance stroke volume.

Dopamine is a naturally occurring catecholamine with alpha-adrenergic, beta-adrenergic, and dopaminergic activity. When given in small doses (less than 4 μg/kg/minute), dopamine stimulates the dopaminergic receptors in the renal, mesenteric, cerebral, and coronary vascular beds, which causes vasodilation. The primary result is an increase in renal blood flow ("turn-off" renin-angiotensin response), glomerular filtration rate, and sodium excretion. The alpha- and beta-adrenergic receptors in the vasculature and myocardium are affected with moderate doses of dopamine (4 to 8 μg/kg/minute). The results are increases in heart rate, stroke volume, and cardiac output. Alpha-adrenergic effects, such as intense vasoconstriction, dominate when dopamine is given in doses larger than 8 μg/kg/minute.[18, 59] Although dopamine can effectively improve cardiac output, it may do so at the expense of the myocardium. An increase in heart rate may increase myocardial oxygen demands and decrease myocardial oxygen supply, which can prove costly to the already ischemic myocardium.

Another inotropic agent is dobutamine, a synthetic derivative of dopamine that has strong beta-stimulatory effects within the myocardium; it increases heart rate and produces more myocardial contractility than dopamine. Dobutamine is capable of increasing the cardiac output without increasing the myocardial oxygen demands or reducing coronary blood flow.[59] It has no direct effect on renal perfusion.

Amrinone is also used to increase cardiac output in clients with severe heart failure. In addition to the positive inotropic effects, amrinone increases renal blood flow and glomerular filtration rate.[59]

Reducing Myocardial Workload

Reduce Preload. Diuretic therapy plays an integral part in the successful management of CHF. Diuretics enhance renal excretion of sodium and water, which reduces circulating blood volume, diminishes preload, and lessens systemic and pulmonary congestion.

Although they are effective, diuretics should be administered cautiously because they have side effects. First, diuretics can produce mild to severe electrolyte imbalance.

CRITICAL TO REMEMBER

Hypokalemia, a particularly dangerous problem, potentiates digitalis toxicity and can cause myocardial weakness and cardiac dysrhythmias.

Second, vigorous diuresis may produce hypovolemia and hypotension, jeopardizing cardiac output and causing rebound tachycardia.

Reduce Afterload. Vasodilating agents have become an increasingly important intervention for CHF. Vasodilators vary in their mechanisms of action, which include (1) direct dilation of veins, (2) dilation of arterioles, (3) combined action on veins and arterioles, and (4) inhibition of angiotensin-converting enzyme. The nurse should closely assess the client receiving vasodilators because they can cause rapid drops in blood pressure.

Venous dilators relax venous smooth muscle and increase the capacity of the systemic venous bed; thereby, blood is "trapped" in the veins, and blood

BOX 24–2

Guidelines for Digitalis Preparations

1. Read the labels of all digitalis preparations with care. Digitalis preparations have similar names but different strengths and dosages.
2. Always take the client's pulse for 1 full minute *apically* before giving a dose of digitalis.
3. Carefully note both the rate and rhythm of the pulse and chart them.
4. If the heart beat is below 60, or a change in the rhythm (PVCs, PAT, heart block) occurs, withhold the drug and notify the physician.
5. Observe the client carefully for signs of digitalis toxicity. When severe symptoms present, call the physician before administering the drug.
6. Monitor serum potassium levels and if the client is hypokalemic, withhold the drug and notify the physician.
7. Teach the client and significant others how to monitor the pulse rate daily. Also reinforce the importance of taking prescribed potassium supplements.

return to the heart is decreased. This increased venous capacity reduces preload and decreases cardiac workload. Examples of venous dilators include nitroglycerin and isosorbide dinitrate.

Arteriolar dilators reduce systemic arteriolar tone, which decreases peripheral vascular resistance and afterload. Reduction in afterload reduces the left ventricular workload and increases cardiac output. Improved renal perfusion may initiate diuresis. Hydralazine is the most commonly used arterial dilator. The nurse must be aware that hydralazine may precipitate reflex tachycardia.

Combined venous and arteriolar dilators decrease both preload and afterload. Sodium nitroprusside helps manage severe heart failure. A potent vasodilator, sodium nitroprusside relaxes the smooth muscles of both veins and arterioles. It does not directly affect the heart muscle or heart rate. Prazosin, an oral agent, provides another example of this class of medication. Physicians often prescribe prazosin for clients with advanced, chronic CHF.

Angiotensin-converting enzyme inhibitors such as captopril suppress the renin-angiotensin-aldosterone system; thereby, the production of the potent vasoconstrictor angiotensin II is blocked. This results in an increase in renal blood flow and a decrease in renal vascular resistance, which enhances diuresis. Angiotensin converting enzyme inhibitors have been shown to prolong survival of clients with CHF.[11, 22]

DIETARY MANAGEMENT

The two major objectives in the treatment of CHF are to improve cardiac efficiency and to control sodium-water retention. Sodium restrictions are placed on the diet to prevent, control, or eliminate edema. Diets containing 2 to 4 g of sodium are usually prescribed (Table 24–5).

From the use of some loop diuretics, potassium is lost via the kidneys, which can lead to dysrhythmias and electrolyte imbalances. Hypokalemia sensitizes the myocardium to digitalis and therefore predisposes the client to digitalis toxicity. Potassium supplements and a dietary potassium can keep the client's potassium in balance.

It is usually not necessary to restrict fluid intake in clients with mild or moderate heart failure. However, with more advanced failure, it is beneficial to limit water to 1000 mL or less daily. The reason for this restriction is that excessive water intake tends to dilute the amount of sodium in the body fluids and may produce a low-salt syndrome (hyponatremia).

OTHER MEASURES

In addition to improving ventricular pump performance and reducing myocardial workload, the client also needs to reduce physical and emotional stress. The client must rest both physically and mentally. Rest can promote diuresis, slow the heart rate, and relieve dyspnea, all of which allow more conservative use of pharmacologic agents (e.g., digitalis, diuretics, and vasodilators).

TABLE 24–5 Sodium Content of Selected Foods

Foods Low in Sodium	
Dairy products	Skim milk, eggs, cottage cheese, cream cheese, ice cream
Meats*	Turkey, chicken, veal, lamb, liver, fresh fish, tuna packed in water (meats should be unprocessed)
Fruits and vegetables*	Any fresh or frozen food in this group
Beverages	Any juice (except tomato or V-8), coffee, tea, Perrier water
Breads	Some breads and cereals
Seasonings	Garlic, onion, bay leaf, pepper, dill, nutmeg, rosemary, allspice, thyme, sage, caraway, cinnamon, almond and vanilla extract, fresh dried herbs
Fats	Margarine, oils, shortening, unsalted salad dressings
Desserts	Sherbet, fruit ice, gelatin, fruit drinks
Miscellaneous	Unbuttered, unsalted popcorn; unsalted nuts; vinegar
Foods High in Sodium	
Milk and dairy products	Aged, hard cheese; pasteurized-processed cheese; buttermilk
Meats	Sausage, wieners, ham, bacon, corned beef; all smoked, pickled, or cured meats; canned meats, "TV dinners," salami, most luncheon meats, beef jerky
Fruits and vegetables	Pickled or canned fruits and vegetables, olives, sauerkraut, pickles
Breads and cereals	Salted crackers, macaroni (in macaroni-and-cheese dinners), pretzels, rye rolls, pizza, commercial pancake mixes
Beverages	Tomato juice, V-8 juice, beef broth, bouillon
Fats	Commercial salad dressings, dips and party spreads, peanut butter
Seasonings	Garlic, celery, or onion salt; Accent, monosodium glutamate (MSG), meat tenderizer, soy sauce, catsup, steak sauce, mustard, canned soup
Desserts	Fruit pies, doughnuts, cake, commercial puddings
Miscellaneous	Baking soda, baking powder, salted popcorn, salted nuts, potato chips

* Food sources high in potassium.

Whether the physician prescribes bed rest or a program of modified bed rest depends on the seriousness of the client's condition. Clinicians may use the functional and therapeutic classifications of heart disease as a guide for activity prescription (Box 24–3).

The physician may prescribe a mild sedative or small doses of barbiturates and tranquilizers to promote rest and overcome problems of restlessness, insomnia, and anxiety.

The client may also be at risk for injury, particularly venous thrombi, due to immobility. The client

BOX 24-3

Functional and Therapeutic Classification of Heart Disease

CLASS I

No limitation on physical activity. Ordinary physical activity does not cause undue fatigue, palpitations, dyspnea, or anginal pain.

CLASS II

Slight limitation of physical activity. Comfortable at rest, but ordinary physical activity results in fatigue, palpitations, dyspnea, or anginal pain.

CLASS III

Marked limitation of physical activity. Comfortable at rest, but less than ordinary physical activity causes fatigue, palpitations, dyspnea, or anginal pain.

CLASS IV

Unable to carry on any physical activity without discomfort. Symptoms of cardiac insufficiency or of the anginal syndrome may be present even at rest. If any physical activity is undertaken, discomfort is increased.

Classifications by the Criteria Committee, New York Heart Association.

should be confined to bed only long enough to regain cardiac reserve, but not so long as to promote the complications of immobility.

Surgical Management

The use of a variety of drugs is typically the mode of therapy for CHF. However, attempts are under way to provide respite for the heart in acute failure, for example, after MI. The common feature of the different approaches is to unload the heart for hours to days while it is recuperating. All methods aim to reduce the external work of the heart and the tension that it develops during systole and to decrease myocardial oxygen consumption at the same time as coronary arterial perfusion is improved. This is done with a mechanical device that diverts blood to an external pump or with a counterpulsation device (internal balloon).

When the heart is irreversibly damaged and can no longer adequately function and the client is at risk of dying, cardiac transplantation and the use of an artificial heart to assist or replace the failing heart are also being pursued as last measures for heart failure. One-year survival rates after transplantation are greater than 85 per cent.[57]

Nursing Management

Assessment

The nurse should assess the client for the clinical manifestations of CHF, especially in the high-risk client.

Nursing Diagnosis, Planning, and Implementation

Nursing Diagnosis: Cardiac Output, Decreased R/T heart failure and/or dysrhythmias.

Planning: Expected Outcomes. The client will have increased cardiac output, as evidenced by regular cardiac rhythm, heart rate within normal limits, and hemodynamic parameters within normal limits.

Implementation. The nurse assesses vital signs and heart rhythm every 15 minutes to 1 hour, depending on the stability of the client's vital signs. Tachycardia is a common compensatory mechanism, but it further taxes the myocardial oxygen supply. The nurse monitors dysrhythmias hourly. Most intensive care units have a central area of monitors for all clients in the unit. Common dysrhythmias include premature atrial contractions, premature ventricular contractions, and paroxysmal atrial tachycardia.

CRITICAL TO REMEMBER

Dysrhythmias reduce ventricular filling time, decrease myocardial contractility, and increase myocardial oxygen demands.

All of these conditions further compromise cardiac output. Respirations are usually rapid and labored, and the client is orthopneic. Hypotension, if present, is due to decreased perfusion, vagal stimulation, and dysrhythmias. Hypertension is usually due to pain, anxiety, or previous history of hypertension.

The nurse monitors lung and heart sounds every 2 to 4 hours. Crackles are common, and respirations may be wet and frothy as pulmonary congestion develops. Heart sounds may be distant and include an S_3 or S_4 as filling and ejection times are delayed. The nurse administers oxygen as prescribed to improve tissue hypoxia.

The nurse monitors urine output hourly, noting changes in color and volume of output. Oliguria may reflect decreased renal perfusion. Diuresis is expected and promoted once the client is digitalized and given diuretics. Fluid balance and left ventricular function for many clients are managed with a pulmonary artery catheter. The catheter and nursing responsibilities are discussed in Chapter 23.

The nurse assesses for changes in mental status every 4 hours. Adequate cerebral perfusion requires adequate cardiac output. The client may exhibit changes in problem solving as an early indicator of cerebral hypoxia.

The nurse feeds the client small meals and provides a rest period after meals. Large meals increase myocardial workload and cause vagal stimulation, which results in bradycardia. If caffeine causes tachycardia or ectopic beats, it should be avoided.

Nursing Diagnosis: Fluid Volume Excess R/T reduced glomerular filtration, decreased cardiac output, increased antidiuretic production, and sodium-water retention.

Planning: Expected Outcomes. The client will have an adequate fluid balance, as evidenced by output exceeding intake if on diuretics, clearing breath sounds, stable vital signs, decreasing weight, and resolving edema.

Implementation. The nurse monitors intake and output every hour during acute phases of CHF. Fowler's position is maintained to facilitate breathing. The nurse provides frequent oral care, at least every 4 hours or more often if breathing through the mouth occurs, and weighs the client daily to monitor response to diuretic therapy. Body weight is a more sensitive indicator of fluid balance than is intake and output.

The nurse monitors for signs of increasing peripheral edema and assesses jugular neck vein distention, peripheral edema in the legs or sacrum, and hepatic engorgement or pain in the right upper quadrant.

The nurse provides the client with a low-sodium diet. Physicians commonly order a 2 to 4 g diet. Fluid restrictions may also be used until diuresis is achieved.

Nursing Diagnosis: Gas Exchange, Impaired R/T fluid in alveoli.

Planning: Expected Outcomes. The client will have improved gas exchange, as evidenced by vital signs within normal limits for client's age and condition, skin and mucous membranes without cyanosis or pallor, decreased dyspnea, and arterial blood gases within normal limits.

Implementation. The nurse auscultates breath sounds every 2 to 4 hours, noting adventitious sounds, which indicate congestion. The nurse encourages the client to turn, cough, and deep breathe to clear the airway and to facilitate oxygen delivery. Fowler's position is maintained to facilitate diaphragmatic expansion and ventilation. The nurse administers oxygen as ordered to improve tissue oxygenation and monitors arterial blood gas results. Arterial blood gas results may reveal severe hypoxia or acidosis. If respiratory failure develops, the client will require intubation and continuous mechanical ventilation.

Nursing Diagnosis: Peripheral Tissue Perfusion, Risk for Decreased R/T decreased cardiac output and vasoconstriction.

Planning: Expected Outcomes. The client will have adequate peripheral tissue perfusion, as evidenced by warm, dry skin, peripheral pulses present, and rapid blanching (capillary refill).

Implementation. The nurse monitors the client's peripheral pulses every 4 hours and notes the color and temperature of the skin. The nurse keeps the extremities warm to promote vasodilation to decrease preload and remains alert for the development of thrombophlebitis, because the legs are commonly kept flat or dependent to decrease venous return. The nurse encourages active range of motion or provides passive range of motion to decrease venous pooling. Clinical manifestations of thrombophlebitis include unilateral swelling, calf pain, and pallor. Homans' sign, which is pain in the calf with dorsiflexion of the foot, is not a reliable indicator of thrombophlebitis.

Nursing Diagnosis: Activity Intolerance, Risk for R/T decreased cardiac output.

Planning: Expected Outcomes. The client will have improved tolerance of activity, as evidenced by having increased levels of activity without dyspnea.

Implementation. Nursing care activity is interspersed with rest periods. The nurse monitors the client's response to each activity, noting the development of dyspnea, tachycardia, angina, hypotension, diaphoresis, and dysrhythmias. Vital signs are assessed prior to any major activity (i.e., getting into a chair, walking), immediately after, and 3 minutes later. The length of time required for vital signs to return to baseline indicates the degree of cardiac deconditioning. Activity levels are increased according to the orders of the cardiac rehabilitation nurse or the physician.

The nurse instructs the client to avoid activities that increase cardiac workload during acute stages of care. Activities that precipitate fatigue may demand more cardiac output than the ailing heart can supply.

During the acute stages of CHF, the nurse provides all self-care activity for the client and allows the client to participate as dyspnea allows.

Nursing Diagnosis: Skin Integrity, Impaired, Risk for R/T decreased peripheral tissue perfusion and immobility.

Planning: Expected Outcomes. The client will maintain intact skin as evidenced by no breaks in skin and no reddened or abraded areas.

Implementation. If possible, the nurse turns the client from side to side every 2 hours. If the client is too dyspneic to turn, a pressure reduction mattress is provided. Heel protectors are used, or the client's calf is elevated. The nurse washes the lower legs carefully, and applies lotion to maintain skin integrity.

Collaborative Problem: Risk for digitalis toxicity R/T impaired drug excretion form hepatic and renal involvement.

Planning: Expected Outcomes. The nurse will monitor the client for signs of digitalis toxicity.

Implementation. The nurse assesses the client for decreased heart sounds, hypokalemia, PVC, and first-degree heart block. He or she monitors serum digitalis levels and potassium.

Nursing Diagnosis: Anxiety, Risk for R/T to decreased cardiac output, hypoxia, and fear of death or serious consequences.

Planning: Expected Outcomes. The client will have few signs of anxiety, as evidenced by being able to rest calmly in bed, being able to ventilate fears, and vital signs becoming stable.

Implementation. The nurse provides for psychological rest by maintaining a calm environment; anxiety is contagious. The nurse explains in advance the routine regimens and management strategies and encourages the client to ask questions.

Intervention for CHF involves a long, often difficult period of adjustment. The initial fear of death, brought on by the dramatic symptoms of acute heart failure, can evolve into a long-term strain on coping resources. The nurse should remember that anxiety and fear further tax the client's failing heart. He or she should take time to talk about the client's concerns and anxieties. Many clients with CHF fail to cope with their condition. They need the nurse's skill and emotional support as well as the additional support of a cardiovascular clinical specialist, counselor, social worker, religious leader, or other appropriate person.

Evaluation

The client will often make initial strides once diuresis begins, being able to breathe more easily. But the disorder is usually chronic, and much more time is required for complete resolution. Many times, the eventual goal must be accepted as less than full resolution.

Modification of Plan of Care for the Elderly

The incidence of heart failure increases with age. Cardiac decompensation can be triggered by seemingly minor illnesses and dietary indiscretions.

Medications commonly used by the elderly may have an impact on heart performance even though they pose little risk of interaction with cardiovascular medications. Nonsteroidal anti-inflammatory agents tend to worsen heart disease because they promote sodium retention; tricyclic antidepressants and neuroleptic agents lead to orthostatic hypotension. Conversely, cardiac performance can also have an impact on the medication's action. The development of right ventricular failure can markedly increase the prothrombin time and thereby increase the action of anticoagulants.

The frail elderly are at risk to develop digitalis toxicity because of decreased lean body mass and age-associated decreased glomerular filtration rate. Serum potassium is closely monitored. The combination of hypokalemia and digitalis therapy can lead to lethal dysrhythmias.

Sodium is controlled in the diet, whereas the intake of cholesterol in the elderly usually is not reduced. Trace elements lost in diuresis are usually replaced with a multivitamin.

Posthospital Care

When the client leaves the health-care facility and returns home, the client needs to pace activities and allow for rest. With growing strength and improvement, the client may gradually undertake a progressive exercise program. Exercises, when performed sensibly, can strengthen the body and decrease cardiac workload. The client will need instruction before discharge on measures to prevent the recurrence of CHF. Such measures include

- Taking digitalis and all other medications exactly as prescribed
- Adhering to the program of diuretic therapy
- Staying on the sodium-restricted diet
- Treating all infections promptly

Medical follow-up should be scheduled as ordered, usually every 2 weeks until the client's health is stable

Dysrhythmias

The heart has its own intrinsic conduction system that allows the orderly depolarization of cardiac muscle tissue. Normal conduction and depolarization via this system result in adequate cardiac output and tissue perfusion. Also, this normal pattern of depolarization produces normal sinus rhythm.

Dysrhythmias, also called arrhythmias, are disorders of the heart rate and rhythm caused by disturbances in the conduction system. Dysrhythmias can lead to dramatic changes in circulatory dynamics, such as hypotension, heart failure, shock, and cardiac arrest.

Incidence

Dysrhythmias are common in clients with cardiac disorders but also occur in other clients with normal hearts. The most serious complication of dysrhythmias is sudden death. It is estimated that there are 300,000 deaths from dysrhythmias in the United States each year. Sixty per cent of deaths in the first hour after an MI are the result of dysrhythmias.

Etiology

Dysrhythmias are caused by

- the abnormal rhythmicity of the sinus node (the internal pacemaker) of the heart
- a shift of the pacemaker function from the sinus node to another part of the atrium
- a block in transmission of the impulse through the heart
- abnormal pathways of conduction through the heart
- the spontaneous generation of impulses from any place along the conduction system

ABNORMAL RHYTHMICITY OF THE SINUS NODE

Rhythms that begin in the sinus node can have normal rates, that is, between 60 and 100 beats per minute, or the rate can decrease or increase.

Tachycardia, a rate above 100 beats per minute, has transmission of impulse through the conduction system that is normal, except that there is a shortened time between each QRS complex. Tachycardia can result from increased metabolic demands that occur with fever, sympathetic stimulation, and toxic conditions. When the myocardium is weakened, such as with MI or CHF, tachycardia also occurs because the heart is not effective as a pump. Blood flow to the extremities is decreased, and this triggers reflexes to increase heart rate.

Bradycardia, a heart rate below 60 beats per minute, occurs normally in athletes because their hearts are effective pumps with a greater than normal stroke volume. Because cardiac output is the product of stroke volume and heart rate, the heart rate decreases and yet cardiac output is adequate. Bradycardia can also occur from vagal nerve stimulation.

The sinus node can also be affected by respiration. During inspiration, venous return to the right atrium is delayed because of increased intrathoracic pressure. In quiet respiration, the heart rate can decrease about 5 per cent. It can decrease up to 30 per cent with deep respiration.

SHIFT OF THE PACEMAKER FUNCTION TO ANOTHER PART OF THE ATRIUM

Although the sinus node in the right atrium is the usual impulse generator, impulses can develop in other points along the atrium, within the AV junction, or even within the ventricular conduction systems. Atrial conduction changes most commonly occur from localized re-entry phenomena, which are discussed under pathophysiology.

BLOCK IN TRANSMISSION OF THE IMPULSE THROUGH THE HEART

Blocks that slow or stop an impulse can occur in the atrium, in the AV junction, or within the Purkinje fibers of the ventricles. Blocks develop as a result of

- ischemia of the tissues
- scarring of conduction pathways
- compression of the AV bundle by scar tissue
- inflammation of the AV node
- extreme vagal stimulation of the heart
- electrolyte imbalances
- increased atrial preload
- digitalis toxicity
- beta-blocking agents
- impaired cellular metabolism
- MI (especially inferior)
- valvular surgery

ABNORMAL PATHWAYS OF CONDUCTION THROUGH THE HEART

The pathway of conduction can be altered by the size of the heart, blocks in transmission, ischemia, and hyperkalemia and in response to various medications such as epinephrine. The alteration of pathways in the heart can cause serious dysrhythmias and is more fully explained under pathophysiology.

SPONTANEOUS GENERATION OF IMPULSES FROM ANY PLACE ALONG THE CONDUCTION SYSTEM

The entire conduction system is capable of generating impulses for causing the heart to contract. These impulses occur when the heart is ischemic; has areas of calcification along different points in the heart; or has toxic irritation of the AV node, Purkinje system, or myocardium from drugs, nicotine, or caffeine.

Risk Factors

Dysrhythmias can occur from a primary problem within the heart or a secondary response to systemic disorders, electrolyte disorders, or drug toxicity.

Pathophysiology

Re-entry and abnormal automaticity are the pathophysiologic mechanisms that lead to tachydysrhythmias. Conduction disorders lead to bradydysrhythmias.

RE-ENTRY MECHANISMS

Normally, when the cardiac impulse has traveled throughout the heart, it has no place to go, so it simply dissipates. Then the heart remains quiet until a new impulse begins in the sinus node.

There are some circumstances in which this mechanism does not occur. Instead, the impulse travels around and around in the cardiac muscle without stopping. This phenomenon is called re-entry and sometimes circus movement. Because re-entry can cause serious dysrhythmias, it is important to understand the problem fully.

An impulse can be imagined to occur in a circle. If the impulse starts at the top of the circle and travels around, it will stop when it reaches the top again. In the heart, the cardiac muscle is the circle, and it is refractory to further stimulation during repolarization. Three conditions impair this process and allow the impulse to re-enter the circle.

First, if the length of the pathway is long, by the time the impulse returns to the top, the muscle will no longer be in a refractory state. Therefore, the impulse can travel around the circle again.

Second, if the distance is the same but the velocity is slowed, there will be an increased time interval, and the impulse can re-enter the circle.

Third, if the refractory time for the cardiac cell is shortened, the impulse can re-enter it.

All three conditions occur in clients. Clients with dilated hearts can have elongated pathways. Clients with hyperkalemia, ischemia, and blockage of the Purkinje fibers have slowed velocity. Finally, various medications, such as epinephrine, cause shortened refractory times. Clinical problems such as fibrillation and flutter are due to re-entry phenomena.

ABNORMAL AUTOMATICITY

Normal automaticity occurs in specialized cells in the AV node and Purkinje fibers. Once the action potential of the cell is reached, the muscle fiber contracts, and the wave of depolarization spreads over the myocardium.

Abnormal automaticity develops when the resting potential of the cell membrane is reduced, making the membrane unstable and subject to abnormal conduction patterns and ectopic beats. Abnormal automaticity is commonly caused by ischemia, hyperkalemia, hypoxia, or medications.

CONDUCTION DELAYS

Delay in the transmission of impulse can occur in the AV node or within the bundle of His and Purkinje fibers in the ventricle. Blocks can produce slowed rhythms because of a reduction in the action potential amplitude and excitability at long diastolic intervals. Blocks can also be progressive (e.g., Mobitz type II). In this type of block, the properties of the impulse-carrying fiber change along its length, so that the action potential loses its efficacy as a stimulus to excite the fiber ahead of it.

Clinical Manifestations

The clinical manifestations of dysrhythmias include palpitations, anginal pain, fainting, shortness of breath, and swelling of the extremities. Physical assessment findings may reveal a heart rate below 50 or above 100 beats per minute; an extremely irregular heart rhythm or pulse; a first heart sound that varies in intensity; sudden appearance of symptoms of CHF, shock, and angina pectoris; and a slow, regular heart rate that does not change with activity.

DIAGNOSTIC ASSESSMENT

Dysrhythmias are diagnosed with the ECG recording (see ECG, Chap. 23).

BOX 24-4
Interpretation of Dysrhythmias from the Electrocardiogram

These seven basic steps assist in the identification of dysrhythmias. The electrocardiogram should be studied in an *orderly* fashion in the following manner.

STEP 1

Calculate the heart rate. The simplest method for obtaining the rate is to count the number of R waves in a 6-inch strip of the electrocardiographic tracing (which equals 6 seconds). Multiply this sum by 10 to get the rate per minute. Because the electrocardiographic paper is marked into 3-inch intervals (at the top margin), the approximate heart rate can be rapidly calculated.

Another method is to count the number of large squares between R waves. Find an R wave crossing a large square. Count the number of large squares until the next R wave. The approximate heart rate is

1 large square = 300 beats per minute
2 large squares = 150 beats per minute
3 large squares = 100 beats per minute
4 large squares = 75 beats per minute
5 large squares = 60 beats per minute
6 large squares = 50 beats per minute
7 large squares = 43 beats per minute
8 large squares = 37 beats per minute
9 large squares = 33 beats per minute
10 large squares = 30 beats per minute

STEP 2

Measure the regularity (rhythm) of the R waves (ventricular rhythm). This can be done by gross observation or actual measurement of the intervals (R-to-R). If the R waves occur at regular intervals (with a variance of less than 0.12 second between beats), the ventricular rhythm is normal. When there are differences in R-to-R intervals (greater than 0.12 second), the ventricular rhythm is said to be irregular. The division of ventricular rhythm into regular and irregular categories assists in identifying the mechanism of many dysrhythmias.

Note atrial regularity and measure the atrial rate. Measure the regularity (rhythm) of the P waves (P-to-P). Use the above method, but calculate the distance between the same point on two consecutive P waves.

STEP 3

Examine the P waves. If P waves are present and precede each QRS complex, the heart beat originates in the sinus node, and a sinus rhythm exists. The absence of P waves or an abnormality in their position with respect to the QRS complex indicates that the impulse started outside the sinoatrial node and that an ectopic pacemaker is in command.

STEP 4

Measure the PR interval. Normally, this interval should be between 0.12 and 0.20 second. Prolongation or reduction of this interval beyond these limits indicates a defect in the conduction system between the atria and the ventricles.

STEP 5

Measure the duration of the QRS complex. If the width between the onset of the Q wave and the completion of the S wave is greater than 0.12 second (three fine lines on the paper), an intraventricular conduction defect exists.

STEP 6

Examine the ST segment. Normally this segment is isoelectric, meaning it is neither elevated nor depressed because the positive and negative forces are equally balanced during this period. Elevation or depression of the ST segment indicates an abnormality in the onset of recovery of the ventricular muscle, usually because of injury (e.g., acute myocardial infarction).

STEP 7

Examine the T wave. Normally the T wave is upright and one third the height of the QRS complex. Any condition that interferes with normal repolarization (e.g., myocardial ischemia) may cause the T waves to invert. An abnormally high serum potassium level will cause the T wave to become very tall—sometimes the height of the QRS complex.

A normal sinus rhythm is a heart rhythm that begins in the sinoatrial (SA) node and is between 60 and 100 beats per minute, with normal intervals and no aberrant or ectopic beats. Assessment of the ECG is described in Box 24–4.

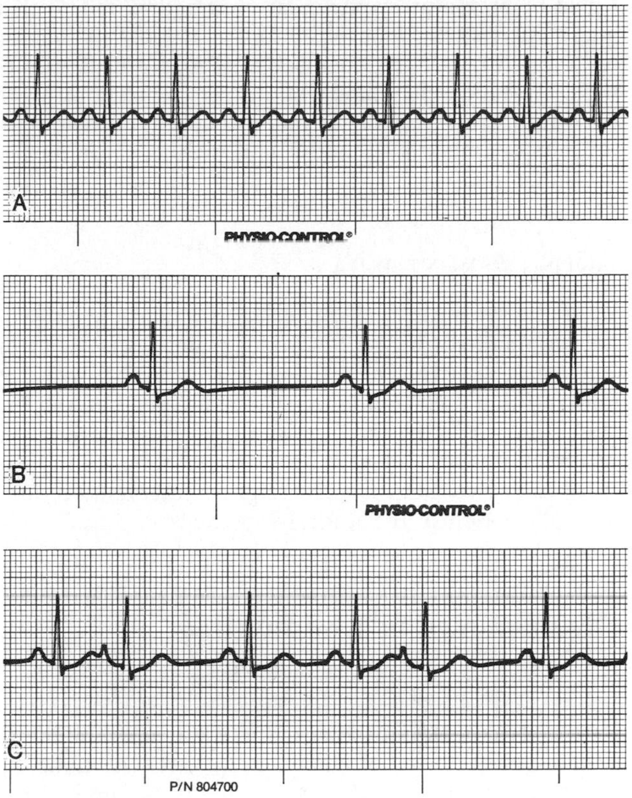

Figure 24–6
Electrocardiographic strips of disorders due to disturbances in atrial automaticity. *A*, Sinus tachycardia. *B*, Sinus bradycardia. *C*, Premature atrial contractions.

MANAGEMENT OF DISORDERS ARISING IN THE ATRIA

Disturbances in Automaticity

SINUS TACHYCARDIA

Sinus tachycardia is characterized by a rapid, regular rhythm at a rate of 100 to 180 beats per minute with a normal P wave and QRS complex (Fig. 24–6*A*). Causes of sinus tachycardia include fever; emotional and physical stress; heart failure; hyperthyroidism; hypercalcemia; medications including caffeine, atropine, nitrates, epinephrine, isoproterenol, and nicotine; and exercise. Most clients do not experience symptoms except for occasional palpitations. Those with underlying heart disease may experience signs of decreased cardiac output and angina pectoris.

Management focuses on alleviating the underlying cause, i.e., replacing volume. If necessary, the physician may prescribe digitalis, beta-adrenergic inhibiting agents (e.g., propranolol), calcium channel blockers, or vagolytics. The client is placed on bed rest to reduce metabolic demand. Oxygen may be prescribed to supply the myocardium adequately.

SINUS BRADYCARDIA

Sinus bradycardia occurs when the SA node fires at a rate less than 60 times per minute. There is a normal P wave and QRS complex (Fig. 24–6*B*). A heart rate that falls below 40 beats per minute could indicate an SA block. Sinus bradycardia usually results from increased vagal tone such as occurs with Valsalva's maneuvers (e.g., straining at stool). Other causes of sinus bradycardia include drugs (especially digitalis, quinidine, procainamide, and beta-adrenergic inhibitors), MI (most often inferior MI), hyperkalemia, and various diseases such as hypothyroidism, myxedema, and obstructive jaundice. Athletes may also manifest sinus bradycardia because of their improved stroke volume.

Sinus bradycardia may be asymptomatic. In symptomatic clients, a subsequent fall in cardiac output may precipitate fatigue, lightheadedness, or syncope. The slowed rate of SA discharge may force junctional or ventricular pacemakers to take over, thereby producing ectopic beats.

Intervention focuses on relief of symptoms and aims to correct the underlying causes of sinus bradycardia. The goal of intervention is to increase the heart rate just enough to relieve symptoms but not enough to cause tachycardia. Beta-adrenergic agonists (isoproterenol) and vagolytics (atropine) may be used, or a temporary transvenous pacemaker may be used.

PREMATURE ATRIAL CONTRACTIONS

Premature atrial contractions (PACs) most often result from enhanced automaticity of the atrial muscle. They occur in normal and diseased hearts. PACs are associated with stress, fatigue, alcohol, smoking, coronary artery disease, cardiac ischemia, heart failure, cardioactive medications (digitalis, quinidine, procainamide), pulmonary congestion, and pulmonary hypertension. Frequent PACs may mark the onset of atrial fibrillation, CHF, and atrial irritability.

Premature atrial contractions cause P waves that occur early (premature P waves) and differ from the normal sinus P wave in direction, size, shape, or a combination of these. Also, a noncompensatory pause usually follows a PAC (Fig. 24–6*C*). To determine the noncompensatory pause, the clinician compares two uninterrupted normal sinus intervals with the P-to-P intervals between two normal sinus beats containing the PAC. The P-to-P interval will be shorter than two normal sinus intervals.

For detecting PACs, one palpates the pulse and auscultates the heart. An early beat will be heard or felt, but it may be difficult to differentiate a PAC from premature beats of other origins (e.g., premature junctional or premature ventricular contractions). The client who experiences numerous PACs may note palpitations or "missed beats." By themselves, PACs are usually benign. However, the client should seek evaluation of the condition. Intervention usually focuses on correcting the underlying cause and may include quinidine or procainamide.

SINUS DYSRHYTHMIA

Sinus dysrhythmia is characterized by phasic changes in the automaticity of the SA node, which cause it to fire at varying speeds. The ECG has a normal P wave, PR interval, and QRS complex. Considered a normal variant, sinus dysrhythmia most frequently develops in conjunction with alterations in vagal tone. Sinus dysrhythmia does not usually require intervention other than alleviation of the underlying cause.

Disturbances in Conduction

SINOATRIAL CONDUCTION DEFECTS

Under certain circumstances, the impulse from the SA node is either (1) not generated in the SA node (SA arrest) or (2) not conducted from the SA node (sinus exit block). Causes of SA node conduction abnormalities include conditions that increase vagal tone, CAD, MI, digitalis and quinidine toxicity, and hypertensive disease. These dysrhythmias may also occur from tissue hypoxia, scarring of intra-atrial pathways, or electrolyte imbalances.

During SA arrest, neither the atria nor the ventricles are stimulated, which produces a pause in the rhythm. After the pause, a new pacer paces the heart at its inherent rate, which is usually slower than the original SA node rate. The most likely new pacer site is another atrial focus, but the junction or ventricle can also escape to assume pacing responsibility.

In sinus exit block, there is a conduction delay between the sinus node and the atrial muscle. Sinus arrest differs from SA exit block in that the SA node intermittently fails to fire at all. The ECG displays normal sinus rhythm that is intermittently interrupted by pauses.

With SA conduction abnormalities, the clinician can palpate or auscultate an irregular pulse.

The client usually remains asymptomatic, depending on the duration and frequency of the pauses. However, lengthy pauses can cause lightheadedness or syncope.

Intervention is unnecessary unless the client becomes symptomatic and exhibits signs of decreased cardiac output. Intervention may include administration of vagolytics (atropine) or sympathomimetics (isoproterenol) to increase the rate of the SA node firing. If pharmacologic measures fail, a pacemaker may be required. Finally, the physician needs to determine and treat the underlying cause of the dysrhythmia.

Disturbances in Impulse Generation

Atrial dysrhythmias are caused by ectopic foci that develop in one of the atrial walls and act to "take over" pacemaker function from the SA node.

Atrial and junctional dysrhythmias are sometimes called supraventricular dysrhythmias because the abnormal foci for ectopic beats originate at a site above the ventricles. An atrial focus may release an impulse before the SA node is due to discharge its normal impulse. This single premature impulse produces a PAC. On the other hand, an atrial ectopic focus may become so irritable that it produces impulses in rapid succession, thereby totally taking over the role of pacemaker. Such rapid rates of impulse formation occur in paroxysmal atrial tachycardia, atrial flutter, and atrial fibrillation.

PAROXYSMAL ATRIAL TACHYCARDIA

Paroxysmal atrial tachycardia (PAT) is the sudden onset of a rapid firing from an ectopic atrial pacemaker. PAT is caused by the re-entry phenomenon.

Clinicians identify atrial tachycardia by three or more consecutive atrial ectopic beats occurring at a rate of 160 to 230 beats per minute alternating with normal sinus rhythm (Fig. 24–7A). Rapid atrial rates may overcome the conduction limits of the AV node, causing varying degrees of AV block. Atrial tachycardia with 2:1 block (that is, two P waves for every QRS complex) most often results from digitalis toxicity.

Whereas PAT occasionally appears in clients with normal hearts, it most often develops in clients with cardiac disease. Cardiac problems precipitating PAT include MI, cardiomyopathy, and pre-excitation syndromes. Other precipitating causes involve extreme emotions, caffeine ingestion, fatigue, smoking, and excessive alcohol intake. PAT decreases ventricular filling time and mean arterial pressure. PAT also increases myocardial oxygen demand.

Management of PAT varies with the severity of symptoms. Clients experiencing this dysrhythmia may note palpitations and lightheadedness. Clients with extremely rapid heart rates or significant underlying cardiovascular disease may develop syncope, heart failure, and angina. The client's heart rate must be immediately reduced. Any maneuver that stimulates the vagus nerve can successfully terminate PAT or increase AV block. Vagotonic maneuvers include carotid sinus massage and Valsalva's maneuvers (bearing down as with bowel movements). Useful pharmacologic agents include propranolol, edrophonium, and verapamil. Sedatives may also be used to reduce sympathetic stimulation. The physician may also employ synchronous cardioversion as an effective means of terminating PAT if medications and vagal stimulation are not effective.

ATRIAL FLUTTER

Atrial flutter is an accelerated rhythm resulting from rapid firing of an ectopic atrial focus. Atrial flutter differs from PAT in that it produces a much more rapid

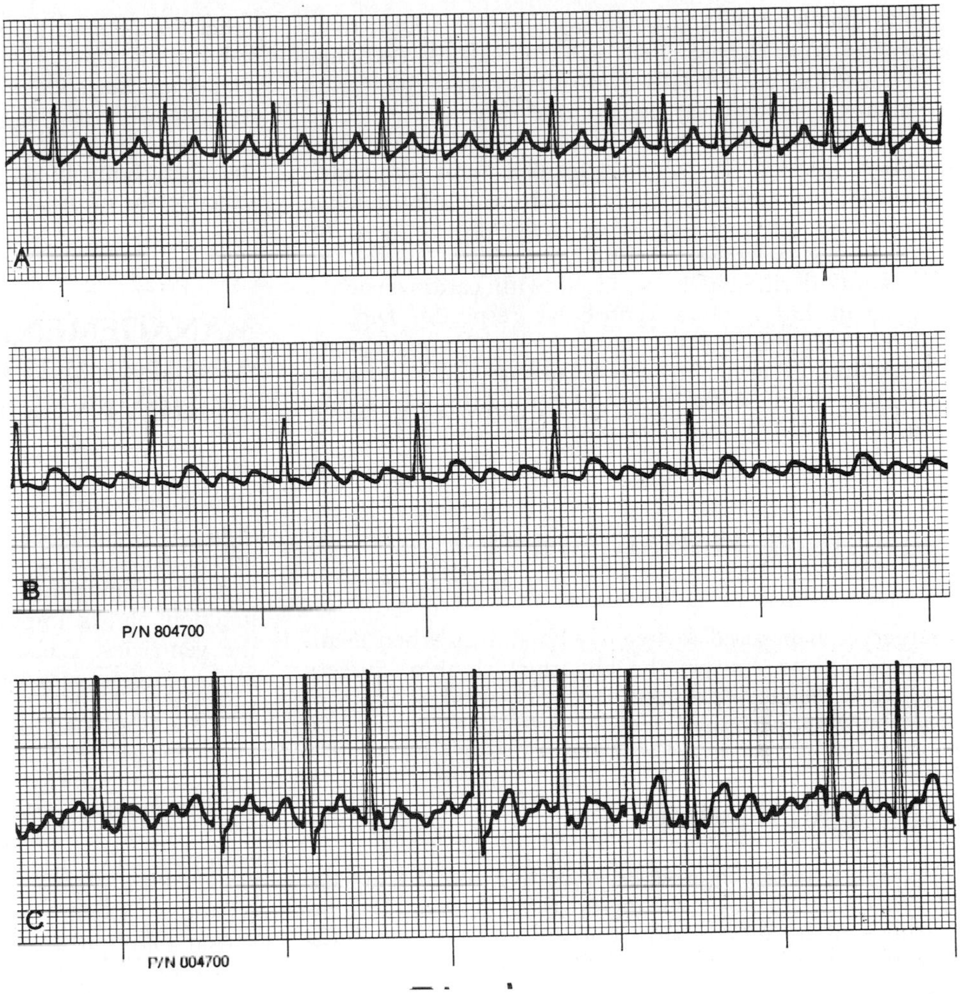

Figure 24–7
Disturbances in atrial impulse generation. *A*, Paroxysmal atrial tachycardia. *B*, Atrial flutter (note saw-toothed pattern of P waves). *C*, Atrial fibrillation (note irregularly occurring R waves).

atrial rate. The P waves are actually inverted or bidirectional, producing a "picket fence" or "saw-toothed" pattern of "flutter waves" (Fig. 24–7*B*). Atrial rate generally ranges from 250 to 350 beats per minute. The AV node cannot conduct all of the atrial impulses that bombard it; that is, it cannot produce a 1:1 conduction. Therefore, the ventricular rate will always be slower than the atrial rate. Thus, the pulse, which reflects ventricular rate, may be normal even though the atrial rate is quite rapid.

The ratio of atrial to ventricular beats may be constant (2:1, 3:1, 4:1, 7:1, and so forth), or it may vary. A variable degree of block produces an irregular pulse.

Atrial flutter most commonly occurs in association with organic diseases such as CAD, mitral valve disease, pulmonary embolus, and hyperthyroidism. In addition, it may follow cardiac surgery. The client may sense occasional palpitations and chest pain, especially when rapid ventricular rates exist.

Intervention aims at controlling rapid ventricular rates. Cardioversion is used. Medications used to treat atrial flutter include digitalis, quinidine, verapamil, propranolol, and procainamide, especially if cardioversion is not successful. Carotid sinus massage helps temporarily slow the ventricular response so that flutter waves can be identified.

ATRIAL FIBRILLATION

Atrial fibrillation is characterized by rapid, chaotic atrial depolarization. The atrial tissue responds to impulses of more than 500 per minute. Atrial fibrillation is a disorder caused by the re-entry phenomenon. However, at extremely rapid rates, the entire atrium may not be able to recover from one depolarization wave before the next begins. This results in mechanical and electrical disorganization of the atria. The ventricular rate ranges from less than 50 to more than 200 per minute. Examination of the ECG reveals erratic or no P waves and a baseline that appears to be irregular and undulating (Fig. 24–7*C*).

Atrial fibrillation most often affects older clients. The causes are similar to those of atrial flutter and include CHF, restrictive pericarditis, organic heart disease, and cor pulmonale. Clients may be asymptomatic, or they may note an irregular pulse and palpitations. The client may have a pulse deficit between apical and radial pulses. Because of atrial disorganization, there is no "atrial kick." This can decrease cardiac output by as much as 20 to 30 per cent. With increasing ventricular rates, cardiac output falls even further and may result in angina pectoris, heart failure, and shock.

Mural thrombi formation can severely complicate atrial fibrillation. Blood pools in the "quivering" atria because of lack of adequate contraction of atrial muscle. This blood can clot, which increases the potential for cerebral and pulmonary vascular emboli.

Atrial fibrillation is managed with cardioversion if the client has a rapid ventricular response. Digoxin, calcium channel blockers, quinidine, and procainamide are commonly used. The physician may order anticoagulants to decrease the threat of mural thrombi formation.

SURGICAL MANAGEMENT

Surgery can be used to treat dysrhythmias when medications fail to convert the abnormal rhythm. Surgery includes chemical ablation and mechanical ablation of the abnormal pathway.[45, 77]

Chemical Ablation

Alcohol or phenol is inserted into involved areas of the myocardium through an angioplasty catheter. Test injections with saline or lidocaine are given to determine whether the dysrhythmia ceases prior to the final injection. Postoperative care is the same as that for angioplasty.

Mechanical Ablation

The abnormal pathway is surgically dissected or treated with a cryoprobe to interrupt its effect on heart rhythms. Supraventricular tachycardia, atrial fibrillation, atrial flutter, and Wolff-Parkinson-White syndrome are dysrhythmias that may be treated with this method when they fail to respond to medication. Prior to surgery, the myocardium is mapped to determine whether other forms of surgery (e.g., coronary bypass grafting or valve replacement) may correct the dysrhythmia. The mapping also isolates the area to be treated. Mechanical ablation with laser is currently under investigation. Surgery may be performed through open heart or closed heart methods. Postoperative care is the same as for other forms of open heart surgery (see Chap. 25).

MANAGEMENT OF DISORDERS ARISING WITHIN THE ATRIOVENTRICULAR JUNCTION

Two major types of dysrhythmias arise in the AV junction: (1) disturbances in automaticity, that is, the AV junctional tissue assumes the role of the pacemaker; and (2) disturbances in conduction, that is, the AV junction blocks impulses journeying from the atria to the ventricles. Causes include ischemia, trauma (after MI or cardiac surgery), digitalis toxicity, and hyperkalemia.

Disturbances in Automaticity

JUNCTIONAL RHYTHMS

Junctional rhythms are characterized by the upward spread of impulses from the AV junction to the atria rather than the normal downward transmission of impulses from the SA node to the AV junction. The PR interval shortens to less than 0.12 second.

The major junctional dysrhythmias are premature junction contractions, junctional escape rhythm, and junctional tachycardias.

The single, early firing of a junctional ectopic focus is called a premature junctional contraction (Fig. 24–8). It has a significance similar to that of a PAC. The inherent rate of the AV junction is 40 to 60 impulses per minute. In the event that the SA node experiences decreased automaticity and fails to function in the role of pacemaker, a junctional escape rhythm will take over and pace the heart at its own inherent rate. A junc-

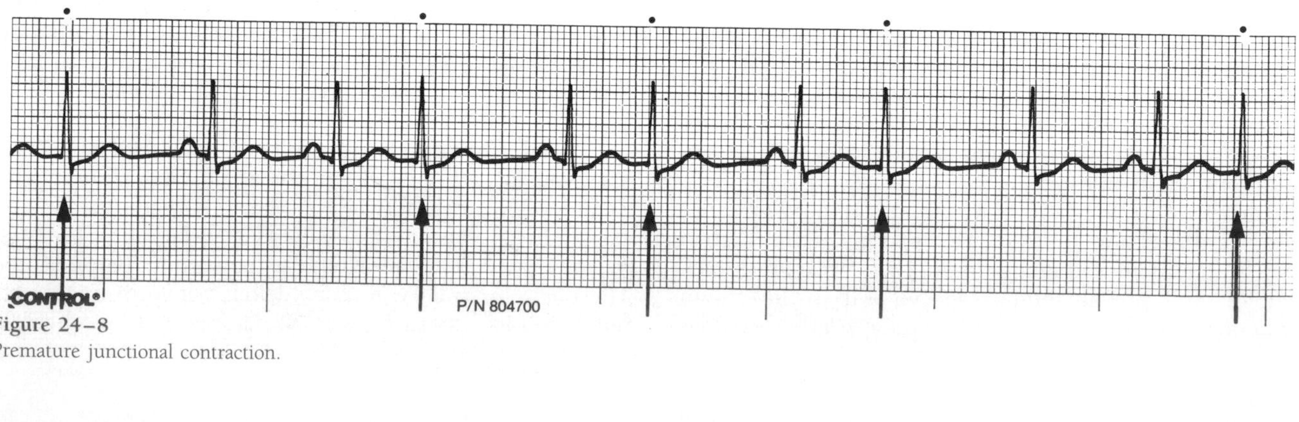

Figure 24–8
Premature junctional contraction.

tional rhythm with a rate that exceeds 60 beats per minute is termed a junctional tachycardia.

Management for rapid junctional rhythms centers on pharmacologic agents and electrical cardioversion. Clients with a junctional escape rhythm do not require intervention unless they are symptomatic for low cardiac output. Then, heart rate may be boosted with the administration of atropine or pacemaker insertion. Premature junctional contractions may be treated with quinidine.

Disturbances in Conduction

ATRIOVENTRICULAR BLOCK

AV block comprises the second group of disturbances arising in the area of the AV junction. Impulses passing through the AV junction are blocked in varying degrees. Therefore, the conduction of impulses from the atria to the ventricles slows or stops entirely, depending on the degree of the AV block. Normally the impulse coming from the SA node is delayed at the AV junction for less than 0.20 second before traveling on to the bundle of His. However, when the AV junction has been damaged by ischemia, rheumatic fever, or drug toxicity, impulses are delayed at the AV junction for abnormally long periods of time.

First-Degree AV Block. This disturbance occurs when conduction in the AV node slows so that the PR interval is longer than 0.20 second (Fig. 24–9*A*). This block is often associated with CAD, increased vagal tone, and congenital anomalies. It may also result from digitalis administration.

First-degree AV block, existing alone as the only abnormal feature of a client's ECG, produces no symptoms and requires no intervention. If the block is caused by digitalis, the medication may be discontinued.

Second-Degree AV Block. This dysrhythmia indicates increased conduction disruption at the AV junction. An intermittent block of supraventricular impulses at the AV junction delays or prevents the depolarization wave through the bundle of His. This results in intermittently dropped QRS complexes. Atrial depolarization continues without disturbance, and normal-appearing P waves occur at regular intervals. The degree of AV block and the number of dropped QRS complexes vary. Every second, third, or fourth (or more) impulse from the atria may be fully blocked, with the creation of a discrepancy between the atrial and ventricular rates. Second-degree AV block does not usually affect conduction through the ventricles, and QRS complexes appear normal in configuration.

Second-degree AV block occurs with CAD, digitalis toxicity, rheumatic fever, viral infections, and inferior wall MI.

The two recognized subdivisions of second-degree heart block are Mobitz type I and Mobitz type II. Mobitz type I (Wenckebach's phenomenon) is composed of recurrent cycles in which the PR interval becomes progressively prolonged until no QRS complex follows the P wave. The client may be asymptomatic or show signs of decreased cardiac output. Intervention is usually not required.

A Mobitz type II block is characterized by a PR interval that remains constant in length until suddenly a ventricular beat is dropped. Mobitz type II block is considered more serious because it often progresses to a block of a higher degree and to life-threatening dysrhythmias.

Clients with second-degree AV block require close ECG monitoring for possible progression to complete heart block (third-degree). Intervention includes (1) administration of atropine and isoproterenol (which speed the rate of impulse conduction), (2) insertion of a temporary or permanent pacemaker, and (3) withholding cardiac depressant drugs (e.g., digitalis). Second-degree

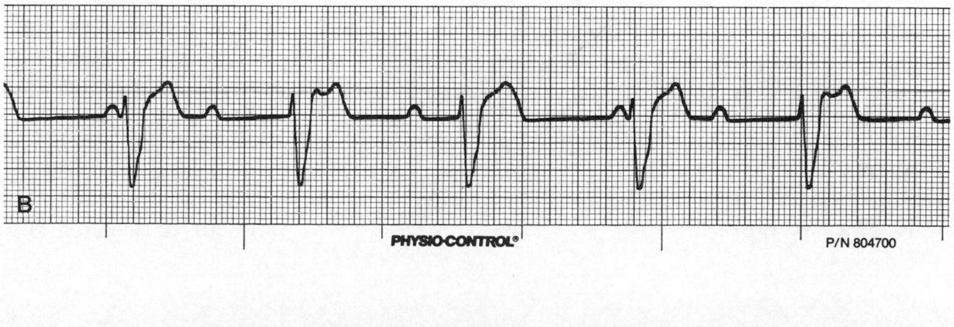

Figure 24–9
Disturbances in junctional conduction. *A*, First-degree atrioventricular block. *B*, Third-degree atrioventricular block (note the variable PR interval and the lack of association of the P wave with the QRS complex).

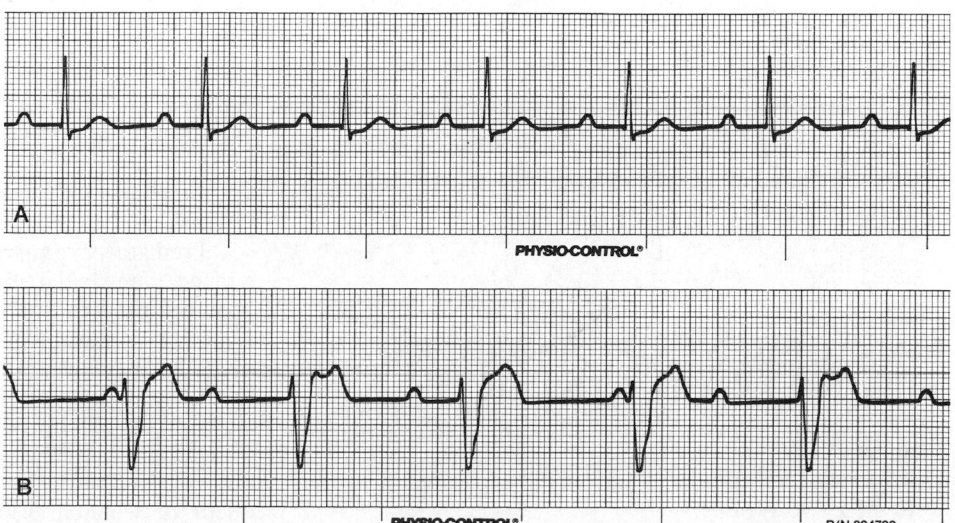

block, which occurs after MI, particularly an inferior MI, may be reversible as the injury of ischemia heals.

Third-Degree AV Block. In third-degree heart block, all impulses from the atria are blocked, and the action of the atria and the ventricles becomes completely disassociated; that is, the atria and the ventricles each have their own pacemaker and beat completely independently of each other (Fig. 24–9*B*). The site of block may occur in the AV node or in the bundle branches.

Less commonly, the block may occur within the His bundle. When third-degree block develops, there may be a pause in the rhythm before a lower pacemaker within the ventricles or junctional tissues begins to produce impulses (escape rhythm). Once the lower pacemaker takes over, the heart rate and QRS duration will differ according to the site of the pacemaker. If a junctional escape rhythm occurs, the ventricular heart rate will be 40 to 60 per minute and the QRS complex will appear normal. If a ventricular escape rhythm occurs, however, the heart rate will range between 20 and 40 per minute and the QRS complex will widen. Other features of the ECG in third-degree heart block include regular P-to-P intervals, regular R-to-R intervals, no meaningful or consistent PR intervals, and normal-appearing P waves.

Third-degree AV block results from a variety of causes including fibrotic or degenerative changes within the conduction system, MI (especially anterior wall MI), congenital anomalies, cardiac surgery, myocarditis, and drug toxicity (digitalis, procainamide, quinidine, verapamil), and trauma.

The slow ventricular rate that develops once the lower pacemaker takes over impulse formation may lead to decreased cardiac output and circulatory impairment. Clients may experience hypotension, angina pectoris, and heart failure.

For management of complete heart block, transvenous-demand pacemakers are inserted while permanent pacemaker insertion is awaited. Isoproterenol may also be used to accelerate ventricular rate. The greatest danger inherent in third-degree AV block is ventricular standstill or asystole, characterized by the Stokes-Adams attack. If a focus in the ventricles does not initiate a heart beat, asystole will lead to immediate loss of consciousness and even death.

CRITICAL TO REMEMBER

Cardiopulmonary resuscitation (CPR) must be instituted immediately when asystole occurs.

MANAGEMENT OF DISORDERS ARISING IN THE VENTRICLES

Disorders of ventricular origin can be divided into the following two groups:

- dysrhythmias that result from ventricular ectopics or a ventricular escape rhythm
- disturbances of impulse conduction through the ventricles as a result of injury to either the right or left bundle branches or pre-excitation syndrome

Disturbances in Ventricular Automaticity

Ventricular dysrhythmias arise below the level of the AV junction. These dysrhythmias are characterized by ectopic impulses, which result from either myocardial irritability or the phenomenon of re-entry. The three ventricular dysrhythmias are premature ventricular contractions, ventricular tachycardia, and ventricular fibrillation.

Ventricular dysrhythmias are generally more serious and life-threatening than are atrial or junctional dysrhythmias. This is because ventricular dysrhythmias more often develop in association with intrinsic heart disease. Conversely, atrial dysrhythmias frequently arise in normal hearts affected by emotions, fatigue, and so forth. Also, ventricular dysrhythmias usually cause greater hemodynamic compromise (e.g., hypotension, heart failure, and shock). The independent contraction of the ventricles results in a reduced stroke volume and therefore a reduced cardiac output. Rapid ventricular rates prevent optimal filling of the ventricular chambers and reduce stroke volume even further. At rates less than 40 per minute, cardiac output is simply not sufficient to support the body's vital functions.

The ECG tracing of ventricular dysrhythmias reveals wide and bizarre QRS complexes. Normally, impulses traverse the ventricles via the shortest, most efficient route. This normal pathway results in a narrow QRS complex. When an impulse originates in the ventricles, however, the impulse follows an abnormal pathway through the ventricular muscle tissue. This abnormality appears as a wide (greater than 0.10 second) complex on the ECG.

PREMATURE VENTRICULAR CONTRACTIONS

Premature ventricular contractions, also called ventricular premature beats, are the most common of all dysrhythmias other than those of the sinus node. They are usually caused by the firing of an irritable focus in the ventricle. A ventricular impulse forms before the next expected impulse from the SA node and takes the place of the normal beat. On the ECG, a wide and bizarre QRS appears, interrupting the underlying rhythm (Fig. 24–10*A*).

Premature ventricular contractions result from enhanced ventricular automaticity or re-entry. Factors promoting PVCs include hypoxia, hypokalemia, hypocalcemia, acidosis, CAD, heart failure, toxic agents (e.g., digitalis, tricyclic antidepressants), exercise, hypermetabolic states, and intracardiac catheters. Also, prolonged sinus arrest or sinus bradycardia may invite the formation of ventricular ectopy. PVCs are innocuous and do not require intervention as long as they remain infrequent or isolated. PVCs are dangerous when they are

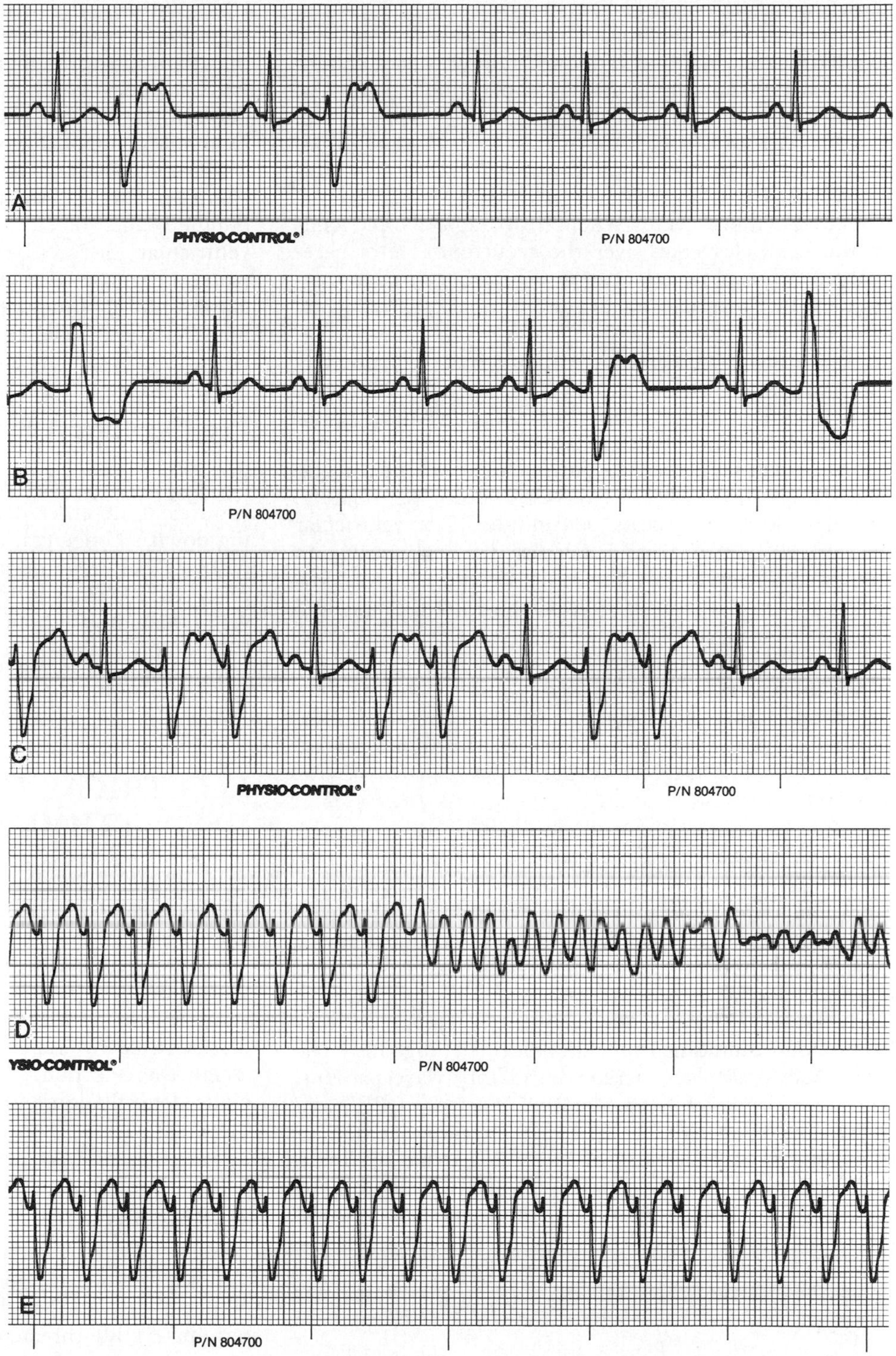

Figure 24–10
Disorders arising in the ventricles. *A*, Unifocal premature ventricular contractions (PVCs). *B*, Multifocal PVCs. *C*, Trigeminal PVCs. *D*, R-on-T phenomenon leading to ventricular fibrillation. *E*, Ventricular tachycardia.

- frequent (more than six per minute)
- coupled with normal beats (bigeminy)
- multiform (Fig. 24–10*B*)
- occurring in pairs (Fig. 24–10*C*)
- occurring as a result of acute MI
- falling on the T wave

Clinicians refer to "falling on the T wave" as the R-on-T phenomenon. The downward slope or the T wave is the most vulnerable period of the cardiac cycle. If the heart is stimulated at this time, it often cannot respond to the stimulus in an organized fashion because the muscle fibers are in various stages of repolarization. Therefore, PVCs occurring during this vulnerable period can precipitate the more life-threatening dysrhythmias of ventricular tachycardia and ventricular fibrillation (Fig. 24–10*D*). Intervention for dangerous PVCs involves administration of antidysrhythmic agents that have myocardial depressant actions. In acute situations, the clinician may administer class I and class II antidysrhythmic agents intravenously, followed by a continuous intravenous drip. Table 24–6 describes a variety of antidysrhythmic agents.

VENTRICULAR TACHYCARDIA

This dysrhythmia occurs when an irritable ectopic focus in the ventricles takes over the recurrent role of pacemaker. All factors that cause PVCs can initiate ventricular tachycardia, but it develops most frequently after MI.

Ventricular tachycardia is characterized by rapidly occurring series of PVCs (three or more) with no normal beats in between (Fig. 24–10*E*). P waves are absent, and PR interval is absent. QRS complex is wide (greater than 0.12 second) and bizarre. The ventricular rate ranges between 100 and 250 beats per minute, usually 130 to 170 beats per minute. The ventricular rhythm is slightly irregular. Ventricular tachycardia, an extremely dangerous dysrhythmia, produces a very low cardiac output that can quickly lead to cerebral and myocardial ischemia. At any time, ventricular tachycardia can develop into ventricular fibrillation.

Ventricular tachycardia that causes loss of consciousness must be terminated immediately with electroshock therapy. The physician may also order intravenous administration of antidysrhythmic agents, usually lidocaine.

VENTRICULAR FIBRILLATION

Ventricular fibrillation is characterized by extremely rapid, erratic impulse formation and conduction. It usually results from severe myocardial damage, hypothermia, R-on-T phenomenon, hypoxia, contact with high-voltage electricity, electrolyte imbalance, and toxicity from quinidine, procainamide, or digitalis. The ECG tracing displays bizarre, fibrillatory wave patterns, and it is impossible to identify P waves, QRS complexes, or T waves (Fig. 24–10*D*). Ventricular fibrillation may be either coarse or fine. This lethal dysrhythmia causes abrupt cessation of effective blood flow. Death results within minutes without immediate intervention.

CRITICAL TO REMEMBER

When ventricular fibrillation appears, the clinician must immediately initiate CPR and defibrillation.

The physician may prescribe epinephrine for fine ventricular fibrillation in order to increase myocardial responsiveness to intervention.

Disturbances in Conduction

BUNDLE BRANCH BLOCK

Bundle branch block means that conduction is impaired in one of the bundle branches (distal to the bundle of His), and thus the ventricles do not depolarize simultaneously. In bundle branch block, the abnormal conduction pathway through the ventricles causes a wide and notched QRS complex. The defect may result from myocardial fibrosis, chronic CAD, MI, inflammation, pulmonary embolism, or congenital anomalies.

Disturbances of conduction through the ventricles result in either a right bundle branch block or a left bundle branch block. Because of its association with left ventricular disease, left bundle branch block has a worse prognosis than does right bundle branch block. No specific treatment exists; in severe cases, the client may require a pacemaker.

Pre-Excitation Syndrome

Pre-excitation syndromes occur when part or all of the ventricle is re-entered by a depolarization wave traveling down a congenital or acquired accessory conducting pathway between the atrium and ventricles (for example, Wolff-Parkinson-White syndrome). If clients develop tachydysrhythmias, the physician may elect to use vagotonic maneuvers, cardioversion, or propranolol administration.

ELECTRICAL MANAGEMENT OF DYSRHYTHMIAS

Dysrhythmias are electrical disturbances within the heart muscle and conduction system. These disturbances can often be effectively managed with exogenously delivered currents of electricity. Electrical intervention can (1) bring abrupt order to erratic electrical discharge or (2) reinstate the flow of electrical current where there is none. Methods of electrical therapy include defibrillation and synchronous countershock (cardioversion).

Defibrillation

Defibrillation is an emergency procedure in which the clinician delivers an electrical current to the heart to terminate a life-threatening dysrhythmia.

CRITICAL TO REMEMBER

The most crucial element for survival after cardiac arrest is the time interval from collapse to care, especially defibrillation.

If ventricular fibrillation is reversed with defibrillation in 6 minutes, the client is three times more likely to survive than if care is delayed.

Defibrillation delivers an electrical current (shock) of preset voltage to the heart through paddles placed on the chest wall (closed chest procedure). This causes the

TABLE 24–6 Medications Used to Manage Dysrhythmias

CLASS	EXAMPLE	ACTION	COMMON SIDE EFFECTS	NURSING IMPLICATIONS
Class IA antidysrhythmics	Quinidine	Prolongs refractoriness and slows conduction velocity Decreases membrane responsiveness by increasing effective refractory period in Purkinje fibers to decrease automaticity and re-entry disturbances Used in treatment of atrial fibrillation, PVCs, and ventricular tachycardia	Prolongs QRS complex or QT interval, which increases vulnerable period in ventricle Can cause tinnitus, vertigo, visual disturbances, loss of hearing, confusion, delirium, and gastrointestinal symptoms May also cause sinus arrest, SA block, and AV block	Monitor vital signs and ECG, especially QT interval Give with meals Monitor plasma levels Avoid excessive citrus fruits, which increase urine pH and decrease excretion
Class IB antidysrhythmics	Lidocaine (Xylocaine)	Depresses the phase 4 stage of the action potential and increases the ventricular fibrillation threshold In the Purkinje fibers, action potential, effective refractory period, and automaticity are decreased Used in treatment of re-entry disturbances, including PVCs and ventricular tachycardia	Because lidocaine is an anesthetic, it can cause paresthesias, numbness, agitation, and disorientation May lead to hallucinations, decreased hearing, twitching, seizures, confusion, and respiratory arrest	Monitor vital signs and ECG continuously Therapy usually initiated with a bolus and then maintained with an IV infusion Common infusion rate is 1–4 mg/min Monitor kidney and liver function tests
Class IC antidysrhythmics	Flecainide acetate (Tambocor)	Depresses sinus node automaticity and prolongs conduction in the atria, AV node, ventricle, and Purkinje fibers	Can aggravate existing dysrhythmias and precipitate new ones May lead to dizziness, visual disturbances, headache, fatigue, palpitations, chest pain, and gastrointestinal distress	Monitor vital signs and ECG continuously Use cautiously in clients taking digitalis and propranolol Usual blood level is 0.2–1 mg/mL
Class II antidysrhythmics	Propranolol (Inderal)	Blocks sympathetic stimulation at the sinus node Reduces automaticity in Purkinje fibers Used to treat atrial fibrillation, atrial flutter, and supraventricular tachycardia	Can cause bronchospasm Contraindicated in bronchial asthma, bronchospasm, and chronic obstructive pulmonary disease	Monitor vital signs and ECG Administer with food
Class III antidysrhythmics	Bretylium tosylate (Bretylol)	Increases action potential duration and refractory period in Purkinje fibers Increases threshold for developing ventricular fibrillation	Hypotension, nausea, and vomiting Neurologic symptoms	Monitor vital signs and ECG closely Potentiates effects of digoxin and warfarin Hypotension more common in clients receiving quinidine or procainamide Monitor liver enzymes Clients on amiodarone need pulmonary function tests with diffusion capacity
Class IV antidysrhythmics	Verapamil (Calan)	Blocks slow calcium channel and has slight nonspecific sympathetic depressant effect Increases relative refractory period through AV node Interferes with re-entry of impulses at AV node Used in treating paroxysmal supraventricular tachycardia, atrial fibrillation, and atrial flutter	Hypotension, syncope, peripheral edema, constipation, bradycardia, AV blocks May precipitate or worsen congestive heart failure Reduces clearance of digitalis	Monitor vital signs and heart rhythm Monitor lung sounds and liver function tests Administer with food Monitor blood pressure and PR interval

Table continued on following page

TABLE 24–6 Medications Used to Manage Dysrhythmias *Continued*

CLASS	EXAMPLE	ACTION	COMMON SIDE EFFECTS	NURSING IMPLICATIONS
Anticholinergics, which compete with receptors for acetylcholine at the para-sympathetic neuronal terminals; this increases the sympathetic tone	Atropine	Accelerates impulse formation in the sinus and AV nodes by inhibiting vagal tone Used to treat SA block, Mobitz I, and complete heart block	Vasodilation; may allow the emergence of junctional pacemakers Depresses exocrine glands (salivary, bronchial mucosa, and sweat glands) Inhibits motor tone of the viscera, leading to distention of the gastrointestinal tract and urinary bladder, dilation of the pupils, and cerebral excitability at high doses and cerebral depression at toxic levels	Monitor vital signs and heart rhythm closely Common rate of administration is 0.4–1 mg every 1–2 hr
Beta-adrenergics (catecholamines); these medications stimulate the heart; they bind to specific receptor sites on the membrane of excitable cells and act directly on automatic and conducting cells by augmenting their sympathetic tone	Isoproterenol (Isuprel)	Stimulates impulse formation and conduction Augments myocardial contraction Produces vasodilation Used to manage symptomatic sinus bradycardia, to increase impulse conduction in SA or AV block, to stimulate escape pacemaker activity in complete AV block	Increases myocardial oxygen demands Generates ectopic beats, especially PVCs Causes central nervous system excitation, facial flushing Action potentiated by antihistamines, tricyclic antidepressants, and thyroid hormone	Assess vital signs closely Common rate of administration is 1–2 mg of a 1 : 5000 solution via an infusion pump Used as a temporary measure with atropine
	Norepinephrine (Levophed)	Stimulates automatic and conductive myocardial fibers (beta-adrenergic) Also has alpha-adrenergic properties, which cause powerful vasoconstriction of the skin, skeletal muscles, kidneys, liver, and intestinal tract Increases heart rate, myocardial contraction, and blood pressure	Ischemia of the splanchnic organs or digits Cardiac and central nervous system effects, like isoproterenol	Assess vital signs closely Common rate of administration is 0.5–3 mL/min in a 0.004 mg/mL dextrose solution Monitor closely for extravasation
	Epinephrine	Like isoproterenol and norepinephrine, it increases heart automaticity, conductivity, and contractility Causes dilation of skeletal muscle blood vessels and constriction of the vessels in the skin, mucous membranes, and splanchnic bed Stimulates breakdown of glycogen to raise blood sugar Inhibits histamine release from mast cells, relaxes smooth muscle in the larynx and bronchial tree	Hypoglycemia/hyperglycemia, dangerously high blood pressure, mental excitation Ischemia of the splanchnic organs or digits	Assess vital signs closely Usual dose is 0.1 mg IV or transbronchially

TABLE 24–6 Medications Used to Manage Dysrhythmias *Continued*

CLASS	EXAMPLE	ACTION	COMMON SIDE EFFECTS	NURSING IMPLICATIONS
	Dopamine hydrochloride (Intropin)	The immediate chemical precursor to the natural production of norepinephrine, it triggers the release of norepinephrine and therefore produces the same effect as norepinephrine Dilates renal vessels through specific receptors in the kidney, uniquely responsive to dopamine (this is an advantage over norepinephrine)	See norepinephrine, except that renal perfusion remains intact	Monitor vital signs closely Infuse by pump with microdrip Usual rate of infusion is 0.5–2.0 μg/kg/min; may be increased to 20 μg/kg/min Monitor neurovascular status of extremities Contraindicated in hypovolemia
	Dobutamine (Dobutrex)	Synthetic catecholamine that acts like dopamine except that it produces a more potent effect on myocardial contractility, a lesser effect on increasing sinus node function, and a slight constriction of peripheral vessels Reduces ventricular preload and afterload Does not increase myocardial oxygen demand as much as the other adrenergics Used in left ventricular failure and cardiogenic shock	Increases ventricular ectopy	Same as dopamine Usual dose is 2.5–2.0 μg/kg/min

AV, atrioventricular; ECG, electrocardiogram; IV, intravenously; PVCs, premature ventricular contractions; SA, sinoatrial.

entire myocardium to completely depolarize at the very moment of shock. It may also allow restoration of organized cardiac action. Defibrillation is always indicated in ventricular fibrillation. It is also used in ventricular tachycardia when the client is unconscious and pulseless. Specially trained nurses, emergency medical technicians, and physicians perform this procedure in emergency settings. Computer-driven defibrillators are now available that automatically interpret the rhythm and advise the clinician whether electroshock is needed. An algorithm for ventricular fibrillation is shown in Figure 24–11.

BEFORE DEFIBRILLATION

Immediately before defibrillation, the nurse should do the following:

- Check the ECG to verify the presence of ventricular fibrillation or tachycardia on the ECG.
- Check the client's pulse.
- Remove any topical nitroglycerin patches (causes a burn).

On confirmation of the emergency, the code alarm is given over the health-care facility intercom system to summon the emergency team (e.g., "Code 99," "Dr. Blue"). In the meantime, CPR measures are started by the first person on the scene.

Open chest defibrillation occurs in an operating room setting where electrical current may be applied directly to the heart.

DURING DEFIBRILLATION

When ventricular fibrillation develops, clinicians must attempt defibrillation at the earliest opportunity. The person performing defibrillation:

- lubricates the paddles to enhance conduction and prevent skin burns (paste should not extend beyond the paddles)
- turns the defibrillator on and confirms that the synchronizer switch is off
- charges to 200 to 300 joules
- assures proper placement of the paddles with 25 to 30 pounds of pressure

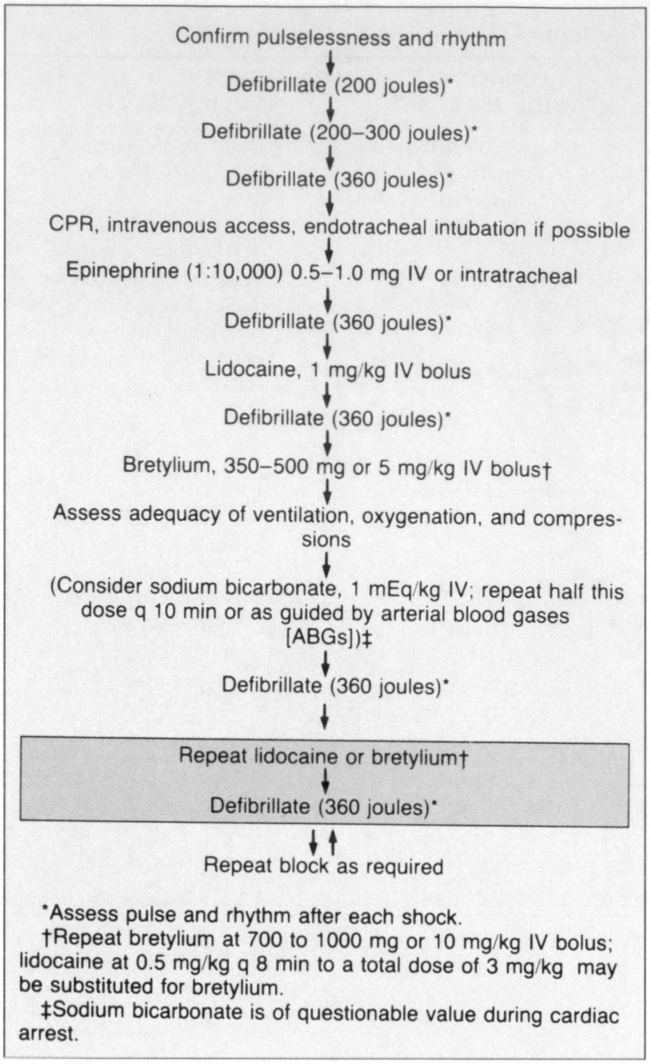

Confirm pulselessness and rhythm
Defibrillate (200 joules)*
Defibrillate (200–300 joules)*
Defibrillate (360 joules)*
CPR, intravenous access, endotracheal intubation if possible
Epinephrine (1:10,000) 0.5–1.0 mg IV or intratracheal
Defibrillate (360 joules)*
Lidocaine, 1 mg/kg IV bolus
Defibrillate (360 joules)*
Bretylium, 350–500 mg or 5 mg/kg IV bolus†
Assess adequacy of ventilation, oxygenation, and compressions
(Consider sodium bicarbonate, 1 mEq/kg IV; repeat half this dose q 10 min or as guided by arterial blood gases [ABGs])‡
Defibrillate (360 joules)*
Repeat lidocaine or bretylium†
Defibrillate (360 joules)*
Repeat block as required
*Assess pulse and rhythm after each shock.
†Repeat bretylium at 700 to 1000 mg or 10 mg/kg IV bolus; lidocaine at 0.5 mg/kg q 8 min to a total dose of 3 mg/kg may be substituted for bretylium.
‡Sodium bicarbonate is of questionable value during cardiac arrest.

Figure 24–11
Algorithm for ventricular fibrillation and ventricular tachycardia. Pulseless ventricular tachycardia is treated identically to ventricular fibrillation. (From Rakel, R. E. [1992]. *Conn's current therapy*. Philadelphia: W. B. Saunders.)

- calls for all personnel to stand back from the bed to prevent accidental shock
- depresses the buttons on the paddles and delivers a shock while standing back from the bed

Two paddle positions are recommended. For the anteriolateral position, one paddle is placed at the second intercostal space, at the right of the sternum, and the other paddle is positioned at the fifth intercostal space, anterior axillary line (Fig. 24–12*A*). For the anteroposterior position, if it is convenient, clinicians may attempt placing the paddles in an anteroposterior position. Because electricity is carried along metal devices and the client, all personnel, including the clinician administering the shock, must stand back from the bed.

AFTER DEFIBRILLATION

The clinician immediately assesses the pulse and ECG after defibrillation. If the first countershock is unsuccessful, then the client must be immediately defibrillated again. Defibrillators are frequently equipped with paddles capable of monitoring the ECG. If left in place after the shock has been delivered, the cardiac response can be quickly evaluated.

A successful response is indicated by cessation of fibrillation, restoration of sinus rhythm, and palpation of a regular pulse. After successful defibrillation, the client requires continuous ECG monitoring. The nurse must also continually assess vital signs along with neurologic status.

In documenting the outcome of defibrillation, the nurse must record the following points:

- preprocedure rhythm
- times and voltage of shocks delivered
- postdefibrillation rhythm pattern
- names, times of administration, and doses of administered medications
- other hemodynamic data available before, during, and after the defibrillation

TERMINATION OF RESUSCITATION

In general, if an organized rhythm and pulse have not returned after 15 to 20 minutes of CPR and advanced cardiac life support, success with further treatment is extremely unlikely. Many times the client has other noncardiac disorders that make resuscitation attempts futile. Only the physician can terminate resuscitation attempts.

ADVANCES IN DEFIBRILLATION

Automatic Implantable Cardioverter Defibrillator. The automatic implantable cardioverter defibrillator (AICD) is a device surgically implanted in clients who have an episode of sudden death and fail drug tests in electrophysiologic testing. It is a system that consists of a pulse generator and a sensor that continuously monitors the heart rhythm. When it detects a dysrhythmia, it automatically delivers a countershock. For ventricular fibrillation, the AICD will give an electrical countershock within 15 to 20 seconds. It can also detect and treat ventricular tachycardia with cardioversion. This implanted system does not require as much energy as external defibrillation does because less energy is lost when the impulse is directly applied to the heart. The AICD is implanted surgically into a pouch into the abdominal wall through a thoracotomy incision.

Clients who require AICDs have a great deal of anxiety. Anxiety can develop from past episodes of near-death as well as from feelings of not ever being able to die. Other patients fear that the AICD will not be able to reverse their dysrhythmia. The nurse is sensitive to these thoughts and facilitates their discussion.

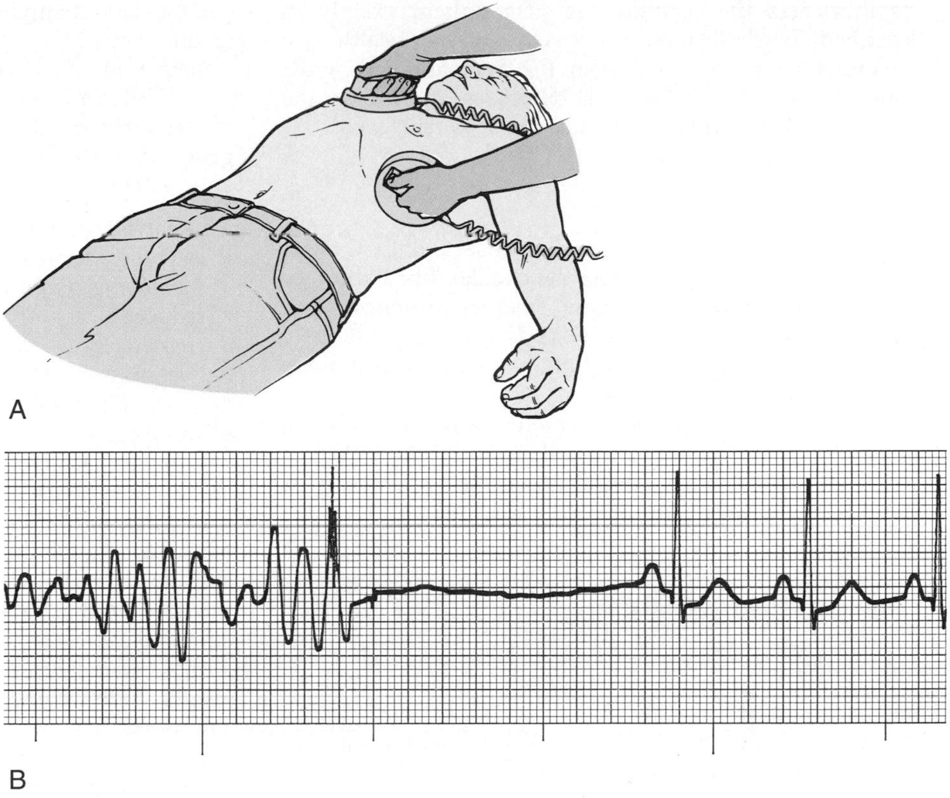

Figure 24–12
A, Anterolateral paddle placement for external countershock. External paddles are placed at the second right intercostal space and at the anterior axillary line in the fifth left intercostal space. *B*, Ventricular fibrillation converted to normal sinus rhythm with external countershock.

Cardioversion

Cardioversion, most often an elective procedure, is the use of electricity to convert a cardiac dysrhythmia to a normal sinus rhythm that is capable of sustaining improved cardiac output. Cardioversion is not used for ventricular fibrillation. The cardioverter (or defibrillator) delivers an electrical current to the heart. The electrical discharge is synchronized with or triggered by the client's QRS complex for avoidance of accidental discharge during the repolarization phase when the ventricle is vulnerable to the development of ventricular fibrillation. Cardioversion can terminate potentially dangerous or exhausting dysrhythmias that have been refractory to pharmacologic intervention. Indications for cardioversion include tachycardias developing in atrial, junctional, or ventricular tissue. A QRS complex must be present for successful conversion of the dysrhythmia. Only specially trained physicians can perform this procedure.

BEFORE CARDIOVERSION

The physician evaluates the ECG to diagnose the type of dysrhythmia present. In a nonemergency situation the client signs an informed consent, and then the intervention is scheduled for a specified hour. The client and family must receive a full explanation of cardioversion.

Cardioversion can be performed at the bedside or in a laboratory setting. However, in case the client develops a life-threatening dysrhythmia after cardioversion, emergency equipment and trained clinicians must be in the room.

If the client has been taking a digitalis preparation, the drug should be held for 2 days before the procedure. Digitalis may predispose the client to the development of ventricular dysrhythmias during cardioversion. A low serum potassium level also increases the risk of lethal dysrhythmias. Therefore, the nurse administers potassium replacement therapy as prescribed before cardioversion. The client is premedicated with prescribed antidysrhythmics to ensure maintenance of postconversion rhythms. The nurse administers oxygen, if prescribed, before cardioversion and discontinues it afterward. The client should receive nothing by mouth for several hours before cardioversion. An intravenous line is started. To reduce fear and promote amnesia, the nurse administers diazepam (Valium) intravenously as prescribed.

DURING CARDIOVERSION

The physician (1) sets the machine within a range of 50 to 200 watt-seconds (more or less voltage depending on the underlying circumstances); (2) turns on the synchronizer switch to deliver the shock during the QRS complex and not on the downslope of the T wave;

(3) lubricates the paddles and places them exactly as described for defibrillation; (4) calls for all health-care personnel to stand back from the bed; and (5) while standing back from the bed, depresses and holds the buttons on the paddles until the shock is delivered.

AFTER CARDIOVERSION

Clinicians immediately assess the pulse and ECG after cardioversion. In some cases, ventricular fibrillation or tachycardia occurs, demanding emergency action. The nurse monitors the client's ECG rhythm continuously for at least 2 hours and carefully assesses for complications.

A successful response to cardioversion resolves the dysrhythmia and restores normal sinus rhythm. With a good response and no complications, the client can be discharged the following day.

Nursing Management

Assessment

The nurse assesses the client for subjective clinical manifestations of dysrhythmias. These include palpitations, angina, shortness of breath, fatigue, and syncope. The client may also feel anxiety about the heart disorder and express nervousness, fear, sleeplessness, uncertainty, or hopelessness. Objective clinical manifestations may include diaphoresis, pallor or cyanosis, variations in radial and apical pulse such as bradycardia or tachycardia, rhythm changes, hypotension, crackles, or decreased mental acuity. The client may be demanding of the nurse and exhibit a fear of being left alone. The client is placed on a monitor, and heart rhythm is monitored continuously. Rhythm strips are examined at least every shift.

Nursing Diagnosis, Planning, and Implementation

Nursing Diagnosis: Decreased Cardiac Output R/T alterations in rate and rhythm of the heart.

Planning: Expected Outcomes. The client will have an adequate cardiac output, as evidenced by heart rate and rhythm and blood pressure returning to baseline; level of consciousness returning to baseline; skin is warm and dry; lung sounds are clear; no S_3 or S_4 and no dysrhythmias.

Implementation. The nurse monitors heart rate and rhythm and vital signs continuously, many times with the aid of the computer. Skin temperature, lung sounds, heart sounds, and peripheral pulses are assessed every 4 hours. Laboratory studies are monitored, especially if the client is suspected of having an MI. Antidysrhythmic medications are given according to orders. Blood levels can be used as a guide for dosages. Many medications, especially antidysrhythmics, can rise to toxic levels, especially if the client has pre-existing liver or renal disorders.

The nurse maintains a quiet atmosphere and administers analgesics to control pain. Stimulation can lead to increased levels of catecholamine release and trigger tachycardias and increased oxygen demand.

Oxygen is applied with nasal prongs to supplement serum levels. Hypoxia can lead to further myocardial ischemia and dysrhythmias.

If life-threatening dysrhythmias develop, many nurses are trained to defibrillate the client. Other emergency interventions include CPR, various medications, and preparation of the client for pacemaker insertion.

Nursing Diagnosis: Anxiety R/T sudden onset of life-threatening disorder and risk of death.

Planning: Expected Outcomes. The client will have a reduced level of anxiety, as evidenced by stating a decreased level of anxiety and discussing feelings of helplessness or hopelessness; increased ability to sleep or rest; return of heart rate to baseline; and reduction of dyspnea.

Implementation. The nurse identifies the client's anxiety and assists the client in discussing sources of fear. Misconceptions are clarified. Commonly, the client or a member of the family has had a heart condition, and the client's ability to cope may be directly influenced by that experience. The nurse also explains the equipment present in the room. Most rooms are stocked with various equipment, and its presence does not always indicate the severity of the client's condition. The nurse remains with the client and explains all procedures and routines. Finally, the nurse explores the usual coping methods with the client. Positive coping methods are usually supported; maladaptive coping mechanisms are discussed, and substitutions are suggested. For example, smoking may be a common coping mechanism, but it is not permitted with cardiac disorders, nor is it permitted in most hospitals. Therefore, if smoking is the client's coping mechanism when stressed, a substitution will need to be found such as nicotine patches or chewing gum.

Evaluation

The degree of expected outcome attainment is assessed hourly (or more often) if the client has life-threatening dysrhythmias. Anxiety can sometimes be abated quickly, but commonly it requires several days for abatement. Some clients remain anxious for their entire hospital stay.

Posthospital Care

Clients who have experienced cardiac dysrhythmias while at a health-care facility may be apprehensive about leaving the facility. Clients with recurring life-threatening dysrhythmias such as ventricular tachycardia will require comprehensive and specialized attention. These clients may have experienced many frightening events in the course of their hospitalization. Teaching about the nature of the disorder is done several times, because the client may have an attention span that is shorter than normal as a result of severe anxiety as well as a physical illness. Discharge instructions about antidysrhythmic agents include

- name of medication
- indication and importance
- administration

TABLE 24–7 Indications for Artificial Pacemakers

Dysrhythmias from depressed impulse formation
Asystole
Sick sinus syndrome
Sinus arrest
Symptomatic sinus bradycardia
Dysrhythmias from blocked conduction
Third-degree AV block with slow ventricular rate or syncope (Stokes-Adams attack)
Mobitz II AV block in a client with an MI
Right bundle branch block with left hemiblock
New left bundle branch block in a client with an MI
Dysrhythmias from re-entry phenomenon
Atrial tachydysrhythmias
Ventricular tachydysrhythmias
Atrial fibrillation with a slow ventricular rate
Prophylactically before surgery in clients with a history of cardiac arrest or AV blocks
Prophylactically after heart surgery

AV, atrioventricular; MI, myocardial infarction.

- dosage
- side effects and what to do if they occur
- what to do if dose is missed

When a client is at risk of developing a life-threatening dysrhythmia, members of the client's household and significant others need to know CPR. The nurse should refer these individuals to community agencies that provide CPR training (e.g., the American Heart Association, the American Red Cross, local fire departments, and some local hospitals).

Sometimes clients with serious, chronic, or potential dysrhythmias use portable telemetry units for monitoring themselves at home after discharge. This allows the resumption of daily activities while providing continuous 24-hour surveillance of cardiac rhythm. Nurses are often responsible for instructing clients in the use of these units. The nurse should ask these clients to keep a diary of their daily activities so that clinicians can correlate factors in the client's life that may be contributing to the development of rhythm disturbances.

Finally, the nurse instructs clients concerning the importance of regular medical follow-up. Also, the client and significant others should know how to obtain emergency medical attention if necessary.

Living under the constant threat of sudden death provokes anxiety, depression, and alterations in family and individual coping. The nurse should assess for problems and refer clients and significant others to appropriate counseling services when needed.

Pacemakers

A pacemaker is a device that delivers battery-supplied electrical stimuli over leads with electrodes in contact with the heart. A pacemaker initiates the heartbeat when the heart's intrinsic conduction system fails or is unreliable. Problems with the conduction system develop when (1) the SA node is damaged and unable to promote a reliable rhythm; (2) impulses from the SA node and atria are not adequately transmitted through the AV junction to the ventricles; or (3) dysrhythmias from ectopic foci are present.

Sophisticated pacemakers use computers that allow multiple programs. They can send out appropriately timed signals, sense cardiac activity, and preserve normal atrial and ventricular sequence (synchrony). Future pacemakers will be able to respond, as the heart does, to changing metabolic requirements by responding to changes in blood pH, oxygenation, respirations, temperature, or muscle activity.[33] The artificial pacemakers control the heart beat by means of direct electrical stimulation of the ventricles or atria. Table 24–7 outlines the indications for pacemaker insertion.

ARTIFICIAL PACEMAKER DESIGN

Whereas there are numerous pacemaker models, each with unique capabilities, every pacemaker consists of a pulse generator and a lead-electrode system.

The pulse generator is essentially the pacemaker's power source. It houses the electronic circuitry responsible for sending out appropriately timed signals and for sensing cardiac activity. The output circuit controls the current pulse delivery rate, pulse duration, and refractory period. The sensing circuit is responsible for identifying and analyzing any spontaneous intrinsic electrical activity and responding appropriately.

The pulse generator can be external or internal (Fig. 24–13). The external unit is designed for temporary pacing, primarily for support of critical bradycardias. A permanent pacemaker has the pulse generator (the size of a stethoscope head) surgically implanted through a small incision made in the anterior chest

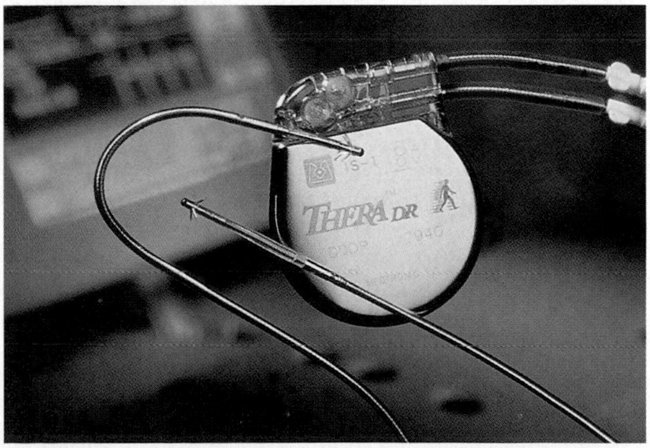

Figure 24–13
Permanent pacemaker (pulse generator). (Courtesy of Medtronic, Inc.; Minneapolis, MN)

TABLE 24–8 Pacemaker Classification System

	RATIONALE	LETTER CODE
1st letter	Denotes chamber to be paced	Atrium (A), ventricle (V), or both (dual) chambers (D)
2nd letter	Denotes chamber to be sensed	Atrium (A), ventricle (V), dual (D), or none
3rd letter	Indicates the type of response to occur	Impulse to be triggered (T), inhibited (I), or both (D)
4th letter	Reflects programmability and rate modulation	The 4th and 5th letter codes are infrequently stated in practice, except for R (to indicate a rate-adaptive pulse generator driven by a sensor)
5th letter	Reflects antitachydysrhythmic functions	

wall. The pacemaker can be reprogrammed with a magnet after insertion.

The lead delivers the electrical impulse from the pulse generator to the myocardium. The electrode is the end of the lead that delivers the impulse directly to the myocardial wall. Not only does this system deliver electrical impulses, but it relays information about spontaneous intracardiac signals back to the sensing circuit within the pulse generator.

Types of Pacemakers

Pacemakers are classified by uniform codes according to a letter-code classification system (Table 24–8).

PACING MODES

Asynchronous (Fixed Rate) Pacing

The earliest form of pacemakers delivers an electrical impulse to the heart at a preset fixed rate regardless of intrinsic cardiac pacemaker action. Because there is no sensing mechanism, the pacing mechanism virtually ignores the client's own intrinsic heart rhythm. Although infrequently used today, this mode of pacing is appropriate for clients with a natural heart rate below 60 beats per minute and without a tendency to develop dysrhythmias. Its circuitry is simpler than others, which reduces the chance of pacemaker failure. The major disadvantages of fixed rate pacing use are

- Potential for tachycardia
- Atrial and ventricular asynchrony
- Risk of ventricular fibrillation if the pacemaker fires during the vulnerable period
- Heart unable to adjust rate to accommodate variations in client's activity level

Noncompetitive (Demand) Pacing

With demand pacing, the pacemaker fires only on demand or when needed to stimulate atrial or ventricular contraction. Demand pacemakers are advantageous in clients with AV block, SA arrest, severe sinus bradycardia, or dysrhythmias requiring electrical overdrive.

To set up demand pacing, the physician must first preset a heart rate into the unit that is suitable for the client. For example, the clinician may program a preset rate of 60 into the demand pacemaker unit. When the client's heart rate falls below 60 beats per minute, artificial pacing ensues. If the natural heart rate increases to greater than 60 beats per minute, the unit will not fire a stimulus.

ATRIAL DEMAND PACING

The atrium is paced and the ventricle is allowed to depolarize following the usual pathways (AV node, Purkinje fibers). Atrial demand pacing is used for clients with symptomatic sinus bradycardia.

VENTRICULAR DEMAND PACING

The ventricle is paced in clients with AV block. The pacemaker senses for ventricular depolarization. When it does not occur at a preset rate, the pacer fires. A disadvantage of this mode is that atrial and ventricular contractions are not synchronous. This loss of "atrial kick" filling the ventricles may lead to hypotension, chest pain, and CHF (called pacemaker syndrome).

Synchronous Pacing

Synchronous pacing operates in a manner similar to that of the demand mode. In synchronous pacing, the sensing electrode is placed in the atrium and the pacing electrode is placed in the ventricle. Thus, the pacemaker unit senses atrial activity and elicits a stimulus to prompt a ventricular depolarization. A major benefit is that it permits the heart rate to vary, and atrial-ventricular synchrony occurs, depending on the physiologic demands of the body. A built-in safety mechanism causes ventricular depolarizations to occur at a fixed rate should atrial rates become too fast.

Atrioventricular Sequential Pacing

In this mode of pacing, the ventricle is sensed and the atrium is paced. If the ventricle does not depolarize after a preset interval, it is also paced. If the pacemaker does not fire, the ventricle depolarizes on its own. Because there is no sensing of atrial activity, the paced atrial impulse is preset at a specific interval to follow a sensed or paced QRS complex. The atrium is paced regardless of its own intrinsic activity; therefore, competition may occur, leading to atrial fibrillation.

Universal Atrioventricular Pacing

Universal or physiologic pacemakers are the most sophisticated pacemakers currently available. They consist of both atrial and ventricular circuits that sense and pace their respective chambers. This type of pacing is used in the management of clients with atrial bradydysrhythmias with or without abnormal AV node conduction and in normal sinus node function with AV block. The advantage of this mode of pacemaker is that it more closely mimics the normal heart. Atrial kick occurs, which increases cardiac output by 30 per cent, and the heart rate can be changed to meet metabolic demands. The major risk of this mode of pacing is the development of pacemaker-induced tachycardia. If a skeletal muscle activity is sensed, a ventricular beat may be triggered.

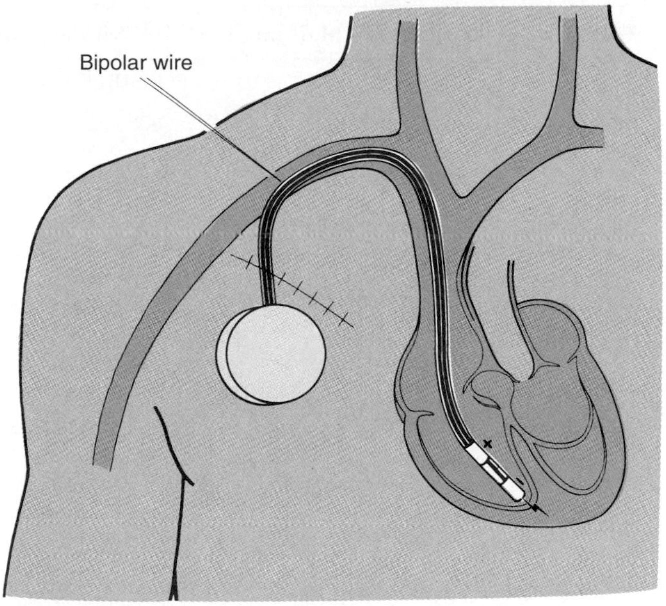

Figure 24–14
Transvenous catheter placement, dual-chamber pacing. Separate electrodes in the atrium and ventricle allow synchronized contraction, and thus stroke volume is improved. (From Phillips, R. E. & Feeney, M. K. [1990]. *The cardiac rhythms: A systematic approach to interpretation.* [3rd ed.]. Philadelphia: W. B. Saunders.)

Temporary Pacing

Temporary pacing may be used in emergency or elective situations that require limited, short-term pacing (less than 2 weeks). In this form of pacing, the pulse generator is external. The unit is the size of a small transistor radio and operates by dry-cell batteries. The unit has dials for adjusting both power and rate of discharge.

Transvenous (Endocardial) Pacing

Transvenous pacing provides the most common means for pacing the heart in emergency situations. The surgeon (1) inserts the pacing electrode via the transvenous route (via the antecubital, femoral, jugular, or subclavian veins) and (2) threads the electrode into the right atrium or right ventricle so that it comes into direct contact with the endocardium. This procedure can be done at the bedside under fluoroscopic control or in a cardiovascular laboratory. Major drawbacks include thrombophlebitis, infection at the insertion site, sepsis from unsterile technique, increased chance of lead displacement as the client changes position, and the discomfort of having the extremity nearest the insertion site immobilized (Fig. 24–14).

Nursing Management

Before the procedure, the nurse explains the purpose of the temporary pacemaker to the client and significant others. The nurse ascertains that a permit for the procedure has been signed and that all questions have been answered. Necessary equipment is gathered, and the functioning of the external generator is checked (battery and sense and pace modes). The client's vital signs are assessed, and a rhythm strip is obtained.

During the procedure, the nurse reassures the client while monitoring the ECG and vital signs continuously. The stimulus and sensitivity settings are maintained according to the physician's orders. The electrode is taped or sutured at the insertion site.

After the procedure, the vital signs are assessed routinely along with heart rhythm and emotional reactions to the procedure and pacing. All connections are secured and routinely checked. Battery and control settings are also monitored. The incision site is cleaned and dressed according to protocols. The nurse keeps the generator dry and the controls protected from mishandling. The client must be protected from electromicroshocks and electromagnetic interference. There are several interventions that protect the client. Exposed wires are covered with rubber gloves or electrical tape. The pulse generator is enclosed in a rubber glove to keep it dry. Rubber gloves are worn when exposed wires are handled. Electrical equipment is checked for adequate grounding.

In addition to protecting the client from injury, the nurse monitors the pacemaker function. The location and type of pacing lead, along with rhythm strips, is documented. The pacing mode, stimulus threshold, sensitivity setting, pacing rate and intervals, and intrinsic rhythm are noted.

Pacemaker complications can occur from insertion. They include phlebitis at the site, pneumothorax, atelectasis, pericardial fluid accumulation, diaphragmatic stimulation (seen as hiccupping or twitching at the pacemaker site), and dysrhythmias. Complications can also occur from malfunctioning of the pacemaker (Table 24–9).

TABLE 24–9 Pacemaker Malfunctions and Nursing Interventions

PROBLEM	POSSIBLE CAUSE	NURSING INTERVENTIONS*
Failure to Pace Properly		
Intermittent or complete absence of pacing artifact Rapid, inappropriate firing of pacemaker (pacemaker-mediated tachycardia)	Battery failure A break or loose connection anywhere along the system Pulse generator failure Circuitry failure "Oversensing" or "undersensing" by the pacemaker	Replace pulse generator Replace battery unit Check and tighten all connections between pulse generator and leads Reduce or increase sensitivity threshold of pacemaker unit Assess client's tolerance of pacemaker failure; have emergency drugs on hand; perform CPR as indicated
Failure to Capture		
Pacing artifact present but is not followed by a QRS complex or P wave	Decreased conductivity by the myocardial tissue due to electrolyte imbalance, infarction, drug toxicity, perforation, or excessive fibrosis of tissue at electrode site Lead displacement due to migration, or idle manipulation of pulse generator ("twiddler's syndrome")	Increase voltage by 1–2 mA (temporary pacemaker) Increase amplitude of pacemaker output (and/or pulse width) Reposition client to either side in attempt to improve contact of electrode with endocardium; in temporary pacemaker, try moving arm if lead wire is inserted in antecubital area Obtain chest film to determine pacemaker position Have emergency drugs on hand; initiate CPR if necessary
Failure to Sense		
Pacing artifact present despite the presence of QRS complexes and P waves A competitive rhythm may develop	Sensitivity threshold set too low Intrinsic beats are of too-low voltage and go undetected by pacemaker's sensing mechanism Dislodged or fractured lead Circuitry failure Electromagnetic interference	Increase sensitivity threshold on pulse generator Reposition client If client's intrinsic rhythm/rate is adequate, turn off pacemaker Increase pacing rate to overdrive client's intrinsic heart rate Give antidysrhythmics to decrease ectopy Notify physician Obtain chest film to determine electrode placement
Oversensing		
Pacemaker senses electrical activity within the myocardium (which should be ignored) or myopotentials	Sensitivity threshold set too high T wave sensing myopotentials Electromagnetic interference Two leads touching	Decrease sensitivity threshold Correct conditions that produce large T waves

* For all problems, document malfunction by an electrocardiogram. If pacemaker is programmable, have reprogramming machine available. Monitor client's tolerance to pacemaker malfunction (vital signs, chest pain).
From Huang, S. H, et al. (1989). *Coronary care nursing* (2nd ed.). Philadelphia: W. B. Saunders.

Permanent Pacing

Permanent pacing is indicated in long-term management of symptomatic or life-threatening dysrhythmias. The surgeon inserts the pacing electrode either via the transvenous route or by direct application to the epicardial surface during thoracotomy. The surgeon places the permanent pulse generator into a small tunnel burrowed within the subcutaneous tissue below the right clavicle or, less often, the left clavicle. The pulse generator is a small, hermetically sealed (to prevent ingress of body fluids) lithium battery.

THE USE OF PERMANENT PACEMAKERS

The client and family are taught about the purpose for the pacemaker and the experience of having a pacemaker inserted. Most permanent pacemakers are in-

CLIENT EDUCATION GUIDE

Permanent Pacemaker

The nurse should give the client the following instructions:

WOUND CARE

- Assess the wound daily; report any signs of inflammation (redness, tenderness, discharge) to the physician.
- Avoid wearing constrictive clothing (e.g., tight bra straps), which puts excessive pressure on the wound and the pulse generator.
- Avoid extensive "toying" with the pulse generator; this could cause pacemaker malfunction.

PACEMAKER MANAGEMENT

- Take your pulse daily, either radial or carotid (as demonstrated by the nurse).
- Notify the physician if your pulse is slower than the set rate; also report excessive palpitations, vertigo, or fainting.
- Avoid engaging in activity that can cause blunt trauma over the pulse generator; such activities would include playing football or firing a rifle with the butt end against the affected shoulder.
- Avoid areas with high voltage, magnetic force fields, or radiation; these can cause pacemaker malfunction. Things to avoid include large running motors (gas or electric), standing near high-tension wires, power plants, radio transmitters, large industrial magnets, and arc welding machines. Riding in a car is safe, but avoid bringing the pacemaker within 6 inches of the distributor coil of a running engine. Contact with such equipment can cause a sudden return of prepacemaker symptoms.
- Airport and other metal detectors may be triggered by the pacemaker's metal casing and the programming magnet. This should be mentioned to the security guards. (The metal detector itself will not harm the pacemaker.)
- Some stores have antitheft devices that may affect pacemaker function. If symptoms suddenly arise, move away from the area and notify the store clerk about your pacemaker.
- If radiation therapy has been prescribed to the area in which the pulse generator was implanted, a relocation of the pulse generator will be necessary.
- Carry a pacemaker identity card (along with programming information—the pacemaker manufacturer and emergency phone numbers) at all times; a special ALERT bracelet is also recommended.

ACTIVITY LEVELS

- Avoid vigorous movement of the arms and shoulders and lifting weights greater than 5 to 10 pounds for the first 6 weeks after surgery; this could increase risk of electrode dislodgement.
- Normal activities can be resumed in 6 weeks, including sexual activity.

MEDICATIONS

- Make sure that you understand the purpose, dose, schedule, and possible side effects of all prescribed medications; ask for written information sheets if these are available.

FOLLOW-UP CARE

- Understand the importance of regular physician or clinic visits for evaluation of pacemaker function and possible reprogramming; keep all scheduled appointments.
- Special telephone monitoring of your electrocardiogram may be done from time to time on an outpatient basis. This provides information regarding the pacemaker function. If this is to be done, make sure that you understand the procedure.

serted transvenously. A preoperative ECG is obtained, and a patent intravenous line is maintained. Prophylactic antibiotics may be given.

After the insertion, the nurse monitors vital signs and pacemaker function. Pain can usually be managed with oral analgesics if the transvenous approach was used. Initially the client is taught to avoid excessive extension or abduction of the arm on the operative side. The nurse performs passive range-of-motion exercises on the arm.

Paced and nonpaced ECGs are obtained. A magnet may be placed over the pulse generator, converting it to a fixed rate pacing mode, so that the client's intrinsic rhythm can be determined. The location of the pacemaker electrodes is determined by x-ray examination. The model and serial numbers of the pulse generator and leads are recorded along with the date of implantation and programmed functions of the initial implant.

The client and significant others are taught how to care for the pacemaker and precautions to follow (see the Client Education Guide: Permanent Pacemaker).

DEFIBRILLATING PACEMAKER CLIENTS

Because pacemakers are vulnerable to extraneous electromagnetic interference, newer models possess components to suppress input. These safety mechanisms may fail, however. Therefore, during defibrillation, certain precautions are taken:

- Use anteroposterior type paddles if available.
- Place anterior paddles at least 4 to 5 inches away from the pulse generator and leads.
- Use the lowest defibrillator current possible (following the standard for advanced cardiac life support).
- If a temporary pacing system is in use, disconnect the pacing lead from the pulse generator immediately before defibrillation and reconnect it after the shock.
- A pacemaker programmer-analyzer should be readily available to examine the pacing system for damage and erroneous reprogramming after defibrillation.
- Monitor for pacemaker malfunction for at least the next 24 hours.[35]

ELECTROCARDIOGRAM OF PACED BEATS

The ECG of a paced rhythm appears different from that of a normal sinus rhythm. A pacing artifact is seen. With atrial pacing, a P wave follows the artifact but may be hidden in some leads. Leads II and V_1 are best for deciding whether a P wave follows a pacer spike. The QRS complex appears normal with atrial pacing; the impulse travels through usual conduction systems.

The ECG with ventricular pacing shows an abnormal QRS complex, because the impulse begins in the ventricle.

The specially trained nurse assesses the ECG strip for pacer spikes followed by the expected appearance of a P wave or QRS complex. Spikes not followed by depolarization waves or paced beats that appear too early or too late may signal pacemaker failure.

PACEMAKER FAILURE

Pacemakers can develop malfunctions in the sensor or pulse generator:

- Failure to sense is the inability of the sensor to detect intrinsic beats, and the pacemaker sends out impulses too early (Fig. 24–15*A*).
- Failure to pace is a malfunction of the pulse generator. The ECG shows a lack of any impulse (Fig. 24–15*B*).
- Failure to capture is a disorder in the pacemaker electrodes; the impulse does not generate depolarization (Fig. 24–15*C*.

Clinical manifestations include syncope, bradycardia or tachycardia, and palpitations. The malfunctioning leads or pacemaker is replaced.

Cardiac Arrest and Cardiopulmonary Resuscitation

When cardiac or respiratory arrest occurs, prompt action is necessary to provide oxygen to the brain and heart until advanced cardiac life support (ACLS) can restore normal cardiac and respiratory function. All nurses need to be trained in CPR. (This is best accom-

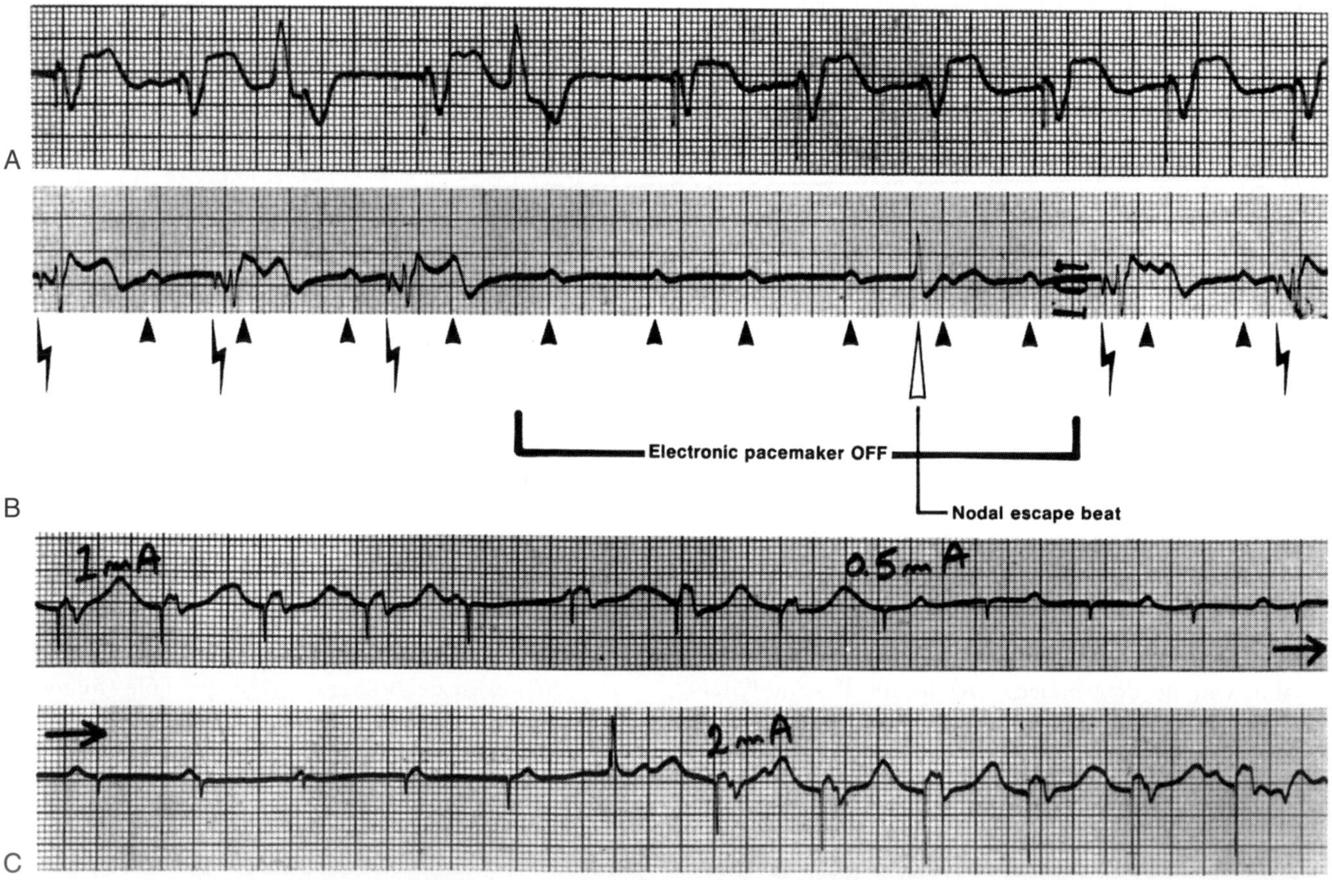

Figure 24–15
Pacemaker failures. *A*, Failure to sense. *B*, Failure to pace. *C*, Failure to capture. (From Phillips, R. E., & Feeney, M. K. [1990]. *The cardiac rhythms: A systematic approach to interpretation.* [3rd ed.]. Philadelphia: W. B. Saunders.)

plished through a CPR course offered by the American Heart Association or the American Red Cross.)

In cardiopulmonary arrest, the client's heart, circulation, and respiration suddenly cease.

Clinical manifestations of cardiopulmonary arrest are as follows:

- abrupt and complete unconsciousness (no response to tap or gentle shaking while asking, "Are you OK?")
- apnea or gasping (agonal) respirations
- absence of heart beat (no carotid, femoral, or radial pulsations) and blood pressure
- ECG reveals asystole or ventricular fibrillation
- development of pallor or cyanosis

DEFINITIVE THERAPY

Definitive therapy commences once a special resuscitation team has arrived to take over CPR. Typically, a nurse from the coronary care unit, the emergency room physician, a respiratory therapist, an intravenous nurse, and a pharmacist make up the core of the resuscitation team. In the community, this team may include emergency medical personnel in contact with the hospital emergency department.

The resuscitation team addresses the following questions:

- What is the underlying cause of the cardiac arrest, and can it be corrected?
- What type of arrest has occurred (cardiac, respiratory, or both)?
- What is the underlying heart rhythm?
- What intervention should be instituted?

The resuscitation team makes every effort to limit the number of times CPR must be interrupted to perform emergency procedures. Two team members must continue to administer CPR while some resuscitation team members do the following:

- Apply a cardiac monitor to the client and identify the rhythm.
- Record electrocardiac events that occur during resuscitation.
- Immediately administer defibrillation in the event of ventricular fibrillation or ventricular tachycardia.
- Quickly attend to the client's airway and oxygenation.
- Insert an oral (artificial) airway to maintain the tongue in a forward position.
- Administer 100 per cent oxygen.
- Insert an endotracheal tube as soon as possible to achieve maximal airway clearance and oxygenation.
- Suction the client as necessary to maintain a patent airway. Nasogastric suction can also facilitate gastric decompression if the stomach fills with air during artificial ventilation. A distended abdomen may compromise respirations.
- Start an intravenous line for administration of resuscitation medications. Large-bore catheters are preferable, because they allow more rapid infusion rates. Two or more lines help ensure access to the circulation and allow simultaneous administration of medications or solutions that are incompatible.
- Administer medications to (1) stimulate myocardial contraction, (2) suppress ventricular ectopy, (3) accelerate cardiac rate, and (4) correct metabolic acidosis. Table 24–10 lists the more commonly used medications.
- Prepare for transthoracic or transvenous pacing in the event of asystole, severe bradycardia, or complete heart block.

TABLE 24–10 Resuscitation Medications

MEDICATION	INDICATIONS
Oxygen	Hypoxemia
Intravenous fluids	Expansion of circulating blood volume
Morphine sulfate	Pain of acute myocardial infarction
Lidocaine	Ventricular ectopy, including ventricular tachycardia and fibrillation
Procainamide hydrochloride	Ventricular ectopy and ventricular tachycardia when lidocaine is contraindicated or has failed to suppress ventricular ectopy
Bretylium tosylate	Resistant ventricular tachycardia and ventricular fibrillation
Beta-adrenergic receptor blocking medications	Reduce rate of nonfatal infarction and recurrent ischemia after thrombolytic therapy
Atropine sulfate	Symptomatic sinus bradycardia
Isoproterenol hydrochloride	Bradycardia that is refractory to atropine and torsades de pointes
Verapamil/diltiazem	Re-entrant dysrhythmias that use atrioventricular nodal conduction
Adenosine	Re-entrant dysrhythmias
Magnesium	Dysrhythmias due to hypomagnesemia
Epinephrine hydrochloride	Increases myocardial and cerebral blood flow
Norepinephrine	Severe hypotension and low peripheral resistance
Dopamine hydrochloride	Severe hypotension with bradycardia
Dobutamine hydrochloride	Heart failure
Amrinone	Heart failure
Calcium	Hyperkalemia, hypocalcemia, or calcium channel block toxicity
Digitalis preparations	Atrial flutter, atrial fibrillation, or paroxysmal supraventricular tachycardias
Nitroglycerin	Heart failure or unstable angina
Sodium nitroprusside	Heart failure, hypertension, and angina
Sodium bicarbonate	Severe acid-base imbalance
Diuretics	Cerebral edema or acute pulmonary edema
Thrombolytic agents	Coronary artery occlusion

Data from Guidelines for cardiopulmonary resuscitation (CPR) and emergency cardiac care (ECC) (1992). *Journal of the American Medical Association, 268(16)*, 2205–2211. Copyright 1992, American Medical Association.

Certain activities, although not directly related to saving the client's life, can improve the efficiency of the resuscitative efforts. The team must perform the following ancillary measures as soon as possible:

- Document the resuscitation. The nurse or another team member must keep an accurate, ongoing record, documenting all procedures and medications given during the resuscitative effort. Most institutions use a flow sheet. This document should be kept as a permanent record of the event.
- Provide information. The client's record (if there is one) and the primary care giver, who either knows the client or has witnessed the precipitating event, should remain close by to provide information to the resuscitation team.
- Reduce environmental overcrowding. If appropriate, ask people to leave the room.
- Reassure individuals nearby. When possible, remove roommates from the area or pull curtains and have available health-care providers sit with that client. People in the immediate vicinity are usually aware of the gravity of the situation and will appreciate an honest, reassuring manner.
- Notify significant others of the critical nature of events if they are not present at the time of the emergency. Arrange to have a nurse meet them when they arrive and inform them of changes in the client's condition. The client's spiritual adviser may also be notified to render additional support.

FOLLOW-UP INTERVENTION

Diagnostic tests are often made during and after resuscitation to determine precipitating causes, evaluate the effectiveness of resuscitation, and detect complications. Tests commonly performed are (1) chest radiograph, (2) ECG, (3) hemodynamic monitoring, and (4) laboratory studies (including arterial blood gases, electrolytes, blood urea nitrogen, creatinine, blood glucose, and cardiac enzymes). Table 24–11 summarizes post-resuscitation complications.

Clients who survive cardiopulmonary arrest are admitted to a critical care unit, where they receive contin-

TABLE 24–11 POSTRESUSCITATION COMPLICATIONS

COMPLICATIONS	ETIOLOGY	CLINICAL MANIFESTATIONS
Trauma		
Fractured ribs and sternum	Improper chest compressions (increased risk in elderly and those with chronic lung disease)	Chest pain that increases with inspiration; asymmetric chest wall movement; crepitus noted over fracture site; "floating" sternum
Pneumothorax	Improper chest compressions; improper central venous line insertion	Chest pain; dyspnea, hypoxemia, cyanosis, decreased or absent breath sounds over affected area, tracheal deviation (tension pneumothorax); noted on chest film
Ruptured spleen	Improper chest compressions	Upper left quadrant pain, hypotension, failing hematocrit
Aspiration pneumonia	Vomiting by a client who is in a semiconscious state	Respiratory distress, hypoxemia, tracheal suctioning of gastric contents; noted on chest film
Anoxic encephalopathy	Prolonged cerebral hypoperfusion during time of unattended arrest or from poorly managed resuscitation	Prolonged coma; confusion; short-term memory lapses; behavioral changes
Renal failure	Prolonged hypoperfusion of kidneys causing acute tubular necrosis	Within 24 hours after resuscitation, urine output will fall below 30 mL/hr; elevated BUN (>20 mL/100 mL) and creatinine (>1.5 mg/100 mL)
Congestive heart failure	Overly vigorous use of sodium bicarbonate and intravenous fluids during resuscitation	Increased heart rate, increased respiratory rate; heart gallops; pulmonary crackles (rales), increased pulmonary artery wedge pressure; noted on chest film
Cardiac tamponade	Perforation of cardiac structures from intracardiac injections or transvenous/transthoracic pacemaker lead insertion	Dyspnea; distended neck veins; narrowing pulse pressure; decreased blood pressure, pulsus paradoxus >10 mm Hg
Skin burns	Repeated defibrillation or delivery of high voltages	Erythema and blistering of skin beneath site of defibrillator paddle placement
Oral, tracheal, and laryngeal damage	Improper or repeated endotracheal intubation causing breakage of teeth and soft tissue injury	Broken teeth, bloody mouth, respiratory distress, hoarseness, stridor
Cervical neck injury	Hyperextension of neck during attempts to open airway can result in cervical nerve trauma	Decreased sensory or motor movement below level of cervical injury

BUN, blood urea nitrogen.

uous cardiac monitoring and have vital signs taken every 15 minutes until stable. Post-resuscitation assessment provides important information regarding the effectiveness of the resuscitation. Common disorders include recurrent dysrhythmias, coma, other neurologic disorders, and renal failure.

After the client regains consciousness, profound anxiety often appears. The nurse should remember that clients need psychological support when they have undergone such a catastrophic physiologic event. Many clients have a very clear recall of the events surrounding the resuscitation, including the verbal communication that occurred. For this reason, members of the resuscitation team should be careful about what they say.

The nurse should take time to assess the client's coping mechanisms. Dismay at perceived betrayal by the body and fear of sudden death can bring on overdependency, withdrawal, and anger. The nurse should encourage expression of such feelings and concerns, not only by the client but by significant others who are equally stressed by the sudden, serious nature of the disorder. Clear explanations and clarification of misconceptions about what has happened help move the client forward to optimal physiologic and psychological recovery.

STUDY QUESTIONS

1. Which of the following factors is not a modifiable risk factor for coronary artery disease?
   A. Smoking
   B. Hyperlipidemia
   C. Diabetes mellitus
   D. Sedentary life-style

2. When caring for a client with a myocardial infarction, the nurse documents the following: blood pressure 90/60, heart rate 110, respiratory rate 25, jugular vein distention, inspiratory crackles, and urine output of 20 mL per hour for 2 hours. Based on this assessment data, the appropriate nursing intervention is to:
   A. Place the client in Sims position.
   B. Allow a rest period after lunch.
   C. Hold the client's dose of oral digoxin.
   D. Ambulate the client in the hall per cardiac rehabilitation protocols.

3. Which of the following pieces of information should be taught to a client who is discharged on sublingual nitroglycerin?
   A. Carry the pills next to the body at all times.
   B. Keep the pills in the original container.
   C. Call the doctor immediately after taking the nitroglycerin.
   D. Take the pill with water when angina occurs.

4. A client presents at the emergency department with chest pain of 45 minutes duration and radiating down the left arm. The pain is unrelieved by nitroglycerin. The client also is exhibiting palpitations, tachycardia, and diaphoresis. Which of the following is most consistent with the diagnosis of myocardial infarction?
   A. Angina radiating down the left arm, tachycardia
   B. Angina radiating down the left arm, tachycardia, palpitations
   C. Angina radiating down the left arm for 45 minutes, unrelieved by three nitroglycerin tablets
   D. Tachycardia, palpitations, diaphoresis

5. A client admitted to the hospital with a permanent ventricular pacemaker in place is showing signs and symptoms of congestive heart failure. The physician has scheduled the client for insertion of a new atrioventricular physiologic pacemaker. The client asks why this is necessary. The best response by the nurse is:
   A. "The physician thinks you need a modern pacemaker because yours is old-fashioned."
   B. "Your current pacemaker only paces the left ventricle and the new one will pace both the ventricle and the atrium. This is closer to the natural heart beat."
   C. "The new pacemaker will speed up when you exercise. This is more like the natural heart beat."
   D. "Pacemakers like yours malfunction more often and the doctor is being cautious."

6. A client is told she has ventricular hypertrophy and asks the nurse to explain what has happened to her heart. The best response by the nurse is:
   A. "Your heart has enlarged to meet the demands of your life-style."
   B. "Now that your heart is larger, it won't have to work so hard."
   C. "The walls of the heart chamber have thickened and your heart is working harder."
   D. "The term hypertrophy means that there is extra growth of tissue around the heart muscle."

7. Which one of the following medications reduces myocardial workload?
   A. Digitalis
   B. Furosemide
   C. Dopamine
   D. Dobutamine

8. Dysrhythmias are caused by:
   A. Disturbances in the conduction system of the heart.
   B. Changes in the fluid balance in the body.
   C. Decreased blood flow to the coronary arteries.
   D. Hereditary factors that influence the age when dysrhythmias occur.

CRITICAL THINKING EXERCISES

SCENARIO A

A 65-year-old active male client has a car accident following an episode of heart block with syncope. Following the insertion of a permanent pacemaker, the client is preparing for discharge. The client states that his children want him to sell his car since he can no longer drive.

Write discharge instructions pertaining to activity restrictions for the client and address the issue of driving.

SCENARIO B

A 60-year-old black male client is seen in the outpatient hypertension clinic. He gives a history of recent episodes of shortness of breath while mowing the lawn. This was accompanied by palpitations. The symptoms abated when he stopped. Medical history is significant for diabetes mellitus, hypertension (controlled), smoking, and hyperlipidemia.

What aspects of the client history are indicative of coronary artery disease? What actions should the nurse take during this clinic visit?

BIBLIOGRAPHY

1. ACC/AHA Task Force Report (1990). Guidelines for the early management of patients with acute myocardial infarction. *Journal of the American College of Cardiology, 16(2),* 249–292.
2. Allard, K. S. (1992). Current trends in defibrillation. *Med-Surg Nursing Quarterly, 1(1),* 27–43.
3. Allen, J. K. (1990). Physical and psychosocial outcomes after coronary artery bypass graft surgery: Review of the literature. *Heart and Lung, 19(1),* 49–54.
4. American Heart Association. *1994 Heart and stroke facts.* Dallas, TX: American Heart Association.
5. American Heart Association. *Heart and stroke facts: 1994 statistical supplement.* Dallas, TX: American Heart Association.
6. American Heart Association (1994). *Instructor's manual: Advanced cardiac life support.* Dallas, TX: American Heart Association.
7. Baas, L. S. (1992). Nursing responsibilities during CPR. *Med-Surg Nursing Quarterly, 1(1),* 1–26.
8. Becker, D. M., et al. (1989). Cholesterol: Interpreting the new guidelines. *American Journal of Nursing, 89(12),* 1621–1633.
9. Berry, S. L., & Schleicher, C. A. (1992). Adjusting the beat: What to teach about antiarrhythmics. *American Journal of Nursing, 92(6),* 28–33.
10. Biggers, V. T. (1992). Codes for a code. *American Journal of Nursing, 92(5),* 56–61.
11. Borek, M., et al. (1989). Angiotensin-converting enzyme inhibitors in heart failure. *Medical Clinics of North America, 73(2),* 315–338.
12. Boykoff, S. L. (1989). Strategies for sexual counseling of patients following a myocardial infarction. *Dimensions of Critical Care Nursing, 8(6),* 368–373.
13. Burke, M., & Walsh, M. (1992). *Gerontology nursing: Care of the frail elderly.* St. Louis: Mosby-Year Book.
14. Calhoun, D. A., & Oparil, S. (1990). Treatment of hypertensive crisis. *The New England Journal of Medicine, 323(17),* 1177–1183.
15. Canobbio, M. (1990). *Cardiovascular disorders.* St. Louis: Mosby-Year Book.
16. Chatterjee, K. (1989). Digitalis and non-ACE inhibitor vasodilators in heart failure. *Cardiology Clinics, 7(1),* 99–118.
17. Cimini, D. M. (1992). Indium-111 antimyosin antibody imaging. *Critical Care Nurse, 12(6),* 44–51.
18. Colucci, W. S. (1989). Positive inotropic/vasodilator agents. *Cardiology Clinics, 7(1),* 131–144.
19. Dimsdale, J. E. (1988). A perspective on type A behavior and coronary disease. *New England Journal of Medicine, 318(2),* 110–112.
20. Drew, B. J. (1992). Using cardiac leads: The right way. *Nursing 92, 22(5),* 50–54.
21. Dunn, F. G. (1990). Prevention of sudden cardiac death. *Cardiovascular Clinics, 20(3),* 95–109.
22. Dzau, V. J., & Creager, M. A. (1989). Progress in angiotensin-converting enzyme inhibition in heart failure. *Cardiology Clinics, 7(1),* 119–130.
23. Eysmann, S. B., & Douglas, P. S. (1992). Reperfusion and revascularization strategies for coronary artery disease in women. *Journal of the American Medical Association, 268(14),* 1903–1907.
24. Faxon, D. P. (1991). Percutaneous coronary angioplasty in stable and unstable angina. *Cardiology Clinics, 9(1),* 99–113.
25. Fleury, J. (1992). The application of motivational theory to cardiovascular risk reduction. *IMAGE: The Journal of Nursing Scholarship, 24(3),* 229–239.
26. Folta, A., & Metzger, B. L. (1989). Exercise and functional capacity after myocardial infarction. *Image, 21(4),* 215–219.
27. Gawlinski, A. (1989). Saving the cardiogenic shock patient. *Nursing 89, 19(12),* 34–41.
28. Gifford, R. W. (1991). Management of hypertensive crises. *Journal of the American Medical Association, 266(6),* 829–835.
29. Gleeson, B. (1991). Loosening the grip of anginal pain. *Nursing 91, 21(1),* 33–40.
30. Gortner, S. R., et al. (1992). Elders after CABG. *American Journal of Nursing, 92(8),* 44–49.
31. Grines, C. (1994). Treating myocardial infarction: Importance of early reperfusion. *The Lancet 344(8921),* 490–491.
32. Gruppo Italiano per lo Studio della Streptochinasi nell'Infarto Miocardico (GISSI) (1986 Feb 22). Effectiveness of intravenous thrombolytic treatment in acute myocardial infarction. *The Lancet, 1(8748),* 397–401.
33. Hayes, D. L. (1992). The next 5 years in cardiac pacemakers: A preview. *Mayo Clinic Proceedings, 67(4),* 379–384.

34. Henneman, E. A., & Henneman, P. L. (1989). Intricacies of blood pressure measurement: Reexamining the rituals. *Heart and Lung, 18(3),* 263–271.

35. Higgins, C. A. (1990). The AICD: A teaching plan for patients and families. *Critical Care Nurse, 10(6),* 69–74.

36. Hix, C. (1993). Magnesium in congestive heart failure, acute myocardial infarction and dysrhythmias. *Journal of Cardiovascular Nursing, 8(1),* 19–31.

37. Holmes, D. R., & Bresnahan, J. F. (1991). Interventional cardiology. *Cardiology Clinics, 9(1),* 115–134.

38. Hopson, J. R., et al. (1989). The role of energy and current in successful defibrillation and cardioversion. *Cardiology Board Review, 6(5),* 31–45.

39. Huang, S., et al. (1989). *Coronary care nursing* (2nd ed.). Philadelphia: W. B. Saunders.

40. Hudak, C., & Galb, B. (1994). *Critical care nursing: A holistic approach* (16th ed.). Philadelphia: J. B. Lippincott.

41. Jessup, M., et al. (1992). CHF in the elderly: Is it different? *Patient Care, 26(18),* 40–61.

42. Jessup, M., et al. (1992). Managing CHF in the older patient. *Patient Care, 26(18),* 65–88.

43. Johnson, J. L., & Morse, J. M. (1990). Regaining control: The process of adjustment after myocardial infarction. *Heart & Lung, 19(2),* 126–135.

44. Kannel, W. B. (1989). Epidemiological aspects of heart failure. *Cardiology Clinics, 7(1),* 1–9.

45. Kater, K. M., et al. (1992). Corralling atrial fibrillation with "maze" surgery. *American Journal of Nursing, 92(7),* 34–38.

46. King, K. B., et al. (1992). Patient perceptions of quality of life after coronary artery surgery: Was it worth it? *Research in Nursing & Health, 15(5),* 327–334

47. Lehne, R. (1994). *Pharmacology for nursing care* (2nd ed.) Philadelphia: W. B. Saunders.

48. Letterer, R. A., et al. (1992). Learning to live with congestive heart failure. *Nursing 92, 22(6),* 34–42.

49. Mailis, A., et al. (1989). Chest wall pain after aortocoronary bypass surgery using the internal mammary artery graft: A new pain syndrome? *Heart & Lung, 18(11),* 553–558.

50. Manson, J. E., et al. (1990). A prospective study of obesity and risk of coronary heart disease in women. *The New England Journal of Medicine, 322(13),* 882–889.

51. Meek, J. (1991). The dreaded defibrillator. *American Journal of Nursing, 91(5),* 32–33.

52. Miller, P., et al. (1990). Marital functioning after cardiac surgery. *Heart & Lung, 19(1),* 55–61.

53. Moss, A. J., & Benhorin, J. (1990). Prognosis and management after a first myocardial infarction. *The New England Journal of Medicine, 322(11),* 743–752.

54. Nara, A. R., et al. (1989). *Biophysical measurement series: Blood pressure.* Redmond, WA: SpaceLabs Inc.

55. Niemann, J. T. (1992). Cardiopulmonary resuscitation. *The New England Journal of Medicine, 327(15),* 1075–1080.

56. Packa, D. R. (1989). Quality of life of cardiac patients: A review. *The Journal of Cardiovascular Nursing, 3(2),* 1–11.

57. Pifarre, R., et al. (1989). Cardiac transplantation. *Cardiology Clinics, 7(1),* 183–194.

58. Rakel, R. E. (Ed.) (1995). *Conn's current therapy 1995.* Philadelphia: W. B. Saunders.

59. Sanders, M. J., et al. (1989). The use of inotropic agents in acute and chronic congestive heart failure. *Medical Clinics of North America, 73(2),* 283–314.

60. Serruys, P., et al. (1994). A comparison of balloon-expandable stent-implantation with balloon angioplasty in patients with coronary artery disease. *The New England Journal of Medicine. 331(8),* 489–495.

61. Shah, P. K. (1991). Pathophysiology of unstable angina. *Cardiology Clinics, 9(1),* 11–26.

62. Sica, D. A., & Gehr, T. (1989). Diuretics in congestive heart failure. *Cardiology Clinics, 7(1),* 87–97.

63. Sirles, A. T., & Selleck, C. S. (1989). Cardiac disease and the family: Impact, assessment, and implications. *The Journal of Cardiovascular Nursing, 3(2),* 23–32.

64. Sommers, M. S. (1992). The near-death experience after cardiopulmonary arrest. *Med-Surg Nursing Quarterly, 1(1),* 55–62.

65. Sommers, M. S. (1992). Preventing complications of CPR. *Med-Surg Nursing Quarterly, 1(1),* 44–54.

66. Spaniol, S., et al. (1994). Patients' reactions to angioplasty: Realistic or not? *American Journal of Critical Care. 3(5),* 368–373.

67. Standards and guidelines for cardiopulmonary resuscitation (CPR) and emergency cardiac care (ECC) (1992). *Journal of the American Medical Association, 268(16),* 2171–2302.

68. Stewart, S. L. (1992). Acute MI: A review of pathophysiology, treatment, and complications. *The Journal of Cardiovascular Nursing, 6(4),* 1–25.

69. Stokes, J. 3d (1990). Cardiovascular risk factors. *Cardiovascular Clinics, 20(3),* 3–20.

70. Stuart, J. V., & Sheehan, A. M. (1991). Permanent pacemakers: The nurse's role in patient education and follow-up care. *The Journal of Cardiovascular Nursing, 5(3),* 32–43.

71. Sytkowski, P. A., et al. (1990). Changes in risk factors and the decline in mortality from cardiovascular disease. *The New England Journal of Medicine, 322(23),* 1635–1640.

72. Waller, B. F. (1989). Atherosclerotic and nonatherosclerotic coronary artery factors in acute myocardial infarction. *Cardiovascular Clinics, 20(1),* 29–104.

73. Wolfe, C. L. (Ed.) (1989). Cardiac imaging: Diagnosis and assessment of cardiac disorders. *Cardiology Clinics, 7(3),* 483–737.

74. Wolfensperber Bradford, C. (1994). When a patient survives sudden cardiac death. *RN, 57(4),* 34–37.

75. Wright, S. M. (1990). Pathophysiology of congestive heart failure. *The Journal of Cardiovascular Nursing, 4(3),* 1–16.

76. Yusuf, S., et al. (1994). Effect of coronary artery graft surgery on survival: Overview of 10 year results of randomised trials by the Coronary Artery Bypass Graft Surgery Trialist Collaboration. *The Lancet, 344(8922),* 563–569.

77. Zipes, D. P. (1992). Management of cardiac arrhythmias: Pharmacological, electrical and surgical techniques. In Braunwald, E., (Ed.) *Heart disease* (4th ed.) Philadelphia: W. B. Saunders.

Chapter 25

Nursing Care of Clients with Cardiac Structure Disorders

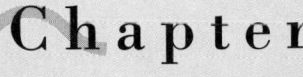

Learning Outcomes

After completing this chapter, the learner will be able to:

1. Assess the client for clinical manifestations of cardiac structure disorders.
2. Teach the client about the etiology, risk factors, basic pathophysiology, and clinical manifestations of cardiac structure disorders.
3. Explain the client's role in medical and surgical management of cardiac structure disorders.
4. Develop plans of care for the prevention of illness, management, and rehabilitation of clients with cardiac structure disorders.
5. Implement nursing interventions that optimize the quality of life for clients with cardiac structure disorders.
6. Evaluate planned client outcomes, using outcome criteria developed in the planning phase of care.

Bacteria and other microbes are found in abundance in our environment. The heart can become infected by these microbes, and an inflammatory response can be initiated. Involvement of the heart can be lethal during the acute stage or lead to structural damage that can impair heart function.

INFECTIVE ENDOCARDITIS

Endocarditis is an inflammatory process of the endocardium, especially the valves. This disorder was once lethal, but morbidity and mortality have been greatly reduced with the use of antibiotics and advanced diagnostic procedures.

Infective endocarditis can be defined or classified as subacute bacterial, acute bacterial, native valve, prosthetic valve, or nonbacterial thrombotic.

- Subacute bacterial endocarditis develops gradually over several weeks or months and is usually caused by organisms of low virulence, such as *Streptococcus viridans,* which has a limited ability to infect other tissues. It is most commonly diagnosed in clients with previously damaged hearts.
- Acute bacterial endocarditis develops over days or weeks with an erratic course and earlier development of complications. It is frequently caused by *Staphylococcus aureus,* which is capable of infecting other body tissues. Acute bacterial endocarditis most often affects people with normal hearts.[44]
- Native valve endocarditis is an infection of a previously normal or damaged valve.
- Prosthetic valve endocarditis is an infection of an artificial valve.
- Nonbacterial thrombotic endocarditis is caused by sterile thrombotic lesions (frequently aggregates of platelets), which may develop in clients with malignancies or other chronic diseases.

Incidence

Changes in the susceptible population are currently altering the classic picture of endocarditis. The proportion of acute cases is rising. Five of every 1000 patients admitted to a hospital have endocarditis. Overall mortality is 20 to 30 per cent and as high as 70 per cent in

CLINICAL MANIFESTATIONS

Subacute Bacterial Endocarditis

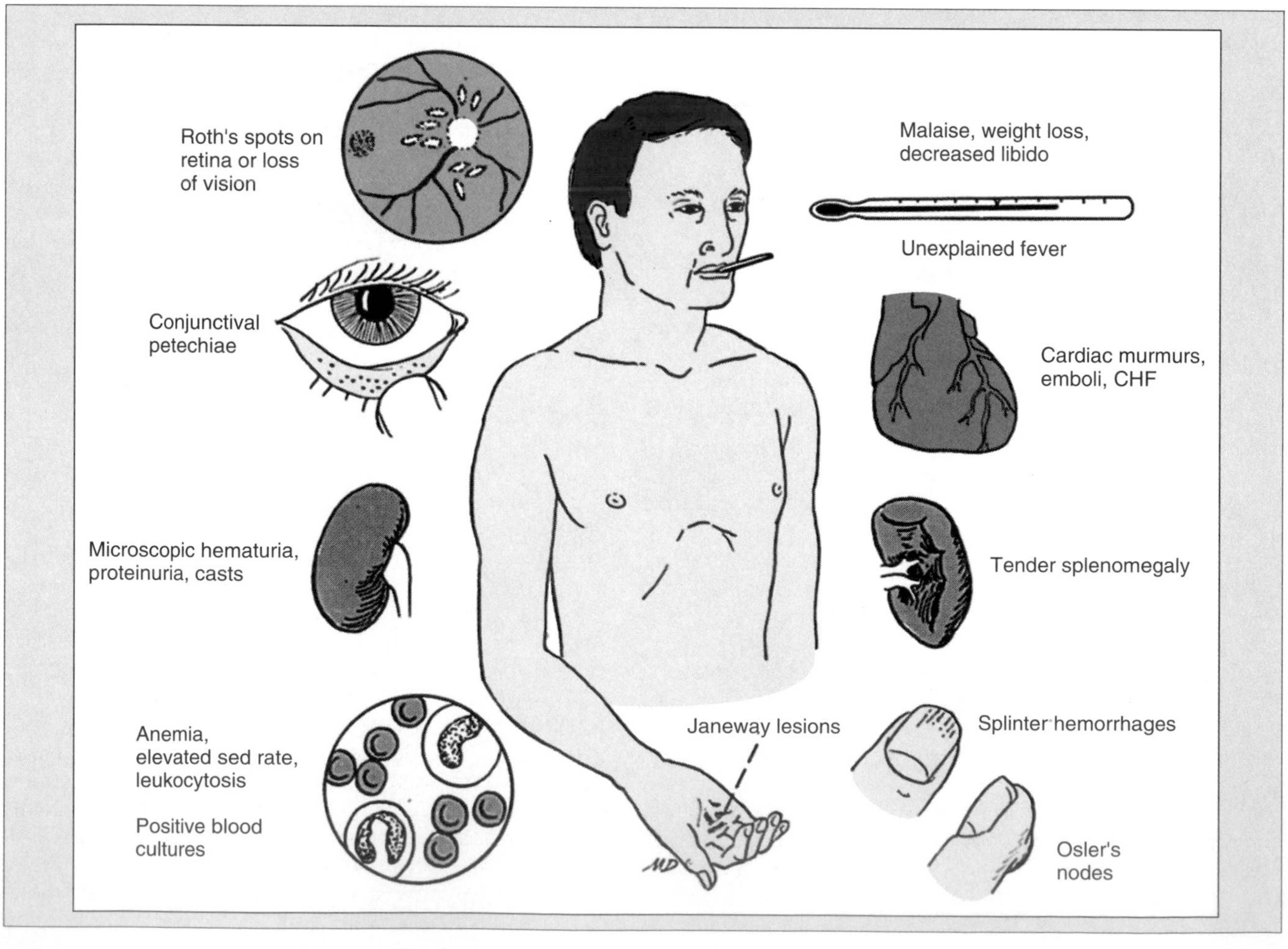

the elderly population.[36] Fewer patients are developing the classic physical signs of advanced endocarditis, such as Osler's nodes, finger clubbing, or Roth's spots (see Clinical Manifestations: Subacute Bacterial Endocarditis). The proportion of cases caused by streptococci has fallen slightly. The proportion of cases caused by gram-negative bacilli, fungi, and other unusual microbes is increasing.

The increase in the incidence of endocarditis caused by yeasts and fungi is attributable to the increased number of clients with valve prostheses, increased number of clients addicted to intravenous drugs, and increasing use of long-term antimicrobial and immunosuppression therapy.

A decreased incidence of rheumatic fever (a delayed response to a group A beta-hemolytic streptococcus that can lead to valve destruction) lowers the incidence of endocarditis, whereas the number of children surviving congenital heart disease raises the incidence of endocarditis. The growing elderly population also has contributed to the increased incidence of endocarditis.

Etiology

Circulating microorganisms in the bloodstream attach to the endocardial surface and multiply. Usually the multiplication of these organisms requires a rough or abnormal endocardium. Intravenous drug abusers may be injecting particulate matter into the bloodstream, which damages the previously normal endocardium and allows the organisms to adhere, thereby initiating acute bacterial endocarditis.

Defective heart valves that cause changes in blood flow and pressures encourage the proliferation of vegetation. Surgical replacement of damaged valves with prosthetic valves also increases the risk of endocarditis.

Risk Factors

Most clients who develop endocarditis have a pre-existing heart condition, but some develop endocarditis in the absence of known heart disease. Acquired valvular disease (especially mitral valve prolapse) and heart valve prostheses can lead to infective endocarditis. In some cases, endocarditis follows an invasive procedure, such as minor surgery, dental procedures, or insertion of renal shunts, urinary catheters, or long-term indwelling catheters (for dialysis, hemodynamic monitoring, or hyperalimentation). Factors that place clients at high risk are listed in Box 25–1.

Secondary prevention in high-risk clients includes the use of prophylactic antibiotics in an attempt to prevent bacterial endocarditis. Bacteremias frequently occur during dental or surgical procedures. Clients at risk (those with a previous case of endocarditis and those with congenital heart defects or prosthetic valves) should follow a specific antibiotic regimen before certain dental or surgical procedures. Tertiary prevention (the reduction of complications) is discussed in the text.

BOX 25–1

Factors That Place Clients at High Risk for Infective Endocarditis

- Congenital heart disease
- Rheumatic heart disease
- Degenerative heart disease
- Mitral valve prolapse
- Cardiac structural and valve lesions
- Heart valve replacement
- Cardiac surgery
- Chronic debilitating disease
- Intravenous drug abuse
- Immunosuppression related to cancer
- Collagen vascular disease
- Hepatitis
- Burn injury
- Diabetes mellitus
- Radiation therapy
- Prolonged drug therapy (antibiotic, cytotoxic, or steroid medications)
- Invasive procedures

Adapted from Guzzetta, C., & Dossey, B (1984). *Cardiovascular nursing*. St. Louis: C. V. Mosby.

Pathophysiology

Microorganisms are able to enter the bloodstream in many ways. Once the colonization process begins on the endothelium, replication occurs, and bacterial colonies form within layers of platelets and fibrin. As the colonies become entangled within the tight layers of fibrin and platelets, they become less and less vulnerable to the body's defense mechanisms and form friable lesions called infective vegetations. It is not uncommon for these vegetations to form thromboses and to then travel to other organs, forming abscesses (Fig. 25–1).

The vegetative lesions can severely damage heart valves by perforating and deforming the valve leaflets. Vegetative lesions on the valve leaflets turn into scar tissue that deforms the shape of the valve. If the valve leaflets do not approximate, then valvular insufficiency occurs. If the leaflet edges fuse, then valvular stenosis develops. Although all four valves are at risk, the mitral and aortic valves are most often affected. Intravenous drug abusers are predisposed to tricuspid valve destruction.[47]

Extensions of the bacterial colonies may invade the aorta or pericardium. The amount of damage depends on the type and virulence of organisms causing the infection.

There are many possible complications. Congestive heart failure may develop because of structural valvular damage. Arterial emboli can occur from the vegetations. Systemic embolization occurs in 30 per cent of clients with left-sided infective endocarditis (Fig. 25–2). Common infarction sites are the kidney, spleen, and brain. Pulmonary embolus is associated with right-sided infective endocarditis. Emboli can also travel to the brain

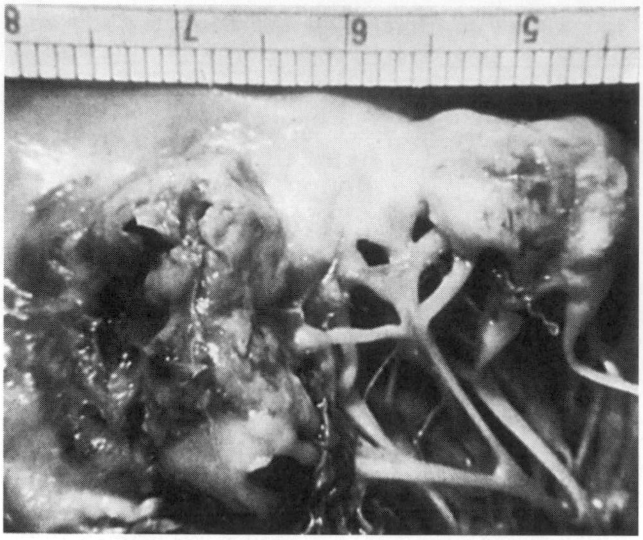

Figure 25–1
Infective endocarditis can lead to vegetation of the heart valve. This client had extensive vegetation of the mitral valve leaflets. (From Braunwald, E. [1992]. *Heart disease: A textbook of cardiovascular medicine* [4th ed.]. Philadelphia: W. B. Saunders.)

and produce a myriad of symptoms. Occasionally, a client will develop renal disease in the form of immune complex glomerulonephritis. Renal function will usually return to normal after the infection has been controlled.

Clinical Manifestations

The clinical presentation of infective endocarditis varies among the different types of the disorder, depending on the

- infecting organism,
- presence of pre-existing heart disease, and
- source of infection.[43]

Clients with subacute bacterial endocarditis often feel as if they have the flu. In those with acute bacterial endocarditis, clinical manifestations occur more quickly and are more severe. Clients appear very ill; fever, rigors, and prostration are commonly so severe that clients seek hospitalization within a few days.

In clients with valve damage, a heart murmur is auscultated. Symptoms of cardiac failure may develop suddenly in either acute or subacute endocarditis (see discussion of congestive heart failure). Mechanical complications include perforation of a valve leaflet, rupture of one of the chordae tendineae, or development of a functional stenosis from obstruction of blood flow by a large vegetative lesion. Myocardial infarction may develop as a result of coronary artery embolism.[8]

Unusual physical examination findings once attributed to embolism may in fact be of immunologic origin.[35] These include splinter hemorrhages, Osler's nodes, Janeway lesions, finger clubbing, ocular changes, and

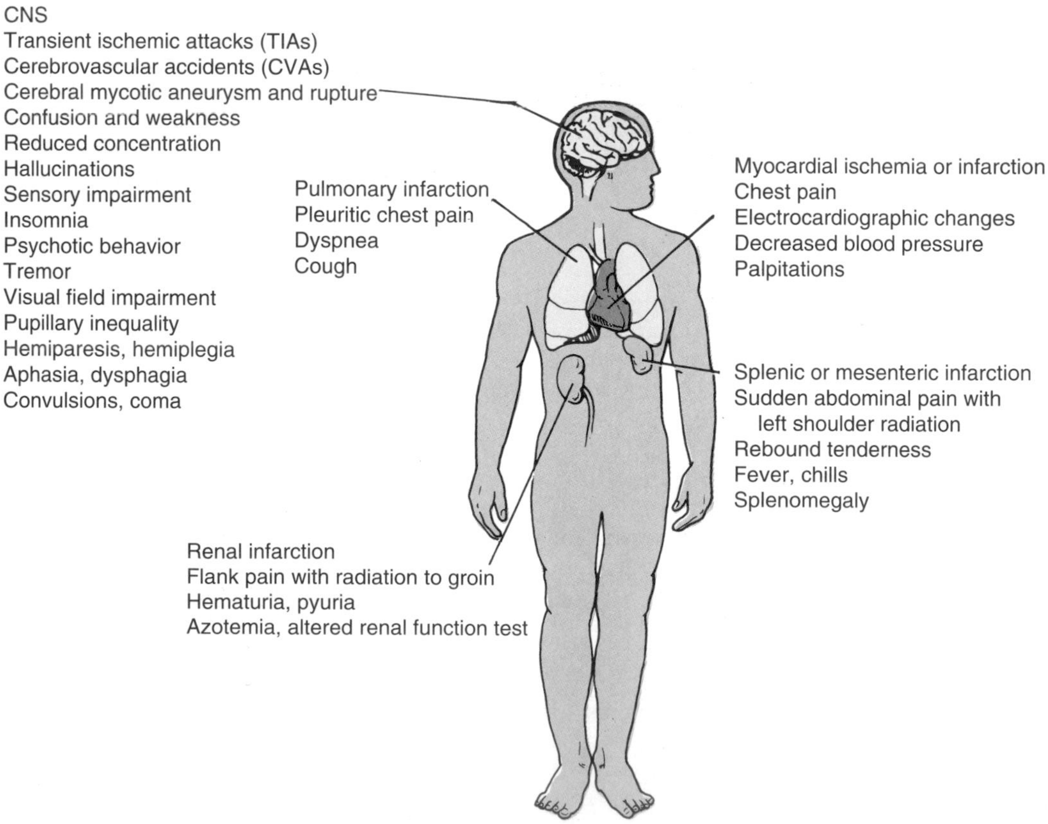

Figure 25–2
Locations and clinical manifestations of emboli of infective endocarditis. (Data from Guzzetta, C., & Dossey, B. [1984]. *Cardiovascular nursing*. St.Louis: C. V. Mosby.)

splenomegaly (see Clinical Manifestations: Subacute Bacterial Endocarditis).

Splinter hemorrhages are characterized by linear subungual hemorrhages appearing like tiny splinters under the nail. Osler's nodes are painful, erythematous, pea-sized nodules in the skin of the extremities, usually on the fingertips. Janeway lesions appear as flat, small, nontender red spots on the palms and soles.

Finger clubbing is found less frequently now but is common in long-standing infective endocarditis. The pathogenesis remains unclear.

Possible ocular signs include

- conjunctival petechiae—small, bright red hemorrhages easily seen when the upper and lower eyelids are everted
- Roth's spots, seen on funduscopic examination as a white or yellow center surrounded by a bright red, irregular halo
- vision loss, which can occur during the course of endocarditis from embolization to the brain or to the retinal artery.

DIAGNOSTIC ASSESSMENT

Diagnosis is made on the basis of the clinical signs and symptoms and laboratory findings. A series of three to six blood cultures obtained over 1 to 4 days is the most important diagnostic test. A positive throat culture for *streptococcus* associated with fever, rash, and elevated erythrocyte sedimentation rate are suggestive of rheumatic fever. Blood cultures should be obtained for all clients who have a fever and heart murmur.

Electrocardiograms (ECGs) should be taken to identify dysrhythmias or concurrent heart ischemia. An echocardiogram is taken to identify valve damage and vegetative lesions. Because the valvular structures are not easily identified, a transesophageal echocardiogram gives a higher quality picture of heart structures and may be useful in the diagnosis of endocarditis. A negative echocardiogram does not rule out endocarditis. Chest radiography is useful for determining early congestive heart failure.

Medical Management

The chief aims of management are to identify and eradicate the infecting organism and to treat complications. Antimicrobial therapy has changed infective endocarditis from a disease that was almost always fatal to one that is rarely fatal. The choice of antibiotic depends on the organism involved. Penicillin plus streptomycin is commonly used. Therapy is usually continued intravenously for 4 to 6 weeks. It is usually begun in the hospital and continued at home with extensive discharge planning and education.

Congestive heart failure is treated with digoxin and diuretics. Anti-inflammatory agents, such as salicylates and corticosteroids, also may be prescribed. Occasionally, the client needs heart valve replacement for reversal of newly developed congestive heart failure.

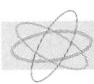

To prevent recurrence, long-term (3 to 5 years) antibiotic therapy may be prescribed, along with lifelong antibiotic prophylaxis (see Client Education Guide: Infective Endocarditis).

Nursing Management

Assessment

In infective endocarditis, nursing assessment focuses on gathering data about the client's

- clinical manifestations
- risk factors
- hemodynamic stability (particularly the presence of a new heart murmur and embolic complications)
- level of comfort

CLIENT EDUCATION GUIDE

Infective Endocarditis

The nurse should plan to begin discharge teaching well in advance of the anticipated discharge date. Teaching should include the following:

- The cause of infective endocarditis.
- Self-administration of intravenous antibiotics with the help of a significant other.
- The purpose of long-term antibiotic administration and the importance of completing the full course of therapy.
- An activity program that will allow a gradual resumption of the client's former lifestyle. Clinicians usually recommend about a month of convalescence at home before a full schedule is resumed.
- Compliance with life-long antibiotic prophylaxis when dental or surgical procedures become necessary, and the need to inform dentists and physicians of the client's endocarditis.
- The importance of careful oral hygiene to help prevent bacteremia and further endocarditis. Suggest daily flossing and use of a soft toothbrush. The client's dentist should be consulted before water-jet devices are used, because they may cause gum bleeding.
- The importance of ongoing assessment to determine the efficacy of treatment.
- Self-monitoring for the manifestations of endocarditis. The client should monitor temperature daily for a month and document it, and should report fever, chills, malaise, anorexia, weight loss, and increased fatigue to the physician.

- coping ability
- support from significant others, support systems
- potential for self-care

Nursing Diagnosis, Planning, and Implementation

Nursing Diagnosis: Activity Intolerance R/T reduced cardiac reserve and enforced bedrest.

Planning: Expected Outcomes. The client will demonstrate progression toward an optimal level of physical activity tolerance, based on underlying cardiovascular status and psychosocial readiness, as evidenced by ability to pace activity without chest pain or ECG changes while heart rate remains under 90 beats per minute, to verbalize decreased fatigue, and to express acceptance of any imposed activity restrictions.

Implementation. Bedrest is important in the acute phase because it reduces myocardial oxygen demand. Bedrest usually continues until the following criteria are met:

- Temperature remains normal without the use of salicylates.
- Resting pulse rate remains under 100.
- ECG tracing is stable.
- Erythrocyte sedimentation rate returns to normal.
- Pericardial friction rub is absent.

The nurse should encourage progressive increase in activity and assess the client's stamina and response to exercise. Vital signs are measured before and after exercise, and then again after 3 to 5 minutes of rest. The client should decrease or discontinue activity if chest pain, vertigo, dyspnea, confusion, decreased blood pressure, or irregular pulse is present. The duration of activity restriction depends on the extent of permanent heart damage. Restrictions may be permanent in severe cases.

Nursing Diagnosis: Nutrition, Altered: Less than Body Requirements R/T fever and infection associated with endocarditis.

Planning: Expected Outcomes. The client will maintain or restore adequate nutritional balance, as evidenced by attainment of ideal weight, no further weight loss, normal serum albumin level, and a positive nitrogen balance.

Implementation. A high-protein, high-carbohydrate diet helps maintain adequate nutrition in the presence of fever and infection. Hypermetabolic states (fever and infection) can induce a catabolic state, which delays healing. Vitamin and mineral supplements may also benefit the client. Oral hygiene every 4 hours, small attractive meal servings, and foods that are not overly rich, sweet, or greasy promote a good appetite. Adequate fluid intake prevents dehydration due to fever. If the client develops congestive heart failure, sodium and fluids must be restricted. Daily weights can serve as an indication of fluid status and effectiveness of nursing interventions.

Nursing Diagnosis: Pain R/T fever and malaise.

Planning: Expected Outcomes. The client will exhibit optimum comfort, as evidenced by reports of restful sleep, demonstration of behavior associated with comfort and relaxation, decreased use of analgesia, and reports of reduced discomfort after comfort measures.

Implementation. The nurse administers antibiotics intravenously as prescribed. Antibiotics will relieve most discomfort within a few days. Fever can be treated with rest, cooling measures, forced fluids, and sometimes salicylates. The nurse should encourage the client to rest mentally and physically.

Nursing Diagnosis: Decreased Cardiac Output R/T cardiac valve dysfunction.

Planning: Expected Outcomes. The client will exhibit restoration and maintenance of hemodynamic status, as evidenced by stable blood pressure and pulse; adequate urine output (>30 mL/hr); no new heart murmur development; clear lung fields with no reports or evidence of dyspnea; and increased activity tolerance, alertness, and orientation.

Implementation. The nurse auscultates for heart murmurs every 8 hours and assesses for rapid pulse, easy fatigability, dyspnea, restlessness, signs of heart failure, and embolic manifestations. The nurse documents these manifestations if they occur and reports them to the physician.

When the client's condition improves, the nurse plans and implements a progressive activity schedule (see under Nursing Diagnosis: Activity Intolerance).

Evaluation

The degree of goal attainment is evaluated. Revisions in the plan of care may be required.

Posthospital Care

The client is discharged when he or she is alert, cooperative, and hemodynamically stable. The full course of intravenous antibiotic therapy will be continued at home. Before discharge, the client or significant other must demonstrate the knowledge and technique required for antibiotic administration. Home health-care nurses often monitor the client's progress. (See Client Education Guide: Infective Endocarditis.)

Modification of Plan of Care for the Elderly

Elderly persons are susceptible to endocarditis because of age-related degenerative changes in the heart valves. In the elderly, the source of infection is often gastrointestinal, genitourinary, or integumentary. The aortic valve is most often affected.

Diagnosis in the elderly client may be difficult because of vague symptoms or concurrent pathology. Subacute bacterial endocarditis should be suspected in an elderly client who presents with:

- fever of unknown origin and a new murmur
- embolism to any system without previous symptoms
- unexplained renal failure and heart murmur[35]

Diagnosis is confirmed with blood cultures and echocardiography. Treatment typically comprises long-term intravenous antibiotic therapy (usually penicillin) plus an aminoglycoside. Age-related renal changes necessitate careful monitoring of peak and trough blood levels of the prescribed antibiotic.

MYOCARDITIS

An acute or chronic inflammation of the myocardial wall, myocarditis affects clients of all ages. An immune-deficient client is at greater risk for myocarditis. Frequently, the inflammation is not limited to the myocardium itself but extends to the pericardium, resulting in associated pericarditis. The incidence of myocarditis is impossible to ascertain; it varies with the age of clients and various etiologic agents.

In the United States, most cases of myocarditis are caused by viral infections. Viruses associated with this disorder include coxsackieviruses A and B, mumps, influenza groups A and B, rubella, rubeola, adenoviruses, echoviruses, variola, cytomegalovirus, and Epstein-Barr virus.[31] Other causes of myocarditis include bacterial infections, hypersensitive immune reactions, toxins and chemicals, drugs, radiation exposure, and parasitic infections.

Myocardial damage from acute myocarditis typically results from the direct invasion by or the toxic effects of the microorganism in cardiac myocytes. Actual virus is only rarely isolated from human hearts in acute myocarditis. This does not prevent the infection from becoming subacute or chronic or from causing dilated cardiomyopathy.[59] Myocarditis usually involves both ventricles.

Clinical manifestations of myocarditis vary widely. The client may be asymptomatic or may report fatigue, dyspnea, palpitations, and chest pain. The health history may reveal a recent upper respiratory infection, a viral pharyngitis, or tonsillitis. The client often experiences chest pain as a mild continuous pressure or soreness in the chest. Thus, the chest pain of myocarditis can be distinguished from the effort-induced pain of angina pectoris. Tachycardia, if present, may be disproportionate to the degree of fever, exertion, or illness. Dysrhythmias can also occur, sometimes producing decreased cardiac output or fatal circulatory collapse. There may be a pericardial friction rub if the client has pericarditis.

In most cases, myocarditis is self-limiting and uncomplicated. If myocardial involvement becomes extensive or prolonged, myofibril degeneration can impair ventricular contractility, resulting in increased ventricular diastolic pressure and decreased stroke volume. This can lead to heart failure with pulmonary congestion, dyspnea, neck vein distention, peripheral edema, and cardiomegaly. Recurrent myocarditis can produce cardiomyopathy. A ruptured myocardial aneurysm may cause sudden death.

Chest x-ray may show an enlarged cardiac silhouette because of ventricular enlargement or pericardial effusion. Routine blood tests may reveal moderate leukocytosis and elevated cardiac enzymes. Echocardiography is helpful in determining heart chamber size and ventricular functioning. Gallium scan shows regional wall abnormalities, dilated ventricles, and hypokinesis of the left ventricle. In addition to tachycardia, ECG may show a bundle branch block or complete atrioventricular heart block.

Medical Management

Medical management begins with specific therapy for the underlying infection. Bed rest is suggested to decrease cardiac work. Dysrhythmias are treated appropriately. Supplemental oxygen may be prescribed for clients with low cardiac output or dysrhythmias. Immunosuppressive therapy is currently being investigated; initial reports are favorable in the treatment of myocarditis.[59] Antipyretic agents are helpful for the fever and the hemodynamic effects of fever that increase myocardial work. Clients who remain at home may use telemetry (Holter) monitoring of the heart.

The outlook for clients with myocarditis is generally good. Most patients recover rapidly; however, some have recurrent or chronic myocarditis, and some become very ill and die.

Nursing Management

Nursing management for clients with myocarditis is essentially the same as that for clients with infective endocarditis. The reader is advised to review those sections in this chapter.

Client teaching begins when acute symptoms have subsided and the client has demonstrated physical and emotional readiness. (See Client Education Guide: Myocarditis.)

Nursing Diagnosis, Planning, and Implementation

Nursing Diagnosis: Anxiety R/T sudden acute illness and potential for lethal arrhythmias.

CLIENT EDUCATION GUIDE

Myocarditis

Discharge teaching should include the following:

- Report sudden changes in heart rate, rhythm, or palpitations.
- Continue self-monitoring after the infectious process resolves:
  Taking own pulse
  Avoiding exposure to risks
  Following correct medication regime
- Keep all scheduled follow-up appointments.
- Encourage family members to take cardiopulmonary resuscitation training.

Planning: Expected Outcomes. The client will describe personal anxiety and coping patterns, report improved psychological comfort, and use effective coping mechanisms, as evidenced by reports of no insomnia, effective ability to solve problems, decreased somatic complaints, and decreased agitation.

Implementation. The nurse determines with the client and significant others the specific focus of anxiety and clarifies any misconceptions that arise. The nurse should speak slowly and calmly and focus on the present situation, giving feedback about current reality. He or she should encourage the use of relaxation techniques and schedule activities around undisturbed sleep. The nurse should encourage cardiopulmonary resuscitation training for significant others.

PERICARDITIS

Acute pericarditis is a syndrome caused by inflammation of the parietal and visceral pericardium. This inflammatory process may develop either as a primary condition or secondary to a number of diseases and circumstances (Box 25–2).

Pericarditis may be either acute or chronic (recurring). The chronic pericarditis is usually called constrictive pericarditis. Chronic constrictive pericarditis is present when a fibrotic, thickened, and adherent pericardium restricts diastolic filling of the heart.[41] This eventually results in cardiac failure.

Acute pericarditis may be either dry (fibrinous) or exudative. The exudate present in acute pericarditis may be serous, purulent, or hemorrhagic. When exudate accumulates in the pericardial sac, cardiac tamponade develops. Without prompt treatment, shock and death can result from decreased cardiac output.

In dry pericarditis, delicate adhesions form within the pericardial space along with serous fibrin deposition, hemorrhage, and calcification. Adhesions may eventually obliterate the pericardial sac. Inflammation of the pericardium frequently penetrates the myocardium to some degree, which produces myopericarditis.

The cardinal signs and symptoms of acute pericarditis are precordial pain, pericardial friction rub, and S-T segment elevation on the ECG. The nature of the precordial pain varies with the client; it may mimic myocardial infarction or pleurisy. The pain is exacerbated by respiration and trunk rotation but usually does not radiate to the arms. Sitting up may relieve the pain.

Pericardial friction rub is a classic sign of acute pericarditis. The rub is produced by inflamed, roughened pericardial layers that create friction as their surfaces rub together during heart movement. Auscultation over the precordium reveals a scratchy, leathery, or creaky sound that is heard anywhere over the precordium but most frequently at the left mid to lower sternal border. The rub is best heard with the diaphragm of the stethoscope and with the client holding his or her breath. In some clients, it is best heard with the client sitting up. Pericardial friction rubs vary with intensity from hour to hour and from day to day.

In addition to S-T segment elevation, the ECG may show decreased amplitude and T wave changes.[31] Other clinical findings may include fever, chills, malaise, nausea, anorexia, weight loss, joint pain, and anxiety. Dyspnea and chest pain can potentiate anxiety. The client's increased heart rate usually corresponds to the degree of his or her fever and anxiety.

Laboratory studies show an elevated erythrocyte sedimentation rate and possibly an elevated white blood cell count. Cardiac enzymes are usually normal but may be elevated.

BOX 25–2

Causes of Pericarditis

INFECTIONS

- Viral: coxsackie, influenza
- Bacterial: tuberculosis, staphylococcus, streptococcus, meningococcus, pneumococcus
- Parasitic
- Fungal

MYOCARDIAL INJURY

- Myocardial infarction (Dressler's syndrome)
- Cardiac trauma: blunt or penetrating
- After cardiac surgery

HYPERSENSITIVITY

- Collagen diseases: rheumatic fever, scleroderma, systemic lupus erythematosus, rheumatoid arthritis
- Drug reaction: procainamide, methysergide, hydralazine
- Radiation therapy
- Cobalt therapy

METABOLIC DISORDERS

- Uremia
- Myxedema
- Chronic anemia

NEOPLASM: LYMPHOMA

AORTIC DISSECTION

Management

When acute pericarditis is of known etiology, treatment of the underlying cause is indicated. If no causal agent is known, symptomatic intervention for acute dry pericarditis will be provided. Aspirin is the drug of choice for relieving pain and fever. Nonsteroidal anti-inflammatory agents or colchicine may be prescribed. Severe pain may require morphine sulfate.

The focus of nursing care for a client with pericarditis is the same as that described for the other inflammatory cardiac diseases discussed in this chapter. Nursing assessment of the client with pericarditis also includes scrutiny for signs of pericardial tamponade (pulsus paradoxus, distended neck veins). Vigilant assessment is necessary, as is reassurance concerning the disorder's temporary nature.

ACUTE PERICARDITIS WITH EFFUSION

Acute pericarditis with effusion results when fluid accumulates within the pericardial sac. Rapid or excessive fluid accumulation may compress the heart and reduce ventricular filling and cardiac output. When fluid accumulates slowly, the fibrous pericardium is better able to stretch and accommodate its presence. From 1 to 2 liters of fluid can be tolerated without an increase in intrapericardial pressure if accumulation is slow. However, the normal unstretched pericardial sac can accommodate the rapid addition of only 80 to 200 mL of fluid without a resultant decrease in cardiac output.

Pericardial effusion may be asymptomatic. If dry pericarditis precedes the condition, the friction rub will often disappear. Fever may develop. Heart sounds may be muffled because the pericardial fluid further separates the stethoscope and the heart chambers.

Pulsus paradoxus can be present. If the client has normal breathing and a systolic difference of greater than 10 mm Hg, evaluation for cardiac compression and possibly cardiac tamponade should be done.[16]

Echocardiography is the most accurate technique for evaluating pericardial effusion. The test is sensitive enough to detect as little as 20 mL of pericardial fluid.[31, 41] Pericardiocentesis is not indicated unless there is evidence of cardiac compression caused by cardiac tamponade[31] (see the next section).

Management

Care of the client with pericardial effusion is similar to that of the client with dry pericarditis. Bed rest, analgesia, and proper positioning can help alleviate symptoms. Psychological support is very important for client and significant others.

CARDIAC TAMPONADE

A life-threatening complication, cardiac tamponade exists when accumulated fluid in the pericardial cavity restricts diastolic ventricular filling. This fluid can be blood, pus, or air in the pericardial sac that accumulates fast enough and in sufficient quantity to compress the heart and restrict blood flow in and out of the ventricles. **This situation is a cardiac emergency.** Large or rapidly accumulating effusions raise the intrapericardial pressure to a point at which venous blood cannot flow into the heart, which decreases ventricular filling. As a result, venous pressure rises, and cardiac output and arterial blood pressure fall.

BOX 25-3

Pathophysiologic Changes and Clinical Manifestations in Cardiac Tamponade

IMPAIRED RIGHT-SIDED CARDIAC FILLING

- Elevated venous pressure (increased central venous pressure)
- Distended neck veins
- Kussmaul's sign (distended neck veins on inspiration)

DISTENDED PERICARDIAL SAC

- Muffled heart sounds
- Pulsus paradoxus
- Decreased friction rub
- Decreased QRS voltage and electrical alternans
- Enlarged cardiac contour on chest film

REDUCED CARDIAC OUTPUT

- Hypotension
- Narrowed pulse pressure
- Tachycardia
- Dyspnea
- Restlessness, anxiety

A narrowing pulse pressure signals cardiac tamponade. The heart attempts to compensate by beating rapidly (tachycardia). Tachycardia cannot sustain the cardiac output for very long. Prompt intervention is necessary to prevent shock and death.

Pathophysiologic changes and clinical manifestations of cardiac tamponade are listed in Box 25–3. The client may be comfortable and quiet one minute and then very restless with a feeling of impending doom the next minute. Clients may panic when fluid accumulates rapidly. Slowly developing tamponade resembles congestive heart failure.

Management

Cardiac tamponade requires immediate intervention. The emergency intervention of choice is pericardiocentesis, which involves aspirating the fluid or air from the pericardial sac (Fig. 25–3). This procedure relieves the pressure on the heart, thereby improving cardiac function and perhaps saving the client's life.

CHRONIC CONSTRICTIVE PERICARDITIS

This chronic inflammatory condition usually begins with an initial episode of acute pericarditis characterized by fibrin deposition, often with pericardial effusion. In most cases, the visceral and parietal layers become completely fused. Constrictive pericarditis is usually symmetric scarring that causes uniform con-

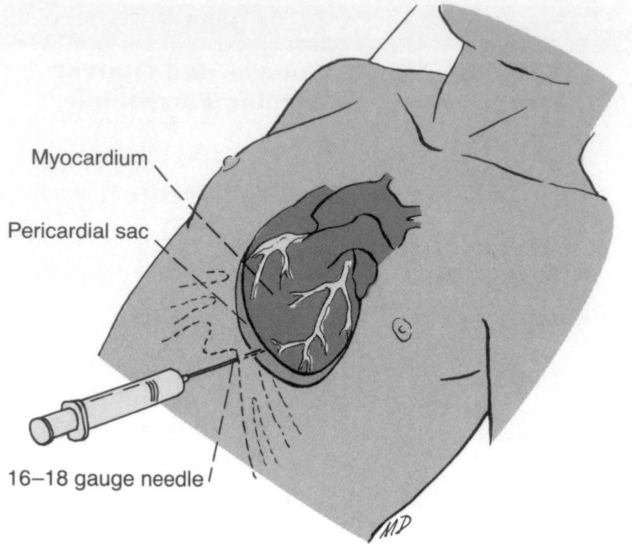

Figure 25–3
Subxiphoid approach to pericardiocentesis.

striction of all heart chambers. The heavily fibrosed pericardium restricts diastolic filling in all chambers and decreases cardiac output. Cardiac failure eventually results from the slow compression of the chambers.

Clinical manifestations begin with right ventricular failure and progress to decreased cardiac output as the left ventricle fails. This is manifested by leg edema, ascites, distended neck veins, dyspnea, fatigue on exertion, diminished pulse pressure, and delayed capillary refill.

Management

Constrictive pericarditis is a progressive disease without spontaneous reversal of symptoms. A minority of clients survive for many years with minor symptoms. Most clients become progressively more disabled over time. Treatment is both surgical and medical. Medical treatment includes digitalis and diuretic therapy and sodium restriction to relieve symptoms of ventricular failure. Surgical intervention involves the excision of the damaged pericardium (pericardiectomy), ideally performed early in the course of the disease.[31, 51]

Structural Abnormalities of the Heart

Structural abnormalities of the heart may be either congenital or acquired. Congenital heart disorders result from faulty development of the heart's structures in utero. Acquired defects arise from disease processes that develop after birth. Congenital disorders include septal defects, vessel stenosis, abnormally positioned vessels, and postnatal patency of the ductus arteriosus. Cardiomyopathies are acquired disorders in which disease of the cardiac muscle fibers reduces myocardial contractility or distensibility. Valvular disorders may be either congenital or acquired.

CARDIOMYOPATHY

Cardiomyopathy is a heart muscle disorder of unknown etiology (idiopathic). The dominant feature of cardiomyopathies is the involvement of the heart muscle itself. The definition excludes structural and functional abnormalities caused by valvular disorders, coronary artery disease, and systemic and pulmonary vascular disorders.[59] Idiopathic cardiomyopathies can be classified according to the ventricular changes they cause (Fig. 25–4).

The three major classes of idiopathic cardiomyopathy are

- idiopathic dilated (congestive) cardiomyopathy
- idiopathic hypertrophic cardiomyopathy (also called idiopathic hypertrophic subaortic stenosis)
- idiopathic restrictive cardiomyopathy.

Table 25–1 compares diagnostic data for these three classes. The incidence of cardiomyopathies has not been recorded.

Etiology

DILATED CARDIOMYOPATHY

Dilated cardiomyopathy may be associated with pregnancy. There may be spontaneous rapid improvement in some women, but early fatality in others. Other etiologic factors are listed in Box 25–4.

HYPERTROPHIC CARDIOMYOPATHY

Hypertrophic cardiomyopathy appears to be a genetically transmitted disease of the heart muscle, but its exact cause remains a mystery. It occurs most often in young adults, both men and women.[27]

Its predominant feature is unexplained myocardial hypertrophy, which typically appears as disproportionate thickening of the interventricular septum compared with the free wall of the ventricle. The term asymmetric septal hypertrophy is sometimes used to describe the disorder. About 50 percent of clients die from sudden death, whereas others exhibit relatively few symptoms.[9]

RESTRICTIVE CARDIOMYOPATHY

Any infiltrative process of the heart that results in fibrosis and thickening can cause restrictive cardiomyopathy, the least common type. The most common associated disorder is amyloidosis (deposition of eosinophilic fibrous protein in the heart).

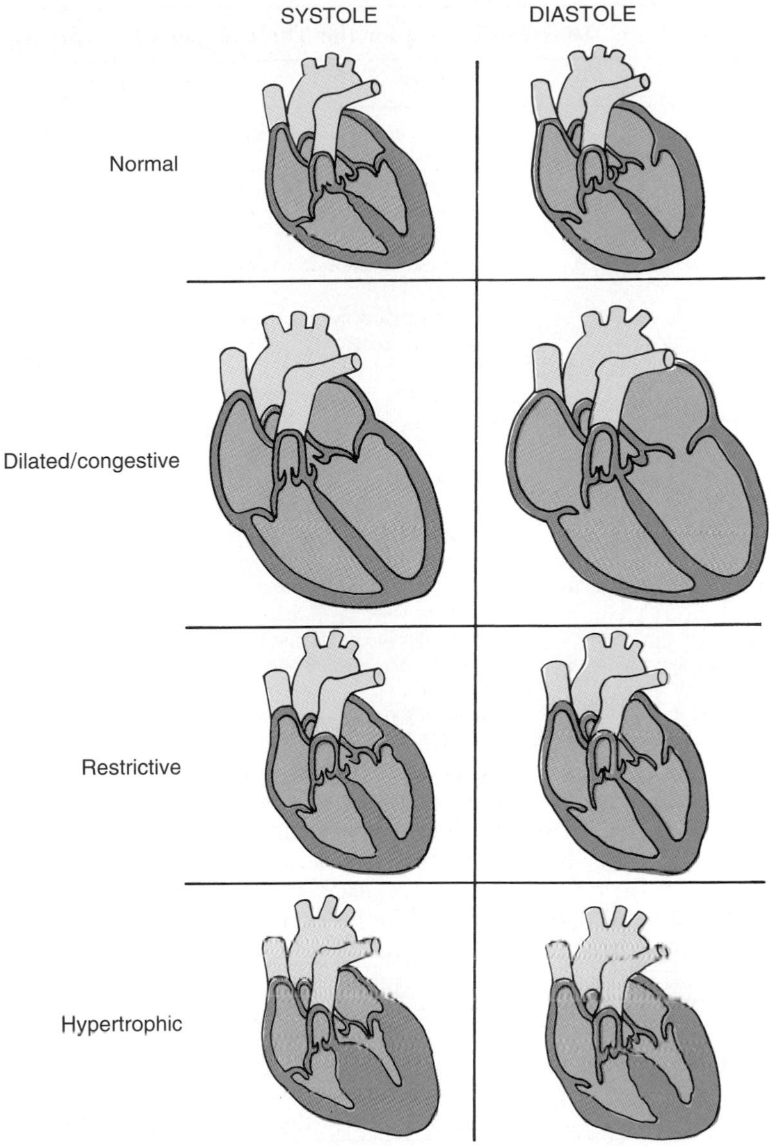

Figure 25–4
Types of cardiomyopathy.

Risk Factors

Four conditions seem to lower the threshold for the development of cardiomyopathy:

- chronic alcohol ingestion
- pregnancy
- systemic hypertension
- various infections.

Pathophysiology

DILATED CARDIOMYOPATHY

Whatever its cause, congestive cardiomyopathy results in a diffuse degeneration of myocardial fibers. Enlargement and dilation of all four chambers occurs. The initial abnormality is ventricular enlargement, followed by impaired ventricular contractility. This eventually leads to congestive heart failure.

HYPERTROPHIC CARDIOMYOPATHY

In this disorder's severest form, the left ventricular myocardium reaches tremendous dimensions and encroaches on the left ventricular chamber, which becomes small and elongated. Disproportionate thickening of the interventricular septum occurs, compared with the free wall of the ventricle. Septal hypertrophy may obstruct the left ventricular outflow tract during systole. Frequently, diastolic dysfunction occurs in the form of stiffness of the left ventricle during diastolic filling. This stiffness raises left ventricular end-diastolic pressure, which eventually results in elevation of left atrial, pulmonary venous, and pulmonary capillary pressures. These clients are at risk for infective endocarditis.

RESTRICTED CARDIOMYOPATHY

In restrictive cardiomyopathy, the ventricular walls are excessively rigid and impede ventricular filling. Myocardial contractility with systole is usually unaffected. Fi-

TABLE 25–1 Diagnostic Data for the Three Types of Cardiomyopathy

	DILATED	RESTRICTIVE	HYPERTROPHIC
Symptoms	Congestive heart failure, particularly left-sided Fatigue and weakness Systemic or pulmonary emboli	Dyspnea, fatigue Right-sided congestive heart failure Signs and symptoms of systemic disease: amyloidosis, iron storage disease, etc.	Dyspnea, angina pectoris Fatigue, syncope, palpitations
Physical examination	Moderate to severe cardiomegaly: S_3 and S_4 Atrioventricular valve regurgitation, especially mitral	Mild to moderate cardiomegaly: S_3 or S_4 Atrioventricular valve regurgitation; inspiratory increase in venous pressure (Kussmaul's sign)	Mild cardiomegaly Apical systolic thrill and heave; brisk carotid upstroke, S_4 common Systolic murmur that increases with Valsalva's maneuver
Chest roentgenogram	Moderate to marked cardiac enlargement, especially left ventricular Pulmonary venous hypertension	Mild cardiac enlargement Pulmonary venous hypertension	Mild to moderate cardiac enlargement Left atrial enlargment
Electrocardiogram	Sinus tachycardia Atrial and ventricular arrhythymias ST-segment and T-wave abnormalities Intraventricular conduction defects	Low voltage Intraventricular conduction defects Atrioventricular conduction defects	Left ventricular hypertrophy ST-segment and T-wave abnormalities Abnormal Q waves Atrial and ventricular arrhythmias
Echocardiogram	Left ventricular dilation and dysfunction Abnormal diastolic mitral valve motion secondary to abnormal compliance and filling pressures	Increased left ventricular wall thickness and mass Small or normal-sized left ventricular cavity Normal systolic function Pericardial effusion	Asymmetric septal hypertrophy Narrow left ventricular outflow tract Systolic anterior motion of the mitral valve Small or normal-sized left ventricle
Radionuclide studies	Left ventricular dilation and dysfunction (RVG)	Infiltration of myocardium (^{201}Tl) Small or normal-sized left ventricle (RVG) Normal systolic function (RVG)	Small or normal-sized left ventricle (RVG) Vigorous systolic function (RVG) Asymmetric septal hypertrophy (RVG or ^{201}Tl)
Cardiac catheterization	Left ventricular enlargement and dysfunction Mitral and/or tricuspid regurgitation Elevated left- and often right-sided filling pressures Diminished cardiac output	Diminished left ventricular compliance "Square root sign" in ventricular pressure recordings Preserved systolic function Elevated left- and right-sided filling pressures	Diminished left ventricular compliance Mitral regurgitation Vigorous systolic function Dynamic left ventricular outflow gradient

RVG, Radionuclide ventriculogram; ^{201}Tl, thallium-201.
From Braunwald, E. (1992). *Heart disease: A textbook of cardiovascular medicine* (4th ed.). Philadelphia: W. B. Saunders Co.

brotic infiltrations into the myocardium, endocardium, and subendocardium cause the ventricles to lose their ability to stretch. The tight heart muscle hampers ventricular diastolic filling. Filling pressures increase, and cardiac output diminishes. Eventually, cardiac failure and mild ventricular hypertrophy occur.

Clinical Manifestations

DILATED CARDIOMYOPATHY

Clinical manifestations usually develop gradually in clients with congestive cardiomyopathy. Fatigue and weakness are common. Chest pain may be present and may be associated with ischemic heart disease. Right-sided heart failure is a late and ominous sign.

Systemic blood pressure is usually normal or low. Symptoms often reveal signs of congestive heart failure. An S_4 gallop often precedes the development of congestive heart failure and an S_3 gallop generally occurs with heart failure.

A systolic murmur of mitral or tricuspid insufficiency may be detected, because ventricular dilation prevents sufficient closure of those valves. Pulmonary crackles become audible as heart failure progresses. Three fourths of patients with dilated cardiomyopathy die within 5 years of the onset of symptoms.[61]

Diagnostic tests including electrocardiography, echocardiography, chest radiography, and blood chemistries are useful for the physician's diagnosis. Electrocardiographic findings include sinus tachycardia, ventricular dysrhythmias, ST-segment changes, and left bundle branch block.

BOX 25-4

Etiology of Cardiomyopathy and Myocarditis

INFLAMMATORY

Infective

- Viral
- Rickettsial
- Bacterial
- Mycobacterial
- Fungal
- Parasitic

Noninfective

- Collagen diseases
- Granulomatous disorders
- Kawasaki's disease

METABOLIC

Nutritional

- Thiamine
- Scurvy
- Obesity
- Carnitine deficiency

Endocrine

- Acromegaly
- Thyrotoxicosis
- Myxedema
- Uremia
- Cushing's disease
- Pheochromocytoma
- Diabetes mellitus

Altered metabolism

- Gout
- Electrolyte imbalance

Toxins

- Cobalt
- Alcohol
- Bleomycin and doxorubicin
- Phenothiazines and antidepressants
- Carbon monoxide
- Lead
- Chloroquine
- Lithium
- Cyclophosphamide
- Hydrocarbons
- Catecholamines
- Phosphorus
- Insect stings and snake bites
- Reserpine
- Corticosteroids
- Cocaine

Infiltrative

- Amyloidosis
- Hemochromatosis
- Neoplastic disorders
- Glycogen storage disorders
- Sarcoidosis

Fibroplastic

- Endomyocardial fibrosis
- Endocardial fibroelastosis
- Carcinoid

Hematologic

- Sickle cell anemia
- Polycythemia vera
- Thrombotic thrombocytopenic purpura
- Leukemia

HYPERSENSITIVITY

- Hypersensitivity to medications
- Giant cell myocarditis
- Cardiac transplant rejection

GENETIC

Hypertrophic Cardiomyopathy

- With gradient
- Without gradient

Neuromuscular

- Duchenne's muscular dystrophy
- Kearns-Sayre syndrome
- Nemaline cardiomyopathy
- Multicore cardiomyopathy

MISCELLANEOUS ACQUIRED

- Postpartum cardiomyopathy
- Obesity

IDIOPATHIC

- Idiopathic dilated cardiomyopathy
- Idiopathic restrictive cardiomyopathy
- Idiopathic hypertrophic cardiomyopathy
- Idiopathic right ventricular cardiomyopathy

PHYSICAL AGENTS

- Heatstroke
- Hypothermia
- Radiation
- Tachycardia

Modified from Braunwald, E. (Ed.). (1992). *Heart disease: A textbook of cardiovascular medicine* (4th ed.). Philadelphia: W. B. Saunders.

HYPERTROPHIC CARDIOMYOPATHY

Signs and symptoms of hypertrophic cardiomyopathy most commonly appear in late adolescence or early adulthood, but may appear at any age. Many clients with hypertrophic cardiomyopathy are asymptomatic and often have relatives with incapacitating symptoms of the disease. Sadly, sudden death is frequently the first clinical manifestation of the disease in asymptomatic clients. Sudden death may follow physical exertion.

The most common symptom is dyspnea caused by the high pulmonary pressures produced by the elevated left ventricular end-diastolic pressure. Other common symptoms include angina pectoris, fatigue, and syncope. Cardiac dysrhythmias frequently occur. Many clients complain of dizzy spells. Exertion tends to worsen most symptoms.

Physical examination findings may be normal in asymptomatic clients. The appearance of a fourth heart sound may be the only sign of the disease. Electrocardiography, chest radiography, echocardiography, and radionuclide scanning aid the physician's diagnosis.

RESTRICTIVE CARDIOMYOPATHY

Manifestations of restrictive cardiomyopathy are related to decreasing cardiac output. As cardiac output falls and intraventricular pressures rise, signs of congestive heart failure appear. The earliest signs may include exercise intolerance, fatigue, and shortness of breath. In severe or end-stage disease, the clinical manifestations of restrictive cardiomyopathy are indistinguishable from those of chronic constrictive pericarditis. (See the preceding text for a more complete discussion of pericarditis.) Cardiac murmurs are usually minimal or absent. Congestive heart failure without cardiac enlargement indicates restrictive cardiomyopathy.

Medical Management

DILATED CARDIOMYOPATHY

Because the cause of idiopathic dilated cardiomyopathy is not known, there is no specific therapy. Treatment is similar to that for congestive heart failure. Only transplantation and specific vasodilator therapy (hydralazine plus nitrates) have prolonged life.[50, 59, 61]

Rest improves cardiac function and reduces heart size. Most clients experience severe activity intolerance during the later stages of the disease. The nurse should advise clients that physical and emotional stress exacerbates the disease. Because alcohol depresses myocardial contractility, the client should abstain from drinking alcoholic beverages.

Pharmacologic intervention focuses on controlling congestive heart failure by enhancing myocardial contractility and decreasing cardiac workload. Digitalis preparations, vasodilators, diuretics, and sodium-restricted diets are the primary interventions used to achieve these objectives. Antiarrhythmic agents may help suppress ventricular irritability. In appropriate candidates, the implantation of the automatic internal cardiac defibrillator may be used to prevent sudden cardiac death.[37, 61] (See Chap. 24.)

The combined problem of ventricular dilation and ineffective myocardial contractility also increases the risk of pooled blood within the heart and subsequent clot formation. Therefore, the physician may prescribe anticoagulants to help prevent clots and emboli.

HYPERTROPHIC CARDIOMYOPATHY

Goals of intervention are to reduce ventricular contractility and to relieve left ventricular outflow obstruction. Beta-adrenergic blocking agents, such as propranolol, provide the mainstay of medical intervention for hypertrophic cardiomyopathy. These medications reduce myocardial contractility and the incidence of chest pain. With decreased vigor of ventricular contraction, outflow obstruction diminishes. Beta-adrenergic blockade also reduces heart rate (which further reduces myocardial workload) and prevents arrhythmias. Calcium channel blocking agents, such as verapamil, are also being used to relieve symptoms and improve exercise tolerance. Nitroglycerin and digoxin are contraindicated in clients with hypertrophic cardiomyopathy because they may increase outflow obstruction.[9]

RESTRICTIVE CARDIOMYOPATHY

Currently there are no specific interventions for restrictive cardiomyopathy. Intervention aims at diminishing congestive heart failure. Diuretics, vasodilators, and salt restriction help accomplish this goal. Digitalis may help in some forms of restrictive cardiomyopathy. Because clients with this condition are prone to digitalis toxicity, they require close monitoring of serum blood levels.

Death due to dysrhythmia from restrictive cardiomyopathy may occur suddenly, or a more progressive course may be followed with eventual, intractable heart failure. The prognosis largely depends on the underlying cause. Unfortunately, intervention for these clients rarely brings about long-term improvement.

Surgical Management

Surgical intervention for hypertrophic cardiomyopathy may become necessary if medical management proves ineffective. Several surgical procedures have been developed to reduce the outflow gradient. The most popular surgical treatment, myotomy (or myectomy), involves excising a portion of the hypertrophied septum. Percutaneous laser myopathy is an experimental therapy for clients who are not candidates for invasive surgical techniques.[9]

The excision of fibrotic endocardium is successful in a limited number of clients with restrictive cardiomyopathy. Cardiac transplantation is becoming increasingly common for clients with dilated cardiomyopathy. Valve replacement may also be required, but it is not commonly performed. Cardiac surgery is discussed later in this chapter.

Nursing Management

Assessment

Nursing assessment for cardiomyopathy focuses on

- the duration and extent of symptoms
- limitations on activity and lifestyle
- the client's and significant others' coping strategies
- the client's and significant others' understanding of, perception of, and reaction to the illness
- genetic counseling

Nursing Diagnosis, Planning, and Implementation

Nursing management of clients with cardiomyopathy is outlined in the Care Plan. In addition, clients who are acutely or chronically ill with cardiomyopathy require strong psychosocial support.

Even though the prognosis for these clients is often poor, the nurse can help them maintain hope and dignity. Encouragement, a caring touch, a listening ear, and attainable goals can promote a high quality of life. The nurse should create an environment in which clients can openly express concerns and acknowledge fears. Acceptance, empathy, and kindness can help these clients adopt more successful coping strategies and maintain a realistic level of health. (See Client Education Guide: Cardiomyopathy.)

VALVULAR HEART DISEASE

The four heart valves maintain the one-way flow of blood. When the valves are healthy, the blood flows through the heart and lungs in a unilateral direction. Dysfunction occurs when the heart valves are unable to fully open or fully close. A stenosed valve may impede the flow of blood from one chamber to the next. An insufficient valve may allow blood to regurgitate back into the chamber from which blood is being pumped.

MITRAL VALVE DISEASE

Disorders of the mitral valve obstruct the flow of blood from the atrium to the ventricle (stenosis) or allow blood to leak back from ventricle to atrium (regurgita-

CLIENT EDUCATION GUIDE

Cardiomyopathy

Before discharge, all clients with cardiomyopathy should be taught the following:

- disease causes and the rationale for treatments
- signs and symptoms of worsening heart failure
- administration route, dosage schedule, and side effects of prescribed medications
- the need to pace activity and get adequate rest.

Clients with hypertrophic cardiomyopathy should also be taught to:

- avoid strenuous activity such as running or active sports
- take prophylactic antibiotics before any dental or surgical procedures and inform health care providers of the cardiomyopathy
- encourage significant others to learn cardiopulmonary resuscitation

Clients with restrictive cardiomyopathy should also be taught:

- signs and symptoms of digitalis toxicity.

All clients should be taught when to seek health care.

tion). Mitral regurgitation overworks the left atrium and left ventricle; mitral stenosis overworks the left atrium.

AORTIC VALVE DISEASE

Aortic valve disease is far less common than mitral valve disease. However, it often occurs in conjunction with mitral disease. Aortic stenosis obstructs the forward flow of blood from the left ventricle into the aorta and systemic circulation. Aortic regurgitation allows blood to leak back from the aorta into the left ventricle. Both aortic stenosis and regurgitation overwork the left ventricle.

Incidence

Valvular heart disease remains fairly common in the United States (see the discussion of infective endocarditis). Mitral valve prolapse syndrome is one of the most common cardiac abnormalities; as much as 5 to 18 per cent of the population is affected.[49] The incidence of the other forms of valvular heart disease is not known.

Etiology

MITRAL STENOSIS

This disorder involves a blockage of blood flow resulting from an abnormality of the mitral valve leaflets. Possible causes include infective endocarditis, calcification of valve leaflets, and systemic disorders, such as lupus erythematosus and rheumatoid arthritis.

MITRAL REGURGITATION

Mitral valve prolapse, coronary artery disease, and infective endocarditis are the most common causes of mitral regurgitation.[44] Regurgitation can occur even in a structurally sound valve from left ventricular failure and dilation, causing an enlargement of the valve orifice. It also can occur with mitral stenosis.

MITRAL VALVE PROLAPSE

In most clients, mitral valve prolapse is a benign disorder, but some clients report a wide variety of cardiac and noncardiac symptoms. This disorder most commonly affects young women.[49] It appears to be caused by connective tissue abnormalities in the valve leaflets that allow one or both valve leaflets to bulge into the left atrium during systole. Mitral valve prolapse can also occur in clients with other disorders, such as Marfan's syndrome and Ehlers-Danlos syndrome, systemic lupus erythematosus, atherosclerosis, muscular dystrophy, acromegaly, and cardiac sarcoidosis. There may be a genetic component.

AORTIC STENOSIS

This disorder can be caused by several congenital defects of the aortic valve. It can also be caused by two degenerative processes: calcification of the valve in elderly persons, or retraction and stiffening of the valve from infective endocarditis. The aging U.S. population has led to an increased incidence of aortic stenosis from calcification.[22, 45]

AORTIC REGURGITATION

The most common cause of aortic regurgitation is an infectious disorder, such as rheumatic fever, syphilis, or infective endocarditis. Aneurysm of the ascending aorta is another possible cause. Connective tissue disorders can also lead to aortic regurgitation.

TRICUSPID AND PULMONIC VALVE DISEASE

Pure lesions of the tricuspid valve are rare; tricuspid disorders usually develop in combination with other structural disorders of the heart. Intravenous drug users are at increased risk for tricuspid valve disorders. Pulmonic valve disorders are commonly caused by congenital defects; few lesions develop after birth. Pulmonary hypertension, caused by mitral stenosis, pulmonary emboli, or chronic lung disease, can precipitate functional regurgitation.

Risk Factors

Factors leading to acquired valvular disease include acute rheumatic fever and infectious endocarditis. Rheumatic heart disease, the most common cause of valvular heart disease, is preventable with early detection and treatment of beta-hemolytic streptococcal infections (the precursor to rheumatic heart disease).

CARE PLAN: The Client with Cardiomyopathy

Nursing Diagnosis/ Collaborative Problem	Planning: Expected Outcomes	Implementation: Nursing Interventions	Rationales
Congestive Heart Failure, Risk for R/T mechanical dysfunction of the heart	The nurse will monitor for clinical manifestations of CHF: • Peripheral edema • Pulmonary edema • Decreased renal perfusion • Decreased CO • Diaphoresis • Dyspnea/orthopnea • Anxiety • Frothy, pink sputum • Presence of S_3	Assess the client every 4–8 hours for • Neck vein distention • Peripheral edema • Altered lung sounds • Dyspnea or orthopnea • Hypoxia • Tachycardia • Hypotension • Confusion • Urine output > 30 mL/hr • Absence of extra heart sounds	To detect early signs of CHF; as the heart muscle fails to pump effectively, falling cardiac output stimulates the adrenergic system and the renin-angiotensin-aldosterone system. These changes lead to tachycardia and oliguria. Increased preload and afterload lead to neck vein distention, peripheral edema, altered lung sounds, dyspnea and orthopnea. Hypoxia may lead to confusion
		Monitor BUN, bilirubin, liver enzymes, and creatinine levels	Abnormal laboratory studies indicate liver failure from congestion of blood
		Monitor fluid balance and electrolyte levels every 8–24 hr Daily weights	Clients are treated with potent diuretics to reduce pulmonary and peripheral edema. Accurate assessment of fluid balance, serum electrolyte levels, and weight assist in determining the effectiveness of the treatment
Decreased Cardiac Output R/T alterations in cardiac structure and function	The client will demonstrate improved cardiac output, as evidenced by • Clear lung sounds • Vital signs within normal limits • Warm, dry skin • Normal sinus rhythm • Absence of S_3 or S_4 • Stable body weight • Urine output > 30 mL/hr • Decreased peripheral edema, neck vein distention, and ascites • Absence of mental confusion	Monitor for clinical manifestations of decreasing CO	Early detection of decreasing CO improves treatment options
		Encourage bed rest during acute phase, limit self-care	Decreases oxygen consumption and demand on myocardium
		Avoid Valsalva's maneuvers (with hypertrophic cardiomyopathy)	Valsalva's maneuvers decrease the inflow of venous blood and impair outflow
		Observe and record dysrhythmias every 4–8 hr	Dysrhythmias may further impair CO
		Monitor intake and output every 1–8 hr	Fluid retention may occur with decreased CO and CHF
		Restrict intravenous and oral fluids as ordered	Decreases the amount of circulating fluids

Pathophysiology

Acquired valvular dysfunction is usually caused by inflammation of the endocardium as a result of acute rheumatic fever or infectious endocarditis. The inflammation causes fibrotic changes in the valve leaflets and chordae tendineae, shortening of the chordae tendineae, and narrowing of the outflow tract (see Pathophysiology: Cardiac Valve Disorders).

If valvular stenosis occurs, the valve orifice narrows and the valve leaflets (cusps) may fuse or thicken; thus, the valve cannot open freely. If valvular insufficiency develops, scarring and retraction result in incomplete closure.

Either problem increases the heart's workload. Valvular stenosis subjects the chamber behind the stenotic valve to greater stress (e.g., the left ventricle in aortic stenosis). This is because the heart must generate more pressure to force blood through the narrowed opening. In valvular insufficiency, the chambers both in front and behind the valve are taxed.

The aortic and mitral valves, on the heart's left side, become dysfunctional more often than the pulmonary and tricuspid valves on the right side of the heart do. This change occurs because the left side of the heart is a system of higher pressures; the right side of the heart is exposed to the lower pressures of the pulmonary circulation.

CARE PLAN: The Client with Cardiomyopathy *Continued*

Nursing Diagnosis/ Collaborative Problem	Planning: Expected Outcomes	Implementation: Nursing Interventions	Rationales
	• Increase activity tolerance • Absence of angina	Administer unloading and inotropic agents as ordered	Used to improve ejection, reduce preload, and improve contractility
		Administer calcium antagonists as ordered	Decreases LV outflow obstruction and increases LV compliance to improve ventricular filling
		In hypertrophic: avoid nitrates, beta-adrenergics, and cardiac glycosides	These agents increase contractility and increase obstruction
		Hemodynamic monitoring: monitor arterial pressure, RAP, PAP, PAWP, CO/CI every 2–4 hr as indicated	Monitors the degree of CHF and the response to therapy
Activity Intolerance R/T mechanical dysfunction of the heart and decreased cardiac reserve	The client will have an improved activity tolerance, as evidenced by	Assess tolerance to activities in bed before ambulating	Provides a baseline to plan activity
	• Demonstrating a progression of activity appropriate to the disorder	During activity, monitor pulse, respirations, color, and ECG	Provides early detection of orthostatic changes as well as data on the ability of the diseased myocardium to meet oxygen demand
	• Showing a willingness to combine rest and activity • Demonstrating minimal change in pulse or BP during activities	Discontinue activity if chest pain, dyspnea, cyanosis, dizziness, hypotension, sustained tachycardia, or dysrhythmias develop	Evidence of myocardial hypoxia
	• Demonstrating minimal fatigue after activity	Monitor pulse, respirations, and BP 3 minutes after activity	Evaluate tolerance of activity
	• Having pulse, respirations, and BP return to normal range within 3 minutes of activity • Accepting any imposed restrictions	Explore which sedentary activities client may enjoy	May provide diversion, if activity is not permitted; these activities do not place a demand on the diseased myocardium

BP, blood pressure; BUN, blood urea nitrogen; CHF, congestive heart failure; CO, cardiac output; CO/CI, cardiac output/cardiac index; ECG, electrocardiogram; LV, left ventricular; PAP, pulmonary artery pressure; PAWP, pulmonary artery wedge pressure; RAP, right atrial pressure.

For a time, the heart may be able to compensate for the additional strain through dilation and eventual hypertrophy. However, if valvular damage worsens, without intervention the heart will eventually fail.

MITRAL STENOSIS

As the valves become calcified and immobile, the valvular orifice narrows, which prevents normal passage of blood from the left atrium to the left ventricle. The valve orifice normally is 4 to 6 cm². When it is mildly stenosed, the orifice is reduced to 2 cm². This mild stenosis allows blood to flow from the left atrium to the left ventricle only if increased pressure is generated. In critical mitral stenosis, the valve opening is reduced to 1 cm². The obstruction of blood flow across the mitral valve during diastolic filling creates a pressure gradient between the left atrium and the left ventricle of approximately 20 mm Hg in critical stenosis.[4] Therefore, the pressure in the left atrium is elevated to approximately 25 mm Hg. The elevated left atrial pressure in turn raises the pulmonary venous and pulmonary capillary pressures. The left atrium hypertrophies to accommodate the increase in pressure and volume, and the right ventricle hypertrophies because of the chronic pulmonary hypertension. Right ventricular failure can result,

PATHOPHYSIOLOGY

Cardiac Valve Disorders

These illustrations show what happens in mitral stenosis *(A)*, mitral insufficiency *(B)*, aortic stenosis *(C)*, and aortic insufficiency *(D)*.

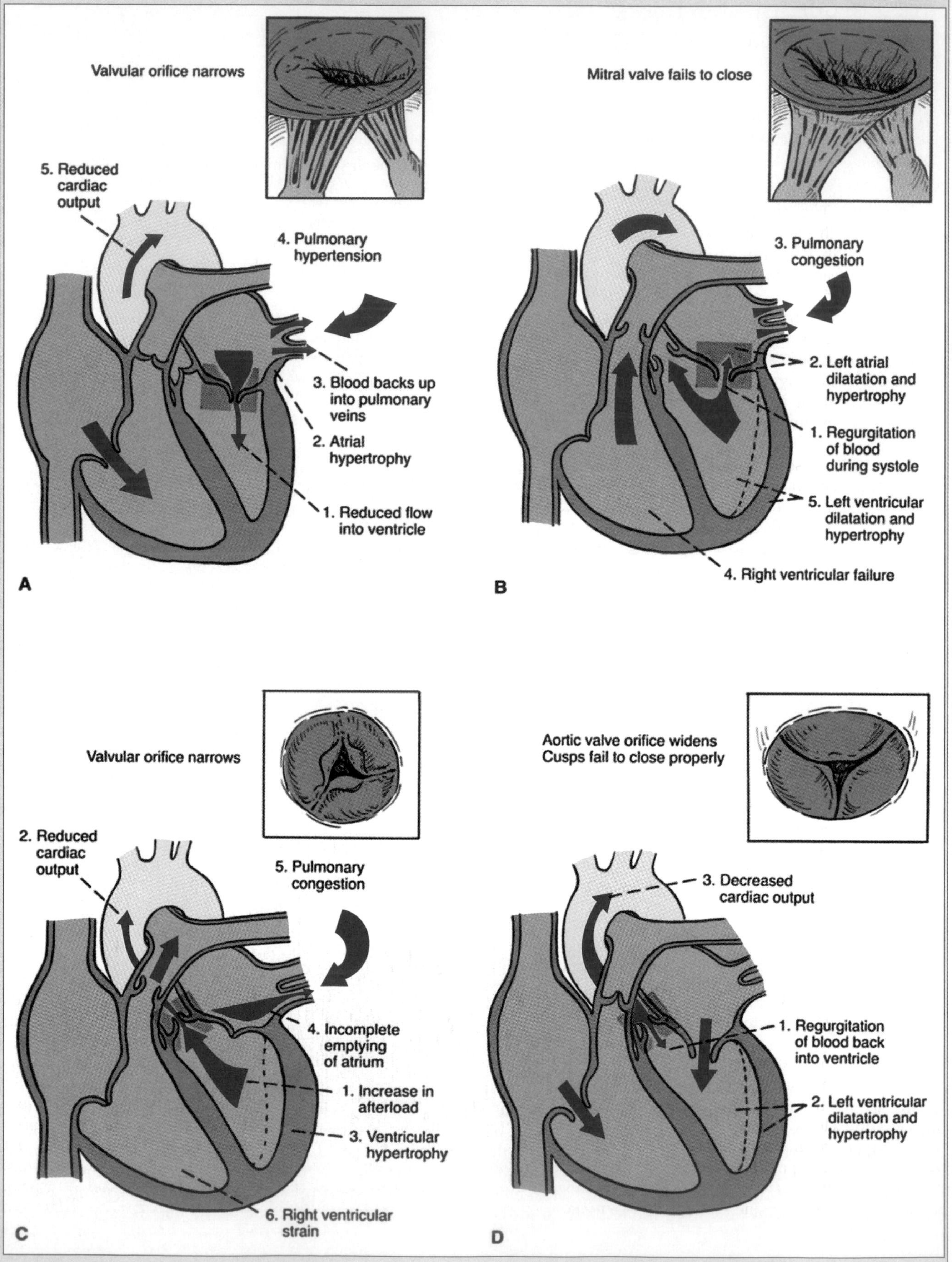

and inadequate filling of the left ventricle (preload) can result in reduced cardiac output.[44]

MITRAL REGURGITATION

Mitral regurgitation occurs during systole. Incompetency of the valve results from

- shortening, rigidity, deformity, and retraction of one or both cusps of the mitral valve
- shortening and fusion of the chordae tendineae and papillary muscles

During systole, much pressure is generated within the left ventricle. The blood in the left ventricle is ejected forward into the aorta and also backward into the left atrium through the mitral valve that is not completely closed. The backward flow of blood causes left atrial and left ventricular enlargement. The left atrium responds to the large volume of blood it is receiving during systole, causing dilation and hypertrophy. The left ventricle responds to the large amount of blood lost to the left atrium by trying to pump harder to preserve the cardiac output. This causes hypertrophy of the left ventricle and eventually left ventricular failure.

Over time, the increased blood flow to the left atrium causes a rise in left atrial pressure. This pressure is reflected backward into the pulmonary venous and arterial system. With continued high pressures, right-sided heart failure can develop.

Trauma, infection, or myocardial infarction can cause acute mitral damage. In acute mitral regurgitation, there is no time for the compensatory mechanisms of hypertrophy and dilation to occur. Cardiac output falls suddenly, followed by cardiogenic shock and pulmonary edema.[22]

MITRAL VALVE PROLAPSE

In mitral valve prolapse, the anterior and posterior cusps of the mitral valve billow upward into the atrium during systolic contraction. The chordae tendineae can be lengthened, which allows the valve cusps to stretch upward. The cusps may be enlarged and thickened. If blood leaks backward into the atrium during systole, mitral regurgitation is present.

AORTIC STENOSIS

In aortic stenosis, the orifice of the aortic valve becomes narrowed, which causes a decrease in the blood flow from the left ventricle into the aorta. The pressure within the left ventricle rises as the blood is ejected through the narrowed opening. A pressure gradient develops between the left ventricle and the aorta. The elevation of the pressure in the left ventricle during systole causes the ventricle to hypertrophy. Dilation of the left ventricle occurs over time when the contractility of the hypertrophied muscle deteriorates. Eventually, the dilated and hypertrophied left ventricle is unable to maintain adequate cardiac output. The rise in left ventricular end diastolic and increased pulmonary hypertension eventually are manifested as congestive heart failure and pulmonary edema.

AORTIC REGURGITATION

In this diastolic event, blood that is propelled forward into the aorta is allowed to regurgitate backward into the left ventricle through an incompetent valve. This causes abnormal filling and a volume overload of the left ventricle. The magnitude of the overload depends on the severity of the incompetence.

To compensate for the decrease in systemic circulation, the left ventricular stroke volume increases to produce an effective forward-moving blood volume into the aorta. A compensatory dilation occurs in the left ventricle, but only a minimal increase in left ventricular end-diastolic pressure develops.[45] As much as 60 per cent of the stroke volume can be regurgitated, markedly increasing left ventricular workload. The compensatory mechanisms of dilation and hypertrophy help maintain adequate cardiac output. However, as the condition progresses and the contractile state of the myocardium declines, cardiac output diminishes.

TRICUSPID AND PULMONIC VALVE DISEASE

Because the tricuspid valve is on the right side of the heart, the major hemodynamic alterations with tricuspid stenosis are decreases in cardiac output and increases in right atrial pressures. The inability of the right atrium to propel blood across the stenosed valve explains these changes. Likewise, with tricuspid regurgitation, the pressures in the right atrium are elevated. In this situation, however, the elevation is due to regurgitation of the blood volume in the right ventricle back into the right atrium during systole.

Pulmonic stenosis and regurgitation lead to decreased cardiac output, because blood does not reach the left side of the heart in adequate supply for metabolic demands. Right-sided heart failure can also develop.

Clinical Manifestations

MITRAL STENOSIS

The symptoms of mitral stenosis may appear gradually or suddenly (see Clinical Manifestations: Valvular Heart Disease).

Auscultation reveals a loud first heart sound and then an opening snap that ushers in a low-pitched, rumbling diastolic murmur. Atrial fibrillation is a common finding. During episodes of atrial fibrillation, the pulse becomes irregular and faint, and the blood pressure often drops.

Up to 20 per cent of clients with mitral stenosis will develop systemic embolization.[44] Ineffective atrial contractions allow some stagnation of blood in the left atrium and encourage the formation of mural thrombi. These thrombi easily break away and travel as emboli throughout the arterial system, causing tissue infarction.

CLINICAL MANIFESTATIONS

Valvular Heart Disease

VALVE DISORDER	CLINICAL MANIFESTATIONS	DIAGNOSTIC ASSESSMENT FINDINGS
Mitral stenosis	Diastolic, rumbling, low-pitched murmur—at apex (bell of stethoscope)[2] Loud snapping S_1—at apex (diaphragm of stethoscope)[2] Fatigue Palpitations Narrowed pulse pressure Hoarseness Left ventricular failure: dyspnea, orthopnea, PND, pulmonary crackles, cough, hemoptysis Right ventricular failure: neck vein distention, peripheral edema	**Chest Film** Left atrial enlargement Pulmonary venous congestion Right ventricular enlargement **Electrocardiogram** Left atrial hypertrophy P-mitrale (prolonged, notched P wave) Right ventricular hypertrophy Atrial fibrillation **Echocardiogram** Thickened mitral valve with diminished movement of leaflets Left atrial enlargement Right ventricular enlargement **Cardiac Catheterization** ↑ Pressure gradient across mitral valve ↑ Left atrial pressure ↑ Pulmonary vascular resistance ↑ LVEDP, ↑ PAWP ↓ Cardiac output
Mitral regurgitation (insufficiency)	Pansystolic, blowing, high-pitched murmur—at apex, radiating to axilla S_1 diminished Split S_2 Weakness, fatigue Left ventricular failure: dyspnea, orthopnea, PND, pulmonary crackles, S_3 and S_4 Palpitations Right ventricular failure: neck vein distention, peripheral edema, hepatomegaly	**Chest Film** Left atrial and ventricular enlargement Pulmonary vascular congestion **Electrocardiogram** Left atrial hypertrophy P-mitrale Atrial fibrillation Left ventricular hypertrophy **Echocardiogram** Bizarre motion of mitral leaflets Hyperdynamic left ventricle Enlarged left atrium and ventricle **Cardiac Catheterization** ↑ Left atrial pressure ↑ Amount of regurgitant flow Rule out prolapse and congenital disorders ↑ LVEDP (preload), ↑ PAWP ↓ Cardiac output
Aortic stenosis	Systolic, harsh, crescendo-decrescendo murmur—right sternal border radiating to neck, early ejection click, palpable thrill at second right intercostal space Diminished S_2 S_3 and S_4 Fatigue Vertigo and syncope Chest pain Ventricular tachycardia Bradycardia Low pulse pressure Left ventricular failure: dyspnea, orthopnea, PND, pulmonary edema	**Chest Film** Calcification of aortic valve Left ventricular enlargement Prominent ascending aorta **Electrocardiogram** Left ventricular hypertrophy Sinus tachycardia, atrial fibrillation Atrioventricular conduction delay Left and right bundle branch block **Echocardiogram** Limited aortic valve movement Thickened left ventricular wall **Cardiac Catherization** ↑ Pressure gradient in systole across aortic valve ↓ Size of aortic orifice ↑ LVEDP

CLINICAL MANIFESTATIONS *Continued*

Valvular Heart Disease

VALVE DISORDER	CLINICAL MANIFESTATIONS	DIAGNOSTIC ASSESSMENT FINDINGS
Aortic regurgitation (insufficiency)	Diastolic; soft, high-pitched blowing, decrescendo murmur—second right intercostal space, radiating to the left sternal border, increases with inspiration Large and diffuse diastolic thrill, left sternal border Loud S_2 Fatigue, weakness Syncope Palpitations (water-hammer pulse) Sinus tachycardia, PVCs Wide pulse pressure Right ventricular failure: neck vein distention, ankle edema, hepatomegaly, ascites Left ventricular failure: dyspnea, orthopnea, PND, pulmonary crackles, S_3 and S_4	**Chest Film** Calcification of aortic valve Left ventricular enlargement Dilation of ascending aorta **Electrocardiogram** Left ventricular hypertrophy Sinus tachycardia, PVCs **Echocardiogram** Dilated and hyperdynamic left ventricle Enlargement of aortic root and left atrium Early closure of mitral valve Diastolic fluttering of aortic valve **Cardiac Catheterization** ↓ Aortic diastolic pressure ↑ LVEDP ↑ Regurgitant flow Reflux through aortic valve
Tricuspid stenosis	Diastolic; rumbling murmur—left sternal border, increases with inspiration Signs of right ventricular failure; neck vein distention, peripheral edema, hepatomegaly, right upper quadrant pain	**Chest Film** Right atrial enlargement **Electrocardiogram** Tall, peaked P wave in leads II, III, aV—right atrial hypertrophy Atrial arrhythmias **Echocardiogram** Thickening and abnormal motion of tricuspid valve **Cardiac Catheterization** ↑ Pressure across tricuspid valve
Tricuspid regurgitation (insufficiency)	Diastolic, holosystolic—left sternal border Signs of right-sided failure	**Chest Film** Right atrial and ventricular enlargement **Electrocardiogram** Tall, peaked P wave Right ventricular hypertrophy **Echocardiogram** Right ventricular dilation Paradoxic septal motion Tricuspid valvular thickening and abnormal motion

LVEDP, left ventricular end-diastolic pressure; PAWP, pulmonary artery wedge pressure; PND, paroxysmal nocturnal dyspnea; PVCs, premature ventricular contractions.

MITRAL REGURGITATION

Clients with mitral regurgitation may be asymptomatic, but if cardiac output diminishes, symptoms will develop. Fatigue and dyspnea are typically the first symptoms. Later, orthopnea, paroxysmal nocturnal dyspnea, and peripheral edema may occur. When the right side of the heart is affected, symptoms are similar to those of mitral stenosis.

Vital signs are usually normal except in severe mitral regurgitation. Atrial fibrillation is common; however, emboli and hemoptysis occur far less often than in mitral stenosis.

MITRAL VALVE PROLAPSE

Many clients with mitral valve prolapse are completely asymptomatic; others report only vague symptoms. In healthy clients, physical examination may reveal a regurgitant murmur or a midsystolic click on auscultation. Symptoms that may appear include tachycardia, lightheadedness, syncope, fatigue, weakness, dyspnea, chest discomfort, anxiety, and palpitations related to dysrhythmias.[39] Mitral valve prolapse has recently been associated with an autonomic dysfunction in which large quantities of catecholamines are produced, with or without adrenergic stimulation. This may help explain the vague and variable symptoms.[49] Only minimal morbidity and mortality are associated with mitral valve prolapse. Clinically, clients have no physical limitations.[39]

AORTIC STENOSIS

Symptoms of aortic stenosis tend to occur gradually and late in the course of the disease. There is usually a long latent period in which the client is asymptomatic. Symptoms begin to appear as the obstruction and ventricular pressure increases to critical levels. Hypertrophy of the left ventricle increases myocardial oxygen consumption; at the same time, cardiac output drops and coronary artery perfusion decreases. The result is exertional angina in about 60 per cent of clients.[46]

Syncope, another common symptom, occurs during exertion because the cardiac output is fixed and unable to meet increased systemic demands. Decreased cerebral perfusion results in syncope.[4, 22] Syncope at rest may be caused by arrhythmias.

In severe aortic stenosis, additional symptoms may include palpitations, fatigue, and visual disturbances. Sudden death occurs in 15 to 20 per cent of symptomatic clients as a result of dysrhythmias and myocardial ischemia.[45]

AORTIC REGURGITATION

Clients with chronic severe aortic regurgitation may have a long asymptomatic period. During this time, the left ventricle gradually enlarges. Clients may complain of an uncomfortable awareness of the heart beat and palpitations. These symptoms are due to the large left ventricular stroke volume with rapid diastolic runoff. This is also apparent with prominent pulsations in the neck and even head bobbing with each heart beat. Sinus tachycardia or premature ventricular contractions may make palpitations more pronounced.

Physical examination may detect elevated systolic blood pressure due to the large stroke volume and decreased diastolic blood pressure due to the regurgitation and distal runoff (increased pulse pressure). Carotid artery pulsations may be exaggerated. This may be noted as a sudden sharp pulse, followed by a swift collapse of the diastolic pulse (Corrigan's or water-hammer pulse).

TRICUSPID AND PULMONIC VALVE DISEASE

Clinical manifestations of tricuspid stenosis include dyspnea and fatigue, pulsations in the neck, and peripheral edema. Physical assessment reveals prominent waves in the neck veins as the atrium is vigorously contracting against the stenotic valve.

Tricuspid insufficiency causes hepatic congestion and peripheral edema. The client often has atrial fibrillation and evident jugular waves.

Pulmonic regurgitation may lead to dyspnea and fatigue. The characteristic murmur is a high-pitched diastolic blowing heard along the left sternal border. No significant ECG changes occur. Pulmonic stenosis produces similar manifestations, except that the murmur is often a crescendo-decrescendo type.

Diagnostic Assessment

Various diagnostic studies are used to detect valvular lesions or structural heart changes. These include echocardiography, transesophageal echocardiography, chest radiography, and cardiac catheterization. The Clinical Manifestations box summarizes diagnostic assessment findings for valvular disorders.

Medical Management

MITRAL STENOSIS

Untreated mitral stenosis can progress from mild disability to severe disability in about 5 years.[44] Improvement of symptoms can be achieved with oral diuretic therapy and a sodium-restricted diet. Digitalis is useful in slowing the ventricular heart rate in clients with atrial fibrillation. Beta-blockers may decrease the heart rate and thus increase exercise tolerance. Anticoagulants are helpful in clients who are not anticipating surgical intervention.

MITRAL REGURGITATION

Symptom reduction is the aim of nonsurgical treatment of mitral regurgitation. The client should restrict physical activities responsible for producing fatigue and dyspnea. Reducing sodium intake and promoting sodium excretion with diuretics will lessen cardiac workload. Nitrates and angiotensin-converting enzyme inhibitors have produced hemodynamic improvement and symptom relief in clients with chronic regurgitation.[64]

MITRAL VALVE PROLAPSE

Treatment of mitral valve prolapse depends on the client's symptoms. Beta-blockers may help relieve severe symptoms of syncope, palpitations, and chest pain. To prevent infective endocarditis, antibiotics are given prophylactically before any invasive procedures. (See Client Education Guide: Mitral Valve Prolapse.)

AORTIC STENOSIS

Noninvasive assessment should be made with the use of Doppler echocardiography. Clients with known or suspected critical aortic valve obstruction should be instructed to avoid vigorous athletic and physical activity.

CLIENT EDUCATION GUIDE

Mitral Valve Prolapse

Before discharge, the client should be taught the following:

- If palpitations occur, exercise moderately; the increased heart rate will override the extra beats.
- If you experience shortness of breath, perform deep inhalation and slow pursed-lip exhalation.
- If chest pain occurs, lie down, bend your legs to a 90-degree angle, and push your feet against a wall for 3 to 5 minutes.
- Maintain an aerobic exercise program in consultation with your physician.
- Decrease caffeine intake, eat a healthy diet, and drink eight 8-ounce glasses of water per day.
- Decrease stress and practice relaxation techniques.
- Tell your dentist of your condition before dental work.

Clients with mild obstruction may continue activity as tolerated.

Prophylactic antibiotics should be given before invasive medical or dental procedures to prevent infective endocarditis. Digitalis and diuretics, commonly used for ventricular failure, will not help in aortic stenosis, because they will not help reduce the mechanical obstruction to outflow.[39] Beta-blockers usually are not used because they can depress myocardial function and induce left ventricular failure. Cardiac dysrhythmias should be treated pharmacologically.

AORTIC REGURGITATION

Medical intervention for aortic regurgitation is the same as for aortic stenosis, aimed at relieving the manifestations of congestive heart failure and preventing infection of the already deformed aortic cusps.

TRICUSPID AND PULMONIC VALVE DISEASE

Tricuspid stenosis usually responds well to diuretic and digitalis therapy. If the leaflets are severely stenotic, surgery may be necessary. However, concurrent mitral valve stenosis may have a higher surgical priority. Treatment of pulmonic valve disorders is usually symptom-based; again, surgery may be required.

Surgical Management

When conservative medical intervention fails to improve hemodynamics in valvular disorders, surgical intervention is indicated. Valve repair or replacement is commonly indicated for severe valvular defects accompanied by left ventricular dysfunction and heart failure. These interventions are not considered curative but can provide long-lasting palliation. Cure is usually unachievable because of the client's preoperative condition.

Valve repair or reconstruction is most often performed on the mitral valve and is most successful in treating mitral insufficiency. Reconstruction has gained popularity because it eliminates the need for anticoagulation therapy, decreases the risk of thromboembolism, decreases the risk of endocarditis, decreases the need for repeat surgery, and increases survival. Aortic valve reconstruction is considered experimental at this time.[22]

Valvular surgery must be performed at an appropriate time during the course of the disease before left ventricular function deteriorates with associated irreversible damage. The projected natural history of the condition, the degree of impact on the client's life-style, and the projected performance of the repaired or replaced valve are factors that the surgeon and the client must consider before valvular surgery is performed. See Box 25–5 for a description of artificial valves.

BOX 25–5

Artificial Heart Valves

Artificial heart valves are continuing to show improvements in design, safety, function, and durability. Mechanical and tissue prosthetic valves are currently available. Tissue valves are of two types:

- xenografts, from porcine and bovine sources
- autografts, from human cadavers

The type of valve prosthesis used is based on a number of considerations. Mechanical valves are very durable but require life-long anticoagulation therapy; tissue grafts may not require anticoagulation but are less durable. The surgeon considers primarily the client's tolerance of anticoagulation and the durability of the valve. For instance, for a client with a preoperative history of bleeding or noncompliance with prescribed pharmacologic therapy, the surgeon may decide to use a tissue valve. Some physicians generally recommend mechanical valves in clients under age 65 or 70 and tissue valves in clients age 70 and older.[4]

Potential complications of heart valves include a risk of thrombus formation, especially in mechanical valves. Newer types of heart valves have reduced rates of thrombus. The major risk with tissue valves is durability. The leaflets of these valves may degenerate, calcify, or develop structural abnormalities. Mitral valves tend to fail most often because of the higher stress on the valve. The rate of xenograft valve failure is 2 to 5 per cent for the first 6 years, and then the rate accelerates. Durability of autografts has not been established.[62] Almost every client with a tissue valve will require replacement eventually.[62] To prevent infective endocarditis, valve replacement clients require life-long antibiotic prophylaxis for dental work and surgical procedures.

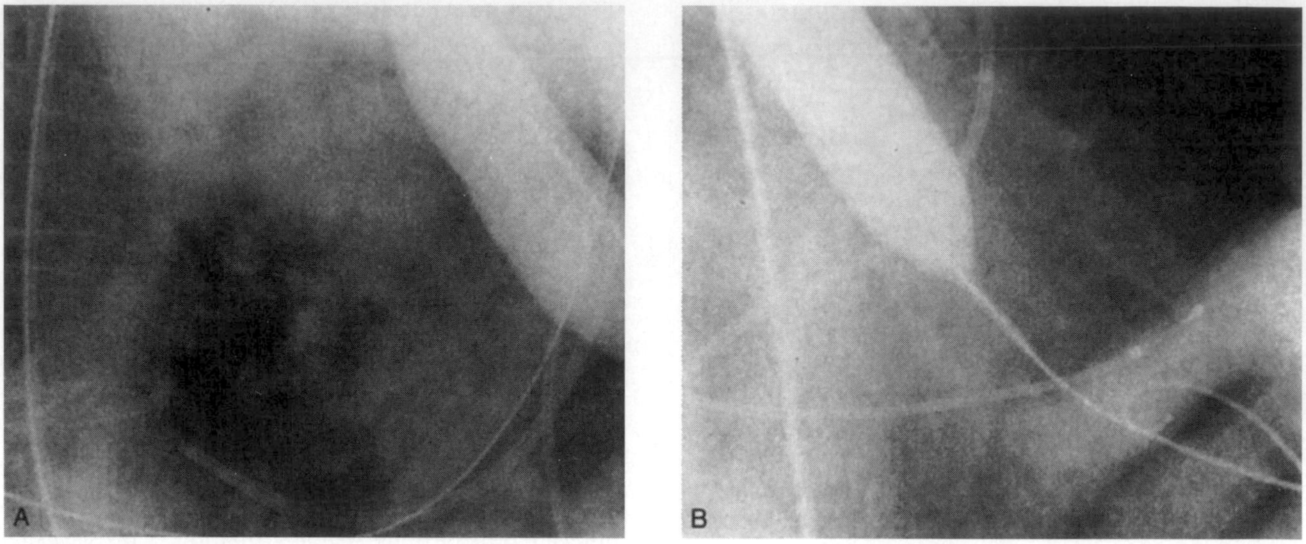

Figure 25–5
A, Valvuloplasty balloon inflated across the aortic valve. Note the indentation ("waist") in the balloon. *B,* Valvuloplasty balloon inflated across the aortic valve after dilation. Note the disappearance of the indentation seen in part *A.* (From Barden, C., et al. [1990]. Balloon aortic valvuloplasty: Nursing care implications. *Critical Care Nurse, 10*(6), 26.)

MITRAL STENOSIS

Because medical management cannot reduce the obstruction through the valve in mitral stenosis, surgery is frequently the treatment of choice. Mitral commissurotomy (surgical division of fused leaflets and release of shortened chordae) is the reconstructive procedure of choice if the mitral valve is pliable; if the valve is not pliable, mitral valve replacement is indicated.

MITRAL REGURGITATION

Surgical intervention should be undertaken before severe left ventricular dysfunction develops. Acute mitral regurgitation in a client who is hemodynamically unstable requires immediate surgical intervention. Reconstruction of the mitral valve is the treatment of choice if the natural valve is not thickened, severely deformed, or calcified.[4, 7, 32] The valve leaflets are surgically drawn together, and the chordae tendineae may be shortened. The circumference of the mitral annulus can be reduced (annuloplasty) with the use of sutures or a flexible ring sewn into the valve.

AORTIC STENOSIS

Surgical intervention should be considered for aortic stenosis when the pressure gradient is greater than 50 mm Hg or the valve orifice is smaller than 0.8 cm^2. Clients with symptomatic aortic stenosis have a poor prognosis without surgical intervention. There is an increase in sudden death once myocardial failure develops. Surgical techniques include valve replacement (see Box 25–5) and balloon aortic valvuloplasty, which uses a catheter with a balloon to dilate the valve orifice (Fig. 25–5).[1]

AORTIC REGURGITATION

Surgical replacement of the incompetent valve provides the only effective long-term intervention for aortic regurgitation. In clients with acute, severe aortic regurgitation and left ventricular failure, early valve replacement can be life-saving. A high percentage of patients with aortic regurgitation and aortic stenosis show striking clinical improvement with valve replacement.[4]

TRICUSPID AND PULMONIC VALVE DISEASE

Intervention for tricuspid valve disorders involves correction of the valvular deformity, usually with annuloplasty and alleviation of the heart failure. Interventions for pulmonic valve disease focus on ameliorating the underlying cause and the presenting signs of right-sided heart failure.

Nursing Management

Assessment

Nursing assessment involves gathering subjective and objective data on:

- type, severity, and progress of the disorder
- degree of heart failure present
- client's tolerance to activity
- client's available support systems
- client's and significant others' understanding of the disorder's nature and the rationale for intervention.

Nursing Diagnosis, Planning, and Implementation

Nursing Diagnosis: Decreased Cardiac Output R/T valvular abnormalities and arrhythmias.

CLIENT EDUCATION GUIDE

Valvular Heart Disease

Teaching should include the following:

- Disease process: factors contributing to symptoms, symptom management, clinical course
- Medications: rationale for use, dosage schedule, administration route, side effects, toxic effects
- The need for antibiotic prophylaxis before any dental or surgical procedures and for informing health care providers of the valve disorder
- The importance of maintaining the prescribed exercise program as tolerated. (Note: Exercise is contraindicated in congestive heart failure; strenuous exercise is contraindicated in aortic stenosis.)
- The need to pace activities and comply with activity restrictions to avoid fatigue, chest pain, or shortness of breath
- The importance of following prescribed dietary restrictions: e.g., restricted-calorie diet for a client who needs to lose weight, low-sodium diet and fluid restrictions for a client with left ventricular failure
- The importance of notifying the physician if new onset of chest pain, palpitations, shortness of breath, peripheral edema, or signs or symptoms of pharyngitis (streptococcal infection) occur.

Planning: Expected Outcomes. The client will maintain or restore normal cardiac output, as evidenced by clear lungs on auscultation, maintenance of stable weight, urine output averaging greater than 30 mL/hr, no reported (or observed) dyspnea or orthopnea, vital signs within normal limits, regular heart rhythm, absence of S_3 and S_4 heart sounds, and decreased or absent peripheral edema.

Implementation. To evaluate the effectiveness of therapeutic interventions, the nurse performs ongoing hemodynamic assessment and monitors vital signs closely every 1 to 4 hours. A decrease in cardiac output is manifested in a compensatory increase in heart rate, decrease in blood pressure, decrease in urine output, and decrease in level of consciousness. The nurse carefully auscultates the chest to identify the presence of adventitious breath sounds (crackles, rhonchi) or heart gallops (S_3, S_4) every 4 hours.

Nursing Diagnosis: Individual Coping, Ineffective R/T chronic nature of valvular disease and activity limitations.

Planning: Expected Outcomes. The client will use adaptive coping strategies, as evidenced by the ability to recognize personal coping patterns and identify appropriate support systems and personal strengths.

Implementation. Valvular heart disease requires life-long management. The disorder's chronicity and potential complications can create an atmosphere of uncertainty, fear, and frustration. The nurse should take time to help the client identify support persons, personal strengths, and coping strategies. The nurse assesses how the client handles frustration or anger and what activities are particularly relaxing. The nurse should address the client's fears and misconceptions. In some instances, counseling referrals may help. The importance of follow-up physical examinations and intervention should be stressed.

Evaluation

The degree of attainment of expected outcomes should be evaluated on an ongoing basis. Because valvular disorders are chronic, extended time frames may be needed for goal attainment. Revisions in the plan of care may be required.

Discharge Teaching

Valvular heart disease is chronic. Treatment may be complex and changeable as the disease progresses and new symptoms arise. The client and significant others need ongoing education and support. (See Client Education Guide: Valvular Heart Disease.)

CARDIAC SURGERY

Cardiac surgery is performed when the probability of survival with a useful life is greater with surgical treatment than with nonsurgical treatment. The first heart surgery, repair of a stenosed mitral valve, was performed in 1923 by Cutler and Levine.[19] Since that time, heart surgery has been revolutionized by the development of cardiopulmonary bypass. Open heart techniques allow the surgeon to directly view the heart structures. The preoperative condition of the client's heart and other body systems greatly influences the results of cardiac surgery. The median sternotomy is the most commonly used surgical approach for heart surgery.

Types of Heart Surgery

There are three types of cardiac surgery: reparative, reconstructive, and substitutional. Reparative surgeries are likely to produce cure or excellent and prolonged improvement. These operations include closure of patent ductus arteriosus, atrial septal defect, and ventricular septal defect; repair of mitral stenosis; and simple repair of tetralogy of Fallot.

Reconstructive procedures are more complex. They are not always curative procedures, and reoperation may be needed. Reconstructive procedures include coronary artery bypass grafting and reconstruction of an incompetent mitral, tricuspid, or aortic valve.

Substitutional surgeries are not usually curative because of the preoperative condition of the client. Examples of substitutional surgeries include valve replacement, cardiac replacement by transplantation, ventricular replacement or assistance, and cardiac replacement by mechanical devices.

Management of the client after heart surgery is discussed later in this section, and a sample clinical pathway for clients undergoing heart surgery is presented in Appendix C.

Heart Transplantation

Cardiac transplantation is now a standard and effective treatment for clients with end-stage cardiac disease. The survival rate for clients who have undergone heart transplantation has improved dramatically as a result of advances in technique and better control of the rejection process. At Stanford University, the mean life expectancy for clients awaiting transplantation (surgery not performed) is about 3 months. More than 80 per cent of clients who receive transplanted hearts survive for at least 1 year; approximately 60 per cent of these clients are alive at 5 years. Another important statistic is that 85 per cent of those 1-year survivors have been rehabilitated and have returned to work or school.[25]

TECHNIQUE

The current orthotopic technique for heart transplant retains a large portion of the recipient's right and left atria and implants the donor heart to the atria (Fig. 25–6*A,B,C*). Cardiopulmonary bypass is used during the operation (see later discussion). Temporary pacemaker wires and chest drainage catheters are inserted.

Another type of heart transplant is the heterotopic transplant. In this form the donor heart is placed parallel to the recipient's heart (Fig. 25–6*D*). The right side of the client's heart can continue to function while the dysfunctional left side of the heart is bypassed.

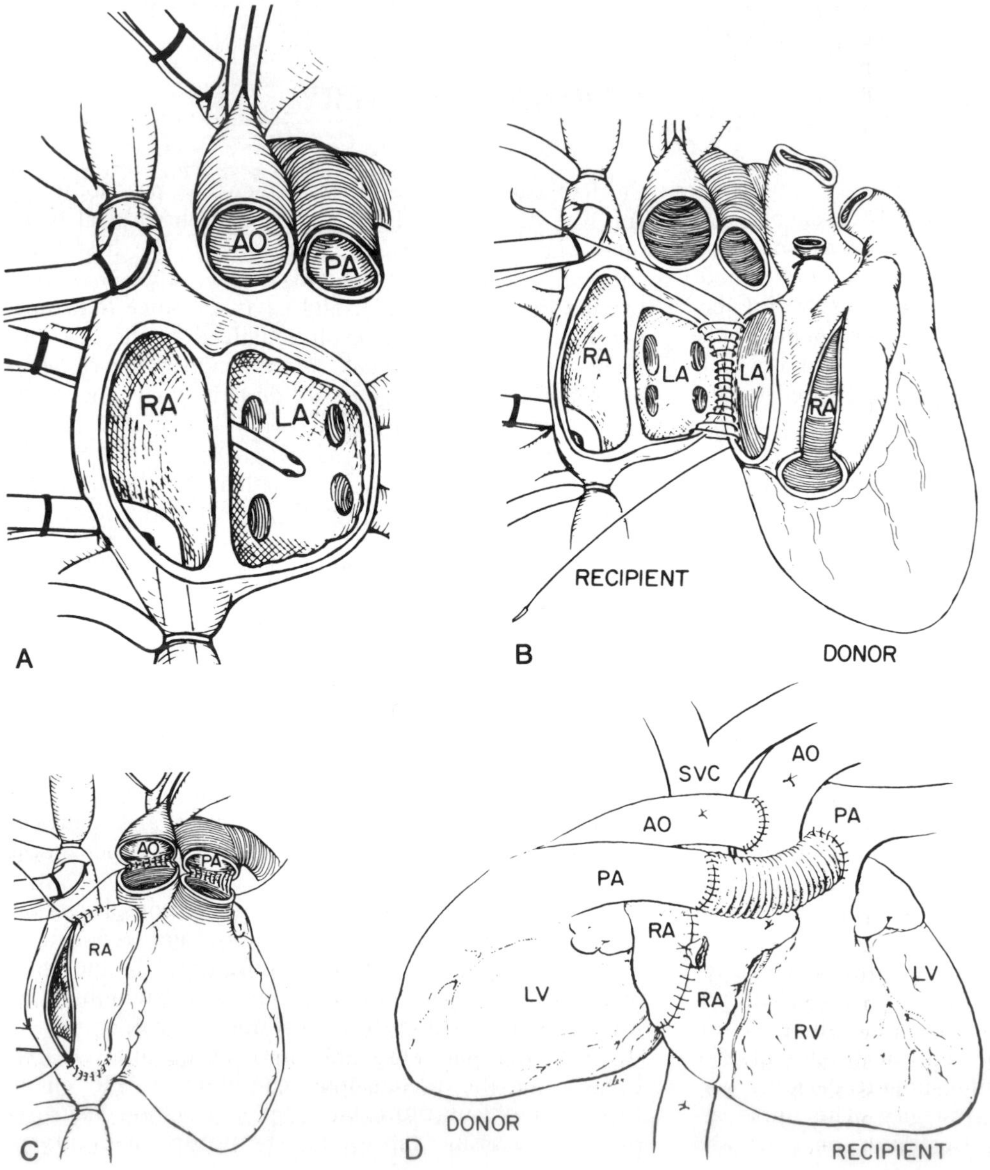

Figure 25–6
Cardiac transplantation. *A* to *C*, Orthotopic transplantation. *D*, Heterotopic transplantation. AO, aorta; LA, left atrium; LV, left ventricle; PA, pulmonary artery; RA, right atrium; RV, right ventricle; SVC, superior vena cava. (From Bolman, R. M. [1990]. Cardiac transplantation: The operative technique. In M. E. Thompson [Ed.], *Cardiac transplantation.* Philadelphia: F. A. Davis.)

THE ARTIFICIAL HEART

The artificial heart is a commercially made device implanted in place of the failing heart. These hearts are made of rubber, silicone, and Teflon and are air-powered through a life-support console. The artificial heart is attached surgically in an operation similar to that described in the heart transplant procedure. Major complications (i.e., hemorrhage, infection, acute tubular necrosis, neurologic disturbances) frequently occur, and the permanent use of the artificial heart is currently not recommended. There is some use of the artificial heart as a bridge to transplantation, helping clients survive until a donor heart can be transplanted.

POSTTRANSPLANTATION CARE

The greatest single problem in performing heart transplants is not the surgical procedure itself but the rejection process by which the client's body rejects the donor heart. Allograft rejection, discussed in Chapter 9, remains poorly understood. The recipient forms antibodies against the foreign heart tissue, which leads to an antigen-antibody reaction. As a result, the heart's lining hemorrhages, the walls thicken, and the myocardium assumes a mottled appearance. Because of the rejection, the new heart fails to function, and circulatory collapse ensues.

Transplantation clients require lifelong immunosuppressive drugs to minimize rejection of the donor heart. Infection is the leading cause of death in these clients.

Transplantation clients demonstrate unique characteristics related to the severing of nerves (denervation) that occurs during transplantation:

- lack of chest pain with myocardial ischemia
- loss of sympathetic stimulation
- orthostatic hypotension
- resting heart rate of 90 to 110 beats/minute.[22]

Medical Management

Stable clients entering the health care facility for elective heart surgery may be admitted the morning of surgery. Thorough medical evaluation will be done on an out-patient basis. Unstable clients may experience angina as the first symptom of coronary artery disease and enter the facility through the emergency department. These clients require extensive psychological support.

Preoperative laboratory tests include urine tests and blood electrolyte, cardiac and liver enzymes, and coagulation studies. Important diagnostic studies that give valuable information about cardiac status include the ECG, phonocardiogram, echocardiogram, vectorcardiogram, chest x-ray films, and cardiac catheterization.

Any physiologic imbalance or problem in cardiac or respiratory status is corrected when possible by means of rest, diet, medication, or other appropriate therapy. Physiologic baselines should be established for postoperative comparison of vital signs, weight, and laboratory values.

Nursing Management

Preparation for surgery is discussed in Chapter 5. However, the client undergoing the stress of heart surgery needs some special preparation and instruction.

Assessment

Data to collect during the initial assessment include

- the primary cardiovascular problem that requires surgical correction and its duration
- the purpose of the surgery and the risk involved
- past cardiopulmonary illnesses that may predispose the client to postoperative complications (e.g., bacterial endocarditis, pulmonary embolus, allergy, abnormal bleeding)
- the degree of cardiac impairment (e.g., does the client have symptoms when at rest or only during exertion?)
- the types of medications and interventions that the client has received or is currently receiving (e.g., digitalis, quinidine, oxygen)
- client's and significant others' understanding of the disease process and surgical intervention.

Psychosocial Assessment: The nurse should note the client's psychosocial readiness for surgery and reactions to the need for heart surgery.

Nursing Diagnosis, Planning, and Implementation: Psychological Preparation

Nursing Diagnosis: Anxiety, Risk for R/T lack of knowledge about the surgery and regarding the health care facility, and possible fear of outcome.

Planning: Expected Outcomes. The client will exhibit or verbalize decreased anxiety, as evidenced by expressing an understanding of immediate postoperative care in the critical care unit (CCU), usual interventions (e.g., ventilator), visiting hours, and probable discharge plans.

Implementation. Psychological preparation of the cardiac surgery client is very important. Preoperative education programs that reduce client and family anxiety are essential. To reduce this preoperative anxiety, such a program should include a thorough explanation of the perioperative procedures. The nurse should give verbal and written information concerning health care facility services, rules, and regulations; visiting hours; the chaplain's name and visitation hours (if appropriate); and names of clinical nurse specialists and other health care professionals who can be contacted for information.

Most clients benefit from a tour of the recovery room and coronary care unit (CCU). This should include the sounds of ECG and respirator alarms. (If the client is not physically able to participate in a tour, audiovisual material is helpful.)

The nurse should allow clients to express in their own words their concerns about their heart problem and the surgery. He or she can correct any misconceptions, using pictures and a model of the heart. Clients tend to ask the greatest number of questions about what will happen to them in the recovery room and CCU. The nurse should prepare them to awaken from anesthesia with a chest tube in place and should also discuss the ventilator that will assist the client's breathing for the first 8 to 24 hours. The nurse should remind clients that during this time they will be unable to talk, but that the nursing staff will observe them constantly. He or she should explain that multiple intravenous lines for fluid or blood will be inserted in the arm, neck, or chest and various equipment that continuously monitors vital signs will be attached to the skin. Clients should also be reassured that lights and alarm noises are part of the critical care environment and do not indicate that something is wrong.

The nurse should emphasize that although the client will experience pain, the pain will be swiftly relieved by medication and comfort measures.

Finally, the nurse should explain that the client will be awakened frequently in the CCU for vital nursing assessments and interventions. He or she can give examples of scheduled activities: vital signs every 15 minutes; temperature every 2 hours; frequent turning, coughing, and deep breathing; blood samples for tests every morning.

Clients also need information concerning discharge from the CCU and health care facility. The nurse explains the average length of stay in the CCU, the room to which the client will return from the CCU, the average length of stay in the health care facility, and the diet and activities permitted once the client is back home. The discussion should be general. The nurse must remember that many unforeseen events can arise and greatly alter the postoperative course.

Preoperative Nursing Care

Preparation the evening before and the day of surgery is essentially the same as the preparation of clients for any thoracic surgery (see Chap. 22). The client may often take several showers with an antimicrobial soap; skin prep (shaving) for a thoracotomy is performed in the operating room. If the surgeon plans a coronary artery bypass graft, the legs may also be prepared in the operating room (see Chap. 5).

Intraoperative Nursing Care

Cardiopulmonary Bypass: Cardiopulmonary bypass is used during cardiac surgery to divert the client's unoxygenated blood and to return reoxygenated blood to the client's circulation. This technique is called extracorporeal circulation (ECC) and is accomplished with a pump oxygenator (heart-lung machine). Through a chest incision, catheters are attached to the superior and inferior vena cava. Blood is diverted from the heart to the pump oxygenator. The diversion of the client's blood allows the surgeon to visualize the heart directly during the operation. The pump oxygenator, more than any other device, has made sophisticated open-heart surgery possible.

The four purposes of the pump oxygenator are to:

- divert circulation from the heart and lungs, providing the surgeon with a bloodless operative field
- perform all gas exchange functions for the body while the client's cardiopulmonary system is at rest (heart not beating and lungs not expanding)
- filter, rewarm, or cool the blood
- circulate oxygenated, filtered blood back into the arterial system.

Although the pump oxygenator is considered safe, it does have risks. The pump can crush and destroy blood cells; sludging of cells can lead to thrombus formation; or air emboli can form. Other complications related to ECC are shock, hemorrhage, hemolysis, and kidney or lung damage.

The extracorporeal membrane oxygenator is a more expensive but improved method of ECC. The advantages include decreased trauma to blood cells and prolonged pump time (up to several days). However, the clinical benefits are still being evaluated.[24]

Hypothermia. During heart surgery, when the client is on cardiopulmonary bypass, the heart and other organs are at risk to develop ischemia. To prevent cardiac damage the heart is cooled to lower than oxygen need. The client is generally systemically cooled to lower than 32 degrees C. This decreases metabolic rate, decreases oxygen demand, and helps preserve major organs.

Postoperative Assessment

The most reliable measures of cardiovascular function and tissue perfusion are the vital signs, including arterial blood pressure, pulses, venous and left heart filling pressures, and temperature. Heart sounds and continuous ECG monitoring are also performed. Stabilization of vital signs after heart surgery usually indicates adequate cardiovascular function. Conversely, severe deviations indicate complications such as hemorrhage, shock, cardiac tamponade, or infection. The normal ranges for each vital sign after cardiac surgery and the meaning of deviations follow.

Most monitors are able to monitor the pulmonary artery, arterial pressures, and ECG tracing simultaneously. This assists in determining the effect that the surgery may have had on hemodynamic status and cardiac output. It can also demonstrate the effect a dysrhythmia, medication, or body temperature change may have on cardiac output.

Arterial Blood Pressure: To obtain a continuous, accurate blood pressure reading postoperatively, the physician places a catheter intra-arterially, usually into the radial artery, and attaches this catheter to a transducer connected to an electronic pressure monitor and oscilloscope. The monitor provides numerical pressure readings and produces a continuous tracing of the arterial pressure waveform as shown in the Bridge to Critical Care. The arterial line is usually irrigated (continuously or at intervals) with heparinized water or saline. The arterial line is often used as a route for obtaining blood for laboratory studies.

In general, the physician will request that the blood pressure be maintained between 20 mm Hg above and

BRIDGE TO CRITICAL CARE

Intra-Aortic Balloon Pumping (IABP)—Counterpulsation

When the left ventricle fails to support adequate circulation and perfusion, intra-aortic balloon pumping can be used in both medical and surgical settings to support the injured or ischemic myocardium. The device consists of a polyethylene balloon that is inserted via the femoral artery into the descending thoracic aorta distal to the left subclavian artery and is connected to an external pneumatic pumping system.

The pump inflates the balloon with helium or carbon dioxide during diastole, and deflates it during systole. The inflation-deflation cycle is triggered by the client's electrocardiogram, specifically, the R wave to signal the beginning of systole. Balloon inflation during diastole augments coronary artery filling. Systolic balloon inflation decreases afterload.

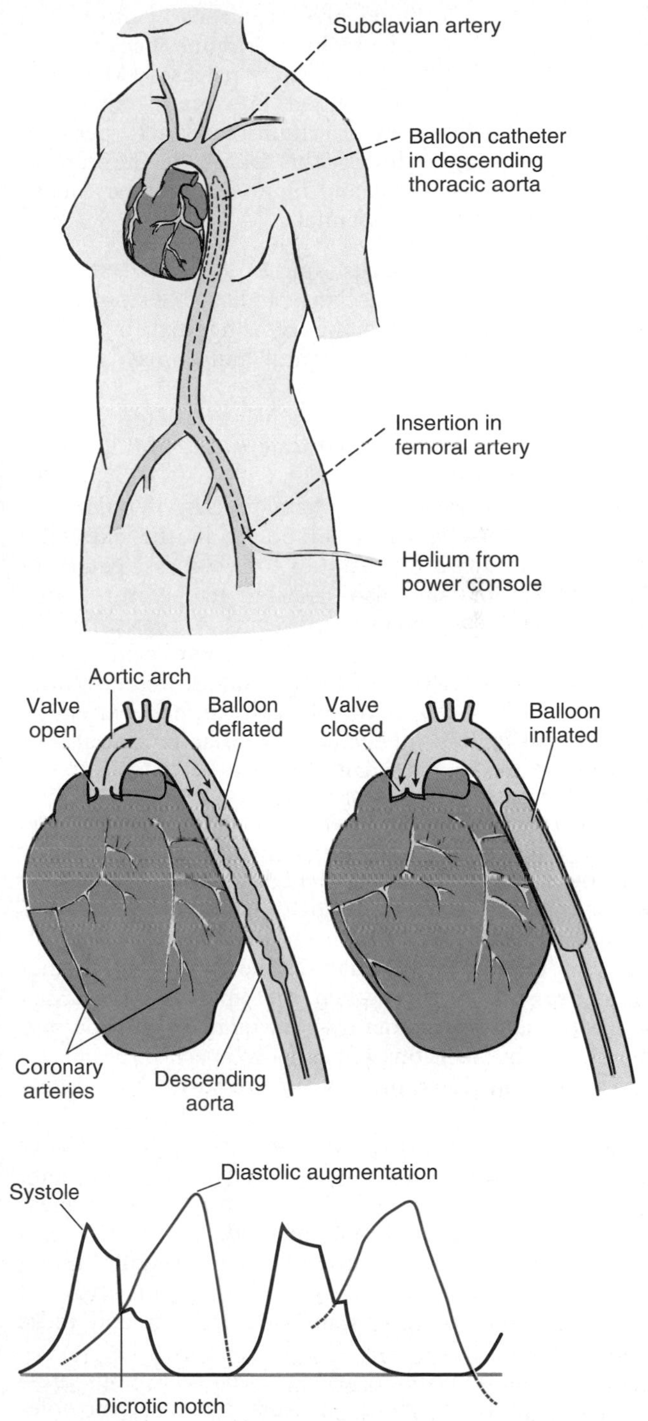

IABP inflating at end of systole (dicrotic notch)
Blood pressure waves

GUIDELINES FOR MANAGEMENT OF IABP

Major Goals

- Aids left ventricular ejection
- Improves cardiac output by reducing myocardial (ventricular) workload
- Increases coronary artery perfusion, decreasing myocardial ischemia
- Reduces the amount of myocardial damage
- Provides hemodynamic stability until definitive treatment can be initiated

Indications for Use

- Complications of acute myocardial infarction
- Cardiogenic shock
- Papillary muscle rupture or dysfunction with severe mitral valve regurgitation
- Refractory ventricular arrhythmias related to ischemias
- Left ventricular failure
- Unstable angina refractory to medications
- Preoperative open heart surgery or cardiac transplantation
- Prophylaxis, noncardiac surgeries, high-risk percutaneous transluminal coronary angioplasty
- Septic shock
- Low cardiac output syndromes

Complications

- On insertion, dissection of the arterial system (femoral, iliac, aorta)
- Dislodgement of plaque, causing embolization
- Balloon rupture
- Arterial occlusion
- Mechanical destruction of red blood cells
- Inability to wean from IABP
- Hematoma at insertion site

Side Effects Requiring Nursing Precautions

- Alterations in tissue perfusion
- Impaired physical mobility
- Risk for alterations in cardiac output
- Anxiety (family)
- Risk for sensory perceptual overload
- Risk for infection
- Risk for bleeding
- Risk for sleep deprivation

Contraindications

- Aortic aneurysm
- Aortic insufficiency
- Central or peripheral atherosclerosis
- Severe left ventricular dysfunction
- Multisystem failure
- Chronic debilitating disease
- Bleeding disorder
- History of emboli

20 mm Hg below the baseline blood pressure. After mitral and aortic valve surgery, clients may tolerate a low systolic blood pressure of 90 mm Hg without difficulty. After surgery on coronary arteries, clients may not tolerate systolic blood pressure drops of more than 10 mm Hg below preoperative baseline because the myocardium may not be adequately perfused. Maintaining a sufficient diastolic blood pressure is also very important because the myocardium receives 70 per cent of its blood supply during this phase of the cardiac cycle. Careful assessment and monitoring of the client's hemodynamic status is essential.

Pulses: The nurse checks apical pulse for rate and rhythm. Rapid apical pulse may indicate dysrhythmias, pain, shock, fear, fever, hypoxia, congestive heart failure, or hemorrhage. Slow apical pulse may indicate heart block or severe anoxia.

The nurse checks apical-radial pulse for a pulse deficit. Pulse deficit may indicate atrial fibrillation, a frequent complication of mitral stenosis.

The nurse assesses peripheral pulses. If pulses are absent, the nurse assesses all pulses in the extremity and check the lower extremities for coldness, pallor, or cyanosis. He or she also assesses temperature, vital signs, and filling pressures. Absence of bilateral pedal pulses may indicate hypothermia or poor cardiac output. Unilateral absence of peripheral pulses may indicate emboli blocking a blood vessel in the extremity. Suspicion of emboli or decreased cardiac output should be reported to the physician immediately.

Venous and Left Heart Filling Pressures: The central venous and pulmonary artery pressures are usually monitored postoperatively. A higher-than-normal pressure may be acceptable after open-heart surgery. This is because a heart that has been diseased and then is subjected to surgical trauma is weak and needs a higher filling pressure to strengthen the force of myocardial contraction and to maintain an adequate cardiac output. Therefore, the surgeon will usually specify parameters for venous and pulmonary artery pressures that address this problem.

If the client has a pulmonary artery (Swan-Ganz) catheter in place, a pulmonary artery wedge pressure (PAWP) can be obtained and a cardiac output measured by the thermodilution method. The PAWP is a reflection of the left ventricular end-diastolic filling pressure. (See the Bridge to Critical Care in Chap. 23 for a discussion of the Swan-Ganz catheter and these parameters.)

Causes of abnormally elevated central venous pressure and left heart filling pressure include hypervolemia, hypothermia, pain, and ineffective myocardial contractions. Abnormally decreased central venous pressure and left heart filling pressure result from hypovolemia, vasodilation, and decreased preload.

Body Temperature: Initially, the client has a low temperature of 35° to 36° C (95° to 96.8° F) because of hypothermia induced during surgery. With careful warming in a heating blanket, the client may reach a normal temperature within 4 hours. The nurse should be aware that the blood pressure and filling pressures may drop dramatically as body temperature elevates.

The temperature may rise 1° to 1.5° C (2° to 3° F) above normal during the first or second day postoperatively and may remain elevated for 3 to 4 days. The nurse should treat this with acetaminophen suppositories as prescribed and minimal bed covering. For persistent elevations, ice bags can be applied or a hypothermia blanket used, if prescribed.

Abnormally low temperatures ranging from 34.4° to 36° C (94° to 96.8° F) result from shock or cardiac decompensation. The physician may order a warming blanket to increase temperature.

Respirations: To assess respiratory function, prevent respiratory complications, and provide appropriate intervention, the nurse should closely monitor the rate and depth of respirations, presence of dyspnea, and presence of wheezing or crackles.

The nurse should make certain that the ventilator is set at a rate that adequately ventilates the client and delivers an appropriate tidal volume and oxygen percentage. A conscious client may initiate respirations in addition to those delivered by the ventilator (usually the assist light will come on). Adjustments are usually determined by arterial blood gas analysis and the assessments by the physician and the nurse.

Assessment of depth of respiration may reveal shallow respirations, which may be due to pain. The nurse can give a prescribed narcotic analgesic, provided that vital signs are stable.

Assessment of dyspnea may reveal that the client is "fighting" the ventilator, in other words, breathing against instead of with the machine. This can lead to inadequate ventilation, and the client may feel short of breath. Airway obstruction (possibly due to excessive secretions), pain, fear, anoxia, acidosis, hemorrhage, and improper placement of the tube may cause the client to have difficulty in breathing and must be investigated immediately. The physician usually orders arterial blood gas studies and a chest film. The ventilator settings may need adjustment, and the client may require sedation. (See the Bridge to Critical Care for ventilators in Chap. 20.)

CRITICAL TO REMEMBER

While the client is on the ventilator, the nurse must make sure that the ventilator alarms are functioning. The alarms should never be turned off, not even during suctioning.

Wheezing or crackles result from pulmonary edema, bronchospasm, or airway obstruction. They may be treated with bronchodilators, diuretics, or suctioning.

The nurse assesses color and amount of pulmonary secretions and accompanying signs of retained secretions: apprehension, perspiration, rapid pulse, dyspnea, cyanosis, gurgling respirations, and triggering of the high pressure alarm on the ventilator.

Assessment of respiration in the pre-extubation period involves drawing blood for arterial blood gas analysis and measuring respiratory parameters including inspiratory effort and tidal volume. The client is ready for extubation if these values are within normal limits.

Respiratory assessment in the postextubation period begins with careful assessment of clinical manifestations of respiratory distress. The nurse checks the rate, depth, and character of respirations frequently and notes the client's skin color and vital signs; changes may indicate inadequate ventilation and the need for reintubation. Arterial blood gases should be analyzed for determining whether the client is breathing adequately after extubation.

Heart Sounds: For the first two days postoperatively, the nurse assesses heart sounds at least every 4 hours. Pericardial rubs are commonly caused by the irritation and inflammation from surgery. A new murmur may indicate valve problems. The nurse should notify the physician if one develops. A gallop probably indicates heart failure. (See cardiovascular assessment in Chap. 23.)

Electrocardiogram Tracings: The nurse monitors electrical activity of the client's heart continuously for at least 3 or 4 days after surgery and observes carefully for abnormal ECG tracings. Heart block, ventricular tachycardia, and atrial fibrillation commonly complicate open-heart surgery. These are treated pharmacologically or with electric shock. The physician requests 12-lead ECGs preoperatively, immediately postoperatively, and before discharge to observe for signs of perioperative infarction.

Often the surgeon implants atrial or ventricular pacing wires during surgery. These are small wires that lead from the myocardium through the chest wall. They can be connected to an external pacemaker and used to treat bradycardias or heart blocks. These wires should always be insulated. When connecting them to a pacemaker, the nurse should wear rubber gloves. Microshocks to these wires could result in atrial or ventricular fibrillation.

Chest Drainage: The nurse checks chest drainage from chest tubes. The surgeon inserts chest tubes to drain air and fluid from the pleural cavity, thereby allowing the lungs to reexpand after surgery. Chest tubes can also drain the pericardial sac. These tubes are referred to as mediastinal tubes.

The nurse measures and observes chest drainage by collecting drainage in a calibrated cylinder. Findings are measured and recorded hourly. Up to 100 mL of drainage may be lost during the first hour postoperatively as a result of re-expansion of the lungs, which forces drainage through the chest tube. There will be approximately 500 mL of drainage over the first 24 hours. Large gushes of drainage are sometimes expelled when the client coughs or turns. Drainage, usually dark red during the early postoperative phase, gradually becomes more serous as time passes. Some facilities use autotransfusions from chest tube drainage to replace the client's blood loss.

Fluid Balance: The nurse carefully measures and records intake and output and obtains daily weights to determine whether the client is retaining fluids within tissues or losing excessive fluid rapidly. Significant fluctuations in weight act as a guide to fluid replacement.

Renal Function: The nurse measures volume hourly for the first 8 to 12 hours after surgery. The client almost always has an indwelling urinary catheter. Normal output is greater than 30 mL/hr. Urine may be bloody as a result of hemolysis of erythrocytes during ECC.

The specific gravity should be assessed. Normal findings are 1.015 to 1.020. Specific gravity may rise because of oliguria or presence of red blood cells. Lowered specific gravity results from overhydration or inability of kidney tubules to filter waste products.

Electrolyte Balance and Blood Studies: Daily electrolyte studies are performed to determine blood levels of sodium, potassium, and chloride. The physician replaces electrolytes parenterally if they are deficient. When diuretics are given to reduce volume overload, the nurse monitors potassium closely and replaces as prescribed. The heart may be particularly sensitive to hypokalemia soon after surgery. The nurse obtains hematocrit, hemoglobin, and prothrombin time daily to determine the extent of blood loss or hemorrhage.

Pain Management: Postoperatively clients must participate in activities that enhance positive outcomes. These include position changes, coughing, early ambulation, incentive spirometry.[33] Postoperative pain can inhibit these activities and have a negative effect on vital signs, rest, and mental status. Pain is typically managed with incremental doses of intravenous morphine sulfate and oral medications such as acetaminophen, nonsteroidal anti-inflammatory drugs, and codeine.

Neurologic Response: After heart surgery, the nurse carefully observes the client's level of consciousness, pupil size and reaction, orientation, and ability to move extremities.

The client should awaken within 1 to 2 hours after surgery. Failure to awaken may result from embolization of air, calcium, fat, or thrombotic particles to the brain. Slow return to consciousness (over 2 to 4 days) may result from a diffuse neurologic deficit because of poor cerebral capillary perfusion during ECC.

The nurse checks pupils hourly during the early postoperative period for size, equality in size, and reaction to light. Sluggish pupillary response may indicate neurologic damage.

Disorientation and restlessness may indicate anoxia or embolization to the brain. Also, fatigue, pain, or fear can produce mental confusion.

Hemiplegia, inability to move an extremity, or extreme weakness of an extremity may indicate embolization to the motor area of the brain.

After cardiac surgery, clients may become disoriented, delusional, and psychotic. Severe depression is not uncommon. Causes of confusion, hallucinations, and psychotic behavior include isolation within the intensive care unit, sensory deprivation, sleep deprivation, fear and anxiety, an impersonal environment if care providers are preoccupied with monitors and machines, and desynchronization of circadian rhythm (CCUs are active and well-lighted 24 hours a day). Causes of postoperative depression include fatigue and debility after surgery and resumption of responsibilities.

Nursing Diagnosis: Decreased Cardiac Output, Risk for R/T heart failure, metabolic acidosis, weakening of the left ventricle, dysrhythmias, and cardiac tamponade.

Planning: Expected Outcomes. The client will have improved cardiovascular function, as evidenced by adequate tissue perfusion, stabilization of vital signs, clear lung sounds on auscultation, stable body weight, adequate urine output (30 mL/hour or greater), no reported or observed dyspnea or orthopnea, regular heart sounds without S_3 or S_4, and decreased or absent peripheral edema (blood pressure within 20 mm Hg of baseline values).

Implementation. Intervention for a failing heart muscle often involves administration of blood products or inotropic agents (e.g., dopamine, isoproterenol, or epinephrine), which increase cardiac contractility. Inotropic agents should be administered cautiously, because they also increase the work of the heart and its need for oxygen.

Complications resulting from persistent hypotension are cerebral ischemia, renal shutdown, myocardial infarction, and shock. To correct these complications, the surgeon may use some mechanical device to support the failing heart if medications are unsuccessful.

The intra-aortic balloon pump is a counterpulsation device that supports the failing heart by increasing coronary artery perfusion and reducing afterload. It consists of a sausage-shaped balloon catheter that is passed through the femoral artery and positioned in the descending thoracic aorta just distal to the subclavian artery. This catheter is attached to a power console that inflates and deflates the balloon in time with the heart. The balloon is inflated during diastole; blood is pushed back into the aorta, and coronary artery perfusion is improved. The balloon is deflated during systole; systemic vascular resistance is decreased, and thereby the workload of the heart is reduced (see the Bridge to Critical Care). A registered nurse with specific education in the use of the balloon pump is assigned to care for the client in this situation. Timing the pulsation to the contraction of the heart, monitoring the effects of the pumping on the client's vital signs, and careful assessment of the extremity distal to the pump require special skills.

Collaborative Problem: Hypertension R/T epinephrine release and hypothermia.

Planning: Expected Outcomes. The nurse will monitor the client for hypertension, as evidenced by blood pressure 20 mm Hg over baseline for sustained periods.

Implementation

CRITICAL TO REMEMBER

Hypertension is dangerous in a client who has undergone a coronary artery bypass graft, because the high blood pressure may cause the new graft to break loose or leak.

Pain and anxiety can increase blood pressure. The nurse should use comfort techniques, explain all procedures (even to the unconscious client), and administer pain medications. Vasoactive medications can be used to improve cardiac functioning (e.g., vasodilators such as sodium nitroprusside).

Nursing Diagnosis: Airway Clearance, Ineffective, Risk for R/T retained secretions.

Planning: Expected Outcomes. The client will exhibit improved airway clearance, as evidenced by clear lung sounds, afebrile state, strong nonproductive cough, and arterial blood gas values within normal limits.

Implementation. The nurse should frequently turn and suction the intubated client and help the nonintubated client turn, take deep breaths, and cough every 1 to 2 hours; the trachea should be suctioned if the temperature rises above 38.5° C (101° F) and the client is coughing ineffectively. In addition, the client can wear a high-humidity oxygen mask after removal of the endotracheal tube for help in loosening secretions. Chest physiotherapy can be used to loosen secretions. Early ambulation is encouraged. Complications of retained secretions include atelectasis, pneumonia, and subsequent inadequate oxygenation of the tissues. The physician orders portable chest films daily until the lungs have re-expanded.

Collaborative Problem: Dysrhythmias, Risk for R/T potassium imbalance, trauma to the conduction system during surgery, hypoxia, decreased cardiac output, or acidosis.

Planning: Expected Outcomes. The nurse will monitor the client for dysrhythmias, as evidenced by changes in heart rhythm on the ECG.

Implementation. Most dysrhythmias can be effectively treated with antiarrhythmic medications. These medications are listed in Chapter 24. Some life-threatening dysrhythmias require defibrillation or cardioversion (see Chap. 24).

Collaborative Problem: Hemorrhage R/T surgical trauma or slipped ligature.

Planning: Expected Outcomes. The nurse will monitor the client for amounts of drainage in excess of 2 mL/kg body weight/hour or a sustained period of bleeding through the chest tube (over 1 minute).

Implementation. The physician should be notified immediately, because the client may need to be returned to the operating room for repair of the bleeding sites.

The nurse replaces blood by transfusion as prescribed. If the client's hematocrit level is adequate, albumin or high-molecular-weight plasma expanders, such as hetastarch, may be prescribed in place of blood.

Collaborative Problem: Cardiac Tamponade R/T occlusion in the pericardial drainage system.

Planning: Expected Outcomes. The nurse will monitor the client for sudden cessation of chest drainage with an increase in venous pressure, pulsus paradoxus, dyspnea, oliguria, distant or inaudible heart sounds, or lowered left atrial pressure.

Implementation. Gentle milking of the chest tube

to express clots that could block drainage may be performed. If clots cannot be removed by gentle milking of the tube, the physician may need to declot the tube using a long catheter with an inflatable balloon on the end. The client may need to be returned to the operating room or have a pericardial tap for removal of fluid.

Collaborative Problem: Renal Failure, Risk for R/T hypovolemia, decreased cardiac output, or hemolysis of erythrocytes during cardiopulmonary bypass.

Planning: Expected Outcomes. The client will have urinary output greater than 30 mL/hour.

Implementation. A client with decreased urine output may be treated with extra fluids (sometimes called a fluid challenge) if dehydration is the probable etiologic factor. Other interventions may include correcting shock or low output failure and administering a diuretic (e.g., furosemide) intravenously. The client who develops renal failure may require peritoneal dialysis or hemodialysis.

Nursing Diagnosis: Tissue Perfusion, Altered Cerebral, Risk for R/T surgical procedure and hemodynamic stability.

Planning: Expected Outcomes. The client will demonstrate adequate cerebral tissue perfusion, as evidenced by continuous progress toward an alert level of consciousness.

Implementation. To prevent mental confusion, undue fear, anxiety, and tension, the nurse should:

- Always address the client by name and introduce himself or herself by name.
- Place a calendar and clock at the bedside to orient the client to the date and time of day.
- Take an interest in the client. Do not ignore the client while working with monitors and equipment.
- Position the cardiac monitor so that it is out of the client's view. Many clients are nervous when watching their own heart action.
- Schedule the day so that periods of nursing intervention alternate with periods of rest and relaxation.
- Encourage the client to freely discuss fears and anxieties.
- Prepare significant others for changes in the client's sensorium after surgery. Before visiting times, warn visitors if the client is hallucinating or is severely depressed so that they know what to expect.
- Explain all interventions to the client and allow time for questions.

Nursing Diagnosis: Physical Mobility, Impaired, Risk for R/T prolonged bed rest after surgery.

Planning: Expected Outcomes. The client will demonstrate postoperative mobility, as evidenced by having mobility that is equal or greater than preoperative mobility.

Implementation. Prolonged periods of bed rest after heart surgery (or any surgery) may cause weakness, pooling of respiratory secretions, atelectasis, thrombophlebitis, osteoporosis, urinary retention, renal calculi, a negative nitrogen balance, and depression. Planned activity is the most important single factor in preventing the complications of bed rest. The type and amount of activity allowed for each client depend on the type of surgery and the client's general postoperative condition.

Turning and Exercising. If the client is stable, the nurse can turn him or her from side to side at intervals for back care. Valve replacement clients may have turning restrictions. The nurse performs passive exercises and leg flexion every 2 hours to prevent thrombosis of lower extremities.

Typical Ambulation Schedule. In a stable client, progression ambulation begins the day after surgery, the client usually dangles her or his legs over the side of the bed for a short period. That evening or on the second postoperative day, the client usually sits in a chair for a brief time. The client progresses to ambulating in the hall by the third postoperative day. Cardiac telemetry monitors are used to evaluate the client's response to increasing activity. Vital signs are taken before, during, and after exercise. Authorities recommend a rise no more than 20 beats per minute in the immediate postoperative period.

It usually takes 8 to 10 weeks for clients to fully regain strength after surgery. The client is discharged with a progressive walking program and may be referred to a cardiac rehabilitation out-patient clinic. (See Phase II Cardiac Rehabilitation, Chap. 24.) The client may be evaluated with a stress test at approximately 6 weeks postoperatively to establish an exercise prescription. The client usually returns to work 2 months after surgery.

Collaborative Problem: Rejection of the Transplanted Heart R/T immune reaction after surgery.

Planning: Expected Outcomes. The nurse will monitor for clinical manifestations of rejection, as evidenced by decreases in oxygenation, fever, malaise, anxiety, and infiltrates on chest film.

Implementation. Rejection and infection are the most common complications of cardiac transplantation. The prevention of rejection with immunosuppression is continually being examined (Box 25–6). Cyclosporine has been helpful in preventing rejection but is quite toxic. Renal failure, hypertension, liver toxic effects, and neurologic disturbances are not uncommon.

Nursing Diagnosis: Infection, Risk for R/T loss of primary defenses and use of immunosuppressive agents in clients with transplant.

Planning: Expected Outcomes. The client will exhibit no clinical manifestations of infection, as evidenced by remaining afebrile and having white blood cell levels within normal limits, no malaise, healed surgical incision, and no abnormal heart sounds.

Implementation. Infection remains the major cause of death in the early postoperative period as well as a major cause of death after 1 year. Clients are treated prophylactically with antibiotics. Nonhealing sternal wounds are promptly treated. Omental grafts may be required.

Evaluation

The degree of expected outcome attainment should be examined frequently. Some of the problems discussed in

BOX 25-6

Stanford University Immunosuppressive Protocol for Heart Transplantation—1988

CYCLOSPORINE

Loading dose 2–8 mg/kg 2–3 hours preoperatively (dose according to preoperative renal function)

Target serum level (first month) 100–150 ng/mL
Target serum level (thereafter) 50–150 ng/mL

STEROIDS

Methylprednisolone 500 mg intraoperatively
Methylprednisolone 125 mg intravenously every 8 hours × 3
Prednisone beginning 0.6 mg/kg/day + tapering

AZATHIOPRINE

Loading dose 4 mg/kg intravenously 2–3 hours preoperatively (to white blood cell tolerance)

Maintenance 1–2 mg/kg/day (to white blood cell tolerance)

OKT_3

5 mg intravenously every day × 14 days beginning postoperative day 1

From Hurst, J. W. (1990). *The heart* (7th ed.). New York: McGraw-Hill.

the care of the client after heart surgery require prompt treatment (e.g., dysrhythmias); others can be evaluated over longer periods of time. Revisions in the plan of care may be required.

Discharge Teaching

Clients are discharged to home as early as 1 week after surgery. The client and significant others need written instructions to follow at home. The instructions should include information about the occurrence of postoperative depression. The client requires information on activity, diet, wound care, and medications. (See Client Education Guide: Post–Heart Surgery.)

Modification of Plan of Care for the Elderly

Age is not a contraindication to heart surgery. Previously fit elderly persons tolerate surgery well.[35] Elderly clients often have many other disorders that interfere with or delay their ability to respond to the hemodynamic changes with surgery and during recovery. Elderly clients are also more prone to problems with skin breakdown and renal impairment. Statistically they require longer ventilator support. Early ambulation and resumption of activity improves functional capacity at the time of discharge.[35] Fluids must be closely titrated.

THE ADULT CLIENT WITH A SURGICALLY CORRECTED DEFECT

Because of the dramatic advances in surgical treatment of children with congenital heart defects in the 1960s, many of these children are living into adulthood. Many of these clients have residual or potential problems, sequelae, or complications that may require medical care. There are also unavoidable consequences of some successful surgical repairs.[38] The only surgery that is not likely to have any long-term problems is the repair of a patent ductus.

There may be only a minor problem that remains after surgical repair. A residual murmur may be found. Proper assessment is crucial for proper diagnosis. Noninvasive diagnostic procedures like color-flow Doppler echocardiography are helpful.

The risk of infective endocarditis is increased in those with artificial valves or with suture repair of atrial septal defect.

CLIENT EDUCATION GUIDE

Post–Heart Surgery

Discharge teaching should include the following instructions to the client:

- In the 6 weeks that it takes for the sternum to heal, do not drive, do not lift anything weighing more than 5 pounds, and do not use your arms to push out of bed or a chair.
- During prescribed progressive exercise, count your pulse rate to monitor your exercise tolerance. (Refer the client to the cardiac rehabilitation clinic.)
- Follow a healthy cardiac diet: low cholesterol and low sodium. (Refer the client to the dietitian.)
- Inspect the surgical wound daily. After showering, may apply povidone-iodine and a dressing to oozing areas. Report any change in drainage from serous to purulent and any new opening in the wound.
- Follow the prescribed dosage schedule for all medications; report any untoward side effects.
- Make sure that a significant other knows how to apply your antiembolism stockings.
- Notify the physician of signs and symptoms of infection (fever, increased tenderness, redness or swelling of incision), palpitations or tachycardia, dizziness or fatigue, sudden weight gain or peripheral edema, shortness of breath, or chest pain.
- Monitor character of stools. May be discharged on stool softeners. Do not strain to evacuate the bowel.
- Keep follow-up appointments.

It is not uncommon for a client with a repaired coarctation of the aorta to find that the aorta has gradually become narrowed again. Frequently, these clients may develop idiopathic hypertension.

Clients who have had cyanotic defects repaired as children are likely to have sequelae and complications in adulthood.[38] There may be some degree of exercise intolerance that can be better managed after proper stress testing.

Arrhythmias frequently present a life-long complication. Clients who have had intraventricular repairs may present with ventricular arrhythmias or complete heart block. A 24-hour Holter monitor and stress testing may help evaluate the client's activity tolerance.

STUDY QUESTIONS

1. Which of the following clients is at greatest risk to develop infective endocarditis?
   a. An elderly client with a mitral murmur scheduled to have a proctoscopy.
   b. A 55-year-old client undergoing dental surgery 2 years after coronary artery bypass graft surgery.
   c. A pregnant woman having dental surgery.
   d. An intravenous drug user.
   A. a & b
   B. a & d
   C. b & d
   D. b & c
2. In evaluating discharge teaching with a client recovering from acute bacterial endocarditis, which of the following statements best displays client understanding?
   A. "I can never get this disease again."
   B. "I will call the doctor if I start to feel sick again, develop a fever, or feel that my heart is racing."
   C. "When I feel better, I can stop the antibiotics."
   D. "I won't see my grandchildren–they might catch this."
3. Mitral insufficiency is commonly associated with:
   A. Increased afterload
   B. Left atrial hypertrophy
   C. Angina and syncope
   D. Systemic hypertension
4. When assessing a client with aortic stenosis, the nurse would expect to see all of the following clinical findings except:
   A. Dyspnea
   B. Activity intolerance
   C. Systolic murmur in the second intercostal space radiating to the neck
   D. Pansystolic murmur at the apex
5. Following mitral valve replacement surgery, a client's vital signs are: heart rate, 110; blood pressure, 90/60; pulmonary artery wedge pressure, 4; urine output, 15 mL for 2 hours. The client is alert, and the pedal pulses are palpable. The nurse should anticipate administration of:
   A. IV fluids to replace volume
   B. Inotropic medications
   C. Pain medication
   D. Intravenous nitroprusside drip
6. A client is admitted to the CCU with the medical diagnosis of dilated cardiomyopathy with left ventricular failure. On physical examination, the nurse detects dyspnea, an S_3 heart sound, and inspiratory crackles. What action(s) should the nurse take?
   a. Place the client in high Fowler's position.
   b. Monitor fluid intake and output.
   c. Administer digoxin and furosemide as ordered by the physician.
   d. Have the client ambulate to help mobilize secretions.
   A. a
   B. a & b
   C. a, b, & c
   D. All of the above

CRITICAL THINKING EXERCISES

SCENARIO A

A previously active 70-year-old client develops acute bacterial endocarditis following a proctoscopy. The physician recommends mitral valve replacement to correct symptomatic mitral insufficiency. What type of clinical course would you anticipate for this client?

SCENARIO B

Heart transplantation is the only option for survival for clients with end-stage cardiomyopathy. Availability of organs remains a problem. Is it the nurse's role or responsibility to approach families of clients declared brain dead as possible organ donors?

BIBLIOGRAPHY

1. Barden, C., et al. (1990). Balloon aortic valvuloplasty: Nursing care implications. *Critical Care Nurse, 10(6),* 22–30, 86.
2. Bates, B. (1991). *A guide to physical examination and history taking* (5th ed.). Philadelphia: J. B. Lippincott.
3. Blanche, C., et al. (1990). Technical aspects of cardiopulmonary bypass. In R. J. Gray & J. M. Matloff (Eds.), *Medical management of the cardiac surgery patient.* Baltimore: Williams and Wilkins.
4. Braunwald, E. (1992). Valvular heart disease. In E. Braunwald (Ed.), *Heart disease: A textbook of cardiovascular medicine* (4th ed.). Philadelphia: W. B. Saunders.

5. Carpenito, L. J. (1993). *Nursing diagnosis: Application to Clinical Practice* (5th ed.). Philadelphia: J. B. Lippincott.
6. Cerney, M. (1993). Solving the organ donor shortage by meeting the bereaved family needs. *Critical Care Nurse, 13(1),* 32–38.
7. Craver, J. M. (1990). Surgical reconstruction for regurgitant lesions of the mitral valve. In J. W. Hurst (Ed.), *The heart.* New York: McGraw-Hill.
8. Durack, D. T. (1990). Infective and non-infective endocarditis. In J. W. Hurst (Ed.), *The heart.* New York: McGraw-Hill.
9. Enfanto, P., et al. (1994). Percutaneous laser myopathy: Nursing care implications. *Critical Care Nurse, 14(3),* 94–100.
10. Fitzgerald, C. A. (1993). Current perspective on prosthetic heart valves and valve repair. *AACN Clinical Issues in Critical Care Nursing, 4(2),* 228–243.
11. Fragomeni, L. S., et al. (1990). Donor identification and organ procurement for cardiac transplantation. In M. E. Thompson (Ed.), *Cardiac transplantation.* Philadelphia: F. A. Davis.
12. Friedman, W. F. (1992). Congenital heart disease in infancy and childhood. In E. Braunwald (Ed.), *Heart disease* (4th ed.). Philadelphia: W. B. Saunders.
13. Grover, F., et al. (1994). Determinants of the occurence of and survival from prosthetic valve endocarditis: Experiences of Veterans Affairs Cooperative Study on Valvular Heart Disease. *Journal of Thoracic and Cardiovascular Surgery, 108(2),* 207–214.
14. Guzzetta, C. E. (1984). The person with infective endocarditis. In C. E. Guzzetta & B. M. Dossey (Eds.), *Cardiovascular nursing.* St. Louis: C. V. Mosby.
15. Guzzetta, C. E., et al. (1989). *Clinical assessment tools for use with nursing diagnosis.* St. Louis: C. V. Mosby.
16. Guzzetta, C. E., & Dossey, B. M. (1990). Cardiovascular assessment. In B. M. Dossey et al. (Eds.), *Essentials of critical care nursing.* Philadelphia: J. B. Lippincott.
17. Guyton, A. C. (1991). *Textbook of medical physiology* (8th ed.). Philadelphia: W. B. Saunders.
18. Guyton, R. A., & Hatcher, C. R. (1990). Techniques of valvular surgery. In J. W. Hurst (Ed.), *The heart.* New York: McGraw-Hill.
19. Hancock, E. W. (1984). Congenital heart disease. In E. Rubenstein (Ed.), *Scientific American Medicine.* New York: Scientific American.
20. Hastillo, A., & Hess, M. L. (1990). Selection of patients for cardiac transplantation. In M. E. Thompson (Ed.), *Cardiac transplantation.* Philadelphia: F. A. Davis.
21. Huang, S., et al. (1989). *Coronary care nursing* (2nd ed.). Philadelphia: W. B. Saunders.
22. Hudak, C., & Gallo, B. (1994). *Critical care nursing: A holistic approach* (6th ed.). Philadelphia: J. B. Lippincott.
23. Hurst, J. W. (Ed.) (1994). *New types of cardiovascular diseases: Topics in clinical cardiology.* New York: Igaku-Shoin.
24. Ingram, R. H., & Braunwald, E. (1992). Pulmonary edema: Cardiogenic and noncardiogenic. In E. Braunwald (Ed.), *Heart disease* (4th ed.). Philadelphia: W. B. Saunders.
25. Johnston, J. (1991). A new beginning: Current trends in pediatric heart transplantation. *Focus on Critical Care, 18(1),* 23–28.
26. Kaplan, E. L. (1990). Acute rheumatic fever. In J. W. Hurst (Ed.), *The heart* (7th ed., p. 1524). New York: McGraw-Hill.
27. Kereiakes, D. J., et al. (1983). Apical hypertrophic cardiomyopathy. *American Heart Journal, 105(5),* 855–856.
28. Kirklin, J. W., et al. (1992). Cardiac surgery. In E. Braunwald (Ed.), *Heart disease* (4th ed.). Philadelphia: W. B. Saunders.
29. Lee, M. E., & Gray, R. J. (1990). Low output states following cardiac surgery. In R. J. Gray & J. M. Matloff (Eds.), *Medical management of the cardiac surgery patient.* Baltimore: Williams & Wilkins.
30. Lee, R. E., & Ramos, R. (1990). Nursing care of the cardiac surgical patient. In R. J. Gray & J. M. Matloff (Eds.), *Medical management of the cardiac surgery patient.* Baltimore: Williams & Wilkins.
31. Lorell, B. H., & Braunwald, E. (1992). Pericardial disease. In E. Braunwald, (Ed.), *Heart disease* (4th ed.). Philadelphia: W. B. Saunders.
32. Magilligan, D. J. (1987). Advantages and disadvantages of tissue valves. In P. J. Starek (Ed.), *Heart valve replacement and reconstruction.* Chicago: Year Book Medical Publishers.
33. Maxam-Moore, V., Wilkie, D., & Woods, S. (1994). Analgesics for cardiac surgery patients in critical care: Describing current practices. *American Journal of Critical Care, 3(1),* 31–38.
34. McCoy, L., & Bell, S. (1994). Organ donation and the rural critical care nurse. *American Journal of Critical Care Nurses, 3(6),* 473–475.
35. Messerti, F. (Ed.). (1993). *Cardiovascular disease in the elderly.* Boston: Kluwer Academic Publishers.
36. Monahan, R., Drake, T., & Neighbors, M. (1994). Adults with circulatory dysfunction. In Monahan, T., et al. (Eds.). *Nursing Care of Adults.* Philadelphia: W. B. Saunders.
37. Miller, D., & Borer, J. (1983). Cardiomyopathies: A pathophysiologic approach to therapeutic management. *Archives of Internal Medicine, 143,* 2157–2162.
38. Nugent, E. W., et al. (1990). The pathology, abnormal physiology, clinical recognition, and medical and surgical treatment of congenital heart disease. In J. W. Hurst (Ed.), *The heart* (7th ed.). New York: McGraw-Hill.
39. Parker-Cohen, P. D., et al. (1994). Alterations of cardiovascular function. In K. L. McCance & S. E. Huerther (Eds.), *Pathophysiology* (2nd ed.). St. Louis: Mosby-Year Book.
40. Penderson, A., Groves, R., Coleman, B., Gresov, G., Shaeffer-McCall, G., & Staring, S. (1993). Intramuscular administration of RATG in heart transplant patients. *Critical Care Nurse,* 13(1), 22–31.
41. Permanyer-Miralda, G., et al. (1985). Primary acute pericardial disease: A prospective series of 231 consecutive patients. *American Journal of Cardiology, 56(10),* 623–630.
42. Pietus, F., Widderhouse, T., Gerardy, A., Geskes, G., Chieriex, E., & Wellens, H. (1993). Risk of aortic dissection after aortic valve replacement. *The American Journal of Cardiology,* 72(1), 1043–1047.
43. Porth, C. (1994). Alterations in oxygenation of tissues. In C. Porth, *Pathophysiology: Concepts of altered health states* (4th ed.). Philadelphia: J. B. Lippincott.
44. Rackley, C. E., et al. (1990). Mitral valve disease. In J. W. Hurst (Ed.), *The heart* (7th ed.). New York: McGraw-Hill.
45. Rackley, C. E., et al. (1990). Aortic valve disease. In J. W. Hurst (Ed.), *The heart* (7th ed.). New York: McGraw-Hill.
46. Raymond, M., et al. (1984). Coping with transient intellectual dysfunction after coronary bypass surgery. *Heart and Lung, 13(5),* 531–539.

47. Relf, M. (1993). Surgical intervention for tricuspid valve endocarditis: Vegetectomy, valve excision, or valve replacement? *Journal of Cardiovascular Nursing, 7(2),* 71–79.

48. Scheld, W. M., & Sande, M. A. (1994). Endocarditis and intravascular infections. In G. L. Mandell, et al. (Eds.), *Principles and practice of infectious diseases* (4th ed.). New York: John Wiley and Sons.

49. Scordo, K. (1992). Mitral valve prolapse syndrome, *Nursing 92, 22(10),* 34–37.

50. Seifert, F. C., et al. (1985). Surgical treatment of constrictive pericarditis: Analysis of outcome and diagnostic error. *Circulation, 72, (Suppl. II),* 264–273.

51. Shapiro, B. A., et al. (1991). *Clinical application of respiratory care* (4th ed.). St. Louis: Mosby-Year Book.

52. Stovsky, B., & Dehner, S. (1994). Patient education after valve surgery. *Critical Care Nurse, 14(2),* 117–123.

53. Stollerman, G. H. (1992). Rheumatic and heritable connective tissue diseases of the cardiovascular system. In E. Braunwald (Ed.), *Heart disease* (4th ed.). Philadelphia: W. B. Saunders.

54. Thompson, M. E. (Ed.). (1990). *Cardiac transplantation.* Philadelphia: F. A. Davis.

55. Turina, J., Hess, O. M., Turina, M., & Krayenbuehl, H. P. (1993). Cardiac bioprosthesis in the 1990s. *Circulation, 88(2),* 775–779.

56. Vaupel-Suart, S., Enzweiller, K., & Bolten, P. T. (1993). Management of intraoperative right ventricular failure with pulmonary balloon counterpulsation. *Clinical Issues in Critical Care Nursing, 4(4),* 645–653.

57. Villaire, M., & Gul, B. (1993). Helping nurses to help families make end-of-life decisions. *Critical Care Nurse, 13(1),* 84–87.

58. Wackowski, C., & Bierman, P. (1995). Dual chamber pacing in patients with hypertrophic obstructive cardiopathy: A case study. *American Journal of Critical Care, 42(2),* 165–168.

59. Wenger, N. K., et al. (1990). Cardiomyopathy and specific heart muscle disease. In J. W. Hurst (Ed.), *The heart* (7th ed.). New York: McGraw-Hill.

60. Wojner, A. (1994). Assessing the five points of the intra-aortic balloon pump waveform. *Critical Care Nurse, 14(3),* 48–51.

61. Wynne, J., & Braunwald, E. (1992). The cardiomyopathies and myocarditides. In E. Braunwald (Ed.), *Heart disease* (4th ed.). Philadelphia: W. B. Saunders.

62. Zimoek, R. (1993). Current perspective on prosthetic heart valves and valve repair. *AACN Nursing Scan in Critical Care, 3(6),* 20–21.

Chapter 26 Nursing Care of Clients with Peripheral Vascular Disorders

Learning Outcomes

After completing this chapter, the learner will be able to:

1. Assess the client for clinical manifestations associated with peripheral vascular disorders.
2. Teach the client about the etiology, risk factors, basic pathophysiology, and clinical manifestations of peripheral vascular disorders.
3. Explain the client's role in medical and surgical management of peripheral vascular disorders.
4. Develop plans of care for the prevention of illness, management, and rehabilitation of clients with peripheral vascular disorders.
5. Implement nursing interventions that optimize the quality of life for clients with peripheral vascular disorders.
6. Evaluate planned client outcomes, using outcome criteria developed in the planning phase of care.

Assessment of the Peripheral Vascular System

Peripheral vascular disease is common in elderly persons and persons with diabetes. It is characterized by disturbances of blood flow through the peripheral vessels. These disturbances eventually result in damage to tissues of the extremities and organs as a result of ischemia and excessive accumulation of waste and fluid caused by venous or lymphatic stasis.

CRITICAL TO REMEMBER

Any factor that narrows, obstructs, or damages blood vessels and thus impedes blood flow is dangerous.

When the blood flow slows, tissue nutrition decreases, cellular waste products accumulate, ischemia develops, and the danger of thrombus and embolus formation escalates. Without intervention, tissue damage may advance to the point of ulceration or gangrene. Limb amputation may be necessary.

Nursing assessment of the peripheral vascular system includes the collection of data through history and physical examination of the arterial and venous circulation.

HEALTH HISTORY

When obtaining a health history, the nurse should be alert for risk factors for cardiovascular disease (see Chap. 24). In addition, the nurse should ask the client about the use of any medications that increase the risk of vascular disease (e.g., birth control pills) as well as medications for circulatory disorders (e.g., vasodilators).

Chief Complaint

When assessing for vascular disease, the nurse elicits specific data to determine whether the client has arterial or venous disease and to characterize the frequency and duration of clinical manifestations. Vascular changes may be associated with extremity discomfort of varying character and intensity (Box 26–1).

With arterial disorders, the chief complaint is usually leg pain with walking, called intermittent claudication. The nurse questions the client about the sequence, duration, and persistence of the discomfort; manner of onset; associated symptoms; and the amount of activity required to cause pain, referred to as claudication distance. The extensiveness of the disease can be gauged by the distance the client can walk without pain. For example, one client may experience claudication after walking one block, whereas another can walk six blocks before pain develops. (See Chronic Arterial Occlusion, Clinical Manifestations, later in this chapter.)

BOX 26–1

Effects of Vascular Changes in Extremities

- Pain, burning, and stinging
- Cramping and numbness
- Intolerance to local heat and cold
- Inability to sense temperature changes
- Decreased touch sensation
- Decreased proprioception
- Edema
- Color changes (dependent rubor, pallor, or cyanosis)
- Lesions
- Poor healing

Clients may also report impotence. Aortoiliac disorders can lead to impotence. If aortoiliac disease is suspected, the nurse asks about sexual changes.

Pain in clients with chronic venous disease, by contrast, has a slow onset and is not associated with exercise or rest. These clients have typically worked at a job involving many hours of standing in one place, had multiple pregnancies, or have abdominal obesity. In these situations, the leg veins have been subjected to increased pressure gradients and obstruction to the return of venous blood. The vein wall eventually loses its competency, and leg edema and ulcerations develop. The client may also have varicose veins and a history of phlebitis. The client will often report feeling heaviness in the legs, aching pain when the legs are dependent, and nighttime cramping. Exercise and elevation generally relieve the pain and swelling as venous return is improved.

Clinical Manifestations: Arterial and Venous Disorders compares the major signs and symptoms of arterial and venous disorders.

History

Any medical history of vascular impairment is noted. The nurse asks specifically whether the client has had a history of hypertension, phlebitis, extremity blood clots, pulmonary emboli, cerebrovascular accidents, diabetes mellitus, edema, varicose veins, stasis ulcers, leg cramps, or extremities that are cold, pale, or blue. The client is asked about any past medical tests, surgery, or treatments involving the cardiovascular system.

The nurse assesses for proper dietary intake, including cholesterol and sodium. A social history is taken to determine use of tobacco, alcohol, and drugs.

Occupational history should be recorded, including the number of hours in various positions (e.g., standing, walking).

A family history of diabetes, hypertension, coronary artery disease, and known peripheral vascular disease is obtained.

The client's activity, rest, and sleep habits are assessed. The nurse also assesses the degree to which symptoms interfere with the client's activities of daily living. Obtaining information about the frequency and

CLINICAL MANIFESTATIONS

Arterial and Venous Disorders

MANIFESTATION	ARTERIAL DISORDERS	VENOUS DISORDERS
Pain	Intermittent claudication Cramping Worse with elevation Aggravated by walking	Slow onset Aching pain Exercise improves pain Better with elevation Nocturnal cramping Pruritus, paresthesias Heaviness in the legs at end of day Positive finding of Homans' sign common
Skin	Absence of hair Small, painful ulcers on pressure points, especially lateral malleolus; delayed healing; gangrene Thin, shiny skin Thick toenails	Broad, shallow, painless ulcers of the ankle and lower leg Normal toenails
Color	Pale, dependent cyanosis or rubor	Brown discoloration Dependent rubor or cyanosis
Temperature	Cool	May be warm if thrombophlebitis is present
Sensation	Decreased; sometimes itching, tingling numbness, paresthesias	Pruritus
Pulses	Decreased to absent Possible systolic bruit over involved arteries	Usually unaffected but may be difficult to palpate if legs edematous
Edema	May be present	Present, worse at end of day, improved with elevation
Muscle mass	Reduced, tissue atrophy	Unaffected

duration of symptoms, precipitating factors, and the symptoms' impact on the client's daily life enables the nurse to understand the severity of the disease. It is also important to assess the client's stress level and emotional state.

The nurse is sensitive to the emotional impact of peripheral vascular disorders. Clients with lesions in visible areas may fear embarrassment. Fear of amputation of the involved limb can generate significant stress.

PHYSICAL EXAMINATION

Physical examination of the peripheral vascular system for discovering signs of vascular disorders involves three techniques: inspection, palpation, and auscultation. The client should be examined in a warm, well-lighted room to minimize cutaneous and small artery vasoconstriction.

Inspection

The nurse observes the client's extremities, noting skin color, hair distribution, venous pattern, and any swelling or atrophy. Lack of hair growth may indicate inadequate circulation to an area. Varicosities indicate venous insufficiency. Angiomas (benign tumors of blood and lymph vessels) and petechiae (small, purplish, hemorrhagic spots on the skin from several causes, including hemorrhage) are also noted. Atrophy may indicate long-standing arterial insufficiency; if atrophy is suspected, the nurse measures the muscle circumference and compares it with the opposite side. Any skin lesions, ulcerations, or scar tissue indicating healed ulcers are also noted; ischemic fissures of the feet and ulcers of ankles and heels are reliable signs of arterial insufficiency. Scars indicating healed ulcers over the medial malleolus can indicate chronic venous insufficiency.

CAPILLARY REFILL

The capillary bed is the portion of the vascular system farthest from the heart. Capillary refill time is an evaluation of peripheral perfusion and cardiac output. This assessment is usually completed while pulses are assessed. The nurse depresses the nail bed of the client's toe or finger until it blanches (becomes pale) and then releases pressure. The nurse notes and documents the time it takes for the usual skin color to return. Normal capillaries refill in a fraction of a second, but "normal" findings include up to 3 seconds. With diminished blood flow, the return to normal color is delayed, and a refill time of more than 3 seconds is sometimes called "sluggish." Note whether the environment is cold, because external temperatures can delay capillary refill.

EDEMA

The nurse assesses for edema of the leg by pressing on the skin over the edematous area for 5 seconds and then releasing. Edematous skin may leave an indentation called a pit; thus, the term pitting edema. The degree of edema is often graded; a commonly used scale is as follows:

0: no edema
1+: barely detectable depression accompanied by normal foot and leg contours
2+: a deeper depression (less than 5 mm) accompanied by normal contours
3+: deep depression (5–10 mm) accompanied by foot and leg swelling
4+: an even deeper depression (more than 1 cm) accompanied by severe foot and leg swelling

The nurse notes and documents the degree of edema and its anatomical location.

Edema resulting from cardiac disease is generally bilateral and occurs in dependent areas: the legs when the client is ambulatory and the sacrum if the client is bedridden. Edema tends to be unilateral in a client with chronic venous obstruction, traumatic injury, or lymphatic obstruction. This type of edema is hard and nonpitting and is called brawny edema.

ELEVATION PALLOR

In clients with arterial occlusion, the foot becomes gray and pale when elevated. When the leg is placed in a dependent position, it becomes dusky and red over 30 to 60 seconds. The changes in color result from a loss of vasomotor tone as a result of tissue hypoxia; the arterial system cannot pump adequate blood into the capillary system through the arterial blockages against gravity. The degree of pallor is tested by elevating the leg 30 to 45 degrees and observing for pallor over 60 seconds. The results can be graded as follows:

0: no pallor in 60 seconds
1: definite pallor in 60 seconds
2: definite pallor in 30 seconds
3: definite pallor in less than 30 seconds
4: definite pallor with leg flat in bed

Because the leg elevation with this test can cause the client pain from further decrease of arterial supply to the leg, it should be performed only as needed. The nurse notes the degree of pallor at rest and uses the test only to assist with determining the severity of ischemia.

CLUBBING

Clubbing is a condition in which the nail bed angle increases to 180 degrees or more. It is related to a long-standing lack of oxygen to the peripheral tissues and is commonly associated with pulmonary disease. The nurse assesses the nail bed angle by inspecting the nails. Clubbing is classified as early, late, or prolonged, as described in Chapter 19.

TRENDELENBURG'S TEST

Superficial varicose veins are usually easy to recognize. They appear as dilated, tortuous (twisting) veins. At times, however, the client may have dilated veins from other causes, and further assessment is needed. The client lies down with the leg elevated until the veins are empty. A tourniquet is applied at midthigh, snugly enough to occlude the superficial veins. With the tourniquet in place, the client stands. The nurse then notes the time required for the veins to fill from below. Normally, veins fill in about 35 seconds. The tourniquet should be released after 60 seconds. The vein normally fills from below; a varicose vein fills from above because of incompetent valves.

Palpation

TEMPERATURE

The nurse palpates the temperature of the extremities with the dorsal surface of the hand. Upper extremities are compared with the lower extremities and left to right. The temperature and vascular tone should be the same in all extremities. Vasoconstriction produces cold, pale, moist skin with collapsed superficial veins. Bilateral vasoconstriction may be due to environmental factors such as smoking, room temperature, apprehension, or generalized arterial disease. Unilateral or localized vasoconstriction indicates peripheral vascular disease.

Skin turgor also may be noted at the time skin temperature is being assessed.

PULSES

The nurse palpates carotid, axillary, brachial, radial, and ulnar pulses (upper extremities) and femoral, popliteal, posterior tibial, and dorsalis pedis pulses (lower extremities) (Fig. 26–1). Pulses should be palpated bilaterally and simultaneously except for the carotid pulse. Carotid pulses should be palpated sequentially to avoid stimulation of the carotid sinus, which could produce bradycardia or sinus arrest. The temporal pulse is usually assessed as part of the head and neck examination (see Chap. 21). Ulnar pulse assessment is performed during Allen's test (see following).

The nurse must always note rhythm, amplitude, and symmetry of pulses. Peripheral pulses should be compared for rate, rhythm, and quality. Pulses may be graded as follows:

1: absent
+1: weak and thready
+2: normal
+3: full and bounding

The nurse records the scale used to assess pulse quality.

The nurse notes whether a pulse is absent or feels unequal bilaterally. The dorsalis pedis pulse is congenitally absent in approximately 10 to 17 per cent of the normal adult population. The posterior tibial pulse is absent congenitally in 9 per cent of the black adult population.

ALLEN'S TEST

Allen's test is used to assess the patency of the radial and ulnar arteries distal to the wrist. It is a common

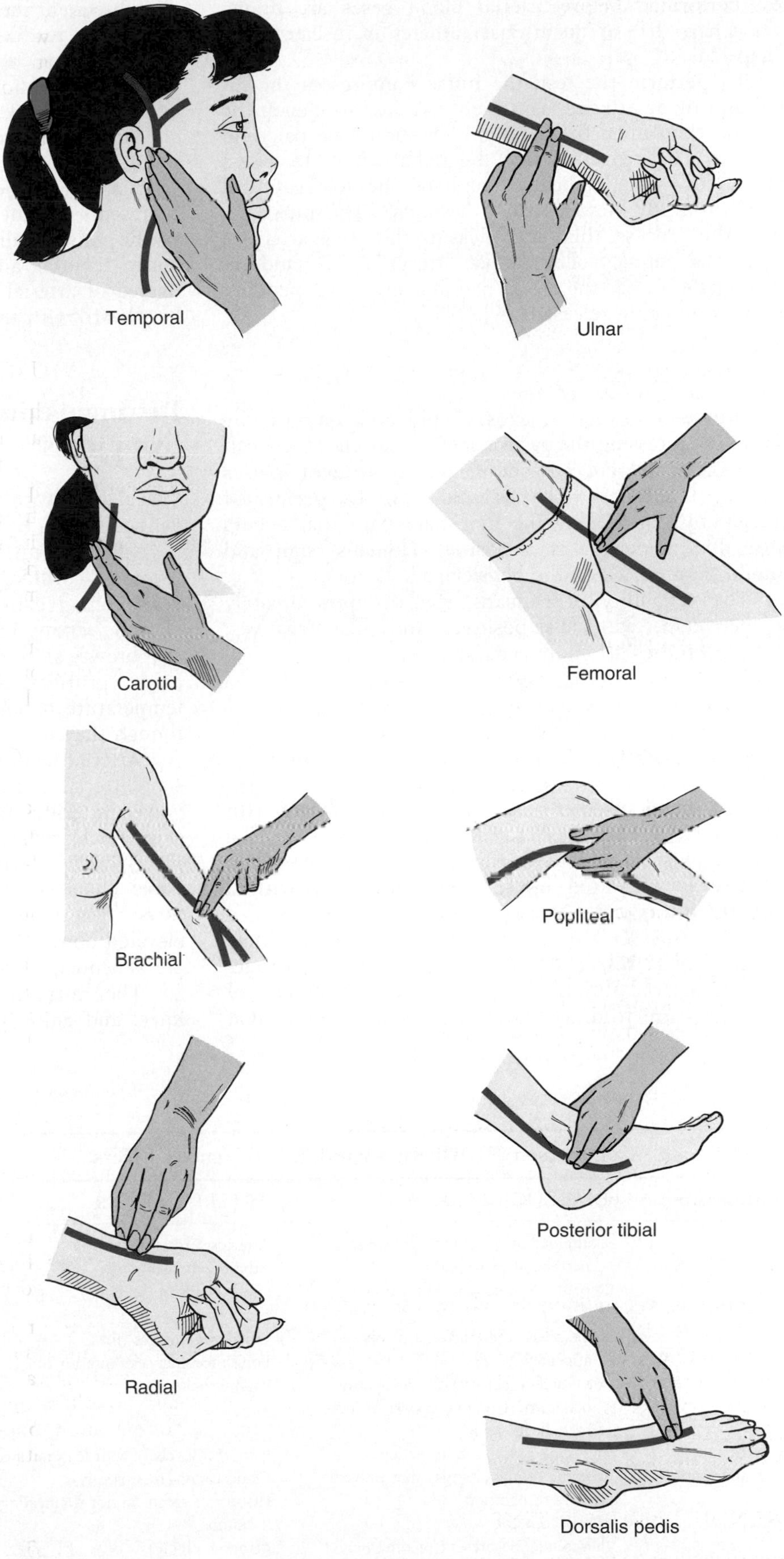

Figure 26–1
Peripheral pulses are assessed bilaterally from head to toe and rated for amplitude, rhythm, and symmetry.

test performed before arterial blood gases are drawn (see Chap. 19) or an arterial catheter is inserted (see Chap. 24).

To perform the test, the nurse compresses the radial and ulnar arteries. The client is asked to clench the fist and then open the hand, which should be pale and mottled. The nurse releases the radial artery to assess patency of the radial artery. The hand should regain full color promptly (fewer than 6 seconds). The nurse repeats the process, this time releasing the ulnar artery to assess the patency of the ulnar artery. If the hand remains pale, either the radial or ulnar artery (depending on the one being released) is possibly occluded.

HOMANS' SIGN

The nurse assesses for signs of phlebothrombosis by gently compressing the gastrocnemius muscle of the calf and asking the client whether this movement causes pain or tenderness. The test can also be performed quickly by dorsiflexing the foot. Calf pain that occurs with this maneuver is a positive Homans' sign and should be reported to the physician.

The reliability of Homans' sign is approximately 50 per cent, with false-positives and false-negatives. Doppler studies are more accurate.

Auscultation

The peripheral vascular system may be auscultated with a stethoscope, but best results are obtained with a Doppler ultrasonographic flowmeter. Arterial blood pressure is measured by sphygmomanometry with a properly fitting cuff. Measurement should be recorded in both arms. Differences in extremity readings may indicate aortic dissection, subclavian artery atherosclerosis, or arterial thromboembolic events. Asymmetry of blood pressure readings should be documented so that all subsequent measurements are made on the arm with the higher reading. The blood pressure is measured in supine, sitting, and standing positions, when possible, and documentation should include position of the client and the site used.

Auscultation over each pulse point should be done to assess for the presence of a bruit. A bruit is described as a "whooshing" sound, soft or loud in pitch; it represents turbulent blood flow caused by irregularities in the vessel wall. Bruits usually occur in the carotid, aortic, femoral, and popliteal arteries and indicate some degree of arterial narrowing. These arterial sounds are best heard with the bell of the stethoscope.

Distinguishing Arterial and Venous Symptoms

Vascular disease in the extremities may affect the venous system or the arterial system.

Clients with venous disease present with dilated, tortuous, cordlike superficial veins. Assessment also reveals aching pain when the legs are dependent. With chronic venous insufficiency, edema, dependent cyanosis, brown skin discolorations, possible ulcers of the ankle, pruritus, and paresthesia will be noted. Skin temperature remains normal and pulses are present, although they may be hard to palpate through the edema.

Arterial insufficiency is marked by decreased or absent arterial pulses; a possible systolic bruit over involved arteries; muscular atrophy; thin, shiny, hairless skin; thick, ridged toenails; cool skin temperature; and ulcers on pressure points of the feet. Table 26–1 compares characteristics of diabetic, arterial, and venous ulcers. The skin color is pale gray when the legs are elevated above the heart level and dusky red after they are dependent. Edema, if present, is mild and brawny.

The nurse assesses range of motion of the hip, knee, and ankle joints. For checking muscle strength,

TABLE 26–1 Comparison of Diabetic, Arterial, and Venous Ulcers

VARIABLE	DIABETIC ULCER	ARTERIAL ULCER	VENOUS ULCER
Cause	Combination of arterial disease and peripheral neuropathy Repetitive unrecognized trauma	Arteriosclerosis obliterans Atheroembolism (Both result in ischemia)	Valvular incompetency Incompetent perforators History of deep vein thrombosis Venous hypertension
Location	Same areas where arterial ulcers appear Areas where peripheral neuropathy occurs (i.e., plantar aspect of foot, toes, heels)	Distal appendages (toes) Bone prominences (anterior tibial) Lateral malleolus	Medial aspect of distal third of lower extremity Behind medial malleolus
Clinical manifestations	Pain caused by sensory deficit Diabetic retinal changes that prevent early recognition Sepsis common Pulses may be present or diminished (arteries become calcified)	Painful, especially with legs elevated Claudication, rest pain History of recent minor nonhealing trauma Atrophic changes Pulses poor quality or absent	Not often painful Dark pigmentation Eczema or stasis dermatitis Edema Comfortable with legs elevated Normal arterial pulses

the nurse places the hands against the client's lower legs and asks the client to flex or extend the knees against opposition from the nurse's hands.

DIAGNOSTIC TESTS

Noninvasive Techniques

Noninvasive diagnostic techniques have assumed an increasingly important role in the management of clients with vascular disease. These techniques provide reliable and relevant data to assess such variables as

- The amount of blood flow through the affected limb
- Abnormal compared with normal blood flow
- Some measure of the degree of functional limitations
- The extent of the disease process

LIMB BLOOD PRESSURE

Blood pressure measurement is the most common noninvasive test of cardiovascular function. It may be the best single indicator of how well perfusion is being maintained. Acute and chronic arterial occlusion produce regional (e.g., one arm) hypotension.

ANKLE-BRACHIAL INDEX

The ankle-brachial index (ABI) is the most commonly used parameter for overall evaluation of extremity status. Ankle pressure is normally the same or higher than brachial systolic pressure. Normal foot arteries have an index of 1.0 to 1.2. An ABI of 0.8 to 1.0 suggests mild obstruction; 0.5 to 0.8, moderate obstruction; below 0.5, severe obstruction.

DOPPLER ULTRASONOGRAPHY

Hand-held Doppler instruments permit assessment of peripheral arterial disease by audible evaluation of arterial signals or measurement of limb blood pressures (Fig. 26–2). This test is simple and inexpensive, but the technique may not detect minor disease and is less accurate than duplex scanning.

Brightness mode ultrasonography is the creation of a two-dimensional image from ultrasound waves. It can be used to assess vein size, compressibility, flow patterns, thrombus formation, and valve function.

ULTRASONIC DUPLEX SCANNER

Ultrasonic duplex scanners are used to localize the site of vascular disease and to estimate its hemodynamic significance. The technique is the most sensitive and specific noninvasive modality for detecting deep vein thrombosis (DVT). This device provides both an ultrasonographic image of the vessel and a Doppler signal characterizing the flow pattern at a given site. The anatomic data allow more specific localization of the level of stenosis than is possible with simple pressure or waveform techniques. The major limitations to these devices are their cost, complexity, and lack of portability.

PLETHYSMOGRAPHY

A plethysmograph records biologic changes in volume in a portion of the body associated with cardiac contractions or respirations or in response to pneumatic venous occlusion. This instrument detects and quantifies vascular disease on the basis of changes in pulse wave contour, blood pressure, or arterial or venous blood flow.

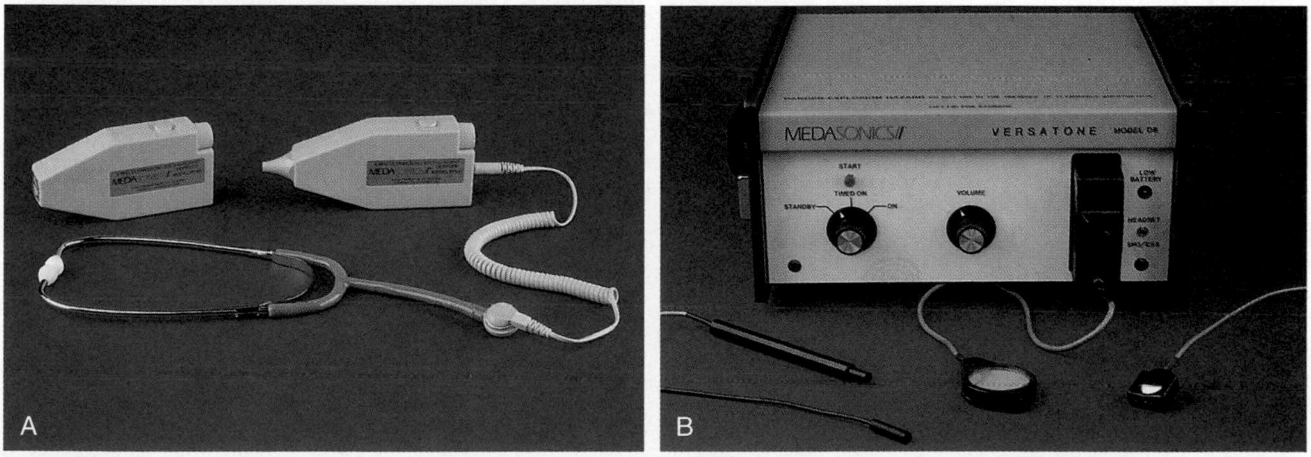

Figure 26–2
The Doppler ultrasonographic flowmeter detects blood flow. *A,* Ultrasonographic stethoscope. *B,* Multipurpose ultrasonographic instrument with interchangeable probes. (Courtesy of Medasonics, Inc., Fremont, CA.)

COMPUTED TOMOGRAPHY

Computed tomography (CT) allows visualization of the arterial wall and its structures. Computed tomographic scans can be used in the diagnosis of abdominal aortic aneurysms and postoperative complications, such as graft infection, graft occlusion, hemorrhage, and abscess.[24] Clients must lie still while a long tube passes over them. If the client cannot lie still or is claustrophobic, sedation may be necessary.

MAGNETIC RESONANCE IMAGING

Magnetic resonance imaging (MRI) uses magnetic fields, rather than radiation, to obtain cross-sectional images. MRI is used to detect deep vein thrombosis from the pelvic iliac veins and leg veins. Clients with implanted metal devices, such as aneurysm clips or iron or steel in their body (e.g., shrapnel), cannot undergo MRI. The client is placed in a long magnetic tube. Clients who cannot lie still or have claustrophobia may require sedation.[24]

It is likely that, in the future, MRI technique will supply much of the information currently available with invasive angiography.

IMPEDANCE PLETHYSMOGRAPHY

This technique is also used to measure venous blood volume changes in the extremities and to diagnose deep vein thrombosis. During the procedure, electrodes from a plethysmograph are applied to a limb along with a pressure cuff. As pressure is increased, electrical resistance is increased; thus, the quality of venous blood flow is indicated.

The client is informed about the purpose of the procedure, that a technique similar to blood pressure measurement will be used, and that the procedure lasts 30 to 60 minutes. The client must be able to assume a supine position with the involved extremity elevated above the level of the heart.

EXERCISE TESTING

Exercise testing provides an objective measurement of the severity of intermittent claudication and how much it interferes with the client's life-style. The most commonly used method for stress testing is the treadmill exercise test. The treadmill test is similar to that used for coronary clients, except that walking speed is usually 1.5 to 2 miles per hour, with a grade elevation of 10 to 20 per cent and a time limit of 5 minutes. If a client can walk 5 minutes, he or she is considered mildly symptomatic; walking times of 1 minute represent severe disease. Test performance is also gauged by measurement of ankle systolic pressure. In normal clients, the time required for return to pre-exercise ankle pressure is usually less than 3 minutes with a 20 per cent (or less) drop from baseline. In clients with intermittent claudication, the recovery time is longer; ankle pressure is usually less than 50 mm Hg and may be unrecordable during recovery. The client should also know that exercise will be stopped at the maximal level of exertion or when symptoms become disabling. (See Client Education Guide: Stress Testing [Chap. 23].)

Invasive Techniques

CONTRAST ANGIOGRAPHY AND VENOGRAPHY

Contrast angiography is the most invasive of the diagnostic procedures for arterial disorders and has the greatest risk for the client. It is frequently performed before vascular surgery and can be used intraoperatively to evaluate an operation. The procedure involves injecting contrast medium into the arterial system and performing radiographic studies. Nursing care and education of a client before and after contrast angiography is described in Chapter 23. Most angiograms take 30 to 90 minutes.

Venography is performed in a similar manner except that the venous system is examined. Venograms can be used to detect deep vein thrombosis or other abnormalities such as incompetent valves.

Complications of angiography besides allergic reaction to the contrast media include thrombi, perforation of the vessel, emboli, and renal failure. Creatinine levels should be monitored. Pseudoaneurysm is a significant complication that may extend the client's hospital stay. Pseudoaneurysm is a contained arterial wall outpouching with persistent communication between the artery and the fluid component of an adjacent mass. Pseudoaneurysms generally result from arterial trauma (after arterial puncture) or occur at the surgical site. They are a site of infection, a source of emboli, and associated with intravascular thrombosis. They can enlarge, compress an adjacent structure, and even rupture, although rupture is rare.

Vascular Endoscopy (Angioscopy). This technique permits imaging of intra-arterial disease in color and in three dimensions with use of fiberoptic technology. The angioscope's major asset is to permit visualization of the surface of the vessel for identifying thrombus, plaque, hemorrhage, ulceration, or embolus. Angioscopes can be used to remove debris from a vessel and to check the integrity of an anastomosis from within a vessel. They may also be used to remove the valves from veins to prepare them for use as bypass grafts. Complications are rare but may include intimal damage, vessel spasm, thrombosis or embolism, perforation, and fluid overload. The incidence of infection is also very low.

Intravascular Ultrasonography. Intravascular ultrasonography provides information about the atherosclerotic intima beneath the luminal surface. It can thus determine the thickness of the arterial wall and distinguish thrombus and calcium from vascular tissue, allowing more exact removal of lesions. One current limiting factor is the need for specialized interpretation of the scans.

Hypertension

Arterial hypertension, or high blood pressure, is generally defined as a persistent elevation of systolic blood pressure above 140 mm Hg and of diastolic pressure above 90 mm Hg. The last two decades have brought remarkable changes in the control of hypertension.[1, 48] The public is more knowledgeable about high blood pressure, more likely to visit a physician for hypertension, and more likely to follow medical advice. These practices have contributed to a 50 per cent decrease in the national age-adjusted stroke mortality and a 35 per cent decline in coronary artery disease mortality since 1972. Nonetheless, hypertension remains a major contributor to morbidity and mortality in our society because, of those clients with high blood pressure,

- 35 per cent are not diagnosed,
- 51 per cent are not receiving therapy, and
- 28 per cent are receiving inadequate therapy.[1]

Classification of Hypertension

Hypertension may be classified according to type (systolic and diastolic), cause, and degree of severity.

SYSTOLIC AND DIASTOLIC HYPERTENSION

Systolic hypertension refers to systolic pressure exceeding 140 mm Hg; diastolic hypertension, to diastolic pressure exceeding 90 mm Hg. For clients older than 65 years, systolic hypertension is defined as systolic pressure exceeding 160 mm Hg and diastolic hypertension is defined as diastolic pressure exceeding 95 mm Hg.

PRIMARY AND SECONDARY HYPERTENSION

Primary hypertension, also known as essential or idiopathic hypertension, constitutes more than 90 to 95 per cent of all cases of hypertension. The cause of primary hypertension is multifactorial. Characteristics include either a gradual onset and prolonged course (benign hypertension) or an abrupt onset and a short, dramatic course that proves rapidly fatal without swift intervention (malignant or accelerated hypertension). Secondary hypertension results from an identifiable cause. Various specific disease states or problems may be responsible. Five to 10 per cent of the hypertensive population have secondary hypertension. When secondary hypertension is identified, the disorder creating the hypertension may be corrected with medications or surgery.

BORDERLINE HYPERTENSION

Borderline, or labile, hypertension is defined as intermittent elevation of blood pressure interspersed with normal readings. Clients with borderline hypertension carry an increased risk of acquiring primary hypertension and cardiovascular disease.

MALIGNANT HYPERTENSION

Malignant hypertension is a syndrome of markedly elevated blood pressure (diastolic pressure exceeding 140 mm Hg) associated with papilledema. Accelerated hypertension is a syndrome of markedly elevated blood pressure with retinal hemorrhage and exudate. Accelerated hypertension presumably develops into malignant hypertension if not well managed.

BENIGN HYPERTENSION

Benign hypertension is a term used to describe uncomplicated hypertension, usually of long duration and mild to moderate severity. Benign hypertension may be primary or secondary.

WHITE COAT HYPERTENSION

White coat hypertension is defined as hypertension in a population of clients who have normal blood pressures except when measurements are taken by a health-care professional, especially a physician. The cause of this response is thought to be anxiety. It is unknown whether white coat hypertension is insignificant or a variant form of hypertension.[56]

Incidence

Arterial hypertension affects nearly 50 million clients, or one in four adults, in the United States.[1] Prevalence of hypertension increases with advancing age, and blacks are affected more often than whites.

CRITICAL TO REMEMBER

Hypertension is the most common public health problem in the United States and the single most important predictor of cardiovascular risk.

The severity of hypertension is proportional to the severity of atherosclerosis, stroke, nephropathy, peripheral vascular disease, aortic aneurysms, and congestive heart failure.

Etiology

Primary hypertension has no single or specific cause but is multifactorial. It develops in response to increased cardiac output or to a rise in peripheral resistance. Factors that affect these two forces include the following:

- Genetic propensity to a heightened neurologic response to stress or to a defect in renal excretion or cellular transport of sodium

TABLE 26–2 Causes of Secondary Hypertension

Renal	Mineralocorticoids: licorice
Renal parenchymal disease	Sympathomimetics
Acute glomerulonephritis	Tyramine-containing foods
Chronic nephritis	and monoamine oxidase
Polycystic disease	inhibitors
Connective tissue diseases	Coarctation of the aorta
Diabetic nephropathy	Pregnancy-induced
Hydronephrosis	hypertension
Renovascular	Neurologic disorders
Renin-producing tumors	Increased intracranial
Renoprival	pressure
Primary sodium retention	Brain tumor
Endocrine	Encephalitis
Acromegaly	Respiratory acidosis
Hypothyroidism	Sleep apnea
Hyperthyroidism	Quadriplegia
Hypercalcemia	Acute porphyria
Adrenal	Familial dysautonomia
Cortical	Lead poisoning
Cushing's syndrome	Guillain-Barré syndrome
Primary aldosteronism	Acute stress, including surgery
Congenital adrenal hyper-	Psychogenic hyperventilation
plasia	Hypoglycemia
Medullary: pheochromo-	Burns
cytoma	Pancreatitis
Extra-adrenal chromaffin	Alcohol withdrawal
tumors	Sickle cell crisis
Carcinoid	Postresuscitation
Exogenous hormones	Postoperative
Estrogen	Increased intravascular volume
Glucocorticoids	Alcohol, drugs, and so on

Adapted from Braunwald, E. (1992). *Heart disease: A textbook of cardiovascular medicine* (4th ed.). Philadelphia: W. B. Saunders.

- Obesity associated with high levels of insulin (hyperinsulinemia) that lead to elevated blood pressure
- Environmental stress
- Loss of elastic tissue and arteriosclerosis of aorta and other large arteries
- Cigarette smoking

Secondary hypertension can result from a variety of identifiable primary causes (Table 26–2).

Risk Factors

PRIMARY PREVENTION

Prevention of hypertension involves identifying nonmodifiable risk factors and identifying and managing modifiable risk factors. A client's relative risk for hypertension depends on the number and severity of modifiable risk factors.

Nonmodifiable Risk Factors

Family History. Genetic predisposition makes certain families more susceptible to hypertension. Clients with parents who have or had hypertension are at a greater risk for hypertension at a younger age. This has not been demonstrated to be solely genetic; environmental factors may also be involved.

Age. The incidence of hypertension increases with age: 50 to 60 per cent of clients older than 50 years have blood pressure exceeding 140/90 mm Hg. However, epidemiologic studies have shown a poorer prognosis in clients whose hypertension began at a young age.

Gender. Men experience hypertension at higher rates and at an earlier age than women until after age 60. Men also have a greater risk of cardiovascular morbidity and mortality. After age 50, hypertension is more prevalent in women. The reasons for this are not clear.

Ethnic Group. Hypertension is the most serious health problem for blacks in the United States. Hypertension is more prevalent in blacks, and, at any given blood pressure, blacks have a greater mortality rate than whites. The reason for the increased prevalence of hypertension among blacks is unclear, but it has been attributed to heredity, greater salt intake, and greater environmental stress.

Modifiable Risk Factors. These include the following:

- Stress
- Obesity
- Diet
- Cigarette smoking

These are discussed later in this chapter (see Nonpharmacologic Intervention).

Prevention in the Community. The incidence of hypertension presents a national problem that individual interventions alone cannot counter. Prevention of hypertension and early discovery of new cases depend on a national public health effort that enlists governmental support and involves such nationwide structures as business and industry, labor organizations, health-care institutions, voluntary associations, and local communities.

Although the exact cause of primary hypertension remains unknown, several risk factors associated with the development of hypertension are known. Once high-risk clients are identified, clinicians can teach these persons how to modify certain risk factors such as diet, smoking, sodium intake, exercise, and so forth.

Hypertensive clients usually find out about their condition through incidental screening in health-care facilities or organized community screening in public settings (e.g., shopping malls, schools, work place).

In addition to identifying undiagnosed or inadequately controlled hypertensive clients, screening programs provide an opportunity to educate the public. It is particularly important to screen high-risk "target groups," such as black and elderly populations. Community services need to keep target groups in mind when choosing settings for blood pressure screenings. Those who take blood pressure readings need to inform clients in writing of their blood pressure, its significance, and, if necessary, the importance of follow-up evaluation.

SECONDARY PREVENTION

Because the beginnings of adult hypertension often lie in childhood and adolescence, children older than 3 years need yearly blood pressure assessment. Asymptomatic youngsters who exhibit elevated blood pressure readings on three separate occasions require a careful work-up and follow-up program.

Childhood obesity is on the rise in the United States. Obese children and teenagers are at increased risk for adult obesity, which is associated with hypertension.

TERTIARY PREVENTION

Once diagnosed, hypertension requires ongoing management despite the absence of symptoms. The many sequelae of unmanaged hypertension (i.e., stroke and myocardial infarction) can be prevented or reduced through proper management. Unfortunately, however, because of the cost of antihypertensive agents, side effects of these agents, and the lack of symptoms, many clients do not manage the disorder well.

Pathophysiology

PRIMARY (ESSENTIAL) HYPERTENSION

Any factor producing an alteration in peripheral vascular resistance, heart rate, or stroke volume affects systemic arterial blood pressure.

Four control systems play a major role in maintaining blood pressure:

- The arterial baroreceptor system
- Regulation of body fluid volume
- The renin-angiotensin system
- Vascular autoregulation

It is probable that no single defect causes essential hypertension in all clients.

Baroreceptors monitor the level of arterial pressure and counteract elevations through vagally mediated cardiac slowing and vasodilation with decreased sympathetic tone. The role of the arterial baroreceptors in hypertension is not well understood. Arterial baroreceptors are found in the carotid sinus and wall of the ventricle.

An abnormality in the transport of sodium in the renal tubules may cause essential hypertension. An excess of sodium and water increases total blood volume, thereby elevating blood pressure. In functional kidneys, a rise in pressure leads to diuresis. Pathologic changes that alter the pressure threshold at which kidneys excrete salt and water alter systemic blood pressure. In addition, the overproduction of sodium-retaining hormones has been implicated in hypertension.

Renin and angiotensin play a role in blood pressure regulation. Renin is an enzyme produced by the kidneys that catalyzes a plasma protein substrate to split off angiotensin I, which is removed by a converting enzyme to the lung to form angiotensin II and then angiotensin III (Fig. 26–3). Angiotensin II and III act as vasoconstrictors and control aldosterone release. With increased sympathetic nervous system activity, angiotensin II and III also seem to inhibit sodium excretion, which results in elevated blood pressure. Increased renin secretion has been investigated as a cause of increased peripheral vascular resistance in primary hypertension.

Clients may also acquire hypertension from deficiencies in vasodilators, such as prostaglandins, or from congenital abnormalities in resistance vessels.

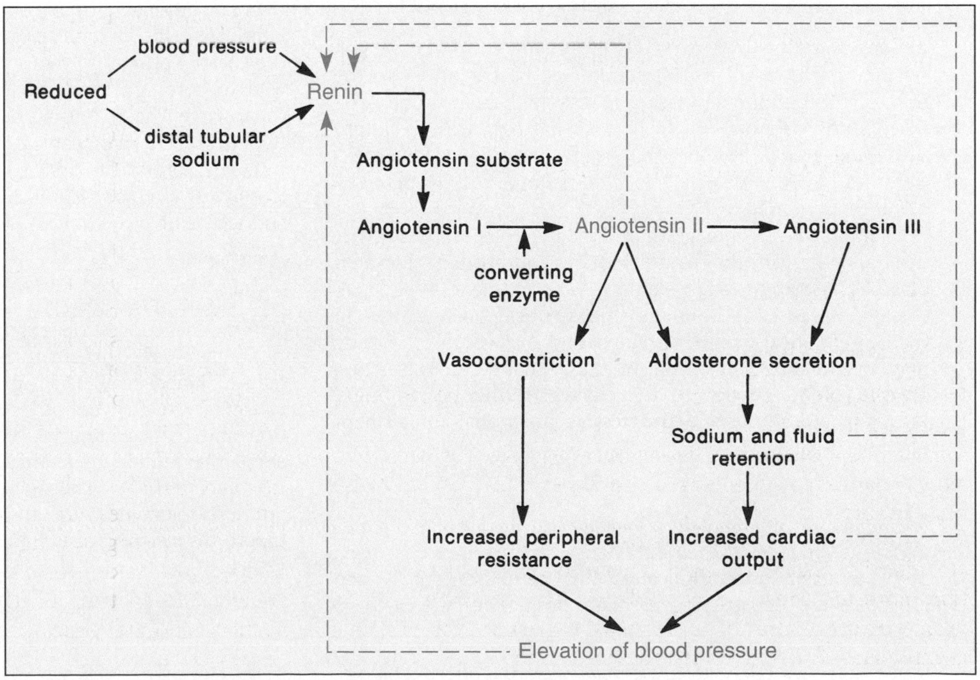

Figure 26–3

Role of renin-angiotensin-aldosterone system in regulation of blood pressure. *Solid lines* represent positive interactions; *broken lines* show negative interactions or feedback inhibition. (From Kumar, V., Cotran, R. S., & Robbins, S. L. [1992]. *Basic pathology* [5th ed.]. Philadelphia: W. B. Saunders.)

SECONDARY HYPERTENSION

The primary mechanisms involved in producing secondary hypertension include the following:

- Increased secretion of catecholamines (e.g., pheochromocytoma)
- Increased release of renin (e.g., renal artery stenosis)
- Expansion of sodium and blood volume (e.g., Cushing's syndrome)

The use of estrogen-containing oral contraceptive pills remains the most common cause of secondary hypertension. Most women who use these drugs demonstrate a slight elevation in blood pressure, and approximately 5 per cent experience hypertension that persists after discontinuation of the pill.

Renal parenchymal disease, mainly chronic glomerulonephritis, is the next most common cause of secondary hypertension.

Adrenal gland dysfunction can cause secondary hypertension as a result of primary excesses of aldosterone, cortisol, and catecholamines. Pheochromocytoma, a small tumor of the adrenal medulla, can cause hypertension as a result of the release of excessive amounts of epinephrine and norepinephrine. Excess aldosterone causes renal retention of sodium and water, expands blood volume, and elevates blood pressure. Other adrenocorticol problems can result in excess production of cortisol (Cushing's syndrome).

VESSEL CHANGES

Early in the course of primary or secondary hypertension, there may be no obvious pathologic changes in the blood vessels and organs. Slowly, widespread pathologic changes occur in both the large and small blood vessels and in the heart, kidney, and brain (see Pathophysiology: Cardiovascular Changes in Hypertension).

Clinical Manifestations

The early stages of hypertension produce no clinical manifestations other than elevations in blood pressure. This unfortunate fact means that there are no signs or symptoms to lead a person to seek health care. As hypertension advances, without treatment clients may report morning occipital headache, fatigue, dizziness, palpitations, flushing, blurred vision, and epistaxis.

Prognosis

The advent of effective antihypertensive agents has dramatically reduced the mortality rate associated with hypertension. Still, if untreated, nearly one half of hypertensive clients die of heart disease, a third die of stroke, and the remaining 10 to 15 per cent die of renal failure. Hypertension may also be a silent factor in many deaths attributed to stroke or heart attacks. When hyperten-

PATHOPHYSIOLOGY

Cardiovascular Changes in Hypertension

VESSEL CHANGES

In long-standing hypertension, eventually the large vessels—such as the aorta, coronary arteries, basilar artery to the brain, and peripheral vessels in the limbs—become sclerosed and tortuous. Their lumens narrow, with resultant decreased blood flow to the heart, brain, and lower extremities. As the damage continues, large vessels may occlude or hemorrhage.

Small vessel damage, equally dangerous, causes structural changes in the heart, kidneys, and brain. Elevated diastolic blood pressure damages the intima of the small vessels. Because of intimal damage, fibrin accumulates in the vessels, local edema develops, and intravascular clotting may occur. The net result of these changes involves decreased blood supply to the tissues of the heart, brain, kidneys, and retina and progressive functional impairment of these organs.

CARDIAC CHANGES

In the development of hypertensive cardiovascular disease, a vicious circle of pathologic changes occurs in which each new manifestation complicates other manifestations. When arterioles are constricted, cardiac contractility increases to maintain normal cardiac output and overcome elevations in afterload. This chronic overwork leads to hypertrophy of the heart, primarily the left ventricle. Hypertrophy may lead to coronary insufficiency and myocardial infarction if the enlarged heart muscle outgrows its blood supply. If the hypertrophied heart cannot maintain sufficient cardiac output, left ventricular failure ensues. Left ventricular hypertrophy is a major risk factor for cardiac arrhythmias and sudden death.

OTHER SEQUELAE

As diastolic pressure rises in the failing left ventricle and atrium, the congestion extends back to involve the entire pulmonary tree; this, in turn, may lead to right ventricular failure. Blood may back up into the systemic circulation, causing systemic venous pressure to rise. Venous congestion and reduced arterial blood flow decrease renal perfusion. The kidneys may then fail, which further aggravates the hypertension. The increased arterial pressure in the arteries, coupled with arteriosclerotic weakening of the blood vessels, can cause aneurysms to develop and blood vessels to rupture.

BOX 26–2

Guidelines for Blood Pressure Measurement

- Seat the client with the arm to be used for measurement bared, supported, and positioned at heart level. The client should not have smoked tobacco within the past 15 minutes or ingested caffeine within the past hour.
- Begin measurement after the client has rested quietly for 5 minutes. Make sure the client's back is supported and both feet are flat on the floor with the legs uncrossed. Instruct the client to not speak while blood pressure is being monitored.
- Use the appropriate cuff size to ensure an accurate measurement. The rubber bladder should encircle at least two thirds of the client's arm; the bladder's width should be one third to one half of the arm's circumference. If the cuff is too wide, the blood pressure reading will be falsely low, and if the cuff is too narrow, the reading will be falsely high. Inaccurate cuff size is the most common error made in blood pressure measurement.
- Ensure that the mercury sphygmomanometer, aneroid manometer, or electronic device is in good repair and calibrated in accordance with manufacturer recommendations.
- Measure and record both the systolic and diastolic blood pressures. Use the disappearance of sound (phase V) for the diastolic reading.
- Average two or more readings to obtain the reading that you record. If the first two readings differ by more than 5 mm Hg, obtain additional readings.

sion arises as a secondary process, death usually results from the primary disease.

Medical Management

DIAGNOSIS OF HYPERTENSION

The diagnosis of hypertension in the adult is determined when the average of two blood pressure readings (taken on a least two separate occasions at least 2 weeks apart) produces a diastolic reading of 90 mm Hg or higher or a systolic reading exceeding 140 mm Hg. Because blood pressure is variable and can be affected by multiple factors, measurement techniques should ensure that readings are representative of the client's usual readings (Box 26–2).

Clients should be informed of their blood pressure reading and advised of the need for periodic remeasurement. When working with lay clients, the examiner should refer to hypertension as "high blood pressure" to help allay confusion. The term "high blood pressure" more accurately conveys the nature of the health problem.

Categorization of Severity. The 1988 Joint National Committee on Detection, Evaluation and Treatment of High Blood Pressure developed a classification of diastolic and systolic blood pressure readings (Table 26–3). Clinicians can use this classification to categorize blood pressure readings and to diagnose hypertension in clients aged 18 years or older. Risk related to hypertension continues to increase as systolic and diastolic pressures rise. The 1984 Joint National Committee used these same classifications to develop follow-up criteria for first-occasion measurement (Table 26–4).

TABLE 26–3 Classification of Blood Pressure in Adults Aged 18 Years or Older*

RANGE (mm HG)	CATEGORY†
Diastolic	
<85	Normal BP
85–89	High-normal BP
90–104	Mild hypertension
105–114	Moderate hypertension
≥115	Severe hypertension
Systolic, when Diastolic is <90	
<140	Normal BP
140–159	Borderline isolated systolic hypertension
≥160	Isolated systolic hypertension

* Classification based on the average of two or more readings on two or more occasions.
† A classification of borderline isolated systolic hypertension (SBP 140–159 mm Hg) or isolated systolic hypertension (SBP ≥160 mm Hg) takes precedence over high-normal BP (DBP 85–89 mm Hg) when both occur in the same client. High-normal BP (DBP 85–89 mm Hg) takes precedence over a classification of normal BP (SBP <140 mm Hg) when both occur in the same client.
BP, blood pressure; DBP, diastolic blood pressure; SBP, systolic blood pressure.
From Joint National Committee (1989). The 1988 report of the Joint National Committee on detection, evaluation, and treatment of high blood pressure. *Archives of Internal Medicine, 148,* 1023. ©1989, American Medical Association.

TREATMENT OF HYPERTENSION

The goal of treating clients with hypertension is to prevent associated morbidity and mortality. Studies consistently reinforce that treatment of even mild hypertension (diastolic pressure 90–104 mm Hg) significantly reduces the risk of cardiovascular disease.[48] The objective is to achieve and maintain arterial blood pressure below 140/90 mm Hg, if possible.

Normalizing high blood pressure may involve psychosocial and economic stressors for the client. These stressors are considered when intervention is initiated. As mentioned, most hypertensive clients do not have symptoms and are not aware that they have hypertension. The long-term nature of intervention, along with the high costs and untoward side effects of pharmacologic interventions, promote poor compliance with therapeutic regimens. Poor compliance has great negative impact on the effectiveness of intervention.

TABLE 26–4 Follow-up Criteria for First-Occasion Measurement

RANGE (mm Hg)	RECOMMENDED FOLLOW-UP
Diastolic	
<85	Recheck within 2 years*
85–89	Recheck within 2 years
90–104	Confirm promptly (not to exceed 2 months)
105–114	Evaluate or refer promptly to source of care (not to exceed 2 weeks)
≥115	Evaluate or refer immediately to source of care
Systolic, when Diastolic is ≤90	
<140	Recheck within 2 years*
140–199	Confirm promptly (not to exceed 2 months)
≥200	Evaluate or refer promptly to source of care (not to exceed 2 weeks)

* Rechecking within 1 year is recommended for clients at increased risk of progressing to higher blood pressures (family history of hypertension, cardiovascular event, weight gain, obesity, black race, use of an oral contraceptive, or excessive ethanol consumption).

From U.S. Department of Health and Human Services (1988). *The 1988 Report of the Joint National Committee on detection, evaluation, and treatment of high blood pressure.* (NIH Publication No. 88–1088). Washington, DC: U.S. Government Printing Office.

Intervention for secondary hypertension rests on treating the underlying disorder, whereas intervention for primary hypertension aims directly at reducing blood pressure. Careful differential diagnosis of primary versus secondary causes of high blood pressure must precede any intervention.

Nonpharmacologic Intervention. Nonpharmacologic intervention is widely advocated as initial therapy for most clients, at least for the first 3 to 6 months after initial diagnosis. This therapy may be effective for many of the 40 per cent of clients with mild hypertension (diastolic levels between 90 and 94 mm Hg). For other clients with hypertension, nonpharmacologic therapy may aid in reducing blood pressure so as to decrease the need for drug therapy.[48]

Weight Reduction. The relationship between obesity—particularly excessive abdominal fat—and high blood pressure has been clearly established. Weight reduction to within 15 per cent of ideal body weight is recommended for all obese hypertensive clients, but even moderate weight reduction of 6.6 to 11 pounds (3 to 5 kg) is associated with reduced blood pressure.[48] Those who are able to maintain weight loss usually achieve significant blood pressure reduction.

Diet Modification. Studies demonstrating the antihypertensive efficacy of moderate sodium restriction (to approximately 1 to 2.5 g of sodium or 4 to 6 g of salt daily) have been reported since the early 1970s. Not using a salt shaker at the table may have more benefits than a severely salt-restricted diet.[48] These studies also demonstrate the ability of most clients to adhere to such a regimen. Moderate sodium restriction is not hazardous and may reduce the degree of potassium depletion accompanying diuretic therapy. Maintaining daily recommended levels of dietary potassium, calcium, and magnesium help maintain normotension.[48]

Modifying dietary fat intake by decreasing the proportion of saturated fat and increasing the proportion of polyunsaturated fat may decrease blood pressure and will decrease cholesterol level, which is an important risk factor for coronary artery disease.

The consumption of more than 1 to 2 ounces of alcohol per day is associated with a higher prevalence of hypertension, poor adherence to the antihypertensive therapy, and, occasionally, refractory hypertension. Alcohol intake should be limited to fewer than 1 to 2 ounces of ethanol per day. (There is 1 ounce of ethanol in 2 ounces of 100-proof whiskey, 8 ounces of wine, or 24 ounces of beer).

Although ingestion of caffeine may temporarily raise blood pressure, long-term moderate caffeine ingestion appears to have no significant permanent effect on blood pressure. Clients should be encouraged to limit daily caffeine intake to 250 mg (the amount in two to three cups of brewed coffee) to prevent activating the sympathetic nervous system. This sympathetic response particularly affects those not used to drinking coffee.

Stress Reduction. Stress elevates blood pressure in some clients by increasing peripheral vascular resistance, increasing cardiac output, and stimulating the sympathetic nervous system. Therapy to reduce the stress response is beneficial in certain clients; such therapies may include transcendental meditation, yoga, biofeedback, and psychotherapy.

Smoking Cessation. For clients who smoke, the most important nonpharmacologic intervention is enrolling in a smoking-cessation program.[48] Nicotine increases heart rate and produces peripheral vasoconstriction, causing transient elevation in arterial pressure. Smokers appear to have a higher frequency of malignant hypertension and subarachnoid hemorrhage. In addition, risk reduction brought about by antihypertensive therapy may not be as great in smokers as in nonsmokers. Smoking cessation greatly reduces the risk of cardiovascular disease, pulmonary disease, and cancer.

Exercise. A regular program of aerobic (isotonic) exercise facilitates cardiovascular conditioning, can aid weight reduction, can raise levels of high-density lipoproteins relative to total blood cholesterol, and may provide some benefit in reducing blood pressure. Heavy isometric exercises, such as weightlifting, may be harmful to the hypertensive client; blood pressure often rises to very high levels because of vasovagal reflexes that occur during an isometric contraction. Hypertensive clients should be advised to initiate exercise programs gradually and receive ongoing professional surveillance of their condition.

Pharmacologic Intervention. Once a decision has been made to use pharmacologic intervention, one of several drugs can be used. If therapy is chosen carefully, mild hypertension can be controlled with a single drug in more than half of clients, and more than 90 per cent of clients can achieve control with no more than two drugs. Long-term compliance has emerged as an essential element in reducing morbidity and mortality associated with hypertension. Several factors related to specific drug use, including side effects, interference with life-style, cost, and inconvenience of use, play an important role in noncompliance. Thus, drug selection is a critical part of the management of the client with hypertension. The ultimate factors in determining whether a correct choice has been made are that the medication controls the blood pressure, is tolerated, is safe, and is a drug that the client is willing to take for the long term.

Antihypertensive medications can be classified by mode of action into the following categories:

- Diuretics
- Adrenergic inhibitors
- Vasodilators
- Angiotensin-converting enzyme (ACE) inhibitors
- Calcium antagonists

Table 26–5 outlines major antihypertensive agents.

Historically, diuretics have been used to initiate antihypertensive therapy. Thiazide diuretics have been used for more than 30 years in the treatment of hypertension. However, an increasing number of hypertensive clients are initially treated with beta-blockers, calcium channel blockers, or ACE inhibitors.

Stepped-Care Approach. The goal of antihypertensive therapy is to control blood pressure with a minimum of side effects. The Joint National Committee on Detection, Evaluation and Treatment of Hypertension has recommended the stepped-care approach to the treatment of hypertension (Table 26–6). The 1988 report expands the pharmacologic choices available for initial and subsequent therapy and encourages substituting drugs as well as adding or reducing drugs to improve blood pressure control or reduce side effects.

Step-Down Therapy. Once a client with mild hypertension has achieved control for 1 year or longer, medications can be titrated down slowly. Regular follow-up is essential.

Combination Therapy. Clients with mild hypertension who do not obtain adequate control with one drug require combination therapy. The combination of a diuretic with a beta-adrenergic blocker or other adrenergic inhibitor has proven effective in many clients who do not respond well to the individual drugs given separately. The combination of diuretic and ACE inhibitor is synergistic because diuretics create high-renin hypertension, a milieu in which ACE inhibitors are effective. Orthostatic hypotension can be a problem, especially in older clients or those with acute volume depletion. The combination of a diuretic and calcium channel blocker has additive effects on blood pressure.

Complication: Malignant Hypertension

Malignant (accelerated) hypertension is a medical emergency. Presenting characteristics are as follows:

- Diastolic pressures exceeding 120 mm Hg
- Retinal hemorrhage
- Rapid vascular deterioration

(See Clinical Manifestations: Malignant Hypertension.)

Malignant hypertension has a peak incidence at age 40 to 50 years; its occurrence in clients younger than 30 years or older than 60 years should raise the suspicion of a secondary cause of hypertension. Without treatment, malignant hypertension results in a 90 per cent mortality rate within 1 year secondary to renal or congestive heart failure, cerebrovascular accident, myocardial infarction, or aortic dissection. Adequate blood pressure control reduces the risk of these complications.

The most common cause of malignant hypertension is untreated hypertension. Other causes include eclampsia, dissecting aortic aneurysms, pyelonephritis, revascular hypertension, glomerulonephritis, sudden catecholamine release (from pheochromocytoma), drug or toxic substance ingestion or exposure, or drug-food interactions (e.g., monoamine oxidase inhibitors and aged cheeses).

MANAGEMENT

Malignant hypertension constitutes a true medical emergency, and any delay in initiating intervention can be catastrophic. The seriousness of the crisis correlates not so much with the level of blood pressure elevation as with the extent of target organ damage. Intervention relies almost entirely on parenteral administration of medications, such as intravenous nitroprusside.[39] Most often, the physician orders concurrent administration of two or three agents (Table 26–7). If possible, blood and urine samples should be obtained before initiating pharmacologic therapy to aid diagnosis of the underlying cause.

These clients require monitoring in an intensive care unit. Parameters requiring close scrutiny include urinary output, blood pressure (monitored via an intra-arterial catheter), central venous pressure, pulmonary capillary wedge pressure, and electrocardiographic (ECG) waveforms.

CLINICAL MANIFESTATIONS

Malignant Hypertension

- Diastolic pressure exceeding 120 mm Hg
- Retinal hemorrhage
- Rapid vascular deterioration
- Papilledema
- Renal insufficiency or acute renal failure (marked by proteinuria, hematuria, casts in urine)
- Encephalopathy (marked by restlessness, decreased level of consciousness, lethargy, dizziness, coma, seizures, nausea, vomiting)
- Left ventricular failure
- Pulmonary edema
- Hemolytic anemia
- Severe headache (occipital or anterior location, steady and throbbing, worse in the morning)
- Visual blurring, reduced acuity, or blindness

TABLE 26–5 Antihypertensive Medication Therapy

MEDICATION	ACTIONS	COMMENTS	CONTRAINDICATIONS	SIDE EFFECTS	NURSING CONSIDERATIONS
Diuretics					
Thiazide and Related Sulfonamides					
Bendroflumethiazide (Naturetin) Benzthiazide (ExNa, Aquatag) Chlorothiazide (Diuril) Chlorthalidone (Hygroton) Hydrochlorothiazide (Esidrex, Hydro-Diuril, Oretic) Methyclothiazide (Naturon) Polythiazide (Renese) Trichlormethiazide (Metahydrin, Naqua) Metolazone (Zaroxolyn) Quinethazone (Hydromox)	Promote renal excretion of sodium, water, and potassium Blood volume and cardiac output are decreased at first; with continued therapy, levels rise to normal Peripheral vascular resistance is increased at first, then drops below normal	All thiazides have a comparable effect on blood pressure, differing mainly in potency and duration Alone, thiazides can control hypertension in 40% of clients; in combination, they permit smaller doses of other antihypertensive agents Inexpensive	Known sensitivity to sulfonamide-derived drugs; renal insufficiency or failure; hepatic disease; lactation; blood urea nitrogen 40% or higher	Hypokalemia, hyperglycemia, hyperuricemia, hypercalcemia, lethargy, dry mouth, thirst, restlessness, muscle cramps, hypotension, polyuria, fatigue, tachycardia, gastrointestinal disturbances, vertigo, gout, leukopenia, and agranulocytosis Sexual dysfunction may occur May increase cholesterol, low-density lipoprotein, and triglyceride levels	Warn client that orthostatic hypotension may be potentiated by alcohol, barbiturates, and narcotics Monitor serum electrolytes, blood urea nitrogen, uric acid Teach client which foods are high in potassium and low in sodium Daily weight monitoring Resulting hypokalemia can potentiate digitalis toxicity Monitor diabetic clients closely
Loop Diuretics					
Furosemide (Lasix) Ethacrynic acid (Edecrin) Bumetadine (Bumex)	Comparable to thiazides Act on loop of Henle to minimize sodium and water reabsorption	Drug of choice in clients with renal failure	Comparable to thiazides; not recommended in pregnant women	Same as thiazides, hyponatremia, plus dehydration, vascular thrombosis, and embolism in elderly Can cause side effects, oral and gastric burning, and a sweet taste	Comparable to thiazides May avoid taking drug before bedtime to prevent frequent urination and loss of sleep May need to increase dose of hypoglycemic agents
Potassium-Sparing Diuretics					
Spironolactone (Aldactone) Triamterene (Dyrenium)	Block action of aldosterone in distal loop, promoting excretion of sodium and water and retention of potassium Action of triamterene is unknown	These are weak diuretics that potentiate other antihypertensive drugs	Acute renal insufficiency, rapidly progressing impaired renal function, and hyperkalemia Avoid concomitant use with calcium channel–blocking agents	Hyperkalemia, hyponatremia, elevated blood urea nitrogen, gynecomastia, menstrual irregularity, hirsutism, headache, urticaria, impotency, and ataxia (with spironolactone) Blood dyscrasias with triamterene	Administer after meals to reduce nausea Potassium supplementation not required Closely monitor potassium, especially in those with renal insufficiency

TABLE 26–5 Antihypertensive Medication Therapy *Continued*

MEDICATION	ACTIONS	COMMENTS	CONTRAINDICATIONS	SIDE EFFECTS	NURSING CONSIDERATIONS
Vasodilators					
Hydralazine (Apresoline)	Direct action on smooth muscle walls of arterioles causing arteriolar vasodilation Cardiac output increases initially, then returns to normal Peripheral vascular resistance is decreased There is also some vasodilation	Most commonly used in combination with a beta-blocking agent and a diuretic with good results. Antihypertensive effects can be counteracted by the increase in cardiac output	Coronary artery disease, mitral valvular rheumatic heart disease, and hypersensitivity to drug	Minimal side effects Headache, palpitation, flushing, dyspnea, angina pectoris, and lupus-like syndrome (after prolonged use)	Monitor for reflex tachycardia Treat headache with acetaminophen, cold packs, or relaxation techniques
Adrenergic Inhibiting Agents					
Beta-Adrenergic Inhibitors (Beta-Blockers)					
Propranolol (Inderal) Metoprolol (Lopressor) Nadolol (Corgard) Atenolol (Tenormin) Timolol (Biocadren) Pindolol (Visken) Labetalol (Trandate, Normodyne)	Block beta-receptors in the heart and peripheral vessels to reduce peripheral vascular resistance	These agents vary in their effects on beta-receptors: some (i.e., propranolol) affect $beta_1$- and $beta_2$-receptors; others (e.g., atenolol, metoprolol, and pindolol) are cardioselective, affecting only $beta_1$-receptors	Bronchial asthma, allergic rhinitis, chronic obstructive pulmonary disease, bradycardia, heart block, pulmonary hypertension, and congestive heart failure Do not give with (or less than 2 weeks after) therapy with monoamine oxidase inhibitors	Bradycardia, congestive heart failure, bronchospasm, hypoglycemia, fatigue, vivid and colorful dreams, insomnia, Raynaud's phenomenon, depression, nausea, vomiting, diarrhea, fluid retention, and (rarely) impotence	Avoid use in clients with bronchial asthma Assess for signs of heart failure Instruct client to take own pulse daily for evidence of bradycardia or irregularity Warn diabetics that these medications may mask signs of hypoglycemia Do not stop abruptly; this may exacerbate myocardial ischemia Toxic effects are reversed with isoproterenol or dopamine
Alpha-Adrenergic Inhibitors					
Prazosin hydrochloride (Minipress)	Vasodilation occurs with a decrease in peripheral vascular resistance Cardiac output and heart rate are usually unchanged	Most effective in combination with a diuretic or other sympatholytic agent	Not recommended for pregnant women	First-dose syncope; postural hypertension, dizziness, light-headedness, headache, drowsiness, nausea, lethargy, palpitations, rash, nervousness, diaphoresis, impotence, urinary frequency, and depression	Monitor closely after drug administration (especially first dose) because postural hypotension and syncope may occur 30 to 90 minutes after dose is initiated Used cautiously in the elderly because postural hypotension is more pronounced

Table continued on following page

TABLE 26–5 Antihypertensive Medication Therapy *Continued*

MEDICATION	ACTIONS	COMMENTS	CONTRAINDICATIONS	SIDE EFFECTS	NURSING CONSIDERATIONS
Central-Acting Adrenergic Inhibitors					
Clonidine (Catapres)	Suppress central nervous system sympathetic outflow Cardiac output decreases at first, then returns to normal Peripheral vascular resistance and heart rate decrease	An extremely effective medication, especially in clients with severe hypertension or renin-dependent disease	Not recommended for pregnant women Tricyclic antidepressants may block drug's effect	Dry mouth, sedation, dizziness, constipation, headache, fatigue, bradycardia, some sodium and water retention (transient), and hyperglycemia	Action potentiated by alcohol, sedatives, digitalis, propranolol, and guanethidine Diabetics may require more insulin Drug should be discontinued over 2–4 days to prevent rebound hypertension Recommended periodic eye examinations Chewing gum or hard candy may relieve dry mouth
Calcium Channel–Blocking Agents					
Nifedipine (Procardia) Verapamil hydrochloride (Calan, Isoptin) Ditiazem (Cardizem) Nicardipine (Cardene)	Block entry of calcium into smooth muscle cells and may interfere with the intracellular release of calcium Cause arteriolar vasodilation and decreased peripheral vascular resistance	Nifedipine has the most potent vasodilating effect Nifedipine and diltiazem are preferred agents in this group	Severe congestive heart failure, sick sinus syndrome, or progressive heart block Avoid use with beta-blocking agents	Headache, dizziness, palpitations, weakness, nausea, flushing, hypotension, arrhythmia, constipation, diarrhea, rash, fluid retention, and edema Verapamil can cause bradycardia	Watch for sudden hypotension, especially with the administration of nifedipine; this can occur 5 minutes after sublingual administration and 20 minutes after the oral route Monitor pulse for bradycardia with use of verapamil May exacerbate asthma, peripheral vascular disease, and diabetes
Angiotensin-Converting Enzyme Inhibitors					
Captopril (Capoten) Enalapril (Vasotec) Lisinopril (Zestril, Prinivil)	Inhibits conversion of angiotensin I to angiotensin II May also inactivate the vasodepressor bradykinin Reduces peripheral vascular resistance without changing cardiac output	Extremely effective in clients with high-renin, severe hypertension Most effective when given in conjunction with a diuretic	Use with caution in clients with preexisting renal insufficiency and renal artery stenosis	Fever, rash, stomatitis, taste loss, tongue ulceration, hyperkalemia, granulocytopenia, hemolytic anemia, and renal damage with proteinuria	Monthly urine protein analysis recommended along with a leukocyte count to detect renal damage Taste loss is a frequent side effect and may decrease desire for eating Hypotension may accompany first dose
Peripheral-Acting Adrenergic Inhibitors					
Reserpine (Serpasil)	Depletes brain and peripheral nerve tissues of norepinephrine Decreases peripheral vascular resistance, heart rate, and standing blood pressure	Has same actions as other rauwolfia alkaloids Seldom used alone but in combination with a diuretic or other sympatholytic agent	Mental depression, especially with suicidal tendencies; peptic ulcer disease; and ulcerative colitis	Depression, weight gain, nasal stuffiness, peptic ulceration, postural hypotension, drowsiness, constipation, bizarre dreams, bradycardia, and impotence	Observe for signs of depression; instruct client to notify physician or nurse if "low mood" sets in Depletes catecholamines, so stop reserpine 2 weeks before elective surgery Concurrent use with digitalis and quinidine may potentiate arrhythmias

TABLE 26–6 Stepped-Care Approach to Drug Therapy of Hypertension

Step 1	The physician starts with less than a full dose of a thiazide diuretic, beta-blocker, calcium channel blocker, or angiotensin-converting enzyme inhibitor and adjusts the dosage as necessary.
Step 2	If blood pressure control is not obtained, the physician increases the dose of the first drug or adds a drug of a different class.
Step 3	If blood pressure control is not obtained, the physician substitutes a second drug or adds a third drug of a different class.
Step 4	If blood pressure control is not obtained, the physician adds a third or fourth drug and evaluates further.

From U.S. Department of Health and Human Services. (1988). *The 1988 Report of the Joint National Committee on detection, evaluation, and treatment of high blood pressure* (NIH Publication No. 88–1088). Washington, DC: U.S. Government Printing Office.

The goal of treatment is to reduce blood pressure. However, as blood pressure drops, evidence of target organ impairment (especially of the kidneys) may appear. Consequently, blood pressure reduction must be done slowly, decreasing the diastolic blood pressure 25 per cent or to 100 mm Hg while maintaining urine output greater than 20 mL/hr.[34,48] Once the client is out of immediate danger, oral medications are administered while vital signs are continuously monitored. The physician typically prescribes a combination of a diuretic, a beta-blocker, and hydralazine. With better surveillance and control of hypertensive clients, hypertensive crisis is becoming less common.

Nursing care of a client with malignant hypertension involves closely monitoring blood pressure (taking readings every 15 minutes) and urine output, titrating the medications to manage blood pressure, and taking steps to reduce the client's anxiety. The client's head is raised to decrease the risk of cerebral bleeding.

TABLE 26–7 Parenteral Drugs for Treatment of Hypertensive Emergency (in Order of Rapidity of Action)

DRUG	DOSAGE	ONSET OF ACTION	ADVERSE EFFECTS
Vasodilators			
Nitroprusside (Nipride, Nitropress)	0.25–10 μg/kg/min as IV infusion	Instantaneous	Nausea, vomiting, muscle twitching, sweating, thiocyanate intoxication, hypotension
Nitroglycerin	5–10 μg/min as IV infusion	2–5 min	Tachycardia, flushing, headache, vomiting, methemoglobinemia, hypotension
Diazoxide (Hyperstat)	50–100 mg/IV bolus repeated, or 15–30 mg/min by IV infusion	2–4 min	Nausea, hypotension, flushing, tachycardia, chest pain
Hydralazine (Apresoline)	10–20 mg IV 10–50 mg IM	10–20 min 20–30 min	Tachycardia, flushing, headache, vomiting, aggravation of angina
Enalaprilat (Vasotec IV)	1.25–4 mg every 6 hr	15 min	Precipitous fall in blood pressure in high renin states; response variable
Nicardipine (Cardene)	5–10 mg/hr IV	10 min	Tachycardia, headache, flushing, local phlebitis
Adrenergic Inhibitors			
Phentolamine (Regitine)	5–15 mg IV	1–2 min	Tachycardia, flushing
Trimethaphan (Arfonad)	O.5–5 mg/min as IV infusion	1–5 min	Paresis of bowel and bladder, orthostatic hypotension, blurred vision, dry mouth
Esmolol (Brevibloc)	500 μg/kg/min for 1 min then 50–300 μg/kg/min IV for 4 min; if effect inadequate, repeat loading dose and increase dose of maintenance infusion	1–2 min	Hypotension
Propranolol (Inderal)	1–10 mg load; 3 ng/hr	1–2 min	Beta-blocker side effect (e.g., bronchospasm, decreased cardiac output)
Labetalol (Normodyne, Trandate)	30–80 mg IV bolus every 10 min 2 mg/min IV infusion	5–10 min	Vomiting, scalp tingling, burning in throat, postural hypotension, dizziness, nausea

IM, intramuscularly; IV, intravenously.
From Kaplan, N. M. (1992). Hypertension. In R. E. Rakel (Ed.). *Conn's current therapy 1992.* Philadelphia: W. B. Saunders.

Nursing Management

Assessment

Assessing the client with hypertension involves three main objectives:

- To determine the extent of target organ involvement
- To ascertain the presence of other cardiovascular risk factors
- To identify symptoms associated with primary or secondary hypertension

The nurse can obtain information relevant to these areas from the history, physical examination, and laboratory studies.

History: The nurse notes the following points when interviewing a hypertensive client:

- Previous documentation of high blood pressure, including age of onset, currently prescribed medical regimen, and compliance with this regimen
- Results and side effects of previous antihypertensive therapy
- Clinical manifestations of cardiovascular disorders, such as angina, dyspnea, and claudication
- Presence of other cardiovascular risk factors, including smoking, obesity, hyperlipidemia, and sedentary life-style
- History of any disease or trauma to target organs
- History of all prescribed and over-the-counter medications (medications that may either raise blood pressure or interfere with the effectiveness of antihypertensive medications include oral contraceptives, steroids, nonsteroidal anti-inflammatory agents, cold remedies, appetite suppressants, cyclosporine, tricyclic antidepressants, and monoamine oxidase inhibitors)
- Psychosocial and environmental factors (e.g., emotional stress, cultural food practices, and economic status) that may influence blood pressure control
- Family history of hypertension, diabetes mellitus, or cardiovascular disease

Physical Examination: Physical assessment should include determination of blood pressure as well as evaluation of target organs. Evaluation of target organs typically includes the following data:

- Funduscopic examination for retinal arteriolar narrowing, hemorrhages, exudates, and papilledema
- Examination of the neck for distended veins, carotid bruits, and enlarged thyroid
- Examination of the heart for increased heart rate, arrhythmias, enlargement, precordial impulses, murmurs, and S_3 and S_4 heart sounds
- Examination of the abdomen for bruits, aortic dilation, and enlarged kidneys
- Examination of extremities for diminished or absent peripheral pulses, edema, and bilateral inequality of pulses
- Neurologic evaluation for signs of cerebral thrombosis, hemorrhage, or encephalopathy

The nurse should be especially alert for assessment findings suggesting secondary hypertension. These include the following:

- Headache, palpitations, and excessive perspiration (suggesting pheochromocytoma)
- Leg claudication and diminished or absent lower extremity pulses (suggesting aortic coarctation)
- Truncal obesity with pigmented striae (suggesting Cushing's syndrome)
- Polyuria, fatigue, and muscle cramps (suggesting hyperaldosteronism)

Laboratory Studies: A few general laboratory tests are usually done before intervention begins. These tests provide useful information in determining the severity of vascular disease, the extent of target organ damage, and the possible causes of hypertension. Studies used in the routine evaluation of hypertension include the following:

- Complete blood count
- Urinalysis
- Serum potassium and sodium
- Fasting blood glucose
- Serum cholesterol
- Blood urea nitrogen
- Serum creatinine
- ECG
- Chest x-ray

Clients with the potential for secondary hypertension may need more extensive studies.

Nursing Diagnosis, Planning, and Implementation

Nursing Diagnosis: Health Maintenance. Altered R/T knowledge deficit about the disease process, its consequences, and the rationale for intervention and proper administration of prescribed medications.

Planning: Expected Outcomes. The client and significant others will demonstrate knowledge required for self-care, as evidenced by their ability to describe the disease process, factors contributing to its symptoms and risks, and reasons that management of this disease is important; their ability to describe the proper administration of prescribed medication therapy, including drug name, rationale for use, dosage, frequency, potential side effects, and measures to minimize side effects; use of proper blood pressure measurement technique for home blood pressure monitoring; and their ability to discuss the importance of lifelong medical follow-up for hypertension control.

Implementation. Because of the chronicity of hypertension and its dangerous complications, clients with this condition need clear, practical, and realistic learning guidelines concerning effective handling of high blood pressure. Guidelines should include information concerning the disease and its management. The nurse uses written materials with clear illustrations to introduce the subject of hypertension to the newly diagnosed client. One must teach the client to monitor and record his or her own blood pressure at home at least once a week and record the findings in a diary.

Nursing Diagnosis: Nutrition, Altered: More than Body Requirements R/T high sodium, calorie, and fat intake.

Planning: Expected Outcomes. The client will demonstrate knowledge of and adherence to the nutritional regimen by describing specific dietary modifications including sodium, fat, and calorie restrictions and their rationale; listing common foods to be avoided; reduced levels of urine sodium and blood cholesterol; and weight loss.

Implementation. The two most important aspects of dietary intervention for hypertension are weight reduction (for overweight clients) and mild to moderate sodium restriction. It is important, therefore, to advise the client with hypertension to eat a diet with no added salt, low in cholesterol and saturated fat, and with adequate calories. The nurse must discuss the prescribed diet with those in the household who prepare food. If possible, enlist the aid of a dietitian to provide detailed dietary instruction. A highly individualized approach to dietary counseling is critical.

Sodium. Sodium is a hidden ingredient in many processed foods, beverages (including water), and over-the-counter drugs (particularly antacids, cough remedies, and laxatives). It cannot be seen and is often not tasted. Whereas the average adult daily intake of salt is 5 to 15 g, the therapeutic effects of sodium reduction on blood pressure do not occur until salt intake is reduced below 5 g/day. Low-salt diets can be very difficult to adhere to, at least initially. The nurse can reassure the client that it becomes easier as the palate adjusts to decreased salt over a period of several weeks to months. When someone becomes fully accustomed to the low-salt diet, unsalted foods usually cease to taste bland.

Calories and Weight. Ideally, weight loss should be no more than 0.5 kg (1 pound) a week. Reduction of fat to less than 30 per cent of total daily caloric intake has proven effective in decreasing weight and helping maintain weight reduction. The overall goal should be achievement and maintenance of a weight that is within 15 per cent of desirable weight.

Guidelines for teaching clients about sodium, fat, and cholesterol reduction are presented in the Client Education Guides: Low-Sodium Diet and Low-Fat, Low-Cholesterol Diet.

Nursing Diagnosis: Health Maintenance, Altered R/T lack of exercise regimen.

Planning: Expected Outcomes. The client will begin and maintain an appropriate exercise program, as evidenced by self-report, demonstration of ability to monitor heart rate during exercise, sensation of reduced physical and emotional stress, and reduced blood pressure.

Implementation. A modest but consistent exercise program provides greater benefits than do spurts of strenuous activity mixed with periods of inactivity. A gradually increasing program of aerobic activity such as walking, jogging, or swimming can thus be recommended. Some clients benefit from a monitored cardiac rehabilitation outpatient program. Current recommen-

CLIENT EDUCATION GUIDE

Low-Sodium Diet

The nurse should instruct the client as follows:

Avoid foods high in sodium:

- Read labels of foods carefully for "sodium," "Na^+," "salt," "NaCl," "bicarbonate of soda," and "MSG" because these are all sources of sodium. If these words appear in the first four to five ingredients listed on the package, avoid the food item.
- Know that sodium is present in large amounts in common commercial preparations such as baking powder, baking soda, monosodium glutamate, meat tenderizer, and soy sauce.
- Be aware that sodium is often added in canned, boxed, and some frozen foods. (Frozen fruits and vegetables are okay.)
- Avoid eating canned, smoked, pickled, or cured meat and fish products (canned tuna in water is okay). Pickled or preserved vegetables always contain salt.
- Keep in mind that not all dietetic foods are sodium free.
- In restaurants, choose foods that are baked, broiled, boiled, or roasted and without salted gravies or juices. Avoid soups and salted or cheesy dressings. Carry your own salt substitute if desired. "Fast foods" also tend to be high in sodium.
- Be aware that light salt has half the sodium of table salt per unit. Nonsodium salt substitutes have a high potassium content and may be used to help prevent potassium deficiency if the client is taking a thiazide diuretic.

Prepare low-sodium meals:

- Do not add salt at the table.
- Use no salt during food preparation (2-g sodium diet); or use only half the salt called for in the recipe (4-g sodium diet).
- Prepare canned vegetables (if they are to be eaten at all) by draining off the canned liquid and heating the food in tap water.
- Natural spices, herbs, and condiments like pepper, parsley, chili, horseradish, lemon, and cloves contain negligible amounts of salt. These can be used liberally. Onion or garlic powder (dehydrated or pulverized) is also useful in low-salt cooking. Steak sauce, catsup, marinade, and soy sauce are all high in sodium.
- Avoid herb salts (celery, onion, garlic), which contain sodium.
- Low-sodium cookbooks are available in bookstores and from heart associations.
- Foods high and low in sodium are listed in Chapter 3.

CLIENT EDUCATION GUIDE

Low-Fat, Low-Cholesterol Diet

The nurse should teach the client tips to reduce intake of saturated fats and cholesterol, including:

- Use margarine and vegetable oils instead of butter.
- Avoid gravies, creams, and cheese sauces.
- Avoid fried foods; broil, bake, or boil instead.
- Use skim or low-fat milk or milk products.
- Choose lean cuts of meat. Trim off all visible fat. Remove all poultry skin.
- Use a wire rack when roasting, broiling, or baking meats so that the fat can drip off.
- Fish, poultry, and veal have lower fat content. Breast of chicken and turkey are the leanest poultry available. Avoid duck and goose. Haddock, cod, and water-packed tuna are the leanest fish available.
- Use Teflon-coated pans to reduce the need for cooking oil.
- Prepare meat stews, soups, and gravies in advance, chill until the fat hardens, and then skim off the fat.
- Eat no more than three egg yolks per week. Egg whites are low in cholesterol, as are many egg substitutes.
- Limit the consumption of organ meats and shellfish.

dations include aerobic exercise, maintaining 70 to 80 per cent of maximal heart rate for 20 to 30 minutes, three times a week. Maximal heart rate is calculated by subtracting age from 220. The client should be instructed, however, to avoid heavy weightlifting and other isometric exercises. (See cardiac rehabilitation after a myocardial infarction, Chap. 24).

Nursing Diagnosis: Noncompliance, Risk for R/T lack of understanding about the seriousness of high blood pressure, cost of therapy, side effects of medications.

Planning: Expected Outcomes. The client will demonstrate understanding of the seriousness of high blood pressure and accept the treatment plan, as evidenced by active participation in creating treatment plan, description of underlying causes of hypertension and self-care strategies, adherence to scheduled follow-up appointments, description of actions and side effects of current medications, and expression of commitment to and self-responsibility for controlling hypertension.

Implementation. Nursing interventions for promoting compliance with the antihypertensive treatment regimen include individualizing care, ensuring adequate follow-up, communicating often with the client, and teaching the client and family (see Ethical Issues in Nursing). Clients should be active partners in their care. They are encouraged to discuss medication side effects with care providers and not simply to stop taking medication. Compliance usually improves dramatically when the client understands the causative factors underlying hypertension as well as the consequences of inadequate intervention and health maintenance. Teaching hypertensive clients the importance of proper medication administration is vital. Health-care professionals must reinforce that medications are to be taken. If side effects or intolerable symptoms occur, the client should continue taking the medications and consult the health-care professional.

Antihypertensive medications may cause emotional lability, sleep disturbances, and sexual changes, including impotency. The nurse must discuss these potential problems with the hypertensive client and significant others. Multiple medication combinations are available that can produce adequate blood pressure control with minimal side effects.

ETHICAL ISSUES IN NURSING

What Is the Responsibility of Health-Care Providers in the Care of Noncompliant Hypertensive Clients?

Hypertension is a major predisposing factor to heart disease. Although many times it can be easily treated with medication, many clients are not aware that they have high blood pressure. There are many behavioral activities one can practice to safeguard against hypertension, including exercise; eating a low-fat, low-sodium diet; limiting alcohol consumption; and avoiding high-stress activities. Sometimes clients need medication along with their healthy life-style adjustments to keep their hypertension under control.

Teaching hypertensive clients the importance of proper medication use is vital. Often, because they may not feel any physical symptoms of hypertension, clients may forget to take their medication or feel that there is no need to take it regularly. Reinforcement from health-care providers that medications must be taken as ordered no matter what symptoms they may or may not have is vital. It is also very important for health-care providers to teach clients about behavioral changes as described. What do health-care providers do with clients who, even after the most intense teaching has been done, are not compliant with their treatment? Should the nurses and physicians give up treating such clients? What is the responsibility of hypertensive clients regarding the following of their treatment guidelines? If such noncompliant clients receive public funds for their health care, should they have to pay back the public programs for treatments rendered as a result of their noncompliance?

Because hypertension is often not indicated by physical symptoms, clients with hypertension can easily ignore their treatment regimen. Not until their high blood pressure causes more severe cardiac and peripheral vascular problems do clients realize the negative aspects of their noncompliance. Not all hypertensive clients, of course, are noncompliant. It is the noncompliant clients, however, who present great challenges to the nursing staff. Again, client teaching is one of the greatest services nurses can offer their clients with high blood pressure.

Evaluation

The nurse evaluates the attainment of expected outcomes. Hypertension is a long-term disorder, and goal attainment should be evaluated after several months and on an ongoing basis.

Modification of Plan of Care for the Elderly

The incidence of hypertension in persons older than 65 years is approaching 50 per cent. Elderly clients with essential hypertension display predominately systolic hypertension.[45] Historically, systolic hypertension in the elderly was considered a normal aging process and a physiologic compensatory mechanism to maintain organ blood flow.[45, 48] However, several studies have shown that untreated systolic hypertension in the elderly is associated with increased morbidity and mortality related to cardiovascular disease (e.g., stroke, myocardial infarction, congestive heart failure, and dissecting aneurysm). Older adults are also more likely to experience adverse reactions to antihypertensive drugs, especially orthostatic hypotension and decreased renal blood flow with decreased urine output.[48]

Because many frail elderly clients have decreased appetites and decreased taste sensation, dietary restrictions may lead to poor nutritional status. Exercise may not be an option because of concurrent disease (e.g., arthritis, congestive heart failure).[11] Although controversy does exist, most elderly clients seem to tolerate ACE inhibitors and calcium channel blockers in combination with thiazide diuretics.[11, 45]

Blood pressure readings in older adults may show greater variability from one reading to the next than readings in younger clients. The examiner must thus guard against making a diagnosis on the basis of too few readings.[12] Close monitoring is important.

Nursing Care of Clients with Arterial Disorders

CHRONIC ARTERIAL OCCLUSION

Peripheral arterial occlusive disorders involve narrowing of the arterial lumen or damage to the endothelial lining. These disorders are sometimes classified according to duration as either acute or chronic.

Peripheral arterial occlusive diseases can be caused by atherosclerosis, embolism, thrombosis, trauma, vasospasm, inflammation, and autoimmunity. The cause of some disorders remains unknown.

Most pathologic changes that occur in peripheral arterial occlusive disease are due to atherosclerosis. Atherosclerosis is discussed in detail in Chapter 24.

The peripheral arterial system delivers oxygen-rich blood to the peripheral vascular beds. Any alteration in blood flow will disrupt the balance between oxygen supply and demand. Prolonged reduction in blood flow or the involvement of large areas of decreased perfusion initiates the compensatory mechanisms of vasodilation, collateralization, and utilization of anaerobic pathways to meet metabolic demands.

These compensatory mechanisms are useful in protecting the blood supply to the peripheral vascular bed but are limited by certain factors. Vasodilation has a limited effect because arteries that become oxygen deprived quickly dilate fully. The diffuse network of collateral vessels needed to protect blood supply develops slowly over time. Cellular anaerobic metabolism tries to meet the basic requirements, but the waste products of lactic acid and pyruvic acid build up quickly, are extremely toxic, and are excreted slowly. Significant increases in these two acids will change the body's acid-base balance. As the compensatory mechanisms prove inadequate to meet peripheral vascular needs and without medical or surgical intervention, the eventual result is peripheral gangrene.

Clinical Manifestations

Clinical manifestations of chronic arterial occlusion resulting from peripheral vascular disease may not appear for 20 to 40 years. The legs are far more susceptible to arterial occlusive disorders and atherosclerosis than are the arms. The most common locations for stenosis in the leg are the aortoiliac bifurcation and the femoral bifurcation (Fig. 26–4). These lesions cause narrowing

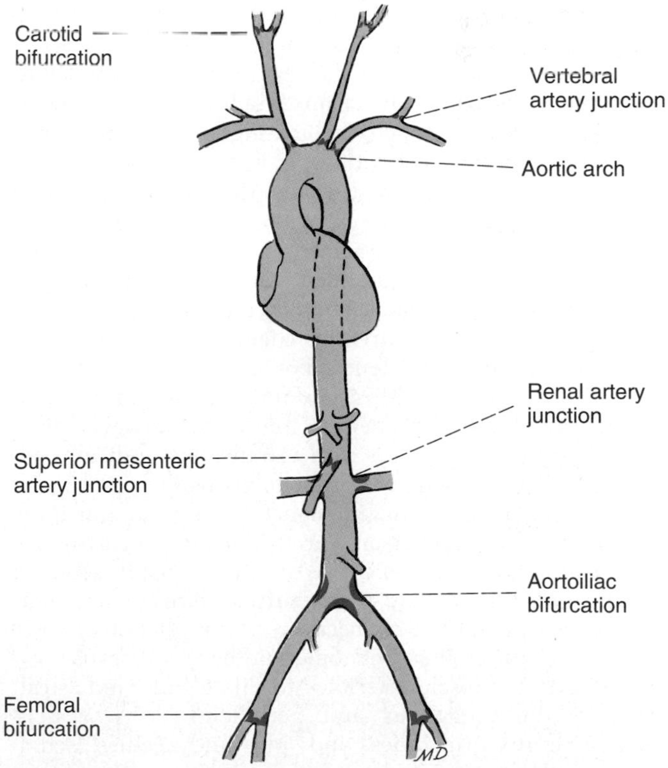

Figure 26–4
Major sites of peripheral atherosclerotic occlusive disease.

BOX 26–3

Intermittent Claudication

A client with chronic arterial occlusive disease will typically complain of pain, described as tightening pressure in the calves, thighs, or gluteal muscles or a sharp, cramplike sensation that occurs during walking and disappears quickly with 1 to 2 minutes of rest. Location of the pain depends on the location of the occlusive process. This pain, known as *intermittent claudication,* is influenced by the speed, incline, or surface of the walk. The client's exercise tolerance decreases over time; episodes of claudication occur more frequently with less exertion. One classic characteristic of intermittent claudication is that it is reproducible; that is, the same situation produces the same response almost every time.

Intermittent claudication occurs when a muscle is forced to contract without an adequate blood supply to meet the metabolic needs of exercise. It is a pathologic process similar to angina. The only specific symptom of peripheral arterial disease, it results from muscular hypoxia and metabolite accumulation.

of the arterial lumen and critically reduce blood flow, possibly producing thrombosis or aneurysm.

The most important manifestations of chronic arterial occlusive disease are intermittent claudication (see Box 26–3) and pain at rest. Nearly half of clients who experience claudication have associated severe coronary artery disease. Claudication, usually insidious in onset, generally occurs in men, although incidence increases in women after menopause. Usually, claudication strikes males in their sixth or seventh decade of life.

The development of pain at rest, usually occurring at night when the client lies supine, indicates progressive disease. Elevation of the legs decreases blood flow and increases pain. This pain, resulting from ischemia of the nerves, is called lancinating or shooting pain. Usually described as a dull aching in the toes or forefoot, this sensation may awaken the client from sleep and cause him or her to hang the foot over the side of the bed or get up and walk around for relief. As symptoms progress, the client may start to sleep in a chair with the legs dependent. This often results in a moderate degree of lower extremity edema. The affected foot usually exhibits dependent rubor.

Other, nonspecific symptoms of arterial insufficiency involve the cutaneous circulation; however, their presence in combination with claudication indicates advanced disease. Skin and subcutaneous tissues require little blood flow for maintenance of normal nutrition. Coldness of the feet is an unreliable sign, but a sudden onset of coldness is indicative of arterial insufficiency or occlusion. Paresthesias with exertion indicate ischemia of the peripheral nerves because of the phenomenon of "arterial steal." This phenomenon occurs because hypoxia causes muscle arterioles to dilate fully and "steal" blood from cutaneous and peripheral nerve vessels, which results in coldness and "pins and needles" sensation.

Aortoiliac disorders are a form of chronic arterial occlusive disease characterized by aortoiliac stenosis and occlusion.

A femoropopliteal disorder refers to an occlusion in the chief arteries of the proximal leg or thigh. Other nonarterial diseases producing similar extremity pain include arthritis, lumbar disc protrusion, neuritis, venous stasis, and muscle cramps.

Diagnostic Assessment

Noninvasive diagnostic tests include ankle/arm blood pressure index, segmental Doppler systolic blood pressures, and pulse waveform analysis, via plethysmography, and MRI. Arteriography, an invasive test, is the definitive examination when surgery is being considered. Arteriography reveals the lumen of the blood vessels; it does not measure actual blood flow like the noninvasive tests.

Medical Management

Medical management of clients with chronic arterial occlusive disease is recommended for those with intermittent claudication and, in general, mild to moderate disease. Surgical intervention has been reserved for clients who experience pain at rest, nonhealing ulcers, or disabling claudication.

CRITICAL TO REMEMBER

Smoking cessation is strongly recommended because cigarette smoking is highly correlated with chronic arterial occlusive disease. Clients who stop smoking exhibit improved treadmill walking distances.

VASCULAR REHABILITATION

Daily walking has proven beneficial for clients with intermittent claudication, although the mechanism by which it improves symptoms is controversial. It probably combines a "training effect" and an increase in collateral blood supply to the extremity. Many clients can significantly increase their walking distance, and most can avoid surgery if they exercise regularly and stop smoking.

DIETARY MANAGEMENT

Interventions for lowering blood lipid levels are recommended for those clients with hyperlipidemia. The initial steps in lowering cholesterol involve dietary intervention. For obese clients, the first step is to reduce the total dietary fat intake to 30 per cent or less of total calories and to reduce the total caloric intake to achieve ideal body weight. In particular, saturated fat intake should be reduced. The most common sources of saturated fat in the American diet are red meats, fried foods, and dairy products, especially whole milk and cheese.

Fast foods, snack foods, and restaurant dining account for a large amount of Americans' excessive fat intake. Substituting fish and poultry for red meat and changing to skim milk and nonfat cheese may be sufficient to meet saturated fat recommendations.

The next goal is to reduce intake of foods high in cholesterol, including egg yolks, organ meats, shellfish, and animal meats. Increasing dietary fiber, especially soluble fiber such as that found in oats, lentils, and beans, has a beneficial effect on lipid levels. Dietary counseling by a registered dietitian is a helpful intervention in helping clients and families change eating habits.

PHARMACOLOGIC MANAGEMENT

Pharmacologic intervention may be needed for those clients with hyperlipidemia and for those in whom dietary changes have been less than successful. The major drug groups include nicotinic acid, fibrin acid derivatives, bile acid resins, meglutol, coenzyme A-reductase inhibitors, and probucol. These medications have varying degrees of effectiveness, and each has important side effects.

Vasodilators have been popular in the past, although there are no convincing studies to support their use. Pentoxifylline (Trental) has been shown to be effective in some clients in combination with conditioning exercises. Pentoxifylline is reported to act by reducing blood viscosity and enhancing oxygen delivery to the muscle of the affected limb. The major side effect is gastrointestinal upset, which may be avoided by taking the medication with meals.

ENDOVASCULAR INTERVENTIONS

The 1980s brought an entirely new field of treatment for atherosclerotic vascular disease: endovascular interventional therapies. This multidisciplinary field applies recently innovated techniques of angioscopy, intraluminal ultrasonography, balloon angioplasty, laser, mechanical atherectomy, thrombolytic therapy, and stents. This field can be defined as a diagnostic and therapeutic discipline that uses catheter-based systems to treat vascular disease. The goal is to operate from within the artery to remove partial or total blockages. Most of the procedures can be done percutaneously or through a small incision and are performed in the radiology department or cardiac catheterization suites. Additional benefits of these therapies include the following:

- A puncture wound instead of a long incision
- Significant reduction in postoperative care
- Reduction in cardiac and pulmonary complications from general anesthesia, because most of these procedures are performed under local or regional anesthesia
- Reduction in hospital costs and length of hospital stays

Percutaneous Transluminal Angioplasty. This technique, also known as balloon angioplasty, uses a catheter with a distal inflatable balloon to dilate vessel stenoses mechanically. Percutaneous transluminal angioplasty (PTA) causes controlled injury to the vessel wall by stretching the artery. Observation of a segment of an arterial wall that has undergone PTA reveals rupture of the plaque at the thinnest place, stretching of the artery wall away from the plaque, and rupture of the media, with the lumen of the artery being maintained by the adventitia. The enlarged vessel's new dimensions are maintained by the hydrostatic pressure of the increased luminal blood flow.

Percutaneous transluminal angioplasty has been used with varying degrees of success to treat hemodynamically significant stenoses in the coronary, aortic, iliac, femoral, popliteal, tibial, mesenteric, and renal circulations as well as stenoses in arteriovenous shunts for dialysis (see the more detailed discussion of percutaneous transluminal coronary angioplasty in Chap. 24).

Possible complications of PTA include bleeding, hematoma, thrombus formation, perforation, dissection of the artery, and acute reocclusion occurring over a longer period (as a result of intimal hyperplasia). Postprocedure nursing care is the same as that after cardiac catheterization (see Chap. 23).

Clients undergoing PTA take aspirin or dipyridamole for the long term. Clients are encouraged to continue exercise, smoking cessation, and a low-cholesterol diet to slow the progress of the disease.

Laser-Assisted Balloon Angioplasty. This technique uses laser energy and balloon catheters to reverse ischemia by reforming the diseased artery. After access is gained to the artery in the same fashion as for PTA, the laser probe or fiber is advanced to the obstructing lesion under fluoroscopy. The catheter tip is placed as close to the center of the occlusion as possible. Very gentle pressure is applied to the catheter until the occluding lesion has been crossed. Standard balloon angioplasty is then used to enlarge the channel to its full diameter. After the procedure is completed, antiplatelet or anticoagulant therapy is given.

Laser-assisted balloon angioplasty carries a higher incidence than PTA of arterial wall perforation or dissection. Nursing responsibilities are much the same as in the care of the client after PTA.

Peripheral Atherectomy. Atherectomy selectively removes atheroma from atherosclerotic diseased arteries. The advantages of this technique over PTA are decreased risk of arterial rupture, because the vessel is not stretched as much, and decreased risk of thrombus formation, because the arterial surface is smoother after the procedure.

The plaque is pulverized by various high-speed drills or blades into small particles. Particles are retrieved, which allows examination for determining whether the occlusion was plaque or thrombus. Atherectomy devices require fluoroscopy and contrast for visualization of the lesion. The restenosis rate is about the same as for angioplasty. The major complications are perforation and arterioembolization.

Nursing care for the atherectomy client is the same as that for an angioplasty client.

Intravascular Stents. The recognized problem of restenosis after PTA has led to the development of intravascular stents. Stents are designed to provide a "scaffold" to maintain the intraluminal structure and patency of the artery after balloon angioplasty. After a stent has been in place for about 8 months, it becomes covered by a thin neointimal layer. After the procedure, clients are treated with aspirin and dipyridamole.

Nursing care includes client education regarding medications as well as information about the procedure and the stent.

Thrombolytic Therapy. Thrombolytic therapy is an important aspect of management of extensive venous or arterial thrombosis. Streptokinase and urokinase are used to treat acute arterial emboli and arterial graft occlusion. Contraindications to therapy are listed in Chapter 24. Thrombolytic agents are given through a peripheral vein or through an intra-arterial catheter. Major adverse reactions include hemorrhage, allergic reactions, and fever.

Nursing management is related to the stage of fibrinolytic therapy:

- Before infusion, the client is monitored closely (commonly in the intensive care unit). Baseline values are obtained for partial thromboplastin time (PTT), prothrombin time (PT), thrombin time, platelet count, hematocrit, and white blood cell count. Because of the risk of hemorrhage, the physician is notified if data reveal a bleeding disorder. A history of recent streptococcal infection may diminish the drug's effects. Baseline pulses and assessments are performed in each extremity, using Doppler ultrasonography if needed. Peripheral pulses should be marked with a pen and data are documented.
- During infusion, vital signs, pulses, skin color, movement, and sensation are assessed frequently. The nurse also assesses for clinical manifestations of bleeding and hematoma formation.

CRITICAL TO REMEMBER

If bleeding does occur, the nurse should stop the infusion, notify the physician, and apply direct pressure when appropriate.

- Streptokinase is administered from glass bottles because it is inactivated by plastic containers. Administration is regulated by a volume-control pump. Bleeding typically is from the gastrointestinal or genitourinary tract, intramuscular, intracerebral, or retroperitoneal.
- After infusion, no intramuscular injections are given for 24 hours, and any medications that have side effects of bleeding are used with caution. There is also a chance that a partially lysed thrombus will embolize. After infusion, pressure is applied on the puncture site. The involved extremity is positioned in straight alignment to facilitate perfusion, and the client is protected from falls and other injury. The client's access limb remains immobile. Heparin therapy in low doses is begun following the procedure.

Nursing Management

Assessment

The client with arterial disorders should be assessed for a history of arterial problems, surgery, medications, and ulcerations. Because of the chronic nature of the problem, a psychosocial assessment should also be performed. Feelings of powerlessness may exist.

Nursing Diagnosis, Planning, and Implementation

Nursing Diagnosis: Tissue Perfusion, Altered Peripheral R/T interruption of blood flow secondary to arterial occlusion.

Planning: Expected Outcomes. The client will maintain normal peripheral tissue perfusion to affected extremities, as evidenced by warm, dry skin with normal peripheral pulse, color, temperature, motor and sensory function, and capillary filling.

Implementation

Position the Client. For safely positioning a client with peripheral vascular disease, the nurse must first learn whether the disorder is arterial or venous in nature.

Because blood flows to dependent parts of the body (i.e., parts lower than the heart), clients with arterial disease must be positioned so that blood flows toward their legs and feet. One must remind clients with arterial insufficiency to avoid raising their feet above heart level unless the physician has specifically prescribed this as an exercise. Authorities vary in their opinion as to the best position for enhancing arterial flow to the feet.

Provide Warmth. Warmth can be both a blessing and a curse for clients with vascular disease. Warmth is beneficial for clients only when it acts as insulation against cold and chilling. For example, the nurse should encourage the client with vascular disease to set the thermostat at home at about 70° F to 72° F (21° C–22° C). If possible, the client's room must be kept comfortably warm. The client must be taught to enter an automobile after it has been warmed in the winter.

Applying any source of heat directly to the extremities is dangerous, especially for diabetics with peripheral neuropathies and paraplegics, because decreased sensation leads to burn injury.

Prevent Vasoconstriction. Factors that cause vasoconstriction include nicotine and caffeine (cause vasospasm), high emotion (stimulates the sympathetic nervous system), and chilling.

The nurse can help clients avoid the damaging effects of prolonged vasoconstriction in the following ways:

- Explain the dangers of smoking to the client who uses tobacco. Encourage the client to stop smoking completely.
- Protect the client whenever possible from upsetting, emotionally charged situations. Encourage the client to try to relax, both mentally and physically. Counseling services may be indicated for highly anxious clients.
- Prevent the client from becoming chilled, using the methods previously described.

Nursing Diagnosis: Skin Integrity, Impaired, Risk for R/T decreased peripheral circulation.

Planning: Expected Outcomes. The client will maintain intact skin surfaces, as evidenced by healed skin surfaces, freedom from signs of infection, and signs of wound healing.

Implementation

Arterial Ulcers. Because of poor circulation, clients with chronic ischemic limbs are highly prone to ulcerations and infection of the extremities. Moreover, once a lesion develops, it tends to heal poorly or not at all (especially in diabetics). Eventually, the client may be forced to undergo limb amputation.

Although skin grafting may ultimately be required to cover the site of arterial ischemic leg ulcers (once the ulcerated area is free from infection and granulation tissue is evident), it should be remembered that intervention for the skin lesion does not cure the underlying disease. Most ulcers require revascularization to heal.

General intervention involves keeping the area of ulceration clean and free from pressure and irritation. Bedrest reduces the oxygen needs of the impaired tissues. Debridement followed by application of wet-to-damp saline dressings is a standard intervention for leg ulcers. Whirlpool treatments provide good debridement. If the ulcer does not become infected, granulation then is enhanced with wet-to-wet dressings or a moist occlusive dressing such as DuoDerm.

Foot Care. Lesions resulting from peripheral artery disease increase the danger of injury to the extremities. Prevention of injury to the extremities, particularly the feet, is an important component of care. Excellent foot care should be an integral part of the daily routine of clients with peripheral vascular disorders because prevention is easier to initiate and maintain than correction.

Important points concerning foot care include the following:

- There are no minor foot problems for clients with peripheral vascular disease, especially clients with diabetes mellitus.
- Care must be taken when referring clients to a podiatrist. Not all podiatrists are vascular specialists.
- The nurse should refer the client with corns, calluses, and ingrown toenails to a physician who specializes in peripheral vascular disease.

See the Client Education Guide: Foot Care for Clients with Vascular Disorders.

Nursing Diagnosis: Pain R/T ischemia.

Planning: Expected Outcomes. The client will experience abatement or absence of pain, as evidenced by self-report and demonstrated knowledge of pain relief measures, both pharmacologic and nonpharmacologic.

Implementation. Any measure that increases circulation to the extremities will help alleviate ischemic pain (e.g., warmth, proper positioning, vasodilators, tobacco avoidance, and bypass surgery). Whereas pain can also be subdued by analgesics, interventions that augment circulation are best. Clients may benefit from a bed cradle to keep pressure of bed sheets off the painful extremity.

When strong analgesics such as morphine are necessary "around the clock," the client may come to accept amputation. Amputation can improve the quality of life by diminishing pain and improving mobility with a prosthesis.

Nursing Diagnosis: Health-Seeking Behaviors, R/T exercise, weight reduction, and smoking cessation.

Planning: Expected Outcomes. The client will begin and maintain the chosen health-promotion program, as evidenced by demonstrated knowledge of the specific activities of the program, regular evaluation of goals against performance, and verbalized feelings of increased well-being.

Implementation

Exercise. Several studies have shown that clients involved in an exercise program generally feel better and can slowly improve their walking distance. A prescribed moderate program of exercise and rest helps increase circulation. Clients with leg or foot ulcers should not exercise. The nurse should inspect extremities before recommending an exercise program. A popular form of exercise for clients with vascular disorders is the Buerger-Allen routine. These exercises are divided into three parts, as shown in Figure 26–5. For obese and chronically ill clients, it is important that an exercise program be individually tailored to clients' abilities, goals, interests, and resources and that the program be written with specific instructions[20] (see the Client Education Guide: Exercise Guidelines for Clients with Vascular Disorders).

Some clients are not aware of chest pain, shortness of breath, or fatigue because their attention is focused on leg discomfort. The nurse takes a careful history and performs a physical assessment to establish a cardiopulmonary profile. Medical or surgical intervention may reduce pain and thus improve walking ability.

Weight Reduction. Obesity is a risk factor in arterial disorders. Although there is no evidence that a special diet will alter the course of atherosclerosis once it has appeared, the nurse should encourage clients to adhere to a low-fat, low-cholesterol diet with increased intake of fruits and vegetables. Weight management and dietary reduction of fat and cholesterol are included in the discussion of hypertension (see earlier).

Smoking Cessation. Cigarette smoke is a potent vasoconstrictor. Clients who stop smoking and start exercising may improve their walking capacity as well as decrease the risk of all cardiovascular disease.

Nursing Diagnosis: Activity Intolerance, Risk for R/T pain (intermittent claudication).

Planning: Expected Outcomes. The client will tolerate appropriate levels of activity with a tolerable level of pain while being free from excess fatigue, as evidenced by normal vital signs, statement of tolerable

CLIENT EDUCATION GUIDE

Foot Care for Clients with Vascular Disorders

The nurse should instruct the client in **daily hygiene,** as follows:

- Do not soak; use mild soap and a washcloth.
- Dry well between toes.
- Check water temperature with a bath thermometer or elbow, not toes, to prevent burns; 32.2° C to 35° C (90° F–95° F) is safe.
- Gently rub corns or calluses. Avoid cutting, digging, or using harsh commercial products.

The nurse should instruct the client in **daily inspection and lubrication,** as follows:

- Use good lighting.
- Put on your eyeglasses, if you wear them.
- Inspect for and promptly report ulcerations, redness, calluses, blisters, cracking of skin on the feet, thickening of nails, and so on.
- Rub soothing lotions and lanolin on hands, feet, legs, and arms to prevent dryness.
- Do not use lotion on sores or between toes.
- Do not use perfumed lotions.
- Dust feet lightly with cornstarch if they sweat.

The nurse should instruct the client in **care of toenails,** as follows:

- Use clippers, not scissors or razor blades.
- Cut nails straight across.
- Avoid "bathroom surgery."
- If your eyesight is poor or you are unable to reach your toes, find qualified assistance.
- Use lamb's wool between overlapping toes.

The nurse should instruct the client regarding **proper shoes and socks,** as follows:

- Never go barefoot, not even at the beach or in the home.
- Avoid high heels and shoes with pointed toes.
- Make sure nothing is in your shoes before putting them on your feet.
- Avoid tight socks and shoes.
- Wear cotton socks for absorbency. Change socks daily.
- Alternate between several pairs of comfortable, firm, well-made shoes during the week.
- Avoid shoes that cause feet to perspire (canvas shoes do).
- Make sure shoes and slippers fit well and are sturdy enough to prevent foot injury.

The nurse should instruct the client regarding **safety,** as follows:

- Avoid sunburn.
- Avoid scratching insect bites on legs to prevent creating open lesions.
- Do not use heating pads.
- Wear adequate foot protection on cold days.
- Turn lights on in dark hallways and rooms when entering to reduce the risk of injury.
- Avoid sitting with your legs crossed.
- Use a cane or walker, if indicated.
- When in doubt, ask for help. Keep telephone numbers handy.

The nurse should instruct the client regarding **activity,** as follows:

- Walking is good, but check with your physician first.
- Do not walk if you have any open ulcerations.
- Walk until pain begins, stop and rest, and then begin again.
- Elevate your feet if they swell.
- Find a nurse and a physician who will get to know you and your feet and will take the time to talk with you when you need help.

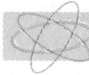

CLIENT EDUCATION GUIDE

Exercise Guidelines for Clients with Vascular Disorders

The nurse should instruct the client as follows:

- Walk or ride a stationary bike for a short period, rest, and then resume; gradually increase the duration of exercise.
- Exercise every day.
- Walk indoors (e.g., in a shopping mall) in cold or hot and humid weather.
- Use your pain as a guide to determine the amount of activity that you can tolerate (pain equals ischemia); stop exercising when pain becomes severe.
- Wear sturdy shoes to help prevent foot trauma.
- Never exercise if leg or foot ulcers are present; exercise uses oxygen necessary for healing.
- Stop smoking.
- If chest pain, shortness of breath, or extreme fatigue occurs, stop exercising immediately and notify the physician.

level of pain, and verbalized understanding of benefits of gradual increase in activity and exercise.

Implementation. Although exercise helps most clients with vascular disorders, it is contraindicated in some clients (e.g., clients with leg ulcers, pain at rest, cellulitis, deep vein thrombosis [see later], or gangrene). Exercise and activity increase the metabolic needs of tissues and, consequently, tissue requirements for oxygenated blood. For this reason, clients with tissue breakdown or necrosis must remain on complete bedrest for a prescribed period. Even minimal activity raises these clients' tissue oxygen requirements beyond that which their damaged arteries can provide.

Evaluation

The nurse monitors the attainment of expected outcomes. The care of the client is long term, and adequate time should be allowed for goal attainment.

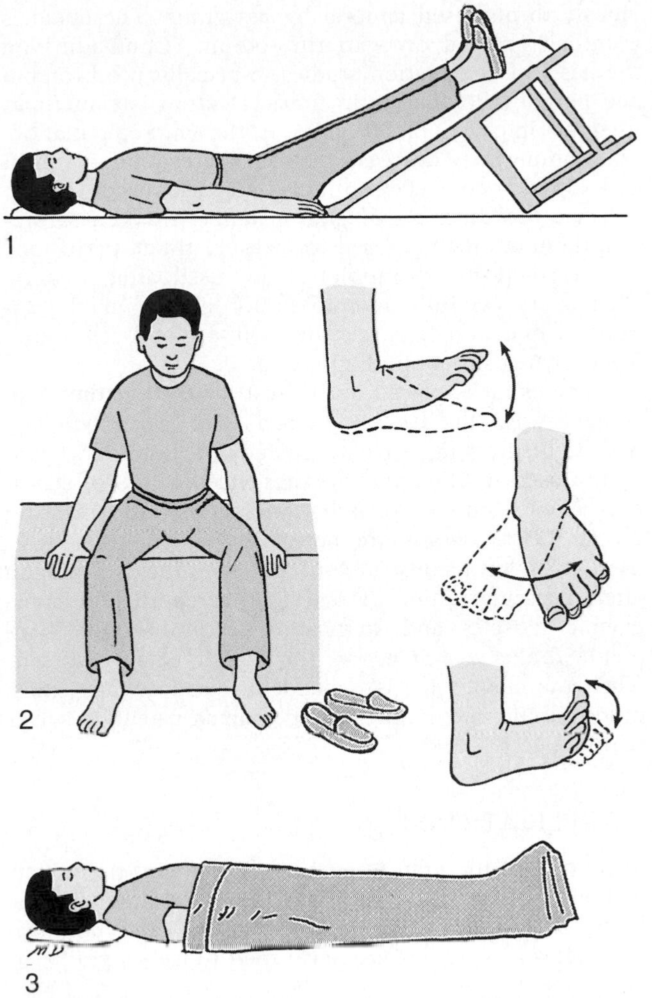

Figure 26–5
Buerger-Allen exercises: instructions for the client. *1,* Elevate feet on padded chair or board for $\frac{1}{2}$ to 3 minutes. *2,* Sit in relaxed position while you flex and extend, then pronate and supinate each foot for 3 minutes. Your feet should become entirely pink. If feet are blue or painful, elevate them and relax as necessary. *3,* Lie quietly for 5 minutes, keeping legs warm with a blanket.

CLIENT EDUCATION GUIDE

Enhancing Circulation

The nurse should instruct the client as follows:

- Elevate the head of the bed to promote flow to the legs.
- Avoid standing in one position for more than a few minutes.
- Avoid crossing the legs at the knees and wearing constrictive clothing (e.g., garters, girdles, tight socks).
- Seek the most comfortable position when sitting and lying down.
- Report new occurrence or worsening of edema or cyanosis.
- Exercise daily.
- Stop smoking.
- Maintain body weight within recommended range.

Modification of Plan of Care for the Elderly

Age-related changes and impairment of physiologic function concomitant with arterial disease will affect the nursing diagnoses of activity intolerance (possibly increased), altered peripheral tissue perfusion (possibly reduced), and pain. An elderly client's recognition of pain may be complicated by physical or cognitive impairments, ongoing drug therapy, and psychosocial factors such as depression or social isolation.[42]

Posthospital Care

The client with intermittent claudication caused by arterial disease should have a checkup at least every 3 months. At this time, the nurse should assess and document the following:

- Extent of claudication
- Impact on life-style
- Manifestations of ischemia
- Pulses
- Ankle-arm indexes
- Condition of the feet
- Venous filling time to determine improvement, stability, or progression of the disease
- Client's understanding of the disease process (see the Client Education Guide: Enhancing Circulation)

Surgical Management

Obstructed arteries can be reconstructed with bypass operations. Various locations along the arterial system can be reconstructed. If the aortoiliac segment is obstructed, clients can have aortofemoral bypass grafting or axillofemoral reconstruction. If the client is a good surgical risk, the option of choice is aortofemoral bypass (Fig. 26–6). The operative mortality is 1 per cent. The patency rate of aortofemoral grafts ranges from 80 to 90 per cent at 5 years.

Axillofemoral grafts have a higher incidence of occlusion than aortofemoral grafts and carry a mortality rate of 4 to 5 per cent, but the necessary anesthesia time is greatly reduced. The patency rate ranges from 60 to 70 per cent at 5 years in part because thrombi are easily removed from axillofemoral grafts. Almost all clients will take one aspirin every day after surgery to help prevent platelet reformation.

The femoral artery can be bypassed with grafts anastomosed (surgically connected) to any one of three lower leg arteries: posterior tibial, anterior tibial, or peroneal artery.

The success of bypass grafts of the legs depends largely on the material used for grafting. The client's own saphenous vein remains the most successful graft-

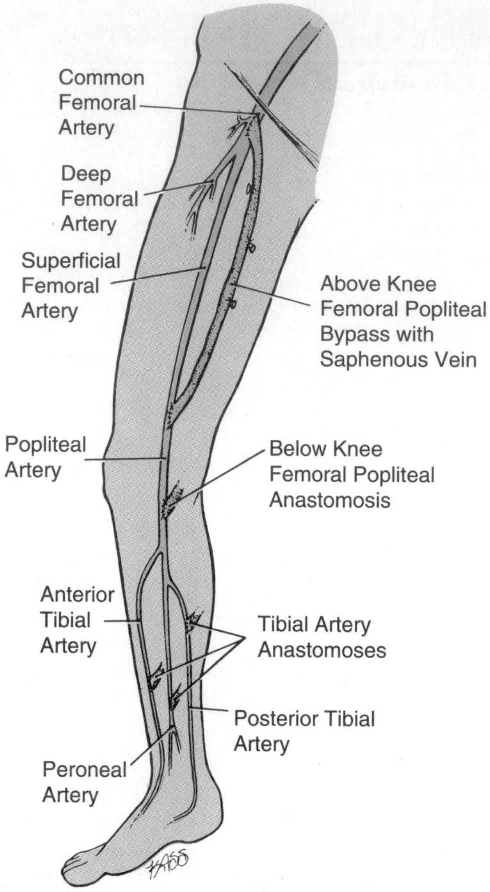

Figure 26–6
Femoral artery bypass grafts. The anastomosis can be to any one of three tibial arteries. (From Fahey, V. A. [1988]. *Vascular nursing.* Philadelphia: W. B. Saunders.)

ing material used today. Seventy-five per cent of saphenous vein grafts are patent after 5 years; in contrast, only 12 per cent of synthetic material (polytetrafluoroethylene) is patent after the same time. (Gore-Tex is a common brand name for this material.) In situ grafts can also be used for reconstruction. In situ grafts use the client's own vein to bypass the artery. A section of vein is anastomosed proximally and distally and then stripped of its valves. The vein then becomes an artery for the client.

PREOPERATIVE CARE

Preoperatively, adequate circulating blood volume must be maintained to permit good perfusion throughout the arterial repair operation. Broad-spectrum antibiotics are usually prescribed 48 hours preoperatively. The client is carefully assessed for infection (e.g., tooth abscess, urinary tract infection, pulmonary infection). Just before surgery, arterial and pulmonary artery catheters may be inserted.

POSTOPERATIVE CARE

Postoperatively, care includes administration of anticoagulants (heparin sodium) in clients who have had previously thrombosed femoral bypass grafts. The client is eventually placed on warfarin sodium (Coumadin) on the basis of coagulation studies, especially prothrombin and partial thromboplastin times. Dextran is sometimes used to improve blood flow in the microcirculation. Medications that decrease platelet aggregation—aspirin and dipyridamole (Persantine)—are also used to help increase the duration of graft patency. Oxygen saturation monitors may be used to measure tissue perfusion.

Broad-spectrum antibiotics are used after surgery. Clients are carefully monitored for clinical manifestations of infection (e.g., elevated white blood cell count, fever, changes in wound appearance).

The client is placed on bedrest for the evening after surgery, with the leg flat in bed. The leg is wrapped with light dressings or a vascular boot. Boots are commonly used in clients who experienced a loss of sensation before surgery or who are at risk for pressure ulcers. Elastic wraps are not used if vein grafts have been used for reconstruction. Leg swelling is common after revascularization related to the reperfusion of ischemic muscles and surgical dissection around lymphatic drainage systems in the leg. If edema worsens when the client's leg is dependent, elastic wraps and a mild diuretic may be prescribed. Edema usually resolves within 4 to 8 weeks.

COMPLICATIONS

Reclotting of the graft is possible. Peripheral tissue perfusion is assessed by neurovascular assessment of the limbs or Doppler ultrasound flowmeter, and noninvasive follow-up studies are performed to assess graft patency.

Infection can occur when synthetic grafting material is used. Because infection in a synthetic graft requires its removal, infection often results in the loss of a limb. Poorly nourished clients appear to be at highest risk of infection and delayed healing.

Bleeding may develop along the suture line and can indicate a disruption in the suture line, pseudoaneurysm formation, or a slipped ligature (suture). These problems require additional surgery.

Compartment syndrome may also develop from swelling around the fascial compartments of the leg. Besides loss of sensation and function, muscle cells can die and release myoglobin, which can cause acute tubular necrosis in the kidney.

Nursing Management

Preoperative Preparation

The nurse teaches the client and significant others the various procedures involved as well as postoperative pulmonary care measures and also offers psychological support.

Preoperatively, the nurse obtains baseline vital signs and documents the character of peripheral pulses comparing one side with the other. One must know exactly which pulses are palpable and which pulses can be assessed only with the Doppler device. The nurse must mark with ink the sites where peripheral pulses can be palpated to assist with postoperative assessment.

Before surgery, the nurse also commonly weighs the client, begins intravenous fluid infusion, and inserts a urinary catheter.

As with any preoperative assessment, for this client careful cardiac, renal, and pulmonary evaluation is vital. Even though the incision for a femoral artery bypass is peripheral and major complications are infrequent, one must remember that the client probably has other manifestations of atherosclerosis (such as heart and kidney disease) that may complicate the surgery. Nutritional status and presence of infections are documented. If the operation is not an emergency, malnutrition can be reversed and open wounds cleaned.

Postoperative Management

Postoperative care of the client after bypass surgery is described in the Care Plan.

Discharge Planning

Most clients are discharged to home. Because activity was limited as a result of claudication before surgery, the client needs to begin regular permissible exercise, including climbing stairs and walking outdoors. The client should be taught that swelling of the operative leg is normal. Elastic wraps can be used when walking but should not be worn continuously. Elastic wraps are usually not permitted on clients with in situ grafts.

Injury to the foot must be avoided, and daily foot inspection is performed. Clothing that constricts blood flow, especially tight socks and garters, must be avoided. (See Client Education Guide: Foot Care.)

ACUTE ARTERIAL OCCLUSION

Acute occlusion of a limb's main artery may be caused by trauma, embolism, or thrombosis and may occur in a healthy or diseased artery. About 90 per cent of acute arterial occlusions occur in the lower limbs.

It is important to differentiate between arterial thrombosis and arterial embolism. Acute arterial thrombosis is usually due to arterial obstruction by a blood clot that forms in an artery damaged by atherosclerosis. Arterial thrombosis may also develop in an arterial aneurysm, especially one that forms in the popliteal artery.

In arterial embolism, the wall of the artery is often healthy; the obstruction arises most frequently from a thrombus within the heart. Causative factors include atrial fibrillation, myocardial infarction, prosthetic heart valves, and rheumatic heart disease. Sometimes portions of a blood clot, such as platelet emboli, form at points of turbulence, lodge at a bifurcation, and initiate a thrombus. Atheromatous emboli sometimes block small arteries. In the lower extremity, more than half of the emboli lodge in either the superficial femoral or the popliteal artery. Other noncardiac causes of emboli include abdominal aortic aneurysm, peripheral aneurysm, and diabetes mellitus. Most of these emboli lodge in the legs; about 15 per cent travel to the arms.

The classic manifestations of acute ischemia resulting from thrombus or embolism are known as *the six Ps* (see Clinical Manifestations: The Six Ps of Acute Ischemia).

> **CLINICAL MANIFESTATIONS**
>
> **The Six *Ps* of Acute Ischemia Resulting from Thrombus or Embolism**
>
> - **Pain** or loss of sensory nerves secondary to ischemia
> - **Paresthesias** and loss of position sense (the client is unable to detect pressure or sense a pinprick and cannot tell whether toes are flexed or extended)
> - **Poikilothermic** (body temperature that varies with environment)
> - **Paralysis**
> - **Pallor** resulting from empty superficial veins and no capillary filling (pallor can progress to a mottled, cyanotic, cadaverous cold leg)
> - **Pulselessness**

Muscle necrosis may start as early as 2 to 3 hours after occlusion. Complete paralysis with stiffness of muscles and joints (rigor mortis) indicates irreversible damage. The leg must be amputated to prevent systemic reaction to the products of massive muscle destruction and systemic sepsis.

Management

Surgery for thrombosis usually involves an arterial reconstructive procedure for revascularization of the leg. Arterial emboli can be removed by an embolectomy.

If the decision is made to remove the occluding embolus or thrombus, surgery should be performed as quickly as possible, generally under local anesthesia. If hours have elapsed since the occlusion occurred, the viability of the limb will determine whether embolectomy should be attempted.

While decisions about surgery are being made, the client should be put to bed in a comfortable, warm room. The limb must be protected from pressure and other trauma and kept at room temperature, neither warm nor chilled. The best position for the limb is level or slightly dependent.

If medical intervention is selected, anticoagulants are generally started. Heparin is usually continued for a minimum of 2 to 7 days, after which a change to an oral anticoagulant may be made. The prevailing practice is to treat all clients who have a definite source of embolism and who have satisfactorily recovered from the acute episode of occlusion with long-term anticoagulant therapy. Thombolytic agents may be used to dissolve a thrombus or embolus.

CARE PLAN: The Client Undergoing Arterial Bypass Surgery of the Lower Extremity

Nursing Diagnosis and Collaborative Problem	Planning: Expected Outcomes	Implementation: Nursing Interventions	Rationales
Fluid Volume Deficit, Risk for R/T hemorrhage, hematoma, third spacing of fluid, or diuresis from contrast given during angiography	Client will maintain adequate vascular fluid volume as evidenced by hemodynamic stability; urine output > 30 ml/hr; warm, dry skin; alert, awake; no excess drainage on dressings; intake equals output; stable hemoglobin and hematocrit.	Observe for signs of hypovolemia: increase in pulse, decrease in blood pressure, anxiety, restlessness, pallor, cyanosis, thirst, oliguria, clammy skin, venous collapse, and level of consciousness.	Hemorrhagic shock can develop from surgical or postoperative blood loss.
		Check dressings for excessive drainage.	Incision drainage first appears on dressings.
		Assess pulmonary artery pressures and cardiac output if parameters are available.	Pulmonary artery pressures and cardiac output parameters are reliable indicators of hemodynamic stability.
		Check daily weights; monitor intake and output closely.	Intake should equal output. Weight is a reliable indicator of fluid balance.
		Check lab values (i.e., hematocrit, hemoglobin) and notify physician if abnormal.	Hematocrit and hemoglobin normally fall slightly because of surgical blood loss. Transfusion may be required.
		Check creatinine level after angiography.	Contrast is excreted by kidneys; fluids assist in excretion of dye.
		Encourage fluids unless contraindicated.	
Tissue Perfusion, Altered, R/T graft thrombosis, compartment syndrome, progressive arterial disease, or inadequate anticoagulation	Client will maintain adequate tissue perfusion to lower extremities, as evidenced by full pedal pulses, capillary refill WNL, intact sensory and motor function, minimal swelling, and warm extremities.	Check pedal pulses every hour for 24 hours, then every shift, unless otherwise ordered. Obtain Doppler pressures per physician's orders.	Pedal pulses indicate graft patency.
		Check sensory and motor function of extremities.	Compartment syndrome may develop because of bleeding.
		Check capillary refill and temperature of extremities.	
		Check leg for hematoma or severe swelling.	Severe swelling may impede flow through graft.
		Monitor CPK levels when appropriate.	Enzymes are released from ischemic muscle.
		Observe for change in color and presence of red blood cells in urine.	Change is due to release of myoglobin, secondary to ischemic muscle.
		Avoid raising knee gatch and placing pillows under the knees.	Pressure may increase possibility of thrombosis.
Skin Integrity, Impaired, Risk for R/T altered circulation, altered nutritional state, presence of infection, or multiple surgical procedures	Client will maintain adequate skin integrity.	Inspect lower extremities on daily basis.	Early detection of ulcerations will improve chances of healing.
		Provide proper skin care using lanolin creams.	Soft skin does not crack open.
		Protect lower extremities from trauma.	Tissue perfusion is decreased; injured sites heal poorly.
		Use sheepskin, bed cradle, or heel protectors when appropriate.	These are devices used to protect the skin from breakdown.

CARE PLAN: The Client Undergoing Arterial Bypass Surgery of the Lower Extremity *Continued*

Nursing Diagnosis and Collaborative Problem	Planning: Expected Outcomes	Implementation: Nursing Interventions	Rationales
		Check sensory and motor function of extremities.	Compartment syndrome may develop because of bleeding or edema.
		Avoid tape on the skin below the knee.	Tape burns from tape removal may be slow to heal.
		Monitor nutritional status and albumin level. Obtain dietitian consultation, if necessary.	Malnutrition is the most common cause of delayed healing.
		Observe strict aseptic technique during dressing changes.	Aseptic technique reduces risk of infection.
		Monitor for low-grade fever, elevated white blood cell count, any drainage from wound, and graft exposure each shift.	These are clinical manifestations of wound infection.
		Apply 4-inch elastic bandages below the knee to the affected extremity when out of bed, if ordered.	Edema can inhibit wound healing.
Physical Mobility, Impaired, R/T surgical procedure, pain, or nerve injury, secondary to ischemia	Client will maintain intact motor function, avoid potential complications of immobility, and demonstrate use of adaptive devices to increase mobility.	Assess causative factors for immobility and client's range of motion and ability to ambulate.	Mobility can be facilitated once cause is known.
		Encourage progressive ambulation and range of motion while in bed.	These activities promote venous return and muscle strength.
		Request physical therapy consult when appropriate.	
		Encourage independence in activities of daily living.	
Pain R/T surgical incision	Client verbalizes or demonstrates increased level of comfort.	Assess client's level of pain: type, duration, and location.	Provides baseline data to evaluate effectiveness of treatment.
		Provide comfort measures and means of distraction.	Distraction is a nonpharmacologic method of pain management.
		Medicate with prescribed analgesics as needed.	
		Evaluate effectiveness of pain medication after each administration.	Evaluation determines adequacy of analgesics.
Body Image Disturbance, R/T change in body image from surgery	Client demonstrates movement toward reconstruction of altered body image.	Establish a trusting relationship with client.	This is the initial step of therapeutic communication.
		Encourage client to verbalize feelings.	This allows unexpressed concerns to be addressed.
		Promote social interaction.	This encourages client to return to previous life-style.
		Make appropriate referrals if indicated.	

WNL, within normal limits; CPK, creatinine phosphokinase.
Adapted from Fahey, V. A. (1988). *Vascular nursing*. Philadelphia: W. B. Saunders.

Objective signs of successful therapy include the following:

- Return of pulse
- Return of normal color, sensation, and warmth of limb
- Elevated ankle-arm index
- Reduction or elimination of pain

ANEURYSMS

An aneurysm may be defined as a permanent localized dilation of an artery. A 50 per cent increase in the size of a vessel is the usual criterion. Once initiated, an aneurysm tends to enlarge gradually, and this, along with the thrombus that develops within the aneurysm, leads to the usual complications of aneurysms: rupture, pressure on surrounding structures, thrombosis, or distal embolization.

Incidence

Atherosclerotic aneurysms occur about 10 times more often in men than in women, most commonly after 50 years of age.

Etiology

The most common cause of arterial aneurysm is atherosclerosis. Less common causes include congenital defects of the arterial wall (e.g., Marfan's syndrome), trauma (both blunt and penetrating types), infection (including syphilis), polyarteritis, and hereditary abnormalities of connective tissue. Hypertension seems to enhance aneurysm formation.

A combination of factors, such as "wear and tear" and impaired nutrition, eventually results in weakening of the arterial wall. This weakening leads to tortuosity, dilation, and aneurysm formation in atherosclerotic arteries. Atherosclerotic aneurysms tend to develop in areas where the artery is not supported by skeletal muscle or is subject to frequent bending with physical activity. The most common locations include the thoracic and abdominal aortas, the iliac arteries, and the femoral and popliteal arteries.

Classification

Aneurysms may be classified according to location, cause, and appearance.

LOCATION

Aneurysms are designated as either venous or arterial. They are also described according to the specific vessel in which they develop (e.g., aortic, iliac artery) and, more precisely, according to the exact area of the vessel that they affect (e.g., thoracic aortic aneurysm, abdominal aortic aneurysm).

ETIOLOGY

Aneurysms can be classified according to the cause, such as atherosclerotic aneurysm, mycotic aneurysm (resulting from bacterial infection), hypertensive aneurysm, or syphilitic (luetic) aneurysm.

GROSS APPEARANCE

Classification of aneurysms is sometimes based on their shape, anatomic features, and size (see Fig. 26–7).

Abdominal Aortic Aneurysm

Abdominal aortic aneurysms (AAAs) occur about four times more often than thoracic aneurysms. The natural course of an untreated AAA is to expand and rupture.

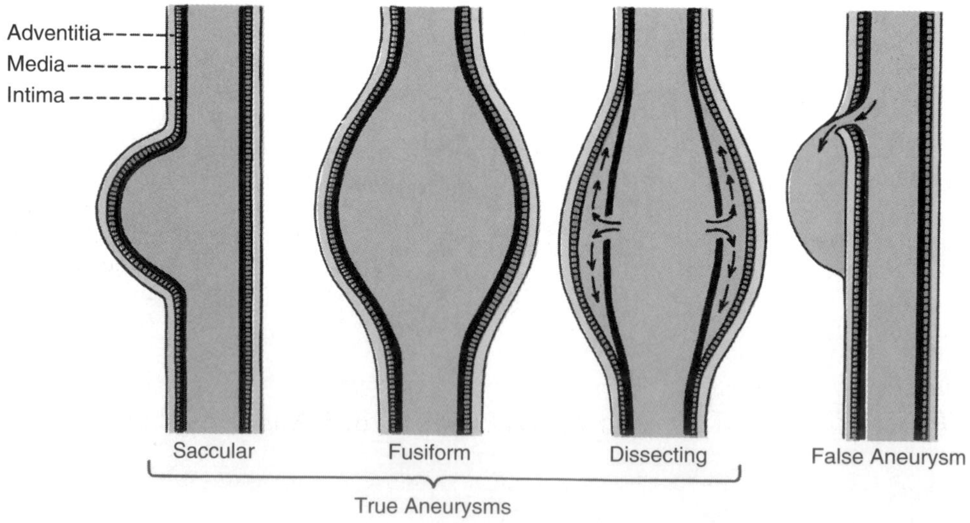

Figure 26–7
Classification of aneurysms. In a true aneurysm, layers of the vessel wall dilate in one of the following ways: *saccular,* a unilateral outpouching; *fusiform,* a bilateral outpouching; or *dissecting,* a bilateral outpouching in which layers of the vessel wall separate, with creation of a cavity. In a false aneurysm, the wall ruptures, and a blood clot is retained in an outpouching of tissue.

The aorta is under greater stress than the rest of the arterial system because of its large diameter and its exposure to high pressure during each systolic ejection of blood. Abdominal aneurysms may extend into the iliac arteries. When the aneurysm reaches about 5 cm in diameter, it can usually be palpated. An abdominal aneurysm 6 cm or greater in diameter has a 20 per cent chance of rupturing within 1 year.

CLINICAL MANIFESTATIONS

The most common symptoms are awareness of a pulsating mass in the abdomen, with or without pain, followed by abdominal pain and back pain. Groin pain and flank pain may be experienced because of increasing pressure on other structures. However, most abdominal aneurysms are asymptomatic.

The most frequent complication of AAA is rupture, which occurs most often in aneurysms 5 cm in diameter or greater. Manifestations of ruptured AAA appear later in this chapter.

Although 90 per cent of large abdominal aneurysms can be diagnosed on physical examination, ultrasonography and CT scanning are the most accurate diagnostic tools. Abdominal aortography is not essential for making the diagnosis but helps identify circulatory anomalies that may be important if resection is planned.

Surgery is usually not performed on clients with an asymptomatic AAA smaller than 4 to 5 cm. Every 6 months, an ultrasonographic examination is indicated to determine whether there is any change in the size. Antihypertensives are usually prescribed.

SURGICAL MANAGEMENT

Surgical management of an aneurysm may be performed as an emergency or an elective procedure. Elective resection and graft replacement has a surgical mortality of less than 5 per cent; emergency surgery after aneurysm rupture has a much higher mortality.

The surgical technique involves exposure of the aneurysm, application of clamps just above and below the aneurysm, excision of the aneurysm, and replacement of the excised segment with a Dacron graft. An abdominal aneurysm is excised through a midline incision that extends from the xiphoid process to the symphysis pubis.

Complications of Abdominal Aortic Aneurysm Surgery

Besides general postoperative complications, specific complications may arise after AAA surgery. Generally, these problems are due to underlying coronary artery disease and chronic and obstructive pulmonary disease. Before elective surgery, proper preoperative screening with stress testing and pulmonary function testing help reduce the incidence of these complications, which may include:

- Acute myocardial infarction (to reduce the risk of this complication, many clients with coronary artery disease undergo coronary artery bypass before aneurysm repair)
- Changes in sexual functioning: retrograde ejaculation in about two thirds of clients and impotency in about one third
- Renal failure, which may develop when the kidney sustains ischemia from decreased aortic blood flow, decreased cardiac output, emboli, inadequate hydration, or the need for clamps on the aorta above the renal arteries during surgery
- Emboli in the arteries of the legs or mesentery; clinical manifestations include those of acute occlusion in the leg (see acute arterial occlusion); bowel necrosis is exhibited as fever, leukocytosis, ileus, diarrhea, and abdominal pain
- Spinal cord ischemia (most common in ruptured AAA), resulting in paraplegia, rectal and urinary incontinence, or loss of pain and temperature sensation

Respiratory, cardiac, and renal complications discussed earlier cause additional problems for the person with a ruptured AAA. Other complications are common to abdominal surgery and include bleeding, infection, and rupture of the suture line.

Nursing Management

Preoperative

Preoperative assessment includes detection of concurrent coronary artery, cerebrovascular, pulmonary, and renal disease. The nurse must assess, mark with ink, and document all peripheral pulses for baseline comparison postoperatively. If dissection or rupture has occurred, the client may receive intravenous fluids (often in large volumes) for maintenance of tissue perfusion. The client and significant others require psychological support and preoperative teaching. When possible, this should include a tour of the intensive care unit.

Postoperative

The care of the client after AAA repair is similar to that for clients who have undergone other abdominal surgery. The client is generally admitted to a critical care area for 24 to 48 hours, where clinicians monitor vital signs and other hemodynamic parameters, manage fluid and electrolytes, obtain daily weights, and monitor pulmonary status. Clients are often maintained on a ventilator, at least overnight, to facilitate respiratory exchange. The nurse assesses circulation at least hourly, with assessment of pulses distal to the graft site. Any signs of occlusion below the graft, including changes in pulses, severe pain, cool to cold extremities, and pale or cyanotic extremities, are reported to the physician immediately.

Ruptured Abdominal Aortic Aneurysm

Possible areas of abdominal aneurysm rupture include the following:

- Into the peritoneal cavity (usually with fatal results)
- Into the mesentery
- Behind the peritoneum (the most common type of rupture with the best prognosis)
- Into the inferior vena cava (which results in shock and heart failure caused by massive arteriovenous fistula)
- Into the duodenum or rectum, causing severe gastrointestinal hemorrhage

CRITICAL TO REMEMBER

Ruptured AAA typically presents with a triad of clinical manifestations:

- Abdominal pain combined with intense back and flank pain and possible scrotal pain
- A pulsating abdominal mass
- Shock, with hypotension, tachycardia, and decreased urine output

Other manifestations include ecchymosis in the flank and perianal area, lightheadedness, and nausea. In addition, the red blood cell count falls and the white blood cell count rises. There are also the signs of a ruptured postoperative abdominal bypass graft.

After the initial rupture comes a phase in which the blood is walled off in the retroperitoneal space, or tamponaded. If the ruptured AAA can be identified during this phase, the client has a much greater chance of survival. Once the aorta ruptures anteriorly into the peritoneal cavity, death is almost certain.

Emergency surgery is the only intervention for clients with ruptured AAA. The operative mortality rate for repair of ruptured abdominal aneurysms may be as high as 35 per cent.

Discharge Planning

The client who has undergone aneurysm repair is taught routine postoperative care, including the following:

- Activity restriction: no lifting greater than 10 to 15 pounds, no driving, and no pushing, pulling, or straining for 6 to 12 weeks
- Wound care
- Pain management
- Dietary modification
- Risk factor modification for atherosclerosis
- Risk factor modification for hypertension
- Referral for follow-up care of sexual dysfunction

THROMBOANGIITIS OBLITERANS (BUERGER'S DISEASE)

Thromboangiitis obliterans is a vasculitis of small and medium-size veins and arteries in the extremities of young adults. The disease process starts distally and progresses upward, involving both upper and lower extremities. It occurs in second through fourth decades of life and is seen predominantly in men, although the incidence in women is increasing.

The cause of Buerger's disease remains unknown. Almost all clients are moderate to heavy smokers. Many clients have a hypersensitivity reaction to intradermal injection of tobacco products. Therefore, the probable cause is an exaggerated autoimmune reaction.

Pain is the outstanding symptom. Intermittent claudication is a common problem that occurs in almost all clients at some stage of the disease. It is often the first symptom noted by the client, usually in the arch of the foot. It is somewhat less common in the calf of the leg but may be noted bilaterally. Rest pain with persistent ischemia of one or more digits and coldness or cold sensitivity may be early symptoms. Various types of paresthesias may occur. Pulsations in the posterior tibial and dorsalis pedis arteries are weak or absent. In advanced cases, the extremities may be abnormally red or cyanotic, particularly when dependent. Advanced forms of the disorder occur when color or temperature changes involve only one extremity, only certain digits, or only portions of digits.

Ulceration and gangrene are common complications and may occur early in the course of the disease. These lesions can appear spontaneously but often follow trauma. Gangrene usually occurs in one extremity at a time. Edema of the legs is fairly common in advanced cases. Changes in the nails and skin appear, and segmental thrombophlebitis affects the smaller veins in about 40 per cent of clients. The primary diagnostic study is leg arteriography. Biopsy may also be used; inflammatory lesions are usually noted.

Thromboangiitis is usually not life threatening. It does, however, result in disability from pain and possible amputation.

Management

Intervention is generally the same as for atherosclerotic peripheral arterial disease and involves the following:

- Arresting progress of the disease (smoking cessation)
- Producing vasodilation (calcium channel blockers or prazosin; regional sympathetic ganglionectomy)
- Relieving pain
- Providing emotional support

Amputation should be deferred until conservative interventions have failed. However, it is unwise to delay amputation of the leg when gangrene extends well into the foot, pain is severe and cannot be controlled, or severe infection or toxic effects occur. Amputation above the knee is seldom necessary.

RAYNAUD'S DISEASE

The term *Raynaud's phenomenon* refers to intermittent episodes during which small arteries or arterioles in extremities constrict, causing temporary pallor and cyanosis of the digits and changes in skin temperature. These episodes occur in response to cold temperature or strong emotion. As the episode passes, the color changes give way to redness. These local changes are not necessarily related to the status of the peripheral vascular system as a whole.

In contrast, *Raynaud's disease* is a primary vasospastic disorder. Criteria for diagnosing primary Raynaud's disease include the following:

- Intermittent attacks of pallor or cyanosis of the digits by exposure to cold or from emotional stimuli
- Bilateral or symmetric involvement
- No evidence of occlusive disease in the digital arteries or of any systemic disease that might be causing the changes
- Gangrene, which (when it occurs) is limited to the skin of the fingertips
- A history of manifestations for at least 2 years

Raynaud's disease appears to be caused by cold hypersensitivity of digital arteries, release of serotonin, and congenital predisposition to vasospasm. Eighty per cent of clients with Raynaud's disease are women between the ages of 20 and 49 years. Primary Raynaud's disease rarely leads to tissue necrosis.

If the disorder is secondary to another disease or underlying cause, the term *Raynaud's phenomenon* is used. Secondary Raynaud's phenomenon is often associated with connective tissue or collagen-vascular diseases such as scleroderma, systemic lupus erythematosus, or rheumatoid arthritis. Raynaud's phenomenon may occur after trauma or may be related to various neurogenic lesions and certain occlusive arterial diseases.

The typical progression of Raynaud's phenomenon is pallor in the digits followed by cyanosis accompanied by feelings of cold, numbness, and occasionally pain, and finally intense redness accompanied by tingling or throbbing. The pallor is caused by vasoconstriction of the arterioles in the extremity, which leads to decreased capillary blood flow. Blood flow becomes sluggish, and cyanosis appears. The intense redness, or rubor, results from the end of vasospasm and a period of hyperemia as oxygenated blood rushes through the capillaries.

Management

Conservative measures will be helpful for most clients with primary or secondary Raynaud's disease. These measures include keeping hands and feet warm and dry; protecting all parts of the body from cold exposure to prevent reflex sympathetic vasoconstriction of the digits; and cessation of tobacco use. Biofeedback has been of help to some clients.

Pharmacologic management is begun when the vasospastic attacks interfere with the client's ability to work or perform activities of daily living or when trophic lesions develop. The aim of drug therapy is to induce smooth muscle relaxation, to relieve spasm, and to increase arterial flow. Drugs used include calcium antagonists, alpha-adrenergic receptor blockers, vasodilators, and agents that interfere with sympathetic nerve activity.

Sympathectomy is sometimes performed in primary Raynaud's disease and lower extremity disease. The long-term results of sympathectomy are disappointing, however. The duration of benefit is limited as peripheral nerves regenerate.

The symptoms of Raynaud's phenomenon may be alarming, so the nurse must reassure the client that the condition is not likely to lead to a serious disability. The client must be advised to stay warm by wearing wool gloves and turtleneck sweaters, turning up the thermostat at home if necessary, and staying out of drafts. Central heating is important to prevent chilling and the shunting of blood from the extremities to the trunk. The client must be encouraged to limit intake of caffeine or chocolate and to stop smoking to control the disease. Stress can also bring on vasospasm, so stress management workshops and biofeedback programs may prove beneficial. The nurse also teaches the client about any prescribed medications.

THORACIC OUTLET SYNDROMES

Thoracic outlet syndromes produce symptoms affecting the neck, shoulder, and upper extremities through compression or mechanical irritation of the brachial plexus, subclavian artery, or subclavian vein as these structures pass through the thoracic outlet.

There are three types of syndromes.

- Neurologic (50 per cent occur following hyperextension injury of the neck or upper back): aching, throbbing pain, and paresthesias of the neck and upper limbs
- Arterial thoracic (chronic compression of the subclavian artery); embolization leads to severe ischemia of the upper extremity
- Venous thoracic (external compression of the axillo-subclavian vein): thrombosis followed by sudden swelling, pain, and cyanosis of the upper extremity

Intervention for neurologic outlet syndrome is usually nonsurgical and involves physical therapy. Some clients will be managed with the surgical removal of the first rib, but this intervention is controversial. Arterial thoracic syndrome requires surgical repair and embolectomy; venous thoracic outlet is treated with thrombolytic or anticoagulant therapy or thrombectomy.

Nursing Care of the Client Undergoing Amputation

Extremity amputation is the surgical removal of all or part of a limb. Clients with peripheral vascular disease are the most frequent candidates for amputation of the lower extremities. Diabetes mellitus is a major cause of arterial occlusion and has been associated with more than 50 per cent of major amputations in clients with lower extremity occlusive disease.

Amputations are classified as primary or secondary. Primary amputations are undertaken as definitive surgical treatment for lower extremity ischemia. Secondary amputations follow a previous vascular reconstructive procedure. Amputations may also be required for acute limb-threatening conditions, mainly trauma, and for malignant tumors and congenital deformities.

ASSESSMENT BEFORE AMPUTATION

Before amputation, the surgeon and rehabilitative team consider:

- The client's physical condition
- The type of amputation to be performed (i.e., closed or open)
- The level of amputation required
- Peripheral vascular function test results
- The client's general attitude toward amputation
- The client's rehabilitation potential
- The type of postoperative prosthetic-fitting and rehabilitative program

Client's Physical Condition

The following physical conditions may determine the need for amputation: ischemic gangrene, rest pain, infection, and massive injury.

Type of Amputation

There are two types of amputation procedure: the open, or guillotine, amputation and the closed, or flap, amputation (Fig. 26–8). The major indication for open amputation is infection. In open amputation, the surgeon does not close the stump with a skin flap immediately but leaves it open, allowing the wound to drain freely. The infected wound is treated with antibiotics and bedrest. Once the infection is completely eradicated, the client undergoes another surgery for stump closure.

In a closed amputation, the surgeon closes or covers the stump with a flap of skin sutured over the end of the stump. This type of amputation is performed when there is no evidence of infection and, consequently, no need for open drainage. However, the surgeon may insert small drains to promote wound healing.

Ongoing advances in vascular surgery have provided outstanding examples of long-term limb salvage in clients who, in the past, would have required amputation. Current data indicate that revascularization should be the first option considered in clients with critical limb ischemia.

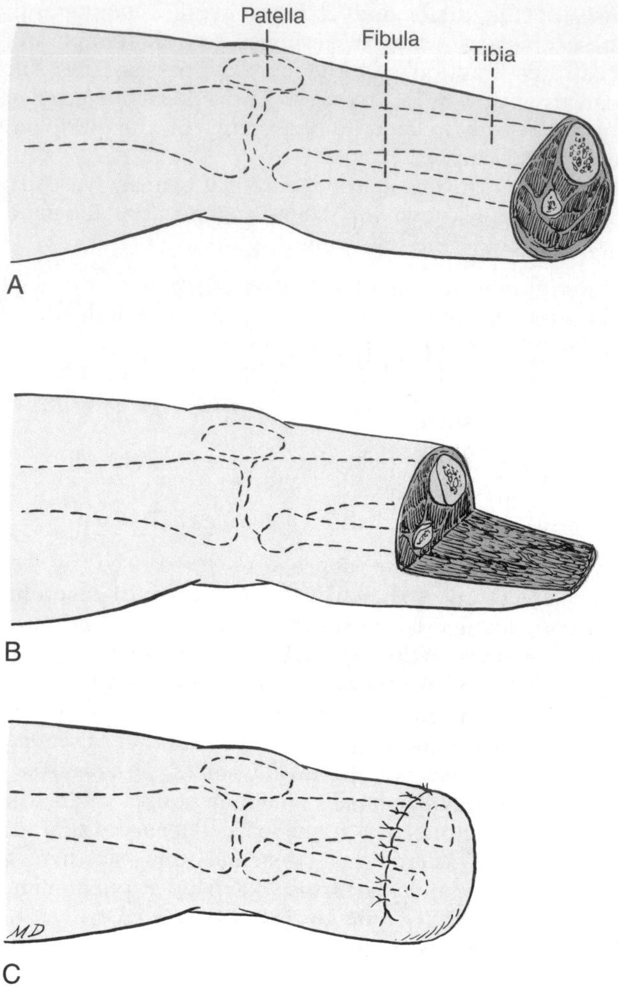

Figure 26–8
Open and closed amputations. *A,* Step 1 of open amputation. This technique is used when infection complicates amputation. *B,* Closed amputation (or step 2 of open amputation, performed when infection has resolved). *C,* Stump closure.

Levels of Amputation

The level of amputation for any extremity should be as distal as possible. Clients with below-the-knee amputations (even bilateral) generally have more success in achieving independent function with a prosthesis than do those with above-the-knee amputations.

Diagnostic Assessment

Angiography is the most common diagnostic study used to determine vascular patency. It commonly reveals a range of problems, from marked reduction in blood flow to the absence of blood flow.

Client's Attitude Toward Amputation

Attitude toward amputation depends largely on the client's age and maturity. Young clients may resist amputation even though it would greatly improve their function. For some, the thought of amputation dramatically conflicts with their ideal self-image.

Conversely, some clients who suffer from the agonizing pain of chronic ischemia may welcome amputation. These clients are more concerned with removing the source of their pain and improving their health status than they are with altering their body image or function.

Evaluation of Rehabilitative Potential

Most clients should attain independent function with the use of a prosthesis. However, prosthetic rehabilitation requires cooperation, commitment, good coordination, and a tremendous amount of energy.

Not all amputees are candidates for prostheses, however. General contraindications may involve concurrent medical conditions (e.g., chronic and progressive mental deterioration, advancing neurologic problems, chronic obstructive pulmonary disease, cardiac disease with congestive heart failure, and angina). Using a prosthesis increases energy requirements and cardiac workload. Rehabilitation requires a team approach, including the client, significant others, physician, nurse, physical therapist, and prosthetist.

Postoperative Prosthetic Fitting and Rehabilitative Program

Clients are fitted with a prosthesis either immediately after surgery or 1 or 2 weeks later when the stump wound has healed and the sutures have been removed. The surgeon decides on the type of prosthetic fitting before surgery. Ideally, the client facing amputation goes to surgery expecting some functional restoration of the limb. Carefully describing the prosthesis to the client helps pave the way to successful rehabilitation.

IMMEDIATE POSTOPERATIVE PROSTHESIS FITTING

Application of the total-contact rigid dressing to the stump in the operating room is one of the most important aspects of immediate prosthetic fitting. The rigid dressing protects the stump from injury and prevents swelling by gently compressing the tissues. Controlling edema enhances wound healing, comfort, and freedom of movement. In below-the-knee amputations, the surgeon immobilizes the knee, thereby eliminating joint flexion.

The rigid dressing is usually changed three to four times before the application of a permanent prosthesis. Cast changes are necessary because the stump tends to shrink as it heals and, consequently, is no longer compressed by the original cast.

DELAYED PROSTHESIS FITTING

Immediate prosthetic fitting is not always possible. However, anyone with a new amputation who is capable of ambulating should receive a temporary prosthesis as soon as possible after surgery. When a conventional delayed prosthesis fitting is anticipated, the client returns from surgery with the stump dressed and covered with elastic bandages or stump socks.

When the sutures are removed 2 to 3 weeks after surgery, the surgeon or prosthetist fits the client with a provisional temporary prosthesis made of plaster of Paris or plastic.

NURSING MANAGEMENT OF CLIENTS UNDERGOING A LOWER EXTREMITY AMPUTATION

Preoperative

The nurse should establish open, honest communication. One must allow the client to freely express fears and negative feelings about the loss of a limb. The client should be encouraged to explore feelings about changes in body image and life-style. The nurse should ask significant others how they feel about the amputation and how they perceive the client is responding. The social worker or psychologist may need to be involved if the client is responding poorly.

The client may also be anxious about unknown consequences and sensations after the amputation. Nursing intervention includes giving and reinforcing information. Most clients feel less anxious when they know what to expect on awaking from surgery.

The nurse must prepare the client for "phantom limb" sensation. Most clients with new amputations experience the peculiar sensation that their missing limb is still present. This sensation, which may be painful or painless, is due to intact peripheral nerves proximal to the amputation site that are used to carrying messages between the brain and the now-amputated part. It may either disappear within hours after surgery or persist for years.

The nurse must also establish expectations. Clients want to know what to expect after surgery and what health-care professionals will expect of them. It should be emphasized that the client is the most important member of the rehabilitation team. To achieve independence, the client will need to

- Exercise several times a day
- Strictly limit weightbearing (if the client is losing part of a leg) until instructed otherwise
- Learn all the intricacies of stump and prosthesis care
- Master the use of the prosthesis

Clients with diabetes mellitus are a high-risk surgical group and require careful preoperative assessment of their metabolic status. Clients with ulcerated legs or osteomyelitis may be treated with antibiotics and bedrest. Debilitated clients need nourishment with foods high in protein. They also may benefit from vitamin and mineral supplements. Dehydration, electrolyte imbalance, or anemia, if present, should be corrected preoperatively.

The client may experience very severe to moderate pain before surgery. The nurse must intervene with supportive measures (e.g., use a footboard and a bed cradle to avoid pressure on injured or ischemic limbs). Also the nurse must administer prescribed analgesics as necessary to relieve pain.

Postoperative

IMMEDIATE POSTOPERATIVE CARE

After an amputation, in addition to routine postoperative care, special attention is given to the following aspects:

- Bleeding: The nurse must look for signs of obvious bleeding or oozing and outline the drainage, including the time, on the pylon (adjustable rigid support) or soft dressing
- Edema, which should be controlled by elevating the stump for the first 24 hours after surgery and then placing the stump flat on the bed to reduce hip contracture.
- Healing: The nurse should assess the incision for indications of healing or infection; the incision should be dry, slightly red along the suture line, and intact.

The nurse must examine the stump carefully for signs of pressure, especially after the application of a new prosthesis.

PSYCHOLOGICAL ASPECTS

After surgery, several psychological responses can be noted. Clients with unrelenting pain before surgery may feel relief that the pain is finally gone. For clients with a chronic disorder, such as diabetes, the amputation may signal a further loss in the battle against the disease. These clients may express anger openly or covertly.

Many clients experience depression after amputation. The client may cry easily, eat little, sleep poorly, sleep more, or avoid interactions with others. Often depression is a reaction to the fear of never walking again; thus, early ambulation is often therapeutic.

Phantom limb sensation may increase clients' anxiety after surgery. As discussed earlier, this sensation is normal, and clients should be prepared for it.

The nurse should encourage all clients who have undergone amputation to verbalize their feelings about the procedure and the anticipated impact on their lifestyle.

REHABILITATION AND PROSTHESIS TRAINING

The most common prosthesis for clients with a below-the-knee amputation is a patellar tendon-bearing limb prosthesis. The interior of the prosthesis contacts all surfaces of the stump and weightbearing is on several areas. Clients with above-the-knee amputation are fitted with either a quadrilateral socket or ischial containment prosthesis. Weight is borne on the ischial tuberosity and soft tissues of the proximal stump, respectively.

Prostheses for the upper extremity consist of a hook or hand device, a harness to supply force to the hand, and a socket for attachment.

Cosmetic prostheses are used primarily to enhance self-esteem and make re-entry into society minus a limb more tolerable for clients who are not candidates for a functioning prosthesis. Because the construction of cosmetic prostheses does not allow weightbearing, clients must be cautioned to never attempt transfers or ambulation with a cosmetic prosthesis of the leg or foot.

ADJUSTMENT TO A PROSTHESIS

After lower limb amputation, clients need teaching on how to care for the stump and prosthesis both in the health-care facility and at home (see the Client Education Guide: Stump and Prosthesis Care).

Clients coping with a new amputation must adjust to the prosthesis physically as well as psychologically. Physically, they need to increase strength and endurance with regularly scheduled exercise, control weightbearing until the wound completely heals, and practice ambulating with the new prosthesis until a skillful, automatic gait is developed.

Physical mobility will be compromised immediately after amputation. Amputating a limb displaces the center of gravity, normally located just below the umbilicus. Clients coping with an amputation must relearn balance because the prosthesis, however similar, will not be an exact replica in weight and movement of the lost limb. Adapting to a change in the center of gravity occurs slowly but progressively until the conscious effort of maintaining balance comes under unconscious control.

Clients coping with an upper extremity amputation must be highly motivated to master the prosthesis and achieve independence. For successful rehabilitation, clients must integrate the prosthetic arm and hand into the total body image.

When the prosthesis is not worn (e.g., during the night), turning also requires a readaptation in body balance. Consequently, clients may need assistance while turning until the new center of gravity is comfortable.

Psychologically, these clients must integrate the new prosthesis into their self-image if they are to become truly independent again. Psychological adjustment to a prosthesis is often more difficult and may take longer than physical adjustment. Some clients may benefit from talking with others who have mastered the use of their prostheses and have attained independent function. Support groups may be helpful in this endeavor.

DISCHARGE PLANNING AND SELF-CARE

When making discharge plans for clients with a new amputation (and probably a prosthesis), the nurse

CLIENT EDUCATION GUIDE

Stump and Prosthesis Care

The nurse should instruct the client in **stump care,** as follows:

- Inspect the stump daily for redness, blistering, or abrasions.
- Use a mirror to examine all sides and aspects of the stump. Skin breakdown on the stump is extremely serious because it interferes with prosthesis training and may prolong hospitalization and recovery. Clients with diabetes mellitus are particularly susceptible to skin complications, because changes in sensation may obliterate the awareness of stump pain.
- Perform meticulous daily stump hygiene. Wash the stump with a mild soap, and then carefully rinse and dry it. Apply nothing to the stump after it is bathed. Alcohol dries and cracks the skin, whereas oils and creams soften the skin too much for safe prosthesis use.
- Wear woolen stump socks over the stump for cleanliness and comfort. To maintain the size and shape of woolen socks, wash them gently in cool water with mild soap and dry flat on a towel.
- Replace, do not mend, torn socks; mending creates wrinkles that irritate the skin.
- Put on the prosthesis immediately when arising and keep it on all day (once the wound has healed completely) to reduce stump swelling.
- Continue prescribed exercises to prevent weakness.

The nurse should instruct the client in **prosthesis care,** as follows:

- Remove sweat and dirt from the prosthesis socket daily by wiping the inside of the socket with a damp, soapy cloth. To remove the soap, use a clean damp cloth. Dry the prosthesis socket thoroughly.
- Never attempt to adjust or mechanically alter the prosthesis. If problems develop, consult the prosthetist.
- Schedule a yearly appointment with the prosthetist.

needs to consider their ambulatory level and the tasks with which they may need help. Frequently, clients are discharged home with multiple needs for assistance in daily living and without the informed and professional advice that can prepare them for their altered lives. Home visits from community health-care nurses should be scheduled until such clients have adjusted to their new situation and feel reasonably comfortable and confident in their ability to provide self-care.

Nursing Care of Clients with Venous Disease

Venous disorders can be separated into acute and chronic conditions. Chronic venous disorders can be further classified as varicose vein formation or chronic venous insufficiency. Acute venous disorders include thromboembolism.

ACUTE VENOUS DISORDERS

Acute venous disorders result from thrombus (clot) formation. Thrombus formation obstructs venous flow. Blockage may occur in both the superficial and deep veins.

SUPERFICIAL THROMBOPHLEBITIS

Usually easily diagnosed, this condition is often iatrogenic, resulting from careless insertion of intravenous catheters or inattentive care of intravenous sites. Symptoms are local and include a raised, red, slightly indurated, warm, tender cord along the course of the involved vein. Comfort is promoted, and symptoms are relieved by applying moist heat.

DEEP VEIN THROMBOSIS

Thrombophlebitis of the deep veins permanently damages the veins and valves and increases the risk for another deep vein thrombosis, pulmonary embolism, and venous stasis ulcers.

Incidence

Deep vein thrombosis is a common disorder, more common in adult women than in men and children. It is particularly common among hospitalized clients. Approximately one third of clients older than 40 years who have either undergone major surgery or sustained an acute myocardial infarction experience deep vein thrombosis.[58]

Etiology

Thrombus formation is usually attributed to

- Venous stasis, caused by any condition that results in immobility or absence of the calf muscle pump
- Hypercoagulability, caused by any condition that raises the platelet count, decreases fibrinolysis, increases the clotting factors, or increases the viscosity of the blood
- Injury to the venous wall, caused by trauma initiated by intravenous injections, fractures and dislocations, and agents that are introduced into the blood stream (e.g., certain antibiotics, sclerosing agents)

It is thought that two of these three conditions (collectively known as Virchow's triad) must be present for thrombi to form.

Risk Factors and Prevention

Common clinical risk factors for venous thrombosis and pulmonary thromboembolism are presented in Table 26–8. In addition to those listed, varicose veins (see later) seem to be associated with the development of thrombosis.

Prevention is geared toward promoting venous return, avoiding injury to the endothelial wall, and maintaining normal coagulability. Prevention methods generally used for the high-risk hospitalized client have included mechanical methods such as devices that elevate the foot of the bed, compression stockings, motorized foot movers, and intermittent calf muscle compressors. Pharmacologic prevention includes warfarin, platelet antiaggregation agents (aspirin being the most common), heparin, and dextran.

Nursing measures generally recommended for prevention of venous stasis include the following:

- Facilitating scheduled active and passive range-of-motion exercises for postoperative, postpartum, and immobilized clients (e.g., dorsiflexion of feet against footboard, foot circles, and isometric flexion and relaxation of calf and thigh muscles)
- Monitoring early ambulation, especially for postoperative and postpartum clients
- Warning against crossing the legs in bed
- Applying antiembolism stockings or pneumatic vascular compression leggings, as ordered
- Encouraging postoperative deep-breathing exercises to promote thoracic pumping action
- Avoiding placing pillows under the legs postoperatively to facilitate venous return
- Warning against sitting or standing in one position for prolonged periods

Nursing interventions to help prevent hypercoagulability include the following:

- Administering prophylactic, preoperative, low-dose heparin therapy for elderly clients with hip fractures, obese clients undergoing surgery, all clients undergoing major surgery, and clients on bedrest
- Teaching clients about risk of oral contraceptives and estrogen and progestin replacement therapy
- Maintaining adequate hydration

Nursing interventions for preventing injury to the vein wall include the following:

- Avoiding infiltration during intravenous therapy
- Using heel cushions during surgery to elevate the calves, thereby avoiding damage to the intima of the vein

TABLE 26–8 Common Conditions Associated with Venous Thrombosis and Pulmonary Thromboembolism

Surgery, especially orthopedic surgery, gynecologic cancer surgery, major abdominal surgery, coronary artery bypass grafting, renal transplantation, and splenectomy
Congestive heart failure, myocardial infarction, and cardiomyopathy
Immobolization (bedrest, stroke, prolonged travel, and so forth)
Malignancy
Previous deep vein thrombosis
Pregnancy, particularly in the puerperium and after cesarean section
Trauma
Estrogen or progestin therapy or oral contraceptives
Age over 50 years
Obesity

Pathophysiology

Thrombus development is a local process. It begins by platelet adherence to the endothelium. Where the platelets adhere to collagen, adenosine diphosphate is released. Adenosine diphosphate is also released from the damaged tissues and disrupted platelets. Adenosine diphosphate produces platelet aggregation, which results in a platelet plug.

Newly formed venous thrombi may become pulmonary emboli. Probably 24 to 48 hours after formation, thrombi undergo lysis or become organized and adhere to the vessel wall. This diminishes the risk of embolization.

As thrombi increase in diameter and length, they obstruct the veins. The resulting inflammatory process can destroy the valves of the veins, thus initiating venous insufficiency and postphlebitic syndrome.

If a thrombus occludes a major vein (e.g., femoral, vena cava, axillary), the venous pressure and volume rise distally. Conversely, if a thrombus occludes a deep small vein (e.g., tibial, popliteal), collateral venous channels usually relieve the increased venous pressure and volume.

COMPLICATIONS

CRITICAL TO REMEMBER

Pulmonary embolism, most commonly arising as a thrombus in the large deep veins of the legs, is an acute and potentially lethal complication of deep vein thrombosis.

Pulmonary embolism is discussed in Chapter 22.

Clinical Manifestations

The most common signs and symptoms are pain, described as a dull ache in the region of the thrombus, and unilateral swelling distal to the site. The pain may increase with ambulation. Other manifestations may include redness or warmth of the leg, dilated veins, and low-grade fever. Unfortunately, however, the first clinical manifestation may be pulmonary embolism (Table

TABLE 26–9 Clinical Assessment of Thrombophlebitis

VEINS	CAUSATIVE FACTORS	CLINICAL MANIFESTATIONS	EDEMA	PULMONARY EMBOLISM	CHRONIC VENOUS INSUFFICIENCY OR POSTPHLEBITIC SYNDROME
Superficial					
Saphenous, median cephalic, median basilic	Varicose veins, intravenous injections, Buerger's disease, blood dyscrasias, cancer	Tender, indurated, red, visible, palpable cord along vein Ovoid nodules in skin	Rare	Rare	Rare
Deep Veins					
Femoral, iliac, axillary, subclavian, superior and interior vena cava, tibial, and popliteal	Immobility, congestive heart failure, blood dyscrasias, cancer, oral contraceptives, fractures, dislocations, obesity, dehydration	Increased muscle turgor and tenderness over affected vein Possible superficial venous distention Deep muscle tenderness, increased warmth in affected limb, occasionally with fever (rarely higher than 38.3° C or 101° F) Positive finding of Homans' sign Cyanosis of occlusion is severe	Common	Possible	Possible; deep vein thrombosis is leading cause of pulmonary embolism and postphlebitic syndrome

26–9). Frequently, clients have thrombi in both legs even though the symptoms are unilateral. About one half of clients are symptomatic.

Homans' sign—discomfort in the upper calf during forced dorsiflexion of the foot—is commonly assessed during physical examination. Unfortunately, this test is insensitive and nonspecific. Homans' sign is present in less than one third of clients with documented deep vein thrombosis, and more than half of all clients with a positive Homans' sign do not have venous thrombosis.

Diagnostic Assessment

NONINVASIVE TECHNIQUES

The Doppler ultrasonographic flowmeter determines blood flow in the larger blood vessels as well as the patency of vessels. This device's reliability is directly related to the skill of the examiner. Moreover, its accuracy is impaired by its inability to detect partially or totally occluded veins, the inaccessibility of deep pelvic and thigh veins, and its inability to distinguish collateral circulation from native veins.

Venous duplex scanning has become the primary diagnostic test of deep vein thrombosis because it allows visualization of the vein, which provides an extremely reliable diagnosis of venous thrombus.

Plethysmographic examination of the venous system entails the recording of volume changes in a limb during venous filling and emptying and is also a very good indicator of deep vein thrombosis.

Plethysmography may produce false-negative results if the client cannot sustain deep inspiration long enough to cause pooling of blood in the deep veins, is unable to lie flat and laterally rotate the hip and bend the knee, has congestive heart failure, or has peripheral arterial occlusion. The client must lie perfectly still during plethysmography; any movement can cause distortion and false readings.

INVASIVE TECHNIQUES

Venography, discussed earlier under assessment of the peripheral vascular system, was once the diagnostic standard but is now being replaced with duplex scanning. Venography is still performed on most clients before vascular surgery. Complications of this procedure include thrombophlebitis and clot formation.

Ventilation-perfusion scanning or pulmonary artery arteriography may be used to assess pulmonary embolism.

Medical Management

Superficial thrombophlebitis can be managed with local measures, such as warm, moist packs and extremity elevation. Sometimes, anti-inflammatory medications are required. Bedrest with leg elevation is usually prescribed for clients with deep vein thrombosis until local signs of inflammation subside. After 7 to 15 days, the client is usually allowed to ambulate wearing elastic stockings.

PHARMACOLOGIC MANAGEMENT

Anticoagulant therapy is based on the premise that the initiation or extension of thrombi can be prevented by inhibiting the synthesis of clotting factors or by accelerating their inactivation. The anticoagulants heparin and warfarin do not induce thrombolysis but effectively prevent clot extension.

Heparin. The drug of choice for treating acute thromboembolic disease, heparin prevents the activation of clotting factor IX and inhibits the action of thrombin in forming fibrin threads. An intravenous bolus of 5000 to 10,000 U is followed by continuous intravenous infusion. Heparin's effect is measured by PTT levels monitored every 4 to 6 hours until therapeutic range is established. Therapeutic PTT values are usually 2 to 2.5 times normal control levels.

The specific antidote to heparin is protamine sulfate. Unfortunately, an excessive protamine dose may actually prolong clotting. Heparin is contraindicated in the following conditions: severe hypertension; cerebrovascular hemorrhage; active gastrointestinal ulceration; overt bleeding from the gastrointestinal, genitourinary, or respiratory tract; recent neurosurgery; and heparin allergy.

Coumarin Derivatives. Used to prevent and treat venous thrombosis, coumarin derivatives inhibit hepatic synthesis of vitamin K–dependent clotting factors. The most commonly used coumarin derivative is warfarin sodium (Coumadin).

The effect of the coumarin derivatives is determined by measuring PT. Prothrombin time must be measured every day before the drug is administered until a therapeutic dose is established. Generally, a PT of 1.5 to 2 times the normal reading is desired. The antidote for the coumarin derivatives is vitamin K (Mephyton). If bleeding occurs, the physician will discontinue the medication for a period.

The coumarin derivatives require 1 to 5 days to take effect. Therefore, heparin, which is fast acting, is usually initiated before coumarin. Both drugs are given until the coumarin takes effect (as determined by PT levels); then heparin is discontinued. Anticoagulation is usually continued about 3 to 6 months after an acute venous thrombosis and after pulmonary embolism.

Fibrinolytic Agents. Fibrinolytic medications (e.g., streptokinase, urokinase) dissolve thrombi by stimulating the conversion of plasminogen to plasmin, an enzyme that decomposes fibrin. Fibrinolytic therapy was discussed earlier in this chapter.

Surgical Management

Surgical measures for deep vein thrombosis fall into two categories:

- Intervention for the thrombus itself
- Surgical prophylaxis against pulmonary embolism involving ligation or interruption of the inferior vena cava with a filter or an "umbrella"

Venous Thrombectomy. The direct removal of venous thrombi is rarely performed because of the high incidence of recurrent postoperative thrombosis.

Umbrella Procedure. During this procedure, a filter on an umbrella is inserted in the vena cava to trap large emboli. Some types of umbrellas can be inserted under local anesthesia by threading the device through the femoral or jugular vein. A rare complication of this technique is the migration of the filter into the iliac vein, renal vein, right atrium, right ventricle, or pulmonary artery. Such migrations may be fatal.

Nursing Management

Goals of nursing management are to prevent existing thrombi from becoming emboli and to prevent new thrombi from forming. When caring for the client with deep vein thrombosis, the nurse must

- Protect the client from thromboemboli and bleeding resulting from anticoagulant therapy
- Teach the client about deep vein thrombosis and anticoagulation therapy
- Provide analgesia
- Assess for pulmonary embolism
- Reduce anxiety
- Promote risk factor modification to prevent future thrombi formation

Bedrest. Bedrest is maintained during the acute phase to prevent emboli. Bedrest also prevents pressure fluctuations in the venous system that occur with walking or sitting. The client should be instructed to not massage the affected limb. The client should be maintained in good body alignment and logrolled from side to side.

Because the client with thrombi will be on bedrest for about 5 to 7 days, the nurse must provide an orthopedic bed frame and trapeze, a pressure-reduction mattress, and heel protectors. One must remember to keep the nightstand, over-the-bed table, call light, and telephone within easy reach. Stool softeners and coughing and deep-breathing exercises are also recommended. Once the threat of embolization is over, walking and exercises in bed to decrease venous pressure and to promote blood flow should be scheduled.

Elastic Support Hose. Increased venous pressure on the tissues of the leg can be counteracted by the compression provided by elastic support hose. The hose are applied before the client gets out of bed. Ideally, the support they provide should just balance the increased venous pressure; thus, the hose should be fitted indi-

CLIENT EDUCATION GUIDE

Anticoagulant Therapy

The nurse must teach the following to the client receiving anticoagulant therapy:

- Name of the prescribed medication, method of administration, and dosage schedule.
- Complications to report immediately: blood in urine or stool, bleeding gums, bruising, flank pain.
- Rationale for blood sampling.
- The importance of keeping all appointments for blood monitoring.
- Tips on avoiding injury (e.g., always wear protective footwear and gloves when operating machinery) and how to apply direct pressure to any cut to stop bleeding.
- To use an electric razor and soft toothbrush.
- To wear a Medic-Alert bracelet identifying that the client is taking anticoagulants.
- Inform dentists and other health-care professionals of anticoagulation therapy before undergoing any invasive procedures.
- To avoid taking any over-the-counter medication without the approval of a health-care professional.

vidually to the client's legs. Measurements of the ankle and calf circumference and from 1 inch below the knee or 1 inch below the groin to the bottom of the foot are taken, after the client has been recumbent and leg edema is minimal. Stockings that extend above the knee often bind the popliteal space and act as a tourniquet, especially when the knee is bent; knee-length elastic stockings are preferable. Jobst stockings are specially fitted elastic hose; the client needs to be measured by the manufacturer's representative.

After thrombosis of a deep calf vein, clients should wear elastic support for at least 6 to 8 weeks and probably for life. Elastic support compresses the superficial veins when the client walks and, with walking, increases blood flow in the veins while keeping venous pressure to a minimum.

Elevation of Legs. Elevating the legs above the level of the heart facilitates blood flow by the force of gravity. The increased blood flow helps prevent venous stasis and the formation of new thrombi. Leg elevation also decreases venous pressure, thus relieving edema and pain. The foot of the bed should be elevated 6 inches (Trendelenburg's position), with a slight knee bend to prevent popliteal pressure. The veins of the legs should be level with the right atrium. The head of the bed may be raised to facilitate eating and bathing. Elastic wraps must be applied snugly from toe to groin. (The nurse must rewrap them every 4 to 8 hours or apply properly fitting elastic stockings.) Calf circumference should be measured and documented daily.

Continuous Warm Packs. The nurse may administer warm moist packs around the involved area. The heat relieves venospasm, produces analgesia, and hastens resolution of inflammation.

Relieve Discomfort. Bedrest, leg elevation, and warm packs usually relieve discomfort. Some clients may need a mild sedative or analgesic as well.

Managing Anticoagulant Therapy. Intravenous heparin followed by oral anticoagulation decreases the risk of new thrombi. The nurse assesses for effectiveness by monitoring the PT and PTT. The nurse monitors for manifestations of excess anticoagulation: bleeding, evidenced by blood in the urine, stool, or along the gums or teeth; subcutaneous bruising; petechiae; and flank pain. The nurse should avoid giving injections when possible and apply direct pressure to all venipuncture and injection sites for a minimum of 5 minutes or until bleeding stops. When invasive studies (e.g., venogram, arterial blood gases) are necessary, pressure is applied to the puncture site for 30 minutes after the puncture. The client is encouraged to use an electric razor and a soft toothbrush) (see Client Education Guide: Anticoagulant Therapy).

Monitor for Development of Pulmonary Embolism. As discussed earlier, pulmonary embolism is an acute and potentially lethal complication of deep vein thrombosis. Care of the client with a pulmonary embolism is discussed in Chapter 22.

Client Teaching

When teaching clients about deep vein thrombosis, one must first assess their learning abilities. Many clients with thrombophlebitis are older and may suffer from sensory loss or limited mobility.

The nurse begins teaching the first day of heparinization, discussing reasons for anticoagulants and bedrest. Prevention is the key to deep vein thrombosis. (See Client Education Guide: Thrombophlebitis.)

CLIENT EDUCATION GUIDE

Thrombophlebitis

The nurse should include the following in client teaching about thrombophlebitis:

- Follow health-care providers' recommendations for risk factor modification (e.g., weight reduction if obese).
- Avoid sitting or standing for long periods; walk every 2 hours or perform calf and leg exercises when traveling.
- Do not cross your legs when sitting or lying down.
- Avoid sitting in chairs too high for your feet to touch the floor or too deep, which will press on the popliteal area.
- Avoid wearing constrictive clothing (e.g., garters, girdles).
- Maintain adequate fluid intake to prevent dehydration.
- Understand the risks associated with oral contraceptives and estrogen and progestin replacement therapy.
- Apply antiembolism stockings before standing.
- Report any signs and symptoms of recurrence: pain, inflammation, swelling, skin changes.
- Understand that you will need periodic examination by a health-care provider for the rest of your life.

CHRONIC VENOUS INSUFFICIENCY

Chronic venous insufficiency, also known as postphlebotic syndrome, is marked by the following:

- Chronic swollen limbs
- Thick, coarse, brownish skin around the ankles (referred to as the "gaiter" area)
- Venous stasis ulceration

This disorder results from dysfunctional valves that reduce venous return, which increases venous pressure and causes venous stasis. Skin ulcerations also occur.

Chronic venous insufficiency follows most severe cases of deep vein thrombosis but may take as long as 5 to 10 years to manifest. Clients with a history of deep vein thrombosis must be monitored periodically for life. However, about 20 per cent of clients with chronic venous insufficiency have no history of deep vein thrombosis. Once the skin is broken and a venous ulcer develops, the client faces a frustrating chronic problem. Venous stasis ulcers do not heal well.

Management

Goals of management are to increase venous blood return and to decrease venous pressure. Antigravity measures increase blood return to the heart. They include elevating the legs above the heart level and avoiding prolonged standing or sitting. (See Client Education Guide: Enhancing Circulation.) In addition, clients should sleep with the foot of the bed elevated 6 inches and the feet and legs elevated above the heart for 8 of every 24 hours.

VENOUS STASIS ULCERATION

Venous stasis ulcer represents the end stage of chronic venous insufficiency. Over a period of years, the excess venous pressure causes small skin veins and venules to rupture, with creation of stasis ulcers, characteristically located in the malleolar area. Once the skin is broken, infection occurs, usually from either *Staphylococcus* or *Streptococcus*.

Management

When ulcers are present, cultures are taken. Antibiotics may be required to treat infection or cellulitis. Local wound care begins. Some ulcers require debridement of eschar, whereas others require protection. Transparent moisture-permeable dressings are used to promote epithelialization. Solutions such as povidone-iodine (Betadine) can be used to control infection, but it is important to realize that any solution other than normal saline retards healing. Skin grafting may be necessary to achieve healing. Surgery to remove incompetent, varicose veins or improve perfusion may also be necessary. Once the ulcer has healed, the client is measured for elastic stockings and taught the precautions discussed in the previous section on chronic venous insufficiency.

An Unna boot is a permeable dressing that can be applied directly over skin ulcers, thereby allowing drainage of exudate. It creates a moist, warm interface between the ulcerated skin and the bandage. It can be changed on a weekly or biweekly basis, which forces the client to wear it without interruption and thereby improves compliance.

VARICOSE VEINS

Varicose veins are a common complaint of clients with venous insufficiency. The loss of valvular competence and the constant elevation of venous pressure cause distention and tortuosity of the superficial veins. The greater and lesser saphenous veins and perforator veins in the ankle are common sites of varicosities.

Varicose veins may be either primary or secondary. Primary varicose veins often result from a congenital or familial predisposition that leads to loss of elasticity of the vein wall. Secondary varicosities occur when trauma, obstruction, deep vein thrombosis, or inflammation damages valves.

Clients with varicose veins often complain of aching, heaviness, itching, moderate swelling, and unsightly appearance of the legs. Severity of discomfort is difficult to assess and does not seem related to the size of varicosities. Superficial inflammation may develop along the path of the varicosed vein and may be associated with complaints of fever and malaise.

To assess for varicose veins, the nurse carefully examines both legs in good lighting. Varicosities appear as dilated, tortuous skin veins. Vein patency can be assessed using a Doppler flowmeter.

Incompetency of the deep and superficial veins can be diagnosed by noting venous pressure changes during walking and performing Trendelenburg's test, phlebography, Doppler flowmeter examination, and plethysmography. (See assessment section in this chapter.)

Surgical Management

Sclerotherapy involves the injection of a sclerosing agent into varicosed veins. The agent damages the vein and endothelium, causing an aseptic thrombosis that closes the vein. Sclerotherapy is palliative, not curative, and is usually performed for cosmetic reasons. Within minutes after injection of the sclerosing agent, elastic compression and active walking should commence. Elastic bandages are worn for about 6 weeks.

Surgical management of varicose veins involves ligation (tying off) of the greater saphenous vein with its tributaries at the saphenofemoral junction, combined with saphenous vein stripping and ligation of incompetent perforator veins. Vein removal is performed through multiple, short incisions.

Elastic compression bandages are applied from foot to groin. The client is usually hospitalized overnight. Complications are rare but may include the usual surgical complications, bleeding, infection, and nerve damage. Hemorrhage occurs most commonly at the surgical wound site in the groin. Bleeding comes primarily from the stripped canal.

Saphenous nerve damage may occur with surgery. In the distal third of the leg, the saphenous nerve runs close to the saphenous vein. Thus, risk of nerve injury increases when the distal part of the vein is involved.

Postoperative Nursing Management

Three important postoperative nursing objectives are to

- Maintain firm elastic pressure over the whole limb
- Promote regular movement and exercise of the legs
- Elevate the foot of the bed 6 to 9 inches so that the legs are above the heart when the client is in bed

The client will be instructed to ambulate for short periods, starting 24 to 48 hours after surgery. The nurse should instruct the client to walk rather than to stand or sit. After the client ambulates, the legs should be elevated again.

The nurse must assess for complications after varicose vein surgery. Major problems to watch for include hemorrhage, infection, nerve damage, and deep vein thrombosis.

Nursing Care of Clients with Lymphatic Disorders

LYMPHEDEMA

Lymphedema is swelling caused by impaired transcapillary fluid transport and lymph transport. Failure of lymph transport allows the plasma proteins in the interstitial fluid to accumulate. As the lymph channels dilate, valves become incompetent. The fluid seeks new pathways through the tissues, causing inflammation, lymphatic thrombosis, and eventually fibrosis.

Lymphedemas are classified into primary and secondary forms.

PRIMARY LYMPHEDEMA

Primary lymphedema may be classified according to age of onset: congenital (present at birth), praecox (early in life), or tardive (late in life). Congenital and familial lymphedema is also called Milroy's disease. It is inherited as an autosomal dominant trait.

Of the primary forms, lymphedema praecox is the predominant type; it peaks in the second decade of life and is more common in females than in males. The edema usually appears spontaneously and without known cause (Fig. 26–9).

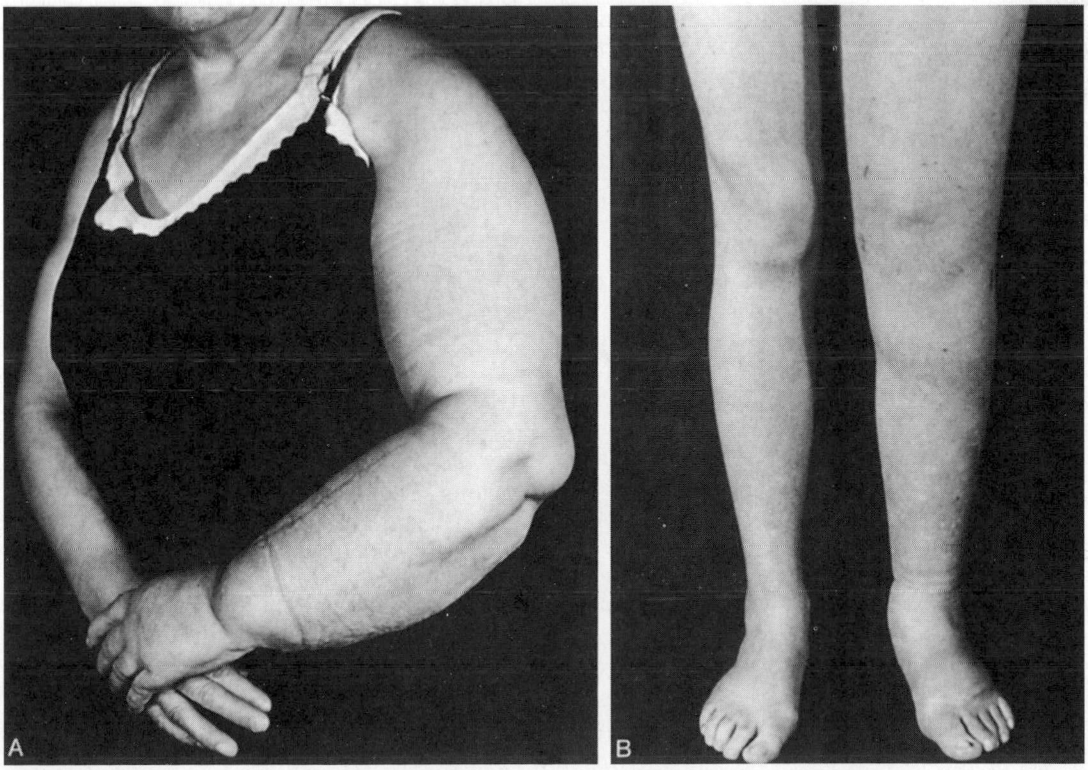

Figure 26–9
Types of lymphedema. *A,* Secondary lymphedema of the arm following mastectomy. *B,* Primary lymphedema.

SECONDARY LYMPHEDEMA

Secondary lymphedema occurs because of some damage or obstruction to the lymph system by another disease process or as a result of trauma, neoplasms (primary or metastatic), filariasis, inflammation, surgical excision, or high doses of irradiation.

Postsurgical lymphedema usually occurs after surgical excision of axillary, inguinal, or iliac nodes, commonly done as a prophylactic or therapeutic measure for metastatic tumor. For example, lymphedema of the arm may develop after mastectomy (see Fig. 26–9).

Prevention

Clients at high risk for lymphedema require elevation of the extremity to improve lymphatic drainage. Range-of-motion exercises also decrease edema by activating the muscle pump.

Clinical Manifestations

Primary lymphedema presents as

- Bilateral mild edema of ankles and legs in females at puberty or shortly after
- Unilateral edema of the entire leg in men and women (see Fig. 26–9)
- Bilateral edema present at birth or a young age

The skin of clients with congenital lymphedema contains vesicles (blisters) filled with lymph.

A dull, heavy sensation is present, but actual pain is absent. Elevation of the limb and bedrest may reduce but not eliminate the edema. Smooth skin becomes roughened; the edema is nonpitting. The limb becomes greatly enlarged, uncomfortable, and disfigured.

Lymphedema can be diagnosed with isotopic lymphography, lymphangiography, and phlebography.

Management

There is no known cure for lymphedema once the swelling appears. The goal of treatment is to remove as much fluid as possible from the affected extremity and to maintain as normal appearing an extremity as possible.

Physical therapy for arm or leg lymphedema involves a mechanical or manual squeezing of the tissue to press the stagnant lymphatic fluid to the proximal part of the limb. This is followed by specific active and passive exercises to transport the lymph farther into the lymphatic system and finally into the blood stream. A number of pneumatic pumping devices for intermittent compression are available. Diuretics may also be prescribed. Elastic stockings are used to maintain the effects of the pneumatic pump.

SURGICAL INTERVENTION

When lymphedematous limbs are massively swollen to the point that compression devices or stockings are no longer beneficial, surgery may be required. The most common surgical procedure for lymphedema is excision, in which all skin, subcutaneous tissue, and deep fascia in the leg are removed. The leg is covered with skin grafts. Scarring is evident, and the cosmetic appearance may not be acceptable to all clients. Another surgical approach involves removal of the bulk edematous tissues. This form of surgery is not curative, but the final appearance may be more acceptable to the client.

Nursing Management

The client with lymphedema is at high risk for infection. Clients are advised to avoid injury (e.g., wear gloves for gardening). The nurse monitors the affected extremity for clinical manifestations of infection, such as redness, warmth, pain, and fever. Meticulous skin care to the extremity is provided using mild soaps and lotions. Nails are kept trimmed.

To reduce swelling, the extremity is elevated above the right atrium. Pneumatic pumps may be used to reduce the extremity size. Activity such as walking should be promoted and sitting and standing discouraged. For bedridden clients, the nurse teaches bed exercises to promote venous and lymphatic return and to maintain muscle strength.

Clients with lymphedema may suffer from self-concept disturbance because of the visibility of their deformity. Variations in clothing style may be suggested to disguise the deformity, and verbalization of feelings should be encouraged.

LYMPHADENITIS

Lymph nodes act as defense barriers and are secondarily involved in virtually all systemic infections and in many neoplastic disorders arising elsewhere in the body. Generalized lymphadenopathy (enlargement of two or three regionally separated lymph node groups) is usually due to inflammation, neoplasm, or immunologic reactions.

Lymphadenitis can be classified as acute or chronic.

Acute Lymphadenitis

Acutely inflamed lymph nodes are most common locally in the cervical region in association with infections of the teeth or tonsils, and in the axillary or inguinal regions, secondary to infections of the extremities. Clinically, in acute lymphadenitis, the lymph nodes are enlarged, tender, warm, and reddened.

Chronic Lymphadenitis

In the course of long-standing infection, the lymph nodes frequently become scarred with fibrous connective tissue replacement. Clinically, these nodes are enlarged, firm to palpation, and not tender or warm. Management of lymphadenitis focuses on treating the underlying disorder.

STUDY QUESTIONS

1. A 50-year-old client has blood pressure readings on three separate occasions over 1 month as follows: 150/92, 148/92, 154/94, respectively. History and physical examination data include the following: client 20 pounds over ideal weight, cholesterol high-normal range, client enjoys swimming but does not have time to exercise on a regular basis. No additional risk factors for cardiovascular disease exist. Which of the following would be the *initial* intervention implemented by the nurse?
   A. Assist the client to develop a weight reduction program plan by decreasing fat to less than 30% of total calories.
   B. Assist the client to develop an exercise plan to incorporate aerobic swimming for 30 minutes three times per week.
   C. Teach the client self-assessment of blood pressure.
   D. Send the client to a dietitian for a no-salt diet.

2. Pertinent assessment of the client with peripheral vascular disease would include which of the following data: (1) palpable peripheral pulses; (2) Doppler ultrasonography assessment of peripheral pulses; (3) capillary refill in seconds; (4) presence of paresthesia and absence of proprioception.
   A. 1
   B. 1 and 2
   C. 1, 2, and 3
   D. All of the above

3. An elderly client states he cannot avoid high-salt canned foods because his daughter can only take him to the store once a month. The nurse should (1) explore access to Meals-on-Wheels with the client; (2) discuss using frozen foods to replace canned foods; (3) call the daughter after client leaves the clinic to discuss weekly frequent shopping trips; (4) reteach the client about low-sodium diet.
   A. 1
   B. 1 and 2
   C. 1, 2, and 3
   D. All of the above

4. A client who underwent aortofemoral bypass graft surgery 3 hours before has the following assessment findings in the operative leg: absence of palpable politeal and pedal pulse, absence of pulse with Doppler ultrasonography, cyanotic calf and foot, and complaints of increased pain. The nurse should
   A. Immediately notify the physician
   B. Administer pain medication and elevate the leg
   C. Check vital signs every 15 minutes
   D. Wrap the leg in warm blanket to improve collateral circulation

5. The client had a below-the-knee amputation in the morning. The client states that "it feels just like my foot is still there." The nurse's *best* response is
   A. "This is called phantom pain and is very rare after an amputation."
   B. "This is phantom pain and is common after an amputation."
   C. "This is phantom pain and will go away in a day or two."
   D. "This is phantom pain and I will give you a shot of morphine to relieve it."

CRITICAL THINKING EXERCISES

SCENARIO A

A client is seen in the clinic with a blood pressure of 180/110 mm Hg. The client states that the physician prescribed a "water pill" 1 year ago but he does not take it any more. After the initial therapy to decrease the blood pressure, what nursing interventions should the nurse implement?

SCENARIO B

The nurse admits a client to the recovery room after abdominal aortic aneurysm repair. The client does not have a bilateral palpable pedal pulse. What priority activity should the nurse perform?

BIBLIOGRAPHY

1. American Heart Association. (1994). *1994 Heart and stroke facts.* Dallas, TX: American Heart Association.
2. Baker, J. D. (1991). Assessment of peripheral arterial occlusive disease. *Critical Care Nursing Clinics of North America, 3(3),* 493–498.
3. Barnes, R. W. (1991). Noninvasive diagnostic assessment of peripheral vascular disease. *Circulation, 83 (Suppl. I),* I20–I27.
4. Beal, K., & Danzig, B. (1990). Lasers in vascular surgery, *Nursing Clinics of North America, 25(3),* 711–717.
5. Becker, G. J., et al. (1991). High-tech options for leg ischemia. *Patient Care, 25(11),* 61–68.
6. Bergan, J. J., & Yao, J. S. T. (1991). *Venous disorders.* Philadelphia: W. B. Saunders.
7. Beven, E. G. (1991). Thoracic outlet syndromes. In J. R.

Young, et al. (Eds.), *Peripheral vascular disease* (pp. 497–510). St. Louis: Mosby-Year Book.

8. Blank, C. A., & Irwin, G. H. (1990). Peripheral vascular disorders. *Nursing Clinics of North America, 25(4),* 777–794.
9. Braunwald, E. (1992). *Heart disease: A textbook of cardiovascular medicine* (4th ed.). Philadelphia: W. B. Saunders.
10. Bright, L. D., & Georgi, S. (1992). Peripheral vascular disease: Is it arterial or venous? *American Journal of Nursing, 92(9),* 34–43.
11. Burke, M., & Walsh, M. (1994). *Gerontologic nursing care of the frail elderly.* St. Louis: Mosby-Year Book.
12. Chenitz, W. C., et al. (1991). *Clinical gerontological nursing: A guide to advanced practice.* Philadelphia: W. B. Saunders.
13. Chobanian, A. V., & Gavras, H. (1991). Hypertension. *Clinical Symposia, 42(5),* 2–32.
14. Cisar, N. S., & Pifarre, R. (1990). Traumatic descending thoracic aneurysms: Discussion and nursing care. *Progress in Cardiovascular Nursing, 5(1),* 13–20.
15. Coffman, J. D. (1991). Raynaud's phenomenon: An update. *Hypertension, 17(5),* 593–602.
16. Collins, J. W. (1991). The treatment of mild to moderate hypertension in patients with diabetes mellitus. *Nurse Practitioner, 16(6),* 28–40.
17. Creamer-Bauer, C., & Webber, M. (1990). Patient teaching strategies for peripheral laser procedures. *Progress in Cardiovascular Nursing, 5(2),* 50–58.
18. Dantzger, D. (1991). *Cardiopulmonary critical care* (2nd ed.). Philadelphia: W. B. Saunders.
19. Dennis, K. E., et al. (1991). Beta-blocker therapy: Identification and management of side effects. *Heart and Lung, 20(5),* 459–463.
20. Edmunds, M. W. (1991). Strategies for promoting physical fitness. *Nursing Clinics of North America, 26(4),* 855–866.
21. Eells, M. A. W. (1991). Strategies for promotion of avoiding harmful substances. *Nursing Clinics of North America, 26(4),* 915–927.
22. Eton, D., & Ahn, S. S. (1991). Trends in endovascular surgery. *Critical Care Nursing Clinics of North America, 3(3),* 535–547.
23. European Working Group on Critical Leg Ischaemia. (1991). Second European consensus document on chronic critical leg ischaemia. *Circulation, 84(Suppl. I),* I1–I22.
24. Fahey, V. A. (1993). *Vascular nursing* (2nd ed.). Philadelphia: W. B. Saunders.
25. Fellows, E., & Jocz, A. M. (1991). Getting the upper hand on lower extremity arterial disease. *Nursing 91, 21(8),* 34–42.
26. Fuster, V., & Verstraete, M. (1992). *Thrombosis in cardiovascular disorders.* Philadelphia: W. B. Saunders.
27. Gold, M. E. (1991). Pharmacology of the nitrovasodilators: Antianginal, antihypertensive and antiplatelet actions. *Nursing Clinics of North America, 26(2),* 437–450.
28. Graor, R. A. (1991). Deep vein thrombosis. In J. R. Young, et al. (Eds.), *Peripheral vascular disease* (pp. 403–422). St. Louis: Mosby-Year Book.
29. Hall, L. T. (1990). Endovascular surgery: An overview. *Progress in Cardiovascular Nursing, 5(2),* 43–49.
30. Herron, D. G. (1991). Strategies for promoting a healthy dietary intake. *Nursing Clinics of North America, 26(4),* 875–884.
31. Hickey, A. (1994). Catching deep vein thrombosis in time. *Nursing 94, 24(10),* 34–41.
32. Hockenberry, B. (1991). Multiple drug therapy in the treatment of essential hypertension. *Nursing Clinics of North America, 26(2),* 417–436.
33. Houston, M. C. (1989). New insights and new approaches for the treatment of essential hypertension: Selection of therapy based on coronary heart disease risk factor analysis, hemodynamic profiles, quality of life, and subsets of hypertension. *American Heart Journal, 117(4),* 911–943.
34. Houston, M. C. (1989). Pathophysiology, clinical aspects and treatment of hypertensive crises. *Progress in Cardiovascular Diseases, 32(2),* 99–148.
35. Huber, C., et al. (1992). Postoperative pulmonary embolism after hospital discharge. *Archives of Surgery, 127(3),* 310–313.
36. Itskovits, H. D. (1991). The role of adrenergic drugs in antihypertensive therapy. *Cleveland Clinic Journal of Medicine, 58(1),* 79–92.
37. Joint National Committee. (1988). The 1988 report of the Joint National Committee on detection, evaluation and treatment of high blood pressure. *Archives of Internal Medicine, 148,* 1023–1038.
38. Kaplan, N. (1991). Long term effectiveness of non-pharmacological treatment of hypertension. *Hypertension, 18(3),* I153–I160.
39. Kaplan, N. (1994). Management of hypertensive emergencies. *Lancet, 344(8933),* 1335–1338.
40. Leon, A. S. (1991). Recent advances in the management of hypertension. *Journal of Cardiopulmonary Rehabilitation, 11(3),* 182–191.
41. Mahan, L. K., & Arlin, M. (1992). *Krause's food, nutrition and diet therapy* (8th ed.). Philadelphia: W. B. Saunders.
42. Mancia, G., & Parati, G. (1990). Clinical significance of "white coat" hypertension. *Hypertension, 16(6),* 624–626.
43. Mannick, J., et al. (1991). Aortofemoral bypass for atherosclerotic aortoiliac disease. In C. B. Ernst & J. C. Stanley (Eds.), *Current therapy in vascular surgery* (pp. 391–393). Philadelphia: B. C. Decker.
44. Markel, A., et al. (1992). Pattern and distribution of thrombi in acute venous thrombosis. *Archives of Surgery, 127(3),* 305–309.
45. Messerti, F. (Ed.). (1993). *Cardiovascular disease in the elderly.* Boston: Kluwer Academic Publishers.
46. Monreal, M., et al. (1992). Deep venous thrombosis and the risk of pulmonary embolism. *Chest, 102(3),* 677–681.
47. Moore, W. S. (1991). *Vascular surgery: A comprehensive review* (3rd ed.). Philadelphia: W. B. Saunders.
48. Rubenstein, E., & Federman, D. (1993). High blood pressure. In E. Rubenstein & D. Federman (Eds.), *Scientific American medicine* (pp. 1–22). New York: Scientific American.
49. Schumann, D. (1991). Sublingual nifedipine controversy in drug delivery. *Dimensions of Critical Care Nursing, 10(6),* 314–320.
50. Schwartz, G. L. (1990). Initial therapy for hypertension—individualizing care. *Mayo Clinic Proceedings, 65,* 73–87.
51. Schwartz, L. L., et al. (1991). Hypertension: Role of the nurse-therapist. *Mayo Clinic Proceedings, 65(1),* 67–72.
52. Setara, J. F., & Black, H. R. (1991). Refractory hypertension. *New England Journal of Medicine, 327(8),* 543–547.
53. Stason, W. B. (1991). Opportunities to improve the cost-effectiveness of treatment for hypertension. *Hypertension, 18(3),* I161–I165.

54. Thacker, H. L., & Jahnigen, D. W. (1991). Managing hypertensive emergencies and urgencies in the geriatric patient. *Geriatrics, 46(10),* 26–36.

55. Ting, M. (1991). Wound healing and peripheral vascular disease. *Critical Care Nursing Clinics of North America, 3(3),* 515–522.

56. Weber, M., Neutel, J., Smith, D., & Ceraettinger, W. (1994). Diagnosis of mild hypertension by ambulatory blood pressure monitoring. *Circulation, 90(5),* 2291–2297.

57. Winer, N. (1990). Hypertensive crisis. *Critical Care Nursing Quarterly, 13(3),* 23–33.

58. Wyngaarden, J. B., et al. (1992). *Cecil textbook of medicine* (19th ed.). Philadelphia: W. B. Saunders.

59. Young, J. R., et al. (1991). *Peripheral vascular diseases.* St. Louis: Mosby-Year Book.

UNIT 8

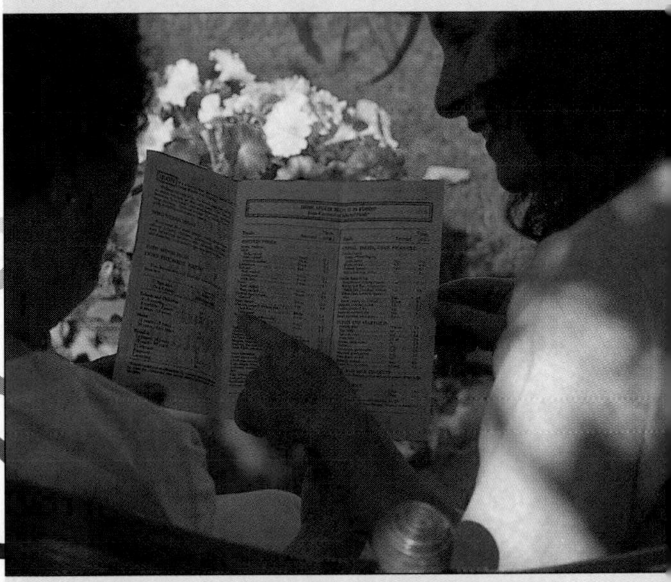

Hematologic Disorders

Within each of us, a sea of fluid bathes, nourishes, and protects our internal environment. Moreover, an internal river—a river of blood with a million tributaries—branches through every organ and tissue, transporting life-sustaining fluid to and from each cell. Disorders of the blood affect the entire body, resulting in tissue hypoxia, infection, or hemorrhage.

This unit introduces basic concepts of hematology and then provides a discussion of the care of clients with hematologic disorders. After a concise review of the components, functions, characteristics, and formation of blood, Chapter 27 presents an overview of hematologic abnormalities, the problems these abnormalities create, and assessment of clients with hematologic disorders. This chapter also discusses the various blood types and the exacting procedures that underlie safe blood administration. This information will help the nurse develop skill in administering blood and blood products and in assessing clients for transfusion reaction and other complications.

The second chapter in this unit includes information on disorders of red and white blood cells and platelets. Disorders such as anemia, leukemia, lymphoma, infectious mononucleosis, polycythemia, and clotting disorders are described, and the nursing care of clients with these problems is discussed.

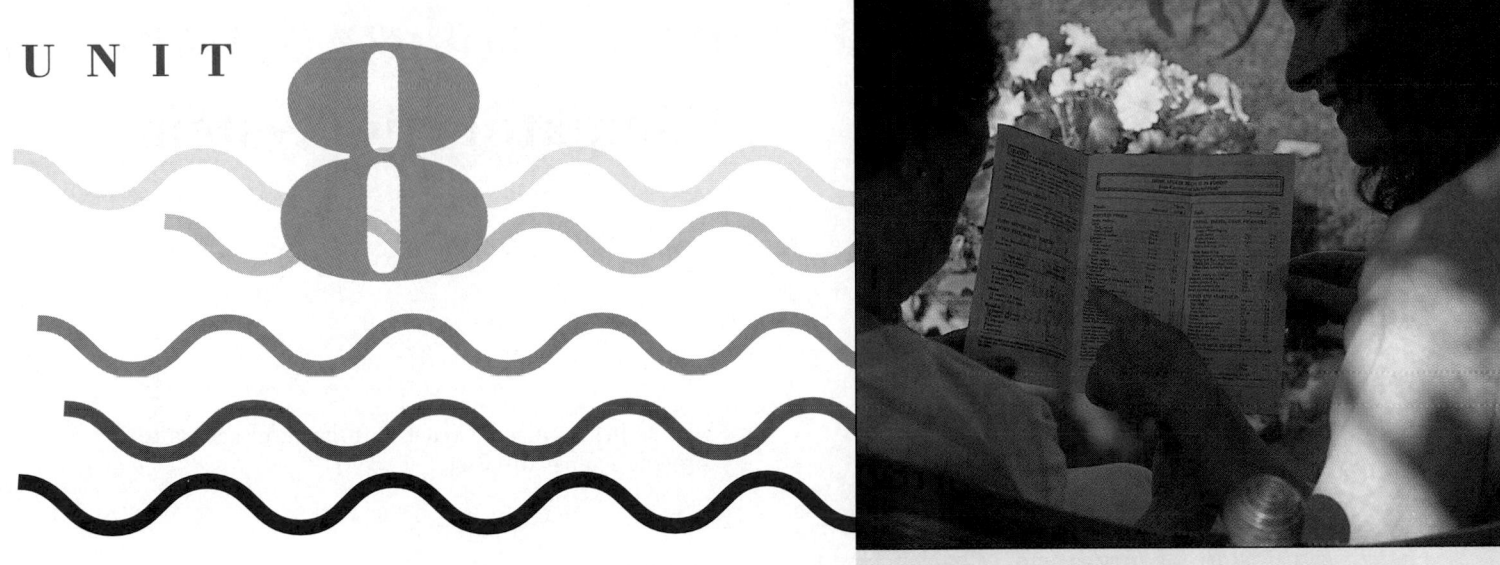

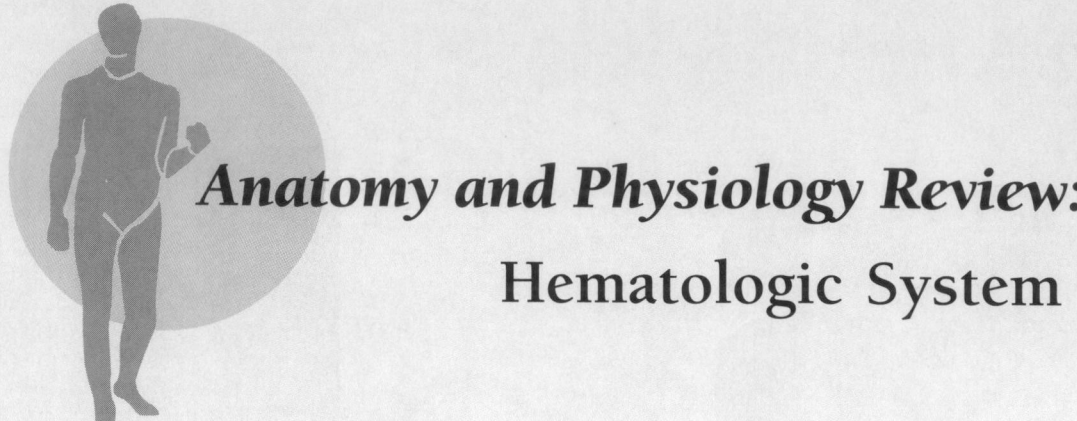

Anatomy and Physiology Review: Hematologic System

CHARACTERISTICS AND FUNCTIONS

Blood is a mixture of plasma and cells that circulates continuously through the heart and vessels. It accounts for approximately 8 per cent of the body weight and has the following characteristics:

- Color. Arterial blood is bright red owing to the oxygen bound to hemoglobin molecules; venous blood is dark red because it has less oxygen content.
- Viscosity. Blood is approximately four times more viscous than water.
- Specific gravity. 1.048 to 1.066.
- pH. 7.35 to 7.45.
- Volume. 70 to 75 mL per kilogram body weight, which is equivalent to 4 to 5 L of blood in the average human body.

As blood circulates throughout the body, it performs many functions, including transportation, regulation, and protection:

Transportation

- Carries oxygen and nutrients to the cells
- Transports carbon dioxide and nitrogenous wastes from the tissues to the lungs, kidneys, and skin for removal
- Carries hormones from the endocrine glands to the target tissues

Regulation

- Helps regulate body temperature by heat transfer
- Helps regulate fluid and electrolyte balance with salts and plasma proteins
- Helps regulate pH through the action of buffers in the blood

Protection

- Clotting mechanisms reduce fluid loss through hemorrhage
- Phagocytic cells destroy microorganisms
- Antibodies in plasma react with harmful agents to protect against disease

COMPOSITION

The liquid portion of blood is plasma, which makes up about 55 per cent of the volume. Blood cells and platelets are solid particles suspended in the plasma and make up the remaining 45 per cent of the volume.

Plasma

Plasma is about 90 to 92 per cent water and 8 to 10 per cent solutes. Because plasma is a transport medium, its solutes are continuously changing as substances are added or removed by the cells. With a healthy diet, plasma is normally in a state of dynamic balance that is maintained by various homeostatic mechanisms. Most of the solutes, about 99 per cent, are plasma proteins, which include albumins, globulins, and fibrinogen. Less than 1 per cent of the solutes are nutrients, metabolic wastes, respiratory gases, enzymes, hormones, and inorganic salts that are being transported in the blood.

Formed Elements

The formed elements of the blood are cells and cell fragments suspended in the plasma. The three classes of formed elements are the erythrocytes, or red blood cells; the leukocytes, or white blood cells; and the thrombocytes, or platelets.

Hematopoiesis. The production of formed elements is called hematopoiesis. Before birth, hematopoiesis occurs primarily in the liver and spleen, but some cells develop in the thymus, lymph nodes, and red bone marrow. After birth, most production is limited to specific regions of red bone marrow, but lymphocytes are pro-

Plasma Proteins and Their Functions

PROTEIN	TOTAL PLASMA PROTEIN, %	FUNCTION
Albumin	60	Maintains blood osmotic pressure
Globulin	36	
α		Transport of lipids and fat-soluble vitamins
β		Transport of lipids and fat-soluble vitamins
γ		Immunity; these are the antibodies
Fibrinogen	4	Blood clotting

duced in lymphoid tissue from precursor cells that migrated there from the bone marrow. The seven types of formed elements develop from a single precursor, or stem, cell type called a hemocytoblast. A specific growth factor controls the development of each formed element.

Erythrocytes

Characteristics. Erythrocytes, or red blood cells (RBCs), are biconcave discs about 7.5 μm in diameter. The shape of the RBC provides a combination of flexibility for moving through tiny capillaries with a maximum surface area for diffusion of gases. Mature cells are filled with hemoglobin and have no nucleus.

Functions. The most important function of RBCs is oxygen transport. Hemoglobin combines chemically with oxygen in the lungs to form oxyhemoglobin. The bond between hemoglobin and oxygen is loose and easily reversed. In the tissues, where the pH is lower, the reaction reverses and oxygen dissociates from the hemoglobin to the tissues. A second function of RBCs is carbon dioxide transport. Hemoglobin combines with carbon dioxide in the tissues and transports it to the lungs, where it is released and exhaled. Transportation of oxygen and carbon dioxide is noncompetitive because the elements bind at different places on the hemoglobin molecule. A third gas that readily combines with hemoglobin is carbon monoxide. This reaction forms a strong bond so that carbon monoxide remains bound to the hemoglobin and is competitive with oxygen. Hemoglobin combined with carbon monoxide cannot transport oxygen to cells and tissues. Consequently, carbon monoxide poisoning of the blood results in tissue hypoxia.

Formation of Erythrocytes. The production of erythrocytes is called erythropoiesis. Mature RBCs cannot undergo mitosis because they have no nucleus; consequently, new cells develop from precursor stem cells (hemocytoblasts) in the bone marrow. Normal production depends on three factors:

- Genetically normal precursor cells
- Functioning red bone marrow
- Adequate iron, vitamin B_{12}, folic acid, protein, pyridoxine, and traces of copper

If any of these factors is missing, erythrocytes may be fragile, misshapen, abnormally large or small, deficient in hemoglobin, or too few in number.

Iron is essential for the synthesis of normal hemoglobin, which is critical for oxygen transport. Hemoglobin holds nearly two thirds of the iron in the body.

Formed Elements in the Blood

FORMED ELEMENT	DESCRIPTION	NUMBER	FUNCTION
Erythrocytes	Biconcave disc; no nucleus; 7–8 μm in diameter	4.5–6.0 million/mm³	Transport oxygen and some carbon dioxide
Leukocytes	Nucleated cells	5000–9000/mm³	Part of the body's defense against disease
Neutrophils	Nucleus with 2 to 5 lobes; indistinct granules in the cytoplasm; 12–15 μm in diameter	60–70% of total WBCs	Phagocytosis
Eosinophils	Nucleus bilobed; red-staining granules in the cytoplasm; 10–12 μm in diameter	2–4% of total WBCs	Counteract histamine in allergic reactions; destroy parasitic worms
Basophils	Nucleus U-shaped or bilobed; granules in cytoplasm stain blue; 10–12 μm in diameter	Less than 1% of total WBCs	Release histamine and the anticoagulant heparin; called mast cells in the tissues
Lymphocytes	Agranulocyte; small cell with large round nucleus; 6–8 μm in diameter	20–25% of total WBCs	Produce antibodies; function in immunity
Monocytes	Large cells with bean-shaped nucleus; may be 20 μm in diameter	3–8% of total WBCs	Phagocytosis; engulf relatively large particles; called macrophages in the tissues
Thrombocytes	Cell fragments of megakaryocytes; 2–5 μm in diameter	250,000–500,000/mm³	Help control blood loss by forming platelet plug and releasing factors necessary for blood clotting

WBCs, white blood cells.
Modified from Applegate, E. J. (1995). *The Anatomy and Physiology Learning System Textbook.* Philadelphia: W. B. Saunders Co.

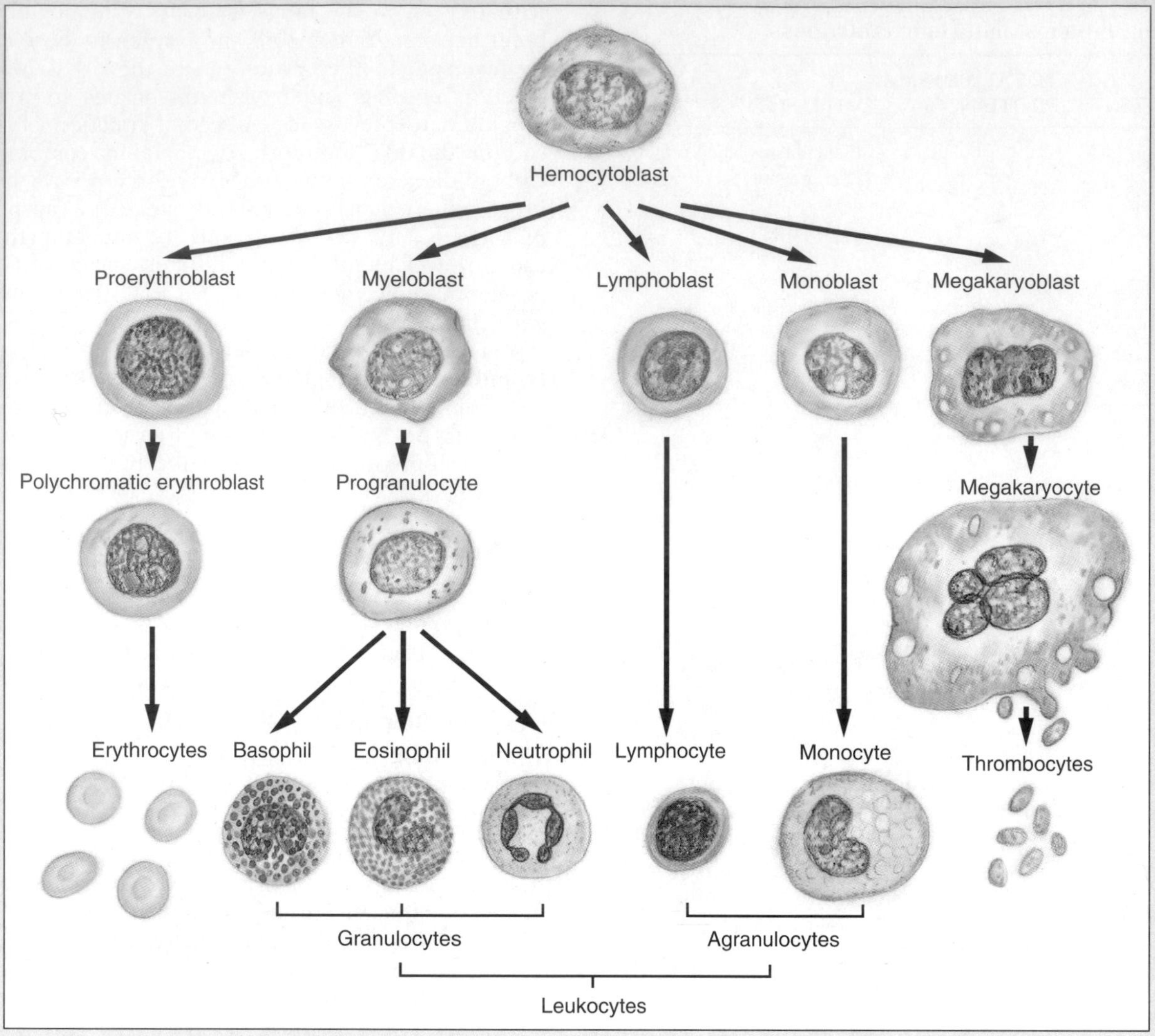

Development of the formed elements.

This is called essential iron. The other one third is found in the bone marrow, spleen, liver, and muscle. If an individual develops an iron deficiency, the nonessential iron is depleted first, followed by a reduction in the essential iron contained in hemoglobin.

Erythrocyte production is regulated by a negative feedback mechanism that uses the hormone erythropoietin. The liver produces erythropoietin in an inactive form and secretes it into the blood. In response to a low concentration of oxygen in the blood, the kidneys

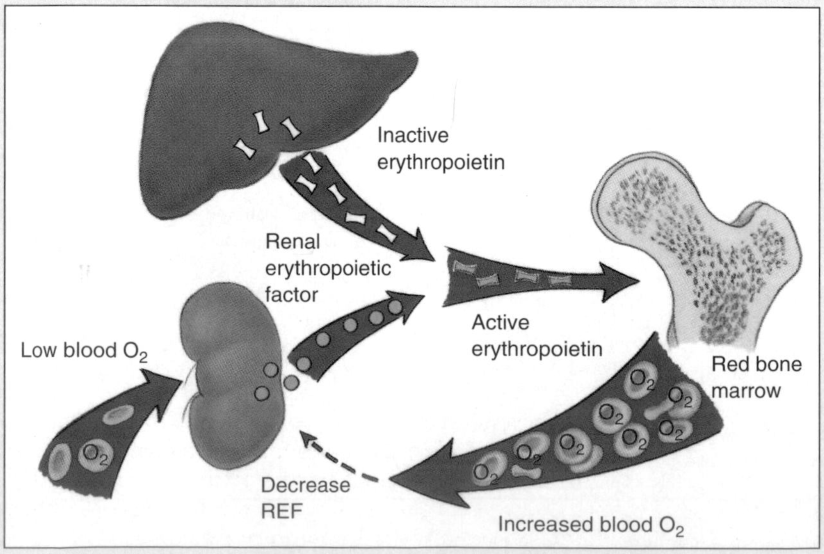

Regulation of erythrocyte production.

Life cycle of red blood cells and breakdown of hemoglobin.

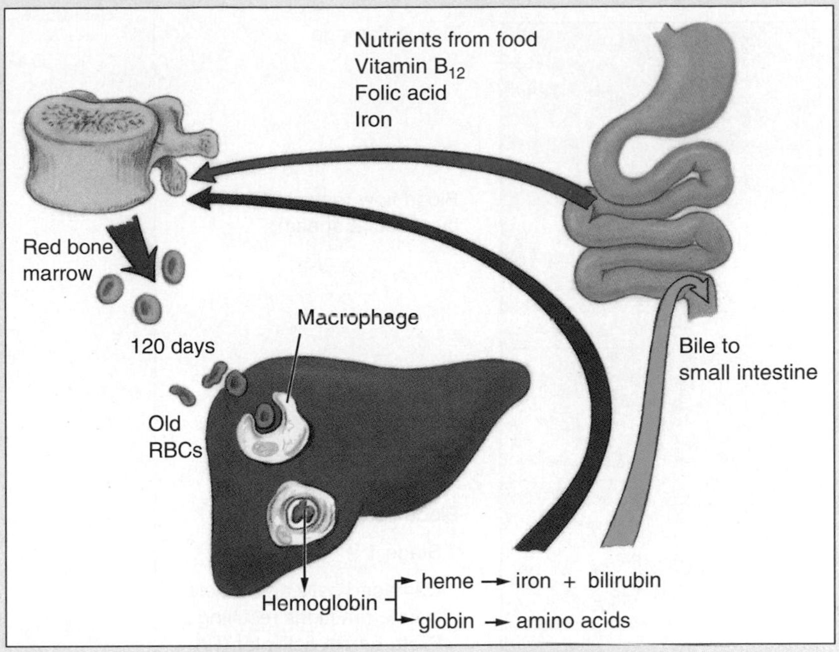

produce a renal erythropoietic factor, which activates the erythropoietin. The erythropoietin stimulates the red bone marrow to produce RBCs, which combine with oxygen to increase the blood oxygen concentration. Young cells leave the bone marrow and enter the general circulation as reticulocytes. These develop into mature erythrocytes during the first 2 to 4 days in the bloodstream.

Destruction of Erythrocytes. Normal erythrocytes live and circulate through the body for about 120 days. As erythrocytes age, their membranes lose elasticity and become fragile. Macrophages in the liver and spleen remove the worn-out RBCs from circulation, and they are replaced by an equal number of new cells. Under typical conditions, over 2 million erythrocytes are destroyed and replaced every second! Hemoglobin from the destroyed cells is separated into its heme and globin components. The protein portion is broken down into its constituent amino acids, which are available for synthesizing new proteins. The iron is removed from the heme and added to the iron stores in the body. The remainder of the heme is converted to bilirubin and secreted into bile to be excreted from the body in the feces and urine.

HEMOSTASIS

Normal hemostasis is a process that reduces blood loss and tissue damage when blood vessels are injured. It includes three separate but interrelated phases:

- Vascular constriction. Initial reflex response of smooth muscle in vessel walls that restricts flow of blood and decreases blood loss; lasts only a few minutes but allows time for other aspects of hemostasis to begin; serotonin prolongs vasoconstriction.
- Platelet plug. Obstructs the opening in an injured vessel to reduce blood loss; collagen in damaged vessels attracts platelets, which become sticky and adhere to each other to form a plug.
- Blood clot or coagulation. Third and most effective mechanism in hemostasis; involves a complex series of chemical reactions and includes numerous clotting factors that are present in the plasma; summarized in three steps as (1) formation of prothrombin activator, (2) formation of thrombin, (3) formation of fibrin, which is the foundation of the clot; platelets, vitamin K, and all the necessary clotting factors must be available for successful clot formation.

Blood contains procoagulants that promote clotting and anticoagulants that inhibit clotting. Normally, anticoagulants predominate so the blood remains fluid. When vessels are damaged, procoagulants increase their activity. After a clot has formed, the fibrin strands contract. This pulls the edges of the wound closer together for healing, reduces blood loss, and reduces probability of infection. Within 24 hours after clot formation, fibrinolysis (clot dissolution) begins. The breakdown of fibrin produces degradation products that act as anticoagulants to return blood flow to normal.

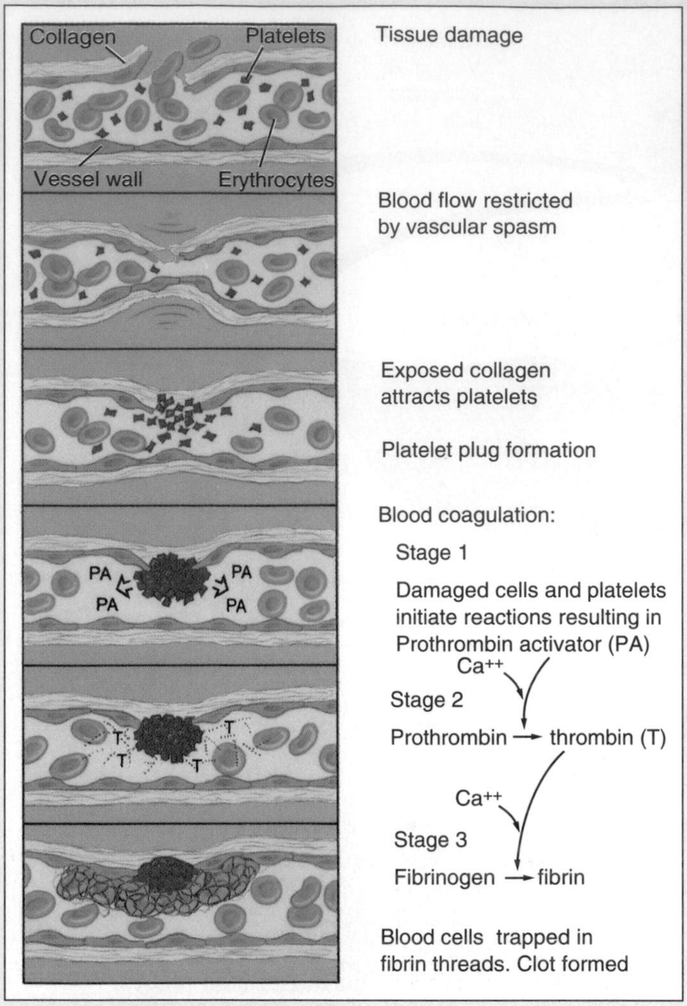

Collagen
Platelets
Tissue damage
Vessel wall
Erythrocytes
Blood flow restricted
by vascular spasm
Exposed collagen
attracts platelets
Platelet plug formation
Blood coagulation:
Stage 1
Damaged cells and platelets
initiate reactions resulting in
Prothrombin activator (PA)
PA
Ca++
Stage 2
Prothrombin → thrombin (T)
T
Ca++
Stage 3
Fibrinogen → fibrin
Blood cells trapped in
fibrin threads. Clot formed

Hemostasis.

BLOOD GROUPS AND TYPING

Agglutinogens and Agglutinins

Human RBCs display antigens, called agglutinogens, on the surface of the cell membrane. There are more than 400 blood group antigens, which are inherited from parents, but fewer than a dozen attract frequent clinical attention. Of these, only the ABO and Rhesus (Rh) are major determinants in compatibility testing. Antibodies called agglutinins are proteins that develop after birth and are found in the plasma. Combining an antigen with an antibody initiates a series of immune responses, called agglutination, that result in the destruction of erythrocytes.

ABO Blood Groups

Blood is typed according to the antigen found on the RBC. Within the ABO system, the antigens are A and B, and the antibodies are antiA and antiB. These antibodies develop within the first 3 months after birth. An individual may have either antigen, both antigens, or neither antigen to give type A, type B, type AB, or type O blood.

In a mismatched transfusion, the antibodies of the recipient react with the antigens of the donor blood to cause agglutination and hemolysis.

The ABO Blood Group System

BLOOD TYPE	FREQUENCY IN THE UNITED STATES, %	AGGLUTINOGENS ON THE RED BLOOD CELL	AGGLUTININS IN THE PLASMA
A	41	A	antiB
B	10	B	antiA
AB	4	Both A and B	Neither antiA nor antiB
O	45	Neither A nor B	Both antiA and antiB

Modified from Applegate, E. J. (1995). *The Anatomy and Physiology Learning System Textbook.* Philadelphia: W. B. Saunders Co.

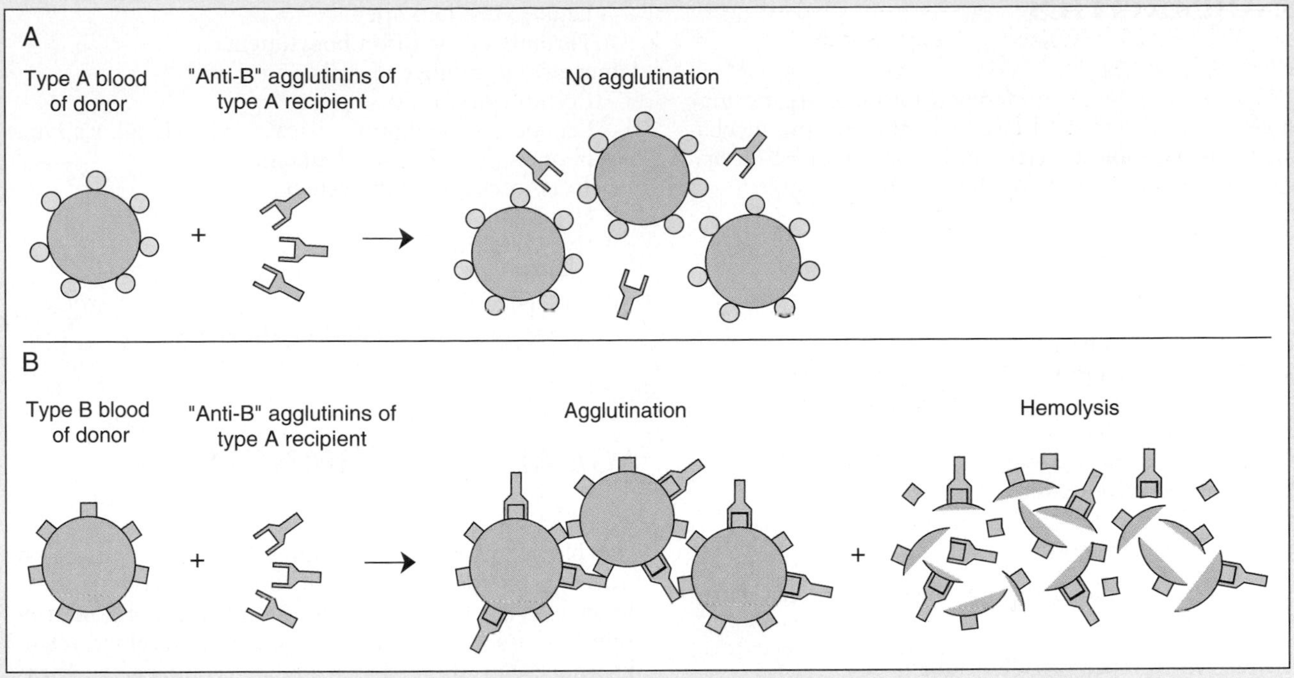

Agglutination reactions.

Rh Groups

The Rh blood groups are nearly equal in clinical importance to the ABO groups. The term Rh positive means the person has the Rh (also called D) antigen on the RBC. The Rh-negative person has no Rh (D) antigen. In the Rh system, antiRh (antiD) antibody formation is never spontaneous. Instead, the antibodies develop after an initial exposure to the Rh antigen. This means that an Rh-negative person does not experience an agglutination reaction upon first exposure to Rh-positive blood, but some degree of RBC destruction is likely to occur with subsequent exposures because antibodies developed after the first exposure. This is particularly significant in pregnancies in which the maternal blood type is Rh-negative and the fetal blood type is Rh-positive. If antiRh antibodies from the mother enter the fetal blood, destruction of fetal RBCs occurs. A single injection of RhoGAM (antiRh antibodies) usually prevents antibody formation after exposure to Rh-positive blood.

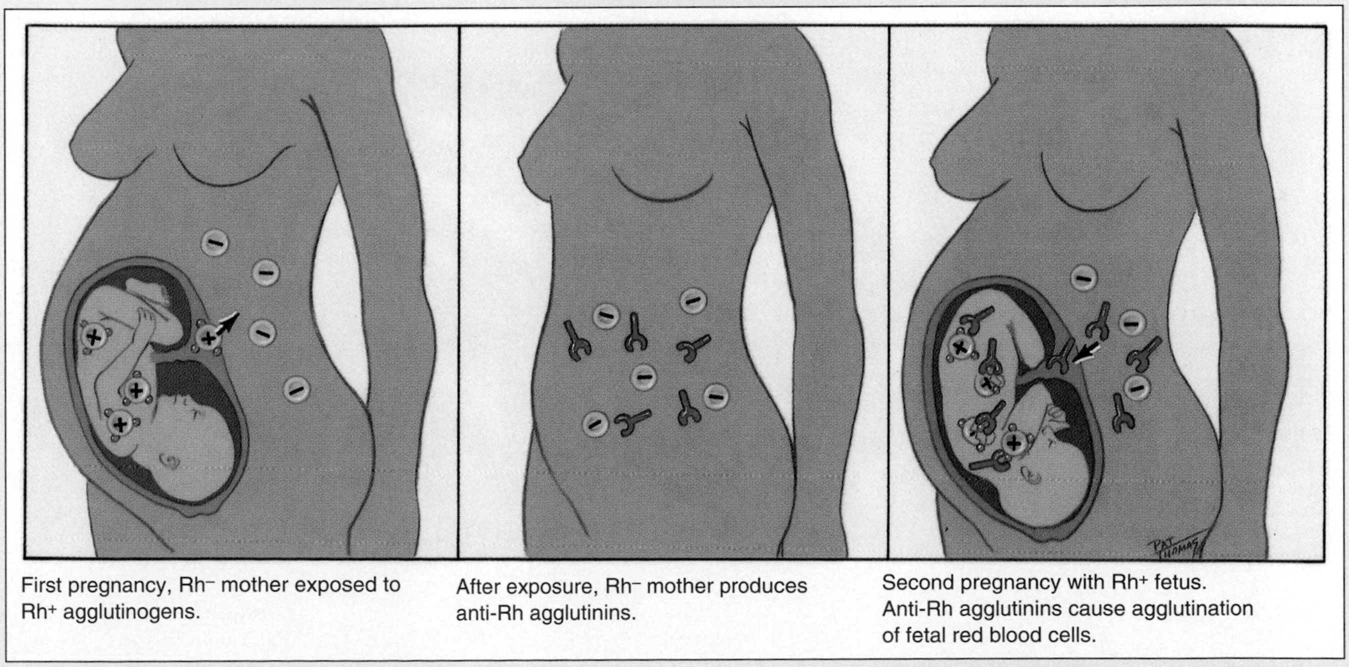

First pregnancy, Rh$^-$ mother exposed to Rh$^+$ agglutinogens.
After exposure, Rh$^-$ mother produces anti-Rh agglutinins.
Second pregnancy with Rh$^+$ fetus. Anti-Rh agglutinins cause agglutination of fetal red blood cells.

Development of hemolytic disease in the newborn.

ABNORMALITIES

Disorders of the blood and blood-forming organs may involve any of the formed elements, the clotting mechanism, or hematopoiesis. General factors involved as primary or secondary causes of the disorders include:

- Hemorrhage
- Genetic predisposition
- Increased destruction
- Radiation
- Malabsorptive disorders
- Metabolic disturbances
- Dietary deficiencies
- Immunologic defects
- Drug and chemical toxicity
- Malignant overproduction
- Infections
- Autoimmune response

Disorders are divided into four groups based on their pathophysiology:

- Decrease in number of cells
  - Erythrocytes: anemia
  - Leukocytes: leukopenia
  - Thrombocytes: thrombocytopenia
- Increase in number of cells
  - Erythrocytes: polycythemia
  - Leukocytes: Hodgkin's disease, non-Hodgkin's lymphomas, lymphocytic leukemia
- Defects in coagulation system
  - Hemophilias
  - Hypoprothrombinemia
  - Disseminated intravascular coagulation
- Disorders of the spleen
  - Excessive destruction of erythrocytes

AGE-RELATED CHANGES

The blood appears to be rather resistant to the aging process, and there are few, if any, clinically significant direct effects of aging on the blood and bone marrow. Aging is associated with an increase in blood-related disorders, but these are usually secondary to disease processes elsewhere in the body.

Chapter 27

Assessment of Clients with Hematologic Disorders

Learning Outcomes

After completing this chapter, the learner will be able to:

1. Explain to a client the vital function of blood.
2. Teach a client about blood groups and blood typing.
3. Conduct a nursing history and physical assessment of a client with an actual or a potential hematologic disorder.
4. Teach a client about diagnostic studies used to detect hematologic disorders.

Understanding the structure, function, and assessment of the hematologic system will help the nurse provide complete care for clients with any of the widely varying disorders affecting this highly complex system.

HISTORY

A complete health history is required when assessing the hematologic system. It includes not only information on the present condition but also a medical history, including use of medications, exposure to chemicals or radiation, family history, psychosocial history and life-style data, and review of systems.

Chief Complaint

Clients present with many vague and nonspecific symptoms, including chills, fever, chronic fatigue, weight loss, and physical discomfort. The nurse conducts a symptom analysis to determine whether the onset was sudden or gradual and whether it was associated with trauma or a known disease. Disorders of the hematologic system often affect all organs and tissues throughout the body, resulting in widespread pathophysiologic manifestations.

Medical History

MAJOR ILLNESSES AND HOSPITALIZATION

The nurse asks the client about previous hematologic problems that may provide clues for the current problem. This entails inquiring about problems such as anemia, recurrent infections, delayed wound healing, thrombophlebitis, deep vein thrombosis, liver disease, or excessive bleeding. Has the client been diagnosed previously with a hematologic disorder?

Surgical procedures that may affect the hematologic system include splenectomy, tumor removal, cardiac valve replacement, and resections of the gastrointestinal tract. For example, loss of duodenal tissue results in decreased iron absorption, partial or total gastrectomy reduces intrinsic factor production and vitamin B_{12} absorption, and loss of the terminal portion of the ileum leads to inability to absorb vitamin B_{12}.

The client is asked whether he or she has received a blood or blood product transfusion. If so, what was the reason for the transfusion? Were there any problems or reactions to the blood or blood products? Does the client know his or her blood type, including Rh factor? This information is particularly important for the client who may be pregnant and is Rh negative (see earlier discussion of the Rh system).

The nurse asks the following questions when assessing the client with a bleeding disorder.

- How long has the client had a bleeding problem? Was it present in childhood, or has it appeared only recently? Do any members of the family have a history of bleeding disorders?
- Is the bleeding linked with any specific event or procedure? For example, does severe bleeding occur with menses or after minor trauma, a tooth extraction, minor surgery, shaving, or participation in contact sports? Does the client have frequent nosebleeds (epistaxis)? Is there a history of bleeding into the joints or cavities? Does the client bruise easily? Does the client report petechiae?
- How severe are any bleeding episodes, and what is their duration? More precisely, is there prolonged oozing of blood from a site or sudden massive bleeding? (Sudden bleeding is far less common than prolonged slow hemorrhage.)
- Does the client have a history of hepatic, splenic, or renal disease? These three conditions are often characterized by hemorrhagic manifestations. Has the client recently taken either anticoagulants or medications that may suppress the bone marrow activity (e.g., chloramphenicol or antineoplastic agents) or medications that interfere with platelet functions?

MEDICATIONS

The nurse asks the client what medications are being used, as a treatment for either a hematologic condition or some other disorder. This includes over-the-counter medications; for example, aspirin or aspirin-containing compounds can interfere with platelet aggregation and cause prolonged bleeding.

ALLERGIES

The nurse specifically inquires about known allergies and allergic reactions, particularly anaphylaxis. If not previously determined, the client is asked for a history of blood or blood product transfusions as well as any complications from the transfusions such as fever, chills, back or flank pain, shock, wheezing, headache, vomiting, or urticaria (hives).

FAMILY HISTORY

A family history of bleeding disorders can be important. A family history of jaundice, anemia, bleeding disorders (hemophilia or polycythemia), malignancies, or congenital blood dyscrasias, such as sickle cell disease, is investigated.

Psychosocial History and Life-Style

Hematologic disorders can result in many physiologic changes that affect the client's psychosocial status and ability to perform activities of daily living (ADLs). Areas to assess are discussed next.

OCCUPATION

The nurse asks the client about previous exposure to toxic chemicals or radiation as a result of occupational exposure or as a treatment. Radiation and chemicals such as benzene, lead, and phenylbutazone can increase the incidence of hematologic problems, particularly anemia. Does the client have sufficient energy to perform ADLs and occupational tasks? Are there problems with fatigue, dyspnea, or other symptoms that interfere with a productive life-style? Has the client missed time from work or school, resulting in financial loss or other economic concerns, such as health or life insurance eligibility?

HABITS

Nutritional habits have a significant effect on the hematologic system. The nurse carefully explains to the client the importance of asking about the use or abuse of alcohol and other recreational drugs. Chronic substance abuse is often accompanied by malnutrition and vitamin deficiency. Many substances, most notably alcohol, damage the structure and function of liver cells, resulting in decreased clotting factor production and increased bleeding tendencies.

A dietary history also is important when assessing whether there may be any vitamin deficiencies causing anemia. Weight loss may indicate hematologic alterations or deficits in nutrients. The nurse asks the client whether he or she is eating foods that contain iron, folic acid, and vitamin B_{12}, all necessary for the development of red cells.

Review of Symptoms

Symptoms related to disorders of the hematologic system can be general as well as specific. The nurse conducts a symptom analysis and a focus assessment for all reported symptoms.

General symptoms include fatigue, apathy, lethargy, malaise, weakness, heat intolerance (anemia), chills, fever, night sweats (infection, particularly recurrent infections), and delayed wound healing (leukopenia).

Integumentary symptoms may be pruritus (Hodgkin's disease and lymphoma), jaundice (hemolytic anemia and pernicious anemia resulting in bile pigment accumulation), pallor, flushing (iron deficiency anemia), petechiae, ecchymoses, and prolonged bleeding (thrombocytopenia and clotting disorders).

Delayed wound healing, lymph node swelling, and infections (leukopenia) may be immunologic manifestations.

Sensory effects on the eyes include visual disturbances (anemia and polycythemia), blindness (thrombocytopenia and retinal hemorrhage related to anemia), and yellowed sclera (jaundice). Regarding effects on the ear, the client might experience vertigo or tinnitus (severe anemia). Symptoms affecting the nose include epistaxis (thrombocytopenia and clotting disorders). Oral manifestations include smooth tongue (pernicious anemia, iron deficiency anemia, and nutritional deficiencies), gingival bleeding (thrombocytopenia and clotting disorders), sores, and ulcerations (leukemia and neutropenia).

The client may exhibit neck lymphadenopathy, particularly if painful (lymphoma).

Respiratory symptoms include fatigue, dyspnea, and orthopnea (anemia).

Cardiovascular symptoms include tachycardia; palpitations (compensatory mechanism to increase cardiac output secondary to anemia); murmurs, particularly systolic (increased volume and velocity of blood through valves related to anemia); and angina (decreased oxygen supply to the heart related to rapid-onset anemia).

The client's gastrointestinal system may be affected by dysphagia (mucous membrane atrophy related to iron deficiency anemia), abdominal pain (intestinal obstruction related to lymphoma, retroperitoneal bleeding, acute hemolysis, allergic purpura, and sickle cell disease), hepatomegaly, splenomegaly (hemolytic anemia resulting in increased need for removal of erythrocytes), hematemesis, and melena (thrombocytopenia and clotting disorders).

Urinary symptoms include hematuria (hemolysis and clotting disorders).

Reproductive symptoms are amenorrhea and menorrhagia (iron deficiency and clotting disorders).

The client may experience musculoskeletal back pain (hemolysis), sternal tenderness (leukemia and sickle cell disease), bone pain (blast crisis in leukemia and multiple myeloma resulting in pathologic fractures), and joint pain (hemarthroses or bleeding into joints, often related to hemophilia).

Systemic neurologic symptoms are confusion (severe anemia and malignant process or infections in the brain), headache (anemia, polycythemia, invasion or compression of brain related to leukemia, lymphoma, infection, or brain hemorrhage related to thrombocytopenia or clotting disorder), syncope (severe anemia and polycythemia), and paresthesias (peripheral neuropathy secondary to pernicious anemia or hematologic malignancy and side effect of vincristine therapy). In addition, the client may experience mental depression (hematologic disorders resulting in fatigue, discomfort, and acute and chronic problems related to disease process or coping difficulties related to a diagnosis of cancer).

PHYSICAL EXAMINATION

The physical examination for the hematologic system can entail both a complete head-to-toe examination and examinations of specific systems, depending on the nature of the client's problem. For example, the client who presents with abdominal pain and absent bowel sounds related to intraluminal hemorrhage needs a complete gastrointestinal examination as well as a hematologic assessment. Similarly, the client with hemarthrosis needs a complete examination of the affected joint as well as a hematologic assessment.

The portions of the physical examination specifically related to the hematologic system include the lymphatic system, liver, and spleen. Lymph node assessment is discussed in Chapter 8, and assessment of the liver and spleen is described in Chapter 36. Findings from the history and physical examination are supplemented by laboratory tests and specific diagnostic studies.

DIAGNOSTIC TESTS

Diagnosis of a blood disorder depends primarily on laboratory analysis. Although dozens of specific tests are used to diagnose individual disorders, all cases generally call for (1) a complete blood count (CBC) to determine the number of leukocytes and erythrocytes; (2) a total differential count to indicate the relative percentages of the different leukocytes; (3) coagulation studies such as prothrombin time (PT) or partial thromboplastin time (PTT) and bleeding time; (4) a bone marrow aspiration and biopsy to determine both the cellularity of the bone marrow and the morphology of the cells present; and (5) a peripheral blood smear (a study of the morphology of blood cells to help differentiate various anemias and blood dyscrasias). The results of laboratory tests also guide therapy for, for example, the client receiving chemotherapy or radiation therapy.

TABLE 27–1 Normal Values for Adult Complete Blood Counts

MEASURE	VALUE*
Erythrocytes	
Hemoglobin (oxygen-carrying pigment of the RBCs)	Women: 12.0–15.5 g/dL of blood Men: 13.0–16.5 g/dL of blood
RBC count	Women: 4.0–5.0 million/mm^3 of blood Men: 4.8–5.5 million/mm^3 of blood
Hematocrit (% volume of RBCs in whole blood)	Women: 37–45% of blood volume Men: 40–45% of blood volume
Leukocytes	
WBC count	4–9 thousand/mm^3 of blood
Differential count	
Granulocytes	
Neutrophils	60–70% of total WBCs
Eosinophils	0–5% of total WBCs
Basophils	0–3% of total WBCs
Agranulocytes	
Lymphocytes	30–40% of total WBCs
Monocytes	0–5% of total WBCs
Thrombocytes	
Platelets	150–450 thousand/mm^3 of blood

* Normal values may differ significantly between laboratories.
RBC, red blood cell; WBC, white blood cell.

Hematologic Tests

COMPLETE BLOOD COUNT

The CBC includes the red blood cell (RBC) count, hemoglobin, hematocrit, red cell indices, white blood cell (WBC) count with or without differential, and platelet count. Table 27–1 present the normal values for the CBC. Table 27–2 reviews the effects of blood dyscrasias on the CBC.

RED BLOOD CELL COUNT

The RBC count measures the number of RBCs per cubic millimeter of blood. These values are useful in verifying findings from other hematologic tests used to diagnose anemia and polycythemia. Normal values vary with age and sex.

HEMOGLOBIN

The hemoglobin determination evaluates the hemoglobin content of erythrocytes by measuring the number of grams of hemoglobin per 100 ml of blood. This measurement helps indicate anemias and polycythemia in clients. Normal hemoglobin levels vary with age and sex.

HEMATOCRIT

Often used in place of the RBC count, hematocrit measures the per cent volume of RBCs in whole blood. This test is useful in the diagnosis of anemia, polycythemia, and abnormal hydration states. The hematocrit value is roughly three times the hemoglobin concentration. Normal values also vary with age and sex.

RED BLOOD CELL INDICES

RBC indices measure erythrocyte size and hemoglobin content. These values derive from the RBC count and hemoglobin level. The three RBC indices—mean corpuscular volume, mean corpuscular hemoglobin, and mean corpuscular hemoglobin concentration—are helpful in assessing the various anemias.

WHITE BLOOD CELL COUNT

The WBC count measures the number of WBCs in a cubic millimeter of blood. It helps detect infection or inflammation and is useful in monitoring a client's response to chemotherapy or radiation therapy.

WHITE BLOOD CELL DIFFERENTIAL

This test determines the proportion of each of the five types of WBCs in a sample of 100 WBCs. To figure the actual (absolute) number of a specific cell, the percentage of the cell is multiplied by the total WBC count. The differential helps in evaluating the body's capacity to resist and overcome infection and in detecting and identifying leukemias.

TABLE 27–2 How Blood Dyscrasias Affect the Complete Blood Count

INCREASED BY	DECREASED BY
Red blood cell count	
Polycythemia vera, cardiac and pulmonary disorders characterized by cyanosis, dehydration, acute poisoning	Anemia, fluid overload, recent hemorrhage, leukemia
Hemoglobin	
Hemoconcentration from polycythemia or dehydration	Hemodilution (fluid overload), anemia, recent hemorrhage
Hematocrit	
Hemoconcentration from loss of fluid, dehydration, polycythemia	Hemodilution, anemia, acute massive blood loss
Mean corpuscular volume	
Pernicious anemia, macrocytic anemia, folic acid or vitamin B_{12} deficiency anemias	Microcytic anemia, iron deficiency anemia, hypochromic anemias, thalassemia, lead poisoning
Mean corpuscular hemoglobin	
Macrocytic anemia	Microcytic anemia
Mean corpuscular hemoglobin concentration	
Spherocytosis	Microcytic, hypochromic anemia, thalassemia, iron deficiency anemia
White blood cell count	
Infection, leukemia, tissue necrosis	Bone marrow depression
Neutrophils	
Inflammatory disease or response, tissue necrosis (burns, myocardial infarction), granulocytic leukemia and other malignancies, acute stress response, bacterial infection	Bone marrow depression, viral diseases, drugs (chemotherapy, some antibiotics, psychotropics)
Eosinophils	
Allergic reactions, parasitic infestations, skin diseases, neoplasms, pernicious anemia	Stress response, Cushing's syndrome
Basophils	
Leukemia, some hemolytic anemias, polycythemia vera	Corticosteroids, allergic reactions, acute infections (note: decline is unlikely to be detected because normal count is 0–2%)
Lymphocytes	
Viral infections (infectious mononucleosis, pertussis, tuberculosis), lymphocytic leukemia, chronic bacterial infections	AIDS, adrenal corticosteroids, immunosuppressive drugs
Monocytes	
Infections (tuberculosis, malaria, Rocky Mountain spotted fever), collagen-vascular diseases, monocytic leukemia	Drug therapy, prednisone
Platelet count	
Malignancies, polycythemia vera, splenectomy	Idiopathic thrombocytopenia purpura, viral infection, AIDS, anemias, hemolytic disorders, chemotherapeutic drugs or radiation, hypersplenism or splenomegaly, infiltrative bone marrow disease, disseminated intravascular coagulation

AIDS, acquired immunodeficiency syndrome.

PLATELET COUNT

The platelet count evaluates thrombocyte (platelet) production, which has a role in blood clotting. The count is valuable in assessing the severity of thrombocytopenia (abnormally low platelet count), which could result in spontaneous bleeding.

PERIPHERAL BLOOD SMEAR

A peripheral blood smear is an examination of the peripheral blood to determine variations and abnormalities in erythrocytes, leukocytes, and platelets. Cells of normal size and shape are termed normocytes. Cells of normal color are called normochromic. Abnormalities of erythrocyte size, shape, and color usually indicate some form of anemia.

DIRECT AND INDIRECT ANTIGLOBULIN TESTS

Direct antiglobulin test (Coombs' test) is used to detect certain antigen-antibody reactions between serum antibodies and RBC antigens, differentiate between various forms of hemolytic anemia, determine unusual blood types, and test for hemolytic diseases in newborns. The direct antiglobulin test examines erythrocytes for the presence of antibodies (agglutinins) that damage erythrocytes without causing clumping or hemolysis. It is used to crossmatch blood for blood transfusions, test umbilical cord blood for erythroblastosis fetalis, and diagnose acquired hemolytic anemia.

The indirect antiglobulin test identifies antibodies to erythrocyte antigens in the serum of clients who have a greater than normal chance of experiencing transfusion reactions. Both tests are agglutination procedures that use a suspension of RBCs.

RETICULOCYTE COUNT

A reflection of RBC production, the reticulocyte count measures the responsiveness of the bone marrow to a diminished number of circulating erythrocytes. Specifically, this test measures the number of reticulocytes released from the bone marrow into the blood. An increase in the reticulocyte count indicates an increase in erythrocyte production, probably resulting from excessive RBC destruction (e.g., hemolytic anemia) or loss (e.g., hemorrhage). A decrease in the reticulocyte count may indicate bone marrow failure or pernicious anemia. In addition, it is used to evaluate the effectiveness of therapy for pernicious anemia and bone marrow failure.

BONE MARROW ASPIRATION

This important procedure is used to assess and diagnose most blood dyscrasias (e.g., aplastic anemia, the leuke-

TABLE 27–3 Laboratory Tests Used in the Diagnosis of Hemorrhagic Disorders

NAME OF TEST	PURPOSE	NORMAL VALUES	INTERPRETATION OF FINDINGS
Bleeding time	Measures the ability to stop bleeding after a small puncture wound	3–8 min in adults (varies with test method)	Prolonged bleeding time occurs in vascular maladies and after aspirin ingestion
Platelet count	Measures number of circulating platelets in venous or arterial blood	150,000–450,000	Low count results in prolonged bleeding time and impaired clot retraction; diagnostic of thrombocytopenia
Partial thromboplastin time	Complex method for testing normalcy of intrinsic coagulation process; used to identify deficiencies of coagulation factors, prothrombin, and fibrinogen; monitoring heparin therapy	25–38 sec	Prolongation of time indicates coagulation disorder (caused by deficiency of a coagulation factor); not diagnostic for platelet disorders
Prothrombin time	Determines activity and interaction of factors V, VII, X, prothrombin, and fibrinogen; used to determine dosages of oral anticoagulant drugs	11–15 sec (one stage)	Prolongation of time indicates person receiving anticoagulants; abnormally low fibrinogen concentration; deficiencies of factors II, V, VII, and X; presence of circulating anticoagulants as seen in lupus erythematosus; impaired prothrombin activity
Activated clotting time	Crude measure of coagulation process in venous blood; used to control heparin therapy; commonly used during cardiovascular surgery and in ICU	7–120 sec (depends on type of activator used)	Prolonged time occurs in severe coagulation problems; therapeutic administration of heparin
Thrombin time	Measures functional fibrinogen available, as shown by time needed to form fibrin clot after thrombin is added	10–15 sec	Prolonged time indicates DIC or hypofibrinogenemia; presence in blood of excess heparin or other anticoagulants
Thromboplastin generation test	Measures generation of thromboplastin; if result abnormal, second stage is done to identify missing coagulation factor	12 sec or less (100%)	Abnormal values found in hemophilia
Fibrinogen level	Measures level of fibrinogen	200–400 mg/100 mL	Abnormally low values may indicate liver disease, congenital or acquired afibrinogenemia, DIC
Clot retraction	Indicates function and number of platelets; measures time needed for contraction of an undisturbed clot	50–100% in 24 hr	Clot retraction retarded in thrombocytopenia; clot is small and soft in thrombasthenia (functional disturbance of platelets)
Capillary fragility test (Tourniquet test, Rumpel-Leede test)	Crude test of vascular resistance and platelet number and function; done by placing blood pressure cuff on arm for 5 min and then counting petechiae	No petechiae	Petechiae appear in thrombocytopenia and vascular purpura
FSP test	Measures the products that result from the breakdown of fibrin clots	Screening assay < 10 μg/mL of FSP Quantitative assay < 3 μg/mL	Abnormally high levels helpful in diagnosis of DIC; monitoring of fibrinolytic therapy

ICU, intensive care unit; DIC, disseminated intravascular coagulation; FSP, fibrin split products.

mias, pernicious anemia, and thrombocytopenia). Examination of the bone marrow reveals the number, size, and shape of the red cell, white cell, and platelet precursors. Hematologists study the marrow cells for various maturational abnormalities. Bone marrow samples are most commonly taken from the posterior iliac crests. Other possible sites for sampling include the sternum and the anterior iliac crests. To prepare the client for a bone marrow aspiration, the nurse

- explains the purpose and procedure of the examination
- makes sure the client has signed an informed consent form before aspiration
- obtains an order for sedation if the client is extremely apprehensive
- positions the client according to health-care facility policy

The procedure for a bone marrow aspiration is detailed in Box 27–1.

After the procedure, the nurse applies pressure until the bleeding stops. Most clients require only a small bandage over the site because there is usually minimal bleeding. However, many clients who require bone marrow aspiration are thrombocytopenic and may need a longer period of pressure to stop bleeding. A pressure dressing and sandbag also may need to be applied in these cases. The nurse observes the site frequently on the day of the procedure and for several days thereafter for clients with an increased risk of bleeding. There may be some discomfort or pain that requires a mild analgesic.

A biopsy of the bone may be taken at the time of marrow aspiration. This bone specimen is ejected into a jar containing a preservative and is sent to the laboratory with the marrow.

BOX 27–1

Bone Marrow Aspiration

The procedure for bone marrow aspiration involves the following steps:

- The nurse cleanses the skin with an antiseptic solution such as povidone-iodine (Betadine).
- The physician anesthetizes the skin and subcutaneous tissue down to the periosteum with a local anesthetic.
- A short, sharp, beveled needle containing a stylus is inserted through the bone cortex into the marrow space. Once the needle is in the marrow space, the stylus is removed. A syringe is then attached to the needle and about 1 mL of marrow is withdrawn. Because the marrow space itself cannot be anesthetized, removal of the marrow usually produces moderate to severe pain of short duration. It stops as soon as suction on the marrow space is stopped.
- The marrow is ejected onto slides.
- Slides must be labeled and sent to the laboratory immediately.

Coagulation Screening Tests

Laboratory studies provide the most crucial evidence for pinpointing the type and cause of a bleeding disorder (Table 27–3). Initially, four basic laboratory tests are performed to discern whether the bleeding problem is due to a vascular, coagulation, or platelet defect. These tests include bleeding time, PT, platelet count, and PTT. Ninety-nine per cent of all bleeding disorders are diagnosed by the PT and PTT.

STUDY QUESTIONS

1. Vitamin B_{12} is essential for
   A. Red cell formation and maturation
   B. Red cell maturation and nervous system function
   C. The production of hemoglobin
   D. Stimulation of erythropoietin
2. A person with AB blood type
   A. Has major antibodies in the red cell
   B. Has antigens A and B present in the red cell
   C. Can safely receive blood of any type
   D. Has one of the more common blood types
3. During a nursing history, a client shares that he does not eat many fruits and vegetables but does eat dairy products, grains, and red meat. The nurse should be alert for symptoms of
   A. Folic acid deficiency
   B. Altered coagulation
   C. Vitamin B_{12} deficiency
   D. Recurrent infections
4. To prepare the client for a bone marrow aspiration, the nurse should explain that the test
   A. Requires the use of general anesthesia
   B. Is done specifically to obtain a biopsy specimen
   C. Requires written consent from the client
   D. Consists of scraping the bone for a specimen

CRITICAL THINKING EXERCISES

The nurse in the hematology clinic is conducting a nursing history and physical assessment of an elderly client.

1. Why does the nurse ask about previous surgeries?
2. Why is a diet history important?
3. Would an occupational history be of importance?
4. What makes the review of all body functions of critical importance?
5. What general symptoms would alert the nurse to a possible disorder of the hematologic system? What implication does this have for the elderly client?

BIBLIOGRAPHY

1. Alkire, K., & Collingwood, J. (1990). Physiology of blood and bone marrow. *Seminars in Oncology Nursing, 6,* 99–107.
2. Baldwin, J. G. (1988). Hematopoietic function in the elderly. *Archives of Internal Medicine, 148,* 2544–2546.
3. Belsky–Lohr, L., & Copstead, L. C. (1995). Lymphoproliferative Disorders. In L. C. Copstead (Ed.), *Perspectives on Pathophysiology.* Philadelphia: W. B. Saunders.
4. Carlson, K., & Golub, A. (1987). *Autologous and directed blood programs.* Arlington, VA: American Association of Blood Banks.
5. Corbett, J. V. (1992). *Laboratory tests and diagnostic procedures with nursing diagnoses.* East Norwalk, CT: Appleton & Lange.
6. DiJulio, J. (1991). Hematopoiesis: An overview. *Oncology Nursing Forum, 18,* 3–6.
7. Duguid, J. K. M. (1990). Developing techniques in blood transfusion. *Bailliere's Clinical Haematology, 3(1),* 999–1017.
8. Ganong, W. F. (1993). *Review of medical physiology* (16th ed.). Norwalk, CT: Appleton & Lange.
9. Hoffbrand, A. V., & Brenner, M. K. (Eds.) (1992). *Recent advances in hematology* (6th ed.). Edinburgh: Churchill Livingstone.
10. Hoffbrand, A. V., & Pettit, J. E. (1992). *Essential hematology.* Cambridge, U.K.: Blackwell Scientific Publications.
11. Hoffman, R., et al. (Eds.) (1991). *Hematology: Basic principles and practice.* Edinburgh: Churchill Livingstone.
12. Jandel, J. H. (1991). *Blood: Pathophysiology.* Cambridge, U.K.: Blackwell Scientific Publications.
13. Melillo, K. D. (1993). Interpretation of laboratory values in older adults. *Nurse Practitioner: American Journal of Primary Health Care, 18(7),* 59–67.
14. Perez, W. E., & Viets, J. L. (1990). Transfusion and coagulation: An overview and recent advances in practice modalities. *Nurse Anesthetist, 1,* 149–161.
15. Read, E. J., & Klein, H. G. (1986). Hematological effects of aging: Considerations for clinical trials. In N. R. Cutler & P. K. Narang (Eds.), *Drug studies in the elderly* (pp. 123–144). New York: Plenum.
16. Salmon, C., et al. (1984). *The human blood groups.* New York: Masson.
17. Sherman, J. L., & Fields, S. K. (1988). *Guide to patient evaluation: History taking, physical examination, and the nursing process* (5th ed.). New York: Elsevier.
18. Welte, K. (1994). Matched unrelated transplants. *Seminars in Oncology Nursing, 10(1),* 20–27.
19. Williams, W. J. (1990). *Hematology* (4th ed.). New York: McGraw-Hill.

Chapter 28 Nursing Care of Clients with Hematologic Disorders

Learning Outcomes

After completing this chapter, the learner will be able to:

1. Assess the client for clinical manifestations of hematologic disorders.
2. Teach the client about the risk factors, basic pathophysiology, and clinical manifestations of hematologic disorders.
3. Explain the client's role in medical and surgical management of hematologic disorders.
4. Develop plans of care for the prevention of illness, management, and rehabilitation of clients with hematologic disorders.
5. Implement nursing interventions that optimize the quality of life for clients with hematologic disorders.
6. Evaluate planned client outcomes, using outcome criteria developed in the planning phase of care.

This chapter discusses disorders affecting red blood cells (erythrocytes), white blood cells (leukocytes), primarily the lymph system and spleen, and platelets and clotting factors.

Red blood cell disorders include anemias and polycythemias. Major disorders that affect white blood cells are (1) the leukemias (acute and chronic), (2) agranulocytosis, and (3) multiple myeloma (plasma cell myeloma). Disorders primarily affecting the lymph nodes and spleen are the lymphomas, classified as either (1) Hodgkin's disease or (2) non-Hodgkin's lymphoma. Disorders affecting platelets and clotting factors include (1) hemorrhagic disorders, (2) purpura, and (3) coagulation disorders.

Disorders Affecting Red Blood Cells

The Anemias

Anemia is a reduction in red blood cells (erythrocytes), which in turn decreases the oxygen-carrying capacity of the blood. Not a disease in itself, anemia reflects an abnormality in red blood cell number, structure, or function.

Anemia is the principal manifestation of many abnormal conditions, such as (1) deficiency states caused by a dietary lack of iron, vitamin B_{12}, and folic acid; (2) hereditary disorders of red blood cells; (3) disorders involving the hematopoietic tissues (bone marrow damage or a hyperactive spleen); and (4) bleeding from the gastrointestinal tract or any organ secondary to cancer or trauma. Increased destruction of red blood cells can also result from extrinsic sources, physical causes such as prosthetic heart valves, or thrombotic thrombocytopenic purpura. It can also result from antibodies, as in immune thrombotic thrombocytopenia; from infectious agents and toxins; or from other causes, such as hypersplenism, vasculitis syndromes, or osmotic and physical injury.

Incidence and Etiology

Studies suggest the prevalence of anemia increases with age; an estimated average of 20 per cent of the elderly are anemic.[6] However, anemia cannot be assumed to be caused simply by aging without the exclusion of reversible causes. The elderly client should be fully assessed for an underlying cause of anemia.

Major causes of anemia are (1) excessive blood loss, (2) deficiencies and abnormalities of red blood cell production, and (3) excessive destruction of red blood cells.

Pathophysiology

Two basic pathophysiologic alterations underlie all red blood cell disorders:

1. a decrease in the hemoglobin concentration or the number of functional red blood cells (anemia) due to one or more of the following:
   - insufficient production of red blood cells by the bone marrow
   - defective synthesis of red blood cells due to the absence of an essential factor
   - increased destruction of red blood cells caused by hereditary factors or an acquired condition
   - increased loss of red blood cells caused by acute or chronic bleeding
2. an increased number of circulating red blood cells (polycythemia) due to one of the following:
   - a disorder of unknown etiology, similar to cancer
   - a compensatory mechanism that develops in response to tissue hypoxia (secondary polycythemia)

Anemias are classified according to either the morphologic features of the red blood cells (e.g., normocytic, microcytic) or the cause of the condition (e.g., hemolytic, hemorrhagic). It is important to be familiar with the more accurate and commonly used morphologic classification system. However, it is more practical to relate nursing assessment, diagnosis, and treatment of an anemia to the classification in Table 28–1 than to its cellular characteristics. Table 28–1 divides the anemias into acquired (common to uncommon), anemias due to excessive blood loss, and congenital categories.

Clinical Manifestations

Symptoms accompanying anemia differ, depending on the severity and chronicity of the anemia, the age of the client, and the presence of other disorders.

CRITICAL TO REMEMBER

Tissue hypoxia is the underlying cause of all symptoms accompanying anemia.

Respiratory and cardiovascular compensatory mechanisms produce many of the symptoms. Clients with mild anemia (hemoglobin of 10 to 12 g/100 mL) are usually asymptomatic. If symptoms do occur, they typically follow strenuous exertion.

Signs and symptoms of anemia associated with specific systems include

- *integumentary:* pallor (particularly of palm lines, nail beds, conjunctiva, and circumoral area), delayed wound healing, sore mouth and tongue, sensitivity to cold, jaundice, spider angiomas
- *respiratory:* shortness of breath, dyspnea on exertion, orthopnea

TABLE 28–1 Classification of Anemias

Acquired Anemias
Anemias resulting from reduced red blood cell production
Anemias due to deficiencies of factors necessary for red blood cell production
Iron deficiency anemia
Anemias due to deficiencies of vitamin B_{12} and folic acid (megaloblastic anemias)
Pernicious anemia
Other anemias due to vitamin B_{12} deficiency
Anemia due to folic acid deficiency
Anemias of bone marrow failure
Aplastic anemia
Hemolytic anemias
Anemias resulting from excessive red blood cell destruction
Hemolysis due to trauma
Hemolysis due to chemical agents and medications (toxic hemolytic anemia)
Hemolysis due to infectious agents
Hemolysis due to systemic diseases (secondary hemolytic anemia)
Hemolysis due to isoimmune hemolytic reactions
Hemolysis due to autoimmune disorders
The paroxysmal hemoglobinurias
Secondary anemias
Anemias Due to Excessive Blood Loss
Acute posthemorrhagic anemia
Anemia due to chronic blood loss
Congenital Anemias
Hemoglobinopathies
Sickle cell anemia and sickle cell trait
Thalassemia
Hemolytic anemias due to intrinsic red blood cell defects
Glucose-6-phosphate dehydrogenase deficiency
Hereditary spherocytosis

- *cardiovascular:* palpitations, angina, tachycardia, cardiomegaly, claudication, dependent edema, bruits, tachypnea, fatigue, weakness
- *gastrointestinal:* anorexia, nausea, dietary change (clay-eating, pica), tarry stool, constipation, diarrhea, hemorrhoids, hematemesis, weight loss
- *genitourinary:* hematuria, menstrual irregularity, loss of libido, impotence
- *neurologic:* headache, dizziness, sternal tenderness, numbness, tingling of extremities, irritability, paralysis
- *general:* chronic fatigue, malaise

DIAGNOSTIC ASSESSMENT

The diagnosis of anemia relies on blood tests, physical assessment and examination, psychosocial assessment, and the health history. The red blood cell count, hemoglobin level, and hematocrit confirm the presence of anemia.

Medical Management

The goals of care for clients with anemia include (1) alleviating or controlling the causes, (2) relieving the symptoms, and (3) preventing complications.

Management of the anemias ranges from specific treatments to symptomatic care. Treatment also varies in intensity and duration because some anemias resolve within a few weeks or months whereas others require lifelong intervention.

The anemias caused by deficiency states respond best to specific intervention. For example, iron preparations and diet can cure iron deficiency anemia; injections of vitamin B_{12} control pernicious anemia.

Other anemias (e.g., aplastic anemia due to bone marrow failure and some of the acquired hemolytic anemias) can be successfully treated by stopping a cytotoxic medication or avoiding a dangerous chemical agent.

Oxygen therapy may be prescribed for clients with severe anemia, because their blood has a reduced capacity for oxygen. Oxygen helps prevent tissue hypoxia and lessens the workload of the heart as it struggles to compensate for the lower hemoglobin levels.

Blood transfusions are valuable in treating anemia caused by acute blood loss. They may also benefit clients with severe chronic anemia (hemoglobin less than 6 g/100 mL) who have responded poorly to other forms of therapy. Transfusion therapy, in which the specific blood components required are transfused, supports clients until they spontaneously recover or respond to treatment.

PHARMACOLOGIC MANAGEMENT

Iron, folic acid, and vitamin B_{12} can be given when the client has anemia caused by deficiency of these elements.

DIETARY MANAGEMENT

When the anemia is related to poor nutrition, or when the cause is blood loss, proper nutrition can improve red blood cell production. A diet high in iron, vitamin B_{12}, and folic acid will help increase red blood cell production if a deficiency of these nutrients is present.

Acquired Anemias

As stated in Chapter 27, effective erythropoiesis depends on the adequate intake and proper assimilation of iron, vitamin B_{12}, folic acid, protein, pyridoxine, and traces of copper. The most common deficiency state is iron deficiency. In addition, deficiencies of vitamin B_{12} and folic acid are prevalent. Protein deficiency is also frequently seen. Pyridoxine (vitamin B_6) and copper deficiencies occur infrequently in humans.

IRON DEFICIENCY ANEMIA

Iron deficiency is defined as anemia associated with either inadequate absorption or excessive loss of iron; it is chronic, microcytic, hypochromic anemia.

Incidence

The worldwide incidence of iron deficiency anemia is high. It is common in countries where nutrition is poor; it is also prevalent in tropical zones and in the southern United States, Mexico, and Puerto Rico, where bloodsucking parasites such as the hookworm are endemic. The poor of all nations suffer far more frequently from iron deficiency than do the middle and upper classes.

Menstruating women and young children also are vulnerable to iron deficiency, whereas adult men and postmenopausal women rarely develop this problem. Iron deficiency anemia also occurs with chronic blood loss.

Etiology

Menstruating and pregnant women, adolescents, children, and infants must have a higher daily intake of iron for prevention of deficiency. Economic constraints, poor dentition, and lack of interest in food preparation commonly lead to iron deficiency in elderly clients.

Menstruation is the most common cause of iron deficiency in women. Gastrointestinal tract bleeding is a common etiologic factor in men; it may result from peptic ulcers, hiatal hernia, gastritis, cancer, hemorrhoids, diverticula, ulcerative colitis, or salicylate poisoning.

Bleeding from the gastrointestinal tract is usually chronic and occult (obscure or not readily apparent). A chronic blood loss of as little as 2 to 4 mL/day can result in iron deficiency anemia, because every 2 mL of blood contains 1 mg of iron.

Pathophysiology

Iron deficiency anemia is caused by an inadequate supply of iron needed to synthesize hemoglobin. This results in a decreased supply to the developing red blood cells of a crucial component of hemoglobin—iron—essential to the oxygen-carrying function of heme. When these disorders of heme synthesis become severe, the marrow produces red blood cells that are deficient in hemoglobin concentration and that are hypochromic and microcytic.

Risk Factors

The major risk factor for iron deficiency anemia is inadequate nutrition. An adequate intake of iron, with normal absorption of the iron, should prevent the disorder.

Clinical Manifestations

In mild cases of iron deficiency anemia, the client is asymptomatic. However, in more severe cases, assessment reveals the general symptoms of anemia (e.g., palpitations, dizziness, and sensitivity to cold).

Later during the disease, hair and nails usually become brittle. In severe cases, dysphagia (difficulty in swallowing), stomatitis (inflammation of the mucosa of the mouth), and atrophic glossitis (tongue is inflamed and smooth owing to atrophy of papillae) may appear. Despite the weakness and discomfort associated with iron deficiency anemia, death rarely occurs unless severe cardiac complications develop.

DIAGNOSTIC ASSESSMENT

Examinations of the blood and bone marrow form the basis for diagnosing iron deficiency anemia. Because they are deficient in hemoglobin, the red blood cells are small (microcytic) and pale (hypochromic), a morphologic characteristic of iron deficiency. Other characteristics of anemia are hemoglobin level decreased to as low as 3.6 g/100 mL; total red blood cell count moderately reduced, rarely dropping below 3 million cells/100 mm^3; mean cell volume, mean cell hemoglobin, and mean cell hemoglobin concentration reduced; serum iron level (normally between 50 and 150 μg/100 mL of blood) may be decreased to 10 μg; total iron-combining capacity elevated to 350 to 500 μg/100 mL (normal is 250 to 350 μg/100 mL); hemosiderin (an insoluble form of storage iron) completely absent from the bone marrow; immunoradiometric serum ferritin assay below normal.

Once the diagnosis of iron deficiency anemia is confirmed, studies are conducted to find the cause of the anemia.

Medical Management

Therapeutic goals for clients with iron deficiency anemia are to (1) diagnose and correct the underlying cause of the anemia and (2) correct the iron deficit through diet and supplemental iron preparations.

PHARMACOLOGIC MANAGEMENT

Supplemental iron is usually administered to increase iron available in the blood. The medications of choice are ferrous sulfate (Feosol), 0.2 g orally, three times a day, with meals; ferrous gluconate (Fergon), 0.3 g orally, twice a day; and iron-dextran (Imferon), 100 to 250 mg intramuscularly. Clients usually receive iron supplements for at least 6 months for repletion of the body stores.

Parenteral iron therapy is administered to clients who (1) have an intolerance to oral iron preparations,

(2) habitually forget to take their medications, or (3) continue to suffer blood losses. Iron-dextran is the parenteral drug of choice. The client typically feels more energetic and has an increased appetite within 48 hours. Peak reticulocytosis occurs about day 10. Red blood cell indices and hemoglobin content gradually return to normal.

Nursing Management

Assessment

Nursing assessment for iron deficiency anemia focuses on data collection of causative factors and risk factors, dietary history, family history, psychosocial problems, and medications. Common physical symptoms are stomatitis, smooth red tongue, cold sensitivity, brittle hair, and spoon-shaped brittle nails (integumentary); dyspnea on exertion (respiratory); tachycardia (cardiovascular); and dizziness, dysphagia, numbness, tingling, decreased concentration, headache, and fatigue (neurologic).

Nursing Diagnosis, Planning, and Implementation

Nursing Diagnosis: Nutrition, Altered: Less than Body Requirements R/T lack of knowledge of adequate nutrition.

Planning: Expected Outcomes. The client will have nutritional deficiencies corrected and optimal nutrition will be achieved, as evidenced by blood tests reaching normal range, activity tolerance improved, and anemia resolved.

Implementation. The nurse should teach basics of good nutrition and encourage diet high in protein, iron, and vitamins with frequent small meals. The nurse should encourage foods cooked in iron pots and ingestion of foods such as liver (the richest source), oysters, lean meats, kidney beans, whole wheat bread, kale, spinach, egg yolk, turnip tops, beet greens, carrots, apricots, and raisins. The nurse should document the client's weight and encourage good oral hygiene.

Nursing Diagnosis: Knowledge Deficit R/T iron preparations.

Planning: Expected Outcomes. The client will verbalize correct dosage of, route of, and indications for iron preparations, as evidenced by correct administration of iron medications and no complications developing.

Implementation. The nurse should teach the client that iron salts are gastric irritants and should always be taken after meals. Liquid iron preparations should be well diluted and taken through a straw (undiluted liquid iron stains teeth). Constipation, commonly seen during iron therapy, is avoided by a high-fiber diet and use of stool softeners or laxatives as required.

The nurse administers parenteral iron medications as ordered. Iron-dextran causes darkening and discoloration of the skin around the injection site unless it is administered properly (Z-track technique).

Evaluation

The nurse must evaluate client outcomes on the basis of the established plan of care. If these goals have not been achieved, the plan and interventions must be revised to meet the client's needs.

Megaloblastic Anemias

Anemias caused by deficiencies of vitamin B_{12} and folic acid are called megaloblastic anemias because they are characterized by the appearance of megaloblasts (large primitive red blood cells) in the blood and bone marrow.

Other common features of the megaloblastic anemias are leukopenia and thrombocytopenia (decrease in platelets); oral, gastrointestinal, and neurologic symptoms; and favorable response to injections of either vitamin B_{12} or folic acid.

PERNICIOUS ANEMIA

Pernicious anemia is anemia caused by decreased absorption of vitamin B_{12}.

Incidence and Etiology

Pernicious anemia is the most prevalent form of vitamin B_{12} deficiency in the United States and Canada. The most common megaloblastic anemia, pernicious anemia, occurs in only 0.1 per cent of the population. It mainly strikes men and women over the age of 50 years and primarily affects people of northern European origin.

This chronic, progressive, megaloblastic anemia of adults is caused by a deficiency of intrinsic factor. Lack of intrinsic factor due to atrophy of the stomach's glandular mucosa is the basic defect in pernicious anemia.

Risk Factors

One major risk factor for the development of pernicious anemias is gastric resection. The parietal cells in the stomach secrete the intrinsic factor required for vitamin B_{12} absorption. The disease can also be congenital as a result of absence of the intrinsic factor.

Pathophysiology

The four major characteristics of pernicious anemia are

- abnormally large red blood cells (macrocytic anemia)
- hypochlorhydria (deficiency of gastric hydrochloric acid)
- neurologic and gastrointestinal symptoms
- a fatal outcome unless the client receives life-long injections of vitamin B_{12}

Pathologic consequences of vitamin B_{12} deficiency are macrocytic anemia and gastrointestinal disorders. Both problems respond to injections of vitamin B_{12}. Clients with pernicious anemia have a high incidence of benign gastric polyps and gastric carcinoma; they require routine assessment for gastric bleeding and tumor growth obstruction. Untreated pernicious anemia causes death; delayed intervention results in permanent disabilities.

Clinical Manifestations

Diagnosis of pernicious anemia is based on the presence of anemia, gastrointestinal symptoms, and neurologic disorders; laboratory blood and bone marrow tests; the absence of gastric hydrochloric acid; and a favorable response to vitamin B_{12} "therapeutic trial."

Low hemoglobin levels and consequent hypoxemia may trigger congestive heart failure because of increased demands on the heart to transport oxygen to the tissues. Angina pectoris also may develop from insufficient oxygenation of the myocardium.

DIAGNOSTIC ASSESSMENT

Laboratory findings that confirm a diagnosis of pernicious anemia include the following:

- Red blood cells are usually reduced to fewer than 3 million/mm^3; mean cell volume and mean cell hemoglobin concentration are likely to be elevated, with white blood cells and mean cell hemoglobin decreased.
- On peripheral blood smear, red blood cells are oval, macrocytic, and hyperchromic.
- Schilling test measures the absorption of orally administered, radioactive vitamin B_{12} (tagged with cobalt-60) before and after parenteral administration of the intrinsic factor. This procedure detects lack of intrinsic factor and is the definitive test for pernicious anemia.

Medical Management

CRITICAL TO REMEMBER

Clients with pernicious anemia need both immediate care and life-long therapy with maintenance vitamin B_{12}.

During the acute phase of illness, the client can be treated with vitamin B_{12} injections.

The response to vitamin B_{12} injections is usually quick and dramatic, often occurring within 24 to 48 hours. Within 72 hours, reticulocytes begin to increase; by the end of the first week, the total red blood cell count rises significantly. Cardiovascular involvement usually lessens with improved hematopoiesis. Although peripheral nerve function may improve with treatment, spinal cord and brain damage usually persist.

PHARMACOLOGIC MANAGEMENT

Prescribed medications may include vitamin derivatives (to correct nutritional or metabolic deficiency): cyanocobalamin (Berubigen, Cyanabin, vitamin B_{12}, and others); and folic acid (Folvite).

Nursing Management

Once the acute stage of the illness is past, the client with pernicious anemia must undertake a life-long program of maintenance therapy. Monthly injections of vitamin B_{12} are needed to avoid relapse. The nurse plays a vital role in educating clients with this disorder about the importance of continuous care.

If therapy remains adequate and uninterrupted, the client with pernicious anemia can expect a life free of anemic symptoms, without further symptoms of neuropathy.

ANEMIA DUE TO FOLIC ACID DEFICIENCY

Anemia associated with folic acid deficiency is very common. Usually, folic acid deficiency results from a poor diet lacking in such foods as green leafy vegetables, liver, citrus fruits, and yeast. Clients with chronic alcoholism, because of their typically inadequate diets, are particularly susceptible to this problem. High levels of alcohol in the blood also partially block the response of the bone marrow to folic acid, which thereby interferes with erythropoiesis.

Folic acid, like vitamin B_{12}, is necessary for DNA synthesis. Both vitamin B_{12} and folic acid deficiencies cause symptoms of megaloblastic anemia (fatigue, cardiac symptoms, slight jaundice) and gastrointestinal tract disturbances (e.g., dyspepsia; smooth, beefy tongue). However, unlike pernicious anemia, a folic acid deficiency does not cause neurologic manifestations.

Anemia due to folic acid deficiency has a slow and insidious onset. The client, often thin and emaciated, usually appears quite ill. The client's malnourished and debilitated state frequently leads to other deficiencies, for example of iron, protein, minerals, and other vitamins.

The megaloblastic anemia caused by folic acid deficiency is the same as that seen in pernicious anemia. It is diagnosed by blood smear and bone marrow examinations. In folic acid deficiency, the serum folate level is less than 4 ng (normal is 7 to 20 ng); Schilling test results are normal; hydrochloric acid is probably present in the gastric juice; neurologic symptoms are absent; and the client responds favorably to a therapeutic trial of 50 to 100 μg of folic acid administered intramuscularly daily for 10 days.

For correction of anemia due to folate deficiency, the client receives oral doses of folic acid (0.1 to 5 mg) daily until the blood picture improves or until the cause of intestinal malabsorption is corrected.

Folic acid is administered intramuscularly in the form of leucovorin calcium (Folinic Acid). Additionally, vitamin C is sometimes prescribed because it increases the role of folic acid in promoting erythropoiesis.

ANEMIAS OF BONE MARROW FAILURE

The anemias of bone marrow failure have several names, each of which is descriptive of some aspect of the disease: aplastic, hypoplastic, regenerative, or primary refractory anemia. Aplastic anemia, the most commonly used term, describes bone marrow that is severely hypoplastic ("empty"), that is, devoid of erythroid, myeloid, and megakaryocytic cell lines. Hypoplastic bone marrow results in anemia, leukopenia, and thrombocytopenia. When all three cellular elements are suppressed, the condition is known as pancytopenia.

Incidence and Etiology

Pancytopenia affects clients of all ages, and both sexes are equally susceptible. The incidence of aplastic anemia is about four cases per million population.

In about one half of cases, the cause of aplastic anemia is unknown. Acquired aplastic anemia may result from either an autoimmune mechanism or a direct injury by myelotoxins (such as medications that cause aplastic anemia as a side effect).

Risk Factors

Clients treated with the myelotoxins are at increased risk of developing aplastic anemia. If clients are receiving any of these agents, they must have their blood count monitored at frequent intervals.

Pathophysiology

The etiologic agents cause the bone marrow to stop producing blood cells when radiant energy inhibits mitosis, or cell division, and antimetabolites used in cancer therapy block the synthesis of purines or nucleic acids. Usually, however, the exact mechanism of marrow failure from these agents is unknown.

The onset of aplastic anemia may be insidious or rapid. In idiopathic or hereditary cases, the onset is usually gradual. When bone marrow failure results from a myelotoxin, however, the onset may be explosive, with quickly developing symptoms. If the condition does not reverse itself when the offending agent is removed, the condition can prove to be fatal.

Clinical Manifestations

Symptoms of pancytopenia are particularly severe. Not only does the red blood cell count fall, but so do the leukocyte and platelet counts. The client consequently develops the following three conditions: normocytic anemia, granulocytopenia, and thrombocytopenia.

NORMOCYTIC ANEMIA

The red blood cell count is usually below 1 million/mm^3, with a low reticulocyte count. The client reports progressive fatigue, lassitude, and dyspnea.

GRANULOCYTOPENIA

The leukocyte count may be less than 2000/mm^3 (normal is 6000 to 9000/mm^3). The client, therefore, suffers from an increased susceptibility to infection, because without leukocytes, the body cannot adequately battle bacteria and other invading organisms. If the granulocyte count drops below 500/mm^3, the client may develop a fulminating bacterial infection.

THROMBOCYTOPENIA

The platelet count may fall below 20,000/mm^3 (normal is 150,000 to 450,000/mm^3), which usually causes bleeding into the skin and mucous membranes. If the platelet count is severely reduced, the client will hemorrhage.

DIAGNOSTIC ASSESSMENT

The diagnosis of aplastic anemia and pancytopenia is based on the differential blood count, the client's symptoms, history of exposure to a myelotoxin, and bone marrow examination. In pancytopenia, the bone marrow is fatty and contains very few developing blood cells.

Medical Management

The client with pancytopenia is often critically ill. Prompt medical attention and skillful nursing care are necessary. The first step in halting the process of aplastic anemia is immediate withdrawal of an offending agent or drug.

If aplastic anemia develops from a suspected myelotoxic agent, blood transfusions are the mainstay of therapy until bone marrow activity signals recovery. If the marrow fails to recover and long-term red blood cell support is required, iron overload often results. This complication was a leading cause of death before iron chelating therapy became available.

Bone marrow transplantation is now the treatment of choice for aplastic anemia when (1) an autoimmune phenomenon is suspected or (2) the bone marrow fails to regenerate after discontinuation of myelotoxic agents. Currently, transplantation can take place only if the client has a human leukocyte antigen (HLA) identical donor.

PHARMACOLOGIC MANAGEMENT

Corticosteroids and androgens are sometimes prescribed to stimulate bone marrow activity; unfortunately, these drugs often fail to work as desired.

Nursing Management

Preventing and treating complications resulting from pancytopenia is of major importance in caring for the client with aplastic anemia. The two main complications of this anemia are infection and bleeding.

HEMOLYTIC ANEMIA

Major hallmarks of hemolytic anemia are

- a shortening of the red blood cell life span
- an abnormal increase in the number of red blood cells destroyed by macrophages
- failure of the bone marrow to replace destroyed red blood cells

Hemolytic anemia may be acute or chronic. Severe, acute episodes of hemolysis, known as hemolytic crises, punctuate some chronic forms of hemolytic anemia. The client with hemolytic anemia suffers from all the general manifestations of anemia discussed earlier (lassitude, fatigue). The specific signs and symptoms that characterize hemolytic anemia are jaundice, splenomegaly, hepatomegaly, and cholelithiasis. Renal failure may be a complication of severe hemolysis. It is caused by excretion of an increased load of red blood cell degradation products.

Laboratory findings indicative of hemolytic anemia usually include normocytic anemia, reticulocytosis due to increased efforts of the bone marrow to compensate for excessive erythrocyte destruction, increased red blood cell fragility, shortened erythrocyte lifespan, hyperbilirubinemia, increased fecal and urinary urobilinogen, and (in cases of massive intravascular hemolysis) hemoglobinema.

HEMOLYSIS DUE TO TRAUMA

When red blood cells are exposed to excessive turbulence in the circulation, they may fragment. Fragmented erythrocytes (schistocytes) are quickly destroyed by phagocytes, which results in anemia.

Hemolytic anemia may develop after external trauma or severe burns. In addition, hemolysis sometimes occurs after prosthetic cardiac valve replacement or cardiac septal defect repair.

Clinical findings include hemoglobinemia, hemoglobinuria, and a drop in the erythrocyte count. Treatment is directed toward correcting the underlying problem.

TOXIC HEMOLYTIC ANEMIA (HEMOLYSIS DUE TO CHEMICAL AGENTS AND MEDICATIONS)

Chemicals and medications can cause hemolysis. Hemolytic reactions are usually the result of the oxidant effects of the medication or chemical or an immune reaction caused by the medication.

Chemical oxidants vary in their potency and in their ability to destroy red blood cells. Potent oxidants cause hemolytic reactions in every client exposed to a sufficient amount (e.g., benzene, phenylhydrazine, nitrites, potassium chlorate, arsenic, colloidal silver, and lead). These powerful compounds can damage the red blood cell membrane, resulting in a fragile cell that is quickly destroyed.

A common example of hemolysis caused by contact with a chemical agent is lead poisoning (plumbism). Lead poisoning causes characteristic changes in the brain, nervous system, spinal cord, and digestive tract.

Researchers estimate that 1.5 million Americans are exposed to potentially dangerous levels of lead while on the job. Clinicians have also discovered that blood lead levels once thought safe and even normal are dangerous and result in many metabolic and neurologic disorders. A lead level higher than 40 μg/100 mL in adults and 25 μg/100 mL in children now is considered unsafe.

Treatment of this condition usually involves the administration of chelating agents such as calcium disodium edetate.

An immune response, the second major cause of toxic hemolysis, is the result of an antigen-antibody reaction (see Chap. 9). Medications that can precipitate antigen-antibody reactions in susceptible clients are quinine, quinidine, methyldopa, sulfonamides, phenacetin, and penicillin.

Finally, certain snake and spider venoms as well as some vegetable poisons (e.g., some mushrooms) cause hemolytic reactions that frequently are fatal.

Secondary Anemias

The secondary anemias, as the name implies, arise in association with other conditions, such as

- chronic systemic diseases (e.g., rheumatoid arthritis, malnutrition, leukemia)
- the lymphomas and multiple myeloma
- chronic infections (lung abscess, empyema, pelvic inflammatory disease)
- acute and chronic renal disease complicated by uremia
- cirrhosis of the liver

- endocrine disorders (myxedema)
- cancer

The anemia accompanying cancer results from chronic blood loss, cell hemolysis, or the development of space-occupying lesions within the bone marrow (myelophthisic anemia).

Although the cause of the secondary anemias varies with the underlying condition, all have two factors in common: the red blood cells have a shortened lifespan, and the bone marrow fails to produce enough red blood cells to compensate for losses.

The anemia that develops in these conditions may be moderate to severe, depending on the underlying cause. Treatment involves correcting the underlying condition. Packed red blood cell transfusions are sometimes given when hemoglobin levels fall below 8 to 9 g/100 mL.

Anemias Resulting from Excessive Blood Loss

ACUTE POSTHEMORRHAGIC ANEMIA

Acute posthemorrhagic anemia is a normocytic, normochromic anemia that develops after the rapid loss of red blood cells during a massive hemorrhage.

Etiology

Common causes of acute bleeding are severed blood vessels due to trauma, spontaneous rupture of an aneurysm, hemorrhagic disorders, and erosion of an artery by a cancerous growth or ulcerative lesion.

Pathophysiology

The adverse effects of acute hemorrhage result from a rapid decrease in blood volume and red blood cells; thereby, the oxygen-carrying capacity of the blood is reduced. The severity of symptoms of and the prognosis for acute hemorrhage depend on (1) the rate of bleeding, (2) the site of the hemorrhage, and (3) the volume of blood lost. A gradual loss of even a large amount of blood is usually less threatening than is the rapid loss of a smaller volume.

Clinical Manifestations

Signs and symptoms of acute blood loss are restlessness, dizziness, syncope, thirst, pallor, diaphoresis, rapid thready pulse, a dramatic drop in blood pressure, rapid deep respirations that later become shallow, and disorientation or coma that is indicative of cerebral anoxia.

In addition to these symptoms, internal hemorrhage into body organs and tissues causes fever, pain in the area of bleeding due to distention of tissues, and symptoms of organ displacement (e.g., hemothorax can result in a mediastinal shift). If internal or external hemorrhage remains uncontrolled, the blood pressure continues to drop, and hypovolemic shock develops (see Chap. 56).

DIAGNOSTIC ASSESSMENT

After hemorrhage, red blood cell count and hematocrit and hemoglobin results may be high (although they are actually low) because of vasoconstriction and loss of plasma volume. These test results return to normal levels after infusion of intravenous fluid and restoration of intravascular volume from extracellular fluids.

ANEMIA DUE TO CHRONIC BLOOD LOSS

Chronic blood loss causes a chronic, microcytic, hypochromic anemia. The major causes of chronic blood loss are bleeding peptic ulcers, prolonged or excessive menses, bleeding hemorrhoids, and cancerous lesions within the gastrointestinal tract.

The results of chronic bleeding are (1) continuous loss of small numbers of erythrocytes, usually replaced by the bone marrow, and (2) continuous loss of iron, which results in a total depletion of iron stores.

Because of this iron loss, the anemia of chronic bleeding closely resembles iron deficiency anemia. Correction of the anemia involves locating and controlling the site of bleeding and replacing iron with a proper diet and iron supplements.

Signs and symptoms of anemia secondary to chronic blood loss are the same as those associated with iron deficiency anemia. In mild cases of anemia, the client is asymptomatic. However, in more severe cases, assessment reveals the general symptoms of anemia (palpitations, dizziness, and sensitivity to cold).

Medical treatment includes modalities generally recommended for anemia. Surgery may be needed to correct chronic blood loss.

Congenital Anemias

THE THALASSEMIAS

The thalassemias are a group of inherited, chronic, hemolytic anemias. These anemias predominantly affect clients of Mediterranean or southern Chinese ancestry; they were first discovered among people living around the Mediterranean Sea, hence the name *thalassos*, meaning "sea." Other names are Mediterranean anemia and Cooley's anemia. The thalassemias also affect African Americans and people from central Africa and southern Asia.

The production of extremely thin, fragile erythrocytes called target cells characterizes the thalassemias.

Pathophysiology

The severity of the anemia produced by the thalassemias depends on whether the afflicted client is homozygous or heterozygous for the thalassemia trait. Thalassemia major and intermedia, both characterized by a profound anemia, appear in homozygotes. Thalassemia minor, characterized by a mild anemia, develops in heterozygotes.

The outlook for clients with thalassemia major is usually poor. Children are retarded in their growth and development. Many fail to live through puberty. Thalassemia minor, on the other hand, does not affect life expectancy.

Clinical Manifestations

The symptoms of thalassemia major resemble those of other hemolytic anemias (e.g., jaundice, cholelithiasis, leg ulcers, and enlarged spleen). In addition, thalassemia is characterized by a pronounced bone hyperactivity that causes a thickening of the cranium and a mongoloid appearance of the facies.

Thalassemia minor is usually asymptomatic, except for a mild anemia. Blood smears of clients with this condition contain small, defective red blood cells.

DIAGNOSTIC ASSESSMENT

Laboratory findings in thalassemia (β form) reveal target cells (abnormally thin, fragile cells) and other bizarrely shaped red blood cells in the circulation, and serum bilirubin and fecal and urinary urobilinogen levels that are elevated because of the severe hemolysis of abnormal cells.

Medical Management

Transfusion therapy is the only treatment available. Clients with thalassemia major receive packed red blood cells, which may be given (1) on a monthly or bimonthly basis (regular transfusion regimen), (2) whenever the hemoglobin falls below 3 to 4 g/100 mL (nonsystemic transfusion), or (3) every 15 days to maintain the hemoglobin at 12 to 15 g/100 mL (hypertransfusion regimen). When it becomes clear that transfused cells are being rapidly destroyed by the spleen (causing a severe hemolytic anemia), splenectomy is necessary.

Thalassemia minor is usually so mild that treatment is not required. However, clients who carry the thalassemia trait need genetic counseling.

Hemolytic Anemias Resulting from Intrinsic Red Blood Cell Defects

GLUCOSE-6-PHOSPHATE DEHYDROGENASE DEFICIENCY

Glucose-6-phosphate dehydrogenase (G6PD) is an important red blood cell enzyme. G6PD deficiency can be classified as an enzymopathy, a genetic defect that involves the partial or complete deficiency of certain essential enzymes.

A deficiency of G6PD makes red blood cells more susceptible to hemolysis after ingestion of medications and foods classified as chemical oxidants.

Incidence

An inherited sex-linked disorder, G6PD deficiency is a common problem affecting at least 100 million people in the world. Among Americans, G6PD deficiency affects about 20 per cent of blacks and about 1 to 2 per cent of whites. It is common among Sephardic Jews, Greeks, Italians, and Arabs.

Pathophysiology

The enzyme G6PD helps use about 10 per cent of the glucose metabolized by red blood cells. When exposed to oxidative medications and foods, red blood cells require even more glucose for energy. If a G6PD deficiency exists, the red blood cells cannot adequately metabolize more glucose and so cannot cope with the oxidative effects of certain substances. As a result, hemolysis occurs. Because young, newly released red blood cells contain a large amount of G6PD, only aging red blood cells are destroyed upon exposure to oxidative agents.

Clinical Manifestations

Clients with this enzymopathy may remain completely asymptomatic throughout their lives. Typically, symptoms develop only after a stressor, such as viral or bacterial infection or certain medications or toxins. Occasionally, however, spontaneous attacks of hemolytic anemia develop that are not precipitated by a known external factor.

More than 40 oxidative medications and foods produce hemolytic anemia in clients with G6PD deficiency (e.g., primaquine, quinine, aspirin, sulfonamides, phenacetin, vitamin K derivatives, chloramphenicol, thiazide diuretics, and fava beans). After exposure to any of these agents, the client with G6PD deficiency develops acute intravascular hemolysis lasting about 7 to 12 days. During this acute phase, the client suffers from anemia and jaundice.

DIAGNOSTIC ASSESSMENT

Laboratory findings include moderate hemoglobinemia and hemoglobinuria, an elevated serum bilirubin, reticulocytosis, and the appearance of Heinz bodies (small particles of oxidized hemoglobin) within the red blood cell.

Medical Management

Correcting the anemia primarily involves identifying and removing the medication or food precipitating the hemolytic reaction. Care of the client during the time of acute hemolysis is purely symptomatic (rest, fluids, and nutritious diet).

HEREDITARY SPHEROCYTOSIS (CONGENITAL HEMOLYTIC JAUNDICE, CONGENITAL SPHEROCYTIC ANEMIA)

Hereditary spherocytosis is a common form of chronic hemolytic anemia found in all races and ages. A simple mendelian dominant trait, spherocytosis can be inherited even if only one parent carries the abnormal gene. In about 20 per cent of cases, hematologic abnormalities are absent in other family members, which suggests that a spontaneous mutation in the client caused the illness.

Pathophysiology

The two most distinctive characteristics of hereditary spherocytosis are (1) the appearance of large numbers of spherical red blood cells (spherocytes) and (2) an enlarged spleen. Spherocytosis develops because the red blood cells have a defective cellular membrane that is extremely permeable to the influx of sodium ions. To curtail the flow of sodium ions through its defective membrane, the red blood cell must increase its metabolic work and, so, its use of glucose.

When glucose and cellular energy become depleted, sodium ions flow through the cellular membrane without resistance. Thus, the red blood cell interior becomes hypertonic; water is drawn into the cell, which causes the red blood cell to swell and become spherical. Spherocytes, thick and rigid, are easily trapped within the splenic venous sinusoids, where they are devoured by phagocytes. As a result, the spleen becomes enlarged, and the client suffers from anemia and jaundice because of the massive red blood cell hemolysis within the spleen.

Clinical Manifestations

Symptoms of hereditary spherocytosis are the same as symptoms of hemolytic anemia discussed earlier (e.g., malaise, mild anemia, jaundice, gallstones, and splenomegaly). Splenomegaly is particularly pronounced, and clients may experience left upper quadrant fullness and abdominal pain. In the presence of systemic infection, the hemolytic rate may increase, inducing further splenic enlargement. Occasionally, acute abdominal pain results from splenic infarction. Such severe hemolytic crises are sometimes fatal.

DIAGNOSTIC ASSESSMENT

Laboratory findings are distinctive and include spherocytes in the blood smear; reticulocytosis; lowered red blood cell count and hemoglobin values; positive direct antiglobulin test; and increased osmotic fragility.

Surgical Management

Although blood transfusions may benefit a client in hemolytic crisis, the only treatment indicated in all cases of hereditary spherocytosis is splenectomy. Ninety per cent of clients who undergo splenectomy experience complete reversal of symptoms. Although spherocytes continue to circulate, these misshapen cells usually have a longer lifespan once the spleen is removed.

Nursing Management

Assessment

See each section under anemia for the appropriate assessments.

Nursing Diagnosis, Planning, and Implementation

Collaborative Problem: Alteration in oxygen-carrying capacity of blood R/T anemia.

Planning: Expected Outcomes. The client will have maintained adequate organ oxygenation, as evidenced by limiting activities or by receiving supplemental agents to enhance red blood cell function, production, or replacement.

Implementation. The nurse administers blood according to policy and teaches indications and possible side effects (see section on blood transfusions). The nurse instructs the client in the cause of anemia, preventive and treatment measures, diet therapy, and proper administration of iron supplements and their effect on stools. The nurse provides oxygen therapy if ordered and paces activities and schedules rest periods to prevent fatigue.

Nursing Diagnosis: Tissue Perfusion, Altered R/T deficit or malfunction of red blood cells.

Planning: Expected Outcomes. The client will experience optimal peripheral tissue perfusion, as evidenced by warm, rapid capillary refill; adequate pulses noted in extremities; and no complaints of tingling or numbness.

Implementation. The nurse monitors for signs of oxygen deprivation: increased pulse and respirations, decreased blood pressure, and shortness of breath. He or she reports symptoms immediately to the physician and starts appropriate medical support. The nurse should keep the extremities warm to prevent vasoconstriction and bathe the client in warm, *not* hot, water.

Nursing Diagnosis: Nutrition, Altered: Less than Body Requirements R/T anorexia, stomatitis, knowledge deficit, and inability to get proper foods (physical/financial problems).

Planning: Expected Outcomes. The client will maintain proper nutrition, as evidenced by maintenance of or increase in body weight and improved intake of proper nutrients.

Implementation. The nurse assesses the client's usual diet and eating pattern, making referrals when necessary (e.g., social worker, dietitian, home health care aide). The nurse provides symptom management for anorexia and administers vitamin B_{12} and other medication as ordered. He or she encourages a diet high in iron, protein, and vitamins.

Nursing Diagnosis: Individual Coping, Ineffective, Risk for R/T chronic status of disease.

Planning: Expected Outcomes. The client will cope effectively with the chronic nature of the illness, as evidenced by client's statements and demonstration of effective coping behaviors such as maintaining usual activities and ability to establish positive relationships.

Implementation. The nurse provides the client with opportunities to express concerns, fears, feelings, and expectations. He or she encourages the client to develop realistic goals and activity levels and instructs the client in the need for rest periods and adequate diets. The nurse collaborates with the client to establish follow-up appointments that enable the client to lead a more normal life. Other resource persons may be used, such as support systems, clinical specialists, social workers, and psychiatric liaison personnel.

Evaluation

The nurse must evaluate client outcomes on the basis of the established plan of care. If these goals have not been achieved, the plan and interventions must be revised to meet the client's needs.

Modification of Plan of Care for the Elderly

The nursing care plan for the aged client should include consideration of problems related to poor dentition, economic constraints, and lack of interest in food preparation.

Polycythemias (Overproduction of Red Blood Cells)

Polycythemia is defined as an increase in both the number of circulating erythrocytes and the concentration of hemoglobin within the blood. Red blood cells may number as high as 8 to 12 million/mm^3, and the hemoglobin concentration rises to 18 to 25 g/100 mL.

POLYCYTHEMIA VERA

Polycythemia vera is classified as a myeloproliferative disorder (meaning overgrowth of bone marrow). It usually develops in middle age. Although the precise cause remains unknown, it is possibly a form of malignancy similar to leukemia and is often considered a premalignant condition.

Pathophysiology

The three major hallmarks of the condition are (1) relentless, unrestrained production of erythrocytes; (2) production of excessive myelocytes (leukocytes within the bone marrow); and (3) overproduction of platelets.

The inordinate mass production of these three cell lines results in the following pathologic consequences: (1) an increase in the blood viscosity; (2) an increase in the total blood volume, which may be twice or even three times greater than normal; and (3) severe blood congestion of all tissues and organs.

Clinical Manifestations

The client may exhibit hypertension, distended superficial blood vessels, epistaxis, headache, redness of the skin, bleeding tendencies, and ecchymosis. The liver and spleen are enlarged. The disease may result in complications such as myocardial infarction, cerebrovascular accident, or hemorrhage.

Diagnostic Assessment

Laboratory findings include red blood cell count as high as 8 to 12 million/mm^3; hemoglobin level of 18 to 25 g/100 mL; hematocrit level greater than 54 per cent in men and greater than 49 per cent in women; platelet count usually increased in polycythemia vera; normal arterial blood gases; hyperplastic bone marrow; and serum uric acid level three to four times normal.

SECONDARY POLYCYTHEMIA

When the body's demand for oxygen increases for any reason, the bone marrow must produce more red blood cells in order to prevent tissue hypoxia. This compensatory response to tissue hypoxia is called secondary polycythemia.

Hypoxia that is sufficiently prolonged to cause polycythemia results from chronic lung disease (particularly emphysema), congenital heart disease, and prolonged exposure to altitudes of 10,000 feet or more. People who live in mountainous areas are not hypoxic because their blood has "thickened." These mountain dwellers produce high numbers of red blood cells, which increases the oxygen-carrying capacity of their blood and enables them to live at an altitude that would incapacitate a newcomer.

The symptoms and laboratory findings for clients with secondary polycythemia are the same as those for clients with polycythemia vera, except the white blood cell and platelet counts are normal and splenic enlargement is absent.

Medical Management

POLYCYTHEMIA VERA

The goals of care in polycythemia vera are twofold: (1) reduction of blood volume and viscosity and (2) reduction of bone marrow activity. These are accomplished through phlebotomy, the administration of myelosuppressive agents, and radiation therapy.

Phlebotomy. Emergency treatment involves removing 500 to 2000 mL of blood until the hematocrit level reaches 45 per cent. Once the hematocrit level has been reduced, subsequent phlebotomies should be carried out as frequently as necessary for maintaining the hematocrit at about 45 per cent. As iron deficiency supervenes, red blood cell production will be retarded, so that clients managed by phlebotomy alone may require as few as two or three phlebotomies a year.

Myelosuppressive Agents. These include radioactive phosphorus, the administration of which sometimes produces remissions that last from 6 months to 2 years (see Chap. 7). Other drugs useful for combating polycythemia are chlorambucil, busulfan, and hydroxyurea.

Radiation Therapy. Radiation therapy may be used to decrease the production of red blood cells in the marrow.

Thrombotic complications claim the lives of about 30 per cent of those affected with polycythemia vera; another 10 to 15 per cent die from hemorrhage. Finally, for obscure reasons, about 15 per cent die from either myelogenous leukemia or myelofibrosis accompanied by pancytopenia. Prognosis depends on age at diagnosis, treatment used, and complications.

SECONDARY POLYCYTHEMIA

Medical management for secondary polycythemia involves treating the underlying disease or condition that causes hypoxia.

Nursing Management

Assessment

In its early stages, polycythemia usually remains asymptomatic (an increased hematocrit level may be an incidental finding). However, as altered circulation secondary to increased red blood cell mass leads to hypervolemia and hyperviscosity, the client may complain of a feeling of fullness in the head, dizziness, headache, tinnitus, visual disturbances, and other symptoms, depending on the body system affected. Symptoms include ruddy complexion and dusky, red mucosa (integumentary); hypertension (with dizziness, headache, and a sense of fullness in the head), congestive heart failure (shortness of breath, orthopnea), which causes increased clotting leading to cerebrovascular accident, myocardial infarction, or peripheral gangrene, and bleeding (hemorrhage in capillaries, venules, and arterioles), which causes rupture of vessels (cardiovascular function); enlargement of liver and spleen, peptic ulcer (gastrointestinal function); and gout (painful swollen joints, usually big toe) secondary to increased uric acid (skeletal).

Nursing Diagnosis, Planning, and Implementation

Nursing Diagnosis: Tissue Perfusion, Altered R/T hypervolemia and hyperviscosity.

Planning: Expected Outcomes. The client will experience optimal peripheral tissue perfusion, as evidenced by rapid capillary refill; adequate pulses noted in extremities; and no complaints of tingling or numbness.

Implementation. The nurse administers medications as prescribed and monitors vital signs and breath sounds. He or she should notify the physician immediately if any signs of a thrombotic event are present. For reducing the blood viscosity, the nurse encourages intake of oral fluids and monitors intake and output. The nurse administers anticoagulants as ordered and monitors for signs of bleeding. The nurse monitors blood studies. For preventing the development of thrombi from circulatory stasis, the client should be encouraged to ambulate if possible, elevate the feet when seated, and wear support hose. The nurse should turn bedridden clients frequently and provide passive exercise to their extremities. Clients undergoing phlebotomy should be cautioned to avoid foods high in iron (clams, oysters, liver, legumes), because a high iron intake somewhat counteracts the therapeutic effects of phlebotomy.

Evaluation

The nurse must evaluate client outcomes on the basis of the established plan of care. If these goals have not been achieved, the plan and interventions must be revised to meet the client's needs.

Disorders Affecting White Blood Cells

White blood cells (leukocytes) are divided into two groups: granulocytes (polymorphonuclear leukocytes) and agranulocytes (mononuclear cells). Granulocytes, in turn, are divided into three groups: neutrophils, basophils, and eosinophils. The three names derive from the color of these cells after staining.

Agranulocytes include lymphocytes (B and T) and monocytes. Plasma cell, or plasmacyte, is another name for B lymphocyte. Plasma cells, formed within the bone marrow and lymph nodes, are probably the primary producers of immunoglobulins (antibodies). Pathologic conditions involving plasma cells are called plasma cell dyscrasias.

Major defects that affect leukocytes and plasma cells are (1) the leukemias, acute and chronic; (2) agranulocytosis; and (3) multiple myeloma (plasma cell myeloma).

THE LEUKEMIAS

Leukemia is a malignant disease of the blood-forming organs.

Incidence

Leukemia accounts for 8 per cent of all human cancers and is the most common malignancy in children and young adults. One half of all leukemias are classified as acute, with rapid onset and progression of disease resulting in 100 per cent mortality within days to months without appropriate therapy. The remaining leukemias are classified as chronic, which have a more indolent course.

Etiology

Although the exact cause of leukemia is unknown, there are several host factors associated with leukemia. These include exposure to radiation and chemicals, congenital abnormalities (i.e., Down syndrome), presence of primary immune deficiency, and infection with the human leukocyte virus HTLV-1.

Acute leukemia is caused by the neoplastic proliferation of large numbers of abnormal, immature leukocytes in the bone marrow that infiltrate the lymph nodes, liver, spleen, and eventually all body systems. In addition, the production of other blood cells (i.e., red blood cells, platelets, neutrophils) is inhibited by a mechanism not clearly understood, which results in inadequate oxygen transport, thrombocytopenia, and immune system malfunction.

Chronic leukemias have a gradual onset and a more protracted course than do the acute forms. In some cases, the client lives for 5 or more years, with or without treatment. The white blood cells produced are more mature and thus can better defend the body against invading microorganisms. Chronic leukemia occurs in clients between the ages of 25 and 60 years.

Risk Factors

Overexposure to radiation is a major risk factor for the development of leukemia, often years after the initial exposure. Alkylating agents used to treat other cancers, especially in combination with radiation therapy, also increase the client's risk for the development of leukemia. Care in the client's exposure to radiation can help decrease the risk.

Pathophysiology

ACUTE LEUKEMIA

There are two major forms of acute leukemia: *lymphocytic leukemia* (ALL), which involves the lymphocytes and lymphoid organs; and *nonlymphocytic leukemia,* which involves hematopoietic stem cells that differentiate into myeloid cells: monocytes, granulocytes, erythrocytes, and platelets. ALL presents most often in children 2 to 10 years of age. Advances in therapy during the last several decades have significantly improved the chances for remission and even a cure. However, the prognosis for clients with ALL is less favorable if any of the following factors exist:

- presentation in younger or older age groups
- male sex
- high leukocyte count (over 100,000) at time of diagnosis
- central nervous system involvement
- chromosomal abnormalities
- some cell subclass types (i.e., T-cell ALL, pre–B cell ALL)

ALL was one of the first human cancers to be cured by combination chemotherapy.

Acute nonlymphocytic leukemia (formerly known as acute myelogenous leukemia) is characterized by aberrations in the growth of megakaryocytes, monocytes, granulocytes, and erythrocytes. The prognostic factors are less clearly defined in acute nonlymphocytic leukemia, and long-term prognosis is usually poor. Bone marrow transplantation is currently the best treatment option.

CHRONIC LEUKEMIA

Chronic leukemia is classified as chronic myelogenous leukemia (CML) or chronic lymphocytic leukemia. CML originates in the pluripotent stem cell. After a relatively slow course for a median of 4 years, the client with CML invariably enters a blast crisis that resembles acute leukemia.

Chronic lymphocytic leukemia is a form of leukemia characterized by the proliferation of early B lymphocytes. It is an indolent form of leukemia most often seen in men over 50 years of age. It is also the only leukemia with a possible genetic predisposition. It is usually discovered when the complete blood count (CBC) is performed as part of a routine physical examination. Peripheral blood smear reveals increased mature and slightly immature lymphocytes.

As the disease progresses, lymphocytes infiltrate the lymph nodes, the liver, the spleen, and ultimately the bone marrow. A staging system has been developed that correlates stage with the extent of lymphocyte infiltration. Progression of the disease may take as long as 15 years.

Blast crisis results in the death of more than 70 per cent of clients with CML. During this phase, increasing numbers of blasts (immature myeloid precursor cells, especially myeloblasts, the most primitive granulocyte precursors) proliferate in the blood and bone marrow. Increased fibrotic tissue in the marrow is another sign of blast crisis. Leukopenia, thrombocytopenia, and anemia are also evident. Death usually occurs within 6 months of onset.

Clinical Manifestations

CRITICAL TO REMEMBER

The signs and symptoms of all types of leukemia are similar. The clinical history will usually reveal symptoms characteristic of anemia, thrombocytopenia, and leukopenia.

Clients often complain of fatigue, weakness, easy bruising, bleeding gums, epistaxis, fever, headache, and generalized pain. In some types of leukemia (most frequently CML), the client may have the feeling of abdominal fullness and early satiety as a result of splenomegaly. On physical examination, pallor, scattered petechiae and ecchymoses, generalized lymphadenopathy, hepatosplenomegaly, bone and joint pain, and fever may be found (see Clinical Manifestations: Leukemia).

DIAGNOSTIC ASSESSMENT

A comprehensive evaluation of all body systems is necessary for establishing the treatment plan. Tests most often included in the initial evaluation are CBC values, bone marrow aspiration, lumbar puncture, radiographic tests, and lymphangiograms.

Complete Blood Count Values. CBC values vary greatly. The total white blood cell count may be normal, abnormally low (less than 1000/mm^3), or extremely high (greater than 200,000/mm^3). The differential may reveal that one type of leukocyte is overwhelmingly predominant. There may be abnormal leukocytes, including immature blast forms, noted on the peripheral smear. The platelet count and hemoglobin level are usually low.

Bone Marrow Aspiration. Bone marrow aspiration or biopsy is a key diagnostic tool for confirming the diagnosis and identifying the malignant cell type. If an adequate sample of marrow cannot be obtained by aspiration, a fragment of bone can be removed for a bone marrow biopsy. Typical findings on the bone marrow aspirate and biopsy are an overall increase in the number of marrow cells with an increase in the proportion of earlier forms.

Lumbar Puncture. Lumbar puncture determines the presence of blast cells in the central nervous system; 5 per cent of cases present with this abnormality.

Radiographic Tests. Radiographic tests may include radiographs of the chest and skeleton; magnetic resonance imaging and computed tomography scans of the head and body detect lesions and sites of infection.

Lymphangiogram. Lymphangiogram or lymph node biopsy may be performed to locate malignant lesions and accurately classify disease.

Medical Management

ACUTE LEUKEMIA

The treatment plan for leukemia is determined by disease classification, presence or absence of prognostic factors, and disease progression. See Appendix C for a sample clinical pathway for clients with acute leukemia.

Radiation therapy may be administered as an adjunct to chemotherapy when leukemic cells infiltrate the central nervous system, skin, rectum, and testes or when a large mediastinal mass is noted at diagnosis (as may occur in ALL).

Current treatment modalities for acute leukemia destroy both normal and aberrant cells. Therapy aims to prevent and resolve complications of acquired and induced pancytopenia: anemia, bleeding, and infection. Transfusions of red blood cells and platelets are required until the marrow can produce mature ones.

Reduced exposure to microorganisms helps prevent infection, but laminar flow rooms and reverse isolation

CLINICAL MANIFESTATIONS

Leukemia

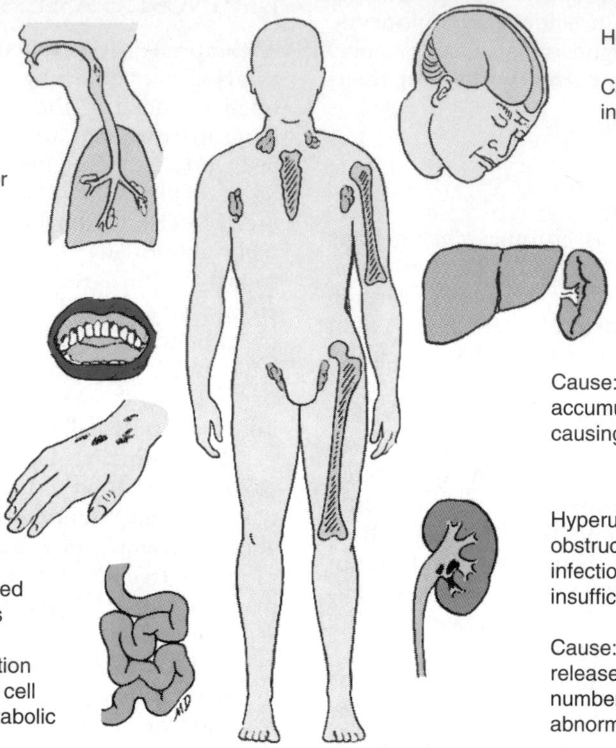
Severe infections (pneumonia, septicemia), ulcerations of mouth and throat
Cause: High numbers of immature or abnormal leukocytes unable to fight and destroy microorganisms
Anemia accompanied by pallor, fatigue, malaise, hypoxia, and hemorrhage (gum bleeding, ecchymoses, petechiae, retinal hemorrhage)
Cause: Rapidly proliferating development of leukocytes inhibiting erythrocytes and thrombocytes
Increased metabolic rate accompanied by weakness, pallor, and weight loss
Cause: Increased leukocyte production requiring large amounts of nutrients; cell destruction increases amount of metabolic wastes
Headache, disorientation
Cause: Abnormal white cells infiltrating central nervous system
Enlarged organs (splenomegaly, hepatomegaly) exerting pressure on adjacent organs
Cause: High numbers of white cells accumulating within liver and spleen, causing distention of tissues
Hyperuricemia causing renal pain, obstruction (from stone formation), and infection; a late development is renal insufficiency with uremia
Cause: Large amounts of uric acid released as a result of destruction of great numbers of leukocytes; in late stages, abnormal leukocytes infiltrate kidneys
Lymphadenopathy and bone pain
Cause: Excessive numbers of white cells accumulating in lymph nodes and bone marrow

have minimal benefits. The client must be watched closely for signs of infection, which may be inhibited because of the severely compromised state of the immune system. Therefore, administration of broad-spectrum antibiotics and antifungals must be started at the first signs of infection.

It is important to note that if the client requires intravenous infusions of red blood cells and amphotericin B, an antifungal agent, they should be separated by at least 1 hour so that serious pulmonary complications are prevented.

CHRONIC MYELOGENOUS LEUKEMIA

The goal of therapy in the chronic phase of CML is to control leukocytosis and thrombocytosis. Leukapheresis can be performed to lower an extremely high peripheral leukocyte count quickly and prevent acute tumor lysis syndrome, but results are temporary. Likewise, thrombocytosis as high as 2 million may require plateletpheresis. Apheresis is usually performed with the use of automated blood cell separators designed to selectively remove the desired blood element and return remaining cells and plasma to the client. If painful splenomegaly develops, irradiating or removing the spleen relieves this symptom.

CHRONIC LYMPHOCYTIC LEUKEMIA

The goal of therapy in chronic lymphocytic leukemia is palliation. Total body irradiation or local radiation to the spleen may also be given as a palliative treatment to reduce complications. Two complications seen during later stages are hemolytic anemia due to autoimmune disorder and hypogammaglobulinemia that further increases susceptibility to infection. Antibiotics, transfusions of red blood cells, and injections of gamma globulin concentrates may be required for these clients.

PHARMACOLOGIC MANAGEMENT

Acute Leukemia. The treatment protocol for acute leukemia involves three phases: induction, consolidation, and maintenance.

Induction. During the induction phase, the client receives an intensive course of chemotherapy designed

TABLE 28–2 Chemotherapeutic Agents Commonly Used to Treat Leukemia

TYPE OF LEUKEMIA	AGENT
Acute nonlymphocytic	Cytarabine in combination with 6-thioguanine or mercaptopurine; with vincristine, prednisone, and cyclophosphamide; with daunorubicin and 6-thioguanine; or with doxorubicin or daunorubicin
Acute lymphocytic	Vincristine, prednisone, L-asparaginase, cyclophosphamide, and daunorubicin
Chronic lymphocytic	Chlorambucil, prednisone, cyclophosphamide, and vincristine
Chronic myelogenous	Busulfan, hydroxyurea, cytosine arabinoside, daunorubicin, methotrexate, prednisone, vincristine, and L-asparaginase
Hairy cell	Chlorambucil, zorubicin, cytarabine, cyclophosphamide, and large-dose methotrexate with folinic acid–"leucovorin rescue"

to induce a complete remission of the disease. Once remission is achieved, the consolidation phase begins.

Consolidation Phase. During the consolidation phase, modified courses of intensive chemotherapy are given to eradicate any remaining disease.

Maintenance Phase. During the maintenance phase, small doses of different combinations of chemotherapeutic agents are given every 3 to 4 weeks. This phase may continue for a year or more and is, therefore, structured to allow the client to live as normal a life as possible.

Table 28–2 lists the various chemotherapeutic agents used to treat leukemia. Note that these drugs are also used in the treatment of Hodgkin's disease and other lymphomas.

If the white blood cell count is high when chemotherapy is initiated, rapid cell lysis can increase uric acid in the blood, which can lead to renal failure; increased levels of serum phosphate, uric acid, and potassium; and decreased serum calcium. This can lead to acute tumor lysis syndrome, which can be prevented by increasing intravenous hydration and administering allopurinol (Zyloprim).

Chronic Myelogenous Leukemia. The most widely used medications are busulfan (Myleran) and hydroxyurea, which are given orally. A blast crisis requires intensive chemotherapy with those agents employed in acute leukemia. These drugs can destroy leukemic blast cells, transform them into normal granulocytes, or prevent leukemic cells from inhibiting formation of normal granulocytes. Unfortunately, they have been ineffective in achieving long-term remission.

Chronic Lymphocytic Leukemia. Chlorambucil (Leukeran) or cyclophosphamide (Cytoxan) may be given orally to decrease symptoms. Chemotherapy is generally given for 2 weeks of every month (i.e., the client is on the medication for 2 weeks and off the medication for 2 weeks). When anemia (stage III) and thrombocytopenia (stage IV) develop, daily oral prednisone is given as an adjunct to the alkylating agents. Prednisone has a marked lymphocytolytic effect and may stimulate the production of red blood cells and platelets.

Surgical Management

ACUTE LEUKEMIA

Bone marrow transplantation presents a treatment option for clients under about 40 years of age who have a suitable HLA-matched donor. Studies indicate that transplant performed during the first remission has a higher success rate than does transplant performed during repeat remissions or the blast phase of chronic leukemia. See Chapters 7 and 9 for a detailed discussion of this aggressive form of therapy.

CHRONIC MYELOGENOUS LEUKEMIA

Bone marrow transplantation before blast crisis offers the best treatment option.

CHRONIC LYMPHOCYTIC LEUKEMIA

Splenectomy is an option if marked splenomegaly and thrombocytopenia present a serious risk of hemorrhage.

Nursing Management

The treatment of all classifications of leukemia is targeted at destroying neoplastic cells and maintaining a sustained remission. During each phase of therapy, the medical treatment may vary, but the basic nursing principles are the same.

Assessment

Nursing care for leukemia focuses on

- obtaining a thorough health history to aid in diagnosis and treatment
- recognizing, preventing, and treating complications of ablative chemotherapy and radiation therapy
- teaching in order to increase understanding of disease and compliance with treatment
- supporting psychosocial needs of clients with a life-threatening illness

It is imperative to obtain a thorough health history from the client and family members. A family history of exposure to chemical toxins (e.g., benzene and arsenic), viral infection (Epstein-Barr, HTLV-1), chromosomal abnormalities, use of medications such as phenylbutazone and chloramphenicol, chemotherapy, or radiation therapy may provide key information regarding the type of leukemia. The severity and longevity of the signs and symptoms of leukemia previously described are also important facts to obtain and document.

The nursing role during the acute phases of leukemia is extremely challenging because the client will have many physical and psychosocial needs. Modern therapy offers hope for remission and possibly cure for some clients with leukemia, but it is still a diagnosis equated with pain, expensive long-term therapy, and potential death.

Nursing Diagnosis, Planning, and Implementation

Collaborative Problem: Sepsis, Risk for R/T neutropenia or leukocytosis secondary to leukemia or treatment.

Planning: Expected Outcomes. The health-care team will prevent infection or will diagnose infection early and treat it effectively, as evidenced by neutrophil count greater than 1000/mm^3, no evidence of fever or respiratory difficulty, and decrease of symptoms and increase of neutrophil count with treatment.

Implementation. The nurse should institute good hand-washing technique for everyone coming in contact with the client. The client should be in a private room with reverse isolation or laminar flow if the neutrophil count is less than 500/mm^3. Visitors with possible communicable diseases should be limited.

The client should be on a low-bacteria diet that excludes raw fruits and vegetables. The nurse should assist the client with a daily bath using antimicrobial soap. The client, or nurse if the client is unable, should practice meticulous oral hygiene several times a day.

Female clients should douche per physician orders and avoid the use of tampons. Daily stool softeners are ordered to reduce the risk of anal fissures. Rectal suppositories, rectal temperature taking, and other invasive procedures should be avoided whenever possible.

The nurse should provide meticulous skin decontamination before venipunctures. Maintain sterile occlusion of central venous catheters and perform routine dressing care according to institutional policy. Intravenous tubing should be changed daily.

Oral temperature should be taken every 4 hours and the physician notified of a temperature over 38° C (100° F). The nurse should help assess the cause of fever before initiation of therapy by obtaining cultures of blood, urine, central line sites, and other potential sources of infection. The nurse administers antibiotics as ordered. Therapy usually consists of multiple broad-spectrum antibiotics administered intravenously on alternating schedules. The nurse administers antipyretics as ordered for relief of discomfort, avoiding aspirin if the client is thrombocytopenic.

The nurse monitors the client closely for signs and symptoms of fungal or viral infections (i.e., increased respirations, crackles, dyspnea, changed oral mucosa). He or she monitors respiratory rate and auscultates breath sounds regularly. Viral and fungal pneumonias are a common cause of death in the neutropenic client (see Client Education Guide: The Immunosuppressed Client).

Collaborative Problem: Bleeding, Risk for R/T thrombocytopenia secondary to either leukemia or treatment.

Planning: Expected Outcomes. Bleeding as a result of injuries such as falls, punctures, cuts, or other environmental hazards, will be prevented or will be diagnosed and treated successfully, as evidenced by absence of bleeding and platelet count greater than 30,000/mm^3.

Implementation. The nurse should institute bleeding precautions:

- Use cotton swabs or sponges for oral hygiene, avoiding flossing or hard toothbrushes.

CLIENT EDUCATION GUIDE

The Immunosuppressed Client

The home environment can often be safer and easier to control than that of the hospital, and it provides the client with a feeling of participation rather than isolation. Identifying sources of infection and practicing infection control in the home can allow the immunosuppressed client to remain independent. The client and significant others should be taught the following:

- To wash hands before preparing or eating meals and after elimination to prevent the spread of infection. Use of antibacterial soap is preferred. Daily bathing and oral hygiene are important. Use of a soft toothbrush and lotion will prevent skin complications.
- That a diet high in protein will promote the client's ability to fight infection and increase energy levels. Fresh fruits and vegetables that harbor bacteria must be avoided. All meat must be cooked for removal of microorganisms.
- To balance activity with periods of rest to avoid fatigue and lowered resistance.
- To alter the home environment to eliminate sources of infections. Contact with family and friends should be monitored and those who are infectious should be avoided. The client should wear a mask in public because crowds are a common source of infection.
- That animals, including household pets, carry many types of germs. The client should avoid close contact with pets because animal licks, bites, and scratches are all sources of infection. A person other than the client should be responsible for care of the pet because birdcages, litter boxes, and fish tanks all harbor bacteria.
- To remove additional sources of bacteria in the home including standing water, such as that found in fish tanks, flower vases, plants, and humidifiers. If these items are present in the home, the client should avoid them. In the case of furnaces and air conditioners, the filters should be changed weekly.
- To recognize signs and symptoms of infection and report them to the appropriate caregiver.

- Instruct the client to avoid blowing or picking the nose, straining at bowel movements, douching or using tampons, or using razors.
- Do not give any injections, intramuscularly or subcutaneously, or insert rectal suppositories.
- Do not give aspirin or medications containing aspirin. Instruct the client not to take these products.
- Avoid catheters whenever possible. If catheters must be inserted, lubricate them well and insert them gently. Avoid mucosal trauma during suctioning.
- Pad the bed rails and remove all hazards and sharp objects from the environment.
- Use an air mattress and turn the client frequently to avoid pressure areas. Use bed cradles to protect extremities.
- Avoid overinflation of the blood pressure cuff and rotate cuff to different sizes. Avoid prolonged use of tourniquets.
- Use only paper tape, avoiding all strong adhesives.

The client and significant others should be taught to institute bleeding precautions during periods of thrombocytopenia.

The nurse should monitor the client every 4 hours for signs of bleeding, such as ecchymoses, petechiae, epistaxis, gingival bleeding, hematuria, occult positive stools, enlarged abdominal girth, disorientation, confusion, and changes in level of consciousness. All urine, stool, and emesis should be tested for blood. The nurse should routinely take and record vital signs, noting symptoms of altered tissue perfusion related to anemia (increased respirations and pulse; decreased blood pressure).

The nurse should check the platelet count, hemoglobin level, and hematocrit level daily. A hemoglobin level of less than 10 g/100 mL and platelet count of less than 20,000/mm^3 should be reported. The nurse administers packed red blood cells and platelet concentrates as ordered. A current blood sample should be kept in the laboratory for crossmatching if needed in an emergency.

Nursing Diagnosis: Nutrition, Altered: Less than Body Requirements R/T gastrointestinal tract effects of radiation therapy and chemotherapy.

Planning: Expected Outcomes. The client will maintain body weight and adequate nutritional status, as evidenced by stable weight, adequate caloric intake, and maintenance of fluid and electrolyte balance.

Implementation. The nurse administers antiemetics as ordered for nausea and vomiting and premedicates the client before meals to encourage food and fluid intake. The nurse administers local and intravenous analgesics as ordered to relieve pain caused by mucositis. The client should be allowed to make food selections. Small, frequent feedings may be tolerated better than three large meals a day. The nurse monitors weight daily. If the client cannot tolerate food for an extended period, the nurse should begin total parenteral nutrition as ordered and monitor intake.

Nursing Diagnosis: Body Image Disturbance R/T alopecia, weight loss, and fatigue.

Planning: Expected Outcomes. The client will not develop disturbance of body image, as evidenced by client's understanding of disease condition and temporary nature of changes in body image and energy.

Implementation. The nurse informs the client of the potential for hair loss before treatment and encourages the use of scarves, hats, or wigs as desired. He or she should explain the temporary nature of alopecia and the potential for the hair to be a different color or texture when it returns.

The nurse encourages the client to balance rest with exercise and activities so that muscle tone can be maintained without the client's developing severe fatigue. He or she discusses daily dietary requirements with the client and provides high-carbohydrate meals and oral supplements.

Evaluation

The nurse must evaluate client outcomes on the basis of the established plan of care. If these goals have not been achieved, the plan and interventions must be revised to meet the client's needs.

Modification of Plan of Care for the Elderly

Elderly clients, as stated earlier, are more prone to chronic leukemia. The use of chemotherapy is less vigorous than with acute leukemia. Bone marrow transplantation is not an option with the elderly client.

BONE MARROW TRANSPLANTATION

In the last 25 years, bone marrow transplantation has progressed from a treatment of last resort to a viable therapeutic modality for a variety of hematologic, malignant, and nonmalignant disorders. Whereas the basic procedures involved in transplantation are well established, many of the techniques used to purify bone marrow to decrease complications and improve prognosis are still investigational.

Indications

Bone marrow transplant may be considered the treatment of choice for clients with the following conditions:

- aplastic anemia
- malignant disorders, specifically leukemia (certain types of acute, chronic, and preleukemic states), lymphoma, multiple myeloma, neuroblastoma, and selected solid tumors (metastatic breast cancer, small cell lung cancer, advanced ovarian cancer, poor-risk germ cell tumors)
- nonmalignant hematologic disorders, such as Fanconi anemia, thalassemia, and sickle cell anemia

- immunodeficiency disorders, such as severe combined immunodeficiency disease and Wiskott-Aldrich syndrome

Bone Marrow Harvesting

HISTOCOMPATIBILITY TESTING

Immunologic recognition of the differences in HLA antigens is the first step in host transplant rejection. As described in Chapters 8 and 9, the HLA system antigens are a complex set of protein structures found on the surface membrane of all human nucleated cells, solid tissues, and circulating blood cells except red blood cells. This genetically inherited mixture of antigens is considered representative of the tissue type of each client.

Siblings have a one in four chance of having identical sets of HLA antigens. This would provide the optimally matched allogeneic bone marrow donor. Because of the complexity of the HLA system, nonrelated clients have less than a 1 in 5000 chance of having identical HLA types. The establishment of the National Bone Marrow Donor Registry in 1987 has given hope to many clients who do not have a compatible relative donor.

SOURCES OF BONE MARROW

There are three classifications of bone marrow donors: allogeneic, syngeneic, and autologous.

Allogeneic Bone Marrow. Allogeneic bone marrow is obtained from a relative or unrelated donor who has an identical HLA type. This has been the most common type of marrow transplant, but it has the highest rate of morbidity and mortality because of complications of incompatibility such as graft-versus-host disease (GVHD) (see later discussion).

Syngeneic Bone Marrow. Syngeneic marrow is donated by an identical twin. Although syngeneic marrow is a perfect HLA match, which eliminates the risks of marrow rejection, the incidence of leukemic relapse is higher than when an allogeneic donor is used.

Autologous Bone Marrow. Autologous marrow is removed from the intended recipient during the remission phase to allow another course of ablative therapy to be given if a relapse occurs. Whereas autologous marrow eliminates the risk of adverse immunologic responses such as GVHD and graft rejection, relapse after autologous bone marrow transplant is a frequent occurrence. This may be due to contamination of the harvested bone marrow by malignant cells.

DONOR PREPARATION

An extensive work-up is performed to ensure compatibility and the mental and physical well-being of the prospective donor. This evaluation includes histocompatibility testing, medical history and physical examination, chest film, electrocardiogram, laboratory evaluation (CBC, chemistry profile, viral testing, RPR [syphilis], ABO and Rh, coagulation studies, cytomegalovirus status), and psychological evaluation (may include psychiatric consultation).

Before marrow harvest, an informed consent, including teaching about potential donor complications (pain, fever, hematoma), must be obtained.

MARROW COLLECTION

The donor is given general or spinal anesthesia in the operating room. The marrow is obtained from the marrow spaces of the posterior and, occasionally, anterior iliac crests and sternum. A total of 400 to 800 mL of marrow is obtained. The blood is placed in heparinized tissue culture media and filtered for removal of fat and bone particles. Marrow can be infused immediately or frozen in a solution containing dimethyl sulfoxide, which preserves stem cells in the frozen state.

The Transplant

RECIPIENT PREPARATION

The physical and psychological evaluation of the recipient is similar to that of the donor. Additional testing may be required to stage the existing disease accurately. The recipient must receive immunoablative therapy before transplant.

Common protocols combine total body irradiation and very high doses of a single chemotherapeutic agent or fractionated doses of multiple agents. A small catheter is inserted to provide suitable access for marrow infusion as well as for antibiotics, blood products, hyperalimentation, and frequent blood sampling.

BONE MARROW INFUSION

The infusion of the marrow is often anticlimactic after the client has undergone the rigorous preparatory chemotherapy and radiation therapy. The marrow is usually administered immediately after the conditioning regimen is complete. Marrow is administered from a large blood infusion bag equipped with a standard blood filter. Small volumes may also be prefiltered and given by intravenous push by a physician.

Potential immediate adverse reactions are allergic (urticaria, chills, fever), volume overload, and pulmonary complications secondary to fat emboli. The period immediately after transplant is critical. Multisystem failure related to the ablative therapy is common, as are immune reactions caused by the transplanted cells.

CRITICAL TO REMEMBER

The most common and potentially disastrous complication of bone marrow transplant is GVHD, which may occur acutely 7 to 30 days after the infusion of viable lymphocytes.

The exact mechanism of GVHD is not clearly understood, but it appears that T lymphocytes from the donor attack and destroy vulnerable host cells. Once the engrafted cells mount this immune response against the host, little can be done to alter the course. The most likely organs to be affected are skin, gut, and liver. Localized skin involvement may resolve without treatment. Systemic complications may be treated with immunosuppressive drug therapy. There is no effective therapy for severe GVHD.

Diagnosis of chronic GVHD is confirmed by skin and oral mucosal biopsy. Chronic GVHD appears approximately 100 days after transplantation; it may affect the liver, gastrointestinal system, oral mucosa, and lungs as well as the skin.

Nursing Management

The client will remain pancytopenic until the transplanted stem cells make their way to the medullary cavities, where subsequent growth and reconstitution of the marrow are confirmed. Indications of successful engraftment are an increase in platelets and red blood cells in the peripheral blood count. This may occur as early as 14 days after marrow infusion. Each day that recovery is delayed places the client at added risk. Graft rejection is evident if the bone marrow fails to produce peripheral blood cells after several weeks.

Nursing management of bone marrow transplant clients follows the plan of care for any completely immunosuppressed client. In addition, those receiving allogeneic transplant must be closely observed for signs of GVHD. Because no therapy effectively prevents or treats this complication, nursing care focuses on symptom management, pain relief, and emotional support.

AGRANULOCYTOSIS

Agranulocytosis (granulocytopenia, malignant neutropenia) is an acute, potentially fatal blood dyscrasia characterized by profound neutropenia. Neutropenia is a reduction in the number of circulating neutrophils. Because neutrophils make up roughly 93 per cent of all granulocytes, the terms neutropenia and agranulocytosis are often used interchangeably.

Incidence

Agranulocytosis is a rare condition. For unknown reasons, women are much more susceptible to this condition than are men. However, even among females, agranulocytosis is relatively rare.

Etiology

The most common cause of agranulocytosis is drug toxicity or hypersensitivity. Two groups of agents are capable of suppressing granulocyte production:

- agents that always produce neutropenia when given in sufficiently large doses over time, such as many cancer chemotherapeutic agents, ionizing radiation, and benzene.
- agents that produce neutropenia only in clients particularly sensitive to the drug, such as tranquilizers (chlorpromazine), antithyroid agents (propylthiouracil), anticonvulsants (phenytoin), antibiotics (chloramphenicol), and phenylbutazone

Risk Factors

Exposure to any of the etiologic factors increases the client's risk of developing agranulocytosis. Avoidance of these agents, whenever possible, helps prevent the development of the condition.

Pathophysiology

Agranulocytosis results either from the failure of neutrophil production to keep pace with destruction of the cells or from increased destruction of neutrophils, which removes them from circulation. Chemotherapy, radiation, and aplastic anemia all decrease or stop neutrophil production through interference with granulopoiesis.

Agranulocytosis may reverse when the cause is removed, or the client will require a bone marrow transplant for survival.

Clinical Manifestations

The symptoms of agranulocytosis result from the neutropenia. Neutrophils constitute a swift and powerful defense against invading microorganisms. Consequently, decreases in their number result in a greater susceptibility to bacterial invasion, especially when the client's white blood cell count drops below 500/mm^3. The mucous membranes of the throat and mouth are particularly vulnerable.

Typically, the onset of this acute disease is rapid. For the first 2 or 3 days, there is severe fatigue and weakness. Next, the client develops a sore throat, ulcerations of the pharyngeal and buccal mucosa, dysphagia, high fever, weak and rapid pulse, and severe chills. Without prompt antibiotic treatment, the disorder usually causes death within a week.

Medical Management

Treatment for clients with agranulocytosis involves eliminating potentially toxic agents that may be responsible for marrow suppression. Agranulocytosis caused by toxic substances usually reverses within 2 to 3 weeks after their elimination.

Surveillance cultures of blood, throat, sputum, urine, and stool should be taken at frequent intervals for monitoring the status of infections.

Granulocyte transfusions may be done if the client develops antibiotic-resistant sepsis. Once removed from the client or an HLA-matched donor (ideally an identical twin), the cells are treated or altered and then reinfused.

PHARMACOLOGIC MANAGEMENT

Pharmacologic treatment includes antimicrobial therapy in the event of positive cultures, fever, or signs and symptoms of impending shock. Combinations of broad-spectrum antibiotics are usually administered until the offending organism is identified. Untreated infectious processes in this situation carry a mortality rate of 80 per cent. Treatment includes marrow stimulation with daily dosage of oxymetholone or lithium carbonate.

Nursing Management

Assessment

Physical assessment should include vital signs with attention paid to a high fever or a weak, rapid pulse. Any complaints of a sore throat, dysphagia, or mouth sores should be examined. The client's history should include names of all drugs the client has taken or is presently taking (prescription or nonprescription).

Nursing Diagnosis, Planning, and Implementation

Nursing Diagnosis: Knowledge Deficit R/T toxic agents that cause agranulocytosis.

Planning: Expected Outcomes. The client will understand the cause of agranulocytosis, as evidenced by the client's verbalization of understanding of the cause of the disorder, the need to avoid self-medication, and the importance of follow-up examinations.

Implementation. An important aspect of nursing management is to prevent agranulocytosis by providing clients with teaching regarding potentially dangerous medications and chemicals. To enhance awareness, the client should be encouraged to avoid self-medication without a physician's order, to schedule frequent follow-up by a physician when medications known to cause granulocytopenia are prescribed, and to realize that repeated exposure to toxic chemicals such as benzene may cause agranulocytosis.

MULTIPLE MYELOMA (PLASMA CELL MYELOMA)

Multiple myeloma is a neoplastic condition characterized by abnormal malignant proliferation of plasma cells.

Incidence

The condition commonly occurs in clients over 40 years of age; the average age is 60 years. It is more common in men and people of African descent. Multiple myeloma is considered a lymphoid malignancy. Its incidence is about 1 per cent of all malignant diseases.

Etiology and Risk Factors

No particular etiologic factors or risk factors have been identified for multiple myeloma.

Pathophysiology

Multiple myeloma is characterized by an abnormal proliferation of plasma cells. With this overproduction of plasma cells, bone destruction also occurs. Multiple myeloma is also characterized by disruption of red blood cell, leukocyte, and platelet production, which results from plasma cells crowding the bone marrow. Impaired production of these cell forms causes anemia, increased vulnerability to infection, and bleeding tendencies, respectively.

Complications of multiple myeloma include hypercalcemia, renal problems, and neurologic disorders. Hypercalcemia resulting from the release of calcium during bone destruction is present in 30 per cent of newly diagnosed clients with multiple myeloma. It causes confusion, anorexia, nausea, vomiting, constipation, abdominal pain, ileus, and impairment of renal concentrating mechanisms that can eventually lead to irreversible renal failure. In addition, renal disease results from particles of coagulated protein that block the convoluted tubules. The major neurologic complications entail compression of the spinal cord, sometimes followed by paraplegia.

Clinical Manifestations

The onset of multiple myeloma is usually gradual and insidious. Most clients pass through a long presymptomatic period that lasts 5 to 20 years. The client is usually asymptomatic; only 10 per cent of clients will be diagnosed at this stage.

Once symptoms appear, they typically involve the skeletal system, particularly the pelvis, spine, and ribs. Some clients have backache or bone pain that worsens with movement. Others suffer sudden pathologic fractures accompanied by severe pain. Drainage of calcium and phosphorus from damaged bones eventually leads to the development of renal stones, particularly in immobilized clients.

DIAGNOSTIC ASSESSMENT

Diagnosis of multiple myeloma rests on x-ray studies, bone marrow biopsy, and blood and urine examination. X-ray studies reveal diffuse lesions in the bone, widespread demineralization, and osteoporosis. The bone marrow is found to contain large numbers of immature plasma cells. Another diagnostic sign of multiple myeloma is the appearance of light-chains from the abnormal immunoglobulin in the urine called Bence Jones protein.

Medical Management

Not all clients diagnosed with multiple myeloma should be treated. Symptoms, physical findings, and laboratory data must be considered. In some cases, treatment might be withheld, and the client is re-evaluated in 2 to 3 months. If overt symptoms are present, chemotherapy is the preferred initial treatment. Palliative radiation should be limited to clients with disabling pain from a well-defined location that has not been responsive to chemotherapy.

PHARMACOLOGIC MANAGEMENT

There is some controversy over the most effective chemotherapy regimen. Melphalan and prednisone or a combination of alkylating agents have both shown objective responses. Prednisone and melphalan given orally for a period of 7 days and repeated at 6-week intervals produces positive results in 50 to 60 per cent of the clients. Leukocyte and platelet counts should be monitored regularly and doses adjusted until modest cytopenia occurs. Combination chemotherapy, commonly melphalan, cyclophosphamide (Cytoxan), carmustine (BCNU), vincristine (Oncovin), and prednisone, has shown a 70 to 75 per cent response rate. This therapy may continue for 1 to 2 years, but relapse almost always occurs when chemotherapy is discontinued. Interferon appears to be beneficial in prolonging the duration of remission.

In addition, the nurse should be alert to the possibility of spinal cord compression, another complication of multiple myeloma. Treatment usually consists of radiation therapy and large doses of steroids, although a laminectomy may be indicated.

Nursing Management

Clients with multiple myeloma must be closely assessed for the development of hypercalcemia. The client will need sufficient fluid to dilute the calcium overload and prevent protein from precipitating in the renal tubules. The client will usually require about 3 L of fluid per day. The client's pain should also be monitored so that ordered analgesics can be administered. The safety of the client should be maintained as pathologic fractures may occur.

Disorders of the Lymphoidal System

Lymphoma is a diverse group of lymphoid neoplasms that results in uncontrolled proliferation of lymphocytes. It arises in the lymphoid tissues, that is, lymph nodes, thymus, spleen, and lymphoid tissue of the gastrointestinal tract. Lymphomas include a number of diseases that have different manifestations, treatments, and prognoses, depending on the lymphocyte type and stage of differentiation. Lymphomas are classified as either (1) Hodgkin's disease or (2) non-Hodgkin's lymphoma. Lymphomas that contain the Reed-Sternberg cell (multinucleated giant cells) are termed Hodgkin's disease; those without it are called non-Hodgkin's lymphoma.

HODGKIN'S DISEASE

Hodgkin's disease is a chronic, progressive, neoplastic disorder of lymphatic tissue characterized by the painless enlargement of lymph nodes with progression to extralymphatic sites such as the spleen and liver. The pathologic involvement of tissues and organs throughout the body follows.

Incidence

A disorder of young adults, Hodgkin's disease principally occurs between the ages of 20 and 40 years. Among those affected, men outnumber women, and boys are stricken five times more often than are girls.

Etiology

The cause of lymphoma is unknown. However, clients who develop long-term immunosuppression due to illness, therapeutic treatment, or drug abuse suffer an increased incidence of the disease. There appears to be a higher risk of Hodgkin's disease in clients with high titers of Epstein-Barr virus or a history of mononucleosis.

Risk Factors

Immunosuppression due to therapy or as a result of disease is a major risk factor for the development of Hodgkin's disease. This risk is usually not preventable, so clients should be carefully monitored for the development of this disease. Drug abuse is the most preventable cause of the disease.

Pathophysiology

The exact mechanism of growth and spread of Hodgkin's disease remains unknown. Hodgkin's disease involves the proliferation of abnormal histiocytes called Reed-Sternberg cells, which are part of the tissue macrophage system. As these atypical glial cells multiply, they replace other cellular elements normally found within the lymph nodes.

Hodgkin's disease is divided into categories or stages according to the microscopic appearance of the

TABLE 28–3 Modified Ann Arbor Staging Classification

STAGE	
I	Involvement of a single lymph node region (I) or of a single extralymphatic organ or site (I_E)
II	Involvement of two or more lymph node regions on the same side of the diaphragm (II) or localized involvement of an extralymphatic organ or site and of one or more lymph node regions on the same side of the diaphragm (II_E)
III	Involvement of lymph node regions on both sides of the diaphragm (III), which may also be accompanied by involvement of the spleen (III_S) or by localized involvement of an extralymphatic organ or site (III_E) or both (III_{SE})
III_1	Involvement limited to the lymphatic structures in the upper abdomen, that is, spleen or splenic, celiac, or hepatic portal nodes or any combination of these
III_2	Involvement of lower abdominal nodes, that is, para-aortic, iliac, inguinal, or mesenteric nodes, with or without involvement of the splenic, celiac, or hepatic portal nodes
IV	Diffuse or disseminated involvement of one or more extralymphatic organs or tissues, with or without associated lymph node involvement

E, extralymphatic site; S, splenic involvement.
From Glick, J. H. (1992). Hodgkin's disease. In J. B. Wyngaarden, et al. (eds.), *Cecil textbook of medicine* (19th ed.). Philadelphia: W. B. Saunders.

involved lymph nodes, the extent and severity of the disorder, and the prognosis. Table 28–3 shows one method of staging.

The complete remission rate for clients with Hodgkin's disease is 75 to 90 per cent. The recurrence rate varies with the stage of disease and is 10 to 20 per cent. When untreated, clients with Hodgkin's disease have a life expectancy of 5 years.

Clinical Manifestations

Hodgkin's disease usually presents as a painless enlarged lymph node, often in the cervical region. The client may experience unexplained fevers, night sweats, and weight loss. Many clients also experience pruritus. Hepatosplenomegaly may be present, although it usually does not cause symptoms. Likewise, although disease may be present in the bone marrow, it often does not cause pancytopenia. The Clinical Manifestations Box outlines the major assessment data for Hodgkin's disease.

DIAGNOSTIC ASSESSMENT

Lymph node biopsy provides a definitive test for diagnosing Hodgkin's disease. With peripheral lymph node enlargement, one entire node is removed and examined for the presence of Reed-Sternberg cells. Also, because of immune system disturbances, clients with Hodgkin's disease usually react abnormally to tuberculin skin testing.

Medical Management

Treatment for Hodgkin's disease varies according to its stage at diagnosis. Stage I and stage II are treated with radiation therapy and supplemental chemotherapy. Clients with stage III disease may receive radiation coupled with an aggressive multiagent chemotherapy regimen.

PHARMACOLOGIC MANAGEMENT

In stage IV disease, a multiagent drug regimen is the treatment of choice. MOPP, a combination of chemotherapeutic agents, is the most widely used regimen (Table 28–4). Other chemotherapeutic regimens have also been used with success.

The most distressing and immediate side effect of the chemotherapeutic agents used to treat Hodgkin's disease is severe nausea and vomiting. Symptoms may be severe enough to force a client to discontinue therapy. Pancytopenia, a toxic effect of these agents, usually occurs 10 to 14 days after intravenous therapy. Any degree of anemia, leukopenia, or thrombocytopenia indicates that treatment must be delayed or the medication dosage adjusted.

Nursing Management

Caring for the client with Hodgkin's disease revolves around control of complications associated with the client's pancytopenia. Supportive measures to prevent or control bleeding and infection are important. If these complications can be avoided during the treatment regimen for Hodgkin's disease, the client has a good chance for long-term survival.

NON-HODGKIN'S LYMPHOMA

Non-Hodgkin's lymphomas are a group of lymphoid disorders. Involvement of the disease starts in the lymph nodes, although a significant number arise outside the lymphatic system more than in Hodgkin's disease. Non-Hodgkin's lymphoma is more common in adults in their middle and older years; it is more common in males than in females in a ratio of 5 to 3. Many classification systems are used to differentiate non-Hodgkin's lymphoma according to histologic type and cytologic characteristics. Treatment protocols and prognosis for clients with non-Hodgkin's lymphoma vary greatly. Without effective treatment, non-Hodgkin's lymphomas are very quickly fatal.

Treatment consists of radiation therapy, chemother-

CLINICAL MANIFESTATIONS

Hodgkin's Disease

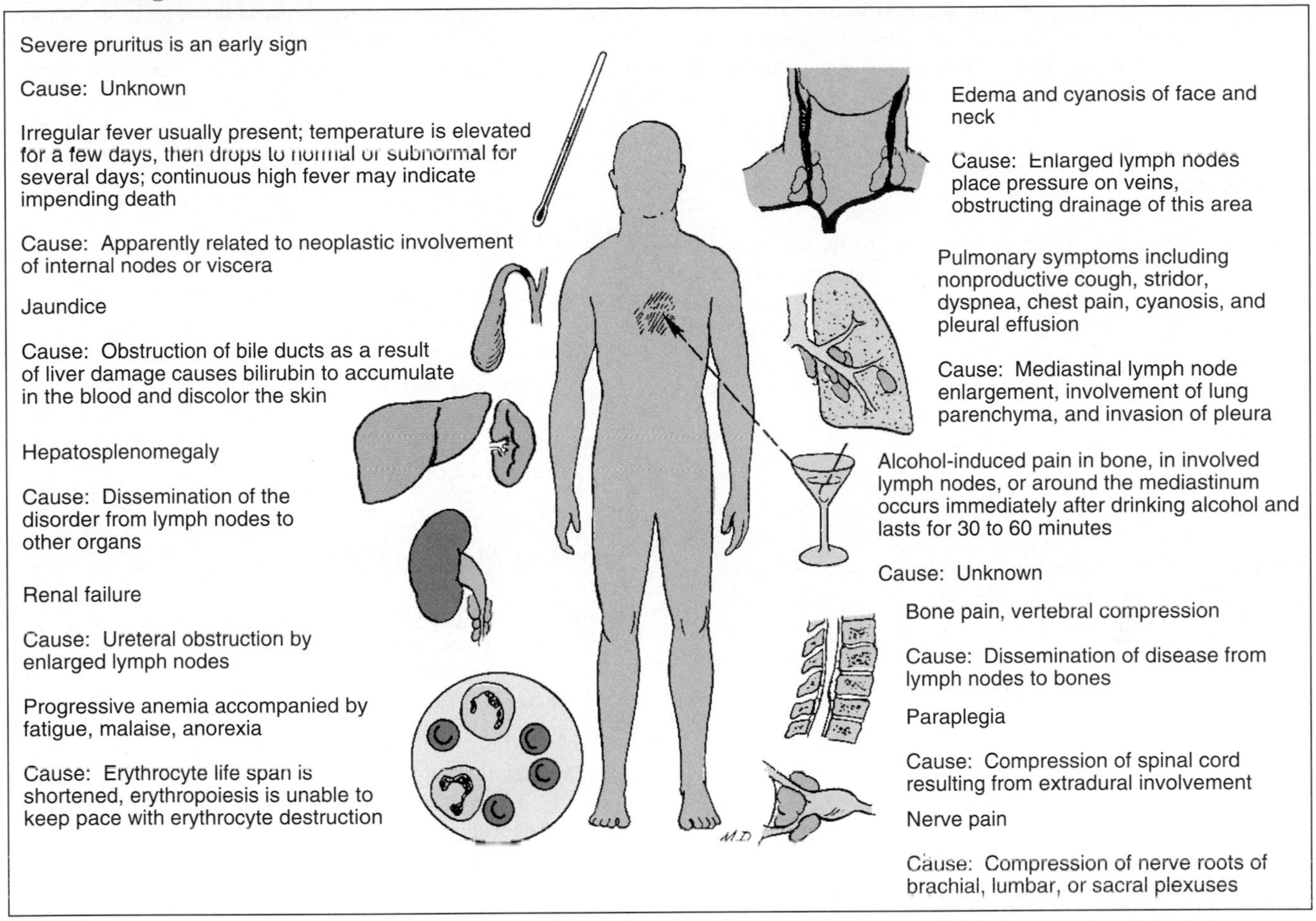

Severe pruritus is an early sign
Cause: Unknown
Irregular fever usually present; temperature is elevated for a few days, then drops to normal or subnormal for several days; continuous high fever may indicate impending death
Cause: Apparently related to neoplastic involvement of internal nodes or viscera
Jaundice
Cause: Obstruction of bile ducts as a result of liver damage causes bilirubin to accumulate in the blood and discolor the skin
Hepatosplenomegaly
Cause: Dissemination of the disorder from lymph nodes to other organs
Renal failure
Cause: Ureteral obstruction by enlarged lymph nodes
Progressive anemia accompanied by fatigue, malaise, anorexia
Cause: Erythrocyte life span is shortened, erythropoiesis is unable to keep pace with erythrocyte destruction
Edema and cyanosis of face and neck
Cause: Enlarged lymph nodes place pressure on veins, obstructing drainage of this area
Pulmonary symptoms including nonproductive cough, stridor, dyspnea, chest pain, cyanosis, and pleural effusion
Cause: Mediastinal lymph node enlargement, involvement of lung parenchyma, and invasion of pleura
Alcohol-induced pain in bone, in involved lymph nodes, or around the mediastinum occurs immediately after drinking alcohol and lasts for 30 to 60 minutes
Cause: Unknown
Bone pain, vertebral compression
Cause: Dissemination of disease from lymph nodes to bones
Paraplegia
Cause: Compression of spinal cord resulting from extradural involvement
Nerve pain
Cause: Compression of nerve roots of brachial, lumbar, or sacral plexuses
M.D.

apy, or a combination of both. Overall, the prognosis of non-Hodgkin's lymphoma is poorer than that of Hodgkin's disease.

The cure rate for aggressive tumors with treatment is significantly better than for the slower-growing, low-grade type, presumably because rapidly growing cells are more susceptible to chemotherapy and radiation therapy. In some clients with large masses, surgical removal or debulking of the mass may be required before chemotherapy or radiation therapy begin.

TABLE 28–4 MOPP Combination Chemotherapy Regimen for Hodgkin's Disease*

	M	O	P	P
DAY OF CYCLE	MUSTARGEN (NITROGEN MUSTARD)	ONCOVIN (VINCRISTINE)	PROCARBAZINE	PREDNISONE†
1, 8	IV	IV	PO	PO
2, 9			PO	PO
3, 10			PO	PO
4, 11			PO	PO
5, 12			PO	PO
6, 13			PO	PO
7, 14			PO	PO

*Therapy consists of at least six 14-day cycles with 14 days' rest between cycles. Intravenous (IV) or oral (PO) medication doses are adjusted according to laboratory test results of white blood cells and platelets.
† In first and fourth cycle only.

INFECTIOUS MONONUCLEOSIS

Infectious mononucleosis (also known as glandular disease and the "kissing disease") is a self-limiting condition characterized by painful enlargement of the lymph nodes, lymphocytosis, sore throat, and fever.

Incidence

Primarily a disease of the young, infectious mononucleosis usually strikes children between the ages of 3 and 5 years and young adults between the ages of 15 and 25 years. The greatest incidence occurs among college students, medical students, and nurses. Although this disease usually occurs sporadically, epidemic forms may sweep through colleges and children's homes.

Etiology

The cause of infectious mononucleosis is a herpesvirus, the Epstein-Barr virus. Although the exact mode of transmission remains unknown, the disease may be transmitted through the oropharyngeal route during close contact, such as with kissing.

Pathophysiology

Infectious mononucleosis is a relatively mild disorder but has widespread effects on the body. For example, the lymph nodes enlarge, lymphocytosis occurs, the spleen may swell to two to three times its normal size, liver function is sometimes impaired, and both peripheral and central nervous system involvement can develop.

Clinical Manifestations

The onset of infectious mononucleosis follows an incubation period of 2 to 6 weeks. Before frank clinical symptoms present, the client may experience fatigue, headaches, malaise, and myalgias. Subsequently, assessment reveals temperatures up to 39° C (102.2° F), pharyngitis, and lymphadenopathy that is more pronounced in the cervical regions. Ten to 15 per cent of those affected develop a maculopapular rash that closely resembles the rash of rubella. Splenic enlargement causes left upper quadrant pain. Nervous system involvement may lead to severe headache.

DIAGNOSTIC ASSESSMENT

The diagnosis of infectious mononucleosis is based on three criteria: clinical manifestations, laboratory tests, and a positive heterophil or Monospot test.

Laboratory Tests. The white blood cell count usually ranges from 12,000 to 20,000/mm^3, of which 50 per cent are lymphocytes and monocytes, and 10 to 20 per cent are large, atypical lymphocytes.

Positive Heterophil (Monospot) Test. The blood of clients with infectious mononucleosis contains heterophil antibodies that agglutinate the red blood cells of sheep. Human beings normally do not produce agglutinins against sheep erythrocytes. Clients usually test positive within 5 to 7 days of acute onset. However, positive tests sometimes occur in other conditions.

Medical Management

No specific intervention either mitigates or shortens the disease process. Because infectious mononucleosis must simply run its course, treatments are directed at symptom control. Bedrest is recommended until fever is resolved. Salicylates, cool sponge baths, and a large fluid intake help control fever. Warm saline throat irrigations may relieve the sore throat.

Nursing Management

In addition to providing symptomatic relief, the nurse works toward preventing complications and administering treatment. When caring for clients with infectious mononucleosis, the nurse should do the following:

- Caution the client against engaging in excessive activity, especially contact sports, for a period of at least 1 month, which could result in splenic rupture or lowered resistance to infection.
- Watch closely for and report the two signs of splenic rupture: abdominal pain and shock.
- If throat pain worsens, report it immediately so that appropriate antibiotic therapy can be started.

Although complications sometimes develop, the prognosis for clients with infectious mononucleosis is generally excellent. The febrile phase of this disorder typically lasts 2 to 4 weeks. During the long convalescence, the client slowly regains strength and energy.

SPLENECTOMY

Despite the important functions of the spleen, it can be removed (splenectomy) without harm in adults. Its role can be taken over completely by other organs (e.g., liver, lymph nodes, and bone marrow). The most frequent indication for splenectomy is rupture of the spleen complicated by severe hemorrhage. Splenic irradiation may achieve a reversal in cytopenia without the risk of surgery.

In hypersplenism, which is a second important indication for splenectomy, the spleen destroys one of the blood cell types in excessive numbers (i.e., erythrocytes, leukocytes, or platelets). Signs of hypersplenism include moderate to massive splenomegaly, anemia, leukopenia, or thrombocytopenia and a compensatory increase in the production of the affected cell line by the bone marrow. Overactivity of the spleen develops either as a primary condition of unknown origin or as a condition secondary to another disease.

Primary hypersplenism occurs in idiopathic thrombocytopenic purpura and congenital spherocytosis. Some etiologic factors associated with secondary hypersplenism include lymphomas (including Hodgkin's disease), leukemias, polycythemia vera, acute infections (including infectious mononucleosis), chronic infections, malaria, syphilis, the hemoglobinopathies, and cirrhosis of the liver.

Primary hypersplenism can be alleviated by splenectomy. Splenectomy is only palliative for clients with secondary hypersplenism, because the surgery has little or no effect on the course of the primary illness. When hypersplenism is diagnosed, it is important to teach the client to prevent complications associated with the specific cytopenia.

Laboratory indications for splenectomy include granulocytopenia of less than 500/mm^3 and thrombocytopenia of less than 20,000/mm^3. The surgery itself is relatively simple unless the spleen is greatly enlarged or surrounded by adhesions.

Adults are at increased risk of infection, especially during the first 3 years after surgery. The splenectomized client should be advised to seek medical treatment at the earliest signs of infection.

Nursing Management

Assessment

The unique functions performed by the spleen will eventually be taken over by other organs. However, the loss of the spleen due to cessation of function or splenectomy does require the client to be monitored for potentially serious complications. The nursing care of the client undergoing splenectomy is generally the same as that discussed in Chapter 5.

Disorders of Platelets and Clotting Factors

Disorders of hemostasis affecting platelets and clotting factors include (1) hemorrhagic disorders, (2) purpura, and (3) coagulation disorders. The three components of the hemostatic mechanism are the blood vessels, platelets (thrombocytes), and coagulation factors.

Hemorrhagic Disorders

The four basic problems underlying hemorrhagic (bleeding) disorders are

- weak, damaged vessels that rupture easily or spontaneously
- platelet deficiency (thrombocytopenia) due to hypoproliferation, excessive pooling of platelets in the spleen, or excessive platelet destruction
- deficiency or total lack of one of the clotting factors
- excessive or insufficient fibrinolysis

Disorders of hemostasis fall into two major categories: purpura and coagulation disorders. Table 28–5 outlines the types of bleeding disorders in these two categories.

TABLE 28–5 Classification of Disorders of Hemostasis

Purpura
Vascular defect purpura
Familial hemorrhagic telangiectasia
Anaphylactoid purpura (allergic purpura)
Toxic purpura
Platelet disorder purpura
Idiopathic thrombocytopenic purpura
Secondary thrombocytopenias
Coagulation Disorders
Hemophilia
Hypoprothrombinemia
Disseminated intravascular coagulation

The diagnosis of hemorrhagic disorders depends on a complete health and family history, physical examination, and laboratory tests for platelet and clotting defects. The history usually offers numerous clues to the type of bleeding problem and its cause.

If the history indicates a bleeding disorder, the nurse should examine the client for overt signs of bleeding. Petechiae (tiny hemorrhagic spots caused by intradermal or submucosal bleeding) are usually present in vascular and thrombocytopenic purpuras. The presence of ecchymoses (large, blotchy, subcutaneous hemorrhagic areas), hematomas (subdermal hemorrhage), and hemarthrosis (blood within the joints) points to hemophilia. However, ecchymoses may develop in any hemorrhagic disorder. Clients who hemorrhage severely from several areas during childbirth or a major surgical procedure may have a fibrinogen deficiency. In addition to any evidence of bleeding, the nurse should search for signs of hepatic cirrhosis (hepatomegaly, jaundice, and so forth) and splenomegaly.

Laboratory studies provide most crucial evidence for pinpointing the type and cause of a bleeding disorder (see Table 27–3).

Clients with hemorrhagic disorders need to understand (1) why they are at risk of bleeding, (2) the signs and symptoms of bleeding, and (3) preventive measures to avoid bleeding. Those who can be managed by home health care should be referred to appropriate health-care agencies. Clients with bleeding disorders should carry an identification card at all times that indicates their diagnosis, name of physician or health-care agency, and blood type. It is important to assess each client before even minor invasive procedures, such as dental extractions, to rule out a history of bleeding disorders.

Purpura

IDIOPATHIC THROMBOCYTOPENIC PURPURA

Purpura is defined as the extravasation of small amounts of blood into the tissues and mucous membranes. Bleeding results from either vessel damage (vascular purpura) or a platelet deficiency (thrombocytopenic purpura).

The term thrombocytopenia means a reduction in platelets below 100,000/mm^3. The two major problems that characterize thrombocytopenia are (1) spontaneous bleeding into any part of the body (such as the central nervous system, muscle, joints) when the platelet count is less than 20,000/mm^3 and (2) prolonged oozing from sites despite local measures to curtail bleeding. The two principal types of thrombocytopenia are idiopathic thrombocytopenic purpura (ITP) and secondary thrombocytopenia. ITP refers to thrombocytopenia caused by an unknown, possibly autoimmune cause.

Incidence

Ninety per cent of adults with ITP are under 40 years of age; the ratio of women to men is 3 to 4 to 1. In children with ITP, 85 per cent of whom are under 8 years of age, the disease is self-limiting.

Etiology and Risk Factors

Childhood ITP is usually acute and follows recovery from a viral infection. In adults, the onset of ITP is usually gradual, without a preceding illness and with a chronic course. In a small percentage of adult cases, the disease has an acute onset.

Pathophysiology

This disorder is characterized by the premature destruction of platelets. Normally, platelets survive 8 to 10 days within the circulation. However, platelet survival in ITP is as brief as 1 to 3 days or less.

The condition is an autoimmune bleeding disorder characterized by the development of antibodies to one's own platelets, which are then destroyed by phagocytosis in the spleen and, to a lesser extent, in the liver.

In adults, indications for treatment depend on severity of bleeding and the degree of thrombocytosis.[94]

Clinical Manifestations

In most cases, ITP takes a course of remissions and exacerbations that, in untreated cases, may continue for years. Assessment reveals petechiae, ecchymosis, epistaxis, bleeding from the gums, and easy bruising. Women may have extremely heavy menses or bleeding between periods.

Complications of ITP include cerebral hemorrhage, which proves fatal in 1 to 5 per cent of clients with ITP; severe hemorrhages from the nose, gastrointestinal tract, and urinary system; bleeding into the diaphragm, which can result in pulmonary complications; and nerve pain, extremity anesthesia, or paralysis resulting from the pressure of hematomas on nerves or brain tissues.

DIAGNOSTIC ASSESSMENT

Laboratory findings that confirm the presence of ITP include (1) a platelet count below 100,000/mm^3, (2) prolonged bleeding time with normal coagulation time (all coagulation factors are present and normal), (3) increased capillary fragility as demonstrated by the tourniquet test, (4) positive platelet antibody screening, and (5) bone marrow aspirate containing normal or increased megakaryocytes.

Clients with ITP have a good prognosis: 80 per cent of children and 10 to 20 per cent of adults recover spontaneously without treatment.

Medical Management

The three basic interventions for ITP are steroid therapy, splenectomy, and platelet transfusions.

PHARMACOLOGIC MANAGEMENT

Clients suffering from severe bleeding of short duration receive steroids (such as prednisone). The purpose of steroid therapy in ITP is to suppress the phagocytic response of splenic macrophages. However, steroids rarely produce a permanent cure. Clients also receive steroids before splenectomy. Plasmapheresis is sometimes used as short-term therapy until the steroid therapy takes effect. Intravenous infusion of gamma globulin in combination with plasmapheresis is under investigation for clients whose condition is refractory to other treatments. Danazol (Danocrine) has recently been used with success in some clients. Immunosuppressive therapy used in refractory cases includes vincristine (Oncovin), vinblastine (Velban), azathioprine (Imuran), and cyclophosphamide (Cytoxan).

Surgical Management

The treatment of choice for clients with ITP is splenectomy (see earlier discussion). In 60 to 80 per cent of cases, removal of the spleen results in complete and permanent remission. The effectiveness of the splenectomy is believed to be related to the removal of the site of premature destruction of the antibody-sensitized platelets. Because young children often recover spontaneously from ITP, pediatricians do not usually recommend splenectomy until the child is over 6 years of age.

Nursing Management

Assessment

Clients with ITP usually present with easy bruising, petechiae, and purpura. Platelet counts are well below normal limits.

During the acute phase, the nurse should teach the client oral hygiene measures to prevent gum bleeding. The client should not use a hard toothbrush and should refrain from flossing during this phase.

CRITICAL TO REMEMBER

The client should not receive any injections, aspirin, or nonsteroidal anti-inflammatory drugs during the acute phase of ITP.

The nurse should monitor the client's platelet count, vital signs, and signs of bleeding or increased intracranial pressure and teach the client to avoid Valsalva's maneuver and to use stool softeners.

The nurse can apply an ice bag or manual pressure over any bleeding site to promote hemostasis. He or she should teach the client and significant others to implement bleeding precautions when the platelet count is low and how to institute immediate medical care for hemorrhage.

The client should be taught about long-term steroid therapy. It is important that the client learn methods to avoid bleeding. The client who has had a splenectomy should be taught to avoid close contact with people with infections.

Modification of Plan of Care for the Elderly

Elderly clients are less likely to develop ITP. When they do develop it, bleeding can be more severe because of their already fragile capillaries. Steroids are used, and surgery is avoided unless necessary.

Coagulation Disorders

The coagulation disorders stem from a defect in the clotting mechanisms. One or more of the clotting factors is depleted or absent. The three important coagulation disorders discussed here are hypoprothrombinemia, disseminated intravascular coagulation, and the hemophilias (see section on congenital conditions).

HYPOPROTHROMBINEMIA

The term hypoprothrombinemia refers to a deficient amount of circulating prothrombin. Prothrombin is a protein produced in the liver and normally found in the blood. For prothrombin synthesis to take place, vitamin K (a fat-soluble vitamin) must be present in the liver to act as a catalyst. Hypoprothrombinemia develops from a vitamin K deficiency or liver disorder or from an overdose of aspirin, coumarin, or coumarin-derivative anticoagulant (such as warfarin), which antagonizes the action of vitamin K.

Dicumarol is an effective anticoagulant used to reduce clot formation in clients with heart disease and peripheral vascular disorders. It acts by interfering with vitamin K in prothrombin synthesis. In excessive doses, the prothrombin time is prolonged (usually below 40 or 50 per cent). If the prothrombin time drops below 10 to 15 per cent, the danger of bleeding or spontaneous hemorrhage increases.

The major manifestations of hypoprothrombinemia are ecchymosis after minimal trauma, epistaxis, postoperative hemorrhage from the incision, hematuria, gastrointestinal tract bleeding, and prolonged bleeding from a venipuncture. The outstanding laboratory finding is a prolonged prothrombin time.

Treatment for hypoprothrombinemia aims at the underlying cause. For example, vitamin K deficiency resulting from malabsorption is corrected through intramuscular or intravenous administration of vitamin K, such as menadione sodium bisulfite (Hykinone) or menadiol diphosphate (Synkayvite).

If overdosage with a coumarin anticoagulant is the underlying problem, anticoagulant therapy is stopped. In order to normalize the prothrombin time, phytonadione (fat-soluble vitamin K) is administered orally for minor bleeding problems or intravenously for hemorrhage.

Finally, if prothrombin deficiency results from liver disease, concentrates of prothrombin or of prothrombin and factors VII, IX, and X may be transfused.

DISSEMINATED INTRAVASCULAR COAGULATION

The term disseminated intravascular coagulation (DIC) means diffuse or widespread coagulation within arterioles and capillaries all over the body.

Etiology

The condition of DIC is a complex and important coagulation disorder characterized by two apparently conflicting manifestations: (1) diffuse fibrin deposition within arterioles and capillaries all over the body, with resultant widespread clotting, and (2) hemorrhage from

TABLE 28–6 Conditions That May Precipitate Disseminated Intravascular Coagulation

Shock
Cirrhosis
Purpura fulminans
Glomerulonephritis
Acute fulminant hepatitis
Acute bacterial and viral infections
Conditions that may cause the release of platelet factor III
  Fat emboli
  Snake bites
  Hemolytic processes due to

- infection
- transfusion reactions
- immunologic disorders

  Tissue damage due to

- trauma
- heat stroke
- extensive burns
- transplant rejections
- surgery—particularly if extracorporeal circulation was used

Conditions that may cause the release of thromboplastin from the tissues
  Neoplastic growths

- acute leukemias
- prostatic cancer
- bronchogenic cancer
- giant cavernous hemangioma

  Obstetric conditions

- abruptio placentae
- retained dead fetus
- amniotic fluid embolism

the kidneys, brain, adrenal glands, heart, and other organs.

The causes of DIC are many, and there is considerable overlap among syndromes that precede its occurrence. Four categories of causative factors are (1) introduction of tissue coagulation factors into the circulation, (2) damage to vascular endothelium, (3) stagnant blood flow, and (4) infection.

Risk Factors

Table 28–6 lists conditions that may precipitate DIC. The nurse should be alert for signs of DIC when caring for clients with any of these conditions.

Pathophysiology

The pathologic chain of events characterizing DIC is detailed in the Pathophysiology box.

The prognosis for clients with DIC varies. The condition may be self-limiting; on the other hand, hemorrhage, organ damage, or even death may occur within a few days.

PATHOPHYSIOLOGY

What Happens in Disseminated Intravascular Coagulation

1. Certain disease states (see Table 28–6) cause the release of thromboplastin substances that result in activation of thrombin, which in turn activates fibrinogen and results in deposition of fibrin throughout the microcirculation.
2. Platelet aggregation or adhesiveness is increased; this enables fibrin clots to form and microthrombi to form in the brain, kidneys, heart, and other organs, causing microinfarcts and tissue necrosis.
3. Red blood cells become trapped in the fibrin strands and are destroyed (hemolysis). The resultant sluggish circulation of blood reduces the flow of nutrients and oxygen to the cells.
4. Platelets, prothrombin, and other clotting factors are consumed in the process, which compromises coagulation and predisposes to bleeding.
5. Excessive clotting activates the fibrinolytic mechanism, which causes the production of fibrin split products.
6. Fibrin split products act to inhibit platelet clotting functions, which causes further bleeding.
7. Ultimately, with clots being lysed and clotting factors being depleted, the blood loses the ability to clot.

Clinical Manifestations

The onset of DIC is usually acute and develops within days to hours after an initial assault to the body system, such as shock syndrome. Subacute DIC may not be apparent initially but may fulminate as the clinical course progresses. Chronic cases of DIC characteristically develop in clients with cancer or in pregnant women carrying a dead fetus. Manifestations may be mild or extremely severe.

Assessment of clients with DIC reveals purpura, petechiae, and ecchymoses on the skin, mucous membranes, heart lining, and lungs; prolonged bleeding from a venipuncture; severe, uncontrolled hemorrhage during surgery or childbirth; oliguria and acute renal failure; and convulsions and coma, which may terminate in death.

DIAGNOSTIC ASSESSMENT

Laboratory findings in severe cases of DIC indicate that the hemostatic mechanism has failed totally. A prolonged prothrombin time, very low platelet count, and incoagulable blood are typical findings. Table 28–7 lists the laboratory tests used in the diagnosis of DIC.

Medical Management

The treatment of DIC is currently under investigation as researchers attempt to validate the most suitable means of managing this dangerous syndrome. To prevent DIC

TABLE 28–7 Laboratory Tests Used in Diagnosis of Disseminated Intravascular Coagulation

TEST	RESULTS
Prothrombin time	Prolonged
Partial thromboplastin time	Usually prolonged
Thrombin time	Usually prolonged
Fibrinogen level	Usually depressed
Platelet count	Usually depressed
Fibrin split products	Elevated
Protamine sulfate test	Strongly positive
Factor assays II, V, VII	Reduced

successfully, clinicians must correct the basic problem (such as shock, delivery of a fetus, surgery, or irradiation for cancer), reverse the pathologic clotting, control bleeding and shock, detect occult bleeding, prevent further bleeding, accurately measure blood loss, administer blood products and medication as prescribed, and observe for and report transfusion reactions and medication side effects.

PHARMACOLOGIC MANAGEMENT

Cryoprecipitate is given for depletion of factors V and VIII. Administration of antithrombin III (in fresh frozen plasma) shortens the course of the disorder and decreases the complications of DIC. In cases in which bleeding cannot be controlled with heparin, aminocaproic acid (Amicar) is given. Cardiac, renal, and electrolyte studies should be followed closely during its use.

Several new agents to control bleeding and reverse laboratory signs of DIC are being studied. Protease inhibitors gabexate and aprotinin (Trasylol) have been used with some success. These drugs are still considered investigational.

Nursing Management

It is important to assess all body systems for the effect DIC has had: bleeding or oozing of blood from venipuncture sites or mucosal surfaces and wounds, pallor, petechiae, ecchymoses, and hematomas (integumentary); tachypnea, hemoptysis, orthopnea, and basilar rales (respiratory); tachycardia and hypotension (cardiovascular); abdominal distention, guaiac-positive stools or nasal aspirate (gastrointestinal); hematuria and oliguria (genitourinary); and vision changes, dizziness, headache, changes in mental status, and irritability (neurologic).

Nursing care of clients with DIC will vary, depending on the severity of the process. Generally, the goal of care is to monitor and quantify blood loss and provide supportive therapy with blood components in order to resolve symptoms of hemorrhage and control further bleeding. The nurse must monitor appropriate laboratory values to determine treatment effectiveness and observe for signs of thrombosis. For avoidance of further complications, the nurse should avoid injections, apply pressure to bleeding sites, and turn and reposition the client frequently and gently. This condition sometimes results in overt bleeding from body orifices and other clinical symptoms that are very frightening to the client and significant others. They will all require strong emotional support.

Congenital Conditions in Which Survival into Adulthood Is Expected

SICKLE CELL ANEMIA AND SICKLE CELL TRAIT

Sickle cell anemia (Hb SS disease) is a chronic hereditary hemolytic disorder.

Incidence

Sickle cell anemia primarily affects the world's black population (Fig. 28–1). In Nigeria, up to 30 per cent of the population carries the sickle trait.

Etiology and Risk Factors

As shown in Figure 28–1, whether a client will have sickle cell anemia, sickle cell trait, or neither depends on the genes for hemoglobin inherited from each parent.

Pathophysiology

In sickle cell anemia, the red blood cells contain an abnormal hemoglobin, that is, hemoglobin S (Hb S) instead of hemoglobin A (Hb A). These abnormal cells assume a sickle, or crescent, shape when oxygen in the blood decreases (Fig. 28–2). Once they "sickle," the red blood cells become rigid and may obstruct capillary blood flow, causing further hypoxia and, consequently, more sickling.

Sickle cell trait, generally a relatively mild condition, may produce few or no symptoms. It is present in clients who are heterozygous for sickle cell hemoglobin.

The exact mechanisms that precipitate the various forms of sickling crises or "attacks" remain somewhat unclear. However, two major factors are definitely linked with the sickling of cells: (1) hypoxia, due to low oxygen tensions, and (2) an increased blood viscosity, due to an increased concentration of sickled cells.

Exposure to low oxygen tensions (as a result of climbing to high altitudes, flying in nonpressurized

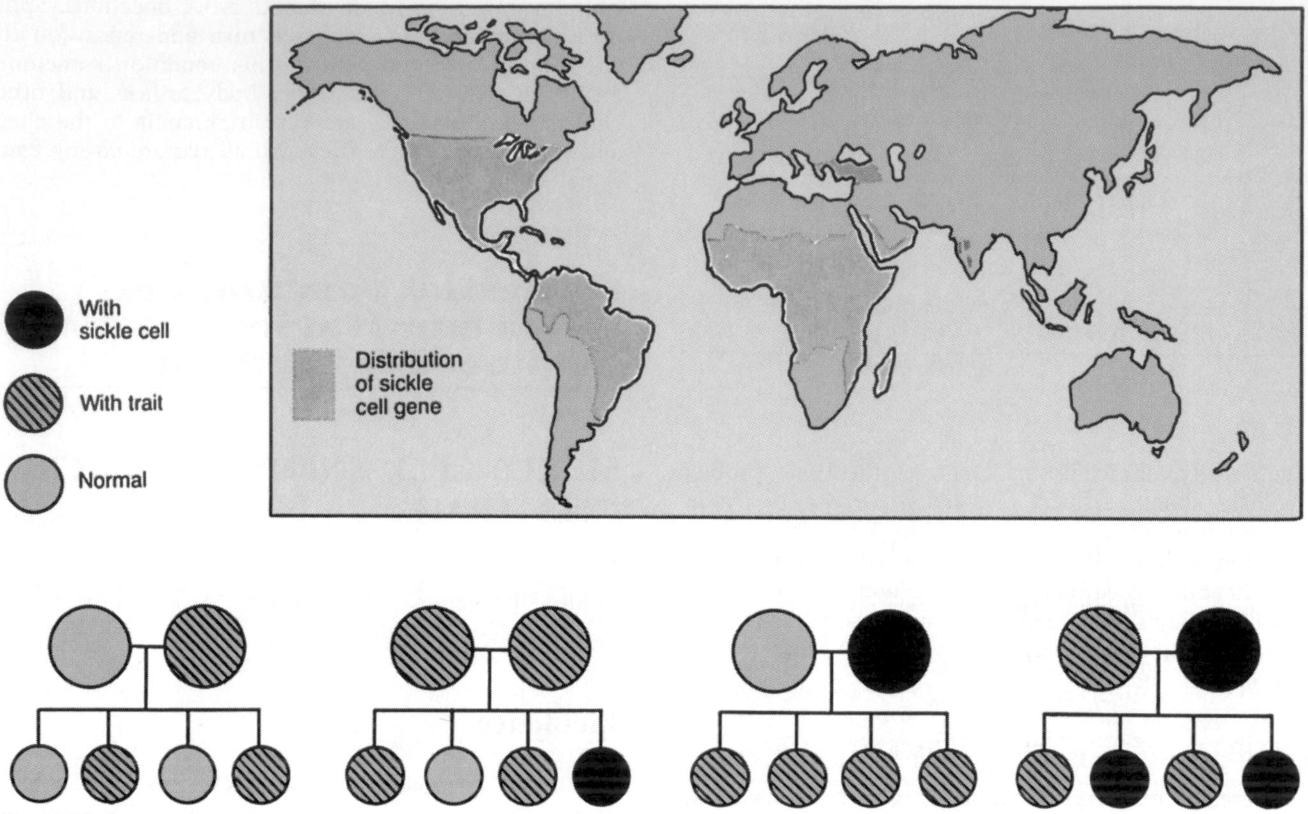

Figure 28–1
Geographic distribution and inheritance pattern of the sickle cell gene. (Redrawn from Page, J., et al. [1981]. *Blood: The river of life.* Washington, DC: Torstar Books.)

planes, exercising strenuously, or undergoing anesthesia without receiving adequate oxygenation) results in hypoxia.

When normal hemoglobin gives up its oxygen, it becomes only half as soluble as when it is oxygenated, whereas sickle cell hemoglobin becomes 50 times less soluble. The decreased solubility of Hb S causes it to crystallize, thereby deforming the cell's shape. The heavy concentration of misshapen cells during a sickling crisis makes the blood abnormally viscous, which results in an extremely sluggish circulation. The pathologic situation is compounded if dehydration is present.

Owing to the increased viscosity and the irregular shape of the cells, the sickle cells tend to pack together or "log jam" within the smaller blood vessels. Occlusion of the microcirculation increases hypoxia, which causes

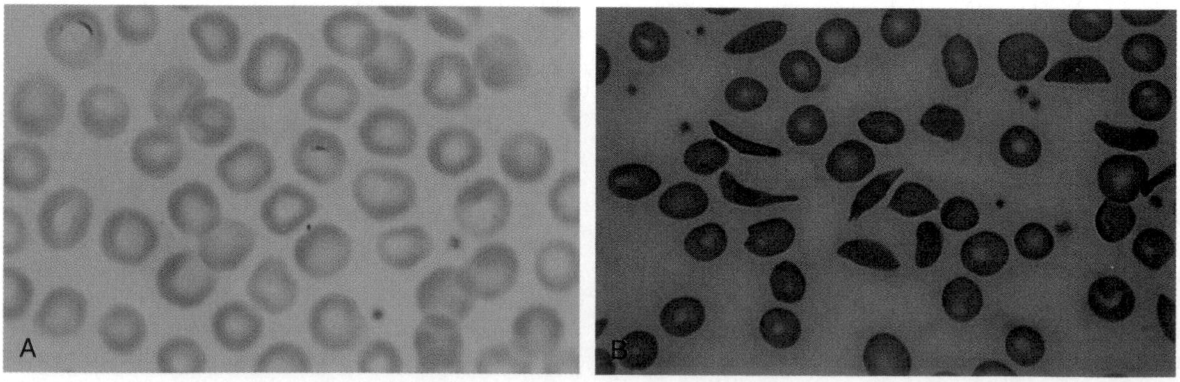

Figure 28–2
Erythrocytes. Comparison of normal red blood cells *(A)* and sickled cells *(B)*. (From Rodak, B. F. [1995]. *Diagnostic hematology.* [pp. 83 & 257]. Philadelphia: W. B. Saunders.)

more erythrocytes to sickle. Thus, a vicious cycle ensues. The organs most vulnerable to infarction and necrosis are the brain and kidneys, because of their constant demand for oxygen, and the bone marrow and spleen, because of their normally sluggish circulation.

Clinical Manifestations

Sickle cell anemia usually manifests itself during childhood but occasionally does not appear until adulthood. Young children who develop the disease fail to grow properly. They typically have spindly legs, a short trunk, and a tower-shaped skull because of bone marrow hyperactivity.

Symptoms, whenever they occur, are due to three underlying factors:

- hemolytic anemia from the destruction of sickle cells; hemoglobin values usually lie in a range of 7 to 10 mg/100 mL
- thrombosis and infarction from the occluded microcirculation
- an elevated bilirubin from the released hemoglobin that may result in gallstone formation (cholelithiasis)

These three problems profoundly affect all organs and tissues with severe, often fatal consequences. Infarctions in the spleen are so common that, after childhood, the spleen of most sickle cell anemia clients is small and scarred.

Other clinical manifestations include necrosis of the head of the femur possibly leading to osteomyelitis, necrotic bone marrow with development of infection, renal medullary ischemia resulting in diminished capacity to concentrate urine, priapism, pulmonary infarctions, myocardial infarctions, and cerebrovascular accidents. Leg ulcers are found in about 75 per cent of older children or adults with the disease.

Thrombotic episodes often cause moderate to severe pain of the extremities, joints, and abdomen. Proliferation of the bone marrow, in an attempt to compensate for the chronic anemia, leads to osteoporosis and, later, osteosclerosis. These are only a few of the possible complications of sickle cell anemia.

DIAGNOSTIC ASSESSMENT

Four laboratory procedures currently indicate the presence of sickle cell hemoglobin in either homozygous or heterozygous carriers: stained blood smear; sickle cell slide preparation; sickle-turbidity tube test (Sickledex); and hemoglobin electrophoresis.

Stained Blood Smear. A stained blood smear is examined for the presence of sickle cells.

Sickle Cell Slide Preparation (Sickle Prep). A blood specimen is observed for the sickling phenomenon after deoxygenation of the blood. This test is accurate but time-consuming.

Sickle-Turbidity Tube Test (Sickledex). This is an excellent mass screening test that detects sickle cell hemoglobin. After a finger prick, blood is mixed with Sickledex solution in a test tube. Five minutes later, the specimen is observed for cloudiness, which demonstrates the presence of Hb S. Solutions mixed with normal hemoglobin remain clear. Although indicative of Hb S, this test does not differentiate between sickle cell disease and the trait.

Hemoglobin Electrophoresis. Hemoglobin electrophoresis differentiates between sickle cell anemia and sickle cell trait.

Many people who carry the sickle cell trait are unaware that they do and that they can transmit this trait to their offspring. Consequently, researchers are perfecting mass screening tests for the detection of Hb S among the black population. Clients who have only the sickle cell trait may never be detected unless they are exposed to extremely low oxygen tensions (e.g., mountain climbing or flying in a nonpressurized plane), extremely hard work or exercise, or pregnancy.

> **CRITICAL TO REMEMBER**
>
> When exposed to extreme stressors, the client with the trait may develop symptoms of sickle cell disease.

Medical Management

Treatment for sickle cell anemia consists chiefly of supportive care (e.g., rest, oxygen, intravenous administration of fluids and electrolytes to ensure adequate hydration, sedation, and the prescription of analgesics).

In some cases, the slow administration of packed red blood cells or partial exchange transfusion helps relieve severe anemic symptoms. During episodes of increased risk (e.g., surgery, pregnancy), some clients benefit from hypertransfusion (transfusions until more than 50 per cent of the circulating red blood cells are of donor origin).

PHARMACOLOGIC MANAGEMENT

Anticoagulants, steroids, and cobalt treatments have all been used to reverse the sickling process without success. Clients with sickle cell disease have an increased need for folic acid and therefore usually receive a daily oral supplement to prevent increased anemia from folate deficiency.

Nursing Management

Assessment

Assessment findings include jaundice or pallor and ulceration (integumentary); joint swelling, disproportionately long arms and legs, fragility, and bone pain (skeletal); delayed sexual maturity and retarded growth (developmental status); enlargement of liver and spleen (gastrointestinal); and self-esteem disturbance, ineffective family coping, altered family processes, anticipatory grieving, noncompliance with health regimen, powerlessness, hopelessness, self-care deficit in activities of daily living, and altered thought processes (psychoemotional status).

Assessment findings during sickle cell crisis include systolic murmurs, arrhythmias, and enlargement (cardiac function); dyspnea and acute respiratory distress, that is, shortness of breath, chest pain, and cyanosis (respiratory); signs and symptoms of increased intracranial pressure due to cerebral hemorrhaging (sensory and motor function); and signs and symptoms of uremia, such as decreased urinary output and edema (renal function).

Nursing Diagnosis, Planning, and Implementation

Nursing Diagnosis: Pain R/T sickling crisis.

Planning: Expected Outcomes. The client will have pain relieved, as evidenced by verbalization of pain relief.

Implementation. The nurse assesses for pain every 2 to 4 hours and administers analgesics as needed according to orders; he or she monitors for effectiveness of analgesia. The nurse applies heat to joints as ordered, provides rest periods, and administers fluids to prevent dehydration and recurrence of pain crisis. Oral fluid intake should be increased. The nurse monitors intake and output. He or she provides the client with information on how to prevent crises, such as (1) avoiding high altitudes and flying in nonpressurized planes, because oxygen tension is lowered under these conditions; and (2) avoiding becoming dehydrated. The client should be advised to call a physician if vomiting, diarrhea, high fever, or any other cause of water loss develops.

Nursing Diagnosis: Knowledge Deficit R/T disease, treatment, and prevention of crises.

Planning: Expected Outcomes. The client will understand the disease, treatment, and prevention of crises, as evidenced by client's statements and absence of crises.

Implementation. When teaching clients about sickle cell anemia or sickle cell trait, the nurse should include the following points in the discussion:

- Explain the nature of the disease, and give the client a chance to express feelings and ask questions.
- Encourage parents of black African heritage to have themselves and their children tested for the presence of Hb S.
- Encourage the client to have routine medical examinations that include a red blood cell count.
- Encourage young adults who carry Hb S to ask their physician for genetic counseling before marrying or having children.
- Warn young women with sickle cell anemia that pregnancy carries a very high risk for them. They may develop pulmonary or renal complications, or both.

HEMOPHILIAS

There are three major types of hemophilia: A (classic hemophilia), B (Christmas disease), and von Willebrand's disease. Their major characteristics are compared in Table 28–8. Because classic hemophilia makes up 80 per cent of all hemophilias, the discussion of symptoms and treatment refers only to this type.

Incidence

The hemophilias are relatively common disorders. Within the United States alone, an estimated 25,000 clients are afflicted with a form of hemophilia. The hemophilias are characterized by prolonged bleeding, particularly after accidental, surgical, or dental trauma.

Etiology

Hemophilia is genetically transmitted in a sex-linked (X chromosome) recessive pattern. Females usually transmit the defective gene, but males develop the bleeding disorder. Females rarely have hemophilia. Female he-

TABLE 28–8 Comparison of the Three Forms of Hemophilia

FORM OF HEMOPHILIA	ETIOLOGY	TRANSMISSION	MAJOR LABORATORY FINDINGS
Hemophilia A (classic hemophilia)	Inherited factor VIII (antihemophilic globulin) deficiency	Transmitted as sex-linked recessive trait; transmitted by females; occurs in males and, rarely, homozygous females	Coagulation time prolonged but bleeding time normal; factor VIII missing from plasma
Hemophilia B (Christmas disease)	Inherited factor IX (plasma thromboplastin component) deficiency	Transmitted as sex-linked recessive trait; transmitted by females; occurs in males and, rarely, homozygous females	Laboratory findings and symptoms same as in hemophilia A; factor IX missing
Von Willebrand's disease	Inherited factor VIII deficiency and defective platelet dysfunction	Transmitted as autosomal dominant trait to both sexes; occurs in both males and females	Both coagulation time and bleeding time prolonged; low factor VIII levels; platelet adhesiveness decreased

mophilia carriers transmit the gene to half of their daughters. They transmit the disorder to half of their sons. Males with hemophilia transmit the gene to all of their daughters but to none of their sons.

Risk Factors

Because this is a hereditary disease, the only way to control the risk is through genetic testing and counseling for decreasing the transmission.

Pathophysiology

Hemophilia A, the most common of the congenital coagulation disorders, is caused by a deficiency in the procoagulant protein factor VIII.

Clinical Manifestations

Hemophilia may be mild or severe, depending on the level of factor VIII or IX coagulant activity. Usually diagnosed in childhood, this disorder is manifested in the following ways: slow persistent bleeding from cuts, scratches, and other minor traumas; delayed hemorrhage that follows minor injuries—bleeding may not start from a site until hours or even days after the moment of trauma; severe hemorrhaging from the gums after dental extraction or even brushing the teeth with a hard toothbrush; severe, sometimes fatal, epistaxis after injury to the nose, overwhelming gastric hemorrhage, which may be linked with gastric disorders such as ulcers; recurrent hematoma formation in the deep subcutaneous tissue, in the intramuscular tissues, and around the peripheral nerves. If nerves are compressed by hematomas, the client suffers severe pain, anesthesia of the innervated part, nerve damage, and paralysis. In addition, muscular atrophy sometimes results. Finally, there is recurrent hemarthrosis (bleeding into the joints), which is common in untreated cases and may result in serious joint deformity and permanent crippling. Hemarthrosis affects the knees, ankles, elbows, wrists, fingers, hips, and shoulders, in that order. All of this bleeding can be controlled with the administration of the missing factor (VIII or IX).

DIAGNOSTIC ASSESSMENT

Platelet function, platelet count, bleeding time, and prothrombin time are normal. The activated partial thromboplastin time will be prolonged. Quantitative assays for factor VIII will determine the severity of the disease.

Medical Management

The goals of care for clients with hemophilia are to stop topical bleeding as quickly as possible; to raise the level of antihemophilic factor (AHF) in the plasma, thereby temporarily supplying the missing factor causing hemorrhage; and to prevent complications leading to and caused by bleeding.

Immediate transfusion of factor VIII or IX concentrate is the primary treatment. Because the procoagulant activity of AHF disappears rapidly, clients need transfusions every 12 hours until bleeding stops.

Transfusion of packed red blood cells or white blood cells are used only to replace blood volume when there has been severe loss. Prophylactic transfusion of factor VIII to a level of 50 per cent above normal is recommended in cases of minor injury, surgery, and dental extractions.

Topical bleeding can usually be temporarily controlled by applying pressure to the injured site, packing the area with a fibrin foam, and applying topical hemostatics such as thrombin.

Hemarthrosis may be controlled if the client receives AHF in the early stages of bleeding. Joint immobilization and local chilling (such as packing ice around the joint) may bring relief.

The prognosis for clients with hemophilia has greatly improved since the discovery of AHF. Home infusion of AHF ensures that treatment is instituted at the first sign of bleeding, and complications are thus prevented.

PHARMACOLOGIC MANAGEMENT

Analgesics and corticosteroids often reduce joint pain and swelling. In mild hemophilia, the use of intravenous desmopressin may eliminate the need for AHF. Desmopressin acts by causing an increase in plasma factor VIII activity.

Nursing Management

Assessment

Although most clients with hemophilia are successfully maintained with home health care, they may be seen in the hospital during acute bleeding episodes or for nonrelated treatments.

CRITICAL TO REMEMBER

If even a minor invasive procedure is planned, it is crucial to assess the factor VIII level and administer a sufficient quantity of factor concentrate before the procedure.

During routine medical examinations, these clients should be assessed for frequency of bleeding episodes and effectiveness of home therapy. The nurse should examine joints for signs of bleeding and related atrophy.

Nursing Diagnosis, Planning, and Implementation

Nursing Diagnosis: Knowledge Deficit R/T potential for bleeding.

Planning: Expected Outcomes. The client will understand how to prevent or immediately treat bleeding, as evidenced by the client's ability to describe precautions and absence of injury or rapid treatment of unavoidable injury.

Implementation. The nurse provides teaching about bleeding precautions for prevention of injury or trauma that may precipitate a bleeding episode. Effective and prompt administration of factors to reduce the incidence of bleeding episodes and resultant complications, such as joint atrophy, is a priority. The client should avoid activities that may induce bleeding. Genetic counseling (if the client has the hereditary form of hemophilia) and education of the client and significant others should be given.

During client teaching, the nurse should review routine situations that increase the client's risk of bleeding, such as contact sports, minor invasive procedures, falls, and cuts. The client should be taught to recognize early symptoms and why it is critical to intervene with treatment immediately. The nurse and client should discuss situations that require medical consultation. The client should wear a bracelet to alert medical personnel to the presence of hemophilia.

Evaluation

The nurse must evaluate client outcomes on the basis of the established plan of care. If these goals have not been achieved, the plan and interventions must be revised to meet the client's needs.

Blood Transfusions

Hematologic disorders or the aggressive ablative therapy used to treat some hematologic diseases can require acute or chronic support with a variety of blood components. Technologic advances to improve the quality and safety of transfusions have caused a revolution in blood banking. This field has evolved into a broader specialty of transfusion medicine wherein the administration of blood components is considerably more complex and tightly regulated. The Joint Commission on Accreditation of Healthcare Organizations requires that all blood transfusions be evaluated in order to confirm that clear medical indications for the transfusion exist and that the client responds as expected. The transfusionist plays a critical role in this process. It is the nurse's responsibility to administer appropriate blood components in a manner that will ensure safety and efficacy.

PREPARING FOR TRANSFUSION

Assessment of the Client

The physician's order for transfusion should specify blood component, volume, and rate of infusion. However, as with all potentially hazardous biologics, the nurse must confirm that the drug being given is safe and appropriate in the present clinical situation. Table 28–9 describes each blood component, appropriate uses, and other pertinent information.

Informed Consent and Client Teaching

In recent years, failure to disclose information and obtain consent for transfusion has resulted in litigation when transfusion complications occurred. Informed consent involves explaining medical indications for transfusion, benefits, risks, and alternatives.

Two alternatives to homologous (random) blood transfusion should be considered: autologous and directed (or designated) donation. Clients who do not have leukemia or bacteremia should be offered the option of donating their own blood before a scheduled surgical procedure if there is a reasonable expectation that blood will be required.

Autologous donations can be made every 3 days if the donor's hemoglobin remains at or above 11 g/100 mL. For the blood to be maintained in a liquid state, donations should begin within 5 weeks of the transfusion date. Donations should cease at least 3 days before the date of transfusion.

Another frequently used method of autologous blood collection is intraoperative, postoperative, or post-traumatic blood salvage. This procedure involves suctioning blood from body cavities, joint spaces, and other closed operative or trauma sites. Tissue debris and other sterile contaminants may necessitate special processing such as washing. Salvaged blood must be reinfused within 6 hours of collection.

A second option is for transfusion recipients to designate their own donors. Directed donations have not been shown to decrease the risk of contracting human immunodeficiency virus (HIV). It is essential to discuss all of these options with the client in sufficient time for permitting donation and blood testing.

Documentation of informed consent may consist of a form in the medical record stating that this information was presented in a manner understandable to the client (that is, "Risks of and alternatives to blood transfusion were explained, and the client consented"). If the client is clinically unable to consent to transfusion, a reasonable effort should be made to secure consent from a family member. If no family member is available or time does not allow, a note to this effect should be placed in the chart. Institutional policy will vary regarding who is permitted to obtain consent.

It is the transfusionist's responsibility to describe the details of the transfusion procedure. Venous access, length of transfusion, and expected outcomes should be explained. The client should be informed of normal physiologic responses to transfusion and symptoms to be reported immediately. Clients released from care after transfusion should be given written information, including the name and phone number of a contact person.

TABLE 28–9 Blood Components

	WHOLE BLOOD	RED BLOOD CELLS	PLATELET CONCENTRATES	FRESH FROZEN PLASMA	CRYOPRECIPITATE	GRANULOCYTE CONCENTRATES	PLASMA DERIVATIVES	COAGULATION FACTOR CONCENTRATES
Composition	RBC, plasma, plasma proteins (globulins, antibodies), 63 mL of anticoagulant-preservative	RBC with CPDA-1 solution (anticoagulant-preservative only), final hematocrit no higher than 80% (80% RBC, 20% plasma) RBC with 100 mL additive solution, final hematocrit about 55–60%	Single-unit platelets contain a minimum of 5.5 × 10^{10} (1 unit) platelets in 50–70 mL of plasma obtained by separating platelet-rich plasma from 1 unit of fresh whole blood; 6–10 units may be pooled for 1 transfusion Single-donor platelets contain a minimum of 3.0 × 10^{11} platelets (6 units) obtained from single donor by use of automated cell separator during apheresis; recipient exposed to fewer donors, which decreases complications	91% water, 7% protein (globulin, antibodies, clotting factors), and 2% carbohydrates Freezing within 8 hr of collection preserves all clotting factors	Each unit contains about 80–120 units of factor VIII (antihemophilic factor) that represents 50% of antihemophilic factor originally present in unit, von Willebrand's factor, 250 mg of fibrinogen, and 20–30% of factor XIII present in a unit of whole blood, suspended in 10–20 mL of plasma	Unit obtained by granulocytapheresis contains a minimum of 1.0 × 10^{10} granulocytes, variable amounts of lymphocytes (usually < 10%), 30–50 mL of RBC and 100–400 mL of plasma, and 6–10 units of platelets; the platelets can be separated from the unit if the granulocyte recipient is not thrombocytopenic	*Albumin:* 96% albumin, 4% globulin and other proteins extracted from plasma; available as a 5% solution, oncotically equivalent to plasma, and also a concentrated 25% solution *Plasma protein fraction:* 83% albumin and 17% globulins extracted from plasma; less pure than albumin and has higher degree of contamination with other plasma proteins; in 5% solution only	*Factor VIII:* Lyophilized concentrate containing large quantities of factor VIII; prepared from large pools of donor plasma, but heat treatment during fractionation process significantly reduces risk of transmitting viral disease *Factor IX:* Lyophilized concentrate containing large quantities of factor IX; also contains factors II, VII, and X; product prepared from large pools of donor plasma, but heat treatment during fractionation process significantly reduces risk of transmitting viral disease
Volume	500 mL/unit	250–350 mL/unit 350–400 mL/unit	50–70 mL/unit 200–400 mL/unit	200–250 mL	5–10 mL/unit	200–400 mL with platelets 100–200 mL without platelets	Albumin: 250 and 500 mL (5%); 50 and 100 mL (25%)	Multiple-dose vial

Table continued on following page

TABLE 28–9 Blood Components *Continued*

	WHOLE BLOOD	RED BLOOD CELLS	PLATELET CONCENTRATES	FRESH FROZEN PLASMA	CRYOPRECIPITATE	GRANULOCYTE CONCENTRATES	PLASMA DERIVATIVES	COAGULATION FACTOR CONCENTRATES
Use	Acute, massive blood loss with hypotension, tachycardia, shortness of breath, pallor, and low hemoglobin/hematocrit	Acute or chronic blood loss with tachycardia, shortness of breath, pallor, low hemoglobin/hematocrit, and fatigue	To control or prevent bleeding associated with deficiencies in platelet number or function Used prophylactically for platelet counts $< 10{,}000$–$20{,}000/mm^3$ Administered if evidence of bleeding with platelet count $< 50{,}000/mm^3$	To increase level of clotting factors in clients with demonstrated deficiency If PT and PTT are < 1.5 times normal, FFP is rarely indicated	To correct deficiencies of factor VIII (hemophilia A), von Willebrand's factor, factor XIII, and fibrinogen Occasionally used to control bleeding in uremic clients	To treat clients with acquired neutropenia or congenital WBC dysfunction, who have serious infections unresponsive to conventional antibiotics Granulocytes are not currently licensed by FDA Long-term therapeutic benefit of granulocyte transfusion still questionable and continues to be evaluated	To provide volume expansion in situations in which crystalloid solutions are not adequate, such as plasma exchange, shock, and massive hemorrhage Also used for treatment of acute liver failure, burns, and hemolytic disease of the newborn	*Factor VIII:* To treat moderate to severe congenital factor VIII deficiency (hemophilia A) *Factor IX:* To treat factor IX deficiency (hemophilia B or Christmas disease); may be used to treat congenital factor VII or factor X deficiency
ABO/Rh Compatibility	The ABO type of the donor should be identical with the recipient's Rh− blood can be given to an Rh− or Rh+ recipient	A can match with A or O; B can match with B or O; O can match only with O; AB can match with A, B, or O Rh− blood can be given to either Rh+ or Rh− recipient	Although platelets have no ABO or Rh antigens, they are suspended in 200–400 mL of plasma containing donor antibodies and a small number of RBC There is evidence that platelet survival decreases if donor plasma is incompatible, and large volumes of incompatible plasma may cause a positive direct Coombs' test result It is also possible for even a small number of Rh+ RBC to stimulate anti-D in an Rh− recipient; therefore, plasma ABO and Rh compatibility is recommended	A can match with A or AB; B can match with B or AB; AB can match only with AB; O can match with A, B, AB, or O Rh− and Rh+ can be given to either Rh+ or Rh− recipient	Cryoprecipitate contains no RBC and a small volume of plasma ABO crossmatching not needed, and plasma compatibility preferred but not required	Granulocytes contain a significant number of RBC and plasma; therefore, ABO of donor should be identical with recipient's Rh− components may be transfused to an Rh+ recipient	Antibodies destroyed during processing; therefore, compatibility not a factor	Antibodies destroyed during processing, so compatibility not a factor

Expected Outcomes	Prevention or resolution of hypovolemic shock and anemia In a nonbleeding adult, 1 unit of whole blood should increase hematocrit by 3% and hemoglobin by 1 g/100 mL	Resolution of symptoms of anemia In a nonbleeding adult, 1 unit of RBC should increase hematocrit by 3% and hemoglobin by 1 g/100 mL	Prevention or resolution of bleeding due to thrombocytopenia or platelet dysfunction 1 unit should raise peripheral platelet count 5000 to 10,000/mm^3 if underlying cause is resolved or controlled Efficacy of platelet transfusion can be determined by obtaining platelet counts at 1 hr and 18–24 hr after infusion	Treatment effectiveness is assessed by monitoring coagulation function that is measured by the PT and PTT or by specific factor assays	Correction of factor VIII, von Willebrand's factor, factor XIII, and fibrinogen deficiency; cessation of bleeding in uremic clients Laboratory values required to assess effectiveness of treatment	Improvement in or resolution of infection No increase in peripheral WBC count usually seen after granulocyte transfusion in adults, although increase may be seen in children An improvement in clinical condition due to resolving infection is the only measure of treatment effectiveness	The client will acquire and maintain adequate blood pressure and volume support	The client will develop hemostasis due to increased levels of factor VIII and factor IX activity

FFP, fresh frozen plasma; PT, prothrombin time; PTT, partial thromboplastin time; RBC, red blood cells; WBC, white blood cells.

Pretransfusion Testing

In today's climate, the client's major concern is likely to be the safety of the transfusion, specifically the risk of contracting AIDS. The transfusionist should dispel misconceptions and provide factual information. Prospective donors are asked two categories of questions: those intended to protect the donor from possible risks of donation, and those intended to protect the recipient from risks of transfusion.

In order to decrease the risk of HIV transmission to blood recipients, there has been a marked increase in the second group of questions. In addition, donors are required to read information about behaviors known to increase the risk of HIV infection and, in most collection centers, they are questioned directly about their involvement in such activities.

In addition to obtaining a thorough donor history, many serologic and infectious disease tests are routinely performed on the donor's blood. The donor's blood is screened for syphilis, hepatitis C, hepatitis B, and the antibodies to HIV and human T-cell lymphotrophic virus type I.

When a need for blood is identified, several tests are done to confirm that the client's blood is compatible with that of the donor. First, the recipient's ABO and Rh type are identified. To determine the presence of antibody other than anti-A or anti-B, an antibody screen is performed. This test is done by adding the recipient's serum to donor red blood cells known to have a certain set of minor blood group antigens.

Blood products containing red blood cells may be further tested for compatibility to crossmatch testing. For this procedure, donor red blood cells are combined with the recipient's serum and Coombs' sera. After an inoculation period, the results are viewed microscopically. If no red blood cell agglutination has occurred, the crossmatch is compatible.

Samples must be labeled at the bedside after asking clients to state their name and comparing it with that on the identification bracelet. If clients are unable to state their name, identity should be confirmed by a family member or other familiar person whenever possible. The date and initials of the phlebotomist must be written on the sample label. Many institutions have adopted a secondary identification system. Several commercial systems are available; each is designed to ensure that the sample used for crossmatch has been drawn from the client who receives the transfusion.

OBTAINING VENOUS ACCESS

Suitable venous access for transfusion varies with the product being infused. When packed red blood cells weighing less than 300 g are infused, a 19-gauge or larger needle will be needed to achieve maximal flow rate. If a smaller gauge needle must be used, the red blood cells can be diluted with 0.9 per cent saline.

CRITICAL TO REMEMBER

No solution other than normal saline should be added to blood components.

Components containing a significant volume of plasma or other diluent can be safely infused at a rapid rate through smaller gauge needles or catheters. A central catheter is an acceptable venous access option for blood transfusion. Experience indicates that the circulation achieved through a blood vessel suitable for central line placement results in rapid mixing of fluids. As a result, no harmful effects have been reported.

Requesting Blood Release

Blood banking regulations state that refrigerated components may not be returned to inventory if they have been warmed to more than 10° C (50° F).

CRITICAL TO REMEMBER

Most transfusion medicine services consider 30 minutes to be the maximal allowable time out of monitored storage.

To avoid delays that may result in the waste of a scarce commodity, certain procedures should be performed before blood is requested.

An intravenous catheter appropriate for transfusing the requested component should be functional, flushed with normal saline, and maintained at a keep-vein-open (KVO) rate. Vital signs should then be taken and recorded. Fever may be a cause for delaying the transfusion. In addition to masking a possible symptom of an acute transfusion reaction, fever can also compromise the efficacy of platelet transfusions.

Premedication may also be required if the client has a history of adverse reactions. In many cases, febrile reactions can be prevented by administering acetaminophen or diphenhydramine hydrochloride (Benadryl). Steroids have been used to avoid severe fever, rigors, and chills that accompany granulocyte transfusions. A history of allergic reactions may require prophylactic administration of antihistamines. For effectiveness to be ensured, oral medication should be administered 30 minutes before the transfusion is started. Intravenous medication may be given immediately before the transfusion is initiated. Medications are never added to blood or blood products.

Blood should be released from the blood bank only to adequately trained personnel. The name and identification number of the intended recipient must be provided and a permanent record of this information maintained in the blood bank. So that delivery to the wrong client is avoided, blood should be transported to only one client at a time.

BEGINNING THE TRANSFUSION

Confirming Blood Acceptability

The most critical phase of transfusion is confirming product compatibility and verifying client identity.

Before going to the client's bedside, the nurse should verify ABO and Rh compatibility. This can usually be done by comparing the bag label with the medical record and forms issued from the blood bank. The bag label should also be checked to ensure that the correct component has been issued and for date of expiration. Components expire at midnight of the day marked on the bag unless otherwise specified.

The nurse should inspect the unit for leaks, abnormal color, clots, excessive air, and bubbles.

At the bedside, the nurse should ask clients to state their name and compare it with the name on the identification bracelet. As with sample collection, clients unable to state their name should be identified by a person who knows them well. The name and number on the identification bracelet should be compared with the tag on the blood bag. If applicable, the secondary identification system should be checked. The American Association of Blood Banks recommends that two qualified individuals perform this critical step.

Blood Infusion Equipment and Devices

Most blood products should be infused through administration sets designed specifically for this use. The set usually contains a 170 μm filter designed to trap fibrin clots and other debris that accumulate during blood storage. Most standard filters have a four-unit capacity. Tubing is available in two basic configurations: straight or Y-type. The use of Y-type tubing simplifies the process of adding normal saline to red blood cells and provides ready access to a saline flush if the transfusion must be interrupted.

Many devices are available to increase the safety of the transfusion. Special filters, electromechanical devices, and blood warmers are frequently used at the bedside. The transfusionist should be familiar with how and why special equipment is used.

Nonstandard Filters

The physician or nurse may determine that the standard 170 μm filter is not adequate in certain clinical situations. The transfusion medicine service may also recommend the use of a nonstandard filter in order to decrease the risk of transfusion complications. It is critically important to follow the manufacturer's instructions exactly.

Electromechanical Infusion Devices

Several types of infusion devices are available to regulate and monitor the flow of intravenous solutions. There are basically two types: infusion controllers, which monitor flow by gravity, and infusion pumps, which deliver solutions under pressure. Infusion controllers may be used with all blood products if they are designed to function with opaque solutions.

It is imperative that machines tested and approved for the infusion of red blood cells be used exactly as recommended by the manufacturer.

If manual pressure cuffs are used to increase red blood cell flow rate, the pressure should not exceed 300 mm Hg. Standard sphygmomanometers should not be used for this purpose because they do not exert uniform pressure against all parts of the bag.

Blood Warmers

Blood warmers can be used to prevent hypothermia, which can be induced by rapid infusion of large volumes of refrigerated blood. Neonatal exchange transfusion, plasma exchange, surgery, and trauma are all clinical situations that may require the use of a blood warmer.

Two types of devices are approved by blood bank regulatory agencies for warming blood. For dry heating, a bag is placed between two aluminum heating plates, or a disposable cuff-style bag is wrapped around a cylindric aluminum heating element. A second type uses warm water to increase the temperature of the blood. Water baths containing water warmed to 37° C (98.6° F) may be used only if they have been specifically designed for warming blood. The blood bag should never be fully immersed in water.

DURING TRANSFUSION

Monitoring the Client and Documenting Signs and Symptoms of Transfusion Reaction

CRITICAL TO REMEMBER

The first 10 to 15 minutes of any transfusion are the most critical. If a major ABO incompatibility exists or a severe allergic reaction such as anaphylaxis occurs, it is usually evident within the first 50 mL of the transfusion.

It is recommended that the transfusion begin slowly, under close observation of medical personnel. If no evidence of a reaction is noted within the first 15 minutes, flow can be increased to the prescribed rate. Be-

BOX 28–1

Possible Signs and Symptoms of a Transfusion Reaction

GENERAL

- Fever (rise of 1° C or 2° F)
- Chills
- Muscle aches, pain
- Back pain
- Chest pain
- Headache
- Heat at site of infusion or along vein

NERVOUS SYSTEM

- Apprehension, impending sense of doom
- Tingling, numbness

RESPIRATORY SYSTEM

- Respiratory rate
  - Tachypnea
  - Apnea
- Dyspnea
- Cough
- Wheezing
- Rales

GASTROINTESTINAL SYSTEM

- Nausea
- Vomiting
- Pain, abdominal cramping
- Diarrhea (may be bloody)

CARDIOVASCULAR SYSTEM

- Heart rate
  - Bradycardia
  - Tachycardia
- Blood pressure
  - Hypotension, shock
  - Hypertension
- Peripheral circulation
  - Color cyanosis, facial flushing
  - Temperature: cool/clammy; hot/flushed/dry
  - Edema
- Bleeding
  - Generalized (DIC)
  - Oozing at surgical site

RENAL SYSTEM

- Changes in urine volume
  - Oliguria, anuria
  - Renal failure
- Changes in urine color
  - Dark, concentrated
  - Shades of red, brown, amber
  - May indicate the presence in urine of red blood cells (hematuria) or of free hemoglobin (hemoglobinuria)

INTEGUMENTARY SYSTEM

- Rashes, hives (urticaria), swelling
- Itching
- Diaphoresis

DIC, disseminated intravascular coagulation.

fore leaving the client unattended, the nurse should instruct the client to report anything unusual immediately. It is advisable to take and record vital signs before the transfusion begins, after the first 15 minutes, and every hour until 1 hour after the transfusion has been discontinued. The vital signs should be checked immediately if the client displays any untoward symptoms.

Regulatory agencies require complete documentation of the transfusion, including identification of personnel starting and ending the transfusion, unique product number, and outcome (that is, "no reaction noted"). If an adverse reaction does occur, the symptoms, actions taken, and future recommendations should also be recorded in the client's medical record.

Nursing Management

Exposure to foreign blood elements may mediate immunologic and nonimmunologic reactions affecting all major body systems as described in Box 28–1. Any unusual sign or symptom occurring during or immediately after a transfusion should be considered a potential reaction. Unconscious clients should be monitored closely because signs of a reaction may be inhibited in the unconscious state (Box 28–2). The most frequently seen acute reactions are described in Table 28–10.

BOX 28–2

Signs of Transfusion Reaction in an Unconscious Patient

- Weak pulse
- Fever
- Hypotension
- Visible hemoglobinuria
- Increased operative bleeding (oozing at a surgical site)
- Vasomotor instability (tachycardia, bradycardia, or hypotension)
- Oliguria/anuria

Whereas treatment may vary depending on the signs and symptoms, certain standard procedures should be followed.

CRITICAL TO REMEMBER

When a reaction is suspected, the nurse should stop the transfusion and keep the intravenous line open with normal saline.

TABLE 28–10 Acute Transfusion Reactions

REACTION	CAUSE	CLINICAL MANIFESTATIONS	MANAGEMENT	PREVENTION
Immunogenic				
Allergic Incidence: 1%	Sensitivity to foreign proteins in plasma	Urticaria, hives, flushing, itching (no fever)	Administer antihistamines as directed If symptoms mild and transient, transfusion may resume	Treat prophylactically with antihistamines
Febrile, nonhemolytic Incidence: 0.5–1.0%	Sensitization to donor white blood cells, platelets, or plasma proteins	Sudden chills and fever (rise in temperature of more than 1° C, 1.8° F), headache, flushing, anxiety, muscle pain	Give antipyretics as prescribed; avoid aspirin in thrombocytopenic clients	Consider leukocyte-poor blood products (filtered, washed, or frozen) if fever occurs more than once
Acute hemolytic Incidence: 1 : 25,000 Fatal: 2 : 1,000,000	Infusion of ABO incompatible red blood cells	Chills, fever, low back pain, flushing, tachycardia, tachypenia, hemoglobinuria, hemoglobinemia, hypotension, vascular collapse, bleeding, acute renal failure, shock, cardiac arrest, death	Treat shock Maintain blood pressure with IV solutions Give diuretics as prescribed to maintain urine flow Insert indwelling catheter or measure hourly output Dialysis may be needed	Meticulously verify recipient from sample collection to transfusion
Anaphylactic Incidence: 1 : 150,000	Infusion of IgA proteins to IgA-deficient recipient who has developed anti-IgA antibodies	Anxiety, urticaria, wheezing progressing to cyanosis, shock, and possible cardiac arrest	Initiate CPR if indicated Have epinephrine ready for injection (0.4 mL of a 1 : 1000 solution subcutaneously)	Give blood components from IgA-deficient donors or remove all plasma by washing
Nonimmunogenic				
Circulatory overload Estimated Incidence: 1 : 10,000 (not usually reported to blood bank)	Infusion of blood at a rate too rapid for the size, cardiac status, or clinical condition of the recipient	Cough, dyspnea, pulmonary congestion (crackles), headache, hypertension, tachycardia, distended neck veins	Place client in upright position with feet in dependent position Administer diuretics, oxygen, and morphine as prescribed Phlebotomy may be required	Adjust transfusion volume and flow rate on basis of client size and clinical status If slow transfusion will exceed 4 hr, request that unit be divided into smaller aliquot volumes
Septicemia Incidence: very rare	Transfusion of component contaminated with microorganism	Rapid onset of chills, high fever, vomiting, diarrhea, marked hypotension and shock	Treat symptoms and administer antibiotics, IV fluids, vasopressors, and steroids as directed Obtain culture of client and blood containers	Collect, process, store, and transfuse blood according to industry standards Infuse within 4 hr of starting time

IV, intravenous; CPR, cardiopulmonary resuscitation.

Life-threatening symptoms, such as respiratory or circulatory failure, must be treated immediately. The nurse contacts the client's physician and the blood banks and, according to institutional policy, obtains appropriate laboratory samples. Samples used to evaluate a reaction include blood and urine. Free hemoglobin found in either indicates that red blood cells have hemolyzed, the most serious serologic finding. After laboratory testing, a physician specialized in transfusion medicine will evaluate the clinical and laboratory evidence to determine whether the client's symptoms were caused by the transfusion. The physician may then make recommendations for reducing the risk of complication in the future.

DELAYED TRANSFUSION COMPLICATIONS

Complications can occur days to years after a transfusion. Fever, mild jaundice, and decreased hematocrit may indicate a delayed hemolytic reaction. Hemolysis of red blood cells may occur 3 days to several months after the transfusion if an antibody was undetected during crossmatch testing and red blood cells containing that antigen were transfused. Usually no medical treatment is required.

Iron overload may occur in clients receiving more than 100 units of blood over a period of time, such as in clients with aplastic anemia. Clinical manifestations are congestive heart failure, arrhythmias, impaired thyroid and gonadal function, diabetes, and cirrhosis. Deferoxamine (Desferal), which chelates and removes accumulated iron via the kidneys, may be administered intravenously or subcutaneously to prevent this potentially fatal complication. Posttransfusion GVHD can occur if donor lymphocytes engraft and divide in the marrow spaces of an immunocompromised recipient. Symptoms are fever, rash, diarrhea, and hepatitis. This frequently fatal complication can be prevented by irradiation of all cellular components.

Many diseases can be transmitted through blood transfusion. The most common is hepatitis C. Although symptoms are milder than those seen with hepatitis B, chronic liver disease and cirrhosis may develop. Hepatitis B should be considered if the recipient develops anorexia, malaise, nausea, vomiting, dark urine, and jaundice within 4 to 6 weeks of transfusion.

On rare occasions, HIV-1 is transmitted from an infected donor to a blood recipient. The client may be asymptomatic for several years or develop flulike symptoms in 2 to 4 weeks. Other infectious diseases that may be transmitted through blood transfusion are HIV-2, HTLV-1, Chagas' disease, Lyme disease, babesiosis, syphilis, Epstein-Barr virus, cytomegalovirus, and malaria. Blood donors are questioned or tested for potential exposure to these diseases.

STUDY QUESTIONS

1. A client with severe iron deficiency anemia should be assessed for:
   A. Gastritis
   B. White-coated tongue
   C. Difficulty in swallowing
   D. Large (macrocytic) red blood cells
2. The client with pernicious anemia should be taught that:
   A. Vitamin B_{12} therapy must be continued for life
   B. Packed red blood cells should be transfused at least once a month
   C. The anemia responds to a diet that includes dark green leafy vegetables
   D. The disease was caused by exposure to toxic chemicals in the environment
3. The person with sickle cell anemia should be taught to expect hypoxia as a result of which one of the following?
   A. Driving a car
   B. Drinking fluids
   C. Eating fatty foods
   D. Exercising strenuously
4. A female African American who has sickle cell anemia should:
   A. Plan on completing a family before age 30
   B. Have a red blood cell count done every 6 months
   C. Seek genetic counseling before beginning a family
   D. Remain on anticoagulant therapy during her working years
5. The plan of care for a client with leukemia should include which one of the following? The client will be:
   A. Placed in respiratory isolation
   B. Assessed for temperature elevation once a day
   C. Monitored closely for signs and symptoms of infection
   D. Placed on a diet high in fiber-rich fresh fruits and vegetables
6. Five minutes after a blood transfusion is started the client states, "It's hard for me to breathe." The nurse should:
   A. Increase the infusion rate of the normal saline
   B. Check the unit of blood to ascertain the correct unit is infusing
   C. Retake the vital signs and compare them to the baseline set taken earlier
   D. Stop the transfusion and keep the intravenous line open with normal saline
7. A client with disseminated intravascular coagulation (DIC) has just had blood drawn for several lab studies. The nurse should:
   A. Administer vitamin K immediately
   B. Expect prolonged bleeding from the site
   C. Assess the site for development of ecchymotic areas
   D. Apply pressure to the venipuncture site for 5 minutes
8. As a result of discharge teaching for the client with idiopathic thrombocytopenic purpura (ITP), the nurse should expect that the client will:
   A. Refrain from brushing the teeth more than once a day
   B. Take nonsteroidal anti-inflammatory medication every 4 hours
   C. Use the Valsalva maneuver to assist in evacuating the bowels
   D. Apply an ice bag over small bleeding sites to promote hemostasis

CRITICAL THINKING EXERCISES

SCENARIO A

An elderly client is newly diagnosed with iron deficiency anemia. She lives with her husband, who was diagnosed with chronic myelogenous leukemia (CML) about 5 years ago.

1. Why are the elderly at risk for iron deficiency anemia?
2. How does iron deficiency anemia affect activities of daily living for the elderly client?
3. How would an iron-rich diet help the client's spouse?
4. What teaching should the nurse give to enhance the client's compliance with the recommended treatment of dietary changes and daily intake of iron supplements?
5. How does CML differ from iron deficiency anemia? Are there any similarities?
6. What teaching will help the spouse optimize his functioning?

SCENARIO B

An African American woman has sickle cell trait. Her brother has sickle cell anemia. Both are in their 20s, employed, and soon to be married.

1. How does the sickling of cells affect the body?
2. Why are the brain, kidneys, bone marrow, and spleen the organs most affected by sickling of cells?
3. Which of the siblings should receive genetic counseling in preparation for starting a family?
4. How effective is the Sickledex test in diagnosing sickle cell anemia?
5. Of the two siblings, which one is more likely to develop sickle cell crisis?
6. What events cause sickle cell crisis?

BIBLIOGRAPHY

1. Afessa, B., et al. (1992). Outcome of recipients of bone marrow transplants who require intensive-unit care support. *Mayo Clinic Proceedings, 67,* 117–122.
2. Alexanian, R., & Barlogie, B. (1990). New treatment strategies for multiple myeloma. *American Journal of Hematology, 35,* 194–198.
3. Anderson, K. C., & Braine, H. G. (1990). Specialized cell component therapy. *Seminars in Oncology Nursing, 6,* 140–149.
4. Asimacopoulos, P. J., Skoumas, I. N., Yawn, D. H., Sakellariouiu, G. A., & Verani, M. S. (1994). *Chest: The Cardiopulmonary Journal, 105(3),* 653–654.
5. Baldwin, J. G. (1988). Hematopoietic function in the elderly. *Archives of Internal Medicine, 148,* 2544–2546.
6. Bell, T. (1990). Disseminated intravascular coagulation and shock. *Critical Care Nursing Clinics of North America, 2,* 255–268.
7. Bertero, C., & Ek, A. (1993). Quality of life of adults with acute leukemia. *Journal of Advanced Nursing, 18(9),* 1346–1353.
8. Brandy, B. (1990). Nursing protocol for the patient with neutropenia. *Oncology Nursing Forum, 17,* 9–15.
9. Brunner, L., & Suddarth, D. (1991). *The Lippincott manual of nursing practice* (5th ed.) (pp. 270–275). Philadelphia: J. B. Lippincott.
10. Buchsel, P. C., & Keller, J. (1989). Bone marrow transplantation. *Nursing Clinics of North America, 24,* 907–938.
11. Cain, J., et al. (1991). Myelodysplastic syndromes: A review for nurses. *Oncology Nursing Forum, 18,* 113–117.
12. Carpenito, L. J. (1991). *Nursing care plans and documentation: Nursing diagnoses and collaborative problems.* Philadelphia: J. B. Lippincott.
13. Dech, Z. F. (1994). Blood conservation in the critically ill. *AACN Clinical Issues in Critical Nursing, 5(2),* 169–177.
14. Dicke, K. A. (1990). Modern trends in the treatment of multiple myeloma. *Current Opinion in Oncology, 2,* 277–284.
15. DiJulio, J. (1991). Hematopoiesis: An overview. *Oncology Nursing Forum, 18,* 3–6.
16. Dolan, J. T. (1991). *Critical care nursing: Clinical management through the nursing process.* Philadelphia: F. A. Davis.
17. Duguid, J. K. M. (1990). Developing techniques in blood transfusion. *Bailliere's Clinical Haematology, 3(1),* 999–1017.
18. Ellenberger, B. J., Haas, L., & Cundiff, L. (1993). Thrombocytopenia purpura: Nursing during the acute phase. *Dimensions of Critical Care Nursing, 12(2),* 58–65.
19. Epstein, C., & Bakanauskas, A. (1991). Clinical management of DIC: Early nursing interventions. *Critical Care Nursing, 11,* 42–54.
20. Erickson, J. M. (1994). Update on Hodgkin's disease. *Nurse Practitioner: American Journal of Primary Health Care, 19(11),* 63–64, 66–68.
21. Flyge, H. A. (1993). Meeting the challenge of neutropenia. *Nursing '93, 23(7),* 61–64.
22. Folkes, M. E. (1990). Transfusion therapy in critical care nursing. *Critical Care Nursing, 13,* 15–28.
23. France-Dawson, M. (1994). Painful crises in sickle cell conditions. *Nursing Standard, 8(45),* 25–28.
24. Franco, T., & Gould, D. A. (1994). Allogeneic bone marrow transplantation. *Seminars in Oncology Nursing, 10(1),* 3–11.
25. Freedman, S., et al. (1990). Nursing considerations in the administration of blood component therapy. *Seminars in Oncology Nursing, 6,* 155–162.
26. Freireich, E. H., et al. (1978). *Leukemia and lymphoma.* New York: Grune and Stratton.
27. Froberg, J. H. (1989). The anemias: Causes and courses of action. *RN, 52(1),* 24–30.
28. Fuller, A. K. (1990). Platelet transfusion therapy for thrombocytopenia. *Seminars in Oncology Nursing, 6,* 123–128.
29. Galloway, R., & McGuire, J. (1994). Determinants of compliance with iron supplementation: Supplies, side effects, or psychology? *Social Science and Medicine, 39(3),* 381–390.

30. Garry, P. J., et al. (1991). A prospective study of blood donations in healthy elderly persons. *Transfusion, 31,* 686–697.
31. Gilyon, K., & Kuzel, T. (1991). Cutaneous T-cell lymphoma. *Oncology Nursing Forum, 18,* 901–908.
32. Gloe, D. (1991). Common reactions to transfusions. *Heart and Lung, 20,* 506–512.
33. Gobel, B. H. (1990). Plasma and plasma derivative therapy for coagulation disorders. *Seminars in Oncology Nursing, 6,* 129–135.
34. Goodnough, L. T., et al. (1989). Red cell mass in autologous and homologous blood units. *Transfusion, 29,* 821–824.
35. Graham, D. L., et al. (1992). Cytogenetic and molecular detection of residual leukemic cells after allogeneic bone marrow transplantation in chronic granulocytic leukemia. *Mayo Clinic Proceedings, 67,* 123–127.
36. Greifzu, S. (1991). Helping cancer patients fight infection. *RN, 54,* 24–29.
37. Griffin, K. B. (1990). Postoperative bleeding, current nursing management. *Critical Care Nursing Clinics of North America, 2,* 549–557.
38. Grindel, C. G. (1994). Fatigue and nutrition. *MEDSURG Nursing, 3(6),* 475–481, 499.
39. Guyatt, G. H., et al. (1990). Diagnosis of iron-deficiency anemia in the elderly. *American Journal of Medicine, 88,* 205–209.
40. Hahn, K. (1989). Monitoring a blood transfusion. *Nursing 89, 19,* 20–22.
41. Harmening, D. (1992). *Clinical hematology and fundamentals of hemostasis.* Philadelphia: F. A. Davis.
42. Hoffman, R., et al. (1991). *Hematology: Basic principles and practice.* New York: Churchill Livingstone.
43. Huff, N. L. (1990). Sickle cell anemia: An IV nursing challenge. *Journal of Intravenous Nursing, 12,* 245–250.
44. Illott, S. (1990). Infection control in general practice. *Nursing Standards, 5,* 25–28.
45. Iserson, K. V., & Huestis, D. W. (1991). Blood warming: Current applications and techniques. *Transfusion, 31,* 558–568.
46. Kelleher, J. (1994). Issues for designing marrow transplant programs. *Seminars in Oncology Nursing, 10(1),* 64–71.
47. King, C. R., & Hoffart, N. (1992). Acute renal failure in bone marrow transplantation. *Oncology Nursing Forum, 19(9),* 1327–1335.
48. Kotwas, L., et al. (1990). Blood collection techniques. *Seminars in Oncology Nursing, 6,* 109–116.
49. Lawrence, J. (1994). Critical care issues in the patient with hematologic malignancy. *Seminars in Oncology Nursing, 10(3),* 198–207.
50. LePage, E. (1993). Using a ventricular reservoir to instill amphotericin B. *Journal of Neuroscience Nursing, 25(4),* 212–217.
51. Letendre, L., et al. (1992). Mayo Clinic experience with allogeneic and syngeneic bone marrow transplantation, 1982 through 1990. *Mayo Clinic Proceedings, 67,* 109–116.
52. Litwack, K. (1991). Bleeding and coagulation in the PACU. *Critical Care Nursing Clinics of North America, 3,* 121–127.
53. Litwack, K. (1992). Practical points for transfusion therapy. *Journal of Post Anesthesia, 2,* 257–261.
54. Lundquist, D. M. (1994). An update on non-Hodgkin's lymphomas. *Nurse Practitioner: American Journal of Primary Health Care, 19(10),* 41, 45, 49–50.
55. Maloney, P. A., & Ryan, L. (1990). Hyperviscosity-polycythemia syndrome: A case study. *Journal of Perinatology Neonatal Nurse, 4,* 64–70.
56. Mansouri, A. (1990). Acquired hemostatic abnormalities in the elderly. *Journal of the American Gerontologic Society, 38,* 809–816.
57. Martinelli, A. M. (1991). Sickle cell disease. *AORN Journal, 53,* 716–724.
58. McVay, P. A., et al. (1991). Probable reasons that autologous blood was not donated by patients having surgery for which crossmatched blood was ordered. *Transfusion, 31,* 810–813.
59. Meyer, C. (1991). New drugs: The class of 1991. *American Journal of Nursing, 91,* 40–43.
60. Napier, J. (1987). *Blood transfusion therapy: A problem-oriented approach* (pp. 54–66). New York: John Wiley and Sons.
61. Neumann, M., & Urizar, R. (1994). Hemolytic uremic syndrome: Current pathophysiology and management. *ANNA Journal, 21(2),* 137–145.
62. Oniboni, A. C. (1990). Infection in the neutropenic patient. *Seminars in Oncology Nursing, 6,* 50–59.
63. Parsons, L., & Klopovich, P. (1990). Immune globulin therapy. *Seminars in Oncology Nursing, 6,* 136–139.
64. Pavel, J. (1990). Red blood cell transfusions for anemia. *Seminars in Oncology Nursing, 6,* 117–122.
65. Pavel, J. N., et al. (1990). *Transfusion therapy guidelines.* Bethesda, MD: National Blood Resource Education Program, NHLBI, NIH.
66. Perez, W. E., & Viets, J. L. (1990). Transfusion and coagulation: An overview and recent advances in practice modalities. *Nurse Anesthetist, 1,* 149–161.
67. Picard, V. T., et al. (1990). Transfusion therapy: Associated risks and alternative approaches. *American Nephrology Nurses' Association, 17,* 457–464.
68. Price, C. A., & McCarley, P. B. (1994). Physical assessment for patients receiving therapeutic plasma exchange, Part 2. *ANNA Journal, 21(4),* 149–154, 201.
69. Querin, J. J., & Stahl, L. D. (1990). 12 simple, sensible steps for successful blood transfusions. *Nursing 90, 20,* 68–81.
70. Rahr, V., & Tucker, R. (1990). Non-Hodgkin's lymphoma: Understanding the disease. *Cancer Nursing, 13,* 56–61.
71. Rayfield, S., & Theriot, B. L. (1990). Maximizing safe blood transfusions. *Advances in Critical Care, 5,* 17–19.
72. Rieger, P. T., & Haeuber, D. (1995). A new approach to managing chemotherapy-related anemia: Nursing implications of epoetin alfa. *Oncology Nursing Forum, 22(1),* 71–81.
73. Rivers, R., & Williams, N. (1990). Sickle cell anemia: Complex disease nursing challenge. *RN, 53,* 24–29.
74. Rostad, M. (1990). Management of myelosuppression in the patient with cancer. *Oncology Nursing Forum, 17,* 4–8.
75. Rosvoll, R. V., et al. (1990). *Accreditations requirements manual* (pp. 4–59). Arlington, VA: American Association of Blood Banks.
76. Rutman, R., et al. (1990). The transfusion service and nursing. *Seminars in Oncology Nursing, 6,* 152–154.
77. Rutman, R., et al. (1990). Home transfusion for the cancer patient. *Seminars in Oncology Nursing, 6,* 163–167.

78. Sander, S. G., et al. (1987). Alternative approaches to transfusion: Autologous blood and directed blood donations. *Progress in Hematology, XV,* 183–219.

79. Sauvage, D., & Saltissi, D. (1993). The comparative efficacy of three regimens of parenteral iron erythropoietin. *Renal Educator, 13(3),* 47.

80. Sazama, K. (1990). Reports of 355 transfusion-associated deaths: 1976–1985. *Transfusion, 30,* 583–590.

81. Scherer, J. C. (1991). *Introductory medical-surgical nursing* (5th ed.). Philadelphia: J. B. Lippincott.

82. Schlossberg, D. (Ed.) (1989). *Infectious mononucleosis* (2nd ed.). New York: Springer-Verlag.

83. Shulman, I. A. (1989). Adverse reaction to blood transfusion. *Blood Transfusion, 85,* 35–42.

84. Swearingen, P. L., & Keen, J. H. (1995). *Manual of critical care: Applying nursing diagnoses to adult critical illness* (3rd ed.). St. Louis: Mosby–Year Book.

85. Tucker, R., & Rahr, V. (1990). Nursing care of the patient with non-Hodgkin's lymphoma. *Cancer Nursing, 13,* 229–234.

86. Urden, L. D., et al. (1992). *Essentials of critical care nursing.* St. Louis: Mosby–Year Book.

87. Urlich, S. P. (1987). Preventing post splenectomy complications. *Nursing 87, 17,* 98–100.

88. Watne, K., & Donner, T. A. (1995). Distinguishing between life-saving and life-sustaining treatments: When the physician and spouse disagree—the ethical case . . . ethical analysis. *Dimensions of Critical Care Nursing, 14(1),* 42–47.

89. Welte, K. (1994). Matched unrelated transplants. *Seminars in Oncology Nursing, 10(1),* 20–27.

90. Whedon, M., & Ferrell, B. R. (1994). Quality of life in adult bone marrow transplant patients: Beyond the first year. *Seminars in Oncology Nursing, 10(1),* 42–57.

91. Widmann, F. K., et al. (1992). *Standards for blood banks and transfusion services* (pp. 1–58). Arlington, VA: American Association of Blood Banks.

92. Wood, L., & Jacobs, P. (1989). Myeloma—the integral role played by the professional nurse. *Curationis, 12,* 67–71.

93. Wyngaarden, J. B., et al. (1992). *Cecil textbook of medicine* (19th ed.). Philadelphia: W. B. Saunders.

94. Yap, P. L. (1990). Transfusion transmitted viral infections—recent developments in blood donor screening. *Postgraduate Medical Journal, 66,* 906–909.

95. Yardley, J. (1989). Multiple myeloma. *Nursing 89, 3,* 4–7.

96. Yeager, K. A., & Miaskowski, C. (1994). Advances in understanding the mechanisms and management of acute myelogenous leukemia. *Oncology Nursing Forum, 21(3),* 541–548.

97. Yeomans, A. C., & Harle, M. T. (1990). Myelodysplastic syndromes. *Seminars in Oncology Nursing, 6,* 9–16.

98. Young, L. M. (1990). DIC: The insidious killer. *Critical Care Nursing, 10,* 26–33.

UNIT 9

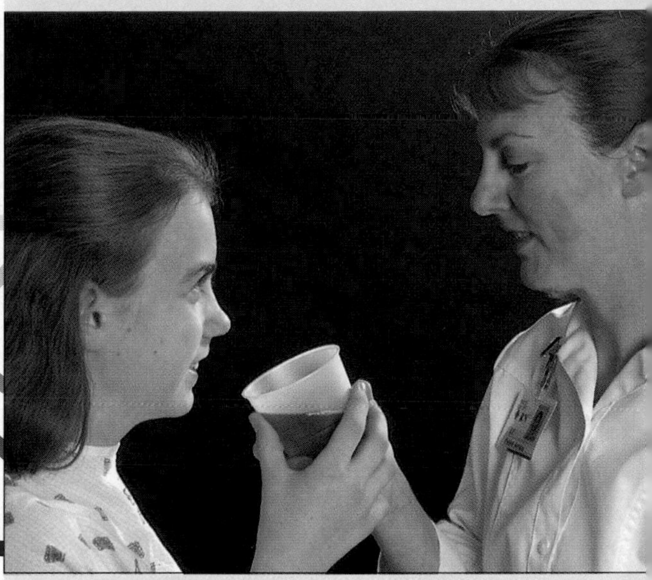

Urinary Disorders

Proper kidney function is vital, and because the bladder is connected to the kidneys, skillful care is crucial for both upper and lower urinary tract disorders. The acute care of clients with short-term, easily managed urinary disorders such as bladder infections is as important as the maintenance care of clients with long-term or terminal disorders such as chronic renal failure.

The nurse must remember to include the client's significant others in care planning to help ensure continuity of care between the health-care facility and the client's home. This is particularly important for clients with long-term urinary problems. Total care planning requires considering the client's and significant others' physical, sexual, emotional, social, spiritual, and cognitive needs, as well as drawing on all resources of the health-care team, the health-care facility, and the community.

This unit comprises three chapters. Following a concise review of urinary system structure and function, Chapter 29 describes the assessment of clients with urinary disorders. Specific disorders of the ureters, bladder, and urethra are discussed in Chapter 30, and disorders of the kidneys are covered in Chapter 31.

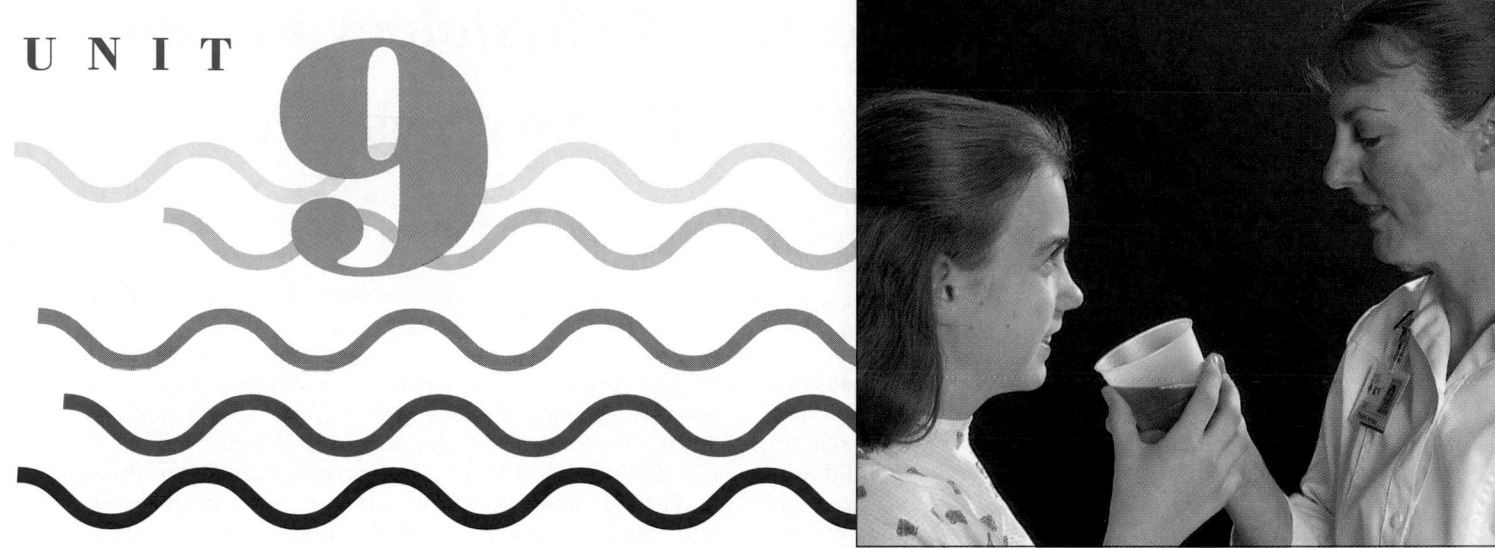

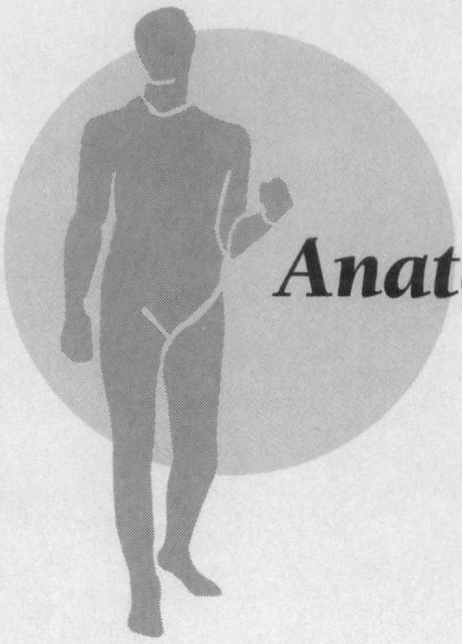

Anatomy and Physiology Review: Urinary System

The urinary system plays a major role in homeostasis by maintaining body fluid composition and volume. Through the formation of urine, the kidneys remove waste products from the body and regulate fluid volume, electrolyte concentration, blood pressure, and pH within the body. The ureters, bladder, and urethra transport and excrete the urine after it is formed.

COMPONENTS OF THE URINARY SYSTEM

Kidneys

The paired kidneys are located between the twelfth thoracic and third lumbar vertebrae, one on each side of the vertebral column. The right kidney usually is slightly lower than the left because the liver displaces it downward. The kidneys are retroperitoneal and lie against the muscles of the posterior abdominal wall. In the adult, each kidney is approximately 3 cm thick, 6 cm wide, and 12 cm long. It is roughly bean-shaped with an indentation, called the hilum, on the medial side. The renal artery, renal vein, lymphatics, and nerves pass through the hilum.

A tough white fibrous capsule surrounds the parenchyma of the kidney. The outer region, next to the capsule, is the cortex. This surrounds the medulla, which consists of a series of renal pyramids. The central region is the renal pelvis, which collects the urine as it is produced. The papillae of the pyramids project into cup-like extensions of the pelvis called calyces.

Each kidney contains over a million microscopic functional units, called nephrons. A nephron consists of two parts, the renal corpuscle and the renal tubule. The renal corpuscle consists of a cluster of capillaries, called the glomerulus, surrounded by a double-layered epithelial cup, called the glomerular capsule or Bowman's capsule. The renal tubule, which carries fluid away from the glomerular capsule, has three regions; the proximal convoluted tubule, the nephron loop (Henle's loop), and the distal convoluted tubule. Urine passes from the renal tubules into collecting ducts, then into the calyces.

In the region of contact between the ascending limb of the nephron loop and the glomerular afferent arteriole, the cells of the ascending limb are modified to form the macula densa, and those in the afferent arteriole are modified to form the juxtaglomerular cells. The macula densa and juxtaglomerular cells, together, make up the juxtaglomerular apparatus. The macula densa monitors sodium chloride in the urine and influences the juxtaglomerular cells, which produce the enzyme renin. Renin has a role in the regulation of blood pressure.

Blood flows through the kidneys at an approximate rate of 1200 mL/minute, which is 20 to 25 per cent of the cardiac output under resting conditions. Blood flow through the kidney follows the sequence of renal artery, segmental artery, interlobar artery, arcuate artery, interlobular artery, afferent arteriole, glomerulus, efferent ar-

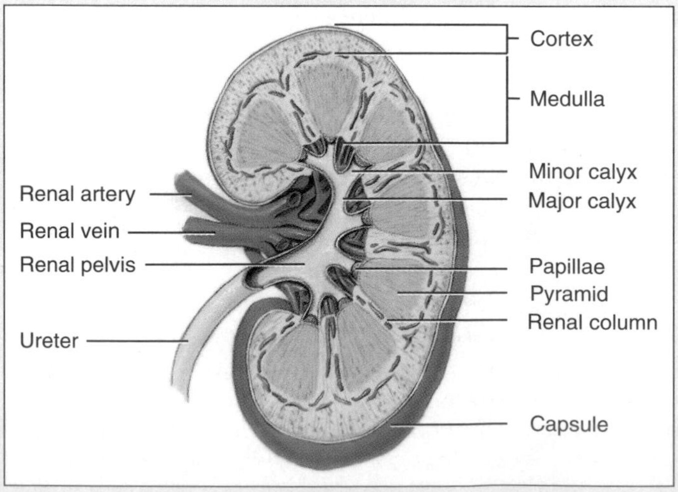

Macroscopic structure of the kidney.

Regions of a nephron.

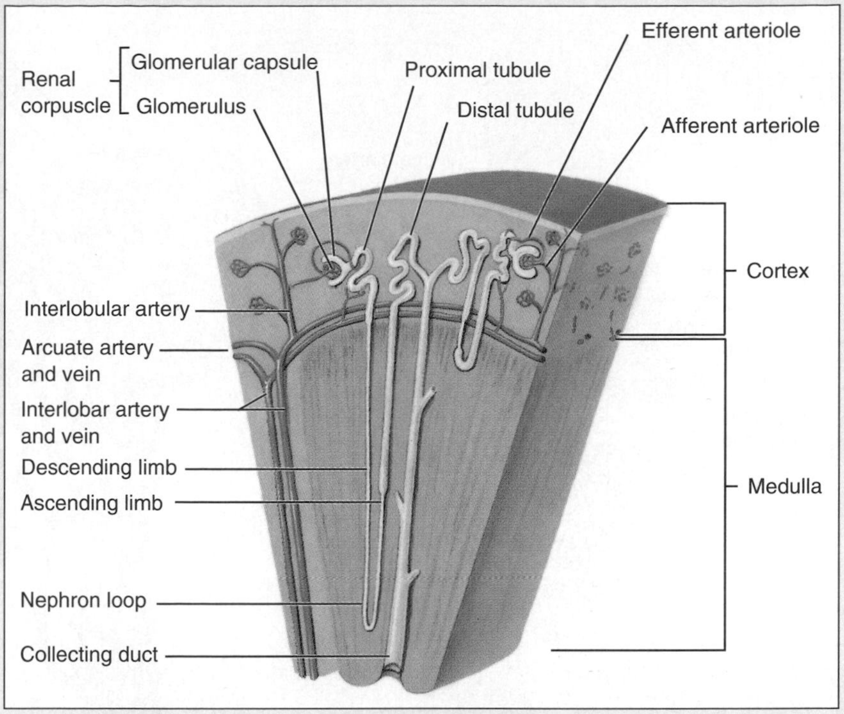

teriole, peritubular capillaries, interlobular vein, arcuate vein, interlobar vein, segmental vein, renal vein, inferior vena cava.

Nerves to the kidney enter the hilum and contain both sympathetic and parasympathetic components. The nerves terminate primarily on the walls of the blood vessels rather than in the tubules and appear to have a vasomotor function. A completely denervated kidney continues to form urine.

Ureters

Each ureter is a small tube, about 25 cm long, that carries urine from the renal pelvis, along the posterior abdominal wall, behind the parietal peritoneum, and into the urinary bladder on the posterior inferior surface. There are three regions where the lumen of the ureter narrows and there are potential points of obstruction:

- Where the ureter leaves the pelvis of the kidney
- Where the ureters cross the iliac arteries at the pelvic brim
- Where the ureters enter the urinary bladder

Renal calculi typically lodge in these regions because it is difficult for them to pass through the narrow passageway. The muscle arrangement in the wall allows urine to be propelled by peristaltic action. Blood is supplied by numerous vessels that run longitudinally along the tube.

Urinary Bladder

The urinary bladder is a temporary storage reservoir for urine. It is located in the pelvic cavity, posterior to the symphysis pubis, and below the parietal peritoneum. The size and shape vary with the amount of urine it contains and with pressure from surrounding organs. The muscular layer of the bladder wall contains smooth muscle fibers interwoven in all directions, and collectively, these are called the detrusor muscle. Contraction of this muscle expels urine from the bladder. A band of the detrusor muscle encircles the opening into the urethra to form the internal urethral sphincter. The trigone is a triangular region in the floor of the bladder that is outlined by the openings for the two ureters and the internal urethral orifice.

Urethra

The final passageway for the flow of urine is the urethra, a thin-walled tube that conveys urine from the floor of the urinary bladder to the outside of the body. The beginning of the urethra, where it leaves the urinary bladder, is surrounded by the smooth (involuntary) muscle that forms the internal urethral sphincter. The external urethral sphincter is skeletal (voluntary) muscle and encircles the urethra where it goes through the pelvic floor. These two sphincters control the flow of urine through the urethra. The female urethra is approximately 4 cm in length and opens to the outside

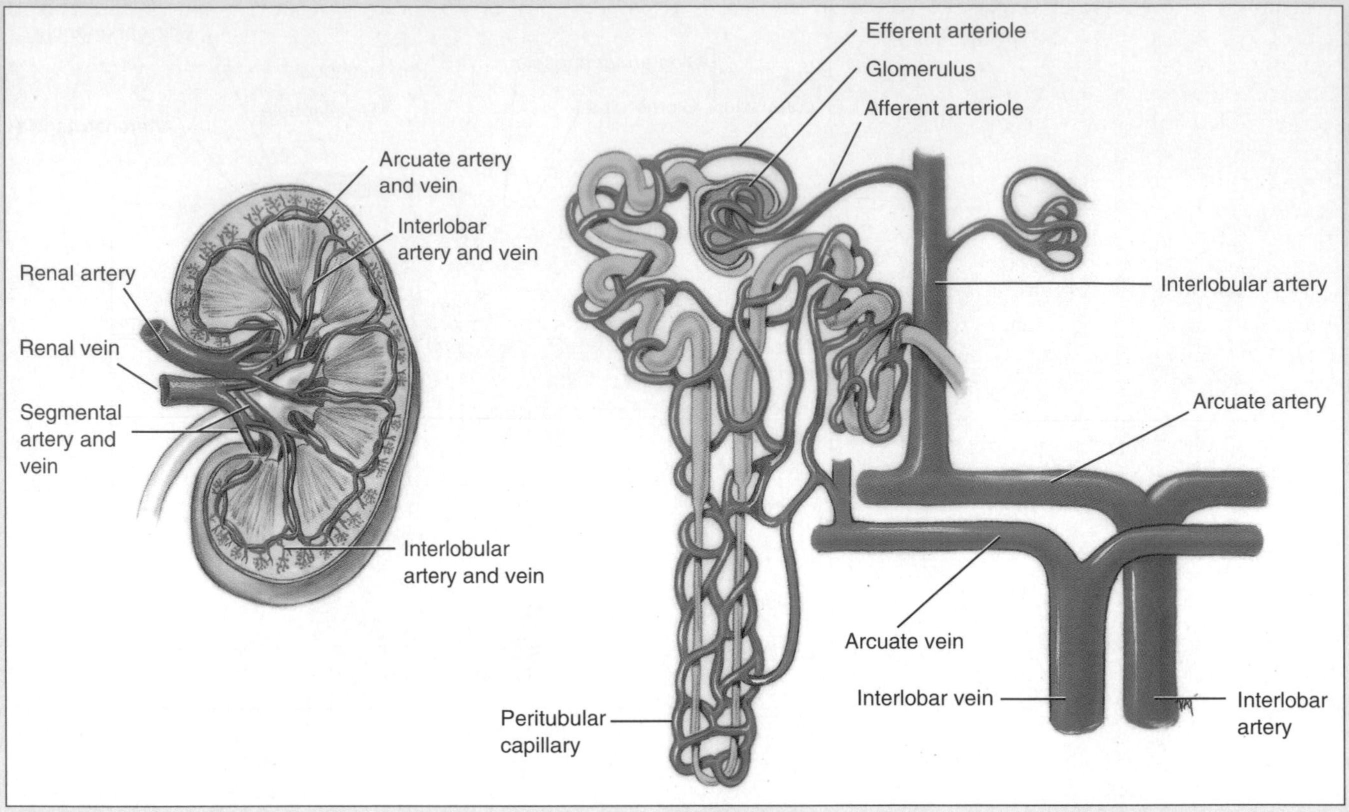

Blood flow through the kidney.

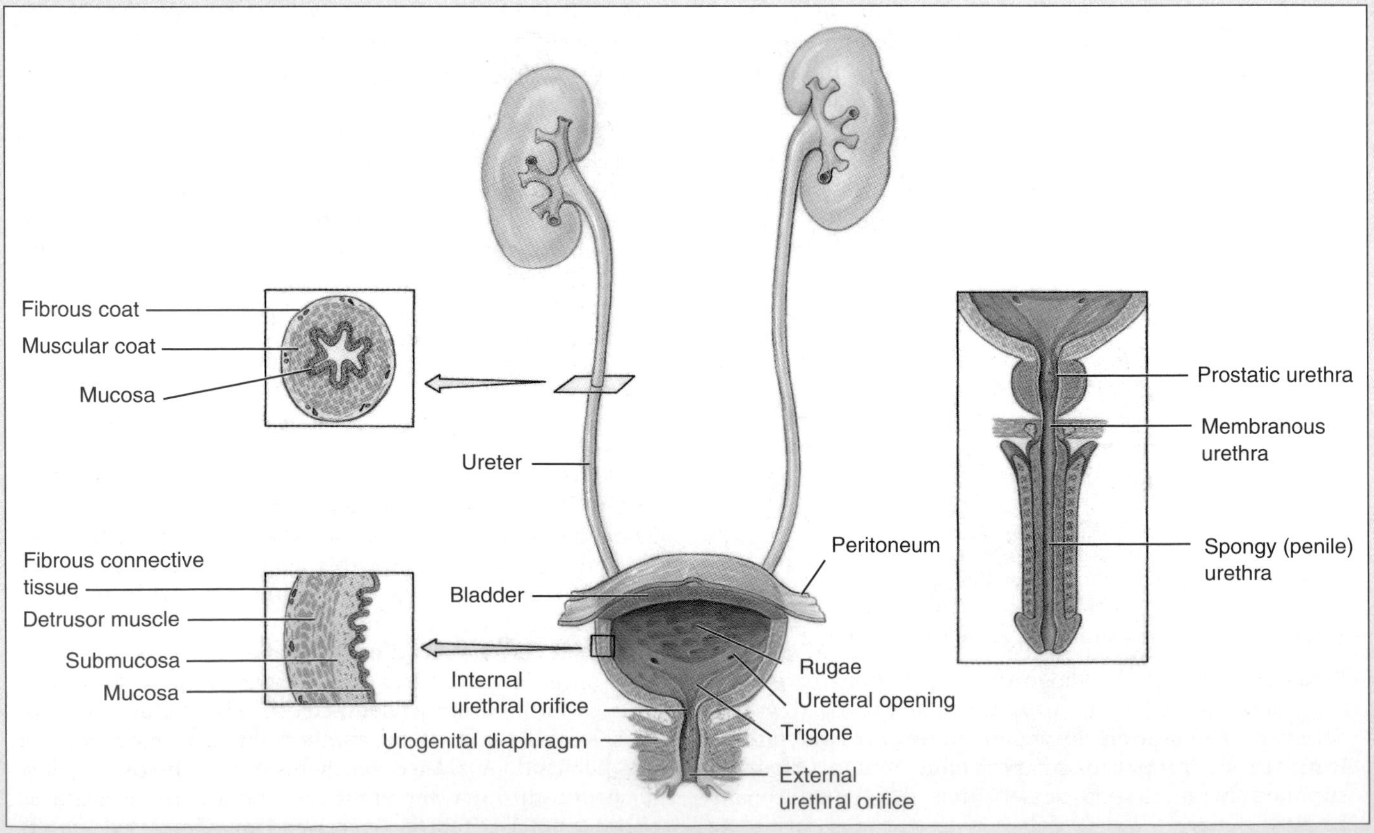

Ureter, urinary bladder, and urethra.

just anterior to the vaginal orifice. The male urethra is about 20 cm long and is anatomically connected to the reproductive system; it transports both urine and semen. The first part of the male urethra, next to the urinary bladder, passes through the prostate gland and is called the prostatic urethra. The prostate gland, although not a part of the urinary system, is a major cause of urinary dysfunction in men. The short middle region, the membranous urethra, passes through the pelvic floor and enters the penis. The third region, the spongy or penile urethra, extends the entire length of the penis, and the external urethral orifice (meatus) opens at the tip of the penis.

URINE FORMATION

The formation of urine in the kidneys involves three basic steps:

- Glomerular filtration
- Tubular reabsorption
- Tubular secretion

Glomerular Filtration

During the process of glomerular filtration, water and solutes move from the blood in the glomerular capillaries into the glomerular capsule. The force that moves the fluid is filtration pressure, and the fluid that enters the capsule is the filtrate. Normally, the filtrate in the glomerular capsule is similar in composition to blood plasma, except that the filtrate lacks plasma proteins. The composition is approximately 94 per cent water and 6 per cent solutes. In a diseased kidney, the filtration membrane may become too porous and may allow blood cells and proteins to pass through, which then appear in the urine. The glomerular filtration rate (GFR) is the amount of filtration that occurs within a given period of time. The GFR for a normal adult male of average size is approximately 125 mL/min, or 180 L/day. Several factors can influence the GFR, including:

- Pressure gradients:
  - Hydrostatic pressure in glomerular capillaries (systemic blood pressure)
  - Hydrostatic pressure in the glomerular capsule (renal edema)
  - Osmotic pressure in glomerular capillaries (due to plasma proteins)
- Rate of renal blood flow
- Permeability of glomerular membrane
- Changes in total surface area of glomerulus

Tubular Reabsorption

Tubular reabsorption is the movement of substances from the filtrate in the kidney tubules into the blood in the peritubular capillaries. Only about 1 per cent of the filtrate remains in the tubules and becomes urine. In general, water and other substances that are useful to the body are reabsorbed. Waste products, such as urea, phosphate, sulfate, uric acid, nitrate, and phenols, are poorly reabsorbed and remain in the filtrate to be excreted. Water is reabsorbed by osmosis, while most solutes are reabsorbed by active transport.

Tubular Secretion

Tubular secretion transports substances from the blood into the renal tubules. Potassium and hydrogen are the two primary ions eliminated from the body by this mechanism, although ammonia and uric acid are also included. Some drug metabolites, such as acetaminophen, probenecid, and penicillin, are excreted by this mechanism.

MICTURITION

Micturition, commonly called urination or voiding, is the act of expelling urine from the bladder. The bladder can hold up to a liter of urine, but normally when it contains 200 to 400 mL, stretch receptors in the bladder wall trigger impulses that initiate the micturition reflex. This is an automatic and involuntary response that is coordinated in the spinal cord. Then, impulses are transmitted along parasympathetic nerves to the detrusor muscle. Even though the micturition reflex is involuntary, it can be inhibited or stimulated by higher brain centers.

THE ROLE OF KIDNEYS IN REGULATING BODY FLUID COMPOSITION

Feedback systems between the nephrons and the body fluids alter filtration, reabsorption, and secretion to regulate the body fluid volume and composition.

Fluid Volume

Assuming that the renal blood flow is adequate, the fluid volumes are maintained principally through the action of antidiuretic hormone (ADH) in the collecting ducts. A solute concentration gradient is maintained throughout the interstitium of the medulla, with a low concentration near the cortex and a higher concentration near the renal pelvis. The collecting ducts progress through this concentration gradient. If ADH is present, the collecting ducts are permeable to water and water is reabsorbed to retain fluid and increase body fluid volume. If ADH is not present, the collecting ducts are not permeable to water, and excess fluids are removed in a dilute urine. A related mechanism that helps regulate fluid volume involves stretch receptors in the atria of the heart. When these receptors are stimulated by in-

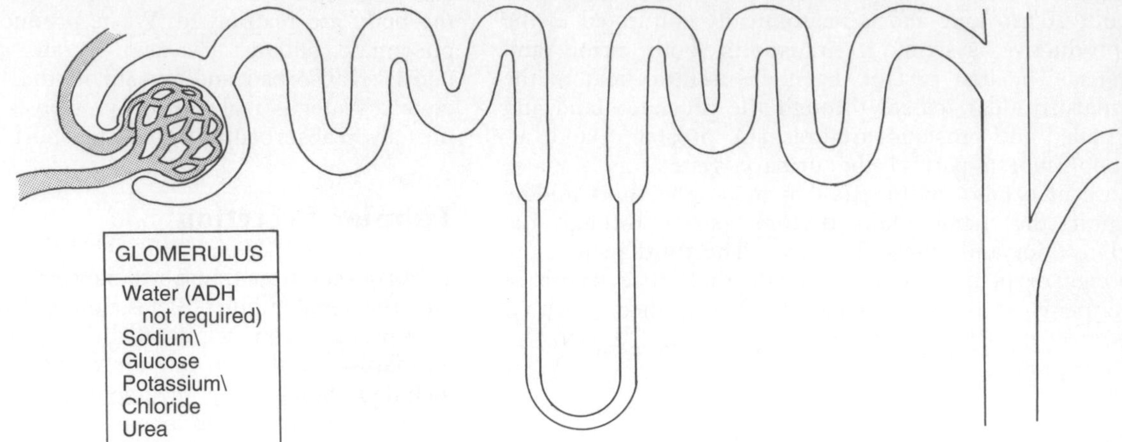

	GLOMERULUS	PROXIMAL TUBULE	LOOP OF HENLE	DISTAL TUBULE	COLLECTING DUCT
GLOMERULAR FILTRATION (from blood into filtrate)	Water (ADH not required) Sodium\ Glucose Potassium\ Chloride Urea Urate Uric acid Proteins Amino acids Bicarbonate Creatinine Phosphate Inulin* PAH*	Isotonic filtrate	Hypertonic filtrate	Isotonic or hypotonic filtrate	Hypertonic or hypotonic filtrate
TUBULAR REABSORPTION (from filtrate into blood)		Water (ADH not required) Sodium Glucose Potassium Chloride Urea Urate Uric acid Proteins Amino acids Carbon dioxide	Water Sodium Chloride Urea Urate Carbon dioxide	Water (ADH required) Sodium Chloride Urea Urate Carbon dioxide	Water (ADH required) Sodium Chloride Urea Urate Carbon dioxide
TUBULAR SECRETION (from blood into filtrate)		Creatinine Hydrogen PAH*		Potassium Uric acid Hydrogen	Potassium Hydrogen

Processes in urine formation. *Although inulin and para-aminohippuric acid (PAH) are not normally present, they are important test substances. (From Black, J. M., & Matassarin-Jacobs, E. [Eds.]. [1993]. *Luckmann and Sorensen's Medical-Surgical Nursing: A Psychophysiologic Approach* (4th ed.). Philadelphia: W. B. Saunders Co.)

creased venous return and pressure due to increased fluid volume, certain cells in the heart release atrial natriuretic hormone. This hormone inhibits the secretion of ADH.

Electrolyte Concentration

Electrolyte concentration and fluid volume are interrelated because the electrolytes are dissolved in the body fluids, and when fluid volume changes, the concentration of the electrolytes also changes. The primary regulation of electrolyte balance is through active reabsorption of positive ions. The negative ions follow by electrochemical attraction. Because sodium and potassium are the predominant cations, they are the most important ones to be regulated. Aldosterone, acting on the kidney tubules, regulates sodium and potassium levels by stimulating the reabsorption of sodium ions from the filtrate into the blood and the secretion of potassium ions in the urine.

Hydrogen Ion Concentration

In the presence of acid-base imbalances, the kidneys excrete either hydrogen or bicarbonate ions to restore balance. Normally, the cells of the renal tubules secrete equivalent amounts of hydrogen and bicarbonate. In acidosis (decreased pH), excess hydrogen ions are secreted into the nephron tubules and collecting ducts and excreted in the urine. When needed, the kidneys can also regenerate new bicarbonate by the following reaction:

$$CO_2 + H_2O \longrightarrow H_2CO_3 \longrightarrow H^+ + HCO_3^-$$

The hydrogen ion is excreted in the urine and the bicarbonate is reabsorbed into the interstitial fluid, which helps to increase pH back toward normal. With alkalosis (increased pH), the kidneys stop excreting hydrogen ions and may actually excrete bicarbonate ions in the urine to restore normal pH.

Regulation of fluid volume.

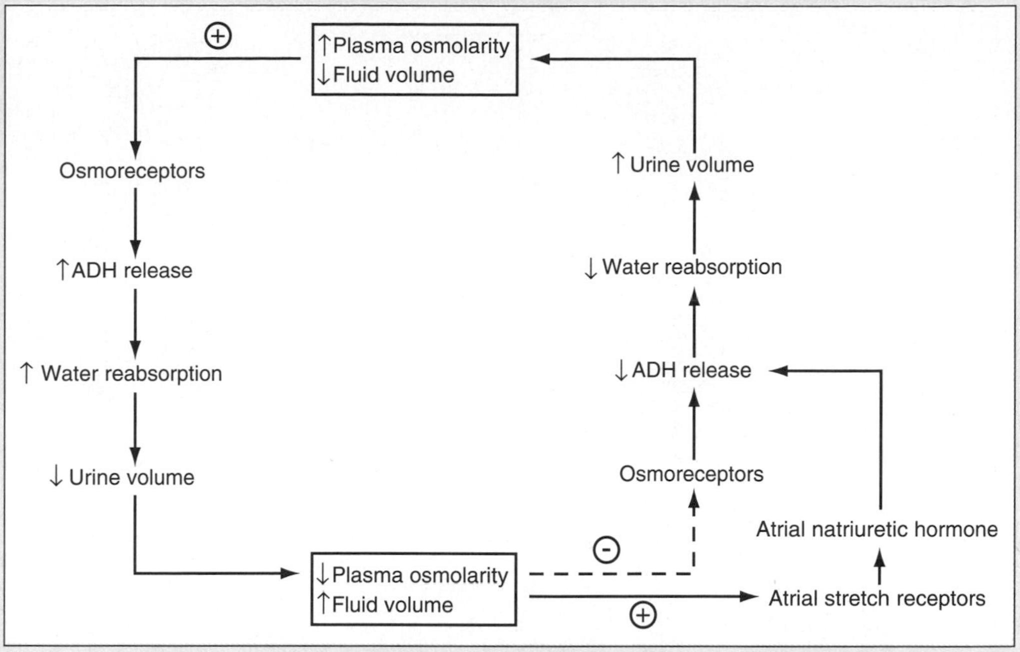

THE ROLE OF KIDNEYS IN THE REGULATION OF BLOOD PRESSURE

The kidneys have a role in the regulation of blood pressure primarily through the renin-angiotensin-aldosterone system. When arterial blood pressure drops, renal blood flow decreases, which stimulates the release of renin from the juxtaglomerular cells. Renin acts on angiotensin substrates in the blood to cause the formation of angiotensin II, which is a powerful vasoconstrictor. Vasoconstriction increases peripheral resistance, which increases the blood pressure toward normal. Angiotensin also stimulates aldosterone secretion from the adrenal cortex. Aldosterone facilitates the reabsorption of sodium and water from the nephron tubules, which results in increased blood volume and increased blood pressure.

METABOLIC AND ENDOCRINE FUNCTIONS OF THE KIDNEYS

In addition to the production of renin, the kidney has several other metabolic and endocrine functions:

Age-Related Change in the Kidney

STRUCTURAL CHANGE	FUNCTIONAL MANIFESTATION
Atrophy and modification of glomeruli	Decreased glomerular filtration rate
Thickening of tubule walls	Less able to reabsorb water, glucose, and sodium; less effective tubular secretion of hydrogen ions and drugs
Weakening and decreased elasticity of detrusor muscle	Reduces capacity of bladder and makes it more difficult to completely empty it
Increased irritability of bladder wall	Adds urgency to normal desire to void
Weakening of external urethral sphincter	Incontinence

- **Synthesis of 1,25-dihydroxycholecalciferol**, a hormone derived from vitamin D. It facilitates the absorption of dietary calcium from the intestine and works with parathyroid hormone to maintain calcium homeostasis.
- **Biogenesis of erythropoietin**, a glycoprotein that stimulates the production of red blood cells in the bone marrow.
- **Degradation of insulin**, a hormone secreted by the pancreas that regulates carbohydrate metabolism. About 20 per cent of the insulin is removed from circulation and broken down by the kidneys.
- **Synthesis of prostaglandins**, derivatives of arachidonic acid that have actions similar to hormones. Prostaglandins have localized effects and act on kidney components to regulate renal function. It appears that they are not essential for renal function in healthy people, but their actions become important when renal function is compromised.
- **Production of energy**, necessary to maintain active transport mechanisms in the kidney. The reabsorption of sodium by active transport is the primary cause for energy use in the kidney and requires that more energy be produced. The provision of this energy is the major metabolic activity of the kidney.

AGE-RELATED CHANGES

Several structural changes occur in the urinary system as a person ages. These changes are reflected in the related functions. Because of these changes, elderly persons may have problems with incontinence, frequency, retention, and dysuria. They are able to maintain relatively stable balances in the blood and body fluids under normal conditions; however, their ability to compensate for drastic changes and abnormal conditions is diminished.

Chapter 29 Assessment of Clients with Urinary Disorders

Learning Outcomes

After completing this chapter, the learner will be able to:

1. Teach the client about the normal structure and function of the urinary system.
2. Explain to the client abnormalities of urinary structure and function.
3. Conduct a nursing history and physical assessment of the client with actual or potential disorders of the urinary system.
4. Teach the client about diagnostic studies common to the urinary system.

The physical examination and specific diagnostic studies used to assess urinary function can be distressing. For example, providing a urine specimen may be embarrassing, especially if the client has to carry the full container down the hall or bring it from home. Some studies require the client to urinate in front of others as with a voiding cystogram or urinary flow rate. When assessing the client, the nurse must keep in mind the client's likely embarrassment or discomfort and be understanding. The nurse should provide as much privacy as possible.

Use of good communication skills is the key to obtaining complete and accurate information. The nurse should allow the client to express anxiety and, in turn, try to make the client comfortable and at ease. The nurse must be aware of what the client communicates nonverbally, because subtle clues may be crucial to diagnosing the client's problem.

HISTORY

As with other systems, history taking is probably the most important part of the assessment process. Most problems usually are discovered at this point. A urologic history consists of the chief complaint and current health history, past medical history, family history, psychosocial history and life-style, and review of symptoms. If the client reports urologic symptoms, a detailed symptom analysis is performed.

Chief Complaint

Common major symptoms in urologic disorders include a change in the usual patterns of voiding, pain, and associated gastrointestinal symptoms. More than one symptom may be present, and each is explored with the client.

CHANGE IN URINARY PATTERNS AND CHARACTERISTICS

The client is asked to describe his or her usual patterns of voiding, including frequency, amount, and usual times of the day or night. The nurse should ask if there are any particular methods the client uses to stimulate urination, such as listening to running water, applying pressure over the lower abdomen, or performing the Valsalva maneuver. The nurse should ask the following questions: Does the client experience difficulty starting or maintaining the urine stream (hesitancy)? Has there been a change in the force or shape of the stream? Does the client have feelings of urgency or difficulty controlling the process of urinating? If so, is the urgency associated with a known factor such as consuming caffeine or, for women, following pregnancy and vaginal delivery? Older men may report gradually diminishing urine stream force and hesitancy if they have enlargement of the prostate gland.

Changes in urine characteristics are explored in detail. The nurse should ask the client what the urine usually looked like before symptoms were present; what the usual color and odor were; what the color and odor are now; whether the urine is clear or cloudy; and whether there are particles present, such as clots, mucus, or shreds of tissue? Infection of the urinary tract results in inflammation so that the urine becomes cloudy with debris.

URINE INCONTINENCE

Urine incontinence is the loss of control over the release of urine from the bladder. The nurse asks the client to describe the onset and associated symptoms that occur with incontinence. The following questions should be asked: How often does it occur? Is there dribbling of urine between voidings? If so, how much? Does incontinence occur at predictable times, such as with coughing, sneezing, and laughing? Does the client have an awareness of the need to void prior to incontinent episodes? How long has the client had difficulty with incontinence? Is the problem getting worse? What methods does the client use to cope with incontinence? The client may have concerns about strike-through wetness on clothing or odor being noticeable to others and may resort to using pads or shields for protection.

PAIN

The client is asked to describe any pain associated with the urinary tract, including its location, type, severity, and duration. The client is also asked whether the pain is getting worse or better; whether he or she is able to relate factors that may have precipitated the pain; what makes the pain better; what makes it worse; whether the pain is accompanied by uncomfortable or painful urination (dysuria) and, if dysuria is present, when during voiding it occurs.

A careful description of any pain may help pinpoint the source of the problem. Kidney pain, which is usually caused by sudden distention of the renal capsule, produces a dull, constant ache in the costovertebral angle.

Ureteral pain is exhibited as back pain from capsular distention and as colicky pain caused by spasm of the renal pelvis and ureteral muscle. It radiates from the costovertebral angle down across the abdomen to the genital area.

The most common bladder discomfort arises from overdistention and is felt in the suprapubic area. Bladder infection causes urgency spasms or a burning pain or both during micturition in the distal urethra for females and in the prostatic urethra for males. Urethral pain is usually felt along the course of the urethra or meatus.

Determining precisely when during the act of micturition burning occurs helps differentiate between bladder and urethral origins. Burning at the beginning of urination (as the bladder contracts the inflamed tissue where the bladder drains into the urethra) indicates urethritis. Bladder infection should be suspected when the burning occurs during and after the voiding process.

GASTROINTESTINAL SYMPTOMS

Urinary tract disorders may be accompanied by gastrointestinal symptoms, such as anorexia, nausea, vomiting, diarrhea, or a metallic taste in the mouth. The unpleasantness of these symptoms may lead the client to alter the amount and type of fluids consumed. The nurse should ask the client to describe the amounts and types of fluids consumed in a day. The nurse determines how the fluid intake compares with the urinary output; whether the client has unusual fluid loss from diarrhea, vomiting, or excess perspiration; and whether there have been weight changes (loss or gain) of 2 pounds or more within a 24-hour period. Such weight fluctuations are usually related to a change in fluid balance.

The anatomic proximity of the kidneys and gastrointestinal structures may mean that intestinal disturbances will mimic renal disorders. This partially explains why clients experience nausea and vomiting, anorexia, diarrhea, and abdominal discomfort concomitantly with urinary tract symptoms. Renal inflammation may also produce signs of peritoneal irritation.

Past Medical History

The past medical history explores the client's experiences with disorders of the urinary tract. These data may be linked to current health problems or may be associated with increased risk for the client to develop urinary tract disorders. A childhood history of problems with urination should be included; such problems often recur during adulthood.

MAJOR ILLNESSES AND HOSPITALIZATIONS

The client is asked about previous hospitalizations or treatment for urinary problems. The nurse determines the date of illnesses or hospitalization, the specific urinary problem, medical treatment (including surgery or manipulation of the urinary tract such as catheterization), and the present status of the problem. The nurse should ask whether the client has undergone diagnostic studies of the urinary tract such as an intravenous pyelogram (IVP) or cystogram. Results of these studies can provide baseline data for assessment of the current problem.

The nurse should ask the client whether there has been trauma to the urinary tract such as a direct blow to the flank or falls with resulting contusion over the lower posterior thorax. He or she should specifically inquire about how the problem was treated and what the result was and should inquire about specific surgical procedures that involve urinary diversion. The nurse should ask: Why was the surgery necessary? Is the diversion temporary or permanent? How does the client manage the diversion or are there problems with its management?

Major illnesses and disease that are linked to urinary tract problems include hypertension, diabetes mellitus, gout, and connective tissue disorders (e.g., scleroderma, systemic lupus erythematosus). The nurse should ask the client about problems with urinary tract stones (calculi) as well as urinary tract infections and systemic infections.

MEDICATIONS

A complete medication history is obtained, including past use, because many drugs are nephrotoxic. The nurse determines the quantity and length of use for medications, because the nephrotoxic effects of certain drugs are dose-specific. Diuretics alter the quantity of urine output. Phenazopyridine (Pyridium) and nitrofurantoin (Macrodantin) alter urine color. Anticoagulants may cause hematuria. Other medications that can affect the urinary tract include antibiotics, narcotics, cholinergics, rifampin, aminophylline, and oncologic agents. Over-the-counter medications that can affect the urinary tract include nonsteroidal anti-inflammatory agents (ibuprofen) and salicylates.

ALLERGIES

The nurse asks the client about allergies to foods, dyes, and medications. Specifically, he or she should inquire about allergies to shellfish, seafood, and iodine. The client should be asked whether he or she has ever had a diagnostic test in which a contrast medium was used and what the result was.

Family History

A family history of certain renal and urinary disorders increases the risk of the client developing similar problems. In addition to asking about hypertension, diabetes mellitus, gout, and recurrent urinary tract infections, the nurse should ask about congenital urinary tract disorders, polycystic kidney disease, nephritis, and urinary calculi.

Psychosocial History and Life-Style

Urinary tract disorders affect many aspects of the client's life, including his or her psychological, social, and occupational life, as well as physical factors.

PSYCHOSOCIAL FACTORS

Psychological Factors. The nurse should assess the client's emotional reaction to the history-taking process and to the physical examination. Just as people are emotionally affected by the performance of the urinary system, so is the urinary system affected by emotions in a number of ways, such as by (1) past experiences, (2) the power of suggestion, (3) anxiety and fear, (4) depression, (5) changes in body image, and (6) the fear of death.

Past Experiences. A client's past experiences produce various effects on the process of voiding. Cultural teachings lead most people to consider the act of micturition a private matter.

Experiences linked with childhood toilet training can have long-lasting effects. A client's negative or positive attitudes toward bladder elimination can sometimes be traced back to this developmental period. The guilt or shame from prolonged enuresis (involuntary discharge of urine, usually during sleep at night or bedwetting) may cause voiding dysfunction long after the enuresis has been cured.

Power of Suggestion. The micturition control center is connected to the various sensory portions of the brain, allowing micturition to be initiated by any number of auditory, visual, or somesthetic stimuli, such as running water in a sink. In fact, the mere act of thinking about voiding may be enough to stimulate the reflex.

Anxiety and Fear. Anxiety may stimulate or hinder micturition. The most noticeable effect of anxiety is to increase the frequency of voidings and produce urgency. Anxiety also may intensify the manifestations of urinary tract disorders and make pain seem worse.

Changes in Body Image. Many urinary disorders necessitate a change in body image and life-style, which, in turn, may lead to anxiety, depression, or anger. Changes that affect body image include an inability to control body functions such as urination, a dependence on others, and a dependency on machines or devices. Anatomic alterations that alter the way urine leaves the body are sometimes surgically created. If the client is unable to produce urine at all, dialysis must be performed. These dramatic and often permanent alterations can destroy a client's healthy body image.

Fear of Death. The possibility of impending death is a real concern for clients with urinary tract problems because most realize that a functioning urinary system is necessary for life. Urinary tract cancers and renal failure are problems that are most likely to cause fear of death. Whether the problem is large or small, it is always possible that a urinary disorder may become terminal.

The nurse must learn as much as possible about the client's psychological disposition. He or she should carefully listen to conversation and observe behavior patterns and look for indirect cues in the way the client answers questions or initiates conversation. Subtle cues may be camouflaged in seemingly unconscious statements.

Whatever communication techniques the nurse uses, the nurse should consciously assess the client's emotional state to provide appropriate referrals and supportive care.

LIFE-STYLE

Urinary problems may cause a change in life-style. To assess the kind and extent of changes that may occur, baseline data are collected in the following areas:

- living conditions
- support systems
- financial status
- occupation
- hobbies and leisure activities
- habits

PHYSICAL EXAMINATION

The physical examination is based on the information obtained during the history-taking process. Although most of the data needed come directly from examining the urinary system, consider other systems, too.

Urinary Tract Organs

KIDNEYS

The nurse inspects for masses in the upper abdomen and flank areas. Typically, because of the location of the kidneys, only the lower poles of the right kidney can be felt on deep palpation done by nurse clinicians and physicians.

Depending on the size of the client and the skill of the examiner, it may be possible to outline both kidneys anteriorly and posteriorly by percussion. This technique is particularly helpful when pain and muscle spasm prevent proper palpation. The nurse can assess costovertebral angle tenderness by placing the left hand over the area and striking it with the right fist. Ordinarily, this percussion would produce a dull sound and no discomfort. With inflammation, there is exquisite tenderness.

BLADDER

As the bladder distends, it rises out of the pelvic cavity above the pubic symphysis. In a very thin client or one with a very distended bladder, it may be visible on inspection and palpated. When a distended bladder is palpated, it is felt as a smooth, round, and rather tense mass. The adult bladder can be percussed if it contains at least 150 mL of urine. Percussion is accomplished in the normal manner, with the sound of bowel often being hollow and the sound of the distended bladder being duller. The bladder can be outlined and may extend as high as the umbilicus. After the initial assessment, the client should void and then the nurse should palpate and percuss again to distinguish the bladder from a possible mass. Residual urine also could be measured at this point. This test is discussed later in this chapter.

URETHRA

Urethral examination primarily involves inspecting the external meatus and the perineal area for signs of discharge, abnormal tissue growth, cleanliness, and anatomic integrity. Aberrant location of the meatus should be noted. The nurse should palpate the penis for masses along the distal portion of the male urethra, and palpate the perineal area for tenderness. In the female, the posterior urethra is examined vaginally for masses, tenderness, or expressed discharge from the urethra.

The size and patency of the meatus and the urethra can be evaluated by the urologist by passing instruments of varying diameter through the urethra. This evaluation is performed with different sizes of rubber or plastic catheters or, if preferred, special urologic instruments.

ALTERNATIVE URINARY OUTLET

The client who has had a urinary diversion procedure, such as an ileal conduit or continent urinary reservoir, will have an opening in the abdominal wall. The nurse should assess this stoma and note its location, size, shape, color, intactness, and odor and observe the quality and quantity of the drainage. In addition, the nurse evaluates the condition of the periostomal skin for color, cleanliness, intactness, and the absence of lesions such as maceration and irritation. For the client with the ileal conduit, the nurse observes the cleanliness and appropriateness of the urine collection system to assess the client's teaching and learning needs. Finally, the client's responses during this part of the examination may indicate the client's acceptance of the altered urinary function.

The client may have a catheter that partially or completely drains the urine from the body. The catheter may be inserted into the bladder, ureter, or a kidney, and may come out of the body through the urethra, the abdomen, or flank wall. The nurse should inspect these catheters during the examination, checking them for patency, location, and cleanliness. The nurse should palpate the tubing for sedimentation by rolling it between the thumb and fingers and feeling for a sandy or gritty sensation. The tissues around the catheter where it enters the body should be observed for cleanliness and the absence of lesions such as inflammation and ulceration. The nurse should discuss the self-care methods that are being used by the client.

Related Body Systems

Selected information from other body systems is crucial for correctly assessing urinary tract problems and planning interventions.

FLUID STATUS

Accurate intake and output measurements help determine the client's fluid status. Intake or output of disproportionate amounts of fluid may indicate volume excess or depletion. Keeping track of intake and output helps identify the presence of important signs of abnormal kidney function, such as oliguria, anuria, and polyuria.

BOX 29-1

Urine Output Abnormalities

- *Oliguria* refers to significantly decreased urine volume, usually 400 mL in 24 hours (134 mL in 8 hours).
- *Anuria* is the absence of urine production (or less than 100 mL in 24 hours). Anuria and oliguria may indicate shock, poisoning, or any other process that would interfere with urine formation in the kidney. Anuria would, of course, be a normal finding in clients undergoing renal dialysis.
- *Polyuria* refers to significantly greater than normal urine output. It can be caused by disorders such as acute or chronic renal failure, diabetes mellitus, and diabetes insipidus, or by interventions such as diuretic administration.

The normal adult on a regular diet who takes in about 1200 to 1500 mL of measurable fluids daily should excrete 1200 to 1500 mL of urine plus insensible fluid loss in a 24-hour period. When determining the presence of oliguria, anuria, or polyuria, the nurse must remember that the output is in relation to normal intake (Box 29–1).

Body weight is a good indicator of fluid gains and losses, provided it is carefully measured daily and compared with previous findings. A gain or loss of more than 2 pounds in 24 hours is considered related to fluid loss or retention.

CRITICAL TO REMEMBER

Dry mucous membranes may signal volume depletion, whereas the presence of edema may be a sign of volume excess.

In assessing edema, it is important to determine its progresssion or recession. Measuring the girth of edematous parts daily provides accurate, objective documentation.

NEUROLOGIC STATUS

The urinary tract depends on an intact nervous system in order to carry out its main function: removing waste from the body. Any abnormality in nervous stimulation to the urinary organs or their surrounding tissue interferes with the propulsion and expulsion of urine. Other tests evaluating relevant neurologic activity are described in this chapter.

INTEGUMENTARY STATUS

The nurse should note the color of the skin when assessing renal dysfunction. For instance, erythropoietin deficiency anemia may cause pallor. Deposits of a carotene-like substance, caused by renal excretion failure, may give the skin a yellowish gray cast. Dry skin may indicate chronic renal failure and may also suggest volume depletion. Bruises or petechiae may represent bleeding tendencies. Crystal deposits on the skin (found primarily in areas of concentrated perspiration) is a secondary sign of severe, prolonged renal failure.

MUSCULOSKELETAL STATUS

Specific muscle groups involved in micturition are the perineal and abdominal muscles. To assess their strength, the nurse should have the client consciously contract or tighten the perineal and abdominal muscles. The ability to purposely interrupt the flow of urine midstream by perineal muscle contraction also indicates adequate perineal musculature.

CARDIOVASCULAR STATUS

Monitoring the cardiovascular system can identify fluid and electrolyte imbalances. Most specific to the urinary tract is blood pressure measurement. Hypertension is a finding in many renal diseases and may result from fluid volume overload or disturbance of the reninangiotension system.

CRITICAL TO REMEMBER

Increasing hypertension can possibly lead to irreversible renal shutdown, and thus requires immediate medical action.

RESPIRATORY STATUS

To some extent, the quality of respirations reflects the client's fluid and acid-base balances. Respiratory assessment is discussed further in Chapter 19. In addition, during renal failure, the breath may have an odor of urine or fruit-flavored gum, which is the result of toxins built up in the bloodstream.

OTHER SYSTEMS

A vaginal and rectal examination are routinely performed to assess urinary problems. If appropriate, the nurse should inspect and palpate these two orifices to help identify fistulas, masses, prolapses, and diverticula. In the male, because of the proximity to the rectum, the posterior lobe of the prostate can be examined for enlargement, tenderness, or masses. In the female, a vaginal examination can detect prolapse of the bladder.

DIAGNOSTIC TESTS

A number of diagnostic tests are available to evaluate the status of the urinary system. They include laboratory tests; x-ray, ultrasonographic, and radioisotope studies; pressure profiles; and surgical exploration. The history, physical examination, and results of previous studies determine which procedures to use.

Laboratory Tests

URINE STUDIES

Collection of Specimens. The nurse and appropriate others—the individual, people in the household, laboratory personnel—all share responsibility for collection of specimens.

The types of urine specimens include random, clean-catch (midstream), catheter, 12-hour, and 24-hour.

Random Specimens. A random specimen is one that can be collected at any time. However, an early morning specimen gives more definitive results for some values. Generally, the client needs no special preparation, although a female client may be asked to wash the perineal area to clean away any collected debris. The specimen is then collected in any clean container. This type of specimen cannot be used for culture and sensitivity tests, because the lack of specific perineal cleaning and the use of an unsterile container contaminate the specimen.

Clean-Catch Specimens. The goal of a clean-catch, or midstream, specimen is to reduce as much as possible the contamination of the specimen by external organisms. This type of specimen is usually collected if the urine is to be cultured. Uncircumcised men are asked to withdraw the foreskin before voiding to decrease the risk of contamination.

Catheter Specimens. A catheterized specimen may be used for culture. This procedure should be avoided when possible because of the increased risk of introducing organisms into the urethra or bladder during the catheterization. In renal failure especially, there may not be enough urine produced to wash out these bacteria, thus increasing the risk of urinary tract infection.

A specimen also may be collected from an indwelling catheter. Urine standing in the collection bag undergoes several chemical changes, may be contaminated with bacteria, and does not reflect the client's current urinary status. For these reasons, it should never be used for urine specimens. Instead, the specimen should be obtained from the catheter or drainage tubing. Opening the drainage system to the air can introduce microorganisms. Most urinary drainage systems have a specimen collection port built into the top of the drainage tubing. This self-sealing rubber-covered area is cleansed, and the urine is aspirated with a sterile needle and syringe. The tubing may need to be clamped for 15 to 20 minutes below the port to allow enough urine to build up.

12-Hour or 24-Hour Specimens. A 12-hour or 24-hour specimen is usually collected in one large container. Some of the specimens may need a chemical preservative in the container and refrigeration during the collection process. If appropriate refrigeration is not available, the specimen container may be packed in ice or insulated ice packs. In this case, the nurse should make sure the cooling agent is replaced frequently enough to maintain the specimen at the necessary temperature. When the specimen collection begins, the client voids and this specimen is discarded. All urine voided in the next 12 or 24 hours, as appropriate, is placed in the container. Twelve or 24 hours from the time of the first voiding, the nurse instructs the client to void again and add this urine to the specimen. One of the major needs during this collection process is careful communication among all persons involved. If any single urine specimen is inadvertently discarded, the entire procedure must begin again.

Examination of the Urine. The urine can be examined by direct visualization, microscopy, or laboratory tests. The results of these examinations may indicate pathologic changes in the urinary tract as well as in other parts of the body.

Routine Urinalysis. A routine urinalysis is usually performed on a single, random specimen, although a midstream or catheter specimen may be used. Table 29–1 summarizes the usual observations made during this test and the normal findings.

Color. The color of urine normally ranges from pale yellow to deep amber, depending on its concentration. Some color changes occur because of medications or food ingested, whereas other colors may indicate pathologic processes. Foods that often cause red urine include blackberries, rhubarb, beets, and foods containing red dyes. Ingesting large amounts of carotene causes a bright yellow urine. Table 29–2 shows some common medications that produce urinary color changes.

The most common significant color change indicating a pathologic disorder results from bleeding in the urinary tract. Bleeding in the upper tract produces dark red or smoky gray urine, whereas bleeding in the lower tract appears as red urine. Other color changes from pathologic conditions include red-brown or tea-colored urine, due to the release of myoglobin from severely damaged muscle tissue, dark yellow or green urine indicating the presence of urobilinogen or bilirubin, and green urine produced by *Pseudomonas* organisms.

Opacity. Freshly voided urine is normally transparent. Increases in opacity denoting a pathologic condition usually result from the presence of bacteria, crystals, or other foreign material in the urine.

TABLE 29–1 Normal Findings in a Routine Urinalysis

COMPONENT	NORMAL VALUES
Color	Pale yellow to deep amber
Opacity	Clear
Specific gravity	1.002–1.035
Osmolality	275–295 mOsm/L
pH	4.5–8.0
Glucose	Negative
Ketones	Negative
Protein	Negative
Bilirubin	Negative
Red blood cells	None to 3
White blood cells	None to 4
Bacteria	None
Casts	None
Crystals	None

TABLE 29–2 Common Medications that Produce Urinary Color Change

MEDICATION	COLOR CHANGE IN URINE
Amitriptyline	Blue
Anthraquinone laxatives	Reddish brown in acid urine; red in alkaline urine
Chloroquine	Rusty-yellow
Chlorzoxazone	Orange or purple-red
Levodopa or methyldopa	Red or brown in hypochlorite toilet bleach
Methylene blue	Green
Multiple vitamins (with riboflavin)	Bright yellow
Phenazopyridine	Orange-brown, orange-red, or red
Phenolphthalein	Pink-red in alkaline urine
Phenothiazines	Red, red-brown, or pink
Phenytoin	Red, red-brown, or pink
Rifampin	Bright orange-red
Sulfasalazine	Orange-yellow

Specific Gravity. Specific gravity indicates the concentration of the urine. Because one of the major functions of the kidney is to maintain fluid balance, typically the more concentrated the urine, the more fluid-depleted the person. Conversely, well-hydrated clients have more dilute urine, with specific gravities as low as 1.005.

Osmolality. Urine osmolality is a more precise way to measure the concentrating ability of the kidneys than is specific gravity. This is because the latter is a constant weight-to-weight relationship and is not unduly affected by the presence of glucose or protein. Urine osmolality increases with hypernatremia, acidosis, and shock. It decreases with diabetes insipidus, hypercalcemia, excessive fluid intake, renal tubular acidosis, severe pyelonephritis, and sometimes hyperglycemia.

pH. Urinary pH usually reflects the plasma pH and the body's acid-base balance. Metabolic alkalosis, low-protein diets high in vegetables and citrus fruits, alkalinizing medications such as bicarbonate of soda and acetazolamide, and ammonia-splitting bacteria all produce alkaline urine. Low urinary pH also indicates renal tubular acidosis in which tubular reabsorption is impaired. Strongly acid urine results from metabolic acidosis, metabolic alkalosis in potassium deficiency, a high-protein diet, uncontrolled diabetes, and some medications, such as ammonium chloride and mandelic acid.

Ketones. Ketones are found in the urine when the body's fat stores are metabolized for energy, thus producing an excess of metabolic end products. This occurs with uncontrolled diabetes and other states of altered carbohydrate metabolism, fasting, pregnancy and lactation, excessive lipid metabolism, and severe infections accompanied by vomiting and diarrhea. False-positive findings may be caused by medications such as levodopa and phenolphthalein.

Protein. The protein usually measured during a routine urinalysis is albumin. Although frequently a benign finding, proteinuria can denote abnormal glomerular permeability, decreased tubular reabsorption, or an overflow of protein in the plasma. Factors that influence glomerular basement membrane permeability include exercise, vasoactive substances such as norepinephrine, and diseases that hinder normal renal microarchitecture. Examples of systemic diseases that may cause proteinuria are diabetes mellitus, systemic lupus erythematosus, lymphoma, solid tumors, hypertension, pre-eclampsia, hepatitis, sickle cell disease, secondary syphilis, febrile diseases, and stress such as trauma or surgery. Medications may cause a false-positive result or a false-negative result.

One of the proteinurias not attributed to albumin is Bence Jones protein, which is found in multiple myeloma. Bence Jones protein is not included in a routine urinalysis but is detected either by heating the specimen or by electrophoresis. Other protein components may be found in macroglobulinemia and various tubular defects.

Pathologic proteinuria usually indicates serious renal disease. In the absence of other abnormal findings, the follow-up of an isolated instance of proteinuria may consist of serial urinalysis to make sure the proteinuria does indeed disappear. However, if proteinuria persists, there may be further evaluation of the urinary system.

Bilirubin. Bilirubinuria usually indicates extrahepatic biliary tract obstruction. Other causes include hepatitis, portal inflammation, and hepatocellular damage. A fresh urine specimen must be used for this test. When a urine specimen containing bilirubin is shaken, a yellow foam is produced. A false-positive finding may occur in a person taking chlorpromazine.

Red Blood Cells. Hematuria, or the presence of red blood cells, can be either microscopic (seen only under the microscope) or gross (obviously bloody). Hematuria is sometimes accompanied by other symptoms. Asymptomatic hematuria often presents a challenging diagnostic problem and requires meticulous evaluation. The cause may be benign or may indicate a pathologic condition. Although the cause of the hematuria may never be found, rigorous investigation is required. Hematuria is always considered to be a sign of urinary tract carcinoma until proved otherwise.

Hematuria also may appear in renal tuberculosis, sickle cell anemia (or sickle cell trait), IgA and IgG nephropathy, systemic lupus erythematosus, and polyarteritis nodosa.

Hemolytic anemia and hemolytic transfusion reactions produce detectable hemoglobin in the urine. Anticoagulants and the use of analgesics leading to papillary necrosis also can produce red blood cells in the urine. Hematuria following trauma, especially in the abdominal and pelvic area, may indicate injury to the urinary tract. Long-distance runners frequently exhibit hematuria (often with clots), which disappears as they recover from the run.

When collecting urine from a woman, the nurse should note whether she is menstruating, because contaminating the specimen with menstrual blood will give a false-positive result. Povidine-iodine washed into the urine specimen will give a false-negative result for occult blood. As with proteinuria, asymptomatic hematuria probably will be monitored initially with repeat urinalyses to determine whether or not the finding is indeed transient. If bleeding persists, further evaluation is necessary.

White Blood Cells. White blood cells in the urine usually designate an infectious process somewhere in the urinary tract. When accompanied by casts, renal epithelial cells, a few red blood cells or bacteria, the leukocytosis is usually the result of a kidney infection.

Pyuria means pus, or a large collection of white blood cells, in the urine. A quantitative determination of more than 5 clumps of white blood cells per high powered field indicates urinary pathogens. A large collection of pus may make the urine turbid and foul smelling.

Bacteria. Because urine is normally sterile, bacteriuria represents infection within the urinary tract or contamination of the specimen. Bacteria in the urine, whether or not accompanied by physical signs and symptoms of urinary tract infection, needs further evaluation with urine cultures.

Casts. Casts are formed elements organized in the nephrons (especially the tubules) by agglutination of protein. They most likely are formed in the distal tubules and the collecting ducts. Casts usually indicate tubular or glomerular disease. There are several varieties of casts and the identification of the specific type helps pinpoint the contributing problem.

Crystals. Crystalluria may or may not indicate disease. Common findings are calcium oxalate, uric acid, and urate crystals in acid urine, and phosphate, carbonate, and amorphous crystals in alkaline urine. The presence of crystals in the urine is an important predisposing factor in calculus formation.

Bacteriologic Studies. Because the kidneys, ureters, and bladder normally are sterile, the urine formed and transported in them also is sterile. Organisms typically colonize the distal portion of the urethra, but these bacteria ordinarily do not reach further up the urinary tract. Therefore, the presence of organisms in the urine is an abnormal finding. Any signs and symptoms reported by the client and/or the presence of significant bacteriuria or urinary leukocytosis indicate the need to examine the urine further.

Significant bacteriuria initially can be determined by using dipsticks that measure leukocyte esterase (an enzyme released by leukocytes); any positive findings need to be confirmed by culture of the specimen.

Pathogens in the urine are most specifically determined by culture. The urine specimens used for this testing are collected by catheterizing the bladder or by obtaining a clean-catch specimen, as described previously.

Many authorities suggest that this specimen should be obtained early in the morning to allow adequate accumulation of organisms within the urine being cultured. Once the specimen is received, it should be immediately transported to the laboratory. If the urine will not be examined within 30 minutes, it should be refrigerated because the bacteria will multiply more rapidly at room temperature.

Frequently, the first screening test performed is a Gram stain in the uncentrifuged urine. This is done so if any organisms are found, this stain will differentiate between the broad classifications of gram-positive and gram-negative organisms. Whether or not a Gram stain is performed, identifying the specific pathogens must be done by culturing the urine.

The urine is swabbed onto media plates or onto agar-coated paddles that are placed into an appropriate growth environment for 24 to 72 hours. Any colonies present are studied further to name and quantify the specific organisms present. Merely finding organisms does not signify clinical infection. Concentrations of 100,000 organisms per mL generally constitute significant infection. If the client is symptomatic, however, a culture of a single organism at a level of 10,000 organisms per mL may be significant and require treatment.

Once the causative organisms are identified, sensitivity tests are performed to designate the proper antibiotics to combat their growth. Once the urine has been obtained for the culture and sensitivity, the client may be started on a broad-spectrum antibiotic until the final sensitivity report is available. The determination of sensitivity tests is becoming even more important as the number of resistant organisms increases.

Clearance Studies. Although direct examination of the urine gives a gross estimate of renal function, more definitive measures such as clearance studies sometimes are necessary. Clearance is defined as the amount of plasma totally cleared of a given substance in 1 minute.

The kidneys clear the blood of certain substances by means of filtration and excretion. Clearance studies determine the glomerular filtration rate and tubular excretory ability by measuring clearance rates of creatinine, urea, inulin, para-aminohippuric acid, phenolsulfonphthalein, and radioactive isotopes.

Creatinine clearance is currently the most accurate measure of glomerular filtration rate. Virtually all formed creatinine, a product of muscle metabolism, is filtered by the glomerulus, and as the glomerular filtration rate falls, the serum creatinine rises. Urine for this test is collected over a 12-hour or 24-hour period, although a 24-hour specimen is preferred.

Urea clearance is used sometimes. Because the rate of tubular secretion varies with the rate of urine flow, it is not as useful as creatinine clearance.

Phenolsulfonphthalein is secreted by the proximal tubule at a rate proportional to the renal blood flow. In this test, the phenolsulfonphthalein is injected intravenously and urine specimens are collected at specified intervals. The nurse should inform clients that the dye may turn the urine red and reassure them that they are not bleeding. The dye begins to appear in the bladder 3 to 6 minutes after its administration; 20 to 30 per cent of it is excreted in 15 minutes, and 65 to 75 per cent is excreted within an hour. Chlorothiazide, penicillin G, and hypoproteinemia may cause false-positive findings.

Radioisotopes frequently are used to determine clearance rates. This procedure, called a renogram, involves the intravenous injection of a minute amount of a radioactive compound. The test does not require special preparation or follow-up care of the client. Also, because the dose of radioactivity is so low, there are no special precautions to observe in caring for the client or the urine specimen.

This test measures renal blood flow and active tubular transport, glomerular filtration, tubular secretion, and excretion. Each kidney can be compared with the other in terms of these measurements.

Other techniques using radioisotopes to measure renal function use blood determination to calculate clearance rates; for example, a radioisotope is injected and plasma samples are drawn to determine the amount of remaining isotope.

Concentration and Dilution. The loss of the kidney's ability to concentrate and dilute urine indicates significant renal tubular damage. Normally, as the body becomes depleted of fluid, larger volumes of water are reabsorbed, resulting in more concentrated urine with a specific gravity over 1.020. Conversely, with increased fluid intake, more water is excreted, causing more dilute urine with a specific gravity often as low as 1.005. One of the first kidney functions to be lost is this ability to concentrate and dilute urine. In severe renal damage, the specific gravity may become fixed at a level of 1.008 to 1.012, regardless of the amount of fluid intake.

Several tests can be performed to evaluate the concentration and dilution aspect of renal function.

Cytologic Examination. Examining cells exfoliated from the urinary tract can be useful in diagnosing cellular problems. The specimen needs good cellular content, so an early morning specimen is preferred. Usually, three random specimens are collected for cytologic evaluation and compared before concluding the presence or absence of disease in the urinary tract. The three specimens may be obtained from three different times within one day, three days in a row at the same time, or three times in the course of a month.

Cytologic examination may help in identifying and monitoring the progress of inflammatory processes resulting from chemical toxins, autoimmune disease, or bodily substances (e.g., hemoglobin and myoglobin); infectious processes (including bacterial, fungal, and viral); and neoplastic disease. Although it is not effective in the early detection of renal neoplasms, cytologic examination is very accurate in identifying urinary tract malignancies below the renal parenchyma, frequently demonstrating the presence of tumors before they are visible endoscopically.[10]

BLOOD STUDIES

Blood Chemistry. Measuring selected components in the blood aids in evaluating renal function. Probably the most frequently used determinant is the blood urea nitrogen (BUN) level. Urea is the end product of protein metabolism and is normally excreted from the body through the kidneys. Therefore, any renal function impairment causes an increase in the plasma urea level. The BUN level starts to rise when the glomerular filtration rate falls below 40 to 60 per cent. Unfortunately, the BUN level also can be elevated by such nonrenal factors as hypovolemia, excessive protein intake, starvation, bleeding into the gut, surgery or trauma, fever, exertion, or corticosteroids. Therefore, this single value must be evaluated very cautiously.

The serum creatinine level usually is measured along with the BUN level. Because creatinine also is excreted through the kidney, increased serum levels indicate decreased renal function. Creatinine excretion is not affected significantly by dietary or fluid intake, and it is thought to be a more accurate indicator of renal function than the BUN level. A rising serum creatinine level indicates nephron loss.

A BUN-creatinine ratio is used as a renal function indicator, with the normal ratio being 20/1. BUN elevations in relation to serum creatinine denote renal impairment due to prerenal causes such as blood loss, severe diarrhea, heart failure, and liver disease.

Hematology. Inspecting a random blood sample provides some data about renal function as well as the progress of disease processes within the urinary tract. Decreased red blood cells, hemoglobin, and hematocrit may indicate bleeding from the urinary tract or may signal reduced erythropoietic function by the kidney. An increased white blood cell count with increased neutrophils may denote an infectious process, whereas a return to normal values represents recovery from infection.

Radiologic Studies

In most diagnostic protocols, examining the urinary tract by x-ray study is the next step in identifying actual or potential malfunction. These studies may be performed with or without the use of contrast material and may involve static or dynamic films, or both. Because these examinations are performed in the x-ray department, the nurse's primary responsibility is to adequately prepare the client physically and mentally for the procedure. This helps ensure accurate results.

KIDNEYS, URETERS, AND BLADDER

An x-ray study of the kidneys, ureters, and bladder (KUB) is a simple film of the lower abdomen. It involves no contrast medium, poses no risk to the client, and can be performed without considering the remaining kidney function. The outline of these organs demonstrates their size, shape, and location. This helps identify soft-tissue masses, malformations, and radiopaque calculi.

INTRAVENOUS PYELOGRAM

An intravenous pyelogram involves the intravenous injection of a radiopaque contrast medium that is filtered by the kidney and excreted through the urinary tract. This examination helps identify the absence or presence, location, size, and configuration of the kidneys, ureters, and bladder. The IVP also helps determine filling of the renal calices and pelvis. A post-voiding film is obtained to assess the efficiency of bladder emptying. If bladder emptying is incomplete, a voiding cystourethrogram would help determine the cause of retention.

Physical preparation of the client for an IVP generally involves restricting fluids and cleaning out the bowel. Food and fluids are withheld after midnight before the examination. This relative fluid depletion allows the radiopaque contrast medium to be more concentrated when it enters the kidney, thus providing clearer films. If the client is receiving intravenous fluids, the infusion rate may be slowed for several hours before the study. Fluid depletion is contraindicated in clients with multiple myeloma, severe diabetes mellitus, or uric acid nephropathy. These conditions can seriously compromise the renal function of these clients, with reduced renal perfusion due to decreased renal blood flow, predisposing the client to the development of acute renal failure. If these clients must have an IVP, they should be well hydrated.

Because the kidneys are located retroperitoneally, the bowel must be cleared of gas and fecal material that may partially or totally obscure the kidneys. Cathartics are usually administered the evening before the examination. This part of the preparation, however, may be omitted in clients with suspected or known inflammatory bowel disease, or when vigorous colonic activity is otherwise contraindicated. If cathartics were not effective or not given for any reason, enemas or a rectal suppository can be administered early in the morning before the x-ray study.

During the examination, the client is placed supine on the x-ray table. Initially, a KUB film is taken. This helps to ensure the bowel is clear enough to continue with the procedure. It also screens for calculi in the renal collecting system. Because the contrast medium in the collecting ducts is the same density as any calcification in this area, some types of stones can be missed easily during the IVP. The radiopaque contrast medium is injected intravenously as a bolus or through an infusion drip. The contrast medium normally produces a flushed face, a warm feeling in the body, nausea, and a salty taste in the mouth. These are transitory effects and do not mean the study should be stopped.

The iodine in the substance, however, may cause severe allergic reactions in hypersensitive clients. Before the examination begins, the nurse should carefully question the client about any allergic history. A known sensitivity to iodinated contrast media is an absolute contraindication to continuing the procedure unless the client has been premedicated with a steroid infusion. If the client is unsure about an iodine allergy, ask the client about an allergy to shellfish. The presence of allergy to shellfish requires skin testing before intravenous injection.

A negative skin test or history, however, does not guarantee there will be no reaction. If any signs of allergic responses such as itching, hives, wheezing, or other signs of respiratory distress appear, the nurse should call for immediate discontinuation of the injection. Antihistamine, epinephrine, vasopressors, oxygen, and cardiopulmonary resuscitation equipment must be available to halt anaphylactic response.

In addition to possible anaphylactic reactions from the contrast medium, cases of acute renal failure following injection of the contrast medium have been documented.

After the contrast medium is injected, films are taken at regular intervals. Sometimes, with delayed renal functioning, additional x-ray studies may be needed 1 to 2 hours later.

RETROGRADE PYELOGRAPHY

A retrograde pyelogram involves passing a small-caliber catheter through a cystoscope into the ureters and into the renal pelvis. (Cystoscopy is described later in this chapter.) A small amount of contrast medium is injected into the kidney through the catheters, and x-ray films are taken to delineate the collecting system. The client may feel some discomfort in the kidney region when the contrast medium is injected, but there is no actual pain unless the renal pelvis has been overdistended. As the catheters are withdrawn, more contrast medium is injected, and films are taken to record the outline of the ureters. Preparing and caring for the client during and after this procedure is the same as that for the client undergoing an IVP and a cystoscopy.

Performing a retrograde pyelogram is indicated when the renal collection system or ureters have not been satisfactorily visualized during the IVP. It is also helpful in assessing the degree of ureteral obstruction. It can be used in clients who are hypersensitive to intravenous contrast media because the contrast medium is not absorbed through the mucous membranes.

There are no particular contraindications to this procedure, although it does carry some risk. Entering the urinary tract occasionally causes primary urinary tract infection or aggravates pre-existing infections. Manipulating the ureters also may cause edema, resulting in temporary obstruction to urine flow.

COMPUTED TOMOGRAPHY

This procedure involves an x-ray beam sweeping around the body and taking multiple, thin, cross-sectional pictures of the internal structure. This procedure allows measurement of various tissue densities. The computer then uses these density readings to reconstruct visual images of the body structures. Intravenous administration of contrast medium, using either bolus technique or intravenous infusion, may be used to enhance the image. This contrast medium is the same as that used in the intravenous pyelogram, so the potential for anaphylactic reaction or for acute renal failure exists. Other than preparing for potential complications, there is no special preparation or post-procedure care for the client.

There are several indications for computed tomographic scanning. These include examining the renal and urinary tract when excretory urogram and ultrasound have been unsatisfactory; characterizing renal retroperitoneal and pelvic masses; staging and monitoring renal tumors; evaluating a nonfunctioning kidney, urinary tract trauma, a transplanted kidney, suspected renal calculi, or gas-forming infections; and computed tomography–guided procedures.

CYSTOURETHROGRAPHY

X-ray examination of the bladder and urethra can be performed separately or together. During cystography, contrast medium is injected into the bladder through a catheter. When the bladder is full, films are taken to profile the size and shape of the bladder and to detect the presence of any vesicoureteral reflux. The client is frequently asked to void, and a follow-up x-ray is performed to measure the amount of residual urine.

URETHROGRAPHY

Urethrography outlines the inner size and shape of the urethra and checks for extravasation and strictures. In males, x-ray studies are performed after a thick, jelly-like radiopaque substance is injected via a wide-mouth syringe into the urethral meatus. This material usually reaches only as far as the urogenital diaphragm. In females, the procedure requires a less viscous contrast medium and a special catheter.

VOIDING CYSTOURETHROGRAPHY

Voiding cystourethrography provides visualization of urethral lesions, vesicoureteral reflux, and bladder and urethral obstructions. The radiopaque material is instilled into the bladder through a urethral catheter. The catheter is removed and the client is asked to void. Films are taken during the voiding process to observe the contrast medium flow. The micturition process may be recorded on film to better visualize the movement of the contrast medium. Voiding in the presence of other people can be very embarrassing for the client and may even interfere with the ability to void. Giving emotional support and judiciously placing screens may help put the client at ease.

RENAL ANGIOGRAPHY

Renal angiography makes it possible to visualize renal vasculature. It is used to (1) diagnose renal artery stenosis or renal vein thrombosis, (2) study renovascular hypertension, (3) demonstrate vascular damage after trauma, (4) investigate causes of acute renal failure, and (5) differentiate highly vascular tumors from avascular cysts.

Renal angiography involves injecting a radiopaque contrast medium into the renal vascular tree and taking serial x-ray films to outline blood vessels. Access to the circulation is usually through the femoral artery. Once the contrast medium has been injected, films are taken at the rate of two to three per second for several seconds to show filling and emptying of the renal artery tree. Delayed films are usually performed to visualize the function of the renal veins.

Pre-examination preparation is the same as for the IVP, including testing the client for hypersensitivity to the contrast medium. This procedure is usually performed under local anesthesia, although pre-procedure sedation frequently is given.

In addition to anaphylactic reactions and possible renal damage due to the radiopaque contrast medium, several other serious potential complications may result from this procedure.

CRITICAL TO REMEMBER

Hemorrhaging along the route of the vessel puncture may occur.

Vascular injury may occur at the puncture site or anywhere along the path of the guide wire and catheter. Thrombosis or embolism can occur as a result of plaque dislodging from the vessel walls during the procedure.

Pressure dressings are applied over the puncture site immediately after the catheter is removed. The nurse should observe the area frequently for several hours for signs of fresh bleeding. The client usually is placed on bedrest for several hours to allow complete sealing of the puncture site.

RENAL PHLEBOGRAPHY

One way to study the venous system of the kidneys is renal phlebography. Because of the small caliber of the renal artery and the copious blood flow in the renal veins, renal arteriography is often inadequate to satisfactorily visualize these vessels. During renal phlebography, the femoral vein is punctured and a catheter is threaded through the inferior vena cava and into the renal veins. The rest of the procedure, as well as caring for the client, is the same as for renal arteriography.

Radioisotope Studies

In addition to renal function tests performed with radioisotopes as described earlier, radioactive compounds can be used to evaluate renal structures, ureters, and the bladder. For renal studies, as with clearance studies, a radioisotope is injected intravenously and a scintillation camera or probe and/or computer is used to record the size and shape of the kidneys. The isotope compounds used are retained in the kidneys for several hours or days. Lesions in the kidney, such as tumors or infarcts, do not absorb the radioactivity and thus appear as "cold" or "blank" spots on the scanner. In this case, the diagnostician needs to investigate further to determine the actual cause of the cold spot. Indications for this procedure include renal hypertension, renal masses, trauma, obstruction, and evaluating transplanted kidneys.

Ultrasonography

Ultrasonography projects high-frequency waves into the abdomen. These waves are reflected back from the surfaces of retroperitoneal structures and converted into electrical energy that is shown on an oscilloscope. Instant-developing pictures are taken of the oscilloscope image to record the outline of the structures. The client lies on a table, and a lubricant, such as mineral oil, is applied to the skin over the area to be examined. This oil promotes good contact between the skin and the transducer used to administer and receive the ultrasonic waves.

Ultrasonography of the kidneys has many uses. Its prime value may well be in differentiating between fluid-filled cysts and solid masses. Other applications include localizing and mapping out the kidney before biopsy by percutaneous aspiration, evaluating transplanted kidneys, determining hydronephrosis in nonfunctioning kidneys, demonstrating papillary necrosis, identifying calculi, describing diverticula, estimating residual urine, determining post-void residuals, and demonstrating changes resulting from urinary tract infections.

Urodynamic Studies

Urodynamic studies are a series of procedures that evaluate the motor and sensory functioning of the bladder and the efficiency of micturition. These tests are used primarily to diagnose voiding problems or loss of bladder control, such as with incontinence, and to evaluate the effectiveness of reconstructive bladder surgery. A series of measurements provide diagnostic information about bladder capacity, pressure profiles before and during micturition, and the dynamics of the urinary system.

UROFLOWMETRY

Uroflowmetry is a simple, noninvasive procedure in which the client voids into a special commode chair equipped with a mechanism that measures weight over time and records the findings on graph paper. This information can be used to calculate the urine flow rate. The client should have a full bladder for the test or, if this is not possible, a catheter can be inserted and the bladder filled. The client is then asked to void and the measurements are retaken.

A residual urine test may be performed after voiding. A residual urine test is obtained by having the client attempt to empty the bladder completely. The client can then be catheterized, with the amount of urine obtained recorded as the residual volume. More recently, bladder ultrasonography has been performed to determine residual urine after measurement of the urinary flow rate so that this urodynamic procedure may remain totally noninvasive.

CYSTOMETROGRAPHY

A cystometrogram measures bladder pressure during filling and voiding. No preprocedure preparation is needed other than client teaching.

Figure 29–1

Equipment for manual cystometrography. A pressure transducer can be used in place of the water manometer.

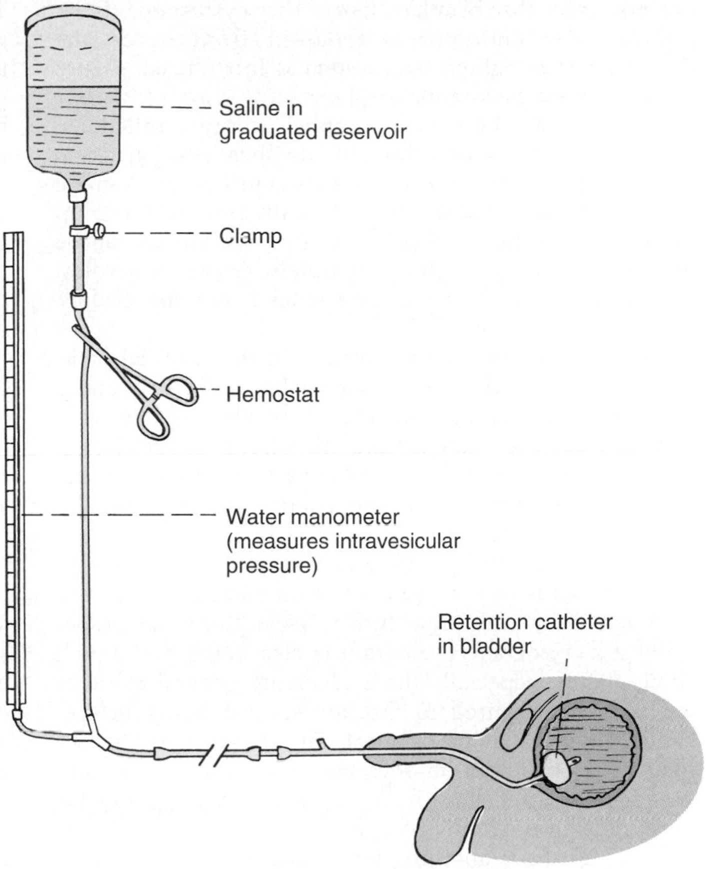

In some institutions, at the beginning of the examination, the client voids while the examiner notes (1) the time and effort needed to initiate voiding; (2) size, force, and continuity of the stream; and (3) whether dribbling occurs after voiding ceases. A catheter is then passed into the bladder, usually through the urethra. Any residual urine is removed and measured. The distal end of the catheter is attached to an apparatus that will deliver saline or carbon dioxide to the bladder while measurements of the intravesical pressures are recorded. Figure 29–1 illustrates one type of set-up of this equipment (special equipment is also used to perform the test).

The client may be asked to cough or perform other maneuvers at specified points during the examination to evaluate the resulting pressure changes. Bladder filling also may be repeated in several different positions in order to reproduce the client's symptoms, including sitting or standing. When filling has been completed, the catheter is removed and the client allowed to empty the bladder while the examiner makes the same observations as during the initial voiding. The amount of residual urine is again determined. To measure bladder pressure during voiding, a tiny urethral catheter may be inserted and left in place during voiding. Intra-abdominal pressure can be measured using a small rectal catheter.

After the procedure, the client is monitored for the development of a urinary tract infection. The nurse also should monitor the client's voiding to make sure that the client does not develop urinary retention.

Direct Visualization

RIGID CYSTOSCOPY

The oldest method of direct visualization of the urinary tract is cystoscopy, which involves inserting a cystoscope into the bladder via the urethra. This procedure may be useful for diagnostic as well as therapeutic purposes. Its five major diagnostic uses include (1) directly inspecting the bladder, making it possible to see tumors, calculi, ulcers, or other defects; (2) collecting urine directly from the renal pelvis and separately from each kidney; (3) x-ray visualization through retrograde pyelography, as described earlier; (4) measuring bladder capacity and evidence of vesicoureteral reflux; and (5) biopsy of the ureters, bladder, and urethra. It also provides endoscopic access to the upper urinary tract. The cystoscope is used in intervention to (1) resect tumors, (2) remove stones and foreign bodies, (3) fulgurate bleeding areas, (4) dilate the ureters, (5) empty the renal pelvis, and (6) implant radium seeds.

Today's rigid cystoscope consists primarily of a sheath and an optical lens system. The sheath is a solid metal tube which, when the obturator (a core that prevents trauma) is in place, can be passed through the urethra into the bladder. Once the cystoscope is in position, the obturator is removed from inside the sheath and the lighted lens system is introduced. Figure 29–2 shows a cystoscope in place.

Several attachments accomplish various functions. Forceps may be passed through the sheath to get tissue samples for biopsy or to remove foreign bodies. A guide can be used to help direct small catheters into and up the ureters to the renal pelvis so that specimens can be obtained from each kidney separately. Scissors, needles, and electrodes also may be introduced into the bladder or urethra as needed.

Cystoscopy may be performed in the hospital or in the physician's office. It also may be performed under local or general anesthesia. The client must remain very still during the examination to avoid urinary tract trauma. Therefore, the type of anesthesia used may depend on whether or not the client can maintain the necessary position.

Physiologic and psychosocial preparation is needed before a cystoscopy. Cathartics or enemas, or both, may be given before the procedure to clear the bowel, especially if a retrograde pyelogram is also being performed. Some clients, especially those receiving general anesthesia, may be required to fast for several hours beforehand. Clients having a local anesthesia may be instructed to maintain an adequate fluid intake to ensure an effective urine flow for specimen collection and for retrograde pyelography, if it is to be performed. Clients who cannot have anything by mouth may receive intravenous fluids. A sedative or narcotic, and sometimes an anticholinergic, is usually administered before the procedure.

As with any procedure, effective teaching helps to alleviate anxiety and ensure optimum cooperation. This is particularly important if the cystoscopy is performed under local anesthesia. Because the procedure is usually performed with the client in the lithotomy position, it can be very tiring and uncomfortable, but it is essential that the client remain still throughout the examination. The nurse can help the client with deep breathing and general relaxation exercises to decrease discomfort as the cystoscope is introduced. The desire to void will be pronounced as the cystoscope passes the neck of the bladder and when bladder capacity is measured by filling it with fluid. The nurse also should warn the client that this procedure is performed with the room lights off so the physician can better visualize the internal bladder.

Sudden pelvic or lower abdominal pain may indicate perforation of the urethra, bladder, or ureters. Cardiac complications have been documented. Consequently, the nurse should monitor high-risk clients continuously during the cystoscopy and make certain that emergency equipment and medications are available to reverse dysrhythmias.

Care after a cystoscopy may include bedrest for a short time. If general anesthesia is used, the client needs the usual postanesthetic monitoring (see Chap. 5). Even if the procedure was performed on an ambulatory basis under local anesthesia, the client should not stand immediately after removing the legs from the stirrups, because sudden circulatory change may cause dizziness and syncope. This is especially true for elderly clients.

Pink-tinged urine is common after cystoscopy, but any bright red bleeding or clots in the urine should be reported to the physician. The nurse should advise the client that the urine may have an unusual color if a contrast medium such as methylene blue was used. Back pain, bladder spasms, fullness and burning in the bladder, and severe burning on urination also may be experienced. Warm tub baths and mild analgesics usually bring sufficient relief. Belladonna and opium (B & O) suppositories or antispasmodics such as propantheline bromide (Pro-Banthine) may relieve bladder spasms.

Urinary retention sometimes occurs from edema following the instrumentation. Men with benign prostatic hyperplasia are at particularly high risk. Hot sitz-

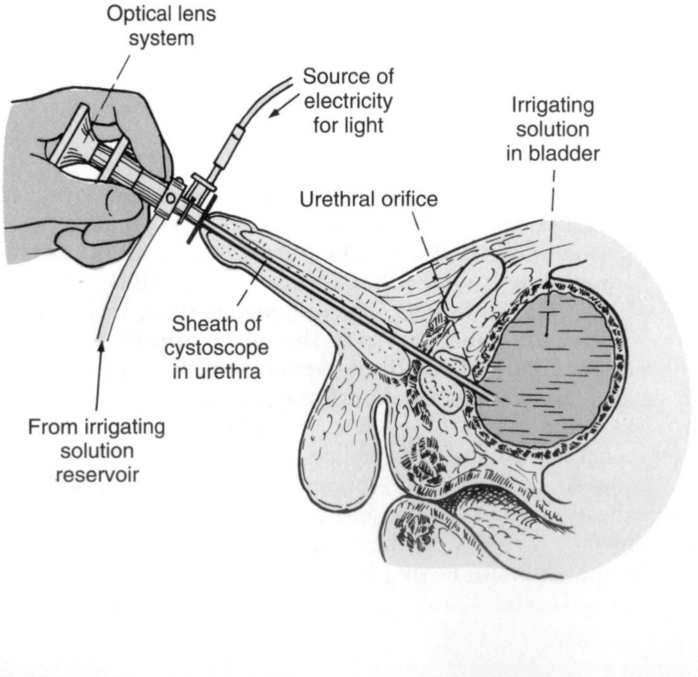

Figure 29–2
Cytoscope in the male bladder.

baths and relaxants often relieve the problem, although catheterization may be necessary. The nurse should encourage the client to drink large amounts of fluids after the procedure. Diluting the urine in this way will help prevent further tissue irritation and will decrease the burning sensation when the client voids. Some chilling and a rise in temperature often occur following cystoscopy. If these symptoms do not subside readily after providing extra warmth and offering frequent fluids, the nurse should investigate the client's condition further. Cystoscopy may spread infection in the urinary tract and can cause bacteremia. Although the method is controversial, some authorities recommend using prophylactic antibiotics after urinary tract instrumentation because of the risk of infection.

Clients are often discharged almost immediately or within several hours after cystoscopy. The nurse should give the client written instructions as well as verbal instructions, to assist clients in remembering the instructions later.

Flexible Fiberoptic Cystourethroscopy

The rigidness of the standard cystoscope often prevents the examiner from visualizing some parts of the bladder. The evolution of flexible endoscopic instruments has helped solve this problem. The client being examined may be positioned supine or prone.

Ureteroscopy and Nephroscopy

Ureteroscopes have been developed to examine the ureter and kidneys. Ureteroscopy evaluates tumors, obstruction, calculi, and the presence of foreign bodies. General or regional (spinal or epidural) anesthesia is used for these procedures because the dilation of the ureteral orifice causes considerable discomfort.

Performed under strict aseptic technique, nephroscopy allows the physician to observe the renal pelvis, calices, fundus, and collecting system. It can be performed to (1) locate and remove calculi; (2) diagnose the cause of hematuria; and (3) biopsy, fulgurate, and resect tumors. Nephroscopy is a safe procedure that is not associated with any significant complications except possible infection. Nursing care for the client before and after the procedure is similar to care needed by clients who undergo a renal biopsy.

Renal Biopsy

A renal tissue specimen for biopsy can be obtained using an open or closed technique. For open biopsy, the surgeon performs a nephrostomy. This incision through the flank allows direct visualization of the kidney, and the tissue obtained is adequate 100 per cent of the time. However, the procedure has a prolonged recuperation period, and therefore, it increases direct costs and time lost from work. Chapter 31 discusses caring for the client who has a renal biopsy.

One method of closed biopsy is the retrograde renal and ureteral brush procedure. This technique collects tissue specimens from the renal pelvis and ureters.

Postoperatively, the client may be given intravenous fluids at a rapid rate to reduce the possibility of clots forming at the biopsy site and to foster specimen collection. Some oozing of blood can be expected for 24 to 48 hours. Moreover, some people experience severe renal colic, which is usually relieved by narcotics and fluids.

The percutaneous renal biopsy is perhaps the most frequently used procedure. During this examination, a specially designed needle pierces the skin and enters the kidney to obtain a small sample of tissue. Fluoroscopy and ultrasonographic techniques allow more precise localization of the biopsy needle.

This important diagnostic tool is helpful either as a one-time examination or when performed serially to monitor the progress of a disease, especially in any disease process that is evenly distributed throughout the kidney. Contraindications to percutaneous biopsy include a single functioning kidney, infection, tumors (because of the danger of dissemination), hydronephrosis, severe hypertension, coagulation disorders, and an uncooperative client. Severe renal failure has previously been regarded as a contraindication. However, better procedures for localizing the kidney have reduced the dangers associated with this technique. Pregnancy usually is considered a contraindication because of the high doses of radiation that may be necessary during localization of the needle. Using ultrasonography instead eliminates this risk.

The procedure usually is performed under local anesthesia with little or no premedication. The client is placed in a prone position with a firm pillow or sandbag under the abdomen to straighten the spine's natural lordosis. The kidney to be biopsied is located with ultrasonography or fluoroscopy, or both, and a contrast medium is injected intravenously. After careful skin preparation, the skin is infiltrated with the anesthetic. The client is instructed to take in as deep a breath as possible and to hold it. The probe needle then is inserted through the skin, midway between the last rib and iliac crest (Fig. 29–3), and positioned inside of the renal (fibrous) capsule. After the correct position of the distal end of the needle has been confirmed, the probe needle is removed and the biopsy trocar inserted. The client may now be allowed to breathe normally, but he or she must inspire deeply each time a tissue specimen is taken. When enough tissue is obtained, the trocar is removed and firm pressure is immediately applied to the site. After several minutes, a pressure dressing is applied.

Complications include microscopic hematuria, pain, fever, or extravasation of the contrast medium. An increased heart rate and hypotension occasionally develop during the procedure. This problem probably is the result of sympathetic stimulation by the needle or pressure of the pillow or sandbag against the abdominal vessels or sympathetic nerves. The condition is transient, and vascular stability is usually restored as soon as the client moves into a supine position.

Hemorrhage is a major complication. It may be suggested by gross or microscopic hematuria, flank or

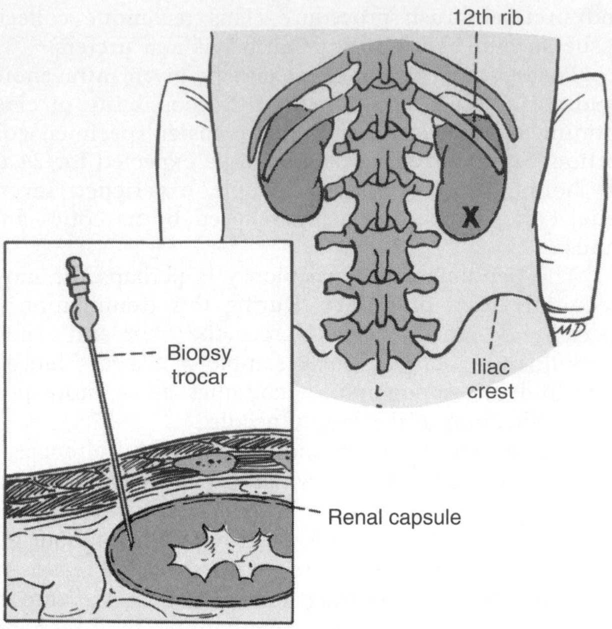

Figure 29–3
Percutaneous renal biopsy showing trocar location.

abdominal pain, hypotension, and a decreasing hematocrit level. However, low hematocrit and hypotension alone are not sufficient indicators of hemorrhage, because some people develop these conditions without significant bleeding. Hemorrhage may occur because of hemodilution or as a result of massive sympathetic stimulation caused by penetration of the needle. Other complications include infection, trauma, and laceration or perforation of the kidney or adjacent structures.

The client may remain prone for approximately 30 minutes or immediately be turned onto the back after the procedure is completed. The nurse monitors vital signs and the puncture site every 5 to 10 minutes. The client then may be transferred to bed and should remain on bedrest and avoid straining for at least 24 hours. The nurse should check vital signs and the puncture site regularly during this time. The nurse obtains serial urine tests, keeping a sample of each voiding in consecutive order to permit comparison and to evaluate bleeding. Dipsticks are used to determine the presence of hematuria, and the nurse sends specimens to the laboratory to more precisely determine the amount of bleeding. The client should be encouraged to drink large amounts of fluid to avoid clot formation and retention, which could obstruct urine flow. The period of bedrest will likely be extended in the presence of continued hemorrhage. A hematocrit and hemoglobin study is usually performed within 8 to 10 hours to test for anemia. The client may also need emotional support while waiting for the diagnosis and its implications.

On discharge, the nurse should advise the client to avoid strenuous activity for approximately 2 weeks. He or she should also instruct the client about the signs of hemorrhage and what to do if hemorrhage occurs. Bleeding may develop several days after the biopsy.

STUDY QUESTIONS

1. When teaching about the urethra, the nurse should include which one of the following statements?
   A. "The female urethra is 15 to 20 cm in length."
   B. "The urethra connects the kidney to the bladder in both sexes."
   C. "The reproductive system is anatomically connected to the urinary tract in males."
   D. "Peristaltic action causes the urine to move through the urethra to the outside of the body."
2. Trauma to the abdomen may result in:
   A. Anuria
   B. Pyuria
   C. Polyuria
   D. Hematuria
3. The client with an iodine allergy is definitely scheduled for an intravenous pyelogram (IVP). Which one of the following will be done as a precautionary measure?
   A. Premedication with a steroid infusion
   B. Restriction of iodine-rich foods in the diet prior to the test
   C. Withholding all medication for a week period prior to the test
   D. Administration of oral rather than intravenous iodine-based medication
4. Which of the following statements indicates that a client is experiencing ureteral pain?
   A. "I feel a burning sensation when I urinate."
   B. "My pain is a dull, constant pain in my side."
   C. "I can feel the pain coming down into my genital area."
   D. "It's like a cramping, squeezing feeling over my bladder."
5. The client who states that his urine has a smoky gray color most likely has:
   A. Bleeding in the upper urinary tract
   B. Bleeding in the lower urinary tract
   C. Urobilinogen or bilirubin in the urine
   D. Absence of urobilinogen or bilirubin in the urine
6. A client with a urinary tract infection is started on a broad-spectrum antibiotic. The nurse should monitor which one of the following diagnostic studies?
   A. Urinalysis
   B. Clearance studies
   C. Cytologic examinations
   D. Culture and sensitivity

CRITICAL THINKING EXERCISES

SCENARIO A

Complete an assessment of urinary function in two adults: one an older male and the other a young male.

1. What differences might you expect in urinary function between males of these two age groups?
2. Would urinalysis indicate any differences that could be related to age?
3. Why are questions about major illnesses and hospitalizations important in the client with a possible urinary disorder?

SCENARIO B

For each of the following diagnostic studies, indicate any potential problems the nurse must assess. Use the following key:

A = Allergy/Anaphylaxis
B = Bleeding/Hemorrhage
TE = Thrombosis/Embolus
UTI = Urinary Tract Infection
N = None
BS = Bladder Spasms
ARF = Acute Renal Failure

1. KUB ______
2. IVP ______
3. Retrograde pyelogram ______
4. CT scan ______
5. Renal angiography ______
6. Ultrasonography ______
7. Cystometrogram ______
8. Rigid cystoscopy ______
9. Renal biopsy ______

BIBLIOGRAPHY

1. Andreesen, G. (1989). A fresh look at assessing the elderly. *RN, 52(6)*, 28–40.
2. Baldwin, K. M. et al. (1995). *Davis's manual of critical care therapeutics.* Philadelphia: F. A. Davis.
3. Bates, B. (1991). *A guide to physical examination and history taking* (5th ed). Philadelphia: J. B. Lippincott.
4. Beck, L. H. (1990). Kidney function and disease in the elderly. *Hospital Practice, 26,* 75–90.
5. Bower, A., & Thompson, J. (1992). *Clinical manual of health assessment (3rd ed.).* St. Louis: C. V. Mosby.
6. Brown, W. W. (1989). Geriatric nephrology and urology–1989. *Peritoneal Dialysis International, 9,* 27–28.
7. Brundage, D. (1992). *Renal disorders.* St. Louis: Mosby-Year Book.
8. Carnevali, D. L., & Patrick, M. (Eds.) (1993). *Nursing management for the elderly* (3rd ed). Philadelphia: J. B. Lippincott.
9. Cella, J. H., & Watson, J. (1989). *Nurse's manual of laboratory tests.* Philadelphia: F. A. Davis.
10. Chadwick, A. T. (1989). BV 2000: A noninvasive technique to assess bladder function. *Journal of Neuroscience Nursing, 21,* 256–257.
11. Chmielewski, C. (1992). Renal anatomy and overview of nephron function. *American Nephrology Nurses' Association Journal, 19(1)*, 34–38.
12. Cooper, C. (1993). What color is that urine specimen? *American Journal of Nursing, 93(8)*, 37.
13. Copstead, L. C. (1995). *Perspectives on pathophysiology.* Philadelphia: W. B. Saunders Co.
14. Davidson, R. A., & Wilcox, C. S. (1992). Newer tests for the diagnosis of renovascular disease. *Journal of the American Medical Association, 268(23),* 3353–3358.
15. Fischbach, F. (1992). *A manual of laboratory and diagnostic tests.* Philadelphia: J. B. Lippincott.
16. Fritz, M. (1988). Noninvasive bladder volume measurement. *Urologic Nursing, 9,* 8–9.
17. Groer, M. W., & Shekleton, M. E. (1989). *Basic pathophysiology: A holistic approach* (3rd ed.). St. Louis: C. V. Mosby.
18. Guyton, A. C. (1991). *Textbook of medical physiology* (8th ed.). Philadelphia: W. B. Saunders.
19. Holochek, M. J. (1992). Glomerular filtration and renal hemodynamics. *American Nephrology Nurses' Association Journal, 19(3),* 237–245.
20. Jarvis, C. (1992). *Physical examination and health assessment.* Philadelphia: W. B. Saunders Co.
21. Karlowicz, K. A. (1995). *Urologic nursing: Principles and practice.* Philadelphia: W. B. Saunders Co.
22. Kee, C. C. (1992). Age-related changes in the renal system: Causes, consequences, and nursing implications. *Geriatric Nursing, 13(2),* 80–83.
23. King, B. A. (1994). Detecting acute renal failure. *Nursing 94, 24(3),* 34–40.
24. Lewandowski, J. (1993). Issues in renal nutrition. *Nephrology Nursing Today, 3(4),* 1–8.
25. Mackety, C. J. (1990). Lasers in urology. *Nursing Clinics of North America, 25,* 697–709.
26. Massery, S. G., & Gassock, R. J. (Eds.) (1988). *Textbook of nephrology.* Baltimore: Williams & Wilkins.
27. Matteson, M. A., & McConnell, E. S. (1988). *Gerontological nursing: Concepts and practice.* Philadelphia: W. B. Saunders Co.
28. McCance, K. L. & Huether, S. E. (1990). *Pathophysiology: The biologic basis for disease in adults and children.* St. Louis: C. V. Mosby.
29. Murray, R., & Zentner, S. (1993). *Nursing assessment and health promotion through the life span.* (5th ed.). Norwalk, Connecticut; Appleton & Lange.
30. Neuman, D. K., et al. (1991). Restoring urinary continence. *American Journal of Nursing 91(12),* 44–45.
31. Pagana, K. D., & Pagana, T. J. (1992). *Mosby's diagnostic and laboratory test reference.* St. Louis: Mosby-Year Book.
32. Porcush, J. G., & Faubert, P. F. (1991). *Renal disease in the aged.* Boston: Little, Brown & Co.

33. Porth, C. (1990). *Pathophysiology* (3rd ed.). Philadelphia: J. B. Lippincott.

34. Powers, I., & William, D. (1992). Urinary incontinence. *Nursing 92, 22(12),* 46–47.

35. Preisig, P. (1992). Urinary concentration and dilution. *American Nephrology Nurses' Association Journal, 19(4),* 351–354.

36. Rebensen-Piano, M. (1989). The physiologic changes that occur with aging. *Critical Care Nursing Quarterly, 12(1),* 1–14.

37. Resnick, B. (1993). Retraining the bladder after catheterization. *American Journal of Nursing 93(11),* 46–49.

38. Resnick, N. M. (1989). Diagnosis and treatment of the institutionalized elderly. *Seminars in Urology, 7,* 117–123.

39. Sabiston, D. C. (1991). *Textbook of surgery: The biological basis of modern surgical practice.* Philadelphia: W. B. Saunders Co.

40. Schrier, R., & Gottschalk, C. (1988). Diseases of the kidney (4th ed.). Boston: Little, Brown & Co.

41. Walsh, P. C., et al. (Eds.) (1992). *Campbell's urology* (6th ed.). Philadelphia: W. B. Saunders.

42. Watson, J., & Jaffe, M. S. (1995). *Nurse's manual of laboratory and diagnostic tests* (2nd ed.). Philadelphia: F. A. Davis.

43. Wyngaarden, J. B., & Smith, L. H. (1988). *Cecil textbook of medicine* (18th ed.). Philadelphia: W. B. Saunders Co.

Chapter 30

Nursing Care of Clients with Disorders of the Ureters, Bladder, and Urethra

Learning Outcomes

After completing this chapter, the learner will be able to:

1. Assess the client for clinical manifestations associated with lower urinary tract disorders.
2. Teach the client about the etiology, risk factors, basic pathophysiology, and clinical manifestations of disorders of the lower urinary tract.
3. Explain the client's role in the medical and surgical management of disorders of the lower urinary tract.
4. Develop plans of care for the prevention of illness, management, and rehabilitation of clients with lower urinary tract disorders.
5. Implement nursing interventions that optimize the quality of life for clients with lower urinary tract disorders.
6. Evaluate planned client outcomes, using outcome criteria developed in the planning phase of care.

The principal function of the ureters, bladder, and urethra is to transport urine from the kidneys. The bladder, urethra, and, sometimes, ureters are called the lower urinary tract. The ureters are sometimes classified, with the kidneys, as the upper urinary tract. Anything that obstructs the flow or interferes with the neuromuscular ability to move and expel urine reduces the ability of these organs to fulfill their role. A disorder can cause psychosocial as well as physiologic problems, which then influence the severity of the disorder and healing progress. The nurse must consider both realms in identifying problems and implementing interventions to solve these problems.

URINARY TRACT INFECTION

Urinary tract infection (UTI) refers to an infection within the lower urinary tract. The infection can affect the bladder *(cystitis)*, the urethra *(urethritis)*, and the ureters *(ureteritis)*.

Incidence

Urinary tract infections are a very common problem. The bladder is the most frequent site of infection within the urinary tract. Studies show that at least 25 per cent of all women experience UTI or cystitis sometime in their lives. Men rarely experience UTIs before the age of 50 years because of the length of their urethra and the antibacterial properties of prostatic fluid.

Etiology

The most common UTI-causing organisms are *Escherichia coli, Enterobacter, Pseudomonas,* and *Serratia.* These organisms, normally found in the gastrointestinal tract, contaminate the urine because of the proximity of the urethral orifice and the anus in women. *E. coli* itself is responsible for about 90 per cent of UTIs in women. *Staphylococcus saprophyticus* especially affects young women, occurs most often in the summer and early autumn, and has a high propensity for ascending into the upper urinary tract.

Candida, another cause of UTIs, is associated with sepsis and death, especially in debilitated clients.

Risk Factors

There are many risk factors associated with UTIs. These include the location of the female meatus, which makes contamination by vaginal and anal organisms likely; sexual intercourse (during coitus, organisms can move up the urethra to the bladder); urinary stasis and reflux in pregnant women caused by pressure on the ureters and hormonal changes; tight or synthetic clothing (causes irritation); and presence of an indwelling catheter. Preventive methods include the following:

- Wiping from meatus back toward the anus (in females)
- Taking showers versus baths (a bath is more likely to cause irritation and contamination of the urethra)
- Avoiding bubble baths, another cause of irritation
- Wearing cotton underpants
- Avoiding wearing pantyhose with slacks
- Washing the perineal area before intercourse and voiding immediately after
- Drinking adequate amounts of fluid, especially those that acidify the urine (e.g., cranberry juice)
- Voiding every 2 hours during pregnancy and increasing fluid intake

In addition, the nurse should remember to use appropriate technique when caring for clients with indwelling catheters.

Pathophysiology

Factors that contribute to the development of UTIs include the following:

- Loss of integrity of mucosal lining (can be caused by an indwelling catheter, a tumor, calculus, or parasites)
- Decreased resistance to invading organisms
- Retention of urine in the bladder
- Undertreated cystitis

When the lining of the urinary tract is invaded by organisms, cellular damage and inflammation occur. Distention of the bladder leads to many UTIs. As the bladder wall expands, blood flow decreases. Ischemic tissue becomes more vulnerable to organism invasion.

Clinical Manifestations

The cardinal symptoms of a bladder infection (cystitis) include the following:

- Burning on urination
- Frequency
- Urgency
- Inability to void
- Incomplete emptying of the bladder
- Voiding in small amounts

Further assessment may reveal the following:

- Low back or suprapubic pain
- Hematuria
- Cloudy urine
- Abdominal and flank pain
- Malaise
- Chills
- Fever
- Incontinence

Most of the symptoms are due to the irritation of the bladder and urethral mucosa. The bacteriuria causes the inflammation, fever, and chills. If the ureters become inflamed also, abdominal symptoms may occur.

DIAGNOSTIC ASSESSMENT

Definitive diagnosis is usually based on a urine culture. However, the dipstick test for leukocyte esterase activity is increasingly used to determine bacteriuria early so interventions can begin promptly.

A urine culture is essential for positive diagnosis because dipsticks alone can give false-positive results. The specific causative organism must be accurately identified. Follow-up cultures are also used to determine the effectiveness of medications used to treat the infection. Sensitivity tests are also done routinely on the urine specimens for identifying the antibiotics that can be used to treat the infection successfully.

In some cases of severe or recurrent cystitis, an intravenous pyelogram (IVP), retrograde pyelogram, or cystoscopy might be done to detect any abnormalities. Congenital anomalies, foreign bodies, calculi, and tumors can be detected as well as abnormalities the repeated infections may have caused. These tests will also detect obstruction within the urinary tract; a common cause of UTI, especially in older men.

Medical Management

Management of UTI is multifaceted, and an initial, acute infection may be treated differently from recurrent infections. The principal intervention of an initial infection is the administration of antibiotics specific to the causative organisms.

PHARMACOLOGIC MANAGEMENT

Pharmacologic intervention begins with a broad-spectrum antibiotic even before the culture and sensitivity results are known, because medication should start as soon as possible. Later, on the basis of sensitivity reports, the exact medication for this infection can be given. Commonly used pharmacologic agents are presented in Table 30–1.

For pregnant women, certain medications must be avoided because of the risk to the fetus. Do not administer trimethoprim-sulfamethoxazole (Bactrim) or sulfonamides in the last trimester of pregnancy. Tetracycline should not be given at all during pregnancy or to children younger than 12 years because developing teeth may be discolored. Care must also be taken in treating the elderly because many suffer from compromised renal function.

The typical course of antibiotic therapy is 10 to 14 days. However, a single large dose, although not accepted by all authorities, is effective in many clients, especially women with an initial uncomplicated infection of the lower urinary tract. Large single-dose therapy does not suppress the client's normal flora to the same degree as does long-term therapy and reduces the development of resistant organisms.[25]

For some clients, frequent recurrent infections are a frustrating problem. Three or more UTIs a year is considered frequent, whether they involve the same or different organisms. Each infection period must be treated with antibiotics. The client must be cautioned against self-diagnosis and treatment of recurrent UTIs. Each infection requires culture and sensitivity and specific treatment.

Treating the client with asymptomatic bacteriuria is yet another problem. In general, physicians currently suggest that an asymptomatic infection be treated only if it is certain that intervention will prevent further morbidity.

Antibiotics can cause some problems. They have the potential for destroying the normal flora, which leads to problems such as vaginal yeast infections in women. There is also the possibility that resistant organisms can develop.

Complications can also occur if the infection is not completely eradicated. An ascending infection can migrate from the bladder to the kidneys, resulting in the development of pyelonephritis. Recurrent pyelonephritis can predispose the client to the development of chronic renal failure if the damage to the kidneys is severe enough.

DIETARY MANAGEMENT

Acidifying the urine decreases the rate of bacterial multiplication. Traditionally, cranberry juice and ascorbic acid (vitamin C) have been used to do this. However, current studies indicate that neither adequately reduces the urinary pH and, therefore, is not as reliable as was previously thought. Although cranberry juice can acidify the urine, commercial products do not contain a sufficiently high concentration of pure juice to reduce the pH unless the client can drink a prodigious amount.

An acid-ash diet is more effective in acidifying the urine (Box 30–1). A diet of meats, eggs, cheese, prunes, cranberries, plums, and whole grains should be encouraged. The client should avoid carbonated beverages and caffeine.

Fluid intake should also be increased to at least 2 to 3 L/day so that a good output is ensured. The increased fluid is extremely important when the client is taking sulfa drugs because these can form crystals in concentrated urine.

Surgical Management

Surgery is performed to treat any anomalies that are causing the repeated infections. Bladder neck strictures and ureteral pelvic junction abnormalities are the most common problems. Benign prostatic hyperplasia (BPH), the common cause of cystitis in older men, can also be treated surgically. Urinary calculi may also require surgical intervention. Once these disorders are corrected, the infections should stop.

TABLE 30–1 Medications Used to Treat Cystitis and Other Urinary Disorders

AGENT	ACTION	DOSAGE	SIDE EFFECTS	NURSING IMPLICATIONS
Urinary Antiseptics				
Cinoxacin (Cinobac)	Effective against *Escherichia coli, Klebsiella, Enterobacter, Proteus, Serratia,* and *Citrobacter*	1 g daily in two to four divided doses for 7–14 days	Dizziness, headache, photosensitivity, nausea and vomiting, abdominal pain, diarrhea, rash	Contraindicated in clients who are hypersensitive to nalidixic acid; warn client about photophobic effect; give with meals to decrease gastrointestinal side effects
Nalidixic acid (NegGram)	For acute and chronic UTIs, especially gram-negative bacterial infections	1 g qid for 7–14 days for acute or 2 g daily for long-term use	Drowsiness, weakness, headache, photophobia, diplopia, abdominal pain, nausea and vomiting, rash, angioedema	Use with caution in clients with liver or renal disorders; contraindicated in clients with a history of convulsions; instruct client to report visual disturbances; encourage fluids and closely monitor output; avoid sunlight
Norfloxacin (Noroxin)	For complicated and uncomplicated UTIs caused by gram-negative organisms, including *Pseudomonas;* especially useful for clients allergic to penicillin, cephalosporin, and sulfa drugs	400 mg PO bid for 7–10 days for mild infections and for 10–21 days for severe infections	Fatigue, somnolence, headache, nausea, constipation, elevated liver function tests, rash	Encourage high fluid intake to ensure high urine output; advise client to take medication 1 hr before or 2 hr after meals because food may hamper absorption
Nitrofurantoin (Macrodantin)	To treat acute and chronic UTIs in clients with adequate creatinine clearance	For acute UTI, 50–100 mg PO qid for 10–14 days, after meals Chronic therapy, 50–100 mg PO as needed; IV, 180 mg bid for adults over 120 lb	Nausea and vomiting, gastrointestinal upset, diarrhea, rash, asthma, peripheral neuropathies, anaphylaxis, dizziness, hypotension	Maintain adequate intake and output; use cautiously in clients with anemia, diabetes, vitamin B deficiency, electrolyte imbalances, or debilitating diseases; watch for hypersensitivity; keep urinary pH in acid range with vitamin C and cranberry juice; give with food; warn client that drugs may discolor urine
Methenamine mandelate (Mandelamine)	Effective in acid urine against gram-positive and gram-negative organisms for chronic UTIs	1 g PO qid after meals	Nausea and vomiting, diarrhea, elevated liver enzymes, rash, dysuria, and frequency in large doses	Contraindicated in clients with renal or hepatic disease or severe dehydration; maintain high urine output; warn client to limit intake of alkaline foods and increase intake of cranberry juice and foods that acidify urine; administer with food or after meals, but avoid antacids

TABLE 30–1 Medications Used to Treat Cystitis and Other Urinary Disorders *Continued*

AGENT	ACTION	DOSAGE	SIDE EFFECTS	NURSING IMPLICATIONS
Sulfonamides				
Co-trimoxazole, sulfamethoxazole-trimethoprim (Bactrim, Septra)	To treat acute UTIs	160 mg trimethoprim/800 mg sulfa or double with double-strength tablet for 10–14 days	Gastrointestinal distress, agranulocytosis, allergic reactions, headache, glossitis, stomatitis, hepatitis, pruritus, photosensitivity, arthralgia, peripheral neuritis, hearing loss, crystalluria, hypoglycemia	Administer with large amounts of fluid; monitor serum glucose levels; monitor for allergies, which occur more commonly in AIDS clients; maintain alkaline pH—more soluble in alkaline urine
Sulfisoxazole (Gantrisin)	To treat acute UTIs	Initially 2–4 g PO, then 1–2 g qid for 10–14 days	Agranulocytosis, aplastic anemia, headache, depression, nausea and vomiting, diarrhea, toxic nephrosis, crystalluria, erythema multiforme, epidermal necrolysis, exfoliative dermatitis, hypersensitivity, anaphylaxis, serum sickness	Monitor closely for allergy; give each dose with full glass of water; maintain high fluid intake; monitor intake and output; more soluble in alkaline urine; monitor CBC; instruct client to take full dose; if Azo Gantrisin is given, urine will be dark brown to red in color
Urinary Analgesics				
Phenazopyridine (Pyridium)	To treat pain of urinary tract irritation or infection	100–200 mg PO tid until pain disappears, usually about 2–3 days	Nausea, headache, vertigo	Warn client that urine will be red to orange in color; contraindicated in clients with renal or hepatic disease; always given with antibiotic—does not treat infection, only pain
Cholinergics				
Bethanechol chloride (Urecholine)	To treat acute postoperative or other nonobstructive urinary retention and for neurogenic atony of bladder with retention	2.5–10 mg SC, never IM or IV; 10–30 mg PO tid or qid; all doses should be individually determined	Cardiac arrest and vascular collapse if given IM or IV, headache, hypotension, abdominal cramps, diarrhea, nausea and vomiting, urinary urgency, flushing, bronchoconstriction	Never used in clients with any possibility of bladder obstruction; never give IM or IV, can lead to circulatory collapse; watch closely for cholinergic overdose; atropine antidote; have bedpan readily available, works within 15 min after injection or 60 min after oral dose; given on empty stomach to decrease nausea and vomiting

Table continued on following page

TABLE 30–1 Medications Used to Treat Cystitis and Other Urinary Disorders *Continued*

AGENT	ACTION	DOSAGE	SIDE EFFECTS	NURSING IMPLICATIONS
Anticholinergics				
Propantheline bromide (Pro-Banthine)	To decrease bladder muscle spasms	Up to 60 mg PO qid	Palpitations, blurred vision, confusion in elderly clients, dry mouth, constipation, urinary hesitancy and retention, decreased sweating	Do not use in clients with narrow-angle glaucoma, obstructive uropathy or gastrointestinal disease, or ulcerative colitis; monitor urine output closely; provide gum or hard candy for dry mouth
Antibiotics				
Ciprofloxacin (Cipro)	To treat severe or complicated UTIs	250 mg PO every 12 hr	Headache, restlessness, tremor, lightheadedness, seizures, nausea, diarrhea, vomiting, oral candidiasis, crystalluria	Contraindicated in clients allergic to quinolone antibiotics, in pregnancy, and in children; give 2 hr after meals; may cause nervous system stimulation and seizures; have client drink plenty of water with medication; prolonged use may result in overgrowth of resistant organisms
Cephalexin monohydrate (Keflex)	To treat genitourinary infections	250 mg to 1 g PO every 6 hr	Transient neutropenia, anemia, pseudomembranous colitis, nausea, anorexia, diarrhea, dyspepsia, urticaria, hypersensitivity	Use carefully in clients with a history of renal insufficiency, previous hypersensitivity to penicillin or cephalosporins; prolonged use may lead to overgrowth of resistant organisms; take with food to decrease gastrointestinal distress; be sure client takes full dose of medication; obtain cultures before starting medication

AIDS, acquired immunodeficiency syndrome; bid, twice daily; CBC, complete blood count; IM, intramuscularly; IV, intravenously; PO, orally; qid, four times daily; SC, subcutaneously; tid, three times daily; UTIs, urinary tract infections.

Nursing Management

Assessment

The nurse should start by assessing the client's risk factors for the development of cystitis. This involves obtaining a detailed history and physical examination.

The nurse must also collect the necessary urine culture and sensitivity specimen. The nurse should instruct the client on the proper procedure for collection so that contamination from other organisms is minimized.

Nursing Diagnosis, Planning, and Implementation

There are several appropriate nursing diagnoses for the client with UTI.

Nursing Diagnosis: Urinary Elimination, Altered (a variety of specifiers such as retention, urgency, and so on) R/T irritation of the bladder mucosa.

BOX 30–1

Acid-Ash Diet

FOODS ALLOWED

Meat, fish, poultry, shellfish, cheese, and eggs
Grains: bread, cereals, crackers, rice, whole grain, pasta, and corn
Vegetables: corn and lentils
Fruits: cranberries, prunes, plums, and their juices
Foods with large amounts of chlorine, phosphorus, and sulfur

FOODS PROHIBITED (BASIC FOODS)

All milk and milk products
All vegetables except corn and lentils
All fruits except cranberries, plums, and prunes
Foods containing large amounts of potassium, sodium, calcium, and magnesium

NEUTRAL FOODS

Coffee and tea
Butter, margarine, oils
White sugar and honey
Cornstarch and tapioca
All pure fats
All pure carbohydrates

Planning: Expected Outcomes. The client will have urinary elimination return to normal within 3 days of the start of treatment, as evidenced by absence of fever, normal white cell count, and absence of pain, burning, frequency, and urgency.

Implementation. The nurse should monitor the client's voiding, noting problems such as frequency, urgency, retention, and dysuria. The symptoms need to be treated immediately so the client can return to normal urinary function.

Nursing Diagnosis: Pain, Acute R/T irritation of bladder and urethral mucosa.

Planning: Expected Outcomes. The client will be able to urinate without discomfort within 24 hours of treatment, as evidenced by verbalization of absence of pain and burning on urination.

Implementation. The nurse should administer any medications prescribed specifically to treat pain, such as phenazopyridine (Pyridium or Azo Gantrisin). Again, increasing fluids will also help relieve the pain by diluting the urine and making it less irritating to the mucosa. A warm sitz bath may also help the pain, especially if the urethra is also irritated. Baking soda can be added to the water to produce a greater soothing effect. Some clients find that a heating pad applied to the suprapubic area helps reduce bladder spasms and suprapubic pain.

Nursing Diagnosis: Infection, Risk for R/T urinary stasis, pregnancy, or other risk factors.

Planning: Expected Outcomes. The client will not acquire UTI or will have infection treated effectively, as evidenced by negative urine culture, absence of fever, and normal white blood cell count.

Implementation. The nurse can help the client to re-establish a normal urinary pattern. One of the best ways to do this is through administration of the prescribed anti-infective agents listed in Table 30–1. The problems of urgency, frequency, and possible incontinence will decrease within 24 hours of beginning the medication. The nurse should also check the culture and sensitivity report to be sure that the proper anti-infectives are being administered.

Nursing Diagnosis: Knowledge Deficit R/T prevention, medications, hygiene, and fluid intake.

Planning: Expected Outcomes. The client will be able to describe ways to prevent UTI, the correct method for taking medication, the proper way to wipe after voiding, and the required fluid intake.

Implementation. The nurse can do much to help the client learn to prevent cystitis. Before discharge, the nurse should teach clients to maintain a high daily fluid intake of at least 2000 mL (eight 8-ounce glasses) a day unless otherwise contraindicated. The nurse should remind the client to void at the first urge (unless the bladder program is planned otherwise) and at least every 2 to 3 hours during the day and one or two times at night to prevent bladder distention. Women should be encouraged to void immediately after sexual intercourse and to drink at least two glasses of water as soon as possible. The nurse should also recommend that women use a position for sexual intercourse that minimizes pressure on the anterior vaginal wall. The nurse should emphasize the need for women to maintain good perineal hygiene and teach them to wipe the perineum from front to back. Women should be advised to use tampons rather than sanitary pads. Women should also be taught to wear cotton underwear and to shower instead of taking tub baths.

The nurse should teach all high-risk clients the signs and symptoms of cystitis, pointing out that the client should seek health-care assistance as soon as possible if these occur. When administering medication, one must make sure that the client understands the drug and its side effects, emphasizing the importance of taking the full course of the drug, even if the symptoms of infection disappear.

Finally, because of the high risk for more serious or recurrent infection and the possible need to begin further intervention early, one must emphasize the importance of complying with the recommended schedule of follow-up urine cultures.

Evaluation

The nurse can evaluate the effectiveness of the interventions on the basis of the expected outcomes identified for this client. If interventions were not successful, the goals and interventions should be modified so that goals can be met.

Modification of Plan of Care for the Elderly

In older adults, cystitis may occur more often, but for different reasons. In older women, the changes in the aging vagina and bladder increase the risk for cystitis. The atrophy of the vagina, decreased vaginal secretions, and muscle weakness in the vagina and bladder predispose this group to infection. In older men, BPH is one of the main risk factors for UTI, and the incidence of BPH increases with age.

The causes of UTIs in this group will alter both prevention and treatment. In men, the best treatment for recurrent UTI is to treat the BPH. Once this problem is eliminated, the infections should be eliminated. In women, use of vaginal lubricants before intercourse can help decrease infections. The Kegel exercise, which helps tighten the vaginal and bladder muscles, is also helpful in women, particularly if women practice these exercises routinely throughout their lives. If the weakness in the muscles is severe, surgery such as an anterior colporrhaphy and bladder suspension can be done.

Sudden confusion and incontinence may be the initial symptoms in the elderly.

When administering medications used to treat UTIs to older adults, the nurse must consider the renal and hepatic function of the client.

INTERSTITIAL CYSTITIS

Cystitis may also be noninfectious. Interstitial cystitis (IC) can be caused by chemical agents, such as medications like cyclophosphamide. Other causes can include radiation therapy and possibly autoimmune responses. This disorder is also called painful bladder disease (PBD). If it is associated with hemorrhage, it is called hemorrhagic cystitis.

This disorder occurs mainly in women (90–95%). Although at one time it was considered a disease of menopause, it actually occurs more frequently in younger women.

Interstitial cystitis is a poorly understood disorder with an unclear pathophysiology. One factor that is clear, however, is that, in spite of the symptoms, the urine is sterile. There seems to be some change in the permeability of the glycosaminoglycan layer of the bladder mucosa, which is usually impermeable to urea and other substances.

The clinical manifestations of PBD are severe lower abdominal or pelvic pain, urgency, frequency (up to 60 times a day in some clients), nocturia, and, in some women, dyspareunia. Some clients may exhibit only the frequency and pain; others will have all the symptoms.

Because this problem is not caused by infection, the prevention and treatment are different from those of infective cystitis. Antibiotics may actually cause further bladder irritation. The treatment for IC is controversial, with no one accepted treatment. Drugs such as anti-inflammatories, antispasmodics, tricyclic antidepressants, and antihistamines are used, as well as tranquilizers and occasionally narcotics.

Other treatments include instillation of a variety of agents into the bladder to promote healing and pain relief. These include agents such as sodium oxychlorosene (Clorpactin), silver nitrate, and dimethyl sulfoxide (DMSO). Oral sodium pentosan polysulfate (Elmiron), a heparin analogue, is given possibly to create a mucin layer in the bladder.

The major nursing responsibility associated with this syndrome is supporting the client through diagnosis and treatment.

Alterations in Urinary Patterns

URINARY INCONTINENCE

Incontinence has been defined by the International Continence Society for the Standardization of Terminology as "a condition in which involuntary loss of urine is a social or hygienic problem and is objectively demonstrable."[25] There are a number of different types of incontinence, such as enuresis, stress, urge, paradoxical (overflow), reflex, environmental, and psychological (Table 30–2).

TABLE 30–2 Types of Incontinence

TYPE OF INCONTINENCE	DESCRIPTION
Stress	Increased intra-abdominal pressure caused by activities such as coughing, laughing, sneezing, walking, or running leads to an involuntary loss of urine; the intravesicular pressure increases to overcome the resistance of the internal sphincter in the urethra
Enuresis	Nighttime incontinence or "bed-wetting" is usually associated with childhood, although the problem can extend into adulthood
Urge	Inability to hold back the flow of urine when feeling the urge to void; spasmodic bladder contractions accentuate the problem
Overflow (paradoxical)	Retention with overflow of small amounts of urine; occurs when the intravesicular pressure exceeds maximal urethral pressure without detrusor activity
Reflex	Abnormal activity of the spinal cord reflex leading to involuntary loss of urine
Psychological	Client aware of need to urinate but unable to respond appropriately to urge because of dementia or confusion
Environmental	Client aware of need to urinate but physically unable to either reach the toilet on own or receive adequate assistance to do so

Incidence

Wide ranges of figures are available on the prevalence of incontinence. These estimates range from about 10 per cent to more than 30 per cent of all older clients with stress and urge incontinence, both alone and combined, seemingly the most common. There are few accurate estimates of the incidence of this problem in adults other than the elderly.

Etiology

Anatomic and physiologic incontinence results from sphincter weakness or damage, urethral deformity, alteration of the urethrovesical junction, detrusor instability, and weak abdominal and perineal muscle tone.

Sphincter weakness or damage is often caused by obstetric trauma, postoperative weakness, and congenital weakness. In men, a prostatectomy may cause temporary or permanent incontinence.

Urethral deformity is often caused by recurrent UTIs, previous gynecologic surgery, trauma, and estrogen deficiency vulvitis.

Alteration of the urethrovesical junction occurs in women. This angle, between the bladder and the posterior proximal urethra, is important to continence in women (Fig. 30–1). Common causes of the loss of this angle include multiple pregnancies, aging, and surgical procedures resulting in abdominal perineal weakness.

Detrusor instability is commonly caused by

- Bladder lesions (e.g., infection, neoplasms, and senile trigonitis)
- Lower motor neuron lesions (e.g., tumor, prolapsed disc, complication of pelvic surgery, and osteoarthritis of the spinal cord)
- Upper motor neuron lesions (e.g., tumor, cerebrovascular accident, multiple sclerosis, and transection of the spinal cord)
- Large bowel diseases, spastic colon, and diverticulosis

Weak abdominal and perineal muscle tone is caused by obesity, lack of exercise, and loss of tone after childbirth or prostatectomy.

Physical causes of incontinence are those independent of the urinary tract. These include physical immobility (e.g., cerebrovascular accident [CVA], fracture, weakness) and failing vision.

Psychosocial causes of incontinence can be related to an unawareness of the need to void or being unable to know what to do when the urge to void is felt. Other possible causes include regression, dependence, rebellion, insecurity, attention-seeking behavior, and sensory deprivation.

Various medications also contribute to incontinence, especially overflow incontinence. These include

- Narcotics, tranquilizers, sedatives, and hypnotics, all of which affect bladder fullness cues and the ability to respond to them
- Alcohol
- Rapid-acting diuretics
- Antihistamines
- Atropine and atropine-like substances
- Hypotensives
- Alpha-adrenergic blockers
- Beta-adrenergics
- Ganglionic blockers

Other factors contributing to the development and maintenance of incontinence include fecal impaction, bladder scarring, urethral adhesions, diabetes mellitus, and obesity. Incontinence may also be a sign of "giving up." Frequent voiding by clients who fear "accidents" leads to decreased bladder capacity, increased detrusor tone, and thickening of the bladder wall, which results in a vicious circle of dysfunction.

Risk Factors

The risk factors for each type of incontinence vary and are shown in Box 30–2.

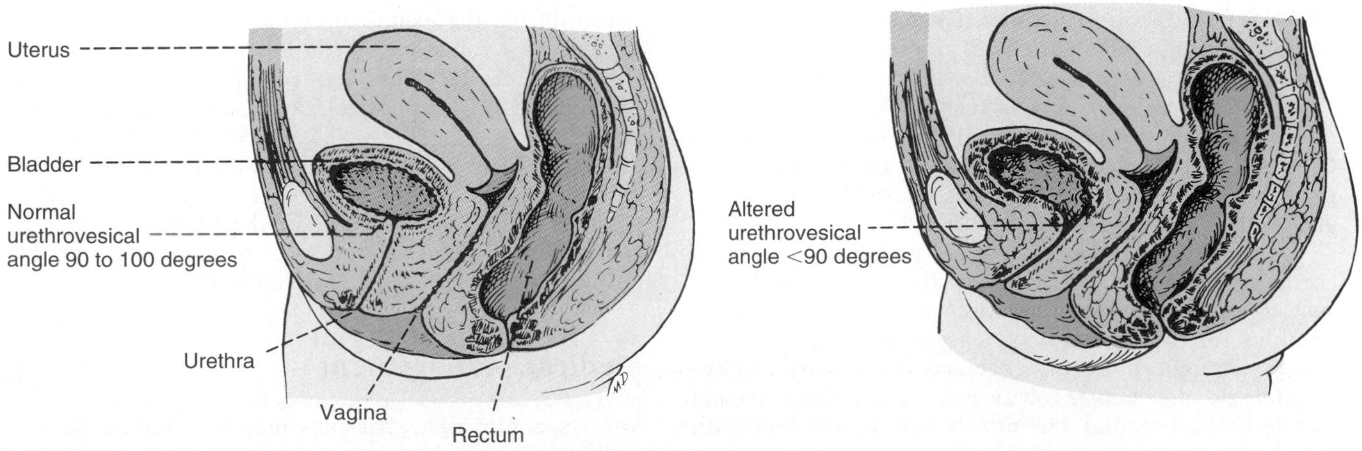

Figure 30–1
Alteration in the normal urethrovesical angle contributes to incontinence in women. *A*, Normal angle. *B*, Altered angle.

BOX 30-2

Risk Factors for Incontinence

TYPE OF INCONTINENCE	FACTORS	PATHOPHYSIOLOGY
Stress	Loss of urethrovesical angle in women Urethral irritation from infection, radiation, damage to the bladder, and injury from prostatectomy in men	Increased pressure overcomes urethral musculature, often associated with coughing, laughing, and sneezing
Urge	Muscle spasms as in multiple sclerosis Recurrent urinary tract infections Strokes Changes in mobility with medications such as hypnotics, tranquilizers, sedatives, and diuretics	Uninhibited muscle contraction, decreased mobility from an upper motor neuron lesion with an inability to stop voiding when an impulse is felt
Overflow	Retention with bladder distention related to, for example, a nervous system lesion, fecal impaction, or benign prostatic hyperplasia	Bladder overdistends and urine overflows
Reflex	Spinal cord injury	Abnormal spinal cord activity associated with the absence of sensation to void
Psychological	Altered mental states	Altered mental states
Environmental	Changes in mobility	Impaired mobility, for example, may cause urinary stasis, resulting in an infection

Pathophysiology

The pathophysiologic changes associated with incontinence are related to the specific causes. Stress incontinence occurs when the intravesical pressure exceeds the maximum urethral pressure in the absence of detrusor activity. This increased vesical pressure is often associated with activities such as sneezing, coughing, and laughing. There may be some weakness in the urethral sphincter or, in women, changes in the urethrovesical angle. Normally, in the first stage of voiding, the urethrovesical angle is lost as the bladder descends. With the loss of the angle, there is descent and funneling of the bladder neck with the bladder rotating down and back. This places them in the anatomic position for the first stage of voiding, so any activity that causes downward pressure on the bladder leads to voiding. In men, the pathophysiologic change is usually BPH, causing retention, overflow, and stress incontinence.

Urgency incontinence is associated with several pathophysiologic changes. One problem is uninhibited detrusor contraction associated with motor disorders.

Overflow incontinence is related to a problem with retention and overdistention of the bladder with an overflow of the excessive amount of urine. The pathophysiologic cause of the retention is usually obstruction at the bladder outlet such as with BPH.

Reflex incontinence is related to abnormal spinal cord activity associated with the absence of the sensation to void. Bladder contraction occurs without direct stimulus for the central nervous system.

Psychological incontinence has as its basic pathophysiologic mechanism changes in the client's mental status; environmental incontinence is a problem with impaired mobility.

The physical complications of incontinence include infection, skin breakdown, and permanent bladder changes.

Clinical Manifestations

The major symptom of incontinence is stated in the definition, that is, involuntary loss of control of voiding. If it is urge incontinence, it may be associated with bladder spasms. The amount of urine expelled can help differentiate whether it is overflow or stress incontinence, because these usually produce small amounts of urine.

DIAGNOSTIC ASSESSMENT

Urodynamic evaluation is the major diagnostic test for incontinence. To determine the precise cause of the client's incontinence, the incontinence should be reproduced during the examination. These tests can also assess detrusor function and the likelihood that treatment will be successful. The degree of pelvic floor prolapse can be assessed by physical examination and radiologic tests.

The variety of urodynamic examinations, including cystometrogram and electromyogram, are described in Chapter 29. Ultrasonography of the bladder or kidneys can detect residual urine. A cystoscopy with cystography may also be useful in diagnosing this problem.

Medical Management

Various noninvasive therapies may be effective in controlling some types of incontinence. Pelvic muscle exercises, the Kegel exercises designed for postpartum women, have been used to improve control in males and females. Reports of success range from 30 to 90 per cent with their use. Use of the Femina cones has improved the success of these exercises. These cones are weighted and inserted into the vagina. Correct muscle contraction is required to keep them in place. Early reports are that they dramatically improve the effectiveness of pelvic muscle exercises.

Behavioral techniques to increase the client's awareness of the need to void can also be initiated. Biofeedback has been used with clients experiencing stress or urge incontinence.

Bladder training is another approach that is used for incontinence. With this technique, the client first voids at short intervals throughout the day, usually hourly or less if necessary. The client then tries to lengthen the time between voiding to intervals up to 3 hours.

Institutionalized clients can also use a form of bladder training. With these clients, health-care workers check the clients at hourly intervals, urging use of the bedpan and praising success. The time between voiding can often be increased to every 2 hours with success. With this technique, it may take 2 or 3 months for progress to show.

Urinary tract infections must be eliminated for irritation to the detrusor muscle to be reduced. In the case of stress incontinence, it is important to suppress a chronic cough.

A variety of medications have been tried to control incontinence. Table 30–3 summarizes these medications. Medications are used mainly with urge incontinence to relax the bladder and possibly increase bladder capacity and sometimes stress incontinence. These medications are contraindicated in clients with bladder outlet obstructions or weak detrusor muscles.

DIETARY MANAGEMENT

The major nutritional alteration involves controlling fluid intake especially after dinner, to reduce incontinence during the night. For obese clients, weight reduction programs may help decrease stress incontinence. The client should avoid bladder stimulants such as alcohol, chocolate, and coffee.

Surgical Management

Electrical inhibition of the reflex to void is a surgical intervention for incontinence. Through the use of electrical stimulation, the client can activate the system to relieve incontinence.

The implantation of an artificial urinary sphincter may help some clients achieve continence. This surgical procedure is usually reserved until after all else has failed. Figure 30–2 shows a sphincter device consisting of an inflatable cuff, a reservoir, and a control pump. The surgeon implants the cuff around the bladder neck or urethra, a deflation (or control) pump in the scrotum or labia, and a fluid reservoir in the abdomen.

Other surgical procedures are used to correct or compensate for anatomic defects contributing to incontinence. The most common surgical procedures are intended to restore the normal urethrovesical angle or to lengthen and support the urethra. Re-establishing the urethrovesical angle allows the internal sphincter to function normally. Lengthening the urethra increases its resistance.

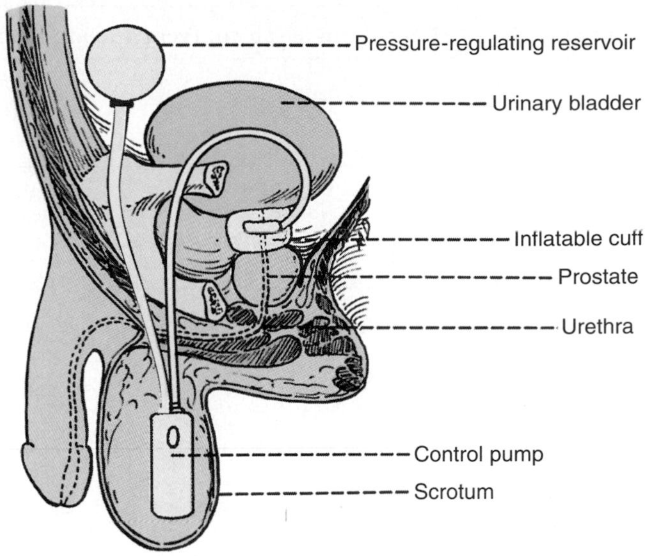

Figure 30–2
Artificial urinary sphincter. This surgically implanted urethral sphincter restores continence. To urinate, the client deflates the cuff around the bladder neck by squeezing the control pump within the scrotum. The cuff reinflates automatically.

In the Marshall-Marchetti-Krantz procedure, the bladder neck and urethra are sutured to the perichondrium of the symphysis pubis or the periosteum of the superior pubic ramus. Procedures such as the Raz are now being done transvaginally. This repair process involves elevation and suspension of the bladder with the use of tissue or inorganic materials for support. Postoperatively, clients undergoing this surgery need a suprapubic or urethral catheter for 5 to 8 days. During this time, they require a high fluid intake to prevent infection. Also, the drainage system must always be patent because the pressure of a filling bladder inhibits the healing process.

Once healing occurs, a reconditioning or clamp and release program is then initiated to help the detrusor muscle regain tone. One must clamp the catheter for lengthening intervals while urine collects in the bladder. If the client begins to experience severe pressure, the catheter should be unclamped immediately. Otherwise, the catheter is unclamped periodically to empty the bladder. If a suprapubic catheter is used, the client should try to void when the bladder is filled; then, if the client is unable to void, the catheter can be emptied. After voiding, measure the residual urine to determine the effectiveness of bladder emptying.

Other surgical procedures aim to provide an intact, patent route for the transport of urine. Scar tissue that interferes with normal bladder neck function must be removed. If urethral or sphincter narrowing contributes to the problem of incontinence, it must be dilated.

TABLE 30–3 Medications Used to Treat Incontinence

AGENT	ACTION	DOSAGE	SIDE EFFECTS	NURSING IMPLICATIONS
Propantheline bromide (Pro-Banthine)	Anticholinergic that inhibits detrusor contraction and may increase bladder capacity; delay and decrease in amplitude of involuntary contractions	15 mg orally tid; larger doses produce too much drying	Dry mouth, dry eyes, constipation, confusion or excitement in elderly; precipitation of glaucoma, blurred vision, mydriasis, palpitations, urinary retention	Do not use in clients with narrow-angle glaucoma, obstructive uropathy or obstructive gastrointestinal disease, ASHD, hypertension, hiatal hernia, and hepatic or renal disease; monitor vital signs and urinary output; use gum or hard candy to alleviate dry mouth
Oxybutynin chloride (Ditropan)	Direct smooth muscle relaxant that works directly on bladder muscle; helps with detrusor instability	Up to 5 mg orally qid	Drowsiness, dry mouth, palpitations, tachycardia, blurred vision, mydriasis, constipation, urinary hesitancy or retention	Contraindicated in clients with myasthenia gravis, gastrointestinal obstruction, obstructive uropathy; use cautiously in elderly; stop therapy at intervals to see whether problem has resolved; rapid onset of action, peaks at 3–4 hr and lasts 6–10 hr; monitor with periodic cystometry; store in tightly closed container
Verapamil hydrochloride (Calan)	Depressant effect on bladder muscles; use for incontinence not well documented	80 mg orally tid	Dizziness, hypotension, heart failure, constipation, nausea, urinary retention, peripheral edema	Use with incontinence not well studied; use cautiously in elderly and clients with existing heart disease; monitor urinary output; check pulse and blood pressure regularly

Nursing Management

Independent nursing interventions for incontinence include weight reduction, establishment of an exercise program, and institution of a bladder-training program. Weight reduction, if necessary, and pelvic exercises not only help regain bladder control but may prevent recurrence of the problem.

Kegel exercises strengthen the pubococcygeal muscle and resolve stress incontinence. To teach Kegel exercises, the nurse asks the client to stop urine flow several times during voiding. Once there is full awareness of the muscles needed to do this, the client should contract these muscles three to four times a day for 5- to 10-minute sessions each. If back pain occurs during the exercises, the client is probably contracting the wrong muscles and thus needs to go back to step 1 of the exercise program.

A successful bladder-training program requires a great deal of patience on everyone's part. The first step in instituting the program is to discuss all procedures and the expected outcome with the client. The sensitive nurse tries to inspire a sense of hope and the knowledge that something indeed can be done about incontinence.

Many clients suffering from incontinence reduce their fluid intake, thinking this will decrease urine production and result in better control. Actually, adequate urine production is necessary to stimulate the micturition reflex. Therefore, unless it is contraindicated by the client's physical status, a daily fluid intake of 2000 to 2500 mL must be encouraged. These fluids must be carefully spaced throughout the day and limited in the evening to allow longer sleep periods at night. The client should avoid beverages containing caffeine because they contribute to bladder irritability.

TABLE 30–3 Medications Used to Treat Incontinence *Continued*

AGENT	ACTION	DOSAGE	SIDE EFFECTS	NURSING IMPLICATIONS
Imipramine hydrochloride (Tofranil)	Anticholinergic and direct relaxant effect on detrusor and contracting effect on bladder outlet (alpha-adrenergic effect)	25–75 mg orally daily	Drowsiness, dizziness, orthostatic hypotension, tachycardia, urinary retention, sweating, blurred vision, mydriasis	Do not use in clients recovering from myocardial infarction, with BPH, or with history of glaucoma or seizure disorders; decrease dose in elderly or debilitated clients; monitor for urinary retention or constipation; warn client to avoid alcohol
Phenylpropanolamine hydrochloride (Acutrim)	Alpha- and beta-adrenergic antagonist used to treat stress incontinence; produces smooth muscle contraction at bladder outlet	25 mg orally every 4 hr	Hypertension, tachycardia, palpitation, insomnia, nervousness, restlessness	Monitor effectiveness; check blood pressure frequently; warn against use of over-the-counter drugs that may interact, especially pseudoephedrine; maintain in light-resistant, tight container
Estrogens	For postmenopausal women with urge incontinence, but ineffective against stress incontinence	Dosage varies with particular agent used	Headache, increased risk of thromboembolism, nausea and vomiting, breakthrough bleeding, hyperglycemia, hypercalcemia, urticaria	Do not use in clients with history of thromboembolic disease of any kind; monitor effectiveness in reducing incontinence; warn client about possible increased risks of cancer

ASHD, arteriosclerotic heart disease; BPH, benign prostatic hyperplasia; qid, four times daily; tid, three times daily.

Meanwhile, a voiding schedule should be developed with the client. The nurse must determine how often the client urinates during the day by maintaining a voiding record. The nurse must check frequently for wetness and document results. Depending on the voiding pattern, the client must be brought to the toilet or commode every 30 minutes to 2 hours. As the program progresses, the client must be encouraged to hold the urine longer and thus increase voiding intervals.

Biofeedback and behavior modification may be included in this bladder-training program. Biofeedback techniques must be used to help the client regain control over the external urethral sphincter and pelvic floor musculature. As the client contracts the perianal muscles, lights indicate the strength or duration of the muscle contraction. Thus, the lights give immediate feedback concerning progress. The device can be used at home.

Behavior modification is a variation of the voiding schedule. This program conditions the bladder to empty when the client sits on the toilet or commode. The theory is that by placing the client on the commode or toilet, micturition will be stimulated. Once a stimulus-response pattern has been established, it can help achieve continence throughout the day. Programs are more successful when bladder capacity is at least 150 to 200 mL. With a capacity below this level, the client voids too frequently to achieve an optimal outcome.

Psychotherapy and hypnosis also help manage incontinence. Psychotherapy may aid clients whose incontinence has a psychogenic origin as well as assist clients in dealing with embarrassment, increased dependence, and self-image problems that may accompany incontinence.

Sometimes none of these measures is effective. Nursing intervention must then be aimed at protecting the clients' skin, clothing, bed linen, and so on. Adult-sized disposable pads or briefs help protect and increase the social mobility of clients experiencing chronic incontinence. If the skin does become wet, it must be meticulously cleaned and dried to prevent serious rashes and skin breakdown resulting from maceration and ammonia production. Indwelling catheters should be used to drain urine only as a last resort because they contribute to UTIs.

External condom drainage involves putting a thin rubber or plastic sheath over the penis and connecting it to either a leg bag or a bedside drainage bag. Problems with this system include leakage (with or without detachment of the condom), twisting of the condom, and stasis of urine, which can macerate the penis. The condom sheath should be attached so that it stays in place without compromising circulation to the distal penis. Many commercially prepared condom systems contain a double-sided adhesive liner that is applied to the penis before the condom. Many newer devices are self-adhesive. When rolling the condom sheath over the penis, one must take care to allow at least 1.5 cm between the distal end of the penis and the internal end of the sheath. This will reduce skin irritation. One must also make sure the foreskin is over the glans. Only elastic tape should be used (to allow expansion or erections). This tape is applied in a spiral only to avoid impaired circulation.

The nurse must monitor the patency of the system frequently and remove the condom at least daily to clean and dry the skin. It is important to teach the client and significant others about incontinent care at home before discharge (see Client Education Guide: Urinary Incontinence).

CLIENT EDUCATION GUIDE

Urinary Incontinence

Before discharge, the nurse must teach the client and significant others the following:

- The symptoms of recurrent urinary bladder incontinence
- How to perform Kegel exercises
- How to maintain a toileting schedule
- Why fluid intake is important and to avoid a decrease in fluid intake
- How to space fluid intake throughout the day and limit intake in the evening
- How to care for the skin and apply and change adult briefs, when indicated
- Application and care of a condom catheter in male clients, when indicated
- The necessity of a bedside commode if the client cannot reach the toilet in time
- Regarding the availability of continence clinics in the area
- Information about Help for Incontinent Persons, which publishes a newsletter containing important information for the incontinent client and significant others
- Regarding the availability of psychological help when the client has problems with self-image, isolation, and helplessness.

Modification of Plan of Care for the Elderly

Incontinence is a common problem among the elderly. They can be treated with any of the previously mentioned treatments. The elderly are more sensitive to many medications, so care should be used when administering them to older adults. The nurse should also remember that muscle weakness, with external factors such as decreased mobility and dependency, is a major cause of incontinence.

URINARY RETENTION

Urinary retention means that the urine is retained in the bladder. Urine production continues, but accumulated urine is not released.

Etiology

Obstruction at or below the bladder outlet is the most common cause of urinary retention. This retention can be caused by a variety of disorders, including BPH, urethral strictures, urethral valves (now considered to be congenital diaphragms in the urethra), phimosis, meatal stenosis, fibrosis, calculi, blood clots, tumors, and bladder neck contractures.

Retention may also be caused by decreased sensory input to and from the bladder, muscle tension, and anxiety. Surgery has traditionally been a factor; spinal anesthesia causes retention more than does general anesthesia.

Other causes include medication and neurologic injuries caused by diabetes, strokes, and spinal cord injuries that may interfere with the micturition reflex. Anorectal problems predispose to retention by applying pressure on the urethra. Decreased intake can also lead to retention through slowed production of urine and failure of normal detrusor reflexes.

Pathophysiology

Retention is a hazardous condition because the resulting urinary stasis contributes to the evolution of UTI and stone formation. There is also the potential for long-term structural damage in the bladder, ureters, or kidneys. Continued bladder distention may lead to loss of bladder tone. The potential effects of a urinary tract obstruction are listed in Pathophysiology: Urinary Tract Obstruction.

Medications, such as opiates, sedatives, antispasmodics, antiparkinsonians, beta-adrenergic blockers, and psychotropic agents, can interfere with normal

PATHOPHYSIOLOGY

Urinary Tract Obstruction

The pathologic effects of any obstruction produce a snowballing effect, as shown in the illustration. Retained urine increases hydrostatic pressure against the bladder wall. This results in hypertrophy of the detrusor muscle, formation of trabeculae (development of connective tissue in the bladder wall), or development of diverticula.

At the same time, peristalsis in the ureteral musculature increases against the pressure of the accumulating urine. The ureter eventually becomes elongated, tortuous, and fibrotic.

The increasing pressure is also transmitted through the renal pelvis and calices into the renal parenchyma. The resulting hydronephrosis also exerts pressure on the blood vessels, causing ischemia and adding to the renal damage. If the process is not interrupted, it can proceed to renal failure and death.

Even after the retention is relieved, in later stages of pressure-related damage, permanent damage may result.

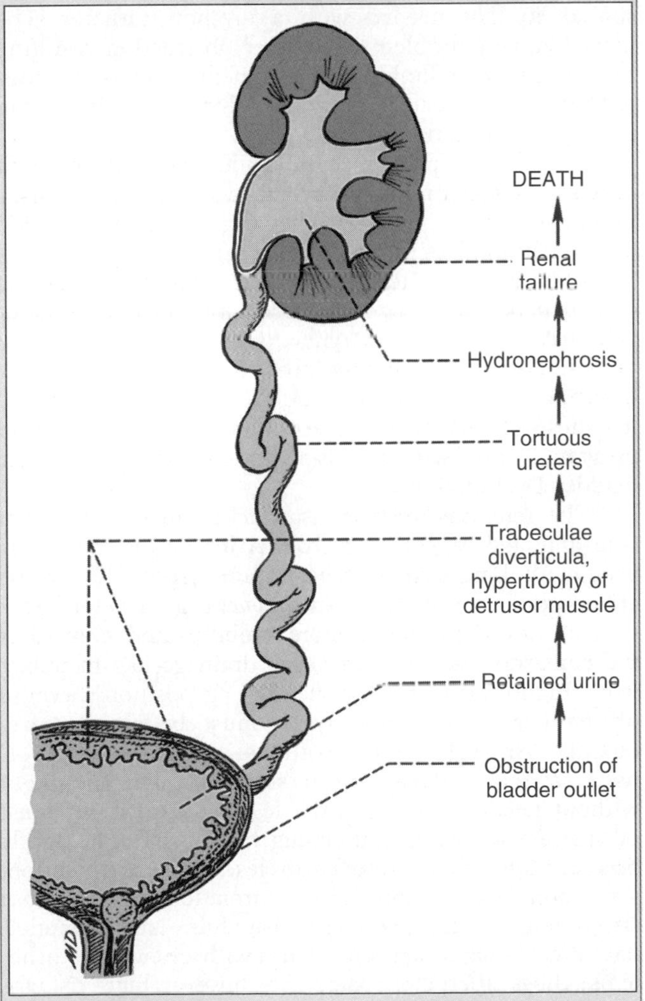

neurologic function and the micturition reflex. Diseases with neurologic impact, such as diabetes mellitus, tabes dorsalis, and spinal cord lesions, also interfere with the micturition reflex.

Decreased fluid intake, either oral or intravenous, reduces glomerular filtration rate, and very slow urine production causes the bladder to fill slowly. This may allow the detrusor muscle to accommodate the increased volume until the muscle's fibers are stretched beyond their ability to contract. When this happens, micturition cannot occur.

Retention with overflow results from the following events. As the bladder continues filling, the intravesical pressure rises. Eventually, this pressure overcomes the restraint of the sphincter. Urine flows out of the bladder until it reduces the intravesical pressure, but only to the level at which the external sphincter can again control the flow of urine. The client reports that the bladder does not feel really empty. The bladder overfills again, and the cycle is repeated.

Clinical Manifestations

The primary manifestation of urinary retention is a distended bladder and the client's inability to void. A high fluid intake but low urinary output record documents that fluid either is not being converted to urine (oliguria or anuria) or is being retained in the bladder.

If the client voids more than once per hour, and releases only 25 to 50 mL at any one time, the problem may be retention with overflow.

DIAGNOSTIC ASSESSMENT

The major diagnostic test for retention is catheterization. If there is more than 250 to 500 mL of urine in the bladder and the client has not been able to void, retention is present. If the cause is thought to be an obstruction, cystoscopy may be performed to determine the cause of that obstruction.

Medical Management

If obstruction causes the urinary retention, the urethra will need to be dilated or the occlusion removed for long-term relief. For dilation of the urethra, progressively larger indwelling catheters may be inserted each day. The urethra can be dilated more quickly with size-graded sounds, filiforms, followers, or other dilating instruments, usually under local or sometimes general anesthesia.

Urinary catheterization with either a straight catheter or a retention catheter is commonly used to treat retention.

PHARMACOLOGIC MANAGEMENT

Cholinergic medications help stimulate bladder contraction, but these drugs must never be used if a mechanical obstruction is present. Although their effect is somewhat controversial, bethanechol (Urecholine) and neostigmine (Prostigmin) are often administered. Bethanechol improves detrusor tone but also increases bladder outlet and urethral resistance. To counteract this, it is sometimes combined with phenoxybenzamine (Dibenzyline), prazosin (Minipress), and terazosin (Hytrin), potent alpha-adrenergic blockers.

Surgical Management

Surgical intervention may be necessary for obstructions below the bladder. If the bladder neck becomes rigid, cystoplasty may be performed to insert an elastic wedge into the area. A transurethral incision of the bladder neck might also be done. Excising urethral strictures, sometimes with plastic repair of the urethra (urethroplasty), helps return it to proper functioning. A meatotomy may be performed to open the urethral meatus better.

Suprapubic catheterization is sometimes used to relieve urinary retention, especially in instances in which urethral catheterization is difficult or dangerous, such as with severely enlarged prostates, with urethral strictures, or in quadriplegics. The suprapubic catheter is inserted by the physician, often under local anesthesia and frequently in the client's room. General anesthesia may be used if another surgical procedure is also performed. To facilitate proper placement of the catheter, the bladder must be distended with fluid before the catheter is inserted. If the bladder is insufficiently distended with urine, additional fluid is instilled through a catheter or cystoscope.

When the suprapubic catheter is removed, the muscle layers of the bladder immediately contract over the puncture site and shrink the surface wound, precluding any need for sutures.

Advantages of the suprapubic over the urethral catheter include a lower rate of UTIs, ease in evaluation of the client's ability to void normally, and increased comfort.

Potential complications of the suprapubic catheter include dislodgement of the catheter, hematuria (especially after the use of a large bore catheter), bowel perforation during insertion, and failure of the wound to close with the development of a urinary fistula.

Nursing Management

It is important for the nurse to distinguish retention from oliguria and anuria. Oliguria means that the kidneys are producing less than 400 mL of urine per 24 hours, whereas anuria means that the kidneys are producing less than 100 mL of urine per 24 hours. In urinary retention, the kidneys are producing a normal amount of urine, but it is not voided. Thus, the bladder fills with urine and is raised above the level of the pubic symphysis, sometimes being displaced to either side of midline. The nurse must palpate above the pubic symphysis for a full bladder. Any percussion over the bladder produces a "kettledrum" sound. The client may experience increasing discomfort and the need to urinate. Assessment may reveal restlessness and diaphoresis.

Nursing interventions may be used initially to treat retention. The nurse should provide privacy, warm the bedpan, and place the client in a normal sitting or standing position, using gravity and increased intra-abdominal pressure to help relieve the problem. The nurse can make use of the "power of suggestion" by running water or flushing the toilet within earshot of the client. Tape-recorded aquatic sounds may be effective. A warm bath or pouring warm water over the perineum often promotes muscle relaxation. Immersing the hands in water sometimes works, as does blowing bubbles with a straw in a glass of water. Applying ice to or stroking the inner thigh with light pressure will stimulate trigger points that may activate the micturition reflex. Anal dilation with a gloved finger is sometimes helpful. If the client is very tense and anxious, any measure that induces relaxation may aid in relieving the situation (e.g., a backrub or soothing music).

The client with a suprapubic catheter requires care similar to that needed with a urethral catheter. The most frequent problem is catheter obstruction resulting from twisting or kinking, or sediment or clots. Disconnecting the catheter from the drainage tubing can disrupt the siphon drainage.

When the suprapubic catheter is removed, frequent dressing changes may be needed to control the urinary leakage from the site. As the site of the suprapubic catheter heals, less drainage will occur.

A straight catheter can be used to drain the bladder and then be removed. A retention, or indwelling, catheter may be inserted to relieve retention over a longer period. The nurse must use strict aseptic techniques for insertion. One exception is the use of a clean technique for those clients on an intermittent self-catheterization program. (See further discussion under Neurogenic Bladder Dysfunction.)

The retention catheter is attached to either a bedside drainage bag or a leg bag. A leg bag is frequently used with long-term catheterization, especially for the client going home with an indwelling catheter. This device allows the client more mobility and eliminates the embarrassment of carrying a drainage bag in public view. Figure 30–3 shows a leg bag in position. Because of the bag's small capacity, it must be emptied frequently. At night, a conventional drainage system is used so that the client can sleep through the night without needing to empty the leg bag. The client must be instructed to avoid attaching the leg bag too tightly because the rubber straps can lead to skin irritation, thrombophlebitis, and ulcer formation. Even loose straps tend to tighten as the bag fills. Newer models have Velcro leg straps for clients with circulatory problems, those allergic to latex, or those at high risk for skin breakdown. Meticulous skin care and periodic removal of the bag help prevent these problems. Cleanliness and odor control are managed by washing the apparatus with soap and water and soaking it in a 1 per cent acetic acid (white vinegar) solution overnight.

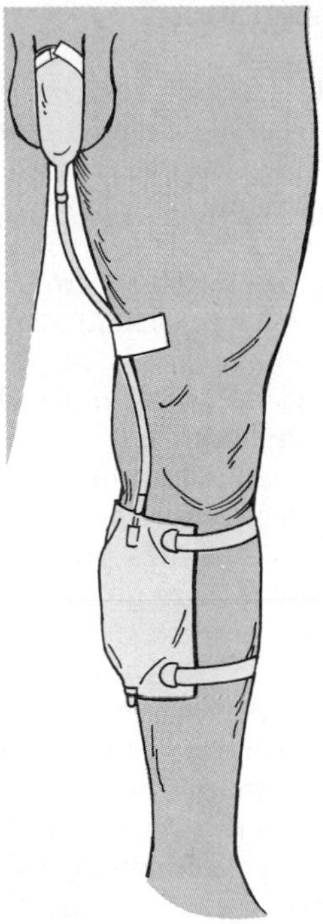

Figure 30–3
Condom drainage and leg bag. The bag may be attached to the calf of the leg, as shown, or to the thigh.

Using indwelling catheters involves several physical hazards, including UTI and tissue trauma. More than 80 per cent of people in whom nosocomial UTIs develop have undergone urologic instrumentation of some kind. Organisms may enter the urinary drainage system when it is opened for any reason, or they may intrude via the thin layer of fluid and exudate that forms around the exterior of the catheter. The development of and intervention for UTI are discussed in this chapter.

Probably the most important weapon in preventing infection is conscientious hand washing before and after any handling of the catheter or drainage system.

To aid in preventing infection

- Maintain a closed drainage system
- Avoid backflow of urine (e.g., keep drainage bag below level of the bladder)
- Avoid unnecessary manipulation of the catheter during perineal cleansing
- Prevent microbial invasion and colonization in the urine collection bag
- Maintain patency of the catheter
- Encourage a high fluid intake
- Provide urine acidification

Because of the potential development of resistant organisms and possible adverse reactions, antibiotics should not be used prophylactically to prevent bacteriuria.

The client who goes home with an indwelling suprapubic or urethral catheter needs to know how to care for the catheter at home. The family and significant others should learn the proper ways to empty the drainage bag and ways of preventing infection, such as encouraging fluids and an acid-ash diet. They should also be taught the signs and symptoms of UTI and instructed to call the physician if one occurs.

The client who goes home with a catheter in place will need to be seen later for removal of the catheter; this varies depending on the cause of the retention. The nurse should check with the physician for the timing of a follow-up visit.

Modification of Plan of Care for the Elderly

The older clients are more prone to retention because of chronic decrease in bladder tone. Retention leading to infection may also be worse in older clients. The treatments, however, remain the same.

URINARY REFLUX

Urinary reflux, or the backward flow of urine within the urinary tract, usually begins at the vesicoureteral junction so urine flows back into the ureter and frequently upward into the renal pelvis.

Etiology

Reflux can be caused by congenital malformations and by infectious processes in which edema and fixation of the intramural ureter and urethra interfere with normal flow. Neuromuscular malfunctions may contribute to reflux, as can bladder neck obstruction, which builds up intravesical pressure until it finally overwhelms the resistance of the ureteral sphincters.

Risk Factors

Risk factors for reflux include any disorder that causes obstruction. Chronic UTIs increase the risk of scarring and, therefore, obstruction. Bladder neck contracture after prostatectomy (see Chap. 52) is another risk factor, as is BPH itself. There is no primary prevention, but those clients with obstructive disorders should be closely checked for reflux.

Pathophysiology

If there is urethral obstruction, the main result is an ever-present residual urine that often leads to the development of UTIs. The continual presence of urine can also change detrusor tone, thereby increasing the bladder's capacity and raising the threshold required to initiate the micturition reflex.

Renal damage and infection are the two primary problems resulting from vesicoureteral reflux. Because the capacity of the renal pelvis is only 5 mL, any larger amounts of urine can cause renal tissue destruction, which can lead to end-stage renal disease. With reflux any pathogens in the bladder are carried through the ureters to the kidney. This problem leads to repeated pyelonephritis (kidney infection), which eventually causes chronic renal failure.

Clinical Manifestations

The major symptoms exhibited by these clients are obstruction and retention. The bladder will be distended if the obstruction is in the bladder neck but not if the obstruction is in the vesicoureteral junction or higher. If the obstruction is higher, then the client may exhibit signs and symptoms of renal failure.

DIAGNOSTIC ASSESSMENT

The major diagnostic studies are cystoscopy to look for signs of obstruction, ureteroscopy to look at the vesicoureteral junction, and IVP to look at the entire collecting system. Blood studies such as blood urea nitrogen and creatinine determinations are performed to assess renal function.

Medical Management

There are few medical treatments for urinary reflux; the primary treatment is surgical.

Surgical Management

The presence of renal damage, from the reflux, usually calls for surgical intervention. Surgery is also indicated for obstruction at the ureteropelvic junction, for intractable infection, and if the problem is not resolved by maturation. Because the most common causes of reflux are ureteral defects, surgical procedures that focus on correcting reflux involve the ureter (e.g., reimplantation of the ureter).

Postoperatively, a urethral or suprapubic catheter keeps the bladder empty to reduce tension on the suture line. A ureteral catheter will also be inserted into each ureter involved in the surgical procedure. This tiny, semirigid catheter is inserted into the ureter with its tip frequently placed in the renal pelvis. The distal end extends through the bladder and out through the urethra or through an abdominal incision. A ureteral catheter splints the ureter to facilitate healing, prevents obstruction from edema after surgery or other trauma in the area, and drains urine.

The major complications to monitor for are problems associated with the ureteral catheters postoperatively. They can clog or become dislodged prematurely. Ureteral catheters are rarely irrigated by the nurse.

Nursing Management

The nurse should carefully assess clients who are at high risk for obstruction for any signs or symptoms of urinary reflux. The client who is being diagnosed for urinary reflux will require support during this diagnostic process.

Preoperative preparation for ureteral surgery is similar to that required by any client requiring surgery (see Chap. 5).

Postoperatively, the nurse must closely monitor the output of the ureteral catheter. Because the renal pelvis holds only 5 mL, ureteral catheters must be kept patent. One must never clamp them! Any unexpected reduction in urine flow requires prompt intervention.

Several conditions can interfere with the flow of urine through these catheters. The catheters are easily plugged with mucous shreds, blood clots, and chemical sediment. Also, ureteral peristalsis occasionally pushes the catheters out of the ureter into the bladder.

One must monitor the output from these catheters closely. Each catheter, ureteral and urethral, should drain into its own collection bag so the source of the reduced flow will be noticed immediately.

If catheter irrigation is ordered by the physician, the nurse must use strict aseptic technique. A maximum of 5 mL of irrigating solution, usually normal saline, should be allowed to flow in by gravity or irrigated with very gentle force. One must never irrigate this catheter with use of force. If patency cannot be established, the physician should be notified immediately.

One must take special care not to dislodge the catheter accidentally. If the catheter is not sutured in place, it should be secured carefully to the skin with tape.

The color of the urine should be assessed frequently. One must expect that the color will progress from bright red to clear yellow over a matter of days. If the urine does not clear, further investigation may be necessary.

Posthospital Care

Discharge teaching depends on a variety of factors, including the cause of the reflux, the treatment done, and the amount of renal damage that occurred.

If reflux is caused by BPH, the probable treatment would be prostatectomy and the discharge instructions would be based on the exact type of surgery done (see Chap. 52). If the cause is a problem with the vesicoureteral junction, then the teaching will possibly include information about catheter care at home, because these clients have a catheter in place longer.

If there is permanent renal damage, then the teaching will be similar to that given to a client with chronic renal failure (see Chap. 31).

The client with renal involvement should have renal function closely monitored, at regular intervals, for about 1 year so that any changes could be detected early.

Modification of Plan of Care for the Elderly

There are no specific modifications for the older client, although men with BPH are in the higher risk group.

BLADDER NEOPLASMS OF THE LOWER URINARY TRACT

Incidence

Bladder cancer is the most frequent neoplasm of the urinary tract. It accounts for approximately 3 per cent of all deaths caused by cancer. It occurs most frequently in the fifth to seventh decades. Also, it appears in men two to three times more often than in women, although the incidence in women is rising. This cancer is now the fifth most common cancer in men and the tenth most common cancer in women. It affects whites twice as often as blacks. It is more common in people living in the northern United States as opposed to those living in the southern states.

Etiology

Although the cause of bladder cancer is uncertain, there are risk factors that are related to increased incidence in males and females.

Risk Factors

The major risk factor for bladder cancer is exposure to cigarette smoke. The best method of preventing bladder cancer is to avoid cigarette smoke, through either smoking or second-hand smoke.

Pelvic radiation, the use of cyclophosphamide (Cytoxan), chronic cystitis, bladder calculus disease, schistosomiasis, and a large phenacetin intake are all predisposing factors in the development of bladder cancer. Many of these are not amenable to primary prevention, but clients who are exposed to these factors should be monitored closely for the development of bladder cancer.

Pathophysiology

Cigarette smoking, either active or passively receiving second-hand smoke, may result in carcinogenic metabolites produced by abnormal tryptophan metabolism.

Most bladder cancers start as papillomas that undergo malignant changes. Nodular tumors occur less frequently but may also invade the bladder wall. Cellular proliferation is chiefly in the transitional epithelium (90 per cent), although squamous cell (6 per cent) or adenocarcinoma (2 per cent) may occur.

Staging of the tumor indicates the depth of penetration into the bladder wall and its degree of metastasis. Staging must be done before selection of the treatment mode. Figure 30–4 illustrates the usual staging schema:

- Stage 0 (T_0,N_0,M_0) tumor is limited to the mucosa.
- Stage A (T_1,N_0,M_0) tumor indicates invasion no farther than the submucosa.
- Stage B_1 (T_2,N_0,M_0) tumor extends not more than halfway through the muscle layer.
- Stage B_2 (T_{3a},N_0,M_0) tumor penetrates more deeply into the muscle layer but not into the fat.
- Stage C (T_{3b},N_0,M_0) tumor has infiltrated beyond the muscle layer but is not metastatic, nor is it invading adjacent structures.
- Stage D_1 (T_{4a},N_{1-3},M_0) tumor metastasizes to the pelvic lymph nodes.
- Stage D_2 (T_{4a},N_4,M_1) tumor metastasizes beyond the pelvis.

Common sites for metastasis include liver, bones, and lungs. As the tumor progresses, it extends into the rectum, vaginal and soft tissue, and retroperitoneal structures. The prognostic "dividing line" lies between

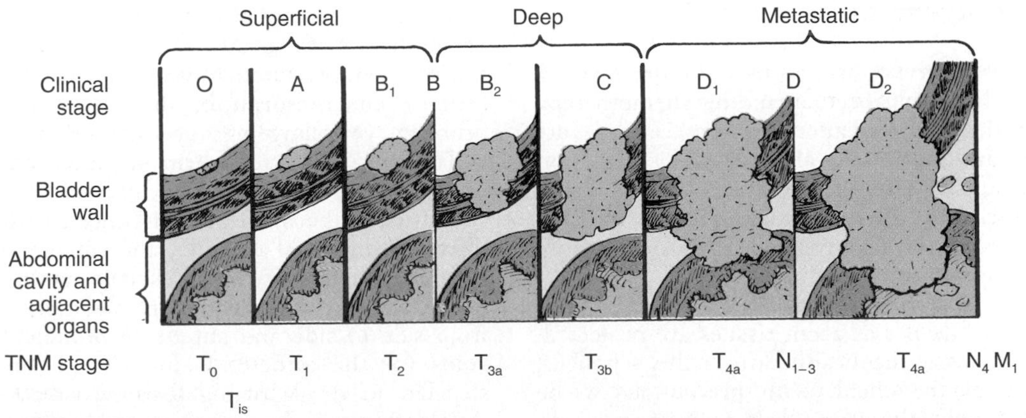

Figure 30–4
The Jewett-Marshall clinical staging of bladder cancer. Diagram shows degree of tumor infiltration at each stage and compares it with the tumor-node-metastasis (TNM) system.

B_1 and B_2; tumors staged C or D on the scale have a much poorer prognosis. Superficial tumors have a good chance of being eradicated or stabilized, although recurrence is frequent. Less than 25 per cent of clients with deeply invasive tumors have a 5-year survival rate; aggressive adenocarcinoma results in an average survival rate of 21 months.

Clinical Manifestations

Painless hematuria is most frequently the first sign of bladder cancer, and it occurs in 75 per cent of all cases. Unfortunately, the bleeding is initially intermittent, which often causes a delay in seeking health-care diagnostic services. As the disease progresses, the client may experience frequent bladder irritability with dysuria. Finally, gross hematuria, an obstruction, or development of a fistula may force the client to seek help.

DIAGNOSTIC ASSESSMENT

The most basic test for bladder cancer is urinalysis. The presence of blood in the urine, especially if no other cause is apparent, warrants further tests. Cystoscopy should be done to visualize the tumor directly and to biopsy the lesion for cytologic study. Flow cytometry can be done to examine the deoxyribonucleic acid content of the urine cells. Cytology on a total voided urine specimen, obtained in the late morning and sent immediately to the laboratory, is done to check for the presence of malignant cells. Cytology can also be done on specimens obtained during cystoscopy. The specimen is obtained when the bladder is irrigated with a solution of Ringer's lactate solution.

Another examination is the IVP, which evaluates not only the bladder but also the ureters and kidneys. Computed tomography, magnetic resonance imaging, and ultrasonography may also be done to assess the bladder and surrounding structures, such as the rectum or uterus, possible sites of metastasis. A tumor marker, the carcinoembryonic antigen level, can also be evaluated.

Medical Management

Several forms of intervention are used in the medical management of bladder cancer, including chemotherapy and radiation therapy. Radiation therapy is more accepted for advanced disease, although it is used on early tumors outside the United States and is being studied for such use in the United States. Bladder cancers are poorly radiosensitive and, therefore, require high doses of radiation.

Intracavitary radiation applies radiation to the bladder malignancy while the adjacent tissues are protected. The nurse must learn the health-care facility's policies about isolation of the client, with precautions to be taken. In general, clients with radium seed implants are in a private room with limited visiting times (see Chap. 7 for more information).

External supervoltage radiation, rather unsuccessful by itself, is effective when used in combination with surgery or chemotherapy. Hyperbaric radiation therapy increases the oxygen tension of the tumor cells and, therefore, radiosensitivity. Palliative radiation may be used to relieve pain, bowel obstruction, and leg edema secondary to venous or lymphatic obstruction or to control bladder hemorrhage.

Several interventions are now being tried to treat bladder cancer. One such intervention is the use of hematoporphyrin derivative, which selectively goes to malignant cells, making them more photosensitive. Phototherapy or laser therapy is then used to destroy tumor cells.

The most frequent complications for the client receiving radiation therapy include severe cystitis and proctitis causing dysuria, frequency, urgency, nocturia, and diarrhea. Delayed adverse effects, such as ileitis, colitis, persistent cystitis, and bladder ulceration and hemorrhage, may occur as late as 6 to 12 months after radiation.

Radiation therapy also increases the risk of fistula formation. A fistula is an abnormal passage between two organs or between an organ and the skin. This allows intercommunication of secretions and other substances. After radiation to the bladder, a vesicovaginal fistula (in women) or a colovesical fistula (in men) may develop.

A fistula is suspected when urine leaves the body from an unnatural site such as the vagina, when fecal material or air appears in the urine, or when the client suffers from recurrent UTIs. Diagnosis is confirmed by IVP, cystoscopy, or sigmoidoscopy.

Before surgical repair of the fistula is undertaken, the client must maintain a continuous flow of urine from the kidney through temporary urinary diversion, either externally or with catheters. Surgical repairs often require multiple stages. The primary goal is to excise the fistula and re-establish tissue integrity.

PHARMACOLOGIC MANAGEMENT

Pharmacologic agents can be administered preoperatively, postoperatively, or instead of surgery. Antineoplastic chemotherapy is administered both topically and systemically. Intravesical instillation of an alkylating chemotherapeutic agent is the most common method; it provides concentrated topical treatment with relatively little systemic absorption. Thiotepa, mitomycin C, doxorubicin (Adriamycin), cyclophosphamide (Cytoxan), and bacille Calmette-Guérin are all used for this purpose.

Usually, the medication is injected into the bladder through a urethral catheter, the catheter is clamped or removed, and the client is asked to retain the fluid for 2 hours and possibly to change position every 2 hours from side to side and supine to prone. The client then voids (or the catheter is unclamped) and is then instructed to drink two glasses of water to help flush the bladder. These treatments are typically repeated weekly for 4 to 8 weeks and then monthly for varying periods.

Systemic agents include cisplatin (Platinol), doxorubicin (Adriamycin), methotrexate, cyclophosphamide (Cytoxan), and pyridoxine. These agents have proved effective in prolonging life, even for metastatic disease.

The major side effects of chemotherapy include hemorrhagic cystitis and bladder irritation. Local application of formalin may control bladder hemorrhaging that results from the cancer or the treatments.

DIETARY MANAGEMENT

There is no particular diet modification associated with treatment of bladder cancer. If the client acquires radiation proctitis, a low-residue diet is ordered.

Surgical Management

Surgical therapy is commonly used to treat bladder cancer. Surgical intervention ranges from local resection and fulguration of the tumor to total cystectomy, which also requires diversion of normal urinary flow. Table 30–4 lists the types of surgical management used. Figure 30–5 shows different types of urinary diversions.

Nephrostomy is insertion of catheters into the renal pelvis by surgical incision or a percutaneous puncture procedure. It is important to stabilize the tube to prevent dislodgement. Figure 30–6 shows a percutaneous nephrostomy tube in place and a suggested method for stabilization.

If the nephrostomy tube is used to divert urine flow while the ureters are repaired, it may be temporary. It is more often permanent, especially if the ureters are removed as part of a cystectomy. Because of the high risk of infection and calculus formation, nephrostomy is a last resort and considered only a palliative measure. Other complications include erosion of the collection system by the catheter, hemorrhage, mucosal edema, obstruction of the catheter, and perforation of the calix during catheter insertion.

An ileal conduit, also called ureteroileostomy, ileal bladder, or Bricker's procedure, is the most common urinary diversion. Using a segment of the intestine as a

TABLE 30–4 Surgical Management of Bladder Cancer

TYPE OF SURGERY	DESCRIPTION
Transurethral resection and fulguration	Done early, it includes tissue destruction by electrical current via fulguration
Segmental partial cystectomy	Up to half of the bladder may be removed; decreased bladder capacity results initially
Total cystectomy, radical cystectomy with urinary diversion	In women, removal of the bladder and urethra, as well as uterus, ovaries, fallopian tubes, and part of the anterior vaginal wall; in men, removal of bladder, prostate and seminal vesicles, ampullary portion of the vas deferens
Urinary diversion	Necessary after removal of the bladder and urethra (see Fig. 30–6)
Cutaneous urostomy	Attaches the ureter to the surface of the abdomen

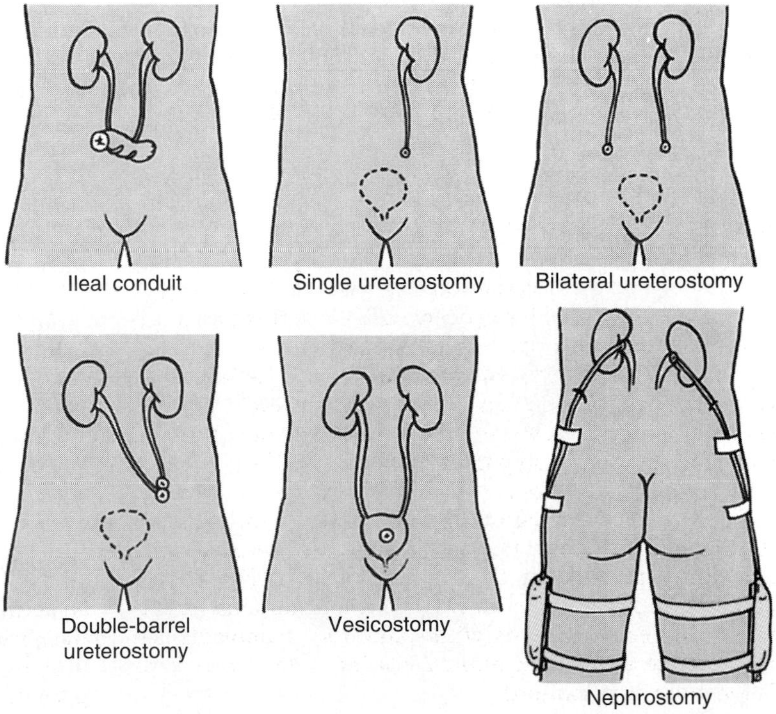

Figure 30–5
Surgical alternatives for urinary diversion.

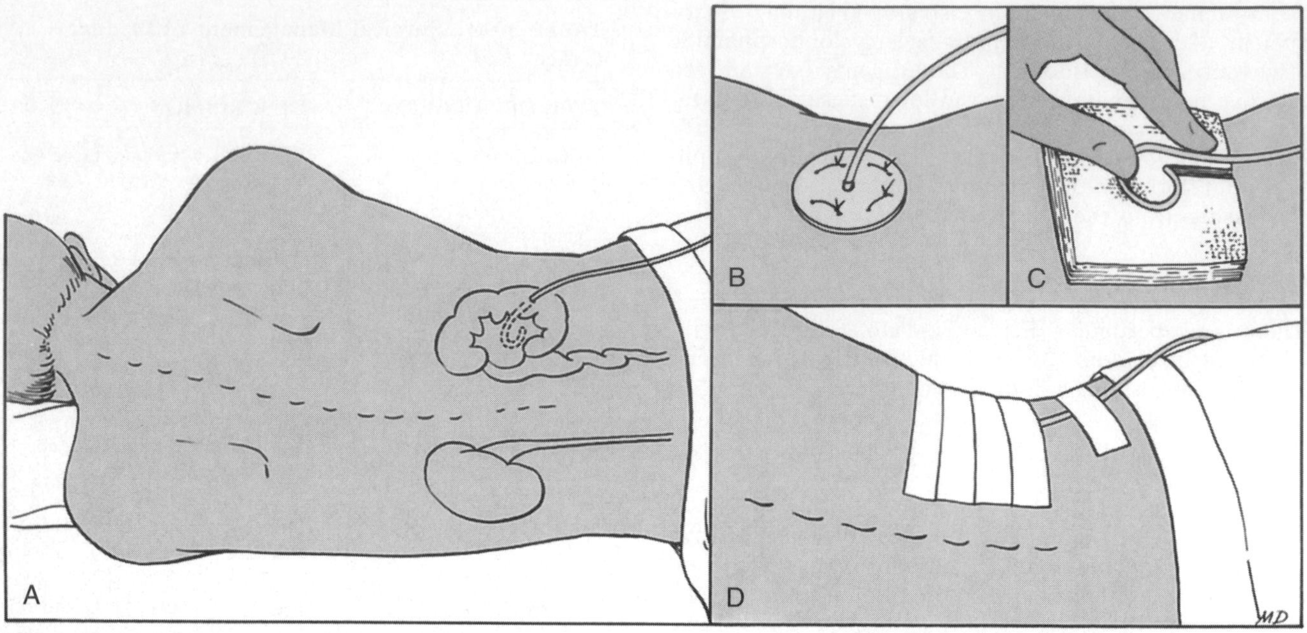

Figure 30–6
Percutaneous nephrostomy tube and suggested method for stabilization. *A*, Insertion point in kidney. *B*, Secure nephrostomy tube to skin with sutured disc. *C*, Snip 4 × 4 pad with sterile scissors, cover disc with pad as shown, and loop tubing. *D*, Cover entire area with tape. (Adapted from Cain, L., & Bigongiari, L. [1982]. The percutaneous nephrostomy tube. *American Journal of Nursing,* 82:296.)

conduit, this procedure constructs a system so that urine is emptied through an opening in the skin. Usually, a portion of the terminal ileum that has the least reabsorptive power is isolated for the diversion. Portions of the sigmoid colon and jejunum can also be used for this procedure. An ileal conduit requires the client to wear an appliance for collecting urine.

A newer procedure is the Kock pouch or continent internal ileal reservoir. The Kock pouch is created from a segment of ileum that has been made into a reservoir (Fig. 30–7). Once the reservoir has been created, the ureters are implanted into the side of the reservoir. A special nipple valve is then constructed and used to attach the reservoir to the skin. The client is then

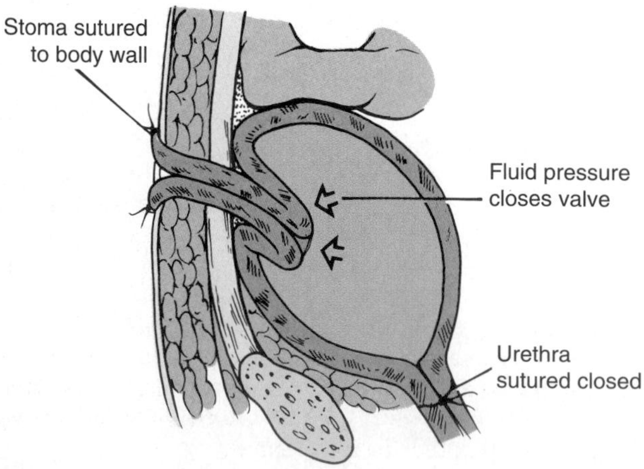

Figure 30–7
A continent vesicostomy.

taught to use a catheter at regular intervals to drain the pouch and achieve continence.

An even newer procedure, similar to the Kock pouch, is the Indiana pouch. During this procedure, a reservoir is created from the ascending colon and terminal ileum, making a larger pouch than the Kock pouch (Fig. 30–8). Clients learn how to catheterize themselves and empty the pouch at 4- to 6-hour intervals. There are other continent reservoir surgeries, varying slightly in surgical technique and the portion of the colon and ileum used. The pouches can store up to 800 mL inside the body.

The most common complication of the ileal conduit is the late development of obstruction at the ureteroileal anastomosis. Other complications include pyelonephritis, leakage at the anastomosis site, stenosis anywhere along the system, hydronephrosis, calculi, peristomal hernia, uremia, skin irritation, ulceration, and stomal defects.

The complications of a Kock pouch or an Indiana pouch include incontinence, difficult catheterization, urinary reflux and possible pyelonephritis, obstruction, bacteriuria, electrolyte imbalances, or absorptive problems.

Nursing Management

Assessment

The nurse should begin the assessment of the client being evaluated for bladder cancer with a careful history, looking especially for exposure to known risk factors.

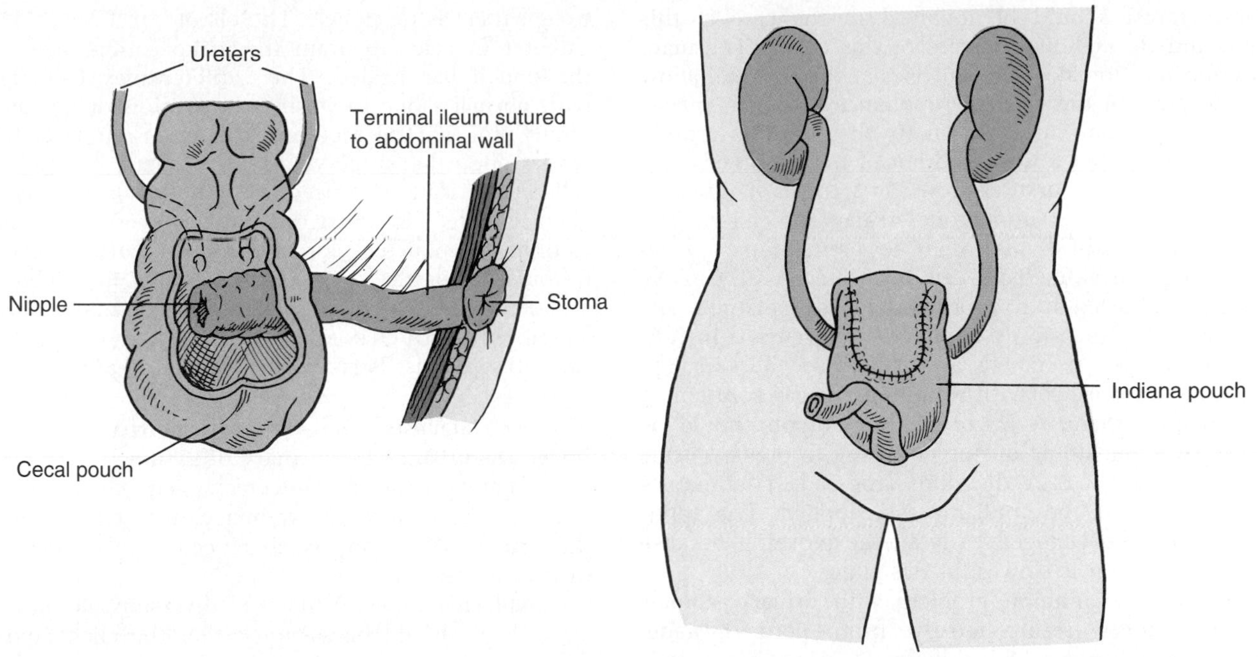

Figure 30–8
Indiana pouch procedure.

The nurse should also question the client about changes in the urine or in urination, noting changes in color, frequency, and amounts of urine. The presence of hematuria should always be investigated further.

Nursing Diagnosis, Planning, and Implementation

Nursing Diagnosis: Injury, Risk for R/T radiation therapy and chemotherapy.

Planning: Expected Outcomes. The client will not experience problems related to radiation therapy or chemotherapy, as evidenced by absence of hemorrhagic cystitis.

Implementation. Intervention for the side effects of radiation therapy includes administering antispasmodics, increasing the client's fluid intake, and administering urinary tract antiseptics for the cystitis. The client with proctitis requires a low-residue diet and agents to decrease intestinal motility. Complete information on nursing care for clients receiving radiation therapy is covered in Chapter 7.

Nursing care for the client receiving chemotherapy is covered in Chapter 7. If the client has intravesical chemotherapy, the nurse should remember to treat the urine as a biohazard, the same as any other chemotherapy that needs to be disposed of properly.

Nursing Diagnosis: Urinary Elimination, Altered (Dysuria) R/T presence of tumors.

Planning: Expected Outcomes. The client will have tumors diagnosed early to eliminate the dysuria, as evidenced by actions taken to seek health care.

Implementation. Nursing care after transurethral resection (TUR) is covered in detail in Chapter 52. The client will have some hematuria and, until the bleeding ceases, an indwelling urethral catheter. Sometimes the catheter will be attached to a continuous or intermittent closed bladder irrigation system to prevent blood clots. Nursing intervention is similar to that after a cystoscopy or TUR of the prostate. This includes adequate intake of fluids, analgesics, and antispasmodics as needed.

Nursing care for the client who has had segmental resection centers on maintaining constant urinary drainage so the bladder does not become distended, straining the suture line. The client usually has both a urethral catheter and a suprapubic catheter. The suprapubic catheter is usually left in for 2 weeks, until complete healing has occurred, so the client will be discharged with the catheter in place.

Nursing Diagnosis: Knowledge Deficit R/T diagnostic tests, surgery, and care of urinary diversion.

Planning: Expected Outcomes. The client will understand the diagnostic tests, surgery, and care of the urinary diversion, as evidenced by client's statements and demonstration of ability for self-care.

Implementation. Preoperative preparation of clients undergoing diversionary surgery includes teaching guidelines concerning urinary diversion and encouraging acceptance of the fact that diversion results in the elimination of urine through the skin, rectum, or specially constructed stoma and not through the urethral meatus as was once "normal."

In addition to general physical and emotional preparation, the client's bowel may need the following special attention: a nonresidue diet for several days, sterilization of the bowel with neomycin, and bowel cleansing with cathartics or enemas.

If the surgeon plans to construct a stoma, the site is selected during the preoperative period. An enterostomal therapist should be involved in the care at this point and throughout the care of this client. The main criterion for stomal placement is that the site will allow the faceplate of the drainage appliance to bind securely to the abdominal surface. Usually the stoma is created in the right or left lower quadrant of the abdomen.

Skin irritation or breakdown is a constant threat to the client who has undergone urinary diversion. The nurse should advise the client to prevent urine from contacting the skin. This can be achieved in part by using a well-fitted and properly attached appliance. The application of an ostomy appliance is discussed in fundamentals texts. If crystals are present on the skin, the skin must be washed with a diluted vinegar solution to help remove them. A gauze pad or tampon should be placed over the stoma during cleansing to prevent urine from flowing out over the skin. This pad or tampon is removed just as the appliance is reapplied. The appliance should be changed early in the morning because urine production is slowest at this time.

Odor is a common problem with urinary stomas. Noxious odors result mostly from poor hygiene, alkaline urine, normal breakdown of urine (ammonia), and the ingestion of certain foods, such as asparagus. Although permanent appliances are rarely used today, to control odors in them, reusable appliances must be washed thoroughly with soap and lukewarm water. The pouch can also be soaked in dilute white vinegar or in a commercial deodorant product for 20 to 30 minutes. The nurse should rinse the pouch and allow it to dry.

For all appliances, deodorant tablets are available that can be placed in the pouch while it is being worn. Ingestion of methionine can alleviate the smell of ammonia, and acidifying the urine reduces odor. Because diluted urine is less odoriferous, adequate fluid intake is most helpful in preventing odor.

Care for the client with a Kock or Indiana pouch is similar to that of any client with a urinary diversion, except there is no pouch. The client will have a Medina catheter in place to drain the urine continuously until the pouch has healed. The catheter may be irrigated with normal saline to wash out any clots or mucus that might plug it. The Medina catheter is removed 3 to 4 weeks after the surgery, and the client is taught the self-catheterization procedure. At the beginning, the client is taught to insert the catheter every 2 to 3 hours to drain the pouch. Later, the interval can be every 4 to 6 hours during the day and once during the night.

Before discharge, the client and significant others should be instructed about care at home. (See Client Education Guide: Post-Urinary Diversion Surgery.)

Nursing Diagnosis: Self-Esteem Disturbance and Body Image Disturbance R/T urinary diversion.

Planning: Expected Outcomes. The client will have a normal self-concept, body image, and self-esteem after the urinary diversion, as evidenced by the client's return to normal life.

Implementation. Whatever diversion alternative is selected, it should be assumed that the client and significant others will need a great deal of emotional support. Changing the normal route of urine flow and the client's usual micturition pattern will change the client's self-image, including alterations in emotional, psychosocial, and perceptual reactions. Preoperative counseling should fully explain the expected anatomic and physiologic alterations, including their possible effect on the client. Counseling should also present ways to maintain the client's current life-style. Community associations and their resources, such as the United Ostomy Association and the American Cancer Society, are a tremendous help to the client undergoing diversion. The nurse may need to restrict teaching content to essentials and frequently repeat instructions before learning actually takes place. Postoperatively, the client and significant others may need help to look at the stoma and to accept it as part of the total self.

CLIENT EDUCATION GUIDE

Post-Urinary Diversion Surgery

Clients who have undergone urinary diversion need the enterostomal therapist's and the nurse's help and encouragement to regain their independence and accept their new body image. The nurse must include both the client and significant other(s) in the teaching before discharge. The nurse must

- Help the client organize the equipment and procedures necessary for stomal care at home and explain where stomal supplies may be purchased in the community
- Arrange for the client to demonstrate removal and reapplication of the appliance, emptying the appliance or pouch, and attaching it to a night drainage system
- Discuss adaptations that may need to be made while traveling
- Discuss selection of new clothing that will not constrict the urine collection device
- Teach the importance of daily fluid intake of at least 2000 mL
- Teach the client how to select proper foods and fluids
- Give clear, written instructions regarding when to contact the physician (e.g., changes in color or quantity of urine output, cloudy or foul-smelling urine, or stomal color changes)
- Teach the client with a suprapubic catheter or Medina tube appropriate care, when indicated; the client will wear a urinary pouch until the surgically created pouch completely heals
- The client with bladder cancer should be taught to continue follow-up appointments to assess for recurrence of the cancer

Nursing Diagnosis: Injury, Risk for R/T postoperative complications such as hemorrhage, paralytic ileus, stomal ischemia, and blocking of ureteral catheters.

Planning: Expected Outcomes. The client will not experience postoperative injury, as evidenced by vital signs within preoperative norms, presence of active bowel sounds within 3 to 4 days postoperatively, pink stoma, and at least 30 to 60 mL urine output via ureteral catheters.

Implementation. Postoperative nursing management of the client includes routine monitoring of the vital signs, inspection of the incision, and other postoperative intervention as described in Chapter 5. The client often has a nasogastric tube in place, because postoperative ileus is a common complication. If the client has nephrostomy tubes, they are connected to a bedside drainage system. The nurse must keep tubing patent to prevent obstruction to the free flow of urine. Also the drainage system must be kept closed to help prevent pyelonephritis. If the client has a stoma, there will be a temporary, clear plastic pouch over the stoma that connects to a gravity drainage system. Sometimes ureteral catheters are used to splint the ureters while they heal. These catheters, usually removed before the client is discharged, may extend through the stoma but are ordinarily visible just inside the stomal opening. Other specific postoperative nursing interventions for clients with urinary diversions are listed in Box 30–3.

Stenosis of the stoma may occur from scarring during stomal maturation. If the opening on the faceplate is too large, epithelial hyperplasia, or thickening of the peristomal skin, may contract the stoma. Clients with urinary diversion are also prone to uric acid and calcium stone disease. The onset of urinary stone development usually occurs at least 2 years postoperatively and sometimes as long as 5 to 10 years later. UTI is a perpetual threat because of the exposure of the urinary tract. Obstruction anywhere in the urinary tract will interfere with normal urine flow.

Nursing Diagnosis: Skin Integrity, Risk for Impaired R/T irritation of peristomal skin.

Planning: Expected Outcomes. The client will not develop an altered skin integrity or irritation of peristomal skin, as evidenced by intact, clear skin.

Implementation. Intervention for any skin irritation must begin promptly. The nurse must check the pH of the urine; strongly alkaline urine irritates the skin and facilitates crystal formation. If urine cultures identify UTI, it must be treated. The appliance should be checked carefully to find any leakage and to determine whether the skin is sensitive to anything used in the process of application. Skin irritation may also result from changing the pouch too frequently. A general recommendation is that the pouch be left in place as long as it is not leaking. During changes of the appliance, the nurse must leave the skin open to the air as much as possible. When the appliance is reattached, the skin is dusted with Stomahesive powder and a pouch applied with a Stomahesive skin barrier. Karaya cannot be used with urinary pouches because urine corrodes the karaya.

Skin irritation around the stoma is often caused by a yeast infection. Nystatin creams or powders are used to treat this. Nystatin powder is applied directly over the irritated skin area and then sealed to the skin with a liquid skin barrier.

Nursing Diagnosis: Sexuality Patterns, Altered R/T potential postoperative impotence in men after radical cystectomy.

Planning: Expected Outcomes. The client will discuss alternative methods of sexual expression as evidenced by client's statements.

Implementation. Male clients have a high risk of impotence after a radical cystectomy related to the extent of the resection. It is important for them to receive counseling both before and after the surgery so they can begin to adjust to any alterations. Chapter 52 discusses alterations in male sexuality in detail.

BOX 30–3

Nursing Intervention for Clients After Urinary Diversion Surgery

For all postoperative clients after diversion, nursing intervention includes the following actions:

- Measure urine output every hour for the first 24 hours and afterward at least every 8 hours.
- Check the ostomy bag for leaks and the skin under it for irritation every 4 hours initially and then every 8 hours.
- Inspect the stoma every hour for the first 24 hours after surgery. This will give you a baseline from which you can quickly detect deviations. Then, if there are no problems, extend intervals to every 4 hours and then every 8 hours.
- Note the stoma's size, shape, and color. An edematous stoma is expected in the immediate postoperative period. However, other changes may indicate complications, warranting action from the physician. A dusky or cyanotic color of the stoma may denote an insufficient blood supply and the onset of necrosis. This is an emergency! Other complications with the stoma include prolapse (protrusion from the skin) or retraction into the abdomen beneath the skin.
- Watch for signs of peritonitis, because leakage at the site of the anastomosis or ureteral separation from the conduit causes urine to seep into the peritoneal cavity.
- Observe for bleeding. Although bleeding from the stoma may indicate a surgical defect, it is also common for the intestinal mucosa, which is very fragile, to bleed during a change of appliance or because of a poorly fitted collection pouch.

Evaluation

To evaluate the care that has been given, the nurse formulates outcome criteria. If the goals were not met, alterations in the plan and interventions will be needed. The nurse must continually evaluate the outcomes and modify the interventions as needed.

Modification of Plan of Care for the Elderly

The major modification for older clients with urinary diversion focuses on possible difficulties they may have with self-care of the appliance. Changing the appliance requires some degree of dexterity, and older clients are more likely to have arthritis and other disabilities that limit their ability to manipulate the pouches. They may require assistance or modification of teaching so they can retain some independence.

NEUROGENIC BLADDER DYSFUNCTION

The term "neurogenic bladder" refers to several bladder dysfunctions, all of which are caused by lesions of the central or peripheral nervous systems. Their manifestations depend on the site of the lesion.

There are five major types of neurogenic bladder dysfunction (Fig. 30–9): uninhibited, sensory paralytic (detrusor muscle hyperreflexic), motor paralytic (detrusor muscle areflexic), autonomous, and reflex.

Incidence

The incidence of neurogenic bladder dysfunctions is dependent on the incidence of the various neurologic injuries or disorders that cause these problems.

Etiology

Causes of neurogenic bladder include

- Lesions in the corticoregulatory tracts (e.g., cerebrovascular accidents, multiple sclerosis)
- Interruption in the lateral spinal tracts (e.g., tabes dorsalis, diabetic neuropathy, and pernicious anemia)
- Lesions in the motor outflow from sacral vertebrae 2 to 4 (S2–S4) (e.g., poliomyelitis, tumor, trauma, and infection)
- Destruction of all nerve connections between the bladder and the central nervous system at S2, S3, or S4 (e.g., trauma, inflammatory processes, spinal anesthesia, or malignancy)
- Transection of the spinal cord above the sacral segments

Pathophysiology

Lesions at the lower motor neuron level of the spinal cord often directly interfere with interpretation of nerve impulses. When the bladder fills, the message is transmitted through afferent fibers to the brain cortex. The injury, however, keeps these impulses from being correctly interpreted, leading to no impulse for micturition. A flaccid bladder with urinary retention is the result.

With upper motor neuron lesions, impulses are not transmitted to or from the lower spinal areas to the cortex. When the client's bladder distends, no sensation is transmitted. Because the lower cord is intact, however, activity of the reflex arc can occur, and the client will have reflex incontinence of urine.

When the damage is to the cortical area itself, such as with a stroke or trauma, the client cannot correctly interpret the impulses that are being transmitted.

The client with a dysfunctional bladder is more likely than normal to experience serious UTIs, skin breakdown associated with incontinence, and even renal disease caused by chronic overdistention of the bladder.

Clinical Manifestations

The major clinical manifestation of neurogenic bladder dysfunctions is either retention or incontinence. The client may or may not feel a need to void or may not even feel a sense of bladder distention. The diagnosis is often made from the type of neurologic dysfunction that has occurred.

DIAGNOSTIC ASSESSMENT

Urodynamic studies including an electromyogram may be done to help determine the extent to neurologic involvement in the retention or incontinence.

Medical Management

If possible, some form of bladder training is attempted for the client with neurogenic bladder dysfunction. This includes a bladder-training program with or without intermittent catheterization, pharmacologic therapy, and sometimes surgical intervention.

Autonomic dysreflexia or hyperreflexia is a serious, potentially life-threatening complication that can affect spinal cord–injured clients during a bladder-training program or if their urinary system becomes obstructed. This condition results from excessive autonomic response to normal stimuli and affects primarily clients with upper motor neuron lesions. The most frequent cause is bladder distention, although autonomic dysreflexia can be triggered by visceral distention or stimulation of pain receptors in the skin. Its most common manifestations are hypertension, bradycardia, throbbing headache, flushing, diaphoresis above the level of the lesion, blurred vision, nasal congestion, nausea, and pi-

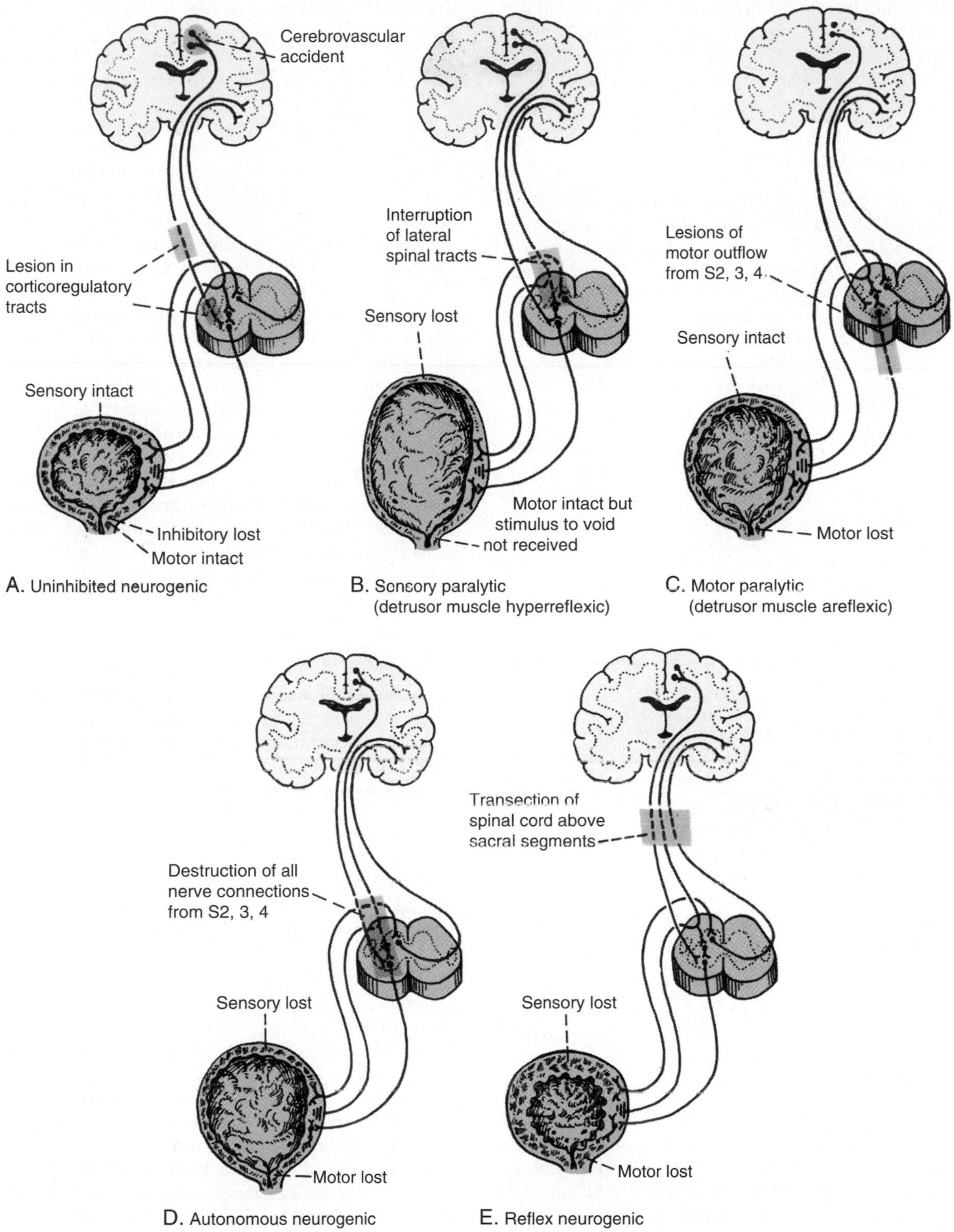

Figure 30–9
Types of neurogenic bladder dysfunction.

lomotor spasm ("goose bumps"). If left untreated, this problem can lead to retinal hemorrhage, seizures, or stroke. The nurse teaches the client to recognize its earliest symptoms and summon help immediately because this is a medical emergency.

PHARMACOLOGIC MANAGEMENT

A number of medications are used to treat neurogenic bladder dysfunction (see Tables 30–1 and 30–3). Antispasmodics and anticholinergics (e.g., dicyclomine, propantheline, and flavoxate) are given to relieve uninhibited or reflex bladder contractions. Phenoxybenzamine and other alpha-adrenergic blocking agents may be used. Bethanechol chloride may help stimulate an atonic bladder.

DIETARY MANAGEMENT

There are no particular nutritional needs for clients with neurogenic bladder dysfunction; however, they should be encouraged to maintain a high fluid intake of at least 3000 mL a day. They also should be encouraged to drink fluids that promote an acidic urine, which helps prevent UTIs in these clients.

Surgical Management

If the conservative measures are ineffective in treating the neurogenic bladder, surgical intervention may be necessary. External sphincterotomy or incision of the bladder neck may restore normal bladder emptying. Interrupting innervation to the bladder reflex can aid an uninhibited bladder. Injection of alcohol into the subarachnoid space or rhizotomy (cutting) of the sacral nerves increases bladder capacity by inhibiting reflex bladder contractions, without interfering with normal sphincter function. Sometimes the physician will do a temporary sacral nerve block before surgery to evaluate the potential candidate. Also, electrodes may be implanted in the thoracic or cervical levels of the spinal epidural space and then attached to a percutaneous stimulator. As soon as the client learns to regulate the electrical stimulation properly, the device can be used to interfere with the reflex bladder contractions. Finally, only if all else fails, urinary diversion may be performed to provide the client with a more manageable urinary system.

Surgery is not always successful in alleviating the problems associated with neurogenic bladder dysfunction. Some clients cannot be helped surgically; therefore, learning other methods of bladder control is important.

Nursing Management

Neurogenic bladders are difficult to control, so the nurse will need to teach many clients with this problem how to stimulate the micturition reflex and maintain urination. The client can be assisted by providing external pressure on the abdomen, which helps contract the detrusor muscle. The client should lean forward or try pushing on the abdomen with the hand or arm. The nurse has the client breathe deeply to force the diaphragm downward. In addition, wearing a corset or girdle provides an extra source of external pressure.

Another method to help the client learn to empty the bladder is the Credé maneuver. The Credé maneuver involves placing the fingers over the bladder and pressing down slowly. Pressure is exerted downward toward the symphysis pubis as though "milking" the urine out of the urinary system.

CRITICAL TO REMEMBER

The nurse or client should use caution when performing this technique. If the client suffers from sphincter dyssynergia (failure of muscular coordination) or if the sphincter does not readily relax, the Credé maneuver can lead to sphincter damage. This maneuver also could result in ureteral reflux if there is any obstruction of outflow.

The client can use several other methods to initiate and maintain micturition. The nurse should locate trigger points on the body (e.g., lower abdomen, inner thighs, and pubic area) and explain how to stimulate them by stroking, pinching, or applying ice. Stretching the anal sphincter also relaxes the reflexes of the external urethral sphincter because they are both innervated by the pudendal nerve. The client leans forward while sitting on the toilet and inserts two gloved fingers into the anus. The fingers are then either widened apart or pulled posteriorly. The male must be careful to avoid touching the glans penis, which stimulates the bulbocavernosus reflex, contracting the external sphincter.

CRITICAL TO REMEMBER

The nurse should always be prepared for the development of autonomic dysreflexia. If the client suddenly experiences symptoms of severe hypertension (sometimes >300/180), flushing, and a pounding headache, the nurse must act immediately.

Nursing interventions involve removing the triggering stimuli, for example, re-establishing urine flow or removing fecal impaction if necessary. A fecal impaction should be removed only after a topical anesthetic has been inserted into the rectum for avoiding further stimulation. In addition, a catheter may be necessary, or if one is already in place, patency of the system must be restored by irrigating or removing kinks and obstructions in the system. Vital signs must be monitored every 5 minutes and the head of the bed raised to semi-Fowler's position. Medications, such as diazoxide (Hyperstat), phenoxybenzamine hydrochloride (Dibenzyline), guanethidine sulfate (Ismelin), propantheline bromide (Pro-Banthine), phentolamine mesylate (Regitine), and mecamylamine hydrochloride (Iversine), relieve both acute symptoms and the chronic recurrence of episodes. Intrathecal administration of tetracaine hydrochloride may block nerve conduction.

For the treatment of long- or short-term bladder atony, an intermittent catheterization program is an alternative to long-term indwelling catheterization. This program consists of inserting a straight urethral catheter into the bladder at specified intervals, draining the urine, and removing the catheter. The catheter may be inserted by the client (self-catheterization), by a significant other, or by anyone properly trained. See Client Education Guide: Urinary Self-Catheterization.

CLIENT EDUCATION GUIDE

Urinary Self-Catheterization

The client and significant others should be taught the following:

- Self-catheterization is an alternative to long-term indwelling catheterization.
- While done as a sterile procedure in the hospital (because of the risk of nosocomial infection), catheterization can be done at home using clean technique. The nurse must teach the client to wash hands thoroughly before and after the procedure.
- To reduce the risk of bacteriuria, urinary antiseptics and acidification or bladder irrigations with antibiotics may be given with each catheterization.
- The catheter should be washed thoroughly after each use with soap and water and stored in a plastic bag or other clean container. Certain catheters may be boiled periodically.
- The client should sit or stand during the catheterization. The female can keep one foot on the floor while placing the other foot on a chair or the toilet lid. The female meatus should be located by touch. (When first learning, a mirror may help with locating the meatus.) A person with physical limitations can be taught to perform the procedure while lying in bed, even though complete emptying may not be achieved.
- Catheterization must be carried out over a 24-hour period. The average interval is 4 hours, but the client usually starts at 2- to 3-hour intervals.
- The client should drink small amounts of fluid (250 mL or less) within 2 hours of catheterization, unless there is a fluid restriction. Ingestion of large amounts of fluid within a short period can cause bladder distention and reflux.
- Poor technique can cause urinary tract infections (UTIs), urethral trauma, and stricture.
- The client should have urinary function monitored at intervals, as suggested by the physician. The client should call the physician at the first sign of a UTI or other urinary problem.

The nurse should ask the client to demonstrate self-catheterization before discharge from the hospital.

Sterile catheterization technique is necessary in health-care facilities because of the high risk for nosocomial infections. However, authorities recommend that clean, rather than sterile, technique be used for catheterization outside health-care facilities. Studies show no increase in the rate of UTIs in comparing clean with sterile technique. Clean technique is also easier and less expensive for the client.

Two main parameters indicate success of an intermittent catheterization program: a catheter-free bladder and absence of bacteriuria. These results may be due to several factors, including intermittent bladder distention, which stimulates the normal micturition reflex, and reactivation of the bladder's normal antibacterial properties.

Intermittent catheterization is not a panacea, however. The program requires that the client assume a great deal of personal responsibility. Some clients are not sufficiently motivated to fulfill the responsibilities involved in self-catheterization. Also, problems can occur when the client is away from home, for instance, at a movie, in a restaurant, or without access to facilities in which the catheterization can be easily performed, such as on a plane. Poor technique can cause UTI, urethral trauma, and stricture. Bladder calculi may result from pubic hairs inadvertently pushed into the bladder by the catheter, where they become the nidus for stones. Also, some people experience a silent hydronephrosis secondary to obstruction, infection, or reflux caused by abnormally high resting bladder pressures. This condition is discovered only with an IVP and monitoring of renal function, both of which should be done frequently. Silent hydronephrosis can be reversed by inserting an indwelling catheter and lowering the bladder pressure.

Modification of Plan of Care for the Elderly

Older clients are more likely to have other problems that may interfere with their ability to use the self-catheterization program to control bladder dysfunction. They may still be able to use this method if they have a significant other who can help with the catheterization process. The nurse must be careful, however, not to force the older client into a dependent state if this is inappropriate.

BLADDER TRAUMA

Bladder trauma is defined as a blunt or penetrating injury to the bladder that may or may not cause bladder rupture. It is often related to automobile accidents, when the seat belt compresses the bladder; it is a fairly common problem. The bladder may also be punctured by bullets, knives, bony splinters from a fractured pelvis, or internal instruments such as a catheter, sound, or cystoscope.

When the bladder ruptures, whatever the cause, urine spills into the peritoneal cavity and continues to leak while the bladder is not intact. Urine leaking into the peritoneal cavity causes peritonitis or pelvic cellulitis to develop.

Bladder injuries usually produce a pain low in the abdomen or pain referred to the shoulder and hematuria. If the client has a history of an injury or blow to the abdomen, this should arouse suspicion of bladder injury. The client may also demonstrate difficulty voiding (e.g., small amounts of bloody urine or inability to void at all).

Diagnostic tests to assess bladder trauma include cystography and a voiding cystourethrogram. This allows assessment of both the intactness of the bladder and the bladder's ability to empty.

Medical Management

The first treatment for suspected bladder injury is insertion of a Foley or suprapubic catheter to monitor for hematuria or a complete lack of urine and to divert urine away from the site of injury. Any injury, other than a simple contusion or very small perforation, will require surgical repair. If blood is coming from the meatus, urethral disruption may be present. In this case, the client should not be catheterized until it is determined whether the urethra is disrupted.

Surgical Management

Bladder injuries usually require surgical interventions. After a urethral or suprapubic catheter has been inserted, surgical repair of the damaged bladder wall is done. The extravasated urine in the perivesical space should be drained. If the pelvis is fractured, this is repaired before the bladder to prevent further injury.

The major complication after bladder repair occurs if urinary drainage is not maintained. Healing will be delayed, and fistulas or leakage may develop.

Nursing Management

Assessment of the client at high risk for bladder injury is very important. The nurse should closely monitor the client's urine output for both amount and the presence of hematuria. The nurse should report any anuria to the physician immediately.

Postoperatively, the nurse must maintain urinary drainage to prevent tension on the sutures in the bladder. The nurse may also have to change dressings around a Penrose drain left in to allow any urine remaining in the pelvis to drain.

Posthospital Care

Because the client may be discharged with an indwelling or suprapubic catheter, it is important the client and significant others be taught how to care for this catheter. The client's self-care abilities should be assessed for the possible need for assistance at home. If the client or significant others are unable to care for the catheter, a visiting nurse must be arranged.

The client will need to be seen by the physician after discharge for assessment of healing and to have the catheter removed. A suprapubic catheter allows the client to begin to void normally before the catheter is removed. If the client has a urethral catheter, this will have to be removed before the client can begin to void normally. If clients do not void within 8 hours of removal of the catheter, they will have to have the catheter reinserted.

Modification of Plan of Care for the Elderly

There are no specific modifications for the aged client, only the modifications associated with surgery covered in Chapter 5.

Urethral Disorders

URETHRITIS

Urethritis is inflammation of the urethra. It is a common problem associated with venereal disease (see Chap. 54 for incidence) and may be seen with cystitis.

Any irritant in contact with the urethra has the potential of causing urethritis. In men, prevention of gonorrhea is the primary way to prevent urethritis. In women, avoidance of perfumed toilet paper and sanitary napkins and of feminine hygiene sprays helps prevent the development of urethritis. If the woman uses spermicidal jelly, she should be aware of the risk of developing urethritis. Sexual intercourse itself has not been shown to cause urethritis.

As with cystitis, assessment reveals burning on urination, frequency, and nocturia. In women, a history reveals exposure to the causative agents. The client may also complain of very low abdominal or perineal pain or discomfort. Pus may be present in the urine (pyuria) even without the presence of bacteria in the urine. Male clients frequently exhibit a discharge, but not females.

Culture and sensitivity testing of the urine may be negative. If the cause is venereal disease, then tests for this are positive. The diagnosis is often made on the basis of the client's history and symptoms.

Management of urethritis includes removing its cause and, if it is caused by micro-organisms, administering systemic and topical antibiotics. Sitz baths, especially with baking soda in the water, and high fluid intake are also helpful. The client should be told to avoid sexual intercourse until the symptoms subside. Although sexual intercourse has not been shown to cause urethritis, the use of lubricants with intercourse seems to decrease irritation in women who have had frequent attacks. Refer to Table 30–1 for common medications. The physician may also prescribe topical estrogens.

This problem is usually not treated surgically. If strictures occur, then the urethra is dilated with sounds. If there is scarring at the meatus, a meatotomy may be done.

URETHRAL TRAUMA

The urethra, as well as the bladder, may be injured in pelvic fractures. Falling astride an object, such as the bar on a boy's bike, with sudden force to the groin may cause urethral contusion and laceration. Injury may occur during medical or surgical interventions or be self-inflicted. Penetrating wounds also cause urethral damage.

Urethral damage is indicated if the client is unable to partially or totally pass urine through the urethra. Even if the client can pass some urine through the urethra, voiding will cause urinary extravasation. Extravasation results in increased swelling of the scrotum or inguinal areas, which can result in sepsis and necrosis. Bleeding may occur at the external meatus, and blood may also extravasate into the surrounding tissues, giving the area an ecchymotic appearance.

Proper management of urethral injuries is controversial. Clinicians generally agree that urinary drainage must first be established with either a urethral or suprapubic catheter; some physicians suggest an immediate primary surgical repair of the urethra, whereas others prefer to wait 2 to 3 weeks to see whether the urethra will heal itself without surgery. During any waiting period, the client must be monitored for signs of developing sepsis and continuing extravasation of urine.

STUDY QUESTIONS

1. A client who is discharged on nitrofurantoin (Macrodantin) should be taught that
   A. Sunlight should be avoided
   B. The urine may be discolored
   C. Fluids should be restricted to 1000 mL/day
   D. The medication should be taken for at least 5 days
2. Which of the following statements indicate the client's understanding of Kegel exercises?
   A. "My fluid intake is 2000 mL per day."
   B. "I stop my urine flow while voiding."
   C. "I use biofeedback four times a day."
   D. "It helps to wait 2 hours before I void."
3. Which of the following assessments indicate the presence of cystitis?
   A. Inability to void
   B. Painless hematuria
   C. Bladder retention
   D. Pain referred to the shoulder
4. Which of the following is a risk factor for the development of a bladder neoplasm?
   A. Smoking
   B. Diet high in calcium
   C. Recurrent cystitis
   D. Painless hematuria
5. A client has had the bladder and urethra removed. Which behavior indicates that discharge teaching has been successful?
   A. The client maintains a high-protein diet.
   B. The client discusses adaptations associated with traveling.
   C. The client controls urinary relaxation by stimulating the micturition reflex.
   D. The client uses Credé's maneuver to empty the bladder at timed intervals.

CRITICAL THINKING EXERCISES

SCENARIO A

A client is ready for discharge after a total cystectomy with urinary diversion to a Kock pouch.

1. What teaching will the client need regarding sexual function?
2. What should the client be taught about emptying the pouch?
3. What type of clothing should the client be encouraged to wear?

SCENARIO B

An elderly female client has a history of recurrent urinary tract infections (UTIs). The present infection has cultured *Escherichia coli* from the urine specimen. The client needs assistance with toileting because she has a recent fractured hip repair and a history of syncope.

1. What has contributed to the client's history of recurrent UTIs?
2. What unhealthy hygiene measure contributed to the infection with *E. coli?* How can the client use the correct measure to prevent recurrence of the UTI?
3. Can clients be expected to observe for the symptoms of a UTI and medicate themselves on the basis of their own observation?
4. How does fluid balance affect urine production? What does the elderly person need to know about fluid balance?

BIBLIOGRAPHY

1. Adams, M. C., et al. (1992). Conversion of an ileal conduit to a continent catheterizable stoma. *Journal of Urology, 147(1),* 126–128.
2. Ahlering, T. E., et al. (1991). A comparative study of the ileal conduit, Kock pouch and modified Indiana pouch. *Acta Urology Belgium, 59(2),* 303–313.
3. Babaian, R. J., & Smith, D. B. (1991). Effect of ileal conduit on patients' activities following radical cystectomy. *Urology, 37(1),* 33–35.
4. Bernstein, I. T., et al. (1991). Bricker's ileal conduit urinary diversion with a simple non-refluxing uretero-ileal anastomosis. *Scandinavian Journal of Urology and Nephrology, 25(1),* 29–33.
5. Blaivas, J. G. (1990). Diagnostic evaluation of urinary incontinence. *Urology, 36(Suppl.4),* 11–20.
6. Burgers, J. K., et al. (1990). Improved technique for creation of ileal conduit stoma. *Journal of Urology, 44(5),* 1188–1191.
7. Burns, P. B., & Swanson, G. M. (1991). Risk of urinary bladder cancer among blacks and whites: The role of cigarette use and occupation. *Cancer Causes and Control, 2(6),* 371–379.
8. Choi, B. C., & Nethercott, J. R. (1991). A proportionate mortality study on risk of bladder cancer among rubber workers. *Cancer Detection and Prevention, 15(5),* 403–406.
9. Chyou, P. H., et al. (1992). A prospective study of the attributable risk of cancer due to cigarette smoking. *American Journal of Public Health, 82(1),* 37–40.
10. Costello, A. J., & Bowsher, W. G. (1992). Radiotherapy as a treatment for bladder cancer. *Australia and New Zealand Journal of Surgery, 62(1),* 81–83.
11. Czarapata, B. J. R. (1994). Clinical highlights: Management of interstitial cystitis. *Urologic Nursing, 14(3),* 145–148.
12. Eure, G. R., et al. (1992). Bacillus Calmette-Guérin therapy for high risk stage T1 superficial bladder cancer. *Journal of Urology, 147(2),* 376–379.
13. Faro, S. (1992). New considerations in treatment of urinary tract infections in adults. *Urology, 39(1),* 1–11.
14. Felsen, D., et al. (1991). Inflammatory mediators and interstitial cystitis. *Seminars in Urology, 9(2),* 102–107.
15. Frye, K. (1993). Understanding interstitial cystitis. *Journal of Urological Nursing, 12(1),* 367–371.
16. Ghoneim, M. A., et al. (1992). Further experience with the urethral Kock pouch. *Journal of Urology, 147(2),* 361–365.
17. Gleeson, M. J., & Griffith, D. P. (1990). Urinary diversion. *British Journal of Urology, 66(2),* 113–122.
18. Hanno, P. M., & Wein, A. J. (1991). Conservative therapy of interstitial cystitis. *Seminars in Urology, 9(2),* 143–147.
19. Hermann, G. G., et al. (1992). Recombinant interleukin-2 and lymphokine-activated killer cell treatment of advanced bladder cancer: Clinical results and immunological effects. *Cancer Research, 52(3),* 726–733.
20. Herzog, A. R., & Fultz, N. H. (1990). Epidemiology of urinary incontinence: Prevalence, incidence, and correlates in community populations. *Urology, 36(Suppl. 4),* 2–10.
21. Hooton, T. M., et al. (1991). Single-dose and three-day regimens of ofloxacin versus trimethoprim-sulfamethoxazole for acute cystitis in women. *Antimicrobial Agents and Chemotherapy, 35(7),* 1479–1483.
22. Jeter, K., Faller, N., & Norton, C. (1990). *Nursing for continence.* Philadelphia: W. B. Saunders.
23. Jolleys, J. V. (1991). Factors associated with regular episodes of dysuria among women in one rural general practice. *British Journal of General Practice, 41(347),* 241–243.
24. Karlowicz, K. A. (1995). *Urologic nursing: Principles and practice.* Philadelphia: W. B. Saunders Co.
25. Krieger, J. N. (1990). Urinary tract infections in women: Causes, classification, and differential diagnosis. *Urology, 35(Suppl. 1),* 4–7.
26. Matsuura, T., et al. (1991). Assessment of the long-term results of ileocecal conduit urinary diversion. *Urology International, 46(2),* 154–158.
27. Mizutani, Y., et al. (1992). Effects of bacille Calmette-Guérin on cytotoxic activities of peripheral blood lymphocytes against human T24 lined and freshly isolated autologous urinary bladder transitional carcinoma cells in patients with urinary bladder cancer. *Cancer, 69(2),* 537–545.
28. Moore, K. N., Kelm, M., Sinclair, O., & Cadrain, G. (1993). Bacteriuria in intermittent catheterization users: The effect of sterile versus clean reused catheters. *Rehabilitation Nursing, 18(5),* 306–309, 355–366.
29. Moore, S., et al. (1993). Treating bladder cancer: New methods, new management. *American Journal of Nursing, 93(5),* 32–39.
30. Nordstrom, G. M., & Nyman, C. R. (1991). Living with a urostomy: A follow up with special regard to the peristomal-skin complications, psychosocial and sexual life. *Scandinavian Journal of Urology and Nephrology (Suppl.), 138,* 247–251.
31. Nurse, D. E., et al. (1991). Problems in the surgical treatment of interstitial cystitis. *British Journal of Urology, 68(2),* 153–154.
32. Oliver, J. R., et al. (1991). Correction of incontinent ileocolic urostomy with Kock's nipple valve. *Gynecology Oncology, 43(2),* 178–181.
33. Perry, J. D., & Hullett, L. T. (1990). The role of home trainers in Kegel's exercise program for the treatment of incontinence. *Ostomy Wound Management, 30,* 46–48, 50–51, 53–57.
34. Pow-Sang, J. M., et al. (1992). Conversion from external appliance wearing or internal urinary diversion to a continent urinary reservoir (Florida pouch I and II): Surgical technique, indications and complications. *Journal of Urology, 147(2),* 356–360.
35. Razor, B. R. (1993). Continent urinary reservoirs. *Seminars in Oncology Nursing, 9(4),* 272–285.
36. Samodai, L., et al. (1991). The efficacy of intravesical BCG in the treatment of patients with high risk superficial bladder cancer. *International Urology and Nephrology, 23(6),* 559–567.
37. Seidman, A. D., & Scher, H. I. (1991). The evolving role of chemotherapy for muscle infiltrating bladder cancer. *Seminars in Oncology, 18(6),* 585–595.
38. Skinner, D., et al. (1984). Techniques of creation of a continent internal ileal reservoir (Kock pouch) for urinary diversion. *Urologic Clinics of North America, 11,* 741.
39. Spinelli, J. J., et al. (1991). Mortality and cancer incidence in aluminum reduction plant workers. *Journal of Occupational Medicine, 33(11),* 1150–1155.

40. Stone, A. R., et al. (1991). Role of the immune system in interstitial cystitis. *Seminars in Urology, 9(2),* 108–114.

41. Webster, D. (1990). Comparing patients' and nurses' views of interstitial cystitis: A pilot study. *Urology Nursing, 10(3),* 10–15.

42. Webster, D. C., & Brennan, T. (1994). Use and effectiveness of physical self-care strategies for interstitial cystitis. *Nurse Practitioner: American Journal of Primary Health Care, 19(10),* 55–61.

43. Wishnow, K. I., et al. (1992). Stage B (P2/3A/NO) transitional cell carcinoma of bladder highly curable by radical cystectomy. *Urology, 39(1),* 12–16.

Chapter 31 Nursing Care of Clients with Renal Disorders

Learning Outcomes

After completing this chapter, the learner will be able to:

1. Assess the client for clinical manifestations associated with renal disorders.
2. Teach the client about the etiology, risk factors, basic pathophysiology, clinical manifestations, and life-style changes associated with renal disorders.
3. Explain the client's role in maintaining homeostasis.
4. Develop plans of care for clients with prerenal, renal, and extrarenal disorders.
5. Implement nursing interventions that optimize the quality of life for clients with renal disorders.
6. Evaluate planned client outcomes, using outcome criteria developed in the planning phase of care.

By producing urine, the kidneys regulate the body's fluid, electrolyte, and acid-base balances while removing toxic substances from the blood. The kidneys play a significant role in erythropoietin and prostaglandin synthesis, in insulin degradation, and in the renin-angiotensin-aldosterone system.

This chapter identifies the common disease processes and injuries that interfere with normal renal function. Although the effects of extrarenal influences on the kidneys are briefly described, the primary purpose of this chapter is to discuss specific renal pathologic processes. Because of the potential seriousness of any renal problem, the client and significant others will have physical as well as psychosocial needs. Nurses should know about both aspects and be constantly aware of the need for appropriate intervention.

Renal Disorders Associated with Extrarenal Conditions and Nephrotoxins

Many conditions primarily located in other parts of the body affect the kidneys. Examples of these include sepsis, hypertension, and diabetes mellitus. The renal implications of these conditions are listed in Table 31–1. For further discussion, see Chapters 3, 26, 40, and 56.

NEPHROTOXINS

Nephrotoxins are substances that have specific, destructive effects on renal cells. They can cause five types of renal injury: (1) acute tubular necrosis, (2) defects in the tubular transport system, (3) interstitial nephritis, (4) vasculitis, and (5) nephrotic syndrome. Many substances in the environment can cause kidney destruction. Box 31–1 lists some of the common nephrotoxic agents. Kidney damage can also result from prescribed medications.

BOX 31–1

Nephrotoxins

ANTIBIOTICS
- Aminoglycosides
- Tetracyclines
- Amphotericin B
- Cephalosporins
- Sulfonamides (co-trimoxazole)
- Bacitracin
- Polymyxin
- Colistin

HEAVY METALS
- Lead
- Mercury
- Arsenic
- Copper
- Gold
- Lithium

POISONS
- Mushrooms
- Insecticides
- Herbicides
- Snake bites

ANESTHETICS

CONTRAST DYES

ORGANIC SOLVENTS
- Glycols
- Gasoline
- Kerosene
- Turpentine
- Tetrachloroethylene

OTHER DRUGS
- Heroin
- Dextran
- Mannitol
- Interleukin-2
- Cisplatin
- Amphetamines

The two most common medications that cause renal damage are antibiotics and certain analgesics. Because the kidneys are the major route of excretion for many antibiotics, renal tissue is directly exposed to these compounds. The longer the exposure to nephrotoxins, the higher the risk of renal toxic effects. Careful monitoring of renal function tests identifies early nephrotoxic reactions so medications can be discontinued or the dose decreased. Besides using these medications as briefly as possible, maintaining a high fluid intake and carefully maintaining only a therapeutic blood level may prevent nephrotoxic effects. A high urine output keeps the medication diluted within the kidneys and helps prevent any crystallization of the compound.

The risk of renal damage from excessive use of certain analgesics has received more attention in recent years. Salicylates, acetaminophen, and non-steroidal

TABLE 31–1 Extrarenal Conditions That May Cause Renal Problems

CONDITION	EFFECT ON KIDNEYS
Diabetes mellitus	Progressive scarring within the kidneys occurs, followed by ischemia, necrosis, and tissue sloughing. As kidney function decreases, the client requires less insulin (kidney metabolizes 30–40% of insulin).
Hypertension	Sustained systemic hypertension can cause nephrosclerosis. There is a direct relationship between the duration of hypertension and the degree of elevated blood pressure and the severity of renal vascular disease.
Hypotension	Decreased renal blood flow results from hypotension. The body is able, with medical treatment, to return blood flow to normal.
Cardiovascular disease	Decreased cardiac output and circulating blood volume along with hormonal changes may decrease the kidney's ability to excrete sodium and water.

anti-inflammatory drugs are the most common causative agents. Short-term overdose or long-term consistent use of these medications may cause acute tubular necrosis or chronic renal failure.

Acquired Disorders

PYELONEPHRITIS

Pyelonephritis is an inflammation of the renal pelvis caused by a bacterial infection.

Etiology

Infection of the renal pelvis is usually secondary to a bladder infection. Two types of pyelonephritis can be differentiated by their clinical picture and long-term effects:

- Acute: often occurs after contamination of the urethra after procedures such as catheterization or cystoscopy.
- Chronic: usually occurs after chronic obstruction of the urethra.

Risk Factors

Risk factors associated with pyelonephritis include

- history of diabetes
- hypertension
- chronic renal calculi
- chronic cystitis
- structural abnormalities of the urinary tract
- presence of stones or tubes
- mechanical drainage

Pathophysiology

Pyelonephritis occurs when bacteria enter the kidney. The inflammatory response occurs, causing edema. After treatment, the kidney tissue may be affected by scarring, which can lead to decreased function and renal failure.

Acute pyelonephritis has a shorter course than chronic pyelonephritis. It can reoccur as a relapse or as a new infection.

Clinical Manifestations

Acute Pyelonephritis. Acute pyelonephritis is characterized by enlarged kidneys, abscess formation, and accumulation of lymphocytes around and within the renal tubules. It may cause minimal symptoms or may be asymptomatic. Typically, however, the client seems in acute distress and appears toxic.

Assessment reveals high fever, chills, nausea, flank pain on the affected side, headache, muscular pain, and general prostration. The pain often radiates down the ureter or toward the epigastrium and may be colicky if the infection is complicated by calculi or sloughed renal papillae. Percussion or deep palpation over the costovertebral angle elicits marked tenderness. Frequently the client has experienced dysuria, frequency, urgency, and other signs of cystitis for several days. The urine may be cloudy or bloody, is foul-smelling and demonstrates a marked increase in white cell casts and white blood cells.

Chronic Pyelonephritis. This disease has no specific symptoms of its own. Thus, it is frequently diagnosed incidentally when the client is being evaluated for hypertension or its complications. Hypertension itself is the most frequent manifestation of the disease.

DIAGNOSTIC ASSESSMENT

Acute Pyelonephritis. Urine culture and sensitivity studies are the primary diagnostic tests with a physical examination. Studies may be done for calculi, especially with recurrent infections, because calculi may cause reinfection, particularly with *Proteus.* X-ray studies, such as of the kidney, ureter, and bladder (KUB), and intravenous pyelography (IVP) are also done. A cystourethrogram is often done, especially after an initial episode of pyelonephritis, to look for underlying defects, particularly any cause of reflux. Magnetic resonance imaging or computed tomography (CT) can also be used to evaluate the kidney size or to detect the presence of other problems.

Chronic Pyelonephritis. Abnormal laboratory studies may show azotemia, pyuria, anemia, acidosis, and proteinuria. They may also demonstrate a poor concentrating ability.

Medical Management

Acute Pyelonephritis. Urine culture and sensitivities will specify causative organisms and antibiotics to be used. Medical care also includes prevention and treatment of underlying causes, e.g., calculi.

Chronic Pyelonephritis. Treatment focuses on preventing further renal damage. This is accomplished via antibiotics and control of hypertension.

PHARMACOLOGIC MANAGEMENT

Antibiotics specific to the bacteria present are given to treat pyelonephritis (see Table 30–1). Although they may be administered orally or by use of the single large-dose method, the usual method involves parenteral antibiotics for 3 to 5 days until the client has been afebrile for 24 to 48 hours; oral administration follows for 2 to 4 weeks. The client must understand that prolonged antibiotic therapy suppresses recurrent infections, so completing therapy is of vital importance.

DIETARY MANAGEMENT

Nutrition is not used to treat pyelonephritis directly, unless renal failure has occurred. The causes, however, may require dietary alterations. For example, if the cause is related to calculi, the dietary management discussed in Chapter 30 would be appropriate. If the client suffers from recurrent urinary tract infections, then the acid-ash diet discussed in Chapter 30 would be appropriate.

Surgical Management

Surgery is done only to correct any underlying defects that might have caused the pyelonephritis, such as obstruction, reflux, or calculus.

Nursing Management

Assessment

Assessment of the client with pyelonephritis begins with a thorough history and physical examination, with close attention paid to the presence of risk factors, hypertension, and costovertebral angle tenderness. The nurse should look for the presence of the signs and symptoms of pyelonephritis as well as visual observation of urine and monitoring of intake and output.

Nursing Diagnosis, Planning, and Implementation

Nursing Diagnosis: Fluid Volume Deficit, Risk for R/T fever, nausea, vomiting, and possible diarrhea.

Planning: Expected Outcomes. The client will not develop fluid volume deficit, as evidenced by balanced intake and output, maintenance of adequate hydration, and no signs of dehydration.

Implementation. The nurse should prepare the client for the diagnostic tests and probable antibiotic therapy. Clients with severe nausea and vomiting may require intravenous fluids. Overhydration may dilute antimicrobials, diminishing the effectiveness of these drugs. Refer to Chapter 30 for specific information on the nursing care of the client with cystitis.

Nursing Diagnosis: Pain R/T inflammation and/or obstruction.

Planning: Expected Outcomes. The client will have no pain or have pain controlled, as evidenced by client's statement.

Implementation. Medications can be given to control the pain caused by calculi that may have precipitated the problem. The tenderness in the costovertebral angle should decrease as the antibiotics control the infection. Medication for nausea can be given as needed with antipyretics for high fevers. The urinary symptoms subside quickly once antibiotic therapy is begun.

Nursing Diagnosis: Urinary Elimination, Altered R/T dysuria, pyuria, and frequency.

Planning: Expected Outcomes. The client will return to normal urinary elimination, as evidenced by the absence of dysuria, pyuria, and frequency.

Implementation. Adequate treatment of the infection quickly reverses the dysuria, pyuria, and frequency. Urinary analgesics described in Chapter 30 can also help the client with these problems.

Nursing Diagnosis: Knowledge Deficit R/T recurrent infections.

Planning: Expected Outcomes. The client will understand how to prevent recurrent infections, as evidenced by client's statements and no recurrence of infection.

Implementation. The preventive measures for acute and chronic pyelonephritis are similar to those for cystitis (see Chapter 30). It is important to prevent permanent renal damage.

When the acute infection subsides, the nurse instructs the client to continue to follow-up care. This includes completing the full course of antibiotic therapy and repeating urine cultures. The nurse also teaches ways of preventing further infections anywhere in the urinary tract (see Chap. 30).

No specific home health care is needed unless the client develops renal failure. This is discussed later in this chapter.

It is vital for the client to return for follow-up urine cultures and possibly for other diagnostic tests if the cause of the pyelonephritis is not clear. The client needs to understand the importance of follow-up cultures because bacteriuria may be present but asymptomatic. The client must also be told to report any signs of recurrence immediately so retreatment can be initiated.

Evaluation

The nurse will evaluate whether the expected outcomes have been met. If they were not, the plan and interventions will be altered to better meet the client's needs.

Modification of Plan of Care for the Elderly

The major difference for older clients is that their kidneys may be less able to recover from a severe infection. Antibiotic therapy should be monitored closely, because the older adult's sensitivity and response to the medication may vary. Older adults may also have altered blood levels of antibiotics because perfusion changes with age.

ACUTE GLOMERULONEPHRITIS

Glomerulonephritis is a term that encompasses a variety of diseases which are caused by changes in the immune system that cause changes in the glomerular portion of the kidney.

Incidence

Although the exact incidence of acute glomerulonephritis is unknown, it is twice as common in men as in women.

Etiology

Classically, the causative factor is a beta-hemolytic streptococcal infection elsewhere in the body, although other organisms may be responsible. Typically, it occurs about 21 days after a respiratory or skin infection.

Postinfectious glomerulonephritis is primarily a disease of children, 95 per cent of whom recover fully. It does, however, sometimes occur in adults.

Infectious glomerulonephritis is also associated with bacterial, viral, or parasitic infections elsewhere in the body. It differs from postinfectious glomerulonephritis in that it occurs during or within a few days of the original infectious process.

Risk Factors

Glomerulonephritis is an immunologic disorder that occurs in response to either endogenous (those already in the body) or exogenous (those associated with infections) causes. Prompt and complete treatment of strep throat may decrease risk. An intact, well-functioning immune system and stress reduction may minimize renal involvement as a sequela to infections.

Pathophysiology

Glomerulonephritis is an immunologic disorder that results in inflammatory and proliferative changes within the glomerulus. Because the primary function of the glomerulus is to filter blood, most cases of glomerulonephritis result from trapping of circulating antigen-antibody complexes within the glomerulus. This causes inflammatory damage and impedes glomerular function, reducing the glomerular membrane's capacity for selective permeability. The source of the antigens may be either exogenous (e.g., poststreptococcal infection) or endogenous (e.g., systemic lupus erythematosus). Evidence also indicates that some antigen-antibody complexes may form in situ within the kidney.

In addition to this immune complex nephritis, glomerulonephritis may also be produced by the fixing of antibodies to the glomerular basement membrane. An example of this is Goodpasture's syndrome, which involves pulmonary hemorrhage and glomerulonephritis.

Acute glomerulonephritis can become a fulminant process, proceeding quickly to uremia or to chronic glomerulonephritis. However, most clients start to recover within 14 days. Most clinical signs return to normal within several weeks, although the hematuria and proteinuria may be present for longer periods. If complete recovery does not occur within 2 years, it probably will not occur at all.

Clinical Manifestations

The development of acute glomerulonephritis may be insidious or sudden. Classic signs of sudden onset include hematuria with red cell casts and proteinuria. Fever, chills, weakness, pallor, anorexia, nausea, and vomiting may be present. Generalized edema, particularly facial and periorbital swelling, is a typical finding. The client may have ascites, pleural effusion, and congestive heart failure.

The client frequently has headache and moderate to severe hypertension. Visual acuity may be reduced owing to retinal edema. Abdominal or flank pain, probably caused by kidney edema and distention of the renal capsule, may be present. Oliguria, and even anuria, may be present for several days; the longer this persists, the more irreversible the kidney damage.

In contrast, the disease may be so mild that the client reports only vague weakness, anorexia, and lethargy.

DIAGNOSTIC ASSESSMENT

Diagnosis is usually based on the presence of an underlying infection and an elevated antistreptolysin O titer. The disease, however, may even be discovered on the basis of a routine urinalysis that reveals red blood cells, protein, low pH, and specific gravity in the mid- to high-normal range.

Other studies also assist in diagnosis. Serum urea nitrogen and creatinine levels will be elevated, and creatinine clearance rates will be down. C-reactive proteins and antistreptolysin O titer are usually elevated. Hematocrit and hemoglobin studies indicate anemia.

Medical Management

Medical intervention aims to eliminate antigens, to alter the client's immune balance, and to inhibit or alleviate the inflammation for prevention of further renal damage and improvement of kidney function.

PHARMACOLOGIC MANAGEMENT

Antibiotic therapy (e.g., penicillin for streptococcal organisms) is used to treat the predisposing infections. Volume overload and hypertension are treated with diuretics, antihypertensives, and restriction of dietary sodium and water. Corticosteroids and immunosuppressive agents (e.g., azathioprine and cyclophosphamide) may be used.

DIETARY MANAGEMENT

A low-sodium diet is used to treat the hypertension and fluid overload. If renal failure develops, then protein and other nutrients and electrolytes will be controlled.

Complications

Common complications are congestive heart failure with pulmonary edema, and increased intracranial pressure. Renal failure may develop. Appropriate monitoring, including vital signs, intake and output, and weights, is essential. Recognizing complications early facilitates prompt medical intervention.

Surgical Management

Surgery is not used to treat glomerulonephritis. If the kidney is abscessed or completely destroyed, a nephrectomy may be performed.

Nursing Management

Assessment

A comprehensive history should be taken from the client with suspected glomerulonephritis related to recent upper respiratory tract or skin infections or a history of glomerulonephritis. The client should also be questioned about any systemic disorders that might be present, such as lupus. Any recent invasive procedures should also be noted.

Physical examination may reveal ascites, pleural effusion, and signs of congestive heart failure with pulmonary edema. The urine should be closely examined for color, amount, and presence of any abnormal substances. The vital signs should be closely checked, especially the blood pressure.

Nursing Diagnosis, Planning, and Implementation

Nursing Diagnosis: Nutrition Less than Body Requirements: Altered R/T anorexia and altered renal function.

Planning: Expected Outcomes. The client will maintain adequate nutritional intake, as evidenced by no weight loss, absence of a negative nitrogen balance, and normal electrolytes.

Implementation: It is important to protect the kidneys while they are recovering their function. The diet prescribed by the physician is generally high-calorie and controlled protein. This diet avoids protein catabolism and allows the kidney to rest because it handles fewer protein molecules and metabolites. The degree to which protein is controlled depends on the amount excreted in the urine and the client's individual requirements. Sodium is also restricted, depending on the amount of edema present. Anorexia, nausea, and vomiting may interfere with adequate intake, requiring creative intervention on the part of the nurse. A dietitian can help plan the client's diet around these restrictions.

Nursing Diagnosis: Fluid Volume Excess R/T decreased fluid excretion by the kidney.

Planning: Expected Outcomes. The client will maintain balanced intake and output, as evidenced by no signs of edema or fluid overload.

Implementation. Appropriate fluid balance is important. Careful monitoring of daily weights and intake and output helps determine the progress of the edema and thus provides an estimate of renal function. Daily measurement of edematous parts (e.g., legs and abdomen) also provides useful, objective data. The client's allowable fluid intake is based on the results of these measurements. Fluid intake is usually restricted. Thirst may be relieved by sucking on hard candies or lemon slices or by using ice chips rather than a glass of water. The nurse should assist the client to "plan" fluid distribution during the day (e.g., with meals).

Nursing Diagnosis: Activity Intolerance R/T fatigue.

Planning: Expected Outcomes. The client will obtain an adequate balance of rest and activity, as evidenced by absence of fatigue.

Implementation. Rest is essential, both physical and emotional. There is a direct correlation between activity and the amount of hematuria and proteinuria. Exercise also increases catabolic activity. The allowable amount of activity depends on the results of serial urinalyses. Bedrest followed by a period of very limited activity may continue for several weeks to months. Therefore, the client may need assistance in arranging personal matters, such as family, home, job, finances, and community responsibility. The nurse should encourage the client to talk about any fears or concerns and, if necessary, help the client deal with the emotional reactions expected during a long-term illness with a questionable prognosis. Only after handling these problems will the client be able to rest emotionally. Appropriate diversionary activities may help the client cope with prolonged physical immobility.

Nursing Diagnosis: Skin Integrity, Risk for Impaired R/T edema and decreased activity.

Planning: Expected Outcomes. The client will not develop skin breakdown, as evidenced by continued intact skin.

Implementation. Edema interferes with cellular nutrition, which makes the client more susceptible to skin breakdown. Therefore, the nurse should take precautions to prevent this complication. Interventions include good hygiene, massage, and position changes as well as the use of other prophylactic measures, such as mattress devices. The nurse can use research-based tools to assess the client's risk of breakdown.

Nursing Diagnosis: Infection, Risk for R/T altered immune response secondary to treatment.

Planning: Expected Outcomes. The client will not develop an infection, as evidenced by normal temperature.

Implementation. Glomerulonephritis markedly diminishes a client's natural defenses to infection, especially to streptococcal organisms. Moreover, immunosuppressives and corticosteroids further reduce host resistance. Although isolation is not necessary, the nurse should take care to protect the client from others with obvious infectious processes. General supportive measures help boost the client's defense mechanisms. The nurse should also teach the client appropriate ways to avoid infections.

Evaluation

The nurse must evaluate client outcomes based on the established plan of care. If these goals were not achieved, the plan and interventions must be revised to meet the client's needs.

Modification of Plan of Care for the Elderly

The older client is at greater risk for renal damage because of the pre-existing effects of age on the kidneys. The older client is also more likely to have concurrent chronic diseases that may have affected the kidneys. Treatment is the same, however.

Posthospital Care

The client's learning needs will depend on the amount of renal damage done by the disease. If it is minimal, the client will need to be told to avoid infections and avoid any stressors on the kidneys.

If the client develops renal failure, teaching will have to be much more involved. If the client develops renal failure and requires dialysis, a great deal of teaching will be necessary. This information is covered later in this chapter.

The level of home health care follow-up that a client needs correlates with the degree of renal damage, he or she has sustained. The client's renal function will be assessed at frequent intervals to monitor the status of the kidneys.

CHRONIC GLOMERULONEPHRITIS

Chronic glomerulonephritis has multiple causes. Acute forms may progress to the chronic state. It may also be first seen as a chronic disease. Onset of the disease is often slow and silent, with signs and symptoms not occurring until years later. These include malaise, weight loss, edema, increasing irritability and mental cloudiness, metallic taste in the mouth, polyuria and nocturia, headache and dizziness, and gastrointestinal upset.

Hypertension is a cardinal sign of chronic glomerulonephritis. Associated manifestations may include epistaxis, arteriosclerosis, cardiomegaly, edema, and hemorrhage into the kidneys, lungs, retina, or cerebrum.

Chronic glomerulonephritis progresses over an extended period, often as long as 30 years. When it progresses to end-stage renal failure, dialytic therapy must be instituted or the client will die.

Medical treatment involves dialysis, transplant, and control of the accompanying symptoms. Chemotherapy with anti-inflammatory agents and anticoagulants may be used. Controlling edema and hypertension with diet and decreased fluid intake is imperative.

Nursing interventions focus on the need for consistent monitoring, symptomatic relief, education of the client about the disease and its management, and helping the client and significant others cope with a long-term illness.

RAPIDLY PROGRESSIVE GLOMERULONEPHRITIS

Rapidly progressive glomerulonephritis is a fulminant variation of the disease. Its stimulus may be a streptococcal, staphylococcal, pneumococcal, or viral infection or collagen disease—or something thus far unidentified. More frequent among men, it strikes at any age but has a peak incidence between the ages of 40 and 60 years. It often begins insidiously and, without effective intervention, relentlessly progresses to renal failure and death within a period of weeks to months.

Initial symptoms include hematuria, edema, hypertension, nausea, vomiting, abdominal pain, diarrhea, proteinuria, oliguria or anuria, and acidosis. Nursing interventions are similar to those for other forms of glomerulonephritis.

IDIOPATHIC MEMBRANOUS GLOMERULONEPHRITIS

Idiopathic membranous glomerulonephritis is primarily a disorder of adults; peak onset is between the ages of 40 and 70 years. Most clients present with asymptomatic proteinuria or nephrotic syndrome, and at least half of them have impaired renal function when the disease is first identified through renal biopsy. The prognosis for these clients is mixed: approximately 25 per cent experience spontaneous remission, 25 per cent have a persistent nephrotic syndrome, 25 per cent have persistent proteinuria, and 25 per cent progress to renal failure despite all treatment. Later stages of this disease become indistinguishable from chronic glomerulonephritis.

TUBULOINTERSTITIAL DISEASES (INTERSTITIAL NEPHRITIS)

Traditionally, the term "interstitial nephritis" has been used to designate a category of renal disease characterized by the presence of inflammatory cells in the spaces between the renal tubules. However, not all disease processes included in this classification are inflammatory. Therefore, the term "tubulointerstitial disease" is being advocated as the label for this category of renal disorders.

Classification

Tubulointerstitial diseases are commonly classified as either acute or chronic.

ACUTE TUBULOINTERSTITIAL DISEASE

The acute form usually represents an allergic reaction and has a rapid onset. Assessment findings typically are the result of tubular injury. Symptoms often include fever, skin rash, eosinophilia, oliguric renal failure, and occasionally gross hematuria. The disease may progress along any of three courses: complete recovery, rapid progression to renal failure and death, or movement to the chronic form. Although corticosteroids are frequently used, their value is unclear. Treatment is similar to that for acute renal failure.

CHRONIC TUBULOINTERSTITIAL DISEASE

In chronic tubulointerstitial disease, there is progressive interstitial fibrosis and usually chronic inflammatory cell infiltration with tubular atrophy.

Pathophysiology

This disease involves progressive changes within the kidney. These changes include interstitial edema, cellular infiltration of interstitium, tubular cellular atrophy, and interstitial fibrosis. These processes affect kidney function beyond the tubules as it progresses. The multiple potential causes of tubulointerstitial disease include acute pyelonephritis, analgesic abuse, systemic lupus erythematosus, and medication hypersensitivity (for example, rifampin, penicillin, and lithium).

Clinical Manifestations

An early sign of tubulointerstitial disease is a sudden, unexplained decrease in renal function that may be mild to severe. Specifically, there is decreased urine concentration, loss of sodium, increased pH of the urine leading to metabolic acidosis, sediment in the urine, and systemic hypertension.

IMMUNOGLOBULIN A NEPHROPATHY

Immunoglobulin A nephropathy, also called Berger's disease, was first described in 1968. It is a focal proliferative process occurring most frequently in children and young adults. There is still much to learn about this disease. Originally, it was believed to be relatively benign because of its seemingly nonprogressive nature. However, evidence suggests it may be chronic; approximately 25 per cent of clients demonstrate deteriorating renal function. The effectiveness of various treatments is still being studied.

NEPHROTIC SYNDROME

The nephrotic syndrome is a set of clinical symptoms arising from protein-wasting because of diffuse glomerular damage.

Incidence

Because of the multiple causes of this syndrome, it is a frequent sequela of both renal disorders and systemic diseases such as diabetes and lupus.

Etiology and Risk Factors

The causes of nephrotic syndrome are numerous; the most common is glomerulonephritis. Predisposing factors include allergic reactions; medication and drug reactions; renal vein thrombosis; sickle cell disease; and congestive heart failure.

Pathophysiology

The pathophysiologic mechanism of this disorder is the abnormal permeability of the glomerular basement membrane to protein molecules, particularly albumin. These proteins are excessively filtered into the tubules and excreted into the urine. This results in pressure changes within the kidney that cause edema.

Potential complications include the effects of extracellular fluid accumulation and the progressive development of renal failure. The client may also experience severe hypovolemia, thromboembolism, secondary aldosteronism, abnormal thyroid function, and increased susceptibility to infections. Osteomalacia may also occur.

Clinical Manifestations

On the basis of this pathophysiologic mechanism, the clinical picture of nephrotic syndrome presents a classic constellation: proteinuria, hypoalbuminemia, and edema. Edema is usually the client's chief problem. Although its onset may be insidious, it becomes massive, and complications of the swelling may be seen. The skin frequently has a characteristic waxy pallor due to the edema rather than to the anemia. Other symptoms include anemia, anorexia, malaise, irritability, and amenorrhea or abnormal menses. The amount of proteinuria may account for losses of 4 to 30 g daily. Serum albumin concentrations may drop as low as 1 to 2.5 g/100 mL. The urine typically contains granular and epithelial cell casts and fat bodies. Some hematuria may be present.

DIAGNOSTIC ASSESSMENT

The urinalysis is the main diagnostic test; high amounts of protein are found in the urine.

Medical Management

The primary aim of medical treatment is to stop loss of protein in the urine. The cycle of edema would then be broken. Much of the intervention concentrates on decreasing the client's edema.

Unless the client is hyponatremic, fluids are not usually restricted. The client's fluid balance should, however, be carefully monitored via daily weights, girth measurements, and intake and output determinations. These data are important because weight loss may represent true tissue loss from protein rather than from lost fluid.

PHARMACOLOGIC MANAGEMENT

Steroids are successful with some clients, depending on the cause of their disease. Cytotoxic agents such as cyclophosphamide and chlorambucil, indomethacin, anticoagulants, and antiplatelet agents may be used.

Loop diuretics, such as furosemide, are typically included in the medication regimen. Plasma volume expanders, such as salt-poor albumin, plasma, and dextran, may be administered to pull fluid from the extracellular spaces, making it available for kidney filtration. Diuresis in elderly clients must be handled with particular caution because of their reduced capability to tolerate sudden shifts in intravascular volume.

There is a significant incidence of renal vein thrombosis among clients with nephrotic syndrome. Because of this, some clients are placed on long-term anticoagulation. The client needs to know how to monitor for possible hemorrhage and should be encouraged to carry identification describing medications being taken.

DIETARY MANAGEMENT

A daily protein intake of 1 to 1.5 g/kg body weight daily with over 35 kcal/kg/day for prevention of further protein breakdown is generally recommended.[6]

Because the kidneys have a reduced capacity to excrete sodium, a mild sodium restriction is usually instituted.

Nursing Management

Nursing interventions are designed to help the client maintain health, manage the edema, cope with long-term illness, and learn about the disease and its treatment.

In addition to helping the client comply with the medication regimen, nursing interventions assist the client to achieve and maintain maximal health. Much of this is accomplished through presenting learning materials to the client and significant others. For example, the nurse should teach the client that the amount of exercise allowed is based, at least in part, on the severity of the edema. Bedrest is imposed only during severe edema, and as the fluid level moves toward normal, the client is allowed more activity.

Because edema interferes with cellular nutrition, skin care is vital. During acute stages, the client and significant others may need help dealing with the accompanying malaise, anorexia, and depression. The nurse should also assess for signs and symptoms of electrolyte imbalance associated with the aggressive diuresis that is required for the client with central edema.

HYDRONEPHROSIS

Hydronephrosis is the distention of the renal pelvis and calices by an obstruction of normal urine flow. Urine production continues, and the urine is trapped proximal to the obstruction. The cause of the occlusion may include calculus, tumor, scar tissue, or a kink in the ureter. In addition to the pressure-related problems, pyelonephritis is always a risk because of urinary stasis.

Medical treatment aims to relieve the obstruction permanently and prevent infection. After the obstruction is relieved, postobstructive diuresis occurs, possibly leading to fluid and electrolyte imbalances including dehydration. The kidney will gradually begin to concentrate urine appropriately. Diuresis can, however, lead to fluid depletion if it continues.

Potential fluid volume deficit related to increased urine output is the most important nursing problem.

CRITICAL TO REMEMBER

Because of the dangers involved in postobstruction diuresis, it is crucial to monitor the client closely after an obstruction is released.

The nurse must make frequent assessments, including hourly outputs; daily weights; vital signs every 30 minutes for the first 4 hours and then every 2 hours; urine for specific gravity, albumin, and glucose; and edema. Periodic serum electrolyte and glucose determinations should be made as well. The nurse should consider the expected presence of severe fatigue caused by urinary losses and the need for frequent observations. Fluid management during this period is crucial; hourly fluid replacement is based on the previous hour's output.

UREMIC SYNDROME

Uremia literally means "urine in the blood." This term and the term "uremic syndrome" describe a set of symptoms that result from loss of renal function. This loss may be sudden or may develop over a long period. It may be self-limiting or irreversible. Sudden loss of kidney function, such as occurs in damage from trauma, shock, toxins, or acute glomerulonephritis, brings on uremia rapidly and usually causes a severe deterioration of the client's condition. Gradual loss of kidney function over an extended period may occur with glomerulonephritis, hypertension, chronic pyelonephritis, and other diseases.

Because the kidneys perform a wide variety of functions, the effects of uremia occur not only within the kidneys themselves but also within other organ systems. Because of the time factor, chronic renal failure produces more degenerative changes in the body than does acute uremia. However, both types have many of the same consequences, and unless the process can be halted, coma, convulsions, and death result.

ACUTE RENAL FAILURE

Acute renal failure (ARF) refers to the abrupt loss of kidney function. Over a period of hours to a few days, the glomerular filtration rate (GFR) falls, accompanied by concomitant rise in serum creatinine and urea nitrogen levels. A healthy adult eating a normal diet needs a minimum daily urine output of approximately 400 mL to excrete the body's waste products through the kidneys. An amount lower than this indicates a decreased GFR. Oliguria refers to daily outputs of urine between 100 and 400 mL; anuria refers to outputs less than 100 mL in 24 hours.

Incidence

The incidence of ARF will depend on the underlying cause. The most common causes of ARF are hypotension and prerenal hypovolemia.

Etiology

The numerous causes of ARF can be categorized into three major areas: prerenal, renal, and postrenal (Fig. 31–1).

PRERENAL CAUSES

Prerenal causes interfere with renal perfusion. The kidneys depend on an adequate delivery of blood to be filtered by the glomeruli. Therefore, a reduced renal blood flow obviously decreases the GFR. Conditions that contribute to decreased renal blood flow include:

- decreased circulating blood volume (diarrhea, hemorrhage, etc)
- fluid volume shifts (vasodilation, gram-negative sepsis)
- decreased cardiac output
- increased vascular resistance
- vascular obstruction

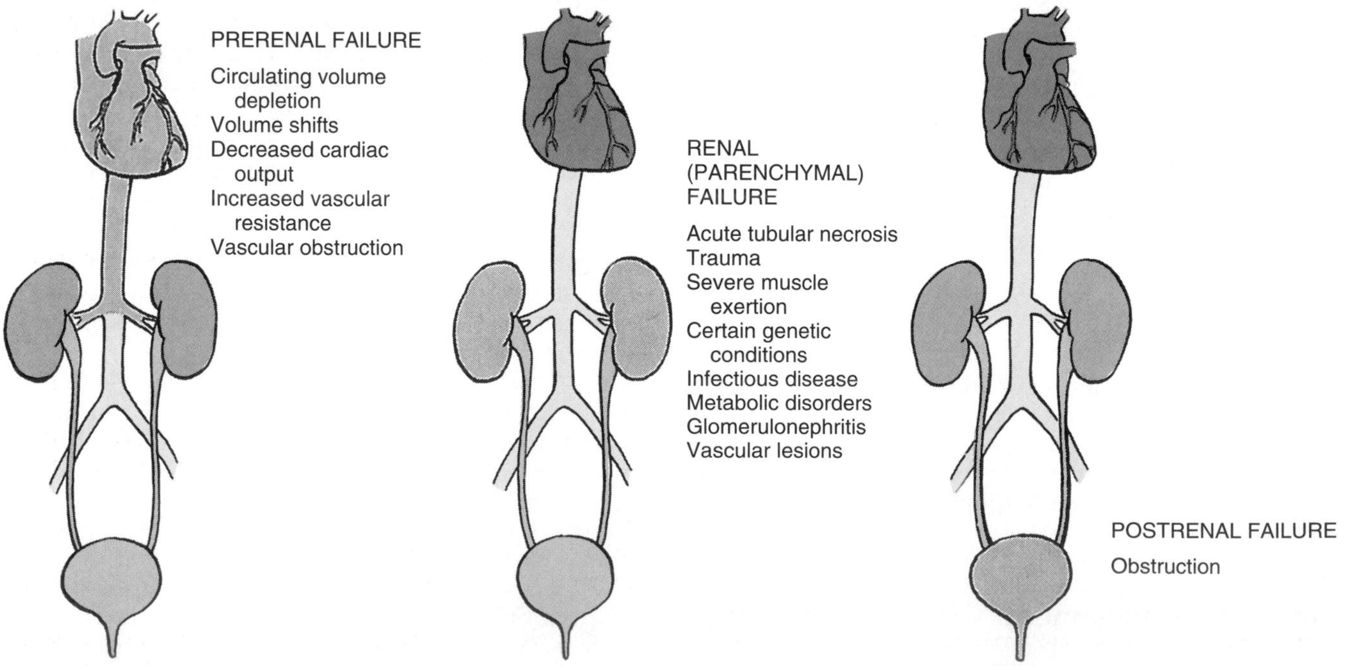

Figure 31–1
Causes of acute renal failure: prerenal, renal, and postrenal.

RENAL CAUSES

Renal causes refer to parenchymal changes from disease or nephrotoxic substances. Acute tubular necrosis is the most frequent renal cause of ARF. This destruction of the tubular epithelial cells is the result of impaired renal perfusion or direct damage from nephrotoxins. In addition to the nephrotoxins described previously, acute tubular necrosis may also be caused by the presence of heme pigments, such as myoglobin and hemoglobin, which are liberated from damaged muscle tissue. This release may result from trauma such as surgery, crush injury, and electric shock or from nontraumatic conditions such as severe muscle exertion, genetic conditions (e.g., diabetes mellitus and malignant hyperthermia), infectious disease, and metabolic conditions (e.g., hypokalemia, phosphatemia, and heatstroke).

Additional renal causes of ARF include glomerulonephritis; thrombosis; vasculitis; scleroderma; trauma; atherosclerosis; and tumors.

POSTRENAL CAUSES

Postrenal causes leading to ARF arise from obstruction in the urinary tract, anywhere from the tubules to the urethral meatus. Common sources of obstruction include prostatic hyperplasia, calculi, invading tumors, surgical accidents, and retroperitoneal fibrosis.

In managing the client with ARF, it is important to determine whether the disorder originates in the prerenal, renal, or postrenal area before intervention begins. Appropriate interventions require determining the origin of the disorder.

Risk Factors

This condition may be preventable with close monitoring by the nurse of the client at risk. Because hypotension and hypovolemia are two causes with the highest mortality rate, early diagnosis and reversal of these problems can save the client's life. The nurse must carefully monitor the vital signs and urine output of clients at risk for the development of ARF.

Nephrotoxic agents are another risk factor for this condition. The nurse should always be aware of the action and potential side and toxic effects of any medication administered to the client.

Pathophysiology

The causes of ARF are not clear. Theories range from damaged tubules not conserving sodium to obstruction of the tubules with cellular and protein debris.

The clinical course of ARF is marked by several phases. The *onset,* or *initiating, phase* covers the period from the precipitating event to the development of renal symptoms. Symptoms may begin immediately or a week after the precipitating event. The oliguric-anuric or nonoliguric phase lasts 1 to 8 weeks. The longer the persistence, the poorer the prognosis. Dialytic therapy may be required during the oliguric-anuric phase.

A gradual or abrupt return to glomerular filtration and leveling of the blood urea nitrogen (BUN) signals the *diuretic phase.* Urine output may be 1000 to 2000 mL/day, which may lead to dehydration; 25 per cent of the deaths from acute renal failure occur during this phase.

The *recovery phase* lasts 3 to 12 months. During this time, the client often returns to a prerenal failure activity level. In actuality, mild tubular abnormalities, including glycosuria and decreased concentrating ability, may continue for years, and the client will continually be at risk for fluid and electrolyte imbalance, especially during times of stress.

The effects of ARF are widespread. The major consequences include:

- fluid and electrolyte imbalances (fluid overload or depletion, hyperkalemia, hyponatremia, hypocalcemia, and hypermagnesemia)
- acidosis
- increased susceptibility to secondary infections
- anemia
- platelet dysfunction
- gastrointestinal complications (anorexia, nausea, vomiting, diarrhea or constipation, and stomatitis)
- increased incidence of pericarditis
- uremic encephalopathy characterized by apathy, defective recent memory, episodic obtundation, dysarthria, tremors, convulsions, and coma

Wound healing is impaired. Other symptoms are usually a result of these sequelae.

Clinical Manifestations

The most common overall sign of ARF is alteration in the expected urine output. Usually this is oliguria or anuria, but polyuric ARF may occur.

There are two varieties of ARF: nonoliguric and oliguric.

Nonoliguric Renal Failure. Although nonoliguric, or polyuric, ARF is being recognized more often, whether it is an entity in and of itself or a phase of oliguric ARF remains controversial. Clients with nonoliguric renal failure may excrete as much as 2 L/day, and this needs to be recognized as a possible sign of ARF. The urine produced is dilute. Hypertension and tachypnea, with signs of fluid overload, are frequently found.

Oliguric Renal Failure. In oliguric ARF, urine production usually falls below 400 mL/day. However, it must be remembered that the aging kidney normally loses its concentrating ability, and the renal function becomes more susceptible to insult. Therefore, the older client may have developed oliguria at urine volumes of 600 to 700 mL/day.

The clinical manifestations of oliguric ARF depend on the cause. In prerenal failure, urine findings include elevated specific gravity and osmolality, mild or no proteinuria, and high BUN-to-creatinine ratio. Intrinsic renal failure indicators include

- edema,
- weight gain,
- hemoptysis,
- weakness
- hypertension

Urinalysis will reveal a fixed specific gravity, high sodium concentration, and proteinuria. If tissue damage is involved, elevations in serum creatinine, phosphokinase, and potassium occur.

Urine produced in postrenal failure may have fixed specific gravity and elevated sodium concentration with little or no proteinuria. Urine sediment is generally normal. The most definitive signs are those indicating obstruction, as described with calculi and neoplasms. Wide fluctuations between anuria and polyuria may indicate intermittent urinary tract obstruction.

DIAGNOSTIC ASSESSMENT

Urinalysis, urine specific gravity and sodium levels, and serum creatinine and urea nitrogen are common diagnostic tests for ARF. The amount of urine in relation to intake is also important in formulating the diagnosis. To measure the exact amount of urine output or obtain a specimen for culture and sensitivity, a straight catheter may need to be inserted.

Medical Management

The medical management of ARF is largely based on preventing and treating its effects. As with any disease process, prevention is the primary intervention. Attaining and maintaining adequate hydration and diuresis in high-risk clients is crucial, as is the prevention of contributing factors. Once ARF has developed, prompt recognition and action facilitate restoration of optimal renal function. Correction of the underlying condition may be all that is necessary in ARF due to prerenal disorders. Postrenal causes must be rectified. Treatment involves dialysis and early identification and treatment of infection (indwelling catheters are avoided for this reason).

Due to the severity of ARF and its influence on other body systems, a critical care unit is preferred for treatment.

PHARMACOLOGIC MANAGEMENT

Fluid replacement must be done very carefully to prevent fluid overload. Fluid replacement volumes are usually calculated on the basis of some fraction of the previous day's urine output plus an amount (e.g., 400 mL) to account for the usual insensible loss that occurs during a 24-hour period. Losses from other sources, such as vomiting and diarrhea, are added to the daily allotment. Unless the client is on total parenteral nutrition, some physicians use a daily weight loss of 0.2 to 0.5 kg/day as a measure of the success of the fluid replacement program. This represents usual daily weight loss from catabolism and loss of lean body mass.

Diuretic therapy may be used, although it remains controversial. Furosemide and mannitol, the most commonly used pharmacologic agents, must be administered cautiously.

Electrolyte replacement is based primarily on urine and serum electrolyte concentrations. Hyperkalemia is probably the most dangerous imbalance because of its contribution to cardiac arrhythmias and arrest.

Metabolic acidosis usually results from the accumulation of acid waste products. Sodium bicarbonate, sodium lactate, or sodium acetate may be used on a short-term basis to correct this condition. Dialysis is usually used for severe acidosis.

DIETARY MANAGEMENT

Proper nutrition is crucial. A high-calorie, low-protein diet is usually prescribed. It may also be low in sodium and potassium. The protein must contain the essential amino acids to reduce the nitrogenous waste products. Adequate carbohydrate intake reverses the process of gluconeogenesis. During the acute phases, intake should be 135 to 150 nonprotein kilocalories for each 6.25 g of protein ingested to prevent protein catabolism. Low-potassium liquid supplements may also be used. If oral intake is not sufficient to meet requirements, tube feedings or total parenteral nutrition may be instituted.

Nursing Management

Assessment

The nurse should assess the client for the presence of risk factors for the development of ARF. The nurse must carefully monitor the client for the development of ARF. Because hypovolemia is a common cause, the nurse must assess the client closely for this problem. The most important assessment the nurse can make, therefore, is fluid balance.

Once the client has been diagnosed with ARF, the nurse must carefully assess the client for the development of complications such as pleural effusion, pericarditis, acidosis, and uremia.

Nursing Diagnosis, Planning, and Implementation

Nursing Diagnosis: Fluid Volume Deficit R/T hypovolemia, followed by Fluid Volume Excess R/T inability of kidneys to produce urine secondary to ARF.

Planning: Expected Outcomes. The client will not develop fluid volume deficit and ARF; if ARF does occur, the client will not develop fluid volume excess or will have it managed with dialysis, as evidenced by return to balanced intake and output.

Implementation. Careful monitoring of fluid balance indicators is crucial to the management of ARF. Accurate intake and output measurements guide the fluid replacement regimen. It is important to compare these values, looking for 24-hour to 48-hour trends. Vital signs, including postural blood pressures, apical pulses, skin turgor, and mucous membranes, are checked approximately every 4 hours, depending on the severity of the illness. Daily weights are carefully obtained. Internal blood pressure measurements may be done. Urine specific gravity, usually an indication of fluid balance, may be negated by intrinsic renal disease. Heart sounds, lung sounds, and mental status changes may indicate the presence of fluid imbalances.

The nurse helps the client stay within the prescribed restriction with careful oral hygiene, judicious use of ice chips, lip ointments, and appropriate diversionary activities. Placing the allotted water in a spray bottle may help to spread out the amount taken. Fluid from nutrition must be taken into account. To conserve fluids for the client, the nurse can administer medications with meals, if possible.

Nursing Diagnosis: Nutrition: Less than Body Requirements, Altered R/T anorexia secondary to renal failure or dietary restrictions.

Planning: Expected Outcomes. The client will maintain adequate nutrition, as evidenced by sufficient intake to prevent protein catabolism.

Implementation. The client frequently experiences anorexia, nausea, and stomatitis accompanying renal failure. That combined with the general unpalatability of the diet makes adequate nutrition a challenge for the nurse and client. Working with the client to plan a diet that is most acceptable is important. The therapeutic dietitian is a good resource. The nurse should provide a pleasant environment at mealtime. Food prepared in an attractive manner and presented in small amounts may help. Medications to alleviate the discomfort of nausea and stomatitis are useful. Total parenteral nutrition may be instituted if the client's nutritional status cannot be maintained with oral intake.

Nursing Diagnosis: Skin Integrity, Risk for Impaired R/T poor cellular nutrition.

Planning: Expected Outcomes. The client will not develop impaired skin integrity, as evidenced by intact skin.

Implementation. The poor systemic nutrition and edema accompanying renal failure may cause skin breakdown. Meticulous skin care, frequent turning, and special mattresses are very important. Range-of-motion exercises facilitate movement and increase circulation.

Nursing Diagnosis: Infection, Risk for R/T lowered resistance.

Planning: Expected Outcomes. The client will not develop infection, as evidenced by normal vital signs and white blood cell count.

Implementation. The client with ARF is immunocompromised and very susceptible to secondary infections, which represent a stress that the kidneys cannot handle. Urethral catheters are avoided if possible. If they must be used, provide meticulous catheter care. Nursing intervention must be designed to prevent infection in the usual high-risk sites (e.g., respiratory tract, wounds, central catheters, and mouth). The nurse must also be alert to early signs of infection so aggressive medical treatment may be instituted.

Nursing Diagnosis: Anxiety R/T unknown outcome of disease process.

Planning: Expected Outcomes. The client will not exhibit signs of anxiety, as evidenced by calmness and ability to focus on disease and its outcomes (within the limits of altered mental status related to elevated BUN).

Implementation. Because the client's physical needs are so obvious, it is easy to forget that the client, as well as significant others, will be anxious and frightened. The nurse should give frequent, careful explanations and remain cognizant of the need for emotional and psychosocial support. The nurse should be aware that the client may be mechanically ventilated and not able to articulate feelings and fears.

Evaluation

The evaluations of outcomes of client goals must be made continually. If the goals have not been met, the nurse must revise the interventions to meet those needs.

Posthospital Care

The client and significant others will require a great deal of teaching about renal function, the signs and symptoms of renal failure, and the possible need for ongoing treatment. (See Client Education Guide: Acute Renal Failure.)

Modification of Plan of Care for the Elderly

The major difference with older clients is their increased risk for developing ARF because of their cardiovascular instability. The older adult has more difficulty maintaining a homeostatic fluid balance. There is

CLIENT EDUCATION GUIDE

Acute Renal Failure

The nurse should teach the client and significant others the following:

- Basic facts about renal function (use drawings and give printed material)
- Importance of watching for and reporting signs and symptoms that indicate further renal damage
- The possibility that chronic renal failure may develop
- The need to monitor body functions by weighing and measuring intake and output
- The reason for compliance with dietary restrictions
- The value of seeking visiting nurse follow-up after discharge
- The need for close follow-up by a nephrologist for at least 1 year after the condition is reversed so that deterioration of renal function can be monitored

also a greater likelihood that older clients have some pre-existing renal damage, especially men, related to benign prostatic hyperplasia and the obstruction it causes.

CHRONIC RENAL FAILURE

Chronic, or irreversible, renal failure (CRF) is a progressive reduction of functioning renal tissue such that the remaining kidney mass can no longer maintain the body's internal environment. It can develop insidiously over many years or can occur as a result of an episode of ARF from which the client fails to recover.

Incidence

As the life expectancy increases and medical science is able to prolong life, the incidence of CRF will continue to increase.

Hypertension and diabetes are the most common causes of CRF, accounting for over 60 per cent of the clients seen on dialysis. Men and women are equally affected by the problem; the incidence is highest among middle-aged clients.

Etiology

The causes of CRF are numerous. Throughout this section, various injuries and disease processes that may potentially end in renal failure have been discussed.

The most common causes of CRF are diabetic and hypertensive nephropathy, glomerulonephritis, chronic pyelonephritis, and then other disorders.

Risk Factors

Clients with a variety of renal and systemic diseases are at risk for CRF. These include diseases such as glomerulonephritis, obstructions, ARF, hypertension, diabetes mellitus, and lupus.

To decrease the risk that these diseases will lead to CRF, clients should be closely followed and receive adequate treatment to control or slow the progress of these problems before they progress to end-stage renal failure. Some conditions, such as lupus and diabetes, however, can progress to failure despite close treatment.

Pathophysiology

The pathogenesis of CRF involves deterioration and destruction of nephrons with progressive loss of renal function (see Pathophysiology: Chronic Renal Failure).

As renal damage advances and the number of functioning nephrons declines, the total GFR decreases further. Thus, the body becomes unable to rid itself of water, salt, and other waste products through the kidneys. When the GFR is less than 10 to 20 mL/min, clinical uremia is evident. The body becomes increasingly toxic.

The result of CRF is uremia and death, unless treatment with dialysis or transplantation is initiated. The introduction of Medicare funding to pay for dialysis in 1973 opened the option of dialysis to clients suffering from CRF.

PATHOPHYSIOLOGY

Chronic Renal Failure

Total glomerular filtration rate decreases (reduced clearance)

↓

Serum creatinine and nitrogen levels increase

↓

Nephrons work harder to eliminate creatinine and nitrogen

↓

Decreased urine concentration results

↓

Urine production increases

↓

Tubules decrease reabsorption of electrolytes

↓

Sodium loss may occur (can result in polyuria)

↓

Renal damage progresses

Clinical Manifestations

Because of the wide diversity of contributing elements and disease processes, the early stages of renal failure are varied. However, as the destruction of nephrons progresses to its end stage, the manifestations become very similar and are classified as uremic syndrome (see Clinical Manifestations: Irreversible Renal Failure).

The clinical manifestations of CRF—with its retention of nitrogenous waste products; changes in fluid, electrolyte, and acid-base balances; and loss of normal kidney functions—are present throughout the body. No organ system is spared. Renal alterations (described previously) include the kidney's inability to concentrate urine and regulate electrolyte excretion. Polyuria progresses to anuria, and the client loses normal diurnal

CLINICAL MANIFESTATIONS

Irreversible Renal Failure

The projected clinical course of irreversible renal failure is as follows:

- Normal functioning.
- Reduced renal reserve, in which the blood urea nitrogen level may be high-normal, but there are no clinical symptoms. Normal functioning is evident as long as the client is not exposed to unusual physiologic or psychosocial stress.
- Renal insufficiency demonstrates a more advanced pathologic process with mild azotemia when the client is on a general diet. Impaired urine concentration with nocturia and mild anemia are common findings. Renal function is easily impaired by stress.
- Renal failure causes severe azotemia, acidosis, impaired urine dilution, severe anemia, and a number of electrolyte imbalances, such as hypernatremia, hyperkalemia, and hyperphosphatemia.
- Finally, end-stage renal disease is characterized by two groups of clinical symptoms: deranged excretory and regulatory mechanisms; and a distinctive grouping of gastrointestinal, cardiovascular, neuromuscular, hematologic, integumentary, skeletal, and hormonal symptoms.

patterns of voiding. In addition, all normal functions of the kidney become curtailed and are eventually lost.

Electrolyte Imbalances. Although many clients maintain a normal serum sodium level, electrolyte balances may be upset by impaired excretion and utilization. The salt-wasting properties of some failing kidneys, in addition to vomiting and diarrhea, may cause hyponatremia. Apparent hyponatremia may be a dilutional effect of water retention. Late in the disease, the problem becomes hypernatremia, and the salt and water retention often contribute to hypertension and congestive heart failure.

Because the kidneys are very efficient potassium excretors, potassium levels usually remain within normal limits until late in the disease. However, hyperkalemia then becomes a challenging problem. Catabolism, potassium-containing medications, trauma, blood transfusions, and acidosis contribute to potassium excess.

Hypocalcemia and hyperphosphatemia occur. This combination stimulates the parathyroid glands to secrete parathyroid hormone in an attempt to facilitate phosphate excretion and raise the serum calcium level by the resorption of calcium from bone. Osteomalacia, osteitis fibrosa, and osteosclerosis are commonly seen in CRF clients as a result of these metabolic alterations.

Mildly elevated serum magnesium levels are found early in the disease. However, these do not usually reach a dangerous level unless the client is receiving magnesium-containing laxatives or antacids.

Metabolic Changes. In advancing renal failure, BUN and serum creatinine levels rise as waste products of protein metabolism accumulate in the blood. The proteinuria accompanying renal disease and inadequate dietary intake of proteins often cause hypoproteinemia, which decreases the intravascular oncotic pressure. Serum uric acid is often high but is not commonly associated with signs of gout.

Carbohydrate intolerance results from impaired insulin production and metabolism. Special care is needed in adjusting insulin doses for clients with diabetes mellitus complicated by renal failure. Results of glucose tolerance tests must be carefully interpreted.

An elevated triglyceride level is almost a universal finding. This type IV hyperlipidemia is thought to be caused by increased production of lipids by the liver in response to the elevated blood glucose and insulin levels.

Metabolic acidosis occurs because of the kidney's inability to excrete hydrogen ions as a result of decreased reabsorption of sodium bicarbonate and decreased formation of dihydrogen phosphate and ammonia. This condition accentuates hyperkalemia and the reabsorption of calcium from the bones.

Hematologic Changes. The primary hematologic effect of renal failure is anemia, usually normochromic and normocytic. Frequently, it is the fatigue, weakness, and cold intolerance accompanying the anemia that initiate the evaluation leading to a diagnosis of renal failure. The mild anemia found in the early stages is usually due to reduced erythropoiesis. Later, hemolysis, gastrointestinal losses, and clotting abnormalities may add to the severity of the condition. Occasionally, the client will be iron- or folate-depleted from nutritional deficiencies. Bleeding tendencies become apparent as the disease progresses. Platelet abnormalities are the primary defect responsible for bleeding in the uremic client. The accumulation of uremic toxins interferes with platelet adhesiveness.

Gastrointestinal Changes. The entire gastrointestinal system is affected. Transient anorexia, nausea, and vomiting are almost universal. Clients often experience a constant bitter, metallic, or salty taste, and their breath commonly smells fetid, fishy, or ammoniacal. Stomatitis, parotitis, and gingivitis are common problems resulting from poor oral hygiene and the formation of ammonia from salivary urea. Accumulations of gastrin (due to increased secretion abnormalities of gastric acid physiology) may be a major cause of ulcer disease. Esophagitis, gastritis, colitis, gastrointestinal bleeding, and diarrhea may be found. Serum amylase levels may be increased, although they may not indicate actual pancreatitis.

Constipation is a common problem. It is often the result of phosphate-binding agents; restriction of fluids and high-fiber foods, many of which are potassium- and phosphorus-rich; and decreased activity. Constipation provides a particular challenge, because the usual interventions for prevention and treatment are contraindicated in the client with renal failure.

Immunologic Changes. Impairment of the immunologic system makes the client very susceptible to infection. Immunosuppression is an important part of the medical management of CRF.

Cardiovascular Changes. At least 50 to 65 per cent of deaths occurring during chronic renal failure result from cardiovascular complications.[29] The most frequent clinical manifestation is hypertension produced through (1) the mechanisms of volume overload; (2) stimulation of the renin-angiotensin system; (3) sympathetically mediated vasoconstriction, e.g., increased levels of dopamine beta-hydroxylase; and (4) the absence of prostaglandins. Any of the many systemic complications of prolonged high blood pressure may be found.

The effects of volume overload on the heart are seen, including left ventricular hypertrophy and congestive heart failure. Arrhythmias may be caused by hyperkalemia, acidosis, hypermagnesemia, and decreased coronary perfusion.

Atherosclerosis is accelerated because of (1) abnormal carbohydrate and lipid metabolism; (2) impaired fibrinolysis, which leads to the development of microemboli; and (3) hyperparathyroidism.

Respiratory Changes. Some of the respiratory effects, such as pulmonary edema, can be attributed to fluid overload. Pleuritis is a frequent finding, especially when pericarditis develops. A characteristic condition called uremic lung is a type of pneumonitis that responds well to fluid removal.

Musculoskeletal Changes. The musculoskeletal system is affected fairly early in the disease process, and bone reabsorption found on x-ray examination may be the first sign of renal failure in some clients. The most prevalent problem, affecting up to 90 per cent of clients with CRF, is renal osteodystrophy. The development of this manifestation results from interrelationships between the kidney-bone-parathyroid and calcium-phosphate–vitamin D connections. As the GFR decreases, phosphate excretion decreases, and calcium elimination increases. The abnormal levels of calcium and phosphate stimulate the release of parathyroid hormone, which mobilizes calcium from the bones and facilitates phosphate excretion.

As the renal failure progresses, demineralization of the bones frees more calcium and phosphorus into the blood. The parathyroid gland may become unresponsive to the normal feedback system and continue to produce parathyroid hormone, causing acceleration of renal osteodystrophy. A partial parathyroidectomy is the treatment of choice when hypercalcemia and high plasma levels of parathyroid hormone cannot be controlled with medication.

In addition to bone demineralization, this process also leads to calcification deposits in the subcutaneous, vascular, and visceral tissues throughout the body. In the advanced stages of this process, joint pain is severe. The client may also report diffuse and generalized bone and muscle pain. Bone deformities and frequent fractures are common.

Integumentary Changes. Integumentary problems are particularly uncomfortable for some clients with CRF. Severe and intractable pruritus may result from secondary hyperparathyroidism and calcium deposits in the skin. The skin is also often very dry because of atrophy of the sweat glands. Pruritus can lead to excoriated skin because of continued scratching.

Several color changes are found in renal failure. The bleeding tendencies often result in increased bruising, petechiae, and purpura. These do not usually cause problems themselves, but their presence may be alarming to the client. The pallor of anemia is evident. The cause of retained urochrome pigments, making the skin orange-green or gray in color, is not clear.

Hair is brittle and tends to fall out, and nails are thin and brittle. Characteristic red bands that develop on the nails are called Muercke's lines. Another nail pattern that has been observed is a "half-and-half" nail with the proximal half normally white and the distal portion brown.

Neurologic Changes. Although dialysis has reduced the incidence of neurologic changes, some clients experience these problems early in the disease process. Peripheral neuropathy causes many symptoms such as burning feet, inability to find a comfortable position for the legs and feet ("restless legs syndrome"), gait changes, footdrop, and paraplegia. These symptoms move up the extremities and may extend to include the upper extremities. Initially, it is primarily a problem of the sensory system, but if left untreated, it may progress to the motor system. Nerve conduction becomes slower, and deep tendon reflexes and vibratory sense are diminished.

Central nervous system involvement is demonstrated through forgetfulness, inability to concentrate, short attention span, impaired reasoning ability and judgment, increased nervous irritability, nystagmus, twitching, dysarthria, seizures, central nervous system depression, and coma. Involvement of the cranial nerves may alter any of the senses. Hearing threshold levels show a definite high-frequency deficit early in the disease, and hearing progressively deteriorates.

Reproductive Changes. Reproductive system changes can be very alarming. Women often experience menstrual irregularities, particularly amenorrhea, and infertility. However, there have been women with CRF who have conceived and successfully carried their pregnancies to term. Men frequently report impotence resulting from both physiologic and psychosocial causes. They may also experience testicular atrophy, oligospermia, and reduced sperm motility. Both sexes report decreased libido, which may be due to both physiologic and psychosocial factors.

Endocrine Changes. CRF also affects the endocrine system. The effect on insulin utilization has been discussed earlier, as has parathyroid function. Pituitary hormones, such as growth hormone and prolactin, may be increased in some people. The levels of luteinizing hormone and follicle-stimulating hormone vary greatly from client to client. Thyroid-stimulating hormone is usually at a normal level, but it may be decreased.

Psychosocial Changes. Psychosocial changes occur, probably as the result of both the physiologic alterations and the extreme stress placed on the client by the presence of a chronic, life-threatening disease. Behavior changes are greatly influenced by the client's personality. Expected alterations include marked personality changes, labile emotions, increased demand on others, withdrawal, depression, agitation, delusions, and psychosis.

Changes in Medication Metabolism. Finally, renal failure has a serious effect on medication metabolism. The uremic client is at very high risk for medication toxicity owing to the effect of renal changes on the pharmacokinetics (absorption, distribution, metabolism, and excretion) of otherwise therapeutic medications. There are various tables and formulas that help guide dosage decisions. The nurse must remember that medication dosages must be altered and that the usual dosage ranges in the medication literature are not safe for the client with CRF. The client should be assessed carefully for toxic reactions.

DIAGNOSTIC ASSESSMENT

Many laboratory tests are performed, including serum sodium, potassium, urea nitrogen, creatinine, phosphorus, creatinine clearance, calcium, and pH levels; urinalysis and urine creatinine clearance; and complete blood count. The normal ratio of BUN to creatinine is 20:1. This ratio remains the same as both the creatinine and BUN levels rise.

A KUB is usually done first to determine whether there is a problem with the structure of the renal system. An IVP and CT scan can be done to assess renal structure and function. Renal angiography may also be done to assess the blood supply to and through the kidneys.

Medical Management

Conservative intervention does not cure the disease but may retard its progress. Eventually, most clients will require renal replacement therapy. However, even successful dialysis and transplant do not preclude the potential for death from complications of renal failure or its treatment.

After the correction of contributing factors, control of blood pressure and fluid and dietary adjustments are the mainstays of conservative intervention for the client with CRF. The five goals of medical management are to (1) preserve renal function, (2) delay the need for dialysis or transplant as long as feasible, (3) improve body chemistries, (4) alleviate other associated symptoms, and (5) provide an optimal quality of life for the client and significant others.

Pruritus can be very aggravating. Many interventions have been tried, including topical emollients and lotions, antihistamines, intravenous lidocaine, and ultraviolet B light, but relief has been inconsistent and often temporary. Subtotal parathyroidectomy has helped some clients, but there have been reports of recurrence. Dialysis seems to relieve the symptoms effectively for many clients.

Neurologic manifestations require safety measures to protect the client from injury. Anticonvulsants and sedatives may be used. Phenothiazines are potentiated by uremia and should be avoided. Reduction in mental function, related to the rising BUN level, requires more patience in explaining and re-explaining things to the client.

DIALYSIS

There are two types of dialysis: peritoneal dialysis and hemodialysis. Each may be used to relieve symptoms of renal failure temporarily until the client regains kidney function or to sustain life in the client with irreversible kidney disease. In the latter case, the dialysis must continue for the rest of the client's life unless a successful kidney transplantation is done. Dialysis is also used to control uremia and to physically prepare the client to receive a transplanted kidney. Dialysis is frequently necessary to keep the client alive until a suitable donor kidney is found. If the transplanted kidney does not immediately function adequately, dialysis may help prevent uremia until the kidney functions sufficiently.

Dialysis is usually accomplished through both ultrafiltration and diffusion. When dialysis is used as a substitute for kidney function, the semipermeable membrane used is either the peritoneal membrane (for peritoneal dialysis) or an artificial membrane (for hemodialysis). This membrane must have pores large enough to allow the passage of electrolytes, urea, and creatinine but too small to allow passage of blood cells and other protein molecules. A specially prepared electrolyte solution called dialysate is placed in a compartment on one side of the membrane while the client's blood is on the other side.

Goals of Dialysis Therapy

The four basic goals of dialysis therapy are to

- remove the end products of protein metabolism, such as urea and creatinine, from the blood
- maintain a safe concentration of serum electrolytes
- correct acidosis and replenish the blood's bicarbonate buffer system
- remove excess fluid from the blood

Peritoneal Dialysis

Peritoneal dialysis involves repeated cycles of instilling dialysate into the peritoneal cavity, allowing time for substance exchange, and then removing the dialysate. The procedure is useful for both ARF and CRF and for fluid and electrolyte imbalances. One of the primary advantages of peritoneal dialysis is its relative ease, which allows it to be used in community health-care facilities without all the sophisticated equipment needed for hemodialysis. It can be easily managed at home and often provides the client more independence and mobility than hemodialysis does.

Peritoneal dialysis may be used for clients with severe cardiovascular disease, especially those whose problems would be worsened by the rapid changes in urea, glucose, electrolytes, and fluid volume that occur during hemodialysis. Some physicians prescribe peritoneal dialysis for their diabetic patients for reducing the risk of retinal hemorrhage from the heparin used during dialysis treatment. Peritoneal dialysis is the dialytic treatment of choice for children.

Contraindications to peritoneal dialysis include hypercatabolism, in which peritoneal dialysis is unable to adequately clear uremic toxins, and poor condition of the peritoneal membrane due to adhesions and scarring. Certain other conditions may be relative contraindications to peritoneal dialysis; these include obesity, history of ruptured diverticuli, abdominal disease, respiratory disease, recurrent episodes of peritonitis, abdominal malignancies, severe vascular disease, and extensive abdominal surgery with drains or tubes that may increase risk of infection.

Types of Peritoneal Dialysis. There are three types of peritoneal dialysis: continuous ambulatory, continuous cycle, and intermittent.

Continuous Ambulatory Peritoneal Dialysis (CAPD). In CAPD, the dialysate is instilled into the abdomen and left in place for 4 to 8 hours. The empty dialysate bag is folded up and carried in a pouch or pocket until it is time to drain the dialysate. The bag is later unfolded and placed lower than the insertion site so the fluid drains by gravity flow. When full, the bag is changed, and new dialysate is instilled into the abdomen as the process continues. In CAPD, there are usually four dialysis cycles every 24 hours, including an 8-hour dwell time overnight. There are two major advantages to this procedure: (1) because there is no need for machinery, electricity, or a water source, the client can go about almost any desired activity during dialysis; and (2) because the continuous exchange process closely resembles normal renal function, the body more easily maintains homeostasis, and there are fewer dietary and fluid restrictions. For diabetic management, insulin can be added to the dialysate.

Continuous Cycle Peritoneal Dialysis (CCPD). CCPD is similar to CAPD in that it is a continuous dialysis process but different in that it requires a peritoneal cycling machine. In this procedure, there are usually three cycles done at night and one cycle with an 8-hour dwell done in the morning. The advantage of this procedure is that the peritoneal catheter is opened only for the on and off procedures, which reduces the risk of infection.

Intermittent Peritoneal Dialysis (IPD). IPD is not a continuous dialysis procedure like CAPD and CCPD. Dialysis is performed for 10 to 14 hours, three to four times a week, with use of the same peritoneal cycling machine as in CCPD. Hospitalized patients may be dialyzed up to 24 to 48 hours at a time if they are catabolic and require additional dialysis time. There are variations in scheduling IPD, such as nightly tidal peritoneal dialysis, in which treatment is performed for 8 to 12 hours each night with no daytime dwells.

Dialysis Procedure. The dialysate is usually allowed to run into the peritoneal cavity by gravity flow. The dialysate is warmed to prevent chilling of the client and to dilate the peritoneal blood vessels, thus facilitating substance exchange. Two liters are usually instilled in adults, although smaller amounts may be needed at first until the client adjusts.

"Dwell time" is the period during which the dialysate is left in the cavity. In IPD, equilibrium between the dialysate and the body fluids usually occurs within 15 to 30 minutes, with the maximum exchange happening within the first 5 minutes. Therefore, the solution is typically left in place 30 to 45 minutes for manual dialysis or 10 to 20 minutes when an automatic cycler is used. The fluid is then allowed to run out through the catheter by gravity. In CAPD and CCPD procedures, the dwell time is prolonged to 4 to 8 hours

BOX 31-2

Complications of Peritoneal Dialysis

PERITONITIS

Peritonitis is the major concern. Manifestations include fever, rebound tenderness, nausea, malaise, and a cloudy dialysate output. If peritonitis develops, appropriate antibiotics are added to the dialysate; in addition, systemic antibiotics may be used. Bacteria may enter the peritoneal cavity through contaminated dialysis fluid, a contaminated catheter lumen, or the catheter insertion site.

CATHETER-RELATED COMPLICATIONS

Catheter problems include displacement and plugging. Obstruction may be due to malposition, adherence of the catheter tip to the omentum, or infection. Constipation can reduce catheter flow, possibly because peristalsis facilitates outflow. A bisacodyl suppository may be used prophylactically even if the client is not constipated. Fluid leakage may indicate improper catheter function, incomplete healing of the insertion site, or excessive instillation. Especially in the early stages, it is sometimes necessary to use small-volume instillations. Bloody effluent is usually insignificant and will disappear spontaneously. However, it may indicate bowel perforation, which is most likely to occur in cachectic clients or where there are abdominal adhesions. Fecal material returned in the dialysate or massive diarrhea after instillation may also signal perforation. Bladder perforation can also occur if the bladder has not been emptied before catheter insertion.

DIALYSIS-RELATED COMPLICATIONS

Pain during dialysis may result from rapid instillation, incorrect dialysate pH or temperature, dialysate accumulation under the diaphragm, or excessive suction during outflow. Some pain is expected in the early stages but should disappear after 1 to 2 weeks. Low back pain may develop with continuous dialysis procedures because of the abdominal weight affecting posture; appropriate exercises help relieve this problem. Hernia formation may occur. Systemic cardiovascular and neurologic effects are usually the result of fluid and electrolyte imbalances. Hyperglycemia may occur in diabetic clients as a result of absorption of glucose from the dialysate and electrolyte changes. These clients require extra insulin. Respiratory difficulties may occur during dwell time because of pressure on the diaphragm.

with a solution that allows continuous exchange and better clearance of certain elements.

The number of dialysis cycles depends on the normalization of body fluids and blood chemistries, as indicated by laboratory studies. Peritoneal clearance is influenced by several factors, including the size of the membrane area, blood flow to the peritoneum, and alterations in the permeability of the peritoneal membrane.

Complications of Peritoneal Dialysis. Although peritoneal dialysis is considered a safe procedure, there are a number of complications that can be attributed to it (see Box 31–2).

Hemodialysis

Hemodialysis is used for clients with acute or irreversible renal failure and fluid and electrolyte imbalances. It is usually the treatment of choice when toxic agents, such as barbiturate overdose, need to be removed from the body quickly.

Dialysis Procedure. The procedure for hemodialysis involves diverting toxin-laden blood from the client into a dialyzer and then returning the clean blood to the client. Figure 31–2 schematically illustrates a typical hemodialysis system. While the blood is within the dialyzer, the dialysis fluid is delivered by a mechanical pump to flow on the other side of the membrane. Toxins diffuse across the membrane from the blood to the dialysate. Strict asepsis must be maintained throughout the procedure.

One of the vital aspects of hemodialysis is the establishment and maintenance of adequate blood access. Without it, hemodialysis cannot be performed. The major routes of access are external arteriovenous shunts and subclavian catheters for acute dialysis and internal arteriovenous fistulas and grafts for chronic dialysis.

The external arteriovenous shunt requires the surgical placement of two cannulas into the forearm or leg. This access can be created quickly and so is particularly suited to situations in which dialysis must be started immediately. Infection at the site of insertion and clotting are frequent complications that often necessitate moving the cannula sites. Other problems that occur with shunts are accidental dislodgement, hemorrhage, and skin erosion.

The internal arteriovenous fistula is the access of choice for chronic dialysis clients. The fistula is created through a surgical procedure in which an artery in the arm is anastomosed to a vein in an end-to-side, side-to-side, side-to-end, or end-to-end fashion (Fig. 31–3*A*). This creates an opening or fistula between a large artery and a large vein. The flow of arterial blood into the venous system causes the veins to become engorged (Fig. 31–3*B*). These fistulas require 2 to 6 weeks to mature before they can be used. Subclavian catheters can be used while the fistula is maturing.

The internal arteriovenous graft is used primarily for chronic dialysis. This access uses an artificial graft made of Gore-Tex or a bovine carotid artery to create

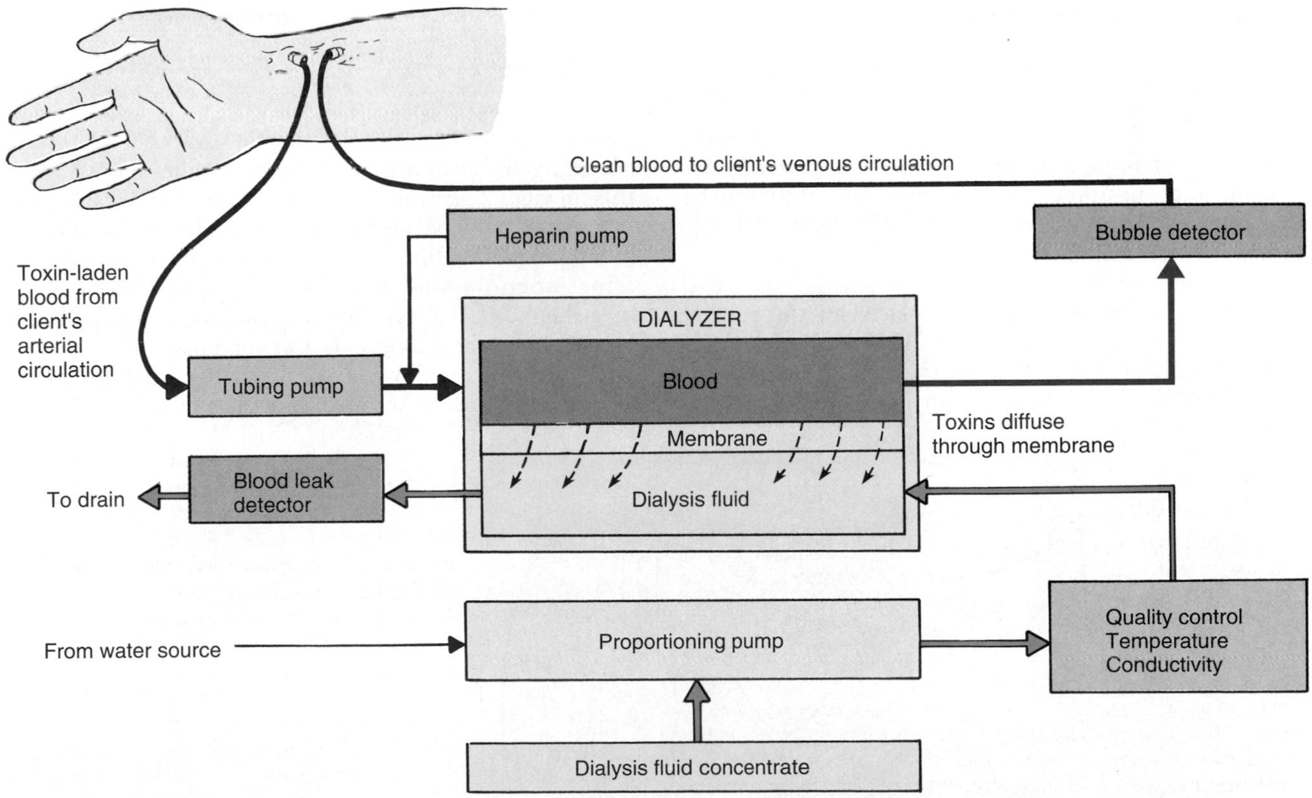

Figure 31–2
Typical hemodialysis system. Toxin-laden blood from client diffuses across membrane within dialyzer into dialysis fluid. Clean blood is returned to client.

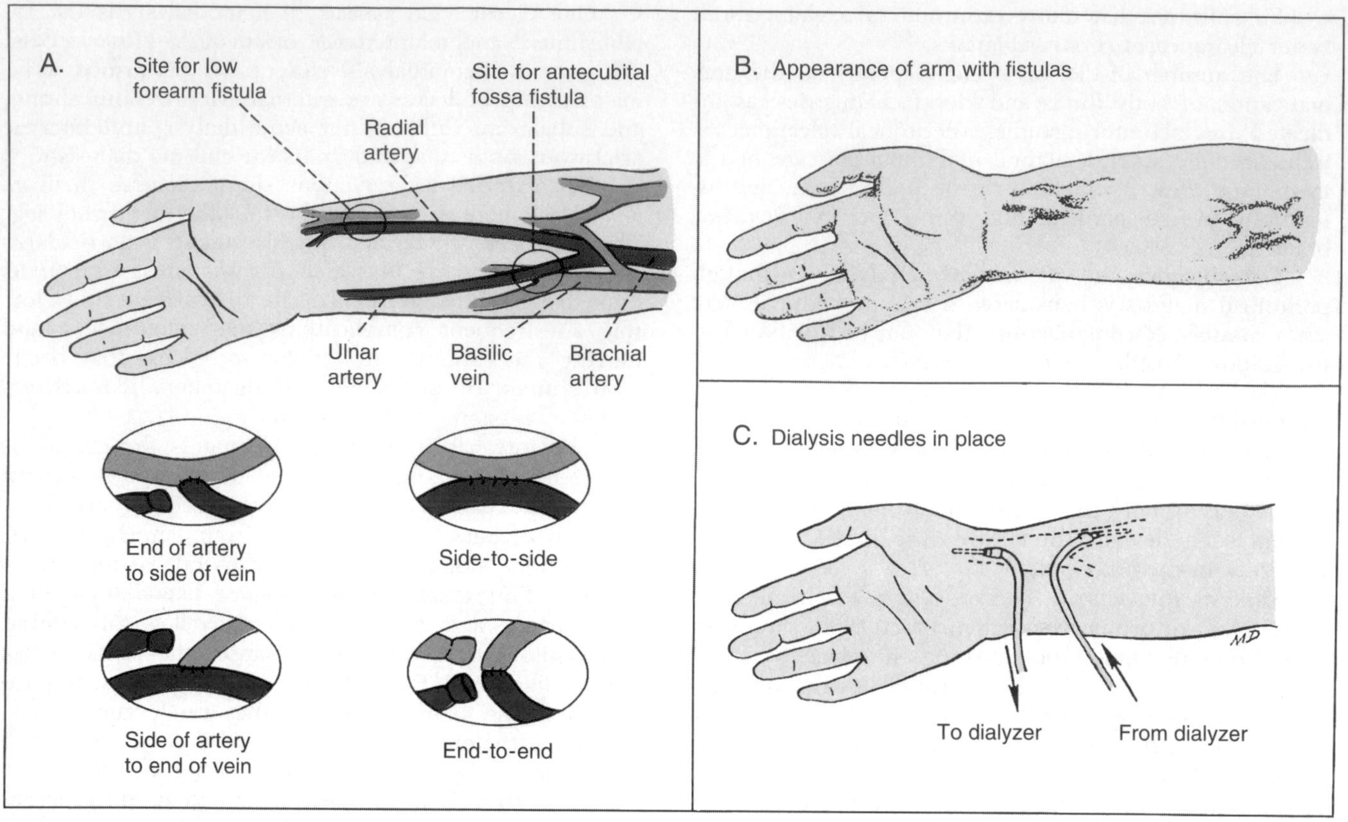

Figure 31–3
Internal arteriovenous fistula. Surgical creation of an arteriovenous anastomosis provides easy access to blood for hemodialysis. This method reduces the risk of infection and makes external shunts unnecessary except during hemodialysis. The internal fistula must be created 2 to 6 weeks before it can be used. Note that in this illustration, arteries, not veins, are colored.

an artificial vein for blood flow. One end of the artificial graft is anastomosed to an artery, tunneled under the skin, and anastomosed to a vein. The graft can be used 2 weeks after insertion. Complications include clotting, aneurysms, and infection.

Once the access is placed and ready for use, two 15-gauge or 16-gauge needles are placed in the vein at each dialysis treatment (Fig. 31–3C). A pump pulls arterial blood out of the vein by way of the fistula and into the hemodialyzer. Blood returns to the client by a tube connected to the other needle. Another method of accessing the fistula is with single-needle dialysis. With this device, only one puncture is required each time, but there may be significant recirculation of dialyzed blood, meaning that clearance rates are decreased. Internal arteriovenous accesses may cause hand swelling or ischemia ("steal syndrome"), carpal tunnel syndrome, hemorrhage, thrombosis, and aneurysms.

Figure 31–4 shows two alternative sites for hemodialysis, the subclavian area and the thigh.

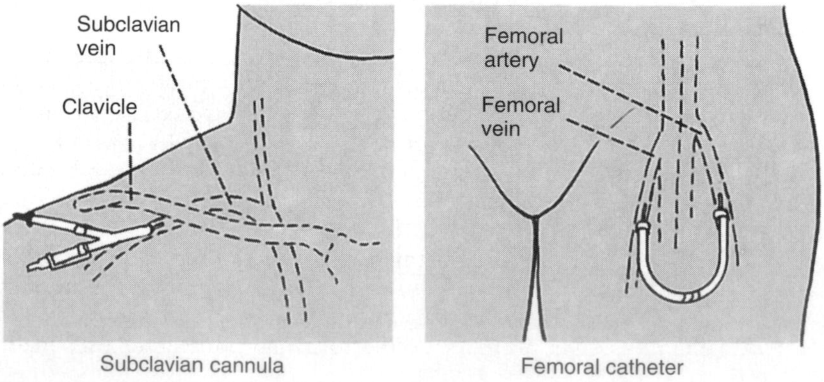

Figure 31–4
Alternative access areas for hemodialysis: clavicle and thigh.

Subclavian and femoral catheters can be inserted at the bedside for use as a vascular access. Subclavian catheters can be used as a temporary or permanent access for hemodialysis. Permanent catheters are surgically placed in the operating room and have Dacron cuffs that are implanted under the skin to anchor the catheter in place. Femoral catheters are always a temporary source of blood flow and must be replaced frequently to prevent infection.

Hemodialysis Schedules. Hemodialysis as a treatment for irreversible renal failure must be continued intermittently for the client's lifetime, unless a successful kidney transplant is done. A typical schedule would be 3 to 4 hours of treatment 3 days per week. This schedule will vary with the size of the client, the type of dialyzer used, the rate of blood flow, the personal preference of the client, and other factors.

Therapeutic Effects of Hemodialysis. The overall therapeutic effect of hemodialysis is to clear waste products from the body; restore fluid, electrolyte, and acid-base balances; and reverse some of the untoward manifestations of irreversible renal failure. The removal of fluids and waste products is temporary. Success is varied.

The usual effect of hemodialysis on serum concentration of medications is increased clearance. This is therapeutic in the case of overdose. Dosage schedules are altered to prevent dialysis loss of medications as much as possible. Timing of medications in relationship to dialysis helps to maintain therapeutic levels.

Complications of Long-Term Hemodialysis. In addition to therapeutic effects, a number of complications are involved with chronic hemodialysis. These include technical problems as well as muscle cramps, a result of hyponatremia or hypo-osmolality. Infection is a significant complication, with hepatitis B being most common. Frequent infectious processes include local access infection, bacteremia, and infectious endocarditis.

Dialysis disequilibrium syndrome is a complication that can occur particularly during the client's first few dialysis episodes. It is characterized by mental confusion, deterioration of the level of consciousness, headache, and seizures and may last for several days. Many dialysis centers avoid this complication by first-time dialyzing for shorter time periods at a reduced blood flow rate.

Aluminum intoxication occurs because of aluminum accumulation from phosphate binders. It leads to mental cloudiness, dementia, and infiltration of the bone with aluminum, leading to significant pain. Aluminum chelating agents may be administered so that aluminum is freed and dialyzed from the body.

PHARMACOLOGIC MANAGEMENT

Diuretics may be used early to stimulate excretion of water by the kidneys. The appearance of edema indicates fluid overload, but some physicians prefer to see a little edema at the end of the day as evidence that fluid depletion is not a danger. Thirst is not a reliable indicator; if thirst were used as a guide, fluid overload would be inevitable. As the failure progresses, it usually become necessary to restrict fluid intake. Although authorities differ in their exact amounts, daily fluid allowances may be 400 to 1000 mL plus measured output.

Water-soluble vitamin supplements (e.g., folic acid, pyridoxine, ascorbic acid) are usually given because controlled-protein diets are typically deficient in these. Fat-soluble vitamins may need to be replaced in clients on dialysis therapy. Vitamin A supplements should be avoided unless total parenteral nutrition is to be used exclusively for several weeks. Vitamin D supplements may be necessary. Work is being done to determine the efficacy of replacing trace elements, such as iron and zinc.

Iron sulfate and folic acid are used only if the anemia is caused by a deficiency of the respective factor. Parenteral iron is frequently given rather than the oral form. Transfusions may be used if the client is symptomatic and the hematocrit level is low.

The primary treatment for anemia in CRF clients is erythropoietin, a hormone produced in the kidney to stimulate red blood cell production. Erythropoietin has been produced by recombinant DNA and is available for intravenous administration.

Much of the treatment for renal osteodystrophy involves dietary and medication regulation of calcium, phosphorus, and acidosis, as directed. The parathyroidism must also be brought under control. Vitamin D in its active form may be used, although it must be administered with care because of its severe side effects from metastatic calcifications. Calciferol helps promote bone mineralization by increasing the intestinal absorption of calcium and decreasing circulating parathyroid hormone and alkaline phosphatase. Some physicians advocate subtotal parathyroidectomy if all other methods fail.

Fluid and sodium regulation are the major interventions for congestive heart failure. Other cardiovascular manifestations are managed much the same as for those clients without CRF, but diuretics are not used except in the very early stages of conservative management. Hypertension must be aggressively controlled with stronger medications. Antihypertensive drugs are administered as necessary in relation to renal function and nephrotic response. Pericarditis may be managed with nonsteroidal anti-inflammatory agents but may require pericardial aspiration or pericardiectomy. Tamponade (fluid in the pericardium) necessitates pericardial drainage.

DIETARY MANAGEMENT

Dietary adjustment is dictated by many components of CRF, including accumulation of nitrogenous waste products, impaired excretion of electrolytes, vitamin deficiencies, and continued catabolism. The wasting syndrome is a major problem. The client with renal failure constantly loses body weight, muscle mass, and adipose tissue.

Specific adjustments of the dietary elements often depend on the results of blood chemistries. Although there is some debate concerning whether and how to restrict proteins, studies are now indicating that maintaining a daily intake of high biologic value protein below 50 g may slow the progression of renal failure. Generally, recommendations range from no restriction other than avoiding high-protein fad diets to restrictions of 1 g/kg/day.

It is also important to provide adequate nonprotein calories to prevent or reduce catabolism. One recommendation is 40 to 50 kcal/kg/day of carbohydrates and fats.

Dietary electrolytes may be encouraged or restricted. The regulation of sodium is a delicate matter. At times the kidneys are salt-wasters, and sodium must be encouraged to replace what is lost. More frequently, however, the kidneys retain sodium and some physicians feel that there should be a moderate restriction of dietary intake with careful monitoring of urinary sodium excretion as a guideline. Serial monitoring of data indicating fluid status also gives important information about sodium needs. Many regimens are used.

Potassium is frequently restricted. Clients must be reminded not to use salt substitutes because they contain potassium chloride. When hyperkalemia becomes evident, restriction of potassium in food and fluids is instituted. In an emergency situation, when the serum potassium is above 7.0, intravenous glucose (50 per cent dextrose in water [$D_{50}W$]), insulin, and calcium gluconate or oral or rectal sodium polystyrene sulfonate (Kayexalate), a cation-exchange resin, may be given. Dissolving the resin in ginger ale helps to (1) prevent it from sticking to the teeth and (2) mask its gritty texture. Sorbitol is usually given with the resin to avoid constipation and counteract the sodium retention that can occur. Dialysis is also effective in removing potassium from the blood.

If serum calcium levels are low, adequate calcium intake is important. Dietary sources may be supplemented with calcium carbonate, calcium lactate, or calcium gluconate. Supplements are definitely needed for clients receiving dialysis therapy. However, if serum calcium levels are high, dietary restriction may be recommended. Phosphorus is restricted. In addition, phosphate-binding gels such as aluminum hydroxide, aluminum carbonate, and calcium carbonate may be used to further reduce phosphorus levels. These agents must be administered cautiously in clients who have had a parathyroidectomy for secondary hyperparathyroidism, because aluminum deposition on bony surfaces is enhanced. Aluminum intoxication also leads to encephalopathy and osteomalacia. Finally, a mild magnesium restriction may be imposed.

Surgical Management

Kidney transplantation, the surgical implantation of a human kidney from one person to another, is performed for clients with irreversible kidney failure. Appendix C presents a sample clinical pathway for clients undergoing kidney transplantation.

The primary limiting factor in the number of transplants done is the availability of kidneys. The Uniform Anatomical Gift Act allows clients to give permission before their own death for the use of their organs for transplantation after their death (requires family consent at the time of potential donation). In 1992, Required Request legislation was passed, which mandates that hospitals ask family members of dying clients who may be suitable organ donors if they would consider donation. There are also regional and national networks known as Organ Procurement and Transplant Networks (OPTN) and the United Network of Organ Sharing (UNOS) that have been organized to coordinate the recovery and distribution of organs and tissue for transplantation.

Selection of a transplant recipient is based on careful evaluation of the client's medical, immunologic, psychosocial, and social statuses. The decision is usually made by the client, significant others, and physician working together. Recipient selection is usually from the group less than 70 years of age who have an estimated life expectancy of 2 years or more and in whom the transplant will improve the quality of life.[43] Important psychosocial concerns include the client's (1) feelings about transplant, (2) understanding and acceptance of the risks and chances of graft survival, and (3) family and social obligations. See Chapter 9 for further discussion of issues associated with transplantation.

The transplanted kidney is surgically placed extraperitoneally in the iliac fossa. The renal artery is anastomosed to the recipient's hypogastric artery and the renal vein to the recipient's iliac vein (Fig. 31–5).

Usually the kidney begins to function immediately. Sometimes adequate functioning is delayed a few days. Hemodialysis may be performed until good function is established.

COMPLICATIONS

Graft Rejection. Except for identical twin donor and recipient, the major postoperative complication is graft rejection. This is an immunologic attack against the foreign donor organ that the body has recognized as foreign tissue.

The signs of transplant rejection include fever, graft tenderness, anemia, and malaise. Urography, renal scan, ultrasonography, and CT scan are among the diagnostic tools used, mainly to rule out other causes of the symptoms.

Antirejection therapy revolves around the use of immunosuppressive drugs, which block the body's normal immune responses. A combination of azathioprine, cyclosporine, and prednisone is used most frequently for maintenance.

Immunosuppressive therapy has three potential serious consequences: (1) increased susceptibility to infection, (2) increased risk of malignancy, and (3) degenerative bone disease often necessitating total hip or knee replacements. These sequelae account for many of the short- and long-term complications of renal transplant. Balancing immunosuppressive therapy to reduce the risk of infection while preventing rejection is the primary goal of post-transplant care.

Infection. Mortality rates for infectious disease in

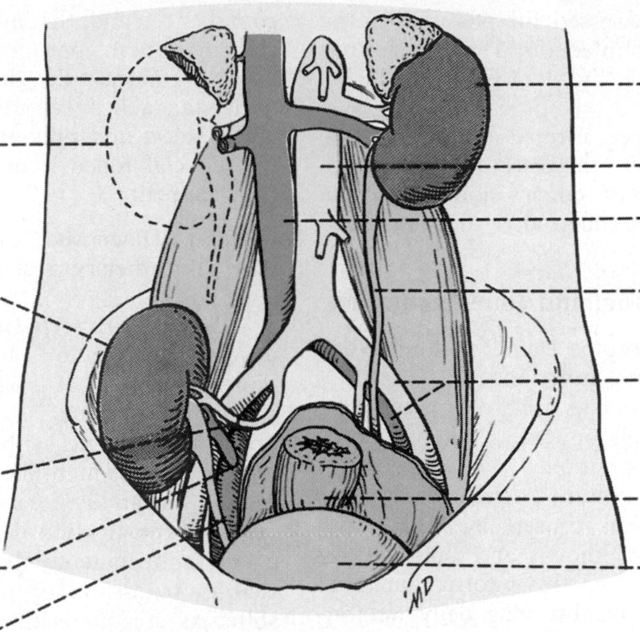

Figure 31–5
Transplanted kidney placement.

renal transplant clients have decreased dramatically in recent years. However, infection remains a potential problem and represents the most serious life-threatening complication in the early transplant period. Urinary tract infections, pneumonia, and sepsis are most commonly seen. Causative agents include bacteria (especially in the early postoperative period), viruses, and fungi. Viral and fungal complications include herpes and, more commonly, cytomegalovirus infection, which can occur in more than 50 per cent of clients who receive transplants. Immunosuppressive drugs can mask early signs of infection, so by the time infections are recognized, they may be well advanced. Sometimes immunosuppressive therapy is reduced for a short time while the infection is brought under control.

Other Complications. Complications after transplant can affect urinary, cardiovascular, respiratory, gastrointestinal, integumentary, and musculoskeletal functions. Serious complications can result in death.

Nursing Management

Assessment

When the client is suspected of having CRF, the nurse must take a complete history, paying close attention to the presence of risk factors. It is important to question clients about past and present medications, diet and weight changes, energy levels and the presence of unexplained fatigue, and the pattern of urinary elimination.

The nurse assesses the client for the presence of the multiple effects of CRF on all body systems, such as the presence of cardiovascular or respiratory abnormalities, neurologic changes, gastrointestinal problems, or skin changes.

The nurse also assesses the client's understanding of CRF, the diagnostic tests that will be done, and the possible treatment regimens. The client's level of anxiety and ability to cope with this chronic disease should be assessed. The nurse should also involve the client's significant others in the assessment to determine their ability to cope with the client's disease and treatments.

When the client has been diagnosed with CRF and is being treated with peritoneal dialysis, the nurse must assess the client's and significant others' understanding of the treatment regimen. The client and significant others, the nephrologist, and the nephrology nurse discuss the use of peritoneal dialysis and decide which type most meets the client's needs. The client's understanding of the treatment is also important to assess, as is the client's ability to cope with the treatment regimen. The significant others' ability to cope and their ability to support the client is also vital to assess.

Once the client has begun peritoneal dialysis, the priority assessment for the nurse is the presence of an infection. The insertion site should be carefully inspected for redness or other signs of infection. The nurse should also carefully assess the effluent after it is drained for the presence of cloudiness, fibrin streaks, or blood. The vital signs and weight are monitored closely.

CRITICAL TO REMEMBER

If the client is undergoing hemodialysis, the priority assessment becomes the patency of the venous access site.

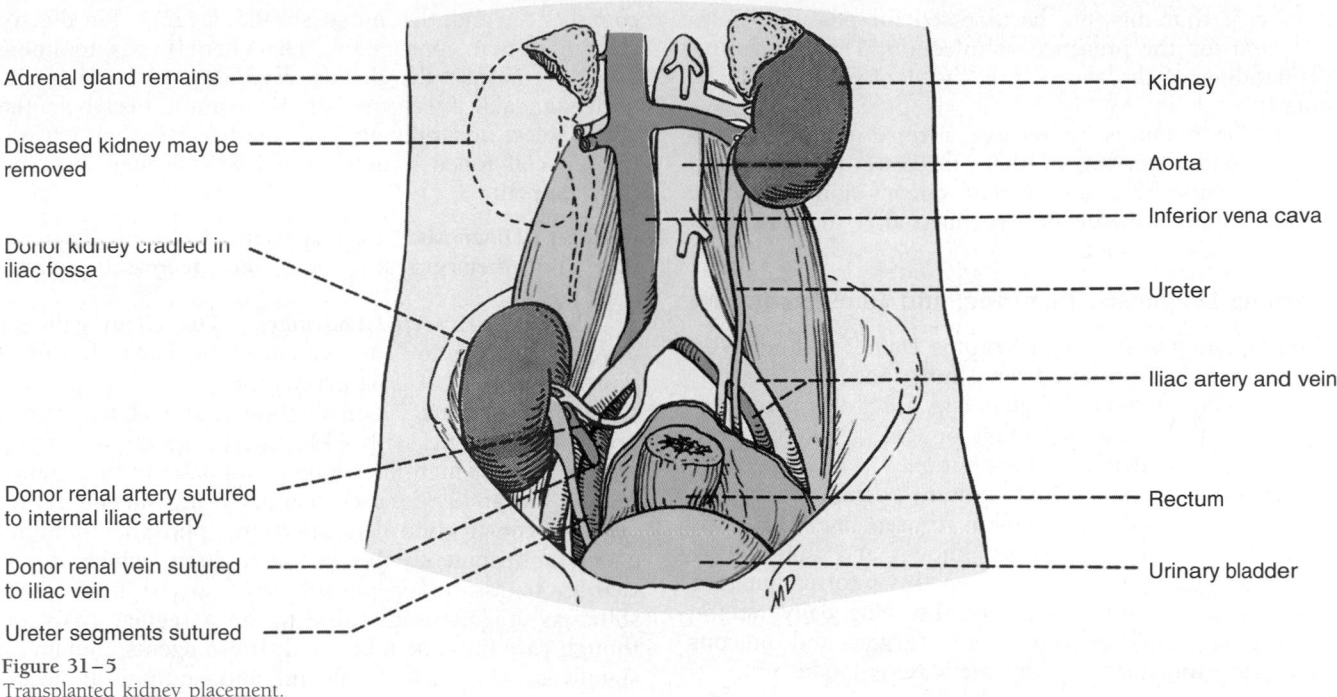

It is vital that this site be assessed for possible occlusion and for the presence of infection. The client's understanding of the access site and care of it should be noted.

If the client is to receive a renal transplant, the client's understanding of the procedure and follow-up regimen must be assessed. The client's ability to cope with a complex medication regimen after the transplant must also be assessed.

Nursing Diagnosis, Planning, and Implementation

Nursing Diagnosis: Fluid Volume Deficit or Fluid Volume Excess R/T impaired renal function.

Planning: Expected Outcomes. The client will not develop a fluid volume deficit or excess, as evidenced by no signs of edema or dehydration.

Implementation. Fluid volume deficits or overloads are a cardinal problem caused by CRF. The current fluid status must be known and fluid intake carefully regulated, depending on this information. The nurse monitors fluid status by observing daily weight, orthostatic blood pressure, skin turgor, and mucous membrane moistness and by meticulous intake and output comparisons. The nurse should give learning guidelines to clients being followed on an ambulatory basis concerning (1) how to weigh themselves and (2) how to interpret the relationship of daily weight loss or gain to their need for sodium and water. The nurse can help clients understand that vomiting, diarrhea, and working or playing in a hot environment may cause excessive fluid loss and must be prevented or controlled. He or she should teach clients how to take their blood pressure.

Once the fluid allowance for the day has been determined, the nurse helps the client follow the recommendation. The assistance needed usually concerns restricting fluid intake. The nurse can offer suggestions about reducing thirst and moistening dry mucous membranes with lip balms, frequent oral hygiene, ice chips, or spray bottles. Fluid intake should be spread out over a longer period of time. If intravenous fluids are used, the nurse should carefully attend to them to ensure proper administration rates.

Nursing Diagnosis: Nutrition: Less than Body Requirements, Altered R/T anorexia, nausea, and dietary restrictions secondary to renal failure.

Planning: Expected Outcomes. The client will maintain adequate nutrition, as evidenced by maintenance of weight without loss of muscle mass.

Implementation. Dietary management is vital in the conservative management of CRF. Anorexia results from many of the manifestations of irreversible renal failure, emotional depression, and a frequently unpalatable diet. Thus, a major nursing challenge is helping the client take in adequate nutrition while minimizing uremic toxicity. This problem grows as the disease progresses and clients tend to develop an aversion to meat and other sources of protein. To help stimulate the client's appetite, the nurse must take measures to relieve nausea and vomiting, stomatitis, and other gastrointestinal manifestations. Diet counseling is essential for compliance, and the nurse should arrange for dietary consultation if appropriate. The client needs to know how to translate the dietary regimen into a palatable, understandable food program. The nurse may help the client select and prepare foods and learn where to obtain special foods if necessary. Exercise may also improve appetite.

Nursing Diagnosis: Constipation R/T medications, fluid and dietary restrictions, and decreased activity level.

Planning: Expected Outcomes. The client will not develop constipation, as evidenced by client having a bowel movement at least every other day.

Implementation. Constipation is almost a universal problem for clients with CRF. Fluid restrictions, inability to eat most high-fiber foods, and activity intolerance reduce the ability to use customary measures for preventing constipation. In addition, phosphate-binding agents contribute to this problem. Bran, which is not rich in potassium or phosphorus, can be used. Stool softeners are often administered on a regular basis, although care must be taken with those agents containing significant amounts of calcium and sodium. If necessary, bulk laxatives (e.g., psyllium hydrophilic mucilloid) may be given. It is important that the recommended amount of fluid be taken with the powder, and this amount must be subtracted from the day's fluid allotment. Stimulant and lubricant laxatives should be used only if necessary, especially compounds containing magnesium or phosphorus. If none of these measures is effective, small-volume, gentle-stimulant enemas may be used sparingly, but large-volume enemas must be avoided because of possible fluid and saline absorption. Renal failure clients are at risk for the development of diverticular disease.

Nursing Diagnosis: Knowledge Deficit R/T disease process and its treatment.

Planning: Expected Outcomes. The client will understand disease process and treatment regimen, as evidenced by client's ability to describe disease and treatment and to participate in treatment regimen.

Implementation. Teaching is a crucial part of the nursing management plan. Most of the time, the client will be followed on an ambulatory basis and will be responsible for following the recommended treatment regimen. The client and significant others must know about normal renal function and how the disease has altered it, the details of the management protocol and how to follow it, a number of self-assessment skills as described earlier, and when to seek professional consultation about possible complications.

Although clients with renal disease need to learn about their disorder, they may not always be ready to learn. Anxiety itself interferes with learning. In addition, the disease retards normal mental functioning; memory deficits and a short attention span may require simple presentations and frequent repeating of information. Retained learning must be continually evaluated.

Significant others may be especially frustrated during teaching sessions by the client's inability to grasp the concepts being presented. The client often seems out of touch with reality. Significant others need reassurance that this is an effect of the disease itself and that the client will become more capable of learning, especially after institution of dialysis.

With the exception of insertion and removal of the peritoneal catheter, peritoneal dialysis is primarily a nursing intervention. The nurse monitors the client, plans care, and, in many instances, teaches the client how to do the procedure independently.

Nursing Diagnosis: Infection, Risk for R/T presence of indwelling peritoneal catheter and instillation of dialysate.

Planning: Expected Outcomes. The client will not develop an infection, as evidenced by normal white blood cell count, absence of fever, and clear dialysate.

Implementation. Because peritonitis is the main complication of peritoneal dialysis, aseptic technique must be used throughout the procedure. Masks are worn by the nurse and client anytime the peritoneal dialysis circuit is opened. Sterile gloves are worn by anyone touching the catheter during all connection and disconnection procedures. The catheter is soaked before and after these procedures in a povidone-iodine solution. Dressing changes are ordered per specific unit protocol. Dressings must be kept dry at all times.

Nursing Diagnosis: Pain, Risk for R/T instillation of dialysate.

Planning: Expected Outcomes. The client will have pain controlled, as evidenced by client's statement.

Implementation. If discomfort is present, it can be relieved in several ways, including slowing the rate of flow, elevating the head, massaging the abdomen, or having the client move around. Analgesics may be necessary. If eating makes the client uncomfortable, the nurse can serve small meals frequently and also try to coordinate the meals with drainage periods.

Nursing Diagnosis: Breathing Pattern, Ineffective R/T pressure of dialysate.

Planning: Expected Outcomes. The client will have an effective breathing pattern, as evidenced by absence of shortness of breath.

Implementation. Because of pressure on the diaphragm by the dialysate, its full excursion may be reduced. The immobilized client may be at risk for the development of respiratory problems. The nurse should encourage the client to cough and deep-breathe regularly. The client also needs to be alert for early signs of compromised respiratory function.

Nursing Diagnosis: Knowledge Deficit R/T peritoneal dialysis and its impact.

Planning: Expected Outcomes. The client will understand peritoneal dialysis and its impact, as evidenced by client discussion.

Implementation. The client and significant others may have significant levels of anxiety and many concerns about peritoneal dialysis and its impact on their lives. Therapeutic communication by the nurse helps them cope with these concerns. If the client will be undergoing long-term dialysis, the client and significant others may have a prolonged relationship with the nurse, and the nurse should be constantly working to establish and maintain a supportive, therapeutic rapport with them. If the client is immobilized during the day for treatment, the nurse may need to help the client develop appropriate diversionary activities.

The client and significant others need to know about peritoneal dialysis and how to work with its ramifications. Because so many clients continue this treatment mode in their homes, this knowledge needs to be complete and detailed. They require a complete training program so they can handle the entire dialysis process independently.

Most of the care required by the client during and after hemodialysis falls within the realm of nursing. Providing this care requires specialized training.

Continuous monitoring during dialysis provides vital information about the progress of the treatment and allows early diagnosis of potential complications. There should be a well-organized plan for observing and recording vital signs, dialysate composition and temperature, functioning of the entire dialysis system, blood flow, and clotting times. The nurse should also be alert to early signs of potential complications as listed earlier. The nurse often serves as case manager and coordinates the services provided by the nephrology team that includes the physician, nurses, social worker, and dietitian.

Nursing Diagnosis: Injury, Risk for R/T trauma to hemodialysis venous access site.

Planning: Expected Outcomes. The client will not suffer injury to venous access site, as evidenced by continued patency of site.

Implementation. Careful attention to the access site is important to its life expectancy. Care of the access site is designed to prevent infection and clotting. A dressing is used to protect cannulas and subclavian catheters from infection. The access must also be protected from trauma that could cause clotting, bleeding, or physical disruption of the access. Blood pressure measurement should not be taken on, or blood drawn from, the limb containing the access. Between dialysis periods, the skin over the fistula or graft requires only routine care with soap and water.

Nursing Diagnosis: Knowledge Deficit R/T nutritional needs during dialysis.

Planning: Expected Outcomes. The client will understand nutritional needs during dialysis and possible home dialysis program, as evidenced by discussion with client.

Implementation. Providing adequate nutrition is often easier during dialysis and for a time afterward. Dialysis usually relieves many of the gastrointestinal problems that frequently interfere with adequate intake. Food and fluid restrictions are sometimes liberalized just before dialysis but are reimposed afterward. As a result, sodium and water are metabolized and ready to be dialyzed during actual dialysis.

Dietary noncompliance remains a major problem during maintenance dialysis, and it may require all the nurse's knowledge and creativity to help the client follow the recommended regimen.

Nursing Diagnosis: Individual Coping, Ineffective R/T effects of long-term hemodialysis.

Planning: Expected Outcomes. The client will cope effectively with effects of long-term hemodialysis, as evidenced by client's ability to look at alternatives and discuss plans.

Implementation. Much of the care required by clients on chronic hemodialysis and significant others revolves around psychosocial aspects of dialysis. Clients on maintenance dialysis often have ambivalent feelings. On one hand, they realize that hemodialysis is their tie with life. Yet, the many restrictions and life-style changes imposed on them make continuation of the program extremely difficult. Clients often report that they feel in limbo between the worlds of life and death.

The process of adaptation to a loss is a part of adjustment. It is not uncommon for clients to feel quite grateful and optimistic at the start of their dialysis treatments. Usually they have felt ill for some time, and they view the intervention as a route to survival and a hope for feeling well again. It takes a few days or weeks for them to fully realize the permanent place of dialysis in their lives. Depression during this period is expected. The suicide rate among clients on dialysis has been estimated at 100 times that of the general population.

Assistance for the client and significant others must begin before dialysis is started. They need to fully understand the intervention and its implications. The nurse should encourage them to discuss their feelings. It is often difficult for clients to voice concerns about continuing dialysis because of its significance. These feelings are often, albeit subconsciously, supported by the nurses; it is sometimes difficult for care providers to accept a client's decision to stop treatment and choose ultimate death instead. The nurses, who often become a kind of "family" to the client, must provide a continued, unified, supportive approach and be ready to accept the whole gamut of reactions to dialysis by the client and significant others. It is helpful to know the client's usual patterns of response to stress. If clients have sound psychosocial coping mechanisms and help from those around them, they usually accommodate themselves to the situation and plan their lives realistically. Clients who handle stress poorly or who have little support from others may never make an adequate adjustment. Active participation by clients in their care is a valuable tool in helping to meet several of the needs identified here.

Nursing Diagnosis: Family Coping, Ineffective R/T chronic treatment and possible home dialysis program.

Planning: Expected Outcomes. The client will cope with chronic treatment, as evidenced by family's ability to work with client and offer support.

Implementation. The number of clients availing themselves of home dialysis is about 15 per cent of all clients receiving dialytic therapy. The cost of this type of program is less than in-center dialysis, and usually the client's quality of life is improved. Home dialysis offers the client more access to significant others and greater feelings of independence and control. However, this type of treatment also produces stress on personal relationships, especially to the person who becomes the "dialyzer helper." Some spouses have voiced concern about the lack of free time and increased responsibility; others see it as an opportunity to give something back to their spouse or loved ones. Some states have funding available to pay for a non-family member to serve as dialysis helper. In some instances, this may reduce tension and improve the quality of life for the family.

Nursing Diagnosis: Knowledge Deficit R/T renal transplant and therapeutic regimen.

Planning: Expected Outcomes. The client will understand the transplant and therapeutic regimen, as evidenced by discussion with client.

Implementation. The donor and recipient must be prepared for postsurgical psychological reactions. Strong emotional ties often develop between the donor and recipient during the evaluation period, and the donor frequently feels responsible for the success or failure of the graft postoperatively. Graft rejection is usually devastating to these clients. Also, the need to protect the remaining kidney may give rise to later feelings of anger. Postoperative traumatic reactions by the donor are less likely in clients who have good inner resources, flexible defense mechanisms, and good mental health. Another source of postoperative stress for the donor is the fact that families tend to pay more attention to the recipient because of the continued possibility of graft rejection. The donor often feels abandoned. However, strong, long-lasting, positive effects include identification of a source of inner strength, a more positive self-image, and a general "sense of feeling good" about saving someone's life.

The donor may be assured that the remaining kidney will assume adequate total renal functioning. The renal blood flow and GFR of the remaining kidney have been reported to increase to 70 to 80 per cent of the preoperative levels of both kidneys together. Within 2 to 6 years, the 24-hour creatinine clearance levels often recover 85 to 87 per cent.

Nursing Diagnosis: Infection, Risk for R/T immunosuppressive therapy.

Planning: Expected Outcomes. The client will not develop an infection, as evidenced by absence of fever and no signs of infection (may be masked by steroids).

Implementation. Much of nursing management is aimed at prevention, early recognition, and treatment of complications plus measures to facilitate maximal renal function and help the client attain an optimal quality of life. Immediate postoperative care of both the donor and recipient encompasses the care required by anyone having surgery, as described in Chapter 5. Care of the donor resembles that of anyone undergoing a nephrectomy. The additional care required by the recipient is partially suggested by the potential complications. The nurse must be constantly aware of the signs and symptoms of these sequelae. Hand washing and universal precautions are measures taken to protect the client from potential sources of infection within the environment.

Because of the high incidence and seriousness of pneumonia to the client with a renal transplant, preventive respiratory treatment is essential. Coughing and deep-breathing exercises are started immediately. These exercises are painful, and the nurse can use analgesics judiciously and put external pressure over the incision to help the client cough and breathe more effectively.

Wound care must be performed with the strictest aseptic technique because the client does not have much resistance to bacterial invasion. Delayed wound healing makes the client susceptible to dehiscence longer than usual. If the client has a fistula or graft for hemodialysis, it will be left in place in case dialysis is needed postoperatively.

Oral hygiene is important because of the high incidence of stomatitis and bacterial and fungal infections. Antifungal mouthwashes may be used. Oral fluids are usually instituted after 12 to 24 hours.

Evaluation

The nurse must evaluate whether the established goals have been met. If they were not, the nurse must alter the plan and interventions to ensure that the client's needs are met.

Modification of Plan of Care for the Elderly

One of the major modifications for an older client is the possible limit of options available for treatment. Renal transplant is not routinely done on elderly clients. Clients over age 60 years are evaluated on an individual basis; clients as old as 75 years have successfully undergone transplantation. The types of dialysis will be evaluated on the basis of the presence of other chronic disorders the client may have that would limit the ability to comply with any treatment.

Older clients may have had multiple abdominal surgeries with the development of adhesions that will limit the usefulness of peritoneal dialysis. They are more likely to have pre-existing cardiovascular problems that may limit the usefulness of many venous access sites.

Posthospital Care

Clients with CRF have a wide variety of learning needs. They and their significant others must understand the disease, its outcome, and the treatment regimen. Diet teaching is important with all the possible treatment regimens and medications that the client will need for the rest of life (see Client Education Guide: Chronic Renal Failure). If clients are on home dialysis, they will need more assistance at home with both the set-up and the maintenance of their dialysis.

The nurse can help the client arrange activities and life-style to avoid highly stressful situations. Additionally, the client may need job retraining. In essence, the client and significant others require the nurse's knowledge and assistance in adjusting to a life-long chronic illness, often with complex, continuous therapy.

Long-term care usually continues throughout the client's lifetime. Clients need continued physical and psychosocial support. The importance of complying with recommended medical management regimens and follow-up evaluation schedules must be emphasized and periodically reinforced.

CLIENT EDUCATION GUIDE

Chronic Renal Failure

The nurse should teach the client and significant others about:

- Medications—purpose, dosage, administration, side effects, and toxic effects
- Manifestations of infection, venous access blockage, or graft rejection
- How to avoid infections and how to manage them when they occur
- The dietary regimen and its preparation
- Information about the transplant that must be given to dentists and other physicians
- The importance of an exercise program to help maintain body function and to maintain muscle mass despite steroid therapy

RENAL CALCULI

Although calculi can form anywhere in the urinary tract, the most frequent site is in the kidney. These stones may travel down the urinary tract with or without resultant damage, may lodge anywhere along the tract, or may stay within the kidney.

Etiology

A number of etiologic factors influence renal stone formation. Development of urinary lithiasis is probably the result not of any one factor but of multiple phenomena. One of the questions still unanswered is why some clients form stones whereas others do not. This problem is particularly important with recurrent "stoneformers."

Risk Factors

Risk factors for stone formation include anything that causes either stasis or supersaturation (increased concentration) of the urine. This includes stressors such as immobility, which increases stasis; dehydration, which leads to supersaturation; and an increase in calcium or other ion in the urine. Another major risk factor is having had urinary calculi previously.

The prime risk factor for uric acid stones is an alteration in purine metabolism as seen with gout. Controlling the production and excretion of uric acid can help prevent these.

Pathophysiology

Regardless of the specific type of calculus, the process of stone formation is one of crystallization. Generally, crystal growth involves nucleation, in which crystallites are formed from supersaturated urine. Growth proceeds by aggregation to form larger particles.

Renal calculi may be of one crystalline type only or a combination of types. Approximately 80 per cent of all urinary tract stones contain calcium, usually as calcium phosphate or calcium oxalate. Calcium stones may range from very small particles, often called sand or gravel, to giant staghorn calculi, which may fill the entire renal pelvis and extend up into the calices (Fig. 31–6). They have a peak onset in the third decade and primarily afflict men.

The second most frequent crystal to cause stones is oxalate, which is relatively insoluble in urine. Its solubility is only slightly affected by changes in urinary pH. The mechanism for oxalate availability is unclear but may be closely related to diet. The disease is most common in areas where cereals are a major dietary component and least common in dairy farming regions.

Struvite stones, also called triple phosphate, are composed of calcium, magnesium, and ammonium phosphate. Their cause is certain bacteria, usually *Proteus*. The stones form staghorn calculi (see Fig. 31–6). Abscess formation is common, sometimes the result of erosion into the perinephric space. These stones are particularly difficult to eliminate because the hard stone forms around a nucleus of bacteria, protecting them from antibiotic therapy. Any small fragment left after surgical removal of the stone begins the cycle again.

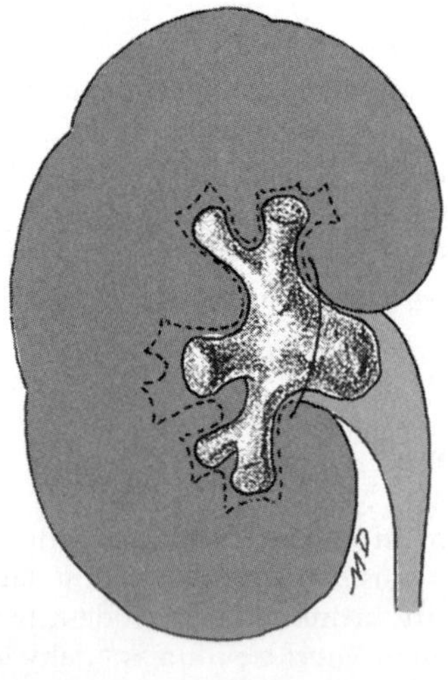

Figure 31–6
Staghorn calculus.

Uric acid stones are caused by increased urate excretion, fluid depletion, and a low urinary pH. Hyperuricuria is the result of either increased uric acid production or the administration of uricosuric agents. A high dietary intake of purine-rich foods may predispose susceptible clients to uric acid stone formation.

Despite the type of stone that forms, the potential damage is essentially the same: pain, obstruction, and tissue trauma with secondary hemorrhage and infection.

Clinical Manifestations

The most characteristic symptom of renal or ureteral calculi is a sharp, severe pain with a sudden onset. Depending on the site of the stone, this pain may be called either renal colic or ureteral colic. Renal colic originates deep in the lumbar region and radiates around the side and down toward the testicle in the male and the bladder in the female. Ureteral colic radiates toward the genitalia and thigh. When the pain is severe, the client will usually exhibit nausea, vomiting, pallor, and diaphoresis and be quite anxious. Urinary frequency may occur. The pain lasts for minutes to days and can be somewhat resistant to narcotic intervention. Pain may be intermittent, which usually means that the stone has moved. Physicians hypothesize that the ureter dilates just proximal to the calculus, which allows urine to pass, relieving the ureteral distention. Then, as the stone moves and sets up a new obstruction site, the pain returns. The pain subsides when the stone reaches the bladder.

Pain caused by renal stones is not always severe and colicky in nature. In fact, it may be a dull, aching, or heavy feeling. This is particularly true during the early stages of hydronephrosis. Sometimes, there may be no sensation, and the first clue the client has is when a "clink" sounds against the toilet when the stone passes.

DIAGNOSTIC ASSESSMENT

The major diagnostic test is a KUB or flat plate of the abdomen to visualize the stone. An IVP is also done to determine if any obstruction is present and, if so, how severe it is.

Medical Management

MECHANICAL INTERVENTION

If it is decided that the stone will not pass before complications occur, mechanical intervention may be used. Depending on the position of the calculus, cystoscopy may be done. Additionally, one or two ureteral catheters may be inserted past the stone. From this point, several different interventions are appropriate. The catheters may be left in place for 24 hours. Their presence drains the urine trapped proximal to the stones and dilates the ureter, which may prompt spontaneous movement of the calculus. Otherwise, the catheters may mechanically guide the stones downward as they are removed. A continuous chemical irrigation may be established to dissolve the stone. Finally, an attempt may be made to manipulate or to dislodge the stone. A variety of special catheters with loops and expanding baskets may be inserted through the cystoscope and used to snare the stone. The postprocedure care of these clients is the same as that following cystoscopy (see Chap. 29). Chapter 30 describes the care of a client with indwelling catheters.

A noninvasive mechanical procedure for breaking up stones so they can pass spontaneously or be removed by other methods is extracorporeal lithotripsy. Figure 31–7 shows how this procedure works. The client is placed in a specially designed tub with the trunk submerged in water. Then, an underwater electrode generates shock waves via a reflector that fragments kidney stone. The client is strapped to a frame and may be sedated during the procedure, because it usually lasts for 30 to 40 minutes and immobility is essential. After the procedure, the client may experience some renal colic that needs spasmolytics. Early ambulation and adequate diuresis are important to fully "wash out" the stone fragments.

PREVENTION

Another aspect of intervention is preventing stone recurrence. Stone recurrence usually happens within a 2- to 3-year period, but may occur as long as 20 years later. As the number of recurrences increases, the interval between the formation of stones tends to become shorter. Thus, prevention is a life-long program.

Two objectives are essential to the total preventive regimen. First, any underlying contributing problem must be corrected (e.g., metabolic and anatomic). Parathyroidectomy may be performed in the case of intractable hypercalcemia. Second, infection must be avoided or aggressively treated for all stone types because it places additional stress on the kidneys.

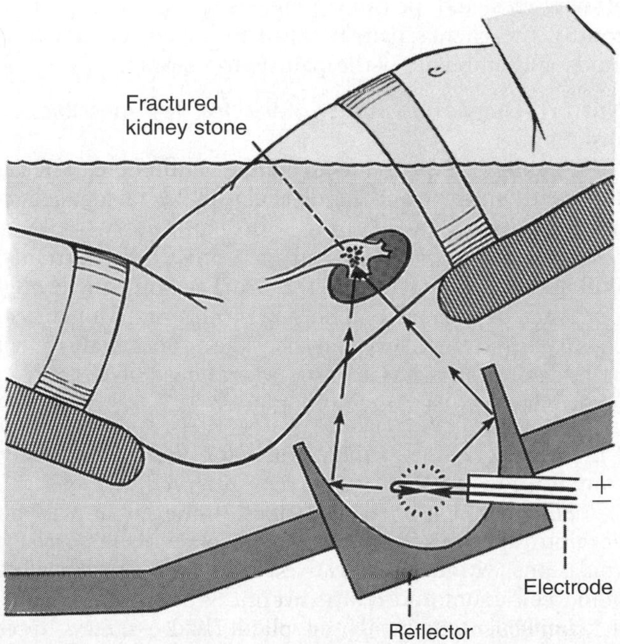

Figure 31–7
Extracorporeal lithotripsy. Electrically generated shock waves fracture kidney stones.

PHARMACOLOGIC MANAGEMENT

There are no particular medications used to treat calcium stones. If the client has uric acid stones, medications to lower uric acid such as allopurinol (Zyloprim) should be given. The client is treated with narcotics and antispasmodics.

DIETARY MANAGEMENT

Once the components of the stone have been identified, diet modification will be used to help prevent recurrence. A low-calcium, low-oxalate diet is used to prevent calcium or oxalate stone recurrence, and a low-purine diet is used to prevent uric acid stone recurrence.

Surgical Management

Percutaneous lithotripsy is an invasive procedure in which tubes are inserted in the area of stone formation. Contrast dye is injected, and forceps are used to remove the stones. If the stones are too large to remove with forceps, ultrasonic waves can be used to break up the stones for easier removal.[6]

Surgical intervention may be performed through a percutaneous approach or by open procedures. The development of advanced fiberoptic equipment has made the percutaneous route the most common. Figure 31–8 shows a nephroscope in place. The stone may be removed by alligator forceps or a stone basket. Irrigation to flush the stone out of its resting place may be done.

After the procedure, a nephrostomy tube remains in place for 1 to 5 days. The client may be sent home with the nephrostomy tube. A nephrotomogram is then done to determine whether all stone fragments were removed. If the kidney is clear, the tube will be removed and a bulky dressing placed over the site. The nurse must be certain that a high fluid intake is maintained during the post-procedure period to flush out any fragments. Recommended daily amounts are 3000 to 4000 mL. The nurse monitors for, or teaches the client to monitor for, complications such as infection, hemorrhage, and extravasation of fluid into the retroperitoneal cavity.

If these procedures do not successfully remove the stone, an open surgical procedure may be required. A stone lodged in the ureter will require a ureterolithotomy, which involves incision into the affected ureter. The approach may be through a lower abdominal or flank incision. The stone is removed, any strictures are repaired, and the incision is closed.

If constricted or tortuous ureters cause recurrent calculi, one of two procedures may be used to correct the problem. An ileal ureter, using a segment of the ileum between the renal collecting system and the blad-

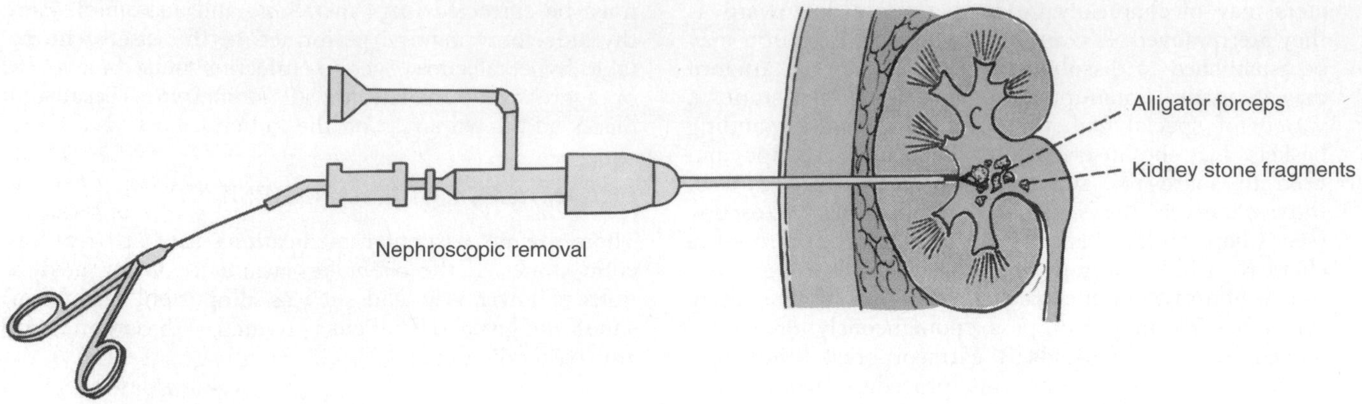

Figure 31–8
Surgical techniques for the removal of kidney stones.

der, may be constructed. This creates a wide-bore passage that replaces the original ureter. A renal autotransplant may also be performed. Here the kidney is transplanted to the ipsilateral or contralateral pelvis. A flap of bladder tissue is raised, formed into a large-caliber tube, and anastomosed to the renal pelvis. The bladder wall is then sutured to re-establish its continuity. These procedures are used very selectively.

The physician may decide that a partial or total nephrectomy is necessary because of extensive kidney damage, overwhelming renal infection, or severe ureteropelvic junction obstruction or, in the case of abnormal renal parenchyma, to prevent stone recurrence. This procedure is used much less now than in the past and is usually considered a "last resort" intervention.

Possible complications after lithotripsy include hemorrhage, urinary retention, infection, and possible stone recurrence.

Nursing Management

Assessment

As with any disease, the history the client gives is very important in identifying the problem. Full information about the onset of symptoms and the pattern of pain is vital. Family history of calculi is suggestive. Recent dietary habits should be evaluated. For instance, a large intake of purines may be significant, and drinking large amounts of fruit juices or tea facilitates oxalate precipitation. The client should be asked about recent medications and the presence of any contributing factors, such as urinary tract infection, immobility, or gout.

Physical findings primarily center on two things: the urine and x-ray studies. Material strained from the urine can be sent to a laboratory for analysis. Urine should be monitored for hematuria. A routine urinalysis gives important information about the pH, the specific gravity, and the presence of red blood cells, white blood cells, crystals, and casts. The nurse should collect 24-hour urine specimens, if necessary, to determine the daily output of possible causative crystals. A urine culture will help identify urinary tract infection. Blood levels of constituent elements, such as calcium, phosphorus, and uric acid, may be determined. Stones containing calcium and cystine are radiopaque and will show up on a KUB x-ray film. IVP and retrograde pyelography are an important part of the evaluation process.

Nursing Diagnosis, Planning, and Implementation

Nursing Diagnosis: Pain R/T irritation from stone movement.

Planning: Expected Outcomes. The client will have pain relieved or controlled, as evidenced by client's statement.

Implementation. Controlling the client's pain is a primary objective of nursing intervention. Large doses of narcotics and possibly antispasmodics are given to control the client's pain because the client cannot force fluids and ambulate if the pain is too severe.

Nursing Diagnosis: Injury, Risk for R/T possible obstruction.

Planning: Expected Outcomes. The client will not suffer an injury from an obstruction, as evidenced by normal output.

Implementation. All urine must be strained. Whenever the client voids, the urine is strained through a strainer or a gauze pad so any stones or sediment can be saved and sent for analysis. The stone analysis will help determine what measures are needed to prevent recurrence.

Nursing Diagnosis: Injury, Risk for R/T postoperative complications.

Planning: Expected Outcomes. The client will not develop injury, as evidenced by absence of hemorrhage, vital signs within preoperative limits, and normal white blood cell count and temperature.

Implementation. If the client had surgery to remove the stone, then postoperative nursing interventions will depend on the incision's location and the type of drainage tubes present. With a flank incision, care is similar to that needed after nephrectomy. The client with an abdominal incision, however, requires the same care as anyone having major abdominal surgery (see Chap. 5).

The nurse needs to know that the incision probably will drain large amounts of urine for days to weeks after surgery. Intervention includes frequent dressing change around the Penrose drain and protection of the skin against the urinary drainage. A nephrostomy tube may be left in place attached to a drainage bag. Care should be taken to ensure a free flow of urine. Sterile technique is always used to prevent infection.

Nursing Diagnosis: Knowledge Deficit R/T fluid requirements, dietary restrictions, and medications.

Planning: Expected Outcomes. The client will understand fluid requirements, dietary restrictions, medications, and preventive measures as evidenced by discussion with client.

Implementation. The three main components of a preventive regimen are fluids, diet, and medications.

The client's fluid intake should be high enough to ensure 2500 to 3000 mL or more of urine output per day. This will require at least 3000 to 4000 mL of fluid daily; more will be needed under certain situations (e.g., hot weather, fever, diarrhea). The increased urine volume resulting from this high fluid intake decreases the concentration of solutes and alleviates urinary stasis. The kind of fluid the client drinks depends on dietary restrictions. At least half of the fluid should be water, which usually has a low calcium content. The fluid intake needs to be as consistent as possible throughout the 24-hour period. Clients are usually advised to drink one glass every hour during the day and two large glasses just before going to bed. This will usually mean that they will need to void about midway through the night, when they can drink another glass of water. These clients will probably need help adjusting their life-styles to accommodate the need for frequent bathroom breaks.

There is some controversy regarding dietary restrictions because of the uncertain therapeutic effectiveness of and problems in long-term compliance with this regimen.

For planning recommended dietary restrictions, the results of a stone analysis are essential. Some stone constituents require specific diet adjustments in order to avoid stone formation. Hypercalciuria may be controlled by limiting excessive calcium intake. Clients with oxalate stones should avoid high-oxalate foods: tea, instant coffee, cola drinks, beer, rhubarb, beans, asparagus, spinach, cabbage, chocolate, citrus fruits, apples, grapes, cranberries, peanuts, and peanut butter. Megadoses of vitamin C increase oxalate excretion in the urine.

If the stone is composed of uric acid, the client should be on a low-purine diet. This limits foods such as aged cheeses, wine, and organ meats.

Medications may also be used to reduce the incidence of recurrent calculi. The nurse should teach the client about these agents and the need for long-term administration. Medications frequently used to control calcium stone formation may include phosphates, thiazide diuretics, and allopurinol. Phosphates reduce urinary calcium and increase the excretion of pyrophosphate, which is responsible for inhibiting crystal formation. Methylene blue may decrease calcium oxalate crystal formation. Clients with these conditions should also avoid calcium-containing antacids.

Cholestyramine, an anion-exchange resin, binds oxalate and promotes its excretion by the intestine. It does have the potential side effect of severe vitamin K deficiency. Because pyridoxine (vitamin B_6) deficiency increases crystal excretion, B_6 may be given to clients who have oxalate stones. Magnesium oxide also decreases oxalate excretion, and isocarboxazid apparently blocks the metabolism of oxalate. Allopurinol, a xanthine oxidase inhibitor, may be used to prevent oxalate and uric acid stone formation. Uricosuric agents should be avoided; they increase uric acid excretion in the urine, thus increasing the solute concentration.

One of the most frequent components of the medication regimen for triple phosphate or struvite stones is long-term antibiotics as an attempt to control the infection. Acidification of the urine, administration of phosphate-binding gels, and dietary restrictions of phosphate are also used. Cystine stone-formers are treated with D-penicillamine or mercaptopropionylglycine, which transform L-cystine into a water-soluble disulfide derivative. Clients treated with these medications usually need supplemental vitamin B_6.

Adjusting the urinary pH as a means to control precipitation of crystals is a possible treatment. An acidic urine, with a pH below 6, is used to prevent possible calcium and triple phosphate or struvite stones. Chapter 30 describes methods for acidifying the urine. Additionally, methionine or ammonium salts may be used. Uric acid and xanthine stones are inhibited in alkaline urine; alkalinization of the urine is usually accomplished with sodium bicarbonate, citrate, or acetazolamide.

The client must be taught methods to avoid recurrence or to at least detect the stones early if they recur. This includes teaching the client to increase fluid intake; void every 2 hours; maintain an acidic urine pH (unless the stones are uric acid); change diet to low-calcium, low-phosphate with calcium stones or low-purine with uric acid stones; and take medications to improve excretion of uric acid with uric acid stones. The client should also be taught to recognize any signs of recurrence.

The client should be followed at intervals for signs of recurrent calculi. Follow-up urinalysis and blood measures for the presence of the stone-causing agents are done at intervals.

Evaluation

The nurse should evaluate whether the established goals have been met for this client. If the goals were not met, the nurse must alter the plan of care and interventions so that the client's needs are met.

Modification of Plan of Care for the Elderly

There are no specific modifications for the older client except recognition of the increased risk of complications of surgery associated with aging (see Chap 5).

RENAL CANCER

Benign kidney tumors are rare. Classifications include lymphangioma, lipoma, medullary fibroma, adenoma, leiomyoma, and oncocytoma. When large tumors occur, it is relatively impossible to distinguish them from malignant tumor by x-ray examination. If other diagnostic tests are also inconclusive, nephrectomy may be performed.

Incidence

At least 85 per cent of all renal tumors are malignant. There are approximately 5000 to 7000 deaths yearly as a result of adult kidney cancer. The figure represents 1 to 3 per cent of all malignancies. The tumors are most frequently found between the ages of 50 and 70 years. They affect men more frequently than women.

Etiology

The exact cause of renal tumors is unknown. Some links have been established between kidney cancer and tobacco, lead, cadmium, and phosphates. A genetic link has also been postulated.

Pathophysiology

Renal cell carcinoma, or adenocarcinoma, is the most frequent type of tumor; it accounts for 90 per cent of all kidney neoplasms. Tumor growth begins in the renal cortex and usually continues for some time before it produces symptoms. It can grow very large and tends to compress adjacent renal parenchyma rather than infiltrate it. The tumor, usually avascular, tends to surround blood vessels and stenose them. The lungs and mediastinum are the most frequent metastatic sites for this tumor. Liver, bone, skin, spleen, renal vein, and brain are other common sites.

Other types of renal cancer include nephroblastoma, sarcoma, and epithelial tumors within the renal pelvis. Nephroblastoma, or Wilms' tumor, is primarily a childhood disease, although it occasionally occurs in adults.

Staging of the tumor helps delineate the appropriate treatment to be used. Figure 31–9 illustrates the typical staging system for renal carcinoma.

Spontaneous regression of renal adenocarcinoma reportedly occurs in fewer than 1 per cent of all cases. Most of these regressions developed after nephrectomy and involved metastatic areas. However, authorities consider these episodes as more evidence that the disease has a definite immunologic or hormonal link. The prognosis depends partially on the stage at time of treatment.

Clinical Manifestations

Symptoms of renal malignancies vary, and tumor growth may advance significantly before the disease is discovered. It is not uncommon for the client to demonstrate signs and symptoms not apparently related to renal disease. Frequently, a palpable abdominal mass found during a routine physical examination arouses the first suspicion. Painless hematuria is a classic sign. The average time between the onset of hematuria and the onset of pain is 9 months, and 14 months between the initial pain and diagnosis. Many times, extrarenal manifestations are found before a diagnosis of renal cancer is confirmed. As many as 35 per cent of all clients have metastasis when the final diagnosis of a renal neoplasm is made.

The common triad of symptoms includes hematuria, flank pain, and a palpable abdominal or flank mass. The hematuria is usually gross and intermittent, which helps explain the client's delay in seeking medical advice. The clinical picture also contains a combination of the following frequent assessment findings: fever, weight loss and cachexia, fatigue, hypertension, amyloidosis, thrombophlebitis, anemia, erythrocytosis, hypercalcemia, abnormal serum liver profile, and an elevated sedimentation rate.

DIAGNOSTIC ASSESSMENT

Several diagnostic tests help confirm a diagnosis of renal cancer. IVP is probably the most helpful in identifying a space-occupying lesion. Ultrasonography helps differentiate between a cyst and a solid mass. Other noninvasive procedures include CT scan, nephrotomography, and radioisotope studies. Arteriography evaluates the renal vascular system. Renal biopsy, usually done percutaneously, provides definitive data about the lesion.

Medical Management

Radiation therapy may be used in adjunction with chemotherapy and surgery. Irradiation is most useful in preoperative preparation of the tumor. It is sometimes also used postoperatively to (1) destroy residual or recurrent tumor cells, (2) treat lymphatic involvement, and (3) treat metastatic sites, such as the bones, palliatively.

PHARMACOLOGIC MANAGEMENT

Clinical investigation continues to search for an effective chemotherapeutic regimen. Medroxyprogesterone

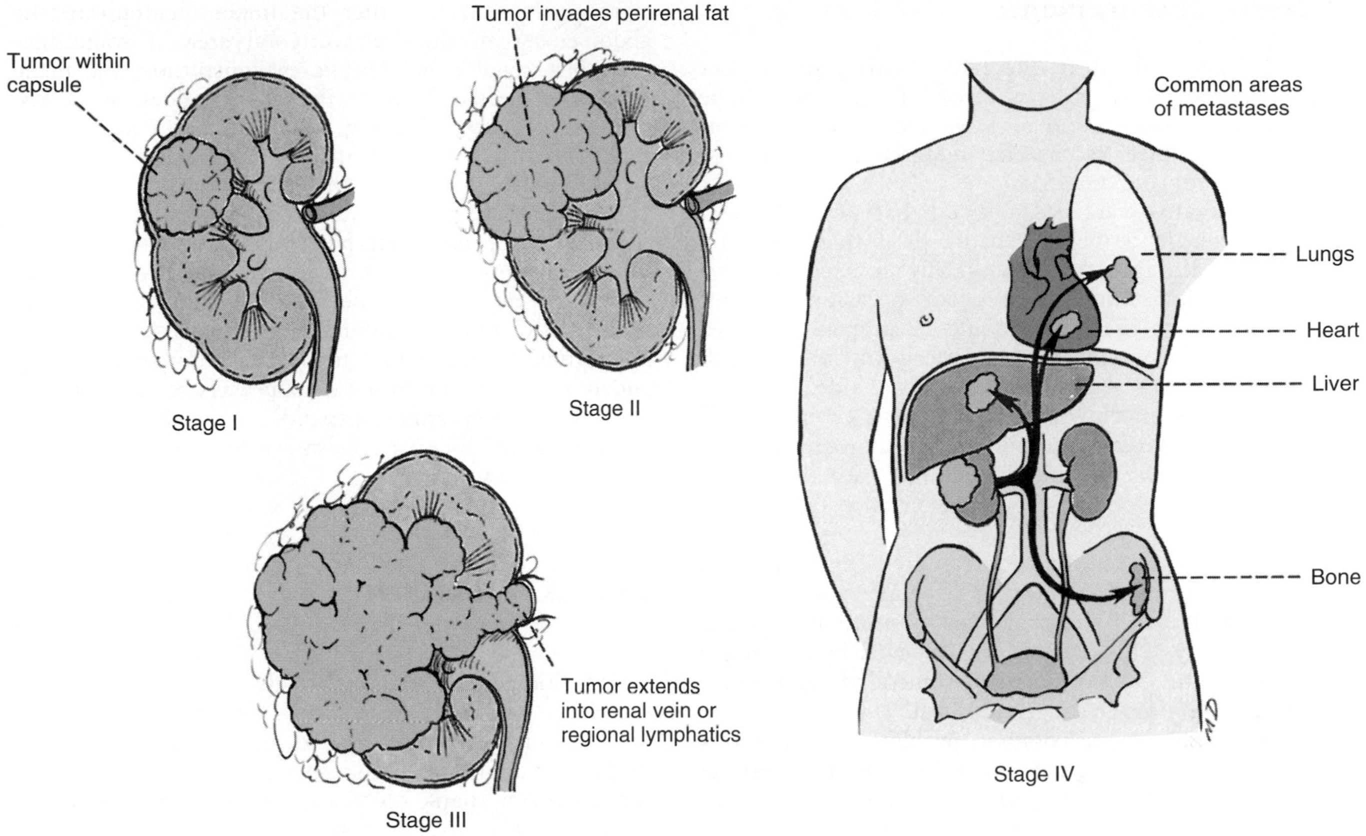

Figure 31–9
Staging system for renal carcinoma. Stage I tumor is confined within renal capsule; stage II tumor extends beyond renal capsule, with invasion of local perinephric fat, but no metastasis; stage III tumor extends into the renal vein or involves local lymphatics; and stage IV tumor has metastasized to other parts of the body.

and testosterone have been used as hormonal therapy, but their effectiveness has been short-lived. Vinblastine seems the most effective single agent, with response rates of 25 per cent. Attempts with combination regimens seem to raise toxic effects without improving response rates. Many agents are being studied, but renal cancer cells seem insensitive to chemotherapeutic or hormonal agents, possibly because of their slow growth rate.

Surgical Management

The conventional and principal intervention for renal cancer is nephrectomy. Radiation and chemotherapy may be part of the medical regimen but are usually adjuncts to surgical kidney removal. For renal cell carcinoma, the surgical procedure of choice is generally radical nephrectomy, including removal of the kidney, the adrenal gland, and perinephric fat with the retroperitoneal lymphatics. Lymphadenectomy remains controversial. When the tumor is located in the renal pelvis, a nephroureterectomy is usually performed because of a tendency for transitional cell cancer to "seed" down the ureter into the bladder. With nephroureterectomy, a cuff of the adjacent bladder is removed. Even in advanced cases, when prognosis is poor, nephrectomy may be done to relieve pain and for hematuria. If the neoplastic disease is bilateral, or if there is a solitary functioning kidney, a partial nephrectomy may be done on at least one kidney, leaving enough renal tissue to support life without long-term dialysis. If partial nephrectomy is not possible in either instance, the entire kidney will be removed and the client placed on dialysis. These clients may be candidates for renal transplant, but they are usually maintained on dialysis for about a year in order to observe for recurrence of the disease.

Preoperative intervention may help shrink the tumor, making it easier to resect during surgery. Irradiation helps reduce the size of the tumor, although slowly.

Preoperative preparation of the client having renal surgery includes general guidelines as described in Chapter 5. Fluid intake should be increased if indicated to ensure adequate excretion of waste products before surgery. The nurse should give emotional support because the client may be anxious, not only about the surgery but about the prospects for adequate postoperative urinary function. If the remaining kidney functions adequately, the client can be assured this kidney will fully meet the body's elimination needs.

Nursing Management

Nursing management of the client with renal cancer must include general aspects of care for any neoplastic disease (see Chaps. 6 and 7). Most specific to the client with kidney cancer is the care required after nephrectomy and nephroureterectomy.

Postoperative care is similar to that for abdominal surgery. One of the biggest challenges is re-establishing effective breathing patterns. Surgically induced or spontaneous pneumothorax does occur occasionally after nephrectomy, so the nurse should be prepared for this possibility by assessing for sudden shortness of breath and loss of breath sounds on the affected side.

Careful monitoring of urine output is essential. The nurse should measure output hourly to identify renal failure as early as possible. Meticulous catheter care is necessary to prevent postoperative urinary tract infection.

The incision used for nephrectomy is extensive and causes significant discomfort. Muscular pain may develop as a result of the prolonged position maintained during surgery. This pain may be relieved by analgesics (including the use of patient-controlled analgesia), proper positioning, massage, and heat.

Paralytic ileus is a common problem. Interventions include carefully assessing the client's gastrointestinal status postoperatively, beginning oral intake only after adequate bowel function has been established, and early exercise (i.e., ambulation).

The skin impairment depends on the size and location of the surgical incision and the number and type of drains present. Wound care is routine; dressing changes are performed as needed for the amount of drainage.

To help reduce feelings of anxiety, the nurse should continue to keep the client and significant others informed about the progress made. All should be encouraged to express their concerns and to talk with one another. The need for this support will continue throughout the follow-up period.

Posthospital Care

The major follow-up depends on the stage of cancer and the need for further treatment.

RENAL ABSCESS

A renal abscess (or renal carbuncle) is a localized infection within the cortex of the kidney. It is usually secondary to urinary tract infection with enterobacteriaceae, often complicated by renal calculi and obstruction. Other organisms, coming from extrarenal sites, may also cause this infectious process. For example, the client will frequently give a history of recent cutaneous furuncles.

Clients with renal abscess typically have high fever and moderate to severe pain. This pain is usually constant and is felt in either the upper quadrant of the abdomen or in the costovertebral area; it sometimes resembles renal colic. Unlike pyelonephritis, the urine is usually sterile, because the abscess does not reach into the urinary collecting system. Other symptoms of this infectious process include weakness, anorexia, weight loss, night sweats, and leukocytosis.

Medical and nursing interventions for renal abscess resemble those for acute pyelonephritis. Aggressive antibiotic therapy is usually successful. A needle aspiration of the abscess may be done for culture and sensitivity study on the contents. This helps pinpoint the appropriate antimicrobial to be used. Surgical incision and drainage of the abscess sometimes is necessary. If so, nursing intervention expands to include postoperative care of the incision. A drain will be left in place for some time.

RENAL TRAUMA

Serious kidney injury is relatively rare because of the protection afforded by the rib cage, the back's heavy muscles, and the tough capsule surrounding the kidney. Traffic accidents and falls wherein the client lands on the abdomen, flank, or back are the most common cause of injury, usually resulting in blunt trauma. Kidney lacerations are also associated with fractures of the spine and ribs as well as penetrating injuries from bullets and knives.

Assessment

The type of injury the client has suffered gives the first real key to identifying renal trauma. There frequently are multiple serious injuries, and renal trauma may not be immediately apparent. Hematuria (gross or microscopic) is a cardinal sign and is found in approximately 80 per cent of cases. It must be remembered, however, that serious renal injury can occur without hemorrhage, so clear urine should not negate a possible diagnosis. Other findings include shock, flank pain, and the development of a palpable mass in the affected flank area or over the eleventh or twelfth rib. Paralytic ileus may also occur. Grey Turner sign refers to bruises over the flank and lower back secondary to retroperitoneal hemorrhage. A KUB, IVP, retrograde pyelography, renal scan, ultrasonography, CT scan, and renal arteriography all help confirm the kind and amount of kidney injury.

Complications

In addition to the immediate problems of hemorrhage and loss of functioning renal tissue, kidney trauma makes the client highly susceptible to a number of other problems. Even in closed injuries, there is a high risk for sepsis leading to the development of kidney and perinephric abscesses. Secondary hemorrhage is not uncommon. Other complications include hypertension due to fibrosis and ischemic kidney; renal artery thrombosis; arteriovenous aneurysms; fistula formation due to extravasation of urine; and the development of urinomas and pseudocysts.

Management

Intervention for renal trauma is controversial and centers on whether to pursue a conservative or a surgical path. Most physicians agree that kidney contusion calls for conservative treatment. Other minor injuries, such as small hematomas and minor lacerations without extravasation, may also be better followed conservatively. Major injuries may require surgical exploration. Possible indicators for exploration include continued moderate to severe hemorrhage and continued urine extravasation. Urine extravasation itself is not definite grounds for surgery, because sterile urine usually resolves or encapsulates spontaneously. However, it sometimes produces severe tissue reaction and causes fistula formation. The pocket of extrarenal urine may also become obstructive.

CONSERVATIVE MANAGEMENT

Conservative treatment, which primarily involves waiting and watching, is possible because the retroperitoneal space allows tamponade. In the absence of other injuries, a client with microscopic hematuria and normal IVP may be followed on an ambulatory basis with careful instructions about activity restrictions and the need for adequate hydration. If there is gross hematuria, the client is placed on bedrest until the urine clears. Serial observations of the urine, hematocrit, and vital signs are made to watch the progress of the hemorrhage. Sequential urine specimens may be collected to compare current and previous urine color and turbidity. Even if replacement fluids are not needed, a prophylactic intravenous line may be established, and a type and crossmatch for blood may be done. If a hematoma is present or the IVP demonstrates extravasation of the urine, the client may receive antibiotics to prevent sepsis. The physician prescribes blood transfusions if the hematocrit is low. After the urine is cleared, the client will be allowed to be more active. After discharge from the health-care facility, the client needs follow-up blood pressure checks and IVPs to rule out the development of secondary hypertension and anatomic derangement of the renal system.

SURGICAL MANAGEMENT

The greatest diversity of opinion concerns proper handling of the renal damage discovered during exploration. When the other kidney is functioning effectively, some physicians recommend free use of nephrectomy to avoid later sequelae, whereas others feel the goal should be salvaging maximal renal function. The latter group advocates giving the conservative approach a fair trial and, if surgery is necessary, attempts to repair the kidney before deciding to remove it. With renal vascular injury, fewer than 50 per cent of kidneys can be salvaged if the injury is 18 hours old; there is virtually no chance of renal recovery after 24 hours.

Nursing interventions during conservative treatment center on monitoring urinary elimination patterns and helping the client to cope and to comply with the medical regimen. Anxiety is common and requires supportive intervention on the part of the nurse. Imposed activity restrictions may result in problems with bowel elimination and adequate fluid intake, circulation, and respiratory function. The client being followed on an ambulatory basis needs an appropriate teaching plan covering health maintenance activities and the need for a follow-up program.

Renal Vascular Abnormalities

The kidneys depend on adequate blood circulation to nourish tissues and to provide blood for filtration so they can perform their intended functions. Anything that interferes with the normal circulatory flow significantly reduces renal capabilities.

RENAL ARTERY DISEASE

Ninety per cent of all renal artery disease is caused by one or two progressive disease processes: atherosclerosis or fibromuscular dysplasia. Atherosclerosis affects men more often than women and usually involves the proximal third of the artery. Fibromuscular dysplasia is an alternating stenosis and dilation; arteriographic studies demonstrate a "string-of-beads" appearance in the artery. This condition affects women four to five times as often as men; its exact cause is unknown.

There are several other less common causes of renal artery disease. Neoplasms may obstruct the vessels. Embolism or thrombosis can cause acute obstruction. Trauma, as described earlier, can interrupt blood flow. The renal artery may be purposely occluded to produce a "medical nephrectomy" or total renal infarction; this may be done preoperatively in the case of renal adenocarcinoma or to control proteinuria or hypertension. Shredded Gelfoam may be used, or a liquid substance that polymerizes instantly when it contacts blood may be injected into the renal artery. A dissecting aneurysm in the renal artery may also interrupt renal circulation.

The end result of any of these conditions, if severe enough, is reduced renal blood flow. This, in turn, causes renal parenchymal ischemia and, finally, renal atrophy. The role of renal artery disease in renovascular hypertension is also well documented, and it alone may indicate treatment of the condition.

Because of the kidney's compensatory mechanisms, the gradual development of renal artery stenosis from atherosclerosis and neoplasms may give rise to very few symptoms, at least until the resulting hypertension and decreasing renal function become evident. However, acute obstruction makes itself known relatively quickly. Symptoms of this sudden episode include flank pain over the affected kidney or abdominal pain and fever. Atrial arrhythmias are a frequent finding, although because they often alternate with periods of normal sinus rhythm this symptom can be missed. Urinalysis may be normal, and blood chemistries may show an elevated aspartate aminotransferase and lactic dehydrogenase. An IVP will demonstrate a nonfunctioning kidney, and a renal scan will show no arterial blood flow.

RENAL TUBERCULOSIS

Tuberculosis of the kidney, which affects men more frequently than women, occurs when the causative organism, *Mycobacterium tuberculosis,* reaches the kidney via the bloodstream from another source in the body, usually the lungs. Once the organism arrives at the kidney, it may become dormant for many years. By the time it again becomes active, the original infection is often well healed. Frequently, the primary tubercular site was asymptomatic, which makes it difficult to identify renal tuberculosis on the basis of history.

The clinical course of renal tuberculosis is generally very slow, and clinical signs and symptoms often do not become evident until the later stages of the disease.

When renal tuberculosis becomes evident, assessment findings are often nonspecific. Renal symptoms may be preceded by general malaise, weight loss, low-grade fever, and night sweats, but these are not as frequent as with pulmonary tuberculosis. Symptoms of cystitis, as described in Chapter 30, are often the presenting indications. Flank pain may be present, and hematuria and pyuria are common. Males frequently have signs and symptoms of epididymitis. A culture of *Mycobacterium tuberculosis* grown from the urine helps confirm a definitive diagnosis of renal tuberculosis. The specimens for culture are collected on at least three successive mornings. Because tubercle bacilli shed intermittently, three to 12 negative cultures are needed to exclude the diagnosis of active renal tuberculosis absolutely.

Chemotherapy with antitubercular agents has reduced the need for surgical intervention. Multiple therapy that typically combines several medications (rifampin, ethambutol, isoniazid and pyridoxine, streptomycin, cycloserine, and sodium para-aminosalicylate) is the most common intervention. Because tubercle bacilli divide slowly, the medications are usually given in a single daily dose. However, if side effects develop, the day's dose may be divided. See Chapter 22 for further information on antitubercular medications.

Surgical intervention includes total or partial nephrectomy or cutaneous ureterostomy. Permanent urinary diversion may be necessary if strictures are severe or bladder damage is irreparable. Indications for surgery include persistent infection that does not respond to chemotherapy, intractable pain, hemorrhage, uncontrollable hypertension, renal malignancy, and progressive strictures.

If surgery is needed, preoperative and postoperative nursing interventions will be similar to those for any client having major surgery (see Chap. 5).

During the acute phase, nursing interventions involve assisting with diagnostic procedures, protecting against the spread of the causative organisms, providing symptomatic relief for the client, and assisting the client with the medication regimen. Because tuberculosis arouses a great deal of fear and a feeling of social isolation, nursing diagnoses will probably include fear and anxiety for the client as well as for the significant others. The nurse should help these clients to discuss and work through their feelings, listen to their concerns, and help them seek additional counseling if necessary.

Renal tuberculosis is a prolonged illness that requires long-term care and support. Because the client is usually followed on an ambulatory basis, instruction in self-care frequently is the primary nursing intervention. One of the biggest problems with clients recovering from renal tuberculosis is continued compliance with the prescribed medical and nursing regimens, especially when the client begins to feel better. The nurse must help the client understand the need for continuous medication therapy and continuing follow-up examinations. The client must also understand the importance of maintaining general good health, such as proper nutrition, adequate rest, and good hygiene. During recovery, the nurse should give the client positive feedback for adhering to the regimens, if appropriate. If not, the nurse can use problem-solving techniques to help the client re-establish compliance with the regimens.

In response to reduced renal circulation, collateral circulation helps preserve the kidney if sufficient development takes place before the total obstruction. Collateral circulation, in addition to a marked reduction in filtration, renal work, and oxygen requirements, allows the kidney to tolerate ischemic periods for up to several weeks.

Treatment of the ischemic kidney usually involves surgical revascularization. Arterial endarterectomy may be done with follow-up anticoagulant or antiplatelet therapy. Percutaneous transluminal renal angioplasty is a procedure in which the vessel is reamed out with the use of a balloon catheter. If the vessel cannot be recanalized, a renal artery resection with end-to-end anastomosis or an aortorenal bypass graft procedure may be performed.

In the postoperative period after an aortorenal bypass graft procedure, the client may experience an initial exacerbation of hypertension. The cause of this development is unclear, but researchers believe it is related to systemic vasoconstriction secondary to general anesthesia and intraoperative hypothermia, severe pain, or transient renin secretion caused by the clamping of the aorta and manipulation of the kidney. This episode usually lasts no more than 48 hours, but it can be significant and may require medical intervention. Nurses must monitor the blood pressure frequently.

RENAL VEIN DISEASE

The primary process involving the renal vein is thrombosis. Obstruction in venous drainage increases interstitial pressure, which reduces renal function. Assessment findings of this condition include severe lumbar pain, renal enlargement, proteinuria, and hematuria. If the obstruction is bilateral, oliguria and azotemia will occur. Contributing factors include diabetic nephropathy, chronic glomerulonephritis, renal amyloidosis, collagen vascular disease, hypercoagulable states, pregnancy, use of oral contraceptives, and nephrotic syndrome.

Kidney survival depends, in large part, on the degree of collateral circulation development before the vessel was totally occluded. Embolectomy or ligation of the renal veins may be done, and anticoagulants may be prescribed. Intravenous streptokinase is used to lyse the occluding clot. If enough renal damage has occurred, nephrectomy is an option.

Congenital Disorders

Renal congenital anomalies usually refer to the number, position, form or size, and structure of the kidneys. There may be an abnormal blood supply, although malformations that significantly affect renal function are rare. Anomalies of the ureteropelvic junction usually obstruct at that point and result in hydronephrosis. Typically, this situation is diagnosed and treated during childhood.

Congenital Anomalies Involving Cystic Disease

A congenitally abnormal kidney structure usually denotes the presence and progression of cysts within the renal tissue. This disorder ranges from a simple, solitary cyst to almost complete replacement of the functioning renal structures by cystic tissue. A simple renal cyst commonly originates superficially within the renal parenchyma. It is slow-growing and usually produces no symptoms until adulthood, when it may cause a heaviness and pain in the abdomen and may become a palpable mass. Diagnosis may be complicated because renal cysts closely resemble malignant tumors; differentiation between the two is vital. As long as a simple renal cyst remains asymptomatic, intervention usually is unnecessary. If needed, the cyst may be aspirated with a needle, or a partial nephrectomy to surgically remove the cyst may be performed.

POLYCYSTIC KIDNEYS

Polycystic disease of the kidney is a hereditary disorder in which grapelike cysts containing serous fluid, blood, or urine replace normal kidney tissue (Fig. 31–10). The condition may strike during childhood or adulthood. In infancy, the disease usually results in death within days, although in milder forms the disease will not appear until childhood. Adult polycystic disease has an incidence rate of 1 per 250 to 1 per 5000 and accounts for about 10 per cent of the clients receiving dialysis or transplantation. It is inherited as an autosomal dominant trait. It usually appears after 40 years of age, although it may begin as early as age 20 years or as late as age 80 years.

Adult polycystic disease displays diverse manifestations. The most common manifestations are dull, aching lumbar or flank pain, which may be colicky in nature, and hematuria. Other common urinary tract findings are proteinuria, palpable kidney masses, pyuria, calculi, and uremia. Early in the disease, the ability to concentrate urine decreases. Hypertension with resultant cardiac enlargement and heart failure are classic findings.

The kidney can become so enlarged that it causes severe pressure on other organs, with production of additional extrarenal symptoms. The ultimate result of this disease is renal failure. As the disease slowly progresses, renal nephrons are destroyed, renal function deteriorates, and uremia ultimately results.

There is no known way to arrest the progress of the destructive cysts, so conservative medical treatment deals with preserving kidney function. Urinary tract infection is the most common complication because of the distorted renal architecture, and chronic infection may occur because of the development of resistant bacteria. Aggressively controlling hypertension is essential.

Unlike clients with increasing creatinine clearance rates caused by other kidney diseases, those with polycystic kidney disease seem to waste rather than retain sodium. Thus, they need an increased sodium and

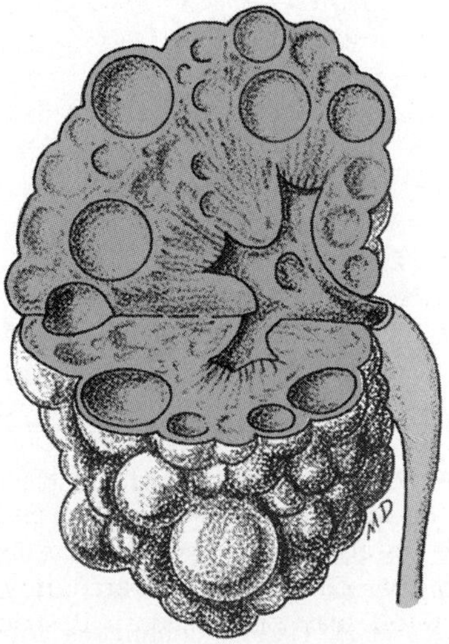

Figure 31–10
Polycystic kidney disease.

water intake. Percutaneous cyst puncture may bring palliative relief of obstruction or aid in draining an abscess. Once end-stage renal disease develops, hemodialysis or renal transplantation may be used. Nursing interventions for clients with renal failure are discussed earlier in this chapter.

Genetic counseling is advisable because of the hereditary nature of the disease. This is particularly recommended if the disease is diagnosed during the childbearing years. However, because the disease typically appears after the childbearing period, the likelihood of transmitting the disease to another generation is greatly increased. Therefore, counseling the extended family is essential once the disease has been identified.

STUDY QUESTIONS

1. When taking a client history of an acute renal failure client, the nurse should pay special attention when the client discusses the prior use of:
   A. Antacids
   B. Sedatives
   C. Anti-ulcer agents
   D. Antibiotics

2. Which one of the following statements indicates client understanding of interventions for chronic renal failure?
   A. "I use salt substitutes."
   B. "My fluid intake is controlled."
   C. "As long as I don't eat protein, I'll be okay."
   D. "Since I'm on dialysis, I can eat anything I want."

3. Which one of the following is not likely to be noted on assessment of the client with extrarenal disorders?
   A. Renal cancer
   B. Hypertension
   C. Recurrent urinary tract infections
   D. Glomerulonephritis

4. When teaching the client about the changes in chronic renal failure it should be noted that sodium intake is usually:
   A. Limited
   B. Unchanged
   C. Increased
   D. Decreased

5. Postoperative evaluation of the client after surgical removal of a kidney stone with a flank incision would reveal:
   A. An indwelling catheter
   B. Use of peritoneal dialysis
   C. Large amounts of urine drainage
   D. Impaired urine drainage from the affected kidney

6. A kidney stone is composed of oxalate. Which one of the following foods should the client avoid?
   A. Cola
   B. Bread
   C. Chicken
   D. Lettuce

CRITICAL THINKING EXERCISES

SCENARIO A

A client with chronic renal failure is on a special diet. For each of the following, show whether an increase, decrease, restriction, or no change occurs and why:

1. Protein __________.
2. Sodium __________.
3. Calcium __________.
4. Potassium __________.
5. Magnesium __________.
6. Phosphorus __________.
7. Fluid intake __________.

SCENARIO B

Outline the pathophysiological changes associated with glomerulonephritis as if you were teaching a client about the disease.

BIBLIOGRAPHY

1. Almond, P. S., et al. (1992). Renal transplant function after ten years of cyclosporine. *Transplantation, 53(2),* 316–323.
2. Baer, C. L., & Lancaster, L. E. (1992). Acute renal failure. *Critical Care Nursing Quarterly, 14(4),* 1–21.
3. Bellomo, R., et al. (1991). Continuous arteriovenous haemodiafiltration in the critically ill: Influence on major nutrient balances. *Intensive Care Medicine, 17(7),* 399–402.
4. Blaivas, J. G. (1990). Diagnostic evaluation of urinary incontinence. *Urology, 36*(Suppl 4), 11–20.
5. Bratton, L. B., & Griffin, L. W. (1994). A kidney donor's dilemma: The sibling who can donate—but doesn't. *Social Work in Health Care, 20(2),* 75–96.
6. Brenner, B. M., & Rector, F. C. (Eds.) (1990). *The kidney* (4th ed.). Philadelphia: W. B. Saunders.

7. Brundage, D. (1992). *Renal disorders.* St. Louis: Mosby-Year Book.

8. Brunier, G. M. (1994). Calcium/phosphate imbalances, aluminum toxicity, and renal osteodystrophy. *ANNA Journal, 21(4),* 171–179.

9. Burrowes, J. D., Alto, A., & Kaufman, A. M. (1993). Intradialytic parenteral nutrition: A practical approach—the malnourished patient undergoing maintenance hemodialysis. *ANNA Journal, 20(6),* 671–677.

10. Cecka, J. M., et al. (1992). Analyses of the UNOS Scientific Renal Transplant Registry at three years—early events affecting transplant success. *Transplantation, 53(1),* 59–64.

11. Chambers, J. K. (1993). Renal insufficiency: Implications for care of the medical-surgical patient. *MEDSURG Nursing, 2(1),* 33–40.

12. Courts, N. F. (1994). Psychosocial interventions for patients receiving hemodialysis. *Urologic Nursing, 14(3),* 79–81.

13. Cunningham, N., & Smith, S. L. (1990). Postoperative care of the renal transplant patient. *Critical Care Nursing, 10(9),* 74080.

14. Dolleris, P. M. (1992). Diuretic and vasopressor usage in acute renal failure: A synopsis. *Critical Care Nursing Quarterly, 14(4),* 28–31.

15. Duffy, M., & Uber, L. (1994). Immunosuppressive medications. *Dialysis and Transplantation, 23(6),* 303–305.

16. Dunn, S. A. (1993). How to care for the dialysis patient. *American Journal of Nursing, 93(6),* 26–33.

17. Erickson, P. (1993). Idiopathic glomerulonephritis: Is it IgA nephropathy? *ANNA Journal, 20(2),* 127–134, 153.

18. Fouque, D., et al. (1992). Controlled low protein diets in chronic renal insufficiency: A meta-analysis. *British Medical Journal, 304(6821),* 216–220.

19. Giorgianni, R., Sanchez, D. L., & Murtha, D. G. (1994). Management of the peritoneal dialysis patient receiving radioactive iodine 131. *ANNA Journal, 21(6),* 364–365.

20. Gjertson, D. W., & Terasaki, P. I. (1992). The large center variation in half-lives of kidney transplants. *Transplantation, 53(2),* 357–367.

21. Gleeson, M. J., & Griffith, D. P. (1990). Urinary diversion. *British Journal of Urology, 66(2),* 113–122.

22. Haddad, A. (1995). Ethics in action: What would you do? *RN, 58(1),* 21–23.

23. Hartshorn, J, et al. (1993). *Introduction to critical care nursing.* Philadelphia: W. B. Saunders Co.

24. Herzog, A. R., & Fultz, N. H. (1990). Epidemiology of urinary incontinence: Prevalence, incidence, and correlates in community populations. *Urology, 36(Suppl 4),* 2–10.

25. Higashihara, E., et al. (1992). Clinical aspects of polycystic kidney disease. *Journal of Urology, 147(2),* 329–332.

26. Hill, M. N., et al. (1991). Changes in causes of death after renal transplantation, 1966 to 1987. *American Journal of Kidney Disease, 17(5),* 512–518.

27. Hricik, D. E., et al. (1992). Withdrawal of steroids after renal transplantation—clinical predictors of outcome. *Transplantation, 53(1),* 41–45.

28. Karlowicz, K. A. (1995). *Urologic nursing: Principles and practice.* Philadelphia: W. B. Saunders Co.

29. Kerman, R. H., et al. (1992). Influence of race on crossmatch outcome and recipient eligibility for transplantation. *Transplantation, 53(1),* 64–67.

30. King, C. R., Hoffart, N., & Murray, M. E. (1992). Acute renal failure in bone marrow transplantation. *Oncology Nursing Forum, 19(9),* 1327–1335.

31. Korber, K. E. (1994). Impaired renal function and dietary protein manipulation. *Physician Assistant, 18(5),* 71–73, 76–78, 92–93.

32. Krieger, J. N. (1990). Urinary tract infections in women: Causes, classification, and differential diagnosis. *Urology, 35(Suppl 1),* 4–7.

33. Kroniewicz, D. M., & O'Brien, M. E. (1994). Evaluation of a hemodialysis patient education and support program—including commentary by Starzomski, R. with author response. *ANNA Journal, 21(1),* 33–39.

34. Levy, F. L. (1993). Nephrolithiasis: Newer management strategies—recertification series. *Physician Assistant, 17(2),* 29–31, 34–36, 41–42.

35. Lewandowski, J. (1993). Issues in renal nutrition. *Nephrology Nursing Today, 3(4),* 1–8.

36. Liu, P. L., et al. (1992). Renal function in unilateral nephrectomy subjects. *Journal of Urology, 147(2),* 337–339.

37. Ludlow, M. (1993). Renal handling of potassium. *ANNA Journal, 20(1),* 52–56.

38. Martinelli, A. M. (1993). Organ donation: Barriers, religious aspects. *AORN Journal, 58(2),* 236–252.

39. Navarro, M., et al. (1991). Anemia of chronic renal failure: Treatment with erythropoietin. *Childhood Nephrology and Urology, 11(3),* 146–151.

40. Neumann, M., & Urizar, R. (1994). Hemolytic uremic syndrome: Current pathophysiology and management. *ANNA Journal, 21(2),* 137–145.

41. Northsea, C. (1994). Using urokinase to restore patency in double lumen catheters. *ANNA Journal, 21(5),* 261–264, 273.

42. Oberley, E. T., & Compton, A. (1994). Nursing interventions for rehabilitating renal patients. *ANNA Journal, 21(7),* 407–411.

43. Pirsch, J. D., et al. (1992). The effect of donor age, recipient age, and HLA match on immunologic graft survival in cadaver renal transplant recipients. *Transplantation, 53(1),* 55–59.

44. Porcush, J. G., & Faubert, P. F. (1991). *Renal disease in the aged.* Boston: Little, Brown & Co.

45. Premminger, G. M. (1992). Renal calculi: Pathogenesis, diagnosis, and medical therapy. *Seminars in Nephrology, 12(2),* 200–216.

46. Pudelski, B., & Bednarz, D. (1992). Nursing intervention to improve dialysis adequacy of intensive care patients in acute renal failure. *ANNA Journal, 19(2),* 163.

47. Rubin, R., Kaplan, R., & Bank, N. (1991). Assessment of the patient with renal disease. In D. Z. Levine (Ed.), *Care of the renal patient.* Philadelphia: W. B. Saunders Co.

48. Rutecki, G. W., & Whittier, F. C. (1993). Kidney disease: A guide to early detection and long-term care. *Consultant, 33(12),* 26–28, 38–39.

49. Sanai, T., et al. (1991). Effect of different doses of aluminum hydroxide on renal deterioration and nutritional state in experimental chronic renal failure. *Mineral and Electrolyte Metabolism, 17(3),* 160–165.

50. Schrier, R. W. (1992). *Renal and electrolyte disorders,* 4th ed. Boston: Little, Brown & Co.

51. Shapiro, R. S., Deshetter, N., and Stockand, H. E. (1994). Fluid overload again! A technique to enhance fluid compliance. *Dialysis and Transplantation, 23(10),* 571–574.

52. Shoop, K. L. (1994). Pruritus in end stage renal disease. *ANNA Journal, 21(2),* 147–153.

53. Smith, S. H. (1993). Uremic pericarditis in chronic renal failure: Nursing implications. *ANNA Journal, 20(4),* 432–438, 508.

54. Stark, J. (1994). Acute renal failure in trauma: Current perspectives. *Critical Care Nursing Quarterly, 16(4),* 49–60.

55. Starzomski, R. (1994). Ethical issues in palliative care: The case of dialysis and organ transplantation. *Journal of Palliative Care, 10(3),* 27–34.

56. Steen, G. (1993). Maintaining near-normal life style for ESRD patients. *ANNA Journal, 20(5),* 593–594.

57. Stein, J. H. (1992). Acute renal failure: Lessons from pathophysiology. *Western Journal of Medicine, 156(2),*176–182.

58. Stein, P. (1994). Perioperative considerations of vascular access for dialysis. *AORN Journal, 60(6),* 947–949, 951–952, 955–956.

59. Strohschein, B. L., Caruso, D. M., & Greene, K. A. (1994). Continuous venovenous hemodialysis. *American Journal of Critical Care, 3(2),* 92–101.

60. Twardowski, Z. J., Nolph, K. D., & Khanna, R. (1990). *Peritoneal dialysis: New concepts and applications.* New York: Churchill Livingstone.

61. Wahrenberger, A. (1992). Differences in immunosuppressant agents. *American Nephrology Nurses' Association Journal, 19(6),* 566–567.

62. Webster, D. (1990). Comparing patients' and nurses' views of interstitial cystitis: A pilot study. *Urologic Nursing, 11,* 10–13.

63. Wood, J. M., & Bosley, C. L. (1995). Acute postrenal failure: Reversing the problem. *Nursing '95, 25(3),* 48–50.

UNIT 10

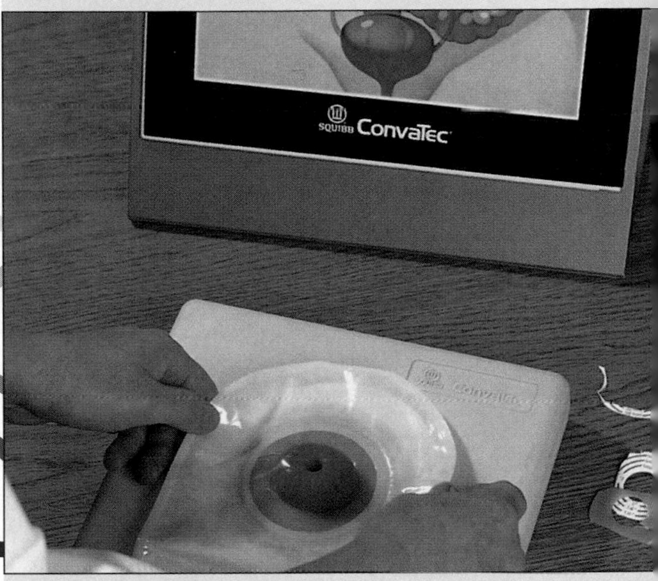

Gastrointestinal Disorders

A functional gastrointestinal (GI) tract is necessary for health and, in most cases, for life itself. However, the GI system is subject to many disorders that can interfere with normal ingestion of foods, absorption of nutrients, and elimination of waste products produced by these processes.

This unit focuses on the nursing care of clients with GI disorders. Chapter 32 provides a basis for a thorough assessment of the GI tract. Chapter 33 covers ingestive disorders; Chapter 34, gastric disorders; and Chapter 35, intestinal disorders.

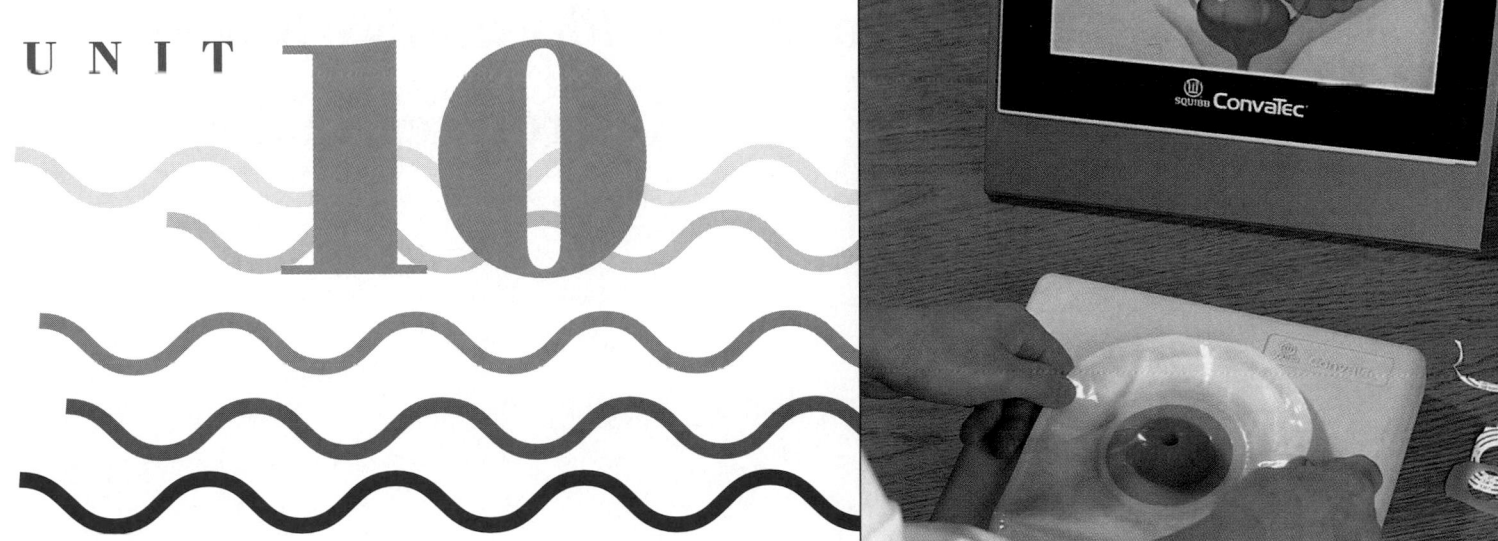

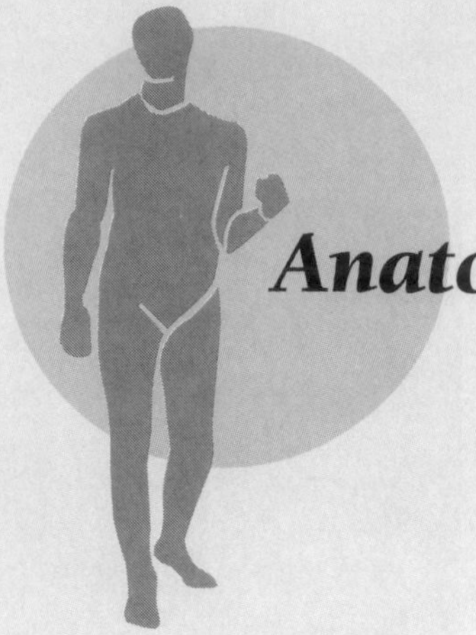

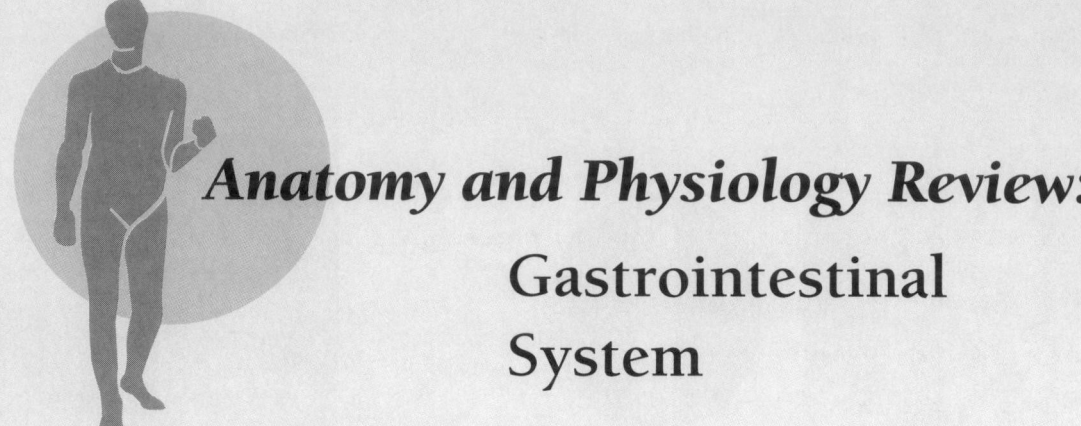

Anatomy and Physiology Review: Gastrointestinal System

The gastrointestinal (GI) tract, also called the digestive tract or alimentary canal, is a hollow muscular tube that extends from the mouth to the anus. Its principal function is to provide the body with nutrients, fluid, and electrolytes. The major activities of the GI tract are:

- Ingestion—to take in food through the mouth.
- Movement of ingested products—includes deglutition (swallowing), mixing movements in the stomach, and peristalsis through the intestines.
- Secretion of electrolytes, hormones, and enzymes—

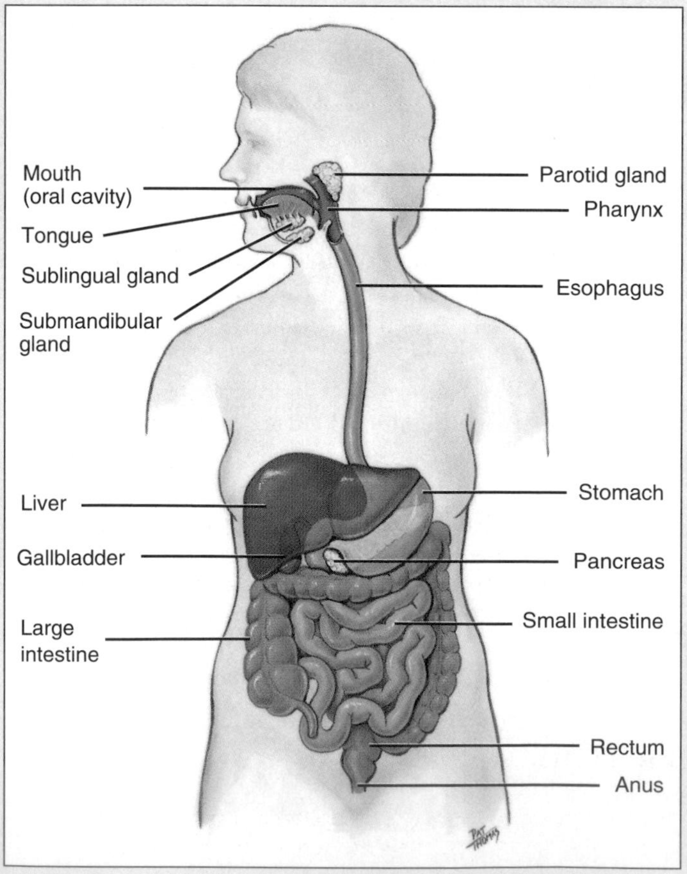

Components of the gastrointestinal tract.

used in the breakdown of ingested material. Mucus is secreted to protect and lubricate the walls of the tract.
- Digestion—includes breaking large pieces of food into smaller ones (mechanical digestion) and breakdown of complex molecules into simple molecules through hydrolysis (chemical digestion).
- Absorption—simple molecules that result from chemical digestion pass through cell membranes into the blood or lymph capillaries for transport and utilization.
- Elimination—ingested material that is not digested is removed from the body.

GENERAL STRUCTURE OF THE GASTROINTESTINAL TRACT

The basic structure of the wall of the tube that makes up the GI tract is the same throughout its entire length, although there are slight variations in each region. The wall of the GI tract has four layers:

- Mucosa—the innermost lining; consists of epithelium, loose connective tissue, and a thin layer of smooth muscle.
- Submucosa—thick layer of loose connective tissue that surrounds the mucosa; contains blood and lymphatic vessels, nerves, and glands.
- Muscular layer—smooth muscle external to the submucosa; muscle fibers are separated into an inner circular layer and an outer longitudinal layer with a nerve plexus between the two layers.
- Serosa—outermost layer surrounding the tube; consists of connective tissue covered by epithelium and secretes serous fluid for lubrication. Above the diaphragm, the epithelium is lacking and this layer is called adventitia.

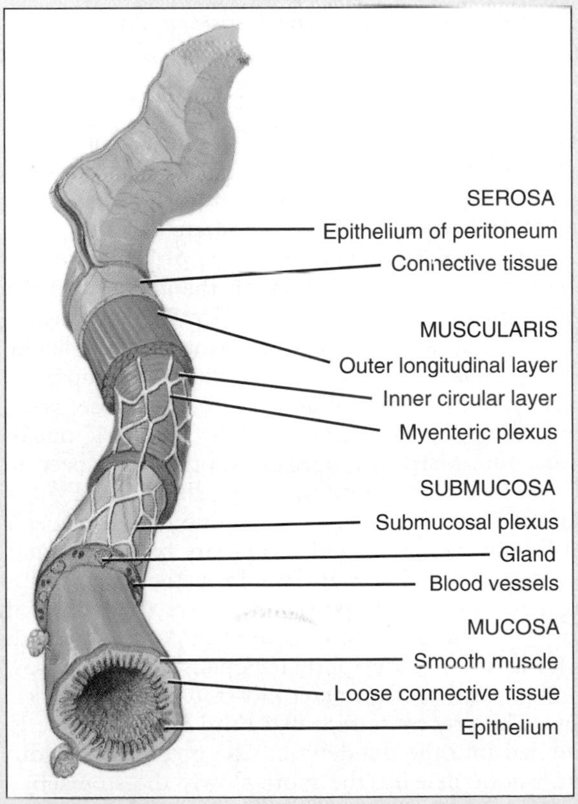

Layers in the wall of the gastrointestinal tract.

MOUTH

Structure

The mouth, also called the oral or buccal cavity, is formed by the cheeks, the hard palate, and the soft palate; the muscular tongue is in the floor of the cavity. The lips are folds of tissue that surround the opening of the mouth.

Function

- Mastication, also called chewing, begins mechanical digestion by breaking foods into smaller pieces to provide more surface area for enzyme action. The smaller pieces also make the food smoother to help prevent trauma to the mucous lining of the esophagus.
- Secretion of saliva from the parotid, sublingual, and submandibular glands provides a liquid medium to dissolve certain components of food, which stimulate the taste buds. Saliva also lubricates and softens the food mass. Saliva contains the enzyme amylase (ptyalin), which begins chemical digestion by breaking down starches to maltose.
- Deglutition, also called swallowing, is a reflex action that moves the food in the mouth, called a bolus, through the pharynx into the esophagus.

ESOPHAGUS

Structure

The esophagus is a hollow muscular tube that lies posterior to the trachea and larynx. It connects the pharynx with the stomach and serves as a passage for the bolus from mouth to stomach. The esophageal wall has the four layers characteristic of the GI tract; however, the muscular layer contains skeletal muscle in addition to smooth muscle. At the distal end of the esophagus, there is a lower esophageal sphincter, also called the cardiac sphincter. This is not a distinctive muscular sphincter but is a zone of increased pressure that provides a physiologic barrier to prevent backflow of stomach contents (gastric reflux). Excessive sphincter pressure may cause difficulty in swallowing (dysphagia), whereas decreased pressure may cause gastric reflux and indigestion.

Function

The esophagus receives a bolus from the pharynx, transports the bolus along its length by peristalsis, pro-

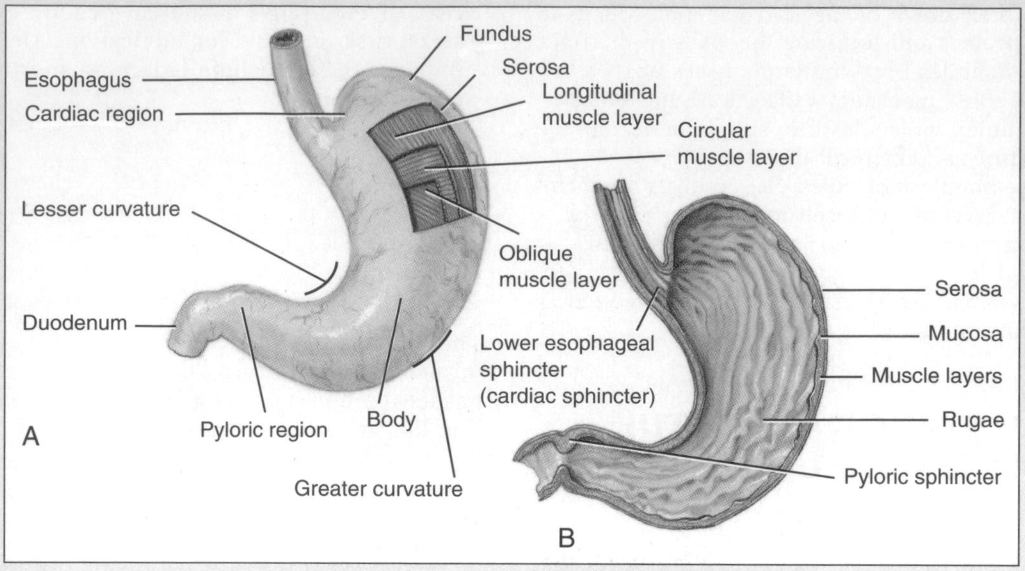

Features of the stomach. **A**, External view. **B**, Internal view.

pels the bolus into the stomach when the lower esophageal sphincter opens, provides a barrier to gastric reflux, and acts as a vent for increased intragastric pressure.

STOMACH

Structure

The stomach is located in the upper left quadrant of the abdomen and has a capacity of about 1500 mL. The lower esophageal sphincter separates the esophagus from the stomach. The stomach region adjacent to the sphincter is the cardiac region, and the fundus lies above and to the left of the sphincter. The central area is the body, and the lower portion is the antrum or pyloric region, which terminates in the pyloric sphincter.

The muscular region of the wall has an additional oblique layer that provides another dimension to the churning and mixing movements of the stomach. The mucosal lining contains many microscopic glands, which secrete gastric juice.

Secretions of Gastric Glands

CELL TYPE	SECRETION	FUNCTION
Mucous cells	Mucus (thick alkaline)	Protects stomach lining
	Mucus (thin, watery)	Medium for chemical reactions
Parietal cells	Hydrochloric acid	Kills bacteria; activates pepsinogen
	Intrinsic factor	Absorption of vitamin B_{12}
Chief cells	Pepsinogen (active form is pepsin)	Begins digestion of proteins into polypeptides
Endocrine cells	Gastrin (a hormone)	Stimulates gastric gland secretion

Function

The functions of the stomach include:

- Mechanical digestion: storage, mixing, and liquefaction of bolus of food into a semifluid mixture called chyme.
- Secretion. Glands in the mucosa secrete 1500 to 3000 mL of gastric juice per day. The major components are mucus, hydrochloric acid, pepsinogen, and water. Gastrin is also secreted, but this is a hormone and is secreted directly into the bloodstream.
- Chemical digestion. The first stage of protein digestion begins in the stomach with the action of pepsin, which breaks proteins into polypeptides; amylase from the salivary glands is inactivated by the acidity of the stomach so carbohydrate digestion stops.
- Absorption, minimal. Water, alcohol, glucose, and some drugs are absorbed through the gastric mucosa.
- Protection. Many microorganisms that have been ingested are destroyed by the hydrochloric acid.
- Controls passage of chyme into duodenum: depends on fluidity of chyme and receptivity of duodenum. When chyme is ready to pass from the stomach into the duodenum, slow peristaltic waves travel from the fundus to the pylorus. Pressure builds up within the pylorus, the pyloric sphincter opens, chyme passes through, and the sphincter closes to prevent backflow. The process is repeated until all the chyme is emptied into the duodenum. The greater the acidity and caloric density, the more slowly the stomach empties. Fats move more slowly than other nutrients.

SMALL INTESTINE

Structure

The small intestine is about 2.5 cm in diameter and 6 m long. It extends from the pyloric sphincter to the ileocecal valve, where it empties into the large intestine. The small intestine is divided into the duodenum, jejunum, and ileum. The duodenum is the first 25 cm, the jejunum is the middle 2.5 m, and the ileum is the final region, about 3.5 m long.

The wall has the four layers that are characteristic of the GI tract, but a few distinctive features are present. The mucosa and submucosa are arranged in folds (plicae circulares) that increase the surface area for absorption. Finger-like extensions of the mucosa, called villi, project from the folds and further increase the surface area. Each villus surrounds a capillary network and a lymph channel, called a lacteal. The lacteals absorb fats and fat-soluble vitamins. The capillary network absorbs other nutrients and water. Microvilli, processes on the surface of the epithelial cells, further increase the surface area for absorption. The microvilli are also known as the brush border. Collections of lymphoid in the submucosa are called Peyer's patches.

Function

The functions of the small intestine include:

- Mucus secretion. Goblet cells and duodenal (Brunner's) glands secrete mucus to protect the mucosa.
- Secretion of enzymes. Brush border cells secrete sucrase, maltase, lactase, and enterokinase that act on disaccharides to form monosaccharides; peptidase that acts on polypeptides; and enterokinase that activates trypsinogen from the pancreas.
- Secretion of hormones. Endocrine cells secrete cholecystokinin, secretin, and enterogastrone that control the secretion of bile, pancreatic juice, and gastric juice.
- Chemical digestion. Enzymes from the pancreas and bile from the liver and gallbladder enter the duodenum and, with the intestinal enzymes, complete the digestion of chyme. Chemical digestion occurs primarily in the jejunum and produces the simple molecules that are ready for absorption into the blood cap-

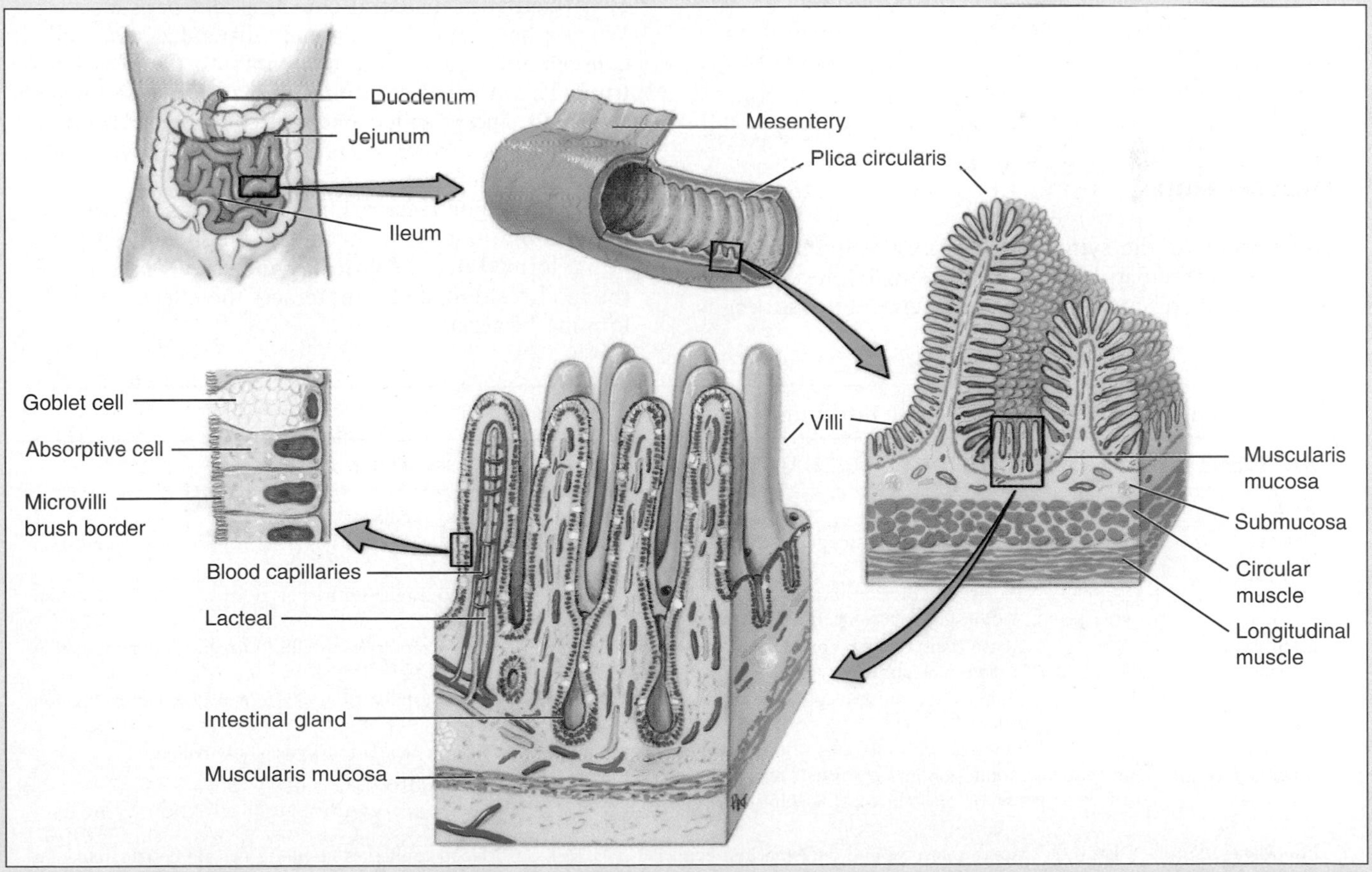

Wall of the small intestine.

illaries and lacteals of the villi. The following equations summarize chemical digestion.

$$\text{Carbohydrates} \xrightarrow[]{\text{salivary \& pancreatic amylase}} \underset{\text{sucrose, maltose, lactose}}{\text{Disaccharides}} \xrightarrow[]{\text{sucrase, maltase, lactase}}$$

Monosaccharides
glucose + fructose
glucose + glucose
glucose + galactose

$$\text{Proteins} \xrightarrow[]{\text{pepsin (stomach), trypsin (pancreas)}} \text{Peptides} \xrightarrow[]{\text{peptidase (small intestine)}}$$

Amino acids

$$\text{Fats} \xrightarrow{\text{bile}} \text{Emulsified fats} \xrightarrow{\text{lipase}}$$

Monoglycerides and free fatty acids

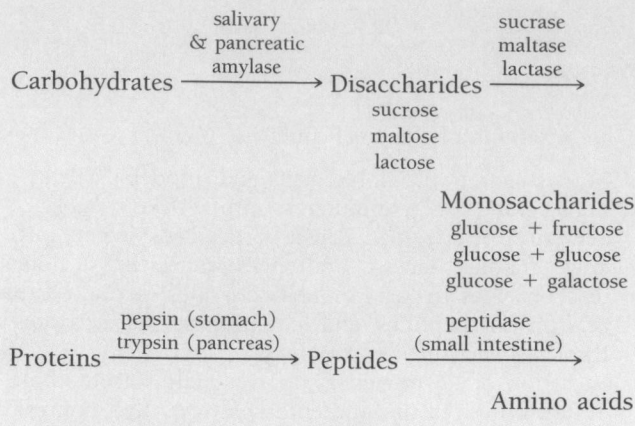

- Absorption. Nutrients and water move from the lumen of the small intestine into the blood capillaries and lacteals in the villi. Approximately 10 L of food, beverage, and secretions enter the digestive tract every day. Of this, about 9 L are absorbed and only 1 L enters the large intestine. Absorption is by active transport, by osmosis, and by simple diffusion.
- Motor activities: mixing (or segmental) contractions and peristalsis. Mixing movements, caused by contraction of circular muscle fibers, bring the chyme into close contact with the secretions involved with digestion and with the villi for absorption. Peristalsis propels the chyme through the tract at a rate of 1 to 2 cm per minute. Chyme remains in the small intestine 3 to 10 hours, and then the residue moves into the large intestine.

Innervation

Stimulation by the sympathetic system inhibits the motility and secretory activity of the small intestine. The parasympathetic system, primarily through the vagus nerve, increases intestinal muscle tone, motility, and digestive processes.

LARGE INTESTINE

Structure

The large intestine extends from the ileocecal valve to the anus and is approximately 1.5 m long. It is divided into the cecum, colon, and rectum, but these parts are not separated by valves or sphincters. The longitudinal muscle layer in the wall is incomplete and is collected into three longitudinal bands, called taeniae coli, that extend the entire length of the large intestine.

The cecum is the first 5 to 6 cm of the large intestine and extends below the ileocecal valve. Relaxation of the cecum allows contents of the ileum to enter the large intestine. The vermiform appendix is attached to the distal end of the cecum. The middle and longest portion of the large intestine is the colon, which is divided into ascending, transverse, descending, and sigmoid sections. The final segments of the large intestine are the rectum and the anus. Internal and external sphincters control the opening of the anus.

Function

The major functions of the large intestine include:

- Motor activities: haustral churning and peristalsis. When a haustrum is completely distended, the walls contract and squeeze the contents into the next haustrum. This process continues, moving residue through the colon, and is called haustral churning. Mass peristalsis involves slow, forceful waves that move residue out of the colon.
- Secretion: major secretory product is mucus. Mucus protects the mucosa from injury, binds fecal particles into a formed mass, lubricates and allows passage of the fecal residue, and counteracts the effects of acid-forming bacteria.

Absorption of Nutrients in the Small Intestine

NUTRIENT	ABSORPTIVE MECHANISM	TRANSPORT ROUTE
Water	Osmosis	Blood capillaries in villi
Glucose and galactose	Active transport into epithelial cells, then diffusion into capillaries	Blood capillaries in villi to hepatic portal circulation
Fructose	Facilitated diffusion into epithelial cells, then simple diffusion into capillaries	Blood capillaries in villi to hepatic portal circulation
Amino acids	Active transport into epithelial cells, then simple diffusion into capillaries	Blood capillaries in villi to hepatic portal circulation
Short-chain fatty acids	Simple diffusion into epithelial cells, then into capillaries	Blood capillaries in villi to hepatic portal circulation
Long-chain fatty acids, monoglycerides, and fat-soluble vitamins	Combine with bile salts to form micelles, then simple diffusion into epithelial cells; within the cell they form chylomicrons, which diffuse into lymph capillaries	Lymph capillaries (lacteals) of a villus
Electrolytes	Active transport and diffusion into epithelial cells, then into blood capillaries	Blood capillaries in villi to hepatic portal circulation
Water-soluble vitamins	Most are absorbed by diffusion into epithelial cells, then into blood capillaries; vitamin B_{12} requires intrinsic factor	Blood capillaries in villi to hepatic portal circulation

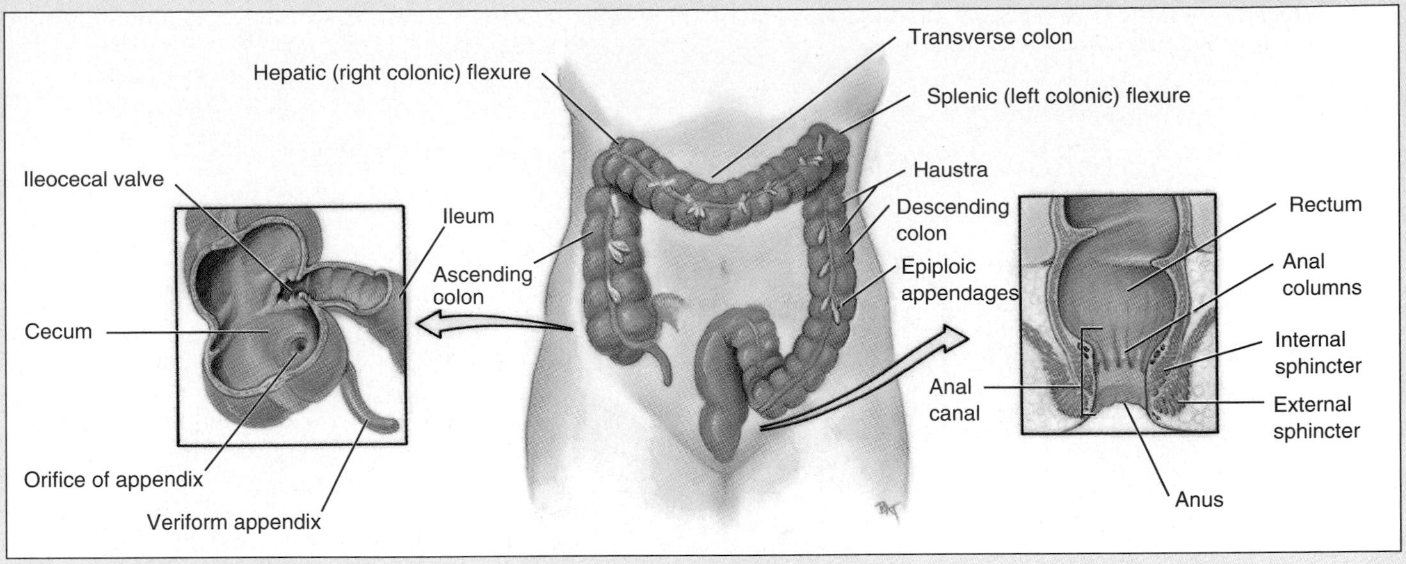

Features of the large intestine.

- Absorption of water, sodium, and chloride. The colon is capable of absorbing 90 per cent of the water and sodium it receives. This reduces the volume of residue and is critical to maintaining fluid and electrolyte balance.
- Vitamin synthesis. Bacteria in the large intestine synthesize vitamin K, thiamine, riboflavin, vitamin B_{12}, folic acid, biotin, and nicotinic acid.
- Formation of feces. Fecal material is three quarters water and one quarter solid material. Solid matter includes food residues and dead cells. Mucus helps hold the material together. Bile pigments give the feces color. Substances that absorb water or prevent the movement of water form a soft bulky mass of fecal material and stimulate colonic movement.
- Defecation: act of expelling feces from the body. When feces and gas are propelled into the rectum, pressure within the rectum increases, distention initiates the defecation reflex, and the internal and external sphincters relax. Voluntary suppression of defecation is achieved by contracting the striated muscles of the external sphincter and the pelvic floor. When this occurs, the rectum relaxes and the desire to defecate disappears.

Innervation

Nerve plexuses within the wall of the large intestine maintain the continuous muscular tone of the large intestine and stimulate movements. Parasympathetic impulses from the vagus nerve stimulate the proximal colon, while the remainder of the large intestine is controlled by the sacral nerves of the parasympathetic system. Sympathetic innervation comes from thoracic and lumbar nerves. In general, sympathetic stimulation reduces peristaltic action and increases the tone of the sphincters.

AGE-RELATED CHANGES

Structural and physiologic changes in the GI tract occur as part of the normal aging process. In the mouth, teeth may loosen from the loss of supporting gums and bone. Decreased output of the salivary glands leads to drying of the mucous membranes (xerostomia). Thus, food is not adequately moistened for chewing and swallowing and there is decreased stimulation of the taste buds. In the stomach, atrophy of the mucosa leads to a decreased secretion of hydrochloric acid, enzymes, and intrinsic factor. This may result in a proliferation of bacteria, gastric disturbances, and anemia from lack of vitamin B_{12} absorption. In the small intestine, mucosal atrophy may lead to fewer enzymes and shorter villi; however, this does not appear to impair digestion and absorption in healthy people. The wall of the large intestine becomes thinner and weakens, resulting in decreased peristalsis and increased susceptibility to diverticulosis. These changes can result in a decreased urge to defecate and an increased incidence of constipation.

Chapter 32

Assessment of Clients with Gastro-intestinal Disorders

Learning Outcomes

After completing this chapter, the learner will be able to:

1. Teach the client about the normal structure and function of the mouth, esophagus, stomach, and intestines.
2. Explain to the client the abnormalities of structure and function of the mouth, esophagus, stomach, and intestines.
3. Conduct a nursing history and physical assessment of the client with actual or potential disorders of the mouth, esophagus, stomach, and intestines.
4. Describe changes in the gastrointestinal tract that occur with aging.
5. Teach the client about diagnostic studies common to mouth, esophagus, stomach, and intestinal function.

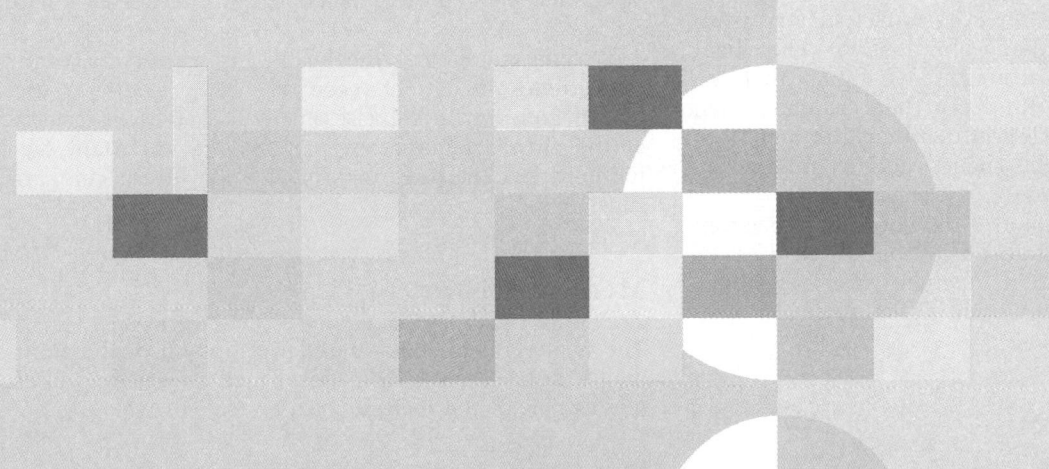

Assessment of the gastrointestinal (GI) tract involves a detailed health history as well as a comprehensive physical examination of the client's oral cavity and abdomen.

HISTORY

Demographic Data

A review of demographic data about the client, such as age, gender, and religion, are helpful when assessing the GI tract. Many GI disorders are associated with age and gender. For example, some GI cancers occur more frequently in the elderly and more frequently in males, whereas others are more common in women. Ulcerative colitis occurs more frequently in young and middle-aged adults and in clients of Jewish descent.

PERSONAL AND FAMILY HISTORY

To continue the history, the nurse should note the client's general health status as well as previous GI disorders and surgery. The nurse should question whether the client currently has or previously has had a change in bowel habits, GI bleeding, jaundice, ulcers, colitis, or unexplained weight loss. Any medications taken routinely such as aspirin, vitamin supplements, laxatives, enemas, or antacids may be important. For example, large doses of aspirin can contribute to ulcer disease. Long-term use of laxatives or enemas could cause bowel dependency.

A family history of many GI disorders may influence a client's risk level. The nurse should ask the client whether any family member has had ulcers, colitis, or GI cancer. Many of these diseases have a higher incidence within families.

Diet History

When assessing GI tract function, a diet history is an essential component of the health history. The client should describe the usual foods and fluids that are typically consumed. The nurse can then evaluate, often with the assistance of a clinical dietitian, the quality of the foods ingested and the client's understanding of a balanced diet.

The nurse should explore the relationship between food intake and GI symptoms. The nurse should assess the client's usual and current appetite. Other symptoms, such as nausea and vomiting and difficulty swallowing, should be noted.

Chief Complaint

A thorough assessment of the client's current health problem is necessary and often a key component of the health history. The nurse should ask the client the following questions about the chief complaint and present illness when conducting a symptom analysis.

Onset. When was the problem first noted? Was the onset gradual or sudden? What was the client doing when the problem was first noticed?

Duration. How long does the problem last? Does it occur occasionally, or is it persistent? Is there a pattern to the problem? If the problem is pain, the nurse should note whether the pain is continuous or intermittent.

Quality and Characteristics. The nurse should ask the client to describe the problem. If the problem is diarrhea, the client should describe the stool's appearance.

Severity. The nurse can ask the client to describe, on a scale of 1 to 10, how severe the problem is. Does it interfere with his or her ability to perform usual daily activities?

Location. Where does the client feel the problem occurs? Does the pain spread to other areas of the body? What happens to the client when the symptoms occur?

Precipitating Factors. Is there anything that seems to bring on the problem? Does anything make it worse or better? When does it occur? Is it related to eating, drinking, or activity?

Relieving Factors. Is there anything the client can do to relieve the problem? Has he or she tried medications, position changes, or anything else for relief?

Associated Symptoms. Are there any other symptoms that bother the client when the problem is present? Does the client lose appetite, get nauseated, vomit, or have diarrhea?

Common GI symptoms include nausea, vomiting, stomach pain, abdominal pain, diarrhea, constipation, abdominal distention, flatulence, dysphagia, heartburn, and indigestion (dyspepsia). The client may also report symptoms such as dry mouth, halitosis, sore mouth, difficulty chewing or swallowing, food intolerance, vomiting of blood (hematemesis), belching, bloody stool (melena), abdominal cramping, anal pruritus or burning, and rectal bleeding. Symptoms associated with the hepatic, biliary, and pancreatic systems may also occur and be reported as GI disturbances (see Chap. 36).

While conducting the health history interview, the nurse notes the client's general health status. A diet history and nutritional assessment as well as assessment of the client's elimination patterns are important data for both baseline information and for future comparisons.

Medical History

The nurse collects data about previous hospitalizations, major illnesses, surgeries, use of medications, and allergies as part of the medical history.

MAJOR ILLNESSES AND HOSPITALIZATIONS

The nurse asks the client about past problems with the GI system. Has the client been hospitalized or treated for peptic ulcer, anemia, hiatal hernia, jaundice, gallbladder disease, colitis, cancer, or a change in bowel habits? Has the client ever had surgery of the oral cavity, throat, stomach, abdomen, or rectal area? If so, the nurse must determine dates and outcomes of the procedures and ask whether the client has had diagnostic tests involving the GI system, such as a barium swallow, upper GI studies, or x-ray studies of the lower GI tract.

MEDICATIONS

The nurse must obtain detailed information about prescribed and over-the-counter medications, both currently used and previously taken. Does the client take antacids? If so, the type and the frequency taken must be determined. Over-the-counter preparations for indigestion often contain sodium bicarbonate (baking soda), which is readily absorbed and may lead to metabolic alkalosis if ingested in sufficient quantities. Also, the nurse must ask about the use of aspirin and aspirin compounds, which may contribute to gastritis and gastric bleeding. Does the client take a vitamin or mineral supplement? Does the client take laxatives or use enemas to aid elimination? Long-term use of laxatives and enemas can cause dependence.

ALLERGIES

The nurse inquires about allergies to foods, taking care to distinguish between actual allergic responses and client dislikes of certain foods. If the client reports food allergies, one must determine what GI symptoms result, such as cramping, flatulence, diarrhea, or other symptoms such as hives or dyspnea.

Family History

A family history of certain GI problems may influence a client's current and past health problems. The nurse asks the client whether any family members have had cancer, ulcers, or colitis. Many of these diseases have a higher incidence within families, for example, ulcerative colitis and Crohn's disease. Duodenal ulcers also occur more frequently in clients with blood group O, suggesting a genetic cause.

Other disorders to inquire about include jaundice, alcoholism, hepatitis, cancer of the colon, intestinal polyps, obesity, peptic ulcers, and irritable bowel syndrome.

Psychosocial History and Life-Style

Sociologic and psychological factors as well as the physical environment can affect health.

OCCUPATION

The nurse should ask the client about his or her occupation. Are there agents present that are toxic if ingested or absorbed such as arsenic, mercury, or carbon tetrachloride? Does the client travel as part of his or her job requirements, which can lead to exposure to unfamiliar foods, pathogens, or parasites?

SOCIAL

Stress-provoking situations, whether at home or in the work environment, may affect the GI system. Can the client relate his or her GI symptoms to stressful situations? Does he or she experience epigastric pain, nausea, diarrhea, or peptic ulcers? Alcohol and nicotine are known irritants to the GI system. Alcohol can cause gastritis if used excessively, and nicotine irritates the GI mucosa.

PHYSICAL EXAMINATION

Assessing the Oral Cavity

The nurse must begin the GI physical assessment with the oral cavity. Assessment of the oral cavity involves inspection and palpation. The nurse puts on gloves, faces the client, and begins by inspecting the lips. The lips are inspected for abnormal color, lesions, nodules, and symmetry.

After applying gloves, the examiner asks the client to remove any dentures or partial appliances to visualize all areas of the mouth better. The oral assessment begins at the left side of the client's mouth and continues in a clockwise fashion. The oral mucosa is inspected for redness, pallor, swelling, ulcers, or leukoplakia. The gums are inspected for redness, pallor, recession, ulcers, and bleeding. Examine the teeth for evidence of dental caries, and dentures and missing or broken teeth. The tongue is inspected for color, ulcers, abnormal coatings, swelling, or a deviation to one side. Using the tongue blade or gauze as a retractor, the examiner moves the tongue to inspect the mucous membranes. The client is instructed to protrude the tongue and move it from side to side and upward and downward. This allows the examiner to observe the tongue for voluntary or involuntary movement. Abnormal tongue movement may be due to infiltration of muscle or nerve by tumor or nerve entrapment. While depressing the tongue, the examiner asks the client to say "ah." The nurse examines the pharynx for any tonsil abnormalities, lesions, ulcers, uvular deviations, and any unusual mouth odor. The lips, gingiva, buccal mucosa, and tongue are palpated, and the area is checked for any masses, swellings, or tenderness.

Assessing the Abdomen

To assess the client's abdomen, the client is placed in a supine position with the arms at the side. Bending the knees slightly helps to relax the abdominal muscles. The nurse begins in the right upper quadrant and proceeds in a clockwise manner (Fig. 32–1). When assess-

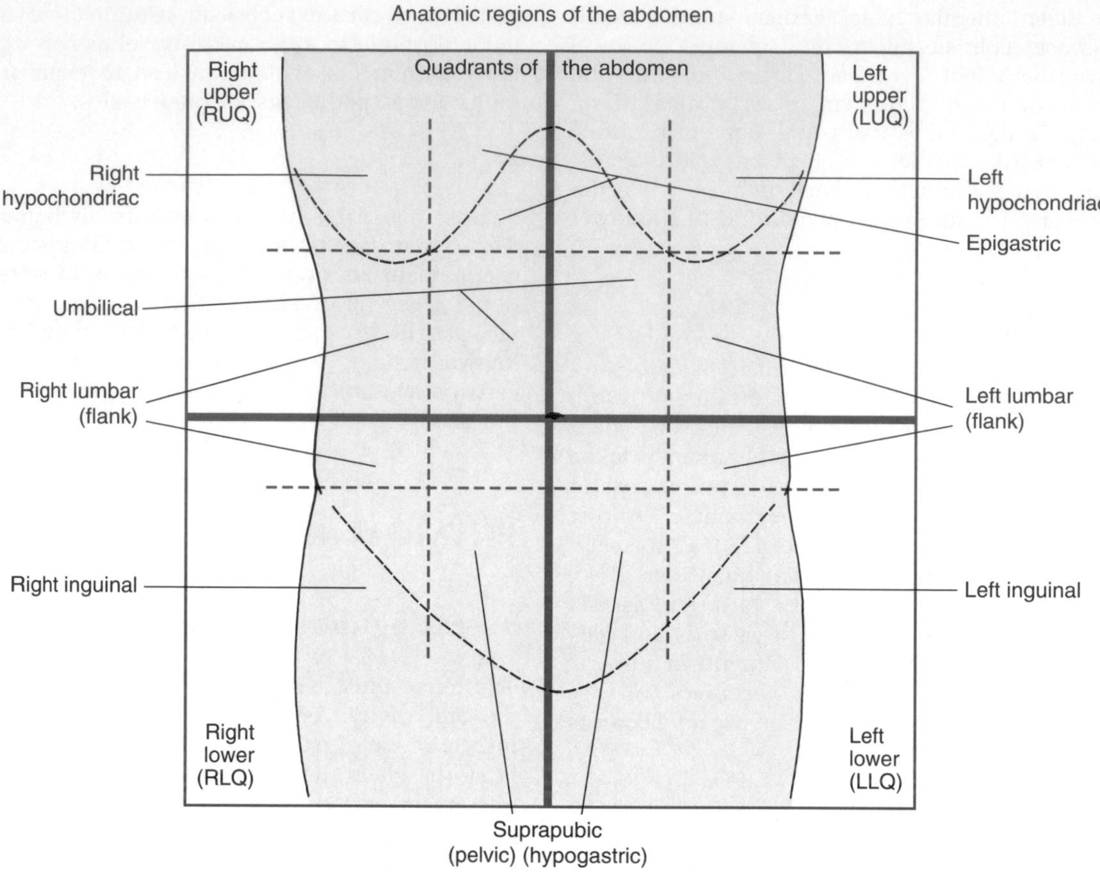

QUADRANTS OF THE ABDOMEN AND THEIR UNDERLYING ORGANS*

Right Upper Quadrant (RUQ)
- Adrenal gland (right)
- Colon (hepatic flexure and portions of ascending and transverse)
- Duodenum
- Kidney (portion of right)
- Liver (right lobe)
- Gallbladder
- Pancreas (head)
- Pylorus

Left Upper Quadrant (LUQ)
- Adrenal gland (left)
- Colon (splenic flexure and portions of transverse and descending)
- Kidney (portion of left)
- Liver (left lobe)
- Pancreas (body)
- Spleen
- Stomach

Right Lower Quadrant (RLQ)
- Appendix
- Bladder (if distended)
- Cecum
- Colon (portion of ascending)
- Kidney (lower pole of right)
- Ovary (right)
- Salpinx (uterine tube; right)
- Spermatic cord (right)
- Ureter (right)
- Uterus (if enlarged)

Left Lower Quadrant (LLQ)
- Bladder (if distended)
- Colon (sigmoid and portion of descending)
- Kidney (lower pole of left)
- Ovary (left)
- Salpinx (uterine tube; left)
- Spermatic cord (left)
- Ureter (left)
- Uterus (if enlarged)

* Small intestine loops in all quadrants.

ANATOMIC REGIONS OF THE ABDOMEN AND THEIR UNDERLYING ORGANS

Right hypochondriac
- Right lobe of liver
- Gallbladder
- Portion of duodenum
- Hepatic flexure of colon
- Portion of right kidney
- Adrenal gland (right)

Epigastric
- Pyloric end of stomach
- Duodenum
- Pancreas
- Portion of liver

Left hypochondriac
- Stomach
- Spleen
- Tail of pancreas
- Splenic flexure of colon
- Upper pole of left kidney
- Adrenal gland (left)

Right lumbar
- Ascending colon
- Lower half of right kidney
- Portion of duodenum and jejunum

Umbilical
- Omentum
- Mesentery
- Lower duodenum
- Jejunum and ileum

Left lumbar
- Descending colon
- Lower half of left kidney
- Portions of jejunum and ileum

Right inguinal
- Cecum
- Appendix
- Ileum (lower end)
- Right ureter
- Right spermatic cord
- Right ovary

Suprapubic
- Ileum
- Bladder
- Uterus (in pregnancy)

Left inguinal
- Sigmoid colon
- Left ureter
- Left spermatic cord
- Left ovary

Figure 32–1
Quadrants and anatomic regions of the abdomen and their underlying organs.

ing the abdomen, the nurse proceeds in the following sequence: inspection, auscultation, percussion, and palpation.

CRITICAL TO REMEMBER

Auscultation is performed in the abdomen before percussion and palpation. This is because percussion and palpation can increase intestinal activity and, therefore, alter bowel sounds.

The nurse must be knowledgeable about the underlying structures of the abdomen for accurate assessment. Figure 32–1 shows abdominal landmark mapping.

INSPECTION

The nurse begins by inspecting the client's abdomen, noting the condition of the skin and the contour of the abdomen. The skin should be smooth and intact, with varying amounts of hair. The nurse assesses for the presence of rashes, discolorations, scars, petechiae, striae (stretch marks), and dilated veins. The contour of the abdomen is flat, concave, rounded, or distended, depending on the client's body type. An irregular contour should be noted and could be due to a hernia, tumor, or previous surgeries. The umbilicus is inspected for shape, position, and color. It should be concave, located at the midline, and the same color as the abdominal skin. The nurse also assesses for bulging flanks and glistening, taut skin.

Abdominal movements are noted. The nurse observes the abdomen for pulsation, especially by the abdominal aorta, and for peristalic movement. Normally, peristalic movements are not visible and should be reported.

AUSCULTATION

Auscultation of the abdomen begins by listening with the diaphragm of the stethoscope and provides information on bowel and vascular sounds. The stethoscope is lightly pressed on the abdominal wall in all four quadrants. As air and fluid move through the GI tract, soft clicks and gurgles can be heard every 5 to 15 seconds. The frequency and character of bowel sounds should be noted with a normal frequency rate of 5 to 35 bowel sounds per minute. Bowel sounds may be irregular. Rapid, high-pitched, loud bowel sounds are hyperactive and may occur normally in a hungry client or in a client with gastroenteritis. Hypoactive bowel sounds occur at a rate of one every minute or longer and can be seen in clients with a paralytic ileus or after bowel surgery. To determine the absence of bowel sounds, the nurse must listen in each quadrant for at least 5 minutes. The nurse must make sure the bladder is empty because a full bladder can interfere with sounds.

PERCUSSION

Abdominal percussion is used to determine the size and location of abdominal organs and to detect fluid, air, and masses. The nurse percusses in all four quadrants of the abdomen and compares sounds. Normally, percussion sounds over the abdomen are tympanic (high-pitched, loud, musical over air) or dull (thudlike sound over fluid or solid organs). Percussion is used to determine the size and position of the liver and spleen and also can be used to assess the level of a distended bladder. Abdominal percussion is contraindicated in clients with suspected abdominal aneurysms and in those clients with abdominal organ transplants.

PALPATION

To palpate the abdomen, the nurse starts by lightly depressing (1–2 cm) the abdomen in a systematic quadrant-to-quadrant manner. The nurse assesses for masses, rebound tenderness, and areas of direct tenderness. Any areas of tenderness are cautiously examined last with deep palpation. Areas of abdominal involuntary rigidity are noted. Deep palpation is used next to determine the size and shape of abdominal organs and masses. Deep palpation should be performed cautiously by a skilled nurse.

DIAGNOSTIC TESTS

Diagnostic measures are performed to locate the nature and level of the problem associated with diseases of the GI tract. The general methods of diagnosis include

- Laboratory tests (Table 32–1)
- Radiographic tests
- Endoscopy
- Gastric analysis
- Cytologic studies
- Magnetic resonance imaging

Laboratory Tests

CARCINOEMBRYONIC ANTIGEN

Carcinoembryonic antigen (CEA) is a glycoprotein normally produced during the first or second trimester of fetal life. Normally, production is halted before birth. Increased CEA levels in clients other than neonates may indicate the presence of colorectal or other cancer. This test is not useful as a screening tool because increased CEA levels are also seen in cirrhosis, hepatic disease, and alcoholic pancreatitis and in clients who smoke heavily. The test is used to assist in preoperative staging of colorectal cancer, monitor the effectiveness of cancer therapy, and test for recurrence of colorectal and other cancers. It is referred to, therefore, as a tumor marker. CEA levels usually return to normal within 6 weeks of successful treatment. A continued elevation suggests residual or recurrent tumor.

Client Preparation. This laboratory test requires a venipuncture. Heparin should be withheld, if possible, for 2 days before the test because it may interfere with test results.

TABLE 32–1 Normal Findings and Significance of Abnormal Findings in Common Laboratory Tests Used to Assess GI Function

VARIABLE	NORMAL FINDING	SIGNIFICANCE OF ABNORMAL FINDINGS
Complete Blood Count		
Red blood cells	4.2–5.4 million/mm³ (women) 4.5–6.2 million/mm³ (men)	Decreased values indicate possible anemia or hemorrhage
Hemoglobin	12–16 g/dL (women) 14–18 g/dL (men)	Increased values indicate possible hemoconcentration, caused by dehydration
Hematocrit	38–46% (women) 42–54% (men)	
Electrolytes		
Potassium	3.5–5.0 mg/L	Decreased values indicate possible GI suction, diarrhea, vomiting, intestinal fistulas
Calcium	8.0–10.5 mg/dL	Decreased values indicate possible malabsorption
Sodium	135–145 mg/L	Decreased values indicate possible malabsorption and diarrhea
D-Xylose	Blood levels peak (25–40 mg/dL) 2 hours after ingestion 80–95% excreted in 5 hours	Decreased values indicate possible malabsorption
CEA	Less than 5 ng/mL (nonsmokers)	Increased values indicate possible colorectal cancer and inflammatory bowel disease
Fecal Analysis		
Stool for occult blood	Negative	Presence indicates possible peptic ulcer, cancer of the colon, ulcerative colitis
Stool for ova and parasites	Negative	Presence indicates infection
Stool cultures	No unusual growth	Presence of pathogens may indicate shigella, salmonella, *Staphylococcus aureus,* or *Bacillus cereus*
Stool for lipids	2–5 g/24 hr (normal diet)	Increased values indicate possible malabsorption syndrome and Crohn's disease

CEA, carcinoembryonic antigen; GI, gastrointestinal.

FECAL ANALYSIS

Stool examinations that may aid in the diagnosis of GI tract disorders include stool for occult blood, stool for ova and parasites, stool cultures, and stool for lipids.

Stool for Occult Blood

Stool can be examined for occult blood to detect GI bleeding and aid in the early diagnosis of colorectal cancer. The guaiac or orthotoluidine test is commonly used.

Client Preparation. If the orthotoluidine test is used, the client may be instructed to eat a high-fiber diet for 48 to 72 hours before the collection of the stool specimen. Red meats, poultry, fish, turnips, and horseradish should be avoided. Other tests for occult blood do not require dietary restrictions. The following medications should be withheld for 48 hours before the test: iron preparations, bromides, rauwolfia derivatives, steroids, indomethacin, and colchicine.

Procedure. The nurse or the client usually collects a total of three stool specimens (over 3 successive days). The nurse should wear gloves while performing the test. A wooden applicator is used to apply the stool to one side of guaiac paper. After applying the required developing solution, color is immediately noted. A positive result, which is blue coloration, should be reported. There is no follow-up care for this procedure.

Stool for Ova and Parasites

Stool for ova and parasites is collected to detect intestinal infections caused by parasites and their ova (eggs).

Client Preparation. The client should be instructed to avoid drugs such as castor oil, mineral oil, or antidiarrheal compounds, all of which may alter the feces. The client should be informed that the test usually requires three stool specimens, one taken every other day or every third day.

Procedure. The nurse should collect the stool and send it immediately to the laboratory. The nurse should wear gloves when obtaining the specimen. Fresh, warm stool is required. If it cannot be examined within 30 minutes, the nurse should place the specimen in a preservative per hospital protocol. There is no follow-up care for this procedure.

Stool Cultures

Stool cultures are performed to identify pathogenic organisms in the GI tract. If a stool culture shows no pathogens, detection of viruses can be performed by immunoassay or electron microscopy, which may help in the diagnosis of nonbacterial gastroenteritis.

Client Preparation. The nurse should report whether the client is or has been taking any antibiotics recently.

Procedure. Stool should be collected using sterile technique and a sterile stool container. The stool may be collected for 3 consecutive days. There is no follow-up care.

Stool for Lipids

Stool can also be examined for lipids. Normally, dietary lipids are almost completely absorbed in the small intestine. Excessive secretion of fecal fats (steatorrhea) may occur in various digestive and absorptive disorders.

Client Preparation. The client should be instructed to eat a high-fat diet and refrain from alcohol for 3 days before the test and during the collection period. The client should avoid drugs that interfere with the test such as mineral oil, neomycin, and potassium chloride.

Procedure. The nurse should collect a 72-hour stool specimen, storing it on ice. There is no follow-up care.

Radiographic Tests

FLAT PLATE OF THE ABDOMEN

A flat plate of the abdomen is an x-ray study performed to visualize abdominal organs. This test can reveal abnormalities such as tumors, obstructions, abnormal gas collections, and strictures.

Client Preparation. For this procedure, the client should be dressed in a hospital gown without any belts or jewelry. There is no follow-up for this procedure.

UPPER GASTROINTESTINAL SERIES (BARIUM SWALLOW)

An upper GI series permits radiologic visualization of the esophagus, stomach, duodenum, and jejunum. It can aid in the detection of strictures, ulcers, tumors, polyps, hiatal hernias, and motility problems.

Client Preparation. The client should be maintained on nothing by mouth orders (NPO) for 6 to 8 hours before the test. The nurse should instruct the client about the procedure and about the barium ingestion.

Procedure. The client drinks a radiopaque contrast medium (barium) while standing in front of a fluoroscopy tube. The client may be asked to move to other positions, such as lying on the x-ray table.

Follow-Up Care. A laxative is ordered after the procedure to help expel the barium and prevent a fecal impaction. The nurse should assess the abdomen for distention and bowel sounds. The nurse should also observe the stool to determine whether the barium has been completely eliminated. Initially, the client's stool is white in color, but it should return to its normal brown color within 72 hours. Constipation with a distended abdomen may indicate a barium impaction.

LOWER GASTROINTESTINAL SERIES (BARIUM ENEMA)

A lower GI series is performed to visualize the position, movements, and filling of the colon. This test can aid in the detection of tumors, diverticuli, stenosis, obstructions, inflammation, ulcerative colitis, and polyps.

Client Preparation. In this procedure, adequate bowel preparation is essential and varies among institutions. The nurse should instruct the client when preparation for the procedure is completed at home. A typical preparation for most adults includes placing the client on a low-residue or clear liquid diet for 2 days before the test. The client usually receives a potent laxative and an oral liquid preparation for cleansing the bowel the day before the test. The client receives a clear liquid diet the morning of the test. The morning of the examination, a suppository or a cleansing enema may be administered. If ultrasonograms, abdominal scans, or colonoscopy are also indicated, they should be performed first because the barium will interfere with these tests.

Procedure. During a lower GI series, a radiopaque contrast medium (barium) is instilled rectally and radiographs are taken with or without fluoroscopy. The client is then placed in various positions to aid barium movement through the colon. Air contrast studies can also be used for more detail. The procedure is often uncomfortable and can be very tiring, especially for the elderly. A barium enema should be completed before an upper GI series is done.

Follow-Up Care. A laxative or cleansing enema is often given after the test to empty the large bowel and prevent barium impaction. Stools are white for 24 to 72 hours after the examination. The client should increase the intake of liquids to prevent a fecal impaction. The client should report any pain, bloating, absence of stool, or bleeding.

COMPUTED TOMOGRAPHY

Tomography uses a beam of radiation to detect density differences in tissue. The computerized data are visualized as cross sections of the body. Computed tomography (CT) is used mainly to identify masses such as neoplasms, cysts, focal inflammatory lesions, and abscesses of the liver, pancreas, and pelvic areas. Computed tomography aids in evaluation of local tumor spread, especially if barium studies suggest the presence of tumor growth beyond the bowel wall (Fig. 32–2). Although CT has the advantage of providing a three-dimensional image, other diagnostic procedures are more valuable for most disorders of the gut. To distinguish normal bowel from abnormal intraperitoneal masses, dilute oral barium or other contrast media may be administered.

Client Preparation. The client receives a clear liquid diet the morning of the test. If a contrast medium will be used, the client should remain NPO for 2 to 4 hours before the procedure. In addition, if contrast media are to be used, the nurse should ask the client about an allergy to iodine.

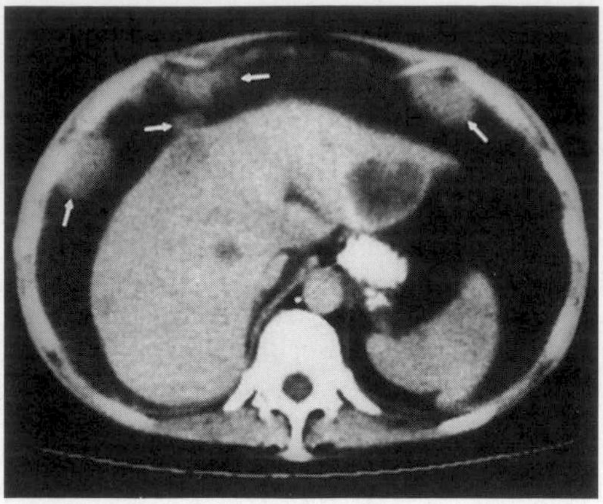

Figure 32–2
Computed tomography of metastatic colon cancer. Scan of the upper abdomen shows ascites, peritoneal implants *(arrows)*, and hepatic metastases. The metastatic lesion in the left lobe of the liver has undergone partial necrosis. Its central necrotic cavity has a low density similar to that of the ascitic fluid. A thick, irregular margin of solid tumor tissue surrounds the cavity. (From Berk, J. E., et al. [1985]. *Bockus' gastroenterology* [4th ed.]. Philadelphia: W.B. Saunders.)

Procedure. A radiation detector is used to visualize three-dimensional images of abdominal structures. The client will have to lie still and hold his or her breath when asked. No follow-up care is needed. If contrast is used, the client should be instructed to increase oral fluid intake (if allowed) to facilitate renal excretion of the material.

Endoscopy

Endoscopy is the direct visualization of the GI tract by means of a lighted, flexible tube. It is more accurate than radiologic examination because the physician can directly observe sources of bleeding and surface lesions and determine the status of healing tissues. Endoscopic procedures require a signed consent.

UPPER GASTROINTESTINAL ENDOSCOPY

Upper GI tract endoscopy includes esophagoscopy, gastroscopy, and esophagogastroduodenoscopy (EGD). These procedures are useful for examining clients with acute or chronic GI bleeding, pernicious anemia, esophageal injury, dysphagia, substernal pain, and epigastric discomfort. Upper GI endoscopy should not be performed on clients with severe cardiovascular disease.

Client Preparation. To prevent aspiration of the stomach contents into the lungs, the client is NPO for 8 hours before the procedure. The client may receive an anticholinergic medication to decrease oropharyngeal secretions and to prevent reflex bradycardia. Sedatives, narcotics, or tranquilizers such as diazepam (Valium) or meperidine (Demerol) also may be given before the procedure to help relax the client. The client's dentures and any removable bridges should be removed before the procedure to prevent dislodgement. The client's oral cavity also should be carefully assessed for the presence of infection or any lesions.

A local anesthetic is sprayed on the posterior pharynx to ease the discomfort and prevent gagging when the tube is inserted. This anesthetic often tastes unpleasant and makes the tongue feel swollen. The client should not swallow saliva after the throat has been anesthetized.

The nurse must provide complete preprocedure teaching because learning about the endoscopy enhances the client's cooperation. The client must be instructed not to drive a motor vehicle for at least 12 hours after the test if sedation was used during the procedure.

Procedure. After being medicated, a flexible, fiberoptic endoscopy tube is passed orally into the esophagus, stomach, and pylorus and duodenum. Some endoscopes are equipped with a camera to enable the physician to obtain color photographs. Other endoscopic tubes have equipment for performing a biopsy or securing cells for cytologic examination if cancer is suspected. Single polyps are sometimes removed via an endoscope.

Follow-Up Care. Vital signs are checked frequently as ordered. The client is also placed on one side to prevent aspiration while the sedation and local anesthesia wear off. The client is NPO until the gag reflex returns (2–4 hours). Many endoscopic procedures are performed on an outpatient basis. The physician may order anesthetic throat lozenges or normal saline gargles for throat irritation or hoarseness.

The nurse must assess the client after an endoscopy for signs of perforation, which include bleeding, fever, and dysphagia. The client with cervical perforation has crepitus (crackling) in the neck from the leakage. Neck and throat pain, aggravated by swallowing or moving, may also occur. Midesophageal perforation can result in referred substernal or epigastric pain. Also, the nurse must assess for cyanosis, pleural effusion, and back pain. Distal esophageal perforation may result in shoulder pain, dyspnea, or symptoms similar to those of perforated ulcer.

LOWER GASTROINTESTINAL ENDOSCOPY (COLON ENDOSCOPY)

Direct visualization of the bowel through a proctoscope, sigmoidoscope, or colonoscope is called colon endoscopy. This procedure is used when a client has a history of constipation, diarrhea, or lower GI bleeding. Colonic endoscopy is useful in diagnosing cancer, strictures, polyps, and ulcerative or inflammatory bowel lesions. Colon endoscopy is contraindicated in clients with inflammatory bowel disease, toxic megacolon, or strictures. This procedure sometimes is complicated by rectal bleeding and, rarely, bowel perforation.

PROCTOSIGMOIDOSCOPY

Proctosigmoidoscopy is the endoscopic examination of the distal sigmoid colon, the rectum, and the anal canal.

This test helps diagnose malignant and benign neoplasms and detect hemorrhoids, polyps, fissures, fistulas, and abscesses within the anal canal and rectum. Health professionals recommend this procedure for clients older than 40 years on an annual or biennial basis because this examination helps diagnose malignancy at an early stage.

Client Preparation. To prepare the client for proctosigmoidoscopy, the nurse must clearly explain the preparation for the procedure, the position for examination (knee chest or left lateral), and the discomfort that may accompany passage of the scopes.

When the entire colon is to be examined, the client usually receives a clear liquid diet 24 hours before the test, takes a cathartic the night before the procedure, and receives a cleansing enema the morning of the test to cleanse the bowel. If bleeding or severe diarrhea is present, examination may be carried out without bowel preparation. To promote visualization, the client is placed in an inverted position (knee chest) that allows the sigmoid colon to straighten. A left lateral Sims' position is suitable for clients who are aged, weak, or very ill.

Procedure. A rigid proctoscope and a sigmoidoscope (rigid or flexible) are used to examine the bowel. Flexible fiberscopes decrease the possibility of perforation and permit examination above the rectosigmoid junction.

Follow-Up Care. The client is observed for signs of perforation, such as bleeding, pain, and fever. Any specimens obtained during the test must be labeled and sent to the laboratory immediately. After the procedure, the client can rest for a few minutes in the supine position before standing up to avoid postural hypotension and fainting. For discomfort, a sitz bath may be ordered.

COLONOSCOPY

If a client has a history of unexplained constipation or diarrhea, rectal bleeding, or lower abdominal pain, and if results from a barium enema and proctosigmoidoscopy are inconclusive, the physician may perform a colonoscopy. Colonoscopy provides visualization of the lining of the large intestine through a flexible endoscope, which is inserted rectally.

Procedure. For colonoscopy, the client is usually sedated and placed on the left side with the knees flexed. Once the lubricated colonoscope is inserted into the anus, a small amount of air is instilled to help the physician visualize the bowel lumen. When the colonoscope reaches the sigmoid junction, the client may be moved to the supine position, making it easier to advance the colonoscope past the splenic flexure. During the test, the nurse should encourage the client to relax. Vital signs should be monitored throughout the procedure; the nurse must watch for a vasovagal response leading to hypotension and bradycardia.

Follow-Up Care. The nurse monitors vital signs as ordered. The nurse should assess for signs of perforation, such as abdominal pain, bleeding, or fever.

Exfoliative Cytology

Exfoliative cytology, developed by George Papanicolaou, is the study of cells that have sloughed off from a tissue. This procedure is used to distinguish between benign and malignant lesions. Malignant cells, which exfoliate more readily than normal cells, are collected by lavage and sent to the laboratory for analysis. Cells of the esophagus, stomach, small intestine, and colon can be examined.

Client Preparation. A written consent is obtained. The client is placed on a liquid diet. For colon studies, laxatives and enemas are administered. The nurse should explain the procedure to the client.

Procedure. In this procedure, cells are obtained from saline lavage through a nasogastric tube, from a proctoscope, or during an endoscopy.

Follow-Up Care. The client is allowed to rest and resume an appropriate diet.

Gastric Analysis

Gastric analysis is performed to measure secretions of hydrochloric acid and pepsin in the stomach. It can aid in the diagnosis of duodenal ulcer, Zollinger-Ellison syndrome, gastric carcinoma, and pernicious anemia. There are two tests performed in gastric analysis: the basal cell secretion test and the gastric acid stimulation test.

Client Preparation. The client is NPO 12 hours before the test. A nasogastric tube is inserted, and any contents left in the stomach are removed. The client should avoid taking drugs that interfere with gastric acid levels (e.g., cholinergics, antacids).

Procedure. The client's nasogastric tube is attached to suction, and stomach contents are collected every 15 minutes for 1 hour. The nurse must properly label the specimens with the time and volume. If the basal secretion test suggests abnormal gastric secretion, a gastric acid stimulation test is usually performed immediately.

The gastric acid stimulation test measures the amount of gastric acid for 1 hour after subcutaneous injection of a drug that stimulates gastric acid secretion (pentagastrin, beta zole [Histalog]). If abnormal results occur, usually radiographic studies or endoscopy are performed to determine the cause.

Follow-Up Care. If the nasogastric tube is left in place, it should be clamped or attached to low intermittent suction if ordered.

Ultrasonography

Ultrasonography is a noninvasive diagnostic procedure during which sound waves are passed into the body to produce an image or photograph of an organ or tissue on an oscilloscope.

Diagnosticians use ultrasonography on the GI system to identify pathophysiologic processes in the pancreas, liver, gallbladder, spleen, and retroperitoneal tissue. Ultrasonography can identify fluid, masses (e.g., tumors), adipose tissue, and hematoma. Diagnosis of an abdominal abscess can be made with ultrasonography. Ultrasonography enhances the physical examination because palpable masses and areas of tenderness can be correlated with anatomic structures while the person is on the examining table. Gas in the abdomen may interfere with ultrasound waves.

Client Preparation. The client may be required to be NPO for 8 to 12 hours before the procedure to reduce bowel gas. The nurse can reassure the client that the test is painless and safe.

Follow-Up Care. There are no specific precautions or observations related to ultrasonography.

Magnetic Resonance Imaging

Magnetic resonance imaging (MRI) is a noninvasive test that can be used in addition to other GI diagnostic tests. An MRI produces cross-sectional images of soft tissue and blood vessels by using magnetic fields. The test is used to study blood flow and identify tumors, infections, and other decreased tissue. The test is contraindicated in clients with pacemakers, aneurysm clips, or orthopedic screws because of the magnetic field.

Client Preparation. The client may not receive anything by mouth for 6 hours before the procedure. The client should be instructed that the test requires that the client lay still during the procedure, which can take from 60 to 90 minutes. All jewelry and metal should be removed.

Procedure. The client lies on a narrow table that slides into a magnetic body scanner. A strong magnetic field is created around the client, which allows the image of tissue to be produced. The client will hear a clanging noise during the procedure. There is no follow-up care.

STUDY QUESTIONS

1. Which one of the following changes is likely to cause problems in the elderly client?
   A. Bacterial activity in the gut decreases.
   B. Hydrochloric acid secretion increases.
   C. Secretion of the salivary glands decreases.
   D. Secretion of digestive enzymes and bile increases.
2. The esophagus is located
   A. In the upper portion of the abdomen
   B. Above and to the left of the cardiac sphincter
   C. At the pyloric valve of the stomach
   D. Posterior to the trachea and larynx
3. The end products of digestion are absorbed by diffusion and active transport in the
   A. Mouth
   B. Esophagus
   C. Stomach
   D. Small intestine
4. Elderly clients are at risk for anemia. Why is this true?
   A. Elderly clients experience a decrease in hydrochloric acid secretion in the stomach.
   B. Elderly clients have decreased salivation in the mouth.
   C. Elderly clients have a decrease in bile secretion in the small intestine.
   D. Elderly clients have decreased peristalsis in the large intestine.
5. After client teaching about upper gastrointestinal (GI) endoscopy, the nurse would know the teaching was effective if the client stated,
   A. "I will be under general anesthesia during the procedure"
   B. "I won't be able to eat or drink anything afterward until I'm sure I can swallow without choking"
   C. "I may eat breakfast the morning of the test but have nothing by mouth after that"
   D. "I will probably have bleeding from my mouth and run a fever after the test"

CRITICAL THINKING EXERCISES

SCENARIO A

A middle-aged man is complaining of epigastric pain that wakens him at night. He states that it is relieved by taking three doses of antacid. He has come to the clinic for diagnosis.

1. What components of the health history contribute to identifying his diagnosis?
2. Which subjective assessment data are pertinent?
3. A diagnostic study commonly used to diagnose upper gastrointestinal abnormalities is the barium swallow. What should the nurse teach the client about this test?

An elderly client has complaints of constipation. She tells the nurse that she never used to have this problem when she was younger. They discuss possible reasons for constipation and suggestions for management.

1. Identify important assessment data for elderly clients with complaints of constipation.
2. What are some physiologic changes in the elderly that may contribute to constipation?
3. What dietary changes can assist the client in managing constipation?

BIBLIOGRAPHY

1. Achker, E., et al. (Eds.). (1992). *Clinical gastroenterology* (2nd ed.) Philadelphia: Lea & Febiger.
2. Barkin, J., & Rogers, A. (Eds.). (1994). *Difficult decisions in digestive diseases* (2nd ed.) St. Louis: Mosby-Year Book
3. Bayliss, T. M. (Ed.) (1994). *Current therapy in gastroenterology and liver disease* (Vol. 3, 3rd ed.). St. Louis: Mosby-Year Book.
4. Beck, M. L. (1989). Percutaneous endoscopic gastrostomy. *American Journal of Nursing, 89,* 76.
5. Bongiovanni, G. L. (Ed.). (1988). *Essentials of clinical gastroenterology* (2nd ed.). New York: McGraw-Hill.
6. Britton, A., et al. (1994). Screening for GI tract malignancy. *Medicine North America, 17,* 247–251.
7. Bullock, G. R. (1989). *Techniques in diagnostic pathology.* San Diego: Academic Press.
8. Cotran, R. S., et al. (Eds.) (1994). *Robbins' pathologic basis of disease* (5th ed.). Philadelphia: W. B. Saunders.
9. Fishbach, F. (1992). *A manual of laboratory diagnostic tests* (4th ed.). Philadelphia: J. B. Lippincott.
10. Gitnick, G., et al. (Eds.). (1994). *Principles and practice of gastroenterology and hepatology* (2nd ed.). Norwalk, CT: Appleton & Lange.
11. Gore, R. M., et al. (1994). *Textbook of gastrointestinal radiology.* Philadelphia: W. B. Saunders.
12. Greenberger, N. J. (1989). *Gastrointestinal disorders: A pathophysiologic approach* (4th ed.). St. Louis: Mosby-Year Book.
13. Gschwantler, M., et al. (1994). Detection of colorectal adenomas by fecal occult blood tests. *Gastroenterology, 106,* 278–280.
14. Guyton, A. C. (1991). *Textbook of medical physiology* (8th ed.). Philadelphia: W. B. Saunders.
15. Haubrich, W. S., et al. (1995). *Bockus gastroenterology* (5th ed.). Philadelphia: W. B. Saunders.
16. Hollander, D., & Tarnawski, A. S. (Eds.). (1989). *Gastric cytoprotection.* New York: Plenum.
17. Isselbacher, K. J. (Ed.). (1994). *Harrison's principles of internal medicine* (13th ed.). New York: McGraw-Hill.
18. Jarvis, C. (1992). *Physical examination and health assessment.* Philadelphia: W. B. Saunders.
19. Johnson, L. R., et al. (1994). *Physiology of the gastrointestinal tract* (3rd ed.). New York: Raven.
20. Kee, J. L. (1995). *Laboratory and diagnostic tests with nursing implications* (4th ed.). Norwalk, CT: Appleton & Lange.
21. Kirsner, J. B., & Shorter, R. G. (Eds.). (1995). *Inflammatory bowel disease.* Baltimore: Williams & Wilkins.
22. Kotler, D. P. (Ed.). (1991). *Gastrointestinal and nutritional manifestations of the acquired immunodeficiency syndrome.* New York: Raven.
23. Miller, C. A. (1994). Alleviating the discomfort of gastroesophageal reflux disease. *Geriatric Nursing, 15,* 171–172.
24. Nickl, N. J., & Cotton, P. B. (1990) Clinical application of endoscopic ultrasonography. *American Journal of Gastroenterology, 85,* 675–682.
25. Overholt, B. F. (1993). Office endoscopy or an endoscopic ambulatory surgery center. *Gastroenterologist, 2,* 91–110.
26. Regezi, J. A., & Sciubba, J. (1993). *Oral pathology* (2nd ed.). Philadelphia: W. B. Saunders.
27. Rush, C. (1994). Gut reactions: Calls for patients with GI bleeds needn't turn into messy nightmares. *Emergency Medical Services, 23,* 35–41.
28. Sabiston, D. C. Jr. (1991). *Textbook of surgery: The biologic basis of modern surgical practice* (14th ed.). Philadelphia: W. B. Saunders.
29. Shaffer, E., & Thomson, A. B. R. (1989). *Modern concepts of gastroenterology.* New York: Plenum.
30. Sleisenger, M. H., & Fordtran, J. S. (Eds.). (1993). *Gastrointestinal disease: Pathophysiology, diagnosis and management* (5th ed.). Philadelphia: W. B. Saunders.
31. Snape, W. J., Jr. (Ed.). (1989). *Pathogenesis of functional bowel disease.* New York: Plenum.
32. Snody, H. (1994). Role of endoscopic ultrasonography in diagnosis, staging, and outcome of gastrointestinal diseases. *Gastroenterologist, 2,* 279–280.
33. Society of Gastroenterology Nurses and Associates. (1993). *Gastroenterology nursing: A core curriculum.* St. Louis: Mosby-Year Book.
34. Soderman, W. A., et al. (1989). *Geriatric gastroenterology.* Philadelphia: W. B. Saunders.
35. Swartz, M. H. (1994). *Textbook of physical diagnosis* (2nd ed.). Philadelphia: W. B. Saunders.
36. Wang, J. Y., et al. (1994). Value of carcinoembryonic antigen in the management of colorectal cancer. *Diseases of the colon and rectum, 37,* 272–277.
37. Williams, S. R. (1993). *Nutrition and diet therapy* (7th ed.). St. Louis: Mosby-Year Book.
38. Wyngaarden, J. B., et al. (Eds.) (1992). *Cecil textbook of medicine* (19th ed.). Philadelphia: W. B. Saunders.
39. Yamada, T., et al. (Eds.) (1991). *Textbook of gastroenterology.* Philadelphia: J. B. Lippincott.

Chapter 33 Nursing Care of Clients with Ingestive Disorders

Learning Outcomes

After completing this chapter, the learner will be able to:

1. Assess the client for clinical manifestation of infections and inflammatory and swallowing disorders of the oral cavity and esophagus.
2. Teach the client about the etiology, risk factors, basic pathophysiology, and clinical manifestations of ingestive disorders.
3. Explain the client's role in medical and surgical management of ingestive disorders.
4. Develop plans of care for the prevention of illness, management, and long-term care of clients with ingestive disorders.
5. Implement nursing actions that optimize the quality of life for clients with ingestive disorders.
6. Evaluate planned client outcomes, using outcome criteria developed in the planning phase of care.

People depend on their mouths for the ingestion of food and fluids, the pleasures of taste, and the ability to communicate verbally. Nevertheless, the oral cavity is subject to many disorders, such as tooth decay, periodontal disease, and tumors, that sometimes destroy vital oral structures. Disorders of the oral cavity threaten the client's general health (especially nutrition and fluid and electrolyte balance), communication, and life-style. Assessment, preventive care, and early intervention help clients maintain optimal oral health.

Oral Disorders

Stomatitis

Stomatitis is an inflammation of the oral cavity. It may be of infectious origin or a symptom of a systemic condition. It may be caused by mechanical or chemical trauma. Jagged teeth, cheek biting, and mouth breathing may result in mechanical trauma. Certain foods and drinks, medications, and sensitivity to mouthwashes or dentifrices may produce chemical trauma.

The inflammatory sloughing of tissue allows organisms to multiply; thus, stomatitis may lead to infection by viruses, bacteria, yeasts, or fungi.

Stomatitis is classified as primary or secondary depending on the cause. Primary stomatitis includes aphthous stomatitis, herpes simplex, and Vincent's angina. Secondary stomatitis is caused when the client's resistance is lowered and an opportunistic infection results. Secondary stomatitis can be caused by local and systemic disorders, such as allergies, bone marrow disorders, nutritional disorders, or disorders resulting from immunosuppressive therapy or immunodeficiency.

HERPES SIMPLEX

Herpes simplex is a form of inflammation and ulceration caused by a viral infection.

Incidence

By the age of 5 years, 90 per cent of the population has had an infection, usually asymptomatic, of primary herpes simplex. Secondary herpes is often seen in clients receiving immunosuppressants and in those with human immunodeficiency virus (HIV) or acquired immunodeficiency syndrome (AIDS).

Etiology

Stomatitis caused by the herpes simplex virus (HSV) can occur as a primary or secondary infection. Primary HSV infection occurs as a result of the initial exposure to the virus and is often asymptomatic. Secondary HSV infection takes the form of herpes labialis (fever blister, cold sore). The current theory is that respiratory infections, sunlight, a fever, or emotional stress can reactivate the virus.

Risk Factors

Age is one of the risk factors for primary herpes because it is most common in children. Immunosuppression is the highest risk factor for secondary herpes. There are no preventive measures for either of these factors.

Pathophysiology

When the client is first infected with the primary herpes virus, lesions appear in the oral cavity. These vesicles, which appear throughout the oral cavity, rupture to form ulcerated areas that resemble canker sores and heal within several weeks. The client's tongue appears heavily coated with a characteristic white coating. The infection may produce symptoms of generalized infection in the client.

Secondary herpes is a recurrent infection that appears to lie dormant after the primary herpes infection. Any infection, especially upper respiratory infections, fever, or even sunlight can reactivate the virus.

Clinical Manifestations

Assessment reveals clear, vesicular lesions, most often appearing at the mucocutaneous junction of the lips and face. The lesions are contagious, last about 1 week, and heal without scarring (Fig. 33–1). Later in the course of the infection, the tongue may appear coated, and the client may complain of a foul breath odor.

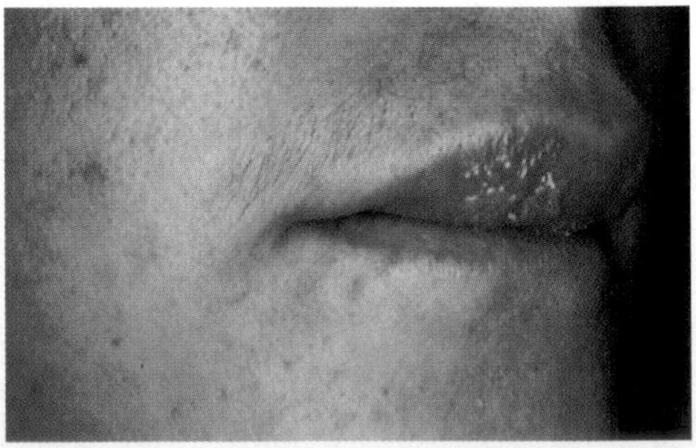

Figure 33–1
Herpes simplex of the lip. (From Hurwitz, S. [1981]. *Clinical pediatric dermatology* [p. 268]. Philadelphia: W. B. Saunders.)

Medical Management

PHARMACOLOGIC MANAGEMENT

General pain may be treated with analgesics. Unless the ulcer is secondarily infected, antimicrobial treatment does not affect the progress of the ulcer. Local ointments and anesthetics may soothe lesions. Clients who are immunocompromised are started on intravenous acyclovir (Zovirax). Clients with competent immune systems also may be given acyclovir but in oral or topical forms.

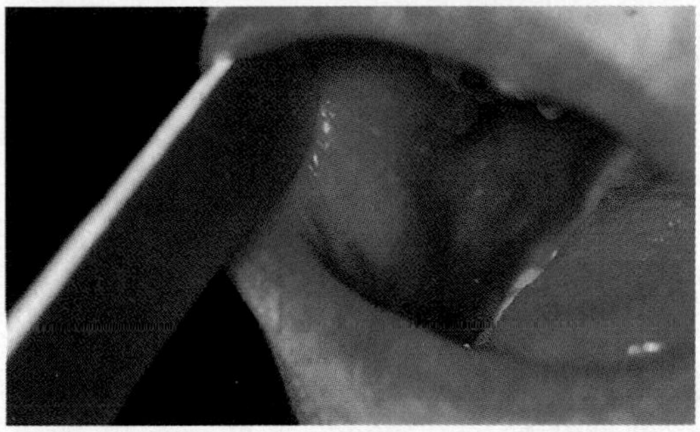

Figure 33–2
Candidiasis. Note the small white patches on the buccal mucosa. (From Moschella, S. L., & Hurley, H. J. [1992]. *Dermatology* [3rd ed.] [p. 231]. Philadelphia: W. B. Saunders.)

Other Oral Disorders

CANDIDIASIS (MONILIASIS)

Candidiasis (thrush) is caused by the organism *Candida albicans*, which is part of the normal flora of the oral cavity.

Incidence

Candidiasis of the oral cavity is commonly seen in clients who are immunosuppressed, such as those receiving chemotherapy or clients with HIV infection or AIDS. There is also a higher incidence in clients with diabetes mellitus and those who are pregnant, under stress, on high doses of or prolonged antibiotic therapy, or on prolonged periods of tube feeding.

Etiology

When the client becomes immunosuppressed or has a decrease in some of the normal oral flora, an overgrowth of the normal flora *Candida* can occur.

Risk Factors

The major risk factors are immunosuppression and the prolonged use of antibiotics that disrupts the normal flora. Clients with either risk factor should be monitored closely, and often prophylactic treatment is started for these high-risk clients.

Pathophysiology

Candidiasis is a secondary infection resulting from either an immunodeficiency or prolonged use of antibiotics. When the normal flora is disrupted, an overgrowth of the *Candida* organism may occur.

Clinical Manifestations

Assessment reveals white patches on the tongue, palate, and buccal mucosa (Fig. 33–2). These lesions adhere firmly to the tissues and are difficult to remove. The lesions are often referred to as milk curds because of their appearance. Clients will often describe the lesions as dry and hot. Clients who have recurrent candidiasis infections should be examined for a possible systemic cause.

Nursing Management

Assessment

The nurse should assess whether the client has pain, tenderness, bleeding in any part of the oral cavity, or any febrile episodes. The client should be questioned about a history of infection elsewhere in the body and the use of any medications such as antibiotics. The client also should be questioned about a history of treatment with radiation or chemotherapy because both can affect the oral mucosa.

The nurse should inspect the oral cavity, noting any areas of inflammation and whether vesicular eruptions, ulcers, white patches, or erythematous gingivae exist. The client should be examined by a dentist to rule out infection of dental origin.

Nursing Diagnosis, Planning, and Implementation

Nursing Diagnosis: Pain R/T altered oral mucous membrane and ulcerations.

Planning: Expected Outcomes. The client will verbalize pain relief and the ability to maintain normal nutrition.

Implementation. The nurse must assess for oral pain and administer analgesics, such as aspirin or acetaminophen, as ordered. Topical agents and topical swishes often provide pain relief. A change in diet to liquid or pureed foods may ease the discomfort of eating. The client should avoid spicy foods, citrus juice, and hot liquids.

Clients with painful lesions cannot tolerate commercial mouthwashes because of the high alcohol concentration of these products. A solution of warm water, half-strength hydrogen peroxide, or mouthwash formulas specific to many institutions are better tolerated and may promote healing.

Nursing Diagnosis: Risk for Infection R/T altered oral mucous membrane, ulcerations, and decreased resistance.

Planning: Expected Outcomes. Infection will not develop or will be controlled, as evidenced by healing of lesions, absence of fever or elevated WBC, and no evidence of secondary infection.

Implementation. If painful oral lesions are present, the nurse may suggest modifications in the client's oral hygiene regimen. Gauze pads may replace toothbrushes, and oral rinses may be needed to cleanse the area of debris and promote healing. Oral pharyngeal cultures should be taken if infection is suspected. Antibiotics and antifungal agents may be used when positive cultures are found. Antifungal agents are frequently given as oral liquids to swish and swallow.

Evaluation

The nurse must evaluate client outcomes based on the established plan of care. If these goals were not achieved, the plan and interventions must be revised to meet the client's needs.

Client Teaching

On discharge, the client should be given oral and written instructions regarding a dental hygiene regimen, diet, medications, and signs and symptoms of complications. The client should demonstrate to the nurse proper techniques of dental hygiene.

Minimal home health-care preparation is required unless the client requires alternate feeding routes. If the client is receiving tube feedings, referral to a home health-care agency may be appropriate to assist with obtaining specialized equipment. The community health nurse may be consulted to assess the client's home environment and to help determine the need for other referrals.

Tumors of the Oral Cavity

Benign Tumors of the Oral Cavity

The most common benign tumors of the mouth are fibromas, lipomas, neurofibromas, and hemangiomas. As with benign tumors in other parts of the body, oral tumors cause problems primarily by occupying space and causing pressure. Benign tumors are usually excised if they cause functional or cosmetic problems.

Premalignant Tumors of the Oral Cavity

LEUKOPLAKIA

Leukoplakia is a potentially precancerous, yellow-white or gray-white lesion. It may occur in any region of the mouth. The size and shape of lesions vary, but they are usually elevated with a roughened or leathery surface and have clearly defined borders (Fig. 33–3).

Incidence

Leukoplakia is a common disorder of the oral mucous membranes, usually seen in the fifth decade of life. Men are twice as often affected as women; however, the incidence in women is increasing.

Etiology

Leukoplakia results from chronic irritation of the mucosa by physical, thermal, or chemical factors. It also sometimes arises from systemic factors, such as poor nutrition or syphilis.

ERYTHROPLAKIA

Erythroplakia is a red, velvety-appearing patch that is often indicative of early squamous cell carcinoma.

Incidence

Erythroplakia occurs most frequently in the sixth and seventh decades of life, with men and women equally affected.

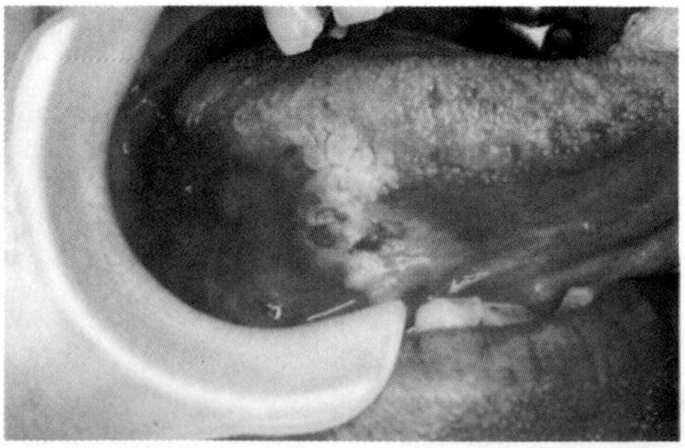

Figure 33–3
Leukoplakia of the lateral edge of the tongue. The lesion shown is associated with squamous carcinoma. (From Sleisenger, M.H., & Fordtran, J.S. [1989]. *Gastrointestinal disease: Pathophysiology, diagnosis, and management* [4th ed.]. Philadelphia: W.B. Saunders.)

Malignant Tumors of the Oral Cavity

Cancers of the oral cavity account for less than 5 per cent of total cases of body malignancies. Cancers in this area most frequently are seen in the fifth and sixth decades of life, affecting men more frequently than women. Cancers of the oral cavity are most often associated with alcohol consumption or tobacco use. With the increase in tobacco use in the younger age groups, especially the use of smokeless tobacco, and by women, the age and sex ratios are changing.

BASAL CELL CARCINOMA

Basal cell carcinoma of the oral cavity occurs primarily in the lips. It starts as a small scab that develops into an ulcer with a characteristic pearly border.

Incidence

Cancer of the mouth accounts for about 4 per cent of all cancers. Basal cell carcinoma is the second most common oral cancer.

Etiology

Basal cell carcinoma primarily occurs as a result of excessive exposure to sunlight. It tends to occur more commonly in fair-skinned individuals who are exposed to sunlight.

SQUAMOUS CELL CARCINOMA

Squamous cell carcinoma is a malignant growth arising from tiny flat squamous cells that line mucous membranes.

Incidence

Squamous cell carcinoma is the leading type of oral cancer. Most tumors occur in clients older than 45 years. Common sites of squamous cell carcinoma include the lower lip and the tongue. Approximately 95 per cent of cancers found on the tongue are squamous cell carcinomas. Malignancies of the tongue represent 1 to 1.5 per cent of all malignancies in the United States.

Etiology

The primary cause of squamous cell carcinoma is chronic irritation of the mucous lining of the mouth and oral cavity. Overuse of alcohol and tobacco is the primary cause of oral irritation. In combination, tobacco and alcohol are extremely destructive to the oral mucosa.

Risk Factors

There are a number of risk factors associated with squamous cell carcinoma of the oral cavity. Tobacco and alcohol are the primary risk factors, and primary prevention is simple if excessive use of these substances is avoided. Other risk factors include poor oral hygiene with bacterial irritation; physical trauma, as from jagged teeth or improperly fitting dentures; chemical and thermal trauma from tobacco, alcohol, oral tobaccos and snuff, or hot or spicy foods or drinks; malnutrition; syphilis or cirrhosis of the liver; and a family history of oral cancer.

Pathophysiology

Squamous cell carcinoma develops from tiny cells that line the oral cavity. It can occur on the lips, buccal mucosa, tongue, floor of the mouth, and tonsils (Fig. 33–4). Squamous cell carcinoma is usually well differentiated and has a less than 10 per cent metastasis rate. Cells metastasize by direct infiltration of local lymph nodes and can extend into the buccal fat and even to the mandible.

Clinical Manifestations

Symptoms of squamous cell carcinoma may include the presence of a sore or lesion in the oral cavity. Red-ap-

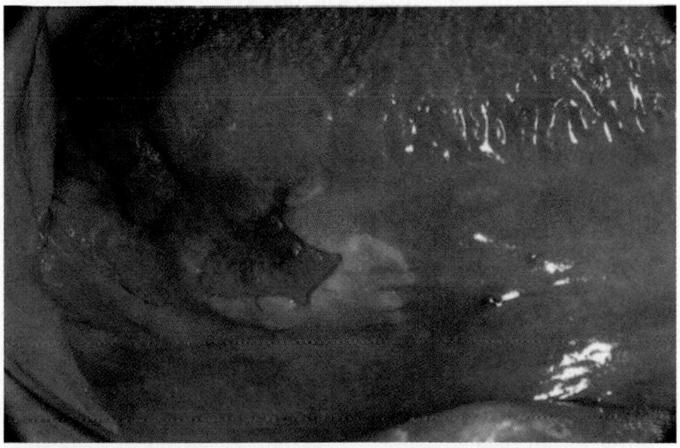

Figure 33–4
Oral squamous carcinoma. Ulcerated lesion with surrounding leukoplakia on the posterior lateral and ventral tongue. (From Neville, B. W., et al. [1995]. *Oral and maxillofacial pathology*. Philadelphia: W. B. Saunders.)

pearing (erythroplakia) squamous cell carcinomas may not be well delineated and often bleed easily. Because squamous cell carcinomas usually grow slowly, they may be large before symptoms are detected. Other symptoms can include a mild irritation of the tongue, sore throat, trouble with wearing dentures, or pain in the tongue or ear.

Diagnostic Assessment

Only biopsy of lesions positively confirms a diagnosis of oral cancer. Cytologic examination of suspicious mucosa, although valuable in screening, unfortunately is not used widely enough to reduce the mortality rate. To be a valuable diagnostic aid, cytologic examination must be followed by biopsy when questionable cells are found.

Medical Management

The survival rate for clients with oral cancer depends on the site and staging of the tumor. Cancer of the lip has one of the highest cure rates of oral cancers. Squamous cell carcinoma of the tongue has the poorest prognosis because of the tongue's extensive vascular and lymphatic supply. Management of oral cancers includes radiation therapy, chemotherapy, and surgery and again depends on the site and staging of the tumor.

PHARMACOLOGIC MANAGEMENT

The effectiveness of chemotherapy for the treatment of oral cancers remains to be determined. Several chemotherapeutic agents are used to treat clients with head and neck cancers (Box 33–1).

Surgical Management

Surgical management of oral cancers can range from local excision of small tumors to extensive surgery for invasive tumors. Small tumors can be treated in outpatient facilities by local excision, radiation, or laser therapy.

BOX 33–1

Chemotherapeutic Agents Used to Treat Head and Neck Cancers

Bleomycin
Cisplatin
Cyclophosphamide
Doxorubicin (Adriamycin)
5-Fluorouracil
Hydroxyurea
Methotrexate
Vincristine

Invasive tumors require extensive surgical excision that usually involves removal of associated lymph nodes. Depending on the location, procedures may include a glossectomy (removal of the tongue), mandibulectomy (removal of the mandible), or hemiglossectomy (removal of part of the tongue). A radical neck dissection is an extensive procedure that involves removal of all tissue under the skin, from the jaw down to the clavicle and from the anterior border of the trapezius muscle to the midline.

Nursing Management

Assessment

The nurse should carefully question the client about his or her symptoms. A common finding is that of a painful ulcer. The client should also be assessed for difficulty in swallowing, white or red patches on the oral mucosa, bleeding in the mouth, lumps in the neck, pain referred to the ear, foul odor, and hoarseness. The nurse should question the client concerning the use of alcohol and tobacco, oral hygiene habits, and exposure to the sun. The nurse must also assess the rehabilitative needs of the client. Surgery can result in disfigurement and alterations in speech and can cause the client to experience depression related to a change in body image.

Nursing Diagnosis, Planning, and Implementation

Nursing Diagnosis: Knowledge Deficit R/T prevention of oral lesions and treatment of lesions should they occur.

Planning: Expected Outcomes. Client will understand and comply with measures to maintain oral mucosa, as evidenced by statements of understanding of substances and activities to avoid, no evidence of lesions, and verbalization of understanding of treatment regimen, including surgery.

Implementation. The nurse should teach the client about the disease itself and treatment protocols.

The best intervention for oral cancers is prevention. The nurse must advise clients to

- Avoid chemical, physical, and thermal oral trauma
- Perform careful, frequent oral hygiene, preferably three times daily
- See a dentist if they have ill-fitting dentures
- See a physician for any mouth lesion that does not heal in 2 to 3 weeks
- Maintain a well-balanced diet

If the client is receiving radiation or chemotherapy, the nurse should instruct the client about possible side effects of these forms of treatment. The nurse should provide the client with comfort measures to minimize the side effects, such as using antiemetics to prevent nausea and vomiting.

If the client is scheduled for a surgical resection, the nurse should ensure that the client understands the procedure to be performed and all implications (such as a temporary or permanent tracheostomy). The client should receive adequate support before surgery to help the client cope with a possibly radically altered appearance. Instructions regarding postoperative procedures will depend on the extent of the surgical resection. Clients should be instructed on the need for frequent vital signs, intravenous fluid therapy, the availability of analgesics for pain, and oxygen therapy after surgery. The purpose and care involved with a feeding tube also should be explained. (See the Client Education Guide: After Oral Surgery.)

Nursing Diagnosis: Nutrition, Altered: Less than Body Requirements R/T oral pain, difficulty eating and swallowing, and altered oral mucosa and surgical procedure.

Planning: Expected Outcomes. The client will maintain weight or show weight gain before surgery, as evidenced by an increase in intake, weight remaining stable, or weight gain of 1 pound per week preoperatively.

Implementation. The location, size, and pain associated with a tumor often interfere with the client's ability to eat. Small, frequent feedings often promote intake. Administering an analgesic 30 to 45 minutes before a meal often decreases pain associated with eating. The nurse should provide oral care before and after meals to remove oral odors and debris.

Unfortunately, treatments such as radiation alter salivation and taste perception. Xerostomia (dryness of the mouth) usually improves with the use of pilocarpine and artificial saliva. The nurse should suggest that the client chew sugarless gum or suck on sugarless candy drops to increase moisture. The client should perform frequent oral rinses with cool water to reduce dryness.

Immediately after surgery, the nurse should monitor intravenous hydration. Bowel sounds should be assessed every shift. The return of bowel sounds is often an indication to begin tube feedings. Before each tube feeding, the nurse should properly assess the client for proper tube placement (see Chap. 34). Nutritional supplements may be administered by pump or bolus feedings.

Once the edema has subsided, adequate healing has occurred, and the tracheostomy tube has been removed, the client may be restarted on oral feedings. The client should be cautioned about a decrease in sensation in the oral cavity after surgery. Swallowing should be carefully assessed before the client begins to eat, and the client should be taught to avoid putting food directly on the surgical resection site. After meals, the client should always perform good oral hygiene.

Nursing Diagnosis: Injury, Risk for R/T surgical procedure, including hemorrhage, ineffective airway clearance, and possible wound infection.

Planning: Expected Outcomes. The client will not experience injury, as evidenced by absence of excessive bleeding, maintenance of a patent airway, and wound healing without signs of infection.

Implementation. The extent of nursing care required by the client after surgery depends on the extent of the procedure. After local excisions, the nurse teaches the client how to perform hygiene gently. If a dressing and packing are in place, the nurse monitors the amount of drainage. After the dressing and packing are removed, the client should rinse the oral cavity with a mild half-strength solution of hydrogen peroxide and water or saline solution every 4 hours to remove debris and promote healing.

With more extensive surgery, the suture lines must be protected from trauma. Oral hygiene and oral suctioning are usually not implemented until healing has begun and the physician decides this type of cleaning can be performed.

Hemorrhage can occur at any time, from the first few hours after surgery to several days after surgery. Hemorrhage can be massive because of the large vessels that supply the mouth and oral area. Should bleeding occur, apply local pressure on the site until the physician can be notified. Surgical repair may be required. If an extensive resection was performed requiring skin grafts, the nurse should monitor the site every shift for drainage and for signs of infection.

The most critical postoperative intervention is to maintain a patent airway. If the surgical procedure has been extensive, there is usually a tracheostomy in place, which helps prevent respiratory difficulty arising from edema of the oral and pharyngeal structures. Clients at risk for ineffective airway clearance should be in semi- to high-Fowler's position after surgery to promote venous lymphatic drainage. The client may have a dusky appearance about the face from venous congestion. Pulse oximeter readings also should be used to determine whether or not the client is sufficiently oxygenated.

For the client with a tracheostomy, some blood-tinged mucus is normal in tracheal secretions for the first 48 hours after surgery. Bright red bleeding from the tracheostomy tube or site is a sign of hemorrhage.

CLIENT EDUCATION GUIDE

After Oral Surgery

On discharge, the nurse should supply the client and significant others with complete instructions regarding diet, medications, signs and symptoms of complications, and any treatments such as wound or tracheostomy care.

Clients who have undergone extensive surgery may need a referral to a home health-care agency for possible assistance with respiratory support, nutritional support, and wound care. Respiratory support may include home oxygen, oral suctioning, or tracheal suctioning. Nutritional support may involve total parenteral nutrition, nasogastric tube feedings, or maintenance of a soft diet. The dietitian should be consulted for meal planning. Wound care involves cleaning the suture line and observing for signs and symptoms of infection, such as swelling, redness, drainage, or fever. When financial concerns exist, a social worker should be consulted.

The client will need to be seen by the physician after discharge to ensure complete healing of any extensive surgical wounds. Tracheostomies may be permanent or may be closed at a later date.

Nursing Diagnosis: Impaired Verbal Communication R/T presence of tracheostomy.

Planning: Expected Outcomes. Client will be able to communicate using alternate forms of communication, as evidenced by ability to continue communication with staff and significant others.

Implementation. The nurse should help clients who cannot communicate verbally to express their needs, concerns, and feelings. The nurse should assess the client's literacy and then provide paper for the client to write on as a substitute for talking or provide the client with a picture board to use for communicating any needs. The nurse should check on the client frequently to reduce any anxiety and loneliness. The nurse also should place the call light within easy reach and respond to the light in person promptly.

The client should be allowed to communicate by gestures or written notes if this approach puts the client at ease. Most important, the nurse's manner should communicate acceptance, compassion, and caring. It is common to treat clients who cannot talk as though they cannot hear or understand. The nurse must be alert to any tendency to treat these clients as though they were mentally incompetent or deaf. The nurse should help the client avoid social isolation.

Evaluation

The nurse must evaluate client outcomes on the basis of the established plan of care. If these goals were not achieved, the plan and interventions must be revised to meet the client's needs.

Disorders of the Salivary Glands

INFLAMMATION

Parotitis, also known as surgical mumps, involves inflammation of the parotid glands. It is the most common inflammatory condition affecting the salivary glands. Inflammation probably results from inactivity of the gland caused by certain medications, such as diuretics, and lack of oral intake, such as that seen in postoperative clients. As secretions of the salivary glands diminish, oral bacteria have an opportunity to invade the gland and multiply. Interventions involve

- Administering frequent oral hygiene to keep the bacterial count of the mouth low
- Keeping the client well hydrated
- Suggesting that the client use sugarless hard candies or chew sugarless gum to stimulate secretions of the glands

CALCULI

Stones, or calculi, form in the salivary glands when the glands are inactive and the client has a metabolic condition favoring the precipitation of salts. A focus, or nidus, is necessary for stimulating salt precipitation. Assessment reveals that irritation from the stones causes local inflammation, swelling, and pain when the gland is stimulated to secrete, as during chewing. Intervention requires local excision.

TUMORS

Most tumors in the salivary glands are benign. Tumors of the submaxillary glands are more likely to be malignant.

Tumors are characterized by enlargement. Pain occurs when expansion within the capsule of the gland creates pressure on sensory nerves. The treatment of choice for both benign and malignant tumors is usually surgical excision. If the tumor has recurred or is highly malignant, radiation therapy may be used.

Disorders of the Esophagus

DYSPHAGIA

Dysphagia, or difficulty with swallowing, can be caused by any esophageal disorder. Specific causes include

- Neuromotor malfunction
- Mechanical obstruction
- Cardiovascular abnormalities
- Neurologic diseases

Mechanical Obstruction

Mechanical obstructions causing dysphagia include congenital defects, carcinoma, and acquired conditions such as hiatal hernia. When an obstruction narrows the esophageal lumen, clients first experience dysphagia only with solid foods. Later, dysphagia becomes associated with semisolid foods and liquids. Finally, these clients are unable to swallow their own saliva. Obstructive disorders, particularly esophageal carcinoma, may be accompanied by weight loss and cachexia.

Cardiovascular Abnormalities

Dysphagia also may result from cardiovascular abnormalities, particularly in the elderly. Specific conditions that cause vascular dysphagia include an enlarged heart,

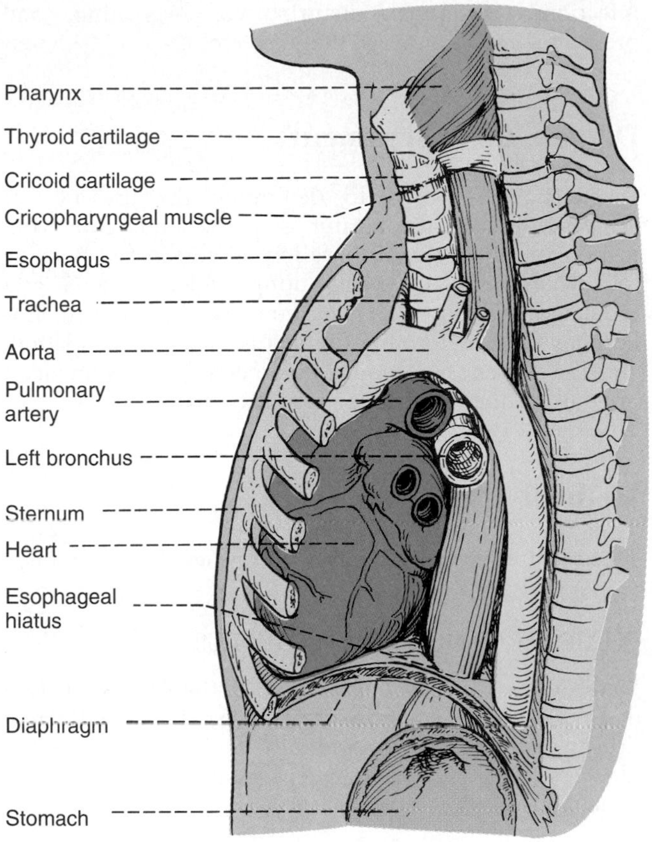

Figure 33–5
Relationship of the heart and great arteries to the esophagus.

an aortic aneurysm, and calcification of the descending aorta. Figure 33–5 shows the relationship of the heart and great arteries to the esophagus.

Neurologic Diseases

Dysphagia also may be caused by certain neurologic diseases such as cerebrovascular accidents, multiple sclerosis, poliomyelitis, and amyotrophic lateral sclerosis.

Other Causes

Dysphagia can be experienced after swallowing if food gets caught in the esophagus. Relief may be obtained by drinking liquids to force the impacted bolus through the narrow segment, or retching may dislodge the food.

REGURGITATION

Regurgitation is the ejection of small amounts of chyme or gastric juice from the mouth without antecedent nausea. It is usually caused by an incompetent lower esophageal sphincter (LES). Regurgitation occurring immediately after swallowing results from structural or motor abnormality in the LES. Stooping or lying down facilitates the flow of gastric contents into the esophagus, thus exacerbating regurgitation.

PAIN

Pain, which sometimes is constant or may occur only with swallowing, suggests diffuse esophageal spasm. Pain may result from alterations of the mucosa caused by reflux disease, radiation, or viral infection. Pain that affects the esophageal mucosa and occurs with swallowing is called odynophagia. The client usually describes the pain as sharp, constricting, sticking, crushing, stabbing, or knifelike. Odynophagia is usually severe, quite distressing, and often associated with a deep and long-lasting pain.

HEARTBURN

Heartburn (pyrosis, indigestion, or dyspepsia) is another common manifestation of esophageal disease. Generally, it is a painful sensation of warmth and burning in the lower retrosternal midline. Clients may use the term "heartburn" to describe very different sensations. Therefore, the nurse must find out exactly what this term means to the client experiencing the symptom. Heartburn usually means substernal, midline burning, which tends to radiate, generally in waves, upward to the neck because of abnormalities of the LES. Clients often describe this discomfort as cramping or knotting. Heartburn is often experienced with postural changes such as bending, stooping, or lifting as well as when someone gulps food or liquids or ingests alcohol. Symptoms often are relieved by standing. Heartburn also arises in the presence of refluxed gastric or duodenal contents. Disorders most commonly associated with heartburn are reflux esophagitis, hiatal hernia, achalasia, and gastric stasis. Heartburn is common in clients with pyloric or duodenal ulcers and LES disorders.

There are many pathologic conditions of the esophagus. Achalasia, diffuse spasm, gastroesophageal reflux disease, hiatal hernia, diverticula, and esophageal neoplasms are discussed in the following sections.

ACHALASIA

Achalasia is a disorder characterized by progressively increasing dysphagia, with the client eventually having great difficulty swallowing and expressing the feeling that "something is stuck in the throat."

Incidence

Achalasia commonly occurs in the third to fourth decades of life and appears with equal incidence in men and in women.

Etiology

Achalasia is a chronic, progressive disease that is considered idiopathic in origin. Occasionally, the client can relate the onset to an episode of acute dysphagia, but usually achalasia has an obscure onset and is only noticed when the dysphagia becomes severe.

Risk Factors

Because achalasia is an idiopathic condition, there are no identified risk factors. It is believed there may be a familial incidence of achalasia.

Pathophysiology

Achalasia is characterized by impaired motility of the lower two thirds of the esophagus. The LES fails to relax normally with swallowing. Inadequate functioning occurs because either nerve impulses are unable to pass through the esophagus or sympathetic receptors are absent from the LES. There also may be degeneration of the ganglion cells or impairment of impulses from Auerbach's plexus. Impaired propulsion and a constricted LES result in accumulation of food and fluid within the lower esophagus. When hydrostatic pressure exceeds the force of resistance of the LES, the contents pass into the stomach.

Complications

Complications of achalasia include esophagitis with resultant ulceration. Aspiration of regurgitated esophageal contents may result in atelectasis and other pulmonary problems.

Clinical Manifestations

The initial symptom of achalasia is dysphagia. Food and fluid do not pass through the region of the LES. In the early stages of achalasia, the client also may have substernal pain resulting from spasms of the esophagus or may be unable to belch. The client may regurgitate undigested food eaten many hours earlier as well as large amounts of mucus that have been stimulated by esophageal irritation. As achalasia progresses, symptoms increase in frequency and severity. Upper respiratory infections, emotional disturbances, overeating, and pregnancy may aggravate the problem.

Diagnostic Assessment

Diagnostic tests used to determine the presence of achalasia include the barium swallow, endoscopy, and manometry. The barium swallow is considered positive for achalasia if it reveals nonpropulsive waves and esophageal dilation. Also, barium may be retained. Endoscopy helps determine the status of the LES, dilation, and the presence of food. Manometry (measurement of pressure in the esophagus) confirms the diagnosis.

Medical Management

Treatment of achalasia is aimed at relieving symptoms.

PHARMACOLOGIC MANAGEMENT

Medications have been investigated that relax the LES or lower esophageal pressures, such as anticholinergic drugs, gastrointestinal hormones, and calcium channel blockers. Pain is controlled with non-narcotic and narcotic analgesics.

DIETARY MANAGEMENT

Changes in diet can often ease the pressure and reflux in the client with achalasia. Small, frequent feedings ease the passage of food, and semisoft, warm foods are better tolerated than cold, hard foods. The client should avoid hot, spicy, and iced foods as well as alcohol and tobacco. All foods should be chewed thoroughly to add saliva to the mixture, providing lubrication and allowing the bolus to pass more easily from the esophagus to the stomach. The client should experiment with different positions to reduce pressure while eating. To prevent nocturnal reflux of food, the client should sleep with the head of the bed elevated.

Surgical Management

Surgical management of achalasia can involve dilating the esophageal sphincter (esophageal dilation) or enlarging the sphincter (esophagomyotomy). Esophageal dilation or bougienage forcefully dilates the lower esophagus and sphincter (Fig. 33–6). It is used to help correct not only achalasia but also esophageal spasms and strictures. Vigorous dilatation has a 75% success rate. This procedure is performed with local anesthesia under radiologic guidance.

A more complex procedure, esophagomyotomy (Heller's procedure) may have to be performed. In this procedure, the surgeon enlarges the vestibule by incising the circular muscle fibers down to the mucosa.

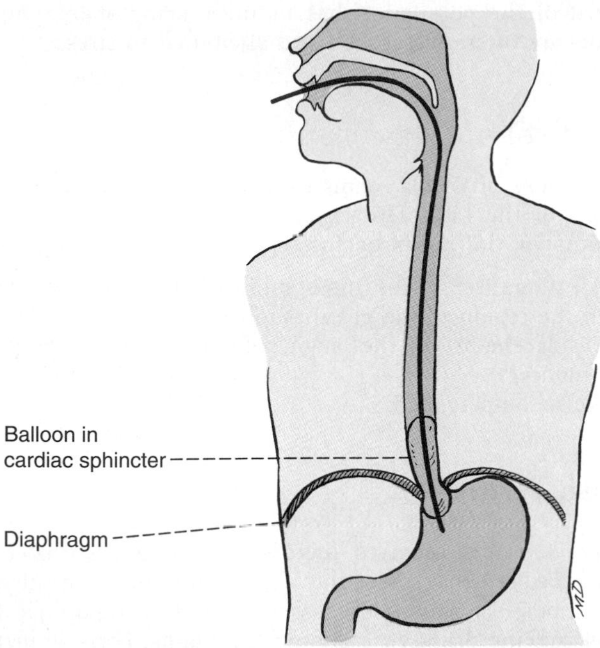

Figure 33–6
Bougienage relieves dysphagia by dilating the lower esophageal sphincter.

Complications of esophagomyotomy include reflux esophagitis and restenosis. If a client cannot swallow for long periods, a gastrostomy tube may be inserted.

Nursing Management

Assessment

The nurse obtains a history, noting the symptoms the client is experiencing. The onset and duration of symptoms with factors that aggravate symptoms should be assessed. The nurse should note any methods the client uses for relief.

Respiratory symptoms also should be assessed because the respiratory tract can be affected with reflux or regurgitation. The nurse should assess the client's nutritional status, noting any weight changes and the effects of esophageal symptoms on dietary habits and the client's respiratory status.

Nursing Diagnosis, Planning, and Implementation

Nursing Diagnosis: Nutrition, Altered: Less than Body Requirements R/T dysphagia.

Planning: Expected Outcomes. The client will maintain an adequate nutritional intake, as evidenced by maintenance of ideal body weight or gaining back any weight lost at a rate of 1 pound per week.

Implementation. The nurse should consult with the client concerning dietary habits and assess the client's intake of nutrients daily. A baseline weight should be obtained, and the client should be weighed daily. The nurse should teach the client about changes in dietary habits that may relieve symptoms.

CLIENT EDUCATION GUIDE

Esophageal Reflux and Aspiration

The client should receive written and oral instructions regarding diet, medications, and symptoms of respiratory complications related to esophageal reflux and aspiration.

- Clients who have undergone an esophagomyotomy should be instructed to sleep with the head of the bed elevated and to recognize signs and symptoms of respiratory complications.
- The client should be instructed about signs and symptoms of infection and esophageal perforation and to notify the physician if any of these problems occur.
- A home health-care agency should be consulted to assist the client with any needs related to medications, wound care, and diet and to provide an ongoing evaluation of the client's condition.
- A referral to a social worker also might be needed to assist the client with financial issues, counseling, and specialized equipment.

Nursing Diagnosis: Pain, Acute and Chronic, R/T episodes of gastric reflux.

Planning: Expected Outcomes. The client will experience a decrease in pain or absence of pain, as evidenced by the client verbalizing a decrease in or absence of pain and the client's ability to maintain oral intake.

Implementation. As stated, pain can be decreased or relieved through the use of medications, dietary changes, and repositioning the client. The nurse should assess the client every shift to determine whether or not the use of medications, changes in diet, and positioning were effective in controlling or relieving pain.

Nursing Diagnosis: Knowledge Deficit R/T preoperative preparation and discharge.

Planning: Expected Outcomes. The client will understand and be adequately prepared for surgery, as evidenced by client questions and statements of understanding.

Implementation. Clients undergoing esophageal dilatation should be told that they will be awake during the procedure. A local anesthetic will be sprayed on the throat, and the client may receive an analgesic or tranquilizer. The client should take long, slow breaths during the passage of the bougies. As the balloon is inflated, the client may feel a brief feeling of discomfort. Esophageal dilatation is often performed on an outpatient basis.

Esophagomyotomy is a more complex procedure. The client will require a general anesthetic and remain hospitalized for several days. The nurse should instruct the client undergoing an esophageal procedure about all usual preoperative procedures, such as taking nothing by mouth after midnight, intravenous fluids, and preoperative medications. The nurse should also discuss pain control, chest tubes, drains, surgical dressings, and the presence of a nasogastric or gastric tube. (See Client Education Guide: Esophageal Reflux and Aspiration.)

Collaborative Problem. Risk for Injury R/T surgical procedure and presence of chest tubes.

Planning: Expected Outcomes. Injury will be prevented, as evidenced by absence of hemorrhage, no signs of perforation, normal temperature, and absence of signs of problems associated with the chest tubes such as respiratory distress.

Implementation. After esophageal dilatation, the nurse should monitor the client for signs of perforation, such as elevated temperature, chest or shoulder pain, and subcutaneous emphysema. If any of these manifestations are noted, the nurse should notify the physician immediately. The client will require an x-ray study to determine whether or not air is in the mediastinum, indicating perforation.

After an esophagomyotomy, the client will have a thoracotomy incision and chest tubes in place. The nurse will need to maintain chest tube drainage and the nasogastric or gastric drainage system and manage the client's pain. (See Chap. 22 for care of the client with chest tubes.)

Evaluation

The nurse must evaluate client outcomes based on the established plan of care. If these goals were not achieved, the plan and interventions must be revised to meet the client's needs.

Modification of Plan of Care for the Elderly

In older adults, an attempt is made to treat the client with less invasive measures (pain medications, positioning, and dietary modification) and, possibly, esophageal dilatation.

GASTROESOPHAGEAL REFLUX DISEASE

Esophageal reflux is defined as the backward flow of gastric contents into the esophagus. Gastroesophageal reflux disease (GERD) is a term used to describe a syndrome resulting from esophageal reflux. Reflux exposes the esophageal mucosa to the gastric contents and gradually breaks down the esophageal mucosa. This condition is sometimes referred to as reflux esophagitis. This reflux is often associated with a sliding hiatal hernia. However, reflux causing complications can occur without a hiatal hernia, and clients with a hiatal hernia may not have symptoms of reflux.

Incidence

Gastroesophageal reflux disease can occur in any age group. It is estimated that 10 per cent of the population has daily symptoms from GERD and as much as one third of the population has monthly symptoms. Symptoms are often overlooked and attributed to stress.

Etiology

The cause of GERD seems to be an inappropriate relaxation of the LES. The exact cause of the relaxation is unknown, but reflux occurs when there is

- An alteration in the innervation of the pressure zone in the region of the gastroesophageal sphincter
- Displacement of the angle of the gastroesophageal junction
- An incompetent LES

Risk Factors

Several factors seem to increase the occurrence of reflux. Factors that affect the LES include nicotine; high-fat foods; xanthine derivatives, including theophylline and caffeine drinks; ganglionic stimulants; beta-adrenergic agents; and high levels of estrogen and progesterone.

Pathophysiology

Normally, a high-pressure zone exists in the region of the gastroesophageal sphincter. High pressure prevents reflux but permits the passage of food and liquids. When there is an alteration in this region, reflux occurs.

Reflux esophagitis also may occur with gastric or duodenal ulcer and after esophageal or gastric surgery, prolonged vomiting, and prolonged gastrointestinal intubation. The reflux most often consists of hydrochloric acid or gastric and duodenal contents containing bile acid and pancreatic juice. Frequent or prolonged reflux results in inflammation of the esophageal mucosa (esophagitis). The degree of reflux esophagitis present depends on the

- Frequency of the reflux
- Contents of the gastric reflux
- Buffering ability of the saliva and mucus secretion
- Rate of gastric emptying

Clinical Manifestations

Clients with GERD may experience a sudden or gradual onset of symptoms. The client may complain of heartburn, odynophagia, dysphagia, acid regurgitation, water brash (the release of salty secretions in the mouth), or eructation. Pain in GERD is typically referred to as a burning sensation that moves up and down. If the condition is severe, the pain may radiate to the back, neck, or jaw. Pain usually occurs after meals and is relieved with antacids or fluids. Discomfort sometimes accompanies activities that increase intra-abdominal pressure, such as lifting or straining. The client may express

TABLE 33–1 Pharmacologic Management in Gastroesophageal Reflux Disease

MEDICATION	MECHANISM OF ACTION	NURSING IMPLICATIONS
Antacids Aluminum-magnesium (Mylanta) Magnesium salts (Maalox)	Conversion of gastric acid to neutral salts	Administer 30 mL 1 hour before and 2 hours after meals
Histamine receptor antagonists Ranitidine (Zantac) Famotidine (Pepcid)	Suppression of acid secretion by blocking H_2 receptors on the parietal cells	Administer with meals and hour of sleep
Parasympathomimetic Bethanecol (Urecholine)	Increases LES pressure and prevents reflux	Give in conjunction with antacids and H_2 receptor antagonists; administer before meals
Gastrointestinal stimulant Metoclopramide (Reglan)	Increases LES pressure by stimulating the smooth muscle of the GI tract and increasing the rate of gastric emptying	Administer before meals

GI, gastrointestinal; H_2, histamine; LES, lower esophageal sphincter.

discomfort when lying supine or when the stomach is distended. Discomfort may be relieved by standing and walking. Dysphagia resulting from edema, spasm, or a narrowed lumen is intermittent and worse at the beginning of meals. Responses to pain-relieving measures (e.g., nitroglycerin) help to differentiate between esophagitis and problems of cardiac origin (e.g., angina pectoris).

Diagnostic Assessment

Diagnosis rests on the demonstration of reflux. Barium swallow, esophageal manometry, esophagoscopy, esophageal biopsy, cytologic examination, analysis of gastric secretions, and acid perfusion tests confirm the diagnosis of GERD (see Chap. 32).

Medical Management

PHARMACOLOGIC MANAGEMENT

Drug therapy for GERD is outlined in Table 33–1.

DIETARY MANAGEMENT

In mild cases of GERD, diet changes may be sufficient to relieve symptoms. The prescribed regimen of therapy should include having the client

- Restrict the diet to small, frequent feedings (4–6 per day)
- Drink adequate fluids at meals to assist food passage
- Eat slowly and chew thoroughly to add saliva to the food
- Avoid extremely hot or cold foods as well as spices, fats, alcohol, coffee, chocolate, and citrus juices
- Avoid eating and drinking for 3 hours before retiring to prevent the common problem of nocturnal reflux
- Elevate the head of the bed 6 to 8 inches to prevent nocturnal reflux
- Lose weight if overweight to decrease the gastroesophageal pressure gradient
- Avoid tobacco, salicylates, or phenylbutazone, which may aggravate esophagitis

Surgical Management

Surgery is used with clients who do not respond to medical management. Any one of three different procedures may be used. They are the Nissen fundoplication, Hill's operation, or Belsey's repair. The Nissen fundoplication is most frequently used and involves a gastric wraparound (Fig. 33–7).

Hill's operation narrows the esophageal opening and anchors the stomach and distal esophagus to the median arcuate ligament (posterior gastropexy). The Belsey (Mark IV) repair consists of plicating the anterior and lateral aspects of the stomach onto the distal esophagus. Clients undergoing a surgical procedure are encouraged to follow the antireflux medical regimen because the recurrence rate is significant.

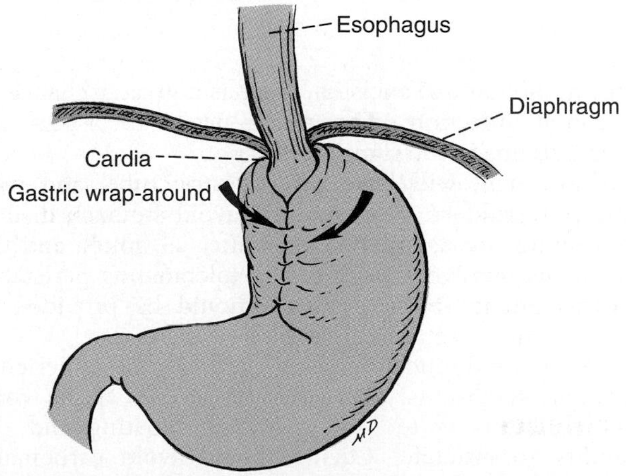

Figure 33–7
Nissen fundoplication for hiatal hernia. The gastric fundus is wrapped around the distal esophagus and sutured to itself.

Nursing Management

Assessment

The nurse should identify what symptoms the client has been experiencing. The nurse should note when symptoms started, their frequency and severity, and the relationship of symptoms to food and various food products. The nurse also should assist in maintaining the client's general appearance and nutritional status.

Nursing Diagnosis, Planning, and Implementation

Nursing Diagnosis: Pain R/T irritation of the esophagus caused by gastric reflux.

Planning: Expected Outcomes. The client's pain will decrease or be absent, as evidenced by the client verbalizing that the pain is decreased or absent.

Implementation. The nurse should teach the client about the prescribed diet regimen and evaluate both the client's understanding and the effectiveness of the treatment. The nurse should administer medications ordered for the pain and document the effectiveness of the medications.

Collaborative Problem: Risk for Injury R/T surgical procedure and presence of chest tubes.

Planning: Expected Outcomes. Injury will be prevented, as evidenced by absence of hemorrhage, no signs of infection, normal temperature, and absence of signs of problems associated with the chest tubes such as respiratory distress.

Implementation. Preoperative care is basically the same as for other surgeries. If a thoracic approach is used, the client should be instructed on the purpose and care associated with chest tubes (see Chap. 22 for the care of the client with a chest tube). Clients may have a nasogastric tube in place after surgery to prevent stomach distention. The client should be taught the purpose and care associated with a nasogastric tube.

CRITICAL TO REMEMBER

The client must cough and deep breathe to avoid respiratory complications, even though postoperative breathing can be painful.

With an abdominal incision, there is a greater chance of a wound infection. The nurse needs to assess the wound drainage for signs of infection.

The client will have a nasogastric tube, and tube patency should be maintained to avoid stomach distention. Fluids are usually resumed after 24 hours, and the diet is progressively advanced as tolerated as peristalsis returns. Small, frequent meals should be provided to avoid overloading the stomach.

After fundoplication, the client could experience gas-bloat syndrome. This condition occurs if the wrap of the fundus is too tight, causing bloating and the inability to eructate. Clients should avoid carbonated beverages, drinking with a straw, and gas-producing foods. Ambulation can assist peristalsis in removing air from the gastrointestinal tract. The condition is usually temporary. Clients should be instructed to report dysphagia, epigastric fullness, bloating, and excessive rumbling to their physician.

Evaluation

The nurse must evaluate client outcomes based on the established plan of care. If these goals were not achieved, the plan and interventions must be revised to meet the client's needs.

HIATAL HERNIA

A hiatal hernia, also referred to as a diaphragmatic hernia, is a condition in which the cardiac sphincter becomes enlarged, allowing the stomach to pass into the thoracic cavity. There are two types of hernias: sliding hernias (type I) and rolling or paraesophageal hernias (type II). In a sliding hernia, the upper stomach and the gastroesophageal junction are displaced upward into the thorax (Fig. 33–8*A*). Sliding hernias account for approximately 90 per cent of the total cases of esophageal hiatal hernias.

With a rolling hernia, the gastroesophageal junction stays below the diaphragm, but all or part of the stomach pushes through into the thorax (Fig. 33–8*B*).

Incidence

The incidence of hiatal hernia is estimated as 5 per 1000 in the general population and may be as high as 60 per cent in clients older than 60 years. Women tend to be more affected than men, and the incidence increases significantly with age. Sliding hiatal hernias may be noted in infants, but they usually do not produce symptoms until the person reaches middle age.

Etiology

Hiatal hernias are related to muscle weakness in the esophageal hiatus, which loosens the esophageal supports and allows the lower portion of the stomach to rise into the thorax. As with other hernias, the muscle weakness is caused by a variety of conditions, such as aging, congenital muscle weakness, trauma, surgery, or anything that increases intra-abdominal pressure.

Risk Factors

Risk factors for the development of hiatal hernias are any factors that lead to weakness of the diaphragmatic muscle and increase intra-abdominal pressure. The pressure may be increased by conditions such as obesity, pregnancy, or ascites.

Primary prevention of the hiatal hernia can be accomplished, or at least delayed, by losing weight and

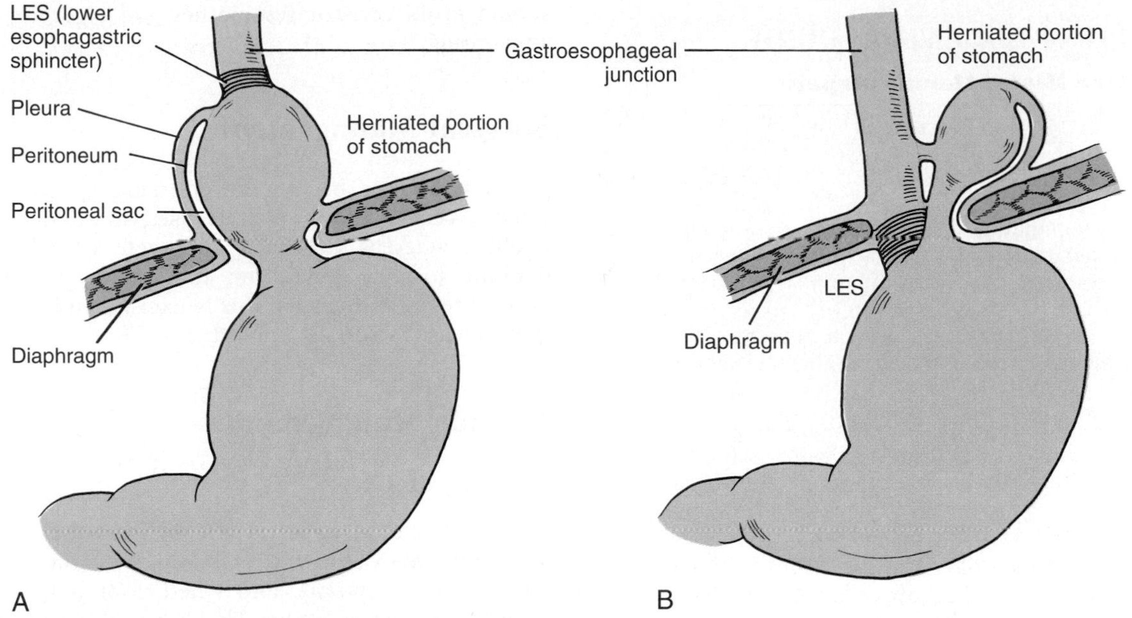

Figure 33–8
A, Sliding and *B*, rolling hiatal hernias.

avoiding any activities that increase intra-abdominal pressure. Other than these measures, hiatal hernias are not preventable.

Pathophysiology

A hiatal hernia involves the herniation of part of the stomach through a weakness in the diaphragm. The resulting regurgitation and motor dysfunction cause the major manifestations of hiatal hernia. With a sliding hernia, reflux appears to be caused by the exposure of the LES to the low pressure in the thorax. The major problem associated with a sliding hernia is the development of reflux.

With a rolling hernia, the LES remains below the diaphragm so reflux is not a problem. Complications of a rolling hiatal hernia include obstruction, strangulation, and the development of a volvulus.

Clinical Manifestations

Manifestations of hiatal hernia vary in kind and severity. In sliding hiatal hernias, clients may have heartburn 30 to 60 minutes after meals. In addition, reflux may result in substernal pain.

The client with a rolling hiatal hernia does not have symptoms of reflux. The client may complain of a feeling of fullness after eating or have difficulty breathing. Some clients experience chest pain similar to anginal pain. Pain is usually worse when the client assumes a recumbent position.

Medical and Surgical Management

The medical management for the client with a hiatal hernia is the same as that for the client with GERD. The client who does not respond to medical treatment may be treated surgically, the same as the client with GERD.

DIAGNOSTIC ASSESSMENT

Hiatal hernias are diagnosed by a barium swallow, with fluoroscopy, showing the position of the stomach in relation to the diaphragm.

Nursing Management

The nursing care of the client with a hiatal hernia is the same as that for a client with GERD. As with GERD, the most common nursing diagnosis is pain related to irritation of the esophagus caused by gastric reflux. (See the Client Education Guide: After Hiatal Hernia Repair.)

DIVERTICULA

Diverticula in the esophagus are saclike outpouchings in one or more layers of the esophagus. As food is ingested, it becomes trapped in the diverticulum and can later be regurgitated. The most common type of esophageal diverticula is esophageal pulsion diverticulum (Zenker's diverticulum).

CLIENT EDUCATION GUIDE

After Hiatal Hernia Repair

The client should be taught the following:

- The appropriate diet modifications, drug therapy, and positioning.
- To avoid straining the incision for at least 6 weeks after surgery. Stair climbing is usually restricted for the first few days at home, and lifting of heavy objects should be avoided.
- To inspect the incision for signs and symptoms of infection, including redness, tenderness, drainage, and swelling.

There are few dietary restrictions, but an eating pattern of several small meals rather than three large meals is better tolerated. The client who smokes or is overweight can reduce the risk of relapse by participating in a smoking-cessation or weight loss support group.

Incidence

Esophageal diverticula are considered rare. Zenker's diverticulum occurs three times more frequently in men than women.

Etiology

The cause of esophageal weakness could be a congenital defect, esophageal trauma, scar tissue, or inflammation.

Clinical Manifestations

Initially, the client usually complains of difficulty swallowing. Other symptoms may include belching, regurgitation of undigested food, halitosis, and a sour taste in the mouth. Coughing also may occur because of irritation of the trachea from regurgitated food or from pressure on the trachea from distention of the diverticulum.

Diagnostic Assessment

A barium swallow is performed to locate diverticulum. Endoscopy is usually contraindicated because the diverticulum may be perforated by the endoscope.

Medical Management

Medical management of symptoms from a diverticulum is achieved through dietary management and positioning. Small, frequent feedings of semisoft foods often facilitate passage of food. The client should note what foods relieve or exacerbate the symptoms.

To prevent reflux of food, the client should have the head of the bed raised for 2 hours after meals. Nocturnal reflux can often be prevented by sleeping with the head of the bed elevated. The client also should avoid constrictive clothes and vigorous exercise after eating.

Surgical Management

When symptoms become severe, surgery may be indicated. A cervical approach is used for Zenker's diverticulum, whereas a thoracic approach is used for diverticulum located lower in the esophagus. In both procedures, the diverticulum is excised and the esophageal mucosa is reanastomosed.

Nursing Management

Assessment

The nurse should obtain a history from the client, noting symptoms. The nurse should note the onset and duration of symptoms, and whether or not they occur at mealtimes or at night. The nurse also should assess the client's respiratory status because regurgitation can cause respiratory complications.

Nursing Diagnosis, Planning, and Implementation

Nursing Diagnosis: Pain R/T dysphagia.

Planning: Expected Outcomes. The client will have a decrease in pain or an absence of pain, as evidenced by the client verbalizing that the pain is decreased or absent and by the client's ability to maintain oral intake.

Implementation. The nurse should teach the client about the necessary changes in diet and how positioning can control symptoms. The nurse should encourage the client to try various foods and various positions to evaluate which are most effective.

Collaborative Problem: Risk for Injury R/T surgical procedure and possible chest tubes.

Planning: Expected Outcomes. Injury will be prevented, as evidenced by absence of hemorrhage, no signs of infection, normal temperature, and absence of signs of problems associated with the chest tubes such as respiratory distress.

Implementation. The nurse should discuss the normal preoperative routines. The client should be told he or she will not be permitted to take anything by mouth after surgery and will have a nasogastric tube. If a thoracic approach is used, the preoperative and postoperative nursing care is similar to that for clients having thoracic surgery and chest tubes (see Chap. 22 for the care of the client after a thoracotomy and with chest tubes).

After surgery, the client's nasogastric tube will be attached to low suction.

CRITICAL TO REMEMBER

The nurse should assess the amount and color of the drainage during each shift and check for continued bloody nasogastric drainage as well as for signs of external bleeding.

Small amounts of bloody drainage may appear for up to 12 hours after surgery. The nurse should not irrigate or reposition the nasogastric tube unless specifically ordered by the physician.

The client will receive intravenous fluids until tube feedings are begun. Once fluids and supplemental feedings are begun, the nurse should record the client's response. The nurse should assess the client for signs of esophageal perforation, such as chest pain, elevated temperature, and subcutaneous emphysema.

The nurse should assess the client's pain and administer analgesics as ordered. After surgery, the head of the bed should be elevated 30 degrees to decrease edema. Frequent practice of oral hygiene increases the client's comfort.

Evaluation

The nurse must evaluate client outcomes based on the established plan of care. If these goals are not achieved, the plan and interventions must be revised to meet the client's needs.

Modification of Plan of Care for the Elderly

Older adults are treated more conservatively, using diet and positioning rather than surgery. Surgery may entail too much risk for the older client.

Client Teaching

The client who had surgery may be discharged with a nasogastric or a gastrostomy tube in place to allow for esophageal healing. The client should have written and verbal instructions about tube feedings, diet, and positioning. Also, the client should be instructed regarding signs and symptoms of infection, perforation, and hemorrhage.

A nurse from a home health-care agency should see the client at home to ensure that the tube feedings are being tolerated well. The client who has had surgery will need to be seen at intervals until the feeding tube can be removed.

ESOPHAGEAL NEOPLASMS

Cancer of the esophagus takes the form of either squamous cell carcinoma or adenocarcinoma of the esophageal mucosa.

Incidence

In the United States, the incidence of squamous cell cancer of the esophagus is 4 per 100,000 males. The incidence is twice as high in men as in women, and it is higher in black, Japanese, and Chinese males than in white males. Adenocarcinoma of the esophagus occurs less often than squamous cell cancer and develops primarily in the distal esophagus.

Etiology

The cause of esophageal neoplasms is unknown, but researchers are studying environmental differences between locations with a low and a high incidence. In the Western world, evidence points to heavy smoking, nutritional deficiencies, and habitual ingestion of alcohol, hot foods, and hot drinks as underlying etiologic factors.

Chronic irritation from other esophageal problems such as achalasia, hiatal hernia, and stricture play a minor role in the development of esophageal cancer.

Risk Factors

The major risk factors are long-term use of alcohol and tobacco combined with poor nutrition. The presence of achalasia, hiatal hernia, reflux, stricture, or poor oral hygiene increases the risk for esophageal cancer. These are very preventable causes.

Pathophysiology

Malignant tumors of the esophagus begin as slow-growing benign tissue changes. Esophageal tumors expand locally and very rapidly, and early spread to the lymph nodes is common. Because the esophagus has no serosal layer to limit its extension, the tumor spreads rapidly. The rich lymphatic supply to the mucosa provides an excellent means for the tumor to metastasize widely.

The disease is progressive and almost always fatal. As it progresses, most clients experience some pulmonary complications because of the formation of tracheoesophageal fistulas that result in aspiration.

Clinical Manifestations

Typically the first symptoms are dysphagia or odynophagia. By the time the client becomes aware of a swallowing problem and seeks medical care, the tumor frequently has invaded the deeper layers of the esophagus and, sometimes, adjacent structures such as the bronchus.

At first, dysphagia is usually mild and intermittent, occurring only after ingestion of solid food (especially meat). Soon, dysphagia becomes constant, and signs of esophageal obstruction appear. These signs include an increase in salivation and mucus in the throat, nocturnal aspiration, regurgitation, and inability to swallow even liquids.

Diagnostic Assessment

The diagnosis is confirmed by barium swallow, endoscopy, cytologic examination, and direct biopsy. Computed tomography scans provide an excellent definition of the size of the primary lesion and the extent of nodal involvement.

Medical Management

Treatment of esophageal cancer depends on the location, size of the tumor, metastases, and the condition of the client.

Radiation therapy is often used alone or in conjunction with surgery. Radiation provides palliation by reducing the tumor size and slowing tumor growth. High-dose radiation therapy may cause stenosis of the esophagus, so radiation treatments are usually administered over a 6- to 8-week period to minimize this effect.

DIETARY MANAGEMENT

Maintaining nutrition is a major goal for the client with esophageal cancer. If necessary, a feeding gastrostomy or jejunostomy may be created. Short-term total parenteral nutrition (TPN) may be used to improve the client's nutritional status before surgery.

CRITICAL TO REMEMBER

Proper positioning after meals is necessary in the client with frequent regurgitation as well as in the client with a prosthesis. The head of the bed should always be elevated 30 degrees.

Surgical Management

Esophageal dilatation may be necessary throughout the course of the disease to treat strictures and tumor obstruction. The treatment should be performed by the physician as often as needed to relieve dysphagia.

Surgery may be performed for cure or palliation, depending on the extent of the disease. Three surgical procedures can be performed. An esophagectomy is the removal of all or part of the esophagus. The resected esophagus is replaced with a Dacron graft. The esophagogastrostomy involves resecting the lower portion of the esophagus and anastomosing the remainder to the stomach, brought up into the thorax. The third procedure, esophagoenterostomy (also known as a colon interposition), involves resecting the esophagus and replacing it with a segment of the descending colon.

Nursing Management

Assessment

The nurse needs to obtain data concerning the client's nutritional status. Most clients complain of dysphagia that is both persistent and progressive.

A careful assessment of dysphagia is important. Other symptoms such as odynophagia, regurgitation, chronic cough, increased secretions, and hoarseness (caused by involvement of the larynx) also are important to assess.

Nursing Diagnosis, Planning, and Implementation

Nursing Diagnosis: Nutrition, Altered: Less than Body Requirements R/T client's inability to swallow.

Planning: Expected Outcomes. The client will maintain an adequate nutritional status, as evidenced by maintenance of stable body weight or slowed weight loss.

Implementation. The nurse must monitor the client's nutritional status throughout treatment. Daily weight, intake and output, and calorie intake are carefully monitored. In the beginning, the nurse should teach the client about diet changes that can make eating easier.

As the disease progresses, the nurse may have to provide tube feedings. The nurse must assess skin around the gastrostomy openings for impairment of skin integrity resulting from leakage of gastric juices. The skin around the opening should be washed with a gentle soap and thoroughly dried twice daily or as needed. Protective ointments such as zinc oxide or Karaya may be applied to the skin for further protection.

Specific nutritional support may include high-calorie, high-protein oral feedings, soft foods in small frequent meals, nasogastric tube feedings, or TPN. Clients are taught to remain upright after meals and to elevate the head of the bed on blocks. Recurrence of symptoms may mean development of an esophageal stricture or tumor regrowth.

Nursing Diagnosis: Swallowing, Impaired, Risk for R/T esophageal obstruction from tumor.

Planning: Expected Outcomes. The client will not experience impaired swallowing, as evidenced by absence of choking and maintenance of patent airway.

Implementation. Many problems arise when the client is unable to swallow. The client can easily choke on saliva and mucous secretions and must spit frequently or drool. Constant wiping of saliva from the lips can cause irritation, cracking of the skin, and open lesions. Because it is impractical to collect this quantity of secretions in tissues, the client should carry a receptacle to receive the saliva. To prevent oral lesions and infections, and to provide comfort, the nurse should administer or assist with frequent oral care.

Nursing Diagnosis: Individual Coping, Ineffective, Risk for R/T changes in body image and potentially terminal prognosis.

Planning: Expected Outcomes. The client will effectively cope with the alterations in body image and potentially terminal prognosis, as evidenced by client's maintenance of activities and continued social interaction by the client.

Implementation. In addition to meeting the client's physical needs, the nurse must provide emotional support. The gastrostomy tube may cause an alteration in body image and increased dependency. The drooling or need to spit constantly also may cause the client a great deal of emotional distress.

The poor prognosis of esophageal cancer necessitates psychological support and interventions aimed at helping the client and significant others prepare for the client's peaceful death.

Collaborative Problem: Risk for Injury R/T surgical procedure.

Planning: Expected Outcomes. Injury will be prevented, as evidenced by absence of atelectasis, fever, wound infection, or problems associated with the chest tubes.

Implementation. Before surgery, clients usually require 2 to 3 weeks of nutritional support. Often, this support includes tube feedings or hyperalimentation. Oral care should be performed four times a day to help prevent infection postoperatively. If an esophagoenterostomy is performed, a complete bowel preparation is performed before surgery.

After surgery, respiratory care is a high priority. The client may be placed on a ventilator (see Chap. 20 for care of a client receiving mechanical ventilation) in a critical care unit. Otherwise, the client must turn, cough, and deep breathe every hour. Supplemental oxygen is administered. Pain medication must be administered frequently, and the nurse should assist the client in splinting the incision while coughing. The client is placed in a semi-Fowler's position to prevent reflux. The nurse should continually monitor the chest tube drainage for amount, color, and patency.

The nurse must assess the client's fluid and electrolyte status. The drainage from the nasogastric, gastric, and all other drainage tubes should be monitored at least every shift. The client will not be permitted to take anything by mouth for 4 to 5 days until peristalsis returns.

CRITICAL TO REMEMBER

During the first 24 hours after surgery, nasogastric or gastric drainage is bloody but should then change to a greenish-yellow color. If bloody drainage continues, it could indicate bleeding at the suture line and should be reported.

Leakage at the site of anastomosis may appear about 5 to 7 days after surgery. The nurse must assess the client for signs and symptoms of postoperative complications (see Chap. 5).

The client should be started on small sips of water. If this intake is tolerated, the quantity is slowly increased. The nurse must supervise the client, making sure the client stays in an upright position, and monitor for signs of leakage at the anastomosis site. If this is tolerated, the client gradually progresses to pureed and semisolid foods. The client must be taught the importance of small, frequent feedings and always sitting upright with meals and for 1 hour after meals to prevent overdistention of the stomach and reflux.

The client should be taught about possible wound and respiratory complications and symptoms that should be reported immediately.

The nurse should make appropriate referrals to community agencies. Most clients need a significant amount of assistance at home. Significant others should be given information about services offered from the American Cancer Society and local hospice care.

Evaluation

The nurse must evaluate client outcomes based on the established plan of care. If these goals were not achieved, the plan and interventions must be revised to meet the client's needs.

VASCULAR DISORDERS

The principal vascular disorder of the esophagus is varices. Because esophageal varices result from portal hypertension, this condition is discussed with liver disorders in Chapter 37.

TRAUMA

Major traumatic conditions of the esophagus include chemical burns (from ingestion of acids or alkalis), presence of foreign bodies, and injuries from external forces, such as endoscopic equipment. Trauma can cause esophageal perforation with resultant contamination of the mediastinum and stricture formation as healing occurs.

Treatment for esophageal strictures involves dilatation of the esophagus or surgical excision of the diseased portion and reanastomosis or interposition of a piece of gut from the stomach or colon (see the section on esophageal neoplasms).

STUDY QUESTIONS

1. In caring for the postesophageal surgery client, the priority nursing assessment is
   A. Fluid balance
   B. Respiratory status
   C. Swallowing ability
   D. Level of consciousness
2. A client has been diagnosed with oral candidiasis. A change in diet is recommended to improve comfort with eating. Which of the following should the nurse encourage?
   A. Orange juice
   B. Hot tea

C. White wine
D. A vanilla milkshake

3. A client is scheduled for local resection of an oral tumor. Which statement made by the client indicates an understanding of preoperative teaching?
A. "I'll have a permanent tracheostomy in place when I wake up."
B. "I'll have pain medication ordered postoperatively."
C. "I won't be able to perform oral hygiene measures for 7 days postoperatively."
D. "I will remain on bedrest for 7 days postoperatively."

4. A nurse is discussing medication scheduling with a client who has been prescribed an antacid medication (Mylanta) and ranitidine. Which statement by the nurse is correct?
A. "Take the medications at the same time."
B. "Take the medications 30 minutes apart."
C. "Take the medications 3 hours apart."
D. "Take the medications on alternate days."

5. Life-style management is important in the discharge planning of a client with gastroesophageal reflux disease (GERD). Which of the following risk factors should be eliminated or reduced in the client's life-style?
A. Smoking two packs of cigarettes per day
B. Playing tennis three times per week
C. Alcohol consumption at social gatherings
D. Acetaminophen for headache

CRITICAL THINKING EXERCISES

SCENARIO A

A 70-year-old woman has been diagnosed with hiatal hernia. She complains of heartburn an hour after meals. She is overweight and drinks alcohol occasionally at social functions. After repair of the hernia, she prepares for discharge from the hospital.

1. What activities should the client avoid during the initial 6-week recovery period?
2. What implications regarding medication therapy with ranitidine and antacids should the client be taught?
3. What dietary restrictions should the client observe?

SCENARIO B

A 40-year-old Chinese man is concerned about his risk of esophageal cancer. He grew up in Northern China and has lived in the United States for 10 years. He began smoking when he came to the United States. His father died of esophageal cancer at age 55 years.

1. What etiologic factors should be considered when counseling the client?
2. How can the client modify his life-style to decrease his risk of esophageal cancer?
3. What early symptoms of the disease should he be taught?

BIBLIOGRAPHY

1. American Cancer Society (1995). *Cancer facts and figures—1995.* New York: Author.
2. Andreoli, T. E., et al. (Eds.). (1993). *Cecil essentials of medicine* (3rd ed.). Philadelphia: W. B. Saunders.
3. Armstrong, D. (1994). Reflux disease and Barrett's oesophagus. *Endoscopy, 26,* 9–19.
4. Baird, S. B., et al. (1991). *Cancer nursing: A comprehensive textbook.* Philadelphia: W. B. Saunders.
5. Barkin, J., & Rogers, A. (Eds.). (1994). *Difficult decisions in digestive diseases* (2nd ed.). St. Louis: Mosby-Year Book.
6. Bates, B. A. (1991). *A guide to physical examination and history taking* (5th ed.). Philadelphia: J. B. Lippincott.
7. Bayliss, T. M. (Ed.). (1994). *Current therapy in gastroenterology and liver disease* (4th ed.). St. Louis: Mosby-Year Book.
8. Beahrs, O. H., et al. (Eds.). (1992). *Manual for staging of cancer* (4th ed.). Philadelphia: J. B. Lippincott.
9. Blot, W., et al. (1991). Rising incidence of adenocarcinoma of the esophagus and gastric cardia. *JAMA, 271,* 1287–1294.
10. Boring, C. C., et al. (1992). Cancer statistics, 1992. *CA, 42,* 19–43.
11. Cameron, J. L. (Ed.). (1992). *Current surgical therapy* (4th ed.). St. Louis: Mosby-Year Book.
12. Cumming, C. W., et al. (1993). *Otolaryngology—head and neck surgery* (2nd ed.). St. Louis: Mosby-Year Book.
13. Davis, J. H., et al. (Eds.). (1994). *Surgery: A problem-solving approach* (2nd ed.). St. Louis: Mosby-Year Book.
14. Frank-Stromberg, M. (1989). The epidemiology and primary prevention of gastric and esophageal cancer. *Cancer Nursing, 12,* 53–64.
15. Gaynor, E. B. (1991). Otolaryngologic manifestations of gastroesophageal reflux. *American Journal of Gastroenterology, 86,* 801–808.
16. Gitnik, G., et al. (Eds.). (1994). *Principles and practice of gastroenterology and hepatology* (2nd ed.). Norwalk, CT: Appleton & Lange.
17. Greenberger, N. J. (1989). *Gastrointestinal disorders: A pathophysiologic approach* (4th ed.). St. Louis: Mosby-Year Book.
18. Groenwald, S. L., et al. (Eds.). (1991). *Cancer nursing: Principles and practice* (2nd ed.). Boston: Jones & Bartlett.
19. Guyton, A. C. (1991). *Textbook of medical physiology* (8th ed.). Philadelphia: W. B. Saunders.

20. Haubrich, W. S., et al. (1995). *Bockus gastroenterology* (5th ed.). Philadelphia: W. B. Saunders.

21. Huber, D., et al. (1994). GI nursing: The community health aspect. *Gastroenterology Nursing, 16,* 219–223.

22. Hurwitz, S. (1993). *Clinical pediatric dermatology: A textbook of skin disorders* (2nd ed.). Philadelphia: W. B. Saunders.

23. Isselbacher, K. J. (Ed.). (1994). *Harrison's principles of internal medicine* (13th ed.). New York: McGraw-Hill.

24. Johnson, L. R., et al. (1994). *Physiology of the gastrointestinal tract* (3rd ed.). New York: Raven.

25. Kitchin, L. I., et al. (1991). Rationale and efficacy of conservative therapy for gastroesophageal reflux disease. *Archives of Internal Medicine, 151,* 448–454.

26. Kotler, D. P. (Ed.). (1991). *Gastrointestinal and nutritional manifestations of the acquired immunodeficiency syndrome.* New York: Raven.

27. Lang, C. A., et al. (1994). Fecal occult blood screening for colorectal cancer. *JAMA, 271,* 1011–1013.

28. Lehne, R. (1994). *Pharmacology for nursing care* (2nd ed.). Philadelphia: W. B. Saunders.

29. Mashberg, A., & Samit, A. M. (1989). Early detection, diagnosis and management of oral and oropharyngeal cancer. *CA, 39,* 67–88.

30. Moschella, S. L., & Hurley, H. J. (1992). *Dermatology* (3rd ed.). Philadelphia: W. B. Saunders.

31. Payne, W. S., & Ellis, F. H., Jr. (1994). Esophagus and diaphragmatic hernias. In S. I. Schwartz, et al. (Eds.), *Principles of surgery* (6th ed.). New York: McGraw-Hill.

32. Rabeneck, L., et al. (1990). Acute HIV infection presenting with painful swallowing and esophageal ulcers. *JAMA, 263,* 2318–2311.

33. Sabiston, D. C., Jr. (1991). *Textbook of surgery: The biologic basis of modern surgical practice* (14th ed.). Philadelphia: W. B. Saunders.

34. Sacher, R. A., & McPherson, R. A. (1991). *Widmann's clinical interpretation of laboratory tests* (10th ed.). Philadelphia: F. A. Davis.

35. Shaffer, E., & Thomson, A. B. R. (1989). *Modern concepts of gastroenterology.* New York: Plenum.

36. Shklar, G. (1994). The oral cavity, jaws, and salivary glands. In R. S. Cotran, et al. (Eds.), *Robbins pathologic basis of disease* (5th ed.). Philadelphia: W. B. Saunders.

37. Sleisenger, M. H., & Fordtran, J. S. (Eds.). (1993). *Gastrointestinal disease: pathophysiology, diagnosis, and management* (5th ed.). Philadelphia: W. B. Saunders.

38. Sloan, S., & Kahrilas, P. J. (1991). Impairment of esophageal emptying with hiatal hernia. *Gastroenterology, 100,* 596.

39. Society of Gastroenterology Nurses and Associates. (1993). *Gastroenterology nursing: A core curriculum.* St. Louis: Mosby-Year Book.

40. Wyngaarden, J. B., et al. (Eds.). (1992). *Cecil textbook of medicine* (19th ed.). Philadelphia: W. B. Saunders.

41. Yamada, T. (Ed.). (1991). *Textbook of gastroenterology.* Philadelphia: J. B. Lippincott.

Chapter 34

Nursing Care of Clients with Gastric Disorders

Learning Outcomes

After completing this chapter, the learner will be able to:

1. Assess the client for clinical manifestations of gastric disorders.
2. Teach the client about the etiology, risk factors, basic pathophysiology, and clinical manifestations of major gastric disorders.
3. Explain the client's role in medical and surgical management of gastric disorders.
4. Develop plans of care for the prevention of illness, management, and rehabilitation of clients with gastric disorders.
5. Implement nursing interventions that optimize the quality of life for clients with gastric disorders.
6. Evaluate the client outcomes using criteria developed in the planning phase of care.

Digestion, which starts in the mouth, continues in the stomach. Protein breakdown and the secretion of gastric juices begin this next phase of digestion. The chief functions of the stomach are to mix and liquefy the bolus of food into chyme and to regulate the flow of gastric contents into the upper intestine. The rate of gastric emptying depends on the volume of food ingested, the size of the particles, the amount of acid production, and the nature of the ingested food. Very little absorption takes place within the stomach. However, the stomach does absorb alcohol, small quantities of water, glucose, and some medications such as acetylsalicylic acid.

GENERALIZED CLINICAL MANIFESTATIONS

Manifestations of gastric dysfunction are caused by excessive gastric secretions that feed on stomach mucosa, excessive motility, or retention of gastric contents. The most prominent symptoms are pain, acid eructation, anorexia, belching, nausea, vomiting, hemorrhaging, and diarrhea.

Pain, the most characteristic symptom, usually results from chemical irritation of nerve endings. Nerve irritation develops when acid comes into contact with the eroded stomach mucosa. It also results from stretching and contracting of the stomach, caused, in turn, by increased motility and increased smooth muscle tension, as is found in an obstruction.

Anorexia, persistent loss of appetite, is often experienced by clients with malignancy or various other disorders. Hunger is normally caused by a number of stimuli, including contraction of the empty stomach. When the stomach empties slowly or there is gastric stasis because of a gastric disorder, anorexia can result.

Nausea is a result of conditions that increase tension on the walls of the stomach, duodenum, or lower end of the esophagus. Unpleasant stimuli or distention, gastritis, and carcinoma of the stomach can produce nausea. Vomiting may follow nausea or occur without it. Recall from Chapter 32 that vomiting is caused by stimulation of the emetic center.

Bleeding results from local trauma or irritations that cause erosion or ulceration of the GI mucosa. The disorders involved include stomach neoplasms, gastric ulcer, gastritis, anastomotic (marginal) ulcers, and duodenal ulcers. Up to three quarters of all cases of upper GI tract bleeding result from esophagogastric varices (venous), hemorrhagic gastritis (capillary), or peptic ulcer.

Diarrhea can be caused by increased peristalsis resulting from an increased gastrocolic reflex or from the effort of the stomach and intestines to eliminate a local irritant.

Belching and *flatulence* result predominantly from swallowed air. Frequently, clients attempt to belch to relieve a vague feeling of distress in the stomach caused by swallowed air.

Dyspepsia (indigestion) can be caused by such factors as strong emotions, GI tract disease, eating too rapidly, inadequate chewing, gas-forming foods (e.g., beans and cabbage), or food allergy.

NUTRITIONAL SUPPORT

Nutritional support is commonly required for clients with gastrointestinal problems. Two types of nutritional support commonly used are enteral nutrition and parenteral nutrition.

Enteral Nutrition

Enteral nutrition is nutrients (containing needed fats, carbohydrates, and proteins) that the client takes in via the gastrointestinal tract. This nutrition can be supplemental to the general diet or can replace oral intake totally.

All kinds of intestinal tubes exist for the administration of enteral feedings in clients who are unable to take them orally. There are nasogastric, gastric, duodenal, and jejunal tubes. Tube feedings are administered either as a bolus feeding or by continuous infusion. The feeding can be administered by bolus push, gravity drainage, or infusion pump. The choice of the type of infusion and method of delivery will depend on the disease and the client's ability to tolerate the feedings.

Gastrointestinal feedings have a number of advantages over parenteral nutrition. There are many physiologic benefits associated with enteral feedings. They help to maintain GI structure (villi height and number) and the mucosal barrier. They also help maintain GI motility, which discourages bacterial overgrowth.

Problems associated with tube feedings include a variety of fluid and electrolyte disturbances. The client's fluid and electrolyte status is monitored closely, and the make-up of the feeding is altered to accommodate any disturbances. Diarrhea is also a common but controllable problem associated with these feedings. Usually decreasing the concentration of the feeding or slowing the rate of administration controls the problem.

When the client is receiving tube feedings via a nasogastric or gastrostomy tube, an important nursing function is to check tube placement before each feeding, before medication administration, or at least every 4 hours. Tube placement can be assessed by either aspirating tube contents for the presence of gastric contents or injecting air with a syringe while listening over the stomach for the movement of the air. This client should also be carefully positioned to prevent aspiration. When the feedings are administered, the client should be in semi- or high-Fowler's position on the right side (see Client Education Guide: Nasogastric Feeding).

Another important nursing intervention is to check for residual after the feedings. Either at regular intervals or usually 1 hour after bolus feedings, the nurse aspi-

CLIENT EDUCATION GUIDE

Nasogastric Feedings

The nurse must teach the client and significant others to perform the following:

- Maintain tube patency; consistently flushing the tube after each feeding with water followed by cola prolongs tube life
- Secure the tube firmly to the client's nose or to either side of the face in a position of comfort
- Always determine whether the tube is in the correct position before starting any infusion
- Follow the physician's, nurse's, and dietitian's recommendations for the tube feeding preparation and the rate and frequency of infusion
- Have the client sit at a 45-degree angle or greater to improve toleration of feedings
- Consult with a home care agency to provide an important resource; they can contact the agency if the tube is accidentally removed or if other difficulties occur, such as tube displacement or client symptoms such as cramping, nausea, and diarrhea.

rates the tube to assess the amount of feeding left in the stomach. If the residual is high, then problems may exist at the gastric outlet and the risk for aspiration increases. The nurse should manage a high residual according to agency protocol, that is, stop the feeding for the specified time and notify the physician.

Parenteral Nutrition (Total Parenteral Nutrition)

Two types of solution are administered when the client receives total parenteral nutrition: amino acid–dextrose solutions and fat emulsions. The amino acid–dextrose solution can contain additives such as electrolytes, sodium, potassium, chloride, calcium, magnesium, phosphate, and trace elements (zinc, copper, chromium, and manganese).

Many clients with GI tract disorders are unable to ingest, digest, or absorb sufficient nutrients to maintain themselves in a state of anabolism or positive nitrogen balance. Total parenteral nutrition (TPN) may also be used to rest the GI tract when there is a fistula or inflammatory bowel disease or after an intestinal obstruction is removed. TPN is most commonly administered through an indwelling subclavian catheter into the superior vena cava (Fig. 34–1). TPN is usually administered in a large vein because solutions used for TPN are hypertonic. Most fat emulsions, however, are isotonic.

Major complications of TPN therapy are infection, hyperglycemia, hypoglycemia, and other electrolyte imbalances.

Clients receiving TPN are very susceptible to infection, especially *Candida* septicemia. Glucose solutions are a medium for infection.

CRITICAL TO REMEMBER

The nurse must exercise stringent surgical asepsis in hanging TPN solutions, assisting with catheter insertion, or changing solutions or dressings.

A filter is used in the intravenous tubing to trap bacteria and particles. The solution and administration equipment must be changed every 24 hours. Dressing changes are done every 48 to 72 hours on the basis of hospital policy. Povidone-iodine (Betadine) or an antibiotic ointment is often applied to the catheter insertion site with each dressing change, and an occlusive dressing is applied. Unused solution is always discarded. The only solution that should be infused in the same line as TPN is lipids. Medication is never administered in a TPN line.

When the rate of glucose infusion is faster than the rate of glucose metabolism, hyperglycemia results. The nurse must check the infusion rate every hour. Blood sugar is usually monitored every 6 hours. Even with steady rates, the client's blood sugar may be elevated because of the high levels of glucose being administered. The physician will often order a varying amount of regular insulin to be given, which is based on the client's blood sugar levels.

One of the body's major responses to high blood glucose levels, such as those found in clients receiving TPN, is increased insulin output from the pancreas. When a hypertonic glucose infusion is abruptly interrupted, insulin levels remain high while glucose levels decline, which results in rebound hypoglycemia.

Venous thrombosis is another possible complication. It is characterized by neck vein distention (unilateral); unilateral edema of the arm, neck, or face; and shoulder pain. If this is suspected, notify the physician immediately.

When caring for clients receiving total parenteral nutrition, the nurse must monitor vital signs and espe-

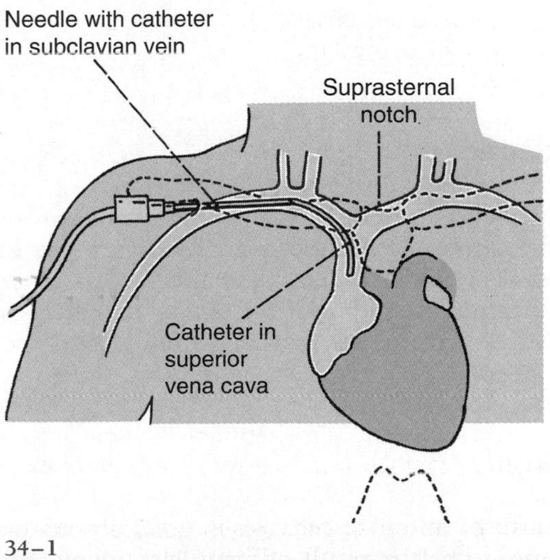

Figure 34–1
Insertion of catheter into superior vena cava via right subclavian vein. Once in place, this catheter may be used for the administration of total parenteral nutrition.

cially note an increase in temperature (a possible sign of infection). The nurse also monitors the intake and output, closely assessing for signs of dehydration or overhydration. Nutritional status must be monitored with daily weights, biochemical blood tests such as blood urea nitrogen (BUN), creatinine, electrolytes, and minerals. The infusion site should be checked for signs and symptoms of infection or inflammation. The nurse should use appropriate techniques to administer TPN, including the following:

- Always use an infusion pump.
- Always start TPN at a slow rate (usually 1 L over 24 hours).
- Do not abruptly discontinue TPN. If TPN stops or the next bottle is unavailable, administer a 10 per cent dextrose solution until the correct fluid can be obtained.

Eating Disorders

Over the past several decades, eating disorders have become of increasing concern to nurses and other health-care professionals. Anorexia nervosa and bulimia are now recognized as potentially life-threatening problems.

ANOREXIA NERVOSA

Anorexia nervosa is a loss of at least 15 to 25 per cent of ideal body weight as a result of voluntary restriction of food intake. Clients with anorexia nervosa experience severe weight loss, related physiologic changes associated with starvation, and a complex of distorted mental perceptions such as alterations in body image, weight phobia, and obsessive self-starvation associated with the fear of being fat.

Incidence

The incidence of anorexia nervosa is increasing; the high-risk group is American girls between the ages of 12 and 18 years. It most commonly occurs in females from the middle and upper class in the Western culture. Males account for approximately 5 to 10 per cent of the population with anorexia nervosa.

Etiology

The cause of anorexia nervosa is not fully understood. It appears to be the result of many factors interacting in a vulnerable client. The importance of each factor to a client can vary.

Risk Factors

Young women with low self-esteem seem to be the highest risk group because they see thinness as a way to improve their self-confidence. The culture in this country that seems to worship the thin model encourages young girls to try to match this appearance.

Pathophysiology

The obvious pathologic changes associated with anorexia nervosa are physiologic, but the real disorder is psychological. The pathophysiologic changes include changes associated with the effects of starvation.

Untreated, this disorder can be fatal when life-threatening fluid and electrolyte imbalances occur because of the limited intake.

Clinical Manifestations

Clients usually seek medical attention when weight loss is apparent. Other symptoms, probably caused by the state of starvation, include amenorrhea, cachexia, constipation, fine hair over the body, dry and sandpaper-like skin, bradycardia, periods of hyperactivity, hypothermia, and hypotension. The blood pressure may be as low as 60/40. To induce weight loss, anorexics often subsist on fewer than 600 calories/day, or if they eat more, they vomit. Eventually, severe dieting causes extreme wasting and cachexia. The facial puffiness, caused by parotid hypertrophy, contrasts with the wasting of the rest of the body.

Clients usually deny the existence of any problem, except a feeling of being fat. They seem to enjoy losing weight as evidence that they are achieving their goals. They often exhibit bizarre rituals associated with food.

DIAGNOSTIC ASSESSMENT

Clients often suffer from profound anemia and electrolyte abnormalities. If the client is dehydrated, the BUN may be elevated. Often serum cholesterol levels are elevated, although the reason for this is not fully understood. Other diagnostic tests may include a chest radiograph and electrocardiogram. Often, psychological testing is done by a psychiatrist as part of the diagnostic process.

Medical Management

Nutritional rehabilitation and improvement of self-image are necessary for the client with anorexia. Intervention must first focus on improving the state of nutrition so the client can undertake psychotherapy for the underlying problem. Eating is the preferred method of achieving weight gain, but sometimes the client refuses to comply. In this case, the physician may institute tube feedings. In addition, the client may receive a combined program of psychotherapy and behavior modification. Intervention normally involves the client's significant others.

BULIMIA NERVOSA

Bulimia, also known as compulsive eating with self-induced vomiting, is another nutritional disorder. Bulimia can overlap with anorexia nervosa; that is, anorexic clients may have bulimia episodes.

Incidence

Bulimia is a common problem, especially among young women during late adolescence and young adulthood. Clients are typically normal weight and from middle- to upper-class socioeconomic background. Most clients with bulimia maintain their weight but weigh less than the norm for their age and height.

Etiology

As with anorexia nervosa, no one knows exactly what causes bulimia. One theory is that bulimia is a primary neurologic dysfunction, an electrical disorder, similar to epilepsy. Another is that the disorder is caused by a disturbance in the appetite-satiety center of the hypothalamus. Some researchers believe bulimia is learned behavior for dealing with stress and unpleasant feelings. Onset of the disorder can sometimes be traced to the young woman having been on a strict weight loss diet.

Risk Factors

The major factor, as with anorexia, is based on the societal image of the thin woman. These clients often have a history of poor family relations with low self-esteem and a history of poor impulse control.

Pathophysiology

Clients often binge after some psychological-emotional factor such as depression, anxiety, anger, or even boredom. Bulimics ingest tremendous amounts of food during these binges without extremes of hunger as the trigger. They may feel some hunger as a trigger; however, the intake of food is out of proportion to the hunger being felt.

Bulimics often do experience weight gains on low-calorie diets and may have a history of being overweight. When they restrict their intake, they may have difficulty losing weight. They find that a large intake of food followed by purging controls their weight.

Clients are aware that the eating pattern is abnormal and they fear they will lose complete control and be unable to stop eating at all. Other types of excessive behavior may be exhibited, such as alcohol or drug abuse or sexual promiscuity. The client has poor impulse control resulting in overindulgence in many aspects of life.

Clinical Manifestations

Assessment reveals a history of repeated binge-eating episodes (rapid consumption of a large amount of food in 2 hours or less), with an awareness of abnormality and a fear of being unable to stop eating. Eating binges are followed by a depressed mood and self-deprecating thoughts. Manifestations of bulimia include consumption of high-calorie and easily ingested foods, inconspicuous eating, abdominal pain, excessive sleeping, self-induced vomiting, repeated attempts to lose weight, and frequent weight fluctuations of 10 pounds or more.

Vomiting, the primary method of purging, decreases the physical pain of abdominal distention. Some clients use laxatives or severely restrictive diets after a bulimia episode. Amphetamines, diuretics, fasting, and excessive exercise may also be used to avoid gaining weight. Other psychological symptoms include impaired impulse control, fear of obesity, and low self-esteem. Bulimics, unlike clients with anorexia, report a strong appetite and usually binge several times a day.

Depression, marked by feelings of gloom, suicidal thoughts, irritability, and impaired concentration, is common. Clients with long-term bulimia also report loneliness, boredom, and anger. Except for frequent weight fluctuations, there are no known clinical signs of bulimia. Chronic vomiting, however, can lead to tooth damage (erosion of the enamel), irritation of the throat and esophagus, swelling of the salivary glands (caused by acidic reflux and constant stimulation), fluid and electrolyte imbalances, and occasionally fistulas of the upper GI tract. Laxative abuse may further aggravate fluid and electrolyte imbalance and may cause rectal bleeding.

Medical Management

Intervention for bulimia has two goals: to interrupt the binge-purge cycle by helping the client gain control of eating habits and to change attitudes toward food, eating, body size, and self. Intervention for bulimia includes pharmacotherapy, aversion therapy, and psychotherapy; sometimes a monoamine oxidase inhibitor medication (tranylcypromine sulfate) may be ordered to decrease the client's urge to binge. The most widely used modes of treatment are individual psychotherapy and self-help groups. Family therapy is also recommended to improve family interactions. Clients are encouraged to strengthen and explore relationships with family members.

OBESITY

Obesity is defined as weight 20 per cent or greater than the desirable weight for adults of a given sex and height.

Etiology

Obesity is usually caused by a caloric intake that exceeds the energy expenditure. When food intake equals metabolic needs, weight remains fairly constant throughout life. A weight gain sometimes accompanies aging because the client does not adjust food intake to lowered metabolism and diminished activity.

Complications

Atherosclerosis and its associated ischemic heart disease are caused by the altered metabolism of obesity. Hypertension and left ventricular hypertrophy occur because blood must be pumped through an enlarged vascular bed. Diabetes mellitus is four times more common in the obese client. Also, studies indicate a link between obesity and breast, endometrial, and ovarian cancer.

Medical Management

Activity increases both the energy output and the caloric deficit of a client after a weight loss diet. Thus, it is an excellent intervention. Any obese client on a calorie-restricted program should also have a planned, gradually increasing exercise program to help with weight loss and muscle tone.

The best intervention for obesity is appetite re-education, in which the client learns to eat and be satisfied with nutritious, well-balanced foods that are low in calories. Other support staff, such as the dietitian, is used to provide teaching about nutrition. Support groups such as Take Off Pounds Sensibly (TOPS), a nonprofit organization, Overeaters Anonymous, and Weight Watchers help some clients. Because weight tends to be self-sustaining, vigilance and continued support are needed to maintain weight losses. No approach will work, however, unless the client is motivated to lose weight.

Surgical Management

Clients who do not respond to dietary methods of weight loss may require surgical procedures to lose weight. A number of surgical procedures can help the obese client. Many surgical approaches are designed to reduce the ability of the body to ingest or absorb ingested nutrients.

Food intake can be reduced by jaw wiring. Subcutaneous fat can be excised in a procedure called lipectomy. Both have advantages and disadvantages and do not always cause permanent weight reduction.

There are more permanent surgical approaches to weight loss. The surgical procedure currently done is the gastroplasty or gastric stapling. A small opening left in the line of staples allows food to enter the rest of the stomach slowly. Depending on the size of the pouch created, the client can eat only about 30 mL of food every 5 minutes until satisfied. Before surgery, the client should receive psychiatric evaluation and begin participation in a support group. Because these clients are high surgical risks, an extensive preoperative assessment should be conducted. Postoperatively, special care must be taken with the nasogastric tube for preventing disruption of the suture line. Pulmonary complications often occur with gastric stapling.

Nursing Management of Eating Disorders

Assessment

A thorough history is necessary to differentiate the type of eating disorder from other illnesses. The nurse should carefully collect demographic data such as age and sex and obtain a thorough medical history. The nurse should note the client's weight history, including the onset of the weight loss or weight gain and the reason for the change in weight. Information about the client's attitude and behavior related to food and weight are important.

CRITICAL TO REMEMBER

The client should describe his or her typical pattern of eating and be asked about the use of any appetite-suppressing medication, laxatives, and self-induced vomiting.

Exercise patterns can also be important. A sexual history, including a menstrual history, should be taken; it should be noted whether amenorrhea is present.

Nursing Diagnosis, Planning, and Implementation

Nursing Diagnosis: Nutrition, Altered: Less than Body Requirements R/T inadequate food intake (anorexia nervosa).

Planning: Expected Outcomes. The client will maintain body weight within normal limits for client, as evidenced by steady weight gain of 2 to 4 pounds/week until ideal weight is reached.

Implementation. When caring for a client with anorexia nervosa, the nurse should help the client select foods from all five food groups. The client is usually allowed to refuse a specific number of foods, such as two or three, so some sense of control is felt. The client must eat only those foods provided by the dietary department and must eat all the meal.

CRITICAL TO REMEMBER

Someone should remain with the client, talking, for at least 1 hour after meals so the client is supported and purging is prevented.

The nurse should maintain an accurate calorie count on the client. The diet should allow the client to gain 2 to 4 pounds/week. The client must be weighed at regular intervals.

The nurse can help prevent the development of anorexia nervosa through education. By helping the public learn about the disease and its causes and manifestations, the nurse can help prevent its development.

Nursing Diagnosis: Nutrition, Altered: More than Body Requirements R/T increased food intake (bulimia nervosa, obesity).

Planning: Expected Outcomes. The client will achieve body weight within normal limits for client, as evidenced by steady weight loss of 2 pounds/week until ideal weight is reached.

Implementation. The nurse must teach the client how to select a healthy diet with portions that are the correct size. Clients should be encouraged to eat slowly and to develop a regular exercise pattern. Exercise is important, especially in bulimics and the obese, because it allows increased calorie intake.

The nurse needs to help the client learn to eat a balanced diet from the five basic food groups, learn to choose proper foods in the right portions, and provide supervision and emotional support for the client to overcome stressful periods and break the binge-purge cycle.

Collaborative Problem: Cardiac Output, Risk for decreased R/T alterations in rhythm caused by hypokalemia (anorexia nervosa and bulimia).

Planning: Expected Outcomes. The client will maintain normal cardiac output, as evidenced by absence of cardiac dysrhythmias and adequate tissue perfusion.

Implementation. The nurse must monitor the client's serum potassium at regular intervals. If the potassium is low, potassium supplements must be administered as ordered. The client's potassium should return to normal once the diet is normalized and the condition controlled. A dietitian can provide valuable nutritional teaching.

Nursing Diagnosis: Body Image Disturbance R/T misconception of body size or negative feelings (all disorders).

Planning: Expected Outcomes. The client will develop a more normal image of self, as evidenced by client's statements concerning self and by client's ability to overcome eating disorder.

Implementation. The nurse needs to recognize that clients suffering from eating disorders often have low self-esteem. These clients see the regulation of food and exercise of self-control in eating patterns and amounts as ways to prove themselves successful. Clients with anorexia nervosa or bulimia nervosa must have inpatient or outpatient therapy before discharge. If the client does not follow the treatment regimen, referral to a facility specializing in eating disorders may be necessary.

Evaluation

The nurse must evaluate whether the client has been able to achieve the goals. If the goals were not achieved, the nurse must revise the plan and interventions to meet the client's needs.

Inflammatory and Neoplastic Disorders

ACUTE GASTRITIS

Gastritis is inflammation of the gastric mucosa. Gastritis is classified as either acute or chronic.

Incidence

The incidence of gastritis is highest in the fifth and sixth decades of life; men are more frequently affected than are women. There is greater incidence in clients who are heavy drinkers and smokers.

Etiology

The acute form of gastritis usually stems from the ingestion of a corrosive, erosive, or infectious substance.

Disorders linked with acute gastritis include uremia, shock, central nervous system lesions, hepatic cirrhosis, portal hypertension, and prolonged emotional tension. Acute gastritis is usually of short duration unless the gastric mucosa has suffered extensive damage.

Risk Factors

Ingestion of gastric irritants is a major risk factor. These include aspirin, alcohol, caffeine, and other irritants. Gastritis may also occur secondary to a variety of diseases, or it may follow treatments such as chemotherapy and radiation therapy.

Pathophysiology

The mucosal lining of the stomach normally protects it from the action of the gastric acid. This mucosal barrier is composed of prostaglandins. If this barrier is penetrated, gastritis will occur, with resultant injury to the mucosa. When hydrochloric acid comes into contact with the mucosa, injury to small vessels occurs with edema, hemorrhage, and possible ulcer formation. The damage associated with acute gastritis is usually limited.

Clinical Manifestations

Assessment typically reveals epigastric discomfort, abdominal tenderness, cramping, eructation, severe nausea and vomiting, and sometimes hematemesis. Sometimes GI bleeding is the only symptom. When contaminated food is the cause of gastritis, the client usually experiences diarrhea within 5 hours of ingestion of the offending substance.

DIAGNOSTIC ASSESSMENT

Diagnosis is based on a detailed history of food intake, medications taken, and any disorders related to gastritis. Also, the physician may perform a gastroscopic examination with a biopsy.

Medical Management

Intervention involves removing the cause or treating the condition symptomatically. Vomiting frequently responds to medications of the phenothiazine group; pain responds to antacids or H_2 antagonists. Initially, foods and fluids are withheld until nausea and vomiting subside. Once the client can tolerate foods, the diet includes decaffeinated tea, gelatin, toast, and simple, bland substances. The client should avoid spicy foods, caffeine, and large, heavy meals. In the continued absence of nausea, vomiting, and bloating, the client can slowly return to a normal diet.

CHRONIC GASTRITIS

This condition appears in three different forms:

- *Superficial gastritis,* which causes a reddened, edematous mucosa with hemorrhages and small erosions
- *Atrophic gastritis,* which occurs in all layers of the stomach
- *Hypertrophic gastritis,* which produces a dull and nodular mucosa with irregular, thickened, or nodular rugae; hemorrhages occur frequently

Etiology

Peptic ulcer disease or gastric surgery may lead to chronic gastritis. Other risk factors are similar to those for acute gastritis. Chronic gastritis is associated with atrophy of the gastrin glands. After gastric resection with a gastrojejunostomy, bile and bile acids may reflux into the remaining stomach, causing the condition.

Risk Factors

The risk factors for chronic gastritis are similar to those for acute gastritis. *Helicobacter pylori* infection can lead to chronic atrophic gastritis, which predisposes to the development of gastric cancer. Age is also a risk factor; chronic gastritis is more common in older adults.

Pathophysiology

The initial pathophysiologic changes associated with chronic gastritis are the same as with acute gastritis. Deterioration and atrophy lead to loss of function of the parietal cells. When the acid secretion decreases, the source of the intrinsic factor is lost, which results in the inability to absorb vitamin B_{12}; this leads to the development of pernicious anemia.

Chronic gastritis usually heals without scarring but can cause hemorrhage and ulcer formation. The atrophic changes eventually result in a minimal amount of acid being secreted into the stomach. This achlorhydria is a major risk factor for the development of gastric cancer.

Clinical Manifestations

Symptoms are vague and may be absent. Assessment may reveal anorexia, a feeling of fullness, dyspepsia, belching, vague epigastric pain, nausea and vomiting, and intolerance of spicy or fatty foods.

Medical Management

Intervention begins once the physician rules out cancer as a causative factor. Discomfort may lessen with a bland diet, small frequent meals, antacids, anticholinergics, sedatives, and avoidance of foods that cause symptoms. Sometimes the physician prescribes corticosteroids in the hope of inducing some parietal cell regeneration. Administer vitamin B_{12} if the client has pernicious anemia.

CRITICAL TO REMEMBER

The client with chronic gastritis should be seen by the physician at regular intervals and tested for the development of gastric cancer.

This is particularly important for the client diagnosed with *H. pylori* infection and atrophic gastritis because these are closely related to gastric cancer.

If conservative measures have not controlled bleeding, surgery may be necessary. These procedures are discussed in the section on peptic ulcer disease.

Nursing Management of Acute and Chronic Gastritis

Assessment

When assessing the client with gastritis, the nurse should carefully focus on risk factors. The client's diet, patterns of eating, use of prescription and over-the-counter drugs, and life-style, including the use of alcohol and cigarettes, are assessed.

Nursing Diagnosis, Planning, and Implementation

Nursing Diagnosis: Pain R/T irritation of the gastric mucosa.

Planning: Expected Outcomes. The client will experience relief of discomfort by removing irritating agents, as evidenced by client's statement of pain relief.

Implementation. The nurse should focus on teaching the client about the causes of gastritis and foods that may aggravate the disease. The nurse should help the client assess factors that increase symptoms, such as stress or fatigue, and assist the client with techniques to reduce the discomfort.

Nursing Diagnosis: Nutrition, Altered: Less than Body Requirements R/T decreased appetite, nausea and vomiting, and pain.

Planning: Expected Outcomes. The client will experience improved nutritional intake by eating a balanced diet, as evidenced by weight gain or cessation of weight loss.

Implementation. If the nausea and vomiting are severe, the client may be given nothing by mouth until these problems decrease in severity. Once the pain and nausea associated with gastritis have subsided, the client is usually willing to follow a prescribed, well-balanced diet. The nurse can help the client identify foods and beverages that stimulate the development of gastritis and encourage the client to avoid these agents.

Evaluation

The nurse must always evaluate the degree to which the goals have been achieved. If they were not completely achieved, the nurse must re-examine the nursing care plan and revise goals and interventions as needed.

PEPTIC ULCER DISEASE

Peptic ulceration is a break in continuity of esophageal, gastric, or duodenal mucosa. It may occur in any part of the GI tract that comes into contact with gastric juices. The ulcer may be found in the esophagus, stomach, duodenum, or (after gastroenterostomy) jejunum.

Incidence

The incidence of peptic ulcer disease occurs in approximately 10 per cent of the population. Gastric ulcers are more likely to occur during the fifth and sixth decades of life; duodenal ulcers more commonly occur during the fourth and fifth decades for men. For women, the occurrence is about 10 years later in life. Men are more likely to experience both gastric and duodenal ulcers.

Etiology

Peptic ulceration depends on the defensive resistance of the mucosa relative to the aggressive force of secretory activity. Ulceration occurs when aggressive factors exceed the defensive ones. The aggressive nature of the gastric juice may be the result of hypersecretion of gastric juices, increased stimulation of the vagus, decreased inhibition of gastric secretions, increased capacity or number of the parietal cells to secrete acid, or increased response of the parietal cells to stimulation.

Risk Factors

Smoking is a major risk factor associated with peptic ulcer disease, as are ulcerogenic agents such as steroids, aspirin, caffeine, and alcohol. Stress has also been shown to increase the risk, especially of duodenal ulcers, because they are more likely to be associated with an increase in acid secretion. The presence of Crohn's disease, Zollinger-Ellison syndrome, and hepatic and biliary disease also increases the risk of ulcer formation.

Pathophysiology

Adrenocorticosteroids may increase the susceptibility of the mucosa, or they may reduce the rate of renewal of mucosal cells and the formation of granulation tissue. When clients undergo stress reactions, the sympathetic nervous system causes the blood vessels in the duodenum to constrict, which makes the mucosa more vulnerable to trauma from gastric acid and pepsin secretion. On activation of the adrenal cortex, mucus production decreases, and gastric secretion increases. Together, these factors result in an increased vulnerability of the client to ulceration. Prolonged stress from burns, severe trauma, and so forth can produce "stress ulcers," or stress erosive gastritis, within the GI tract.

An infection with *H. pylori* may contribute to ulceration and may affect persons who have a history of chronic gastritis.

Certain medications may contribute to gastroduodenal ulceration by altering gastric secretion, producing localized damage to mucosa, interfering with the reparative process, or delaying the healing process. Antiinflammatory agents, aspirin, caffeine, chemotherapeutic agents, and alcohol are related to mucosal damage.

Zollinger-Ellison syndrome is a condition characterized by abnormal secretion of gastrin by a rare islet cell tumor in the pancreas. Pathophysiologic changes associated with this syndrome include hypergastrinemia and

TABLE 34–1 Classification of Peptic Ulcers

ASSESSMENT DATA	DUODENAL ULCERS	GASTRIC ULCERS
Location of ulcer	¼ to 1 inch from pylorus	Junction of fundus and pylorus, some in antrum
Acid secretion	Increased	Normal to decreased
Serum pepsinogen I	Increased	Normal
Serum gastrin		
Fasting	Normal	Elevated
Postprandial	Elevated	
Blood group	Most frequently type O	No difference
Age of onset	25–50 years	Peaks 45–54 years
Gender predominance	Men to women, 4 : 1	Men to women, 2 : 1
Associated gastritis	None	Common and increased
Pain	Occurs on empty stomach, 2 to 3 hr after meals or in middle of night; relieved by food and antacids	Variable pain pattern; may be made worse by food; antacids ineffective
Nutritional status	Usually well nourished	Probably malnourished
Malignancy potential	Rare, no increase in incidence	Occurs in approximately 10% of clients
Bleeding pattern	Melena more common than hematemesis	Hematemesis more common than melena
Recurrence	May occur as marginal ulcers after surgery	Recurrence unlikely after surgery

diarrhea secondary to fat malabsorption from decreased duodenum-inactivating pancreatic lipase or from acid-induced injury of the villi. Besides gastric secretion, there is hyperplasia of the gastric mucosa induced by the trophic effects of gastrin. Treatment of the Zollinger-Ellison syndrome is aimed at suppression of acid secretion.

Critically ill clients are susceptible to stress ulcers. Stress ulcers manifest with superficial gastric erosions, often accompanied by painless massive gastric hemorrhage. The mechanism causing stress ulcerations is unknown but probably involves ischemia. In the presence of acid, ischemia can produce erosive gastritis and ulcerations. Increased hydrogen ion back-diffusion and decreased mucosal perfusion may also contribute to stress ulcer formation. Low gastric pH (high acidity) is necessary for stress ulcer development.

Table 34–1 distinguishes the types of peptic ulcers.

DUODENAL ULCERS

Duodenal ulcers, which have a higher incidence than gastric ulcers, usually occur within 1.5 cm of the pylorus. They are usually characterized by high gastric acid secretion. Clients with duodenal ulcers have more rapid gastric emptying. Combined with hypersecretion of acid, rapid emptying of food from the stomach reduces the buffering effect of food and results in a large acid load in the duodenum. Within the duodenum, inhibitory mechanisms and pancreatic secretion may be insufficient to control the acid load.

GASTRIC ULCERS

Gastric ulcers, which tend to heal within a few weeks, form within 1 inch of the pylorus of the stomach in an area of gastritis. Gastric ulcers are probably caused by a break in the "mucosal barrier." Decreased blood flow to the gastric mucosa may also alter the defensive barrier. Decreased blood flow may make the duodenum more susceptible to gastric acid and pepsin trauma. The recurrence rate in gastric ulcer is lower than in duodenal ulcer.

STRESS (STRESS-EROSIVE GASTRITIS) AND DRUG-INDUCED ULCERS

Besides peptic and gastric ulcers, acute gastric erosion, frequently called stress ulcers or stress-erosive gastritis, can occur after an acute medical crisis. Six major assaults can give rise to gastroduodenal ulcerations:

- Severe trauma or major illness
- Severe burns (sometimes called Curling's ulcers)
- Head injury or intracranial disease (frequently called Cushing's ulcers)
- Drug ingestion (e.g., aspirin and alcohol) that acts on the gastric mucosa
- Shock
- Sepsis

Clinical Manifestations

PAIN

The principal symptom experienced by the client with ulcers is an aching, burning, cramplike, gnawing pain. The pain has a definite relationship to eating. With gastric ulcers, food may cause the pain, and vomiting may relieve it. Clients with duodenal ulcers have pain on an empty stomach, and discomfort may be relieved by the ingestion of food or antacids. Gastric ulcer pain often occurs in the upper epigastrium, with localization to the left of the midline, whereas duodenal pain is in the right epigastrium. Ulcer pain also varies with the site, size, or penetration of the ulcer or the amount of surrounding fibrotic tissue.

In duodenal ulcers, steady pain near the midline of the back between the sixth and tenth thoracic vertebrae with radiation to the right upper quadrant may indicate perforation of the posterior duodenal wall. Fullness or hunger may also be present. Distention of the duodenal bulb produces epigastric pain, which may radiate to the back and thorax. Hydrochloric acid secretion may produce edema and inflammation, with resultant pain, or may activate motor changes, with increased spasm, intragastric pressure, and increased motility, also with resultant pain. In addition, ulcer pain tends to occur within distinct periods (periodicity).

NAUSEA AND VOMITING

Clients with duodenal ulcer usually have a normal appetite unless pyloric obstruction is present. Carcinoma, gastric ulcers, or gastritis may be associated with anorexia, weight loss, and dysphagia. Vomiting occurs more often with gastric ulcer than with uncomplicated duodenal ulcer. It also occurs more frequently when the ulcer is in the pylorus or antrum. Vomiting usually results from gastric stasis or pyloric obstruction. The client with a gastric ulcer or pyloric obstruction typically vomits undigested food. Severe retching and vomiting may suggest an esophageal tear.

BLEEDING

Clients with ulcers often bleed when the ulcer erodes through a blood vessel. Bleeding may occur as massive hemorrhage or may be occult from slow oozing. Approximately 25 per cent of clients with gastric ulcers may experience bleeding.

DIAGNOSTIC ASSESSMENT

Ulcers are diagnosed on the basis of symptoms, x-ray evidence, and endoscopy. The history and physical examination do not yield much significant data in an uncomplicated peptic ulcer. A complete blood count with decreased hematocrit and hemoglobin values may indicate bleeding. Stool for occult blood might also be positive, if bleeding is present.

The major diagnostic tests are an upper GI tract series and esophagogastroduodenoscopy (EGD). The EGD has several advantages. It allows the physician to take tissue specimens and treat the ulcer with either multipolar electrocoagulation or heater-probe therapy (see Medical Management). A test for *H. pylori* may be completed during a gastroscopy.

Medical Management

The primary objective of intervention for peptic ulcer is to provide stomach rest. This may include such approaches as neutralizing or buffering hydrochloric acid, inhibiting acid secretion, and decreasing the activity of pepsin and hydrochloric acid. Specific measures include medications, physical and emotional rest, dietary management, and stress reduction.

Response to the therapeutic program will vary with the client's perception of his or her health status and the degree to which life-style influences the ulcer disease.

PHARMACOLOGIC MANAGEMENT

Medications are prescribed for clients with peptic ulcer for three major reasons: to reduce secretions, to neutralize acid, and to protect the mucosal barrier (Table 34–2).

DIETARY MANAGEMENT

In uncomplicated ulcer disease, few physicians favor strict dietary changes. There is little evidence that diet treatment promotes or accelerates healing. Foods known to increase gastric acidity or cause discomfort should be avoided, such as coffee, alcohol, and milk.

COMPLICATIONS

Hemorrhage. Hemorrhage varies from minimal, manifested by occult blood in the stool (melena), to massive, in which the client vomits bright red blood (hematemesis). The usual symptom of GI tract bleeding is either the vomiting of coffee ground–colored material or the passing of tarry stools. Hemorrhage tends to occur more often with gastric ulcers, especially among the elderly. Although the onset of hemorrhage may be associated with fatigue, nervous tension, upper respiratory tract infection, dietary indiscretion, alcoholism, or irritating drugs, there may be no known precipitating factor.

Symptoms depend on the severity of the hemorrhage. In mild bleeding, the client may experience only slight weakness and diaphoresis. Severe blood loss of more than 1 L per 24 hours may cause manifestations of shock, such as hypotension, weak thready pulse, chills, palpitations, and perspiration.

Intervention for massive bleeding aims to treat hypovolemic shock, prevent dehydration and electrolyte imbalance, and stop the bleeding. The client, who should be fasting, receives intravenous fluids until the bleeding subsides. The nurse or physician may insert a nasogastric tube in the presence or absence of blood in the stomach to assess the rate of bleeding, to prevent gastric dilation, to administer saline lavage, and to check gastric pH.

Arterial administration of vasopressin (via an infusion pump) can also successfully control acute hemorrhage. Vasopressin has few complications if given intravenously for less than 36 hours to control the bleeding.

Another approach to the control of bleeding is selective arterial embolization via angiography. The client must remain on absolute bedrest for several days after bleeding has subsided. Rest decreases blood pressure and GI tract activity. When bleeding stops, the client is allowed bathroom privileges.

During the first few days of hemorrhaging, gastric pH should be maintained between 5.5 and 7.0. To accomplish this, the nurse must administer ranitidine intravenously as prescribed and monitor gastric pH at least each shift. Anticholinergics are not recommended

TABLE 34–2 Medications Commonly Used to Treat Peptic Ulcers

MEDICATION	ACTION	SIDE EFFECTS	NURSING IMPLICATIONS
Hyposecretory Agents			
Histamine (H_2)-Receptor Antagonists			
Cimetidine (Tagamet)	Same action as Zantac	Fever, rash, headache, dizziness, somnolence, confusion (especially in elderly), hypotension, diarrhea, neutropenia, gynecomastia, and impotence	Monitor mental status of elderly; do not take antacids within 1 hr of Tagamet; take with meals and at bedtime; interacts with theophylline, phenytoin, warfarin, and beta-blockers; continue treatment for at least 8 weeks to ensure healing
Ranitidine hydrochloride (Zantac)	Inhibits gastric acid secretion by blocking H_2 receptors on parietal cells	All side effects rare, including nausea, constipation, bradycardia, increased liver enzymes, and headache	Give antacids at least 1 hr before or 2 hr after Zantac; can be given in single bedtime dose; use cautiously in clients with liver or renal disorders; absorption not affected by food; interacts minimally with other drugs
Famotidine (Pepcid)	Same action as Zantac	Headache, diarrhea, constipation, nausea, flatulence, increased blood urea nitrogen and creatinine, and rash	Should not be taken longer than 8 weeks without physician's specific order; may be given with antacids; can be given in single bedtime dose; has no significant drug interactions
Nizatidine (Axid)	Same action as Zantac	Diarrhea, rash, bronchospasms, somnolence, joint pain, and sweating	Give as single bedtime dose or, if given twice a day, one dose at bedtime; assess for excessive drowsiness; monitor and record stools; do not give antacids within 1 hr of Axid; must be taken 4 to 8 weeks for ulcer healing; notify physician if somnolence or rash develops
Prostaglandin Analogs			
Misoprostol (Cytotec)	Suppresses secretion of gastric acid and stimulates production of cytoprotective mucus	Diarrhea, nausea, abdominal discomfort, headache, and dizziness	Cannot be used in pregnancy because it stimulates uterine contractions; use for treatment in peptic ulcer disease currently under investigation; considered equivalent to cimetidine in ability to heal duodenal ulcers; useful in treating gastric ulcers also; recommended for clients on long-term aspirin or nonsteroidal anti-inflammatory drug therapy
Anticholinergics			
Dicyclomine hydrochloride (Bentyl)	Muscarinic antagonist; inhibits secretion of gastric acid in large doses	Headache, palpitations, dizziness, constipation, paralytic ileus, urinary hesitancy and retention, and dry mouth	Do not use in clients with obstructive uropathy, gastrointestinal obstruction, ulcerative colitis, unstable cardiovascular status, or toxic megacolon; use carefully in clients with narrow-angle glaucoma, hyperthyroidism, hiatal hernia, congestive heart failure, hepatic or renal disease; give $\frac{1}{2}$ hr before meals and at bedtime; monitor vital signs and urine output; report blurred vision; maintain good fluid intake

TABLE 34–2 Medications Commonly Used to Treat Peptic Ulcers *Continued*

MEDICATION	ACTION	SIDE EFFECTS	NURSING IMPLICATIONS
Antacids			
Aluminum hydroxide (Amphojel)	Buffers and neutralizes acid in gastrointestinal tract	Constipation, anorexia, intestinal obstruction, and hypophosphatemia	Give 1 to 2 hr after meals and at bedtime; do not give within 1 to 2 hr of H_2 receptor antagonists, enteric-coated drugs, or tetracycline; monitor and treat constipation; shake suspension well before use; follow tablets with water; contains salt, so contraindicated in large doses or long-term use with clients on sodium-restricted diets; used in clients with renal failure
Magnesium oxide (Mag-Ox)	Increases gastric pH to reduce pepsin activity; strengthens gastric mucosal barrier and esophageal sphincter tone	Diarrhea, nausea, and hypermagnesemia	Do not use in clients with renal disease; monitor for development of symptoms of hypermagnesemia; alter with aluminum or combination product if diarrhea occurs; do not give within 1 to 2 hr of H_2-receptor antagonists, tetracycline, or enteric-coated tablets
Aluminum-magnesium combinations (Riopan, Maalox, Mylanta, Gelusil)	Increases gastric pH to reduce pepsin activity; strengthens gastric mucosal barrier and esophageal sphincter tone	Mild constipation or diarrhea	Do not use in clients with renal disease; monitor bowel movements and signs of hypermagnesemia; Riopan low in sodium; do not give within 1 to 2 hr of H_2-receptor antagonists, tetracycline, or enteric-coated tablets
Calcium carbonate (Tums, Titralac)	Increases gastric pH to reduce pepsin activity; strengthens gastric mucosal barrier and esophageal sphincter tone	Constipation, gastric distention, rebound hyperacidity, hypercalcemia, and hypophosphatemia	Do not use in clients with renal disease; do not give with milk; monitor for symptoms of hypercalcemia and constipation; do not give within 1 to 2 hr of H_2-receptor antagonists, tetracycline, or enteric-coated tablets
Mucosal Barrier Fortifiers			
Sucralfate (Carafate)	In presence of mild acid condition, forms viscid and sticky gel and adheres to ulcer surface, forming a protective barrier	Dizziness, constipation, sleepiness, nausea, and gastric discomfort	Best on an empty stomach, 1 hr before meals and at bedtime; monitor for constipation; pain and ulcer symptoms may subside, urge client to take entire prescribed regimen; drug minimally absorbed, so few adverse reactions

for treatment of gastric hemorrhage. Antacids should be administered for 1 week to complement the ranitidine.

If bleeding continues beyond 48 hours, recurs, or is associated with perforation or obstruction, surgery may be indicated. Increased surgical risk is associated with prolonged bleeding, multiple transfusions, debilitation, electrolyte imbalances, and increased age.

Blood volume depletion presents a major problem for the client who has severely hemorrhaged. For those who have suffered a massive upper GI tract hemorrhage, a primary objective of intervention is to replace blood volume. Restlessness and tachycardia are the earliest symptoms of hypovolemia. The client will also have a greatly decreased urine output, which should be monitored via an indwelling catheter and tested for specific gravity every 8 hours. See Appendix C for a sample clinical pathway for clients with GI hemorrhage.

Perforation. Perforation is usually a surgical emergency. When the ulcer perforates, gastroduodenal contents empty through the anterior wall of the stomach into the peritoneal cavity, resulting in chemical peritonitis, bacterial septicemia, and hypovolemic shock. Peristalsis diminishes, and paralytic ileus develops.

Perforation occurs most frequently with duodenal ulcers. Perforation develops when an ulcer erodes through the tunica muscularis. The client experiences sudden, sharp, severe pain beginning in the midepigastrium. As peritonitis develops, the pain spreads over the entire abdomen, which then becomes tender, hard, and rigid. (See discussion of peritonitis in Chap. 35.)

The degree of pain depends on the amount and type of contents spilled. Characteristically, the pain causes the client to bend over or draw the knees up to the abdomen in an effort to decrease the tension on the abdominal muscles. If the perforation occurs on the posterior gastric wall, however, it may erode through to adjacent organs and become sealed, causing few symptoms. Manifestations of pancreatitis usually develop when a perforation erodes into the pancreas.

If perforation occurs, the client needs immediate replacement of fluid, blood, and electrolytes and administration of antibiotics. Nasogastric suction should be instituted to drain gastric secretions and thus prevent further peritoneal spillage. A small perforation that closes immediately by adhering to the adjacent tissues usually causes only a small loss of gastric contents. In this instance, the client may recover without surgery.

If surgery is necessary, antibiotics should be administered to combat peritonitis. The nasogastric tube remains in the stomach until peristalsis returns. Postoperative complications include subphrenic abscess, hemorrhage, duodenal or gastric fistula, atelectasis, or pneumonia.

Obstruction. Long-standing ulcer disease causes scarring from repeated ulcerations and healing. Scarring at the pylorus frequently causes pyloric obstruction manifested most often by pain at night when the stomach cannot be emptied by peristalsis. Pyloric obstruction can also lead to vomiting. Surgery, a pyloroplasty, is usually required to correct the problem.

Surgical Management

Most chronic, recurring ulcers are eventually treated surgically. Emergencies such as acute obstruction, perforation, and acute intractable hemorrhage are usually treated by surgical intervention immediately. Hemorrhage sometimes responds to medical management, but when medical approaches do not stop the bleeding, emergency surgery is required to save the client's life.

The surgical approaches for reducing acidity of the stomach are as follows: severing nerves that stimulate the acid-secreting cells (vagotomy) and removing the acid-secreting portions of the stomach (antrectomy).

SUBTOTAL GASTRECTOMY

Subtotal gastrectomy, a generic term referring to any surgery that involves partial removal of the stomach, may be formed by either a Billroth I or a Billroth II procedure (Fig. 34–2).

In a *Billroth I* procedure, the surgeon removes a part of the distal portion of the stomach, including the antrum. The remainder of the stomach is anastomosed to the duodenum. This combined procedure is more properly called gastroduodenostomy. It decreases the

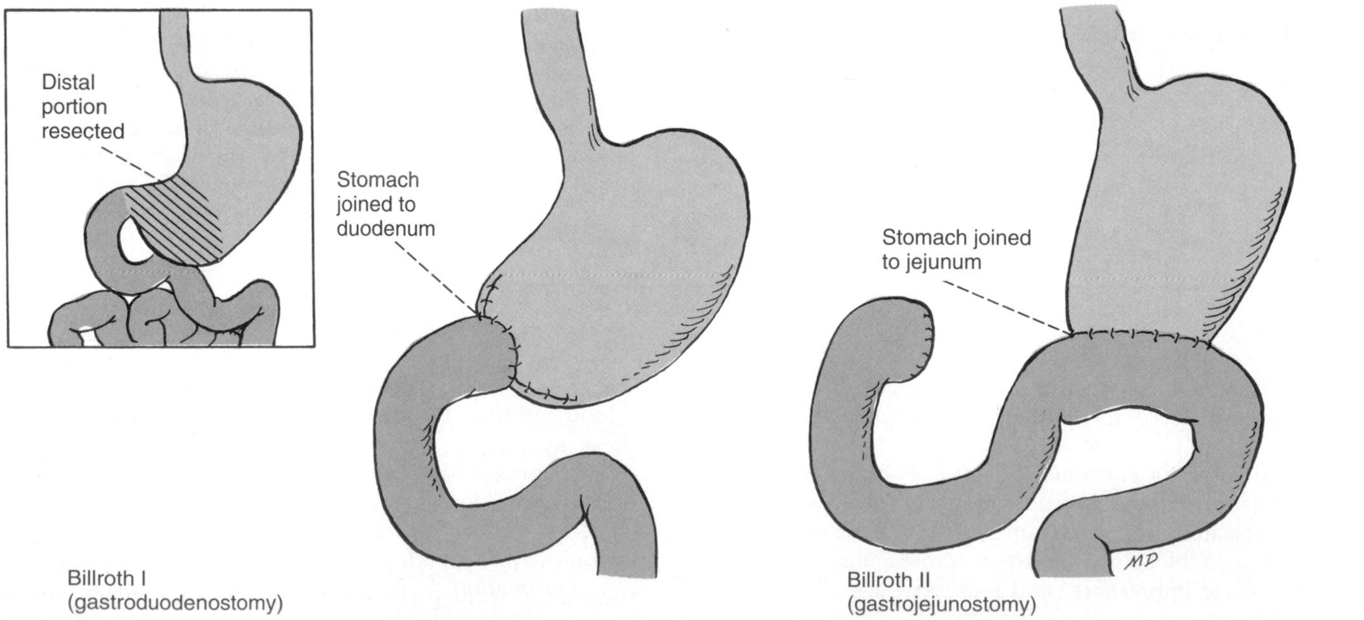

Figure 34–2
Subtotal gastrectomy removes acid-secreting portions of the stomach. After removing the distal stomach *(inset)*, a surgeon sutures the remaining portion of the stomach to the duodenum (Billroth I procedure) or to the proximal jejunum (Billroth II procedure).

incidence of dumping syndrome, which often occurs after a Billroth II procedure.

A *Billroth II* resection involves reanastomosis of the proximal remnant of the stomach to the proximal jejunum. Pancreatic secretions and bile continue to be secreted into the duodenum even after gastrectomy. Because these secretions are necessary for digestion, a route to the intestine must be preserved for them. Recurrent ulceration develops less frequently with this procedure.

TOTAL GASTRECTOMY

Total resection of the stomach is the principal intervention for extensive gastric cancer. This surgery involves removal of the stomach, with anastomosis of the esophagus to the jejunum (esophagojejunostomy) (Fig. 34-3). To perform total gastrectomy, the surgeon enters the chest; thus, the client returns to the recovery room with chest tubes.

COMPLICATIONS

Marginal Ulcers. A marginal ulcer can develop where gastric acids contact the operative site, either at the site of the anastomosis or in the jejunum. This ulceration may cause scarring and obstruction of the passages. Hemorrhage and perforation can also occur.

Hemorrhage. The reported incidence of hemorrhage after gastric surgery is 1 to 3 per cent. It is usually caused by a splenic injury or slippage of a ligature. The nurse must assess the client postoperatively for signs and symptoms of bleeding and intraperitoneal hemorrhage.

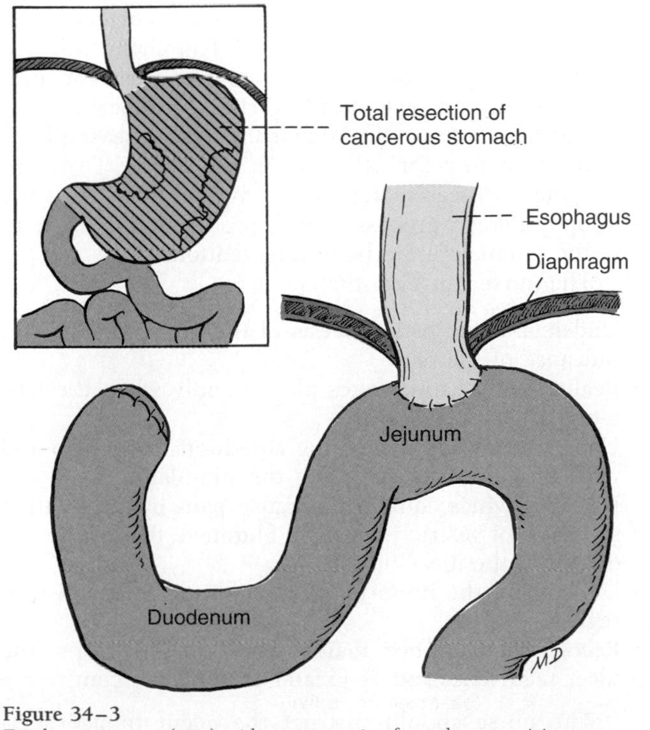

Figure 34–3
Total gastrectomy (*inset*) with anastomosis of esophagus to jejunum (esophagojejunostomy) is the principal intervention for extensive gastric cancer.

Alkaline Reflux Gastritis. Alkaline reflux gastritis resulting from duodenal contents occurs after gastric surgery in which the pylorus has been bypassed or removed. It also occurs after pyloroplasty and gastrojejunostomy. An associated vagotomy has usually been performed.

Acute Gastric Dilation. In the immediate postoperative period, distention of the stomach produces epigastric pain, tachycardia, and hypotension. The client complains of a feeling of fullness, hiccups, or gagging. This situation rapidly improves after insertion of a nasogastric tube or clearing of a plugged nasogastric tube. These symptoms must be reported to the physician immediately.

Nutritional Problems. Nutritional problems common after stomach removal include vitamin B_{12} and folic acid deficiency, calcium metabolism disorders, and reduced absorption of calcium and vitamin D. Such problems result from a shortage of intrinsic factor and inadequate absorption caused by rapid entry of food into the bowel.

Dumping Syndrome. This postprandial problem occurs after gastric resection because ingested food rapidly enters the jejunum without proper mixing and without the normal duodenal digestive processing. It usually subsides in 6 to 12 months. Early manifestations, which occur 5 to 30 minutes after eating, involve the vasomotor disturbances of vertigo, tachycardia, syncope, sweating, pallor, palpitation, diarrhea, and nausea with the desire to lie down. The client's blood pressure and pulse may either rise or fall. Intestinal manifestations of dumping include epigastric fullness, distention, discomfort, abdominal cramping, nausea (with only occasional vomiting), and borborygmi (rumbling in the bowel). The client may experience tenesmus (a desire to defecate). Pain is not present.

Early manifestations are probably due to rapid movement of extracellular fluids into the bowel to convert the rapidly entering hypertonic bolus into an isotonic mixture. This rapid fluid shift decreases the circulating blood volume. A jejunum distended with food and fluid increases intestinal peristalsis and motility.

Late manifestations, which occur 2 to 3 hours after eating, are a result of the rapid entry of high-carbohydrate food into the jejunum, a rise in blood sugar, and excessive insulin.

Management of dumping syndrome involves decreasing the amount of food taken at one time and maintaining a high-protein, high-fat, low-carbohydrate, dry diet. Gastric emptying can be delayed by eating in a recumbent or semirecumbent position, lying down after meals, increasing the fat content in the diet, and not taking fluids 1 hour before, with, or 2 hours after meals.

Gastrojejunocolic Fistula. This postoperative complication follows recurrent peptic ulcer disease. The fistulas arise from perforation of a recurrent ulceration at the gastrojejunal anastomosis site. The perforation forms a fistula between the ulcer and adjacent bowel. Symptoms are variable but include fecal vomiting, diarrhea, weight loss, and anorexia. Belching of gas that has a fecal odor may also occur. The symptoms are caused by bacterial overgrowth in the small intestine.

Pyloric Obstruction. Pyloric obstruction, manifested by vomiting, occurs at the pylorus and is due to scarring, edema, inflammation, or a combination of these. When vomiting persists, the client is apt to experience alkalosis because large quantities of acid gastric juice are vomited (see Chap. 4). A client who vomits persistently is usually hospitalized to receive intravenous fluids fortified with electrolytes. Pyloroduodenal obstruction can cause gastric dilation, gastritis, and gastric stasis. These mechanisms create symptoms that gradually make it more difficult for the stomach to empty. The nurse must assess the client for feelings of fullness, distention, or nausea after eating, with a loss of appetite and weight loss.

Management of obstruction focuses on restoring fluid and electrolytes and decompressing the dilated stomach; if necessary, surgical intervention is instituted.

Nursing Management

Assessment

Nursing assessment involves gathering both psychosocial and pathophysiologic data concerning the client.

CRITICAL TO REMEMBER

To assess psychosocial aspects associated with ulcer disease, the nurse should ask the client about

- Familial incidence of ulcer
- Ingestion of medications causing gastric irritation
- Cigarette smoking
- Alcohol intake
- Stressors
- Coping patterns

Questions about life-style, occupation, work, and leisure can yield valuable information. Physical assessment includes accurately observing and immediately reporting symptoms, including pain, vomiting, and occasionally bleeding and changes in appetite. The nurse should always obtain a complete history of ulcer attacks, including frequency, duration, manifestations, and response to intervention.

Assessment also involves describing the bleeding, including hematemesis and melena; note is made of such factors as the color, amount, consistency, and frequency. Bright red blood usually signifies new bleeding, whereas dark red blood indicates old bleeding. In severe bleeding, the nurse should always maintain an accurate and up-to-date record of the client's hemoglobin, hematocrit, red cell count, and fluid intake and output.

Nursing Diagnosis, Planning, and Implementation

For the client treated medically for peptic ulcer disease, the plan of care is as follows.

Nursing Diagnosis: Pain R/T gastric mucosal injury.

Planning: Expected Outcomes. The client will have pain relieved, as evidenced by healing of gastric or duodenal mucosal injury and client's statement.

Implementation. The nurse should administer medications as ordered and must assess the effectiveness of the medication on the client's pain.

Avoidance of strenuous physical activity decreases gastric secretions and peristalsis. Thus, a primary nursing goal is to promote recovery by helping the client achieve rest, both physically and mentally. The nurse must be alert for factors that interfere with the client's rest. The environment should be arranged to encourage relaxation. If certain visitors or telephone calls agitate the client, these visits or calls should be discouraged until the client improves.

Clients who attempt to carry on their normal work routine (despite prescribed rest) should be encouraged to schedule physical and mental relaxation. The nurse should explore ways, with the client and significant others or coworkers, to reduce work responsibilities temporarily.

The diet must meet basic nutritional needs.

CRITICAL TO REMEMBER

Because an empty stomach stimulates gastric acid secretion, the nurse should advise the client to eat small amounts at frequent, regular intervals.

Ingestion of alcohol, cola, tobacco, caffeine, milk, and foods that cause discomfort should be discouraged. The client may drink decaffeinated beverages.

Nursing Diagnosis: Knowledge Deficit R/T cause of ulcer and measures to treat and prevent recurrence.

Planning: Expected Outcomes. The client will understand the cause of ulcer and how to treat and prevent recurrence, as evidenced by client's statements.

Implementation. Treatment for ulcer disease places the responsibility for self-care on the client. To maintain good self-care, the client must understand the pathophysiologic process underlying ulcer development and the rationale underlying intervention.

The nurse can help the client to

- Understand the pathogenesis of the ulcer and the significance of the pain
- Realize that healing takes place rapidly when the irritating effect is removed
- Understand what caused the condition to develop and what must be done to lessen the stimulation
- Discover which substances cause pain by stimulating secretion of gastric juices and eliminate them from the diet until the ulcer heals
- Understand the importance of continuing the medical regimen
- Recognize that once maintenance therapy stops, the ulcer recurrence rate is greater than 50 per cent

The nurse should instruct the client to use acetaminophen instead of aspirin preparations. The client must be taught to examine the labels of all nonprescription medications, particularly cold remedies, for aspirin (acetylsalicylic acid), other salicylates, or ibuprofen. If any of these medications must be taken, the nurse must advise the client to check with the physician first, eat between meals, and use prescribed H_2-receptor antagonists or antacids.

Helping clients with ulcers cope with psychosocial problems is a vital part of intervention. The nurse should take time to learn about their stressors. Discussing coping and relaxation techniques may enable clients to better deal with their problems.

Collaborative Problem: Injury, Risk for R/T complication (e.g., hemorrhage, perforation, obstruction).

Planning: Expected Outcomes. The client will not suffer any injury, as evidenced by the absence of hemorrhage, perforation, or obstruction.

Implementation. The nurse must monitor for the development of complications of ulcers including hemorrhage, perforation, or obstruction. The nurse should monitor vital signs closely for the development of symptoms of shock that might occur if bleeding is present. The nurse must document and report the occurrence of melena or hematemesis. If hemorrhage occurs, treatment to stop hemorrhage and prevent shock should be implemented immediately (see Chap. 56).

The nurse must monitor the client for the development of perforation. The abdomen should be assessed for pain, tenderness, or rigidity. Suspected perforation should be reported to the physician immediately and the client prepared for possible surgery. The client should also be monitored for the development of gastric obstruction. If the client vomits, the nurse should record the frequency and consistency (digested or undigested food or hematemesis) of the vomitus. If pyloric obstruction is present, the client will require a nasogastric tube and intravenous fluids until the problem is corrected surgically.

For the client undergoing surgery for peptic ulcer disease, the plan of care is as follows.

Nursing Diagnosis: Knowledge Deficit R/T preoperative preparation, postoperative care, diet, and long-term prevention of recurrence.

Planning: Expected Outcomes. The client will understand preoperative preparation, postoperative care, diet, and long-term prevention of recurrence, as evidenced by client's statements and no recurrence of ulcer disease.

Implementation. Surgical intervention for gastric and duodenal conditions may be either a planned procedure or an emergency. When emergency surgery is required (e.g., for acute obstruction, perforation, or hemorrhage), the client is very ill and usually frightened. The nurse should provide calm, efficient, knowledgeable care and explain what is being done and note and respond to the client's nonverbal behavior. The nurse should also help significant others provide the client with empathy and emotional support.

When cancer is suspected, the client may want to talk about fears and concerns. The nurse should listen to the client carefully, respond to cues, and offer support and understanding. The client may wish to attend to personal matters before surgery (e.g., check a will, see a minister).

When elective surgery is done, the client will probably have an extensive series of preoperative examinations, such as a GI tract series, endoscopy, and perhaps acid-secretion studies (see Chap. 32). These may be done on an outpatient basis.

Preoperative teaching should include an explanation of what surgery generally involves. The nurse explains that the client will have either a nasogastric tube or possibly a gastrostomy tube and suction and intravenous infusion in the hand or arm for fluids until the surgical site heals. The importance of deep-breathing exercises must be thoroughly demonstrated and discussed. The high incision increases the risk of respiratory complications.

Postoperatively, some clients need help to reduce the number of stressors in their lives. Strategies for altering life-style may be an important part of the rehabilitation and recovery plan. Most clients can learn to control symptoms and lead a fairly normal life.

Collaborative Problem: Injury, Risk for R/T postoperative complications (immediate and delayed).

Planning: Expected Outcomes. The client will not suffer injury related to postoperative complications (immediate and delayed), as evidenced by decreasing bloody drainage from nasogastric tube, absence of abdominal distention, and normal breath sounds.

Implementation. Nursing care after gastric surgery is the same as postoperative care for any client recovering from major abdominal surgery. In addition to general postoperative care, the nurse should

- Check the drainage from the nasogastric tube
- Ensure that the tube is attached to suction, as ordered
- Assess the operative site for excessive drainage; too much fluid in the remaining gastric stump could cause increased pressure and injury
- Note the color and consistency of drainage from the operative site and report bleeding or hemorrhaging

Immediate complications after gastric surgery include gastric dilation, obstruction, hemorrhage, and disruption of the suture line. Also, the nurse should observe for general surgical complications such as shock, hemorrhage, pulmonary problems, thrombosis, evisceration, and infection. Nausea and vomiting should not occur if the nasogastric tube is patent.

CRITICAL TO REMEMBER

Carefully measure and document intake (oral and intravenous) and output (urine, suction, and wound drainage).

The client will return from surgery with a nasogastric or gastrostomy tube for preventing the retention of gastric secretions. The nurse should carefully assess for abdominal distention. The nasogastric or gastrostomy tube should not be repositioned after gastric surgery and should be irrigated gently, *only* if specifically ordered.

The color of the drainage in the nasogastric tube may be bright red during the early hours after surgery but should become dark red by the end of 24 hours.

The client should be kept comfortable with liberal administration of pain medications. This helps the client to cooperate more fully during deep-breathing and coughing exercises. Fluids must be administered by intravenous infusion as ordered until edema and swelling have diminished enough to allow fluids to pass the operative area (seen as a decrease in the gastric tube output).

Nursing Diagnosis: Nutrition, Altered: Less than Body Requirements R/T decreased nutrient absorption secondary to dumping syndrome.

Planning: Expected Outcomes. The client will maintain adequate nutrition, as evidenced by client's ability to maintain weight at normal level and no evidence of dumping syndrome.

Implementation. When healing has occurred, oral intake can begin by giving the client clear water, usually 30 mL at a time. The tube should be aspirated an hour or so later to see whether the fluid has been retained. When GI function has returned (e.g., active bowel sounds, passing flatus) and the client tolerates clear water, the nasogastric tube is usually removed and the diet progressed. Next, progress to soft foods and eventually to a regular diet of five or six small meals a day. The diet should not begin too early or progress too rapidly. The client may experience discomfort, at first, if too much food is taken at one time.

Clients need to know that convalescence after gastric surgery tends to be slow. It may be 3 months before clients regain strength and even partial ability to eat in a more normal manner. It may take a year or so before they can eat three normal meals a day. The nurse should observe the client postoperatively for persistent gastric disturbances.

Evaluation

The nurse must evaluate the degree to which the goals and outcomes have been achieved. If the client's goals have not been met, the plan and interventions must be revised so they can be met.

GASTRIC CANCER

Gastric cancer refers to the malignant neoplasms found in the stomach, usually adenocarcinoma, although they may be malignant lymphomas.

Incidence

The incidence of gastric cancer in the United States has decreased dramatically during the past 40 years. Despite the reduced incidence, this is the sixth most common cause of death from cancer in the United States.

Although little is known of the cause, it is known that stomach cancer is twice as common in men as in women, more common in American whites, and more frequent in clients who have pernicious anemia. It often develops in conjunction with atrophic gastritis and affects individuals who have a low socioeconomic status, live in an urban area, eat smoked fish, or are exposed to background radiation or trace metals in the soil. The presence of *H. pylori* in the stomach increases the incidence of gastric cancer.

Etiology

Although there are no specific etiologic factors associated with gastric cancer, several factors do seem associated with the development of the disease. These include chronic atrophic gastritis, achlorhydria, and pernicious anemia. The changes in the mucosa may lead to an increase in the absorption of carcinogens from the diet, such as pickled foods, salted fish, and nitrates. Smoking also appears to be associated with an increased incidence of gastric cancer. There may also be a genetic factor because it does seem to run in families.

Risk Factors

Metal crafts workers, coal miners, bakers, and those working in dusty, smoky, and sulfur dioxide–containing environments are at greater risk. Wood or tobacco smoke, nitrite food preservatives, and overheated fat products may predispose clients to stomach cancer.

Pathophysiology

Gastric cancer most often arises from the mucous lining of the stomach. The majority of these cancers occur in the lesser curvature of the stomach in the pyloric and antral regions.

Most carcinomas of the stomach develop in its lower half. Stomach cancer spreads by direct extension into the pancreas, the lymphatics, or hematogenous infiltration of the liver, lungs, and bones.

The disease is resectable in early stages before it has invaded the wall of the stomach. The 5-year survival rate is about 90 per cent for local disease; this rate drops to less than 10 per cent for stage III disease.

Clinical Manifestations

Because the symptoms occur late, stomach cancer is seldom diagnosed in an early stage. Furthermore, unless hemorrhage or perforation occurs, manifestations are vague and indefinite. The presence of a palpable mass, ascites, or bone pain from metastasis may be the first symptom. Symptoms vary, depending on the location of the tumor in the stomach. If the neoplasm grows near the cardia, the client may experience dysphagia from early involvement of the esophagus. If the neoplasm is near the pylorus, symptoms may occur from obstruction.

Assessment reveals weight loss, a vague indigestion, anorexia, or a feeling of fullness or mild discomfort so insidious that the client does not recognize it as abnormal or seek medical assistance. Discomfort may be brought on or relieved by food. Anemia from blood loss commonly occurs, and occult blood may be present in the stool. The presence of lactic acid and a high lactate dehydrogenase level in the gastric juice suggests carcinoma.

DIAGNOSTIC ASSESSMENT

Upper GI tract x-ray examination and gastroscopy enable diagnosis of gastric cancer. Gastroscopy allows the lesion to be viewed directly. Cytologic brushing and biopsy can be used to diagnose cancer cells.

Medical Management

There is little effective medical treatment for gastric carcinoma. Clients may receive chemotherapy and radiation therapy, but the primary treatment for this condition is surgical resection.

At present, best results are achieved with multiple drug combinations. The combination of radiation and chemotherapy may be done after surgery.

Total parenteral nutrition is a method for providing nutrition to the client.

Surgical Management

Surgery is the only intervention that effectively treats stomach cancer. Unfortunately, because the diagnosis is usually late, surgery is more often palliative than curative. Gastrectomy, either partial or complete, depending on tumor location, is the usual procedure. Ideally, the surgeon removes all local growth and the associated lymph nodes. When an extensive tumor makes resection impractical or impossible and the pylorus is obstructed, the surgeon may perform a palliative gastroenterostomy (surgical creation of a passage between the stomach and small intestine). Chemotherapy and, less often, radiation may be used with surgery.

Nursing Management

Assessment

As mentioned, the symptoms associated with gastric cancer are usually vague. Clients may present with symptoms similar to ulcer disease, but often symptoms are not present until the tumor is advanced.

CRITICAL TO REMEMBER

The nurse should note on the client's history any risk or predisposing factors to the development of gastric carcinoma. These include a history of chronic gastritis, pernicious anemia, gastric surgery, or smoking.

The nurse should also note in the client history whether the client ingests large amounts of nitrates, smoked fish, salty foods, or pickled foods.

Nursing Diagnosis, Planning, and Implementation

Nursing Diagnosis: Pain, Acute R/T gastric erosion; and Pain, Postoperative R/T high surgical incision.

Planning: Expected Outcomes. The client will have pain controlled or experience a reduction in pain, as evidenced by client's statements.

Implementation. It is very important that the client receive pain relief. Pain that is not controlled can interfere with sleep and eating and contribute to overall physical and mental deterioration.

Nursing Diagnosis: Nutrition, Altered: Less than Body Requirements R/T decreased appetite, pain, possible gastric obstruction, and nausea and vomiting.

Planning: Expected Outcomes. The client will maintain nutritional intake to meet metabolic requirements, as evidenced by maintenance of normal body weight.

Implementation. Nutritional therapy is a very important aspect of management of the client with gastric cancer. TPN or jejunostomy tube feedings may be used postoperatively (or for inoperable clients) to maintain the nutritional status.

Nursing Diagnosis: Fear R/T knowledge deficit, treatment, and life-threatening illness.

Planning: Expected Outcomes. The client will have fear reduced or controlled, as evidenced by client's ability to understand and discuss disease and treatment options.

Implementation. The client needs an explanation of the disease and all treatment options. The nurse needs to reinforce information to the client as needed. The client also needs to have preoperative teaching concerning operative procedures (nothing by mouth; holding area; intravenous infusions). Information will help decrease the client's fear.

Postoperative complications include hemorrhage, obstruction, anemia, nutritional deficiency, dumping syndrome, duodenal stump leakage, gastric dilation, and delayed gastric emptying.

Evaluation

The nurse must evaluate the degree to which the goals and outcomes have been achieved. If the client's goals have not been met, the plan and interventions must be revised so they can be met.

STUDY QUESTIONS

1. When collecting subjective data from a client with peptic ulcer disease, the nurse should ask which of the following?
   A. "Are you vomiting bloody secretions?"
   B. "Are you having abdominal pain?"
   C. "Are your stools tarry black?"
   D. "Are you having diarrhea stools?"
2. After administration of an intermittent tube feeding, which of the following implications should the client be taught?
   A. Lie flat for 45 minutes to 1 hour.
   B. Assess the tube for patency.
   C. Check placement in the stomach.
   D. Sit upright for 1 hour.
3. Which of the following foods should the client with acute gastritis include in the diet?
   A. Gelatin and toast
   B. Chocolate and coffee
   C. Pepperoni pizza and Diet Coke
   D. Burritos with hot sauce and milk
4. Medications that neutralize gastric acid secretions are known as
   A. H_2-receptor antagonists
   B. Anticholinergics
   C. Antacids
   D. Mucosal barrier protectors
5. Perforation, a complication of ulcer disease, manifests as
   A. A dull ache in the left lower quadrant
   B. Scar tissue at the pylorus
   C. Substernal pain
   D. Severe epigastric pain

CRITICAL THINKING EXERCISES

SCENARIO A

A middle-aged man is seen in the clinic with complaints of epigastric pain and malaise. The physician recommends antacids for relief of pain and an upper gastrointestinal x-ray film to rule out duodenal ulcer.

1. What risk factors should the nurse assess for when taking a client history?
2. Identify implications for client teaching when taking antacids.
3. What dietary restrictions are recommended for the client with duodenal ulcer?
4. What complications can occur with duodenal ulcer?

SCENARIO B

An elderly woman with the diagnosis of cerebrovascular accident is unable to swallow. After discharge from the hospital, the woman's daughter will be administering bolus enteral feedings through a nasogastric tube. Her daughter is learning the procedure while the client is still hospitalized.

1. What should the nurse teach the daughter about maintaining tube patency.
2. What problems should the daughter observe for?
3. How should the daughter check for tube placement?

BIBLIOGRAPHY

1. Akridge, K. (1989). Anorexia nervosa. *Journal of Obstetric, Gynecologic, and Neonatal Nursing, 18,* 25–30.
2. American Cancer Society (1995). *Cancer facts and figures—1995.* New York: Author.
3. Baird, S. B., et al. (1991). *Cancer nursing: A comprehensive textbook.* Philadelphia: W. B. Saunders.
4. Barkin, J., & Rogers, A. (Eds.). (1994). *Difficult decisions in digestive diseases* (2nd ed.). St. Louis: Mosby-Year Book.
5. Beahrs, O. H., et al. (Eds.). (1992). *Manual for staging of cancer* (4th ed.). Philadelphia: W. B. Saunders.
6. Correa, P. (1991). Is gastric carcinoma an infectious disease? *New England Journal of Medicine, 325 (16),* 1170–1171.
7. Cotran, R. S., et al. (Eds.) (1994). *Robbins pathologic basis of disease* (5th ed.). Philadelphia: W. B. Saunders.
8. Esberger, K. K. (1991). Guide to gastrointestinal problems of elders. *Geriatric Nursing, 12,* 74–75.
9. Flood, M. (1989). Addictive eating disorders. *Nursing Clinics of North America, 24,* 45–54.
10. Frank-Stromberg, M. (1989). The epidemiology and primary prevention of gastric and esophageal cancer. *Cancer Nursing, 12 (2),* 53–64.
11. Gilinsky, N. H. (1990). Peptic ulcer disease in the elderly. *Gastroenterology Clinics of North America, 19,* 255–268.
12. Graham, D. Y., & Go, M. F. (1993). Helicobacter pylori: Current status. *Gastroenterology, 105,* 279–282.
13. Greenberger, N. J. (1989). *Gastrointestinal disorders: A pathophysiologic approach* (4th ed.). St. Louis: Mosby-Year Book.
14. Groenwald, S. L., et al. (1990). *Cancer nursing: Principles and practice* (2nd ed.). Boston: Jones & Bartlett.
15. Guyton, A. C. (1991). *Textbook of medical physiology* (8th ed.). Philadelphia: W. B. Saunders.
16. Haubrich, W. S. (1995). *Bockus gastroenterology* (5th ed.). Philadelphia: W. B. Saunders.
17. Kandel, G. (1990). Management of nonvariceal upper GI hemorrhage. *Hospital Practice, 25,* 167–184.
18. Kirsner, J. B., & Shorter, R. G. (Eds.). (1995). *Inflammatory bowel disease.* Baltimore: Williams & Wilkins.

19. Kohn, C. L., & Keithly, J. K. (1989). Enteral nutrition: Potential complications and patient monitoring. *Nursing Clinics of North America, 24,* 339–351.
20. Kopeski, L. M. (1989). Diabetes and bulimia: A deadly duo. *American Journal of Nursing, 89,* 482–485.
21. Lehne, R. (1994). *Pharmacology for nursing care* (2nd ed.). Philadelphia: W. B. Saunders.
22. Levinson, M. (1989). Gastric stress ulcer. *Hospital Practice, 24,* 59–67.
23. Marble, D., & Ward, J. (1989). Managing NSAID-induced peptic ulcer. *Drug Therapy, 19,* 34–45.
24. Meize-Grochowski, A. R. (1991). When the DX is Crohn's disease. *RN, 54,* 52–55.
25. NIH Consensus Development Panel on *Helicobacter Pylori* in Peptic Ulcer Disease: *Helicobacter pylori* in peptic ulcer disease. (1994). *JAMA, 272(1),* 65–69.
26. Parrsonett, J., et al. (1991). *Helicobacter pylori* infection and the risk of gastric carcinoma. *New England Journal of Medicine, 325(16),* 1127–1136.
27. Prevost, S. S., & Oberle, A. (1993). Stress ulceration in the critically ill patient. *Critical Care Nursing Clinics of North America, 5,* 163–169.
28. Sabiston, D. C., Jr. (1991). *Textbook of surgery: The biologic basis of modern surgical practice* (14th ed.). Philadelphia: W. B. Saunders.
29. Sleisenger, M. H., & Fordtran, J. S. (Eds.). (1993). *Gastrointestinal disease* (5th ed.). Philadelphia: W. B. Saunders.
30. Society of Gastroenterology Nurses and Associates. (1993). *Gastroenterology nursing: A core curriculum.* St. Louis: Mosby-Year Book.
31. Williams, S. G., & Dipalma, J. A. (1992). Medication-induced digestive system injury in the elderly. *Geriatric Nursing, 13,* 39–42.
32. Wyngaarden, J. B., et al. (Eds.). (1992). *Cecil textbook of medicine* (19th ed.). Philadelphia: W. B. Saunders.

Chapter 35

Nursing Care of Clients with Intestinal Disorders

Learning Outcomes

After completing this chapter, the learner will be able to:

1. Assess the client for clinical manifestations of intestinal disorders.
2. Teach the client about the etiology, risk factors, basic pathophysiology, and clinical manifestations of major intestinal disorders.
3. Explain the client's role in medical and surgical management of intestinal disorders.
4. Develop plans of care for the prevention of illness, management, and rehabilitation of clients with intestinal disorders.
5. Implement nursing interventions that optimize the quality of life for clients with intestinal disorders.
6. Evaluate the client outcomes using criteria developed in the planning phase of care.

GENERALIZED CLINICAL MANIFESTATIONS

Manifestations of intestinal disorders vary according to which function (motility, digestion, or absorption) is disturbed and the cause of this disturbance. The major manifestations of dysfunction are hemorrhage, pain, tenderness, distention, vomiting, malabsorption, constipation, diarrhea, abdominal masses, and abnormal fecal contents.

Hemorrhage

Bleeding may be caused by trauma, ulceration, inflammation, or a growth that erodes through a blood vessel (Fig. 35–1). The usual manifestation is blood in the stool (melena). The amount of bleeding varies from a minute quantity that is invisible except by testing (occult blood) to large quantities that cause the stools to be bright red to tarry black. Because color comes from the digestive processes acting on the blood, the examiner can use the amount of color change to determine the level of the bowel in which bleeding occurs. The rapidity with which the chyme passes through the bowel also affects stool color passed in a certain period and what color changes occur. For instance, slow bleeding from the duodenum may not increase peristalsis and may produce a tarry stool. If the rate of bleeding or of peristalsis increases, subsequent stools may become brighter in color.

Pain

Pain results from stimulation of nerve endings in the muscular or submucosal layers of bowel wall and from increased tension when the bowel is distended. Discomfort occurs in various places, including the involved portion of the bowel, another previously diseased area, or a nearby somatic portion of the body (referred pain). Previous surgical procedures influence the location at which pain is felt.

Obstruction of blood supply to the intestine also can cause pain. Acute or partial occlusion of the mesenteric artery causes intermittent pain during digestion because of the increased need for blood at that time.

Nausea and Vomiting

In intestinal disorders, nausea results from distention of the duodenum. If vomiting occurs and is fecal in nature, it originates from the bowel and is usually due to a high small intestinal obstruction.

Malabsorption

Malabsorption is a defect in the mechanism by which food is absorbed by the small intestinal mucosa. In the intestinal phase of absorption, the intestinal villi secrete enzymes that stimulate intestinal motility and facilitate absorption. Abnormalities may result from:

- Loss of ileal function
- Decreased production of pancreatic enzyme, especially inadequate secretion of lipase
- Inflammation of the intestinal mucosa
- Any surgical loss of absorptive mucosa, such as gastric, small bowel, or colon resection

Diarrhea

Rapid propulsion of intestinal contents through the small bowel usually results in diarrhea.

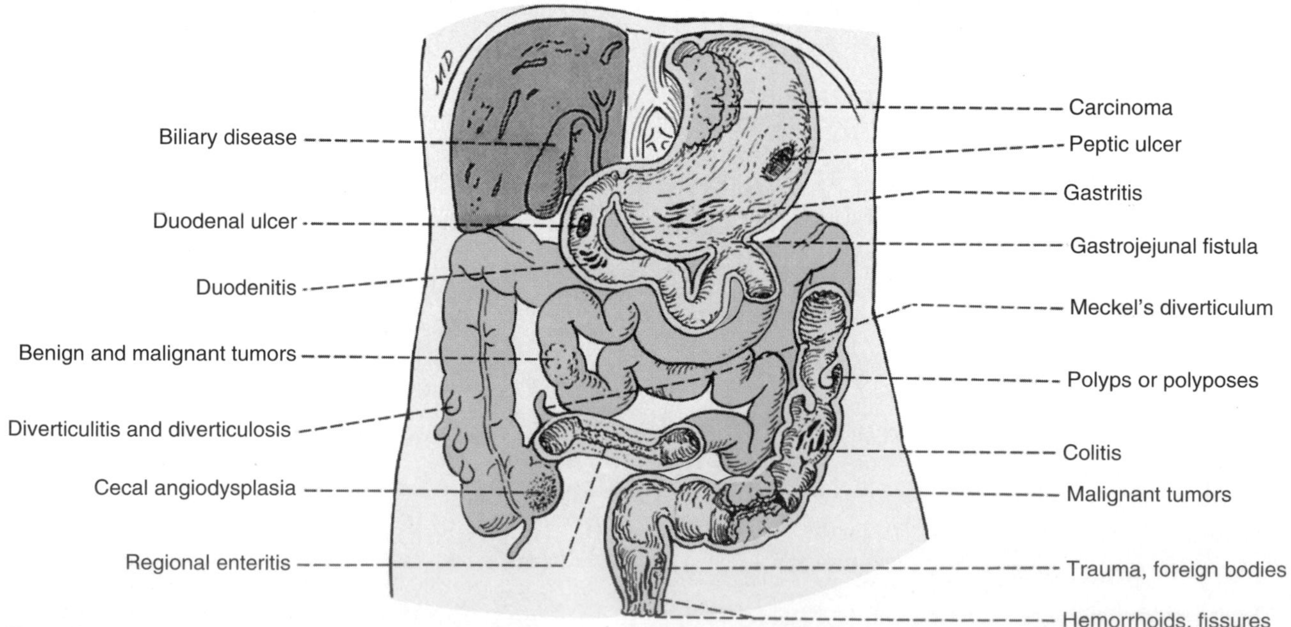

Figure 35–1
Causes of gastrointestinal bleeding.

Constipation

Constipation, a very common symptom, can be caused by inadequate fluid or bulk, mechanical blockage of the passage of intestinal contents (by a tumor), or slow peristalsis.

Abnormalities in Fecal Content

The presence of fats or other abnormal constituents normally absorbed from the stool indicates malabsorption. Other fecal abnormalities that may aid in diagnosis are bacteria, parasites, pus, blood, and abnormal quantities of mucus from the colon.

GASTROINTESTINAL INTUBATION

Gastric and intestinal tubes are inserted for several purposes: decompression, lavage, gastric analysis, and tube feedings. Decompression relieves the pressure caused by gastrointestinal (GI) contents and gases that remain in the stomach or bowel because of some obstruction. Long intestinal tubes are sometimes used to dilate or release an obstruction. Postoperative decompression removes secretions that cannot pass through the GI tract because of edema and decreased gastric motility. Intubation helps prevent vomiting, distention, and obstruction.

Lavage is the irrigation or washing out of an organ. Gastric lavage washes out the stomach. It is used most frequently as an emergency treatment in poisoning. Lavage is also used for exfoliative cytology.

Tube feeding, or *enteral nutrition,* is a method of giving clients fluids and nutrients via a tube when oral intake is inadequate or impossible.

Types of Tubes

Two types of tubes are used for decompression. Short nasogastric tubes are used for the stomach and long tubes for the rest of the GI tract (Table 35–1).

SHORT TUBES

These include the Levin and Salem sump tubes. Short tubes are long enough to extend into the stomach but not into the bowel. These tubes are attached to intermittent suction.

LONG TUBES

The long tubes extend into the small bowel, sometimes for its entire length. They are between 6 and 10 feet long and are used to prevent gas and fluid accumulation in the intestine, which is usually due to intestinal obstruction. The more common long tubes are the Miller-Abbott, Cantor, and Harris tubes.

Suction

When suction is applied to a GI tube to remove accumulated gas and fluid, it is important to ensure that the GI mucosa is not traumatized. Excessive negative pressure causes the mucosa to be sucked into the openings on the tube, impairing the effectiveness of the suction and injuring the mucosa. Intermittent suction is commonly used to avoid this problem. Because mucus tends to plug the openings of these tubes, the nurse must irrigate the tubes as ordered to maintain or check their patency.

Nursing Management

It is very important to maintain the client's comfort while the tube is in place. Some helpful nursing interventions are outlined in Box 35–1.

Placement of the tube in the throat may result in cricoid chondritis (irritation of the cricoid cartilage of the larynx) and laryngeal injuries. Presenting symptoms include localized odynophagia, pain radiating to the ears, sore throat, stridor, bloody sputum, and mild hoarseness. The nurse must assess for these potential complications and report the observations immediately. The physician may order anesthetic lozenges or gargles to relieve the symptoms.

The nurse must frequently assess the material aspirated via the tube for color, odor, and quantity. Any

TABLE 35–1 Gastric and Intestinal Tubes

TUBE TYPE	LENGTH	SIZE (FRENCH)	LUMEN	OTHER CHARACTERISTICS
Short				
Levin type (plastic or rubber)	125 cm (50″)	12, 16, 18	Single	Removes fluid or gas
Salem sump	120 cm (48″)	12, 14, 16, 18	Double	Sump-type suction; decompresses the stomach
Long				
Cantor	300 cm (10′)	16	Single	Mercury weighted; used for suction
Harris	180 cm (6′)	14, 16	Single	Mercury weighted; used for suction
Miller-Abbott	300 cm (10′)	12, 14, 16, 18	Double	Mercury weighted; used for aspiration of contents

BOX 35-1

Comfort Measures for Clients With a Gastrointestinal Tube

The nurse should implement the following comfort measures:

- Gently clean and lubricate the external nares. They may become sore from crusted secretions around the tube.
- Tape the tube in a manner that prevents irritation to the nares.
- Administer frequent oral hygiene to remove debris, increase comfort, maintain a healthy oral cavity, and stimulate saliva secretion. The client's mouth is usually dry because the absence of chewing prevents the normal stimulus to salivary secretions and because mouth breathing results from the presence of the tube.
- If possible, let the client chew gum or suck on sour candies or ice chips to help stimulate salivation.
- Brush the client's teeth or assist the client to do so.
- Request an order for anesthetic mouth rinses or lozenges because clients frequently suffer sore throats from the presence of the tube.

changes should be reported to the physician. Samples of these secretions may need to be sent to the laboratory for analysis. The nurse must measure contents of the suction bottles to maintain an accurate record of GI losses. Metabolic alkalosis may result from a major loss of water and electrolytes.

The nurse must remember that the irrigating solution instilled into a GI tube is counted as intake. Accurate records must be kept of the amount instilled and the amount aspirated from the tube during irrigations. Normal saline is often the irrigating solution of choice because water, a hypotonic solution, increases electrolyte loss through osmotic action if the tube is irrigated often.

Disorders of the Large and Small Bowel

Inflammatory Disorders

Inflammation can occur in any portion of the bowel and can be caused by

- Organisms
- Toxins produced by organisms
- Infiltration of the bowel wall by granulomatous processes
- Injury from radiation
- Medications

All types of organisms, from viruses to large parasites, can cause inflammation.

VIRAL AND BACTERIAL INFECTIONS: GASTROENTERITIS AND DYSENTERY

Gastroenteritis is an inflammation of the stomach and intestinal tract that primarily affects the small bowel. It is associated with abdominal cramps, diarrhea, vomiting, and fever.

Dysenteries are inflammatory conditions affecting the colon. They are exhibited by severe bloody diarrhea and abdominal cramping.

Incidence

Viral gastroenteritis occurs throughout the world and is common. It often occurs in epidemic outbreaks.

Dysenteries caused by *Escherichia coli* and *Shigella* also occur worldwide. *Shigella* occurs more frequently in children younger than 10 years and in homosexual populations. Salmonella, also referred to as food poisoning, may cause dysentery.

Infection with *Clostridium difficile,* also known as pseudomembranous colitis, is a bacterial dysentery commonly seen in clients who have been receiving large doses of antibiotics or who have taken antibiotics for a long period of time. The condition is becoming increasingly common in the hospitalized population. Careful assessment of these individuals for continued need for these medications is important.

Etiology

The cause of gastroenteritis is usually a virus or bacteria. The virus varies and is often referred to as the "flu." In staphylococcal food poisoning, the bacteria produce a toxin when infected foods are allowed to remain warm for a time before being eaten.

Amebic and bacterial organisms such as *Entamoeba histolytica, Shigella bacilli, Escherichia coli,* or *Salmonella* cause most dysenteries. Cholera also causes dysentery-like symptoms.

Risk Factors

Viral gastroenteritis is often associated with crowds and frequently occurs more in the fall and winter months. The risk factors for gastroenteritis caused by food poisoning are improper handling and storage of foods or food handling by infected individuals.

The risk factors for dysentery include overcrowding, (2) poor sanitary conditions, and (3) food remaining at a temperature high enough for organisms to incubate and colonize easily. The major risk factor for gastroenteritis caused by *Clostridium difficile* is the use of antibiotics, either for long periods or in high doses.

Pathophysiology

If *Staphylococcus* organisms multiply sufficiently, they can cause a violent gastroenteritis to develop in 2 to 4 hours. Bacterial or viral food poisoning usually develops within 16 hours after ingestion of contaminated food.

CRITICAL TO REMEMBER

Gastroenteritis temporarily disables people, but the condition is of short duration and usually is not serious, except in infants, the very elderly, and weakened or debilitated individuals. These clients are at risk for life-threatening fluid and electrolyte imbalances.

Diarrhea associated with dysentery is caused, in part, by the inflammatory action of the organisms on the lining of the bowel. The organisms can invade and actually destroy the mucosal lining of the bowel, leading to fluid leaking into the bowel.

Endotoxins produced by the infective organisms stimulate the mucosal cells lining the bowel, leading to further diarrhea. These mucosal cells increase secretion of water and electrolytes into the intestinal lumen. The active secretion of chloride and bicarbonate ions in the small bowel leads to the inhibition of sodium reabsorption. To balance the excess sodium, large amounts of protein-rich fluids are secreted into the bowel, overwhelming the large bowel's ability to reabsorb the fluid.

Dysentery can prove fatal in the debilitated, aged, and very young persons. Early detection and intervention with fluids and electrolytes are critical to prevent death or disability.

Clinical Manifestations

Assessment reveals vomiting, profuse diarrhea, and resultant severe fluid and electrolyte loss. Varying amounts of blood may be present in the stool, and the client may experience a mild-to-severe temperature elevation, depending on the causative organism.

Management

Management of gastroenteritis includes resting the GI tract and replacing fluids. The client must rest with nothing by mouth until the vomiting has stopped. If the client has fluid depletion, an intravenous infusion is administered. A potassium supplement may be ordered if the client's serum potassium level is low.

The client is started on small amounts of clear liquids, as tolerated. The client may be given Gatorade or other electrolyte replacement beverage. The diet is advanced after 24 hours, as tolerated. In gastroenteritis, the infecting agents need to be eliminated, so drugs that decrease intestinal motility are not administered.

If the infecting organism is *Shigella,* an anti-infective agent such as sulfamethoxazole with trimethoprim (Bactrim, Septra) is administered. In the case of prolonged diarrhea in which the stool is leukocyte positive, antibiotics are given.

PROTOZOAL INFECTION: AMEBIASIS

Amebiasis produces diarrhea when a protozoan (*Entamoeba histolytica)* invades the lining of the colon. Symptoms include rectal inflammation and blood, pus, and amoebae in the stool. Metronidazole (Flagyl) is the drug of choice to treat this condition.

PARASITIC INFESTATIONS

The intestinal tract may be infested with any of several species of parasitic worms, including *Ascaris* (roundworms), *Enterobius* (pinworms), *Trichinella spiralis* (which causes trichinosis), and various species of tapeworms. Worms also may cause urinary tract infections or pruritus ani. Fortunately, most of these parasites are susceptible to medications such as mebendazole and pyrantel pamoate. Piperazine and quinacrine hydrochloride also may be used, but they produce more side effects. Treatment for all household members may reduce reinfection.

Schistosomiasis is caused by a blood fluke (a parasitic worm). It is prevalent worldwide. The cercariae of the parasite penetrate the skin, migrate to the liver via the lungs, and remain in intrahepatic portal venules while the worm matures. The mature worm, which does not multiply within humans, then moves into its final habitat, where it lays eggs. These eggs, which form pseudotubercles, are commonly found in the liver and veins of the abdomen and lungs but have been identified in every system of the body, including the nervous system. Some eggs are excreted in the urine or feces.

In humans, schistosomiasis may have no symptoms. It may be mild or severe, depending on the species of worm involved and the number present. The prognosis is usually good, although there is an increase in the incidence of bladder cancer in clients with this parasite.

Schistosomiasis begins with dermatitis at the site of penetration, followed by a fever in 20 to 60 days, and later by symptoms from the extrusion of eggs. Laboratory studies must examine the eggs or worms and identify the species before pharmacologic treatment can begin. Medications of choice include oxamniquine, metrifonate, praziquantel, and niridazole.

Nursing Management of Intestinal Infections and Infestations

Assessment

Most clients present with an acute onset of diarrhea. The nurse must carefully note a description of the diarrhea, including onset, number of stools, color, consistency, and accompanying symptoms such as nausea and vomiting. The nurse should ask the client about recent foreign travel, eating habits, and antibiotic use.

The nurse should assess the abdomen. Examination may reveal hyperactive bowel sounds, distention, and tenderness. Dehydration may be present depending on the amount of fluids lost. Metabolic alkalosis from bicarbonate loss is also a potential problem.

Nursing Diagnosis, Planning, and Implementation

Nursing Diagnosis: Diarrhea R/T intestinal hypermotility.

Planning: Expected Outcomes. The client will have cessation of diarrhea, as evidenced by a decrease in the number of stools and the solid consistency of feces.

Implementation. The nurse must carefully examine all stool for blood and mucus and must accurately record intake and output. The nurse must examine the anal area for irritation. After cleaning the area, a moisture barrier (e.g., petroleum jelly, zinc oxide) can be applied.

The nurse administers medications to treat the specific cause of the diarrhea, such as antibiotics and antiparasitics. Antidiarrheals also may be ordered if the diarrhea is uncontrollable.

Nursing Diagnosis: Fluid Volume Deficit, Risk for R/T GI fluid and electrolyte losses.

Planning: Expected Outcomes. The client will have return of normal fluid and electrolyte balance as evidenced by normal serum electrolytes and balanced intake and output.

Implementation. If the client shows signs of fluid and electrolyte imbalance, intravenous fluids may have to be started until oral fluids are tolerated. Clear liquids with electrolytes are then started in small amounts until the client can tolerate the diet advanced to include toast and saltines. If this diet is tolerated, the diet is usually advanced to a bland diet and then a general diet as tolerated.

Evaluation

The nurse must evaluate client outcomes based on the established plan of care. If these goals were not achieved, the plan and interventions must be revised to meet the client's needs.

APPENDICITIS

Appendicitis is an inflammation of the vermiform appendix that develops most commonly in adolescents and young adults.

Incidence

Appendicitis can occur at any age but is rare in clients younger than age 2 years and reaches a peak incidence in clients between ages 20 and 30 years. It is not common in older adults, but when it does occur in this age group, rupture is more common.

Etiology

Appendicitis can be caused by:

- A fecalith (a fecal calculus or stone) that occludes the lumen of the appendix
- Kinking of the appendix
- Swelling of the bowel wall
- Fibrous conditions in the bowel wall
- External occlusion of the bowel by adhesions

Risk Factors

There are no particular risk factors for appendicitis. It is not preventable, so early detection of the condition is important.

Pathophysiology

When the appendix becomes obstructed, the intraluminal pressure increases, leading to decreased venous drainage, thrombosis, edema, and bacterial invasion of the bowel wall. With continued obstruction, perforation will result.

After the initial obstruction, the appendix becomes increasingly hyperemic, warm, and covered with exudate, progressing to gangrene and perforation.

Clinical Manifestions

The classic manifestations begin with acute abdominal pain, which comes in waves. At first, the pain may be perceived merely as discomfort that makes the client feel that passing flatus or having a bowel movement will bring relief. Unfortunately, many clients take a laxative during this period, which may lead to rupture of the appendix and peritonitis. The pain typically starts in the epigastrium or periumbilical region. It then shifts to the right lower quadrant as the inflammatory process spreads to involve the serosal layers of the bowel, thereby bringing the inflammatory process into contact with the peritoneum. The pain becomes steady rather than intermittent, and the client often guards the area by lying still and drawing the legs up to relieve tension on the abdominal muscles. Assessment also may reveal vomiting that begins after the pain starts, loss of appetite, low-grade fever, coated tongue, and bad breath.

DIAGNOSTIC ASSESSMENT

Mild leukocytosis is usually present, with the white cell count between 10,000 and 15,000. Physical findings confirm the diagnosis. Pain at McBurney's point, which lies midway between the right anterior superior iliac crest and the umbilicus, may be diagnostic.

Medical Management

There is no medical treatment as such for appendicitis. Until surgery can be performed, intravenous fluids and antibiotics are administered.

Surgical Management

Surgical intervention involves removing the appendix (i.e., appendectomy) within 24 to 48 hours of onset of the symptoms. Delay usually causes rupture of the organ and resultant peritonitis. Surgery is frequently delayed, however, because the diagnosis is difficult to make and clients often seek medical aid belatedly. Older clients may have very few symptoms and do not seek aid until after perforation has occurred.

Diagnosis also can be difficult in very young children. Numerous diseases mimic appendicitis. The client will require antibiotics and possibly surgical drainage if perforation occurs.

Nursing Management

The client is usually admitted with severe abdominal pain. The nurse should carefully assess the pain, especially to determine its location. The client also should be assessed for the presence of peritonitis (see section on Peritonitis). The nurse must carefully assess the client's vital signs, fluid and electrolyte status, and laboratory data. The client with appendicitis should fast in preparation for surgery.

Nursing Diagnosis, Planning, and Implementation

Nursing Diagnosis: Pain, Acute R/T inflammation.

Planning: Expected Outcomes. The client will understand why pain medication is held preoperatively and have pain controlled postoperatively, as evidenced by client verbalization.

Implementation. The client will have pain medication withheld until the diagnosis is confirmed. Sometimes, pain medication will not be given until the client is actually ready for surgery.

CRITICAL TO REMEMBER

The nurse should never give an enema or a laxative or apply heat to the abdomen of the client with appendicitis because these actions could lead to perforation.

An abrupt change in the character of the pain preoperatively could indicate perforation. Postoperatively, pain control should be practiced.

Nursing Diagnosis: Fluid Volume Deficit, Risk for R/T vomiting.

Planning: Expected Outcomes. The client will have fluid and electrolyte balance maintained, as evidenced by balanced intake and output and electrolytes within normal limits.

Implementation. As soon as the client is admitted, intravenous fluids are started to maintain fluid balance, with electrolytes added as needed. If the client is vomiting, a nasogastric tube is inserted. Intake and output should be carefully measured and discrepancies reported to the physician.

Nursing Diagnosis: Risk for Infection R/T rupture of appendix.

Planning: Expected Outcomes. The client will not acquire an infection or will have rupture diagnosed early, as evidenced by removal of appendix before rupture or prompt treatment.

Implementation. The client's vital signs must be checked regularly, monitoring closely for an increase in temperature and a change in pulse and blood pressure that may signify a ruptured appendix. The client's pain also should be closely monitored. If the pain becomes generalized throughout the abdomen and the abdomen becomes rigid and boardlike, rupture may have occurred.

If a rupture of the appendix is suspected, the symptoms should be reported to the physician immediately so the client can be prepared for surgery. Preoperative antibiotics are usually administered to decrease the infection.

After surgery, the nurse will monitor vital signs, urine output, level of consciousness, and intravenous therapy, and assess the client's respiratory status and the surgical wound. The client may have a drain, and if the appendix ruptured, packing may be present. The nurse must assess the dressings, provide wound care, reposition the client, and adequately manage the client's pain.

Evaluation

The nurse must evaluate client outcomes based on the established plan of care. If these goals were not achieved, the plan and interventions must be revised to meet the client's needs.

Posthospital Care

The client with uncomplicated appendicitis should resume normal activity in 2 to 4 weeks. Discharge teaching and posthospital care for the client with a routine appendectomy are the same as for any client after surgery.

If the client had a ruptured appendix with an infected wound, the client will have to be taught the proper way to care for the wound. Wound care usually includes irrigation of the wound with sterile saline and application of a sterile dressing several times a day.

The nurse should assess the client's ability to function at home and to care for the wound. A home health-care referral may be needed to assist the client with physical needs.

The client with a ruptured appendix may have to return for surgery after the abscess has walled off. The client with an infected wound will have to be seen at intervals to ensure that the wound is healing properly.

PERITONITIS

Peritonitis is the inflammation of the peritoneal membrane. Because it is well supplied with somatic nerves, stimulation of the parietal peritoneum that lines the abdominal and pelvic cavities causes sharp, well-localized pain. The visceral peritoneum is relatively insensitive.

Incidence

The incidence of peritonitis caused by perforation or rupture of abdominal viscus is hard to determine. Data usually relate to the underlying cause.

Etiology

Peritonitis can be primary or secondary and acute or chronic. The major sources of inflammation are from the gastrointestinal tract, from the external environment, and through the blood stream. The peritoneum is able to produce an inflammatory reaction and wall off a localized process to combat an infection, if the stimulus is not too massive or the source of infection does not continue.

Specific causes of peritonitis are listed in Box 35–2.

Normal bacterial flora of the intestine become a source of infection when they enter the sterile peritoneal cavity. The most common organism is *E. coli,* although *streptococci, staphylococci,* and *pneumococci* also may be involved.

BOX 35–2

Causes of Peritonitis

- Gangrenous cholecystitis
- Ruptured gallbladder
- Perforated carcinoma of the stomach
- Perforated gastric or duodenal ulcer
- Ruptured spleen
- Acute pancreatitis
- Penetrating wound of the gastrointestinal tract
- Ulcerative colitis
- Gangrenous obstruction of the small bowel resulting from (1) adhesions, (2) carcinoma, (3) volvulus, or (4) intussusception
- Perforation of Meckel's diverticulum
- Mesenteric thrombosis
- Perforation of a diverticulum
- Regional ileitis
- Appendicitis with perforation
- Ruptured retroperitoneal abscess
- Strangulated hernia
- Puerperal infection
- Salpingitis
- Septic abortion
- Ruptured bladder
- Iatrogenic perforation
- Result or complication of peritoneal dialysis

Risk Factors

There are no specific risk factors for peritonitis because the condition is a result of another problem. The major preventive measure to consider with this disorder is early diagnosis of clients at risk for the condition secondary to one of its many causes. Early diagnosis and the initiation of early treatment help to prevent spread of the infection.

Pathophysiology

Peritonitis creates severe systemic effects. Circulatory alterations, fluid shifts, and respiratory problems can cause critical fluid and electrolyte imbalances. The circulatory system undergoes great stress from several sources. The inflammatory response shunts extra blood to the inflamed area of the bowel to combat the infection. Peristaltic activity of the bowel ceases. Fluids and air are retained within its lumen, raising pressure and increasing fluid secretion into the bowel. Thus, the circulating blood volume diminishes.

The inflammatory process increases oxygen requirements at a time when the client's ability to ventilate has been reduced. The client has difficulty ventilating because of abdominal pain and increased abdominal pressure, which elevates the diaphragm.

Clinical Manifestations

Manifestations of peritonitis vary depending on the cause. Pain may be either localized or generalized. Well-localized pain that causes rigidity of abdominal muscles and pain that increases with any pressure or motion of the abdomen is characteristic of peritonitis. Also, the client usually experiences nausea, vomiting, and possibly a low-grade fever. Assessment reveals absence of bowel sounds and shallow respirations because the client is trying to avoid the pain caused by body movement.

DIAGNOSTIC ASSESSMENT

The client with peritonitis commonly has an elevated white cell count (20,000/mm^3) with a high neutrophil count. Abdominal x-rays studies are performed, which may show dilation and edema of the intestines, or free air or fluid in the abdominal cavity. If the client is vomiting, signs of altered fluid and electrolyte balance also may be present.

Medical Management

If peritonitis is advanced and surgery is contraindicated because of shock and circulatory failure, oral fluids are prohibited and intravenous fluids are necessary for replacement of electrolyte and protein losses. Usually, a long intestinal tube is inserted through the nose into the intestine to reduce pressure within the bowel. Once the infection has become walled off and the client's condition improves, surgical drainage and repair can be attempted.

The other major treatment for peritonitis is intravenous antibiotic therapy with potent broad-spectrum agents.

Surgical Management

Surgery may be performed to prevent peritonitis, such as with an appendectomy for an inflamed appendix or a colon resection for inflamed diverticula. If the perforation is not prevented, then the major surgical intervention is incision and drainage of the abscess once it is walled off.

Nursing Management

Assessment

The nurse must obtain a thorough history, including specific information about the client's pain. The nurse should assess the abdomen, noting the presence of bowel sounds. The abdomen should be palpated, noting if the abdomen is firm, distended, or rigid. Areas of tenderness should be noted.

CRITICAL TO REMEMBER

The nurse also should assess for the presence of rebound tenderness.

The client probably has a high fever, indicating peritonitis.

Nursing Diagnosis, Planning, and Implementation

Nursing Diagnosis: Injury and Infection, Risk for R/T possible perforation and ischemia.

Planning: Expected Outcomes. The client will not acquire an infection or complications of peritonitis or will have infection and complications adequately treated, as evidenced by normal vital signs, no sign of inflammation, absence of shock, renal failure, adult respiratory distress syndrome (ARDS), or sepsis.

Implementation. Clients with peritonitis are acutely ill. They are started on broad-spectrum antibiotics immediately on admission to the hospital.

Surgery is usually performed to repair the perforated organs as soon as clients are stable enough to withstand the stress of surgery.

CRITICAL TO REMEMBER

Postoperatively, the nurse must carefully monitor clients for the development of postoperative complications such as ARDS, sepsis, and shock.

The vital signs should be closely monitored and any signs of sepsis, such as a drop or increase in temperature or drop in blood pressure, reported immediately.

Nursing Diagnosis: Fluid Volume Deficit, Risk for R/T vomiting.

Planning: Expected Outcomes. The client will maintain normal fluid volume, as evidenced by adequate output, good skin turgor, moist mucous membranes, and absence of vomiting.

Implementation. Intravenous fluids are administered along with antibiotic therapy. In the client with peritonitis, the nurse must maintain the nasogastric tube (see Gastrointestinal Intubation). The nurse also must monitor the client's fluid balance by assessing vital signs, urine output, skin turgor, intravenous fluid replacement, weight, and mucous membrane integrity.

Evaluation

The nurse must evaluate client outcomes based on the established plan. If these goals were not achieved, the plan and interventions must be revised to meet the client's needs.

INFLAMMATORY BOWEL DISEASE

Inflammatory bowel disease (IBD) includes two chronic inflammatory disorders: Crohn's disease (regional enteritis) and ulcerative colitis. Both diseases are characterized by periods of exacerbation and remission. These chronic, recurrent diseases predominantly affect younger people. Treatment is symptomatic and responses are often unpredictable. Frequently, clients with IBD require surgery, which may be followed by recurrence. Because of the similarities between Crohn's disease and ulcerative colitis, we compare and contrast these two conditions throughout the following discussion of IBD (Table 35–2).

Crohn's Disease. Crohn's disease (regional enteritis) is a chronic relapsing disease that may develop discontinuously in any segment of the alimentary tract. The most common location is the terminal ileum. Crohn's disease more characteristically involves the entire thickness of the bowel wall (transmural) but particularly the submucosa. The mortality rate is not high, but recurrences and complications can result in disability.

Ulcerative Colitis. This is a disease that spans the entire length of the colon and involves only the mucosa and submucosa. The disease usually starts in the rectum and distal colon and spreads upward beyond the rectosigmoid valve to involve most of the sigmoid and descending colon.

Ulcerative colitis causes inflammation, thickening, congestion, edema, and minute lacerations that ooze blood and eventually develop into abscesses. The edema may lead to extreme friability of the mucosa, so bleeding occurs from any minor trauma.

Incidence

Crohn's Disease. This disease is more common in whites and among Jewish people. There is an increased

TABLE 35–2 Differentiation Between Crohn's Disease and Ulcerative Colitis

CHARACTERISTIC	REGIONAL ENTERITIS (CROHN'S DISEASE)	ULCERATIVE COLITIS
General Description		
Age at onset	Young	Young to middle
Pathology and Anatomy		
Depth of involvement	Transmural (all layers of submucosa)	Mucosa and submucosa
Rectal involvement	50%	95%
Right colon involvement	Frequent	Occasional
Small bowel involvement	Involved, ileum narrow	Usually normal
Distribution of disease	Segmental	Continuous
Inflammatory mass	Chronic and extensive	Rare (crypt abscess)
Cobblestone-like mucosa and granuloma	Common	Absent
Mesentery lymph involvement	Edema and hyperplasia	Not involved
Toxic megacolon	Occasional	Occasional
Steatorrhea	Frequent	Absent
Malignancy results	Rare	After 10 years
Fibrous stricture	Common	Absent
Clinical		
Course of disease	Slowly progressive	Remissions and relapses
Rectal bleeding	Occasional	Common (90–100%)
Abdominal pain	Colicky (45%)	Predefecation (60–70%)
Hematochezia	Unusual or absent	Almost always present
Diarrhea	Present (65–85%)	Early and frequent (80–95%)
Vomiting	Present (35%)	Present (15%)
Nutritional deficit	Common	Common
Weight loss	Present (60–70%)	Present (20–50%)
Fever	Present (35%)	Present (10%)
Anal abscess	Common (75%)	Occasional (10%)
Fistula and anorectal fissure fistula	Common (80%)	Rare (10–20%)
Systemic Manifestations		
Arthritis	20%	Uncommon (10%)
Peripheral sacroiliitis	18%	18–20%
Hepatobiliary involvement	Uncommon	15% cholestatic dysfunction 19–38% fatty liver 30–50% pericholangitis
Skin: erythema nodosum, pyoderma grangrenosum	Common	Present (5–10%)
Nephrolithiasis	Occasional	Rare

incidence within families. It occurs at all ages but more often in the third decade of life. Both sexes are affected equally.

Ulcerative Colitis. This is more common than Crohn's disease. It occurs at all ages but has a higher incidence among young adults, women, and Jewish people. It has demonstrated a familial tendency.

Etiology

Crohn's Disease. The cause of Crohn's disease is unclear, although the literature suggests there is some genetic or hereditary basis. The disease is also considered autoimmune in nature.

Ulcerative Colitis. Several theories have attempted to explain the cause of ulcerative colitis. These include

- Bacterial origin
- Allergic reaction
- Altered immunity
- Destructive enzymes and a lack of protective substances in the bowel wall.

An emotional disturbance can precipitate an exacerbation or prolong an attack of the disorder, but it is not the primary cause.

Risk Factors

Crohn's Disease. The only risk factors identified for Crohn's disease are genetic ones. There are no preventive measures that can be taken.

Ulcerative Colitis. There are no preventable risk factors associated with ulcerative colitis. Once the client has the disease, controlling stress can help keep the disease in remission.

Pathophysiology

Crohn's Disease. Lesions typically develop in several separated segments of bowel. They are grossly visible and examination of the bowel tissue by oscopy reveals edematous, heavy, reddish purple areas. Granular spots also may be present. Enlarged lymph nodes appear in the submucosa, and Peyer's patches are seen in the intestinal mucous membrane. These areas undergo small superficial ulceration with granulomas and fissures. Fissures may completely penetrate the bowel wall, leading to fistulas and abscesses. Collections of lymphocytes throughout the mucosa, submucosa, and serosa are the only microscopic features of Crohn's disease. The small bowel wall becomes congested and thickened, and the lumen narrows. The mucosa has an erythematous, cobblestone-like appearance. In later stages of the disease, the intestinal wall becomes permanently fibrosed, thickened, and narrowed.

Small bowel–related complications of Crohn's disease include malabsorption, kidney stones, gallstones, and hydronephrosis. Anorectal problems include internal fistulas and abscesses. Nephrolithiasis, hydronephrosis, and growth retardation are other complications. Fissure in ano is the most common lesion and is directly related to the severity of the diarrhea, which produces ulceration of the perianal skin. Pain commonly accompanies defecation.

Assessment may reveal an area of induration, swelling, and redness. Internal fistulas characterize Crohn's disease of the ileum and right colon. Rectovaginal fistulas may occur in women. Incontinence is common owing to breakdown in the relatively thin rectovaginal septum. Fistulas into the bladder precipitate recurrent urinary infections and, in some instances, even fecaluria. Treatment may include either drainage to control infection or excision.

Arthritis is a transient, acute, painful swelling present in 20 per cent of clients with Crohn's disease.

Toxic megacolon is an extreme dilatation of a segment of the diseased colon (often the transverse) that results in complete obstruction. Toxic megacolon usually occurs during an acute exacerbation and may follow hypokalemia, a barium enema, or the use of anticholinergics, narcotics, corticosteroids, or antibiotics. Bacterial overgrowth contributes to the development of toxic megacolon.

Assessment reveals paralytic ileus, dehydration, fever, tachycardia, lethargy, leukocytosis, decreased serum protein and albumin levels, anxiety, and prostration. In addition, perforation and peritonitis may complicate toxic megacolon.

Ulcerative Colitis. The appearance of the colon depends on the stage, activity, and severity of the disease. The most characteristic lesion of ulcerative colitis is an inflammatory infiltrate called crypt abscess. This abscess consists of polymorphonuclear leukocytes, lymphocytes, red cells, and cellular debris appearing at the base of the glandular crypts. The crypt abscess secretions result in purulent discharge. The abscesses may become necrotic and may ulcerate.

Infections secondary to ulcerative colitis produce further inflammatory reactions in the mucosa and submucosa. When the inflammatory lesions heal, scarring and fibrosis, with narrowing, thickening, and shortening of the colon and loss of haustral folds, may follow.

Cancer of the colon is more common among clients with ulcerative colitis than among the general population.

Complications of ulcerative colitis vary with its severity and location. Ankylosing spondylitis and clubbing of the fingers are found in a few clients. Anemia and nutritional deficiency may occur, causing dry skin that lacks turgor. In addition, assessment reveals erythema pustules, abscesses, and neurodermatitis.

Toxic megacolon occurs during an acute exacerbation and is described under Crohn's Disease.

Clinical Manifestations

Crohn's Disease. This disease may have acute manifestations, but the condition is usually slow and unaggressive. The client may be treated for mild and intermittent symptoms months before the diagnosis of Crohn's disease is made.

Assessment typically reveals abdominal pain, diarrhea, and weight loss as a result of nutritional deficits. The pain is usually intermittent. Terminal ileum involvement produces pain in the periumbilical region. The client experiences jejunal pain in the upper and left midabdomen. Pain of the ileum is intermittent and is felt in the lower right quadrant. A constant aching, soreness, or tenderness usually indicates advanced disease. The client may experience relief of discomfort after passing stool or flatus.

Diarrhea is usually less severe than that associated with ulcerative colitis. Stool consistency is typically soft or semiliquid. Malabsorption, associated with steatorrhea, may develop. If so, stools may be foul smelling and fatty. Urgency to expel stools may awaken the person at night. In contrast to ulcerative colitis, the client rarely passes gross blood.

Passage of blood indicates ulceration. The client with severe steatorrhea, diarrhea, or long-standing enteritis may have associated nutritional deficits, weight loss, anorexia, pain, anemia, debility, fatigue, and metabolic disturbances. Nutritional deficits arise from

- A reduction in the intestinal absorptive surface
- Impaired absorption of fat, vitamin B_{12}, folic acid, iron, calcium, and vitamins A, C, D, E, and K
- Malabsorption of protein and carbohydrates

Alterations in bile salt and vitamin metabolism may result from surgery or mucosal defects. Metabolic requirements increase because of the inflammatory process and infection, decreased food intake, and nutrients lost in the feces owing to rapid GI transit time. Electrolytes lost from diarrhea include sodium, potassium, chloride, the trace elements (magnesium, zinc, copper), and minerals.

Nitrogen excretion remains normal if there is no loss of protein from the inflammatory exudate.

Temperature elevation may occur with acute inflammation; associated fistulas, abscesses, or sinus tracts; or rheumatoid manifestations. Sudden, severe, right lower quadrant pain, leukocytosis, and tenderness accompany the elevated temperature. Nausea and vomiting are rare unless there is a small bowel obstruction.

Additional acute inflammatory symptoms include pain in the lower right quadrant, cramping, tenderness, flatulence, nausea, and diarrhea. Borborygmus and increased peristalsis also may develop. Pain sometimes mimics acute appendicitis or bowel perforation, and symptoms may be confused with those of ulcerative colitis. If anal disease occurs, fissures, fistulas, skin tags, ulcers, and strictures may be present.

The client may experience periods of remission interrupted by exacerbations of active Crohn's disease. Because exacerbations often follow dietary indiscretions, emotional upsets, or illness, the nurse should inquire into the client's life events at the time of the exacerbation.

Ulcerative Colitis. The predominant symptom of ulcerative colitis is rectal bleeding. Clients often experience diarrhea, possibly 20 or more stools per day. A sense of urgency and cramping abdominal pain may occur with the diarrhea. The client typically experiences colicky pain in the lower left quadrant.

Nausea, vomiting, anorexia, weight loss, and decreased serum potassium may occur with severe disease. In addition, the client loses plasma proteins, prothrombin, and fluids. The development of anemia depends on the degree of blood loss, severity of the illness, and dietary iron intake.

When the disease is acute, the client experiences fever. Severe diarrhea or vomiting may cause metabolic acidosis. Physical findings include tenderness in the lower left quadrant, guarding, and (in severe ulcerative colitis) abdominal distention. After remissions, ulcerative colitis may recur after bouts of emotional stress, dietary indiscretion, or the ingestion of irritants such as laxatives or antibiotics. Physical exertion, respiratory infections and overfatigue also may cause an attack. As in Crohn's disease, it is important to inquire into the client's life events prior to recurrences.

DIAGNOSTIC ASSESSMENT

Physical assessment may reveal certain characteristic manifestations. The general appearance of clients with IBD varies from reasonably healthy to wasted, drawn, and malnourished, with varying degrees of pallor. Some clients have a fever and tachycardia. They usually report a steady and progressive weight loss. Inspection reveals a flat or concave shape of the abdomen, with visible peristaltic activity. Palpation of the abdomen reveals tenderness over the area of inflamed bowel. Increased bowel sounds are heard on auscultation. The rectal sphincter is found to be tight, the rectum empty, and the anal area irritated. Hemorrhoids and, in Crohn's disease, perianal abscess, fistula, or ulcers may be apparent.

Decreased levels of hematocrit and hemoglobin are usually noted. A barium enema study with air contrast is often performed to differentiate between ulcerative colitis and Crohn's disease. The client with suspected IBD routinely undergoes colonoscopy. Biopsy and cytologic studies also help distinguish between carcinoma, ulcerative colitis, and Crohn's disease.

Medical Management

Medical treatment, which primarily aims to control the symptoms, is similar for ulcerative colitis and for Crohn's disease. Because the inflammatory process in Crohn's disease involves deeper layers of the bowel wall and is more chronic, healing may occur more slowly than in ulcerative colitis. Thus, anti-inflammatory therapy, including steroids, is required for longer periods in Crohn's disease than in ulcerative colitis.

Fluids, electrolytes, and blood are replaced as needed to maintain the client's homeostasis. Physical activity should be kept to a minimum during the acute attack to decrease intestinal motility. The client with mild attacks may work but needs extra rest. The client with fever, toxemia, frequent bowel movements, bleeding, or pain sometimes requires bedrest. Failure of the inflamed colonic mucosa to reabsorb water and electrolytes, bile salts, and lactose interferes with control of diarrhea. The extent of large bowel involved in the disease influences the severity of diarrhea. The client should keep a record of the number of stools, their consistency and color, and the presence of blood.

PHARMACOLOGIC MANAGEMENT

Antidiarrheal preparations may provide symptomatic benefit (Table 35–3). Loperamide (Imodium) is superior to diphenoxylate (Lomotil) in controlling diarrhea of Crohn's disease, with fewer side effects. Opiates for diarrhea control may cause distention and megacolon. Hydrophilic mucilloids, such as psyllium or methylcellulose, may improve the consistency of stools and rectal continence. Antispasmodic medications such as belladonna extract, propantheline bromide, glycopyrrolate, or dicyclomine hydrochloride may reduce postprandial pain and diarrhea.

Diarrhea associated with IBD may be treated successfully by antimicrobial agents such as sulfasalazine. In an attempt to control diarrhea, tincture of opium and paregoric are sometimes given. Bowel rest and total parenteral nutrition may result in restored immunocompetence, greater resistance to infection, correction of nutritional deficiencies, and relief of edema and bowel inflammation.

TABLE 35–3 Drugs Used in the Treatment of Diarrhea

DRUG	DAILY DOSAGE	NURSING INTERVENTION
Diphenoxylate hydrochloride with atropine sulfate (Lomotil)	5 mg, four times daily (altered doses for elderly are not specifically established)	1. Assess number of stools and consistency throughout treatment 2. Assess fluid and electrolyte balance 3. Assess for dry mouth, tachycardia, rash, and urinary retention 4. May be administered with food if GI irritation occurs 5. Assess for abdominal distention, pain, and fever
Loperamide hydrochloride (Imodium)	4 mg initially, then 2 mg after each loose stool; maximum dose, 16 mg daily	1. Assess number of stools 2. Assess for drowsiness, dry mouth, N/V, constipation 3. Assess for abdominal distention, pain, and fever
Opium preparations (opium tincture, paregoric)	Paregoric: 5 to 10 mL, one to four times daily Tincture: 0.6 mL, four times a day	1. Assess for N/V 2. Dilute opium tincture in 15 to 30 mL of liquid 3. Assess for abdominal distention, pain, and fever

GI, gastrointestinal; N/V, nausea and/or vomiting.

Clients who fail to respond to general supportive measures may require anti-inflammatory medications. Adrenal steroids and corticotropin may be used with other therapy to reduce the body's response to inflammation. Steroids do not cure IBD, but by reducing inflammation, they may modify its course. The systemic effects of IBD also respond to steroids.

Antacids or histamine receptor antagonists should be given during steroid therapy to prevent gastric ulceration. Steroids decrease adrenal function and may impair resistance, causing defective healing of abscesses and fistulas. Corticosteroids interfere with intestinal absorption of calcium.

6-Mercaptopurine, an immunosuppressive agent, is used when other treatment modalities fail and can be effective against chronic, unrelenting Crohn's disease and many of its complications. The medication should be used during the chronic phase. To be effective, therefore, the client must receive steroids or corticotropin beforehand.

During acute exacerbations, the client is given anticholinergic medications to relieve abdominal cramps and help control diarrhea. Anticholinergics, antidiarrheal agents, and antispasmodics allow the colon to rest and decrease the gastrocolic reflex. Anticholinergics may decrease muscle spasm and discomfort but have little effect on diarrhea. These medications should be withheld if there are signs of obstruction. Treatment with these agents may cause further iatrogenic problems.

Medications commonly used to prevent or control infections include the sulfonamides and antibiotics. If antibiotic therapy is effective, you will note a decrease in temperature, number of stools, and bleeding. Antibiotics may be given to control secondary bowel inflammation and infection.

DIETARY MANAGEMENT

Total parenteral nutrition is indicated for the client who fails to respond to medical intervention, is being prepared for surgery, or has had an intestinal resection. This feeding method provides bowel rest by removing all stimulation of secretion and by decreasing fecal bulk. When oral food and fluids are resumed, they should be chemically and mechanically nonirritating and high in calories, protein, and minerals. Foods such as cocoa, chocolate, citrus juices, cold or carbonated drinks, nuts, seeds, popcorn, and alcohol should be excluded.

Elemental diets provide nutritionally balanced meals. They are residue free, low in fat, and digested mainly in the upper jejunum.

Anemia and vitamin B_{12} deficiencies should be corrected nutritionally. Folate deficiency, which may be due to therapeutic use of sulfasalazine, may be prevented by increasing dietary intake of folate, giving sulfasalazine between meals, or supplementing the intervention regimen with folic acid.

A diet high in protein and calories is given in an attempt to restore normal nutritional levels but is not always well tolerated. Eating tends to increase diarrhea and anorexia, and nausea and vomiting are often present.

COMPLICATIONS

Nutritional deficiencies are the most common complications of IBD. These deficits derive from

- Decreased intake
- Increased nutritional requirements
- Increased losses
- Side effects of certain medications

Therapeutic interventions such as special diets, antibiotic agents, and anti-inflammatory medications, also may cause anorexia or stomatitis. Specific nutritional and metabolic problems caused by IBD include diminished absorption of vitamin B_{12} and trace metals including zinc, calcium, and magnesium and decreased reabsorption of bile salts.

Extraintestinal manifestations occur frequently in clients with IBD and complicate its management. Manifestations involve the joints (most common symptom), skin, eyes, and mouth. The major skin manifestations are erythema nodosum and pyoderma gangrenosum. Local tissue involvement can cause rectal complications, such as anal fissures, and bowel complications, such as local abscesses, perforation, and stenosis from healing lesions. Infrequent nonspecific manifestations include osteoporosis, liver disease, peptic ulceration, and amyloidosis.

Surgical Management

Surgery is commonly used to treat ulcerative colitis, but not Crohn's disease, except to treat complications.

Possible procedures that may be performed to treat ulcerative colitis include a total proctocolectomy with a permanent ileostomy (Fig. 35–2) and restorative procedures such as an ileorectal anastomosis (Fig. 35–3), an ileoanal reservoir (Fig. 35–4), and a Kock pouch (Fig. 35–5).

This continent ileostomy, or Kock pouch, has advantages because the client does not need to wear an external pouch, has minimal skin problems, and usually has no leakage of stool or flatus. The client drains the pouch several times per day using a catheter, usually when a feeling of fullness occurs.

After the formation of the Kock pouch, suture line leakage with local or generalized peritonitis (the most frequent complication with the reservoir) may occur in the early postoperative period. Other complications, including fistula formation, sliding of the valve, and obstruction with food residue, may occur later in the recovery period.

In Crohn's disease, surgery is used only to treat the complications, because even when the diseased portion is removed, there is a 50 per cent incidence of recurrence. The physician may prescribe antibiotics to control infection. During surgical resection for Crohn's disease, attempts are made to preserve as much of the small intestine as possible.

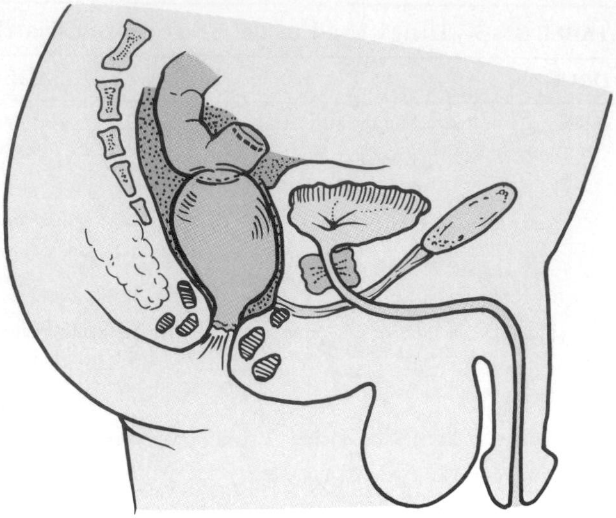

Figure 35–3
Ileorectal anastomosis following subtotal colectomy. This operation eliminates proctectomy with its attendant complications but does not provide definitive treatment for ulcerative colitis.

COMPLICATIONS

For 1 to 3 weeks after extensive small bowel resection, the client may be unable to tolerate oral intake and may have further losses in body protein or lean body mass. Total parenteral nutrition is given until oral intake can be resumed. Diarrhea usually occurs during the first 6 weeks after surgery. Anemia (from iron deficiency, steatorrhea, or decreased protein absorption) also may ensue. Paralytic ileus is another possible complication.

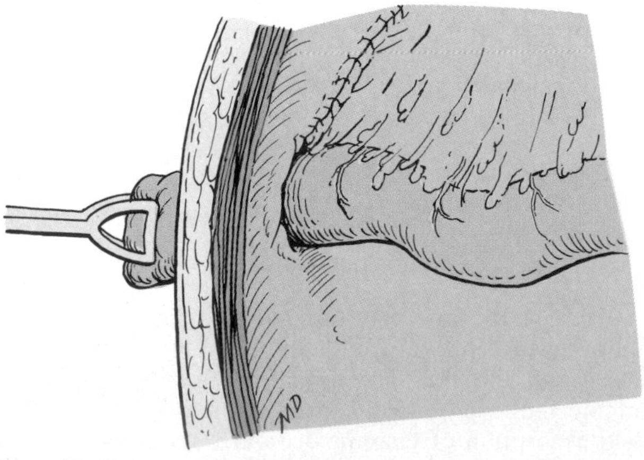

Figure 35–2
Ileum being drawn through abdominal wall to form ileostomy stoma.

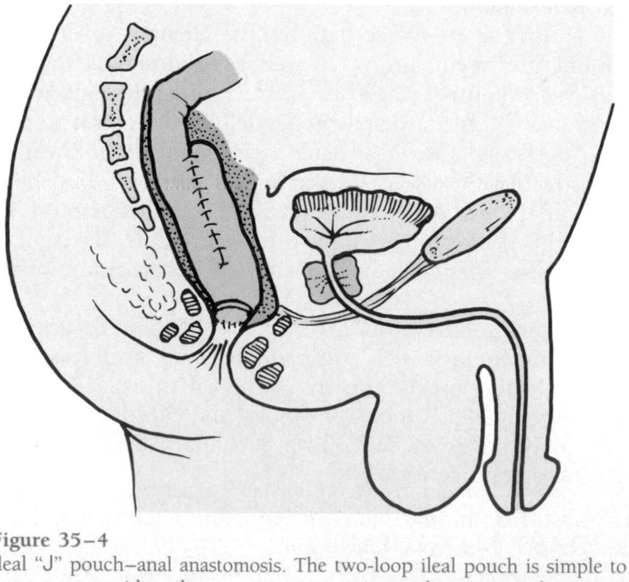

Figure 35–4
Ileal "J" pouch–anal anastomosis. The two-loop ileal pouch is simple to construct, provides adequate storage capacity, and is evacuated spontaneously and fully.

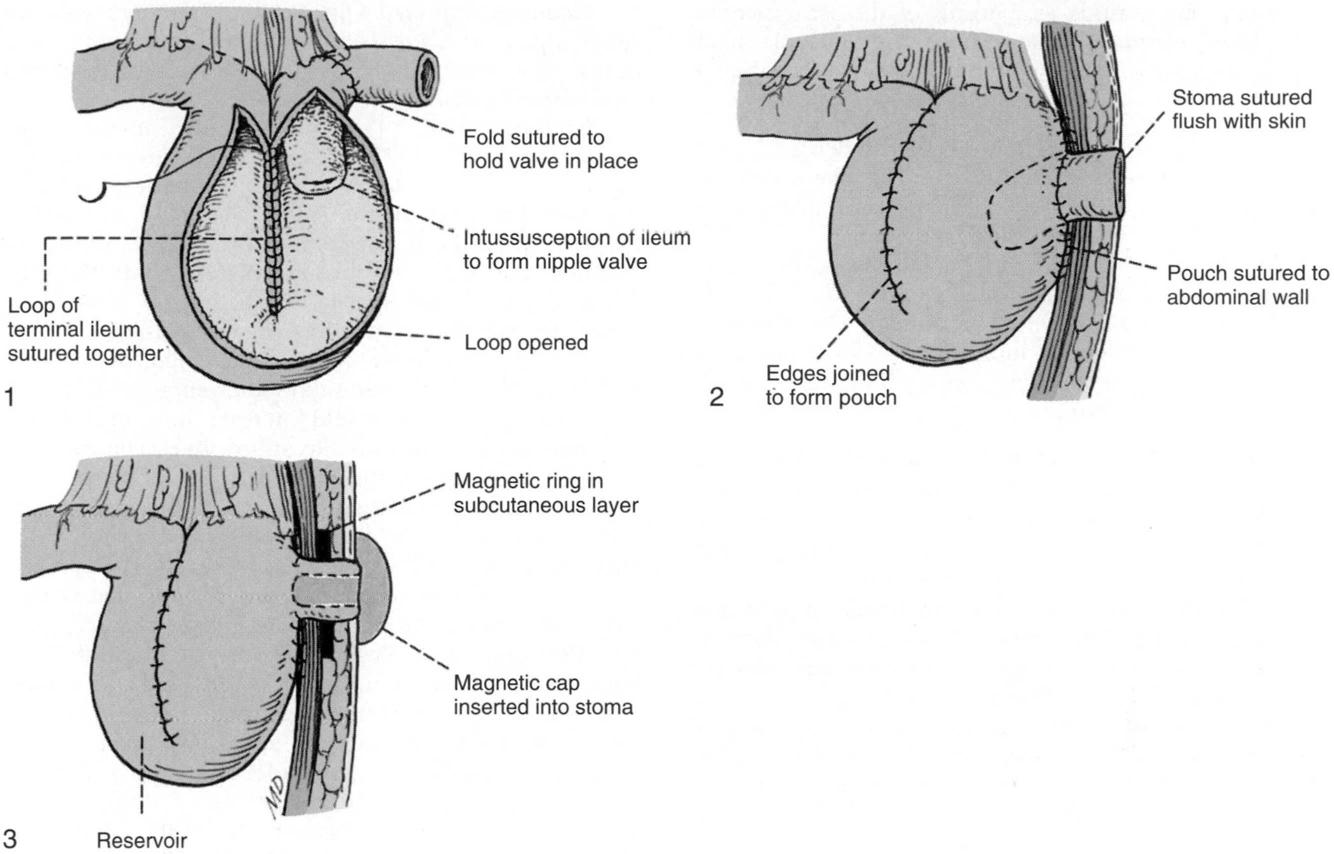

Figure 35–5
Continent ileostomy (Kock pouch) with magnetic ring device. *1,* Loop of terminal ileum is sutured together and cut open. Using forceps, the surgeon intussuscepts the distal ileum to form a nipple valve. *2,* Free edges sutured together to form reservoir; stoma sutured flush with skin, and pouch sutured to abdominal wall. *3,* Magnetic ring is implanted in subcutaneous layer and stoma closed with magnetic cap.

Nursing Management

Assessment

The nurse should assess the client's bowel elimination pattern, noting the number of stools, color, and consistency as well as the presence of blood or steatorrhea. The nurse also should assess the abdomen, noting bowel sounds and the location of pain.

Nursing Diagnosis, Planning, and Implementation

Nursing Diagnosis: Diarrhea R/T inflamed intestinal mucosa.

Planning: Expected Outcomes. The client will experience a decrease in diarrhea, as evidenced by a decreased number of stools and increased consistency of stools.

Implementation. Antidiarrheal medications are commonly administered to control the client's diarrhea. See Table 35–3 for a summary of drugs commonly used to treat diarrhea. The nurse should closely monitor the number and consistency of stools.

Perianal excoriation often occurs with diarrhea. After every bowel movement, the nurse should gently cleanse the skin with warm water and apply a protective moisture barrier product.

Nursing Diagnosis: Altered Nutrition: Less than Body Requirements R/T diarrhea and malabsorption.

Planning: Expected Outcomes. The client will increase nutritional intake to meet metabolic requirements, as evidenced by weight stabilization and, possibly, weight gain.

Implementation. The nurse must monitor the client's nutritional intake. The type of diet ordered depends on the condition of the client. If the client can tolerate food, intake of fluids and food must be encouraged. Because eating stimulates the gastrocolic reflex and the urge to defecate, many people are afraid to eat. Small servings may allow the client to avoid this problem. Foods should be bland and easily digested to promote absorption during the short time the food remains in the bowel.

Clients with Crohn's are often on home total parenteral nutrition because they are unable to tolerate foods for long periods as a result of disease exacerbation. These clients also may have had multiple small bowel resections, resulting in problems of malabsorption.

Nursing Diagnosis: Pain R/T inflamed mucosa.

Planning: Expected Outcomes. The client will experience a relief in abdominal pain, as evidenced by client's statement of pain relief.

Implementation. The nurse must assess the client's pain and give pain medications as ordered. The nurse should note any changes in the client's complaints of pain, because they may indicate the development of complications. Narcotics are generally used sparingly because they mask symptoms.

Nursing Diagnosis: Ineffective Individual Coping, Risk for R/T stress of disease and exacerbations R/T stress.

Planning: Expected Outcomes. The client will cope effectively with the disease, as evidenced by fewer exacerbations and client's improved coping style.

Implementation. Although emotional factors may not contribute to the cause of the disease, they do influence its course. Prolonged stress often precedes the onset of IBD and exacerbations. The nurse should recommend that the client schedule a follow-up physical examination and colonoscopy every 1 to 2 years, depending on the duration of bowel disease symptoms and previous findings.

Nursing Diagnosis: Knowledge Deficit R/T surgical procedure and possible ileostomy or other bowel resection.

Planning: Expected Outcomes. The client will understand surgical procedure and implications of bowel resection, as evidenced by client's ability to verbalize the procedure and demonstrate ileostomy care.

Implementation. If the client is scheduled for an ileostomy, then ostomy surgery, a procedure that may provoke a life crisis, must be fully explained to the client. In some instances, a preoperative visit from a member of an ostomy association may be helpful. An enterostomal therapist should assist with the preoperative preparation. Before surgery, the site of the ileostomy is selected, consideration being given to the location of the disease, body contours, convenience, and the type of clothing the client wears. If an ostomy pouch is indicated, the client may wear the pouch for 1 to 2 days before surgery to ensure comfort with the site selected. To provide assistance and support, the nurse must assess the client's body image and feelings about loss of a major body part.

If the client is not having an ileoproctectomy, but one of the continence-sparing surgeries, extensive teaching is still required. The client needs to understand the type of bowel resection to be performed and the implications of this surgery.

Nursing Diagnosis: Injury, Risk for R/T postoperative complications such as stomal cyanosis, distention, intestinal obstruction, and fluid and electrolyte imbalances.

Planning: Expected Outcomes. The client will not suffer injury, as evidenced by minimal distention, rapid return of normal peristalsis, and absence of fluid and electrolyte imbalance.

Implementation. The nurse must monitor the stoma after surgery. The nurse should ensure there is no pressure on the stoma that could interfere with circulation. The color of the stoma should be assessed at frequent intervals. If the color becomes pale, dusky, or cyanotic, the nurse should immediately notify the physician. If the blood supply to the stoma is compromised, the stoma may require surgical revision.

A nasogastric, gastrostomy, or jejunostomy tube will be in place for several days after surgery to remove gases and fluids that would increase intestinal distention and put pressure on the suture line. The drainage must be accurately noted. The passage of flatus indicates return of peristalsis. As bowel sounds return, the nurse must clamp the tube as prescribed and give the client ice chips and water. When the client has tolerated this for a minimum of 24 hours, the tube is usually removed and clear liquids are given.

Although most ileostomies are uneventful postoperatively, several complications can occur. The most common is an intestinal obstruction that may be caused by lumen obstruction, adhesions, food, or stomal edema. Early signs include anorexia, abdominal cramps, no ileostomy drainage, or a foul, brown, watery discharge in the pouch, or visible peristalsis. Other early postoperative complications include hemorrhage, hypoxia, and fluid and electrolyte imbalance. If there are severe or prolonged problems with absorption, an elemental diet or parenteral nutrition may be necessary.

Nursing Diagnosis: Ineffective Individual Coping R/T disturbance of body image and self-concept secondary to ostomy.

Planning: Expected Outcomes. The client will experience a positive body image and self-concept, as evidenced by the client's statements and ability to care for his or her own ostomy without embarrassment.

Implementation. A few days after surgery, the client needs to begin to confront the stoma and to begin integrating its function and appearance into his or her body image. The nurse must help the client look at and touch the stoma as soon as possible. The nurse should always use proper terms for the stoma and equipment.

Clothing can be a concern for the client with an ostomy, and clothing options need to be discussed with the client. The client should be discouraged from wearing a tight waistband that might rub on the stoma. The client should be encouraged to try on various outfits to ensure that the stoma and pouch are invisible.

Encourage the client to verbalize feelings about the stoma and its appearance. The client may be very accepting of the stoma because the illness (ulcerative colitis) is now gone and the client's life may be more normal and productive than it had been with the disease. Young men and unmarried women may express the greatest concern about body image.

The client needs to be aware of the nearest ostomy supply center so equipment will be easy to obtain. Clients may want to join the local ostomy association for emotional support. This organization often helps clients regain lost self-esteem and improves their self-concept and body image.

Nursing Diagnosis: Knowledge Deficit R/T ileostomy care, care following ileorectal anastomosis, care of an ileoanal reservoir, or care of a continent ileostomy.

Planning: Expected Outcomes. The client will understand proper care of an ileostomy, an ileorectal anastomosis, ileoanal reservoir, or a continent ileostomy, as evidenced by ability to apply own appliance correctly, without leakage, and to empty pouch appropriately, absence of perianal breakdown, absence of fecal leakage, or ability to empty reservoir correctly and absence of leakage.

Implementation. Ileostomy. The client must soon begin to master the skills needed to provide self-care. Initially, the client can simply observe the care of the stoma. Stoma care is the area of greatest concern to the client with an ileostomy. The nurse can begin by telling the client what the stoma looks like; that it extends 1 to 2 cm beyond the abdominal wall and is very red and swollen at first. The client must be assured that permanent changes in stoma size usually occur within the first 3 to 4 months after surgery when the swelling subsides, with the stoma shrinking to a slightly smaller permanent size.

When changing the pouch, the client should learn to check the size and color of the stoma and the odor of the drainage. Also, the nurse should check the stoma for signs of irritation or cyanosis.

When the ileostomy begins to function, the output is minimal. As the client takes in more food, the drainage becomes thicker in consistency and has a weak odor. The discharge is irritating to the skin because of the alkaline contents of the effluent. Because an ileostomy drains continuously, a pouch must be worn and the stoma must be covered with gauze when the pouch is being changed.

If skin irritation does occur, the nurse should first check the fit of the pouch. The best initial treatment for this problem would be to reapply the ostomy appliance (one with a karaya or hydrocolloid skin barrier), ensuring a proper fit and seal. The skin should be washed and rinsed thoroughly between pouch changes. The skin barrier of the appliance is usually sufficient to protect and heal the skin. If this method does not work, other barriers must be used. A wide variety of skin care products are available. If the problems continue, an enterostomal therapist should be consulted for further assistance.

Skin infection also can occur. *Candida* is the most common cause. The peristomal skin takes on a rashlike appearance. An antifungal powder such as nystatin should be applied directly to the affected skin area. The barrier can then be applied over the powder.

The frequency with which the ileal pouch needs to be emptied varies with each client. It should be emptied when the pouch is approximately one third to one half full. The client should be taught to empty the pouch during times of low output, usually before meals, at bedtime, and on arising in the morning.

When changing the pouch, all equipment should be ready before the old one is removed. The old pouch must be removed carefully. A piece of gauze may be held over the stoma until the new pouch is attached. The client should be encouraged to inspect and touch the stoma at this time. The nurse should remind the client with a new ileostomy to take ostomy supplies along when traveling. The client may want to keep supplies handy in a shaving or cosmetic case instead of a suitcase.

Many different types of pouches are available. Clients should try to find the best pouch for their needs. Small ileostomy drainage pouches are available for small adults and children. Foods such as eggs, fish, onions, cabbage, or greens cause stool odor; therefore, deodorizing solutions and tablets may be placed in the pouch. Spinach, parsley, yogurt, and buttermilk decrease drainage odor.

The client also needs special instructions regarding prescription and over-the-counter medications. Enteric-coated tablets, such as iron preparations, vitamins, and hormones, multilayer tablets, time-release capsules, and gelatin capsules may not be absorbed in the small intestine. The client should note whether any medications are obvious in the pouch drainage. The physician will need to prescribe different medications or different forms of the medication.

The client who has had an ileostomy needs to pay close attention to fluid intake. It is very easy for this client to become dehydrated. The approximate output from an ileostomy is 1200 or 1500 mL per day. The client must monitor this output for any increase that could lead to severe fluid and electrolyte imbalance.

A low-residue diet that is high in protein, carbohydrates, and calories is recommended after the surgery. Supplemental vitamins A, D, E, K, and B_{12} may be needed. Berries, whole-grain cereals, and raw fruits and vegetables can cause problems for clients with an ileostomy. Foods that cause discomfort or diarrhea should be omitted. Ingested foods will pass through the ileostomy within 4 to 6 hours. It is not advisable to eat a large meal close to bedtime.

Ileostomy clients must learn to chew their food well because the shortened bowel transit time means that poorly chewed food will be passed undigested. High-fiber and high-cellulose foods may absorb excessive moisture, leading to swelling and possibly constipation or even obstruction. Foods that should be avoided or limited include popcorn, peanuts, tough fibrous meats, skinned vegetables, rice, bran, and coconuts.

Some clients with ileostomies tend to acquire calcium oxalate, uric acid, or urinary calculi. Uric acid stones tend to form when urine volume is low and the urine is persistently acidic. Ingestion of sodium bicarbonate or potassium citrate will alkalinize the urine.

Allopurinol may be used if uric acid levels remain elevated. Fluid intake should be at least 1500 mL per day.

Ileorectal Anastomosis. The client with an ileorectal anastomosis does not have to learn about stoma or pouch care. The major goal of teaching centers on the importance of defecating before the rectum becomes overly distended. Most clients find that they have four to five stools per day once their bodies have adjusted to the surgical alteration.

The feces in these clients is often described as pasty in consistency and appears to contain fewer electrolytes than the drainage from a traditional ileostomy. It may take up to 1 year for the client's altered bowel to adapt.

Clients having the ileoanal anastomosis must understand the importance of follow-up meetings with the physician. They must understand that the remaining mucosa can become diseased with ulcerative colitis or Crohn's disease, requiring further resection and possibly formation of an ileostomy. They also need to know that they are at an increased risk for the development of rectal cancer. These clients have to receive regular proctoscopic examinations after their surgery.

The client should learn to avoid foods that may have caused diarrhea in the past. It is best to try new foods one at a time so the effect can be determined. The diet is usually not limited; however, it should include adequate fluids to avoid dehydration.

Ileoanal Reservoir. The client with the ileoanal reservoir also has no need to learn about stoma or pouch care. The client will learn to respond to the sensation to defecate so spillage does not occur. After the bowel adapts to the surgical alteration, the stool becomes more formed and many clients will have only two to four stools per day. The client should maintain an adequate fluid intake.

Continent Ileostomy, or Kock Pouch. During the surgical formation of the Kock pouch, an evacuation catheter is inserted. A skin barrier and special gauze dressing are then applied. These hold the catheter in an upright position to avoid stress on a healing nipple valve. It is imperative to avoid distention of the ileostomy reservoir in the early postoperative period because of the pressure it would cause on the suture line. Thus, it is emptied every 2 hours for about 2 weeks.

The nurse carefully observes for the start of ileal drainage, which usually occurs 3 to 4 days postoperatively. About 2 weeks after surgery, the catheter is removed from the pouch. The marked catheter may then be used to drain the pouch. The intervals between drainings are gradually increased each week until the ileostomy is emptied two to four times per day but not at night.

To empty the reservoir, the client should sit up. The catheter is lubricated with a water-soluble lubricant and inserted into the stoma through the valve. Contents are allowed to drain by gravity through the catheter into the toilet, with complete drainage occurring in 3 to 5 minutes. A small gauze dressing is then applied over the stoma. The equipment is cleaned with mild soap and rinsed and can be carried in a plastic case.

The reservoir volume continues to increase to a maximum of about 600 mL in 6 months. The client needs an oral intake of at least eight 8-oz glasses of fluid per day. No long-term restrictions are placed on physical activities. The nurse should instruct the client to wear a Medic Alert identification bracelet and to carry a brief description of the pouch and drainage procedure in case of emergency.

The client needs to learn about dietary restrictions associated with a continent ileostomy. Foods that could cause a blockage of the valve and the stoma need to be avoided. These include foods such as mushrooms and nuts. All foods need to be chewed thoroughly so partly digested food will not occlude the stoma. Refer to Client Education Guide: Inflammatory Bowel Disease.

Nursing Diagnosis: Sexual Dysfunction R/T concern about ileostomy.

Planning: Expected Outcomes. The client will not experience a sexual dysfunction, as evidenced by client's ability to return to preillness sexual functioning and role.

Implementation. The ileostomy may cause concern about sexual activity and pregnancy. The nurse should encourage the client to express any such concerns and to discuss them with the sexual partner. Impotency is uncommon, and psychological reasons should be explored if it does occur. Pregnancy and normal vaginal delivery are possible. The United Ostomy Association has a wide variety of booklets available for individuals with an ostomy. Topics include "Sex, Pregnancy and the Female Ostomate," "Sex, Courtship and the Single Ostomate," "Sex and the Male Ostomate," and "Insight into the Emotional Aspects of Ileostomies and Colostomies." The American Cancer Society also has resources available.

The client and sexual partner should be encouraged to discuss sexuality and to verbalize any fears. Clients

CLIENT EDUCATION GUIDE

Inflammatory Bowel Disease

Before discharge, the nurse should educate the client about the following:

- Availability of support groups such as the Crohn's and Colitis Foundations of America and the ileostomy associations associated with the American Cancer Society; encourage the client to join one of these support groups
- Care of the stoma or diversion; include the enterostomal therapist in teaching sessions
- Purchase of equipment available in the community
- Dietary implications such as limiting gas-producing foods; the client should also be taught about daily fluid intake
- The importance of follow-up appointments to ensure that healing has occurred; the client with Crohn's disease will need to be monitored for disease recurrence
- A follow-up appointment with an enterostomal therapist to ensure that the appliance fits well and that there are no problems with stoma care
- Written instructions, including the brand name, order number, size of pouch, skin barrier, and pouch deodorants, as well as the name, address, and telephone number of a local medical supply facility

can be taught activities to lessen the intrusiveness of the pouch such as emptying it before intercourse, wearing a soft flannel pouch cover, and being open to using different positions for intercourse. If there are problems, a sexual therapist should be consulted for further information and assistance.

Evaluation

The nurse must evaluate client outcomes based on the established plan of care. If these goals were not achieved, the plan and interventions must be revised to meet the client's needs.

Modification of Plan of Care for the Elderly

Crohn's disease and ulcerative colitis occur less often in the older age groups. The treatment, however, when it does occur in this age group is the same as for the younger client.

If the aged client has an ileostomy or other diversion, teaching may take a little longer, but most older clients can learn to care for themselves without difficulty. If the client has an ileostomy, issues such as eyesight and dexterity are important. Sometimes the older client cannot manipulate the clamp used to close the pouch. If the client is unable to manipulate the equipment, a family member may have to assume that responsibility. The nurse should carefully assess the older client's ability to care for self and the appliance.

Neoplastic Disorders

BENIGN TUMORS

Various kinds of benign tumors are found in the bowel. Polyps are the most commonly found benign tumor of the large bowel. A polyp is a lesion that projects into the lumen of the bowel. Some polyps have stems (pedunculated), whereas others do not (sessile). Polyps are usually benign lesions, but some types are precursors of cancer (i.e., premalignant tumors). Polyps are dangerous in two ways: They can mask the presence of a malignant tumor, and they may serve as the focus for bowel obstruction or intussusception. Benign bowel tumors produce manifestions similar to those of malignant tumors. Some benign tumors bleed profusely and cause abdominal discomfort. Bleeding benign tumors are usually removed surgically.

CANCER OF THE SMALL BOWEL

Only about 1 per cent of all GI cancers involve tumors of the small bowel. Symptoms are vague and nonspecific and include weight loss, pain, anemia, nausea, vomiting, obstruction, palpable mass, and hemorrhage. Surgery is the only intervention that offers hope of cure.

COLON CANCER

Cancers of the colon are usually adenocarcinomas.

Incidence

In both sexes, colonic and rectal cancer is the second most frequent cause of death from cancer in the United States. It ranks just behind lung cancer as cause of cancer deaths in the United States. It occurs with the same frequency in men and women. Most tumors are found in the distal portion of the large bowel, from the sigmoid colon to the anus. In recent years, the incidence of carcinoma of the right colon has increased, whereas that of the rectosigmoid area has decreased.

Etiology

The cause of colon cancer is not definitely known. There are identifiable predisposing factors, however. There also seems to be a familial tendency for colon cancer.

Risk Factors

There are a number of known risk factors for colon cancer. These include

- Family history of colon cancer
- Previous colon cancer
- Age greater than 40 years
- Ulcerative colitis
- High-fat, low-residue diet that is high in refined foods
- Familial polyposis
- Adenomatous polyps
- Living in highly industrialized, urban societies

Many of these risk factors have no primary prevention, so early detection is more important. Early detection includes yearly digital rectal examinations for adults older than 40 years, proctoscopic examination after age 50, and stool guaiac after the rectal examinations. Reducing the amount of fats and refined foods and increasing the amount of fiber in the diet may help reduce the risk of colon cancer.

Pathophysiology

The majority of malignant tumors (at least 50 per cent) occur in the rectal area; another 20 to 30 per cent are found in the sigmoid and descending colons. The remainder are found in the transverse and ascending colons.

Cancers of the colon almost always develop from adenomatous polyps. As this tumor becomes malignant, it increases in size within the lumen and begins to invade the bowel wall.

Malignant bowel tumors spread by direct extension to a nearby organ, as to the stomach from the transverse colon; lymphatic and hematogenic channels, usually to the liver; and seeding or implanting of cells into the peritoneal cavity.

Clinical Manifestations

Symptoms of carcinoma vary according to the area in which the tumor is found and the type of tumor involved. Symptoms of colon cancer include rectal bleeding, changed bowel habits, intestinal obstruction, abdominal pain, weight loss, anorexia, nausea and vomiting, anemia, and palpable mass (see Clinical Manifestations: Colon Cancer). Bleeding is the symptom that often alerts the client to seek health care. When the tumor occludes the bowel, obstructive symptoms result.

DIAGNOSTIC ASSESSMENT

One third of malignant tumors of the distal colon and rectum can be felt with the examining finger. A stool guaiac test is done to test for GI bleeding. Carcinoembryonic antigen may be elevated in colon cancer and aids in determining the progress of the disease. X-ray studies of the colon may show either a filling defect or a stricture. Ultrasonography and computed tomography (CT) help establish tumor size and metastasis. A sigmoidoscopy can identify more than one half of the tumors. Flexible fiberoptic scopes permit better visualization into the right colon, extend the diagnostic capabilities of the procedure, and allow biopsy (see Chap. 32).

Medical Management

The primary treatment for colon cancer is surgery; however, medical treatment is used as an adjunct to improve survival in tumors that cannot be completely removed. Radiation therapy is often given before surgery in the hope that the malignant cells will not metastasize and to reduce the size of the tumor and thus make it more resectable.

Local interventions at the tumor site after surgery include the implantation of isotopes into the tumor area and electrocoagulation. Interstitial implant includes radium, cesium, or cobalt. Iridium has been used in the rectum.

Chemotherapy has had limited success, although 5-fluorouracil has produced some positive results. Chemotherapy may be used to reduce metastasis and control symptoms of metastasis. In clients with liver metastasis, intrahepatic arterial chemotherapy may be administered.

CLINICAL MANIFESTATIONS

Colon Cancer

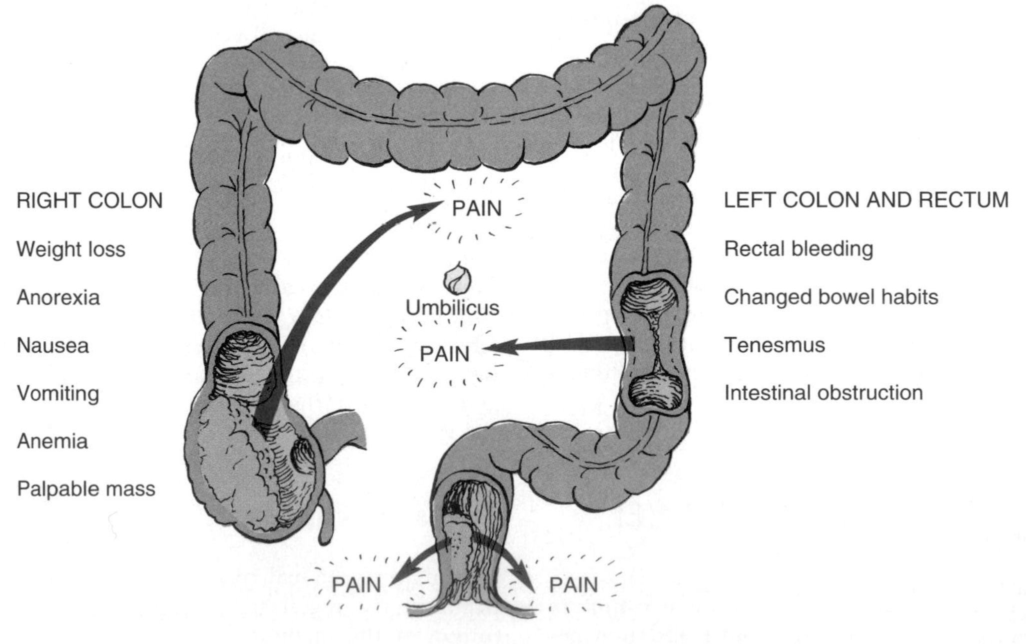

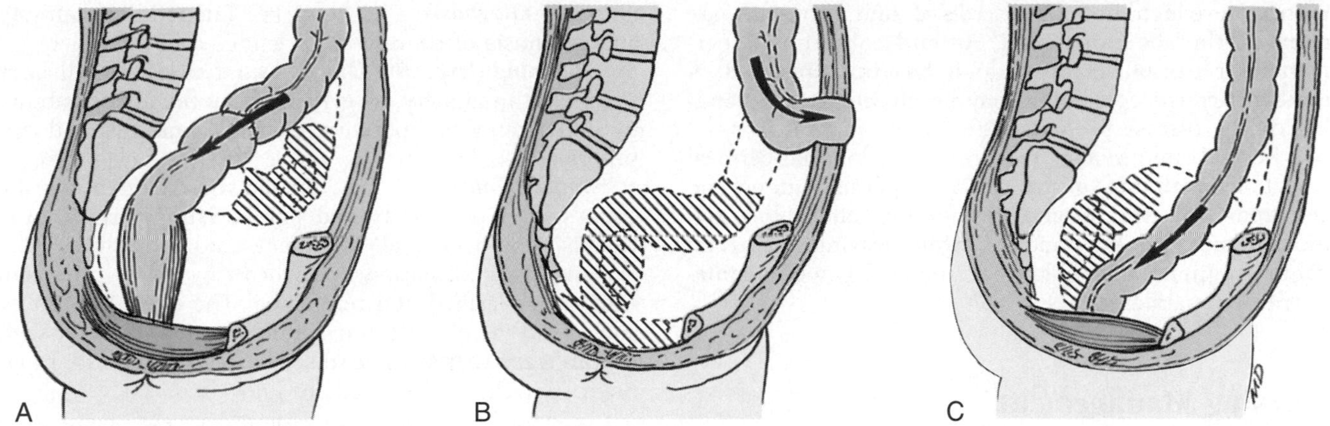

Figure 35–6
Resecting malignant tumors in rectosigmoid segment of bowel. *A*, Anterior resection with primary anastomosis is used for cancer at any point in the bowel except the terminal rectum. Associated lymph nodes are resected. *B*, Abdominoperineal (anteroposterior) resection with formation of permanent colostomy (Miles operation) for cancer involving the anus and terminal portion of the rectum. *C*, Proctosigmoidectomy with "pull-through" and preservation of external sphincter muscles is appropriate when the tumor is in the proximal rectum and unlikely to metastasize further.

Surgical Management

Intervention depends on the type of tumor, its location and stage, and on the client's general condition. A variety of surgical procedures are performed to treat colorectal cancer (Figs. 35–6 and 35–7). All procedures entail colon resection. The tumor is removed with several inches of colon on either side of the tumor. An end-to-end anastomosis is performed, if possible.

A colostomy may have to be performed. This procedure involves creating an opening between the colon and abdominal wall, from which fecal contents will pass. A colostomy can be located in the ascending, transverse, descending, or sigmoid colon. A colostomy can be permanent or temporary. A temporary colostomy allows the bowel to rest and later may be reanastomosed. The temporary colostomy also can be used to treat inoperable bowel cancer, with the ostomy placed proximal to the cancer. Because the main function of the large bowel is to absorb water, the colostomy is easier to manage nearer the sigmoid colon than in the transverse or right colon because the stool is formed.

A colostomy may also be single or double barreled. When only one loop of bowel is opened onto the abdominal surface, it is called an end colostomy; the client has only one stoma. A double-barreled colostomy

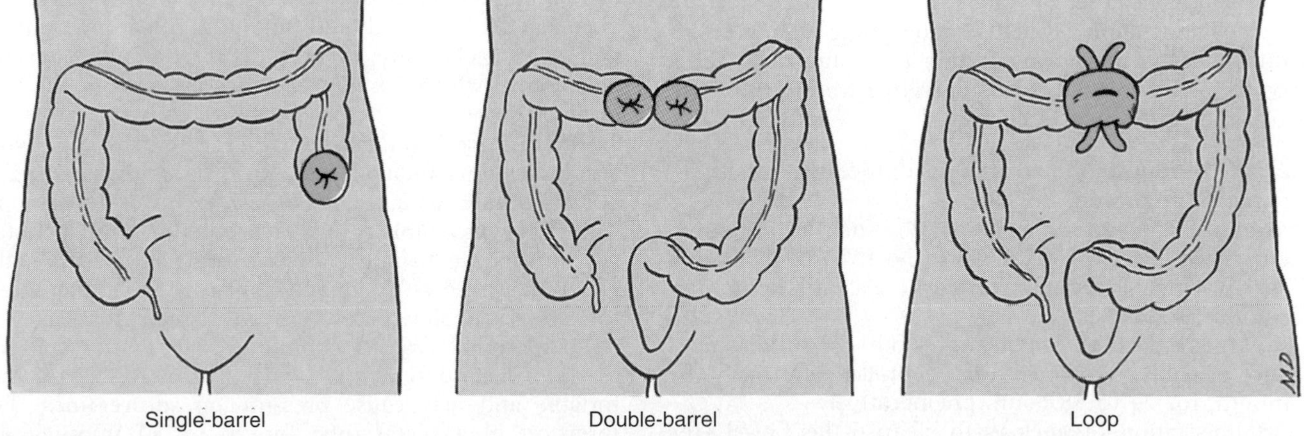

Figure 35–7
Types of colostomies. Single-barrel colostomies are usually permanent. Double-barrel colostomies are usually temporary and stomas may be adjacent or several inches apart. Loop colostomies are temporary and formed by bringing a loop of colon through the abdominal wall and supporting it with a plastic brace.

is one in which both loops, distal and proximal, are open on the abdominal wall. An end colostomy is permanent if the bowel distal to it has been resected. A double-barreled colostomy may be closed later depending on the disease present.

Rectal tumors may require an abdominal-perineal resection, with the formation of a permanent or end colostomy. Newer surgical techniques allow low sigmoid tumors to be removed while leaving the rectal sphincter intact. This allows for normal bowel elimination to be maintained.

Nursing Management

Assessment

The client often presents with weight loss and a change in bowel habits. The nurse should obtain accurate descriptions of symptoms as well as assess major risk factors, such as a family history of colon cancer, ulcerative colitis, or familial polyposis. The nurse should assess the abdomen, noting any abnormalities such as pain and distention, and check for any masses.

Nursing Diagnosis, Planning, and Implementation

Nursing Diagnosis: Altered Nutrition: Less than Body Requirements R/T nausea and anorexia.

Planning: Expected Outcomes. The client will attain an optimal level of nutrition, as evidenced by weight gain (or absence of weight loss), and normal serum electrolytes and protein levels.

Implementation. Preoperatively, a diet high in calories, protein, and carbohydrates but low in residue may be given to provide nutrition and decrease peristalsis. Total parenteral nutrition may be required to provide the nutrients and vitamins the client requires.

Nursing Diagnosis: Infection, Risk for R/T contamination from the bowel during surgery.

Planning: Expected Outcomes. The client will not develop a postoperative wound infection, as evidenced by absence of fever or elevated white cell count and good wound healing.

Implementation. Clients undergoing a bowel resection need a bowel preparation to minimize bacterial growth in the bowel and postoperative wound infection. This preparation usually includes

- A low-residue or liquid diet to reduce the fecal contents of the bowel
- Administration of cathartics orally such as polyethylene glycol-electrolyte solution (Go-LYTELY) or other agent, which is usually started at least 24 hours preoperatively
- Administration of antibiotics, such as sulfonamides and possibly neomycin and cephalexin, usually by mouth, for 24 to 48 hours preoperatively
- Administration of enemas to cleanse the bowel (the inside of the bowel lumen should be as clean and bacteria free as possible)
- Blood transfusions to correct severe anemia

Nursing Diagnosis: Anxiety R/T impending surgery and diagnosis of cancer.

Planning: Expected Outcomes. The client will have a decrease in anxiety, as evidenced by the client's ability to understand preoperative teaching and respond appropriately.

Implementation. The nurse should identify the client's level of anxiety and provide supportive efforts. Clients should have all treatments and procedures fully explained. Information provided by the physician should be clarified and reinforced. The client should be allowed to ventilate feelings and have time to meet with health team members to discuss treatments and prognosis. The client also needs to know

- What to expect after the operation
- What measures are necessary to prevent complications, such as deep breathing and leg exercises
- The type of anesthetic to be used
- Whether a nasogastric tube will be in place after surgery

If a colostomy will be performed, an enterostomal therapist should be consulted to teach the client about the ostomy, answer questions, and advise on optimal placement of the stoma. If an enterostomal therapy nurse is not available, the nurse must assume the responsibility for teaching the client about the stoma. The client may be concerned with sexual dysfunction after surgery. The physician should explain this risk to the client, and the nurse should provide support to the client.

Nursing Diagnosis: Injury, Risk for R/T postoperative complications, including infection, hemorrhage, wound disruption, thrombophlebitis, and abnormal stomal function.

Planning: Expected Outcomes. The client will not experience an injury, as evidenced by absence of signs of infection, no bleeding, and no evidence of wound disruption, thrombophlebitis, stomal ischemia, or bowel spillage.

Implementation. Immediate postoperative interventions are the same as those used for any major abdominal surgery. Additionally, if a colostomy was created, the nurse should monitor colostomy output and use special care to keep fecal contents from the colostomy (which contain bacteria) away from the surgical incision.

The nurse should assess for the return of peristalsis. Indications include passage of flatus and return of bowel sounds, which can be heard with a stethoscope. The client may remain on gastric suction until peristalsis returns. It usually takes several days before the client can receive food and fluids and, as the client tolerates food, slowly advance to a regular diet.

Abdominal cramps commonly occur after surgery, as does distention of the bowel. Distention is uncomfortable and may cause pressure on suture lines. The insertion of a rectal tube for 20 to 30 minutes per physician order will help if the rectum contains gas.

Postoperatively, if an abdominal-perineal resection with creation of an end colostomy was performed, the nurse must assess not only the abdominal wound but a large draining perineal wound. Drains are often left in the incision and may be attached to a suction device such as a Hemovac. When suction is not used the nurse may need to change the client's dressing.

CRITICAL TO REMEMBER

The nurse should assess the character, volume, and odor of the drainage. Should the drainage in any way suggest a developing infection, the nurse should take a culture of the wound to identify the organism.

In the immediate postoperative period, sump drainage is often placed in the perineal wound. The sump tube is attached to suction, allowing the wound to heal from its deepest portion without forming an abscess. If a Penrose drain is used, rectal dressings will need to be changed frequently because the large, deep wound drains profusely. It will take several weeks to months for the wound to heal completely because of its size. The client should be prepared to wear a rectal dressing throughout the healing period.

The perineal wound can be very painful, and the client should receive sufficient pain medication to control the pain. Once the packing is removed, the wound is irrigated and the client should take a sitz bath three to four times a day. The client will find a side-lying position much more comfortable.

CRITICAL TO REMEMBER

The client's stoma must be assessed closely for the presence of stomal ischemia. The stoma should be very red and moist. If it becomes dark or dusky, the nurse must immediately report this to the surgeon.

Clients may have a colostomy pouch over the stoma. The nurse must ensure that this pouch is not applying any pressure to the stoma, interfering with its blood supply. When the pouch is changed or emptied, one must prevent contamination of the surgical wound by fecal discharges. The return of bowel function should be monitored by observing the type and quantity of discharges from the stoma.

The high lithotomy position associated with the abdominal-perineal resection is associated with an increased risk of the development of postoperative phlebitis. The nurse should monitor the client for the development of symptoms of thrombophlebitis, such as redness, swelling, or the presence of Homans' sign.

Nursing Diagnosis: Ineffective Individual Coping, Risk for R/T disturbance in self-concept.

Planning: Expected Outcomes. The client will adjust to changes in body image, as evidenced by the client's ability to identify and use effective coping methods in dealing with disease and losses experienced.

Implementation. The nurse must provide emotional support while the client begins the process of adjusting to the colostomy. It is also important to provide extensive teaching regarding how to care for the colostomy.

Some clients refuse to look at the stoma and find it very difficult to accept its presence, whereas others begin to participate in stoma care almost immediately. The nurse's reactions and manner toward the client and the care required can affect the client's adjustment. For some clients, the colostomy represents a "cure," whereas for others, it is merely palliation, as for those with extensive cancer.

The client's significant others also must adjust to the colostomy. Nurses help significant others by listening to their reactions and interpreting the client's problems to them.

Continuing sexual relationships are one major concern for clients with colostomies and their significant others. There is no physical reason the client cannot enjoy normal sexual relationships, although a small number of men become impotent after a radical perineal dissection. If this complication occurs, the physician may recommend a urology consultation to discuss treatment options for impotence. Psychological barriers may cause problems. With love, patience, understanding, and good hygienic practices, there should be no problem. However, it may take several months after surgery before a couple manage to re-establish a satisfactory sexual relationship.

Nursing Diagnosis: Knowledge Deficit R/T end colostomy care, irrigation, and possible complications associated with colostomies.

Planning: Expected Outcomes. The client will understand care of the end colostomy, as evidenced by the client's ability to apply the pouch; care for peristomal skin, irrigate colostomy, if applicable, and prevent or treat any associated problems.

Implementation. The nurse should carefully assess the client's physical condition and emotional and mental attitude toward the colostomy before attempting to teach ostomy self-care. The teaching must be paced to the client's level of acceptance of the colostomy and ability to manage it.

The client should be taught how to apply the pouch to the stoma correctly. The client first should be taught to examine the stoma. A healthy stoma is red and slightly raised. The skin around the stoma should be clear, without evidence of irritation. The skin around the stoma should be cleaned well with a mild soap and water and dried well before the new pouch is applied. The skin should be treated with a skin barrier and the new pouch applied, cut about 1/16 to 1/8 inch larger than the stoma. The pouch should be changed about every 4 to 5 days or more often if leakage occurs. If it is changed after the bowel has evacuated, there will be less risk of spillage during the change.

The client also should be taught how to empty the pouch when it is about one half full. The client should be shown how to clean out the pouch when emptying it. The client should demonstrate the ability to empty and change the pouch independently before discharge. See the section on ileostomy care for further information.

The client must regularly cleanse the skin around the stoma to prevent irritation. Excoriation resulting from the constant presence of moisture can usually be prevented or healed with a light dusting of karaya or other powder. Too much powder will prevent the pouch from sticking, however.

Clients with end colostomies can be taught to regulate the colostomy by increasing dietary fiber and maintaining a daily exercise program. Clients who are able should be given the option of learning to irrigate the colostomy. Some clients, in spite of irrigation, may never gain regularity. If they have not become regulated within 6 months, they probably will not.

Irrigation is taught in much the same way the nurse would teach clients to self-administer an enema. (See the Client Education Guide: Colostomy Irrigation.) The best time for irrigation is when the client formerly had a daily bowel movement, because the bowel is already 'trained' to evacuate at this time.

Clients find that by irrigating the bowel daily or every other day, the bowel evacuates after the irrigation and then does not empty until it is irrigated again.

If there is difficulty inserting the catheter, the client can let a little solution flow in and rotate the catheter. If it will not go in, the client must be taught to apply gloves or a finger cot, lubricate the finger, and gently pass it into the stoma. This method will often dislodge any feces that may be near the stoma. If the client cannot pass a catheter and no obstruction is felt digitally, the client should notify the physician.

CLIENT EDUCATION GUIDE

Colostomy Irrigation

The nurse must teach the client to perform the following:

1. Assemble all the irrigation equipment and pouch, skin care products, and new colostomy pouch.
2. Remove and discard the old pouch.
3. Clean the peristomal skin.
4. Apply the irrigating sleeve and close off the distal end or place it into the toilet.
5. Using 500 to 1000 mL of warm tap water, suspend the solution container about 18 inches above the stoma, clear the air from the irrigation tubing, insert the lubricated catheter (water-soluble lubricant) 2 to 4 inches into the stoma **(never force the catheter),** and allow the solution to flow gently into the colon.
6. Once all solution has been instilled, either allow the majority of the stool to pass into the toilet and then close off the pouch for another 30 to 45 minutes or simply close off the end of the pouch until the bowel evacuates.
7. Once the bowel has emptied, simply remove the sleeve, clean the stoma, and cover it with a small pouch or a gauze pad.

If cramping occurs, the client should stop the solution temporarily, take a few deep breaths, and restart the solution slowly.

The client should be told never to use more than 1000 mL, irrigate more than once a day, or irrigate if diarrhea is present.

If there is no return after irrigation, the client should ambulate, gently massage the abdomen, and try drinking some warm water. If there is still no return, the client should apply a pouch and try the irrigation again the next day. If there is no return, the physician must be contacted.

Diarrhea is a serious problem for clients with colostomies. Medications to slow the motility of the bowel should be prescribed by the physician. Two problems can result from diarrhea: excoriation of skin from digestive juices that have not been reabsorbed and electrolyte imbalance when the condition persists. The client should be encouraged to drink water, broth, and plain tea; no solid food should be ingested until bowel motility returns to normal.

When hard stools are present, the client has difficulty evacuating the bowel and irrigating the colostomy. Fecal impactions also can occur. Sometimes the physician prescribes a stool softener such as dioctyl sodium sulfosuccinate (Colace). The client also needs to reevaluate the diet and increase the amount of fruit, vegetables, fiber, and water if constipation persists.

Flatus is an embarrassing problem because clients may have no control over its passage and no sensations to indicate when it is about to pass. The noise of the passage of gas can make clients avoid social situations. Clients can be taught how to muffle the passage of gas from their colostomies. Women may hold their purses or arms over the colostomy and men may hold their folded jackets or hats over the stoma to disguise the noise. Odor-proof pouches and those with charcoal filter discs are commonly available, but the most satisfactory way to control flatus is by proper diet. Because every client is different, clients have to learn by trial and error which foods cause gas. In general, nuts, cabbage, sauerkraut, broccoli, corn, cauliflower, and legumes are gas-forming foods. Swallowing air by eating too rapidly, chewing gum, and drinking carbonated beverages also cause intestinal gas.

Strictures of the stoma may occur after some surgeries because the rectus muscles of the abdominal wall tend to close over the artificial opening made through them. Some clients, especially those who do not irrigate, may be taught to dilate their stoma with a gloved, lubricated finger. This is usually not a problem in clients who irrigate because the irrigation nipple dilates the stoma.

Evaluation

The nurse must evaluate client outcomes based on the established plan of care. If these goals were not achieved, the plan and interventions must be revised to meet the client's needs.

Other Disorders of the Large and Small Bowel

HERNIATIONS

A hernia is the abnormal protrusion of an organ, tissue, or part of an organ through the structure that normally contains it. Hernias most frequently occur in the abdominal cavity as a result of a congenital or acquired weakness of abdominal musculature.

Incidence

Hernias can occur at any age and in either sex. Indirect inguinal hernias are the most common type and typically occur in men. Direct hernias are found more commonly in older adults. Incisional or ventral hernias occur most often in clients who had poor wound healing after surgery. Obese or pregnant clients are more likely to acquire umbilical hernias.

Etiology

Two factors must be present for a hernia to occur: a defect in the integrity of the muscular wall and increased intra-abdominal pressure.

Risk Factors

Congenital muscle weakness is one risk factor combined with the factors that increase intra-abdominal pressure.

Pathophysiology

Defects in the muscular wall may be congenital owing to weakened tissue or a wide space at the inguinal ligament, or they may be caused by trauma. Intra-abdominal pressure most commonly increases as a result of pregnancy or obesity. Heavy lifting also causes increased pressure, as do coughing and traumatic injuries from blunt pressure. When two of these factors coexist, with some tissue weakness, the person may acquire a hernia. Increased pressure without a weakness is not likely to cause a hernia. Weakness, in addition to being present from birth, is acquired as part of the aging process. As clients age, muscular tissues become infiltrated and are replaced by adipose and connective tissues.

When the contents of the hernia sac can be replaced into the abdominal cavity by manipulation, the hernia is said to be reducible. Irreducible and incarcerated are terms that refer to a hernia that cannot be reduced or replaced by manipulation. When pressure from the hernia ring (the ring of muscular tissue through which the bowel protrudes) cuts off the blood supply to the herniated segment of bowel, the bowel becomes strangulated. Incarcerated hernias usually become strangulated. This situation is a surgical emergency because unless the bowel is released, it soon becomes gangrenous owing to a lack of blood supply.

Hernias may penetrate through any defect in the abdominal wall, through the diaphragm, or through some internal structure within the abdominal cavity (Fig. 35–8). For this discussion, only the more common types of hernias are covered. The most common hernias are the inguinal (both indirect and direct), femoral, umbilical, and incisional. (Hiatal hernia was discussed in Chap. 33).

INDIRECT INGUINAL HERNIA

This herniation occurs through the inguinal ring and follows the spermatic cord through the inguinal canal. It is more common in males than in females because of the space allowed for the testicles to descend. These hernias can become extremely large and often descend into the scrotum.

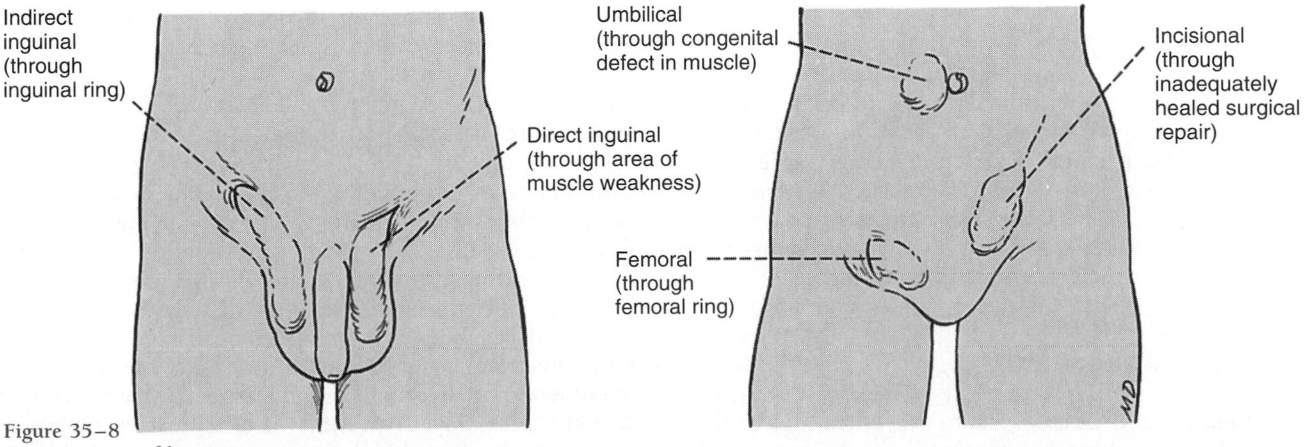

Figure 35–8
Common types of herniation.

DIRECT INGUINAL HERNIA

This hernia passes through the abdominal wall in an area of muscular weakness, not through a canal as do indirect inguinal and femoral hernias. It is more common in the elderly. Direct inguinal hernias gradually develop in an area that is weak because of congenital deficiency in the number of fibers it contains.

FEMORAL HERNIA

A femoral hernia occurs through the femoral ring and is more common in females than in males. It begins as a plug of fat in the femoral canal that enlarges and gradually pulls the peritoneum, and almost inevitably the urinary bladder, into the sac. There is a high incidence of incarceration and strangulation with this type of hernia.

UMBILICAL HERNIA

Umbilical herniation in the adult is more common in women and is due to increased abdominal pressure. It usually occurs in obese clients and in multiparous women.

INCISIONAL OR VENTRAL HERNIA

This type of hernia occurs at the site of a previous surgical incision that has healed inadequately because of postoperative problems such as infection, inadequate nutrition, extreme distention, or obesity.

Medical Management

Hernias that are not strangulated or incarcerated can be mechanically reduced. A truss also can be used to keep the hernia reduced. A truss is a firm pad held in place by a belt. The pad is placed over the hernia after it has been reduced and left in place to prevent the hernia from recurring. The client is taught to apply the truss daily before arising. The client should carefully inspect the skin under the truss for any sign of breakdown.

Surgical Management

A hernia repair is performed using a small incision directly over the weakened area. The intestine is then returned to the perineal cavity, the hernia sac excised, and the muscle closed tightly over the area. Many hernia repairs are now performed as outpatient procedures. Clients with difficult repairs are usually hospitalized for 1 to 2 days to receive prophylactic antibiotics.

Nursing Management

The nurse should make certain the client voids after surgery because urinary retention is a common problem, especially in male clients. The client must return to a general diet as soon as the client tolerates food. The nurse should assure the client that during the immediate postoperative period the hernia will not recur. Some clients hesitate to become active because of this fear.

After an inguinal hernia repair, an ice pack is usually applied to the incisional area to control pain and decrease swelling. In male clients, the scrotal area should be carefully assessed for swelling. An ice pack also can be applied to the scrotal area. To decrease scrotal swelling, the scrotum should be elevated and a scrotal support worn when the client is up.

The client should be told not to engage in heavy lifting from 4 to 6 weeks after surgery.

DIVERTICULAR DISEASE

Diverticular disease is the term used to describe diverticulosis and diverticulitis. Diverticulosis refers to the presence of noninflamed outpouchings of the intestine. Diverticulitis is inflammation of a diverticulum. A diverticulum is a blind outpouching or herniation of intestinal mucosa through the muscular coat of the large intestine, usually the sigmoid colon.

Incidence

Diverticular disease is common in men and women older than 45 years and in the obese. It is present in approximately one third of the population older than 60 years. It is more common in the United States, the United Kingdom, Australia, and France.

Etiology

The causes of diverticulosis include atrophy or weakness of the bowel muscle increased intraluminal pressure, obesity, and chronic constipation.

Diverticulitis occurs when undigested food blocks the diverticulum, leading to a decrease in the blood supply to the area and predisposing the bowel to invasion of bacteria into the diverticulum.

Risk Factors

The highest risk factor for the development of diverticulum is chronic constipation. A low-fiber diet is one of the leading causes of chronic constipation. The major risk factor for the development of diverticulitis is the ingestion of indigestible roughage, such as corn, popcorn, and tomatoes or cucumbers with seeds, in clients with diverticulosis because these foods can block the opening of the diverticulum and trigger inflammation.

The best way to prevent diverticulosis is to maintain adequate bowel habits by consuming a high-fiber diet that helps prevent constipation. Once the condition has developed, avoiding indigestible bulk may help prevent inflammation of the diverticula.

Pathophysiology

Diverticula have narrow, flasklike necks, which communicate with the bowel lumen. Weak points in the bowel muscularis exist where branches of the blood vessels penetrate the colonic wall. These weak points create areas for bowel protrusion when there is increased intraluminal pressure.

Diverticula frequently develop in the sigmoid colon because of the high pressures in this area required to move the stool into the rectum.

Diverticulitis may be acute or chronic. If the diverticulum is not infected (diverticulosis), these lesions cause few problems. However, when fecaliths do not liquefy and drain from the diverticulum, they may become trapped and cause irritation and inflammation (diverticulitis).

The inflamed area becomes congested with blood and may bleed. Diverticulitis can lead to perforation when the trapped mass in the diverticula erodes the bowel wall. Chronic diverticulitis can result in increased scarring and, eventually, narrowing of the bowel lumen, potentially leading to obstruction.

Clinical Manifestations

Symptoms produced by diverticulitis depend on the extent of the inflammation and the site of occurrence. Discomfort includes episodic, dull, or steady left-quadrant or midabdominal pain. Assessment also reveals alteration in bowel habits (constipation, diarrhea, or both), increased flatus, anorexia, and low-grade fever.

Rectal bleeding occurs in about 15 per cent of clients. Stools also may contain mucus. Urinary frequency can occur if the inflammation is in the proximity of the bladder. Straining, coughing, or lifting causes an increase in intra-abdominal pressure and symptoms. The clinician may palpate a tender mass on digital and rectal examinations.

Medical Management

Asymptomatic diverticular disease requires no specific therapy other than modification of the client's diet. Mild disease can be treated by adherence to a high-fiber diet and prevention of constipation with bran and bulk laxatives (hydrophilic colloids). One must advise clients to notify the physican of any change in bowel movement pattern (constipation or diarrhea) and character (presence of mucus or blood) and when fever, abdominal pain, or urinary symptoms develop.

Diverticulitis may be treated conservatively with medical intervention by allowing the colon to rest. Clients with acute diverticulitis are not permitted anything by mouth, may have a nasogastric tube, and receive parenteral fluids until pain, inflammation, and temperature decreases. When the acute episode begins to subside, they can ingest oral liquids and, later, a progressively more inclusive diet.

Intervention also aims to control inflammation. The nurse must administer prescribed antibiotics and advise the client to

- Avoid activities that increase intra-abdominal pressure, such as bending, lifting, stooping, coughing, or vomiting
- Drink at least eight glasses of water every day
- Reduce weight if client is obese

Surgical Management

Surgery is indicated for clients in whom complications develop, such as hemorrhage, obstruction, abscesses, or perforation. Further information on the care of these clients is discussed in the section on colon resections.

MECKEL'S DIVERTICULUM

Meckel's diverticulum is an outpouching of the bowel, a vestige of embryonic development found on the ileum within 10 cm of the cecum. The pouch may be lined with gastric mucosa or may contain pancreatic tissue. The gastric mucosal lining sometimes ulcerates and bleeds or perforates. In addition, the diverticulum may become inflamed and mimic appendicitis. Meckel's diverticulum is sometimes attached to the umbilicus by a fibrous band and may be the focus around which the bowel twists, causing obstruction. Treatment involves surgical excision of the diverticulum.

OBSTRUCTION

Partial or complete impairment of the forward flow of intestinal contents is known as an intestinal obstruction. Most obstructions occur in the small bowel, especially in the ileum, the narrowest segment. Obstructions of the small intestine are a common surgical emergency. Obstruction produces nausea, vomiting, dehydration, and severe pain. Intestinal obstruction has a high mortality rate if it is not diagnosed and treated promptly.

Incidence

The incidence of obstruction depends on its cause.

Etiology

Obstruction of the small intestine may be caused by narrowing of the intestinal lumen as a result of inflammation, neoplasms, adhesions, hernia, volvulus, intussusception, food blockage, or compression from outside the intestine. Paralytic ileus, vascular problems such as mesenteric embolus or thrombus, or hypokalemia from diuretics or antihypertensive agents also may result in small bowel obstructions. Infections of the abdomen and sometimes of the thoracic cavity, such as lobar pneumonia, peritonitis, or pancreatitis, frequently produce an ileus of infectious origin.

Cancer accounts for approximately 80 per cent of obstructions of the large intestine, with most occurring in the sigmoid colon. Other causes include diverticulitis and ulcerative colitis. Factors causing intestinal obstructions may be mechanical, neurogenic, and vascular.

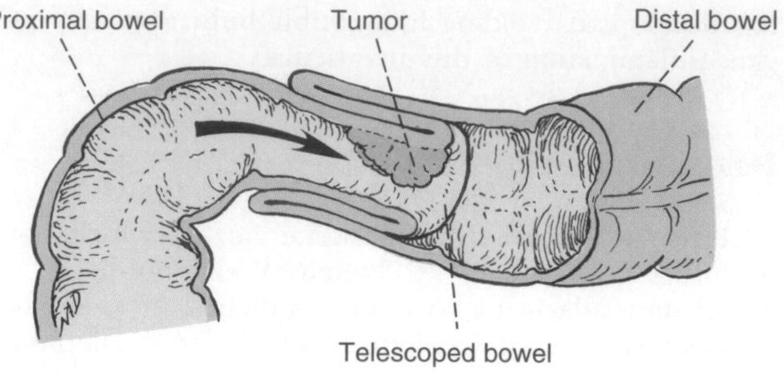

Figure 35–10
Intussusception. Portion of bowel telescopes into adjacent (usually distal) bowel.

Risk Factors

MECHANICAL FACTORS

Adhesions. Adhesions are probably the most common cause of obstruction in the small and large intestines combined. Adhesions form after abdominal surgery, and for unknown reasons some clients acquire massive adhesions. Irritants that remain in the abdomen following surgical procedures enhance the formation of adhesions. These fibrous bands of scar tissue can become looped over a portion of the bowel. The presence of multiple adhesions increases the risk of obstruction.

Hernia. An incarcerated hernia may or may not cause obstruction, depending on the size of the hernia ring. However, the potential for obstruction is always present in any hernia. A strangulated hernia is always obstructed, because the bowel cannot function when its own blood supply is cut off.

Volvulus. Volvulus is a twisting of the bowel that frequently occurs about a stationary focus (e.g., tumor or Meckel's diverticulum) in the abdominal cavity (see Fig. 35–9). It can cause infarction of the bowel and can occur in either the large or small bowel. Volvulus can sometimes be corrected without surgical intervention. Successful decompression of the bowel with a long tube releases pressure against the proximal end of the loop, thus allowing a small bowel volvulus to relax.

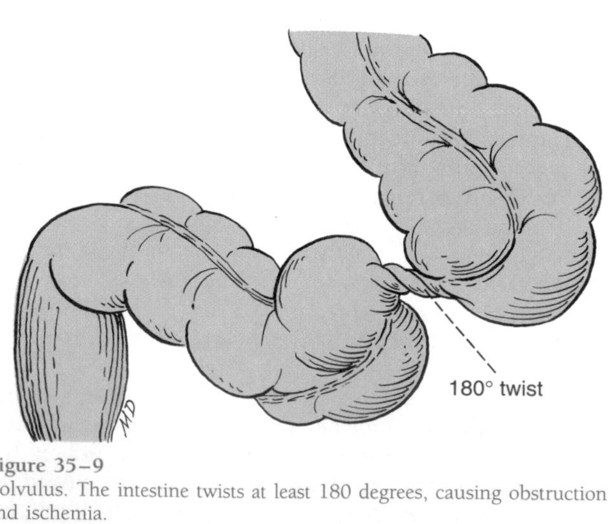

Figure 35–9
Volvulus. The intestine twists at least 180 degrees, causing obstruction and ischemia.

Intussusception. Intussusception, which sometimes complicates IBD, is a telescoping of the bowel on itself (Fig. 35–10). The condition is often associated with tumor of the large bowel. Peristaltic action telescopes the proximal bowel into the bowel distal to it. Intramural lesions often cause intussusception.

Tumors. In the large bowel, tumors are the chief cause of obstruction. The process develops slowly. In the small bowel, obstructive symptoms are frequently the first sign of a tumor. Even though the lumen of the small bowel is smaller, manifestations still do not occur early in the process because the intestinal contents are liquid.

NEUROGENIC FACTORS

An adynamic (or functional) obstruction, sometimes called a "paralytic ileus," is caused by a lack of peristaltic activity. Paralytic ileus commonly occurs after abdominal surgery. The bowel ceases to function for a few hours to several days. Procedures in which the surgeon handles the bowel extensively and procedures in the retroperitoneal area may cause a postoperative neurogenic problem. Treatment involves aspiration of the secretions by gastric suction until the bowel begins to function.

VASCULAR FACTORS

When the blood supply to any part of the body is interrupted, the part ceases to function and pain occurs. Obstruction of blood flow can arise as a result of complete occlusion (mesenteric infarction) or partial occlusion (abdominal angina).

Complete Occlusion (Mesenteric Infarction). Any occlusion of arterial blood supply to the bowel, as in mesenteric thrombosis, effectively stops bowel function. The usual cause is an embolus.

An acute occlusion, at its onset, causes intense abdominal pain, usually without any signs of advanced intestinal obstruction. This is because the pain results from ischemic tissue rather than from obstruction. As the process advances, fever, leukocytosis, shock, and other symptoms of bowel gangrene develop. Acute mesenteric obstruction constitutes a surgical emergency and carries a high mortality rate (approximately 75 per cent).

Partial Occlusion (Abdominal Angina). This condition usually results from atherosclerosis of the mesenteric arteries. It is a common although often asymptomatic problem.

Symptoms arise only when interruption of blood supply is sufficient to compromise bowel function. At this time, in addition to pain after eating, assessment reveals

- A change in bowel habits
- Nausea and vomiting
- Weight loss resulting from restriction of intake by the client because of discomfort experienced when eating

Pathophysiology

Normally, 7 to 8 L of electrolyte-rich fluid are secreted by the bowel, and most of it is reabsorbed. When the bowel is obstructed, this fluid is partially retained within the bowel and partially eliminated by vomiting, causing severe reduction in circulating blood volume, resulting in hypotension, hypovolemic shock, and diminished renal and cerebral blood flow. Because fluid is lost but blood cells are not, the hematocrit and hemoglobin increase, thus increasing the potential for vascular occlusive disorders such as coronary, cerebral, and mesenteric thrombosis.

For instance, with the onset of an obstruction, fluids and air collect proximal to the site of the problem, causing distention. Manifestations occur sooner and are more intense in a small bowel blockage because the small bowel is narrower and normally more active. The large volume of secretions from the small bowel adds to the distention. The only significant secretion from the large bowel is mucus.

Distention causes a temporary increase in peristalsis as the bowel attempts to force the material through the obstructed area. Within a few hours, the increased peristalsis ends and the bowel becomes flaccid, thus decreasing pressure within the lumen and slowing the process caused by the obstruction. Increased pressure within the bowel reduces its absorptive ability, which increases the fluid retention still further. Soon the intraluminal pressure reduces venous return, which increases venous pressure, congestion, and vessel fragility. This process, in turn, raises the capillary permeability and allows plasma to extravasate into the bowel lumen and into the peritoneal cavity. The bowel wall becomes permeable to bacteria, and bowel organisms enter the peritoneal cavity. Increasing pressure in the bowel wall soon slows arterial blood flow, causing necrosis and, in some cases, toxemia and peritonitis.

Strangulation of the bowel results in decreased arterial blood supply. Necrosis and perforation may force intestinal contents into the peritoneal cavity, causing peritonitis. Bacteria proliferate in the strangulated bowel and may form an endotoxin. When the endotoxin is released into the peritoneal cavity or systemic circulation, there is rapid circulatory collapse with endotoxic shock, accounting for the high mortality rate associated with this condition. These complications are especially likely to occur in elderly persons, who tend to have atherosclerotic narrowing of these vessels, making thrombosis more likely.

Clinical Manifestations

Manifestations of intestinal obstruction depend on

- The level and length of bowel involved
- The degree to which the obstruction interferes with blood supply
- The completeness of the obstruction
- The type of lesion producing the obstruction

The client with small bowel obstruction typically experiences abdominal pain in rhythmically recurring waves. The pain results from distention and the small intestine's peristaltic efforts to push its contents past the obstruction. Small intestine pain is felt in the upper and midabdomen, whereas colonic pain is experienced in the lower abdomen. Soon after the small intestine becomes distended, the nurse can see the peristaltic waves and hear accompanying high-pitched tinkling sounds. The client usually becomes nauseated and vomits, which brings some relief from the pain, provided the obstruction is high or proximal to the ileum.

If the obstruction lies below the ileum, vomiting fails to empty the bowel completely, allowing the accumulation of fluids, residue, and gases. As the muscles become atonic, loops of the small bowel dilate, compounding the problem of distention. Eventually, severe distention may raise the diaphragm, thereby inhibiting respirations. Hypoxia (resulting from inadequate respirations and decreased circulating blood volume and hypotension) often develops. Vomiting is more severe if the obstruction is located high in the small bowel. At first, vomitus is composed of semidigested food and chyme and, later, becomes watery and contains bile. Finally, the client vomits dark fecal material owing to bacterial growth in the fluid that has stagnated in the obstructed bowel.

When the colon is obstructed, the competent ileocecal valve prevents regurgitation and the pressure within the lumen increases, resulting in distention. In some cases, the cecum may perforate. Obstruction of the colon results in altered bowel habits, lower abdominal pain, a desire to defecate, distention, and borborygmi. Vomiting is not a common symptom because of the competent ileocecal valve. In the presence of an incompetent ileocecal valve, distention progresses to the small intestine. Vomiting that accompanies large intestine obstruction is a very late symptom and occurs only secondarily to a distended small intestine.

Clients with vomiting may experience severe fluid and electrolyte imbalances. They lose not only water but also sodium, chloride, potassium, and bicarbonate. The result is an acute extracellular volume deficit (dehydration), which, in turn, decreases the circulating blood volume. Hydrogen ion imbalances frequently occur in intestinal obstructions, with metabolic acidosis being the most common problem.

DIAGNOSTIC ASSESSMENT

Specific diagnostic tests include flat plate x-ray studies, which will show gas shadows; barium or radiopaque x-ray studies; and complete blood studies. Increased hemoglobin and hematocrit values may indicate dehydration. Leukocytosis may point to a strangulated bowel. A decrease in sodium, potassium, and chloride levels and a rise in the nonprotein nitrogen and blood urea nitrogen levels may indicate small bowel obstruction.

Medical Management

The major treatment for an intestinal obstruction is the insertion of an intestinal tube (see the section on intestinal tubes). Often, an intestinal tube both decompresses the bowel and breaks up the obstruction.

In adynamic ileus, the best intervention is rest and prevention of distention by gastric suction. Medications are not effective in stimulating bowel activity. The bowel will respond when it completely recovers from the effects of obstruction.

Surgical Management

If intestinal intubation does not relieve the obstruction, surgery is the only remaining option. The major objective in treating bowel obstruction is to relieve the cause and thus eliminate the problem.

In the majority of vascular and mechanically caused obstructions, surgical excision of the cause is the only intervention. Surgery relieves the obstruction and removes any ischemic bowel. Relieving the obstruction should re-establish bowel patency. The type of surgery depends on the location and type of obstruction. The surgeon may perform bowel resection, colostomy, or a bypass procedure.

Nursing Management

Assessment

The nurse should obtain a complete history of the onset of symptoms, eating patterns, food tolerance, vomiting episodes, stools (number per day and appearance), and distention.

During physical assessment, one must note the following:

- Abdominal distention
- Quality of bowel sounds
- Presence and extent of dehydration
- Muscle guarding or signs of abdominal pain

A lack of bowel sounds indicates peritoneal irritation or adynamic ileus. Usually, in the case of bowel obstruction, auscultation reveals high-pitched peristaltic rushes with high, metallic tinkling sounds.

Nursing Diagnosis, Planning, and Implementation

Nursing Diagnosis: Fluid Volume Deficit R/T vomiting, decreased intestinal reabsorption of fluid, and decreased intestinal secretions.

Planning: Expected Outcome. The client will maintain fluid balance, as evidenced by balanced intake and output, no signs of dehydration and blood pressure within the client's normal range.

Implementation. The nurse must maintain good fluid balance in the client with an obstruction by carefully replacing fluids and electrolytes. The nurse administers parenteral fluids with sodium chloride, bicarbonate, and potassium added as ordered.

One must maintain an intestinal tube attached to suction to relieve the vomiting and distention (see the section on care of a client with intestinal tubes). If the obstruction is not mechanical, an intestinal tube can achieve decompression. If the obstruction is due to adhesions, hernia, or tumors, the tube stops at the point of obstruction and keeps the bowel decompressed above the obstruction.

Nursing Diagnosis: Altered Gastrointestinal Tissue Perfusion, Risk for R/T intestinal obstruction.

Planning: Expected Outcomes. The client will not experience an alteration in tissue perfusion to the bowel, as evidenced by the return of normal peristalsis and usual bowel elimination.

Implementation. The client will have the intestinal tube inserted to help relieve the obstruction. The nurse must recognize and immediately report to the physician symptoms such as emesis, increasing distention and pain, and temperature elevation, all of which are signs of bowel strangulation.

If the blood supply becomes impaired, the client will require emergency surgery. The nurse must prepare the client for this procedure. Antibiotics are often given before surgery. The nurse must be careful about administering narcotics because these medications may mask symptoms of increasing obstruction or impaired blood flow.

The client with a bowel obstruction with impaired tissue perfusion requires an emergency bowel resection. (See the section on care of a client after a bowel resection with or without a colostomy.)

Evaluation

The nurse must evaluate client outcomes based on the established plan of care. If these goals were not achieved, the plan and interventions must be revised to meet the client's needs.

Posthospital Care

The learning needs of the client depend on the resolution of the obstruction. If the obstruction was relieved without surgery, the client needs to learn ways to prevent recurrence and maintain bowel elimination. The client needs to maintain an adequate nutritional intake so lost weight can be regained.

If the client had surgery, the learning needs vary on the basis of the surgical procedure performed. The client with a temporary colostomy needs to learn to care for the colostomy.

The client needs to be seen at intervals after the obstruction is relieved to ensure that it has not recurred. The client's nutritional status also should be monitored to ensure that adequate nutrition is maintained.

IRRITABLE BOWEL SYNDROME

Irritable bowel syndrome (IBS) is a functional disorder of motility in the small and large intestines. It develops without organic disease or anatomic abnormality. Other descriptive names for this condition are spastic colon, irritable colon, nervous indigestion, functional dyspepsia, pylorospasm, spastic colitis, intestinal neuroses, and laxative or cathartic "colitis."

Incidence

Irritable bowel syndrome is the most common gastrointestinal disorder in Western society, accounting for 50 per cent of subspecialty referrals. It is more common in women than men and occurs during middle age.[35]

Etiology

Several factors appear to be involved in the pathogenesis of IBS:

- Prediverticular disease characterized by increased width of the sigmoid circular muscles, increased segmentation, and nonpropulsive intraluminal pressures
- Psychologic stress
- A low-residue diet
- Lactose intolerance

Risk Factors

Risk factors associated with IBS include diets high in rich foods such as creams and fats. Other foods such as fresh fruits also seem to trigger the diarrhea. Gas-producing foods such as carbonated beverages and beans cause severe bloating. Alcohol and smoking, both gastric stimulants, increase gastric stimulation and increase the diarrhea.

Stress is another factor that increases the incidence of IBS. Alterations in sleep and rest may precipitate the problem.

Pathophysiology

Irritable bowel syndrome appears to be a disorder of GI motility; this motility may be altered by any number of factors, including diet and emotions. The alteration in the motility can cause diarrhea, constipation, or alternating diarrhea and constipation. The structure of the bowel mucosa is not altered, although the disease continues whenever the client is exposed to the causative agents. The causative agents vary among clients; however, most clients can clearly identify their agents.

Clinical Manifestations

The client with IBS is usually found to have some combination of the following symptoms: abdominal pain, altered bowel function, constipation or diarrhea, hypersecretion of colonic mucus, dyspeptic symptoms (flatulence, nausea, anorexia), and some degree of anxiety or depression. Symptoms vary in intensity. Roughage, fruits, alcohol, and fatigue aggravate or precipitate symptoms.

Symptoms may mimic various organic and systemic diseases. Pain may be steady or intermittent, and there may be a dull, deep discomfort with sharp cramps in the morning or after eating. The typical pattern consists of lower left quadrant abdominal pain, constipation, and diarrhea. There may be tenderness over the sigmoid area.

Diarrhea tends to be the major problem but not usually at night. Nocturnal diarrhea tends to be associated with organic disease of the bowel. Examination of the stool reveals mucus but not blood. Eating may aggravate pain and defecation, and passing flatus or stool may provide temporary relief. Spastic contractions sometimes occur with stools that are small, dry, hard, and pellet like. Other symptoms include abdominal disturbances such as nausea, distention, dyspepsia, eructation (belching), and borborygmus resulting from aerophagia and decreased gas motility. Anorexia, foul breath, sour stomach, flatulence, and cramps also may be present. Associated behavioral disturbances are anxiety, tension, nervousness, depression, sleep disturbances, weakness, or difficulty concentrating.

DIAGNOSTIC ASSESSMENT

Because there are no confirmatory diagnostic tests or histologic features for IBS, diagnosis generally is made by excluding other diseases. Diagnostic techniques, therefore, must eliminate the possibility that the client has organic GI disease.

When functional bowel disease develops, the client usually gives a history of nervousness and emotional disturbances. The client also may be conscious of the bowel and frequently use cathartics and enemas. Palpation may demonstrate abdominal tenderness, particularly along the course of the colon.

Sigmoidoscopy or colonoscopy may reveal spasm and mucus in the colonic lumen. A barium enema is usually performed. A complete blood count and stool examination is needed to rule out the presence of occult blood, ova, parasites, and pathogenic bacteria.

Medical Management

Treatment is palliative and supportive. The nurse should advise the client to limit responsibilities, seek rest, and adopt measures to decrease stress. The client can control symptoms through diet, medication, and regular physical activity. The client must continue with routine follow-up assessment and care.

PHARMACOLOGIC MANAGEMENT

Sedative and antispasmodic medications may help the client feel more relaxed. Taking vegetable mucilages such as psyllium hydrophilic mucilloid (Metamucil) can increase stool bulk.

DIETARY MANAGEMENT

Increased fiber in the diet helps control IBS through the production of bulkier stools and reduction of tension in the walls of the sigmoid colon.

Sources of fiber include unprocessed Miller's bran, packaged bran cereals, whole wheat, and fresh vegetables. Clients should drink six to eight glasses of water daily because increased water helps regulate stool consistency and frequency. If diarrhea is a problem, the client needs to avoid foods that may cause diarrhea, such as cold drinks, and drink liquids between meals rather than at mealtime.

Nursing Management

The nurse should reinforce the physician's explanation of the nature of the disorder, the intervention plan, and the prognosis. The nurse must make it clear to the client that the bowel responds to stress, foods, and medications. The importance of regular hours, nourishing meals, and adequate sleep, exercise, and recreation must be stressed. The nurse should help the client reestablish a regular bowel routine.

The nurse should reinforce diet teaching to the client and advise the client with diarrhea to

- Limit foods that are normally gas producing or irritating
- Avoid caffeinated beverages, alcohol, and foods containing nondigestible carbohydrates, such as beans
- Exclude milk and milk products

Disorders of the Anorectal Area

The major function of the rectum is to store feces until evacuation. When feces enter the rectum, peristalsis occurs. Many disorders in the rectal area result from constipation or failure to empty the rectum when peristalsis occurs.

Lesions of the external anal canal are very painful. The two most common symptoms are bleeding and pain. Drainage of mucus and fecal matter and irritation of the skin from organisms can cause intense itching.

Hemorrhoids and skin tags may protrude from the anal opening, and there may be drainage of pus from abscesses. Bright red blood per rectum usually indicates a lesion of the left colon or anorectal region. Blood on the toilet paper alone usually indicates perianal disease, whereas blood on the surface of a formed stool may suggest a polyp or carcinoma of the left colon or rectum. Blood mixed with the stool suggests IBD or carcinoma of the proximal colon. Blood in the toilet bowl after the passage of formed stool suggests hemorrhoidal bleeding. All rectal bleeding must be evaluated by a physician.

HEMORRHOIDS

Hemorrhoids are perianal varicose veins. Hemorrhoids may be internal or external (Fig. 35–11). Internal hemorrhoids are varicosities of the superior hemorrhoidal plexus occurring above the mucocutaneous border (pectinate line) and are covered by mucous membrane and innervated by the autonomic nervous system.

External hemorrhoids are dilatations of the inferior hemorrhoidal plexus and are covered by anal skin. As these vessels dilate, they stretch the overlying mucous membrane and skin and eventually protrude down the anal canal. This bulging plexus may be traumatized or pushed outside the anus by the passage of hard stool.

Incidence

Hemorrhoids are a common disorder, affecting both men and women of any age, but the incidence is increased in clients between 20 to 50 years. Enlargement of hemorrhoids is caused by increased intraabdominal pressure. Pregnancy, congestive heart failure, prolonged sitting or standing, and cirrhosis with portal hypertension also increase the incidence of hemorrhoids.

Etiology

Both internal and external hemorrhoids may result from the many anastomoses between the plexuses and the lack of valves in the veins of the superior hemorrhoidal plexus, which leads into the portal vein. Internal hemorrhoids are frequently caused by portal hypertension. Several causes contribute to acute enlargement of hemorrhoids, including constipation, diarrhea, and prolonged straining. Congestive heart failure also can cause hemorrhoids.

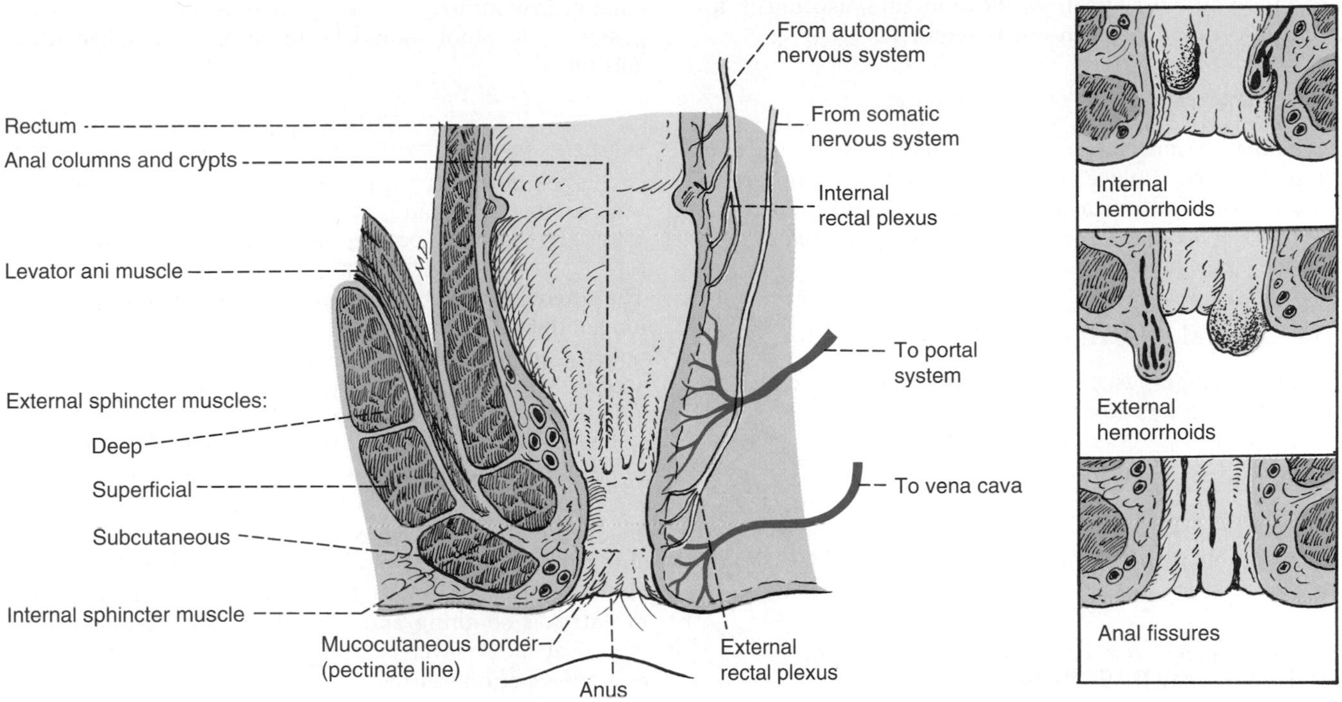

Figure 35–11
Common anal disorders: internal hemorrhoids, external hemorrhoids, and anal fissures.

Risk Factors

Any condition that increases the constipation, intra-abdominal pressure, and hemorrhoidal venous pressure increases the risk of the development of hemorrhoids. Prevention of constipation through increased roughage in the diet is an excellent measure to decrease the risk of hemorrhoid development.

Pathophysiology

Straining during a bowel movement increases intra-abdominal and hemorrhoidal venous pressures, leading to distention of the hemorrhoidal veins. When the rectal ampulla is filled with formed stool, venous obstruction is believed to occur. As a result of the repeated and prolonged increase in this pressure and the obstruction, permanent dilation of the hemorrhoidal veins occurs. As a result of the distention, thrombosis and bleeding also may occur.

Clinical Manifestations

The major symptom of external hemorrhoids is an enlarged mass at the anus. Internal hemorrhoids are characterized by bleeding and prolapse. Other symptoms include rectal itching and constipation. Pain may be present if there is associated thrombosis. The blood is bright red and may be seen in the stool or on the toilet tissue. A prolapse may occur in severe cases after exercise or after prolonged standing. Hemorrhoids may prolapse during defecation and spontaneously return, or the client may need to replace them manually. In some clients, hemorrhoids are prolapsed at all times.

DIAGNOSTIC ASSESSMENT

External hemorrhoids are diagnosed by visual examination; internal hemorrhoids are diagnosed through history, digital palpation, and proctoscopy. Asking the client to strain during assessment causes the veins to enlarge, thus aiding diagnosis.

Complications

Primary complications of hemorrhoids are bleeding, thrombosis, and hemorrhoidal strangulation. Severe bleeding from prolonged trauma to the vein during defecation can cause iron deficiency anemia. Blood oozes or may even spurt out after a bowel movement. Thrombosis within the hemorrhoids can occur at any time and is manifested by intense pain. Strangulated hemorrhoids, prolapsed hemorrhoids in which blood supply is cut off by the anal sphincter, can result in thrombosis when blood within the hemorrhoid clots.

Medical Management

Medical therapy is used only for small, uncomplicated hemorrhoids with mild symptoms. Treatment involves reducing pressure by treating the constipation and relieving pain with heat application and astringent lotions. No other intervention is required.

PHARMACOLOGIC MANAGEMENT

Constipation unrelieved by diet may require use of a stool softener (Colace) or a hydrophilic psyllium preparation. Use of a topical anesthetic or steroid preparation such as lidocaine (Xylocaine) or steroid creams also reduces pain or itching.

DIETARY MANAGEMENT

Dietary changes used to treat constipation include increasing fluid and fiber in the diet.

PAIN MANAGEMENT

For pain, an initial application of cold packs, followed by warm sitz-baths, three to four times a day should help.

Surgical Management

A number of surgical procedures are used to treat hemorrhoids. A common procedure for internal hemorrhoids, ligation is performed in the physician's office. The client can usually carry on normal activities immediately after the treatment. Unfortunately, the procedure cannot be used for external hemorrhoids and may be only temporarily effective.

Cryosurgery, freezing of the hemorrhoids, is performed less commonly today. It is also an outpatient procedure. The freezing of the tissue leads to necrosis and sloughing of the hemorrhoids.

Laser removal is the newest procedure. This also is performed on an outpatient basis. The hemorrhoid is burned off with the laser. There is minimal bleeding, although the procedure causes some pain.

With a hemorrhoidectomy, the vein is excised and the area is either left open to heal by granulation or sutured closed. The open method is very painful but has a high rate of success. The sutured method, although far less painful, is more likely to cause infection and result in poor healing.

COMPLICATIONS

Complications include infection, stricture formation as the lesion heals, and hemorrhage. Hemorrhage may occur immediately after surgery or about 10 days later as a result of sloughing of tissue. Also, bleeding may not be evident because it can occur in the rectum and not pass immediately.

Nursing Management

The client should take measures to avoid constipation. The anal area is very painful, and the client may avoid defecating, resulting in hard stool or fecal impaction. The nurse should encourage the client to take bulk laxatives or mineral oil as prescribed to promote stool passage. The stool should be monitored for consistency and blood.

CRITICAL TO REMEMBER

The nurse should teach the client to consume fiber-containing foods and ample fluids to prevent straining and to avoid laxatives, when possible.

The client should be reminded not to sit on the toilet longer than necessary to have a bowel movement. This position impairs blood flow and puts added pressure on anal vessels.

After the client has had any of the procedures to remove the hemorrhoids, the nurse should stress the importance of keeping the area clean and the stool soft but formed to help prevent strictures. The nurse should encourage the client to wash the area after defecation and pat it dry. Local moist heat, applied with a washcloth or piece of cotton to the anal opening for a few minutes, is soothing and cleansing and promotes healing. Heat must never be applied in the immediate postoperative period because of the increased risk of hemorrhage. Most physicians prescribe sitz baths three or four times a day or as the client desires, beginning 12 hours after surgery.

Postoperative complications requiring nursing assessment include hemorrhage and urinary retention. The proximity of the bladder and tenderness in the area sometimes makes urination difficult.

Postoperative pain can be controlled with parenteral and then oral analgesics. The client must be warned to avoid vigorous perianal wiping during the immediate postoperative period. The client is usually given a stool softener and mineral oil to soften and lubricate the first stool. The nurse should warn clients that fainting can occur, through pain and vagal stimulation, during the first postoperative bowel movement.

PILONIDAL CYST

A pilonidal cyst occurs at the base of the sacrum, usually contains hair, and becomes infected, forming an abscess and then a sinus tract.

Acute pain and swelling result, followed by a discharge. Treatment involves surgical excision of the abscess. Healing is slow, and if the infectious process is not completely removed, the condition may recur. The client also may receive antibiotics.

RECTAL FISSURE (FISSURE IN ANO)

A rectal fissure is an ulceration or tear of the lining of the anal canal, usually on the posterior wall. An acute fissure occurs as a result of excessive tissue stretching

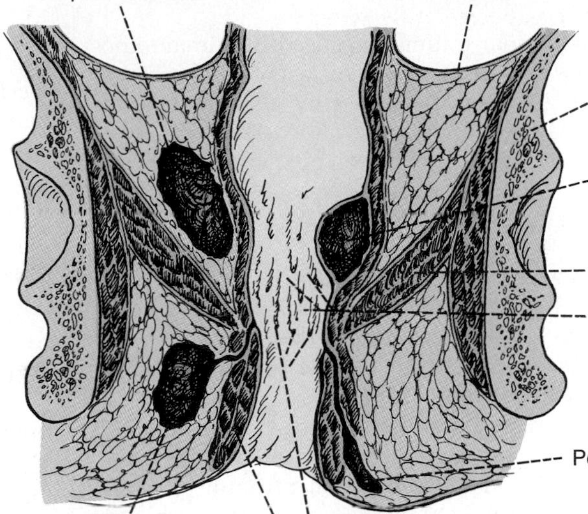

Figure 35–12
Abscesses of the anorectal area.

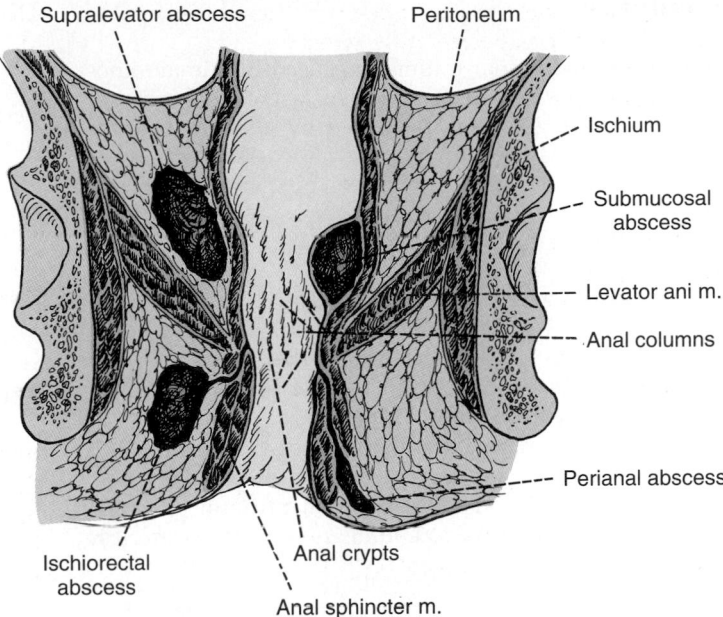

and possibly from passage of a hard or large stool through the area. The skin tear is very tender and tends to reopen at subsequent periods of defecation.

The nurse should advise the client to

- Keep the stool soft with Metamucil, mineral oil, or Colace as prescribed
- Have a bowel movement daily
- Clean the area after defecation, preferably with warm water

Sitz-baths aid healing and may relieve pain. Suppositories with a local anesthetic may help constipation.

RECTAL FISTULA (FISTULA IN ANO)

A fistula is a sinus tract that develops between two body cavities or between a body cavity and the external environment. A rectal fistula is a tract that leads from the anal canal to the skin outside the anus or from an abscess to either the anal canal or the perianal area. It usually is preceded by an abscess. A fistula may heal over temporarily and then open and drain periodically.

This is a chronic condition for which surgery is the only cure. The surgeon excises the tract and cleans the area, leaving it open to heal by granulation. It may heal very slowly and be very painful. The nurse should advise the client to keep the area clean, especially after a bowel movement.

RECTAL ABSCESS

Rectal abscesses form in several locations; Figure 35–12 illustrates the common ones. Most abscesses begin as cryptitis, with the formation of cysts that extend through the tubular ducts into the submucosal spaces. They also may originate from abrasions of the local tissues, with the entry of a virulent organism.

Treatment involves draining the abscess and surgical excision of any associated fistulas. It may take two stages of surgery to accomplish the needed resection.

TUMORS OF THE RECTUM

Carcinoma and melanoma both can occur at the anus but are rare, constituting less than 5 per cent of rectal cancers. They spread by local extension into the perirectal spaces and then to the inguinal nodes. Surgical intervention involves excision of the anus with an abdominoperineal resection. Preoperative irradiation and chemotherapy are other modes of intervention for anal cancer. Regional intra-arterial infusion of 5-fluorouracil as palliative therapy can relieve pain and improve the quality of life for the client with rectal cancer.

Abdominal Trauma

BLUNT OR PENETRATING TRAUMA OF THE ABDOMEN

Blunt or penetrating trauma to the abdomen refers to the accidental or intentional trauma causing internal injuries.

Incidence

Most blunt abdominal trauma is caused by the automobile steering wheel or pedestrian accidents, whereas most penetrating trauma is caused by gunshot wounds or stabbings.

Etiology

Almost any kind of injury can cause blunt trauma to the abdomen. In automobile accidents, rapid, uncontrolled deceleration is the force that produces the trauma when the client's body hits the steering wheel or some other object.

Penetrating trauma commonly results from gunshot wounds, which cause a great deal of internal damage. Stabbings are the next most common cause of penetrating abdominal wounds, although these wounds are less traumatic.

Risk Factors

Trauma is the leading cause of death for adults younger than 40 years and the third leading cause of death for all adults. Although not all of these cases of trauma are abdominal trauma, abdominal injuries are common with motor vehicle accidents.

One method of prevention is wearing seat belts, which could decrease abdominal trauma in case of accidents.

Pathophysiology

Blunt trauma to the abdomen can cause shearing, crushing, or compressing forces that can cause rupture of bowel and other abdominal structures.

Gunshot wounds have the potential of damaging every structure in the abdomen. The gunshots may perforate the stomach or bowel, causing peritonitis and sepsis.

Stab wounds produce less trauma to internal abdominal structures because the abdominal organs have more time to shift out of the way of the penetrating instrument.

Clinical Manifestations

Assessment of the client first involves obtaining a thorough history of the accident so the degree of blunt trauma can be estimated. For penetrating trauma, careful assessment of the position of entry and possibly exit wounds is vital.

The client may show signs of an acute abdomen with either type of trauma. With both injuries, either internal or external hemorrhage may occur. If the bowel is ruptured, signs and symptoms of peritonitis are present. All abdominal drainage is closely assessed for the presence of bowel contents.

DIAGNOSTIC ASSESSMENT

Abdominal lavage is commonly used to assess the presence of bleeding in all abdominal wounds. This involves performing paracentesis after the instillation of a crystalloid solution into the peritoneal cavity.

A CT scan of the abdomen is now considered the base assessment of intra-abdominal injury. Angiography, intravenous pyelography, and other studies may be performed to assess different organs and the degree of trauma suffered.

Medical Management

If minimal blunt trauma was sustained without severe injury to any abdominal organs, the client may simply be observed for problems once the diagnostic tests have been conducted. Penetrating trauma always requires some type of surgical intervention.

PHARMACOLOGIC MANAGEMENT

The client's pain is treated conservatively until the degree of trauma has been determined. If the bowel has been ruptured, large doses of intravenous antibiotics are given to control infection. If hemorrhage and shock are present, intravenous fluids, colloids, and vasopressors may be used.

DIETARY MANAGEMENT

The client receives nothing by mouth until the abdomen has been assessed and found to be intact.

COMPLICATIONS

The major complications of trauma are hemorrhage, shock, peritonitis, and sepsis.

Surgical Management

The treatment of choice for abdominal trauma with injury to the abdominal contents is an exploratory laparotomy. Depending on the exact injury found, the surgery may be as simple as a closure of tears or as complex as a bowel resection and even a temporary colostomy.

Nursing Management

Careful assessment of the client's injury is vital. The nurse must often prepare the client for immediate emergency surgery. The nurse must prepare the client as quickly as possible, knowing that postoperatively, much more teaching and support will be required.

STUDY QUESTIONS

1. The client most likely to be diagnosed with appendicitis is
   A. A 22-year-old college student
   B. A 6-month-old infant
   C. A 60-year-old retiree
   D. A 79-year-old grandparent
2. In a client with suspected peritonitis, it is important for the nurse to assess the presence of
   A. Nausea
   B. Vomiting
   C. Pain
   D. Diarrhea
3. A client with Crohn's disease may exhibit which of the following characteristics?
   A. Chronic constipation
   B. Cobblestone appearance of the bowel
   C. Absence of blood in the stool
   D. Sudden weight gain
4. After dietary instruction of the client at risk for diverticular disease, the nurse would know he understood the teaching if he stated which of the following?
   A. "I'll eat a low-residue diet."
   B. "I'll take a laxative daily."
   C. "I'll maintain a high-fiber diet."
   D. "I'll reduce daily fluid intake."
5. A hernia that cannot be reduced or replaced by manipulation is
   A. Indirect
   B. Direct
   C. Femoral
   D. Incarcerated

CRITICAL THINKING EXERCISES

SCENARIO A

A young man is diagnosed with Crohn's disease. He complains of intermittent abdominal pain, diarrhea, and weight loss. His nutritional status is compromised, and diet teaching is required.

1. What factors influence nutritional status in a client with Crohn's disease?
2. What type of diet is recommended for a client with Crohn's disease?
3. Which foods should be avoided and why?

SCENARIO B

An elderly man has undergone a bowel resection with placement of a temporary transverse colostomy for treatment of colon cancer. He lives with his wife of 40 years, who will be caring for him after his discharge from the hospital. The nurse develops and implements a plan for discharge teaching.

1. What foods should clients with a colostomy avoid?
2. What interventions will help to decrease the odor from a colostomy?
3. What is the appearance of a healthy stoma and of healthy skin around the stoma?

BIBLIOGRAPHY

1. American Cancer Society. (1995). *Cancer facts and figures—1995*. New York: Author.
2. Bartlett, J. G. (1991). *1991 Pocketbook of infectious disease therapy*. Baltimore: Williams & Wilkins.
3. Bates-Jensen, B. (1989). Psychological response to illness: exploring two reactions to ostomy surgery. *Ostomy/Wound Management, 23,* 24–30.
4. Bragg, V. (1989). Continent intestinal reservoir: Ileostomy option. *Ostomy/Wound Management, 23,* 32–41.
5. Braun, J., et al. (1991). Anal sphincter function after intersphincteric resection and stapled ileal pouch–anal anastomosis. *Diseases of the Colon and Rectum, 34(1),* 8–16.
6. Boarini, J. (1990). Gastrointestinal cancer: Colon, rectum and anus. In S. L. Groenwald, M. M. Frogge, M. Goodman, & C. H. Yarbro (Eds.), *Cancer nursing: Principles and practice* (2nd ed., pp. 792–805). Boston: Jones & Bartlett.
7. Cotran, R. S., et al. (Eds.) (1994). *Robbins pathologic basis of disease* (5th ed.). Philadelphia: W. B. Saunders.
8. Eisenberg, P. (1989). Enteral nutrition: Indications, formulas and delivery techniques. *Nursing Clinics of North America, 24,* 315–338.
9. Gitnick, G., et al. (Eds.). (1994). *Principles and practice of gastroenterology and hepatology* (2nd ed.). Norwalk, CT: Appleton & Lange.
10. Greenberger, N. (1989). *Gastrointestinal disorders: A pathophysiologic approach* (4th ed.). St. Louis: Mosby-Year Book.
11. Guyton, A. C. (1991). *Textbook of medical physiology* (8th ed.). Philadelphia: W. B. Saunders.
12. Hampton, B. G., & Bryant, R. A. (1992). *Ostomies and continent diversions: Nursing management.* St. Louis: Mosby-Year Book.
13. Hallgren, T., et al. (1990). The stapled ileal pouch–anal anastomosis: A randomized study. *Scandinavian Journal of Gastroenterology, 25(11),* 1161–1168.
14. Hocking, M. P., & Vogel, M. P. (1991). *Woodward's postgastrectomy syndromes* (2nd ed.). Philadelphia: W. B. Saunders.

15. International Association of Enterostomal Therapy. (1989). *Standards of care: Patients with colostomy.* Irvine, CA: Author.
16. Isselbacher, K. J. (Ed.). (1994). *Harrison's principles of internal medicine* (13th ed.). New York: McGraw-Hill.
17. Kelman, G., & Minkler, P. (1989). An investigation of quality of life and self-esteem among individuals with ostomies. *Journal of Enterostomal Therapy, 16,* 4–11.
18. Kirsner, J. B., & Shorter, R. G. (1995). *Inflammatory bowel disease* (4th ed.). Baltimore: Williams & Wilkins.
19. Krasner, D. (1990). What's wrong with this stoma? *American Journal of Nursing, 90(4),* 46–47.
20. Lehne, R. (1994). *Pharmacology for nursing care* (2nd ed.). Philadelphia: W. B. Saunders.
21. Madda, M. A. (1991). Helping ostomy patients manage their medications. *Nursing, 21(93),* 47–49.
22. Porter, J. A., et al. (1989). Complications of colostomy. *Diseases of the Colon and Rectum, 32,* 299–303.
23. Rakel, R. E. (Ed.). (1995). *Conn's current therapy 1995.* Philadelphia: W. B. Saunders.
24. Sabiston, D. C. Jr., (1991). *Textbook of surgery: The biological basis of modern surgical practice* (14th ed.). Philadelphia: W. B. Saunders.
25. Sachar, D. B. (1990). The problem of postoperative recurrence of Crohn's disease. *Medical Clinics of North America, 74,* 183–188.
26. Schroeder, S. A., et al. (1991). *Current medical diagnosis and treatment.* Norwalk, CT: Appleton & Lange.
27. Sleisenger, M. H., & Fordtran, J. S. (Eds.). (1993). *Gastrointestinal disease: Pathophysiology, diagnosis, and management* (5th ed.). Philadelphia: W. B. Saunders.
28. Smith, L. E. (1989). Surgical therapy in ulcerative colitis. *Gastroenterology Clinics of North America, 18(1),* 99–110.
29. Society of Gastroenterology Nurses and Associates. (1993). *Gastroenterology nursing: A core curriculum.* St. Louis: Mosby-Year Book.
30. Sodeman, W. A., et al. (1989). *Geriatric gastroenterology.* Philadelphia: W. B. Saunders.
31. Sparks, S. M., & Taylor, C. M. (1991). *Nursing diagnosis reference manual.* Springhouse, PA: Springhouse.
32. Way, L. W. (1991). *Current surgical diagnosis and treatment.* Norwalk, CT: Appleton & Lange.
33. Williams, S. (1993). *Nutrition and diet therapy* (7th ed.). St. Louis: Mosby-Year Book.
34. Wyngaarden, J., et al. (Eds.). (1992). *Cecil textbook of medicine* (19th ed.). Philadelphia: W. B. Saunders.
35. Yamada, T. (Ed.). (1991). *Textbook of gastroenterology.* Philadelphia: J. B. Lippincott.

UNIT 11

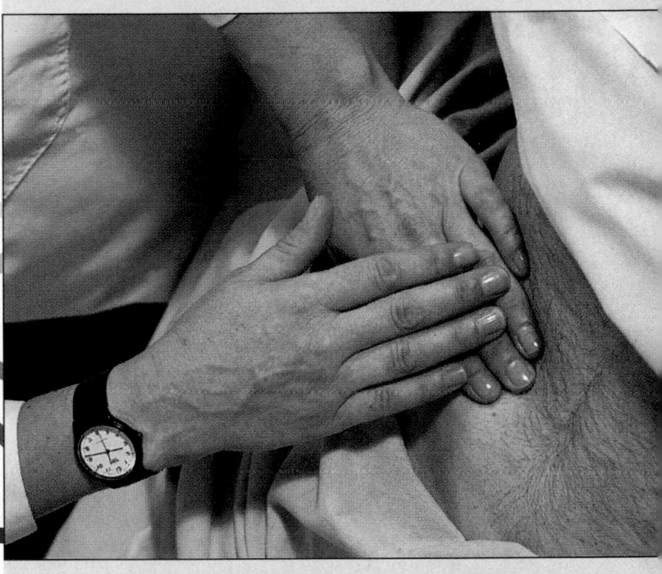

Hepatic, Biliary Tract, and Exocrine Pancreatic Disorders

The liver, biliary tract, and exocrine pancreas are located together in the upper abdominal cavity, where they facilitate digestion and metabolism. The liver also detoxifies chemicals, destroys bacteria in the blood, synthesizes blood-clotting factors, and assists in regulation of blood volume.

Chronic, progressive disorders of the liver, biliary tract, and exocrine pancreas require long-term assessment and management. Severe hepatic and pancreatic damage demands intensive, complex nursing interventions. When these disorders are caused by drug or alcohol dependence, the client's life-style may be in conflict with traditional cultural values. In these situations, the nurse must care for the client and meet the client's needs without allowing preconceived ideas to influence the care.

Acute, episodic problems of the gallbladder may necessitate surgery. The client requires careful attention during the immediate postoperative period, but with appropriate care planning, no long-term difficulties should arise.

This unit explores assessment of the liver, biliary tract, and exocrine pancreas. It identifies disorders related to one or common to all, and discusses current medical treatment and nursing management.

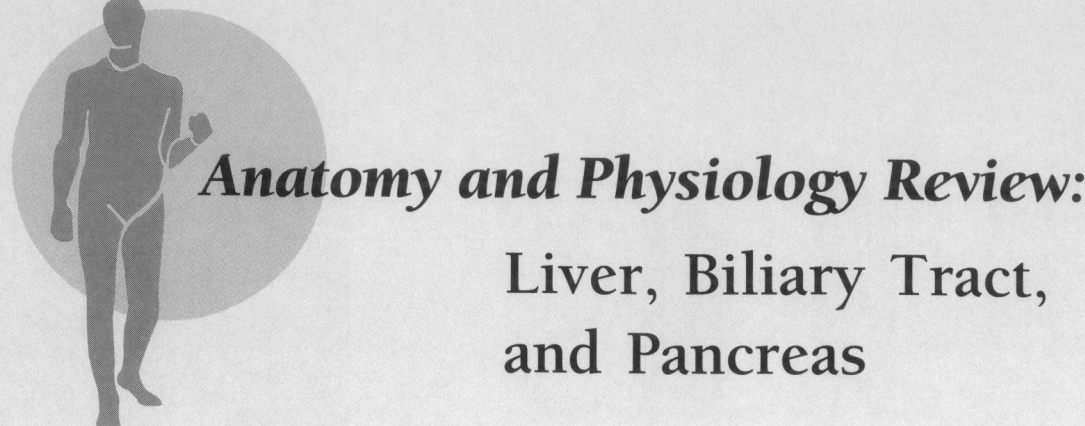

Anatomy and Physiology Review: Liver, Biliary Tract, and Pancreas

LIVER

Structure

The liver is a large reddish-brown organ that weighs about 1.5 kg. It is located in the upper right quadrant of the body, just below the diaphragm. The rib cage encloses and protects the liver, except for the lower margin. The substance of the liver is divided into functional units called liver lobules. A liver lobule consists of plates of cells called hepatocytes that radiate outward from the central vein. The channels between the plates are sinusoids.

One third of the blood supply to the liver is oxygen-rich blood brought by the hepatic artery. The other two thirds is nutrient-rich venous blood from the gastrointestinal tract that is carried by the portal vein. The blood from these two sources mixes together as it flows through the sinusoids to the central vein, and many substances are exchanged between the blood and the hepatocytes. Phagocytic cells lining the sinusoids remove bacteria and other particles from the blood as it passes through the sinusoids. Bile is formed in the hepatocytes, is secreted into the bile canaliculi, and then travels through the hepatic and bile ducts to the gallbladder.

Function

The liver has a wide variety of functions, many of which are vital to life. Hepatocytes perform most of the functions attributed to the liver, but the phagocytic Kupffer cells that line the sinusoids are responsible for cleansing the blood. Liver functions include:

- Secretion. The liver produces and secretes about 1 L of bile each day.
- Synthesis of bile salts. Bile salts are cholesterol derivatives that are produced in the liver and facilitate fat digestion and the absorption of fats and fat-soluble vitamins.
- Synthesis of plasma proteins. The liver synthesizes albumin, fibrinogen, globulins except immunoglobulins, and clotting factors.
- Storage. The liver stores glucose in the form of glycogen, iron, and vitamins A, B_{12}, D, E, and K.
- Detoxification. The liver alters the chemical composition of toxic compounds, such as ammonia, to make them less harmful. It also changes the configuration of certain drugs, such as penicillin, and excretes them in the bile to remove them from the body.
- Excretion. Hormones, drugs, cholesterol, and bile pigments from the breakdown of hemoglobin are excreted in the bile.
- Carbohydrate metabolism. The liver has a major role in maintaining blood glucose levels through (1) glycogenesis, the conversion of glucose to glycogen; (2) glycogenolysis, the breakdown of glycogen to glucose; (3) storage of glycogen; (4) conversion of galactose and fructose to glucose; and (5) gluconeogenesis, the conversion of amino acids to glucose.
- Lipid metabolism. The liver is responsible for a major part of the metabolism of fats. Activities of the liver in relation to fat metabolism are (1) oxidation of fatty acids for energy; (2) formation of most lipoproteins; (3) synthesis of cholesterol and phospholipids; and (4) synthesis of fat from proteins and carbohydrates.
- Protein metabolism. Although carbohydrate and fat metabolism are important, human survival depends on the liver's role in protein metabolism. The primary activities of the liver in relation to protein metabolism are (1) deamination of amino acids; (2) transamination of amino acids to create needed amino acids from others that are available; (3) formation of urea for the removal of ammonia from the body; and (4) formation of plasma proteins.
- Filtering. The phagocytic Kupffer cells that line the sinusoids remove bacteria, damaged red blood cells, and other particles from the blood.

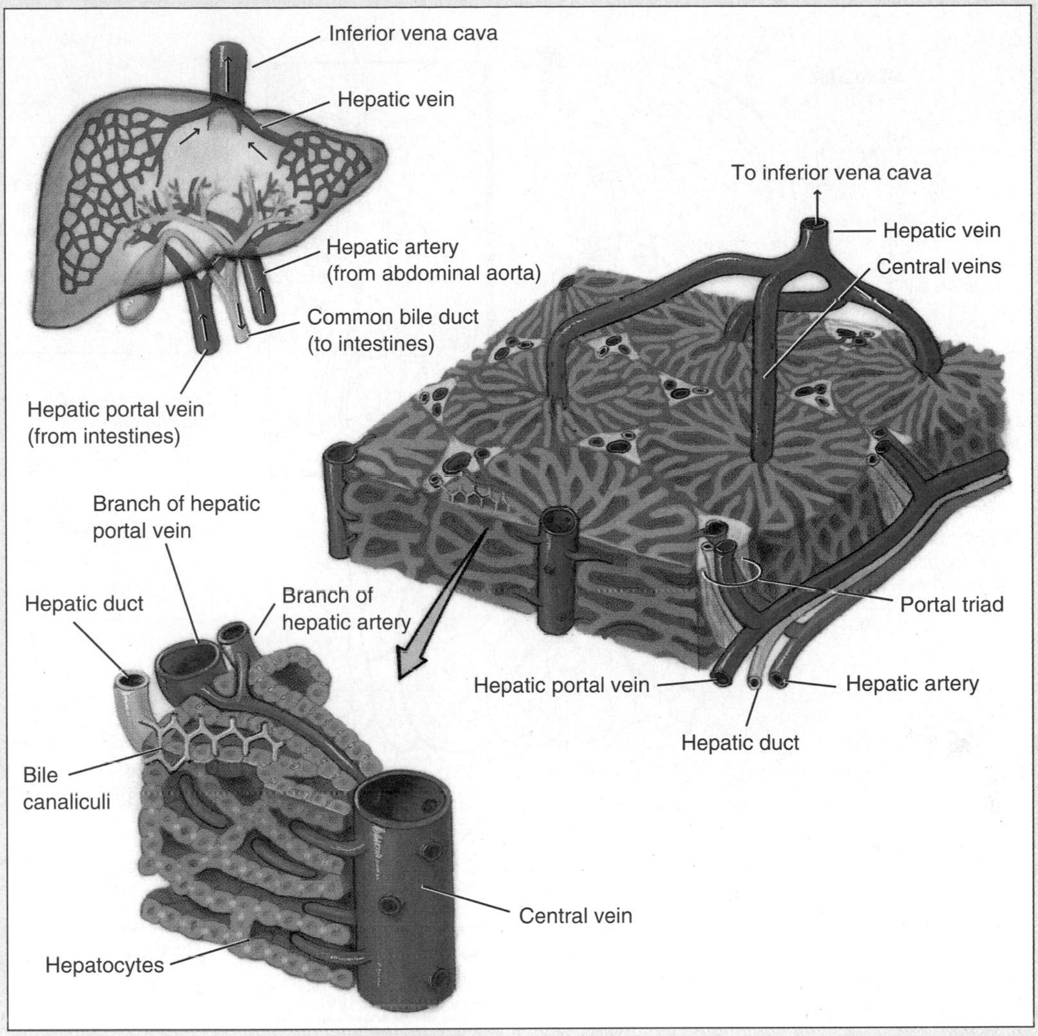

Liver lobules.

Bile

Bile is a slightly alkaline fluid (pH 7.6 to 8.6) that helps neutralize the acid chyme in the duodenum. The basic components of bile are water, bile salts, bile pigments (primarily bilirubin), cholesterol, fatty acids, lecithin, and electrolytes. The liver continuously secretes bile, which is then stored in the gallbladder until it is needed in the duodenum for digestion. When the gallbladder concentrates the bile, a large portion of the water and electrolytes is reabsorbed by the gallbladder mucosa.

Although they are not enzymes, bile salts have a function in the digestion of fats. They act as emulsifying agents that break large fat globules into tiny fat droplets to increase the surface area for enzyme action. Bile salts also help in the absorption of fatty acids, other lipids, and fat-soluble vitamins from the small intestine. Bilirubin, the principal bile pigment, is produced in the breakdown of hemoglobin from damaged red blood cells and is excreted in the bile. It is responsible for the color of urine and feces. Cholesterol is supplied in the diet and also synthesized in the liver as a product of lipid metabolism. It is highly insoluble in water and requires bile salts to keep it in suspension. When the balance of cholesterol and bile salts is disturbed, the cholesterol may precipitate and form gallstones.

BILIARY TRACT

Structure

The biliary tract consists of the gallbladder and the ducts associated with it. The gallbladder is a small, pear-shaped sac that is attached to the visceral surface of the liver by the cystic duct and can hold approximately 100 to 150 mL of bile. Bile, which is produced in the liver, flows from the bile canaliculi into the right and left hepatic ducts, then into the common hepatic duct. The cystic duct from the gallbladder joins the common hepatic duct from the liver to form the common bile duct, which empties into the duodenum of the small intestine.

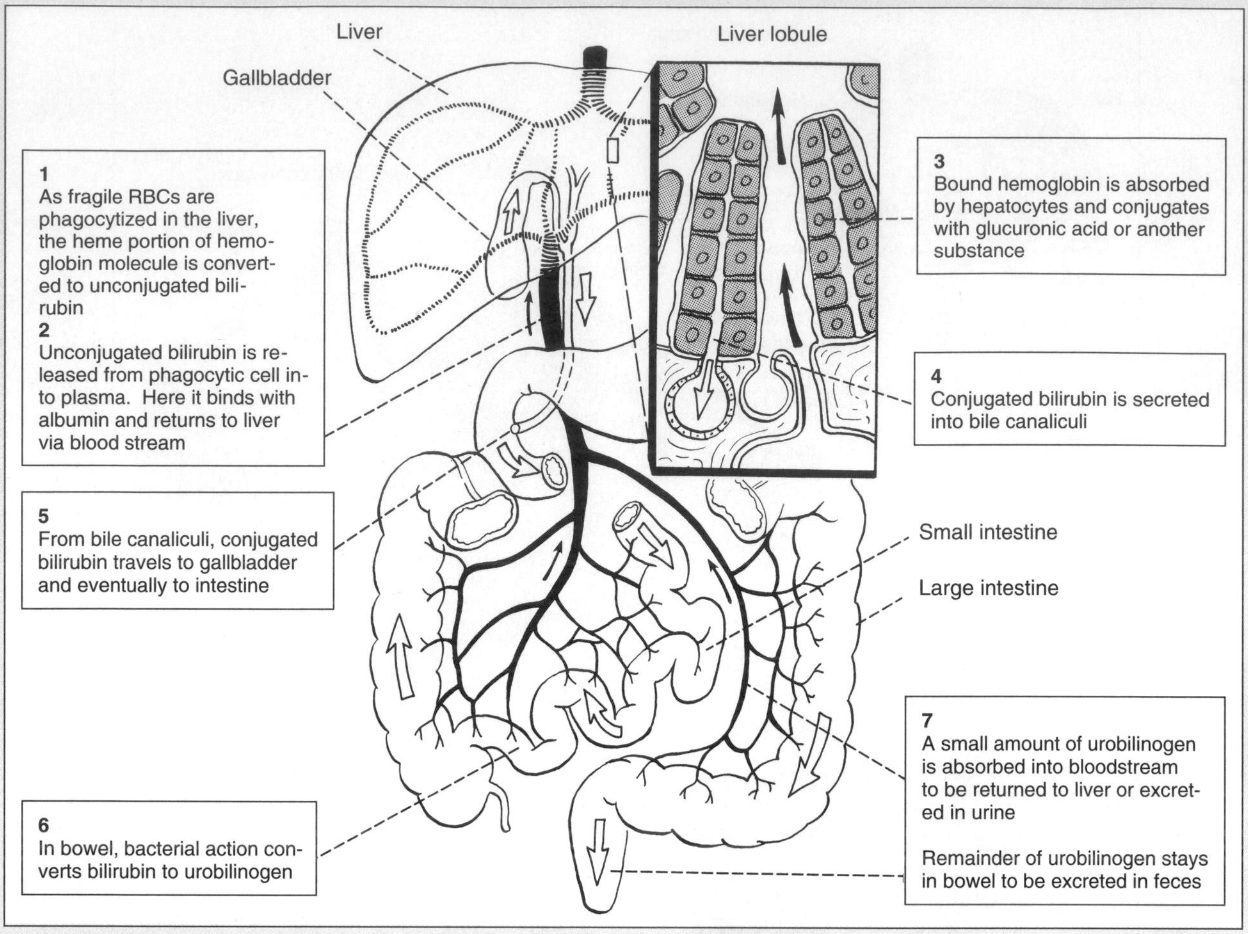

Liver
Liver lobule
Gallbladder
1
As fragile RBCs are phagocytized in the liver, the heme portion of hemoglobin molecule is converted to unconjugated bilirubin
2
Unconjugated bilirubin is released from phagocytic cell into plasma. Here it binds with albumin and returns to liver via blood stream
3
Bound hemoglobin is absorbed by hepatocytes and conjugates with glucuronic acid or another substance
4
Conjugated bilirubin is secreted into bile canaliculi
5
From bile canaliculi, conjugated bilirubin travels to gallbladder and eventually to intestine
Small intestine
Large intestine
7
A small amount of urobilinogen is absorbed into bloodstream to be returned to liver or excreted in urine
Remainder of urobilinogen stays in bowel to be excreted in feces
6
In bowel, bacterial action converts bilirubin to urobilinogen

Bile formation, metabolism, and excretion. (From Black, J. M., & Matassarin-Jacobs, E. [1993]. *Luckmann and Sorensen's medical-surgical nursing: A psychophysiologic approach* [4th ed.]. Philadelphia: W. B. Saunders Co.)

Function

The principal functions of the gallbladder are to store and to concentrate bile, which is necessary for the digestion of dietary fat. The common bile duct enters the duodenum at the sphincter of Oddi. When chyme with fatty content enters the duodenum, the hormone cholecystokinin stimulates the gallbladder to contract and the sphincter to open. This permits bile to enter the duodenum. When there is no fat present, the sphincter remains closed and bile backs up into the gallbladder where it is stored. Following surgical removal of the gallbladder, the bile ducts act as small reservoirs, but the ability to secrete large quantities of bile after the ingestion of a fatty meal is lost.

PANCREAS

Structure

The pancreas is an elongated and flattened organ that is located along the posterior abdominal wall behind the parietal peritoneum and posterior to the greater curvature of the stomach. One end of the pancreas, the head, is on the right side, enclosed by the curve of the duodenum. The other end, the tail, is on the left side next to the spleen. The aorta, inferior vena cava, portal vein, and hepatic artery are in the immediate vicinity of the pancreatic head, which greatly complicates extensive surgery in this area.

The major part of the pancreas is exocrine in nature and consists of pancreatic acinar cells that secrete digestive enzymes into tiny ducts interwoven between the cells. These tiny ducts merge to form the main pancreatic duct, which extends the full length of the gland. The pancreatic duct usually joins the common bile duct to form a single point of entry into the duodenum. Both ducts are controlled by the sphincter of Oddi (hepatopancreatic sphincter).

Function

The pancreas normally produces 1200 to 3000 mL of a clear pancreatic juice daily. Pancreatic juice has a high concentration of bicarbonate ions and contains digestive enzymes that act on carbohydrates, lipids, and proteins.

Features of the biliary tract and pancreas.

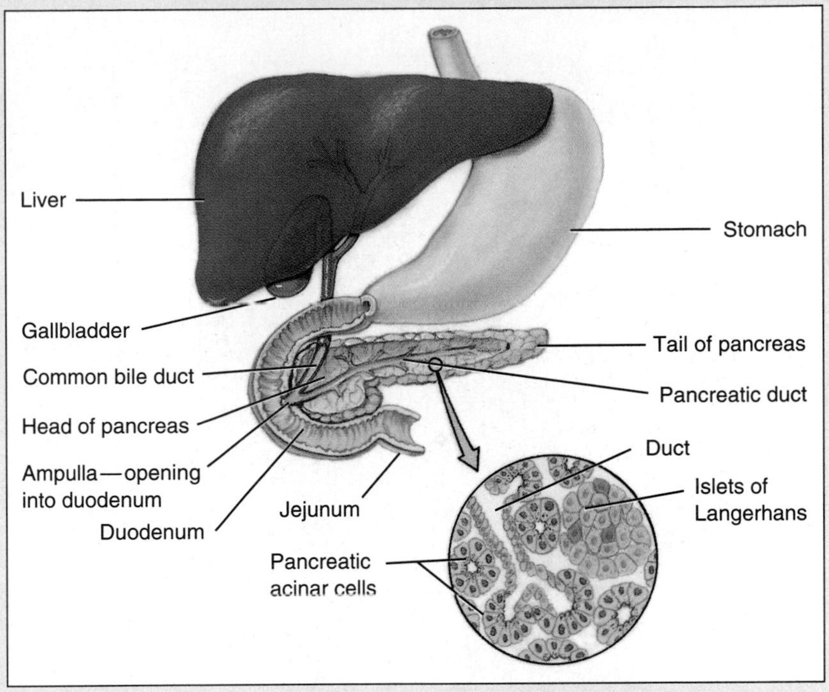

Pancreatic juice travels through the pancreatic duct to the duodenum, where it acts on the chyme. The active components of pancreatic juice are

- *Bicarbonate ions* to neutralize the acidity of the chyme.
- *Amylase* to split carbohydrates into disaccharides.
- *Lipase* to hydrolyze fats into glycerol and fatty acids.
- *Protease enzymes* to split proteins into amino acids. These include trypsin, chymotrypsin, and carboxypeptidase.

When acid chyme enters the duodenum, cells in the intestinal mucosa secrete the hormone secretin, which stimulates the pancreas to produce a fluid that is rich in bicarbonate ions to neutralize the acidity of the chyme. This is necessary because pancreatic enzymes require an alkaline environment to function. Proteins and fats in the chyme cause the intestinal mucosa to secrete cholecystokinin, which stimulates the pancreas to produce a fluid that has a high concentration of the digestive enzymes. Acetylcholine from the parasympathetic vagus nerve endings and gastrin from the stomach also stimulate the secretion of an enzyme-rich pancreatic juice.

AGE-RELATED CHANGES

The aging process leads to a decrease in the number and size of hepatic cells and an increase in the amount of fibrous tissue. This results in decreased liver mass and function and diminished ability to synthesize proteins and cholesterol. These changes reduce the liver's ability to detoxify drugs, which increases the risk of toxic amounts of a variety of medications accumulating in elderly people.

In the pancreas, advanced age brings calcification of the pancreatic vessels and alterations in the size of the ducts. A decrease in the production of lipase results in diminished fat digestion and absorption and an increase in the amount of fat excreted through the feces. Absorption of fat-soluble vitamins also may be affected.

Chapter 36

Assessment of Clients with Hepatic, Biliary Tract, and Exocrine Pancreatic Disorders

Learning Outcomes

After completing this chapter, the learner will be able to:

1. Teach the client about the normal structure and function of the liver, biliary system, and exocrine pancreas.
2. Explain to the client the abnormalities of structure and function of the liver, biliary system, and exocrine pancreas.
3. Conduct a nursing history and physical assessment of the client with actual or potential disorders of the liver, biliary system, and exocrine pancreas.
4. Teach the client about diagnostic studies common to liver, biliary system, and pancreatic function.

Assessment of the liver, biliary tract, and exocrine pancreas may reveal inflammation, fibrosis, lithiasis, or neoplasms. Underlying causative factors may include poor dietary habits, substance abuse, or environmental problems. Bacteriologic, biochemical, radiographic, and surgical diagnostic procedures provide only partial assessment data. For thorough assessment, the client's presenting symptoms, nutritional status, life-style, activities of daily living, and health history must be examined.

HISTORY

A thorough history includes an account of (1) the present illness and presenting symptoms, (2) recent skin or mucous membrane disruption, and (3) psychosocial history and life-style patterns, including environmental and occupational history.

During collection of historical data, the nurse can help the client recall experiences and onset of symptoms by placing them in a time sequence. Linking events and disease manifestation helps establish the diagnosis and, in some cases, can even predict the course of the disease.

Chief Complaint

Thorough investigation of the client's chief complaint is necessary for accurate assessment. Common symptoms related to the hepatic, biliary, and pancreatic systems include problems associated with the gastrointestinal, neurologic, genitourinary, integumentary, or cardiovascular systems (see Box 36–1).

Past Medical History

MAJOR ILLNESSES AND HOSPITALIZATIONS

The client is asked to describe past problems with jaundice, hepatitis, abdominal pain, gallbladder disease, anemia, or changes in bowel elimination such as diarrhea, clay-colored stools, and melena. The nurse should ascertain whether the client has ever been hospitalized for any of these problems or ever had surgery of the liver or gallbladder. The client is asked to recall if diagnostic procedures such as a gallbladder x-ray study, liver biopsy, or ultrasonographic examination of the gallbladder have ever been performed, or whether he or she has ever received a transfusion of blood or blood products.

Recent Skin or Membrane Disruption. Blood tests, transfusion of blood products, dental procedures, ear piercing, tattooing, and any intravenous injection with a potentially contaminated needle are important to assess. The nurse should note any unexplained puncture holes. Such breaks in the skin may be the route of entry for hepatitis virus (types B or C) or other pathogens.

Medications. The nurse should inquire specifically about medications the client is taking currently or took previously, including over-the-counter drugs. Many drugs and chemicals are potentially hepatotoxic, such as allopurinol, alcohol, gold compounds, mercury, phosphorus, anabolic steroids, acetaminophen, isoniazid,

BOX 36–1

Common Signs and Symptoms of Hepatic, Biliary, and Exocrine Pancreatic Disorders

GASTROINTESTINAL

- Abdominal pain (Right upper quadrant discomfort suggests gastrointestinal dysfunction)
- Nausea
- Vomiting
- Anorexia and weight loss
- Chronic indigestion (may be a sign of cholecystitis)
- Fatty food intolerance (another possible sign of cholecystitis)
- Constipation or diarrhea
- Melena (blood in the stool)
- Clay-colored stools
- Steatorrhea (bulky, fatty, foul-smelling stools)

NEUROLOGIC

- Mild depression
- Clouded sensorium
- Irritability
- Drowsiness (Dramatic neurologic symptoms can signal the onset of hepatic encephalopathy)

GENITOURINARY

- Dark yellow or tea-colored urine

INTEGUMENT

- Jaundiced skin (Jaundice first appears on the hard palate)
- Yellowed sclerae
- Pruritus

CARDIOVASCULAR

- Bleeding tendencies, e.g., nosebleeds
- Easy bruising
- Hemorrhoids
- Ascites
- Edema of limbs
- Spider angiomas

GENERAL

- Fatigue
- Fever
- Intolerance to alcohol
- Intolerance to medications

halothane, sulfonamides, arsenic, thiazide diuretics, and anti-cancer drugs such as methotrexate. Other medications to ask about are oral contraceptives, anesthetic agents, and antipsychotic drugs, which may also cause liver damage.

Family History

The nurse asks the client if any family members have had cancer (especially of the bowel or liver), jaundice, hepatitis, alcoholism, obesity, or gallbladder disease. Incidence of these problems in family members increases the client's risk status for their occurrence.

Psychosocial History and Life-Style

Assessment of the client's psychosocial history and life-style patterns provide data about his or her physical and psychological status. The nurse should include questions about the client's occupation, environment, and habits.

OCCUPATIONAL AND ENVIRONMENTAL FACTORS

The nurse should ask about the client's occupation and work environment and whether any factors are present that are known to cause liver damage. For example, heavy metals, such as mercury and lead, and chemicals, such as carbon tetrachloride, are known hepatotoxins. The nurse should ask whether the client engages in activities that increase the risk of exposure to substances that cause hepatitis or pancreatitis, for instance:

- Any close contact with hazardous waste or polluted water
- Travel in hepatitis or pancreatitis endemic areas
- Consumption of raw or steamed shellfish from polluted water
- Contact with hepatitis-infected animals or people
- Ingestion of mushrooms that were not purchased in a store
- Exposure to dry-cleaning fluids

HABITS

The nurse asks the client about eating patterns and the use of alcohol and other recreational substances, such as illicit drugs.

Eating patterns are important. The nurse should investigate

- Food preferences
- Daily consumption of proteins, carbohydrates, fats, and sodium
- Changes in eating patterns, including onset of changes
- Meal preparation—by whom, style of preparation
- Recent development of food intolerances

The nurse should carefully explore the client's use of alcohol and other mind-altering substances, paying attention to alcohol use patterns, because alcoholism often accompanies liver and pancreatic disease, such as fatty infiltration of the liver.

The nurse should be alert to whether the client provides confusing or conflicting data and whether the client's behavior alters in any way as the assessment proceeds. For example, does the client become angry, silent, or tearful? If significant others are present, do they corroborate the client's story? The client who does not acknowledge a substance abuse problem may not provide reliable information regarding usage.

PHYSICAL EXAMINATION

Physical assessment for liver, biliary, or pancreatic dysfunction involves careful exploration of the entire body.

The nurse should begin by assessing the client's general appearance and health status. For instance: Is there yellowing of the client's sclerae and integument? (See section on jaundice.) Does the client appear acutely or chronically ill? Does the client exhibit a tense facial expression or fidgety movement, indicating discomfort or pain?

The nurse should assess the client's nutritional status, weigh the client, and determine the amount of subcutaneous fat and muscular development. Obesity may accompany gallbladder disease. Malnutrition may exist in clients with a substance abuse history or cirrhosis. Ascites may account for recent rapid onset of weight gain with accompanying loss of muscle mass.

Next, the nurse assesses the abdomen. Prior to examination, the nurse should ask the client to point to any painful area and examine that section last. As stated earlier, hepatic and biliary pain is often located in the right upper quadrant. Pain that is dull and difficult to localize or describe may arise from an organ (viscera). Somatic pain is sharp, bright, easy to localize, and arises from nerve endings in the peritoneum.

The nurse should inspect the abdomen for ascites (fluid-filled abdomen) and prominent venous collateral networks common to cirrhosis. Characteristics of ascites include a distended abdomen with tight and glistening skin, bulging flanks, and prominent abdominal veins. Palpation is used to assess for muscle guarding or tenderness.

Percussion is used to assess the presence of ascites in the abdomen by observing for a fluid wave. The client is supine. Two nurses are needed to perform this assessment maneuver. One nurse places the edges of his or her hands on the client's abdominal midline to stabilize the abdominal wall. The second nurse places one hand on one side of the client's abdomen while briskly tapping the opposite side of the abdomen with the other hand. The second nurse feels for the movement of a fluid wave against the palpating hand opposite to the side percussed.

In addition to assessment of the abdomen, the nurse observes for systemic signs suggestive of hepatic, biliary, or pancreatic dysfunction. Such signs include jaundice, purpura, hair loss, weight loss, gynecomastia, spider angiomas, and reddened palms (palmar erythema).

While taking the history and performing physical assessment, the nurse should continue assessment of the client's mental and neurologic status. He or she should informally observe the client's verbal and nonverbal behavior, and notice facial expressions at rest and while talking, and try to assess the client's mood. For example, is there evidence of anxiety, depression, apathy, anger, exhaustion, or hostility? If possible, the nurse should directly question the client regarding sensorium, and note the presence of confusion, disorientation, or lethargy. The nurse should question the client's use of alcohol or other drugs. Since handwriting deteriorates with diminishing liver function, a handwriting sample should be recorded for subsequent comparison, should the client develop progressive hepatocellular damage (see also Chap. 37).

DIAGNOSTIC TESTS

A client with dysfunction of the liver, biliary tract, or pancreas frequently requires multiple diagnostic measures. No single laboratory test, radiographic study, or surgical procedure yields sufficient data to confirm a diagnosis or establish the degree of malfunction. The nurse should afford the individual a sense of self-worth and understanding during repeated diagnostic procedures. This helps gain the person's cooperation and also reduces the fatigue and anxiety that frequently accompany these experiences.

Laboratory Studies

The nurse should become familiar with common laboratory tests of liver, biliary, and pancreatic function. Table 36–1 is a summary of these tests.

Ultrasonography

Ultrasonography uses high-frequency sound waves to examine the interior of the body. In abdominal ultrasonography, the examiner passes a transducer over the abdomen. The technique proceeds rapidly and requires little or no preparation. Depending on the area to be examined, the client may or may not fast prior to the procedure. Ultrasonography is noninvasive and generally accurate. Because it does not involve x-rays, it is safe for pregnant women.

Ultrasonographic examination provides valuable diagnostic information for liver, pancreatic, and biliary tract conditions. It is a valuable diagnostic tool for presence of tumors as well as patency of vessels.

Radiologic Studies

Many of the procedures used to diagnose disorders of the liver, pancreas, and biliary tract involve the use of x-rays. Plain x-ray films of the abdomen may show diaphragm elevation caused by hepatic enlargement or calcification in the abdominal organs. Upper or lower gastrointestinal series using barium contrast medium also provide important information about the accessory organs of digestion, that is, the liver, gallbladder, and pancreas.

Radiologic studies using iodinated contrast media permit visualization of tubes or vessels. Before all of these procedures, the nurse should question the person about known hypersensitivity to iodine or seafood.

ORAL CHOLECYSTOGRAPHY (GALLBLADDER SERIES)

This examination is an x-ray test for gallbladder or cystic duct disease. The evening before the examination, the client ingests a radiopaque dye determined by the fat content of the evening meal. If the client has a regular or low-fat dinner, the client may receive sodium ipodate (Oragrafin). After a high-fat dinner, the client must be given iopanoic acid (Telepaque). These dyes contain iodine.

CRITICAL TO REMEMBER

The nurse must carefully observe the client for allergic reactions to the dye, even when the health history reveals no known allergies to iodine or seafood.

Possible hypersensitive reactions include nausea and vomiting, diarrhea, abdominal pain, rash, and anaphylaxis.

Conjugation of the dye occurs in the liver. The nurse should be aware that these dyes are potentially toxic to the liver and kidneys. This is especially true in clients with pre-existing hepatic or renal failure.

Following excretion of the opaque medium into the bile, the gallbladder concentrates the contrast medium.

During the test, radiography permits visualization of the gallbladder. When contraction of the gallbladder is desirable, the client consumes a high-fat meal during the procedure. Following an oral cholecystogram, some people experience burning on urination because of the presence of the dye in the urine. Forcing fluids decreases this problem.

Poor or no visualization of the gallbladder indicates gallbladder disease, presumably because biliary obstruction prevents passage of the dye. Occasionally, stones can be visualized as shadows within the opaque medium. The test results are accurate only when gastrointestinal and liver function allow absorption and conjugation of the dye.

CHOLANGIOGRAPHY

A cholangiogram or cholangiopancreatogram allows visualization of the bile ducts. Following administration of an organic iodine dye called iodipamide meglumine (Cholografin), x-ray filming begins.

Again, the nurse should assess for iodine allergies. Possible allergic reactions include dyspnea, tachycardia, sweating, nausea, vomiting, and chills.

TABLE 36–1 Laboratory Tests of Liver, Biliary, and Pancreatic Function

MEASUREMENT	NORMAL VALUE*	PROCEDURE	INTERPRETATION
Biliary Excretion			
Serum bilirubin Direct (conjugated) Indirect (unconjugated) Total	 0.1 to 0.3 mg/100 mL 0.2 to 0.8 mg/100 mL 0.1 to 1.0 mg/100 mL	Blood drawn without special preparation; protect sample from ultraviolet light	Direct bilirubin increased with impaired biliary excretion, causing conjugated fraction to accumulate in plasma Indirect bilirubin increased with excessive erythrocyte hemolysis Total bilirubin measures direct and indirect levels together
Urine bilirubin	0	Urine collection (urine appears smoky or tea-colored); protect from light	Urine bilirubin measures conjugated bilirubin only; increased with impaired bile excretion
Urine urobilinogen	0 to 4 mg/24 hr or 0.1 to 1.0 Ehrlich unit	24-hr or 2-hr afternoon collection placed in brown refrigerated bottle with sodium carbonate	Urine urobilinogen decreased with impaired bile excretion; increased with erythrocyte hemolysis
Fecal urobilinogen	40 to 280 mg/24 hr	Entire stool to laboratory	Fecal urobilinogen decreased with impaired bile excretion; increased in erythrocyte hemolysis
Serum cholesterol	150 to 250 mg/100 mL	Blood drawn after low-cholesterol diet for 12 hours	Cholesterol elevated when excretion blocked by bile duct obstruction, but reduced when severe liver damage reduces ability to synthesize it
Carbohydrate Metabolism			
Serum amylase Serum pancreatic isoamylase Urine amylase	80 to 150 Somogyi U/100 mL or 56 to 190 IU/liter (depends on test used)	Blood drawn without special preparation 2-, 12-, or 24-hour urine collection with no preservative unless specified	Pancreatic digestive enzyme released with breakdown of acinar cells; serum levels increase 2 to 3 hr after pain onset with pancreatitis and return to normal in 24 to 48 hr; elevations not directly correlated with severity; amylase test measures both pancreatic and salivary amylase; pancreatic isoamylase is a more specific test; urinary levels elevated longer with pancreatitis
Protein Metabolism			
Total protein	6 to 8 gm/100 mL	Blood drawn without special preparation	Less plasma protein synthesized in liver damage (albumin, α and β globulins); γ globulins produced by plasma cells, not liver
Serum albumin	3.5 to 5.5 gm/100 mL		
Serum globulin include α_1, α_2, β, γ	2.5 to 3.5 gm/100 mL		
A/G ratio (albumin/globulin)	1.5/1 to 2.5/1	Blood drawn without special preparation	A decrease in the ratio may indicate chronic liver disease
Blood ammonia	<75 μg/100 mL	Blood drawn without special preparation	Reduced synthesis of urea from body ammonia in severe hepatocellular damage produces elevated blood ammonia
Methemalbumin	Absent	Fluid from peritoneal or pleural tap analyzed	Product of hemoglobin digestion elevated when blood released into body fluids, as in hemorrhagic pancreatitis
Fat Metabolism			
Serum lipase	0 to 1.5 U	Blood drawn from fasting person	Pancreatic digestive enzyme released with breakdown of acinar cells

Table continued on following page

TABLE 36–1 Laboratory Tests of Liver, Biliary, and Pancreatic Function *Continued*

MEASUREMENT	NORMAL VALUE*	PROCEDURE	INTERPRETATION
Metabolism of Foreign Substances			
Bromsulphalein (BSP) excretion	< 5% retention in 1 hr	Control blood taken after fasting for 12 hr BSP given, blood drawn at intervals	Dye retained with diminished hepatocellular ability to remove it from blood and excrete it; infrequently used
Serum Enzymes†			
Aspartate aminotransferase (AST) (formerly SGOT) Alanine aminotransferase (ALT) (formerly SGPT) Lactate dehydrogenase (LDH)	5 to 40 U/mL 5 to 35 U/mL Varies with units used	Blood drawn without special preparation	Serum aspartate aminotransferase, alanine aminotransferase, and lactic dehydrogenase released from damaged liver, heart, kidney, and muscle cells; levels not directly correlated with degree of damage; elevations above 400 U accompany acute hepatocellular alteration
Alkaline phosphatase (ALP)	Varies with method and age of person	Blood drawn without special preparation	Increase in biliary obstruction; produced by cells lining the biliary tract; this enzyme is also found in bone, intestine, and placenta
Serum 5′-nucleotidase	0.3 to 3.2 Bodansky units	Blood drawn without special preparation	Enzyme located mainly in liver and confirmation of liver disease occurs if ALP and this both elevated
Serum gamma-glutamyl transpeptidase (GGTP)	< 65 IU/liter	Blood drawn without special preparation	Enzyme located in liver and kidney; elevation of GGTP and ALP significant indication of liver disorders
Hepatitis Antigens and Antibodies			
Hepatitis A, hepatitis B, and hepatitis C viruses	Negative for antigens Positive or negative for antibodies, depending on history	Blood drawn without special preparation	Antigens indicate hepatitis; antibodies indicate past or present hepatitis or immunization (hepatitis B)
Hemostatic Function			
Prothrombin time (PT)	12 to 15 sec	Blood drawn without special preparation	Assesses function of extrinsic pathway in clotting process (factors I, II, V, VII, X) PT prolonged with (1) decreased synthesis due to liver cell damage or (2) decreased vitamin K absorption due to bile duct obstruction Vitamin K necessary for liver to synthesize prothrombin (factor II)
Partial thromboplastin time (PTT)/Activated partial thromboplastin time (APTT)	30–45 sec. (PTT) 35–45 sec. (APTT)	Blood drawn without special preparation	Assesses function of intrinsic pathway and the coagulation pathway
Platelets	150,000 to 400,000/mm^3	Blood drawn without special preparation	May fall when spleen is enlarged in portal hypertension
Exocrine Pancreatic Function			
		Oral bentiromide given after overnight fast; urine is collected for 6 hr	Pancreatic chymotrypsin splits bentiromide; para-aminobenzoic acid (PABA), a breakdown product, is excreted in urine; less PABA is excreted with pancreatic insufficiency

TABLE 36–1 Laboratory Tests of Liver, Biliary, and Pancreatic Function *Continued*

MEASUREMENT	NORMAL VALUE*	PROCEDURE	INTERPRETATION
Antigens Associated with Cancer			
Alpha-fetoprotein (AFP)	< 10 ng/mg	Blood drawn without special preparation	AFP is synthesized by fetus but not by healthy adult; AFP level > 1000 ng/mL usually indicates hepatocellular carcinoma

* Normal values may differ significantly between laboratories.

† Trends in elevation are of particular importance in predicting the rapidity with which the liver is failing. If levels rise, fall, then rise again, liver failure may be occurring.

Also, to prevent renal damage, the nurse should instruct the client to drink ample amounts of fluid following administration of the dye.

There are four types of cholangiography.

- Intravenous cholangiography is used for common bile duct visualization. The radiopaque dye burns intensely upon injection.
- Percutaneous cholangiography involves injecting the dye directly into the ductal system, directly through the skin via a long, slender needle.
- Retrograde cholangiography involves passage of an endoscope through the mouth into the duodenum. After location of the ampulla of Vater, the examiner passes a catheter into the common bile duct and, possibly, the pancreatic duct. Dye is injected through the catheter into the duct.
- T-tube cholangiography involves injecting dye into the pre-existing bile drainage tube.

In all four types of cholangiography, failure of the opaque dye to pass through the bile ducts provides evidence of duct obstruction.

ANGIOGRAPHY

Angiography is helpful in the study of the pancreas, spleen, and portal system. This x-ray procedure allows visualization of the visceral vessels in order to identify abnormalities of vascular structure and function, observe masses, and note sites of bleeding. A contrast medium is injected through the femoral artery.

Following angiography, the nurse assesses the needle insertion site for signs of bleeding, because with liver conditions clients often have concurrent clotting disorders.

COMPUTED TOMOGRAPHY

Computed tomography (CT) is another radiologic technique used to diagnose and evaluate liver, biliary tract, and gallbladder disease. A CT scan is performed by rotating a finely focused x-ray beam around the client. A computer then assembles data from the detector and provides an image.

Radionuclide Scanning

Radionuclide scanning, or scintigraphy, involves the intravenous infusion of gamma-emitting isotopes. Following infusion, a scintillation detector passes over the abdomen. This procedure investigates biliary duct patency and indicates whether a tumor or abscess is present in the liver, gallbladder, or pancreas.

Paracentesis

The purpose of paracentesis, or peritoneal tap, is to extract fluid accumulations in the peritoneum (ascites) to relieve intra-abdominal tension, which can impair the client's respiratory status, or to obtain the fluid to send for culture. The nurse actively participates in this procedure, which usually takes place at the bedside. Beforehand, the nurse reinforces teaching about the purpose of the procedure and the steps involved, and checks that written consent has been obtained. The client is asked to void immediately prior to the procedure to decrease the risk of bladder puncture. The nurse has the client sit upright on the edge of the bed, with feet resting on a stool and back well supported. Following cleansing of the skin and infiltration with a local anesthetic, the physician, using sterile technique, inserts a long aspirating needle with a syringe to collect a fluid specimen. To drain ascitic fluid (if desired), the physician inserts a trocar aseptically through a small stab wound below the umbilicus. This allows fluid (usually several liters) to drain slowly through a catheter into a collection bottle.

The major complication of paracentesis is hypovolemia and shock secondary to fluid drainage from the peritoneum, and the resulting fluid shift from intravascular to interstitial space as well as the sudden change in intra-abdominal pressure on the vessels. This fluid shift is exacerbated by hypoalbuminemia.

The nurse assesses vital signs and peripheral circulation every few minutes during and immediately following paracentesis. He or she should observe for hypovolemic shock: pallor, tachycardia, decreased blood pressure, and oliguria and dyspnea.

Hepatic encephalopathy due to reduced tissue perfusion is another complication arising from drainage of ascitic fluid. Because of the high protein concentration of ascitic fluid, the physician may prescribe albumin infusions for 24 hours following paracentesis to compensate for protein losses. Potassium depletion may occur following multiple paracentesis procedures. Infection, peritonitis, and bleeding due to vessel trauma occasionally complicate paracentesis.

The nurse should carefully assess for abdominal pain following paracentesis. Monitoring the site for persistent leakage of ascites is also important.

Peritoneoscopy

Insertion of a peritoneoscope through an abdominal stab wound permits direct visualization of the liver and peritoneum. Visualization of structural changes aids in the diagnosis of cirrhosis and cancer. During peritoneoscopy, the examiner may take photographs and perform a biopsy.

Peritoneoscopy is relatively safe and simple. Contraindications include infections of the abdominal cavity, clotting disorders, or intestinal obstruction. In addition, the client must be able to cooperate throughout the procedure. Obesity and ascites interfere with test results. Box 36–2 lists the steps in preparing a client for peritoneoscopy.

When peritoneoscopy includes liver biopsy, 24 hours of bed rest follow the procedure. If biopsy is not performed, the client resumes activity following recovery from effects of medication. Complications are uncommon and more often occur secondary to biopsy.

Possible post-peritoneoscopy complications are pneumothorax, subcutaneous emphysema, air embolism, bile peritonitis, perforation of a hollow organ, and shoulder or abdominal pain.

Biopsy

Biopsy is the single most valuable diagnostic study to the physician. It involves the removal of a sample of living tissue for analysis. Biopsies may be open or closed procedures. An open biopsy necessitates a general anesthetic and a major abdominal incision. A client may have an open biopsy at the time of a concurrent operative procedure. An advantage of the open biopsy is that the surgeon can observe the entire liver, identify grossly altered tissue, and remove the biopsy specimen for study.

A closed biopsy or percutaneous liver biopsy is a simpler procedure than open biopsy. It involves aspiration of a core of tissue via needle for histologic study.

Contraindications to percutaneous liver biopsy are severe thrombocytopenia, local infection of lung base, prolonged prothrombin time, peritonitis, massive ascites, an uncooperative client, and extrahepatic obstructive jaundice, especially with an enlarged gallbladder. The client with cancer or amyloidosis has an increased risk of post-procedure hemorrhage. Also, if the client is unable to remain still and cooperate during the procedure, an organ could be accidentally punctured.

To prepare for percutaneous liver biopsy, the client fasts for at least 6 hours before the test. The procedure is usually performed at the bedside using a local anesthetic. The nurse places the client either in the supine position or in a lateral position with the upper arm elevated. Less frequently, the nurse may ask the client to assume a prone position. During insertion of the needle, the nurse has the client exhale and then hold the breath on expiration for 5 to 10 seconds to avoid puncturing of the diaphragm (Fig. 36–1).

BOX 36–2

Preparing a Client for Peritoneoscopy

To prepare a client for peritoneoscopy, the nurse should follow these steps:

- Check that written consent has been obtained.
- Check the laboratory record to make certain the client has normal or adequate clotting factors. If not, inform the physician.
- Check the client and health care record for contraindications to preprocedural medications.
- Inquire as to whether the client is sensitive to local anesthetics.
- Prepare the skin and administer preprocedural medication when appropriate.
- Instruct the client to take nothing by mouth and to empty the bowel and bladder just before the procedure begins.
- Provide adequate teaching before and during the actual procedure.
- Explain that it may be difficult to breathe when CO_2 is placed into the abdominal cavity.
- Instruct the client to elevate the abdominal wall by holding the breath to protect major organs during needle insertion.

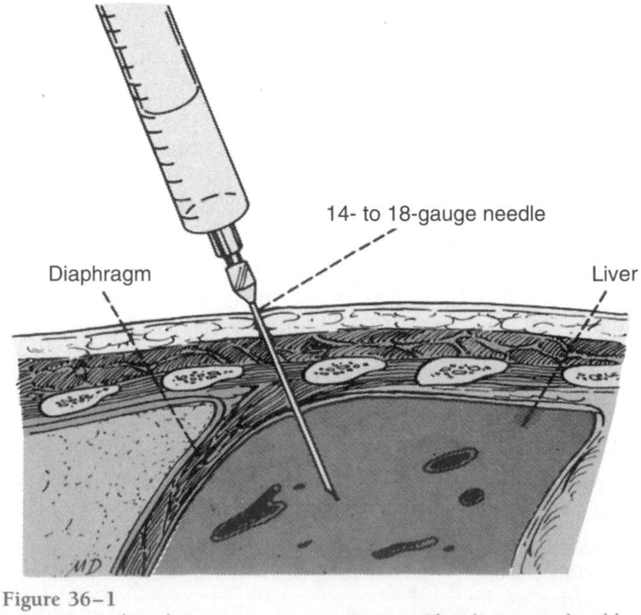

Figure 36–1
Percutaneous liver biopsy requires cooperation. The client must be able to lie quietly and hold his or her breath after exhaling.

BOX 36–3

Nursing Care after Percutaneous Liver Biopsy

For care of a client after percutaneous liver biopsy, the nurse should undertake the following measures:

- Monitor vital signs for the first 8 to 12 hours.
- Carefully assess for tachycardia and decreasing blood pressure, which may indicate hemorrhage.
- Observe for pain in the right upper quadrant of the abdomen due to a subcapsular accumulation of blood or bile, or at the right shoulder as a result of blood on the undersurface of the diaphragm.
- Maintain the client on bed rest for 24 hours following the procedure. The right side-lying position for the first 1 to 2 hours decreases the risk of hemorrhage and bile leakage.
- Administer postprocedure medications on an individual basis, depending on the client's physical status.
- Give vitamin K if prescribed.
- Assess respiratory status for signs of dyspnea.

Following percutaneous liver biopsy, the nurse performs the nursing assessments and interventions listed in Box 36–3.

Inherent risks following biopsy include hemorrhage and puncture of adjacent organs or structures. Hemorrhage, the most serious complication, may result from penetration of the arterial tree or a distended vein radicle. Hemorrhage may occur during the first 24 hours after the biopsy procedure. The risk of hemorrhage is increased if vascular channels are distended or if the client breathes during needle insertion into the liver. Puncture of a lung can cause pneumothorax. A large biopsy needle (14- to 18-gauge) can penetrate a dilated intrahepatic duct in a person with obstructive jaundice. Bile leakage and resultant peritonitis can develop. Bile peritonitis is treated with surgical decompression. Cross-contamination may occur following puncture of an adjacent organ. Clients with potentially effusive conditions (e.g., ascites, chronic lung disease) in addition to liver abnormality are at great risk for cross-contamination.

Fine-needle aspiration biopsy, often performed when a suspicious area of the liver is localized, helps diagnose malignancy. This approach is ideal when only a few cells are necessary for cytologic study. The risks of fine-needle aspiration biopsy are far less than guided regular biopsy, since the tissue sample is much smaller. Also, this procedure greatly reduces any risk of tumor metastasis along the needle track.

There are few contraindications to the guided regular or fine-needle aspiration biopsy procedures. Clients with impaired coagulation associated with liver disease, however, may not be appropriate candidates for the closed procedure.

Portal Pressure Measurements

Measurements of portal pressure and flow help to (1) diagnose portal hypertension, (2) indicate the severity of portal hypertension, and (3) guide decisions as to appropriate intervention, which may include surgery.

Portal pressure measurements are minor surgical procedures that are performed in the operating room or a special studies laboratory. Often, the surgeon concurrently injects contrast media. These measures require standard preoperative and postoperative care, with special postoperative assessment of the incision site for hematoma formation.

The client should be instructed to hold his or her breath during needle insertion and passage. The nurse carefully observes for bleeding or pneumothorax afterward.

STUDY QUESTIONS

1. Of the following liver functions, which is the most important to human survival?
   A. Carbohydrate metabolism
   B. Fat metabolism
   C. Protein metabolism
   D. Fluid and electrolyte reabsorption
2. Disease of the pancreas may cause which one of the following?
   A. Dyspnea
   B. Cyanosis
   C. Neck vein engorgement
   D. Left lower quadrant pain
3. When a client experiences pancreatic disease, the nurse must assess which of the following intake of dietary components?
   A. Fats
   B. Proteins
   C. Carbohydrates
   D. Fats, proteins, and carbohydrates
4. A client asks the nurse how the body uses bile. The best response is:
   A. "Protein and fat breakdown occur when bile is released."
   B. "Bile is used to break down fat when it reaches the duodenum."
   C. "Carbohydrate molecules are processed by the bile in the gallbladder."
   D. "Bile is used to break down undigested materials in the small intestine."
5. After the client returns from a percutaneous liver biopsy, the nurse should assess him or her for:
   A. Pain in the pelvic area
   B. Signs and symptoms of hemorrhage
   C. Ability to walk unassisted the first 12 hours
   D. Knowledge of liver disease, diagnostic studies, and treatments

CRITICAL THINKING EXERCISES

SCENARIO A

A client is admitted to the hospital with severe pain in the epigastric area. The pain has been present for 24 hours and the client is exhausted.

1. What admission assessment should be completed for the client?
2. What information regarding family history of disease is important?
3. How would you assess the abdomen for the possibility of ascites?
4. If a cholangiogram is ordered, what should you teach the client regarding anticipated results?

SCENARIO B

A client is scheduled for a liver biopsy in the morning and the nurse is teaching him about expectations for care following the biopsy:

1. What should the client be taught if he is scheduled for a closed biopsy?
2. What risks are inherent in any client who has a liver biopsy?

BIBLIOGRAPHY

1. Arias, I. M., et al. (1988). *The liver: Biology and pathobiology.* New York: Raven Press.
2. Axon, A. T. (1989). Endoscopic retrograde cholangiopancreatography in chronic pancreatitis: Cambridge classification. *Radiologic Clinics of North America, 27(1),* 39–50.
3. Balthazar, E. J. (1989). CT diagnosis and staging of acute pancreatitis. *Radiologic Clinics of North America, 27(1),* 19–37.
4. Bayless, T. M. (1989). *Current therapy in gastroenterology and liver disease* (vol. 3, 3rd ed.). St. Louis: The C.V. Mosby Co.
5. Bongiovanni, G. L. (Ed.) (1988). *Essentials of clinical gastroenterology* (2nd ed.). New York: McGraw-Hill.
6. Clouse, M. E. (1989). Current diagnostic imaging modalities of the liver. *Surgical Clinics of North America, 69(2),* 193–234.
7. Copstead, L. C. (1995). *Perspectives on pathophysiology.* Philadelphia: W. B. Saunders.
8. Ebersol, P., & Hess, P. (1994). *Toward healthy aging: Human needs and nursing response* (4th ed.). St. Louis: C. V. Mosby.
9. Fischbach, F. (1992). *A manual of laboratory & diagnostic tests* (4th ed.). Philadelphia: J. B. Lippincott.
10. Gitnick, G. (Ed.) (1989). *Modern concepts of acute and chronic hepatitis.* New York: Plenum Publishing Corp.
11. Gitnick, G. (1994). *Principles and practice of gastroenterology and hepatology* (2nd ed.). Norwalk, CT: Appleton & Lange.
12. Guyton, A. C. (1991). *Textbook of medical physiology* (8th ed.). Philadelphia: W. B. Saunders.
13. Holland, P., & Hussain, I. (1989). Biliary lithotripsy: Nonsurgical treatment of gallstones. *Society of Gastrointestinal Assistants Journal, 3,* 158–162.
14. Isselbacher, K. J. (Ed.) (1994). *Harrison's principles of internal medicine* (13th ed.). New York: McGraw-Hill.
15. Jarvis, C. (1992). *Physical examination and health assessment.* Philadelphia: W. B. Saunders.
16. Jeffery, R. B. (1989). Sonography in acute pancreatitis. *Radiologic Clinics of North America, 27(1),* 5–17.
17. Marta, M. R. (1987). Endoscopic retrograde cholangiopancreatography: Its role in diagnosis and treatment. *Focus on Critical Care, 14(5),* 62–63.
18. McCance, K. L., & Heuther, S. E. (1994). *Pathophysiology: The biologic basis for disease in adults and children* (2nd ed.). St. Louis: C. V. Mosby.
19. Mosley, J. W., et al. (1990). Non-A, non-B hepatitis and antibody to hepatitis C virus. *JAMA, 263,* 77–78.
20. Pagana, K. D., & Pagana, T. J. (1994). *Diagnostic testing and nursing implications: A case study approach* (4th ed.). St. Louis: C. V. Mosby.
21. Rakel, R. E. (1995). *Conn's current therapy 1995.* Philadelphia: W. B. Saunders.
22. Rector, W. G., Jr. (1992). *Complications of chronic liver disease.* St. Louis: C. V. Mosby.
23. Sabiston, D. C., Jr. (1991). *Textbook of surgery: The biologic basis of modern surgical practice* (14th ed.). Philadelphia: W. B. Saunders.
24. Sacher, R. D., et al. (1991). *Widmann's clinical interpretation of laboratory tests* (10th ed.). Philadelphia: F. A. Davis.
25. Schiff, L., & Schiff, E. R. (1993). *Diseases of the liver (7th ed.).* Philadelphia: J. B. Lippincott.
26. Seeff, L. B., & Lewis, J. H. (Eds.) (1989). *Current perspectives in hepatology.* New York: Plenum.
27. Septimus, E. J. (1984). Seroprevalence of hepatitis B markers in health care workers at a teaching medical center at two community hospitals. *Advances in Therapy, 1,* 215.
28. Setchell, K. D. R., et al. (Eds.) (1988). *The bile acids.* New York: Plenum.
29. Shaffer, E., & Thomson, A. B. (Eds.) (1992). *Modern concepts of gastroenterology, Vol. 3.* New York: Plenum.
30. Sleisenger, M. H., & Fordtran, J. S. (Eds.) (1993). *Gastrointestinal disease: Pathophysiology, diagnosis, and management* (5th ed.). Philadelphia: W. B. Saunders.
31. Soloway, R. D. (Ed.) (1983). *Chronic active liver disease.* New York: Churchill Livingstone.
32. Swartz, M. H. (1994). *Textbook of physical diagnosis: History and examination* (2nd ed.). Philadelphia: W. B. Saunders.
33. Swenson, S. A. (1984). Diagnosis: hepatic neoplasms. *Hospital Medicine, 20,* 190.

34. Thomson, J. C. (Ed.) (1990). *Gastrointestinal endocrinology.* New York: Academic Press.

35. Tierney, L. M., Jr., et al. (1994). *Current medical diagnoses and treatment.* Norwalk, CT: Appleton & Lange.

36. VanSonneberg, E., et al. (1989). Imaging and interventional radiology for pancreatitis and its complications. *Radiologic Clinics of North America, 27(1),* 65–72.

37. Watson, J., & Jaffe, M. S. (1995). *Nurse's manual of laboratory and diagnostic tests* (2nd ed.). Philadelphia: F. A. Davis.

38. Wilkinson, M. (1990). Nursing implications after endoscopic retrograde cholangiopancreatography. *Gastroenterology Nursing,* 13(2), 105–109.

39. Williams, J. W. & Simel, D. L. (1992). Does this patient have ascites? How to define fluid in the abdomen. *Journal of the American Medical Association, 267(19),* 2645–2648.

40. Witkin, G. B., et al. (1987). Choosing liver function tests. *Emergency Medicine, 19(20),* 22–46.

41. Wyngaarden, J. B., Smith, L. H., & Bennett, J. C. (Eds.) (1992). *Cecil textbook of medicine* (19th ed.). Philadelphia: W. B. Saunders.

42. Yatto, R., & Siegel, J. (1984). Cholestasis: an alternative to surgery in older patients. *Geriatrics, 39,* 113.

43. Zakim, D., & Boyer, T. D. (Eds.) (1990). *Hepatology: A textbook of liver disease* (2nd ed.). Philadelphia: W. B. Saunders.

Chapter 37

Nursing Care of Clients with Hepatic Disorders

Learning Outcomes

After completing this chapter, the learner will be able to:

1. Assess the client for clinical manifestations of infectious or inflammatory and obstructive hepatic disorders.
2. Teach the client about the etiology, risk factors, basic pathophysiology, and clinical manifestations of major hepatic disorders.
3. Explain the client's role in medical and surgical management of hepatic disorders.
4. Develop plans of care for the prevention of illness, management, and rehabilitation of clients with hepatic disorders.
5. Implement nursing interventions that optimize the quality of life for clients with hepatic disorders.
6. Evaluate planned client outcomes using outcome criteria developed in the planning phase of care.

TABLE 37–1 Types of Jaundice (Icterus)

	CAUSES	ASSESSMENT	CONJUGATED (DIRECT) BILIRUBIN (0.1–0.3 mg/ 100 mL)	UNCONJUGATED (INDIRECT) BILIRUBIN (0.2–0.8 mg/100 mL)
Prehepatic jaundice	Excessive hemolysis caused by transfusion reactions, hemolytic disease of newborn, severe burns, bacterial toxins, venoms, hypotonic parenteral solutions, etc; defective albumin binding	Liver function usually normal; compensates for ↑ bilirubin by ↑ metabolism of bilirubin	Normal	↑
Hepatic jaundice	Liver's inability to conjugate or transport bilirubin to canaliculi for excretion caused by hepatitis, liver congestion, cirrhosis, metastatic cancer, prolonged use of medications metabolized by liver, etc	Liver may be enlarged Abdomen may be tender May have bruising or bleeding resulting from vitamin K malabsorption†	↑	Normal or slight ↑
Posthepatic jaundice (obstructive)	Blocked flow of bile into duodenum resulting from inflammation, scar tissue, stones, or tumors in liver, biliary, or pancreatic system	↑ Level of unconjugated bilirubin if liver cell function is diminished May have bruising or bleeding as a result of vitamin K malabsorption (bile is necessary for vitamin K absorption)† Abdomen may be tender Stools are clay colored (bile gives stool its dark color) Urine is brown or foamy (conjugated bilirubin is excreted in urine)	↑	Normal or ↑

* Normal values will vary among laboratories.
† Parenteral vitamin K will improve prothrombin time only if jaundice is due to posthepatic cause.
SGOT, serum glutamic-oxaloacetic transaminase; SGPT, serum glutamic-pyruvic transaminase.
Adapted from Gannon, R. B., & Pickett, K. (1983). Jaundice. *American Journal of Nursing, 83,* 404.

Hepatic Disorders

Jaundice

Jaundice, or icterus, is the yellow pigmentation of the sclerae, skin, and deeper tissues as a result of excessive accumulation of bile pigments in the blood. Bilirubin (bile pigment), a product of red cell breakdown, is deposited in the skin and excreted in the urine when present in the blood in excessive amounts (hyperbilirubinemia). This characteristic makes jaundice a valuable indicator for a variety of disorders involving either hemolysis or biliary obstruction. When there is an obstruction blocking the flow of bile into the intestine, jaundiced individuals may have clay-colored stools as a result of the lack of bilirubin and its metabolites in the intestine. For a description of normal bilirubin metabolism, see Figure 36–4.

Etiology

Jaundice can be classified according to the location of the pathologic change. Jaundice may occur because of a problem in the blood before reaching the liver (prehepatic jaundice), within the liver itself (hepatic jaundice), or after the bilirubin leaves the liver (posthepatic or obstructive jaundice). The pathologic causes underlying these three types of jaundice are outlined briefly here and in more detail in Table 37–1.

PREHEPATIC JAUNDICE

Prehepatic jaundice results from excessive red cell destruction. Excessive red cell destruction may occur from transfusion reactions, hemolytic anemia, severe burns, or defective albumin binding. The liver normally compensates for the increased unconjugated bilirubin it receives by increasing its rate of bilirubin conjugation. The excess can then be excreted in the urine and feces.

LABORATORY TESTS

TOTAL BILI-RUBIN (0.1–1.0 mg/100 mL)	URINE BILIRU-BIN (0)	URINE URO-BILINO-GEN (0–4 mg/d)	FECAL UROBILIN-OGEN (40–280 mg/d)	ASPARTATE AMINO TRANSFER-ASE (SGOT) (5–40 U/mL)	ALANINE AMINO-TRANSFER-ASE (SGPT) (5–35 U/mL)	PARTIAL THROM-BOPLAS-TIN TIME (30–40 sec*)	PRO-THROM-BIN TIME (12–15 sec)
↑	None	↑	↑	Normal	Normal	Normal	Normal
↑	↑	↑ ↓	↓	↑	↑	Prolonged	Prolonged
↑	↑	↓	Absent or ↓	Normal or ↑	Normal or ↑	Prolonged	Prolonged

Prehepatic jaundice disappears once the rate of hemolysis slows.

HEPATIC JAUNDICE

Hepatic jaundice is due to defective uptake, conjugation, or transport of bilirubin within the liver. Liver cell dysfunction or necrosis caused by hepatitis, for example, or defective bile transport in the bile canal and small bile duct can cause hyperbilirubinemia. Unknown channels absorb the pooled bile components into the blood stream. Although "obstructive jaundice" usually refers to posthepatic jaundice, an obstruction within the liver can make this term appropriate for hepatic jaundice as well.

POSTHEPATIC (OBSTRUCTIVE) JAUNDICE

Posthepatic (obstructive) jaundice results from impaired bilirubin transport and excretion in the biliary system. In this case, the problem arises from obstruction of an extrahepatic bile duct, for example, occlusion of the common duct by gallstones.

Clinical Manifestations

Manifestations of jaundice include yellow sclerae, yellowish orange skin, clay-colored feces, tea-colored urine, pruritus, fatigue, and anorexia.

Diagnostic Assessment

The following diagnostic test results are consistent with jaundice:

- Increased levels of direct (conjugated) serum bilirubin (>0.4 mg/100 mL) because bilirubin returns to the plasma when it cannot be excreted
- Increased indirect (unconjugated) serum bilirubin values (>0.8 mg/100 mL)

- Absence of bilirubin in the urine (unconjugated bilirubin is not water soluble)
- Increased urine urobilinogen (>4 mg/24 hr)
- Reduced fecal urobilinogen (<40 mg/24 hr) because it does not reach the intestine
- Increased alkaline phosphatase and cholesterol serum levels because they cannot be excreted into the bile as normal
- In extreme cases of fulminant liver failure, unusually low cholesterol level, indicating the liver's inability to synthesize it at all
- Increased serum bile salts with consequent deposition in the skin, causing pruritus
- Prolonged prothrombin time (>40 seconds) owing to reduced absorption of fat-soluble vitamin K

Medical Management

Treatment for jaundice aims to resolve the underlying disease. See Chapter 28 for a discussion of interventions in hemolytic anemia (prehepatic anemia). Time and rest compose the primary treatment for resolution of jaundice in hepatitis. Treatments for hepatic jaundice are discussed later. Treatments for posthepatic jaundice include dissolution therapy and surgical removal of the obstruction.

Surgical Management

Surgical exploration of the common bile duct (choledochostomy) enables the diagnostician to differentiate between choledocholithiasis (stone in the common bile duct) and tumor. If carcinoma (usually of the pancreas head) is discovered during exploration, the surgeon may perform a palliative anastomosis of the gallbladder to the jejunum to bypass the common bile duct (see Chap. 38).

Nursing Management

Assessment

The client should be closely observed for the development of jaundice. Often, the first symptom the client notices is a change in taste, manifesting as a distaste for a food or drink the client liked, such as coffee.

CRITICAL TO REMEMBER

Because the hard palate is the first place that jaundice will appear, this area should be assessed first. (Scleral color may be deceptive, especially in nonwhite clients.)

Pruritus is another early sign of developing jaundice.

Nursing Diagnosis, Planning, and Implementation

Nursing Diagnosis: Skin Integrity, Impaired R/T pruritus.

Planning: Expected Outcomes. The client will maintain skin integrity, as evidenced by client's statements of relief, decreased dryness of skin, and a decrease in scratching by the client.

Implementation. Pruritus is probably caused by an accumulation of bile salts in the skin, resulting from obstructed biliary excretion. Some clients experience only mild itching, whereas others suffer such extreme itching that it causes them to tear at their skin or scratch in their sleep.

Oral cholestyramine resin provides some relief by binding bile salts in the intestine so they can be excreted. Antihistamines also may relieve the itching. Phenobarbital has been effective in some cases because of its ability to enhance bile flow.

Nursing Diagnosis: Self-Esteem Disturbance R/T yellowing of skin and sclerae.

Planning: Expected Outcomes. The client will cope with self-esteem disturbance, as evidenced by the client's not isolating him- or herself and being able to discuss feelings associated with jaundice.

Implementation. A highly visible sign of illness, jaundice may have a considerable emotional impact and may impair body image. Jaundice and its manifestations can dominate the client's feelings and require ongoing emotional support and information to reduce unfounded fears.

Nursing Diagnosis: Knowledge Deficit R/T cause of jaundice.

Planning: Expected Outcomes. The client will acknowledge the cause of jaundice, as evidenced by the client's statements and ability to redefine illness.

Implementation. Clients often wonder why they are jaundiced, how long the condition will last, and how to cope with the problem. The nurse should take the time to explain the condition in a manner appropriate to the client's knowledge base and desire to learn about the illness.

Jaundice usually begins to disappear within 4 to 6 weeks. The return of normal stool and urine colors is an indication of resolution.

Evaluation

The nurse must evaluate client outcomes on the basis of the established plan of care. If these goals were not achieved, the plan and interventions must be revised to meet the client's needs.

Hepatitis

Simply stated, hepatitis is inflammation of the liver. This inflammation may be caused by a virus, bacteria, or toxic substance. Jaundice usually develops, and the liver is tender. Other systemic manifestations depend on the causative agent and the degree of organ disruption.

There are several different types of hepatitis. These include viral, toxic, chronic, and alcoholic hepatitis.

VIRAL HEPATITIS

There are five major types of identified viral hepatitis: hepatitis A, hepatitis B, hepatitis C, delta hepatitis, and hepatitis E. Although the symptoms are similar, each of these conditions is caused by a different virus and differs in incubation, period, mode of transmission, and severity (Table 37–2).

Previously, when a client had a viral hepatitis that was unidentified, the condition was termed non-A, non-B hepatitis. Now that hepatitis C has been identified, all unidentified strains of hepatitis are referred to as non-A, non-B, non-C hepatitis.

Two other types of viral hepatitis have been identified: delta hepatitis and hepatitis E.

Etiology

Agents that may cause viral hepatitis include hepatitis A virus (HAV), hepatitis B virus (HBV), Epstein-Barr virus (infectious mononucleosis virus), cytomegalovirus, rubella virus, herpes simplex virus, varicella virus, retrovirus, yellow fever virus, coxsackievirus, adenovirus, and Marburg virus.

Hepatitis A. Hepatitis A, also known as short incubation hepatitis, infectious hepatitis, and MS_1 hepatitis, is caused by a ribonucleic acid (RNA) virus of the enterovirus family.

Causes of epidemics include infected water, milk, and food, especially raw shellfish from contaminated waters. In the general population, those younger than 15 years are at the most risk.

Hepatitis B. The major sources of this infection are carriers and clients with the acute process. Contact with the serum of an infected client is the major mode of transmission. The virus also may be transmitted by other body fluids, such as saliva and semen. Hepatitis B virus can survive on environmental surfaces for at least a week.

Hepatitis C. Hepatitis C is transmitted parenterally through the blood, by personal contact, and possibly by the fecal-oral route. In contrast to hepatitis A, but similar to hepatitis B, hepatitis C may be spread by carriers.

Delta Hepatitis. Delta hepatitis is transmitted only through blood contact, so it is seen most commonly in clients exposed to blood and blood products, such as hemophiliac individuals and intravenous drug users.

Hepatitis E. Hepatitis E is transmitted by the fecal-oral route, contaminated water, and poor sanitation. It is seen in Asia, Africa, and Mexico but is not common in the United States.

TABLE 37–2 Comparison of Four Types of Viral Hepatitis

FACTOR	HEPATITIS A	HEPATITIS B	HEPATITIS C	DELTA HEPATITIS
Incidence	Endemic in areas of poor sanitation Common in fall and early winter	Worldwide, especially in intravenous drug users and clients and others exposed to blood and blood products Occurs all year	Post-transfusion Those working around blood and blood products Occurs all year	Found in conjunction with hepatitis B (must have HBV to be infected with HDV)
Incubation period	15–45 days	28–180 days	7–8 weeks	Same as hepatitis B
Risk factors	Close personal contact Handling feces-contaminated wastes	Health-care workers in contact with blood and blood products Hemodialysis and post-transfusion clients Homosexually active males and intravenous drug users	Same as for hepatitis B	Same as hepatitis B
Mode of transmission	Infected feces, fecal-oral route May be airborne if copious secretions Shellfish from contaminated water Also parenteral	Parenteral Sexual contact Fecal-oral route	Contact with blood and body fluids	Coinfects with hepatitis B, close personal contact
Severity	Usually not fatal	More serious; may be fatal	Not known	Increased mortality with hepatitis B
Diagnostic tests	IgM positive in acute infection IgG positive after infection	HB_sAg, HB_cAg, and HB_eAg positive	Anti HCV	Anti-HDV IgM (current infection) Anti-HDV IgG (postinfection)
Vaccine	Vaccine under development	Hepatitis B vaccine	None	Same as for hepatitis B

HB_cAg, hepatitis B core antigen; HB_eAg, hepatitis B e antigen; HB_sAg, hepatitis B surface antigen; HBV, hepatitis B virus; HCV, hepatitis C virus; HDV, delta hepatitis virus; IgG, immunoglobulin G; IgM, immunoglobulin M.

Risk Factors

Hepatitis A. Hepatitis A spreads from person to person by close contact or by the handling of feces-contaminated articles. Because the infected client's feces contain the virus before the onset of manifestations, the remaining household members are at risk.

People who work with animals imported from areas where hepatitis A is endemic are at increased risk, as are individuals who eat raw or steamed shellfish.

This problem also may spread in an institution such as a day-care center, prison, or facility for developmentally disabled people.

Hepatitis B. Health-care workers are at high risk for hepatitis B because of their close contact with the blood of carriers. Clients who have multiple blood transfusions or dialysis are also vulnerable to this infection. Other high-risk populations are homosexually active males, morticians, persons who undergo tattooing, parenteral drug abusers, and sexual partners of infected heterosexual persons.

Hepatitis C. Because hepatitis C is also parenterally transmitted, the risk factors are similar to those for hepatitis B.

Delta Hepatitis. The risk factors for delta hepatitis are the same as for hepatitis B.

Hepatitis E. The risk factors for hepatitis E are similar to those associated with hepatitis A.

To a great extent, viral hepatitis can be prevented by proper controls within the home, community, and health-care facility setting.

PREVENTION

Health education is the greatest weapon in the prevention of all types of viral hepatitis.

Hepatitis A

Personal Hygiene. Because transmission of hepatitis A and possibly C is by the fecal-oral route, good personal hygiene is important. Food handlers must wash their hands thoroughly. In some facilities, the disease is present because residents are unable to care for themselves properly. Care providers must supervise handwashing by ambulatory residents. Personnel in day-care centers need to wash their hands carefully after changing diapers.

Water Supply. Treatment of municipal water supplies prevents transmission of HAV. Private water supplies can be sources of contamination and need to be under government or some other type of control. Shellfish that come from polluted waters can be a major source of hepatitis A.

Restaurants. Local health authorities need to monitor eating establishments via serologic screening of food handlers for hepatitis A, which reduces its transmission. Because the disease can be transmitted via food, a client with active hepatitis A should not work in food services.

Animal Care. Isolating newly imported animals for a 2-month period reduces the incidence of hepatitis A among people who handle them. If isolation is impossible, these individuals need to wear protective clothing and use good hand-washing technique.

Passive Immunization. Physicians may prescribe standard immunoglobulin. Immune globulin is helpful prophylaxis both before and after exposure. Immune globulin (gamma globulin, Gammar) is administered intramuscularly after exposure but not after the development of clinical symptoms. Clients who live in or visit areas of high risk for hepatitis A can be protected for about 2 months by immune serum. The earlier in the incubation period that the prophylactic immune serum is given, the greater the protection. Adverse effects of intramuscular injection include pain, tenderness, and at times hematoma formation.

Hepatitis B

Control of Blood, Blood Products, and Skin-Piercing Instruments. Hepatitis B is transmitted by the serum of the infected client; thus, blood, blood products, and instruments that pierce the skin and contact the vascular system are all potential sources of contamination. Some donor-related precautions that decrease the incidence of hepatitis B are screening of donors' blood for HBV surface antigen (HB_sAg), use of volunteer rather than paid donors, registration of carriers, and sharing of accurate records among institutions. It is possible to reduce the transfusion recipient's exposure to hepatitis B by using blood products only when necessary, using only the necessary amount of blood or blood products, cross-checking laboratory data to reduce errors of reported results, and encouraging clients who are having elective surgery to donate their own blood (autologous transfusions).

Many health-care facilities use disposable equipment, especially needles and syringes, to reduce hepatitis transmission. Nondisposable equipment must be sterilized to prevent virus transmission.

Personal Hygiene. Good personal hygiene by clients with hepatitis B or hepatitis B carriers also reduces transmission. Such clients should not share razors, toothbrushes, washcloths, cigarettes, or other personal items with others.

Passive Immunization. Standard immune globulin may contain antibodies against hepatitis B. However, another preparation called specific hepatitis B immune globulin contains much higher levels of antibody. The preparation is usually given in three doses. The second and third doses are given 1 month and 6 months after the initial dose. Physicians may prescribe hepatitis B immune globulin or standard immune globulin for post-exposure prophylaxis when there has been percutaneous exposure to blood that contains HB_sAg.

Active Immunization. Hepatitis B vaccine may provide active immunization before exposure to HBV. The injection is best given into the deltoid muscle. Authorities recommend this killed virus vaccine for persons in the high-risk categories for hepatitis B. It may be used in conjunction with specific hepatitis B immune globulin after documented exposure to hepatitis B.

Hepatitis C. Transmission of hepatitis C is similar to that of hepatitis B. Therefore, many of the same measures are probably useful in its prevention. Physicians sometimes prescribe standard immune globulin

TABLE 37–3 Immunizations for Hepatitis A, B, C, E and Delta Hepatitis

IMMUNIZATION TYPE	HEPATITIS TYPE				
	A	B	C	DELTA	E
Active	Vaccine under development	Hepatitis B vaccine (killed virus) Before exposure	No vaccine	No vaccine	No vaccine
Passive	Standard immunogobulin Before and after exposure	Specific hepatitis B immunoglobulin (preferred) Standard immunoglobulin After exposure	Standard immunoglobulin (of questionable value) After exposure	Standard immunoglobulin (of questionable value) After exposure	Not available in United States

for postexposure passive immunization to hepatitis C. However, this intervention has not yet been well documented and needs further research. As with hepatitis A, there is no vaccine for active immunization against hepatitis C.

Delta Hepatitis. Because delta hepatitis must coexist with hepatitis B, the hepatitis B vaccine can help prevent delta hepatitis also. The precautions that help prevent hepatitis B also are useful in preventing delta hepatitis.

Table 37–3 summarizes the immunizations for hepatitis A, hepatitis B, hepatitis C, delta hepatitis, and hepatitis E.

Pathophysiology

The physical manifestations of viral hepatitis reflect liver cell damage. Hepatocytes are damaged by the body's immune response to the virus, which alters cellular function. The degree of functional impairment depends on the amount of hepatocellular damage. Vascular and ductule tissues undergo inflammatory changes. The hepatocytes generally heal in 3 to 4 months.

HEPATITIS A

Antibodies to hepatitis A are of two types. The immunoglobulin M antibody develops soon after infection and remains in the body for 6 to 8 weeks; it is, therefore, an indicator of current infection. The immunoglobulin G antibody against hepatitis A develops several weeks after infection and persists for years, providing immunity against the disease; it is, therefore, an indicator of past infection.

Clients who are otherwise healthy usually recover from hepatitis A without major sequelae. Although hepatitis A has a low mortality rate, fulminant hepatitis A may result. The fulminant form resembles acute liver failure. It causes severe illness and even death. It should be noted that there is no active immunization for HAV infection.

HEPATITIS B

The hepatitis B virus is a deoxyribonucleic acid (DNA) virus that has an inner core and a surface envelope. The body forms antibodies to HBV core antigen (HB_cAg) and HB_sAg. The presence of HB_sAg in the blood denotes a previous or resolving infection with hepatitis B; a continuing chronic infection; or immunization with immunoglobulin or hepatitis B vaccine.

Acute HBV infection may result in death in severe cases. Up to 10 per cent of persons affected become chronic carriers and may be at risk for cirrhosis, liver cancer, and death. Anyone with hepatitis B is at risk for delta hepatitis.

HEPATITIS C

Little specific information is available about hepatitis C. Neither a specific antigen nor antibody has been found.

DELTA HEPATITIS

The delta hepatitis virus is a defective RNA virus, requiring the helper function of hepatitis B virus. An antigen, HD Ag, and an antibody, anti-HD, have been identified.

HEPATITIS E

Hepatitis E has an incubation period of 15 to 64 days (average, 26–42 days in different epidemics). It may be similar to hepatitis A in infectiousness. Serologic tests are currently under development. Full recovery is likely with no chronic carrier state.

Typically, clients with viral hepatitis completely recover from the illness in 3 to 16 weeks. Mortality from hepatitis A is low, except for the fulminant form. Clients with hepatitis B tend to develop more complications. One in 10 clients acquires chronic active hepatitis as a result of hepatitis B, often leading to destruction of the liver. Cirrhosis may follow a severe case of hepatitis B or chronic active hepatitis. Primary hepatocellular carcinoma is a potential complication of chronic hepatitis.

Clinical Manifestations

Clients with viral hepatitis all experience liver inflammation and other sequelae that are similar. Hepatitis B and delta hepatitis are usually the most severe, although they may be asymptomatic in some clients. The onset of manifestations varies according to the incubation period and the degree of infectivity.

Symptoms of viral hepatitis are systemic and vary from client to client. Symptoms might include jaundice, lethargy, irritability, myalgia, arthralgia, anorexia, nausea, vomiting, abdominal pain, diarrhea or constipation, fever, and other flulike symptoms (see Clinical Manifestations: Hepatitis). Pruritus (itching) is typically mild and transient and may be more intense at its onset and termination. Jaundice is first seen on the hard palate and then in the sclerae of the eyes and mucous membranes. Anicteric (without jaundice) hepatitis may or may not precede jaundice. Children with hepatitis are usually anicteric. Adults often note the appearance of darker urine and clay-colored stools a few days before clinical jaundice develops. The other symptoms often abate when jaundice appears, but they also may worsen.

If irritability and drowsiness become severe, the nurse assesses for the possibility of hepatic encephalopathy. Deterioration of handwriting is an early sign of hepatic encephalopathy; thus, clients should be asked to write their name each shift, and their writing should be observed closely for changes. Asterixis, an abnormal muscle tremor sometimes called liver flap, may accompany encephalopathy. This sign is easily elicited by applying a blood pressure cuff and noting whether the flapping is present when the cuff is released. Mild depression is not uncommon, owing to the nature of the illness (weakness, jaundice, itching, and nausea), its length and cost, confinement, and forgetfulness and the inability to concentrate on completion of activities of daily living (ADLs).

Anemia may occur because of the decreased lifespan of erythrocytes. Erythrocyte destruction results from liver enzyme alterations. A transient hyperglycemia sometimes develops, and a client with diabetes may need to increase insulin dosage at this time. The liver is larger than normal with hepatitis and tender on palpation. Some people experience spider angiomata, palmar erythema, and gynecomastia, which disappear during the recovery period. A small percentage (5–15 per cent) of clients experience splenomegaly or enlargement of the posterior cervical lymph nodes. Occasionally, hepatitis B is accompanied by arthralgias, rash, vasculitis, or glomerulonephritis.

Other clients may manifest fulminant viral hepatitis. This life-threatening form resembles acute liver failure with manifestations of encephalopathy (increased excitability, insomnia, somnolence, and impaired mentation). The liver rapidly decreases in size. Other problems include gastrointestinal bleeding, disseminated intravascular coagulation, fever with leukocytosis and neutrophilia, hepatorenal problems of oliguria and azotemia, edema and ascites, hypotension, respiratory failure, hypoglycemia, bacterial infection of the respiratory or urinary tract, and thrombocytopenia and coagulopathy. The prognosis is poor, and death may occur before jaundice appears. A liver transplant may be performed to save the client's life.

CLINICAL MANIFESTATIONS

Hepatitis

Assessment Data	Pathophysiologic Bases
Jaundice, clay-colored stools (no pigment); ↑ serum bilirubin; darkened urine (bilirubin and urobilin)	Impaired excretion of conjugated bilirubin Urobilin in blood excreted through kidneys instead of bowel
Pruritus	Bile salt accumulation in skin
Abdominal pain in right upper quadrant	Stretching of Glisson's capsule (surrounding liver) as a result of inflammation
Fever	Release of pyrogens in inflammatory process
Fatigue and weakness	Reduced energy metabolism by liver
Anorexia, nausea, vomiting	Changes in stomach or bowel
Bleeding tendencies	Reduced prothrombin synthesis by injured hepatic cells Reduced fat-soluble vitamin K absorption as a result of reduced bile in intestine
Anemia	Decreased red cell life caused by liver enzyme alterations, hemorrhage

DIAGNOSTIC ASSESSMENT

The serologic markers of viral hepatitis are presented in Table 37–4. Presence of HB_sAg in the blood usually indicates that the individual is infectious. HB_sAg is sometimes called the Australian antigen. Another antigen, hepatitis B e antigen, is often associated with the progression from acute hepatitis to chronic hepatitis and indicates a highly infectious state.

The serum aminotransferases first elevate and then begin to fall as the bilirubin starts to increase. Levels that rise, peak, drop, and then rise again indicate severe liver damage and a poor prognosis. Jaundice occurs as bilirubin rises above 2.5 mg/100 mL. Bilirubin that rises above 20 mg/100 mL and remains elevated for a long period may indicate severe liver necrosis, which has a poor prognosis. Mild prolongation of the prothrombin time sometimes occurs. The gamma globulin fraction and alkaline phosphatase elevate in some clients. If hepatitis B is responsible, detection of HB_sAg is possible even before the level of aspartate aminotransferase (formerly serum glutamic-oxaloacetic transaminase) rises.

TABLE 37–4 Laboratory Tests for Viral Hepatitis

HEPATITIS TYPE	LABORATORY TEST
A	Anti-HAV IgM (indicates current infection) Anti-HAV IgG (indicates past, resolved infection)
B	HB_sAg (indicates current or chronic infection) HB_eAg (a marker for increased infectivity) Anti-HB_c (a marker for infection at some time) Anti-HB_e (a marker for decreased infectivity) Anti-HB_s (a marker for immunity and the antibody produced in response to the HBV vaccine)
C	Anti-HCV (a marker for infection with HCV virus)
D	Anti-HDV IgM (indicates current infection) Anti-HDV IgG (indicates past infection)
E	Serologic tests are currently under development

Note: All tests are done on blood serum.
Anti-, antibody; HAV, hepatitis A virus; HB_c, hepatitis B core; HB_e, hepatitis B e; HBeAg, hepatitis B e antigen; HB_s, hepatitis B surface; HB_sAg, hepatitis B surface antigen; HCV, hepatitis C virus; HDV, delta hepatitis virus; IgG, immunoglobulin G; IgM, immunoglobulin M.

Medical Management

Five important interventions for clients with viral hepatitis are:

- Rest
- Proper diet
- Emotional support
- Relief of pruritus
- Correction of knowledge deficits regarding the disease

PHARMACOLOGIC MANAGEMENT

If given early, standard immune globulin (proteins capable of acting as antibodies and formerly termed immune serum globulin) can prevent hepatitis A or decrease the severity of symptoms. The HAV does not remain in the blood long; therefore, there is no healthy carrier state for hepatitis A, as there is for hepatitis B.

Few medications are available for treating viral hepatitis. Antibiotics are not prescribed. Immunoglobulin, although not used to treat viral hepatitis, does provide prophylactic assistance for family members. High-titer immune globulin (hepatitis B immune globulin) can also be given to reduce the risk of HBV infection.

CRITICAL TO REMEMBER

Antiemetics decrease nausea and vomiting; phenothiazines should not be used because they are biotransformed in the liver and, therefore, potentially toxic.

The corticosteroids are not necessary in uncomplicated cases of acute viral hepatitis, and authorities question their use in several cases.

Estrogens can raise serum bilirubin levels. Therefore, clinicians need to evaluate the use of oral contraceptives during acute viral hepatitis.

The administration of cholestyramine or ursodiol can relieve the pruritus associated with severe cholestatic liver disease. These medications act by bonding bile salts in the intestine.

All in all, clinicians administer very few medications to clients with hepatitis. Medications such as chlorpromazine, aspirin, acetaminophen, and a variety of sedatives are given as infrequently as possible because they all have the potential to damage an already damaged liver.

DIETARY MANAGEMENT

A diet high in carbohydrates and calories with moderate amounts of fat and protein is recommended. Meals should be given in small portions and given four to six times daily. The client's food preferences should be accommodated.

Nursing Management

Assessment

The nurse always begins by questioning the client about possible exposure to risk factors to assess the type of hepatitis present. The presence of common symptoms, especially jaundice, is assessed, as are signs of progression of the disease, such as hepatic encephalopathy (see section on hepatic encephalopathy). Liver function studies are monitored to assess the progression of the disease.

Nursing Diagnosis, Planning, and Implementation

Nursing Diagnosis: Activity Intolerance R/T extreme fatigue.

Planning: Expected Outcomes. The client will maintain adequate rest to conserve energy, as evidenced by compliance with activity restrictions and a gradual increase in activity to preillness level.

Implementation. Fatigue associated with hepatitis may interfere with ADLs. Most clients experience the greatest fatigue during the anicteric phase and begin to feel stronger during the icteric phase. Fatigue may persist, however, even after the jaundice clears. During the period of severe fatigue, the client should be advised to rest in bed. Most clients who feel capable of being up and around can do so without any harm, if they rest after meals and do not engage in any activity to the point of being overly tired. Because prolonged bed rest itself can lead to weakness, a reasonable activity level is more conducive to recovery than enforced bed rest.

ADLs such as bathroom privileges, personal hygiene, and feeding should be encouraged unless they cause excessive fatigue. The client should be advised to plan rest periods while jaundiced, especially after meals. Clients who engage in excessive activity too early in the recovery phase sometimes experience a relapse, possibly leading to liver failure.

Nursing Diagnosis: Physical Mobility, Impaired R/T prolonged bed rest.

Planning: Expected Outcomes. The client will regain mobility without complications, as evidenced by increasing mobility and the absence of complications.

Implementation. In very severe cases of hepatitis, the client may need to remain in bed for a prolonged period. In this case, the nurse needs to intervene to prevent the complications of prolonged immobility (e.g., pressure sores, contractures, anorexia, and depression). For detailed information on preventing problems due to immobility, see Chapter 44.

Nursing Diagnosis: Nutrition, Altered: Less Than Body Requirements R/T anorexia, nausea, bile stasis, and altered absorption and metabolism.

Planning: Expected Outcomes. The client will maintain an intake of the required calories to maintain weight, as evidenced by no weight loss and possible weight gain.

Implementation. To help the client meet the nutritional requirements associated with hepatitis, the nurse should

- Provide a nutritious breakfast. Anorexia usually worsens during the day, so breakfast may be the best-tolerated meal.
- Encourage the client to avoid heavy, greasy food, which can induce nausea.
- Devise a dietary plan for a diet high in protein (75–100 g) and carbohydrates (300–400 g) and moderate in fat (60–100 g). This diet is optimal to allow recovery of injured liver cells. The amounts of protein and fat are decreased only if there is a problem with their digestion and metabolism. If the client has no problem with protein metabolism, a normal intake is helpful for tissue repair. However, clients with very severe hepatitis who are in danger of experiencing hepatic encephalopathy require a diet low in protein (because of the buildup of ammonia in the blood). Alterations in fat metabolism differ according to the degree of interruption in bile production and excretion.
- Suggest multiple small meals. This allows the client with anorexia to ingest a diet of 2500 to 3000 calories more comfortably. Also, candy, juice, sweetened tea, and carbonated drinks can supply calories when nausea is a problem.
- Remind the client to avoid alcohol because it is an extremely hepatotoxic agent.
- Tell the client that vitamin supplements are not generally necessary in uncomplicated hepatitis, provided the diet is adequate in nutrition. Vitamin K supplements as ordered may be administered if the prothrombin time is longer than normal.

Clients who experience severe nausea and vomiting may obtain relief from antiemetics. However, before these medications are administered, their effect on liver functions should be reviewed. Phenothiazines such as chlorpromazine (Compazine) are usually contraindicated. Clients who are unable to tolerate any oral intake may require intravenous nutrition.

Nursing Diagnosis: Tissue Integrity, Impaired R/T pruritus.

Planning: Expected Outcomes. The client will maintain skin integrity, as evidenced by the client's statements of comfort and the absence of scratching.

Implementation. Clients with severe jaundice may suffer pruritus. See section on jaundice for a discussion of nursing interventions for itching.

Nursing Diagnosis: Knowledge Deficit R/T the disease and its course.

Planning: Expected Outcomes. The client will understand the disease and its treatment, as evidenced by the client's ability to state the causes of the disease and rationales for treatment.

Implementation. Teaching for the client with hepatitis varies with the causative agent. In addition to teaching how to prevent recurrence and spread, the nurse instructs the client to return to former activity levels slowly to avoid a relapse. Instructions concerning the diet need to be clear.

Evaluation

The nurse must evaluate client outcomes on the basis of the established plan of care. If these goals were not achieved, the plan and interventions must be revised to meet the client's needs.

Modification of Plan of Care for the Elderly

Older clients are at higher risk for liver damage because they are more likely to have already had some changes in the liver. They are at greater risk for experiencing complications.

Client Teaching

HEALTH PROMOTION AND ILLNESS PREVENTION

Clients who are at risk because of compromised health status, age, or environmental and occupational exposure should be provided with current, relevant facts on viral hepatitis. Education should include preventive measures and risk factors.

All health assessments should include questions about health practices, living conditions and travel inside and outside the person's native country.

DISCHARGE AND HOME HEALTH TEACHING

Complications from hepatitis, although rare with HAV infection, can occur. The HBV, hepatitis C virus, and delta hepatitis virus forms all can lead to complications and death. Nurses must be able to provide information on life-style changes, medications, and treatments that fit each client. Family members or significant others should be included in the teaching sessions.

Discharge teaching in the hospital or clinic is not sufficient. Provisions should be made for follow-up contact with the health department, home health agency, or other outreach health-care professionals.

TOXIC HEPATITIS

Toxic hepatitis occurs after exposure to hepatotoxins. These substances cause liver alterations by initiating either drug-induced hepatitis or drug-induced cholestasis. Either of these responses may be dose related and predictable or idiosyncratic and unpredictable, depending on the chemical nature of the hepatotoxin or the genetic make-up of the individual. Idiosyncratic hepatotoxicity is often due to hypersensitivity (immune response). Some substances cause liver damage because they are converted to toxic metabolites. Table 37–5 lists some hepatotoxic agents. Liver necrosis occurs within 2 or 3 days after acute exposure to a hepatotoxin with dose-related toxicity. However, several weeks may pass before manifestations of idiosyncratic reactions appear. Clients with either process experience abnormal reactions to liver function tests.

Clients who are repeatedly exposed to some hepatotoxins in minimal amounts but over long periods of time may acquire cirrhosis. Individuals experiencing a hypersensitivity reaction may demonstrate eosinophilia, fever, arthralgia, and sometimes xanthomatosis (an excessive accumulation of lipids brought about by faulty lipid metabolism).

Nursing intervention consists of removal of the causative agent, rest, alleviation of side effects (e.g., cholestyramine for pruritus), high-calorie diet with fats if tolerated, high-protein diet if there is no evidence of impending hepatic encephalopathy, and steroids for hypersensitivity reactions.

Renal failure sometimes appears as a complication of toxic hepatitis. Assessment and interventions for renal failure are discussed in Chapter 31.

CRITICAL TO REMEMBER

Nurses should be careful to review laboratory protocols for drug therapy, especially in elderly clients. Although toxic hepatitis may not be totally preventable, the incidence can be decreased.

TABLE 37–5 Substances Known to Be Hepatotoxic

	TYPE OF LIVER ALTERATION	
VARIABLE	HEPATITIS	CHOLESTASIS
Dose related	Acetaminophen *Amanita phalloides* (mushroom) Aspirin Benzene Carbon tetrachloride Chloroform Methotrexate Tetracyclines	Oxymetholone
Idiosyncratic	Alpha-methyldopa Sulfasalazine Halothane Isoniazid Nitrofurantoin Phenytoin Quinidine	Allopurinol Anabolic steroids Carbamazepine Chlordiazepoxide Chlorpromazine Chlorpropamide Diazepam Erythromycin estolate Flurazepam Oral contraceptives

CHRONIC HEPATITIS

Chronic hepatitis exists when liver inflammation continues beyond a period of 3 to 6 months. This disease process may manifest as chronic persistent hepatitis (CPH) or chronic active hepatitis (CAH). CPH is usually benign and seldom progressive. CAH is more serious and differential diagnosis is of utmost importance. (see Clinical Manifestations: Chronic Active Hepatitis [Idiopathic]). Definitive diagnosis and decisions regarding appropriate intervention depend on liver biopsy findings.

Nursing intervention involves assessing the client's reactions to medications as well as supportive management. It is important to discontinue medications that may be causing inflammatory changes. The physician may prescribe steroids for a period of 3 to 5 years. Clients who cannot tolerate large doses of steroids may benefit from azathioprine and smaller steroid doses. Clinicians generally do not recommend steroid therapy for asymptomatic CAH, especially in elderly clients. In addition to pharmacologic intervention, bedrest is encouraged during the active phase of the disease. The client usually remains at home to convalesce. There may be periods of remission, but liver necrosis continues.

With steroid therapy, fatigue and anorexia resolve in a few days or weeks. Laboratory values return to normal within weeks or months. The physician reduces the dose of steroids in small increments to prevent a relapse and allow the adrenal glands time to resume normal secretion.

Untreated CAH has a high mortality rate. Death results from hepatic failure, bleeding varices, hepatic encephalopathy, or primary hepatocellular carcinoma.

Liver transplantation is a consideration for those individuals with end-stage liver disease that can no longer be medically managed.

ALCOHOLIC HEPATITIS

Alcoholic hepatitis is either an acute or a chronic inflammation of the liver. It is caused by parenchymal

CLINICAL MANIFESTATIONS

Chronic Active Hepatitis (Idiopathic)

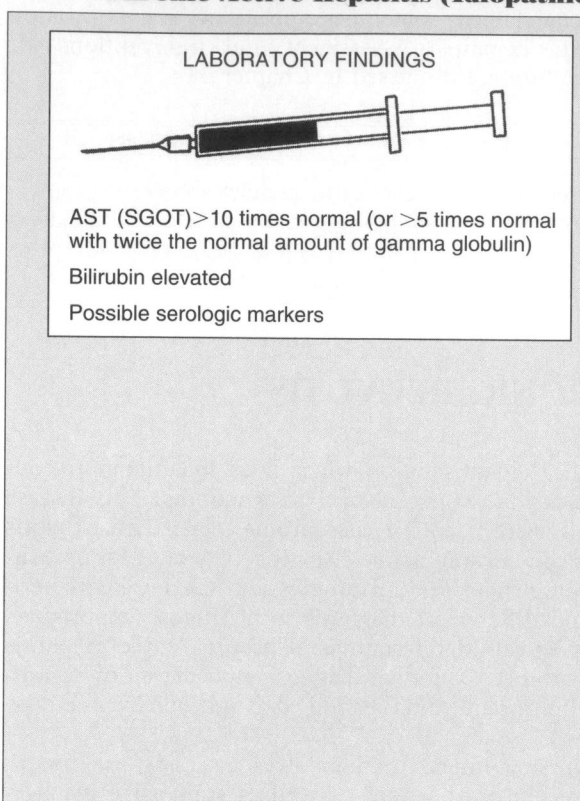

LABORATORY FINDINGS

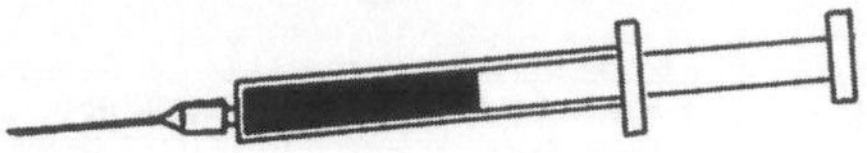

AST (SGOT)>10 times normal (or >5 times normal with twice the normal amount of gamma globulin)

Bilirubin elevated

Possible serologic markers

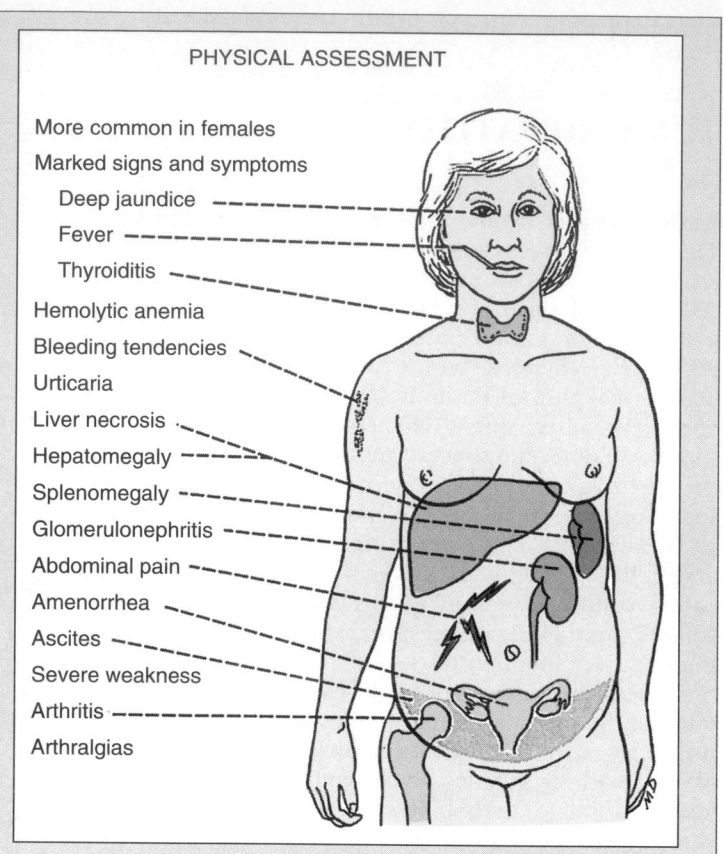

PHYSICAL ASSESSMENT

More common in females

Marked signs and symptoms

- Deep jaundice
- Fever
- Thyroiditis

Hemolytic anemia

Bleeding tendencies

Urticaria

Liver necrosis

Hepatomegaly

Splenomegaly

Glomerulonephritis

Abdominal pain

Amenorrhea

Ascites

Severe weakness

Arthritis

Arthralgias

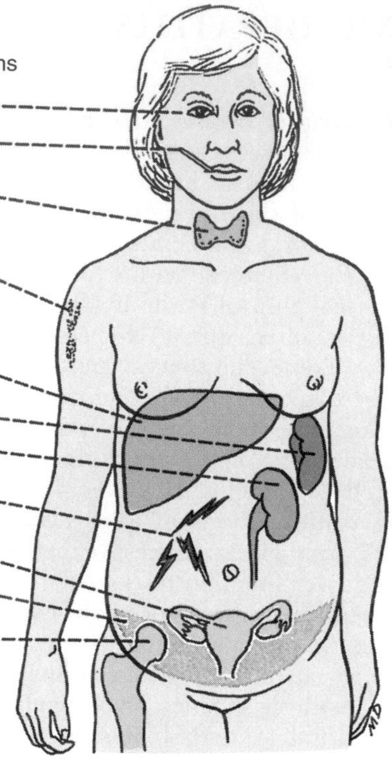

AST, aspartate aminotransferase.

necrosis resulting from heavy alcohol ingestion. Although sometimes reversible, this condition is the most frequent cause of cirrhosis. This fact is important because cirrhosis of the liver is a common cause of death among adults in the United States.

Clinical manifestations of alcoholic hepatitis usually develop after a bout of heavy drinking. Assessment reveals anorexia, nausea, abdominal pain, splenomegaly, hepatomegaly, jaundice, ascites, fever, and encephalopathy. Laboratory studies typically show anemia, leukocytosis, and an elevated serum bilirubin.

Nursing intervention includes monitoring and teaching the client about a high-vitamin, high-carbohydrate diet; folic acid supplements; and parenteral fluids. Steroids sometimes have a beneficial effect, although their use remains controversial.

Hepatitis resulting from excessive alcohol intake has a poor prognosis, particularly if the client continues to use alcohol.

Cirrhosis

Cirrhosis occurs when the normal flow of blood, bile, and hepatic metabolites is altered by fibrosis and changes in the hepatocytes, bile ductules, vascular channels, and reticular cells.

There are four major types of cirrhosis: Laënnec's (micronodular), postnecrotic (macronodular or toxin induced), biliary, and cardiac (Table 37–6). The two major clinical problems in cirrhosis are decreased liver function and portal hypertension. The latter develops in severe cirrhosis.

Incidence

Only 10 to 15 per cent of clients with chronic alcoholism acquire cirrhosis; however, more than 65 per cent of all cases of cirrhosis are related to alcohol ingestion. Laënnec's cirrhosis is, therefore, the most common type. Men are more likely than women to develop Laënnec's cirrhosis. Cirrhosis is the fourth leading cause of death in clients between 35 and 54 years of age. It is the ninth leading cause of death overall in the United States and may occur at any age.

Worldwide, postnecrotic cirrhosis is the most common type of cirrhosis. It is also more common in women. Mortality is higher from all types of cirrhosis in men and nonwhites.

Etiology

The exact causes of cirrhosis have not been clearly identified. Genetic predisposition with a familial tend-

TABLE 37–6 Comparison of Macronodular, Biliary, and Cardiac Cirrhosis

DEFINITION	ETIOLOGY	PATHOLOGY	ASSESSMENT DATA	DIAGNOSIS AND PROGNOSIS	INTERVENTION
Macronodular Cirrhosis (Postnecrotic)					
Most common worldwide form Massive loss of liver cells, with irregular patterns of regenerating cells	Postacute viral (types B and C) hepatitis Postintoxication with industrial chemicals Some infections and metabolic disorders	Liver small and nodular	Similar to Laënnec's except less muscle wasting and more jaundice	Needle biopsy of liver establishes pathologic process Within 5 years 75% die of complications ↑ Serum aminotransferases ↑ Gamma globulins	Treat complications as needed
Biliary Cirrhosis					
Bile flow is decreased with concurrent cell damage to hepatocytes around bile ductules	*Primary:* chronic stasis of bile in intrahepatic ducts; cause unknown; autoimmune process implicated *Secondary:* obstruction of bile ducts outside of liver	Early-stage biopsy reveals inflammatory process with necrosis of cells and ducts Hepatocytes are lost and scar tissue remains End stage similar to postnecrotic	Generalized pruritus Dark urine Pale stools Jaundice Impaired bile flow Steatorrhea ↓ Absorption of fat-soluble vitamins ↑ Serum lipids ↑ Cholesterol deposits in subcutaneous tissues Signs of portal hypertension	↑ Serum bilirubin levels Early: 3–10 mg/100 mL Late: >50 mg/100 mL High elevations of alkaline phosphatase ↑ Gamma globulins ↑ Blood lipids Presence of lipoprotein X ↑ Serum bile salts Hypoprothrombinemia ↑ Antimitochondrial antibody in primary cases ↑ Serum copper in primary cases	*Primary:* treatment is symptomatic (e.g., high-calorie diet; lower intake of fats by 30–40 g/day if problems develop); cholestyramine for pruritus; supplement of fat-soluble vitamins *Secondary:* treatment to relieve mechanical obstruction
Cardiac Cirrhosis					
Chronic liver disease associated with severe right-sided long-term congestive heart failure (fairly rare)	Atrioventricular valve disease Prolonged constrictive pericarditis Decompensated cor pulmonale	*Early:* dark colored liver enlarged by blood and edema fluid *Late:* liver capsule thickens and nodular scarring occurs	Slight jaundice, enlarged liver, and ascites in person with severe cardiac impairment over 10-year span RUQ pain during acute congestion Cachexia Fluid retention Circulatory problems	↑ Conjugated bilirubin in serum ↑ Bromsulphalein ↓ Albumin in serum ↑ Serum aminotransferases ↑ Alkaline phosphatase Liver biopsy	Cause of chronic congestive failure is treated if possible

RUQ, right upper quadrant.

ency as well as a hypersensitivity to alcohol is seen in alcoholic cirrhosis.

Laënnec's or micronodular cirrhosis is most commonly found in clients who chronically abuse alcohol. However, it is also found in nondrinkers.

Any chemical or organism that causes liver destruction predisposes a client to cirrhosis. In Laënnec's cirrhosis, it is the hepatotoxic nature of alcohol that causes the damage. If the client is in a poor nutritional state, the damage is more likely and more severe.

Risk Factors

The primary risk factor for cirrhosis is alcohol ingestion, especially in the absence of proper nutrition. Any client with a family history of alcoholism should avoid alcohol because of the increased risk.

Viral hepatitis is the primary risk factor for postnecrotic cirrhosis, and thus it is very important for the client with hepatitis to avoid any other stressors and allow the liver to heal completely without further insult. Clients with hepatitis must avoid any exposure to other hepatotoxins.

Avoidance of industrial or chemical compounds by working in well-ventilated areas and taking other safety measures decreases the risk from these toxins. Prompt treatment of biliary disorders helps decrease the risk of biliary cirrhosis. Adequate treatment of congestive heart failure can help prevent cardiac cirrhosis.

Pathophysiology

Cirrhosis is the final stage in many types of liver insults.

Portal hypertension develops in severe cirrhosis. Recall that the portal vein receives blood from the intestines and spleen. Thus, an increase of pressure in the portal vein causes

- A reverse flow of blood and enlargement of the esophageal, umbilical, and superior rectus veins, which may result in bleeding varices
- Ascites (fluid accumulation in the peritoneum)
- Incomplete clearing of metabolic wastes, leading to hepatic encephalopathy

Continuation of the process from unknown causes or from alcohol abuse usually results in death from hepatic encephalopathy, bacterial infection (gram negative), peritonitis (bacterial), hepatoma (liver tumor), or complications of portal hypertension.

Clinical Manifestations

Cirrhosis initially progresses slowly. Thus, people with cirrhosis often discover they have the condition when they are seeking health care for other problems. In the early stages of cirrhosis, assessment findings include hepatomegaly (enlarged liver), vascular changes, and abnormal laboratory tests. Palpation reveals a firm (scarred), lumpy (nodular), usually enlarged liver (although the liver becomes hard and shrunken in late cirrhosis) (see Clinical Manifestations: Liver Cirrhosis).

In advanced cirrhosis, assessment reveals severe complications such as ascites, gastrointestinal bleeding from varices, or encephalopathy. Splenomegaly (enlarged spleen) indicates severe portal hypertension. Anemia, leukopenia, or thrombocytopenia may result from splenomegaly.

DIAGNOSTIC ASSESSMENT

Laboratory results reveal impaired hepatocellular function: elevated liver serum enzymes, reduced Bromsulphalein dye excretion, hypoalbuminemia, and elevated prothrombin time. Liver biopsy provides a definitive diagnosis and its sequelae.

Medical Management

Three goals guide the medical management of a client with cirrhosis:

- Maximize liver function. This goal is accomplished by minimizing trauma risk and promoting a nutritious diet and adequate rest.
- Prevent infection. This goal is accomplished by adequate rest, diet, and environmental control.
- Control disabling complications. Ascites, bleeding esophageal varices, and hepatic encephalopathy are discussed in depth later in this chapter. They are the most feared complications of cirrhosis. Renal failure (hepatorenal syndrome) and infection also are deadly.

Management of all forms of cirrhosis is essentially the same.

PHARMACOLOGIC MANAGEMENT

Corticosteroids may be used for postnecrotic cirrhosis to reduce manifestations of cirrhosis and improve liver function. The B vitamins and fat-soluble vitamins (vitamins A, D, E, and K) are commonly given to clients with Laënnec's cirrhosis. Other medications may be used to treat the complications, such as diuretics for ascites (discussed later in this chapter).

DIETARY MANAGEMENT

A nutritious diet is recommended for clients with cirrhosis. The diet should be high in protein (as long as the blood ammonia levels are normal) and calories. Fat intake need not be restricted.

Nursing Management

Assessment

Because the symptoms of cirrhosis are sometimes vague and nonspecific, the client may not be aware of the disease's early symptoms. The nurse closely assesses the client for the presence of any of the early symptoms, such as hepatomegaly, and carefully checks the laboratory data for any indication that cirrhosis is present.

As the disease progresses, the nurse should assess for symptoms of complications of cirrhosis, such as ascites, portal hypertension, or hepatic encephalopathy. These are discussed later.

When a client with cirrhosis is hospitalized, the nurse uses laboratory data and the client's physical and psychosocial assessment data to guide care planning.

Nursing Diagnosis, Planning, and Implementation

Nursing Diagnosis: Nutrition, Altered: Less Than Body Requirements R/T anorexia, impaired liver function,

CLINICAL MANIFESTATIONS

Liver Cirrhosis

Assessment Data	Pathophysiologic Bases	Assessment Data	Pathophysiologic Bases
Emaciation, ascites	Malnutrition, portal hypertension, hypoalbuminemia, and hyperaldosteronism	Anemia	Gastrointestinal blood losses; erythrocyte destruction in enlarged spleen; folic acid deficiency resulting from inadequate diet
Splenomegaly	Portal hypertension		
Lower leg edema	Hypoalbuminemia, hyperaldosteronism, and pressure of massive ascites obstructing venous return from legs	Renal failure	Rapidly failing hepatic function; occasionally precipitated by volume depletion; hepatorenal syndrome
Prominent abdominal wall veins (caput medusae)	Collateral vessels bypass scarred liver to carry portal blood to superior vena cava; portal hypertension causes dilation	Infections	Leukopenia caused by enlarged, overactive spleen; bacteria in portal blood bypass liver, so not removed by Kupffer cells
Internal hemorrhoids	Superior rectal veins dilate with pressure of portal hypertension	Encephalopathy	Ammonia, no longer removed by liver, accumulates to levels toxic to brain
Palmar erythema, spider nevi, altered hair distribution; amenorrhea, atrophy of testicles, gynecomastia	Probably decreased hormone metabolism in liver, resulting in manifestations of estrogen excess	Initial or recurrent symptoms of hepatitis (jaundice)	Chronic viral, toxic, or alcoholic hepatitis progressing to cirrhosis may have inflammatory exacerbations
Bleeding tendency, especially gastrointestinal	Hypoprothrombinemia, thrombocytopenia; portal hypertension and esophageal varices; peptic ulcers common in alcoholism	Esophageal varices	Collateral veins in esophagus bypass scarred liver to carry portal blood to superior vena cava; portal hypertension causes dilation

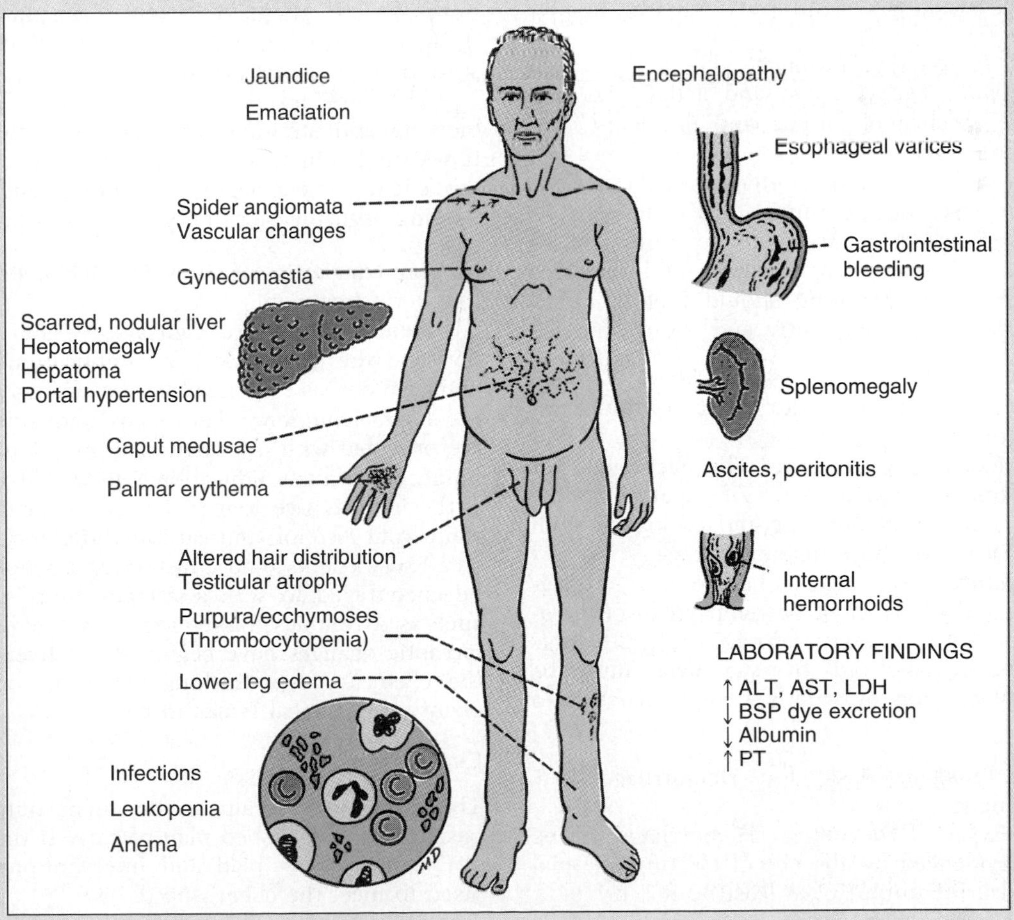

ALT, alanine aminotransferase; AST, aspartate aminotransferase; BSP, Bromsulphalein; PT, prothrombin time.

decreased absorption of fat-soluble vitamins, and diarrhea.

Planning: Expected Outcomes. The client will take in adequate nutrition, as evidenced by no weight loss and no signs of malnutrition.

Implementation. The diet should provide ample protein to rebuild tissue but not enough protein to precipitate hepatic encephalopathy. The diet should supply sufficient carbohydrates to maintain weight and spare protein. Fat restriction is not necessary. Total daily calories should range between 2000 and 3000. The client is placed on daily weight, intake and output, and calorie counts to assess fluid and nutritional balance. The laboratory and nutritional panels are closely monitored for signs of improvement or further deterioration.

If the client has ascites or edema, sodium and possible fluids should be restricted in the diet. Small, frequent meals will make it easier for clients with anorexia to ingest enough food. Adequate rest and a stable environmental temperature should be ensured to allow optimal use of calories.

The physician usually prescribes a maintenance multivitamin preparation and administers therapeutic levels of vitamins in severe malnutrition. Also, vitamins A, D, E, and K are supplied if fat malabsorption is present. The client with severe malabsorption may require intravenous vitamins with calcium gluconate supplementation.

Nursing Diagnosis: Activity Intolerance R/T bedrest, lack of energy, and altered respiratory function (ascites pressing on fluid).

Planning: Expected Outcomes. The client will maintain a balance between rest and activity, as evidenced by the absence of fatigue and problems associated with immobility.

Implementation. Clinicians often prescribe rest for clients with cirrhosis, but how much rest is necessary is debated. During periods of acute malfunction, rest reduces metabolic demands on the liver and increases circulation. Long-term planning should include counseling the client to rest frequently and avoid unnecessary fatigue.

Nursing Diagnosis: Risk for Injury R/T continued intake of hepatotoxins.

Planning: Expected Outcomes. The client will not suffer injury from continued intake of hepatotoxins, as evidenced by cessation of drinking and avoidance of all medications that might cause further damage.

Implementation. All known hepatotoxic medications (including alcohol) must be removed from therapeutic regimens. In addition, dosages of all drugs thought to be metabolized by the liver must be lowered. Administration of sedatives and opiates is to be avoided.

Collaborative Problem: Risk for Hemorrhage R/T bleeding tendencies.

Planning: Expected Outcomes. Hemorrhage will be prevented, as evidenced by absence of bleeding, normal vital signs, and urine output of at least 30 mL/hr.

CLIENT EDUCATION GUIDE

Cirrhosis

The nurse should initiate discharge teaching as soon as possible. The client and significant others should be included so that, by the time of discharge, they can verbalize the following:

- The need to avoid hepatotoxins, especially alcohol.
- The value of seeking help (e.g., Alcoholics Anonymous) with alcohol abstinence.
- The need for a nutritious diet that is rich in vitamins with sufficient calories and protein. If encephalopathy is present, protein intake may be limited. The client must be given a printed list of permitted foods.
- A low-sodium diet if edema is present. If fluid restrictions are indicated, the nurse must teach the client how to measure and record all fluid intake.
- Signs of complications such as ascites, portal hypertension, or hepatic encephalopathy. For example, bleeding from varices or a decrease in the level of consciousness would require immediate medical attention.
- The need for periodic blood tests to assess liver damage.

Implementation. The nurse monitors the client for bleeding gums, purpura, melena, hematuria, and hematemesis. The nurse protects the client from physical injury resulting from falls or abrasions and gives injections to the client only when absolutely necessary, using only small-gauge needles. The nurse should be sure to apply gentle pressure after an injection.

The nurse teaches the client to avoid vigorous nose blowing and straining with bowel movements. Sometimes stool softeners may be ordered. The nurse advises the client to use a soft toothbrush and refrain from flossing until the bleeding problem has improved.

Nursing Diagnosis: Knowledge Deficit R/T disease and long-term treatment.

Planning: Expected Outcomes. The client will understand the disease and the implications of long-term management, as evidenced by the client's statements.

Implementation. The client and significant others are provided with information in preparation for care at home (see Client Education Guide: Cirrhosis). Clients with cirrhosis live longer if they get adequate rest, abstain from alcohol, and eat nutritious meals.

Those clients with a history of alcohol abuse should be encouraged to seek assistance from support groups such as Alcoholics Anonymous to stop drinking. Even if cirrhotic changes have begun in the liver, it is vital for the client to stop drinking before irreparable damage occurs (see Ethical Issues in Nursing).

Evaluation

The nurse must evaluate the client outcomes on the basis of the established plan of care. If these goals were not achieved, the plan and interventions must be revised to meet the client's needs.

ETHICAL ISSUES IN NURSING

Do Nurses Have an Obligation to Care for a Client with a Life-Style Disease?

Cirrhosis of the liver can be a very serious and often deadly condition. Although cirrhosis may be caused by several different sources, alcohol abuse accounts for a large percentage of such disease. Cirrhosis can affect both men and women and does not discriminate by age. The end stages of liver cirrhosis are uncomfortable for the client as well as for those who care for him or her.

Health-care workers who have not received specialized education about substance abuse often care for those persons who have abused alcohol or other pharmacologic substances. These clients appear in all nursing care settings (e.g., medical-surgical, intensive care, obstetric-gynecologic, and home health care). Because many nurses have not had formal training in the care of substance abusers, it is easy to misunderstand these clients. Caring for a person who has destroyed his or her liver through years of alcohol abuse is difficult with the knowledge that the problems were purely self-induced. When care givers see these clients and their families go through such an emotional experience because the clients could not control their alcohol consumption, it is easy to judge the clients harshly. For example, if the client becomes demanding, requiring more nursing time, it is easy to think unkindly of him or her, figuring that, after all, had the client not abused him- or herself, the client would not be in this situation.

It is difficult not to prejudge persons with conditions brought about by their own substance abuse. Health-care providers, although they may not approve of such abuse, have a responsibility to assist in the care of those who are in need. In the case of the alcoholic client with liver cirrhosis, the nurse can refer the client or family to a substance abuse center or other such services. Nurses who have the potential for caring for substance abusers on an ongoing basis should receive special training in the care of such persons. It is natural to feel that those who abuse anything should more or less receive whatever comes from such activity; however, health-care workers must look beyond the abusive personality and treat the person holistically.

Complications of Cirrhosis

PORTAL HYPERTENSION

Portal hypertension occurs when there is a persistent increase in the pressure in the portal venous system as a result of increased resistance or obstruction of the blood flow through the portal venous system.

Incidence and Etiology

Most cases of portal hypertension in the United States relate to cirrhosis. The portal vein is likely to be obstructed by a thrombus; a tumor is the next most common cause.

Pathophysiology

The normal flow to and from the liver depends on proper functioning of the portal vein, the hepatic artery, and the hepatic veins. Disease processes that damage or alter the flow of blood through the liver or its major vessels are responsible for the development of portal hypertension. The amount of liver dysfunction varies with the initial process, the length of the process, and individual differences.

The spleen and other organs that empty into the portal system also begin to undergo the effects of congestion. Eventually, clinical manifestations arise.

Clinical Manifestations

In clients with portal hypertension, assessment reveals

- Slightly tortuous epigastric vessels that branch off the area of the umbilicus and lead toward the sternum and ribs *(caput medusae)*
- An enlarged, palpable spleen
- Internal hemorrhoids
- Bruits, which may be heard over the upper abdomen
- Ascites, which typically appears when there is concurrent liver disease

DIAGNOSTIC ASSESSMENT

The diagnosis of portal hypertension often relies on indirect measurements of portal pressure—liver scans, splenoportography, abdominal angiography, liver biopsy, and other laboratory data (see Chap. 36). Radiography and endoscopy procedures may be used to differentiate variceal hemorrhage from other types of gastrointestinal bleeding.

Complications

Hemorrhage constitutes the major life-threatening complication of portal hypertension. As portal pressure rises, the superior rectal veins, abdominal wall veins, and esophagogastric veins dilate and distend. These swollen, dilated veins are called varices. Various factors can contribute to the rupturing of varices: a sharp rise in portal pressure, increased intrathoracic pressure (coughing and straining at stools), irritation by food or alcohol, and erosion by gastric juices. Veins of the stomach and esophagus are most subject to rupture.

Another mechanism that leads to hemorrhage involves the spleen. The splenic vein merges with the superior mesenteric vein to form the portal vein. When pressure increases in the portal system, damage to the spleen occurs. Damage to the spleen is not proportional to the increase in portal pressure. As the spleen enlarges, it tends to destroy blood cells, and especially platelets, which then increases the risk of hemorrhage and anemia.

Hepatic encephalopathy is an extremely dangerous complication of portal hypertension. This problem usually arises after a period of bleeding into the gastrointestinal tract. Digestion of this blood takes place in the intestines. Because blood is a protein substance, this process increases ammonia in the gut and bloodstream. In turn, the excessive ammonia disturbs brain function. Hepatic encephalopathy is discussed later in this chapter.

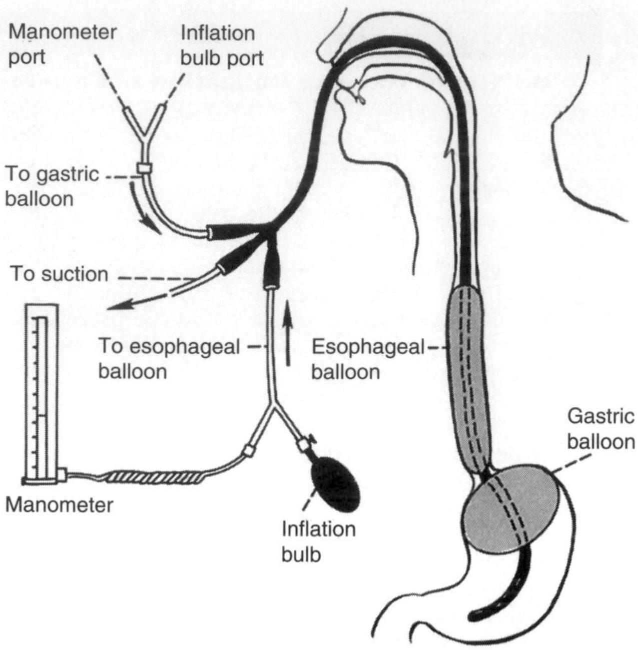

Figure 37–1
A Sengstaken-Blakemore tube can be used to control ruptured esophageal varices, a potential complication of portal hypertension.

Medical Management

Nonsurgical approaches to treat varices include the administration of propranolol and sclerotherapy. To perform sclerotherapy, the physician passes an endoscope into the esophagus and injects a sclerosing agent (e.g., morrhuate sodium) that flows into the varices. The sclerosing agent initially causes inflammation of the vein wall and then fibrosis. The physician may give repeated injections over a period of weeks until the varices are no longer prominent.

Death often follows rupture of esophageal varices. To stop hemorrhage, health practitioners perform emergency measures: administration of vasopressin, balloon tamponade, injection sclerotherapy, direct ligation of the bleeding varices, transhepatic embolization of the left gastric vein, or even urgent portacaval shunt surgery. Cold saline lavage is probably ineffective but is done while the client is awaiting transport to surgery or the gastrointestinal laboratory. Fluids, especially volume expanders and blood products, are administered to maintain volume. Vital signs should be closely monitored throughout this period. This is a very critical time for nursing intervention and can be a very stressful time for the client, family, and the nurse.

Applying pressure to ruptured varices via balloon tamponade may stop the hemorrhage. For this intervention, the clinician inserts a Sengstaken-Blakemore or Minnesota tube into the stomach and inflates the esophageal and gastric balloons (Fig. 37–1). The pressure of the balloon against the varices may stop the bleeding. It is important to release this pressure periodically to prevent tissue necrosis. The esophageal balloon is not left inflated for more than 24 hours. Also, it is important to remove secretions and saliva that accumulate above the balloon to prevent aspiration. The Minnesota tube actually has a fourth port for aspiration of secretions above the esophageal balloon.

PHARMACOLOGIC MANAGEMENT

Propranolol (Inderal) reduces portal pressure. Administered on a long-term basis, it appears to decrease the risk of bleeding from esophageal varices. Propranolol is a beta-blocker; therefore, it reduces the heart rate and masks the early manifestation of hypoglycemia should it occur.

Administration of vasopressin (Pitressin) achieves temporary lowering of portal pressure. These agents reduce portal blood flow by constricting afferent arterioles. Direct infusion of vasopressin into the superior mesenteric artery is most effective. Sometimes vasopressin is administered intravenously. Systemic side effects include hyponatremia, myocardial ischemia, and stimulation of uterine and gastrointestinal contractions (cramping and diarrhea).

Surgical Management

Several surgical approaches reduce the danger of hemorrhage from varices caused by portal hypertension. Surgical approaches include a variety of portosystemic shunt procedures to reduce portal pressure.

Surgical creation of a portosystemic shunt reduces portal hypertension by sending portal blood directly into the inferior vena cava, bypassing the liver. Such a procedure decreases portal hypertension and thus the risk of rupturing esophageal varices. The process increases the incidence of hepatic encephalopathy, however, because the shunted blood is not cleared of toxic substances. For this reason, clinicians usually reserve

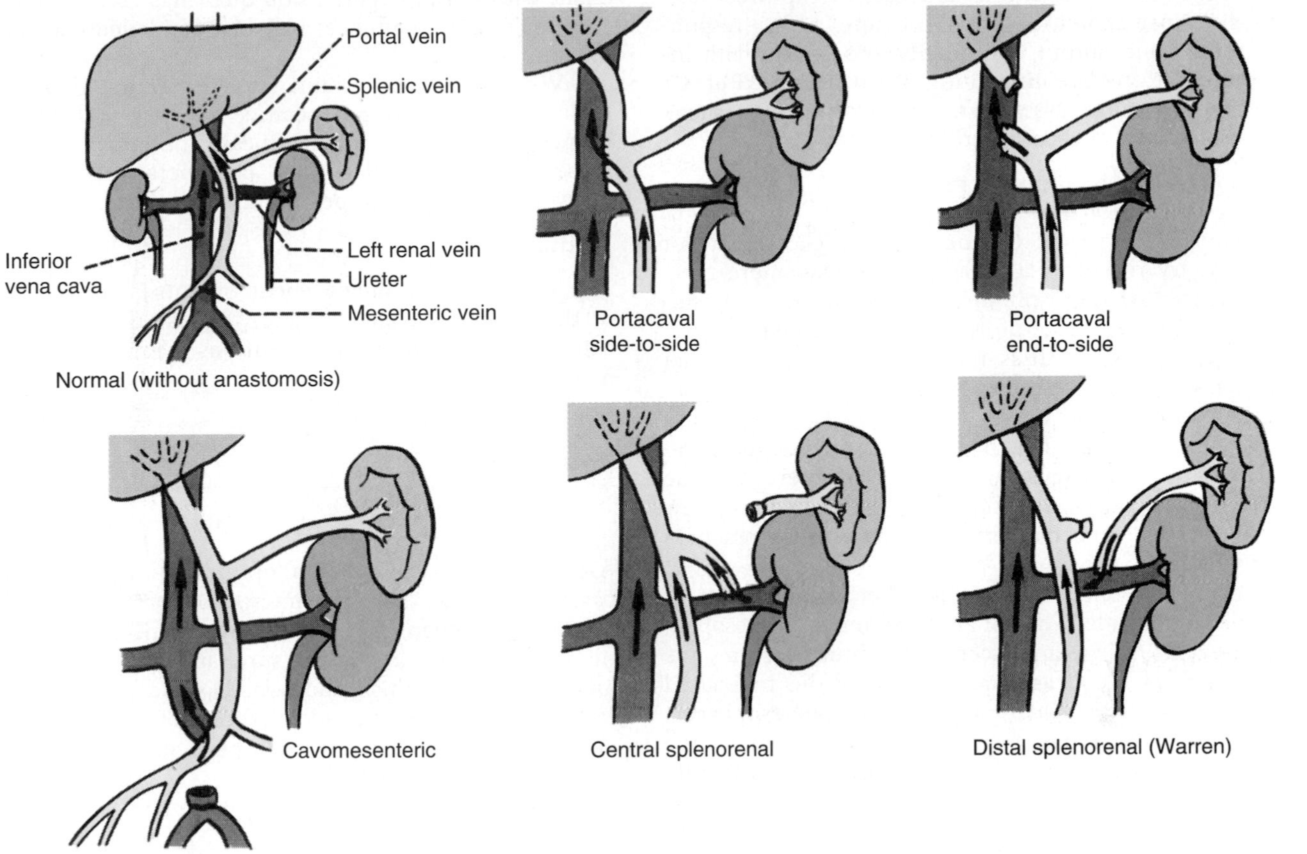

Figure 37–2
Some types of portacaval shunt procedures used to reduce portal hypertension.

portosystemic shunt procedures for clients who have had one or more episodes of bleeding varices.

Figure 37–2 illustrates some of the many portacaval shunt procedures possible. The goal of these procedures is threefold:

- To reduce portal blood flow enough to prevent variceal hemorrhage
- To preserve enough blood inflow to the liver to prevent hepatic encephalopathy and hepatic failure
- To increase client comfort (this is a palliative procedure)

Achievement of these goals requires a delicate balance between the reduction of expendable blood flow and the preservation of essential blood flow.

Nursing Management

Assessment

The major assessment for the nurse to make is for the presence of hemorrhage. The other important assessment is the client's condition after any interventions to treat the hemorrhage, such as the functioning of the Sengstaken-Blakemore tube. The client's vital signs are continuously assessed for any significant changes.

Nursing Diagnosis, Planning, and Implementation

Collaborative Problem: Decreased cardiac output R/T blood volume loss secondary to rupture of esophageal varices and resultant hemorrhage.

Planning: Expected Outcomes. An adequate cardiac output will be maintained as evidenced by the return of vital signs to normal and no further bleeding.

Implementation. The client can learn activities to help decrease the risk of rupture of esophageal varices. The nurse should teach the client to

- Avoid straining maneuvers that increase intrabdominal or intrathoracic pressure.
- Avoid rough foods that may traumatize the esophagus or spicy foods that may irritate the esophageal mucosa.
- Develop an emergency plan if the client has severe esophageal varices that may rupture. Included in this plan should be a list of all emergency telephone numbers. The plan should be discussed with both the client and significant others.

If hemorrhage occurs as a result of ruptured varices, the nurse monitors blood pressure, pulse, respiration, and urine output continually and assists with interventions to restore circulating blood volume. Further information on the assessment and treatment of shock and hemorrhage can be found in Chapter 56.

Nursing Diagnosis: Injury, Risk for R/T the presence of Sengstaken-Blakemore tube.

Planning: Expected Outcomes. The client will not suffer injury related to the Sengstaken-Blakemore tube, as evidenced by no respiratory distress, absence of aspiration, and no evidence of esophageal ischemia.

Implementation. It is important to remember that the pressure of the esophageal balloon on the esophagus not only stops hemorrhage but also may cause esophageal necrosis. The nurse must release the pressure on the esophagus periodically to prevent tissue damage. The physician should be consulted on how often to release the balloon pressure because practices vary widely.

Aspiration pneumonia is another complication of balloon tamponade. The inflated balloon in the esophagus prevents saliva and secretions from reaching the stomach. The nurse ascertains whether the tube used for tamponade has a suction port above the esophageal balloon. If not, a nasogastric tube is inserted to the upper balloon level or suctioning performed frequently to remove accumulating fluid.

Tubes inserted through the nose may cause erosion of the nares, especially if traction is applied to the tamponade (practices differ). To prevent this complication, the nurse cleans and lubricates the external nares. Padding is provided if necessary.

The last complication of balloon tamponade is airway obstruction. This occurs when the gastric balloon deflates or breaks and the traction on the tube pulls the esophageal balloon up into the oropharynx. Scissors should be kept at the bedside in case this emergency arises. The nurse cuts the tube and pulls it out to restore airway patency. To prevent this complication, the nurse may label each port of the tube to prevent accidental deflation of the gastric balloon.

Nursing Diagnosis: Thought Processes, Altered, R/T development of hepatic encephalopathy secondary to shunt procedure.

Planning: Expected Outcomes. Hepatic encephalopathy will be prevented or will be diagnosed early, after the shunt surgery, as evidenced by no decreased level of consciousness and no increase in blood ammonia level.

Implementation. If the client with portal hypertension undergoes portosystemic shunt surgery, the nurse provides postoperative care as described in Chapter 5. In addition, the client is assessed for hepatic encephalopathy (see the section on clinical manifestations of hepatic encephalopathy). If portal hypertension is due to liver disease, the nurse carefully monitors for postoperative hemorrhage, because bleeding tendencies often arise from liver cell malfunction. Because the shunt increases venous return to the heart, cardiovascular function must be assessed carefully. Recall that the client with portal hypertension often has ascites, hepatic encephalopathy, jaundice, bleeding tendencies, or alcoholism.

When emergency shunt surgery occurs, there may be little time to give preoperative teaching and information to the client and significant others. The nurse presents careful explanations postoperatively to compensate for the lack of preoperative teaching.

Evaluation

The nurse must evaluate client outcomes on the basis of the established plan of care. If these goals were not achieved, the plan and interventions must be revised to meet the client's needs.

Ascites

Ascites is the accumulation of fluid in the peritoneal cavity. It results from the interaction of several pathophysiologic changes. Portal hypertension, lowered plasma colloidal osmotic pressure, and sodium retention all contribute to this condition. Disease processes that lead to these events include cirrhosis of the liver, right-sided heart failure, tuberculous peritonitis, cancer, and complications of pancreatitis.

Pathophysiology

Any process that blocks the flow of blood through the liver sinusoids to the hepatic veins and vena cava causes an increase in hydrostatic pressure in the portal venous system. Most commonly, this problem develops in cirrhosis of the liver or right-sided heart failure.

Three mechanisms that underlie ascites formation are

- Portal hypertension resulting in increased plasma and lymphatic hydrostatic pressures
- Hypoalbuminemia resulting in decreased colloid osmotic pressure
- Hyperaldosteronism resulting in renal sodium and water retention

Clinical Manifestations

Ascitic fluid typically produces abdominal distention, bulging flanks, and a protruding (downward) umbilicus. Figure 37–3 depicts a client with ascites before therapy. Although large accumulations of ascitic fluid are obvious, small or moderate amounts may be more difficult to diagnose.

DIAGNOSTIC ASSESSMENT

Diagnostic tests to confirm the presence of ascites include paracentesis, abdominal x-ray studies, ultrasonography, and computed tomographic scan. These tests may locate fluid in the peritoneal cavity. A paracentesis

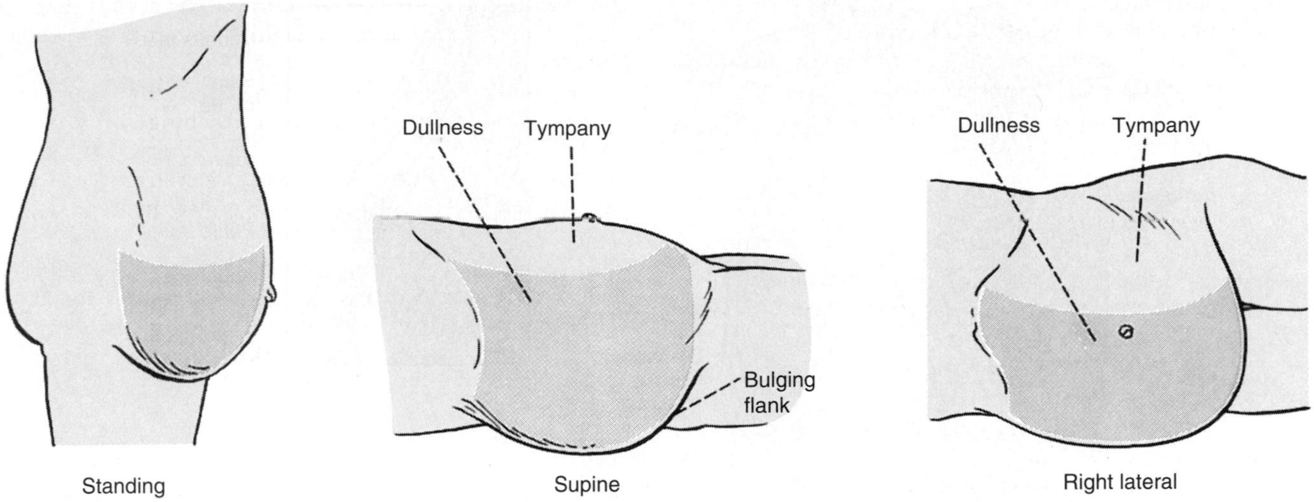

Figure 37–3
Assessing fluid levels in ascites.

provides samples of fluid for analysis. Findings help determine the source of the ascites, such as the finding of malignant cells.

Medical Management

The goal of intervention for ascites is to correct fluid and electrolyte imbalances by improving renal sodium excretion and restricting sodium and water intake. This involves discontinuing medications that inhibit prostaglandin synthesis (e.g., aspirin and indomethacin) and thus impair renal sodium excretion.

The use of repeated paracenteses for removal of ascitic fluid has fallen into disfavor. Repeated removal of fluid, protein, and electrolytes from the body causes severe disturbances of homeostasis.

PHARMACOLOGIC MANAGEMENT

Diuretics, especially spironolactone, are useful in decreasing fluid retention. In addition, the physician may prescribe intravenous administration of albumin.

DIETARY MANAGEMENT

The diet is a low-sodium diet with restriction of fluids. Protein intake is moderate unless the client has signs of hepatic encephalopathy.

Surgical Management

The client with refractory and disabling chronic ascites may obtain relief from the insertion of a peritoneovenous shunt (e.g., LeVeen or Denver shunt). As Figure 37–4 shows, a properly functioning shunt moves fluid from the peritoneal (abdominal) cavity into the venous blood of the superior vena cava. Resolution of ascites may be dramatic after implantation of a peritoneovenous shunt.

Complications of shunt implantation include infection, disseminated intravascular coagulation, congestive heart failure, and shunt clotting.

Nursing Management

Assessment

Some simple assessments that can be performed at the bedside are as follows:

- Percuss the abdomen. If the client has ascites, the sound will be dull.
- Turn the client laterally and percuss the abdomen (see Fig. 37–3). Because ascitic fluid flows to the lowest point in the abdomen, it will move downward when the client turns. This causes a shift in the area where dullness is heard.
- Tap the abdomen to elicit a fluid wave.

The amount of distress that the ascites is causing also should be assessed. The nurse assesses whether the fluid is interfering with sleeping, eating, and breathing.

Nursing Diagnosis, Planning, and Implementation

Collaborative Problem: Fluid volume excess in third space combined with fluid volume deficit in intravascular space R/T fluid shifts secondary to portal hypertension, hypoalbuminemia, and hyperaldosteronism.

Planning: Expected Outcomes. A normal balance of fluid between the intracellular and extracellular spaces will be maintained, as evidenced by absence of hypovolemia, normal serum albumin, decreased abdominal girth, and normal blood pressure.

Implementation. The client is on a fluid restriction that must be strictly followed. To better space the fluids, the nurse may give medications with meals, if

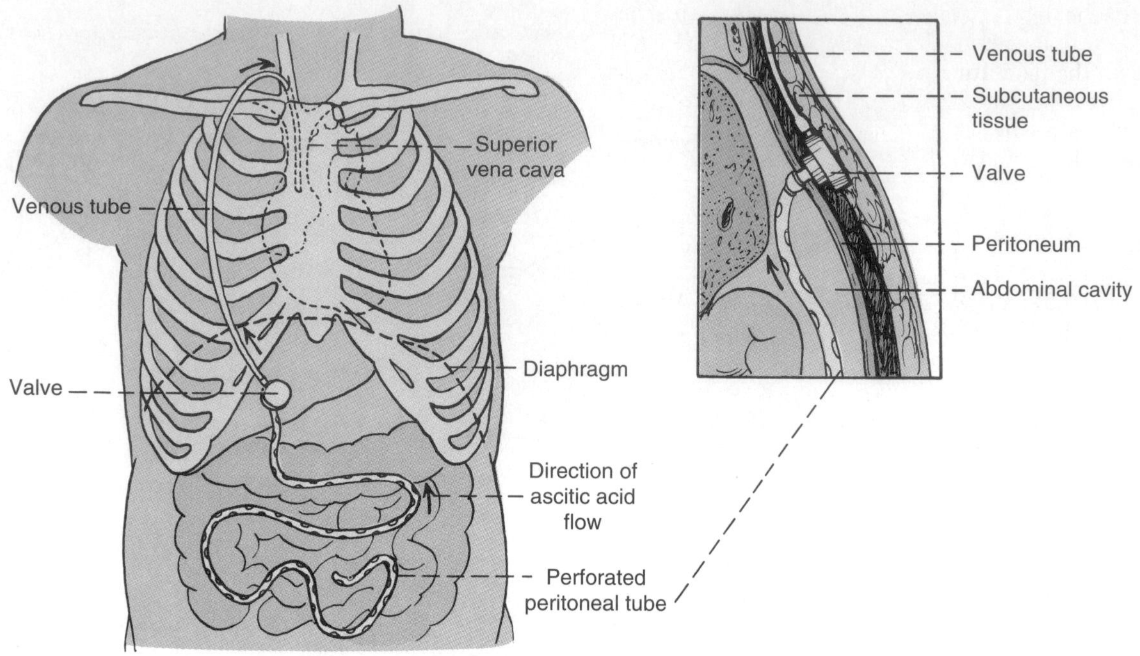

Figure 37–4
LeVeen peritoneovenous shunt for chronic ascites moves fluid from the peritoneal (abdominal) cavity into the superior vena cava.

possible, so these fluids can be used to take the medications. The abdominal girth should be measured daily and sometimes twice a day, and daily weights should be taken. Aspirin should be avoided because it stimulates prostaglandin secretion.

The client is monitored closely after a paracentesis. The nurse checks vital signs frequently to ensure that the client tolerated the procedure well and checks the dressing carefully to ensure that excessive amounts of fluid are not lost.

Nursing Diagnosis: Breathing Pattern, Ineffective R/T increased intra-abdominal pressure on diaphragm.

Planning: Expected Outcomes. The client will maintain an effective breathing pattern, as evidenced by the absence of shortness of breath and the presence of normal respiratory excursion.

Implementation. The nurse positions the client in high Fowler's position to facilitate breathing and monitors the client's respiratory status for the development of atelectasis or pneumonia. The client is asked to cough and take a deep breath hourly to maintain adequate respiratory function. The client may need to use an incentive spirometer or receive ultrasonic treatments if the cough is ineffective.

Nursing Diagnosis: Skin Integrity, Impaired, Risk for, or Actual Impaired R/T immobility, edema, and pressure from the abdomen.

Planning: Expected Outcomes. The client will maintain skin integrity, as evidenced by intact skin.

Implementation. The nurse turns the client frequently, providing adequate support for the distended abdomen. If the client is on bedrest, a specialty mattress is used to prevent skin breakdown. The client's skin is carefully inspected daily, and lotions and creams are used if necessary.

Nursing Diagnosis: Knowledge Deficit R/T ascites, treatment, and self-care after discharge.

Planning: Expected Outcomes. The client will understand ascites, its treatment, and self-care after discharge, as evidenced by the client's statements and compliance with the treatment regimen and abstention from alcohol.

Implementation. The nurse discusses the causes of ascites with the client, making sure that the client understands ways to slow the recurrence. The nurse ensures that the client understands the need for dietary modifications, fluid restrictions, and home health-care needs. The client must be helped to understand that all alcohol intake must be stopped. Refer the client to Alcoholics Anonymous for assistance with abstinence if necessary.

Evaluation

The nurse must evaluate client outcomes on the basis of the established plan of care. If these goals were not achieved, the plan and interventions must be revised to meet the client's needs.

Hepatic Encephalopathy

Hepatic encephalopathy encompasses a spectrum of central nervous system (CNS) disturbances. These disturbances may appear in conjunction with severe liver injury, liver failure, or portal shunt. The cause of this disorder is the liver's inability to metabolize ammonia to form urea that is then excreted. Ammonia is a CNS depressant. Changes during the initial stages of hepatic encephalopathy include reduced mental alertness, confusion, and restlessness. Loss of consciousness, seizures, and irreversible coma occur in the terminal stage.

Pathophysiology

Hepatic encephalopathy is characterized by elevation of ammonia levels in the blood and cerebrospinal fluid.

Normally, the liver converts ammonia into glutamine, which is stored in the liver and later converted to urea and excreted through the kidneys. Blood ammonia rises when the liver cells are unable to perform this conversion.

Any process that increases protein in the intestine, such as increased dietary protein or gastrointestinal bleeding, causes elevated blood ammonia levels and possibly signs of hepatic encephalopathy in clients with hepatocellular failure or portal shunt.

Although intervention usually alleviates hepatic encephalopathy, the client may succumb to circulatory or respiratory complications, infection, or delirium and convulsions. Mortality is high among clients who progress into coma with hepatic failure. Health-care practitioners often use dramatic measures to reduce toxic levels of ammonia in the blood. Such measures include peritoneal dialysis and exchange transfusions, which involve removal and replacement of approximately 80 per cent of the client's blood. A liver transplant may be performed for cases of fulminant liver failure.

Clinical Manifestations

Manifestations of hepatic encephalopathy progress from mild mental confusion to deep coma. Hepatic encephalopathy impairs memory, attention, concentration, and rate of response. Sleep pattern reversal often occurs, with the client awake at night and sleepy during the day. The nurse evaluates handwriting and speech for significant changes. Asterixis (liver flap) may be present. Some clients with hepatic encephalopathy experience hyperventilation with respiratory alkalosis. The presence of methylmercaptan causes a characteristic odor on the breath called fetor hepaticus.

As the syndrome progresses, the client's level of consciousness slowly diminishes, and confusion becomes more severe. However, the level of CNS depression commonly fluctuates.

Coma may eventually ensue, deepening until there is no pain response and the reflexes, including corneal, are completely absent. Table 37–7 lists the stages of hepatic encephalopathy.

TABLE 37–7 Stages of Hepatic Encephalopathy

Stage 1	
	Fatigue Restlessness Irritability Decreased intellectual performance Decreased attention span Diminished short-term memory Personality changes Sleep pattern reversal
Stage 2	
	Deteriorated handwriting Asterixis Drowsiness Confusion Lethargy Fetor hepaticus
Stage 3	
	Severe confusion Unable to follow commands Deep somnolence, but arousable
Stage 4	
	Coma Unresponsive to painful stimuli Possible decorticate or decerebrate posturing

DIAGNOSTIC ASSESSMENT

Laboratory results show elevated blood ammonia and cerebrospinal fluid glutamine. Although findings help to confirm the diagnosis of encephalopathy, they are not specific to this entity.

The nurse monitors serum ammonia levels, electrolytes, blood gases, and hepatic function tests (bilirubin, albumin, prothrombin, and enzymes) throughout the course of this syndrome. These clinical findings help determine the degree of imbalance and the extent of hepatic injury and malfunction (see Chap. 36).

Medical Management

The goals of intervention for clients with hepatic encephalopathy are to control or reduce further degenerative processes, correct present metabolic imbalances, and preserve remaining physiologic functioning.

Five principles guide intervention in hepatic encephalopathy:

- Reduce protein in the intestine. Reducing dietary protein serves to reduce protein in the intestine. If no other precipitating factors are present, this alone may eliminate symptoms.
- Prevent gastrointestinal bleeding, or, if it occurs, quickly remove the blood from the gastrointestinal tract with lactulose enemas.
- Reduce bacterial production of ammonia. Neomycin and lactulose are useful pharmacologic agents for this purpose.

- Eliminate fluid and electrolyte imbalances, hypoxia, infection, and sedation.
- Maintain safety and function in the unconscious client. The immobile client who lacks reflexes is vulnerable to numerous complications.

PHARMACOLOGIC MANAGEMENT

Neomycin and lactulose are given to reduce the bacteria in the intestinal tract. Because neomycin is not absorbed into the circulation, it exerts a powerful effect on the intestinal bacteria responsible for ammonia production. Undesirable side effects result from the depletion of intestinal flora (e.g., diarrhea and vitamin K deficiency). Because neomycin is ototoxic and nephrotoxic, its use in clients with renal insufficiency should be avoided.

DIETARY MANAGEMENT

Protein might be totally eliminated from the diet, with an intake of fruit juices and intravenous fluids, although this radical restriction leads to catabolism of the client's own protein stores. The usual protein restriction is to 20 to 40 g/day. The client with chronic hepatic encephalopathy may need to adjust to a long-term, low-protein diet (50 to 60 g/day), which can be difficult.

Nursing Management

Assessment

When working with a client susceptible to hepatic encephalopathy, the nurse uses interviewing and assessment techniques to evaluate psychophysiologic status. For example, has the client's normally neat handwriting become sloppy and difficult to read? Is speech slow and slurred? The nurse observes for personality changes with labile feeling states and elicits flapping tremor (asterixis or liver flap) by asking the client to dorsiflex the hand with the rest of the arm resting on the bed. The hand cannot be held steady.

The nurse, who is with the client over time, is often the best person to assess a change in level of mental functioning. Early detection of a depressed or confused level of consciousness greatly improves the client's chances of recovery. To make nursing progress notes relevant, the nurse should describe behavior vividly and objectively ("States pigeons are pecking at his bedclothes") rather than offer interpretations that may have a different meaning for each reader ("Seems more confused"). As the client progresses into coma, the nurse makes ongoing neurologic checks to determine the level of consciousness. See Unit 4 for neurologic assessment of comatose clients.

Nursing Diagnosis, Planning, and Implementation

Nursing Diagnosis: Knowledge Deficit R/T reduction in protein in the diet and long-term pharmacologic intervention with neomycin.

CLIENT EDUCATION GUIDE

Complications of Cirrhosis

The nurse should plan to initiate discharge teaching well in advance of the anticipated discharge date. By the time of discharge, the client and significant others should be able to verbalize the following:

- Signs and symptoms of possible complications
- Importance of a low-protein diet to reduce the protein in the intestine
- Medications such as neomycin and lactulose to reduce the bacteria in the intestinal tract
- Altering the home setting to accommodate limitations in mobility and prevent injury
- Locating the bedroom near a bathroom if diuretics are taken
- Calling the physician if changes requiring medical attention occur (this might include new symptoms or worsening of present symptoms)
- Follow-up appointments for diagnostic testing to monitor the status of the liver

Planning: Expected Outcomes. The client will understand and comply with the reduction in protein in the diet and long-term pharmacologic intervention with neomycin, as evidenced by the client's following a low-protein diet and stating reasons why neomycin should be taken.

Implementation. It is important that the client understand the importance of the protein-reduced diet to have the motivation to remain on this diet (see Client Education Guide: Complications of Cirrhosis).

In addition to ensuring a low-protein diet, the nurse assesses for signs of gastrointestinal bleeding, checking for bright blood in the stool or for black, tarry stools. Bleeding results in protein accumulation in the gastrointestinal tract, which exacerbates hepatic encephalopathy. To reverse the progression of symptoms, constipation must be prevented. Cathartics and enemas hasten the exit of protein material from the intestine.

Nursing Diagnosis: Diarrhea R/T laxative action of lactulose.

Planning: Expected Outcomes. The client will have diarrhea controlled, as evidenced by a decrease in the number of diarrheal stools.

Implementation. Intervention for severe hepatic encephalopathy commonly combines neomycin therapy with protein restriction and bowel cleansing. The physician may prescribe maintenance doses of neomycin and a low-protein diet for clients with chronic hepatic encephalopathy. Lactulose is a combination of galactose and fructose that passes through the intestine unchanged. The physician may prescribe lactulose to decrease ammonia by trapping ammonium ions in the bowel. The appropriate lactulose dosage causes two to three soft stool evacuations daily. Diarrhea may be a side effect. The physician may reduce the dosage to prevent further electrolyte imbalance.

Nursing Diagnosis: Fluid Volume Deficit R/T bleeding, decreased intake, and ascites.

Planning: Expected Outcomes. The client will maintain a balanced fluid volume, as evidenced by normal blood pressure, absence of edema, absence of ascites, and balanced intake and output.

Implementation. Hypovolemia often precipitates hepatic encephalopathy by reducing hepatocellular perfusion. Fluid balance must be achieved, maintained, and monitored to prevent further hepatic injury and reduced renal perfusion. Intravenous fluids are delivered evenly over time. Vital signs and central venous pressure are monitored frequently. If necessary, urine output is measured hourly.

Electrolyte and acid-base disturbances may precipitate hepatic encephalopathy or develop during its course. Laboratory tests indicate what replacement therapy is necessary.

Collaborative Problem: Injury, Risk for R/T loss of protective mechanisms secondary to hepatic coma.

Planning: Expected Outcomes. Injury or complications of immobility will be prevented or diagnosed early, as evidenced by absence of corneal abrasions or problems related to immobility.

Implementation. Hypoxemia may precipitate hepatic encephalopathy by damaging the hepatic cell. To prevent and treat hypoxemia, the nurse attends to respiratory interventions (e.g., maintaining a patent airway).

Concurrent infection, with protein accumulating from tissue catabolism, requires rapid intervention. The client is particularly vulnerable to nosocomial infections. Nurses should wash their hands thoroughly and take other measures to prevent cross-contamination.

The nurse must be alert to possible harmful accumulations of ammonia resulting from diuretic therapy. Hypokalemia from the use of diuretics contributes to hepatic encephalopathy by increasing ammonia production in the kidney.

Finally, depressants may precipitate coma. Their use should be avoided. If agitation occurs in early encephalopathy, agents that are excreted partially through the kidney instead of the liver (e.g., phenobarbital) are administered. Phenobarbital should be administered with caution! The nurse should know which narcotics, tranquilizers, and sedatives are biotransformed by the liver. They are often contraindicated in clients with decreased hepatic function.

The immobile client who lacks reflexes is vulnerable to numerous complications. Preventing complications requires intensive nursing intervention. Pneumonia and skin breakdown may be prevented by turning the client frequently and promoting lung aeration.

Physiologic agitation may appear as the body accumulates metabolic substances. Therefore, the client should be protected from self-injury (i.e., by lowering the bed and padding the side rails). See Unit 4 for further discussion of the comatose client and the client with neurologic disturbances.

Evaluation

The nurse must evaluate client outcomes on the basis of the established plan of care. If these goals were not achieved, the plan and interventions must be revised to meet the client's needs.

Liver Neoplasms

Tumors of the liver are either primary or metastatic in origin. Primary liver tumors may arise from hepatocytes, connective tissue, blood vessels, or bile ducts. These tumors are either benign or malignant.

Metastatic malignant tumors arise from the gastrointestinal tract (particularly the colon), the breasts, and the lungs.

PRIMARY LIVER NEOPLASMS

Adenomas

Adenomas are benign hepatic cell tumors. The incidence of this type of tumor is increasing. Researchers postulate that there is an association between some adenomas and either oral contraceptives used by women or androgens used by men.

Although these tumors are classified as benign, they are nevertheless dangerous because of their vascularity. A benign adenoma may rupture, with consequent hemorrhage. Hepatic arteriography is a valuable early diagnostic test for this condition. Liver biopsy is helpful but poses a danger because of the problem of possible hemorrhage. Other liver function tests usually reveal normal findings.

Intervention for benign adenomas depends on the cause. Simply discontinuing oral contraceptives or androgens when a tumor appears to be hormone dependent may correct the condition. Otherwise, treatment may include surgical excision of the involved liver segment. If acute hemorrhage precipitates surgery, the surgeon may perform a hepatic lobectomy.

Primary Hepatocellular Carcinoma

Primary hepatocellular carcinoma (malignant hepatoma) occurs more frequently in men. Etiologic factors that may contribute to hepatoma are hepatitis B, chronic liver disease, hemochromatosis, certain mycotoxins (aflatoxins), anabolic steroid use, polyvinylchloride, nitrosamines, and long-term androgen therapy.

Primary hepatocellular carcinoma is the main cause of death from cancer in many areas of the world.

Benign hepatic tumors have an excellent prognosis if they can be removed surgically before they rupture and cause death from hemorrhage.

After the diagnosis of liver cancer and if intervention fails to terminate the tumor process, the individual usually dies of hepatic failure within 4 to 6 months.

METASTATIC TUMORS

Metastatic tumors of the liver are tumors that began elsewhere in the body and have spread to the liver. The liver is one of the common sites of metastasis for all cancers. In the United States, metastatic tumors of the liver are more common than primary liver tumors.

Etiology and Risk Factors

The liver is a common site of metastatic tumors because of a variety of anatomic factors. Melanomas and tumors from the gastrointestinal tract, lung, and breast lead to liver metastasis more frequently than do tumors of the prostate, skin, or thyroid.

Pathophysiology

The liver is a common site of metastasis because of the liver's high rate of blood flow, size, and portal drainage from the major abdominal organs. Metastatic tumors spread to the liver by direct extension from adjacent organs (stomach and gallbladder) or via the hepatic arterial system or the portal venous system. Also, as a result of cell migration, the surface of the liver may become seeded with metastatic cells.

Unfortunately, these metastatic tumors may be far advanced before clinical manifestations or laboratory findings indicate their presence. For this reason, this condition usually carries a poor prognosis. Interventions with radiotherapy and chemotherapy may be only palliative.

Clinical Manifestations

Clients with primary (benign and malignant) and secondary (metastatic) tumors often present with similar signs and symptoms. Early indicators of liver neoplasm are usually vague. The client may report minor temperature elevation and gastrointestinal symptoms. Common manifestations include right upper quadrant distress and tenderness, abdominal distention, diarrhea or constipation, and nausea. Diagnostic studies and physical examination may reveal the following:

- Hepatomegaly
- Liver mass
- Friction rub or bruit over the liver
- Positive angiography
- Hypoproteinemia
- Blood-tinged ascites
- Decreased liver function
- Elevated alkaline phosphatase and reversal of albumin-globulin ratio

Some clients also may experience metabolic derangement such as polycythemia, blood sugar disorders, and high levels of calcium. Other clients may present with high leukocytosis and anemia. Jaundice occurs more often when the bile ducts are the primary site or the tumor mass obstructs a major outflow duct. Still other manifestations may be present, but they vary according to the concurrent pathologic condition. At times, the tumor process causes elevation of the diaphragm and some respiratory problems.

Although neoplasms of the liver create numerous clinical manifestations, many of these manifestations may not occur until the tumors have grown quite large. Malignant tumor cells may have replaced as much as 90 per cent of normal liver tissue before liver insufficiency becomes clinically evident.

DIAGNOSTIC ASSESSMENT

In primary hepatocellular cancers, diagnostic tests often reveal high levels of alpha-fetoprotein (AFP). This substance is sometimes present in clients who have metastatic tumors, but levels rarely match those found in clients with primary tumors.

The physician usually orders isotope scans of the liver. Findings from the scans, along with those of ultrasonography or computed tomography, may help to locate liver tumors. Blood tests for liver cancer are under development.

Liver biopsy is very helpful in diagnosis. The route of access may be percutaneous, direct via laparotomy, or through a peritoneoscope. Each method has its limitations. Percutaneous procedures may cause seeding of tumor cells along the exit pathway. Laparotomy requires anesthesia and therefore may be too dangerous. Peritoneoscopy may be impossible if there are extensive adhesions. Because all of these biopsy procedures require membrane puncture, the nurse must be sure the client has an acceptable prothrombin time.

Medical Management

Dearterialization of the liver by hepatic artery ligation or occlusion decreases oxygen supply to the liver. As a result, tumor cells undergo a reduction in number and activity. Although the portal vein carries a sufficient oxygen supply to nourish the hepatocytes, the client should be observed carefully for signs of liver failure. The physician may prescribe a combination of chemotherapy and dearterialization.

Irradiation of liver tumors may provide temporary relief. Percutaneous biliary drainage or the internal placement of a biliary drain helps increase the passage of bile into the duodenum and decrease jaundice and discomfort.

Post-intervention, it is important to monitor the AFP levels in clients with primary liver tumors to assess their progress.

PHARMACOLOGIC MANAGEMENT

Regional perfusion of the liver via the hepatic artery helps relieve pain or slow tumor growth. During surgery, the surgeon may implant a chemotherapy infusion pump. Such pumps, filled percutaneously, deliver medication continuously into the hepatic artery. In metastatic growths, the physician may prescribe systemic chemotherapy to reduce tumor size and pain.

Surgical Management

For tumors that are small and confined to one liver segment or lobe, the surgeon may perform resection of the segment or lobe if the client is able to withstand the stress of surgery.

Nursing Management

Nursing diagnoses and interventions for clients with liver neoplasms vary according to the amount of liver dysfunction. The nurse should plan to assess the client for metabolic malfunctions, bleeding problems, ascites, edema, inability to biotransform endogenous and exogenous (drug) wastes, hypoproteinemia, jaundice, and endocrine complications.

The nurse takes time to prepare the client in the diagnostic stage for the various procedures and assesses carefully for postprocedure complications. See Chapters 6 and 7 for detailed discussion of nursing care of clients with malignant tumors.

Liver Transplant

Liver transplant is now considered a feasible intervention for various end-stage liver diseases, including

- Primary biliary cirrhosis (adult)
- Hepatitis—chronic or fulminant (usually adult)
- Sclerosing cholangitis (adult)
- Biliary atresia (pediatrics)
- Alpha$_1$-antitrypsin deficiency (usually pediatric)
- Confined hepatic malignancy (adult or pediatric)
- Wilson's disease
- Budd-Chiari syndrome (hepatic vein obstruction)

There are two general approaches to liver transplant: *orthotopic* (the diseased liver is removed during transplant) and *heterotopic* (the diseased liver is left in during transplant). Orthotopic transplant is by far the more common of the two.

As with other forms of transplant, immunosuppressive therapy (cyclosporine and newer experimental medications) prevents the rejection of the transplanted liver. Matching proper organ size and blood and tissue type is the most crucial factor in finding suitable donors.

The appropriate candidate for liver transplant is younger than 55 years and not suffering from life-threatening complications such as bleeding varices, advanced cardiac disease or severe hypertension, advanced catabolism, active alcoholism, or metastatic malignancy. The client must be stable psychologically and should have good support systems for the complex postoperative course.

Surgery can last anywhere from 6 to 20 hours. The surgery involves anastomosis of veins, arteries, and biliary ducts. Postoperative complications include infection, rejection, hemorrhage, atelectasis, and acute renal failure. Rejection most commonly occurs between the fourth and tenth postoperative days. Symptoms of acute rejection include fever, tachycardia, right upper quadrant or flank pain, and increasing jaundice. Steroids are used to attempt to stop the rejection; otherwise, rapid deterioration of liver function occurs.

The nurse must closely monitor the client during the postoperative period. Table 37–8 lists the postoperative nursing assessments and interventions and explains the rationale for each. The other major nursing function is teaching the client and significant others about long-term care (see Client Education Guide: After Liver Transplant).

Liver Abscess

Liver abscess usually develops after one of the following three conditions:

- *Bacterial cholangitis,* which results from obstruction of the bile ducts by stone or stricture
- *Portal vein bacteremia,* which may develop following bowel inflammation or organ perforation
- *Amebiasis* (infestation with amebae from tropical or subtropical areas)

Other predisposing factors are diabetes mellitus, infected hepatic cysts, metastatic liver tumors with secondary infection, and diverticulitis.

The client commonly reports right-sided abdominal and tight shoulder pain. Assessment also reveals liver enlargement, tenderness, nausea, vomiting, weight loss, fever, and diaphoresis. At times, the client may experience a right pleural effusion. The liver's proximity to the base of the right lung contributes to this process.

Liver scans are extremely valuable in diagnosis. Other useful diagnostic measures include ultrasonography, computed tomography, and arteriography. Laboratory data reflect slight to marked elevations of aminotransferase, alkaline phosphatase, and bilirubin. High levels indicate the presence of concurrent obstruction. A positive blood culture occurs in some cases.

Intervention for hepatic abscess consists of percutaneous drainage of the abscess with antimicrobial therapy, surgical drainage of large abscesses with postoperative antimicrobial therapy, or antimicrobial therapy without drainage for a few months. Any concurrent problem disposing the client to abscess requires attention as well. These clients are very ill. Early diagnosis

TABLE 37–8 Postoperative Liver Transplant Nursing Assessment, Interventions, and Rationales

ASSESSMENT-INTERVENTION	RATIONALES
Observe for signs of respiratory compromise.	Client may be on a ventilator for 24 to 48 hours postoperatively. Incision under diaphragm limits excursion owing to pain and edema; may have chest tube in place.
Monitor fluid and electrolyte status.	Client is somewhat fluid overloaded from receiving extensive volumes of blood products administered during the long surgical procedure. This overload could lead to pulmonary edema and congestive heart failure.
Monitor for signs of bleeding.	Coagulopathy and thrombocytopenia may persist into the early postoperative period. The transplant procedure itself consists of several vascular anastomoses that may be source of hemorrhage.
Monitor blood pressure, pulse, central venous pressure, and pulmonary artery pressures.	Correlation of these factors can help diagnose early changes in the cardiac and circulatory status.
Follow immunosuppressive protocols.	The amount of immunosuppressant varies for each client. Maintaining proper levels of immunosuppressive drugs helps prevent rejection.
Monitor wound drains and bile drains for patency.	Obstruction of wound drains causes increased intra-abdominal pressure from accumulation of ascites and blood. Obstruction of bile flow can cause damage to the liver and the biliary system.
Keep the client and significant others informed of changes and requirements	The level of acuity may be alarming to both the client and significant others; in addition, the client is likely to have difficulty expressing concerns because of grogginess and the presence of an endotracheal tube.
Teach the client and significant others about the procedures required postoperatively.	Both the client and significant others require education about procedures such as cholangiography, liver biopsy, and abdominal ultrasonography. Much of the teaching is done preoperatively unless the client required emergency transplant as a result of fulminant liver failure.

and intervention reduce mortality from liver abscess to about 10 per cent.

Abscesses resulting from amebic infestation (e.g., *Entamoeba histolytica*) are similar to other liver abscesses. The major difference in intervention is that physicians prescribe metronidazole (Flagyl) or chloroquine phosphate (Aralen) instead of broad-spectrum antibiotics.

CLIENT EDUCATION GUIDE

After Liver Transplant

Discharge teaching should include the following topics:

- **Medication management.** Explain to client why each medication is important as well as when to take each and what to do if medication is forgotten and not taken on time.
- **Dietary management.** Although most clients do not go home with dietary restrictions, some clients may require a low-sodium diet. All clients need a nutritious diet to help with healing.
- **Signs of infection.** Explain what to do when fever, cough, malaise, nausea-vomiting, headache, or other untoward symptoms are present. Include the importance of avoiding self-medication with over-the-counter drugs and when to call the physician.
- **Signs of rejection.** The client should be told to report any changes in liver function, such as jaundice, to the physician. The client needs to know that any changes in liver function tests may indicate rejection.
- **Activity and exercise.** The client should resume activities slowly. Although there are very few limitations on normal physical activities, more vigorous ones may require the physician's permission.

CRITICAL TO REMEMBER

It is important to dispose of feces carefully and wash hands to prevent transmission of *Entamoeba histolytica.*

When caring for the client with liver abscess, the nurse assesses vital signs regularly. High temperature and rapid pulse may indicate the presence of general sepsis, a likely complication. Movement, coughing, and deep breathing should be encouraged to prevent or limit pulmonary complications related to hepatic abscess. The client's fluid is increased, and skin care is provided in the event of hyperpyrexia.

The nurse helps the client's significant others accept the seriousness of the condition and provides a supportive environment that allows close associates to express fears and concerns.

Liver Injuries

Liver injury usually results from a penetrating injury or blunt trauma. Either may lead to laceration and hemorrhage.

Penetrating injuries are usually knife or missile wounds (gunshot), whereas blunt trauma injuries occur from an impact from a steering wheel or a fall.

Intervention for hemorrhage constitutes the major immediate problem after injury. The nurse monitors victims of trauma carefully for the falling blood pressure and tachycardia that may indicate hemorrhage. The problem is more difficult when the liver's blood vessels or bile ducts receive damage as well. Later complications include bile peritonitis and abscess formation.

Intervention for liver injuries consists of hemorrhage control, debridement, and drainage. It may be necessary to remove liver lobes, but more often the major goal is to control hemorrhage. When a damaged blood supply causes sloughing of a hepatic segment, hemorrhage follows as a late problem.

Common postoperative problems include pulmonary infections and abscess formation. Clients are assessed postoperatively for manifestations of infection (e.g., fever, chills, difficulty breathing). Interventions to prevent pneumonia are performed. For information on preventing postoperative complications, review Chapter 5.

STUDY QUESTIONS

1. To gather subjective data from a client with hepatic jaundice, which one of the following questions should the nurse ask?
   A. "Is your urine yellow?"
   B. "Are your stools clay colored?"
   C. "Does your breath have a strong odor?"
   D. "Are you having diarrhea stools?"
2. A mode of transmission for hepatitis A is
   A. Shellfish from contaminated water
   B. Sexual contact
   C. Contact with blood and body fluids
   D. Coinfection with hepatitis B
3. A client has severe, long-standing heart failure that has resulted in a diagnosis of cardiac cirrhosis. He has been placed on restricted fluids. To provide the client with a choice of appropriate fluids, which one of the following should the nurse encourage?
   A. Milk shakes made with skim milk and egg substitute
   B. Low-fat chicken or beef broth
   C. Vegetable juice
   D. Fruit juice
4. A nurse is performing a health assessment on a client with suspected hepatitis of unknown cause. Which one of the following questions would be appropriate when gathering data?
   A. "Describe your activities of daily living."
   B. "Describe your living environment."
   C. "Have you been visiting outside the country lately?"
   D. All of the above
5. When evaluating the outcome of client goals for a client who has undergone liver transplantation, the nurse would expect a successful outcome if
   A. The client could state why most of the medications were important
   B. The client could relate the reasons for a high-protein diet
   C. The client could explain what to do when a fever, nausea, or a headache occurs
   D. The client resumes exercise slowly and carefully

CRITICAL THINKING EXERCISES

SCENARIO A

A young woman has been diagnosed with hepatitis A. She complains of extreme fatigue and anorexia. She must depend on her husband to prepare her meals. Because her husband is away from home during the day, he must prepare all of her meals before he leaves for work. At the time of her diagnosis, the young woman weighed 200 pounds.

1. What are the major components of a dietary plan for a client with hepatitis?
2. What would you teach the client's husband about preparing his wife's diet?
3. The husband tells the nurse he wants his wife to lose weight so he plans to decrease her caloric intake by preparing a high-fiber, low-fat diet. How would you respond?
4. How would you modify your dietary teaching if the young woman was also a diabetic?

SCENARIO B

A middle-aged client is diagnosed with primary biliary cirrhosis. He is hospitalized with esophageal varices. The initial treatment is intravenous vasopressin (Pitressin) drip. Intravenous nitroglycerin (Nitrostat) is given simultaneously.

1. Why are vasopressin and nitroglycerin used simultaneously? What other drug could be prescribed to constrict the vessels in the client's gastrointestinal tract?
2. The nurse is responsible for detecting cardiac side and toxic effects. What observations would be noted if there were side and toxic effects?
3. The client becomes very agitated. How should the nurse decrease his anxiety?

BIBLIOGRAPHY

1. Adams, L., & Soulen, M. C. (1993). TIPS: A new alternative for the variceal bleeder . . . transjugular intrahepatic portosystemic shunt. *American Journal of Critical Care, 2(3),* 196–201.
2. American Cancer Society. (1995). *Cancer facts and figures—1995.* Atlanta: Author.
3. Bayless, T. M. (1994). *Current therapy in gastroenterology and liver disease* (4th ed.). St. Louis: Mosby-Year Book.
4. Benning, C. R., & Smith, A. (1994). Psychosocial needs of family members of liver transplant patients. *Clinical Nurse Specialist, 8(5),* 280–288.
5. Boone, P., Kelly, S., & Smith, C. D. (1992). Liver transplantation: Living-related donations. *Critical Care Nursing Clinics of North America, 4(2),* 243–248.
6. Brown, B. R. (1989). The patient with an abnormal liver function study. *Current Reviews for Post Anesthesia Care Nurses, 11(11),* 82–88.
7. Bryden, G., & Raine, R. (1993). Liver transplantation: The surgical ICU experience, General Division, the Toronto Hospital. *CACCN, 4(1),* 28–33.
8. Budinger, J. M., & Donnelly, S. (1994). Nursing care protocols for the kidney/islet/islet cell transplant recipient. *ANNA Journal, 21(2),* 123–128.
9. Butler, R. (1994). Managing the complications of cirrhosis. *American Journal of Nursing, 94(3),* 46–49.
10. Chiu, I. (1990). Infection control in patients infected with hepatitis C virus. *Infection-Control-Canada, 5(3),* 9–11.
11. Ebersol, P., & Hess, P. (1994). *Toward healthy aging: Human needs and nursing response* (4th ed.). St. Louis: Mosby-Year Book.
12. Eyster, M. E., & Silva, E. (1994). Impact of HIV and its treatment on chronic hepatitis C in hemophiliacs. *Aids Patient Care, 8(Suppl 1),* 6–9.
13. Gitnick, G. (Ed.). (1989). *Modern concepts of acute and chronic hepatitis.* New York: Plenum.
14. Grimson, A. E. S., et al. (1986). A randomized trial of vasopressin and vasopressin plus nitroglycerin in the treatment of acute variceal hemorrhage. *Hepatology, 6,* 410–413.
15. Guyton, A. C. (1991). *Textbook of medical physiology* (8th ed.). Philadelphia: W.B. Saunders.
16. Hedges, C. B. (1994). Recognizing the patient at risk for opportunistic infections. *Medical-Surgical Nursing, 3(6),* 445–452.
17. Jackson, R. (1994). Viral hepatitis: Anatomy of a diagnosis. *American Journal of Nursing, 94(3),* 43–48.
18. Kaplan, M. M. (1993). Hepatitis B: Twelve questions physicians often ask. *Consultant, 33(3),* 145–147, 151–152.
19. Kelso, L. A. (1992). Fluid and electrolyte disturbances in hepatic failure. *AACN Clinical Issues in Critical Care Nursing, 3(3),* 681–687.
20. Kelso, L. A. (1994). Alcohol-related end-stage liver disease and transplantation: The debate continues. *AACN Clinical Issues in Critical Care Nursing, 5(4),* 501–506.
21. Kerber, K. (1993). The adult with bleeding esophageal varices. *Critical Care Nursing Clinics of North America, 5(1),* 153–162.
22. Labovich, T. M. (1994). Selected complications in the patient with cancer: Spinal cord compression, malignant bowel obstruction, malignant ascites, and gastrointestinal bleeding. *Seminars in Oncology Nursing, 10(3),* 189–197.
23. Lieber, C. S., & Guadagnini, K. S. (1990). The spectrum of alcoholic liver disease. *Hospital Practice, 25(2A),* 51–55, 59–64, 66–69.
24. Lisanti, P., & Talotta, D. (1994). An overview of viral hepatitis: A through E. *AORN Journal, 59(5),* 997–998, 1000–1005.
25. Maddeux, M. S. (1989). The pharmacology and complications of immunosuppressive therapy. *Problems of General Surgery, 6(2),* 85–96.
26. Margolis, H. S. (1993). Prevention of acute and chronic liver disease through immunization: Hepatitis B and beyond. *Journal of Infectious Disease, 168(1),* 9–14.
27. Mayo Clinic Health Letter. (1994). Immunizations: They're not just for kids. *Mayo Clinic Health Letter. 12(10),* 6–7.
28. Meissner, J. E. (1994). Caring for patients with cirrhosis. *Nursing, 24(9),* 44–45.
29. Mosley, J. W., et al. (1990). Non-A, non-B hepatitis and antibody to hepatitis C virus. *Journal of the American Medical Association, 263,* 77–78.
30. Mudge, C., & Carlson, L. (1992). Hepatorenal syndrome. *AACN Clinical Issues in Critical Care Nursing, 4(1),* 131–148.
31. Muir, T. W. (1994). Exposure control plans define risks for bloodborne pathogen infections. *Occupational Health and Safety, 63(4),* 75–76.
32. Oberfield, R. A., et al. (1989). Liver cancer. *Ca: A Journal for Clinicians, 39,* 206–218.
33. Pons, P. T., & MacMath, T. L. (1984). Alcohol and the gastrointestinal and biliary systems. *Topics in Emergency Medicine, 6(2),* 58–65.
34. Quinless, F. W. (1985). Severe liver dysfunction: Client problems and nursing actions. *Focus on Critical Care, 12(1),* 24–32.
35. Ronk, L. L., & Girard, J. J. (1994). Risk perception, universal precautions compliance: A descriptive study of nurses who circulate. *AORN Journal, 59(1),* 253–254, 256–258.
36. Rosman, A. S., et al. (1993). Hepatitis C virus antibody in alcoholic patients: Association with the presence of portal and/or lobular hepatitis. *Archives of Internal Medicine. 153(8),* 965–969.
37. Sabiston, D. C., Jr. (1991). *Textbook of surgery: The biologic basis of modern surgical practice* (14th ed.). Philadelphia: W.B. Saunders.
38. Schiff, E. R. (1993). The patient with chronic hepatitis C . . . including commentary by Greenberger. *Hospital Practice, 28(8),* 25–33.
39. Smith, S. L., & Ciferni, M. L. (1992). Liver transplantation. *Critical Care Nursing Clinics of North America, 4(1),* 131–148.
40. Trifon, C. (1990). Importance of diagnosing alcoholic hepatitis. *Journal of The American Academy of Physicians Assistants, 3(4),* 243–252.
41. Vargo, R. L., & Rudy, E. B. (1989). Infection as a complication of liver transplant. *Critical Care Nurse, 9(4),* 52–62.

42. Werzberger, A., et al. (1992). A controlled trial of a formalin-inactivated hepatitis A vaccine in healthy children. *New England Journal of Medicine, 327*(7), 453–457.

43. Williams, B. A. H., et al. (1991). *Organ transplantation: A manual for nurses.* New York: Springer.

44. Wilson, B., et al (1994). *Nurses drug guide.* Norwalk, CT: Appleton & Lange.

45. Wyngaarden, J. B., et al. (Eds.). (1992). *Cecil textbook of medicine* (19th ed.). Philadelphia: W.B. Saunders.

46. Zakim, D., & Boyer, T. D. (Eds.). (1990). *Hepatology: A textbook of liver disease* (2nd ed.). Philadelphia: W.B. Saunders.

Chapter 38

Nursing Care of Clients with Biliary and Exocrine Pancreatic Disorders

Learning Outcomes

After completing this chapter, the learner will be able to:

1. Teach the client about the etiology, risk factors, pathophysiology, and clinical manifestations of abnormal biliary and exocrine pancreatic functions.
2. Explain to the client the differences between medical and surgical management of biliary and exocrine pancreatic disorders.
3. Explain the client's role in the medical and surgical management of biliary and exocrine pancreatic disorders.
4. Develop plans of care for the prevention of illness, management, and rehabilitation of clients with biliary and exocrine pancreatic disorders.
5. Implement nursing interventions that optimize the health status of clients with biliary and exocrine pancreatic disorders.
6. Evaluate planned client outcomes, using outcome criteria developed in the planning phase of care.

Biliary Disorders

CHOLELITHIASIS (GALLSTONES)

The biliary system is composed of the gallbladder, bile ducts, and the cystic duct. The cystic duct (from the gallbladder) joins with the hepatic duct (from the liver) to form the common bile duct. The function of the biliary system is to transport bile (secreted by the liver) from the gallbladder (where it is stored) into the duodenum.

Disorders of the gallbladder and ducts are extremely common. The two most common conditions are cholelithiasis (presence of gallstones) and associated cholecystitis (inflammation of the gallbladder). Approximately 98 per cent of clients who present with symptomatic gallbladder disease have gallstones. Malignancies and congenital anomalies of the biliary system are relatively uncommon.

The terms that are used in association with biliary tract conditions are presented in Table 38–1.

Incidence

It is estimated that 20 million people in the United States have gallstones, and that 475,000 cholecystectomies are performed every year. Studies show that the incidence of gallstones increases with age, as do the risks associated with cholelithiasis. Women account for nearly 70 per cent of those treated for gallstones, although studies have suggested that the mortality rate is higher in men. Twice as many white Americans are affected as black Americans.

Etiology

The etiology of gallstone disease is not well understood. Based on various theories, there are four possible explanations of stone formation.

TABLE 38–1 Biliary Tract Terminology

TERM	DEFINITION
Chole-	Pertaining to bile
Cholangi(o)-	Pertaining to bile ducts
Cholangiography	X-ray study of bile ducts
Cholangitis	Inflammation of bile duct
Cholecyst-	Pertaining to gallbladder
Cholecystectomy	Removal of gallbladder
Cholecystitis	Inflammation of the gallbladder
Cholecystography	X-ray study of gallbladder
Cholecystostomy	Incision & drainage of gallbladder
Choledocho-	Pertaining to common bile duct
Choledocholithiasis	Stones in common bile duct
Choledochostomy	Exploration of common bile duct
Cholelith-	Pertaining to gallstones
Cholelithiasis	Presence of gallstones
Cholescintigraphy	Radionuclide imaging of biliary system

First, bile may undergo a change in composition. Studies of clients with cholesterol gallstones indicate that their bile is supersaturated with cholesterol but deficient in bile salts. The cholesterol saturation of bile seems to increase with age. Changes in bile composition, however, do not completely explain why gallstones form.

Second, gallbladder stasis may lead to bile stasis. Bile stasis may (1) change bile composition, (2) supersaturate bile with cholesterol, and (3) precipitate some bile constituents. Gallbladder stasis may result from decreased contractility of the gallbladder and spasm of the sphincter of Oddi. Total parenteral nutrition without oral intake for longer than 1 month is associated with gallbladder sludge formation and cholelithiasis. Delayed emptying of the gallbladder may correlate with hormonal factors. This may explain why gallstones seem to be associated with pregnancy.

Third, infection may predispose a person to stone formation. Inflammatory debris can form a nidus (point of origin) for stone growth.

Finally, genetics also seems to play some role in stone formation, as evidenced by the prevalence of the condition in the Pima and Chippewa Indians.

Risk Factors

Conditions that predispose clients to gallstone formation include

- Diabetes mellitus
- Multiple pregnancies
- Vagotomy, a surgery that results in decreased gallbladder motility
- Ileal disease or resection, which results in bile salt depletion
- Long-term parenteral nutrition, which results in decreased gallbladder motility
- Cirrhosis of the liver
- Chronic hemolytic disorders, which result in increased bile pigments
- Obesity
- Exogenous estrogen administration
- Pancreatitis
- Caloric restriction with certain diets
- Clofibrate therapy (for treating hyperlipidemia)
- Cholestyramine therapy

Pathophysiology

Gallstones are generally divided into the following three groups: (1) cholesterol stones, (2) pigment stones, and (3) mixed stones. The incidence of a pure stone formation is rare, so stones are generally classified by the predominant constitution.

Cholesterol stones are the most common; the incidence of cholesterol stones increases with age and is greater in women. The stones are usually smooth and are whitish yellow to tan in color. *Pigment stones* are present in about 30 per cent of the clients with cholelithiasis in the United States. In these clients, the bile contains an excess of unconjugated bilirubin. *Mixed stones* may be a combination of cholesterol and pigment stones or either of these stones with some other substance. Calcium carbonate, phosphates, bile salts, and palmitates constitute the more common minor constituents of stones. Most gallstones are formed in the gallbladder but may also form in the common duct or hepatic ducts of the liver. Some stones do not cause symptoms and pass through the ducts into the bowel unnoticed.

Once a client becomes symptomatic, treatment and follow-up are essential to prevent progression to a more severe, and sometimes fatal, complication of gallbladder disease. Approximately one third of these complications are due to free perforation, which occurs when a gangrenous area becomes necrotic and bile breaks into the peritoneal cavity, causing peritonitis. Pericholecystic abscess accounts for 50 per cent of the complications and is the least severe, with a mortality rate of approximately 15 per cent. Abscess formation occurs while the perforation is walled off by omentum or adjacent organs such as the colon, stomach, or duodenum.

Clinical Manifestations

Manifestations of biliary system disorders are similar to those of a number of other conditions. Box 38–1 lists some of the more common diseases that must be differentiated from acute and chronic cholecystitis.

Fewer than half of the clients with gallstones report any distress, because gallstones cause no symptoms unless complications develop. The primary symptom is pain or biliary colic. This pain usually follows the temporary obstruction of the gallbladder outlet. Characteristically, the pain starts in the upper midline area. It may radiate around to the back and right shoulder blade, although some clients complain that it passes straight through to the back and substernal areas.

The client is often restless, changing positions frequently to relieve the pain's intensity. Pain may persist for only a few hours or several days and the interval between attacks is variable.

Jaundice only appears when common duct obstruction is present. If the stone is blocking the cystic duct, the client may develop signs of acute cholecystitis (see the section on acute cholecystitis). If the stone lodges in the common duct, gallstones may be complicated by cholangitis (inflammation of the bile ducts) and pancreatitis.

Nausea and vomiting may occur, and occasionally, self-induced vomiting alleviates the symptoms. Assessment may further reveal a history of flatulence, bloating, dyspepsia, belching, an intolerance of fatty foods, and vague upper abdominal sensations. Often, clients who have these problems still have them after cholecystectomy.

Assessment of these clients becomes important in light of the fact that symptoms of biliary colic and coronary artery disease are remarkably similar. Considering the prevalence of both these problems, accurate diagnosis is essential.

Many times, the diagnosis is made based on the symptoms alone. Physical findings are present only during an attack with pain, with pain being the cardinal symptom. The right upper quadrant or epigastric area is tender to palpation with voluntary muscle guarding, but signs of peritonitis are absent. The gallbladder is not palpable, and the temperature is normal.

BOX 38–1

Disorders with Symptoms Similar to Those of Chronic and Acute Cholecystitis

CHRONIC CHOLECYSTITIS

- Angina pectoris
- Chronic pancreatitis
- Esophagitis
- Hiatal hernia
- Peptic ulcer
- Pyelonephritis
- Spastic colitis

ACUTE CHOLECYSTITIS

- Acute appendicitis
- Acute hepatitis
- Acute myocardial infarction
- Acute pancreatitis
- Acute pyelonephritis
- Intercostal neuritis
- Intestinal obstruction
- Perforated ulcer
- Pleurisy
- Renal calculus
- Right lower lobe pneumonia

DIAGNOSTIC ASSESSMENT

Blood test results are unremarkable. Jaundice is not present unless there is common duct obstruction. Diagnosis of cholelithiasis may involve abdominal ultrasonography, computerized axial tomography, cholescintography, cholangiography, cholecystography, or rarely, biliary drainage examination.

Current trends, however, point to the use of endoscopic retrograde cholangiopancreatography and endoscopic retrograde catheterization of the gallbladder in diagnoses. Refer to Chapter 36 for a discussion of these procedures. Biliary ultrasonography (cholecystosonography) may be the initial study because it is accurate and safe, does not use radiation, and can be performed without preparation.

Medical Management

For clients with symptomatic cholelithiasis, treatment is dictated by the severity of symptoms. An oral analgesic may be prescribed, and the client may be instructed to avoid those foods that precipitated the attack. It may mean hospitalization and

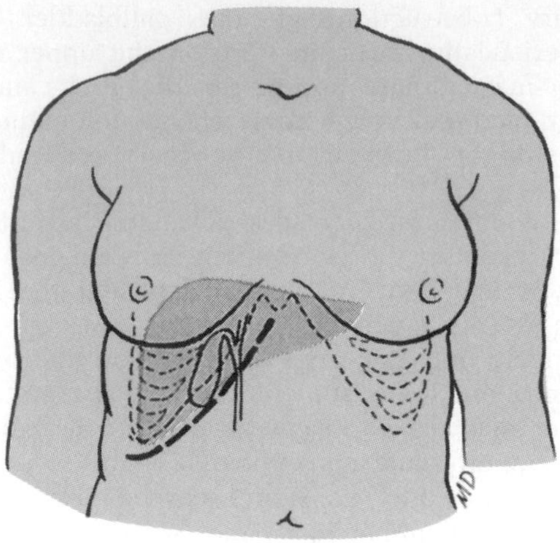

Figure 38–1
Right subcostal incision.

- administration of parenteral analgesics for the discomfort of biliary colic (nitroglycerin may reduce colic as well)
- insertion of a nasogastric tube for the symptomatic relief of vomiting or for those who have probable pancreatitis
- maintenance of fluid and electrolyte balance with intravenous fluids
- monitoring for progression of abdominal complications, which may include bile duct obstruction, cholangitis, pancreatitis, acute calculous cholecystitis, and subsequent sepsis and death

Retrograde endoscopy for stone removal is an important nonsurgical alternative. To remove a gallstone from the common bile duct, the physician passes an endoscope through the throat into the duodenum, then passes a wire snare into the common bile duct through the ampulla of Vater, securing and removing the obstructing stone. If stones remain in the common bile duct after cholecystectomy and a T-tube is still in place, the physician may pass a stone-retrieving basket or other device through the T-tube tract to remove the stone.

Another important nonsurgical intervention is the use of oral administration of dissolution agents for cholesterol gallstones. Ursodeoxycholic acid (ursodiol) has become widely used because it is effective and produces no side effects. It acts by reducing the amount of cholesterol in bile.

Surgical Management

Whether or not to operate on a client with asymptomatic cholelithiasis (silent gallstones) is another area for debate and involves the question of when prophylactic gallbladder removal is appropriate. The potential for serious complications (e.g., acute cholecystitis; choledocholithiasis, sepsis) can pose a significant risk. Elderly clients and people with insulin-dependent diabetes have a high incidence of gallstones. Because such people are at high risk during acute biliary attacks and emergency procedures, surgeons recommend that they undergo elective cholecystectomy to avoid later emergency surgery.

CHOLECYSTECTOMY

Cholecystectomy consists of excising the gallbladder through a right subcostal incision (Fig. 38–1). Common duct exploration may also occur through this incision site, if necessary. When stones are suspected in the common duct, an operative cholangiography may be performed (if it was not ordered preoperatively). Also, the surgeon may dilate the common duct if it is not already dilated as a result of a pathologic process. This facilitates stone removal. The surgeon passes a fine instrument into the ducts to collect the stones, either whole or after crushing them.

Following exploration of the common duct, the surgeon usually inserts a T-tube to ensure adequate bile drainage during duct healing. The T-tube also provides a route for postoperative cholangiography or stone dissolution, when appropriate. Inserting a T-tube also prevents bile from spilling into the peritoneal cavity and maintains patency of the duct (Fig. 38–2). T-tubes can be attached to continuous-gravity drainage bags or to collapsible bags in the dressing site.

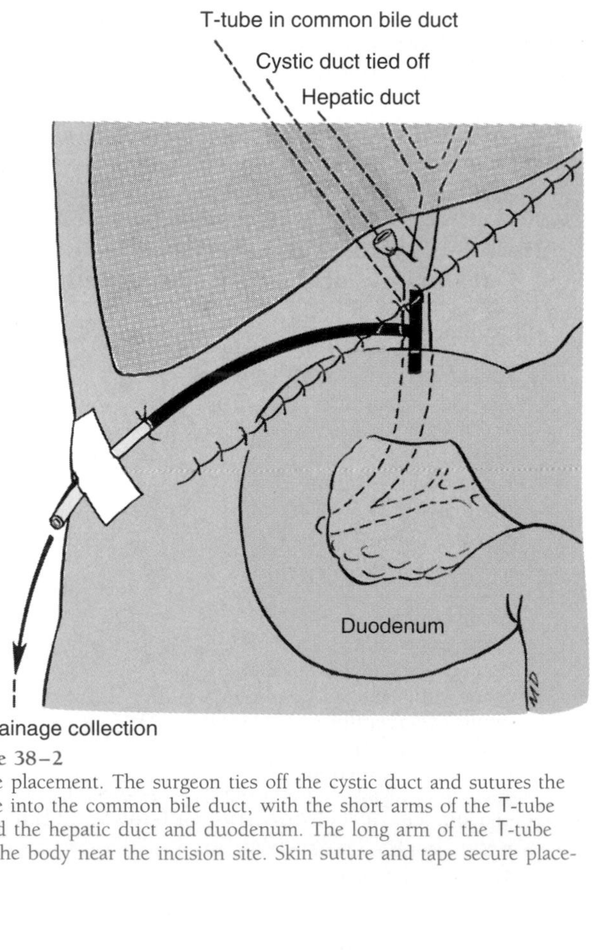

Figure 38–2
T-tube placement. The surgeon ties off the cystic duct and sutures the T-tube into the common bile duct, with the short arms of the T-tube toward the hepatic duct and duodenum. The long arm of the T-tube exits the body near the incision site. Skin suture and tape secure placement.

Following cholecystectomy, the client should be monitored for the usual postoperative complications, such as hemorrhage, pneumonia, thrombophlebitis, urinary retention, and ileus. The risk of bile leakage into the abdominal cavity is more specific for surgeries that involve the gallbladder. With hemorrhage and bile leakage, the client feels severe pain and tenderness in the right upper quadrant, abdominal girth increases, bile or blood may leak from the wound, blood pressure drops, and tachycardia develops.

Cholecystectomy is the most common surgical intervention for gallstones. However, changes in medical care reimbursement have initiated the innovation of laparoscopic cholecystectomy. Certain criteria are used to determine which clients are good candidates for the procedure. Clients are usually admitted for a 23-hour stay.

Risks from this procedure include hemorrhage, bile duct injury, and injury to other organs. However, the advantages of small scars and a short hospital stay have influenced the increased use of this procedure. Although the possible postoperative complications are the same as with traditional cholecystectomy, clients who undergo this procedure are at lesser risk because they are ambulatory sooner and usually require only oral analgesia.

EXTRACORPOREAL SHOCK WAVE LITHOTRIPSY

Extracorporeal shock wave lithotripsy may be used in a selected group of clients. Minor complications may include ecchymosis over the area of entry of the shock waves, gross hematuria through microscopic hematuria because of the close proximity of the right kidney, and biliary pain when large fragments pass through the cystic duct.

PERCUTANEOUS CHOLECYSTOLITHOTOMY

With a percutaneous cholecystolithotomy, surgeons extract stones using cystoscopes, stone baskets, and instruments designed for nephrolithotomy. Stones too large to extract manually can be fragmented using a lithotriptor or laser fiber. General anesthesia is not necessary for this procedure.

Nursing Management

Assessment

The nurse's assessment should focus on collecting subjective and objective data and noting the client's response to ordered therapeutics (i.e., analgesics). The client's knowledge of the diagnostic process also should be assessed.

The client should be closely monitored for symptoms of obstruction from the gallstones. Vital signs should be checked at regular intervals to note inflammation associated with the stones.

Generally, surgical management for cholelithiasis is elective and is not performed in an emergency situation, unless obstruction has occurred. The client should be assessed, however, for knowledge of preoperative and postoperative care.

Nursing Diagnosis, Planning, and Implementation

Nursing Diagnosis: Pain R/T biliary spasms.

Planning: Expected Outcomes. The client will demonstrate an absence or a decrease in pain, as evidenced by verbalizing that pain is absent or decreased and by resting quietly.

Implementation. The nurse should administer pain medications as ordered and document and report effectiveness of the medication. Meperidine (Demerol) is the drug most frequently ordered. Nitroglycerin may be ordered sublingually to relax smooth muscle and, thereby, decrease colic.

Other comfort measures may be helpful. Providing a quiet environment and using relaxation techniques such as a backrub or positioning may promote rest and enhance the effects of the analgesics given.

Nursing Diagnosis: Fluid Volume Deficit, Risk for R/T vomiting and nasogastric suctioning.

Planning: Expected Outcomes. The client will maintain adequate hydration, as evidenced by normal skin turgor, moist oral mucous membranes, and urinary output equal to or greater than 30 mL/hr.

Implementation. If the client continues vomiting, the nurse should obtain an order for a nasogastric tube with a suction attachment to relieve distention and vomiting. Suction also removes the gastric juices that stimulate cholecystokinin, which causes painful contractions of the gallbladder.

The nurse should administer intravenous fluids as ordered and assess and document intake and output, communicating discrepancies to the physician. The nurse assesses the client for signs of dehydration, such as dry mucous membranes, poor skin turgor, and urinary output less than 30 mL/hr. For a detailed discussion of fluid and electrolyte imbalances and nasogastric suction, see Chapters 3 and 32.

Nursing Diagnosis: Knowledge Deficit R/T treatment modalities and diagnostic procedures.

Planning: Expected Outcomes. The client will indicate understanding of therapeutics and diagnostics, as evidenced by verbalizing understanding and decreased anxiety.

Implementation. The nurse must consider the client's pain and give explanations that are simple and direct when the client is the most comfortable, if possible. The nurse should provide simple and concise written information or films as well as verbal instruction, if appropriate.

Nursing Diagnosis: Knowledge Deficit R/T surgery and recovery.

Planning: Expected Outcomes. The client will indicate understanding, as evidenced by ability to verbalize information regarding the surgical procedure; ability to demonstrate accurate coughing, deep breathing, and leg exercises; and ability to verbalize information given regarding immediate postoperative course.

Implementation. The nurse should reinforce information given to the client regarding the surgical procedure. Verbal instruction and demonstration are necessary to ensure that the client can perform postoperative exercises (turning, coughing, deep breathing, and wound splinting) accurately as well as understand their importance.

The client also needs to have some knowledge of what to expect postoperatively (e.g., intravenous fluids; T-tube placement and drainage, if applicable; and pain control and activity).

Collaborative Problem: Injury, Risk for R/T postoperative complications of hemorrhage, infection, fluid and electrolyte imbalance, pulmonary changes (atelectasis, pneumonia), urine retention, ileus, decreased gastrointestinal (GI) motility.

Planning: Expected Outcomes. The client will receive appropriate assessments and interventions for early detection and prevention of injury from postoperative complications, as evidenced by stable vital signs; normal pulmonary function; normal GI function; laboratory values within normal limits; normal urinary function, which returns within 6 to 8 hours postoperatively; an intact incision that does not exhibit redness, odor, or purulent drainage; and no signs of thrombus or embolus.

Implementation. When a T-tube has been inserted, the nurse measures the drainage from it. The T-tube usually drains 300 to 500 mL in the first 24 hours. This amount decreases to less than 200 mL after 3 to 4 days. The nurse records the color and the volume of the drainage. Excessive drainage may indicate obstruction. Excessive bile losses may necessitate recycling the client's bile drainage. The bile can be returned through a nasogastric tube or orally in a medium such as fruit juice.

After a few days, the nurse will probably clamp the T-tube during meals to aid fat digestion. When a T-tube cholangiogram indicates an absence of obstruction, the surgeon may decide to remove the T-tube. If a retained stone is discovered, the client may go home with the T-tube in place with removal planned for a later date.

Nursing Diagnosis: Pain R/T surgical procedure and incision.

Planning: Expected Outcomes. The client will verbalize feelings of comfort, have blood pressure and heart rate within normal limits, and show ability to tolerate postoperative exercises and activities.

Implementation. The nurse should assess and document the level, location, and type of pain, as well as the client's response to pain medication. It may be necessary to administer medication to coincide with activity to keep the client active. Nonpharmacologic comfort measures are helpful as well. The nurse must be sure to assist the client in splinting the incision and to instruct the client on the best way to get out of bed and lie down (see Client Education Guide: Cholelithiasis).

CLIENT EDUCATION GUIDE

Cholelithiasis

PREVENTION OF CHOLELITHIASIS

- Consider risk factors (diet, weight, multiple pregnancies, diseases that affect gallbladder function)
- Maintain weight reduction and control
- Adopt a low-fat diet (avoid fried foods, meats, dairy products, and dessert foods)

DISCHARGE TEACHING

After an episode of cholecystitis, the nurse should teach the client about:

- etiology of the inflammation and what the client can do to avoid future episodes; e.g., lose weight and increase exercise
- action, doses, and expected side effects of prescribed medications (such as antibiotics or analgesics)
- signs and symptoms of recurrence and the need to report jaundice, dark-colored urine, pale-colored stools, and pruritus

After a laparoscopic cholecystectomy, the nurse should teach about:

- the need for rest and sleep
- activity progression (such as how soon driving and physical exercise may be resumed)
- the possibility of some fat being tolerated; the client may be able to tolerate certain foods and not others; the response is highly individual
- comfort measures for pain (such as a quiet, dim environment, small frequent meals, avoidance of constipation, sleep position, etc.)
- wound care: how to change a dressing, if indicated; progress of healing
- signs and symptoms of infection (fever, malaise, redness, drainage, odor in the area of the wound)
- the importance of follow-up care via postoperative appointment with the physician

After an abdominal cholecystectomy, the nurse should teach:

- all of the above, along with dressing changes and T-tube care: why the T-tube is retained, how to care for the site, how to observe the drainage (include color, amount, odor), and who to call for questions during recovery.

Nursing Diagnosis: Oral Mucous Membranes, Altered R/T NPO status, intubation, and nasogastric suctioning.

Planning: Expected Outcomes. The client will maintain normal oral mucosa, as evidenced by intact, moist oral cavity and verbalizing of decreased or absent discomfort.

Implementation. Oral care should be offered at least every 2 hours while the client is taking nothing by mouth (NPO). The oral mucous membranes should be assessed at least every 8 hours for their integrity, color, and moistness. While the client is NPO, it may be helpful to place a wet washcloth over the lips to humidify the air as he or she breathes. Ice chips or sips of liquid as soon as allowed will also provide much relief.

Evaluation

The client will be evaluated based on the expected outcomes. If the outcomes are not achieved, the plan and implementations should be revised.

Modification of Plan of Care for the Elderly

CRITICAL TO REMEMBER

Gallstones in the elderly may not cause pain, fever, or jaundice. Mental confusion, shakiness, and an elevated alkaline phosphatase may be the only manifestations.

Nonsurgical decompression techniques may be preferred in high risk elderly clients.

When the older client has a cholecystectomy, he or she is at greater risk for injury related to anesthesia, pain medications, and sometimes, the response to the trauma of surgery. Postoperative care should be modified to prevent this injury. Especially in the immediate postoperative period, the side rails should be up, the bed in low position, and the call light within easy reach.

Depending on the older client's response to anesthesia and pain medication, frequent reorientation to the environment and circumstances may be necessary. The nurse should remind the older client how to summon help and why it is important that he or she does not get up alone. The nurse should be sure that all intravenous lines and drain tubes are secure to prevent the client from inadvertently disconnecting or dislodging them.

In particular, older adults have a tendency to become confused following surgery (especially at night), so the nurse must be alert to this possibility and may need to take precautions, such as use of soft wrist or vest restraints or a device such as a bed-check machine, which is placed under the client and sounds an alarm if it senses that weight is no longer on it.

ACUTE CHOLECYSTITIS

Acute cholecystitis is acute inflammation of the gallbladder wall.

Incidence

There is an increased incidence of cholecystitis in clients who are overweight, especially those with sedentary lifestyles. Certain ethnic groups, including Chinese, Jews, and Italians, also have a higher rate of the disease.

Etiology

The exact etiology of cholecystitis is unknown. Gallstones are a major cause of acute cholecystitis along with anything that affects normal gallbladder function or affects the blood supply to the organ. Anatomic abnormalities such as kinking or twisting of the bile ducts can lead to acute disease.

Risk Factors

The major preventable risk factors are sedentary lifestyle and obesity. If the client increases his or her level of activity and maintains a low-fat diet, the risk of cholecystitis can be reduced.

Pathophysiology

Acute calculous cholecystitis is a common complication of cholelithiasis. In fact, calculous cholecystitis accounts for 95 per cent of all cases. It appears to be caused by obstruction of the cystic duct, which, in turn, causes distention of the gallbladder. Subsequently, (1) venous and lymphatic drainage is impaired, (2) proliferation of bacteria occurs, (3) localized cellular irritation and/or infiltration takes place, and (4) areas of ischemia may develop. The inflamed gallbladder wall is edematous and thickened, and may have areas of gangrene or necrosis.

Complications of untreated acute cholecystitis are usually associated with septic complications. Others are consequences of ischemia and gangrene: perforation, pericholecystic abscess, and fistula.

Acalculous cholecystitis (cholecystitis without stones) is far less common than cholecystitis due to gallstones.

Clinical Manifestations

Inflammation of the gallbladder may be an acute or a chronic process. The most common and reliable finding on physical examination is tenderness in the right upper quadrant, epigastrium, or both.

Pain in acute cholecystitis may be located in the epigastric, subscapular, or right upper quadrant area. Sometimes, the pain is referred to the right scapula. The pain usually starts suddenly, steadily increases, and reaches a peak in about 30 minutes. During examination of the abdomen, extreme tenderness often causes the client to guard the upper right quadrant. When palpating the right subcostal area, the nurse should ask the client to take a deep breath. If the client experiences extreme tenderness and stops breathing on inspiration, Murphy's sign has been elicited. About 75 per cent of clients with acute cholecystitis have experienced biliary colic episodes in the past.

In addition to pain, assessment of clients with acute cholecystitis reveals the following problems:

- Nausea and vomiting occur in 60 to 70 per cent of the clients.
- Approximately 80 per cent of all clients have an elevated temperature, but this may be absent in the elderly, immunocompromised clients, and those on steroidal therapy.
- Mild jaundice occurs in only 10 per cent of the cases.

See the Clinical Manifestations box for a summary of assessment data for cholecystitis and cholelithiasis.

DIAGNOSTIC ASSESSMENT

Diagnostic examinations for acute cholecystitis include the following:

- Biliary ultrasonography is often the initial diagnostic procedure that may reveal abnormalities of the structure of the biliary system or cholelithiasis.
- Aminotransferase, alkaline phosphatase, and sulfobromophthalein parameters may be slightly abnormal.
- An abdominal x-ray study occasionally reveals the enlarged gallbladder.
- Radionuclide imaging (cholescintigraphy) can provide additional information (when the diagnosis is clinically obscure) by pinpointing cystic duct obstruction. Confirmation is based on nonvisualization of the gallbladder.
- The white blood cell count is elevated in 85 per cent of clients, with the exception of the elderly or those on steroidal therapy.

Refer to Chapter 36 for a discussion of other diagnostic techniques.

Medical Management

Clients suspected of having acute cholecystitis should be hospitalized, and initial management should include administration of antibiotics effective against organisms found in the bile in approximately 80 per cent of the clients. These organisms include both gram-positive and gram-negative aerobes and anaerobes: *Escherichia coli, Klebsiella aerogenes, Streptococcus faecalis, Clostridium welchii, Proteus* species, *Enterobacter* species, and anaerobic streptococci.

Further medical management is the same as for symptomatic cholelithiasis (see the section on cholelithiasis).

Surgical Management

Once the diagnosis of acute cholecystitis is made, the decision for early or delayed cholecystectomy depends on the risk factors, for example, the presence of diseases such as unstable angina, significant carotid artery disease, congestive heart failure, and cirrhosis.

Cholecystectomy for acute cholecystitis is more difficult than elective surgery because of the distended gallbladder. Usually, the gallbladder must be decompressed first to allow complete visualization of all surrounding structures and avoid injury to the extrahepatic bile ducts.

Cholecystotomy is usually performed only when cholecystectomy is too dangerous given all the risk factors. The treatment of the complications of cholecystotomy is usually cholecystectomy.

Nursing Management

Assessment of these clients becomes extremely important because several other disease entities may produce the same symptoms (see Table 38–1). The nurse collects subjective and objective data and notes the client's response to ordered therapeutics. The nursing care plan is the same as for medical management of cholelithiasis

CLINICAL MANIFESTATIONS

Cholecystitis and Cholelithiasis

Assessment Data	Pathophysiologic Basis
Abdominal pain, most commonly right upper quadrant or epigastric; often radiates to back	In cholelithiasis, ductal spasm when a stone moves from gallbladder into ducts may cause waves of pain (biliary colic) In cholecystitis, pain may be steady (because of inflammation) and increases in severity with peritoneal extension
Nausea and vomiting	Distention of bile ducts initiates impulses to vomiting center
Fat intolerance	Contraction of inflamed gallbladder to release bile to digest fat often precipitates pain
Fever and leukocytosis	Response to inflammation
Jaundice	In cholelithiasis, obstruction to common bile duct causes increased serum bilirubin In cholecystitis, edema sometimes obstructs the duct enough to increase bilirubin levels

except that it is certain these clients will receive a course of antibiotics. The client should be observed for the development of complications. For more information on nursing management, see the section on nursing management for surgical intervention in cholelithiasis.

ACUTE ACALCULOUS CHOLECYSTITIS

Acute acalculous (absence of stones) cholecystitis accounts for approximately 4 to 8 per cent of all cases of acute cholecystitis. Although pain is the cardinal symptom in the calculous type, it may be obscured or absent in acalculous cholecystitis because of narcotic administration, decreased level of consciousness, or abdominal pain from an incision or other disease process. Significant physical findings are the same as those of acute calculous cholecystitis, and the same diagnostic procedures are used.

The standard treatment is emergency cholecystectomy because of the increased risk of gangrene and perforation.

CHRONIC CHOLECYSTITIS

Chronic cholecystitis sometimes arises as a sequela to acute cholecystitis. Typically, however, it develops independently of acute cholecystitis. In addition, it is almost always associated with gallstones. Chronic cholecystitis principally affects middle-aged and older obese women. The female-to-male ratio is 3 : 1.

Assessment data for chronic cholecystitis are similar to those for acute cholecystitis with certain exceptions. In chronic states, (1) the pain is less severe, (2) the temperature is not as high, and (3) the leukocyte count is lower. Vague symptoms of dyspepsia, fat intolerance, heartburn, and flatulence accompany chronic cholecystitis. The client has usually experienced these manifestations for a long time as well as repeated attacks (mild or severe) of acute cholecystitis. Eventually fibrous tissues begin to replace the normal muscle and mucosal tissues of the gallbladder. As a consequence, the gallbladder loses its ability to concentrate bile.

Diagnosis of chronic cholecystitis largely depends on ultrasonography. Other diagnostic procedures provide supplementary information. Diagnostic findings include

- Cholelithiasis
- Gallbladder wall thickening (greater than 3 mm)
- Delayed visualization or nonvisualization of the gallbladder on radionuclide scanning. Scarring from chronic inflammation may partially or completely obstruct the cystic duct and thus account for this delay.

It may be difficult to differentiate chronic cholecystitis from other disorders. Conditions that mimic the manifestations of cholecystitis (acute and chronic) appear in Table 38–1. The diagnostic process serves to rule out these conditions.

Conservative interventions include a low-fat diet, weight reduction, and administration of anticholinergics, sedatives, and antacids. When medical intervention is ineffective, cholecystectomy may be the treatment of choice. About 90 per cent of clients obtain relief of symptoms after cholecystectomy. Ninety-five per cent of removed gallbladders contain stones.

CARCINOMA OF THE GALLBLADDER

Although cancer of the gallbladder is the most common malignant lesion of the biliary tract, it accounts for only 5 per cent of all cancers at the time of autopsy. Of all clients who develop this malignancy, 91 per cent are over the age of 50 and the incidence in women is three to four times that in men. However, the incidence of bile duct cancer is higher in men. Native Americans, Hispanics, Inuit, northeastern Europeans, Israelis, and Japanese immigrants to the United States are at greatest risk of developing cancer of the gallbladder. At least 70 per cent of these clients have gallstones. Adenocarcinoma accounts for 82 per cent of all cases.

The clinical presentation differs depending on the stage of the disease. There is no distinct pattern because the symptoms are dependent on the site of the lesion, its extent, and the presence or absence of pre-existing biliary symptoms.

The prognosis of cancer of the gallbladder is poor. About 88 per cent of clients die within the first year, and only about 4 per cent are alive within 5 years. Treatment varies from radical resection, to palliative relief of duct obstruction, to chemotherapy or radiation.

Disorders of the Exocrine Pancreas

A client with a pancreatic disorder may have problems with both digestion and glucose use. The following sections include a discussion of exocrine illness. See Chapter 39 for coverage of hormonal disorders. Measures used to diagnose disorders of the pancreas include various laboratory and radiographic studies.

ACUTE PANCREATITIS

Acute pancreatitis is an inflammation of the pancreas that may result in autodigestion of the pancreas by its own enzymes.

Incidence

Pancreatitis, or inflammation of the pancreas, may be acute or chronic. Acute pancreatitis is a fairly common but potentially lethal inflammatory process that results in varying degrees of pancreatic edema, fat necrosis, and hemorrhage. Typically, the manifestations of acute pancreatitis disappear once causative factors are eliminated. Nine out of ten clients experience the disease with mild to moderate symptoms and improve with supportive care. Conversely, in one out of ten clients, the condition evolves into a severe life-threatening form of acute pancreatitis. Studies have revealed that the late complication of multisystem organ failure and pancreatic abscess contributed to most of the deaths. Pulmonary edema and congestion are also contributory factors to the mortality rate.

Etiology

In 90 per cent of the cases of acute pancreatitis, the cause is related to excessive alcohol intake or biliary tract disease. Alcohol abuse is the major cause of acute pancreatitis in urban areas of the United States. In other areas of the United States, Asia, and Europe, gallstone-associated pancreatitis is predominant.

Risk Factors

Alcohol abuse is a high-risk factor for the development of pancreatitis. Avoidance of alcohol is the best way to decrease the risk of the disease. The other major risk factors are cholecystitis and cholelithiasis.

Pathophysiology

The precise mechanism that causes pancreatic damage remains unclear. The pathologic changes occurring in the pancreas may be due to premature activation of proteolytic and lipolytic pancreatic enzymes. These enzymes are normally activated in the duodenum. In pancreatitis, however, the activation of the proteases and lipases occurs prior to secretion into the intestine. This causes tissue damage in the pancreas.

Exactly how the enzymes become active in the pancreas is unknown, but they may be triggered by reflux of bile from the duodenum into the pancreatic duct or by pancreatic duct obstruction. The net effect of this enzymatic activation is autodigestion of the pancreas. Once pancreatic inflammation begins, a vicious circle continues the process of further tissue damage and enzyme activation. As the process becomes chronic, destruction of pancreatic parenchyma occurs.

The clinical course of up to 90 per cent of clients with acute pancreatitis follows a self-limited pattern. However, in 10 to 15 per cent of clients, a severe form of illness develops that requires a lengthy hospitalization, complications, and significant rates of morbidity and mortality. These clients present a major medical challenge by requiring an intensive care setting, hemodynamic monitoring, and frequent laboratory and radiographic evaluation.

Clinical Manifestations

Symptoms in clients presenting with acute pancreatitis can vary from mild nonspecific abdominal pain to profound shock with coma and ultimate death. The predominant clinical feature is abdominal pain, which normally begins in the midepigastrium and achieves maximal intensity several hours into the illness. In most clients, the pain has a penetrating quality, which radiates to the back (see Clinical Manifestations: Acute Pancreatitis).

Physical examination typically reveals fever, tachycardia, epigastric tenderness, and abdominal distention. Severe hemorrhagic pancreatitis may produce two dis-

CLINICAL MANIFESTATIONS

Acute Pancreatitis

Assessment Data	Pathophysiologic Basis
Extreme epigastric or umbilical pain, extending into back and flank	Edematous distention of pancreatic capsule; local peritonitis due to enzyme release into peritoneum; ductal spasm, or pancreatic autodigestion stimulated by increased enzyme secretion while eating
Persistent vomiting	Pain stimulates vomiting center; intestinal peristalsis reduced because of localized peritonitis
Abdominal distention, fever	Paralytic ileus of small bowel loop due to localized peritonitis
Shock and cardiac dysfunction	Release of pyrogens by tissue breakdown
	Hypovolemia caused by the loss of fluid into the retroperitoneal space and decreased preload into the heart, the release of kinins that cause peripheral vasodilation and increased vascular permeability and toxemia
Hypocalcemia, usually mild, although tetany is possible	Calcium may be deposited in areas of fat necrosis; undigested intestinal fat traps calcium in feces
Impaired glucose tolerance	Some degree of islet involvement
Jaundice	Common bile duct obstruction by pancreatic edema
Pleural effusion	Spread of inflammation into surrounding tissues

tinctive signs: Turner's sign (bluish discoloration of the left flank) and Cullen's sign (bluish discoloration of the periumbilical area).

Clients with severe pancreatitis may exhibit severe circulatory complications such as hypotension, hypovolemia, hypoperfusion, and obtundation. As many as one third of the clients have evidence of left pleural effusion or left hemidiaphragmatic elevation.

Other clinical findings include subcutaneous fat necrosis and cerebral abnormalities such as belligerence, confusion, psychosis, and coma. It is speculated that the cerebral abnormalities are caused by hyperosmolality, hypoperfusion, hypoxia, cerebral fat embolism, or disseminated intravascular coagulopathy. Transient hyperglycemia is found in 50 per cent of the clients, probably as a result of damage to the islets. Hypocalcemia occurs in up to 30 per cent.

DIAGNOSTIC ASSESSMENT

Serum amylase is the most widely used test in the diagnosis of pancreatitis; however, the absence of hyperamylasemia does not exclude the diagnosis. The absence of hyperamylasemia may reflect extensive pancreatic necrosis or the failure of a chronically diseased gland. In most cases, hyperamylasemia is seen within 24 hours of the onset of symptoms and resolves within 7 days. If hyperamylasemia persists, it may indicate the development of complications.

The measurement of urinary amylase has been indicated as a sensitive index of the disease. Urinary amylase elevations persist for a longer period of time. Again, however, hyperamylasuria is not a true indicator of acute pancreatitis.

The elevation of serum lipase is a more accurate indicator of acute pancreatitis because lipase is solely of pancreatic origin. Also, the duration of hyperlipasemia often exceeds that of hyperamylasemia. However, hyperlipasemia may be seen in perforated peptic ulcer, acute cholecystitis, and intestinal ischemia.

Serum lipase is one of the most specific tests for acute pancreatitis. Serum lipase may be elevated in clients with hereditary hyperlipidemia-associated pancreatitis or in alcohol-induced pancreatitis.

Additionally, a white blood cell count above 10,000 cells/mm^3 is common; also, hyperglycemia, mild azotemia, abnormal liver function tests, and hypocalcemia may be present.

Chest film findings are supportive but not specific for acute pancreatitis.

Although no findings on upper GI series are specific for acute pancreatitis, the studies may reveal widening of the duodenal loop and anterior displacement of the stomach.

Ultrasonography can be used to detect pancreatic edema and acute peripancreatic fluid collections but may be limited by the presence of air and fluid-filled loops of bowel.

Nearly all acute pancreatitis clients have some abnormality on computed tomographic (CT) scan. Pancreatic changes include parenchymal enlargement, edema, or necrosis. A CT scan is also helpful in identifying other structural changes that develop, such as pancreatic pseudocyst, abscess, or phlegmon. A magnetic resonance imaging study reveals the same information as computed tomography.

Medical Management

Acute pancreatitis is commonly associated with massive fluid isolation. Fluids can accumulate in the bowel secondary to ileus or in the peripancreatic region because of edema. Fluids also can be lost in the form of emesis. Therefore, an essential first step in the management of these clients is replacing lost body fluids, correcting hypovolemia, and restoring electrolyte balance. In clients with pre-existing cardiac, pulmonary, or renal disease, or in clients with severe pancreatitis, invasive monitoring, including urinary catheterization, central venous pressure monitoring, or monitoring of cardiac output and filling via a Swan-Ganz catheter, is indicated.

Those with severe hemorrhagic pancreatitis may require blood transfusions or transfusion of clotting factors to correct abnormal coagulation problems.

Often, a variety of electrolyte abnormalities are encountered. Clients with severe and persistent vomiting may require saline solutions containing potassium chloride. Serum calcium may be depressed secondary to hypoalbuminemia.

Respiratory complications may require supportive measures such as oxygen administration and physical therapy, or the lesser supportive measures such as endotracheal intubation and positive pressure ventilation.

Treatment may involve attempts to suppress pancreatic exocrine function. Therapy to decrease these enzymes may include nasogastric suction, or administration of histamine H_2-receptor antagonists, antacids, anticholinergics, glucagon, calcitonin, somatostatin, and proglumide.

It may be necessary to perform peritoneal dialysis to rid the peritoneum of potentially toxic compounds commonly found in exudate from acute pancreatitis.

PHARMACOLOGIC MANAGEMENT

Pain is usually treated with administration of narcotic analgesics, with meperidine being the drug of choice. Morphine is contraindicated because it may cause spasm of the sphincter of Oddi, which could then potentiate ongoing pancreatic parenchymal injury.

Antibiotics, in theory, are not necessary in most mild to moderate cases. However, prophylactic antibiotics may be ordered, particularly in the more severe cases of pancreatitis.

DIETARY MANAGEMENT

Oral intake is prohibited initially but generally can be resumed once abdominal pain and tenderness have improved. Caution must be taken because premature return to oral intake has been associated with the development of pancreatic abscess and reactivation of pancreatic inflammation. Clients with severe cases may need to be supported nutritionally by the parenteral route. Administration of carbohydrate-based and amino acid–based solutions along with lipids as a source of calories may be necessary.

Surgical Management

Operative intervention is indicated in four specific circumstances:

- uncertainty of diagnosis
- treatment of pancreatic sepsis
- correction of associated biliary tract disease
- progressive clinical deterioration despite optimal supportive care

Following pancreatic excision, the nurse should find out how much pancreatic tissue was removed. When there is a decrease in endocrine tissue, control of blood sugar with insulin and diet becomes necessary. Exocrine loss does not pose immediate postoperative problems but will necessitate life-long enzyme replacement when the client returns to oral food ingestion.

COMPLICATIONS

It was discussed previously how difficult it may be to diagnose acute pancreatitis and to exclude other potentially fatal diagnoses. When such a condition exists, exploratory laparotomy is indicated to eliminate processes such as perforated viscus or acute mesenteric ischemia. Then if uncomplicated acute pancreatitis is present, no manipulation is needed and the surgery is terminated.

Treatment of pancreatic abscess combines antibiotic therapy and surgical drainage. Operative débridement is necessary to remove the thick, debris-filled, pastelike collections of infected necrotic material.

Correction of Associated Biliary Tract Disease. Formerly, biliary tract surgery for gallstone-associated pancreatitis was deferred for up to 8 weeks. However, up to 50 per cent of clients awaiting elective surgery had a recurrence of pancreatitis. Now, most surgeons proceed with surgery as soon as the initial symptoms of pancreatitis resolve.

When clients with severe pancreatitis do not respond to medical management, operative intervention may be indicated to débride necrosis, or again to exclude other possible diagnoses as causative factors.

Nursing Management

Assessment

Until a confirmed diagnosis is made, nursing should concentrate on treating the symptoms and preparing clients for diagnostic procedures. The nurse should keep in mind that the degree of nursing intervention is directly related to the severity of illness and the client's overall condition.

Nursing Diagnosis, Planning, and Implementation

Nursing Diagnosis: Pain R/T inflammation of the pancreas and surrounding tissue, biliary tract disease, obstruction of pancreatic ducts, and interruption of the blood supply.

Planning: Expected Outcomes. Client will demonstrate absence or decrease in pain, as evidenced by verbalizing that pain is absent or decreased and resting quietly.

Implementation. The nurse should assess the location, severity, and character of the pain as well as the onset, duration, and precipitating or relieving factors. This assessment should be documented, and significant changes should be reported. The nurse should evaluate the client's response to pain and the therapies used to decrease discomfort.

Not allowing the client to take anything by mouth not only rests the GI tract but also decreases pancreatic stimulation. The nurse must keep in mind that even ice chips can stimulate enzymes and increase pain. Nasogastric suctioning helps decrease distention and, thereby, promote comfort. The system should be checked frequently to ensure that the nasogastric suction is functioning properly to avoid pooling and stimulation of enzyme secretion.

The nurse must be sure to administer pain medications in a timely manner and remember that opiate narcotics may stimulate spasm of the ducts and increase pain. Demerol is usually the drug of choice. Other drugs may be ordered (such as anticholinergics) to quiet the pancreas and decrease enzyme secretion.

Positioning (side-lying, knee-chest position with a pillow pressed against the abdomen or a sitting position with the trunk flexed may be helpful), back rubs, relaxation techniques, and providing a quiet environment all help promote comfort and rest.

Collaborative Problem: Fluid Volume Deficit and Electrolyte Imbalance R/T vomiting, nasogastric suctioning, NPO status, shifting of body fluids, fever, and diaphoresis.

Planning: Expected Outcomes. The client will receive appropriate assessments and interventions for early detection or prevention of fluid and electrolyte imbalance.

Implementation. The nurse monitors vital signs for changes in pulse and blood pressure (fluid volume changes) and respirations (acid-base imbalance). If the client is in the intensive care setting, hemodynamics should be assessed for changes in fluid status (see Chap. 3), and heart monitor rhythm changes may be a first indication of electrolyte imbalance (see Chap. 3). The nurse should check laboratory values as they are ordered for significant changes and observe for physical symptoms indicating hyperglycemia, hypocalcemia, and hypokalemia. The nurse should monitor the client's response to fluid administration and blood products by checking for edema, lung sounds, skin turgor, and mucous membranes, and monitoring the intake and output. Significant changes should be reported promptly because these clients are at increased risk.

Nursing Diagnosis: Breathing Pattern, Ineffective R/T abdominal distention or ascites, pain, or respiratory complications.

Planning: Expected Outcomes. The client will maintain an effective breathing pattern, as evidenced by a respiratory rate within normal limits, relaxed respiratory effort, absence of cyanosis, and clear lungs.

Implementation. The nurse should assess the client's respirations for rate and effort. Assessments should include lung auscultation for decreased lung sounds (potential for atelectasis), rales or rhonchi (potential for pneumonia and pleural effusion), and cyanosis. Many times, these clients are on bed rest, which precludes the need for prophylactic nursing interventions of pulmonary hygiene (e.g., turning, coughing, deep breathing, and incentive spirometry). Keeping the client comfortable with the administration of pain medications enhances full inspiration and normal breathing patterns. Positioning, such as placing the client in semi-Fowler's or a side-lying position, may facilitate normal respirations.

Nursing Diagnosis: Nutrition, Altered: Less than Body Requirements R/T nausea and vomiting, NPO status, and nasogastric suctioning.

Planning: Expected Outcomes. The client will maintain adequate nutritional status, as evidenced by maintaining normal body weight, keeping blood sugar within normal limits, and finding no evidence of muscle wasting.

Implementation. Again, depending on the severity of illness, these clients may take nothing by mouth for an extended length of time. When extended fasting is necessary, nutrition is provided through hyperalimentation and lipids (see Chap. 34). Nursing assessment should include the overall nutritional status of the client by checking daily weights, tissue integrity, and the presence of adequate body fat and muscle mass.

Acute pancreatitis clients are allowed to have an oral diet when all abdominal pain and tenderness have resolved. However, if oral intake is resumed too soon, re-exacerbation of symptoms may occur. Therefore, the nurse should monitor the client's response to oral intake carefully and begin intake slowly with liquids and progress to a normal diet. It may be necessary to administer antispasmodics, anticholinergics, and antacids to reduce gastric and pancreatic secretions. Also, if the pancreas has been severely damaged, it may be necessary to give replacement pancreatic enzymes to replace enzyme deficit and aid in digestion. The nurse then must monitor the effects of these drugs.

Nursing Diagnosis: Knowledge Deficit R/T causes of pancreatitis, treatment, possible complications, and home health care.

Planning: Expected Outcomes. The client and significant others will accurately verbalize home health-care needs, as evidenced by being able to verbalize an understanding of diet; list medications, including indications, dosage, frequency, and side effects; and list signs and symptoms of recurrence.

Implementation. The nurse should begin preparing clients for discharge by assessing their level of understanding and learning needs. The medication regimen, including the medication's purpose, dosage, frequency, and possible side effects, should be discussed. The client may require an insulin supplement because of pancreatic damage. Teaching should begin as soon as possible to ensure that the client and significant others are fully prepared to deal with glucose monitoring, diet, and insulin administration (see Chap. 40 for Diabetic Teaching). The nurse should instruct the client about dietary restrictions, such as restricting alcohol, tea, coffee, spicy foods, and heavy meals that stimulate pancreatic secretions and attacks of pancreatitis. Clients should understand the benefit of eating small, frequent meals that include high-protein, low-fat, and moderate- to high-carbohydrate foods. The nurse should ensure that the client is aware of which symptoms may indicate that pancreatitis is recurring and understands the importance of reporting these symptoms immediately. These symptoms include steatorrhea (fatty-looking stools); severe back or epigastric pain; persistent gastritis, nausea, and vomiting; weight loss; elevated temperature; and symptoms of hyperglycemia.

Nursing Diagnosis: Injury, Risk for R/T malfunction of pancreatic drains or loss of endocrine and exocrine function secondary to removal of the pancreas.

Planning: Expected Outcomes. The client will be free from injury, as evidenced by proper draining of pancreatic drains and no symptoms of hypoglycemia or digestive disorders related to absence of exocrine enzymes.

Implementation. The nurse should assess for placement of drains, the location of the drains (internal or external), and proper function and patency of the drains. If the drains do not appear to be functioning, the physician should be notified immediately.

If the client has lost all endocrine function, he or she will require insulin (see Chap. 40). The nurse continues to monitor the client for signs of hypoglycemia.

With the loss of exocrine function, replacement of pancreatic enzyme function with medications such as pancrelipase (Pancrease) will be necessary. When the client begins to eat, the nurse should watch for the development of diarrhea and steatorrhea, which indicates that insufficient pancreatic enzymes are present.

Nursing Diagnosis: Knowledge Deficit R/T care, postoperative nutritional needs, diabetic care, and pancreatic enzyme replacement.

Planning: Expected Outcomes. The client will understand discharge instructions, as evidenced by the ability to describe and demonstrate appropriate wound care, diet, proper diabetic care, and correct administration and side effects of medication regimen.

Implementation. The nurse assesses the knowledge of the client and significant others before providing appropriate learning guidelines prior to discharge. The nurse provides instructions for wound care. The client will require alterations in his or her diet to reflect the new status as a diabetic. The nurse provides teaching guidelines regarding nutritional needs and appropriate low-fat, diabetic diet (see Chap. 40).

The nurse provides the client with important information concerning diabetes, including information about hyperglycemia (polyuria, polydipsia, and polyphagia) and information about hypoglycemia. See Chapter 40 for further information on diabetic teaching.

The nurse provides the client with information about pharmacologic therapy (pancreatic enzymes), including the medication action, side effects, and when to notify the physician.

Nursing Diagnosis: Individual Coping, Ineffective R/T alcohol abuse.

Planning: Expected Outcomes. The client will learn to cope with life more effectively, as evidenced by admitting alcohol is a problem, seeking help with alcohol abstinence, and seeking long-term support to develop more effective coping strategies.

Implementation. The client must be encouraged to face the problem that alcohol ingestion is causing. The nurse should spend time with the client and encourage verbalization of problems. The nurse facilitates counseling for alcohol abuse by recommending groups such as Alcoholics Anonymous to the client and supporting the client's decision to join such a program. The nurse discusses supportive services available as necessary with the client and significant others.

Evaluation

The client will be evaluated based on the expected outcomes. If the outcomes are not achieved, the plan and the interventions should be revised.

Modification of Plan of Care for the Elderly

The older client may be less able to survive the life-threatening effects of pancreatitis. Treatment is the same as for younger clients, although surgery may not be performed unless the condition becomes life-threatening.

Posthospital Care

DISCHARGE TEACHING

CRITICAL TO REMEMBER

The client with loss of pancreatic endocrine function requires extensive teaching regarding diabetes and diabetic care (see Chap. 40).

All clients require teaching on good nutrition to maintain adequate output. The client will need to understand and follow a nutritious, low-fat diet.

Avoidance of alcohol is another area of postoperative teaching for these clients. The client needs to understand the problems that alcohol is creating and the need to stop drinking before irreversible damage is done.

HOME HEALTH-CARE NEEDS

The client should probably be seen by a visiting nurse after discharge to assess the client's ability to follow the postoperative regimen.

FOLLOW-UP CARE

The client will need to be seen at regular intervals to ensure that the postoperative regimen is being followed. The client's ability to abstain from alcohol should be carefully assessed, and further counseling provided.

CHRONIC PANCREATITIS

Chronic pancreatitis is a progressive, inflammatory, destructive disease of the pancreas. The incidence of chronic pancreatitis in the United States is about four cases per 100,000 population. Chronic pancreatitis involves progressive fibrosis and degeneration of the pancreas.

Characteristically, the pancreas is progressively destroyed by repeated flare-ups of usually mild attacks of pancreatitis.

CRITICAL TO REMEMBER

After repeated attacks of acute pancreatitis, the inflammatory process results in scarring and calcification of pancreatic tissue. The damage is irreversible, affecting both endocrine and exocrine pancreatic functions.

Within the United States (and other industrialized countries), chronic alcoholism is the most frequent cause of chronic calcifying pancreatitis.

In chronic pancreatitis, as in acute pancreatitis, dull pain alternates with severe pain, vomiting, fever, and jaundice. When sitting in bed with knees flexed and pressing a pillow to the abdomen, the client may experience some pain relief. The client generally experiences more pain when lying supine.

Because food may aggravate the pain, the client usually decreases food intake, resulting in weight loss. Reduction in digestive enzyme secretion eventually causes malnutrition and contributes to this weight loss.

Eventually, because of involvement of the islet tissue, the client develops hyperglycemia with manifestations of diabetes. Insulin-dependent diabetes mellitus occurs in up to one third of clients.

The client also suffers from abdominal distention with flatus and cramps and frequent passage of foul, fatty stools (steatorrhea). Thus, the clinical group of symptoms that serves as a classic presentation of chronic pancreatitis is abdominal pain, weight loss, diabetes, and steatorrhea.

Additionally, many clients present with a history of narcotic analgesic abuse because of efforts to control pain.

Pain or digestive disturbance may motivate a person with chronic pancreatitis to seek help.

Because of a reduced amount of functioning tissue in chronic pancreatitis, pancreatic enzyme analysis may be normal. Blood studies may reveal a mild leukocytosis. X-ray studies may show reduced bowel motility, calcifications, and adhesions. Both ultrasonography and the more expensive CT study provide useful diagnostic data. Angiography indicates vascular changes. Cholangiography and cholecystography show biliary alterations, which may be either a cause or a consequence of the pancreatic disorder.

Pancreatitis frequently reveals bloody fluid that is high in amylase and methemalbumin from hemoglobin digestion. Other studies may be in order, especially when the diagnosis is obscure.

The three areas that are treated medically are (1) control of pain, (2) treatment of endocrine insufficiency, and (3) treatment of exocrine insufficiency.

The control of pain can be a major problem and is generally the sole indication for surgical intervention. For alcohol-related pancreatitis, total abstinence from alcohol is imperative and sometimes successful in itself in pain relief. Control of diet may decrease painful stimulation of pancreatitis enzyme secretion. Attempts to control pain pharmacologically should begin with non-narcotic analgesics and progress to narcotic analgesics, if needed.

Exogenous insulin therapy may be necessary because of destruction of islet tissue. Exocrine insufficiency is treated with exogenous pancreatic enzyme therapy. This therapy may include lipase, trypsin, or histamine H_2 receptor antagonists.

The three major goals of surgical intervention for chronic pancreatitis are to (1) correct the primary tract disease (ampullar procedure), (2) relieve ductal obstruction (ductal drainage), and (3) relieve pain (ablative procedure). Several surgical approaches are available.

The prognosis in chronic pancreatitis is good if acute attacks decrease in frequency. Replacement therapy for chronic fat indigestion permits a fairly normal life. If the client continues to drink alcohol, the prognosis is poor. Repeated attacks eventually cause death from shock or renal failure.

PANCREATIC CANCER

There are approximately 28,000 cases of cancer of the pancreas in the United States each year. It is the fifth most common cause of cancer death, exceeded only by lung, colorectal, breast, and prostate cancer. Ninety per cent of pancreatic cancer clients die within the first year after diagnosis. Cancer of the pancreas is more common in blacks than in whites, smokers than nonsmokers, and males than females.

It appears to be linked to diabetes mellitus, use of alcohol, history of previous pancreatitis, and the ingestion of a high-fat diet.

Duct cell adenocarcinoma accounts for over 90 per cent of malignant pancreatic exocrine tumors. The most common site of origin is the pancreatic head.

Periampullary adenocarcinomas originate in the region of the ampulla of Vater. Clients typically present with jaundice, weight loss, and abdominal pain. The majority of clients are managed operatively by either resection or palliative therapy.

Carcinomas of the tail and body of the pancreas represent up to 30 per cent of pancreatic carcinomas. Clients usually present with significant weight loss and abdominal pain. Because of their location, these tumors generally grow to a large size before symptoms occur and the diagnosis is made. Therefore, the resectability rate is low (less than 7 per cent), and the prognosis is poor (5 to 6 month mean survival).

PANCREATIC TRAUMA

The pancreas is injured in less than 2 per cent of clients with abdominal trauma. Two thirds of pancreatic injuries are associated with penetrating abdominal trauma, and the rest are due to blunt trauma. Clients with penetrating abdominal trauma show signs of hemorrhage, progressive peritonitis, and hypovolemia.

Treatment involves surgery to control hemorrhage, débride nonviable tissue, preserve viable tissue, and provide drainage of pancreatic secretions.

CYSTIC FIBROSIS

Cystic fibrosis (CF) is a hereditary, chronic disease characterized by abnormal secretions of the exocrine glands. It is genetically transmitted as an autosomal recessive trait. Approximately 4 to 5 per cent of the population are carriers, and the incidence in the United States is about 1 in every 1600 to 2000 births of white people.

Pancreatic exocrine function is affected by decreased lipase released into the bowel. This results in malabsorption of lipids and causes blockage of the pancreatic ducts with thick mucus. Pancreatic degeneration, fibrosis, and atrophy of tissues follow, with eventual development of fatty infiltration and loss of function. The intestines have thick, viscous mucus, which may cause a thick mass within the bowel. The lack of pancreatic enzymes causes steatorrhea.

Pulmonary complications are the most physically visible. These clients have obvious respiratory compromise, with frequent bronchopneumonia and chronic bronchitis.

Recent improvements in the management of infants and children with CF have led to a greater number of adults with CF. Typically, these clients have a small stature and appear somewhat emaciated. They are barrel-chested and have clubbed fingers.

Because the digestive problems encountered with CF are generally managed with diet and oral administration of pancreatic enzymes and fat-soluble vitamins, these clients are hospitalized for treatment of respiratory complications rather than for intestinal problems. The current trend is to hospitalize the client routinely for thorough pulmonary hygiene with a full course of intravenous antibiotics (with emphasis on antifungals) and respiratory therapy.

Nursing diagnoses that may apply to people with CF include

- Ineffective Airway Clearance R/T thick, viscous, mucous secretions from the submucosal glands of the respiratory tract
- Altered Nutrition: Less than Body Requirements R/T lack of pancreatic enzymes
- Knowledge Deficit R/T dietary management of CF

Interventions for clients with CF include

- Prophylactic pulmonary support—expectorants, postural drainage, antibiotics, and exercise
- Administration of pancreatic enzymes
- Dietary management—high-protein, high-calorie, high-salt, and low-fat diet
- Replacement of fat-soluble vitamins

STUDY QUESTIONS

1. A client is scheduled for a cholecystectomy and a choledochostomy. The surgeon plans to remove the gallbladder and:
   A. Drain the gallbladder
   B. Open the common bile duct
   C. Excise the common bile duct
   D. Insert a T-tube in the common bile duct
2. A client is admitted with acute cholecystitis and asks the nurse, "Why won't the doctor take my gallbladder out?" The best response is:
   A. "You need your gallbladder as the body can't function without it."
   B. "The doctor believes that this attack will soon be over and you can go home."
   C. "If your gallbladder is removed, you can never eat fatty or fried foods again."
   D. "Antibiotic medication is usually ordered for someone like you who has an acute infection."
3. The client is taught to follow a low-fat diet. Which of the following menu choices are appropriate for the client's lunch?
   A. Lean roast beef and corn on the cob
   B. Cheese omelet and chocolate pudding
   C. Chicken salad and fresh tropical fruit cup
   D. Ham salad hoagie and strawberry ice cream
4. The plan of care for the client scheduled for an abdominal cholecystectomy should include which of the following teaching?
   A. The removal of the gallbladder causes bleeding tendencies so extra care must be given when injury occurs.
   B. A T-tube may be inserted during the surgery so that extra blood and plasma can drain from the cavity left by the missing gallbladder.
   C. Reduce stress in daily life because the loss of the gallbladder causes abdominal cramping when life becomes too stressful.
   D. Fatty and fried foods may be eaten to tolerance because the bile still flows into the duodenum and helps digest the fat.
5. The most accurate diagnostic study for the presence of acute pancreatitis is:
   A. Serum lipase
   B. Serum amylase
   C. Creatinine clearance
   D. Complete blood count
6. A client with pancreatitis is NPO. The family is questioning this order because the client is thirsty and asking for water. Teaching by the nurse should include which one of the following statements?
   A. "Oral intake of food or fluids stimulates pancreatic enzymes and increases the pain."
   B. "A nasogastric tube will be inserted to remove gastric secretions and help alleviate the thirst."
   C. "The replacement of pancreatic enzymes is the only intake permitted by mouth for 48 hours."
   D. "The client is permitted to have as many ice chips as desired to help decrease thirst and moisten the oral mucosa."
7. The plan of care for a client who is diagnosed with pancreatitis should include which one of the following?
   A. Prevention of falls
   B. Glucose monitoring
   C. Promotion of weight loss
   D. Regulation of fluid intake
8. Which client statement helps the nurse evaluate teaching about causes of recurrence of pancreatitis?
   A. "I will follow a high-fat diet faithfully."
   B. "I'm willing to try to stop drinking alcohol."
   C. "I will decrease my intake of high-protein products."
   D. "I will be careful about exposing myself to infection."

CRITICAL THINKING EXERCISES

SCENARIO A

A middle-aged female client is diagnosed with cholecystitis. She resides with her husband and four children in a small home they recently purchased. She prides herself on her ability to provide a nutritious diet while struggling to make mortgage payments on the new house. The diet is high in fatty foods; the client and two of the children, aged 12 and 14, are each about 15 pounds overweight. The client does everything for her family and the nurse discovers they are not willing to change their life-style to accommodate her illness.

1. What teaching should be done with the client's husband and children?
2. How should the nurse teach the client about low-fat food purchasing and cooking?
3. If surgery is indicated, what additional teaching and modifications in life-style must be considered as part of client education?

SCENARIO B

An elderly client is living with his son, daughter-in-law, and two grandchildren. His problems with pancreatitis have caused much concern among family members. The family was not aware of his alcohol intake until his third experience with pancreatitis.

1. What are the implications for the client who continues to ingest alcohol?
2. How should the family support the client so that he can abstain from alcohol intake?
3. What kind of teaching is needed if pancreatic enzyme replacement is ordered?
4. How will you respond to the statement "If I refuse surgery to remove my pancreas, I won't need to take enzymes."
5. What information should be taught regarding medical treatment of chronic pancreatitis?

BIBLIOGRAPHY

1. Abbott, J. T. (1994). Problems in the pregnant abdomen. *Emergency Medicine, 23(7)*, 54–58, 62, 65–67.
2. American Cancer Society. (1995). *Cancer facts and figures 1995*. Atlanta: Author.
3. Babb, R. R. (1993). Managing gallbladder disease with prostaglandin inhibitors. *Postgraduate Medicine, 94(1)*, 127–128, 130, 203–205.
4. Brodrick, R. L. (1991). Preventing complications in acute pancreatitis. *Dimensions of Critical Care Nursing, 10(5)*, 262–270.
5. Brown, A. (1991). Acute pancreatitis: Pathophysiology, nursing diagnosis, and collaborative practice. *Focus on Critical Care, 18(2)*, 121–130.
6. Cappell, M. S. (1991). Hepatobiliary manifestations of the acquired immune deficiency syndrome. *American Journal of Gastroenterology, 86*, 1.
7. Collins, A. S. (1990). Gastrointestinal complications in shock. *Critical Care Nursing Clinics of North America, 2(2)*, 269–277.
8. Dudley, S. L., & Starin, R. B. (1991). Cholelithiasis: Diagnosis and current therapeutic options. *Nurse Practitioner, 16(3)*, 13–18, 23–24.
9. Fair, J. A., & Amato-Vealey, E. (1988). Acute pancreatitis: A gastrointestinal emergency. *Critical Care Nursing, 8(6)*, 47–63.
10. Fulton, J. S., & Johnson, G. B. (1993). Using high dose morphine to relieve cancer pain. *Nursing, 23(2)*, 34–40.
11. Gauwitz, D. F. (1990). Endoscopic cholecystectomy: The patient-friendly altervative. *Nursing, 20(12)*, 58–59.
12. Giger, J. N., & Davidhizar, R. E. (1994). *Transcultural nursing: Assessment and intervention* (2nd ed.). St. Louis: Mosby-Year Book.
13. Greifzu, S., & Dest, V. (1991). When the diagnosis is pancreatic cancer. *RN, 54(9)*, 38–45.
14. Groer, M. W., & Shekleton, M. E. (1989). *Basic pathophysiology: A holistic approach* (3rd ed.). St. Louis: Mosby-Year Book.
15. Guyton, A. C. (1991). *Textbook of medical physiology* (8th ed.). Philadelphia: W. B. Saunders.
16. Holland, P., & Hussain, I. (1989). Biliary lithotripsy: Nonsurgical treatment of gallstones. *Society of Gastrointestinal Assistants Journal, 3*, 158–152.
17. Jurf, J. B., et al. (1990). Cholecystectomy made easier. *American Journal of Nursing*, 38–40.
18. Kohn, C. L., et al. (1993). Nutritional support for the patient with pancreatobiliary disease. *Critical Care Nursing Clinics of North America, 5(1)*, 37–45.
19. Levitt, M. D. (1992). Pancreatitis. *In* J. B. Wyngaarden et al. (Eds.), *Cecil textbook of medicine* (19th ed.). Philadelphia: W. B. Saunders.
20. McCance, K. L., & Huether, S. E. (1994). *Pathophysiology. The biologic basis for disease in adults and children* (2nd ed.). St. Louis: The C. V. Mosby Company.
21. Ritchie, A. C. (1990). *Boyd's textbook of pathology* (9th ed.). Philadelphia: Lea & Febiger.
22. Sabiston, D. C. Jr. (Ed.). (1991). *Textbook of surgery. The biological basics of modern surgical practice* (14th ed.). Philadelphia: W. B. Saunders.
23. Schade, R. R., & Cattano, C. J. (1992). Trends in gallbladder disease and its treatment, part 2. *Hospital Medicine, 28(11)*, 30, 32, 37–40.
24. Smith, A. (1991). When the pancreas self-destructs. *American Journal of Nursing, 91(9)*, 38–48.
25. Willis, D. A., et al. (1990). Gallstones: Alternatives to surgery. *RN, 53(4)*, 44–51.

UNIT 12

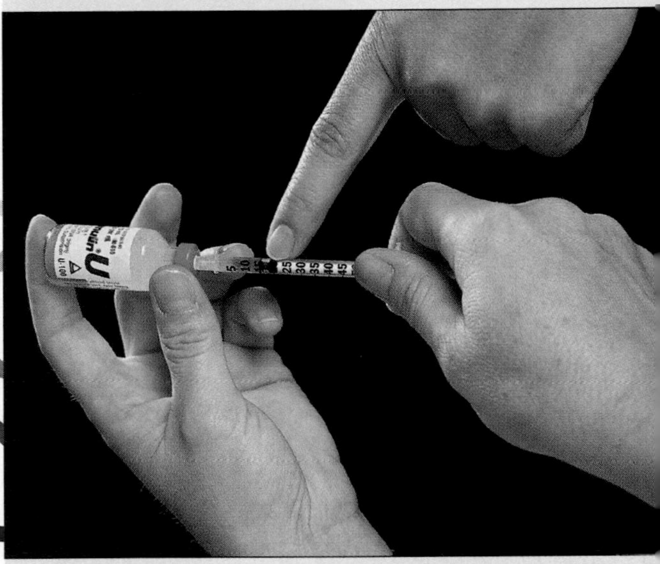

Metabolic Disorders

The endocrine system often is considered one of the body's most complex systems. Only recently has its function been well understood and well defined. With the advent of endocrinology and the increased understanding of the system, nurses have found themselves deeply involved in the care of clients with endocrine disorders.

Nurses play a major role in the care of clients with endocrine disorders, both in assessment of these disorders and in client care during treatment. Many of these disorders require minimal hospital care, usually only at initial diagnosis and if severe complications occur. The clients typically remain at home, seeking health care only at periodic intervals. After extensive client teaching, these disorders are usually well controlled by the clients themselves.

The chapters in this unit cover assessment of the endocrine system and all its potential disorders, along with nursing care of clients with specific disorders of the pituitary gland, endocrine pancreas, thyroid gland, parathyroid glands, adrenal glands, and gonads.

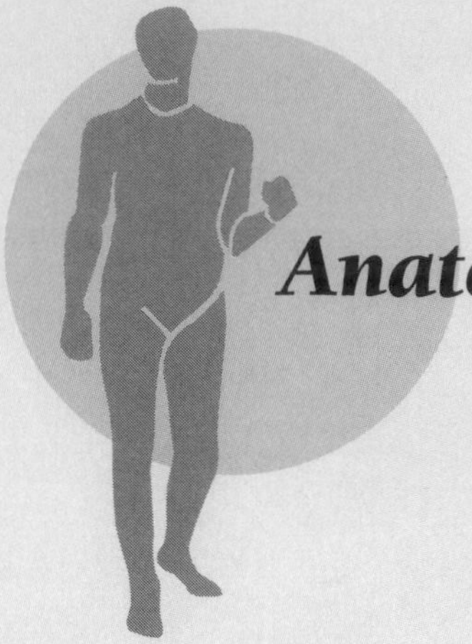

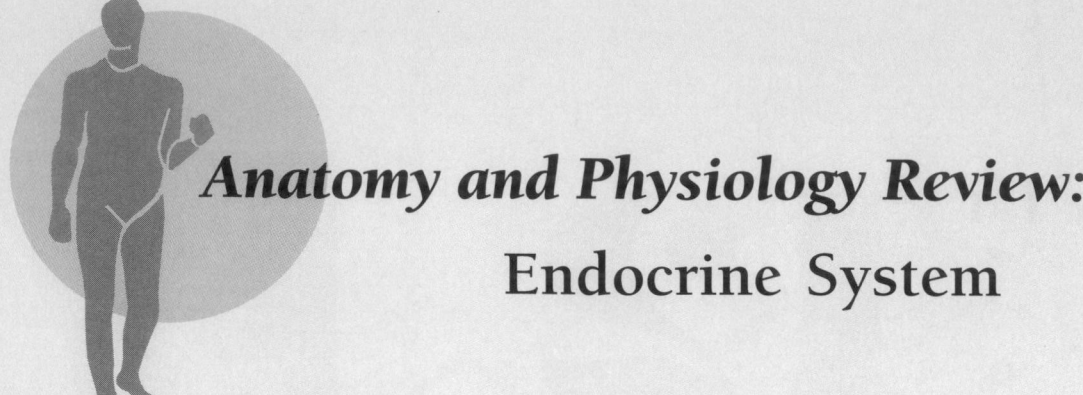

Anatomy and Physiology Review: Endocrine System

COMPARISON OF THE ENDOCRINE AND NERVOUS SYSTEMS

The endocrine system, along with the nervous system, functions in the regulation of body activities. These two systems work together to maintain homeostasis. Although closely related in their functions, they differ in certain characteristics.

CHARACTERISTIC	NERVOUS SYSTEM	ENDOCRINE SYSTEM
Mediator	Nerve impulses and neurotransmitters	Chemical messengers called hormones
Response	Rapid onset	Slower onset
Duration	Short duration	Longer duration
Extent	Selective, localized	More general, widespread
Effector	Muscles and glands	Growth, development, metabolic activities

COMPARISON OF EXOCRINE AND ENDOCRINE GLANDS

There are two types of glands in the body: exocrine and endocrine. Exocrine glands have ducts that carry the secretory product to a surface. These include the sweat glands, salivary glands, lacrimal glands, acinar cells of the pancreas, and others located throughout the body. In contrast, endocrine glands do not have ducts. Instead, they release their secretions, called hormones, directly into the blood, which transports the hormones throughout the body.

HORMONES

General Functions

The word hormone is derived from a Greek word that means to set in motion, arouse, or excite. Hormones set into motion metabolic processes that govern life and maintain homeostasis. Five general types of hormone functions are:

- Maintenance of optimal internal environment
- Coordination of the reproductive systems
- Stimulation of growth processes in appropriate sequence
- Differentiation of reproductive and nervous systems in the fetus
- Initiation of adaptive responses to stressors

Characteristics

Each hormone produced in the body is unique. Each one is different in its chemical composition, structure, and action. In spite of the differences, all hormones have the following characteristics:

- Secreted in one of three patterns. (1) Diurnal secretion is a pattern that rises and falls within a 24-hour period. For example, cortisol levels rise in the morning and fall by evening. (2) Pulsatile and cyclic secretions rise and fall along another time frame, such as monthly. Estrogen is an example of this secretion pattern. (3) Variable secretion depends on levels of other substances in the blood. For example, parathyroid hormone is secreted in response to serum calcium levels.
- Operate within a feedback system for control of secretion.
- Control the rate of cellular activity. Hormones do not initiate biochemical changes.

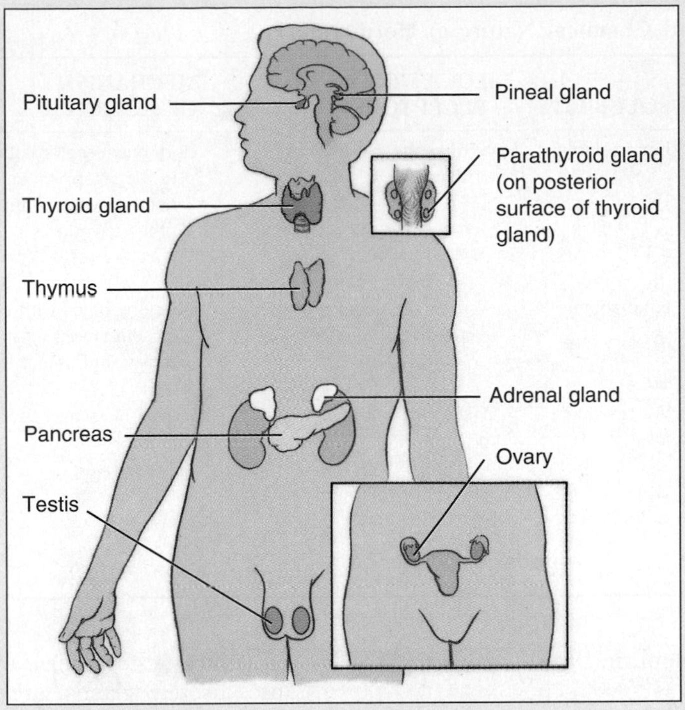

Endocrine glands

- Affect only cells that contain the appropriate receptors.
- Have both independent and interdependent functions. Some hormones act independently, while others depend on other hormones to trigger their release.
- Constantly deactivated by the liver or other cellular mechanisms and excreted by the kidney.

Mechanism of Action and Chemical Nature

Hormones are carried by the blood throughout the entire body, yet they affect only certain cells. The specific cells that respond to a given hormone have receptor sites for that hormone. These receptor sites may be located on the surface of the cell membrane, within the cytoplasm of the cell, or within the chromosome material in the nucleus. The reaction between a hormone and its receptor initiates events that bring about changes attributed to the hormone action. Three different mechanisms of action correspond to the three different types of receptor sites:

- Second messenger mechanism. (1) The hormone binds with the receptor on the membrane surface; (2) this activates adenyl cyclase, which diffuses into the cytoplasm; (3) adenyl cyclase causes formation of cyclic AMP (or some other second messenger) within the cytoplasm; (4) cyclic AMP activates a cascade of enzymes within the cytoplasm to bring about the hormone action.
- Steroid action. (1) The hormone binds with the receptor in the cytoplasm; (2) the receptor/hormone complex enters the nucleus; (3) the combination binds to DNA strands and activates formation of messenger RNA; (4) the messenger RNA enters the cytoplasm and initiates protein synthesis.
- Thyroid hormone action. (1) The hormone binds with the receptor within the chromosome complex of the nucleus; (2) the reaction activates genetic mechanisms that are responsible for the formation of hundreds of proteins that promote enhanced intracellular metabolic activity in nearly all cells.

Control of Hormone Action

Most endocrine activity is controlled either directly or indirectly by the hypothalamus, which links the nervous system to the endocrine system. This usually is accomplished through a negative feedback mechanism involving both the hypothalamus and the pituitary gland. In response to input from other areas of the brain or from hormones in the blood, the hypothalamus secretes releasing and inhibiting hormones. These hormones act on specific cells in the pituitary gland that regulate the secretion of pituitary hormones, which cause the secretion of hormones from other glands.

Blood levels of substances other than hormones can also trigger hormone secretion and are controlled through a negative feedback system. For example, the release of insulin from the pancreatic islets is stimulated by elevated blood glucose levels. Parathyroid hormone is secreted in response to low blood calcium levels. Another mechanism, direct nerve stimulation, stimu-

Mechanism of Action and Chemical Nature of Hormones

CHEMICAL NATURE	SOLUBILITY	LOCATION OF RECEPTORS	MECHANISM OF ACTION	EXAMPLES
Steroids: derivatives of cholesterol	Lipid soluble	Within the cytoplasm of the cell	Hormone/receptor complex in the cytoplasm enters nucleus where it initiates protein synthesis	Hormones from the ovaries, testes, placenta, and adrenal cortex
Derivatives of amino acid tyrosine				
Thyroid hormones	Lipid soluble	Within the nucleus of the cell	Hormone binds with chromosome receptor and activates protein synthesis	Thyroxine and triiodothyronine from the thyroid gland
Catecholamines	Water soluble	Surface of cell membrane	Second messenger mechanism	Epinephrine and norepinephrine from the adrenal medulla
Proteins and peptides	Water soluble	Surface of cell membrane	Second messenger mechanism	Hormones from the anterior pituitary, posterior pituitary, parathyroid, and pancreas

lates the release of epinephrine and norepinephrine from the adrenal medulla.

PROSTAGLANDINS

Prostaglandins, all derivatives of arachidonic acid (an essential fatty acid), are potent chemical regulators that are similar to hormones but different enough that they are not classified as hormones. Prostaglandins are produced by cells that are widely distributed throughout the entire body, have a localized effect on or near the cell in which they are made, have an effect that is immediate and short term, are readily inactivated, and cannot be stored but must be synthesized on demand. In contrast, hormones are produced by cells collected into discrete glands, are transported in the blood and may have an effect distant from their origin, are slower to act, and have longer-lasting effects.

Numerous and varied effects are attributed to prostaglandins. Some modulate hormone action; others affect smooth-muscle contraction; still others are involved in blood clotting mechanisms. Prostaglandins foster many aspects of the inflammatory process, including the development of fever and pain. They also appear to inhibit the gastric secretion of hydrochloric acid. Drugs, such as aspirin, ibuprofen, and acetaminophen, that inhibit prostaglandin synthesis, will reduce the inflammation of rheumatoid arthritis, bursitis, and other inflammatory disorders. These drugs may make an individual susceptible to peptic ulcers by increasing hydrochloric acid secretion.

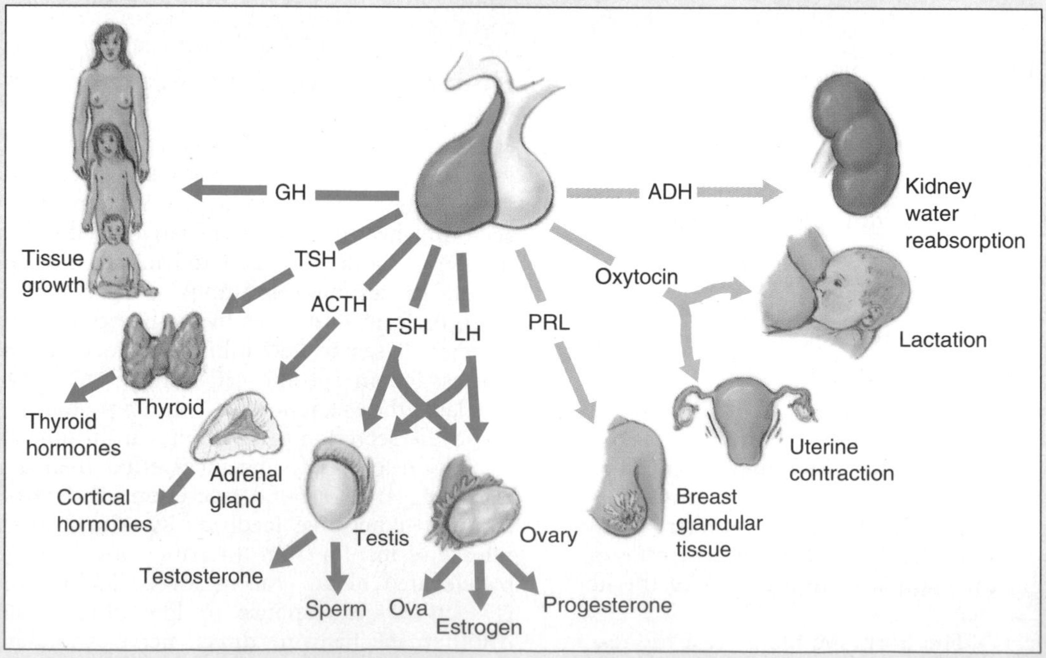

Effects of hormones from the pituitary gland

SPECIFIC HORMONE ACTIONS

The Principal Endocrine Glands and Their Hormones

GLAND	HORMONE	TARGET TISSUE	PRINCIPAL ACTIONS
Hypothalamus	Releasing and inhibiting hormones	Anterior lobe of pituitary gland	Stimulates or inhibits secretion of specific hormones
Anterior lobe of pituitary	Growth hormone (GH)	Most tissues in the body	Stimulates growth by promoting protein synthesis
	Thyroid-stimulating hormone (TSH)	Thyroid gland	Increases secretion of thyroid hormone; increases the size of the thyroid gland
	Adrenocorticotropic hormone (ACTH)	Adrenal cortex	Increases secretion of adrenocortical hormones, especially glucocorticoids such as cortisol
	Follicle-stimulating hormone (FSH)	Ovarian follicles in the female; seminiferous tubules of testis in the male	Follicle maturation and estrogen secretion in the female; spermatogenesis in the male
	Luteinizing hormone (LH); also called interstitial cell–stimulating hormone in males	Ovary in females; testis in males	Ovulation; progesterone production in female; testosterone production in male
	Prolactin (PRL)	Mammary gland	Stimulates milk production
Posterior lobe of pituitary	Antidiuretic hormone (ADH)	Kidney	Increases water reabsorption (decreases water lost in urine)
	Oxytocin	Uterus; mammary gland	Increases uterine contractions; stimulates ejection of milk from mammary gland
Thyroid	Thyroxine and triiodothyronine	Most body cells	Increases metabolic rate; essential for normal growth and development
	Calcitonin	Primarily bone	Decreases blood calcium by inhibiting bone breakdown and release of calcium; antagonistic to parathyroid hormone
Parathyroid	Parathyroid hormone or parathormone	Bone, kidney, digestive tract	Increases blood calcium by stimulating bone breakdown and release of calcium; increases calcium absorption in the digestive tract; decreases calcium lost in urine
Adrenal cortex	Mineralocorticoids (aldosterone)	Kidney	Increases sodium reabsorption and potassium excretion in kidney tubules; secondarily increases water retention
	Glucocorticoids (cortisol)	Most body tissues	Increases blood glucose levels; inhibits inflammation and immune response
	Androgens and estrogens	Most body tissues	Secreted in small amounts so that effect is generally masked by the hormones from the ovaries and testes
Adrenal medulla	Epinephrine, norepinephrine	Heart, blood vessels, liver, adipose tissue	Helps cope with stress; increases heart rate and blood pressure; increases blood flow to skeletal muscle; increases blood glucose level
Pancreas (islets of Langerhans)	Glucagon	Liver	Increases breakdown of glycogen to increase blood glucose levels
	Insulin	General, but especially liver, skeletal muscle, adipose tissue	Decreases blood glucose levels by facilitating uptake and utilization of glucose by cells; stimulates glucose storage as glycogen and production of adipose
Testes	Testosterone	Most body cells	Maturation and maintenance of male reproductive organs and secondary sex characteristics
Ovaries	Estrogens	Most body cells	Maturation and maintenance of female reproductive organs and secondary sex characteristics; menstrual cycle
	Progesterone	Uterus and breast	Prepares uterus for pregnancy; stimulates development of mammary gland; menstrual cycle
Pineal	Melatonin	Hypothalamus	Inhibits gonadotropin-releasing hormone, which consequently inhibits reproductive functions; regulates daily rhythms such as sleep and wakefulness
Thymus	Thymosin	Tissues involved in immune response	Immune system development and function

Modified from Applegate, E. J. (1995). *The anatomy and physiology learning system textbook.* Philadelphia: W. B. Saunders Co.

AGE-RELATED CHANGES

With age, most endocrine glands show some degree of glandular atrophy, with increased amounts of fibrous tissue and fat deposits. However, in general, the glands remain responsive to stimulation and secrete adequate amounts of hormones. There is no evidence that age-related structural changes in the endocrine glands have serious functional significance or contribute to the overall aging process. Possible age-related changes in the endocrine system include:

- Loss of self-regulation, leading to autoimmune or immunodeficiency disorders such as diabetes.
- Target organs may lose some of their ability to respond to hormones.
- Hypothalamus and pituitary gland may be affected by changes in neurotransmitters.

Chapter 39

Assessment of Clients with Metabolic Disorders

Learning Outcomes

After completing this chapter, the learner will be able to:

1. Assess clients for clinical manifestations of hyper- or hypofunction of the endocrine system.
2. Explain the incidence, etiology, and risk factors to clients with disorders of the endocrine system.
3. Explain the client's role in diagnostic tests specific to disorders of the endocrine system.
4. Evaluate possible endocrine imbalances or disorders in light of a nursing assessment.

The endocrine system works in unison with the nervous system to maintain homeostasis. There are two types of glands: endocrine, which release hormones into the blood, and exocrine, which release hormones into ducts. Endocrine glands include the pancreas, gonads, adrenal, thyroid, parathyroid, and thymus glands. Assessment of the client includes the usual history and physical examination. Blood levels of the various hormones can be determined.

Assessment of the endocrine system is often difficult because of the variety of symptoms that may occur. Each body system is affected by hormones; thus, clinical signs and subjective symptoms may be specific or nonspecific. Additionally, symptoms may be related to causes other than endocrine disorders. Thorough health history interviewing and physical examination assist in the diagnostic process.

HISTORY

Throughout the history interview, the nurse gathers information about the client's present condition and previous medical history. The history begins with the biographic data and proceeds to the chief complaint, including a symptom analysis. Additional subjective data are collected about the client's past medical history, family history, psychosocial history and life-style, and a review of systems.

Biographic Data

The nurse notes the client's age, because the endocrine system is affected by the aging process. Fewer hormones may be produced, or their effect on the target organs is decreased. For example, the incidence of Type II diabetes mellitus increases with age.

Chief Complaint

The client's presenting symptoms may be specific or nonspecific. Common nonspecific symptoms include fatigue and depression, often accompanied by altered alertness, decreased energy, sleep pattern disturbances, weight changes, altered mood and affect, changes in the condition of the skin and hair, altered general appearance, and sexual dysfunction. Some symptoms are specific for certain endocrine disorders, as listed in Box 39–1.

Past Medical History

The client's past medical history is explored to determine whether there have been previous endocrine disorders. The nurse specifically inquires about patterns of growth and development, head trauma, and general health status. The client is asked to identify changes that have occurred in his or her health status, either in general or more specifically.

GROWTH AND DEVELOPMENT

The nurse should ask the client (or the client's significant others) whether there have been noticeable delays or accelerations in growth and development. For example, does the client have a history of being small or large for his or her chronologic age and ethnic background? The nurse also asks about family members' growth patterns so that valid comparisons are made.

The client is asked about changes in body size that may have occurred since physical maturation. Have there been changes in the size of the hands, feet, or head circumference? For example, has the client had to get shoes in a larger size? gloves? rings? hats? Similarly, the nurse asks the client about changes in secondary sex characteristics. For example, has there been increased amounts of facial hair (women) or decreased amounts (in men, thus less need for shaving)? For both men and women, the nurse asks whether there have been changes in pubic or axillary hair such as the amount and its distribution and whether the female client has problems with menstruation, infertility, or pregnancy.

MAJOR ILLNESSES AND HOSPITALIZATIONS

The nurse asks the client to identify whether there is a history of head trauma such as a forceful blow. Trauma can lead to hypopituitarism. The nurse should ask whether the client has been hospitalized for surgery to the head or neck and whether there is a history of chemotherapy or radiation therapy to the head or neck. Specific disorders to ask about include primary brain tumors, metastatic tumors, meningitis, brain infarctions, diabetes mellitus, diabetes insipidus, hypertension, and goiter.

MEDICATIONS

All medications, past and current, are included for identification. The nurse specifically asks about use of hormones and steroids, including name, dose, and duration of use, and whether the client has a history of using anabolic steroids.

FAMILY HISTORY

When assessing a client with an endocrine disorder, the nurse should inquire into the family history. A number of endocrine disorders are inherited or at least associated with a familial trend.

The nurse asks whether there are family members who have or have had problems similar to those of the client. Disorders to inquire about include growth and development problems, obesity, goiter, hypothyroidism or hyperthyroidism, hypertension, hypotension, diabetes mellitus, diabetes insipidus, autoimmune diseases (e.g., Addison's disease), and problems with the adrenal gland (e.g., pheochromocytoma).

BOX 39-1

Common Signs and Symptoms of Endocrine Disorders

MENTAL STATUS CHANGES

The client may report increased nervousness, lability of mood, mental confusion, and depression. Extreme alterations in consciousness such as coma may occur in uncontrolled diabetes mellitus.

CHANGES IN VITAL SIGNS

Body temperature and pulse rate may be elevated due to hyperthyroidism. Kussmaul's respirations (deep rapid breathing) are a classic sign of diabetic ketoacidosis. Tumors of the adrenal glands, causing increased secretion of epinephrine (e.g., pheochromocytoma), can result in hypertension. Insufficient antidiuretic hormone from the pituitary gland can cause dehydration, whereas oversecretion can cause excessive retention of body water.

PALPITATIONS

Increased heart rate with sweating and flushing can occur in hyperthyroidism and also in pheochromocytoma.

TREMORS

Uncontrolled tremors can be a possible indication of hyperthyroidism.

FATIGUE

May signify emotional stress and/or pathophysiologic changes.

WEAKNESS

Weakness may be generalized or localized. Localized weakness often indicates a neurologic problem, which can be a complication of an endocrine disorder.

APPETITE CHANGES

The client may report polyphagia (excessive hunger) associated with diabetes mellitus or anorexia (lack of appetite).

WEIGHT CHANGES

Eating more but losing weight may indicate diabetes mellitus or hyperthyroidism. Clients with hypothyroidism may gain weight.

POLYDIPSIA AND POLYURIA

Abnormal thirst plus passage of large amounts of urine may indicate diabetes mellitus.

CHANGES IN BOWEL STATUS

Frequent loose stools are a sign of hyperthyroidism, while constipation can indicate hypothyroidism.

ABNORMALITIES INVOLVING THE SEXUAL ORGANS AND LIBIDO

Menstrual cycle irregularities (including amenorrhea), loss of libido, loss or premature development of secondary sexual characteristics, impotence, and infertility are sexual changes characteristic of endocrine disorders.

UNTOWARD CHANGES IN APPEARANCE

Acromegaly produces enlargement of the hands and feet and a coarsening of the facial features.

ADRENOCORTICAL HYPERFUNCTION (CUSHING'S SYNDROME)

Adrenocortical hyperfunction is manifested in moon facies, thin extremities, and truncal obesity.

GROWTH ABNORMALITIES

Growth may be delayed, stunted (dwarfism), excessive (gigantism), or inappropriate (acromegaly).

SKIN AND TISSUE CHANGES

Hyperpigmentation occurs in chronic adrenocortical insufficiency (Addison's disease). Areas of hypopigmentation (vitiligo) may indicate other endocrine disorders. Delayed tissue healing and susceptibility to infection are associated with diabetes mellitus. Hard, nonpitting edema occurs in adult hypothyroidism (myxedema).

HAIR

Excessive hair (hirsutism) in women may indicate ovarian or adrenocortical disorders. Axillary and pubic hair loss may indicate a pituitary disorder. Hair feels soft and silky in hyperthyroidism and coarse, dry, and brittle in hypothyroidism.

EYES

Exophthalmos (bulging eyes) is an important characteristic of hyperthyroidism. A pituitary tumor may cause partial or total loss of vision. Diabetes may cause temporary blurred vision or permanent blindness.

BONE AND JOINT PROBLEMS

Clients with hyperparathyroidism often develop bone pain, cysts, and fractures. Cushing's syndrome produces a rapid breakdown of bone.

RENAL COLIC AND STONES

Renal problems such as stone development may follow the bone disorders found in hyperparathyroidism.

TETANY, PARESTHESIAS, AND MUSCLE CRAMPS

These manifestations may develop in clients with insufficient parathyroid hormone.

Psychosocial History and Life-Style

The nurse inquires about the client's stress tolerance and coping patterns. Stressors can be either physiologic (illness) or emotional. The nurse should ask about job-related stressors such as amount of time spent on the job both in the work setting and at home. For example, are there strained interpersonal relationships among workers or management that contribute to increased stress levels? Are there opportunities for the client to retreat from the work place and engage in recreational activities? The nurse should also ask about the home environment and family interpersonal relationships and obligations. The nurse should ascertain what the client's support systems are and whether the client can say that current coping strategies are effective. If possible, the nurse asks family members or significant others to corroborate or help identify behavior changes.

The nurse considers other aspects of life-style and coping and asks the client about habits such as smoking, exercise, diet, and sleep patterns. The client should be asked to describe the usual patterns as well as changes that may have occurred.

Review of Systems

A careful review of systems is important if an endocrine problem is suspected. All body systems are reviewed because endocrine disorders can affect the entire body with multisystem effects.

PHYSICAL EXAMINATION

Physical examination of the endocrine system is integrated throughout the interaction with the client, beginning with the history interview. As the client responds to questions, the nurse observes the client's level of consciousness (orientation, alertness), memory, affect, and speech patterns. Signs of anxiety or nervousness are noted.

General Appearance. The nurse should observe the client's state of dress, growth and development, level of consciousness, orientation, body size. Height and weight are measured and compared to published norms. Extremities are observed for proportion to the rest of the body.

Vital Signs. The nurse should measure and assess vital signs. The temperature will be elevated in hyperthyroidism or may be low normal or below normal in hypothyroidism. The nurse observes respirations for change in rate and rhythm. Blood pressure changes include hypotension, hypertension, widening pulse pressure, and orthostatic changes along with pulse changes.

Integument. The nurse should observe hair texture and distribution over body surfaces, noting brittleness or alopecia. The nurse inspects the skin for color, pigmentation, striae, ecchymosis and palpates the skin for texture, thickness, moisture, diaphoresis. The nails are inspected and palpated for color, texture, brittleness, ridges, peeling.

Head. The nurse should inspect head contour and shape, noting symmetry of facial features. He or she should observe skin color for erythema or a rash over the cheeks and observe the client's facial expression for anxiety.

Eyes. The nurse should inspect and palpate the eyebrows, noting hair distribution. He or she observes eye position, symmetry, shape, and lid lag, assesses visual acuity, extraocular movements, and visual fields, and inspects for lens opacity and eye edema.

Nose. The nurse should inspect mucosa for swelling and color and listen for noisy breathing.

Mouth. The nurse should note the size and shape of the jaw. He or she inspects oral mucosa color and condition of teeth (mottling), noting malocclusion. The nurse observes tongue size and activity for fasciculations.

Neck. The nurse should listen to the client's voice for hoarseness or huskiness and note speech clarity, pitch, and volume. The nurse should ask the client to swallow and observe for difficulty swallowing or pain, repeating this maneuver with the neck hyperextended. The neck is inspected for symmetry, alignment, thickness or bulging over the thyroid gland, and midline position of the trachea. The presence of hyperpigmentation should be noted. The nurse observes for forceful pulsations over the carotid arteries.

Extremities. The nurse should examine the arms and legs for size, shape, symmetry, and their proportion to the trunk. The distance from the symphysis pubis to the heel is usually about half of a body's total height. The nurse should note peripheral edema, palpate and rate peripheral pulse amplitude, and assess deep tendon reflexes and observe their relaxation time (see Chap. 12).

Upper Extremities. The nurse should ask the client to extend the hands with palms down and observe for fine tremors. The nurse should inspect for thenar wasting, Dupuytren's contracture, and nail clubbing (see Chap. 19) and assess grip strength and muscle strength of the fingers and arms (see Chap. 43).

Lower Extremities. The nurse should note the color and distribution of hair and assess the size of the feet in proportion to the rest of the client's body. He or she inspects for corns and calluses, separating the toes and observing for deformities and skin changes such as thickening, fissures, or nail thickening. The nurse palpates and rates pedal pulses and assesses leg muscles for weakness (see Chap. 43).

Thorax. The nurse should inspect for gynecomastia in males and auscultate for extra heart sounds, such as a systolic murmur (see Chap. 23).

Abdomen. The nurse should note areas of hyperpigmentation such as in scars or striae. When lightly palpating the abdomen, the nurse observes the client for signs of pain.

Genitalia. The nurse should observe the pattern of pubic hair distribution, particularly in female clients. A diamond-shaped (male) pattern is indicative of a masculinizing tumor. The nurse should note the size of the testes and the clitoris for comparison to expected norms.

The remainder of endocrine assessment is with diagnostic studies, as the only endocrine glands accessible to physical examination are the thyroid and gonads. Assessment of the gonads is discussed in Chapter 51.

DIAGNOSTIC TESTS

Tests of the endocrine system involve several general types of clinical evaluations. Blood levels of the various hormones are obtained through radioimmunoassay and enzyme immunoassay. Radioimmunoassay is a technique in which antibodies to the hormone and radioactively tagged hormones are placed in a test tube with untagged hormones. The two types of hormones compete for sites on the antibodies. If most of the radiotagged hormone is bound to the antibody, there is a decreased amount of client hormone. Enzyme immunoassay is performed like the radioimmunoassay, except that enzymes are used instead of radioisotopes. This method allows hormones, such as thyroid hormone, to be tested in small amounts.

Pituitary Function

The structure of the pituitary gland can be assessed with skull x-ray study, computed tomography, or magnetic resonance imaging. Tumors of the pituitary may be visualized with these studies.

Growth hormone is secreted in a diurnal pattern, and its level can be assayed. It is usually drawn in the morning to determine basal levels; usual levels are 3 μg/mL. Growth hormone can be stimulated with levodopa (500 mg orally), insulin (0.1 units/kg intravenously), or bromocriptine (5 mg orally). Following the stimulus, blood is drawn at intervals up to 120 minutes. Growth hormone levels usually peak 60 minutes after the stimuli.

An absence of antidiuretic hormones leads to diabetes insipidus. To diagnose diabetes insipidus, the

TABLE 39–1 Thyroid Function Tests

Test	Preparation	Procedure	Normal Findings	Significance of Abnormal Findings
Serum thyroxine (T_4) or triiodothyronine (T_3)	No food or water restrictions. Question client concerning medications recently taken	Sample of venous blood drawn and sent to laboratory	4.5–11.5 μg/100 mL of serum (adults)	Low concentration of thyroxine or triiodothyronine indicates hypothyroidism. Excessive concentrations of thyroid hormones indicates hyperthyroidism
Serum thyroid-stimulating hormone (TSH)	No restrictions	Sample of venous blood drawn and sent to laboratory	1 to 10 μ units/mL	Elevated levels indicate primary hypothyroidism
Radioiodine uptake test (^{131}I uptake)	No food or water restrictions. Reassure client that doses of radioiodine used for tests are extremely small and not harmful. Notify physician of recent ingestion of seafood and iodine-containing medication or recent x-ray studies	Client receives tracer dose of ^{131}I. 24-hour urine specimen is started at time of drug administration. After 24 hours, scintillation counter is placed over thyroid gland to measure exact amount of radioactivity emitting from gland. 24-hour urine specimen is labeled and sent to lab for analysis.	15 to 35% uptake. Urine excretion: 40 to 80% ^{131}I within first 24 hours	*Uptake results:* early high peak in ^{131}I uptake indicates hyperthyroidism. Persistent low ^{131}I uptake indicates hypothyroidism. *Urine excretion:* excretion less than 40% indicates hyperthyroidism. Excretion greater than 80% indicates hypothyroidism
Triiodothyronine (T_3) resin uptake	No food and water restrictions. No special preparation	Blood sample drawn from client and sent to laboratory for incubation with T_3 and resin particles	Standardized in each laboratory	Depression of resin uptake of T_3 may indicate hypothyroidism. Elevation of resin uptake of T_3 may indicate hyperthyroidism.
Thyrotropin-releasing hormone (TRH) stimulation test	No restrictions	Client receives intravenous TRH. Serum TSH is measured in serum drawn before and 30 min after TRH injection	Increase in TSH	No rise in TSH in pituitary disease (secondary hypothyroidism) or hyperthyroidism

client is given a water deprivation test. Water is withheld for 4 to 18 hours, and during this time, the client's vital signs, urine output, and urine specific gravity are assessed hourly. Hypovolemic shock can develop from dehydration. In a client without diabetes insipidus, urine output decreases and urine osmolarity increases. The client with diabetes insipidus is not able to respond and continues to produce high volumes of dilute urine (low osmolarity).

Thyroid Function

A number of tests are available to assess thyroid function. The most important tests are outlined in Table 39–1.

Serologic Tests. Many thyroid disorders are presumed to have an autoimmune basis, such as Hashimoto's thyroiditis, some types of myxedema, and Graves' disease (a form of hyperthyroidism). Consequently, serologic tests may be performed to determine if the person's blood contains any antithyroid antibodies.

Adrenal Function

Adrenal function tests are divided into medullary and cortical types. Adrenal hormones include cortisol, aldosterone, and adrenocorticotropic hormone (ACTH). Medullary hormones include the catecholamines.

Cortisol is secreted in a diurnal pattern, and levels are assessed at 8:00 AM and 8:00 PM. A cortisone suppression test is the suppression of the pituitary ACTH with dexamethasone. Normally after administration of dexamethasone, 24-hour levels of ketosteroid in the urine drop 50 per cent. Dexamethasone can also be given at midnight, and then serum cortisol assessed at 8:00 AM. In clients with increased adrenocortical stimulation, there will be no decrease in ketosteroid production in urine or serum levels of cortisol.

Plasma levels of aldosterone, angiotensin II, and renin can be measured at any time. Plasma levels of aldosterone can be increased by giving potassium, restricting sodium, or having the client assume an upright position. Plasma levels of aldosterone can be decreased by infusing saline.

Serum levels of ACTH can be assessed after the infusion of synthetic ACTH. Urine levels of ketosteroid would be expected to rise to 25 mg/24 hours; plasma levels of cortisol should rise to 10 to 40 μg/100 mL. Urine levels of ketosteroid can be measured with 24-hour urine specimens. These substances are metabolites of the hormones produced by the adrenal cortex. A preservative is required for the collection bottle, and if the client has an indwelling catheter, the bag is placed on ice.

The adrenal cortex can be assessed for tumors by x-ray study, computed tomography, and magnetic resonance imaging.

The function of the adrenal medulla can be assessed through urine levels of catecholamines and their metabolites (vanillylmandelic acid). A 24-hour urine sample is collected and assayed. The medulla can be suppressed with the administration of ganglionic blocking agents. These agents normally decrease the urine levels of catecholamines. In clients with pheochromocytoma, a tumor of the adrenal medulla, there is a negligible effect.

Pancreatic Function

Diagnostic assessment of pancreatic function is discussed in Chapters 36 and 40.

STUDY QUESTIONS

1. A client who has an endocrine disorder involving an increase in cortisol production should exhibit which change in vital signs?
   A. Decrease in temperature
   B. Increase in pulse
   C. Decrease in respiration
   D. Increase in blood pressure
2. The etiology of disorders of carbohydrate metabolism are affected by all of the following hormones except which one?
   A. Aldosterone
   B. Insulin
   C. Glucagon
   D. Epinephrine
3. While doing a physical examination on a client with a suspected endocrine disorder, the nurse observes that the client exhibits exophthalmos. The nurse should assess for further signs of:
   A. Addison's disease
   B. Hyperthyroidism
   C. Acromegaly
   D. Diabetes mellitus
4. A client is scheduled for a radioactive iodine uptake test. The nurse knows that his or her teaching has been effective when the client verbalizes that:
   A. He must stay in the hospital overnight because he will be radioactive.
   B. He must not eat or drink anything before the test.

C. He must notify the physician of recent ingestion of seafood.
D. There are no restrictions on him before the test.

5. A client with a known endocrine disorder comes to the clinic complaining of increased thirst. During the nursing assessment, the nurse notices that the client is dehydrated. Which of the following hormones might be responsible for these signs and symptoms?
A. Antidiuretic hormone (ADH)
B. Melanocyte-stimulating hormone (MSH)
C. Luteinizing hormone (LH)
D. Follicle-stimulating hormone (FSH)

CRITICAL THINKING EXERCISES

SCENARIO A

A client is scheduled for a radioactive iodine uptake test (^{131}I) of the thyroid gland.

1. What is the purpose of the ^{131}I test?
2. This procedure may be used with other diagnostic tests in the evaluation of what clinical states?
3. What signs and symptoms would a client manifest who is a candidate for this test?
4. What factors can interfere with the results of this test?

SCENARIO B

A client with an endocrine disorder is placed on a glucocorticoid to be taken three times a day.

1. What is the major glucocorticoid in humans?
2. What effects does cortisol have on the following:
   a. Glucose metabolism
   b. Protein metabolism
   c. Fluid and electrolyte balance
   d. Inflammation and immunity
   e. Stressors
3. What nursing assessments in the area of glucose metabolism are warranted for a client on cortisol therapy?
4. What nursing assessments are warranted for a client on cortisol therapy to monitor the antianabolic effects of the drug?
5. Why is it necessary to stop the treatment of cortisol gradually?

BIBLIOGRAPHY

1. Applegate, E. (1995). *The anatomy and physiology learning system textbook.* Philadelphia: W. B. Saunders.
2. Bates, B. (1991). *A guide to physical examination* (5th ed.). Philadelphia: J. B. Lippincott.
3. Corbett, J. (1991). *Laboratory tests and diagnostic procedures with nursing diagnoses* (3rd ed.). Norwalk, CT: Appleton & Lange.
4. Fischbach, F. (1992). *A manual of laboratory and diagnostic tests* (4th ed.). Philadelphia: J. B. Lippincott.
5. Jarvis, C. (1992). *Physical examination and health assessment.* Philadelphia: W. B. Saunders.
6. McCance, K., & Huether, S. (1994). *Pathophysiology: The biological basis for disease in adults and children* (2nd ed.). St. Louis: Mosby-Yearbook.
7. Price, S., & Wilson, L. (1992). *Pathophysiology: Clinical concepts of disease processes* (4th ed.). St. Louis: Mosby-Yearbook.
8. Sheldon, H. (1992). *Boyd's introduction to the study of disease* (11th ed.). Philadelphia: Lea & Febiger.
9. Solomon, E., et al. (1990). *Human anatomy and physiology* (2nd ed.). Philadelphia: Saunders College Publishing.
10. Wilson, J., & Foster, D. (1992). *Williams textbook of endocrinology* (8th ed.). Philadelphia: W. B. Saunders.

Chapter 40 Nursing Care of Clients with Endocrine Disorders of the Pancreas

Learning Outcomes

After completing this chapter, the learner will be able to:

1. Assess the client for clinical manifestations of IDDM (Type I) and NIDDM (Type II).
2. Describe the incidence, etiology, risk factors, and basic pathophysiology of diabetes mellitus to the client.
3. Explain the client's role in the assessments utilized in the diagnosis of diabetes mellitus.
4. Develop a plan of care based on dietary management, pharmacologic intervention, and a modification of lifestyle for the client with diabetes mellitus.
5. Implement nursing interventions to promote health maintenance for clients with diabetes mellitus through health education.
6. Teach the client about acute and chronic complications of diabetes mellitus and the appropriate health care interventions.
7. Evaluate planned client outcomes utilized for planning the care of a client with diabetes mellitus.

Diabetes Mellitus

Diabetes mellitus is a heterogeneous group of disorders characterized by glucose intolerance. It is a disease caused by an imbalance between insulin supply and insulin demand. In diabetes mellitus, either there is not enough insulin or the insulin that is produced is ineffective, resulting in high blood glucose levels. Diabetes mellitus also causes disturbances of protein and fat metabolism. These abnormalities are associated with microvascular, macrovascular, and neuropathic changes.

There are two main types of diabetes mellitus: insulin-dependent diabetes mellitus (IDDM or Type I) and non–insulin-dependent diabetes mellitus (NIDDM or Type II) (Table 40–1).

Incidence

Approximately 12 to 14 million Americans have diabetes, and approximately 6 million of these are undiagnosed. About 600,000 new cases of diabetes are reported in the United States each year. Twice as many black Americans between the ages of 45 and 65 years have diabetes than do whites, and Hispanics are three times as likely to develop diabetes mellitus. Native Americans have the highest rate of NIDDM in the world. Nearly one third of clients with diabetes mellitus are over the age of 60 years.

Most clients in the United States (85 to 90 per cent) who develop diabetes mellitus are non–insulin-dependent. Approximately 10 per cent are insulin-dependent, and about 2 per cent of diabetes is secondary to other causes (i.e., medications, receptor problems, genetic disease, hormonal changes). Gestational diabetes develops in about 2 to 5 per cent of all pregnancies.

Diabetes, with its complications, is the fourth leading cause of death by disease in the United States; 160,000 clients will die from diabetes mellitus and its complications this year. Even when diabetes does not kill, it can produce major permanent disabilities. Diabetes mellitus is

- the leading cause of new blindness in adults
- the leading cause of new cases of renal failure (one fourth of all clients requiring dialysis have diabetes)
- responsible for 50 to 70 per cent of all nontraumatic amputations in the United States
- responsible for an increased risk of coronary artery disease and strokes. Clients with diabetes are twice as likely to have coronary artery disease and three times as likely to suffer a stroke

Over the previous decades, the incidence of diabetes in the United States has steadily increased. Diabetes mellitus is becoming more frequent for a number of reasons:

- longer life expectancy
- obesity
- children of diabetic parents who themselves develop diabetes

Etiology

INSULIN-DEPENDENT DIABETES MELLITUS

Both genetic and environmental factors seem to precipitate IDDM. Because the highest incidence of new cases of IDDM occurs during seasonal variations, it is believed that environmental factors have a role in the development of diabetes. In clients who are predisposed to the development of diabetes, infection with certain viruses and organisms, such as coxsackievirus B and streptococcus, is an etiologic factor. These viruses and organisms attack the islet cells of the pancreas, which renders them useless for producing insulin.

It appears also that there is some autoimmune response in the development of IDDM. Apparently, some trigger causes the body to develop islet cell antibodies and anti-insulin antibodies. These antibodies attack the beta cells of the pancreas and also the insulin molecules themselves. Circulatory islet cell antibodies are found in approximately 85 per cent of all newly diagnosed IDDM clients.

Heredity is also believed to play a role in the development of IDDM. Siblings of clients with diabetes have 10 times the risk of developing diabetes over the general population. Certain human leukocyte antigens

TABLE 40–1 Comparison of Dietary Interventions for Insulin-Dependent and Non–Insulin-Dependent Diabetes

INTERVENTION	INSULIN-DEPENDENT (NONOBESE CLIENT)	NON–INSULIN-DEPENDENT (OBESE CLIENT)
Calories	No special caloric restrictions	Restrict calories; weight loss often decreases blood sugar level to within normal limits
Size and frequency of meals	Routine (e.g., 3 meals/day) with regular and appropriate snacks	Optional, but total calories/day should provide for 0.5–1 kg (1–2 lb) weight loss/week
Hypoglycemia	Prevent by increasing calories during increased exercise or stress; intervene with foods high in simple sugars (orange juice, hard candy)	Prevent by regular, reasonable diet; provide strategies for regulating meal plans
Exercise	Exercise planned with appropriate insulin and glucose adjustments	Exercise usually needed to promote weight loss

on specific chromosomes appear to predispose clients to the development of IDDM.

NON–INSULIN-DEPENDENT DIABETES MELLITUS

Viruses and human leukocyte antigens do not appear to play a role in the development of NIDDM. Heredity, however, does have a major role. Research also indicates that obesity is one of the most important determinants for the development of NIDDM. Approximately 80 per cent of all clients with NIDDM are obese (20 per cent over ideal body weight). Overweight clients require more insulin for metabolizing the food they eat. Hyperglycemia develops when the pancreas cannot secrete enough insulin to match the body's needs or when the number of insulin receptor sites is decreased or altered (as often occurs with obesity). Increasing age may also be a risk because the pancreas becomes more sluggish with age in clients who are already predisposed to diabetes.

Risk Factors

Clients with a family history of diabetes are at far greater risk for developing diabetes, especially NIDDM. Primary prevention of NIDDM centers on maintaining as ideal a body weight as possible. Secondary prevention is the initiation of weight reduction measures and exercise programs by dietitians, nurses, and exercise physiologists or physical therapists.

Because diabetes cannot always be prevented, health agencies strive to diagnose diabetes in its early stages, often before clients are aware of the symptoms. Screening is a form of secondary prevention.

The nurse should suspect diabetes in anyone who (1) is obese; (2) suffers from excessive thirst, hunger, urination, and weight loss; (3) has given birth to a baby over 9 lb; (4) has a family history of diabetes; or (5) is over the age of 40 years. Anyone who is found to have an elevated blood glucose level during screening should be referred to a physician for more conclusive tests.

Pathophysiology

Insulin-dependent diabetes mellitus is associated with inflammation of the islets of the pancreas and appears to be an autoimmune response. Infection with coxsackievirus B has been shown to be the likely trigger of the autoimmune response, although other etiologic factors may also exist, such as inherited susceptibility. After infection with the virus, the beta cells inappropriately express an antigen. The antigens on the beta cells are recognized and destroyed by circulating T cells. The process of cellular destruction is marked by the appearance of islet cell antibodies. Islet cell antibodies occur in up to 85 per cent of newly diagnosed insulin-dependent diabetics.

Sometimes the pancreas will attempt to produce near-normal or normal levels of insulin during a "honeymoon phase," usually noted after initial diagnosis. This phase may last 6 months or longer, but eventually, in true diabetes, the client will develop signs of hyperglycemia again.

A refractoriness to insulin in the cell membrane receptor causes NIDDM. The development of this form of diabetes is consistent with all the pathophysiologic changes seen in long-term obesity, with one exception. In obesity, insulin resistance is compensated by increased insulin production. In diabetes, the pancreas cannot compensate for problems in the receptors by increasing insulin production. Some newer theories suggest that over time, the high levels of circulating insulin that occur with obesity "insulinize" the cells, making them more resistant to the action of insulin.

METABOLIC EFFECTS OF DIABETES

Without insulin, three major metabolic problems occur: decreased utilization of glucose, increased mobilization of fat, and increased utilization of protein.

Decreased Glucose Utilization. In diabetes, cells that require insulin as a carrier for glucose can take in only about 25 per cent of the glucose they require for fuel. The skeletal and cardiac muscles and adipose tissues rely on insulin for glucose transport. Glucose remains in the blood, and blood glucose levels rise (hyperglycemia). The glucose level continues to rise because the liver cannot store glucose as glycogen without insulin.

In an attempt to restore balance and normal levels of glucose, the kidney excretes the excess glucose. Sugar appears in the urine (glucosuria). Glucose excreted in the urine acts as an osmotic diuretic and causes excretion of increased amounts of water. This process results in fluid volume deficit.

Increased Fat Mobilization. Fortunately, the body can rely on fat stores for energy when glucose is not available. Unfortunately, the process of fat metabolism leads to the formation of breakdown products called ketones. Ketones accumulate in the blood and are excreted through the kidneys and lungs. Ketone levels can be measured in the blood and urine and can serve as an indicator of diabetes. Ketones interfere with acid-base balance by producing hydrogen ions. The pH can fall, and the client can develop metabolic acidosis. In addition, when ketones are excreted, sodium is also eliminated, which results in sodium depletion and further acidosis. When ketones are excreted, they also increase osmotic pressure and cause increased fluids to be lost.

When fats are used as the primary source of energy, the body lipid level can rise to five times normal. This elevated level can lead to atherosclerosis.

Increased Protein Utilization. Lack of insulin also causes protein wasting. Normally, proteins are constantly being broken down and rebuilt. Without insulin to stimulate protein synthesis, the balance is altered, and there is increased catabolism. Amino acids are converted to glucose in the liver, which further compounds the elevated glucose levels. Untreated, the diabetic individual appears thin and emaciated.

Clinical Manifestations

CARDINAL SIGNS OF DIABETES

The excretion of glucose and ketones leads to increased urine output and thirst. Extra food is eaten but cannot be metabolized, which leads to hunger, and the client loses weight. These processes result in the four cardinal signs of diabetes:

- polyuria
- polydipsia
- polyphagia
- weight loss

(See the box, Clinical Manifestations: Cardinal Signs of Diabetes.)

The client with IDDM usually presents with the cardinal signs and symptoms and sometimes already has complications.

Clients with NIDDM may also develop the cardinal signs and symptoms; however, these symptoms usually develop more slowly in NIDDM because many of these clients are elderly and may not recognize the abnormal thirst or frequent urination as abnormal for their age. More commonly, they may only experience visual blurring, neuropathic complications (such as pain in the feet), or infections. NIDDM is commonly diagnosed while the client is hospitalized for another problem.

DIAGNOSTIC ASSESSMENT

Blood Glucose (Blood Sugar). A blood sample for determination of glucose level may be drawn at any time and requires no preparation of the client. The results should be within normal limits for both nondiabetics and diabetics in good control. Elevated blood glucose levels may occur after meals, after stressful events, if the sample was drawn from above an intravenous site, or in clients with diabetes.

Elevated blood glucose levels (hyperglycemia) warrant investigation if the client is not a known diabetic. Fluctuations in blood glucose over 24 hours in a client with uncontrolled diabetes mellitus are shown in Figure 40–1.

Hypoglycemia also warrants investigation in the nondiabetic.

Fasting Blood Sugar. For fasting blood sugar tests, the client may not eat for 4 hours, but water intake may continue. If the client is being infused with a dextrose intravenous solution, the results of the test will not be accurate. If the client is a known diabetic, food and insulin are withheld until after the specimen is drawn. Average normal values for adults are 70 to 110 mg/100 mL but vary with age. As a general rule, in an adult, a fasting blood sugar level over 140 mg for two to three consecutive tests may indicate diabetes.

Postprandial Blood Sugar. These blood glucose levels are tested after meals. Sometimes the client is given a standard amount of glucose, but most commonly the sample is drawn after a standard meal. The purpose of the meal is to determine how well the carbohydrates are digested. After 2 hours, the blood sugar level should return to normal. Nurses accurately record the meal eaten and ascertain that the sample was drawn 2 hours after eating. This test is usually used as a mass screening effort in communities, and the results may not be accurate because of self-reporting by the client of the meal eaten.

Blood Glucose Finger Sticks. The invention of self-monitoring devices for blood sugar has revolutionized diabetes care. These new machines use reagent strips and a photometer and have a digital readout of blood sugar values. There are two major drawbacks to this method: the need to stick oneself; and the cost of the monitor, strips, lancets, and wipes.

Blood glucose monitoring tests must be performed with extreme care and accuracy. The Joint Commission on Accreditation of Hospitals and other regulating bodies dictate the procedure and frequency for quality control of meters. Most devices have some type of con-

CLINICAL MANIFESTATIONS

Cardinal Signs of Diabetes

Clinical Manifestations	Pathophysiologic Bases
Polyuria (frequent urination)	Water not reabsorbed from renal tubules because of osmotic activity of glucose in the tubules
Polydipsia (excessive thirst)	Polyuria causes severe dehydration, which causes thirst
Polyphagia (excessive hunger)	Tissue breakdown and wasting cause a state of starvation that compels the client to eat excessive amounts of food
Weight loss (primarily in insulin-dependent diabetes)	Glucose not available to cells; thus, the body breaks down fat and protein stores for energy

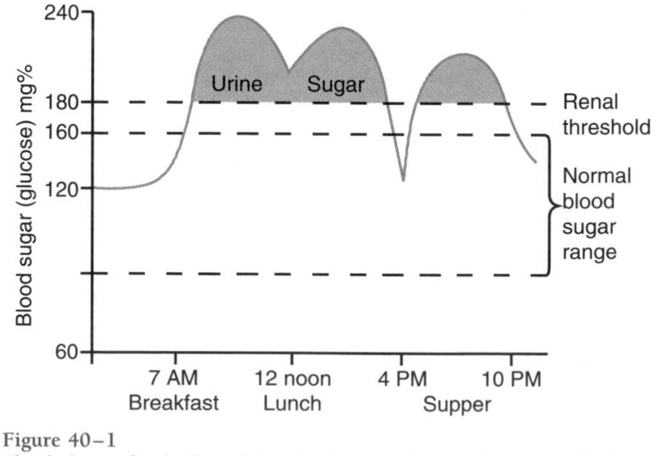

Figure 40–1
Blood glucose levels throughout the day in a client with uncontrolled diabetes mellitus. Sugar appears in the urine when blood glucose exceeds 180 mg/100 mL (renal threshold). (Adapted from Kozak, G. P. [1982]. *Clinical diabetes mellitus.* Philadelphia: W. B. Saunders.)

trol process for determining accuracy of the machine. Manufacturers' instructions must be followed exactly because test results are used to adjust insulin or oral hypoglycemic dosages, exercise regimens, and dietary management. The devices are technique-dependent, and because treatment is based on results, accuracy is a major concern.

Self-monitoring of blood glucose is recommended for all clients with IDDM, clients with NIDDM who require insulin, pregnant women, clients who have an insulin pump, and clients who have widely fluctuating blood glucose levels.

Glycosylated Hemoglobin. Glucose normally attaches itself to the hemoglobin molecule on a red blood cell. Once attached, it cannot dissociate. Therefore, the higher the blood glucose levels have been, the higher are the glycosylated hemoglobin results. Glycosylated hemoglobin is the average of blood glucose control over the previous 3 months—the lifespan of a red blood cell.

Glycosylated hemoglobin can be sampled at any time during the day, in contrast to a fasting blood sugar specimen, which is drawn before breakfast. This allows the test to be done during a client's initial visit to a physician in order to obtain a more accurate assessment of the client's compliance with the prescribed plan of care, evaluate a client with wide fluctuations in blood glucose levels, or manage blood glucose levels during pregnancy.

Glucose Tolerance Test. The oral glucose tolerance test is considered one of the best methods of diagnosing diabetes. However, because there are so many factors that render the test invalid, many hospitalized clients are diagnosed by fasting blood sugar levels. Bed rest, infection, trauma, medications, and stress can alter the test results.

The client needs to be on a normal diet for several days before the test is done. The test is usually done in the morning so that the client is in a fasting state. At the start of the test, a blood sample for fasting blood glucose level and a urine sample for glycosuria are taken. The client is then given 100 g of glucose to drink. Blood and urine samples are taken at 1-, 2-, and 3-hour intervals afterward. The client cannot eat after the glucose ingestion but can drink water to stimulate urine production.

The results of the samples are plotted on a graph to see how long it takes blood glucose to return to normal levels. Diabetics either take longer to return to normal or never return to normal. In a client below the age of 55 years, the blood sugar should return to normal in 2 hours, with a peak of 120 to 160 mg. In clients over 55 years, the peak may be as high as 200 mg, and normal values may not return for over 3 hours.

Criteria for diagnosis of diabetes are listed in Box 40–1.

BOX 40–1

Criteria for Diagnosis of Diabetes Mellitus

DIABETES MELLITUS (ADULT)

- Elevation of plasma glucose (≥200 mg/100 mL) and classic symptoms of diabetes, including polydipsia, polyuria, polyphagia, and weight loss
- Fasting plasma glucose >140 mg/100 mL on two consecutive occasions or oral glucose tolerance test values >200 mg/100 mL at 2 hours and at one intervening point between 0 and 2 hours

IMPAIRED GLUCOSE TOLERANCE

- Fasting blood glucose <140 mg/100 mL *and*
- 2-hour blood sugar level ≥140 and <200 mg/100 mL *with*
- one intervening blood sugar level ≥200 mg/100 mL after a 75 g glucose load

GESTATIONAL DIABETES MELLITUS

Diagnosis is confirmed when two or more of the following blood sugar levels are met or exceeded when a 100 g glucose load is used rather than 75 g

- Fasting blood sugar ≥105 mg/100 mL
- 1 hour ≥190 mg/100 mL
- 2 hour ≥165 mg/100 mL
- 3 hour ≥145 mg/100 mL

Medical Management

To date, there is no known cure for diabetes. Consequently, the overall goal of care for clients with diabetes is control or regulation of blood glucose levels rather than cure. When diabetes is successfully regulated, the client may avoid the complications of hyperglycemia and hypoglycemia, with minimal disruption to a normal lifestyle. Unfortunately, clients with diabetes may develop complications despite their own vigorous efforts to carefully control their disease.

Diabetes control depends on the proper interaction of three factors: (1) diet, (2) insulin or oral medication to lower blood glucose, and (3) exercise.

The intervention planned for the treatment of diabetes must be individualized. It needs to be based on the client's age, life-style, nutritional needs, maturation, activity level, occupation, and ability to independently perform the skills required by the treatment plan (i.e., monitoring of blood glucose levels, insulin injection).

CRITERIA FOR GOOD CONTROL OF DIABETES

Diabetes is generally considered under control when the following conditions are met:

- The client's weight is within recommended medical limits and the client enjoys good health.
- Glycosylated hemoglobin is in normal range (normal values vary between laboratories).
- Fasting blood glucose level is under 140 mg/100 mL
- Blood glucose level is no higher than 180 mg/100 mL 1 to 2 hours after meals.

DIETARY MANAGEMENT

Dietary management is discussed first, because diet is considered the cornerstone of diabetic management.

The balanced nutritional plan for clients with diabetes has a twofold purpose: (1) to discourage the ingestion of foods with high sugar and fat content and (2) to correct or avoid obesity. Table 40–1 outlines the contrasting strategies that clinicians use for regulating the diet of clients who are either obese but not insulin-dependent or not obese but insulin-dependent.

Some of the nutritional goals for clients with diabetes are to (1) achieve normoglycemia, as possible, (2) maintain lipids within a normal range (cholesterol, low-density lipoproteins, high-density lipoproteins, triglycerides), (3) prevent wide swings in the blood glucose levels, (4) have normal growth and development in children and adolescents, and (5) meet individualized weight loss goals (usually 1 to 2 lb per week as appropriate). It is now known that hyperglycemia and hyperlipidemia promote the complications of diabetes. Therefore, the emphasis for clients with diabetes is on controlling concentrated sweets and fat intake.

The current recommendations for the distribution of calories are

- 55 to 60 per cent carbohydrates
- 30 per cent fats
- 12 to 20 per cent proteins

The current recommendations from the American Dietetic Association and the American Diabetes Association call for less fat in the meal plan than was previously allowed because of the known increased risk for myocardial infarctions, strokes, and other blood vessel diseases in clients with diabetes.

Carbohydrates should be mostly complex, including foods high in soluble fiber such as corn, oats, peas, apples, potatoes, broccoli, carrots, and dried beans. In addition to being filling, these foods lower glucose and cholesterol levels and insulin requirements. Fats should be primarily polyunsaturated or monounsaturated. Proteins should come from low-fat sources too.

Recent research has indicated that clients with diabetes may not have to eliminate all simple sugars from their diets. Concentrated sweets should be avoided, but 5 per cent of the diet can be sucrose as long as it is eaten at intervals and with other foods.

Overweight NIDDM clients should remain on a weight-loss diet until they reach a medically recommended weight. Weight reduction slows the release of glucose into the bloodstream and increases the number of insulin receptor cells, with lessening of the defects that might impair normal use of glucose. Blood glucose levels begin to improve with as little as a 5- to 10-lb weight loss. Carbohydrate exchanges are shown in Box 40–2.

BOX 40–2

Carbohydrate Food Exchange List

CARBOHYDRATE REPLACEMENT

Fruit exchange = 15 g carbohydrate
Bread/starch exchange = 15 g carbohydrate
Milk exchange = 12 g carbohydrate

THE FOLLOWING CONTAIN APPROXIMATELY 15 g CARBOHYDRATE

½ c applesauce
½ banana
15 grapes
¾ c mandarin oranges
⅓ c pineapple
⅛ c peaches, pears, cherries
¾ c dry cereal (except bran)
½ c bran cereal, Shredded Wheat
½ c corn, peas, potato, lima beans
1 slice bread
3 c popcorn
3 graham cracker squares
½ c diet pudding, custard
½ c pasta
⅓ c rice
6 saltine crackers
½ c sherbet (½ of container)
½ c vanilla ice cream
6 vanilla wafers
1 c milk
1 c plain yogurt
½ c apple, orange, pineapple, grapefruit juices
⅓ c regular cranberry, grape, prune juices

PHARMACOLOGIC MANAGEMENT

Oral Hypoglycemic Agents

Some clients with NIDDM may require oral hypoglycemic agents for lowering blood glucose levels. Oral hypoglycemic agents are *not* insulin. They lower the blood glucose in part by stimulating the pancreatic beta cells to release insulin. They also appear to make target tissues more sensitive to the effects of insulin by increasing the number of receptor sites and by enhancing insulin's action at the postreceptor sites. Some of them also work to decrease glucose production (gluconeogenesis) in the liver.

Oral hypoglycemic agents currently available in the United States are the sulfonylureas (Table 40–2).

The average candidate for the oral hypoglycemic agents (1) is over the age of 40 years, (2) has no history of ketosis, (3) is not pregnant, (4) is on less than 40 units of insulin per day, and (5) has mild to moderate symptoms of hyperglycemia.

Oral hypoglycemic agents are contraindicated in clients with IDDM, pregnant or breastfeeding women, children, surgery clients, and those with allergies to sulfa.

Side effects of the oral hypoglycemic agents include hypoglycemia, especially in the elderly; and a disulfiram-like effect in about 35 per cent of all clients taking chlorpropamide. These symptoms include a severe flushing, nausea, and vomiting. Chlorpropamide also has a long half-life (up to 36 hours) and should be discontinued 24 to 48 hours before surgery because of its potential for causing hypoglycemia during surgery. As a result of its long half-life, it should also be used with caution in the elderly.

TABLE 40–2 Oral Hypoglycemic Agents

AGENT	STARTING DOSE	MAXIMAL DOSE	DURATION OF ACTION	FREQUENCY	METABOLISM
First-Generation					
Tolbutamide (Orinase)	0.5 g	2.0–3.0 g	6–12 hr	1–3/day	By liver to inactive product
Tolazamide (Tolinase)	100 mg	1.0 g	12–24 hr	1–2/day	By liver to active and inactive products requiring renal route
Acetohexamide (Dymelor)	250 mg	1.5 g	12–18 hr	1–2/day	Same as tolazamide
Chlorpropamide (Diabinase)	100–250 mg	0.5 g	60 hr	1/day	Approximately 70% by liver to less active products but renal route imperative
Second-Generation					
Glyburide (DiaBeta; Micronase)	1.25–5.0 mg	20 mg*	16–24 hr	1–2/day	By liver to mostly inert products
Glyburide (Glynase)	1.5–3 mg	12 mg*	24 hr	1–2/day	By liver to inert products
Glipizide (Glucotrol)	2.5–5.0 mg	40 mg*	12–24 hr	1–2/day	By liver to inert products

* Lower levels of glyburide and glipizide have been effective in reducing blood glucose by 25 per cent at 15 mg/day.

Glipizide should be administered about one half hour before a meal because its absorption is retarded by food. Both glipizide and glyburide have fewer side effects and less drug interaction with other medications than do the other oral hypoglycemic agents.

Insulin Therapy

All clients with IDDM must inject insulin daily to survive. Some clients with NIDDM may require insulin if diet, exercise, and oral hypoglycemic agents are ineffective. Some medications such as prednisone may elevate blood glucose levels and necessitate insulin injections for a time.

Insulin lowers blood glucose by (1) promoting the transport of glucose into the cells and (2) inhibiting the conversion of glycogen and amino acids to glucose. There are several different types of insulin. They are grouped according to speed of action in the body: (1) rapid-acting, (2) intermediate-acting, and (3) long-acting. Table 40–3 compares and contrasts these insulins. Whereas all types of insulin have the same basic action (i.e., the reduction of blood glucose), they differ in onset, peak, and duration of hypoglycemic effect and thus in the time period in which an insulin reaction is likely to occur.

If blood glucose is difficult to control, two different insulins can be mixed and administered as a single injection. For example, neutral protamine Hagedorn (NPH) and regular insulin can be mixed to provide for both the immediate and day-long insulin needs. Lente, Semilente, and Ultralente insulins can be mixed with each other. When regular insulin is mixed with Lente or Ultralente, the zinc in the intermediate- and long-acting insulin can cause prolonged actions of the regular insulin.

The absorption and duration of insulin varies by anatomic site. Insulin injected into the abdomen is absorbed fastest, and as a consequence, the duration is shortest. Moving the injection site to the arm, leg, or buttocks progressively slows absorption and lengthens duration.[1]

Insulin Sources. There are three sources of insulin: beef, pork, and "human." If the source is not specified on the bottle, the bottle contains a mixture of beef and pork. Pork insulin most closely resembles human insulin and is considered the least antigenic animal insulin. Human insulin is produced commercially by recombinant DNA technology. Human insulin is also produced by chemically modifying porcine insulin. Human insulin has less antigenicity than animal insulin. Human insulin may have a shorter duration and onset of action than beef or pork insulin. The peak may also be affected in intensity. Human insulin dosages may need to be reduced, therefore, if a client changes from animal-source insulin to human insulin. Clients should not change insulin sources on their own, but only under the direction of a physician.

Insulin Dosage. Insulin dosage varies greatly. Two major considerations determine insulin dosage.

Requirements of the Client. The insulin requirement usually increases when a client (1) is seriously ill, (2) develops an infection, (3) undergoes surgery, (4) suffers trauma, or (5) is going through puberty.

Client's Response to Insulin Injections. Because clients with diabetes vary widely in their response to insulin, the process of regulating insulin dosage may require several weeks. The starting dose of insulin is usually determined to be between 0.5 and 1 unit/kg body weight/day. Clients will optimally monitor their blood glucose at home, and physicians will regulate insulin on the basis of blood glucose level, diet, exercise, and other factors such as stress. Many clients are now initiated on insulin therapy as outpatients because metabolic demands may be quite different when the client is in the hospital than when he or she is at home.

TABLE 40–3 Types of Insulin

PREPARATION	SOURCE	APPEARANCE	ACTION IN HOURS: ONSET	PEAK	DURATION
Short					
Injection: Regular insulin		clear	½–1	2–4	6–8
Iletin I Regular*	beef/pork	clear	½–1	2–4	6–8
Iletin II Regular*	pork	clear	½–1	2–4	6–8
Humulin R*	human	clear	½–1	2–4	6–8
Novolin R†	human	clear	½–1	2–4	6–8
Velosulin human†	human	clear	½–1	2–4	6–8
Purified pork R†	pork	clear	½–1	2–4	6–8
Zinc suspension: Semilente insulin		cloudy	½–1	2–8	8–16
Intermediate					
Isophane suspension: NPH insulin†	beef	cloudy	1–2	6–12	18–26
Iletin I NPH*	beef/pork	cloudy	1–2	4–12	24–28
Iletin II NPH*	pork	cloudy	1–2	4–12	24–28
Humulin N*	human	cloudy	1–2	4–12	24–28
Novolin N†	human	cloudy	1–2	4–12	24–28
Purified pork N†	pork	cloudy	1–2	4–12	24–28
Zinc suspension: Lente insulin†	beef	cloudy	1–3	6–12	18–26
Iletin I Lente*	beef/pork	cloudy	1–3	6–15	24–28
Iletin II Lente*	pork	cloudy	1–3	6–15	24–28
Humulin L*	human	cloudy	1–3	6–15	24–28
Novolin L†	human	cloudy	1–3	6–15	24–28
Purified pork Lente†	pork	cloudy	1–3	6–15	24–28
Long					
Protamine zinc suspension: Protamine zinc insulin‡		cloudy	4–6	18–24	28–36
Extended zinc suspension: Ultralente insulin	beef	cloudy	4	10–30	36
Humulin U	human	cloudy	6–10	none	20–30
Premixed					
Humulin 50/50 (50% NPH, 50% regular)	human	cloudy	½	2–8	18–24
Humulin 70/30 (70% NPH, 30% regular)	human	cloudy	½	2–12	18–24
Novolin 70/30 (70% NPH, 30% regular)	human	cloudy	¼–1	2–8	24

NPH, neutral protamine Hagedorn.
* Manufactured by Eli Lilly, Indianapolis, IN.
† Manufactured by Novo Nordisk, Princeton, NJ.
‡ Seldom used.
Data from Schlafer, M., & Marieb, E. (1989). *The nurse, pharmacology, and drug therapy.* New York: Addison-Wesley Publishing Co.; and *Medical management of insulin-dependent (type I) diabetes.* (2nd ed). (1994). Alexandria, VA: American Diabetes Association Clinical Education Series.

Insulin Pumps. Small portable pumps for the continuous administration of regular insulin are now sometimes used (Fig. 40–2). The small pump, worn externally, injects insulin subcutaneously into the abdomen through an indwelling needle site that is usually rotated every 2 to 3 days. Insulin is normally infused at a low, "basal" rate (i.e., a rate that matches the client's basal metabolic needs), with additional infusion of larger amounts (boluses) of insulin before meals.

Insulin pumps often improve blood glucose control by means of continuous subcutaneous insulin infusion. However, they do not have a built-in feedback mechanism for monitoring blood glucose levels. To benefit from an insulin pump, the client must comply with

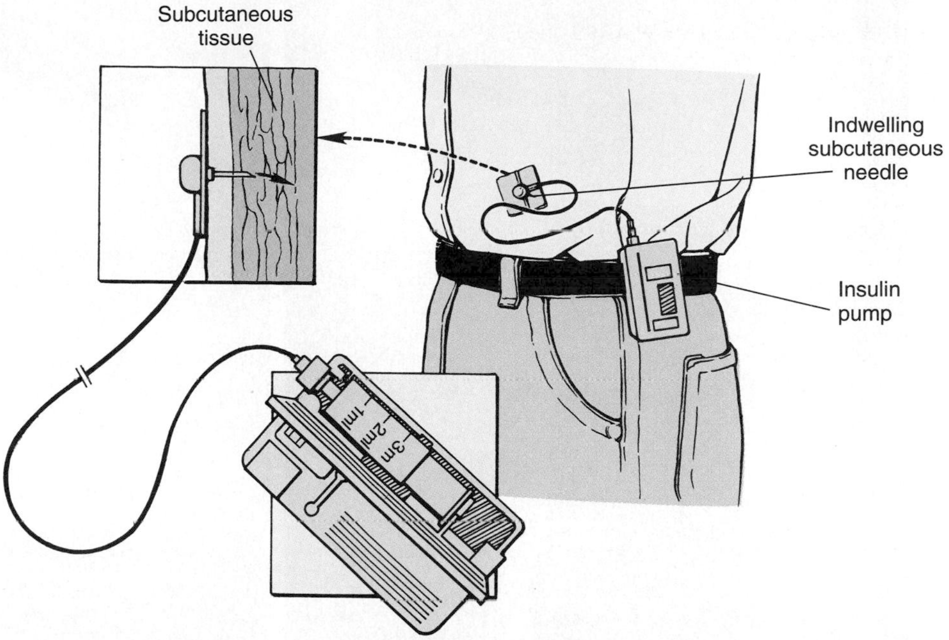

Figure 40–2
Insulin pump is worn externally with an indwelling subcutaneous needle usually placed in the abdomen.

dietary requirements and usually must deliver the correct premeal bolus of insulin. Clients must also monitor their blood glucose levels four to six times a day and make decisions regarding dosages based on the results.

These pumps store insulin either in syringes or in a disposable reservoir.

> **CRITICAL TO REMEMBER**
>
> Only regular insulin is used with the pump.

Disposable or rechargeable batteries power the pumps. Some of the newer pumps are no larger than a credit card.

Complications arising from use of insulin pumps include

- local infection at the injection site
- hypoglycemia due to error in calculating insulin dosage or to pump malfunction
- diabetic ketoacidosis due to injection of insufficient insulin to meet regular or increased metabolic needs or to pump malfunction

For initiation of insulin pump therapy, the client must be carefully supervised in either an inpatient or outpatient setting. During this time, the clinician adjusts the pump for basal and bolus doses before meals according to the client's usual diet and exercise regimen and previous insulin requirements.

Some clinicians and clients may decide to use an intensive insulin therapy program rather than insulin pump therapy. In intensive insulin therapy, the client must be willing to monitor blood glucose levels four to six times day and inject insulin three to five times a day. Throughout the initiating period of the pump or intensive insulin therapy, the nurse should assess the client's knowledge concerning (1) the meal plan, (2) monitoring techniques, (3) management goals, and (4) symptoms of and interventions for hyperglycemia and hypoglycemia. The client also needs to be made aware of the extra financial and emotional burdens. The family and significant others need to be involved in the teaching process. Finally, the client needs to know that there are no guarantees currently that either protocol will definitely prevent long-term complications.

Complications of Insulin Therapy

Insulin therapy may be complicated by one or more of the following conditions: hypoglycemia; tissue hypertrophy, atrophy, or both at the site of injection; erratic insulin action; insulin allergy; and insulin resistance.

Hypoglycemia. Clients usually experience symptoms of hypoglycemia (such as altered consciousness, tachycardia, or increased perspiration) when the blood glucose level drops to 60 mg/100 mL or less. In diabetes, an overdose of insulin, late or skipped meals, or overzealous exercise may cause hypoglycemic reactions. Hypoglycemia is discussed later in this chapter.

Tissue Hypertrophy or Atrophy. Tissue hypertrophy (lipohypertrophy) involves thickening of the subcutaneous tissues at injection sites (Fig. 40–3*A*). Tissue atrophy (lipoatrophy), in contrast, involves a loss of subcutaneous fat at the injection site. A hypertrophied area may feel lumpy and hard or spongy and soft. Tissue changes due to atrophy may be slight, causing only a dimpling of the tissues, or they may be extensive, causing large "craters" (Fig. 40–3*B*).

Erratic Insulin Action. Some clients respond erratically to insulin (i.e., with periods of hypoglycemia followed by periods of hyperglycemia). Box 40–3 lists the important causes of erratic insulin action.

Insulin Allergy. Clients who develop allergies during insulin therapy are usually sensitive to the insulin itself. Most insulin manufactured today, however, is extremely pure.

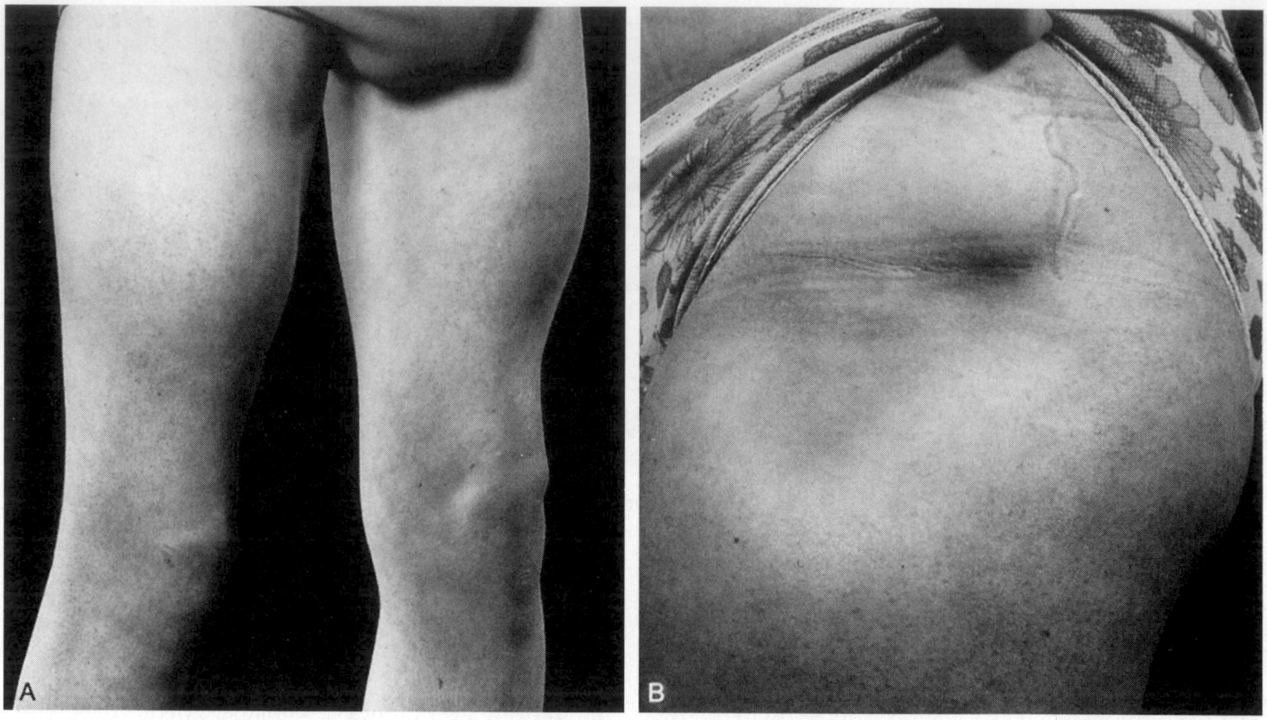

Figure 40–3
A, Lipohypertrophy at insulin injection sites, a consequence of the lipogenic effect of insulin. *B,* Lipoatrophy at insulin injection sites, caused by high circulating levels of insulin antibody. (From Besser, G., et al. [1988]. *Clinical diabetes: An illustrated text.* London: Gower Medical Publishing.)

BOX 40–3

Causes of Erratic Insulin Action

DIETARY

- Overeating
- Irregular meals
- Omission of snacks

INSULIN TECHNIQUE ERRORS

- Inaccurate measurement (visual problems)
- Failure to rotate injection sites
- Injecting insulin at sites of lipodystrophy
- Inadequate mixing
- Frozen or outdated insulin
- Improper dosage adjustment

PSYCHOLOGICAL ERRORS

- Deliberate omission or overdosage of insulin
- Inaccurate blood or urine tests
- Feigned insulin reactions
- Marital or parental tensions

CHRONIC OVERDOSAGE OF INSULIN (SOMOGYI EFFECT)

INTERMITTENT USE OF HYPER- OR HYPOGLYCEMIC DRUGS

(aspirin, phenylbutazone, steroids, birth control pills, alcohol, beer, cough syrups, thiazides, nicotinic acid, etc.)

IRREGULAR EXERCISE OR REST PERIODS

Insulin Resistance. The client who is insulin-resistant requires more than 200 units of insulin per day. Insulin resistance may be caused by specific insulin antagonists within the blood or by circulating antibodies that link to insulin, making it unavailable to the target tissue.

To treat insulin resistance, the clinician may first attempt to give the client human insulin. If human insulin fails, the clinician must then order as high a dosage of insulin as is needed to control the client's diabetes. Consequently, dosages may range from as low as 80 units/day to as high as thousands of units per day. There are special preparations of U-500 insulin available for those clients who require high insulin dosages.

SOMOGYI EFFECT

The Somogyi effect (also known as rebound hyperglycemia) is a rapid decrease in the blood glucose that generates the release of counter-regulatory hormones (epinephrine, cortisol, glucagon). Glucose is then released from muscle and liver cells, which causes a rapid rise in blood glucose. The hypoglycemia may be caused by (1) autonomic neuropathy, which results in no early warning signs of hypoglycemia; (2) inappropriate timing of insulin; the client's insulin may be peaking at 2:00 to 3:00 AM when blood glucose levels may be lower because of decreased metabolism; (3) exercise without adequate caloric intake; or (4) excessive insulin treatment, in which the client has consistently high glucose in the morning. Checking the glucose around 3:00 AM should help in differentiating the cause. Clients may interpret the hyperglycemia as a worsening of their condition and thus increase their insulin dose, which leads to perpetuation of the Somogyi effect. Therapy is aimed as gradual reduction of the insulin dose.

DAWN PHENOMENON

The dawn phenomenon is an early-morning (5:00 to 6:00 AM) increase in the blood glucose levels that is usually associated with the release of growth hormone. Monitoring the blood glucose at 3:00 AM should help to differentiate whether the hyperglycemia is related to the release of nocturnal growth hormone. If the 3:00 AM blood glucose level is normal and the 8:00 AM blood glucose level is elevated, the cause is probably the dawn phenomenon. To correct this, the clinician may change the time the evening insulin is given. For example, intermediate insulin may be given at 10:00 PM, which would peak around the same time as the release of growth hormone.

"HONEYMOON" PHASE

Shortly after a client with IDDM is newly diagnosed, the few remaining islet cells can "kick in," resulting in an apparent disappearance of symptoms. The nurse should warn clients and their significant others that the honeymoon phase happens and that diabetes does not go away. This phase can last up to 6 months or longer. The client may need very little or no insulin during this time.

EXERCISE

A program of planned exercise can greatly benefit the client with diabetes. Exercise (1) lowers the blood sugar by increasing carbohydrate metabolism, (2) facilitates weight reduction and proper weight maintenance, (3) increases high-density lipoproteins and decreases triglycerides, (4) decreases blood pressure, and (5) decreases stress and tension.

Goals of Exercise. The goals of planned exercise are as follows:

- Exercise to 60 to 75 per cent of the maximal heart rate for the client's age. This is determined by subtracting present age from 220 and multiplying by 60 to 75 per cent. Thus, a client 20 years old could exercise to a heart rate of 120 to 150 beats per minute, but a client 60 years old could exercise only to a heart rate of 96 to 120 beats per minute.
- Exercise for a period of 20 to 45 minutes at the desired heart rate.
- Exercise a minimum of three times a week.

CRITICAL TO REMEMBER

Clients with diabetes must consult their clinician before starting an exercise program.

Many clients with diabetes may not be able to exercise intensely to a calculated heart rate because of pre-existing heart conditions, age, or joint problems. The client should be helped in choosing an exercise and setting reasonable goals, because any increase in activity level is beneficial. Walking is usually well tolerated. Using an exercycle or swimming is possible when foot problems exist. Clients with diabetes must start any new activity at a well-tolerated intensity level and duration, gradually (over a period of weeks or months) increasing the activity until they reach their exercise goals. They should have warm-up and cool-down periods before and after the exercise. It is best to exercise at the same time of day, when possible. Because regular exercise is so important, the client should plan an alternative activity in case environmental or other factors make the usual exercise difficult. Unplanned exercise can be dangerous for clients taking insulin or oral hypoglycemic agents. During periods of exercise, the muscles are stimulated to take up glucose. Therefore, blood glucose levels can abruptly fall.

CRITICAL TO REMEMBER

Clients with blood glucose levels at or near 300 mg/100 mL should *not* exercise because vigorous activity can also raise the blood glucose level by releasing stored glycogen.

Surgical Management

PANCREAS TRANSPLANTS

Today, most pancreas transplants are done in clients who have IDDM and who have had a kidney transplant. This is usually because the antirejection medications (e.g., cyclosporine) have such severe side effects, which include hyperglycemia and nephrotoxicity. The client's own pancreas is left intact (98 per cent of its function is exocrine), and the new pancreas is usually anastomosed to the iliac artery and vein, where insulin can enter the systemic pathway. The exocrine secretions of the new pancreas drain into the bladder and are not absorbed. The client survival rate is 98 per cent after transplant; the pancreas remains functional in 60 per cent of clients.[31] Research is being conducted on the use of transplanted pancreatic islets rather than the entire pancreas.[33]

Nursing Management

Assessment

The assessment of the client with diabetes depends on the situation under which the condition was diagnosed. Some clients are admitted with the classic symptoms of IDDM that has advanced to ketoacidosis. Clients with NIDDM are frequently diagnosed during the treatment of hypertension, visual changes, or urinary tract, vaginal, or skin infection.

All clients with diabetes need (1) a health history, including family history, diet, and educational level; (2) a complete physical examination focused on the common acute and chronic manifestations of diabetes; (3) laboratory findings for diagnostic assessment; (4) a complete evaluation of home life, daily schedule, and life-style; and (5) consideration of health beliefs.

Clients with newly diagnosed diabetes need extensive education for self-management. Long-term diabetics also need to have their management of diabetes reviewed. Many times, the nurse can discover some errors in their self-care or introduce them to newer technologies.

As in all chronic disorders, the client's physical condition, age, and basic personality must be considered when interventions are planned.

The nurse should investigate the client's habits and attitudes toward the illness before deciding on a plan of intervention and teaching.

CRITICAL TO REMEMBER

The client should always be included in the planning of his or her treatment.

The plan should be tailored as much as possible to the client's personality and life-style.

Nursing Diagnosis, Planning, and Implementation

Nursing Diagnosis: Health Maintenance, Altered R/T lack of knowledge about diabetes mellitus.

Planning: Expected Outcomes. The client will relate the basic pathophysiologic mechanism of diabetes mellitus; explain the need for insulin, exercise, and diet in the treatment; and list the clinical manifestations of acute and chronic complications.

Implementation. The nurse or diabetes educator explains the basic pathophysiologic mechanism of diabetes to the client and family. Sometimes the information is given through classes or by videotape. The client should also be given some form of written information, tailored to his or her individual plan, for reinforcement of the material. If the client is newly diagnosed with diabetes, ample time must be given for questions. In addition, the nurse monitors for possible denial or anger about the diagnosis as part of a coping response. These coping responses are accepted and discussed with the client.

If the client has had diabetes for a while, the nurse assesses for the need for refresher material. The client is asked whether he or she wishes to review material on diabetes and is asked to relate some basic pathophysiology. If the nurse notices a deficiency, the client is encouraged to review the disease once again.

Nursing Diagnosis: Health Maintenance, Altered R/T blood glucose and urine ketone testing.

Planning: Expected Outcomes. The client will state personal goals for urine ketone and blood glucose testing parameters; demonstrate correct techniques for blood glucose tests (including timing of tests); demonstrate correct technique for urine ketone test (including timing of test); test blood glucose at regular times, including when ill and when traveling; prick the side of the finger, because there are fewer nerve endings there and more blood is available; test urine for ketones when glucose is high (over 250 mg/100 mL) or when ill; keep a record of all tests performed and bring this record to regular, scheduled follow-up visits; and store testing materials away from heat, light, and moisture.

Implementation. All clients with newly diagnosed diabetes mellitus require teaching about blood glucose monitoring. Even clients with diabetes who are admitted for other reasons may require review or update of information for self-care.

Newer, easier, and more accurate blood glucose meters are constantly being made available. Only the basics are covered in this discussion, so the nurse must keep up-to-date on each meter's advantages and disadvantages.

Glucose meters are available for the visually impaired that give audio commands to use the device and announce the blood glucose measurement.

In addition to demonstrating the techniques of blood glucose self-monitoring, the nurse should discuss the normal blood glucose range, individualized goals for good control, when to test, how to record test results, and what to do for abnormal results. The nurse can consult a diabetes educator for assistance in helping the client choose the right meter.

Some clients visually read blood glucose strips when they are not able or willing to purchase a meter. The nurse must make sure that the client is not colorblind, or these results will be inaccurate. The client's results should be routinely compared with a blood glucose meter to check for accuracy.

With some meters and strips there is a 15 per cent difference between capillary blood and venous blood glucose levels. The capillary blood reading will be lower. When insulin is being adjusted, this difference must be accounted for. As long as there is a consistent source of blood, no adjustment of this sort will be required.

Quality control of glucose monitors is a constantly changing area; nurses and clients must keep updated.

Urine testing for glucose is rarely done now. Urine, however, can be tested for ketones. These substances appear in the urine of (1) clients who are fasting, (2) clients with IDDM who are insulin-deficient, and (3) clients with IDDM or NIDDM who have a secondary illness.

Nursing Diagnosis: Health Maintenance, Altered R/T lack of knowledge about dietary management of diabetes.

Planning: Expected Outcomes. The client will state the relationship of dietary management to blood glucose control; choose foods that meet the caloric needs and offer a well-balanced diet; recognize the times when it is necessary to substitute a food to maintain blood glucose levels; discuss with the health-care team difficulties seen in compliance with plans for diet; maintain blood glucose and weight within preset parameters.

Implementation. A balanced nutritional plan is important for all clients whether they have diabetes or not.

CRITICAL TO REMEMBER

The nurse must emphasize to the client and significant others that they are not eating a diabetic diet but rather a balanced meal plan.

A registered dietitian (preferably a certified diabetes educator) should always be consulted for initial evaluation and teaching of any client with a new diagnosis of diabetes. Each client should receive an individualized meal plan based on ethnic, religious, and cultural background; eating, cooking, and work habits; and food preferences.

Ideally, the nurse and dietitian working together will develop teaching goals for the nutritional plan. All clients need to know the basics, which will include the following:

- Avoid adding sugar to coffee, cereal, and so forth.
- Avoid foods sweetened with sugar or honey (e.g., jellies, jams, cakes, ice cream).
- Check blood glucose levels regularly.
- Keep periodic appointments with health-care providers for evaluation of blood glucose control.
- Be consistent regarding amount, distribution, and timing of nutrients.
- Increase amount of carbohydrate in the meal before sustained exercise.
- Limit intake of saturated fat and cholesterol.

Some clients will need or want more specific information about the exchange diet and how to measure or weigh foods until the portion size can be accurately estimated. Again, the dietitian should instruct the client and significant others on this. The nurse can reinforce and answer questions as appropriate.

Practical examples that can be used in food preparation to help decrease the fat and caloric content are listed in the Client Education Guide.

The client with diabetes who requires strict dietary control and insulin or oral hypoglycemic agents should be advised as follows:

- Eat all of the food prescribed; if a meal cannot be finished, always compensate for the uneaten portion of food by eating a comparable amount of calories and nutrients as a snack later in the day.
- Eat meals and snacks at regular times; if a meal is delayed, drink a glass of milk or eat a cracker while waiting in order to avoid an insulin reaction.
- Never skip a meal, but take the carbohydrate portion of the meal in the form of soup, regular soda, or juice when there is loss of appetite.
- Take precautions to avoid hypoglycemic reactions during periods of prolonged or unusual exercise by increasing caloric intake as needed. Clients on insulin therapy should eat 10 to 15 g of carbohydrate before exercising. Clients on oral hypoglycemic agents usually do not have to increase their carbohydrate intake.

CLIENT EDUCATION GUIDE

Food Preparation Techniques

- Use only water-packed fruits and artificially sweetened gelatin desserts, beverages, and so forth. If foods are bought that are packed in heavy syrup, rinse well with water before eating.
- Oils and margarines that are liquid at room temperature are better than those that are hard (e.g., shortening).
- Include foods high in fiber such as whole grains, vegetables, legumes, and fresh fruits.
- When dining out, order standard foods (e.g., broiled fish, baked potato); avoid casseroles, gravies, fried foods, and sweetened desserts.
- Avoid alcohol if possible. Limit alcohol to 2 ounces or less daily taken with meals or snacks. Alcohol should never be drunk on an empty stomach because of its ability to cause hypoglycemia if the client takes insulin or oral hypoglycemic agents. Use water or nonsweetened mixes if desired.
- Use noncaloric sweeteners and fat substitutes.
- Carefully read all food labels.

The obese client with NIDDM may not require insulin or oral hypoglycemic agents if adequate weight control is maintained. Sometimes the promise that insulin injections can be avoided is enough of an impetus for clients to lose weight.

The client with NIDDM is usually over 40 years of age and has a life-long history of eating habits. The nurse should set goals with this in mind. If the client normally eats three eggs and four pieces of bacon for breakfast, the nurse will need to set realistic goals that may include having the client eat only one egg per day and two pieces of bacon. Then the goal of no bacon and three eggs per week can be gradually obtained. Many clients also associate food with love, memories of childhood, religious rituals, ethnic holidays, and special personal occasions such as birthdays, weddings, and the like. The nurse should collaborate with the dietitian, client, and significant others to allow certain foods to be eaten at certain times. For example, for a birthday, angel food cake without icing might be an alternative to cake with frosting.

The nurse can evaluate whether the client's needs were met by (1) evaluating blood glucose results, (2) evaluating client's weight loss or gain, and (3) evaluating lipid levels.

It is important to work with the client, significant others, and dietitian to arrange a meal plan that is practical and relevant for each client.

Nursing Diagnosis: Health Maintenance, Altered R/T insulin injections.

Planning: Expected Outcomes. The client will state that insulin lowers blood glucose, state the type or types of insulin prescribed and the onset, peak, and duration of each; take injections at regular times, 30 to 60 minutes before meals, every day, even when ill; wash hands before preparing insulin injection; demonstrate proper mixing of insulin; withdraw prescribed dosage using sterile technique; when on two types of insulin, withdraw the prescribed dosage of each insulin into one syringe without contaminating either bottle (regular insulin is drawn up first); demonstrate the correct technique of insulin injection; rotate injections according to a definite plan; store at least one extra bottle of insulin in the refrigerator and not use insulin past the expiration date; purchase insulin syringes before all of current supply has been used; wear a Medic Alert bracelet or necklace, or carry an identification card; state symptoms and treatment of hypoglycemia; and always carry something for treatment of hypoglycemia.

Implementation.

Insulin Administration. Administered correctly, insulin acts as a life-saving medication for the insulin-dependent client. Administered incorrectly, insulin may cause complications ranging from tissue damage to lethal hypoglycemia (insulin shock). To administer insulin properly, the client must be familiar with information about insulin concentrations, syringes, storage, preparation for injection, site selection and rotation, and techniques for self-injection.

Insulin Concentrations. Insulin is prescribed in units. Thus, pharmaceutical companies prepare types of insulin (NPH, regular, Lente) in 10-mL glass vials that contain 100 units/mL. U-100 insulin contains 100 units of insulin per milliliter. Some clients who require very large doses of insulin (i.e., over 150 units/day) may require U-500 insulin. Insulin is available only in glass vials because it adheres to plastic.

Insulin Syringes. U-100 syringes are available for the administration of insulin. At home, clients can reuse syringes up to four times. In order to reuse a syringe, after injecting, the client expels any remaining insulin in the syringe and recaps the needle. The entire syringe is then refrigerated.

Insulin Storage. Insulin should never be frozen or kept at temperatures over 80° F. Insulin can be kept at room temperature for 1 month. If it is not used in 1 month, it should be refrigerated; there is some deterioration of insulin potency when it is not refrigerated.

CRITICAL TO REMEMBER

Clients should be instructed never to leave their insulin in a car or in the baggage compartment of an airplane because of possible temperature alterations.

Preparation and Injection of Insulin. The client needs to learn to draw up insulin into a syringe and obtain an accurate dose. The client should be taught how to maintain sterility while working with the syringe, how to recap the needle safely, and how to dispose of used syringes. If the client has lost vision, visiting nurses can prepare the syringes for the client in advance.

If clients must mix two insulins in the same syringe, the regular insulin should be drawn up first. Then it can be given immediately or within 24 hours.

Site Selection and Rotation. Over time, the repeated use of an injection site can result in either atrophy or hypertrophy of the tissues. These abnormal tissue changes may cause decreased absorption of the injected insulin with consequent loss of control. For prevention of tissue changes, the client must choose the injection site carefully and rotate sites systematically. The sites for injections should be (1) easily accessible (use thighs, upper arms, abdomen, and lower back; Fig. 40–4), (2) relatively insensitive to pain (avoid the midline of the body where there are numerous nerve endings), and (3) relatively normal in appearance and to touch.

Insulin absorption varies from site to site.

CRITICAL TO REMEMBER

To avoid dramatic changes in daily insulin absorption, the client should give injections in one site, about an inch apart, until the whole area has been used, then change to another site.

The client should be instructed to avoid sites above muscles that will be exercised heavily that day, because exercise increases the rate of absorption. The client who is on two injections daily may use one site for the morning injection and another site for the evening injection. Some clinicians instruct their clients to use only the abdomen because of its more even absorption. The nurse should emphasize to the diabetic client the importance of adhering to a definite injection plan to avoid tissue damage.

Techniques for Self-Injection. The majority of clients who take insulin learn to give their own injections. It is primarily the nurse's responsibility to instruct clients with diabetes in the technique of preparing insulin and giving injections to themselves. The amount of teaching needed depends on the client's familiarity with insulin and the injection equipment. Teaching guidelines for clients with IDDM are discussed later in this chapter.

Equipment that the client must purchase for home use includes (1) insulin of the type prescribed, (2) absorbent cotton, (3) approved syringes with needles, and (4) 70 per cent ethyl or 91 per cent isopropyl alcohol.

Although the prospect of daily injections for life is far from pleasant, the client's attitude toward this intervention may be largely influenced by the nurse. A compassionate but matter-of-fact attitude helps the client understand and accept responsibility for self-care. The nurse should schedule a teaching/learning session for self-injection techniques. Some clients find it difficult to insert the needle into their own skin. For these clients, the nurse might select the site and insert the needle. Then, as the first step in self-injection, the client can push in the plunger and remove the needle. As the client gains confidence, self-injecting will seem less traumatic.

Use of Oral Hypoglycemic Agents. The nurse should warn clients not to ingest a large number of aspirin (i.e., over 12 to 14) when taking the sulfonylureas because aspirin tends to increase the hypoglyce-

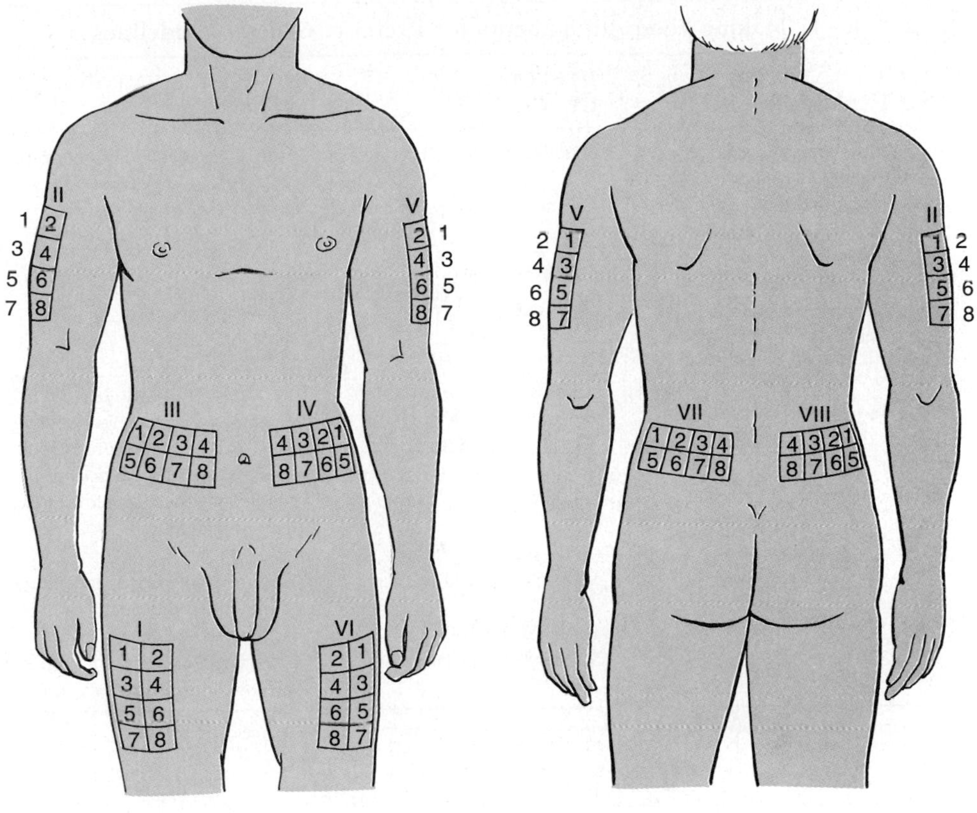

Figure 40–4
Insulin injection sites. To avoid overuse of injection sites and dramatic changes in daily insulin absorption, an approved method of site rotation should be used. One method is to begin with site I (right thigh), give injections consecutively at points 1 to 8, then move to site II (right arm) (e.g., a client on a regimen of one injection daily would inject insulin into the right thigh for 8 days, then into the right arm for 8 days).

mic effect of these agents. Other agents that may increase the hypoglycemic effect of the sulfonylureas include alcohol, dicumarol, sulfonamides, and acetaminophen.

The nurse should also instruct clients taking oral hypoglycemic agents to notify the physician at once if they develop an infection or febrile illness. Clients have a greater need for insulin when ill. Consequently, they may need temporary insulin injections until they recover.

Nursing Diagnosis: Health Maintenance, Altered R/T exercise.

Planning: Expected Outcomes. The client will follow a normal activity schedule so that diet and insulin dosage are in balance with the regular activity level while interventions are being planned; eat additional food if exercising more than usual (generally, the equivalent of a bedtime snack is adequate for preventing hypoglycemia); monitor glucose levels before and after activities; relate that the effects of exercise can be felt up to 12 to 24 hours later, including effects on hypoglycemia; and recognize that time and practice will be needed to learn how much energy is expended in various activities and be able to regulate the diet accordingly. The client will state that insulin is injected in sites away from the exercising lines of the body; for example, insulin should not be injected in the thighs shortly before riding a bike. The client should exercise with someone else who is familiar with the symptoms of hypoglycemia and its treatment. The client should state that if a hypoglycemic reaction is experienced (even a mild one) after eating a snack, more food is needed before that particular activity. If, on the other hand, blood glucose is elevated, more food than necessary has been eaten for that activity.

Implementation. The insulin-dependent client must regulate activity so that the rate of energy expenditure balances the amount and type of insulin and food intake. Because glucose can enter the cell without insulin during exercise, the client needs a lighter diet or more insulin when exercising less than usual. If exercising more than usual, the client needs either to eat more food or to lower the insulin dosage. Any variation in one factor necessitates adjustment of the other two factors. The nurse should encourage the non–insulin-dependent client to exercise in order to foster weight loss, improve blood glucose control, and burn excess calories.

Table 40–4 describes various exercises (including their intensity and duration) and corresponding suggested dietary adjustments.

Evaluation

The degree of expected outcome attainment (stable blood glucose levels) is evaluated on an ongoing basis. A few days are required for many of the teaching goals for the newly diagnosed diabetic to be accomplished.

Modification of Plan of Care for the Elderly

A client with diabetes over the age of 65 years who has had diabetes mellitus for a period of time will probably

TABLE 40–4 Making Food Adjustments for Exercise: General Guidelines

TYPE OF EXERCISE AND EXAMPLES	IF BLOOD GLUCOSE IS:	INCREASE FOOD INTAKE BY:	SUGGESTIONS OF FOOD TO USE
Exercise of short duration and of low to moderate intensity (walking a half mile or leisurely bicycling for less than 30 minutes)	Less than 100 mg/100 mL	10–15 g of carbohydrate per hour of exercise	1 fruit or 1 starch/bread exchange
	100 mg/100 mL or above	Not necessary to increase food	
Exercise of moderate intensity (1 hour of tennis, swimming, jogging, leisurely bicycling, golfing)	Less than 100 mg/100 mL	25–50 g of carbohydrate before exercise, then 10–15 g per hour of exercise	½ meat sandwich with a milk or fruit exchange
	100–180 mg/100 mL	10–15 g of carbohydrate	1 fruit or 1 starch/bread exchange
	180–300 mg/100 mL	Not necessary to increase food	
	300 mg/100 mL or above	Do not begin exercise until blood glucose is under better control	
Strenuous activity or exercise (about 1 to 2 hours of football, hockey, racquetball, or basketball; strenuous bicycling or swimming; shoveling heavy snow)	Less than 100 mg/100 mL	50 g carbohydrate; monitor blood glucose carefully	1 meat sandwich (2 slices of bread) with a milk and fruit exchange
	100–180 mg/100 mL	25–50 g carbohydrate, depending on intensity and duration	½ meat sandwich with a milk or fruit exchange
	180–300 mg/100 mL	10–15 g carbohydrate	1 fruit or starch/bread exchange
	300 mg/100 mL or above	Do not begin exercise until blood glucose is under better control	

From Franz, M. J., & Norstrom, J. (1990). *Diabetes actively staying healthy (DASH): Your game plan for diabetes and exercise.* Minneapolis: International Diabetes Center.

experience some complications. The normal changes of aging will only compound these problems and make self-care more difficult. Some elderly clients may lack the dexterity or the ability to monitor their blood glucose levels or inject their own insulin. They may need to have a family member or significant other do this.

Clients who are elderly and are newly diagnosed with diabetes mellitus may find it very difficult to change or alter their life-long eating habits. If they are not used to a regular exercise program, this may also be difficult to implement because of cardiovascular concerns or other disorders (such as arthritis).

The quality of life is essential. Optimal blood glucose levels may not be possible for some in this group. It is important to remember, however, that some clients *will* be able to perform the skills necessary for good blood glucose control. The nurse should discuss with the client and significant others what their optimal blood glucose control is.

Client Teaching

Before discharge, the client and significant others must have a full understanding of diabetes and its management with blood glucose monitoring, insulin injections, dietary management, and exercise. Because diabetes is a chronic disorder, the client needs time to adapt as well as to learn about the many changes occurring. Discussions should be held about the potential compliance with any regimen. The client should be encouraged to anticipate a usual day at work, school, or home and taught how and when insulin would be given, how blood glucose would be monitored, and what type of foods would be eaten.

Diabetic clients need ongoing monitoring of their self-care ability. Glycosylated hemoglobin levels are usually checked, as is the client's log of daily glucose levels and insulin. Female clients will need to increase their insulin during menses.

The chronic changes that occur from diabetes are also assessed on an ongoing basis. The client's vision, kidney function, degree of neuropathy, hypertension, and condition of the skin (particularly the feet) are assessed (see Box 40–4).

If the client is elderly or debilitated, visiting nurses may be an excellent asset for the client. A referral to the visiting nurses should be started before discharge.

Acute Complications of Diabetes Mellitus

HYPERGLYCEMIA AND DIABETIC KETOACIDOSIS

Hyperglycemia is an elevated blood glucose level over 120 mg/100 mL. Hyperglycemia results when glucose cannot be transported into the cells because of a lack of insulin. Without available carbohydrates for cellular fuel, the liver converts its glycogen stores back to glucose (glycogenolysis) and increases the biosynthesis of

BOX 40-4

Foot Care for the Diabetic Client

Normal foot care activities can be a real difficulty for the diabetic client. These clients may have diminished vision and difficulty reaching their feet because of their diabetes or other chronic diseases. Peripheral vascular complications, other circulatory problems, and the decrease of sensation and lack of healing in extremities can combine to make even routine foot care a hazard. These hazards have been noted among the home visit and health maintenance population, especially when the clients are elderly.

The home health-care nurse completes an initial assessment and evaluates the client's mobility, gait, hygiene, hydration, color, temperature, edema, pain, and sensation. Circulation is checked by palpating pedal pulses and blanch/return time of nail beds. The nails are evaluated for thickness and discoloration due to possible fungal infection. The nurse needs to ask, "Who has been cutting your nails?" When the nurse plans to trim toenails for a diabetic client, he or she should check for physician's orders.

Toenails are easiest to cut after they are soaked in warm, soapy water or just after bathing. It is important that the nurse be able to see both sides of the cutting instrument before cutting, and then to protect the eyes from "flying" toenail pieces. The nail should be cut to follow the curve of the toe: not so straight across that edges are created that cause pressure on adjacent toes, and not so rounded or short that tissue is left unprotected. The nail should be filed with an emery board to smooth the edges and prevent clothing snags and nail damage. If nails have not been cut for an extended time, the nurse should not try to remove too much of the nail. A manicure stick can be used to gently push the cuticle back under the nail. The nurse should tell the client that he or she will trim a portion of the nail today; then ask the client to soak the feet daily and return in 2 weeks for further trimming. If the nails are so thick that they cannot be cut with a nipper or clipper, the client should be referred to a podiatrist.

glucose (gluconeogenesis). Unfortunately, however, these responses aggravate the situation by raising the blood glucose even higher.

In IDDM, as the need for cellular fuel grows more critical, the body begins to draw on its fat and protein stores for energy. Excessive amounts of fatty acids are mobilized from adipose tissue cells and transported to the liver. The liver, in turn, accelerates the rate at which it produces ketone bodies (ketogenesis) for catabolism by other body tissues, particularly muscle. As fat metabolism increases, the liver may produce too many ketone bodies. Ketone bodies accumulate in the blood (ketosis) and are excreted into the urine (ketonuria). Metabolic acidosis develops from the acidic (pH lowering) effect of the ketones, acetoacetate, and beta-hydroxybutyrate. This condition is called diabetic ketoacidosis. Severe acidosis may cause the diabetic client to lose consciousness, a condition often called diabetic coma.

Incidence

Diabetic ketoacidosis is a fairly common complication of diabetes and a common cause of hospital admission.

Etiology

Diabetic ketoacidosis is primarily a complication of IDDM, although non–insulin-dependent clients can also develop ketoacidosis during periods of extreme stress. Causes of diabetic ketoacidosis commonly include (1) taking too little insulin; (2) omitting doses of insulin; (3) failing to meet an increased need for insulin due to surgery, trauma, pregnancy, stress, puberty, or infections; and (4) developing insulin resistance owing to insulin antibodies.

Risk Factors and Prevention

Primary prevention of diabetic ketoacidosis is through client education. Clients with diabetes should learn to

- Take insulin as discussed.
- Monitor blood glucose frequently (at least before each meal and at bedtime).
- Monitor urine ketones when blood glucose levels rise (above 250 mg/100 mL).
- Schedule regular appointments with the physician for regular review of blood glucose results, weight gain or losses, and general health and well-being.
- Recognize signs and symptoms of infection (a major cause of diabetic ketoacidosis). The first sign of an infection in a foot or leg—or upper respiratory, urinary tract, or vaginal infection—should be reported immediately to the physician. Other stressors, such as family or emotional problems, can also precipitate diabetic ketoacidosis.

The physician should be called if any of the following develops:

- Anorexia, nausea, vomiting, or diarrhea
- Ketonuria persisting for more than 8 hours
- A febrile illness or infection
- Any sign or symptom of acidosis

The nurse should emphasize to the client that the greatest weapons against diabetic ketoacidosis are (1) regular, daily self-monitoring of blood glucose; (2) adherence to the diabetes management program; and (3) early recognition of and intervention for mild ketosis.

Pathophysiology

In diabetic ketoacidosis, there is a relative or absolute lack of insulin. Insulin may be present, but there is not a sufficient amount for the increased need for glucose due to the stressors present (i.e., infections).

When the body lacks insulin and cannot use carbohydrates for energy, it resorts to fats and proteins. Ketosis and metabolic acidosis represent the final stages in

PATHOPHYSIOLOGY

Diabetic Ketoacidosis

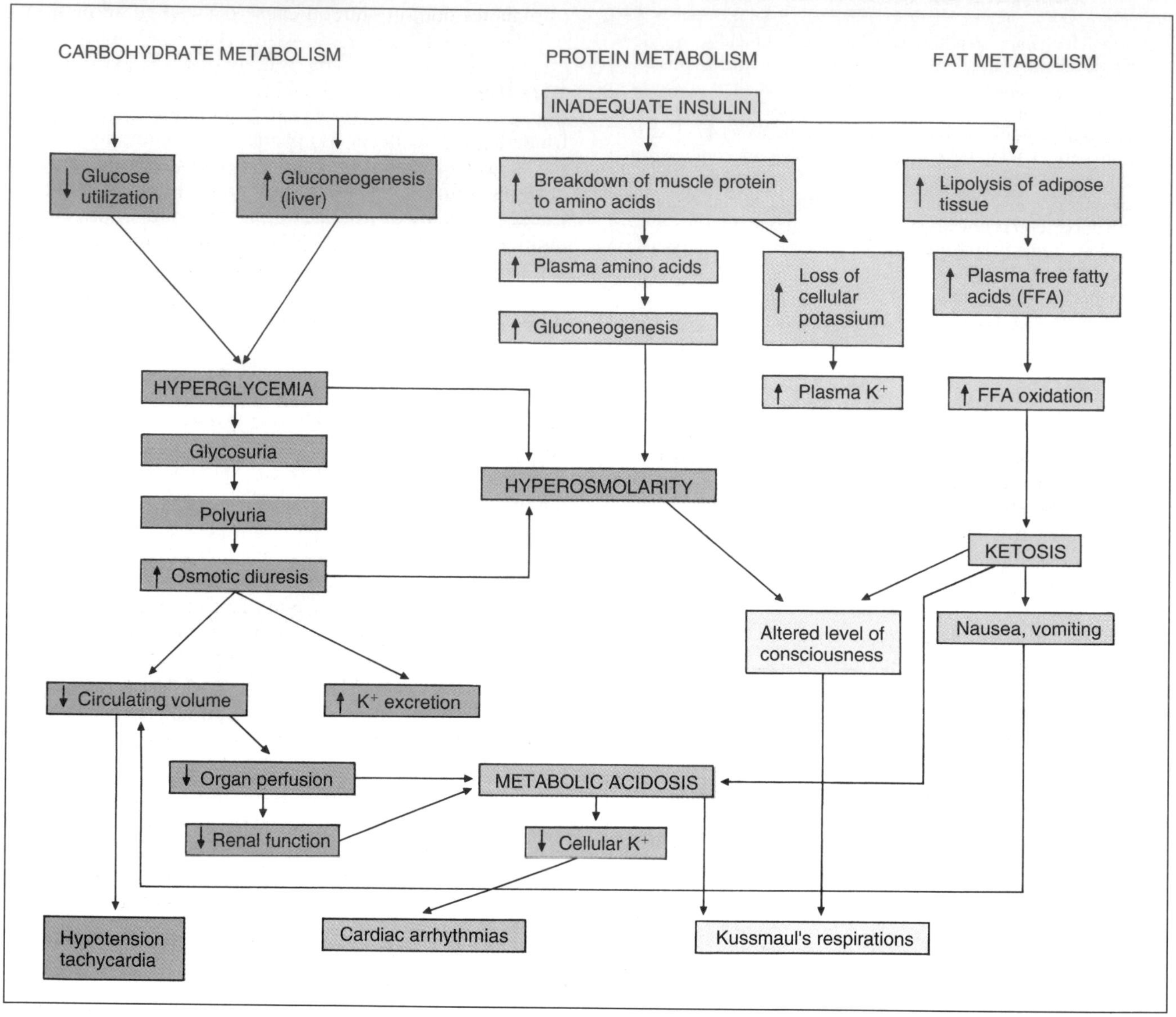

the body's struggle for fuel. (See Pathophysiology: Diabetic ketoacidosis.)

DEHYDRATION

Clients with ketoacidosis lose fluids from several sources. They excrete large amounts of urine in an attempt to eliminate excessive glucose and ketone bodies. Second, acidosis can cause severe nausea and vomiting, with resultant further losses of fluid and electrolytes (notably sodium and chloride). Finally, water is lost in the breath as the body attempts to rid itself of excessive acetone and carbon dioxide. Typically, clients in diabetic coma lose an amount of water equivalent to 15 per cent of body weight and approximately 40 g of sodium. Severe dehydration resulting from these fluid losses may be followed by hypovolemic shock and lactic acidosis.

LACTIC ACIDOSIS

When water losses are critical, blood volume falls, which results in hemoconcentration. Hemoconcentration in turn impedes blood circulation, causing a severe, generalized tissue anoxia accompanied by the production of large amounts of lactic acid. The rise in lactic acid within the blood adds more hydrogen to the body's already overwhelming acid load.

ELECTROLYTE IMBALANCE

As the pH of the blood decreases (acidosis), the accumulating hydrogen moves from the extracellular fluid to

CLINICAL MANIFESTATIONS

Diabetic Ketoacidosis

- Polyuria (early sign)
- Thirst (early symptom)
- Sunken eyeballs
- Acetone breath odor
- Dry mucous membranes, cracked lips, hot, flushed skin
- Electrocardiographic changes due to potassium imbalance
- Kussmaul's respiration
- Nausea and vomiting
- Hypotension (shock is a late sign)
- Abdominal pain and rigidity
- Paresthesias, weakness, paralysis
- Oliguria or anuria (late sign)
- Stupor or coma (late sign)

the intracellular fluid. If the client becomes severely dehydrated, hemoconcentration and oliguria may cause the serum potassium levels to rise still higher.

In addition to potassium losses, the client in metabolic acidosis loses excessive amounts of sodium, phosphate, chloride, and bicarbonate in the urine and vomitus.

Signs and symptoms of diabetic ketoacidosis are listed in the Clinical Manifestations box.

Collaborative Management

Dehydration resulting in hypovolemic shock, acute tubular necrosis, and uremia are major causes of death in untreated diabetic ketoacidosis. Diabetic ketoacidosis is an emergency. Rapid medical care and nursing intervention are essential.

Management goals in diabetic ketoacidosis are to

- correct fluid and electrolyte imbalances
- restore normal circulating blood volume
- shift from a state of fat catabolism to a state of carbohydrate catabolism by providing insulin
- identify and correct those factors that precipitated the ketoacidosis

Intravenous infusions of isotonic saline (0.9 per cent sodium chloride) are started immediately. Usually, the client receives 1000 mL of isotonic solution intravenously during the first hour, followed by 2000 to 8000 mL more of solution over the next 24 hours. Clients with compromised cardiovascular function may require slower intravenous fluid replacement.

Hemodynamic readings, vital signs (including blood pressure, pulse, and respirations), and level of consciousness need to be assessed frequently (every 1 to 2 hours initially). The development of crackles in the lung may indicate overhydration. Dehydration and hemoconcentration can lead to thrombus formation. Unilateral leg edema or shortness of breath or other signs of a pulmonary embolus or a deep vein thrombus need to be reported immediately.

A nasogastric tube may be necessary if the client is comatose or is vomiting and is likely to aspirate. The client's mouth may be dry because of the nasogastric tube and dehydration. Frequent oral care is important.

The nurse should assess weight, skin turgor, and hematocrit level for the client in diabetic ketoacidosis. When the client is sufficiently hydrated, skin turgor improves, weight increases, and the hematocrit drops to normal levels.

Bowel sounds should be assessed frequently for changes. Once the client can tolerate fluids, fluid intake is encouraged. Drinking broth is beneficial because it contains needed sodium chloride. Intake and output are recorded accurately. Most clients require a urinary catheter, but because clients with diabetes are more prone to infection, aseptic catheter care is essential.

REVERSING SHOCK

See Chapter 56 for a discussion of the treatment of shock.

RESTORING POTASSIUM BALANCE

Potassium leaves the cells in untreated ketoacidosis, and transient hyperkalemia develops. However, once intervention begins, the client may develop dangerous hypokalemia with weakness, extreme dyspnea, and even cardiac arrest. Hypokalemia occurs because potassium re-enters the cells (along with glucose) with insulin administration, and potassium is excreted in the urine with rehydration and renal function restoration. General agreement exists on the following points of assessment and nursing intervention.

- Frequently assess and measure urine output. Do not administer potassium to a client with low urine output; dangerous hyperkalemia may develop. Notify the physician promptly if the urine output falls dramatically or is less than 30 mL/hr.
- Assess the client continuously for signs of hyperkalemia (bradycardia, cardiac arrest, weakness, flaccid paralysis, oliguria) or hypokalemia (weakness, flaccid paralysis, paralytic ileus, cardiac arrest). Hyperkalemia may be present during the first 4 hours of intervention. Hypokalemia usually develops 4 to 24 hours after the initial intervention.
- Carefully monitor the client's electrocardiogram. Flattening or inversion of the T wave and prolonged QT intervals indicate hypokalemia. Peaking of T waves, loss of P wave, and a disrupted QRS complex indicate hyperkalemia (see Chap. 3).
- Plan to begin potassium administration 2 hours or more after the client's admission to the health-care facility and after adequate urine output is ensured.
- When the client has recovered sufficiently to resume eating and drinking, give foods and liquids high in potassium such as orange juice or bananas.

Sodium chloride and phosphate levels also need to be closely monitored. Sodium is replaced as described in the preceding. Phosphate levels can vary the same as potassium does and can be replaced intravenously.

Sometimes the physician will alternate potassium chloride with potassium phosphate in the intravenous fluid.

CORRECTING pH

Clinicians usually administer sodium bicarbonate only to clients with a pH of 7.1 or below. Such replacement therapy partially corrects the metabolic acidosis. As the client's condition improves, normal body mechanisms restore the blood pH to normal (see Chap. 4).

Low-dosage insulin therapy (5 to 10 units/hr) will be ordered for the client in diabetic ketoacidosis. The client in ketoacidosis may receive an initial bolus of regular insulin (0.3 to 0.4 units/kg) in the emergency room. Before starting an infusion of insulin, the nurse should ask whether the client has already received insulin that day. Insulin should never be given subcutaneously to someone in diabetic ketoacidosis because the subcutaneous tissues are dehydrated and poorly perfused with blood from dehydration and hypovolemic shock. Insulin can be given intramuscularly, but blood glucose levels are much easier to control if it is given intravenously through an infusion pump.

Blood glucose levels need to be monitored every 1 to 2 hours initially, preferably with a blood glucose meter. Rapid blood glucose results allow the nurse to adjust the insulin infusion rapidly and correctly. Dextrose is usually added to the intravenous solution when the blood sugar reaches 250 mg/100 mL for preventing hypoglycemia.

HYPERGLYCEMIC, HYPEROSMOLAR, NONKETOTIC COMA

Hyperglycemic, hyperosmolar, nonketotic coma (HHNK) is another acute complication of diabetes. It is a variant of diabetic ketoacidosis. HHNK is characterized by extreme hyperglycemia (800 to 2000 mg/100 mL), mild or undetectable ketonuria, and the absence of acidosis. HHNK is most commonly seen in older clients with NIDDM.

The precipitating factors of HHNK may be the same as those precipitating diabetic ketoacidosis, such as infections, medications (i.e., thiazide diuretics, steroids, and phenytoin), or stress. For some clients, HHNK is their first indication of having diabetes. Total parenteral nutrition (hyperalimentation) and dialysis may also precipitate HHNK if the client receives solutions containing large amounts of glucose.

The major difference between HHNK and diabetic ketoacidosis is the lack of ketonuria with HHNK. Because there is some residual ability to secrete insulin in NIDDM, the mobilization of fats for energy is avoided.

When there is an absence of adequate insulin, blood becomes concentrated with glucose. Glucose is too large to pass into cells; therefore, osmosis of water occurs from the interstitial spaces and cells to dilute the glucose in the blood. Osmotic diuresis occurs. Eventually, the cells become dehydrated.

The client's fluid intake can initially balance the loss of fluid and glucose through the urine. The imbalance gradually becomes more severe as the client cannot match intake to output. In time, the client becomes obtunded and unable to respond to thirst. At this point, the process is self-perpetuating.

Clinical manifestations of HHNK are polyphagia, polydipsia, polyuria, glucosuria, dehydration, abdominal discomfort, hyperpyrexia, hyperventilation, changes in sensorium and coma, hypotension, and shock. Lactic acidosis can develop.

Management

This type of coma is treated with vigorous fluid replacement. A common intervention is to infuse 2 L of hypotonic saline solution (0.45 per cent) over a 2-hour period. As in diabetic ketoacidosis, potassium, sodium, chloride, and phosphates are administered intravenously. Insulin is given via an infusion pump but usually at lower dosages because the client is producing some insulin. Dextrose is added to the intravenous fluid when the blood sugar reaches around 250 mg/100 mL to prevent hypoglycemia. Because many clients in HHNK are elderly and have other cardiovascular or renal disorders, fluid volume and electrolyte changes must be carefully assessed.

As the population ages, an increasing number of clients will experience HHNK, and nurses need to be alert for its signs and symptoms. Before discharge, the nurse reviews the causes of HHNK with the client and family, including insulin injection and blood glucose testing techniques. The nurse helps the client understand how serious these acute complications are and how to prevent them in the future.

HYPOGLYCEMIA (INSULIN REACTION)

Hypoglycemia is defined as a blood glucose level less than 60 mg/100 mL. Most clients who take insulin experience a hypoglycemic reaction at some time. Hypoglycemic reactions result from (1) an overdose of insulin or, less commonly, a sulfonylurea; (2) omitting a meal or eating less food than usual; (3) overexertion without additional carbohydrate compensation; (4) nutritional and fluid imbalances due to nausea and vomiting; and (5) alcohol intake.

Low blood glucose levels trigger an adrenergic response that stimulates the liver to convert glycogen (stored glucose) into glucose. In addition, the reticular activating system is stimulated to a state of wakefulness and alertness. When the liver's supply of glycogen is exhausted and glucose is not replaced, brain damage can occur.

Untreated prolonged hypoglycemia can result in coma. When the brain is deprived of glucose, brain cells are destroyed, which can cause permanent brain damage; memory loss, decreased learning ability, and even paralysis can result.[5] Brain damage develops when the brain is deprived of needed glucose after a drastic drop in blood sugar. In this respect, hypoglycemic shock is more dangerous than diabetic ketoacidosis.

CRITICAL TO REMEMBER

Some medications, such as propranolol and sulfamethoxazole, can mask the symptoms of hypoglycemia, and clients may not know they are having a reaction.

The time period during which the client is most likely to experience an insulin reaction depends on (1) the type of insulin given, (2) the client's response to that type of insulin, and (3) the timing of the insulin injection. When insulins are given in the morning, short-acting preparations tend to produce reactions before lunch; intermediate-acting insulins, 2 or 3 hours before dinner; and long-acting insulins, between 2:00 AM and breakfast. NPH or Lente insulin injected before dinner (5:00 PM) can cause hypoglycemia around 2:00 AM when the normal blood glucose level is lowest because of the decrease in metabolism.

Early clinical manifestations of an insulin reaction (hypoglycemia) include headache, weakness, irritability, lack of muscular coordination, and apprehension. Because epinephrine is released when the blood glucose drops abnormally low, the client usually becomes diaphoretic. In addition, these clients may behave as if they are drunk or psychotic. Some clients may become combative, and others may stare at the wall and become unresponsive to verbal commands.

Clinical manifestations of hypoglycemia at night may include bizarre nightmares, restlessness, diaphoresis, sleeplessness, or confusion. These symptoms can be misinterpreted as "sundown syndrome" in the elderly. If the client exhibits these symptoms or complains of a headache when arising, blood glucose levels should be checked the next morning around 3:00 AM.

Management

Management of hypoglycemia depends on the severity of the reaction. For reversal of mild hypoglycemia, the client is instructed to drink a glass of orange juice or to eat hard candy. This should be followed by a small snack of carbohydrate and protein such as half a sandwich or graham crackers and milk. A blood glucose test (with a glucose meter) should be performed as soon as the symptoms are recognized for determining the blood glucose level. If a meter is not available, it is safer to assume and treat hypoglycemia. The nurse retests the blood glucose in 15 to 30 minutes and treats again if the blood glucose is not over 100 mg/100 mL. Testing should continue until the blood glucose level goes above 100 mg/100 mL. Some clients who have had high blood sugar levels (over 250 mg/100 mL) for a long period of time may experience signs and symptoms of hypoglycemia even if their blood glucose level is 110 to 120 mg/100 mL. They have become accustomed to high glucose levels and perceive normal blood glucose levels as too low.

As an alternative to orange juice or candy, some clients purchase glucose tablets or a glucose gel. Clients who are tempted by candy to go off their diet may prefer commercial products such as the gel.

An unconscious or semiconscious client should never be forced to drink liquids because fluid may be aspirated into the lungs. The unconscious client with severe hypoglycemia needs glucagon or intravenous glucose immediately. Significant others of clients with diabetes can administer glucagon at home in the event of a serious hypoglycemic reaction. Glucagon, administered intramuscularly or subcutaneously, may eliminate the need for emergency department intervention.

The client who experiences severe hypoglycemia in the hospital usually receives 20 to 50 mL of 50 per cent glucose by intravenous push. Once the client fully regains consciousness, orange juice is given, followed by a longer-acting carbohydrate and protein snack.

Because insulin reactions are so common, newly diagnosed diabetic clients must understand (1) why reactions occur, (2) when reactions are most likely to occur, (3) early clinical manifestations of hypoglycemia, (4) the danger of severe or repeated reactions, (5) the importance of early intervention, and (6) how to prevent insulin reactions. Whenever a client is begun on insulin or an oral hypoglycemic agent, teaching must include clinical manifestations and management of hypoglycemia.

Once a client develops and then fully recovers from an episode of hypoglycemia, the nurse needs to thoroughly reassess the intervention program. In some cases, insulin reactions develop because the client carelessly prepares insulin dosages, fails to eat, or exercises excessively. The nurse must talk to the client who is careless about the dangers of repeated insulin reactions and stress the importance of conscientious adherence to the therapeutic program.

In other cases, hypoglycemia develops because the prescribed insulin dosage is too large or the client's dietary intake is too small. The nurse should instruct the client to record the time and probable cause of any hypoglycemic episodes on the blood test record. The health-care team can then evaluate the record together, making appropriate changes. The nurse teaches the client with IDDM to adjust diet and insulin by monitoring results. Finally, the nurse must be certain that the client with diabetes obtains a diabetic identification tag or bracelet and an identification card from the clinician or the local diabetes association. Sometimes, clients who are suffering an insulin reaction behave as if they were intoxicated or mentally disturbed. By carrying proper identification, the client can avoid being arrested at a time when emergency care is desperately needed. Table 40–5 compares the data and interventions for diabetic ketoacidosis, HHNK, and hypoglycemia.

As with many chronic disorders, the client needs to develop a positive self-concept and a feeling of control. The nurse should help the client and significant others understand the complications associated with diabetes. Equally important, the nurse should assist the client to develop and maintain interventions that meet emotional and social needs as well as physical ones.

TABLE 40–5 Acute Complications of Diabetes

	DIABETIC KETOACIDOSIS (DKA)	HYPERGLYCEMIC, HYPEROSMOLAR, NONKETOTIC COMA (HHNK)	HYPOGLYCEMIA
Type of diabetes	Insulin-dependent	Non–insulin-dependent, nondiabetic client	Insulin-dependent or non–insulin-dependent
Clinical manifestations	History of warm and dry skin, nausea, vomiting, flushed appearance, dry mucous membranes, soft eyeballs, Kussmaul's respirations or tachypnea, abdominal pain, alterations in level of consciousness, hypotension, tachycardia, acetone breath Polyuria (early) Oliguria/anuria (late)	Same as DKA except Kussmaul's respirations and acetone breath usually not present Alterations in level of consciousness Nausea and vomiting not present	Cool and moist skin or diaphoresis, pallor Tachycardia, thready pulse Nausea, loss of appetite, hunger, malaise Visual disturbances, headache Alterations in level of consciousness: memory loss, confusion, hallucinations, generalized or focal seizures, status epilepticus, primitive movements (sucking, smacking lips, picking or grasping, Babinski's reflex) may be present
Precipitating factor	Undiagnosed diabetes Skipping insulin dose Puberty Infection Cardiovascular disorder Other physical or emotional stress such as pregnancy or surgery	Undiagnosed diabetes Infection or other stress Medications: Dilantin, thiazide diuretics, mannitol steroids Dialysis Hyperalimentation Acute pancreatitis Central nervous system disorders Major burns rehydrated with high volumes of glucose	Delay or omission of meal Insulin overdosage Excessive exercise
Onset of symptoms	Slow (hours to days)	Slow (hours to days)	Rapid (minutes to hours)
Laboratory findings			
Blood glucose	300–1500 mg/100 mL	600–3000 mg/100 mL	60 mg/100 mL or less
Serum sodium	Normal or decreased	Elevated	Normal
Serum potassium	Normal or elevated at first, then decreased	Same as DKA	Normal
Blood urea nitrogen	Elevated	Elevated	Normal
Serum ketones	Elevated	Normal	Normal
White blood cells	Elevated	Elevated	Normal or elevated
Hematocrit	Elevated	Elevated	Normal
Urine glucose	Elevated	Elevated	Normal
Urine ketones	Elevated	Normal	Normal
Arterial blood gas	Metabolic acidosis with compensatory respiratory alkalosis	Normal (metabolic acidosis of shock is profound and prolonged)	Normal or slight respiratory acidosis
pH	Less than 7.3	Usually normal or slightly decreased	
Osmolarity	300–350 mg/100 mL	Usually over 350/100 mL	
Intervention	Insulin IV fluids such as normal saline, possibly half normal saline Potassium when urine output is adequate Sodium bicarbonate if pH is less than 7.0	Insulin IV fluids such as half normal or 0.45% normal saline Potassium when urine output is adequate	Candy, glucose gel or tablets, orange juice if awake 50% dextrose IV push, 5–10% D/W IV drip, or glucagon if unconscious Follow with a complex carbohydrate and protein (e.g., cheese and crackers)

D/W, dextrose in water; IV, intravenous.

HYPERFUNCTION OF THE ISLETS OF LANGERHANS (HYPERINSULINISM)

Hyperinsulinism is excessive secretion of insulin by the pancreas. It is either organic or functional in origin. Organic hyperinsulinism is usually caused either by hyperplasia (overgrowth) of the islets or by an adenoma of the pancreas that secretes excessive amounts of insulin.

Functional hyperinsulinism develops with far greater frequency than does the organic form. In this case, the exact cause of insulin hypersecretion remains unknown. However, functional hyperinsulinism frequently strikes tense, anxious clients who also have various manifestations of autonomic nervous dysfunction (e.g., neurocirculatory asthenia and excessive diaphoresis). Second, this disorder may be a forerunner of diabetes mellitus. Finally, functional hyperinsulinism sometimes follows gastrectomy. After removal of the stomach, ingested carbohydrates pass directly into the small bowel (the "dumping syndrome") and are absorbed. The sudden, resultant hyperglycemia causes excessive insulin release, with symptoms of hypoglycemia appearing 1 to 2 hours later (see Chap. 33).

Because oversecretion of insulin causes an abnormally low blood glucose level, manifestations of hyperinsulinism are identical to those of hypoglycemia previously discussed (e.g., hunger, weakness, tremor, sweating, personality changes). The client and significant others are taught the usual clinical manifestations of, interventions for, and preventive measures for hypoglycemia. Repeated or prolonged attacks may ultimately result in progressive and irreversible neuropathy, retinal hemorrhages, cerebrovascular accidents, permanent personality changes, and intellectual damage.

Management

The goals of intervention in functional hyperinsulinism are to control and to prevent the symptoms of hypoglycemia. Interventions include psychological counseling, diet, medications, and follow-up care.

Emergency intervention for acute hypoglycemic attacks is the same as that for an insulin reaction, that is, immediate administration of a simple carbohydrate in any quickly digested form (orange juice). However, for permanently alleviating organic hyperinsulinism, surgery is required. The operation involves either removing the insulin-secreting tumor or resecting hyperplastic pancreatic tissue.

Clients who are anxious may find relief by learning to relax more fully and more frequently. The help of a psychiatrist may be needed in extreme cases. Sedation may help the anxious client relax. Anticholinergic medications may help control the "dumping syndrome."

Most authorities recommend a diet of normal composition but with no large meals or concentrated sweets. Six small meals rather than three large meals may also be helpful. The client should ingest carbohydrates of the slowly assimilated variety (e.g., starches and vegetables).

The nurse should advise clients with functional hyperinsulinism to schedule periodic physical examinations so they can be assessed for the signs of overt diabetes mellitus.

Chronic Complications of Diabetes Mellitus

Unfortunately, the long-term complications of diabetes are relentless. They can be divided into those resulting from disorders of the microcirculation (neuropathy, retinopathy, and nephropathy) and of the macrocirculation (peripheral vascular lesions, coronary artery disease, stroke, hypertension, and infection). They are summarized in Table 40–6.

Most of the long-term complications of diabetes mellitus are related to the cell's inability to receive nutrition and rid itself of waste because of the thickened membrane. Unfortunately, the process may start as early as 2 years after the onset of diabetes.

The widespread effects of microangiopathy can be disastrous. The eyes and kidneys are the organs most seriously affected. Vascular degeneration within the retina can cause microaneurysms, retinal hemorrhages, and eventual blindness. Small vessel changes within the kidney eventually result in intercapillary glomerulosclerosis and renal failure.

NEUROPATHY

Neuropathy is the most common chronic complication of diabetes. Even though nerve fibers do not have their own blood supply, they depend on the diffusion of nutrients and oxygen across the membrane. When axons and dendrites are not nourished, their transmission of impulses slows. In addition, sorbitol accumulates in nerve tissue, further diminishing both sensory and motor function. Clients with diabetes may develop both temporary and permanent neurologic problems during the course of their illness. Identified causes of diabetic neuropathy include vascular insufficiency, chronic elevations in blood glucose levels, hypertension, cigarette smoking, and increasing age. Clients may present with mononeuropathy or polyneuropathy and may have sensory or motor impairment, depending on which nerves are involved.

Peripheral Nerve Degeneration

This common form of diabetic neuropathy tends to develop in stages. During its earliest stage, the affected

TABLE 40–6 Long-term Complications of Diabetes

COMPLICATION	CLINICAL MANIFESTATIONS	PREVENTION	INTERVENTION
Vascular Changes			
Macroangiopathy (atherosclerosis)		Control blood sugar levels	
Coronary artery disease	Angina pain	Control hypertension Diet low in cholesterol and saturated fat	Medical management Surgical intervention when necessary
Cerebrovascular disease	Fainting episodes Paralysis		
Peripheral vascular disease	Intermittent claudication	Avoid cigarette smoking Regular exercise program Daily foot inspection and foot care aimed at prevention and early intervention	
Microangiopathy			Photocoagulation
Retinopathy	Advanced stages lead to blindness	Regular eye examinations every 6 months to 1 year Control hypertension Control blood sugar levels	Vitrectomy
Nephropathy	Fluid accumulation Fatigue Increased incidence of hypoglycemia	Prompt, vigorous treatment of urinary tract and kidney infections Low-protein diet	Hemodialysis Peritoneal dialysis Renal transplantation Decrease insulin dose
Neuropathy			
Peripheral neuropathy	Numbness, tingling, or pain in extremities	Daily foot inspection and foot care aimed at prevention and early intervention	Tricyclic antidepressants Pentoxifylline (Trental) Capsaicin
Autonomic neuropathy	Nausea, vomiting, and abdominal discomfort from delayed emptying of gastric contents	Maintain blood sugar near normal levels	Metoclopramide 3 or 4 times a day before meals
	Diarrhea or constipation		
	Urinary retention or incontinence		Bladder training using Credé's and other techniques
	Decreased sweating		Metoclopramide Self-catheterization 9-Fluorohydrocortisone Support stockings
	Fainting episodes		Metoclopramide
	Male impotence		Implantation of penile prosthesis if desired
	Vaginal dryness		Lubrication jelly during intercourse
	Silent myocardial infarction		Medical or surgical intervention

client usually suffers from temporary episodes of pain and tingling in the extremities (particularly in the feet). Later, the pain may grow more nagging and constant. Discomfort becomes particularly troublesome at night. Finally, in the months or years after development of diabetes, the client may experience a painless neuropathy characterized by an inability to perceive pain. Painless neuropathy is a dangerous condition. Clients may be totally unaware of injury, particularly of the lower extremities.

Atherosclerosis results in reduced blood supply to the feet, which causes intermittent claudication, cold feet, paresthesias, infections, delayed healing of foot lesions, ulceration, and gangrene of the extremities. Clients with diabetes are five times more likely than the general population to develop gangrene. Lesions of the extremities may become so severe that the client faces amputation of the toes, foot, or leg. To decrease the risk of foot infections, clients with diabetes are taught the principles of good foot care (see Client Education Guide: Foot and Skin Care).

POLYNEUROPATHY

Polyneuropathy is damage to a variety of nerves with resultant weakness, pain, various paresthesias, sensory loss, and decreased or absent reflexes. Amyopathy is wasted muscle mass and decreased response to infection due to nerve damage leading to weakness in the pelvic girdle and legs.

CLIENT EDUCATION GUIDE

Foot and Skin Care

GENERAL

- Do not soak feet unless directed to do so
- Use mild soap and a washcloth to clean between toes
- Check water temperature with an elbow or thermometer and not with the toes (32.2° to 35° C [90° to 95° F] is safe)
- Always do foot care at the same time each day as a memory aid

FOR DAILY CARE

- Use good lighting
- Use a mirror to see bottom of feet if necessary or have a significant other look at feet daily
- Do not use lotion between toes
- Use lotion (preferably containing lanolin) on bottom of feet, especially if feet are cracked from dry skin
- Use powder if feet perspire
- Do not use harsh chemicals (povidone-iodine, corn removers, peroxide) on the feet

CARE OF TOENAILS

- Use clippers or scissors with rounded edges
- Cut nails straight across and not at an angle (nails may be slightly rounded at the edges)
- Trim nails after a shower or bath
- See a podiatrist if the nails are thick (i.e., from an infection) or are difficult to see or cut
- Do not cut corns or calluses or use commercial preparations on them

SAFETY

- Do not go barefoot or wear shoes without socks
- Do not use hot water bottles, heating pads, or electric blankets
- Wear adequate foot protection on cold days; wear cotton socks to keep feet warm
- Guard against frostbite
- Turn lights on in dark hallways and rooms
- Do not sit with legs crossed

FOOTWEAR

- Shop for shoes in the afternoon when feet are a little swollen
- Buy shoes with thick rubber soles and soft tops and ones that have plenty of room for toes
- Check insides of shoes before dressing for stones, pins, and the like
- Leather shoes are usually best to protect one's feet because they allow the feet to "breathe"; rubber and plastic cause the feet to perspire
- Avoid shoes with thick seams or bindings that can cause blisters
- Avoid high heels and shoes with pointed toes
- Avoid tight socks and shoes
- Change socks daily; observe socks for any signs of infections (e.g., bleeding, pus); cotton and wool absorb perspiration best; do not wear mended socks

INFECTIONS

- Be alert for signs of infection: redness, swelling, drainage, pain, foul odors; even slight injuries can become infected
- Notify a physician immediately at the first sign of an infection
- Carefully cleanse areas that are slightly injured with soap and water; do not use antiseptics that contain phenol, povidone-iodine, or salicylic acid because these substances can burn the skin; after cleansing, apply a sterile gauze bandage; avoid using adhesive tape because it irritates the skin
- Remove socks and shoes at every office visit and have the feet inspected by the nurse and physician

Autonomic Neuropathy

Autonomic neuropathy causes a variety of problems seen in the autonomic nervous system. Gastroparesis is slowed digestion. Clients experience bloating and feelings of fullness. Because digestion is slowed, dietary regulation of blood glucose is also impaired. Gastroparesis may be diagnosed when the client is having increasing problems with self-regulation. Other clinical manifestations of autonomic nerve damage include diarrhea or constipation, urinary incontinence or retention, decreased sweating, orthostatic hypotension, and impotence in men. Also, clients with diabetes depend on an intact autonomic nervous system to signal development of hypoglycemia. Clients with damaged autonomic nerves may find it difficult to recognize when they are becoming hypoglycemic. The nurse should be sure to alert clients to this problem when teaching the management of hypoglycemia.

Some clients with autonomic neuropathy may also have "silent myocardial infarctions" without angina. The first symptom may be shortness of breath due to congestive heart failure. Clients may also experience no increase in heart rate with stress or exercise because of the decrease in innervation to the heart.

OCULAR DISORDERS

Diabetes is the leading cause of new cases of blindness in adults in the United States today. The most common eye complications include blurred vision, diabetic retinopathy, and cataracts.

Blurred Vision

Blurred vision usually results from an abnormally elevated blood glucose level. Consequently, once the client's diabetes is under control, vision often clears. Clients should wait at least 6 weeks until blood glucose control is established before obtaining new prescription lenses.

Diabetic Retinopathy

Diabetic retinopathy is a major cause of blindness among clients with diabetes. Diabetes may be severely complicated by microangiopathy or vascular degeneration of the small vessels supplying the eyes and kidneys. The retina, which is the most essential structure of the eye, has the highest rate of oxygen consumption of any tissue in the body. Consequently, if the retina is deprived of oxygen-carrying blood from the destruction of its capillaries, tissue anoxia swiftly develops. Background retinopathy is the early phase of retinopathy. Microaneurysms (outpouching) develop and allow fluid to leak. Vision is not usually affected in this stage. In proliferative retinopathy, the weakened, damaged vessels may rupture, causing retinal hemorrhage and exudates. Hemorrhage is followed by the growth of new capillaries into the vitreous, called neovascularization, and by retinal scar tissue formation. Contraction of this scar tissue can result in retinal detachment.

Although many clients develop some degree of retinopathy, most do not suffer visual impairment. When retinopathy does occur, it tends to develop slowly and insidiously.

Unfortunately, to date there is no cure for this condition. Diabetic retinopathy may progress to permanent blindness, either partial or total. The progress of diabetic retinopathy can sometimes be slowed by maintaining good blood glucose control. Hypertension, if present, must also be controlled.

The most common intervention for diabetic retinopathy is photocoagulation, a procedure that destroys retinal tissue or blood vessels. The physician performs photocoagulation with a laser beam or xenon arc. Another intervention involves the actual removal of vitreous hemorrhages, which thereby minimizes tension on the retina by a procedure called vitrectomy (see Chap. 17).

Clients should have their eyes checked, preferably by an ophthalmologist, every 6 to 12 months. Many clients with retinopathy have no signs or symptoms, so routine examination by a qualified professional is essential.

Cataracts

A cataract is an opacity of the lens. Fortunately, surgical removal of the cataracts or use of glasses or implanted lenses helps restore vision in the majority of clients.

Clients who are visually impaired may continue to give their own insulin injections by using syringe magnifiers or other available devices. In some cases, the nurse may need to plan for a family member or home health-care nurse to draw up the insulin for the client. Self-monitoring of blood glucose may be done with a special device that announces the result or with the help of another person. The Association for the Blind provides training that enables many visually impaired clients to maintain independence in daily living. Strenuous exercise increases intraocular pressure in the eye, as does heavy lifting, so the nurse should warn the client with severe retinopathy against these activities.

KIDNEY DISEASE

Pyelonephritis

Clients with diabetes are susceptible to kidney infections, particularly recurrent pyelonephritis. Females are most susceptible to renal and bladder infections. Approximately one half of all women who have diabetes for 10 or more years have developed at least one kidney or bladder infection during that time. Fortunately, sulfonamides, antibiotics, and the urinary antiseptics successfully treat the majority of renal infections.

Diabetic Nephropathy

A second and far more devastating form of kidney disease is diabetic nephropathy. A consequence of microangiopathy, nephropathy involves damage and eventual obliteration of the capillaries that supply the glomerulus of the kidney. Damage of the glomerular capillaries in turn leads to a complex of pathologic changes and symptoms (intercapillary glomerulosclerosis, nephrosis, gross albuminuria, and hypertension). Some clients now check their microalbumin levels at home. This test can detect very small quantities of urinary albumin, which can indicate very early renal disease. With worsening of the nephrosis, chronic renal failure ensues. Unless the client can be maintained with hemodialysis or receives a renal transplant, uremia eventually causes death (see Chap. 30).

Clients with nephropathy monitor their blood sugar levels and blood pressure at home. They are taught to eat a low-protein diet and avoid nephrotoxic drugs (like gentamicin). If the client must have a contrast dye for radiographic study, mannitol may be ordered, but the client must drink fluids after the test to clear the dye from the kidneys.

Like diabetic retinopathy, diabetic nephropathy cannot be cured. However, prompt and adequate intervention for renal and bladder infections can prevent these causes of renal failure. Control of hypertension and efforts to normalize the blood glucose can contribute to a delay in the development of nephropathy or a decrease in its progression.

INFECTIONS

Clients with diabetes are susceptible to infections of many types. Infections, once they occur, are difficult to treat. Infected areas heal slowly because the damaged vascular system cannot carry sufficient oxygen, white blood cells, nutrients, and antibodies to the injured site. Infections increase the need for insulin and the possibility of ketoacidosis. Areas of the skin particularly subject to local infection by yeast organisms include the neck, axillae, and groin. In addition, obese women may develop raw, infected areas under their breasts.

The nurse should teach clients to prevent severe foot problems by instructing them to visually and manually inspect their feet for blisters, sores, cuts, and ingrown nails. It should be emphasized to older clients that their ability to perceive pain may be diminishing and that they must rely on their senses of touch and sight to protect themselves from injury. The nurse should also point out that even trivial injuries (particularly of the feet) require immediate intervention for preventing the development of severe complications.

Special Situations in the Care of Diabetics

SURGICAL CARE OF CLIENTS WITH DIABETES MELLITUS

Surgery interrupts the client's usual therapeutic regimen; the diet must be temporarily changed, and the dosage of insulin or oral hypoglycemic agent readjusted; the stress of surgery raises serum glucose level as a result of an increase in the level of stress hormones (epinephrine, norepinephrine, glucagon, cortisol, and growth hormone); the client is prone to infection; and the surgical incision itself becomes a new portal of entry for infectious agents. Furthermore, postoperative healing in these clients may be slow, owing to vascular disease.

Preoperative and Intraoperative Management

The goal of preoperative care for clients with diabetes is thorough regulation of blood glucose levels before surgery. Clients with IDDM will need to be closely monitored for several days or even weeks before elective surgery in order to stabilize their condition and thereby decrease surgical risk. Sometimes a poorly controlled insulin-dependent client requires emergency surgery. In this situation, the surgeon must make the critical decision between operating on a hypoglycemic or hyperglycemic client and postponing an emergency operation until the diabetes is controlled. In either case, the client will need constant monitoring of vital signs, frequent laboratory and bedside glucose meter studies, and vigilant nursing intervention.

In contrast to clients who have IDDM, clients with well-controlled NIDDM usually undergo surgery with only slightly more risk than the general population. Typically, preoperative preparation for clients with diabetes includes

- preoperative laboratory tests, including (1) fasting and preprandial blood glucose levels; (2) glycosylated hemoglobin; (3) electrolytes, blood urea nitrogen, and creatinine; (4) complete blood count; (5) electrocardiogram and cardiac enzymes; and (6) chest radiograph
- early morning scheduling of the surgery so that the client's diet and insulin regimen undergo as little disruption as possible
- omission of food, water, and oral hypoglycemic agents on the morning of surgery. One long-acting hypoglycemic agent, chlorpropamide, should be discontinued 1 to 2 days before surgery because of its long half-life.
- beginning an intravenous infusion of insulin for those clients who are insulin-dependent or insulin-requiring. Glucose (5 per cent) is usually also administered to prevent the possibility of hypoglycemia. If the surgery is relatively minor (i.e., cataract removal), the surgeon may order a 5 per cent dextrose solution infusion begun and one half the usual intermediate-acting insulin administered. The anesthesiologist in the operating room can monitor blood glucose levels.
- a blood glucose determination performed and reported to the physician within 1 hour before the operation for ensuring that the client (NPO since midnight) will not develop hypoglycemia while in surgery

Once the client arrives in surgery, management again depends on the severity of the diabetes and the extent of the surgery. Regular insulin, based on the client's blood glucose levels according to a sliding scale or an insulin protocol, can be given intravenously. Subcutaneous insulin should not be given intraoperatively because its absorption is affected by body temperature, circulatory blood volumes, and certain types of anesthetics.

Postoperative Management

After surgery, the goals of postoperative management are to stabilize the client's vital signs, correct fluid and electrolyte imbalances, re-establish control of the diabetes, prevent wound infection, and promote wound healing. The following are important postoperative nursing interventions:

- Administer prescribed intravenous infusions and regular insulin until the client is able to take oral nourishment.
- Once the client is able to tolerate fluids, offer fluids that contain calories for prevention of hypoglycemia. Once the client can eat, an American Diabetes Association diet, which consists of three meals a day with between-meal snacks, should be provided. Discuss the client's caloric level with a registered dietitian so that enough calories for postoperative wound healing are being provided.
- Obtain blood glucose level four to six times daily.
- Resume the client's prescribed preoperative insulin type (e.g., NPH, Lente) and dosage once blood glucose control is re-established.
- Observe for signs of hypoglycemia after surgery. These may include a decrease in the blood pressure or an increase in the heart rate in a client who is still unresponsive from anesthesia.
- Avoid catheterization if at all possible to help prevent bladder infections.
- Change wound dressings with meticulous sterile technique for prevention of wound infection.
- Observe for signs of skin breakdown and treat, especially if peripheral vascular disease or neuropathy is present.
- Assess the client's wound and incision frequently for signs of infection. Be alert for abnormal amounts of drainage or foul-smelling drainage.

ETHICAL ISSUES IN NURSING

How Do Nurses Teach Compliance to Diabetic Clients?

With proper care, people with diabetes have a very good chance of living their lives to the fullest with few complications. However, there are complications that may arise no matter how meticulous a client is regarding the diabetic treatment plan. Even so, the best defense against long-term complications is to follow one's prescribed diabetic treatment plan closely.

Diabetic clients are seen in all different health-care settings. They may be seen in an office setting for high blood pressure or at a clinic for an eye examination. In other words, nurses will see clients with diabetes for reasons other than primarily their diabetes. Many times, these other reasons are adversely affected by diabetes (as in hypertension, glaucoma, and weight gain). It is important that nurses in all settings speak to their diabetic clients about their disease (no matter what the presenting problem is). Because diabetes requires daily behavioral restrictions, predominantly dietary, diabetic clients may need more reinforcement than other clients do. If a nurse sees a client with high blood pressure who is also a diabetic, the nurse can take an opportunity to do some teaching. Noncompliance among diabetics is high, most probably because the disease touches on so many aspects of their lives.

Diabetic education is important not only for the new-onset diabetic but also for the long-term diabetic. Health-care providers should take advantage of every opportunity to assess their diabetic client's level of understanding and feelings about the disease. It is through this education that diabetic clients are given their best defense against the complications of their disease.

TRAVEL

All clients with diabetes face special challenges when they travel. They may travel across different time zones, and their mealtimes will probably be altered. The nurse should discuss with the client how to accommodate diabetes when traveling. Most airlines now offer special meals that are well balanced. Insulin should never be packed in the luggage; it should be carried on board.

CLIENT EDUCATION GUIDE

Sick Days

With a short-term illness (usually less than 72 hours), most diabetics will not eat anything and not take their insulin and end up in ketoacidosis. The nurse must teach the client to:

- Never omit insulin: infection is a stressor that causes a release of epinephrine, which causes glycogen to be converted to glucose.
- Go to bed and keep warm: have someone stay with you if possible.
- Test blood glucose and urine ketones every 3 to 4 hours.
- Take liquids every hour: keep a record of all food and fluid taken and retained and report this information to the physician; fluids should contain sodium (e.g., broth) to replace sodium lost through vomiting and diarrhea.
- If unable to eat prescribed diet, replace carbohydrates with liquid or semiliquid foods (e.g., gingerale, eggnog, sherbet) 6 to 8 times per day.
- If still unable to eat the prescribed diet after replacing 4 to 5 meals with liquids, call the physician.

SICK DAY GUIDELINES

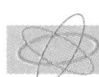

Clients should be taught never to skip their insulin or oral hypoglycemic agent when they are experiencing an acute illness (see the Client Education Guide: Sick Days).

FORMAL DIABETES INSTRUCTION

Learning to live with diabetes requires that the client (1) grasp unfamiliar factual material (e.g., the nature of diabetes and insulin), (2) learn to perform certain diagnostic procedures (e.g., blood testing), and (3) permanently change certain behavior patterns such as eating habits and recreational activities (see Ethical Issues in Nursing). Like any student, the client with diabetes needs scheduled classes, planned instruction, appropriate reading materials, demonstrations of new procedures (e.g., blood tests and insulin preparation), and the opportunity to perform these procedures with supervision.

Clients with diabetes can be instructed either individually or in groups, depending on the policy of the individual health-care facility and the number of staff members available for teaching. Group instruction offers the advantage of bringing clients with diabetes together to discuss common problems and share feelings.

The nurse needs to plan the client's course of instruction. Many hospitals and outpatient clinics employ certified diabetes educators who can help the nurse implement teaching; the nurse should refer to the institution's standardized teaching program for ensuring that all important points are discussed and reinforced by the nurse and the diabetes educator. Teaching should be integrated throughout the day. For example, basic foot care can be taught while the nurse is helping clients with their bath. The nurse should have a checklist with spaces for recording the date when instruction has taken place as well as the dates for retesting to measure how well the client has learned the material. Information for establishing quality diabetes programs can be obtained from the American Association of Diabetes Educators and the American Diabetes Association. Lists of names for cookbooks and free diabetes client education information can also be obtained from them.

The client may not learn everything while in the hospital. Some clients will need continual training in an outpatient setting. Sometimes the nurse can only provide the basic information that clients will need to know for preventing acute problems. The outpatient classes or instructions can provide them with more detailed information on sick day guidelines, exercise, and the like. The nurse should be careful not to overwhelm the client by giving all the information in 1 to 2 days. Teaching should be prioritized.

The nurse must remember that clients will go through the phases of grief (fear, denial, anger, bargaining, depression, and acceptance) when learning they have diabetes. The nurse should listen and observe for cues about what the client and significant others are saying and doing. If they are denying the client has diabetes, they probably will not listen to discussion about the complications of diabetes or how to draw up insulin. The nurse must help them deal with their denial and their feelings and move on from there.

Diabetes affects the whole family, not just the client. The nurse should include the client's significant others as much as possible in discussions. The interdisciplinary team can be utilized to provide a balanced approach to diabetes teaching and support. The social worker, nurse, dietitian, and physician are all valuable members of the diabetes teaching team, and a plan of care should be developed that involves them also.

A poor self-image may result in a client's wondering if insulin injections, blood glucose monitoring, and dietary restrictions are worth the effort. The client's and significant others' attitudes can affect their compliance with and adherence to the diabetes regimen. Counseling may be necessary for obtaining good diabetes control.

STUDY QUESTIONS

1. Which of the following symptoms is an early sign of hypoglycemia if manifested by a client with Type I diabetes?
   A. Feeling of nervousness
   B. Flushing of face and neck
   C. Sudden onset of fatigue
   D. Feeling of thirst
2. All of the following have been implicated in the etiology of diabetes mellitus except:
   A. Environmental factors
   B. Viral attack of the islet cells of the pancreas
   C. High consumption of refined carbohydrates
   D. Hereditary
3. A 40-year-old diabetic client takes NPH Humulin 16 units and Regular Humulin insulin 4 units every morning before breakfast. An hour before dinner, the client calls the nurse and demands that the nurse come to her room. Upon entering the room, the nurse finds the client pale and perspiring. The nurse's initial action should be to:
   A. Take the client's blood pressure
   B. Give the client a glass of orange juice
   C. Obtain a urine specimen from the client
   D. Give the client her regular insulin as ordered
4. The nurse instructs a diabetic client on the use of the American Diabetes Association exchange lists when planning a diet. The nurse explains that within this system, foods are grouped according to:
   A. Total calories in each food group
   B. Total carbohydrates in each food group
   C. Glucose, carbohydrates, and total calories in each food group
   D. Calories, carbohydrates, fat, and protein in each food group
5. A diabetic client is planning his diet with the use of the American Diabetes Association exchange lists. He is correct in choosing which of the following foods as a 15 g carbohydrate:
   A. 1 teaspoon margarine
   B. 3 ounces lean meat
   C. 1/2 banana
   D. 6 walnuts
6. In reviewing foot care with a diabetic client, the nurse should encourage the client to do which of the following:
   A. Apply alcohol after cleansing feet to prevent infection
   B. Apply lanolin generously between the toes
   C. Cut toenails rounded at the edges and close to the skin
   D. Wear a shoe-type slipper at home

CRITICAL THINKING EXERCISES

SCENARIO A

A business executive has been newly diagnosed with IDDM (Type I). He commutes 2 hours one way by train to his work. His physician has placed him on NPH Humulin insulin 15 units and Regular Humulin insulin 9 units daily with two thirds of the combined dose being given at 7:00 AM and one third of the combined dose being given at 4:00 PM.

1. Why are an intermediate- and short-acting insulin given concurrently? What other intermediate- and short-acting insulins could be used?
2. How should you teach the client to store and administer his insulin?
3. What would you teach the client about his diet relevant to appropriate types and placing of snacks?

SCENARIO B

An elderly woman with Type I IDDM calls the clinic and tells the nurse that she has the "flu." She tells the nurse that she usually takes Humulin N 15 units and Humulin R 10 units every morning, but she did not take it this morning because she was nauseated and vomiting and did not eat. She tells the nurse that she lives alone. What advice should the nurse give to the client about:

1. Her omitted morning insulin?
2. Her food and fluid intake?
3. Her daily routine?

BIBLIOGRAPHY

1. Albisser, A. M., & Sperlich, M. (1992). Adjusting insulins. *The Diabetes Educator, 18(3)*, 211–219.
2. American Diabetes Association. (1992). *Direct and indirect costs of diabetes in the U.S.* Alexandria, VA: Author.
3. American Diabetes Association. (1993). *Diabetes vital statistics.* Alexandria, VA: Author.
4. American Diabetes Association. (1994). *Medical management of insulin-dependent (type I) diabetes* (2nd ed.). Alexandria, VA: Author.
5. Bischoff, L. C., et al. (1992). Acute and chronic effects of hypoglycemia on cognitive and psychomotor performance. *Nebraska Medical Journal, 77(9)*, 253–263.
6. Campbell, K. (1990). Insulin update. *The Diabetes Educator, 16(1)*, 60–61.
7. Christensen, M. H., et al. (1991). How to care for the diabetic foot. *American Journal of Nursing, 91(3)*, 50–58.
8. Deakins, D. A. (1994). Teaching elderly patients about diabetes. *American Journal of Nursing, 94(4)*, 38–42.
9. Diabetes Update 93. *Nursing 93, 23(8)*, 59–61.
10. Dunning, D. (1989). Diabetes now: Safe travel tips for the diabetic. *RN, 52(4)*, 51–55.
11. Fain, J. A. (Ed.). (1993). Diabetes. *Nursing Clinics of North America, 28(1)*, 1–120.
12. Frantz, M., & Norstrom, J. (1990). *Diabetes actively staying healthy (DASH): Your game plan for diabetes and exercise.* Minneapolis: International Diabetes Center.
13. Galloway, J., et al. (1988). *Diabetes mellitus.* Indianapolis: Eli Lilly & Co.
14. Gavin, J. F. (1988). Diabetes and exercise. *American Journal of Nursing, 88(2)*, 178–180.
15. Glynase PresTab Tablets (glyburide): Clinical Monograph. (1992). Kalamazoo, MI: The Upjohn Company, April.
16. Grundy, S. M. (1991). Diet therapy in diabetes mellitus: Is there a single best diet? *Diabetes Care, 14(9)*, 796–801.
17. Guthrie, D. (1988). *Diabetes education: A core curriculum for health professionals.* Chicago: American Association of Diabetes Educators.
18. Henry, R. R., & Edleman, S. V. (1992). Advances in treatment of type II diabetes mellitus in the elderly. *Geriatrics, 47(4)*, 24–30.
19. Hernandez, C. G. (1989). The pathophysiology of diabetes mellitus: An update. *The Diabetes Educator, 15(2)*, 162–170.
20. Holler, H., & Pastors, J. (1991). Nutrition guidelines and meal planning: A step-by-step teaching process. *Diabetes Spectrum, 4(2)*, 58–61, 104–107.
21. Kestel, F. (1993). Using blood glucose meters: What you and your patient need to know. Part I. *Nursing, 23(3)*, 34–41.
22. Kestel, F. (1993). Using blood glucose meters: What you and your patient need to know. Part II. *Nursing, 23(4)*, 50–53.
23. Kestel, F. (1993). Using blood glucose meters: What you and your patient need to know. Part III. *Nursing, 23(5)*, 51–54.
24. Kopeski, L. M. (1989). Diabetes and bulimia: A deadly duo. *American Journal of Nursing, 89(4)*, 482–485.
25. Krall, L., & Beaser, R. (1989). *Joslin diabetes manual* (12th ed.). Philadelphia: Lea and Febiger.
26. Levin, M. E., et al. (1993). *The diabetic foot.* St. Louis: Mosby-Year Book.
27. Ley, B., & Goldman, D. (1991). Sick day management: Preparing for the expected. *Diabetes Spectrum, 4(3)*, 173–176.
28. Macheca, D. (1993). Diabetic hypoglycemia: How to keep the threat at bay. *American Journal of Nursing, 93(4)*, 26–30.
29. Melillo, K. D. (1993). Interpretation of laboratory values in older adults. *Nurse Practitioner, 18(7)*, 56–67.
30. Nathan, D. M. (1993). Long-term complications of diabetes mellitus. *New England Journal of Medicine, 328(20)*, 1676–1685.
31. Nettles, A. T. (1992). Pancreas transplantation: A University of Minnesota perspective. *The Diabetes Educator, 18(3)*, 232–238.
32. Petersen, A., & Drass, J. (1991). Managing acute complications of diabetes. *Nursing, 21(2)*, 34–39.

33. Pyzdrowski, K. L., et al. (1992). Preserved insulin secretion and insulin independence in recipients of islet autografts. *The New England Journal of Medicine, 327(4)*, 220–226.

34. Robertson, C. (1989). Coping with chronic complications . . . diabetes. *RN, 52(9)*, September, 34–43.

35. Robertson, C., & Cerrato, P. L. (1993). Managing diabetes: A major study injects good news. *RN, 56(10)*, 26–29.

36. Sabo, C., et al. (1989). Managing DKA and preventing recurrence. *Nursing, 19(2)*, 50–56.

37. Saltiel-Berzin, R. (1992). Managing the surgical patient who has diabetes. *Nursing, 22(4)*, 34–42.

38. Saudek, C., et al. (1990). Implanted insulin pumps: a status report. *Practical Diabetology*, 18–20.

39. Steil, C. F., & Deakins, D. (1990). Today's insulins: What you and your patient need to know. *Nursing, 20(8)*, 34–40.

40. Steil, C. F., & Deakins, D. A. (1992). Oral hypoglycemics. *Nursing 92, 22(11)*, 34–45.

41. White, J. R. (1992). Insulin and oral sulfonylureas in the treatment of diabetes mellitus. *American Pharmacy NS, 32(8)*, 39–43.

Chapter 41

Nursing Care of Clients with Thyroid and Parathyroid Disorders

Learning Outcomes

After completing this chapter, the learner will be able to:

1. Assess the client for clinical manifestations of hyperthyroidism, hypothyroidism, goiter, thyroiditis, thyroid cancer, hyperparathyroidism, and hypoparathyroidism.
2. Educate the client about the incidence, etiology, risk factors, and basic pathophysiology of major thyroid and parathyroid disorders.
3. Explain to the client the assessments and diagnostic tests utilized in the diagnosis of thyroid and parathyroid disorders.
4. Develop plans of care for the management and follow-up of clients with thyroid and parathyroid disorders.
5. Implement nursing interventions to restore, maintain, and promote health for clients with thyroid and parathyroid disorders.
6. Teach the client about acute and chronic complications of major thyroid and parathyroid disorders and appropriate health care interventions.
7. Evaluate planned client outcomes utilized for planning the care of clients with thyroid and parathyroid disorders.

Thyroid Disorders

There are many terms to describe normal and abnormal states of thyroid function. *Euthyroid* signifies normal thyroid function and secretion. *Hyperthyroidism* is characterized by overactivity of the thyroid gland, hypersecretion of thyroid hormone, and increased body metabolism and heat production. Hypothyroidism is characterized by underactivity of the thyroid, hyposecretion of thyroid hormone, and decreased body metabolism and heat production.

Enlargement of the thyroid gland (goiter) may or may not be associated with abnormalities of hormone secretion. An enlarged thyroid may result from lack of iodine, inflammation, or benign or malignant tumors. Enlargement may also appear in hyperthyroidism, especially Graves' disease.

The goal of care in hyperthyroidism is to slow the client's racing metabolic state by correcting the thyroid hormone excess. The goal of care in hypothyroidism is to increase the client's metabolism by correcting the thyroid hormone deficiency.

Pathophysiology

Secretion of thyroid hormones depends on endocrine activity in the hypothalamus and the pituitary glands. The regulation of the thyroid hormones is based on a negative feedback mechanism. When the amount of circulating thyroid hormone is low, a message is sent to the hypothalamus to release thyrotropin releasing hormone, which stimulates the pituitary to release thyroid stimulating hormone (TSH), which stimulates the thyroid gland to release the thyroid hormones.

Once a hormone level is sufficient to produce its intended effect, further elevations in the hormone are prevented. Rising levels of hormone negate the initial change that triggered the hormone release (Fig. 22–3).

Insufficient release of thyroid hormones, due to a problem within the hypothalamus, pituitary gland, or thyroid gland itself, results in a slowing of all body processes. This condition is known as *hypothyroidism*.

Excessive release of thyroid hormones due to a problem within the hypothalamus, pituitary gland, or thyroid gland itself stimulates an increase in all body processes. This condition is known as *hyperthyroidism*.

HYPOTHYROIDISM

Hypothyroidism refers to a deficiency of thyroid hormone resulting in slowed body metabolism. Hypothyroidism may occur in children because of congenital absence or atrophy of the gland. Both mental and physical growth are stunted, leading to a condition known as cretinism.

Myxedema is a complication of hypothyroidism characterized by a generalized hypometabolic state. Myxedema coma is a life-threatening situation in which all body systems are severely compromised. The hypometabolic state may lead to a decreased oxygen consumption by the tissues and pronounced personality changes.

Incidence

Hypothyroidism affects women more than men (about 4:1). Although hypothyroidism may be congenital and therefore present at birth, the highest incidence is in people between 30 and 60 years of age. More than 95 per cent of all clients with hypothyroidism have the primary form of the disease. Secondary hypothyroidism, resulting from pituitary or hypothalamic disease, accounts for fewer than 10 per cent of the cases of hypothyroidism. Myxedema is most commonly identified in postmenopausal, hypothyroid women in their 60s.

Etiology

There are three types of hypothyroidism: primary, secondary, and tertiary.

Primary hypothyroidism may be caused by (1) congenital defects of the thyroid (cretinism), (2) defective hormone synthesis, (3) iodine deficiency (prenatal and postnatal), (4) antithyroid drugs, (5) surgery or radioactive therapy for hyperthyroidism, and (6) following chronic inflammatory diseases such as Hashimoto's disease, amyloidosis, and sarcoidosis.

Secondary hypothyroidism develops when there is insufficient stimulation of the normal thyroid gland; consequently, TSH levels are increased. This may start as a malfunction of the pituitary gland or hypothalamus. It may also be caused by peripheral resistance to thyroid hormone.

Tertiary or central hypothyroidism can develop if the hypothalamus fails to produce thyroid-releasing hormone and subsequently does not stimulate the pituitary gland to secrete TSH. This may be due to a tumor or other destructive lesion in the hypothalamic region.

There are two major forms of simple goiter: endemic and sporadic. Endemic goiter is principally caused by nutritional iodine deficiency. It tends to occur in "goiter belts," geographic areas characterized by soil and water deficient in iodine. Major "goiter belts" within the United States are the Midwest, Northwest, and Great Lakes region. Endemic goiter typically occurs in the winter and fall and is twice as prevalent in women as in men.

Sporadic goiter is not restricted to any geographic area. Major causes include

- genetic defects resulting in faulty iodine metabolism
- ingestion of large amounts of nutritional goitrogens (goiter-producing agents that inhibit T_4 production), such as rutabagas, cabbage, soybeans, peanuts, peaches, peas, strawberries, spinach, and radishes, all of which contain goitrogenic glycosides

- ingestion of medicinal goitrogens, e.g., thioureas (propylthiouracil), thiocarbamides (aminothiazole, tolbutamide), and iodine in large doses. Some people take iodine-containing solutions as a tonic.

Risk Factors

Endemic goiter occurs in clients living in areas that are iodine-deficient in the soil and water. The use of iodized salt and food additives has almost eliminated this problem in this country.

Congenital hypothyroidism cannot be prevented, so secondary prevention with early diagnosis is vital if retardation is to be prevented by early intervention.

Clinical Manifestations

The symptoms of hypothyroidism depend on whether it is mild or complicated with myxedema or by myxedema coma. Clients with mild hypothyroidism (the most common form) may be asymptomatic or may experience vague symptoms so ordinary as to escape detection. For example, clients may experience mild sensitivity to cold, lethargy, dry skin or hair, forgetfulness, depression, and some weight gain. On the other hand, clients with the more rare and severe coma develop a multitude of striking symptoms. They slow drastically in both physical and mental reactions and appear abnormally fatigued and apathetic (Table 41–1).

Myxedema is characterized by a dry, waxy type of swelling with abnormal deposits of mucin in the skin and other tissues. The edema is of the nonpitting type and is common in the pretibial and facial areas.

Myxedema coma is characterized by a drastic decrease in the metabolic rate, hypoventilation leading to respiratory acidosis, hypothermia, and hypotension. Myxedema coma may be brought on by stress such as surgery, infection, or noncompliance with thyroid treatment.

Typically, clients with goiter seek medical advice when the goiter grows large enough to distort the appearance of the neck (Fig. 41–1). They may also experience respiratory distress and difficulty swallowing if the goiter is very large. The client with simple goiter rarely has symptoms until the gland enlarges enough to produce normal amounts of T_4.

The client's physical appearance also changes (Fig. 41–2). Often, obesity develops, features become coarse, hair becomes dry and sparse, and the skin feels dry, flaky, and inelastic. In addition, clients with hypothyroidism suffer an intolerance to cold because of a decreased metabolic rate. The client's ability to sweat also diminishes. Constipation and fecal impaction due to slowed peristaltic action and lack of normal physical activity constitute serious problems. Also, there is increased susceptibility to infection. When myxedema develops, the client looks puffy and edematous owing to infiltration of fluid into the interstitial tissues.

The major complication of hypothyroidism is myxedema coma. This is an extremely rare condition.

DIAGNOSTIC ASSESSMENT

Diagnostic tests for hypothyroidism confirm the clinical picture of hypometabolism and depressed thyroid activity (Table 41–2). Serum TSH level is elevated in hypothyroidism as an attempt to compensate for low levels of T_3 and T_4. Radioactive iodide uptake is decreased in hypothyroidism. A tracer dose of ^{131}I is given, and a thyroid scan is done 24 hours later to determine the uptake of ^{131}I.

Clients with myxedema may also have hypercholesterolemia, hyperlipidemia, and proteinemia as a result of T_4 changes on the synthesis, mobilization, and degradation of serum lipids. Elevated lipid levels may be a contributing factor to the later development of cardiac problems. Dilutional hyponatremia may develop as a result of the marked impairment of water excretion related to decreased delivery of sodium and volume to the distal renal tubules as a result of decreased renal blood flow. Elevated creatine phosphokinase, aspartate aminotransferase, and lactate dehydrogenase may also develop secondary to altered metabolism (see Table 41–1).

Diagnosis of simple goiter is confirmed by history and laboratory tests. The client is often euthyroid; the symptoms and diagnostic signs of hypothyroidism are seldom present because the gland enlarges enough to produce normal amounts of T_4.

Medical Management

PHARMACOLOGIC MANAGEMENT

Hypothyroidism. The goals of treatment for hypothyroidism are to correct thyroid hormone deficiency, reverse symptoms, and prevent further cardiac and arterial damage.

For hypothyroidism to be reversed permanently, the client usually needs to take thyroid hormone preparation throughout life (Table 41–3).

Clients with cardiac complications must be started on small doses of thyroid hormone.

CRITICAL TO REMEMBER

Large doses could precipitate heart failure or myocardial infarction by increasing body metabolism, myocardial oxygen requirements, and consequently the workload of the heart.

Once clients have responded to thyroid hormone therapy, they are placed on a life-long maintenance dose of T_4 daily. Clients are also told to stop all pharmacologic goitrogens such as sulfonamides, salicylates, and lithium.

The drug of choice for thyroid replacement is sodium levothyroxine (Synthroid) (see Table 41–3).

Simple Goiter. The goals for treatment of simple goiter are to halt further enlargement of the thyroid gland and to promote regression of the gland.

When enlargement is a compensatory reaction to iodine deficiency and consequent suppression of T_4 se-

TABLE 41–1 Signs and Symptoms of Hypothyroidism and Hyperthyroidism

SYSTEM	HYPOTHYROIDISM	HYPERTHYROIDISM
Cardiovascular	↓ HR + ↓ SV: ↓ CO	↑ HR + ↑ SV: ↑ CO
	Myocardial O_2 demand ↓	↑ O_2 consumption
	↑ Peripheral vascular resistance	Systolic BP ↑ 10–15 mm Hg
	Possible hypertension	Diastolic BP ↑ 10–15 mm Hg
	Hyperlipidemia	Palpitations
	Hypercholesterolemia	Rapid, bounding pulse
	Distant heart sounds	Possible congestive heart failure, edema
	Bradycardia	
Hematologic	Normocytic, normochromic anemia	No specific changes
	Macrocytic anemia (pernicious)	
	Easy bruising	
Respiratory	Reduced hypoxic drive	↑ Respiratory rate and depth
	Hypercapnic ventilatory drive	Shortness of breath
	Respiratory muscle weakness	
	Possible CO_2 retention on ABGs	
	Dyspnea	
Renal	Fluid retention	Fluid retention
	↓ Urinary output	↓ Output
	↑ Total body water	
	Dilutional hyponatremia	
	↓ Production of erythropoietin	
Gastrointestinal	↓ Peristalsis	↑ Peristalsis
	Anorexia	↑ Appetite
	Possible weight gain	Weight loss
	Constipation	Diarrhea
	↓ Protein metabolism	↑ Use of adipose and protein stores
	↑ Serum lipids	↓ Serum lipids
	Delayed glucose uptake	↑ Gastrointestinal secretions
	↓ Glucose absorption	Vomiting, abdominal pain
	Achlorhydria	
Musculoskeletal	Transient pain	Negative nitrogen balance
	Muscle cramps and stiffness	Malnutrition
	Slow movements	Fatigue
	↑ Bone density	Muscle weakness
	↓ Bone formation and resorption	Proximal muscle wasting
		Incoordination due to tremors
Integumentary	Dry, coarse, scaly skin	Profuse sweating
	Hair that falls out	Moist skin
	Thick, brittle nails	Flushed, warm skin
	Expressionless face	Hair: fine, soft, straight, possible hair loss
	Periorbital edema	Heat intolerance
	Thick, puffy skin: face and pretibial areas	
	Cold intolerance	
	Decreased heat production	
Endocrine	Normal to enlarged thyroid	Thyroid usually enlarged
		Bruit over thyroid
Neurologic	↓ Deep tendon reflexes	↑ Deep tendon reflexes
	Muscle sluggishness	Fine tremors
	Fatigue, somnolence	Nervousness, restlessness
	Slow, deliberate speech	Emotional instability: anxiety, worry, paranoia
	Apathy, depression, paranoia	
	Impaired short-term memory	
	Lethargy	
Reproductive	Females: menorrhagia, anovulation, irregular menses, decreased libido	Females: amenorrhea, irregular menses, ↓ fertility, ↑ tendency for spontaneous abortion
	Males: decreased libido, impotence	Males: impotence, decreased libido
		↓ Sexual development prepuberty
Other	Myxedema	Exophthalmos

ABGs, arterial blood gas analyses; BP, blood pressure; CO, cardiac output; CO_2, carbon dioxide; HR, heart rate; O_2, oxygen; SV, venous oxygen.

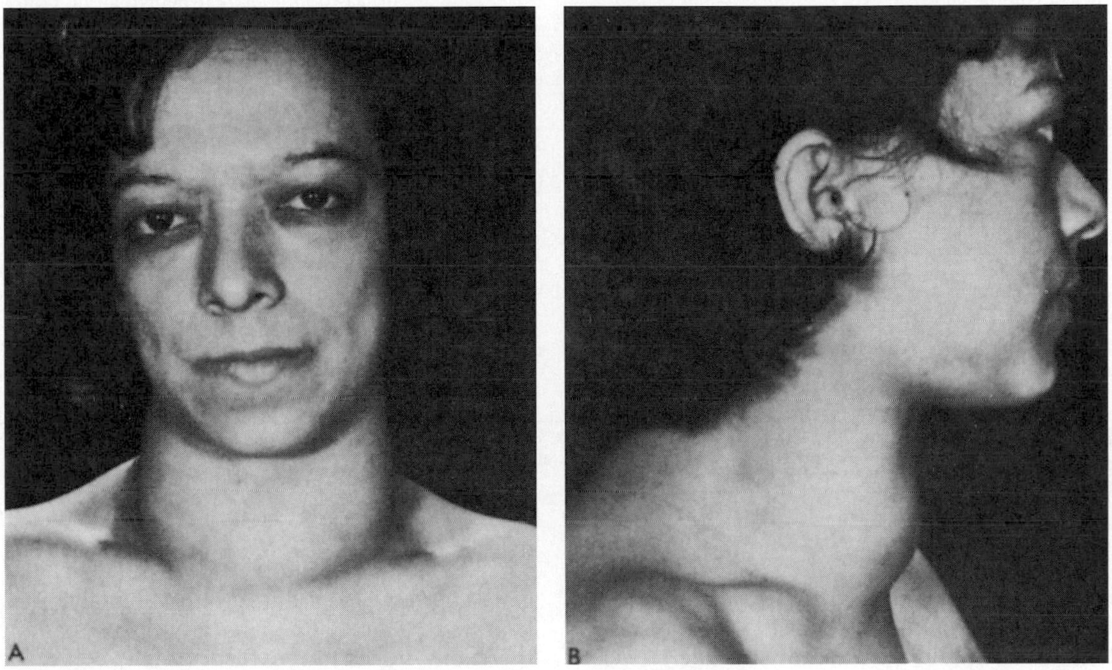

Figure 41–1
Massive thyroid enlargement due to diffuse toxic goiter. *A*, Front view. *B*, Side view. (From Wilson, J. D., & Foster, D. W. [1992]. *Williams textbook of endocrinology* [8th ed.]. Philadelphia: W. B. Saunders.)

Figure 41–2
Typical facial appearance of myxedematous clients. (From Wilson, J. D., & Foster, D. W. [1992]. *Williams textbook of endocrinology* [8th ed.]. Philadelphia: W. B. Saunders.)

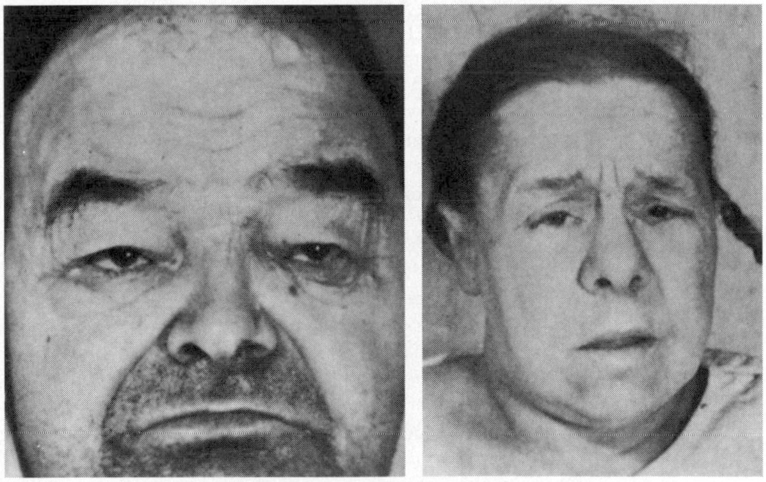

TABLE 41–2 Diagnostic Tests for Hypothyroidism and Hyperthyroidism

TEST	NORMAL VALUE	RESULTS
Thyrotropin releasing hormone stimulation test (TRH)	15–40 IU/mL	Increased in primary hypothyroidism, delayed response in secondary; slightly increased or no response in hyperthyroidism.
Thyroid-stimulating hormone (TSH)	0.5–6 milliIU/L	Increased in primary hypothyroidism: decreased in secondary and tertiary hypothyroidism and hyperthyroidism.
Thyroxine (serum T_4)*	5–12.5 μg/dL (65–155 nmol/L)	Decreased in hypothyroidism, myxedema, cretinism; increased in hyperthyroidism.
Triiodothyronine (serum T_3)*	70–220 ng/dL (1.15–3.10 nmol/L)	Decreased in hypothyroidism; increased in hyperthyroidism.
Free† thyroxine (FT_4)	0.8–2.4 ng/dL (10.3–31.0 pmol/L)	Decreased in primary, secondary, and tertiary hypothyroidism; increased in hyperthyroidism.
Free triiodothyronine (FT_3)	230–660 pg/dL (3.54–10.16 pmol/L)	Decreased in primary and secondary hypothyroidism; increased in hyperthyroidism.
Triiodothyronine by radioimmunoassay (T_3-RIA)	120–195 ng/dL (1.86–3.00 nmol/L)	Normal to decreased in hypothyroidism; increased in hyperthyroidism.
Radioactive iodine up-take test (RAI)		Decreased uptake may be caused by hypothyroidism, but is not diagnostic for it; increased uptake suggests hyperthyroidism.

* Measures free and bound or total serum content.
† Not bound to protein.

cretion, the client can be treated with preparations of iodine and thyroid hormone. However, the availability of iodized salt and thyroid hormones has made replacement therapy with iodine obsolete in the United States.

Myxedema Coma. The goal of treatment for myxedema coma is to reverse the condition to save the client's life. Supportive measures are begun immediately, such as maintaining a patent airway, giving oxygen, and replacing fluids intravenously. The client is kept warm, and vital signs are closely monitored until the client begins to recover from the coma.

Sodium levothyroxine is given intravenously with glucose and corticosteroids. When administering thyroid hormone to a client with myxedema heart disease, the nurse should assess the client carefully for anginal pain, dyspnea, or orthopnea.

TABLE 41–3 Medications Used to Treat Thyroid Disorders

MEDICATION	USE	USUAL DAILY DOSAGE*	SIDE EFFECTS	NURSING IMPLICATIONS
Propylthiouracil (PTU; Propyl-Thyracil)	Antithyroid medication used to treat hyperthyroidism	100 mg PO tid	Nausea, vomiting, diarrhea, loss of taste, skin changes, headache, dizziness, drowsiness, lymphadenopathy, hypersensitivity, agranulocytosis, hypothyroidism	Use carefully in combination with any drug that causes agranulocytosis; observe for sore throat, fever, headache; monitor blood counts; should not be used in the last trimester of pregnancy or during lactation; report any symptoms of infection; give every 8 hr around the clock; urge continued compliance because response is slow
Methimazole (Tapazole)	Antithyroid medication used to treat hyperthyroidism	5–20 mg PO tid	Agranulocytosis, headache, drowsiness, diarrhea, nausea and vomiting, jaundice, urticaria, arthralgia, lymphadenopathy	Use carefully in pregnancy; monitor thyroid function closely; check CBC periodically; watch for signs of hypothyroidism, colds, other infections; stop drug if rash or lymphadenopathy occurs; give with meals to decrease gastrointestinal effects; store in light-resistant containers

TABLE 41–3 Medications Used to Treat Thyroid Disorders *Continued*

MEDICATION	USE	USUAL DAILY DOSAGE*	SIDE EFFECTS	NURSING IMPLICATIONS
Saturated solution of potassium iodide (SSKI)	Antithyroid medication that blocks thyroid hormone production and release; used to treat hyperthyroidism	0.1–0.3 mL tid for 10–14 days before thyroidectomy	Diarrhea, nausea and vomiting, stomach pain, hypothyroidism, hypersensitivity, iodine poisoning, irregular heart beat, productive cough	Use with caution in clients with tuberculosis, hyperkalemia, acute bronchitis, impaired renal function, or cardiac disease; safety not established in pregnancy, lactation, or childhood; give after meals with fruit juice; monitor potassium level; avoid sudden withdrawal; keep in light-protected bottle; avoid use of over-the-counter drugs containing iodine; restrict iodine-rich foods and iodized salts; ensure preoperative compliance
Radioactive iodine (^{131}I)	Antithyroid medication that destroys thyroid tissue; used to treat hyperthyroidism; may be used to treat thyroid cancer	4–10 millicuries PO for hyperthyroidism, 50–150 millicuries for thyroid cancer	Feeling of fullness in neck, metallic taste, hypothyroidism, possible increased risk of leukemia later in life	Contraindicated in pregnancy and lactation for hyperthyroidism; stop all antithyroid medications 1 week before ^{131}I administration; monitor thyroid function closely; give on empty stomach; institute radiation precautions on body secretions for 3 days after ingestion; teach client to avoid close, prolonged contact with children for a week, should also sleep alone for a week; client should not resume antithyroid medications for 6 weeks
Levothroxine sodium (Synthroid)	Thyroid replacement medication T_4 used to treat hypothyroidism	0.2–0.5 mg IV for myxedema coma; initially 0.25–0.1 mg PO daily increased until response to 0.1–0.4 mg PO daily for hypothyroidism	Rare hyperthyroidism, tremors, hunger, palpitations, headache, nervousness, tachycardia, insomnia, heat intolerance, weight loss	Use with caution in clients with acute MIs, hypertension, renal insufficiency, or diabetes and in elderly or pregnant clients; give a single dose in AM; watch for adverse effects early in treatment; do not use to treat depression or obesity; stress need for life-long replacement; toxicity may last for weeks with overdosage; monitor for improvement of symptoms
Liothyronine sodium (Cytomel)	Thyroid replacement medication T_3 used to treat hypothyroidism	For myxedema, 5 μg daily increased to 50–100 μg daily maintenance dose; for thyroid hormone replacement, use 5 μg daily increasing to 12.5–25 μg PO daily	Signs of hyperthyroidism, diarrhea, abdominal cramps, vomiting, tachycardia, weight loss, heat intolerance	Use with caution in clients with acute MIs, hypertension, renal insufficiency, or diabetes and in elderly or pregnant clients; give a single dose in AM; watch for adverse effects early in treatment; smaller doses required for older clients; monitor pulse, blood pressure, and thyroid function.
Propranolol (Inderal)	Effective against sinus tachycardia, persistent atrial systoles, and tachyarrhythmias due to thyrotoxicosis	20–60 mg every 4 hours PO or 1–2 mg IV every 12 hours	Dyspnea, bradycardia, hypotension, agranulocytosis thrombocytopenia, laryngospasm	Assess blood pressure, pulse, respirations during beginning therapy; weigh every day, report gain of 5 pounds or more; monitor echocardiogram, white blood cells and red blood cells; teach client to make position changes slowly; teach client to report signs and symptoms of infection.

* Dosages vary with age and condition.
CBC, complete blood count; IV, intravenously; MIs, myocardial infarctions; PO, orally; tid, three times a day.

DIETARY MANAGEMENT

If the hypothyroidism and goiter are caused by iodine deficiency, the client should be on a diet higher in iodine. This is accomplished simply by switching to iodized salt. Dietary goitrogens such as turnips, soybeans, rutabagas, and to a lesser degree, seafood, green leafy vegetables, carrots, and peanuts should also be avoided.

Surgical Management

Surgery is done for goiter that is very large, not responding to treatment, or putting too much pressure on other structures in the neck. Surgery is discussed in detail under Hyperthyroidism (see later).

Nursing Management

Assessment

The nurse should carefully assess the client for the presence of signs and symptoms of hypothyroidism. He or she should obtain a careful history, looking for the signs and symptoms that reflect a decrease in metabolic functions such as weight gain, excessive sleeping, and generalized fatigue.

The nurse should also take a thorough diet history, looking particularly at the intake of iodine. The clients should also be questioned regarding the intake of goitrogenic substances and residence in a "goiter belt."

The nurse should question the client about other medical conditions that might be present, such as a previous history of hyperthyroidism treated with surgery or radioactive iodine, both of which predispose to hypothyroidism. The nurse should also question the client about the use of medications that may lead to hypothyroidism; lithium, aminoglutethimide, sodium or potassium perchlorate, or cobalt can decrease thyroid metabolism.

The client should be observed for the physical signs of hypothyroidism, such as periorbital and facial edema, a blank facial expression, a thick tongue, and generalized slowing of all muscle movement.

Nursing Diagnosis, Planning, and Implementation

Nursing Diagnosis: Nutrition, Altered: More than Body Requirements R/T slowed metabolic rate.

Planning: Expected Outcomes. The client will return to normal weight, as evidenced by a loss of at least 2 lb/week.

Implementation. When thyroid medication is begun, the client's activity level and decreased edema often lead to significant initial weight loss without alteration of the diet. Typically, however, the appetite also increases as the medication begins to work. It is important, therefore, to provide a low-calorie diet until the weight stabilizes at the ideal body weight.

Nursing Diagnosis: Activity Intolerance R/T weakness and apathy secondary to decreased metabolic rate.

Planning: Expected Outcomes. The client will develop increased tolerance to activity, as evidenced by a return to pre-illness activity levels.

Implementation. Once thyroid hormone replacement is begun, the client returns to a level of physical and mental activity that should gradually improve with the hormone therapy.

Nursing Diagnosis: Constipation R/T decreased peristalsis secondary to slowed metabolic rate and activity intolerance.

Planning: Expected Outcomes. The client will return to a normal pre-illness bowel pattern, as evidenced by a bowel movement at least every other day.

Implementation. The nurse needs to implement measures to prevent constipation and fecal impaction. As the hypothyroidism reverses and cardiac status improves, encourage more activity. Advise the client to drink six to eight glasses of water every day and to eat foods high in fiber such as fresh fruits, vegetables, and grains. If this is ineffective, a stool softener or cathartic may be indicated.

> **CRITICAL TO REMEMBER**
>
> Enemas should not be given in hypothyroidism, as they may produce vagal stimulation that could be hazardous in clients with cardiac pathology.

Nursing Diagnosis: Skin Integrity, Impaired, risk for R/T edema and dryness secondary to infiltration of fluid into interstitial spaces.

Planning: Expected Outcomes. The client will have all skin remain intact, as evidenced by absence of injury and resolution of edema.

Implementation. The nurse must monitor the sacrum, coccyx, elbows, scapula, and other pressure points for signs of redness or tissue breakdown. The nurse must remember that edematous tissues are more prone to decubitus ulcer formation. The client should be placed on a strict turning schedule and on a pressure reduction mattress.

Nursing Diagnosis: Hypothermia R/T slowed metabolic rate.

Planning: Expected Outcomes. The client will maintain a normal body temperature.

Implementation. The nurse provides the client with a comfortable, warm environment, remembering that hypothyroidism sharply increases sensitivity to cold. If necessary, extra clothing and warm blankets should be supplied. The client should not use heating pads or electric blankets, as these may cause peripheral vasodilation, further loss of body heat, and vascular collapse.

Nursing Diagnosis: Social Isolation R/T lethargy, weakness, apathy, and changes in appearance.

Planning: Expected Outcomes. The client will return to a pre-illness level of social interaction, as evidenced by increasing interaction with others and statements of acceptance of reversibility of appearance changes.

Implementation. The nurse must reassure the client and significant others that the client's appearance and energy level will gradually improve with thyroid hormone therapy.

Ongoing assessment of the client undergoing treatment for goiter is necessary because further enlargement or growth of nodules within the tissues may indicate thyroid cancer.

Collaborative Problem: Injury, Risk for R/T hypersensitivity to anesthetics, sedatives, and narcotics secondary to decreased metabolic rate.

Planning: Expected Outcomes. The nurse will prevent injury to the client, as evidenced by normal responses by the client to anesthesics, sedatives, and narcotics.

Implementation. The client should not receive sedatives unless it is absolutely necessary. If a sedative or narcotic must be given, no more than one half to one third the usual dose should be administered, and then the nurse should assess the client carefully for signs of respiratory depression or a decreased level of consciousness.

Collaborative Problem: Decreased Cardiac Output, Risk for R/T sustained bradycardia, edema, and decreased urine output.

Planning: Expected Outcomes. The client will have a normal cardiac output maintained, as evidenced by normal heart rate, evidence of normal perfusion, absence of edema, and urine output of at least 30 mL/hr.

Implementation. As the client takes the hormone replacement, the edema and puffiness will start to lessen. The nurse should continue to monitor intake and output, which become more balanced. Urine output should significantly increase during thyroid therapy. The client's daily weight will be monitored.

To help prevent further strain on the already overburdened heart, the nurse should always help the client to turn so the client is not straining and placing an extra burden on the heart. If any new cardiac symptoms occur, the nurse must notify the physician immediately. Thyroid hormone should not be given until the physician has reappraised the client's condition.

When administering thyroid preparations, the nurse should assess the client carefully for symptoms of thyrotoxicosis (i.e., tachycardia, increased appetite, diarrhea, sweating, agitation, tremor, palpitations, shortness of breath). If any of these symptoms develop during thyroid therapy, the nurse should notify the physician at once so the dosage can be reduced.

Nursing Diagnosis: Knowledge Deficit R/T pharmacologic regimen, nutrition, and follow-up care.

Planning: Expected Outcomes. The client will understand the pharmacologic regimen, nutrition, and follow-up required for control of the condition, as evidenced by the client's statements and compliance with the therapeutic regimen.

Implementation. Once clients are mentally alert, the nurse should evaluate their knowledge level regarding the disorder and the importance of taking thyroid hormone daily for life. The nurse develops and implements a teaching plan based on each client's needs and provides a written list of the symptoms of thyroid deficiency or excess. The nurse should instruct the client and significant others to phone the physician if those symptoms develop.

Endemic goiter can be prevented by the use of iodized salt. Adults require at least 50 μg of iodine per day.

Modification of Plan of Care for the Elderly

Subclinical hypothyroidism is the combination of elevated TSH levels and normal T_3 and T_4 levels without symptoms. Subclinical hypothyroidism occurs in up to 15 per cent of postmenopausal women.

The most common causes of subclinical hypothyroidism are listed in the order of frequency: autoimmune thyroiditis, Hashimoto's thyroiditis, previous thyroid surgery or radioactive treatment, and noncompliance with prescribed T_4 replacements.

Medical treatment is not indicated for those clients who are without symptoms. Those clients with generalized complaints of hypothyroidism may benefit from small doses of T_4, which thus proves that their condition was symptomatic rather than subclinical.

CRITICAL TO REMEMBER

A principal hazard in giving T_4 to an elderly client is the development of ischemic heart disease as evidenced by angina. Client response to therapy and serum levels must be observed closely.

The difficulty in diagnosing hypothyroidism in the elderly is that the symptoms are usually vague and generic to other disease processes. Hypothyroidism must be considered in the differential diagnosis of a variety of conditions affecting the elderly client.

Posthospital Care

The client needs to have thyroid hormone levels checked at intervals until these levels are stabilized and then at regular intervals to be sure that normal levels are being maintained.

HYPERTHYROIDISM

Hyperthyroidism is defined as excessive secretion of thyroid hormone. Thyrotoxicosis is an acute exacerbation of all thyrotoxic symptoms.

Incidence

Hyperthyroidism is a highly preventable endocrine disorder. Like most thyroid conditions, it is predominantly a disorder of women. It affects women four times as often as it does men, especially young women between the ages of 20 and 40 years.

Etiology

Hyperthyroidism may be caused by the overfunctioning of the entire gland or, less commonly, by single or multiple functioning adenomas of thyroid cancer. Also, overtreatment of myxedema with thyroid hormone may result in hyperthyroidism. The most common form of hyperthyroidism is Graves' disease (toxic, diffuse goiter), which has three principal hallmarks: (1) hyperthyroidism, (2) thyroid gland enlargement (goiter), and (3) exophthalmos (abnormal protrusion of the eyes). Graves' disease is likely to be an autoimmune disorder. About 60 to 80 per cent of clients with Graves' disease have circulating autoantibodies that react against thyroglobulin. Also, thyroid-stimulating immunoglobulins (TSIs) are present in the serum of 95 per cent of hyperthyroid clients. Evidently, TSIs are autoantibodies that react against a component of the thyroid cell membranes, stimulating enlargement of the thyroid gland and secretion of excess thyroid hormone. TSIs apparently are not involved in the development of exophthalmos. Also, the severity of the hyperthyroidism cannot be determined by TSI levels in the serum.

Risk Factors

Because the disorder is probably autoimmune in nature, there are no known risk factors or preventive measures.

Pathophysiology

Hyperthyroidism is characterized by loss of the normal regulatory controls of thyroid hormone secretion. Because the action of thyroid hormone on the body is stimulatory, hypermetabolism results, with increased sympathetic nervous system activity.

The excessive amounts of thyroid hormone stimulate the cardiac system and increase the number of beta-adrenergic receptors. This leads to tachycardia and increased cardiac output, stroke volume, adrenergic responsiveness, and peripheral blood flow.

Metabolism increases greatly, leading to a negative nitrogen balance, lipid depletion, and a resultant state of nutritional deficiency.

Hyperthyroidism also results in the alteration of secretion and metabolism of hypothalamic, pituitary, and gonadal hormones. If hyperthyroidism occurs before puberty, sexual development is delayed in both sexes, but after puberty it results in decreased libido in men and women. After puberty, women will also exhibit menstrual irregularities and decreased fertility.

Clinical Manifestations

Because hyperthyroidism is caused by an excess secretion of thyroid hormone, the clinical picture of Graves' disease is in many ways opposite to that of myxedema. Assessment reveals a client who appears extremely agitated and irritable, with a hand tremor at rest. Despite a ravenous appetite, weight loss occurs as a result of the quickened metabolism. Because of the high levels of circulating thyroid hormone, the client's body processes literally "speed up." Manifestations include loose bowel movements, heat intolerance, profuse diaphoresis, tachycardia, and incoordination due to tremor. Also, the skin becomes warm and smooth because of accelerated circulation to the tissues. The hair appears thin and soft (see Table 41–1).

Moreover, the client's emotions are adversely affected by the turbulent activity within the body. Moods may be cyclic, ranging from mild euphoria to extreme hyperactivity or delirium. The excessive hyperactivity in turn leads to extreme fatigue and depression, again followed by episodes of overactivity, and so forth. As a result of the client's chaotic emotional state, interpersonal relationships may deteriorate, further accentuating the emotional disturbance.

Goiter, the second characteristic of Graves' disease, is caused by hyperplasia and hypertrophy of the thyroid cells. The gland may enlarge up to three to four times its normal size. Cellular overgrowth results in the release of excessive amounts of thyroid hormone into the blood.

Exophthalmos is the third major manifestation of Graves' disease. The client who suffers from exophthalmos has protruding eyes and a fixed stare due to the accumulation of fluid in the fat pads and muscles that lie behind the eyeballs. Because the eyes are surrounded by unyielding bone, edema forces them forward out of their sockets, producing the typical facies of exophthalmos (Fig. 41–3).

DIAGNOSTIC ASSESSMENT

Graves' disease is diagnosed on the basis of (1) the client's often striking physical appearance (enlarged neck, protruding eyes, agitated expression); (2) the symptoms of agitation, restlessness, and weight loss; and (3) laboratory findings. The serum thyroid hormone levels are usually all elevated, although they occasionally may be within the normal range (so-called euthyroid Graves' disease). Serum cholesterol levels are usually depressed. Refer to Table 41–2 for usual laboratory findings.

Complications

The three major complications of Graves' disease are (1) exophthalmos, (2) heart disease, and (3) thyroid storm (thyroid crisis, thyrotoxicosis).

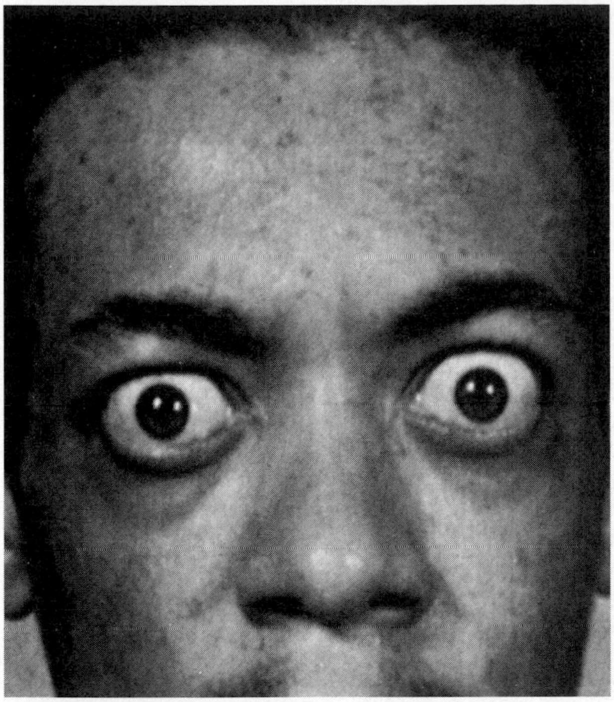

Figure 41–3
Extreme exophthalmos in hyperthyroidism. Because the eyes are surrounded by unyielding bone, fluid accumulation in the fat pads and muscles behind the eyeballs causes protruding eyes and a fixed stare in the client with exophthalmos. Without intervention, the client with severe exophthalmos may be unable to close the eyelids and may develop corneal ulceration or infection. Eventually, this can result in total loss of vision. (From Delp, M. H., & Manning, R. T. [1981]. *Major's physical diagnosis* (9th ed.). Philadelphia: W. B. Saunders.)

EXOPHTHALMOS

Unlike the manifestations of goiter and hyperthyroidism, exophthalmos does not necessarily regress with therapy. Diuretics and glucocorticoids (e.g., prednisone) are sometimes used to reduce edema of the periorbital tissue. Methylcellulose eye drops, 0.25 per cent four times daily, help reduce eye irritation. Radiation therapy to the retro-orbital tissues may help in severe cases. Surgical decompression of the orbits may be performed when all other measures fail to correct the exophthalmos. This procedure may save the client's vision when eye changes are severe.

A number of general nursing interventions also help to reduce eye discomfort and prevent corneal ulceration and infection. The nurse should instruct clients with exophthalmos to wear dark glasses and warn them to avoid getting dust or dirt in their eyes. When they cannot close their eyelids easily or at all, they should wear a sleeping mask (available in drug stores) or lightly tape the eyes shut with nonallergenic tape. The nurse can elevate the head of the bed at night and have the client restrict salt intake to relieve edema.

HEART DISEASE

Heart disease, the second complication of Graves' disease, poses a serious threat. Tachycardia almost always accompanies thyrotoxicosis, and atrial fibrillation may also appear. Congestive heart failure is found among older clients with long-standing thyrotoxicosis. The treatment of these cardiac complications is discussed in detail in Unit 7.

THYROID STORM (THYROTOXICOSIS)

Thyroid storm (thyrotoxicosis) is a sometimes fatal, acute episode of thyroid overactivity characterized by high fever, severe tachycardia, delirium, dehydration, and extreme irritability. It was once a commonly occurring crisis but seldom develops today, thanks to modern intervention techniques.

Because it is an emergency, thyroid storm requires heroic intervention for control. The high fever is treated with hypothermic blankets; dehydration is reversed with intravenous fluids. Treatment of thyroid storm involves suppressing hormonal release, inhibiting hormonal synthesis, blocking conversion of T_4 to the more active T_3, and inhibiting the effects of thyroid hormone on body tissues as well as treating the precipitating cause, if known. Blockade of thyroid hormone release is usually achieved by the administration of iodides such as SSKI (saturated solution of potassium iodide) given orally. Sodium iodide may be given intravenously. Glucocorticoid dexamethasone and propylthiouracil are also commonly used oral drugs. Beta-blockers are given to decrease the effects of sympathetic nervous system stimulation and for treating tachycardia.

CRITICAL TO REMEMBER

Aspirin is not given to reduce the temperature because aspirin has a synergistic effect with thyroxine. It displaces T_4 and T_3 from thyroxine-binding globulin, leading to an increase in free thyroid hormones.

Medical Management

PHARMACOLOGIC MANAGEMENT

The goals of care for clients with Graves' disease are to curtail the excessive secretion of thyroid hormone and to prevent and treat complications. Choice of intervention is based on (1) age, (2) goiter size, and (3) whether other health problems exist.

The three major forms of therapy are (1) antithyroid medication, (2) radioiodine, and (3) surgery.

Antithyroid Medication Therapy. This intervention is recommended for clients under 18 years of age and for pregnant women. The major medications used to control hyperthyroidism include the thioureas, propylthiouracil, and methimazole (see Table 41–3). Adrenergic blocking agents may also be administered as adjunctive therapy.

Propylthiouracil is the most commonly used antithyroid medication. It corrects hyperthyroidism by impairing thyroid hormone synthesis but does not interfere with the release or activity of stored thyroid hormone. Therefore, with the usual dosage regimen, propylthiouracil ameliorates Graves' disease within 4 to 8 weeks. However, several months may pass before symptoms completely abate. Once euthyroid, the client is given a maintenance dose of propylthiouracil, usually three times daily. Propylthiouracil, although an ideal medication in many ways, causes significant side effects in about 9 per cent of clients using it.

Methimazole (Tapazole) acts to block the action of thyroid hormone in the body. Unfortunately, methimazole also produces agranulocytosis in a small percentage of people.

Iodine therapy is prescribed for two reasons: (1) to reduce the vascularity of the thyroid gland before subtotal or total thyroidectomy and (2) to treat "thyroid storm" (see earlier discussion). Iodine preparations temporarily act to prevent release of thyroid hormone into the circulation by increasing the amount of thyroid hormone stored within the gland. However, the stored thyroid hormone is eventually released back into the circulation, once again producing hyperthyroidism. For this reason, iodine preparations are usually given only for a 10- to 14-day period before surgery. If iodine is given for a longer period or if it is given alone (i.e., not in combination with propylthiouracil), the thyroid gland may "escape" before thyroidectomy. "Escape of the thyroid" means that the iodine is no longer capable of maintaining thyroid hormone storage. As a result, thyroid hormone floods the circulation, and hyperthyroidism returns in a more severe form than before.

The iodine medication of choice is SSKI. Lugol's solution is also used but is more expensive than SSKI and tends to inactivate antithyroid preparations within the bowel.

Adrenergic blocking agents (e.g., Inderal, reserpine) are sometimes given as adjunctive therapy to control the activity of the sympathetic nervous system. There is now evidence that these agents are of great benefit to the "hyperthyroid heart," which has an increased sensitivity to catecholamines and an increased number of beta-adrenergic receptor sites. Therefore, these agents help lessen distressing symptoms such as palpitations and tachycardia. Tremor and nervousness may also be alleviated by adrenergic blocking agents.

Radioiodine Therapy. Therapy with ^{131}I is principally prescribed for middle-aged and elderly clients. This intervention offers many advantages: it is economical, is simple to administer, and can be prescribed on an outpatient basis.

The rationale behind ^{131}I therapy for Graves' disease is simple. The thyroid gland is unable to distinguish between regular iodine atoms and radioiodine atoms. Consequently, when the client receives a dose of ^{131}I, the thyroid gland picks up the radioiodine and concentrates it just as it would regular iodine. As a result, the cells that concentrate ^{131}I to make T_4 are destroyed by the local irradiation. Thus, thyroid hormone secretion diminishes, and the signs of hyperthyroidism and goiter disappear. However, because radioiodine destroys thyroid cells, one of the major possible complications of ^{131}I therapy is hypothyroidism. Therefore, the nurse should assess for symptoms of hypothyroidism after ^{131}I therapy.

^{131}I is administered orally dissolved in water. Dosage is determined both by the size of the gland and by the thyroid's uptake of a tracer dose of radioiodine. After receiving the radioiodine, the client may go home unless the dosage is extremely large. In that case, the client must be placed in isolation for several days to prevent radioactive contamination. The symptoms of hyperthyroidism usually subside within 6 to 12 weeks after ^{131}I administration. Sometimes, resistant clients require a second or (in rare cases) third dose of radioiodine. Once they become euthyroid, clients still need regular medical check-ups, because hypothyroidism may develop several years after radiotherapy. Clients who become hypothyroid require life-long hormone replacement with thyroid preparations.

Surgical Management

A thyroidectomy (removal of the thyroid gland) may be total or partial. Total thyroidectomy is performed to remove thyroid cancer. Clients who undergo this operation must take thyroid hormone on a permanent basis. Subtotal thyroidectomy is performed to correct hyperthyroidism and extreme cases of simple goiter. Approximately five sixths of the gland is removed, but because one sixth of the functioning gland is left intact, hormonal replacements may not be necessary.

Preoperative preparation for a subtotal thyroidectomy is extremely important. The client must be euthyroid before the operation, if possible. If the client is not euthyroid, the risk of thyroid storm occurring postoperatively is greatly increased. Therefore, preoperative care for clients with Graves' disease includes administration of (1) antithyroid drugs to suppress secretion of thyroid hormone and (2) iodine preparations to reduce the size and vascularity of the organ, thereby diminishing the chance of hemorrhage. Clients should be adequately rested, at optimal weight, and in good health before entering the operating room. Adequate preoperative preparation may take as long as 2 to 3 months.

Surgical treatment is effective in most people with Graves' disease.

Nursing Management

Assessment

The nurse should begin the assessment by obtaining a complete client history. By asking questions concerning weight, appetite, activity, heat intolerance, and bowel activity, the nurse can assess for the presence of typical signs and symptoms of hyperthyroidism.

The nurse should assess the client for all the typical clinical manifestations associated with Graves' disease. Symptoms of the hypermetabolic state may be obvious with apparent weight loss, and exophthalmos may be readily apparent. The client should also be questioned regarding visual difficulties, fatigue, weakness, tremors, or insomnia.

The nurse should also question significant others about mood alterations experienced by the client. Mood swings, irritability, decreased attention span, and manic behavior may be experienced by the client with hyperthyroidism. Although the client may not be aware of some of the mood changes, the significant others can usually notice the change.

Nursing Diagnosis, Planning, and Implementation

Nursing Diagnosis: Nutrition, Altered: Less than Body Requirements R/T accelerated metabolic rate.

Planning: Expected Outcomes. The client's weight loss will stop, as evidenced by client's ability to take in sufficient calories to return to ideal body weight.

Implementation. The client should be provided with a well-balanced, high-calorie diet (4000–5000 calories per day). Clients with Graves' disease are usually extremely hungry because of the increased metabolism. Six full meals a day may be needed to satisfy their appetite. However, they may lose weight rapidly despite unusually large meals. Also, they usually are in a state of negative nitrogen balance. Therefore, the nurse should encourage them to eat foods that are nutritious and contain ample amounts of protein, carbohydrates, fats, and minerals. The nurse should discourage eating of foods that increase peristalsis and thus result in diarrhea (e.g., highly seasoned, bulky, or fibrous foods). Clients should be weighed daily, and weight losses of more than 2 kg (4.4 lb) should be reported. If they continue to appear malnourished despite an ample diet, supplemental vitamins, particularly vitamin B complex, may be needed.

Nursing Diagnosis: Activity Intolerance R/T exhaustion secondary to accelerated metabolic rate.

Planning: Expected Outcomes. The client will be able to engage in a normal level of activity, as evidenced by client's ability to maintain a proper balance of rest and activity to prevent exhaustion.

Implementation. The nurse should provide the client with an environment that is restful both mentally and physically. It is a challenge to help hyperthyroid clients relax. These clients should be assigned to a private room to promote rest and to prevent them from disturbing others through hyperactivity and restlessness. The nurse should approach the client calmly and unhurriedly. He or she should encourage frequent short walks during the day and maintenance of usual bedtime rituals at night. The client should be instructed to eliminate caffeine (e.g., coffee, tea, cola, chocolate) from the diet.

Collaborative Problem: Injury, Risk for: corneal ulcerations, infection, and possible blindness R/T inability to close eyelids secondary to exophthalmos.

Planning: Expected Outcomes. The nurse will prevent corneal ulceration, infection, or blindness, as evidenced by no further development of exophthalmos.

Implementation. The treatment should be started as soon as possible once the diagnosis is made so exophthalmos can be avoided, because the condition is irreversible. The nurse instructs the client to restrict salt intake to help reduce periorbital edema. The client should be encouraged to elevate the head of the bed at night to promote drainage of fluid from the periorbital area. The client should use artificial tears and eye patches as needed to prevent irritation if the exophthalmos has already occurred.

Nursing Diagnosis: Hyperthermia R/T accelerated metabolic rate.

Planning: Expected Outcomes. The client's temperature will return to normal.

Implementation. The nurse provides the client with a cool environment, remembering that clients with Graves' disease suffer from heat intolerance. Only a lightweight sheet should be used for the top cover, and the client should be given light loose pajamas. If the client is diaphoretic, the nurse may need to bathe the client and change the bedsheets and clothes frequently.

Nursing Diagnosis: Social Interaction, Impaired R/T extreme agitation, hyperactivity, and mood swings.

Planning: Expected Outcomes. The client will be able to interact without difficulty with agitation, hyperactivity, or mood swings.

Implementation. The nurse explains to significant others that any bizarre, difficult behavior is likely to be temporary and should steadily improve with intervention. The nurse should maintain a quiet, understanding manner when caring for clients with Graves' disease and accept their irritation and emotional outbursts as normal expressions of the disease.

Occupational therapy can be incorporated into care planning. The occupational therapist may be able to provide clients with simple activities designed to distract them from focusing on the disorder (e.g., putting together a puzzle with large pieces, molding clay, watching television). For a very restless client, the nurse should discuss with the physician the need for a sedative (such as Valium) or possibly one of the adrenergic blocking agents.

Collaborative Problem: Injury, Risk for R/T preoperative preparation, euthyroid state, and surgical procedure.

Planning: Expected Outcomes. The client will be free from injury, as evidenced by client's statements of understanding of preoperative preparation; euthyroid state preoperatively; and absence of hemorrhage, respiratory distress, loss of voice, hypocalcemia, tetany, or thyroid storm.

Implementation. Clients must be carefully prepared for a thyroidectomy to avoid complications (such as thyroid storm, hemorrhage). Outcomes of successful preparation of clients for thyroid surgery include the following:

- The client is euthyroid before entering the operating room. Tests of thyroid function must be within normal limits.
- Signs of thyrotoxicosis are greatly diminished or absent. The client appears rested and relaxed.
- Weight and nutritional status are normal, and any weight losses suffered earlier have been regained.
- Cardiac problems are under control, pulse rate is normal, and electrocardiographic tracings taken preoperatively show no dangerous arrhythmias.

For help in meeting these outcomes, the client undergoing a thyroidectomy is treated with antithyroid drugs, iodine preparations, bed rest, a nutritious diet, and supplemental vitamins. Thorough preparation may take months. However, once good health has been restored, the client can undergo surgery with confidence that the operation will be successful and the symptoms alleviated.

The immediate goals of postoperative care after a thyroidectomy are to (1) maintain airway patency, (2) decrease the strain in the suture line, (3) relieve discomfort from the sore throat and tracheal irritation, (4) prevent pooling of respiratory secretions, (5) prevent or relieve the complications of thyroidectomy, and (6) maintain laboratory values within normal limits, especially calcium levels.

Typical postoperative orders, their rationale, and important associated nursing interventions are outlined in Table 41–4.

Major complications after a thyroidectomy may include

- respiratory obstruction due to edema of the glottis, bilateral laryngeal nerve damage, or tracheal compression from hemorrhage
- hemorrhage
- weakness and hoarseness of the voice due to trauma or damage of one laryngeal nerve
- hypocalcemia and tetany resulting from accidental removal of one or more parathyroid glands
- thyroid storm
- permanent hypothyroidism

Temporary hoarseness and voice weakness may occur if there has been unilateral injury to the recurrent laryngeal nerve during surgery. To assess the client's voice, the nurse should ask "What is your name?" as soon as full recovery from anesthesia occurs. The nurse should have the client speak every 30 to 60 minutes thereafter, and carefully note any voice changes. If hoarseness or voice weakness is present, the nurse can reassure the client that the problem will probably subside in a few days. Unnecessary talking should be discouraged to minimize hoarseness.

Muscular twitching and hyperirritability of the nervous system may indicate hypocalcemic tetany. Hypocalcemia can develop after thyroidectomy if the parathyroid glands are accidentally removed during surgery. Symptoms may develop 1 to 7 days after surgery. If the client develops numbness and tingling around the mouth, fingertips, or toes; muscle spasms; or twitching, the physician should be called immediately. The nurse must make sure that calcium gluconate ampules are available.

Nursing Diagnosis: Knowledge Deficit R/T medications, eye care, and possible complications.

Planning: Expected Outcomes. The client will understand eye care and possible complications, as evidenced by client's statements and ability to comply with medication regimen.

Implementation. Once the immediate postoperative period and its dangers have passed, the nurse's attention should be turned to teaching. Several important areas should be included. First, the nurse teaches the client how to support the weight of the head and neck when sitting up in bed. He or she can show clients how to place their hands at the back of the head when flexing the neck or moving. Usually, clients are able to perform this maneuver by the first postoperative day. Second, as the wound heals (around the second to fourth postoperative day), the nurse instructs the client in range-of-motion exercises for prevention of contractures. With the surgeon's permission, the nurse teaches clients to flex the head forward and laterally, to hyperextend the neck, and to turn the head from side to side. They should perform these exercises several times every day. Third, if a total thyroidectomy has been performed, the nurse gives instruction concerning self-administration of thyroid medications, as outlined previously under the section on hypothyroidism.

Modification of Plan of Care for the Elderly

Hyperthyroidism in the elderly accounts for 10 to 15 per cent of all thyrotoxic clients. Some clients present with typical symptoms of hyperthyroidism, especially when the diagnosis is Graves' disease. However, hyperthyroidism in the elderly is also notorious for presenting with atypical or minimal symptoms. It is often overlooked because the symptoms and signs are not the usual ones and the symptoms are frequently attributed to aging. Weight loss, lack of eye findings, and normal-sized thyroid glands are frequently found on assessment. Many clients actually appear apathetic instead of hyperactive. Cardiovascular abnormalities such as congestive heart failure, atrial arrhythmias (usually digoxin-resistant), and various degrees of heart block are much more common in the elderly. A relative lack of tachycardia has been documented; approximately 40 per cent of elderly clients have heart rates less than 100.

TABLE 41–4 Postoperative Orders, Rationale, and Associated Nursing Interventions After Thyroidectomy

POSTOPERATIVE ORDER	RATIONALE	ASSOCIATED NURSING INTERVENTIONS
Vital signs every 15 min until stable; then every 30 min for next 12 hours	After thyroidectomy, hemorrhage and respiratory obstruction may develop. Elevated pulse and hypotension indicate hemorrhage and shock. Restlessness is an early sign of hemorrhage. Dyspnea, stridulous respirations, and retraction of neck tissues indicate respiratory obstruction.	Check dressing after checking vital signs. Observe for bleeding at front, sides, and back of neck. Examine back of client's neck and shoulders for bleeding because blood tends to drain posteriorly. Check dressing for tightness; uncomfortable tautness may indicate bleeding into tissues. Loosen dressing and call surgeon immediately.
Semi-Fowler's position when conscious unless client is hypotensive; support head and neck with pillows and sandbags; ambulate second day as tolerated	Immobilization of head and neck is essential to prevent flexion and hyperextension of neck with resultant strain on suture line. Semi-Fowler's position is used for comfort.	Place sandbags on either side of client's head for immobilization and maintenance of good alignment. Warn client not to extend or hyperextend neck; reassure client that sandbags will prevent moving head too much. Gently rub back of client's neck to relieve tension. Support client's head and neck when moving or changing position.
Fluids by mouth as tolerated; if nausea or vomiting, notify surgeon; soft diet on afternoon of second day	Give intravenous fluids if nauseated or vomiting. Otherwise, start oral fluids as soon as client is fully conscious.	Maintain intake and output record for 2 or 3 days. Assess for difficulty swallowing. Normally this problem lasts for only 1 or 2 days postoperatively. Weigh client once a full diet is started; weight lost during early postoperative period should be regained.
Meperidine (Demerol) or morphine sulfate, every 3–4 hr as needed for pain in throat area	Demerol and morphine sulfate are both used during early postoperative period to relieve pain and promote rest.	Do not give narcotics if respirations below 12/min or if respiratory congestion; consult physician for further orders.
Cough and deep breathe every half hour; suction mouth and trachea if necessary	Pooling of mucous secretions in trachea, bronchi, and lungs will cause respiratory obstruction with resultant atelectasis and pneumonia. Secretions must be raised to prevent respiratory complications.	Instruct client to cough and deep breathe as taught during preoperative period. If client cannot raise secretions, gently suction mouth and trachea. Do not oversedate clients with profuse respiratory secretions; give narcotics judiciously.
Tracheostomy set, endotracheal tube, laryngoscope, and oxygen on hand in room	Acute respiratory obstruction due to hemorrhage, edema of glottis, laryngeal nerve damage, or tetany is an emergency. Equipment for establishing an airway and administering oxygen must be available for immediate use.	Continuously assess for signs of airway obstruction, e.g., increasing restlessness, tachycardia, apprehension, cyanosis, stridulous respirations, and retraction of neck tissues. Report any of these signs to surgeon immediately.
Continuous mist inhalation until chest is clear	Humidification of air promotes easier breathing and helps to liquefy mucous secretions.	Keep doors closed so that moist air is retained in room.
Rectal temperature every 4 hr for 24 hr, then orally	One of the first signs of thyroid storm is an elevated temperature.	Carefully assess for signs of thyroid storm: elevated temperature, extreme restlessness, agitation, and tachycardia. Report any elevation over 37.7° C (100° F) rectally or 37.2° C (99° F) orally.

The diagnosis of hyperthyroidism is established by appropriate laboratory tests. It is usual to find an elevated T_4 and a suppressed TSH. Therapy for hyperthyroidism in the elderly is radioactive iodine.

Posthospital Care

The nurse should teach the client the medication regimen and the need for life-long replacement therapy. He or she should make an appointment for the client at the clinic or physician's office after discharge, emphasizing that the client who has had a thyroidectomy must see a physician at least twice yearly to avert possible complications (e.g., hypothyroidism, hypoparathyroidism, or recurrent hyperthyroidism).

The nurse should teach the client how to care for the incision once it has healed with the use of lanolin cream to soften the wound. This will help to lessen the scar.

THYROIDITIS

Thyroiditis simply means inflammation of the thyroid gland. It appears in three basic forms: (1) acute suppurative, (2) subacute granulomatous and lymphocytic, and (3) chronic (Hashimoto's disease).

Etiology

Acute suppurative thyroiditis is an uncommon inflammatory disease usually caused by bacterial invasion of the thyroid gland. Subacute granulomatous thyroiditis is a self-limiting inflammatory condition.

Chronic thyroiditis (Hashimoto's thyroiditis), a long-term inflammatory disorder, is the most common form of thyroiditis. Like Graves' disease, chronic thyroiditis has an autoimmune basis. Genetic predisposition also plays a role in its causation.

Clinical Manifestations

Symptoms of acute thyroiditis include abrupt onset of unilateral anterior neck pain, with possible radiation to the ear or mandible on the affected side. Fever, diaphoresis, and other symptoms of bacterial toxicity may also be present.

Subacute granulomatous thyroiditis is usually painful, whereas subacute lymphocytic thyroiditis is usually painless. Assessment data may include characteristic anterior, unilateral neck pain that may occur with an abrupt onset. Radiation to the ear on the ipsilateral side may occur. Symptoms like viral infection may be present that consist of myalgia, low-grade fever, lassitude, and sore throat.

Subacute lymphocytic thyroiditis is characterized by occasional hyperthyroidism and a painless goiter.

Symptoms of chronic thyroiditis include painless, asymmetric enlargement of the gland, which in turn causes pressure on the surrounding structures and can lead to dysphagia and respiratory distress. Most clients are euthyroid; about 20 per cent are hypothyroid, and less than 5 per cent are hyperthyroid.

Medical Management

The course of Hashimoto's thyroiditis varies. Some clients experience spontaneous remission, whereas others remain stable for years. In approximately one third of the cases, hypothyroidism develops because of gradual atrophy of the gland. Intervention is directed toward reducing the size of the gland and correcting any thyroid function abnormalities.

Acute thyroiditis usually responds to parenteral antibiotic therapy.

Treatment for subacute granulomatous thyroiditis includes salicylates, nonsteroidal anti-inflammatory agents, and oral glucocorticoids such as prednisone.

The treatment goal for subacute lymphocytic thyroiditis is to provide relief of symptoms from the hyperthyroidism with beta-adrenergic blocking agents. Antithyroid medications are not indicated.

Surgical Management

Acute thyroiditis that does not respond to medical treatment may require incision and drainage of the affected gland.

Nursing Management

Nursing care for clients with thyroiditis is usually supportive until the diagnosis is made. The care then, as with other thyroid disorders, revolves around helping the client learn correct medication administration. If surgery is necessary, then care is the same as discussed earlier.

Posthospital Care

As with other clients with thyroid disorders, discharge teaching is centered on making sure that clients understand their medication and how to take it. Clients should have their thyroid functions measured at regular intervals after discharge to monitor the development of hyperthyroidism or hypothyroidism and for testing the effectiveness of medication.

THYROID CANCER

There are four major types of thyroid cancer: papillary adenocarcinoma, follicular adenocarcinoma, medullary carcinoma, and anaplastic carcinoma. Benign adenomas and malignant thyroid tumors constitute the third cause of thyroid enlargement (hypothyrodism and hyperthyroidism constitute the first two causes). Like other benign tumors, most thyroid adenomas are usually well encapsulated and consequently do not spread out or extend into other tissues.

Incidence

Malignant tumors of the thyroid are rare. They account for approximately three to four new cases per 100,000 population per year in the United States. Thyroid

TABLE 41–5 Types of Thyroid Cancer: Incidence, Characteristics, Intervention, and Prognosis

TYPE	INCIDENCE	CHARACTERISTICS	INTERVENTION	PROGNOSIS
Papillary adenocarcinoma	Comprises 60% of thyroid cancers Mainly affects clients in 40s	Slow-growing firm tumor Palpable nodule Spreads to regional nodes in approximately 50% of cases Radiation-related thyroid cancer with 10- to 20-year latency period	Total or near-total thyroidectomy Others recommend lobectomy and isthmectomy	Excellent if cancer restricted to thyroid gland Surgery usually curative
Follicular adenocarcinoma	Comprises 15% of thyroid cancers Mainly affects clients in 50s	Slow-growing nodule with about 15% metastasis to regional nodes at diagnosis Associated with radiation, iodine deficiency, endemic goiter	Total thyroidectomy	Good but inferior to that of papillary adenocarcinoma
Medullary carcinoma	Comprises 5–10% of thyroid cancers Mainly affects clients 40–50s	Tumor is hereditary and familial Tends to secrete adrenocorticotropic hormone, serotonin Metastases to surrounding structures at diagnosis in 50%	Total thyroidectomy Radical neck resection if metastasis	Poor; mean survival = 6.6 years
Anaplastic carcinoma	Comprises 5–15% of thyroid cancers Mainly affects clients 60–70s	Highly malignant Grows rapidly Local and widespread metastasis within 1 year	Combination of thyroidectomy, external radiation therapy, chemotherapy, and tracheostomy as needed	Grave; mean survival = 6.2 months; 5-year survival = 7.1%

cancer accounts for approximately 0.2 per cent of cancer deaths; it develops mainly in women between the ages of 40 and 60 years. Females are affected more than males in a ratio of 2.5:1. The incidence, characteristics, intervention, and prognosis of each thyroid cancer are compared in Table 41–5.

Etiology

Benign adenomas are usually not dangerous, although on rare occasion they grow large enough to cause respiratory symptoms by pressing against the trachea. Occasionally, however, malignant transformation occurs, and the benign nodules become cancerous. Also, malignant transformation of benign nodules can apparently follow prolonged stimulation of the thyroid gland by the pituitary hormone TSH.

Risk Factors

Thyroid carcinoma occurs more frequently among clients who have received large doses of radiation to the head and neck. Prevention centers around avoiding radiation to the area, shielding the thyroid area if possible if radiation is done, and closely following clients who had radiation to that area.

DIAGNOSTIC ASSESSMENT

Thyroid cancer is diagnosed by fine-needle aspiration and biopsy.

Nursing Management

Nursing care for the client with thyroid cancer is similar to the care of any client undergoing a thyroidectomy. The client will also need the support and teaching that a cancer client requires. If the client is to undergo chemotherapy, then additional teaching is needed.

Posthospital Care

If the client has total thyroidectomy, replacement of the thyroid hormone is necessary. Discharge teaching is centered on making sure the client understands the medication and how to take it.

There are no special home health-care needs other than the needs of a client after thyroidectomy or those of a client on chemotherapy or radiation therapy.

Parathyroid Disorders

HYPERPARATHYROIDISM

Hyperparathyroidism is a disorder caused by overactivity of one or more of the parathyroid glands. Hyperparathyroidism is classified as primary, secondary, or tertiary.

Incidence

Hyperparathyroidism usually occurs in clients over the age of 60 years and affects women 2:1 in a population of 1000.

Etiology

Primary hyperparathyroidism develops when the normal regulatory relationship between serum calcium levels and parathyroid hormone (PTH) secretion is interrupted. This occurs when either an adenoma or hyperplasia of the gland exists without an identifying injury.

Secondary hyperparathyroidism occurs when the glands are hyperplastic from malfunction of another organ system. This is usually the result of renal failure but may also occur with osteogenesis imperfecta, Paget's disease, multiple myeloma, and carcinoma with bone metastasis.

Tertiary hyperparathyroidism occurs when PTH production is irrepressible (autonomous) in clients with normal or low serum calcium levels.

Risk Factors

The risk factors vary on the basis of whether the condition is primary, secondary, or tertiary. In the presence of other disorders, the best secondary prevention is early detection in those clients who are at high risk. Screening of the serum calcium level is important in these clients so interventions can be taken early.

Pathophysiology

The normal function of PTH is to increase bone resorption, thereby maintaining the proper balance of calcium and phosphorus ions within the blood. Excessive circulating PTH leads to bone damage, hypercalcemia, and kidney damage.

BONE DAMAGE

Oversecretion of PTH causes excessive osteoclast growth and activity within the bones. When bone resorption is increased, calcium is released from the bones into the blood, causing hypercalcemia. Thus, the bones suffer demineralization as a result of calcium loss. In time, the bones may become so fragile that they cause pathologic bone changes including kyphosis of the dorsal spine and compression fractures of the vertebral bodies. Also, as the uncontrolled osteoclast proliferation continues, the skeleton may develop cystic lesions. If this condition is not corrected, the client eventually may develop a severe bone disease called osteitis fibrosa cystica (Recklinghausen's disease of bone).

HYPERCALCEMIA

An increased serum calcium level is the consequence of bone resorption due to excessive PTH secretion. Hypercalcemia eventually results in hypercalciuria (excessive calcium in the urine). Also, because of the high serum calcium levels, excess calcium may precipitate as calcium phosphate in the kidneys, lungs, muscles, heart, and eyes. Hypercalcemia can stimulate hypergastrinemia, abdominal pain, and peptic ulcer disease. Pancreatitis is also influenced by high serum calcium levels.

KIDNEY DAMAGE

Excessive PTH levels cause hyperphosphaturia. As serum calcium continues to rise in hyperparathyroidism, excessive amounts of both phosphorus and calcium are excreted and lost from the body. Large amounts of both calcium and phosphate are being excreted by the renal system, so calcium phosphate may be deposited within the renal tubules, causing a kidney condition called nephrocalcinosis. Calcium salts are quite insoluble in urine. Thus, kidney stones composed of calcium phosphate may be found in the urine of clients with primary hyperparathyroidism.

If hyperparathyroidism is surgically treated early in its course, the chance of total recovery is good. Bone pain may disappear within 3 days after removal of parathyroid tissue, and bone lesions may heal completely. Unfortunately, serious renal disease may not be reversible by parathyroid surgery.

Clinical Manifestations

Some clients with hyperparathyroidism may be entirely asymptomatic. Others suffer from a myriad of symptoms arising from the skeletal disease, renal involvement, gastrointestinal tract disorders, and neurologic abnormalities (Table 41–6).

Manifestations of bone disease range from backache, joint pain, and bone pain to pathologic fractures of the spine, ribs, and long bones. In long-standing cases, assessment reveals deformity and bending of the bones.

Symptoms of renal involvement include (1) polyuria and polydipsia; (2) the appearance of sand, gravel, or stones within the urine; (3) azotemia; and (4) hypertension due to renal damage. Without intervention,

TABLE 41–6 Characteristics of Hyperparathyroidism and Hypoparathyroidism

HYPERPARATHYROIDISM	HYPOPARATHYROIDISM
Increased bone resorption	Decreased bone resorption
Elevated serum calcium levels	Depressed serum calcium levels
Depressed serum phosphate levels	Elevated serum phosphate levels
Hypercalciuria and hyperphosphaturia	Hypocalciuria and hypophosphaturia
Decreased neuromuscular irritability	Increased neuromuscular activity, which may progress to tetany

renal insufficiency may progress to fatal renal hypertension and uremia.

Hypercalcemia mainly produces gastrointestinal tract manifestations (e.g., thirst, nausea, anorexia, constipation, ileus, and abdominal pain). Often, clients have a history of peptic ulcer or gastrointestinal tract bleeding. Assessment may also reveal psychiatric symptoms. Listlessness, depression, and paranoia are sometimes associated with high levels of serum calcium. Finally, calcium may form calcification within the eyes, impairing vision.

The major complications of hyperparathyroidism are the symptoms associated with hypercalcemia and those associated with treatment such as dehydration, hypocalcemia, and gastrointestinal tract symptoms.

DIAGNOSTIC ASSESSMENT

The diagnosis of hyperparathyroidism mainly rests on laboratory and x-ray findings. Serum calcium is elevated, whereas serum phosphate is depressed; urine calcium and phosphorus are both high. In addition, alkaline phosphatase is elevated among the 25 per cent of affected clients who have associated bone disease. Also, clients with skeletal damage have the following characteristic x-ray findings: diffuse demineralization of bones, bone cysts, subperiosteal bone resorption, and loss of the lamina dura surrounding the teeth (Table 41–7).

Medical Management

The treatment of hyperparathyroidism includes (1) lowering severely elevated calcium levels, (2) increasing urinary calcium excretion with diuretics, and (3) long-term management of hypercalcemia with drugs to increase bone resorption of calcium.

PHARMACOLOGIC MANAGEMENT

Serum calcium levels are lowered by hydration and calciuresis. Hydration may be achieved with a normal saline infusion. Normal saline is the fluid of choice because it both expands the volume and acts in the kidney to inhibit the resorption of calcium. Furosemide (Lasix), a loop diuretic, may also be used to promote calciuresis. Thiazide diuretics are not used because they promote calcium retention in the kidneys.

Drugs that inhibit bone resorption include plicamycin (Mithracin), gallium nitrate (Ganite), phosphates, and calcitonin. Plicamycin is a cancer chemotherapeutic agent that is very effective in lowering serum calcium levels. The hypocalcemic effect is seen after 24 hours and lasts for about 1 to 2 weeks. The dose is about one tenth that used for cancer treatment, so the adverse effects are proportionally lower.

A newer drug, gallium nitrate, is now being used more often because it has even fewer side effects. Glucocorticoids may be used to reduce hypercalcemia by decreasing gastrointestinal absorption of calcium. Etidronate (Didronel) or calcitonin may be used to decrease the release of calcium by bones. Drugs used to treat hypercalcemia are summarized in Table 41–8.

DIETARY MANAGEMENT

The client with hypercalcemia should be on a low-calcium, low–vitamin D diet.

Surgical Management

Definitive treatment of hyperparathyroidism is surgical removal of the gland or glands that cause hypersecretion of PTH. Usually, only the diseased parathyroid glands are resected. However, if all four glands are hyperplastic, three and one-half glands are removed. Fortunately, one half of a parathyroid gland is usually sufficient to maintain normal levels of circulating PTH.

Autotransplantation of the parathyroid glands is a useful modality for the management of clients with certain forms of hyperparathyroidism. After partial parathyroidectomy, it is possible to transplant the remaining healthy parathyroid tissue to a safer location, such as the brachioradialis muscle of the forearm. Reexploration of the neck in the future may cause laryngeal nerve damage and influence complications from the original surgery. Transplants take some time to come to full effect. Clients must be supplemented with calcium and vitamin D for prevention of hypoparathyroidism and hypocalcemia until the transplant matures.

The complications after parathyroidectomy are similar to those after thyroidectomy. Hypocalcemia is a potentially life-threatening complication even if some parathyroid glands are left untouched because edema decreases their function. The client can also develop respiratory distress related to either hemorrhage or recurrent laryngeal nerve damage.

Nursing Management

Assessment

There are no obvious signs or symptoms of hyperparathyroidism and the resultant hypercalcemia. The nurse should elicit a good history from the client to see if any of the risk factors for developing the condition exist.

TABLE 41–7 Diagnostic Test of Parathyroid Function: Purpose, Procedure, Normal Range, and Interpretation of Abnormal Findings

TEST	PURPOSE	PROCEDURE	NORMAL RANGE	INTERPRETATION OF ABNORMAL FINDINGS	REMARKS
Total serum calcium	Measures amount of ionized and nonionized calcium in serum	Venous blood to laboratory	4.8–5.2 mEq/L or 8–11 mg/100 mL	Elevated in hyperparathyroidism; depressed in hypoparathyroidism, tetany, rickets, nephrosis, and osteomalacia	Normally 50% of total serum calcium is ionized; amount of ionized calcium available decreases in alkalosis
Qualitative urinary calcium (Sulkowitch's test)	Measures roughly amount of calcium in urine; used as quick method for diagnosing if tetany is due to hypoparathyroidism	Collect urine specimen and send to laboratory	Fine white precipitate should form when Sulkowitch reagent is added to urine specimen	Absence or decreased density of precipitate indicates low serum calcium and hypoparathyroidism	Medications that elevate serum calcium levels include vitamin D, parathyroid injection, and dihydrotachysterol
Quantitative urinary calcium (calcium deprivation test)	Measures exact amount of calcium in 24-hr urine specimen	Collect 24-hr urine specimen and send to laboratory	75–175 mg calcium per 24 hr	Elevated in hyperparathyroidism; depressed in hypoparathyroidism	Foods high in calcium include milk, cheese, molasses, turnip greens, and dandelion greens
Serum phosphorus	Measures amount of inorganic phosphorus in serum	Venous blood to laboratory	1.3–1.75 mEq/L (2.5–4.5 mg/100 mL) in adults	Elevated in hypoparathyroidism, uremia, and alkalosis; depressed in hyperparathyroidism, rickets, and osteomalacia	There is an inverse relationship between serum calcium and serum phosphorus levels
Serum alkaline phosphatase	Measures amount of alkaline phosphatase in serum; aids in diagnosing bone and liver disorders	Venous blood to laboratory	2.0–5.0 Bodansky units	Elevated in hyperparathyroidism, osteomalacia, rickets, healing fractures, and pregnancy and after ingestion of large amounts of vitamin D	Alkaline phosphatase is an enzyme normally present in small amounts in serum; some medications causing false elevations of alkaline phosphatase levels include allopurinol, some androgens, colchicine, erythromycin, methyldopa, some oral contraceptives, procainamide, and tolbutamide
Parathyroid hormone (PTH) radioimmunoassay test	Measures level of PTH in serum	Venous blood to laboratory	Depends on serum calcium concentration	High concentrations indicate hyperparathyroidism	When evaluated in conjunction with serum calcium levels, this is the most specific test for hyperparathyroidism

TABLE 41–8 Drugs Used to Treat Hypercalcemia

MEDICATION	DOSAGE	SIDE EFFECTS	NURSING IMPLICATIONS
Furosemide (Lasix)	Up to 100 mg IV	Volume depletion and dehydration, orthostatic hypotension, hypokalemia, hypochloremic alkalosis, hyperuricemia, dilutional hyponatremia, hypocalcemia, hypomagnesemia	Monitor intake and output carefully; monitor blood pressure and pulse; give with 0.9% sodium chloride; monitor serum electrolytes, watch calcium level closely
Plicamycin (Mithracin)	25 μg IV daily for 1 to 4 days	Thrombocytopenia, bleeding tendencies, nausea and vomiting, facial flushing, diarrhea; increased BUN and creatinine; decreased serum calcium, potassium, and phosphorus; anorexia	Therapeutic effect in hypercalcemia may not be seen for 24 to 48 hr and may last 3 to 15 days; monitor serum electrolytes, liver enzymes, and BUN and creatinine; monitor platelet count and watch for bleeding; watch for sudden drop in serum calcium; check closely for signs of hypocalcemia; give antiemetics before administration to reduce nausea
Etidronate disodium (Didronel)	5 mg/kg body weight PO daily as single dose 2 hr before meals, up to dose of 20 mg/kg	Diarrhea, nausea, bone pain, increased risk of fractures, elevated serum phosphate	Do not administer with food or antacids; monitor serum phosphate; tell client that onset of therapeutic effect may take several months; do not give for more than 6 months continuously, stop, then restart after 3 months; monitor renal function
Gallium nitrate (Ganite)	100–200 mg/m² daily for 5 consecutive days	Increased BUN and creatinine, hypocalcemia, decreased serum bicarbonate, transient hypophosphatemia, anemia, hypotension, nausea and vomiting	Administer IV with 0.9% sodium chloride; monitor serum calcium, bicarbonate, and phosphate; check blood pressure at intervals; monitor renal function; check for signs of anemia
Calcitonin (Cibacalcin)	0.5–1 mg SC daily or 2 to 3 times a week	Nausea and vomiting, urinary frequency, flushing of face and hands, hypocalcemia	Administer at bedtime to decrease nausea and vomiting; monitor for signs of hypocalcemia; treatment may last for 6 months; monitor serum phosphate; warn client about transient facial flushing

BUN, blood urea nitrogen; IV, intravenously; PO, orally; SC, subcutaneously.

The client may exhibit some psychosocial changes that the nurse could assess, such as lethargy, drowsiness, memory loss, or emotional lability, all signs of hypercalcemia.

Nursing Diagnosis, Planning, and Implementation

Nursing Diagnosis: Injury, Risk for R/T demineralization of bones resulting in pathologic fractures.

Planning: Expected Outcomes. The client will be free from injury, as evidenced by absence of pathologic fractures or hypercalcemia.

Implementation. The nurse protects the client from accidents. If bone involvement exists, the client may develop pathologic fractures from even small bumps or minor falls. The client's bed should be kept the client is weak or has joint or skeletal disease, the nurse assists in ambulation.

Nursing Diagnosis: Urinary Elimination, Altered R/T renal involvement secondary to hypercalcemia and hyperphosphaturia.

Planning: Expected Outcomes. The client will return to a normal urinary output, as evidenced by no development of stones and urine output of 30 to 60 mL/hr.

Implementation. The client should take in at least 3000 mL of fluid a day.

CRITICAL TO REMEMBER

Dehydration is dangerous for clients with hyperparathyroidism because it both increases the serum calcium level and promotes the formation of renal stones.

Cranberry and prune juice may help make the urine more acidic. High urinary acidity helps prevent renal acidic urine than in an alkaline urine.

If the client has a kidney stone, the nurse should strain all urine to detect gravel and stones, saving any specimens of abnormal urine for the physician to examine and for laboratory analysis. Also, the nurse should observe the urine for blood and assess the client for renal colic (see Chaps. 30 and 31).

Nursing Diagnosis: Nutrition, Altered: Less than Body Requirements R/T anorexia and nausea.

Planning: Expected Outcomes. The client will have an adequate intake, as evidenced by absence of nausea and return to or maintenance of ideal body weight.

Implementation. A low-calcium diet to correct hypercalcemia is encouraged. The nurse should explain to from peptic ulcers will need to take antacids or histamine-receptor antagonists.

Nursing Diagnosis: Constipation R/T adverse effects of hypercalcemia on the gastrointestinal tract.

Planning: Expected Outcomes. The client will maintain a normal bowel pattern, as evidenced by a bowel movement that is normal for the client.

Implementation. The nurse must work to prevent constipation and fecal impaction resulting from hypercalcemia. The nurse should help the client to be as active as possible, depending on the extent of bone disease. If constipation continues despite these measures, the nurse should obtain an order for a stool softener or laxative.

Collaborative Problem: Injury, Risk for R/T preoperative drug sensitivities and postoperative complications.

Planning: Expected Outcomes. The client will be free from injury, as evidenced by no medication reactress, hemorrhage, and hypocalcemia after surgery.

Implementation. If the client is on digitalis, the nurse must administer this medication with extreme caution. Clients with hypercalcemia are hypersensitive to digitalis and may quickly develop toxic symptoms.

During the postoperative period, new problems arise, some of which are the reverse of those found preoperatively. During the immediate postoperative period, nursing care is similar to that after thyroidectomy. The nurse should also watch for signs of hormonal imbalance.

Mild tetany caused by the drop in serum calcium is expected after the removal of the parathyroid tissue. Typically, the uncomfortable tingling of the hands and around the mouth that follows parathyroid resection usually disappears without problem. This mild tetany is usually temporary; however, if it persists or is severe, calcium gluconate is administered intravenously to relieve symptoms.

Clients with bone disease require additional therapy after surgery. Removal of the parathyroid glands reduces bone resorption, and because bone rebuilding proceeds at a rapid rate, the client can develop the "hungry bones" syndrome. This is characterized by hypocalcemia and severe tetany resulting from the rapid utilization of calcium by the bones. To prevent low serum calcium levels due to bone recalcification, the nurse should instruct these clients to eat foods high in calcium. Tetany is treated with injections of calcium gluconate. To maintain adequate calcium levels, oral calcium preparations are usually given for months until the skeletal tissues have been rebuilt. Finally, clients are usually encouraged to ambulate as soon as possible after surgery, because weight-bearing speeds the recalcification process.

Modification of Plan of Care for the Elderly

Hyperparathyroidism in the elderly is an overlooked disease. It is estimated that 1 per 1000 men and 2 per 1000 women over the age of 60 years experience hyperparathyroidism. This disease often goes undiagnosed in the elderly because symptoms in the early stages are subtle and attributed to old age, depression, or anxiety. The symptoms only intensify as the level of serum calcium continues to rise and other physiologic and functional changes occur. Laboratory diagnosis is made in the same way as for a client younger than 60 years of age, but treatment may be complicated by medical problems and medication.

Posthospital Care

Clients and significant others need to understand discharge medications that may be needed for continued control of hypercalcemia. The client and significant others should also be taught about any dietary restrictions of calcium or phosphorus.

HOME HEALTH CARE NEEDS

If the client suffered from severe osteoporosis or pathologic fractures, some assistance may be required at home. The client may need a visiting nurse to help assess the current home situation and make recommendations on how it could be made safer. The home will need to be cleared of articles such as throw rugs that might increase the client's risk of falling. The client may also need assistive devices such as a railing in the bathroom, a bedside commode, or a walker.

HYPOPARATHYROIDISM

Hyposecretion of the parathyroid glands produces a syndrome opposite that of hyperparathyroidism. Thus, serum calcium levels are abnormally low, serum phosphate levels are abnormally high, and pronounced neuromuscular irritability (tetany) may develop.

Incidence

Idiopathic hypoparathyroidism strikes children nine times as often as adults and affects twice as many women as men.

Etiology

The causes of hypoparathyroidism are either iatrogenic or idiopathic. Iatrogenic causes of hypoparathyroidism include (1) accidental removal of the parathyroid glands during thyroidectomy, (2) infarction of the parathyroid glands resulting from an inadequate blood supply to the glands during surgery, and (3) strangulation of one or more of the glands by postoperative scar tissue.

Idiopathic hypoparathyroidism, like Graves' disease and Hashimoto's thyroiditis, may be an autoimmune disorder with a genetic basis. This type of hypoparathyroidism is far less common than the iatrogenic form.

Risk Factors

The major risk factor for hypoparathyroidism is thyroid or parathyroid surgery. The only preventive measure is early detection through close monitoring of clients who have had these procedures.

Pathophysiology

When parathyroid secretion is reduced, bone resorption slows, serum calcium levels fall, and severe neuromuscular irritability develops. Somewhat paradoxically, calcifications form in various organs (e.g., the eyes and basal ganglia). Also, without sufficient PTH, fewer phosphorus ions are secreted by the distal tubules of the kidney, renal excretion of phosphate decreases, and serum phosphate levels rise.

The client may fully recover from the effects of hypoparathyroidism if the condition is diagnosed early, before the advent of serious complications. Unfortunately, cataracts and brain calcifications, once formed, and irreversible.

Clinical Manifestations

The symptoms of hypoparathyroidism are mainly caused by low serum calcium levels. They are always more severe in clients who have an elevated serum pH (alkalosis) from any cause (e.g., ingesting antacids, hyperventilation). Symptoms worsen because when the pH of the blood rises, the amount of ionized calcium drops, although total serum calcium remains the same. With less ionized calcium available to the body, the symptoms resulting from hypocalcemia become more severe until the alkalosis is corrected.

Acute Hypoparathyroidism. This condition is caused by accidental damage to parathyroid tissues during thyroidectomy. It is characterized by greatly increased neuromuscular irritability, which results in tetany. Clients with tetany experience painful muscle spasms, irritability, grimacing, tingling of fingers, laryngospasm, and arrhythmias. Assessment also reveals Chvostek's and Trousseau's signs. In some cases, tetany is so severe that a tracheostomy is required to correct acute respiratory obstruction secondary to laryngospasm.

Chronic Hypoparathyroidism. This condition is usually idiopathic. It causes lethargy; thin, patchy hair; brittle nails; dry, scaly skin; and personality changes. Ectopic calcifications may appear in the eyes and basal ganglia. Thus, the client may develop cataracts and permanent brain damage accompanied by psychosis or convulsions. In addition, severe persistent hypocalcemia adversely affects the heart, causing arrhythmias and eventual cardiac failure.

DIAGNOSTIC ASSESSMENT

The diagnosis of hypoparathyroidism is based on

- presence of Chvostek's sign (spasms of facial muscles after a tap on the side of the face, signifying hyperirritability of the facial nerve)
- presence of Trousseau's sign (carpal spasms of the fingers and hand after application of a blood pressure cuff to the arm)
- numbness and tingling around the mouth and fingertips
- laboratory findings of low serum calcium, high serum phosphate, and low or absent urinary calcium
- x-ray studies showing calcification of the basal ganglia
- eye examinations that may reveal the early development of cataracts due to the formation of calcifications within the lens of the eye

Medical Management

Acute hypoparathyroidism (with its major manifestation of acute tetany) is a life-threatening disorder. The three goals of emergency care are to (1) elevate serum calcium levels as rapidly as possible, (2) prevent or treat convulsions, and (3) control laryngeal spasm and consequent respiratory obstruction.

The goal of intervention for clients with chronic hypoparathyroidism is to restore the serum calcium level to normal concentrations. This is done more gradually than with acute hypoparathyroidism.

PHARMACOLOGIC MANAGEMENT

For acute hypoparathyroidism, to elevate the serum calcium levels quickly, the physician will prescribe 10 per cent calcium gluconate solution in an intravenous infusion. While administering the calcium gluconate, the nurse should instruct the client to inhale carbon dioxide by breathing into a paper bag. This causes a mild metabolic acidosis, which serves to elevate the amount of ionized calcium in the blood.

Once the condition has stabilized and the dangers of tetany have passed, the client is given oral calcium salts and vitamin D to maintain normal serum calcium levels.

For chronic hypoparathyroidism, the client is given oral calcium salts (either calcium gluconate, calcium lactate, or calcium chloride) and vitamin D. Commercially available forms of vitamin D include calciferol (vitamin D_2), dihydroxycholecalciferol, and dihydrotachysterol (Hytakerol). Although calciferol is a more reliable and less expensive drug than dihydrotachysterol or dihydroxycholecalciferol, all three forms of vitamin D are effective in correcting hypocalcemia. They are all obtainable as either tablets or oily liquids.

DIETARY MANAGEMENT

The client with hypoparathyroidism should be on a diet high in calcium but low in phosphorus.

Nursing Management

Assessment

The nurse should carefully assess the client at risk for acute hypoparathyroidism, such as the post-thyroidectomy client, for the development of hypocalcemia. The nurse should question the client for any sign of numbness and tingling around the mouth or in the fingertips or toes. The nurse should also check for a positive finding of Chvostek's or Trousseau's sign. It is also important to assess for any sign of respiratory distress secondary to laryngospasm.

In the client with chronic hypoparathyroidism, the nurse should assess the client for the presence of obvious physical changes such as dry skin and hair. The nurse should also assess for the presence of a Parkinson's-like syndrome or the presence of cataracts. The nurse should also assess the teeth because pits may encircle the teeth, indicating enamel hypoplasia.

Nursing Diagnosis, Planning, and Implementation

Collaborative Problem: Injury, Risk for R/T severe tetany secondary to decreased serum calcium levels.

Planning: Expected Outcomes. The client will be free from injury, as evidenced by calcium levels returning to normal range and by normal respiratory rate and blood gases within normal limits.

Implementation. When caring for clients with severe hypoparathyroidism, the nurse should always be ready for the client with tetany to suffer laryngeal spasm and respiratory obstruction. An endotracheal tube, laryngoscope, and tracheostomy set should always be available.

When a client is at risk for sudden hypocalcemia, such as after thyroidectomy, an ampule of intravenous calcium gluconate is usually kept at the client's bedside for immediate use if necessary.

Nursing Diagnosis: Knowledge Deficit R/T diet and medication regimen.

Planning: Expected Outcomes. The client will understand the diet and medication, as evidenced by client's statements and ability to follow diet and medication regimen.

Implementation. Teaching is the priority for the client with chronic hypoparathyroidism because this client will require life-long medication and dietary modification.

When teaching the client about take-home medications, the nurse must make sure the client knows that all forms of the vitamin D, except dihydroxycholecalciferol, are slowly assimilated by the body. The nurse should warn the client that it may take a week or longer for the symptoms to improve.

Posthospital Care

The nurse must teach the client about a diet high in calcium but low in phosphorus and remind the client to omit cheese and milk products from the diet, because these foods have a high phosphorus content.

The nurse should tell the client that calcium supplements may be obtained in either tablet or solution form, depending on the client's preference. Oral calcium administration is usually discontinued once the client responds successfully to the vitamin D preparations.

FOLLOW-UP CARE

The nurse must emphasize the importance of life-long medical care for the client with chronic hypoparathyroidism and instruct the client to have the serum calcium level checked by a physician at least three times a year, every year. Normal blood serum calcium levels must be maintained to prevent complications. If hypercalcemia or hypocalcemia develops, the physician will need to adjust the treatment regimen to correct the imbalance.

STUDY QUESTIONS

1. Of the three hormones secreted by the thyroid gland, which of the following is noniodinated:
   A. Tetraiodothyronine
   B. Thyroxine
   C. Triiodothyronine
   D. Thyrocalcitonin
2. Which one of the following may be a symptom of hypothyroidism?
   A. Constipation
   B. Hand tremor
   C. Weight loss
   D. Profuse diaphoresis

3. Which of the following statements is not true about the incidence of hyperthyroidism?
   A. It is predominantly a disorder of women.
   B. It affects women in their late 60s and early 70s.
   C. It affects women four times as often as men.
   D. It is a highly preventable endocrine disorder.
4. In explaining the diagnostic tests that may be used for hypoparathyroidism, the nurse can inform the client that which of the following results may be indicative of this disorder?
   A. Laboratory findings of high serum calcium, low serum phosphate, and high urinary calcium
   B. X-ray studies showing decalcification of the basal ganglia
   C. Carpal spasms of the fingers and hand after application of a blood pressure cuff to the arm
   D. Drooping of facial muscles after a tap on the side of the face
5. Which of the following medications may be used in the treatment of hypothyroidism?
   A. Tapazole (methimazole)
   B. SSKI (saturated solution of potassium iodide)
   C. Synthroid (levothyroxine sodium)
   D. PTU (propylthiouracil)
6. A client comes to the Emergency Room in thyroid crisis. His pulse is 145 beats per minute, respirations 40 per minute, and temperature of 105.8 degrees Farenheit. All of the following measures are appropriate in an attempt to decrease the client's temperature except:
   A. Cool enemas
   B. Aspirin suppositories
   C. Hypothermia blanket
   D. Ice packs

CRITICAL THINKING EXERCISES

SCENARIO A

A client comes to the clinic with symptoms of weight gain, lethargy, fatigue, and bowel impaction secondary to prolonged constipation. After diagnostic workup, the client is diagnosed with hypothyroidism and placed on Synthroid 0.1 mg every day.

1. What major side effects and adverse reactions should the nurse teach the client about?
2. What data will be used to evaluate the therapeutic response of this client?
3. What general information about the medication should the nurse impart to the client and/or family?

SCENARIO B

A hyperthyroid client is to be scheduled for a subtotal thyroidectomy.

1. What preoperative nursing preparation should the client receive?
2. What possible postoperative complications should the nurse be aware of?
3. What advice should the nurse give to the client for follow-up care?

BIBLIOGRAPHY

1. Aviolo, L. V. (1987). Primary hyperthyroidism recognition and management. *Hospital Practice, 22(9)*, 69–74.
2. Baber, K. H., & Feldman, J. E. (1993). Thyroid cancer: A rereview. *Oncology Nursing Forum, 20(1)*, 95–104.
3. Bagdade, J. G., et al. (1995). *The year book of endocrinology. 1995* St. Louis: Mosby-Year Book.
4. Bayer, M. F. (1992). Effective laboratory evaluation of thyroid status. *Medical Clinics of North America, 75(1)*, 1–26.
5. Bilenikian, J. P. (1994). Primary hyperparathyroidism: Another important metabolic bone disease of women. *Journal of Women's Health, 3(1)*, 21–32.
6. DeGroot, L. J. (Ed.) (1989). *Endocrinology* (2nd ed.) Philadelphia: W. B. Saunders.
7. Gaedeke, M. K. (1993). Evaluating T.S.H . . . thyroid-stimulating hormone. *Nursing, 23(10)*, 72.
8. Greer, M. A. (1990). *The thyroid gland.* New York: Raven Press.
9. Halloran, T. H. (1990). Nursing responsibilities in endocrine emergencies. *Critical Care Nursing Quarterly, 13*, 74–81.
10. Kaye, T. B. (1993). Thyroid function tests: Application on newer methods. *Postgraduate Medicine, 94(1)*, 81–83, 87–88, 90.
11. Kim, T. S. (1994). Primary hyperparathyroidism. *Orthopedic Nursing, 13(3)*, 17–25.
12. Lammon, C. A., & Hart, G. (1993). Recognizing thyroid crisis. *Nursing 93, 23(4)*, 33.
13. Levy, E. G. (1991). Thyroid disease in the elderly. *Medical Clinics of North America, 75(1)*, 151–168.
14. Litwack-Saleh, K. (1992). Practical points in the care of the patient post-thyroid surgery. *Journal of Postanesthesia Nursing, 7(6)*, 404–406.
15. Lyerly, H. K. (1991). Hyperthyroidism. In D. C. Sabiston, Jr. (Ed.), *Textbook of surgery: The biological basis of modern surgical practice* (14th ed, pp. 568–579). Philadelphia: W. B. Saunders.

16. McMillan, J. Y. (1988). Preventing myxedema coma in the hypothyroid patient. *Dimensions in Critical Care Nursing, 7,* 136–145.

17. Piziak, V. K. (1992). Thyroid disease: Some considerations in later life. *Emergency Medicine, 24(5),* 67–8, 73–4.

18. Sherman, J. L. (1991). Patient evaluation: What's causing Jean's sore throat? *Nursing, 21(2),* 32L, 32N, 32P.

19. Shoemaker, W. C., et al (Eds.) (1989). *Textbook of critical care* (2nd ed.). Philadelphia: W. B. Saunders.

20. Spittle, L. (1992). Diagnosis in opposition: Thyroid storm and myxedema coma. *AACN. Clinical Issues in Critical Care Nursing, 3(2),* 300–308.

21. Van Middlesworth, L. (1989). Effects of radiation on the thyroid gland. *Advances in Internal Medicine, 34,* 265–284.

22. Walworth, J. (1990). Parathyroidectomy: Maintaining calcium homeostasis. *Today's OR Nurse, 12(4),* 20–24, 31–33.

23. Wells, S. A., & Ashley, S. W. (1991). The parathyroid glands. In D. C. Sabiston, Jr. (Ed.), *Textbook of surgery: The biological basis of modern surgical practice* (14th ed, pp. 598–615). Philadelphia: W. B. Saunders.

24. Wilson, J., & Foster, D. (Eds.) (1992). *Williams textbook of endocrinology* (8th ed.). Philadelphia: W. B. Saunders.

25. Wyngaarden, J. B., & Smith, L. H. (Eds.) (1992). *Cecil textbook of medicine* (19th ed.). Philadelphia: W. B. Saunders.

Chapter 42 Nursing Care of Clients with Adrenal, Pituitary, and Gonadal Disorders

Learning Outcomes

After completing this chapter, the learner will be able to:

1. Assess the client for clinical manifestations of adrenal, pituitary, and gonadal disorders.
2. Educate the client about the incidence, etiology, risk factors, and basic pathophysiology of major adrenal and pituitary disorders.
3. Explain to the client the assessments and diagnostic tests used in the diagnosis of major adrenal and pituitary disorders.
4. Develop plans of care for the management and follow-up of clients with major adrenal and pituitary disorders.
5. Implement nursing interventions to restore, maintain, and promote health for clients with major adrenal and pituitary disorders.
6. Teach the client about acute and chronic complications of major adrenal and pituitary disorders and appropriate health-care interventions.
7. Evaluate planned client outcomes used for planning the care of clients with major adrenal and pituitary disorders.

Adrenocortical Disorders

Glandular hypofunction and hyperfunction characterize the major disorders of the adrenal cortex.

Adrenal Insufficiency

Hypofunction of the adrenal cortex can originate from a disorder within the adrenal gland itself (primary adrenal insufficiency), or it may be due to hypofunction of the pituitary-hypothalamic unit (secondary adrenal insufficiency). Adrenocortical insufficiency can be either chronic or acute.

CHRONIC PRIMARY ADRENAL INSUFFICIENCY (ADDISON'S DISEASE)

Addison's disease is a condition that occurs as a result of a disorder within the adrenal gland.

Incidence

Addison's disease strikes only 4 of 100,000 persons. Adrenal insufficiency affects all age groups and both sexes.

Etiology

At one time, most cases of Addison's disease were a complication of tuberculosis. Today, 70 per cent are considered idiopathic in origin. Because one half to two thirds of clients with idiopathic Addison's disease have circulating autoantibodies that react specifically against adrenal tissue, this condition may have an autoimmune basis. In addition, a few cases of Addison's disease are caused by neoplasm, amyloidosis, or systemic fungal infections. Sudden cessation of long-term use of exogenous steroids and bilateral adrenalectomy are two other possible causes of Addison's disease.

Risk Factors

The major risk factors for Addison's disease are the diseases listed under the section on etiology. There are no known risk factors for the idiopathic disease.

Pathophysiology

Adrenocortical hypofunction results in decreased levels of both mineralocorticoids (aldosterone), glucocorticoids (cortisol), and androgens.

Aldosterone deficiency causes numerous fluid and electrolyte imbalances. A deficiency of aldosterone causes increased sodium excretion, which results in the following chain of events:

- Water excretion increases.
- Extracellular volume becomes depleted (dehydration).
- Hypotension develops.
- Cardiac output decreases.
- The heart becomes smaller as a result of its diminished workload.

Eventually, hypotension becomes severe and cardiovascular activity weakens, leading to circulatory collapse, shock, and death. Although the body excretes excess sodium, it retains excess potassium. Potassium levels of more than 7 mEq/L result in arrhythmias and, possibly, cardiac arrest.

CRITICAL TO REMEMBER

Clients with high potassium levels may be asymptomatic. Electrocardiogram changes—peaked T waves, absent P waves, and broadened QRS complex—may be the initial sign.

Glucocorticoid deficiency causes widespread metabolic disturbances. Remember that the glucocorticoids promote gluconeogenesis and have an "anti-insulin" effect. Consequently, when glucocorticoids become deficient, gluconeogenesis decreases, with resultant hypoglycemia and liver glycogen deficiency. The client grows weak and exhausted and suffers from anorexia, weight loss, nausea, and vomiting. Emotional disturbances can develop, ranging from mild neurotic symptoms to severe depression. In addition, glucocorticoid deficiency diminishes resistance to stress. Surgery, pregnancy, injury, infection, or salt loss resulting from profuse diaphoresis can cause an addisonian crisis (acute adrenal insufficiency). Finally, cortisol deficiency results in a failure to inhibit anterior pituitary secretion of adrenocorticotropic hormone (ACTH) (see Pathophysiology: Effects of Addison's Disease).

Melanocyte-stimulating hormone stimulates the epidermal melanocytes, which manufacture melanin, a dark pigment. Increased ACTH secretion leads to increased pigmentation of the skin and mucous membranes. Thus, clients with Addison's disease have increased levels of ACTH and a bronzed, or tanned, appearance.

Androgen deficiency fails to produce symptoms in men with Addison's disease because the testes supply adequate amounts of sex hormones. However, women depend on the adrenal cortex for an adequate secretion of androgens.

The hormones secreted by the adrenal cortex are essential to life. Untreated Addison's disease is ultimately fatal.

Clinical Manifestations

The onset of Addison's disease is usually insidious. The client experiences mild fatigue, languor, irritability,

PATHOPHYSIOLOGY

Effects of Addison's Disease

This diagram shows how Addison's disease affects endocrine function. The *dashed arrows* indicate feedback mechanisms. ACTH, adrenocorticotropic hormone; CRH, corticotropin-releasing hormone; Na^+, sodium; K^+, potassium.

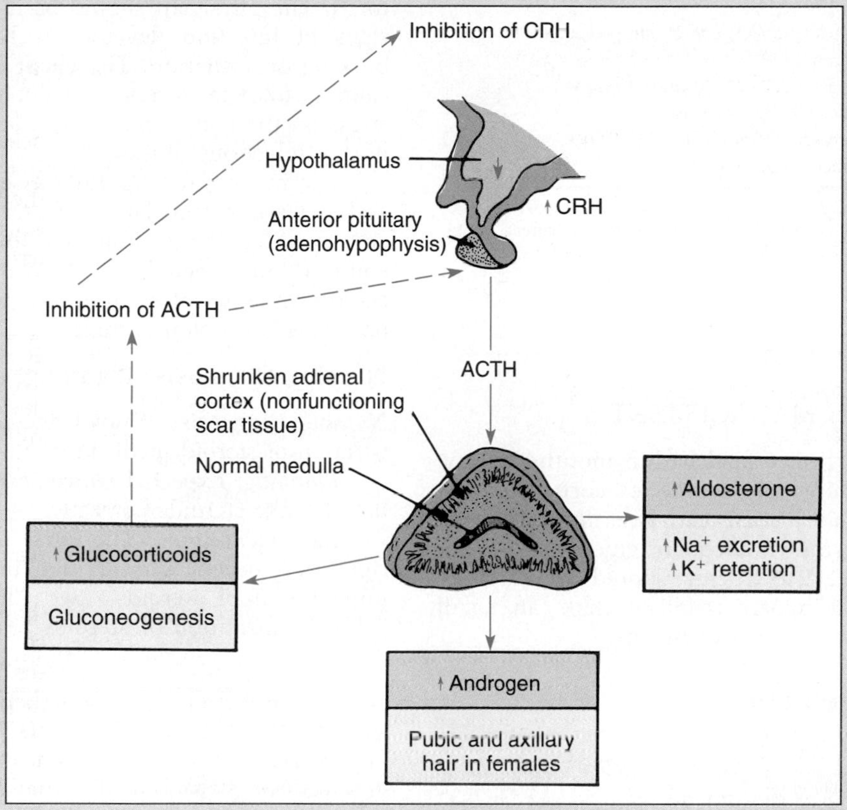

weight loss, nausea, vomiting, and postural hypotension weeks or months before diagnosis of the disease. As the disorder progresses, symptoms intensify. In the 19th century, Addison vividly described the manifestations of this debilitating and potentially fatal condition:

The patient, in most of the cases I have seen, has been observed gradually to fall off in general health; he becomes languid and weak, indisposed to either bodily or mental exertion; the appetite is impaired or entirely lost; . . . the pulse small and feeble . . . excessively soft and compressible; the body wastes . . . slight pain or uneasiness is from time to time referred to the region of the stomach, and there is occasionally actual vomiting . . . it is by no means uncommon for the patient to manifest indications of disturbed cerebral circulation. . . . We have discovered a most remarkable, and, so far as I know, characteristic discoloration taking place in the skin—sufficiently marked indeed as generally to have attracted the attention of the patient himself, or of the patient's friends. . . . It may be said to present a dingy or smoky appearance, or various tints or shades of deep amber or chestnut brown. . . . The body wastes . . . the pulse becomes smaller and weaker, and . . . the patient at length gradually sinks and expires.

For those receiving appropriate intervention, the prognosis is now excellent.

DIAGNOSTIC ASSESSMENT

Diagnosis of Addison's disease depends primarily on blood and urine hormonal assays. Diagnostic tests of adrenocortical function include:

- *ACTH stimulation test.* This is the most reliable screening test for Addison's disease. In the ACTH stimulation test, synthetic corticotropin is administered parenterally. Normally, plasma cortisol levels rise markedly after administration. However, in a client with Addison's disease, the plasma cortisol response is low or absent.
- *Plasma ACTH.* Failing the screening test, plasma ACTH determination will accurately categorize clients with primary (high) and secondary (normal or low) adrenal insufficiency.
- *Serum electrolytes.* Serum sodium level is usually decreased, whereas potassium and calcium levels are usually increased (Table 42–1).

TABLE 42–1 Routine Laboratory Findings Suggesting Addison's Disease

Blood chemistry	Low serum Na^+ (<130 mEq/L)
	High serum K^+ (>5 mEq/L)
	Ratio of serum $Na^+:K^+$ (<30:1)
	Low fasting blood glucose level (<50 mg/100 mL)
	Decrease in CO_2 combining power (<28 mEq/L)
	Elevated BUN (>20 mg/100 mL)
Hematology	Relative lymphocytosis
	Increased eosinophils
	Hemoconcentration

Na^+, sodium; K^+, potassium; CO_2, carbon dioxide; BUN, blood urea nitrogen. Data from Bethune, J. E. (1989). The diagnosis and treatment of adrenal insufficiency. In L. DeGroot (Ed.), *Endocrinology and metabolism* (2nd ed.). Philadelphia: W. B. Saunders.

Medical Management

PHARMACOLOGIC MANAGEMENT

Addison's disease was once fatal within months. Today, with the manufacture of synthetic corticosteroids, clients with Addison's disease can live normal, active lives provided they receive adequate glucocorticoid replacement (Table 42–2). Clients should be carefully assessed for signs of hypercortisolism that can result from excessive long-term cortisol therapy.

Nursing Management

Assessment

The client's vital signs should be monitored closely while the disease is being diagnosed. The nurse must check the pulse carefully, at least every 4 hours, and report drops in blood pressure below the baseline.

The nurse must assess for signs and symptoms of increased physical vitality and emotional well-being. Bony prominences must be assessed to avoid pressure sores in immobilized clients. With therapy, listlessness and exhaustion should gradually lessen and disappear.

Exposure to cold and infections should be monitored. The physician should be informed immediately if signs of infection develop, such as a sore throat or burning on urination. The client with Addison's disease cannot tolerate stress. Infection imposes additional stress on the body, and cortisol levels need to be higher during infectious illnesses.

The nurse must carefully assess for signs of sodium and potassium imbalance. If steroid replacement therapy is inadequate, sodium loss and potassium retention continue uncorrected. If steroid dosage is too high, excessive amounts of sodium and water are retained and potassium excretion is high.

Nursing Diagnosis, Planning, and Implementation

Nursing Diagnosis: Knowledge Deficit R/T self-administration of steroid medications.

Planning: Expected Outcomes. The client will state how to take steroids correctly.

Implementation. The nurse provides the client and significant others with written instructions for self-administration of steroids. (See Client Education Guide: Self-Administration of Steroids.)

CRITICAL TO REMEMBER

The client must be instructed to *NEVER* stop taking prescribed steroid medication on his or her own. Failure to take the prescribed medication may precipitate an addisonian crisis and possible vasomotor collapse and death.

TABLE 42–2 Major Adrenocortical Medications

MEDICATION	ACTION	USES	SIDE EFFECTS
Hydrocortisone	Glucocorticoid, mineralocorticoid, anti-inflammatory, anti-immunologic, antianabolic	Replacement therapy for adrenal insufficiency; control of allergic reactions; suppression of inflammatory reactions; treatment of mesenchymal or collagen disorders	Overdosage produces Cushing's syndrome
Predisone (Deltasone, Meticorlen) Methylpredisone (Medrol, Solu-medrol)	Similar to cortisone but 4 to 5 times more potent glucocorticoid activity	For anti-inflammatory action and to suppress immune system (e.g., after organ transplants)	Similar to cortisone but less mineralocorticoid activity
Dexamethasone	Similar to prednisone but 20 to 25 times more potent glucocorticoid activity	For very potent glucocorticoid effects	Similar to prednisone
Fludrocortisone acetate (Florinef)	Mineralocorticoid	Replacement therapy for adrenal insufficiency	Mineralocorticoid effects: hypertension, edema caused by sodium retention, muscle weakness, and arrhythmias resulting from hypokalemia
Deoxycorticosterone (cortate)	Mineralocorticoid	Replacement therapy for adrenal insufficiency	Mineralocorticoid effects: same as for Florinef

CLIENT EDUCATION GUIDE

Self-Administration of Steroids

Information given to the client and significant others should include

- Actions of prescribed hormones (hydrocortisone, fludrocortisone).
- Importance of taking the medications daily, without fail, exactly as prescribed.
- Principles of self-administration of oral medications (e.g., check the label on the bottle before taking the medication, document when medications are taken and their side effects).
- Signs of over- and underdosage.
- Importance of hydrocortisone self-injection when unable to tolerate oral medication (as a result of nausea-vomiting) and during times of acute stress (auto accident, trauma) because the body is unable to compensate for its need for additional glucocorticoid coverage.
- Need for an intramuscular self-injection kit to be available at all times.
- Client's and significant others' ability to demonstrate ability to prepare medication, draw up medication into syringe, and perform injections (normal saline) before discharge.
- Need for a Medic Alert bracelet, worn to indicate the diagnosis or need for cortisol replacement.
- Need for the client to contact health-care provider if questions arise after discharge from medical center. The nurse must emphasize to clients who take glucocorticoids that they must call the physician to get a dosage increase when experiencing stressful situations (e.g., emotional upheavals, dental extractions, minor surgery, or upper respiratory infections). In addition, temporary mineralocorticoid dosage increases may be indicated if the client experiences profuse diaphoresis, for any reason (strenuous physical exertion, heat spells, fever). Clients should be encouraged to consult their physician for dose adjustment. The medication will need to be administered intramuscularly when nausea and vomiting prevent oral administration.

Finally, clients must be reminded to adhere to semi-annual appointments with their physician, even when they are in good health and the process of self-medication is proceeding smoothly. As in diabetes mellitus, the control of Addison's disease is a lifelong responsibility.

Nursing Diagnosis: Injury, Risk for R/T acute adrenal insufficiency secondary to addisonian crisis (adrenal crisis).

Planning: Expected Outcomes. The client will be free of injury, as evidenced by the absence of hypotension, shock, or other signs of acute adrenal insufficiency.

Implementation. The nurse should closely monitor for signs and symptoms of addisonian crisis, including:

- Sudden profound weakness
- Severe abdominal, back, and leg pain
- Hyperpyrexia followed by hypothermia
- Peripheral vascular collapse
- Coma
- Renal shutdown

The development of an adrenal crisis constitutes a medical emergency that must be treated rapidly and vigorously. The three major goals of intervention are to reverse shock, restore blood circulation (the client usually suffers from a deficit of at least 20 per cent of extracellular fluid [ECF] volume), and replenish the body with essential steroids.

Immediately on admission, a rapid infusion of 1000 mL of normal saline is administered with water-soluble glucocorticoid (hydrocortisone phosphate or hydrocortisone sodium succinate) added. The dosage of the prescribed glucocorticoid is gradually reduced. It is administered intramuscularly or intravenously every 6 hours during the first day of crisis and every 8 hours of the second day and is gradually reduced thereafter.

Plasma, oxygen, and vasopressor medications may be indicated. Antibiotic therapy is appropriate if an infection triggered the crisis. Throughout the emergency period, the nurse must monitor blood pressure, administer intravenous infusion and medications, monitor hourly urine output and report oliguria (a sign of shock), minimize exposure to emotional and physical stress, and observe for symptoms of glucocorticoid overdose and overhydration, such as generalized edema resulting from fluid retention, hypertension, flaccid paralysis resulting from hypokalemia, psychoses, and loss of consciousness.

With rapid, efficient intervention, addisonian crisis usually passes by 12 hours. The client's condition stabilizes, and the convalescent period begins. When the client is able to tolerate food and fluids by mouth, steroid replacement can be administered orally.

After the immediate crisis has passed, the nurse should help the client prevent further development of adrenal insufficiency. Identification bracelets and emergency kits should be obtained for all clients with Addison's disease before their discharge from the hospital. Clients should be instructed to carry these items at all times. The client's name and diagnosis should appear on the identification bracelet, and a wallet card should state that the client receives daily hydrocortisone and that the medication must be administered by injection in any emergency.

Dexamethasone can be kept in a prepared syringe in an emergency kit with sterile alcohol wipes for cleaning the injection site. The kit also should contain written information on the client's diagnosis, medication prescription, dosage schedules, and emergency telephone numbers, including the physician's name and telephone number.

Evaluation

The nurse must evaluate client outcomes based on the established plan of care. If these goals were not achieved, the plan and interventions must be revised to meet the client's needs.

Modification of Plan of Care for the Elderly

When older clients suffer from Addison's disease, the symptoms are often more pronounced because their adrenal function may already be decreased from the aging process. The elderly also may be more sensitive to the side effects of steroid therapy such as osteoporosis, hypertension, diabetes, and so on because these problems may already exist in the client.

Posthospital Care

The client has significant teaching needs before discharge. The client must understand the proper self-administration of steroids, implications of the side effects, and what to do if problems arise. The discharge teaching these clients receive will directly affect their ability for self-care.

The client must be seen at regular intervals so the effects of the medication can be assessed. The client also must be aware of the need to seek medical attention in case of severe stress or illness so the dosage of steroids can be altered by the physician.

SECONDARY ADRENAL INSUFFICIENCY

Secondary adrenal insufficiency is defined as that caused by other conditions outside the adrenals.

Etiology

Causes of adrenocortical insufficiency include

- Bilateral adrenalectomy.
- Hemorrhagic infarction and necrosis of the adrenal glands. Adrenal apoplexy can develop as a complication of meningococcal septicemia or anticoagulant therapy.

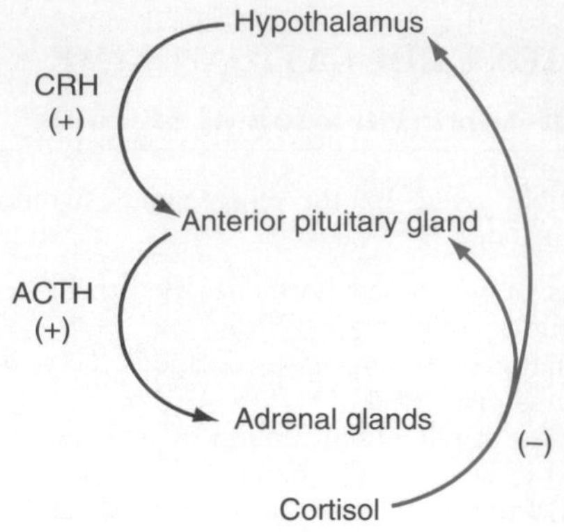

Figure 42–1
The hypothalamic-pituitary-adrenal axis, demonstrating stimulation and feedback between the hypothalamus, anterior pituitary, and adrenal glands.

- Hypopituitarism resulting in decreased secretion of ACTH by the pituitary gland, causing decreased secretion of cortisol and androgens by the adrenal gland (secondary adrenal insufficiency) (see Fig. 42–1, which illustrates the hypothalamic-pituitary adrenal [HPA] axis).
- Suppression of hypothalamic-pituitary secretion of ACTH hypercortisolism caused by either exogenous administration of corticosteroids or by oversecretion of corticosteroids by an adrenal tumor. In both cases, the adrenal glands atrophy and become filled with lipids. Because the circulating levels of corticosteroids remain high, these clients do not experience symptoms of adrenocortical insufficiency unless steroid therapy is discontinued suddenly or the tumor is resected. Fortunately, if corticosteroid drug therapy is terminated by gradually reducing the dosage each day, adrenal gland function usually returns to normal.

Nursing Management

Assessment reveals that clients with secondary adrenal insufficiency experience cortisol deficiency. Aldosterone continues to be secreted in sufficient amounts.

Treatment involves administering glucocorticoids, as in Addison's disease. Mineralocorticoid replacement is unnecessary. Client teaching should include instruction regarding the need to wear an emergency identification bracelet and carry an emergency kit for hydrocortisone injection in case an adrenal crisis occurs.

Adrenocortical Hyperfunction

Hyperfunction of the adrenal cortex can result in excessive production of glucocorticoids, mineralocorticoids, and androgens. The three major conditions of adrenocortical hyperfunction are

- Cushing's syndrome (glucocorticoid excess)
- Conn's syndrome or aldosteronism (aldosterone excess)
- Congenital adrenal hyperplasia (adrenogenital syndrome, androgen excess)

HYPERCORTISOLISM (CUSHING'S SYNDROME)

Cushing's syndrome was first described by Harvey Cushing in 1932. It results from overactivity of the adrenal gland, with consequent hypersecretion of glucocorticoids.

Incidence

Cushing's syndrome is a relatively rare condition. It occurs mainly in women, and the average age of onset is age 20 to 40 years. It can, however, be seen up to age 60 years.

Etiology

Hypersecretion of cortisol can be caused by a cortisol-secreting adrenal tumor (most of which are benign) or by adrenal hyperplasia caused by overproduction of ACTH. The two sources of excessive ACTH secretion are (1) pituitary hypersecretion and benign pituitary tumors and (2) ectopic ACTH secretion. Pituitary hypersecretion of ACTH resulting in glucocorticoid excess is called Cushing's disease. An ACTH-secreting tumor located outside the pituitary gland is a rare cause of Cushing's syndrome.

Additionally, iatrogenic Cushing's syndrome, another form of the disorder, results from exogenous administration of synthetic glucocorticoids.

Risk Factors

One of the major risk factors for increased levels of cortisol is the administration of exogenous steroids. Whenever steroids are administered, a degree of excess is present. Placing the client on the lowest amount of steroids possible can help to control this problem.

Other risk factors are outlined under Etiology. These factors are related to hyperplasia of the adrenal gland, either as a primary disorder or secondary to excessive amounts of ACTH. In the latter case, control of the primary disease decreases the adrenal hyperplasia. There are no particular preventive measures.

Pathophysiology

When Cushing's syndrome develops, the normal function of the glucocorticoids (see Chap. 39) becomes exaggerated and the classic picture of the syndrome emerges. This exaggerated physiologic action of glucocorticoids appears as

- Persistent hyperglycemia ("steroid diabetes").
- Protein tissue wasting, which results in weakness caused by muscle wasting, capillary fragility, resulting in ecchymosis, and osteoporosis caused by bone matrix wasting. Osteoporosis can become so severe that even mild trauma can cause fractures. Compression fractures can develop in the osteoporotic spine, leading to kyphosis and loss of height.
- Potassium depletion, leading to hypokalemia, arrhythmias, muscle weakness, and renal disorders.
- Sodium and water retention, causing edema and hypertension.
- Hypertension, which eventually predisposes the individual to left ventricular hypertrophy, congestive heart failure, and cerebrovascular accidents.
- Abnormal fat distribution (in conjunction with edema), resulting in a moon-shaped face, a dorsocervical fat pad on the neck (buffalo hump), and truncal obesity with slender limbs. Also, pink and purple striae appear on the breasts, axillary areas, abdomen, and legs as a result of thinning of skin. Striking changes occur in appearance after both development and cure of Cushing's syndrome. Old photographs can be useful in recognizing changes over time.
- Increased susceptibility to infection and lowered resistance to stress increase vulnerability to micro-organisms of all types. Because of suppression of the inflammatory response, people with Cushing's syndrome can show few signs of infection. The client also demonstrates poor wound healing.
- Possible increased production of androgens can cause virilism in women. Manifestations of virilism include acne, thinning of scalp hair, and hirsutism (abnormal growth and distribution of hair).
- Mental changes include memory loss, poor concentration and cognition, euphoria, and depression. Some clients experience "steroid psychosis." Depression can predispose the client to suicidal thoughts.

Clinical Manifestations

The typical clinical picture of a client with hypercortisolism is illustrated in Clinical Manifestations: Cushing's Syndrome. The pathophysiology of the disease also provides a clear picture of the client with this disorder.

DIAGNOSTIC ASSESSMENT

Although there is a classic cushingoid appearance to clients with hypercortisolism, it is important to perform diagnostic studies to confirm the diagnosis.

In Cushing's syndrome glucose tolerance decreases and glucosuria appears. The white cell count often rises above 10,000/mm^3, but the total eosinophil count can drop below 50 cells/mm^3. Also, lymphocytes can fall below 20 per cent. Both urinary 17-hydroxysteroids and blood cortisol rise to high levels.

CLINICAL MANIFESTATIONS

Cushing's Syndrome

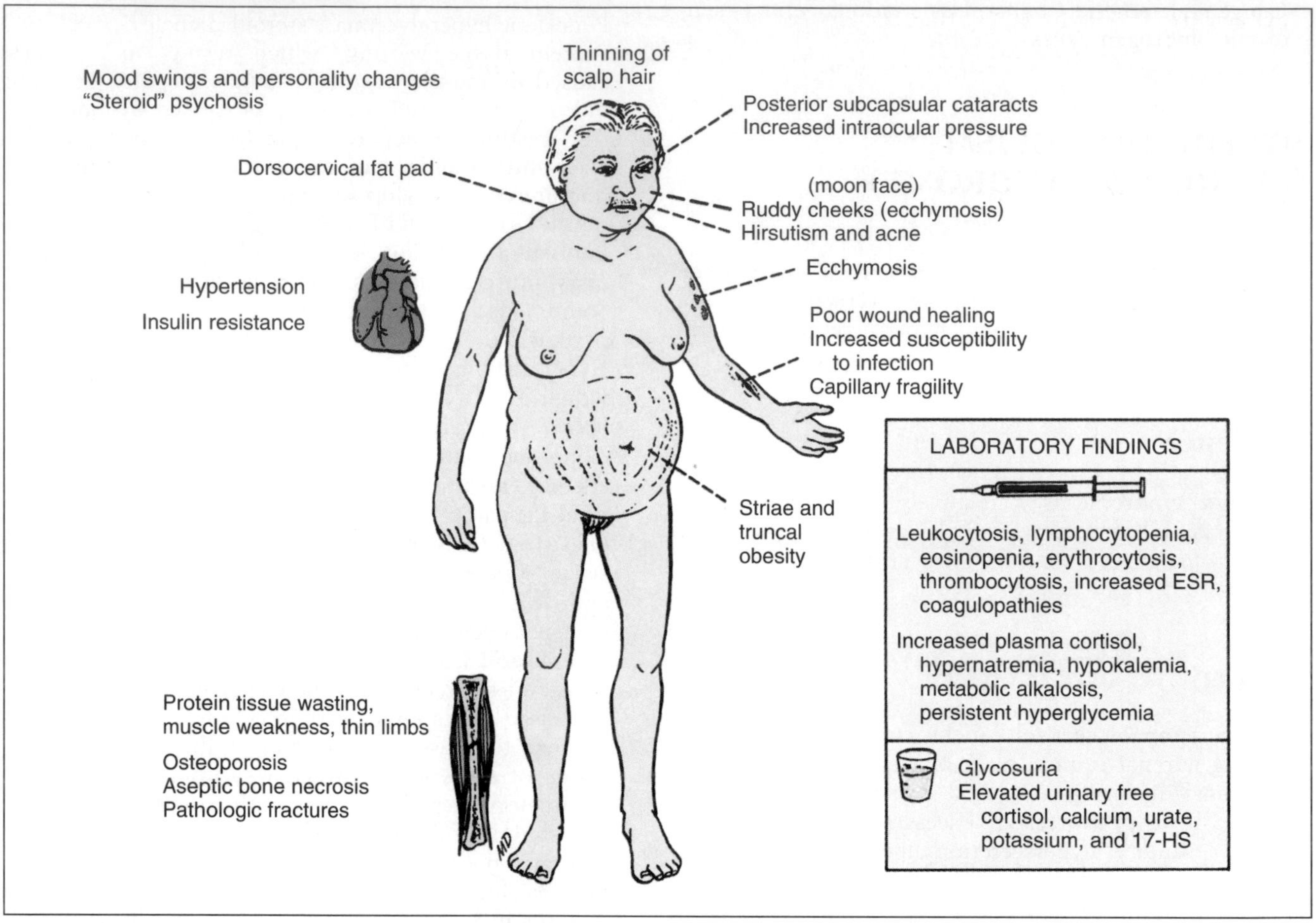

ESR, erythrocyte sedimentation rate; 17-HS, 17-hydroxysteroid.

Normally, plasma cortisol follows a diurnal pattern, rising in the early morning (10 to 25 μg/dL), then gradually falling to less than 10 μg/dL in the evening, and approaching undetectable levels near midnight. Clients with Cushing's syndrome have elevated plasma cortisol levels throughout the day and can demonstrate a loss of diurnal variation.

Urinary free cortisol (UFC) measurement is used as a screening test to identify elevated urinary excretion of free cortisol. Clients with Cushing's syndrome will have UFC levels above 100 μg/day.

The overnight dexamethasone suppression test is often used in the differential diagnosis of Cushing's syndrome. It can be performed on an outpatient basis:

- Day 1: Administer dexamethasone, 1 mg orally at 11 PM.
- Day 2: Draw plasma cortisol level at 8 AM.

The normal range is below 5 μg/dL. Severe stress or depression can cause false-positive results (i.e., plasma cortisol greater than 5 μg/dL despite otherwise normal endocrine function). If dexamethasone fails to suppress the HPA (see Fig. 42–1) axis and the morning cortisol level is greater than 5 μg/dL, an abnormality of feedback is suggested that is compatible with Cushing's syndrome.

The standard dexamethasone suppression test (performed over 6 consecutive days) differentiates Cushing's disease (caused by pituitary oversecretion of ACTH) from other causes of Cushing's syndrome.

The plasma ACTH test demonstrates that low ACTH levels point toward an adrenal tumor as the cause of hypercortisolism. The overproduction of cortisol from the adrenal tumor provides negative feedback to the pituitary gland, which responds by decreasing ACTH release. The high cortisol level also provides feedback to the hypothalamus, which decreases release of cortisol-releasing hormone.

The presence of an ectopic ACTH-producing tumor usually yields a normal or elevated ACTH level. ACTH production from the tumor is independent of pituitary production of ACTH and so despite negative feedback to the hypothalamic-pituitary unit, ACTH levels will remain high.

An adrenal computed tomographic (CT) scan is performed to seek an adrenal mass in the right or left adrenal gland. Contrast dye is used, when possible, to enhance the clarity of the scan.

TABLE 42–3 Therapies Prescribed for Cushing's Syndrome, Cushing's Disease, and Ectopic Adrenocorticotropic Hormone Syndrome

CONDITION	RESPONSIBLE LESION	THERAPIES	REMARKS
Cushing's syndrome	Adrenal tumor (benign or malignant)	Adrenalectomy (surgical excision)	Adrenalectomy for a benign unilateral tumor; usually curative Bilateral adrenalectomy must be followed by lifelong administration of corticosteroids
	Adrenal carcinoma with widespread metastases	Surgery and chemotherapy: o,p'-DDD	Chemotherapy largely unsuccessful
Cushing's disease	Pituitary tumor (or unidentified lesion) that secretes excessive amounts of ACTH	Microsurgical resection of pituitary adenoma	Pituitary surgery is successful in 95 per cent of cases
		Irradiation of pituitary gland	Irradiation successful in 75 per cent of cases; therapeutic effects not apparent for months after initiation of therapy
		Total bilateral adrenalectomy (corrects adrenal hyperplasia resulting from excessive ACTH stimulation)	Total bilateral adrenalectomy must be followed by lifelong replacement therapy with a glucocorticoid and mineralocorticoid
Ectopic ACTH syndrome	Extra-adrenal malignant tumor	Surgical removal of ectopic malignant tumor; chemotherapy used to control hypercorticism and promote remission in individuals with inoperable cancer	Surgery rarely successful because metastasis usually occurs before diagnosis; chemotherapy purely palliative

Medical Management

Although surgery is the usual treatment for primary adrenal hyperplasia, other palliative treatments are available (Table 42–3). Radiation therapy can be used to treat primary pituitary tumors and other ACTH-secreting adenomas. Radiation can be either internally or externally applied to the pituitary gland for tumors. Internally, the radiation is applied through a transsphenoidal implant. Radiation must be used with care because of the proximity of the optic nerve. Radiation is not always effective in even palliative treatment of tumors and may destroy normal tissue. For ACTH-secreting adenomas such as lung tumors, palliation is possible. See Chapter 7 for a discussion of care of the client undergoing radiation therapy.

PHARMACOLOGIC MANAGEMENT

Medications that interfere with ACTH production or adrenal hormone synthesis are available. Mitotane (Lysodren) is a cytotoxic antihormonal agent that inhibits corticosteroid synthesis without destroying cortical cells. Aminogluthethimide (Cytadren) and trilostane (Modrastane) are other cytotoxic agents that block the synthesis of glucocorticoids and adrenal steroids.

Cyproheptadine (Periactin) is used less commonly to treat hypersecretion caused by pituitary abnormalities resulting in increased ACTH levels. This agent appears to interfere with the ACTH production, thereby decreasing the effect on the adrenals.

Surgical Management

The resection of most pituitary tumors causing Cushing's syndrome is performed via transsphenoidal hypophysectomy. Occasionally, large or anatomically complex tumors are excised via a transfrontal approach. (See the section on hypophysectomy.)

For Cushing's syndrome resulting from adrenal tumor (or possibly ectopic ACTH-secreting tumor), an adrenalectomy can be performed to remove the gland containing the tumor. In cases of ectopic ACTH-secreting tumors, the tumor can be difficult to localize. If no source is found, a bilateral adrenalectomy can be performed to interrupt the production of cortisol in response to ACTH produced by the tumor, or the client can be treated with antiglucocorticoids while continuing to search for the tumor.

Nursing Management

Assessment

The nurse begins by collecting a careful history from the client with potential Cushing's syndrome. The client may well exhibit the characteristic clinical manifestations identified previously.

The client will require support during the diagnostic phase of the disease.

During the preoperative phase, the client with Cushing's syndrome requires expert nursing assessment and care.

Nursing Diagnosis, Planning, and Implementation

Collaborative Problem: Infection, Risk for R/T lowered resistance to stress and compromised immune response.

Planning: Expected Outcomes. Infection will be prevented or detected early, as evidenced by absence of leukocytosis, fever, or other signs of infections.

Implementation. The nurse should protect clients from exposure to infectious organisms. Clients must be isolated from health-care personnel and significant others with contagious disorders. Care givers must use careful hand-washing technique before contact with clients.

Because glucocorticoids suppress immune and inflammatory reactions, clients with Cushing's syndrome may experience only mild symptoms, even in the presence of a severe infection. A slight elevation in body temperature may indicate the presence of a severe infection.

Collaborative Problem: Injury, Risk for: fractures, hypertension, or diabetes R/T osteoporosis, sodium and water retention, or the presence of an insulin antagonist.

Planning: Expected Outcomes. Injury will be prevented, as evidenced by absence of fracture, hypertension, or hyperglycemia.

Implementation. The nurse must protect clients against falls and accidents. Clients with Cushing's syndrome have osteoporosis and tend to experience fractures even with mild trauma. The bed must be kept in the lowest position and side rails raised for protection. Clients must be assisted with ambulation to avoid falls.

Vital signs must be monitored at frequent intervals. Clients must be assessed carefully for signs of severe hypertension (e.g., elevated blood pressure [BP], headache, failing vision, irritability, and dyspnea.) The nurse checks for postural hypotension, encouraging slow position change to avoid injury from sudden drop in BP.

The nurse must obtain daily weight in a consistent manner. If sodium intake is reduced, edema and weight should diminish. The nurse must measure daily blood glucose levels via finger stick and test urine for acetone. Positive results may indicate the development of diabetes mellitus (steroid diabetes) resulting from the insulin antagonist action of the excessive cortisol.

Nursing Diagnosis: Activity Intolerance R/T fatigue and muscle weakness from protein wasting, persistent hyperglycemia (and possible diabetes mellitus), and potassium depletion.

Planning: Expected Outcomes. The client will tolerate activity and engage in rest periods.

Implementation. The nurse must promote mental and physical rest for the client with Cushing's syndrome. It is important to minimize stress and confusion so the client can achieve maximal periods of rest.

Nursing Diagnosis: Skin Integrity, Risk for Impaired R/T tissue catabolism (thinning of skin), decreased connective tissue, and edema secondary to sodium and water retention.

Planning: Expected Outcomes. Client will maintain skin integrity.

Implementation. The client's skin should be meticulously monitored for the presence of breakdown. The client is extremely prone to breakdown from the tissue catabolism. The nurse should avoid the use of tape or other irritants that may result in skin tearing or excoriation.

Nursing Diagnosis: Thought Processes, Altered (Memory Loss, Cognitive Impairment, Mood Swings, Euphoria, Depression) R/T increased levels of glucocorticoids and ACTH.

Planning: Expected Outcomes. Client will maintain optimal thought processes, as evidenced by decrease in symptoms of memory loss, cognitive impairment, or mood swings or will have symptoms minimized.

Implementation. The nurse must anticipate clients' mood swings. Clients can become easily upset by changes in their appearance caused by the disease process. They also can become alarmed by the bizarre feelings and emotions they experience. Reassurance should be given, explaining that appearance and moods should gradually return to normal after the disorder is treated unless the treatment requires the client to receive steroid replacement. If clients have to receive steroid therapy, they will continue to experience some side effects.

Nursing Diagnosis: Knowledge Deficit R/T the disease, surgery, and proper diet.

Planning: Expected Outcomes. The client will understand the disease, planned surgery, and proper diet, as evidenced by statements of understanding and ability to choose correct diet.

Implementation. It is important for clients to understand their condition and the proposed treatment. Clients should be given the opportunity to ask questions about the treatment and should be assessed for their understanding of it.

Encourage a diet low in calories, carbohydrates, and sodium but with ample protein and potassium content. Such a diet promotes weight loss, reduction of edema and hypertension, control of hypokalemia, and rebuilding of wasted tissue. The client with diabetes mellitus or gastric ulcers requires a special diet (see Chaps. 40 and 34, respectively).

Collaborative Problem: Injury, Risk for R/T surgical procedure.

Planning: Expected Outcomes. Injury will be prevented or will be detected early, as evidenced by absence of shock, hemorrhage, infection, or addisonian crisis.

Implementation. On the morning of surgery, administer a glucocorticoid preparation (intramuscular or intravenous [IV]) as prescribed. A water-soluble cortisol preparation (diluted in an IV infusion) may be given throughout the surgical procedure. Cortisol protects the client from the development of acute adrenal insufficiency during adrenalectomy. Even if the surgeon plans to remove only one adrenal gland, temporary glucocorticoid support may be needed until the remaining adrenal gland begins to secrete sufficient amounts of cortisol. Because of the excessive secretion of cortisol by the tumorous gland, the healthy gland can atrophy and require time to readjust.

During the immediate postoperative phase, major goals are to

- Prevent shock
- Prevent infection
- Sustain adequate cortisol levels
- Control pain and incisional discomfort

The nurse observes for signs of shock resulting from hemorrhage (hypotension, and rapid, weak pulse). The nurse should document vital signs every 15 minutes and measure urine and record hourly output, observing for oliguria, a sign of shock and renal shutdown. The nurse should administer IV fluids, pressor amines, and corticosteroids as prescribed.

CRITICAL TO REMEMBER

Remember that the signs of addisonian crisis resemble shock.

The client should be closely assessed for the development of this complication, and IV cortisol should be administered in high doses until the symptoms subside. The client will continue to require increased amounts of steroids until the remaining adrenal gland returns to a normal level of functioning and the stress associated with the treatment subsides.

The nurse should encourage clients to cough, turn, and deep breathe to prevent respiratory infections. The nurse should use meticulous sterile technique with wound care to prevent infection. Ileus is less common because the flank approach is usually used.

Nursing Diagnosis: Knowledge Deficit R/T self-administration of replacement hormones.

Planning: Expected Outcomes. Client will understand self-administration of replacement hormones, as evidenced by the client's ability to repeat and comply with instructions, so that the client does not develop addisonian crisis or adrenal insufficiency. (See the discussion of nursing management of Addison's disease for more information.)

Implementation. After bilateral adrenalectomy, lifelong glucocorticoid replacement is essential. If only one adrenal gland has been removed, daily cortisol replacement continues until the remaining gland functions normally (usually 6–12 months later). Before discharge, the client, family, and significant others need instruction on self-administration of replacement hormones (hydrocortisone). The client and significant others should successfully demonstrate the self-injection technique before discharge from the hospital.

CRITICAL TO REMEMBER

A client on lifelong steroid replacement should always wear a Medic Alert identification and carry a prepared syringe of hydrocortisone in case of emergency.

Evaluation

The nurse must evaluate client outcomes based on the established plan of care. If these goals were not achieved, the plan and interventions must be revised to meet the client's needs.

Modification of Plan of Care for the Elderly

Elderly clients may exhibit excessive symptoms from Cushing's syndrome because these clients may already exhibit many of the characteristic manifestations, such as osteoporosis, hypertension, and diabetes. The client also is more prone to the side effects of steroid replacement therapy.

Posthospital Care

The discharge teaching and follow-up care are the same as for the client with Addison's disease (see the section on Addison's disease).

PRIMARY HYPERALDOSTERONISM (CONN'S SYNDROME)

Aldosterone is the most powerful of the mineralocorticoids. Its primary role is to conserve sodium, and it also promotes potassium excretion.

Incidence

The exact incidence of Conn's syndrome is unknown. It strikes females twice as often as males and appears most frequently in middle-aged clients.

Etiology

Hypersecretion of aldosterone caused by an adrenal lesion results in primary hyperaldosteronism. In contrast, secondary hyperaldosteronism arises as a consequence of edematous disorders (cardiac failure, cirrhosis of the liver with ascites, and nephrotic syndrome). It also develops in clients with hypertension resulting from destructive renal artery disease.

The major cause of primary hyperaldosteronism is usually a single benign aldosterone-secreting tumor called an aldosteronoma.

Risk Factors

There are no particular risk factors for primary hyperaldosteronism. The risks for secondary hyperaldosteronism include chronic heart failure, cirrhosis with ascites, nephrotic syndrome, and hypertension resulting from destructive renal artery disease. The preventive measures, therefore, are successful treatment and control of the causative disease process. The more successfully these factors are controlled, the less secondary hyperaldosteronism will be present.

Pathophysiology

Hypersecretion of aldosterone affects the tubular reabsorption of sodium (Na^+) and water and the excretion of potassium (K^+) and hydrogen (H^+) ions in the renal tubular epithelial cells (see Pathophysiology: Effects of Primary Aldosteronism). This leads to the development of hypernatremia, hypervolemia, hypokalemia, and metabolic alkalosis. With the hypervolemia and hypernatremia, the blood pressure increases, often to very high levels, and renin production is suppressed. The hypertension can lead to cerebral infarcts and to renal damage.

Secondary hyperaldosteronism is due to the continuous secretion of aldosterone secondary to the high levels of angiotension II, resulting, in turn, from high plasma renin activity. The decreased renal perfusion resulting from a variety of causes is the underlying mechanism.

PATHOPHYSIOLOGY

Effects of Primary Aldosteronism

Excessive aldosterone secretion causes increased sodium (Na^+) and water (H_2O) retention and increased potassium (K^+) excretion.

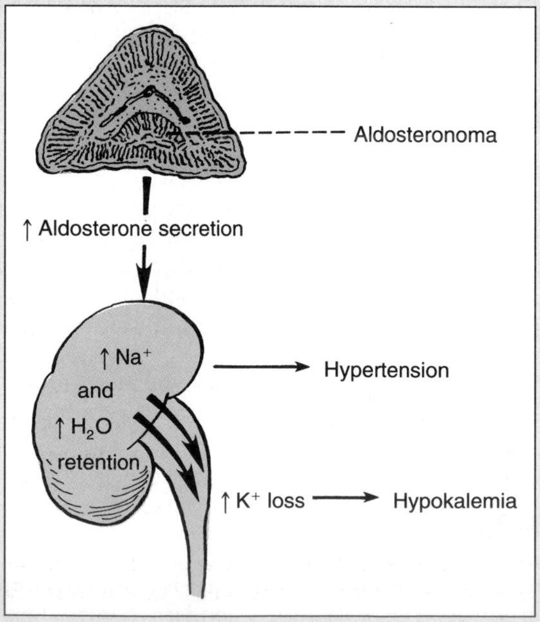

Clinical Manifestations

Clients with primary hyperaldosteronism experience hypertension, hypernatremia, and hypokalemia. Without intervention, they can develop all the complications of chronic hypertension, such as visual disturbances, heart failure, renal damage, and cerebrovascular accident.

Hypokalemia results from excessive urinary excretion of K^+ (see Chaps. 3 and 4). This problem, in turn, causes muscle weakness, paralysis, or cardiac arrhythmias, because K^+ loss reduces normal neuromuscular irritability. In addition, excessive excretion of K^+ results in polyuria. The large urinary output leads to polydipsia (excessive thirst). Finally, hypokalemia leads to metabolic alkalosis from shifting of H^+ into the cells in exchange for K^+ and exchange of H^+ within the tubular cells for Na^+ from the tubular urine. Metabolic alkalosis causes a decrease in ionized calcium levels, which can result in tetany and respiratory suppression (see Chaps. 3 and 4).

Despite sodium retention, clients with hyperaldosteronism rarely experience overt edema. Although ECF increases moderately, excessive water is normally excreted in the urine with potassium ions. Over time, the kidneys tend to adjust physiologically to excessive secretion of aldosterone, so water excretion reaches an equilibrium with sodium intake. The ability of the kidneys to eventually "escape" from the sodium- and water-retaining action of aldosterone is sometimes called the escape phenomenon.

DIAGNOSTIC ASSESSMENT

Diagnosis of primary hyperaldosteronism is based on low serum potassium, alkalosis, and elevated urinary or plasma aldosterone with low plasma renin levels. Additionally, radiographic studies can reveal cardiac hypertrophy resulting from chronic hypertension. Radionuclide scanning techniques using radiolabeled iodocholesterol allow visualization of the tumors.

Medical Management

The three goals of intervention for clients with primary hyperaldosteronism are to reverse hypertension, correct hypokalemia, and prevent kidney damage. In two thirds of the cases, removal of the aldosterone-secreting tumor completely resolves the hypertension. Most clients have normal BP readings by the third postoperative month.

Unfortunately, the renal complications resulting from long-term hypertension tend to be progressive. Therefore, clients with primary hyperaldosteronism need to be diagnosed and treated early in the course of the disease.

PHARMACOLOGIC MANAGEMENT

If clients cannot be treated surgically, they are often given spironolactone (Aldactone), a potassium-sparing diuretic, to increase sodium excretion and to treat the hypertension and hypokalemia. The client's potassium level should be carefully monitored for the development of hyperkalemia, especially if the client has been receiving potassium supplements or has been on a high-potassium diet.

Surgical Management

Surgery is the treatment of choice for primary hyperaldosteronism. A unilateral or bilateral adrenalectomy must be performed. Clients undergoing a unilateral adrenalectomy may need temporary replacement of glucocorticoids, whereas those requiring bilateral adrenalectomies will need permanent replacement (see the section on Addison's disease). Clients usually receive glucocorticoids preoperatively to prevent any adrenal hypofunction.

Nursing Management

The nurse must help prepare the client for the diagnostic assessment so the diagnosis of hyperaldosteronism can be achieved rapidly and treatment performed before permanent damage occurs. The nurse should administer prescribed medications and closely monitor the client for hypertension or renal damage. The preoperative and postoperative management is the same as that described previously under Cushing's syndrome.

Adrenomedullary Disorders

Two important tumors occur in the adrenal medulla:

- Pheochromocytoma, a tumor that results in hyperactivity of the gland
- Neuroblastoma, a malignant tumor made up of cells resembling neuroblast.

PHEOCHROMOCYTOMA

A pheochromocytoma is a catecholamine-secreting tumor of the chromaffin cells usually found in the adrenal medulla.

Incidence

Pheochromocytomas are rare, causing about 0.1 per cent of the cases of hypertension. The condition is slightly more common in women than in men. Although the disease can occur at any age, it is most common in middle age and rarely occurs after age 60 years.

Etiology

The exact cause of pheochromocytomas is unknown. In some cases, pheochromocytomas appear to have a hereditary basis. They often occur in association with neuroectodermal diseases and with medullary cancer of the thyroid gland.

Risk Factors

Pregnancy and stress can precipitate and amplify the manifestations of pheochromocytoma.

Pathophysiology

The pheochromocytoma, usually weighing less than 200 g, is composed of chromaffin cells, so named because they stain a dark color with chromium salts. In 80 to 90 per cent of cases, pheochromocytomas arise within the adrenal medulla. Occasionally, however, they develop from the chromaffin tissues forming the sympathetic paraganglia.

Pheochromocytomas are typically benign; fewer than 10 per cent are malignant. Because of the excessive amounts of epinephrine and norepinephrine they secrete, they can produce severe symptoms and even death (Table 42–4). Without early intervention, the client is at risk for cerebral hemorrhage and cardiac failure. Fortunately, if pheochromocytomas are discovered early in their development, they can usually be eliminated by surgical removal.

Clinical Manifestations

The client with pheochromocytoma can experience symptoms similar to those of diabetes mellitus (elevated blood glucose and glucosuria), essential hypertension (elevated BP, headaches), hyperthyroidism (increased metabolic rate, diaphoresis, agitation, rapid pulse, emotional outbursts), and psychoneurosis (emotional instability).

Hypertension is the principal manifestation of pheochromocytoma and can be persistent, fluctuating, intermittent, or paroxysmal in nature. Typically, the client has episodes of high BP accompanied by pounding headaches. Other manifestations of sympathetic overactivity include sweating, apprehension, palpitations, nausea, and vomiting. The excessive release of catecholamine also results in excessive conversion of glycogen into glucose in the liver. Consequently, hyperglycemia and glucosuria occur during attacks. Such manifestations can develop spontaneously or be precipitated by emotional stress, physical exertion, or change in body position.

Acute attacks can be associated with profuse diaphoresis, dilated pupils, and cold extremities. Severe hypertension can precipitate a cerebrovascular accident or sudden blindness.

TABLE 42–4 Comparative Effects of Epinephrine and Norepinephrine

EPINEPHRINE	NOREPINEPHRINE
Cardiovascular System	
Constricts superficial blood vessels; in small doses, dilates muscle, brain, and coronary vessels, thus shunting blood supply to organs; essential for "fight or flight"	Constricts all blood vessels (especially peripheral), causing increased peripheral resistance
Raises blood pressure	Raises blood pressure greatly
Increases cardiac output	Decreases cardiac output because of increased peripheral resistance
Increases pulse dramatically	Increases pulse moderately
Constricts spleen, shunting stored red cells into general circulation	
Increases coagulability of blood	
Respiratory System	
Increases rate and depth of respirations	
Dilates bronchi	
Nervous System	
Stimulates central nervous system, increasing alertness and producing a feeling of fright, excitation, and impending doom	
Dilates pupils	Dilates pupils
Inhibits gastrointestinal tract	Inhibits gastrointestinal tract
Metabolism	
Increases nonesterified fatty acid level of blood	Increases nonesterified fatty acid level of blood
Promotes conversion of glycogen to glucose	
Increases body metabolism	Increases body metabolism slightly

Data from Campese, V. M., & DeQuattro, V. (1989). Functional components of the sympathetic nervous system: Regulation of organ systems. In L. DeGroot (Ed.), *Endocrinology and metabolism* (2nd ed.). Philadelphia: W. B. Saunders.

DIAGNOSTIC ASSESSMENT

Because pheochromocytoma is curable, early and accurate diagnosis is essential. Current methods of diagnosis include the following:

History and Physical Examination. The client may describe symptomatic attacks over weeks, months, or even years. The BP may change with exertion or emotional upset. In long-standing cases, complications of hypertension (e.g., visual disturbances), symptoms of heart disease (dyspnea, edema), and manifestations of kidney damage (albuminuria, proteinuria, and increased blood urea nitrogen) can exist.

Chemical Tests. Two hormonal assay tests are useful in diagnosing pheochromocytoma:

- Assay of the urinary catecholamines and their metabolites (metanephrines and vanillylmandelic acid [VMA]). The normal range of urinary catecholamines is up to 14 μg/100 mL of urine, with higher levels occurring in pheochromocytoma.
- Determinations of plasma catecholamine concentrations. Assays of urinary VMA levels are performed on 24-hour urine specimens only. Clients must be advised to avoid tea, chocolate, vanilla, and all fruits for at least 2 days before urine collection begins. Also, they must be reminded not to take any medications for 2 to 3 days before the test. Normally, the amount of VMA is less than 7 mg per 24 hours. Urinary VMA rises in clients with pheochromocytoma.

The laboratory also performs a direct assay of catecholamines in the blood. The normal range of catecholamines in the blood is epinephrine, 0.02 to 0.2 μg/L, and norepinephrine, 0.1 to 0.5 μg/L.

X-ray Imaging. Various radiographic techniques can help confirm and identify adrenomedullary tumor location, such as CT scan and magnetic resonance imaging (MRI).

Miscellaneous Nonspecific Laboratory Tests. In the presence of pheochromocytoma, the basal metabolic rate increases, blood sugar rises abnormally, and glycosuria can occur.

Medical Management

PHARMACOLOGIC MANAGEMENT

Alpha-adrenergic blocking agents such as phentolamine (Regitine) can be used in an IV bolus or IV drip for hypertensive crisis. Oral phenoxybenzamine (Dibenzyline) is used preoperatively to control the BP before definitive treatment: surgical removal of the affected gland.

Surgical Management

The primary treatment for a pheochromocytoma is surgical removal of one or both adrenal glands, depending on whether the tumor is unilateral or bilateral. The procedure is the same as that described for treatment of Cushing's syndrome.

Surgical removal can cure the client, provided the growth is discovered before cardiovascular damage becomes permanent. The operation, however, is not without danger. There are two serious hazards. First, excessive discharge of pressor hormones during induction of anesthesia or manipulation of the tumor can cause extreme rises in BP and cardiac arrhythmias. Second, after resection of the tumor, BP can fall precipitously.

Nursing Management

Assessment

It is important to assess and control the client's blood pressure preoperatively. The client must be closely monitored for the development of stressful episodes before treatment has begun. It is also important to assess the client's neurologic status in case the client has a stroke from the extremely elevated BP.

Nursing Diagnosis, Planning, and Implementation

Collaborative Problem: Injury, Risk for R/T excessive release of epinephrine and norepinephrine preoperatively.

Planning: Expected Outcomes. Injury will be prevented or will be detected early, as evidenced by the absence of hypertensive episodes and cardiovascular or cerebral damage.

Implementation. During the preoperative phase, the goal of treatment is to prevent attacks of acute paroxysmal hypertension, thereby decreasing the risk of further damage to the cardiovascular system. Important nursing interventions include (1) promoting rest and relief from stress; (2) administering prescribed sedatives; (3) providing a high-vitamin, high-mineral, and high-calorie diet; (4) prohibiting beverages with caffeine such as coffee and tea; and (5) monitoring vital signs. In most cases, the physician will prescribe an alpha-adrenergic blocking agent such as phenoxybenzamine.

Collaborative Problem: Injury, Risk for R/T post-operative hypotension, hemorrhage, and shock.

Planning: Expected Outcomes. Injury will be prevented or will be detected early, as evidenced by normotensive state and the absence of hemorrhage, shock, or addisonian crisis.

Implementation. The first 24 to 48 hours after surgery is a critical period demanding vigilant nursing assessment and intervention. During the immediate postoperative period, nursing interventions include observation for signs of shock and hemorrhage.

After removal of the tumor, profound shock can develop as catecholamine levels drop. Hypotension can persist for 24 to 48 hours. Hemorrhage can occur as a result of the high vascularity of the adrenal glands. To prevent postoperative shock, the nurse must

- Give IV fluids as prescribed, such as blood, plasma, dextran, or glucose in water to maintain blood volume.
- Administer IV pressors as prescribed at a rate sufficient to maintain BP within a safe range. Check BP as often as is necessary to titrate the medication.
- Carefully measure hourly urinary output. If the client voids less than 30 mL per hour, notify the physician. Oliguria can signify impending shock and consequent renal shutdown.
- Assess the client for signs of hemorrhage. Check the dressing every half hour for bloody drainage. If the client is bleeding internally, an abdominal hematoma can develop, resulting in paralytic ileus. Symptoms of paralytic ileus include abdominal pain, distention, severe nausea, vomiting, and diminished or absent bowel sounds.
- Assess the client closely for signs of adrenal insufficiency if cortical tissue was resected during surgery (see the section on addisonian crisis). If both adrenal glands have been removed, the client must receive cortisol replacement for life.

Nursing Diagnosis: Pain R/T surgery, headache, and other manifestations of pheochromocytoma.

Planning: Expected Outcomes. Client will be without pain, as evidenced by client's statements, normotensive state, and absence of evidence of painful expression.

Implementation. When administering medication for incisional pain, the nurse must monitor BP frequently. The nurse should remember that narcotics, particularly meperidine, produce hypotension as a side effect; however, withholding pain medication also can lead to hypotension and severe pain. It is important to control the pain so the client's level of stress will decrease.

Nursing Diagnosis: Knowledge Deficit R/T self-administration of corticosteroids.

Planning: Expected Outcomes. The client will understand self-administration of steroids, as evidenced by the ability to explain administration and compliance with medication regimen.

Implementation. Once the critical postoperative period is over, most clients pass through an uneventful convalescence. Clients who will be self-administering corticosteroids need instruction concerning the administration and side effects (see the section on Addison's disease).

Evaluation

The nurse must evaluate client outcomes based on the established plan of care. If these goals were not achieved, the plan and interventions must be revised to meet the client's needs.

Modification of Plan of Care for the Elderly

The elderly client is more likely to suffer damage related to any hypertensive episodes associated with the pheochromocytoma because their cardiovascular and cerebrovascular systems are likely to be weaker and prone to damage from the elevated pressure.

Posthospital Care

The discharge teaching and follow-up care for the client on steroids are the same as for the client with Addison's disease (see the section on Addison's disease).

Anterior Pituitary Disorders

Disorders of the pituitary gland occur most frequently in the anterior lobe (Table 42–5 and see Fig. 39–2). Major causes of pituitary disease include

- Functioning tumors
- Nonfunctioning tumors
- Pituitary infarction
- Genetic disorders
- Trauma

The three principal pathologic consequences of pituitary disorders are hyperpituitarism, hypopituitarism, and local compression of brain tissue by expanding tumor masses.

HYPERPITUITARISM

Hyperpituitarism is defined as oversecretion of one or more of the hormones secreted by the pituitary gland. It is primarily caused by a hormone-secreting pituitary tumor, typically a benign adenoma. Syndromes associated with hyperpituitarism are Cushing's syndrome, acromegaly, amenorrhea, galactorrhea, hyperthyroidism, and rarely, hypergonadism in the male.

The diagnosis of hyperpituitarism involves radiologic and laboratory testing. Measurement of plasma levels of hormones such as growth hormone (GH), ACTH, follicle-stimulating hormone, and luteinizing hormone usually establishes the diagnosis of pituitary hormone hypersecretion. CT scan and MRI can allow visualization of pituitary tumors.

Pituitary tumors produce both systemic effects and local manifestations. Systemic effects include

- Excessive or abnormal growth patterns resulting from overproduction of GH
- Abnormal milk secretion (galactorrhea)
- Overstimulation of one or more of the target glands, resulting in the release of excessive thyroid, sex, or adrenocortical hormones

Locally, pituitary tumors produce symptoms because the bony cranium that houses the tumor cannot expand to accommodate a growing mass. Local manifestations include visual field abnormalities, resulting from pressure on the optic chiasma; headaches; and somnolence.

ACROMEGALY

Acromegaly is a disease of adults and develops after closure of the epiphyses of the long bones.

Incidence

There is a low incidence of acromegaly. The acidophilic, GH-producing tumors that cause acromegaly, however, are the second most common type of hyperpituitarism.

Etiology

Acromegaly results from GH-secreting adenomas of the anterior pituitary gland.

Risk Factors

There are no identified risk factors for the development of a GH-producing tumor. Also, there is no familial tendency for development of these tumors.

Pathophysiology

Acidophilic, GH-producing tumors are characterized by an excessive secretion of GH. The increased amounts of GH lead to rapid growth in all body tissues. This increased growth leads to acromegaly, if it occurs after epiphyseal closure.

As the tumor continues to grow, the size often results in destruction of the entire pituitary gland, leading to hypopituitarism. The size of the tumor also can result in pressure on the optic nerve, which crosses directly above the pituitary gland, leading to blindness.

Prognosis depends on the age at which the client experiences an oversecretion of GH and seeks health intervention. Many of the somatic changes are irreversible, and the longer the client is in a hyperpituitary state, the higher the mortality rate. Thus, the earlier the diagnosis, the more likely the client is to benefit from treatment.

TABLE 42–5 Pituitary Hormones

NAME	RELEASING FACTOR	TARGET CELLS	RESPONSE	INCREASED LEVEL	DECREASED LEVEL
GH	GHRH	Bone, muscle	Stimulates growth; promotes active transport of amino acids into cell and influences lipid, CHO, and Ca^{2+} metabolism	Child: gigantism (before epiphyseal closure); child grows very tall Adult: acromegaly (after epiphyseal closure); bones increase in thickness; increase in soft tissue growth	Child: dwarfism Adult: lethargy, increased weight, loss of reproductive function, premature aging
ACTH	CRH	Adrenal cortex	Stimulates adrenal gland secretion of mineralocorticoids and glucocorticoids	Cushing's disease: increased amounts of cortisol and aldosterone	Addison's disease: decreased cortisol and aldosterone, increased MSH
TSH	TRH	Thyroid	Stimulates thyroid to increase secretion of thyroxine (controls rate of most chemical reactions in body)	Goiter; increased BMR; decreased weight; increased cardiac output, HR, and BP; increased cerebration; fine muscle tremors	Reduced thyroid activity; decreased BMR; increased weight; decreased cardiac output, HR, and BP; decreased cerebration; somnolence
Prolactin		Breast	Stimulates breast to lactate	Amenorrhea	Too little milk
FSH	LHRH	Ovaries, testes	Stimulates growth of ovaries and sperm		Late puberty
LH	LHRH	Ovaries, testes	Growth of follicles and increased secretion of estrogen and progesterone; increased testosterone secretion in the male	Excess testosterone, menstrual cycle disturbance	Amenorrhea; diminished progesterone and testosterone
Posterior Pituitary					
Oxytocin	Labor, sucking	Uterus, breasts	Stimulates uterus to contract at childbirth; stimulates lactation	Precipitate childbirth, excess milk	Prolonged childbirth, diminished milk
ADH (vasopressin)	Dehydration	Arterioles, distal renal tubule	Vasoconstriction of arterioles to increase arterial pressure; increased water reabsorption in distal tubules, stimulates smooth muscle of GI tract	Increased BP, decreased urinary output, edema	Diabetes insipidus, dilute urine, increased urinary volume

ACTH, adrenocorticotropic hormone; ADH, antidiuretic hormone; BMR, basal metabolic rate; BP, blood pressure; Ca^{2+}, calcium; CHO, carbohydrate; CRH, cortisol-releasing hormone; FSH, follicle-stimulating hormone; GH, growth hormone; GHRH, growth hormone–releasing hormone; GI, gastrointestinal; HR, heart rate; LH, luteinizing hormone; LHRH, luteinizing hormone–releasing hormone; MSH, melanocyte-stimulating hormone; TRH, thyrotropin-releasing hormone; TSH, thyroid-stimulating hormone.

Adapted from Davis, J., and Mason, C.: *Neurologic critical care.* New York: Van Nostrand Reinhold Co., 1979.

Clinical Manifestations

Clients with acromegaly have a characteristic appearance (see Clinical Manifestations: Acromegaly). The coarsening of the facial features, the prognathism (protrusion of the jaw), and the broad hands with spadelike fingers characterize the disease. In addition, clients with acromegaly experience local manifestations such as headache, diplopia, blindness, and lethargy caused by compression of brain tissue by the tumor. In advanced cases, clients can suffer from associated hormonal disturbances such as diabetes mellitus, goiter, Cushing's disease, changes in libido, and menstrual disorders.

CLINICAL MANIFESTATIONS

Acromegaly

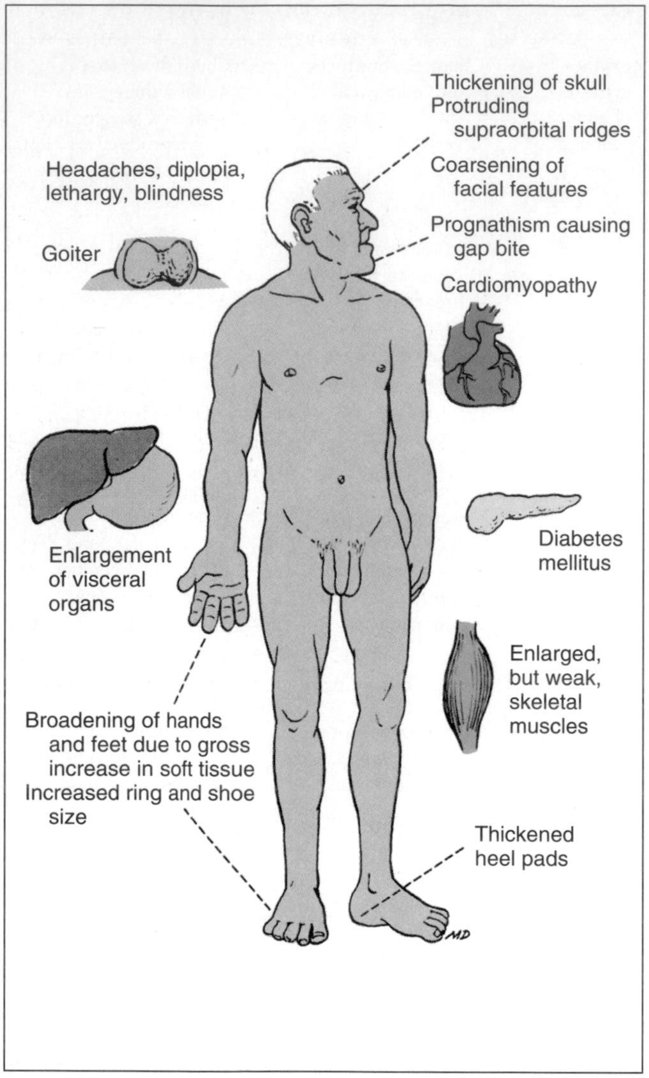

Medical Management

Treatment for pituitary tumors can be accomplished through irradiation of the pituitary gland to destroy the tumor. This is usually performed through a radiation implant via the transsphenoidal approach.

PHARMACOLOGIC MANAGEMENT

Bromocriptine (Parlodel) can reduce the levels of growth hormone and decrease tumor size. This agent can be used if the levels of growth hormone remain high after surgery or until the effects of radiation occur.

Surgical Management

The treatment of choice for acromegaly is a surgical hypophysectomy. Partial or complete removal of the pituitary gland occurs during surgical resection of pituitary tumors.

Surgeons prefer the transsphenoidal route for clients with tumors remaining within the sella turcica or tumors with only moderate suprasellar extension. This approach avoids disturbing the cranium and avoids scarring. Access to the pituitary gland is obtained through an incision made in the upper gum line. Preoperatively, the client's sinuses are cleansed and antibiotic nasal spray is used.

The surgeon, when performing a transsphenoidal hypophysectomy, takes muscle or fat from the thigh and places it in the tumor cavity. The nasal cavities are then packed with Vaseline gauze, and a mustache dressing is applied under the nose. After surgery, the need for cortisone replacement may be permanent.

Nursing Management

Assessment

Most clients are frightened by the prospect of undergoing surgical removal of the pituitary gland. The nurse must provide the client and significant others with emotional support and comfort throughout the preoperative period. The initial symptoms are vague; therefore, clients have often seen many physicians in the past and have had multiple examinations and tests seeking a diagnosis. The client and family might be fearful, skeptical, or relieved at the final diagnosis of a pituitary tumor. The nurse's assessment should include the client's reaction to the diagnosis, expectations of surgery, educational needs related to diagnosis and treatment plan, and available support network after discharge.

The nurse's physical assessment of the client includes baseline vital signs and weight as well as neurologic assessment. These findings are essential to establish a baseline for postoperative comparison. To perform the neurologic assessment, the nurse must check

- pupil equality and reactivity to light
- handgrip for strength, equality, and ability to release on command
- level of consciousness
- orientation to time, place, person, and situation
- appropriate response to stimuli
- visual acuity and visual fields

Nursing Diagnosis, Planning, and Implementation

Nursing Diagnosis: Knowledge Deficit R/T surgery and possible outcomes.

Planning: Expected Outcomes. The client will understand the planned surgery and possible outcomes, as evidenced by client's statements, questions, and ability to describe the procedure and outcomes.

Implementation. The client should have the surgery explained in detail, along with potential outcomes of surgical treatment. The nurse can use drawings of the brain to explain the transsphenoidal approach. The client must be prepared for the presence of an indwelling urinary catheter, IV catheters, and any other catheters or monitors that may be needed after surgery. The client must be notified that vital signs will be closely monitored after surgery.

Preoperative preparation also includes coaching the client in deep-breathing exercises and assisting in keeping records of intake and output.

CRITICAL TO REMEMBER

Clients must be warned to avoid coughing, sneezing, or blowing their nose after surgery.

Collaborative Problem: Injury, Risk for R/T post-operative complications.

Planning: Expected Outcomes. Injury will be prevented after surgery, as evidenced by the absence of addisonian crisis, balanced output, no signs of increased intracranial pressure, normal temperature, and absence of symptoms of cerebrospinal fluid leakage or meningitis.

Implementation. Before surgery, the client usually receives cortisol by injection or intravenously. Glucocorticoids help the client to tolerate the stress of an operation that can result in loss of adrenocortical function.

Management after transfrontal hypophysectomy resembles that for any craniotomy (see Chap. 14). Immediately after surgery, the nurse assesses for signs of cerebral edema and rising intracranial pressure (elevated BP, widened pulse pressure, low pulse rate, pupil changes, altered respiratory pattern).

The pituitary no longer produces tropic hormones; therefore, the nurse must watch for signs of target gland deficiencies, such as adrenal insufficiency and hypothyroidism. In addition, diabetes insipidus can occur temporarily as a result of antidiuretic hormone (ADH) deficiency. Intake and output must be strictly documented. The nurse must notify the physician if urine output is greater than 200 mL/hr with specific gravity of less than 1.005.

The client must be assessed carefully for signs of meningitis, a potential complication of surgery. Any temperature elevation, severe headache, irritability, or nuchal rigidity must be reported.

The client who has undergone transsphenoidal hypophysectomy requires frequent oral hygiene using a gauze sponge, and the lips should be lubricated with petroleum jelly. The client should not brush the teeth for 2 weeks after surgery.

The nasal packing is usually removed in 2 to 5 days. After its removal, the client must be observed for rhinorrhea, which can indicate a cerebrospinal fluid (CSF) leak. The client should report frequent postnasal drainage. The nurse collects any serous drainage and tests it for the presence of CSF (see Chap. 12) or sends it to the laboratory for analysis. It is possible for the muscle or fat graft to dislodge, causing a CSF leak. The client must be instructed to avoid sneezing, coughing, and bending over from the waist to avoid disrupting the graft.

Nursing Diagnosis: Knowledge Deficit R/T self-administration of pituitary replacement hormones.

Planning: Expected Outcomes. The client will understand the self-administration of medication, as evidenced by the client's statements, ability to comply with postoperative medication regimen, and absence of symptoms to hypopituitarism.

Implementation. As stated earlier, people who have undergone complete hypophysectomy must take cortisone replacements for the rest of their lives. These clients should be instructed to avoid gastric irritation by taking cortisone with milk, food, or an antacid. Clients must be advised to notify the physician if frequent gastritis, tarry stools, or frank blood in the stools is noted.

Some clients also may require thyroid or sex hormone replacement. In addition, some will need vasopressin replacement to treat diabetes insipidus. Diabetes insipidus is usually transient after surgery but can persist, indicating the need for chronic hormone replacement.

Evaluation

The nurse must evaluate client outcomes based on the established plan of care. If these goals were not achieved, the plan and interventions must be revised to meet the client's needs.

Posthospital Care

Client teaching must include self-administration of hormones, side effects, and signs of overdosage or underdosage of prescribed hormones.

Because the client is taking many hormones, imbalances can develop as a result of the hypophysectomy. It is important, therefore, to stress the importance of maintaining follow-up appointments. Clients must be advised to obtain a physical check-up at least every 6 months and whenever symptoms of imbalance appear.

SEXUAL DISTURBANCES

Excess prolactin secretion can cause amenorrhea or galactorrhea (excessive flow of milk) in women. Physicians consider surgical removal to be the treatment of choice for radiologically apparent tumors.

Clients with increased prolactin secretion and no radiologic or neurologic evidence of a pituitary tumor often respond to bromocriptine, an ergot-like compound. Clients with prolactinomas can be successfully treated with bromocriptine. Bromocriptine, a dopamine agonist, inhibits prolactin secretion. Surgery is no longer the treatment of choice in most of these cases.

HYPOPITUITARISM

In contrast to hyperpituitarism, hypopituitarism is a deficiency of one or more of the hormones produced by the anterior lobe of the pituitary. When both the anterior and posterior lobes fail to secrete hormones, the condition is called panhypopituitarism.

Incidence

Hypopituitarism and panhypopituitarism are rare disorders.

POSTERIOR LOBE (NEUROHYPOPHYSEAL) DISORDERS

Unlike the adenohypophysis, disease rarely destroys the neurohypophysis. Even if the posterior lobe becomes damaged or is surgically destroyed with the anterior lobe, hormonal deficiencies usually do not develop. This is because the hypothalamus continues to synthesize oxytocin and ADH. On the other hand, if the hypothalamus suffers damage, deficiencies of oxytocin and ADH develop even if the neurohypophysis is healthy and intact.

The major disorder of the posterior lobe is ADH deficiency (diabetes insipidus) (Fig. 42–2). Excessive ADH causes the syndrome of inappropriate ADH secretion (SIADH), which can occur with lung cancer, head injuries, cranial surgery, pituitary tumors, encephalitis, poliomyelitis, and myxedema.

DIABETES INSIPIDUS

Diabetes insipidus is a deficiency of ADH resulting in a physiologic imbalance of water.

Incidence

Diabetes insipidus is a rare disorder.

Etiology

Diabetes insipidus results from a deficiency of ADH. Causes of ADH deficiency are categorized as follows:

- Central or neurogenic diabetes insipidus resulting from (1) abnormalities in the hypothalamus and pituitary gland from familial or idiopathic causes (primary diabetes insipidus), (2) destruction of the gland by tumors in the hypothalamic-pituitary region, trauma, infectious processes, vascular accidents, or metastatic tumors from the breast or lung (secondary diabetes insipidus), and (3) medications such as phenytoin (Dilantin), alcohol, and lithium carbonate, can interfere with the synthesis or release of ADH in some clients.

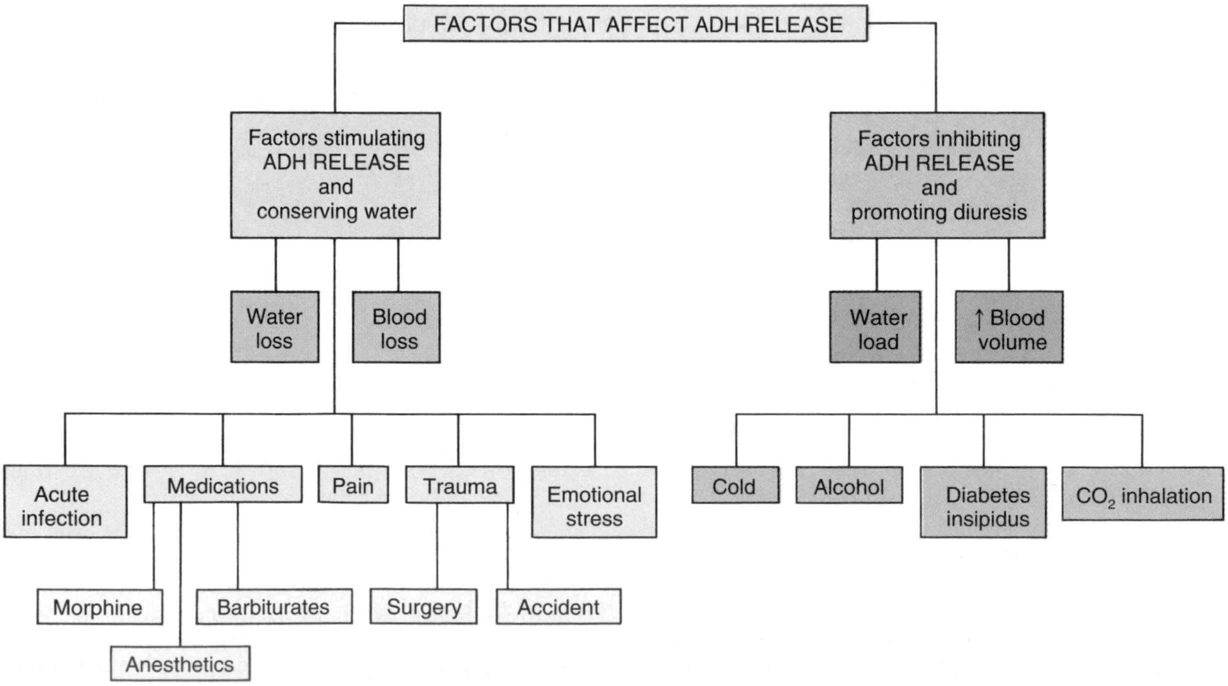

Figure 42–2
Factors that stimulate and inhibit the release of antidiuretic hormone (ADH).

- "Nephrogenic" diabetes insipidus. Owing to an inherited defect, the kidney tubules cannot respond to ADH.

Risk Factors

Risk factors include head injuries, infections, and other factors that lead to destruction of the gland. Certain medications also may lead to the development of diabetes insipidus. Prevention is mainly related to identification of risk factors and early detection.

Pathophysiology

When ADH production decreases excessively, the kidney tubules fail to reabsorb water; consequently, the client excretes large amounts of dilute urine. As in diabetes mellitus, clients with diabetes insipidus excrete excessive amounts of urine. Urine in diabetes mellitus contains large amounts of glucose, whereas urine in diabetes insipidus is highly dilute and contains no glucose.

Clinical Manifestations

Diabetes insipidus can arise slowly or can appear suddenly after injury or infectious disease. Its two major manifestations are polyuria and polydipsia. The thirst mechanism in some clients with diabetes insipidus, however, may not be intact. The client can drink and excrete 5 to 10 L of fluid per day! The urine is very dilute, with a specific gravity of 1.001 to 1.005 (normal specific gravity is 1.001–1.030). The client must drink fluid almost continuously to avoid severe dehydration and hypovolemic shock.

DIAGNOSTIC ASSESSMENT

Diabetes insipidus can be diagnosed by a water deprivation test. The client must be instructed not to drink water to concentrate the urine. Test results are positive for diabetes insipidus if the urine remains dilute. Clients with nephrogenic diabetes insipidus do not respond to ADH injection.

Medical Management

PHARMACOLOGIC MANAGEMENT

Clients with diabetes insipidus often benefit from administration of the benzothiadiazine diuretics either alone or in combination with the sulfonylurea chlorpropamide.

In addition, injection of vasopressin (aqueous Pitressin) can control the symptoms of diabetes insipidus. Vasopressin typically alleviates polyuria, and usually polydipsia, for 24 to 72 hours. The synthetic polypeptide desmopressin acetate (DDAVP) can be insufflated through the nose in the morning and at bedtime. This medication has largely replaced vasopressin tannate for long-term treatment of clients with severe diabetes insipidus.

After administering vasopressin, clients need to be assessed for signs and symptoms of water intoxication, which can lead to fluid overload, cerebral edema, and seizures (see Chap. 3).

Surgical Management

Surgical resection of the tumor can cure clients with diabetes insipidus secondary to a tumor.

Nursing Management

Assessment of the client with suspected diabetes insipidus should center on monitoring of the client's intake and output. The client should be asked about the presence of excessive thirst or urination. The client's fluid and electrolyte balance must be closely monitored. The client also should be assessed for exposure to risk factors.

The nursing interventions center around maintaining adequate hydration and electrolyte balance and preventing complications. The nurse should not only administer the ordered vasopressin or synthetic ADH but also should assess the effectiveness of the medication. The client also must learn self-administration of either the injections or the nasal spray.

If the client undergoes surgical resection of a tumor of the pituitary, one must provide nursing care for the hypophysectomy client (see the section on hypophysectomy).

SYNDROME OF INAPPROPRIATE ANTIDIURETIC HORMONE

The syndrome of inappropriate antidiuretic hormone is a disorder associated with excessive amounts of ADH, resulting in a water imbalance.

Incidence

The syndrome is one of the most common causes of hyponatremia, although the exact incidence of SIADH itself is not known.

Etiology

There are a wide variety of causes of SIADH, including the stress of surgery and many disorders and medications.

Risk Factors

Treatment of diabetes insipidus with vasopressin can lead to SIADH if excessive amounts are administered. Care must be taken when vasopressin is administered so this complication does not occur.

A variety of malignancies are risk factors for SIADH. It is important to monitor the high-risk client for sudden fluid retention or weight gain.

Pathophysiology

This syndrome is the opposite of diabetes insipidus. Instead of large fluid losses, clients with SIADH may have water intoxication resulting from fluid retention. Factors that affect ADH secretion are summarized in Figure 42–2.

Under normal circumstances, ADH regulates serum osmolality. When serum osmolality falls, a feedback mechanism causes inhibition of ADH. This, in turn, promotes increased water excretion by the kidneys to raise serum osmolality to normal. When this feedback mechanism fails and ADH levels are sustained, fluid retention results. Ultimately, serum sodium falls, resulting in hyponatremia and water intoxication.

Clinical Manifestations

Central nervous system (CNS) dysfunction, characterized by alterations in level of consciousness, seizures, and coma, can become evident when serum sodium falls to 120 mEq/L or less.

Hyponatremia can result in diminished gastrointestinal function, and this problem is further complicated by the need for fluid restriction.

DIAGNOSTIC ASSESSMENT

Diagnosis rests on the presence of hyponatremia with a normal or expanded plasma volume.

Medical Management

Treatment for SIADH includes fluid restriction, very careful replacement of sodium chloride, administration of diuretics and demeclocycline (a tetracycline that increases free-water clearance), and correction of the cause, if possible.

The physician also can prescribe cathartics or low-volume, hyperosmolar fluid enemas. In general, administration of tap water or saline enemas should be avoided because the fluid can be absorbed from the bowel and contribute to water intoxication.

Treatment is the same as for any client with dilutional hyponatremia (see Chap. 3).

Nursing Management

Assessment

The client with suspected SIADH should have fluid status and electrolytes closely monitored. The client's cardiovascular status also should be assessed regularly so any alterations are immediately noted.

The client's weight should be recorded, and any gain of more than 2 pounds should be reported to the physician. The client's neurologic status should be monitored so any alterations related to the hyponatremia are immediately diagnosed and treatment can be started.

Nursing Diagnosis, Planning, and Implementation

Nursing Diagnosis: Injury, Risk for R/T to the danger of cerebral edema, water intoxication, and CNS dysfunction.

Planning: Expected Outcomes. The client will be free from injury, as evidenced by absence of signs of increased intracranial pressure, hypertension, altered level of consciousness, and seizures.

Implementation. Nursing care for clients with SIADH includes accurate assessment of fluid balance, daily weights, and careful and frequent assessment of neurologic status.

The client must be positioned so the person's head is flat or raised no more than 5 degrees, unless contraindicated. This position helps prevent possible development or worsening of cerebral edema. It also avoids stimulation of receptors in the atrium of the heart that are sensitive to volume changes and that can increase ADH secretion. See Chapter 13 for further information on cerebral edema.

The nurse should perform frequent neurologic checks and notify the physician if any significant changes occur. The nurse continues to monitor the client's mental status by assessing the client's orientation to person, place, and time.

See Chapter 3 for information on the nursing care associated with dilutional hyponatremia.

Nursing Diagnosis: Fluid Volume Excess R/T excessive secretion of ADH secondary to SIADH.

Planning: Expected Outcomes. The client will maintain optimal fluid balance or will have the excess resolved without injury, as evidenced by return to normal blood pressure, absence of edema, and balanced intake and output.

Implementation. Clients with SIADH will have significant fluid restrictions, often as low as 500 to 600 mL/24 hr. The intake and output and daily weights must be closely monitored. A continued imbalance of intake and output, with intake higher than output, should be immediately reported. If the client's weight increases by 2 pounds or more in a 24-hour period, it may represent fluid retention. The client also will be maintained on a very low sodium intake and diuretics administered.

Once the client has begun to recover, the output should increase significantly, becoming greater than the intake until balance is restored. The client's weight should begin to decrease gradually.

Evaluation

The nurse must evaluate client outcomes based on the established plan of care. If these goals were not achieved, the plan and interventions must be revised to meet the client's needs.

Posthospital Care

If the client's SIADH has not been resolved, the client and significant others will have to understand the continued need for sodium and fluid restrictions. The client also should learn to weigh daily and to report any excessive gain (2 pounds or more a day). Clients should be taught to avoid the use of aspirin or nonsteroidal anti-inflammatory agents because these drugs can increase the hyponatremia.

The client should have access to a scale so his or her weight can be monitored regularly.

The client with chronic SIADH will need to be monitored closely by the physician on a regular basis. The client should be reminded of the need to notify the physician whenever changes in his or her condition occur.

STUDY QUESTIONS

1. Of the hormones secreted by the adrenal cortex, which of the following, if excreted in excess, is responsible for sodium retention and potassium excretion?
   A. Cortisol
   B. Estrogen
   C. Aldosterone
   D. Testosterone
2. Signs and symptoms that a nurse may notice in a client with Addison's disease include all of the following, except
   A. Craving for salt
   B. Hypertension
   C. Personality changes
   D. Hemoconcentration
3. One of the major risk factors for increased levels of cortisol is the administration of exogenous
   A. Estrogens
   B. Aminoglycosides
   C. Oral hypoglycemics
   D. Steroids
4. Diagnostic tests for the client with primary hyperaldosteronism may show which of the following:
   A. Low serum potassium
   B. Acidosis
   C. Decreased urinary aldosterone levels
   D. Elevated plasma renin levels
5. Assessment of the client with diabetes insipidus should focus on monitoring the client for
   A. Intake and output
   B. Blood pressure
   C. Daily weight
   D. Specific gravity of urine

CRITICAL THINKING EXERCISES

SCENARIO A

A client is hospitalized with unexplained fatigue, weight loss, and postural hypotension. After numerous tests, the client is diagnosed with Addison's disease and is placed on long-term steroid therapy of methylprednisolone (Medrol), 8 mg daily. The client is to be discharged tomorrow. What information should the nurse impart to the client?

SCENARIO B

A client is diagnosed as having primary hyperaldosteronism. The physician has placed him on a low-sodium, high-potassium diet. The client is also to take spironolactone (Aldactone), 100 mg twice daily. What information should the nurse teach the client?

BIBLIOGRAPHY

1. Baxter, J. D. (1992). Disorders of the adrenal cortex. In J. B. Wyngaarden et al. (Eds.), *Cecil textbook of medicine* (19th ed., pp. 1271–1290). Philadelphia: W. B. Saunders.
2. Baylis, P. H. (1995). Vasopressin and its neurophysin. In L. DeGroot et al. (Eds.), *Endocrinology* (3rd ed., pp. 406–420). Philadelphia: W. B. Saunders.
3. Becker, K. L. (1990). General principles of endocrinology. In K. Becker (Ed.), *Principles and practice in endocrinology and metabolism* (pp. 2–80). Philadelphia: J. B. Lippincott.
4. Blackman, M. R., et al. (1995). Endocrinology and aging. In L. DeGroot et al. (Eds.), *Endocrinology* (3rd ed., pp. 2702–2730). Philadelphia: W. B. Saunders.
5. Bryce, J. (1994). S.I.A.D.H.: Recognizing and treating syndrome of inappropriate antidiuretic hormone secretion. *Nursing, 24(4)*, 33.

6. Closson, B. L., et al. (1993). Diabetes insipidus and spinal cord injury: A challenging combination. *Rehabilitation Nursing, 18(6),* 368–374, 427–428.

7. Eldar-Geva, T., et al. (1990). Secondary biosynthetic defects in women with late-onset congenital adrenal hyperplasia. *New England Journal of Medicine, 323:*855–863.

8. Epstein, C. D. (1991). Fluid volume deficit for the adrenal crisis patient. *Dimensions of Critical Care Nursing, 10(4),* 210.

9. Epstein, C. D. (1992). Adrenal insufficiency in the critically ill patient. *AACN. Clinical Issues in Critical Care Nursing, 3(3),* 705–713.

10. Findling, J. W. (1992). Cushing syndrome—An etiologic workup. *Hospital Practice, 27(10),* 107–122.

11. Gumoski, J., et al. (1992). Endocrinopathies of hyperfunction: Cushing's syndrome and aldosteronism. *AACN. Clinical Issues in Critical Care Nursing, 3(2),* 331–347.

12. Helmstadter, C., et al. (1991). Nursing care of pituitary surgery: An example of advanced clinical practice. *AXON, 13(1),* 6–12.

13. Imperato-McGinley, J. (1992). Disorders of sexual differentiation. In J. B. Wyngaarden et al. (Eds.), *Cecil textbook of medicine* (19th ed., pp. 1320–1332). Philadelphia: W. B. Saunders.

14. Kaiser, H. R. (1995). Pheochromocytoma and related tumors. In L. DeGroot et al. (Eds.), *Endocrinology* (3rd ed., pp. 1853–1880). Philadelphia: W. B. Saunders.

15. Lee, L. M., & Gumoski, J. (1992). Adrenocortical insufficiency: A medical emergency. *AACN. Clinical Issues in Critical Care Nursing, 3(2),* 319–330.

16. Lindaman, C. (1992). S.I.A.D.H.: Is your patient at risk? *Nursing, 22(6),* 60–63.

17. Loriaux, D. L. (1990). The adrenal glands. In K. Becker (Ed.), *Principles and practice in endocrinology and metabolism.* Philadelphia: J. B. Lippincott.

18. Neiman, L. K., & Cutler, G. B., Jr. (1995). Cushing's syndrome. In L. DeGroot et al. (Eds.), *Endocrinology* (3rd ed., pp. 1741–1769). Philadelphia: W. B. Saunders.

19. Peterson, A., & Drass, J. (1993). How to keep adrenal insufficiency in check. *American Journal of Nursing, 93(10),* 36–39.

20. Robertson, G. L. (1990). The endocrine brain and pituitary gland. In K. Becker (Ed.), *Principles and practice in endocrinology and metabolism.* Philadelphia: J. B. Lippincott.

21. Stoffer, S. S. (1993). Addison's disease: How to improve patients' quality of life. *Postgraduate Medicine, 93(4),* 265–266, 271–276, 278.

22. Young, W. F. (1993). Pheochromocytoma: A brief management guide. *Hospital Medicine, 29(10),* 67–72, 76–79, 98–101.

23. Yucha, C., & Blakeman, N. (1991). Pheochromocytoma: The great mimic. *Cancer Nursing, 14(3),* 136–140.

24. Yucha, C., & Suddaby, P. (1991). David could have died of thirst—yet he never felt thirsty. *Nursing 91, 21(7),* 42–43.

UNIT 13

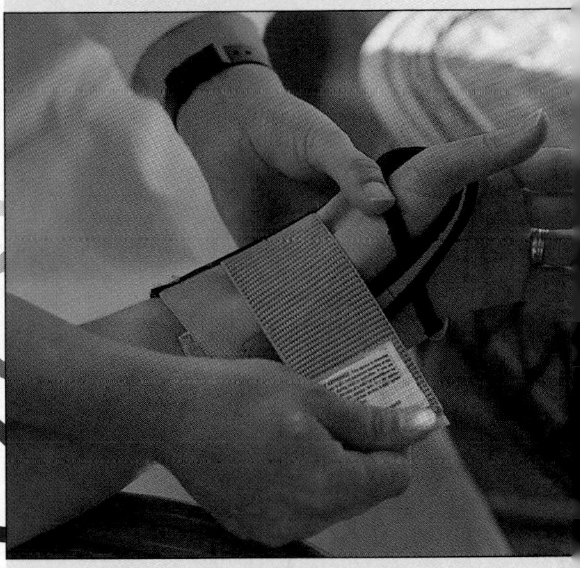

Musculoskeletal Disorders

The ability to move and maintain a desirable position is a basic human need. The bony skeleton provides support and movable parts; the musculature facilitates movement.

Movement serves two general purposes. First, it is necessary to perform normal activities of daily living. Second, it is in itself a source of pleasure. There is increasing interest in performing activities that contribute to physical fitness because such activities promote physical health and because they are pleasurable. People who enjoy exercise programs describe feelings of well-being or a ''high'' that comes from physical exertion.

Musculoskeletal disorders are among the oldest known diseases. Treatment of fractures had reached a sophisticated level by the time of Hippocrates. Arthritis was also common at the time of the Roman era and presumably the reason for extensive bathing pools throughout the empire.

The four chapters in this unit cover nursing and medical assessment and intervention for musculoskeletal problems (Chap. 43); common musculoskeletal interventions, such as rest, physical therapy, assistive devices (e.g., crutches, supports), casts, traction, and surgery (Chap. 44); the care of clients with metabolic musculoskeletal disorders, such as osteoporosis, Paget's disease, bone tumor, osteomyelitis, and carpal tunnel syndrome (Chap. 45); and the care of clients experiencing musculoskeletal injury and overuse problems (Chap. 46).

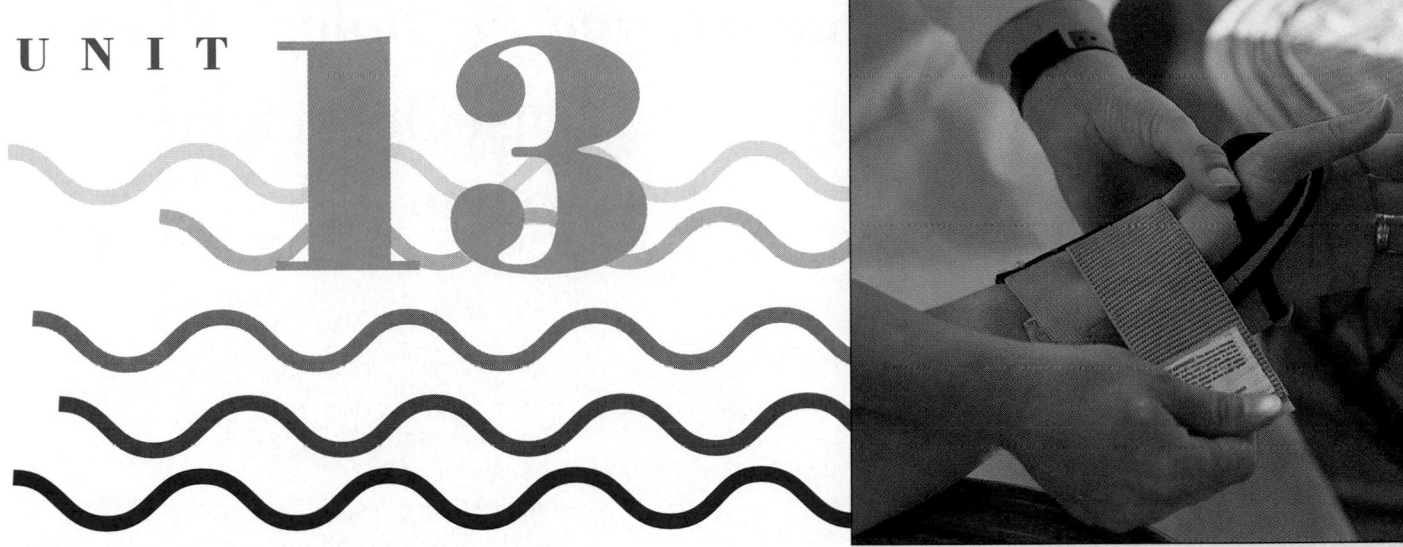

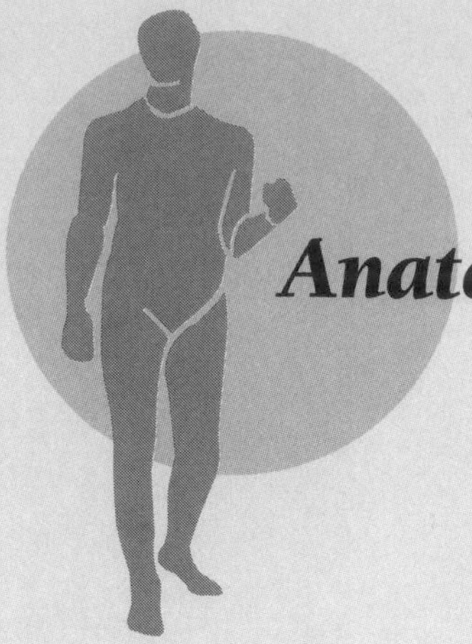

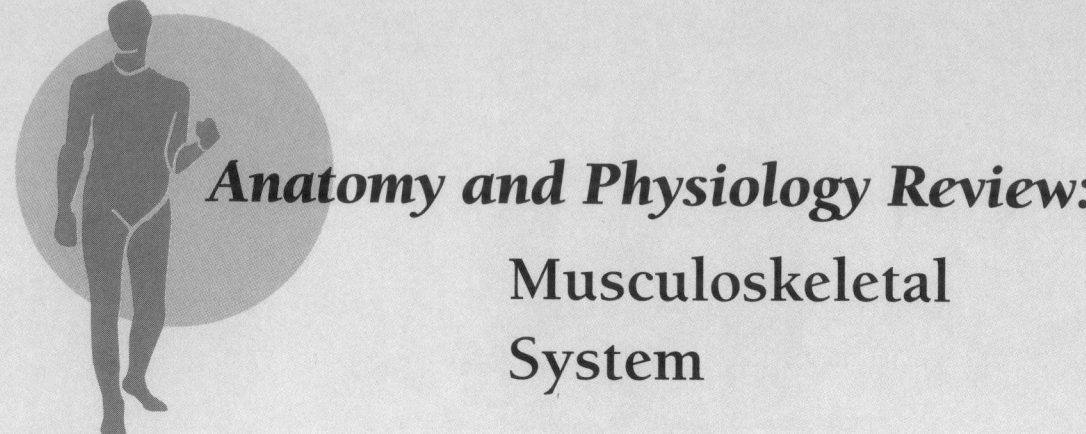

Anatomy and Physiology Review: Musculoskeletal System

THE SKELETAL SYSTEM

Divisions

The body contains 206 named bones, which are divided into the axial and appendicular skeletons. The *axial skeleton* consists of 80 bones, which include the skull, vertebral column, and thorax. The *appendicular skeleton* consists of 126 bones of the legs, arms, shoulder, and pelvis.

Classification of Bones

- *Long bones* are longer than they are wide. They are primarily compact bone but have spongy (cancellous) bone at the ends. Examples include the humerus, femur, radius, and phalanges. Long bones have a shaft, called a diaphysis, that surrounds a medullary cavity. In the adult, the medullary cavity contains yellow bone marrow. At each end is an expanded portion called the epiphysis, spongy bone covered by a thin layer of compact bone. Articular cartilage covers the epiphyses to provide smooth surfaces for movement in the joints. In growing bones, there is an epiphyseal plate of hyaline cartilage between the diaphysis and epiphysis.
- *Short bones* are roughly cube-shaped. They consist primarily of spongy bone covered by a thin layer of compact bone. Examples of short bones include the bones of the wrist and ankle.
- *Flat bones* are thin, flattened, and usually curved. They usually have a layer of spongy bone covered on each side by a layer of compact bone. Most of the bones of the cranium are flat bones.
- *Irregular bones* are those that don't fit any other category. They are primarily spongy bone covered with a thin layer of compact bone and have a variety of shapes. The vertebrae and some of the bones in the skull are irregular bones.
- *Sesamoid bones* are small bones that grow in tendons. Most sesamoid bones are not named, and they vary in location and number. The patella is a large sesamoid bone that is named. Sesamoid bones increase the leverage of muscles.

Function of Bones

Bones give shape and form to the body. They also perform several other functions and play an important role in homeostasis. These functions include:

- Support. Bones provide a rigid framework that supports the soft organs of the body and the body against the pull of gravity.
- Protection. The skeleton protects the soft body parts such as the brain, spinal cord, lungs, and heart.
- Movement. The skeleton contributes to movement by providing attachments for tendons and ligaments.
- Blood cell formation. Red bone marrow functions in the formation of red blood cells, white blood cells, and platelets.
- Storage. Bones store and release minerals, especially calcium, for cellular metabolism. They provide an essential part of mineral balance in the body.

Bone Remodeling

The internal structure of bone is maintained by remodeling, a three-part process by which existing bone is resorbed and new bone is laid down to replace it. Remodeling plays an important role in mineral balance, as calcium is resorbed and replaced in the bone matrix, and in the body's response to changes in gravitational

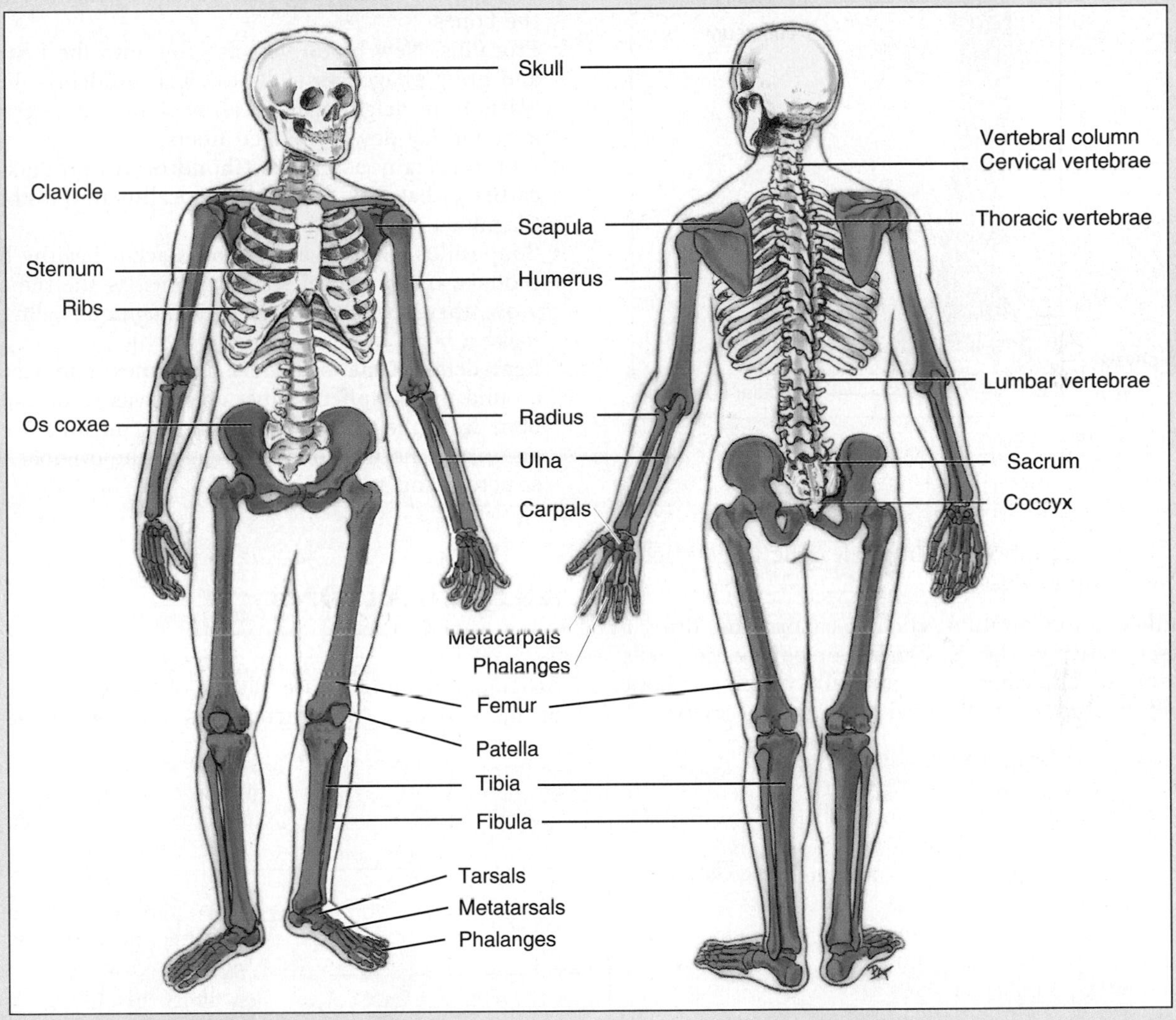

Divisions of the skeleton.

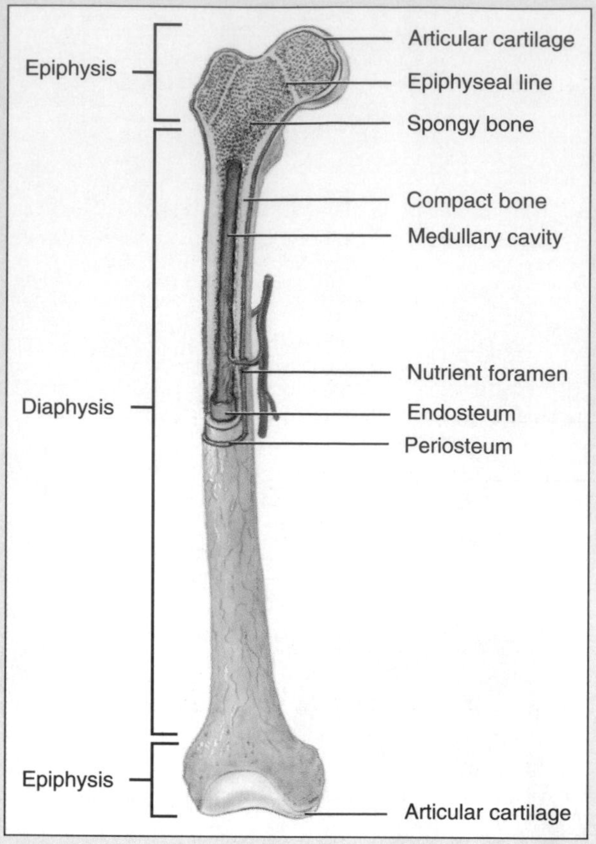

General features of long bones.

forces due to alterations in life-style. The three steps in the remodeling process are:

- Stimulus. Some stimulus, such as a hormone, drug, or stressor, activates the osteoclasts, or bone-eating cells.
- Resorption. The osteoclasts gradually resorb the bone, leaving behind a cavity called a resorption cavity.
- New bone. Osteoblasts lay down new bone, following the path of the osteoclasts to create new haversian systems and trabeculae.

Repair of Fractures

When a bone fracture occurs, a continuum of events takes place that results in the repair of the bone. These events may be grouped into five stages:

- Hematoma. The periosteum and blood vessels that cross the fracture line are torn when a bone breaks. Blood from the torn vessels forms a clot, or fracture hematoma, which plugs the gap between the ends of the bones.
- Procallus. New blood vessels grow into the hematoma and bring phagocytic cells to clean up debris. Fibroblasts from neighboring healthy tissue migrate to the area and lay down collagen fibers.
- Fibrocartilaginous callus. Chondrocytes produce fibrocartilage that transforms the procallus into a fibrocartilaginous callus.
- Bony callus. Osteoblasts from adjacent healthy bone produce trabeculae of spongy bone. As the trabeculae grow, they infiltrate the fibrocartilaginous callus to make a bony callus.
- Remodeling. Osteoblasts lay down new compact bone around the periphery while osteoclasts resorb spongy bone from the inside to form a new medullary cavity and make the new bone similar to the original in structure and strength.

ARTICULATIONS

Articulations (joints) are places of union between two or more bones. Movement does not always occur at

Structure of a synovial joint.

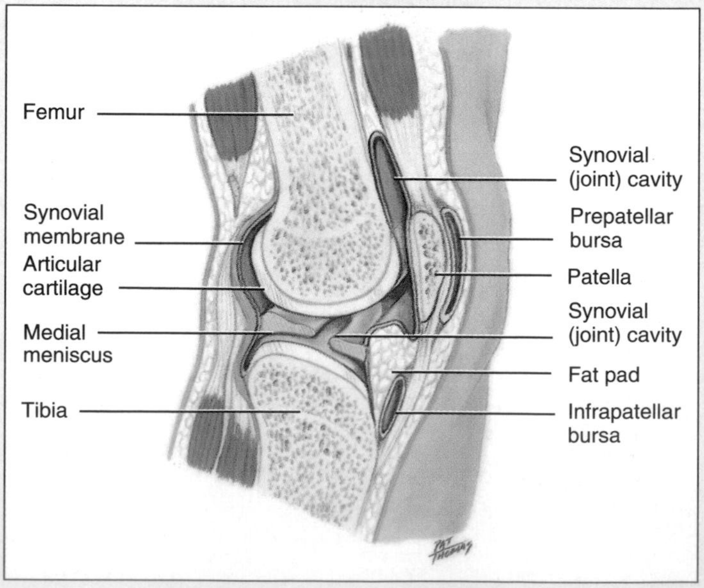

Types of Freely Movable Joints

TYPE	SHAPE OF JOINT SURFACES	RANGE OF MOVEMENT	EXAMPLES
Ball-and-socket	Ball-shaped end of one bone fits into cup-shaped socket of another	Permits widest range of movement in all planes, including rotation	Shoulder, hip
Condyloid	Oval-shaped condyle of one bone fits into elliptical cavity of another	Angular motion but not rotation	Occipital condyles with atlas; metacarpals and metatarsals with phalanges
Saddle	Articulating surfaces of both bones have concave and convex regions; shapes of the two bones complement each other	Permits wide range of movement	Carpometacarpal joint of the thumb is only saddle joint in body
Pivot	Rounded or conical surface of one bone fits into a ring of bone or tendon	Rotation	Joint between the atlas and axis; proximal radioulnar joint
Hinge	Convex projection of one bone fits into concave depression in another	Permits flexion and extension only	Elbow and knee joints
Gliding	Flat or slightly curved surfaces are moving against each other	Sliding or twisting without circular movement	Between the carpals in the wrist and between the tarsals in the ankle

Modified from Applegate, E. J. (1995). *The anatomy and physiology learning system textbook.* Philadelphia: W. B. Saunders Co.

joints. There are three types of joints, classified according to the degree of movement permitted:

- Synarthroses. Immovable joints. Examples include the sutures in the skull and the temporary epiphyseal plate between the epiphysis and diaphysis of a long bone that is still growing.
- Amphiarthroses. Slightly movable joints. Examples include the symphysis pubis and the joints between the vertebrae.
- Diarthroses. Freely movable joints. These are also called synovial joints because they have a joint cavity lined with a synovial membrane. Synovial joints also have a fibrous joint capsule, ligaments that reinforce the capsule, and articular cartilage covering the ends of the opposing bones. Some freely movable joints have bursa, little sacs of synovial membrane filled with synovial fluid, to cushion friction areas. The knee has fibrocartilaginous pads, called the lateral meniscus and medial meniscus, that rest on the tibia to help stabilize the joint and act as shock absorbers. Synovial joints are classified by the shape of the articulating ends of the bones involved.

Movement in diarthrotic articulations is limited only by adjacent structures such as bones, muscles, tendons, ligaments, and the direction of force exerted by the muscles.

THE MUSCULAR SYSTEM

Types of Muscle Tissue

There are three types of muscle tissue in the body; skeletal, visceral, and cardiac. Each type differs from the others in structure, location, and function, but all muscle tissue exhibits characteristics of excitability, contractility, extensibility, and elasticity.

Functions of Skeletal Muscle

Skeletal muscles make up 40 to 50 per cent of body weight. Muscle contraction fulfills four important functions in the body:

- Movement. Nearly all movement in the body is the result of muscle contraction. Exceptions to this are

Summary of Muscle Tissue

FEATURE	SKELETAL	VISCERAL	CARDIAC
Location	Attached to bones	Walls of internal organs and blood vessels	Heart
Function	Produce body movement	Contraction of viscera and blood vessels	Pump blood through the heart and blood vessels
Cell shape	Cylindrical	Spindle-shaped, tapered ends	Cylindrical, branching
Number of nuclei	Many	One	One
Striations	Present	Absent	Present
Type of control	Voluntary	Involuntary	Involuntary

Modified from Applegate, E. J. (1995). *The anatomy and physiology learning system textbook.* Philadelphia: W. B. Saunders Co.

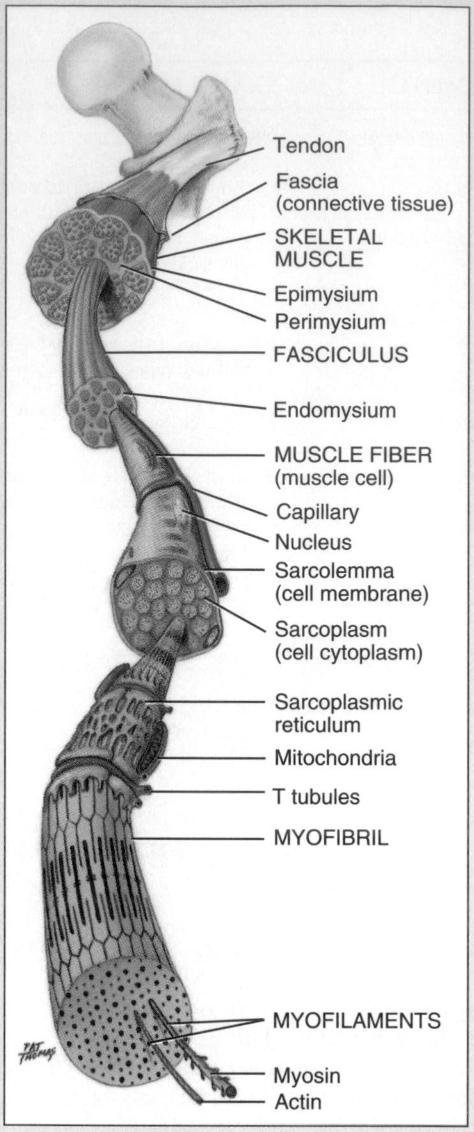

Organization and connective tissue components of skeletal muscle.

the action of cilia and of the flagellum on sperm cells, and the ameboid movement of some white blood cells.

- Posture. The skeletal muscles are continually making fine adjustments that hold the body in position.
- Joint stability. The tendons of many muscles extend over joints and in this way contribute to joint stability.
- Heat production. An important by-product of muscle metabolism is heat production to maintain body temperature. Nearly 85 per cent of the heat produced in the body is the result of muscle contraction.

Organization and Connective Tissue Components of Skeletal Muscle

A whole skeletal muscle is considered an organ of the muscular system. Each organ or muscle consists of skeletal muscle tissue, connective tissue, nerve tissue, and blood or vascular tissue.

An individual skeletal muscle may be made up of hundreds, or even thousands, of muscle fibers bundled together and wrapped in a connective tissue covering. Each muscle is surrounded by a connective tissue sheath called the epimysium. Portions of the epimysium project inward to divide the muscle into compartments, each with a bundle of muscle fibers, called a fasciculus, surrounded by perimysium. Within the fasciculus, each individual muscle fiber (muscle cell) is surrounded by endomysium. The epimysium, perimysium, and endomysium extend beyond the fleshy part of the muscle to form a thick rope-like tendon or a broad, flat sheet-like aponeurosis that forms attachments from muscles to bones or to other muscles. The fixed, or stable, end is called the origin of the muscle, and the more movable attachment is called the insertion.

AGE-RELATED CHANGES

The primary age-related change in the skeletal system is the loss of calcium from the bones in both men and women. Another change is a decrease in the rate of collagen synthesis. This means that the bones have less strength and are more brittle. Bones fracture more readily, and the healing process may be slower or incomplete. Tendons and ligaments are less flexible because of changes in the collagen.

The articular cartilage at the ends of bones tends to become thinner and to deteriorate with age. This leads to joint disorders. People also appear to become shorter as they get older, partially because of loss of bone and muscle mass and partially because of compression of the intervertebral discs.

The loss of muscle mass with age involves a decrease in the number of cells and in the diameter of the remaining fibers. This is accompanied by a corresponding decrease in muscle strength. The decrease in muscle mass and strength varies, depending on the amount of physical activity the person engages in, his or her nutritional state and heredity, and the condition of the motor neurons that supply the muscle tissue. Continued physical activity and good nutrition are probably the best deterrents to age-related changes in the musculoskeletal system.

Chapter 43 Assessment of Clients with Musculoskeletal Disorders

Learning Outcomes

After completing this chapter, the learner will be able to:

1. Assess clients for clinical manifestations of disorders or trauma of the musculoskeletal system.
2. Perform a physical assessment on adult clients appropriate to the musculoskeletal system.
3. Compare assessment findings with the underlying anatomic structures and normal physiologic processes.
4. Use knowledge of diagnostic and laboratory tests when interpreting a client's role in diagnostic and laboratory testing.

Assessment of the musculoskeletal system includes the client's history, physical examination, and diagnostic studies. The health history provides direction for further musculoskeletal system assessment.

HISTORY

The musculoskeletal history includes the client's biographic data, chief complaint (including symptom analysis), medical history, family history, psychosocial history and life-style data, and review of systems. Information is collected to help determine the nature and extent of current disorders. If the client's chief complaint is related to trauma, the history interview is brief and focused on the cause of injury or it may be deferred, depending on the extent of the injury. Once the client's condition is stable, a more complete history is obtained.

Biographic Data

Knowing where the client lives and the kind of transportation used helps the nurse understand the energy expenditure the client needs to keep an appointment. Identifying and getting to know significant others is essential in planning care. The client's age and sex may suggest possible causes for musculoskeletal symptoms.

Chief Complaint

The client is asked to describe the reason for seeking health care. Common symptoms related to the musculoskeletal system include pain, tenderness, muscle tightness, muscle weakness, joint stiffness, cramps, muscle spasms, swelling, redness, deformity, reduced movement or joint range of motion (ROM), sensory changes, and other abnormal sensations. Activities of daily living (ADLs) may be affected. The nurse asks the client and significant others to relate their perceptions of the problem and its cause. Their answers often provide not only information about areas for further assessment but also clues about personal fears and concerns.

PAIN

The client should be asked to point to the pain's exact location. Poorly localized pain is usually associated with blood vessels, joints, fascia, or periosteum. The client should describe the pain. Is it an ache, sharp pain, throbbing? Throbbing pain is usually bone related and aches are often muscular. Sharp pain is associated with fractures and bone infection. The client should describe anything that makes the pain worse, such as temperature changes, movement, lifting, or carrying something heavy. Pain associated with movement is typical of joint problems. Degenerative hip conditions produce pain during weightbearing and during and after walking. Degenerative knee problems produce pain during and after walking. Vertebral disc herniation produces pain on bending or lifting and tends to radiate down one leg or the other. Pain associated with osteoarthritis is worse in cold, damp weather. The client should also be asked whether pain is worse at any particular time of day. For instance, does the pain wake the client up or prevent him or her from sleeping at night? Inflammation of bursae or tendons is worse at night. Degenerative joint pain is often worse at the end of a day. Most musculoskeletal pain is helped by rest. The nurse should determine what medications help relieve the pain. Pain from inflammation is usually helped by aspirin or nonsteroidal anti-inflammatory drugs (NSAIDs). Narcotics are usually required for traumatic injury. The nurse should also ask whether the client has had any recent injuries. Sometimes a client does not relate a fall or other injury with current symptoms. Is the pain associated with chills, fever, rash, or sore throat? Joint pain occurring 10 to 14 days after sore throat may be from rheumatic fever.

JOINT STIFFNESS

The client should be asked to identify the point to which joints are stiff, whether the joints are always stiff, and how long the stiffness lasts. Some conditions, such as ankylosing spondylitis, have remissions and exacerbations. The client should identify what time of day the stiffness is worst. With degenerative joint disease, stiffness is often most severe in the morning after inactivity in bed. The client should describe what relieves the stiffness, such as temperature changes or exercise. Coldness and lack of use generally increase joint stiffness. Heat may reduce muscle spasm. Heat to a recently injured joint may increase stiffness by increasing bleeding into and swelling of the joint. The nurse can ask the client whether the joint locks, and whether the client can hear or feel bones rubbing together. Bone malalignment within a joint causes locking (joint cannot move). Crepitus (sound of bone ends rubbing together) indicates fractures or joint destruction. The client should be asked whether there is pain or weakness in muscles with certain movements. Weakness in muscles may be due to various neuromuscular disorders. It should also be ascertained whether weakness impairs the client's usual activities.

SWELLING

The client should indicate how long the swelling has been present and whether there is also pain. Swelling and pain often accompany bone and muscle injury. With degenerative joint disease, swelling often does not develop for some time, maybe weeks, after pain is present or it may not develop at all. The nurse should determine whether movement is limited by the swelling. Limited movement is associated with soft tissue damage and swelling within a joint. The client should be asked whether rest or elevating the part gives relief. Elevation reduces swelling in acute injuries. The nurse should ask whether the client has had a cast on this body part recently. Removing a cast can precipitate temporary swelling. A casted extremity may have muscle atrophy. The client should also be asked whether the area has been hot or red. Redness and heat indicate inflammation, infection, or recent injury and are not usually present with degenerative conditions.

DEFORMITY AND IMMOBILITY

The nurse should ascertain whether the deformity developed suddenly or gradually, as a gradually developing mass may indicate a tumor. The client should be asked whether movement is limited, whether movement limitation is always present, and whether it is worse after activity. The client should identify any particular body position that makes it worse or better. Immobility from degenerative joint disease varies with the severity of the condition. The client should also describe how the deformity affects his or her daily activities and whether any supportive equipment, such as crutches, a walker, or bandages, are used. Use of such aids indicates the severity of the disability.

SENSORY CHANGES

The client should be asked about a history of back pain or injury. If such a history exists, the client should describe where the pain is located and whether it travels, for example, down the back of the leg. The client should also be asked whether he or she has problems walking, has loss of feeling anywhere, has any tingling or burning sensation, or has loss of feeling associated with pain. Pressure on nerves or blood vessels can occur from swelling, tumors, or fractures, causing sensation loss. Sensory changes may be associated with pain in an arm or hand.

Medical History

CRITICAL TO REMEMBER

The nurse asks the client about a number of past health problems because there are many diseases that can affect the musculoskeletal system.

Both childhood and adult-onset disorders are explored because of the possible long-term effects.

Previous trauma, accidents, or surgery involving bones or joints is carefully assessed. Previous accidents leading to bony fracture may predispose the client to degenerative changes.

CHILDHOOD AND INFECTIOUS DISEASES

Some health conditions affect the musculoskeletal system either directly or indirectly. For example, diabetes may predispose the client to degenerative joint disease. Blood dyscrasias, such as hemophilia, may cause bleeding in joints that produces pain, swelling, tenderness, and deformity. Psoriasis may precede psoriatic arthritis. Trauma producing cartilage damage may precipitate degenerative changes in a relatively young person. The nurse should ask about a history of tuberculosis, poliomyelitis, inflammatory and degenerative arthritis, scurvy, rickets, osteomyelitis, soft tissue infection, fungus infection of bones or joints, and neuromuscular disorders. The nurse should also ask about infections, which can be a source of secondary bacterial infection, such as ears, tonsils, sinuses, genitourinary system, or pelvic inflammatory disease. Detailed information about any of these conditions, if present, should be sought.

IMMUNIZATIONS

CRITICAL TO REMEMBER

The nurse must document the date of the client's last immunizations, especially tetanus and polio. Specifically, the nurse should inquire whether the client has had a tuberculin skin test, the date, and the results.

Some clients may report a history of positive reaction to the purified protein derivative (PPD) test but do not have active tuberculosis. Inoculation with the bacille Calmette-Guérin vaccine usually results in the client having a positive PPD test result from that time on.

MAJOR ILLNESSES AND HOSPITALIZATIONS

In addition to diseases such as diabetes mellitus, tuberculosis, poliomyelitis, and arthritis, the nurse should ask the client about hospitalizations related to musculoskeletal disorders, including trauma. If the client or significant others cannot remember details, the nurse must ask for permission to obtain the medical records. The nurse should ask about past or present minor and major injuries, including the circumstances of the injury, diagnosis of injury, treatment received, duration of treatment, and any current problems resulting from the injury.

Musculoskeletal injury includes fractures, sprains, strains, and joint dislocations. Some injuries are minor and are treated on an ambulatory basis, whereas others are major and require prolonged hospitalization, surgery, or rest and immobilization. The nurse should ask whether the client has any residual impairment from the injury such as a need to use assistive devices (e.g., cane, crutches, or walker) and inquire whether there has been a need to change or adjust ADLs because of lingering limitations.

MEDICATIONS

The client must be questioned carefully about past and present prescription and over-the-counter medications. The nurse should ask the reasons for taking each medication, its dose, frequency, how long it was taken, and any observed side effects. The nurse should ask specifically about medication used for musculoskeletal problems, such as muscle relaxants, salicylates, NSAIDs, and steroids. Some medications affect the musculoskeletal system. For example, corticosteroids can precipitate necrosis of the head of the femur, leading to septic arthritis, and can also precipitate muscle weakness. High doses of anticoagulants can produce hemarthrosis (blood in joints); anticonvulsants may cause osteomalacia; phenothiazines may produce gait disturbances; potassium-depleting diuretics may produce cramps and muscle weakness; and amphetamines and caffeine cause generalized, increased motor activity. For the postmenopausal woman, the nurse should inquire about use of hormone replacement therapy with estrogen, which has been shown to modify the effects of osteoporosis.

FAMILY HISTORY

Genetically related family history is important to identify musculoskeletal problems that have a familial predisposition, such as arthritis, ankylosing spondylitis, gout, Heberden's nodes in osteoarthritis, muscular dystrophy, and scoliosis. Thirty per cent of people with psoriatic arthritis have a family history of psoriasis.

PSYCHOSOCIAL HISTORY AND LIFE-STYLE

The nurse inquires about the client's daily activities and habits. When assessing clients with chronic illnesses and degenerative processes, the nurse asks whether the disorder has affected the client's interactions with others or friends and the client's view of himself or herself. Crippling illnesses often curtail social activity and decrease self-esteem.

DAILY ACTIVITIES

Are there any everyday activities that the client finds difficult or impossible, such as opening containers, pouring liquids, cutting up food; dressing; using zippers; fastening or unfastening buttons, snaps, or hooks; grooming; combing hair; applying make-up; running a bath and testing water temperature; washing the hair; shaving; writing; getting out of the house; climbing stairs; or getting in and out of chairs or cars? The nurse should ask whether there is anything in everyday life the client wants to do that symptoms prevent.

Occupation. The nurse should ask whether a lot of heavy lifting or strenuous activity is typical. This can cause muscle strain, degenerative vertebral disc problems, and other trauma. Low back pain can arise from jobs involving a lot of driving. Habitually carrying heavy objects, such as a mail bag, shoulder bag, attaché case, or other equipment, causes musculoskeletal problems by placing uneven pressure on the spinal column.

Habits. The client's habits and life-style can increase the risk of developing musculoskeletal disorders. Similarly, musculoskeletal impairment affects the ability to perform ADLs. The nurse documents details of the client's typical recreational activities and exercise pattern. Lack of exercise produces poor muscle tone, which leads to muscle strain. Sporadic exercise in poorly toned muscles causes muscle injury and spasm. In addition, the lack of warm-up increases the likelihood of injury. Fractures and other trauma can arise from contact sports, such as football and hockey. Achilles tendon damage can arise from improperly landing on the heels while jogging. Pain in arm joints can arise from racket sports such as tennis and squash, which require a strong grasp, wrist extension, and forearm rotation. The nurse should ask about typical footwear. High-heeled shoes can shorten the Achilles tendons and pitch the center of gravity forward, leading to lordosis.

The nurse should try to ascertain the client's attention to safety by asking about safety practices at work and at home. Does the client use the recommended equipment for recreational activities, such as correct shoes? Does the client wear safety goggles when using power tools or scraping paint?

CRITICAL TO REMEMBER

There is a high incidence of accidental injury among people who pay little attention to safety practices.

Dietary history is important to provide clues to musculoskeletal problems. For example, obesity stresses weightbearing joints and predisposes the client to ligamentous instability, particularly of the lower back. Poor calcium intake can precipitate fractures as a result of bone decalcification. The nurse should ask the client to list foods eaten on a typical day. Dietary history forms help with dietary assessment and teaching. Adequate dietary intake of vitamins A and D, calcium, and protein is important for musculoskeletal health. The nurse should ask about recent major weight changes. Excessive weight gain can place stress on the musculoskeletal system.

Review of Systems

The nurse asks the client about problems such as muscle pain, spasm, or tenderness; joint pain, stiffness, swelling, or redness; weakness; limited movement; clumsiness; crepitus; backache; and changes in joints or bones. Each reported problem is investigated with a symptom analysis as well as an inquiry about the effect the problem has had on the client's ability to perform ADLs.

Assessment findings from other body systems sometimes indicate musculoskeletal problems. For example, (1) pain or burning when urinating is associated with Reiter's syndrome; (2) cardiovascular symptoms such as tachycardia and hypertension may accompany gout; (3) chronic diarrhea may occur when arthritis is associated with colitis or other gastrointestinal problems; (4) conjunctivitis may indicate Reiter's syndrome, and nongranulomatous uveitis may occur with ankylosing spondylitis; (5) skin changes may indicate musculoskeletal problems (e.g., dry skin over thumb and first two fingers with carpal tunnel syndrome); (6) cramping leg pain on activity may signal intermittent claudication; (7) generalized muscle cramping may result from electrolyte imbalances; and (8) joint pain associated with recent chills, fever, or sore throat may be due to rheumatic fever.

PHYSICAL EXAMINATION

During musculoskeletal assessment, the client should sit, stand, and walk (unless any position is contraindicated by the client's condition).

The musculoskeletal assessment includes inspection and palpation of muscle masses for symmetry, involuntary movements, tenderness, tone, and strength; joints for symmetry, crepitus, tenderness or pain, and ROM; and bones for deformity.

General Musculoskeletal Examination

Using inspection and palpation, the nurse should examine each body part. The body must be first examined at rest. Then ROM and muscle strength must be assessed.

First while the client sits on the edge of the examining table, the nurse looks at the client's general appearance and body build and examines the head, neck, shoulders, and upper extremities.

Then with the client standing, the nurse examines the chest, back, and ilium. The nurse should observe posture; body build; body contours; body alignment; and the cervical, thoracic, and lumbar spine. Also the nurse should observe the relationships of various body parts to each other (e.g., relationship of feet to legs, legs to hips, and hips to pelvis). The nurse should ask the client to walk and observe gait, body mobility, joint motion. While observing movement and gait, the nurse watches for gait patterns associated with specific disorders, objective evidence of discomfort, indications of joint stiffness or muscle weakness, lack of coordination, or deformities. The nurse should observe the client's stance and note any spinal deformities (Fig. 43–1), such as (1) kyphosis (abnormally increased roundness of the thoracic curve) (Fig. 43–1*A*); (2) scoliosis (an obvious lateral deformity of the spine) (Fig. 43–1*B*); or (3) lordosis (abnormal increase in the lumbar curve) (Fig. 43–1*C*). Other observable abnormalities include genu varum, that is, "bowed" legs (Fig. 43–1*D*), and genu valgum, that is, "knock-knees" (Fig. 43–1*E*). The terms "varus(-um)" and "valgus(-um)" refer to the direction in which the apex of a deformity lies in relation to the midline. In other words, with a varus deformity the apex of the deformity points away from the midline. With a valgus deformity it points toward the midline. These terms are used to describe the direction of a deformity in any body region.

Last, while the client lies supine, the nurse examines the hips, knees, ankles, and feet.

MUSCLES

The nurse compares each muscle group with its contralateral side. Muscles should be free of *fasciculations* (fine muscle twitches) and smooth, without bulges or lumps. The nurse palpates muscle groups gently, from a proximal to distal direction, feeling the *muscle tone* (i.e., the state of tension in a muscle at rest, which is felt as firmness). Muscles should feel firm, smooth, and bilaterally equal in size and be nontender.

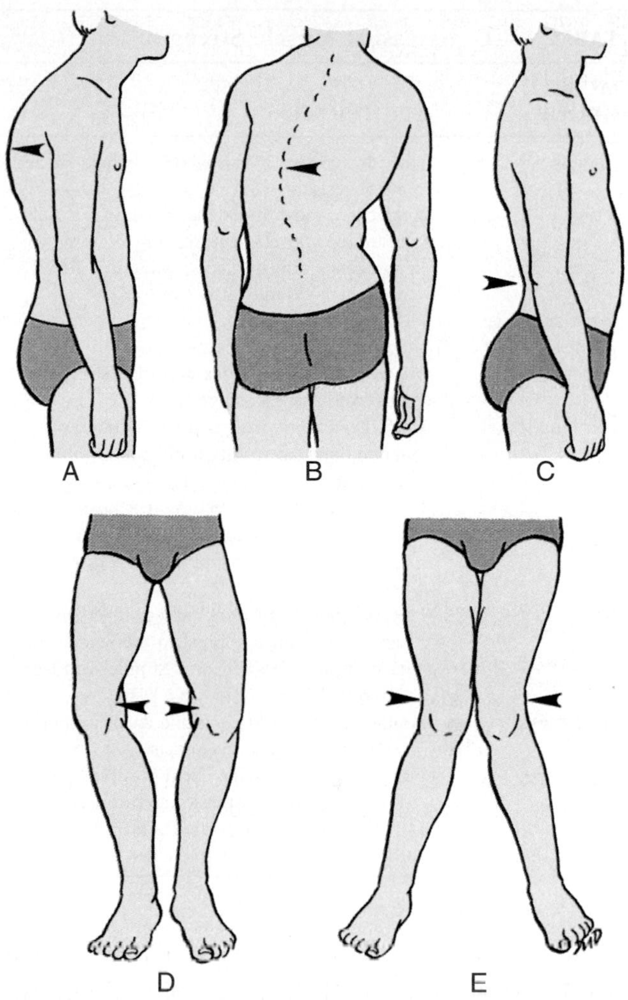

Figure 43–1
Musculoskeletal deformities observable during assessment. *A*, Kyphosis. *B*, Scoliosis. *C*, Lordosis. *D*, Genu varum. *E*, Genu valgum. *Arrowheads* indicate the deformities.

CRITICAL TO REMEMBER

A slight increase in mass or hypertrophy on the dominant side is normal, whereas atrophy, or decreased muscle size, on either side is abnormal.

If muscle groups are noticeably asymmetric in size, a tape measure can be used to assess limb circumference. Differences of 1 cm or less are considered within normal variation.

The nurse should assess *muscle strength* while putting the client's joints through active ROM. If detailed assessment of muscle strength is necessary, each major muscle group can be assessed separately. The nurse should follow the guidelines in Table 43–1. (The sternocleidomastoid and trapezius muscles are tested as part of the head and neck [i.e., cranial nerve] examination and are omitted from the table.) The nurse tests muscle strength by asking the client to repeat ROM

TABLE 43–1 Assessing Muscle Strength

MUSCLE GROUP	TECHNIQUE
Deltoid	Push down client's arm while it is held up and client resists
Biceps	Hold client's arm in extension while it is fully extended and client flexes arm
Triceps	Keep client's arm in flexion while it is flexed and client extends arm
Wrist and finger muscles	Push client's fingers together while client spreads them and resists
Grip strength	Try to pull crossed index and middle fingers out from the client's grasp
Hip muscles	Hold down client's leg while it is fully extended and client lifts it off the table (client is supine)
Hip abduction	Prevent client from spreading legs apart against resistance applied to the lateral surface of the knees (client is supine with legs extended)
Hip adduction	Prevent client from bringing legs together against resistance applied to the medial surface of the knees (client is supine with legs extended)
Hamstrings	Straighten client's knees while client is supine with knees flexed and resists
Quadriceps	Flex client's knee while client is supine with knee partially in extension and resists
Ankle and foot muscles	Dorsiflex client's foot while client resists. Plantar flex client's foot while client resists

while resistance is applied and notes the strength the client uses against the resistance. If there is weakness, the nurse should decrease the resistance. Because the dominant arm is usually stronger, the nurse should ask whether the client is right- or left-handed.

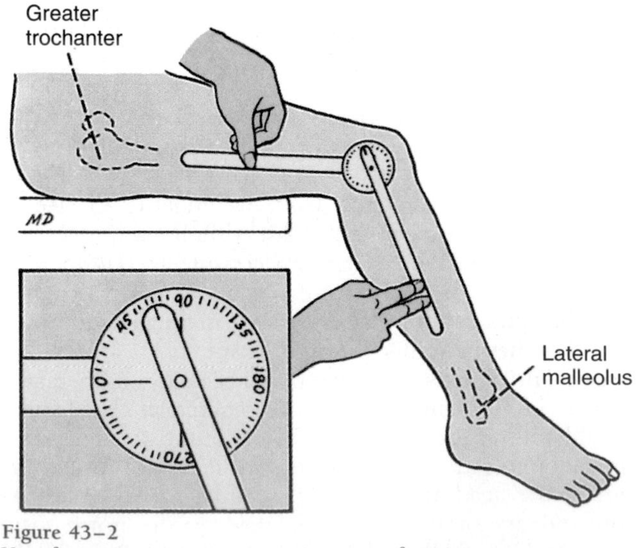

Figure 43–2
Use of a goniometer to measure joint range of motion.

Joints and Bones

The nurse inspects the joints and bones and compares findings bilaterally. They should be symmetric and without redness, swelling, enlargement, or deformity. Each joint and bone is palpated for edema and tenderness, which should be absent. The joints also are palpated as they move for *crepitus* (grating sound or feeling), which is abnormal. Joints should feel smooth as they move, and nodules should not be present. ROM is the maximum amount of movement that a healthy joint is capable of. ROM is measured with a goniometer, which is based on the degrees of a circle (Fig. 43–2). This flexible, protractor type of instrument is placed on a joint to measure the angles created by joint movement. Figure 43–3 displays the joints that are assessed and the types and degrees of ROM possible.

DIAGNOSTIC TESTS

Roentgenography (X-Ray Studies, Radiography)

Roentgenography is the most widely used musculoskeletal diagnostic procedure. X-ray examinations are important to establish the presence of a musculoskeletal problem, follow its progress, and evaluate treatment effectiveness. A plain x-ray film is common, usually from an anteroposterior or lateral view. Common views include a notch (posterior or less commonly anterior) view of the knee in flexion, oblique (45-degree angle) view and a sunrise or patella view of the underside of the patella. The client is asked to remove any radiopaque objects that could appear on the x-ray film, such as jewelry. No additional preparation is needed except possibly analgesics for some clients. If possible, the client may be asked to move into various positions so that x-ray films may be taken from the most useful angles. This may be difficult or painful. X-ray tables are very hard. Analgesia and other pain-relieving interventions may be needed after x-ray.

Studies Using Contrast. Other specialized radiographic procedures allow more precise visualization. An arthrogram is a radiographic examination of soft tissue joint structures. It is used to diagnose trauma to joint capsules or supporting ligaments especially involving the shoulder, wrist, hip, ankle, or knee. Under local anesthesia, a contrast medium or air is injected into the joint cavity using aseptic precautions. The joint is moved through ROM as a series of x-ray films is taken.

The nurse should (1) explain the procedure to the client and significant others and answer their questions; (2) explain that the procedure may take up to an hour (follow-up x-rays are sometimes taken 30 minutes after the injection) and that the client will need to remain as still as possible except when asked to reposition; (3) ask whether the client has any allergies, especially to local anesthetics, iodine, seafood, or contrast; (4) suggest that the client void before the procedure to be

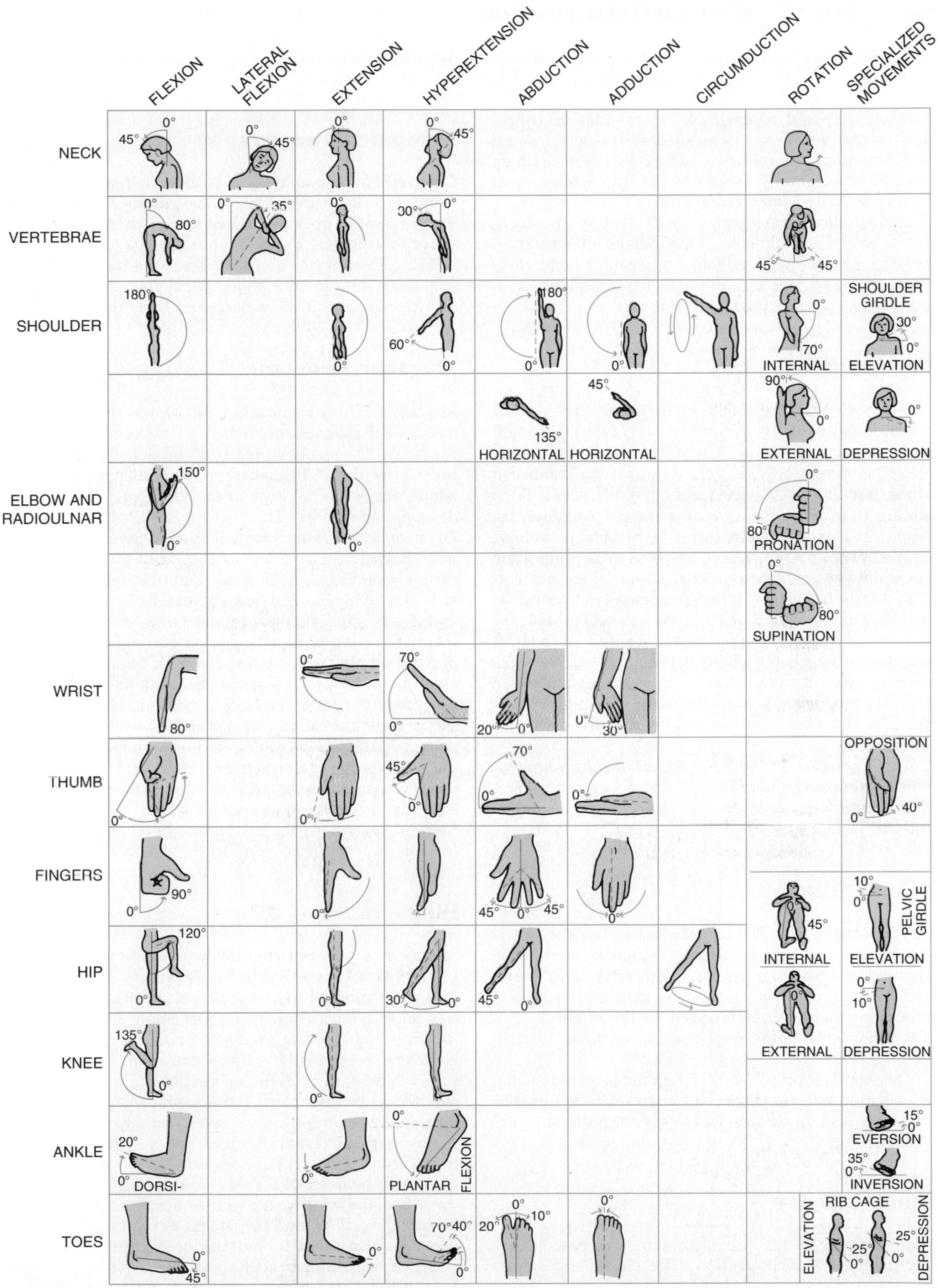

Figure 43–3
Joint range of motion (ROM). All joints are at 0 degrees when in anatomic position. ROM begins at 0 degrees, as shown by solid lines. Attainment of the average ROM is shown by dotted lines and the number of the degrees in the angle formed by the two lines. Shoulder flexion and abduction to 180 degrees include scapular motions. Hip flexion to 120 degrees is with the knee flexed.

comfortable; and (5) advise the client that the joint may be uncomfortable for 1 to 2 days afterward and to avoid strenuous exercise.

Sinography and myelography are similar to arthrograms in that a contrast is injected and x-ray films are taken. Sinography examines sinus tracks (deep draining wounds). Myelography examines the spinal cord so as to detect herniated intervertebral discs.

Tomography. *Tomograms* (body section roentgenograms) are x-ray films showing details of structures otherwise hidden by overlying, radiopaque bone. This technique allows views of tissue at various planes as if slices had been made through the tissue.

Bone Scanning

Radioisotopes that are taken up by bone are injected intravenously (usually technetium ^{99m}Tc). This substance migrates to bone. The whole body is usually scanned, although only an extremity may be scanned if a stress fracture is suspected (i.e., pinhole scan). Bone scanning is used to detect malignancies, osteomyelitis, osteoporosis, and some fractures (especially pathologic fractures). The isotope collects in these areas, indicating abnormal bone metabolism. The isotope does not collect in poorly perfused bone. The nurse (1) explains the procedure to the client and significant others and answers their questions; the procedure takes about 1 hour, during which the client lies supine; (2) reassures the client that the procedure is not painful and there are no harmful effects from the isotopes; and (3) suggests that the client urinate before the procedure for comfort.

After the scan, no special precautions are required. There is minimal radioactivity in the isotope and therefore no hazard to the nurse. The isotope is excreted in urine and feces.

Gallium Scan

Gallium scans are similar to bone scans, but the test is more specific to bone disorders. Gallium is the isotope used, and it also migrates to brain, liver, and breast tissue. Gallium is taken up by bone more slowly than is technetium; therefore, it is given to the client 2 to 3 hours before the scan by a nuclear medicine technician.

The scan requires 30 to 60 minutes to complete. Mild sedation may be needed for clients who are in pain or who are restless or elderly. No special follow-up care is required.

Indium Imaging

Indium imaging is the use of indium tagged to leukocytes to detect bone infection. The clients' leukocytes are separated from a sample of blood and labeled (tagged) with indium. The tagged cells are reinjected. They accumulate in areas of bone infection and can be detected on scanning. No special preparation or follow-up care is necessary.

Computed Tomography

Computed tomography (CT) scans use both x-rays and computers for three-dimensional physical assessment. Images appear on a computer screen in cross-sectional views. A complete examination takes 10 to 30 views or slides. CT scans are useful in assessing some bone and soft tissue tumors and some spinal fractures. This procedure takes about 30 minutes per body part.

Magnetic Resonance Imaging

Magnetic resonance imaging (MRI) is a tissue-imaging device that assesses the density of hydrogen protons in the body. Because bone marrow and soft tissue are high in hydrogen, MRI facilitates the early diagnosis of many conditions, such as knee problems, degenerative bone disease, and tumors. The client is slid inside a horizontal cylinder (a giant solenoid) and exposed to a magnetic field that is roughly 15,000 times greater than the earth's natural magnetic field. Radio waves knock protons out of their polarized alignment. When the radio waves are shut off, the protons swing back into alignment, releasing a measurable amount of energy. This process allows MRI to make rapid, detailed, and efficient pictures of body tissue. The nurse (1) explains the procedure to the client and significant others and answers their questions (they may be anxious about the new procedure; if possible, the nurse should show them the equipment); (2) reassures the client that no discomfort is experienced with this procedure; (3) explains that the procedure takes about 15 to 20 minutes per body part; and (4) suggests that the client urinate before the procedure for comfort.

Biopsy

A biopsy is the removal and histologic examination of tissue for diagnostic purposes. Disorders such as infection and cancer of the bone and atrophy and inflammation of the muscle are detected. Bone or muscle may undergo biopsy during surgery or through a needle or bore not requiring a surgical incision. The latter is called aspiration, punch, or needle biopsy. Sometimes aspiration biopsy with radiographic control is performed. Bone biopsies are taken in the radiology department or an operating room under sterile conditions to prevent osteomyelitis. Local anesthesia is used. Bone or muscle biopsies take about 30 minutes.

After the biopsy the nurse monitors the site for bleeding, swelling, and hematoma development. Because dressings usually surround the biopsy site, assessment is performed through analysis of the client's pain. Mild to moderate discomfort is usual; more severe levels of pain may signal complications. The biopsy site is elevated for 24 hours to reduce edema. Vital signs are monitored every 4 hours for 24 hours. A mild analgesic is usually required. Ongoing assessments of the site for signs of infection are performed by the nurse or client when discharged.

Arthroscopy

Arthroscopy is common and a very useful diagnostic tool. An arthroscope is a small fiberoptic instrument that allows endoscopic examination of various joints, including the hip, knee, shoulder, elbow, and wrist, without making a large incision into the joint. Arthroscopy is usually an outpatient procedure performed under local anesthesia. The client is usually home and returned to work sooner than if an arthrotomy (opening the joint) were performed. Arthroscopy is contraindicated in clients whose joint flexion is less than 50 per cent (e.g., in fibrous ankylosis) or if skin or wound infection is present at the site. Complications are rare but include infection, hemarthrosis (blood in the joint), swelling, synovial rupture, joint injury, or thrombophlebitis.

Nursing Management

The nurse explains the procedure to the client and significant others and answers their questions.

The client is instructed to fast from midnight the night before. The nurse should be sure the client and significant others know where the procedure will be performed and by whom and that appropriate consent forms are understood and signed. If a local anesthetic will be used, the client must be told that there may be mild discomfort as it is administered and a thumping sensation may be felt as the arthroscope is inserted. The nurse teaches the client to watch for indications of postprocedure infection, such as temperature elevation and local inflammation at the incision site, and to report this promptly. The nurse should also ensure necessary pain relief after the procedure. The client should be told that a normal diet may be resumed as soon as desired and advised that, unless surgical excision is performed and the surgeon gives specific instructions, walking is usually permitted after sensation has returned but excessive exercise should be avoided for a few days.

Arthrocentesis

Arthrocentesis is a method of aspirating synovial fluid, blood, or pus via a needle inserted into the joint cavity. It is used to diagnose rheumatoid arthritis and other inflammatory conditions or to remove fluid to relieve pain. The procedure is done under local anesthesia with aseptic precautions. Medication may be instilled into the joint if necessary, such as to alleviate inflammation. A compression bandage is applied after arthrocentesis and the joint is rested for 8 to 24 hours.

Electromyography

Electromyography (EMG) is used to assess lower motor neuron lesions. It measures the electrical potential associated with skeletal muscle contractions. Needles are inserted into muscles. Recordings of muscular electrical activity are then traced on an audiotransmitter, on an oscilloscope, and on recording paper. EMG helps diagnose neuromuscular conditions.

Nurses explain the procedure to the client and significant others, teach that needle insertion is uncomfortable, and instruct the person not to take any stimulants or sedatives for 24 hours before the procedure.

Bone Mineral Content

Methods used to measure bone density are performed to diagnose osteoporosis, because the condition is not

TABLE 43–2 Common Laboratory Studies Used in Diagnosing Musculoskeletal Conditions

TEST/NORMAL VALUE	SIGNIFICANCE OF RESULTS
Erythrocyte sedimentation rate Normal: Westergren's method: men, 0–15 mm/hr women, 0–20 mm/hr Wintrobe's method: men, 0–9 mm/hr women, 0–15 mm/hr	Elevations common in arthritic conditions, infection, inflammation, cancer, cell or tissue destruction
Mineral Metabolism	
Calcium 8.0–10.5 mg/dL or 4.5–5.5 mEq/L	Decreased levels found in osteomalacia, osteoporosis Increased levels found in bone tumors, Paget's disease, healing fractures
Alkaline phosphatase 30–90 IU/L	Elevations found in bone cancer, osteoporosis, osteomalacia, Paget's disease
Phosphorus 2.5–4.0 mg/dL	Increased levels found in healing fractures, osteolytic metastatic tumor diseases
Muscle Enzymes	
Aldolase A 1.3–8.2 U/dL	Elevations in muscular dystrophy, dermatomyositis
Aspartate aminotransferase 10–50 mU/mL	Found in skeletal muscle but primarily heart and renal cells
Creatine phosphokinase 15–150 IU/L	Increased levels found in traumatic injuries, progressive muscular dystrophy, polymyositis
Lactate dehydrogenase (LDH_4, LDH_5) 60–150 IU/L	Elevations in skeletal muscle necrosis, extensive cancer, progressive muscular dystrophy

evident on x-ray study until 30 to 50 per cent of the bone mass is lost. One method of measuring bone mass is the use of single-photon absorptiometry. This technique measures the amount of radioisotopes absorbed by the bone. The radioisotope is passed beneath a bone, usually the forearm, and the amount is read from above the arm by a detector. The test takes about 10 minutes. Several other techniques can detect osteoporosis in other sites, such as the spine and hips. No preparation is required; the client may require teaching about osteoporosis once the findings are known.

Laboratory Tests

Table 43–2 lists the most common laboratory tests for clients with musculoskeletal disorders. Chapter 11 includes laboratory tests specific for rheumatic problems.

STUDY QUESTIONS

1. A client's chief complaint is "swelling of the right elbow." To determine whether or not the client has sustained an acute injury, which of the following questions should the nurse ask?
   A. "Is your movement limited by the swelling?"
   B. "Does keeping the elbow dependent reduce the swelling?"
   C. "Does exercise reduce the swelling?"
   D. "Has the swelling been accompanied by a tingling sensation?"
2. Which of the following physical findings would be considered normal when assessing a client's muscles?
   A. Hypertrophy of the muscles on the client's dominant side
   B. A difference of 2 cm in circumference of muscle groups from one side of the body to the other
   C. Palpable fasciculations in a muscle group
   D. Palpable soft muscle groups
3. Which of the following physical findings would the nurse expect to see when performing a musculoskeletal assessment on clients older than 65 years?
   A. Decreased excursion of the chest wall during inspiration
   B. Elongation of the vertebral column when standing erect
   C. Normal muscle strength in legs, diminished strength in arm muscles
   D. Nodules on metatarsals and metacarpals
4. A client is scheduled to undergo an arthrocentesis. When instructing the client about this procedure, the nurse should teach the client to expect:
   A. Rest of the joint for 48 hours
   B. Moist heat applied to the joint for several days
   C. Compression bandage applied to the joint
   D. Cold compresses for 72 hours
5. A nurse is obtaining a history from a woman who is menopausal. The woman's diet is deficient in calcium, and she is overweight and participates in no regular exercise. Considering her history, the nurse should ask the client whether she is currently taking which of the following drugs that would adversely affect her present condition?
   A. Anticoagulants
   B. Antihypertensives
   C. Antihistamines
   D. Anticonvulsants

CRITICAL THINKING EXERCISES

SCENARIO A

An elderly client who is "hard of hearing" and has diminished eyesight requires an assessment of his musculoskeletal system. He uses a cane because of an unsteady gait.

1. How would you modify your questions when gathering subjective data?
2. How would you modify your physical examination?

SCENARIO B

You belong to a women's health spa. As a health-care professional, you are asked to address the clients concerning healthy exercise and diet habits specific to good muscle and skeletal health. A 40-year-old woman asks you to give her some advice about how to regulate her diet and exercise so that her muscles and joints will remain healthy. What is your advice?

BIBLIOGRAPHY

1. Bryan, V. (1990). Troubleshooting arthroscopic equipment. *Orthopaedic Nursing, 9(1),* 18–25.
2. Jarvis, C. (1992). *Physical examination and health assessment.* Philadelphia: W. B. Saunders.
3. Mourad, L. (1991). *Orthopedic disorders.* St. Louis: C. V. Mosby.
4. Pavlik, M. (1991). Measuring bone mineral content. *Orthopaedic Nursing, 10(2),* 39–42.

5. Peters, V., & Ferkel, R. (1989). Arthroscopic surgery of the ankle. *Orthopaedic Nursing, 8*(5), 12–19.

6. Schoen, D. (1988). Assessment for arthritis. *Orthopaedic Nursing, 7*(2), 31–39.

7. Swartz, M. (1994). *Textbook of physical diagnosis* (2nd ed.). Philadelphia: W. B. Saunders.

8. Williams, M. (1992). *Nutrition for fitness and sport* (3rd ed.). Dubuque, IA: W. C. Brown.

9. Zubay, R. (1988). Understanding magnetic resonance imaging from a nursing perspective. *Orthopaedic Nursing, 7*(6), 17–23.

Chapter 44

Common Musculoskeletal Interventions

Learning Outcomes

After completing this chapter, the learner will be able to:

1. Assess the client for clinical manifestations resulting from common musculoskeletal interventions.
2. Teach the client about the risk factors, basic pathophysiology, and clinical manifestations associated with common musculoskeletal interventions.
3. Explain the client's role in the application of musculoskeletal interventions.
4. Develop plans of care for the prevention of injury and management, and rehabilitation of clients undergoing musculoskeletal interventions.
5. Implement nursing interventions that optimize the quality of life for clients with musculoskeletal interventions.
6. Evaluate planned client outcomes using outcome criteria developed in the planning phase of care.

Orthopedic interventions are some of the oldest recorded areas of medical practice. The nurse treating the client with musculoskeletal disorders is challenged to deal with traditional methods and to stay current with change. All interventions challenge the nurse to plan care that promotes independence and a return to self-care.

Rest

Rest is an essential intervention for many clients with musculoskeletal problems. After trauma or for clients with rheumatic disorders, rest promotes healing and minimizes inflammation, swelling, and pain. Rest is sometimes achieved by immobilizing affected joints with splints or casts. Splints prevent joint deformities and minimize pain by relieving muscle spasms.

Unfortunately, however, bone, joint, and muscle deconditioning occurs. The bone demineralization that occurs with immobility appears to be secondary to decreased stress on bones. Decreased range of motion (ROM) results from an increased density of connective tissue around the joint. Muscle mass is also decreased by immobility. This deconditioning process is normal during prolonged immobilization. Use of physical therapy and nursing interventions are essential to avoid the problems associated with deconditioning.

Traction

Therapeutic traction (pull) is accomplished by exerting a pull (on the head, body, or limbs) in two directions, that is, pull of traction and pull of countertraction. Traction often is produced by weights. Countertraction may be produced with either the person's body weight or other weights. The traction and countertraction must be equal to be therapeutic.

When using traction, it is important to (1) support and stretch the extremity in a direction that properly aligns bone fragments (traction is exerted on the distal fragment to align it with the proximal fragment), (2) not overstretch the limb (overstretching excessively distracts bone fragments), and (3) maintain stretching forces that are constant in amount and direction until bone union occurs.

When traction is properly applied in bed, the person is centered in the bed and the affected part is held aligned by a constant two-way pull. When applied to a long bone, the direction of traction is in line with the bone's long axis. When applied to the head or pelvis, the pull is in line with the person's spinal column. The bed is usually elevated or tilted under the part in traction; for example, the foot of the bed may be elevated when traction is applied to lower extremities. If the bed is not properly tilted, countertraction from the client's body weight is inadequate. Then the person tends to slide in the direction of the traction force. This defeats the purpose of the traction apparatus, and effective traction is not achieved on the injured part. With some types of traction, countertraction is applied with ropes, pulleys, and weights pulling in a direction opposite to that of the traction. The purposes of traction are listed in Box 44–1.

BOX 44-1

Purposes of Traction

- Reduce fractures and dislocations and maintain alignment
- Decrease muscle spasms and relieve pain
- Correct, lessen, or prevent deformities
- Promote rest of an injured part
- Promote exercise

METHODS OF APPLYING TRACTION

Traction may be applied (1) manually, by pulling on the body part with the hands; (2) mechanically, by exerting a pull on the body part with ropes and pulleys; (3) with devices inserted in casts (plaster traction); or (4) with braces (e.g., hyperextension braces).

Major disadvantages of most types of traction are that prolonged hospitalization and bedrest are necessary. Advantages of traction include (1) a greater potential for exercising joints and muscles than is possible with casts and (2) elimination of the need for surgery and its risks.

TRACTION TECHNIQUES

Continuous Versus Intermittent Traction

Traction may be continuous (constant pull) or intermittent (pull periodically relieved by lifting the weights). Continuous traction typically is used to treat some fractures or dislocations. Intermittent traction may be used to treat arthritis (e.g., to reduce flexion contractures) or low back disorders (e.g., to reduce pain and muscle spasm). One must always assume that traction is continuous unless the physician specifically states it should be intermittent.

Running Versus Suspension Traction

Running traction (straight traction) exerts a direct pull on the affected part without a hammock or splint to provide balanced support. It pulls in one plane and may be unilateral or bilateral. Running traction may be applied to the skin (skin traction) or skeleton (skeletal traction).

Suspension traction (balanced traction) exerts a pull on the affected part and also supports the extremity in a hammock or splint held in place by balanced weights attached to an overhead bar (Fig. 44–1). Countertraction is supplied by a system of ropes, pulleys, and weights. With suspension traction, the pull remains the same even when the person moves because countertraction takes up any slack caused by the movement. Thus, suspension traction allows more movement and activity than does running traction.

Suspension traction may be either skeletal or skin and may use any type of splint or hammock. Examples of suspension traction are illustrated in Figure 44–1*B*. The traction must be continuous to be effective.

Skin Traction

Skin traction applies traction to the underlying skeletal system and other structures, such as muscles. It may be applied by using commercially prepared adhesive backed materials or encircling a body part with a halter, corset, or sling. A halter may be used to apply traction to the head, and a corset or sling may be used to apply traction to the pelvis. An anklet or bandage may be used with a splint to apply temporary traction to the ankle. Countertraction is provided by the person's weight when the bed is tilted down toward the head.

Skeletal Traction

Skeletal traction is accomplished by surgically inserting metal wires (Kirchner wires) or pins (Steinmann pins) through bones or by anchoring metal tongs (Crutchfield, Barton, or Vinke tongs) in the skull. The traction apparatus is then attached to the metal insertion. Skeletal traction applied to the skull is discussed in Chapter 16. Kirschner wires and Steinmann pins are round stainless steel rods typically inserted (with a drill) perpendicular to and completely through bones. A traction bow is attached to the wire or pin and the traction force is applied to the bow (also called spreader,

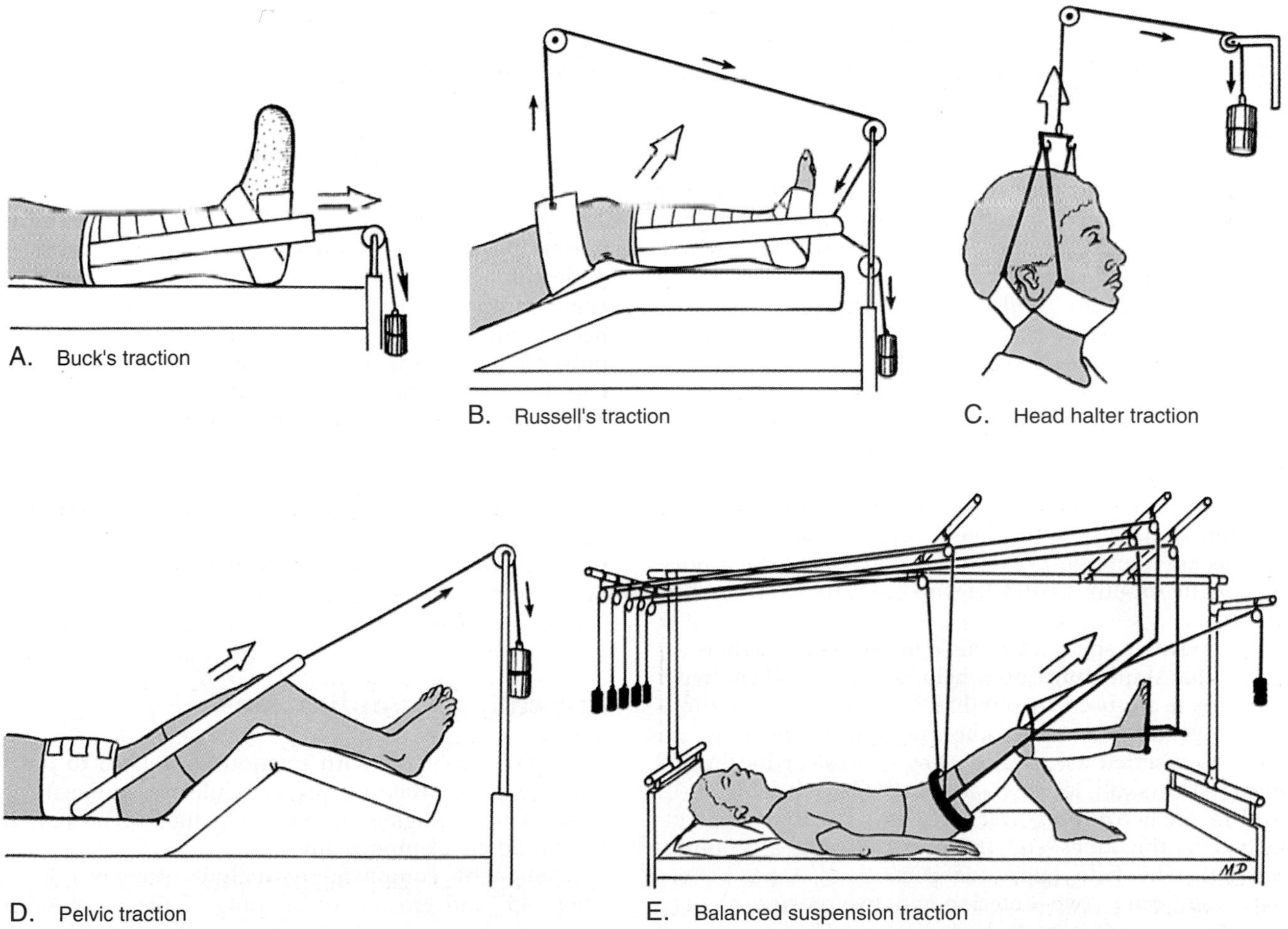

Figure 44–1
Some common types of traction used in treating musculoskeletal problems. Solid arrows show pull on cables; open arrows show traction pull on body.

stirrups, or calipers). The insertion site of pins, wires, or tongs determines the location where traction force is applied.

Wires and pins are not inserted through joints. They are inserted so that they only penetrate skin, subcutaneous tissue, and bone. Joints, muscles, tendons, arteries, and nerves are avoided. Inserting skeletal pins or wires is a sterile procedure performed under local or general anesthesia. Because the skin is opened for the placement of wires and pins, bone infection (osteomyelitis) is a potential complication.

Skeletal traction is used to reduce unstable fractures of long bones until the client is able to undergo more definitive surgical treatment, such as insertion of intramedullary nails and various plates.

TYPES OF TRACTION

Buck's Traction

Buck's traction is a form of skin traction exerted by a straight pull on one or both legs. It may be used to immobilize a limb for a short time (e.g., a fractured hip prior to internal surgical fixation) or to reduce muscle spasm. Buck's extension is contraindicated for people with diabetic gangrene, stasis dermatitis, arteriosclerosis, serious varicosities, or leg ulcers. Buck's traction is applied by using a prefabricated boot. The boot should encase the lower leg to 1 to 2 inches below the knee, and the ankle movement should not be restricted. The client should be able to move his ankle in the boot. The traction should be continuous unless otherwise stated. If the weights must be removed, manual traction should be applied until the weights are replaced.

Cervical Traction

Cervical traction is used to hold the head in extension to treat muscle sprains, strain, and spasm. Cervical traction is usually applied with a head halter. Cervical sprains are common because there are many small muscles with multiple attachments around the cervical spine.

Cervical traction can also be skeletal traction, as used with skull tongs or a halo apparatus. These types of traction are used to stabilize fractures or dislocations of the cervical or upper thoracic spine. The tongs or pins are inserted aseptically using general or local anesthesia. The skull tongs (Gardner-Wells, Crutchfield, or Vinke) are a running traction device with weight attached to the tongs and the client is used as countertraction. The halo apparatus consists of a head piece with four pins (two anterior and two posterior). The headpiece attaches to a body jacket. The purpose of halo traction is immobilization.

Pelvic Traction

Pelvic traction is accomplished with a belt applied just above and encircling the iliac crests. The belt attaches to a spreader bar and pulley system. Traction is applied to the lumbar spine. Some physicians order pillows beneath the legs; others want the foot of the bed elevated. The most desirable position is the Williams position (hips and knees each flexed 30 degrees). An overhead trapeze helps the person lift up off the bed. A snug-fitting pelvic belt ensures adequate traction. Pelvic traction should not increase a person's back or leg pain. If it does so, the nurse must notify the physician. Pelvic traction is most often intermittent but can be continuous.

Russell's Traction

Russell's traction is a modification of Buck's traction. Russell's traction adds a vertical pull by placing a sling under the leg above the knee. Russell's traction can be used for fractures of the tibial plateau in adults or, less commonly, for hip contractures or fractures.

MANAGEMENT

Maintaining Vector of Force

The goal of traction is to return bone fragments to their normal position. Sometimes bones must be turned and pulled into alignment so that they can heal and the client can gain complete function and return to his or her preinjury appearance. To return the bones to the proper position, various forces are applied to the bone. One force pulls the extremity distally (also to counteract muscle spasms), and the countertraction pulls the opposite way. A third force is the position (e.g., flexion of knee and hip). These forces combine to create the exact direction of pull along the long axis of the bone; this process is called the vector of force. It is imperative that the position of the pulleys and the angle of splints not be adjusted without physician direction.

Preventing Complications

Short-term problems with traction are related to immobility (e.g., pneumonia, pressure ulcers) and malalignment of bony fragments. Nurses reduce or prevent the complications of immobility.

Long-term complications include osteomyelitis (see Chap. 45) and erosion or slipping of the pin resulting from excess weight. If the pin moves, it can be reinserted if needed.

Removing Traction

When skeletal traction is to be removed, the nurse must prepare the skin around the pin site according to the physician's instructions. A physician removes the wire. The nurse covers the skin insertion and exit incisions with small sterile dressings. Clients will often be placed in a cast to allow complete bone healing.

Nursing Management

When planning nursing intervention for people in traction, it is important to know (1) the nature of the injury, (2) the purpose of the traction, (3) how the traction device accomplishes its purpose, (4) permitted movements and positions, (5) potential complications associated with traction, and (6) appropriate intervention to prevent complications.

If possible, the nurse must prepare the client physically and psychosocially before using traction. The nurse should explain to the client and significant others the purposes of traction and reasons why specific body positions must be maintained for long periods of time. The nurse should make sure they understand contraindicated movements or positions. Also, the nurse should explain that moving into contraindicated positions defeats the purpose of traction and disrupts healing. Traction helps tight muscles to relax and the client will probably feel more comfortable after a few hours. The physician tells the client how long traction is likely to be maintained.

Neurovascular assessment is essential when applying skeletal traction.

CRITICAL TO REMEMBER

Before a pin is inserted, the nurse must establish neurovascular baseline measurements for later comparison between preinsertion and postinsertion assessment.

Neurovascular assessment includes color, warmth, movement, sensation, pedal pulses, and capillary refill.

The nurse must periodically assess a skeletal traction apparatus. Sometimes the sharp ends of the wires or pins extend beyond the bow. If so, corks or adhesive tape must be placed over these protruding ends to prevent injury to people or damage to clothing. The nurse should frequently inspect skin around pin sites for signs of infection, such as odor, redness, and drainage. Some physicians cover these stab wounds with sterile dressings and do not want dressings disturbed unless there is evidence of infection. Others direct dressings to be changed daily and pin sites to be cleaned with antiseptic solution, followed by application of antibiotic ointment. The nurse should assess wrapped extremities for indications of constriction. Swelling is most likely to occur 24 to 48 hours after injury.

Much nursing intervention is directed at preventing complications from prolonged immobility and the traction equipment itself (see nursing Care Plan).

The affected limb (or limbs) must be covered without interfering with the traction, such as wrapping the limb in a lightweight blanket. The nurse should not allow coverings to press on the footplate of leg traction. Also, the nurse should be sure that ropes and pulleys remain free. Linen should be changed by proceeding from the top to the bottom of the bed. The nurse must be careful not to jerk the client by catching linens in traction equipment.

Once muscle spasms have subsided, about 48 to 72 hours after the application of traction, the client should have only mild discomfort when still. Pain may be reported with movement; adequate analgesia should be used preventively.

A client confined in traction, especially if it continues for some time, may experience a diversional activity deficit. This problem can occur because of inadequate environmental stimulation or lack of variation. It is particularly common in young adults and elderly clients. Appropriate nursing intervention focuses on preventing sensory deprivation.

The nurse should provide normal aids to orientation, such as accurate clock, current calendar and publications, clean glasses, and hearing aids, if worn by the client. Prism glasses may help a person read more easily while lying flat. The radio and television should be clearly tuned, but they must not be left on continuously if the person cannot control them independently. Continuous noise can increase confusion.

Some clients in traction are not able to perform many usual self-care activities independently. The nurse must be aware of which activities a client can and cannot perform, such as washing the feet. The client can also have control of care by being included in scheduling of procedures such as bath or linen changes.

The nurse should use a fracture bedpan (small, flat bedpan with a tapering slope from front to back) for a person in traction. For enemas, a large bedpan can be used, however. Some women prefer a kidney basin for urination. If the client can use a trapeze, the nurse should position and remove a bedpan while the person raises the hips off the mattress.

Immediately after traction removal, a client is often weak and unsteady. If a limb was immobilized, it may have some muscle atrophy. Orthostatic hypotension may occur if the client has been bedridden for several days or more. To combat this problem, the nurse can help the client very gradually resume a sitting (and later standing) position. The head of the bed should be elevated a little at a time to combat orthostatic hypotension. Raising the bed to a full sitting position may require several days. The nurse should have adequate help and provide careful physical support when a client first sits on the edge of the bed or gets out of bed.

CRITICAL TO REMEMBER

Safety precautions are imperative to prevent falls until the nurse is sure the client has secure balance, self-support, and strength.

CARE PLAN: The Client in Skeletal Traction

Nursing Diagnosis/ Collaborative Problem	Planning: Expected Outcomes	Implementation: Nursing Interventions	Rationales
Skin Integrity, Impaired R/T inability to change position secondary to skeletal traction	Client will retain intact skin, as evidenced by • No reddened areas • No abrasions	Assess pressure points (sacrum, heels under ropes and bones) every shift Provide skin care every shift by lifting client Apply therapeutic mattress to bed	Common pressure points for clients in supine position Clients in traction cannot turn Some mattresses (Geomatt) reduce surface pressure
Physical Mobility, Impaired R/T confinement in traction	Client will not experience complications of immobility, as evidenced by • Maintaining preinjury ROM in joints • Not developing thrombophlebitis • Having a bowel movement every other day • Maintaining clear lung sounds	Place all joints (except those immediately proximal and distal to fracture) through ROM every shift Assess lung sounds every shift Teach client to deep breathe and cough every shift Assess for clinical manifestations of thrombophlebitis: unilateral leg edema or pain Do not rely on Homans' sign as an indicator Monitor bowel movement • Encourage fluids and food containing fiber • Administer laxatives as necessary	ROM assists to maintain muscle tone Immobility and use of analgesia may cause hypoventilation and atelectasis Deep breathing and coughing hyperventilate and clear secretions Thrombophlebitis is a complication resulting from immobility Constipation is a side effect of immobility Fiber and fluids assist to add bulk and soften bowel movement, making its passage easier Laxative irritates or stimulates the colon
Injury, Risk for R/T traction	Client will sustain no injury while in traction	Ensure that weights hang freely from pulleys Ensure that knots in the rope do not catch in the pulleys Add and remove weights slowly with physician's order Pin site care per agency policy Adjust the position of the bed	If weights rest on the bed or floor, the traction is not effective Traction is not effective when knots catch in pulleys Slow, steady pull reduces muscle spasms Reduce risk of infection
Compartment Syndrome and Neurovascular Compromise, Risk for	Nurse will monitor for symptoms and signs of compartment syndrome every shift	Monitor color, warmth, movement, and sensation of extremity distal to traction every shift Assess pedal (radial) pulse every shift Monitor reports of degree of pain and relief by analgesia	Signs and symptoms of compartment syndrome include pallor, pulselessness, cool extremities, inability to move, loss of or change in sensation, and pain that is not relieved with usual analgesia

ROM, range of motion.

The nurse should prepare the client for a lack of proprioceptor response (awareness of body position, movement, and posture) after traction removal. The nurse should explain that the client may feel faint or weak and that joints may be stiff or unstable. Weakened limbs may require temporary support at their joints, and crutches may be needed for a while.

Casts

Casts are temporary devices of plaster or fiber glass that immobilize a body part, usually an extremity. However, clients can wear casts over the torso also. The purposes

BOX 44–2

Types of Casts

NAME OF THE CAST	DESCRIPTION
Short arm	Used to treat stable metacarpal, carpal, distal radius, or humerus fractures, or wrist sprains. Cast extends from the palm and thumb to midarm. May include a thumb spica for thumb fractures or may be a hanging cast for humerus fractures.
Short leg	Used to treat fractures of the tibia, fibula, and ankle. Cast extends from the foot to below the knee. May be weightbearing or non-weightbearing.
Long leg	Used to treat unstable fracturs of the femur, tibia, and fibula. Cast extends from foot to hip and holds the knee in flexion if fracture is unstable to prevent weightbearing. If weightbearing is permitted, a cylinder cast is used.
Cast brace	Used to treat a stable distal femur fracture. Cast consists of two parts, above and below the knee, with a hinge at the knee to allow range of motion.

for a cast include (1) immobilization; (2) prevention or correction of deformity; (3) maintenance, support, and protection to realign bone; and (4) promotion of healing, which allows early weightbearing for ambulation. The types of casts are described in Box 44–2 and shown in Figure 44–2.

APPLYING A CAST

Cast Materials

Plaster of Paris bandages are individual rolls of precut crinoline impregnated with plaster. They are available in various sizes. The body part to be casted determines the amount of plaster used.

Synthetic casting materials are made of fabric impregnated with high-density thermoplastic resin or fiber glass. These materials provide strong, lightweight casts that set in about 20 minutes. Unlike plaster of Paris, synthetic casts maintain their shape and firmness even if they become wet. However, if a synthetic cast becomes wet, it must be thoroughly dried to prevent skin maceration. If there is no incision under the cast, a synthetic cast can be dried with a cast dryer.

Procedure

The nurse should explain the procedure to the client and significant others. If a fracture is to be reduced before a cast is applied, the client is usually given an anesthetic. Cast application must be performed quickly. It is helpful to have a nurse present to concentrate on the client's needs. The procedure for skin preparation and casting is the same whatever body part is being casted and whether a plaster or synthetic cast is being applied. Skin preparation includes thoroughly cleaning the skin. The nurse must closely examine the skin while preparing it and document lesions, unremovable dirt, and foreign particles.

After the skin is prepared, it may be covered with stockinette or padding. The nurse should make sure these coverings fit smoothly, without wrinkles. Wrinkles or uneven surfaces can abrade skin and lead to skin breakdown. The tubular stockinette should always be cut longer than the expected finished cast length, so that the excess portions can be pulled. Whether fiber glass or plaster of Paris is used, the area to be casted should be covered with a stockinette and then padding. When the fiber glass material is used, the padding should be of a synthetic material. The padding may be applied more heavily over a bony prominence, but caution must be used because too much padding can cause pressure. When padding is applied, the nurse should make sure it is smooth and even so that it does not cause pressure sores.

Plaster-filled bandages are submerged in a bucket of clean water one at a time, the excess water is removed, and the bandage is applied to encircle the body part. Plaster bandages are applied wetter than are synthetic bandages. If a large plaster cast is being applied, the water in the cast bucket should be changed. Use of clean dipping water speeds up cast setting.

During cast application, an assistant may support the extremity. The extremity should always be supported from underneath in the palms of the hands in such a way that pressure is not applied to any one area. One must not press finger tips into the cast or rest the cast on a hard or sharp surface. Doing so would cause flattening or indentations in the cast, which could result in pressure problems.

One must never empty plaster-laden water into an ordinary sink because plaster sediment will solidify and plug the plumbing. If a sink with a plaster trap is not available, one should wait for sediment to settle into the bottom of the plastic-lined bucket and then drain off the water from the top. The plaster sediment should be scraped off the bottom of the bucket and disposed of in the garbage.

As soon as the casting procedure is complete, the client's skin is cleaned of excess casting material. An x-ray may be performed to verify correct bone alignment.

Drying Casts

Synthetic casts are dry to the touch in a few minutes but take about 20 minutes to set completely. Synthetic casts dry with a thermal reaction and may feel hot. Also, the surface is sticky and should be handled only

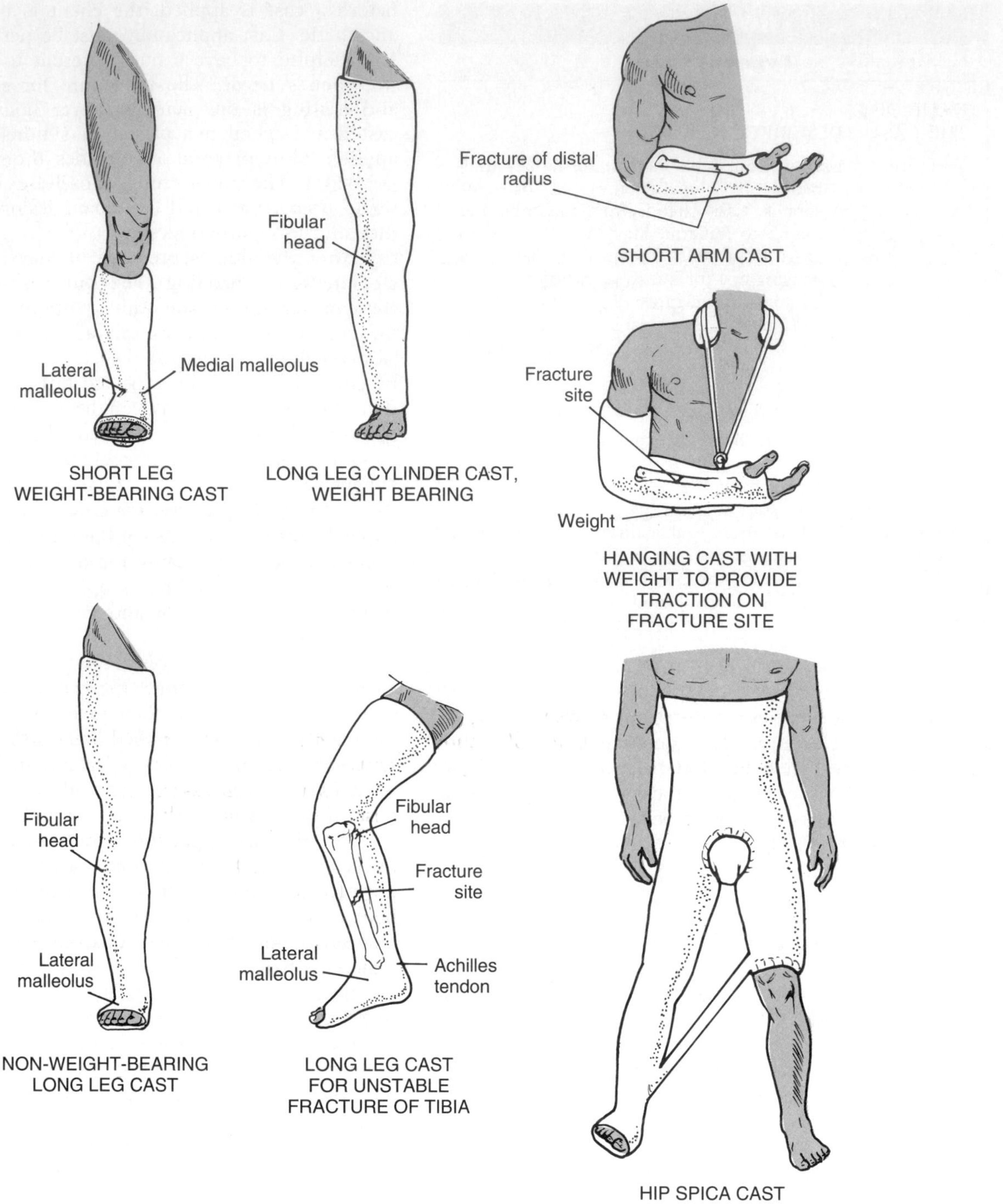

Figure 44–2
Common types of casts for extremity fractures and nursing interventions.

with gloves. Plaster casts set rapidly but take several hours to dry completely (large casts may take several days). The water from a newly applied cast (green cast) eventually evaporates, leaving a mature cast of full strength. Factors influencing the drying time of a plaster cast include (1) the amount of water to be evaporated from the cast; (2) the thickness of the cast, such as the number of layers of plaster bandages; and (3) the surrounding environment, such as humidity, temperature, and air circulation.

The nurse should promote the circulation of warm, dry air around a damp cast to enhance moisture evaporation and speed the drying process. A client being casted should be warned that heat is created during the cast's early setting (hardening) stages (both plaster of Paris and fiber glass generate heat). The sensation of heat under a cast can be frightening if it is not understood. The heat generated in a newly applied cast should be allowed to dissipate into circulating air. During the green period (while the cast is still damp), a casted person may feel cold and chill easily. Adequate covering should be provided while also allowing air to circulate around the cast. If the client has a large cast, the nurse can avoid excessive chilling by covering some parts of the cast for a brief time and rotating the exposed portions.

Unless contraindicated, a person in a green cast should be turned periodically to expose more of the casted area to air. A wet plaster of Paris cast is musty smelling, is dull on percussion, is gray in appearance, and feels cold to the touch. A dry plaster cast is odorless, is resonant when percussed, is white in appearance, and feels similar to the room temperature. Wet, or green, fiber glass casts appear a creamy color and feel hot to the touch. The surface also is sticky. The surface should not be touched without gloves until the cast is "dry" (about 20 minutes). A fiber glass cast should be placed as is a plaster cast. Fiber glass casting material should not be placed over a drainage area containing pads, such as bluepads, because paper and plastics will adhere and become a permanent part of the cast.

The nurse should place new casts on plastic-protected pillows to protect them from pressure and flattening while drying. Once completely dry, a cast can be placed on a hard surface if the person wishes (e.g., a casted arm may rest on a table), but it is usually more comfortable to rest the casted area on pillows.

WINDOWING AND BIVALVING A CAST

Cutting windows in casts and bivalving casts are two techniques commonly used to relieve or prevent excessive pressure in casted body areas or to provide access to or visualization of certain body parts. Windows may be cut (in dried casts) (1) to prevent uncomfortable abdominal distention (e.g., in a body cast or hip spica); (2) to assess a radial pulse (e.g., to check circulation in a casted arm); (3) to inspect areas of discomfort or areas of suspected tissue damage; and (4) to remove drains or care for wounds.

Bivalving a cast means splitting it along both sides (1) to allow tissue swelling, (2) so half of it can be removed to facilitate care and the taking of x-ray films, (3) so the cast can be removed and reapplied while a person is learning to adjust to being without a cast, or (4) to make a half-cast for use as an intermittent splint (e.g., to prevent deformities). Once a cast is bivalved, either half can be removed easily without disturbing alignment. When reapplying a bivalved cast, the client's extremity should be handled carefully, taking care not to pinch skin between the two cast halves. When both halves of the cast are properly fitted, they should be secured with a wrap.

COMPLICATIONS

Although casts are protective and therapeutic, they can also cause serious complications, such as swelling of the casted part, or vascular or nerve damage sustained during injury or treatment, such as from surgery, fracture reduction, or vascular emboli or thrombi. The cast, because it is inflexible and meant to restrict movement, can cause pressure and constriction of the casted limb. Complications can arise from impaired blood flow or innervation, which may lead to paralysis, paresis or paraesthesia, or anesthesia. In extreme cases, amputation may be necessary.

CRITICAL TO REMEMBER

Careful assessment is essential to prevent serious complications.

Clinical manifestations of complications are found in Table 44–1. These complications are discussed in Chapter 45 in the section on complications of fractures.

Nursing Management

Assessment

Thorough assessment and prompt intervention are essential to prevent cast-related complications. The nurse must establish an assessment pattern and always make observations sequentially. For example, in a casted extremity, the nurse should assess (1) color, (2) movement of distal fingers or toes, (3) warmth, (4) sensation, (5) swelling, and (6) pulses distal to cast. Another helpful way of remembering some significant assessment findings with cast-related complications is the 6 *Ps* mnemonic: pain, pallor, paralysis, pulselessness, paresthesia, and poikilothermia (skin cold to the touch). The nurse should document and report any abnormalities.

Skin temperature should be felt in areas distal to the cast, such as the hand, foot, fingers, and toes. Skin temperature on a casted extremity should be compared with the opposite extremity. Arterial insufficiency causes abnormal coolness in exposed fingers and toes. The nurse should feel the surface of the cast by placing the palm of the hand on the cast and moving it over the cast's entire surface. "Hot spots" (areas that feel warmer than other areas) may indicate tissue necrosis or infection under the cast. "Wet spots" may indicate a need for drying or drainage beneath the cast.

When assessing peripheral pulses, the nurse should compare casted and uncasted limbs. Peripheral pulses are absent with impaired arterial blood flow. The nurse must assess the radial pulse at the wrist of a casted arm and the dorsalis pedis pulse on the dorsum of the foot of a casted leg. Occasionally, the client's cast covers the dorsum of the foot and pulses cannot be palpated. In this situation, the nurse must rely on other assessment parameters.

TABLE 44–1 Clinical Manifestations of Complications from Cast Use

Impaired blood flow producing soft tissue ischemia (e.g., caused by pressure in casted extremity). Clinical manifestations may include

- Pulselessness: slow nail bed capillary refill, as evidenced by refill greater than 3 seconds
- Skin pallor, blanching, cyanosis, or coolness
- Pain, swelling, painful edema peripheral to cast
- Paresthesias (tingling, prickling), heightened sensitivity, numbness; hypoesthesia (diminished sensitivity to touch); anesthesia (numbness)
- Motor paralysis of previously functioning muscles

Nerve damage from pressure where a nerve passes over a bony prominence. Clinical manifestations may include

- Increasing, persistent, localized pain
- Hypoesthesia (diminished sensitivity); anesthesia (numbness); paresthesias (tingling, prickling, heightened sensitivity, numbness)
- Feelings of deep pressure
- Motor weakness or paralysis not previously present

Infection, tissue necrosis (e.g., caused by skin breakdown). Clinical manifestations may include

- Musty, unpleasant odor over cast or at ends of cast
- Drainage through cast or cast opening
- Sudden unexplained body temperature elevation
- "Hot spot" felt on cast over lesion

Compartment syndrome, which compromises circulation, viability, and function of tissues within the compartment. Clinical manifestations may include

- A dramatic increase in pain that is no longer controlled by analgesia
- Loss of movement
- Loss of sensation
- Pain with passive motion
- Pulselessness

Cast syndrome occurs with body casts and may be fatal if untreated. Possible assessment findings include

- Prolonged nausea; repeated vomiting
- Abdominal distention; vague abdominal pain

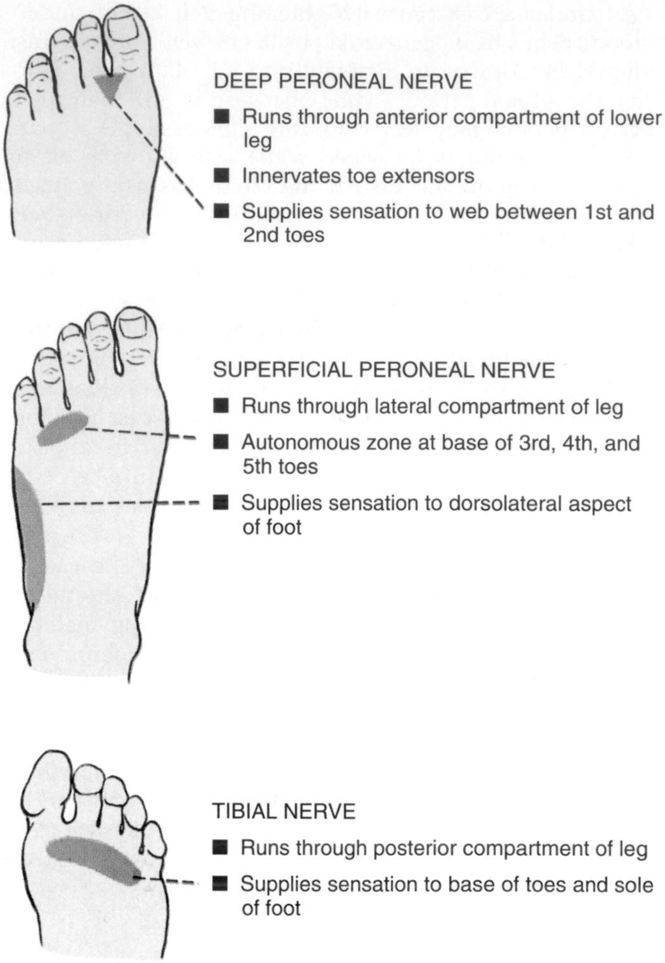

DEEP PERONEAL NERVE
■ Runs through anterior compartment of lower leg
■ Innervates toe extensors
■ Supplies sensation to web between 1st and 2nd toes
SUPERFICIAL PERONEAL NERVE
■ Runs through lateral compartment of leg
■ Autonomous zone at base of 3rd, 4th, and 5th toes
■ Supplies sensation to dorsolateral aspect of foot
TIBIAL NERVE
■ Runs through posterior compartment of leg
■ Supplies sensation to base of toes and sole of foot

Figure 44–3
Nursing assessment of lower extremity nerve function.

The nurse assesses a client's awareness of pinpricks and light touch in areas distal to a cast. Hypoesthesia or anesthesia indicates serious damage to a limb. The nurse should assess for indications of peroneal nerve damage in a casted leg and median, ulnar, or radial nerve damage in a casted arm (Fig. 44–3). When assessing for sensory losses, the client's history must be reviewed to determine whether such losses were present before cast application.

Skin color should be assessed distal to the cast. The nurse should look for indications of circulatory impairment, such as pallor, blanching, and cyanosis. Cyanosis results from impaired venous return, such as that caused by soft tissue constriction.

CRITICAL TO REMEMBER

Cyanosis may be a late indication of impaired circulation.

Pallor or blanching may indicate arterial insufficiency.

A blanching test assesses circulation by observing nail bed capillary refill time. The nurse should compare capillary refill time in the casted limb with that on the unaffected side. However, this is not a conclusive test because nail bed capillary refill can remain fairly normal even though a limb is pulseless.

The client should be asked to move fingers or toes on the casted limb. Movement should be easy and painless, unless the person's injury restricts motion. Motion paralysis of fingers or toes may be due to primary nerve damage, or the person may be unable to move because of pain.

CRITICAL TO REMEMBER

Painful motion usually indicates excessive swelling. A person can wiggle the toes by active flexion, and they will return to neutral position by passive recoil. This indicates complete loss of extensor power. The nurse should document these findings and notify the physician. Moving the fingers or toes (even very gently) of an ischemic limb is extremely painful. Motor paralysis is a late symptom of ischemia.

The nurse assesses skin around cast edges for skin damage or swelling. Injury to an extremity and subsequent treatment (e.g., reduction, surgery) usually produce swelling, which progresses for the first 12 to 24 hours after injury or surgery. Swelling may be greatest for the first 24 to 48 hours. Although mild swelling of exposed fingers and toes is not unusual, moderate or severe swelling associated with pain and discoloration is abnormal. When a casted part swells markedly, structures within the cast are constricted and severe complications result. Swelling may obstruct blood flow.

The nurse should assess the cast surface for indications of wound drainage (stains) or bleeding and closely inspect areas of the cast that cover wounds (e.g., surgical incisions or accidental wounds) and all pressure points (for indications of damage to underlying skin).

CRITICAL TO REMEMBER

When an area of drainage or bleeding becomes visible, one must document the time, date its appearance, and describe the observation.

Drainage on the surface of fiber glass casts may not appear at the area of the wound or incision. Because of the makeup of the cast, the drainage may not wick outward but may wick to the dependent area if the cast is flat, or the drainage may be found posterior and superior if the limb is elevated. The drainage may even seep out of the cast at the posterior and superior aspects of the elevated cast or the distal end of a dependent cast. Continued assessment is, of course, necessary.

The nurse should smell for odors indicative of tissue necrosis and infection. A cast often develops a sour smell after being worn a while from perspiration and normal sloughing of outer skin layers. However, pathologic tissue necrosis emits an easily detectable, musty, strong, offensive odor. If the odor of mildew is present, especially with a fiber glass cast, the cast may have become wet at one time and not thoroughly dried. If this event has occurred, the physician should be notified and the cast will probably be removed.

INTERVENTION

Intervention to prevent or relieve excessive swelling typically includes (1) full-length elevation of the cast higher than the person's heart, (2) exercising the fingers or toes to stimulate circulation, and (3) placing ice bags around the cast. Pressure caused by swelling must be relieved by cutting the cast before irreversible damage occurs. Pressure (without swelling) by the edge of a cast against skin may be relieved by a position change or loosely padding the uncomfortable area.

Positioning. Because a cast is heavy and inflexible, a client wearing a cast can easily lose his or her balance and fall. Safety straps should be used to secure a casted client being transported and to assist with transfer procedures, such as to a cart. Safety straps may be required to make sure that a green cast is handled properly. Footdrop may develop in a casted leg. The foot should be splinted or supported at a 90-degree flexion in the ankle. The nurse should protect the toes of a casted foot from the pressure of bedclothing; stockings may provide warmth.

CRITICAL TO REMEMBER

A casted extremity should be elevated to minimize swelling and promote drainage. This procedure is especially important for the first 24 to 48 hours.

Elevating a casted part stimulates circulation and reduces swelling (and thus pressure within the cast). The nurse should elevate casted extremities on rubber or plastic-protected pillows. A casted arm may be placed in a sling or arm immobilizer when the person is ambulatory. The entire arm, including the elbow, wrist, and hand (wristdrop leads to neurovascular complications), should be supported and the fingers kept higher than the elbow (to minimize swelling). If a sling or immobilization is not used, the person should be encouraged to exercise the uncasted joints such as the shoulder or elbow to prevent complications of disuse. A pillow can be used to elevate the arm while sitting if this position is more comfortable.

The nurse should position the client carefully and comfortably on a fracture bedpan designed for use by clients wearing body casts. The head of the bed should be raised slightly to facilitate elimination and to prevent body excrement from running up under the cast. Raising head and shoulders slightly to use a bedpan is usually allowed unless the client is in shock, is hemorrhaging, or has a spinal injury. Damp, soiled casts become odorous and may mold or break. Dampness also causes skin irritation and may increase the risk of infection if an open wound is present.

Frequent position changes are essential to prevent complications of immobility. A client with a cast often needs help to turn in bed. If possible, give the client turning instructions and encourage practice before the cast is applied. The nurse should always have adequate help to move and position a casted person; that is, to turn a person with a heavy cast, at least one other staff member should help the nurse and one person should always be on each side of the bed. Wet casts are particularly heavy.

People in casts can often bear weight as soon as the cast is dry. Synthetic casts can be walked on immediately after application. Plaster casts require 36 to 48 hours before bearing weight. Weak, aged, and debilitated clients often find the weight of a cast difficult to deal with and may tire rapidly when ambulating for the first few times. They must be observed closely to prevent excessive fatigue and accidents. Pain may be experienced the first few times that a casted leg is lowered to a dependent position. The nurse should prepare the client for this pain by explaining that pain is not unusual and that it occurs as blood rushes into the leg. Initially, the nurse can assist the client in lowering the leg for brief periods and gradually lengthen the time of dependence. Once the client's leg becomes accustomed to the increased blood, pain subsides.

Exercises. The nurse should instruct the client in exercises to stimulate circulation, increase venous return, enhance healing, and facilitate rehabilitation. Usually, exercises are prescribed for the joints above and below the cast. It usually is important to exercise the uncasted shoulder of a casted arm because the shoulder joint can become stiff quickly (this is one reason why a sling may be contraindicated). Also, the shoulder supports the weight of the arm cast. The client should be taught not to hold the shoulder immobile but to periodically lift the casted arm up over the head and to move each finger frequently.

Isometric exercises do not actually move the limb or bend the joints, but they do contract the muscles. Isometric muscle exercises help maintain muscle strength and mass by combating weakness and disuse atrophy. The nurse should begin by teaching isometric exercises on unaffected limbs and then on casted areas.

A client confined to bed may need other exercises, such as gluteal setting, abdominal tightening, and deep breathing, to prevent complications and to prepare for future activities such as crutch walking. The client must be taught full ROM exercises for uncasted structures and joints. Uncasted structures need to be in optimal condition to perform the extra duties necessary to relieve the weight and work of casted areas. The nurse should encourage active exercise several times a day. Self-care activity provides significant indirect exercise.

Nutrition. Increased dietary fiber helps people with reduced mobility maintain normal bowel elimination. A person in a body cast may need to avoid gas-forming foods to prevent abdominal distention. A general, well-balanced diet promotes wound healing.

Client Teaching. The nurse should teach the client and significant others about skin care and how to prevent skin damage, as discussed later. Skin care includes assessing the client's skin condition, washing and drying the skin, applying emollient lotions, and turning frequently. Skin areas subjected to irritation or pressure can rapidly develop into pressure sores. All exposed skin areas and all pressure areas, that is, the back of the head, ears, elbows, iliac crests, sacrum, and heels, should be inspected frequently, especially around the edges of the cast. The nurse should look for friction rubs, swelling, irritation, or discoloration, such as redness, blanching, cyanosis. The physician should be notified of any indications of skin problems, including irritation or pressure. See Client Education Guide: The Client with a Cast.

Follow-Up Care

Cast changes are often necessary when a cast no longer fits because of weight changes or muscle atrophy. Sometimes, cast changes are necessary for additional treatment or so the area can be inspected. During cast

CLIENT EDUCATION GUIDE

The Client with a Cast

Client Teaching. The nurse must teach the client and significant others the following:

- The cast will be warm at first when it is setting; if warm areas continue after the cast has dried, infection may be present. Notify the physician at once if infection is suspected.
- Watch for increased pain or soreness, especially around the wrist or ankle.
- Check the skin for color and temperature several times a day. When checking circulation in a toe or finger, pinch the tip and check to see whether color returns after 2 to 4 seconds. If color does not return or if the color is red, blue, or pale, *notify the physician.*
- Any of the following should be brought to the physician's attention *immediately:*

  Increased swelling
  Tingling or burning sensation
  Inability to move muscle around the cast
  Foul odor around cast edges
  Drainage, especially that which shows through the cast
  Cracks or breaks in the cast

Regarding care of the cast, the nurse must instruct the client and significant others as follows:

During the first 24 hours after the cast has been applied

- Avoid overhandling.
- Use palms of hands to move cast.
- Dry with a fan placed 18 to 24 inches from the cast.
- Keep cast and extremity above heart level for 48 hours. Prop on pillow.
- Place ice directly over the fracture. Place ice in plastic bag.
- Move parts of body, above, and below cast regularly to heighten circulation

After the first 24 hours

- Keep the cast dry.
- Protect the cast with plastic when bathing or showering.
- Do not insert objects inside of the cast.
- Do not use powder inside of the cast.
- Use a sling or crutches to enhance comfort, safety, and ambulation.

After the cast has been removed

- Soften and condition skin.
- Use dampened cloth and gentle soap or detergent.
- Rinse well and pat dry.
- Use a mild analgesic to relieve soreness.
- Elevate the limb to reduce any swelling.
- Gradually resume activities, keeping in mind that it will take from 1 to 4 weeks to regain strength in the limb.

changes, the nurse should assess and care for the client's skin.

Cast Removal. The length of time a client wears a cast varies with the type and extent of injury, disease, or surgery and the rate of healing. A cast is usually removed with an electric cast cutter, which resembles a small electric saw with a circular blade. Because of its appearance and noise, a cast cutter is often frightening. The nurse should show the client the cast cutter before using it and explain that it cannot cut skin because the blade does not whirl around and cut like a saw. Rather, it breaks the cast by oscillating or vibrating rapidly back and forth sideways. When a cast cutter is used, the client may feel sensations of heat, vibrations, or pressure. A cast spreader may also be used to spread open a cut cast so that underlying padding material can be cut.

Skin under a casted area often becomes very sensitive and is mottled and covered with yellow-brown scales or crusts of dead skin, oil, and exudate. Muscles under a cast may appear atrophied, and the extremity feels stiff and weak from inactivity. New aches and pains may appear with movement after cast removal, and muscles and tissues are subjected to new stresses and strains. The client's balance is altered, because removing a cast removes weight.

Gentle soaking and washing for a few days after a cast is removed returns skin to its normal appearance. Many clients want to vigorously scrub the skin, but this often causes irritation. After a gentle washing, the skin should be dried and lubricated with cocoa butter, lanolin, or another emollient to promote softening. Because newly uncasted skin is sensitive and can burn easily, the nurse should advise the client to prevent overexposure to the sun.

After cast removal, swelling may develop for a while when the involved limb is dependent. The client should elevate the limb when sitting or lying down. Swelling decreases with increased activity and improved muscle tone and circulation. Sometimes the physician recommends elastic bandages or stockings during ambulation to minimize swelling. Ambulation should be encouraged because intermittent weight bearing acts as an effective venous pump.

Rehabilitation. Rehabilitation instructions are given by the physician according to the client's condition. A physical therapist often participates in rehabilitative care after cast removal. For example, a physical therapist may teach and supervise graded active exercises (to stimulate circulation and increase muscle strength) and joint ROM and perform other prescribed activities such as whirlpool baths to force joints and muscles during recovery (by passive stretching exercises, resistive exercises, or forced movements). Placing excessive demands on stiff, weakened limbs may further impair motion by increasing fibrosis and excessively engorging the area with blood.

External Fixation

An external fixator may be used as an alternative to either a cast or traction or for maintaining bones and surrounding tissues for limb lengthening, such as the Ilizarov procedure. External fixators can be used on arms, legs, and, occasionally, fingers or the pelvis. These devices are made of aluminum, titanium, or nylon. An external fixator is a device consisting of pins that are placed in bone and attached to a rigid external frame. The open pin sites and wound need ongoing assessment and wound care. Usually, the client is ambulatory with a non-weightbearing gait. Care is similar to that used for pin care with skeletal traction.

Musculoskeletal Surgery

Musculoskeletal Surgical Procedures

Musculoskeletal procedures may reconstruct, replace, or remove diseased or injured structures or correct deformities. They may be performed on bone (e.g., bone grafting, osteotomy, total hip and knee replacements, arthrodesis) or soft tissues (e.g., tendon transfer, lateral release, tenotomy, and rotator cuff repair). Common musculoskeletal surgical procedures include arthroscopy, arthroplasty, arthrodesis, osteotomy, tenotomy, and bone grafting.

ARTHROSCOPY

Arthroscopy (see Chap. 44) is used for two purposes: diagnosis and treatment.

Diagnosis is the main purpose. Arthroscopy is also the surgery type of choice for

- Excising tears of the meniscus
- Removing foreign bodies and adhesions
- Biopsy of synovial disorder or partial synovectomy
- Patellar shavings (smoothing knee cartilage) because of arthritis or chondromalacia

Clients undergoing arthroscopy usually have the procedure performed on an outpatient basis. The wounds are usually covered by an elastic bandage. The bandage may be removed within 3 days, and the client returns to normal activity within 3 weeks. Home instructions to the client should include a description of signs and symptoms of infection.

ARTHROPLASTY

Arthroplasty is used to re-establish movement of diseased or painful joints. Common arthroplasties are total hip, knee, shoulder, elbow replacements, or wrist replacements. (See Chap. 11.)

OSTEOTOMY

Osteotomy is a surgical procedure used to realign the bone by removing a wedge from it. The most common disorders behind osteotomies are varus and valgus deformities of the knee resulting from osteoarthritis.

Varus deformities refer to alateral angulation, and valgus refers to a medial deformity. The tibia or femur is wedged so as to realign the knee. The purpose of the surgery is to maintain joint function but also to stabilize the joint and relieve pain. Usually, the client is in the hospital for 3 to 5 days for pain management and gait training.

TENOTOMY

Tenotomy, cutting a tendon, is often used to release contracture related to spasticity such as that which occurs with cerebrovascular accident or cerebral palsy.

BONE GRAFTING

Bone grafting is transplanting pieces of cancellous or compact bone to new locations. Grafts may be (1) autogenous (obtained from the person having the transplant), (2) homogeneous (obtained from another human being), or (3) heterogeneous (obtained from an animal or synthetic material).

PULSING ELECTROMAGNETIC FIELDS

Pulsing electromagnetic fields is a form of treatment used to assist nonunion fractures in long bone fractures, especially in the elderly, who tend to have prolonged healing.[16] The electric current helps to stimulate bone regeneration through an as-yet unknown mechanism.

Nursing Management

Preoperative Management

Musculoskeletal surgical procedures are often elective, allowing time to prepare clients physically and psychosocially.

Preoperative intervention to prevent possible postoperative infection is essential. Bone is more susceptible to infection than soft tissue. Bone infection (osteomyelitis) is difficult to treat and can lead to permanent disability, such as chronic infection or joint stiffness. Bone union will not occur if infection is present. Specific skin preparation for musculoskeletal surgery varies, but the underlying principles are the same. Skin preparation is performed meticulously in a nontraumatic manner. In surgery, open traumatic wounds such as compound fractures are cleaned carefully, because they may be contaminated. Preparation is performed under aseptic conditions and usually by the surgeon.

POSTOPERATIVE MANAGEMENT

Prolonged immobilization is usually necessary for bone healing. As with any type of surgery, postoperative intervention focuses on preventing complications. Possible postoperative complications include shock (see Chap. 56), thrombophlebitis (see Chap. 26), pulmonary embolism (see Chap. 22), and fat embolism (see Chap. 46), and compartment syndrome (see Chap. 45).

General care includes assessment of dressings and drainage. The nurse checks dressings frequently and documents drainage. Using aseptic technique, the nurse reinforces saturated dressings to minimize the introduction of infection by capillary action. Staining of casts from blood seepage or serous or purulent drainage should be documented including the dimensions of stained areas, such as "a circle of bloody drainage about 1 inch in diameter." Measurements should be compared with previous measurements to assess whether or not drainage has stabilized or is increasing. Unusual drainage should be reported.

The nurse positions, turns, and exercises the client postoperatively according to physician's instructions. Frequently, the nurse must assess the person's posture and position to ensure that healing is occurring in correct alignment and to prevent other complications. Operated extremities are usually elevated postoperatively to prevent or minimize swelling. Limbs should be supported along their entire length (e.g., do not place a pillow just under the heel or knee).

After surgery, clients with joint disease should use movement to prevent the joints from becoming stiff and immobile. Early ambulation is desirable but sometimes cannot be started until adequate bone healing has occurred. Soft tissues heal more quickly than bone. Thus, although a skin incision may be healed, the underlying bone may not be. The nurse and client must follow physician's instructions about whether weight may be placed on an affected limb while the client is standing or walking.

Postoperative rehabilitation may include occupational therapy, prosthetics, bracing, and physical therapy (e.g., gait training, muscle reeducation, exercise, heat application, massage). It is important to keep the person mobilized and participating in safe self-care activities.

After discharge from a health-care facility, contact continues with the physician and other health-care professionals, as necessary. Community health nurses may make home visits. Before discharge, learning and teaching sessions are essential to make the client and significant others aware of indicated and contraindicated activities. They also need information about indications of complications.

POSTOPERATIVE REHABILITATION

Therapeutic exercises have many benefits, including maintaining or restoring adequate joint activity, preventing muscular atrophy and other deformities, building or maintaining muscular bulk and strength, maintaining or improving joint ROM, building endurance, and stimulating circulation. Exercises include (1) active or passive joint ROM exercises to preserve joint motion; (2) quadriceps setting exercises to stabilize the knees; (3) gluteal and abdominal muscle tightening to improve trunk stability; (4) lifting exercises to increase biceps strength.

Exercises such as resistive, isometric, and ROM can be performed with the client on bedrest.

Physical therapy and nursing work as a team. Often, the physical therapist sees the client once or twice a day to teach exercises or gait training. The nurse, in turn, takes on the responsibility to reinforce these instructions.

Assistive Devices

CRUTCHES

Two important points about crutch fitting and crutch use are

- *Crutches must be of correct length.* If they are too long, they cause excessive pressure and rubbing in the axilla. Excessive axillary pressure can cause nerve damage (to branches of the brachial plexus) and arm paralysis (crutch palsy or crutch paralysis). Arm paralysis may be evidenced by numbness or wristdrop. If the client is unable to make a fist, he or she may be experiencing wristdrop. Crutches that are too short can slip, and the person may fall.
- *People using crutches are prone to accidents.* Clients must never walk on crutches in stocking feet, slippers, or high-heeled shoes. Accidents can be prevented by (1) teaching people proper crutch walking (see Client Education Guide: Directions for Using Crutches, Walkers, and Canes), (2) pointing out possible hazards, and (3) teaching environmental safety consciousness, such as keeping floors litter free and dry and opening doors carefully.

CANES

The cane needs to be long enough for the person to extend the elbow and bear weight on the hand grasping the cane. For safety, a cane needs a soft, pure rubber suction tip and a curved handle with a comfortable hand grip.

WALKERS

Walkers of different kinds are available. Some people find it helpful to use walkers before trying crutches. Walkers provide better support and stability than crutches. Walkers are useful for older clients and clients who have trouble with balance. The walker should be adjusted so the elbow is slightly bent (30 degrees or less). Exercises to prepare for using a walker include resistance exercises to strengthen triceps muscles (may be performed in bed). Some walkers have underarm supports similar to those used on crutches.

SUPPORTS

Various supports such as braces or straps may be part of the treatment for musculoskeletal disorders. Braces and supports can be used to the back, neck, and any joint of the arm and legs. Braces and supports are a

CLIENT EDUCATION GUIDE

Directions for Using Crutches, Walkers, and Canes

GAITS	
Two point	Some weightbearing is permitted bilaterally. The right leg and left crutch move simultaneously and then the left leg and right crutch simultaneously.
Three point	No weightbearing or partial weight should be allowed on the affected leg. Both crutches and the affected leg move in unison, while the body weight is supported on the unaffected leg. (The affected leg may be used for balance if partial weight is allowed).
Four point	Weightbearing is permitted on both legs. Crutches and feet are moved alternately: left crutch, right foot, right crutch, left foot.
Swing through	No weightbearing should be allowed on the affected legs. Both crutches move forward, and both legs swing through between the crutches, while the weight is borne by the crutches.
Stairs	*Up:* Lead with the unaffected leg; the crutches and affected leg move together. *Down:* The crutches and the affected leg lead.
Walkers	Lift the walker and place it ahead, walk up to the walker. Do not slide the walker. Do not use the walker as a base to come to standing.
Cane	The cane is used on the side opposite of the affected leg. The cane and affected leg move in unison, while weight is borne on the unaffected leg.

common sight in the treatment of musculoskeletal complications, in which the goal is support yet early mobility. Braces or supports to joints are often hinged and can be adjusted to allow controlled ROM during the healing process. Often, a person's appearance and body image are altered by a brace. This factor may be difficult to adjust to.

Supports need careful fitting, application, and maintenance. The client and significant others must be taught to assess the skin frequently for indications of skin damage. A mirror can be used to examine areas that cannot otherwise be seen. If a person has impaired sensation, visual skin inspection is even more important. In a health-care facility, nurses may initially assess the client's skin. Adjustments may be needed to fit the appliance properly.

The client and significant others must be taught how the support works and the reasons for wearing it. Informed and involved clients are more likely to comply with treatment. If used incorrectly, supports may be detrimental to the client's condition. If supports do not fit comfortably and correctly, clients may become discouraged and not wear them, and the condition may worsen.

STUDY QUESTIONS

1. A client will be placed in skeletal traction for treatment of a fractured femur. To assess the client's neurovascular status accurately, the nurse should begin by assessing:
   A. Sensation and movement of the client's leg
   B. Color and warmth of the client's leg
   C. Pedal pulses and capillary refill
   D. Neurovascular status before the pin is inserted
2. An elderly client who has been taking antihypertensives has just been removed from Buck's traction. The nurse has taught the client to observe safety precautions before resuming ambulation. Of the following client responses, which indicates that the client has understood the nurse's instructions?
   A. "I'll perform abduction and adduction exercises before I walk."
   B. "I'll take several deep breaths before I begin to walk."
   C. "I'll sit on the side of the bed for several minutes before attempting to walk."
   D. "I'll drink plenty of water to prevent hypotension when I stand up."
3. A client who has a short arm cast asks the nurse to explain what she should look for if an infection were to develop under her cast. The nurse replies that the client would experience:
   A. Paresthesia in her hand
   B. Edema in her hand
   C. Pale color of her hand
   D. Musty odor over her cast
4. A client with a short arm cast is experiencing swelling of his fingers. The first action the nurse should take is to
   A. Call the physician immediately
   B. Check the color of his fingers and his capillary refill
   C. Elevate his entire arm on pillows, keeping his fingers higher than his elbow
   D. Elevate his lower arm on pillows, keeping his fingers higher than his elbow
5. A nurse has instructed a client on the proper use of a walker. What statement best indicates that the client has learned the proper use of a walker?
   A. "I slide my walker ahead of me and then step up to it."
   B. "I like the fact that my walker can be used to steady me when I get up from my chair."
   C. "I lift my walker, place it ahead of me, and walk up to it."
   D. "I move my right foot and my walker together, then my left foot and the walker."
6. A client with a short arm cast may experience complications of immobility of the casted arm. Which of the following client goals indicates that the nurse and client have developed a plan of care to prevent complications of immobility?
   A. The client will remove the arm sling every 4 hours.
   B. The client will hold his shoulder immobile.
   C. The client will periodically lift the casted arm over his head and move his fingers.
   D. The client will perform isometric exercises with his casted arm.

CRITICAL THINKING EXERCISES

SCENARIO A

A 40-year-old business woman and mother of three teenagers has just had a short leg plaster cast applied for treatment of a compression fracture of the tibia. The physician has instructed the client to elevate her leg as much as possible for the next 48 hours. As the orthopedic nurse, you will be asked to teach the client about monitoring for possible complications and about cast care. The client tells you that she leads a very active life and will have little time to "baby" herself. She sees the fracture as a nuisance.

1. How would you proceed to teach this client?
2. If she calls during the first 24 hours and complains of pain on passive movement of her toes, even after elevating her leg, what would you tell her?

SCENARIO B

An elderly woman is placed in balanced skeletal traction for treatment of a severe fracture of the humerus. The nurse manager tells you to provide routine skin care for the client. "Let her do as much for herself as possible." How would you proceed?

BIBLIOGRAPHY

1. Berg, E. E. (1990). Progress in orthopaedic surgery: The 1980's in review. *Orthopaedic Nursing, 9(5),* 29–31.
2. Evarts, C. M. (1990). *Surgery of the musculoskeletal system* (2nd ed., Vol. 3). New York: Churchill Livingstone.
3. Fecht-Gramley, M. (1994). Emergency! Recognizing compartment syndrome. *American Journal of Nursing, 94(10),* 41.
4. Funk, J. R., et al. (1990). Tibial osteotomy. *Orthopaedic Nursing, 9(2),* 29–34.
5. Hart, K. (1994). Using the Ilizarov external fixator in bone transport. *Orthopaedic Nursing, 13(1),* 35–40.
6. Jones-Walton, P. (1991). Clinical standards in skeletal traction pin site care. *Orthopaedic Nursing, 10(2),* 2–16.
7. Lane, P. L. (1990). Crutchwalking. *Orthopaedic Nursing, 9(5),* 31–37.
8. Mims, B. C. (1989). Fat embolism syndrome: A variant of ARDS. *Orthopaedic Nursing, 8(3),* 22–25.
9. Mourad, L. (1991). *Orthopedic disorders.* St. Louis: Mosby-Year Book.
10. Nance, D. K., & Mardjetko, S. M. (1994). Technical aspects and nursing considerations of limb lengthening. *Orthopaedic Nursing, 13(1),* 21–33.
11. Newschwander, D. E., et al. (1989). Limb lengthening and the Ilizarov external fixator. *Orthopaedic Nursing, 8(3),* 15–21.
12. Olson, B. (1990). Self-care needs of patients in the halo brace. *Orthopaedic Nursing, 9(1),* 27–33.
13. Peters, V. J., et al. (1989). Arthroscopy surgery of the ankle. *Orthopaedic Nursing, 8(5),* 12–18.
14. Ross, D. (1991). Acute compartment syndrome. *Orthopaedic Nursing, 10(2),* 33–38.
15. Schwartsman, V., McMurray, M. C., & Martin, S. N. (1989). The Ilizarov method—the basics. *Contemporary Orthopedics, 19(6),* 628–638.
16. Sneed, N., & VanBree, K. (1990). Treating ununited fractures with electricity: Nursing implications. *Gerontological Nursing, 16(8),* 26–31.
17. Steywood Jones, I. (1990). Making sense of . . . traction. *Nursing Times, 86(23),* 39–41.

Chapter 45 Nursing Care of Clients with Musculoskeletal Disorders

Learning Outcomes

After completing this chapter, the learner will be able to:

1. Assess the client for clinical manifestations resulting from common musculoskeletal disorders.
2. Teach the client about the risk factors, basic pathophysiology, and clinical manifestations associated with common musculoskeletal disorders.
3. Explain the client's role in the prevention and treatment of musculoskeletal disorders.
4. Develop plans of care for the prevention, management, and rehabilitation of clients with musculoskeletal disorders.
5. Implement nursing interventions that optimize the quality of life for clients with musculoskeletal disorders.
6. Evaluate planned client outcomes using outcomes developed in the planning phase of care.

Metabolic Bone Disease

Metabolic bone disease may result from an inappropriate function of the parathyroid gland, vitamin deficiency, estrogen deficiency, and malabsorption syndrome. Osteoporosis, osteomalacia, and Paget's disease can cause severe deformity, significant restriction of activity, lost income, and increased health-care costs.

OSTEOPENIA

Osteopenia is a condition, not a diagnosis, that is common to all metabolic bone diseases characterized by a reduction in bone mass greater than expected for age, race, or sex. The causes of osteopenia include a decrease in bone formation, inadequate bone mineralization, or excessive bone deossification.

OSTEOPOROSIS

Osteoporosis is a common age-related metabolic bone disease in which there is severe general reduction in the skeletal bone mass and an increased susceptibility to fractures, especially in the wrist, hip, and vertebral column. Bone resorption occurs faster than bone formation.

Osteoporosis can be classified into primary and secondary forms. Primary or type I postmenopausal osteoporosis is the most common and cannot be associated with an underlying medical condition. Secondary or type II osteoporosis results from an associated underlying condition, such as hyperparathyroidism, or an iatrogenic cause, such as long-term corticosteroid or heparin administration.

Primary osteoporosis can be divided into two subgroups. The first or type I postmenopausal osteoporosis occurs in women between the ages of 51 and 75 years. The bone loss is primarily in the cancellous bone trabecular network, resulting in fractures of the vertebrae or distal radius (Colles' fracture). Type II senile osteoporosis occurs in those individuals older than 70 years, affecting women twice as often as men. This results in equal trabecular and cortical bone loss; fractures of the hip and vertebrae are most common.

Incidence

In the United States alone, osteoporosis affects 25 million individuals and is responsible for more than 1.3 million fractures each year, most of which occur after 65 years of age.

One third of American women older than 50 years will eventually have a compression or vertebral fracture of the spine. Osteoporosis occurs in about one fourth of all elderly people; the incidence of the disease is greater in women than men (at least 5:1) and white women are affected more often than black women.

Etiology and Risk Factors

The exact cause of osteoporosis is unknown; however, several factors increase the risk that osteoporosis will occur (Box 45–1).

Women are at a high risk for early bone loss related to menopause. In postmenopausal women, estrogen production and bone calcium storage decrease. Estrogen appears to protect against bone loss. Accelerated bone loss also occurs with women who have early or surgically induced menopause or amenorrhea as a result of prolactin-producing pituitary tumors or anorexia

BOX 45–1

Risk Factors for Osteoporosis

- Advanced age
- Hereditary tendencies, including blonde or red hair, freckles, and fair skin
- Northern European ethnic background
- Female
- Postmenopausal
- Thin, small-framed body
- Inactive or bedridden
- Calcium-deficient diet
- Vitamin D deficiency
- Heavy cigarette smoking
- Heavy caffeine intake
- Alcohol consumption to excess
- Long-term corticosteroid use
- Long-term heparin use
- Long-acting psychotropic drugs
- Use of antacids
- Use of laxatives
- Cushing's disease
- Parkinson's disease
- Dementia
- Bilateral oophorectomy
- Endocrine disorders
- Type II diabetes
- Scoliosis
- Rheumatoid arthritis with no disability
- High-protein diet
- Anorexia and bulimia with resultant amenorrhea
- Excessive exercise

nervosa or in those who undertake intense long-distance running associated with undernourishment. These situations are all accompanied by estrogen deficiency, which is likely to be a major determinant of accelerated bone loss. Bone loss also occurs when estrogen therapy is withdrawn.

The susceptibility to fracture may be, in part, hereditary. The presence of the so-called "dowager hump" or collapse and wedging of vertebra in a mother may indicate a risk for her daughters.

PREVENTION

Once the clinical expression of osteoporosis has occurred, treatment is less than satisfactory. Therefore, it is important to identify those individuals at risk early to initiate therapy when it will have maximum efficacy. Strategies for preventing osteoporosis are most efficient when started early in life.

Adequate calcium intake requires consuming more dairy products, which provide about 75 per cent of the calcium in the average diet. Most authorities recommend that women consume 1000 to 1200 mg of calcium per day before menopause. Diets should be rich in dairy products and green, leafy vegetables.

Some individuals have difficulty digesting milk because of a lack of the enzyme lactase, which breaks down the milk sugar lactose. Acidophilus milk, yogurt, and hard cheeses may be tolerated because of the way they are processed.

Vitamin D plays a major role in both calcium absorption and its incorporation into bone. Vitamin D is the key that allows calcium to leave the intestine and enter the blood stream. Vitamin D is formed naturally in the body after exposure to sunlight. Vitamin D supplements may be necessary for the institutionalized or homebound individual.

Common therapeutic modalities may include the administration of vitamin D, calcium, calcitonin (available in parenteral form), and estrogen preparations (available as a transdermal patch). The hormone calcitonin is naturally secreted by the thyroid in response to increased amounts of serum calcium. With aging, the calcitonin level decreases and is less effective in inhibiting bone resorption, so bone mass is lost. Calcitonin therapy must be given parenterally each day for 12 to 18 months, at which time either bone resorption stabilizes or bone mass slightly increases.

Calcium supplements vary (Table 45–1) and may be absorbed differently as well as contraindicated in individuals with a history of renal stones, granulomatous conditions, or hypercalemic conditions. Excessive serum calcium can cause damage to the urinary system; therefore, calcium supplements should be prescribed by a physician or nurse practitioner. A lumbosacral brace for vertebral fractures, surgical repair of fractures when indicated, and pain management are key interventions.

Individuals who exercise regularly generally have a higher peak bone mass because bone responds to exercise by becoming stronger. Weightbearing exercise, such as walking, jogging, or stair climbing, is recommended over non-weightbearing exercise such as cycling or swimming. However, it is important to note that some type of physical activity is better than none.

Pathophysiology

Throughout the lifespan, new bone is formed (osteoblastic activity) while old bone is resorbed (osteoclastic activity). Two major theories have been proposed regarding the development of osteoporosis. The most popular theory suggests an increase in osteoclastic activity causing bone resorption or thinning. The second theory suggests that osteoporosis may result from decreased osteoblastic activity perhaps from less efficient or short-lived bone-forming cells.

Bone mass or density peaks between 30 and 35 years of age. After the peak years, calcium stored in the spongy bone (cancellous mass) leaves the tissue. Bone trabeculae are decreased in numbers and width, while marrow spaces are widened, and the bone mass decreases as calcium leaves the compact bone (cortical mass).

With osteoporosis, the supporting skeletal structures are weak, so even minimal stress can cause fractures. Spinal fractures occurring with osteoporosis are usually "compression fractures" and are very painful. They occur when one or more vertebrae simply collapse from carrying the weight of the upright body.

Clinical Manifestations

Clinical manifestations may reveal shortened stature, difficulty in bending over, marked kyphosis of the thoracic spine (dowager hump), or impaired breathing as a result of deformities of the spine and rib cage (Fig. 45–1).

Back pain and fractures are the most characteristic presenting symptoms. Vertebral compression fractures (often multiple and most commonly T12 to L2), proximal femur fractures (femoral neck and intertrochanteric), distal radius fractures, and pelvic fractures are the most common fracture types. The loss of height secondary to multiple fractures is characteristic of individuals with osteoporosis. Bone loss can occur in the jaw bone, which, along with oral health problems, may lead to tooth loss or improperly fitting dentures. This complication may lead to changes in the appearance of the individual's face. These changes, in addition to the shortened stature and kyphosis associated with osteoporosis, may have a profound negative impact on the individual's self-esteem.

At present, there is no way for individuals to tell whether they have low bone mass from a family or personal history. Medical tests are available that measure bone mass in various sites in the body. With information obtained from bone mass measurements, family history, and risk factor assessment, the individual's likelihood to fracture can be predicted.

No definitive laboratory tests confirm a diagnosis of primary osteoporosis. A battery of tests is performed to rule out secondary osteoporosis or other metabolic bone

TABLE 45–1 Calcium Supplement Types

FORM OF CALCIUM	PER CENT OF ELEMENTAL CALCIUM	DIETARY CHARACTERISTICS	CAUTIONS	SIDE EFFECTS	CONSIDERATIONS
Calcium carbonate	40	Take 1 hour after meals and at bedtime	Do not take with milk or food high in vitamin D_2	Constipation, gastric distention, flatulence, acid-rebound nausea, hypercalcemia, hypophosphatemia, milk alkali syndrome	Avoid if too little or no stomach acid secretions
Calcium lactate	13	Milk and yogurt are main source Powder form = 650 mg/level tsp	Contains lactose	Less constipating; same as above	Avoid if lactose-intolerant; symptoms are: gas, bloating, cramps or diarrhea
Calcium gluconate	9	Sweet		Less constipating; same as above	Must be taken frequently because of low concentration
Chelated calcium					Calcium anchored to a protein or yeast, amino acid not absorbed any better than standard calcium
Calcium levulinate	13	Bitter salty taste			
Calcium chloride	27	Used to pickle foods		Irritates stomach	Tends to irritate stomach
Calcium orate	10				
Bone meal	31		May contain lead	Same as above	Not well absorbed
Dolomite	22		Same as above		

Calcium Supplement Brands

BRAND	MILLIGRAMS/PILL	SOURCE OF CALCIUM
Alka-2 antacid (chewable)	200	Calcium carbonate
Calcet	153	Calcium gluconate, lactate, carbonate
Calcium lactate—Arco	83	Calcium lactate
Chelated calcium—Arco	150	Calcium, amino acid chelate
Caltrate 600 (chewable)	600	Calcium carbonate
Chooz antacid gum (chewable)	200	Calcium carbonate
Dical D capsules (133 IU vitamin D added)	117	Dibasic calcium phosphate
Dical D wafers (chewable, 200 IU vitamin D added)	232	Dibasic calcium phosphate
Os-Cal 250 (125 IU vitamin D added)	250	Calcium carbonate
Os-Cal 500 (high potency)	500	Calcium carbonate
Tums antacid (chewable)	200	Calcium carbonate
Tums E-X (chewable)	300	Calcium carbonate

Prepared by Barbara M. Schultz, RN, BSN, C, patient care and education coordinator at the Veterans Administration Domiciliary, White City, Oregon.
From Urrows, S. T., et al. (1991). Profiles in osteoporosis. *American Journal of Nursing, 91*(2), 36.

diseases. These tests include serum calcium, phosphorus, and alkaline phosphatase, which are normal in this condition. Serum osteocalcin is elevated. Urinary calcium is initially high and then returns to normal.

Bone biopsy may be performed when diagnosis by noninvasive measures is considered unreliable or when there has not been a positive response to therapy.

Medical Management

Intervention in the care of the client with osteoporosis focuses on the symptoms expressed.

Important goals are adequate nutrition, strengthening exercises, mobility in a hazard-free environment, and pain management. Fracture is usually the first

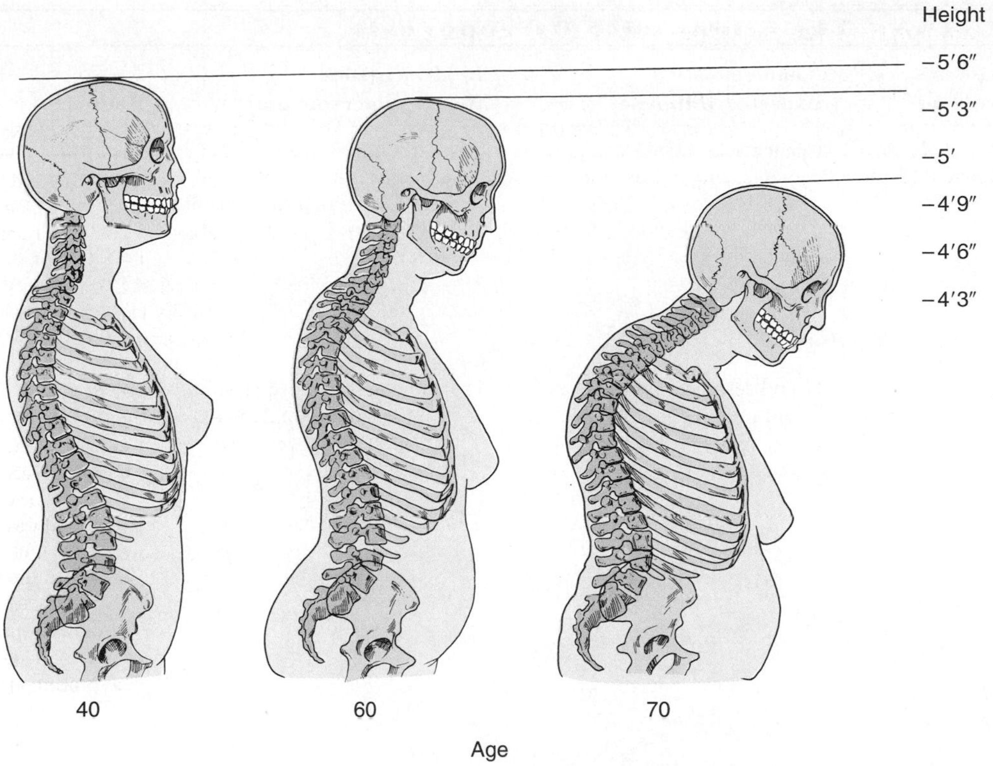

Figure 45–1
Osteoporotic changes. Normal spine at age 40, and osteoporotic changes at ages 60 and 70. These changes can cause a loss of height and can result in the deformity called dowager hump in the upper thoracic spine.

symptom that causes an individual to seek medical intervention; therefore, the plan should include further fracture prevention techniques.

Many of the nonsurgical management interventions are given for the treatment of the disease as well as for the prevention of osteoporosis. These include diet and drug therapy used to slow bone resorption and promote new bone growth.

Nursing Management

Nursing management for the client with osteoporosis is shown in the Care Plan. The teaching plan for the client with osteoporosis includes fall prevention, an exercise program, diet management, and drug therapy (see the Client Education Guide).

PAGET'S DISEASE (OSTEITIS DEFORMANS)

Paget's disease is defined as a disorder of bone architecture characterized by an initial phase of increased rate of bone tissue breakdown by osteoclasts followed by excessive abnormal bone formation by osteoblasts. The diseased bone is structurally weak and prone to fractures. Paget's disease most frequently produces painful deformities of the femur, tibia, lower spine, pelvis, and cranium.

The exact cause of Paget's disease is unknown. Although no definite hereditary pattern has been established, a familial clustering has been reported.

Paget's disease occurs worldwide, but it appears to afflict those of northwestern European extraction in North America. In the United States, 2.5 million people older than 40 years are affected, and it is more common in males than females.

Many individuals are diagnosed because they have experienced some sort of trauma, and their radiographic studies demonstrate the characteristic changes of the disease. Ten to 20 per cent of individuals with the disease are asymptomatic. Before clinical manifestations occur, radiographic studies show increased bone expansion and density.

In symptomatic Paget's disease, the most common presenting complaints include one or more of the following: bone pain, skeletal deformity (barrel-shaped chest or bowing of tibia-femur, or kyphosis), changes in skin temperature, pathologic fractures through diseased bone, and symptoms related to nerve compression. Pressure on the cranial nerves by diseased bone may result in

CARE PLAN: The Client with Osteoporosis

Nursing Diagnosis/ Collaborative Problem	Planning: Expected Outcomes	Implementation: Nursing Interventions	Rationales
Nutrition: Less than Body Requirements, Altered R/T calcium imbalance	Client meets USRDA requirements for calcium and vitamin D. Client describes foods high in calcium.	Teach the importance of diet in further osteoporosis. • Refer to dietitian for consult. • Teach about foods high in calcium.	Dietary calcium is needed to maintain serum calcium levels to maintain bone mass. Foods high in calcium include plain yogurt, dairy products, seafood, sardines, green vegetables, calcium-fortified orange juice, and cereals.
	Client describes types of calcium supplements. Client uses less caffeine and alcohol.	Provide current information about calcium supplements. Teach the need to decrease alcohol and caffeine intake.	Excessive alcohol and caffeine use increase bone resorption.
	Client discusses ways to decrease lactose intolerance.	Teach ways to avoid symptoms of lactose intolerance.	Lactose intolerance is caused by the inability to break down milk sugar lactose. Use of acidophilus milk, as well as commercially prepared lactase, decreases the symptoms of lactose intolerance.
Physical Mobility, Impaired R/T osteoporosis	Client complies with physical mobility plan to level of independent ADLs.	Consult with physical therapy to develop exercise program. • Weightbearing exercises • Strengthening exercises • Discuss benefits of walking at least $\frac{1}{2}$ mile three times a week • Teach the importance of exercise in prevention of osteoporosis	Weightbearing exercises increase bone formation. Strengthening exercises increase muscle tone and circulation. NIH Consensus on Osteoporosis 1984 recommends walking, tennis, hiking, and ballroom dancing.

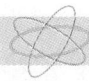

CLIENT EDUCATION GUIDE

The Client with Osteoporosis

The nurse should teach the client and significant others the following:

- Medical treatment will be based on specific client needs depending on age, degree of bone loss, and past or present evidence of fractures.
- Calcium and vitamin D supplements might be prescribed.
- Estrogen or estrogen combined with progesterone may be prescribed.
- Sodium fluoride given with calcium and vitamin D may be prescribed to stimulate bone growth.
- All medications should be monitored by a physician. Make sure you understand the exact dosage, major side effects, and augmental treatments (e.g., exercise, diet, and safety measures).

DIETARY MEASURES

- Eat calcium-rich foods: Yogurt, ice cream, cheese, fish (sardines with bones and salmon), dark green vegetables, and white vegetables, such as bok choy and cauliflower, are rich in calcium.
- Adults should ingest 1000 mg of calcium per day. After menopause, women need 1500 mg/d. Vitamin D is necessary to aid in calcium absorption.
- Limit alcohol intake; avoid smoking, beverages with caffeine, and a diet overly rich in protein.

EXERCISE

- Engage in weightbearing exercises.
- Exercise regularly to build strength and stamina.
- Tailor an exercise program to your age, body build, flexibility, and overall health.

SAFETY MEASURES

- Ensure that the house is hazard-proof.
- Identify and correct household practices that could prove to be safety hazards.

CARE PLAN: The Client with Osteoporosis

Nursing Diagnosis/ Collaborative Problem	Planning: Expected Outcomes	Implementation: Nursing Interventions	Rationales
	Client uses assistive devices to perform independent ADLs.	Assist with ADLs, allowing client to remain independent.	Pain may limit client's ability to perform ADLs.
		Evaluate need for assistive devices for ADLs and home use.	Devices may be needed for independent ADLs.
	Client identifies and avoids potential hazards, thereby avoiding falls and fractures resulting from minimal injury.	Establish a hazard-free hospital environment. • Provide adequate lighting • Adjust bed to lowest position with side rails up, when client is in bed • Place necessary articles within client's reach, including call light, water pitcher, telephone, and eyeglasses • Keep client area free of spills and clutter	Establishment of a hazard-free environment will reduce the risk from falls or minimal injury.
Pain R/T fracture (vertebral, Colles' wrist, hip)	Client experiences pain reduction or relief so client may be independent.	Assess pain medication needs.	Client may not be receiving adequate medication as a result of inadequate dosing, the need for around-the-clock administration, or iatrogenic causes. Therefore, plan medication schedule with client.
	Client uses alternative measures to reduce or alleviate pain.	Teach alternative modalities for pain relief.	Alternative modalities have been found effective in reducing pain. Include comfort measures such as positioning, warm compresses, application of assistive devices, distraction, imagery, biofeedback, and hypnosis.

ADLs, activities of daily living; NIH, National Institutes of Health; USRDA, United States Recommended Dietary Allowance.

vertigo, hearing loss with tinnitus, and blindness. Rheumatoid arthritis, ankylosing spondylitis, gout, and calcific periarthritis are commonly associated with Paget's disease.

An increase in hydroxyproline during a 24-hour urine collection indicates osteoclastic activity. A normal or increased serum calcium, anemia, and increased alkaline phosphatase are indicative of the disease process.

Management

The primary indication for treatment is pain. Analgesics such as aspirin, indomethacin, or ibuprofen may decrease bone pain. Further orthopedic treatment may be indicated for severe disabling arthritis, severe bowing deformities of the femur or tibia, and pathologic fractures. Calcitonin and etidronate, both of which retard bone resorption, may be administered, especially in painful pseudofracture. The cytotoxic antibiotic mithramycin (Mithracin) may be used to decrease serum calcium, urinary hydroxyproline, and serum alkaline phosphatase.

OSTEOMALACIA

Osteomalacia, also known as adult rickets, is a disease in which the bone becomes abnormally soft because of a disturbed calcium and phosphorous balance secondary to a vitamin D deficiency, resulting in marked deformities of the weightbearing bones and pathologic fractures.

Osteomalacia mainly affects women. Occasionally, the disease can be found in strict vegetarians or postgastrectomy patients. Primary hypoparathyroidism, renal tubular disorders, pancreatic insufficiency, hepatobiliary disease, and small intestine disease contribute to the incidence of osteomalacia. Women who have had multiple frequent pregnancies and who have breast-fed their children may have a higher incidence of the disease, as may individuals on long-term anticonvulsants, tranquilizers, sedatives, muscle relaxants, or antidiuretics.

Osteomalacia is always due to an inadequate concentration of calcium or phosphorus in the body fluids. Inadequate calcium or vitamin D in the diet may cause a decrease in the absorption of calcium from the intestine. Increased urinary excretion of calcium or the loss of calcium or phosphorus during pregnancy and lactation may cause osteomalacia.

Osteomalacia is characterized by widespread decalcification and softening of bones, especially in the spine, pelvis, and lower extremities. Bones become bent and flattened as they soften. In the spine, scoliotic and kyphotic deformities are present. Coxa vara deformity of the femoral neck caused by pressure on the femoral neck is common.

Serum calcium and phosphorus levels are reduced, and the alkaline phosphatase level is moderately elevated. Urinary calcium and creatinine excretion levels are low.

Radiographic studies indicate generalized demineralization with trabecular bone loss. Pseudofractures (milkman's fractures) and cyst formation are common. Compression fractures and bowing and bending deformities of the long bones are often present. Biopsy may assist in diagnosis.

Management

Intervention for osteomalacia includes vitamin D administered daily until signs of healing take place when a daily low maintenance dose is continued. Adequate intake of calcium and phosphorus as well as protein should be ensured. Supplemental calcium in the form of lactate or gluconate is administered.

Other Musculoskeletal Disorders

SCOLIOSIS

Scoliosis is defined as a lateral curvature of the spine when viewing from the posteroanterior view. The spine normally appears straight in this plane. Adult scoliosis is a spinal curvature existing after skeletal maturity. A curve may present in any area of the spine: cervical, thoracic, thorocolumbar, and lumbar. There is usually a second compensatory curve in the opposite direction. The most common curve pattern is a right thoracic, which produces a rib prominence.

Adult scoliosis occurs in individuals aged 40 years or older. Most cases are idiopathic and are defined as a structural spinal curvature of unknown cause that arises during adolescence and persists into adulthood. Curves of less than 40 degrees, without symptoms, generally remain stable and do not require intervention. A progressive curve (more than 65 degrees) in the thoracic spine may be responsible for shortness of breath and fatigue. Other symptoms may include back pain, progressive spinal curvature accompanied by decreased height, cardiopulmonary failure, and cosmetic deformity. Evaluating the character, severity, and specific location of back pain helps determine whether or not the pain is caused by scoliosis. A progressive curve in the lumbar spine may be responsible for low back fatigue and pain. Back pain associated with scoliosis is usually located at the apex of the curve on either the convexity or the concavity. Early degenerative changes include spinal stenosis. If nerve root entrapment occurs, surgery is indicated.

Diagnosis is based on radiographic findings of a curvature of greater than 10 degrees, combined with structural changes in the spine, including vertebral rotation. Functional scoliosis occurs as a result of leglength discrepancy or posture.

Management

Surgical procedures for adults include the application of spinal instrumentation either through an anterior or posterior approach. The type of instrumentation used is based on the discretion of the surgeon. Other considerations include diagnosis, magnitude of the curve, flexibility of the curve, inherent strength of the bone, and the individual's ability to wear postoperative immobilization.

Nursing management focuses on education of the client about postoperative care, pain control, providing adequate fluid replacement, and progressive ambulation.[21]

OSTEOMYELITIS

Osteomyelitis is a term used to describe any infection of the bone. Acute osteomyelitis responds to a 4- to 6-week course of intravenous antibiotics, whereas chronic osteomyelitis persists longer than 4 weeks and involves sequestered (necrotic bone that has separated from living tissue) areas of infection.

Osteomyelitis is generally bacterial in origin but may also be caused by viral or fungal infections. *Staphylococcus aureus* is the most common organism, but *Escherícha coli, Klebsiella, Proteus, Pseudomonas,* and *Salmonella* may also cause osteomyelitis. These organisms may be directly introduced into the bone, or they may be spread from adjacent soft tissue infection or travel through the blood to the infected site. The causative bacterial agent is able to multiply readily in bone because bone has a slow circulatory system.

Clinical manifestations of osteomyelitis include fever (temperature usually higher than 101° F [38° C]);

localized pain or tenderness; erythema (redness); heat; and swelling around the affected bone.

CRITICAL TO REMEMBER

Early diagnosis is important to prevent progression of the infection.

Symptoms are based on the area affected. Diagnostic tests include radionuclide bone scans, gallium scans, indium scans, computed tomography, and magnetic resonance imaging. In acute osteomyelitis, radiographic changes are usually not visible until 2 to 3 weeks after onset. Laboratory findings include an elevated white blood cell count, an elevated erythrocyte sedimentation rate, and, if bacteremia is present, a positive blood culture for the organism causing the infection.

Management

Needle aspiration or a percutaneous needle biopsy may assist with the diagnosis of acute osteomyelitis as well as relieve pressure from within the bone. Treatment requires administration of intravenous or intramuscular injection of one of the penicillin type of antibiotics for 4 to 6 weeks.

Chronic osteomyelitis requires sequestrectomy (surgical removal of dead bone) and saucerization (removal of scar or infected tissue, sequestra, and necrotic bone, leaving a saucer-like depression). Intravenous antibiotics are used for 4 to 6 weeks followed by a course of oral antibiotics.

Bone Tumors

PRIMARY BONE TUMORS

Primary bone tumors (those originating in bone) may be benign or malignant. The two major types include chrondrogenic (from cartilage) and osteogenic (from bone). Primary bone tumors are described in Box 45–2.

Management

The treatment of primary bone lesions is radical surgery, combined with radiation or chemotherapy. Radiation and chemotherapy are described in Chapter 7.

SURGICAL MANAGEMENT

The customary treatment of bone and soft tissue sarcomas has been amputation. Over the past 2 decades, much progress has been made in understanding the tumor, chemotherapy, and radiation therapy, thereby enabling salvage of the limb. Research has shown that

BOX 45–2

Primary Bone Tumors

CLASSIFICATION/ NAME	DESCRIPTION
Benign chondrogenic	
Osteochondroma	Most common benign tumor; commonly found in the femur and tibia; about 10 per cent develop into sarcoma
Endochondroma	Common to mature hyaline cartilage in hands, feet, ribs, spine, sternum, or long bones; frequently leads to pathologic fractures
Benign osteogenic	
Osteoid, osteomas	Usually small tumors with clearly outlined area of reactive bone; common to the proximal femur, tibia, scaphoid bone of the wrist, talus, or calcaneus of the foot; causes pain at night
Osteoblastoma	Evolves more rapidly and into a larger tumor than an osteoid osteoma; found in the vertebrae, distal femur, diaphysis of long bones, hands, and feet
Giant cell tumor	Aggressive and extensive lesion; has a tendency to recur and metastasize to the lung; commonly found in the distal femur, tibia, distal radius, sacrum, proximal humerus, and proximal fibula; produces pain, edema, and limitation in movement
Malignant osteogenic	
Osteosarcoma	Most common malignant bone tumor; occurs in the metaphysis of lone bones at the sites of the most rapid bone growth; common to the distal femur, proximal tibia, and proximal humerus; can be induced by ionizing radiation and may follow therapeutic radiation; causes pain, swelling, and pathologic fracture; serum alkaline phosphatase is markedly elevated; prognosis improving with combination therapies, reaching 65 per cent survival
Ewing's sarcoma	Common to young adults and found in the pelvis and lower extremities; metastasizes quickly to the lungs and other bones; clinical manifestations include pain, edema, low-grade fever, leukocytosis, and anemia; improving prognosis with aggressive therapy; 65 per cent survival rate
Chondrosarcoma	Common to the pelvis, ribs, proximal femur, and proximal humerus
Fibrosarcoma	Common to the femur and tibia

clients have the same disease-free survival rate with limb-sparing operations as those who have amputations.[25]

Before surgery, the client undergoes chemotherapy and radiation therapy to decrease the tumor size and treat small metastases. During surgery, the tumor and a margin of normal bone are removed. The defect created by tumor removal is filled in with bone allograft. Bone grafts are usually from cadaveric donors. The recipients of bone allografts do not require immunosuppressive treatment because the bone is frozen after harvesting. Freezing diminishes the immune response of the bone tissue. The bone graft is secured with metallic pastes and screws.

Nursing Management

Before surgery, the health-care team discusses the options with the client and significant others (many clients are adolescents or young adults). Autologous blood donations before surgery are not permitted for tumor resection; therefore, the family or significant others may wish to donate blood.

After surgery, the limb is immobilized and elevated. Pain is usually severe and controlled with narcotic analgesics through epidural or patient-controlled analgesia modes. Postoperative anemia may require transfusion. Complications of the surgery typify other orthopedic surgeries: infection, deep vein thrombosis, and nonunion of the bone grafts. Ambulation is begun the day after surgery, and the client is taught to walk with crutches.[32,43]

METASTATIC BONE TUMORS

CRITICAL TO REMEMBER

Skeletal metastases are the most common form of malignant bone tumors, and virtually every malignant tumor can metastasize to bone.

Evidence suggests that distant metastases seem to develop from tumor seed cells that travel through the lymphatic system, blood vessels, and other surrounding tissues. Primary lesions of the prostate, the breast, the kidney, the thyroid, and the lung most commonly seek to metastasize to bone. The femur, the pelvis, the ribs, and the vertebrae are the most commonly affected bone sites. Pathologic fractures are common especially in the acetabulum and proximal femur. Serum levels of alkaline phosphatase and calcium and sedimentation rate may be elevated.

Pain may occur before changes are detectable on radiographic studies. Diagnosis may be made through radiographic studies, incisional biopsy, or frozen section. Many bone tumors produce typical patterns on radiographic studies. Whenever malignant lesions are suspected, anteroposterior and lateral chest films and computed tomograms of the chest are taken to detect pulmonary metastases. A scintigraphy (bone scan) is performed to locate additional osseous lesions. Computed tomography and magnetic resonance imaging are used to detect soft tissue involvement and the location of tumor and neurovascular structures.

Disorders of the Hand

CARPAL TUNNEL SYNDROME

Carpal tunnel syndrome is a frequently seen painful disorder caused by pressure on the median nerve at the wrist. The exact cause is unknown and is often seen in those with recent fractures, arthritis, lipomas, ganglion, or congenital anomaly. This condition may develop in people with histories of strenuous or repetitive use of the hands.

Early clinical manifestations include burning or tingling pain in the thumb, index, and middle fingers. Aching pain may radiate to the upper extremity and, occasionally, to the shoulder, neck, and chest. Pain may be episodic or constant and exacerbated at night and by movement. The physical examination reveals the presence of Tinel's sign (tingling or shocklike pain) elicited by light percussion over the median nerve, at the wrist. Phalen's sign (hand tingling with acute wrist flexion) may also be present.

Treatment ranges from nonsteroidal anti-inflammatory agents, splints, and steroid injections, to surgical release. The client is advised to limit the specific motion that aggravates carpal tunnel syndrome.

GANGLION

A ganglion is the most common benign soft tissue mass in the hand, consisting of a round cystlike lesion overlying or adjacent to the wrist joint or tendon. The synovium surrounding the tendon degenerates, allowing the tendon sheath to buckle and weaken. The onset may be gradual or sudden, and it may be post-traumatic. Clinical manifestations include localized pain and a freely movable mass. Symptoms are exacerbated by dorsiflexion of the wrist. Treatment includes the aspiration of the ganglion followed by an injection of corticosteroid into the joint. Nonsteroidal anti-inflammatory agents are prescribed. Surgical excision may be necessary if symptoms persist and range of motion is impaired. Ganglion formation may recur in some instances.

Disorders of the Foot

HALLUX VALGUS

The hallux valgus (bunion) deformity is the most common disorder of the foot. Although the terms hallux valgus and bunion are frequently used synonymously, they actually refer to separate elements of the same disorder. It is defined as a painful swelling of the bursa when the great toe deviates laterally at the metatarsophalangeal joint. The problem may be congenital or may be acquired by wearing shoes that are too short or too narrow. Females are affected more frequently than males.

Initial assessment findings include a painful valgus deformity of the great toe and callus formation on the bottom of the feet. Weightbearing radiographic studies of both feet are performed.

Treatment includes suggesting the use of open-toed shoes made with soft leather or sneakers. Metatarsal pads relieve some of the pressure from weightbearing. Intra-articular corticosteroid injections are given for acute bursitis, and analgesics are administered for pain. Simple bunionectomy involves osteotomy (bone resection) of the first metatarsal, removing the bony overgrowth and bursa. Kirschner wires are inserted vertically through the toes and remain in place for 3 weeks postoperatively. Corks are placed on the tips of the wires for protection.

HAMMER TOE

Hammer toe deformity is a flexion contracture of the proximal interphalangeal joint with extension or slight hyperextension of the distal interphalangeal joint. Hammer toe deformity often accompanies hallux valgus deformity.

Clinical manifestations may include a family history of hammer toe, rheumatoid arthritis, and clawfeet. Shoes may fit incorrectly, and there is often pain on walking, with alterations in stride length. Corns may be present on the dorsum of the toe.

Treatment includes the use of pads to cushion the foot from the shoe, removal of corns, and passive stretching exercises. Surgical intervention involves osteotomy of the toe and resection of the proximal phalanx. In the very young child, surgery may consist of transplanting the flexor tendons to the extensor sides of the toes.

MORTON'S NEUROMA (PLANTAR NEUROMA)

Morton's neuroma, also known as a plantar neuroma or plantar digital neuritis, is the thickening of a nerve or the formation of a small tumor, secondary to pressure, in the area around the lateral branch of the medial plantar nerve. Pain is described as a severe, burning sensation, usually occurring in the web space between the third and fourth toes. Treatment is the surgical excision of the neuroma. Palliative measures may include steroid injection and insertion of a metatarsal arch to relieve pressure.

STUDY QUESTIONS

1. A client has difficulty digesting milk products. What dairy products can be consumed for the client who is lactose intolerant?
   A. Buttermilk and cheese
   B. Cheese and skim milk
   C. Cheese and yogurt
   D. Any type of cheese
2. A female client of Mediterranean ancestry comes to a clinic to be screened for osteoporosis. She tells you she is 35 years old, eats a diet rich in calcium and protein, and is essentially healthy. Her weight and height are within the acceptable range for her age and body build. Which of the following is a possible risk for osteoporosis?
   A. Age
   B. Ancestry
   C. Health
   D. Diet rich in protein
3. Which of the following signs or symptoms is not a clinical manifestation of osteoporosis?
   A. Lordosis
   B. Impaired breathing
   C. Back pain
   D. Bone loss in the jaw
4. Which of the following statements made by a sedentary client with a family history of osteoporosis best indicates an understanding of the benefits of exercise in the prevention and retardation of osteoporosis?
   A. "I'll definitely perform isometric exercises."
   B. "I'll cycle for at least 1 hour every day."
   C. "I'll start running up and down the stairs."
   D. "I'll begin walking at least half an hour every day."
5. A client has just undergone surgery to remove a fibrosarcoma of the femur. He is experiencing severe pain that is being managed with epidural analgesia. He is receiving the maximum dose allowed but is still restless. Which of the following interventions should the nurse use?
   A. Give a dose of intravenous narcotic to supplement the epidural.

B. Monitor the client's dressing and neurovascular responses.
C. Raise his leg on pillows above his heart level.
D. Apply warm, wet compresses to the leg.

6. Which of the following client statements best indicates the client has incorporated life-style changes as a result of surgery to correct hallux valgus?
A. "I'll wear shoes two sizes larger than the ones I now wear."
B. "I'll wear open-toed shoes made of soft leather."
C. "I'll wear high heels to prevent the condition from occurring again."
D. "I'll go barefoot as much as possible."

CRITICAL THINKING EXERCISES

SCENARIO A

A middle-aged client is concerned about bone loss resulting from osteoporosis. She tells you that her mother has severe osteoporosis, and she realizes her life-style and family history are positive for osteoporosis. She asks you to develop a life-style plan for her and a preventive life-style program for her teenage daughters.

1. How would you proceed with a plan to decrease bone loss in this client? (Do not include medical therapy).
2. How would you design a prevention plan for her daughters?

SCENARIO B

An elderly female client tells you her physician wants her to eat a diet high in calcium. He tells her he wants her to consume 1500 mg of calcium per day without taking enriched antacids or calcium supplements. She is lactose intolerant and has a hiatal hernia. She is also on a limited income. She asks you to plan a menu for her. How would you proceed?

BIBLIOGRAPHY

1. Ali, N., & Twibell, R. (1994). Barriers to osteoporosis prevention in perimenopausal and elderly women. *Geriatric Nursing, 15(4),* 201–206.
2. Aloia, J. F. (1989). *Osteoporosis: A guide to prevention and treatment.* Champaign, IL: Leisure Press.
3. Barden, R. M., & Sinkora, G. L. (1991). Bone stimulators for fusions and fractures. *Nursing Clinics of North America, 26(1),* 89–103.
4. Bender, L. H. (1991). Osteogenesis imperfecta. *Orthopaedic Nursing, 10(4),* 23–31.
5. Boden, S. D., & Kaplan, F. S. (1990). Calcium homeostasis. *Orthopaedic Clinics of North America, 21(1),* 31–42.
6. Brosnan, H. (1991). Nursing management of the adolescent with idiopathic scoliosis. *Nursing Clinics of North America, 26(1),* 17–31.
7. Carrasco, C. H., & Murray, J. A. (1989). Giant cell tumors, *Orthopaedic Clinics of North America, 20(3),* 395–405.
8. Doheny, M. O., & Sedlak, C. A. (1987). Body image considerations for the adult scoliosis patient having spinal fusion surgery. *Orthopaedic Nursing, 6(6),* 18–22.
9. Doleysh, N., et al. (1991). Neuromuscular disorders. In S. W. Salmond, et al. (Eds.), *Core curriculum for orthopaedic nursing* (2nd ed., pp. 299–303). Pitman, NJ: National Association of Orthopaedic Nurses.
10. Einhorn, T. A., et al. (1990). Nutrition and bone. *Orthopaedic Clinics of North America, 21(1),* 43–50.
11. Fueyo, L. (1991). Hand. In S. W. Salmond et al. (Eds.), *Core curriculum for orthopaedic nursing* (2nd ed., pp. 239–250). Pitman, NJ: National Association of Orthopaedic Nurses.
12. Gagliardi, B. A. (1991). The impact of Duchenne muscular dystrophy on families. *Orthopaedic Nursing, 10(5),* 41–48.
13. Gertner, J. M., & Root, L. (1990). Osteogenesis imperfecta. *Orthopaedic Clinics of North America, 21(1),* 151–162.
14. Gitelis, S., & Schajowicz, F. (1989). Osteoid osteoma and osteoblastoma. *Orthopaedic Clinics of North America, 20(3),* 313–325.
15. Haberman, E. T., & Lopez, R. A. (1989). Metastatic disease of bone and treatment of pathological fractures. *Orthopaedic Clinics of North America, 20(3),* 468–486.
16. Hahn, T. J. (1993). Metabolic bone disease. In W. Kelley et al. (Eds.), *Textbook of rheumatology* (4th ed., pp. 1593–1627). Philadelphia: W. B. Saunders.
17. Hansel, M. J. (1988). Fractures and the healing process. *Orthopaedic Nursing, 7(1),* 43–48.
18. Hay, E. K. (1991). That old hip: The osteoporosis process. *Nursing Clinics of North America, 26(1),* 43–51.
19. Ignatavicius, D. D. (1995). Interventions for clients with musculoskeletal problems. In D. D. Ignatavicius et al. (Eds.), *Medical-surgical nursing: A nursing process approach* (2nd ed., pp. 1411–1447). Philadelphia: W. B. Saunders.
20. Kaiser, J. M., & Piasecki, P. A. (1991). Tumors. In S. W. Salmond et al. (Eds.), *Core curriculum for orthopaedic nursing* (2nd ed., pp. 407–425), Pitman, NJ: National Association of Orthopaedic Nurses.
21. Kanis, J. A. (1990). Editorial: Osteoporosis and osteopenia. *Journal of Bone and Mineral Research, 5(3),* 209–211.

22. Klein, M. J., et al. (1989). Osteosarcoma: Clinical and pathological considerations. *Orthopaedic Clinics of North America, 20(3),* 327–345.

23. Lamphier, P. C. (1985). Primary bone tumors. *Orthopaedic Nursing, 4(5),* 17–23.

24. Lindsay, R. (1989). Osteoporosis: An updated approach to prevention and management. *Geriatrics, 44(1),* 45–52.

25. Lisanti, P., & Tompkins, J. S. (1991). Pain. In S. W. Salmond et al. (Eds.), *Core curriculum for orthopaedic nursing* (2nd ed., pp. 95–107). Pitman, NJ: National Association of Orthopaedic Nurses.

26. Liscum, B. (1992). Osteoporosis: The silent disease. *Orthopaedic Nursing, 11(4),* 21–25.

27. Maier, T., & Pietrocarlo, T. (1991). The foot and footwear. *Nursing Clinics of North America, 26(1),* 223–231.

28. Martin, M. E. (1989). Oral antibiotics for the treatment of patients with chronic osteomyelitis. *Orthopaedic Nursing, 8(3),* 35–38.

29. McCaffery, M., Beebe, A. (1989). *Pain: Clinical manual for nursing practice.* St. Louis: Mosby-Year Book.

30. McMahon, M., Peterson, C. & Schilke, J. (1992). Osteoporosis: Identifying high-risk persons. *Journal of Gerontological Nursing, 18(10),* 19–26.

31. Merkow, R. L., & Lane, J. M. (1990). Paget's disease of bone. *Orthopedic Clinics of North America, 21(1),* 171–189.

32. Mitchell, N. R., et al. (1991). Infection. In S. W. Salmond et al. (Eds.), *Core curriculum for orthopaedic nursing* (2nd ed., 251–263). Pitman, NJ: National Association of Orthopaedic Nurses.

33. Mooney, N. E. (1991). Pain management in the orthopaedic patient. *Nursing Clinics of North America, 26(1),* 81–84.

34. Mosher, C. M. (1991). The Papineau bone graft: A limb salvage technique. *Orthopaedic Nursing, 10(3),* 27–32.

35. Mourad, L. (1991). *Orthopedic disorders.* St. Louis: Mosby-Year Book.

36. National Osteoporosis Foundation. (1991). *Boning up on osteoporosis: A guide to prevention and treatment.* Farmington, CT: University of Connecticut Health Center.

37. Nestle Information Services. (1991). Osteoporosis: The silent thief. *Worldwide, 3(2),* 1–8.

38. Parker, B. C. (1988). Rehabilitative aspects of nerve injuries of the hand. *Orthopaedic Nursing, 7(1),* 29–34.

39. Pavlik, M. (1991). Measuring bone mineral content. *Orthopaedic Nursing, 10(2),* 39–43.

40. Piasecki, P. A. (1991). The nursing role in limb salvage surgery. *Nursing Clinics of North America, 26(1),* 33–41.

41. Prior, J. C., et al. (1990). Spinal bone loss and ovulatory disturbances. *New England Journal of Medicine, 323(18),* 1221–1271.

42. Rodts, M. F. (1987). Surgical intervention for adult scoliosis. *Orthopaedic Nursing, 6(6),* 11–17.

43. Rodts, M. F., & Ruda, S. C. (1991). Spine. In S. W. Salmond et al. (Eds.), *Core curriculum for orthopaedic nursing* (2nd ed., pp. 357–361). Pitman, NJ: National Association of Orthopaedic Nurses.

44. Sauers, K. F. (1991). Self-concept. In S. W. Salmond et al. (Eds.), *Core curriculum for orthopaedic nursing* (2nd ed., pp. 109–115). Pitman, NJ: National Association of Orthopaedic Nurses.

45. Tomaski, A. M., & Dobert, J. H. (1991). Metabolic bone disease. In S. W. Salmond et al. (Eds.), *Core curriculum for orthopaedic nursing* (2nd ed., pp. 265–279). Pitman, NJ: National Association of Orthopaedic Nurses.

46. Urrows, S. T., et al. (1991). Profiles in osteoporosis. *American Journal of Nursing, 91(12),* 32–37.

47. Weinerman, S. A., & Bockman, R. S. (1990). Medical therapy of osteoporosis. *Orthopedic Clinics of North America, 21(1),* 109–119.

48. Zwolski, K., et al. (1991). Miscellaneous disorders. In S. W. Salmond et al. (Eds.), *Core curriculum for orthopaedic nursing* (2nd ed., pp. 430–433). Pitman, NJ: National Association of Orthopaedic Nurses.

Chapter 46

Nursing Care of Clients with Musculoskeletal Trauma or Overuse

Learning Outcomes

After completing this chapter, the learner will be able to:

1. Assess the client for clinical manifestations resulting from common musculoskeletal trauma or overuse.
2. Teach the client about the risk factors, basic pathophysiology, and clinical manifestations associated with common musculoskeletal trauma or overuse.
3. Explain the client's role in the prevention and treatment of musculoskeletal trauma or overuse.
4. Develop plans of care for the prevention, management, and rehabilitation of clients with musculoskeletal trauma or overuse.
5. Implement nursing interventions that optimize the quality of life for clients with musculoskeletal trauma or overuse.
6. Evaluate planned client outcomes using outcomes developed in the planning phase of care.

Musculoskeletal Injuries

Fractures

A fracture is a disruption of normal bone continuity that occurs when more stress is placed on a bone than it is able to absorb. Surrounding soft tissue injury often also occurs. Although some fractures are life threatening (because of associated hemorrhage and shock), most are not.

Classification

FRACTURE PATTERN

Some of the more common types of fractures are illustrated in Figure 46–1. The following terms help establish generally the pattern of a fracture:

- *Closed (simple) fracture.* This is an uncomplicated fracture with intact skin over the fracture site; that is, bone does not protrude through the skin (Fig. 46–1*A*).
- *Open (compound) fracture.* In this type, a break in the skin is present over the fracture site. The wound communicates from the skin (externally) to the fractured bone (internally). Because of this communication with the external environment, an open fracture is always potentially infected (Fig. 46–1*B*). Open fractures are further divided into grades of severity.
- *Complete fracture.* The fracture line extends through the entire bone substance; that is, the periosteum is disrupted on both sides of the bone (Fig. 46–1*C*).
- *Incomplete (partial) fracture.* The fracture line extends part way through the bone; that is, bone continuity is not completely disrupted. This type of fracture is also called a willow, greenstick, or hickory-stick fracture (Fig. 46–1*D*).
- *Displaced fracture.* Bone fragments are separated at the fracture line (Fig. 46–1*E*).
- *Comminuted fracture.* There is more than one fracture line, and bone fragments are crushed or broken into several pieces (Fig. 46–1*F*).
- *Impacted fracture ("telescoped fracture") or compression fracture.* One bone fragment is forcibly driven into another adjacent bone fragment (Fig. 46–1*G* and *I*).
- *Pathologic fracture.* The fracture occurs as a result of underlying bone disorders such as osteoporosis or tumor. It usually occurs with minimal trauma (Fig. 46–1*H*).
- *Greenstick fracture.* This is a fracture in which one side of the bone is broken and the other side is bent (Fig. 46–1*J*).

The just-mentioned terms describing fractures may be used in combination to provide more complete description.

When a fracture of an extremity divides a bone into two fragments, the fragments are referred to as the proximal (uncontrollable) fragment and the distal (controllable) fragment. The proximal fragment is the section of bone nearer the body. This fragment cannot be manipulated or moved when the fractured bones are being set (i.e., therapeutically correctly aligned) because of its muscle attachments and location. The distal fragment (farther away from the body) can be manipulated or moved to realign it with the proximal fragment.

Terms used to describe the direction of fracture line in relation to the affected bone's longitudinal axis include the following:

- *Linear fracture.* The fracture line runs parallel to the bone's long axis.
- *Oblique fracture.* The fracture line is at an oblique angle (see Fig. 46–1*A* and *B*).
- *Longitudinal fracture.* The fracture line extends longitudinally (see Fig. 46–1*D*).
- *Transverse fracture.* The fracture line is straight across the bone (see Fig. 46–1*C*).
- *Spiral fracture.* The fracture line forms a spiral encircling the bone (see Fig. 46–1*E*).
- *Stellate.* There is a central fracture point with several fissures radiating outward.

FRACTURE LOCATION

In long bones fractures are described as being proximal, distal, or midshaft, based on their location on the bone. Other terms include angulation fracture, avulsion fracture, blow-out fracture (results from blow that fractures the floor of the orbit of the eye), compression fracture (see Fig. 46–1*I*), and a fatigue or march fracture (fracture of metatarsals resulting from long marches).

Two common examples named for physicians are

- *Colles' fracture.* This is a common fracture in which the distal radius is fractured within 1 inch of articular surface.
- *Pott's fracture.* This fracture occurs at the medial malleolus of the tibia and fibula and often is associated with rupture of the internal lateral ligament or chipping off of a piece of the medial malleolus, or both.

Fractures involving or close to joints are described as

- *Articular fracture* (joint fracture), which involves a joint surface
- *Extracapsular fracture,* which is near a joint but does not enter the joint capsule.
- *Intracapsular fracture,* which is within a joint capsule.
- *Epiphyseal fracture,* which involves ossification center at the extremity of long bones; these fractures may result in alterations in bone growth

Fractures are also classified according to their causes. For example, a stress fracture may occur in a bone that is subjected to prolonged, unaccustomed muscular action. Pathologic fractures occur in diseased bones (see Fig. 46–1*H*), such as bones with osteoporosis.

FRACTURE DISPLACEMENT

Displacement of the fracture ends and fragments of bone depend on the causative force and degree of

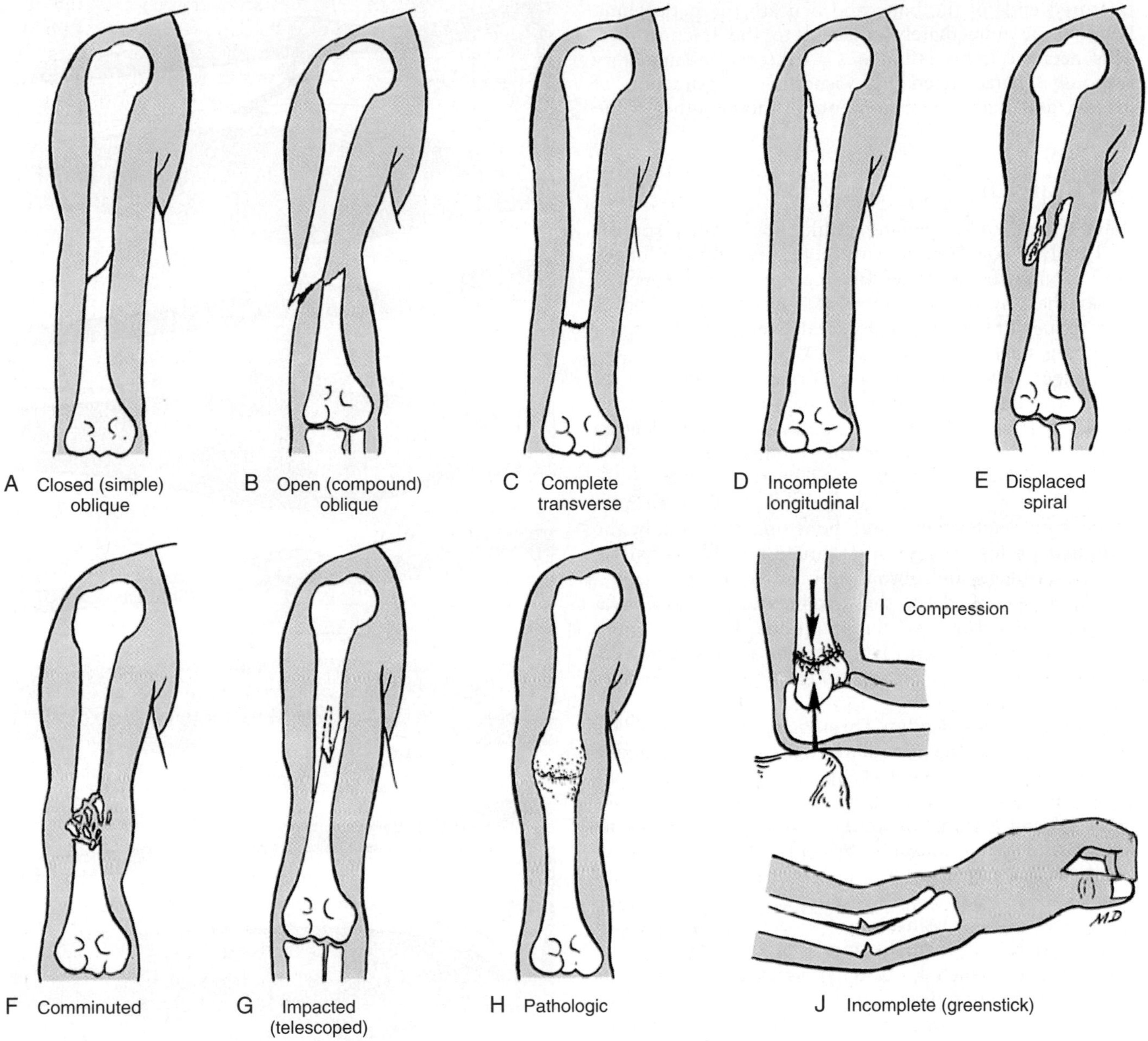

Figure 46–1
Common types of fractures.

spasm in surrounding muscles. Displacement may occur sideways, at an angle (angulated), as an override, rotated, or offset.

Incidence

The incidence of fractures varies with the site of the fracture. Rib fractures are the most common bone fracture in adults. Femoral fractures are most common in young and middle-aged adults. The elderly client often fractures the hip and wrist.

Etiology

The most common cause of fracture is direct trauma to the bone. Motor vehicle accidents and falls are the primary mechanism of injury. In addition, primary bone disease such as osteoporosis or metastatic bone cancer can weaken the bony structure and lead to fracture.

Fractures occur from direct or indirect force and are affected by biologic and behavioral factors. Direct force is the result of a moving object contacting the bone. Indirect force can be caused by contracting muscles exerting a powerful pulling force on the bone.

Pathophysiology

When a bone is broken, the periosteum and blood vessels in the cortex, marrow, and surrounding soft tissues are disrupted. Bleeding occurs from the damaged ends of the bone and from nearby soft tissues (muscles). A hematoma forms in the medullary canal between the fractured ends of the bone and beneath the periosteum. Bone tissue immediately adjacent to the fracture dies. This necrotic tissue stimulates an intense inflammatory response characterized by vasodilation, exudation of plasma and leukocytes, and infiltration of other white cells.

BONE HEALING

Bone is able to regenerate, unlike some other specialized body tissue. Fracture healing occurs by the formation of new bone tissue (to reunite bone fragments) rather than by the formation of nonspecialized fibrous scar tissue. Fractures usually heal over 6 weeks in the following stages (Fig. 46–2).

Stage One—Hematoma Formation. Within 24 hours, the blood clot begins to organize. As the blood in the hematoma clots (coagulates), a loose, delicate mesh of fibrin forms around the fracture site.

Stage Two—Cellular Proliferation. This stage takes place at the fracture site, where torn ends of periosteum, endosteum, and bone marrow supply the cells that proliferate and differentiate into fibrocartilage, hyaline cartilage, and fibrous connective tissues.

After several days, the combination of periosteal elevation and the granulation tissue forms a collar around the end of each fragment. The collars eventually advance, unite, and form a bridge across the fracture site.

Stage Three—Callus Formation. Six to 10 days after the injury, the granulation tissue changes and a provisional callus (procallus) forms. Newly formed cartilage and bone matrix (derived in part from the undamaged periosteum and endosteum of adjacent bone margins) disperse through the soft tissue callus. They increase in number until a provisional callus is established.

Stage Four—Ossification. A permanent callus of true, rigid bone eventually forms by the deposition of calcium salts, which knits the fractured bone ends together. Ossification first forms an external callus (between the periosteum and cortex), next an internal callus (medullary plug), and finally an intermediate callus (between the cortical fragments). During the third to tenth weeks of healing, the callus converts into bone. This formation of bone firmly binds together the fractured ends and completes healing.

Stage Five—Consolidation and Remodeling. At the same time that true bone is forming, the callus is remodeled by osteoblastic and osteoclastic activity. In effect, excess bone is chiseled away and absorbed from the callus. This remodeling process is governed by the stresses imposed on it by muscles and weightbearing.

HEALING TIME

This varies with the type of fracture and type of bone. Spongy bone heals more rapidly than compact bone because of the rich blood supply. Impacted fractures require several weeks to heal, whereas displaced fractures may require months to years for complete healing.

Different bones also heal over different time frames. The bones of the arm may heal in 3 months, whereas

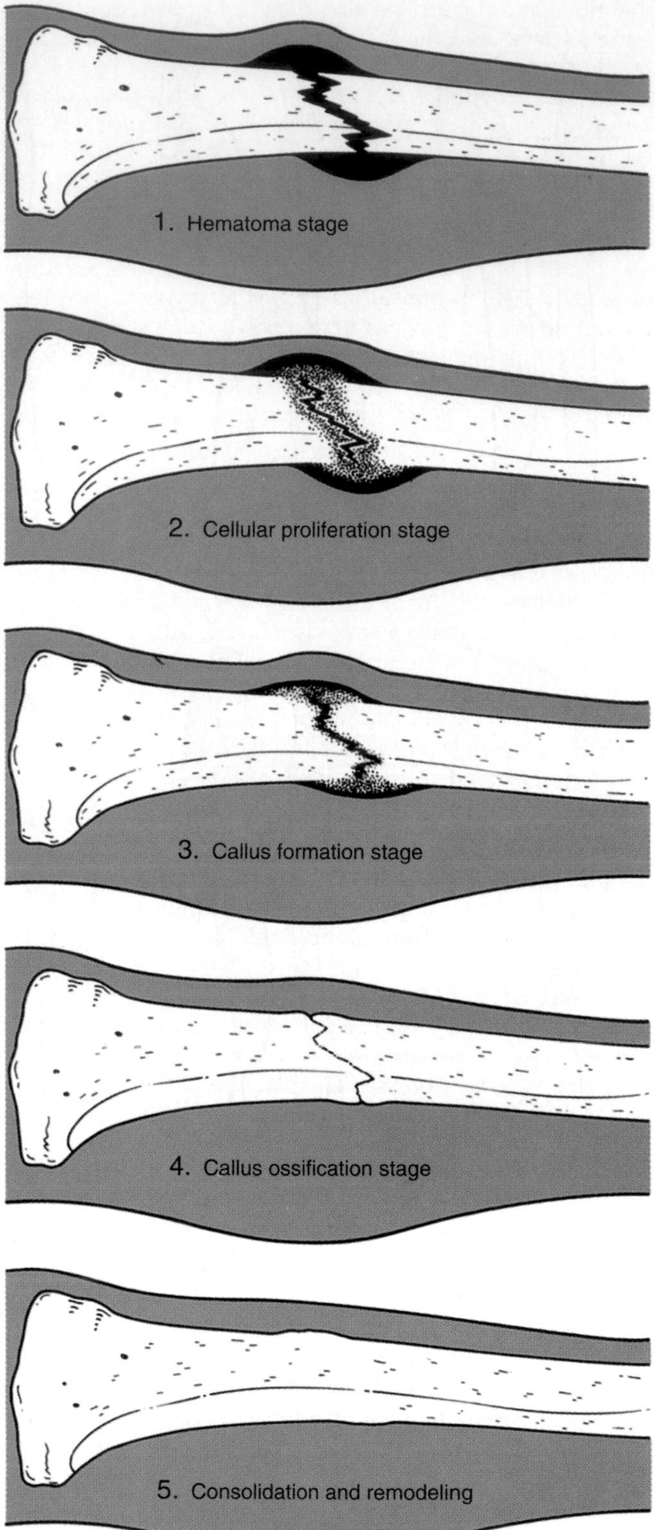

Figure 46–2
Stages of fracture healing. Possible complications during the hematoma stage include prevention of coagulation and loss of hematoma through (a) open fracture, (b) débridement, or (c) action of fibrinolytic synovial fluid. Possible complications during the cellular proliferation phase include interruption of the vascular network by (a) motion or infection; (b) a hostile environment because of an inadequate blood supply; (c) unbridgeable gaps between bone ends; or (d) devitalization of periosteal, intramedullary, or extraosseous mesenchymal tissues from which red blood cells originate. A possible complication during the callus formation stage is that the collagen matrix may be rendered nonossifiable by hypercortisonism or scurvy.

the tibia and femur require 6 months or longer. The more surface area the fracture fragments have, the more rapidly they heal.

Most function returns in 6 months after bony union takes place, but complete function may not be regained for a year or more. In a year, a simple fracture will resume an almost normal appearance if aligned correctly. A fracture that has healed in excellent position may still have some reduced joint motion.

Conditions That Modify Healing. Because healing of fractures is a continuous sequential process, any interruption in the process may result in delayed healing. Bone healing may be delayed by inadequate mobilization of the fragments, decreased blood supply, interposition of soft tissues into the fracture site, or infection.

Clinical Manifestations

Many factors affect the clinical manifestations a fracture may produce, such as site, severity, type of fracture, and amount of damage to other structures. Some fractures produce few clinical manifestations and would not be detected if x-ray films were not taken to assess the injury. Various combinations may be present (see Clinical Manifestations: Fractures).

DIAGNOSTIC ASSESSMENT

Radiology or fluoroscopy is used to confirm the diagnosis of a fracture by showing the location of the fracture and the direction of fracture line. Findings vary according to site and type of fracture. X-ray films of fractured bones are taken in two planes and include the joint above and the joint below the fracture (to identify dislocations or subluxations). Anteroposterior and lateral views are commonly taken before reduction, after reduction, and periodically during the healing process.

Complications

CRITICAL TO REMEMBER

Possible early complications of fractures include arterial damage, compartment syndrome, fat embolism, infection, shock, and Volkmann's ischemic contracture.

Arterial Damage. This may consist of contused, thrombosed, lacerated, severed, or spastic arteries. Arteries may be constricted by bandages or casts that are too tight. Indications of arterial damage include variable or absent pulse, swelling, pallor or patch cyanosis distal to the fracture, continuing blood loss, pain, a large fracture hematoma, poor capillary return, poorly filled veins in a cold extremity, and paralysis or anesthesia distal to the fracture (in the absence of known neurologic injury).

CRITICAL TO REMEMBER

The nurse must promptly report and document assessment findings indicating arterial complications.

Emergency intervention may include splitting or removing tight encircling casts or bandages, elevating or changing the position of the injured part, reducing fractures or dislocations, or surgery.

Compartment Syndrome. This is a serious complication of fractures. Compartments are made up of muscles, bones, nerves, and blood vessels wrapped by a fibrous membrane. A compartment, therefore, is a closed space. After trauma, edema or bleeding can occur within the compartment. Because a compartment is a closed space, the edema or bleeding exerts pressure on the pliable muscles, nerves, and vessels. Compartment syndrome can also develop if external pressure is applied, such as from a cast or tight dressing.

CLINICAL MANIFESTATIONS

Fractures

Signs and symptoms associated with fractures vary widely and may include various combinations of the following:

- *Deformity:* strong muscle pull may cause bone fragments to override; therefore alignment and contour changes occur, such as (1) angulation, rotation, limb shortening; (2) bone depression; and (3) altered curves in the injured site especially when compared with the opposite site
- *Swelling:* edema may appear rapidly from localization of serous fluid at the fracture site and extravasation of blood into adjacent tissues
- *Bruising (ecchymosis),* which occurs from subcutaneous bleeding
- *Muscle spasm* (involuntary muscle contraction near the fracture)
- *Tenderness* over fracture site resulting from underlying injuries
- *Pain* (immediate severe pain at the time of injury; after injury, pain may result from muscle spasm, overriding of the fractured ends of the bone, or damage to adjacent structures)
- *Impaired sensation (numbness),* which may occur from nerve damage or nerve entrapment from edema, bleeding, or bony fragments
- *Loss of normal function,* which may result from instability of the fractured bone, pain, or muscle spasm; paralysis may be caused by nerve damage
- *Abnormal mobility* (movement of a part that is normally immobile caused by instability when long bones are fractured)
- *Crepitus* (grating sensations or sounds felt or heard if the injured part is moved; crepitus results from broken bone ends rubbing together)
- *Hypovolemic shock,* which may result from blood loss or other injuries

Compartment syndrome is managed by removing the cause of the compression. The cast or dressing is loosened or removed. If it is due to edema or bleeding, a fasciotomy (incision into the fascia) is performed. Sometimes the incision is left open until the swelling decreases. If it is left untreated, compartment syndrome leads to a functionless extremity or requires amputation.

Fat Embolism. This is a relatively uncommon but potentially life-threatening complication of long bone and pelvis fractures. Fat embolism syndrome (FES) occurs 24 to 48 hours after injury. The cause of FES includes direct damage to the lung, soft tissue injury, hypotension, and aspiration of blood or gastric contents. The pathophysiology of FES is similar to that of adult respiratory distress syndrome.

Once fat droplets enter the circulation, the fat is too large to pass through pulmonary circulation. They lodge in the capillaries and break down into fatty acids. Free fatty acids are toxic to lung parenchyma, capillary endothelium, and surfactant. The result is pulmonary hypertension.

The nurse must have a high index of suspicion for FES. The classic picture of the client with FES includes altered mental status, tachypnea, tachycardia, hypoxemia, petechiae, and fever. Many times, it is difficult to distinguish FES from pulmonary embolism. The distinguishing features are listed in Table 46–1.

TABLE 46–1 Comparison of Characteristics for Pulmonary Embolism and Fat Embolism Syndrome

CHARACTERISTICS	PULMONARY EMBOLISM	FAT EMBOLISM SYNDROME
Pathophysiology and etiology	Local venous trauma Venous stasis Hypercoagulability	Fat globulin release from long bone or multiple fractures Stress-related release of catecholamines that mobilize lipids from adipose tissues
Risk factors	Immobility Age $>$40 years History of heart disease, especially myocardial infarction or congestive heart failure Prior history of DVT or pulmonary embolus Surgery or trauma to hip, pelvis, or knee Obesity	Hypovolemia/shock Delayed immobilization or surgery Multiple traumatic injuries Joint replacement
Clinical manifestations*	Dyspnea Chest pain Apprehension/anxiety Cough/hemoptysis Tachypnea Localized rales Tachycardia Low-grade fever Thrombophlebitis	Dyspnea Restless, agitated, confused, stuporous Tachypnea $>$30/min Diffuse rales (late) Tachycardia $>$140/min Temperature $>$103° F Petechial skin rash
Diagnostic assessment	ABGs (Po_2 $<$80 mm Hg) Chest radiograph Electrocardiogram Lung scan Pulmonary angiogram	Hypoxemia (Po_2 $<$80 mm Hg) Chest radiograph Electrocardiogram Laboratory Thrombocytopenia ↓Hemoglobin Fat in urine and blood Increased sedimentation rate Increased levels of fibrin split products
Prevention	Early ambulation Leg elevation Elastic stockings Leg exercises Intermittent pneumatic compression Medications Anticoagulants Antiplatelet agents	Immobilize fractures Adequate hydration Oxygen Corticosteroids
Management	Anticoagulation Surgical intervention IVC interruption Embolectomy	Oxygen Fluid replacement Mechanical ventilation with PEEP Corticosteroids Maintain adequate hemoglobin

* Occur within 48 to 72 hours in venous thromboembolism and within 24 to 48 hours in fat embolism.

ABGs, arterial blood gases; DVT, deep vein thrombosis; IVC, inferior vena cava; PEEP, positive end-expiratory pressure; Po_2, partial pressure of oxygen.

Modified from Slye, D. (1991). Orthopedic complications. *Nursing Clinics of North America, 26*(1), 113–132.

Infection. Infection after a fracture may result from contamination of open fractures, or it can be introduced at the time of surgery. Compound fractures may be complicated by tetanus or gas gangrene.

Pseudomonas is another common infectious agent. Any infection can lead to delayed union or osteomyelitis.

Gas gangrene infections may develop in deep, grossly contaminated wounds. Gas gangrene is caused by anaerobic bacteria (various species of *Clostridium*). These organisms produce a characteristic cellulitis in which gas is present under the skin. *Assessment reveals* (1) a precipitous drop in hemoglobin, (2) temperature elevation, (3) rapid pulse, (4) pain, (5) sudden local puffiness (with discoloration of tissues), and (6) thin, watery, extremely foul-smelling exudate. Crepitation may be felt, on palpation of the skin, as a result of the presence of gas bubbles in muscles and subcutaneous tissue. Treatment of gas gangrene involves opening the wound widely to admit air and permit drainage. Generous, multiple incisions are made through the skin and fascia. Sutures and any gangrenous material are removed and the wound is irrigated. Anti-infective agents are administered. If massive gangrene develops, amputation is necessary.

Shock. Most musculoskeletal injuries are not life threatening. However, some are due to shock resulting from blood loss and increased capillary permeability, leading to decreased oxygenation.

Volkmann's Ischemic Contracture. This serious and potentially crippling condition of the hand or forearm arises from a complication of a fracture around the elbow joint or forearm bones. It begins as a compartment syndrome that compromises arterial and venous circulation. If it is not relieved, pressure causes prolonged ischemia and muscle is gradually replaced by fibrous tissue that traps tendons and nerves. The typical end result is a permanent, stiff, clawlike deformity of the arm and hand. Often, anesthesia and paralysis are also present. Volkmann's ischemic contracture most commonly arises after a supracondylar fracture of the humerus. It may also occur after other fractures of the elbow joint and forearm, crushing injuries of the forearm, and excessive use of forearm muscles and from tight bandages or casts.

CRITICAL TO REMEMBER

To avoid permanent deformity, compartment syndromes must be recognized and treated early.

LONG-TERM COMPLICATIONS

Delayed Union. This is the failure of a fracture to consolidate within the time usually required for union. Delayed union is usually due to a retardation of the healing process from the previously discussed factors such as decreased blood supply. Delayed union usually is correctable with additional time and the application of weightbearing to the fracture site.

Nonunion. This is the failure of a fracture site to consolidate and produce a complete, firm, and stable union after 6 to 9 months. Nonunion is characterized by excessive motion in the fracture site, which leads to a false joint or *pseudoarthrosis*. The risk factors to nonunion are the same as those presented earlier. Nonunion is commonly treated with bone grafts.

Malunion. This is the healing of a fracture site with an increased degree of angulation or deformity. Malunion seen early in fracture healing can be corrected with adjustment of traction or reimmobilization. Malunion after healing is usually treated with surgery.

Medical Management

Primary goals of treatment of a fracture are to return an injured limb to maximal function, prevent complications, and obtain the best possible cosmetic result.

The physician may need to manipulate a fracture to restore peripheral pulses distal to the fracture and to reduce normal compression or stretching of nerves. With a displaced fracture, there may be damage to large blood vessels and a hematoma may develop in the soft tissues. Blood loss may be considerable. Massive hemorrhage accompanying a fracture is a surgical emergency. Vital signs are closely monitored, and the client is given nothing by mouth in case surgery is needed.

Fracture reduction restores the injured bone to normal anatomic alignment, position, and length and brings the fractured fragments into close approximation with one another. Fracture reduction is usually painful and requires anesthesia.

Fortunately, not all fractures require reduction. Fractures may be reduced in three basic ways used singly or in combination.

Traction. (See Chap. 44.) With reduction traction, considerable pull is exerted on the distal fragment of a fracture to align it with the less manageable proximal fragment. The amount of traction needed to achieve alignment is usually intense and is applied for just a short time. Once a fracture has been reduced, the amount of weight applied through the traction setup is the smallest amount required to maintain proper alignment and apposition of bone fragments.

Closed Reduction (Manipulation). A physician performs closed reduction by manually applying traction to lock the ends of a fragment together and restore normal bone alignment. A surgical incision is not needed. Three basic maneuvers used for manipulation are traction and countertraction, angulation, and rotation. After a closed reduction, x-ray films are taken and a cast is usually applied.

Open Reduction. An incision is made, and the fracture is aligned during surgery under direct vision. At the time of surgery, various internal fixation devices may be applied to the fractured bone to maintain alignment (e.g., screws, plates, pins, wires, nails), or rods may be placed through bone fragments, fixed to the sides of the bone, or inserted directly into the bone's medullary cavity. For some fractures, open reduction is the treatment of choice, such as for compound fractures that are comminuted and accompanied by serious neurovascular injuries, or fractures with widely separated fragments or soft tissue interposed between bone fragments. Open reduction is usually needed for fractures of the femur and fractured joints. Although internal fixation devices initially help immobilize a fracture and prevent deformity, they are not a substitute for bone healing. If proper bone healing does not occur, the metallic internal fixation devices succumb to stress, loosen, or break.

Management of Specific Fractures

HIP FRACTURES

Hip fractures are generally divided into three types: femoral neck, intertrochanteric, and subtrochanteric (Fig. 46–3). Fractures of the femoral neck and intertrochanteric regions constitute 97 per cent of hip fractures.[15]

Incidence

Hip fractures are the leading traumatic injury in the elderly, and, with degenerative arthritis increasing in frequency with age, hip surgery is a very common orthopedic procedure.

Etiology

Hip fractures result from two major changes seen with aging. The most significant loss in the aged is the loss of postural stability, leading to an increased incidence of falls. The amount of bone mass has been shown to be equal in clients who fall and in age-matched controls. This leads to the conclusion that falling is the more significant cause.

Decreased bone mass does contribute to hip fractures, however. Bone mass decreases linearly with age. The combination of decreased bone mass and tendency toward falls explains why the incidence of hip fracture doubles every 5 years after the age of 50.

Pathophysiology

The pathophysiology of fracture injury was discussed earlier in this chapter.

Femoral neck fractures are often called the unsolved fracture because there is a significant failure rate after primary fixation.[15]

Intertrochanteric fractures are usually comminuted and more osteoporotic, leading to difficulty with good anatomic reduction of the fragments and fixation.

Clinical Manifestations

The client or significant other reports a history of a fall. Even accidents that seem relatively minor, such as slipping out of a chair onto the floor, can produce hip fracture in the aged.

CRITICAL TO REMEMBER

Objective findings include a shortened, externally rotated hip and sometimes deformity along the lateral side of the hip.

There may also be ecchymosis and tissue trauma from the fall. Other sites of tissue trauma may also be present, such as forehead or hand lacerations.

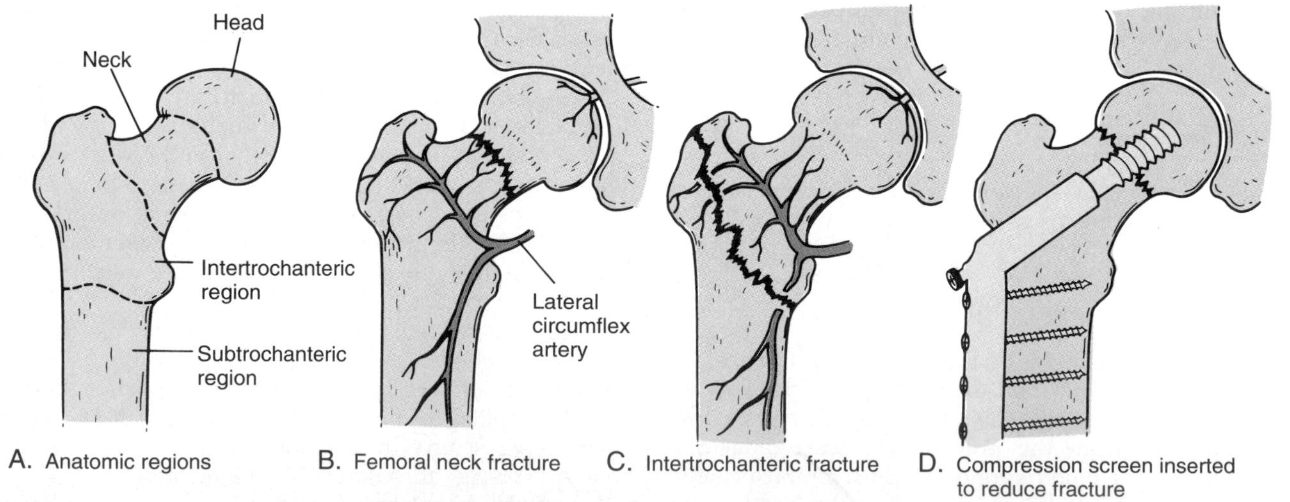

Figure 46–3
A, Normal proximal end of femur. *B*, Intracapsular fracture of proximal end of femur. Note blood supply. *C*, Extracapsular intertrochanteric fracture. Note effect of fracture on blood supply. *D*, Femoral neck fracture with compression screw inserted for reduction.

DIAGNOSTIC ASSESSMENT

Hip fracture is confirmed by x-ray study. Other diagnostic tests may be used to assess the client's readiness for surgery and anesthesia. A complete blood count, electrolyte levels, urinalysis, chest x-ray study, and electrocardiogram are the most common tests.

Medical Management

Treatment plans vary depending on the type of fracture, other injuries sustained during the fall, and concurrent medical conditions. While the client is being stabilized for surgery, perhaps with blood transfusions or correction of underlying disorders such as heart failure, skin traction is commonly applied to the leg (e.g., Buck's traction [see Chap. 44]). Traction assists to realign the fractures and reduce muscle spasms in the extremity. In general, the client is taken for surgical repair quickly because placing an elderly person at bedrest increases the risks of immobility.

The number of disorders the client has (concomitant illnesses) increases the risk of morbidity and mortality with hip fracture. Nursing home residents with hip fractures are at increased risk of perioperative complications. These clients often have preoperative limitations in mobility and can seldom return to any form of ambulation. Because of the limited progress clients can make and their surgical risk, sometimes hip fractures in these clients are not surgically repaired.

Surgical Management

The primary goal of surgery is to provide a solid union of fracture sites to allow for early weightbearing and functional recovery.

Femoral Neck Fractures. Four surgical procedures are common to repair femoral neck fractures:

- Knowles pin
- Jewett nail (Fig. 46–4*A*)
- Sliding nail or compression screw (Fig. 46–4*B*)
- Hemiarthroplasty or total hip arthroplasty

After fixation with a Knowles pin, full weightbearing is not allowed because the pin does not pull the fracture fragments together (a process called compression). The Jewett nail also does not provide compression of the fragments, but it is a stronger device and the client can usually bear weight after surgery. The compression screw is the most commonly used device and has an advantage of drawing the fracture fragments together. The alignment of the fractures increases healing and allows for weightbearing. A hemiarthroplasty, with replacement of the femoral component of the hip with a noncemented metallic prosthesis, can be performed. This procedure allows the client to have full weightbearing. However, when the hip prosthesis is used, there is a risk of postoperative dislocation. Because of the problems with nonunion after hip fracture, a complete hip replacement can also be performed. Total hip arthroplasty is discussed in Chapter 11.

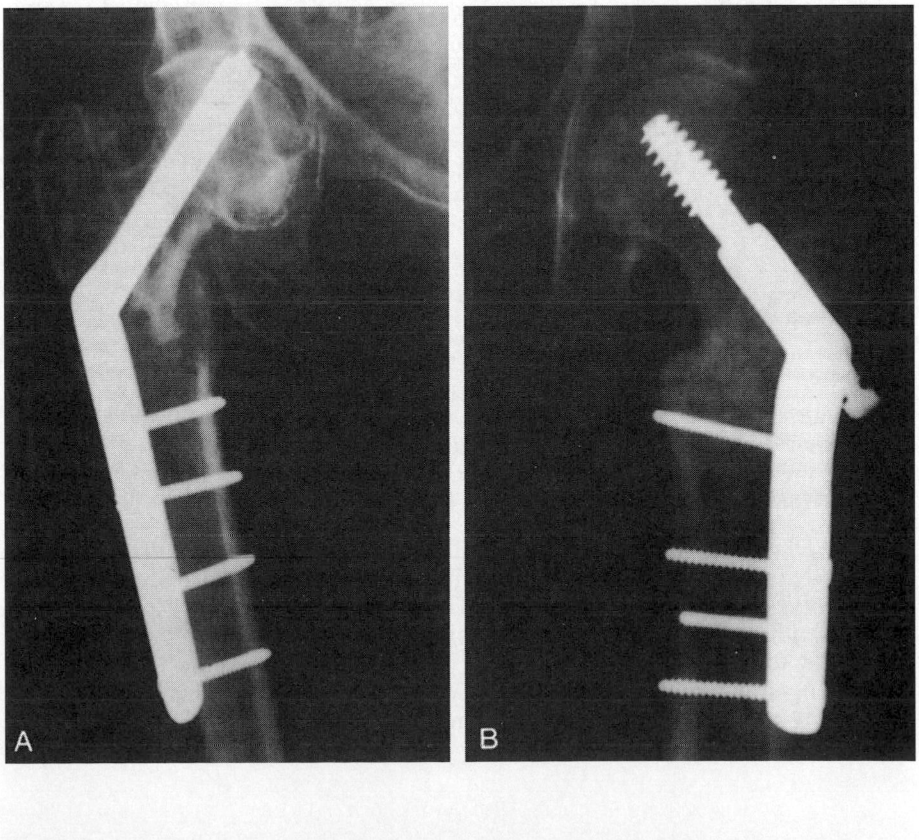

Figure 46–4
A, A single-piece Jewett nail fixation of an intertrochanteric fracture. With medial displacement of the fracture fragments, the rigid nail has penetrated the femoral head, causing pain and limitation of motion of the hip. *B,* Femoral neck fracture repaired with the use of a Richards compression set screw. The screw is driven into the femoral head and locked in place by a set screw on its lateral end. (From Ochs, M. [1990]. Surgical management of the hip in the elderly patient. *Clinics in Geriatric Medicine, 6[3],* 571–587.)

Intertrochanteric Fractures. The most widely used device for repair of intertrochanteric fractures is the sliding nail or compression screw. After surgery, clients cannot bear weight. These clients also have a poorer functional outcome and higher mortality than those with fractures of the femoral neck.

Postoperative Complications. Several complications can result from both the surgery and the postoperative immobility: deep vein thrombosis, pressure ulcers, and delirium.

Deep Vein Thrombosis. Because approximately 20 per cent of clients with deep vein thrombosis experience pulmonary embolus, the prevention of thrombosis is essential. Measures to decrease the risk of deep vein thrombosis include the use of aspirin, heparin, warfarin, low-molecular-weight dextran, and external pneumatic compression devices. Antiembolism stockings are also commonly used.

Pressure Ulcers. Pressure ulcers occur in 20 to 70 per cent of clients after hip fracture. It should be recognized that significant pressure has often been applied to the skin before the client is admitted to the nursing unit, from lying on a hard floor or hard surfaces in ambulances and emergency departments and x-ray departments. Prevention of ongoing ischemia is critical and can be accomplished by decreasing the risk of pressure through the use of therapeutic mattresses, excellent skin care, early ambulation, and elevation of the heels from the bed with rolled towels. High-risk clients can be identified using assessment tools.

Delirium. Postoperative confusion usually occurs in response to systemic stressors rather than the result of central nervous system disorders. Medications, infection, impaction, and hypoxemia are common causes of delirium.

Rehabilitation. Physical therapists teach the client how to ambulate, and most clients are moved to a chair the day after surgery. Eventual recovery of clients after the repair of hip fractures is influenced by premorbid dementia, preoperative immobility, presence of intertrochanteric fracture, and advanced age.[1] Several large series report that, of clients surviving 1 year after a fracture, only 50 per cent achieve prefracture functional status.[15]

Nursing Management

Assessment

On admission, the client is usually weighed before being placed in bed. A complete assessment is performed, including the assessment of abrasions or other injuries from the fall.

Nursing Diagnosis: Mobility, Impaired R/T prescribed limitations in movement and pain.

Planning: Expected Outcomes. The client will maintain adequate strength to regain physical mobility once able to ambulate, by performing exercises while bedridden, transferring to the chair with decreasing need for assistance once ambulatory, and walking with a walker safely.

Implementation. The client is encouraged to perform various exercises for the upper and lower extremities. A trapeze is placed above the bed to facilitate upper arm and shoulder strength. Exercises such as quadriceps setting, gluteal setting, and leg movements up and down in bed maintain some muscle strength. Passive and active range of motion (ROM) exercises should also be implemented.

When the client is allowed to be in the chair, the nurse assists the client to the edge of the bed while keeping the legs abducted. The client is assisted by at least two nurses to stand and then balance with the walker. The degree of weightbearing that the client can safely use must be reinforced as the client stands. If the client is unable to stand, a complete lift is usually performed to assist the client to the chair.

Collaborative Problem: Risk for dislocation of the hip R/T inappropriate stress on the joint and surrounding tissues.

Planning: Expected Outcomes. The nurse will monitor the client for clinical manifestations of hip dislocation and position the client to decrease the risk of dislocation.

Implementation. The operated leg should be handled gently after hip surgery. Before moving the client, the nurse should explain what is going to happen and how the client can help. An overbed trapeze helps with moving. The client should be taught how to use the trapeze and avoid extremes of position after hip surgery. The client should keep the leg abducted (i.e., out to the side) at all times. The leg must never be adducted past the body's midline (e.g., over the other leg), or the head of the femur (or prosthesis) may dislocate out of the acetabulum. A pillow or A-frame must be placed between the client's legs to help maintain abduction and to remind the client not to cross the legs.

CRITICAL TO REMEMBER

One must avoid acute flexion of the operated hip.

This can be caused by excessive elevation of the head of the bed. The nurse should check the physician's instructions about how high the head of the bed can be safely elevated. Some can have the head of the bed raised 35 to 40 degrees. If the head of the bed can be somewhat elevated, the client should be instructed not to lean farther forward because this further flexes the hip and may cause dislocation.

The nurse can prevent external rotation of the leg on the operated side by placing a trochanter roll beside the external aspect of the thigh. Without this intervention, the operated leg may tend to lie slightly externally rotated when the person is supine.

The client should be turned only with the physician's order after hip surgery. Commonly after hip surgery the client can be turned to the unoperated side. After hip pinning, some clients are permitted to turn to either side. However, after other types of hip surgery, such as total hip replacement, turning is not permitted for several days. When helping a client to turn following internal fixation

- Avoid adduction of the operated leg and excessive movement
- Prevent strain on the hip
- Keep the leg and hip in proper alignment

If the client is permitted to turn onto the operated side, the client can be rolled gently toward the nurse after placing pillows between the legs. The bed acts as a splint for the injured leg. If it is not permitted to turn to either side, the client may be able to lift straight up off the bed by using a trapeze for back care and linen changes.

Commonly after an anterior surgical approach, the operated limb is positioned so it is internally rotated and in a neutral or an abducted position. The individual may be permitted to sit up unless the capsule has been removed. With a posterior approach the operated leg is positioned in slight abduction and external rotation (a change from "typical" positioning) and the client lies fairly flat.

The bed should not be positioned too low when a client is getting up after hip surgery. Less hip strain and bending occurs if the bed is somewhat elevated. The nurse should be sure the bed is locked so it will not move while the client is getting up. For the same reasons, elevated toilet seats are needed after hip surgery once the client can go to the bathroom.

Usually when a client first gets up in a chair following hip surgery, the operated leg is kept extended, well supported, and elevated. Once the operated leg may be lowered, the client should sit with hips even with knees. The client must be instructed not to cross the legs but to keep both feet on the floor (see the Client Education Guide: After Hip Surgery). Crossing the legs adducts the operated leg and can dislocate the hip. The first few times the leg is lowered, the nurse should assess for swelling and discoloration.

CLIENT EDUCATION GUIDE

After Hip Surgery

The nurse must teach a client who has undergone surgical repair of the femoral head to:

- Avoid crossing legs while sitting, standing, and lying down
- Avoid putting excess weight on operated leg
- Use supportive devices per orders of physician (canes, crutches, or walker)
- Hazard-proof the home environment
- When riding in a car, stop at least once every hour and walk around to increase circulation
- Perform exercises daily or as ordered by physician
- Eat a diet rich in vitamins and minerals, low in fat, and high in fiber
- Drink plenty of fluids
- Avoid weight gain, because obesity causes stress on the femoral repair
- Use elevated toilet seats

Collaborative Problem: Risk for compartment syndrome R/T leg edema and bleeding.

Planning: Expected Outcomes. The nurse will monitor the client for clinical manifestations of compartment syndrome.

Implementation. The nurse monitors the color, capillary refill, warmth, movement, sensation, pedal pulses, and ability to dorsiplantar flex the operative leg using the nonoperative leg as a control. Clinical manifestations of compartment syndrome include pallor, pulselessness, paresthesias, pain, and paralysis of the leg. These findings must be reported to the physician immediately.

Nursing Diagnoses: Pain R/T trauma and surgical repair of a fractured hip.

Planning: Expected Outcomes. The client will experience improved comfort, as evidenced by less facial grimacing and guarding with movement, ability to transfer to the chair or ambulate without reports of pain, and use of a decreasing amount of narcotics for pain relief.

Implementation. Most surgical and traumatic pain is managed with narcotic analgesics until the pain subsides somewhat. Usually within 3 to 4 days, less potent narcotics and non-narcotic analgesics are used for pain relief.

The treatment of clients with discomfort from lying in one position (supine) can be decreased by placing a small folded bath towel beneath the lumbar spine and by moving the legs slightly in bed.

Epidural Analgesia. Some clients are being pain managed with epidural narcotics. Before ambulating a client with an epidural infusion, the nurse closely assesses for sensation by asking about numbness and by touching the client's legs with an alcohol wipe. The ability to lift the legs from the bed is also assessed. Once the client is moved to the chair, the blood pressure measurement should be reassessed to detect orthostatic hypotension. Clients with epidural anesthetics have decreased venous return as a result of the lack of muscle activity in the legs. They can very quickly experience orthostasis and faint.

Nursing Diagnosis: Constipation, Risk for R/T side effects of narcotics and immobility.

Planning: Expected Outcomes. The client will decrease risk of constipation by consuming high-fiber and bulk foods and adequate fluids and having a bowel movement every 2 to 3 days.

Implementation. The nurse determines the client's usual defecation pattern and monitors for the return of bowel sounds after surgery. Once the client is eating, foods with fiber such as bran and prunes should be encouraged, along with at least 1500 mL of water or other fluids daily. Some clients find that hot fluids such as coffee stimulate the bowels. Bowel programs should be instituted in the morning after breakfast because the gastrocolic reflex is strongest at that time. Docusate sodium (Colace) and other stool softeners are commonly prescribed. In addition, the client may require suppositories or enemas to maintain a normal bowel movement schedule. When possible, the client should be placed on a bedside commode to facilitate moving the bowels.

Evaluation

The degree of expected outcome attainment is assessed frequently, usually daily. Some of the expected outcomes for mobility may require extended periods of time to accomplish, depending on the status of the client before surgery.

FRACTURES OF THE FEMUR SHAFT

Femoral shaft fracture most often results from severe violence and occurs in young or middle-aged people. Fractures of the proximal femur are more common in the elderly. A fractured femur shaft commonly causes marked displacement and deformity and extensive soft tissue damage with swelling. It is essential that the leg be protectively immobilized during transportation, such as with an air splint or Thomas splint. Blood loss at the time of injury is often considerable and the client often experiences shock. If the fracture is relatively simple and the client is in good general condition with no skin damage, treatment by open reduction and internal fixation (ORIF) by intramedullary rod insertion may be used. This allows immediate ambulation (with guarded weightbearing).

Fractures of the distal end of the femur may be reduced by continuous skeletal traction and manipulation or by internal fixation with rods, nails and plates, or screws. A complication of these fractures is tearing or compression of the sciatic nerve or popliteal artery. Care of the client in skeletal traction is discussed in Chapter 44.

FRACTURES OF THE PELVIS

Pelvic fractures occur in nearly 30 per cent of all multiple trauma injuries. Pelvic fractures are associated with injuries to the major arteries, lower urinary tract, uterus, testes, bowel and rectum, abdominal wall, and spine and spinal cord. Pelvic fractures can result in hemorrhage, and usual clinical manifestations include hypotension, pain with pressure applied to the pelvis, and bleeding into the peritoneum or urinary tract.

Management of pelvic fractures depends on the severity of the fracture. Unstable, weightbearing pelvic fractures are treated with external fixation devices and through ORIF. Less severe fractures of non-weightbearing portions can be successfully treated with bedrest and traction.

Nursing management centers on maintaining adequate circulation to the skin because the client in traction can seldom turn. In addition, the client needs adequate pain control, assessment of neurovascular status, and assessment for complications such as thrombophlebitis and fat embolism.

FRACTURES OF THE TIBIA AND FIBULA

Fractures of the lower leg, tibia, and fibula are most commonly casted after reduction. Complex fractures may require traction or external fixation. Open fractures of the distal third of the leg are often slow to heal in many people owing to diminished blood supply from atherosclerosis.

FRACTURES OF THE FOOT

Minimally displaced fractures of the foot are treated with open walking shoes, casts, or braces to reduce direct contact with the fracture site and to splint the area. In fractures with significant displacement, open reduction and casting may be necessary. A Pott's fracture occurs at the medial malleolus of the tibia and fibula.

FRACTURES OF THE UPPER EXTREMITY

Humerus. Fractures of the proximal humerus are common in the elderly. The fracture may be impacted or displaced. Impacted fractures are usually immobilized with a sling. Displaced fractures are treated by surgical open reduction and fixation with pins. Fractures of the dominant arm in elderly clients often make them dependent and immobile. There is also an increased risk of falling because balance is reduced as a result of the loss of the use of the arm.

Fractures of the shaft of the humerus are usually managed with traction via a hanging arm cast or splint. Sometimes, the fracture is surgically reduced and repaired with intermedullary rods or plates and screws (ORIF). Nonunion is a common complication of humeral shaft fractures, and bone grafting may be required.

Fractures of the condyles of the humerus usually occur from a direct blow. These fractures can result in damage to the brachial or median nerves. The fracture is treated with ORIF, although skeletal traction and casts can be used.

Radius and Ulna. Colles' fracture is a fracture of the distal radius resulting from a fall on an outstretched hand. It is most common in women. The distal radius has a large percentage of cancellous bone, the type that is most commonly affected by osteoporosis. These fractures can be treated by ORIF, splints, casts, or external fixation, depending on their severity.

The radius and ulna usually fracture together. The fracture may be treated with ORIF or casted. Closed reduction with casting is the most common form of treatment.

Olecranon. Fractures of the olecranon are common and usually result from a fall onto the elbow. Treatment includes closed reduction and long arm casting. Healing is slow and so is rehabilitation of range of motion in the elbow once the cast is removed. Six weeks to 2 months is the usual length of time the cast is left on, and several months may be required for full return of function.

Wrist and Hand. The most common bone fractured in the hand is the carpal scaphoid, and this injury most often occurs in young men. A fracture of one or more of the bones in the wrist and hand can occur. Closed reduction and casting is the usual treatment. Casts are usually worn for 6 to 12 weeks.

Fractures of the metacarpals and phalanges are seldom displaced. They are immobilized with splints for 10 days for phalangeal fractures and 3 to 4 weeks for fractures of the metacarpals.

Nursing Management

The nurse assesses the client's radial and ulnar arteries as well as color, warmth, movement, sensation, and capillary refill in the fingers. The client's arm should be elevated on two pillows. During the night, the client needs frequent assessment to be certain the arm does not become dependent. The arm can quickly swell and occlude arterial and nerve supply to the hand. Cast care should be taught to the client and significant others (see Chap. 44).

Sports Injuries

OVERUSE SYNDROMES

Overuse syndromes are common sports-related problems. They begin insidiously, and although uncomfortable, they do not completely stop a person's activity. Thus, the person may continue to exercise. However, continuing exercise sets up a cycle that worsens the overuse syndrome. Overuse syndromes relate to specific athletic activities, such as excessive running. Gradually, an overload of stress produces microtrauma, causing inflammation and pain. Stopping the activity that is producing the syndrome usually corrects the problem. Intervention consists of resting the injured part, applying ice, and performing supervised, gradual rehabilitative exercises of the part before returning to athletic activity.

People at greatest risk for overexercising and overuse injury are (1) competitive athletes; (2) first-time athletes; (3) "born-again" athletes, that is, individuals who were once very active and begin exercising again after a decade or so of sedentary living; and (4) people recovering from injury. Some authorities suggest that exercising 5 days a week is beneficial and relatively safe, whereas exercising 6 or 7 days a week greatly increases the risk of injury, including overuse injury. Anatomic variants, that is, bone malalignment, also increase risk for overuse injury.

Overuse syndromes may be prevented by avoiding factors that precipitate overuse injury, such as

- *Training errors,* such as progressing too fast and lack of conditioning
- *Improper technique,* such as arm problems from poor tennis technique
- *Improper equipment,* such as incorrect shoes for the sport
- *Unsafe environmental factors,* such as a slippery surface

Some common overuse syndromes of the leg are described in Box 46–1.

BOX 46–1

Overuse Syndromes of the Leg

- *Patellar tendinitis* ("jumper's knee") is caused by repetitive stress on the patellar tendon during jumping. The person experiences tenderness at the insertion of the patellar tendon on the tibia.
- *Plantar fasciitis* produces heel pain during or immediately after exercise and often on arising in the morning. It is caused by repetitive stress on the long plantar ligament that attaches to the plantar (sole) surface of the calcaneus (heel bone) with its fibers fanning out and attaching to the forefoot.
- *Chondromalacia* is a painful patella caused by repeated quadriceps contractions with the knee semiflexed (e.g., during running, mountain climbing, skiing). Symptoms are usually diffuse aching, worsened by climbing stairs or hills, and weakness of the vastus medialis. Chondromalacia is more common in women athletes than in men.
- *Stress fractures* are partial or complete fractures of bone that are due to recurrent submaximal trauma. They are common in but not confined to the lower limbs. Clinical manifestations include localized swelling and point tenderness across a bone. Most stress fractures are "hairline fractures" of the bone; therefore, it takes several weeks for new bone to be seen. Most stress fractures are preventable with proper preconditioning and preseason training.

Stretching is extremely important before exercise requiring joint flexibility. Flexibility is determined mainly by muscles and much less by capsules and tendons. Stretching exercises affect muscles and are, therefore, important in increasing general flexibility. Stretching exercises also help maintain and increase ROM around a joint. They do not increase endurance or strength. Stretching exercises should be static (i.e., should hold muscles in a stretched position for a few moments rather than repeatedly stretching and relaxing them). Static stretching (1) reduces the danger of overstretching or tissue damage, (2) causes less muscle soreness than a bouncing or ballistic stretch, and (3) relieves muscle soreness when it does occur. Box 46–2 summarizes some ways of preventing injuries in fitness programs.

BOX 46–2

Preventing Injuries in Fitness Programs

Lack of fitness is one of the main causes of sport injury. The nurse must instruct the client about the following:

WARM-UP AND STRETCHING EXERCISES

Always warm up and stretch before strenuous exercises. Warm up means to begin and finish exercises gradually. Stretching exercises increase muscle flexibility.

PACING

Build up an exercise program gradually. It takes at least 6 to 8 weeks to get into strong condition. Add small, gradual increments of exercise. Proceed gradually and do not overdo. Tired muscles are prone to injury.

INTENSITY

When preparing for a specific event, plan training programs accordingly; that is, a marathon demands a more intense training program than does a shorter race.

CAPACITY LEVEL

Exercise to the capacity of physiologic limits.

STRENGTH

Build strength gradually to gain greater endurance, speed, and power.

MOTIVATION

Success in an exercise program depends on individual motivation.

RELAXATION

Relaxation exercises relieve fatigue and tension.

ROUTINE

Regular exercise is more valuable and less likely to lead to injury than bursts of activity followed by long periods of inactivity.

Strains

Strain is trauma to the body of a muscle or attachment of a tendon caused by overstretching, misuse, or overextension. Strains usually arise from twisting or wrenching movements. They may be acute (e.g., occur during unaccustomed vigorous exercise) or chronic (e.g., develop after repetitive muscle overuse). Strains may occur in any age group and in any body part that contains muscles and tendons.

Management

X-ray examination is required to rule out the possibility of fracture. Ecchymosis develops later.

Acute strains require rest, and possibly splinting. The nurse must elevate the injured part. Ice pack applications for the first 24 to 48 hours after injury reduce swelling. Heat may then be prescribed to promote comfort, to encourage reabsorption of blood and fluid, and to promote healing. Surgical repair may be necessary if rupture is present at the tendon-bone interface. During healing (4–6 weeks) movement of the injured part should be minimal. Activity should never be such that it produces symptoms, such as swelling or pain. After mature scar tissue has formed, the part can be gradually and progressively exercised. Avoid overactivity during rehabilitation.

Sprains

A sprain is a ligament injury resulting from overstress causing damage to ligament fibers or their attachment. They commonly result from sudden injury or forced hyperextension. Sprains may be mild (grade 1), moderate (grade 2), or severe (grade 3). A mild sprain tears a few ligament fibers, but there is no loss of function and the ligament is not weakened. Therefore, protection of the ligament is not vital. A moderate sprain tears a portion of a ligament, producing some loss of function. Protection is vital to prevent further tearing. A severe sprain completely tears a ligament either from its attachment or within the ligament body itself. Complete rupture often requires surgical repair. Approximation of the ligament ends is important to ensure strength and stability of the ligament (Fig. 46–5).

Upper extremity sprains often result from overstressing a joint during sports activity, while attempting to break a fall, or while bracing during a motor vehicle accident. Ankle sprains are often the result of missteps, motor vehicle accidents, or sports injuries. Cervical sprains most often result from whiplash injuries.

Clinical Manifestations

On physical examination, the severity of a sprain may not be apparent. With severe sprains the person may say the joint feels loose or like "something coming apart." The person may describe what feels like a snap, pop, or tearing. This usually indicates severe injury. The amount of swelling also indicates severity. Diffuse swelling (grade 1 sprains) results from microscopic ligament tearing, whereas severe swelling (grade 3 sprains) comes from bleeding into the tissues. Ecchymosis does not necessarily indicate either the severity or site of the injury. For example, gravity causes bruising in a part of the foot distal to a sprained ankle.

After a sprain injury, tenderness to palpation develops that is well localized at first and later becomes more diffuse. Other assessment findings include swell-

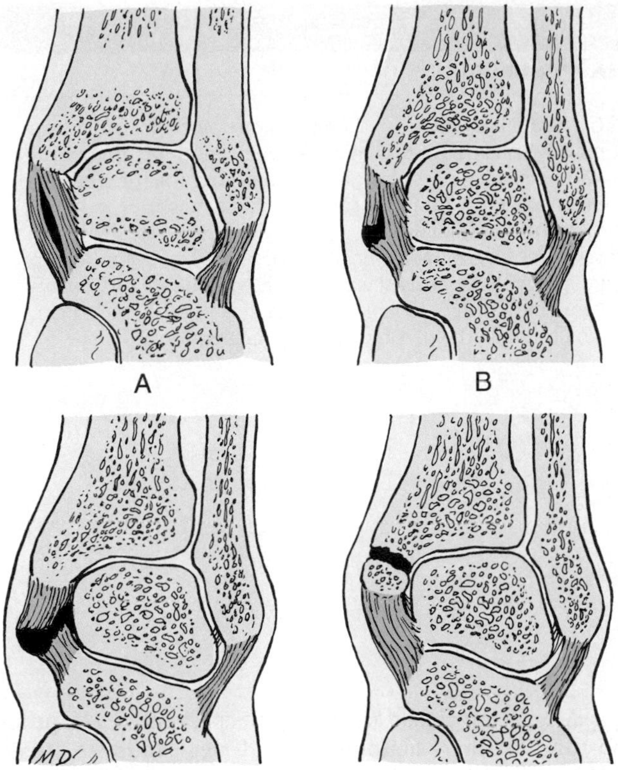

Figure 46–5
Various types of sprain. (This figure shows the ankle.) *A*, Mild (grade 1) sprain. There is a small hematoma in a localized ligament area. A few fibers are separated. *B*, Moderate (grade 2) sprain. More severe fiber tearing than in *A*. No more than half the fibers are torn. *C*, Severe (grade 3) sprain. Tearing is completely through the ligament. *D*, Sprain fracture. Ligament is completely torn off, and a fragment of bone is torn off also.

ing, severe pain, discoloration, decreased motion (limited joint motion and function), and disability. Disability may not be very severe initially but may be extensive after 2 to 3 hours. X-ray study may show soft tissue swelling but no evidence of bone or joint injury.

Management

Immediate intervention includes elevating the injured joint and applying ice. The joint may be immobilized by splinting, casting, or taping. Immobilization may continue from 3 to 4 weeks. Casting helps approximate the ligament ends and alleviates pain. A mature scar forms in connective fibrous tissue in 4 to 6 weeks. After complete healing the person needs a carefully planned exercise program.

Dislocations and Subluxations

Dislocation and subluxation are both displacements of a joint from its normal position. Dislocation is the separation of both articulating surfaces. Subluxation occurs when the articulating surfaces lose partial contact. These injuries usually occur from direct or indirect pressure to the joint. A displaced bone may impede blood supply, tear ligaments, rupture blood vessels, damage nerves, and rupture muscle attachments. Dislocations and subluxations disrupt a joint by tearing the capsule and ligaments. They are often accompanied by a fracture of the joint surface.

Clinical Manifestations

Dislocations and subluxations may or may not produce visible deformity. Dislocation may alter the length of an affected extremity. Localized joint pain and loss of function may occur. A dislocation differs from a fracture in that it partially immobilizes a joint. (A fracture site typically has abnormal free movement.) Before treatment, the nurse must assess and document the neurovascular status of parts distal to the injury. Once diagnosis is confirmed by x-ray examination, the dislocation or subluxation is reduced.

Management

Prompt intervention is essential to prevent complications, that is, ischemia or aseptic necrosis (resulting from impaired blood supply to parts distal to the dislocation) and impaired nourishment of the articulating cartilage in the injured joint. Reduction is usually performed without surgery (closed reduction). Occasionally, surgery (open reduction) is required, that is, for some knee injuries that completely rupture ligaments. Closed manipulation is performed under general anesthesia.

After reduction of a dislocation or subluxation, the joint is immobilized by a splint or cast. Immobilization may be needed for 3 to 6 weeks. The nurse must encourage prescribed active exercise of adjacent nonimmobilized joints. After immobilization is removed, active motion of the injured part, that is, voluntary muscle contraction, must be encouraged. Passive stretching can be harmful.

Low Back Pain

Low back pain occurs in the low lumbar, lumbosacral, or sacroiliac areas. It often relates to degenerative processes and musculotendinous strain caused by stress from the human upright posture. The lumbar area is the most easily injured part of the back and is the most common site of back pain. Back pain can also occur from

- A ruptured vertebral disc or herniation of the nucleus pulposus
- Back or pelvic fractures, tumors, or infection (e.g., osteomyelitis)

BOX 46–3

Specific Back Pain Problems

- *Degenerative changes* (osteoarthritis). Osteoarthritis in intervertebral discs and posterior articulating facets often occurs along with spinal stenosis. These conditions occur mainly in middle-aged people. Assessment findings include early morning stiffness and pain made worse by sitting or standing. Walking usually brings some relief. Spinal stenosis is relieved most by lying down. Sciatic radiation may occur. Symptoms are increased by fatigue, obesity, and muscle tension.
- *Osteoporosis.* Osteoporosis is the most common disorder causing low back pain (see also Chap. 45).
- *Spondylolysis and spondylolisthesis.* The breaking down of a vertebra (spondylolysis) or the forward slipping of a vertebra (spondylolisthesis) often results from stress fractures. Frequently, they involve the fifth lumbar vertebra. These conditions may be asymptomatic or cause low back pain with or without sciatic radiation. Acute symptoms are relieved by bedrest and analgesics.
- *Compression fractures.* Compression vertebral fractures may be caused by minimal trauma. Cancer or osteoporosis is considered as the cause of repeated fractures resulting from only minimal trauma. Stable fractures respond to bedrest and analgesics.
- *Scoliosis.* Degenerative changes develop more rapidly in people with scoliosis than in those without such deformities. Uncorrected scoliosis in adults can cause back pain, which can be helped by surgical intervention.

- Inflammation such as ankylosing spondylitis
- Congenital back deformities
- Muscle spasm associated with strain or sprain
- Back strain from stretched abdominal muscles caused by obesity or pregnancy (see Box 46–3)

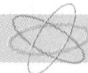

Much low back pain can be prevented by proper posture, strong abdominal and leg muscles, using proper lifting techniques, and keeping oneself in good physical condition (see the Client Education Guide: Techniques for Managing Chronic Back Pain).

CLIENT EDUCATION GUIDE

Techniques for Managing Chronic Back Pain

The nurse should instruct the patient as follows:

WALKING, STANDING, AND SITTING

Maintain erect posture.
Avoid prolonged standing or sitting. Change position frequently.
Avoid cramped, uncomfortable, or tense positions.
Walk, stand, and sit as tall as possible. When walking, hold head erect, chin tucked in slightly, and hold stomach in. The abdominal muscles help support the lower back.
When sitting, use a footstool to keep knees level with hips. Keep both feet on the floor. Keep your back against the chair back (do not slouch). Use a rolled towel as needed to support the lower back.
Stand with lower back as flat as possible. (Avoid "hollow" of the back.) Tuck hips in by tightening abdominal muscles.
Avoid excessive hip and knee extension.
When standing for some time, place one foot on a small stool to relieve lumbar lordosis. Lean body slightly forward and place hands in front of body.
Avoid bending, lifting, twisting at waist level.
Do not wear high-heeled shoes.
Squat with a straight lower back.
Alternate activity with periods of rest.

EXERCISING

Begin a fitness program with the approval of a physician.
Start a fitness program slowly.
Use a program that provides general fitness as well as a specific back-conditioning exercise.
In each session, begin exercises gradually (warm up) and at the end slow down gradually (cool down). Do not start and end exercises abruptly.
Avoid exercises that hyperextend the back (e.g., straight leg sit-ups or back bends).
Avoid exercises that have caused you back pain previously. While standing straight, place your hands on your hips and bend over backward. Hold for 30 to 60 seconds. While sitting, bend at the waist and place your head on your knees. Hold for 2 to 5 minutes. While lying flat on the floor, place your legs on a chair and hold for up to 15 minutes.

Back pain may be relieved by bedrest, local heat, local ice, analgesia (e.g., aspirin), nonsteroidal anti-inflammatory drugs, and muscle relaxants. Traction is occasionally needed to relieve muscle spasm, but bedrest is usually sufficient. After the acute pain is relieved, a lumbosacral corset and muscle-strengthening exercises may be prescribed to strengthen back support structures. Narcotic analgesics should be avoided unless absolutely necessary.

Anterior Cruciate Ligament Injury

The ligaments of the knee stabilize the joint and control into motion. The anterior cruciate ligament (ACL) is the strongest and least compliant ligament within the knee. It functions primarily to prevent anterior displacement of the tibia on the femur as well as to control the rotary stability of the knee joint.

The ACL is susceptible to injury and is the most frequently completely torn ligament of the knee. Two basic mechanisms of injury exist. In the first type of injury, an excessive valgus force is applied to the knee. This type of force damages the medial collateral ligament and the ACL. The second type of injury to the ACL occurs with hyperextension while the leg is internally rotated. This mechanism causes isolated ACL rupture and more subtle symptoms.

At the time of injury, there is a snapping sensation and, at times, a popping noise. Within hours, the knee becomes tense, swollen, stiff, and painful. If it is not treated, the knee will give way, leading to falls. The knee loses support during lateral pivots.

ACL tears can be repaired within several weeks of injury and still allow the return of function and stability. Various devices, including autograft and artificial ligament materials, have been used for reconstruction. Reconstruction after the surgery requires an effective balance between mobilization and immobilization. Some clients are treated with continuous passive motion (CPM) machines. They are placed in the recovery room and provide support to the limb as well as put the knee through preset degrees of passive range of motion. The CPM is used at least 3 hours a day or until full ROM is achieved.

When the CPM is not used, the limb is placed in long leg limb brace set at 40 degrees flexion for 1 week. The client is taught to do isometric quadriceps setting, bent knee-leg raises, and foot exercises. Over the course of the next 4 to 6 weeks, progressive ROM is added to the brace.

A newer form of reconstruction is through artificial grafts to reconstruct the ACL. These clients can undergo rapid rehabilitation, obtaining full ROM in 3 to 4 days most of the time.

STUDY QUESTIONS

1. Arterial damage after a fracture produces which of the following signs or symptoms?
   A. Anesthesia distal to the fracture
   B. Anesthesia proximal to the fracture
   C. Filled veins in a cold extremity
   D. Patch cyanosis proximal to the fracture
2. A nurse is monitoring a client after an open reduction of a fracture of the femoral shaft. The client exhibits the following signs and symptoms:

   Restlessness
   Petechial skin rash
   Respiratory rate of 32 (client norm, 18)
   Temperature of 103.6° F

   The nurse should report these signs to the physician because they are probably indicative of
   A. Pulmonary embolism
   B. Infection of the bone
   C. Fat embolism syndrome
   D. Compartmental syndrome
3. A nurse is teaching a client about appropriate and safe position changes after the client has undergone the insertion of a compression screw to correct a femoral neck fracture. Which of the following client statements indicates the client understands proper positioning?
   A. "I'll avoid sitting straight up in bed."
   B. "I'll turn my operated leg outward when I sit in the chair."
   C. "I'll turn my leg slightly inward when I am in bed or in a chair."
   D. "I'll turn only on my operated leg."
4. A goal for a client having an anterior approach to the surgical repair of a fractured hip would include specific objectives to
   A. Internally rotate the operated hip in a neutral or abducted position
   B. Slightly abduct and externally rotate the operated hip
   C. Internally rotate the operated hip in a neutral or adducted position
   D. Slightly adduct the operated leg and externally rotate it
5. Specific, successful outcomes after surgical repair of an intertrochanteric fracture would include absence of which of the following?
   A. Deep vein thrombosis
   B. Anesthesia of the lower leg
   C. Brachial paralysis
   D. Fat embolism syndrome

CRITICAL THINKING EXERCISES

SCENARIO A

A young adult is injured in an automobile accident. While riding in the front passenger seat of the car, his body is forced into the dashboard when the driver stops quickly to avoid a rear-end collision. On impact, the passenger's knees hit the dashboard, pushing one of his femurs upward and into his pelvis. This maneuver also forces the injured hip to dislocate posteriorly.

1. Why would this type of accident be considered an emergency?
2. Considering the pathophysiology of such a fracture, what would the nurse expect to see for signs and symptoms? How would the signs and symptoms vary if the hip was dislocated anteriorly?
3. What would the nurse's responsibility be in the emergency room?

SCENARIO B

An elderly woman is in a car accident and sustains a femoral shaft fracture. The emergency team learns the woman is a runner who has competed in marathons. Before this accident, she was considered to be in excellent health.

1. What makes this woman at greater risk than a 35-year-old athlete?
2. How should the nurse respond to this client?

BIBLIOGRAPHY

1. Barangan, J. (1990). Factors that influence recovery from hip fracture during hospitalization. *Orthopaedic Nursing, 9(5),* 19–29.
2. Folcik, M. (1988). Winter sports injuries. *Orthopaedic Nursing, 7(6),* 25–28.
3. Folcik, M. (1991). Meniscal injuries. *Nursing Clinics of North America, 26(1),* 181–198.
4. Funk, J., MacBrair, B., & Peterson, A. (1990). Tibial osteotomy. *Orthopaedic Nursing, 9(2),* 29–36.
5. Gross, R. (1991). Initial assessment and management of a patient with a gunshot wound to the femur. *Orthopaedic Nursing, 10(6),* 9–13.
6. Herron, D., & Nance, J. (1990). Emergency department nursing management of patients with orthopedic fractures from motor vehicle accidents. *Nursing Clinics of North America, 25(1),* 71–84.
7. Johnson, L. (1989). Operative management of unstable pelvic fractures. *Orthopaedic Nursing, 8(4),* 21–26.
8. Martin, M. (1989). Oral antibiotics for treatment of patients with chronic osteomyelitis. *Orthopaedic Nursing, 8(3),* 35–40.
9. Mims, B. (1989). Fat embolism syndrome: A variant of ARDS. *Orthopaedic Nursing, 8(3),* 22–27.
10. Mitchell, C. A., Gallo, K., & Turnes, C. (1992). Geriatric trauma: A case study. *Geriatric Nursing, 13(4),* 210–213.
11. Mooney, N. (1991). Pain management in the orthopedic patient. *Nursing Clinics of North America, 26(1),* 73–88.
12. Mourad, L. (1991). *Orthopedic disorders.* St. Louis: Mosby-Year Book.
13. Nelson, L., et al. (1990). Improving pain management for hip fractured elderly. *Orthopaedic Nursing, 9(3),* 79–83.
14. Nussman, D., & Poole, R. (1991). Rescue and recovery in traumatic hip dislocation. *American Journal of Nursing, 91(11),* 34–38.
15. Ochs, M. (1990). Surgical management of the hip in the elderly patient. *Clinics in Geriatric Medicine, 6(3),* 571–585.
16. Pellino, T. (1994). How to manage hip fractures. *American Journal of Nursing, 94(4),* 46–50.
17. Peters, V., & Ferkel, R. (1989). Arthroscopic surgery of the ankle. *Orthopaedic Nursing, 8(5),* 12–20.
18. Ross, D. (1991). Acute compartment syndrome. *Orthopaedic Nursing, 10(2),* 33–38.
19. Rothenberg, J. (1991). Innovations in treating anterior cruciate ligament injury. *Orthopaedic Nursing, 10(2),* 17–26.
20. Shea, K., & Folcik, M. (1989). Water sports injuries. *Orthopaedic Nursing, 8(6),* 11–17.
21. Slye, D. (1991). Orthopedic complications: Compartment syndrome, fat embolism syndrome and venous thromboembolism. *Nursing Clinics of North America, 26(1),* 113–132.
22. Smrcina, C. (1991). Stress fractures in athletes. *Nursing Clinics of North America, 26(1),* 159–166.
23. Wittington, C., & Carlson, C. (1991). Anterior cruciate ligament injuries: Evaluation, arthroscopic reconstruction and rehabilitation. *Nursing Clinics of North America, 26(1),* 149–158.

UNIT 14

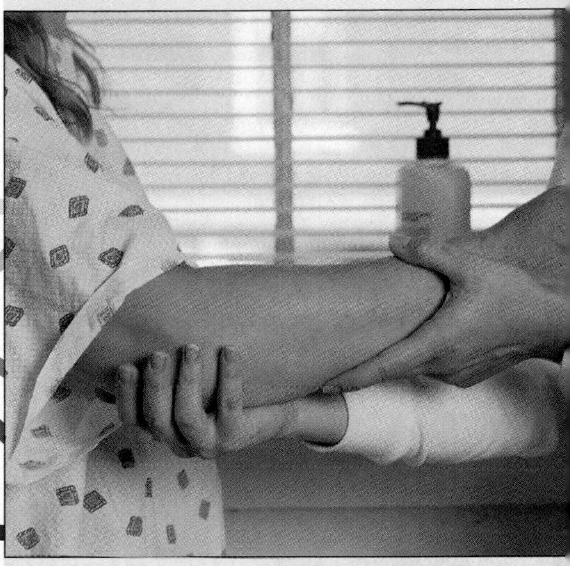

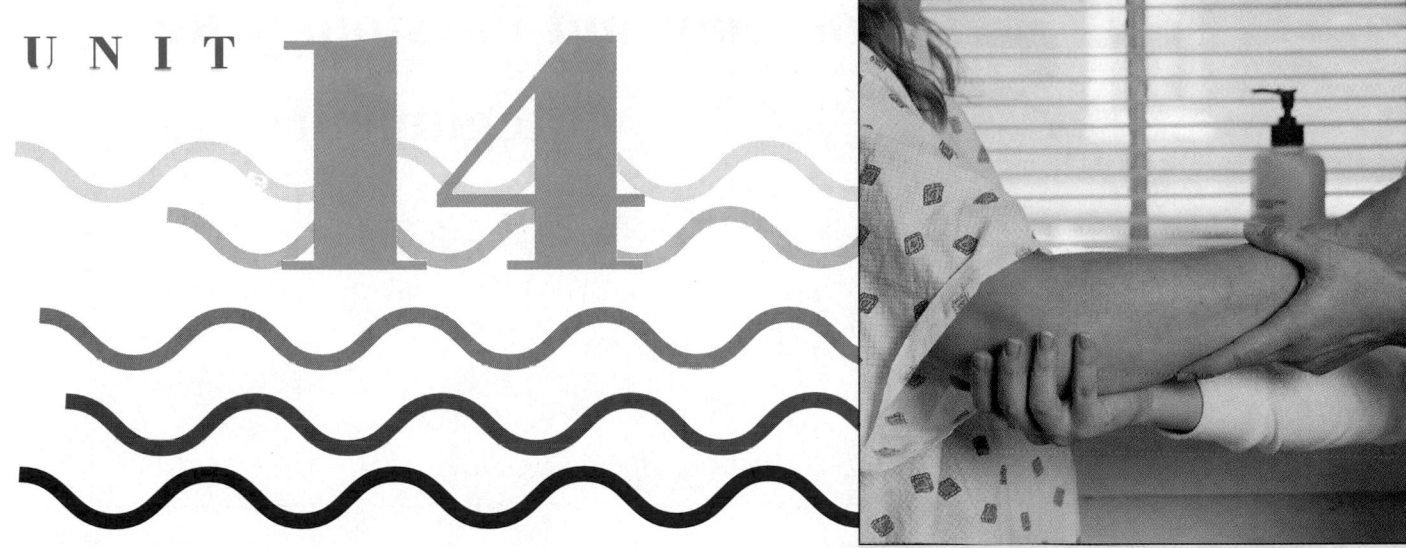

Integumentary Disorders

The body's largest and most visible organ, the skin plays a vital role in physical and mental health. Nurses in both outpatient and inpatient practice settings have a unique opportunity to significantly affect a client's dermatologic care.

Clients should be taught to appreciate the skin's functional importance and to recognize that some skin conditions are indeed life-threatening. For example, forecasts indicate that by the year 2000, as many as 1 in 75 Americans will be afflicted by malignant melanoma, a life-threatening, often fatal skin cancer.

The skin's cosmetic role should not be overlooked. Healthy skin is seen as integral to a positive self-image and good self-esteem. Our society has a long-standing prejudice against imperfect skin that needs to be dispelled. Clients with visible chronic skin problems often experience withdrawal from social situations, altered interpersonal relationships, and increased social isolation. When these clients seek professional care for skin problems, psychosocial as well as physical concerns must be addressed.

The chapters in this unit provide information to help promote optimal nursing care and outcomes for clients experiencing skin disorders, trauma, and surgery.

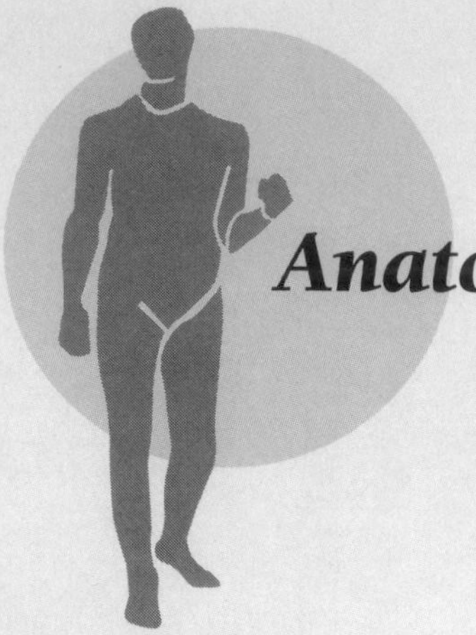

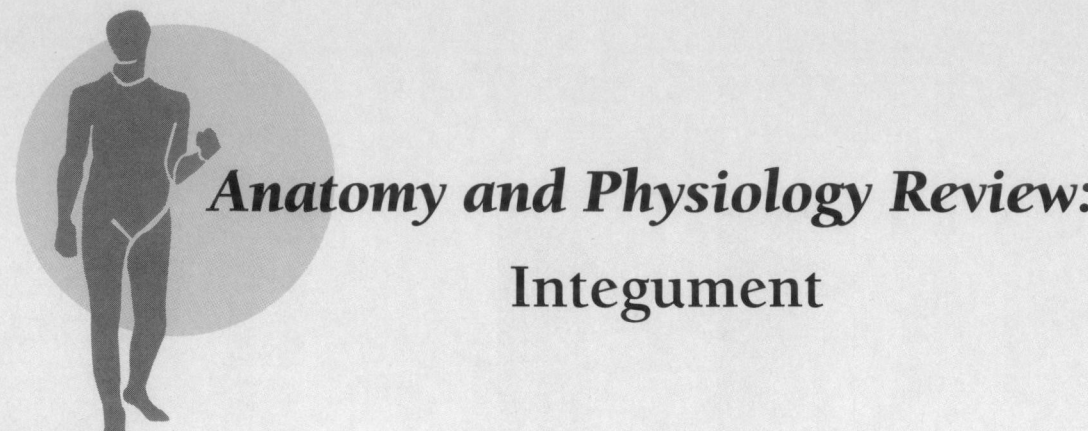

Anatomy and Physiology Review: Integument

STRUCTURE OF THE SKIN

The skin and the glands, hair, nails, and other structures that are derived from it make up the integumentary system. It is the largest body organ and weighs about 10 pounds. The skin, sometimes called the cutaneous membrane, consists of an outer epidermis and an inner dermis. These are anchored to underlying structures by a third layer, the subcutaneous tissue.

Epidermis

The epidermis is stratified squamous epithelium, which varies in thickness from about 0.4 mm on the eyelids to 4 mm on the palms of the hands and soles of the feet. Because it is epithelium, it has no blood vessels and must receive oxygen and nutrients by diffusion from underlying tissues. There are four distinct types of cells in the epidermis:

- *Keratinocytes* comprise about 90 per cent of the epidermal cells and produce the protein keratin that helps waterproof the skin and protects underlying tissues.
- *Melanocytes* comprise about 8 per cent of the cells and produce melanin, a dark brown pigment that contributes to skin color and absorbs ultraviolet light.
- *Langerhans cells* are scattered among the keratinocytes and play a role in the cell-mediated immune reactions of the skin. They are easily damaged by ultraviolet light.
- *Merkel cells* are located in the deepest layer of the epidermis of thick hairless skin and function in the sensation of touch.

The skin covering most of the body has four distinct regions, or layers, in the epidermis. Thick skin has five regions, and each region is thicker than the corresponding region in thin skin. The regions are

- Stratum corneum—outermost region consisting of flattened dead cells; continually sloughed off and replaced by cells from deeper layers.
- Stratum lucidum—present only in thick skin.
- Stratum granulosum
- Stratum spinosum
- Stratum germinativum—innermost or deepest layer, closest to the blood supply; actively mitotic layer.

Dermis

The dermis, or stratum corium, is dense connective tissue that is deeper and usually thicker than the epidermis. It contains both collagenous and elastic fibers to give it strength and elasticity. The fibers also form a framework for the numerous blood vessels, lymphatic vessels, sense receptors, and nerves that are present in the dermis but not in the epidermis. The dermis contains fibroblasts, macrophages, mast cells, and lymphocytes, which help protect against bacterial invasion and promote wound healing. Hair, nails, and certain glands, although derived from the epidermis, are embedded in the dermis.

Subcutaneous Layer

The subcutaneous layer is not actually a part of the skin, but it anchors the skin to underlying organs. Because it is beneath the dermis, it is sometimes called the hypodermis. It is also referred to as the superficial

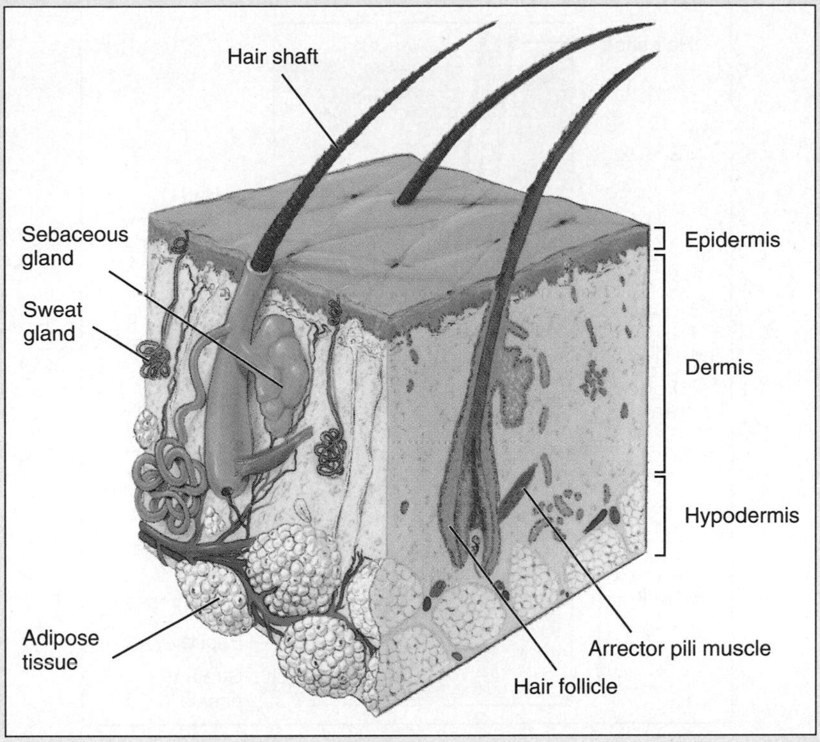

Structure of the skin. (From Jarvis, C. (1992). *Physical examination and health assessment.* Philadelphia: W. B. Saunders Co.)

fascia. The subcutaneous layer consists primarily of loose connective tissue and adipose tissue. The adipose tissue in the subcutaneous layer cushions the underlying organs from mechanical shock and acts as an insulator in temperature regulation. Age, heredity, and other factors influence the thickness of the subcutaneous layer.

Epidermal Derivatives

Epidermal derivatives are extensions of the stratum germinativum into the dermis. These derivatives include the following:

- *Eccrine, or merocrine, sweat glands* are widely distributed throughout the skin. They are most numerous on the palms, soles, and forehead and are absent on the lips, nail beds, glans penis, and labia minora. They have a duct that opens to the surface of the skin through a sweat pore. The secretion is primarily water with a few salts. Eccrine sweat glands play an important role in temperature regulation; their main stimulus for secretion is heat.
- *Apocrine sweat glands* are larger than the eccrine sweat glands and their distribution is limited to the axillae and external genitalia. Their ducts open into the hair follicles in these regions. Their secretion contains water, salts, and organic compounds that are odorless when released but become odiferous when altered by the skin's surface bacteria. These glands become active at puberty and are stimulated by the nervous system in response to pain, emotional stress, and sexual arousal.
- *Sebaceous glands* are associated with hair follicles and are found throughout the skin except on the palms and soles. The oily secretion, called sebum, is transported by a duct into a hair follicle, and from there it reaches the surface of the skin. Sebum functions to keep hair and skin soft and pliable, to inhibit bacterial growth on the skin, and to help prevent water loss. Sebaceous glands are stimulated by sex hormones, so they become highly active during puberty and decrease in activity during old age.
- *Hair* is found on nearly all body surfaces except the palms of the hands and the soles of the feet. All hair has the same structure and consists of a shaft and a root that are composed of dead, keratinized epithelial cells. The root is enclosed in a hair follicle that extends through the epidermis and is embedded in the dermis.
- *Nails* are thin plates of dead stratum corneum that contain a very hard type of keratin. Stratum germinativum from the epidermis grows under the nail body to form the nail bed. This is thickened at the proximal end to form the nail matrix, which is responsible for nail growth. The eponychium, or cuticle, is a fold of stratum corneum that grows over the proximal portion of the nail body. Nails appear pink because of the rich supply of blood vessels in the underlying dermis.

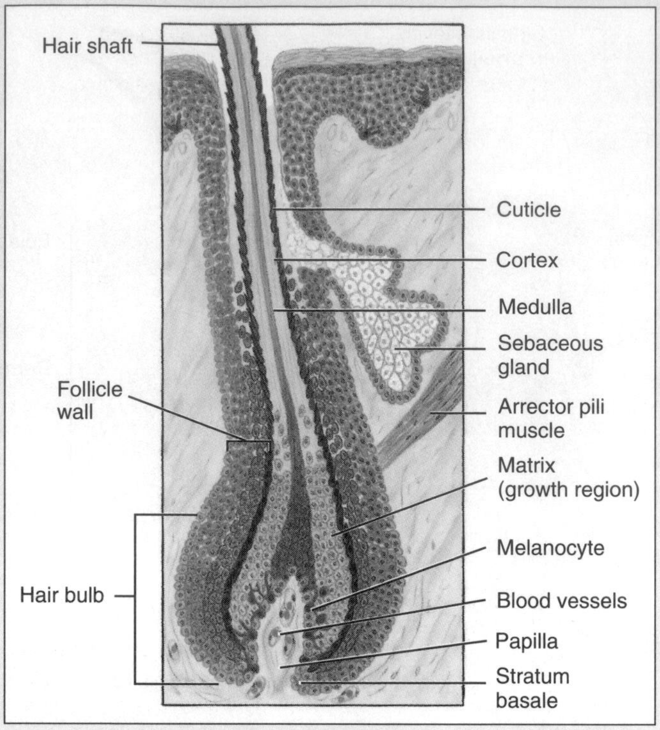

Structure of hair and hair follicles.

FUNCTIONS OF THE INTEGUMENT

Functions of the integument include

- protection
- sensory reception
- homeostasis
- temperature regulation

Protection

The skin forms a protective covering over the entire body. Unbroken skin provides a barrier against bacteria and other invading organisms. The oily secretions of the sebaceous glands are acidic and inhibit bacterial growth. Melanin pigment helps protect underlying tissues from the harmful effects of ultraviolet light. Skin also protects underlying tissues from chemical, thermal, and mechanical injury.

Sensory Reception

The dermis contains sense receptors of heat, cold, pain, touch, and pressure. Different nerve endings are responsible for responding to different stimuli and have varying concentrations over the body. The sense receptors in the skin relay information to the brain so that changes can be made to prevent or minimize injury. Sense receptors also provide a means of communication between individual people.

Homeostasis

The keratin in the skin is a waterproofing substance that helps prevent excessive loss of fluids and electrolytes from the internal environment. The skin also contains molecules that are precursors to vitamin D. When these molecules are exposed to ultraviolet light, they are converted to vitamin D, which is essential for effective calcium and phosphorus absorption in the small intestine.

Temperature Regulation

The skin helps regulate body temperature in two ways, by dilation and constriction of blood vessels and by activity of the sweat glands. Both of these mechanisms are examples of negative feedback in maintaining homeostasis.

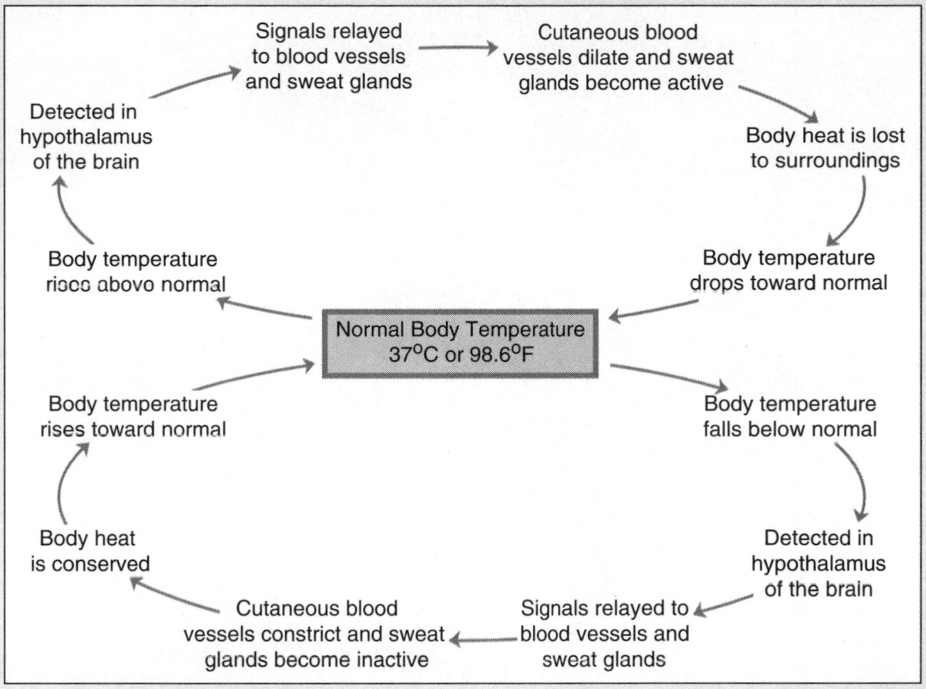

Role of the skin in temperature regulation.

AGE-RELATED CHANGES

The skin undergoes numerous visible changes throughout the lifespan. As the skin ages, the number of elastic fibers decreases and the amount of adipose tissue in the dermis and subcutaneous layer decreases. This causes the skin to sag and wrinkle. There is a reduction in the amount of collagen in the dermis, which reduces the ability of the skin to heal. Mitotic activity in the stratum germinativum decreases, so the skin becomes thinner and more fragile. As aging progresses, there is a reduction in sebaceous gland activity that contributes to difficulties with dry skin and brittle hair. Alterations in sweat gland activity make the glands less effective in temperature regulation, so the aging person is more susceptible to heat and cold.

Chapter 47 Assessment of Clients with Integumentary Disorders

Learning Outcomes

After completing this chapter, the learner will be able to:

1. Teach the client about the normal structure and function of the skin.
2. Explain to the client abnormalities of structure and function of the skin.
3. Conduct a nursing history and physical assessment of the client with actual or potential skin disorders.
4. Teach the client about diagnostic studies common to skin function.

Even though the skin is the largest organ in the body, it is often taken for granted. During the course of a lifetime, gallons of caustic chemicals contact the skin, yet the skin repairs itself quickly. When disorders do occur, the nurse is often the first health-care provider to recognize them. Thorough assessment is important for accurate diagnosis and proper care.

A thorough health history assists in diagnosis of integumentary disorders, such as occupation-related contact dermatitis, or in revealing psychosocial aspects of disease processes. Many medications can cause skin changes as a side effect. The physical examination can confirm integumentary disorders as well as reveal disorders that the client may have omitted during the history.

HISTORY

The history includes asking questions about the chief complaint, past medical history, medications, allergies, family history, psychosocial history and life-style including occupational and travel history, and a review of systems.

The most common problems related to the integument are itching (pruritus), dryness, rashes, lesions, ecchymoses, lumps, and masses. The nurse asks about changes in the skin, hair, and nails.

Past Medical History

Various systemic diseases have cutaneous manifestations. It is important to find out whether the client has other systemic illness relevant to the skin, that is, immunologic, endocrine, collagen, vascular, renal, or hepatic conditions. Information on recent exposure to infectious or childhood diseases is helpful, as is knowing the immunization status. Previous trauma and surgical intervention may give the explanation for unusual lesions or location.

Medications. Prescription as well as over-the-counter medications that the client is currently taking or has recently finished should be noted. History of past allergic reactions to foods or medications is important for avoiding inadvertent reaction through readministration.

Allergies. The nurse asks the client about allergies to medications and foods. Certain foods, when ingested, cause itching, burning, or eruption of skin rashes. Foods high in citric acid and chocolate are common culprits. Fresh fruits that have been treated with pesticides or preservatives may also be problematic, as may prepared foods containing preservatives.

PSYCHOSOCIAL HISTORY AND LIFE-STYLE

Psychosocial factors influencing the dermatologic disorders often play a large role, particularly in long-term and chronic processes. Skin disease can greatly affect life-style and self-image. Cultural and familial influences on how to care for a particular disorder may conflict with prescribed therapies.

Socioeconomic factors cannot be ignored. Compliance with outlined therapies and return for follow-up care are influenced by social expectations or financial ability to pay for medications or treatments.

Habits. The nurse inquires about the client's habits to determine the frequency of hygiene practices, what products are used (e.g., soaps, lotions, abrasives), and whether cosmetics are used. Products used, including brand names, are recorded. The nurse reviews the client's diet history for intake of sufficient nutrients, such as water; protein; vitamins A, D, E, and C; and dietary fat. The nurse should also ask about exercise and sleep patterns, which affect circulation, nourishment, and repair of the skin. Does the client engage in recreational activities that incur prolonged exposure to the sun, unusual cold, or other conditions that may damage the integument?

Occupational and Travel History. Occupational history is significant because a large number of skin problems are caused or worsened by exposure to irritants and chemicals in the home and work environment. It is important to understand what the client comes in contact with and to what extent.

Travel history can be helpful. This is especially true if the travel included hiking or exposure to any variety of outdoor wonders that have resulted in dermatologic disorders such as poison ivy, sumac, and oak or Lyme disease.

Family History

A family history helps determine genetic predisposition to skin disorders as well as predisposition to parasitic or other conditions based on the family's life-style and living environment. Genetically transmitted dermatologic conditions include alopecia (loss of patches of hair), ichthyosis, atopic dermatitis, and psoriasis. Systemic diseases with dermatologic manifestations include diabetes mellitus, blood dyscrasia, and collagen vascular diseases (lupus erythematosus). Other diseases, such as scabies, are likely to passed on to family members because of close and frequent exposure.

Nursing History

A complete history of skin changes is important. The nurse specifically asks about past problems with unusual itching, dryness, lesions, rashes, lumps, ecchymoses, and masses. Has the client had problems with moles or other lesions, especially if they have undergone changes in size, shape, or color?

PHYSICAL EXAMINATION

Examination of the skin is done as thoroughly as the examination of any other body organ. Inspection, palpation, and olfaction are used to assess hair, nails, and skin. Effective assessment requires knowledge, awareness, and practice in describing skin of individuals of all ages and different life-styles and in recognizing normal and abnormal skin changes.

Terminology

The intent of this section is to clarify some of the commonly used dermatology terminology and to assist the nurse in recognizing and describing skin disorders. Table 47–1 is a glossary of commonly used dermatologic terms.

Types of Lesions

Examination and diagnosis of skin disorders depend on identifying skin lesions or changes. Two major types of lesions are distinguished: primary and secondary lesions.

The primary lesion is the first lesion to appear on the skin and has a visually recognizable structure. Figure 47–1 illustrates and describes 10 primary lesions: macule, papule, plaque, nodule, tumor, wheal, vesicle, bulla, cyst, and pustule.

When changes occur in the primary lesion, it becomes a secondary lesion. These changes may be brought about by the client or the client's environment and often occur in the epidermal layer. These changes may result from many factors, including scratching, rubbing, medication, natural disease progression, or processes of involution and healing. Figure 47–2 illustrates and describes the following secondary lesions: scale, crust, erosion, ulcer, scar, lichenification, excoriation, fissure, and atrophy.

Examination Environment

A well-lit, private room with moderate temperature and neutral, white, or cream-colored walls is best for assessment. Excessive warmth can produce changes in skin color (e.g., redness) by causing vasodilation. Colored walls can affect normal skin hue (color). The nurse asks the client to undress for a complete examination; a gown should be provided. The nurse should inform the client that all skin surfaces will be examined and should avoid unnecessary exposure as the examination proceeds.

Depth of Examination

Examination is systematic and as complete as appropriate. A total body skin examination includes hair, scalp, nails, mucous membranes, and the skin. General

TABLE 47–1 Glossary of Dermatologic Terms

Circumscribed	Limited to a certain area by sharply defined border
Coalesce	To merge one with another
Comedo	Plug in a skin duct containing keratin (blackhead)
Dermatome	Area of skin supplied by a single dorsal nerve root
Dermatophyte	Fungus that enters the skin's surface causing infection
Desquamation	Scaling, peeling of epidermis
Discoid	Coinlike
Eczematous	General term for disease process characterized by blisters, weeping, crusting, and inflammation
Erythema	Redness
Exfoliative	Shedding of skin in fairly large quantities
Folliculitis	Hair follicle inflammation
Guttate	Small, water drop–sized lesions, usually widespread
Hives	Spontaneously occurring wheals
Hyperkeratosis	Thickening of stratum corneum, usually from repeated pressure or friction
Hyperpigmentation	Increased or excessive skin pigmentation (melanin) causing an area of skin to be darker than surrounding areas
Hypopigmentation	Decreased pigmentation
Indurated	Hard (tissue)
Intertrigo	Irritation of body areas with opposing skinfolds that are subject to friction
Lesion	Detectable change from normal skin structure
Maceration	Tissue softening or disintegration from excessive moisture
Milia	Small, white papules
Mosaic	Resembling inlaid material
Periungual	Under the nailplate
Pigmentation	Degree of skin or mucous membrane color
Polymorphic	Existing in many forms
Pruritus	Itching
Sclerosis	Hardening or induration of skin
Sebum	Lipid excretion produced by sebaceous glands
Texture	Tactile or visual skin characteristics, e.g., coarseness, dryness
Urticaria	Wheals (hives)
Wheal	Lesion found in hives

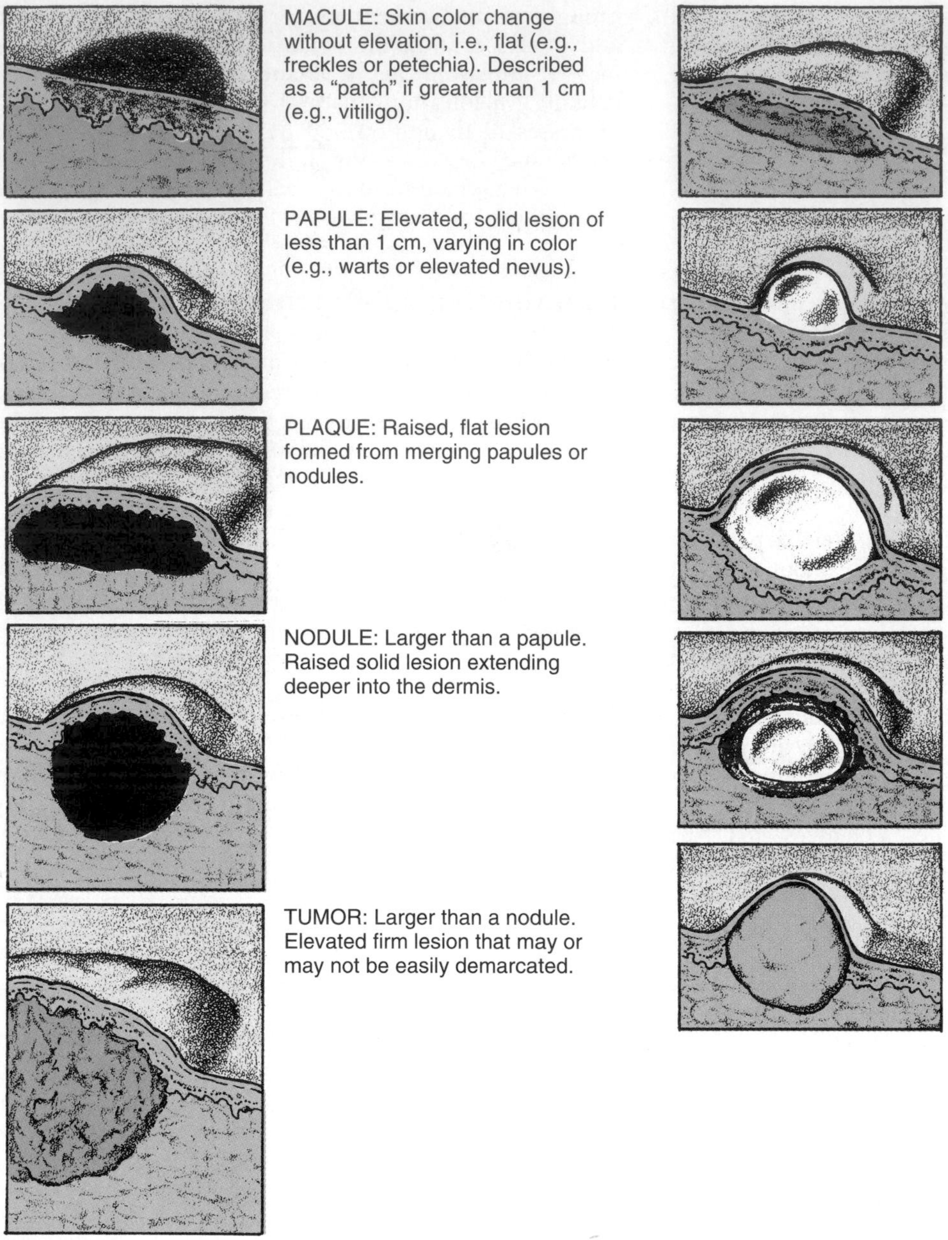
MACULE: Skin color change without elevation, i.e., flat (e.g., freckles or petechia). Described as a "patch" if greater than 1 cm (e.g., vitiligo).
PAPULE: Elevated, solid lesion of less than 1 cm, varying in color (e.g., warts or elevated nevus).
PLAQUE: Raised, flat lesion formed from merging papules or nodules.
NODULE: Larger than a papule. Raised solid lesion extending deeper into the dermis.
TUMOR: Larger than a nodule. Elevated firm lesion that may or may not be easily demarcated.
WHEAL (hive): Fleeting skin elevation that is irregularly shaped because of edema (e.g., mosquito bite or urticaria).
VESICLE (blister): Elevated, sharply defined lesion containing serous fluid. Usually less than 1 cm (e.g., blister, chickenpox, or herpes simplex).
BULLA (plural, *bullae*): Large, elevated, fluid-filled lesion greater than 1 cm (e.g., second-degree burn).
CYST: Elevated, thick-walled lesion containing fluid or semisolid matter.
PUSTULE: Elevated lesion less than 1 cm containing purulent material. Lesions larger than 1 cm are described as boils, abscesses, or furuncles (e.g., acne, or impetigo).

Figure 47–1
Primary lesions: visually recognizable structural changes in the skin that have specific characteristics.

changes can alter total body skin color (i.e., jaundice, cyanosis, pallor), thickness, turgor, temperature, and vascularity (i.e., purpura, petechiae). General findings such as these can suggest systemic disease and may require complete physical examination and appropriate work-up. This discussion is limited to assessment of hair, scalp, nails, and skin lesions.

Assessment of Hair, Scalp, and Nails

HAIR AND SCALP

Hair distribution patterns are examined for symmetry and distribution according to age and sexual development. Fine hair covers much of the body and is of the same color as scalp hair. Increased distribution occurs normally in the axillae and pubic areas. Excess body hair is known as hirsutism.

The hair and scalp are inspected under good light. If the nurse suspects lesions or infestation with lice, gloves are worn. The hair is inspected and palpated for distribution, thickness, texture, lubrication, and signs of infestation or infection. Texture and lubrication are affected by the type of hair care products used (e.g., harsh shampoo, curling irons, or hair dryers) as well as by a protein-deficient diet or health problems such as febrile illness, all of which tend to leave hair dry and brittle. Hair loss or thinning (alopecia) can result from genetic predisposition to baldness or a health problem such as recent chemotherapy.

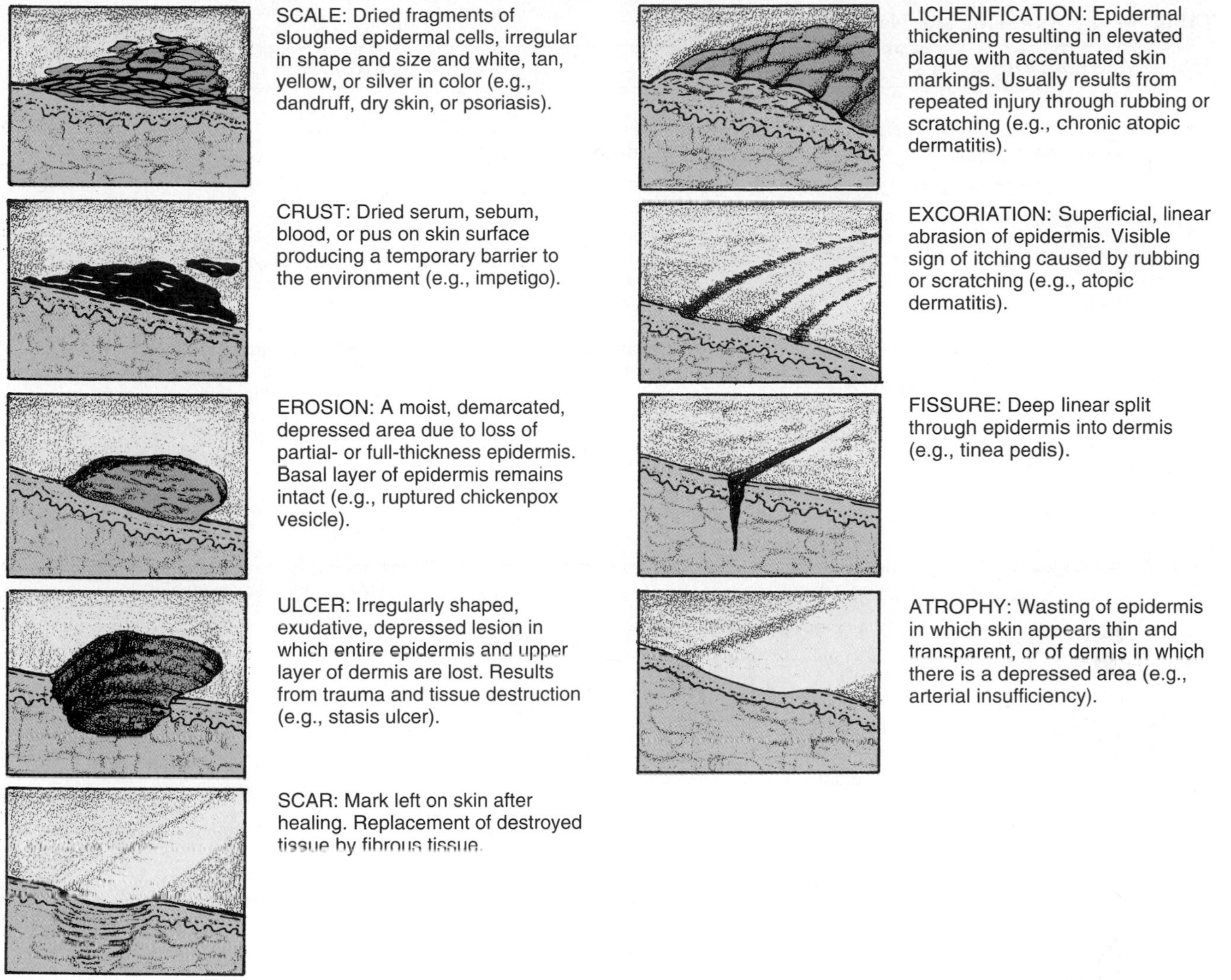
SCALE: Dried fragments of sloughed epidermal cells, irregular in shape and size and white, tan, yellow, or silver in color (e.g., dandruff, dry skin, or psoriasis).
LICHENIFICATION: Epidermal thickening resulting in elevated plaque with accentuated skin markings. Usually results from repeated injury through rubbing or scratching (e.g., chronic atopic dermatitis).
CRUST: Dried serum, sebum, blood, or pus on skin surface producing a temporary barrier to the environment (e.g., impetigo).
EXCORIATION: Superficial, linear abrasion of epidermis. Visible sign of itching caused by rubbing or scratching (e.g., atopic dermatitis).
EROSION: A moist, demarcated, depressed area due to loss of partial- or full-thickness epidermis. Basal layer of epidermis remains intact (e.g., ruptured chickenpox vesicle).
FISSURE: Deep linear split through epidermis into dermis (e.g., tinea pedis).
ULCER: Irregularly shaped, exudative, depressed lesion in which entire epidermis and upper layer of dermis are lost. Results from trauma and tissue destruction (e.g., stasis ulcer).
ATROPHY: Wasting of epidermis in which skin appears thin and transparent, or of dermis in which there is a depressed area (e.g., arterial insufficiency).
SCAR: Mark left on skin after healing. Replacement of destroyed tissue by fibrous tissue.

Figure 47–2
Secondary lesions: primary lesions that have changed owing to the natural progression of the lesion or to physical change (i.e., scratching, irritation, or secondary infection).

The scalp is inspected and palpated for lesions, excoriation (from scratching), lumps, or bruises, which should be absent. Hair shafts are examined for the presence of nits, which are the eggs of the human head louse *(Pediculus capitis)* and appear as particles of oval dandruff. The areas behind the ears and along the back of the neck are where adult lice bite the scalp.

If lesions are seen, the nurse describes them and asks the client about recent trauma or injury to the head. If the client has not already provided information during the health history interview, the nurse conducts a symptom analysis.

NAILS

The nurse inspects the client's nails for color, shape, texture, integrity, and thickness (Table 47–2). The nails reflect the client's overall health, indicating nutrition and respiratory status. The nailplate is usually transparent and colorless and, when viewed from the side, has a convex shape. The vascular bed underlying the nailplate gives the nail its color. In light-skinned clients, the color is pink, whereas it is darker in dark-skinned clients. A deficiency in hemoglobin is seen in the nail bed as pallor, and decreased arterial circulation appears as cyanosis. The nurse performs a blanche test by palpating the nail beds to assess capillary refill. The nail bed is pressed firmly for 5 seconds, then quickly released while the rate of color return to the nail bed is observed. Color return should be immediate within 3 to 5 seconds. When palpated, the nail bed feels firm with no softness (i.e., bogginess) or tenderness.

Texture is smooth; healthy nails are of uniform thickness with no signs of dryness, softness, brittleness, splitting, peeling, ridges, or pitting. The angle formed between the nailplate and posterior nailfold is approximately 160 degrees without separation. Changes in nail shape and nail bed angle can indicate health problems. Clubbing of the nails is an increase of more than 160 degrees in the angle between the nailplate and nail base.

TABLE 47–2 Assessing the Nails

ASSESSMENT FINDING	DESCRIPTION	CAUSES
Normal nail 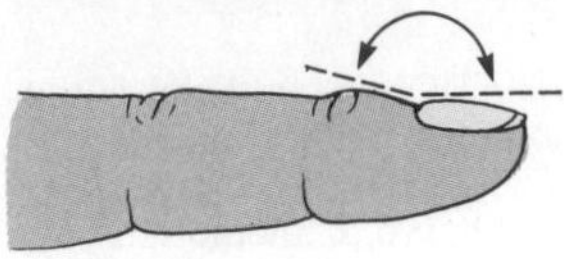	Nail shape is convex, and nailplate angle is approximately 160 degrees	
Beau's line 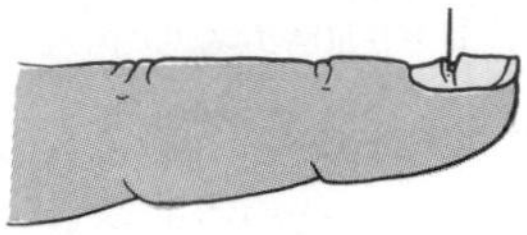	Horizontal depression in nailplate; depressions can occur singly or in multiples	Nail growth is disturbed temporarily; related to systemic illness (e.g., infection) or direct injury to the nail root
Splinter hemorrhages 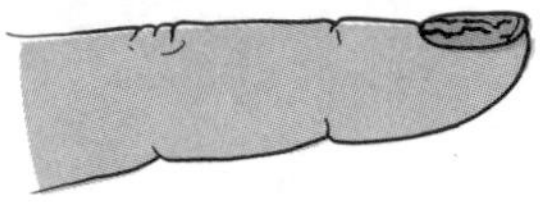	Linear (vertical) red or brown streaks in the nail bed	Minor trauma to the nail bed; subacute bacterial endocarditis; trichinosis
Paronychia 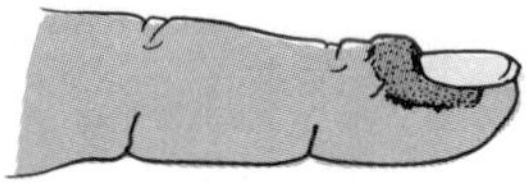	Inflammation of the skinfold at the nail margin	Trauma; skin infection at the nail base
Spoon shape 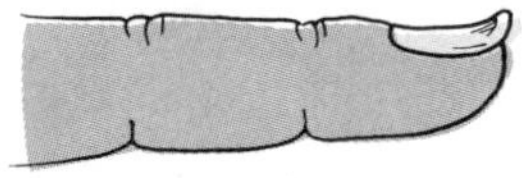	Nail shape is concave as the nail curves upward from the nail bed	Use of strong detergents; iron deficiency anemia; syphilis
Clubbing 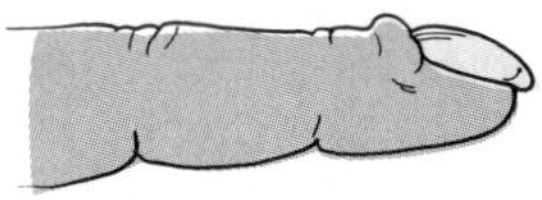	Increased angle between nailplate and nail base	Long-standing hypoxia

The nail base of a clubbed nail is spongy and soft on palpation. These changes result from hypoxia (diminished tissue oxygenation). Nail clubbing commonly occurs in clients with congenital heart defects or chronic lung disease.

The tissue surrounding the nail should appear intact without signs of inflammation, jagged edges (hangnail), or dryness. Inferior or lateral nailfold inflammation is a sign of paronychia (i.e., nailfold infection). If these abnormalities are noted, the nurse asks the client about nail care habits such as biting or cutting cuticles. While examining the fingers and toes, the nurse may note common abnormalities such as calluses or corns. A callus is a flat, painless thickening of a circumscribed area of skin. Calluses usually occur on the hands and feet. A corn is a horny induration and thickening of the skin caused by friction and pressure.

Assessment of Skin

COLOR

Overall skin color is assessed during the health history interview. A more thorough assessment is conducted as the nurse proceeds through the remainder of the physical examination. The nurse observes the client's face and visible skin surfaces for color tones, which should be congruent with the client's stated race. Abnormal findings include pallor (paleness), flushing or a ruddy complexion, cyanosis (blue cast), jaundice (yellow cast), and areas of irregular pigmentation.

Areas that are less pigmented reveal abnormal findings more readily than do heavier pigmented surfaces. For example, pallor is best seen in the buccal (mouth) mucosa, especially in clients with dark skin. Cyanosis is evident more readily in less pigmented areas such as the nail beds, lips, and palms. Jaundice sharply contrasts with the white of the sclera, especially in dark-skinned clients who have more carotene deposits. Jaundice is best assessed in dark-skinned clients by inspecting color changes in the hard palate.

Local areas of color change are examined closely by the nurse. Hyperpigmentation describes areas of increased pigmentation; hypopigmentation describes areas of decreased pigmentation. Skin color also results from the circulation supply; an increased blood supply may result in the redness of inflammation (rubor), whereas extreme pallor may be a result of anemia or impeded arterial circulation to the area.

MOISTURE

Moisture refers to the skin's hydration level for both wetness and oiliness. Overall skin moisture is dry but not excessively so and often reflects ambient temperature and humidity levels. Moistness usually occurs in intertriginous areas such as the axillae and groin. Skin that feels overly moist and cool (i.e., clammy) is abnormal.

TEMPERATURE

Temperature is assessed with the dorsum of the hand. The skin should feel uniformly warm, because it reflects circulation. Areas of hypothermia or hyperthermia are compared with the same area on the opposite side.

TEXTURE

The nurse palpates texture by stroking the skin lightly with the fingertips. The skin should feel smooth, soft, and resilient. There should be no areas of lumps or unusual thickening or thinning (atrophy).

TURGOR

Turgor is the skin's elasticity and is measured by the time it takes for the skin and underlying tissue to return to its original contour after being pinched up. The skin over the forearm is lightly pinched between the nurse's thumb and index finger, then released. If the skin remains elevated (i.e., tented) more than 3 seconds, turgor is decreased. Normal turgor is a return to baseline contour within 3 seconds when the skin is mobile and elastic. Turgor decreases with age as the skin loses elasticity.

EDEMA

The nurse palpates for edema, particularly if areas of taut, shiny skin are noted on inspection. Edematous areas are palpated for consistency, temperature, shape (i.e., extent), tenderness, and mobility. The nurse presses a finger firmly against the edematous area for 5 seconds to assess for pitting edema, that is, a residual indentation left by the finger's pressure when the fluid is displaced from the underlying tissue. The depth of pitting is expressed in millimeters or centimeters. Because of a variation in rating scales, it is more accurate for the nurse to state the depth of pitting rather than to rate it. Areas examined by the nurse for edema include over the sacrum (especially in bed-ridden clients), the feet, ankles, and over the tibia on the shins.

TENDERNESS

Tenderness is an abnormal finding and is elicited as the nurse palpates. There should be no areas of tenderness in a healthy, uninjured client.

ODOR

The skin should be free of pungent odors. Odors, when noted, are usually present in the axillae and skinfolds or open wounds and are related to the presence of bacteria on the skin, inadequate hygiene, or infection.

LESIONS

The nurse inspects the skin for detectable lesions and palpates to determine the characteristics of contour (e.g., flat, raised, or depressed), size, consistency (e.g., firm, soft), mobility, and tenderness. Lesions can be mobile or immobile (fixed to underlying tissue).

Location, Distribution, and Size. Location is described in reference to anatomic landmarks. The nurse measures lesions for size, because this helps to classify their type (e.g., macule, papule). If there are multiple lesions, the distribution pattern could be helpful in determining the diagnosis. Extent of the presence of the lesions is noted. Lesions can be localized (confined to a specific area), regional, or generalized (present over a large surface). The nurse should compare sides bilaterally to determine if lesions are symmetric or asymmetric. Another commonly noted distribution is in sun-exposed areas. Certain diseases have a classic lesion distribution, such as herpes zoster (following along a nerve root dermatome).

Arrangement. The arrangement refers to the pattern of nearby lesions. Two of the typical patterns include "linear" and "satellite," which can also be helpful in confirming diagnosis. Linear lesions are found in a straight line (e.g., in scabies). Satellite lesions are the small peripheral lesions around a central larger lesion (e.g., in diaper candidiasis).

Color. Skin lesions can assume a wide variety of colors; they may be flesh-colored, brown, red, yellow, tan, or blue. Color can be influenced by many factors, including the client's normal skin color, which often makes the lesion's color hard to accurately describe. Slight color changes can best be assessed in areas having the least amount of natural pigmentation and those with superficial capillary beds (i.e., buccal membrane of the mouth, mucosa, lips, nail beds, ocular conjunctiva, palms, and soles). These areas are especially important in assessing darkly pigmented skin.

Configuration. Configuration refers to the shape or the outline of the lesion. Most lesions are circular. The term nummular is used for a circular lesion when it is the diameter of a large coin (e.g., nummular eczema). Annular describes lesions found with an active ring-shaped border and some central clearing (e.g., granuloma annulare).

DIAGNOSTIC TESTS

Before a diagnostic skin procedure (or treatment), the nurse should perform an assessment and document findings. Nursing intervention for diagnostic procedures includes explaining the procedure to the client and significant others, allowing them to ask questions and express concerns. The nurse should teach them appropriate wound care and indications of possible side effects and complications that should be reported, such as prolonged bleeding or infection (indicated by swelling, redness, increased discomfort, temperature elevation). Instructions (preferably written) for follow-up care should be provided as well as a follow-up appointment and telephone number. Documentation of diagnostic procedures (exactly what was done and by whom) and the specific location of the lesion must be completed by appropriate personnel.

Potassium Hydroxide Examination and Fungal Culture

Fungal infection of skin, hair, or nails may be confirmed by microscopic identification and culture of scrapings from the area. Any scaly dermatitis may be scraped for this test. Typical sites are the scalp, intertriginous areas (between the toes, axillae, groin, under or between the breasts, abdominal folds), and the nailfold. The scrapings are examined under the microscope. For a culture, scrapings from a suspicious lesion are obtained and implanted onto the appropriate culture medium. For a nail culture, an altered, dystrophic nail is snipped and implanted into the medium. Debris from the nail's subungual area is less suitable for culture.

Tzanck's Smear

Tzanck's smear is the microscopic assessment of fluids and cells from vesicles or bullae. The presence of multinucleated giant cells establishes a diagnosis of viral infection, such as herpes simplex or herpes zoster.

Scabies Scraping

The test for scabies is most accurate when a papule that has not been scratched is chosen. The most difficult part of this procedure is finding the proper lesion from which to take the specimen, and it often requires several areas being prepped. Local anesthesia is not necessary, and fine bleeding should be expected. There will be some discomfort when the lesion is opened.

Wood's Light Examination

Wood's light examination is assessment with a high-pressure mercury lamp that transmits long-wave ultraviolet light (UVA; 360 nm). It has several diagnostic uses. For example, it (1) detects superficial fungal and bacterial skin infections, (2) delineates pigmentary disorders by highlighting the degree of contrast between lesions and normal skin color, and (3) accentuates the contrast between hypopigmented and totally amelanotic areas. Wood's light ("black light") examination is done in a darkened room. The procedure is painless.

Patch Testing

Patch testing is done to attempt to identify substances that produce allergic skin responses. Patch testing is often done to differentiate between an irritant contact dermatitis and an allergic contact dermatitis. Small amounts of various substances or allergens are applied to the skin on aluminum discs placed on a special tape. Compounds of low concentration are used to prevent possible excessive irritation. Patch testing should not be performed if acute dermatitis is present. The potential allergen could worsen the dermatitis. The tape must be worn for 48 hours without disturbing the patches, and interpretations are made at 48, 72, and 96 hours and sometimes at 1 week. An eczematous response at the test site with erythema, papules, or small vesicles indicates a positive reaction and confirms an allergic contact sensitivity to the substance on the disc.

Biopsy

Skin biopsy is the removal of a skin tissue specimen for histologic (cellular microscopic) assessment. There are three types: shave, dermal punch, and surgical excision. In all three procedures, local anesthesia is used, and small-gauge needles (26 to 30 gauge) are recommended to limit trauma to the skin. Clean or sterile technique as appropriate should be used in dealing with the biopsy site. The specimen is placed in formalin solution, properly identified, and sent for pathologic assessment.

SHAVE BIOPSY

This procedure is performed to obtain tissue for analysis from possibly malignant epidermal growths, except potential melanoma.

PUNCH BIOPSY

A dermal punch biopsy uses a circular instrument with a sharp cutting edge to remove a specimen of skin that includes epidermal, dermal, and subcutaneous tissue. This method is used for biopsy of a well-developed, mature lesion.

SURGICAL EXCISION BIOPSY

This biopsy is used (1) when it is necessary to excise a lesion totally (e.g., when full skin thickness is needed), (2) when a lesion's borders are indistinct from surrounding skin, or (3) when there is a recurrent or aggressive cancer, such as malignant melanoma.

Nursing Management

Depending on the size of the excision, the nurse should instruct the client to avoid the use of aspirin and products containing aspirin for 48 hours before the biopsy to avoid a prolonged postprocedure bleeding time. If the client uses anticoagulants (e.g., heparin or Coumadin), the physician must be notified. If the client has a history of cardiac valve replacement, the nurse should be sure prophylactic antibiotics are prescribed. The client should eat a light meal before the procedure to avoid syncope (fainting episodes).

Following the procedure, the nurse covers all biopsy sites with an antibiotic ointment and a clean or sterile dry dressing and pressure dressings when appropriate. The nurse should remind the client that follow-up assessment is necessary and plan a follow-up appointment for suture removal. The client should be informed of how biopsy results will be reported.

STUDY QUESTIONS

1. Which one of the following are the sweat-producing glands of the body?
   A. Eccrine glands
   B. Apocrine glands
   C. Epocrine glands
   D. Sebaceous glands
2. A client with poison ivy asks the nurse, "How did I get infected with poison ivy?" The best response is:
   A. "This is a disease known as allergic contact dermatitis."
   B. "You caught it when you were walking through the woods."
   C. "Your skin is sensitive to the changes in environmental temperature."
   D. "Can you tell me how long you've had the disease and how you are treating the rash?"
3. The best way to assess a client's skin is to:
   A. Give the client a complete bath
   B. Ask the client about his or her skin condition
   C. Use palpation, inspection, and percussion during the assessment
   D. Read the client's chart, check diagnostic results, and assess the skin under a good light
4. Which one of the following questions is imperative to ask during an assessment completed prior to a client's scheduled biopsy?
   A. "Have you ever had an allergic reaction to anything with iodine in it?"
   B. "Have you taken any aspirin, ibuprofen, or anticoagulants during the past 2 weeks?"
   C. "Do you know how to apply a topical ointment? It will be necessary to do so after the biopsy."
   D. "Do you have someone to drive you home after the biopsy? The anesthetic may cause some drowsiness."

CRITICAL THINKING EXERCISES

SCENARIO A

A 59-year-old male arrived for an appointment at the clinic. He wished to have a "growth" on his scapula checked by the doctor. He had not checked his skin for other lesions and believed he had only one.

1. What teaching does the client need about the function of the skin?
2. What physical examination methods are used to examine the skin?

3. What diagnostic test should the nurse prepare the client for if scabies is suspected?
4. If the doctor decides to perform a biopsy, what preparations should be made?

SCENARIO B

The nurse is preparing to instruct a mentally challenged client to provide skin care for her very dry skin. The client appears to want to understand more about her body. She asks, "Why is my skin dry all the time?"

1. How could the nurse teach the client about the structure and function of the skin?
2. How can the nurse gather more information from the client on which to base hygienic teaching?

BIBLIOGRAPHY

1. Ablon, G. R., & Rosen, T. (1994). Cutaneous signs of systemic disease: A guide to gleaning diagnostic clues from the skin. *Consultant, 34(4),* 495–499, 503–503, 506.
2. Arnold, H. L., Odom, R. B., & James, W. D. (1990). *Andrews' diseases of the skin* (8th ed.) Philadelphia: W. B. Saunders.
3. Bielan, B. (1994). What's your assessment? . . . Many skin diseases manifest nail changes. *Dermatology Nursing, 6(6),* 408–409.
4. Burrage, R., et al. (1991). Physical assessment. An overview with sections on the skin, eye, ear, nose and neck. In W. Chenitz, et al. (Eds.), *Clinical gerontological nursing.* Philadelphia: W. B. Saunders.
5. Caughman, S., et al. (1989). Cutaneous signs of internal cancer. *Patient Care, 23(2),* 28–41.
6. Chapel, T., et al. (1988). Cutaneous signs of infection. *Patient Care, 22(13),* 185–197.
7. Copstead, L. C. (1995). *Perspectives on pathophysiology.* Philadelphia: W. B. Saunders.
8. Dellasega, C., & Burgunder, C. (1991). Perioperative nursing care for the elderly surgical patient. *Today's OR Nurse, 13(6),* 12–17.
9. Eaglstein, W. H., McKay, M., & Pariser, D. M. (1994). The problems that plague aging skin. *Patient Care, 28(7),* 89–92, 95–96, 101–107.
10. Fitzpatrick, T. B., & Eisen, T. B. (1992). *Dermatology in general medicine.* Hightstown, NJ: McGraw-Hill.
11. Jarvis, C. (1992). *Physical examination and health assessment.* Philadelphia: W. B. Saunders.
12. Hill, M. J. (1994). From the editor. Stop, look, and listen . . . Too often, nurses become very shortsighted in their observations. We tend to look for what we know and recognize, rather than questioning what we see and don't understand. *Dermatology Nursing, 6(6),* 392
13. Jaubovic, H., & Ackerman, A. (1992). Structure and function of the skin. In S. Moschella & H. Hurley (Eds.), *Dermatology* (3rd ed., vol. 1). Philadelphia: W. B. Saunders.
14. Kreisberg, S., et al. (1989). Skin signs of endocrine disease. *Patient Care, 23(6),* 73–86.
15. Pogue, S. (1992). Nursing assessment of the elderly for dermatologic procedures. *Dermatology Nursing, 4(1),* 15–23.
16. Rudy, S. (1991). From conception to birth: The development of the skin and nursing implications. *Dermatology Nursing, 3(6),* 381–392.
17. Watson, J., & Jaffe, M. S. (1995). *Nurse's manual of laboratory and diagnostic tests.* Philadelphia: F. A. Davis.

Chapter 48 Nursing Care of Clients with Integumentary Disorders

Learning Outcomes

After completing this chapter, the learner will be able to:

1. Assess the client for clinical manifestations of common integumentary disorders.
2. Teach the client about the etiology, risk factors, basic pathophysiology, and clinical manifestations of selected integumentary disorders.
3. Explain the client's role in medical and surgical management of integumentary disorders.
4. Develop plans of care for the client with actual and potential integumentary disorders.
5. Implement nursing interventions that optimize the quality of life for clients with integumentary disorders.
6. Evaluate planned outcomes using outcome criteria developed in the planning phases of care.

General Principles of Dermatologic Nursing

Many effective treatments are available for skin problems. Some are specific to certain conditions. Some treatments are directed at skin cellular metabolism; these include altering skin temperature, reducing or increasing blood flow, adapting delivery of oxygen to and from skin tissue, altering inflammatory responses, and adapting absorption of toxins and mediators. Dermatologic intervention includes topical medications, soaks and wet wraps, protective dressings, skin lubricants, and ultraviolet light (UVL) therapy.

TOPICAL MEDICATIONS

Pharmacologic Therapy

Topical therapy can be used to

- Restore hydration
- Alleviate symptoms
- Reduce inflammation
- Protect the skin
- Reduce scale and callus
- Cleanse and débride
- Eradicate causative organisms

Topical medications are chosen both for the action of the active ingredients (which are delivered directly to the skin surface) and for the vehicle (base in which the medication is suspended). Topical medications have many different actions and cover a large spectrum of drug categories, including antibacterial, antifungal, and antipruritic (Table 48–1).

Topical Vehicles

Examples of various topical vehicles include ointments, creams, gels, aerosols, lotions, powders, and pastes. The various ingredients used to formulate the different bases may be irritating to individual clients, and care must be taken in recommending any product. Both the active ingredient and the vehicle must be appropriate for the condition being treated. For acute dermatosis (i.e., weeping, blistering lesions), a water-based compound provides a drying effect. An ointment-based vehicle has the opposite effect; it promotes lubrication and occlusion and can help treat the dryness and scaling caused by chronic dermatitis.

Differences in skin permeability also influence the effectiveness of topical medications. For example, absorption increases in inflamed skin. Depending on the medication and the specific condition, topical medication may be specifically applied to localized lesions or to larger skin surfaces. When increased absorption of the medication is needed, topical medication may be prescribed for application under an occlusive dressing (Table 48–2). Ointments, creams, and gels have greatly increased absorption if they are applied to skin that is wet.

Topical Corticosteroids

Corticosteroids are the most commonly used topical medication. A large selection of topical steroids, ranging from very low potency to extremely high potency, is available today. Clients should be informed of what strength topical steroid they are given and the potential side effects. The lowest potency corticosteroid that is effective should be used. Rebound (exacerbation or worsening) of the condition can occur if treatment is stopped abruptly.

Clients must clearly understand how, when, and where to use topical steroids. Properly applying the medication evenly and sparingly one or two times daily to the affected areas can eliminate many potential problems. It is rarely helpful to apply the topical corticosteroid more than twice per day. This increases the chance of side effects, makes the therapy more costly, and does not increase effectiveness. As the skin disorder improves, the frequency of use may be changed or a less potent topical corticosteroid prescribed. When the skin disease disappears or comes under good control, a tar preparation, moisturizer, or other topical preparation may be substituted.

SOAKS AND WET WRAPS

Soaks can be done in a variety of ways and serve several purposes. A wet environment softens dry epidermis and aids in removal of crusts. Removal of cellular skin debris promotes healing and improves absorption of topical medication. The risk of infection is decreased by the removal of necrotic tissue and occlusive crusts. Cooling also results from the gradual evaporation of water and acts as an anti-inflammatory, thus reducing itching.

Wet wraps used immediately after soaking and occlusion can optimize hydration and topical therapy; this also promotes cooling of the skin. Wet wraps and occlusion can be done in a variety of ways. The location and severity of lesions often determine the choices.

PROTECTIVE DRESSINGS

Dressings and bandages allow control of the affected skin's environment and remain important in the treatment of wounds, ulcers, and recalcitrant dermatitis. Protection is the primary function of the dressings. Dressings limit the exposure of injured skin to dirt, mechanical trauma, and irritants. Ulcers and denuded

TABLE 48–1 Dermatologic Medications

CATEGORY	EXAMPLE	ACTION	NURSING INTERVENTION
Acne products	Benzoyl peroxide (Benzagel, Benzamycin, Desquam, Panoxyl, Xerac)	Keratolytic Bacteriostatic Decreases production of irritant-free fatty acids in follicle	Applied once or twice a day after washing area Observe for dryness or redness
	Tretinoin (Retin-A)	Vitamin A acid Decreases cohesiveness of epithelial cells, increasing cell mitosis and turnover; an irritant causing desquamation	Applied once daily at bedtime, 20 minutes after washing area Instruct client to expect some redness and peeling within a week, lasting 3–4 weeks Flare-up of acne may occur in first 2–4 weeks before improvement Clearing of acne requires 2–3 months Client must avoid excessive sun exposure, use sunscreen daily, keep agent away from eyes
Antibacterials	Bacitracin ointment Polysporin ointment	Alter chemistry of micro-organism's structure: denature proteins, increase cell wall permeability, and interfere with metabolism	Clean skin of adherent crust and debris before application Apply ointments frequently (two to three times daily), as prescribed
Antibiotics	*Topical* Erythromycin (T-Stat, Erycette, Benzamycin) Clindamycin (Cleocin-T) Mupirocin (Bactroban)	Suppressive effects on inflammatory response; effective on papular and pustular lesions	Apply as prescribed Observe for redness, itching, or burning
Antifungals	*Topical* Nystatin (Mycostatin) Clotrimazole (Lotrimin) Oxiconazole (Oxistat) Naftifine (Naftin)	Alter cell wall permeability	A 2- to 3-week course of twice daily application is necessary for adequate treatment Overapplication can irritate sensitive, damaged skin
Antimetabolites	5-Fluorouracil (Efudex, Fluoroplex)	Interfere with DNA synthesis Inhibit thymidylate synthetase activity Effective in treating large areas of sun-damaged skin having premalignant or malignant lesions (e.g., basal cell epithelioma)	Apply medication with gloved hand, avoiding mucous membranes and eyes Describe to the client expected response to the medication (e.g., a brisk inflammatory response with burning and itching) Advise client to avoid sun exposure, which can increase the intensity of reaction to medication
Antiparasitics	Permethrin (Nix) Lindane (Kwell) Permethrin (Elimite)	Unknown	Avoid getting in eyes Observe for signs of reinfestation Observe for side effects (e.g., rash, redness, itching, burning, tingling) Full course of therapy needs to be completed Wash clothing in hot water or dry-clean Seal clothing that cannot be washed or dry-cleaned in plastic for 30–35 days All sexual contacts must also be treated

Table continued on following page

TABLE 48–1 Dermatologic Medications *Continued*

CATEGORY	EXAMPLE	ACTION	NURSING INTERVENTION
Antipruritics	*Lotions/Pastes* Phenol (0.5–2%) Menthol (0.1–2%) Camphor (1–3%) Calamine lotion Baths/cornstarch Oatmeal Aveeno	Antihistamine effect, blocking histamine and serotonin effects Cool and soothe skin	Apply frequently to reduce discomfort, unless medication contains an anesthetic ingredient (e.g., lidocaine); avoid the eyes If it contains anesthetic ingredient, apply as prescribed (two to four times daily)
	Wet Dressings Potassium permanganate (1:4000–1:16,000) Aluminum acetate Burow's solution (1:10–1:40) Boric acid (1 tablespoon in 1 L of water) Normal saline (2 teaspoons salt in 1 L of water) Magnesium sulfate (8 teaspoons in 1 L of water) Silver nitrate 0.25%	Cool and soothe Some germicidal activity	Assess for contact sensitivity Instruct client to use caution when entering and exiting tub; most solutions are slippery Protect linens from stains with wet dressings
Antiseptics	Chlorhexidine gluconate (Hibiclens)	Effective against staphylococci, streptococci, and gram-positive bacteria	Use for irrigating and cleansing wounds but not for packing because it may cause dermatitis
	Acetic acid (0.25%) solution	Effective against *Pseudomonas*	Protect healthy skin with a layer of petrolatum because it excoriates the skin
	Hydrogen peroxide (3%)	Breaks up necrotic tissues	Use to irrigate and clean necrotic tissues from wounds Inhibits tissue formation, so avoid use in healing wounds
Corticosteroids	Hydrocortisone (Hytone) Alclometasone (Aclovate) Triamcinolone (Kenalog) Fluocinolone (Synalar) Mometasone (Elocon) Halcinonide (Halog) Betamethasone (Diprosone) Diflorasone (Psorcon) Clobetasol (Temovate)	Reduce blood flow by vasoconstrictive effects Antimitotic effect; slow epidermal cell production Reduce erythema and itching by anti-inflammatory action *Note:* Potent corticosteroids should be avoided in treating face, neck, and intertriginous sites because increased side effects may occur	Apply in even amounts Monitor length of prescribed topical administration to avoid long-term side effects Use care in clients with systemic bacterial, fungal, or viral infections May be applied to hydrated skin or with occlusive dressings to increase penetration
Dressings	DuoDerm Tegasorb Op-Site Zinc oxide in Unna's boot	Physical protectants	Physical skin protectants should be used according to manufacturer's direction
Emollients/protectants	Vaseline Aquaphor ointment Eucerin cream Moisturel cream Neutrogena emulsion	Emollients provide a temporary barrier, protecting and softening skin Protectants cover skin and alleviate irritation	Apply evenly and smoothly; most useful when applied immediately after bathing Reapplication is required to provide protection when product has been absorbed or has worn off
Keratolytics	Salicylic acid (DuoFilm, DuoPlant, Occlusal, Ionil shampoo, T/Sal shampoo, Meted shampoo, Keralyt gel) Lactic acid (DuoFilm, LactiCure lotion)	Soften keratin and loosen cornified epithelium of the stratum corneum Débride excessive scale Used in varying concentrations to treat conditions ranging from dry, ichthyotic scalps or skin to warts	Apply only to involved area; can produce irritation and erythema in normal skin If prescribed for scale débridement, discontinue as soon as scale disappears If erythema and irritation occur, seek physician's approval to reduce frequency of use

TABLE 48–1 Dermatologic Medications *Continued*

CATEGORY	EXAMPLE	ACTION	NURSING INTERVENTION
Sunscreens	PABA PABA esters Cinnamates Salicylates Anthranilates Benzophenone	Provide protection through absorption, reflection, and scattering of ultraviolet radiation	Instruct client to apply liberally 30 minutes to 1 hour before sun exposure and to reapply after swimming or sweating or with prolonged ultraviolet exposure
Tars	*Coal Tar Products* PsoriGel T-Derm Estar gel	Keratolytic Keratoplastic Photosensitizing Antipruritic	May be applied locally to specific lesions or widely to skin Do not apply to face or intertriginous sites Explain drug's photosensitizing properties to client

DNA, deoxyribonucleic acid; PABA, para-aminobenzoic acid.

skin heal more quickly when kept damp by an occlusive or semiocclusive dressing because regenerating epithelium migrates more easily across a moist surface. These wounds are less painful when kept damp, and enhanced absorption of topical medications will occur. Occlusive or semiocclusive dressings range from adhesive strips, nonstick gauze (Telfa), and petrolatum-impregnated gauze to dressings such as DuoDerm and OpSite. Snug dressings such as elastic wraps over the lower legs effectively reduce edema and decrease healing time in stasis ulcers.

Finally, Unna's boot, a dressing designed to be removed only by medical personnel at a later visit, can be extremely useful for treatment of stasis ulcers that have venous insufficiency or when there is a concern about client compliance, scratching (neurodermatitis), or even self-injury. Unna's boot is a fixed, protective dressing that stimulates granulation tissue and restores epithelial growth. Unna's boot is removed weekly for assessing damaged skin and cleaning normal skin.

Ideally, the area of damaged skin decreases, granulation tissue forms, and signs of chronic inflammation are reduced. Treatment continues for weeks until improvement occurs. It is important to explain to the client and significant others to keep the dressing dry and intact and that the Unna's boot needs to be removed if there is excessive drainage or localized pain (signs of infection). Routine follow-up is very important.

SKIN LUBRICANTS

Agents to hydrate the skin play an important therapy in many xerotic, pruritic, and inflammatory skin disorders. Measures to prevent skin dryness include elimination of drying compounds, which may include soaps and solvents, and use of emollients such as humectants, occlusive agents, and keratin-softening agents.

Skin is dry not because it lacks oil but because it lacks water. The primary means of correcting dryness is to add water to the skin and then apply a hydrophobic occlusive substance to retain the absorbed water. To seal in the water, the use of occlusives such as white

TABLE 48–2 Occlusive Dressings

PURPOSE/DESIRED EFFECT	NURSING IMPLICATIONS
Produces airtight barrier, usually with plastic film Enhances absorption of topically applied medication (e.g., corticosteroids, keratolytics) by preventing evaporation Increases stratum corneum rehydration Softens hyperkeratotic areas by moisture retention	Clean skin site of debris and "old" medication before applying prescribed topical medication Apply topical medication while skin is still damp Apply plastic film (Saran wrap) snugly Use plastic bags for feet, polyethylene gloves for hands, plastic shower caps for scalp Press air out; seal borders with paper tape Leave dressing intact for 2–12 hours (as prescribed); then remove and gently clean the site Observe and document complications (e.g., maceration, oozing, signs of secondary fungal or bacterial infection, and folliculitis) When occlusive dressings are used in conjunction with topical corticosteroids, frequent, prolonged use can result in permanent skin changes; these include striae, nonhealing ulcerations, telangiectasias, erythema, and skin atrophy

petrolatum (Vaseline), Aquaphor ointment, or Crisco is very effective.

Frequent use of emollients should be encouraged. If emollient products are not successful, it may be necessary to try more potent agents. Humectants are substances such as urea (Aquacare 10 per cent, Carmol 20 per cent) that attract and hold water, which results in transepidermal water migration. The alpha-hydroxy acids such as lactic acid (LactiCare) or ammonium lactate (Lac-Hydrin) may be tried; these hold moisture and decrease the rough scale that creates the sensation of dryness. Also popular with clients are additives such as aloe, vitamin E, jojoba, elastin, and collagen. No scientific evidence has shown that these have special, intrinsic properties beyond their minimal lubricating effects.

ULTRAVIOLET LIGHT THERAPY

Artificially reproduced forms of UVL are used therapeutically with topical or systemic photosensitizing drugs to cause desquamation (shedding or peeling of epidermis). UVL also temporarily suppresses mitosis of the basal cell layer by inhibiting deoxyribonucleic acid (DNA) mitosis. Ultraviolet A and ultraviolet B are used to treat diseases responsive to UVL, such as psoriasis, vitiligo, cutaneous T-cell lymphoma, uremic pruritus, chronic eczematous eruptions, and, more rarely, acne vulgaris.

Every client must have a complete history and physical examination before initiation of any UVL therapy for assessment of multiple factors. The nurse should record highlights of the client's history, taking care to include complete medication history because the client could be taking one or more of the many photosensitizing drugs (i.e., thiazide diuretics, tetracyclines). Clients should also be asked specifically about previous herpes simplex infections because these can be stimulated by UVL. Pretreatment assessment includes identifying solar-induced skin malignancies, cataracts, or lupus erythematosus. Clients with a history of basal cell or squamous cell epitheliomas are at risk for additional neoplastic changes with this treatment. Thus, potential benefit is weighed against potential risk. A complete ophthalmologic examination is important before treatment is started and yearly thereafter during long-term treatment. A history of cataract formation is a potential contraindication to psoralen plus UVA (PUVA) therapy. Anyone showing early cataract changes needs extra photoprotective measures (e.g., the complete occlusion of goggles or PUVA glasses) and more frequent ophthalmologic assessments (every 3–6 months). The skin changes of clients with lupus erythematosus are aggravated by sun exposure, so photochemotherapy is contraindicated. Before therapy is initiated, an antinuclear antibody test should rule out this condition.

The nurse must be aware that because treatments to the face and genitalia increase risk for cumulative effect of UVL, minimal exposure is indicated. Periodic assessments must be done throughout the course of therapy for signs of actinic damage (e.g., severe wrinkling, "tissue paper" transparency) or cutaneous malignancy. Post-therapy clients must be observed for potential side effects, including dry skin, pruritus, and potential delayed (36–48 hours after exposure) phototoxic reaction (such as erythema, vesicles, and pain).

PSYCHOSOCIAL ASPECTS OF SKIN DISORDERS

Anger, frustration, and anxiety are commonly experienced by clients with skin disorders, which often exacerbates the condition. Clients with underlying skin disease are more likely to respond to stress, frustration, embarrassment, or any emotionally upsetting event with itching and scratching. Excitability and arousal of the central nervous system from an emotional upset can intensify the vasomotor and sweat responses in the skin and lead to the itch-scratch cycle (see Pruritus).

Learning about the acute or chronic nature of the given disorder, the exacerbating factors, and the management measures that can control it is important for both the client and significant others. Maintaining a healthy outlook is important. Counseling and other psychosocial intervention is often very helpful for dealing with the frustrations of skin disease. It is especially helpful to adolescents and young adults, who may consider the lesions disfiguring or unattractive.

The client education needs of those affected by skin disease are vast. Health-care providers need to consist-

CLIENT EDUCATION GUIDE

Skin Care

The nurse must include the following points in client teaching:

- The skin is a protective organ and is the body's first line of defense against infection.
- Inspect skin for changes at frequent intervals. Observe and inspect the skin for edema, redness, abrasions, skin tears, and skin wounds. Report any changes to the physician.
- Apply prescribed topical medications as ordered. Be aware of expected side effects, including photosensitivity and other skin-related effects. A light layer of medication is adequate.
- Understand the relationship of a well-balanced diet and hydration to healthy skin. Hydration is especially important because it provides the skin tissues with moisture from within. Moist skin is not as prone to skin damage (dryness, tearing) as dry skin.

CLIENT EDUCATION GUIDE

Skin Self-Examination

The nurse must teach the client the following:

WHAT YOU WILL NEED

A bright light
Full-length mirror
Hand-held mirror
Two chairs or stools
A blow-dryer
Body maps
Pencil

HOW TO PROCEED

- Examine your face, especially the nose, lips, mouth, and ears (front and back) (A). Use one or both mirrors to obtain a clear view.
- Thoroughly inspect your scalp, using a blow-dryer and mirror to expose each section to view (B). Ask a friend or family member to help.
- Check your hands carefully: palms and backs, between the fingers, and under the fingernails (C). Continue checking up the wrists to examine both front and back of your forearms.
- Standing in front of the full-length mirror, begin at the elbows and scan all sides of your upper arms (D). Do not forget the underarms.
- Next focus on the neck, chest, and torso (E). Women should lift breasts to view the underside.
- With your back to the full-length mirror, use the hand mirror to inspect the back of your neck, shoulders, upper back, and any part of the back of your upper arms you could not view previously (F).
- Still using both mirrors, scan your lower back, buttocks, and backs of both legs (G).
- Sit down; prop each leg in turn on the other stool or chair. Use the hand mirror to examine the genitals (H). Check front and sides of both legs, thigh to shin, ankles, tops of feet, between toes, and under toenails. Examine soles of feet and heels.

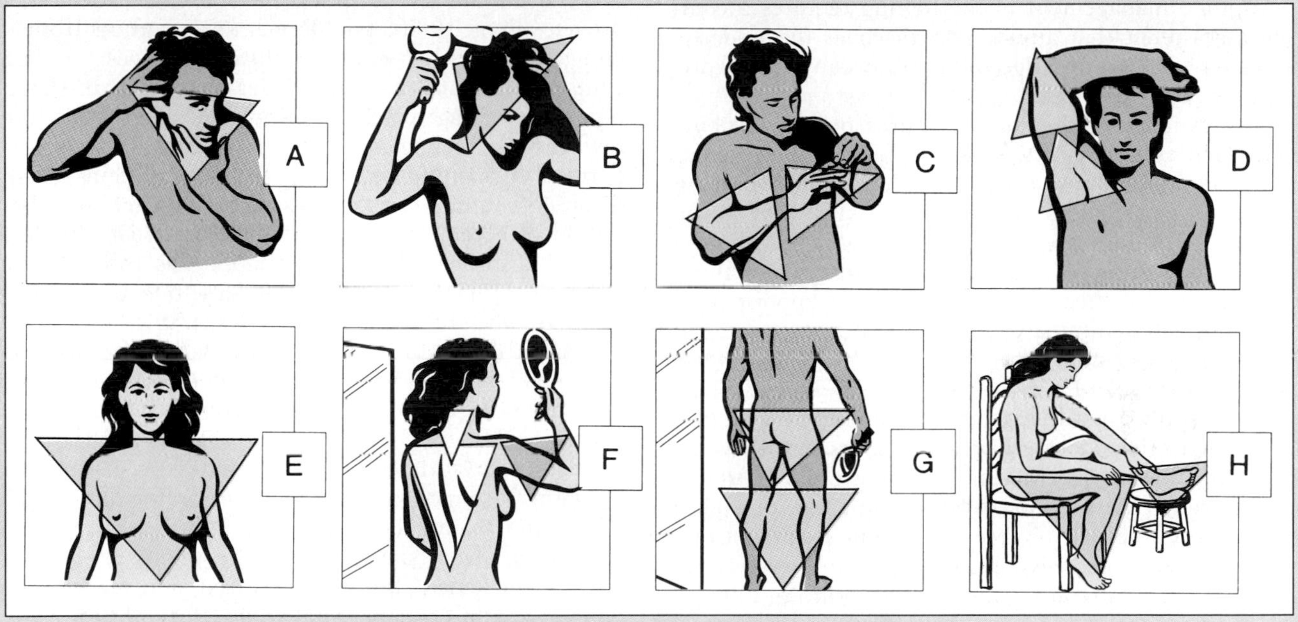

Adapted from The Skin Cancer Foundation. (1992). *Skin cancer: If you can spot it, you can stop it.* New York: Author.

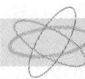

ently provide information that includes detailed skin care plans, general disease information, and availability of client-oriented support organizations as well as updates on hopeful research results. Most clients will forget or confuse the important skin care recommendations without written instructions. Clearly outlining the skin care recommendations to the client in both a verbal and written manner is essential for good outcomes (see the Client Education Guides: Skin Care and Skin Self-Examination). Client education pamphlets are available through a variety of sources, including the many dermatologically oriented client support groups, professional dermatology agencies such as the Dermatology Nurses' Association, and the American Academy of Dermatology.

Common Skin Disorders

PRURITUS

Pruritus (itching) is one of the most common manifestations of skin problems; it is a symptom, not a disease. Pruritus has been defined as an unpleasant skin sensation producing a strong desire to scratch, localized to or generalized over a body area. It can lead to damage if scratching injures the skin's protective barrier, possibly with resultant infection and scarring.

Pruritus can be a secondary symptom of conditions

ranging from dry skin to carcinoma. Systemic diseases that can cause generalized and severe pruritus include chickenpox, severe liver disease, diabetes mellitus, uremia resulting from chronic renal failure, drug hypersensitivities, intestinal parasites, and neoplastic conditions (i.e., leukemia and lymphoma).

Stimulation of itching can be initiated by almost any chemical or physical substance, especially if skin is damaged. Once the itch sensation is established, the client has an almost uncontrollable urge to scratch. Scratching leads to further skin damage and increased inflammation. Pruritus therefore increases, and so does the urge to scratch. Thus, the itch-scratch-itch cycle develops. To minimize skin trauma caused by scratching, fingernails should be kept short. Relieving this symptom, especially for chronically ill clients, is a nursing challenge because of its common occurrence and the major effect it may have on a client's quality of life.

Management

Appropriate management of the itching requires a complete assessment that attempts to discover the underlying cause and knowledge of appropriate therapeutic modalities for treatment.

Dry skin may either be the source of or contribute to pruritus, and it is often helpful to use good hydration in addition to any other topical therapy. One bath or shower per day for 15 to 20 minutes with warm water and a mild soap should be immediately followed by the application of an emollient, with or without other topical medications, to prevent evaporation of water from the hydrated epidermis. Other topical medications are often added to emollients to help alleviate itching. (See Table 48–1 for examples of antipruritics.) Topically applied antihistamines and anesthetics are relatively ineffective and are best avoided because they can be potent allergic sensitizers. This is especially true if these products are used on inflamed skin. Use of topical corticosteroids should be reserved for the treatment of a specific steroid-responsive dermatosis. Long-term application of topical steroids, especially on skin not affected with an eczematous condition, may result in thinning of the skin, striae, telangiectasias, and easy bruising.

Systemic antihistamines may be prescribed. They are most helpful in disorders in which histamine is the principal mediator but may be of benefit through sedative or even placebo effect. A trial of H_1-blocker antihistamine (hydroxyzine, diphenhydramine, chlorpheniramine) is appropriate either on a regular schedule or as indicated for itching. Tricyclic antidepressants (doxepin hydrochloride, amitriptyline hydrochloride) have a high binding capacity for histamine H_1 receptors and may be helpful for clients who would benefit from their antidepressant as well as antipruritic effect.

Modification of Plan of Care for the Elderly

Elderly clients often have difficulty in following through with frequent bathing or showering because of decreased mobility. In this situation, when hydration cannot precede the application of moisturizers, more frequent application and use of more hydrating products may be needed. Additionally, the elderly may have difficulty being able to apply the needed topicals properly, and assistive personnel may be required to offer the client proper therapy. Antihistamine therapy should be administered carefully with use of small doses initially because many elderly have a very low tolerance and may experience severe drowsiness, especially at therapy initiation.

Eczematous Disorders

Eczema is not a specific disease. Dermatitis and eczema are terms that may be used interchangeably to describe a group of disorders with a characteristic appearance. A few examples of eczema or dermatitis (and abbreviated definitions) include allergic contact dermatitis (eruptions from allergy to poison ivy, sumac, or oak or proven allergen); irritant dermatitis (eruption from direct contact with cosmetics, chemicals, dyes, or detergents); nummular eczema (appearance of coin-shaped, oozing, crusting patches); seborrheic dermatitis (yellowish-pink scaling of scalp, face, and trunk); stasis dermatitis (eruption resulting from peripheral venous disorders); and atopic dermatitis (characteristic distribution of eczema in clients with a family history of an allergic disorder). Eczema-dermatitis has three primary stages; eczema may manifest in any one of the three stages, or the three stages may coexist.

Acute dermatitis is characterized by extensive erosions with serous exudate or by intensely pruritic, erythematous papules and vesicles on a background of erythema. *Subacute dermatitis* is characterized by erythematous, excoriated, scaling papules or plaques that are either grouped or scattered over erythematous skin. Often, the scaling is so fine and diffuse that the skin acquires a silvery sheen. *Chronic dermatitis* is characterized by thickened skin and increased skin marking secondary to rubbing and scratching (lichenification); excoriated papules, fibrotic papules, and nodules (prurigo nodularis); and postinflammatory hyper- and hypopigmentation.

ATOPIC DERMATITIS

Atopic dermatitis is a common, chronic, relapsing, pruritic type of eczema. The word "atopic" refers to a group of three associated allergic disorders: asthma, allergic rhinitis (hay fever), and atopic dermatitis.

Incidence

According to several studies, 75 to 80 per cent of clients with atopic dermatitis have a personal or family history of allergic disorders. Atopic dermatitis is a common disorder affecting 0.5 to 1 per cent of the people in all parts of the world.

Etiology and Risk Factors

The exact cause of atopic dermatitis is unknown. Xerosis is usually worse during periods of low humidity; winter in northern latitudes may aggravate pruritus.

Pathophysiology

Compared with normal skin, the dry skin of atopic dermatitis has a reduced water-binding capacity, a higher transepidermal water loss, and a decreased water content. Water loss leads to further drying and cracking of the skin, which leads to more itching. Rubbing and scratching of itchy skin are responsible for many of the clinical changes seen in the skin.

Clinical Manifestations

Atopic dermatitis begins in many clients during infancy. Also called acute dermatitis, it first appears as a red, oozing, crusting rash. As the child grows, the skin shows the chronic form of dermatitis, with thickened, dry texture, brownish gray color, and scaling. The rash tends to become localized to the large folds of the extremities as the client becomes older. It is found mainly on elbow bends, backs of knees, neck, sides of the face, eyelids, and the backs of hands and feet. Hand and foot dermatitis becomes a significant problem in some clients.

Pruritus is the major symptom of atopic dermatitis and causes the greatest morbidity. The urge to scratch may be mild and self-limiting, or it may be intense, leading to severely excoriated lesions, infection, and scarring.

Complications

Clients with atopic dermatitis have a tendency to contract viral, bacterial, and fungal skin infections. The most common viral infection is herpes simplex, which tends to spread locally or become generalized.

Medical Management

The goal of therapy is to break the inflammatory cycles that cause excess drying and cracking as well as the itching and scratching. Primary prevention begins with daily skin care that hydrates and lubricates the skin. The health-care team's understanding of each client's disease pattern and the discovery and reduction of exacerbating factors are crucial to effective management of this chronic disorder. Other factors that must be considered include irritants, allergens, physical environment, and emotional stresses.

Hydration is the key to management but is often difficult to achieve. Soaks followed by application of occlusive substances are usually prescribed (see Soaks and Wet Wraps).

PHARMACOLOGIC MANAGEMENT

Occlusives, moisturizers, topical corticosteroids, and tar preparations can all be used topically in various combinations to control atopic dermatitis. Topical steroids are a very important component of therapy in treating eczema (see Topical Corticosteroids). All of these preparations will be best absorbed into hydrated skin or by using wet wraps and occlusion. Topicals containing chemicals or drugs that would cause skin eruptions themselves are avoided.

Systemic medications may include antibiotics and antihistamines. The use of a systemic corticosteroid is rarely warranted in atopic dermatitis.

When a short-term course of oral steroid therapy is given, it is important to taper the dosage as it is discontinued. Intensified skin care should also be instituted during the taper to suppress flaring of the dermatitis.

DIETARY MANAGEMENT

Dietary management of atopic dermatitis has continued to be a controversial subject. The significance of food allergies is not known in the causation of atopic dermatitis or what percentage of atopic dermatitis clients have food allergies. The most common allergens that appear to be important are eggs, cow's milk, soy, wheat, nuts, and fish. Known allergens are avoided. Care must be taken to avoid inadvertent malnutrition when any type of restrictive diet is used.

Nursing Management

The client with atopic dermatitis should be assessed for present hygienic habits (e.g., does the client bathe with soap and hot water?), present medication regimen, exposure to known allergens, environmental exposure, and history of skin eruptions.

Nursing management of the client with atopic dermatitis is presented in the nursing Care Plan.

Modification of Plan of Care for the Elderly

Dermatitis is a common skin disorder in the elderly. It may be caused by hypoproteinemia, venous insufficiency, allergens, irritants, or underlying malignancy such as leukemia or lymphoma. Because the elderly client often takes multiple medications, dermatitis from drug-drug interaction is considered. The fragility of the skin should be considered in planning any form of treatment. Most aged clients do not need a daily bath and should avoid hot water for bathing as well as soap. Tepid water and nondrying bath agents should be used.

CARE PLAN: The Client with Atopic Dermatitis

Nursing Diagnosis/ Collaborative Problem	Planning: Expected Outcomes	Implementation: Nursing Interventions	Rationales
Skin Integrity, Impaired R/T cutaneous dryness	The client will maintain skin that has good hydration and reduced inflammation, as evidenced by • Verbalization of increased skin comfort • Decreased flaking and scaling • Decreased redness • Decreased excoriations from scratching • Healing of previous areas of breakdown	Bathe at least once every day for 15–20 minutes. Immediately on leaving the bath, apply an appropriate emollient or prescribed topical. Bathe more often when signs and symptoms increase.	Soaking saturates the stratum corneum. Application of an occlusive moisturizer 2–4 minutes after the bath is critical for preventing evaporation of water from the hydrated epidermis
		Use warm water, not hot.	Hot water causes vasodilation, which increases pruritus.
		Use superfatted soaps (i.e., Dove or Basis) or soaps for sensitive skin (i.e., Neutrogena, Moisturel, Aveeno, Oilatum, Purpose). Avoid bubble baths.	The use of drying soap may compound the problem. Superfatted soaps are less alkaline and less drying to the skin.
		Apply occlusive topical emollient or prescribed topical preparation two to three times per day.	Ointments and creams seal in water and thereby hydrate the skin. The particular emollient selected depends mostly on client preference and whether the ingredients in the base are irritants.
Skin Impairment, Risk for R/T exposure to allergens	The client will maintain skin integrity as evidenced by avoidance of allergens	Teach the client to avoid or decrease exposure to known allergens.	Avoidance of allergens will decrease the incidence of allergic responses.
		Read labels on prepackaged food or prepare all food from scratch when food is an allergen.	Avoidance of allergens will reduce the incidence of reaction related to ingestion, inhalation, or contact with allergens.
		Avoid pets.	If allergic to animal dander, avoid pets or restrict the pet to certain areas of the home.
		Use air conditioning whenever possible in the home and work place.	Air conditioning helps reduce exposure to certain allergens present in the environment.
Alteration in comfort, R/T pruritus	The client will experience a decrease in pruritus, as evidenced by • Decrease in observed and reported scratching • Decreased excoriations from scratching • Decreased restlessness during sleep • Verbalization of increased skin comfort	Explain the itching symptom as it relates to cause (i.e., dryness of the skin) and the principles of the selected therapy (i.e., hydration) and the itch-scratch-itch cycle.	Understanding the physiologic or psychological process and principles of itching and its treatment increases cooperation.
		Wash all new clothes before wearing for removal of formaldehyde and other chemicals, and avoid use of fabric softeners.	Pruritus is often precipitated by irritant or allergic effects of certain chemicals or components of fabric softeners.
		Change to a milder detergent and add a second rinse cycle to ensure removal of soap.	Residual laundry detergent in clothing may be irritating. The actual laundry soap that is used is not the key, but rather that all soap is rinsed out so that an irritant effect is avoided.

CARE PLAN: The Client with Atopic Dermatitis *Continued*

Nursing Diagnosis/ Collaborative Problem	Planning: Expected Outcomes	Implementation: Nursing Interventions	Rationales
		Wear open-weave, loose-fitting, cotton-blend clothing. Avoid overdressing, rough or wool fabrics, and tightly woven fabrics.	Light cotton-blend clothing allows air circulation and minimizes perspiration, which intensifies itching.
		Work and sleep in comfortable surroundings with a fairly constant temperature (68–75° F) and humidity level (45–55 per cent). Air conditioning in the home, particularly the bedroom, may be beneficial.	Extremes of temperature cause pruritus frequently secondary to vasodilation and increased cutaneous blood flow. In addition to providing a cooler environment, air conditioning will decrease aeroallergen exposure.
		Keep fingernails very short, smooth, and clean.	Trimmed nails prevent damage and infection to the skin.
		Appropriate use of antihistamines may reduce itching to some degree.	Histamine is the most commonly known itch mediator. The sedating antihistamines also provide relief.
		Use sunscreen on a regular basis.	Sunburn may cause flare-up of dermatitis.
		Immediately after swimming, take a shower or bath, washing with a mild soap from head to toe, and then apply an appropriate moisturizer.	Residual chlorine or bromine on the skin after swimming in a pool may be irritating.
Infection, Risk for R/T • Skin excoriation • Decreased resistance to cutaneous viral, fungal, and staphylococcal organisms	The client will be free of infectious lesions, as evidenced by absence of pustules, exudate, or crusting	Explain to client the signs of infection and be sure the client understands that presence of these signs indicates need for medical intervention.	Infections are a potentially serious complication of disorders of open skin.
			Leftover medications may be outdated and may be inappropriate treatment.
		Ensure that the client understands the importance of not self-treating with leftover medication at home.	Medications can become contaminated and lead to infection or lose their potency.
		Emphasize that it is important to take the antibiotic on schedule and the entire course.	This will ensure complete eradication of the infectious organism.
Body Image Disturbance R/T • Skin lesions • Response of significant others to appearance	The client will exhibit a positive self-concept, as evidenced by • Engaging in social activities • Expressing feelings of importance, self-worth • Enjoying interpersonal interactions	Encourage client to teach others that eczema is not contagious unless severely infected.	Eczema can be mistaken for impetigo or as an indication of uncleanliness, causing social isolation.
		Encourage client and significant others to share feelings with each other regarding the client's appearance and the chronic nature of eczema.	Unidentified fears and concerns may hinder interpersonal relationships.
		Reinforce client's sense of identity and personal competence. Encourage self-management of eczema and understanding that controlling scratching will greatly reduce lesions.	Allowing client to determine need for various treatment modalities, such as when to initiate wet wraps or minor alterations in topical therapy, promotes positive self-concept.

XEROTIC ECZEMA (DRY SKIN)

Xerotic (dry) skin is dehydrated, erythematous, scaling, and finely cracked. Xerosis occurs in patches and may involve any skin surface. It is common in elderly clients. If xerosis is severe, the skin is tight, itchy, and painful. In low humidity, which is especially prevalent in artificially heated rooms in wintertime, excessive water is lost from the stratum corneum. Water loss causes xerotic chapping. The problem is accentuated by use of drying skin cleansers, soaps, disinfectants, and solvents and infrequent use of moisturizers.

The treatment of xerotic skin consists primarily of correcting dryness and avoiding irritating factors. Teaching the client correct daily skin care is essential in treating this condition.

STASIS DERMATITIS

Stasis dermatitis is the development of areas of very dry skin and sometimes shallow ulcers on the lower legs primarily as a result of venous insufficiency. The process of dermatitis begins with edema of the leg caused by slowed venous return. The client commonly has a history of varicose veins or deep vein thrombosis. As the venous stasis continues, the tissue becomes hypoxic from inadequate blood supply. As the blood pools, hemoglobin is released from the red cell and deposited in the tissues. This poorly nourished tissue begins to necrose. The clinical manifestations include itching, a feeling of heaviness in the legs, brown-stained skin, and open shallow lesions. The lesions are very slow to heal because of the lack of oxygenated blood.

Management

The legs need improved venous return. This can be accomplished with leg elevation and support hose. Clients should be instructed to raise the legs during the day, especially if they are employed at a job in which they stand still in one area for long periods of time (e.g., cashier). Stasis ulcers are treated with wet-to-dry dressings for débridement of the area, Unna's boots, and skin grafts.

CONTACT DERMATITIS

Contact dermatitis is an inflammatory response of the skin to chemical or physical allergens. *Irritant contact dermatitis* is due to exposure to a chemical or physical irritant. Clinical manifestations range from mild erythema to vesicles to ulceration. *Allergic contact dermatitis* is a delayed hypersensitivity reaction from contact with an allergen. This response is due to action of the T lymphocyte. Clinical manifestations begin at the site of exposure with itching, stinging, erythema, and edema but then extend to more distant sites.

Management

Management of contact dermatitis begins by determining the causative agent. Determining the agent usually begins by interviewing the client for recent exposure to chemicals, metals, and the like. Patch testing is done to determine the specific agent, if necessary. Pain and itching may be controlled with topical medications or wet dressings. Antihistamines and steroids may be required.

PSORIASIS VULGARIS

Psoriasis vulgaris is a chronic, recurrent, erythematous, inflammatory disorder involving keratin synthesis. Pruritus can be severe. The term "vulgaris" means common. Psoriasis occurs in both sexes, usually commencing in early adulthood.

The cause of psoriasis vulgaris is unknown. However, alterations in cyclic nucleotides, and possible immunologic abnormalities have been noted. Genetic predisposition is also possible.

Rapidly proliferating epidermal cells form small, scaly patches of skin that develop into erythematous, dry, scaling patches of various sizes. The course of psoriasis vulgaris is prolonged and unpredictable. Anxiety and stress often precede flare-ups. Exacerbations and remissions are common. It usually recurs at intervals and lasts for increasingly longer periods. Spontaneous clearing is uncommon. Psoriatics have greater than normal colonization of *Staphylococcus* on plaques. Psoriatics who are human immunodeficiency virus (HIV) positive are at high risk for infection from self-inoculation.

Psoriatic patches are covered with silvery white scales. The eruptions (usually symmetric) commonly occur on the scalp, elbows, knees, and sacral regions.

Medical Management

Mild psoriasis may be treated locally with natural sunlight or topical therapy, including tar preparations and topical corticosteroids (see Topical Corticosteroids) or intralesional corticosteroids. Injecting small, diluted amounts of corticosteroids (e.g., triamcinolone acetonide) into or just below a lesion gives a high drug concentration to a localized site. Potential localized side effects include atrophy, hypopigmentation, infection, and, rarely, ulceration. Keratolytic agents (e.g., salicylic acid) may remove scale and allow greater penetration of topical agents.

Anthralin is an effective topical therapy for psoriasis with widespread discrete lesions consisting primarily of thick plaques. There are varying methods of application of this topical. With all methods, it is important to apply medication only to the affected lesions, avoiding contact with normal surrounding skin. The client should wash hands immediately after application, leave medication on for the prescribed period of time, and then remove it by showering or bathing. Anthralin products have the potential to stain fabric, hair, skin, nails, furniture, and bathroom fixtures. For avoidance of excessive staining, it is recommended that medication be carefully applied and that as much medication as possible be removed with tissue or a previously stained towel before bathing.

Scalp care with psoriasis consists of removing scales and treating inflammation. Tar shampoos with keratolytic agents, followed by topical corticosteroid lotions, are useful. It is often necessary to use steroids under occlusion (under dressings) for percutaneous absorption to be enhanced. There is no consistently effective treatment of psoriatic involvement of the nails. Usually, the scalp and nails improve with remission of psoriasis on the body surface.

Widespread involvement may require whole-body irradiation with UVL (see earlier).

Systemic treatment is sometimes prescribed for widespread psoriasis. The vitamin A derivative etretinate (Tegison) has been shown to be useful in pustular and erythrodermic psoriasis but not as useful in chronic plaque-type psoriasis. The side effects of etretinate are similar to those of the oral retinoid isotretinoin (see Acne Vulgaris). Because of the teratogenicity of the drug and the extremely long half-life, its use in women of childbearing age is unwarranted.

Antimetabolites (e.g., methotrexate) in small doses are useful for inhibiting DNA synthesis. Methotrexate is a folic acid antagonist used to treat psoriasis that is unresponsive to all topical therapies; it is reserved for the most severe cases.

Nursing Management

Although the physician orders the medical regimen for the client, the nurse and the physician collaborate in the ongoing assessment of the client's response to treatment and the development of new lesions.

The nurse's role in client care centers on teaching the client about the UVL treatments and medications. In addition, the nurse should assist the client in coping with an altered self-concept. The appearance of skin lesions may make the client feel "dirty" or untouchable. In addition, the smell of the tar preparations and the stain may add to the psychological reaction. The client is also at high risk for secondary infection in the open lesions. The client should be taught to keep the creams or ointments on and keep the areas clean and dry.

To keep psoriasis in remission, the client needs to control the causative factors. Adequate rest, nutrition, and exercise promote health. Stress should be minimized and illness and infection treated early.

ACNE VULGARIS

Acne is a common, self-limiting, multifactorial disorder. One of four clients affected has enough significant disease to seek professional treatment. Potential facial disfigurement is a major concern. Acne requires active treatment for control until it spontaneously resolves.

The most common lesion is a comedo (hair follicle filled with debris; plural, comedones). It is either a blackhead (open follicle) or a small, flesh-colored papule (with a closed follicular orifice). Erythematous papules and pustules occur at the inflammatory stage of the closed comedones. Cysts (actually deep nodules) may produce scarring (deep triangular pits).

Acne is initiated by androgenic hormones that activate sebaceous glands. Sebum production increases, which encourages colonization by anaerobic diphtheroids (*Corynebacterium acnes*). The irritant effect of bacterial by-products and excessive follicle keratinization block follicle patency. There is no scientific evidence that factors such as chocolate, nuts, or fatty foods affect acne. However, exacerbations coinciding with the menstrual cycle result from hormonal activity. Heat, humidity, and excessive perspiration also have a role in increased acne.

Management

Treatment depends on the severity of acne. To prevent scarring, it is important to suppress inflammation. See Table 48–1 for further discussion of acne medications.

Failure of response to topicals indicates needed evaluation for addition of oral antibiotics (tetracycline or erythromycin). Tetracycline or erythromycin administered over an extended period (e.g., several months) suppresses *C. acnes* and decreases inflammation. Long-term systemic antibiotics can cause monilial vaginitis and gastrointestinal symptoms, and clients should be taught how to monitor for these and what interventions to take. Improvement may not be apparent for 4 to 6 weeks.

Hormone therapy may be indicated for severe cystic acne. Medication containing estrogens suppresses sebaceous gland activity. Estrogenic therapy requires treatment through a minimum of three to four menstrual cycles.

In severe cystic acne resistant to standard management, isotretinoin (Accutane) is used to inhibit inflammation. Dosage is determined by body weight and is taken in divided, daily doses for several months. The drug has many side effects and requires frequent follow-up visits and laboratory evaluations. Adverse effects include elevated triglycerides, skin dryness, cheilitis (lip inflammation), and eye discomfort (i.e., dryness, burning). Isotretinoin is a teratogen; thus, this drug should not be used in women without strict and adequate contraception throughout the course of therapy and for a determined period after therapy. The nurse must reinforce the fact that close medical follow-up is needed and that dry skin and cheilitis can be decreased by

TABLE 48–3 Common Skin Infections

NAME	ORGANISM	CLINICAL MANIFESTATIONS	MANAGEMENT
Parasitic			
Scabies	*Sarcoptes scabiei*	Multiple straight or wavy threadlike lines beneath the skin, itching.	Application of a scabicide with retreatment of the residual eggs in 1 week. All clothing and linen should be washed and dried in hot cycles or dry-cleaned.
Lice	*Pediculus humanis/ Phthirus pubis*	Intense itching, scratch marks may be evident.	Application of pediculicides. For head lice, the shampoo should be worked into dry hair until it is saturated. A fine-toothed comb should be used to remove the dead lice and nits. Brushes and combs should be washed in the pediculicide also. For body lice, a pediculicide lotion is applied to involved body areas. Clothing should be washed and dried in hot cycles or dry-cleaned. Family members or close contacts should be treated also.
Bacterial			
Impetigo	Streptococcus A	Pruritic vesicle or pustule that breaks and leaves a thick honey-colored crust.	Antibiotics until cultured include erythromycin or dicloxacillin. Use of mupirocin being studied. Teach control of contagiousness; infection is contagious as long as skin lesions are present. Thorough hand washing, separate laundry for client's linens, separate washing of client's dishes.
Folliculitis, furuncles, carbuncles	*Staphylococcus aureus*	White pustules on forehead, chest, upper back, neck, thighs, groin, and axillae. Furuncles are deeper inflamed nodules. Carbuncles are interconnected furuncles. Often rupture expelling purulent, foul smelling thick drainage.	Localized folliculitis is treated with warm compresses, gentle washing, and topical antibiotics. Furuncles are treated as folliculitis and are incised and drained (I&D) to avoid rupture. Carbuncles are treated with systemic antibiotics and I&D. Teach men to use disposable razors. Reduce spread of infection by careful hand washing and separate laundry of linens.
Fungal			
Candidiasis	*Candida albicans*	Appearance depends on location. In the mouth, it is called thrush, and appears as white plaques with an underlying red base with	Eliminate or control the predisposing factors such as antibiotics (which alter the flora), malnutrition, diabetes, immunosuppression, pregnancy, or use of birth control pills. Use topical antifungal powders and creams. Keep the skin dry, keep the environment cool.

emollients and lip balms. Any vitamin A supplements must be discontinued during this treatment.

There is no convincing evidence that dietary management, mild drying agents, abrasive scrubs, oral vitamin A, cryotherapy, or incision and drainage have any beneficial effects in the management of acne. Some may notice an improvement in the summer months as a result of additional UVL exposure.

It is important to explain the mechanism of acne and the treatment plan and to set goals of therapy. The client should understand that improvement is not usually seen for 4 to 8 weeks. The nurse must assess the client's skin care practices and reinforce compliance with topical or systemic therapy and appropriate skin cleansing methods, with special emphasis on not scrubbing the face and using only the agreed-on topicals. Areas of self-induced skin damage should be noted, and the client must be instructed not to squeeze, prick, or pick at lesions.

ACNE ROSACEA

This chronic, inflammatory eruption, characterized by erythema, papules, pustules, and telangiectasis, occurs on the face, especially the nose. Acne rosacea has an insidious onset, usually between ages 30 and 50 years, and affects women more frequently than men. It is more common in fair-skinned clients with a history of easy facial flushing. Precipitating factors that appear to make the flushing worse include consumption of tea, coffee, alcohol (wine), caffeine-containing products, and

TABLE 48–3 Common Skin Infections *Continued*

NAME	ORGANISM	CLINICAL MANIFESTATIONS	MANAGEMENT
Fungal *Continued*			
		fissures on corners of the mouth. Skin lesions are pruritic, red, and moist with eroded scales. Skin lesions are common to the axilla, gluteal, perianal, and interdigital folds. Vaginal thrush causes intense itching and a cheesy drainage.	
Tinea (several locations) Tinea corporis (ringworm) Tinea capitis (on scalp) Tinea cruris (jock itch) Tinea pedis (athlete's foot)	Variety of dermatophytes	Tinea capitus presents as patchy hair loss, inflammation, scales, and folliculitis. Tinea corposis appears as round red macules and papules with scales. They have advancing borders and healing centers. Tinea cruris appears as red lesions with raised borders. Tinea pedis causes scaling, maceration, pain, and vesicles.	Infection is controlled with antifungal solutions and creams. Acute lesions may require wet dressings, keratolytic agents, or both to remove the scales. Client is taught to reduce risk by thoroughly drying after a bath or shower, wearing absorbent underwear and socks, applying talc to intertriginous areas, and wearing open shoes during warm weather.
Viral			
Herpes simplex	Herpes simplex virus	Vesicles preceded by sensation of itching or burning. Clear exudate from vesicles, followed by crusting. Common to the nose, lips, cheeks, ears, and genitalia.	No cure available today. Treatment includes pain relief and topical anesthetics. Acyclovir, an antiviral drug, may decrease viral shedding and hasten healing. Avoiding the sun or using sunscreens reduces recurrent lesions on the lips. Reduce contagiousness by frequent hand washing, not picking at lesions, avoiding intercourse and kissing while lesions are active, and not sharing lipsticks. Try to identify (and avoid or control) personal triggers for lesions.
Warts	Human papilloma virus	Rough, flesh, or gray-colored skin protrusion.	Numerous therapies, some over-the-counter. May require electrodesiccation or cryosurgery. Intralesional injections of cytotoxic drugs may also be used.

spicy foods; exposure to sunlight and extremes of hot and cold; and emotional stress. Sebaceous hyperplasia of the nose (rhinophyma) is often associated with years of chronic acne rosacea resulting in a "W. C. Fields nose." This results from chronic inflammation and increased connective tissues and may be mistaken for an indication of excessive alcohol consumption. Ocular changes such as eyelid inflammation and conjunctivitis may occur.

Avoidance of the stimuli that trigger acne rosacea may be sufficient for mild disorders. Clients should be instructed to avoid factors that provoke their facial vasodilation, such as caffeine, excessive sunlight, alcohol (especially wine), temperature extremes, hot liquids, and spicy foods. Systemic antibiotics usually are necessary. The nurse should remind the client that improvement with systemic antibiotics will be gradual. Antibiotics are given in small, usually tapered doses for long periods. Relapse is common in clients who discontinue therapy. Topical therapy with nonfluorinated topical corticosteroid cream can be used to reduce inflammation.

Bullous Disorders

PEMPHIGUS

Pemphigus is a chronic disorder that results in the development of blisters (called bullae). It is fairly uncommon in the general population but has an increased incidence in the Jewish and Mediterranean peoples. There are several types of pemphigus: pemphigus vulgaris, pemphigus foliaceus, and pemphigus erythematosus. This discussion focuses on pemphigus vulgaris, the most common type.

Pemphigus is an autoimmune disease caused by circulating immunoglobulin G autoantibodies. These autoantibodies react with the intracellular cement or the substance that holds epidermal cells together. The reaction causes intraepidermal blister (bulla) formation and acantholysis (loss of cohesion between epidermal cells).

Clinical manifestations include flaccid bullae that rupture easily, emitting a foul-smelling drainage and leaving crusted, denuded skin. The lesions are common on the face, back, chest, groin, and umbilicus. Even slight pressure on an intact blister causes it to spread to adjacent skin, which is called Nikolsky's sign.

Management includes large doses of steroids and immunosuppressives. Plasmapheresis has had some success with pemphigus. If the client has a large portion of denuded skin, the management is similar to that for a burn client. The client is at increased risk for infection, fluid and electrolyte imbalance, and stress response complications (i.e., stress ulcers, body system failure). In addition, nursing management focuses on self-concept and pain management. Potassium permanganate baths may be used to reduce the risk of infection, control the odor of the drainage, and ease the pain.

Infectious Disorders

Several organisms lead to skin infections. Common skin infections are described in Table 48–3. A few are discussed in detail in the text.

ERYSIPELAS AND CELLULITIS

Erysipelas is an acute, superficial, rapidly spreading inflammation of the dermis and lymphatics. The usual causative agent is beta-hemolytic streptococcus group A. The organism enters tissue via an abrasion or wound. Fever and leukocytosis (elevated white cell count) are present. The skin is elevated beginning with a small, bright red area. The involved area spreads peripherally to become a plaque with sharp, indurated borders. Lesions are most common on the face and extremities. Recurrence in the same area is common, possibly because of underlying lymphatic obstruction.

Cellulitis is a suppurative inflammation of the dermis and subcutaneous tissues without sharp, indurated borders that spreads widely through tissue spaces. The skin is erythematous, edematous, tender, and sometimes nodular. *Streptococcus pyogenes* is the usual cause of this infection; however, other pathogens may be responsible. Lymphangitis may occur; if cellulitis is untreated, gangrene, metastatic abscesses, and sepsis result.

Clients at increased risk for erysipelas and cellulitis include the elderly and clients with lowered resistance from diabetes, malnutrition, steroid therapy, and the presence of wounds or ulcers. Other predisposing factors include the presence of edema or other cutaneous inflammation or wounds (e.g., tinea, eczema, burns, trauma). There is a tendency for recurrence, especially at sites of lymphatic obstruction.

Management

Erysipelas and cellulitis are treated by systemic antibiotics; penicillin is the antibiotic of choice. Before antibiotics are administered, a culture and sensitivity test of the wound should be taken, although it is usually difficult to yield an organism on culture. Soaks may reduce edema and inflammation. The enzymes that facilitate a rapid spread of infection also seem to produce other significant manifestations such as high fever, tachycardia, confusion, and hypotension; appropriate interventions should be taken if these occur. One must monitor the client's temperature and administer prescribed antipyretic medication. Cross-contamination must be prevented by teaching the client careful hand washing and careful disposal of linen, clothing, dressings, and so forth. Universal precautions should be used as appropriate.

HERPES ZOSTER

Herpes zoster or shingles is an infection caused by the same virus that causes varicella (chickenpox). Although herpes zoster is much less communicable than is varicella, clients who have not had varicella may contract it after exposure to a client with herpes zoster. An increased incidence of herpes zoster occurs in clients with lymphoma, leukemia, and acquired immunodeficiency syndrome (AIDS), probably because of their decreased immunologic response. Diagnostic tests are often not necessary because of the specific characteristics of herpes zoster. A Tzanck smear will demonstrate multinucleated giant cells (see Chap. 47).

In herpes zoster, clusters of grouped vesicles appear unilaterally along cranial or spinal nerve dermatomes after 1 to 2 days of pain, itching, and hyperesthesia. Because they follow nerve pathways, the lesions do not cross the body's midline; however, the nerves of both sides may be involved. Herpes zoster lesions evolve into crusts on the skin and ulcers on the superficial mucous membrane.

The eruption clears in about 2 weeks unless the period between the pain and the eruption is longer than 2 days. In the latter situation, a prolonged convalescence may be expected. Residual pain, postherpetic neuralgia, and itching are the major problems with herpes zoster. The pain may be constant or intermittent and vary from light burning to a deep visceral sensation. The duration of the pain can be weeks or months to years. Unfortunately, in the elderly, the pain generally lasts months to years. Another potential complication is trigeminal herpes zoster involving the facial and acoustic nerves; ophthalmic involvement requires close medical attention for avoidance of ocular complications.

Management

Treatment for herpes zoster is acyclovir (Zovirax) given in a large dose orally or a smaller dose intravenously five times daily. Acyclovir, when started early in the course of the disease, reduces acute pain as well as accelerates healing. The role of acyclovir in preventing postherpetic neuralgia remains unclear. Use of systemic corticosteroids appears to decrease the incidence of postherpetic neuralgia in clients older than 50 years. Analgesics and sedatives are prescribed for pain relief.

Topical therapy is primarily symptomatic: applications of cool compresses, use of cooling antipruritic preparations (see Table 48–1), and measures to prevent secondary infection. If pain is present, the client's normal pain tolerance and current pain level must be assessed. Systemic analgesics and occasionally narcotics are usually required; however, in chronic pain, these may be addictive alternatives. The nurse should assess the effectiveness and side effects of prescribed analgesics. Because postherpetic neuralgia can last a long time, the client and significant others need continued intervention and support. Chronic pain management may include use of tricyclic antidepressants, phenothiazines, and other local physical modalities.

Cancer of the Skin

Precursors to Cancer

Precursors to cancer of the skin include recurrent skin trauma (sunburn) and various skin lesions. To understand the role of prevention of skin cancer, they are discussed here.

SUNBURN

Sunburn is an acute inflammatory skin response that occurs as a reaction to excessive exposure to sunlight. Dermatopathologic changes include the production of epidermal cells that have cytoplasmic and nuclear changes. These changes are cumulative over the lifespan and lead to an increased incidence of skin cancer.

Prevention is obviously the best therapy for sunburn. Client teaching emphasizing sun protection should never be omitted when caring for the sunburned client (see Client Education Guide: Simple Guidelines for Protection Against the Damaging Rays of the Sun).

CLIENT EDUCATION GUIDE

Simple Guidelines for Protection Against the Damaging Rays of the Sun

The nurse should instruct the client in the following:

- Minimize sun exposure during the hours of 10 AM to 2 PM (11 AM to 3 PM daylight saving time), when the sun is strongest. Try to plan your outdoor activities for the early morning or late afternoon.
- Wear a hat, long-sleeved shirt, and long pants when out in the sun. Choose tightly woven materials for greater protection from the sun's rays.
- Apply a sunscreen before every exposure to the sun and reapply frequently and liberally, at least every 2 hours, as long as you stay in the sun. The sunscreen should always be reapplied after swimming or perspiring heavily, because products differ in their degrees of water resistance. Sunscreens with a sun protection factor of 15 or more printed on the label are recommended.
- Use a sunscreen during high-altitude activities such as mountain climbing and skiing. At high altitudes, where there is less atmosphere to absorb the sun's rays, your risk of burning is greater. The sun is also stronger near the equator, where the sun's rays strike the earth most directly.
- Do not forget to use your sunscreen on overcast days. The sun's rays are as damaging to your skin on cloudy, hazy days as they are on sunny days.
- Clients at high risk for skin cancer (outdoor workers, those who are fair skinned, and those who have already had skin cancer) should apply sunscreens daily.
- Photosensitivity—an increased sensitivity to sun exposure—is a possible side effect of certain medications, drugs and cosmetics, and birth control pills. Consult your physician or pharmacist before going out in the sun if you are using any such products. You may need to take extra precautions.
- If an allergic reaction develops to your sunscreen, change sunscreens. One of the many products on the market today should be right for you.
- Beware of reflective surfaces! Sand, snow, concrete, and water can reflect more than half the sun's rays onto your skin. Sitting in the shade does not guarantee protection from sunburn.
- Avoid tanning parlors. The ultraviolet light emitted by tanning booths causes sunburn and premature aging and increases your risk for skin cancer.
- Keep young infants out of the sun. Begin using sunscreens on children at 6 months of age, and then allow sun exposure with moderation.
- Teach children sun protection early. Sun damage occurs with each unprotected sun exposure and accumulates over the course of a lifetime.

Adapted from The Skin Cancer Foundation, New York.

Treating sunburn involves decreasing inflammation and rehydrating the damaged skin. For localized, first-degree sunburn, cool tap water soaks must be applied for 20 minutes or until the skin is cool. This limits skin destruction, prevents edema, and potentially reduces blisters. Tepid tap water baths are indicated for large sunburned areas. After a bath or soak, apply water-based emollients, preferably refrigerated for an additional cooling effect. Emollients should also be applied throughout the day to soothe and relieve dryness. Lotions or foams containing camphor or menthol (e.g., Sarna) can also be beneficial.

For second-degree sunburn, continuous cool, normal saline soaks or soaking baths should be applied to reduce oozing and edema. The nurse should aspirate very large blisters and apply sterile dressings. Débridement should be avoided unless there is evidence of secondary bacterial infection. Silver sulfadiazine may be prescribed. The use of over-the-counter remedies containing local anesthetics (benzocaine, Nupercaine, or Xylocaine) should be avoided because they are rarely effective and have the potential of contact sensitivity.

Prostaglandin inhibitors (aspirin, indomethacin) may be used to reduce the erythema and inflammation. Topical corticosteroids may be prescribed to be used sparingly in nonocclusive vehicles (i.e., cream or lotion) for their vasoconstrictive effects. Systemic corticosteroids are prescribed only for clients with very extensive, painful burns, but their use has declined in favor of prostaglandin inhibitors.

ACTINIC KERATOSIS

Actinic keratosis, the most common epithelial precancerous lesion among whites, is caused by sun exposure. It affects nearly 100 per cent of the elderly white population. There is a small but definite risk of malignant degeneration and subsequent metastatic potential in neglected lesions.

Topical application of 5-fluorouracil (5-FU, Efudex), a topical antimetabolite, is presently one of the best approaches to treatment of widespread actinic damage with multiple lesions. The advantage of 5-FU is that large areas of widespread disease can be treated at the same time. Use of 5-FU not only removes the majority of premalignant and superficial malignant lesions that can be seen but also will uncover and destroy clinically undetectable lesions of this type.

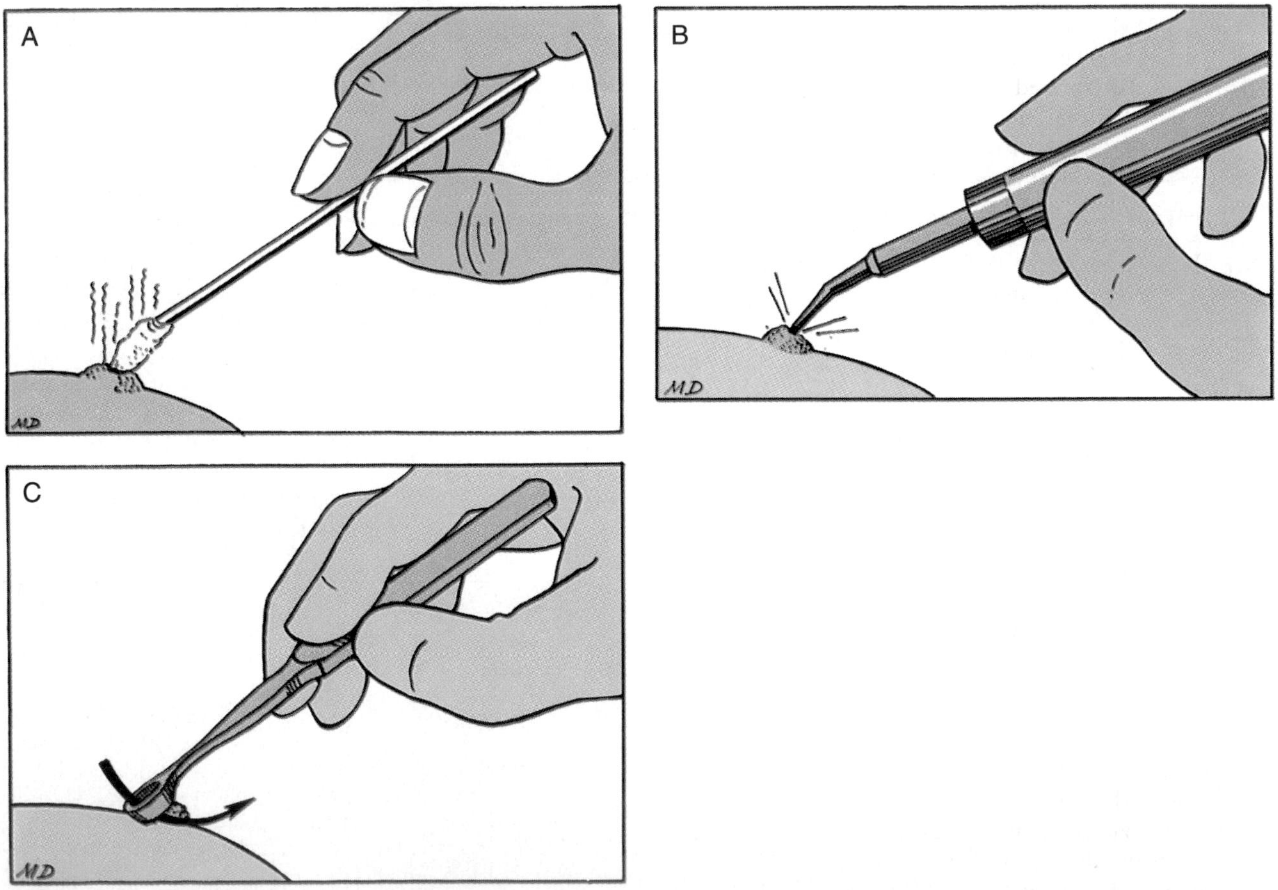

Figure 48–1
Methods for destroying skin lesions. *A*, Cryotherapy. Liquid nitrogen is applied with a saturated cotton-tipped applicator directly to the lesion or sprayed on. This causes tissue destruction by freezing. *B*, Electrodesiccation. Tissue is destroyed by heat from an electrical current; note gloved hand. *C*, Curettage. A curet (cutting instrument) removes tissue by scraping or scooping; note gloved hand.

Surgical management consists of cryotherapy, electrodesiccation and curettage, and shave or excisional biopsy.

Liquid nitrogen is usually applied with a cotton applicator or spraying device and requires no local anesthetic (Fig. 48–1*A*). The client does note a small amount of discomfort at the time of freezing, which may linger afterward.

Electrodesiccation produces superficial destruction through bursts of electrical current and is usually done under local anesthesia (Fig. 48–1*B*). The tissue is destroyed by mechanical disruption of cells and heat. The tissue is removed by scraping or scooping with a loop-shaped instrument called a curet (Fig. 48–1*C*). This method does provide tissue for histologic diagnosis if needed.

Shave or excisional biopsy is indicated on lesions that are large or hypertrophic or have other characteristics of a cutaneous malignancy (induration, erythema, erosion). It is often difficult to distinguish a large or hypertrophic actinic keratosis from a squamous cell carcinoma without histologic diagnosis.

Skin Cancer

Definition and Incidence

Skin cancer is the most common cancer in the United States. Skin cancer is a malignant condition caused by uncontrolled growth and spread of abnormal cells in a specific layer of the skin. The several different kinds of skin cancer are distinguished by the types of cells involved. Basal cell carcinoma, squamous cell carcinoma, and malignant melanoma are the three most common types of skin cancer. More than 90 per cent of all skin cancers fall into the first two classifications. Both basal cell carcinoma and squamous cell carcinoma are slow-growing tumors that have a cure rate of 95 per cent or greater with early treatment.

Etiology and Risk Factors

The cause of skin cancer is well known.

CRITICAL TO REMEMBER

Prolonged or intermittent exposure to UVL radiation from the sun, especially when it results in sunburn and blistering, plays a key role in the induction of skin cancer, especially malignant melanoma.

The majority of all nonmelanoma skin cancers occur on parts of the body unprotected by clothing (face, neck, forearms, and backs of hands) and in clients who have received considerable exposure to sunlight. All clients are at risk for skin cancer regardless of skin tone and hair color; however, some clients are at much greater risk than others. In general, clients with red, blond, or light-brown hair with light complexions or freckles, many of Celtic or Scandinavian origin, are most susceptible; blacks and Asians are least susceptible.

Danger signals in moles are presented in Box 48–1. Suspicious lesions should be examined by a physician.

The history of a client's pattern of reaction to acute sun exposure is correlated with the client's tendency to acquire actinic keratosis and skin cancer. Those who never tan and always burn after 1 to 2 hours of midday summer sun are most susceptible. Those who burn once or twice at the beginning of summer and then tan are somewhat less susceptible. Those who never burn and always tan are the least susceptible. The most severely affected clients usually have a history of long-term occupational (farmers, construction workers, surveyors, sailors) or recreational (swimmers, skiers, surfers, sunbathers) sun exposure.

Clinical Manifestations

BASAL CELL CARCINOMA

Basal cell carcinoma, the most common form of skin cancer, is a malignant epithelial tumor of the skin that arises from the basal cells contained in the epidermis.

The tumor is usually painless and slow growing, generally appearing on sun-exposed skin, face, ears, head, neck, or hands. Occasionally, basal cell carcinoma may appear on the trunk, especially the upper back and chest. The majority are caused by chronic overexposure to UVL radiation, and only a few cases can be linked to arsenic, burns, scars, exposure to radiation, or genetic predisposition. Clinical and histologic findings are used to identify the tumor.

The most common clinical presentation of basal cell carcinoma is the nodular lesion (Fig. 48–2). This is a dome-shaped papule with a well-defined border containing a classic "pearly" texture. Basal cell carcinoma has this flesh-colored "pearly" or shiny appearance because it does not keratinize. Telangiectatic vessels frequently overlie the lesion. As the lesion enlarges, the

BOX 48–1

Danger Signals Suggestive of Malignant Transformation in Pigmented Nevi

- *Change in color,* especially red, white, and blue; sudden darkening; mottled shades of brown or black
- *Change in diameter,* especially sudden increase
- *Change in outline,* especially development of irregular margins
- *Change in surface characteristics,* especially scaliness, erosion, oozing, crusting, bleeding, ulceration, development of a mushrooming mass on the surface of the lesion
- *Change in consistency,* especially softening or friability
- *Change in symptoms,* especially pruritus
- *Change in shape,* especially irregular elevation from a previously flat condition
- *Change in surrounding skin,* especially "leaking" of pigment from the lesion into surrounding skin or pigmented "satellite" lesions

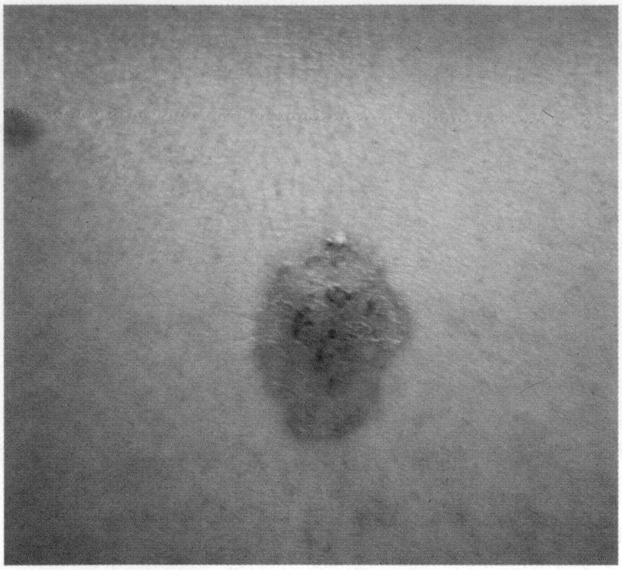

Figure 48–2
Basal cell carcinoma of the back. (Courtesy of University of Nebraska Medical Center, Biomedical Communications.)

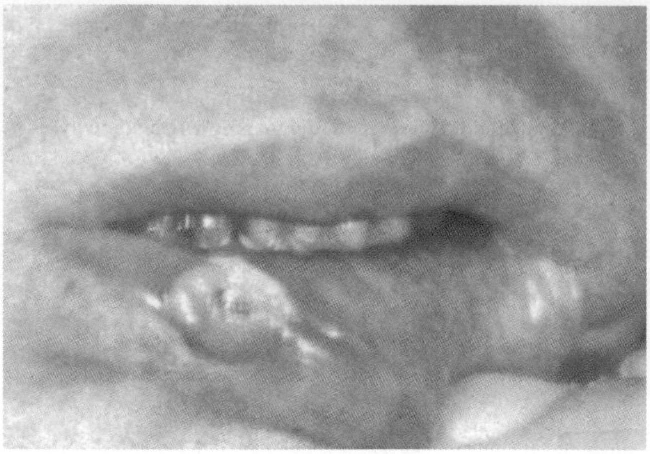

Figure 48–3
Squamous cell carcinoma of the lip. (From Wenig, B. M. [1993]. *Atlas of head and neck pathology*. Philadelphia: W. B. Saunders.)

center may flatten or ulcerate; however, the border will still be raised and give a "rolled" appearance.

Basal cell carcinomas almost never metastasize. They can, however, be locally destructive and invasive through tissue. This is particularly true on the face, where a lesion can invade deep structures with resultant loss of an eye, ear, or nose. If untreated, the tumor can invade through bone and brain. However, if the tumor is identified and treated early, local excision or even nonexcisional destruction is usually curative.

Clients who have had one basal cell carcinoma are at greater risk for acquiring others. Recurrences of previously treated basal cell carcinomas are also possible but more unusual. The possible recurrence generally occurs within the first 2 years after removal or therapy.

SQUAMOUS CELL CARCINOMA

Squamous cell carcinoma is the second most common skin cancer in whites. It is a tumor of the epidermal keratinocytes and rarely occurs in dark-skinned clients. It is found on areas often exposed to the sun, typically the rim of the ear, the face, the lips and mouth, and the dorsa of the hands. Squamous cell carcinoma is more difficult to characterize than is basal cell carcinoma. These tumors are poorly marginated; the edge often blends into surrounding sun-damaged skin. Squamous cell carcinoma may present as an ulcer, flat red area, cutaneous horn, indurated plaque, or hyperkeratotic papule or nodule (Fig. 48–3). Often they present as a red- to skin-colored papule surmounted by varying amounts of scale. These lesions grow more rapidly than does a basal cell carcinoma. These tumors are potentially dangerous because they may infiltrate surrounding structures, metastasize to lymph nodes, and be subsequently fatal.

MALIGNANT MELANOMA

Malignant melanoma is a cancer of melanocytes; it is the deadliest form of skin cancer. The incidence and death rate from melanoma are rising worldwide. In countries populated with fair-skinned whites, the incidence of melanoma and mortality have risen by 7 to 15 per cent per year, more than doubling over the past decade. Whites have 10 times the incidence that blacks do.

UVL continues to be one of the most important causes of malignant melanoma. However, melanoma can appear anywhere on the body, not just on sun-exposed areas. The majority of malignant melanoma appears to be associated with the intensity rather than the duration of sunlight exposure, in contrast to basal cell and squamous cell carcinomas. Melanoma tends to be observed more often in whites who move to sunny climates, or in professionals who take short vacations with intense sun exposure, than in clients who suffer from chronic sun exposure. The suspicion of melanoma is based on history as well as clinical appearance (Figs. 48–4 and 48–5). The tumor can metastasize, usually to the brain, lungs, bones, liver, and skin, and is ultimately fatal. The prognosis of melanoma has become more predictable. Clinically, metastatic melanoma is universally fatal. Prognosis and mortality of melanoma that is not clinically metastatic at presentation depend critically on the depth of the lesion at the time of excision. The more superficial or "thin" the tumor, the better the prognosis.

Medical Management

Medical management begins by having a high index of suspicion for any type of skin cancer but specifically melanoma. The need for early detection cannot be overstressed in dealing with malignant melanoma. Any indication, whether it is a high-risk client or a suspicious lesion, is adequate reason for referral.

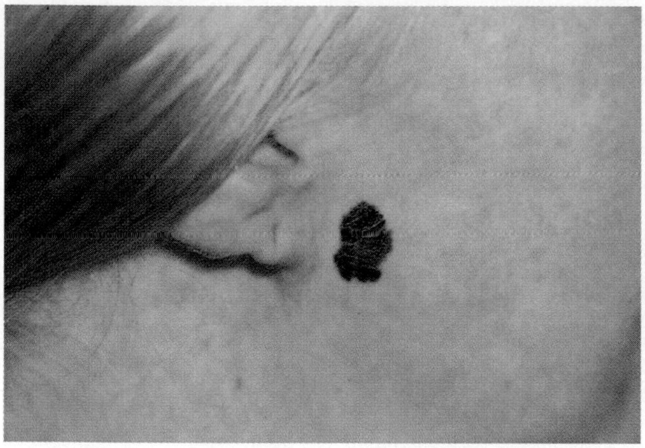

Figure 48–4
Superficial spreading melanoma.

Surgical Management

Treatment of any and all skin cancer requires removal of the lesion. The tumor removed needs to have a specified margin free of tumor (differs depending on type of skin cancer) to guarantee full removal of the skin cancer.

BASAL CELL AND SQUAMOUS CELL CARCINOMAS

A special surgery technique primarily used for the removal of skin malignancies such as basal cell and squamous cell carcinoma is Mohs surgery. Mohs surgery is also indicated for primary lesions in areas where preservation of normal skin is necessary (e.g., eyelids, pinna, nasolabial folds). The technique is based on a series of excisions. Careful microscopic tissue assessment "maps" the presence or absence of malignant cells within each specimen. The procedure may be lengthy. After all tumor tissue is removed, the wound is closed with sutures or with a flap (see Chap. 50) or allowed to close by secondary intention.

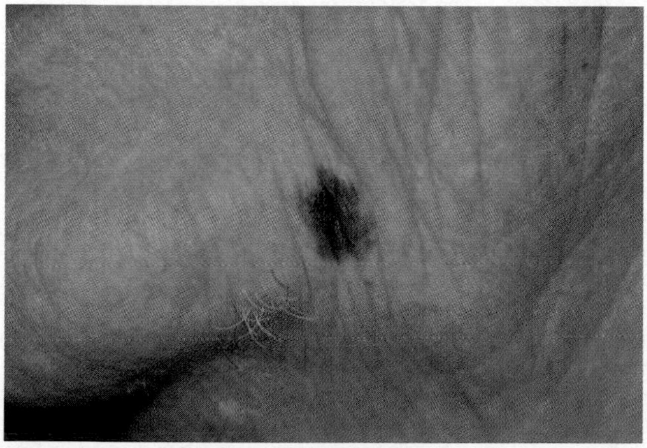

Figure 48–5
Nodular melanoma.

Basal cell and squamous cell carcinoma can also be excised and the area closed primarily or with a skin flap. The advantage of this technique is that it requires much less time, and the scar is controllable as a fine line. The tumor is completely excised with adequate margins of tumor-free tissue. If there is doubt about the adequacy of margins, the specimen is sent for pathologic diagnosis (frozen section). Surgery can be combined with Mohs technique.

MELANOMA

The treatment for malignant melanoma is wide local excision. There is no role at present for chemotherapy or radiation therapy as the initial treatment.

Surgical excision begins with a biopsy for determining the stage of the cancer. Biopsies are performed whenever the client cannot be assured that a lesion is benign. Excisional biopsy is the removal of the lesion and a narrow margin of normal-appearing tissue. This tissue is examined, and the melanoma is staged (Fig. 48–6).

The final excision is usually completed within 1 week of biopsy. Nurses should be aware that although there is theoretic risk of tumor spread during biopsy, there is no convincing evidence that waiting 1 to even 6 weeks after biopsy jeopardizes the outcome. In fact, sometimes the delay allows the client time to prepare for surgery, both physically and psychologically.

Wide excision of the tumor with a 1- to 3-cm margin of normal-appearing skin is the treatment. The margin is based on the type of melanoma. The area is closed in surgery, either primarily (skin edges sewn together) or with grafts of flaps.

Advanced Metastatic Melanoma. The client with advanced metastatic melanoma has a poor prognosis. There is no cure today for metastatic melanoma, but some therapies will improve the quality of life. A treatment plan is arranged on the basis of several factors: site of the tumor, number of metastases, rate of tumor growth, previous treatments, response to treatment, age of the client, general health of the client, and desires of the client.

Some treatments include surgery to remove metastatic lesions, radiation therapy, chemotherapy, and local hyperthermia. Of course, the client can opt for no further treatment. Immunotherapy and hormonal therapy are currently investigational.

Cutaneous T-Cell Lymphoma (Mycosis Fungoides)

Cutaneous T-cell lymphoma (CTCL), also known as mycosis fungoides or Sézary syndrome, is a malignant disease involving the helper T cells. Malignant T cells in the blood migrate to the skin, where they have an affinity for the epidermis. The malignant cells continue to grow and change, eventually moving into the dermis. The cause is not known. This disease has exacerbations

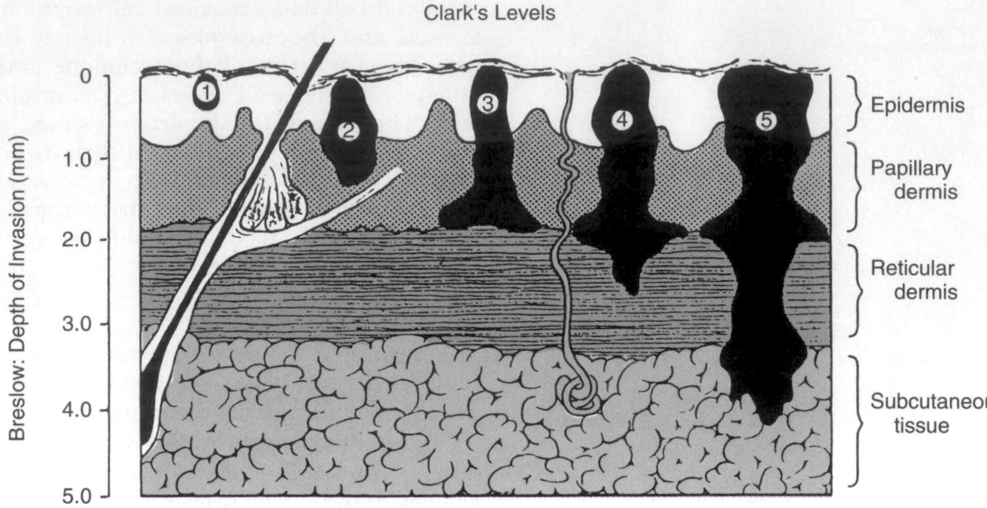

CLARK'S LEVEL OF INVASION	BRESLOW MICROSTAGE	SURVIVAL 10 YEARS
I in situ	less than 0.1 mm.	greater than 95%
II papillary dermis	0.1–0.76 mm.	90%
III papillary & reticular	0.76–1.50 mm.	80%
IV reticular dermis	1.50–3.0 mm.	60%
V subcutaneous	greater than 3.0 mm.	30%

Figure 48–6
The combination of Clark's level of invasion and Breslow's depth of invasion allows prediction of 10-year survival in melanoma. (From Eisenbaum, S. L., & Black, J. M. [1988]. Melanoma. *Plastic Surgical Nursing, 8[2],* 42–47.)

and remissions but is invariably fatal. Median lifespan after tissue biopsy is 5 years. Virtually every organ, especially the liver, spleen, and lungs, may be involved. There seems to be a correlation between high exposure to environmental toxins and this disease.

CTCL is an extremely difficult disorder to diagnose and is often misdiagnosed. In its early stages, CTCL can clinically mimic eczematous processes. Clinical manifestations include eversion of the eyelids and hyperkeratosis of the palms and soles, often with fissuring. Finally, the plaques form tumors that ultimately ulcerate. Tumors can also develop spontaneously in previously unaffected areas, and eventual visceral or organ involvement ensues. Clients often feel desperate by the time diagnosis is confirmed, which adds to the psychological difficulties.

Management

Control of pruritus is essential at all stages and is accomplished by rehydration of the skin, various dry skin therapies, topical corticosteroids, and UVB therapy (see Ultraviolet Light Therapy). Prevention of secondary infections is important. Nitrogen mustard administered topically acts as a cytotoxin. It is applied daily and is often initial treatment. Photophoresis, a treatment involving the removal of small amounts of blood that is irradiated and then returned to the body, is used frequently in more advanced stages. Total-body electron beam therapy with or without adjuvant chemotherapy is a favorably aggressive approach often used. Unfortunately, even if these therapies succeed in clearing the skin, the disorder is still fatal because of systemic involvement.

Kaposi's Sarcoma

Kaposi's sarcoma is a vascular malignancy that presents as a skin disorder. It has a long history. Kaposi's sarcoma used to be a skin disease common in 50- to 60-year-old men of Jewish or Mediterranean descent. It was seen less frequently in clients who were black, homosexual, or immunosuppressed (e.g., renal transplant clients). Recently, Kaposi's sarcoma has been seen in many clients with AIDS.

The cause of Kaposi's sarcoma is not known, although the HIV and cytomegalovirus have been suggested as the cofactors in its development. It is considered to be due to a failure in the immune system, perhaps as a result of frequent or overwhelming infec-

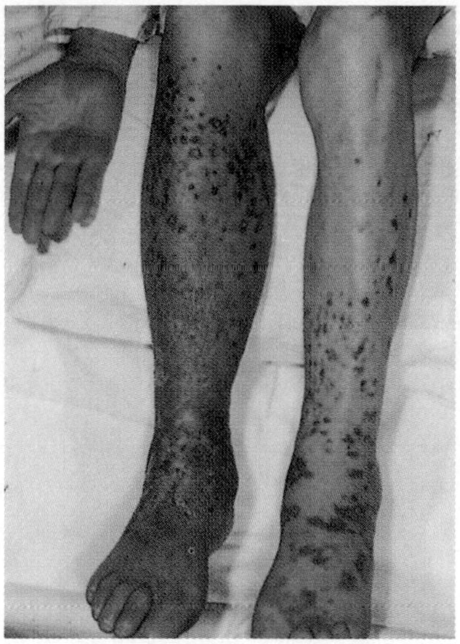
Figure 48–7
Kaposi's sarcoma.

tions. The lesions begin in the mid-dermis and extend upward into the epidermis.

Kaposi's sarcoma lesions begin as red, dark blue, or purple macules on the lower legs that coalesce into larger plaques (Fig. 48–7). These large plaques frequently ulcerate or open and drain. The lesions spread by metastasis through the upper body and then to the face and oral mucosa. About 75 per cent of clients acquire lesions of the lymph nodes, gastrointestinal tract, and lungs.[11] Clients also report pain and itching in the lesions; as Kaposi's sarcoma progresses, the legs become edematous.

Kaposi's sarcoma is diagnosed by skin biopsy, and a high index of suspicion should exist for those clients who are immunosuppressed. Local lesions can be excised. Systemic lesions are treated with a combination of interferon-alpha, cytotoxic agents, and radiation. General response to treatment is poor. A complete discussion of AIDS can be found in Chapter 9.

STUDY QUESTIONS

1. An assessment of the client with atopic dermatitis includes which one of the following?
   A. Skin that is brown stained
   B. Skin reddened from scratching
   C. Skin that has small, scaly patches
   D. A nodular lesion on the skin's surface
2. Which one of the following is a precursor to skin cancer?
   A. Anthralin
   B. Fair skin
   C. Psoriasis
   D. Sunburn
3. Which one of the following statements indicates to the nurse that the client has accepted the treatment recommended for his integumentary disorder?
   A. "I'll do it, but I don't know if it will do any good."
   B. "My physician says I need the surgery to save my life."
   C. "I understand that even with treatment there is no cure."
   D. "I use the prescription cream twice a day and spread it all over my body."
4. The plan of care for a client with pruritus should include teaching about which one of the following?
   A. Self-examination of the skin
   B. Signs and symptoms of an infection
   C. Use of distraction to prevent scratching
   D. Administration of an antianxiety agent to reduce tension
5. Surgical treatment for skin cancer may result in disfigurement. Which nursing intervention would most likely help the client?
   A. The client should be taught about wound care.
   B. The nurse should ask the spouse to touch the scar.
   C. The client should be encouraged to look in the mirror.
   D. The nurse should interact with the client in the usual manner.
6. When evaluating the outcome of client goals for a client who has cancer of the skin, the nurse would expect a successful outcome if the client can
   A. Explain the need for a diet high in calories and vitamin C
   B. Relate the difference between basal cell and squamous cell carcinoma
   C. Explain the reason for changes in the structure and function of the skin
   D. Discuss the need to report changes in the nevi present on the skin's surface

CRITICAL THINKING EXERCISES

SCENARIO A

A young female client arrives at the medical clinic with a severe case of sunburn. She tells the nurse she is cultivating a suntan and plans to spend at least 3 or 4 hours in the sun each day. Her favorite time of day for sunbathing is the middle of the day because "that's when it's the hottest." Her sunburn covers most of her body except where her bikini bathing suit protected her. Her skin is bright red, and she has blisters on the forehead, nose, and shoulders.

She is thinking of using a tanning booth to keep her skin darkened. She gives a history of being on birth control pills.

1. What teaching does the client need before discharge from the clinic?
2. How does culture and society view tanned skin? What are the implications for client teaching?
3. How do birth control medications affect the tanning process?
4. What specific information about the use of tanning booths would help the client make the decision to avoid them?

SCENARIO B

A recently retired gentleman is diagnosed with malignant melanoma. He planned to keep busy during retirement by working on his tennis game. He stated he had a couple of growths on his left ear and cheek for a number of years and believed they were part of the aging process because his father had the same kind of growths when he grew old. He delayed seeking help until some time after the lesions changed in color and increased dramatically in size. He is scheduled for surgery and reports that his ear lobe will be excised and there will be a large scar on his cheek because so much tissue will be removed.

1. Were his beliefs about skin changes associated with the aging process correct?
2. How can people be educated about seeking medical help for changes in their bodies?
3. Is this client the most likely to be at risk for malignant melanoma? What risk factors contributed to the development of the disease?
4. How was the diagnosis determined?
5. How much tissue will be removed during the surgery?
6. How will the disease affect his self-image, his reaction to future health needs, and his life expectancy?

BIBLIOGRAPHY

1. Abel, E. A., et al. (1986). Drugs in exacerbation of psoriasis. *Journal of the American Academy of Dermatology, 15(11),* 1007–1022.
2. Arndt, K. W. (1989). *Manual of dermatological therapeutics* (4th ed.). Boston: Little, Brown.
3. Buller, M. K., Loescher, L. J., & Buller, D. B. (1994). "Sunshine and skin health": A curriculum for skin cancer prevention. *Journal of Cancer Education, 9(3),* 155–162.
4. Clark, R. A. F., & Adinoff, A. D. (1989). Aeroallergen contact can exacerbate atopic dermatitis: Patch tests as a diagnostic tool. *Journal of the American Academy of Dermatology, 2(4),* 863–869.
5. Clark, R. A. F., et al. (1990). Atopic dermatitis. In M. Sams & P. Lynch (Eds.), *Principles and practice of dermatology* (pp. 365–380). Philadelphia: W. B. Saunders.
6. Clark, R. A. F., et al. (1990). Current concepts in the management of the patient with atopic dermatitis. *Modern Medicine, 58(3),* 78–94.
7. Cunliffe, W. J. (1987). Evolution of a strategy for the treatment of acne. *Journal of the American Academy of Dermatology, 16(3),* 591–599.
8. Dunn, M. L., et al. (1988). Treatment options for psoriasis. *American Journal of Nursing, 88(8),* 1082–1087.
9. Eisenbaum, S. L., & Black, J. M. (1988). Melanoma. *Plastic Surgical Nursing, 8(2),* 42–47.
10. Fitzgerald, E., & Kantor, G. R. (1994). Alleviating the pain of herpes zoster. *Emergency Medicine, 26(3),* 34–39.
11. Fitzpatrick, T. B., et al. (1993). *Dermatology in general medicine* (4th ed.). New York: McGraw-Hill.
12. Frank-Stromborg, M., & Rohan, K. (1992). Nursing involvement in the primary and secondary prevention of cancer: Nationally and internationally. *Cancer Nursing, 15(2),* 79–108.
13. Friedman, L. C., et al. (1994). Early detection of skin cancer: Racial-ethnic differences in behaviors and attitudes. *Journal of Cancer Education, 9(2),* 105–110.
14. Gilleaudeau, B., & McClelland, B. (1994). Cyclosporine: A new therapeutic option for severe, recalcitrant psoriasis. *Dermatology Nursing, 6(6),* 395–407.
15. Glizzard, D. (1991). Understanding the pathophysiology of psoriasis. A nursing perspective. *Dermatology Nursing, 3(5),* 305–314.
16. Hussar, D. A. (1994). Drug for psoriasis: Calcipotriene. *Nursing 94, 24(12),* 54.
17. Jenkins, A. P., & Olsen, L. K. (1994). Health behaviors of health educators: A national survey. *Journal of Health Education, 25(6),* 324–332.
18. Loescher, L. J. (1993). Skin cancer prevention and detection update. *Seminars in Oncology Nursing, 9(3),* 184–187.
19. McCance, K., & Heurter, S. (1994). *Pathophysiology* (2nd ed.). St. Louis: Mosby-Year Book.
20. McMahon, M. A. (1994). Herpes zoster and the aging. *Journal of Gerontological Nursing, 20(12),* 42–46.
21. Nicol, N. H. (1987). Atopic dermatitis: The (wet) wrap-up. *American Journal of Nursing, 87(12),* 1560–1564.
22. Nicol, N. H. (1989). Actinic keratosis: Preventable and treatable like other precancerous and cancerous skin lesions. *Plastic Surgical Nursing, 9(2),* 49–55.
23. Nicol, N. H. (1989). Early detection and prevention of skin cancer. *Dermatology Nursing, 1(1),* 11–20.
24. Nicol, N. H. (1989). What's new in sunscreens? Choices, choices, choices. *Pediatric Nursing, 15(4),* 417–418.
25. Nicol, N. H. (1990). Current considerations and management of atopic dermatitis. *Dermatology Nursing, 2(3),* 129–138.
26. Nicol, N. H., & Clark, R. A. F. (1988). Therapy of atopic dermatitis. In E. Farmer & T. Provost (Eds.), *Current therapy in dermatology—2.* Philadelphia: B. C. Decker.
27. Provan, A., & Phillips, T. (1991). An overview of moist wound dressings: The under cover story. *Dermatology Nursing, 3(6),* 393–400.

28. Safai, B., Diaz, B., & Schwartz, J. (1993). Malignant neoplasms associated with human immunodeficiency virus infection. *AIDS Patient Care, 7(5),* 262–274.

29. Salasche, S. J. (1988). Actinic keratosis and keratoacanthoma. In E. Farmer & T. Provost (Eds.), *Current therapy in dermatology—2* (pp. 74–76). Philadelphia: B.C. Decker.

30. Sams, V. M., & Lynch, P. J. (1990). *Principles and practice of dermatology*. New York: Churchill Livingstone.

31. Scotto, J., & Fears, T. R. (1987). The association of solar ultraviolet and skin melanoma incidence among caucasians in the United States. *Cancer Investigation, 5(4),* 275–283.

32. Shelk, J. (1991). Phototherapy: A nursing overview. *Dermatology Nursing, 3(6),* 401–410.

33. Smith, D. P., & Nicol, N. H. (1991). Controlling pruritus. In D. P. Smith (Ed.), *Comprehensive child and family nursing skills: Assessment and intervention* (pp. 503–510). St. Louis: Mosby-Year Book.

34. Stoll, H. L., & Schwartz, R. A. (1987). Squamous cell carcinoma. In T. B. Fitzpatrick et al. (Eds.), *Dermatology in general medicine* (pp. 746–758). New York: McGraw-Hill.

35. Wilkner, N. E., & Weston, W. L. (1988). Skin neoplasms. In R. W. Schrier (Ed.), *Medicine: Diagnosis and treatment* (pp. 513–530). Boston: Little, Brown.

Chapter 49 Nursing Care of Clients with Burn Injury

Learning Outcomes

After completing this chapter, the learner will be able to:

1. Assess the client for risk factors implicated in burn injuries.
2. Discuss the pathophysiologic changes that occur during the emergency, acute, and rehabilitative phases of burn injury.
3. Use the rule of nines to estimate burn area.
4. Assess clients for factors that affect burn severity, management, and recovery.
5. Develop plans of care for the prevention, management, and rehabilitation of clients with burn injuries.

Injuries that result from direct contact or exposure to any thermal, chemical, electrical, or radiation source are termed burns. Burn injuries occur when energy from a heat source is transferred to the tissues of the body. The depth of injury is a function of temperature and the duration of exposure.

Incidence

Burn care has improved in recent decades, resulting in a lower mortality rate for victims of burn injuries. In the United States, two million people seek medical attention every year for injuries caused by burns; of these, 70,000 are hospitalized with severe injuries. Burn injuries are the third leading cause of accidental death in all age groups. Males tend to be injured more frequently than females, except in the elderly population (older than 70 years).

Etiology

Burn injuries are categorized according to their mechanism of injury.

THERMAL BURNS

Thermal burns are caused by exposure to flame, hot liquids, semiliquids (steam), semisolids (tar), or hot objects. Specific examples of thermal burns are those sustained in residential fires, explosive automobile accidents, scald injuries, clothing ignition, and ignition of poorly stored flammable liquids.

CHEMICAL BURNS

Chemical burns are caused by tissue contact with strong acids, alkalis, or organic compounds. Chemical burns can result from contact with certain household cleaning agents and various chemicals used in industry, agriculture, and the military. More than 25,000 products capable of causing chemical injuries have been identified.

ELECTRICAL BURNS

Electrical burns are caused by heat that is generated by the electrical energy as it passes through the body.[22] Electrical injuries can result from contact with exposed or faulty electrical wiring or high-voltage power lines. Individuals struck by lightning also sustain an electrical injury.

RADIATION BURNS

Radiation burns are the least common type of burn injury and are caused by exposure to a radioactive source. These types of injuries have been associated with the use of ionizing radiation in industry or from therapeutic radiation sources in medicine. A sunburn from prolonged exposure to ultraviolet rays is also considered to be a type of radiation burn.

Risk Factors

Data collected from the National Burn Information Exchange reveals that 75 per cent of all burn injuries result from the actions of the victim, with many of these injuries occurring in the home environment. The client over age 70 is at a high risk for burn injury. Risk factors include contact with scalding liquids, clothing ignition during meal preparation, and residential fires. Safety practices in the home are important and should include the installation and maintenance of smoke detectors. Fire extinguishers and instruction in their use are another preventative measure.

Pathophysiology

CUTANEOUS BURNS

The pathophysiologic changes that occur immediately following a cutaneous burn injury depend on the extent or size of the burn. For smaller burns, the body's response to injury is localized to the injured area. However, with more extensive burns, i.e., 25 per cent of the total body surface area (TBSA) or greater, the body's response to injury is systemic and proportional to the extent of the injury. Extensive burn injuries affect all major systems of the body.

Cardiovascular System. Immediately following a burn injury, vasoactive substances (e.g., catecholamines, histamine, serotonin) are released from the injured tissue. These substances initiate changes that cause an increase in capillary permeability, allowing plasma to seep into surrounding tissues. Direct heat injury to vessels further increases capillary permeability. Direct injury to cell membranes permits sodium entry and potassium exit from the cell. The end result of these fluid changes is an increase in intracellular and interstitial fluid and a decrease in intravascular fluid volume (see Pathophysiology: Cardiovascular Changes in Burns).

Renal and Gastrointestinal Systems. The body responds initially by shunting blood from the kidneys and decreasing glomerular filtration rate, causing oliguria. Blood flow to the mesenteric bed is also diminished, leading to the development of intestinal ileus and gastrointestinal dysfunction in clients with burns greater than 25 per cent of TBSA.[43]

Immune System. Immune system function is depressed. Depression of lymphocyte activity, a decrease in immunoglobulin production, suppression of complement activity, and an alteration in neutrophil and macrophage functioning are evident following extensive burn injuries. Together, these changes result in some degree of immunosuppression, increasing the risk of infection and life-threatening sepsis.

Respiratory System. The client may exhibit modest pulmonary artery hypertension, resulting in a decrease in arterial oxygen tension levels and lung com-

PATHOPHYSIOLOGY

Cardiovascular Changes in Burns

Initial cardiovascular changes include:

- Increased capillary permeability that causes a fluid shift to the tissue (generalized edema) from the vascular system
- Release of vasoactive substances and decreased vascular fluid that cause an increased heart rate
- Decrease in vascular fluid causes an increase in the hematocrit level
- Increased evaporative fluid loss that remains elevated until the burn is healed

Further cardiovascular changes include the following:

- Capillary permeability decreases in 18 to 36 hours, but takes an additional 2 to 3 weeks to normalize
- Cardiac output increases to meet the increased metabolic needs of the body approximately 24 hours after the burn
- Hematocrit level decreases to below normal because of red blood cell loss and damage
- The body begins to reabsorb edema, and diuresis begins to rid the body of excess fluid (Fig. 49–1)

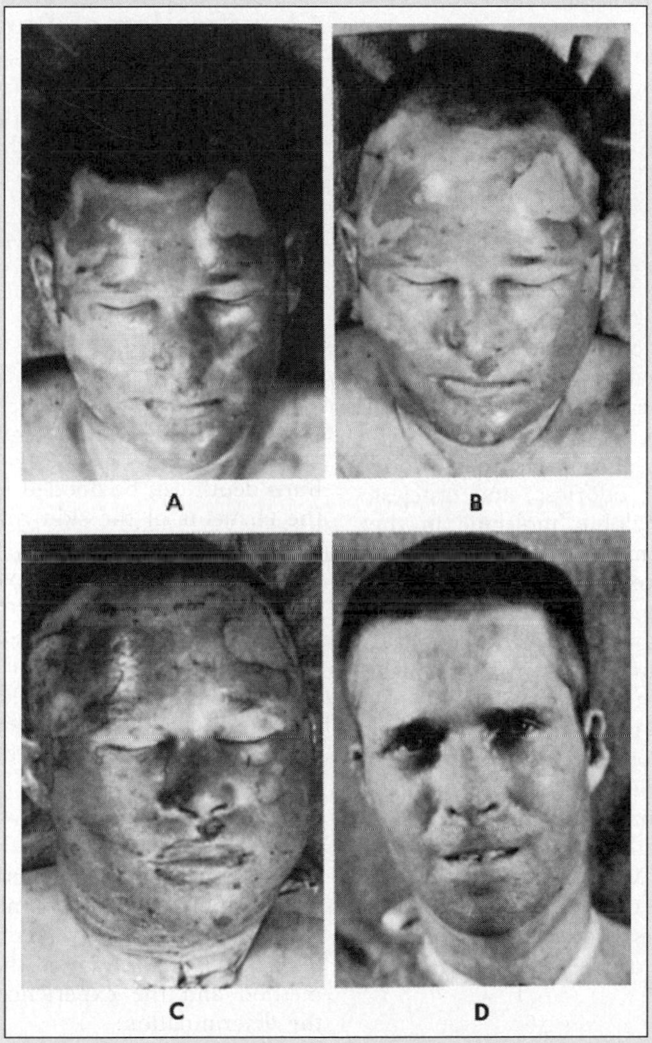

Figure 49–1
Facial edema at various times following a burn injury to the face and neck. Edema worsens over the first 24 to 48 hours following a burn. *A,* 3 hours after burn. *B,* 8 hours after burn. *C,* 24 hours after burn, when the edema has typically maximized. *D,* Complete healing after 40 days. (From Artz, C. P., et al. [Eds.] [1979]. Burns: A team approach. Philadelphia: W. B. Saunders.)

pliance even when the client sustains no inhalation injury.

SMOKE INHALATION

The inhalation of smoke and resulting pulmonary injury are often associated with flame injuries, particularly if the victim was trapped in an enclosed, smoke-filled space (e.g., a residential fire).

Clinical manifestations suggestive of inhalation injury (emergent through acute phase) include

- facial burns
- erythema
- swelling of the oropharynx or nasopharynx
- singed nasal hairs
- agitation or anxiety
- tachypnea
- flaring nostrils
- stridor
- wheezing
- dyspnea
- hoarse voice
- carbonaceous (sooty) sputum
- cough

The pulmonary pathophysiology that occurs with inhalation injury is multifactorial and relates to the severity and type of smoke or gases inhaled.

Carbon Monoxide Poisoning. CO is a common by-product released when organic substances (e.g., wood or coal) burn. It is a colorless, odorless, and tasteless gas that attaches to the hemoglobin molecule in the place of oxygen. When carbon monoxide and hemoglobin combine, the result is carboxyhemoglobin (COHb). Tissue hypoxia occurs from an overall decrease in the blood's oxygen-delivering capability. COHb levels are easily monitored via blood serum levels in the clinical setting. Associated symptoms are listed in Table 49–1.

Smoke Poisoning. Smoke poisoning results from the inhalation of the by-products of combustion: noxious chemicals and particulate matter. The pulmonary response includes a localized inflammatory reaction, a decrease in bronchial ciliary action, and a decrease in alveolar surfactant. Mucosal edema in the smaller airways occurs, leading to audible wheezing on auscultation. After several hours, sloughing of the tracheobronchial epithelium may occur and hemorrhagic tracheobronchitis may develop. If the disease process continues, adult respiratory distress syndrome may follow.

Direct Thermal (Heat) Injury. Thermal burns to the upper airways (mouth, nasopharynx, pharynx, and larynx) are common and generally appear erythematous and edematous with mucosal blisters or ulcerations. The mucosal edema can lead to upper airway obstruction, particularly during the first 24 to 48 hours after the burn. Therefore, all clients with head and neck burns should be suspect for developing an airway obstruction and immediately considered for endotracheal intubation. Thermal burns to the lower airways are rare.

TABLE 49–1 Clinical Manifestations of Carbon Monoxide (CO) Poisoning

CO LEVEL (%)	CLINICAL MANIFESTATIONS
5–10	Impaired visual acuity
11–20	Flushing, headache
21–30	Nausea, impaired dexterity
31–40	Vomiting, dizziness, syncope
41–50	Tachypnea, tachycardia
>50	Coma, death

Adapted from Cioffi, W. G., & Rue, L. W. (1991). Diagnosis and treatment of inhalation injuries. *Critical Care Clinics of North America, 3*(2), 195.

Classification of Burn Severity

The severity of a burn injury is assessed with respect to the risk of mortality and the risk of cosmetic or functional disability. Factors that influence injury severity include:

- Burn depth (Fig. 49–2)
- Burn size (percentage of TBSA)
- Burn location
- Age
- General health
- Mechanism of injury

BURN DEPTH

Burn depth can be divided into four categories based on the elements of the skin that are damaged: (1) superficial, (2) partial thickness, (3) full thickness, and (4) fourth degree. Most burn wounds that require medical intervention are a combination of partial- and full-thickness burns. A partial-thickness burn is shown in Figure 49–3. A full-thickness burn is shown in Figures 49–4 and 49–5. A fourth-degree burn injures and exposes muscle, bone, and tendons. Fourth-degree burns of an extremity may require amputation.

BURN SIZE

The size of a burn is determined by one of two techniques: (1) the rule of nines or (2) the Lund and Browder method. Burn size is expressed as a percentage of TBSA. The accuracy of the calculation varies with the method and the experience of the individual making the determination.

The basis of the rule of nines is that the body is divided into anatomic sections, each of which represents 9 per cent or a multiple of 9 per cent of the TBSA (Fig. 49–6). This method is easy, requiring no diagrams to determine the percentage of TBSA injured. Therefore, it has been used in emergency departments where the initial triage occurs.

The Lund and Browder method modifies the percentages for body segments according to age and provides a more accurate estimate of burn size. It uses a diagram of the body, divided into sections with the representative percentage of TBSA for ages greater than 1 year.

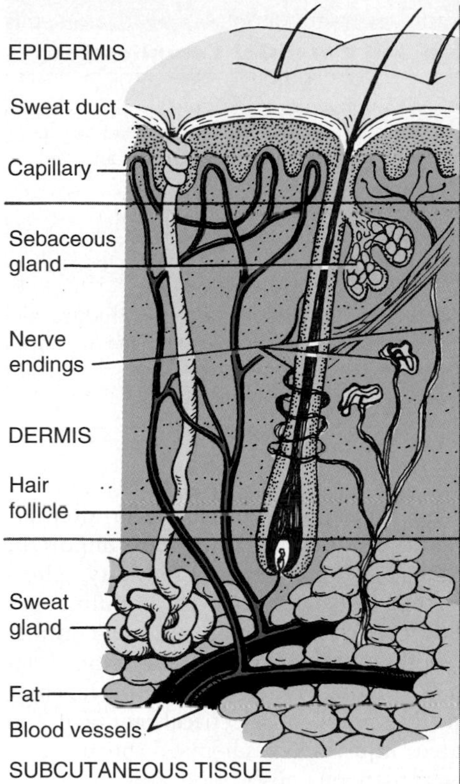

	APPEARANCE	SENSATION	COURSE
SUPERFICIAL BURN	Mild to severe erythema; skin blanches with pressure	Painful Hyperesthetic Tingling Pain eased by cooling	Discomfort lasts about 48 hours Desquamation peeling in 3–7 days
PARTIAL-THICKNESS BURN	Large thick-walled blisters covering extensive area (vesiculation) Edema; mottled red base; broken epidermis; wet, shiny, weeping surface	Painful Sensitive to cold air	Superficial partial-thickness burn heals in 14–21 days Deep partial-thickness burn requires 21–28 days for healing Healing rate varies with burn depth and presence or absence of infection
FULL-THICKNESS BURN	Variable, e.g., deep red, black, white, brown Dry surface Edema Fat exposed Tissue disrupted	Little pain Insensate	Full-thickness dead skin suppurates and liquefies after 2–3 weeks Spontaneous healing impossible Requires removal of eschar and subsequent split or full-thickness skin grafting Hypertrophic scarring and wound contractures likely to develop without preventive measures

Figure 49–2
Burn injury classification according to the depth of injury.

BURN LOCATION

The location of burns is implicated in the potential complications listed in Box 49–1.

AGE

The client's age affects the severity and outcome of the burn. Very young and the elderly people are most at risk. High mortality and morbidity statistics in elderly burn clients result from the combination of functional impairments (slower reaction time, impaired judgment, and decreased mobility), living alone, and environmental hazards.

GENERAL HEALTH

Pre-existing processes may influence the client's response to injury and treatment. Cardiac disorders, diabetes, alcoholism, and renal failure are among the con-

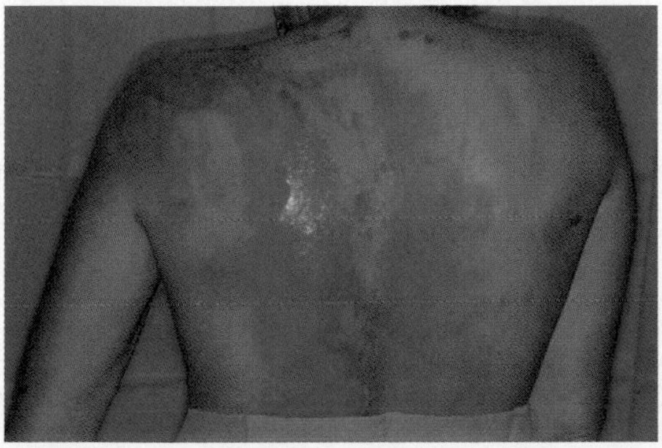

Figure 49–3
Partial-thickness burn injury.

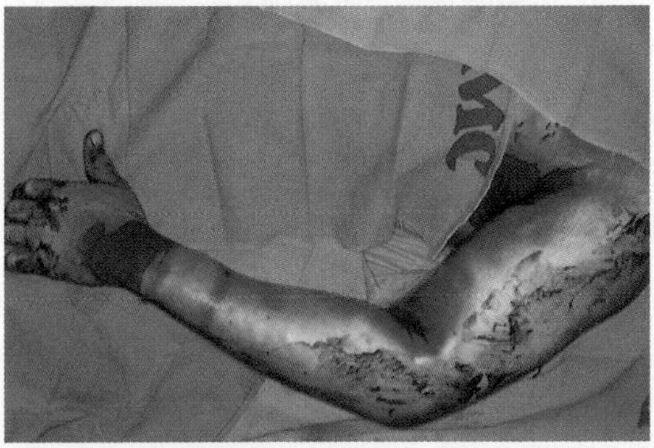

Figure 49–4
Full-thickness burn injury.

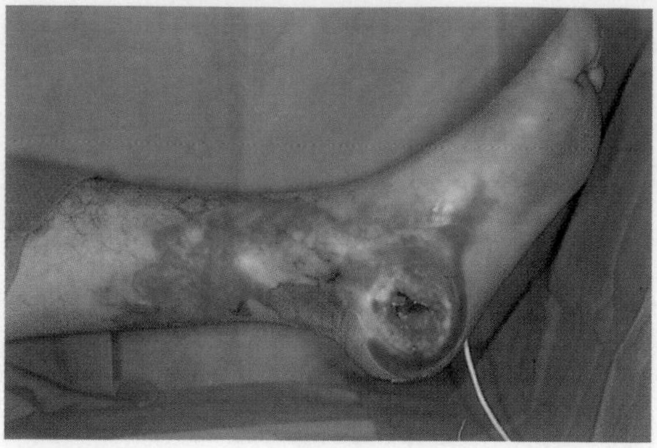

Figure 49–5
Full-thickness burn injury with underlying subcutaneous tissue damage at the heel from contact with an electrical source.

BOX 49–1

Burn Location and Potential Complications

Head, neck, chest	Pulmonary complications Circumferential burns can lead to decreased chest wall expansion and pulmonary insufficiency
Face	Corneal abrasions
Ears	Infection and loss of tissue
Hands, joints	Decreased movement with possible disability (loss of function) Circumferential burns may produce a tourniquet-like effect and lead to impaired circulation
Perineal area	Contamination by feces

ditions that can adversely affect the client's response to injury and treatment.

MECHANISM OF INJURY

The mechanism of injury is another factor used to determine the severity of injury. In general, any burn associated with inhalation injury requires special consideration.

In electrical burns, heat is generated as the electricity travels through the body, resulting in internal tissue damage. The voltage, type of current (direct or alternating), contact site, and duration of contact are important considerations because they may affect morbidity. Alternating current is often associated with cardiopulmonary arrests, ventricular fibrillation, tetanic muscle contractions, and long bone or vertebral compression fractures.[42] In addition, victims of electrical injuries may have fallen from the point of electrical contact and sustained associated injuries. In chemical burns, systemic toxicity from cutaneous absorption may occur.

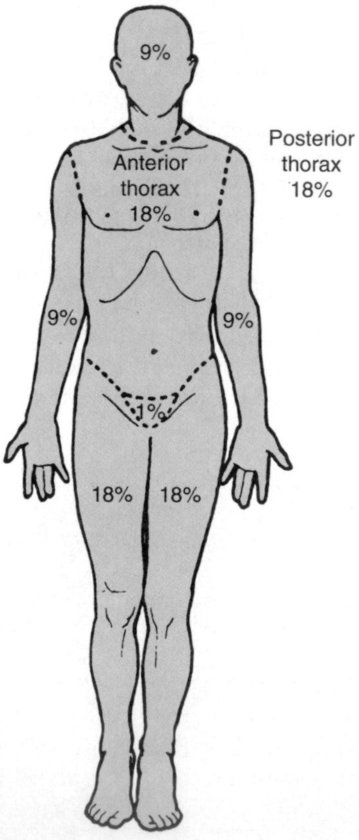

Figure 49–6
The "rule of nines" provides a quick method for estimating the extent of a burn injury.

Management

Nursing diagnoses, related goals, and treatments are presented in the nursing Care Plan, and the phase(s) of recovery in which they are most applicable are specified. The clinical course of the burn client can be divided into three phases: the emergency and resuscitation phase, the acute phase, and the rehabilitation phase.[9]

THE EMERGENCY PHASE

The emergency phase begins at the time of injury and concludes with the restoration of capillary permeability, usually at 48 to 72 hours following the injury.

CRITICAL TO REMEMBER

The primary goal during the emergency phase of recovery is to prevent hypovolemic (burn) shock and to preserve vital organ functioning.

Prehospital care, emergency department management, and the resuscitation period are included within this phase and are discussed separately.

Prehospital Care

Prehospital care of the burn victim begins at the scene of the accident and concludes when institutional emergency medical care is obtained. Prehospital care should begin with removing the victim from the source of the burn and/or eliminating the source of the heat. This action requires some consideration of the mechanism of injury so as to avoid further injury to the victim and injury to the rescuer.

Prehospital care also involves establishing an airway for breathing, assessing circulation, conserving body heat, considering the need for intravenous fluid administration, and preparing for transport.

Emergency Department Management

The care in the emergency department is a continuation of that administered at the scene. If little or inadequate assessment and/or treatment has been done, prehospital care is provided in the emergency department. Treatment of the burn wound (débridement and dressings) should not take precedence over the evaluation and treatment of any associated life-threatening problems.

Data collection in the emergency room should include information about the cause and time of the burn injury, the client's level of consciousness, and the presence of associated trauma. Information concerning the client's past medical history as well as general health should be obtained. Specifically, information regarding any cardiac, pulmonary, endocrine, or renal disease should be obtained because it may have implications for treatment. Known allergies should also be identified as well as the client's current medication regime.

Minor Burns. Care of the client with minor burn injuries is frequently provided on an ambulatory or outpatient basis.

Emergency department care of minor burn wounds includes

- pain management
- tetanus prophylaxis
- initial wound care
- teaching

CRITICAL TO REMEMBER

It is during care in the emergency department that the nurse has a major responsibility for teaching home wound care and the clinical manifestations of infection that would necessitate the client's return to medical care.

Clients who have been immunized against tetanus but not within the past 5 years should receive a tetanus toxoid booster. For clients who are not immunized, tetanus immune serum as well as active immunization with tetanus toxoid is administered.

Other teaching goals include the need to perform active range-of-motion (ROM) exercises to maintain normal joint function and to decrease edema formation and the possibility of scar formation, although it is minimal to nonexistent with minor, superficial burn wounds. The need for any follow-up evaluations or treatments should be confirmed with the client at this time.

Major Burns. For clients with extensive burn wounds, the emergency department management includes

- Re-evaluation of airway, breathing, and circulation (ABCs) and associated trauma
- Initiation of fluid resuscitation
- Placement of indwelling urinary catheter
- Placement of nasogastric tube
- Vital signs/baseline laboratory studies
- Pain management
- Tetanus prophylaxis
- Data collection
- Wound care

The oropharynx is inspected for evidence of erythema, blisters, or ulcerations, and the need for endotracheal intubation considered. If inhalation injury is suspected, administration of 100 per cent oxygen via a tight fitting non-rebreather face mask continues until carboxyhemoglobin levels fall below 15 per cent.[43] Hyperbaric oxygen may also be used.

Fluid Resuscitation

For adults with burn injuries affecting more than 15 per cent of TBSA, intravenous fluid resuscitation is generally required. Peripheral intravenous access or cannulation of a central vein (subclavian, internal or external jugular, or femoral) by a physician may be necessary.

The resuscitation period begins with initiation of fluid resuscitation measures and concludes when capillary permeability returns to near-normal levels and the large fluid shifts have decreased.

The goal of fluid resuscitation is to maintain vital organ perfusion while avoiding the complications of inadequate or excessive therapy.[41] Several formulas are used to calculate fluid requirements. In the calculation of fluid infusion rates, the time of injury, and not the time the fluid resuscitation was initiated, is used. The client's weight and the extent of the burn are taken into consideration when determining the fluid infusion. Also considered are the presence of inhalation injury, delay in the initiation of resuscitation, and deep tissue injury. When these factors are present, the amount of fluid needed for adequate resuscitation may be increased. Generally, the first 24 hours after the burn dictates the infusion of a balanced salt solution; during the second 24 hours, colloid-containing solutions are administered along with 5 per cent dextrose in water in varying amounts.

It is important to remember that all resuscitation formulas serve only as guides and should be adjusted according to the client's physiologic response. Successful or adequate fluid resuscitation in the adult is signaled by stable vital signs, adequate urine output, palpable peripheral pulses and clear sensorium (see the Care Plan).

An indwelling urethral catheter should be placed to measure hourly urine production.

CRITICAL TO REMEMBER

Urine output is the most readily available and reliable indicator for determining the adequacy of fluid resuscitation.[41, 43]

Circumferential burns of the extremities and of the thorax may compromise circulation and respiration, re-

Text continued on page 1378

CARE PLAN: The Burn-Injured Adult Client

Nursing Diagnosis/ Collaborative Problem	Planning: Expected Outcomes	Implementation: Nursing Interventions	Rationales
(E) Fluid Volume Deficit R/T increased capillary leak and large fluid shift from intravascular to interstitial space	Client will have improved fluid balance, as evidenced by urine output of 30–50 mL/hr, clear sensorium, pulse rate < 120 bpm without dysrhythmias, and blood pressure within expected range for age and medical history (pain control achieved).	Assess for hypovolemia every 1 hour for 36 hours.	Fluid shifts lead to hypovolemia.
		Obtain admission weight; weigh client daily.	Weight is an accurate index of fluid balance.
		Monitor and document hourly intake and output.	Urine output is a measure of effectiveness of fluid resuscitation.
		Administer IV fluid and electrolyte replacement per physician's order.	IV fluids are used to restore fluid volume.
		Monitor serum electrolytes and hematocrits.	Hyperkalemia and elevated hematocrit are common findings.
Collaborative Problem (E) Paralytic ileus R/T stress from injury	The nurse will monitor for normoactive bowel sounds, absence of abdominal distention, flatus production, and normal bowel movements.	Assess need for placement of NG tube.	Ileus is common in burns >20–25% TBSA.
		Assess bowel function: • Auscultate bowel sounds every 4 hours. • Observe for abdominal distention. • Monitor gastric output and amount, color, and presence of blood and pH.	Bowel sounds indicate whether peristalsis is present. Abdominal distention indicates ileus. Gastric output may require fluid replacement. Gastric ulcers are common following major burns.
Collaborative Problem (E) Renal failure R/T presence of hemachromagens in the urine due to deep burn and/or crush injury	The nurse will monitor for visible urinary hemachromagens and adequate urine output of 75–100 mL/hr.	Monitor and document hourly urine output and urine color.	Urine is red or dark brown when hemachromagens are present.
		Ensure patency of urinary catheter.	Catheter can become plugged with hemachromagens.
		Administer IV fluids per physician's order.	Hemachromagens are flushed from the body.
		Send urine samples for urine myoglobin/hemoglobin levels per physician's order.	Provides quantitative information on risk of renal failure.
(E, A) Gas Exchange, Impaired R/T carbon monoxide poisoning, smoke poisoning, and heat damage to lungs	Client will have improved gas exchange, as evidenced by unlabored respirations of 16–24/min, $PaO_2 > 90$ mm Hg, $PaCO_2$ 35–45 mm Hg, $SaO_2 > 95\%$, and clear bilateral breath sounds.	Assess for signs of respiratory distress as evidenced by restlessness, confusion, labored breathing, tachypnea, dyspnea, diminished and/or adventitious breath sounds, tachycardia, decrease in PaO_2 and SaO_2 levels, cyanosis.	Impaired gas exchange can lead to respiratory distress from hypoxemia.
		Monitor arterial blood gas and carboxyhemoglobin levels per physician's order.	Provides data on effectiveness of respiration/oxygenation.
		Monitor SaO_2 levels continuously.	Provides noninvasive oxygenation data.
		Administer oxygen therapy as prescribed.	Reduces hypoxemia.
		Instruct client on the use of incentive spirometer.	Encourages deep breathing.
		Elevate head of bed.	Facilitates lung expansion.
		Monitor need for endotracheal intubation.	Intubation may be required to maintain oxygenation.

CARE PLAN: The Burn-Injured Adult Client *Continued*

Nursing Diagnosis/ Collaborative Problem	Planning: Expected Outcomes	Implementation: Nursing Interventions	Rationales
(E, A) Airway Clearance, Ineffective R/T tracheal edema, airway epidermal sloughing, and depressed pulmonary ciliary action from inhalation injury.	Client will have effective airway clearance, as evidenced by clear bilateral breath sounds, clear to white pulmonary secretions, effective mobilization of pulmonary secretions, and unlabored respirations of 16–24/min.	Have client turn, cough, and deep breathe every 1–2 hours for 24 hours, then every 2–4 hours while awake.	Facilitates clearance of upper airways.
		Place oral suction device within client's reach for independent use.	Encourages removal of oral secretions and expectorated sputum.
		Perform endo- or nasotracheal suction as necessary and monitor and document character of sputum.	Removes secretions from upper airway. Sputum color, consistency, odor, and amount may indicate infection.
(E, A) Peripheral Tissue Perfusion, Altered R/T decreased blood flow from constriction due to circumferential burns.	Client will have adequate peripheral perfusion, as evidenced by pulses present by palpation or Doppler, capillary refill of unburned skin <2 seconds, absence of numbness or tingling, and absence of increased pain with active ROM exercises.	Remove all constricting jewelry and clothing.	May compromise circulation as edema ensues.
		Limit use of constricting blood pressure cuffs in affected extremity.	May reduce arterial inflow and venous return.
		Monitor arterial pulses by palpation or ultrasonic flow detector (Doppler) hourly for 72 hours.	Pulses will diminish with circulation impairments.
		Assess capillary refill of unburned skin on affected extremity.	Capillary refill will be prolonged with impaired circulation.
		Assess pain level with active ROM exercises	Ischemic tissues cause pain.
		Elevate affected extremities above the level of the heart.	Reduces dependent edema formation
		Encourage active ROM exercises.	Promotes venous return and reduces muscle atrophy.
		Anticipate and prepare client for escharotomy.	Escharotomy is used to restore circulation to compromised tissues.
		Posteschartomy care: Assess adequacy of circulation: • Check pulses. • Note color, movement, and sensation of affected extremity.	These data indicate adequacy of perfusion.
		Control posteschartomy bleeding with pressure.	Viable tissue beneath eschar bleeds.
(E, A) Hypothermia R/T epithelial tissue loss and fluctuating ambient air temperatures.	Client will achieve normothermia, as evidenced by core body temperature between 99.6° and 101.0° F.	Monitor client's rectal or core temperature as indicated (hourly during the emergency phase and after surgery).	Hypothermia may follow loss of skin as a thermal regulator and with some anesthetics.
		Limit the amount of body surface area exposed during wound care.	Exposure leads to hypothermia. Heat is lost in open wounds and after hydrotherapy by evaporation.
		Limit hydrotherapy treatment sessions to 30 minutes or less with water temperature 98°–102.0° F.	

Care Plan continued on following page

CARE PLAN: The Burn-Injured Adult Client *Continued*

Nursing Diagnosis/ Collaborative Problem	Planning: Expected Outcomes	Implementation: Nursing Interventions	Rationales
		Keep procedure rooms and surgical suites warm.	
		If air-fluidized therapy bed is in use, monitor and maintain appropriate bed temperature and consider reducing the flow of fluidization if hypothermia develops.	Heat is lost due to convection.
Collaborative Problem (E, A) Stress Ulcers R/T stress response from the burn injury	The nurse will monitor for gastrointestinal bleeding and will maintain gastric pH > 5.	Monitor and document gastric pH values and heme content every 2 hours while NG tube is in place.	Acidic gastric secretions may lead to bleeding.
		Administer antacids and/or H_2 receptor antagonists per physician's order.	Reduces gastric acid content.
		Monitor stools for occult blood.	Stress ulcers cause bleeding, which may be excreted in stools.
(A) Nutrition: Less Than Body Requirements, Altered R/T increased metabolic needs for wound healing	Client will have adequate nutrition, as evidenced by maintaining 85–90% of pre-burn weight.	Obtain accurate pre-burn weight.	Caloric needs are based on pre-burn weight.
		Consult dietitician.	Dieticians perform nutritional assessments.
		Assess eating habits/patterns, food preferences, food allergies within 72 hours of admission.	Establishes a baseline.
		Record caloric intake (calorie counts).	Quantitative data on caloric intake.
		Weigh client daily to follow weight trends (exception: if operative procedure limits movement).	Weight should be stable if caloric needs are being met.
		Provide oral hygiene each shift and as necessary.	Prevents stomatitis, enhances appetite.
		Provide an aesthetically pleasing environment.	Conducive to eating.
		Schedule treatments to provide for uninterrupted meal times.	Interruptions may decrease calorie intake.
		Allow a period of rest prior to meal time if the client has endured a painful procedure or treatment.	Pain decreases appetite.
		Provide aids and devices for eating utensils.	Facilitates self-care.
		Encourage significant others to bring favorite foods from home.	Client may be willing to eat familiar foods. Foods must be nutritionally sound.
		Provide nutritious supplements between meals.	Caloric needs are often too high to be eaten in three meals.
		Provide positive reinforcement for eating.	Anorexic clients may believe there is no benefit to eating.
		Consider other methods to meet caloric needs, such as tube feeding, total parenteral nutrition	Oral feeding may not provide adequate calories for healing.

CARE PLAN: The Burn-Injured Adult Client *Continued*

Nursing Diagnosis/ Collaborative Problem	Planning: Expected Outcomes	Implementation: Nursing Interventions	Rationales
(E, A) Infection, Risk for R/T loss of skin barrier, impaired immune response, presence of invasive catheters (indwelling urinary catheter and intravenous catheters), and invasive procedures (venous and arterial blood sampling and bronchoscopy)	Client will have no burn wound microbial invasion, as evidenced by (quantitative wound cultures < 100,000 organisms); core body temperature will maintain 99.6°–101.0° F; will have no swelling, redness, or purulence at invasive line insertion sites; and will have negative blood, urine, and sputum cultures.	Administer tetanus prophylaxis as necessary.	Anaerobic environment beneath eschar may allow tetanus organism to grow.
		Maintain infection control techniques.	Prevent cross contamination.
		Instruct significant others on infection control measures.	Promote compliance.
		Enforce strict hand washing.	Minimize incidence of cross-contamination.
		Assess for clinical signs of infection: discoloration of wounds or drainage, odor, delayed healing; headache, chills, anorexia, nausea; change in vital signs; hyperglycemia; paralytic ileus, confusion, restlessness, hallucinations.	Burn wound is open and client is immunocompromised; therefore, local wound infection or systemic infection is a risk.
		Before reapplying topical cream, cleanse and rinse the burn wound.	To remove wound debris that would prevent cream from adhering to the wound.
		Débride wound of loose, nonviable tissue.	These tissues are a medium for bacterial growth.
		Shave or cut body hair in and around wound margins (exception: eyebrows and eyelashes).	Hair is contaminated and prevents cream adherence.
		Apply topical therapy (antimicrobial agent or temporary wound covering).	Provides wound coverage.
		Assess for signs of infection at catheter insertion site twice a day.	
(E, A, R) Pain R/T burn injury, exposed nerve endings, treatments, and anxiety	Client will have more comfort as evidenced by verbalizing relief or control of pain/discomfort and identifying factors that contribute to pain/discomfort.	Assess client's response to pain with wound care, physical therapy, and at rest (background pain).	Establishes a baseline.
		Medicate prior to painful procedures: 45 minutes for oral, 30 minutes for intramuscular, 5–10 minutes for IV. Do NOT administer intramuscular medications to clients with major burns during the emergency phase.	Adequate time allowed for onset of analgesia. Intramuscular injections are not given because of erratic and diminished circulation impairing absorption.
		Explore relaxation technique, music therapy, guided imagery, distraction, and hypnosis.	Nonpharmocologic analgesics.
		Explain all procedures to the client and allow time for preparation.	To reduce anxiety.
		Talk to the client while providing care and performing procedures.	Promotes client's trust.
		Assess for the need of anxiolytic medications.	Anxiety decreases pain threshold.
		Document the client's response to prescribed medications and nonpharmocologic treatments.	Evaluate effectiveness of interventions.

Care Plan continued on following page

CARE PLAN: The Burn-Injured Adult Client *Continued*

Nursing Diagnosis/ Collaborative Problem	Planning: Expected Outcomes	Implementation: Nursing Interventions	Rationales
(A, R) Self-Care Deficit (Grooming, Bathing, Eating, Elimination) R/T functional deficits resulting from the burn injury, pain, dressings, splints, and enforced immobility	Client will have less self-care deficit as evidenced by increased participation in self-care.	Assess the client's ability to provide self-care.	Provides a baseline.
		Consult with occupational therapy regarding the need for assistive devices.	Promotes self-care.
		Encourage client to participate in self-care tasks.	Helps to motivate client to overcome fear and dependency.
		Ensure that the client has adequate time to accomplish tasks.	Helps establish self-control.
		Provide positive reinforcement when tasks are accomplished.	Promotes independence and motivation.
(E, A, R) Physical Mobility, Impaired R/T edema, pain, dressings, splints, surgical procedures, and wound contractures	Client will have improved physical mobility, as evidenced by returning to maximum activities of daily living with minimal disability and disfigurement.	Assess ROM and muscle strength in burned areas prone to develop contractures every day and as necessary.	Determine baseline.
		Maintain burned areas in position of physiologic function within limits imposed by associated injuries, grafting, other therapeutic devices.	Prevent/reduce contracture development.
		Explain rationale for activities and positioning to client and family. Reinforce as necessary.	Improves compliance.
		Consult physical and occupational therapy for an individualized rehabilitation schedule. Adjust schedule as needed.	Will provide needed devices and teaching for ambulation and ROM.
		Wrap burned legs and/or unburned legs with donor sites with elastic wraps (figure-8 technique) before placing in any dependent position. As healing progresses, other elasticated support bandages can be worn.	Decrease capillary venous stasis, which impairs graft healing.
		Encourage active ROM every 2–4 hours while awake unless contraindicated because of a recent grafting procedure.	Control postresuscitation edema and prevent muscle atrophy, tendon adherence, and joint stiffness.
		Ambulate client to chair or walking (unless contraindicated by a recent grafting procedure or other injuries).	Ambulation promotes muscle strength and cardiopulmonary reserve. After grafting, clients remain on bed rest.
		Provide passive exercise and stretching if client is unable to actively participate (i.e., comatose or paralyzed).	Passive ROM maintains joint motion and muscle tone.

CARE PLAN: The Burn-Injured Adult Client *Continued*

Nursing Diagnosis/ Collaborative Problem	Planning: Expected Outcomes	Implementation: Nursing Interventions	Rationales
(A, R) Self-Esteem Disturbance, Risk for R/T threatened or actual change in body image, physical loss, and loss of role responsibilities	Client will develop improved self-esteem as evidenced by making social contact with others outside of immediate family, developing effective coping mechanisms through the stages of recovery, and verbalizing feelings about self-concept.	Determine previous coping style.	Determine baseline; previous coping styles will be tried by client
		Provide an atmosphere of acceptance.	
		Explain projected appearance of burns and grafts during different phases of wound healing.	Provides information; may reduce misconceptions.
		Allow client to progress at own pace through stages of denial, grief, and acceptance of injury and recovery.	Clients progress at varying rates depending on the degree of injury, perception of injury, support systems, and previous coping styles.
		Assess need for limit setting for maladaptive behavior. Consult with burn team members to establish limits and treatment plan. Explain and assist significant others to maintain same limits.	Maladaptive behavior is harmful and is usually controlled by setting limits for all to follow. A psychiatric consultation may be ordered.
		Promote client's self-confidence:	
		• Ensure continuity of care providers.	Promotes trust.
		• Discuss all activities and procedures prior to initiation.	Reduces anxiety.
		• Support client's role in care and treatment.	Motivates client; reduces fear.
		• Keep client informed of progress.	
		• Provide honest, positive reinforcement.	Do not provide false hope of functional return if there is irreparable damage.
		• Help significant others to interact with client.	Significant others may be fearful and require guidance.
		Encourage interaction with others outside immediate family.	Facilitates societal reintegration.
		Help prepare client for social interactions after discharge by discussing potential situations and how client might deal with them.	Provides rehearsal of events and reduces anxiety.
		Make home health care nurse or physical therapist referral as indicated.	To assess client's adjustment at home, ability to continue with needed therapy, further teaching, and care requirements.
(E, A, R) Family Coping: Ineffective; Risk for R/T the emergency and critical nature of the injury and separation from family/friends	Significant others will have improved coping strategies, as evidenced by verbalizing goals of treatment regimen; emotional stressors, concerns, and behaviors; and understanding and knowledge of available support services.	Prior to significant others' initial visit:	
		• Communicate extent of burn and changes in client's appearance;	Preparation to reduce degree of fright.
		• Provide significant others with information that meets their basic needs.	Common needs of family members.

Care Plan continued on following page

CARE PLAN: The Burn-Injured Adult Client *Continued*

Nursing Diagnosis/ Collaborative Problem	Planning: Expected Outcomes	Implementation: Nursing Interventions	Rationales
		• Provide brief, simple explanations of procedures and equipment.	Simple explanations more readily retained.
		Determine how the client and significant others have coped with past stress.	Provides a baseline.
		Assist client with dealing with stress by providing coping strategies such as diversion and relaxation techniques.	Provides client with new coping strategies
		Allow for uninterrupted visitation during visiting hours if possible.	Assists client to cope.
		Provide significant others with daily updates regarding changes in client's condition.	Maintains realistic perception of client's progress.
		Consult with psychologist, psychiatrist, social worker, or psychiatric clinical nurse specialist as necessary.	These professionals may assist client to improve coping strategies.
		Encourage significant others' attendance at support group meetings.	Provides support and helps to dispel misconceptions.
		For impending client transfer, provide significant others with support services to assist with their travel.	To reduce anxiety during transition.

A, acute phase; TBSA, body surface area; E, emergency phase; IV, intravenous; NG, nasogastric; $PaCO_2$, arterial carbon dioxide tension; PaO_2, arterial oxygen tension; R, rehabilitation phase; ROM, range of motion; SaO_2, arterial oxygen percent saturation.

Data from Dyer, C., & Roberts, D. (1990). Thermal trauma. *Nursing Clinics of North America, 25(1),* 101–115; Burgess, M. C. (1991). Initial management of a patient with extensive burn injury. *Critical Care Nursing Clinics of North America, 3(2),* 175–177; Duncan, D. J., & Driscoll, D. M. (1991). Burn wound management. *Critical Care Nursing Clinics of North America, 3(2),* 202–204; Carlson, D. E., & Jordan, B. S. (1991). Implementing nutritional therapy in the thermally injured patient. *Critical Care Nursing Clinics of North America, 3(2),* 229–231.

spectively. These complications are more likely to occur during resuscitation, when fluid shifts into the interstitial tissues (causing edema) are at their peak. With circumferential burns of the extremities, elevating the extremity above the level of the heart helps reduce dependent edema; however, circulatory compromise may still occur. Frequent assessment of distal extremity perfusion is necessary.

An escharotomy is the appropriate treatment for circulatory compromise due to circumferential burns. The physician makes a lengthwise incision through eschar, relieving the constriction to circulation (Fig. 49–7). It is generally performed at the bedside and without anesthesia because the eschar does not bleed and there is no pain. Viable tissue beneath the burn may bleed, however. The wound created by the escharotomy can be dressed in the usual fashion. If adequate tissue perfusion does not return, a fasciotomy may be necessary. This procedure, in which the fascia is incised, is performed in the operating room under anesthesia.

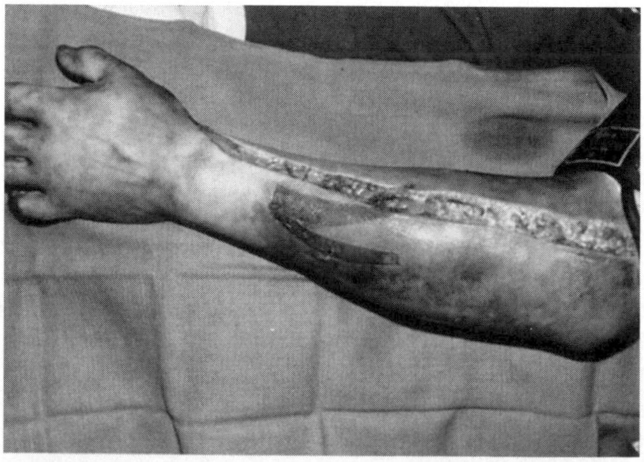

Figure 49–7
Escharotomy. Incision is made through the constricting burn eschar to permit expansion of the underlying subcutaneous tissues as edema forms. (Courtesy of the University of Washington Burn Center at Harborview Medical Center, Seattle, WA.)

Many centers advocate the placement of a nasogastric tube for clients with burns of 20 to 25 per cent or more of TBSA to prevent emesis and reduce the risk of aspiration.[43]

CRITICAL TO REMEMBER

Gastrointestinal dysfunction results from the intestinal ileus that develops almost universally in these clients during the early post-burn period. All oral fluids should be restricted at this time.

Vital signs provide baseline information as well as additional data for determining the adequacy of resuscitation. Diagnostic studies should include the following:

- Baseline blood glucose, blood urea nitrogen, serum creatinine, serum electrolytes, and hematocrit levels
- Arterial blood gas and COHb levels, particularly if inhalation injury is suspected
- A chest x-ray for all clients with extensive burns or inhalation injury
- X-rays to rule out fractures or associated trauma, as indicated
- Alcohol and drug screen, if indicated by circumstances of the injury
- Continuous electrocardiographic monitoring for all clients with major burns and high-voltage electrical injury as well as clients with previous cardiac problems

Pain management is achieved through the administration of intravenous narcotic agents, typically morphine.

CRITICAL TO REMEMBER

Intramuscular and subcutaneous routes for the administration of pain medication are not used because absorption from the soft tissues is unreliable during the period when hypovolemia and large fluid shifts are occurring. The oral route is not used because of the likelihood of gastrointestinal dysfunction.

Tetanus prophylaxis for a client with a major burn is the same as for one with a minor burn (see earlier discussion).[46]

Wound care in the emergency department consists of covering the wound with a clean, dry sheet and blankets to maintain body heat. Clients with burns of the head and face should be positioned with their head elevated and all burned extremities elevated on pillows above the level of the heart. These measures help decrease dependent edema formation. For small burns, application of a cool, sterile compress aids in pain control. Unless transport time to the receiving medical facility is prolonged, no further treatment of the wound is generally necessary.

Consideration of transferral to a specialized burn care facility is appropriate for all clients with major burn injuries. Prompt contact with the receiving burn center is important to facilitate a smooth transfer.

THE ACUTE PHASE

The acute phase of recovery following a major burn begins when the patient is hemodynamically stable, capillary permeability is restored, and diuresis has begun. This is generally considered to be 48 to 72 hours after the time of injury. Many of the same principles of care outlined for the emergency phase apply to the acute phase; however, more emphasis is placed on restorative therapies. The acute phase continues until wound closure is achieved.

Medical management of the client during the acute phase focuses on

- infection control
- wound care
- wound closure
- nutritional support
- pain management
- physical therapy

Infection Control

Sources of infection for the burn-injured client include autocontamination from

- the oropharynx
- fecal flora
- unburned skin and cross-contamination from staff, visitors, and the air[43]

Specific infection control practices and isolation techniques exist for all burn centers. These practices differ and include the use of gloves, caps, masks, shoe covers, scrub clothes, and plastic aprons.

CRITICAL TO REMEMBER

Strict hand washing is stressed to reduce the incidence of cross-contamination between clients.

Staff and visitors are generally prevented from client contact if they suffer from any skin, gastrointestinal, or respiratory tract infections.

Wound Care

Care of the burn wound is ultimately aimed at promoting wound healing. Daily wound care involves cleansing, débridement, and dressing of the burn wound.[51]

Hydrotherapy. The wound is cleansed by the use of hydrotherapy.[50] This is accomplished by immersion (Fig. 49–8*A* and *B*), showering, or spraying (Fig. 49–8*B*). A hydrotherapy session of 30 minutes or less is optimal for clients with acute burns. Longer time periods may increase sodium loss (water is hypotonic) through the burn wound, heat loss, and pain and stress. During hydrotherapy, the wounds are gently washed using a variety of solutions: dilute sodium hypochlorite,[20] dilute povidone-iodine,[18, 21, 23] and dilute chlorohexidine.[14] Care should be taken to minimize bleeding and to maintain body temperature during this procedure. To prevent cross-contamination between clients, single-use, plastic hydrotherapy tub liners are available. Clients excluded from hydrotherapy are generally those

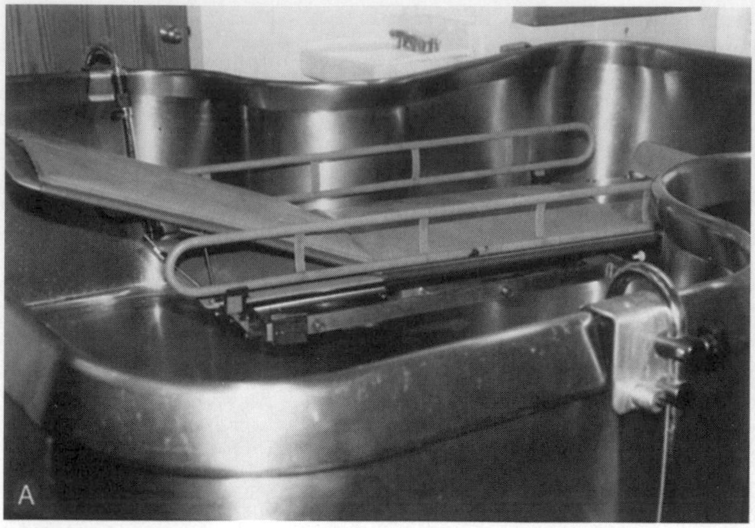

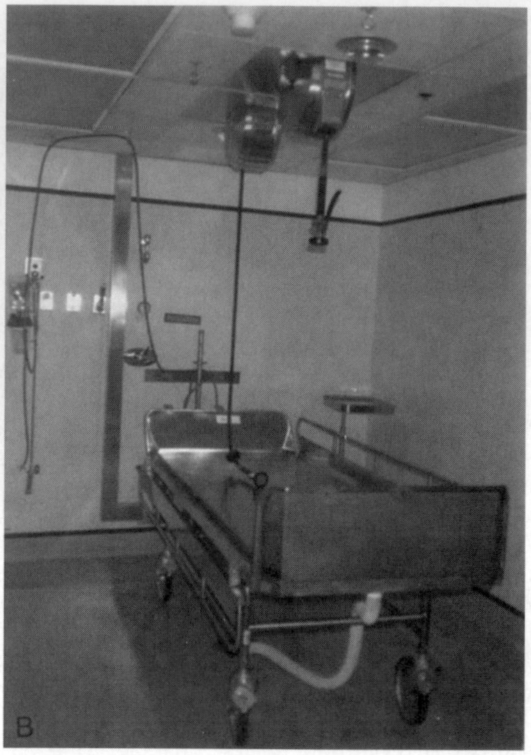

Figure 49–8
A, Hubbard tank used for immersion hydrotherapy treatment of burn wounds. (Courtesy of the Burn Center at the Washington Hospital Center, Washington, DC.) *B,* Spray table used for hydrotherapy treatments of burn wounds. The long, flexible hose allows for ease in washing of the wounds. (Courtesy of the University of Washington Burn Center at Harborview Medical Center, Seattle, WA.)

who are hemodynamically unstable and those with new grafts.[13] If hydrotherapy is not used, wounds are washed and rinsed while the client is in bed prior to the application of antimicrobial agents.

Débridement. Burn wound débridement involves the removal of the eschar. This serves to promote wound healing by preventing bacterial proliferation in and under the eschar.[20] Débridement of the burn wound is accomplished through mechanical, enzymatic, or surgical means.

Mechanical Débridement. Mechanical débridement can be accomplished with the careful use of scissors and forceps to lift and trim away loose eschar. Dressing changes are another effective means of mechanical débridement. This is accomplished by the use of wet-to-dry and wet-to-wet dressings. Mechanical débridement of the burn wound can be extremely painful; therefore, effective pain management is paramount.

Enzymatic Débridement. Enzymatic débridement involves the application of commercially prepared proteolytic and fibrinolytic topical enzymes. These products selectively digest necrotic tissue, facilitating eschar removal. They require a moist environment to be effective and are applied directly to the burn wound. Pain and bleeding are major problems with this treatment and should be assessed continuously throughout treatment.

Surgical Débridement. Surgical débridement of the burn wound involves excision of devitalized tissue. There are different techniques that can be used to surgically remove tissue. The decision is made by the surgeon.

Use of Specialized Wound Coverings. Deep partial or full-thickness burn wounds are treated initially with topical antimicrobial agents. These agents are applied once or twice daily following cleansing, débridement, and inspection of the wound. The nurse assesses for eschar separation, the state of the granulation tissue or the presence of re-epithelialization, and signs of infection. The most commonly used topical antimicrobial agents are listed in Table 49–2. Although no one agent is universally used, many burn centers choose silver sulfadiazine cream as the initial topical treatment for burn wounds.

Open Versus Closed Methods. Burn wounds are treated using either an open or closed dressing technique. For the open method, the antimicrobial cream is applied and then left open to the air without gauze dressings. The agent is reapplied as needed, although formal reapplication occurs every 12 hours due to the agent's duration of activity. The advantages of this method include increased visualization of the wound, easier mobility and joint ROM, and simplicity in wound care. The disadvantages include an increased chance of hypothermia from exposure and the psychological difficulty for the client of continuously viewing the wound.[5]

In the closed method of wound care, gauze dressings of various types are used. Dressings are prepared by applying a 1/16 inch thick layer of cream after hydrotherapy. When applied, the gauze is carefully wrapped from the distal portion of the extremity proximally, to ensure that circulation is not compromised. No two burn surfaces should be allowed to touch, because this could promote webbing of digits, contracture

TABLE 49–2 Topical Antimicrobial Agents Used in Burn Care

AGENT	ANTIMICROBIAL SPECTRUM	APPLICATION	SIDE EFFECTS	NURSING CONSIDERATIONS
Water-Based Creams				
1% Silver sulfadiazine	Broad spectrum, including some fungi and yeast	2 times daily, 1/16-inch thickness Gauze dressing not required	Transient leukopenia typically appearing after 2 or 3 days of treatment Macular rash	Assess for side effects.
Mafenide acetate	Broad spectrum, little antifungal activity	2 times daily, 1/16-inch thickness Gauze dressing not required	Hyperchloremic metabolic acidosis from bicarbonate diuresis due to the inhibition of carbonic anhydrase Pain/burning sensation on application to superficial burns Maculopapular rash	Assess for side effects. Assess adequacy of pain management. If pain and discomfort continue, consider other topical treatments. Use cautiously in clients with acute renal failure.
Solutions				
5% Mafenide acetate	Broad spectrum	Gauze dressing required and moistened with solution for application to the wound	Pain on application Pruritus Skin rash Fungal colonization	Remains investigational and requires informed consent. Assess for side effects. Assess adequacy of pain management.
0.5% Silver nitrate	Broad spectrum, including *Candida* species	Multiple layers of gauze dressing required and moistened with solution for application to the wound	Hyponatremia Hypochloremia Hypokalemia Hypocalcemia	Check serum electrolytes daily. Penetrates eschar poorly. Rewet dressings every 2 hours to avoid wound desiccation. Protect the environment. Stains everything a blackish-brown color.

development, and poor cosmetic outcome. The advantages of the closed method technique are decreases in evaporative fluid and heat loss from the wound surface. In addition, gauze dressings may aid in débridement. The disadvantages of the use of gauze dressings are mobility limitations and a potential decrease in effective ROM exercises. Wound assessment is also limited to the times when dressing changes are performed.

Wound Closure

Temporary Wound Coverings. Temporary wound coverings are frequently used as a kind of wound "dressing." Table 49–3 outlines the most common biologic, biosynthetic, and synthetic wound coverings available today. These products are temporary wound coverings, each having specific indications.

Autografting is the surgical removal of a thin layer of the client's own unburned skin (Fig. 49–9) and application of it to the excised burn wound. This procedure occurs in the operating room while the client receives anesthesia. A split-thickness graft uses a thinner layer of skin than a full-thickness graft. A full-thickness graft involves the epidermis and part of the dermis. For all autografts, the area of the body where the skin was removed is referred to as the donor site.

In addition to routine postoperative nursing care, care of the client following autografting includes:

- Assessment of bleeding from the graft site
- Proper positioning and immobilization of the graft site
- Donor site care
- Care of specialized autografts (e.g., cultured epithelial autografts)

Assessment of Bleeding. Bleeding beneath an autograft may prevent successful adherence of the graft to the excised wound and ultimately result in some degree of graft loss, particularly beneath sheet grafts.

Positioning and Immobilization. Autografts are immobilized following surgery, generally 3 to 7 days. This period of immobilization allows the autograft time to adhere and attach to the wound bed. Immobilization

TABLE 49–3 Temporary Wound Coverings Used in Burn Care

CATEGORY/ EXAMPLES	DESCRIPTION	INDICATIONS	NURSING CONSIDERATIONS
Biologic			
Amnion	Amniotic membranes collected from human placentas	To protect partial-thickness burns To protect granulation tissue prior to autograft application	Cover dressing is changed every 48 hours with amnion.
Allograft homograft	Donated human cadaver skin harvested within 24 hours after death	To débride exudative wounds To cover excised wounds and test for receptivity prior to autograft application To cover and protect meshed autografts	Observe for wound exudate and signs of infection that may be indicative of a wound infection beneath the allograft/xenograft.
Xenograft heterograft	Porcine skin harvested after slaughter	To promote healing of clean, superficial partial-thickness wounds	Xenograft over granulation tissue is changed every 2–5 days. For superficial wounds, ensure that the wound is clean and well rinsed. Apply xenograft with slight overlapping of edges to allow for shrinkage. Trim away xenograft when skin beneath it has healed.
Biosynthetic			
Biobrane (Winthrop Pharmaceuticals, New York City)	Skin substitute made of nylon fabric, silicone rubber membrane and porcine skin products	Donor site dressing Protective cover over meshed autografts To promote healing of clean superficial partial-thickness wounds	Secure to the surrounding intact skin by staples, skin closure strips, tape, or sutures and then wrap with a gauze dressing. This outer dressing can be removed by 48 hours to check for adherence of the Biobrane. Once adherence has occurred, the tape, sutures, and staples can be removed. The Biobrane can then be left exposed to the air. New and healing donor sites of the legs require support during ambulation. The figure-8 elastic wrapping technique is recommended to minimize trauma to newly formed capillaries. Assess for infection beneath the fabric and at wound periphery.
Integra (Marion-Merrell Dow, Inc., Kansas City, KS)	Bilaminate substitute composed of collagen (dermal analog) and a Silastic covering (epidermal analog) The dermal analog is allowed to incorporate into the wound, becoming permanent.	For application to excised wounds	The silastic portion is removed after several days, providing a wound bed for placement of a very thin split-thickness skin graft. Assess for infection. Protect the grafted site from mechanical shearing forces.

can be accomplished in a variety of ways to prevent unwanted movement and shearing of grafts. The nurse also implements various actions to reduce the hazards of immobility.

Donor Site Care. Various types of dressings are used to cover donor sites, depending on the size, location, and condition of adjacent skin or tissue. The donor site may be covered with a special dressing that allows the epithelium to form beneath it. The dressing is peeled away after re-epithelialization occurs (10 to 14 days). A compression bandage covers the donor site dressing for 48 hours after surgery, after which the donor site may be left open to the air.

The donor site wound requires the same meticulous care as other partial-thickness wounds in order for healing to occur and infection to be prevented. If the donor site becomes infected, the dressing should be gently removed or soaked off. The wound can then be thoroughly cleaned and an antimicrobial agent applied. Once the donor site has healed, lubricating lotions can be applied to soften the area and reduce itching. Donor sites can be reused once complete healing has occurred.

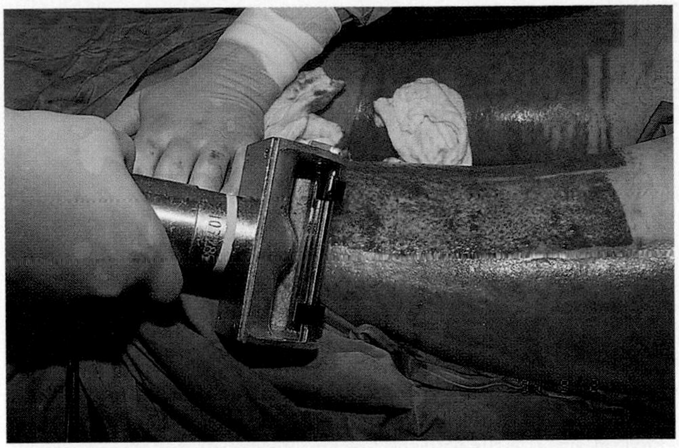

Figure 49–9
The harvesting of donor skin from the anterior-lateral portion of the client's thigh. (Courtesy of the Burn Center at the Washington Hospital Center, Washington, DC.)

Nutritional Support

Maintenance of adequate nutrition during the acute phase is essential in promoting wound healing and in preventing infection. Basal metabolic rates may be higher than normal levels, depending on the extent of the burn. Metabolic rates decrease as wound coverage is achieved. In addition, glucose metabolism is altered following a burn injury, resulting in hyperglycemia.

CRITICAL TO REMEMBER

Aggressive nutritional support is required to meet the increased energy requirements necessary to promote healing and prevent the untoward effects of catabolism.

Formulas are used to estimate energy requirements by factoring several different indices: weight, sex, age, extent of burn, and activity of injury.

$$(25 \text{ kcal} \times \text{body weight [kg]}) + (40 \text{ kcal} \times \% \text{ TBSA burn}) = \text{kcal/day}$$

Aggressive nutritional support is generally indicated for the burn client with any one of the following: 30 per cent or greater TBSA burn, a clinical course requiring multiple operations, the need for mechanical ventilatory support, a compromised mental status, and a poor preburn nutritional state.[12]

Methods for delivering nutritional support include oral diet, enteral tube feedings, peripheral parenteral nutrition, total parenteral nutrition, and a combination of these modalities.

Pain Management

Physiologic factors that have an impact on pain include the depth of injury, extent, and stage of wound healing. Typically, partial-thickness burns and newly harvested donor sites are exquisitely painful due to stimulation of exposed nerve endings. In contrast, full-thickness burns are insensate because the superficial nerve endings have been destroyed. However, nerve endings located at the wound's periphery can be extremely sensitive. It is important to remember that the perception of pain and response to painful stimuli are individual and that the treatment plan should be individualized as well.

The most common approach to pain control is the use of pharmacologic agents. Morphine, codeine, and meperidine are the most commonly used narcotic analgesics to control the pain associated with burn injuries and treatment. Nonsteroidal anti-inflammatory agents are also prescribed for the treatment of mild to moderate pain.

Nonpharmocologic modalities used to treat burn-related pain include hypnosis, guided imagery, art and play therapy, relaxation technique, distraction, biofeedback, and music therapy.[36]

Physical Therapy

Maintenance of optimal physical functioning in the client with a burn injury is a challenge for the entire burn team. Nurses work closely with occupational and physical therapists to identify the rehabilitative needs of burn clients.

Wound contracture and hypertrophic scarring are two major problems for the burn client. Wound contractures are typically more severe with extensive burns. Areas seemingly predisposed to contracture are the hands, head, neck, and axilla.[26]

Measures used to prevent and treat wound contractures include therapeutic positioning, ROM exercises, splinting, and client/family education.

Therapeutic Positioning. Allowing the burn client to assume a position of comfort most often contributes to contracture formation. Therefore, proper positioning should be maintained for the burn client while both in and out of bed. These techniques position the affected area opposite to the anticipated contracture or deformity. (Fig. 49–10 and Table 49–4).

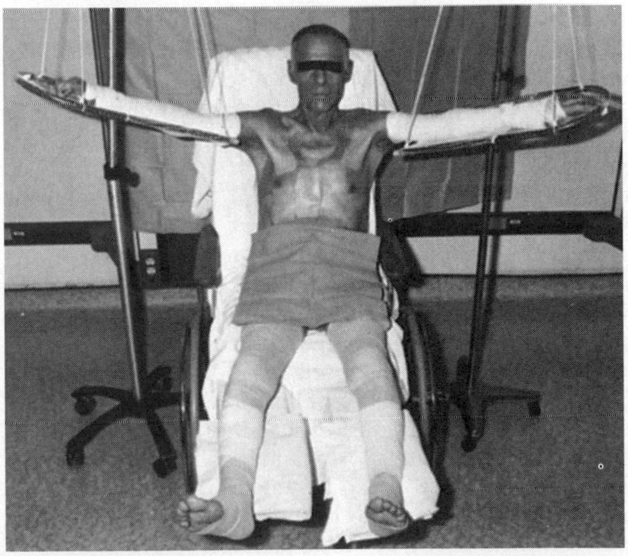

Figure 49–10
Example of therapeutic positioning for a client with extremity burns. Note that the client's arms are abducted and his legs are wrapped with elastic bandages in a figure-8 pattern to reduce dependent edema formation and provide pressure therapy support.

TABLE 49–4 Therapeutic Positioning for the Burn-Injured Client

BURNED AREA	THERAPEUTIC POSITION	POSITIONING TECHNIQUES
Neck		
Anterior	Extension	No pillow Small towel roll beneath cervical spine to promote neck extension
Circumferential	Neutral toward extension	No pillow
Posterior or Asymmetrical	Neutral	No pillow
Shoulder/axilla	Arm abduction to 90–110 degrees	Splinting Arms positioned away from the body and supported on arm troughs
Elbow	Arm extension	Elbow splint Elbows positioned in extension with slight bend at the elbow (no greater than 10-degree elbow flexion)
Hand		Arms supported on arm troughs with the forearm in slight pronation
Wrist	Wrist extension	Hand splint
Metacarpal Interphalangeal Joints (MCP)	MCP flexion at 90 degrees	Hand splint
Proximal and distal interphalangeal joints (PIP/DIP)	PIP/DIP extension	Hand splint
Thumb	Thumb abduction	Hand splint with thumb abduction
Web spaces	Finger abduction	Web spacers of gauze, foam, or thermoplastics to decrease webbing formation
Hip	Hip extension	Supine with the head of bed flat and legs extended Trochanter roll to maintain neutral hip rotation (toes should be pointing toward the ceiling) Prone positioning
Knee	Knee extension	Supine with knees extended (toes should be pointing toward the ceiling) Prone positioning with feet extended over the end of the mattress Sitting in chair with legs extended and elevated Knee splint
Ankle	Neutral	Padded footboard Ankle positioning devices (avoid ankle inversion and eversion positions)

Exercise. Active ROM exercises are prescribed early in the acute phase of recovery to reduce edema and maintain strength and joint function. In addition, activities of daily living can be effective in maintaining function and ROM. Ambulation also maintains strength and ROM of the lower extremities and should be initiated as soon as the client is physiologically stable. Passive ROM and stretching exercises should be included as part of the daily treatment plan if the client is unable to perform active ROM exercises.

Splinting. Splints are used to maintain proper joint positioning and prevent or correct contractures. Two types of splints are frequently used: static and dynamic. A static splint immobilizes the joint. Static splints do not replace exercise and are frequently applied for periods of immobilization, during sleeping hours, and in the client who cannot maintain proper positioning. In contrast, dynamic splints exercise the affected joint. Care must be taken to ensure that all splints fit properly and do not apply pressure that could lead to further tissue or nerve damage.

Education. Education of the client and significant others regarding correct positioning and the need for continued exercise is very important. Written guides and handouts on positioning, splinting, and exercise routines can facilitate learning and cooperation.

Control of Scarring

Hypertrophic scarring results from an overabundant deposition of collagen in the healed burn wound. The severity of hypertrophic scarring depends on several factors: burn depth, race, age, and type of autograft. The nonoperative method for minimizing hypertrophic scarring is pressure therapy (Fig. 49–11).

Several products are commercially available that provide continuous pressure over the healing burn wound. During the early stages of wound healing, elastic wraps and bandages can be used to apply continuous pressure to the healing skin while it is still fragile and vulnerable to mechanical shearing. Ultimately, custom-fit antiburn scar support garments can be ordered and worn 23 hours a day until the burn scar tissue has matured (typically 18 months to 2 years after the burn).

Surgical options for the treatment of wound contractures and hypertrophic scarring include (1) split-thickness and full-thickness skin grafts, (2) skin flaps, (3) Z-plasties, and (4) tissue expansion. These surgical options are discussed in Chapter 50.

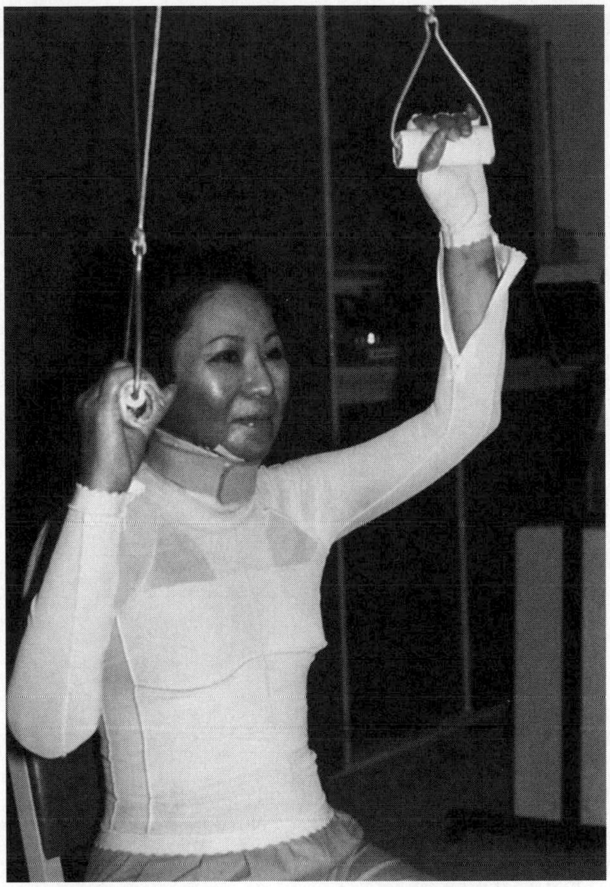

Figure 49–11
Client wearing custom-fit antiscar support garment. When worn 23 hours a day, this garment is effective in providing pressure therapy over healing burn wounds. Pressure therapy helps to minimize the development of hypertrophic scarring.

THE REHABILITATION PHASE

The rehabilitation phase of recovery represents the final phase of burn care (see the Client Education Guide: Post-Burn Care at Home). Although this phase overlaps the acute care phase and lasts well beyond the acute inpatient hospitalization, the goals and principles of physical rehabilitation are similar to those previously described. Ultimately, a burn rehabilitation program is designed for the client to gain independence through achievement of maximal functional recovery. Measures to promote wound healing, prevent or minimize deformities and hypertrophic scarring, increase strength and function, and provide emotional support and education are part of the ongoing rehabilitation process.

Special Considerations

PSYCHOSOCIAL CONSIDERATIONS

Psychological rehabilitation is equally as important as physical in the overall recovery process. A myriad of psychological and emotional responses to burn injuries have been identified, ranging from fear to psychosis. A victim's response is influenced by age, personality, cultural and ethnic background, extent and location of injury, and the resulting impact on body image. In addition, separation from family and friends and the change in the client's normal role and responsibilities affect the reaction to burn trauma. Nursing care should focus on maximizing the client's psychosocial recovery through appropriate interventions (see Care Plan and Ethical Issues in Nursing: Should Severely Burned Clients Be Allowed to Refuse Treatment?).

CLIENT EDUCATION GUIDE

Post-Burn Care at Home

For physical healing of the burn, the nurse should teach the client and significant others that:

- physical therapy will be continued at home or on an outpatient basis to assist in re-establishing or maintaining function
- a high-calorie, high-protein diet is prescribed to facilitate healing
- continued attention to skin care via application of creams or lotions to new skin and scabbed areas is beneficial
- Eucerine cream, Nivea oil (not cream), Keri lotion, or any lanolin-rich lotion may be applied and covered with a dressing of loose gauze or loose cotton underclothing to relieve itching and pain to areas that feel tight and dry while healing

For emotional healing, the following should be discussed:

- The course of rehabilitation (length and type of treatment, expected results, etc.)
- The need to change or adapt to a new life-style and new goals in life and how the adaptation will affect the client and significant others
- The challenges faced by the client and significant others as they leave the security and acceptance of the hospital environment
- Anticipatory guidance and encouragement as the client and significant others cope with public appearances if visible, disfiguring effects remain after healing is complete
- Coping strategies for emotions such as frustration, anger, and depression
- The need to seek and participate in mental health counseling when usual coping strategies are ineffective

ETHICAL ISSUES IN NURSING

Should Severely Burned Clients Be Allowed to Refuse Treatment?

People who have sustained severe burns are perhaps the most fragile of all clients. The road to recovery is long and hard, and full recovery may never occur. In the most severe cases, the treatments for these clients may take months and induce intense pain. Even though months of whirlpool and débridement treatments may be required and the client may be put through severe pain with each treatment, death may be the end result. Even if death does not occur, return to a "normal" life may never happen.

Should the severely burned client be allowed to die without any medical intervention except for pain management? Should there be a set of criteria that a client must meet to determine what treatment options are offered to him or her? These criteria, of course, would be based on the client's best interests, respect for the client's dignity as a person, and the availability of resources. Should clients be allowed to refuse treatments, even if their chance of survival is good, simply because they believe the potential quality of their life will be too low?

Currently there are national statistics based on age, depth of the burns, degree of inhalation damage, and so on that assist caregivers in the burn unit in calculating the potential survival rate of a given burn client. The survival rate does assist in the recommended treatment options, but clients may still choose death over treatment. When in such a physical and mental state, are clients competent to make such a final decision regarding their own survival? There are, undoubtedly, many challenges facing both clients and caregivers in the burn unit setting. Each case should be individually evaluated, and caregivers should always be sensitive to the client and the client's significant others. There are many uncomfortable ethical questions regarding the care of burn clients and the answers are no less comfortable, if the questions are answered at all.

STUDY QUESTIONS

1. Which one of the following clients is most at risk for thermal burn injury?
   A. A 70-year-old male cook
   B. A 39-year-old male nurse
   C. A 47-year-old female machinist
   D. A 25-year-old electrician
2. A client was admitted to the burn unit with second- and third-degree burns about 10 hours ago. His wife is here for her first visit. Which word would prepare her for her husband's appearance?
   A. Scarred
   B. Dyspneic
   C. Edematous
   D. Diaphoretic
3. Use the rule of nines to estimate the total body surface area (TBSA): anterior thorax, head, and the left upper extremity. The percentage of area burned is:
   A. 19%
   B. 27%
   C. 36%
   D. 54%
4. Which of the following would result in information that would best assess burn severity and associated care?
   A. Occupation
   B. Marital status
   C. General health
   D. Home environment
5. A client is scheduled for an allograft and asks the nurse what the graft is made of. The nurse should respond by saying it is:
   A. Cadaver skin
   B. Porcine skin
   C. Amnion membrane
   D. Nylon fabric and silicone
6. A nursing assessment 12 hours after a client has suffered second- and third-degree burns reveals that the client is experiencing moderate pain. Which one of the following interventions is appropriate at this time?
   A. Explanation of all procedures
   B. Administration of oxygen via nasal mask
   C. Application of a topical anesthetic agent
   D. Administration of intramuscular meperidine

CRITICAL THINKING EXERCISES

SCENARIO A

A nurse is invited to present a talk to a senior citizens group on prevention of injury in the elderly. He chooses the prevention of burns as his topic. Answer the following questions as if you are the nurse preparing for the talk.

1. For what reasons are the elderly at high risk for burn injuries?
2. How can the elderly prevent burn injuries in the home?
3. How would an elderly person know a scald injury has occurred?
4. What home remedies might be used by elderly people if burn injury occurs? Are home remedies effective?

SCENARIO B

A female client was cleaning up after a session of laying tile on the basement floor. She was using gasoline to clean the black tar-like substance used to glue the tile to the floor. An explosion occurred and the client's husband summoned an emergency squad. The client was admitted to the Trauma Center with second- and third-degree burns caused by the fire that began after the explosion. The burns were present on her face, neck, and scalp, both arms to the shoulders, the anterior thorax, and scattered first degree burns on the torso and lower extremities. Since she used her hands to try to beat out the flames, the skin of both arms was charred and peeling off.

1. How much TBSA is involved (use the rule of nines)?
2. What are the greatest concerns of the trauma team?
3. When would pain medication be administered?
4. Since the TBSA is so extensive, what other measures might be initiated in the Trauma Center? Why?

BIBLIOGRAPHY

1. Achauer, B. M., & McGuire, A. (1989). Fire safe cigarettes —an update. *Journal of Burn Care & Rehabilitation, 10(2),* 173–174.
2. Adams, L. E., Purdue, G. F., & Hunt, J. L. (1991). Tap-water scald burns. *Journal of Burn Care and Rehabilitation, 12,* 91–95.
3. Bayley, E., et al. (1991). Research priorities for burn nursing: Patient, nurse, and burn prevention education. *Journal of Burn Care and Rehabilitation, 12,* 377–383.
4. Bayley, E. W., et al. (1990). Standards for burn nursing practice. *Journal of Burn Care & Rehabilitation, 10(4),* 362–374.
5. Bayley, E. W. (1990). Wound healing in the patient with burns. *Nursing Clinics of North America, 25(1),* 205–222.
6. Berry, C. C., et al. (1982). Differences in burn size estimates between community hospitals and a burn center. *Journal of Burn Care & Rehabilitation, 3(3),* 176–177.
7. Boots Pharmaceuticals, Inc. (1991). *Travase ointment—indications and usage* (Product Monograph). Lincolnshire, Ill: Author.
8. Briggs, S. E. (1990). Rationale for acute surgical approach. In J. A. Martyn (Ed.). *Acute management of the burned patient.* Philadelphia: W. B. Saunders.
9. Burdge, J. J., et al., (1988). Surgical treatment of burns in elderly patients. *Journal of Trauma, 28(2),* 214–217.
10. Burgess, M. (1991). Initial management of a patient with extensive burn injury. *Critical Care Nursing Clinics of North America, 3(2),* 165–179.
11. Calistro, A. (1993). Burn care basics and beyond. *RN, 56(3),* 26–31.
12. Carlson, D. E., & Jordan, B. S. (1991). Implementing nutritional therapy in the thermally injured patient. *Critical Care Nursing Clinics of North America, 3(2),* 221–235.
13. Carrougher, G., & Marvin, J. (1989). Mechanical débridement: Views from University of Washington Burn Center at Harborview, Seattle, Washington [Editorial]. *Journal of Burn Care & Rehabilitation, 10(3),* 271–272.
14. Cioffi, W. G., & Rue, L. W. (1991). Diagnosis and treatment of inhalation injuries. *Critical Care Nursing Clinics of North America, 3(2),* 191–198.
15. Constable, J. D. (1994). The state of burn care: Past, present and future. *Burns, 20(4),* 316–324.
16. Copstead, L. C. (1995). *Perspectives on pathophysiology.* Philadelphia: W. B. Saunders.
17. Demling, R. H. (1987). Fluid replacement in burned patients. *Surgical Clinics of North America, 67(1),* 15–30.
18. Duncan, D. J., (Ed.). (1991). Burn management. *Critical Care Nursing Clinics of North America, 3(2),* 165–267.
19. Dyer, C., & Roberts, D. (1990). Thermal trauma. *Nursing Clinics of North America, 25(1),* 85–117.
20. Gordon, M. K. (1987). Burn wound care: Silver sulfadiazine application [Editorial]. *Journal of Burn Care & Rehabilitation, 8(5),* 429.
21. Helvig, B., & Curry, V. (1989). Mechanical débridement: Views from Shriners Hospitals for Crippled Children, Burn Unit, Galveston, Texas [Editorial]. *Journal of Burn Care & Rehabilitation, 10(3),* 272–273.
22. Herndon, D. N., et al. (1988). Inhalation injury in burned patients: Effects and treatment. *Burns, 14(5),* 349–356.
23. Jarvis, R., & Weireter, L. J. (1989). Mechanical débridement: Views from Sentara Norfolk General Hospital, Norfolk, Virginia [Editorial]. *Journal of Burn Care & Rehabilitation, 10(3),* 273.
24. Jones, J. D., et al. (1989). Alcohol use and burn injury. *Journal of Burn Care & Rehabilitation, 12(2),* 148–152.
25. Knaysi, G. A., et al. (1968). The rule of nines: Its history and accuracy. *Plastic and Reconstructive Surgery, 41(6),* 560–563.
26. Kraemer, M. D., et al. (1988). Burn contractures: Incidence, predisposing factors, and results of surgical therapy. *Journal of Burn Care & Rehabilitation, 9(3),* 261–265.
27. Kuehn, C. N. (1994). Management of a self-immolation victim: A nursing challenge in burn care. *Critical Care Nursing Clinics of North America, 6(4),* 863–872.
28. Leske, J. S. (1991). Overview of family needs after critical illness: From assessment to intervention. *AACN Clinical Issues in Critical Care Nursing, 2(2),* 220–226.
29. Lillico, S. (1992). *National Burn Awareness.* Encino, CA: The National Burn Awareness Task Force.
30. Linares, A. Z., & Linears, H. A. (1990). Burn prevention: The need for a comprehensive approach. *Burns, 16,* 281–285.
31. Lund, C. C., & Browder, N. C. (1944). The estimation of

areas of burn. *Surgery, Gynecology and Obstetrics 79(4)*, 352–358.

32. Maley, M. P. (1989). Scald burns associated with tap water. *Journal of Burn Care & Rehabilitation, 10(2)*, 172–173.
33. Mancusi-Ungaro, H. R., Van Way, C. W., & McCool, C. (1992). Caloric and nitrogen balances as predictors of nutritional outcomes in patients with burns. *Journal of Burn Care and Rehabilitation, 13*, 695–702.
34. Martyn, J. A. (Ed.). (1990). *Acute management of the burned patient.* Philadelphia: W. B. Saunders.
35. Marvin, J. A. (1991). Infection control. In R. B. Trofino (Ed.), *Nursing care of the burn injured patient.* Philadelphia: F. A. Davis.
36. Marvin, J. (1987). Pain management in the burn patient: Excerpts from a symposium on pain management at Harborview Hospital, Seattle, Washington, July 23, 1986. *Journal of Burn Care & Rehabilitation, 8(4)*, 307–318.
37. McLoughlin, E., & McGuire, A. (1990). The causes, cost, and prevention of childhood burn injuries. *American Journal of Diseases of Children, 144(6)*, 677–683.
38. Molter, N. C., Duncan, D. J., & DePew, C. L. (1993). Burns. In J. Hartshorn, et al., (Eds.). *Introduction to critical care nursing.* Philadelphia: W. B. Saunders.
39. Monafo, W. W. (1992). Then and now: 50 years of burn treatment. *Burns, 18*, S7–S10.
40. Monafo, W. W., Jr. (1971). The treatment of burns: Principles and practices. St. Louis, MO: Warren H. Green.
41. Nebraska Burn Institute. (1990). Advanced burn life support manual. Lincoln, NE: Author.
42. Orr, J., & Hain, T. (1994). Burn wound management: An overview. *Professional Nurse, 10(3)*, 153–156.
43. Pruitt, B. A., Jr., & Goodwin, C. W., Jr. (1990). Burn injury. In E. E. Moore, et al. (Eds.). *Early care of the injured patient* (pp. 286–306). Philadelphia: Decker.
44. Purdue, G. F., et al. (1990). Obesity: A risk factor in the burn patient. *Journal of Burn Care & Rehabilitation, 11(1)*, 32–34.
45. Roa, L., Gomez-Cia, T., & Cantero, A. (1990). Pulmonary capillary dynamics and fluid distribution after burn and inhalation injury. *Burns, 16*, 25–35.
46. Rue, L. W., & Cioffi, W. G., Jr. (1991). Resuscitation of thermally injured patients. *Critical Care Nursing Clinics of North America, 3(2)*, 181–189.
47. Sadowski, D. A. (1989). Smoke inhalation/carbon monoxide poisoning. In M. S. Sommers (Ed.), *Difficult diagnosis in critical care nursing.* Rockville, MD: Aspen.
48. Sadowski, D. A. (1987). Burn wound care: Silver sulfadiazine application: Feature protocol from Shriners Burns Institute. Cincinnati. *Journal of Burn Care & Rehabilitation, 8(5)*, 429–431.
49. Schumann, L. L. (1991). Care of the patient with major burns. In R. B. Trofino (Ed.). *Nursing care of the burn-injured patient.* Philadelphia: F. A. Davis.
50. Thomas, C. L. (Ed.) (1993). *Taber's cyclopedic medical dictionary* (17th ed.). Philadelphia: F. A. Davis.
51. Thomson, P. D., et al. (1990). A survey of burn hydrotherapy in the United States. *Journal of Burn Care & Rehabilitation, 11(2)*, 151–155.
52. Trofino, R. B. (1991). *Nursing care of the burn-injured patient.* Philadelphia: F. A. Davis.
53. Turner, D. G., et al. (1989). Cooking-related burn injuries in the elderly: Preventing the "granny gown" burn. *Journal of Burn Care & Rehabilitation, 10(4)*, 356–359.
54. Van Rijn, O. J. L., et al. (1989). The etiology of burns in developed countries: Review of the literature. *Burns, 15(4)*, 217–221.
55. Ward, R. S. (1991). Pressure therapy for the control of hypertrophic scar formation after burn injury. *Journal of Burn Care and Rehabilitation, 12*, 257–262.
56. Ward, R. S. (1991). The rehabilitation of burn patients. *Critical Reviews in Physical and Rehabilitation Medicine, 2(3)*, 121–138.
57. Williamson, J. (1989). Actual burn nutrition care practices —a national survey (part II). *Journal of Burn Care & Rehabilitation, 10(2)*, 185–194.

Chapter 50 Nursing Care of Clients Undergoing Plastic Surgery

Learning Outcomes

After completing this chapter, the learner will be able to:

1. Assess the client for preoperative and postoperative status related to plastic surgery.
2. Teach the client about the etiology, risk factors, and healing process associated with plastic surgery.
3. Explain the client's role as the recipient of plastic surgery.
4. Develop plans of care for the client who receives plastic surgery.
5. Implement nursing interventions that optimize the quality of life for clients receiving plastic surgery.
6. Evaluate planned outcomes using outcome criteria developed in the planning phases of care.

Plastic Surgery

Plastic surgery is the surgical subspecialty concentrating on the restoration of function and form to body structures damaged by trauma, the aging process, disease processes such as skin cancer, and congenital defects. Plastic surgeons repair defects in skin and underlying tissue, sometimes including the skeletal framework. Plastic surgeons and nurses approach the plastic surgery client as a whole being. They intervene as a team to help the client deal with the psychosocial impact of deformity on body image as well as the physical aspects of surgery.

AESTHETIC AND RECONSTRUCTIVE SURGERY

Plastic surgery can be divided into two major areas: (1) aesthetic (cosmetic) surgery and (2) reconstructive surgery.

Aesthetic plastic surgery alters the appearance of any physical feature that is already within "normal" range. Thus, it is elective and typically not covered by insurance. People seek aesthetic plastic surgery for many reasons (e.g., to look younger, maintain a job, or improve self-image). People often have high expectations of aesthetic plastic surgery and may be dissatisfied with anything but "perfect" results.

Reconstructive surgery attempts to restore an abnormal body part to normal. The abnormality may be due to injured tissue, disease, or missing tissues or may be causing other medical problems. People undergoing reconstructive surgery are typically motivated to try to gain increased function of body parts and improve their appearance. Although they may hope that plastic surgery will make them "normal," they usually know this may be unrealistic.

Initial reconstructive procedures focus on saving a person's life. For example, after a burn injury, skin grafting may be performed to reduce fluid and heat loss and the risk of infection. Later, additional reconstructive surgery is performed to restore physical function and finally to improve the person's appearance. Reconstructive plastic surgery is used to repair or reconstruct traumatic injuries, congenital defects, and acquired deformities such as cancer.

Incidence

The "incidence" of plastic surgery procedures is not recorded. They are becoming quite common, however. Technology and plastic surgery techniques have improved rapidly in recent times. Plastic surgery is able to address successfully many problems (e.g., amputated digits, breast reconstruction after mastectomy, and unsightly birthmarks) that were not repairable just a few years ago.

Etiology

Many disorders may be corrected or improved through plastic surgery. Disorders range from those that are life threatening (e.g., burns) to disorders within the realm of normal but unacceptable to the client. It is a normal desire to want to physically resemble one's peers reasonably closely (e.g., to have acceptably "normal" facial features). The desire to be attractive or beautiful is present in people of all cultures, but the perception of what is attractive varies.

BODY IMAGE

A significant portion of any deformity rests in the client's perception of it. Perceptions develop in part from body image. Body image describes an individual's perception of his or her body—how the *person* thinks he or she looks, rather than an objective assessment of the person's characteristics.

An individual with a physical deformity, real or perceived, can have a severely damaged body image. Even the usual processes of aging can be detrimental to body image. Body image is an important factor in the nursing assessment of the client having plastic surgery.

Prevention

Primary prevention of disorders requiring plastic surgery is directed at reducing congenital disorders through prenatal care and genetic counseling. Plastic surgery is also used in the treatment of malignancies; therefore, primary prevention focuses on cancer detection and treatment. Conditions requiring aesthetic surgery generally are not preventable.

Clinical Manifestations

Most clients with conditions requiring plastic surgery have some degree of deformity. The deformity can be *actual,* that is, objectively measured by others, such as a missing breast or deviated septum. Deformity can also be *perceived,* that is, the client is aware of the deformity, but it may not be noticeable to others. Fine facial wrinkling indicative of aging is an example.

DIAGNOSTIC ASSESSMENT

All clients must be assessed for their physical readiness for surgery. Before a major operation, a complete blood cell count is taken, electrolyte levels are assessed, and a chest x-ray study and electrocardiogram (for clients older than 40 years) are performed. Other diagnostic assessments vary with specific procedures.

Medical Management

In this section, basic principles and practices in plastic surgery are discussed. Specific techniques are discussed later in the chapter.

RECONSTRUCTIVE LADDER

One of the greatest challenges in plastic surgery is reconstructing deformities. The reconstructive ladder is a guide to plan reconstruction. Factors taken into consideration include:

- Amount of missing tissue (e.g., bone, muscle, subcutaneous tissue, or skin)
- Amount of tissue available for repair
- Possible deficit that might result from moving donor tissue
- Use of the simplest method of reconstruction to achieve the desired results (e.g., simple suture, flap, or skin grafting)

MINIMAL SCARRING

Skin Lines. Plastic surgeons strive for minimal postoperative scarring. The quality of scarring is affected by many variables. The client's age, general health, skin type, and healing ability are important. Surgical technique and the quality of wound care also affect the healing process.

Every individual has normal lines and skinfolds. Incisions made perpendicular to these lines result in more obvious scars. Incisions made parallel to the lines heal camouflaged by natural skinfolds. Incisions can also be hidden in the scalp or by the eyebrow or concealed by clothing.

Elliptical Incision. When excising a lesion, the surgeon designs the incision lines longer than the lesion (Fig. 50–1). The resulting defect is elliptical, and the skin edges can be approximated easily. When the defect is round, tissues bunch up at the ends of the incision.

Suturing Techniques. To heal with minimal scarring, the edges of the skin incision must be approximated precisely without undue tension. The suture lifts up the skin edges while it approximates them. Each suture puncture represents a miniature wound, and scar tissue forms at the site of each puncture. Suture lines must be kept clean, or stitch abscesses will develop and increase scarring. Sutures removed within 7 days leave no discernible suture marks or tracks. Unfortunately, the skin on some areas of the body (e.g., the back) is tough and slower to heal and requires that sutures remain for a longer period of time. It is difficult to achieve fine scarring in these areas.

SURGICAL MODALITIES

Flaps and Grafts. Raw or exposed tissue left to its own heals slowly by secondary intention. Skin coverage is managed by approximating skin edges, covering the area with a graft, or transferring a flap. Most plastic surgery procedures are based on the transfer of tissue, either locally or to distant areas of the body.

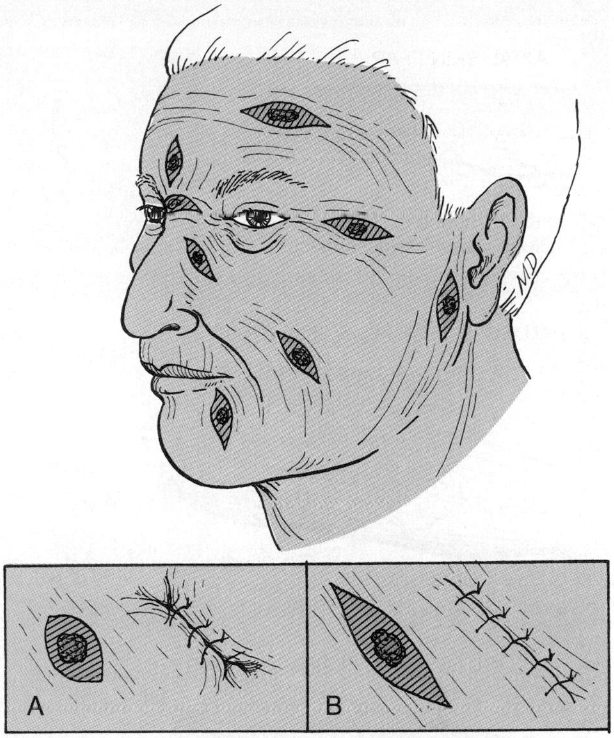

Figure 50–1
Examples of elliptical excisions around skin lesions. Note that the incisions are placed along normal skin lines so that the scars are hidden. The *shaded area* shows the area of tissue removed with each lesion. *A,* If the ellipse is too short, puckers or "dog ears" form at the ends of the incision. This creates an unsightly scar. *B,* Correct length of elliptical incision for minimal scarring. (Redrawn from Grabb, W., & Smith, J. [1979]. *Plastic surgery* [3rd ed.]. Boston: Little, Brown.)

A graft is tissue (e.g., skin, bone, nerve, or vessel) that is harvested without a blood supply from a donor site. It is transferred to a recipient site, where it develops a new blood supply. For the tissue to remain viable, or take, there must be a healthy vascular supply at the recipient site. The graft is anchored in position, and the area is immobilized until a new blood supply to the graft is established. Skin grafts always result in scars.

Skin grafts are used extensively to resurface exposed surfaces. The grafts vary in thickness from very thin split-thickness skin grafts, which contain epidermis and a very thin layer of dermis, to full-thickness grafts, which contain epidermis and all of the dermis.

A flap is tissue that is elevated with its blood supply intact. Local flaps are rotated or advanced to reconstruct an adjacent defect (Fig. 50–2). Free flaps are harvested from one area of the body to reconstruct a defect in a distant area. The donor tissue (skin, muscle, bone, or a combination of these) is detached from its blood supply at the donor site and reattached by microvascular anastomosis to arteries and veins at the recipient site.

Microvascular Surgery. The development of microvascular techniques has made it possible to reconstruct defects that were previously untreatable. For ex-

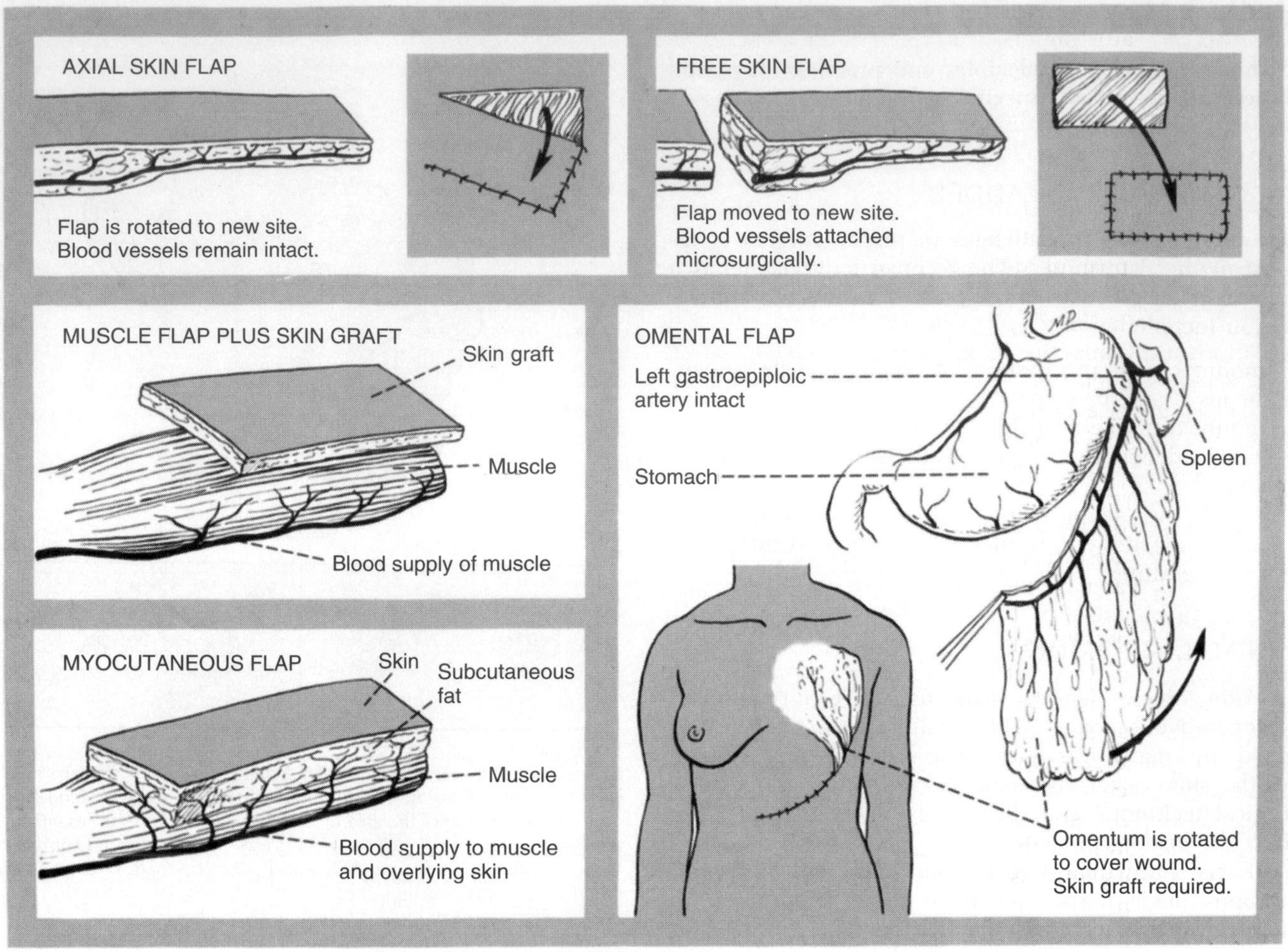

Figure 50–2
Common flaps.

ample, tissue from the forearm can be used in facial reconstruction. In some cases, sophisticated microvascular procedures have replaced less effective reconstructive approaches.

Adequate blood flow may be difficult to maintain in the anastomosed vessels in free flap owing to vasospasm and edema. When the flap becomes engorged with blood, a leech may be used to remove the excess blood. A sterile leech is applied by the surgeon. The leech injects an anticoagulant into the wound and removes blood. The therapy is usually effective in 30 minutes. Because of the anticoagulant in the wound, blood flow usually remains adequate after the leech is removed.

Implants. Implant material can be used to augment or replace tissue in all parts of the body. Polymers such as medical-grade silicone rubber are used most frequently in plastic surgical procedures. Silicone prostheses can be very soft (breast prostheses), flexible (finger and toe joints), or rigid (bones and joints). Stainless steel; Vitallium; and titanium plates, screws, and wire are used to approximate, replace, and stabilize bone fragments. Injectable collagen can be used to fill out skin depressions and fine wrinkles.

Facial structures (including the nose, chin, ears, orbital floor, and malar complex), breasts, bones and joints, and genitalia are often augmented or reconstructed with implant material. Material for implants must be biocompatible and not rejected by body tissues. It must not cause severe foreign body reaction or infection. Implants must be noncarcinogenic, nontoxic, nonallergenic, and sterile when implanted.

In 1991, the use of implants for breast augmentation was placed under strict regulations. The long-term risks of their use are being studied. The nurse caring for clients with breast implants must remain up to date by reading the scientific literature.

Skin Expansion. This is a technique used to increase the amount of local tissue available to reconstruct a defect. An inflatable silicone balloon is placed under the skin or muscle flap adjacent to a defect. The expander is inflated sequentially over several weeks or months to stretch the overlying tissue. When there is sufficient tissue to resurface the adjacent defect, the balloon is removed, and the flap is contoured (shaped) and advanced to cover the defect.

Liposuction. Liposuction, or suction-assisted lipectomy, is a technique used (1) to aspirate fatty tissue from areas resistant to diet and exercise (lipodystrophy), (2) to contour flaps, and (3) to remove lipomas (benign fatty tumors). It is also used adjunctively with other plastic surgical procedures to create better contour and enhance the aesthetic result.

Complications of liposuction include hematoma, skin necrosis, infection, and undesirable scars or skin dimpling.

Many clients expect the results of liposuction to be immediate. Usually up to 6 months is required for final results to be apparent after edema subsides and subcutaneous tissue heals.

Lasers. The laser (acronym for *l*ight *a*mplification by *s*timulated *e*mission of *r*adiation) is a coagulating, vaporizing, and cutting tool used frequently in plastic surgery. A precise beam of laser light is directed onto tissue. The light is converted into heat energy that is absorbed by the cells. Cells heat up, lose their moisture, and are destroyed.

There are different colors and wavelengths of laser light. Each is absorbed differently, depending on cell pigment and water content.

The advantages of laser surgery include precision and accuracy of cell destruction, with reduced bleeding and swelling and sometimes less postoperative pain. Operating time may be longer, but tissue damage is less, and the postoperative infection rate is lower.

Craniofacial Surgery. This is an approach for reconstructing facial bones through an incision on the top of the skull. The skin and muscles over the forehead and face are lifted off the bones and muscles. Once the face is free of its soft tissue drape, bones are rearranged to correct congenital or acquired deformities. Bone grafts from the ribs, iliac crest, or skull may provide bone for reconstruction. Adults likely to undergo craniofacial surgery are those with facial fractures and facial skeletal tumors.

Serious risks accompany craniofacial surgery (i.e., death from increased intracranial pressure, blindness, brain damage, and infections such as meningitis and osteomyelitis of the skull).

Postoperative care focuses on managing intracranial pressure, airway patency, and postoperative edema. The length of hospitalization varies with the underlying cause.

CLIENT SELECTION PROCESS

The success of a plastic surgical procedure is determined by the degree to which it meets the client's expectations. A surgical procedure may produce excellent clinical results, but the client will not consider it a success unless it achieves a specific appearance or level of function. Therefore, it is essential that the surgeon and nurse understand what the client expects and that the client have a realistic view of what can and cannot be accomplished by surgery.

Because most procedures affect appearance, clients make a considerable emotional commitment when they elect to have plastic surgery. Assessing the client's motivation is essential. Plastic surgery does not cure an individual's underlying emotional problems or alleviate major stress. An external change does not make a happy, well-adjusted person out of an individual who is unhappy, poorly adjusted, or excessively stressed.

DOCUMENTATION THROUGH CLINICAL PHOTOGRAPHY

Photographs are used extensively in plastic surgery. It is essential to document the client's condition before any surgical intervention. Once changes have been made in appearance, it is very difficult to remember the details of the original situation. Photographic documentation provides an accurate record.

The client must give written permission for photographs to be taken, especially if they are to be used for teaching purposes in addition to documentation for the medical record.

Nursing Management

Preoperative Care

Because the majority of plastic surgical procedures are not emergencies, there is ample time to be certain the client is physically and psychologically prepared for surgery. Nurses assess the client's physical readiness for surgery. Other disorders, such as diabetes and hypertension, also must be under control before surgery.

Preoperative teaching includes helping the client develop realistic postoperative expectations. The client must understand how the surgery will affect usual routines. Thorough planning ensures minimum disruption in routines. Preoperative teaching must include information about restrictions on activity, the location and extent of scars, and the clinical manifestations of possible complications. Including family members or significant others in the teaching process promotes an effective support system for the client.

The nurse must help clients understand that any incision in tissue results in the formation of scar tissue. It is essential that the client have a realistic expectation of the location and extent of scarring that will result from the surgical procedure. The nurse must remind the patient that a scar matures over a long period of time. Some scars take as long as several years to achieve their final appearance.

Preoperatively, it is essential to reinforce the fact that the body is naturally asymmetric. In preparing the client for realistic postoperative expectations, the surgeon and nurse must reinforce the fact that perfect symmetry is not a realistic expectation.

Survival of tissue that has been manipulated during surgery depends on promoting adequate blood flow. The nurse teaches the client to avoid anything that inhibits blood flow to the tissue. Aspirin and aspirin-containing compounds interfere with platelet agglutination and can promote bleeding and hematoma formation. Nicotine is a potent vasoconstrictor and can interfere with tissue perfusion. Smoking can result in flap necrosis and the loss of a significant amount of tissue. The client is also taught to elevate the surgical site.

Postoperative Assessment

The surgical site is inspected every 2 hours if no dressing is present. Dressings put on by the surgeon are not removed to make assessments. The nurse assesses and documents pain, pressure, bleeding, skin color, temperature, sensation, presence of blisters, presence or absence of edema or seroma (accumulation of serosanguineous drainage), and blanching time.

Any indications of complications at the surgical site are reported to the surgeon, including cool, pale, or cyanotic skin; increased (prolonged) blanching time as compared with preoperative findings; and changes in sensation (e.g., tingling). Abnormal pain, pallor, or cyanosis in transferred skin is immediately reported to the surgeon.

The nurse must assess the surgical site for venous stasis and edema. Either can seriously impair tissue perfusion. Venous stasis increases local tissue hypoxia because metabolic tissue waste is not removed promptly. Local tissue hypoxia can cause tissue necrosis.

CRITICAL TO REMEMBER

Prolonged blanching time is an early assessment finding that indicates venous stasis.

Venous engorgement makes the flap appear blue. Any sign of decreased vascularity (change in color or temperature, size, or tightness) must be reported immediately. Tissue oxygenation monitors may also be used.

Blisters (small blebs of serum) indicate reduced circulation and impaired tissue viability. The nurse documents and reports to the surgeon the presence of blisters. Sometimes, blisters under a skin graft need to be drained.

The amount of pain is assessed. Donor sites commonly are more painful than recipient sites.

The client's ability to cope with a temporary or permanent, perceived or actual, disfigurement is also assessed. The nurse assesses the client's coping mechanisms. The nurse listens to the client, alert for positive and negative statements about the self. The degree of anxiety and fear is noted. The nurse assesses the client's willingness or unwillingness to touch or look at involved body area, and the client's comfort in being near other people.

Nursing Diagnosis, Planning, and Intervention

Nursing Diagnosis: Tissue Perfusion, Altered Peripheral R/T tissue transfer.

Planning: Expected Outcomes. The client will have adequate peripheral tissue perfusion, as evidenced by usual color of skin, no pallor or cyanosis, warm and dry skin, blanching in 3 to 5 seconds, no edema or blebs, intact incisions, and controllable pain.

Implementation

Postoperative Flaps. Many plastic surgical procedures involve flaps. Failure of all or part of the flap can result in significant tissue loss. Flap failure is a devastating experience, physically and emotionally. Not only does the defect remain unrepaired, but the tissue used for the reconstruction is also sacrificed. The client's emotions are also devastated.

Protecting the blood supply to a flap is a primary nursing responsibility. Nursing interventions are designed to avoid factors that can jeopardize blood flow. Tension on the flap can stretch or kink the feeding blood vessels, reducing the flow of blood to the tissues. A blood clot can restrict blood flow.

CRITICAL TO REMEMBER

The first sign of compromised blood flow is pallor.

The nurse positions the client so that he or she is comfortable and the flap is relaxed and elevated. Gravity promotes edema and venous congestion, both of which impede blood flow. Interventions to increase venous return include elevating the involved body part and applying elastic stockings or wraps as prescribed.

A hematoma under a flap can be a severe complication. It can place pressure on vessels and inhibit blood flow. Hematomas can also precipitate an infection and release toxic substances. Increasing swelling and a feeling of tightness and pressure are danger signs. Hematomas can be removed if recognized early. Continued evaluation ensures that any factors inhibiting vascularity are reported and addressed immediately.

Implants. Postoperatively, assessment and intervention focus on

- Preventing displacement of the implant
- Ensuring adequate blood flow to the operative site
- Preventing infection

Implants themselves are not painful, but the surgical procedure causes mild to moderate pain. Infection is a serious complication that could result in having to remove the implant. Excellent wound care is imperative.

CRITICAL TO REMEMBER

The nurse must teach the client to recognize the clinical manifestations of infection so that treatment can be initiated quickly.

Pain that is unrelieved with analgesics must be investigated. Changes in temperature and local changes such as drainage, increasing edema, hyperemia, and increasing skin temperature may indicate a developing infection or implant rejection.

The process of skin expansion involves an extended period of time, commitment, and significant, although temporary, disfigurement. Each expander has an injection site into which a sterile needle is inserted percutaneously. Saline is injected slowly until the tissue is very tight over the expander. Sometimes a small amount of saline needs to be withdrawn to reduce discomfort. The tightness may be uncomfortable for several hours but subsides as the tissue begins to expand.

The nurse teaches the client to keep the incision and the injection site clean and dry to prevent infection. It is important that the client understand that pressure on the expander compromises blood flow and could cause tissue breakdown. Infection is a serious complication and may require that the expander be removed altogether. If the incision line dehisces, exposing the expander, it does not usually result in aborting the treatment. Fluid can be removed from the expander to relieve the tension. When the incision has healed sufficiently, expansion can begin again.

In most cases, the client and nurse can camouflage the expander with clothing. So that no pressure is placed on the expander, the clothing must be loose. The client should sleep in a position that protects the expander from pressure. Those clients with expanders in exposed areas such as the neck or scalp must be able to cope with the temporary physical inconvenience and insult to body image.

Liposuction. Because moderate to large quantities of tissue and fluid can be removed during liposuction, the nurse must assess the client for signs of hypovolemia and electrolyte imbalance (syncope, dizziness, and abnormal blood values). If drains are used, assessing the quantity and quality of drainage is important.

Compression dressings or elastic compression garments may be used to help collapse the tunnels and prevent fluid collection (hematoma and seroma), maintain the desired body contour, and promote healing. Dressings usually remain in place for at least 24 hours.

CRITICAL TO REMEMBER

The nurse must ensure that dressings remain smooth and uniform or contour irregularities can result.

Sometimes the client wears a compression garment for several weeks postoperatively to promote good healing.

After liposuction, clients rest for several hours. They may gradually resume normal activity except for strenuous exercise. It may be 4 to 6 weeks before the client attains the preoperative level of exercise. Resuming activity too rapidly may result in soreness and swelling. Bruising is common after liposuction and may take weeks to disappear completely.

The nurse reinforces that results may not be apparent for 6 months after surgery. This period of time is required for complete resolution of edema and reconnection of soft tissues.

Laser Surgery. Laser energy generates intense heat and clients experience a burning sensation. The tissue reaction can be similar to a first-degree burn with blistering. Ointment applied to the affected area for 2 to 4 weeks keeps the tissue moist until healing is complete. It is also essential that the area treated with laser energy be protected from sun exposure for several weeks.

Craniofacial Surgery. Postoperative care after craniofacial surgery includes elevating the head of the bed to reduce edema. The head can and should be turned while being supported behind the coronal incision line. Care must be taken that no pressure is placed on areas of bone grafts. The client can lie supine or on the nonoperative side but not directly on the operated side of the head or cheek, because pressure on the bony grafts may dislodge them. Neck flexion is permitted. Frequent neurologic assessment is important for increasing intracranial (Chap. 12) and intraocular pressure. Diplopia (double vision) is usually due to edema, is temporary, and may be helped with alternating eye patches. Relatively mild doses of analgesics or narcotics may control discomfort. However, the donor sites for rib or iliac bone grafts are often very painful. Analgesics that contain aspirin are avoided because they increase risk of bleeding.

Care of the client with Body Image Disturbance, R/T perceived or actual disfigurement is discussed in the Care Plan.

Evaluation

The degree of expected outcome attainment is evaluated before discharge from the postanesthesia area, hospital room, or office setting. Because the clinical manifestations of impaired tissue perfusion may develop hours after surgery, the client needs thorough education in order to detect reportable problems. (See the Client Education Guide: The Client Undergoing Plastic Surgery.)

Modification of Plan of Care for the Elderly

Many elderly clients have both aesthetic and reconstructive surgery. The nurse ascertains that the client understands the surgical plans, often by using education forms with large print. Many elderly clients routinely take anticoagulants and, therefore, tend to bleed more easily. Pressure dressings may be required for a longer period of time. Finally, some clients may resist not being independent with driving and self-care. Safety issues must be discussed. For example, the side effects of anesthetics and narcotics as well as facial edema and dressings prohibit driving after facial surgery.

CLIENT EDUCATION GUIDE

The Client Undergoing Plastic Surgery

The nurse should discuss the following with the client and significant others:

- A well-balanced diet that includes the five food groups should be maintained to promote healing.
- Aspirin or analgesics containing aspirin are restricted before and after surgery to decrease the risk of bleeding.
- Keep the incision line clean and dry.
- Observe for and report changes in skin color and sensation. Promptly notify surgeon of any skin changes.
- Follow postoperative activity restrictions to avoid tension on the suture line and promote the healing process.
- Keep in mind that achieving the final desired results takes time; don't be discouraged if progress seems slow.

CARE PLAN: The Client Undergoing Plastic Surgery

Nursing Diagnosis/ Collaborative Problem	Planning: Expected Outcomes	Implementation: Nursing Interventions	Rationales
Body Image Disturbance in Self-Concept, R/T perceived or actual disfigurement	The client will have improved self-image with incorporation of changed body part into body image as evidenced by	Continue to assess apparent self-concept, coping methods, defense mechanisms, degree of anxiety, and fears frequently.	Continued assessment provides data about degree of self-concept.
	• Effective coping and appropriate use of defense mechanisms	Assist client to explore and express feelings.	Allowing the client to express feelings assists client to work through feelings.
	• Verbalizes feelings comfortably and appropriately • Expresses satisfaction with changed body image	Be sensitive to client's feelings and needs.	Sensitivity is imperative to facilitate open communication.
	• Able to verbalize feelings openly • Makes positive statements about self • Normal level of anxiety and normal fears	Acknowledge client's feelings.	Using phrases such as "I know how you feel" builds barriers to communication. "You are angry" or "you seem depressed" identifies the feeling.
	• No indications of depression • Comfortably looking at self in mirror or touching deformed body area, healed surgical site, or other scars • Able to be with others comfortably	Present reality.	Building false hope is detrimental. Reality need not be brutal, however. Healing is unpredictable, questions should be referred to the surgeon.
		Demonstrate appropriate feelings of value and positive regard toward client.	Nurse must believe and respect client to facilitate feelings of self-worth.
		Provide necessary physical care if client is depressed. (Depressed clients may be unable to meet these needs because they lack energy or desire to do so.)	Do not force the client to view or touch self.
		Gently assist client to look at and touch deformity or healed surgical site. (Help incorporate it into client's self-concept and body image.)	Desensitization begins in safe environments and proceeds to new situations. Client is prepared for stares and remarks.
		Encourage client to begin meeting in public to begin desensitization to reactions of others, such as by taking walks in halls.	
		Assist client, as necessary, to be with others, walking in halls.	
		Discuss reaction of others to client. Support grief reactions.	
		Prepare visitors and family members before seeing client if facial deformity is present.	This allows family members time to prepare and control reactions.
		Look for vocal expression or hand gestures if client is facially disfigured.	Facial expression may be limited in clients with extensive facial scars or skin grafting.

Facial Rejuvenating Surgery

In childhood, skin is very elastic and is supported at maximum distension by the adipose tissue (sometimes called "baby fat"). During aging, the skin loses elasticity and the subcutaneous fat diminishes and changes in character. Skinfolds and wrinkles become increasingly noticeable. The tissues around the eyes and jowls sag, producing a drooping, weary, or worried expression.

RHYTIDECTOMY

Rhytidectomy, also called a face lift, removes the larger skin wrinkles and folds from the face and neck. Rhytidectomy may restore a more youthful appearance to the face (perhaps 5–10 years younger) (e.g., by removing wrinkles from the forehead and along the eyes and mouth) (Fig. 50–3).

Rhytidectomy is usually performed on a day surgery basis under general or local anesthesia with intravenous sedation. Incisions are made along the ear and out into the hair-bearing scalp. Through the incisions, excess facial skin is undermined and pulled back toward the ear. On completion of the operation, facial compression dressings are applied.

Before rhytidectomy, the client thoroughly shampoos the hair and washes the face well. Men carefully shave.

Postoperatively, the client is assessed for hematoma development (e.g., increasing facial asymmetry associated with pain or tightness on one side of the face). The nurse reports these findings immediately to the surgeon and makes certain the client understands the importance of also doing so at home. Large hematomas are removed surgically because of potential skin necrosis as a result of pressure from the hematoma on blood vessels nourishing the skin. The nurse also assesses blood pressure and reports elevations, because this increases the risk of bleeding. Antiemetics can be used to reduce nausea and vomiting. Vomiting increases blood pressure and the risk of bleeding. Other common complications of a face lift include hair and skin loss and nerve damage.

The client should be taught to keep the head of the bed elevated for 1 week to minimize edema and to rest the face for 1 week to achieve fine, unnoticeable scars (minimize talking and chewing, i.e., take a soft diet). The surgeon usually removes dressings the morning after rhytidectomy. The face may then be gently washed, and creams and cosmetics applied. However, the suture line should not be touched with soap, water, creams, or cosmetics until healing is complete. Washing the hair is usually postponed for 48 hours. Dandruff shampoo is avoided.

BLEPHAROPLASTY

Blepharoplasty is the surgical removal of excessive tissue from the upper or lower eyelid. If eyelid tissue obstructs vision, blepharoplasty is classified as reconstructive. The aging process causes a loss of elasticity and relaxation of eyelid skin. Excessive eyelid tissue occurring in young and middle-aged people may be inherited, be an allergic reaction, or result from cardiovascular or thyroid disease. Complete medical assessment is essential to rule out these physical causes of excessive eyelid skin.

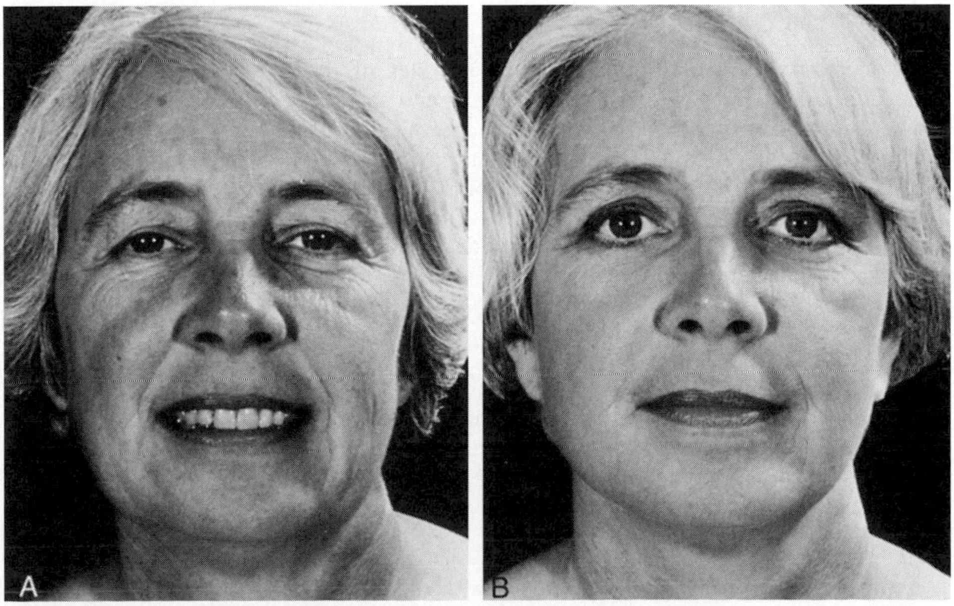

Figure 50–3

Before *(A)* and *(B)* a face lift (rhytidectomy) and blepharoplasty. (From Baptist, G. [1985]. Perioperative nursing roles for the aesthetic surgical patient. *Plastic Surgical Nursing, 5*(3), 86–93.)

Blepharoplasty is usually performed on a day surgery basis. General or local anesthesia can be used. Wide elliptical incisions are made on the eyelid. The excised wedge of excess tissue is lifted off, and herniated fat is removed.

Blepharoplasty can be performed alone or with rhytidectomy (face lift). Complications from blepharoplasty are rare.

Because blepharoplasty clients are not hospitalized, preoperative nursing care is brief. The nurse confirms that the person has taken nothing by mouth since midnight. The presence of food or liquid in the stomach may necessitate postponing the operation. Preoperative near and distant vision is assessed in each eye by asking the person to read from a book as well as from something in the distance with the eye not being examined covered. These baseline data are critical to assess postoperative changes.

Postoperatively, the nurse teaches the client the following:

- Report changing vision or eye pain not relieved by prescribed analgesia immediately to the surgeon.
- Apply cold compresses to the eyes as prescribed (typically for 24–48 hours after surgery). At home, clean washcloths soaked in ice water work well. The cloths should be damp and changed frequently.
- Sleep on the back with the head elevated for the first 48 hours. Lying on one side causes facial edema on that side, increasing tension on the suture lines.
- Avoid bending over from the waist for 48 hours.
- Avoid vigorous activity for 1 month.
- Bruising and swelling are common around the eyes. Hence, the client may want to wear sunglasses. The nurse shows the client how to apply and remove the eyeglasses carefully to avoid bumping the incisions.

ADJUNCTIVE PROCEDURES

Chemical Peel

Rhytidectomy does not remove all the wrinkles of the face. The fine lines around the mouth and at the corners of the eyes can be treated with chemical peel. This process uses a caustic solution containing phenol, which produces a controlled chemical burn of the top layers of skin. Chemical peel is best suited for fair-skinned people because individuals with darker skin tones may experience a change in skin color.

Trichloracetic Acid Peel

Trichloracetic acid is a form of chemical peel. The chemical is brushed on the skin until the skin frosts.

Dermabrasion

Dermabrasion is a process of sanding away the surface layers of skin on cheeks and forehead to remove pitting and surface blemishes, leaving a smoother skin surface. The healing process and nursing care after dermabrasion are similar to those following a chemical peel.

Collagen Injection

Collagen is sometimes injected to fill in small wrinkles or depressed blemishes in the skin.

The client's reaction to collagen is tested before treatment because some individuals experience induration (hard, raised area) and swelling at the injection site. Clients with autoimmune disorders are not candidates for collagen injection.

Other Elective Facial Surgery

RHINOPLASTY

Rhinoplasty is the surgical correction of external nose deformities. Rhinoplasty is frequently performed as day surgery, under local anesthesia and sedation or general anesthesia. Incisions are made inside the nose. Procedures are individualized and may include reshaping the bony dorsum of the nose, the tip of the nose, and cartilage along the nares (nostrils). The nasal bones may be fractured to achieve a desirable result. After surgery, the inside of the nose is packed and an external splint is applied.

Preoperative nursing care focuses on teaching the client to breath through the mouth after surgery and not to touch the nose. Postoperatively, the nurse must assess for bleeding.

CRITICAL TO REMEMBER

While the client is sleepy from the anesthetic, excessive swallowing may be the only sign of bleeding.

The nurse should examine the back of the throat with a flashlight to look for blood. Some bleeding is normal down the back of the throat and on the nasal packs and dressings. The nurse promptly reports excessive bleeding to the surgeon. The head of the bed is kept elevated to control postoperative edema. Nasal packing can be very uncomfortable. Pain management is important and can usually be achieved with oral analgesics (e.g., codeine or acetaminophen). Aspirin is avoided for 1 week before and 3 weeks after surgery.

In preparation for discharge, client education typically includes the following:

- Sleep with the head of the bed elevated for 1 week.
- Do not remove the external splints or nasal packing.
- Do not blow the nose. Sneeze only with the mouth open.
- Remain on a soft diet for 2 days.
- Avoid decongestant nasal sprays because they are va-

soconstrictors and they decrease the blood supply needed for healing.

- After nasal packs and external splints are removed, the nose will remain swollen and bruised for a while. Wait 3 months before judging the final results of the surgery.

Breast Surgery

POSTMASTECTOMY BREAST RECONSTRUCTION

Mastectomy for breast cancer or other breast disease not only disfigures but also causes emotional trauma (Chap. 55). For many women planning to have a mastectomy, the knowledge that breast reconstruction is possible reduces some of their anxiety. It is important that the client realize that the cosmetic results will not match the opposite breast. The reconstructed breast does not feel like a normal breast, but it has distinct advantages over external prostheses in feel and appearance in clothes.

Breast reconstruction can be performed immediately after mastectomy (during the same operation) or many years later. The timing of the reconstruction varies with the woman's preference and the surgeon's opinion. Disadvantages of immediate reconstruction are an increased risk of poor tissue perfusion and hematoma owing to the just-completed mastectomy.

Breast reconstruction is usually a collaborative effort among the general surgeon, the plastic surgeon, and the oncologist. A variety of reconstructive approaches are available and depend on the situation.

- Inserting a tissue expander. A tissue expander is inserted under the chest tissues and expanded slowly, by adding fluid via percutaneous injection. After a few weeks, when the chest tissue has expanded, the expander is removed and an implant inserted. The prosthesis is inserted beneath existing breast tissue through an inframammary (under the breast), transaxillary (through the axilla), or periareolar (around the nipple) incision. Women with little or no breast tissue may have the implant placed beneath the pectoralis muscle (called subpectoral placement) to provide protective tissue over the implant.
- Rotating the latissimus dorsi muscle. This large flat muscle is in the back. The muscle and skin can be lifted up from the back, tunneled through the axilla, and formed into a breast mound on the chest. An implant is then inserted. The incision is positioned so that it can be hidden under the brassiere. Functional loss of strength and shoulder abduction and loss of ability to pull occur after latissimus dorsi breast reconstruction.
- The transverse abdominal musculocutaneous (TRAM) flap is breast reconstruction using abdominal muscle and skin. This form of reconstruction does not usually require a prosthesis. The tissue can be rotated to the chest wall with the blood vessels intact, or the blood vessels can be reattached as a free flap through microsurgery. The donor site in the abdomen is closed as a modified abdominoplasty (Fig. 50–4). Although the contour of the abdomen is improved (flattened), the scar is usually visible.

  To undergo a TRAM flap, the client must have sufficient redundant abdominal tissue. Previous abdominal surgery and smoking can be contraindications if the blood supply to the TRAM is impaired.
- Free flaps, including flaps from the gluteal area and TRAM, have also been used for reconstruction.

The breast reconstruction techniques just discussed rebuild the breast mound. Some women elect to have

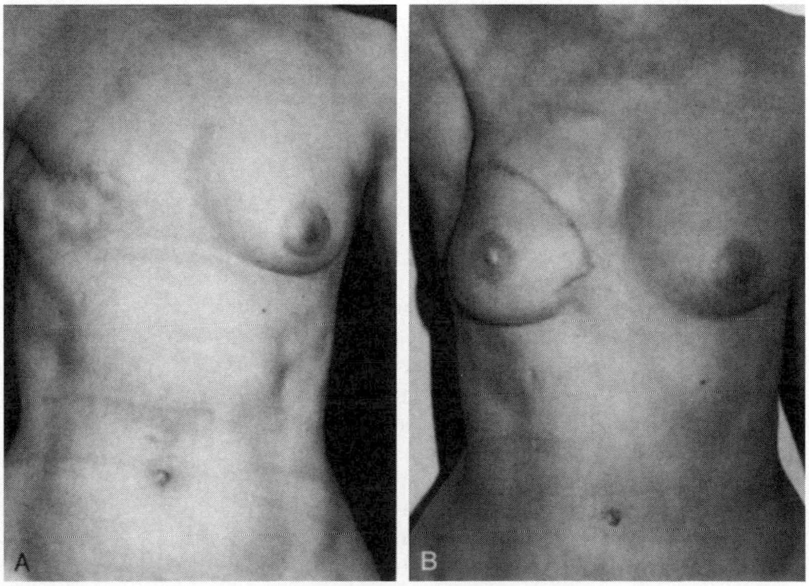

Figure 50–4
Preoperative *(A)* and postoperative *(B)* transverse rectus abdominus myocutaneous reconstruction. (From Lerberg, L., & Prin, J. [1991]. TRAM breast reconstruction. *Plastic Surgical Nursing, 11[2]*, 58–61.)

the nipple-areola complex also replaced. To achieve symmetry, nipple reconstruction may be delayed for several months after breast reconstruction.

Nursing Management

Preoperative nursing care includes reinforcing the surgeon's discussion and teaching the client about the planned procedure and postoperative care. If surgery is being performed for known or suspected cancer, the nurse facilitates the expression of feelings (e.g., powerlessness, disbelief, anger, fear, or depression).

In addition to providing the postoperative nursing care required by any person having surgery (Chap. 5), after reconstructive breast surgery the nurse assesses the flap or breast area, color, temperature, and capillary refill. The nipple-areola complex is also assessed if possible. Dressings are usually cone shaped with the nipple-areola complex open for assessment. A dusky, deep-red, purple, or black-edged areola indicates circulation impairment. The nurse documents assessment findings and immediately reports any that indicate possible complications to the surgeon.

Pain management varies with the type of surgery. Epidural analgesia has been used in breast reconstruction. When epidural analgesia is used, the nurse assesses the respiratory rate, degree of pain relief, and presence of numbness or paralysis in lower extremities every 2 hours. Caution must be used to protect the client from falling when ambulating.

A client with a recent subpectoral implant needs to know that initially the implant feels very firm and is higher on the chest than a normal breast. Over time the muscle stretches, allowing the implant to drop and soften. Women with subpectoral implants do not wear bras, because the implant needs to move into the pocket created in the chest wall. Women having other types of surgery may or may not return from the operating room wearing a bra to support the breasts. A front-closing support bra, without wires, is preferred. Wearing a bra also helps some women feel more normal, encouraging a return to wellness.

OTHER BREAST SURGERY

Reduction Mammoplasty

Reduction mammoplasty surgically reduces the size of large, pendulous breasts. Women usually seek such surgery to reduce the physical and psychosocial discomforts of large breasts, such as back pain, bra strap indentations in the shoulders, inability to wear normal clothing styles, intertriginous dermatitis (skin breakdown under large breasts) from skinfolds resting on each other, and being the subject of jokes or uncomfortable comments about breast size. These procedures may also be performed for men with gynecomastia (breast enlargement).

Subcutaneous Mastectomy

Some women acquire premalignant lesions, have a high risk of breast cancer, have had cancer in one breast, or have multiple suspicious breast nodules. These clients may elect to undergo prophylactic mastectomy (a mastectomy done to prevent cancer) on one or both breasts. One alternative to simple prophylactic mastectomy is subcutaneous mastectomy, during which almost all breast tissue is removed. An implant is inserted immediately, or tissue expanders may be used. This operation reduces the risk of cancer later developing in the operated breast. However, a few women develop tumors in the remaining bit of breast tissue within the nipple.

Traumatic Injury Repair

FACIAL INJURIES

Injuries to the face are a common result of automobile accidents and physical violence. Although they may be serious, facial injuries are seldom fatal. Proper management helps to avoid sensory impairment and permanent disability and can minimize disfigurement.

Lacerations

Facial lacerations can range from very small (0.50 cm) that can be repaired under local anesthesia to extensive lacerations with soft tissue injury requiring repair under general anesthesia. Before closure, wounds are cleansed of debris and devitalized tissue.

Excellent wound care, including cleansing and applying prescribed topical antibiotics, promotes the healing of facial abrasions and lacerations. A client who is taking nothing by mouth (NPO) and has dried blood in the mouth needs frequent oral care. If the client's mouth has sutures, the mouth is simply rinsed with saline. Oral care *must* be performed, however. With severe facial trauma, soft toothbrushes suffice for oral care. Devices that deliver water under pressure may further damage such injuries and are usually contraindicated. The nurse takes measures to prevent aspiration during oral care.

The nurse teaches the client and family or significant others to keep facial incision lines clean by applying a prescribed topical antibiotic. Skin incisions must not get wet (e.g., when showering), because moisture allows bacteria to enter the wound along the sutures. Infected incisions tend to produce more scar tissue.

Facial Fractures

Facial fractures can occur in the individual bones of the face: the nasal orbit, malar prominence, mandible, or maxilla.

The client with facial fractures has often been involved in an automobile accident, an assault, or a sports injury. Pain, improper bite (malocclusion), swelling, bruising, diplopia (double vision), facial asymmetry, enophthalmos (sunken eye), or exophthalmos (bulging eye) are other clinical manifestations of facial fractures. Diagnostic assessment includes x-ray studies. Life-threatening problems such as airway obstruction, hemorrhage, or cervical spine injury that may accompany facial trauma must be managed immediately. Repair of facial fractures can be delayed for up to 3 weeks and still achieve good results.

Nursing Management

The nurse assesses airway patency and breath sounds every 2 hours or more often if bleeding is present. Suction equipment is present at the bedside. The client is taught to breath through the nose. Trying to open the mouth may dislocate the fracture. When the client has intermaxillary wiring, wire cutters should be with the client at all times. If airway problems develop that cannot be managed with suction, the wires should be cut. The nurse and client need to be informed which wires should be cut. There are usually two wires on each side of the mouth, and they are the only wires present that attach the top and bottom teeth.

Facial edema and ecchymosis may be present. The head of the bed is elevated. Liquid tears may be needed if the client has reduced blinking.

The nurse assesses the client for diplopia and blurry vision. When these disorders are present, the nurse assists the client's ambulation to prevent injury.

The client remains on a liquefied diet until the wires are removed. Without adequate nutrition, clients can lose 10 to 20 pounds during convalescence. The client is taught how to blenderize food and maintain adequate balances of carbohydrates, fat, protein, and calories. Milk shakes can be made with a wide variety of foods. High-calorie food supplements can augment the regular diet, and liquid multivitamins may be useful. Alcoholic and carbonated beverages can cause nausea and fizz and foam in the back of the throat, leading to airway problems, and therefore are to be avoided.

The nurse assesses the client for clear rhinorrhea or otorrhea. Rhinorrhea or otorrhea may indicate leaking cerebrospinal fluid (CSF), which must be reported to the physician. With CSF leakage, there is the potential for developing meningitis.

CRITICAL TO REMEMBER

To assess for rhinorrhea or otorrhea, the nurse observes bed linens because CSF dries in concentric, halo-like rings and does not crust.

Initially, the nurse and client must establish a means of communication. Although talking is possible through clenched teeth, hand signals or writing may be most effective initially. Trying to open the mouth may dislocate the fracture. Clients initially require reassurance that they will not choke or suffocate.

Oral hygiene aids in healing of oral wounds, prevents infection and destruction of teeth and gums, increases comfort, and enhances self-esteem. Rinsing the mouth with water or a mouthwash followed by a low pressure rinse with a pressurized water device removes particles from the front of the mouth while the tissues are still tender. Once the initial swelling and tenderness subside, the teeth must be brushed and the mouth rinsed after every meal and at bedtime. Pieces of paraffin wax can be placed on the open ends of the wires if they irritate buccal surfaces.

Before discharge, the client and family or significant others need to be taught about the wires and diet and oral care. Once the incisions have healed, the client can resume normal activities. However, while the jaws are wired, the client must carry a wire cutter and know which wires to cut. A well-balanced blenderized diet and oral care should be continued.

TRAUMATIC AMPUTATIONS

Immediate care of a client after a traumatic amputation, like that of any other injured person, focuses on lifesaving activities (see Chap. 57). Hemorrhage is controlled with direct pressure on the bleeding points. Tourniquets and cautery are not used. They may damage surrounding tissue and prevent replant. All amputated parts, including small pieces of tissue, are sent to the health-care facility with the injured person. As soon as possible (1) these parts are rinsed with sterile normal saline, (2) the parts are wrapped in sterile wet gauze, (3) the parts are sealed in a watertight bag, and (4) the bag is placed in ice. Cooling the amputated part reduces metabolism, increasing the time the part can survive without blood. For example, an amputated finger can survive for 18 hours if effectively cooled. Although the part is rinsed with normal saline, it is never stored or left in normal saline or on dry ice or frozen because this causes extensive cellular damage.

Replantation surgery is performed under regional block or general anesthesia. After surgery, incisions are dressed, the extremity is immobilized with casts or splints, and the entire extremity is elevated.

After replantation, a person requires careful, frequent nursing assessment (every 15 minutes) and documentation of the replanted part's color, temperature, and capillary refill. A reimplanted part may have blocked arterial or venous blood flow, which, if not immediately corrected surgically, will cause the part to die. Toes and finger tips are usually left uncovered for assessment. Doppler assessments help measure pulses in the part. Temperature probes are often placed on the extremity. The surgeon usually states the ideal temperature range for replantations. A temperature decrease of 2° C or more in an hour or a decline to 32° C (89.6° F) demands immediate attention and is promptly reported to the surgeon. Aspirin is usually prescribed to reduce blood-clotting tendencies. A temperature of 34° to 36° C (93.2°–96.5° F) is considered excellent for a replanted finger. Owing to lengthy anesthesia (18–24 hours), nursing care also focuses on monitoring recovery from anesthesia.

An active rehabilitation program usually begins 2 weeks after injury and continues for months. Joint motion initially may be restricted by pins through joints and by bulky dressings. Because peripheral nerves take a long time to regenerate, protective sensation may be absent for months. The person must be careful to avoid injuring the part. Rehabilitation is accomplished through prescribed active and passive range-of-motion exercises several times each day.

Psychosocial adjustment after replantation varies with each person. Grieving over the loss of appearance and function of the extremity (the replant never achieves normal complete function and appearance) is a normal reaction that requires support. Praise and encouragement during rehabilitation are very helpful.

The nurse teaches the person to avoid activities and substances that cause vasoconstriction (which precipitates necrosis) for 2 weeks after surgery (e.g., tobacco, nicotine, cocaine, amphetamines). Air conditioning is harmful. The client is taught to avoid cold and chilling (e.g., by wearing extra clothing and having the car prewarmed before entering to prevent vasoconstriction).

A final indication of the success of replantation is return of sensory-motor nerve function in the reimplanted part.

STUDY QUESTIONS

1. A client is scheduled for plastic surgery. An important nursing action is to
   A. Assess for the presence of a physical deformity
   B. Assess the client's perception of body image
   C. Plan for a set of baseline vital sign measurements
   D. Plan to begin discharge teaching after the client returns from surgery
2. Which statement about scar formation is correct?
   A. Sutures will leave minute scarring after surgical wounds heal.
   B. A scar will fade over a period of time and become invisible to the naked eye.
   C. Incisions are made parallel to the skin lines so that scarring will be camouflaged.
   D. The surgeon will avoid use of an elliptical incision because the skin edges cannot be closely approximated.
3. The client who is receiving a breast implant needs to know that
   A. The body may reject the implant
   B. Infection is a serious complication
   C. The result will be perfectly matched breasts
   D. The implant is placed just under the nipple of the affected breast
4. The nurse is preparing for the arrival from the operating room of a client who has had a repair of a facial fracture. The most important assessment the nurse makes is for
   A. Blood pressure
   B. Blurred vision
   C. Airway patency
   D. Dryness of the eyes
5. The best intervention for the client with the nursing diagnosis of risk for body image disturbance related to actual disfigurement is to
   A. Support the client who wishes to remain in seclusion until healing is more complete
   B. Wait for the client or significant other to initiate questions about the disfigurement
   C. Continue to assess the client for anxiety and fears as well as use of defense mechanisms
   D. Refer the client or significant other to the surgeon for discussion of perceptions of body image
6. As a result of teaching the client about replantation of an amputated finger, the client should be able to state one cause of vasoconstriction that should be avoided postoperatively. Which of the following statements by the client is correct?
   A. "I plan on going skiing as soon as the pain is gone."
   B. "My husband is bringing in my cigarettes. I can't wait to smoke!"
   C. "My husband plans on warming the car for a few minutes so I won't get cold."
   D. "Because the blood vessels are constricted, I won't have any feeling in my reattached finger."

CRITICAL THINKING EXERCISES

SCENARIO A

A young female client is scheduled for a mastectomy and has asked the surgeon to implant a prosthesis during the same surgery. The nurse who completed the preoperative assessment discovered that the client's husband wanted her to have the implant done at the time of surgery because he could not accept her disfigurement. He wanted her to still have a perfect body.

1. What kind of support and teaching should the nurse extend to the client?
2. How should the nurse approach the client's spouse regarding his unacceptance of her disfigurement?
3. What misconceptions does the husband have about symmetry of the body?

SCENARIO B

An elderly female client is recovering from surgery performed to correct trauma inflicted during an attempted robbery. The client was beaten about the face and arms and sustained injuries that necessitated general anesthesia for plastic repair. The client is a widow who lives with her only child and his family.

1. How will the client feel about the change in her body image? How can the nurse help?
2. Will the areas of surgery as well as inflicted trauma heal adequately?
3. How might family and visitors treat the client now that she faces disfigurement as a result of the massive trauma?

BIBLIOGRAPHY

1. American Society of Plastic and Reconstructive Surgical Nurses. (1989). *Core curriculum for plastic and reconstructive surgical nursing*. Pitman, NJ: Author.
2. Baue, A. E. (1994). Breast conservation operations for treatment of cancer of the breast. *Journal of the American Medical Association, 271(15)*, 1204–1205.
3. Belger, D. (1989). A care plan to the patient having hand surgery. *Plastic Surgical Nursing, 9(3)*, 126–128.
4. Black, J. (1990). Complications following blepharoplasty. *Plastic Surgical Nursing, 10(4)*, 151–155.
5. Black, J. (1991). Reconstructive surgery in the elderly. *Plastic Surgical Nursing, 11(4)*, 151–162, 167.
6. Black, J., & Mangan, M. (1991). Body contouring and weight loss surgery for obesity. *Nursing Clinics of North America, 26(3)*, 777–788.
7. Carlsson, M., & Hamrin, E. (1994). Psychological and psychosocial aspects of breast cancer and breast cancer treatment. A literature review. *Cancer Nursing, 17(5)*, 418–428.
8. Chick, K., et al. (1989). Nursing care of adults having craniofacial surgery. *Plastic Surgical Nursing, 9(1)*, 16–19.
9. Cohen, T., et al. (1992). *Wound healing: Biochemical and clinical aspects*. Philadelphia: W. B. Saunders.
10. Daniel, R., & Farkas, L. (1988). Rhinoplasty, image and reality. *Clinics in Plastic Surgery, 15(1)*, 1–10.
11. Dillerud, E. (1990). Abdominoplasty combined with suction lipoplasty: A study of complications, revisions and risk factors in 487 cases. *Annals of Plastic Surgery, 25(5)*, 333–343.
12. Frioch, S., et al. (1990). Ambulatory surgery. A study of patients' and helpers' experiences. *AORN Journal, 52(5)*, 1000–1009.
13. Furnas, H., & Rosen, J. (1991). Monitoring in microvascular surgery. *Annals of Plastic Surgery, 26(3)*, 265–272.
14. Georgiade, G. S., et al. (1992). *Textbook of plastic, maxillofacial and reconstructive surgery* (2nd ed.). Baltimore: Williams & Wilkins.
15. Gilboa, D., et al. (1990). Emotional and psychosocial adjustment of women to breast reconstruction and detection of subgroup(s) at risk for psychological morbidity. *Annals of Plastic Surgery, 25(5)*, 397–401.
16. Goodman, T. (1987). Tissue expansion: A new modality reconstructive surgery. *AORN Journal, 45(2)*, 198–216.
17. Goodman, T. (1988). Flaps and grafts in plastic surgery. *AORN Journal, 48(4)*, 678–690.
18. Hinojosa, R. (1991). Breast reconstruction through tissue expansion. *Plastic Surgical Nursing, 11(2)*, 52–57.
19. Hofer, D., & Wise, L. (1994). Breast cancer therapy update: Controversies, choices, and conclusions. *Consultant, 34(3)*, 385–388, 391–392, 394.
20. Hutcheson, H. (1991). Epidural analgesia in the postoperative patient: A nursing perspective. *Plastic Surgical Nursing, 11(1)*, 6–10, 27.
21. Hutcheson, H., & Bostwick, J. (1989). Nipple and areola reconstruction. *Plastic Surgical Nursing, 9(3)*, 105–109, 119.
22. Hutcheson, H., et al. (1991). Breast reconstruction using the inferior gluteus free flap. *Plastic Surgical Nursing, 11(2)*, 65–71.
23. Ivey, C., & Gordon, S. I. (1994). Breast reconstruction: New image, new hope. *RN, 57(7)*, 48–53.
24. Keene, A. (1991). Perioperative assessment and nursing implications for the elderly. *Plastic Surgical Nursing, 11(4)*, 143–150.
25. Kroll, S., et al. (1990). Long-term survival after chest-wall reconstruction with musculocutaneous flaps. *Plastic and Reconstructive Surgery, 86(4)*, 697–701.
26. Lerberg, L., & Prin, J. (1991). TRAM breast reconstruction. *Plastic Surgical Nursing, 11(2)*, 58–61.
27. McCain, L. (1992). Making a difference in the breast implant issue. *Plastic Surgical Nursing, 12(1)*, 28–30.
28. McCarthy, J. (1991). *Plastic surgery*. Philadelphia: W. B. Saunders.
29. Meland, N., & Weimar, R. (1991). Microsurgical reconstruction: Experience with free fascia flaps. *Annals of Plastic Surgery, 27(1)*, 1–8.
30. Millward, J. (1994). On the receiving end of breast cancer. *Journal of Clinical Nursing, 3(3)*, 134–137.
31. Moncada, G. A., Maksud, D. P., & Jensen, J. (1994). Breast cancer treatment: Issues and controversies. *Plastic Surgical Nursing, 14(3)*, 187–189.
32. Napoleon, A., & Lewis, C. (1990). Psychological considerations in the elderly cosmetic surgery candidate. *Annals of Plastic Surgery, 24(2)*, 165–169.
33. Oberle, K., & Allen, M. (1994). Breast augmentation surgery: A women's health issue. *Journal of Advanced Nursing, 20(5)*, 844–852.
34. O'Hara, M. (1991). Beauty and the beast: Nursing care of the patient undergoing leech therapy. *Plastic Surgical Nursing, 11(3)*, 101–104.
35. Roeder, J., & White, S. (1990). Tissue expansion for the treatment of keloids. *Plastic Surgical Nursing, 10(3)*, 114–117, 125.
36. Rubayi, S., et al. (1990). Myocutaneous flaps: Surgical treatment of severe pressure ulcers. *AORN Journal, 52(1)*, 40–56.

37. Russell, B., & Russell, R. (1990). The role of the plastic surgery nurse collagen specialist. *Plastic Surgical Nursing, 10(2)*, 51–60.

38. Sciartelli, C. H. (1995). Using a clinical pathway approach to document patient teaching for breast cancer surgical procedures. *Oncology Nursing Forum, 22(1)*, 131–137.

39. Smith, J., & Aston, S. (1992). *Grabb and Smith's plastic surgery*. Boston: Little, Brown.

40. Solomon, M., & Garnick, M. (1990). Plastic surgery in the elderly. *Clinics in Geriatric Medicine, 6(3)*, 633–657.

41. Steuer, K. (1991). Facial fractures. *AORN Journal, 54(4)*, 773–795.

42. Teimourian, K. (1989). Complications associated with suction lipectomy. *Clinics in Plastic Surgery, 16(2)*, 385–394.

43. Vander Kam, V., & Achauer, B. (1990). Lasers in plastic surgery: Applications and nursing interventions. *Plastic Surgical Nursing, 10(3)*, 107–111, 125.

44. Walsh, K. (1991). Breast reconstruction using the latissimus dorsi flap. *Plastic Surgical Nursing, 11(2)*, 43–51.

45. Waltman, N. (1994). Treatment options for the patient with breast cancer. *Plastic Surgical Nursing, 14(1)*, 15–26.

46. Watson, D., & James, D. (1990). Intravenous conscious sedation. *AORN Journal, 51(6)*, 1512–1523.

47. Westlake, C. (1991). Commitment to function: Microsurgical flaps. *Plastic Surgical Nursing, 11(3)*, 95–100.

48. Whedon, M. A. (1995). What do you do to expedite discharge after surgery? *Oncology Nursing Forum, 22(1)*, 147–150.

49. Whitman, M. (1994). Breast surgery: Helping patients choose. *Nursing 94, 24(8)*, 25.

50. Williams, L. (1991). Mastopexy. *Plastic Surgical Nursing, 11(3)*, 130–132.

51. Williams, L., & Peters, C. (1989). Blepharoplasty. *Plastic Surgical Nursing, 9(1)*, 28–30.

52. Williams, L., & Peters, C. (1989). Rhinoplasty. *Plastic Surgical Nursing, 9(2)*, 82–85.

53. Williams, L., & Peters, C. (1989). Rhytidectomy. *Plastic Surgical Nursing, 9(4)*, 163–165.

54. Williams, L., & Peters, C. (1990). Reduction mammaplasty. *Plastic Surgical Nursing, 10(2)*, 84–87.

UNIT 15

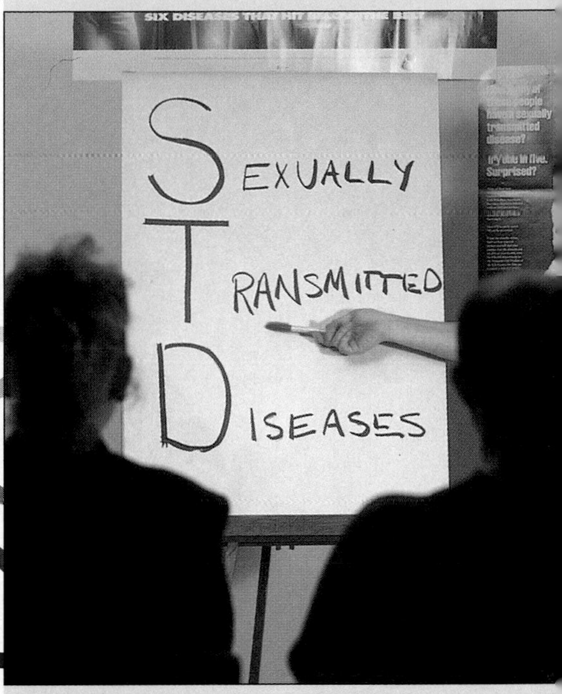

Reproductive Disorders

Clients experiencing disorders of sexual structure and function are often reluctant to tell anyone about their problems because of shyness, embarrassment, and fear that private, sexual aspects of their lives will need to be discussed. Thus, unless symptoms become acute, these clients often put off seeking the help of health professionals.

When helping a client with reproductive and sexually related problems, the nurse must remember to consider the client's psychosocial as well as physical needs. A nurse who cannot discuss reproduction and sexuality openly and nonjudgmentally should refer the client to a health professional who can. Nurses who feel uncomfortable talking about these topics need to find ways to clarify their own feelings and attitudes about sexuality and thus increase their professional competency. Nurses have no business judging clients' sexual behavior, but rather should focus on helping clients achieve satisfactory sexual functioning in ways that each individual client finds comfortable and desirable.

The chapters in this unit cover assessment of female and male sexual and reproductive function and nursing care of clients with reproductive disorders, sexually transmitted diseases, and breast disorders.

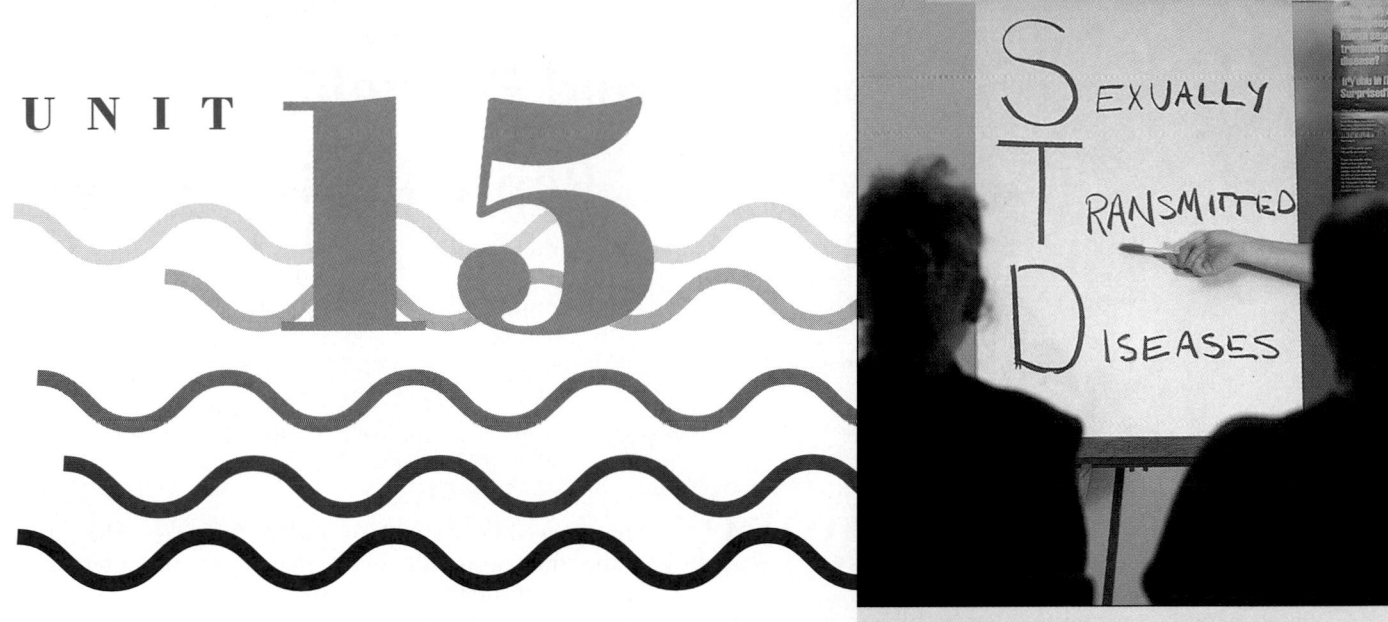

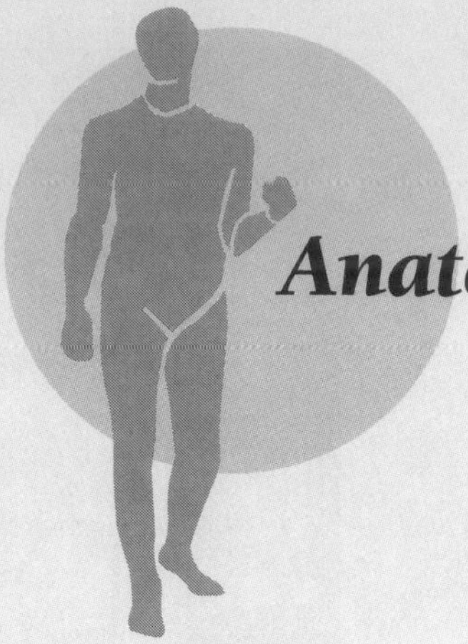

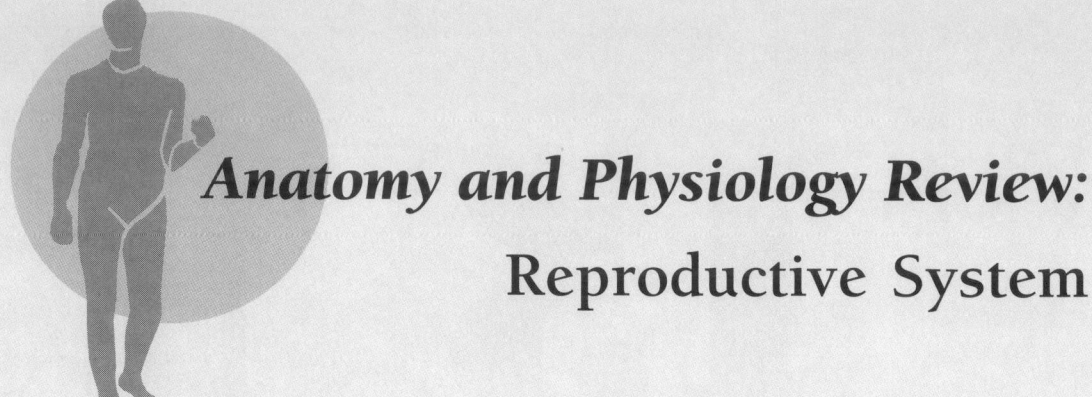

Anatomy and Physiology Review: Reproductive System

FEMALE REPRODUCTIVE SYSTEM

The organs of the female reproductive system produce and sustain egg cells, transport these cells, provide a favorable environment for developing offspring, move the offspring to the outside at the end of prenatal development, and produce the female sex hormones.

Gonads

The female gonads are the ovaries, which produce the female reproductive cells, the ova, and the hormones estrogen and progesterone. The ovaries are about the size and shape of an almond and are located in shallow depressions in the lateral walls of the pelvic cavity. They are held loosely in place by peritoneal ligaments. The substance of the ovaries is indistinctly divided into an outer cortex, which contains ovarian follicles with oocytes in various stages of development, and an inner medulla, which is loose connective tissue with blood vessels, lymphatic vessels, and nerves. All follicles develop before birth and remain dormant until puberty. Thereafter, one or more follicles resume development each month to become mature vesicular (graafian) follicles. A mature follicle ruptures to release its oocyte and a few cells in a process of ovulation. The remaining follicular cells become a glandular structure called the corpus luteum. This eventually degenerates to become scar tissue, the corpus albicans.

Internal Reproductive Tract

The female internal reproductive tract includes the uterine tubes, uterus, and vagina. There are two uterine tubes, also called fallopian tubes or oviducts, one extending laterally from each side of the uterus to the region of the ovary on that side. The end near the ovary expands to form an infundibulum, which is surrounded by finger-like extensions called fimbriae. The uterine tube transports the ovulated cell to the uterus. The journey through the uterine tube takes about 7 days. Because the oocyte is fertile for only 24 to 48 hours, fertilization usually occurs in the tube.

The hollow, thick-walled, muscular uterus looks like an inverted pear. It receives the fertilized ovum and provides an appropriate environment for the developing fetus. The upper, bulging surface of the uterus is the fundus. The large main portion is the body and the narrow region that is directed inferiorly is the cervix. The cervix opens into the vagina through the external os. Normally, the nonpregnant premenopausal uterus is anteverted and anteflexed. The wall of the uterus has three functional layers. The outer layer, the perimetrium, is a thin peritoneal membrane covering of the uterus. The middle layer, the myometrium, forms the bulk of the uterus and is composed of smooth muscle. The mucous membrane lining the inner surface of the uterus is the endometrium. A fertilized ovum implants in the endometrium. When the ovum is not fertilized, the endometrium sloughs off during menstruation.

The vagina is a musculomembranous canal that connects the uterus with the external genitalia. The mucosa of the inner surface of the vaginal wall folds over in small ridges called rugae to add to the vagina's elasticity, making it distensible. The elasticity diminishes with age during the menopausal and postmenopausal years.

External Genitalia

The external genitalia are also referred to as the vulva or pudendum and include the labia majora, mons pubis, labia minora, clitoris, and glands within the vestibule. The labia majora are two large fat-filled folds of skin that enclose the other external genitalia. Anteriorly, the labia majora merge to form the mons pubis, a rounded elevation of fat that overlies the pubic symphysis. After puberty, the mons pubis is covered with hair. The labia

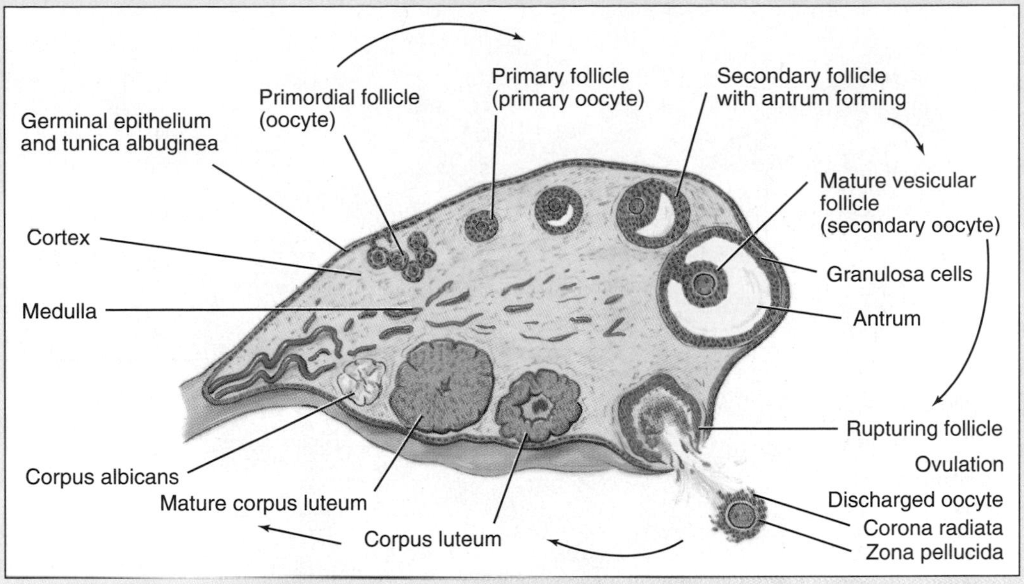

Structure of an ovary, showing stages of follicle development.

minora are two smaller folds of skin medial to the labia majora. The area between the two minora is the vestibule. At the anterior end of the vestibule, there is a small mass of erectile tissue called the clitoris, which is homologous to the male penis and becomes erect in response to sexual stimulation. Posterior to the clitoris, the urethra and vagina open into the vestibule. Openings for paraurethral (Skene's) glands, which secrete mucus, lie on either side of the urethral orifice. Adjacent to the vaginal orifice, the greater vestibular glands (Bartholin's glands) open into the vestibule. These glands produce a mucus-like secretion in response to sexual stimulation.

Breast

The female breast, which contains the mammary glands and varying amounts of adipose, extends from the second to the sixth rib and overlies the pectoralis major muscle. Externally, each breast has a raised nipple surrounded by a circular pigmented area called the are-

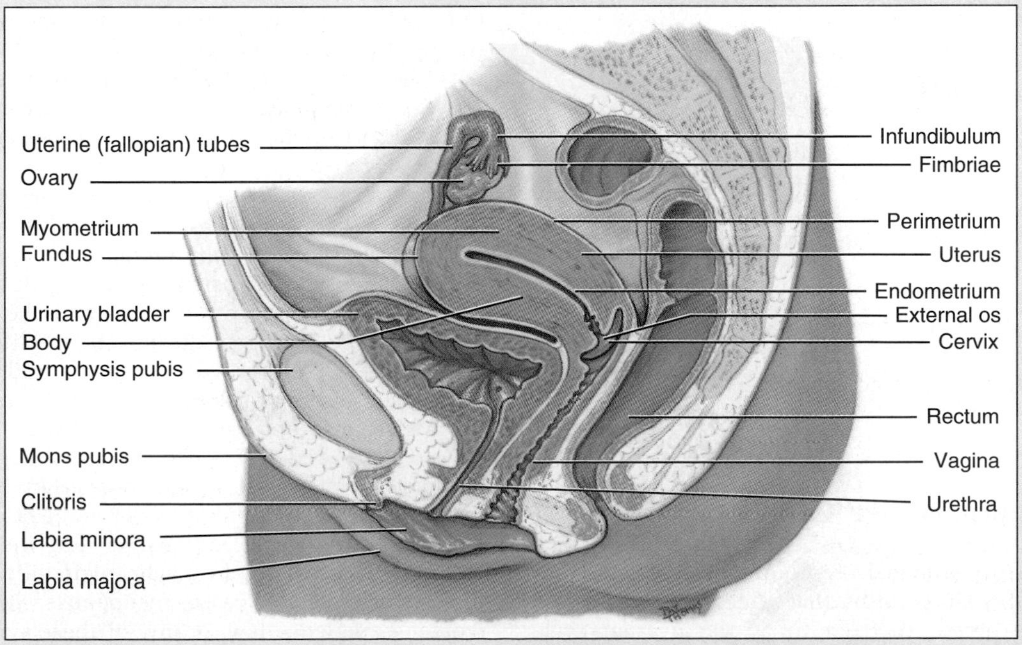

Organs of the female reproductive system.

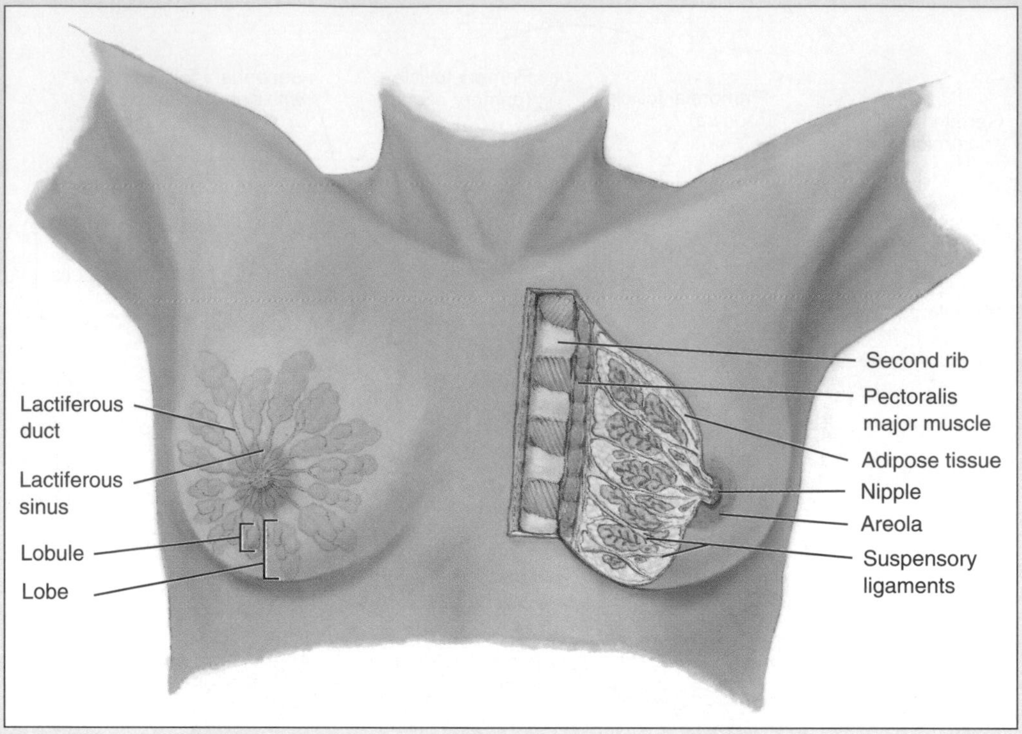

Breast and mammary glands. (From Jarvis, C. [1992]. *Physical examination and health assessment.* Philadelphia: W. B. Saunders Co.)

ola. The mammary glands, located within the breast, consist of lobules of glandular units that produce milk. Lactiferous ducts transport the milk to the nipple. Hormones are responsible for physiologic changes that affect the breast. These changes are related to (1) growth and development, (2) the menstrual cycle, and (3) pregnancy and lactation. Estrogen and progesterone stimulate the development of glandular tissue and ducts in the breast. Prolactin stimulates the production of milk, and oxytocin causes the ejection of milk.

Hormonal Control

The hypothalamus, anterior pituitary gland, and ovaries secrete hormones that have significant roles in the control of reproductive functions. The hypothalamus secretes gonadotropin-releasing hormone (Gn-RH), which stimulates the anterior pituitary gland; the anterior pituitary gland secretes follicle-stimulating hormone (FSH) and luteinizing hormone (LH), which stimulate the development of the ovarian follicles and corpus luteum; and the ovaries secrete the sex hormones estrogen and progesterone.

Female Reproductive Cycles

The secretion of the female reproductive hormones follows monthly cyclic patterns that affect the ovaries and uterus. These cycles, referred to as the ovarian cycle and the menstrual (uterine) cycle begin at puberty when certain unknown stimuli cause the hypothalamus to start secreting Gn-RH. In females, the beginning of puberty is marked by the first period of menstrual bleeding, called menarche. After this the cycles continue, more or less regularly, for about 40 years until they become increasingly irregular and finally stop. Menopause is the cessation of the reproductive cycles.

The ovarian cycle reflects the changes that occur within the ovaries. It begins with follicle development during the follicular phase, continues with ovulation during the ovulatory phase, and concludes with the development and regression of the corpus luteum during the luteal phase. Each of these phases is accompanied by corresponding changes in estrogen and progesterone secretion.

The menstrual (uterine) cycle takes place simultaneously with the ovarian cycle and is the result of estrogen and progesterone secretion by the ovaries. The cycle begins with menstrual bleeding during the menstrual phase, continues with repair of the endometrium stimulated by estrogen during the proliferative phase, and ends with the growth of glands and blood vessels stimulated by progesterone during the secretory phase.

Menopause occurs when the ovaries stop responding to FSH and LH from the pituitary gland. It is marked by decreased levels of ovarian hormones and increased levels of pituitary FSH and LH. The changing hormone levels are responsible for the hot flashes, sweating, depression, headache, irritability, and insomnia often associated with menopause; however, many women experience few, if any, of these symptoms.

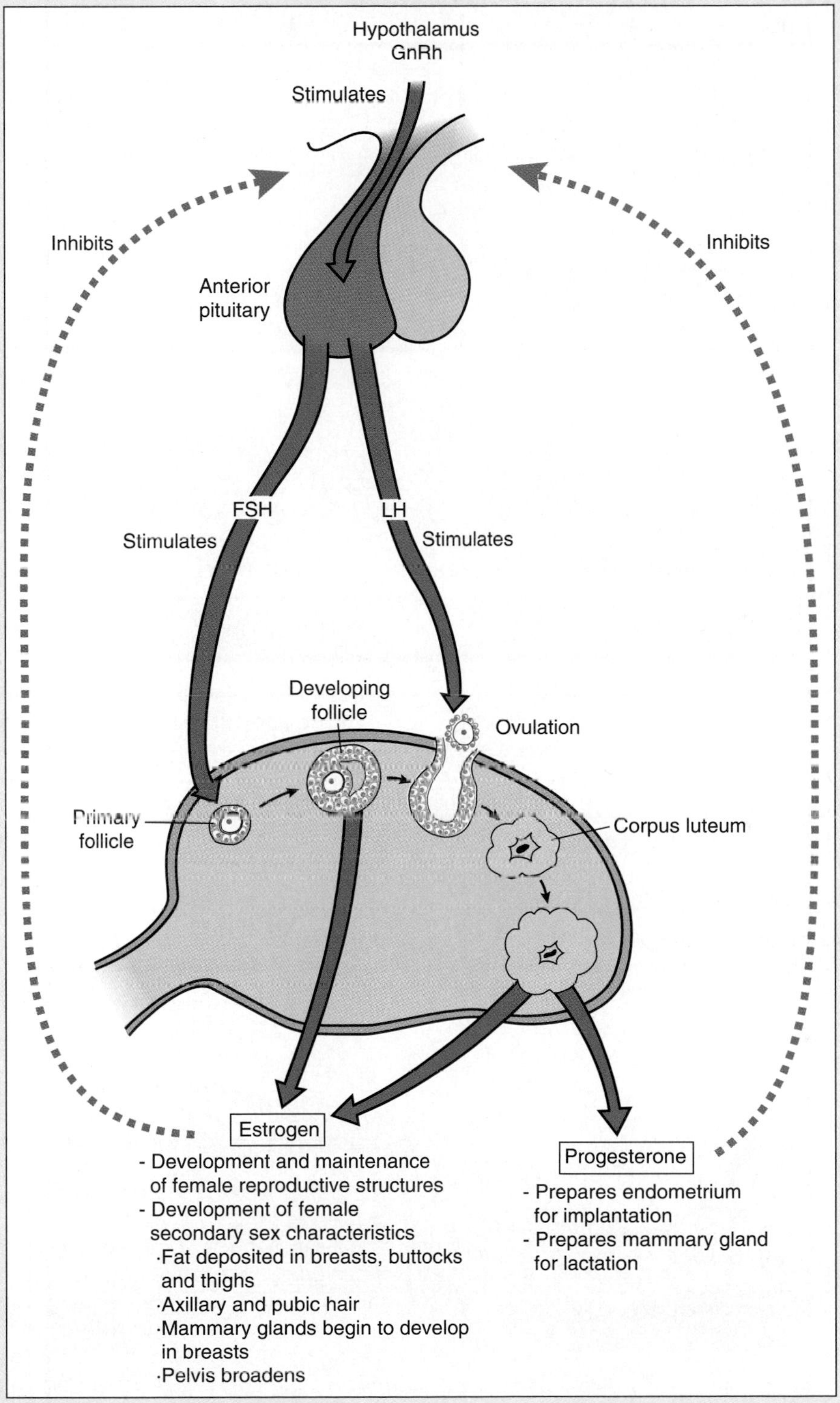
Hypothalamus
GnRh
Stimulates
Inhibits
Inhibits
Anterior
pituitary
FSH
LH
Stimulates
Stimulates
Developing
follicle
Ovulation
Primary
follicle
Corpus luteum
Estrogen
Progesterone
- Development and maintenance of female reproductive structures
- Development of female secondary sex characteristics
·Fat deposited in breasts, buttocks and thighs
·Axillary and pubic hair
·Mammary glands begin to develop in breasts
·Pelvis broadens
- Prepares endometrium for implantation
- Prepares mammary gland for lactation

Hormonal regulation of female reproductive functions.

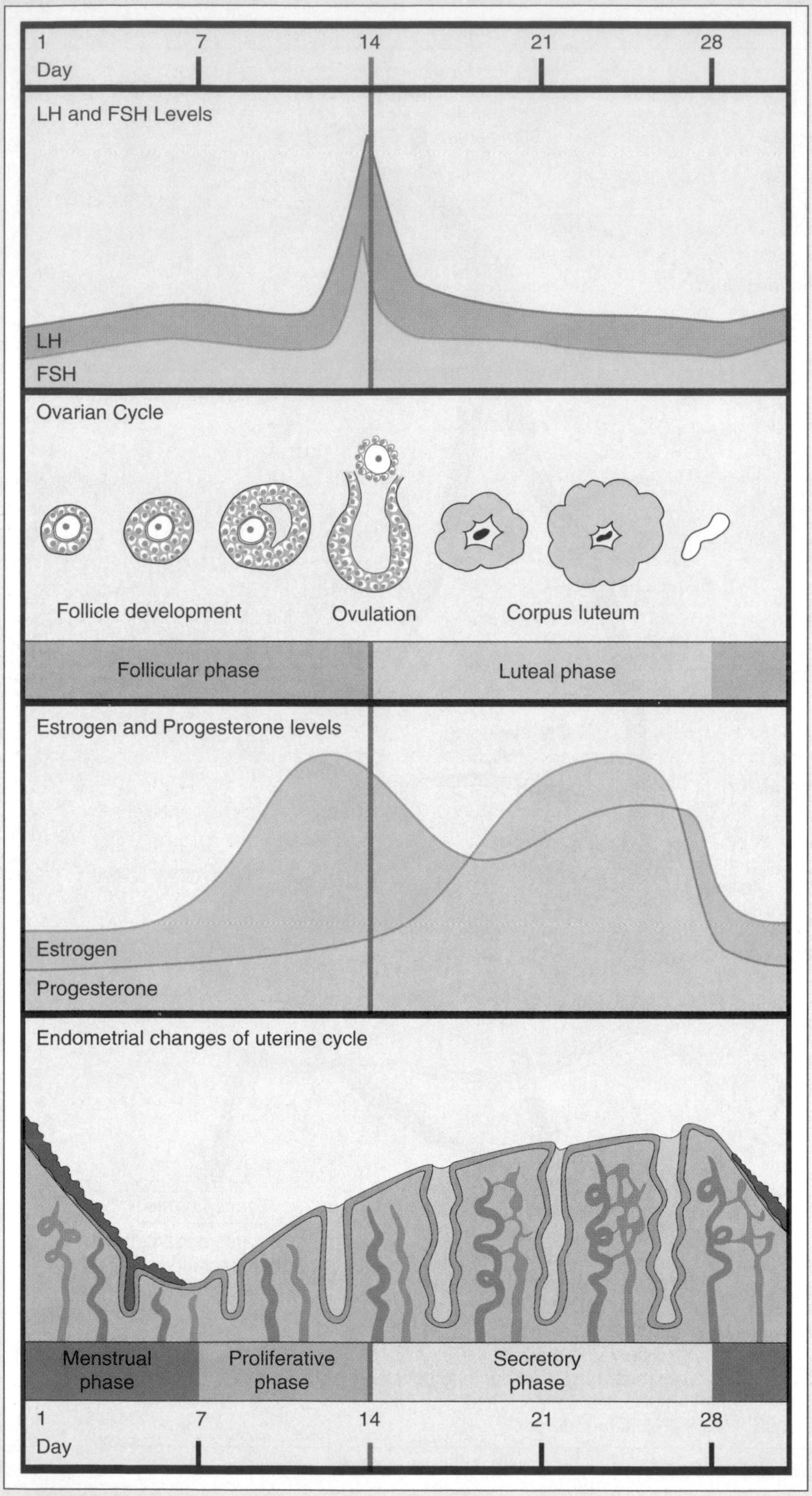

Correlation of events in the ovarian and uterine cycles.

MALE REPRODUCTIVE SYSTEM

The male reproductive system produces, sustains, and transports sperm; introduces the sperm into the female vagina; and produces the male sex hormones.

Gonads

The male gonads are the testes, which produce the male reproductive cells, the sperm, and the male sex hormones, principally testosterone. Shortly before birth, the testes descend from the abdominal cavity, through the inguinal canal, and into the scrotum, a pouch of skin that extends below the abdomen and posterior to the penis. This location provides a temperature about 3° C lower than normal body temperature. The lower temperature is necessary for the production of viable sperm.

The testes are divided into lobules packed with one to four highly coiled seminiferous tubules, where the sperm are produced. Interstitial cells (Leydig's cells), which produce the male sex hormones, are located between the seminiferous tubules within a lobule. Sperm production begins at puberty and continues throughout the life of a male.

Internal Reproductive Tract

The male internal reproductive tract includes the epididymis, ductus deferens, ejaculatory duct, and urethra. Sperm leave the testes through a series of ducts that enter the epididymis, a tightly coiled comma-shaped organ located along the superior and posterior margins of the testes. Here the sperm complete their maturation process, become fertile, and are stored.

The ductus deferens, also called vas deferens, is a fibromuscular tube that begins at the bottom of the epididymis, enters the abdominal cavity through the inguinal canal, passes over the urinary bladder, and descends along the posterior bladder toward the prostate. Just before it reaches the prostate gland, each ductus deferens joins the duct from the adjacent seminal vesicle to form a short ejaculatory duct. Each ejaculatory duct penetrates the prostate gland and empties into the urethra. The male urethra is a passageway for sperm, fluids from the accessory glands, and urine. The urethra is divided into the prostatic urethra, which is within the prostate gland; a short membranous urethra, which passes through the pelvic floor; and the penile (spongy) urethra, which extends the length of the penis.

Accessory Glands

The accessory glands of the male reproductive system are the seminal vesicles, prostate gland, and the bulbourethral glands. These glands secrete fluids that enter the urethra. The paired seminal vesicles are saccular glands posterior to the urinary bladder. The fluid from the seminal vesicles is alkaline, viscous, and contains fructose that provides an energy source for the sperm, prostaglandins that contribute to the motility and viability of the sperm, and proteins that cause slight coagulation reactions in the semen after ejaculation. The prostate gland is a firm, dense structure that is located just inferior to the urinary bladder. The secretions of the prostate are alkaline, thin, and milky-colored. They enhance the motility of sperm. The paired bulbourethral (Cowper's) glands are small and located near the base of the penis. In response to sexual stimulation, they secrete an alkaline mucus-like fluid that neutralizes the acidity of urine residue in the urethra, helps to neutralize the acidity of the vagina, and provides some lubrication for the tip of the penis during intercourse.

Seminal fluid, or semen, is the slightly alkaline (pH 7.5) mixture of sperm cells and secretions from the

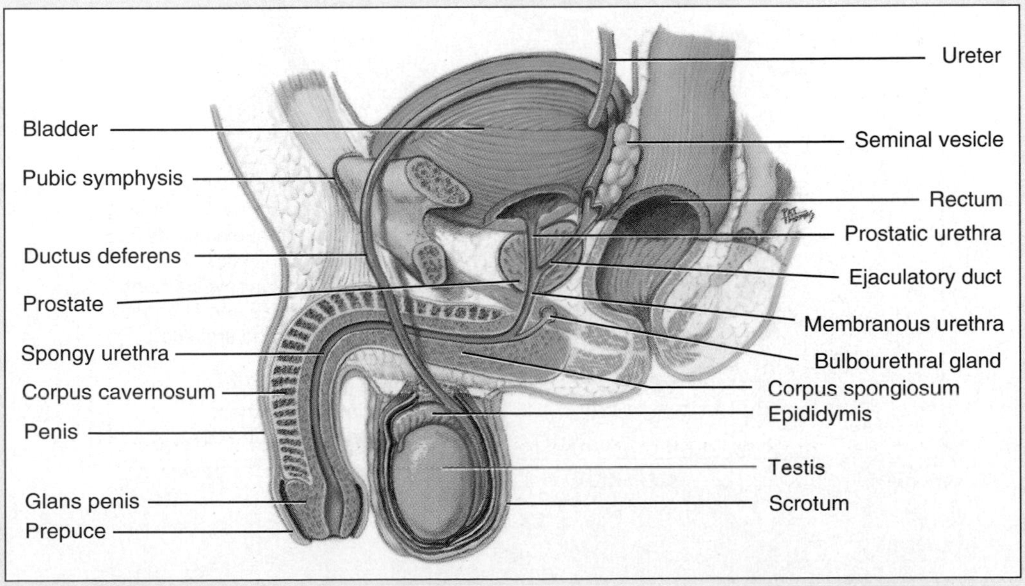

Structures in the male reproductive system.

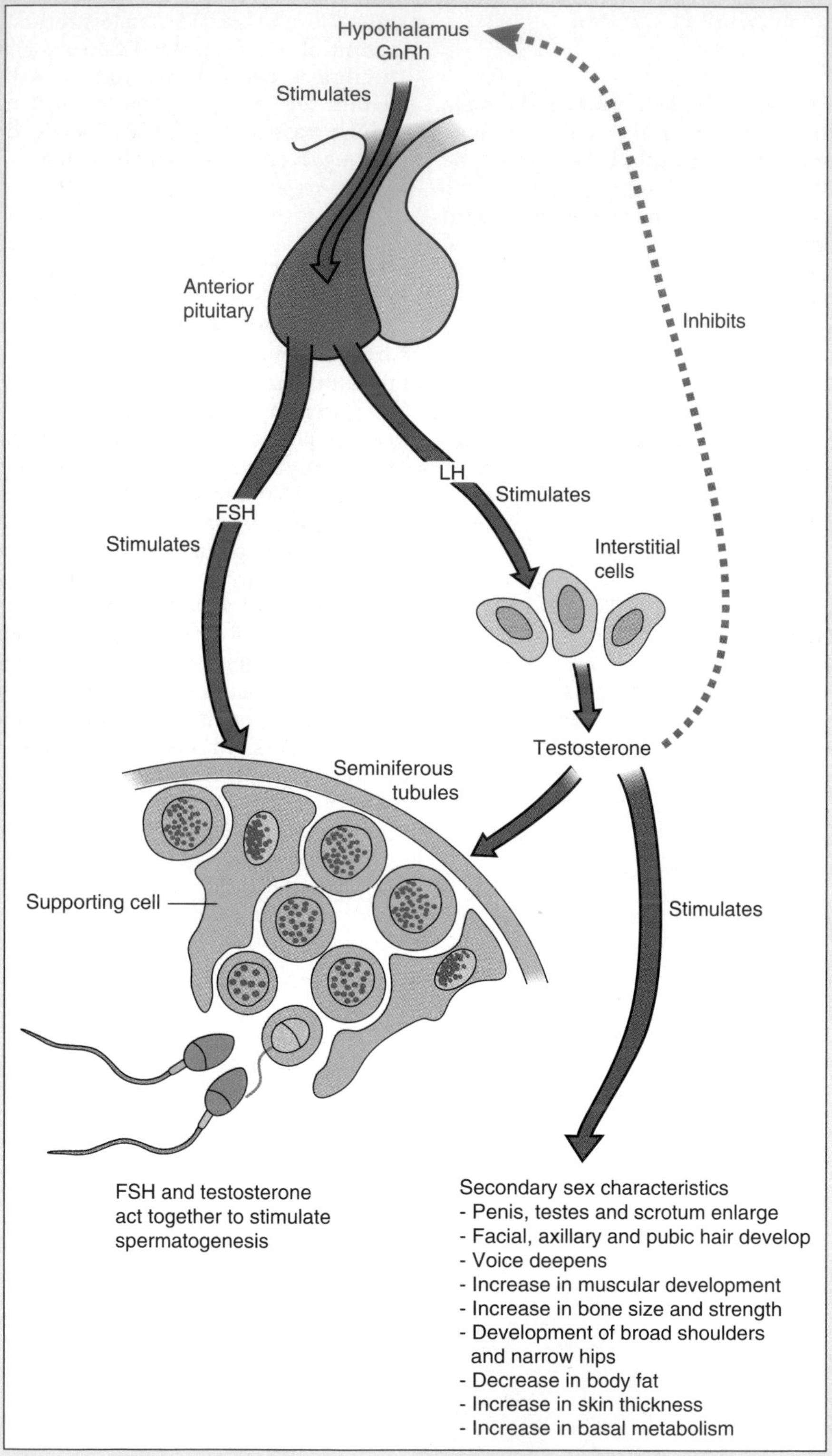

Hormonal regulation of testicular function.

accessory glands. Secretions from the seminal vesicles make up about 60 per cent of the volume; the remainder comes from the prostate gland. Sperm and secretions from the bulbourethral glands contribute very little volume. After ejaculation of seminal fluid, sperm can live within the vagina for 24 to 48 hours.

Penis

The penis, the male copulatory organ, is a cylindrical pendant organ located anterior to the scrotum. It functions to transfer sperm to the vagina. The penis consists of three columns of erectile tissue that engorge with blood under parasympathetic stimulation to produce an erection. The two dorsal columns are the corpora cavernosa, and the single midline ventral column surrounding the penile urethra is the corpus spongiosum. The root of the penis attaches it to the pubic arch, the body is the visible pendant portion, and the distal expanded end of the corpus spongiosum is the glans penis. A loose fold of skin, the prepuce, covers the glans penis.

Hormonal Control

The hypothalamus, anterior pituitary gland, and testes secrete hormones that have significant roles in the control of male reproductive functions. The relationship between these areas is sometimes referred to as the brain-testicular axis. The sequence of events that triggers the onset of puberty is unknown, but it begins when the hypothalamus starts secreting gonadotropin-releasing hormone (Gn-RH), which stimulates the anterior pituitary gland; the anterior pituitary gland secretes follicle-stimulating hormone (FSH) and luteinizing hormone (LH), which stimulate the testes; and the testes secrete androgens, primarily testosterone. Testosterone is responsible for the development and maintenance of male secondary sex characteristics.

AGE-RELATED CHANGES

In women, most of the changes associated with aging are believed to be caused by a reduction in estrogen. The ovaries undergo progressive atrophy. The uterus becomes smaller, and fibrous connective tissue replaces some of the myometrium. The vagina becomes narrower, and its walls become thinner and less elastic. The reduction in estrogen also appears to affect nonreproductive organs, particularly bones and blood vessels, leading to increased incidence of osteoporosis and cardiovascular disease.

Men normally do not experience a sudden decline in reproductive function comparable to menopause in women. Instead, they experience a gradual and subtle decline over many years. There may be some testicular atrophy, partially due to a decrease in the size of the seminiferous tubules and partially due to a reduction in the number of interstitial cells. These changes are accompanied by a decline in sperm and testosterone production. The portion of the prostate gland that surrounds the urethra often enlarges and may constrict the urethra, making urination difficult. Although age-related physical and hormonal changes take place in the reproductive systems of both men and women, studies demonstrate that sexuality remains important to many older people.

Chapter 51 Assessment of Clients with Reproductive Disorders

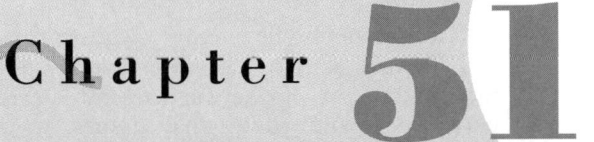

Learning Outcomes

After completing this chapter, the learner will be able to:

1. Establish an effective rapport and an empathetic client approach through an understanding of the special concerns of clients with reproductive disorders.
2. Conduct a systematic assessment of a client with reproductive disorders, including history and physical examination.
3. Teach the client about self-assessment techniques and preventive health maintenance.
4. Make appropriate referrals when manifestations of disorders are found.

Assessing Women Experiencing Gynecologic Conditions

In recent years, there has been an increased emphasis on women's health concerns and on the importance of health promotion activities for women. Because many women receive most, if not all, of their primary health care with reproductive care, nurses participating in this area of health care must focus not only on the gynecologic condition but also on the woman's total health maintenance needs. A thorough assessment includes the usual health history and physical examination as well as a review of the woman's life-style, health habits, self-perception, body image, and developmental stage with consideration of cultural, religious, socioeconomic, and educational factors. These factors influence the woman's health and health-seeking behaviors. A nonjudgmental attitude and respect for the woman's values will allow the nurse to provide more effective care. The woman's cultural or ethnic background, socioeconomic status, or sexual preference should not limit her access to or quality of health care.

Psychosocial Impact of Gynecologic Problems

For many women, the genital organs and reproductive capacity have symbolic significance, affecting their sexuality and sense of femininity. Gynecologic problems may be associated with changes in a woman's self-concept, body image, personal identity, and role performance. Reproductive capabilities and the experience of sexuality and sexual activities may be affected. There may be psychosocial consequences for some women experiencing gynecologic disorders. For this reason, psychological assessment is especially important. A woman's outward reaction to gynecologic problems does not necessarily correlate with either her inner experience or the seriousness of the condition.

Sensitivity is vital in interviewing a woman. Remember that the woman herself may not understand her own responses. Empathetic listening is supportive, often lessening the stress the woman experiences.

Fear may be expressed because of a suspicion the woman holds of unhealthy changes in the genitals or of unwanted pregnancy. Women may consider the pelvic examination unpleasant despite the insignificant risk of injury or physical pain. Other feelings that may be expressed include humiliation, guilt, or anger. In the event of deep, powerful feelings, women may avoid seeking gynecologic care. Many women have never received accurate information about reproductive problems.

Approach to Gynecologic Care

Women have the right to be informed and to participate actively in decisions about their health. A supportive, respectful attitude on the part of the nurse promotes the woman's participation in her care and cooperation. The nurse also is alert for sexist attitudes in the health-care system, which may lead to women's health complaints being ignored or unnecessary prescriptions being written. The nurse can act as an advocate for the woman, positively influencing her perception of health care and the importance of health maintenance. Common misconceptions include the following:

- Surgical removal of the uterus means that menopause will begin
- An extensive hysterectomy (without vaginectomy) ends sexual activity (an extensive hysterectomy removes the top of the vagina, the uterus, and the paracervical and paravaginal tissues; a vaginectomy removes one third to one half of the vagina)
- Removing reproductive organs makes a woman less womanly
- Removing one ovary produces sterility
- A suspicious Papanicolaou (Pap) test always means cancer

Providing privacy and creating an environment that is conducive to the expression of feelings allow a woman to discuss her concerns openly. It is important to assess the woman's understanding of health-care information and to elicit her perception of her needs and problems. The nurse may need to repeat information, especially if the woman is anxious or stressed, for example, when information is received during a pelvic examination. Nurses can provide a sensitive, humane orientation to gynecologic health care.

The annual gynecologic examination provides opportunity for the nurse to discuss health maintenance activities with women. For example, a health visit for a Pap smear is a good time to teach breast self-examination (BSE) as well as self-examination of the external genitalia and to talk about risk factors associated with gynecologic cancer. It also is a good time to provide information about developmental changes such as adolescence, menarche, or menopause and about menstrual hygiene and menstrual symptom management. Information on the ways the woman can promote her health through diet, exercise, adequate sleep and rest, stress management, cessation of smoking, and general risk factor identification also should be discussed. If appropriate, the nurse provides the client with information about protection against sexually transmitted diseases (STDs).

Gynecologic Assessment

After establishing rapport with the woman, the nurse performs a comprehensive gynecologic nursing assessment appropriate to the situation. This information is a basis for nursing intervention.

HISTORY

Chief Complaint

The client is asked to describe her problem in her own words. These data alert the nurse to the possible nature of the client's problem as well as to the level of the client's understanding of the problem. This information provides direction for the nurse during the remainder of the health history interview. The nurse asks the client to relate the history of the problem, including a symptom analysis.

Medical History

The medical health history has many components significant to the reproductive system. These include childhood and infectious diseases, immunizations, major illnesses and hospitalizations, medications, allergies, gynecologic and obstetric history, family history, psychosocial history, and review of systems.

CHILDHOOD AND INFECTIOUS ILLNESSES

The most common childhood infectious illness to affect a woman of childbearing age is rubella. The nurse specifically asks whether the client has had rubella or has been immunized against it.

MAJOR ILLNESSES AND HOSPITALIZATIONS

The nurse asks the client about major illnesses such as diabetes, hypertension, thrombophlebitis, angina, anemia, thyroid disorders, cholecystitis, hepatitis, and migraine headaches. Diabetes is associated with increased morbidity and mortality in women who are pregnant or who take oral contraceptives. Pregnancy and oral contraceptive use also are linked with higher morbidity and mortality rates in women with a history of cardiovascular diseases such as angina, hypertension, and thrombophlebitis. Anemia can result from menstrual disorders such as dysfunctional uterine bleeding, or it can be aggravated even by normal menstruation. Endometrial implants (endometriosis) can cause painful menstruation and fertility problems so that the woman who wishes to become pregnant may need treatment with medication and surgery for the implants to be reduced or removed.

CRITICAL TO REMEMBER

Hypothyroidism and hyperthyroidism affect the menstrual cycle, as can other endocrine disorders.

Renal and urinary tract disorders can interfere with sexual function.

Women with a history of migraine headaches or seizure disorders should avoid oral contraceptives because of an associated increased risk of occurrence with their use. Cholecystitis may be aggravated by oral contraceptives; hepatitis and other liver disorders are a contraindication for taking estrogen because of its route of metabolism.

CRITICAL TO REMEMBER

The progesterones in oral contraceptives thicken respiratory secretions, which complicates the treatment of women with asthma or chronic obstructive respiratory disorders.

The nurse asks the client about surgery involving the reproductive system. The nurse must inquire about interruptions to pregnancies, such as planned or spontaneous abortion.

MEDICATIONS

A complete medication history is obtained for prescription, over-the-counter, and recreational drugs. Diuretics are often prescribed for women who are subject to premenstrual edema. There also are many over-the-counter preparations for premenstrual "bloating." Use of hormones should also be determined, such as thyroid preparations. Recreational drugs including amphetamines, barbiturates, marijuana, and other hallucinogens can affect sexual behavior and physiologic function of the reproductive system.

ALLERGIES

The nurse asks the client specifically about allergies to penicillin, sulfonamides, and latex or rubber. Genitourinary disorders such as vaginitis and urinary tract infections are often treated with penicillin and sulfa compounds. Latex and rubber are used in contraceptive devices such as diaphragms and some condoms; allergy eliminates their use for contraception.

GYNECOLOGIC HISTORY

Adaptations should be made for the woman who has had a hysterectomy or is menopausal.

Breast History. The nurse should ask the client about breast pain or tenderness and its occurrence in relation to the menstrual cycle. Many women experience breast tenderness before menses onset. The nurse should also inquire whether the woman has had or currently has breast lumps or masses. If a lump is present, the woman should be asked to describe its location, onset, and size and whether it is painful. The nurse should determine whether the lump has changed shape, size, consistency, or amount of tenderness since it was first noticed and whether the lump changes during the menstrual cycle. The woman should be asked the date of her last menstrual period to better evaluate a breast lump.

CRITICAL TO REMEMBER

The breasts become more firm and cystic during the luteal phase so that the best time to perform breast palpation is 7 to 10 days after menses onset.

The nurse also asks about discharge from the nipple. Nipple discharge is abnormal in women who are not pregnant or lactating. If discharge is present, color, consistency, amount, and odor must be determined.

The nurse should inquire about the practice of breast self-examination on a monthly basis, asking not only about frequency of performance but also about technique to determine whether the woman could benefit from a review of the procedure and supervised practice. The nurse should note whether the woman includes the axillary nodes as part of her self-examination. Last, she should be asked whether there is a history of breast cancer in blood-related female relatives, such as mother, sister, maternal aunts, or maternal grandmother. Incidence of breast cancer in these relatives increases a woman's risk of breast cancer occurrence.

Menstrual History. The nurse should determine the woman's age at menarche and document the woman's usual duration of menses, amount and type of flow, interval between menses, and any dysmenorrhea, premenstrual symptoms, or menopausal symptoms.

Contraceptive History. The nurse documents the woman's current contraceptive method (if any), her satisfaction with the method, duration of use, any contraceptive problems, and any desire to change methods. She should be asked about previous contraceptive methods, problems encountered, and reason for discontinuation and whether she wants any contraceptive information. For women at risk for pregnancy (those of reproductive age, not sterilized, and heterosexually active), the nurse should determine whether they wish to become pregnant.

Sexual History. After careful psychosocial and environmental preparation, the nurse obtains a sexual history using a direct approach and terms the woman understands. The purpose of a sexual history is to identify sexual problems and give the woman an opportunity to ask questions or express concerns. The nurse begins with general questions about whether the woman is satisfied and comfortable with her current sexual activity. A nonjudgmental approach is essential. The nurse should follow up on any concerns or issues the client raises (Table 51–1).

Obstetric History. If the woman is in her childbearing years, the nurse must ask whether she thinks she may be pregnant. (Pregnancy may contraindicate mammography or other radiologic studies.) If the woman has been pregnant, information about each pregnancy should be obtained, including the delivery and postpartum period. Details of any difficulties or complications (physical or psychosocial) should be documented. Any spontaneous abortions or voluntarily interrupted pregnancies should be recorded. If the woman has never been pregnant or has no living children, the nurse should ask whether children were or are desired. If the woman has relinquished a child for adoption, the nurse should explore her feelings about it.

Gynecologic-Genitourinary History. The nurse asks about previous problems with genitourinary infections and vaginitis. The nurse should determine whether the woman has had a previous pelvic infection and, if so, the treatment prescribed. The woman should be asked whether she previously had an STD and about problems or complications resulting from the disease. The nurse should determine whether the woman experiences urinary incontinence and the circumstances when incontinence occurs. Chapter 29 discusses assessment of urinary incontinence.

Reproductive Health Practices. The nurse seeks information about menstrual, sexual, and gynecologic hygiene. The woman should be asked about the frequency of gynecologic examinations and whether she performs monthly breast self-examination as necessary. The nurse should determine whether the woman protects herself against STDs, if appropriate.

Family History

A number of diseases with a familial tendency can affect the reproductive system. In addition to breast cancer, the nurse asks about other types of cancer, especially of the reproductive organs. Also, the nurse should inquire about diabetes mellitus, hypertension, cerebrovascular accidents (stroke), angina, myocardial infarction, anemia, and endocrine disorders, including hypo- and hyperthyroidism.

Women should be asked whether their mothers had a history of taking diethylstilbestrol (DES) during pregnancy. In utero exposure to DES is associated with increased incidence of cervical adenosis and adenocarcinoma of the cervix and vagina in these women.

Psychosocial History and Life-Style

Many factors in the psychosocial history can have an effect on reproductive function. The nurse assesses the following areas.

OCCUPATIONAL AND ENVIRONMENTAL FACTORS

Many toxic substances are known to affect or are suspected of affecting sexual function and reproductive ability adversely. The nurse must ask about exposure to chemicals and environmental pollutants.

HABITS

The nurse assesses the client's use of caffeine, alcohol, and cigarettes. These substances as well as numerous other drugs can be harmful to a developing fetus (see

TABLE 51–1 Sexual Health Assessment

Sexual health assessment may include consideration of the client's current

- Knowledge about sexuality
- Attitudes about sexuality and toward sexual partner(s)
- Level of comfort and feelings of adequacy regarding own sexuality
- Concerns about sexuality of significant others
- Perception of own sex role and that of sexual partner(s)
- Sexual self-concept as a female or male
- Fears and anxiety about intimacy and other aspects of sexuality
- Self-perception of own body (body image)
- Ability to function sexually (e.g., to obtain an erection and control ejaculation, to please sexual partner, to achieve pain-free orgasm, to reproduce, to obtain adequate contraception, to obtain sufficient vaginal lubrication, to give and receive effective sexual stimulation and pleasure)
- Typical sexual patterns and activities (e.g., partner choice [female, male, spouse, extramarital, multiple, single, same partner, different partners], frequency of sexual activity, type of sexual activity [vaginal, anal, oral, masturbation], partner satisfaction, self-satisfaction)
- Level of interest in sexual activity (sex drive)
- Level of satisfaction regarding current sexual opportunity and activity
- Physical health problems affecting sexuality (e.g., menstrual problems, pregnancy, medication, surgery [colostomy, surgical amputation, recent heart surgery or brain surgery], paralysis, illness [hypertension, diabetes, recent myocardial infarction, "stroke"], injury [recent spinal cord injury, recent head injury, burns, traumatic amputations], sexually transmitted disease, genitourinary problems)

Sexual History

There is no single approach to taking a sexual health history. Information obtained may relate to historical (past) information about the following:

Both Females and Males

- Pregnancies (information about unplanned pregnancies)
- Fertility management
- Genitourinary problems
- Sexually transmitted disease
- Sexual abuse (e.g., incest, rape, pedophilia, battering)
- Relationship-partner history (e.g., number of sexual partners, sexual orientation [bisexual, homosexual, heterosexual])
- First experience of sexual activity
- Early sexual development and influences
- Adolescent sexual experiences
- Sexual techniques used (e.g., masturbation, intercourse [oral, vaginal, anal])
- Role models for sexuality (e.g., peers, parents, guardians, famous people, advertising models)
- Spiritual-philosophical models influencing the client's sexuality

Females

History specific to menstruation, abortion, pregnancy

Males

History specific to impotence, nocturnal emissions

Ethical Issues in Nursing). Cigarette smoking has been linked to increased morbidity in women who also take oral contraceptives. Women who consume a high-fat diet have increased incidence of breast cancer.

Review of Systems

Before the physical examination, the nurse reviews the physical health history, proceeding from head to toe.

PHYSICAL EXAMINATION

A standard gynecologic examination includes the following physical assessment and laboratory data:

- Vital signs (temperature, pulse, respiration, blood pressure)
- Height
- Weight
- Complete blood count (CBC)
- Urinalysis
- Pelvic examination and Pap smear
- Physical assessment of heart, lungs, breasts and axillae, thyroid, and abdomen

Breast and Axilla Examination

The breast and axilla examination is an important part of the annual gynecologic examination. Good lighting is essential. Some examiners complete this portion of the examination before assessing the anterior lungs and heart. Because the breasts are sensitive and closely asso-

ETHICAL ISSUES IN NURSING

Should Pregnant Women Who Engage in Substance Abuse Be Held Liable for Damage to the Fetus?

The rights of procreation are continually challenged as technology allows more and more reproductive options. Much controversy exists around reproductive issues such as abortion, in vitro fertilization, surrogate motherhood, sperm banks, and genetic selection (to name a few). There is, however, controversy surrounding the right to reproduce that does not involve any modern technology. This controversy surrounds the responsibilities of the mother to her unborn baby.

Pregnant women who engage in substance abuse often are directly responsible for physical and mental handicaps with which their infants are born. These infants, who might otherwise have been healthy, will live their lives with disabilities that could have been prevented had their mothers not abused drugs or alcohol. Should such women be legally prosecuted for the harm they have inflicted on their children? Although a woman has a right to do with her own body what she wants, abusing toxic substances does not simply affect her body alone. Should a woman who gives birth to a baby addicted to cocaine and perhaps disabled for life be ordered by the courts not to ever procreate again? Is court-ordered sterilization ever ethically justified? Society has an obligation to help care for its members who are physically and mentally handicapped. Does society also have a responsibility to see that its members (however potential they might be) are not treated in such ways that intentional physical and mental handicaps result in order not to overburden the society? (Intentional means that had substance abuse not occurred, perhaps the handicaps might not have either.)

Nurses who care for infants and children who are handicapped from maternal substance abuse may develop negative feelings for the parents of such infants and children. It is hard to see the innocent suffer, no matter what the cause. It is very important that caregivers in these situations express their concerns and emotions in an arena in which it is safe to do so, for instance, in team care conferences or informal sessions with a peer or social worker.

ciated with sexuality, other nurses delay examining them until there has been more "hands-on" interaction with the client during the lungs and heart assessments and sequence this portion of the physical examination to follow the heart. The nurse instructs the client in this procedure while performing it. (See Chapter 55 for further information in breast self-examination.)

The nurse asks the client when the last menstrual period began. Breasts are usually tender the week before menses onset and the least tender the week after. If the client reports that one breast is tender, the nurse begins palpation with the opposite breast. Thorough examination requires the client to have both breasts exposed for bilateral comparison.

INSPECTION

The nurse begins inspecting the breasts while the client is seated (Fig. 51–1). The breasts are inspected for symmetry, size, shape, contour, skin characteristics, including vascular pattern, and nipple and areola characteristics in all positions.

The breasts are symmetric, although it is not unusual for one breast to be slightly larger than the other. They should point laterally and hang evenly between the third and fourth ribs with the nipples approximately level with the fourth intercostal space when the client sits with arms at the sides. With aging and loss of tissue elasticity, the breasts hang lower. Contour is even without signs of dimpling (retraction), masses, or surface flattening, which are abnormal. Skin color is the same as that of the abdomen. *Striae* (i.e., stretch marks from rapid skin stretching) may be present; recent striae are reddened, but they become paler with time. If venous patterns are noticeable, they should be symmetric. There should be no local areas of hyperpigmentation or edema.

The client is asked to raise the arms over the head while the nurse examines the lateral and under surfaces of each breast. The contraction of the pectoral muscles will emphasize any signs of retraction or skin flattening. Areas of redness or excoriation may be noted in women with large breasts from brassiere rubbing. The breasts should elevate evenly so that the areolae remain at the same level. The client is then asked to put her hands on her hips and press inward firmly while the nurse repeats inspection for masses, retraction, or skin flattening.

The *areolae* and *nipples* are inspected for size, shape and contour, symmetry, surface characteristics, and masses or lesions. *Areolae* are pink in light-skinned people and darker in dark-skinned clients. Slight asymmetry is common, but the nipples should point in symmetric directions. The shape is round or oval. Masses or lesions are abnormal. There may be prominence of *Montgomery's tubercles* around the nipple, which is normal. The *nipples* are round, equal in size, of the same color, soft, and smooth. If one or both nipples are inverted, the nurse asks whether this is a recent occurrence or has been present for a while and for how long. Recent nipple inversion is abnormal, and the client is referred to the physician for follow-up. There should be no rashes, crusts, cracks, or discharge unless the client is in the later stages of pregnancy, when *colostrum* (a yellowish fluid) may leak from the nipples.

The *axillae* are inspected for rashes, masses, and areas of unusual pigmentation, which should be absent. Axillary hair is present unless the client removes it.

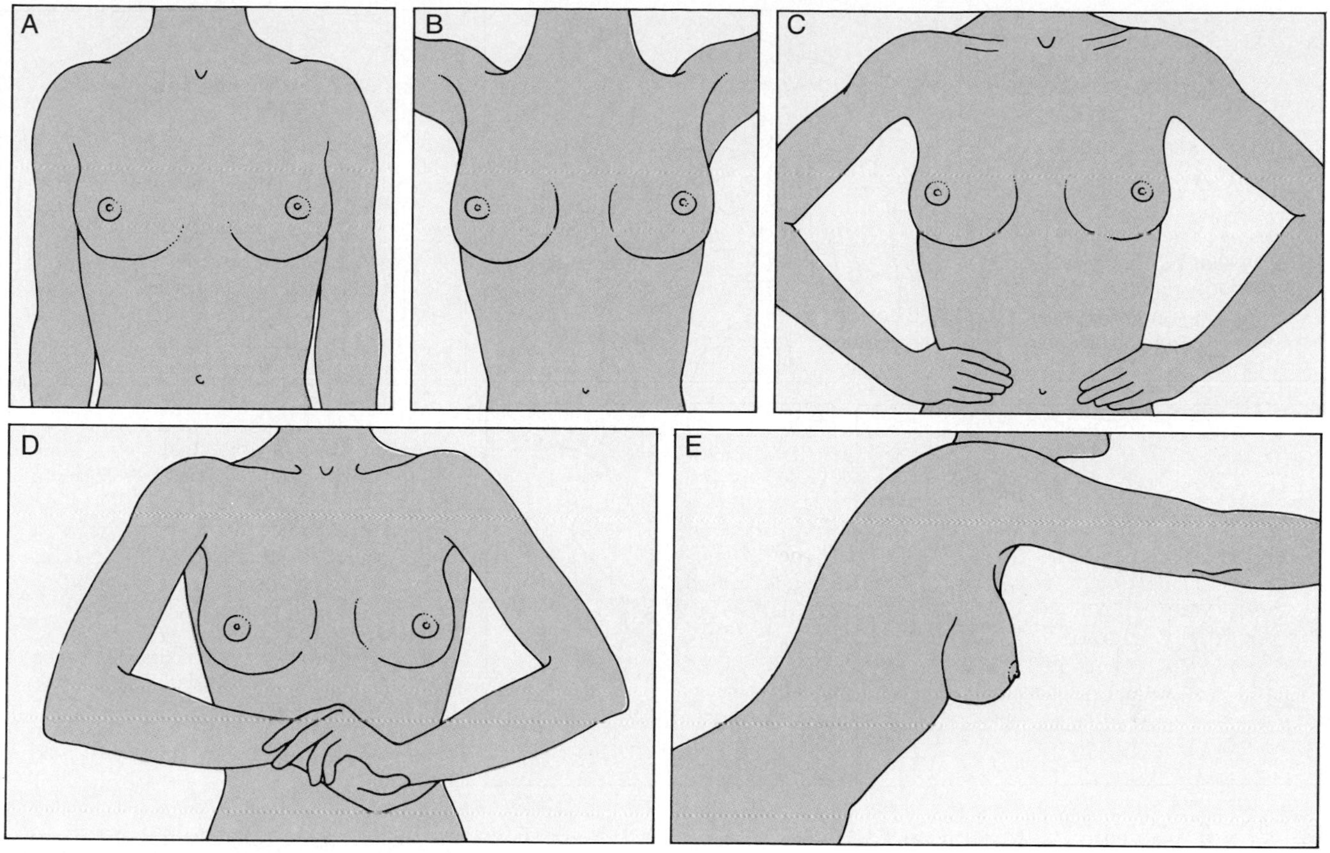

Figure 51–1
Positions for breast examination. *A,* Arms at sides. *B,* Hands raised over head. For tightening pectoral muscles, the examiner asks the client to press hands firmly on hips *(C)* or to press hands together *(D)*. *E,* Breasts can also be examined with the client leaning forward at the waist, allowing the breasts to hang down.

PALPATION

Palpation of axillae and breasts is done while the client is seated, although breast palpation is facilitated with the client supine. Clients with large and pendulous breasts, with a history of breast masses or cancer, or who are at increased risk for breast cancer should have their breasts palpated in both positions.

Palpation of the axillae includes examination of five sets of *lymph nodes,* which are illustrated in Figure 51–2. The client is encouraged to relax the arm, which assists in relaxing the muscles and eases palpation. All nodes should be nonpalpable, although the detection of one or two small, nontender, mobile central nodes is often normal. Abnormal findings include firm, fixed nodes that may or may not be tender. If nodes are palpated, the nurse notes the number of nodes felt, location, size, shape, mobility, tenderness, and consistency.

Breast palpation is conducted systematically so that all breast tissue, including the *tail of Spence* in the upper outer quadrant, is examined. The breast and areola may be palpated in concentric circles, in a wheel-and-spokes pattern, or back and forth from the superior to inferior aspects.

The nurse slides the fingers along the tissue using a rotary motion to press the breast against the chest wall. The fingers remain in contact with the skin surface. The nurse will feel a firm, curved ridge along the inferior breast, which is the *inframammary ridge.* Breast consistency varies from firm and elastic in young women to stringy and nodular in older women. If the client reports a mass, the nurse begins palpation with the unaffected breast so that there is a basis for comparison.

CRITICAL TO REMEMBER

The nurse pays particular attention to the upper outer quadrant and tail of Spence, where most of the glandular tissue is located and 50 per cent of breast lesions are found.

There should be no masses or local areas of increased warmth. If a lump or mass is felt, its characteristics are noted, including exact location (and the position the client is in for the palpation) with the areola for a reference point, size, shape, contour, consistency, mobility, tenderness, and discreteness. The breast can be

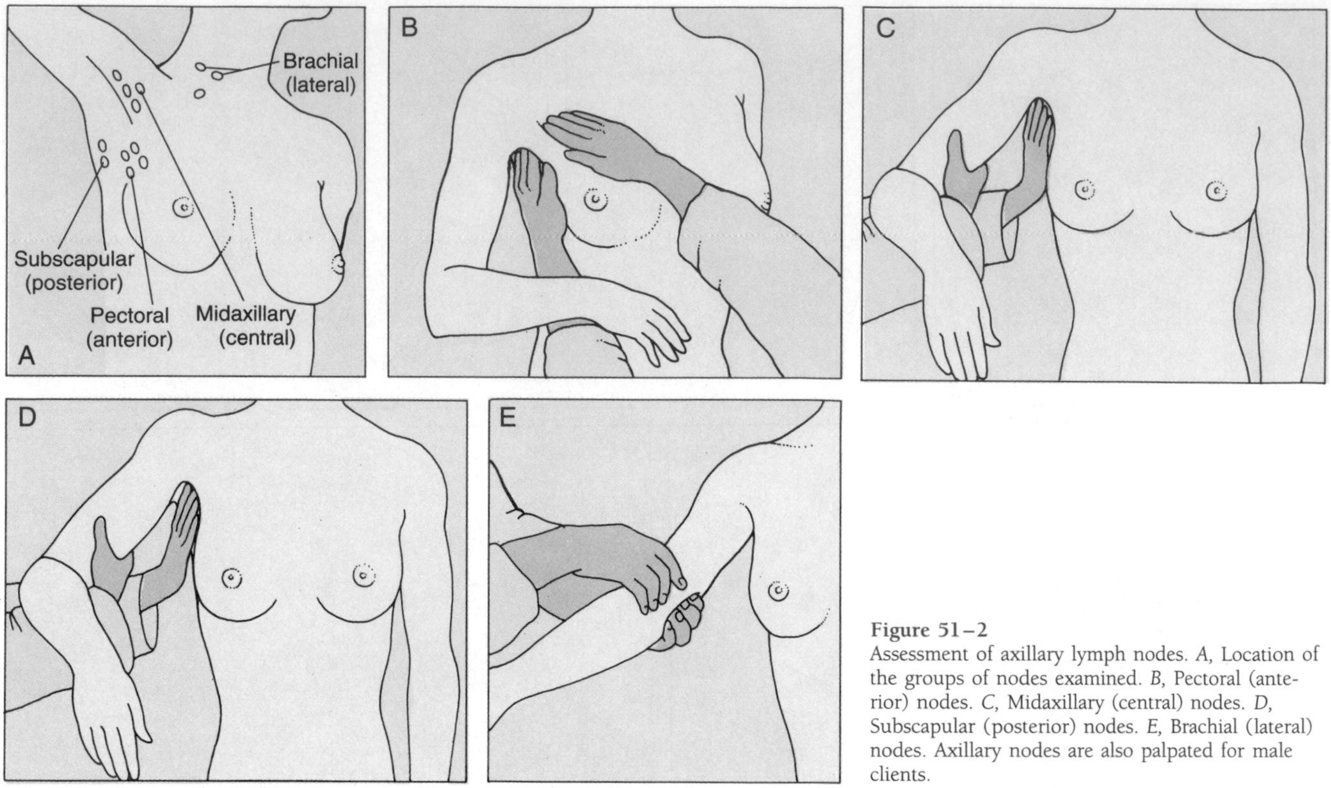

Figure 51–2
Assessment of axillary lymph nodes. *A*, Location of the groups of nodes examined. *B*, Pectoral (anterior) nodes. *C*, Midaxillary (central) nodes. *D*, Subscapular (posterior) nodes. *E*, Brachial (lateral) nodes. Axillary nodes are also palpated for male clients.

visualized as having four quadrants plus the tail; the location of lesions can be diagrammed in the written record.

The *areola* and *nipple* are palpated gently. The nipple is compressed between the thumb and index finger in an attempt to express any discharge, which should be absent. Erection and wrinkling of the nipple with manipulation is normal.

Breast Self-Examination

Breast self-examination is a technique that all women can use to assess their own breasts. The American Cancer Society recommends that all women older than 20 years perform monthly BSE.[1] Teaching the skills of BSE can be life saving and is one of nursing's most important activities. With regular BSE, malignancy may be discovered early and effectively treated. Regular monthly BSE is an essential health maintenance activity.

Women familiar with their own normal breast characteristics can easily notice the development of abnormalities early. Nurses have many opportunities to encourage and educate men and women about this important health maintenance procedure. Individualized instruction in BSE that guides the client in self-examination produces more thorough BSE performance than films, pamphlets, or posters. As with any teaching procedure, it is desirable to allow a return demonstration and time for discussion and questions.

The nurse emphasizes that the breasts easily lend themselves to self-examination by palpation and inspection in a mirror. Sexual partners may help perform breast examinations.

Techniques of BSE for a woman are described in Figure 51–3. As part of BSE instruction, the nurse should teach about the risk factors of breast cancer (see Chap. 55). Each woman should be aware of her own risk factors. The importance of obtaining professional consultation as soon as breast abnormalities are noted should be emphasized. BSE definitely contributes to the early detection and improved survival of clients with breast cancer.

IMAGING TECHNIQUES

Various techniques have been tried in an effort to identify early-stage breast cancer in women accurately and safely when assessment indicates breast lesions. Such techniques are also important to find an effective method to screen women without clinically apparent findings. At present, only mammography has been shown to be effective for widespread use.

Mammography. A mammogram is a soft tissue radiologic breast examination. Two common methods to obtain mammograms are film-screen mammography and xeromammography. Each technique has its own strengths and limitations. Both provide mammograms at acceptably low radiation doses.[34]

With mammography, it is possible to identify some breast cancers before they reach a size that could be detected by palpation.

The American Cancer Society (ACS) recommends a baseline mammogram for all women between the ages

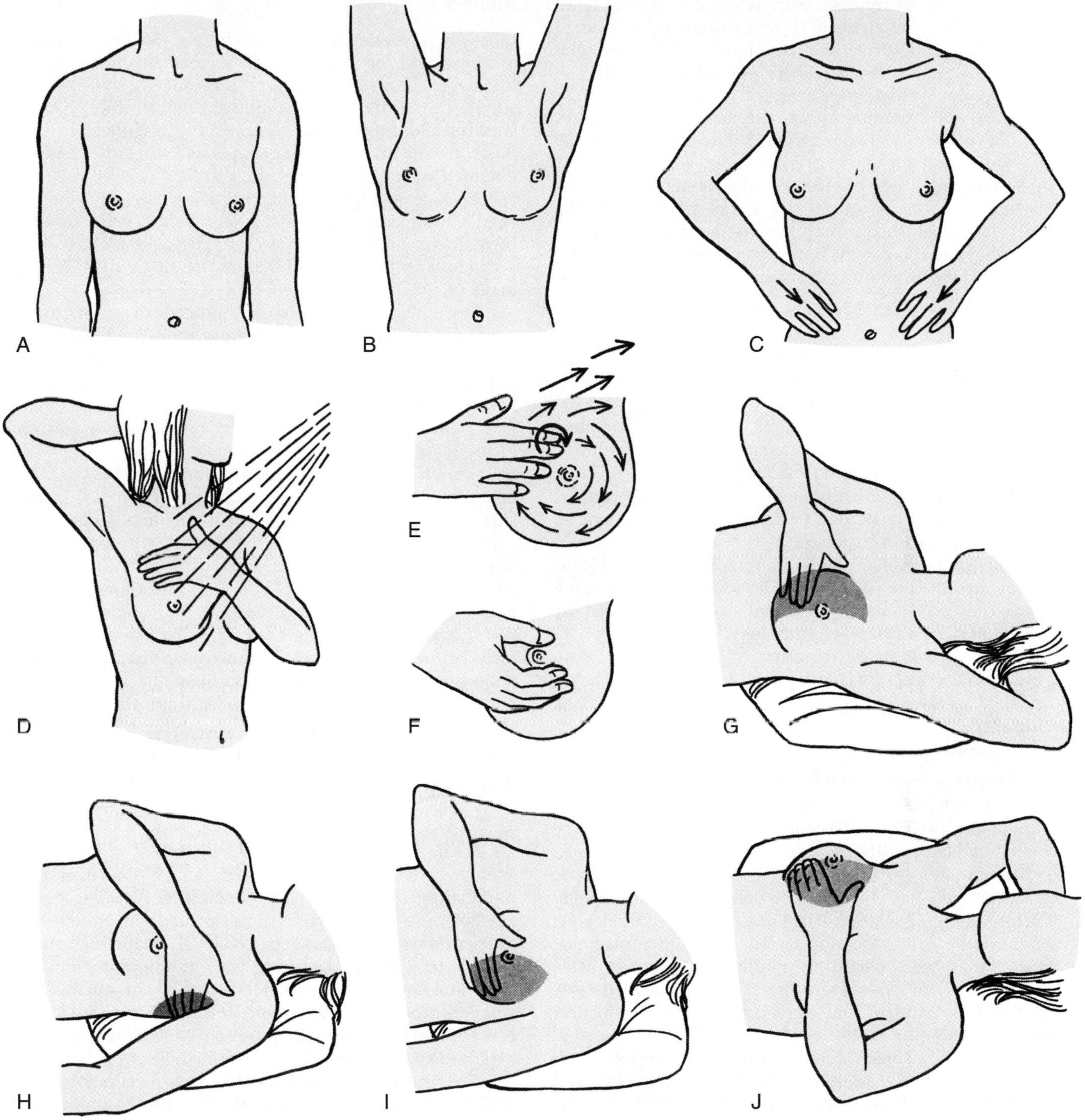

Figure 51–3
Self-examination of female breasts and axillae accomplished by observation and palpation. Various positions are assumed for observation while standing in front of a mirror. The client should be instructed to: *A,* Stand with arms relaxed at sides. Next, lean forward. *B,* Raise arms high overhead. Press arms behind head. *C,* Rest palms on hips and firmly press inward to flex chest muscles. *D,* In shower, examine breast contours. *E,* Method of palpating breast. With fingers flat, gently press in small circular motions around an imaginary clock face, i.e., begin at 12 o'clock. Move an inch at a time toward nipple. *F,* As a final step, squeeze nipple gently between thumb and index finger. Palpation of breast is accomplished while lying down. *G,* Position to examine inner breast. *H,* Position to examine axilla. *I,* Position to examine outer breast. *J,* Entire process is repeated for opposite breast and axilla. (See text for discussion of technique and observations.)

of 35 and 40 years and mammography screening of asymptomatic women aged 40 to 49 years at intervals of 1 to 2 years and annually after 50 years. A woman who is at high risk for breast cancer should follow the recommendations of her physician.

It is not uncommon for the nurse to be asked, "Should I have a mammogram?" The nurse must be able to answer this important question. Women need to know not only the risk factors associated with the development of breast cancer (see Chap. 55) but also the risks and benefits of procedures used for breast cancer screening and detection. Some common questions and possible answers about mammography include:

- *How often should I have a mammogram?* Use the ACS guidelines for the age and risk group.
- *Cost?* Prices vary. Inquire at the facility where the mammogram will be performed. Tell the client it is worthwhile to compare prices.
- *Time involved?* About 15 to 30 minutes to complete the procedure. Results are usually available within 7 to 21 days, depending on the facility.
- *Is there pain?* Some discomfort may be experienced with the pressure needed to flatten the breast (done to decrease radiation exposure).
- *Where is it available?* Mammography is available at most health-care facilities. The nurse should make sure the facility has a dedicated machine certified by the American College of Radiology.
- *Is there a risk in the exposure to the radiation?* The long-term effects of yearly mammography are being studied, although it is thought to be harmless. Both film-screen and xeromammography use the smallest dose possible.

Ultrasonography. Ultrasonography of the breast involves scanning with an automated whole breast scanner and a hand-held real-time sector scanner, very useful in determining the consistency of breast masses. It differentiates cystic (fluid-filled) from solid lesions. It cannot differentiate benign from solid cancerous lesions. Ultrasonography is useful in confirming the fluid consistency of cystic-appearing lesions seen on a mammogram. It is also useful in guiding fine-needle aspiration (FNA) of cysts and other breast masses. Ultrasonography is painless and does not involve a radiation risk.

Computed Tomography Scanning. Computed tomographic (CT) scanning provides cross-sectional images of the breast, mediastinum, axilla, supraclavicular area, and tissue adjacent to the chest wall. CT scanning may be useful in staging breast cancer, but it is currently not in use for routine screening and the diagnosis of breast cancer. Magnetic resonance imaging (MRI), transillumination, and thermography also are not considered useful in detecting breast lesions.

LABORATORY STUDIES

No laboratory tests can screen for breast cancer. Some progress has been made in identifying biologic tumor markers for breast cancer that detect metastatic disease.

BIOPSY

Biopsy is essential to diagnose breast cancer. No treatment should be undertaken without an unequivocal histologic diagnosis of cancer. Core-needle biopsy is a simple procedure that is useful during an office visit to confirm and expedite the diagnosis of a clinically obviously malignant breast mass. A small core of tissue is obtained with a special needle.

FNA is a slightly different procedure in which a needle and syringe are used to aspirate cells from a breast mass or fluid from a cyst. The cells are fixed on a slide (as in a Pap smear), and a cytologic diagnosis is made.

Open biopsy, the biopsy procedure most often used, is performed in an operating room under general or local anesthesia. About 35 per cent of clients requiring an open biopsy for a breast lesion have a malignancy. Excisional biopsy removes the entire mass that was palpated. Incisional biopsy removes only a portion of the mass for histologic assessment.

Percutaneous needle localization may be used to determine the area for an open biopsy if a mass is very small (e.g., those detected by mammograms alone). Localization of the lesion (i.e., locating it accurately) is done in a radiology department. The position of the lesion is confirmed with a repeat mammogram. The needle is taped into place and the woman is taken to the operating room where an open biopsy is immediately performed. A frozen section is a pathologic examination sometimes performed to obtain the results of an open biopsy while the client is still in the operating room.

Pelvic Examination

PSYCHOSOCIAL CARE

Women often find pelvic examinations embarrassing, humiliating, and anxiety producing, especially if the examination is incorrectly performed in rough or hurried ways. Insensitive professional treatment causes damage to women, producing fear, humiliation, submission, and low self-esteem. Memories of an uncomfortable or otherwise unpleasant pelvic examination may make women avoid such examinations. Thus, gynecologic health care may not be obtained.

The nurse must put a woman at ease before and during the pelvic examination. The nurse makes the client more comfortable by being nonjudgmental, relaxed, and competent. All actions are explained before they are performed. Quick movements are avoided because they may cause the client to tense muscles, which results in greater discomfort. Client comfort is enhanced when the nurse examiner is gentle, provides privacy, keeps the woman warm, warms hands and instruments, uses lubricant to ease insertion during invasive maneuvers, and cleans the perineum after the examination. The nurse must scrupulously protect the woman's dignity and communicate comfortably with her before, during, and after the examination. With the use of a mirror during the examination, the nurse should show the woman her anatomy, if she desires, to facilitate the teaching-learning process.

The nurse remains professional and avoids actions or remarks that may be misconstrued by the client as being demeaning or sexually provocative. Some agencies dictate that a male examiner be accompanied by a woman assistant when examining a woman.

PRE-EXAMINATION PREPARATION

The woman must be instructed not to douche, have intercourse, or use any vaginal products for 2 to 3 days before a pelvic examination. Just before the examination, the woman should be asked to empty her bladder and bowels to make the examination more comfortable and accurate. If necessary, a urine specimen should be collected at this time. The woman should remove enough clothing to allow examination of the abdomen and perineal structures. If a breast examination is planned, the woman should disrobe completely and put on a gown. The nurse asks the woman about previous experiences with pelvic examinations and acknowledges any feelings she may have. If this is the client's first examination, the nurse should explain the procedure fully and show the client how the speculum works. All women should be told what examinations will be performed. Telling the woman when she will be touched can help her avoid tensing up, which produces unnecessary discomfort.

EXAMINATION EQUIPMENT

The following equipment is used during a pelvic examination:

- Vaginal speculum (appropriate size)
- Materials for obtaining smears and cultures for cytologic study, such as Pap smear, including sterile cotton-tipped swabs, vaginal spatulas (wooden or plastic) or cytology brush, glass slides and glass cover slides, cytology fixative, and culture plates for gonorrhea screening
- Good light source
- Water-soluble lubricant
- Examination gloves (appropriate size)

EXAMINATION POSITION

The client is assisted in assuming a dorsal recumbent or lithotomy position and kept draped until the examiner is ready to proceed. In a lithotomy position, the woman's buttocks need to be flush with the end of the table. The client does not have to put her feet into stirrups if only the external genitalia are examined. The nurse assists the client to flex and abduct her hips and knees while arms are at the sides or crossed over the chest. The height and distance of the stirrups should be adjusted from the examination table to match the client's height. Being in a lithotomy position with one's perineum exposed is uncomfortable and embarrassing. A client must not be kept exposed any longer than necessary. The client's head may be elevated on a small pillow. Clients who have lower back pain or hip deformity may be unable to assume this position; an alternative position is necessary, such as Sims', or an assistant may be needed to help the client abduct one or both legs. There must be an adjustable light source.

EXAMINATION TECHNIQUE

Two persons should be present during a pelvic examination, and at least one should be a woman. While the examiner is performing the examination, the second person offers the woman emotional support, gives aid during the examination, and protects the examiner against accusations of sexual abuse.

External Genitalia Assessment. The nurse inspects the external genitalia and perineum (Fig. 51–4). The *mons pubis* is a mound of tissue superior to the labia. In adults, it is usually covered by *pubic hair* distributed as an inverse triangle over the mons, anterior perineum, and medial aspects of the upper thighs. The hair is inspected for nits and the skin for parasites, irritation, inflammation, edema, and lesions. There is no offensive odor present. Discharge, if present, is minimal and clear.

Perineal skin is slightly darker than that of the rest of the body. The *labia majora* are symmetric, rounded, and full. If the client has had a previous vaginal delivery, the labia majora gape slightly and the *labia minora* are evident. After menopause, the labia majora slowly atrophy. They are free of edema, inflammation, or lesions. The labia minora are thinner than the labia majora, and one side may be larger than the other.

The clitoris, urethral meatus, hymen (if present), and vaginal orifice (introitus) are inspected and presence is noted of discharge, inflammation, edema, or lesions, which should be absent. The *clitoris* is of the same color as the rest of the vulva. It can be the site of syphilitic chancres in young women and the site of dry, scaly, nodular lesions that are malignant in older women. When examining the *introitus*, the examiner also inspects the *hymen*, which is just inside the introitus. The hymen may be prominent and restrict the vaginal opening in a virgin, or it may be mostly absent in a sexually active client. *Bartholin's glands* are found near the posterior of the introitus and normally are not visualized or palpable. If inflammation and edema are present near the posterior introitus, the examiner palpates each gland between thumb and index finger (Fig. 51–4*A*).

The *urethral meatus* is between the clitoris and introitus and can be difficult to locate, particularly in women who have had a vaginal delivery. It is a small slit just above the vaginal opening and the same color as surrounding tissues. In women who have had several vaginal deliveries, the opening may be located just inside the vaginal orifice. The meatus is free of discharge, inflammation, or swelling. If these are present, the examiner palpates *Skene's glands* (paraurethral glands), which are at both sides of the urethral meatus (Fig. 51–4*B*). They usually are not visualized or palpable. The index finger is drawn along the vaginal wall as it is removed from the vagina so that any discharge is

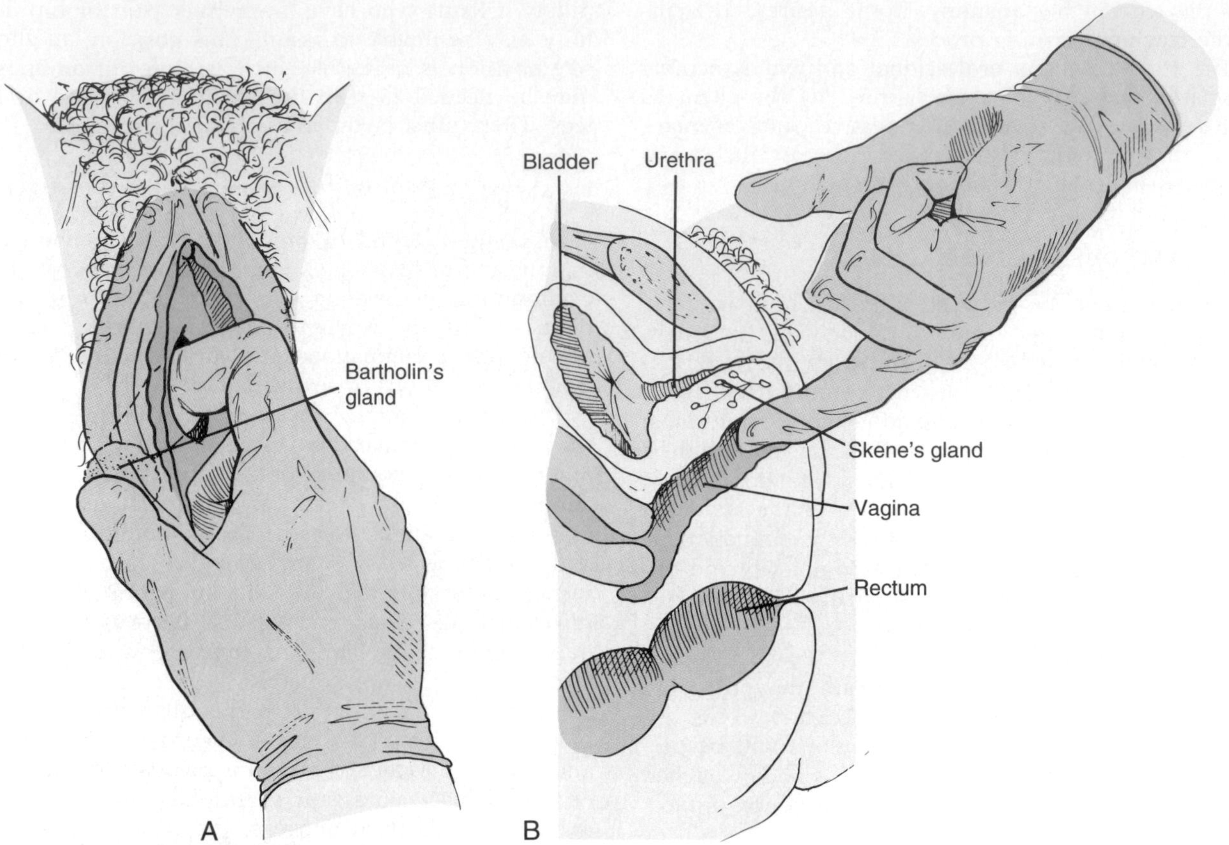

Figure 51–4
A, Palpation of Bartholin's glands. *B*, Palpation of Skene's glands.

"milked" from the glands into the urethra and out the meatus. If discharge is present, the examiner collects a specimen for culture and changes gloves before proceeding further with the examination.

In the final portion of the physical examination of external female genitalia, the examiner assesses the integrity of the *pelvic floor musculature.* If the anterior wall of the vagina bulges, the client probably has a *cystocele* (prolapse of the urinary bladder). A posterior vaginal wall bulge is often a result of a *rectocele* (rectal wall prolapse). Both of these are common in multiparous or obese clients.

Vaginal Speculum Examination. Wearing gloves, the examiner inserts a prewarmed vaginal speculum gently into the vagina (Fig. 51–5) without lubricants (lubricants interfere with the accuracy of the various cytologic examinations, such as the Pap smear). Vaginal speculum insertion is easier and more comfortable for the woman if the speculum is warmed in warm water. If lubricant is used, it is water soluble. The client is asked to bear down while the examiner looks for a cystocele or rectocele.

Vaginal *mucous membranes* are moist and pink, without discharge. If a discharge is present, it should be thin and white to clear in color. Abnormal findings include dry or inflamed mucosa; discharge that may be thick, curdy, yellow, green, odorous, or profuse; ulcers; lesions; masses; and bulges of the vaginal wall (e.g., rectocele, cystocele).

The *cervical os* is usually round but may be irregularly shaped after pregnancy. It is pink and smooth; a discharge is usually present, which varies from thin and clear to thick, white, and stringy, depending on the phase of the menstrual cycle. Abnormal findings include unusual color of the mucosa, abnormal consistency of discharge, ulcerations, growths, masses, nodules, inflammation, and bleeding. If abnormal discharge is present, a culture is obtained.

Before the speculum is removed from the vagina, a Pap smear and culture, if indicated, are obtained. The speculum blades are left slightly open as they are withdrawn for visualizing the vaginal walls.

Bimanual Examination. One or two fingers of the dominant hand are lubricated and inserted gently into the vagina, and the other hand is placed on the lower abdomen (see Fig. 51–6*E*). The pelvic contents are palpated between the fingers in the vagina and the hand on the abdomen. The *cervix* is located and assessed. The size, shape, surface characteristics, consistency, position, mobility, and tenderness of the *uterine body* and *fundus* are assessed. Last, each of the *adnexal areas* (left and right) is palpated. Normal *ovaries* may or may not be palpated, and normal *fallopian tubes* are not palpable. Postmenopausal ovaries should not be palpable.

The uterus is typically in an anterior position. It is normally firm, smooth, mobile, and nontender and is approximately 7.5 cm (3 inches) in length. Abnormal findings include prolapse into the vagina, feeling hard

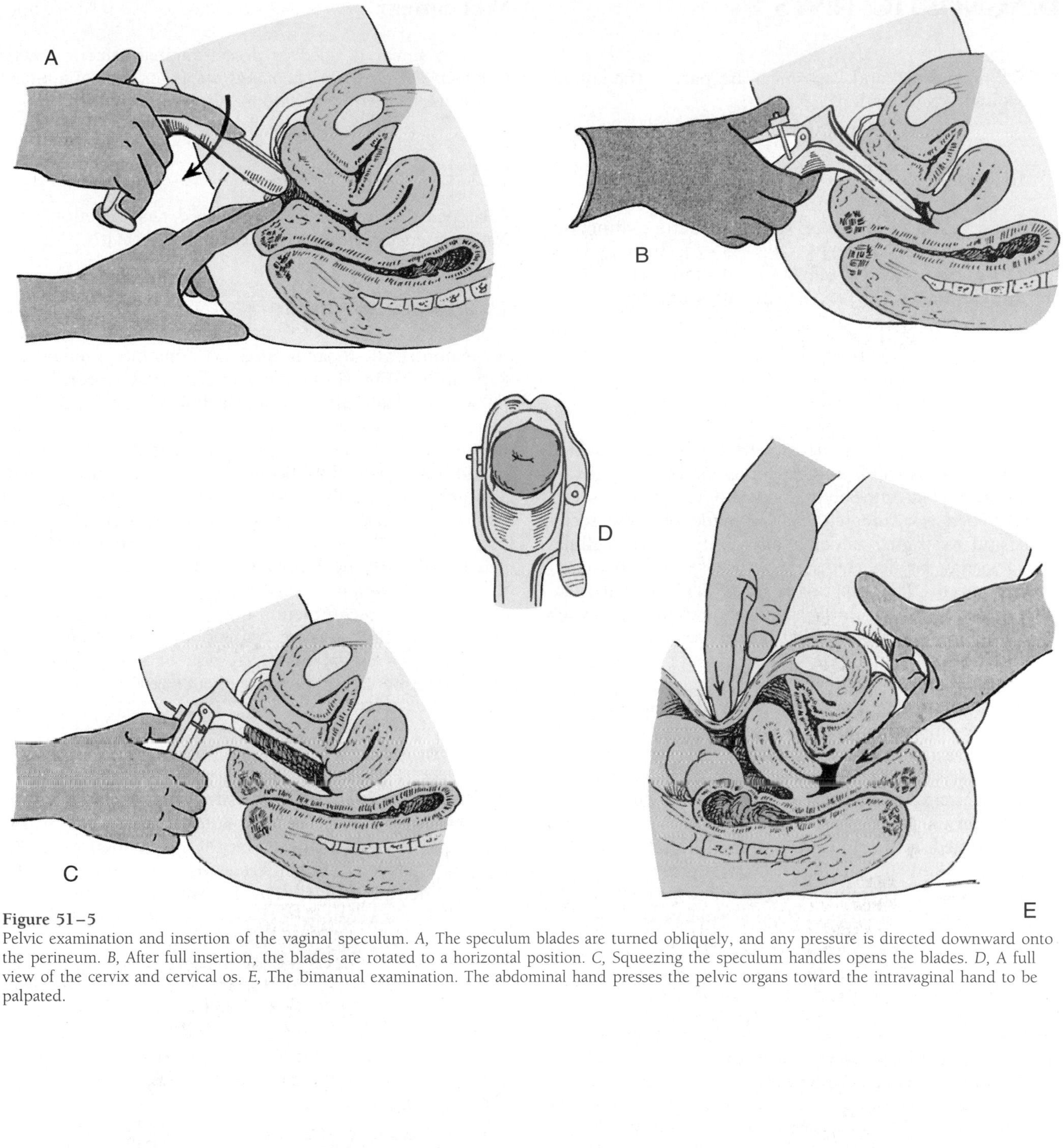

Figure 51–5
Pelvic examination and insertion of the vaginal speculum. *A,* The speculum blades are turned obliquely, and any pressure is directed downward onto the perineum. *B,* After full insertion, the blades are rotated to a horizontal position. *C,* Squeezing the speculum handles opens the blades. *D,* A full view of the cervix and cervical os. *E,* The bimanual examination. The abdominal hand presses the pelvic organs toward the intravaginal hand to be palpated.

or soft, being fixed in position, irregular contour, enlargement, or tenderness.

Slight tenderness on palpation is normal when ovaries are palpated, but uncomfortable tenderness or pain or masses are not.

Rectovaginal Examination. With insertion of one finger into the rectum, the rectal tissues can be assessed for abnormalities, for example, hemorrhoids. Rectal examination also confirms uterine position. Normal pelvic organs can be palpated through the posterior cul-de-sac. Abnormal masses or normal ovaries are often felt in the cul-de-sac.

If a stool specimen is needed for occult blood, it is obtained at this time. When the examination is completed, the nurse assists the client to sit up and offers tissues or wipes for perineal hygiene.

If well performed, a vaginal examination in women who have no pathologic conditions usually causes only minimal discomfort. Some discomfort may occur during palpation of the ovaries during the bimanual and rectal examination. The nurse should acknowledge this, and help the woman relax by asking her to bear down during the rectal examination and to breathe deeply through her mouth during ovary palpation. After the examination is completed, the nurse should give instructions and conduct appropriate health teaching.

DIAGNOSTIC TESTS

A CBC, urinalysis, and Pap smear are part of the annual gynecologic examination.

Cytology

Cytology is the examination of the structure, function, and formation of any cells (Fig. 51–6). In a gynecologic context, cytology refers to a Papanicolaou (Pap) smear. The Pap smear or test identifies preinvasive and invasive cervical cancer.

Papanicolaou Smear

A Pap test is based on the fact that cells (normal and abnormal) are shed from the lining of the uterus and cervix and pass into both cervical and vaginal secretions. When a cytologic smear is made of these secretions and examined under a microscope, early cellular changes may be detected before disease becomes clinically apparent. The Pap test is up to 95 per cent accurate in diagnosing early cervical carcinoma, when correct sampling and handling techniques are used. It is much less accurate (about 40 per cent) in detecting endometrial carcinoma.

Obtaining a Pap smear is usually painless. The ACS[3] currently recommends that women who are or have been sexually active, or have reached age 18 years, should have annual Pap tests and pelvic examinations. After a woman has had three or more consecutive satisfactory normal annual examinations, the Pap test may be performed less frequently at the discretion of her physician. Many physicians, however, continue to recommend annual examinations. The Pap test should be continued after menopause. Vaginal smears are obtained for Pap smear in women who have had a hysterectomy (see Chap. 53).

The nurse must be sure the woman knows when and where she can get the results of her Pap test. Descriptive reports are currently preferred because they are more useful in clinical decision making. Such reports either classify findings as normal or describe more fully the cellular changes seen. Specific infections may also be identified, and hormonal assessment may be done. A Pap test may be used to follow some abnormalities, and women may be taught to get their own specimens.

A suspicious Pap smear does not necessarily mean that the woman has a malignancy. There is about a 5 per cent false-positive or false-negative rate for the Pap test, and this rate may be much higher if the specimen was incorrectly collected or handled. However, having an abnormal Pap smear can be a frightening experience. Careful interpretation of cytologic findings to a woman is very important. She needs ample opportunity to ask questions, to discuss concerns and feelings, and to participate in follow-up care planning.

Wet Smear

The wet smear is used to detect vaginal infection with *Candida albicans, Trichomonas vaginalis,* or organisms that cause bacterial infections.

Cervical Culture

A cervical culture may be done to detect infection with *Neisseria gonorrhoeae* or *Chlamydia trachomatis.*

Endometrial Smear

An endometrial smear is made in a manner similar to a Pap smear (Fig. 51–7). An endometrial smear is obtained by swabbing the uterine lining to get cells and secretions for examination. This test differs from a Pap test in that the cervix must be dilated under sterile conditions to get the specimen. The procedure is usually done during the first 12 hours after the onset of menses, because the cervix is easier to enter at this time. Cervical dilation may cause cramping, which is usually relieved by analgesics and heat application to the lower abdomen.

The ACS[3] recommends that women at high risk for endometrial cancer have an endometrial tissue smear performed at menopause. Subsequent smears are recommended by calculating the client's risk.

Endometrial Biopsy

A sample of endometrial tissue can be obtained for histologic study on an outpatient basis through the technique of endometrial biopsy. Endometrial tissue may be analyzed for menstrual disturbances, infertility, or endometrial cancer. The biopsy is performed after bimanual examination of the uterus. Because the biopsy may cause cramping, the woman may receive a paracervical block to relieve the discomfort. If cramping persists after the procedure, the nurse must administer analgesics as ordered or apply heat to the lower abdomen.

Colposcopy

Colposcopy involves using a magnifying instrument (colposcope) to examine the cervical epithelium, vagina, and vulva. A colposcope is a stereoscopic binocular microscope. Colposcopy is indicated for all women with Pap smears showing dysplasia and may be used to examine any suspicious lesion in the lower genital tract. In this office-clinic procedure, the woman is placed in lithotomy position and her cervix is exposed with a vaginal speculum. A solution of 3 per cent acetic acid (common household vinegar) is applied to remove mucus and debris and to dehydrate the cells slightly on the cervix. The cervix and upper vagina are then inspected with the colposcope. Epithelial abnormalities

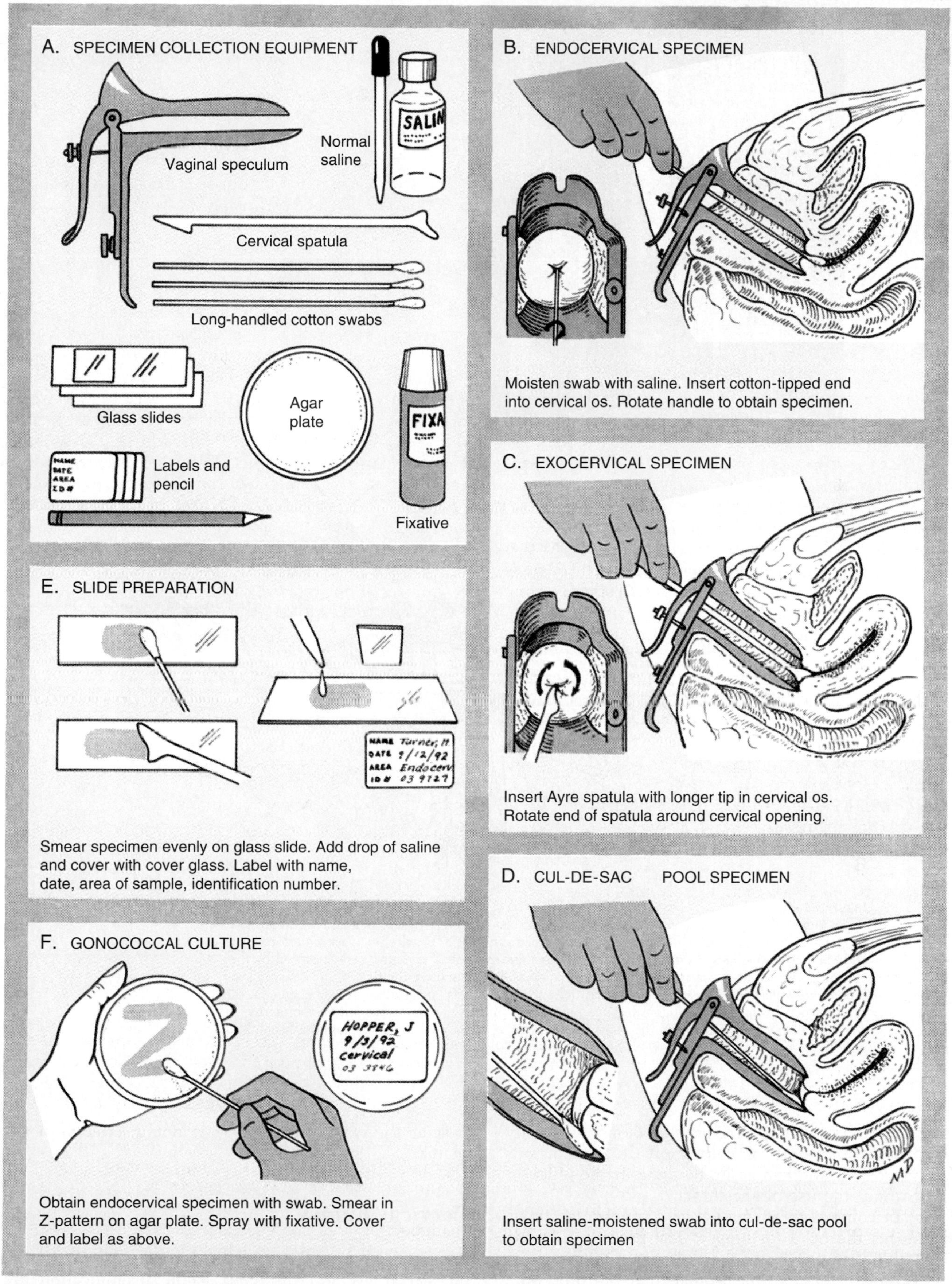
A. SPECIMEN COLLECTION EQUIPMENT
Vaginal speculum
Normal saline
SALIN
Cervical spatula
Long-handled cotton swabs
Glass slides
Agar plate
FIXA
Labels and pencil
NAME
DATE
AREA
ID#
Fixative
B. ENDOCERVICAL SPECIMEN
Moisten swab with saline. Insert cotton-tipped end into cervical os. Rotate handle to obtain specimen.
C. EXOCERVICAL SPECIMEN
Insert Ayre spatula with longer tip in cervical os. Rotate end of spatula around cervical opening.
D. CUL-DE-SAC POOL SPECIMEN
Insert saline-moistened swab into cul-de-sac pool to obtain specimen
E. SLIDE PREPARATION
NAME Turner, H.
DATE 9/12/92
AREA Endocerv
ID# 03 9727
Smear specimen evenly on glass slide. Add drop of saline and cover with cover glass. Label with name, date, area of sample, identification number.
F. GONOCOCCAL CULTURE
HOPPER, J
9/3/92
cervical
03 3846
Obtain endocervical specimen with swab. Smear in Z-pattern on agar plate. Spray with fixative. Cover and label as above.
MD

Figure 51–6
Cervical cytology specimen collection.

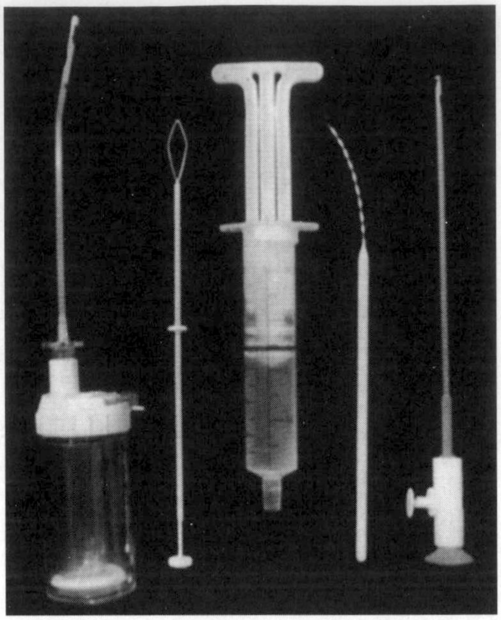

A

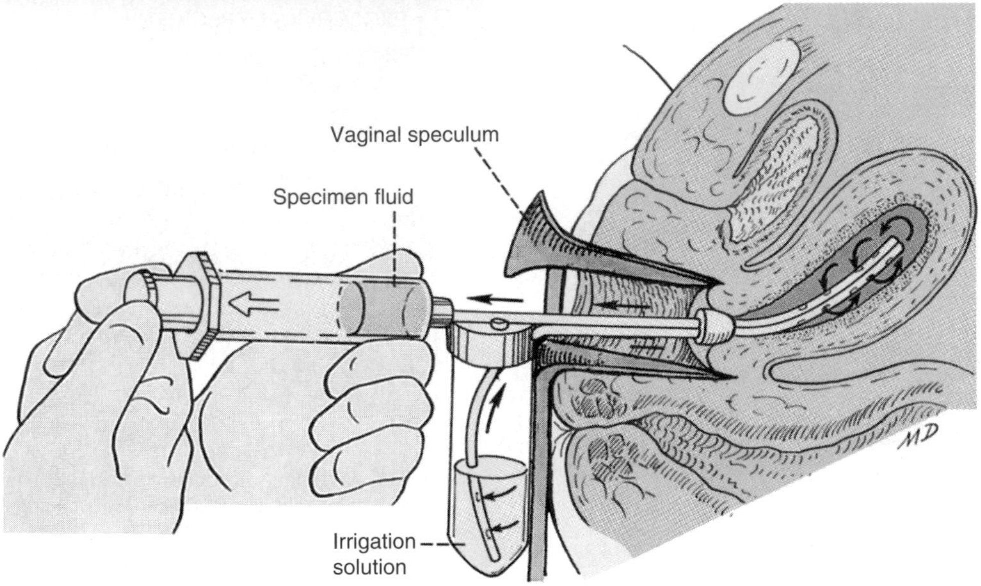

B

Figure 51–7
A, Endometrial sampling devices for uterine cancer screening. *Left to right:* Vakutage, Accurette, syringe for Karman cannula, Mi-Mark helix, and Karman cannula. *B,* Gravlee Jet Washer performing endometrial uterine lavage with sterile normal saline under negative pressure. Cells loosened by the "washing" are obtained for cytopathologic examination. *Arrows* indicate the flow of the irrigating solution and collection of the specimen. Fluid does not enter the fallopian tubes. A rubber plug at the cervical os helps create an airtight, negative pressure within the uterus. *Arrows* within the uterus show circulation of fluids within the uterus. (From Boone, M. I., et al. [1984]. Uterine cancer screening by the family physician. *American Family Physician, 30,* 157.)

can be detected as can specific lesions. Biopsy is usually performed at the time of colposcopy if a suspicious lesion is present and can easily be done in the office or clinic without the use of anesthesia.

Use of colposcopy increases the diagnostic accuracy and reduces the need for biopsy. The procedure is safe and painless and can be done on pregnant women. The nurse should explain to the woman that the procedure is like a pelvic examination and that, when the speculum is in place, a large microscope will be used to look at the cervix. The scope is not inserted into the vagina.

Cervical Biopsy

Biopsies of suspicious cervical lesions identified with the naked eye or with colposcopic magnification are usually performed in the outpatient setting with the use of little or no anesthesia. A solution of 3 per cent acetic acid can be applied to the cervix to identify areas suspicious for dysplasia, metaplasia, or malignancy. These areas undergo a color change and appear white.

A biopsy may be done when a cervical lesion is first noted or delayed until about 1 week after the menstrual period (when the cervix is least vascular). Multiple biopsies are usually obtained at specific sites with biopsy forceps. Hemostasis is achieved with topical application of silver nitrate or Monsel's solution. The biopsies are usually somewhat painful. For ruling out disease in the endocervical canal, endocervical curettage may be performed.

The woman should be allowed to rest for a short time before going home. The nurse should instruct her to avoid activity for the next 24 hours. Although she may note a small amount of blood-tinged vaginal discharge, any excessive bleeding should be reported to the physician immediately. The client should be advised to abstain from vaginal sexual activity, avoid tampons, and avoid douching for several days to achieve hemostasis, lessen trauma, and promote healing.

Cold Knife Conization

Today, colposcopy, biopsy, and endocervical curettage have largely replaced conization, but there are some circumstances in which it is indicated. When the lesion is in the endocervix or when the Pap smear suggests invasive carcinoma, conization may be done. The goal of conization is to excise the cervical lesion entirely by cutting out a cone-shaped section of tissue with an adequate surgical margin. Conization is usually performed in an outpatient room under general or spinal anesthesia. After excision of the conization specimen, curettage of the remaining endocervical canal is usually performed. The carbon dioxide laser can be used in place of cold knife cone biopsy. Laser conization is carried out the same way as the cold knife procedure. Postoperative care is similar to that after dilation and curettage. Vaginal packing may be used to control bleeding for 24 to 48 hours. Immediate complications include intraoperative or postoperative hemorrhage. The nurse should tell the woman that some vaginal discharge (often blood tinged) usually occurs after 3 to 5 days and that her next two to three menstrual periods may be prolonged, heavier than usual, and possibly preceded by a dark-brown premenstrual discharge. Bleeding can occur about 1 week after surgery when the absorbable suture placed in the surgical bed reabsorbs. Complications are rare after conization but include infection, incompetent cervix, or cervical stenosis.

Culdoscopy

Culdoscopy allows visualization of structures in the cul-de-sac through a culdoscope, a lighted hollow tube-like instrument. Laparoscopy has replaced culdoscopy in most settings because it provides superior visualization of the entire pelvis, especially the cul-de-sac, and permits a more complete visualization of the abdominal cavity.

Hysteroscopy

In this technique, the intrauterine cavity is directly viewed through an endoscope called a hysteroscope. Hysteroscopes have a fiberoptic lighting system and use 5 per cent glucose in water, highly viscous dextran solutions, or carbon dioxide as the uterine-distending medium. The hysteroscope is passed into the uterus via the vagina. The uterine cavity is distended and may be rinsed to clear away blood and secretory debris that would obstruct vision. In addition to direct visualization of the uterine cavity, directed biopsies and resections of endometrial abnormalities can be done. The hysteroscope can also be used to deliver a laser beam into the uterus for therapeutic procedures. Hysteroscopy may be used for

- Ruling out organic causes in abnormal uterine or postmenopausal bleeding
- Suspected leiomyomas or polyps
- Removal of intrauterine device with missing string
- Infertility evaluation
- Surgical techniques for uterine abnormalities

Hysteroscopy is contraindicated if the woman has acute pelvic inflammatory disease, recurrent chronic upper genital tract infection, or recent uterine perforation; has or is suspected of having cervical malignancy; or is pregnant. Complications include bleeding, uterine perforation, infection, and perhaps bowel injuries.

Laparoscopy

A laparoscope is a commonly used diagnostic and therapeutic tool (Fig. 51–8). It is a telescope with an illuminated optical system that is inserted into the abdomen through a small incision near the umbilicus. Abdominal and pelvic organs can be visualized through a laparoscope. Laparoscopy is a safe, convenient procedure that can be performed in hospitals or office or clinics equipped for outpatient surgery. The post-procedure recovery period is short, and the scar is small.

Laparoscopy may be performed (1) diagnostically for conditions such as pelvic pain, pelvic masses, infertility, suspected ectopic pregnancy, and endometriosis; and (2) therapeutically for procedures such as tubal ligations for contraceptive purposes and minor surgical procedures. The main contraindication to laparoscopy is serious cardiac or pulmonary disease. Previous lower abdominal surgery is not a contraindication but should be considered.

Preoperatively, a woman scheduled for a laparoscopy should be given a complete explanation of the procedure and how she can expect to feel afterward. She should have someone drive her to the hospital or clinic, because she may not feel like driving if she has local anesthesia and should not drive at all if she has general anesthesia. She will be more comfortable if she

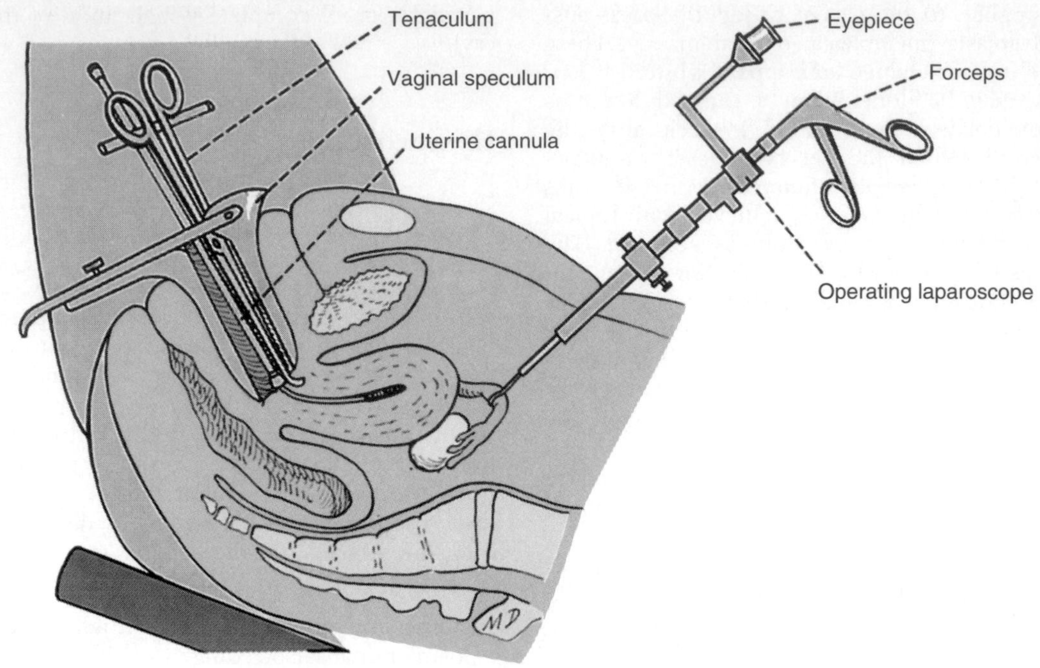

Figure 51–8
Laparoscopy.

wears loose-fitting clothes to the facility, because it will be easier to prepare to go home after the procedure. Typically, women having laparoscopy in a same-day surgical setting can go home 2 to 4 hours after the procedure.

The woman is usually instructed to have nothing by mouth past midnight on the day the laparoscopy is scheduled. Depending on the physician's preference, a cathartic or enema and a partial perineal shave might be required (usually they are not). Abdominal skin preparation (scrubbing and shaving) is done in the operating room.

Postoperatively, the nurse must measure vital signs every 15 minutes for the first hour or until the client is stable. If local anesthesia has been used, the woman can have fluids and a light snack as soon as she wants. After general anesthesia, the woman may have fluids and a light snack as soon as she is fully awake and has no nausea. The nurse should explain to the client that she may experience mild to moderate transient shoulder pain or a feeling of "bloatedness" as a result of the carbon dioxide or nitrous oxide used to distend the abdomen during the procedure (separating the organs and allowing better visualization). The discomfort usually lasts only a few hours and may be relieved by comfortable positioning or mild analgesics. The woman also may experience mild incisional pain or abdominal cramping for the first few hours or days after the procedure, which is usually relieved by rest. If the woman had general anesthesia, she might have a sore throat from intubation or a sore chest from insufflation. These symptoms usually disappear within 48 hours. The client should be taught to keep the incision clean and dry. After it heals, the scar will be barely noticeable. Sexual intercourse can be resumed within a week or less.

Assessing Men with Reproductive-Urinary Tract Disorders

Male reproductive problems are common disorders experienced by men of all ages. Assessing men's reproductive-urinary tract disorders requires expertise on the part of the nurse. This expertise is required in both the history and psychosocial assessment as well as in assisting in the physical examination. The nurse must display sensitivity and tact when working with these clients because men are often uncomfortable discussing issues associated with these disorders.

PSYCHOSOCIAL ASSESSMENT

An overview of assessment areas pertinent to males with reproductive disturbances is presented here. When taking a nursing history for such men, one must consider the following factors. The nurse will probably not be able to obtain detailed information in each of these areas, but the outline will signal areas that will help understand each man and his significant others as individuals and avoid stereotypic and possibly judgmental nursing care.

- *Self-concept*. How has the client's health affected how he feels about himself? How do his partner and significant others feel about him? What is his posture, dress, grooming? What is his emotional response? What is his mood or feeling tone?

- *Role relationships.* Who are the important people to this client? Who accompanied him to the health-care facility? Who does he say is his most significant other? How was the client's health affected? How is he able to carry out his various social roles (e.g., partner, husband, friend, father, worker)? How has his health affected his economic situation and his partner or significant others?
- *Communication.* How does the client communicate both verbally and nonverbally with (1) the nurse, (2) his significant others? Does he maintain eye contact? Does he use gestures or touch? How does he speak (e.g., volume, tone, vocabulary, repetition)?
- *Value-belief system.* What values, opinions, and beliefs does the client hold? What is his predominant lifestyle? What is his cultural or subcultural background?
- *Coping, stress tolerance.* Who supports and nurtures the client? Does he experience a degree of intimacy with anyone? How connected is the client with significant others? What supports and resources does he have? How does he spend his leisure time? To what extent does he engage in physical activity or exercise?
- *Cognitive-perceptual.* What is the client's use of speech and vocabulary? Can he read? What is his level of comprehension? What is his major source of reproductive health information?

HISTORY

A complete health history and physical examination are necessary for men experiencing reproductive problems. A sexual and reproductive history is important. History taking provides an opportunity to

- Give men permission to express sensitive concerns
- Identify myths and misinformation held by the client
- Give health information
- Offer referrals
- Facilitate further communication

Those aspects of history taking that address major risk factors pertinent to men's reproductive health are discussed here.

Chief Complaint

The client may present with problems related to the genitourinary, reproductive, or sexual systems. Areas in a chief complaint may include

- Systemic disturbances, such as weight loss, fever, and malaise
- Voiding disturbances, such as frequency, polyuria, oliguria, nocturia, pyuria, enuresis, dysuria, urgency, or incontinence
- Disturbances in the character of urine, such as hematuria, pyuria
- Gastrointestinal disturbances, such as nausea, vomiting, anorexia, abdominal discomfort, constipation, or diarrhea
- Reproductive disturbances, infertility, history of STDs, genital lesions, or genital discharge in self and partner; genital trauma
- Sexual functioning, whether sexually active or celibate; changes in sexual desire; changes in erectile ability; decreased ejaculatory ability; gynecomastia; effects of symptoms, disability, chronic disease, trauma, surgery, or treatment on sexual functioning

Medical History

Significant medical history for the male reproductive system includes childhood and infectious diseases, immunizations, major illnesses and hospitalizations, medications, allergies, sexual and reproductive history, family history, psychosocial history, and review of systems.

CHILDHOOD AND INFECTIOUS ILLNESSES

The most significant childhood infectious illness to affect male fertility is mumps. Its occurrence in young men is associated with sterility. The nurse asks the client whether he has ever had the mumps or has been immunized against them.

MAJOR ILLNESSES AND HOSPITALIZATIONS

The nurse asks the client about major illnesses such as diabetes, hypertension, cerebrovascular accident (stroke), and myocardial infarction. Men who have diabetes frequently have problems with impotency related to the accompanying neurologic and vascular changes that occur. Hypertension and its serious complication of stroke can cause impotence because of physiologic or psychological factors. Impotence may also occur in men who have had myocardial infarctions because of a fear of precipitating another heart attack as a result of sexual excitement and activity. The nurse is alert to the man's concerns and fears and remains nonjudgmental, offering the support of counseling and referral to peer groups established for this purpose. Renal and urinary tract disorders can interfere with sexual functioning because of the close physiologic and anatomic relationships. Endocrine disorders can also interfere with sexual performance.

The nurse asks the client about surgery involving the reproductive system. Specific surgical procedures include herniorrhaphy, vasectomy, prostatectomy, varicocelectomy, and testicular torsion repair.

MEDICATIONS

The nurse obtains a complete medication history for prescription, over-the-counter, and recreational drugs. Some medications prescribed for hypertension may cause impotence (e.g., methyldopa, clonidine, guanethidine, and hydralazine). Tranquilizers can interfere with sexual performance. Recreational drugs that alter behavior can also affect physiologic reproductive function, for example, marijuana and other hallucinogenics.

ALLERGIES

The client should be asked specifically about allergies to penicillin and sulfonamides and to rubber or latex. Male genitourinary disorders are often treated with these antibiotics, and latex and rubber are ingredients found in condoms as well as in the gloves used by the examiner during the rectal examination.

SEXUAL AND REPRODUCTIVE HISTORY

The sexual and reproductive history for a man includes the following.

Breast History. Data should be collected about the breast and axilla for both men and women. The nurse asks the client about breast pain or tenderness, masses, lumps, and nipple discharge. If any of these symptoms are present, a symptom analysis is performed. The nurse should ask whether the man or his sexual partner has noticed any changes in breast tissue, such as enlargement (*gynecomastia*). Gynecomastia can occur in obese or elderly men.

Contraceptive History. The nurse documents the man's current contraceptive method (if any), his satisfaction with the method, effect of contraception on sexual function, and any desire to change methods. Has the man used contraceptive methods previously, and if so, were there problems leading to their discontinuation?

Sexual History. The nurse inquires about the client's patterns of sexual relationships. Can the man relate the total number of sexual partners he has had and the frequency of sexual activity? Multiple partners and contacts increase the client's risk of STDs as well as human immunodeficiency virus (HIV) infection. Does the man use condoms during sexual intercourse? Does the client engage in homosexual or bisexual relationships, both of which increase the risk of HIV infection?

Does the client have any sexual concerns, such as an inability to attain or maintain an erection? If so, the nurse asks whether this is a problem that occurs frequently or occasionally. Is the client able to discuss sexual concerns with his partner? Have he and his partner developed ways to cope with or adjust to disturbances in sexual function? If sexual dysfunction exists, does the client wish a referral or consultation with a sexual counselor?

Genitourinary History. The nurse should ask about past problems with genitourinary infections, such as prostatitis, and determine whether the client has had a previous pelvic examination. Are there problems with urine incontinence or dribbling, hesitancy, weak urine stream, or other symptoms? Also see Chapter 29 for assessment of the urinary system.

Reproductive Health Practices. The nurse inquires about sexual and reproductive hygiene. How often does the man perform self-examinations of the breast and testes? Does he protect himself against STDs?

Family History

The nurse should ask whether there is a family history of infertility, diabetes, hypertension, cerebrovascular accidents (stroke), or endocrine disorders. Like women whose mothers took DES during pregnancy, men exposed to DES in utero are at increased risk for congenital anomalies, including structural defects of the genitourinary system and decreased semen levels.

Psychosocial History and Life-Style

In addition to those areas previously discussed under Psychosocial Assessment, the nurse assesses the following areas.

OCCUPATIONAL AND ENVIRONMENTAL FACTORS

The nurse determines the type of work and recreational activities of the client for identifying risk of exposure to chemicals, pesticides, heat, heavy metals, hormones, and radiation. These materials can directly affect the number and integrity of sperm and germal tissue.

HABITS

The nurse assesses the client's use of caffeine, alcohol, smoking tobacco, and marijuana. These substances may affect the sperm count, contribute to impotence, or decrease the libido.

Review of Systems

When conducting the review of systems, the nurse should ask specifically about diabetes, hypertension, stroke, myocardial infarction, angina, endocrine disorders, renal disorders, and urinary tract problems.

PHYSICAL EXAMINATION

Skillful history taking can help establish a therapeutic relationship that facilitates successful physical examination. Many men find physical examination for problems of the reproductive system stressful and embarrassing. Genitals are viewed by many as private and even unclean.

Sometimes a man will have an erection during an examination. This possibility is lessened by a kind yet professional manner. If the man does have an erection, the nurse should explain that this is normal and does not have any sexual connotation.

Physical examination for reproductive problems focuses on findings that may be associated with reproductive or sexual problems. These may be

- Inflammatory (e.g., enlarged, tender, movable, or fixed lymph nodes in the inguinal regions)

- Endocrinologic and genetic (e.g., general body appearance for indications of conditions such as Cushing's syndrome or acromegaly; hair distribution; gynecomastia)
- Neurologic (e.g., gross neurologic examination of the lower extremities)
- Vascular (e.g., status of femoral and pedal pulses)
- Traumatic (e.g., hernia)

The examiner follows an orderly approach for the physical examination and teaches the client how to do similar self-examinations regularly. The male breast and axilla are included here as part of the examination of the reproductive system.

Breast Examination

It is important that the nurse examine the breasts of male clients. Although the incidence of breast cancer in men is low, it does occur because men have glandular tissue beneath each nipple. Likewise, the axillary nodes are examined for men.

The nurse should inspect and palpate the breasts and axillae while the man is sitting, following the same guidelines as discussed for the female breast examination. The male breast is flat and symmetric without nodules, edema, or ulceration. Unilateral enlargement that persists past puberty is abnormal. Palpation reveals a small, flat disc of glandular tissue under the areola. There should be no masses or discharge present. Axillary nodes should be nonpalpable (see Fig. 51–2).

Male Genitalia

The nurse ensures that the client's urinary bladder is empty. The client may be supine or lying on his side with legs spread slightly for the first portion of the genitalia examination but will be asked to stand when the examiner assesses for inguinal herniation. An alternative position is to have the client stand for the entire examination of the genitalia while the examiner is seated on a stool. Because the male urethra is the common conduit for both urine and semen, examination of the male reproductive tract also includes assessment of the urinary system.

The examiner inspects the external genitalia and perineum, observing the *pubic hair* and *skin*. The client's general appearance and body build are important. The examiner should notice hair distribution. Pubic hair distribution is triangular, with hair covering the symphysis pubis, base of the penis, and inner aspects of the thighs. Hair distribution may also spread toward the umbilicus in a diamond pattern. Hair is inspected for nits and the skin for parasites, rashes, excoriation, and lesions. Masses, lesions, edema, and offensive odors should be absent. *Scrotal skin* is darker than other skin surfaces, loose, and wrinkled.

The *penis* includes the penile shaft, prepuce (foreskin), glans, and urethral meatus. The examiner inspects and palpates these structures for lesions, nodules, swelling, inflammation, atrophy, and discharge. *Penile skin* in the unerect penis is wrinkled. The *foreskin,* if present, covers the glans. The foreskin is absent in a circumcised client. The examiner instructs the client to retract the foreskin to expose the *glans,* which is easily accomplished. The examiner may note a small amount of cheesy, thick, white, odoriferous *smegma* between the glans and the foreskin, which is normal. If other discharge is noted, the examiner obtains a specimen for culture. The area between the glans and foreskin is a common site for venereal lesions. It is normally free of lesions; if any are present, the examiner palpates them for tenderness, size, shape, and consistency.

Next, the examiner inspects the *urethral meatus,* which is located at the tip of the penis and looks like a slit. Malposition of the meatus on either the underside of the penile shaft *(hypospadias)* or upper side *(epispadias)* is usually a congenital condition. The meatus is pink and without ulcers, scars, inflammation, or discharge. The examiner gently compresses the glans between thumb and index finger to open the meatus and inspects for discharge. If the client reports a urethral discharge, the examiner asks the client to compress the penis from base to tip between his thumb and fingers in an attempt to express a discharge. If one is expressed, a specimen is obtained for culture or microscopic examination.

The *penile shaft* is gently palpated between the thumb and first two fingers. It is smooth and semifirm, and the skin moves easily over underlying structures. The penis is free of nodules, thickened or hard areas, and tenderness.

The *scrotum* is inspected and palpated for symmetry, size, shape, and swelling. The scrotum has a right and left half, each containing a testis, epididymis, and vas deferens. The left testis usually hangs lower than the right. Scrotal size varies with ambient temperature; cold results in contraction, and warmth in relaxation. The examiner asks the client to hold the penis to one side and then the other and to lift the scrotum up while the examiner inspects. The skin is loose, without tenseness. The *testes* are oval. On palpation, they are smooth, firm, and rubbery without nodules, masses, or tenderness. Elderly clients have smaller, less firm testes. In younger, adolescent males, the nurse notes that both testes are present in the scrotum. Testes may temporarily migrate as a result of being touched during examination or from exposure to the cold air. They may be palpable later in the examination when the client is more relaxed. If a testis is not apparent, the femoral and inguinal area should be palpated. A client with an undescended testis is referred to the physician. A small (pea size), hard lump located on either the anterior or lateral aspect of a testis is suggestive of a malignancy, and the client is referred to the physician for follow-up. The testes are compared bilaterally and should be similar.

The examiner then palpates each *epididymis* between thumb and index finger. They are located on the superior aspects of the testes and extend down the posterior surfaces. The epididymis feels soft, resilient, and tender. Swelling and hardness are abnormal. The *vas deferens* (spermatic cord) begins at the superolateral aspect of the testis. The examiner differentiates it from the epididymis by its firmer, tubular feel and compares findings bilaterally. The vas deferens is palpated along its length toward the inguinal canal while the examiner notes any thickening or asymmetry, which is abnormal.

If the examiner finds swelling, nodules, or other abnormal results during the scrotal examination, transillumination of the scrotum is performed. The examiner darkens the room and shines a flashlight through the scrotum from behind the mass. A scrotum filled with serous fluid will transilluminate as a red glow. More solid lesions, such as a hematoma or mass, will not transilluminate and may be seen as a dark shadow. The examiner describes the characteristics of the abnormality, including whether it transilluminates.

Examination of the client for *inguinal herniation* is best performed while the client stands. A *hernia* is a prolapse or protrusion of a loop of intestine through the inguinal wall or canal. A *direct inguinal hernia* enters the inguinal canal behind the external ring because of a weakened abdominal wall; it does not pass through the inguinal canal. An *indirect inguinal hernia* enters the inguinal canal through the internal ring and can remain in the canal or pass down through the external ring and into the scrotum. A *femoral hernia* (more common in women) occurs inferiorly and more laterally than an inguinal hernia; it often has the appearance of an enlarged inguinal lymph node.

The examiner inspects the inguinal areas for bulges while the client stands quietly and again after he is instructed to bear down and strain as though attempting to have a bowel movement. Bulges should be absent. Presence of a *direct hernia* is assessed by the examiner gently inserting an index finger into the loose scrotal skin over the external inguinal ring; the finger does not enter into the external ring. The examiner then instructs the client to bear down while feeling for a bulge, which should be absent (Fig. 51–9*B*). Asking the client to flex the knee on that same side may assist in relaxing the muscles so that the examiner can insert the finger through the external ring and into the inguinal canal. The mass retreats back up the canal when the client relaxes. The examiner palpates the inguinal area directly for a *femoral hernia* while the client is relaxed and again after he is instructed to bear down. A palpable mass should be absent.

After examination of the anterior male genitalia, the examiner assesses the rectum and prostate gland. A rectal-prostatic examination should be performed during physical examination annually for men older than 40 years. This assesses (1) for evidence of STD; (2) the prostate gland for alterations in size, consistency, and evidence of tumors; and (3) for acute and chronic in-

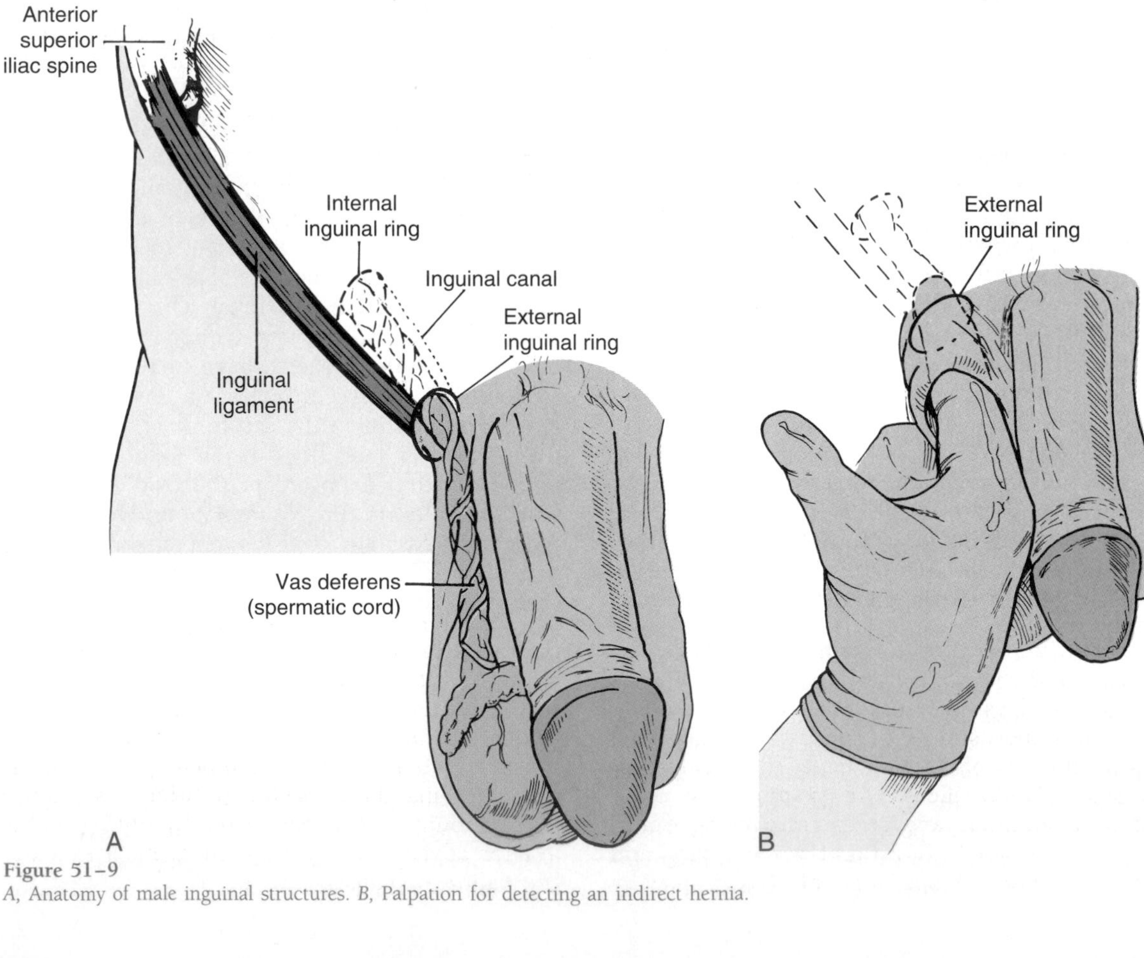

Figure 51–9
A, Anatomy of male inguinal structures. *B*, Palpation for detecting an indirect hernia.

fection. The nurse must impress on the man the importance of regular rectal-prostatic examination as the best way to detect prostatic cancer early enough for effective treatment.

Just before rectal-prostatic examination, the nurse should ask the client to empty his bladder. A urine specimen should be collected at this time if one is needed. The nurse should explain that this makes the examination more comfortable and more accurate and that it is normal to experience sensations of having to urinate or defecate during the examination.

Two possible positions for the client during rectal examinations are (1) knee-chest position with buttocks elevated or (2) bending over from the hip with elbows placed either on the knees or on the examining table.

The perineum and perianal areas are observed for lesions, hemorrhoids, inflammation, or discoloration. The normal prostate is located 2 to 5 cm beyond the anal sphincter along the anterior wall of the rectum. It is normally about 4 cm long and 5 cm wide. The posterior and lateral lobes only can be felt through the rectal wall. The lateral lobes should be symmetric. A normal prostate should feel smooth, rubbery, and firm, rather like the base of the thumb. Benign prostatic hypertrophy feels larger than normal, with a firmer consistency like that of the chin. Tenderness and bogginess (like the cheek of the face) may indicate acute or chronic prostatitis. Carcinoma feels "stony hard" or like a "hard nodule," that is, a circumscribed area of induration. Any induration is abnormal. The seminal vesicles (superior and lateral to the prostate) are normally nonpalpable.

Prostatic massage may be indicated even when the client is asymptomatic, in order to diagnose prostatitis. Resultant meatal secretions should be sent for microscopic examination. Large numbers of pus cells suggest prostatitis. Acid-fast organisms may be identified by staining. Cultures may be needed to identify organisms such as gonococci, chlamydiae, or tubercle bacilli. If a culture is required, the glans of the penis must be cleaned and the bladder emptied to clean the urethra before prostatic massage. Meatal secretions should be collected in sterile culture media.

Anus and Rectum

This portion of the physical examination is a potential source of embarrassment and discomfort to the client. The examiner manipulates tissues slowly to avoid causing unnecessary discomfort and uses a professional, matter-of-fact manner.

The position for rectal examination depends on the circumstances of the examination. If the rectal examination is performed as part of the screening examination, the client stands and leans across the examining table. This position is often used to facilitate palpation of the prostate gland. Clients are examined in Sims' position if only the anus and rectum are being examined. Clients are draped to prevent unnecessary and embarrassing exposure. A specimen of stool is usually obtained for occult blood (guaiac) testing at the time of the examination.

INSPECTION

Perianal skin is darker than the skin of the surrounding buttocks and should be intact. The *anal area* has coarse skin and is moist without hair. The anus is closed without sign of *rectal prolapse* (i.e., protrusion of rectal mucous membrane through the anus). The perianal area is without fissures (cracks), excoriation, rash, inflammation, ulceration, abscess, lumps, fistula openings, or *hemorrhoids.* Hemorrhoids are dilated veins seen as skin protrusions that are reddened.

PALPATION

The client is instructed to bear down. It is normal for the client to feel like having a bowel movement. If insertion is difficult or the examiner meets with resistance or rectal bleeding, the examination is stopped.

The examiner assesses the *anal sphincter tone,* which is normally strong.

The examiner palpates the *prostate gland* through the anterior rectal wall (Fig. 51–10*B*). It is felt as a rounded, heart-shaped structure approximately 2.5 to 4 cm (1–1½ inches) in diameter with discrete borders. The gland is firm, rubbery, nontender, and movable. Enlargement, bogginess, nodules, hardness, or tenderness is abnormal.

The presence of *stool* is noted on the examiner's glove. Feces, if present, is normally brown. Mucus or blood and black, tarry, light tan or gray stool is abnormal. The nurse tests a sample of the stool for *occult blood,* which should be negative. If presence of STD is suspected, the nurse also obtains a rectal culture. The examiner or nurse wipes the perianal area and informs the client that the physical examination is completed.

DIAGNOSTIC TESTS

Various diagnostic tests may be used to assess male reproductive disturbances. Men and their significant others are often anxious about diagnostic tests. The nurse can reduce anxiety by giving careful explanations before and during the tests. It is much less frightening if a client knows what to expect and is included in the process.

The nurse must learn the specific preparation necessary for each test. Sometimes sedation or pain relief is required. Informed consent authorization may be necessary. Physiologic preparations may be required (e.g., fasting, enema). During the test, the client must be kept informed about what is happening. The nurse must help him maintain specific positions as required. The client should be observed carefully during and after the test for adverse reactions, such as pain, excessive anxiety, pallor, or nausea.

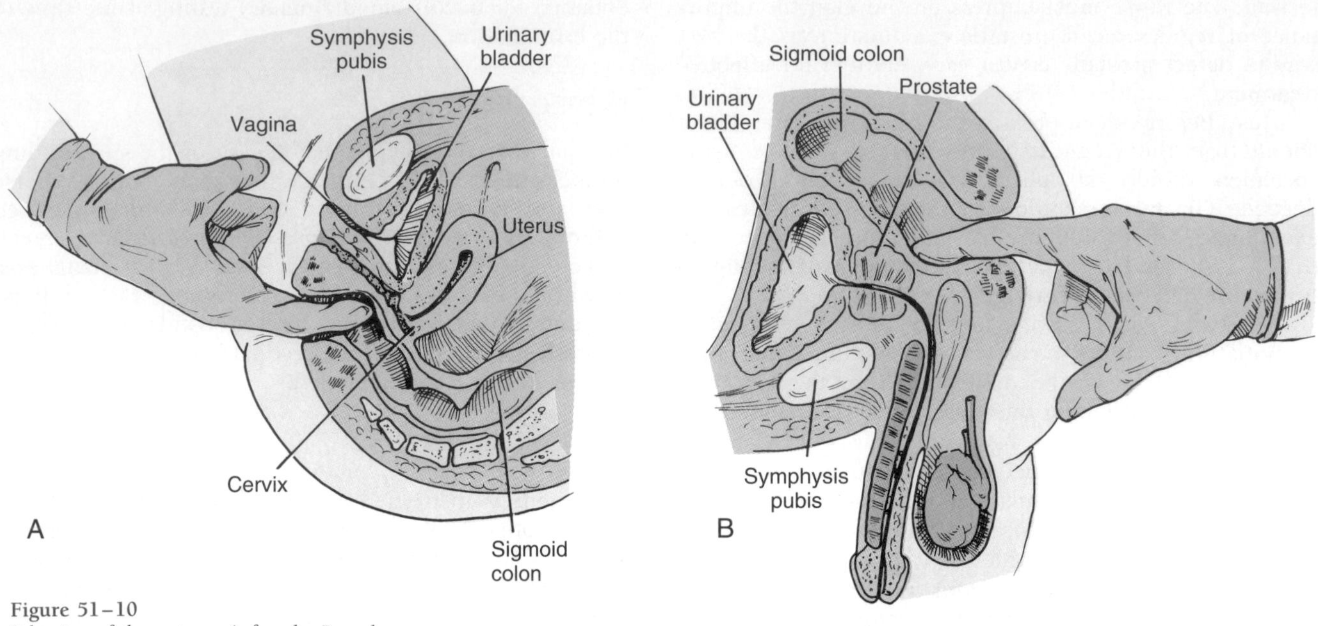

Figure 51–10
Palpation of the rectum: *A*, female; *B*, male.

Cystoscopy

A cystoscope is indispensable in both assessment and treatment of urologic problems. It is a metal instrument with optical systems providing a magnified illuminated image of the bladder. Flexible cystoscopes are also available and make the procedure much more comfortable for the client. Some indications for cystoscopy are (1) to determine the source of urinary bleeding, (2) to determine the cause of unexplained urinary symptoms, (3) to determine the source of pyuria, (4) to catheterize the ureters to localize the infection and subsequent treatment, (5) to obtain biopsy specimens, and (6) for follow-up examinations. A cystoscopy may be done in a urologist's office or (if the client is quite symptomatic) in an operating room before surgery. Inspection of the bladder interior includes looking for trabeculation, diverticula, and bladder neck contracture and checking the size and contours of the prostatic lobes.

Computed Tomography

CT scans are used in the clinical staging of testicular tumors and prostatic cancer. The client lies on an x-ray table, which moves him into various positions while scans are taken at various planes. If an injectable contrast medium is used, the client should be asked about any history of allergies. The procedure takes about 30 minutes.

Ultrasonography

Ultrasonic waves (sound waves too high in frequency for the human ear to hear) are "bounced off" tissue surfaces and produce an electronic image of body structures that can differentiate masses. This technique is used to visualize an enlarged prostate or scrotum. This procedure is done transrectally to help detect prostate lesions.

Magnetic Resonance Imaging

Magnetic resonance images are reflections of hydrogen densities in body tissues induced by a strong magnetic field. This method provides very clear images of soft tissues. MRI may be used to visualize pelvic structures, including the prostate, bladder, seminal vesicles, and penis. The test uses a strong magnetic field, so metallic objects must be kept away from the field to prevent injuries. Clients with pacemakers, metal joint replacements, or surgical clips cannot undergo this study.

Urodynamic Assessment

Urodynamic studies measure (1) pressure (e.g., from the bladder or urethra), (2) urinary flow, and (3) striated muscle activity. Common tests include the uroflowmeter test, cystometrography, electromyography, and urethral pressure profile. They are useful to determine the cause of frequency and decreased urinary stream in men (e.g., prostatic obstruction).

The client should be asked not to empty his bladder before the tests, because he will be asked to pass urine during the tests. Sedatives, analgesics, and cholinergic or adrenergic drugs should be withheld 6 to 8 hours before testing because these may interfere with bladder function. During the tests, the client is asked to void into a funnel or commode connected to a uroflowmeter, which measures voiding patterns (i.e., rate, time, volume, effort needed to initiate stream, strength and continuity of stream). During cystometrography, a urethral or suprapubic catheter is inserted and residual urine measured. Then, 30 mL of saline solution at room temperature is introduced into the bladder, followed by 30 mL of fluid at 110° to 115° F. The client is asked to describe sensations as the bladder fills (e.g., need to void, nausea, flushing, discomfort, temperature). The bladder is drained, the catheter is connected to a cystometer, and normal saline or carbon dioxide is slowly introduced into the bladder. A transducer connected to the catheter records pressure changes in the bladder. The client is asked to report when he first feels the need to void, and then when he feels an urgent need to void. He voids when the bladder reaches its full capacity.

An electromyogram assesses sphincter activity during voiding. A needle electrode is inserted through the perineum into the external sphincter. Normally, sphincter activity ceases during voiding and resumes when the man stops voiding. The urethral pressure profile involves slowly withdrawing a catheter through the urethra.

All these tests may be quite uncomfortable and embarrassing for the client. Intake and output must be documented for 24 hours after the test. Any hematuria should be documented and reported.

Scans

Scans may be used to assess testicular abnormalities (e.g., torsion, epididymitis, abscess, tumors, hydroceles, varicoceles, and spermatoceles). A radioactive substance is administered intravenously, and several scans are taken. Before a scan is taken, the client should be asked whether he has any history of allergies.

Secretion Analysis

Body secretions may be examined for micro-organisms from the throat, penis, and anus or lesions from the oral, pharyngeal, and perineal areas. A sterile applicator with a cotton tip is placed on or in the affected area and transferred to a sterile tube or slide. Care should be taken not to touch any other surface with the applicator.

PREVENTION OF MALE REPRODUCTIVE PROBLEMS

Prevention of a problem before it occurs includes activities such as genetic counseling; immunization against infectious diseases; good nutrition; careful genital hygiene; healthy sexual practices, such as use of condoms to prevent STD; knowing one's partner; avoiding multiple sex partners; and avoiding sex (oral or genital) with a person who has genital lesions.

Self-Examination

Self-examination of the perineal and genital areas, including the penis, scrotum, and testes, is important. The nurse takes every opportunity to talk with men about this part of self-directed health care. Teach self-examination to all males past puberty. Such secondary prevention practices can be taught anywhere, including all health-care settings, schools and colleges, and work place clinics. Self-examination can identify potential problems early when treatment is likely to be more successful; for example, testicular self-examination can detect testicular cancer while it is treatable.

The nurse must explain the procedure carefully and provide opportunities to ask questions and express concerns. Whenever possible, the client should be given literature to take home (the ACS publishes a useful pamphlet on testicular self-examination).

When teaching genital self-examination to men, the nurse should present the following tips:

- Develop a habit of doing self-examination once a month. Connect it in your mind with some other

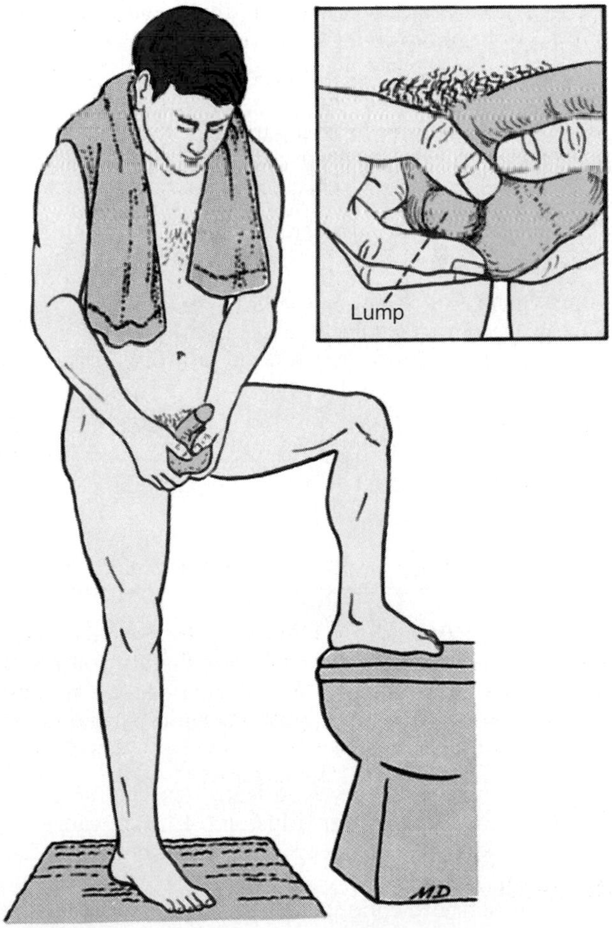

Figure 51–11
Testicular self-examination. See text for details of procedure.

monthly event (e.g., paying bills, receiving the first pay check of the month).

- Use a mirror to check inaccessible places (e.g., buttocks, perianal area, scrotum).
- Look for any changes from normal, such as swelling, lumps, tenderness, lesions, discoloration, asymmetry, or discharge.
- The best time to do a testicular self-examination is after a shower when you are warm, the scrotum is relaxed, and the testicles are easier to examine. When the testicles are cold, the scrotum pulls close to the body, making the testicles hard to feel. The left testicle is usually lower than the right because of a longer cord.
- The technique for testicular self-examination is as follows: Hold the scrotum in the palms of your hands and examine each testicle with thumb and fingers of both hands. Index and middle fingers should be on the underside of each testicle and thumbs on the top. Roll the testicles between your thumb and fingers (Fig. 51–11).
- A normal testicle is shaped like an egg. It feels firm but not hard (rather like an ear lobe), even rubbery, and quite smooth with no lumps.
- Examine the epididymis (a storage tube found on the side, behind the testicles). Each epididymis should feel soft and may be spongy.
- Examine the spermatic cords, which ascend from the epididymis behind the testicles. They are normally firm, smooth, tubular structures.
- Do not hesitate to seek professional assessment and advice about anything unusual you find. It is better to learn that everything is all right than to wait too long.

STUDY QUESTIONS

1. To promote a comfortable setting for the client with reproductive disorders, with which question should the nurse begin the interview?
   A. "Have you ever had an abortion or sexually transmitted disease?"
   B. "Would you like for me to step out while you remove your clothes?"
   C. "Can you tell me something about your usual patterns of health?"
   D. "Is this the first time you have had an exam of your genitals?"
2. Which one of the following findings would be least likely to affect reproductive function?
   A. History of hypertension
   B. Use of oral contraceptives
   C. Family history of obesity
   D. Fear of pregnancy
3. Which of the following would be the most effective sequence for a reproductive assessment?
   A. Medical history, obstetric and menstrual history, physical examination, allergies
   B. Physical examination, sexual history, breast examination, psychosocial assessment
   C. Chief complaint, psychosocial history, gynecologic history, physical examination
   D. Breast examination, physical examination, laboratory studies, medical history
4. Which of the following statements by the nurse would be most effective in encouraging self-assessment?
   A. "With monthly self-checks, you can learn what is normal for you."
   B. "As your nurse, I can show you what is to be included in self-assessment."
   C. "You can save a lot of money by doing this yourself."
   D. "If you don't do self-assessment, you will probably get cancer."
5. A client preparing for a pelvic examination states, "I hate this part. It is so hard to relax." Which action by the nurse would be most helpful?
   A. Provide additional drapes for privacy.
   B. Encourage her to keep her eyes and hands open.
   C. Tell her to bear down as if trying to have a bowel movement.
   D. Explain the procedure.

CRITICAL THINKING EXERCISES

SCENARIO A

A young woman presents to your facility for a routine yearly examination. She is married, has no children, is in her early 30s, and works as a receptionist in a local high school.

1. In your initial history, you learn that she has some concerns about maternal history of breast cancer. How would you proceed with the gathering of data for this client?
2. Suppose she mentions pain during an abdominal assessment. Would you need to obtain any other subjective data related to her complaint of pain?
3. How could you be sure you have gathered all relevant data?

SCENARIO B

A Vietnamese woman presents with her husband for a physical examination. She speaks some English; he almost none. You are ready to perform a pelvic examination.

1. How would you ask the husband to leave?
2. What adjustments in the environment might be helpful?

BIBLIOGRAPHY

1. American Cancer Society. (1995). *Cancer facts & figures—1995.* New York: Author.
2. American Cancer Society. (1992). *Guidelines for the cancer-related check-up.* Atlanta: Author.
3. American Cancer Society. (1989). *Special touch: A personal plan of action for breast health* (Publication No. 87-1MM-Rev. 9/89-No. 2095-LE). Atlanta: Author.
4. Andrist, L. C. (1988). Taking a sexual history and educating clients about safe sex. *Nursing Clinics of North America, 23(4),* 959–973.
5. Bates, B. (1991). *A guide to physical examination and history taking* (5th ed.). Philadelphia: J. B. Lippincott.
6. Champion, V. L. (1991). The relationship of selected variables to breast cancer detection behaviors in women 35 and older. *Oncology Nursing Forum, 18(4),* 733–739.
7. Campion, M. J., & Reid, R. (1990). Screening for gynecologic cancer. *Obstetrics and Gynecology Clinics of North America, 17(4),* 695–727.
8. Chilcote, W. A. (1988). Screening for breast cancer. In S. Grundfest-Broniatowski & C. B. Esselstyn (Eds.), *Controversies in breast disease: Diagnosis and management* (pp. 181–197). New York: Marcel Dekker, Inc.
9. Cooke, B. A., & Sharpe, R. M. (1988). *The molecular and cellular endocrinology of the testis.* New York: Raven Press.
10. DeGroot, L. J., et al. (Eds.). (1995). *Endocrinology* (3rd ed.). Philadelphia: W. B. Saunders.
11. Fogel, C. I., & Lauver, D. (1990). *Sexual health promotion.* Philadelphia: W. B. Saunders.
12. Frankl, G. (1988). Screening and detection of breast cancer. In M. E. Lippman, et al. (Eds.), *Diagnosis and management of breast cancer* (pp. 10–21). Philadelphia: W. B. Saunders.
13. Glenn, B. L., & Moore, L. A. (1990). Relationship of self-concept, health locus of control, and perceived cancer treatment options to the practice of breast self-examination. *Cancer Nursing, 13(6),* 361–365.
14. Gonzalez, J. T. (1990). Factors relating to frequency of breast self-examination among low income Mexican American women: Implications for nursing practice. *Cancer Nursing, 13(3),* 134–142.
15. Gray, M. E. (1990). Factors related to practice of breast self-examination in rural women. *Cancer Nursing, 13(2),* 100–107.
16. Gruhn, J. G., & Kazer, R. R. (1989). *Hormonal regulation of the menstrual cycle.* New York: Plenum.
17. Habegger, D., & Ellerhorst-Ryan, J. M. (1988). Needle localization for nonpalpable breast lesions. *Oncology Nursing Forum, 15(2),* 192–194.
18. Hacker, N. F., & Moore, J. G. (1992). *Essentials of obstetrics and gynecology* (2nd ed.). Philadelphia: W. B. Saunders.
19. Helderman, G., et al. (1990). Comparing two sampling techniques for endocervical cell recovery on Papanicolaou smears. *Nurse Practitioner, 15(11),* 30–32.
20. Helvie, M. A., et al. (1990). Radiographic guided fine needle aspiration of non-palpable breast lesions. *Radiology, 174(3141),* 657–661.
21. Herbst, A. L., et al. (1992). *Comprehensive gynecology* (2nd ed.). St. Louis: Mosby-Yearbook
22. Jarvis, C. (1992). *Physical examination and health assessment.* Philadelphia: W. B. Saunders.
23. Jones, H. W., et al. (Eds.). (1988). *Novak's textbook of gynecology* (11th ed.). Baltimore: Williams & Wilkins.
24. Kaunitz, A. M., & Grimes, D. A. (1988). The woman over 50: Endometrial sampling in older women. *Contemporary Obstetrics and Gynecology, 31(Suppl.),* 85.
25. Kisslo, J., et al. (1988). *Doppler color flow imaging.* New York: Churchill Livingstone.
26. Knobil, E., et al. (Eds.). (1994). *The physiology of reproduction* (2nd ed.). New York: Raven Press.
27. Lee, P., et al. (1988). Accuracy of Papanicolaou smears: Art or science? *Journal of Reproductive Medicine, 33,* 795–798.
28. Lierman, L. M., et al. (1994). Effects of education and support on breast self-examination in older women. *Nursing Research, 43(3),* 158–163.
29. Masood, S., et al. (1989). The potential value of mammographically guided fine-needle aspiration biopsy of nonpalpable breast lesions. *American Surgeon, 55(4),* 226–231.
30. McMillan, S. C. (1990). Nurses' compliance with American Cancer Society guidelines for cancer prevention and detection. *Oncology Nursing Forum, 17(5),* 721–736.
31. Morrison-Beedy, D., & Robbins, L. (1989). Sexual assessment and the aging female. *Nurse Practitioner, 14(12),* 35–45.
32. National Cancer Institute. (1988). *Breast exams: What you should know* (NIH Publication No. 90-2000). Washington, DC: Author.
33. Newton, M., & Newton, E. R. (1988). *Complications of gynecology and obstetric management.* Philadelphia: W. B. Saunders.
34. Pennes, D. R., & Adler, D. D. (1988). Mammography: Changing roles and concepts. In J. K. Harness et al. (Eds.), *Breast cancer: Collaborative management* (pp. 79–95). Chelsea, MI: Lewis Publishers.
35. Pleatman, M. A., & Cardona, R. R. (1990). Detection of breast cancer. *Obstetrics and Gynecology Clinics of North America, 17(4),* 729–740.
36. Saite, A. (1989). Cervical cytology in general practice. *New Zealand Nursing Journal, 82(1),* 18–19.
37. Smith, D. B. (1989). Discussing sexuality. *Oncology Nursing Forum, 16(1),* 106.
38. Soules, M. R. (1989). *Problems in reproductive endocrinology and infertility.* New York: Elsevier.
39. Swartz, M. H. (1994). *Textbook of physical diagnosis* (2nd ed.). Philadelphia: W. B. Saunders.
40. Szydlo, V. L. (1988). Approaching a male adolescent about a pelvic exam. *American Journal of Nursing, 88,* 1052–1056.
41. Walker, R. (1993). Modeling and guided practice as components within a comprehensive testicular self-examination educational program for high school males. *Journal of Health Education, 24(3),* 162–168.
42. Wynn, R. M., & Jollie, W. (Eds.). (1989). *The biology of the uterus* (2nd ed.). New York: Plenum.
43. Yen, S. S. C., & Jaffe, R. (1991). *Reproductive endocrinology: Physiology, pathophysiology, and clinical management* (3rd ed.). Philadelphia: W. B. Saunders.
44. Zuspan, F. P., & Quilligan, E. J. (1994). *Current therapy in obstetrics and gynecology* (4th ed.). Philadelphia: W. B. Saunders.

Chapter 52

Nursing Care of Men with Reproductive and Urinary Disorders

Learning Outcomes

After completing this chapter, the learner will be able to:

1. Assess the client for clinical manifestations of male reproductive and urinary disorders.
2. Teach the client about the etiology, risk factors, basic pathophysiology, and clinical manifestations of common reproductive and urinary disorders of men.
3. Explain the male's role in medical and surgical management of reproductive and urinary disorders.
4. Develop plans of care for prevention, management, and rehabilitation of reproductive and urinary disorders of men.
5. Implement nursing interventions that optimize reproductive and urinary function of men.
6. Evaluate planned client outcomes using outcome criteria developed in the planning phase of care.

Today, men are showing more interest in being actively involved in health maintenance. This is evident in (1) the increasing interest by men in fitness, (2) men's increased attainment of life-style factors related to fitness (such as stopping smoking), and (3) men's increased participation in childbirth and parenting.

PSYCHOSOCIAL FACTORS INFLUENCING REPRODUCTIVE HEALTH

When caring for men who are experiencing sexual, reproductive, or urinary problems, the nurse needs to plan sensitive care to meet the psychosocial and physical needs of men undergoing very personal procedures. In men, the urinary system and reproductive system are the same, so any problem in the urinary system may be seen as a threat to the man's reproductive system and sexuality. Men are often reluctant to ask for help because they see any problem as a potential threat to their sexuality and embarrassing.

There are many stereotypes concerning men's reluctance to seek health care. Some are true, because men are less likely than women to seek health care. What is important for the nurse to remember, however, is that urinary or reproductive problems and sexual preference are very personal, and the client may be very hesitant to talk about these problems (see Ethical Issues in Nursing: Should a Client's Sexual Life-Style Influence His Nursing Care?).

Because men may be reluctant to ask for help, skillful therapeutic interaction is essential to help them express their concerns. The nurse should be very sensitive and give the client permission to talk about his problem. The nurse should be sensitive to the client's discomfort and attempt to put the client at ease. Statements such as "Many men are concerned about how this problem will affect their sex lives," "It is common to worry about how your partner might feel about this problem," and "What are some of your concerns?" may help the client begin to talk about his concerns.

Giving men permission to express their feelings and health-related concerns draws them and their significant others into the process of health care. Teaching men reproductive and urinary health maintenance and self-care contributes to their overall health.

ETHICAL ISSUES IN NURSING

Should a Client's Sexual Life-Style Influence His Nursing Care?

Personal attitudes toward sexuality help make us who we are. Our sexuality is an important part of how we identify with ourselves as well as others. Attitudes toward others who may not view sexuality in the same way influence our relationship with those people.

Homosexuality, especially among men, is a subject that produces various responses. Recently, acquired immunodeficiency syndrome has caused a negative reaction toward gay males because at first the human immunodeficiency virus (HIV) was seen primarily in homosexual men. Although this virus now is seen in heterosexual as well as homosexual populations, a negative association with homosexuals remains.

Health-care providers take care of many kinds of people who are certain to have different attitudes about sexuality. Nurses may or may not be aware of the sexuality of their clients. Those who care for homosexual men need to confront their own feelings about providing such care, which may reflect social discomfort or the fear of contracting HIV. Although this fear is a reality for many health-care professionals, all clients should be treated equally and with respect and dignity. Also, the use of universal precautions may alleviate some of the apprehensions associated with HIV. The sexuality of clients is just as private as the sexuality of caregivers, and the respect shown toward one's own private life-style should be shown equally to others, no matter what personal attitudes are held.

PHYSICAL FACTORS AFFECTING MALE REPRODUCTION

Some men find reproductive assessment difficult and need considerable support. Some men simply refuse to participate, perhaps fearing abnormal results. Masturbation is necessary to obtain a semen sample, and some men find this difficult for personal, cultural, or religious reasons. Some men may be fearful of having an erection during the examination.

Assessment of reproductive problems in men includes (1) careful reproductive history taking of men at risk and their partners, including exposure to hazards from occupations, hobbies, and environment; (2) sexual history of men at risk and their partners; (3) semen analysis; and (4) hormonal studies (e.g., radioimmunoassay for follicle-stimulating hormone [FSH], luteinizing hormone (LH), and testosterone.

Environmental and Occupational Agents

The effects of a variety of chemical agents, such as the pesticide dibromochloropropane (DBCP), on the male reproductive system are well documented. In 1977, the toxicity of the pesticide DBCP was dramatically linked to adverse testicular effects in workers in a California plant manufacturing the chemical.[34] The workers suspected the problem when they realized as a group they had conceived few children. Interesting findings were made: (1) low sperm counts correlating with the length of time men had worked in the plant and (2) higher than normal levels of FSH and LH. Some men's sperm counts improved after they were no longer exposed to the pesticide. DBCP has also been found in community water supplies in California and Arizona. It has since been banned for agricultural use in the United States except on Hawaiian pineapples (little residue having been found on pineapples).[33]

Other agents associated with adverse reproductive effects in men include

- Anesthetic gases used in operating rooms and dentists' offices
- Carbon disulfide from rubber vulcanization
- Estrogen during manufacturing
- The pesticides ethylene dibromide and chlordecone (Kepone)
- Inorganic lead from smelters, painting, and printing
- Inorganic mercury from manufacturing and dental work
- Microwaves leaking from machines
- Neurotoxins from the manufacture of polyurethane foam
- Ionizing radiation from x-rays and gamma-emitting radioisotopes
- Uoulene diamine from chemical manufacturing
- Waste water treatment at petroleum refineries.[33]

Reproductive effects of chemical exposure vary, including abnormal sperm counts, loss of motility, impotence, spontaneous abortion, birth defects, and decreased libido (sex drive).[33]

Pharmacologic Agents

CRITICAL TO REMEMBER

Whenever a man is taking any drug, the possibility of sexual or reproductive health effects should be considered during nursing assessment.

When planning nursing care, the nurse should always review the specific use and action of drugs being taken by clients. Asking a client simply to "tell me about any changes in your sexual activity" can reveal problems that may be corrected by medication changes.

Some drugs may actually enhance sexual and reproductive functioning, such as clomiphene citrate (Clomid), which increases the sperm count. Other drugs depress sexual and reproductive functioning, such as phenytoin (Dilantin), which decreases spermatogenesis. The effects of some drugs are variable, enhancing functioning in one man and depressing it in another. Drugs that delay ejaculation (alcohol, cocaine, and amphetamines) may improve sexual functioning in a man who ejaculates prematurely. However, overuse of such drugs may lead to other problems, such as erectile dysfunction.

Many drugs (prescription, over the counter, and recreational) are known to have sexual and reproductive effects in males. Others may not have been identified yet.

Major sexual and reproductive effects of drugs on men include decreased desire for sex (libido), decreased erectile ability (impotence), decreased ejaculatory ability, decreased sperm quality, and gynecomastia. The following drugs may have one or more of such effects: antihypertensives, antipsychotics, tricyclic antidepressants, monamine oxidase inhibitor antidepressants, hormones, sedative-hypnotics and tranquilizers, stimulants, chemotherapeutic agents, opiates, and recreational drugs.

Many other drugs also have been found to affect sexual or reproductive functioning in males.

Systemic Conditions

Sexual dysfunction and other reproductive problems may be associated with medical or surgical conditions, such as diabetes mellitus, renal disease, prostate surgery, and spinal injury. It is important to assess a man's previous level of sexual functioning. Nurses must be aware of the wide range of normal sexual and reproductive function to reassure clients about their normalcy. What may be normal for one man may be considered abnormal by another and, therefore, a cause for concern.

INFERTILITY

Male infertility is extensive, occurring in 5 to 10 per cent of married men. Ten to 15 per cent of marriages are childless, and another 10 to 15 per cent have fewer children than they would like. In 30 to 50 per cent of such marriages, it is the man who is infertile. However, the two partners are best treated together. Minimal fertility in one partner can be offset by strong fertility in the other. On the other hand, if both are minimally fertile, infertility is more likely.

An awareness of these statistics alerts health-care professionals to clients who may have concerns about infertility but who have difficulty expressing them.

Etiology

Causes of male infertility include

- Pretesticular: endocrinopathy and sexual dysfunction, such as excessive ejaculation frequency
- Testicular: varicocele (varicose testicular vein), failure of testicle to produce sperm because, for example, of the effects of drugs, environmental factors, development of chromosomal abnormalities, mumps orchitis, and spinal cord injury
- Post-testicular: ejaculatory dysfunction, obstruction, such as from trauma, infection, and surgery
- Genitourinary: infection
- Immunologic: sperm antibodies in one or both partners

Diagnostic Assessment

Both the client and his partner may need help and support to express concerns and fears about infertility.

Failure to conceive may make severe demands on the couple, threatening their individual self-concepts, sex roles, relationship, and sexual interaction. Guilt and blame about previous sexual activity, sexually transmitted diseases (STDs), or abortion may come between them. Fear and anxiety may be lessened by taking a thorough nursing history. This also provides the nurse with the opportunity to give support, respond to questions, and explain diagnostic and treatment procedures.

Assessment of male infertility includes obtaining a detailed history (sexual, medical, and reproductive) and a thorough physical examination. Semen analysis includes (1) gross examination, noting volume, viscosity, and color; and (2) pH, concentration, motility, morphology, and sperm agglutination. Other, more specific tests of sperm function include the fructose concentration and the Sims-Huhner test to assess the penetration of cervical mucus by sperm. Additional tests are performed for azoospermia (absence of sperm in the semen) or oligospermia (less than normal number of sperm in the semen). Other studies include tests for sperm antibodies in serum and chromosome karotyping to detect genetic abnormalities.

Endocrinologic studies assess FSH, LH, prolactin, and serum testosterone levels, all of which can help to identify endocrinologic causes of the infertility. A testicular biopsy provides further information about spermatogenesis.

A genitourinary source of infertility can be assessed through a urinalysis, urine culture, serum creatinine, and an examination of prostatic secretions.

Medical Management

Thorough and complete infertility assessment is expensive and often ineffective. It is more effective to prevent infertility from developing. Clients who either want to conceive at present or may want to conceive in the future can try to prevent infertility by

- Avoiding excessive intake of alcohol
- Avoiding tobacco, marijuana, and other recreational drugs
- Decreasing exposure to occupational and environmental hazards, including toxic substances and radiation
- Keeping the scrotum cool (e.g., avoiding excessive heat, hot baths, and tight clothing)
- Avoiding transmission of sexually transmitted organisms by limiting the number of sexual partners and using condoms, contraceptive foam, and other spermicides, especially with new partners (STDs, particularly gonorrhea and those caused by *Chlamydia trachomatis,* may account for up to 30 per cent of cases of infertility in populations at high risk)
- Developing effective means of stress reduction
- Eating a well-balanced nutritious diet

Treatment for pretesticular causes of male infertility varies. No treatment is available for primary testicular failure or hypogonadism. Testosterone may be prescribed to correct low testosterone levels. Hyperprolactinemia may be treated by surgical removal of a pituitary tumor or by administration of bromocriptine (Parlodel).

Treatment of testicular causes of male infertility varies. Reduced spermatogenesis from testicular atrophy caused by infection may be treated by (1) avoiding factors that depress spermatogenesis, such as drugs, heat, alcohol, marijuana; (2) keeping the testes cool by avoiding hot baths and tight clothing, or using a commercially prepared, water-dampened scrotal cooling device (keeping the testes cool seems to improve the sperm count); and (3) good nutrition. Medication, such as human chorionic gonadotropin (hCG) testosterone (DEPO-Testosterone), is sometimes prescribed, with varying degrees of success. Varicocele is treated surgically.

Treatment for post-testicular causes of male infertility involves correcting ejaculatory abnormalities and obstruction. Ejaculatory abnormalities may be corrected by the split-ejaculate technique. The first half of the ejaculate contains more sperm than the second half. This first half may be used for artificial insemination or deposited in the vagina during intercourse, followed by withdrawal of the penis. Absence of ejaculation or retrograde (backward) ejaculation may be treated with drugs such as ephedrine, imipramine, or antihistamines. Artificial insemination may be done using sperm from urine obtained by centrifuge. Obstructive infertility is treated by surgery.

Appropriate antimicrobial drugs are used to treat genitourinary infections. Immunologic causes of male infertility may be treated with steroids and artificial insemination of sperm that have been washed to remove antibodies contained in the sperm.

Referral for counseling or support groups, or both, for infertile couples may be appropriate. A nationally known support group in the United States is RESOLVE, 1310 Broadway, Somerville, MA 02144.

ERECTILE DYSFUNCTION

Erectile dysfunction (impotence) was once thought to be entirely psychogenic in origin. We now know there are physiologic causes in about half the cases. The number is even higher in men older than 50 years.

Psychogenic Dysfunction

Indications of psychogenic erectile dysfunction include

- Normal and sustained erection during foreplay but loss of erection at the moment of intromission (penetration)
- Normal erection with some sexual partners but not with others
- Normal erection with masturbation but not with partners

- Sudden onset of total impotence in a man younger than 40 years
- Alternating periods of normal function and total impotence

ASSESSMENT

Assessment begins with carefully gathering the client's sexual and medical history and physical assessment. Physiologic causes must be eliminated. It is not true that nothing is physically wrong with a man if he can achieve a partial erection. Men with diabetic, vasculogenic, neurogenic, or endocrine pathologic conditions and men using certain drugs (see the section on Infertility) may be able to achieve some erectile activity, especially in the morning. Therefore, all medical possibilities, including drug use, are assessed and documented before an erectile problem is considered psychogenic.

Physical examination includes complete blood count; urinalysis; examination of prostatic secretions; liver function studies; thyroid function tests; assessment for diabetes mellitus; and serum creatine, serum testosterone, LH, and prolactin tests.

Psychometric testing, including the Minnesota Multiphasic Personality Inventory, Derogatis Sexual Function Inventory, or the Walker Sex Form, may be used to assess psychologic functioning.

MEDICAL MANAGEMENT

Treatment for erectile dysfunction of psychogenic causes includes various psychotherapeutic approaches.

Physiologic Dysfunction

ASSESSMENT

As stated previously, there are many tests that can be performed to identify physiologic causes of erectile dysfunction.

MEDICAL MANAGEMENT

Treatment for physiologic erectile dysfunction includes medical treatment, such as discontinuing or modifying the drugs that affect sexual functioning or treating endocrine abnormalities.

SURGICAL MANAGEMENT

Surgical treatment includes the use of penile prostheses, intracavernosal injections (using papaverine or prostin), and penile revascularization. Various penile prostheses are available. There are basically three types: (1) semirigid, (2) self-contained, and (3) inflatable. There are also vacuum erection devices that have been in use the last several years.

The original semirigid penile prosthesis (Small-Carrion) consists of a pair of plastic rods inserted within the corpus cavernosa (Fig. 52–1*A*). Silicone rods with a soft area at the scrotal junction are now available (Fig. 52–1*B*). The penis becomes permanently semirigid. Other semirigid prostheses include the Jonas malleable prosthesis.

A newer variation of this semirigid model is the self-contained prosthesis (Fig. 52-1*C*). Semirigid prostheses can be implanted under local anesthesia and are successful in about 95 per cent of cases. Semirigid penile prostheses are the most commonly used.

Inflatable penile prostheses may be composed of (1) cylinders that are inflatable, with a pump placed within the scrotum and a reservoir in the abdomen (Fig. 52–1*D*), (2) a self-contained unit, with a pump and reservoir within the cylinder; and (3) a partially self-contained unit, with the pump in the cylinder and reservoir in the scrotum. An erection is achieved through digital inflation of the cylinders, and the unit is deflated by a release valve at the side of the pump.

Penile revascularization may be used to correct vasculogenic erectile dysfunction. This surgical approach is still in its infancy. Currently, microsurgical techniques are being tried to revascularize the dorsal or central penile arteries.

Prostate Disorders

BENIGN PROSTATIC HYPERPLASIA

With aging, the prostatic tissue undergoes benign hyperplasia. Benign prostatic hyperplasia (BPH) is one of the most common disorders affecting men. The prostate is the urologic organ most frequently affected by benign and malignant neoplasms.

Incidence

It is estimated that by 50 years of age, 50 per cent of men have some degree of BPH; the incidence increases to more than 75 per cent in men older than 80 years. It is more common in white men.

Etiology

The exact cause of BPH is not known. Because it is a universal disorder in older men, a number of theories concerning the cause have been examined. Factors such as diet, effects of chronic inflammation, socioeconomic factors, heredity, and race have all been considered without definite conclusions. The prevailing theory is that hormonal alteration is responsible. Testicular androgen seems to be the most common hormone suspected as the cause of BPH.

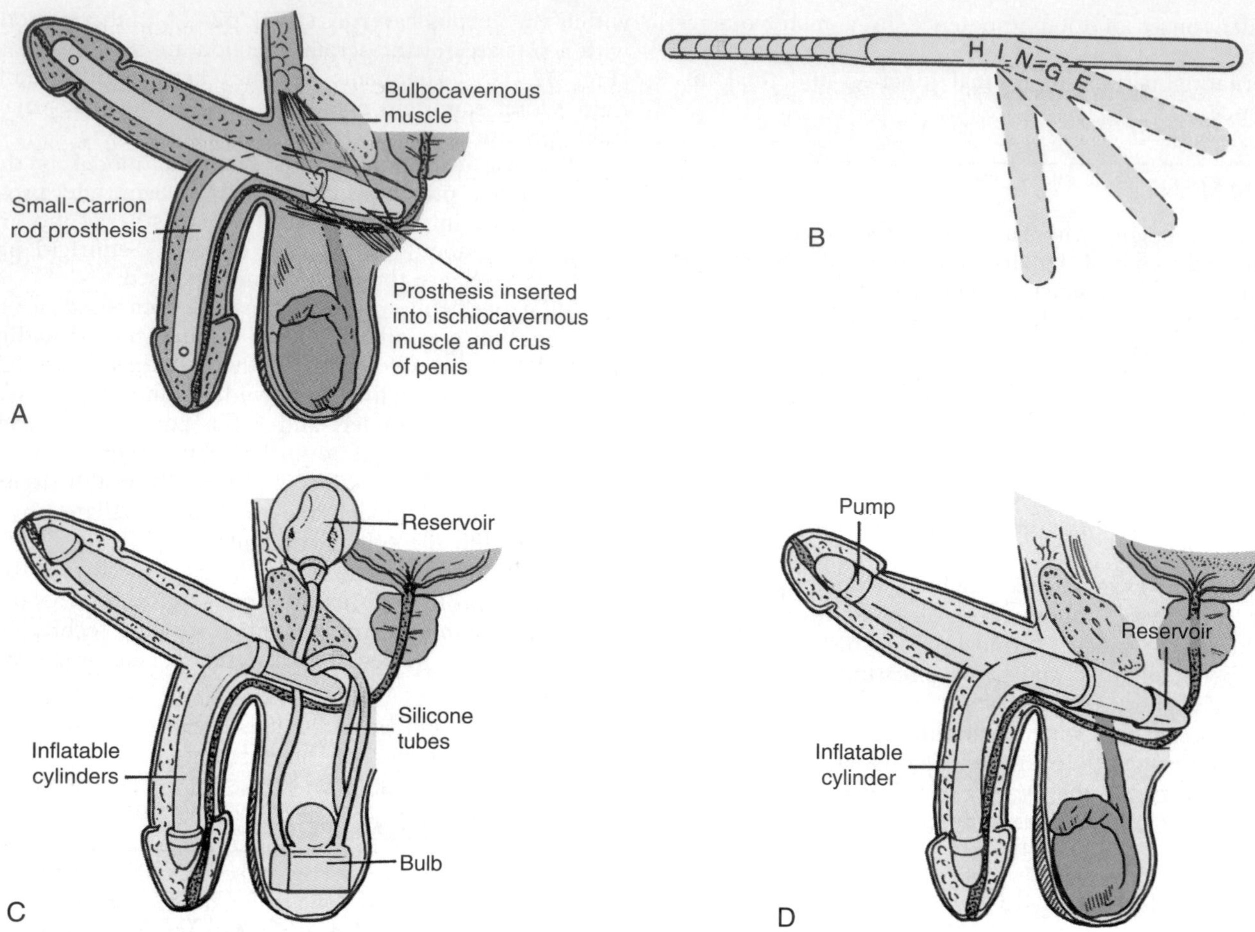

Figure 52–1
Penile prostheses. *A*, Small-Carrion prosthesis consisting of plastic rods. *B*, Flexrod semirigid penile implant. *C*, Inflatable penile prosthesis. *D*, Self-contained penile prosthesis.

Risk Factors

Aging is the major risk factor for the development of BPH, so there are no primary preventions. Early detection is the best secondary prevention available. Early detection can lead to early treatment, which can prevent complications related to urinary obstruction. Examination of the prostate annually for men older than 40 years ensures early detection.

Pathophysiology

Benign prostatic enlargement occurs by an abnormal increase in number of normal cells (hyperplasia) in the prostate, rather than an increase in cell size (hypertrophy). With aging, the periurethral glands undergo hyperplasia. Gradually, they grow and compress surrounding normal prostatic tissue, pushing it toward the gland periphery, forming a false or surgical capsule. Tissue inside the capsule can be shelled out during surgery.

Potential complications of prostatic enlargement (include impeded urinary outflow and urinary reflux (backward flow) because of decompensation of the ureterovesical junction (see Pathophysiology: Complications of Benign Prostatic Hyperplasia). Decompensation results from long-term elevated bladder pressure. Thickening, trabeculation (fibromuscular bands), and bladder wall diverticula may occur. Bladder diverticula may retain urine, causing infection and calculi development. Fishhooking of the ureters entering the bladder is common (i.e., ureters looping downward like a fishhook as they enter the bladder). The ureters may be compressed and obstructed by the thickened bladder wall, causing hydroureter (ureter abnormally distended with urine). A similar situation (hydronephrosis) may develop in the kidneys, because urine flow is obstructed in the ureters and urine backs up. In this situation, the pelvis and renal calyces distend with urine and the renal parenchyma atrophies. Ultimately, prolonged urinary obstruction or reflux can cause renal insufficiency.

Clinical Manifestations

Benign prostatic hyperplasia usually develops slowly and may persist for a long time in a silent state without

PATHOPHYSIOLOGY

Complications of Benign Prostatic Hyperplasia

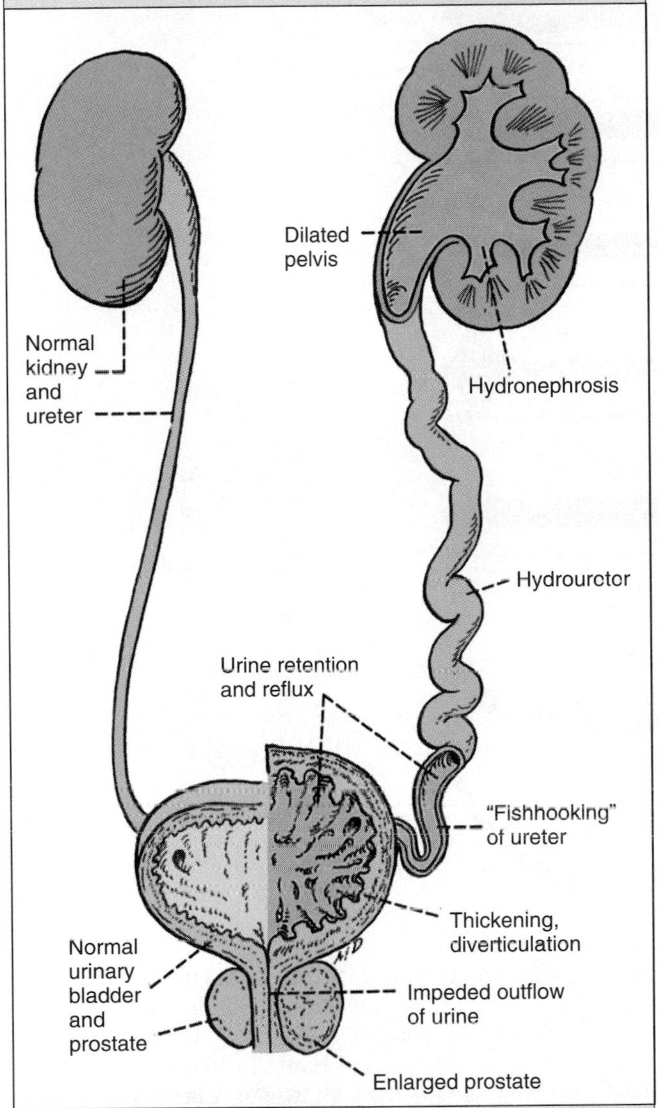

The left side of the illustration shows a normal kidney, ureter, bladder, and prostate. The right side shows potential complications of benign prostatic hyperplasia.

creating a major problem. As the client ages, he may assume that increasing frequency of urination is part of aging. Reduction in both the size and force of urinary stream is abnormal and should be assessed.

With developing BPH, the urinary stream first lacks force and then becomes weak and dribbling. The client feels unable to empty his bladder and either strains to urinate or urinates more frequently. There may be blood in the urine (a symptom more common in benign hypertrophy than in cancer).

As the prostate enlarges, there is a danger of complete urinary obstruction and retention. Retention may be precipitated by (1) the client becoming chilled, (2) drinking alcoholic beverages, (3) an infection, (4) delay in voiding, and (5) bedrest. Some medications may also provoke retention, such as decongestants, anticholinergics, and antidepressants. Obstruction can be a painful emergency requiring catheterization. Figure 52–2 shows various types of urethral catheters.

DIAGNOSTIC ASSESSMENT

Assessment for BPH is by

- A general physical examination, including rectal examination
- Laboratory examination of blood, urine, and renal function
- X-ray examination including intravenous pyelogram and cystography
- Instrumental examination, including catheterization and cystoscopy

The client should be asked about the size and force of the urinary stream. A uroflow test may be performed. Straight catheterization after voiding assesses the amount of residual urine. Other studies used to assess obstruction include urethral pressure profile and electromyelography of the sphincter muscles.

Rectal examination and prostatic massage for a sample of prostatic secretion can be performed. The secretion can be examined under the microscopic for pus cells, which may indicate infection. Urine, obtained before prostatic massage, may be normal in asymptomatic men, or it may show infection by the presence of red or white cells and an alkaline pH.

The enlarged prostate may cause urinary back pressure, leading to renal damage. Assessing for indication of renal problems is, therefore, important, and renal function studies must be included in the assessment.

Medical Management

Some clients find their symptoms considerably relieved by conservative interventions. The client can learn some techniques that will decrease his symptoms and possible complications. The nurse should explain to the client that if his bladder is distended rapidly, it can increase his symptoms and precipitate acute retention; the hyperplastic muscle of the bladder can lose its tone if distended quickly. The nurse should advise the client to void whenever the urge to do so is felt and not put it off, avoid consuming large quantities of fluid over a short period, and avoid alcohol, because its diuretic effect, with the volume of fluid, increases bladder distention. Alcohol intake is the most common precipitating factor for acute urinary retention.

Prostatic massage, sexual intercourse, and hot sitz baths may relieve symptoms by releasing a small amount of prostatic fluid, which reduces the edema. Urinary frequency is then decreased, and stream flow is increased.

Mild or asymptomatic BPH may be associated with prostatitis, which causes increased prostatic swelling

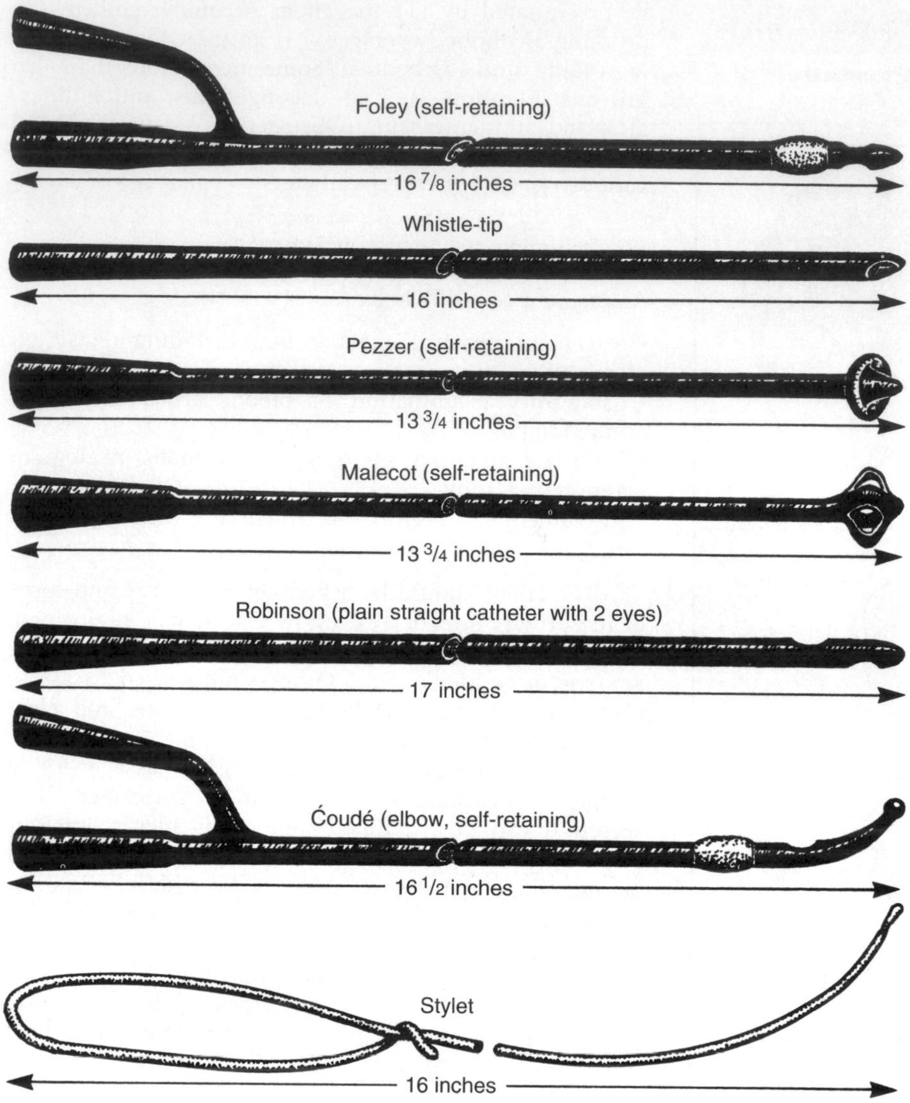

Figure 52–2
Types of urethral catheters and a catheter stylet. (From Smith, D. R. [1984]. *General urology* [11th ed.]. Los Altos, CA: Lange Medical Publications.)

and worsening of symptoms. Antibiotics may relieve acute symptoms and possibly delay surgery. Sympathomimetic drugs such as phenylpropanolamine and phenylephrine, found in common cold and cough remedies, worsen BPH. The nurse must warn the client not to take any of these medications.

Medical treatment (Table 52–1) is aimed at androgen deprivation in efforts to inhibit prostatic hypertrophy, such as prescribing estrogen. Testosterone-sparing agents are also used without the side effects of estrogens or antitestosterones. Alpha-adrenergic blocking agents have also been used to decrease muscle tone and improve voiding.

Surgical Management

Surgery is the most common means of relieving urinary obstruction caused by BPH. The part of the prostate gland causing obstruction is removed (prostatectomy). Indications for prostatectomy include

- Upper urinary tract dilatation (hydroureter, hydronephrosis) and impaired renal function
- Severe discomfort and inconvenience for the client
- Total urinary obstruction
- Vesical (urinary bladder) calculus, indicative of long-standing obstruction associated with BPH and infection
- Long-standing urinary obstruction that impairs renal function
- Severe and prolonged hematuria (recurrent bleeding)
- Chronic urinary retention
- Recurrent urinary tract infections

Enlarged prostate tissue may be removed by various approaches (Fig. 52–3). These approaches include

- Transurethral resection
- Suprapubic prostatectomy

TABLE 52–1 Selected Medications Used to Treat Benign Prostatic Hypertrophy

MEDICATION	ACTION
Testosterone-Ablating Agents	
Diethylstilbestrol Flutamide (Eulexin) Gonadotropin-releasing hormone analog (GnRH) • Nafarelin acetate (Synarel) • Buserelin (Suprefact-investigational) • Leuprolide (Lupron) • Goserelin acetate (Zoladex) Cyproterone acetate (Androcur)	Testosterone-ablating agents decrease the amount of circulating testosterone levels, leading to suppression of prostatic tissue growth. Estrogens inhibit prostatic growth by suppressing release of leuteinizing hormone-releasing agent, leading to a decrease in testosterone. Flutamide is an antiandrogen that competes with testosterone for androgen receptor sites. GnRH inhibits the release of pituitary gonadotropin, preventing testosterone biosynthesis. Cyproterone is a synthetic antiandrogen that acts as an androgen-receptor inhibitor.
Testosterone-Sparing Agents	
Finasteride (Proscar)	A 5-α reductase inhibitor that blocks dihydrotestosterone without suppressing circulating testosterone. Decreases prostatic tissue without affecting potency or libido.
Alpha-Adrenergic Blocking Agents	
Phenoxybenzamide (Dibenzyline) Terazosin (Hytrin) Prozasin (Minipress)	There is abundant autonomic innervation of the bladder neck and prostatic smooth muscle. Prostatic obstruction is due in part to the neurogenic tone of the bladder neck and prostatic smooth muscle. These agents block the alpha receptors, improving urination by decreasing outlet obstruction.

- Retropubic prostatectomy
- Perineal prostatectomy

The method used depends on the size of the prostate and the general health of the client.

Transurethral Resection. Transurethral resection of the prostate (TURP) is the most widely used of all prostatic surgical techniques. TURP is especially suitable for men with relatively small prostatic enlargements or who are poor surgical risks. No incision is made. Repeated TURPs may be needed because of postoperative urethral strictures, bladder neck scarring, and prostatic tissue regrowth.

The technique is performed by inserting a resectoscope through the urethra (Fig. 52–3*A*). The surgeon is able to visualize the inside of the bladder by inserting a telescope through the resectoscope. Bleeding is controlled by cauterization. Irrigating fluid can be passed into and out of the area through the resectoscope, and debris falls back into the bladder and is then washed out. Closed-system, sterile gravity irrigation is used with a solution of isotonic irrigation fluid. Water is never used, because during surgery the client absorbs about 900 mL of irrigating fluid through the tissues and veins at the operative site. Water could precipitate hemolysis and acute renal failure. Surgery must be completed within about 60 to 90 minutes to avoid excessive blood loss and absorption of irrigating fluid. Monitoring fluid and electrolyte balance and renal function before, during, and after surgery is important. Fluid absorption (water intoxication or dilutional hyponatremia) during surgery can produce hypervolemia. Postoperative assessment includes observing for hypertension, bradycardia, weakness, and seizures.

CRITICAL TO REMEMBER

If the client undergoing a transurethral resection (TUR) is elderly, it is especially important to remember that the symptoms of fluid volume excess and electrolyte imbalance include confusion, agitation, decreased mental alertness, and tremor and should not be mistaken for effects of hospitalization. Careful and frequent assessment of vital signs and reporting of significant changes to the client's physician may be life saving.

Suprapubic Prostatectomy. This surgical approach is through a lower abdominal incision (Fig. 52–3*B*). Indications for this procedure include (1) a prostate too large to be resected transurethrally; (2) bladder abnormality (e.g., diverticula or calculi); (3) the presence of large, pedunculated middle lobe or lateral prostatic lobes; or (4) a need to explore the abdomen.

An incision is made into the bladder, and the enlarged tissue is enucleated by blunt dissection. Both suprapubic and urethral catheters are inserted. An advantage of suprapubic prostatectomy is that bladder abnormalities can be treated concurrently, because an incision is made into the urinary bladder. Thorough exploration and complete tissue removal are facilitated. Disadvantages include (1) difficulty in obtaining hemostasis (therefore, assess for shock and hemorrhage);

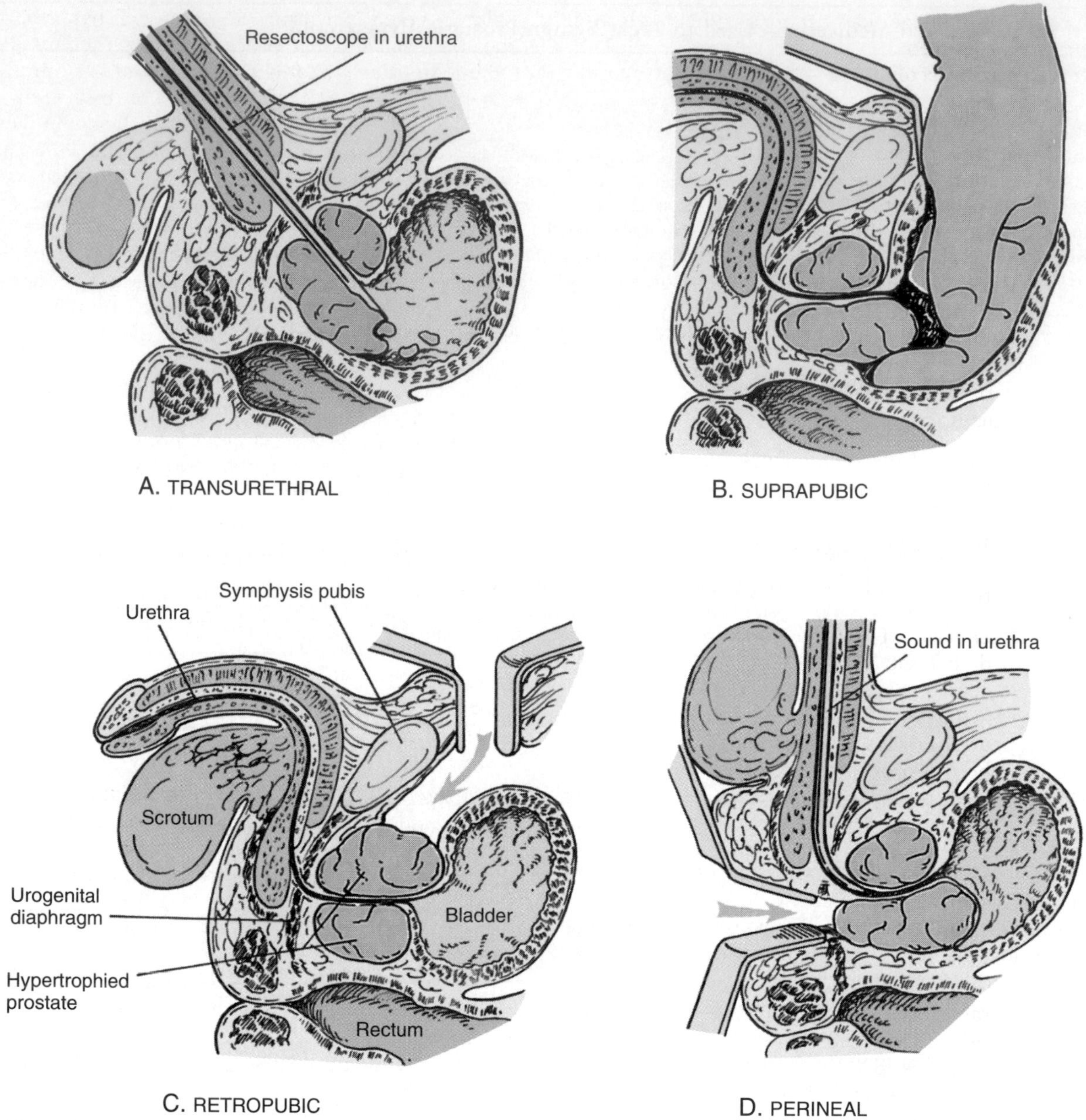

Figure 52–3

Surgical approaches to the prostate. *A*, Transurethral resection prostatectomy is a closed method of treatment, i.e., no incision is made and the hyperplastic prostate tissue is removed through a resectoscope (like a cystoscope) inserted through the penis. *B*, Suprapubic (transvesical) prostatectomy is an open method of treatment in which the hyperplastic prostatic tissue is enucleated through the anterior walls of the abdomen and bladder. *C*, Retropubic (extravesical) prostatectomy is an open method in which a low abdominal incision is made between the pubic arch and the bladder. *D*, Perineal prostatectomy is an open method involving an incision between the anus and the scrotum.

(2) bladder spasms; (3) urinary leakage into an abdominal wound around the suprapubic catheter; and (4) relatively prolonged and uncomfortable convalescence. Incontinence sometimes occurs. A small number of men experience erectile dysfunction after this procedure.

Retropubic Prostatectomy. Retropubic prostatectomy is the most recently developed open method (Fig. 52–3*C*). A low abdominal incision facilitates approaching the prostate without entering the bladder. Indications for use are when the prostate is too large to be removed transurethrally and the presence of severe urethral stricture. Advantages include direct visualization of the prostate and direct hemostasis in the prostatic fossa. A disadvantage is that any associated pathologic condition in the bladder cannot be treated, because the bladder is not entered. Also, osteitis pubis (pubic bone inflammation) may occur. A suprapubic catheter may be inserted to control bleeding, or constant bladder irrigation may be used. Infrequent complications include incontinence and erectile dysfunction (impotence). Postoperative urinary leakage may occur for a few days after the catheter is removed.

Perineal Prostatectomy. An incision is made into the perineum, between the anus and the scrotum (Fig. 52–3*D*). The perineal prostatectomy is performed to treat prostatic cancer. Because of possible postoperative erectile dysfunction, it is not performed to treat BPH.

A subtotal prostatectomy may be performed when enlarged glands are filled with calculi or when abscesses fail to respond to treatment. In a subtotal prostatectomy, the entire gland and capsule are removed, but the seminal vesicles and sections of the vas deferens are left in place. A major disadvantage is that the procedure is carried out in a lithotomy position, which is contraindicated for people with arthritis or cardiopulmonary disease. Complications include

- A stronger likelihood of erectile dysfunction than with other procedures
- Rectourethral fistula
- Urinary tract infections
- Epididymitis
- Urinary retention

Other Procedures. There are other newer surgical procedures used to treat BPH. These include the transurethral incision of the prostate (TUIP), balloon dilation of the prostate, microwave-hyperthermia of the prostate, transurethral laser incision of the prostate (TULIP), and the insertion of prostatic stents.

The TUIP is an option for men with small prostates causing outlet obstruction. This procedure has fewer postoperative complications and can be performed under local anesthesia for high-risk clients. Greater client satisfaction has also been reported with this procedure; many clients have reported no change in ejaculation, making this an excellent procedure for younger men with small glands.

Transurethral balloon dilation of the prostate is another new procedure that has become increasingly popular. The procedure is actually not surgical, but it is invasive. It involves the insertion of a small catheter into the urethra, with the positioning of a balloon within the prostatic urethra and inflating it to apply pressure to the enlarged gland, causing it to dilate. The balloon is carefully placed inside the prostatic urethra in a variety of ways. Care is taken to ensure that the balloon does not migrate downward, damaging the sphincter, or upward into the bladder, negating the effect. The balloon is inflated and left in place for 15 minutes. The client has a urethral catheter overnight.

This surgical procedure can be performed under local anesthesia, and there is no associated blood loss, making it appropriate for many high-risk clients. The hospital stay is short, and there are few postoperative complications. There are two major concerns with this procedure. First, because no tissue is removed, prostatic cancer could be missed. The other concern is the length of time this procedure will be effective. Because it is such a recent innovation, clients have not been monitored long enough to determine whether or not recurrence of the obstruction is common.

Microwave hyperthermia is one of the newest procedures being performed. Microwave hyperthermia is delivered via a rectal probe over a period of 4 to 10 treatments. Each treatment lasts about 60 minutes and is performed without anesthesia on an outpatient basis.

The newest treatment is TULIP. It is similar to the TUIP, but a laser is used to make the incision. The procedure results in minimal blood loss and requires no irrigation, and the client does not need a catheter after surgery.

The remaining new treatment is the insertion of a prostatic stent. This procedure is used for clients who are extremely poor operative risks. This hollow tube can be inserted through an endoscope into the prostatic urethra, where it holds the urethra open mechanically. It is safer than an indwelling urethral catheter because there is no risk of infection. The stent can be left in place for 4 to 6 weeks without problems. If left in place longer than this, epithelial cells will grow over the stent.

The most common early complication is postoperative bleeding. Other complications include

- Retrograde ejaculation (semen passing into the bladder instead of out through the penis) because of bladder neck surgical trauma
- Urethral stricture
- Bladder neck constriction
- Urinary incontinence
- Epididymitis

There is no treatment for retrograde ejaculation. The condition should be explained to clients so they are not frightened by this. The condition will result in sterility because the sperm are ejaculated into the bladder.

Urethral stricture can be treated postoperatively with dilation with urethral sounds. If the stricture is severe, a urethroplasty can be performed. Bladder neck contractures, if severe, also can be treated with surgical reconstruction.

Urinary incontinence is usually caused by trauma to the urinary sphincter. The client can decrease the symptoms by performing perineal exercises to improve muscle control. Kegel exercises are described in Chapter 30.

Epididymitis is a preventable complication if a vasectomy is performed at the same time as the prostatectomy. Tying the vas deferens prevents retrograde bacterial infection or inflammation of the epididymis. If the prostate is removed in its entirety, or is almost completely removed, the client will be sterile anyway.

Other possible complications are urinary tract infection, obstruction, accidental displacement of the catheter, incontinence, impotence, and recurrence of symptoms.

Nursing Management

Assessment

Men often have only a vague understanding about what an enlarged prostate is and may be afraid of the tests and their results. The nurse should carefully explain each part of the assessment process, show the client and significant others a picture of the reproductive organs and prostate, and explain the effects of enlargement on urine excretion.

The client should be asked to describe all urinary symptoms, including the pattern of urination, presence of urgency, frequency, decreased or altered urinary stream, hesitancy, and nocturia. The nurse should question the client about the presence of hematuria.

The ability of the client to empty his bladder also must be assessed. The client's bladder should be palpated for distention. If the client is unable to void, the need for a urethral catheter should be assessed.

Careful preoperative assessment in both physical and psychosocial areas is important. The client's knowledge about the surgery and its outcomes should be assessed. Because so many types of treatment are possible, the client may not understand the implications of the treatment he will be receiving.

Nursing Diagnosis, Planning, and Implementation

Collaborative Problem: Urinary Elimination, Altered Patterns R/T urethral obstruction.

Planning: Expected Outcomes. The client will be free of symptoms of BPH, as evidenced by absence of frequency, urgency, hesitancy, change in stream, incontinence, retention, or nocturia.

Implementation. The client may have preoperative urinary difficulties, such as obstruction, urinary retention, and diminished renal function. These problems may require early admission to the health-care facility for treatment. An indwelling catheter may be inserted, or drainage may be achieved by cystostomy.

A urinary catheter should never be forced. If it cannot be inserted with gentle pressure, the nurse should contact a urologist. Emergency catheterization for complete bladder obstruction requires a urologist's skills and possibly special instruments, such as insertion of a stylet (thin wire) into the catheter lumen, metal catheters, or other firm, specially angled catheters (coudé).

Nursing Diagnosis: Anxiety R/T hospitalization, urinary problems, and treatments.

Planning: Expected Outcomes. The client will state that his anxiety is reduced and he is able to rest quietly.

Implementation. Anxiety may be lessened by taking a nursing history and giving appropriate explanations. The nurse must respond to the concerns of the client and significant others with empathetic listening, accurate information, and ongoing support.

Nursing Diagnosis: Fluid Volume Deficit, Risk for R/T urinary symptoms and self-imposed fluid restriction.

Planning: Expected Outcomes. The client's fluid volume will remain within safe limits, as evidenced by intake of at least 2 L of fluid a day.

Implementation. It is important to improve the client's nutritional status preoperatively, especially fluid balance. Many clients limit their fluid intake to combat the symptoms of frequency and urgency they experience as a result of the prostatic enlargement. Clients increase their risk of urinary tract infection and even renal or cardiovascular dysfunction with this limited intake. The client should maintain, unless otherwise contraindicated, an intake of at least 2500 to 3000 mL/day to correct dehydration and azotemia (nitrogen waste products in the blood).

Nursing Diagnosis: Self-Esteem disturbance, Risk for R/T threats to sexuality from disease and treatment.

Planning: Expected Outcomes. The client will maintain a stable self-concept, as evidenced by client's willingness to discuss sexual issues.

Implementation. Most clients undergoing prostatectomy are older than 50 years. The aging process compounds the psychosocial threat involved in intimate surgery. Such clients may experience disturbing changes in self-concept, including body image, self-esteem, role performance, and personal identity. Sexual concerns may be a part of these changes.

It is usually helpful if the client and significant others can talk about these concerns with a supportive person. They need reassurance that their concerns (including fears of being unable to perform sexually) are common to men who undergo major surgery. Recommendations for any restrictions on sexual intercourse and alternative sexual activity are best given in collaboration with the physician. Clients who leave health-care facilities with incontinence, weakness, pain, and indwelling catheters may have additional concerns and self-doubts.

Significant others also need support after prostatectomy. They may not understand what is happening and may be concerned about potential or actual changes in their relationships.

Collaborative Problem: Fluid Volume Deficit, Risk for R/T postoperative hemorrhage.

Planning: Expected Outcomes. The client will maintain an adequate fluid volume, as evidenced by absence of hemorrhage and maintenance of at least 30 mL of urine output every hour.

Implementation. The nursing assessment described in Chapter 5 should be carried out to identify hemorrhage. In addition, the nurse must observe the wound drains, wound packing, and catheter drainage for excessive bleeding. Wound drains may be in place after perineal, retropubic, or suprapubic prostatectomies. A suprapubic urinary catheter positioned directly into the bladder through the abdominal wall is in place after suprapubic prostatectomies. Sometimes, the balloon of the indwelling catheter (Foley type) is inflated with 30 mL or more of fluid, up to 100 mL (rather than the usual 5 mL) to promote hemostasis at the operative site.

Some hematuria (blood in the urine) is usual for several days after surgery. However, frank bleeding, arterial or venous, may occur during the first day after surgery.

CRITICAL TO REMEMBER

Arterial bleeding is bright red, has numerous clots, and is viscous.

Blood pressure may fall, and emergency surgical intervention may become necessary. Venous bleeding in the prostatic area may be controlled by increasing the pressure (adding fluid) in the ballooned end of the urethral catheter and pulling the catheter tightly so the balloon moves into the prostatic fossa, then taping the catheter to the thigh (called applying traction). Traction is left in place for 24 hours or more and released by the physician when the bleeding has stopped. The physician also can remove fluid slowly from the balloon as the bleeding decreases.

Overdistention of the bladder must be avoided because it can precipitate secondary hemorrhage by placing undue strain on freshly coagulated blood vessels.

Nursing Diagnosis: Pain R/T surgery and bladder spasms.

Planning: Expected Outcomes. The client will report pain relieved or controlled.

Implementation. Pain control after surgery is discussed in Chapter 5. Additional pain can occur after prostatectomy if urinary drainage tubes become obstructed.

CRITICAL TO REMEMBER

The best intervention is to prevent catheters from becoming blocked.

If a client experiences pain after a prostatectomy, the nurse must first assess the drainage apparatus for patency. Relief of obstruction often alleviates pain without the need for analgesics. Clots are often the cause of the obstruction.

Bladder spasms also may occur because of bladder overdistention or irritation from an indwelling catheter balloon. Analgesics and antispasmodics may reduce the discomfort of bladder spasms. Antispasmodic drugs can cause constipation, and straining at stool can precipitate bleeding from the operative site, so stool softeners, such as docusate sodium (Colace) often are given.

Collaborative Problem: Injury, Risk for R/T presence of urinary catheters, irrigation, or suprapubic drains.

Planning: Expected Outcomes. The client will be free from injury such as infection, catheter obstruction, water intoxication, or injury resulting from the catheter, as evidenced by absence of fever; normal white cell count; adequate wound healing; adequate catheter drainage; hyponatremia, hypertension, or other signs of water intoxication; excessive bleeding or trauma from the catheter; urinary retention after catheter removal; or fistula formation.

Implementation. Indwelling catheters (urethral or suprapubic) are generally used to facilitate urinary drainage after all types of prostatectomies (see Fig. 52–3). Various types of catheter irrigation systems may be used with these catheters. Closed irrigation, referred to as a constant bladder irrigation, permits either constant or intermittent irrigation without the hazard of breaking aseptic technique. Continuous irrigation requires enough irrigant to maintain outflow of clear or slightly pink urine. The fluid must be isotonic, because water could lead to a depletion of electrolytes or water intoxication (see Chap. 3).

The nurse must frequently assess drainage from the catheter. Because the client usually receives intravenous fluid postoperatively, urinary catheters should be draining. Accurate records of intake and output must be kept, accounting for the amount instilled with the irrigation.

While a urinary catheter is in place, it must be kept patent (open, clear, and unobstructed). Urinary flow may become obstructed in various ways, such as with blood clots, prostatic chips, mucous plugs, kinked tubing, or tube displacement. The nurse should frequently assess catheter patency to make sure it is draining.

The catheter may become blocked by clots or sediment, leading to complications, such as infections, bladder distention, and painful bladder spasms. Some bladder spasms occur with bladder distention, whereas others are a response to irritation from the catheter balloon (from excessive fluid in the balloon to prevent bleeding).

It is important to prevent bladder overdistention, such as during irrigation or as a result of urinary obstruction. Bladder overdistention can cause hemorrhage by placing undue strain on freshly coagulated blood vessels. The nurse should assess the client for bladder overdistention by shutting off continuous irrigation and palpating the lower abdomen. The surgeon must be contacted for specific orders.

If a catheter cannot be cleared, it may have to be removed and a new one inserted. This procedure is usually performed by the surgeon.

The client may be confused immediately after surgery and may accidentally pull out the catheter. The client must be told repeatedly that he has a tube in his bladder through his penis or abdomen (whichever it is) and reminded not to touch it. A displaced or removed urinary catheter after prostatic surgery is painful and disrupts recovery. If the client does pull the catheter out, the surgeon should be contacted for reinsertion.

The nurse should observe the client carefully for local or systemic indications of infection. Catheters, drainage apparatus, and urine collection should be handled carefully to avoid introducing micro-organisms into the urinary tract. Aseptic technique is especially important after a perineal prostatectomy because of a high possibility of infection in a wound so close to the anal area. Meticulous aseptic technique is also necessary around the area of insertion of a suprapubic catheter.

The surgeon may make the initial dressing change and delegate subsequent wound care to the nurses. The client may be taught to change his own dressing. When a perineal incision is present, a double-tailed T-binder may be used to secure dressings. Wound trauma after perineal surgery must be prevented by avoiding the use of enemas, rectal tubes, or rectal thermometers. The wound must be cleaned thoroughly after each bowel movement.

The length of time urethral catheters are left inserted varies according to surgeon preference, the client's recovery, and the type of surgery. After perineal prostatectomy, a urethral catheter may be left in place for 12 to 14 days to allow for healing of the resected bladder neck and urethra. After a simple TUR, it may be removed after 2 to 3 days if the urine remains clear. Sometimes the catheter is removed early if it is causing problems, such as bladder spasms.

After a urethral catheter is removed (and after a TUR), the nurse should monitor the client closely for signs of urinary retention and urethral strictures. Indications of urinary retention include inability to pass urine and bladder overdistention. Indications of urethral stricture include a small urinary stream, dysuria, and straining to urinate. The nurse should talk to the client and significant others about the importance of urinating when the client first feels a desire to do so. Holding the urine may increase the possibility of retention.

Temporary urinary frequency or incontinence may occur after the catheter is removed. The nurse must be understanding of the client's feelings and keep him dry without embarrassing him. The nurse should keep reminding him and his significant others that these problems are temporary, but that they may take some time to resolve. Urinary control usually returns quickly in young men, whereas in older men, a period of dribbling for up to 3 months is not unusual. Perineal exercises may reduce this problem (see the section on Knowledge Deficit). Additional surgery is sometimes required for persistent incontinence.

Wound drains are usually removed earlier than suprapubic drains. The suprapubic drain is left in place until urinary function has returned. Once the client is voiding well, the suprapubic drain can be removed. If it is removed before the client has returned to a normal voiding, the wound may not heal properly, leading to fistula formation.

Nursing Diagnosis: Knowledge Deficit R/T postoperative exercises and return of urinary function.

Planning: Expected Outcomes. The client will express an understanding of how to perform postoperative exercises and of the return of urinary function.

Implementation. Throughout the postoperative period, the nurse must explain each procedure and expectation, such as not to strain at stool, to the client and encourage his participation. Specific teaching opportunities for the client and significant others are appropriate and include the following categories.

Catheters, Wound Drains, Urinary Drainage, and Irrigation. The nurse should provide information about related procedures and answer questions patiently. The client and significant others must be told that it is important not to touch the equipment, pull out the tubes, or obstruct the drainage. The client must be helped to learn ways of turning and getting out of bed without pulling on the catheter or kinking the drainage tubing. The client must be reminded not to lie on the tubing. The nurse can show the client and significant others how to make sure the tubing always remains above the level of the drainage bag, because if the tubing falls at or below the drainage bag the flow of urine may be impeded and actually pass back into the bladder.

Common Sensations. Common sensations experienced by clients after a prostatectomy are that (1) the ureteral catheter may cause bladder spasms and a sensation of needing to pass urine, and (2) after removal of a catheter, dribbling of urine and a sense of urgency may occur.

Urinary and Wound Drainage. Urinary and wound drainage, such as bloody urine, is not unusual early in the postoperative period.

Permission to Tell Nurses of Concerns or Discomforts. Many men find it difficult to admit to discomfort or pain, such as from bladder spasms. The nurse must ask them frequently about this problem and remind them of the importance of revealing this.

Self-Help Activities. These include drinking increased amounts of fluids while a catheter is in place, performing bed exercises, incorporating early ambulation, and measuring fluid intake and urinary output. Prolonged sitting increases intra-abdominal pressure and may precipitate bleeding. Therefore, the client should avoid sitting except during meals. After he leaves the health-care facility, driving an automobile or taking prolonged automobile rides should be avoided until at least 2 weeks after surgery, when the risk of bleeding lessens. Strenuous exercise is also contraindicated.

The client must be advised not to strain during defecation for at least 6 weeks after surgery, because this can lead to bleeding from the operative site. The surgeon will prescribe appropriate stool softeners or mild laxatives.

Perineal Exercises. These help the client regain urinary sphincter control. From the second or third postoperative day, the client must be taught to breathe normally while contracting abdominal, gluteal, and perineal muscles 12 to 25 times each hour. A good way to describe this action is "Contract your muscles as if you have to pass urine urgently and there is no place to relieve yourself."

Another helpful exercise is to squeeze the rectal sphincter tensely while relaxing other body muscles. The nurse should teach the client to place his hands on his abdomen to assess abdominal tension. The abdomen should not be tense and a Valsalva maneuver should not occur when the exercise is performed correctly. During these exercises, it may help the client concentrate if he says aloud words such as relax and squeeze. The client must be encouraged to establish a planned schedule of exercising during waking hours and continue this routine until complete urinary control is achieved.

Advice on Leaving the Health-Care Facility. The client is usually discharged 2 to 3 days after a TUR and up to 10 days after a radical perineal prostatectomy. The nurse must be sure he knows when and where to contact his surgeon next and how to get in touch with health-care professionals if he has concerns before that time. The nurse must tell the client to be sure to report to his surgeon any bleeding, infection, or obstructed urine flow. However, he must be given support and permission to discuss any concern with a health-care professional.

The nurse should advise the client to avoid strenuous activity for 4 to 6 weeks (e.g., mowing the lawn, lifting more than 20 pounds). He will probably need extra rest while at the same time maintaining a balance of activity with ambulation. He may drive a car when given permission, usually after his first visit to the physician.

The client should be advised to continue a high daily intake of nonalcoholic fluids to minimize clot formation. If he is discharged home with an indwelling catheter, the nurse should provide him and his significant others with appropriate information (see Box 52–1).

Nursing Diagnosis: Sexual Dysfunction R/T removal of prostate, retrograde ejaculation, and sterility.

Planning: Expected Outcomes. The client will be without sexual dysfunction, as evidenced by client statements and the client's ability to discuss fears and concerns with staff.

Implementation. Retrograde ejaculation consists of the ejaculation of semen into the bladder rather than through the urethra. The man experiences erection and orgasm, but normal ejaculation does not occur. Retrograde ejaculation may occur after a prostatectomy because when the prostatic capsule contracts, the semen passes more easily into the bladder rather than through the urethra. Semen passes into the bladder and mixes with the urine, producing cloudy urine. The client must be advised to observe his urine for cloudiness and tell his physician if it occurs.

Erectile dysfunction (impotence) is a rare complication of prostatectomy.

Referral for sexual counseling may be helpful. The client needs to know that he can still please a partner and that sometimes lovemaking techniques other than intercourse may even be necessary. The couple may need information about alternatives to intercourse such as cuddling, stroking, or manual or oral stimulation to orgasm. Talking about options may enhance communications between the client and his partner. A penile implant may be considered (see the section on Erectile Dysfunction).

Evaluation

The nurse must evaluate client outcomes based on the established plan of care. If these goals were not achieved, the plan and interventions must be revised to meet the client's needs.

Client Teaching

As stated previously, the client should be taught about potential urinary incontinence and the exercises that should decrease it. They are also taught about any further need for treatment with some therapies, such as recurrence years after a TUR.

Clients should be taught to maintain a high fluid intake (2000–3000 mL/day) to ensure a good urine output. Clients who had undergone TUR or balloon dilation also must be taught about the possibility of recurrence, because prostatic tissue that is left can continue to hypertrophy.

There are no specific home health-care needs for this client. The only equipment the client may have is a catheter, which should be removed within several weeks of surgery.

The client should be encouraged to discuss any sexual problems that occur after the surgery. If necessary, sexual counseling may be required.

The client should be seen after surgery to be checked for the development of urethral strictures or bladder neck contractures. Clients may need urethral dilation after surgery.

If the entire gland was not removed, clients should continue yearly checkups for the development of prostate cancer.

BOX 52–1

Catheter Insertion in the Home Setting

When inserting a catheter in the home setting, there is rarely the convenience of a hospital bed. Often, the lighting is not ideal. Although supplies may be sent home from the hospital with the client, obtaining the supplies is usually the responsibility of the home health-care nurse.

Male catheters are frequently inserted by the female home health-care nurse. The nurse may want to make a shared visit with an experienced home health-care nurse for the first time or two to achieve a little more confidence. If difficulty is encountered inserting the catheter in a male client, the catheter can be removed and 3 to 5 mL of K-Y gel inserted directly into the meatus by using a sterile syringe without the needle. If the nurse knows the catheter change is going to be difficult, the K-Y gel can be instilled first. Then, when resistance is met, one can use steady, easy pressure and rotate the catheter slowly until it finally slips through the constricture.

Most urologists use lidocaine (Xylocaine) gel for inserting male catheters, so the nurse may request an order from the physician for Xylocaine gel. It is inserted just like the K-Y gel, and a few minutes must pass before the catheter is inserted. This will relieve some of the pain and help the client relax.

Remember that if the client has had a catheter inserted for a long time, an immediate urine return may not be achieved. The person should drink a glass of water and wait 15 to 30 minutes. Because it may be some time before the home health-care nurse returns, it is especially important that the client has been instructed to drink adequate fluids, observe the color and amount of urine, and report changes to the nurse or physician.

PROSTATE CANCER

Incidence

Prostate cancer is the most common cancer among men and the third leading cause of death among men in the United States.[6] Most clients with clinically detectable prostate cancer are older than 50 years; therefore, the man's risk of prostate cancer increases with each decade after age 50. Young men, however, seem to have more aggressive disease and are more likely to have metastasis at time of diagnosis.

Black men have a higher incidence than white men in this country. The condition tends to occur more in certain families regardless of race.

Etiology

The cause of prostate cancer is unknown, but epidemiologic studies suggest several associated factors.

HORMONAL FACTORS

Although exact mechanisms and factors are not known, the incidence of prostate cancer is higher in men (1) who had a late puberty, (2) who have high frequency of sexual experience, (3) with a history of multiple sexual partners, and (4) with higher fertility. Because the risk of prostatic cancer increases with age, it may be associated with the hormonal shifts associated with aging, such as lower amounts of androsterone and higher serum levels of estrogen and estradiol.

DIET

Differences in mortality rates from prostatic cancer between Asians and Caucasians have been associated with dietary differences. High fat consumption (typical of American diets) can alter cholesterol and steroid metabolism, which may increase the risk of cancer. Green and yellow vegetables (typical of Japanese diets) could have a protective effect against prostatic cancer.

CHEMICAL CARCINOGENS

Occupational and environmental hazard exposure to carcinogens may increase the risk of prostatic cancer. There is a higher incidence in urban areas, which suggests air pollution may be a factor. Occupations linked to higher rates of prostatic cancer include employment in fertilizer, textile, and rubber industries; and work with batteries containing cadmium.

VIRUSES

The observation by electron microscopy of virus particles in carcinomatous prostatic tissue suggests that viruses may be associated with the disease. Gonorrhea is also associated with an increased incidence of prostatic cancer, although it is assumed that people with gonorrhea are exposed to a virus concurrently.

It is hoped that late prostatic cancer will become rare as increasing emphasis is placed on early diagnosis through routine rectal examinations, rectal ultrasound studies, measurement of prostate-specific antigen (PSA), and prompt intervention.

Pathophysiology

The appearance of prostatic cancer is variable, adding to the difficulty of diagnosis and staging and grading of the tumor. These tumors are usually adenocarcinomas. The tumor begins in the periphery of the posterior lobe of the gland, whereas BPH occurs centrally and is large by the time it restricts urination. The tumor may appear as a normal prostate, which delays diagnosis.

Clinical Manifestations

CRITICAL TO REMEMBER

There may be no symptoms of prostatic cancer, unless BPH is present at the same time.

The presenting findings are most often those of prostatitis, such as infection. Obstruction is rare unless BPH is present, because the cancer is usually found in the periphery of the posterior lobe. Unfortunately, the tumor may escape detection until the disease is advanced. Also, 15 to 40 per cent of men with prostatic cancer present with late symptoms caused by metastasis, such as hip or back bone pain. Rectal pressure or obstruction from local tumor growth may produce stool changes and painful defecation. Painful ejaculation also may be experienced.

DIAGNOSTIC ASSESSMENT

Early diagnosis is essential. Diagnostic tests include digital rectal examination; laboratory tests such as alkaline and acid phosphatase, radiography, rectal ultrasound, computed tomography (CT) scanning, radionuclide imaging, transrectal and percutaneous needle aspiration and biopsy, and tumor markers such as the PSA.

CRITICAL TO REMEMBER

Annual digital rectal examination is recommended for all men older than 40 years, because colon cancer and prostate cancer can be screened for at the same time.

Examination every 6 months is recommended if (1) the client has a history of continuing urinary symptoms, especially if a blood relative has had prostate cancer, or (2) if he has BPH or has had subtotal prostatectomy. Even so, 10 to 20 per cent of tumors are too small to be determined by rectal examination.

Transrectal ultrasonography is a modality used for early detection of prostatic cancer. This simple diagnostic test is capable of discovering possibly twice as many prostate cancers as digital rectal examination.[6]

Tumor markers are another means of assessment. The serum level of acid phosphatase was the most important biochemical test in diagnosing prostate cancer. The newer and even more specific test is the PSA. The PSA is particularly useful in monitoring clients with prostate cancer; an elevation of the PSA signals that the tumor is growing.

Acid phosphatase is not usually a tumor-specific marker because it is produced in a number of body tissues. High serum levels of prostatic acid phosphatase are associated with metastatic prostate cancer.

Laboratory tests screen for indications of bladder obstruction, tumor obstruction, or metastasis to areas such as the liver and bone marrow. These tests include complete blood count, SMA-12, blood urea nitrogen, creatinine, and liver function studies.

X-ray assessment includes chest radiography, intravenous pyelogram (IVP), and lymphangiography, and is used to screen for obstructive uropathy and metastases in the skeleton and lymph nodes.

Ultrasonography, CT scanning, and magnetic resonance imaging (MRI) assess for the local extent of the tumor. Although CT scanning does not differentiate cancer of the prostate from BPH, it is useful in assessing large tumors. Transrectal ultrasonography is useful in assessing the size and shape of the prostate, locating tumors within the capsule of the prostate, and monitoring tumor response to treatment.

Radionuclide imaging is used to detect bone lesions. Bone metastasis occurs in 75 to 85 per cent of men with prostatic cancer, depending on the stage of the disease. Lesions may be detected by bone scans 6 months or more before abnormalities appear on a bone x-ray film.

Needle aspiration or biopsy is used to confirm suspected malignancy.

GRADING AND STAGING

Grading of prostatic cancer is conducted to try to establish the activity or virulence of the disease. Staging is an attempt to define the extent to which the carcinoma has developed. Refer to Chapter 6 for staging information.

Medical Management

The treatment of prostatic cancer is controversial because of the varied biologic behavior of the disease and staging methods that do not accurately predict malignant potential. Various treatment combinations may be used, depending on the choices of the person and physician, and the stage the condition has reached. For example, if the tumor is well differentiated and of low volume, TUR may be sufficient. However, if extensive metastases have developed by the time a diagnosis is made, palliative treatment may be all that is available.

RADIATION THERAPY

Radiation therapy includes (1) interstitial irradiation, (2) combined interstitial and external-beam irradiation, and (3) external beam megavoltage irradiation (see also Chap. 7). Interstitial irradiation is used to control locally advanced tumors (usually stage B or C). Radioactive metals, such as iodine (^{125}I), are used to destroy tumors directly. One widely used technique is to perform a pelvic lymphadenectomy and implant iodine seeds into the prostate, with needles. Complications include thrombophlebitis, lymphocele formation, edema, and obstructive problems during voiding.

Combined interstitial and external beam irradiation involves implanting gold in the prostate, followed by external beam irradiation. Thus, an effective dose can be delivered in several weeks, followed by external beam full pelvic irradiation over several more weeks. Implanting gold alone would destroy surrounding tissue. Complications include edema of the penis and lower extremities, cystitis, and urethritis. A major advantage of interstitial therapy is preservation of erection for most men treated this way.

External beam megavoltage irradiation is used when tumors are confined to the prostate and surrounding tissue. Surrounding tissue is relatively spared. The result depends on the size and grade of the tumor.

PHARMACOLOGIC MANAGEMENT

Endocrine therapy is used based on an observation that prostate epithelial cells atrophy if they are deprived of androgens. Endocrine therapy is used to (1) remove the source of androgen, (2) suppress pituitary gonadotropin, (3) interfere with androgen synthesis, and (4) interfere with the action of androgen on the tissue.

The first oral androgen blocker, flutamide (Eulexin), is one of the newest medications used to treat prostate cancer. The gonadotropin-releasing hormone analogs leuprolide (Lupron) and goserelin acetate (Zoladex) are also being used. These agents block the action or secretion of androgens, which stimulate tumor growth, without causing the side effects that estrogen does. Finasteride (Proscar) is also used to treat it.

Administration of estrogen (diethylstilbestrol [DES]) suppresses the release of pituitary gonadotropin and reduces serum testosterone levels. Side effects include cardiovascular symptoms and gynecomastia. Gynecomastia can be lessened by giving the client breast radiation before estrogen therapy.

Nonendocrine chemotherapy (either singly or in combination) has been used with prostate cancers to treat or sometimes stabilize the disease. Examples of chemotherapeutic agents sometimes used are cyclophosphamide (Cytoxan), 5-fluorouracil (Fluorouracil), estramustine phosphate (Emcyt), doxorubicin hydrochloride (Adriamycin), and mitomycin-C (Mutamycin).

Surgical Management

Surgical approaches include TURP and radical prostatectomy and cryosurgery. TURP may be used for well-differentiated tumors of low volume or to relieve obstruction in advanced disease. Repeated TURP is sometimes needed to maintain an adequate channel through the prostatic urethra. (See discussion of TURP.)

Radical prostatectomy via a perineal (see Fig. 52–3*D*) or retropubic approach may be performed. Radical surgery involves removing (1) the entire prostate gland (rather than just enucleation), (2) the outer capsule, (3) the seminal vesicles, (4) sections of the vas deferens, and (5) possibly portions of the bladder neck. This surgery may be chosen for clients who have no other serious medical problems, a discrete tumor involving less than one lobe (i.e., stage B-1), and a survival expectation of at least 10 to 15 years. It is sometimes used for clients with stage B-2 or C tumors.

Common side effects of radical prostatectomy are erectile dysfunction (as high as 85–90 per cent) and incontinence (10–15 per cent). Both of these side effects are difficult for a man to experience and discuss. Improved surgical techniques and advances in treating erectile dysfunction and incontinence help many clients overcome these difficulties.

Cryosurgery, an experimental surgery using liquid nitrogen at subzero temperatures inserted via tiny punctures through five probes, may become the preferred treatment for prostate cancer. Although the procedure takes only a few hours and requires only a week's stay in the hospital, complication such as fistula formation are possible.

Artificial urinary sphincters have been surgically implanted for refractory urinary incontinence.

Bilateral orchiectomy is the most effective way to remove the source of androgen. This surgical procedure removes the testicles, which lowers serum testosterone significantly.

Nursing Management

Nursing care of clients with prostatic cancer is essentially the same as that for a client with BPH. Their concerns are often considerable and may include the choices of available treatments, fear of death, anxiety about residual disability and illness, and the possible effects of the illness on people in their social network.

Modification of Plan of Care for the Elderly

Again, prostate cancer occurs most commonly in men older than 50 years, so the older client is the one most likely to develop this disorder. Hormonal manipulation seems to prolong survival significantly for the older client.

Client Teaching

Discharge teaching is similar to that for the client with BPH. If the client is experiencing incontinence, the Kegel exercises will help control this condition. Teaching concerning medication and further therapy also will be needed.

The client will need to be seen by the physician at regular intervals to measure the PSA level. An increase in this antigen indicates further tumor growth and the need for further treatment.

PROSTATITIS

Prostatitis, inflammation of the prostate gland, may be (1) acute bacterial, (2) chronic bacterial, or (3) nonbacterial.

Acute bacterial prostatitis is usually caused by aerobic gram-negative rods, the coliforms (especially *Escherichia coli*) and *Pseudomonas*. Routes of infection include (1) urethral ascent, (2) descent from the urinary bladder or kidneys, (3) direct extension or lymphatogenous spread from the rectum, and (4) hematogenous spread (via blood). Assessment reveals chills and fever, low back and perineal pain, and urinary urgency, frequency, nocturia, and dysuria. Bladder outlet obstruction, myalgia (painful muscles), and arthralgia (painful joints) may occur. On examination, the prostate is extremely tender and swollen, yet it is firm, indurated, and warm to the touch. Acute cystitis (bladder inflammation) is common, with hematuria and cloudy, malodorous urine. Urine cultures identify the infecting organisms. Exudate from prostatic massage (see Chap. 51) can also identify the organism, but this is not usually performed, because such massage is very painful for a client with prostatitis and can precipitate bacteremia. Transurethral instrumentation, including catheterization, is avoided during acute infection, because it can push infection up into the bladder. Intervention includes rest, analgesics, stool softeners (constipation is painful with prostatitis), antimicrobial medication, sitz baths, and increased oral fluids. Occasionally, the inflammation is so severe that the client cannot pass urine, and catheterization is needed.

Chronic bacterial prostatitis is a nonacute infection of the prostate gland. It is most commonly caused by the same organisms that cause acute bacterial prostatitis and has the same routes of infection. Chronic bacterial prostatitis is a less severe inflammation than the acute type. Some clients have no symptoms. A diagnosis may be made after finding bacteriuria (bacteria in the urine) on routine urinalysis. Other clients may experience (1) voiding dysfunction, such as urgency, frequency, nocturia, and dysuria; (2) low back or perineal pain; or (3) occasional myalgia (muscle aches) and arthralgia (painful joints). There may be inflammatory cells in prostatic secretions. If the client has cystitis, organisms may be identified in urine specimens. If urine is not infected, organisms may be identified from midstream urine specimen, urethral specimens, and prostatic massage.

Discomfort and pain may be relieved by sitz baths, anti-inflammatory agents, and anticholinergic drugs. Repeated prostatic massage and ejaculation may be helpful. Surgical intervention is rarely required. Long-term, low-dose antimicrobial drugs may control symptoms.

Nonbacterial prostatitis is the most common form of prostatitis. Its cause is unknown. It has the same symptoms as bacterial prostatitis, but no causative organism is found. On prostatic massage, abnormal numbers of inflammatory cells are noted in the prostatic fluid, but no infectious agent is found.

Assessment findings for nonbacterial prostatitis are similar to those of bacterial prostatitis except that bacteria are not found in the urine or prostatic secretions. Diagnosis is made by systematically ruling out other types of prostatitis. This can be depressing for the client because diagnosis and treatment are not specific. Intervention includes anti-inflammatory agents or short-term antimicrobial medication. Warm sitz baths and normal sexual activity are recommended.

Testicular Disorders and Procedures

TESTICULAR TUMORS

Testicular cancer is the most common and serious solid tumor cancer in men between the ages of 15 and 35 years.

Incidence

Testicular cancer rarely occurs in men younger than 15 years or older than 40 years. Two to 3 cases per 100,000 men are diagnosed in the United States each year.

Etiology

The cause of testicular cancer is unknown. Exogenous estrogen and cryptorchidism are considered possible causes.

Risk Factors

The major risk factor for testicular cancer is cryptorchidism (undescended testicles). It is now recommended that any child born with an undescended testicle have an orchiopexy as soon as possible after birth. It is believed that the longer the testicles are left undescended, the greater the risk of testicular cancer. Performing an orchiopexy, however, does not completely eliminate the risk of cancer.

The male offspring of women who used the drug DES, a synthetic estrogen, during the first trimester of pregnancy (called DES sons) or who were exposed to estrogen-progestin combinations frequently used in diagnostic tests to confirm pregnancy are at greater risk for testicular cancer.

It is now being found that 30 to 70 per cent of DES sons also have genital abnormalities, such as undescended testicles (increased risk of cancer), micropenis, meatal stenosis (narrowing of penile opening), varicocele, hypoplastic (underdeveloped) testicles, and epididymal cysts. DES sons also have an increased risk of infertility and abnormal semen.

There is no primary prevention for testicular cancer, so all men between the ages of 15 and 40 years should practice testicular self-examination on a regular monthly basis.

Pathophysiology

Most of the cases of testicular cancer (97 per cent) are germinal cell tumors, such as seminomas (about 40 per cent of all tumors), teratocarcinomas, embryonal carcinoma, or choriocarcinoma. Seminomas generally have a favorable prognosis of about a 90 per cent 5 year survival rate because they are usually localized and metastasize late. These tumors are usually treated with orchiectomy and radiation therapy. They are usually confined to the testes and retroperitoneal nodes.

Nonseminomatous germ cell tumors are not as sensitive to radiation therapy; however, with the advent of newer chemotherapy regimens after orchiectomy, the cure rate has risen to 95 per cent overall.

Nongerminal tumors make up the remainder of testicular cancers. These tumors arise from interstitial cells or cells that compose the fibrous or vascular networks. They are classified as either interstitial cell tumors or testicular adenomas that are usually benign.

The overall survival rate from all types of testicular cancer is about 89 per cent in whites and 78 per cent in blacks.[29]

Clinical Manifestations

Most commonly, men with testicular tumors experience a painless enlargement, noted as heaviness, in the testicle (about 75 per cent). Some men describe it as a dragging sensation. Pain is rarely felt; however, the tumor is often found after an injury because the testicle is examined as a result of the injury. Hydrocele or hematocele may develop. Some symptoms of testicular cancer resemble the symptoms of varicocele, and some are similar to the symptoms of prostatitis.

Assessment findings suggesting metastasis include back pain, vague abdominal pain, nausea and vomiting, anorexia, and weight loss.

DIAGNOSTIC ASSESSMENT

A thorough physical examination of the scrotum and testicles is the first diagnostic test performed. Unlike a simple hydrocele, a testicular tumor is not translucent to light.

A radical orchiectomy is the major diagnostic tool because the entire testicle is removed for biopsy after a mass has been detected. Any testicular mass is considered malignant until proved otherwise.

Other diagnostic tests used to determine the possible extent of the tumor include (1) a chest x-ray study or CT of the lungs for lung metastasis, (2) an abdominal and pelvic CT scan or MRI for retroperitoneal lymph node involvement, (3) an IVP for urinary tract involvement, (4) a lymphangiogram for retroperitoneal lymph node involvement (performed less frequently because CT and MRI are available), and (5) laboratory studies for serum alpha-fetoprotein and hCG-β as tumor markers.

Medical Management

The primary treatment for testicular cancer is surgical resection of the testicle. Radiation and chemotherapy also may be used.

Seminomas are particularly radiosensitive. The perineum and pelvis and the mediastinal and supraclavicular nodes are also irradiated if the peritoneal nodes are positive. Side effects include common complications associated with pelvic radiation. Radiation is not used for nonseminomatous tumors because they are not very radiosensitive.

Chemotherapy is used for both seminomas and nonseminomatous tumors that have any sign of spread. The major agent used is cisplatin in combination with vinblastine and bleomycin. Cisplatin in combination with other agents dramatically increased the long-term survival rate for men with testicular cancer. These agents in combination with a variety of others have been used to treat metastatic disease or refractory tumors with some success.

Complications of these chemotherapeutic agents are discussed in detail in Chapter 7. The major problem associated with cisplatin is nephrotoxicity; with bleomycin, pneumonitis; and with vinblastine, peripheral neuropathy.

Surgical Management

As discussed earlier, a radical orchiectomy is performed to diagnose testicular cancer, so it also is the primary treatment. The amputated testicle can be replaced with a testicular prosthesis. This reconstructive surgery is recommended to help the young client's self-esteem.

Many surgeons are opting simply for the radical orchiectomy and diagnostic studies of the retroperitoneal lymph nodes without surgical resection.

The group that supports the retroperitoneal node dissection believes that using this approach limits the amount of chemotherapy needed because the extent of the tumor spread can be removed.

The major complication of retroperitoneal node dissection is impotence. If a bilateral orchiectomy is performed, infertility occurs.

Nursing Management

One of the primary activities of the nurse that is used to help with early detection of this treatable cancer is teaching young men testicular self-examination. This procedure is detailed in Chapter 51.

During assessment, the nurse should ask whether his mother took any medication during pregnancy to prevent pregnancy or miscarriage. If he seems at particular risk but does not know these details, it may be necessary to obtain the mother's medical history.

Supportive nursing care is very important for these young men both during diagnosis and treatment. The nurse must be very aware of the threat to sexuality this condition and its treatment have on the young men. Chapters 5 and 7 discuss the care of clients undergoing surgery, chemotherapy, and radiation therapy.

HYDROCELE, HEMATOCELE, AND SPERMATOCELE

Hydrocele (Fig. 52–4*A*) is a painless collection of clear, yellow fluid anywhere along the spermatic cord. The soft intrascrotal mass is translucent to light (see Chap. 51). If complications develop, such as discomfort from enlargement or impaired circulation, aspiration or surgical drainage may be performed.

A hematocele is a collection of blood in the tunica vaginalis. A spermatocele is a dilation, originating in the epididymis, containing a milky fluid and spermatozoa.

VARICOCELE

Varicocele (Fig. 52–4*B*) is a dilation and varicosity of the pampiniform plexus (network of veins supplying the testicles) within the scrotum. Ninety per cent of varicoceles are left sided. They occur in 15 to 20 per cent of men between 15 and 25 years of age. The client may experience a pulling sensation, a dull ache, or scrotal pain. Pain may be relieved by masturbation or sexual intercourse.

On palpation, with the client standing, a varicocele feels like a mass of tortuous veins above and posterior to the testicle. When the client lies down, the mass abates. Although the condition is not clearly understood, varicocele is an important cause of male infertility. Treatment includes the use of a scrotal support, with surgery being performed only if complications

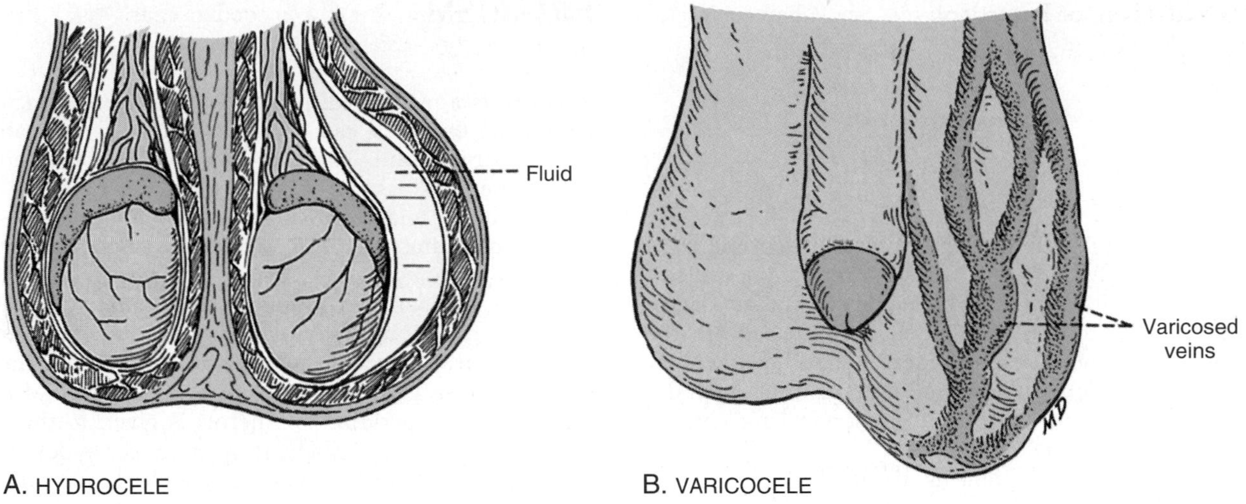

Figure 52–4
Disturbances of the testicles.

occur, such as severe pain, or if the varicocele is thought to contribute to infertility.

VASECTOMY

A vasectomy is an elective surgical procedure performed as a permanent method of contraception (although sometimes a vasectomy can be surgically reversed). This procedure also often is performed after a prostatectomy to prevent retrograde epididymitis.

The surgery is usually performed under local anesthesia in the urologist's office or an outpatient setting. The procedure, performed through a small incision in the scrotum, involves the cutting out of a piece of the vas deferens and folding and ligating the remaining ends (Fig. 52–5).

Postoperatively, slight pain and swelling are easily controlled with an ice bag and mild analgesia such as acetaminophen. A scrotal support also increases client comfort. The client can resume sexual intercourse whenever he finds it comfortable, usually about 1 week after the procedure. The client must continue to practice other means of birth control until the follow-up semen analysis shows azoospermia, because live sperm are left in the ampulla of vas.

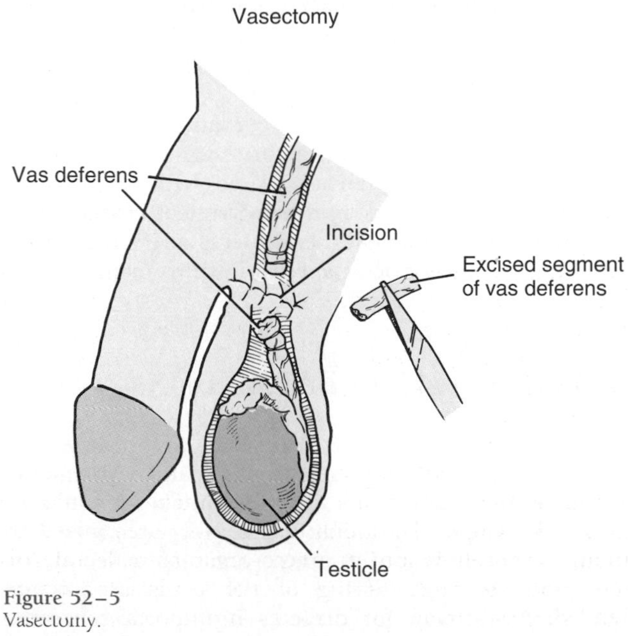

Figure 52–5
Vasectomy.

Penile Disorders

URETHRITIS

Urethritis is an acute urethral inflammation and is discussed under sexually transmitted diseases and urinary disorders (see Chaps. 30 and 54).

URETHRAL STRICTURE

Urethral stricture is caused by urethral scarring or narrowing. It may be congenital or caused by untreated or severe urethritis or urethral injury (including urologic instrumentation, e.g., cystoscopy). Symptoms are caused by obstruction, such as small-caliber urinary stream, hyperdistended bladder, infection, fever, and dysuria. Urethral strictures are released surgically by urethral dilation or urethroplasty. See Chapter 30 for further information.

PHIMOSIS

Phimosis occurs when the penile foreskin (prepuce) is constricted at the opening, making retraction difficult or impossible. It is caused by edema or inflammation and is often associated with poor cleaning beneath the foreskin. Assessment reveals edema, erythema, tenderness, and purulent discharge. Intervention includes controlling infection with local treatment and broad-spectrum antimicrobial drugs.

Effective genital hygiene is essential to prevent acquired penile disorders. In uncircumcised males, the penis is cleaned by pulling the foreskin back gently and washing the area with a washcloth.

Routine circumcision has not been seen as medically necessary according to the American Academy of Pediatrics and many other health professionals and health organizations. Circumcision may be indicated in clients with penile infection, phimosis, or paraphimosis. Potential risks include excessive bleeding, infection, and penile trauma. However, they have reconsidered this decision based on the fact that the rate of penile cancer is almost zero in circumcised men. The nurse must be sure uncircumcised men know how to retract the foreskin daily and clean the smegma from beneath it properly.

PARAPHIMOSIS

Paraphimosis (Fig. 52–6) occurs when a tight foreskin, once retracted, cannot be returned to its normal position. Circulation is thus impeded, and the glans swells rapidly. Paraphimosis sometimes occurs after rigorous cleaning, masturbation, sexual intercourse, or cystoscopy if the foreskin is not returned to its normal position. Manual reduction may be attempted by squeezing the glans for 5 minutes. Surgical incision with local anesthesia may be necessary.

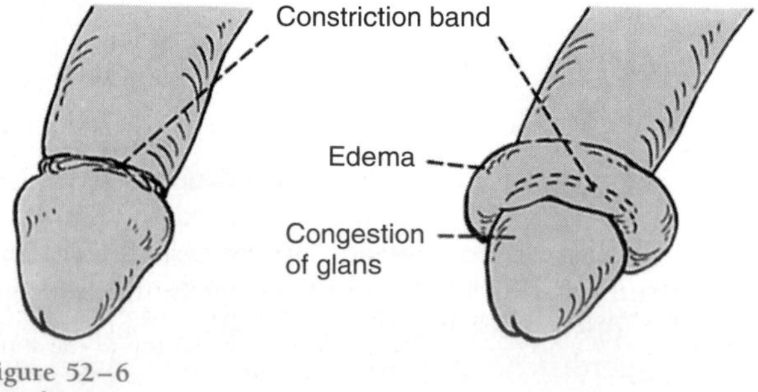

Figure 52–6
Paraphimosis.

PRIAPISM

Priapism is a prolonged, persistent penile erection without sexual desire. It can last hours or even days and is usually very painful. There is no known cause, although it is sometimes associated with leukemia or sickle cell anemia. It also may result from some medications, such as anticoagulants, alcohol, phenothiazines, and marijuana.

This problem is considered an emergency situation because circulation to the penis is usually compromised and the client may be unable to void. Treatment includes bedrest, prostatic massage, and sedation. Medication such as meperidine (Demerol) is given in the hope it will both relax the client and cause hypotension. Warm blankets are sometimes applied to promote venous dilatation. If the client is unable to void, he may have to be catheterized by the physician.

Priapism must be resolved within 24 hours or penile ischemia, gangrene, fibrosis, and even impotence might develop. If the more conservative treatments are unsuccessful in resolving the problem, aspiration with a large-bore needle or incision of the corpus cavernosa may be required. If the cause can be identified, treatment also is directed at preventing recurrence.

The nurse caring for this client must be sensitive to the embarrassing nature of this problem. Men are often reluctant to admit that this problem has occurred and yet are often in severe pain. The nurse must be understanding and attempt to make the client comfortable while decreasing the client's embarrassment over this problem.

PEYRONIE'S DISEASE

Fibrous plaques may develop near the dorsal midline of the penile shaft in middle-aged and older men. A high percentage of older men acquire these plaques. Diagnosis is usually made only if the nurse questions the client about this during the history.

Assessment reveals penile curvature on erection, painful erection, and unsatisfactory vaginal penetration. Peyronie's disease is often associated with Dupuytren's contracture of the hand tendons. Surgical correction is often necessary, but other treatments are often tried, including waiting for spontaneous improvement.

POSTHITIS AND BALANITIS

Posthitis is foreskin inflammation. Balanitis is inflammation of the glans penis and the mucous membrane beneath it. These conditions (Fig. 52–7) are caused by irritation and invasion of micro-organisms. Good hygiene and thorough drying of the penis are recommended. Assessment for diabetes is important because

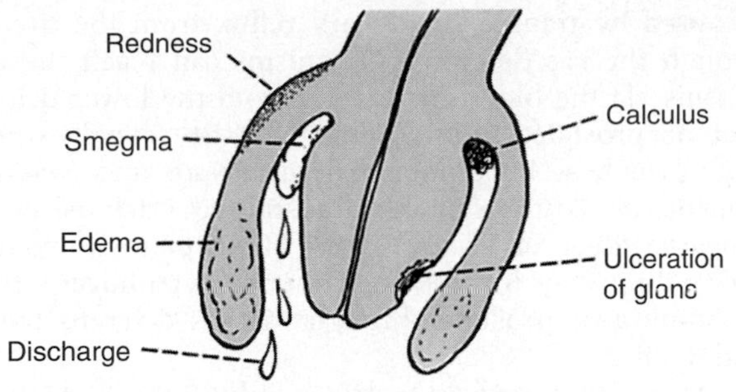

Figure 52–7
Posthitis and balanitis.

diabetes predisposes the client to the development of secondary infection. Antibiotics help control local infection. Circumcision may be necessary.

URINARY EXTRAVASATION

Urinary extravasation is the escape of urine and other fluid into the perineum, scrotum, and penile tissue. It may be caused by trauma or may be secondary to urethral stricture. It is an emergency condition. Assessment reveals discoloration of the tissue, shock, and fever. Emergency intervention consists of alternative drainage of the bladder (urethral or suprapubic catheter) and drainage of the tissues with a Penrose drain.

PENILE INJURY

Penile trauma results in edema, hematoma, bruising, or laceration. Ice packs should be applied to control bleeding and appropriate dressings to reduce the possibility of infection. Urologic consultation is needed. With microsurgical techniques, it may be possible to replant an amputated penis. To facilitate such treatment, an amputated penis should be dampened with a sterile saline solution, kept chilled, and transported with the client for emergency treatment.

Scrotal Disorders

INFECTIONS

Scrotal skin is very thin and is in constant contact with clothes and the thighs. The scrotum has many rugae (folds) that inhibit ventilation. It is, therefore, exposed to moisture and rubbing and is prone to infection. Nonvenereal disorders, such as erysipelas, abscesses, fistulas, and gangrene, may occur. Parasites, such as scabies and lice, and many common skin diseases, such as fungal infections (*Candida,* also known as jock itch), contact dermatitis, drug eruptions, eczema, lichen planus, and psoriasis, may spread to the scrotum. Heat, friction, obesity, and tight clothing aggravate scrotal disorders. Medications (often topical) specific to the infection, good hygiene, and prompt intervention are essential.

INJURY

The most common scrotal injury is tearing when clothes are caught in machinery. Blunt or penetrating trauma also may occur. Saddle injuries also occur to the scrotum and perineum from accidents. First aid intervention includes control of bleeding by applying an ice pack, scrotal support (Fig. 52–8), and rapid transportation to a health-care facility.

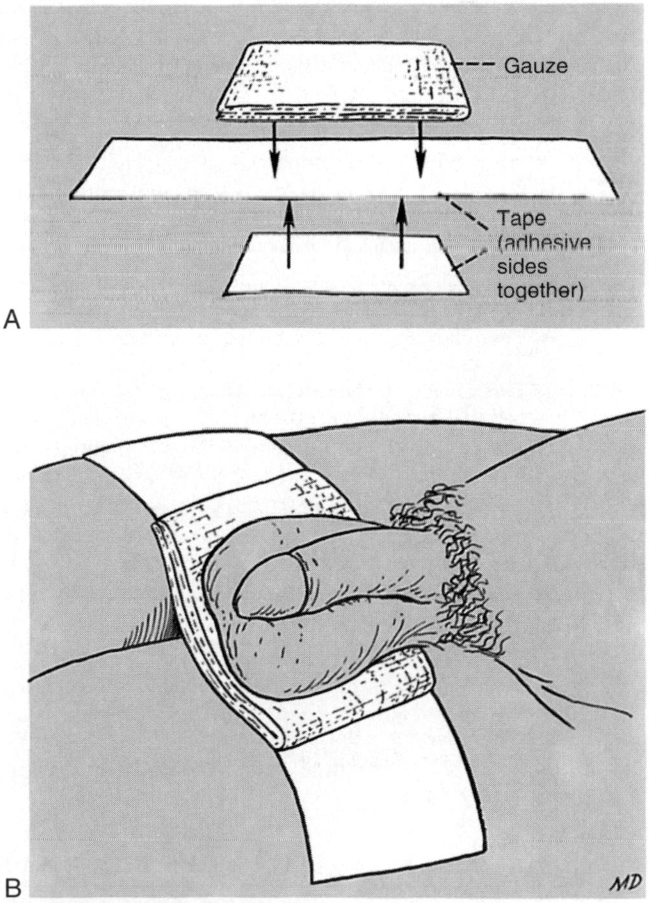

Figure 52–8
Scrotal support (Bellevue bridge type). *A,* Prepare the support by placing two pieces of tape with their adhesive edges together, the smaller piece in the center of the longer piece. This provides a "nonadhesive" section between the client's legs. Place folded gauze on top of the support. *B,* Gently place the support under the scrotum and attach the adhesive ends of the support to the thighs.

EDEMA

Scrotal edema may occur from infection, local irritation, and allergic reactions. It also can follow surgeries such as a hernia repair or a vasectomy. It also may be associated with systemic diseases such as congestive heart failure. Scrotal support, such as a Bellevue bridge, increases comfort for the client (see Fig. 52–8).

Disorders of the Reproductive Ducts

The system of ducts through which spermatozoa pass from the testicles to the urethra includes the epididymis and vas deferens.

Epididymitis is inflammation of the epididymis, most often caused by infection. Sometimes, however, it is caused by trauma or urinary reflux from the urethra through the vas deferens. Organisms can reach the epididymis via the blood or directly from the lower urinary tract or prostate. Epididymitis may be sexually transmitted, such as by *Chlamydia trachomatis* and *Neisseria gonorrhoeae,* or nonsexually transmitted, such as by *Enterobacteriaceae* or *Pseudomonas.* Strain or pressure during voiding may force urine-containing pathogens from the urethra or prostate through the vas deferens to the epididymis.

Assessment reveals acute, painful scrotal swelling, often accompanied by nausea, vomiting, fever, and chills. It is important to distinguish acute epididymitis from testicular torsion. Intervention includes bedrest, scrotal elevation, ice packs, sitz baths, analgesics, and antibiotics. It is important to treat sexual partners also for sexually transmitted forms of epididymitis. Nonsexually transmitted forms can be prevented by treating underlying causes of urinary tract infection and prostatitis. Complications include epididymal abscess (which may extend to the testicles) and chronic epididymitis.

STUDY QUESTIONS

1. To gather objective data from a man with a reproductive or urinary disorder, which one of the following questions should the nurse ask?
   A. "Is urination painful or difficult?"
   B. "How often do you drink excessive alcohol?"
   C. "How often do you get up to go to the bathroom at night?"
   D. "Does your urine have a strong odor?"
2. In teaching the male client about prevention of infertility, which of the following should be included?
   A. The relaxing effect of alcohol and tobacco
   B. The fact that heat increases the motility of sperm
   C. The danger of exposure to environmental and occupational hazards
   D. Tight clothing will improve attractiveness and, therefore, fertility
3. The incidence of benign prostatic hyperplasia is considered to be
   A. Rare
   B. As much as 50% in men older than 50 years
   C. More common in black men
   D. Less common than cancer of the prostate
4. Which of the following client statements demonstrates effective learning?
   A. "There is little point in performing testicular self-examination because testicular cancer usually occurs in men who are of retirement age."
   B. "There is no chance of getting my partner pregnant since my vasectomy last week."
   C. "Because prostate cancer is the most common cancer in men, a yearly checkup is wise."
   D. "Now that I have had my prostate removed, I can enjoy sex with my wife without fear of cancer."
5. An understanding of the risks involved in surgery for benign prostatic hyperplasia is demonstrated by which of the following nursing interventions?
   A. Assessment of intake and output and vital signs every 3 hours after surgery
   B. Restriction of pain medications until the client is well oriented after surgery
   C. Provision of pain medications if bladder overdistension occurs
   D. Assessment of vital signs and mental alertness for signs of fluid and electrolyte imbalance
6. Before removing an indwelling catheter, which of the following should the nurse do?
   A. Determine recent hourly output
   B. Provide extra fluids by mouth
   C. Be sure the client is ambulatory
   D. Check laboratory values for electrolyte balance

CRITICAL THINKING EXERCISES

SCENARIO A

A 63-year-old man presents with complaints of nocturia, urgency, frequency, sensation of full bladder after voiding, and other symptoms of benign prostatic hyperplasia (BPH). Recently retired, he does the housework while his wife continues full-time employment. Both he and his wife are concerned about the implications of the disease on their life-style and relationship.

1. How would a female nurse approach the assessment of his urinary-reproductive function?
2. Cancer of the prostate has been ruled out. How would the nurse advise the client regarding future prevention and detection of prostate cancer?
3. If a conservative approach to treatment has been agreed on at this time, how would you teach the client to manage symptoms?
4. What would the nurse teach the client's wife about her husband's sexual function and restrictions?

SCENARIO B

There are many factors involved in sexual dysfunction in men. A young man asks your advice about erectile dysfunction.

1. How would you begin?
2. What advice would you offer?

BIBLIOGRAPHY

1. Barry, M. J. (1990). Epidemiology and natural history of benign prostatic hyperplasia. *Urologic Clinics of North America, 17(3),* 495–507.
2. Benson, R. C., et al. (1991). Malignant potential of cryptorchid testis. *Mayo Clinic Proceedings, 66,* 3712–3718.
3. Bostwick, D. G. (1989). The pathology of early prostate cancer. *CA: A Cancer Journal for Clinicians, 39(3),* 376–393.
4. Brawer, M. K., & Lange, P. H. (1989). Prostate-specific antigen and premalignant change: Implications for early detection. *CA: A Cancer Journal for Clinicians, 39(3),* 361–375.
5. Cozad, J. (1988). Impotence: Psychosocial aspects, evaluation methods and treatment. *Urologic Nursing, 9(2),* 10–12.
6. Drago, J. R. (1989). The role of new modalities in the early detection and diagnosis of prostate cancer. *CA: A Cancer Journal for Clinicians, 39(3),* 326–336.
7. Gaillard-Moguilewsky, M. (1991). Pharmacology of antiandrogens and value of combining androgen suppression with antiandrogen therapy. *Urology, 37(2, Suppl.),* 5–11.
8. Gershman, S. T., & Stolley, P. D. (1988). A case-controlled study of testicular cancer using Connecticut tumour registry data. *International Journal of Epidemiology, 17,* 738–742.
9. Goodman, M. (1988). Concepts of hormonal manipulation in the treatment of cancer. *Oncology Nursing Forum, 15(5),* 639–647.
10. Hayes, R. B., et al. (1990). Occupation and risk for testicular cancer: A case-control study. *International Journal of Epidemiology, 19(4),* 825–831.
11. Hill, D. J. (1990). The patient with testicular cancer: Nursing management of chemotherapy. *Oncology Nursing Forum, 17(2),* 243–249.
12. Joseph, A. C., & Chang, M. K. (1989). A bladder behavior clinic for post-prostatectomy patients. *Urologic Nursing, 9(3),* 15–19.
13. Karlowicz, K. (1995). *Urologic nursing: Principles and practices.* Philadelphia: W. B. Saunders Co.
14. Klein, L. (1990). Current approaches to balloon dilatation of the prostate. *Astra Urologue, 20(5),* 1–7.
15. Lee, F., et al. (1989). The role of transrectal ultrasound in the early detection of prostate cancer. *CA: A Cancer Journal for Clinicians, 39(3),* 337–360.
16. Lepor, H. (Ed.). (1988). Pharmacologic intervention in benign prostatic hypertrophy. *Urology, 32(Suppl. 6),* 2–31.
17. Loughlin, K. R. (1991). Medical and nonmedical therapy for benign prostatic hypertrophy. *Geriatrics, 46(6),* 26–31.
18. Mallon, D., & Williams, C. F. (1987). A review of patient and partner perspectives of the penile prosthesis. *Journal of Urologic Nursing, 6(1),* 17–26.
19. Matzkin, H., & Braf, Z. (1991). Endocrine treatment of benign prostatic hypertrophy: Current concepts. *Urology, 37(1),* 1–13.
20. Millon, R., & Underwood, S. (1992). Factors influencing early detection of prostate cancer. *Applied Nursing Research, 5(1),* 30–31.
21. Moore, S., et al. (1992). Nerve-sparing prostatectomy. *American Journal of Nursing, 92(4),* 59–64.
22. Murphy, G. P. (1989). Progress against prostatic cancer. *CA: A Cancer Journal for Clinicians, 39(3),* 325.
23. Ofman, U. (1993). Psychosocial and sexual implications of genitourinary cancers. *Seminars in Oncology Nursing, 9(4),* 286–292.
24. Perez, C. A., et al. (1989). Carcinoma of the prostate. In V. Devita, S. Hellman, & S. Rosenburg (Eds.), *Cancer, Principles and practice of oncology* (Vol. 1, 3rd ed.). Philadelphia: J. B. Lippincott.
25. Pollack, A. (1993). Long-term consequences of female and male sterilization. *Contemporary Obstetrics and Gynecology, 38(8),* 41–54.
26. Razanauzskas, M., & Hoebler, L. (1994). Cold comfort: Treating prostate cancer with cryosurgery. *Nursing 94, 20(11),* 66–68.
27. Reddy, E. K., et al. (1990). Testicular neoplasms: Seminoma. *Journal of the National Medical Association, 82(9),* 651–655.
28. Rudolf, V. M., & Quinn, L. M. (1988). The practice of TSE among college men: Effectiveness of an educational program. *Oncology Nursing Forum, 15(1),* 45–48.
29. Silverberg, E., & Lubera, J. A. (1989). Cancer survival rates. *CA: A Cancer Journal for Clinicians, 39,* 3–32.
30. Stepp, C. (1991). Balloon dilatation of the prostate: A historical review. *Urologic Nursing, 5,* 21–24.

31. Walsh, P., et al. (Eds.). (1992). *Campbell's urology* (6th ed.). Philadelphia: W. B. Saunders.

32. Waterhouse, R. L., & Resnick, M. I. (1989). The use of transrectal prostatic ultrasonography in the evaluation of patients with prostatic carcinoma. *Journal of Urology, 141*(2), 233–239.

33. Whorton, M. (1984). Environmental and occupational hazards. In J. Swanson & K. Forrest (Eds.), *Men's reproductive health.* New York: Springer.

34. Whorton, M., et al. (1977). Infertility in male pesticide workers. *Lancet, 2,* 1259.

35. Willis, D. (1992). Overgrown prostate. *American Journal of Nursing, 92*(2), 34–40.

36. Wilson, B., et al. (1994). *Nurses' drug guide.* Norwalk, CT: Appleton & Lange.

Chapter 53

Nursing Care of Women with Gynecologic Disorders

Learning Outcomes

After completing this chapter, the learner will be able to:

1. Assess the client for clinical manifestations of gynecologic disorders.
2. Teach the client about the etiology, risk factors, basic pathophysiology, and clinical manifestations of common gynecologic disorders.
3. Explain the client's role in medical and surgical management of gynecologic disorders.
4. Develop plans of care for the prevention of gynecologic disorders, regular self-examination for gynecologic disorders, and management and rehabilitation of clients with gynecologic disorders.
5. Implement nursing interventions that optimize the quality of life for clients with gynecologic disorders.
6. Evaluate planned client outcomes using outcome criteria developed in the planning phase of care.

Menstruation and childbearing are processes exclusive to women. Historically, these two events have been invested with enormous social significance. Thus, the physical and psychological aspects of menstruation and menstrual disorders are closely interwoven.

In the 19th century, it was a commonly reported medical view that the uterus and ovaries dominated a woman's body. Irrational, hysterical symptoms were thought to arise from a discontented uterus. Women were labeled unreliable and illogical because they were thought to be controlled by raging hormonal cycles. Even in modern times, this view has been used in subtle forms to deny economic, political, and social opportunity to women.

Until recently, the pathophysiologic mechanisms responsible for menstrual dysfunction were poorly understood. Advances in neuroendocrinology, endocrinology, and the biochemistry of gonadal function permit a better understanding of the physiology of menstruation. Research on psychosocial and physical aspects of menstruation is enlarging our understanding of normal and abnormal menstruation. New developments in physical and psychosocial intervention are emerging.

Menstrual Disorders

Women react to menstrual problems in differing, individual ways. Whereas some promptly seek health care, others may not for various reasons. For example, one woman may hesitate and be unable to discuss menstruation because she views it as a personal, intimate problem and does not wish to talk about it. Another woman may accept some menstrual discomfort and inconvenience as inevitable. Yet another may have low self-esteem and dismiss her complaints as unimportant. Some women do not seek help because they believe their problems will go away in time, whereas others question whether relief is actually possible or whether the treatment will be worse than the problem. Thus, many menstrual problems go undetected unless nurses are skillful and sensitive in assessment. Menstrual problems may be discovered by nurses when clients are discussing unrelated concerns such as contraception needs. Some menstrual problems include dysmenorrhea, premenstrual syndrome, and abnormal uterine bleeding.

Dysmenorrhea

Until the early 1970s, dysmenorrhea (painful menstrual flow) was considered by many medical practitioners, as well as the lay public, to be mainly psychosomatic.[32] Women were told by everyone, including health-care workers, it was all in their heads or indicative of their inability to adjust to the feminine role. Thus, most women did not even consider asking for help with this problem. Today, however, dysmenorrhea is taken seriously as a health problem, and new knowledge has provided the basis for useful therapies to relieve the discomfort.

Dysmenorrhea may be primary or secondary. The true incidence and prevalence of women with this condition are unknown, although most women are affected to some degree.[5] Ultimately, this discomfort has the potential to affect women's productivity and increase absenteeism. Dysmenorrhea is a different entity from premenstrual syndrome (PMS) and requires different treatment modalities.[5] However, some women have symptoms of both.

PRIMARY DYSMENORRHEA

Etiology

Research indicates that the mechanisms involved in primary dysmenorrhea include elevated uterine prostaglandin levels as well as endocrine, myometrial, biochemical, and psychosocial factors. It appears that prostaglandin synthesis at the time of menstruation produces strong myometrial contractions. The severe muscle spasms constrict blood vessels supplying the uterus, causing ischemia and pain. The excess prostaglandins in smooth muscle also help explain the presence of gastrointestinal symptoms such as nausea, vomiting, and diarrhea, or headache.

Endocrine factors appear to have a role in primary dysmenorrhea because symptoms occur in ovulatory cycles. Psychosocial factors associated with dysmenorrhea include anxiety, insecurity, immaturity, dependency, rigid conformity, underachievement, and perfectionism.[32] Once menstrual pain has been experienced, women often become anxious as the next period approaches. Thus, the added stress and the expectation of pain may induce more pain.

Pathophysiology

Primary dysmenorrhea characteristically begins 1 to 3 months after menarche in conjunction with ovulatory cycles. Generally, it increases in severity over several years until the mid-20s and then begins to decline. Primary dysmenorrhea often decreases significantly after childbirth. It is often associated with prolonged menstrual flow and is more common in obese, sedentary women.

The discomfort of primary dysmenorrhea commonly begins 1 to 2 days before the onset of menstrual flow. The more severe discomfort is usually experienced during the first 24 hours of flow and typically subsides by the second day. More than half of the women experiencing dysmenorrhea also have systemic symptoms such as nausea, vomiting, diarrhea, syncope, headache, and leg pain.

Medical Management

The traditional therapeutic approach to primary dysmenorrhea was to prescribe narcotics and sedatives. The current approach emphasizes prevention and education, so a client can participate in her own self-care. For clients with mild symptoms who want to avoid medication, nonpharmacologic remedies might be effective. For example, biofeedback, therapeutic touch, or acupuncture might be helpful.

If contraception is desired as well as relief of dysmenorrhea, combination oral contraceptives may relieve menstrual pain. The resulting inhibition of ovulation results in decreased endometrial prostaglandin production and a concurrent reduction of uterine activity. For clients with intrauterine devices (IUDs), removal of the device may lead to relief.

Exercise also has been used as a remedy for dysmenorrhea.[11] Exercise increases blood levels of beta-endorphins, the body's endogenous opiates, making them available for pain relief. However, the exact mechanism responsible for relief is not known.

PHARMACOLOGIC MANAGEMENT

Prostaglandin synthesis inhibitors also may provide relief via decreased prostaglandin activity, even in the presence of ovulatory cycles. Some commonly prescribed medications in this group are ibuprofen (Motrin), mefenamic acid (Ponstel), indomethacin (Indocin), and naproxen sodium (Naprosyn). Ibuprofen is currently available as a nonprescription drug in 200-mg tablet form, which makes it convenient to obtain.

These medications may have gastrointestinal side effects. Other possible side effects are salt and water retention, skin rashes, and potential allergic reactions.

CRITICAL TO REMEMBER

Prostaglandin synthesis inhibitors should not be used by nursing or pregnant women.

Acetaminophen is a satisfactory drug for some women experiencing mild to moderate dysmenorrhea. For maximum effectiveness, the medications should be administered either before or at the onset of menses.

Nursing Management

Education and supportive reassurance are important nursing interventions for women with primary dysmenorrhea. Provide information about the mechanisms involved in dysmenorrhea and the actions and possible side effects of any prescribed medications. The nurse must assess the client's general health status; encourage adequate nutrition and appropriate rest, sleep, and exercise; assess stress and explore methods of stress management.

SECONDARY DYSMENORRHEA

Etiology

Secondary dysmenorrhea may be caused by conditions such as pelvic inflammatory disease (PID), endometriosis, adenomyosis (invasion of uterine myometrium by endometrial tissue), uterine prolapse, uterine myomas, or polyps. Secondary dysmenorrhea is suspected when pain is concentrated in a specific area or only on one side, or when its onset occurs after age 20.

Pelvic inflammatory disease is an infectious process that may involve the fallopian tubes, ovaries, pelvic peritoneum veins, and pelvic connective tissue. The onset of dysmenorrhea associated with PID is usually sudden and acute. Often, dyspareunia (painful intercourse) is present as well. The PID may occur after a bout of gonorrhea. Antibiotic therapy generally provides relief.

Endometriosis is a condition in which endometrial tissue (which responds to hormonal stimulation) is found outside the uterine cavity. Dysmenorrhea associated with endometriosis usually begins after menstrual flow has started and lasts throughout the menstrual period. Pain may be localized at a particular site and often increases in intensity as the menstrual period progresses.

Uterine myomas are benign tumors; polyps are small masses of tissue formed in the uterus (they may protrude from the cervix). Both may cause dysmenorrhea in later reproductive years. Along with menstrual pain, heavy menstrual flow may occur. Myomas and polyps may be found during pelvic examination and confirmed by ultrasonography. Intrauterine polyps are very difficult to detect.

Secondary dysmenorrhea associated with uterine prolapse (downward uterine displacement caused by weakening of support structures) normally appears as premenstrual backache persisting throughout the menstrual period. It may be associated with dyspareunia. Cystocele (bladder herniating into the vagina caused by weakening of the anterior vaginal wall) is often associated with uterine prolapse. Thus, urinary stress incontinence also may be present.

Medical Management

Treatment for secondary dysmenorrhea is directed toward the underlying cause. Antiprostaglandin agents may provide some relief.

Nursing Management

Nursing interventions focus on educational and psychosocial needs of the individual client.

Premenstrual Syndrome (PMS)

Despite its popularization, PMS (first described in 1931) is still not well understood. Much confusion surrounds its diagnosis, treatment, and nursing management.

Incidence

The incidence of PMS is difficult to determine because of the variable symptoms and the lack of a clear understanding about the syndrome. Variable reports in the literature indicate that approximately 70 to 90 per cent of all women experience some form of PMS. Probably only 20 to 40 per cent of these women experience symptoms that disrupt their lives. The relationship between PMS and dysmenorrhea is currently unclear.

Etiology

The etiology of PMS is unclear; however, neuroendocrine mechanisms appear to be involved. It is not clear whether PMS is a single syndrome or a group of separate disorders. Some popular theories are that PMS may be caused by (1) estrogen-progesterone imbalance; (2) fluid retention; (3) estrogen, progesterone, and aldosterone interaction; (4) vasopressin; (5) prolactin; (6) dietary factors such as vitamin B_6 deficiency or hypoglycemia; or (7) endogenous opiates.

Clinical Manifestations

Typically, symptoms of PMS occur during the last few premenstrual days, and sudden relief of symptoms occurs with full menstrual flow. However, symptoms may begin with ovulation and may not be relieved until during or toward the end of menses. Characteristically, symptoms gradually worsen until menses begin.

Various symptoms are attributable to PMS, including altered emotional states, behavioral changes, somatic problems, altered appetite, and motor effects. Different sets of symptoms are experienced by individual women. Commonly, emotional symptoms include tension, depression, irritability, hostility, insomnia, loneliness, crying easily, and indecision. Some of the most common somatic symptoms are bloatedness, headache, breast tenderness, fatigue, and backache. Alterations in appetite include craving alcohol or certain foods (e.g., sweet or salty foods) or avoiding certain foods. Motor effects reported are vertigo, changes in coordination, and clumsiness. Many other symptoms also have been reported.

Because PMS symptoms usually do not occur during the menstrual flow, women may not associate PMS with the menstrual cycle. Also, women may be reluctant to admit the apparently irrational symptoms. Such symptoms may be misdiagnosed as psychological or emotional problems.

DIAGNOSTIC ASSESSMENT

To date, there are no objective methods of diagnosing PMS. Diagnosis is usually made by documenting the cyclic nature of the symptoms on a menstrual calendar. A diagnosis of PMS requires a recurrence of symptoms for a minimum of three menstrual cycles. Diagnosis is made on the timing of symptoms rather than on the presence of particular symptoms.

Medical Management

PHARMACOLOGIC MANAGEMENT

There is no known effective pharmacologic treatment for PMS. Treatment is directed toward relief of symptoms. What helps one client may not be effective for another. A variety of therapies have been used. Daily intake of vitamin B_6 has improved some premenstrual symptoms. Other nonprescription drugs include calcium, vitamin A, magnesium, and trace elements. Essential fatty acid supplements are often recommended.

Prescription medications commonly include vaginal progesterone (Progestasert), oral spironolactone (Aldactone), oral bromocriptine (Parlodel), oral contraceptives, and tranquilizers. Sedatives and analgesics are often useful for symptomatic relief.

Nursing Management

Assessment

Premenstrual syndrome is a significant problem for many women in spite of the confusion surrounding its cause, definition, and management. Nurses are in a key position to help women identify and cope with PMS when it is present.

Nursing Diagnosis, Planning, and Implementation

Nursing Diagnosis: Knowledge Deficit R/T syndrome and symptom management.

Planning: Expected Outcomes. Client will express understanding of PMS and the management of its symptoms.

Implementation. Once the diagnosis of PMS is made, the client needs information about the syndrome and reassurance that there is a physiologic basis for her symptoms, even though the mechanisms are not clearly understood. Clients are often helped by the opportunity to talk about their feelings and experiences with PMS, especially because of the confusion and misconceptions surrounding the syndrome. Significant others also benefit from information and reassurance.

Nursing Diagnosis: Health Maintenance, Altered R/T poor physical health.

Planning: Expected Outcomes. The client will have improved health, as evidenced by improved physical condition and decrease of PMS symptoms.

Implementation. Women who are in poor physical condition may be particularly susceptible to premenstrual difficulties. Thus nursing assessment includes the client's general life-style, sleep and dietary habits, and overall health maintenance.

Suggested dietary modifications include reducing salt and refined carbohydrate intake. Careful attention must be given to stress management and reduction. Adequate physical exercise and weight reduction (if necessary) are very important. It also may be helpful to reduce alcohol and caffeine intake and stop or reduce smoking.

Nursing Diagnosis: Individual Coping, Ineffective, Risk for, R/T distress from symptoms of PMS.

Planning: Expected Outcomes. The client will cope effectively with PMS and its symptoms, as evidenced by client's statements and a decrease in symptoms.

Implementation. Another major nursing responsibility is assisting the client and her significant others to cope with the symptoms of PMS. For example, a reallocation of responsibilities within the family might help to reduce the client's stress. If she prefers to retain her current responsibilities, the nurse might help her learn how to manage them in ways that minimize stress. Support groups or educational sessions may serve as a forum for sharing information, providing mutual support, and discussing feelings. Daily, vigorous exercise has been recommended, both to reduce stress and to increase a sense of well-being.

Evaluation

The nurse must evaluate client outcomes based on the established plan of care. If these goals were not achieved, the plan and interventions must be revised to meet the client's needs.

Abnormal Uterine Bleeding

Abnormal uterine bleeding encompasses a wide variety of menstrual disorders, such as lack of menstrual flow, irregular uterine bleeding, and excessive uterine bleeding. Changes in menstrual patterns can be frightening to the woman and, if they are severe enough, symptoms can disrupt daily living. Sometimes, abnormal uterine bleeding indicates underlying disease conditions. The term *dysfunctional uterine bleeding* means abnormal uterine bleeding for which no organic cause can be found through the usual assessment techniques. Abnormal uterine bleeding always requires careful assessment by a qualified health professional.

AMENORRHEA

Amenorrhea means the absence of menses or skipping periods. Amenorrhea, the absence of cyclic vaginal bleeding, is classified as primary when no menstruation has occurred or as secondary when previous spontaneous menstrual bleeding has occurred before cessation of flow. A diagnosis of secondary amenorrhea also requires a lack of bleeding for 6 months in a woman having regular cyclic bleeding or 12 months in a woman with a history of irregular bleeding.

Incidence

Amenorrhea is common. Many women experience it at some time during their life.

Etiology

Often chromosomal abnormalities or structural genital malformations are discovered in clients with primary amenorrhea, although other factors may be present (Fig. 53–1). Pregnancy is a common physiologic cause of amenorrhea. Excessive exercise, such as occurs with athletes or dancers, can sometimes cause a woman to stop having her periods.

Amenorrhea may signal menopause in a mature woman. The diagnosis can be confirmed by finding elevated luteinizing hormone and follicle-stimulating hormone levels. However, pregnancy testing should be considered in a mature woman as well, because pregnancy may occur after a short period of amenorrhea, if additional ovulatory cycles have occurred.

Some medications may cause amenorrhea (e.g., neuropharmacologic agents such as psychotropics and antihypertensives). Some women experience amenorrhea after discontinuing oral contraceptives.

Weight loss or excessive physical activity and psychosocial stress may be associated with amenorrhea. One hypothesis is that a critical percentage of fat (about 22 per cent of body weight) is necessary to maintain regular menstruation after age 16 years. Thus, a simple weight loss of 10 to 15 per cent of the total body weight might result in amenorrhea. Amenorrhea may be associated with heavy physical exercise, such as jogging, running, and aerobic dancing. Psychosocial stress also may be associated with amenorrhea, although the mechanisms are not well understood. A growing consensus is that the endogenous opioid and dopaminergic systems are probably involved in stress-induced amenorrhea.

Other potential causes of amenorrhea are pituitary, ovarian, and endocrine factors. Hypothyroidism, either from neoplasms or trauma, can result in gonadotropin abnormalities and amenorrhea. Ovarian abnormalities can lead to altered estrogen release, which can result in amenorrhea or abnormal uterine bleeding. Other endocrine abnormalities, such as polycystic ovarian syndrome or Cushing's syndrome, also may lead to amenorrhea.

Medical Management

Treatment for amenorrhea depends in part on the client's needs and desires. Particularly important are her wishes regarding childbearing.

PHARMACOLOGIC MANAGEMENT

If pregnancy is not desired, medroxyprogesterone may be used to produce withdrawal bleeding. If pregnancy is

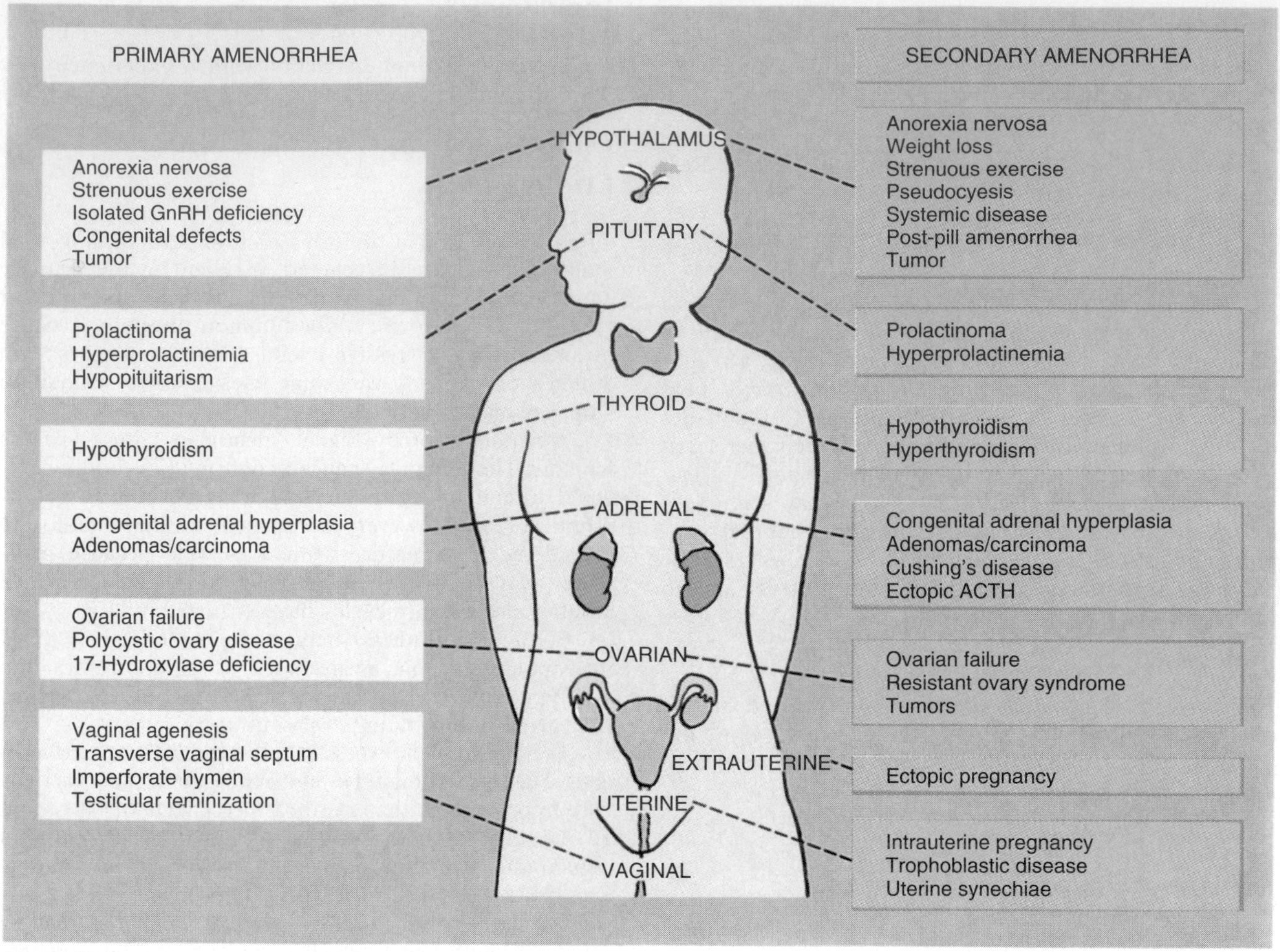

Figure 53–1
Causes of amenorrhea. ACTH, adrenocorticotropic hormone; GnRH, gonadotropin-releasing hormone.

desired, ovulation induction with clomiphene citrate or bromocriptine may be undertaken.

Nursing Management

Absence of spontaneous menstrual flow before age 17 years requires careful assessment, including history and physical examination. Pregnancy also must be ruled out for any woman of childbearing age experiencing secondary amenorrhea.

Teaching opportunities are an important part of nursing care. Depending on the cause of amenorrhea, the client may need help in gaining weight, reducing energy drain from excessive physical activity, and stress reduction. The nurse must assess general health and help the client plan and make changes as indicated.

MENORRHAGIA

The term *menorrhagia* means excessive vaginal bleeding at normal intervals, which can cause women grave distress and inconvenience.

Menorrhagia can have a variety of causes. A single heavy episode of bleeding may indicate spontaneous abortion. Excessively heavy menstrual periods may be associated with IUD use for contraception. Fibroids and adenomyosis also are common causes of menorrhagia. Other potential causes include systemic diseases such as blood dyscrasias and hypothyroidism. Medications such as anticoagulants also have been associated with excessive menstrual flow.

Assessing the actual amount of blood loss can be difficult. The nurse should ask clients to compare the number of pads or tampons used during the abnormal period with the number used during a normal cycle. Also, the usual tests to identify possible anemia may be performed.

Treatment may consist of dilation and curettage (D & C) or administration of medications such as estrogens, progestins (alone or in combination with oral contraceptives), or antifibrinolytic agents, depending on factors thought to be associated with the cause.

During the first few hours after D & C, the nurse should monitor for excessive bleeding, inability to void, or excessive pain. The client usually experiences only minimal uterine cramping postoperatively. Mild analgesics such as acetaminophen and codeine usually relieve any discomfort. The nurse must provide client teaching

CLIENT EDUCATION GUIDE

Procedure After Dilation and Curettage

Follow-up instructions to the client include the following:

- Avoid strenuous activity for about 1 week.
- Avoid douching and vaginal or rectal intercourse until the physician gives permission (usually after about 1 week).
- Expect a small amount of pinkish vaginal discharge followed by dark red or dark brown discharge during the healing process.
- Realize that subsequent menstrual periods may or may not be affected.
- Keep all scheduled follow-up appointments.
- Report any signs and symptoms of complications to the surgeon.

After a D & C, the next period may not occur, may not occur on schedule, or may vary from the usual time of onset. Indications of possible complications include excessive bleeding, excessive pain, or elevated temperature.

(see the Client Education Guide: Procedure After Dilation and Curettage).

An important aspect of nursing care is to provide reassurance because heavy vaginal bleeding can be very frightening.

METRORRHAGIA

Metrorrhagia, or vaginal bleeding between periods, may occur as spotting or outright bleeding. Common causes are similar to those responsible for menorrhagia and also may include ectopic pregnancy, spotting with ovulation, cervical polyps, or breakthrough bleeding that occurs in conjunction with the use of oral contraceptives. For breakthrough bleeding, the dosage of oral contraceptive can be adjusted or a different agent may be prescribed.

MENOPAUSE

Normal menopause is discussed in detail in Chapter 51.

Surgical Menopause

Menopause may be induced at any age by surgical removal of the ovaries or pelvic irradiation. Hysterectomy (removal of the uterus), not including removal of the ovaries, does not cause surgical menopause. However, some symptoms such as hot flashes have been reported after hysterectomy. In these instances, it is possible that blood vessels supplying the ovaries may have been injured, and the resulting loss of blood supply caused the ovaries to atrophy. Another cause of such symptoms could be the hormone imbalance produced by removal of the uterus and its loss as a hormone receptor. Delayed onset of the climacteric (about ages 55–60 years) is associated with a higher incidence of pathologic conditions and requires careful assessment.

Menopausal Difficulties

The most commonly reported menopausal difficulties are vasomotor instability, menstrual irregularities, and atrophic vaginitis. A wide variety of physical and psychosocial symptoms have been attributed to the perimenopausal period, but controversy remains as to whether they are actually related to menopause or to other factors, such as aging or stressful life events.

Symptoms of vasomotor instability, such as hot flashes, night sweats, and occasional palpitations and dizziness associated with menopause, are probably caused by hormonal imbalances. Estrogen appears to exert a protective effect on subcutaneous blood vessels. Lowered estrogen makes many women more sensitive to stimuli that precipitate sweating, skin discoloration, and the sensation of heat loss.

Hot flashes are sudden involuntary waves of heat beginning in the upper chest or neck and proceeding up the face and head. It lasts from a few seconds to several minutes and is aggravated by anything that increases heat production in the body. A hot flash may or may not be accompanied by a hot flush, which is a measurable change in skin temperature, a visible pink to bright red flush in skin color, and perspiration.

Generally, the subjective symptom of the hot flash occurs about 45 seconds before the hot flush. The reported incidence of the hot flash varies for perimenopausal women from 68 to 92 per cent, depending on the age group studied.[13] There is great variance in both the quantitative and qualitative aspects of women's experience of hot flashes.

Many women require detailed information about what menopause is and what is happening to their bodies. The nurse should provide practical suggestions for coping with hot flashes, such as

- Dress in layers so that some clothing can easily be taken off during the sensation and put back on as cooling commences.
- Avoid hot environments and keep the thermostat at about 65° F or lower.
- Avoid getting excited because emotional stress sometimes triggers hot flashes.
- Avoid highly seasoned, spicy foods, coffee, tea, and alcohol if they trigger hot flashes. The nurse will need to ask what spicy foods have an effect for each particular client.
- Keep a record or diary of when you experience hot flashes and try to identify common triggers and work out ways of avoiding them.
- Learn to control your reactions to the hot flash. Guided imagery may prove helpful.
- Use cooling techniques, such as fans, showering, or applying cold cloths or ice cubes to various body parts.

The vaginal mucous membrane is especially responsive to low estrogen levels. When these levels remain low both during and after menopause, vaginal walls become thinner and drier, and susceptibility to infection increases. These changes lead to an increase in vaginitis in menopausal women. Other symptoms may include vaginal irritation, burning, pruritus, leukorrhea, bleeding, and dyspareunia.

Vulvar epithelium loses its elasticity and subcutaneous fat after menopause. Pubic hair may become thinner. As the epidermal layer thins, the labia majora and minora flatten. The urethra may atrophy, and when this occurs, the incidence of cystitis and urethritis increases. Pubococcygeus muscles tend to lose their tone, and stress urinary incontinence also may occur.

Some women experience backache, joint pain, and other symptoms of osteoporosis. Osteoporosis is a skeletal disorder characterized by an increased predisposition to bone collapse or fracture resulting from a reduced amount of bone mass. Estrogen seems to inhibit bone breakdown and loss. A decrease or absence of estrogen may lead to osteoporosis.

Spinal osteoporosis, giving rise to vertebral biconcavity and compression fractures, is particularly common in postmenopausal women. Lower forearm fracture is an osteoporotic syndrome occurring almost exclusively in postmenopausal women. Osteoporosis is more severe among women who are sedentary and who smoke (see Chap. 45).

Many other difficulties can occur that may or may not be related to climacteric changes. Some women report insomnia or other sleep disturbances, headache, forgetfulness, nervousness, apprehension, and irritability. Wardrop and colleagues found a high incidence of oral symptoms such as dryness of the mouth, a burning sensation in the mouth, and altered taste perceptions among perimenopausal clients.[33] Psychosocial stress may affect other menopausal symptoms. The psychosocial changes experienced by some women may result from a combination of hormone imbalance and adjustment to the aging process.

The nursing role in working with menopausal clients and their significant others involves providing support, education, and assistance in moving through this normal life experience as comfortably as possible. Accurate information about menopause and what to expect can be helpful and reassuring. The nurse must tailor assistance in coping with minor discomforts of menopause to the needs of the individual woman (see the Client Education Guide: Coping with Problems of Menopause).

The nurse should remind women experiencing menopause of the value of good health habits. Balanced nutrition and adequate sleep and rest are important. Exercising at least three times per week for 45 minutes will promote cardiovascular health. Nurses can be effective in assisting women to make menopause a positive experience.

CLIENT EDUCATION GUIDE

Coping with Problems of Menopause

A menopausal client may find the following self-care measures useful:

Preventing vaginal dryness. Continued intercourse or masturbation aids circulation and keeps tissues flexible. Use water-soluble jelly for lubrication; use estrogen cream if needed.

Preventing osteoporosis. Engage in regular weight-bearing exercise, such as walking, dancing, bicycling; increase calcium intake; stop smoking; decrease alcohol and caffeine intake.

Preventing urinary tract infection. Void frequently; increase fluid intake; maintain good perineal hygiene; wear cotton underwear.

Promoting pelvic relaxation. Perform Kegel exercises to improve muscle tone (see Chap. 30); lose weight if necessary.

HORMONE REPLACEMENT THERAPY

Hormone replacement therapy (HRT) (estrogen plus progesterone) may be part of the medical management of perimenopausal symptoms. Individuals must be informed of the advantages and potential dangers of HRT in order to make informed safe decisions about treatment. Nurses need up-to-date information about HRT to support clients making this important decision.

It is often difficult for clients to decide about HRT because authorities differ markedly in their advice. HRT can alleviate vasomotor instability, vaginal and urinary tract atrophy, dyspareunia, and a number of affective symptoms.[22] It also has been studied as a preventive measure against osteoporosis and cardiovascular disease, with some researchers claiming a protective effect against breast cancer and others citing it as a risk factor for breast cancer development.[22] In the mid- to late 1970s, evidence for an association between estrogen replacement therapy (ERT) and endometrial cancer was discovered. In subsequent years, this association has been studied extensively, and today estrogen is given with a progestational agent to stimulate the normal menstrual cycle.

It is generally accepted that estrogens should not be given to women with

- Known or suspected breast or uterine cancer or any estrogen-dependent neoplasia (or a strong family history of the same)
- Undiagnosed abnormal uterine bleeding
- Previous or present thrombophlebitis
- Acute liver disease or cerebrovascular disease
- Combined risk factors such as obesity, varicosities, high blood pressure, and heavy smoking

Women with uterine fibromyomas, hyperlipidemia, severe varicose veins, chronic hepatic dysfunction, diabetes mellitus, and severe hypertension require thorough assessment before estrogen is prescribed.

The use of HRT should be individualized according to the client's needs, desires, and individual symptoms and risks. The risk for women with fibrocystic breast disease is unclear, but careful assessment must be made.

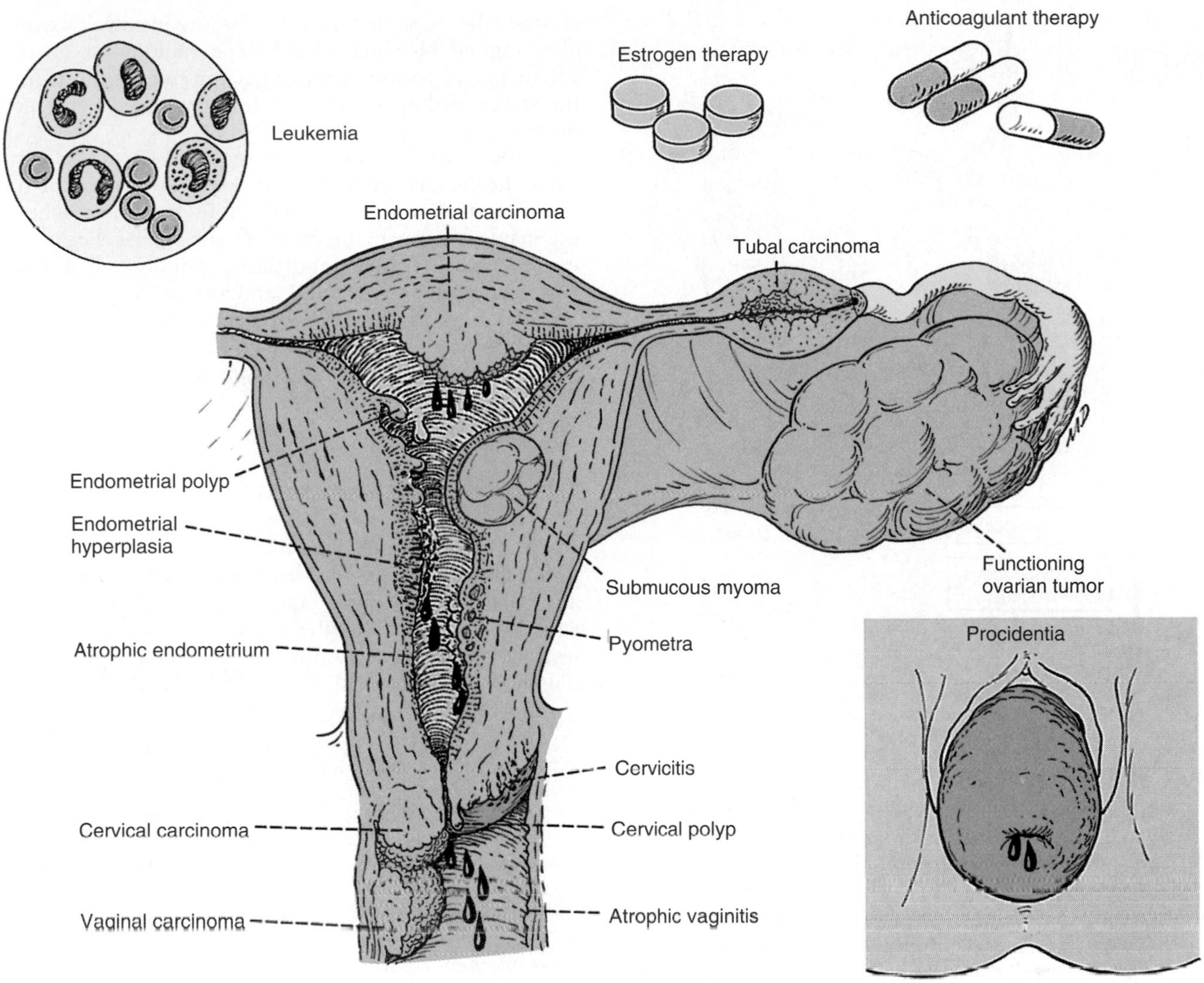

Figure 53–2
Causes of postmenopausal bleeding.

Risks should be assessed for endometrial cancer, osteoporosis, cardiovascular disease, and breast cancer.

At present, the risk from HRT for the development of breast cancer is unclear and further research is needed. When a client decides to use ERT or HRT, she should be carefully monitored for the development of breast cancer and receive breast examinations on a regular basis.

POSTMENOPAUSAL BLEEDING

Postmenopausal bleeding, vaginal bleeding occurring after menopause, is a symptom, not a diagnosis (Fig. 53–2). It requires careful assessment because it may be a symptom of genital tract cancer. Other causes of postmenopausal bleeding include atrophic vaginitis, cervical polyps, fibroids, endometrial hyperplasia, or cervical erosion.

Pelvic Inflammatory Disease

Pelvic inflammatory disease (PID) refers to ascending pelvic infections, that is, those involving the upper genital tract (beyond the cervix).

Etiology

Gonococci, staphylococci, streptococci, and other pus-producing (pyogenic) organisms commonly cause PID.

Pathophysiology

Once an infection is in the upper genital tract, it may travel along several routes (Fig. 53–3).

Gonococcal and staphylococcal organisms spread along the uterine endometrium to the fallopian tubes,

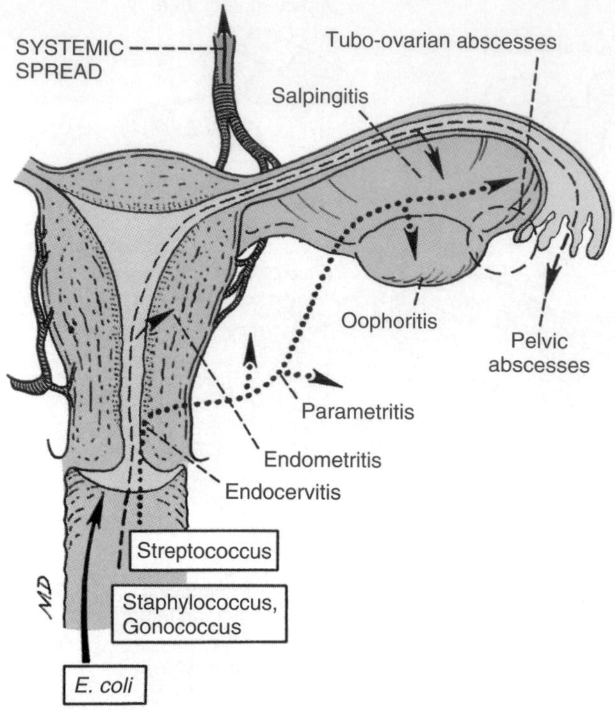

Figure 53–3
Routes of spread of pelvic inflammatory disease.

where they cause an acute salpingitis (inflammation of the fallopian tubes). The tubes become partially occluded and may drain pus, leukocytes, and other debris into the pelvic cavity, causing pelvic peritonitis, or the material may form a pocket around the ovary, causing a tubo-ovarian abscess.

Streptococci spread similarly, except they tend to travel via the uterine or cervical lymphatics across the parametrium to the tubes or ovaries. There they may cause pelvic cellulitis and sometimes thrombophlebitis of the major pelvic veins, with the risk of the development of embolisms.

Another route of spread of infection is from the pelvic cavity itself. Organisms such as *Escherichia coli* may be extruded from a ruptured viscus, causing peritonitis.

Complications from PID may occur. Although septic shock and other severe complications can occur, the most common complication is a pelvic abscess.

Frequently, women with PID are unable to become pregnant after the infection has cleared because the inflammatory process causes scarring and closing of the fallopian tubes.

Clinical Manifestations

Clinical manifestations include signs and symptoms of generalized infection, such as general malaise, fever, chills, anorexia, nausea, vomiting, general aching, and tachycardia. In addition, the woman usually experiences acute, sharp, severe aching on both sides of the abdomen or pelvis. Pain is aggravated by defecation and is accompanied by a heavy, purulent, odoriferous discharge (the odor depends on the organism). Occasionally, vaginal bleeding occurs. The rapidity of onset of PID depends on the virulence of the infecting organism, the status of the woman's pelvic organs, and her general health.

Other helpful clues pointing to PID are obtained from the history. A history of acute lower genital tract infection is significant. It is helpful to know whether the pain accompanying the current illness began during menses (typically indicating gonococcal PID) or between periods (usually nongonococcal infections). Various other data, including a thorough sexual history, are important. Included is a contraceptive history, because the presence of an IUD correlates with a higher incidence of PID.

Diagnostic Assessment

The usual laboratory tests for infection, including multiple cultures, are performed. Some practitioners culture any evident drainage, and obtain specimens from various organs such as the cervix and from a culdocentesis (Fig. 53–4). A sample of peritoneal fluid may be obtained from the cul-de-sac. Additional cultures are helpful because it is not uncommon for several kinds of organisms to be involved or for an organism cultured from the cervix to differ from that found in the upper genital tract. When this situation occurs, several types of antibiotics may be necessary to treat the infection.

Medical Management

Most women are treated as outpatients, receiving antibiotics appropriate to the specific cause of the infection. Women with this condition are cautioned to avoid sexual activity, douches, and other activities that could worsen the infectious process. If the woman's condition improves, she is usually evaluated in about a week to be sure the infection is gone. The nurse should advise the woman treated at home for PID to return for assessment if her condition deteriorates or her symptoms continue. Hospitalization may be necessary. A client requiring hospitalization for PID is usually very ill.

Surgical Management

Some abscesses are treated relatively easily, whereas others require surgical intervention or may rupture, causing peritonitis. The type of surgical intervention and its timing (acute or after a cooling off period) varies somewhat with the health-care provider's philosophy and the presenting problem.

Treatment of some clients with PID requires a laparotomy. Although dead and infected tissue is surgically removed, it also may be necessary to remove the uterus, ovaries, and tubes.

Surgery that is performed while PID is acute increases the client's operative risk. This risk must be

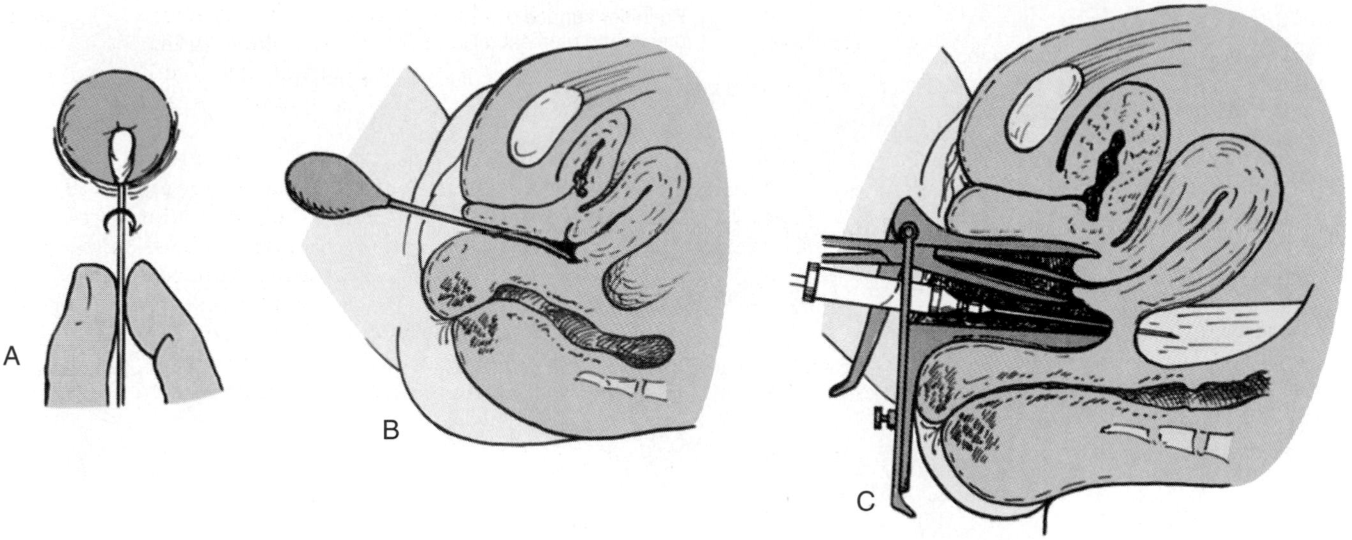

Figure 53–4
Some procedures used to diagnose pelvic inflammatory disease. *A,* Swabs may be obtained from the cervix, urethra, and rectum. *B,* The vaginal pool may be aspirated. *C,* Culdocentesis may be performed. Gram stains of cervical secretions show gram-negative intracellular diplococci. Cultures are placed on Thayer-Martin medium. Negative stains and cultures do not rule out gonococcal disease.

balanced against the risk of continuing unsuccessful medical therapy that can lead to chronic PID.

Nursing Management

Nursing care for women experiencing PID is directed toward providing health information and psychosocial support to the client and her significant others. Because PID is often caused by sexually transmitted diseases, there may be guilt feelings and problems with significant others centered on the client's contracting the infection.

Some women are infertile after PID. This change in fertility may be a difficult loss for the client and her significant other to accept. It is important to plan and provide time for the expression of such feelings.

Education is important for the client with PID. Women with PID can benefit from factual discussion about the infection, how to identify recurrences, and general hygienic measures that may help prevent new infections. The nurse must teach the client to wash her perineal area regularly with soap and water, to wipe from front to back, to change tampons and pads several times a day during menses, and to wash hands before and after changing tampons or pads. Balanced nutrition and rest, sleep, and exercise can improve the client's general health and reduce the risk of infection. These clients need to know when they can resume sexual activity and when other restrictions can be eliminated.

CHRONIC PELVIC INFLAMMATORY DISEASE

Chronic PID can occur if the acute phase of the illness does not respond to treatment or if treatment is inadequate. Clinical manifestations include chronic pelvic discomfort, menstrual disturbances or dysfunctional uterine bleeding, constipation, malaise, or periodic return of acute symptoms. Sterility, one of the more serious complications, results from destruction of part of the fallopian tubes and loss of their patency. Sterility is usually irreversible.

Treatment of chronic PID is aimed at removing the offending organism and improving the client's general health. If treatment is unsuccessful, surgical removal of the pelvic organs may be necessary.

Uterine Disorders

ENDOMETRIOSIS

Endometriosis is an abnormal condition in which endometrial tissue (which normally lines the uterine cavity) is located in other sites.

Incidence

Endometriosis is found most commonly in premenopausal women in their 30s to late 40s. It rarely occurs in women younger than 20 years. Endometriosis appears to be hereditary, occurring more commonly in women whose mothers had the disorder. The highest incidence is in white women who are nulliparous.

Etiology

The exact cause of endometriosis is unknown. Several theories as to the cause of endometriosis have been

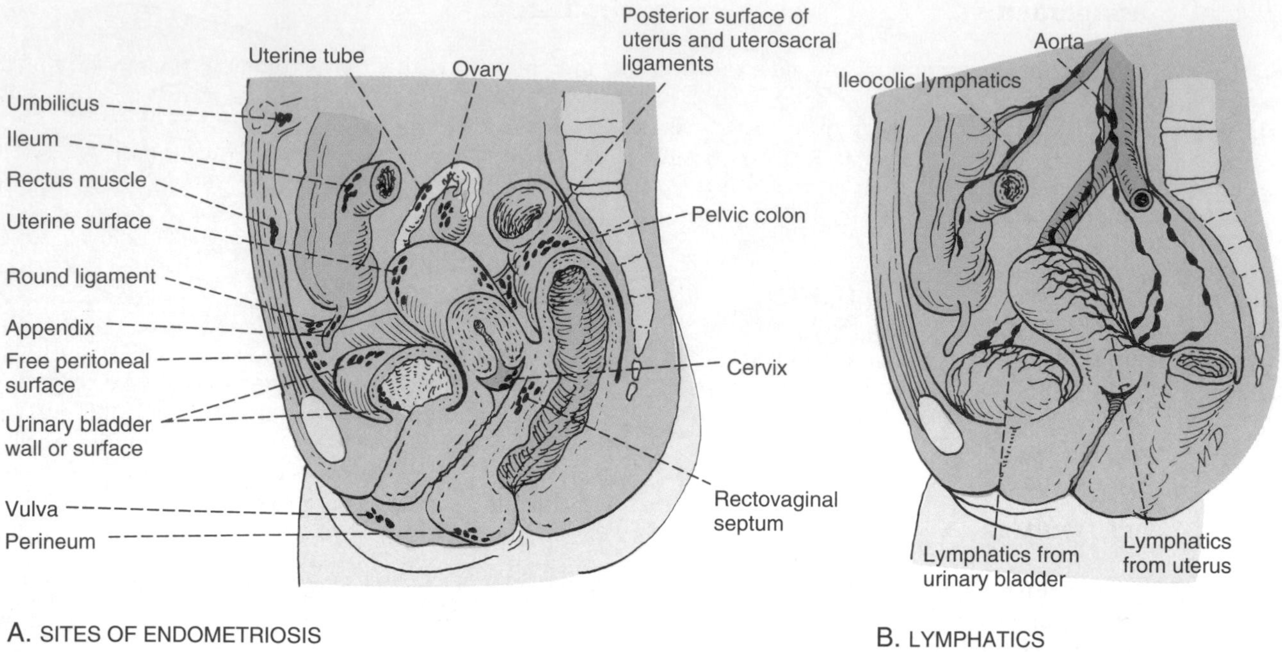

Figure 53–5
Endometriosis. *A*, Sites of endometriosis. Those most frequently affected are the ovaries and the dependent pelvic peritoneum. However, as can be seen, other sites can also be involved. *B*, Pelvic and lymph nodes are important.

proposed. One theory, the implantation theory, suggests that menstrual flow regurgitates through the fallopian tubes and deposits particles of viable endometrial tissue outside the uterine cavity. Spread then occurs via metaplasia (endometrial tissue reproducing itself).

The second theory, the vascular and lymphatic dissemination theory, proposes that spread of endometrial glands occurs through the lymphatic and vascular systems to locations outside the uterus. This may explain some of the distant sites of metastasis, such as the lungs and kidneys.

Pathophysiology

Although this abnormally located tissue is usually confined to the pelvic cavity, it also may occur in many other areas. The most frequent locations are the ovary and the dependent portion of the pelvic peritoneum. Rarely, tissue may be found outside the pelvis, such as in surgical scars, lungs, and extremities. Possible locations of endometriosis are shown in Figure 53–5.

Regardless of the location, this misplaced endometrial tissue responds to hormonal stimulation and bleeds, producing a variety of symptoms. Scarring and inflammation occur at sites of endometriosis. Repeated episodes of interperitoneal bleeding (from hormonal stimulation of the endometrial tissue) cause adhesions. Eventually, one peritoneal surface may become fixed to another.

Infertility is a major complication of endometriosis. Usually, the cause of infertility is unknown; sometimes, however, endometriosis produces tubal obstruction.

Endometrial tissue is hormone dependent; therefore, the tissue atrophies with the normal ovarian regression associated with menopause. It also regresses during pregnancy.

Clinical Manifestations

Symptoms of endometriosis relate more to the location than to the degree of disease present. Pain is the most characteristic manifestation of endometriosis. However, about one quarter of women with this condition are asymptomatic. Pain typically begins before the menstrual period, lasting for the duration of menstruation and sometimes for several days afterward. Pain usually reaches its peak just before the onset of menstrual flow and during the first 1 or 2 days of the menstrual period. The pain may be located in a variety of areas, making the diagnosis more difficult. Unfortunately, some women with endometriosis are erroneously viewed as not having real pain and being neurotic.

Other manifestations of endometriosis include dyspareunia (pain during vaginal intercourse), menstrual irregularities, and infertility in the absence of tubal obstruction. When the condition occurs inside the ovary, it produces a chocolate cyst. Severe pain is associated with rupture of this cyst. Implants on the ureters may obstruct them, whereas those involving the rectum may be associated with bleeding, diarrhea, or obstruction.

DIAGNOSTIC ASSESSMENT

Diagnosis is generally made by history, pelvic examination, and observation of lesions either by laparoscopic examination or pelvic surgery.

Medical Management

Appropriate treatment for endometriosis depends on the client's symptoms, age, and parity. When symptoms are mild, the client is given support, information about the disease, and some guidelines about ways to cope with the pain. Mild analgesics may be helpful. If symptoms become severe, more treatment is generally necessary.

PHARMACOLOGIC MANAGEMENT

Medication may inhibit endometriosis enough to allow pregnancy. Pharmacologic intervention includes inducing a pseudopregnancy with oral contraceptives, progesterone, or both and ovarian suppression or pseudomenopause with danazol (Danocrine).

Surgical Management

Exploratory or therapeutic surgery directed at the endometriosis may make pregnancy possible. Conservative surgical intervention includes restoring normal anatomy and removing or destroying endometriotic foci. A carbon dioxide laser may be used to treat endometriosis by vaporizing adhesions and endometrial implants. Even if the client states that she does not desire future pregnancy, conservative surgery might be used for a woman younger than 35 years in case she changes her mind.

More radical surgery involves removing the uterus, as many implants as possible, and possibly, some ovarian tissue if severely damaged. This procedure is most commonly used in women between ages 35 and 45 years who do not wish to retain their childbearing ability.

Even more radical surgery to treat endometriosis is removal of the uterus, ovaries, tubes, and as many endometrial implants as possible. Disadvantages of this approach include surgically induced menopause and permanent sterility. If the ovaries are normal and do not have endometrial implants, induced menopause often produces severe symptoms. This surgery is generally limited to clients older than 45 years. Conservative surgery is effective for most women. More radical surgery is almost completely effective.

Nursing Management

Nursing care of the client with endometriosis is individualized and depends on the severity of her symptoms, age, and childbearing status. Nursing care includes helping the woman during the diagnostic process as she considers the various treatment options.

BENIGN UTERINE TUMORS (LEIOMYOMAS)

Leiomyomas, also called myomas or fibroids of the uterus, are benign tumors of the uterine muscles.

Incidence

Leiomyomas are the most common tumors of the female genital tract. They occur in more than 20 to 30 per cent of all women during their menstrual years.[16] The incidence of leiomyomas in black women is two to three times greater than in white women.[23] Fibroids are more common in women approaching menopause.

Etiology

The exact cause of leiomyomas is unknown. The growth of the leiomyomas does seem to be related to estrogen stimulation because the fibroids often enlarge with pregnancy and decrease in size with menopause. Leiomyomas begin as simple proliferation of smooth muscle cells. It has been theorized that this proliferation is stimulated by physical or mechanical means and may occur at points of maximal stress within the myometrium. With the multiple points of stress within the uterus as a result of contractions, there are often multiple fibroids (Fig. 53–6).

Pathophysiology

Frequently, leiomyomas are asymptomatic. Symptoms that do appear generally relate to tumor size, location, or number. Additionally, abnormal bleeding, often re-

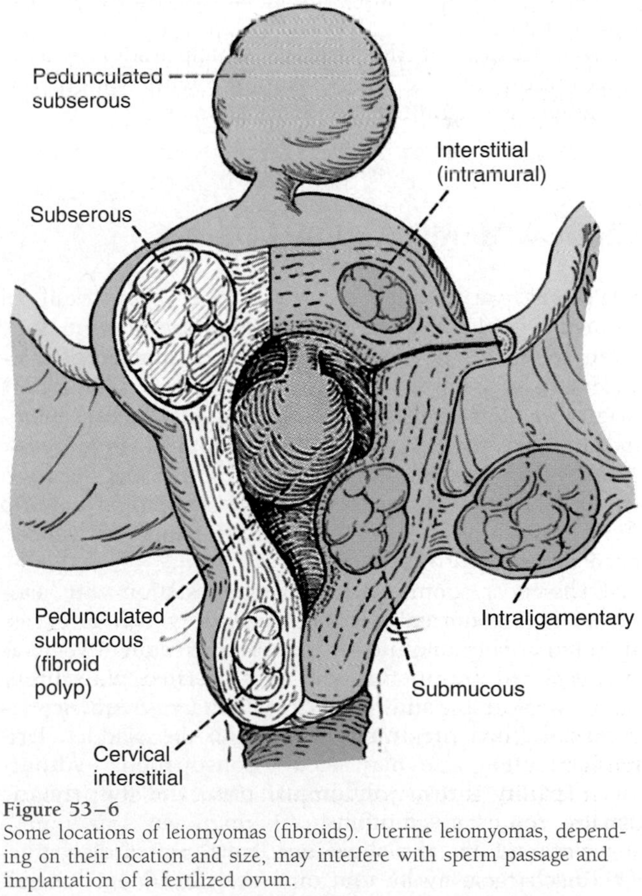

Figure 53–6
Some locations of leiomyomas (fibroids). Uterine leiomyomas, depending on their location and size, may interfere with sperm passage and implantation of a fertilized ovum.

sulting in hypermenorrhea, may be present and is related to the fibroid's hormone dependence.

Leiomyomas are known by various names (some not technically correct) related to the tissue involved (e.g., fibroids, fibromas, fibromyomas, fibroleiomyomas, myomas, and fiber balls). Leiomyomas are composed mainly of muscle and fibrous connective tissue.

Leiomyomas may be classified according to their location. Those occurring in the uterine body are most common (see Fig. 53–6).

SECONDARY CHANGES

Secondary changes can occur in all categories of leiomyomas. These changes include

- Hyaline degeneration, which occurs when the tumor outgrows the blood supply
- Cystic degeneration, which tends to follow hyaline degeneration, when the tumors become liquefied and ultimately cystic
- Calcification, which is more common in large tumors
- Infection, which is more common in submucosal tumors
- Sarcomatous (malignant) degeneration, which is rare and is suspected with rapidly enlarging tumors, recurrent tumors, and when hemorrhage occurs with a known tumor
- Red (cameous) degeneration, which usually occurs during pregnancy with clinical manifestations of an acute abdomen (i.e., acute pain over the area of the leiomyoma, fever, tachycardia, nausea, vomiting, and abdominal rigidity)
- Acute torsion of the pedicle, which leads to acute disruption of the blood supply, with gangrenous changes and symptoms of acute abdomen
- Fatty degeneration, which is rare

Clinical Manifestations

Symptoms vary widely and occur in about half of women with leiomyomas. When they are present, they often relate to the size, location, and number of leiomyomas. The onset of symptoms most commonly occurs in the late 40s and early 50s, just before menopause. Once menopause begins, symptoms often cease. It is rare for symptoms to begin after menopause, when leiomyomas tend to regress. If new symptoms develop during these years, other diagnoses, such as cancer, need to be ruled out.

The most common clinical manifestation with leiomyomas is abnormal uterine bleeding, which is excessive either in amount or duration. Frequently, it is accompanied by anemia and is associated with tiredness, weakness, and lethargy. Urinary frequency is common when the tumor presses on the bladder. Urinary retention also may occur. Constipation, hydroureter, hydronephrosis, abdominal pain, and dyspareunia are less common symptoms.

Occasionally, the client may have vaginal discharge. The discharge may be foul or watery and blood tinged. Abdominal pressure occurs if the leiomyoma is large enough to enlarge the abdomen. The tumor may be palpable. Also, the client may have problems with sterility or a history of one or more spontaneous abortions.

DIAGNOSTIC ASSESSMENT

A characteristic history, confirmed by abdominal and pelvic examination findings, usually establishes the diagnosis. Ultrasonography may indicate an abnormal uterine shape. Various disorders, such as cancer or a problem pregnancy, need to be ruled out before treatment is planned.

Medical Management

A plan of treatment for leiomyomas depends on symptoms, age, location and size of the tumors, onset of complications, and the client's desire to become pregnant. If a woman is nearing menopause and her uterus is smaller in size than that of a uterus at less than 12 weeks' gestation, the physician may assess the woman frequently (every 3–6 months) and hope menopause will alleviate the problem. Although malignant degeneration is rare, if the client experiences rapid increase in the size of the leiomyomas, more definitive therapy is considered.

Surgical Management

Younger, asymptomatic women may require no treatment. However, when definitive treatment is indicated, it typically includes myomectomy (removal of a tumor without removal of the uterus), if the tumor is small, or hysterectomy (removal of the uterus). Uterine leiomyomas are a common indication for a hysterectomy.

Nursing Management

Assessment

Many women may be asymptomatic; however, many will seek medical help because of some form of abnormal uterine bleeding. The nurse must obtain a thorough history from the client, especially concerning when the excessive bleeding occurs; assess the client's knowledge of her condition and the surgery, if one is planned; pay particular attention to any question the client has concerning sexuality after treatment.

Nursing Diagnosis, Planning, and Implementation

Nursing Diagnosis: Knowledge Deficit R/T surgical procedure and possible outcomes of surgery.

Planning: Expected Outcomes. The client will discuss surgery and outcomes.

Implementation. Frequently, a woman experiencing gynecologic surgery needs assistance in understanding her problem and the surgery being performed to correct it, either a myomectomy or a hysterectomy. She

CLIENT EDUCATION GUIDE

Posthysterectomy

Be sure that the client understands the type of surgery she underwent and what follow-up is required. If she had a myomectomy, pregnancy is still an option, and she must continue to receive regular gynecologic examinations. If she had a total abdominal hysterectomy with bilateral salpingo-oophorectomy, menopause and estrogen replacement therapy should be discussed.

Discharge teaching should also include the following instructions:

- Perform prescribed abdominal strengthening exercises to tone muscles affected by surgery.
- Avoid heavy lifting for about 2 months to prevent straining healing abdominal muscles.
- Avoid activities that may increase pelvic congestion (e.g., prolonged standing, dancing, horseback riding) until the surgeon says they are safe.
- Avoid vaginal and rectal sexual intercourse and douching until the surgeon permits. These activities could interfere with healing of the vaginal cuff or other tissues and possibly introduce infection.
- Avoid wearing constrictive clothing for several months.
- Report any bleeding and any abnormal (i.e., other than nonodorous whitish or yellowish fluid) vaginal discharge.
- Return for follow-up care as requested by the surgeon.

needs information as to what to expect postoperatively and how to care for herself (see Client Education Guide: Posthysterectomy).

If the client is going to have a hysterectomy, she needs to understand that her reproductive capacity will be lost. If the woman is near menopause and is also having her ovaries removed, surgical menopause should be discussed with her. It is important to remember, however, that some women are relieved at the loss of the risk of unwanted pregnancy and the disappearance of severe symptoms.

It is particularly important for the client to know that sexual intercourse will be perfectly normal following a hysterectomy. The client should be told that once healing has occurred, intercourse should be pain-free and orgasms are still possible; she has only lost her reproductive capacity. The nurse should answer any questions honestly and encourage the client to express any feelings or concerns about sexuality.

Nursing Diagnosis: Pain R/T dyspareunia and pelvic pain secondary to multiple or enlarged leiomyomas.

Planning: Expected Outcomes. The client will express relief of pain.

Implementation. The client can be taught ways to decrease pain associated with intercourse, such as altering positions, so that the leiomyomas are not pressed on during intercourse, and using water-soluble lubricants with intercourse.

Pain medications can be used for severe pain. Sometimes, sitz baths or the application of heat to the lower abdomen is helpful in relieving pain.

Nursing Diagnosis: Grieving R/T loss of reproductive capacity and perceived loss of femininity.

Planning: Expected Outcomes. The client will go through normal grieving over her loss without developing dysfunctional grieving.

Implementation. When reproductive ability is lost, the client may well experience a grief response. It is important to understand the grieving process and to be able to help the client understand that what she is experiencing is normal. The nurse should support normal grieving, including temporary denial, which is a part of the grieving process. If the client continues to experience grief beyond the normal degree, she may require counseling to help her cope with her loss.

Nursing Diagnosis: Urinary Elimination, Altered R/T infection with frequency and urgency.

Planning: Expected Outcomes. The client will be free of altered urinary elimination with normal output and no evidence of urinary tract infections.

Implementation. The proximity of the bladder to the female reproductive organs increases the risk that urinary problems might occur postoperatively. These problems are even more likely to occur if a vaginal hysterectomy was performed because of the pull on the musculature. A Foley catheter is usually inserted at the time of surgery to prevent bladder distention and injury during surgery. Sometimes, it is left in place for several days postoperatively. Potential problems that might occur postoperatively include urinary tract infection, difficulty urinating after the catheter is removed, and retention.

While the Foley catheter is in place, the nurse must instruct the client to keep the urinary drainage container below the level of the bladder, to drink at least 2 to 4 L of fluid daily, and to report any urinary pain or discomfort. The nurse should check the urinary drainage system closely for leaks, provide complete perineal care every shift, and report any change in color or odor of the urine.

When the catheter is removed, the nurse must observe for the first voiding, frequent voiding in small amounts, severe pain on voiding, inability to void, or hematuria. If the client experiences any of these symptoms, the nurse must report them to the physician so that prompt treatment can begin.

Nursing Diagnosis: Constipation R/T bowel manipulation during surgery.

Planning: Expected Outcomes. The client will be free of constipation and distention.

Implementation. Pain and discomfort after abdominal hysterectomy usually center on the incision and postoperative gas pains. After abdominal hysterectomy, gastrointestinal functioning returns slowly. Uncomfortable gas pains are often experienced during the early postoperative period. Early, frequent ambulation helps improve gastrointestinal function.

If gas pains continue, an enema may be prescribed to facilitate peristalsis and to prevent constipation. The nurse should continue to encourage frequent ambulation to facilitate the return of normal gastrointestinal functioning. Six glasses of warm water a day also help peristalsis to return.

Evaluation

The nurse must evaluate client outcomes based on the established plan of care. If these goals were not achieved, the plan and interventions must be revised to meet the client's needs.

ENDOMETRIAL (UTERINE) CANCER

Incidence

Endometrial cancer is the second most common genital malignancy. It is estimated that 1 in 100 women in the United States will acquire uterine cancer.[1]

Etiology

Endometrial cancer is related to the hormone estrogen because estrogen is the primary stimulant of endometrial proliferation.

Risk Factors

Many risk factors are associated with the development of endometrial cancer. The greatest risk is for women receiving exogenous ERT for long periods without concomitant progesterone therapy. Other risk factors include

- Obesity (increased estrogen production and storage)
- History of pelvic irradiation
- Hyperestrogenism—early menarche, late menopause, dysfunctional uterine bleeding, delayed onset of ovulation
- Old age
- Other reproductive cancer, including breast cancer
- History of infertility or habitual abortion
- Family history
- History of diabetes or hypertension
- White race
- Postmenopausal bleeding

Primary prevention involves life-style changes, such as weight loss and proper use of estrogens. Early detection is very important to increase the rate of survival in patients with endometrial cancer. All women at menopause and older should be encouraged to have a yearly pelvic examination and Papanicolaou (Pap) smear, although these tests are effective in diagnosing endometrial cancer only about 50 per cent of the time. Women at high risk should have an endometrial tissue sample performed at menopause and at regular intervals.

Pathophysiology

The cell type in endometrial cancer is usually adenocarcinoma (involving the glands). An adenocarcinoma is a relatively slow-growing tumor that metastasizes late in its course.

Endometrial cancer tends to spread slowly to other organs. Most commonly, the carcinoma invades the uterus, entering either the uterine cavity or the myometrium. From the uterus, it can spread to other peritoneal structures, including the lymphatics and blood vessels. It can then spread to the vagina, through the lymphatics to other areas, and, occasionally, to distant structures such as the brain and lungs.

Endometrial cancer may extensively invade the uterus, causing uterine enlargement. Extension of the cancerous process may occur along the endometrial surface to the cervix or the ovarian tubes and ovaries. After invading the cervix, further spread resembles that of cervical cancer.

If endometrial cancer is diagnosed early, its prognosis is relatively good. The death rate has decreased over the last 40 years resulting from regular pelvic examination and assessment. Once endometrial cancer has spread to the cervix, significantly invaded the myometrium, increased the size of the uterus, or spread outside the uterus, the prognosis is more serious.

Clinical Manifestations

Currently, there is no practical, accurate method to screen women for endometrial cancer. Thus, the cancer is usually discovered after the first symptoms appear. The most significant symptom is some type of abnormal uterine bleeding, especially postmenopausal bleeding. This occurs relatively late in the disease. Other symptoms relate to invasion, metastasis to other organs, or both (Fig. 53–7).

DIAGNOSTIC ASSESSMENT

A diagnosis of endometrial cancer is usually established by pelvic examination under anesthesia, followed immediately by D & C, which is used to obtain tissues for pathologic analysis. Women at high risk may have periodic sampling via uterine washings. Occasionally, a hysterosalpingography (an x-ray study using a contrast medium to show the uterus and fallopian tubes) or a hysteroscopy (use of an instrument to visualize uterine contents) is used to assist with the diagnosis.

Medical Management

PHARMACOLOGIC MANAGEMENT

Precancerous endometrial changes may be treated with the hormone progesterone.

Chemotherapy and hormonal therapy with estrogen and tamoxifen (Nolvadex) are used to treat late stages of endometrial cancer.

Surgical Management

Endometrial cancer is generally treated with surgery, radiation, or a combination of both. Early endometrial

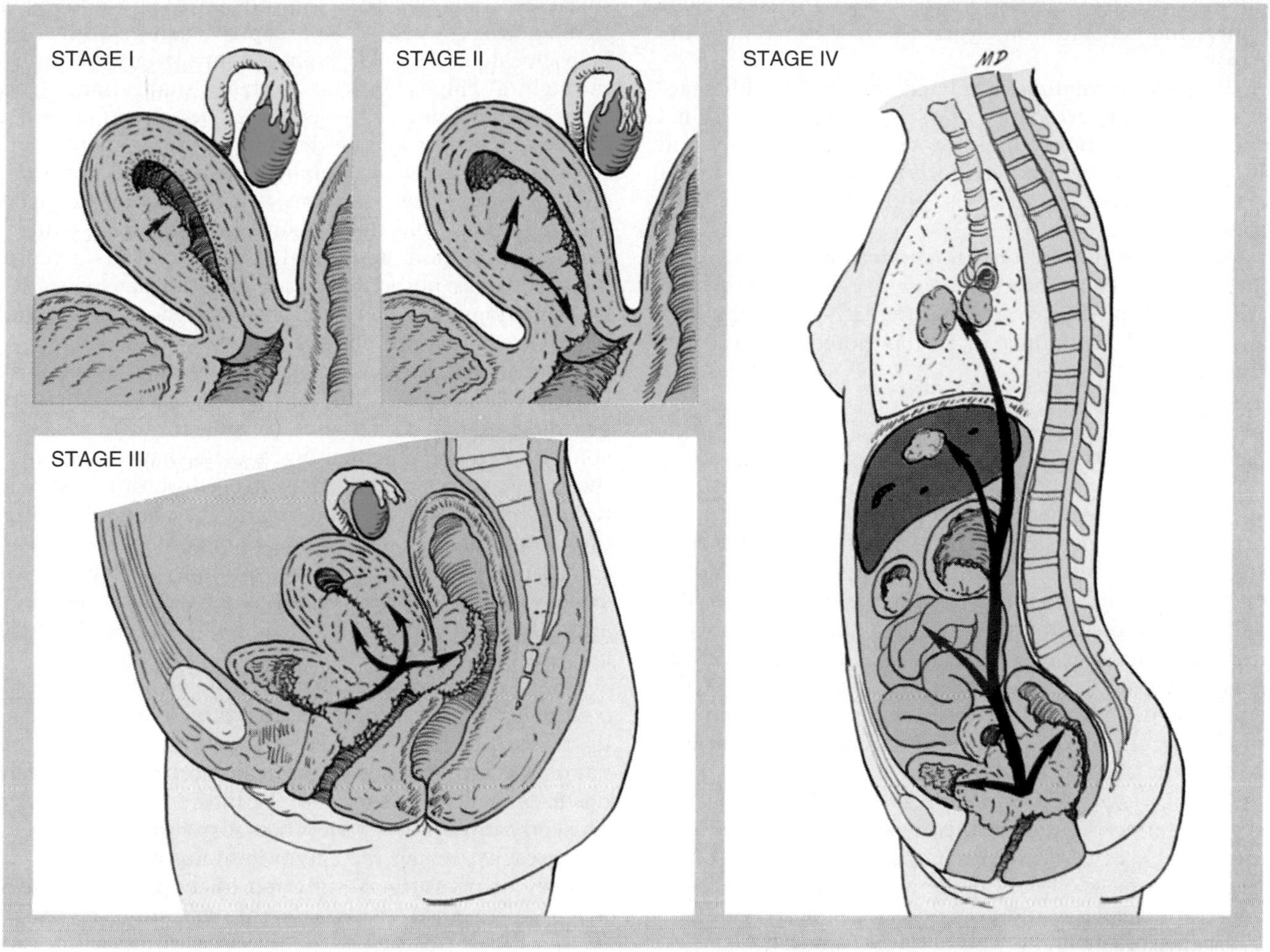

Figure 53–7
Staging uterine cancer. Stage I: Tumor is confined to the uterine corpus. Stage II: The cancer has invaded the cervix also. Stage III: The cancer has spread beyond the uterus but remains confined to the pelvis, such as in the bladder or rectum. Stage IV: Highest level of invasiveness; the cancer has spread beyond the pelvis, causing metastatic disease and large masses, such as in the liver or lungs.

cancer is surgically treated by a total abdominal hysterectomy–bilateral salpingo-oophorectomy (TAH-BSO). Surgery may be preceded or followed by irradiation, either external or internal.

Nursing Management

See the sections on cervical cancer and uterine fibroids for nursing management.

CERVICAL CANCER

Incidence

The incidence of invasive cervical cancer has steadily decreased over the years, whereas that of cervical carcinoma in situ has risen. Death rates for cervical cancer have also dropped 50 per cent over the last 20 years; however, it is still the second most fatal cancer of the reproductive system.

Etiology

The exact cause of cervical cancer is unknown, although chronic irritation is often present before diagnosis of cervical cancer. There is a strong relationship between the presence of the human papillomavirus types 16 and 18 and cervical intraepithelial neoplasia.

Risk Factors

A number of risk factors for the development of cervical cancer have been identified. Blacks, Native Americans, and prostitutes have a higher risk, as do those of lower socioeconomic class. Multiparity, early age of and frequent intercourse with multiple partners, early first pregnancy, postpartal laceration, untreated chronic cervicitis, and sexually transmitted disease are all potential risk factors. Women whose partners have a history of penile or prostate cancer also have a high risk. Jewish women and celibate women have a very low risk of the disease.

Primary prevention is related to good health practices such as the avoidance or early treatment of vaginal or cervical infections, limiting sexual intercourse, and possibly the use of condoms to limit the transmission of sexually transmitted diseases and human papillomavirus.

Secondary prevention for cervical cancer is excellent. Regular Pap smears are an excellent method of early detection. This test is particularly important because cervical carcinoma in situ is potentially 100 per cent curable.

Pathophysiology

Potentially, all women with carcinoma in situ can be cured. Also, 90 per cent of women with nonmetastatic disease can be cured. Five to 10 years may elapse between the preinvasive and invasive stages of cervical cancer. Most cervical cancers are of the squamous cell type. Squamous cell carcinoma usually begins at the squamocolumnar junction near the external end of the cervix. Some cervical adenocarcinomas occur but are more difficult to diagnose. Adenocarcinoma generally involves the endocervical glands.

Cervical dysplasia, the earliest premalignant change noted in cervical epithelium, is now further divided into several levels of cervical intraepithelial neoplasia (CIN): Mild dysplasia is CIN 1, moderate dysplasia is CIN 2, and severe dysplasia and carcinoma in situ are CIN 3.

Spread of squamous cell cervical cancer occurs first by direct extension to the vaginal mucosa, the lower uterine segment, parametrium, pelvic wall, bladder, and bowel. Distant metastasis occurs mainly through lymphatic spread, with some spread occurring through the circulatory system to the liver, lungs, or bones.

Clinical Manifestations

There are no early indications of carcinoma in situ or early cervical cancer. An abnormal Pap smear, however, is an indication for further assessment.

Late assessment findings include the presence of vaginal discharge and bleeding, especially after intercourse. Metrorrhagia (uterine bleeding between normal menses), postmenopausal bleeding, and polymenorrhea (increased frequency of menstrual bleeding) may be present. However, early bleeding also may occur as spotting or contact bleeding from cervical trauma secondary to sexual intercourse or douching. This early minimal bleeding increases in amount and duration as the cancer progresses. It usually indicates that the disease process involves the lymphatics.

DIAGNOSTIC ASSESSMENT

The Pap smear is the primary diagnostic tool for cervical cancer. Further assessment of an abnormal Pap smear typically includes repeated cytologic and pelvic examinations. Also, colposcopic examination often helps locate lesions for biopsy. Biopsies are performed through a colposcope for better visualization. These biopsies are commonly performed as an office procedure and cause moderate discomfort to the client.

Less commonly, a Schiller test may be performed before biopsy. This test consists of cleaning the debris off the cervix and then painting the tissue with an iodine preparation. Abnormal tissue, which is glycogen depleted, does not stain. The biopsy is then performed by removing a bit of tissue from various areas, including all areas that are not stained.

Occasionally, biopsies may be obtained by performing cold conization. This may be performed when colposcopic examination is not considered adequate. Cold conization involves obtaining a cone-shaped section of the cervix with a scalpel. This procedure provides more tissue for analysis, thus increasing the chances of identifying any area of invasive carcinoma, because invasive carcinoma and carcinoma in situ may coexist in the same woman. The procedure is particularly helpful if areas that are not readily visualized, such as the endocervical glands, may be involved.

Sometimes, analysis of the tissue removed during a cold conization demonstrates that a wide area of normal tissue surrounds an excised malignancy. When this situation occurs, conization not only serves as the diagnostic procedure but may be the only treatment needed. This procedure allows the client to maintain reproductive capacity, which may be an important consideration. Cautery or cryosurgery (freezing of the cervical tissues) may be performed instead of cold conization.

It is vital that clients receive careful follow-up care, including serial Pap smears. This is important because conization, cautery, or cryotherapy is not always sufficient treatment.

Medical Management

Irradiation is used as a primary therapy for early cervical cancer (see Chap. 7 for further information of radiation implants). It is usually curative but it induces menopause.

Surgical Management

Treatment ranges from cryosurgery or conization for local Stage 0 tumors to a radical hysterectomy for invasive cervical cancer.

Cryosurgery is the local freezing of abnormal cells and tissues with volatile gases such as nitrous gases (nitrous oxide, Freon, or carbon dioxide). Cell death results from dehydration and cell membrane destruction. Dead tissue then sloughs off.

Conization is the removal of a small cone of tissue with a sharp instrument. Laser therapy also may be performed to remove the abnormal tissue. There is usually minimal bleeding; however, the client may note a slight vaginal discharge.

A total abdominal hysterectomy can be used to treat carcinoma in situ in clients who have finished childbearing. A radical hysterectomy can be used to treat invasive cancer. A pelvic exenteration, an extremely radical procedure, can also be performed. A total pelvic exenteration involves removal of all pelvic organs, including the uterus, tubes, ovaries, vagina, bladder, rectum, and colon. An ileal conduit and ileostomy are formed.

Nursing Management

Care of the client with a hysterectomy is discussed in the section on uterine fibroids. See Chapter 7 for the nursing management of a client receiving an internal radiation implant. For women undergoing a pelvic exenteration, see Chapter 30 for care of the client with an ileal conduit and Chapter 35 for care of a client with a colostomy or ileostomy.

Irradiation thins the vaginal epithelium and reduces vaginal lubrication. It also may cause vaginal adhesions and stenosis. Such changes can make vaginal sexual activities uncomfortable or painful. Vaginal penetration during the course of irradiation and the subsequent months minimizes the possibility of vaginal stenosis and contracture. Depending on personal preference, vaginal penetration and dilation can be accomplished with the woman's own finger, a vaginal dilator, or her sexual partner's fingers or penis.

Nursing preparation of a client for cryosurgery and laser therapy involves clarifying that this procedure is not actual surgery and an incision will not be made. The nurse must explain that the procedure is performed with a vaginal speculum in place, as during a routine pelvic examination. During treatment, a few women experience headaches, dizziness, flushing, and some cramping.

During the procedure, the nurse can provide psychosocial support by

- Staying with the client
- Informing her of what is to be done
- Talking with her, listening to her, and facilitating her expression of concerns
- Continuing to acknowledge the client's presence during the procedure rather than excluding her
- Allowing the client to retain as much self-control as possible (e.g., tell her what she can do during the procedure to help it move along quickly and smoothly); also, the nurse should discuss how she can help manage postprocedure discomfort, such as performing slow, deep breathing.

The client's discomfort during the procedure must be assessed. A mild analgesic may be prescribed for the pain after the procedure. The client should be told what to expect afterward. Mild pain may continue for several days. A clear, watery discharge occurs. For about 14 days, this is followed by discharge containing debris (dead cells) that may be malodorous. If the discharge continues longer than 8 weeks, an infection is suspected.

Meticulous perineal hygiene minimizes the risk of infection and makes the client more comfortable. Healing takes about 10 weeks. Showers or sponge baths should be taken during this period; the client must avoid tub or sitz baths.

All women who have been treated conservatively for cervical cancer need information about recurrence. Women who have been treated for cervical cancer should be encouraged to have frequent health examinations and Pap smears to diagnose a possible recurrence of the cancer early so it can be treated before it spreads.

Modification of Plan of Care for the Elderly

Older clients may have cervical cancer treated by less invasive methods, if possible. The older client undergoing internal radiation treatments should be monitored closely after treatment for the development of fistulas.

UTERINE PROLAPSE

Prolapse, descent, or procidentia of the uterus occurs in three stages (Fig. 53–8).

First Degree. The uterus descends into the vaginal canal, and the cervix reaches but does not go through the introitus (entrance to the vagina).

Second Degree. The body of the uterus is still within the vagina, but the cervix protrudes through the introitus.

Third Degree. The entire uterus and cervix protrude through the introitus, and the vaginal canal is inverted (turned inside out).

Prolapse commonly follows multiple childbirths, childbirth trauma, aging, and failure to maintain the perineal musculature.

The incidence of prolapse has decreased with improved obstetric care (e.g., less use of forceps during delivery and better preparation of women for labor).

Cystocele

A cystocele is a protrusion of part of the urinary bladder through the vaginal wall as a result of weakened pelvic muscles (Fig. 53–9*A* and *B*). Urinary difficulties caused by the cystocele include frequency, urgency, or both; urinary tract infections; difficulty emptying the bladder; and stress incontinence. Mild symptoms may be relieved by pelvic (perineal) strengthening (Kegel) exercises. Kegel exercises may be prescribed to help a client achieve pubococcygeal muscle control. This is a form of conservative treatment for mild stress incontinence. The client must be instructed to practice alternately tightening and relaxing her rectal and vaginal muscles. She should tighten these muscles as if she were trying to hold back a bowel movement or a stream of urine. The nurse should instruct her to hold this

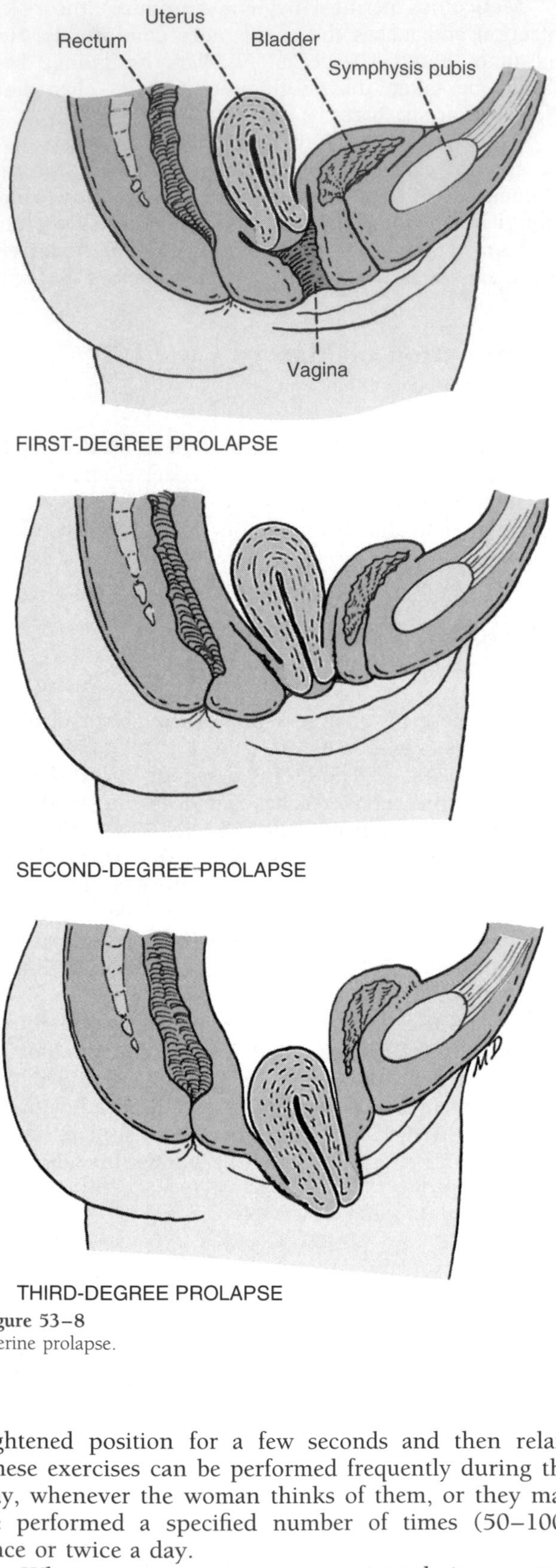

Figure 53–8
Uterine prolapse.

tightened position for a few seconds and then relax. These exercises can be performed frequently during the day, whenever the woman thinks of them, or they may be performed a specified number of times (50–100) once or twice a day.

When symptoms are severe, a cystocele is corrected surgically by tightening the pelvic muscles to provide better bladder support. This type of vaginal surgery is known as an anterior colporrhaphy or anterior repair. Nursing care is the same as for a vaginal hysterectomy.

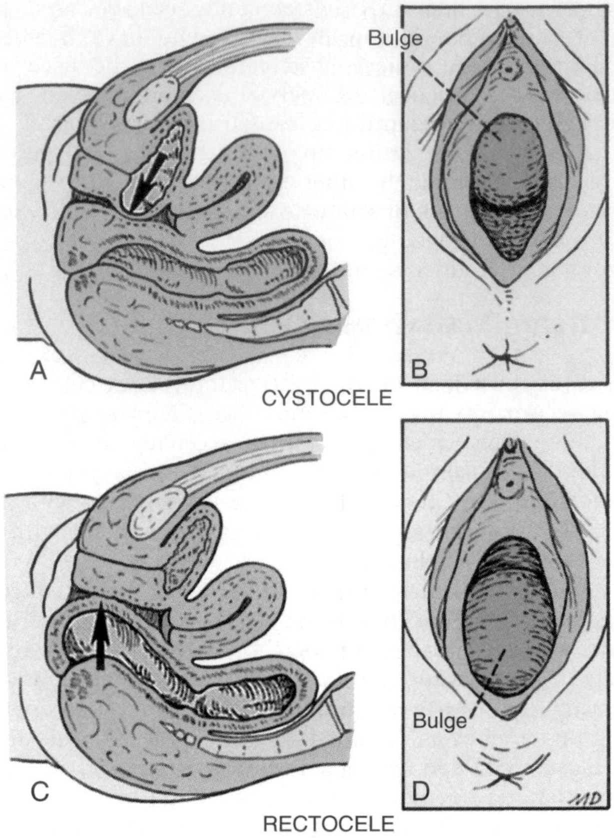

Figure 53–9
A, Cystocele. Note the bulging of the anterior vaginal wall. The urinary bladder is displaced downward. *B,* This pushes the anterior vaginal wall downward into the vagina. *C,* Rectocele. *D,* Note the bulging of the posterior vaginal wall.

Rectocele

A rectocele is the protrusion of a portion of the rectum through a weak place in the vaginal wall musculature (see Fig. 53–9*C* and *D*). A rectocele produces constipation, heaviness, and hemorrhoids. Additionally, a rectocele may be associated with incomplete or complete tearing of the anal sphincter.

Surgical management is used to correct this problem by strengthening the weakened muscles. This is known as a posterior colporrhaphy or posterior repair. Occasionally, this procedure is performed with an anterior repair. It is then called an anteroposterior colporrhaphy or anteroposterior repair. A low-residue diet and a cathartic are used before surgery to empty the bowel. Postoperatively, the client is given a low-residue diet until healing occurs and then stool softeners to prevent straining. The client is warned to avoid constipation, which could cause recurrence.

Complete Uterine Prolapse

Complete prolapse of the uterus usually develops gradually. When it is complete and also involves a cystocele, rectocele, and enterocele, the client is said to have pelvic relaxation. When the cervix protrudes through the vaginal orifice, it is exposed and constantly irritated. Tissue changes occur, and malignant degeneration is possible.

Clinical manifestations experienced by the woman with uterine prolapse do not necessarily correlate with the amount of prolapse present. However, most women with a significant degree of prolapse feel something is descending internally. Other findings include dyspareunia and vague abdominal problems, including feelings of pressure, dragging, and heaviness; backaches; and bowel and bladder symptoms. Stress incontinence also may be present.

Treatment for prolapse is insertion of a pessary or a vaginal hysterectomy. For a vaginal hysterectomy, an incision is made through the vaginal wall into the pelvic cavity. The uterus is removed from its supporting ligaments (broad, round, and uterosacral). The supporting ligaments are attached to the vaginal cuff to maintain the normal vaginal length. Special care is given to the Foley catheter to keep the bladder decompressed and pressure off the anterior vaginal muscles until adequate healing has occurred. When the catheter is removed, the client must be taught to keep her bladder empty by voiding every 2 hours to help prevent recurrence.

Postoperatively, the nurse should monitor the client closely for excessive vaginal bleeding. There is normally a small-to-moderate amount of pink, yellow, or brown serous drainage or even a small amount of frank vaginal bleeding may occur.

CRITICAL TO REMEMBER

If heavy vaginal bleeding is accompanied by a rapidly distending, rigid abdomen, referred shoulder pain, and indications of shock, immediate surgery may be indicated.

Other times of potential bleeding are the fourth, ninth, fourteenth, and twenty-first days after surgery as the sutures dissolve. If vaginal packing, a drain, or both are in place, the surgeon usually removes them in 24 to 48 hours. Often postoperative sitz baths are prescribed, usually beginning the first postoperative day.

POLYPS

Polyps are pedunculated tumors arising from the mucosa and extending into the opening of a body cavity. Genital polyps occur primarily in the uterus and cervix (Fig. 53–10). Uterine polyps may cause hypermenorrhea, intermenstrual bleeding, and postmenopausal bleeding. They occasionally undergo malignant changes, particularly in postmenopausal women. Cervical polyps may bleed after vaginal intercourse and are prone to infection.

If polyps are asymptomatic, they may simply be monitored. Because cervical polyps have a pedicle, they are easily removed by snipping or ligating them. This procedure is usually performed in the physician's office. Uterine polyps are not easily removed because of their location within the uterus.

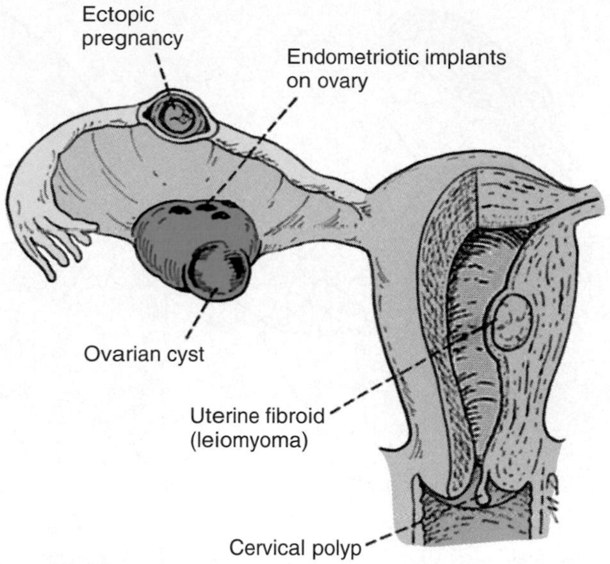

Figure 53–10
Common sites of some benign gynecologic lesions.

UTERINE DISPLACEMENT

The uterus normally lies midline in the pelvis and is symmetric and freely movable (Fig. 53–11*A*). However, variations occur from this typical position, some of which cause symptoms. The most common variation is a posterior displacement, referred to as retroverted (Fig. 53–11*D*). The uterus can also be anteverted (Fig. 53–*B*), anteflexed (Fig. 53–11*C*), or retroflexed (Fig. 53–11*E*). Another common displacement is a downward displacement, or prolapse of the uterus (see Fig. 53–8).

Most women with uterine retrodisplacement are asymptomatic. Diagnostic findings, when present, do not necessarily correlate with the amount of displacement. They may include backache (accentuated by standing a long time or occurring during the menses), secondary amenorrhea, infertility, a feeling of pelvic pressure, and dyspareunia. Pelvic congestion and adhesions may cause some of these symptoms because the uterus is less mobile than normal.

Treatment for uterine retrodisplacement is directed toward the underlying cause, if it can be determined. Some women, particularly those who have recently given birth, may be helped by exercise therapy. Assuming a knee-chest position for a few minutes several times each day may correct mild retrodisplacement.

Ovarian Disorders

BENIGN OVARIAN TUMORS

Benign ovarian tumors are either solid or cystic in nature. Ovarian tumors are often asymptomatic until they

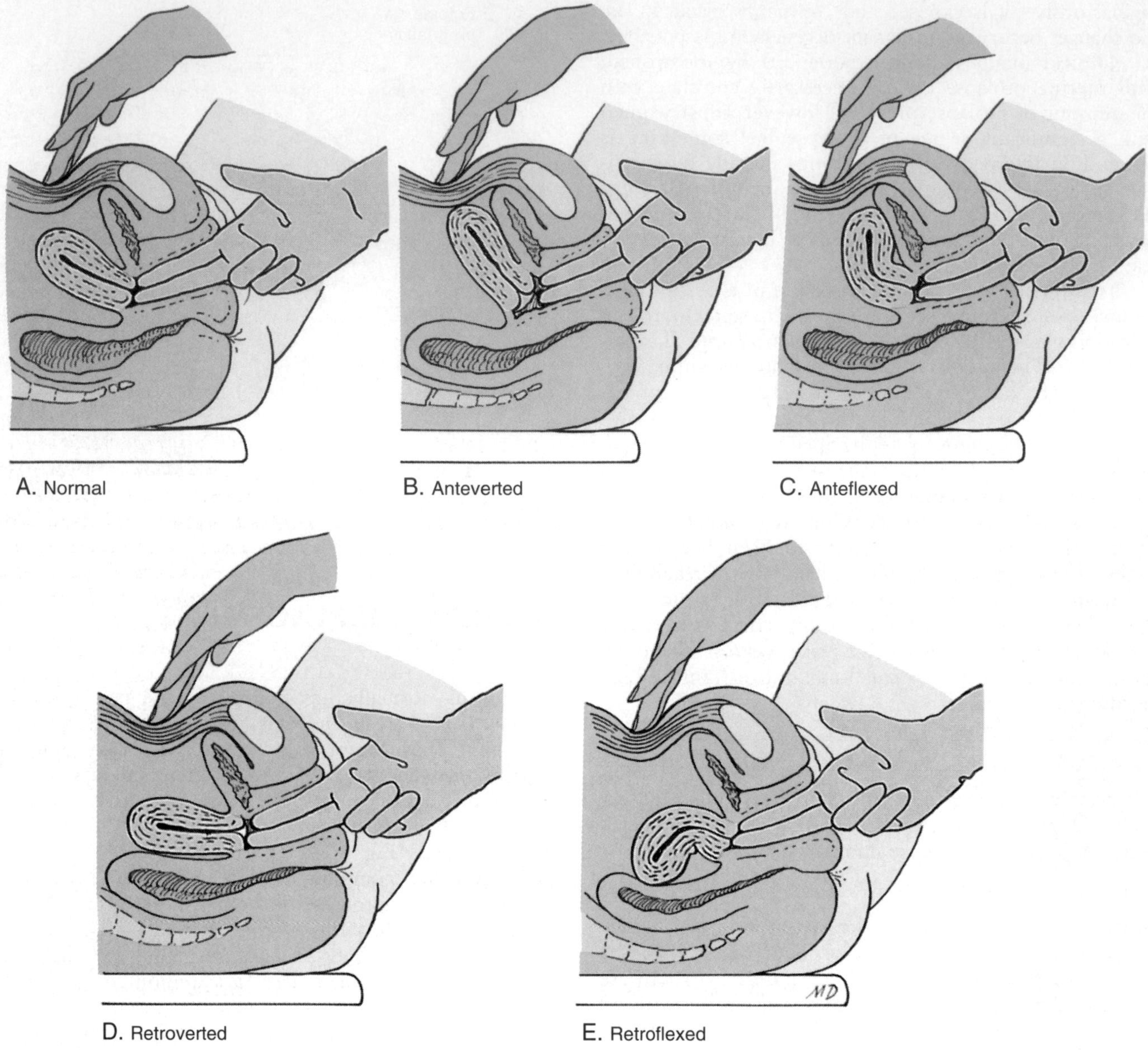

Figure 53–11
Displaced positions of the uterus.

are large enough to cause pelvic pressure. This makes early detection of malignancies difficult. Typical symptoms associated with pressure include constipation, urinary frequency, a full feeling in the abdomen, vague pelvic aching and sensations of heaviness, painful defecation, and dyspareunia. Acute pain may be experienced during menses. Often, the woman's abdominal girth increases and her clothes may not fit as well. Generally, the woman is unable to become pregnant.

Later symptoms include marked abdominal distention with dyspnea, peripheral edema, and anorexia. Pelvic pain may be present as a later symptom if the ovarian tumor is growing rapidly. If the tumor produces hormones, there may be menstrual irregularities and masculinizing or feminizing effects.

Complications from ovarian tumors include

- Hemorrhage into a cyst, with rupture and possible infection
- Torsion of a cystic pedicle
- Malignant changes

Treatment depends on the type of tumor. Tumors are removed surgically, either through a laparoscopy or open surgery, when they are bilateral, growing rapidly, and disrupt function of the pelvic organs or the ovary. Surgery may include removal of only the tumor, the tumor and the ovary or ovaries, or the tumor, both ovaries and tubes and the uterus. The amount of nursing care needed depends on the specific type of surgery performed.

Ovarian cysts are physiologic tumors of ovaries. They are common and may or may not produce symptoms. When symptoms do occur, the client may experience pelvic pain that often is worse on one side, pressure in the lower abdomen, backache, and menstrual irregularities.

OVARIAN CANCER

Incidence

Ovarian cancer is the leading cause of death from reproductive malignancies. The death rates have risen over time, probably because of the lack of early detection methods. Ovarian cancer ranks second to uterine cancer in incidence of female genital cancers. White women have a higher rate of ovarian cancer than black women.

Etiology

The exact cause of ovarian cancer is not known, although there does seem to be a familial association.

Risk Factors

Ovarian cancer usually affects women older than 40 years. Other risk factors include a family history of ovarian cancer, nulliparity, infertility, and a history of heavy menstrual bleeding and dysmenorrhea. Obesity, especially with a diet high in animal fat, is being examined as a possible link.

There is no effective primary prevention for ovarian cancer. All women should have routine pelvic examinations, including a bimanual examination. Women who are considered to be high risk should have a transvaginal ultrasound examination performed as part of their routine pelvic examination, and if this is suspicious, a Doppler study should be done. It has been suggested that women near or postmenopause who require a hysterectomy also undergo an oophorectomy.

Pathophysiology

Most ovarian cancers are epithelial tumors. However, some are adenocarcinomas. Ovarian cancer tends to grow and spread silently (without symptoms) until it causes pressure on adjacent organs or abdominal distention. When these pressure-related symptoms finally appear, the malignancy has usually spread to the fallopian tubes, uterus, and ligaments. Ovarian cancer often spreads to the other ovary and associated structures. The cancer may invade bowel surfaces, the omentum, liver, and other organs. When the pelvic blood vessels become involved, distant metastasis occurs. The usual routes of spread include lymphatic, hematogenic, local extension, and peritoneal seeding.

Clinical Manifestations

Clinical manifestations of ovarian cancer include abdominal distention, urinary frequency and urgency, pleural effusion, malnutrition, pain from pressure caused by the growing tumor, and the effects of urinary or bowel obstruction, constipation, ascites with dyspnea, and ultimately general severe pain. Indications of ovarian cancer do not typically occur until the malignancy is well established, which is often not until it has spread. Unfortunately, unless the malignancy is diagnosed early (e.g., when asymptomatic), most women eventually acquire terminal cancer.

DIAGNOSTIC ASSESSMENT

Palpation of the ovary in postmenopausal women should always be considered an abnormal finding. Identification of a pelvic mass by palpation is usually the first assessment finding. However, detecting such a mass may be difficult in obese women or in those who cannot relax during the examination. When an ovarian mass is suspected, a complete work-up is performed, including an intravenous pyelogram and a barium enema. Ultrasonography may be performed to detect a mass. Generally, following the work-up, exploratory surgery is performed to look directly at the ovaries, and, if the mass is malignant, to resect it.

Medical Management

PHARMACOLOGIC MANAGEMENT

Adjuvant therapy varies with the stage of the disease. With any ovarian cancer, clients typically receive irradiation or chemotherapy after surgery to destroy cancer cells that may have spread into the abdominal cavity. Intraperitoneal and systemic chemotherapy may be done (see Chap. 7).

Surgical Management

The extent of an ovarian malignancy is determined by exploratory surgery. Ovarian cancer is usually treated aggressively. A young client with a borderline malignancy may be treated conservatively with a TAH-BSO. However, generally the surgery of choice is a TAH-BSO, partial or complete omentectomy, and removal of all visible tumor. The less residual tumor left, the better the prognosis.

Some clients with ovarian cancer recover after treatment. Commonly, clients who are clinically free of disease and who have received chemotherapy for 6 to 24 months have a second-look laparotomy to decide whether or not treatment should be continued.

Nursing Management

See the section on nursing care of the client with a TAH-BSO for care of the client with ovarian cancer.

Vaginal Disorders

VAGINAL DISCHARGE AND PRURITUS

The female reproductive tract maintains its integrity through various natural defense mechanisms. Inflammation and infection occur when organisms disrupt or overcome these natural defenses. The resulting symptoms, although not usually life-threatening, can be uncomfortable and annoying. Vaginal discharge and pruritus are among the most frequent problems women mention to health-care providers.

All women have normal, nonbloody, asymptomatic vaginal discharge called leukorrhea. This discharge, secreted by the endocervical glands, is a clear exudate that keeps vaginal mucous membranes moist and clear. As this exudate passes through the vagina, it may become cloudy and acquire a slight odor as desquamated epithelial cells, leukocytes, and normal vaginal flora are added.

The amount of vaginal discharge often varies in relation to the menstrual cycle. It is greatest at ovulation and just before menses. Pregnancy, sexual stimulation, and oral contraceptives tend to increase the discharge. Some women view normal vaginal discharge and odor as offensive and go to great lengths to decrease it. However, excessive douching or using perfumed vaginal deodorants may cause vaginal irritation and infection. The consensus in medical literature is that periodic douching is unnecessary and may be detrimental because it washes away normal protective mucus and bacterial flora of the vagina and may introduce other bacteria.

The most common causes of vaginal discharge and irritation are vaginal infections; parasites, such as pinworms; sexually transmitted diseases (see Chap. 54); and mechanical or allergic irritants. An example of a mechanical irritant is a tampon left in place too long. Some forms of contraceptive creams or foams may be allergic irritants for some women.

Most inflammatory and infectious vaginal problems are accompanied by pathologic vaginal discharge, which may be copious, malodorous, and abnormal in color. It frequently leaks from the vagina, causing itching, irritation, and redness of the vulva and surrounding areas. It may be accompanied by burning and frequency of urination, anal discomfort, and pain in the lower abdominal region.

VAGINITIS

Vaginitis is inflammation of the vagina, a common problem experienced by most women at some time in their life.

Etiology

Vaginitis occurs when (1) there is a change in the normal vaginal flora, (2) vaginal pH becomes more alkaline, (3) virulent organisms invade the vagina, or (4) some combination of these conditions occurs. Vaginitis can be caused by insults such as congestion of pelvic organs, mechanical irritation (e.g., foreign objects such as tampons), chemical irritation (e.g., strong douches), vaginal infection, overmedication, especially with antibiotics (destruction of normal protective flora), and long-term steroid therapy.

Pathophysiology

The vagina is a potential cavity with a normal, protective population of flora, including various bacteria. For example, Döderlein's bacillus apparently helps maintain normal vaginal pH. The adult vagina is normally acidic because of lactic acid formed from the glycogen in desquamating vaginal epithelium. Normal vaginal function depends on a delicate balance between hormone and bacteria. Disturbance of this balance can precipitate infection.

Clinical Manifestations

Vaginitis is typically characterized by a change in vaginal discharge (i.e., it becomes profuse, odoriferous, and purulent).

DIAGNOSTIC ASSESSMENT

Vaginitis is diagnosed with a pelvic examination. This examination may be painful because of the infection and must be performed as gently as possible. Some bleeding may occur during and after the examination. The nurse should tell the client that pain and bleeding may occur and provide her with a perineal pad.

Medical Management

Vaginitis can be a stubborn, discouraging problem. It requires early, vigorous treatment to avoid chronicity. Treatment is aimed at correcting the cause of the vaginitis.

Nursing Management

Attention must also be given to the client's overall health. Rest, sleep, good nutrition, exercise, and meticulous personal (particularly perineal) hygiene all assist treatment. Women should be reminded to wipe the perineum from front to back to avoid spreading bacteria from the anus to the vagina and instructed to change tampons at least three to four times a day during menses and to wash their hands before and after each change. The nurse should warn women that feminine hygiene sprays can irritate the vulva. Soap and water are best for keeping the perineal area clean. Tight-fitting jeans, pants, pantyhose, or any garment restricting perineal ventilation may contribute to vaginitis.

ATROPHIC (SENILE) VAGINITIS

Atrophic (senile) vaginitis occurs in postmenopausal women. Atrophic, thin, vaginal mucosa and watery alkaline vaginal secretions provide an environment conducive to invasion by pyogenic bacteria (as in simple vaginitis). Assessment findings include discharge that may be blood-flecked, a vaginal burning sensation, itching of the vagina and vulva, and dyspareunia. If secondary infection is present, vulvar excoriation and burning with urination typically occur.

Short-term use of diethylstilbestrol suppositories or estrogenic creams is the usual medical treatment. If a secondary infection is present, additional therapy with an appropriate drug is added.

VAGINAL FISTULAS

Fistulas are abnormal tubelike passages from the vagina to the bladder (vesicovaginal), rectum (rectovaginal), or urethra (urethrovaginal) (Fig. 53–12).

Incidence

Fistulas are an extremely distressing and common problem in the genital and urinary tract.

Etiology

Some fistulas are congenital; others result from injury or diagnostic or therapeutic surgery. Causes of vaginal fistulas include

- An abnormal opening between two adjacent organs
- A result of the spread of a malignant lesion
- Irradiation for cancer
- Venereal and other inflammatory diseases (rare)
- Prolonged, difficult labor and delivery

Clinical Manifestations

Urine or flatus and feces leak into the vagina. Excoriation and irritation of the vaginal and vulvar tissues occur. Severe infection may occur. Rectovaginal fistulas may cause an offensive, particularly unpleasant odor. The woman experiences wetness and a sensation of feeling dirty.

In addition to producing unpleasant physical symptoms, vaginal fistulas produce severely distressing psychosocial problems. Women with vaginal fistulas often become social recluses, greatly disrupting their significant relationships and other social activities.

Women often do not seek professional health care until the problem becomes severe. Even then they may be embarrassed and reluctant to discuss it.

DIAGNOSTIC ASSESSMENT

A fistulogram (injection of a dye into the vagina) can be performed to assess the exact location and extent of the fistula.

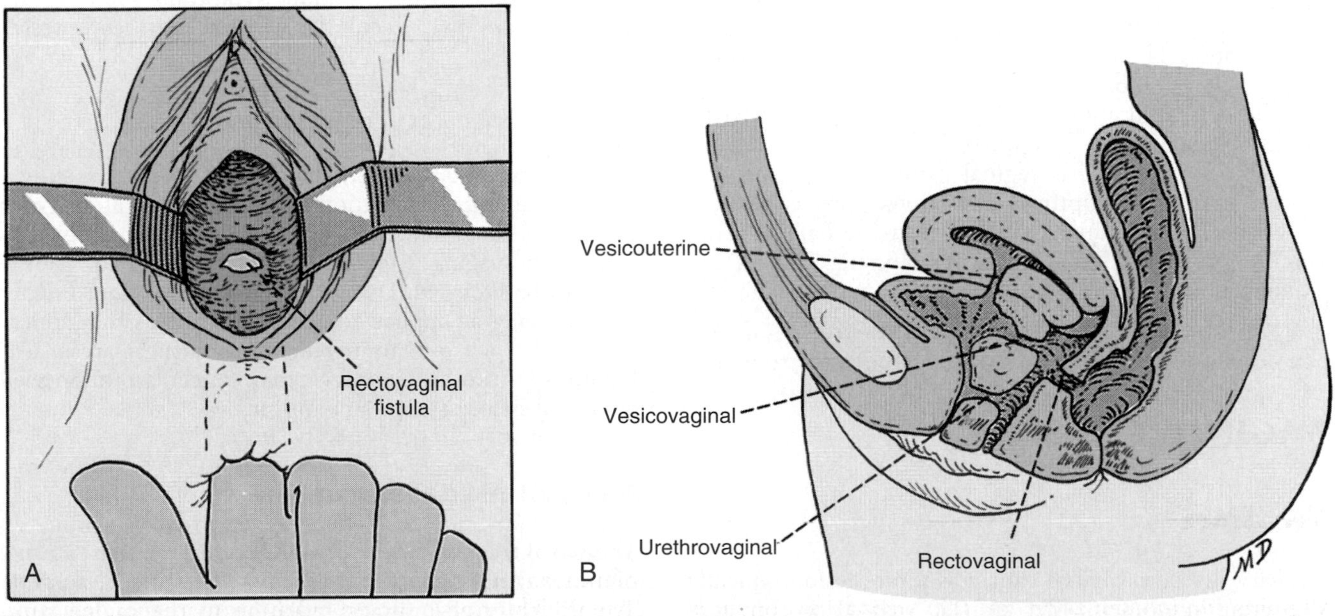

Figure 53–12
Vaginal fistulas. *A*, During examination, a rectovaginal fistula can be seen as the examiner's gloved finger (in the rectum) pushes upward toward the vagina. *B*, Locations of main types of vaginal fistulas.

Surgical Management

The diagnosis and treatment of vaginal fistulas may be difficult. Treatment varies with the fistula's location, extent, and cause and the client's general condition. Small fistulas may heal spontaneously after 1 to 3 months; however, surgical excision is often needed. Surgery is not always successful. For this reason, it is important for the client to be in optimal condition before surgery is attempted.

A waiting period of about 6 months is required before surgery while the inflammation and tissue edema subside. Treatment during this time focuses on preventing infection by performing frequent, thorough perineal hygiene and improving the client's overall health status. A temporary colostomy may be necessary to treat a rectovaginal fistula (see Chap. 35).

Nursing Management

An accepting attitude from health-care professionals toward a woman with a vaginal fistula is essential to help her comfortably accept and follow through with needed treatments.

The nurse must make sure the client understands the importance of increasing her fluid intake to decrease infection. Perineal hygiene measures may include cleaning the perineum every 4 hours (with sterile materials after surgery), sitz baths, douches, and perineal pads (changed frequently). Deodorizing and comforting measures may include using vitamin A and D ointment, deodorant powders, heat lamp, and various types of prescribed weak acid or weak base irrigating solutions (depending on the urine pH). The latter solutions are poured over the perineum.

Postoperatively, care is directed toward avoiding stress on the repaired area and preventing infection. A Foley catheter is used after a vesicovaginal or urethrovaginal fistulectomy to drain the urinary bladder. Careful attention is necessary to keep the catheter patent and draining. Also, the nurse must provide and encourage enough fluid intake for the client so that internal catheter irrigation is accomplished.

Surgical repair of a vaginal fistula may not be successful even under optimal conditions. This is particularly true if a woman has extensive tissue damage from tumors or irradiation. Supportive nursing care is extremely important for clients experiencing this distressing disorder and their significant others.

VAGINAL CANCER

Incidence

Primary invasive vaginal cancer is a rare lesion typically occurring in women older than 50 years. However, it is seen in younger women whose mothers ingested diethylstilbestrol during pregnancy.

Etiology and Risk Factors

Maternal digestion of diethylstilbestrol is associated with clear-cell vaginal adenocarcinoma in female offspring exposed to the drug in utero. Adenocarcinoma develops in these women generally between menarche and age 30 years.

Other possible risk factors include repeated pregnancies, syphilis, uterine prolapse, pessary use, leukoplakia, and leukorrhea. Vaginal cancer is rare in blacks and almost nonexistent in Jewish women.

Pathophysiology

Primary in situ vaginal cancer also is rare; when it occurs, it is usually part of an in situ vulvar lesion. Secondary vaginal cancer is rare, but it may occur from trophoblastic disease.

The staging of vaginal cancer is similar to that used for other pelvic malignancies. The primary lesion and involvement of adjacent structures are considered. Primary invasive cancer tends to involve the anterior or posterior vaginal walls, or both. Complications may involve the urinary bladder or bowel, such as fistula formation.

Despite active treatment, the prognosis for vaginal cancer is generally poor. The overall cure rate reported by the American Cancer Society is about 35 per cent. One-half of the women with vaginal cancer die within 18 months of diagnosis.[1]

Clinical Manifestations

Indications of vaginal cancer include foul vaginal discharge, painless vaginal bleeding, pruritus, pain (not associated with bleeding), and the presence of a vaginal mass or lesion. Urinary bladder symptoms such as pain and frequency may occur if a vaginal mass compresses the bladder.

DIAGNOSTIC ASSESSMENT

Women exposed to diethylstilbestrol in utero should receive careful examination of the cervix, along with cytologic examination of the cervix and any suspicious area in the vagina. Colposcopy may be used to identify areas to be biopsied. During pelvic examination, Lugol's solution may be applied to any vaginal areas that appear abnormal. Lack of staining identifies suspect areas. Unfortunately, the lesions of vaginal cancer are often well advanced before symptoms appear.

Medical Management

The usual treatment for vaginal cancer is either external or intravaginal radiation therapy or, less often, surgery. The difficulty of applying radiation to the vagina without harming adjacent tissues (e.g., bladder, rectum) has led some physicians to prefer surgical intervention.

Surgical Management

For earlier stages, radical hysterectomy, lymphadenectomy, and vaginectomy are used. Vaginectomy refers to removal of the upper one third to one half of the vagina as part of the procedure in a radical hysterectomy. Pelvic exenteration (removal of pelvic organs, creating an ileostomy and an ileal conduit) is used in more advanced cancer when the bladder or rectum or both are involved. Pelvic exenteration is indicated when there are recurrent metastases.

Nursing Management

During assessment, the nurse should ask women about medications their mothers may have taken during pregnancy. All whose mothers took diethylstilbestrol when pregnant with them should have a gynecologic examination at least twice yearly beginning at menarche, or at age 14, whichever comes first.

Vaginal surgery may be anxiety promoting and frightening to a woman. An ostomy (see Chaps. 30 and 35) also may need to be performed, adding to the woman's fears and problems. Postoperatively, vaginal sexual activity is not possible unless vaginal reconstruction is performed.

Sexuality is an important nursing consideration in the care of women with vaginal cancer. The nurse must create a therapeutic environment that allows the client to feel comfortable discussing sexual concerns.

Potential problems include fatigue, pain, dyspareunia (secondary problems to radiation therapy), decreased libido, and altered body image (from surgery, radiation, or chemotherapy). If a partial vaginectomy (one third to one half removed) is performed, the client can probably still enjoy normal vaginal sexual activity, using large amounts of lubricant and modified positioning, because vaginal tissue will stretch.

To cope with fatigue and pain, the nurse can suggest that the client schedule sexual activity after resting and schedule pain medication so that the peak of action coincides with sexual activity. A warm bath, back rub, positioning, or relaxation techniques might also help. The client should be advised to use a water-soluble lubricant during intercourse and, perhaps, a vaginal dilator at other times to prevent vaginal fibrosis and tightening.

Vulvar Disorders

VULVITIS

Vulvitis (inflammation of the vulva) is caused by the direct irritation of vulvar tissues or by the direct extension of irritation of vulvar tissues or by the direct extension of irritation from the vagina to the vulva. Itching and pruritus result.

Etiology

Vulvitis has many causes, including skin disorders, inflammatory problems, infection, vulvar kraurosis (dryness and atrophy of the vulva), vulvar leukoplakia (atrophic disease of the older female's external genitalia, with a white marble appearance of the skin, itching, and excoriation), vulvovaginitis (inflammation of both vulva and vagina), senile atrophy, irritation secondary to vaginitis, uncontrolled diabetes mellitus (with high amounts of sugar in the urine), pediculosis, scabies, allergies, psychological problems, cancer, ulcerative glandular or skin lesions, systemic conditions, urinary incontinence, and poor perineal hygiene.

Medical Management

Medical treatment is based on the specific cause of the condition. Itching (the most common symptom) associated with vulvitis can be severe.

Nursing Management

The nurse can teach the client measures to relieve itching, such as

- Applying calamine lotion and using hot compresses and sitz baths
- Wearing light, nonrestrictive clothing, including well-washed and well-rinsed cotton underpants (synthetic underpants tend to keep the vulval area warm and moist
- Avoiding feminine hygiene sprays
- Applying prescribed hydrocortisone ointment or anesthetic sprays
- Keeping the vulva clean and dry (e.g., cleansing after elimination—washing the vulva with soap and water, wiping with toilet tissue or washcloth from front to back, rinsing and drying well, and applying cornstarch to maintain dryness.

VULVAR CANCER

Incidence

Vulvar cancer occurs mainly in women older than 50 years. It accounts for about 5 per cent of female genital carcinoma.

Etiology and Risk Factors

Risk factors for vulvar cancer include a history of chronic vulvar dystrophies (leukoplakia), sexually transmitted disease, kraurosis (vulvar and mucous membrane skin atrophy, and dryness), diabetic vulvitis, and other primary malignancies, such as cervical cancer.

CRITICAL TO REMEMBER

Early detection of vulvar cancer is very important. Significant changes are detected early by women who practice regular vulvar self-assessment using a mirror. Teaching the importance of such self-assessment is an important nursing activity.

Pathophysiology

Vulvar cancer arises from skin, urethra, glands, or subcutaneous tissues. Approximately 90 to 95 per cent of vulvar cancers are squamous cell. The rest are adenocarcinoma, Paget's disease, malignant melanomas, and sarcomas.

Vulvar cancer has a slow growth rate and remains localized for a long time. Most lesions are located in the labia, primarily the labia majora. Some are on the clitoris. Local spread may occur to the urethra, vagina, anus, and rectum. Lymphatic spread is to the inguinal, femoral, pelvic, and finally, periaortic nodes. The usual causes of death from widespread vulvar cancer are distant metastasis, urethral obstruction, infection, uremia, hemorrhage, and general disability.

The prognosis is poor with vulvar invasive lesions. Five-year survival rates of patients with vulvectomy and lymphadenectomy are approximately 65 per cent. Recurrence as well as distant metastasis may appear in the first 2 years. When lesions are diagnosed in an advanced stage with node involvement, the survival rate is only 8 to 10 per cent.[1]

Clinical Manifestations

Leukoplakia vulvae is characterized by thickened gray patches of epithelium scattered over the vulva and perineum. Cracked areas in these patches provide an ideal medium for infection that can lead to ulceration and maceration. Eventually, these areas may become malignant.

Kraurosis also can become secondarily infected. It is characterized by bright red, smooth, almost transparent vulvar epithelium. Kraurosis is most common in postmenopausal women. With its progression, the vulvar tissues shrink and constrict the vaginal opening.

Both disorders cause itching and soreness or pain, or they may be asymptomatic. Both are diagnosed according to appearance.

Clinical manifestations of early vulvar cancer include pruritus, minimal vulvar soreness, and tissue irritation with some bleeding. The potential seriousness of these relatively mild problems may not be appreciated by women or their health-care providers because the manifestations are similar to those of nonmalignant vulvar lesions.

As the vulvar cancer progresses, clinical manifestations include vulvar edema and pelvic lymphadenopathy. Secondary infection may cause a foul-smelling discharge.

DIAGNOSTIC ASSESSMENT

Diagnosis is made from biopsy of suspicious lesions.

Medical Management

With leukoplakia, a biopsy to rule out cancer is indicated. In both disorders, infection is treated with an appropriate systemic antibiotic. Other manifestations are treated symptomatically.

Irradiation and chemotherapy are used less often than is surgical therapy. Irradiation is not generally used because the involved tissues do not tolerate it well.

PHARMACOLOGIC MANAGEMENT

Chemotherapy is typically given unless greater metastasis has occurred. The agent of choice is then based on the extent of metastasis.

Surgical Management

A simple vulvectomy involves the removal of the labia majora and minora and possibly the glans clitoris. Occasionally, the perineal area is also removed, requiring plastic surgery to cover the vulvar area. However, extensive surgery is avoided if the woman's condition allows a simpler procedure.

A radical vulvectomy includes excision of tissue from the anus to a few centimeters from the symphysis pubis (skin, labia majora and minora, and clitoris). Bilateral dissection of groin lymph nodes also may be performed, such as superficial groin and deep inguinal, femoral, iliac, hypogastric, and obturator nodes.

Nursing Management

For a client undergoing vulvar surgery, psychosocial support is especially important and should begin preoperatively. Some problems the nurse might anticipate are fear of disfigurement, grief over the loss of a body part, fear of death, and sexual concerns.

Preoperative preparation is similar to that for other gynecologic surgeries; however, it will also include an enema, douche, and insertion of a Foley catheter.

BARTHOLINITIS

Inflammation of Bartholin's glands can be caused by various organisms, including gonococci, streptococci, staphylococci, and *Escherichia coli*. The infection involves the duct of the gland, producing edema and, eventually, obstruction. Because the inflamed gland cannot drain, it swells and an abscess forms. Cellulitis develops in the surrounding tissues, producing more pain and systemic symptoms. The abscess may rupture spontaneously or may require incision and drainage.

After the acute episode, occlusion of the duct owing to fibrosis and scarring causes secretion retention and dilation of the duct. It then becomes a palpable, mobile cyst that usually is not painful. Symptoms relate to the size, such as dyspareunia or pain on walking.

Systemic antibiotics specific for the causative organism are prescribed. Local heat with hot packs or sitz baths may help to promote drainage. Surgery may be necessary, such as either an incision and drainage or removal of the gland, if cancer is suspected or for repeated infections with abscess formation.

OTHER VULVAR DISORDERS

Skin disorders of the vulva include many of those mentioned earlier as well as chemical burns, irritation with harsh soaps, genital herpes (generally, herpes simplex virus type II), psoriasis, folliculitis, and eczema. All are treated by removing the cause whenever possible and by the performance of excellent perineal hygiene.

Both the mite *Sarcoptes scabies* and the louse *Phthirus pubis* cause vulvar irritation. They are transmitted during sexual contact with an infested client, from infected bedding, or from toilets. Both the affected client and environment must be treated to get rid of the organisms and their eggs.

Other Gynecologic Disorders

CHORIOCARCINOMA

Choriocarcinoma is an extremely malignant neoplasm of the chorion characterized by its tendency to metastasize early, rapidly, and widely. It develops in about 3 per cent of women having a hydatidiform mole. Metastases occur with choriocarcinoma to the lungs (most common), vagina, brain, or central nervous system (these respond poorly to treatment), liver (responds poorly), kidney, and spleen. Choriocarcinoma responds well to chemotherapy.

The clinical course of choriocarcinoma is capricious. Without intervention, it is rapid and often fatal within 6 to 12 months. A few women experience spontaneous disappearance of the disease without treatment.

Clients with gestational trophoblastic disease (invasive mole or choriocarcinoma) require complex and expert nursing care. The disease process is confusing and frightening for the client and significant others. Because of the rapid progression of the disease, aggressive treatment must be begun quickly. There is generally little time to adapt to what is happening. Often, the client becomes extremely ill because of the toxic effects of the medications used. Clients and their significant others need support, reassurance, information, and meticulous nursing care.

When trophoblastic disease occurs, the pregnancy will be lost, adding additional stress to the woman and significant others. The woman probably has a knowledge deficit about the disease, and also experiences actual normal grieving. The nurse can provide support by allowing the client and her significant others to grieve and by accepting or facilitating grief responses. The nurse can offer reassurance and provide information as the people involved become ready to learn more about what happened.

The prognosis with choriocarcinoma directly relates to the duration of the illness and to the human chorionic gonadotropin titer level at the time of diagnosis. If the duration has been short and the titers are low, and if the client's medication regimen is carefully managed, the prognosis may be excellent.

STUDY QUESTIONS

1. An appropriate opening remark by the nurse to a woman seeking gynecologic screening might be
   A. "You can relax because none of this will hurt."
   B. "You are to be commended for making this appointment today."
   C. "You may call me as soon as you have taken off all your clothes."
   D. "Because you are not having symptoms, this will not take long."
2. The nurse can document learning on the part of the patient if the client makes which of the following statements about the cause of menstrual disorders?
   A. "Because I believe I have problems, I will be okay once I get it out of my mind."
   B. "My mother talked to a witch when she was carrying me, so I will always be cursed."
   C. "If I had stayed married, I would not be suffering these problems."
   D. "If the prescribed medicines help with hormone balance, I should also see some relief of anxiety, which may also help."
3. An understanding of the role of the client in the management of perimenopausal symptoms might lead the nurse to make which of the following statements?
   A. The client should take hormone replacement therapy (HRT) because it will relieve the symptoms.
   B. The client should discuss HRT with her nurse and her physician before she decides.
   C. There is no reason to suffer when HRT is available.
   D. There is still not enough research to make a decision about HRT.
4. In planning care for the client with endometriosis, the nurse should
   A. Recognize the potential for infertility and be prepared to offer support

B. Know that pain is not a common manifestation of endometriosis
C. Be careful not to embarrass the client because she usually has multiple sex partners
D. Realize that most of the symptoms are psychosomatic and make appropriate referrals

5. When pelvic exenteration is performed for treatment of invasive cancer, the nurse must
A. Accept the terminal condition of the client and help her and her family and significant others adjust
B. Provide information and assistance in helping the client redefine her sexuality
C. Use protective isolation because radiation is a threat
D. Be prepared to assist the client in adapting to an iliostomy or other diversion

6. The client undergoing a vulvectomy will demonstrate goal achievement for the nursing diagnosis of body image disturbance when which of the following takes place?
A. She dresses with several layers of clothes to be able to adjust to temperature variations.
B. She is able to prepare a meal for her family.
C. She no longer cries when someone mentions her surgery.
D. She is able to look at her wound in a mirror and express concerns about body function.

CRITICAL THINKING EXERCISES

SCENARIO A

A 49-year-old woman presents to the physician's office for annual gynecologic health screening. The physician, a male, is especially careful to protect the client's modesty. As a matter of fact, you, the female nurse, notice that he appears not to even look at the external genitalia as he performs the pelvic examination. The client is quiet and does not ask questions.

1. What are the nursing responsibilities in relation to the examination?
2. What is the nurse's responsibilities in relation to the physician?
3. What patient education opportunities are noted in this situation?

SCENARIO B

A 45-year-old client is diagnosed with leiomyomas (uterine fibroids) and has been advised to have a hysterectomy. She is very resistant to the idea and asks for a second opinion. She is married and has two children, ages 5 and 11 years, and works as a receptionist.

1. How would you advise this client?
2. What would you do if you believed the hysterectomy is necessary?
3. The laboratory values include hemoglobin of 8.5 and hematocrit of 30. Is this significant to the discussion?

BIBLIOGRAPHY

1. American Cancer Society (1995). *Cancer facts and figures—1995.* New York: Author.
2. Baird, S. B., et al. (1991). *Cancer nursing: A comprehensive text.* Philadelphia: W. B. Saunders.
3. Ball, K. A. (1988). Laser endometrial ablation treatment of dysfunctional uterine bleeding. *AORN Journal, 48,* 1153–1164.
4. Bobak, I. M. (1989). *Maternity and gynecologic care* (5th ed.). St. Louis: Mosby-Year Book.
5. Booten, D. A., & Seideman, R. Y. (1989). Relationship between premenstrual syndrome and dysmenorrhea. *AAOHN Journal, 37(8),* 308–315.
6. Bush, T. L. (1992). Feminine forever revisited: Menopausal hormone therapy in the 1990s. *Journal of Women's Health, 1(1),* 1–4.
7. Charles, A. G. (1989). Estrogen replacement after menopause, when is it warranted? *Postgraduate Medicine, 85(4),* 99–104.
8. Christian, A. (1993). The relationship between women's symptoms of endometriosis and self-esteem. *Journal of Obstetric, Gynecologic and Neonatal Nursing, 22(4),* 370–376.
9. DiSaia, P. J., & Creasman, W. T. (1992). *Clinical gynecologic oncology* (4th ed.). St. Louis: Mosby-Year Book.
10. Ensign, J. E., et al. (1988). Premenstrual syndrome. *AORN Journal, 47(4),* 962–971.
11. Gannon, L. (1988). The potential role of exercise in the alleviation of menstrual disorders and menopausal symptoms: A theoretical synthesis of recent research. *Women & Health, 14(2),* 105–127.
12. Gruhn, J. G., & Kazer, R. R. (1989). *Hormonal regulation of the menstrual cycle.* New York: Plenum.
13. Harper, D. C. (1990). Perimenopause and aging. In R. Lichtman & S. Papera (Eds.), *Gynecology: Well woman care* (pp. 405–424). East Norwalk, CT: Appleton & Lange.
14. Havens, C. (Ed.). (1991). *Manual of outpatient gynecology.* Boston: Little, Brown.
15. Heitkemper, M. N., Shaver, J. F., & Mitchell, E. S. (1988). Gastrointestinal symptoms and patterns across the menstrual cycle in dysmenorrhea. *Nursing Research, 37,* 108–113.
16. Herbst, A. L., et al. (1992). *Comprehensive gynecology* (2nd ed.). St. Louis: Mosby-Year Book.

17. Jenkins, B. (1988). Patients' reports of sexual changes after treatment, for gynecologic cancer. *Oncology Nursing Forum, 15,* 349–354.

18. Jones, H. W., et al. (Eds.). (1988). *Novak's textbook of gynecology* (11th ed.). Baltimore: Williams & Wilkins.

19. Kaunitz, A. M., & Grimes, D. A. (1988). The woman over 50: Endometrial sampling in older women. *Contemporary Obstetrics and Gynecology, 31(Suppl.),* 85.

20. Kjerulff, K. H., et al. (1992). Hysterectomy: An examination of a common surgical procedure. *Journal of Women's Health, 1(2),* 141–147.

21. Lee, P., et al. (1988). Accuracy of Papanicolaou smears: Art or science? *Journal of Reproductive Medicine, 33,* 795–798.

22. Lichtman, R. C. (1991). Perimenopausal hormone replacement therapy; Reviews of the literature. *Journal of Nurse Midwifery, 36(1),* 30–48.

23. Meyers, M. (1986). The enlarged uterus. In C. Havens, N. Sullivan, & P. Tilton (Eds.), *Manual of outpatient gynecology* (pp. 51–56). Boston: Little, Brown.

24. Murata, J. (1989). Primary amenorrhea. *Pediatric Nursing, 15,* 125–129.

25. Newton, M., & Newton, E. R. (1988). *Complications of gynecologic and obstetric management.* Philadelphia: W. B. Saunders.

26. Patsner, B. (1993). Screening for gynecologic malignancies in primary care: Uterine cancer. *Emergency Medicine, 25(4),* 157–158.

27. Rostad, M. E. (1988). The radical vulvectomy patient: Preventing complications. *Dimensions of Critical Care Nursing, 7,* 289–294.

28. Saite, A. (1989). Cervical cytology in general practice. *New Zealand Nursing Journal, 82(1),* 18–19.

29. Sloane, E. (1993). *Biology of women* (3rd ed.). Albany, NY: Delmar.

30. Smith, D. B. (1989). Discussing sexuality. *Oncology Nursing Forum, 16(1),* 106.

31. Soules, M. R. (1989). *Problems in reproductive endocrinology and infertility.* New York: Elsevier.

32. Sullivan, N. (1990). Dysmenorrhea. In R. Lichtman & S. Papera (Eds.), *Gynecology: Well women care* (pp. 345–353). East Norwalk, CT: Appleton & Lange.

33. Wardrop, R. W., et al. (1989). Oral discomfort at menopause. *Oral Surgery, Oral Medicine, Oral Pathology, 67,* 535–540.

34. Wynn, T. M., & Jollie, W. (Eds). (1989). *The biology of the uterus* (2nd ed.). New York: Plenum.

Chapter 54

Nursing Care of Clients with Sexually Transmitted Diseases

Learning Outcomes

After completing this chapter, the learner will be able to:

1. Assess the client for clinical manifestations of sexually transmitted diseases (STDs).
2. Teach the client about the etiology, risk factors, pathophysiology, mode of transmission, and clinical manifestations of common STDs.
3. Develop plans of care for the prevention, medical management, and prevention of transmission of STDs.
4. Implement nursing interventions that maximize the potential for control of the spread of STDs and prevention of complications of STDs.
5. Evaluate planned client outcomes, using outcome criteria developed in the planning phase of care.

The five classic venereal diseases (gonorrhea, syphilis, chancroid, granuloma inguinale, and lymphogranuloma venereum) are now included with such other infectious diseases as trichomoniasis, chlamydial infections, genital herpes, acquired immunodeficiency syndrome (AIDS), and enteric infections in a broader category of diseases called sexually transmitted diseases (STDs) (Box 54–1). The newer term now encompasses the broad range of conditions that are usually or can be transmitted by genital, oral, or anal sexual contact.

Sexually transmitted diseases share several characteristics:

- Despite their biologic differences, they are transmitted by sexual activities (not only by vaginal/penile intercourse but also by other oral and anal sexual activities between same sex or opposite sex partners).
- All sexual partners of the infected client need to be assessed for treatment.
- The diseases frequently coexist in the same client (e.g., a client may have both chlamydial infection and gonorrhea).

The last fact may be responsible for some treatment failures. Current treatment guidelines for STDs are available in the United States from the division of STD, Centers for Disease Control and Prevention (CDC) in Atlanta.

Etiology

Sexually transmitted diseases represent a serious, increasing, broad-range public health problem.. These diseases occur worldwide, have been recognized since the beginning of recorded history, affect all age groups and socioeconomic strata, and are associated with substantial morbidity and in some cases mortality.

BOX 54–1

Sexually Transmitted Diseases

BACTERIA

- Gonorrhea
- Chlamydial infection
- Syphilis
- Bacterial vaginosis
- Nongonococcal urethritis
- Granuloma inguinale
- Chancroid
- Lymphogranuloma venereum
- Sexually transmitted enteric infections

VIRUSES

- Human immunodeficiency virus
- Genital herpes
- Genital (venereal) warts
- Viral hepatitis

PROTOZOA

- Trichomoniasis

FUNGI

- Vulvovaginal candidiasis (only occasionally transmitted sexually)

ECTOPARASITES

- Scabies
- Pediculosis

Incidence

Except for the common cold and influenza, STDs are the most prevalent communicable diseases in the United States. Every year, STDs are diagnosed in more than 10 million people in the United States. Over the past decade, the incidence of STDs has increased dramatically. Most sources describe STD rates as epidemic. Whereas AIDS is probably the most dangerous and best publicized, the most common STDs are chlamydial infection, gonorrhea, syphilis, genital herpes, and venereal warts.

The exact incidence of STDs is unknown. Accurate statistics are difficult to compile for a number of reasons. Reporting to federal and state agencies is required only for AIDs, the five classic STDs (gonorrhea, syphilis, chancroid, granuloma inguinale, and lymphogranuloma venereum), and viral hepatitis. Rates for other STDs are based on estimates derived from local studies and physician reports. These estimates are thought to be low, and even rates developed from mandatory case reporting are also believed to be low because of underreporting.

The age-specific rates for STDs are highest for sexually active adolescents and young adults. All age groups, however, are at risk. Anyone who engages in intimate physical contact can contract an STD and then transmit it to others. No age group is safe simply because of age.

Other factors associated with increased risk include

- lower socioeconomic status
- lower educational level
- limited access to medical care
- drug abuse
- sexual activity with multiple partners

A lower risk of developing STD is found in people who are celibate or engaged in a monogamous sexual relationship.

The estimated increased incidence of STDs worldwide is due to many factors, some of which are only incidentally related. Many societies have become more permissive with increased mobility, sexual freedom, unemployment, and drug abuse. Only recently have the media and concerned organizations begun to present information about sex and STDs in a manner designed to appeal to young people.

Risk Factors

Most STDs are transmitted from person to person almost exclusively by some mode of sexual contact. (The other main exceptions are AIDS and hepatitis, which can be transmitted through the blood of intravenous drug users who share needles.) This is because the etiologic organisms thrive in a warm, dark, moist environment and survive only very briefly outside that environment. It follows that prevention and control must concentrate on breaking the chain of sexual transmission.

According to the CDC, the prevention of STDs should focus primarily on changing the sexual behavior of clients at highest risk. Prevention is based on four major areas:

- education on modes of transmission and methods to reduce transmission
- detection of symptomatic and asymptomatic infected clients
- diagnosis and treatment of infected clients
- evaluation, treatment, and counseling of all sex partners of infected clients

Health education is crucial in the primary prevention of STDs. Education is directed toward informing the public about sexual practices that significantly reduce the risk of STD transmission.

CRITICAL TO REMEMBER

The surest way to prevent STDs is abstinence. There is no such thing as completely safe sex, but certain practices improve safety.

These practices include limiting the number of sex partners, knowing the sexual history of all sex partners, avoiding sexual contact with those who have symptoms of STDs (e.g., genital discharge, lesions), avoiding risky sexual practices such as those that tear mucous membranes, using a male or female condom with any genital contact, and using over-the-counter spermicide in conjunction with mechanical barriers such as condoms and diaphragms.

Nursing Management

Assessment

Nurses need to be well informed about the variety of sexual activities, their effect on the transmission of STDs, and the common symptoms to assess. Educational intervention is necessary to help combat this major health problem while information about safe sexual activity is provided. It is necessary for a health professional to separate a personal view of morality from appropriate nursing activities. At times, this is difficult for some nurses.

There is a social stigma associated with STDs (see Ethical Issues in Nursing). Many clients are ashamed of having an STD and try to keep the diagnosis secret. Many associate STDs with low social status and immorality. Many have misconceptions about the dangers of venereal disease and may be fearful and uninformed about STDs.

Other social problems may surface with the discovery of an STD. For example, a newly infected client may be angry at the responsible sexual partner or be hesitant to identify or inform sexual partners about the STD. When a marital or committed relationship is involved, further problems may develop, such as the client's worrying about potential infertility as a consequence of the disease.

A nonjudgmental attitude on the part of the nurse is essential for providing quality care for a client with an STD.

CRITICAL TO REMEMBER

A moralistic, judgmental attitude may deter clients with suspected STDs from seeking health care.

ETHICAL ISSUES IN NURSING

Does the Right to Privacy of Clients with STDs Supersede the Right to Know of Potentially Infected Partners?

Sexually transmitted diseases (STDs) are a very serious public health matter. Such diseases may predispose one to various cancers and cause sterility and even death. There are ways of decreasing the spread of STDs, and large educational campaigns have been launched as a result of the incidence of AIDS and recent increases in the spread of syphilis and chlamydial infection.

Clients who test positive for certain STDs are reported to the Department of Public Health. This department studies the statistics of such diseases in order to track trends and address educational and treatment needs of the public in general. In many states, the names of clients with syphilis, gonorrhea, and chlamydial infection are reported to the Department of Public Health, and follow-up is initiated for those clients. Follow-up includes the department's notifying the sexual partners of the infected client so treatment may be initiated for them as well. The ethical question here is the right to privacy issue. Does a public health department have the right to know the sexual partners of those with STDs even if it is in the best interest of the public at large? Should the infected client alone be responsible for disclosing such information to his or her partners? Do partners of infected clients have a right to be told of their partner's infection so that they may seek treatment?

Health-care workers who deal with the care of those with STDs have an obligation to secure the privacy of their clients as well as an obligation to assist those who have potentially been infected. Nurses must inform their infected clients of the public health guidelines that must be followed. Information given to public health departments needs to be as honest and concise as possible. Clients do have a right to privacy, but this privacy must be altered when the rights influencing the health of others are involved.

The nurse needs to be very skillful in interpersonal communication to help clients appropriately. The client needs accurate information and support. Moralistic, judgmental attitudes do not change others' sexual behavior. Instead, they may deter clients from seeking adequate care. An accepting professional attitude may ensure treatment and prevent the spread of disease to sexual partners or prenatal and postnatal infants. The nurse must encourage and support the client's seeking treatment.

Treatment can be sought in various facilities, including health department STD clinics, physician offices, Planned Parenthood, and community-based clinics. Such clinics deal with STDs frequently and have staff especially sensitive to clients' needs; complete confidentiality is emphasized.

Nursing Diagnosis, Planning, and Implementation

Nursing Diagnosis: Knowledge Deficit R/T STDs.

Planning: Expected Outcomes. The client will express understanding of the cause, treatment, and prevention of the specific STD.

Implementation. Provide information about the transmission, prevention, and treatment of STDs. When caring for clients with STDs, nurses obtain privileged and private information and conduct teaching activities about these diseases. Both activities require sensitivity and skillful interaction. History obtained from a client often includes sexual activities; sexual partners; previous infections, treatment, and test results; parenteral infections; recent use of antibiotics; allergy to antibiotics (including manifestations); and signs and symptoms of STDs. The nurse should remember that sexual partners may include persons of the same sex.

The many myths about STDs should be corrected. The nurse can supply accurate, factual information to help the client avoid reinfection or infection of others. The following topics should be included in teaching sessions about STDs:

- name, nature, and seriousness of the condition
- mode of transmission
- actions to prevent spread of infection to others
- incubation periods
- indications (signs and symptoms) of infection
- asymptomatic problems
- when and how to seek treatment
- treatment methods
- importance of follow-up care (when and how to obtain it)
- consequences of lack of complete treatment
- risk and consequences of recurrent infections

Box 54–2 offers some examples of questions clients with STDs may ask and some suggested responses by the nurse.

In the United States and other countries, there are a variety of community and national programs in which health-care professionals collaborate with lay people. Nurses play a pivotal role by helping identify and meet public needs.

BOX 54–2

Questions Associated with STDs

EXAMPLES OF QUESTIONS CLIENTS MAY ASK AND SUGGESTED RESPONSES

Q: Will treatment protect me from getting this again?
A: No, immunity to reinfection is rare if it indeed even exists. You may be infected again.

Q: Can I resume my sexual activity?
A: It is better to wait until the tests come back showing no organisms are present. If you wait, you will not be in danger of spreading the infection to your sex partners and possibly reinfecting yourself.

Q: Do I have to come back for more treatment?
A: We would like to see you again (make an appointment) to be sure that you are cured (especially with the resistant strains of gonorrhea).

Q: *(Women)* Since I didn't have any symptoms this time, how will I be able to tell if I have this infection again? *(Men)* How will I know if I have this infection again?
A: *(For women)* When you have your periodic Pap smear, ask your doctor to check for sexually transmitted diseases as well. *(For men)* Watch for the return of symptoms (because men are more likely to have symptoms).

Nursing Diagnosis: Anxiety R/T uncertainty of condition and social stigma.

Planning: Expected Outcomes. The client will demonstrate a decreased level of anxiety by being able to discuss the disease and treatment in a calm, realistic manner.

Implementation. Learning that he or she has an STD can threaten a client's self-concept and pose potential physical problems such as possible infertility or damage to an unborn fetus. Feelings of guilt, apprehension, and rejection by others may be expressed. The nurse should work with the client to reduce anxiety, being warm and supportive. The client must be kept informed of what is happening and what he or she can expect. The nurse can facilitate the client's expression of feelings and help plan and implement effective coping strategies.

It is important that personnel caring for clients with STDs examine their own attitudes toward sexuality and sexual behavior in order to provide nonjudgmental care. Although one's own moral values are important in guiding personal behavior, prejudicial attitudes may interfere with therapeutic professional relationships. Bias and prejudice can be communicated in both obvious and subtle ways that make the affected client feel more uncomfortable, judged, and discounted.

Evaluation

The nurse must evaluate client outcomes on the basis of the established plan of care. If these goals have not been achieved, the plan and interventions must be revised to meet the client's needs.

GONORRHEA

Gonorrhea (common lay terms include white, drips, strain, clap, and dose) can be divided into two groups: local and disseminated infection (Table 54–1).

- *Local infections* involve the mucosal surfaces of the urethra, cervix, rectum, pharynx, and conjunctiva.
- *Systemic infection* involves polyarthritis, dermatitis, endocarditis, or meningitis secondary to bacteremia. Systemic infection is more common in women than in men.

Incidence

Gonorrhea continues to be one of the most common STDs in the United States. Incidence varies with age. Teenagers and young adults are at highest risk; the highest rates occur in the 20- to 24-year-old age group.

Etiology

Gonorrhea is caused by the gram-negative diplococcus *Neisseria gonorrhoeae,* which does not survive for long outside the body. The disease is easily transmitted by sexual contact, and there is a large carrier population (i.e., people who have no symptoms but who carry the organism and can transmit the disease). It has a variable incubation time, usually 3 to 8 days. There is no lasting immunity that prevents reinfection.

Risk Factors

Gonorrheal infection is almost always sexually transmitted, although other current sources point to self-inoculation with contaminated hands. The few rare exceptions are (1) children, who can develop gonorrhea from close contact with the mother's infected areas (vaginal or other mucous membranes), and (2) medical personnel with lacerations, who can develop gonorrhea from contact with infected discharges.

Clinical Manifestations

An initial gonorrheal infection in women may involve the endocervix, vestibular glands, urethra, and anus. Although the vagina is resistant to the infection in adulthood, before puberty it is not. The disease may be asymptomatic in women. Symptoms may include heavy, yellow-green, purulent discharge; a red, swollen, sore vulva; dysuria; and urinary frequency. The most common complication of gonorrhea in women is salpingitis, which can progress to pelvic inflammatory disease (PID). See Chapter 53 for information on PID and salpingitis. Both PID and salpingitis can produce infertility. The first actual symptoms of gonorrhea in women may arise from PID.

In men with gonorrhea, symptoms are usually evident earlier than in women. The infection is principally one of the anterior urethra that produces a purulent discharge, dysuria, and urinary frequency. Complications include epididymitis and prostatitis, but these are not common with early and complete antibiotic therapy.

In addition to the gender-specific manifestations, either sex may have pharyngitis due to orogenital contact (fellatio, cunnilingus) or proctitis from anal contact (sodomy).

Diagnostic Assessment

Diagnosis is made by history, physical examination, identification of the gonococcus on a smear, and culture of exudate from the endocervix, urethra, and other infected areas. All clients with gonorrhea should also be tested for chlamydial infection, syphilis, and other coexisting STDs such as trichomoniasis.

Medical Management

PHARMACOLOGIC MANAGEMENT

Gonorrhea is treated aggressively with antibiotics. The recommended regimen is ceftriaxone sodium (Rocephin), a cephalosporin antibiotic, one dose intramuscularly followed by doxycycline hyclate (Vibramycin Hyclate). For clients who cannot tolerate ceftriaxone sodium, a single intramuscular injection of spectinomycin dihydrochloride (Trobicin) or Cipro 500 mg orally in a single dose can be used. After completion of therapy, a follow-up examination and culture should be done. A positive culture, however, may indicate reinfection rather than treatment failure.

Nursing Management

Clients experiencing gonorrhea must understand information about the disease, how it spreads, and how it is treated. Self-care information is essential. The nurse should discuss the possibility of reinfection and infection of sexual partners and the importance of identifying and treating all sexual partners. The nurse should encourage sexual abstinence or the use of a male or female condom until the infection is cured.

Clients receiving treatment for gonorrhea must understand the importance of taking the complete course of prescribed medications and of returning for follow-up evaluation after completing the medication.

Treatment for gonorrhea is subject to change as organisms become more resistant. Many clients are not aware that the doses of penicillin used to treat gonorrhea are much greater than those used for most other infections and mistakenly think that an antibiotic taken for some other problem (e.g., respiratory infection) will also "cure" gonorrhea. Public education is an essential part of the fight against STDs.

TABLE 54–1 Management of Common Sexually Transmitted Diseases

CONDITION/ CAUSATIVE ORGANISM	DIAGNOSTIC METHODS	MANIFESTATIONS	TREATMENT OF CHOICE*	MANDATORY REPORTING	SEXUAL PARTNER TREATMENT*
Gonorrhea/*Neisseria gonorrhoeae*	Smear culture	Incubation period: 3–8 days Female: asymptomatic or • thick, purulent vaginal discharge • genital irritation • dysuria, urinary frequency • pharyngeal infection • late: pelvic pain (PID) Male: asymptomatic or • urethral discharge • dysuria, urinary frequency • pharyngeal infection • late: scrotal pain (epididymitis) • perineal pain (prostatitis) Disseminated infection, either sex: • bacteremia • arthritis-dermatitis syndrome	Ceftriaxone IM once *plus* Doxycycline PO for 7 days	Yes	All contacts within the preceding 30 days should be examined, cultured, and treated presumptively
Chlamydial infections/*Chlamydia trachomatis*	Culture Antigen-antibody tests Enzyme immunoassay Monoclonal antibody test	Incubation period: 7–21 days Female: asymptomatic or • mucopurulent vaginal discharge • dysuria • abnormal vaginal bleeding • pelvic pain (PID) Male: asymptomatic or • mild dysuria • white or clear urethral discharge • testical pain (epididymitis)	Doxycycline PO for 7 days	No	All contacts within 30 days should be examined and treated

Sexual contact investigation is essential for the prevention and control of gonorrhea. Reporting sexual contacts can be difficult and frightening for an infected client. The nurse should ask for contact information in a positive, nonthreatening, sensitive way. During the initial treatment visit, clients should be asked about sexual contacts. However, this is best asked after the treatment is actually administered so they will not become anxious and possibly avoid necessary care.

TABLE 54–1 Management of Common Sexually Transmitted Diseases *Continued*

CONDITION/ CAUSATIVE ORGANISM	DIAGNOSTIC METHODS	MANIFESTATIONS	TREATMENT OF CHOICE*	MANDATORY REPORTING	SEXUAL PARTNER TREATMENT*
Syphilis/*Treponema pallidum*	Darkfield microscopy (chancre, granulomata lata) Serologic antibody tests • nonspecific, e.g., VDRL • specific, e.g., FTA-ABS	Incubation period: 10–90 days Primary • painless chancre at site of exposure • regional lymphadenopathy Secondary • maculopapular skin rash • generalized lymphadenopathy • mucous patches • condylomata lata • fever, malaise • alopecia Latent • asymptomatic	Early syphilis: benzathine penicillin G IM single dose	Yes	All contacts with early syphilis (primary, secondary, or latent syphilis of 1 year's duration) should be evaluated and treated All contacts within 90 days should be treated presumptively
	Cerebrospinal fluid (late syphilis)	Late • cardiovascular changes, e.g., aortic aneurysm • central nervous system changes, e.g., paresis, tabes dorsalis, dementia	Cardiovascular syphilis: benzathine penicillin G IM weekly for 3 weeks Neurosyphilis: aqueous penicillin IV every 4 hours for 10–14 days	No	
Genital herpes/ *Herpes simplex* virus (HSV) type I or II, primarily type II	Culture Pap smear	Incubation period: 3–7 days Acute phase • paresthesia/burning at site of exposure • painful genital vesicles that ulcerate • fever, chills, muscle aches Latent phase • symptomatic	No cure Acyclovir PO for 5–10 days for acute episodes	No	All contacts of clients with active lesions should be evaluated and, if symptomatic, treated
Genital warts/ Human papillomavirus (HPV)	Pap smear Colposcopy Biopsy	Incubation period: 1–2 months Single or multiple painless genital or anorectal warts	Cryotherapy with liquid nitrogen or cryoprobe	No	All contacts should be evaluated and, if symptomatic, treated

* CDC 1989 sexually transmitted diseases treatment guidelines.
FTA-ABS, fluorescent treponemal antibody absorption test; IM, intramuscularly; IV, intravenously; PID, pelvic inflammatory disease; PO, orally; VDRL, Venereal Disease Research Laboratory test.

CHLAMYDIAL INFECTIONS

Infection with *Chlamydia trachomatis* is the most common STD in the United States today (Table 54–1).

Incidence

The incidence of chlamydial infection is three times that of gonorrhea. The number of new cases per year is estimated to be at least 3 to 4 million. Unlike gonorrhea, the disease is not reportable to the public health department, so the exact incidence is unknown.

Etiology

The etiologic organism, *C. trachomatis,* is a nonmotile, gram-negative bacterium that is most often responsible for what was previously termed nonspecific vaginitis in females and nongonococcal or nonspecific urethritis in males. The incubation period is 7 to 21 days.

Risk Factors

C. trachomatis is always transmitted by intimate sexual contact, never casual contact. Women usually acquire the infection during intercourse with an infected male. Males can also transmit the infection through homosexual contact. The infection does not cross the placenta, but exposure during delivery can cause conjunctivitis and pneumonia in newborns.

Clinical Manifestations

Chlamydial infections primarily affect the urethra, endocervix, and rectum. *C. trachomatis* is found in these areas and the Bartholin glands in women. In many cases, the infection is asymptomatic for an extended period. When present, symptoms resemble those of gonorrhea but are less severe.

In women, the organism produces a friable, edematous cervix that causes a yellow, mucopurulent vaginal discharge that may be accompanied by spotting at menstrual midcycle or with sexual intercourse. With Bartholin's duct involvement, there is a purulent discharge. In both sexes, there is dysuria associated with urethritis.

Diagnostic Assessment

Because there are few or no symptoms, the diagnosis of chlamydial infections is difficult and often missed. Clients tend not to seek medical treatment. Manifestations are often nonspecific and virtually indistinguishable clinically from those of gonorrhea. For this reason, and because these two infections often coexist, it is recommended that diagnostic tests for both be done when either condition is suspected.

The best diagnostic test for chlamydial infections is the tissue culture of cellular material from the urethra, endocervix, or rectum. Rapid nonculture antigen detection tests done on urogenital secretions are also available. These are antigen-antibody tests that use either an enzyme immunoassay or a monoclonal antibody technique. Although slightly less accurate than a culture, these tests hold the advantage of being more convenient, rapid, and less expensive than a culture. These rapid tests are recommended for the screening of asymptomatic high-risk clients in whom chlamydial infections would otherwise go undetected. Priority groups for testing, if resources are limited, are high-risk pregnant women, adolescents, and women with multiple sex partners. The Papanicolaou (Pap) smear has no diagnostic value in the diagnosis or screening of chlamydial infection.

Chlamydial infection is known as "the great sterilizer." Undetected and untreated cases can progress to serious, irreversible consequences. *C. trachomatis* causes an inflammation that leads to scarring and ulcerations of involved tissue. In men, the infection can extend to the epididymis. The ensuing epididymitis can produce sterility or Reiter's syndrome with symptoms of urethritis, arthritis, conjunctivitis, and hyperkeratotic skin lesions. In women, the infection can extend to the endometrium and salpinx; the major consequence is salpingitis with subsequent infertility or placement at high risk for ectopic pregnancy. Secondary extension to the peritoneum can cause PID very similar to that caused by gonorrhea.

Medical Management

All sexual contacts within 30 days before diagnosis should be examined and treated. In clinical settings in which testing for chlamydial infection is not available, treatment is often prescribed on the basis of clinical diagnosis or as cotreatment for gonorrhea.

PHARMACOLOGIC MANAGEMENT

Doxycycline 100 mg two times a day or azithromycin (Zithromax) 1 g in a single dose is the treatment of choice for chlamydial infection. In order to increase the absorption and efficacy of the antibiotic, clients should be instructed to take the medications 1 to 2 hours after meals and to avoid iron, dairy products, and antacids. Clients who are allergic to these preparations are treated with erythromycin orally for 7 days. If salpingitis and the other serious sequelae are to be prevented, it is imperative that treatment be started early and that the entire course of antibiotics be completed. Antichlamydial therapy is almost always effective. To confirm a cure, a repeat culture 4 to 7 days after treatment should be done whenever possible.

Nursing Management

Clients should be instructed about the sexual mode of transmission of chlamydial infection. The increased risk of infection with multiple sex partners should be stressed. Clients should also be informed of the serious danger of sterility. Infected clients should avoid all sexual activity (intercourse, fellatio, cunnilingus, or sodomy) until cured, and both men and women should wear condoms thereafter for prevention of reinfection.

SYPHILIS

Syphilis (street terms include bad blood, lues, pox, and syph), although currently less common than gonorrhea, can progress to blindness, mental illness, paralysis, heart disease, and death (Table 54–1).

Incidence

Syphilis has become dramatically less prevalent since the advent of antibiotics but has not been eradicated. In fact, the number of reported cases has increased in recent years. It is the third most commonly reported communicable disease in the United States. Adolescents, young adults, and homosexual males are at greatest risk.

Etiology

This systemic, infectious disease is caused by the motile spirochete *Treponema pallidum*. Syphilis can occur alone or with other STDs. The incubation period varies from 10 to 90 days, averaging 20 to 30 days.

Risk Factors and Transmission

CRITICAL TO REMEMBER

Although *T. pallidum* cannot survive long outside the body, syphilis is highly infectious. The organism enters the body through intact mucous membranes or abraded skin almost exclusively by direct sexual contact (acquired syphilis).

Sexual transmission requires exposure to the moist mucosal or cutaneous syphilitic lesions. After entry, the organisms multiply locally and disseminate through lymphatics and the bloodstream.

Clinical Manifestations

Syphilis is characterized by well-defined stages that occur over a period of years: primary, secondary, latent, and late. The manifestations vary with each stage.

PRIMARY STAGE

Primary syphilis has two principal symptoms: the appearance of a chancre and lymphadenopathy. Typically, a *chancre* is an oval ulcer with a raised border that does not bleed readily and is painless unless infected.

The chancre is at the site of inoculation, usually the genitalia, anus, or mouth. Usually, a single chancre occurs about 4 weeks after initial infection. Chancres in women are often not noticed. *Lymphadenopathy* occurs as local lymph glands near the chancre swell painlessly. If untreated, a chancre disappears after 4 to 6 weeks. The infected client then is often asymptomatic for a time.

SECONDARY STAGE

The secondary stage begins from 2 weeks to 6 months after the chancre disappears. Indications of the second stage include

- *Generalized skin rash.* Typically a maculopapular and nonpruritic rash appears on the palms (Fig. 54–1) and soles of the feet (few other diseases cause a rash in these locations).
- *Generalized lymphadenopathy*
- *Mucous patches.* Gray, superficial patches occur on the mucous membranes in the mouth and may be accompanied by a sore throat.
- *Condylomata lata.* These are broad-based, flat papules that can usually be easily distinguished from the typical narrow-based, pedunculated growth of condylomata acuminata (venereal warts, see later). They may develop in warm, moist body areas—most commonly on the labia or anus or at the corners of the mouth. Condylomata are highly contagious.
- *General flulike symptoms:* nausea; anorexia; constipation; headaches; muscle, joint, and bone pain; and a chronically elevated temperature.
- *Patchy hair loss* from eyebrows and scalp (alopecia). Secondary stage symptoms usually disappear after 2 to 6 weeks, and a latency period begins.

LATENT STAGE

The latent stage of syphilis typically has no symptoms. The disease is not transmitted by sexual contact during this phase; however, transmission through the bloodstream by blood donation can occur. Serologic testing for syphilis in all prospective blood donors is essential. Latent stage syphilis usually occurs about 2 or more years after the primary lesion and can last as long as 50 years. About two thirds of infected clients remain in

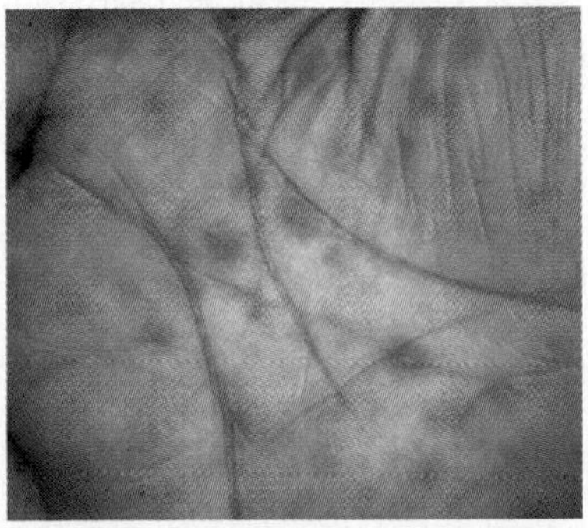

Figure 54–1
Rash seen in secondary syphilis. (From Lockingbill, D. P., & Marks, J. G. [1986]. *Principles of dermatology.* Philadelphia: W. B. Saunders.)

this stage without further problems. Some clients relapse into the primary or secondary stage during the first 2 years of latency.

LATE STAGE

If untreated, about one third of infected clients develop devastating, irreversible complications such as chronic bone and joint inflammation, cardiovascular problems (e.g., valvular involvement, aneurysms), granulomatous lesions (gummas) on any part of the body, and central nervous system problems (including mental illness, slurred speech, ataxic gait, paralysis, judgment loss, and senility). This stage is not infectious but may be terminal if untreated. (Chap. 14 discusses central nervous system manifestations.)

Diagnostic Assessment

The diagnosis of syphilis is based on health assessment and various laboratory studies. The laboratory tests are both direct and indirect. A direct test identifies the causative organism. Indirect tests merely identify antibodies of the causative agent. Primary or secondary stage lesions can be scraped and the causative organism identified with a darkfield microscope technique. Darkfield examination must be done by an expert because other spirochetes are present in the oral and genital areas. This test confirms a diagnosis of syphilis in the primary (when other tests are generally negative) and secondary stages.

Serologic tests for syphilis are indirect tests that detect antibodies that are not present in the serum until 4 weeks *after* the appearance of the chancre. Such tests include the Venereal Disease Research Laboratory (VDRL) and fluorescent treponemal antibody absorption (FTA-ABS) tests.

The VDRL test for nonspecific antibodies is the most commonly used screening test for syphilis. It is negative in the early primary stage before antibodies to *T. pallidum* are formed and are present in the circulation. It is falsely positive with certain viral infections and collagen diseases (e.g., mononucleosis, lupus). Results are given as nonreactive, borderline, weakly reactive, or reactive. Reactive and weakly reactive are considered positive results.

The FTA-ABS serologic test is more specific in that it measures antibodies specific to *T. pallidum*. It is used when the VDRL is positive but the diagnosis of syphilis is still uncertain. This test usually becomes positive 3 to 4 weeks after the infection. Once positive, treponemal antibody tests usually remain positive for life, regardless of treatment or cure. In late neurosyphilis, cerebrospinal fluid may be examined for characteristic findings.

Syphilis often coexists with other general infections. The CDC recommends that all clients with syphilis be counseled on the risks for human immunodeficiency virus (HIV) infection (AIDS) and be encouraged to be tested for AIDS.

Medical Management

PHARMACOLOGIC MANAGEMENT

Penicillin intramuscularly or intravenously is the drug of choice for the treatment of syphilis. All stages of syphilis respond to antibiotic therapy, but the structural changes present in late syphilis are irreversible despite successful treatment. For early syphilis, the treatment of choice is benzathine penicillin G intramuscularly in one dose. The dosage schedule and length of therapy are determined by the stage of the disease and current guidelines for treatment. For clients allergic to penicillin, oral doxycycline or tetracycline may be used, but they are not as effective as penicillin. Treatment failure can occur with any given regimen. Compliance is often a problem; follow-up with repeat VDRL tests or serial cerebrospinal fluid assessment (in late syphilis) is essential to confirm a cure.

Nursing Management

Clients with primary or secondary syphilis should abstain from sexual contact for at least 1 month after treatment. All sexual contacts must be identified and treated. Most practitioners treat contacts as if they have primary syphilis, whether or not infection is evident. When an infected but untreated woman has been in the latency stage for at least a year, she is not considered infectious unless she becomes pregnant, because she can then infect her unborn child. Adequate treatment is curative, but reinfection is possible and can be detected by monitoring serologic titers and by clinical reexaminations.

CRITICAL TO REMEMBER

An infection does not confer lasting immunity to syphilis.

A client with syphilis needs health-care information and psychosocial support. Nurses must provide clients with accurate, individualized information about transmission, reinfection, early detection, treatment, follow-up, proper hygiene, and safe sexual habits.

GENITAL HERPES

Genital herpes is a recurrent, systemic infection (see Table 54–1).

Incidence

Genital herpes is one of the most common STDs and it is the most common cause of genital ulceration. Its peak incidence occurs in the adolescent and young adult.

Etiology

Caused by herpes simplex virus (HSV) type II, the infection is closely related to other herpes infections such as the classic "cold sore" caused by HSV type I. Type I herpes is mainly nongenital, occurring above the waist (often on the lips or nose). Type II herpes occurs primarily below the waist as a sexually transmitted genital infection. It is, however, possible for HSV type I to cause genital infections and for HSV type II to cause oral lesions.

Risk Factors

The HSV organism is present in the exudate of the lesion. The disease can be transmitted while a lesion is present and for 10 days after a lesion has healed. Genital herpes is usually transmitted by direct contact with the exudate during sexual activity, but transmission is possible by fomites such as towels used by an infected client.

Clinical Manifestations

Symptoms of genital herpes usually occur 3 to 7 days after contact. Initially, there is a burning sensation or paresthesia at the site of inoculation. Next, numerous small vesicles with an erythematous border form painful, shallow ulcers that then crust and heal with a scar in about 2 to 4 weeks.

CRITICAL TO REMEMBER

The major problem in HSV infections is recurrence.

About one half to three quarters of infected clients have recurrence within 1 year of the first episode. The herpes virus is believed to lie dormant in the body, probably in the trigeminal ganglion (HSV-I) and sacral ganglion (HSV-II), until it is activated and another episode of genital herpes with the characteristic lesion occurs. Certain situations such as stress, infection, trauma, menses, or sexual intercourse seem to trigger recurrent episodes.

Characteristically, recurrent genital herpes causes local, but not systemic, symptoms. Prodromal sensations of burning or paresthesias may be experienced before the vesicles erupt. The vesicles tend to reappear at the same locations, but previous sites of infection are not always involved. Symptoms are similar to those associated with primary infection although usually less severe. Vesicles rupture in 24 to 48 hours, and the syndrome generally lasts 7 to 10 days.

Potential complications of HSV infections include aseptic meningitis and transverse myelitis. Women are at risk for spontaneous abortions, and there is some evidence that HSV-II predisposes to carcinoma of the cervix.

Diagnostic Assessment

A diagnosis of genital herpes is made by health assessment findings, including history of the symptoms and the presence of vesicles. The diagnosis is confirmed by a viral culture of the exudate from the ulcer. The Pap smear can be done in women. The presence in the Pap smear of multinucleated giant cells with or without inclusion bodies is characteristic of a herpes infection.

Medical Management

PHARMACOLOGIC MANAGEMENT

Genital herpes is a chronic disease. There is no cure. The recommended treatment for primary or recurrent infection or for prophylaxis of active lesions is acyclovir (Zovirax) orally for 5 to 10 days. Palliative measures include keeping the involved area clean and dry, sitzbaths, cool applications, and analgesic medications.

Nursing Management

When the vesicles of active genital herpes rupture, they release a highly contagious exudate. Therefore, clients as well as health-care personnel must observe strict medical asepsis. For avoiding autoinoculation from the genital area to other body sites, clients should be advised to wash their hands thoroughly after any contact with the herpetic lesions. HSV infections of the eye are particularly serious. Infected clients should have separate towels and other personal items. Sexual contact should be avoided during initial and recurrent infections. The use of condoms during latent periods is encouraged because of the possible risk of transmission even when symptoms are not present. Women should be told to have annual pelvic examinations and Pap smears.

Many clients find that coping with genital herpes is emotionally difficult. Tremendous psychosocial stress may develop because the infection cannot be cured and recurrence cannot be predicted. The pain caused by these lesions is especially problematic. Psychosocial support includes providing clients with accurate information about the infection.

GENITAL WARTS (CONDYLOMATA ACUMINATA)

Etiology

Genital warts, the fourth most common STD, are venereal warts caused by the human papillomavirus (HPV);

they are usually transmitted by sexual contact (see Table 54–1).

Typically the warts occur in multiple, painless clusters on the vulva, vagina, cervix, perineum, anorectal area, urethral meatus, or glans penis 1 to 2 months after exposure. Oral, pharyngeal, and laryngeal lesions can also occur. HPV can cause laryngeal papillomatosis in infants born to mothers with vaginal warts.

Diagnostic Assessment

Diagnosis is typically made by observation of the warts. Subclinical warts can be identified by Pap smear and colposcopy of the cervix and vagina. Biopsy of lesions may be done to differentiate venereal warts from condylomata lata lesions of the secondary stage of syphilis or from carcinoma.

Medical Management

PHARMACOLOGIC MANAGEMENT

Topical application of podophyllin in compound with tincture of benzoin or surgical removal is the treatment of genital warts. Recurrence is common. Sexual partners must also be treated. Clients must be seen every 1 to 2 weeks until all warts have disappeared. There is no cure, so treatment only ameliorates the symptoms.

Surgical Management

Warts can also be treated with cryotherapy with liquid nitrogen or a cryoprobe. For extensive warts, carbon dioxide lasers, electrocautery, and surgical excision can be used. Again, it must be remembered that the warts are not cured and recurrence is common.

Nursing Management

The nurse must warn clients with genital warts that they are at increased risk for genital malignancy, such as cancer of the vulva and penis and especially carcinoma of the cervix. All women with anogenital warts should have an annual Pap smear and, when indicated, cervical colposcopy and biopsy. The detection and treatment of subclinical HPV infection in men may be important for the prevention of genital carcinoma in women.

ACQUIRED IMMUNODEFICIENCY SYNDROME

Acquired immunodeficiency syndrome is a viral STD that has reached worldwide epidemic proportions. AIDS is described in detail in Chapter 9.

TRICHOMONIASIS

Trichomoniasis is a protozoal infection causing vulvovaginitis.

Incidence

A common cause of vulvovaginitis is infection with the anaerobic, flagellated, parasitic protozoon *Trichomonas vaginalis.* Although not life-threatening, trichomoniasis has a very high incidence worldwide and remains a major health problem.

Etiology

The organism prefers an alkaline environment (pH 6 to 7), and changes in the vaginal flora make a woman more susceptible to it. Trichomoniasis may be difficult to cure, and recurrence is common. The organism is almost always transmitted sexually from one partner to another, which makes simultaneous treatment of both partners necessary for cure.

Clinical Manifestations

Symptoms may be minor and are usually so in an infected male. In a female, they include a copious, malodorous, yellow-green vaginal discharge. This is irritating to the vulva, causing severe itching and burning and excoriation and maceration of the vulvar tissues. Occasionally, the cervix is covered with punctate hemorrhages ("strawberry cervix"). The vaginal mucosa appears reddened and slightly edematous. Some women experience dyspareunia (pain during vaginal sexual activity). The organism does not affect the uterus and fallopian tubes.

If trichomoniasis extends to the urethra, frequency and burning with urination may occur. This is the most common symptom in a male. Anal involvement may also occur, either asymptomatically or with a slight discharge. Bladder and anal involvement is more common when the infection has become chronic.

Diagnostic Assessment

A diagnosis of trichomoniasis is established by obtaining a fresh, warm, wet mount and identifying the motile trichomonad under the microscope. A wet mount is obtained by placing a drop of the exudate on a glass slide, mixing in a drop of saline, and covering it with a cover slide. Cultures can be obtained to establish the diagnosis, but they are rarely necessary. For the female, the vaginal speculum used to obtain vaginal secretions must be inserted without lubrication to avoid destroying the organism. If possible, the client should be told not to douche before the vaginal examination. Reassurance and a calm attitude can help allay the client's anxiety and minimize any discomfort with the examination.

Medical Management

PHARMACOLOGIC MANAGEMENT

The preferred treatment for trichomoniasis is a single 2-g dose of metronidazole (Flagyl) orally for the client and all sexual contacts. Flagyl should not be taken during pregnancy because it may, especially during the first trimester, adversely affect fetal development. *T. vaginalis* does not affect the fetus. Clients taking metronidazole should be advised not to drink alcoholic beverages (including mouthwash and some cold preparations), so that side effects of nausea, vomiting, and headaches are prevented. Vaginal clotrimazole (Gyne-Lotrimin) cream, although not nearly as effective as metronidazole, is an alternative treatment that can be used during pregnancy. This treatment is now available over-the-counter, which has led to some misuse by women who do not understand the seriousness of the disorder.

Single-dose metronidazole therapy is usually curative, but recurrence is common. Clients should be instructed to seek prompt treatment if symptoms return. Metronidazole may be given in a 7-day regimen for recurrent infection.

Nursing Management

A woman with trichomoniasis should refrain from sexual intercourse or use the female condom, and an infected male should use condoms while the infection remains active. The nurse should emphasize to the client the importance of good perineal hygiene. Treatment should be continued through the woman's menstrual period, because the vagina is more alkaline during this time of the cycle and a flare-up may occur. After therapy has been completed, clients are evaluated and treated again if necessary.

BACTERIAL VAGINOSIS

Bacterial vaginosis is the term now used for what was previously called nonspecific vaginitis. This new term was adopted since *Gardnerella vaginalis* (also known as *Haemophilus vaginalis* or *Corynebacterium vaginalis*) was isolated and usually found to be the causative organism.

Etiology

Bacterial vaginosis can be confirmed by culture in both symptomatic and asymptomatic women. The new name implies there may be multiple etiologic organisms, possibly coexisting anaerobic bacteria; it also indicates that vaginal white blood cells are not the predominant feature in this type of vaginitis.

Clinical Manifestations

The vulvovaginitis produced by *G. vaginalis* is mild or asymptomatic. The most common symptom is a mild to moderate amount of malodorous ("fishy"), gray, homogeneous, thin vaginal discharge accompanied by some vaginal irritation and vulvar pruritus. Symptoms are almost always confined to the vulvovaginal area.

Diagnostic Assessment

Diagnosis is made by a culture positive for *G. vaginalis* or visualization of coccobacilli or clue cells on a saline wet mount preparation of vaginal secretions. Clue cells are desquamated vaginal epithelial cells characteristically stippled by the adherence of coccobacilli to their surfaces. If potassium hydroxide (KOH) is mixed with the vaginal discharge, a fishy odor is elicited (positive "sniff test").

Medical Management

PHARMACOLOGIC MANAGEMENT

The recommended treatment for bacterial vaginosis in nonpregnant women is metronidazole (Flagyl) orally for 7 days. Single-dose regimens can be used to improve compliance, but they are less effective than the 7-day course.

Nursing Management

Clients on Flagyl should be cautioned to abstain from alcohol during and for 3 days after the medication to prevent intense nausea, vomiting, and headache. Treatment of male partners is recommended only with recurrent or resistant infection. Even so, treatment of the male has not been shown to be highly beneficial for either partner. Clients are advised to avoid sexual intercourse during the treatment, and condom use is recommended to prevent recurrence.

CHANCROID

Chancroid is a highly contagious infection caused by the gram-negative *Haemophilus ducreyi* bacillus. The initial papules and pustules produce multiple, painful, irregular, and deep genital ulcers, often accompanied by regional lymphadenopathy. Although chancroid is more common in the tropics, the incidence is increasing in the United States. Outside the United States, chancroid has been associated with increased infection rates for HIV.

Diagnosis is confirmed by a culture positive for *H. ducreyi*. Recommended treatment is oral erythromycin for 7 days or ceftriaxone (Rocephin) intramuscularly in a single dose.

PEDICULOSIS PUBIS AND SCABIES

Cutaneous infestation with pubic lice (pediculosis pubis) or mites (scabies) results either from contact with contaminated objects such as linens or from close physical contact. Because they can be transmitted sexually, these conditions are sometimes included with STDs. (For further discussion, see Chap. 48.)

SEXUALLY TRANSMITTED ENTERIC INFECTIONS

Dysenteries and hepatitis caused by enteric pathogens are typically acquired from food or water contaminated with fecal matter. Since the mid-1970s, it has been recognized that these pathogens can also be transmitted by oral and anal sexual contact. Sexually transmitted enteric infections occur predominantly in homosexual males. The infections include shigellosis, salmonellosis, amebiasis, giardiasis, and hepatitis A. See Chapter 35 for discussion of dysentery and Chapter 37 for discussion of hepatitis A.

HEPATITIS B AND DELTA HEPATITIS

Sexual contact is the most frequently reported mode of transmission of the hepatitis B virus. The extent of sexual transmission for delta hepatitis is uncertain. Clients at high risk for sexually transmitted hepatitis B are homosexual males, sex partners of intravenous drug abusers, and male and female heterosexuals with multiple partners. See Chapter 37 for further discussion of hepatitis B and delta hepatitis.

STUDY QUESTIONS

1. A 25-year-old woman presents with vague complaints of painful urination and midcycle spotting. Although her cervix is slightly edematous, she denies other symptoms. She is anxious and irritable. The nurse should
   A. Reassure the client that she will be fine since she has no apparent genital lesions.
   B. Avoid discussion of sexual partners since she is obviously upset.
   C. Provide support and prepare to test for gonorrhea.
   D. Tell her to list all her sexual contacts for the previous 30 days.
2. Learning can be documented when the client makes which of the following statements?
   A. "There is no cure for syphilis so there is no point in going to the doctor for this sore."
   B. "I will teach my family to avoid using towels or tissues that someone else has just used."
   C. "Genital herpes is nasty but at least it can be cured."
   D. "I can use a lima bean to treat the warts on my 'privates' as my grandmother used to do."
3. A female client is being treated for gonorrhea. Which of the following would be a priority in planning care for your client?
   A. Demonstrating use of condom or diaphragm
   B. Teaching the importance of finishing all prescribed antibiotics
   C. Explaining the necessity of abstinence
   D. Emphasizing the economic costs of STDs worldwide
4. Which response by the nurse would be most likely to encourage responsible behavior in a client at high risk for STDs when that client asks, "Will treatment protect me from getting this again?"
   A. "No. There is no immunity for (this STD). You may be reinfected again."
   B. "No. You will have to change your life-style if you want to stay clean."
   C. "Yes. As long as you keep taking your medicine, you will not get it again."
   D. "Yes, unless you continue to have sex with multiple partners."
5. When evaluating the outcome of client goals for a client who has been treated for genital herpes, the nurse would consider that a goal had been met if:
   A. The woman makes an appointment for an annual Pap smear and pelvic examination.
   B. The client is cured for genital herpes.
   C. The client realizes she can do nothing for the discomfort of the active lesions.
   D. She tells you that sexual contact is the only means of transmission of genital herpes.

CRITICAL THINKING EXERCISES

SCENARIO A

A young woman presents for evaluation for possible STDs. She works as a prostitute in a large city. She is 36 years old, 5′7″ tall, and weighs 135 pounds. She is neat, clean, and well-groomed.

1. What assessment data should you collect?
2. What nursing responsibilities do you anticipate?
3. Discuss teaching needs for this client.

SCENARIO B

A 40-year-old man presents with complaints of dysuria, urinary frequency, and a purulent discharge from the penis. He is found to be positive for gonorrhea and chlamydial infection and trichomoniasis. He is being treated with ceftriaxone sodium (Rocephin) 2 g, followed by doxycycline hyclate 100 mg, orally every 12 hours for 7 days.

1. Why are both drugs being used?
2. What teaching responsibilities are associated with the administration of these drugs?
3. How can the nurse help the client prevent reinfection?

BIBLIOGRAPHY

1. *ACOG guide to preconception care.* (1990). Washington, DC: The American College of Obstetricians and Gynecologists.
2. Andrist, L. C. (1988). Taking a sexual history and educating clients about safe sex. *Nursing Clinics of North America, 23,* 959.
3. Barton, S., & Hunter, J. (1994). New therapies for the treatment of genital warts. *Nursing Times, 90(20),* 38–40.
4. Cates, W., Jr., et al. (1990). Sexually transmitted diseases—overview of the situation. *Primary Care, 17,* 1.
5. Centers for Disease Control and Prevention (1993). Sexually transmitted diseases treatment guidelines. *Morbidity and Mortality Weekly Report, 42*(RR-14), 1–102.
6. Centers for Disease Control and Prevention. (1993). Special focus: Surveillance for sexually transmitted diseases. *Morbidity and Mortality Weekly Report, 42,* 1–39.
7. Cook, L. S., et al. (1994). Circumcision and sexually transmitted diseases. *American Journal of Public Health, 84(2),* 197–201.
8. Custodio, D. E., et al. (1991). Sexually transmitted diseases. *Topics in Emergency Medicine, 13,* 66.
9. Danis, D. M., & Halm, K. (1994). Sexually transmitted disease treatment guidelines revised. *Journal of Emergency Nursing, 20(3),* 238–239.
10. Featherston, W. E. (1990). Sexual identity and practices relating to the spread of sexually transmitted diseases. *Primary Care, 17,* 29.
11. George, J. E., & Quattrone, M. S. (1994). Erroneous reporting of sexually transmitted diseases. *Journal of Emergency Nursing, 20(2),* 148–149.
12. Holmes, K. K., et al. (Eds.), (1990). *Sexually transmitted diseases.* New York: McGraw-Hill.
13. Katner, H. P., et al. (1987). Sexually transmitted diseases in heterosexuals. In F. H. Messerli (Ed.), *Current clinical practice.* Philadelphia: W. B. Saunders.
14. Katz, A. R. (1989). Chlamydia trachomatis: A frequently overlooked public health menace. *Hawaii Medical Journal, 48,* 156.
15. Melvin, S. Y. (1990). Syphilis—resurgence of an old disease. *Primary Care, 17,* 47.
16. Millstein, S. G., et al. (1994). Female adolescents at high, moderate, and low risk of exposure to HIV: Differences in knowledge, beliefs, and behavior. *Journal of Adolescent Health, 15(2),* 133–141.
17. Nettina, S. L., et al. (1990). Diagnosis and management of sexually transmitted genital lesions. *Nurse Practitioner, 15,* 34.
18. Pankey, G. A., et al. (1987). Sexually transmitted infections. In F. H. Messerli (Ed.), *Current clinical practice.* Philadelphia: W. B. Saunders.
19. Progress toward achieving the 1990 objectives for the nation for sexually transmitted diseases. (1990). *Morbidity and Mortality Weekly Report, 39,* 53.
20. Smith, R. E., et al. (1987). Chlamydia. In F. H. Messerli (Ed.), *Current clinical practice.* Philadelphia: W. B. Saunders.
21. Spence, J. R. (1989). Epidemiology of sexually transmitted diseases. *Obstetrics and Gynecology Clinics of North America, 16,* 453.
22. Talashek, M. L., et al. (1990). Sexually transmitted diseases in the elderly—issues and recommendations. *Journal of Gerontological Nursing, 16,* 33.
23. Thomason, J. L., et al. (1989). *Trichomonas vaginalis. Obstetrics and Gynecology, 74,* 536.
24. Vulvovaginitis. *ACOG Technical Bulletin No. 135,* 1989.
25. Wardell, D. W. (1988). Chronic exposure to sexually transmitted diseases. *Nursing Clinics of North America, 23,* 947.
26. Weiss, S. H., et al. (1993). Safe sex? Misconceptions, gender differences and barriers among injection drug users. *AIDS Education and Prevention, 5(4),* 279–293.

Chapter 55 Nursing Care of Clients with Breast Disorders

Learning Outcomes

After completing this chapter, the learner will be able to:

1. Assess the client for clinical manifestations of breast disorders.
2. Teach the client about the etiology, risk factors, basic pathophysiology, and clinical manifestations of breast disorders.
3. Explain the client's role in medical and surgical management of breast disorders.
4. Develop plans of care for the prevention of breast disorders and the management and rehabilitation of clients with breast disorders.
5. Implement nursing interventions that optimize the quality of life for clients with breast disorders.
6. Evaluate planned client outcomes using outcome criteria developed in the planning phase of care.

One of nine women will develop breast cancer in her lifetime.[3] Because breast cancer is such a feared disease, nurses have an important role teaching women about normal breasts; common benign breast problems; breast self-examination and mammography; and risk factors for, incidence of, and treatments for breast cancer.

Many misconceptions exist about breast cancer. In a 1981 National Cancer Institute study, half of those surveyed were incorrect in thinking that a breast injury could cause cancer. Many did not know that nipple changes can be a sign of breast cancer. Also, many did not know about diagnostic procedures for breast cancer or treatment options other than surgery.[35] However, in spite of such misconceptions, there is also a growing public awareness about breast cancer.

Nurses have an educational role concerning breast lesions. By allowing clients to talk about breast cancer, correcting misinformation, and supplying accurate facts when possible, nurses can reduce associated fear, anxiety, and misinformation. Women may then seek earlier assessment, diagnosis, and effective treatment. Factual answers to questions are not always available. However, by maintaining a comfortable therapeutic relationship, nurses can support clients and their significant others.

TABLE 55–1 Causes of Breast Masses for Three Age Groups

Younger than 35 years
Fibrocystic condition
Fibroadenoma
Mastitis
Traumatic fat necrosis
Carcinoma of breast
Between 35 and 50 years
Fibrocystic condition
Carcinoma
Fibroadenoma
Traumatic fat necrosis
Mastitis
Papilloma
Older than 50 years
Carcinoma
Fibrocystic condition
Fat necrosis
Paget's disease of breast
Acute mastitis
Papilloma

Data from Robbins, S. L., et al. (1984). *Pathologic basis of disease* (3rd ed., p. 1190). Philadelphia: W. B. Saunders.

BREAST CANCER

Definition and Incidence

Breast cancer refers to a group of malignant diseases that commonly occur in the female breast and infrequently in the male breast. In 1995, it was estimated that 182,000 new breast cancers would occur in the United States and that about 46,240 deaths would occur from breast cancer.[3] One in every nine women is expected to develop breast cancer. Because of improvements in early detection and treatment, the 5-year survival rate for breast cancer has improved. This has helped stabilize (although not actually decrease) the mortality rates from breast cancer over the past 50 years despite an increasing incidence of breast cancer. Breast cancer, however, is the leading cause of cancer deaths in women between the ages of 14 and 54 years.[3] Lung cancer is now the leading cause of cancer deaths in all women; breast cancer is second.

Breast cancer in men is rare. Approximately 1400 new male breast cancer diagnoses and 240 deaths from male breast cancer are estimated to occur in 1995.[3] Breast cancer is often diagnosed in a more advanced stage in men than in women.

Etiology

The cause of breast cancer has not been definitely established; genetic predisposition and hormonal factors may be involved (Table 55–1).

Risk Factors

Many factors have been associated with a significantly increased risk of breast cancer (Table 55–2). However, many women diagnosed with breast cancer have no risk factors. Most women can identify with at least one risk factor. The factors associated with the highest risk include

- Advancing age
- Mother or sister with breast cancer

TABLE 55–2 Factors Involved in a Significantly Higher Risk of Breast Cancer

Gender	99 : 1 women > men
Age	Growing older
Socioeconomic status	High
Age at first full-term pregnancy	Older than 30 years
Health history	Mammographic pattern of dysplastic parenchyma Past diagnosis of atypism, hyperplasia, or other benign proliferative disease in breast biopsy Large dose of radiation therapy to the chest Previous diagnosis of cancer in one breast
Family history	Mother or sister with history of breast cancer Any first-degree relative with breast cancer

Adapted from Kelsey, J. L., & Gammon, M. D. (1991). The epidemiology of breast cancer. *CA: A Cancer Journal for Clinicians, 41(3)*, 157.

Other important risk factors are

- Previous breast cancer
- Previous radiation to the chest
- Previous diagnosis of proliferative disease
- Mammographic pattern of dysplastic parenchyma
- Age greater than 30 years at the time of first full-term pregnancy
- High socioeconomic status
- Early menarche and late menopause[48, 96]

Risk factors related to ovarian function suggest a hormonal influence. Artificial menopause before the age of 35 years reduces the risk of breast cancer to one third of that experienced by those with natural menopause.[44] Hormonal and other factors associated with a moderate risk include

- Early menarche
- Late menopause
- Nulliparity
- Exogenous estrogen given for menopause symptoms (contraceptives do not seem to produce higher risk)
- History of cancer of the uterus, ovary, or colon

Risk factors under study as possible causes of increased incidence of breast cancer include

- Oral contraceptives
- Exogenous hormones
- Above-average weight and height, especially in postmenopausal women
- Diet high in total fat
- Alcohol consumption
- Ovarian-pituitary dysfunction
- Genetic factors
- Benign breast disease
- Radiation exposure[52, 57, 89]

Factors that may lower a woman's risk of breast cancer include

- Late menarche
- Early menopause
- Oophorectomy premenopausally
- Maintaining a normal or lighter than average weight after menopause

For the best prognosis, it is extremely important for breast cancer to be detected early before metastases occur. Breast self-examination, mammography, and a thorough breast examination by a clinician are important in early detection.

One of the nurse's roles, therefore, is to encourage all women to practice breast self-examination and follow the screening advice of the American Cancer Society (Box 55–1). Nurses also have a role in identifying clients at risk for breast cancer and convincing them of the necessity for appropriate, careful assessment. Unfortunately, currently, little can be done in the way of primary prevention to reduce most risk factors for breast cancer. Exceptions are maintaining normal or lighter than average body weight and reducing dietary fat (e.g., meat, dairy products). Growing evidence suggests that dietary fat promotes carcinogenesis because of its effect on hormone activity (see Client Education Guide: Preventive Breast Care).

BOX 55–1

Important Factors for Successful Breast Self-Examination

The nurse should instruct the client to perform the following:

- Examine the breasts at the same time each month.
- Examine the breasts in a consistent pattern.
- Examine all surface areas: the breast, tail of Spence, and axilla.
- Examine all depth of the tissue: use pads of fingers and press deeply.
- Check for discharge, inspect the breasts visually, and feel for changes.
- Report any changes to the physician.

Pathophysiology

Various histopathologic types of breast cancer exist with various prognoses.[44] These include intraductal carcinoma, infiltrating ductal carcinoma, medullary carcinoma, mucinous or colloid carcinoma, tubular carcinoma, lobular carcinoma in situ, infiltrating lobular carcinoma, inflammatory breast cancer, and Paget's disease (Table 55–3).

Cancer Staging

Numerous staging systems (see Chap. 21) have been developed for cancer. The staging of a cancer is based on (1) size of the primary lesion, (2) extent of the cancer's spread to regional lymph nodes, and (3) presence or absence of metastases. Staging provides prognostic information; Figure 55–1 illustrates breast cancer staging. The commonly used TNM staging system (Table 55–4) groups breast cancers according to the characteristics of the primary tumor (T), regional lymph nodes (N), and distant metastases (M).[6] With breast cancer, subgroup assignments are made according to tumor size, tumor attachment to underlying structure, and other characteristics such as edema.

Several other parameters are useful in determining the prognosis of and treatment for clients with breast cancer.[20, 44, 74, 97] These include multicentricity, estrogen-progesterone receptor status of the tumor, and the immunocompetence of the client. If cancer is found in two or more locations (multicentric) in the breast, the client will probably not be a candidate for lumpectomy or quandrantectomy. If the tumor is estrogen-progesterone receptor positive, she will probably receive antiestrogen hormonal therapy.

Cancer is graded on the cytologic differentiation of tumor cells and the number of mitoses within the tumor. Grading tries to identify some degree of a tumor's malignancy or to estimate its aggressiveness.

CLIENT EDUCATION GUIDE

Preventive Breast Care

- Consideration of how women can prevent and detect early symptoms of any breast disease should be the primary focus of home health-care nursing. First, women need education about their level of risk. Women at high risk include those older than 55 years, never married, older than 30 years at first pregnancy, and with a family history of breast cancer.
- Women can make changes in their life-style to lower their risk for breast disease. Monthly breast self-examinations are essential. Most lumps are found by women themselves. The earlier breast cancer is detected, the greater is the chance of cure. Besides breast self-examination, an examination by a physician should be done every 3 years for women 20 to 40 years of age and every year for women older than 40 years.
- Diet is another area in which women can make sufficient changes for preventing disease. A low-fat diet can play an important part in prevention. Decreasing fat intake to 20 per cent of dietary calories is an admirable goal. Alcohol intake increases risk in relation to the amount of alcohol consumed.
- Certain foods are helpful in decreasing risk. Cruciferous foods (broccoli, cabbage, cauliflower) help convert estrogen to a form less likely to cause cancer. Vitamin A (beta-carotene foods, orange and dark green vegetables) inhibits abnormal cell growth. Soybeans suppress estrogen production.
- Women should be informed about and encouraged to have mammograms. Mammograms can detect very small tumors long before they might otherwise be found by manual breast examination. The recommendations for mammograms are as follows: obtain a baseline at age 35 to 39 years unless high-risk factors exist; repeat every 1 to 2 years for ages 40 to 50 years and yearly for women older than 50.
- The American Cancer Society is an excellent source for further information about the prevention, detection, and treatment of breast cancer. Call 1-800-ACS-2345.

The grading of breast cancer is similar to that of other cancers. Newer studies are closely examining the grade of a breast cancer as a prognostic factor.

Clinical Manifestations

The nurse should be alert for assessment findings indicating breast cancer, although detection may be difficult. Initially, breast cancer typically appears as a unilateral, single mass or thickening most often in a breast's upper outer quadrant (Fig. 55–2). The mass is usually painless, nontender, hard, irregular in shape, and nonmobile. Presentation of 64 to 70 per cent of breast cancers is as a palpable mass found by the client.[26] Four to 30 per cent are found by mammography.

DIAGNOSTIC ASSESSMENT

Pretreatment assessment varies. Chest x-ray examination, complete blood count, liver chemistries, and mammography of the opposite breast are frequently done. Other studies are in question, however. Bone scans or liver scans can give false-positive results and yield little useful information in asymptomatic clients. Some physicians believe scans should be used only for clients with stage III disease or abnormal liver chemistries. Others believe a baseline study, especially a bone scan, is valuable for later comparison.

Tumor markers (substances produced either by the tumor itself or by the body in response to tumor tissue) may be present in the serum of a client with breast cancer. The tumor markers—carcinoembryonic antigen, ferritin, and human chorionic gonadotropin—are easy

TABLE 55–3 Histopathologic Types of Breast Cancer

TYPE	PROGNOSIS	COMMENTS
Intraductal carcinoma	Excellent	A precancerous marker; also known as ductal cancer in situ
Infiltrating ductal carcinoma	Poor	Found in 70% of breast cancers; palpated as a stony-hard lump
Medullary carcinoma	Good	Found in 5–7% of breast cancers; frequently reaches large size
Mucinous (colloid) carcinoma	Good	Found in 3% of breast cancers; slow-growing; can become quite large
Tubular carcinoma	Excellent	Frequently occurs with other types
Lobular carcinoma in situ	Excellent	A precancerous marker lesion
Infiltrating lobular carcinoma	Fair	Found in 5–10% of breast cancers; usually present as area of thickening vs. a lump; may be involvement of the opposite breast; axillary lymph node metastasis common
Inflammatory breast cancer	Poor	Edema, redness, warmth, and induration; distant metastasis common

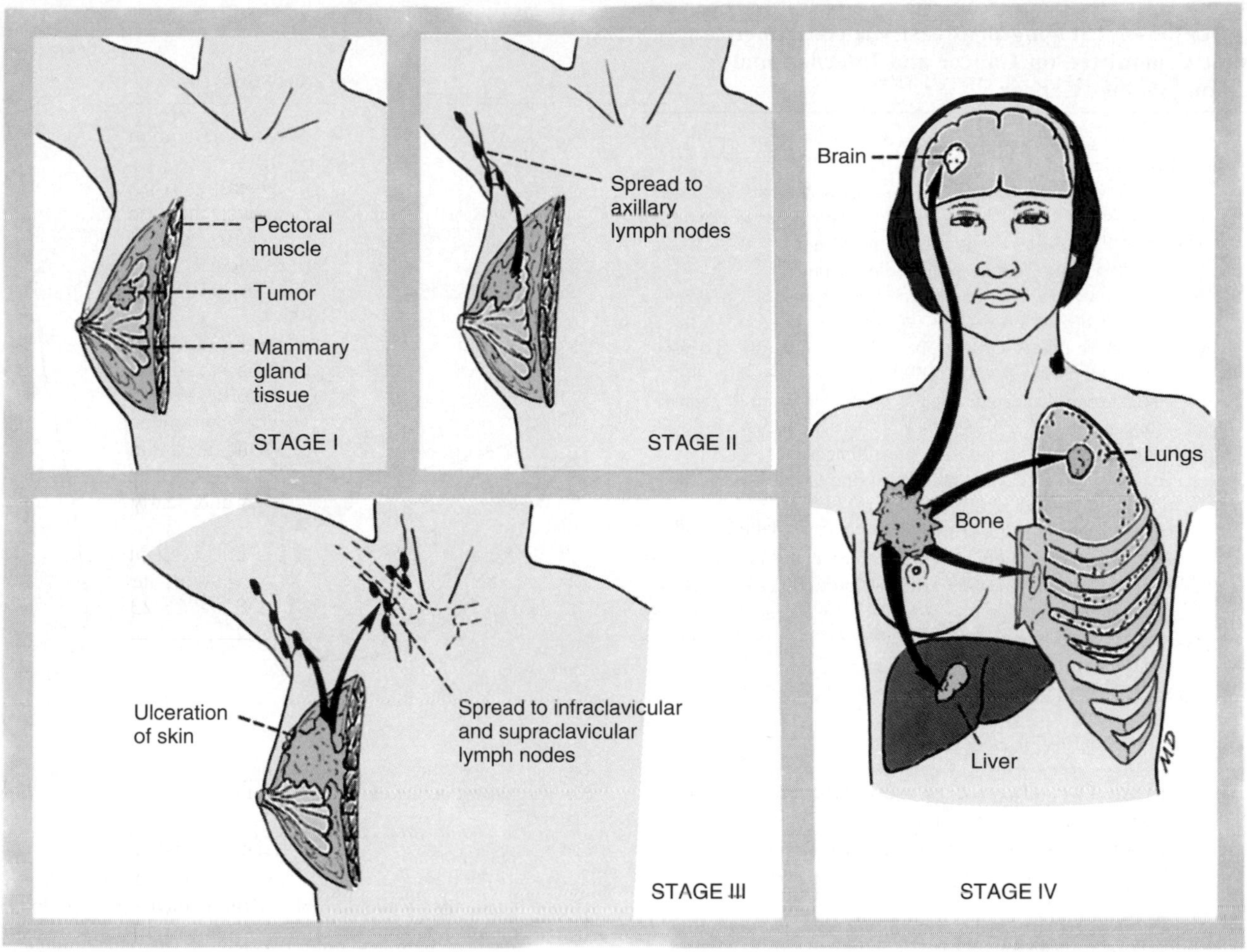

Figure 55–1
Clinical staging of breast cancer. Stage I: tumor less than 2 cm and confined to breast. Stage II: tumor up to 5 cm, or axillary lymph nodes contain early metastasis. Stage III: tumor larger than 5 cm, or extends to chest wall or skin, or involvement of infraclavicular or supraclavicular lymph nodes. Stage IV: distant metastasis such as to brain, bone, or liver.

to obtain, so trying to identify these and to follow them after diagnosis is recommended.

Medical Management

Public knowledge is increasing about treatment options for breast cancer. Nurses must be knowledgeable about recent advances in treatment as well as treatment controversies to support women and their significant others as they make decisions.[47, 80] It is important for the nurse to know that a client diagnosed with early-stage breast cancer may live a long, healthy life and keep her breast.

Because of greater understanding of tumor biology, it is now recognized that breast cancer requires multimodality therapy.[16, 31, 39] Historically, the belief was that cancer spread locally to the lymph nodes in an orderly, defined manner. If this were true, the radical mastectomy should eliminate the disease. It is now known that breast cancer does not spread in an orderly manner and that cancer cells use the blood stream to metastasize to other organs such as bone, lung, brain, and liver. Because of this, less radical surgical procedures are used in combination with radiation therapy, hormonal therapy, or chemotherapy.[49, 75] In 1988, 62 per cent of breast cancer clients had mastectomies, 9 per cent had no surgical procedure, and 25 per cent had only partial mastectomies.[77] Now various treatment combinations are used to cure breast cancer through local, regional, or systemic treatments. Women who have early small breast cancers may be best served by first having a mastectomy or lumpectomy to be followed by radiation therapy, chemotherapy, or hormonal therapy as indicated. Women with locally advanced stage II breast cancer may be better served by having hormonally synchronized chemotherapy shrink the breast cancer before surgery and radiation therapy. Local and regional treatment involves treating the breast and chest wall. Mastectomy or adjuvant radiation therapy in combination with a lumpectomy or a quadrantectomy is used for local control of stage I or stage II breast cancer. Adju-

TABLE 55–4 Staging of Breast Cancer, American Joint Committee on Cancer and International Union Against Cancer

TX	Primary tumor cannot be assessed
T0	No evidence of primary tumor
Tis	Carcinoma in situ: intraductal carcinoma, lobular carcinoma in situ, or Paget's disease* of the nipple with no tumor
T1	Tumor 2 cm or less in greatest dimension
	T1a 0.5 cm or less in greatest dimension
	T1b More than 0.5 cm but not more than 1 cm in greatest dimension
	T1c More than 1 cm but not more than 2 cm in greatest dimension
T2	Tumor more than 2 cm but not more than 5 cm in greatest dimension
T3	Tumor more than 5 cm in greatest dimension
T4	Tumor of any size with direct extension to chest wall† or skin
	T4a Extension to chest wall
	T4b Edema (including peau d'orange) or ulceration of the skin of the breast or satellite skin nodules confined to the same breast
	T4c Both (T4a and T4b)
	T4d Inflammatory carcinoma
NX	Regional lymph nodes cannot be assessed (e.g., previously removed)
N0	No regional lymph node metastasis
N1	Metastasis to movable ipsilateral axillary lymph node(s)
N2	Metastasis to ipsilateral axillary lymph node(s) fixed to one another or to other structures
N3	Metastasis to ipsilateral internal mammary lymph node(s)
MX	Presence of distant metastasis cannot be assessed
M0	No distant metastasis
M1	Distant metastasis (includes metastasis to ipsilateral supraclavicular lymph node[s])

* Paget's disease associated with a tumor is classified according to the size of the tumor.
† Chest wall includes ribs, intercostal muscles, and serratus anterior muscle but not pectoral muscle.
From Beahrs, O. H. (1991). Staging of cancer. *CA: A Cancer Journal for Clinicians, 41(2)*, 122–124.

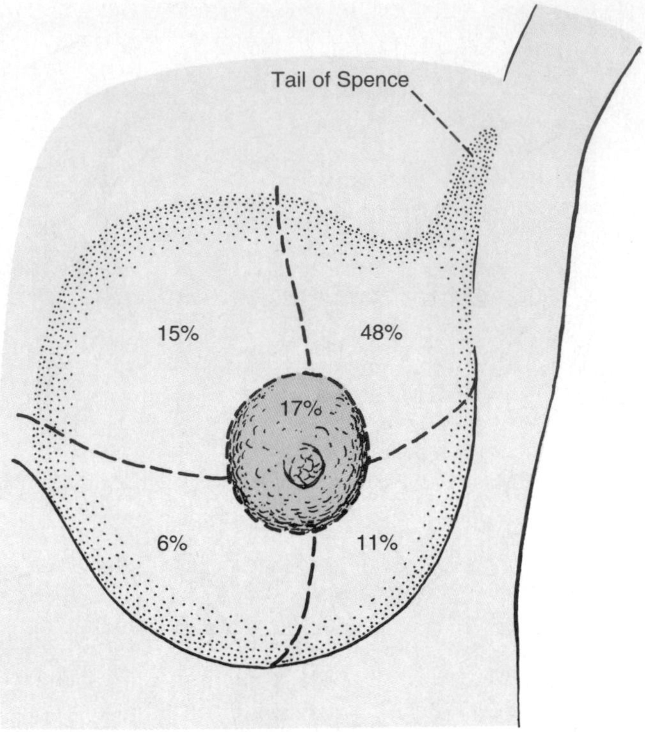

Figure 55–2
Frequency of occurrence of breast cancer according to location. Note that the highest occurrence is in the upper outer quadrant and tail of Spence.

vant (given after surgery) or neoadjuvant (given before surgery) chemotherapy or hormonal therapy may be given to reduce the risk of recurrence. Chemotherapy and hormonal therapy treat potential or known metastatic disease for systemic control. Hormonal therapy is used to treat clients with estrogen and progesterone receptor-positive breast cancer. Chemotherapy is used to treat clients with positive lymph nodes (stage II), locally advanced cancer (stage III), and metastatic breast cancer (stage IV) and even some clients with lymph node–negative (stage I) disease.

To provide multimodality therapy, a multidisciplinary evaluation is needed for determining the best course of treatment. A few major cancer treatment centers provide a consultation appointment at which surgical oncologists, medical oncologists, radiation oncologists, plastic surgeons, gynecologists, pathologists, mammographic radiology specialists, specialized nurses, and social workers are all available at the one appointment to evaluate the client and her disease and to recommend the best treatment combination.[11, 29, 40] The nurse is important in facilitating the multidisciplinary process in both the major treatment centers and in other settings. Whatever the setting, the nurse has a major role in helping the client through all phases of diagnosis and treatment.

Most breast cancer treatment is done on an outpatient basis. Mastectomy and other breast procedures that include an axillary lymph node dissection typically involve only a 2- to 3-day hospital stay. To have continuity of care for the client undergoing multimodality therapy, the nurses in the various treatment disciplines need to collaborate and share assessment information, nursing care plans, and reports on the client's progress.

Women with breast cancer at any stage fear disfigurement and death. Much has been written about the psychosocial impact of breast cancer.[33] Some women choose to have reconstructive surgery to rebuild their breasts and create new nipples. Breast reconstruction helps some women adjust to the loss of their breast.

With more women receiving breast-conserving procedures, it is important for nurses and health professionals to consider the impact of these therapies. A client who has had a lumpectomy and radiation therapy will still have scars and other physical changes of which she will be aware and that will be there to remind her that she has had breast cancer. Because she has kept her breast, she may worry about recurrence or wonder if she should have had a mastectomy. Daily radiation treatments for several weeks may delay resumption of her normal pattern of daily activities. Also, there are the side effects of radiation therapy that the client will have to cope with. Some of the common complaints are tenderness, change in the texture of the breast, and arm or hand numbness.[10]

RADIATION THERAPY

Radiation in combination with lumpectomy or quadrantectomy is an accepted treatment for early stage (e.g., stage I or stage II) breast cancer.[55, 76, 81] An axillary dissection is usually done for staging purposes. Women who are eligible for these treatment choices are women with

- Lesions less than 5 cm
- No large or fixed ancillary nodes
- No demonstrable disease
- Clear surgical margins
- Breasts that can be easily evaluated mammographically

Lumpectomy and quadrantectomy, with dissection of axillary lymph nodes (for staging) and radiation to the breast area, have produced good results. The survival rates and incidence of local and distant recurrence are equal to those from mastectomy.[44] Radiation therapy can be administered through an external beam and via iridium implants.

External beam radiation is administered 5 days a week by a cobalt machine or linear accelerator with use of approximately 5000 rad over 5 weeks.[49] Regional lymph nodes may be treated if they were not removed.

A concentrated boost of radiation is given to the small area where the tumor is located. A radiation boost to only the small area involved reduces the risk of side effects while the area of highest risk of disease is treated. After more than 5000 rad is given to the entire breast, the incidence of side effects increases. However, if the total radiation dose is too low, the risk of recurrence increases. The boost of radiation can be given with several additional linear accelerator treatments by electron beam therapy or via an interstitial iridium implant.

Interstitial implant therapy using iridium (^{192}Ir) is performed over 2 to 3 days as an inhospital procedure. The insertion of the iridium implant may be done with local anesthesia. Stainless steel guide needles are threaded through the tumor area at 1-cm intervals. Flexible plastic tubes are inserted in the guide needles. The guide needles are then removed, leaving the tubing in place. Strands of radioactive iridium seeds are threaded through each tube. The seeds, at 1-cm intervals, form a grid with those above and below to cover the tissues evenly with radiation. At the end of the insertion procedure, a button is attached, and the ends are crimped and then cut to prevent the seeds from falling out. An x-ray film confirms the implant's location. The length of time the implant must remain in place usually is 2 or 3 days. The procedure is mildly uncomfortable. The woman is able to be up and about in her room. Radiation precautions related to time, distance, and shielding are maintained.

Radiation therapy, in combination with lumpectomy or quadrantectomy, effectively treats early-stage breast cancer and avoids the psychosocial trauma of mastectomy. It is surprising to some health professionals that this treatment modality is not used more frequently. Let us consider three objections to the use of radiation for treatment of breast cancer. The first is concern that undetected cancer may remain after the identified tumor is removed by the excisional biopsy. However, several studies show that survival and local control are equal to those achieved with mastectomy.[55, 76, 81] A second objection is the concern that radiation might induce new cancers in the remaining breast or adjacent tissue. However, radiation has been used for more than 30 years, and thus far the incidence of secondary malignancies attributable to radiation therapy for breast cancer is small.[30] The third objection is the thought that the breast may not be cosmetically pleasing after radiation because of fibrosis or pigment changes. However, in most cases, the skin changes are minimal.

Side effects from radiation to the breast include the following:

- Temporary skin changes are common (e.g., itchy, dry, tender, red, swollen, or dry desquamation).
- Fatigue.
- Dry throat (rare) occurring in the later weeks of treatment is due to radiation's effect on pharyngeal mucosa if the supraclavicular area is irradiated. Although often described as a "lump in the throat," it should not interfere with eating.
- Pneumonitis (rare), indicated by dry cough and dyspnea, is due to inflammatory changes in the irradiated underlying lung.
- Arm edema (rare) may occur after axillary irradiation.
- Increased susceptibility to rib fractures occurs in the irradiated field.

Radiation therapy can be a long, difficult process for the client being treated. It is emotionally taxing to receive treatments daily for 5 to 7 weeks. Nursing support is needed during this period. Clients receiving radiation therapy have many of the same fears as those who had a mastectomy: fear of death, fear of mutilation, and feelings of sexual inadequacy. These are compounded by the stress of daily treatments and the fatigue that occurs with radiation therapy.

PHARMACOLOGIC MANAGEMENT

Adjuvant Chemotherapy. Adjuvant chemotherapy is given after surgical removal of any measurable cancer. The goal of adjuvant chemotherapy is to prolong the disease-free survival while helping the client maintain a high quality of life. Before 1988, premenopausal women with breast cancer in their lymph nodes commonly received chemotherapy. It was believed that women with node-negative breast cancer and postmenopausal women with positive lymph nodes would not benefit from chemotherapy. In 1988, a clinical alert was issued from the National Cancer Institute recommending consideration of adjuvant chemotherapy or hormonal therapy for all women with breast cancer. Premenopausal women will probably receive adjuvant hormonal therapy and may or may not receive chemotherapy.[31]

Typically, adjuvant chemotherapy is administered in an ambulatory setting beginning a few weeks after surgery or after the completion of radiation therapy. Various combinations of antineoplastic agents are used.[14, 27, 52, 98, 102] Cyclophosphamide (Cytoxan), 5-fluorouracil (5-FU), and methotrexate make up one of the most frequently used combinations (i.e., CMF).

High-dose chemotherapy with autologous bone marrow transplant has been used to treat women with breast cancer.[1] Bone marrow transplant may be used with stage II, stage III, or stage IV disease. Bone marrow rescue permits larger doses of agents, which otherwise are limited because of their severe myelosuppressive toxicity.

Neoadjuvant Chemotherapy. Neoadjuvant chemotherapy is given to treat locally advanced breast cancer (stage III) before surgical removal of the cancer. The goal of neoadjuvant chemotherapy is to evaluate the response of the measurable cancer to treatment. Clients with a breast cancer tumor greater than 5 cm in the breast or axilla may receive neoadjuvant chemotherapy and hormonal therapy before surgery or radiation therapy.[19, 93] The goal is to shrink the local disease and reduce the risk of systemic spread. Hormonal synchronization with combination chemotherapy has been under investigation.[19, 93] Because it is known that certain cell cycle–specific chemotherapies (e.g., methotrexate and 5-FU) are more effective on growing cells, estrogen is given to stimulate cell growth in order to maximize cell kill.

Systemic Therapy for Metastatic Breast Cancer. When the cancer has spread outside the breast and the ipsilateral axillary regions, systemic therapy is necessary. No one combination offers a clear advantage.

Side Effects of Chemotherapy. Common side effects for most antineoplastic chemotherapy combinations include varying degrees of alopecia (hair loss); constipation; depression of red cells, white cells, and platelets; diarrhea; fatigue; menopausal symptoms; nausea; peripheral neuropathy; photosensitivity; sterility; stomatitis; vaginal dryness; vomiting; and weight gain.[17, 50, 52] Several of the agents have their own specific toxic side effects (see Chap. 7). In addition to these side effects, receiving chemotherapy may reduce the client's social, household, and work-related activities; cause problems in marital, sexual, and family life; and cause a financial burden that can change the client's quality of life.[101] Understanding this can help the nurse plan and provide appropriate support for clients receiving chemotherapy.

Hormonal Therapy. Some breast cancers respond to hormonal therapy because they contain high levels of receptor proteins specific for certain steroids. These receptor proteins are capable of binding estrogen, progesterone, androgen, and corticosteroids. It is standard practice for breast biopsy tissue that is diagnosed as cancer to be sent for estrogen receptor assay and progesterone receptor assay.[44]

It is important to know the estrogen status of breast tumors because estrogen receptor–positive (ER+) tumors are associated with slower growth rates, less aggressive behavior, and longer survival. Both ER+ and progesterone receptor–positive (PR+) results predict tumors that will respond well to hormonal manipulation. Hormonal therapy may successfully treat metastases to bone, lymph nodes, skin, remaining breast tissue, and lung. It is rarely successful in treating brain or liver metastases. Various medical and surgical methods have been used with varying degrees of success.

Antiestrogen. Tamoxifen is the antiestrogen commonly used. Other antiestrogens are under investigation. Tamoxifen is administered orally in the treatment of ER+ breast cancer. Often, it is prescribed for years.[34] It has relatively few side effects, most of which are fairly well tolerated by most clients. Side effects may include hot flashes, vaginal dryness, nausea, vomiting, hypercalcemia, or a flare response (a transient flare of breast cancer symptoms). These side effects often decrease after a few weeks. The nurse needs to help the client cope with side effects, in particular, the menopause type side effects (i.e., hot flashes and vaginal dryness).

Estrogen has been used since 1950 to treat breast cancer in postmenopausal women.[44] The antitumor effect may take several weeks to occur. Side effects commonly include anorexia, nausea, vomiting, sodium and fluid retention, increased libido, withdrawal bleeding, and hypercalcemia. Rarely, a flare response of the disease with increased bone pain may occur. This usually indicates a good response to the therapy.

Androgens are usually less effective than estrogens but may be superior for bone metastases. Side effects include virilization and increased libido. Progesterone, in large doses, is also used for those who have previously responded to other additive hormones.

Aminoglutethimide may be prescribed to inhibit adrenal steroid production in metastatic breast cancer. This therapy is superior to an adrenalectomy. It avoids the need for lifelong replacement therapy, which must be continued after adrenalectomy or hypophysectomy. When aminoglutethimide is used, adrenal suppression leads to a reflex rise in adrenocorticotropic hormone, which can overcome the effect of aminoglutethimide. Therefore, suppressive doses of corticosteroids must be given. However, corticosteroids need to be continued only as long as the aminoglutethimide is used. Possible side effects of aminoglutethimide include lethargy, dizziness, visual blurring, and rash. They are dose dependent and transient.

Surgical Management

Surgery is important in the diagnosis and treatment of most breast cancers. Some breast surgical procedures are very disfiguring (e.g., radical mastectomy and modified radical mastectomy). However, less extensive procedures may be used (e.g., lumpectomy and quadrantectomy).

An axillary lymph node dissection (axillary dissection) is done typically for help in staging the disease. Axillary lymph nodes are not the only site of spread of breast cancer. However, when cancer is found in the nodes (node positive), there is a greater likelihood that there are distant metastases and that systemic therapy, chemotherapy, is needed.

Occasionally, a prophylactic mastectomy is done to prevent breast cancer in women who are at a high risk for breast cancer. This is a controversial surgery. The goal is to decrease the likelihood of development of breast cancer. However, typically a conservative approach involving careful observation is usually recommended for women at high risk.

Possible complications of breast surgery may include lymphedema, infection, seroma, hematoma, and cellulitis. Nurses need to teach clients the signs and symptoms of these problems.

SURGICAL PROCEDURES FOR BREAST CANCER

The lumpectomy, quadrantectomy, modified radical mastectomy, and axillary node dissection procedures are the most frequently used surgical procedures for treatment of breast cancer (Box 55–2).[7]

In postmenopausal women and those who have had surgical or medical oophorectomies, other surgical procedures, such as bilateral adrenalectomy or hypophysectomy (removal of the anterior pituitary), can be used to decrease the remaining low level of estrogen further. If so, daily cortisone replacement is required to prevent adrenal crisis. Fludrocortisone acetate (Florinef) is also required to replace the adrenal salt-regulating hormone.

Hypophysectomy also requires daily replacement of cortisone, thyroid hormone, and posterior pituitary hormones (e.g., vasopressin or antidiuretic hormone), if necessary.

Daily replacement therapy after bilateral adrenalectomy or hypophysectomy is required for life. A medical identification bracelet should be worn at all times after these surgeries. A card indicating the type and dose of necessary replacement medications should also be carried.

BREAST RECONSTRUCTION

Breast reconstruction is an option for clients who have had a mastectomy.[13, 46] Consideration needs to be given to a client's overall health and ability to tolerate a prolonged surgery, the stage of disease, the need for radiation therapy or chemotherapy, and the client's expectations (Fig. 55–3).

New techniques provide clients with choices for the type of reconstruction and when to do reconstruction. Breast reconstruction can be done by use of tissue expanders, implants, latissimus dorsi muscle, transverse rectus abdominis muscle, or gluteus maximus muscle.[23, 45] The nurse needs to know about each of these procedures in order to answer questions. A client may choose to delay reconstruction until after radiation or chemotherapy is completed. Alternatively, she may choose immediate reconstruction to be done at

BOX 55–2

Surgical Procedures for Breast Cancer

Lumpectomy. This procedure involves the removal of the cancerous mass and some normal tissue for clean margins. Frequently, the initial excisional biopsy is the lumpectomy. A re-excision may be needed if the margins are not clean in the original biopsy.

Quadrantectomy. This procedure removes the quadrant of the breast in which the cancer is located. A greater portion of normal tissue surrounding the cancer is removed with some of the overlying skin and underlying muscular fascia to provide a wide margin of cancer-free tissue.

Modified Radical Mastectomy. This procedure involves the en bloc removal of the breast, axillary lymph nodes, and overlying skin. This is the most commonly performed mastectomy.

Axillary Node Dissection. This procedure removes ipsilateral lymph nodes. It is part of the modified radical mastectomy and the standard mastectomy. An axillary node dissection may be the only additional surgical procedure needed by a woman who had an excisional biopsy that diagnosed and removed a small breast cancer with clean margins. The axillar dissection is not usually done to treat the disease, but it stages the disease and determines the need for more chemotherapy.

Total (Simple) Mastectomy. This procedure involves resection of breast tissue and some skin from the clavicle to the costal margin and from the midline to the latissimus dorsi. The axillary tail and pectoral fascia are removed also. Axillary nodes are not removed. This procedure is rarely used to treat diagnosed breast cancer. More frequently, bilateral simple mastectomies or total mastectomies are done to prevent breast cancer in women who are at high risk for having the disease.

Standard Radical Mastectomy. This procedure involves the en bloc removal of the breast, overlying skin, pectoral muscles, and axillary nodes. It removes the local lesion and the axillary nodes with a wide "safety margin" of surrounding tissue. Dissatisfaction with treatment results and morbidity has caused the number of radical mastectomies performed for primary breast cancer to decline sharply.

Extended Radical Mastectomy. This procedure involves the removal of the internal mammary nodes in addition to the structures removed during the standard radical mastectomy. This procedure currently has few advocates because it does not seem to be significantly more effective than irradiation in preventing recurrence from internal mammary metastases.

Surgical Hormonal Manipulation. A bilateral oophorectomy has been used for more than 80 years as a form of hormonal therapy in premenopausal women with advanced breast cancer. Radiation to the ovaries may also be used to achieve medical oophorectomy (stopping the function of the ovaries), but it may take up to 2 months for the therapy to be effective.

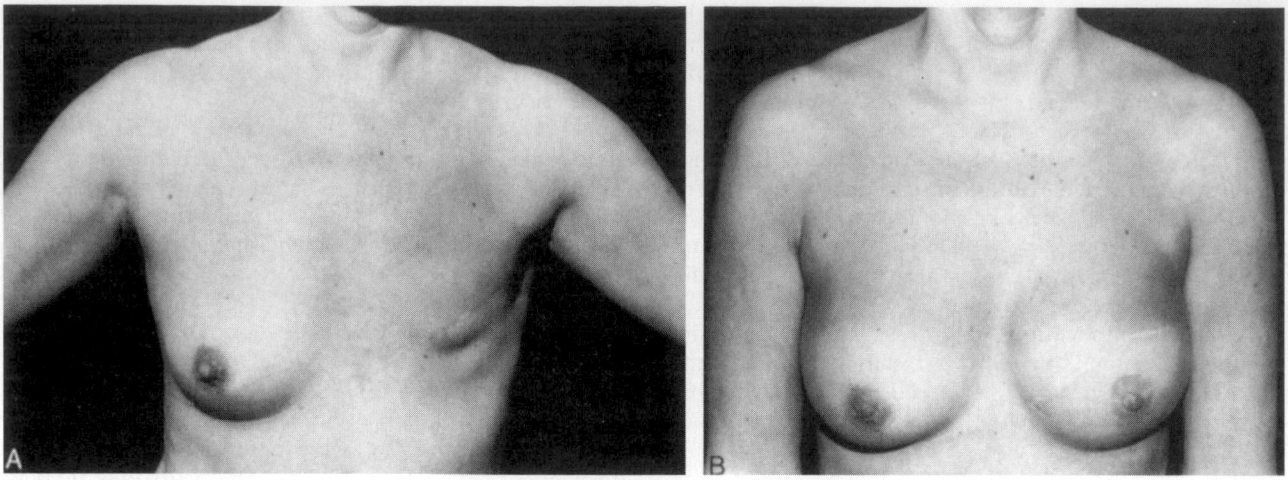

Figure 55–3
Preoperative (*A*) and postoperative (*B*) views of an ideal result from the use of a latissimus dorsi myocutaneous flap and an implant. A subpectoral implant was used in the right breast for symmetry. (From Bland, K. I., & Copeland, E. M. (Eds.) [1991]. *The breast: Comprehensive management of benign and malignant disease.* Philadelphia: W. B. Saunders.)

the same time as the mastectomy so she has a breast when she comes out of the anesthetic.

Breast reconstruction can help restore the woman's balance, symmetry, and body image. The nurse can help the client while she is deciding about reconstructive surgery, while preparing for reconstructive surgery, and while recovering from the surgery (see Chap. 5). Knowing about reconstruction and whether it is an option for her may help a client with breast cancer cope with the need for a mastectomy. The nurse can provide information about reconstruction.

Nursing Management

Assessment

The assessment of the client should begin with assessment of the breasts, identification of the client's risk factors, a description of the lump or problem, and current fears or concerns. It is also important to find out how the client discovered the lump.

The preoperative period before breast surgery for cancer or possible cancer is a very stressful time. Many fears surface, and the lives of the client and significant others are disrupted. A contradiction exists because usually the client feels well in spite of impending surgery. The preoperative period may also be stressful for health professionals. Nurses need an opportunity to explore their personal feelings about breast cancer before they can satisfactorily help others. Nurses providing preoperative care assess the client's and significant others' reactions to the frightening experience. The client and significant others need an opportunity to talk about the surgery and feel that someone cares about them. Nursing assessment focuses on the woman's knowledge level, coping ability, self-concept, and sexual concerns. It helps to include the sexual partner in assessment and planning. Nurses also need to be knowledgeable about all aspects of care and the therapeutic plan for each client so they can accurately discuss questions.

Postoperative assessments should also include the client's psychological reaction to the surgery. Other important assessments include the wound, drains, presence of lymphedema, signs and symptoms of infection, and pain.

Nursing Diagnosis, Planning, and Implementation

Nursing Diagnosis: Knowledge Deficit R/T available options of treatment and surgery (if chosen).

Planning: Expected Outcomes. The client will question and state options concerning available treatment and surgery and will explain her choice.

Implementation. The client should receive information about recommendations and treatment options before surgery or treatment is initiated. The nurse can help clients understand treatment options.[99] Because the typical hospital stay for a modified radical mastectomy or lumpectomy and axillary node dissection surgery is 2 to 3 days, preoperative teaching is done on an outpatient basis. The nurse needs to consider postoperative teaching along with preoperative care.

Nursing assessment provides data about knowledge deficits for use in formulating a teaching plan. This includes preoperative activities, explanations of surgery, postoperative care, discharge planning, and ways in which the client can participate. The client's anxiety level may be so high that new information cannot be remembered, so the nurse must provide written as well as verbal instructions. It is important to evaluate learning and to repeat information as often as necessary.

Nursing Diagnosis: Individual Coping, Ineffective R/T diagnosis of cancer and surgical changes in breast.

Planning: Expected Outcomes. The client will cope with the diagnosis of cancer and surgical changes in the breast, as evidenced by the client's statement of acceptance and decisions about treatment.

Implementation. Preoperatively or before any treatment, the nurse assesses the client's and significant others' coping ability and concerns. The assessment must not be rushed. The nurse should identify the coping mechanisms usually used by the client and significant others. Are there any potentially disabling coping patterns? This information should be used as the basis of support. The client may fear pain, mutilation, death, loss of control, and the hospital environment. These findings can be used to establish a plan of care to help the client use positive growth-producing coping and to avoid disabling coping.

Nursing Diagnosis: Body Image Disturbance R/T impending changes in breast and sexuality.

Planning: Expected Outcomes. The client will develop a positive body image, as evidenced by wearing make-up, own nightgown, and other feminine attire after breast surgery.

Implementation. If the assessment reveals problems with body image or sexuality, the nurse may choose to include other health-care professionals (e.g., social worker, sex therapist) in the plan of care for addressing these needs adequately. It may be helpful for someone who has had a similar surgery to talk with the client preoperatively or postoperatively.

Women who undergo surgery for breast cancer experience a sense of loss; changes in their routine life, social interactions, self-concept, and body image; and the fear of death.[61, 87] Those clients may benefit from opportunities to interact with nurses in ways in which they feel comfortable expressing their fears and problems.

Recovery during the postoperative period after mastectomy takes a lot of energy. A client's usual coping strategies may not be effective. Not everyone perceives or handles stress in the same way. Displacement, projection, denial, hope, prayer, meditation, stoicism, fatalism, or any combination of these reactions may occur. Clients who have surgically lost a breast may adapt in the same way they would to any loss. Phantom breast symptoms are not uncommon in the missing breast.[56]

Effective postoperative care is essential for successful psychosocial and physical rehabilitation. During the 2- to 3-day hospital stay, the focus of nursing care is toward recovery from surgery and anesthesia and aimed at discharge planning for self-care postoperative management. The client's self-image will improve with self-care activities.

Losing a breast or having breast cancer may not make its full impact until the client goes home. Many clients are surprised by events such as the amount of pain and discomfort, marked fatigue, slow incision healing, arm swelling, and jittery feelings. Ordinary things, such as finding a comfortable position in bed, may be difficult and painful. The client has to decide whether to hide the incision from significant others or let it be seen. The defect may be camouflaged for a woman by an appropriately fitted brassiere or a special bathing suit or evening dress, but doubts and fears about her attractiveness may affect even the most secure woman.

Body image is further altered by weight gain and alopecia. If a client wishes, a suitable wig can be obtained before hair is lost. Fatigue, decreased libido, and periods of depression are common in clients receiving chemotherapy and radiation therapy. It may help a client to talk with others who face the same problems. Breast cancer support groups may also be beneficial.

As time passes, there is a reorganization and restructuring of the lives of the client and significant others. During this time, the client resumes her role in society. Significant changes in this role may be necessary. Different women cope differently; feelings of sexual inadequacy, poor body image, and loss of a sense of femininity are common. The client needs to talk with and share concerns. Nurses are often able to offer such support. Nurses can offer understanding and facilitate communication between the client and significant others. Certain events, such as fitting the permanent prosthesis, can cause a breakdown in denial that a client may have been using after a mastectomy. A new lump or any new problem may precipitate aspects of the grieving process (e.g., anger, depression, and regression). Fear of metastases or recurrence of cancer may cause new symptoms to become magnified and every new pain to cause new anxiety.

Breast cancer support groups often provide a place for talking about shared and individual problems. Women encountering similar problems and finding solutions may effectively help each other. It often helps to realize that one is not alone in feelings and problems. The nurse should find out details about such support groups in the community and share this information as appropriate.

Nursing Diagnosis: Skin Integrity, Risk for Impaired R/T surgery or radiation therapy.

Planning: Expected Outcomes. The client will maintain skin integrity after surgery or radiation therapy without redness, infection, hematoma formation, or breakdown.

Implementation. Postoperatively, a pressure dressing is usually used initially. A drain, connected to gentle suction, prevents blood or serum collection in the operative space after a modified radical mastectomy or axillary node dissection. The nurse needs to instruct the client about emptying the drain and recording the amount of drainage; the physician is notified if the drain becomes plugged, is dislodged, or shows signs of infection or if frank bleeding develops.

When the dressing is changed, the nurse should gently encourage the client to look at the incision. Seeing the incision for the first time is often a difficult experience. A matter-of-fact approach by the nurse can help. Future dressing changes can be used to teach methods of cleaning the incision at home and for watching signs of infection.

Scaling, flaking, dryness, itching, erythema, hair loss, rash, or dry desquamation of the involved skin may occur. Careful treatment of the skin is important in minimizing the skin effects of radiation therapy.[65] Nurses need to teach clients how to care for their skin.

Nursing Diagnosis: Injury, Risk for R/T increased risk of infection and lymphedema secondary to axillary node dissection.

Planning: Expected Outcomes. The client will not experience injury, as evidenced by absence of infection or lymphedema.

Implementation. Arm edema (e.g., lymphedema) was a common complication after the standard radical mastectomy. However, with less extensive surgery, it occurs less frequently. Arm edema (on the operative side) can occur immediately postoperatively, or secondary edema may occur months or years after surgery. In the immediate postoperative period, the nurse should encourage arm exercises and should have the client elevate the arm to promote lymphatic drainage and prevent infection. Wearing an elastic bandage or a custom-fitted pressure gradient elastic sleeve may also be helpful. A sign should be placed on the client's bed warning that no blood pressure readings, injections, intravenous catheterizations, or blood draws should be done on the arm on the operative side. These procedures can cause circulatory impairment or infection.

After the client leaves the hospital, burns, cuts, and abrasions are the most frequent sources of infection. After axillary node dissection, secondary edema from infection in the arm may cause some permanent edema. Also, postoperative radiation to the axilla often increases the frequency and degree of arm edema. One must explain that the client is vulnerable to secondary edema in the arm on the operative side for the rest of her life and that any trauma in the arm may lead to edema and infection.

Nursing Diagnosis: Knowledge Deficit R/T postoperative arm exercises and care, breast prosthesis, chemotherapy, and radiation therapy.

Planning: Expected Outcomes. The client will demonstrate postoperative arm exercises and care and knowledge about breast prosthesis, chemotherapy, and radiation therapy.

Implementation. The nurse plans interventions for restoring full hand, arm, and shoulder range of motion. Sometimes a surgeon attempts to enhance mobility by placing the arm on the operative side at a right angle to the chest wall immediately postoperatively.

These early limited postoperative arm exercises are important and usually started within 24 hours after surgery. The client must be taught to perform hand and wrist movements and to flex and extend the elbow hourly. The nurse should encourage self-care activities (e.g., feeding, combing hair, washing face) and other activities that use the arm, with care taken not to abduct the arm or raise the arm or elbow above shoulder height until the drains are removed.

When wound healing is well established and axillary drains are removed, the client should begin abduction and external rotation of the upper arm, including pendulum swings to improve shoulder function, forward and lateral elevation of the arms, overhead pulley suspension to obtain full elevation, and wall climbing and rope running (Fig. 55–4). Exercises may need to be approved by the physician. Arrangements for a physical therapist to assist with range of motion may need to be made at the time surgery is planned because the short hospital stay means that there may not be time postoperatively. It is important for the nurse to provide written and verbal instructions about arm precautions after axillary node dissection (see Client Education Guide: Arm Precautions After Axillary Lymph Node Dissection).

The Reach for Recovery program of the American Cancer Society is a rehabilitation program for women who have had breast surgery. This program is designed to help women meet common psychosocial, physical, and cosmetic needs. With authorization of the physician, volunteers from this program visit the hospital or the home and give the woman information and help, including

- A Reach for Recovery kit, ball, book, rope, and temporary soft cotton prosthesis (for clients who have had a mastectomy)
- Postoperative axillary node dissection exercises
- Discussion of brassiere comfort, various breast prostheses, clothing adjustments, and personal problems as appropriate

Clients who have had a mastectomy may wear a temporary lightweight prosthesis immediately after the sutures and drains are removed. This may help the client's adjustment to the loss of her breast. A soft, cotton breast form may be supplied by the Reach for Recovery visitor. Alternatively, cotton padding inserted into a pocket sewn onto a lightweight brassiere is a good, temporary substitute. A permanent prosthesis should not be purchased until the wound has healed completely, because the incision site may change. Prostheses are expensive. They may be purchased in foundation departments in most large stores or at medical-surgical supply stores that sell durable medical equipment. Most of these stores have fitters to help clients obtain the right fit. It would be helpful for the nurse to learn about suppliers in the local area so she can provide the name to the client. Most private and government insurance plans pay for at least the first prosthesis and brassiere.

Teaching is a major role for the nurse caring for clients receiving radiation therapy. Many clients have misconceptions about radiation. Through assessment, the nurse identifies misconceptions and develops a teaching plan to clarify misunderstandings and meet the client's needs.[18, 64] Two booklets, *Radiation Therapy: A Treatment for Early Stage Breast Cancer* and *Radiation Therapy and You*,[71, 72] may help the client and are obtainable free of charge from the National Cancer Institute by calling 1-800-4-CANCER. See Chapter 7 for further information on radiation therapy.

Nurses are responsible for educating clients who receive chemotherapy. This includes teaching them the names of medications being received, how the medications are administered, expected side effects, side effect management, preventive measures, and complications

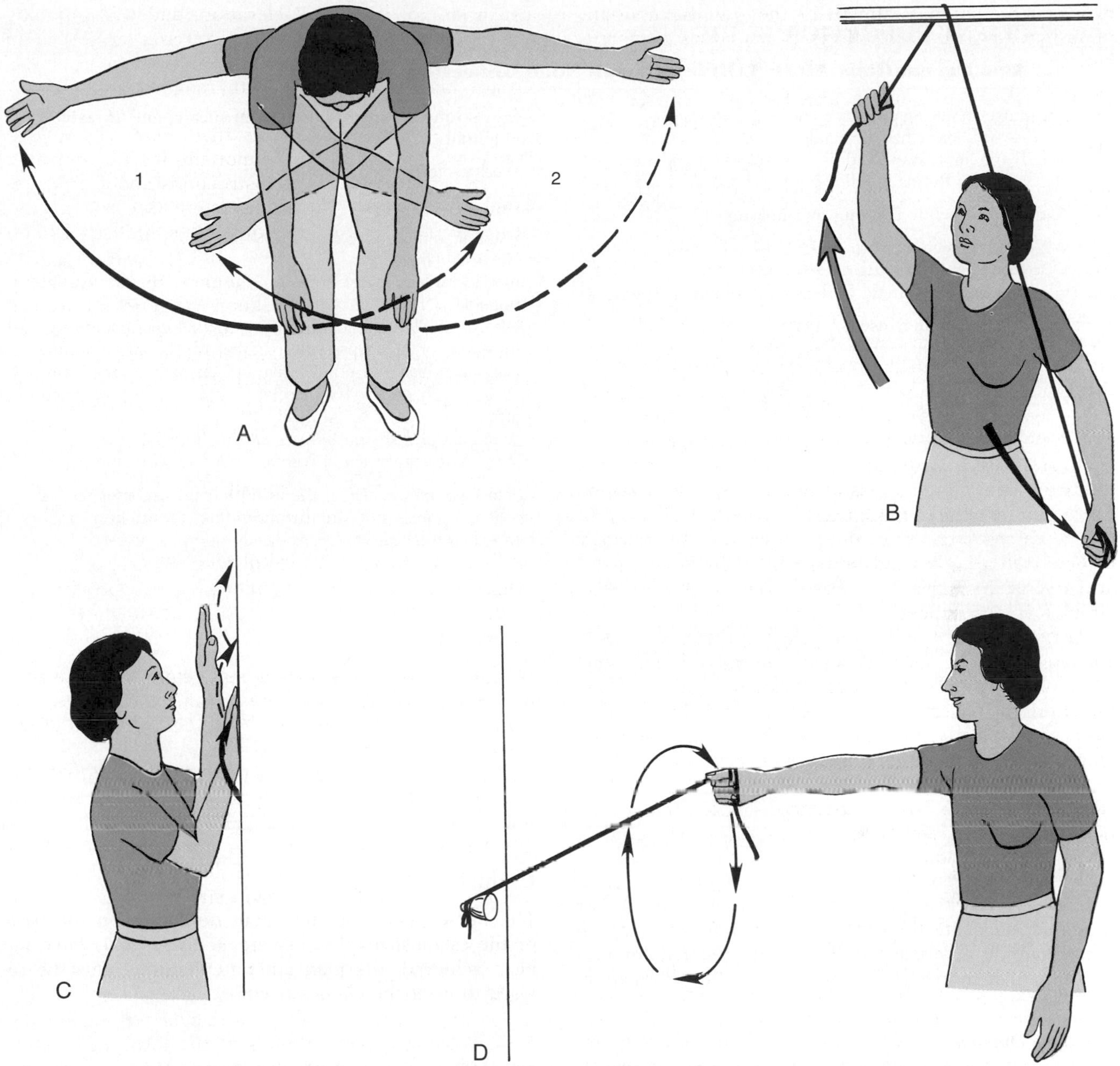

Figure 55–4
The client should be instructed in the following postmastectomy exercises. *A*, Arm swings. Stand with feet 8 inches apart. Bend forward from waist, allowing arms to hand toward floor. Swing both arms up to sides to reach shoulder level. Swing back to center, then cross arms at center. Do not bend elbows. If possible, do this and other exercises in front of mirror to ensure even posture and correct motion. *B*, Pulley motion. Using operated arm, toss 6-foot rope over a shower curtain rod (or over top of a door that has a nail in the top to hold the rope in place for the exercise). Grasp one end of rope in each hand. Slowly raise operated arm as far as comfortable by pulling down on the rope on opposite side. Keep raised arm close to your head. Reverse to raise unoperated arm by lowering the operated arm. Repeat. *C*, Hand wall climbing. Stand facing wall with toes 6 to 12 inches from wall. Bend elbows and place palms against wall at shoulder level. Gradually move both hands up the wall parallel to each other until incisional pulling or pain occurs. (Mark that spot on wall to measure progress.) Work hands down to shoulder level. Move closer to wall as height of reach improves. *D*, Rope turning. Tie rope to door handle. Hold rope in hand of operated side. Back away from door until arm is extended away from body, parallel to floor. Swing rope in as wide a circle as possible. Increase size of the circle as mobility returns.

CLIENT EDUCATION GUIDE

Arm Precautions After Axillary Lymph Node Dissection

The nurse should instruct the client as follows:
Because you have had an axillary node dissection, the affected arm may swell and is less able to fight infections. Use your arm normally following these recommendations.

Avoid burns while cooking or smoking.

- Wear a long-length oven mitt.
- Do not reach into a hot oven with this arm.
- Do not hold a cigarette in the affected hand.

Avoid sunburn and insect bites.

- Wear long-sleeve shirts and gloves.
- Use sunscreen.
- Use insect repellent to avoid bites and stings.

Avoid cuts, pinpricks, and scratches.

- Wear gloves when gardening.
- Do not work near thorny plants or dig with your hands.
- Use a thimble when sewing.
- Use an electric razor with a narrow head for underarm shaving to reduce the risk of nicks or scratches.
- Never cut or pick at cuticles; use hand cream or lotion.
- Wash cuts promptly; treat them with antibacterial medication and cover them with sterile dressing. Check often for redness, soreness, pus, or other signs of infection.

Avoid strong detergents, harsh chemicals, and abrasive compounds.

- Wear protective gloves when doing dishes and cleaning.

Avoid other trauma.

- Use a lanolin hand cream a few times each day.
- Have all injections, vaccinations, blood samples, and blood pressure tests done on the other arm whenever possible.
- Wear a Medic Alert identification tag that cautions no test injections or blood pressure readings on the affected arm.
- Carry handbag and other heavy objects on the other arm.
- Wear watch or jewelry loosely, if at all, on the operated arm.
- Avoid elastic cuffs on blouses and nightgowns.
- Wear an elastic sleeve if recommended by your physician.

Contact your physician if the arm or hand becomes red, is swollen, or feels hot. In the meantime, try to keep your arm over your head and periodically pump your fist.

Adapted from National Cancer Institute. (1990). *After breast cancer: A guide to follow up care* (NIH Publication No. 90–2400). Washington, DC: Author.

that must be reported to the physician or nurse (e.g., infection, fever, bruising, bleeding, or mouth sores). For example, adequate fluid intake is required when cyclophosphamide (Cytoxan) is being administered for prevention of hemorrhagic cystitis. For more information, see Chapter 7.

Nursing Diagnosis: Nutrition: Less than Body Requirements, Altered R/T nausea, vomiting, and stomatitis secondary to chemotherapy.

Planning: Expected Outcomes. The client will take in adequate nutrition without evidence of nausea and vomiting, control of stomatitis, intake of adequate calories daily, and no loss of weight.

Implementation. Nausea, vomiting, anorexia, stomatitis, and taste change are common side effects of chemotherapy. Yet an adequate nutritional intake is essential for providing strength and well-being. Stomatitis may make eating and drinking extremely difficult. Careful oral hygiene and topical analgesics may help. Adequate dosage and timing of antiemetics can control nausea and vomiting. The client may need to try different foods to find ones that taste good to her. The nurse must emphasize the importance of good nutrition by helping the client find high-calorie and high-protein foods that can be tolerated. Weight and dietary patterns must be monitored. Meeting nutritional needs can be difficult and must be individualized.

Evaluation

The nurse must evaluate client outcomes on the basis of the established plan of care. If these goals have not been achieved, the plan and interventions must be revised to meet the client's needs.

Modification of Plan of Care for the Elderly

The care of older clients with breast cancer is similar to that of younger clients. The only difference might be in the extent of treatment. If the older client is not in good health generally, radiation therapy and hormonal manipulation may be all that is recommended.

METASTATIC BREAST CANCER

Metastatic breast cancer is a chronic disease.[44, 52] Metastases have been known to occur up to 25 years after the initial diagnosis of breast cancer. Alternatively, breast cancer can be a rapidly progressing terminal disease. Knowledge of the usual metastatic patterns with breast cancer and common complications can aid early recognition and effective treatment. Metastases usually develop in one or more of the following sites: lymph nodes, skin, remaining breast tissue, bones, lung, pleura, peritoneum, liver, and central nervous system. Women with metastases to the liver or central nervous system have a poorer prognosis.

Treatment of metastatic disease may involve radiation therapy, hormonal manipulation, chemotherapy, or possible surgery. A combination of treatments is usually used. Excellent palliation can be achieved for metastatic breast cancer, which offers longer survival for this disease than for many other types of cancers.

Hypercalcemia is a common complication of metastatic breast cancer. It may be due to bone involvement or hormonal therapy. Prompt treatment includes hydration and diuretics. Mithramycin or a newer drug, gallium citrate, is initiated for severe hypercalcemia.

Spinal cord compression, usually from extradural metastases, is a complication requiring prompt diagnosis and intervention for prevention of paraplegia. Assessment findings such as back pain, leg weakness, and sphincter disturbances indicate possible spinal cord compression. Treatment involves radiation therapy or surgery, often followed by chemotherapy.

Nursing care of clients with metastatic breast cancer involves helping them manage the complications caused by their disease and the side effects caused by treatments. Providing support for the clients and significant others is equally important. Physical symptoms may be difficult to manage.

Currently under investigation is the treatment of clients with metastatic disease using autologous bone marrow transplantation and high-dose chemotherapy.[1] This procedure involves having the client donate her own bone marrow, either through bone marrow aspiration or through peripheral stem cell pheresis. The client is then given very high-dose chemotherapy followed by reinfusion of her own marrow or stem cells to rescue her after the chemotherapy destroys her own marrow. Further information on bone marrow transplantation can be found in Chapters 7 and 9.

Previously established coping mechanisms may falter during this period as hope dwindles and energy is spent coping with pain, physical problems, and fears. Old unresolved issues may resurface. In addition to providing physical care, the nurse must assist the client and significant others to re-establish effective coping mechanisms. Women with breast cancer need a strong support system and people with whom they can comfortably and helpfully discuss their problems. Nurses can help provide this support where it is lacking. Nurses need to identify and reinforce beneficial coping to help the woman with advanced breast cancer live a meaningful life.[4, 21]

MALE BREAST CANCER

Breast cancer in men is rare.[22, 26] The incidence is 1 per cent of that of women. The average age at occurrence is about 60 years (10 years older than the average for women). Factors associated with an increased risk of breast cancer in men include high estrogen levels, obesity, testicular abnormalities or injury, Klinefelter's syndrome, exposure to ionizing radiation, increased prolactin level, use of phenothiazines, and having a first-degree male or female relative with breast cancer.

Assessment findings indicating male breast cancer include a painless lump beneath the areola or, more often, nipple discharge, retraction, crusting, or ulceration. Staging is the same as for women. Biopsy is necessary for diagnosis of male breast cancer. It is as important in men to test for estrogen receptors as it is in women.

Initial treatment consists of a radical or modified radical mastectomy. Postoperative radiation is frequently used. The pattern of metastasis is similar to that in the female, with soft tissue, bone, and visceral site involvement occurring frequently. Hormonal therapy is very important in the treatment of metastasis, because estrogen receptors have been found in 84 per cent of the tumors.

Tamoxifen and an orchiectomy are the primary hormonal therapies used to treat disseminated male breast cancer. Tamoxifen has provided a response rate of 71 per cent in ER+ male breast cancer. Orchiectomy provides a mean response rate of 55 per cent in clients of all ages. Other hormonal manipulations are used in men as in women.

BENIGN BREAST DISEASE

Fibrocystic Breasts

Ninety per cent of all women have cysts. Fibrocystic breasts are not a disease per se even though the label fibrocystic breast disease is often given to the condition.[62, 78] Fibrocystic breasts are the most frequent condition of the female breast. The exact cause is unknown, although some evidence indicates hormonal imbalance may be associated with it. The fibrocystic condition typically improves during pregnancy and lactation. It occurs during the reproductive years and disappears with menopause.

Typical fibrocystic lesions are fluid-filled cysts that are round, well circumscribed, and movable. Depending on the amount of fluid in the cyst, it may feel soft or hard.

Assessment findings may include nodularity and tenderness. Pain occurs frequently and the cysts increase in size premenstrually. Generally, cysts are managed by aspiration rather than by surgical biopsy. However, if there is any question, a biopsy is done. A biopsy is necessary particularly if the cyst keeps recurring after being aspirated.

Once the diagnosis is confirmed, treatment is symptomatic.[78, 84] Conservative measures include breast support with a firm brassiere, local applications of heat or ice bags, mild analgesics, or the occasional use of diuretics. It has been found that reducing methylxanthines (e.g., caffeine and theophylline medications) is associated with symptom reduction.

Medications have been used with some success in treating fibrocystic breasts. Large doses of vitamin E relieve symptoms in some women but may raise cholesterol levels. Danazol, a synthetic androgen, may be used continuously for 3 to 6 months and repeated if symptoms recur. Side effects include menstrual irregularities, fluid retention, acne, muscle cramps, or possible hepatic dysfunction. Danazol should be used only for severe fibrocystic breasts.

Hyperplasia and Atypical Hyperplasia

Ductal hyperplasia is found in 20 per cent of all breast biopsy specimens.[94] Atypical lobular hyperplasia is found in 1 per cent of breast biopsy specimens. Hyperplasia and atypical hyperplasia can be diagnosed only by pathologic examination of breast tissue from a biopsy. Finding hyperplasia or atypical hyperplasia indicates the woman is at increased risk for breast cancer.

Fibroadenoma

Fibroadenoma is a common breast tumor that usually occurs in young women, most frequently between the ages of 15 and 30 years.[91, 94] This tumor is usually a nontender, round, firm, or rubbery mass 1 to 3 cm in diameter. Movability of the adenoma in the breast tissues is one of its most distinctive characteristics. Excision is the only effective treatment.

Papilloma

Intraductal papillomas are lesions growing in the terminal portion of a duct (solitary) or throughout the duct system of a sector of breast (multiple or intraductal). Papillomas typically occur in women in their 40s. A ductogram may help in locating the papilloma.

Solitary intraductal papillomas are usually not precancerous. Multiple papillomas may occasionally be cancerous. Intraductal papilloma is usually indicated by a serous, serosanguineous, or bloody discharge from the nipple. Often no mass is palpable, although a small soft tumor in a central or periareolar portion of the breast is usually present. It is necessary to excise the lesion and have its tissue examined for determining whether it is benign or malignant.

Duct Ectasia

Duct ectasia, a disease of ducts in the subareolar zone, occurs in aging breasts usually in perimenopausal or postmenopausal women. Symptoms may include a palpable dilated duct; a thick, sticky nipple discharge, and burning pain, itching, and inflammation. There appears to be no association with cancer. However, biopsy is performed because on physical examination it is difficult to differentiate duct ectasia from cancer. Recommended treatment is excision of the ducts.

Mastodynia and Mastalgia

Mastodynia and mastalgia[63, 94] refer to breast pain. Breast pain is the most common breast complaint. Pain is not usually associated with breast cancer. Many women have cyclic premenstrual mastodynia. Women with cyclic premenstrual mastodynia usually have lumpy breast (nodularity) and pain for the week before menses. After any other problems have been ruled out, treatment is symptomatic. Wearing a well-fitting bra for support, particularly during jogging and other bouncing exercise, may help. Decreasing salt and caffeine intake may also help.

Gynecomastia

Gynecomastia, hypertrophy of one or both male breasts, is common at puberty and in older men.[8] It occurs 60 to 70 per cent of the time at puberty and typically resolves spontaneously in 1 to 2 years. The hormonal mechanism causing gynecomastia is not well understood, although some suggest it is due to increased estrogen. Careful assessment and follow-up are required to rule out causes such as tumors, thyroid or hepatic problems, or Klinefelter's syndrome.

The client must be assured that the condition is temporary. If the gynecomastia causes severe psychosocial trauma, reduction mammoplasty or medications such as an antiestrogen (e.g., tamoxifen) or a synthetic androgen (e.g., danazol) may be prescribed.

Men aged 50 to 70 years occasionally experience gynecomastia that usually regresses spontaneously after a few months to a year. This is not associated with endocrine abnormality. Because cancer is more common in this age group, any lesions found may require biopsy for differentiation from cancer. Certain medications can cause gynecomastia in any age group.

MAMMOPLASTY

Women who are uncomfortable with the appearance of their breasts often have a poor body image. Some women who have small breasts seek surgical procedures to enlarge their breasts, such as augmentation mammoplasty. Augmentation mammoplasty has been a popular cosmetic procedure that uses implants or myocutaneous tissue to either enlarge underdeveloped breasts or reconstruct breasts after removal of benign or malignant lesions.

Breasts change over time. With advanced aging, the breasts atrophy and lose some glandular tissue. Some women have large, heavy breasts that are uncomfortable. Breast reduction surgery, reduction mammoplasty, may benefit them. Reduction mammoplasty may help alleviate neck pain, backaches, possible curvature of the spine, and painful bra strap irritation.

Augmentation mammoplasty and reduction mammoplasty are discussed in Chapter 50. Women having such surgery believe it increases their attractiveness as perceived by themselves or others. There has been some controversy about the safety of silicone and polyurethane implants.[79] In 1992, the Food and Drug Administration restricted use of these implants because of problems with rupturing of the implants, leaking of silicone, and resultant health problems. Nurses can help clients understand the facts about the risks and benefits of mammoplasty.

STUDY QUESTIONS

1. Your client presents with a watery discharge from her right nipple. What other assessment data would be the most significant?
   A. Presence of any lumps or masses
   B. Support system
   C. Red cell count, hemoglobin, and hematocrit
   D. Discharge from left nipple
2. You can document a client's learning regarding breast cancer risks when the client tells you
   A. "I won't need regular screening for breast cancer because my mother was cured of it 6 years ago."
   B. "Since I had chemotherapy after my standard radical mastectomy, I can enjoy as much sunbathing as I like."
   C. "I intend to cut down on coffee intake in case that might help the symptoms of my fibrocystic breasts."
   D. "Since I am having yearly mammograms, I do not need to do breast self-exams."
3. Which of the following statements by the nurse regarding treatment for breast cancer would be most appropriate?
   A. "You need to trust your physician to decide what to do about cancer treatment."
   B. "You and your significant others should talk about all the options and I will be glad to help clarify any concerns."
   C. "You must not take time for a second opinion because the cancer will grow out of control if you do."
   D. "Because breast cancer is usually curable, you should not have a mastectomy unless another physician tells you to."
4. Which of the following plans would be most helpful for the client who recently underwent a standard radical mastectomy?
   A. Arrange for a pastor to talk about death and other spiritual concerns.
   B. Arrange for significant others to assist with cooking until the client can practice such things as stirring soup with one hand.
   C. Arrange for Meals-on-Wheels or some other agency to provide for the family's nutritional needs.
   D. Arrange for neighbors to screen visitors to prevent emotional upsets.
5. To provide effective nursing care for the client who has been diagnosed with breast cancer, the *first* action the nurse should take is to
   A. Teach the client what to expect postoperatively
   B. Include the client's significant others in the planning phase of care
   C. Maintain radiation precautions according to agency guidelines
   D. Explore his or her own feelings about breast cancer

CRITICAL THINKING EXERCISES

SCENARIO A

A 60-year-old woman is being assessed after a minor injury suffered in an automobile accident. You learn that she has had one mammogram 8 years ago. She stated that "it hurt so I never had it done again."

1. What should the nurse say to her?
2. What teaching needs do you recognize?
3. What is the role of the nurse in relation to health screening?

SCENARIO B

The client is a 55-year-old woman with metastatic breast cancer. Her mother and one sister have died of carcinoma of the breast, and she refuses chemotherapy even though she has undergone modified radical mastectomy 8 months ago. Her husband and two living sisters insist that she submit to chemotherapy or radiation therapy or both.

1. What is the responsibility of the client's nurse in this conflict?
2. What other resources are there for the family?
3. Discuss other areas of concern for the health-care team.

BIBLIOGRAPHY

1. Affronti, M. L., et al. (1990). Autologous bone marrow transplant for the treatment of advanced breast cancer. *Innovations in Oncology Nursing, 6(4),* 2–6, 19–21.
2. American Cancer Society. (1989). *Special touch: A personal plan of action for breast health.* New York: Author.
3. American Cancer Society. (1995). *Cancer facts & figures—*1995. New York: Author.
4. Arathuzik, D. (1991). Pain experience for metastatic breast cancer patients: Unraveling the mystery. *Cancer Nursing, 14(1),* 41–48.
5. Baird, S. B., et al. (1991). *Cancer nursing: A comprehensive textbook.* Philadelphia: W. B. Saunders.
6. Beahrs, O. H. (1991). Staging of cancer. *CA: A Cancer Journal for Clinicians, 41(2),* 121–125.
7. Bland, K. I., & Copeland, E. M. (Eds). (1991). *The breast: Comprehensive management of benign and malignant diseases.* Philadelphia: W. B. Saunders.
8. Bland, K. I., & Page, D. L. (1991). Gynecomastia. In K. I. Bland & E. M. Copeland (Eds.), *The breast: Comprehensive management of benign and malignant diseases* (pp. 135–168). Philadelphia: W. B. Saunders.
9. Blesch, K. S., et al. (1991). Correlates of fatigue in people with breast cancer or lung cancer. *Oncology Nursing Forum, 18(1),* 81–87.
10. Bodner, S., & Flynn, K. T. (1987). Symptom distress of women treated with conservative surgery and primary radiation for carcinoma of the breast (abstract #234). *Oncology Nursing Forum, 14(Suppl.),* 140.
11. Bord, M. A., & Carpenter, L. C. (1990). A coordinated approach to comprehensive breast care. *Innovations in Oncology Nursing, 6(2),* 13–19.
12. Boring, C. C., et al. (1992). Cancer statistics, 1992. *CA: A Cancer Journal for Clinicians, 42(1),* 19–38.
13. Bostwick, J. (1990). Reconstruction after mastectomy. *Surgical Clinics of North America, 70(5),* 1125–1140.
14. Breitmeyer, J. B., & Henderson, I. C. (1990). Adjuvant chemotherapy of breast cancer. *Surgical Clinics of North America, 70(5),* 1081–1113.
15. Brinker, N., & Harris, C. M. (1990). *The race is run one step at a time.* New York: Simon & Schuster.
16. Cady, B., & Stone, M. D. (1990). Selection of breast-preservation therapy for primary invasion breast carcinoma. *Surgical Clinics of North America, 70(5),* 1047–1059.
17. Camp-Sorrell, D. (1991). Controlling adverse effects of chemotherapy. *Nursing 91, 12(4),* 34–41.
18. Cawley, M., et al. (1990). Informational and psychosocial needs of women choosing conservative surgery/primary radiation for early stage breast cancer. *Cancer Nursing, 13(2),* 90–94.
19. Cody, R. L., & Wicha, M. S. (1988). Contemporary chemotherapy. In J. K. Harness et al. (Eds.), *Breast cancer: Collaborative management* (pp. 157–177). Chelsea, MI: Lewis Publishers.
20. Collins-Hattery, A. M., & Blumberg, B. D. (1991). S phase index and ploidy prognostic markers in node negative breast cancer: Information for nurses. *Oncology Nursing Forum, 18(1),* 59–62.
21. Coward, D. D. (1991). Self-transcendence and emotional well-being in women with advanced breast cancer. *Oncology Nursing Forum, 18(5),* 857–863.
22. Crichlow, R. W., & Galt, S. W. (1990). Male breast cancer. *Surgical Clinics of North America, 70(5),* 1165–1178.
23. d'Angelo, T. M., & Gorrell, C. R. (1989). Breast reconstruction using tissue expanders. *Oncology Nursing Forum, 16(1),* 23–27.
24. DeVita, V. T., et al. (Eds.). (1993). *Cancer: Principles and practice of oncology* (4th ed.). Philadelphia: J. B. Lippincott.
25. Donegan, W. L. (1988). Evaluation of breast masses. In J. K. Harness et al. (Eds.), *Breast cancer: Collaborative management* (pp. 3–9). Chelsea, MI: Lewis Publishers.
26. Donegan, W. L. (1991). Cancer of the breast in men. *CA: A Cancer Journal for Clinicians, 41(6),* 339–354.
27. Dorr, F. A., & Friedman, M. A. (1991). The role of chemotherapy in the management of primary breast cancer. *CA: A Cancer Journal for Clinicians, 41(4),* 231–241.
28. Duelberg, S. I. (1992). Preventive health behavior among black and white women in urban and rural areas. *Social Science and Medicine, 34(2),* 191–198.
29. Durant, J. R. (1990). How to organize a multidisciplinary clinic for the management of breast cancer. *Surgical Clinics of North America, 70(4),* 977–983.
30. Findlay, P. A. (1988). Radiation therapy as definitive treatment of breast cancer. In M. E. Lippman et al. (Eds.), *Diagnosis and management of breast cancer* (pp. 155–207). Philadelphia: W. B. Saunders.
31. Fisher, B. (1991). Biological perspective of breast cancer: Contributions of the national surgical adjuvant breast and bowel project clinical trials. *CA: A Cancer Journal for Clinicians, 41(2),* 97–111.
32. Fisher, B., et al. (1989). A randomized clinical trial evaluation sequential methotrexate and fluorouracil in the treatment of patients with node-negative breast cancer who have estrogen-receptor-negative tumors. *New England Journal of Medicine, 320(8),* 473–478.
33. Ganz, P. A., et al. (1987). Rehabilitation needs and breast cancer: The first month after primary therapy. *Breast Cancer Research and Treatment, 10(3),* 243–253.
34. Gibson, D. F. C., & Jordan, V. C. (1990). Adjuvant antiestrogen therapy for breast cancer: Past, present, and future. *Surgical Clinics of North America, 70(5),* 1103–1113.
35. Gordon, R. S. (1981). Survey finds U. S. women knowledgeable about breast cancer. *Journal of the American Medical Association, 245(9),* 918.
36. Grindel, C. G., et al. (1989). Food intake of women with breast cancer during their first six months of chemotherapy. *Oncology Nursing Forum, 16(3),* 401–407.
37. Grundfest-Broniatowski, S., & Bauer, T. W. (1988). Benign breast disease. In S. Grundfest-Broniatowski & C. B. Esselstyn (Eds.), *Controversies in breast disease: Diagnosis and management* (pp. 3–42). New York: Marcel Dekker.
38. Grundfest-Broniatowski, S., & Esselstyn, C. B. (Eds.). (1988). *Controversies in breast disease: Diagnosis and management.* New York: Marcel Dekker.
39. Harness, J. K. (1988). Organizing for collaborative management: What are the options? In J. K. Harness et al. (Eds.), *Breast cancer: Collaborative management* (pp. 3–9). Chelsea, MI: Lewis Publishers.
40. Harness, J. K., et al. (1987). Developing a comprehensive breast center. *American Surgeon, 53(8),* 419–423.

41. Harness, J. K., et al. (Eds.). (1988). *Breast cancer: Collaborative management.* Chelsea, MI: Lewis Publishers.

42. Helvie, M. A., et al. (1990). Radiographic guided fine needle aspiration of non-palpable breast lesions. *Radiology, 174(3141),* 657–661.

43. Henderson, I. C. (1987). Adjuvant chemotherapy and endocrine therapy in patients with operable breast cancer. *Principle and Practice of Oncology Update, 1(3),* 1–14.

44. Henderson, I. C., et al. (1989). Cancer of the breast. In V. T. DeVita et al. (Eds.), *Cancer principle and practice of oncology* (3rd ed., pp. 1197–1269). Philadelphia: J. B. Lippincott.

45. Hutcheson, H. A. (1986). TAIF: New option for breast reconstruction. *Nursing 86, 16(2),* 52–53.

46. Kalinowski, B. H. (1990). Options and decisions: Reconstructive surgery: Rehabilitation after mastectomy. *Innovations in Oncology Nursing, 6(1),* 2–9.

47. Kelly, P. T. (1993). Breast cancer risk: The role of the nurse practitioner. *Nurse Practitioner Forum, 4(2),* 91–95.

48. Kelsey, J. L., & Gammon, M. D. (1991). The epidemiology of breast cancer. *CA: A Cancer Journal for Clinicians, 41(3),* 146–165.

49. Kinne, D. W. (1991). Surgical management of primary breast cancer. *CA: A Cancer Journal for Clinicians, 41(2),* 71–84.

50. Knobf, M. T. (1986). Physical and psychologic distress associated with adjuvant chemotherapy in women with breast cancer. *Journal of Clinical Oncology, 4(5),* 678–684.

51. Knobf, M. T. (1990). Early-stage breast cancer: The options. *American Journal of Nursing, 90(11),* 28–30.

52. Knobf, M. T. (1991). Breast cancer. In S. B. Baird et al. (Eds.), *Cancer nursing: A comprehensive textbook* (pp. 125–451). Philadelphia: W. B. Saunders.

53. Kushner, R. (1984). *Alternatives.* Cambridge, MA: The Kensington Press.

54. Leis, H. P. (1991). Prognostic parameters for breast cancer. In K. I. Bland & E. M. Copeland (Eds.), *The breast: Comprehensive management of benign and malignant disease* (pp. 331–350). Philadelphia: W. B. Saunders.

55. Lichter, A. S. (1988). The treatment of breast cancer with excision followed by radiation therapy. In J. K. Harness et al. *Breast cancer: Collaborative management* (pp. 137–156). Chelsea, MI: Lewis Publishers.

56. Lierman, L. M. (1988). Phantom breast experiences after mastectomy. *Oncology Nursing Forum, 15(1),* 41–44.

57. Lindsey, A. M., et al. (1987). Endocrine mechanism and obesity: Influences in breast cancer. *Oncology Nursing Forum, 14(2),* 47–51.

58. Link, J. S. (1993). Benign breast disease. *Nurse Practitioner Forum, 4(2),* 96–99.

59. Lippman, M. E., et al. (Eds.). (1988). *Diagnosis and management of breast cancer.* Philadelphia: W. B. Saunders.

60. London, S., et al. (1992). A prospective study of benign breast disease and the risk of breast cancer. *Journal of the American Medical Association, 267(7),* 941–944.

61. Loveys, B. J., & Klaich, K. (1991). Breast cancer: Demands of illness. *Oncology Nursing Forum, 18(1),* 75–80.

62. Mack, E. (1990). Most breast lumps aren't cancer! *RN, 53(12),* 20–23.

63. Mansel, R. E. (1988). Diagnosis and treatment of mastalgia. In S. Grundfest-Broniatowski & C. B. Esselstyn (Eds.), *Controversies in breast disease: Diagnosis and management* (pp. 63–77). New York: Marcel Dekker.

64. Mast, D. E., & Mood, D. W. (1990). Preparing patients with breast cancer for brachytherapy. *Oncology Nursing Forum, 17(2),* 267–270.

65. McGowan, K. L. (1989). Radiation therapy: Saving your patient's skin. *RN, 52(6),* 24–27.

66. McGuire, W. L. (1988). Clinical alert from the National Cancer Institute (editorial). *Breast Cancer Research and Treatment, 12(1),* 3–5.

67. Morrow, M. (1990). Management of nonpalpable breast lesions. *Principles and Practice of Oncology Updates, 4(1),* 1–11.

68. Nail, L. M., et al. (1991). *Oncology Nursing Forum, 18(5),* 883–887.

69. National Cancer Institute. (1990). *After breast cancer: A guide to follow up care* (NIH Publication No. 90–2400). Washington, DC: Author.

70. National Cancer Institute. (1990). *Mastectomy: A treatment for breast cancer* (NIH Publication No. 91–658). Washington, DC: Author.

71. National Cancer Institute. (1990). *Radiation therapy and you* (NIH Publication No. 91–2227). Washington, DC: Author.

72. National Cancer Institute. (1991). *Radiation therapy: A treatment for early stage breast cancer* (NIH Publication No. 91–659). Washington, DC: Author.

73. National Cancer Institute. (1991). *Taking time: Support for people with cancer and the people who care about them* (NIH Publication No. 91–2059). Washington, DC: Author.

74. Osborne, C. K. (1990). Prognostic factors in breast cancer. *Principles and Practice of Oncology Update, 4(3),* 1–11.

75. Osbourne, M. P., & Borgen, P. I. (1990). Role of mastectomy in breast cancer. *Surgical Clinics of North America, 70(5),* 1023–1046.

76. Osteen, R. T., & Smith, B. L. (1990). Results of conservative surgery and radiation therapy for breast cancer. *Surgical Clinics of North America, 70(5),* 1005–1021.

77. Osteen, R. T., et al. (1992). Regional differences in surgical management of breast cancer. *CA: A Journal for Clinicians, 42(1),* 39–43.

78. Page, D. L., & Simpson, J. F. (1991). Benign, high-risk, and premalignant lesions of the mamma. In K. I. Bland & E. M. Copeland (Eds.), *The breast: Comprehensive management of benign and malignant diseases* (pp. 113–134). Philadelphia: W. B. Saunders.

79. Pennisi, V. R. (1990). Long-term use of polyurethane breast prostheses: A 14-year experience. *Plastic and Reconstructive Surgery, 86(2),* 368–371.

80. Pierce, P. F. (1988). Women's experience of choice: Confronting the options for treatment of breast cancer. In J. K. Harness et al. (Eds.), *Breast cancer: Collaborative management* (pp. 273–292). Chelsea, MI: Lewis Publishers.

81. Pierce, S. M., & Harris, J. R. (1991). Role of radiation therapy in the management of primary breast cancer. *CA: A Cancer Journal for Clinicians, 41(2),* 85–96.

82. Piper, B., et al. (1989). Fatigue patterns over time in woman receiving CMF chemotherapy for breast cancer (abstract #355). *Oncology Nursing Forum, 16(Suppl.),* 217.

83. Rebner, M., et al. (1989). Breast microcalcifications after lumpectomy and radiation therapy. *Radiology, 170(3),* 691–693.

84. Rogers, K., & Coup, A. J. (1990). *Surgical pathology of the breast.* London: Wright.

85. Russell, L. C. (1989). Caffeine restriction as the initial treatment for breast pain. *Nurse Practitioner, 140(3),* 36–40.

86. Rust, D., & Kloppenborg, E. (1990). Don't underestimate the lumpectomy patient's needs. *RN, 53(3),* 58–64.

87. Schain, W. S. (1988). The sexual and intimate consequences of breast cancer treatment. *CA: A Cancer Journal for Clinicians, 38(3),* 154–161.

88. Schain, W. S. (1990). Physician-patient communication about breast cancer. *Surgical Clinics of North America, 70(4),* 917–936.

89. Schottenfeld, D. (1988). Epidemiology of the breast. In J. K. Harness et al. (Eds.), *Breast cancer: Collaborative management* (pp. 55–68). Chelsea, MI: Lewis Publishers.

90. Schover, L. R. (1991). The impact of breast cancer on sexuality, body image, and intimate relationships. *CA: A Cancer Journal for Clinicians, 41(2),* 112–120.

91. Schydlower, M. (1982). Breast masses in adolescents. *American Family Physician, 25(2),* 141–145.

92. Sheth, S. P., & Allegra, A. C. (1991). Endocrine therapy of breast cancer. In K. I. Bland & E. M. Copeland (Eds.), *The breast: Comprehensive management of benign and malignant diseases* (pp. 937–947). Philadelphia: W. B. Saunders.

93. Sorace, R. A., & Lippman, M. E. (1988). Locally advanced breast cancer. In M. E. Lippmann et al. (Eds.), *Diagnosis and management of breast cancer* (pp. 272–295). Philadelphia: W. B. Saunders.

94. Souba, W. W. (1991). Evaluation and treatment of benign breast disorders. In K. I. Bland & E. M. Copeland (Eds.), *The breast: Comprehensive management of benign and malignant diseases* (pp. 715–729). Philadelphia: W. B. Saunders.

95. Spindler, J. (1991). Seeing through the mask of cancer. *Nursing 91, 12(5),* 37–40.

96. Stoll, B. A. (Ed.). (1989). *Women at high risk for breast cancer.* Dordrecht, Netherlands: Kluwer Academic Publishers.

97. Sunderland, M. C., & McGuire, W. L. (1990). Prognostic indicators in invasive breast cancer. *Surgical Clinics of North America, 70(5),* 989–1004.

98. Walters, P. (1990). Chemo: A nurse's guide to action, administration, and side effects. *RN, 53(2),* 52–67.

99. Ward, S., & Griffin, J. (1990). Developing a test of knowledge of surgical options for breast cancer. *Cancer Nursing, 13(3),* 191–196.

100. Wellisch, D. K., et al. (1989). Psychosocial outcomes of breast cancer therapies: Lumpectomy versus mastectomy. *Psychosomatics, 30(4),* 365–373.

101. Wilson, S., & Morse, J. M. (1991). Living with a wife undergoing chemotherapy. *IMAGE: Journal for Nursing Scholarship, 23(2),* 78–84.

102. Wolmark, N. (1989). 1989: The year of adjuvant therapy in node-negative breast cancer. *Principle and Practice of Oncology Updates, 3(12),* 1–10.

UNIT 16

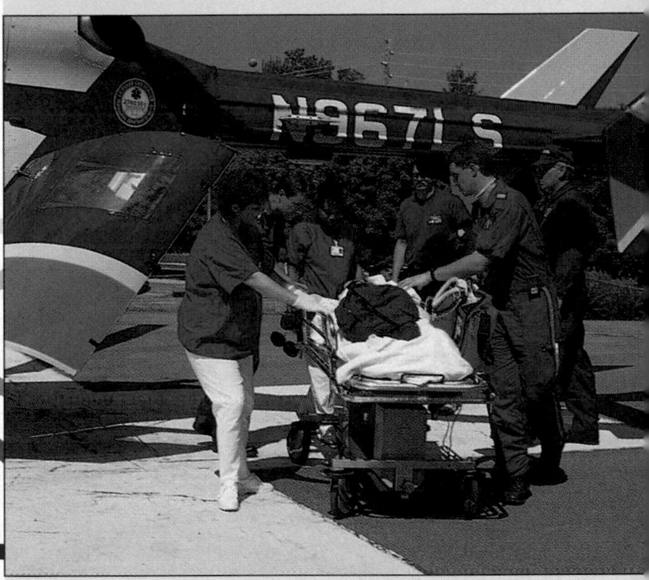

Multisystem Disorders

This final unit focuses on multisystem disorders, highlighting shock and emergency conditions. The term *multisystem* denotes that the physical and psychosocial components of several body systems may be simultaneously involved in the clinical manifestations or management of a particular disorder.

Shock, a life-threatening condition involving generalized circulatory inadequacy, ultimately affects virtually all body systems. Care focuses on restoring optimal tissue perfusion and oxygenation and interrupting the cycle of decompensation that, if uninterrupted, almost invariably results in death.

Clearly, emergency situations can involve any body system. For example, a client seen in an emergency department may have sustained a head injury, may be experiencing myocardial infarction, or may have been sexually assaulted, resulting in both physical and psychosocial injuries. The management of emergency situations revolves around setting priorities and quickly recognizing and intervening for life-threatening situations.

Chapter 56 Shock

Learning Outcomes

After completing this chapter, the learner will be able to:

1. Assess the client for clinical manifestations of hypovolemic, cardiogenic, and distributive shock.
2. Develop plans of care for the prevention and management of shock and for the rehabilitation of clients at risk for or manifesting subjective or objective data indicative of shock.
3. Implement nursing interventions that optimize the quality of life for clients in shock.
4. Evaluate planned client outcomes, using outcome criteria developed in the planning phase of care.

Shock is a complex clinical problem. It is a life-threatening condition associated with generalized circulatory inadequacy.

Shock causes thousands of deaths and unknown numbers of permanent injuries each year. Because shock is potentially lethal, it is essential that nurses be able to identify clients at risk for developing shock, recognize the early assessment findings indicating shock, and initiate prescribed therapy before shock ensues.

Identifying accurate, individualized interventions is paramount to the nursing process and to appropriate care of the client in shock. This chapter discusses three major classifications of shock: hypovolemic, cardiogenic, and distributive.

Shock is defined as inadequate tissue perfusion. Inadequate tissue perfusion can be caused by various disorders that result in decreased oxygenation at the cellular level. This inadequate oxygenation leads to an abnormal physiologic state in which there is inadequate cellular metabolism and accumulated waste products in cells. If the condition is untreated, cell and organ death occurs.

Incidence

The incidence of occurrence among the various forms of shock differs widely. Hypovolemic shock from hemorrhage or dehydration occurs most commonly and develops when the intravascular volume decreases to the point that compensatory mechanisms are unable to maintain adequate tissue perfusion and normal cellular function.

Cardiogenic shock occurs in 15 to 20 per cent of all clients following myocardial infarction (heart attack) and has at least an 80 per cent mortality rate. Cardiogenic shock resulting from direct pump failure may also be caused by cardiac arrest, ventricular dysthythmias, and cardiomyopathies, to name just a few.

Distributive shock, caused by decreased vascular volume or tone, may be neural or chemically induced. A few possible causes are spinal cord injury, pain, anesthesia, anaphylaxis, sepsis, and burns.

Etiology

The three major categories of shock, hypovolemic, cardiogenic, and distributive, are discussed in the following sections.

Risk Factors

Risk factors for the various forms of shock are numerous and varied. Any client experiencing major trauma may be at risk for hypovolemic or neurogenic shock. A client with a history of previous myocardial damage is at risk for cardiogenic shock when conditions that stress the heart occur. The client receiving immunosuppressive therapy, or the client with a disease process that impairs the immune system, is at risk for developing septic shock. Anaphylactic shock would be anticipated in a client exposed to an allergen that previously caused a significant allergy reaction.

Primary prevention is not usually an option for shock, although clients with marked sensitivity to allergens can be desensitized to reduce the risk of an allergic response.

CRITICAL TO REMEMBER

Early recognition is important in any of the shock states.

Early recognition allows earlier treatment, which will decrease the risk of complications and death.

HYPOVOLEMIC SHOCK

The primary event precipitating hypovolemic shock is a decrease in the circulating blood volume so large that the body's metabolic needs cannot be met. Conditions that may cause a reduction in the circulating volume include hemorrhage, burns, and dehydration.

Hemorrhage

Hypovolemic shock develops when there is a significant decrease in a client's intravascular blood volume. Assessment findings indicative of hypovolemic shock may begin to appear with a blood volume deficit of about 500 to 1500 mL in an adult with a normal circulating volume. Shock fully develops if a previously healthy client loses about one third of the normal circulating blood volume.

The loss of smaller amounts of blood may cause shock in clients less able to compensate rapidly (e.g., the elderly with decreased vascular tone and impaired cardiac function). The extent to which a client develops shock after blood loss also depends on the length of time over which the blood loss occurs. Clients with slow blood loss over a period of days or weeks tolerate their blood loss better than do those whose blood loss occurs rapidly over minutes or hours. Hypovolemic shock due to trauma is typically caused by hemorrhage. The classes of hemorrhage and the associated assessment findings are listed in Table 56–1.

Burns

Hypovolemic shock due to burns occurs most often in clients with large partial-thickness or full-thickness burns. It is caused primarily by a shift of plasma from the vascular space into the interstitial space or loss through the surface of the burn wound. Shock related to burns is discussed in Chapter 49.

TABLE 56–1 Management of Hypovolemic Shock

ETIOLOGY	CLINICAL SITUATION	INTERVENTION*
Blood loss	Massive trauma Gastrointestinal bleeding Ruptured aortic aneurysm Surgery Erosion of vessel due to lesion, tubes, or other devices DIC	Stop external bleeding with direct pressure, pressure dressing, tourniquet (as last resort) Decrease intra-abdominal or retroperitoneal bleeding by applying MAST suit Administer crystalloids Transfuse with fresh whole blood, packed cells, fresh frozen plasma, or platelets if significant improvement does not occur with crystalloid administration; administer crystalloids as well Use nonblood plasma expanders (albumin, hetastarch, dextran) until blood is available Autotransfusion if appropriate
Plasma loss	Burns Accumulation of intra-abdominal fluid Malnutrition Severe dermatitis DIC	Administer albumin, fresh frozen plasma, hetastarch, or dextran along with crystalloids
Crystalloid loss	Dehydration (e.g., diabetic ketoacidosis, heat exhaustion) Protracted vomiting, diarrhea Nasogastric suction	Isotonic or hypotonic saline with electrolytes as needed to maintain normal circulating volume and electrolyte balance

* Assumes that airway management and cardiac monitoring are ongoing.
DIC, disseminated intravascular coagulation; MAST, medical antishock trouser.

Other conditions that may produce fluid shifts similar to those in burns include nephrotic syndrome, severe crush injuries, starvation, and conditions causing plasma fluids to accumulate in the abdominal cavity (e.g., cirrhosis of the liver, pancreatitis, and bowel obstruction).

Dehydration

Shock may also occur from either decreased oral fluid intake or significant losses of fluid. Examples of situations in which inadequate oral fluid intake may occur are (1) rigorous exercise causing fluid loss because of both sweating and insensible fluid loss through the respiratory tract and (2) hot environments. Loss of fluid, leading to dehydration-induced hypovolemic shock, may occur in clients with excessive urine output or prolonged vomiting or diarrhea. With a prolonged fluid deficit, all compartments—intravascular, interstitial, and intracellular—are depleted.

CARDIOGENIC SHOCK

Clients with hypovolemic shock may develop cardiogenic shock. This happens because the rapid heart rate initiated to compensate for decreased volume and to increase the cardiac output does not allow time for the coronary arteries to fill with blood, decreasing the oxygen supply to the myocardium. Also, the increased heart rate increases the myocardium's need for oxygen. In addition, the decreased venous return associated with hypovolemia results in decreased coronary artery perfusion and inadequate oxygenation of the myocardium. Finally, shock results in the release of MDF and lactic acid, which decreases myocardial function.

Myocardial Infarction

Impaired heart muscle action is most often caused by myocardial infarction (see Chapter 25). The area of myocardium that normally receives blood through the coronary artery fails to receive enough blood to supply oxygen to the muscle. Necrosis and ischemia of the tissue result. This area of dead or dying tissue impairs contractility of the myocardium, and the cardiac output decreases.

Impaired myocardial contractility also occurs with traumatic cardiac contusion, cardiomyopathy, and congestive heart failure.

Clients with cardiogenic shock may also develop some degree of hypovolemic shock. This is most often caused by therapeutic use of diuretics or edema in interstitial spaces in the extremities or other dependent areas (due to inadequate cardiac pumping activity and venous congestion).

Valvular Insufficiency and Cardiac Dysrhythmias

Other causes of cardiogenic shock include valvular cardiac insufficiency resulting from trauma or disease; myocardial aneurysms (usually due to previous myocardial infarction or congenital abnormalities); rupture of a valvular papillary muscle; rupture of a ventricle; aortic stenosis; mitral regurgitation; cardiac tamponade; or cardiac dysrhythmias.

Obstructive Conditions

Mechanical obstructions to blood flow causing cardiogenic shock include a large pulmonary embolism, pericardial tamponade, and tension pneumothorax.

DISTRIBUTIVE SHOCK

Distributive shock (also sometimes called vasogenic shock) results from inadequate vascular tone. With distributive shock, the blood volume remains normal. However, the size of the vascular space increases dramatically because of massive vasodilation.

After extensive vasodilation, blood pressure, return of venous blood to the heart, and cardiac output are decreased. As with other forms of shock, tissue anoxia and cell destruction result.

The massive vasodilation present with distributive shock can be due to several major causes:

- allergic reactions (anaphylactic shock)
- loss of innervation to blood vessels (neurogenic shock)
- massive sepsis (septic shock)

Each of the three basic types of shock—hypovolemic, cardiogenic, and distributive—has a different primary cause. However, sometimes shock is caused by combinations of problems that do not fit into a single category.

The initial clinical course and initial intervention for the various primary events causing shock differ, depending on the etiologic factor. However, whereas factors that may initiate shock vary, the underlying problem is always inadequate tissue perfusion.

PATHOPHYSIOLOGY

Stages of Shock

Shock is a clinical syndrome that is usually in a constant state of flux. A client in shock may progress through various stages of the condition. These stages are termed compensated, decompensated, and progressive.

COMPENSATED STAGE

During the initial or compensated stage of shock, cardiac output is slightly decreased. The body will, however, attempt to compensate for the decreased cardiac output. During this stage, the body's compensatory mechanisms are able to maintain blood pressure (BP) within a normal to low-normal range and are able to maintain tissue perfusion to the vital organs.

During the compensatory phase, the systemic circulation and microcirculation work together. Both undergo a major readjustment in which their activities are coordinated to preserve the entire system.

Compensation occurs because decreased cardiac output causes decreased blood flow through the capillaries, which results in decreased hydrostatic pressure within the capillaries. As the hydrostatic pressure decreases to a level below that of the surrounding tissues, fluid moves from the higher pressure tissues into the lower pressure vascular system, thereby increasing circulating volume. The decreased cardiac output also stimulates the sympathetic nervous system. The vasoconstriction caused by this stimulation and the accompanying tachycardia further maintain blood pressure.

DECOMPENSATED STAGE

If shock and the compensatory vasoconstriction persist, the body begins to decompensate and the systemic circulation and microcirculation no longer work in unison. As vasoconstriction continues, the microcirculation dilates. This dilation causes decreased venous return and decreased circulation of reoxygenated blood.

Lactic acidosis occurs as a result of anaerobic metabolism from the decreased oxygen delivery, causing increased capillary permeability and relaxation of the capillary sphincters. Relaxation of the sphincters allows increased blood in the capillaries and increased capillary pressure. This increased pressure, along with the increased capillary permeability, allows fluid to move back into the tissues. In doing so, the microcirculation has reversed its pattern and is trying to secure for itself (and the tissue it supplies) more of the limited supply of available blood. Thus, the blood supply is progressively retained in the capillary bed. Because the cells demand greater perfusion time, many or most of the capillaries remain open at any one time. This increases the vascular space in the microcirculation.

Increased vascular capacity, decreased blood volume, or decreased heart action reduces the mean arterial blood pressure. In turn, the pressure gradient for the venous return of blood decreases. This also contributes to venous "pooling" of blood, decreased venous return to the heart, and decreased cardiac output.

Because there are no feedback systems within the body to change this pattern, the events become progressively more severe. Eventually, the circulation is totally disrupted. Once the vascular space enlarges (owing to vasodilation of the microcirculation), even a normal blood volume cannot fill all these small vessels and the larger ones as well. The result is a low central venous pressure and inadequate venous return to the right side of the heart, with a further decrease in cardiac output.

This resultant decrease in circulating volume and capillary flow does not allow adequate perfusion and oxygenation of the vital organs. With the prolonged decrease in capillary blood flow, the tissues become hypoxic. This process is described in Figure 56–1.

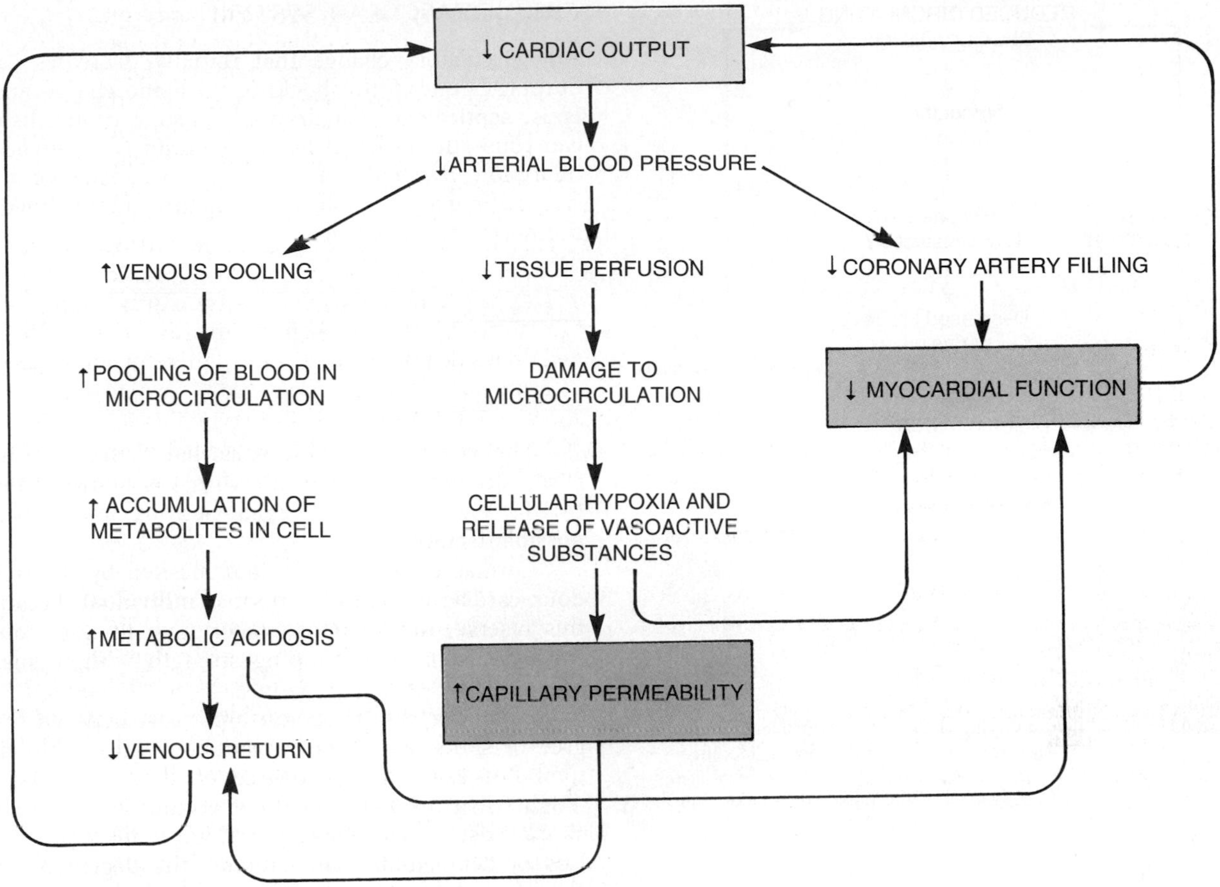

Figure 56–1
Vicious circle of events occurring in shock. The shock syndrome can be initiated anywhere in the circle, depending on the precipitating cause, e.g., impaired myocardial function due to myocardial infarction, blood loss due to trauma, or the release of vasoactive toxins due to sepsis. Hypovolemic shock resulting from blood loss, for example, results in decreased arterial blood pressure, setting in motion a cascade of events that worsen the shock state.

PROGRESSIVE STAGE

The progressive stage of shock occurs if the cycle of inadequate tissue perfusion is not interrupted. The shock state becomes progressively more severe, even though the initial cause of the shock is not increasing in severity. Cellular ischemia and necrosis lead to organ failure and death of the client.

Systemic Effects of Shock

RESPIRATORY SYSTEM

Despite many advances in shock prevention, early recognition, and management, respiratory failure continues to be a major cause of death with shock.

Respiratory Alkalosis/Acidosis. As previously emphasized, shock produces prolonged circulatory insufficiency. This leads to variable and inadequate perfusion of certain organs and tissues, particularly at the microcirculation level. Such circulatory deprivation results in tissue hypoxia and anoxia.

In response to the change in oxygenation, the rate and depth of respirations are increased. This results in respiratory alkalosis. However, the cellular hypoxia is not due to impaired gas exchange but to inadequate tissue perfusion. Therefore, the increased respiratory effort does little to correct the problem.

Hypoxia and anoxia can be tolerated for a short time. However, as the time lengthens, the chances for recovery diminish. A lack of oxygen appears to stimulate the development of the progressive stage of shock. The greater the difference between the amount of oxygen available and the amount needed, the more rapidly progressive shock develops. If sufficient oxygen is available to the cells to meet the body's needs, progressive shock is less likely to occur.

Metabolic Acidosis. To function properly, cells depend on adequate circulation to receive nutrients, electrolytes, and oxygen and to remove waste products. Oxygen and nutrients are essential to life because they make possible complex chemical transformations. Anaerobic metabolism results, producing anaerobic metabolites, such as lactic acid (which causes intracellular

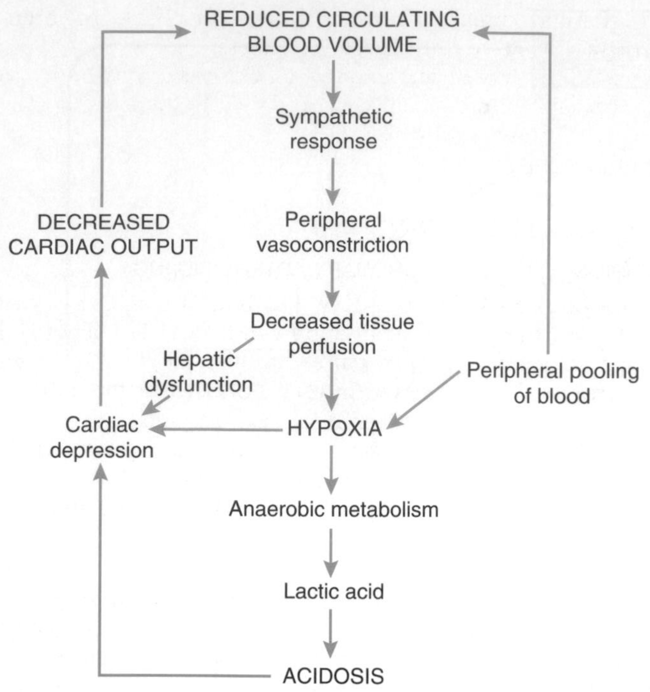

Figure 56–2
Shock leads to tissue hypoxia, with blockage of normal aerobic metabolism. Lactic acid accumulates, resulting in tissue acidosis. (Modified from Condon, R. E., & Nyhus, L. M. [1992]. *Manual of surgical therapeutics* (8th ed). Boston: Little, Brown. © by Robert E. Condon and Lloyd M. Nyhus.)

acidity with consequent cellular damage) and substrates of the adenylic acid system (Fig. 56–2).

Because lactic acid is not exhaled, it accumulates in tissue fluids. This causes them to become increasingly acidic. Eventually, metabolic acidosis is produced. During metabolic acidosis, blood pH, carbon dioxide partial pressure (PCO_2), and bicarbonate fall. Pyruvate, lactate, phosphate, and sulfate rise. Unless circulation is restored, the acidotic reaction resulting from metabolic acidosis ultimately kills the cells.

Respiratory alkalosis or respiratory acidosis (induced by pulmonary ventilatory or diffusion changes) may be superimposed on the metabolic acidosis. As perfusion and oxygen delivery to the tissues decrease, cellular energy production decreases. To compensate, cells increase anaerobic metabolism, which results in the buildup of lactic acid in the cell. As the pH of the cells decreases, lysosomes within the cell explode, releasing powerful, destructive enzymes. These enzymes destroy the cellular membrane and digest the cell contents. Once this process begins, the cellular changes are irreversible. The end result is cellular death.

Some causes of respiratory failure during shock in addition to those discussed earlier are

- Respiratory overload due to fever, infection, or metabolic acidosis
- Cerebral arterial insufficiency, which obtunds the gag and cough reflexes as well as the respiratory center sensitivity, leading to aspiration
- Stupor, coma, or aspiration of gastric contents, causing airway obstruction.

CARDIOVASCULAR SYSTEM

Any circulatory change that initially decreases cardiac output can lead to shock (e.g., hemorrhage, anaphylaxis, septicemia, dehydration). Also, various disorders can cause the heart to fail as a pump (e.g., myocardial infarction, dysrhythmias, cardiac tamponade, or a massive pulmonary embolism obstructing blood flow from the heart's right ventricle).

CRITICAL TO REMEMBER

Cardiac deterioration is one of the major causes of death from shock.

The exact cause of myocardial depression is unclear, although a polypeptide with vasoactive properties (MDF) and myocardial zonal lesions are considered possible factors.

Cardiac depression is often masked by the tremendous cardiac reserve of a normal individual. Because of this reserve, the heart can deteriorate to less than one third of its normal pumping strength without measurable evidence of cardiac failure.

Blood Factors. Relationships exist between the degree of shock and derangements in various blood factors. For example, the degree of shock is more than "slight" if a third of the blood volume is lost. "Severe" shock exists when half of the blood volume is lost. The loss of hemoglobin also parallels the degree of shock. However, the percentage of hemoglobin loss is typically greater than the blood volume loss.

Coagulation. During shock, hypoxia of tissues results from the slow movement of blood in the capillaries. Anaerobic metabolism begins, increasing the production of lactic acid. The slow-moving acid blood is hypercoagulable; however, it will not actually coagulate unless some clot-initiating factor is present. Such factors include bacterial toxins and thromboplastin of red blood cells (liberated by hemolysis). Hemolysis (destruction of red blood cells with the liberation of hemoglobin) accompanies trauma, especially when massive crushing injury occurs. When any of these factors is present, along with the stagnant, acidic blood of shock, widespread intravascular clotting (called disseminated intravascular coagulation [DIC]) may occur in the vessels.

This DIC is associated with multiple thrombi or emboli that are deposited in the microvascular circulation, with resultant organ obstruction and increased tissue ischemia. As blood attempts to flow through partially obstructed vessels, widespread hemolysis may occur. When red blood cells are destroyed, hemoglobin is liberated. Anemia occurs because the liberated hemoglobin is excreted by the kidneys.

As DIC progresses, clotting factors are depleted, causing an inability for normal clot formation in the presence of hemorrhage. Treatment of the precipitating cause and anticoagulant therapy need to be started as soon as possible for maximal effectiveness. DIC is a serious complication of shock and can be fatal.

Carbon Dioxide. Sluggish circulation also results in decreased removal of carbon dioxide (CO_2) from the tissues. Increased CO_2 dilates arterioles located in active tissues and constricts those in nonactive tissues. Because of the heart's increased activity, excessive CO_2 is produced in the myocardium. This directly dilates the coronary arteries leading to the myocardium, which allows the myocardium to receive more arterial blood. CO_2 is also a powerful stimulant of the vasoconstrictor center in the sympathetic nervous system. With vasoconstriction of nonactive tissues, blood is shunted to the more active tissues.

Enzymes. Lysosomal enzymes are released in dead cells undergoing autolysis. They are also released by the liver just before cell death due to cellular anoxia or some other form of injury. This is one mechanism of cell destruction resulting from prolonged shock. The presence of hepatic lysosomal active enzymes in the bloodstream, along with blocking of the reticuloendothelial system (RES), may contribute to death from shock. Blockade of the RES drastically reduces its capacity to clear bacteria from the bloodstream.

Lysosomal enzymes become most active in an acid pH range. During shock, the accompanying metabolic acidosis accelerates the activation of these enzymes in hypoxic tissues.

The activation of lysosomal hydrolases within the cells and their release into the circulation markedly exacerbate the tissue injury that occurs during shock. The release of active lysosomal proteases and other enzymes from damaged tissue into the bloodstream and their action on extracellular and intracellular structures probably contribute to the progression of injury from cell to cell.

Vasoactive Substances. Vasoactive substances are highly variable in promoting vasoconstriction or vasodilation in a client experiencing shock. The influence they exert may be altered by factors such as pH, specific tissue (e.g., heart, lung), presence of drugs or other substances, serum electrolyte levels, and sensitivity of the end organ.

Catecholamines. Epinephrine and norepinephrine are present early in shock. Their general effects are to increase blood flow to the brain, heart, and striated (skeletal) muscle and to decrease blood flow to the skin, kidneys, and splanchnic bed. Sustained vasoconstriction contributes to stagnant hypoxia and cellular death.

Histamine. Histamine causes vasodilation, increased capillary permeability, bronchoconstriction, coronary vasodilation, and cutaneous reactions (flares, wheals). The effects of histamine are especially obvious in anaphylactic and septic shock.

Vasoactive Polypeptides. Bradykinin, angiotensin, and MDF are among the more important vasoactive polypeptides that appear to play significant roles in shock

- *Bradykinin* is known to produce vasodilation, increased capillary permeability, smooth-muscle relaxation, pain, and infiltration of an area with leukocytes. Kinins appear to be most active in late shock.
- *Angiotensin* results from the action of renal renin on angiotensinogen. This potent substance causes vasoconstriction and increased vascular resistance. Although similar to norepinephrine in effect, angiotensin may have fewer negative effects.
- *MDF* is a vasoactive polypeptide that contributes to cardiac failure in clients in shock by depressing cardiac muscle contraction.

NEUROENDOCRINE SYSTEM

Neuroendocrine responses during shock are defensive reactions that occur during the body's stage of resistance in the general adaptation syndrome. The length of the stage of resistance varies among clients and is determined by a body's ability to compensate for its deficiencies. Hence, one client may be able to combat shock longer than another. For example, a previously healthy client may have a longer stage of resistance against shock than will a client who is debilitated before shock develops.

Adrenal Response. Some basic features of the neuroendocrine responses are (1) the release of epinephrine and norepinephrine from the adrenal medulla, which results in increased respiratory and heart rates, increased BP, increased blood flow to organs, and decreased blood flow to peripheral tissues; and (2) the release of mineralocorticoids and glucocorticoids.

Increased production of adrenocortical mineralocorticoid hormones occurs. The main mineralocorticoids, aldosterone and desoxycorticosterone, help to increase intravascular fluid volume by stimulating the kidneys to retain sodium and hence water. The renal tubular conservation of sodium occurs with any type of fluid loss or blood volume depletion. Aldosterone is essential in this conservation of sodium. Because water is retained in the body along with sodium, urine excretion is diminished during shock. This fluid is retained in the bloodstream in an effort to increase the blood volume. Increasing the volume of blood in this way is aimed at increasing venous return, cardiac output, and blood pressure.

Pituitary Response. The blood's osmolality (osmotic concentration) increases with dehydration. This stimulates osmoreceptors in the hypothalamus to release antidiuretic hormone from the posterior pituitary gland. The release of antidiuretic hormone causes the kidneys to conserve water.

The sympathoadrenal response to a major stressor is illustrated in Figure 56–3.

Metabolic Response. Generally, the hormonal response to stress rapidly provides fuel for the body's various tissues, organs, and systems. These fuels (e.g., amino acids, fatty acids, glucose, sodium, and water) are produced by the breakdown of food into sugars, fatty acids, and amino acids. Chemical conversion of these fuels into energy results in adenosine triphosphate, which is the main source of energy produced and used inside the body's cells.

The glucocorticoids, particularly hydrocortisone, mobilize energy stores. During the initial phase of shock, the body's small stores of available carbohydrate are rapidly depleted. Then it becomes necessary to mobilize protein and fat stores to meet the body's energy requirements. Protein catabolism and negative nitrogen

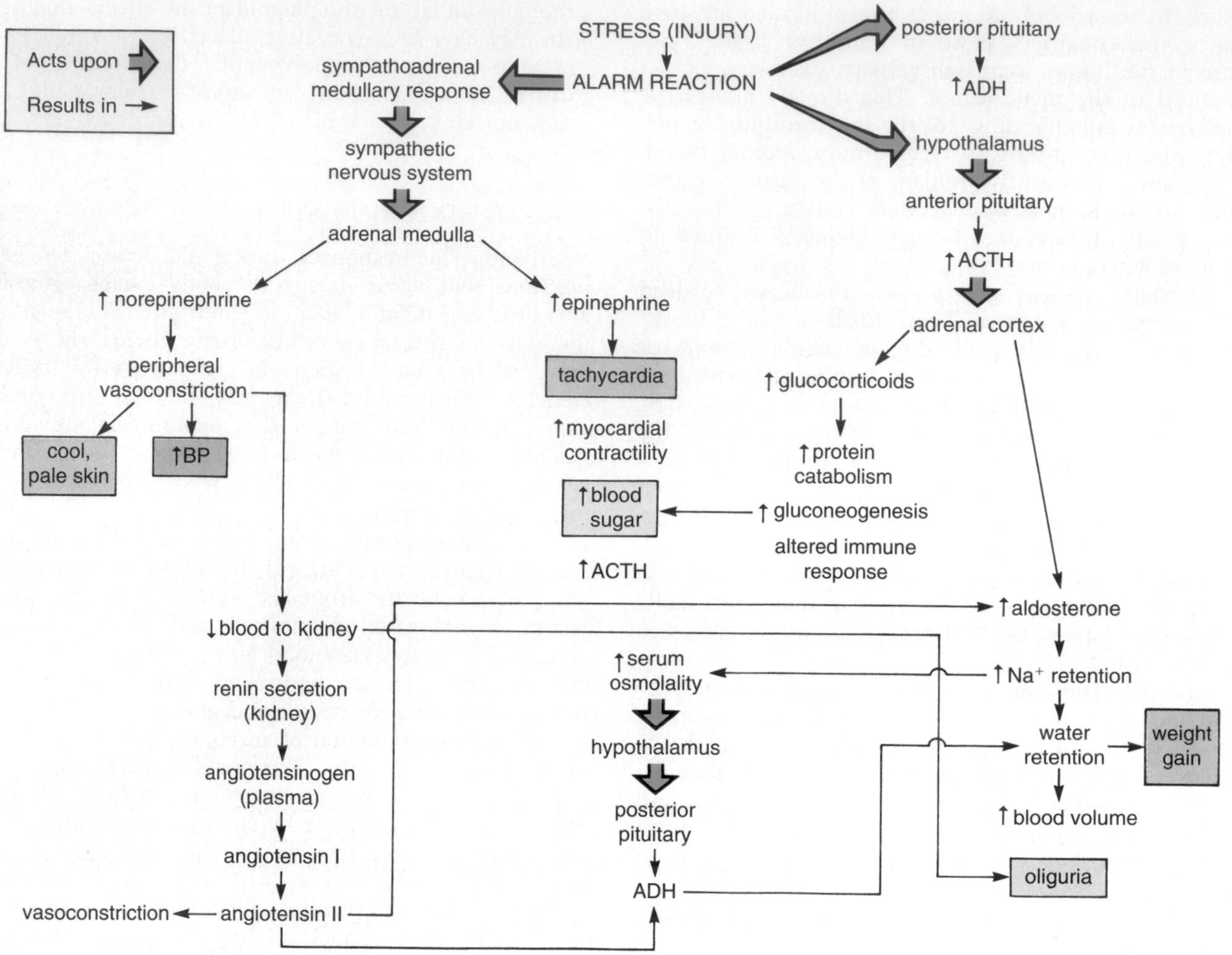

Figure 56–3
Components of the sympathoadrenal response to a major stressor. Readily observed clinical signs as well as laboratory values are indicated by boxes. ACTH, adrenocorticotropic hormone; ADH, antidiuretic hormone; BP, blood pressure.

balance occur as part of the metabolic response, because of gluconeogenesis and starvation.

Neurologic Response. With shock, cerebral blood flow and thereby cerebral metabolism may become insufficient to maintain normal mental functioning and level of consciousness. Brain cells are highly sensitive to a shortage of oxygen and glucose. When the brain becomes hypoxic, the cerebral vessels dilate to restore blood flow. Likewise, blood is diverted to the brain from the other less vital organs.

IMMUNE SYSTEM

All forms of shock severely depress the RES and antibacterial defense mechanisms. The capacity of the RES to remove bacteria and the constantly formed endotoxins from the bloodstream is greatly reduced. Alterations occur in immunologic factors circulating in the bloodstream.

Alterations in the blood itself are partially due to tissue hypoxia and impairment of monitoring activities of the RES. Indeed, the stasis, sludging, tendency to venular thrombosis, impaired capillary permeability, and subnormal vascular reactivity that occur during shock can all be traced to RES dysfunction.

Toxic Agents. The impaired ability of the RES to ward off toxic agents is critical. Reduced blood flow through the intestines during shock impairs the vitality of intestinal tissue so extensively that bacterial products from the intestines gain access to the bloodstream. Further compounding the problem is the fact that the client in a state of shock is more susceptible than normal to bacterial products, particularly bacterial endotoxins.

GASTROINTESTINAL SYSTEM

Because various tissues have differing oxygen requirements, some organs are irreversibly damaged before other tissues reach a stage of destruction. Microcirculatory failure appears greater in abdominal visceral tissues. Yet, even there the changes are not uniform.

Biliary (Liver) Function. Shock causes serious changes in functions of the liver and the intestines. The visceral (splanchnic area) blood vessels are those most strongly constricted by reflex sympathetic nervous system activity and by vasopressor agents. Thus, visceral circulation is highly susceptible to the dangerous effects of prolonged vasoconstriction during shock. The liver and intestines both suffer from this impaired circulation and appear to be sources of toxic materials.

Normally, the liver protectively traps and disposes of toxic materials that are products of bacterial enzyme actions. During shock, the anoxic liver develops metabolic deficiencies and, probably, an impaired ability to detoxify.

The liver plays a key role in visceral circulation. During shock, pooling of blood occurs in the visceral area. Pooling of blood in the liver and portal bed may occur from masses of agglutinated (clotted) blood plugging numerous small hepatic vessels, sinusoids, and intrahepatic radicles of the portal vein and hepatic artery. A prolonged, extreme resistance to portal blood flow may lead to stagnation of blood in the portal system. This presumably results in the backing up of blood into the vessels of the intestines, adding to mucosal congestion and pooling of blood within intestinal capillaries.

The depressed protective action of the RES permits the release of bacterial endotoxins (e.g., *Escherichia coli, Brucella melitensis*). These agents seem to destroy the integrity of the microcirculation.

Gastrointestinal Function. Gastrointestinal changes now appear to have a more vital role in the progression of shock than was previously thought. The submucosa of the intestine becomes ischemic early in shock. If the period of congestion and subsequent stagnant anoxia is prolonged, actual tissue necrosis and loss of integrity of intestinal mucosa occur. The intestinal arterioles and venules seem highly susceptible to the extensive vasoconstriction that occurs during shock. The massive amount of tissue destruction within the intestines that results from vasoconstriction and tissue anoxia is sufficient to cause death even if bacteria are not present. Bacteria and their toxins contribute to shock by escaping into the systemic circulation because of destruction of the intestinal mucosa barrier.

RENAL SYSTEM

Urinary Production and Circulation. Adequate urine output indicates adequate circulation even if the arterial blood pressure is below normal.

During shock, urine output should be measured and compared with normal urine production. The normal rate of urine excretion from the kidneys is 1 mL/min, or 60 mL/hr. A client who becomes acutely hypovolemic or is experiencing a redistribution of circulating volume cannot maintain an hourly output of 40 to 60 mL of urine. Decreased urine output (oliguria) typically occurs in shock. Often during shock, the urine output may stop completely (anuria). When this occurs, the client is said to be in renal shutdown or renal failure.

Capillary Blood Pressure and Glomerular Filtration. Glomerular filtration within the kidneys depends on the pressure at which the blood is circulating through the glomerular capillaries.

During shock, when the blood volume and blood pressure decline steadily, glomerular filtrate is progressively reduced. Because it cannot be excreted by the kidneys, sodium, along with the water, leaves the body through the sweat glands. Damaged kidneys lose their crucial ability to regulate electrolyte and acid-base balance.

Inadequate perfusion of renal capillaries is believed to be the cause of early renal failure in shock. Later, if shock persists, actual renal shutdown occurs from focal tubular necrosis. Unfortunately, vasoconstriction in the kidneys may continue for a long time after the systemic blood pressure is restored to normal levels.

Renal Ischemia. The kidneys may suffer from renal ischemia during shock because microcirculatory failure targets abdominal visceral tissues. When injury to the kidneys is extensive and renal failure ensues, tubular necrosis occurs. With appropriate intervention, including careful fluid administration, the kidneys can repair this condition. Normal kidney function returns after 10 to 14 days.

Oliguria does not contraindicate the administration of large volumes of fluid in the treatment of shock. In fact, restoring renal capillary perfusion along with that of other vital capillaries restores urine volume production as long as tubular necrosis is not already present. Indeed, fluid administration may prevent renal tubular necrosis.

A large amount of tissue damage (e.g., crush injuries) may cause a release of myoglobin from muscle tissue. Because the myoglobin molecule is large, a type of mechanical renal failure may result from attempts to excrete large amounts of the myoglobin.

CLINICAL MANIFESTATIONS

General Signs and Symptoms of Shock

Because the body is made up of many cells, which may function or malfunction at different stages of metabolic impairment, shock causes many diverse signs and symptoms. Subjective complaints are usually nonspecific and may not be particularly helpful to the clinician who is attempting diagnosis and treatment. The individual may report feeling sick, weak, cold, hot, nauseated, dizzy, confused, afraid, thirsty, and short of breath. Observable and measurable signs and symptoms are often conflicting in nature. BP, cardiac output, and urinary output are usually, but not always, decreased. Respiratory rate is usually increased. Variable indicators of shock include alterations of heart rate, core body temperature, skin temperature, systemic vascular resistance, and skin color. Dyspnea, diaphoresis, and altered sensorium may be present.

CRITICAL TO REMEMBER

Early recognition of shock is vitally important. Treatment may become very difficult if shock is not suspected or recognized until the development of overt hypotension, cyanosis, and a clammy, cold skin.

The classic signs and symptoms of hypovolemic shock are illustrated in Clinical Manifestations: Hypovolemic Shock. Assessment findings caused by other types of shock are similar to these; however, specific symptoms of other forms of shock are also discussed.

RESPIRATORY

Rapid respirations (tachypnea) typically occur during shock owing to decreased tissue perfusion. The respiratory rate increases as the blood's oxygen-carrying capacity decreases. Also, the respiratory rate increases because the accumulation of excessive amounts of CO_2 stimulates the respiratory center. As discussed earlier, tachypnea results in respiratory alkalosis.

CARDIOVASCULAR

Pulse. Generally, the pulse rate increases (tachycardia) in shock from increased sympathetic stimulation. This occurs in the body's attempt to maintain adequate cardiac output.

In addition to being increased, the pulse is typically weak and thready. Serial observations of the pulse rate over a period of time are highly useful to (1) assess the client's condition and the direction of the shock state

CLINICAL MANIFESTATIONS

Hypovolemic Shock

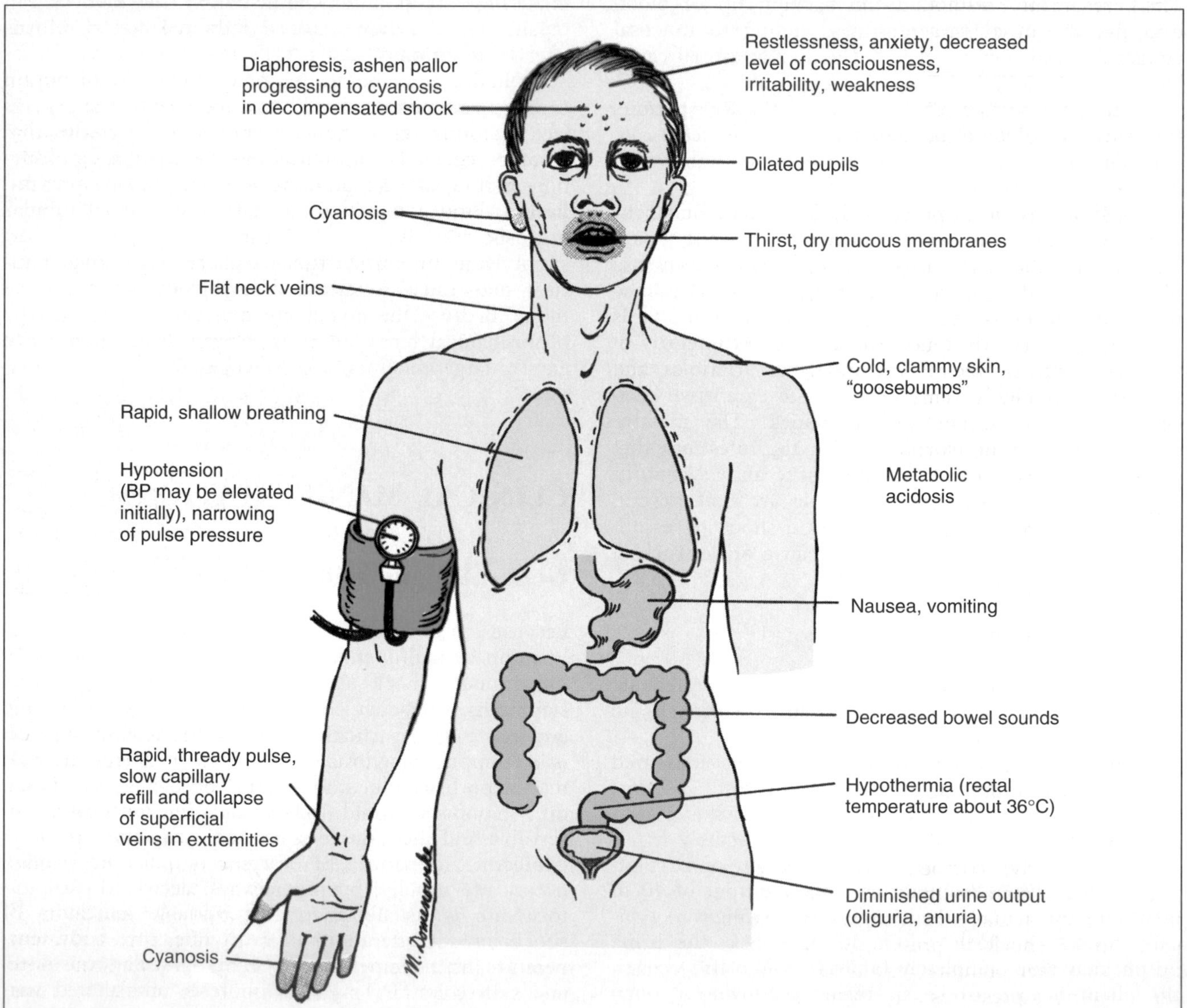

and (2) evaluate the effectiveness of intervention. Elderly clients (with and without various degrees of heart block) are an exception to this. Their heart rates may show little change in spite of the presence of conditions causing circulatory failure (e.g., hemorrhage).

Blood Pressure. The BP relates inversely to the heart rate. Thus, a decreased BP is accompanied by an increased heart rate. The systolic BP indicates the integrity of the cardiac mechanism, the arteries, and the arterioles. The diastolic BP indicates the resistance of blood vessels. The amount of peripheral resistance (or vasoconstriction) is indicated by the level of the diastolic BP.

When the diastolic BP falls significantly, vasoconstriction is being lost as a compensatory mechanism. When vasoconstriction is replaced by marked vasodilation, there is no resistance to the blood flow, and adequate BP is difficult to maintain.

Usually, the BP begins to fall when the total blood volume is decreased by about 15 to 20 per cent. However, some people lose as much as 25 per cent of their total blood volume without showing a fall in BP. This is especially true in young adults.

CRITICAL TO REMEMBER

In young adults, falling BP is a *very* late sign of shock.

Typically, as shock progresses, the systolic and diastolic BPs drop—the systolic pressure dropping more than the diastolic. The pulse pressure also falls, because it is equal to the difference between the systolic and diastolic blood pressures.

During shock, the pulse pressure is actually more significant than is the BP, because it tends to parallel the cardiac stroke volume. The pulse pressure is affected by stroke volume and peripheral resistance. In shock, the pulse pressure may decrease even in the presence of an acceptable systolic BP. This may provide a clue to worsening of the shock. In shock, the pulse pressure is often less than 20 mm Hg.

CRITICAL TO REMEMBER

To supply the myocardium with blood, a minimal systolic BP of 60 to 70 mm Hg is necessary. In interpreting BP readings, the nurse needs to know what the client's BP was previously. When a client is in a supine position, a decline in BP may be a late finding. It is important to note that hypotension by itself (without other abnormal assessment findings) is not shock.

In the early, compensated stages of shock, BP changes are generally unreliable because the arterial pressure may actually be normal or slightly elevated even though shock is present. In fact, blood volume deficits of a liter or more may occur even though arterial and venous pressures are normal or elevated.

When severe vasoconstriction is present, the BP may be normal even though the circulation is actually highly inadequate. Also, conversely, the blood flow may be adequate even though the BP is decreased (e.g., because of mechanisms such as vasodilation).

Valuable information about the level of arterial pressure in vasoconstricted clients can be gained by assessing the strength of the femoral pulses.

Level of Consciousness. Early in shock, hyperactivity of the sympathetic nervous system with increased secretion of epinephrine usually causes the client to feel anxious, nervous, and irritable.

Assessment findings associated with lack of blood to the brain are determined by the suddenness with which the shock develops and by its severity. With sudden, severe shock, the body may not have time to initiate its compensatory adjustment mechanisms. Consequently, the brain is deprived of its blood supply. The client may feel dizzy and faint on sitting up from a horizontal position. Fainting and unconsciousness may occur. If shock develops gradually over a period of hours, early assessment findings may include apathy and confusion, or the opposite, restlessness and unusual alertness.

The systolic BP is important in maintaining blood flow to the brain. Usually, a decrease in systolic BP is accompanied by a reduced flow of blood to the brain. However, the brain's vessels, like those of the heart, are not constricted by the vasoconstrictor center in the medulla oblongata. Thus, blood from the peripheral vessels can be shifted to the brain as an emergency compensatory measure.

A client's level of consciousness decreases as circulation to brain tissue becomes increasingly impaired. Confusion, agitation, and restlessness may occur.

CRITICAL TO REMEMBER

In trauma situations, restlessness can be mistaken for pain. When this happens, if narcotics are given, the client's situation may be worsened.

In decompensated shock, apathy may ensue. Drowsiness and stupor are more likely to occur in shock related to severe infection than in shock caused by trauma and hemorrhage. Ultimately, a comatose condition may be reached.

RENAL

A decreased urine volume often is the earliest sign of developing shock. It may occur even while the arterial BP and pulse remain stable. Urine output is one of the most sensitive indices in shock. However, it should be kept in mind that any form of shock that develops very rapidly (e.g., due to trauma) shows other symptoms before decreased urine output is noticed.

Urine output should be kept above 0.5 mL/kg/hr. If the hourly output diminishes significantly, treatment must be instituted to prevent renal failure. Urine flow of less than 20 mL/hr can cause acute tubular necrosis from inadequate renal circulation.

Signs and Symptoms of Specific Types of Shock

All forms of shock have altered cardiac output and altered tissue perfusion. The mechanism by which these occur may be different. The following is a discussion of some clinical manifestations for each type of shock.

HYPOVOLEMIC

Sympathetic nervous stimulation results in decreased tissue perfusion to the skin, causing the skin to feel cool and clammy and to appear pale. In later stages, diaphoresis occurs because of reduced aldosterone secretion. When aldosterone secretion is decreased, sodium can no longer be retained in the body. Consequently, water cannot be retained, and it leaves the body via the sweat glands.

Cyanosis may indicate either decreased tissue perfusion or decreased oxygenation or both. Cyanosis is a late sign of decreased oxygenation and should not be the principal defining characteristic for diagnosis of decreased oxygenation in any form of shock.

Initially, urine osmolality and specific gravity increase because of sodium and water reabsorption, which attempts to support circulating volume. As altered tissue perfusion and the hypovolemic shock progress, urine osmolality and specific gravity decrease owing to the kidneys' inability to reabsorb sodium and water.

CARDIOGENIC

As in hypovolemic shock, there is stimulation of the sympathetic nervous system due to decreased cardiac output and decreased blood pressure. The sympathetic nervous system causes decreased tissue perfusion to the skin and all of its resultant clinical manifestations.

Because of the impaired muscle action or mechanical obstruction that caused the cardiogenic shock, blood is inadequately pumped through the heart. This results in a "back-up" of blood. When the shock is due to right-sided heart failure, this "back-up" will be evidenced as jugular venous distention.

DISTRIBUTIVE

Anaphylactic. Initially, the client may complain of a vague feeling of uneasiness or a feeling of impending doom. The massive vasodilation that occurs with anaphylaxis may cause complaints of headache as well. This may be followed by severe anxiety, dizziness, disorientation, and loss of consciousness.

Respiratory involvement may be manifested through a variety of symptoms. The initial complaint may be of feeling as though there were a lump in the throat. This is due to laryngeal edema and is followed by hoarseness, coughing, dyspnea, and stridor. Diffuse wheezes and prolonged expiratory phase are heard on auscultation.

Additional complaints may include pruritus and urticaria. Direct observation may also demonstrate edema of the eyelids, lips, or tongue (angioedema).

Neurogenic. In neurogenic shock, interruption or loss of sympathetic innervation is experienced. The result is abnormal distribution of fluid volume. Clinical manifestations of neurogenic shock are basically the same as those for shock in general. Some exceptions are related to heart rate, BP, skin temperature, and skin moisture. Because of loss of sympathetic control, the client experiences bradycardia and hypotension. Below the level of injury, skin temperature takes on the same temperature as the room (poikilothermia). There is also an inability to sweat, so skin feels dry to the touch.

Septic. Several signs and symptoms resulting from septic shock may be misleading, making early detection difficult. Increased permeability of the vasculature permits plasma to seep out of vessels into tissues. Even though a client may be hypovolemic, peripheral edema manifests the picture of fluid overload. Release of cytotoxins produces fever in most but not all individuals and is one of the earliest signs of septic shock. Those who do not develop a fever (the elderly or immunosuppressed clients) have a grave prognosis. Systemic vascular resistance and blood pressure are lowered owing to generalized vasodilatation. These changes may give the impression of adequate tissue perfusion. Neutrophils gather at the site of inflammation to destroy the infecting organism, when the complement system is stimulated. Because the inflammation is so overwhelming, neutrophil aggregation occludes the microvasculature, damaging the endothelium and causing fibrin and platelet clumping. Other more complex factors follow, leading to tissue ischemia.

Diagnostic Assessment

Assessment of respiratory status can be accomplished to some degree by noninvasive procedures. Spirometry measures tidal volume and minute volume. A pulse oximeter assesses arterial oxygen saturation. Corneal oxygen sensors may also be used to assess arterial oxygen saturation. The pulse oximeter does not replace arterial blood gas analysis, which provides information about alveolar oxygen tension (PaO_2), alveolar carbon dioxide tension ($PaCO_2$), and pH. However, it may be valuable in determining when arterial blood gases are needed.

The $PaCO_2$ is measured by arterial blood gas analysis for determining whether the metabolic acidosis that occurs with shock is being effectively combated by hyperventilation. It will also be important to monitor PaO_2 levels to determine whether the client is being adequately oxygenated. (See Chap. 20 for discussion of therapeutic respiratory interventions.)

Central venous pressure (CVP) measurement is one of the first invasive assessments made in the presence of shock. CVP is an important means of estimating fluid loss.

Other noninvasive assessment and monitoring tools are the cardiac monitor and the 12-lead electrocardiogram. Laboratory studies include a complete blood count and chemistries. Other specific studies, such as blood alcohol levels, may be indicated for certain clients.

MEDICAL MANAGEMENT

Treatment should generally be instituted for shock whenever at least two of the following three conditions occur:

- systolic BP of 80 mm Hg or less
- pulse pressure of 20 mm Hg or less
- pulse rate of 120 or more

Methods for treating inadequate tissue perfusion vary according to the specific cause of a client's shock state. Thus, assessment and an accurate differential medical diagnosis, which establish the specific cause of the shock state, form the basis for treatment. The differential medical diagnosis is usually readily made unless the shock is in an advanced stage, in which several specific forms of shock may exist at the same time. Some forms of shock that are usually easily recognized are hypovolemic shock due to extensive burns and cardiogenic shock with severe chest pain and electrocardiographic readings indicating acute myocardial infarction. Septic shock is probably the most difficult shock diagnosis to make because of its insidious onset and confusing symptoms.

Management of the client in shock largely depends on the stage of shock, cause of the shock, and resources available for care. The emphasis here is on treatment of hypovolemic shock, with occasional reference to other forms of shock.

The primary aim in treating shock is to increase tissue perfusion. Unless this is accomplished early, subsequent therapeutic measures are of no avail, and death can be anticipated. Identifying and managing the cause of shock is part of the process in achieving a satisfactory outcome.

Emphasis is placed on adequate fluid resuscitation, positions that do not interfere with pulmonary ventilation, and the use of medications that have both vasoconstrictor and vasodilator effects.

As with many other areas of clinical care, clear-cut and final answers concerning the treatment of shock cannot be presented. As with any care, the nurse must recognize that intervention for shock is individualized and follow specific physician prescriptions or agency guidelines. The management of the client in shock is presented as collaborative management in this section. Nursing management is discussed later in the chapter.

Of central importance in current shock intervention is establishing and maintaining an adequate circulating blood volume. In addition, other treatment adjuncts are necessary. The adjuncts facilitate the distribution of blood to the body and enhance the perfusion and oxygenation of the tissues with the circulating blood.

During shock intervention, all of the basic pathophysiologic changes associated with the development of shock must be corrected. Characteristically, impaired tissue perfusion is correctable during early shock. Before a client's shock state is viewed as probably irreversible, the following therapies must have been attempted:

- Restoration of circulating volume
- Identification and treatment of occult bleeding
- Identification and treatment of any factors interfering with cardiopulmonary functioning
- Identification and treatment of overwhelming infection

Treating the Shock

Treatment modalities discussed in the following pages can be divided into two major categories: (1) those used to treat the shock state itself and (2) those used to prevent or treat complications of shock through early symptom intervention.

RESPIRATORY SUPPORT

A client in shock must be assessed immediately to ascertain that the airway is open and functioning. If necessary, the caregiver must ensure ventilation by resuscitation. Circulatory improvement depends on adequate respiratory function. By increasing the rate of pulmonary ventilation (through spontaneous or mechanical hyperventilation), it is possible to compensate for minor degrees of metabolic acidosis. This increased "blowing off" of carbon dioxide with hyperventilation restores acid-base balance.

Endotracheal intubation or tracheostomy may be performed to rest an exhausted client during severe or prolonged shock and to correct respiratory failure.

In all types of shock, regardless of cause, supplemental oxygen is administered to protect against hypoxemia. Oxygen can be delivered via nasal cannula, mask, high-flow non-rebreathing mask, endotracheal tube, or tracheostomy tube.

For the prevention or treatment of hypoxia, positive end-expiratory pressure may be added when the client is being mechanically ventilated. This assists in preventing atelectasis and provides a higher PaO_2 for the client at a lower oxygen concentration setting.

In addition to the respiratory support measures mentioned, nursing care also includes vigorous pulmonary hygiene and chest physical therapy, including vibration, percussion, and postural drainage.

Sometimes the interventions discussed cannot establish optimal tissue oxygenation. In these instances, hyperbaric oxygenation or extracorporeal membrane oxygenation may be used.

CIRCULATORY ASSIST DEVICES

Mechanical devices that assist circulation or decrease the heart's workload are commonly used as temporary measures in managing clients in shock. Examples of these include the military or medical antishock trouser (MAST suit), intra-aortic balloon pump, and external counterpulsation device. (See Chap. 24 for more information.)

Intra-aortic Balloon Pump (IABP). An IABP is used primarily for individuals with cardiogenic shock and after open heart surgery. The heart's ability to pump blood adequately is augmented by a balloon-tipped catheter placed in the descending thoracic aorta. Details of the IABP are found in Chapter 24.

External Counterpulsation Device. This device uses the same general principles as an IABP but is applied externally to the legs. The legs are encased in air-filled or water-filled tubular bags connected to a pumping unit. Pressure is applied to the legs during diastole and is released in systole.

POSITIONING

A client in shock is usually positioned in a modified shock position with the lower extremities elevated about 45 degrees, knees straight, trunk horizontal or very slightly raised, and neck comfortably positioned with the head level with the chest or slightly higher. This position promotes increased venous return from the lower extremities without compressing the abdominal organs against the diaphragm.

Elevating the legs mobilizes blood that has pooled in the lower extremities. As a result of gravity, the additional circulating blood increases venous return to the heart, thus improving cardiac output. The position is of temporary value in moderate hypovolemia. However, it does not help severe hypovolemia because the extremities have very little blood in them in such a state. Generally, the modified shock position is not used with cardiogenic shock, when there is already circulatory overload.

FLUID THERAPY

All forms of shock involve a decreased effective circulating blood volume.

The mainstay of hypovolemic shock therapy is expansion of circulating blood volume by intravenous administration of blood or other appropriate fluids. Fluid replacement should be administered through large-bore peripheral lines, central venous lines, or both.

Various fluids are given to correct specific problems, such as electrolyte or protein deficiencies or other defects of the blood. However, in treating hypovolemic shock, the immediate results of therapy seem to depend less on the type of fluid administered for fluid replacement than on the amount of fluid administered. Generally, enough fluid is given to exceed the normal blood volume. In part, this "extra" fluid is required because the vascular space is expanded owing to dilation of the microcirculation. Additional fluid is also administered to replace intracellular fluid that was mobilized into the circulation as an early response to the hypovolemia.

In replacing fluids, enough volume must be administered to fill the client's capillaries and run through into the veins. Such fluid replacement maintains the central venous pressure and provides an adequate venous return to the heart. This promotes additional cardiac output. In addition, adequate fluid replacement decreases the blood catecholamine level and thus produces a vasodilation that promotes capillary flow. Adequate flow of fluids in the capillaries in turn perfuses tissues and prevents sludging and coagulation of blood within the vessels.

CRITICAL TO REMEMBER

The nurse must carefully monitor intravenous fluid replacement therapy to prevent circulatory overload. Hypervolemia can be lethal.

Intravenous fluids used in shock management may include crystalloids or balanced salt solutions, colloids, and blood.

Crystalloid or Balanced Salt Solutions. During hypovolemic shock, the loss of circulating blood volume is associated with redistribution of extravascular fluid. Thus, a sizable amount of fluid (about 4 L in moderately severe shock) leaves the interstitial space. This is in addition to fluid lost from the circulating volume. Thus, fluid replacement therapy must replace both blood lost from the circulation and fluid lost from the interstitial space. For a client's estimated blood loss, three times the crystalloid must be administered to volume-resuscitate the person adequately. Crystalloid solutions that may be administered include normal saline, Ringer's lactate, half-normal saline, or 5 per cent dextrose in water (D_5W).

Electrolyte solutions such as Ringer's lactate or saline buffered with bicarbonate help expand extracellular volume, reduce viscosity, and prevent sludging. It is thought, however, that a solution containing lactate might further compound the problem of lactic acidosis.

Abnormalities of electrolyte and acid-base balance are corrected with the specific substance needed. Therapy is gauged by serial arterial blood gas and electrolyte determinations.

Colloid Solutions. Colloid solutions contain molecules large enough to remain in the general circulation. These solutions are used in treating hypovolemic shock when crystalloid solutions fail to maintain an adequate circulating volume. The most commonly used colloid solutions include plasma and its components, plasma substitutes (e.g., dextran), oxygen-carrying solutions other than blood (e.g., perfluorocarbons) and hetastarch. (See discussions of blood and blood transfusions, Chap. 28.)

Plasma is sometimes used in treating clients with low serum protein levels in an effort to control fluid escape from the vascular system. Fresh frozen plasma is the form commonly used to improve serum protein levels. Fresh frozen plasma can be administered after massive transfusions to restore some clotting factors deficient in "banked" blood. Fresh frozen plasma requires 15 to 30 minutes to thaw. Hence, it is not used in initial fluid resuscitation with shock.

Albumin may also be used to achieve adequate osmotic pressure. Occasionally, it is administered when sufficient amounts of other fluids fail to restore an adequate circulating volume. Use of albumin is controversial because it may move into the pulmonary interstitial space, drawing water along with it. Thus, albumin may contribute to the development of adult respiratory distress syndrome.

Dextran may be used in both high- and low-molecular-weight forms. The advantage in using dextran is that it contains large size molecules that should effectively and rapidly expand the intravascular volume.

CRITICAL TO REMEMBER

Dextran can interfere with blood type and crossmatch procedures and with clotting factors.

It should, therefore, be used only after type and crossmatch have been done and until blood is available for transfusion.

New substances have recently been introduced for shock management. Perfluorocarbons such as Fluosol-DA are nonblood, oxygen-carrying solutions that remain in the circulation for about 12 to 24 hours. Major problems associated with use of perfluorocarbons relate to limited immediate availability (the product must be stored frozen) and accumulation of the chemicals in the body. A significant advantage is that Fluosol-DA is acceptable to clients whose religious beliefs prohibit the use of blood products. Fluorocarbons are largely experimental at this time. Hetastarch is another solution with limited use as a volume expander in shock situations.

Blood. When hemorrhage is the primary cause of shock, the rapid administration of large volumes of packed cells may be necessary. Type-specific, crossmatched blood is the most desirable form of blood replacement. However, if the client is hemorrhaging, it may be necessary to administer type-specific, uncrossmatched blood; O-negative blood; or O-positive, low–antibody titer blood.

When shock resulting from hemorrhage is treated, crystalloid is usually given as an initial emergency treatment to sustain blood pressure. Later, the acute anemia resulting from the hemorrhage must be corrected by administration of packed cells for prevention of hypoxemia.

During fluid replacement, a normal red blood cell mass should be maintained. Fluids given in excess of normal volume should be fluids other than blood so that they can be easily removed from the circulation by the kidneys once the shock is corrected. If the normal red blood cell mass is exceeded, it is difficult for the body to get rid of the excess red blood cells after the vascular volume contracts to normal (after adequate perfusion of tissues with blood is achieved).

Autotransfusion. Autotransfusion involves collecting and retransfusing blood into the same client. Autotransfusion is commonly used in the prevention or treatment of existing hypovolemic shock due to hemorrhage.

As mentioned earlier, the volume of fluid given generally exceeds estimates of blood or fluid loss or volume deficit. Sometimes up to 8 to 12 L fluid may be administered in only a few hours.

Often, fluid replacement is the only treatment required for shock. However, it is difficult to evaluate whether fluid replacement is adequate.

Internal losses of circulating fluid volume, including whole blood, into areas of traumatized tissue, infection, and so forth are difficult to estimate. If a vasoconstrictor drug has been administered or if prolonged vasoconstriction occurs, an additional considerable loss of circulating volume may also occur owing to vasoconstriction. Large volumes of intravenous fluid may be administered either until systemic blood pressure, urine volume, and lactate levels become relatively normal or until central venous or pulmonary artery pressures, or both, elevate.

Infusion of blood or other fluids usually continues only as long as the CVP is low, that is, below 10 cm H_2O or 2 mm Hg. Some clients have a normal or low CVP in spite of faulty left ventricular function. They readily develop congestive failure or pulmonary edema. Thus, a low or normal CVP does not always mean that fluid administration is advisable.

Intravenous fluid administration should be stopped before extremely high elevations of pulmonary artery pressure occur if there is an adequate systemic response.

PHARMACOLOGIC MANAGEMENT

Unfortunately, the management of shock easily lapses into treating the client's BP rather than promoting tissue perfusion. Because shock is a complex syndrome with differing causes, various medications may be used.

Vasoactive Medications. As their name implies, vasoactive medications affect blood vessels. Included in this discussion of vasoactive medications are vasoconstrictors, vasodilators, and combination vasoconstrictor-vasodilator medications.

Opinion differs about the use of vasoconstrictors and vasodilators in treating shock. In general, vasoconstrictors increase peripheral resistance, whereas vasodilators decrease peripheral resistance, allowing greater blood flow in tissues.

Vasoconstrictors. Vasoconstrictors elevate the systemic blood pressure. However, the excessive vasoconstriction they cause may actually impede rather than enhance tissue perfusion.

Whereas the use of vasoconstrictors during shock is being critically evaluated, they do favorably increase blood flow to the brain and heart. This may particularly benefit elderly clients who cannot tolerate prolonged, severe hypotension because of arteriosclerotic narrowing of their coronary or cerebral arteries.

Vasoconstrictor agents may be used briefly in shock if compensatory vasoconstriction is unable to maintain blood flow to vital organs. They may also be used to correct hypotension secondary to vasoconstrictor nerve paralysis, as in spinal anesthesia or conditions associated with massive vasodilation. However, vasoconstricting agents should not be used exclusively but should be given concomitantly with intravenous fluids in an attempt to restore adequate circulation and perfusion.

Perfusion of vital organs with blood is impossible when systolic BP is below 50 mm Hg. Usually, the goal of using vasoconstrictors is to achieve and maintain a mean BP of 70 to 80 mm Hg. This maintains a BP level sufficient to perfuse tissues. Generally, attempts to increase the BP beyond this level are not advisable because vasoconstrictors increase the heart's oxygen demand and may cause fatal dysrhythmias.

Major adverse effects of vasoconstrictors include

- Increased myocardial oxygen consumption
- Ventricular dysrhythmias

- Decreased blood flow to kidneys and splanchnic area
- Excessive or sudden rise in arterial BP
- Overloading of the vascular system, because vasoconstricting medications must be diluted before administration
- Pulmonary edema or left ventricular decompensation
- Gangrene of the fingers and toes from prolonged vasoconstriction

The nurse must carefully monitor arterial blood pressure during vasoconstrictor administration, watching for undesirable BP elevations. Carefully adjust intravenous flow to establish and maintain the desired blood pressure. Inspect intravenous sites frequently for evidence of infiltration.

Vasodilators. Agents that induce vasodilation or inhibit vasoconstriction may promote recovery from shock. These include adrenergic blocking agents, ganglionic blocking agents, and direct-acting peripheral vasodilators.

Adrenergic blockade prevents the following harmful effects of prolonged vasoconstriction in shock: increased capillary pressure and decreased blood flow to the splanchnic area, resulting in a decreased exchange of metabolites with tissue cells and a buildup of waste products. Not only does adrenergic blockade prevent these changes in circulation, it may also induce opposite beneficial changes.

Vasodilators may be helpful during shock when vasoconstriction is severe and persistent. Vasodilators may be administered to try to inhibit vasoconstriction so the blood can be redistributed. That is, blood trapped peripherally would become available to enhance tissue perfusion, and the vascular volume increases.

Vasodilation, after an adequate circulating blood volume is restored, may improve capillary flow, tissue perfusion, and cellular metabolism, increasing the client's chances of survival. When shock is caused by hypovolemia, rapid and adequate fluid replacement is essential before vasodilators are used. Vasodilators are dangerous because they lower arterial blood pressure if they are given while circulating blood volume is deficient. This is because while the circulating blood volume is inadequate, the body depends on vasoconstriction to try to maintain arterial pressure. However, when the vascular space is full and cardiac venous return is adequate, vasodilation should open arterioles in the lungs and elsewhere. This lets blood circulate, increasing cardiac output and capillary perfusion without lowering systemic blood pressure. In fact, a vasodilator may produce a dramatic, sustained rise in the systemic arterial pressure.

The nurse should continually monitor blood pressure and CVP when vasodilator drugs are being used. Usually, a mean blood pressure of 70 mm Hg is acceptable. However, if abrupt severe hypotension occurs, administration of the vasodilator is generally stopped and fluid administration increased.

Central venous pressure drops substantially if peripheral resistance markedly decreases. Blood volume needs to be expanded as the vascular space enlarges, and CVP measurements are used to determine the amount of fluid needed to fill the enlarging vascular space. It is serious if the CVP continues to fall in spite of fluid replacement. This means that the rate and volume of fluid replacement are not sufficient to meet the client's physiologic needs.

CRITICAL TO REMEMBER

Clients who are receiving vasodilators should be kept lying relatively flat. Elevation of the head could produce dangerous orthostatic hypotension.

Older clients may have sclerotic blood vessels and may not tolerate the hypotension that may accompany administration of vasodilators. In this situation, a cardiogenic drug (such as dobutamine) may be given with the vasodilator to increase cardiac output. This helps maintain or raise the blood pressure.

Vasoconstrictor medications are sometimes given in combination with vasodilator medications. This may be done to offset the profound effects that may occur with some vasoconstrictors. This may also be done to provide the benefits both types of drugs have to offer.

Other Medications. Included in this section are antibiotics, heparin, steroids, calcium, histamine H_2-receptor antagonists, naloxone, diphenhydramine hydrochloride (Benadryl), narcotics, and cardiotonic medications.

Antibiotics. Antibiotics are essential when shock is caused by infection. If septic shock is suspected, a blood specimen for culture and sensitivity is taken at once, and broad-spectrum antibiotics are started even though the specific infectious organism has not yet been identified. When the blood sample is drawn, samples of urine, sputum, and fluid from draining wounds, sinuses, and so forth are also taken for culture. The antibiotic selected depends on the cause of the infection treatment and should not be initiated until after all cultures have been taken.

Heparin. The anticoagulant effect of heparin may help prevent or treat some complications of shock. Heparin may be used in treating myocardial infarction because of the tendency for small thrombi to form on or near large areas of infarction. These can move and cause systemic emboli. Heparin is also used because of the prolonged immobility often associated with shock. The treatment of DIC may include heparin administration to minimize consumption of clotting factors. Also, heparin may be appropriate for people with adult respiratory distress syndrome if the primary cause of the respiratory insufficiency is believed to be from DIC or massive microembolism.

Steroids. Steroids may be given during shock intervention. Glucocorticoids (e.g., cortisone, hydrocortisone) have an established place in treating some types of shock.

The precise action of steroids is unknown. However, some possible actions include

- Antitoxic effect. In treating shock, steroids may counteract the detrimental effects of gram-negative endotoxins. Steroids may help mobilize the inactive pools of venous blood that reduce cardiac output in toxic shock. If administered early, steroids may improve the survival rate of clients with septic shock.

- Antiplatelet aggregating effect; may help minimize pulmonary damage associated with shock.
- Stabilizing lysosomal membrane and preventing intracellular release of enzymes.
- Increasing blood volume by increasing sodium retention.
- Cardiotonic (e.g., increased cardiac output) as well as vascular effects. Glucocorticoids may counteract the reduced cardiac output and the increased total resistance to blood flow that are the basic hemodynamic problems with shock. Thus, they may be administered for shock to increase blood flow and decrease blood resistance, augmenting the beneficial effects of vasoconstricting medications. In large doses, glucocorticoids may promote a more adequate blood pressure level as a result of improved systemic blood flow. When they are used, it is recommended that glucocorticoids be given early rather than as a last resort.

Some physicians give steroids in combination with vasoconstricting medications to treat shock. Steroids may help clients with protracted hypotension associated with severe allergic (hypersensitivity) reactions.

Complications may accompany steroid therapy in the high dosage ranges used in treating shock.

Calcium. Calcium is needed for normal functioning of the nervous and cardiovascular systems and for blood clotting. The value and dosages of calcium in treating shock are not clear. However, calcium may be administered if impaired cardiac function is evident.

Calcium may precipitate toxic effects in a person who has received digitalis. It is given only with extreme caution to such a person.

Calcium chloride should be given intravenously only. Calcium gluconate may be given intramuscularly but is very irritating to tissues. Whereas calcium chloride and calcium gluconate are both available as 10 per cent solutions, they are not identical in concentration. One should not be substituted for the other.

Indications of hypocalcemia may be subtle. Careful assessment is essential. (See discussions of calcium in Chap. 3.)

Histamine H_2-Receptor Antagonists. Cimetidine, famotidine, and ranitidine are histamine H_2-receptor antagonists, which inhibit gastric acid secretion. Any of them may be administered to a client experiencing shock for preventing stress ulcers, which are often lethal complications of severe illness or injury. They are commonly given intravenously to the client in shock and may be prescribed in combination with oral antacids.

Naloxone (Narcan). This opiate antagonist is commonly used to treat narcotic and synthetic narcotic overdosages. During stress, opiate-like substances known as enkephalins and endorphins are released from the brain. Although the mechanisms of action are not clear, endorphins may play a role in capillary bed vasodilation found in all forms of shock.

Diphenhydramine Hydrochloride (Benadryl). Anaphylaxis or less severe allergic reactions are treated with this antihistamine. This medication acts primarily to relieve symptoms associated with anaphylaxis rather than to stop the release of histamine. Therefore, epinephrine is always administered first in treating anaphylaxis.

Narcotics. The need for pain relief may be obvious in clients experiencing different types of shock. However, the use of narcotics for pain management may unfortunately be dangerous for them. Narcotics interfere with vasoconstriction, and vasoconstriction may be the only way the client's blood pressure is being maintained.

Morphine sulfate, however, causes pooling of blood in the extremities and contributes to the decrease of anxiety. These effects may prove useful for the client in cardiogenic shock.

CRITICAL TO REMEMBER

Do not administer narcotics to a client suffering from acute, multiple trauma without first knowing that the blood volume is adequate.

Narcotic administration causes vasodilation, which results in severe hypotension or shock. Also, if a narcotic is administered intramuscularly to a client in shock, it may not be completely absorbed because of the vasoconstriction that is present. Then, because the client experiences little or no pain relief, a second injection may be given. Once fluid resuscitation is complete and the circulating volume is restored, the client may absorb both doses of the narcotic and go back into shock.

CRITICAL TO REMEMBER

No one in shock should be given intramuscular medications.

When narcotics are appropriate for a client in shock, they are most effective if administered intravenously in small doses. When caring for trauma victims, especially those with massive injury, the nurse should remember that the extent of the injury does not necessarily coincide with the amount of pain being experienced. Careful assessment is necessary once narcotic administration seems safe (in terms of the client's hemodynamic status). The nurse should assess the client's blood pressure more closely after the intravenous administration of narcotics to watch for hypotension.

When caring for clients experiencing shock, the nurse should carefully make diagnoses concerning pain and impaired gas exchange. Restlessness is an assessment finding common to both and can thus be easily misinterpreted. Too often, clients who are restless, especially trauma victims, are given narcotics because their behavior is incorrectly interpreted as resulting from pain. However, the restlessness frequently is actually due to hypoxia, and narcotics worsen the problem. The decision to administer narcotics is often a nursing decision. It is important to assess the need for these medications carefully. Attention to positioning, splinting of injured areas, breathing techniques, and comfort measures may provide safer and more effective pain relief than narcotics will.

Cardiotonic Medications. Medications that improve myocardial contraction are basic in treating those forms of shock that decrease cardiac output (e.g., hypovolemic shock and cardiogenic shock.

- *Digitalis* is often used if there is evidence of cardiac failure. By strengthening and slowing the heart beat, digitalis supports a weakened heart and may reduce the heart rate to a more normal level. It is not given to clients who are already digitalized.
- *Lidocaine, bretyllium, quinidine,* and *procainamide* may treat dysrhythmias that tend to reduce cardiac efficiency. However, these medications do reduce myocardial contractility.
- *Atropine* may treat bradycardias, which predispose clients to cardiogenic shock.

RENAL SUPPORT

Impaired kidney function and acute renal tubular necrosis may result from inadequate renal tissue perfusion as discussed earlier. In an attempt to prevent acute renal damage, the urine output is monitored with an indwelling catheter, and diuretics (e.g., furosemide) may be given. Correcting metabolic acidosis and using other measures to increase blood volume and improve cardiac output also benefit the kidney as well as other tissues. If tubular necrosis is present, peritoneal dialysis or hemodialysis may be needed until regeneration of functioning renal tubular epithelium occurs. (Chap. 31 discusses management of renal disorders in detail.)

THERMOREGULATION

CRITICAL TO REMEMBER

Even though a person in shock may feel cold and may be hypothermic, heat should not be applied to the skin.

Heat application dilates peripheral blood vessels and draws blood away from the vital organs (where it is life-sustaining) into the vessels of the skin. This interferes with the body's initial compensatory mechanism of peripheral vasoconstriction. Also, heat increases the body's metabolism. In turn, this increases the need for oxygen and puts an added strain on the heart.

This does not mean that the person is kept in a cold environment. The environment is kept warm because it is important that the person not become chilled. Chilling and shivering require energy expenditure needed to maintain vital functions. Also, chilling contributes to sludging of blood in the microcirculation. Hypothermia slows the heart, increases the likelihood of ventricular fibrillation, and inhibits the body's reparative processes.

NASOGASTRIC SUCTION

An early physiologic response to shock is a decrease in splanchnic circulation. This reduces blood supply to the stomach and bowel, causing inadequate gastrointestinal tissue perfusion and delayed gastric emptying; thus, vomiting with aspiration of gastric contents into the lung may develop. For this reason and for diagnostic purposes, nasogastric suction is often used during treatment for shock. Continuous suction is used rather than intermittent suction.

The nurse should assess gastric aspirate periodically for blood. Guaiac solution or Hemoccult tablets and reagent check for blood; litmus paper checks the pH to determine the acidity of the stomach. New findings of blood or increases in the amount of blood should be reported promptly. Antacids are commonly instilled through the tube when the pH is acidic in an attempt to minimize the formation of stress ulcers.

It is a nursing responsibility to maintain proper nasogastric suction and to irrigate the tube as prescribed. Periodic assessment of the client's pulmonary system is essential.

The medical management of shock has been discussed in general. Tables 56–1, 56–2, and 56–3 identify some of the specific interventions for hypovolemic, cardiogenic, and distributive shock.

Nursing Management

Assessment

Because a client's condition can change rapidly in shock, frequent nursing assessment is essential. Documentation of progress and response to intervention needs to be concise yet convey the client's status minute by minute.

Noninvasive Techniques: Because nurses often provide health care in settings other than hospitals, it helps to know about assessment and monitoring techniques that do not require sophisticated machinery or invade body tissues or cavities. These noninvasive techniques can be performed rapidly and relatively easily, and they require little equipment and are readily observable.

The first step in assessing a person in shock is a general overview, giving attention as necessary to the ABCs—airway, breathing, and circulation. Once the airway is patent, air exchange is adequate, a pulse is present, and the cervical spine is immobilized (if it is a trauma situation), the nurse performs a rapid, cursory initial head-to-toe physical assessment. The initial assessment goal is to identify major problems and gross abnormalities. Further, detailed attention should be given to specific injuries or problems after shock is stabilized.

With the use of physical assessment skills, the following observations should be made:

- Airway patent; presence of noisy respirations, obstructions
- Breathing; respiratory rate and effort
- Circulation; pulse present; skin color and temperature
- Level of consciousness; orientation ×4 (i.e., person, place, time, and self); ability to move extremities, sensation in all extremities; hand-grasps; response to verbal and painful stimuli; pupil size and reaction to

TABLE 56–2 Management of Cardiogenic Shock

ETIOLOGY	CLINICAL SITUATION	INTERVENTION*
Myocardial disease or injury	Acute myocardial infarction Myocardial contusion Cardiomyopathies	Fluid challenge with up to 300 mL of normal saline solution or Ringer's lactate to rule out hypovolemia, unless congestive failure or pulmonary edema is present Insert CVP or pulmonary artery catheter, monitor cardiac output, pulmonary artery pressure, and pulmonary capillary wedge pressure; administer intravenous fluids to maintain left ventricular filling pressure of 15–20 mm Hg Administer dopamine or dobutamine Vasodilators (e.g., sodium nitroprusside) Diuretics (e.g., mannitol or furosemide) Cardiotonics (e.g., digitalis) Glucocorticosteroids† Rotating tourniquets if pulmonary edema present (rarely done) Intra-aortic balloon pump or external counterpulsation device if unresponsive to other therapies
Valvular disease or injury	Ruptured aortic cusp Ruptured papillary muscle Ball thrombus	Same as above: if rapid response does not occur, provide for prompt cardiac surgery
External pressure on the heart interferes with heart filling or emptying	Pericardial tamponade due to trauma, aneurysm, cardiac surgery, pericarditis	Relieve tamponade with ECG-assisted pericardiocentesis; repair surgically if it recurs
	Massive pulmonary embolus	Thrombolytic (streptokinase) or anticoagulant (heparin) therapy
	Tension pneumothorax	Relieve air accumulation with needle thoracostomy or chest tube insertion
Cardiac dysrhythmias	Tachyarrhythmias Bradyarrhythmias Electromechanical dissociation	Treat dysrhythmias; be prepared to initiate CPR, cardiac pacing

* Assumes that airway management and cardiac monitoring are ongoing.
† Controversial.
CPR, cardiopulmonary resuscitation; CVP, central venous pressure; ECG, electrocardiogram.

light; presence of abnormal posturing; and so on to evaluate neurologic function
- State of hydration and perfusion of the skin (e.g., capillary refill time < 3 seconds); condition of mucous membranes, sclera, and conjunctiva; presence of pallor or cyanosis
- Fullness of neck veins, which may suggest cardiogenic shock
- Position of trachea; tracheal deviation may indicate tension pneumothorax
- Respiratory pattern; chest wall expansion; chest wall bulges or defects
- Heart sounds
- Presence and location of pain
- Abdominal sounds, distention, rigidity
- Circumference of abdomen or extremities
- Peripheral pulses
- Presence of lacerations, contusions, ecchymosis, petechiae, purpura (also check for bruising over flank area)
- Bone deformities
- Presence of medical alert tags or bracelets

After potentially life-threatening problems are treated, the nurse takes complete vital signs. It is important to take postural vital signs if it is safe to do so. The nurse should not take postural vital signs if the client has multiple traumatic injuries; if there is evidence of vertebral, pelvic, or femoral fracture; or if hypotension already exists. Clients with postural hypotension should not be sent to the x-ray department for upright films until they are adequately volume resuscitated. If the x-ray films must be taken, clients require constant attendance by a nurse who monitors vital signs, administers intravenous fluids if necessary, and provides guidance to x-ray department personnel regarding movement, positioning, and timing of studies.

Measurement of postural vital signs is indicated under the following circumstances:

- History or presence of significant blood loss
- Unexplained tachycardia
- History of fluid loss (e.g., diarrhea, vomiting, diuretic therapy, or third space loss)
- Unexplained syncope
- Blunt chest or abdominal trauma
- Abdominal pain
- Unexplained hypotension

Alternative Methods of Obtaining Blood Pressure. Often when a client is in shock it is difficult to

TABLE 56-3 Management of Distributive Shock

ETIOLOGY	CLINICAL SETTING	INTERVENTION*
Anaphylactic shock	Allergy to food, medicines, dyes, insect bites, or stings	Prepare for surgical management of the airway Decrease further absorption of antigen (e.g., stop intravenous fluid, place tourniquet between injection/sting site and heart if feasible) Epinephrine (1 : 1000) 0.3–0.5 mL given intramuscularly, sublingually, or by inhalation, or 0.01 mg/kg *or* Epinephrine (1 : 10,000) 0.5–10 mL given intravenously slowly over 5–10 minutes Intravenous fluid resuscitation with isotonic solution MAST suit may be useful Diphenhydramine hydrochloride 50–100 mg intramuscularly Aminophylline intravenous drip for bronchospasm Steroids Vasopressors (e.g., norepinephrine, metaraminol bitartrate, high-dosage dopamine) Gastric lavage for ingested antigen Ice pack to injection or sting site Meat tenderizer paste to sting site
Septic shock	Often gram-negative septicemia but also caused by other organisms in debilitated, immunodeficient, or chronically ill clients	Identify origin of sepsis Apply MAST suit Vigorous intravenous fluid resuscitation with normal saline, D_5W, or colloids Antibiotic therapy: in initial phase, until sensitivities are reported, broad-spectrum coverage may include a combination of penicillin, aminoglycoside, and clindamycin or chloramphenicol Dopamine or dobutamine, norepinephrine, metaraminol bitartrate, isoproterenol, digitalis, calcium Naloxone Diphenhydramine hydrochloride Steroids (dexamethasone, methylprednisolone) Temperature control (both hypothermia and hyperthermia are noted) Heparin if DIC develops
Neurogenic (spinal) shock	Spinal anesthesia Spinal cord injury	Treat bradycardia with atropine Vasopressors (e.g., norepinephrine, metaraminol bitartrate, high-dosage dopamine, and phenylephrine may be given
Vasovagal reaction	Severe pain Severe emotional stress	Place client in a head-down or recumbent position Give atropine if bradycardia and profound hypotension; eliminate pain

* Assumes airway management and cardiac monitoring are ongoing.
DIC, disseminated intravascular coagulation; D_5W, 5 per cent dextrose in water; MAST, medical antishock trousers.

hear the BP with a standard stethoscope. Two commonly used techniques to obtain BP measurements are palpation of radial or brachial pulse during deflation of the BP cuff and use of a Doppler instrument. When palpation is used, the first palpable pulse noted during deflation of the cuff is the systolic BP. The BP is documented as such (e.g., 90/palp).

For clarity and accuracy, the nurse documents the method by which BP readings are taken (in addition to the readings themselves) and if palpation or a Doppler monitor is used. This is important because these readings may be higher or lower than those obtained in the standard way with a cuff and stethoscope. Likewise, the nurse should document whether readings are obtained by automatic BP machines even though readings from these machines may not differ from those taken in the standard way.

Direct measurement of arterial BP by use of an arterial line often is done during shock. Discussion of arterial lines is found in Chapter 24.

An accurate core temperature measurement is important in assessing a person in shock. Sometimes an indwelling flexible rectal probe connected to a continuous display monitor is more accurate and less traumatic than are intermittent rectal temperature measurements with a standard thermometer. Core temperature can also be obtained if the client has a thermodilution (Swan-Ganz) catheter in place.

Oral temperature measurement is not accurate or safe. During shock, the buccal mucosa is poorly perfused, and the client should be receiving oxygen by mask or nasal prongs.

For assessment and evaluation purposes, electrical activity of the heart needs to be continuously monitored in all clients in shock, regardless of age. Nurses caring for clients experiencing shock need to be able to initiate cardiac monitoring, recognize cardiac dysrhythmias, and initiate treatment for any potentially lethal dysrhythmias that occur (see Chap. 25).

Invasive Techniques: Hemodynamic Monitoring. Measurement of the CVP is one hemodynamic technique that may be used in initial shock management, especially with hypovolemic shock. However, because the CVP is of limited value, peripheral intra-arterial lines or a pulmonary artery catheter is inserted as soon as possible. Peripheral arterial catheters are commonly used in shock to measure arterial BP and mean arterial pressure and to obtain blood samples for chemical and blood gas analysis. These catheters are usually placed in the radial and brachial arteries. Pulmonary artery and pulmonary capillary wedge pressure measurements are monitored to assess left-sided heart function and to guide fluid administration. These pressures are measured through a Swan-Ganz catheter.

Cardiac Output Monitoring. Cardiac output, measured in liters per minute, is the amount of blood pumped by the left ventricle into the aorta each minute. During shock, cardiac output may be decreased because of myocardial damage resulting from a myocardial infarction or, in hypovolemic shock, from inadequate volume replacement.

Because of the widespread use of Swan-Ganz catheters and the ease of performing measurements, cardiac outputs are used in managing all types of shock. These measurements assess overall cardiac function and function of the heart's left ventricle. Factors that may alter cardiac output include heart rate, peripheral resistance, age, body size, exercise, and (in persons with cardiac problems) decreased filling or emptying of the left ventricle.

Cardiac index is the cardiac output divided by the body surface area. Cardiac output as a separate reading does not take into account the amount of tissue that needs to be perfused. By figuring body size into the calculation, a more accurate assessment is obtained.

Urine Output Monitoring. An indwelling urinary catheter is a simple means of monitoring a client during shock. Continuously measuring urine flow provides important information about peripheral blood flow and kidney function. Because the amount of urine excreted during shock is often very small, it is important to have an accurate, calibrated urine collector. In some settings, the catheter may be attached to a urimeter collector or to a more complex electric urimeter.

Urine volume changes can be highly important as an index of the success or failure of therapy. Minimal or absent urine output indicates that treatment is not successful. Increasing urine output is a favorable sign. The nurse should assess the client's urine output routinely and record it at least every hour.

Nursing Diagnosis, Planning, and Implementation

Nursing Diagnosis: Some potential nursing diagnoses for the client in shock are listed in Table 56–4.

TABLE 56–4 Potential Nursing Diagnoses for a Client in Shock

Airway Clearance, Ineffective
Breathing Pattern, Ineffective
Gas Exchange, Impaired
Tissue Perfusion, Altered: cerebral, cardiopulmonary, renal, gastrointestinal, peripheral
Decreased Cardiac Output
Fluid Volume Deficit
Nutrition: Less than Body Requirements, Altered
Constipation
Activity Intolerance
Physical Mobility, Impaired
Injury, Risk for
Sensory/Perceptual Alterations: visual, auditory, kinesthetic, gustatory, tactile
Sleep Pattern Disturbance
Skin Integrity, Impaired
Skin Integrity, Risk for Impaired
Self-Care Deficit: feeding, bathing/hygiene, dressing/grooming, toileting
Body Image Disturbance
Self-Esteem Disturbance
Role Performance, Altered
Personal Identity Disturbance
Anxiety
Fear
Pain
Communication, Impaired Verbal
Spiritual Distress (distress of the human spirit)
Thought Processes, Altered
Family Coping: Compromised, Ineffective
Family Processes, Altered
Grieving, Anticipatory

Planning: Expected Outcomes. Nursing care of the client with shock is complex. Frequent reassessment of the client and nursing activities is essential because the client's status often changes rapidly. Specific nursing and medical interventions vary according to individual needs and the setting in which care is delivered (e.g., emergency room versus intensive care unit). However, four major outcomes of care are desired:

- Tissue perfusion and cellular function return to normal
- Metabolic demands are met
- Further injury is prevented
- Coping of the client and significant others is effective

Implementation. Other nursing considerations in caring for clients in shock include

- Continuous assessment for cardiovascular and respiratory changes. These changes can occur rapidly, and intervention must be promptly adjusted accordingly. Observations should be documented clearly and concisely.
- Helping the client (and significant others) to feel physically and emotionally comfortable. For the client in shock, this helps reduce the physical need for oxygen and nutrients and promotes rest.
- Facilitating the expression of concerns and questions by the client and significant others. For example, the nurse should try to reduce the client's fears and anxieties about what is happening and about the equipment being used.
- Keeping equipment and supplies (e.g., suction, emergency drugs) available and in working order.
- Implementing appropriate, planned nursing interventions to prevent complications that can develop from enforced immobilization.

- Providing adequate pain relief, because pain intensifies shock. This intervention should be based on careful assessment.

A client in shock is extremely ill and may die. In addition, the stress of the situation is compounded by emergency medical treatment with all the people, equipment, and movement this entails.

The nurse must keep the client's significant others informed of what is happening. They need information on which to base decisions. Because of their anxiety, the nurse may need to calmly repeat information several times, remembering that the client and significant others may be experiencing "psychological shock." Often they need (and greatly appreciate) opportunities to discuss with care providers their important concerns.

Loved ones should not be kept away from the client unnecessarily. There may be times when, because of limited space, they have to wait in another room for a while. However, they should not be kept away long. They should not be asked to leave their loved one without being given a reasonable explanation of why it is necessary.

A client experiencing shock requires emotional support. When caught up in the sudden drama of an emergency or critical care, health professionals sometimes forget that the experience and setting are often new and very frightening for the client. Unfortunately, "dehumanization" of the client may occasionally occur during the rush of emergency treatment. Whether a client appears to be conscious or not, the nurse should always explain what is happening. The nurse should keep the atmosphere as quiet and orderly as possible and eliminate unnecessary chatter. Commonly, recovered clients remember hearing what was said and were aware of what happened to them even though they seemed unconscious.

Evaluation

The expected outcomes should be evaluated frequently; revisions in the plan of care may be required hourly to maintain tissue perfusion.

STUDY QUESTIONS

1. A client with a history of myocardial infarction is admitted to the hospital for diagnostic tests. His admitting vital signs are: pulse 96 and blood pressure 122/66 (His blood pressure was 148/86 on his last admission and his pulse was 88.) He states that his doctor has ordered nitroglycerin 0.5 mg SL every 5 minutes for chest pain. Several hours after admission, he calls to tell the nurse he is having chest pain. He requires 3 nitroglycerin tablets over 15 minutes. Which of the following early signs of cariogenic shock should you expect the client to exhibit?
   A. Pulse of 90
   B. Blood pressure lower than 122/66
   C. Blood pressure higher than 122/66
   D. Temperature of 102° F, orally
2. When planning care for clients experiencing cardiogenic and/or hypovolemic shock, the nurse should write nursing orders that include monitoring for which of the following?
   A. Full and bounding peripheral pulses
   B. Urinary output of less than 20 mL per hour
   C. Decreased respiratory rate
   D. Capillary refill of less than 3 seconds
3. The primary goal in treating septic shock is directed toward:
   A. Restoring adequate oxygenation throughout the body
   B. Reducing the level of circulating toxins in the blood stream
   C. Improving cardiac function and blood pressure with fluids
   D. Correcting nutritional imbalances with appropriate nutritional support
4. A client with severe compound fractures of both legs exhibits a blood pressure of 90/50, a pulse of 120 and a temperature of 102.2° F and respiration of 28. He is very restless. The nurse should ask the physician for an order to:
   A. Medicate him for pain
   B. Increase his intravenous fluids
   C. Increase the liter flow for his oxygen mask
   D. Administer vasoactive drugs
5. If hypovolemic shock caused by dehydration is being treated successfully by medical and nursing therapies, the nurse would expect to see which of the following outcomes?
   A. Bounding peripheral pulses
   B. Cool skin temperatures
   C. Increased urine osmolality and specific gravity
   D. Urinary output above 50 mL per hour

CRITICAL THINKING EXERCISES

SCENARIO A

A 25-year-old client is receiving regular doses of corticosteroids for treatment of a collagen disorder (connective tissue disorder). The client is taken to an urgent care center with a fever of 100° F and complaints of severe flank pain and states "there is pus in my urine." Upon further assessment, the nurse records the following vital signs:

- Pulse: 120 (normal for the client is 80)
- Respirations: 28 and rapid (normal for client is 14)

- Blood pressure: 110/60 (normal for client is 130/76)

The client becomes extremely agitated when the physician recommends hospitalization. The diagnosis is pyelonephritis resulting from *Escherichia coli,* a gram-negative bacterium.

1. Why is the client a prime candidate for shock?
2. What type of shock will the client develop and why?
3. Explain the pathophysiology of the client's vital signs
4. What is the nurse's role in relation to maintaining the client's respiratory status and overall systemic functions?

SCENARIO B

Of the following clinical situations, which individual is most at risk for developing shock and why?

1. A 20-year-old person who suffers a loss of 500 mL of blood over 3 days.
2. A 40-year-old life-long long-distance runner who has run a 26-mile marathon in temperatures of 80 to 85° F.
3. An 80-year-old person who has had diarrhea for 2 days and is consuming less than 1000 mL of fluid in 24 hours.

BIBLIOGRAPHY

1. Aguilar, M. M., & Hartley-Winkler, M. (1990). CAVHD during extracorporeal membrane oxygenation. *Dialysis and Transplantation, 19(8),* 436–439.
2. Barone, J. E., & Snyder, A. B. (1991). Treatment strategies in shock: Use of oxygen transport measurements. *Heart and Lung, 20(1),* 81–85.
3. Bell, T. N. (1990). Disseminated intravascular coagulation and shock: Multisystem crisis in the critically ill. *Critical Care Nursing Clinics of North America, 2(2),* 255–268.
4. Blansfield, J. (1990). Emergency autotransfusion in hypovolemia. *Critical Care Nursing Clinics of North America, 2(2),* 195–199.
5. Brown, K. (1994). Septic shock: Stopping the deadly cascade. *American Journal of Nursing, 94(9),* 20–27.
6. Brown, K. (1994). Critical interventions in septic shock. *American Journal of Nursing, 94(10),* 20–26.
7. Burns, K. M. (1990). Vasoactive drug therapy in shock. *Critical Care Nursing Clinics of North America, 2(2),* 167–178.
8. Charette, A. L. (1989). Bridging the gap between hemodynamics and monitoring. *Critical Care Nursing Clinics of North America, 1(3),* 539–546.
9. Collins, A. S. (1990). Gastrointestinal complications in shock. *Critical Care Nursing Clinics of North America, 2(2),* 269–277.
10. Daily, E. K. (1989). Use of hemodynamics to differentiate pathophysiologic causes of cardiogenic shock. *Critical Care Nursing Clinics of North America, 1(3),* 589–602.
11. Gardner, P. E. (1989). Cardiac output: Theory, technique, troubleshooting. *Critical Care Nursing Clinics of North America, 1(3),* 577–587.
12. Gawlinski, A. (1989). Saving the cardiogenic shock patient. *Nursing, 19(12),* 34–41.
13. Goran, S. F. (1989). Vascular complication of the patient undergoing intra-aortic balloon pumping. *Critical Care Nursing Clinics of North America, 1(3),* 459–467.
14. Houston, M. C. (1990). Pathophysiology of shock. *Critical Care Nursing Clinics of North America, 2(2),* 143–149.
15. Hoyt, N. J. (1990). Preventing septic shock: Infection control in the intensive care unit. *Critical Care Nursing Clinics of North America, 2(2),* 287–297.
16. Jillings, C. R. (1990). Shock: Psychosocial needs of the patients and family. *Critical Care Nursing Clinics of North America, 2(2),* 325–330.
17. Karch, A. M. (1992). *Handbook of drugs and the nursing process* (2nd ed.). Philadelphia: J. B. Lippincott.
18. Lancaster, L. E., & Rice, V. (1990). Nurse care planning: Overview and application to the patient in shock. *Critical Care Nursing Clinics of North America, 2(2),* 279–286.
19. Lancaster, L. E. (1990). Renal response to shock. *Critical Care Nursing Clinics of North America, 2(2),* 221–233.
20. Lekander, B. J., & Cerra, F. B. (1990). The syndrome of multiple organ failure. *Critical Care Nursing Clinics of North America, 2(2),* 331–342.
21. Ley, S. J. (1988). Fluid therapy following intracardiac operation. *Critical Care Nurse, 8(1),* 26–36.
22. Lorenz, A. (1989). Lactic acidosis: A nursing challenge. *Critical Care Nurse, 9(4),* 64–73.
23. Martin, E., Harris, A., Johnson, N., et al.: (1989). Autotransfusion systems. *Critical Care Nurse, 9(7),* 65–73.
24. McCormac, M. (1990). Managing hemorrhagic shock. *American Journal of Nursing, 90(8),* 22–27.
25. Mims, B. C. (1989). Physiologic rationale of SvO_2 monitoring. *Critical Care Nursing Clinics of North America, 1(3),* 619–628.
26. Mohrman, D. E., & Heller, L. J. (1991). *Cardiovascular physiology.* New York: McGraw-Hill.
27. O'Neal, Pamela. (1994). How to spot early signs of cardiogenic shock. *American Journal of Nursing, 94(5),* 36–41.
28. Perkins, S. B., & Kennally, K. M. (1989). The hidden danger of internal hemorrhage. *Nursing, 19(7),* 34–41.
29. Phoenix, J. (1990). Low blood pressure: How to investigate this ominous sign. *Nursing, 20(11),* 34–39.
30. Rice, V. (1991). Shock, a clinical syndrome: An update. Part 1. *Critical Care Nurse, 11(4),* 20–27.
31. Rice, V. (1991). Shock, a clinical syndrome: An update. Part 2. The stages of shock. *Critical Care Nurse, 11(5),* 74–82.
32. Rice, V. (1991). Shock, a clinical syndrome: An update. Part 3. Therapeutic management. *Critical Care Nurse, 11(6),* 34–39.

33. Rice, V. (1991). Shock, a clinical syndrome: An update. Part 4. Nursing care of the shock patient. *Critical Care Nurse, 11(7),* 28–40.

34. Roach, A. C. (1990). Antibiotic therapy in septic shock. *Critical Care Nursing Clinics of North America, 2(2),* 179–186.

35. Robins, E. V. (1990). Burn shock. *Critical Care Nursing Clinics of North America, 2(2),* 299–307.

36. Scherer, P. (1989). Shock trauma. *American Journal of Nursing, 89(11),* 1440–1445.

37. Schott, K. E. (1990). Intra-aortic balloon counterpulsation as a therapy for shock. *Critical Care Nursing Clinics of North America, 2(2),* 187–193.

38. Schumann, L. L., & Remington, M. A. (1990). The use of naloxone in treating endotoxic shock. *Critical Care Nurse, 10(2),* 63–71.

39. Siskind, J. (1990). Handling hemorrhage wisely. *Nursing, 20(3),* 137–143.

40. Stroud, M., et al. (1990). Cellular and humoral mediators of sepsis syndrome. *Critical Care Nursing Clinics of North America, 2(2),* 151–160.

41. Summers, G. (1990). The clinical and hemodynamic presentation of the shock patient. *Critical Care Nursing Clinics of North America, 2(2),* 161–166.

42. Teplitz, L. (1989). Clinical close-up on atropine. *Nursing, 19(11),* 44–47.

43. Teplitz, L. (1989). Clinical close-up on dopamine. *Nursing, 19(12),* 50–53.

44. Teplitz, L. (1989). Clinical close-up on epinephrine. *Nursing, 19(10),* 50–53.

45. Vaughan, P., & Brooks, C. (1990). Adult respiratory distress syndrome: A complication of shock. *Critical Care Nursing Clinics of North America, 2(2),* 235–253.

46. Young, L. M. (1990). DIC: The insidious killer. *Critical Care Nurse, 10(10),* 26–33.

Chapter 57 Nursing Care of Clients During Medical-Surgical Emergencies

Learning Outcomes

After completing this chapter, the learner will be able to:

1. Assess the client for clinical manifestations resulting from medical-surgical emergencies.
2. Teach the client about the risk factors, basic pathophysiology, and clinical manifestations associated with medical-surgical emergencies.
3. Explain the client's and family's role in the prevention and treatment of medical-surgical emergencies.
4. Develop plans of care for prevention, management, and treatment in cases of medical-surgical emergency.
5. Implement nursing interventions that optimize the quality of life for clients with medical-surgical emergencies.
6. Evaluate planned client outcomes using outcomes developed in the planning phase of care.

Medical-Surgical Emergencies

An emergency is any sudden illness or injury that is perceived by the client or significant other as requiring immediate intervention. The emergency continues until the condition is stable or no longer threatens the client's integrity or well being.

Emergency situations can occur anywhere. Therefore, it is important for all nurses to have the basic knowledge and skills needed for rapid assessment, intervention, and safe management of emergencies. The focus of this chapter is to identify general principles, priorities, and management of common emergencies encountered by adult clients.

ETHICAL AND LEGAL CONSIDERATIONS

Consent to Treatment

Informed consent to treatment means that clients are knowledgeable of all treatments and procedures and agree to these before implementation. The information must be presented in a language in which the client is fluent and at an appropriate level so the client understands the implications of any treatments. Clients also have the right to refuse any treatments or procedures before they are implemented.

However, informed consent is valid only if the client is of "adult years and sound mind." Not all adult clients are capable of giving informed consent. Clients with emergencies may be hypoxic, be intoxicated, or have an altered level of consciousness.

EMERGENCY DOCTRINE

When a client is unable to give consent or is unconscious, emergency treatment can be provided under the emergency doctrine. This doctrine implies that the client would have consented to treatment if able, because the alternative would have been death or disability. The emergency doctrine removes the need for obtaining informed consent before emergency treatment and care are initiated.

Right to Privacy and Confidentiality

All clients have a right to privacy, and clients with emergencies are no different. This right includes the need for consent to use names and photographs of the client; not allowing unauthorized persons into the client's hospital area; and not disclosing private facts to the public or falsely representing the client to the public. Information about the client's condition, treatments, and outcomes are to be respected and handled with discretion.

CRITICAL TO REMEMBER

Any communication about the client's conditions and treatments and its documentation are confidential and disclosed only with the client's permission.

Mandatory Reporting

Mandatory reporting laws require hospitals, nurses, and physicians to notify the appropriate local, state, or federal agency when certain conditions or incidents occur. These include child, spouse, or elder abuse; motor vehicle crashes; injuries resulting from violence; attempted suicides; animal bites; overdoses; and poisonings. Certain communicable disorders, such as meningitis, sexually transmitted diseases, and food poisonings, are also reportable to the state health department. When injuries are suspected or identified, the nurse must notify the physician in charge of the care and other individuals identified by hospital policy. The appropriate agency must be notified and a report filed.

Physical Evidence and Chain of Custody

Meticulous documentation and handling of evidence are of particular concern in situations in which injury resulted from a violent crime, such as a shooting or sexual assault. All evidence discovered during the examination is recorded. Documentation of samples includes the location from which the sample was obtained and when and to whom it was delivered.

Evidence should be maintained in its original condition. Clothing is stored in a paper bag instead of plastic to prevent decomposition. If clothing needs to be cut off the client, special attention is taken not to destroy evidence inadvertently.

BULLETS

Bullets removed from a client's body or recovered from clothing are handled with great care. The bullet is then placed in a sealed bag, labeled, and given to proper authorities. The bag is sealed so that removal of the seal will be obvious.

SPECIMENS

Specimens obtained for legal purposes, as opposed to clinical purposes, include blood samples for determination of blood alcohol levels and items obtained during the examination of an alleged sexual assault victim. When a blood alcohol determination is desired by either the client or legal authorities, the client's written permission must be obtained before the specimen is drawn. No client may be forced into having a blood sample drawn. In many instances, police officers have a kit with the necessary equipment for drawing the specimen. Isopropyl alcohol or any antiseptic solution containing alcohol must not be used as a skin preparation before a blood alcohol specimen is drawn. These agents may falsely elevate the blood alcohol level and render the test invalid. The nurse must know the laws within the state that identify who may draw blood for alcohol level determinations.

Once the specimen is drawn, it is handed to a police officer, who signs that the specimen has been received. Documentation of the procedure on the client's clinical record, along with the nurse's signature and the name and badge number of the officer, is important.

Transfer Laws

In 1986, Congress passed the Consolidated Omnibus Budget Reconciliation Act (COBRA) in response to inappropriate patient transfers and denial of care. Provisions of the COBRA legislation require treatment for all clients with emergency conditions and pregnant women with active contractions regardless of ability to pay. This includes an appropriate medical screening examination, necessary stabilizing treatments, and appropriate transfer to another facility with consent, if indicated. It is important for emergency nurses to be aware of the hospital guidelines and transfer protocols. Nurses can be active patient advocates and ensure that clients receive necessary emergency treatments. Failure to comply with COBRA legislation may result in substantial fines and penalties.

EMERGENCY NURSING CARE

The Emergency Nurses Association defines emergency nursing care as the "assessment, diagnosis and treatment of perceived, actual or potential, sudden or urgent, physical or psychosocial problems that are primarily episodic or acute. These may require minimal care or life-support measures, client and significant other education, appropriate referral and knowledge of legal limitations."[9]

Because less than 20 per cent of the clients seeking emergency care have life-threatening problems, teaching is a major nursing role. Many emergency departments provide written instructions as well as verbal teaching.

For many, the emergency department may be the usual source of health care, and emergency nurses may be the only contact the client has with the health-care system. Nurses must be aware of clients who frequently return to the emergency department. These clients may have special health needs, have exacerbations of chronic conditions, be victims of abuse, have no primary health-care provider, or have little or no health insurance. Research has shown that clients use emergency departments because they perceive their symptoms as serious, and emergency departments are viewed as faster and more convenient than clinics.[10]

BOX 57–1

Assessment Findings Implying a High Priority for Care

- Significant alteration in vital signs (e.g., hypo- or hypertension, hypo- or hyperthermia, cardiac dysrhythmias, respiratory distress)
- Altered level of consciousness
- Chest pain, especially in clients older than 35 years
- Severe pain
- Bleeding not controlled by direct pressure
- Conditions that will worsen from delay in treatment (e.g., chemical burns, drug or toxic substance ingestion, allergic reaction, impaled objects)
- Sudden vision loss
- Dangerous, aberrant, or disruptive behavior
- Psychologically devastating conditions (e.g., sexual assault, death or near death of a loved one)
- Elderly or very young client
- Symptom that is vague but causes the triage officer (emergency assessor) concern

Initial Assessment

On first being confronted with a seriously ill or injured client, the nurse must gain as much information as quickly as possible from all possible sources. The initial impression is important for early identification of and intervention for life-threatening signs and symptoms (Box 57–1). Historical information provides clues to the urgency of the situation and treatment priorities. Client management consists of a brief history and primary assessment, resuscitation of vital functions, a thorough secondary assessment, and definitive care.

HISTORY

The history provides clues to the priority assessments and interventions. A history should include information about when and where the emergency occurred, what has been done, and whether the client has any known health problems. One way to obtain this information quickly is through the mnemonic AMPLE:

- A Allergies
- M Medications currently prescribed or using
- P Past medical and surgical history
- L Last meal
- E Events preceding the emergency and any care rendered.

Establishing Priorities

The goal of emergency care is prompt, effective resuscitation and stabilization of critically ill or injured clients. The process of organizing client care, controlling traffic, and providing prompt and timely emergency care is called *triage*.

Triage ensures that clients requiring immediate attention for life-threatening emergencies receive it.

TABLE 57–1 Triage Categories

CATEGORY	DEFINITION	EMERGENCY EXAMPLES
Emergent	Life-threatening emergency Usually involves the ABCs The client may die without immediate intervention	Airway obstruction, cardiac arrest, chest pain with dyspnea or cyanosis, shock, coma, open chest wounds, sudden vision loss, and psychologically devastating conditions
Urgent	Emergencies that require intervention within a few hours	Intraperitoneal bleeding, cerebrovascular accident, severe pain, sudden paralysis, persistent nausea, vomiting, or diarrhea
Nonurgent	Not life threatening Interventions may be delayed beyond a few hours	Soft tissue injuries, surface trauma, extremity fractures without circulatory compromise

ABCs, *a*irway, *b*reathing, *c*irculation.

Although triage categories may vary, three common categories are emergent, urgent, and nonurgent (Table 57–1). Because performance of a complete assessment is difficult initially, it is wise to err on the side of assigning a higher triage priority than a lower one. An effective triage nurse possesses three critical qualities: expert assessment skills, nonjudgmental communication and interviewing techniques, and organizational skills to regulate control of traffic flow into the treatment areas.[33]

Because the emergency department may be a place where violent behavior occurs, the triage nurse must be knowledgeable about common responses to crises and able to react quickly and in a calm manner.[22] The ability of the triage nurse to assess, intervene, and communicate effectively helps establish rapport and trust with the client and significant others.

Documentation

Documentation of assessments, interventions, and client responses is essential. Because time is often limited, flow sheets are frequently used. During life-threatening situations, critical data may be recorded on a white board mounted on the treatment wall so that all members of the team are able to visualize important data rapidly. It is desirable for one person to be responsible for documentation.

Priority Nursing Interventions

AIRWAY PATENCY

Common airway obstructions are the tongue and foreign bodies such as food (a "café coronary"), teeth, bone fragments, or blood clots. In a conscious client, the nurse can assist the client to remove the obstruction by initiating an abdominal thrust.

If the airway is open but the client is not breathing, the nurse should begin rescue breathing (see discussion of cardiopulmonary resuscitation [CPR], Chap. 24). The nurse should watch for the rise and fall of the chest during these breaths. If the chest rises and falls, the airway is open. Various artificial airways are used when the airway is not patent or is inadequate (see Chap. 20).

A nasopharyngeal airway can be inserted if the client is semiconscious; an oropharyngeal airway is used if the client is unconscious and without a gag reflex (Fig. 57–1).

In the hospital setting, endotracheal intubation or tracheostomy tubes are preferred. Two cricothyroidotomy procedures are used when endotracheal intubation is impossible or an obstruction is present. Both measures are temporary until tracheal intubation or a tracheotomy can be performed. A cricothyrotomy (coniotomy) involves a transverse incision through the cricothyroid membrane located below the thyroid prominence of the neck. The percutaneous transtracheal ventilation (needle cricothyroidotomy) involves inserting a 14-gauge intravenous catheter with a needle into the trachea through the cricothyroid membrane. Once the catheter is inside the trachea, the needle is removed, and the client is ventilated through the catheter.

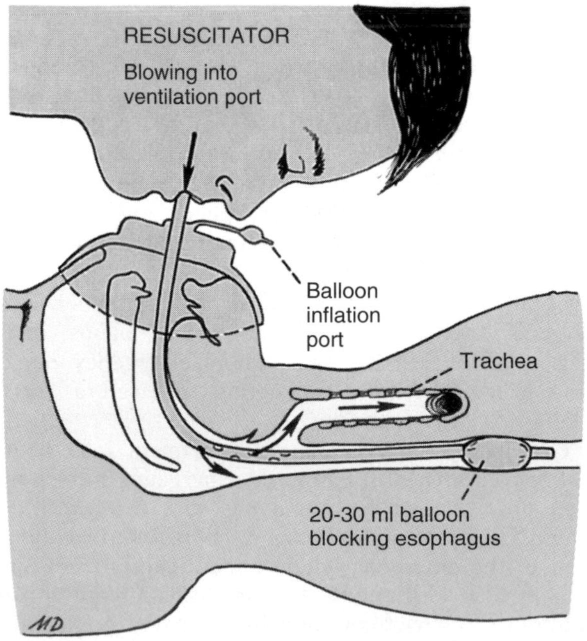

Figure 57–1
Esophageal obturator airway, a ventilatory device used for resuscitation in emergencies. A face mask anchors the airway and seals off the mouth and nose. The lungs are ventilated via openings in a flexible tube at the level of the pharynx. Possible aspiration of gastric contents is minimized by an inflated balloon at the tube's distal end, which blocks the esophagus.

SUPPLEMENTAL OXYGEN

Severe injuries and respiratory distress indicate a need for 100 per cent oxygen for treatment of any resultant hypoxemia. Supplemental oxygen is initiated at 6 to 10 L/min in situations of severe injury or stress such as myocardial infarction, smoke inhalation, or shock. Supplemental oxygen is provided if the client has chest pain, signs and symptoms of poor cardiac output (decreased pulse and blood pressure), signs and symptoms of hypoxemia (confusion, anxiety, or restlessness), profuse bleeding, or nausea. See Chapter 20 for various supplemental oxygen delivery systems.

SPINAL PRECAUTIONS AND IMMOBILIZATION

In a client with a decreased level of consciousness, and if history of or potential for traumatic injury is suspected, the spinal column is immobilized to prevent neurologic injury. The ideal precaution for spinal immobilization includes a cervical collar, two rolled towels or intravenous bags, or a head immobilizer placed on each side of the head and taped securely across the forehead onto a long backboard[9] (Fig. 57–2).

CARDIOPULMONARY RESUSCITATION

The nurse must begin CPR (see Chap. 24), remembering to stabilize the client's head in a neutral, in-line position, if the client is not breathing and has no pulse. CPR aids in perfusing the client's tissues. The nurse should keep in mind that the client needs to have enough blood volume to circulate with CPR. If the client has profuse bleeding, large-bore intravenous catheters need to be inserted immediately to restore intravascular fluid volume with fluids or blood products.

BRIEF NEUROLOGIC EXAMINATION

After the *a*irway, *b*reathing, and *c*irculation (ABCs) are stabilized, the nurse must conduct a brief neurologic assessment. The client's general appearance, mental status, and orientation must be observed and any eye opening, verbal, and motor responses to verbal, tactile, and noxious stimuli noted (see discussion of Glasgow Coma Scale, Chap. 13). The nurse must observe for any posturing and spastic or flaccid extremities and assess for abnormal breath or body odors (e.g., alcohol, gasoline, chemicals, urine, or feces), facial expressions, tremors, asymmetry between sides, or obvious deformities.[8, 9]

Additional Nursing Assessments

One of the most common clinical manifestations of an emergency is pain. Acute pain may result from soft-tissue injury, ischemia, or peripheral nerve damage such as in a crush injury or compartment syndrome. A symptom analysis is performed.

Any loss of sensation should be further assessed. It may be due to spinal cord injury and spinal shock, cerebral hemorrhage, or neurovascular compromise.

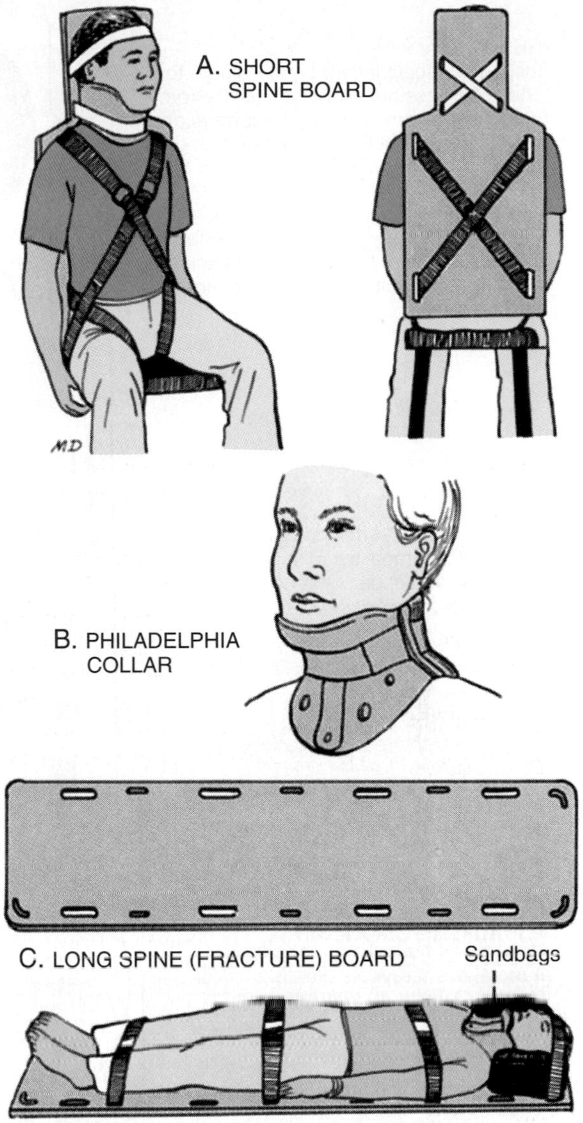

Figure 57–2
Spine immobilization devices. *A*, A short spine board is applied to the client in a seated position (e.g., in an automobile) and is applied, along with a cervical collar, before extrication from the vehicle. *B*, A Philadelphia collar is a two-piece, hard, molded plastic device that can be applied without manipulating the neck and provides better cervical spinal column immobilization. *C*, A long spine (fracture) board is made of wood and contains cut-out sections along the sides for securing restraining straps and for lifting the injured client.

Secondary Nursing Assessment

The secondary assessment involves a complete head-to-toe assessment guided by the client's chief complaint.

Objective physical assessments are performed (Fig. 57–3), concentrating on areas relating to the client's chief complaint. It should be kept in mind that not all of the assessment procedures are performed on every client with an emergency, but these are a guideline for establishing priorities.

Client Teaching

Because of the short time of the interaction, teaching conducted by emergency nurses must be specific to the

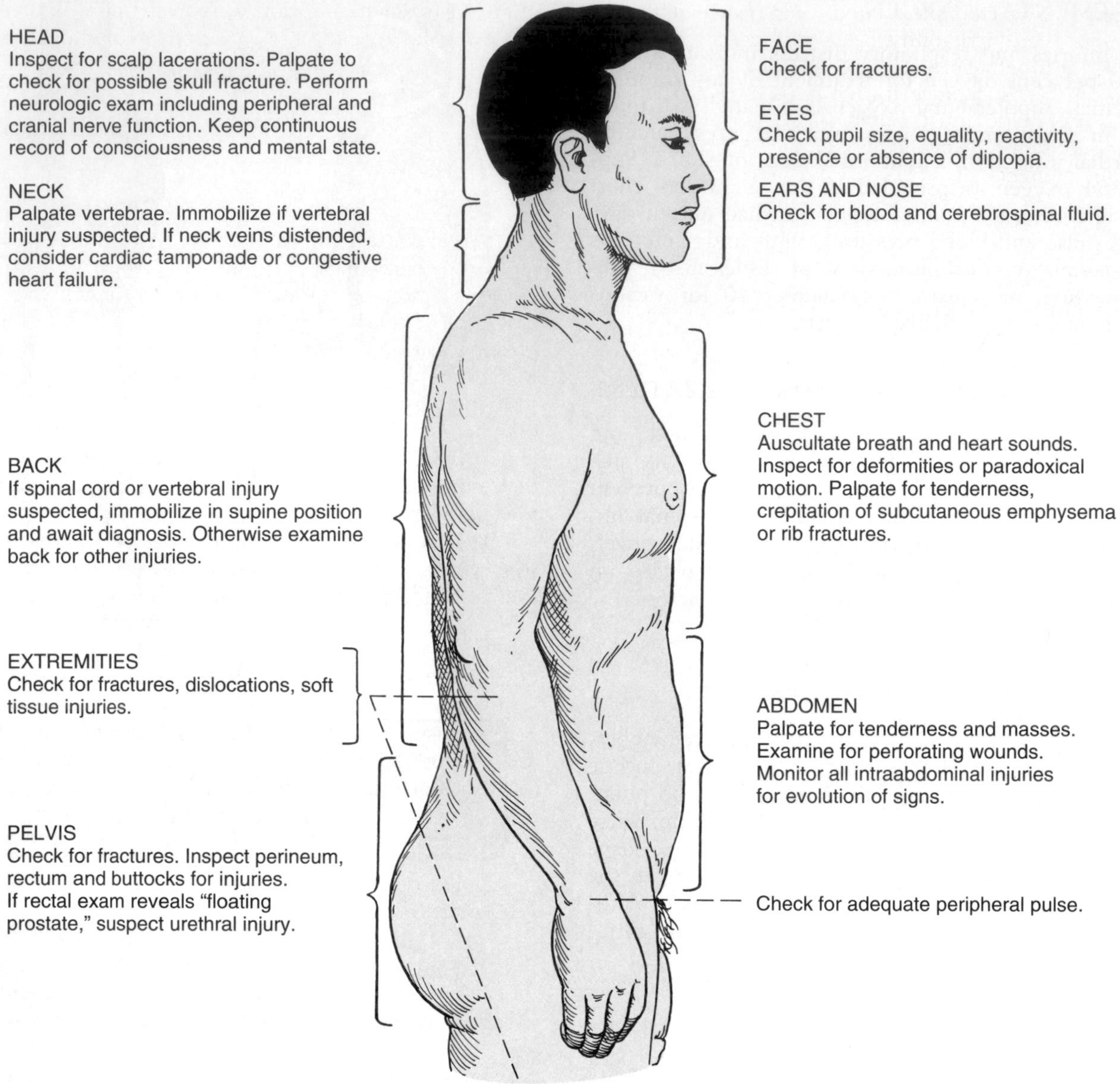
HEAD
Inspect for scalp lacerations. Palpate to check for possible skull fracture. Perform neurologic exam including peripheral and cranial nerve function. Keep continuous record of consciousness and mental state.
NECK
Palpate vertebrae. Immobilize if vertebral injury suspected. If neck veins distended, consider cardiac tamponade or congestive heart failure.
BACK
If spinal cord or vertebral injury suspected, immobilize in supine position and await diagnosis. Otherwise examine back for other injuries.
EXTREMITIES
Check for fractures, dislocations, soft tissue injuries.
PELVIS
Check for fractures. Inspect perineum, rectum and buttocks for injuries. If rectal exam reveals "floating prostate," suspect urethral injury.
FACE
Check for fractures.
EYES
Check pupil size, equality, reactivity, presence or absence of diplopia.
EARS AND NOSE
Check for blood and cerebrospinal fluid.
CHEST
Auscultate breath and heart sounds. Inspect for deformities or paradoxical motion. Palpate for tenderness, crepitation of subcutaneous emphysema or rib fractures.
ABDOMEN
Palpate for tenderness and masses. Examine for perforating wounds. Monitor all intraabdominal injuries for evolution of signs.
Check for adequate peripheral pulse.

Figure 57–3
Checklist for rapid evaluation of the injured client after the immediate treatment priorities have been covered. After initial examination, the state of consciousness and vital signs are monitored frequently while x-ray and laboratory data are being obtained.

client's most pressing problems. Emphasis is placed on return demonstration or verbal understanding. Information includes recognizing the most likely or significant complication, how and when to obtain follow-up care, and what to do if complications occur. A discharge instruction sheet reinforcing this information is given to the client or significant other at discharge, and teaching is documented on the emergency record.

Psychosocial Needs in Emergencies

The psychosocial needs of clients and significant others vary widely during an emergency. A number of factors influence reactions to emergencies. Some of these factors include little or no time to prepare; little experience with the type of stressor; little or no guidance available for what is expected of them; loss of control and feelings of helplessness; the amount of time spent in crisis and its on-again, off-again nature; the disruption to client and family roles, responsibilities, and routines, and the perceived danger to and emotional impact on the client and significant others.

Clients' reactions are unique. Some are anxious, fearful, and occasionally angry. Others experience loss of control, loss of individuality, and possible loss of dignity. The mechanism and strategies used are usually based on past experiences and previous coping styles.

Some behavioral responses may be related to the physiologic process of the emergency and should be considered. For example, anoxia can cause agitation, restlessness, and irritability. In addition, cognitive impairment and behavioral changes may result from head injury, trauma, substance ingestion, and metabolic disorders. The nurse must carefully assess the behaviors and reactions but always keep in mind the potential for physiologic effects.

SIGNIFICANT OTHERS

The needs of significant others require special attention in emergency settings. Unless they accompanied the client, they may be notified by telephone. Advising significant others of the client's presence in the emergency setting by telephone requires tact and sensitivity. The nurse must exercise caution when discussing the urgency of the situation. It is important to advise significant others to have someone else bring them to the hospital.

The nurse must communicate to team members and record on the medical record when significant others have been notified or are present. It is important that the nurse providing the care periodically update significant others with clear explanations regarding the client's condition, treatment, and progress using easily understood language. Significant others need to have opportunities to visit the client as appropriate. Before they visit, the nurse must prepare significant others regarding the client's condition and appearance, being sure to mention the presence of tubes, equipment, bandages, and other devices present. This is particularly important when there is disfigurement or loss of ability to communicate.

A private waiting area may help significant others cope with an emergency.

Selected Emergencies

Shock

Circulatory shock is a profound alteration in tissue perfusion. It occurs from either a decreased cellular perfusion or an inability to use an adequate perfusion. See Chapter 56 for a discussion of shock.

Altered Level of Consciousness

An altered level of consciousness may range from restlessness and disorientation to unconsciousness. The causes of an altered level of consciousness include hypoxic, metabolic, and pathologic conditions of the brain. The mnemonic device "vowel tipps" is a helpful guide for determining the cause of unconsciousness.

- A Alcohol
- E Epilepsy
- I Insulin
- O Opiates
- U Urates
- T Trauma
- I Infection
- P Psychological
- P Poison
- S Shock

Key historical information to be obtained from significant others or prehospital personnel includes any history of trauma; chronic health problems (e.g., diabetes, hypertension, heart or kidney disease); use of prescription, over-the-counter, or street drugs or home remedies; alcohol use; mental health history; general health status; activities when the client was last seen or communicated with; temperature of environment in which the client was found; and clues that may help to determine cause (e.g., medication bottles, incontinence, medical alert tag or card).

The nurse should assess the color of skin, respiratory pattern, pupillary reaction, motor function, odors, nuchal rigidity, and posturing. Measures to stabilize the ABCs should be instituted. Vital signs should be monitored and neurologic status assessed. The nurse must also calculate and document the Glasgow Coma Scale score (see Chap. 13), pupillary responses, and reflexes. An intravenous catheter must be inserted and blood drawn for laboratory work (complete blood count [CBC], glucose, calcium, electrolytes, creatinine, magnesium, drug screen, and alcohol level).

Management

Because the history may be inadequate for determining whether thiamine deficiency is probable, thiamine is routinely administered prophylactically. The nurse must administer intravenous dextrose if the client has a history of hypoglycemia or a low serum glucose. Glucose paste may also be applied sublingually, or intramuscular glucagon may be administered to raise the blood sugar.

Naloxone (Narcan), 2 mg intravenously, may be administered if a narcotic overdose is suspected, and it can be repeated. Caution should be used, however, because if the drug that is reversed by naloxone has a longer half-life, the effect of the drug may last longer than the effect of naloxone, and the client may lapse back into unconsciousness. Observation for several hours is usually indicated for these clients.

Ongoing nursing management includes safety measures. The nurse must manage airways and secretions for prevention of aspiration; position the client on the side while maintaining spine immobilization, and suction as needed; protect the eyes from drying by applying artificial tears and taping the eyelids shut (using cellophane rather than adhesive tape); be sure to check the eyes for contact lenses and remove if present; prevent skin necrosis by position changes and skin care; and protect from falls by raising the side rails, and locking them.

CRITICAL TO REMEMBER

The nurse should minimize the potential for increased intracranial pressure by positioning the client's head in neutral alignment, hyperventilating with 100 per cent oxygen before suctioning, suctioning for short periods, and avoiding restraints if possible.

The nurse can prepare for and assist with diagnostic studies (e.g., computed tomographic [CT] scans or magnetic resonance imaging).

Multiple Trauma

Multiple trauma includes injury to more than one body system. Many different scoring systems are used to categorize and determine severity of injury. One of these is the Champion Trauma Score (Table 57–2). This score uses physiologic measurements (heart rate, respiratory expansion, systolic blood pressure, and capillary return) and the Glasgow Coma Scale. Points are assigned on the basis of the client's responses, and a total score is obtained. Optimally, a client with a Champion Trauma Score of less than 12 should be transferred to a tertiary trauma system. The Champion Trauma Score correlates highly with mortality.

TABLE 57–2 Champion Trauma Score

Glasgow Coma Scale (GCS)		
Eye-opening response	Spontaneous	4
	To voice	3
	To pain	2
	None	1
Best verbal response	Oriented	5
	Confused	4
	Inappropriate words	3
	Incomprehensible sounds	2
	None	1
Best motor response	Obeys command	6
	Localizes pain	5
	Withdraws (pain)	4
	Flexion (pain)	3
	Extension (pain)	2
	None	1
Total	Apply this score to GCS portion of Trauma Score	3–15
Trauma Score		
GCS (total points from above)	14–15	5
	11–13	4
	8–10	3
	5–7	2
	3–4	1
Respiratory rate	10–24/min	4
	25–35/min	3
	36/min or greater	2
	1–9/min	1
	None	0
Respiratory expansion	Normal	1
	Retractive-none	0
Systolic blood pressure	90 mm Hg or greater	4
	70–89 mm Hg	3
	50–69 mm Hg	2
	0–49 mm Hg	1
	No pulse	0
Capillary refill	Normal	2
	Delayed	1
	None	0
Total trauma score		1–16

Trauma score	16	15	14	13	12	11	10	9	8	7	6	5	4	3	2	1
Percentage survival	99	98	96	93	87	76	60	42	26	15	8	4	2	1	0	0

From Moore, E. E., et al. (1990). *Early care of the injured patient.* Philadelphia: B. C. Decker.

Mechanism of Injury

The mechanism of injury helps in estimating the amount of force applied and provides insight into the pattern of injury (Fig. 57–4).

In addition to the mechanism of injury, the type and extent of injury also involve environmental conditions (weather, geographic location) and characteristics of the client such as age, sex, nutrition, underlying disease processes, and any conditions altering cognitive function and judgment (alcohol, drug use, or fatigue).

PENETRATING INJURIES

Penetrating injuries cause a break in the skin integrity. The nurse must remember to consider potential injuries to underlying organs and tissues. A thoracic wound may involve an interruption in the heart, great vessels, or even diaphragm, depending on whether the injured client was inspiring (diaphragm down) or expiring (diaphragm up) at the time of injury. Because of the diaphragm's location, a diagnostic peritoneal lavage is often performed for evaluation of possible abdominal injury by penetrating wounds below the nipple line.[1, 25]

NONPENETRATING (BLUNT) INJURIES

Blunt (nonpenetrating) injuries result in significant injuries that may be more difficult to detect. These involve direct, indirect, and acceleration-deceleration forces. For instance, in a motor vehicle crash, the driver (traveling at the speed of the car) impacts on the steering wheel. The force of the impact is exerted through the chest structures and may result in broken ribs, cardiac or pulmonary contusions, pneumothorax, or ruptured aorta. Alternatively, the client's head may hit the windshield, which causes frontal lobe damage of the brain (coup); as the head falls backward, damage to the occipital lobe can occur (contrecoup). Solid organs are more likely to be crushed or compressed (liver, spleen). Hollow, air-filled organs are more likely to burst when compressed or subject to blast forces (lung, intestines).

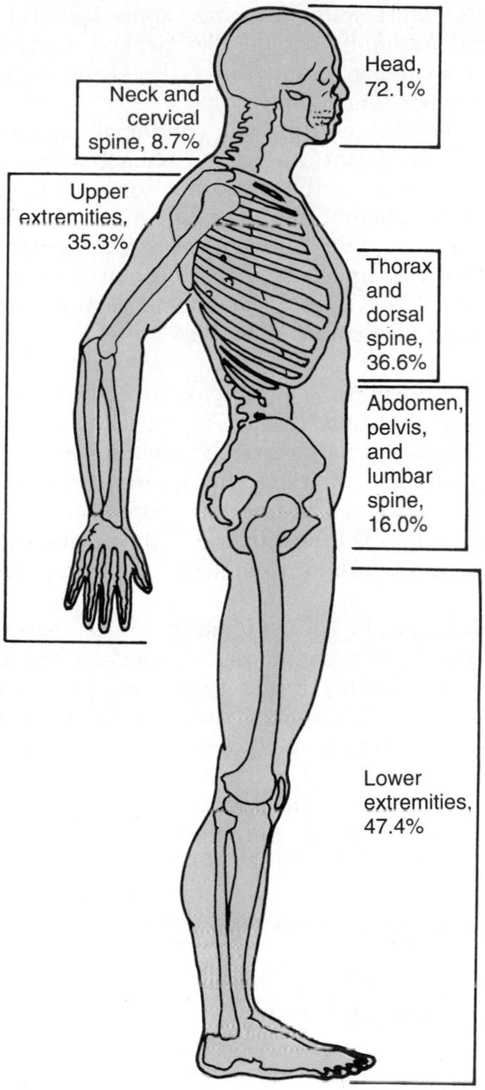

Figure 57–4
Motor vehicle accidents can result in multiple injuries. Two thirds of the victims suffer injuries to the head and facial area. Other anatomic areas also are often involved. (From *Patterns of disease*, a publication of Parke, Davis & Co.)

The history and mechanism of injury constitute vital information and must be obtained promptly. This information helps guide assessment and intervention (Table 57–3). In addition, injuries should be matched to the reported mechanism. Clients and significant others may deny or falsify the history of injury for many reasons.[14]

Management

GENERAL INTERVENTIONS

The nurse must

- Ensure an adequate airway with spinal immobilization
- Ventilate and initiate oxygen therapy
- Insert one or two peripheral intravenous lines
- Initiate cardiac monitoring; obtain a 12-lead electrocardiogram (ECG)
- Insert nasogastric tube
- Insert a urinary catheter if no blood is present at the meatus
- Monitor urine output every 15 to 30 minutes
- Monitor vital signs continuously and document
- Provide continuous psychosocial support to client and significant others

PRIMARY ASSESSMENT AND PRIORITY INTERVENTIONS

With a multiply injured client, time is vital. Priorities are determined by the ABCs, and the general interventions are implemented immediately.

The nurse must control external bleeding by direct pressure, pressure dressing, or rapid fluid replacement if the client is hypotensive (crystalloid or colloid). The client may be in cardiac arrest from shock, chest injuries, or respiratory failure. Two large-bore intravenous catheters must be inserted for rapid infusion of fluids.

The nurse should start CPR immediately if no pulse is present.

TABLE 57–3 Common Associated Injuries

MECHANISM OF INJURY	POTENTIAL ASSOCIATED INJURIES
Adult pedestrian struck by a car	Suspect fractures at 1. Point of impact with the car bumper 2. Point of impact with the car hood 3. Point of impact when adult is thrown Fractures are sustained at the points of impact with the car bumper and hood Disruption of knee ligaments in the opposite knee from excessive stress
Unrestrained driver	Head and facial injuries from windshield impact Fractured ribs and sternum from impact on the steering wheel Cardiac contusions Lacerated solid organs from blunt compression Patellar injury from striking dash, with an associated femur fracture and dislocation
Client falls from a height and lands on the heels	Suspect: 1. Bilateral calcaneal fractures 2. Compression fractures of the vertebrae 3. If the client lands and braces self with the hands, suspect Colles' fractures at both wrists

CRITICAL TO REMEMBER

If the client has lost fluid volume, CPR will not be fully effective until fluid volume is restored.

Blood must be drawn while inserting an intravenous catheter for appropriate studies. Common studies include CBC, electrolytes, blood urea nitrogen (BUN), glucose, amylase, type and crossmatch (T & C), coagulation screen, possible drug and alcohol levels, creatinine if renal trauma is suspected, and arterial blood gases (ABGs). The nurse must prepare for possible blood transfusions.

A full set of vital signs must be obtained every 15 minutes until the client is stabilized and a brief neurologic and mental status examination performed. The nurse must also calculate the Glasgow Coma Scale score and trauma scores. A flow sheet for documentation of assessments, interventions, and client responses must be started.

The nurse must completely undress the client (by cutting off clothes, if necessary) and cover the client with a sheet or blanket. Helmets must be removed carefully to avoid neck flexion. The nurse must ensure that the client's clothes or valuables are safeguarded, and use the proper chain of custody.

SECONDARY ASSESSMENT AND INTERVENTIONS

The nurse proceeds with a complete head-to-toe examination, bearing in mind the possibility of associated injuries and the various internal structures potentially affected by the known injury pattern.

The nurse must obtain a urinalysis after insertion of a urinary catheter, and monitor urine output every 15 to 30 minutes. A nasogastric tube should be inserted, if indicated (nasogastric tubes are not inserted if a basilar skull fracture is suspected because of possible insertion into the cranium; instead, an orogastric tube may be used to decompress the stomach). Gastric aspirant must be tested for blood and connected to suction. The client must be maintained on nothing by mouth (NPO) orders.

Other diagnostic procedures, according to injuries, may include chest tube insertion, needle thoracostomy, or diagnostic peritoneal lavage (see separate discussion). The nurse must prepare for radiographs of the cervical spine, or chest and CT scans or magnetic resonance imaging, as indicated. If a portable x-ray machine is not available, x-ray studies should be coordinated so the client makes only one trip to the radiology department.

A tetanus booster must be administered if wounds are present.

CRITICAL TO REMEMBER

The nurse must avoid moving the client suddenly. Rapid position changes may precipitate cardiovascular collapse.

The nurse must splint fractures, apply ice, and elevate the area. Wounds should be cleaned and dressed. Wounds are repaired only after the client is stabilized or in the operating room.

The nurse should provide emotional support to the client and significant others, and remain with the client during transport to the operating room, radiology department, or nursing unit. The nurse must also provide a verbal report to the nurses assuming responsibility for subsequent care and ensure that written documentation accompanies the client; data about significant others and what information they have received should be included.

Pain medication is commonly not given initially for clients with multiple trauma and cardiovascular instability. Medication may mask the identification of significant injuries and interfere with accurate neurologic assessments. Narcotics, if given, are administered in small intravenous doses. Coordination with the anesthesia department is important if immediate surgery is anticipated.

Elderly clients with traumatic injuries have special needs. The body's compensatory mechanisms may be delayed, and chronic health problems and medications may contribute to complications. For instance, a client with a heart condition who is taking a beta blocker does not present with tachycardia in the presence of shock. Also, abuse of the elderly is an increasing problem that may appear as multiple trauma.[5]

Respiratory Emergencies*

NEAR-DROWNING

Clients who initially survive suffocation after submersion in a water or fluid medium are diagnosed with near-drowning, or immersion syndrome.

Freshwater drowning (e.g., in swimming pools) is more common than saltwater drowning. Alcohol or drug ingestion, overestimation of swimming skills, hypothermia, hyperventilation, and hypoglycemia are risk factors.

Additional injuries may be present, including associated trauma, spinal cord injury from diving, air embolism from scuba diving, and seizures.

Both fresh water and salt water wash out alveolar surfactant. Fresh water also changes the surface tension of surfactant. The loss of surfactant leads to alveolar collapse, intrapulmonary shunting, and hypoxemia. Poor perfusion and hypoxemia result in acidosis and eventual pulmonary edema.

Near-drowning compromises the respiratory system and leads to hypoxia, hypercapnia, cardiac arrest, and severe alterations in fluid-electrolyte balance. Bronchospasm, from aspirating water into the lungs, causes most drowning deaths.

* Written by Sherrill Cronin, RN, MSN.

Management

The nurse obtains a history of the submersion, including the length of submersion, temperature of the water, any associated injuries (possible spinal cord injury from diving), and type of water.

Assessment and interventions should be begun with the ABCs. The nurse notes any respiratory efforts and adventitious sounds; opens the airway while maintaining spinal immobility; assesses the level of consciousness; looks for signs of hypoxia, such as confusion, irritability, lethargy, or unconsciousness; and obtains a complete set of vital signs.

For respiratory insufficiency, intubation and ventilation with 100 per cent oxygen and 5 to 10 cm of positive end-expiratory pressure are initiated to prevent the alveoli from collapsing. If the client is breathing, respiratory support must be provided with a nonrebreather.

The nurse should remove the client's wet clothing and wrap him or her in a warm blanket. Core rewarming may be indicated if the client is hypothermic. The client should be rewarmed slowly to avoid a rapid influx of metabolites that may be trapped in the cold extremities.

Once the vital functions are stabilized, acid-base or electrolyte abnormalities are corrected. Diagnostic studies include ABGs, CBC, electrolytes, appropriate toxicology studies if alcohol or drug ingestion is suspected, and a chest radiograph. Clients with near-drowning emergencies must be observed for at least 24 hours because of the high risk for pulmonary edema. Care must be taken to monitor the neurologic status. A deteriorating level of consciousness may indicate cerebral edema, severe acidosis, or increased hypoxia.

FOREIGN BODY AIRWAY OBSTRUCTION

Foreign body airway obstruction may rapidly lead to cardiopulmonary arrest if it is not dealt with quickly.

Foreign bodies usually enter the right main bronchus because its orifice is slightly wider than that of the left main bronchus. It also lies in a more direct line with the trachea.

Clinical manifestations of an aspirated foreign body include severe dyspnea; hemoptysis (if there has been mechanical trauma to air passages); fever; atelectasis; pulmonary infection; excessive mucus production (if the airways are irritated); harsh, brassy cough; wheezing (if a foreign body passed into the larger airways, i.e., beyond the trachea into the right bronchus); and inspiratory stridor (if the obstruction is at the laryngeal level). If airway obstruction is complete (or nearly complete) and at the laryngeal level, there will be obvious respiratory distress, ineffective ventilation efforts, and inability to speak because it is impossible for air to pass the obstruction. Asphyxia follows rapidly.

Clients may signal airway obstruction resulting from foreign body aspiration by the international sign for distress. They can be helped by the Heimlich maneuver and thrust techniques.

Complete airway obstruction is a life-threatening emergency requiring immediate intervention. Foreign bodies small enough to pass through the glottis seldom lodge in the trachea but pass on into the bronchus. However, those that do lodge in the laryngeal area may be removed with grasping forceps inserted through a laryngoscope under local or general anesthesia.

The client is usually placed in Trendelenburg's position so that the foreign body is prevented from entering the trachea or esophagus. If the foreign object is pushed farther into the airway, a bronchoscope and special grasping forceps are used. (See Chap. 19 for discussion of laryngoscopy and bronchoscopy.) If time permits, a radiograph is taken to confirm the presence and location of the object. If the obstruction is complete, emergency airway maneuvers are necessary.

Chest Trauma

The chest is a large, exposed portion of the body that is very vulnerable to impact injuries. Chest injuries can range from relatively minor bumps and scrapes to severe crushing or penetrating trauma.

Chest injuries often result from falls or the use of machinery or lethal weapons (i.e., knives and guns). Many chest injuries are associated with motor vehicle crashes in which clients are thrown against the steering wheel, dashboard, or front seat.

Chest injuries may be penetrating or nonpenetrating (blunt). *Penetrating chest injuries* (i.e., from bullets, knives, impaled objects, or flying shrapnel or splinters) may cause an open chest wound, permitting atmospheric air into the pleural space and disrupting the normal ventilation mechanism. Penetrating chest injuries may seriously damage the lungs, heart, and other thoracic structures.

Nonpenetrating (blunt) injuries are not as obvious as penetrating wounds and may, therefore, be more difficult to diagnose. Blunt chest injuries are most commonly deceleration injuries associated with motor vehicle crashes. Deceleration injuries occur when a vehicle or body stops abruptly from a relatively high speed. For example, when a car stops suddenly, the body of the client in the car continues forward until it hits the steering wheel, windshield, dashboard, or front seat. Blunt chest trauma may also result from falls or blows to the chest.

Injury to the thoracic cage and its contents can restrict the heart's ability to pump blood or the lungs' ability to exchange air and oxygenate blood. Major dangers associated with chest injuries are internal bleeding and punctured organs.

Initial assessment is directed toward identifying and treating immediate life-threatening conditions. Any client with chest trauma should be considered to have a serious injury until it is proved otherwise. Airway patency, adequacy of breathing, and circulatory sufficiency (to rule out shock) are always of primary concern.

Once initial emergencies have been addressed, the client is assessed more thoroughly (Box 57–2). A medical history helps identify any pre-existing conditions that may further complicate the injury. A thorough physical examination should be performed, with care being taken not to focus only on obvious injuries. Information about the accident (obtained from the injured client or witnesses) assists in the diagnosis of regional as well as anatomic injuries. A chest film and electrocardiogram are obtained for detecting possible pulmonary or cardiac impairment.

Management

Ventilation-perfusion imbalances may result from atelectasis, hemopneumothorax, flail chest, aspiration, or pulmonary contusion. Oxygen or mechanical ventilation may be required. General respiratory status (e.g., rate and depth of respirations, chest movement, spontaneous vital volumes) and ABGs should be monitored closely. Deterioration may indicate previously undetected injury or late-developing complications.

Therapeutic measures such as thoracentesis, chest tube insertion, bronchoscopic aspiration, or thoracotomy (Chaps. 20 and 27) may be indicated. Clients with chest injuries may experience significant hypovolemia. Fluid replacement is with blood and blood products, if indicated, or with crystalloid intravenous solutions (e.g., lactated Ringer's solution, normal saline). The nurse should continually monitor for signs of shock.

Excessive blood loss may further compromise the client's oxygenation. External bleeding should be carefully assessed, and estimated blood loss should be determined. Internal bleeding may result from injuries to the thoracic or abdominal viscera, torn muscles, or fractures. Considerable bleeding (i.e., 2 L or more) into the pleural space may occur. This usually can be quickly detected. Bleeding into areas such as the chest wall (e.g., from torn intercostal muscles) is more difficult to assess. A liter of blood can accumulate between the chest wall muscles without producing much swelling.

A chest-injured client may require large quantities of blood replacement. Until the results of typing and crossmatching are available, the patient is given O-negative blood. The volume of blood replacement is determined through assessment of clinical findings, hemodynamic measurements, and laboratory results (e.g., hemoglobin and hematocrit). When possible, surgery is delayed until the client's blood volume is restored.

Shock often results from hypovolemia, but in the chest-injured client it may also be caused by cardiac tamponade, cardiac contusion, flail chest, or tension pneumothorax. Once the cause of shock is determined, rapid intervention is given (see Chap. 56).

BOX 57–2

Assessment of and Therapeutic Intervention for the Chest Trauma Victim

Maintain airway, breathing, and circulation.
Obtain a quick history.

- What happened?
- What was the mechanism of injury?
- How long ago did it happen?
- Where is the pain? Does it radiate?
- Is there anything that makes the pain better or worse?
- What does the pain feel like?
- How severe is the pain on a scale of 1 to 10?
- Is there any medical history?

Perform a quick (1-minute) evaluation.

- Check for shortness of breath and cyanosis.
- Check vital signs.
- Check skin color and temperature.
- Check wound size and location.
- Check for paradoxical chest movement.
- Check for distended neck veins.
- Listen for respiratory stridor.
- Listen for bilateral breath sounds.
- Look for epigastric and supraclavicular indrawing.
- Give rough estimate of tidal volume.
- Check for tracheal deviation.
- Assess intercostal muscle use.
- Assess accessory muscle use.
- Check for subcutaneous emphysema.
- Look and listen for sucking chest sounds.
- Listen to heart sounds.

Provide therapeutic intervention.

- Maintain airway.
- Ensure adequate air movement.
- Administer oxygen.
- Cover any open chest wound.
- Control flail segment.
- Insert needles or chest tube into anterior chest wall if tension pneumothorax is present.
- Initiate an intravenous line (two or more lines if possible, but do not delay transport to do this).
- Do pericardiocentesis, if indicated.
- Get chest x-ray film if more than three ribs are fractured, because victim is considered multitraumatized and one must search for other associated injuries. It is essential at this time to obtain cross-table lateral cervical spine x-ray film for detection of cervical spine injury before any other diagnostic tests are initiated or the victim is moved.
- Frequently recheck vital signs.
- Monitor for dysrhythmias.

From Sheehy, S. B. (1985). *Emergency nursing: Principles and practice.* St. Louis: C. V. Mosby.

Pain associated with chest injuries may cause the client to breathe rapidly and shallowly, which leads to atelectasis and pooling of tracheobronchial secretions. Analgesics minimize pain and permit periods of rest and relaxation. They also allow the client to cough and take deeper breaths. Administration must be done cautiously to avoid respiratory depression. Intercostal nerve blocks or epidural analgesia may be used in clients with underlying health problems. Splinting the chest may also be helpful.

Complications

Severe chest trauma may produce numerous complications, including

- Pneumothorax
- Tension pneumothorax and mediastinal shift
- Open pneumothorax and mediastinal flutter
- Hemothorax
- Fractured ribs
- Fractured sternum
- Flail chest

PNEUMOTHORAX

Pneumothorax is the presence of air in the pleural space that prohibits complete lung expansion. Air may enter the pleural space directly through a hole in the chest wall (open pneumothorax) or diaphragm. Air may escape into the pleural space from a puncture or tear in an internal respiratory structure (e.g., bronchus, bronchioles, alveoli). This form of pneumothorax is called closed or spontaneous pneumothorax (Fig. 57–5).

Clinical manifestations of moderate pneumothorax include tachypnea; dyspnea; sudden sharp pain on the affected side with chest movement, breathing, or coughing; asymmetric chest expansion; diminished or absent breath sounds on the affected side; hyper-resonance (tympany) to percussion on the affected side; restlessness or anxiety; and tachycardia.

Clinical manifestations of severe pneumothorax include all the preceding and distended neck veins; shift in the point of maximal impulse of the heartbeat; subcutaneous emphysema; decreased tactile and vocal fremitus; tracheal deviation toward the unaffected side; and progressive cyanosis.

Management

If pneumothorax is suspected (but respiratory distress is too severe to permit x-ray confirmation), the physician may perform an emergency thoracentesis. Aspiration demonstrates whether free air is present in the pleural space.

However, most physicians prefer to insert a chest tube immediately into the pleural space via the fourth intercostal space at mid- or anterior axillary line. The chest catheter is connected to closed-chest drainage. (Management of closed-chest drainage is discussed in Chap. 22.) Sometimes thoracotomy (surgical opening into the chest cavity) is done to explore the chest surgically and repair the site of origin of the pneumothorax or hemothorax.

TENSION PNEUMOTHORAX AND MEDIASTINAL SHIFT

Tension pneumothorax is a serious type of pneumothorax in which air enters the pleural space with each inspiration, becomes trapped there, and is not expelled

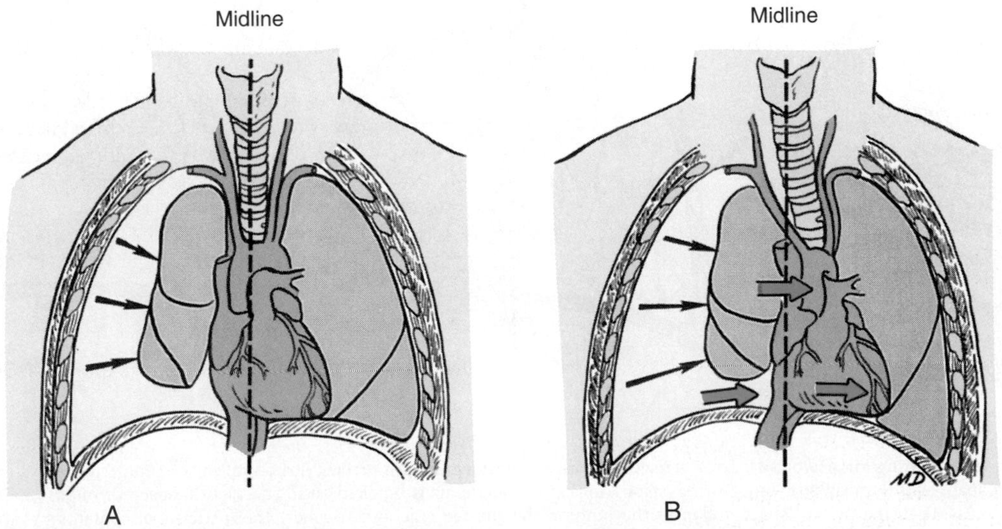

Figure 57–5
A, Pneumothorax. Lung collapses as air gathers in the pleural space. *B*, Mediastinal shift in tension pneumothorax. In addition to collapsed lung, the mediastinal contents are displaced against the unaffected side of the chest.

during expiration (i.e., one-way valve effect). Pressure builds in the chest as the accumulation of air in the pleural space increases. Tension pneumothorax most commonly occurs with blunt traumatic injuries and is frequently associated with flail chest injuries.

If untreated, tension pneumothorax collapses the lung on the affected side as intrapleural pressure or tension increases. It may then cause a mediastinal shift (see Fig. 57–5). This means the contents of the mediastinum (heart, trachea, esophagus, and great vessels) are pushed or "shifted" toward the chest's unaffected side. Mediastinal shift may cause (1) compression of the lung in the direction of the shift (i.e., the lung opposite the pneumothorax) and (2) compression, traction, torsion, or kinking of the great vessels (e.g., vena cava); thus, blood return to the heart is dangerously impaired. The latter causes a subsequent decrease in cardiac output and blood pressure.

CRITICAL TO REMEMBER

Tension pneumothorax produces serious circulatory and pulmonary impairment that can be rapidly fatal. This is a high-priority emergency requiring prompt assessment and intervention.

Clinical manifestations of tension pneumothorax include marked, severe dyspnea; tachypnea; crepitus (subcutaneous emphysema in the neck and upper chest); progressive cyanosis; acute chest pain on the affected side; hyper-resonance (tympany) to percussion on the affected side; tachycardia; asymmetric chest wall movement; diminished or absent breath sounds on the affected side; and restlessness and agitation.

Other clinical manifestations include neck vein distention; laryngeal and tracheal deviation or shift to the unaffected side; feeling of tightness or pressure within the chest; point of maximal impulse shift laterally or medially; severe hypotension leading to shock; and muffled heart sounds.

A suspected mediastinal shift may be confirmed by x-ray study. Laryngeal and tracheal deviation can be detected by gentle palpation and with x-ray study. ABGs demonstrate hypoxia and respiratory alkalosis. When mediastinal shift is severe and not immediately corrected, respiratory acidosis may ensue.

Management

Immediate intervention is to convert tension pneumothorax into open pneumothorax (a less serious disorder). An open pneumothorax is most easily and rapidly created by inserting an 18-gauge needle into the pleural space at the level of the second intercostal space at the midclavicular line. Prompt thoracentesis to remove air may be life saving. As trapped air rushes from a tension pneumothorax, the tension is relieved; the lung re-expands; and if mediastinal shift is present, it corrects itself. After emergency treatment, the physician inserts a chest catheter and connects it to a waterseal drainage system.

OPEN PNEUMOTHORAX

An open pneumothorax occurs with "sucking" chest wounds. With this type of wound, a traumatic opening in the chest wall is large enough for air to move freely in and out of the chest cavity during ventilation (Fig. 57–6). This abnormal movement of air through the

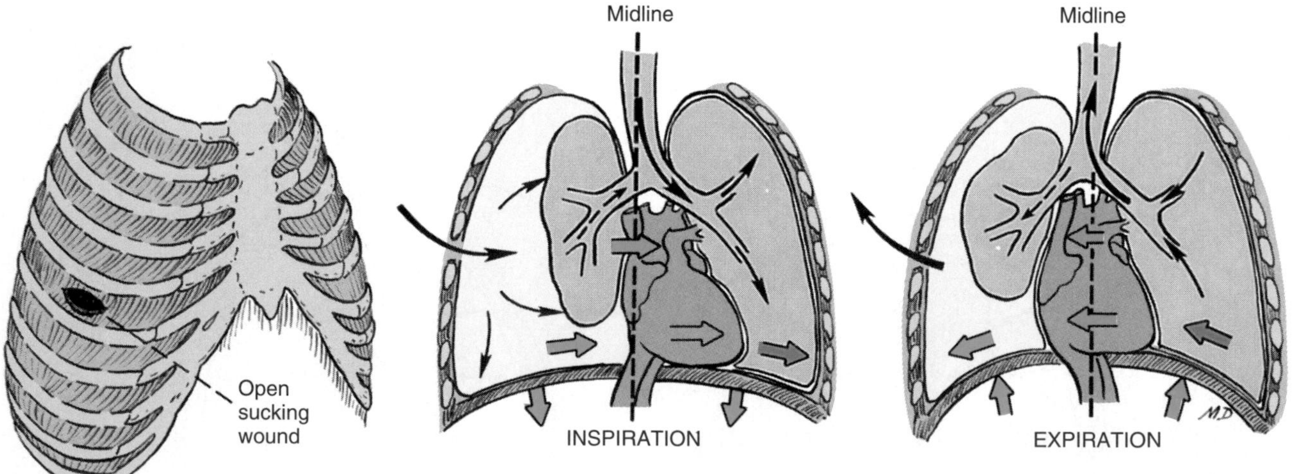

Figure 57–6
Open pneumothorax (sucking chest wound). *Solid arrows* indicate air movement; *open arrows,* structural movement. A chest wall wound connects the pleural space with atmospheric air. During inspiration, atmospheric air is "sucked" into the pleural space through the chest wall wound. Positive pressure in the pleural space collapses the lung on the affected side and "pushes" the mediastinal contents toward the unaffected side. This reduces the volume of air in the unaffected side considerably. During expiration, air escapes through the chest wall wound, lessening positive pressure in the affected side and allowing the mediastinal contents to "swing" back toward the affected side. Movement of mediastinal structures from side to side is called mediastinal flutter.

chest wound produces a "slurping" or "sucking" noise that is audible in a quiet environment.

Open sucking chest wounds may result from accidental injuries or surgical trauma.

Management

When an open sucking chest wound is detected, emergency intervention includes immediately covering the wound securely with anything available. An airtight covering usually prevents tension pneumothorax and preserves ventilation of the opposite lung. The nurse should not waste time looking for a sterile gauze petrolatum dressing (the ideal covering for such a wound) if it is not immediately available.

The nurse must immediately cover the wound with whatever is at hand (e.g., a towel) until someone can bring a sterile petrolatum dressing. When possible, the temporary dressing should be fixed firmly in place with several strips of wide tape.

If the client is conscious and cooperative, the nurse should ask the client to take a very deep breath and then attempt to blow it out while keeping mouth and nose closed. This pushing effort against a closed glottis helps push air out through the chest wound and re-expand the lung. When the client does this, the dressing should be applied before the client can again inhale.

The nurse must stay with the chest-injured client after a dressing has been applied to a sucking wound and assess carefully for indications of tension pneumothorax and mediastinal shift. This may develop if the air leak is in the lung or a bronchus, which permits air to escape into the pleural space. In such a situation, closing the chest wall wound with an airtight dressing prevents the outflow of escaping air. Thus, an open pneumothorax has been accidentally converted into a tension pneumothorax. If tension pneumothorax appears to be developing after the wound is sealed, the seal should immediately be unplugged (Fig. 57–7).

Although it is dangerous to have air moving into and out of the pleural space with each respiration (open pneumothorax), it is far more dangerous when air moves only into the pleural space and cannot move back out (tension pneumothorax).

Closed-chest drainage will be necessary to (1) remove the air from the pleural space and (2) allow the lung to re-expand if collapsed.

HEMOTHORAX

Hemothorax may be present in clients with chest injuries. A small amount of blood (less than 300 mL) in the pleural space may cause no symptoms and may not require intervention (blood will be reabsorbed spontaneously). Severe hemothorax (1400–2500 mL) may be life threatening because of resultant hypovolemia and tension (Fig. 57–8). Clinical manifestations include dullness to percussion on the affected side, tachycardia, hypotension, and shock.

Management

If the client is in severe distress, the physician may aspirate blood from the pleural space by inserting a 16-gauge needle into the fifth or sixth intercostal space at the midaxillary line. To drain intrathoracic accumu-

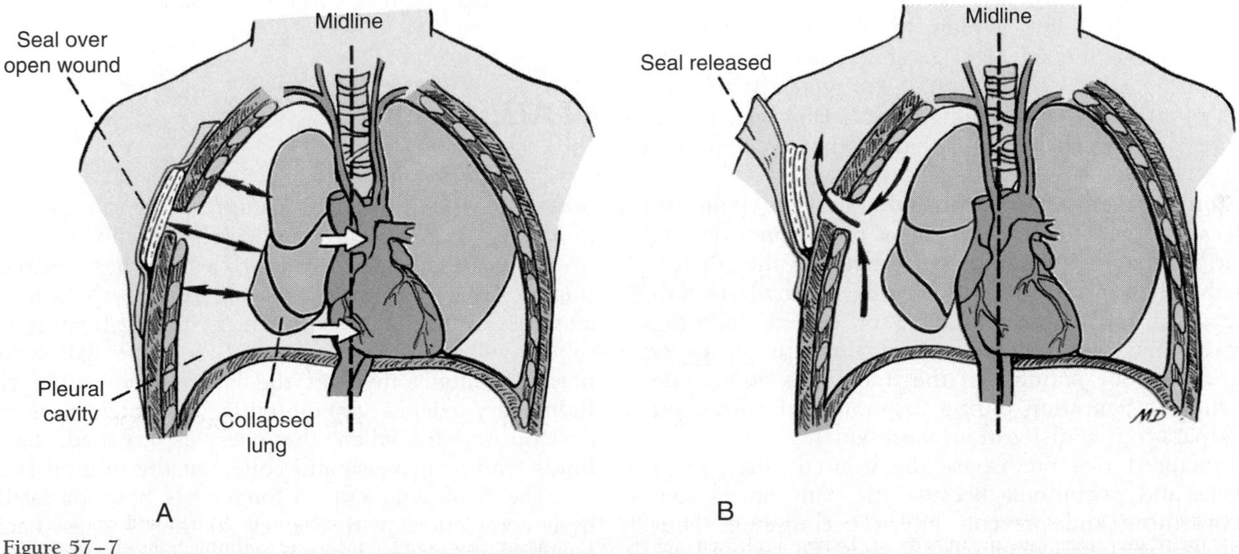

Figure 57–7
Tension pneumothorax. *A*, If an open pneumothorax is covered (e.g., with a dressing), it forms a seal, and tension pneumothorax with a mediastinal shift develops. A tear in lung structure continues to allow air into the pleural space. As positive pressure builds in the pleural space, the affected lung collapses, and the mediastinal contents shift to the unaffected side. *B*, Tension pneumothorax is corrected by removing the seal (e.g., dressing), allowing air trapped in the pleural space to escape.

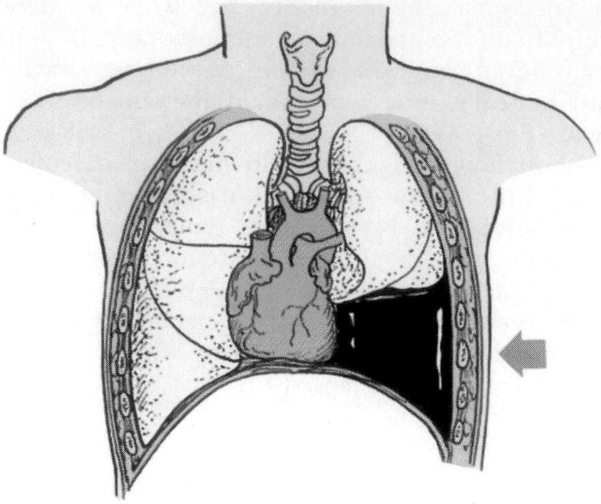

Figure 57–8
Massive hemothorax *(arrow)* below left lung, causing collapse of lung tissue.

lations of blood, the physician inserts a large-caliber (36 French or larger) chest catheter. An initial drainage of 500 to 1000 mL is considered moderate and may not require additional treatment. However, continued large amounts of drainage (200 mL or more per hour) may indicate a need for emergency thoracotomy. Such drainage should be documented and promptly reported to the physician. An initial drainage of 1500 mL or more is an indication for immediate exploratory thoracotomy.

FRACTURED RIBS

Rib fractures are common chest injuries, particularly in the elderly. They are usually associated with a blunt injury, such as a fall, a blow to the chest, or (more frequently) the impact of a steering wheel against the chest during rapid deceleration. A rib typically fractures at the point of maximal applied force. However, it may fracture at its weakest point, that is, the costochondral joint.

Clinical manifestations include localized pain and tenderness over the fracture area on inspiration and palpation; shallow respirations; tendency of the client to hold the chest protectively or breathe shallowly to minimize chest movements; bruising or surface markings (may or may not be present) at the site of injury; protruding bone splinters if the fracture is compound; and clicking sensation during inspiration if costochondral separation or dislocation is present.

Fractured ribs predispose the injured client to atelectasis and pneumonia because the pain causes shallow breathing and prevents effective coughing. Thus, secretions accumulate, which obstruct the bronchi and become a site for infection. Shallow breathing also reduces lung compliance.

Bone splinters from fractured ribs may cause pneumothorax or hemothorax by puncturing the lung and pleura. Bright red sputum may be coughed up if the lung has been penetrated. The nurse should assess the client for signs of pneumothorax or hemothorax and report such findings promptly.

Management

Fractured ribs are generally treated conservatively with rest, local heat, and analgesics. The pain from fractured ribs usually lasts 5 to 7 days. Complete healing occurs in approximately 6 weeks.

If pain is severe enough to impair ventilation significantly, a local anesthetic may be injected at the fracture site itself. Intercostal nerve blocks may also be used. Adequate pain control and splinting of the chest during coughing and deep breathing help the client with rib fractures to carry out these painful but vital activities more comfortably. Hospitalization may be required, especially in the elderly, whose vital capacity may be significantly compromised.

FRACTURED STERNUM

Sternal fractures usually result from blunt deceleration injuries, such as impact from the steering wheel. They are usually accompanied by other major injuries, such as flail chest; pulmonary and myocardial contusions; ruptured aorta, trachea, bronchus, or esophagus; and hemothorax or pneumothorax. Clinical manifestations include sharp, stabbing pain; tenderness, swelling, and discoloration over the fracture site; and crepitus. The main priority is to control associated injuries. A client with a nondisplaced fracture may need analgesics or intercostal nerve blocks for pain relief. Severe sternal fractures may require surgical fixation.

FLAIL CHEST

Severe chest injuries that compress the rib cage often produce a crushed chest in which the ribs are pushed in on lung tissue. By definition, a flail chest consists of fractures of two or more adjacent ribs on the same side and possibly the sternum, with each bone fractured into two or more segments (Fig. 57–9). The flail segment most commonly involves the lateral side of the chest. Pulmonary edema, pneumonitis, and atelectasis often develop rapidly when the chest is crushed, because fluids tend to increase and collect at the injured site.

The "flail" segment no longer has bony or cartilaginous connections with the rest of the rib cage. Lacking attachment to the thoracic skeleton, the flail section "floats," moving independently of the chest wall during ventilation. This disrupts the normal bellows action of the thorax by causing paradoxical motion.

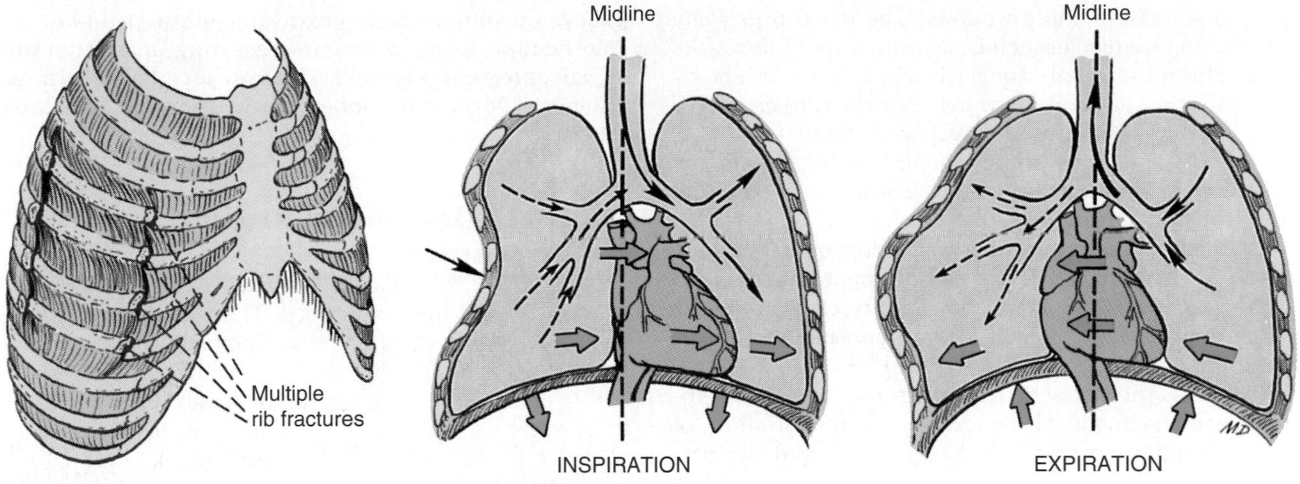

Figure 57–9
Flail chest. *Solid arrows* indicate air movement; *open arrows*, structural movement. *A*, A flail chest consists of fractured rib segments that are unattached (free-floating) from the rest of the chest wall. *B*, On inspiration, the flail segment of ribs is "sucked" inward. The affected lung and mediastinal structures shift to the unaffected side. This compromises the amount of inspired air in the unaffected lung. *C*, On expiration, the flail segment of ribs "bellows" outward. The affected lung and mediastinal structures shift to the affected side. Some air within the lungs is shunted back and forth between the lungs instead of passing through the upper airway.

During paradoxical motion, the flail portion of the chest and its underlying lung tissue are "sucked in" with inspiration, instead of expanding outward as normal, and ballooned out ("blown out") with expiration, instead of collapsing normally inward. This alteration in normal chest wall mechanics diminishes the client's ability to achieve an adequate tidal volume and to produce an adequate cough. Hypoventilation and hypoxemia may result, which leads to respiratory failure without rapid intervention.

In addition, pulmonary contusion results in the underlying lung tissue. This produces an accumulation of fluid in the affected alveoli, which leads to intrapulmonary shunting and further hypoxia.

Furthermore, mediastinal structures tend to swing back and forth (mediastinal flutter) with significant paradoxical motion. These "swings" may seriously affect circulatory dynamics, producing elevated venous pressure, impaired filling of the right side of the heart, and decreased arterial pressure.

The client is typically very anxious, cyanotic, and severely dyspneic. Respirations are usually rapid, shallow, and grunting. Paradoxical movement of the chest wall is usually obvious.

The physiologic abnormalities usually become increasingly serious in the first 48 to 72 hours after injury. Hypercapnia and hypoxia worsen as the effort necessary to breathe further depletes the already diminished oxygen supply.

Management

If severe respiratory distress is present, treatment is usually with intubation and mechanical ventilation. These actions (1) restore adequate ventilation, thus reducing hypoxia and hypercapnia; (2) decrease paradoxical motion by using positive pressure to stabilize the chest wall internally; (3) relieve pain by decreasing movement of the fractured ribs; and (4) provide an avenue for secretion removal. Internal stabilization with continuous ventilation may require 21 days or more. Muscle relaxants or musculoskeletal paralyzing agents (e.g., pancuronium bromide) may be administered to reduce the risk of separation of the healing costochondral junctions.

For the client with adequate pulmonary function, intubation should be avoided. This helps reduce the incidence of infection, a complication associated with higher morbidity and mortality rates in clients with flail chest.[25] Initial treatment in this client is aimed at providing adequate pain relief to prevent splinting, thus enabling the client to deep breathe and clear secretions effectively. Intermittent positive-pressure breathing may be used to enhance lung expansion.

Frequent assessments of blood gases are needed to monitor respiratory effectiveness and detect acidosis. A variety of factors may produce metabolic and respiratory acidosis in chest-injured clients. Chest physiotherapy and postural drainage may be required to facilitate secretion removal. The nurse should assess breath sounds before and after any intervention.

TRACHEOBRONCHIAL TRAUMA

Trauma (rupture, tears) to the tracheobronchial tree may be caused by blunt injury (sternal fracture); caustic ingestion; iatrogenic instrumentation (e.g., it may occur with deep tracheobronchial suctioning or bronchoscopy); or missile or knife wounds. The usual injury site is on the main stem bronchus, within 1 inch above the carina. The most lethal sequela is a tear from the bronchus into the pulmonary veins, which can cause air bubbles to be sent into the systemic circulation. It is particularly dangerous when an air bubble enters the pulmonary vein and goes into a coronary or cerebral vessel, causing cardiac arrest or cerebral air embolism.

Clinical manifestations of tracheobronchial trauma include dyspnea and severe air hunger, hemoptysis (often massive), subcutaneous emphysema into the neck and face, pneumomediastinum, and pneumothorax (simple or tension).

Management of tracheobronchial rupture or tear includes establishment of an airway, administration of high-flow oxygen, closed-chest drainage, and surgical repair.

Chest Pain

Chest pain is one of the most common complaints of clients entering an emergency department. Effective triage is essential for early detection and intervention of life-threatening conditions. There are several causes of chest pain (see Chap. 23, Table 23–1).

Because the pain experience is subjective, careful assessment of the pain is important. The nurse should perform a complete symptom analysis (see Chap. 23).

The nurse proceeds with an objective assessment in the ABC order. Breath sounds should be compared bilaterally for the presence of any rales or wheezing. The nurse should listen to the heart sounds; listen for a friction rub (possible pericarditis) or murmurs (valvular disease or endocarditis); assess for the presence of adrenergic (elevated blood pressure, tachycardia, diaphoresis, dilated pupils, and anxiety) or cholinergic influences (bradycardia, nausea, and vomiting); and determine the level of consciousness. This may be diminished because of hypoxia. A full set of vital signs must be obtained.

Management

Supplemental oxygen via mask or nasal prongs must be provided. The nurse must apply a cardiac monitor for monitoring the heart rate and rhythm and obtain a 12-lead ECG. Any dysrhythmias present must be treated (see Chap. 24). Nitroglycerin is commonly used to treat angina or ischemic pain; this may be sublingual, intravenous, or dermal. The nurse should be sure to monitor blood pressure after the dose because it may cause hypotension. For severe pain, morphine, 2 to 4 mg intravenously, is administered. The nurse should be sure to assess respirations, vital signs, and pain control.

The head of the bed should be positioned for the client's comfort. Ongoing vital signs should be obtained. If dysrhythmias are present, the nurse should provide continual cardiac monitoring. Throughout the emergency, the nurse must provide emotional support and information using a calm, reassuring manner. Additional interventions will depend on the determined diagnosis. Myocardial infarction is discussed in Chapter 24.

Neurologic-Neurosurgical Emergencies

HEAD TRAUMA

Any client with an injury to the head or who has experienced an insult that typically produces head trauma requires a thorough neurologic assessment. This is true even if the client appears to feel "fine" when first evaluated.

The major causes of head trauma are motor vehicle crashes, falls, and assaults. Head trauma may range from minor scrapes and contusions to severe blunt and penetrating injuries. Central nervous system effects of severe head injury and treatment are discussed in Table 57–4. Care of the client with severe head injury is discussed in Chapter 14.

Alcohol is a major risk factor associated with head injury. There is a high correlation between alcohol consumption and motor vehicle crashes, falls, and assaults. Age, sex, stress, drug abuse, and underlying seizure disorders and loss of musculoskeletal control are additional risk factors for head trauma.

CLIENT EDUCATION GUIDE

Head Injuries

Clients who sustain minor head trauma (concussions) may be treated in the emergency department and released. The nurse must be sure to include the following teaching-learning points in the discharge instructions for clients with head injuries and their significant others:

- Wake the client every 2 hours (for the next 8 hours) and check level of consciousness and orientation.
- Give only liquids initially for the first 8 hours and then progress to a regular diet.
- Give acetaminophen for headache. If stronger medication is required, contact a physician. (Note: The nurse must emphasize this because clients often have narcotics from previous illnesses and must understand that narcotics are contraindicated in head injury.)
- Notify a physician or return to the emergency department if any of the following occur: one or both pupils become dilated and nonreactive; the level of consciousness decreases; inability to use an arm or leg develops; seizure is experienced; or there is continued vomiting.
- Provide written as well as verbal instruction and include an appropriate telephone number for additional questions once the client returns home.

TABLE 57–4 Classification of Acute Head Injuries and Treatment Summary

TYPE OF INJURY	CNS EFFECTS AND SIGNS AND SYMPTOMS	TREATMENT
Linear fracture	Variable, from none to both localized and generalized signs because of damage to underlying brain tissue Fractures of temporal bone are of concern because of possibility of epidural hematoma Fractures associated with a scalp laceration are considered open fractures; infection and meningitis are concerns	Observation, possibly at home, unless it is a temporal fracture or is associated with a laceration
Basilar skull fracture	A form of linear fracture occurring at base of skull; dural lacerations may occur, exposing brain to contamination from paranasal sinuses and to loss of CSF; meningitis is a major concern Fracture may be difficult to visualize radiographically; thus, physical findings are used to make the diagnosis: blood behind the tympanic membrane–ruptured tympanic membrane with blood in the ear canal; CSF oto- or rhinorrhea; hearing loss; facial nerve palsy; ecchymosis of mastoid area (Battle's sign); periorbital ecchymosis (raccoon eyes); pneumocephalus	Admission for observation, antibiotics, possible surgery if CSF leak continues or infection ensues
Depressed fracture	Variable, depending on damage to underlying brain tissue	Surgery to elevate bone fragments and to treat hematomas or brain injury
Comminuted fracture	More than one fracture line; symptoms variable	Admit for observation This type of fracture suggests that the magnitude of force was great, predisposing to significant vessel or brain injury
Mild concussion	Temporary alterations in neurologic function without loss of consciousness (e.g., confusion, disorientation without amnesia) Alterations occur immediately after the accident, are momentary, and are associated with no sequelae	Observation, at home with reliable observers, or in the health-care facility
Classic cerebral concussion	Temporary neurologic deficiency associated with temporary loss of consciousness Confusion with amnesia develops 5–10 minutes after accident; permanent amnesia for events immediately preceding the accident Confusion and disorientation usually resolve within a few seconds	Observation, often in the emergency department for several hours or in the health-care facility
Intracerebral hematoma-hemorrhage	Focal or generalized alterations in neurologic function, depending on size and location of injury	Surgical evacuation of hematoma if feasible; ICP monitoring and measures to decrease ICP

CNS, central nervous system; CSF, cerebrospinal fluid; ICP, intracranial pressure.

Management

Clients who sustain minor head trauma (concussions) may be treated in the emergency department and released (see Client Education Guide: Head Injuries).

SPINAL INJURIES

All clients who sustain traumatic injury are at risk for spinal cord injuries. These injuries result in loss of motor or sensory function that may be permanent. Refer to Chapter 16 for further discussion of spinal injuries.

The mechanisms of injury commonly associated with closed spinal injuries involving the cervical area include hyperflexion, hyperextension, flexion compression, and acceleration whiplash (see Chap. 16, Fig. 16–1). In addition to obvious cord injury (complete or partial transection), edema, hemorrhage, and impaired vertebral artery circulation may cause permanent spinal cord damage.

Management

The nurse assesses and maintains the ABCs.

CRITICAL TO REMEMBER

A cervical spine injury must be suspected in all unconscious trauma victims and those with injuries above the clavicle.

The nurse must immobilize the spine before the client is removed from an automobile or the scene (whenever possible) by applying a hard cervical extrication collar or Philadelphia collar and placing the client on a long spine board. When the client has been extricated, the nurse should leave the collar in place, secure the head and neck alignment with towel rolls or a head immobilizer, and secure the client's head to the backboard. The client must be cautioned not to turn or move the head. This instruction must be reinforced frequently, especially if the client is under the influence of drugs or alcohol.

Respiratory insufficiency may be present, especially with a cervical spine injury, because the phrenic nerve (controls the diaphragm during respiration) exits the spinal column at the level of C4. The nurse should keep in mind the risk for hypotension related to neurogenic shock.

The nurse should assess for pain caused by vertebral displacement or spasm of paraspinal muscles.[32] The nurse should note any difficulty moving upper or lower extremities and assess for numbness.

Clients with spinal cord injuries may be fully conscious and aware of motor and sensory losses. Fear and anxiety are often present. The nurse should be sure to communicate with the client and provide information about any treatments and procedures.

Abdominal Emergencies

ACUTE ABDOMEN

Abdominal pain is common; its causes are numerous. Serious emergencies requiring immediate assessment and management must be identified. The term "acute abdomen" is used to describe the condition of a client with a sudden onset of abdominal pain. Most clients with acute abdomens requiring surgery can wait for a more complete evaluation. However, those with intra-abdominal catastrophes like ruptured aortic aneurysm must be identified and managed within minutes. Problems causing an acute abdomen include inflammation with or without perforation, obstruction of a hollow viscus, gastrointestinal hemorrhage, and blunt or penetrating abdominal trauma.

The following specific historical information must be included in the client assessment:

- Assess the pain for location, quality, and duration and ask whether it radiates. Determine whether there is a history of injury.
- Is there a history of nausea, vomiting, or loss of appetite? What is the amount and character of the emesis, if present?
- When was the last bowel movement? Was it normal? What was the character of the stool? When did the client last eat? What did the client eat?
- What medication or remedies have been used in an attempt to relieve the pain? Are any medications, including over-the-counter drugs, taken on a routine basis?
- Determine the menstrual history in all sexually active females of childbearing age.

The nurse must assess the abdomen in order of inspection, auscultation, percussion, and palpation; assess the client's position; assess for distention, masses, umbilical protrusion, and discoloration around the flank (Grey Turner's sign) or umbilicus; look for evidence of blunt or penetrating trauma; auscultate for bowel sounds; and note any abnormal, hyperactive, hypoactive, or absent bowel sounds.

Priorities of care focus on maintaining the ABCs. The nurse must be sure to monitor vital signs for changes. Intravenous access should be initiated as needed for hydration and lactated Ringer's solution or normal saline infused until hypotension or orthostasis is resolved. The client must be kept NPO until the cause of the abdominal pain is identified.

RUPTURED OR DISSECTING AORTIC ANEURYSM

An aneurysm is an outpouching of a vessel wall, usually as a result of arteriosclerotic changes or trauma involving the tunica media (muscular layer of an artery). Aneurysms may be saccular (balloon out) or fusiform (encircle the vessel). Aortic aneurysms may involve the thoracic aorta or abdominal aorta. The abdominal aorta is most commonly affected in males older than 60 years.

CRITICAL TO REMEMBER

Few emergencies require as rapid and efficient recognition and management as does a ruptured or dissecting aortic aneurysm. A ruptured or dissecting aneurysm is a surgical emergency.

In aortic dissection, blood separates the vessel layers, and a larger portion of the vessel may be affected. In an expanding aneurysm, the aneurysm wall is still intact. Symptoms are caused by increased pressure on the surrounding structures. A rupture occurs when the vessel wall loses continuity.

Management

Assessment findings include severe abdominal and back pain if the aneurysm is leaking. Back pain is often due to irritation from blood accumulation in the retroperitoneal space. Extreme pain indicates a catastrophic event. Narcotics may be of no value in pain relief but may be administered liberally. The nurse assesses for an enlarging abdominal girth with a palpable, pulsatile abdominal mass. There may be leg numbness, tingling, or loss of motor function. The nurse assesses for mottled cyanosis below the level of the aneurysm. Profound hypotension is typical, and occasionally initial hypertension occurs. (Note: if the aneurysm is thoracic or dissects into the thoracic aorta, blood pressure may differ significantly on one arm, and chest pain is usually present.) The nurse assesses for diminished distal pulses and monitors urine output for amount and hematuria. The client may be apprehensive, anxious, and restless.

The definitive treatment is surgery. Rapid intervention is vital. The nurse must provide supplemental oxygen; insert two to four large-bore intravenous catheters and infuse Ringer's lactate; monitor the client's fluid response closely to avoid fluid overloading; monitor vital signs continuously, and institute a cardiac monitor. The pneumatic antishock garment (PASG) may be indicated to help tamponade the bleeding. Antihypertensive agents may be used to minimize extension of a dissection. The nurse must obtain blood for laboratory studies (CBC, electrolytes, coagulation screen, and T & C for 10 to 20 units of whole blood); obtain an ECG and portable chest and abdominal films; prepare the client and significant others for emergency surgery; notify the operating room and laboratory of the urgency of the client's condition; and transport the client to the operating room, with resuscitative personnel in attendance and an emergency laparotomy tray on the stretcher. If the client is stable, and the diagnosis unclear, an aortogram may be done. A nurse must be present and provide care during this procedure.

GASTROINTESTINAL BLEEDING

The causes of gastrointestinal bleeding are many. Immediate interventions focus on cardiovascular stabilization, identification of the source of bleeding, and attempts to stop the bleeding. Additionally, psychosocial support for the client and significant others is important. Massive bleeding is frightening, and many procedures that may be uncomfortable are carried out rapidly in the initial phase of care.

Abdominal Injuries

The manifestations of abdominal injuries are often subtle and require astute assessment and intervention.

Abdominal injuries, caused by blunt or penetrating trauma, may result in significant organ injury and shock. Low-velocity trauma (fist) usually results in single-organ injury. High-velocity trauma (motor vehicle crashes) often produces multiple-organ involvement. Once the mechanism of injury is identified, the nurse should keep in mind the potential of associated injuries to underlying organs and tissues. Blunt trauma is more likely to cause injury to the solid organs (spleen, liver, pancreas, or kidneys).

Penetrating abdominal injuries are often caused by gunshot or stab wounds. The underlying injuries will depend on the mechanism of injury, trajectory, and location. Infection (peritonitis) is a common complication with penetrating abdominal trauma, especially if the bowel is ruptured. Hemorrhage and shock may develop if major blood vessels, liver, and spleen are injured. The client with a penetrating abdominal injury will require surgical exploration.

Clinical manifestations include

- Abdominal pain
- Distention
- Rigidity
- Nausea
- Vomiting
- Altered or absent bowel sounds
- Hypotension
- Shock

The nurse should assess for any open wounds. If open wounds are present, evisceration may occur.

CRITICAL TO REMEMBER

Exposure of abdominal contents to air may dry them out and lead to necrosis. An open wound, if found, must be covered with a warm, moist, sterile towel.

The spleen is the abdominal organ most commonly injured by blunt trauma, yet injury may also result from penetrating trauma. (Intense left shoulder pain may be Kehr's sign, which often occurs in splenic rupture.) Small tears may be repaired by a surgical hemostatic agent. For injuries of the left upper quadrant, left lower rib fractures, or left pneumothorax, a spleen injury should be suspected. The nurse should be sure to watch for shock and support the circulatory status.

Liver injury may result from abdominal trauma and should be suspected with right lower rib fractures. The liver is highly vascular, and injury may result in shock and bleeding disorders. Surgical repair through hemostatic agents and repair of blood vessels may be indicated.

Management

The nurse must manage and support the ABCs; provide supplemental oxygen; initiate one to two large-bore intravenous catheters and begin fluid support; obtain serial vital signs; apply PASGs if the client is hypotensive and it is not contraindicated; draw blood for laboratory studies (CBC, T & C, amylase, aspartate aminotransferase); insert a urinary catheter and obtain samples for urinalysis and specific gravity determination; insert a nasogastric tube, test the aspirate for blood, and connect to suction to decompress the stomach; and prepare the client for an intravenous pyelogram if hematuria is present. An ultrasonogram or CT scan of the abdomen may be performed if the client is stable. A culdocentesis may be done on females. The nurse should prepare the client for a diagnostic peritoneal lavage.

A diagnostic peritoneal lavage is performed by a physician to determine the presence of blood in the abdominal cavity (Fig. 57–10). The area below the umbilicus is anesthetized, and a large angiocatheter or peritoneal dialysis catheter is inserted into the abdomen. A syringe is attached to the catheter, and an attempt to aspirate blood is performed. One liter of normal saline is infused into the abdomen and drained by gravity. The fluid is evaluated for gross blood and sent to the laboratory for evaluation. If the finding is positive, one must prepare the client for immediate surgery.

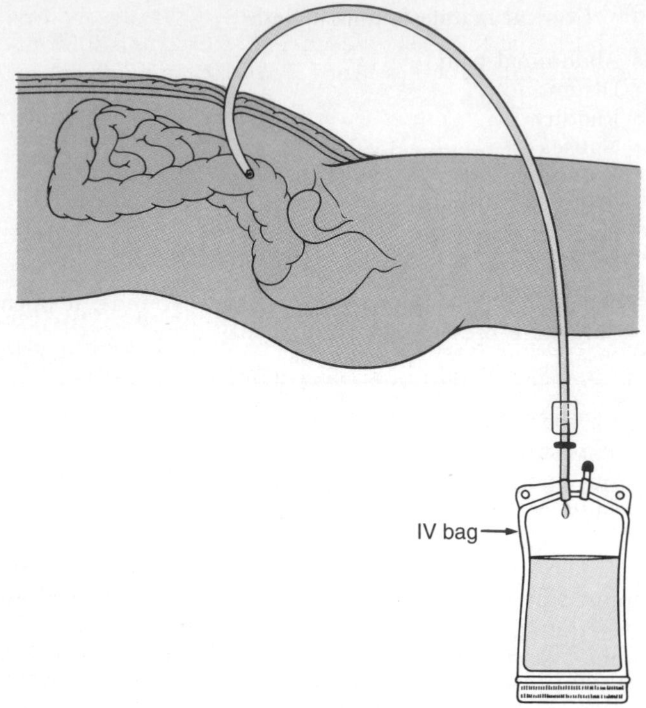

INTERPRETATION OF RESULTS

After blunt injury	
Positive result	Free-flowing blood on aspiration >100,000 RBC/mm³ >500 WBC/mm³ Amylase>serum amylase Bile staining Presence of foreign body material Exit of lavage fluid from urinary or thoracic catheters
Equivocal result	<5 ml bloody aspirate 50,000–100,000 RBC/mm³ 100–500 WBC/mm³
After stab wound	
Positive result	>10,000 RBC/mm³ Amylase>serum amylase Bile staining Presence of foreign material Exit of lavage fluid from urinary or thoracic catheters

Figure 57–10
Diagnostic peritoneal lavage. IV, intravenous; RBC, red blood cell; WBC, white blood cell. (Tabular content from Moore, E. E., et al. [1990]. *Early care of the injured patient.* Philadelphia: B. C. Decker.)

Client Teaching

Many clients with blunt abdominal trauma are assessed and discharged from the emergency department. However, some injuries (delayed rupture of the spleen) may not become apparent for several hours or days. Therefore, it is important to emphasize a need for repeat evaluation, particularly if the following symptoms occur:

- Increased localized or generalized abdominal pain
- Shoulder pain unrelated to shoulder trauma (Kehr's sign, suggestive of diaphragm irritation resulting from fluid or blood in the abdominal cavity)
- Malaise, lethargy, or dizziness suggestive of slow blood loss
- Fever of unexplained origin
- Nausea or vomiting, particularly if persistent
- Hematemesis or melena

Genitourinary Emergencies

ALLEGED SEXUAL ASSAULT

Health-care providers are required to use the term "alleged sexual assault" when caring for clients who may be victims of rape. Rape is a legal term. Although clients who experienced sexual assault may be males, most are female. Victims of sexual assault should be advised that health professionals are required to use the term "sexual assault" rather than "rape." Otherwise, they may understandably become infuriated by the staff's seeming insensitivity and lack of understanding.

Sexual assault victims often experience both acute and long-term physical and psychological trauma. This results from the assault itself and events that follow the assault. The psychological trauma, known as rape-trauma syndrome, may last only a few days to weeks or may last many years.

Lengthy legal proceedings, public humiliation, and destruction of social relationships prolong recovery. Although sexual assault victims may not be physiologically compromised on arrival in the emergency care setting, they are psychologically fragile and should be afforded the highest triage priority.

The goal of emergency care for clients is to provide sensitive, thorough physical care coupled with empathetic psychosocial support and to carefully gather vital information and evidence that is usually legally evaluated. The nurse must expedite the registration process and place the client in a private examination room; privacy must be ensured. If the assault is unreported, the nurse should encourage reporting it to authorities. Information should not be given over the telephone to media or others. The client must be instructed not to wash, gargle, or douche until necessary specimens are obtained. The client must be given an opportunity to bathe after the examination.

A detailed history and physical examination should be obtained after explaining the need for detail. The history must be taken immediately and only once. Sexual assault victims report that giving a history is almost as traumatic as the assault. The history should be recorded in detail, using the client's own words.

Management

The nurse must begin assessments and interventions with the ABCs. Some clients have massive trauma with loss of consciousness. For others, the physical result of the sexual assault may not be obvious. Possible sexual assault should be considered in unconscious clients with traumatic injury when the history is unknown or suspicious. Some common signs include ecchymotic areas, especially of the face or neck, and multiple contusions or lacerations. The nurse assesses for trauma to the larynx and fracture (with or without dislocation) of the mandible. The extent, location, and treatment of all injuries should be recorded. Pictures may be included. In females, a gynecologic examination should be carried out only once, preferably by a practitioner experienced in caring for these clients who will be available for court trial.

Specimens for laboratory study should be obtained, including cultures for gonorrhea; hanging drop analysis and smears for the presence of sperm and their motility; acid phosphatase of vaginal secretions; analysis of foreign pubic hairs by the police laboratory; and serologic fluorescent treponemal antibody studies.

Emotional responses may vary. The nurse must keep in mind the use of defense mechanisms that preserve psychosocial integrity and never assume that a lack of concern or relative calm means that the assault did not occur or the client is handling it well. Feelings of guilt, humiliation (especially after meeting with police), and fear may stop many victims from expressing their feelings. The nurse must provide psychosocial support and clear, understandable explanations; obtain the client's permission to contact sexual assault counselors if they are available and it has not already been done; and suggest that someone stay with the client after the event for support.

The condition of the client's clothing should be noted. Clothes may be stained, torn, or disheveled. However, they may be used as court evidence. The nurse should be sure to handle them carefully. Clothes are often taken by the police as evidence, so arrangements should be made for clean clothes to be brought to the client. Clothes must be placed in a paper bag.

Medications should be administered as ordered. Penicillin, 4.8 million units, is given intramuscularly 30 minutes after 1 g of probenecid (Benemid) is given orally for venereal disease prophylaxis. A short course of contraceptive pills may be used if pregnancy is suspected.

Client Teaching

Teaching includes

- Scheduling of follow-up care in 4 to 6 weeks for test results, pregnancy test, and psychosocial support
- Providing the name and number of someone to contact if the client is unwilling or unable to use counseling resources at the time of the emergency treatment
- Discussing some emotional responses to this type of trauma (rape-trauma syndrome)

The nurse should be sure to document the history, assessments, interventions, and teaching carefully. These hospital records are often placed in a "security file" because of possible use in court. Only the medical records department should release records and information and only to authorities with proper credentials.

Ocular Emergencies

Ocular emergencies, involving the eye and surrounding structures, range from mild corneal abrasions to avulsion of the eye, retinal detachment, and acute glaucoma and receive a high triage priority. All clients with ocular emergencies should be seen by an ophthalmologist.

CHEMICAL EYE BURNS

The nurse determines the history. The conjunctiva is often reddened, and there is severe pain. Copious tearing may be present unless deeper structures are involved. The nurse should be sure to determine what measures, if any, have been taken to relieve the pain or remove the chemical.

The nurse must reassure the client and explain all procedures. The eye must be immediately irrigated copiously with normal saline, water, or other mild solution. The eye's pH may be frequently tested and used to guide irrigation. Irrigation may continue until pH is in the 6 to 7 range. Often it is necessary to use a short-acting local anesthetic to irrigate the eye adequately. Alkali burns may need continuous irrigation for several hours, and special irrigation devices are available. Antibiotic drops, ointments, or irrigants may be used. Pain is often due to blepharospasm, and a mydriatic (homatropine, cyclopentolate [Cyclogyl]) may relieve the pain. Both eyes should be patched if necessary to immobilize the affected eye. If the burn is significant, the client is usually referred to an ophthalmologist or admitted.

OCULAR FOREIGN BODY

Ocular foreign bodies include surface, imbedded, and impaled objects. The client will complain of "something in the eye." Often the history is compatible with a foreign body. Pain and tearing may be present.

The nurse must be sure to remove any contact lenses, if present, and place in sterile saline solution. Contact lenses may become dislodged, which makes removal by the client difficult. The lenses are often found under the upper eyelid.

Small foreign bodies should be removed with a moistened cotton-tipped applicator. If they are not able to be removed after a few tries, attempts should be stopped. Impaled objects are left intact until they are removed by an ophthalmologist. The object should be stabilized by applying dressings (moistened with normal saline) around the base of the object and securing the object to the head. The nurse should avoid exerting pressure on the globe, and immobilize the head.

CRITICAL TO REMEMBER

The nurse must not attempt to stop bleeding from the eye or eyelids with direct pressure. This can cause further injury.

After removal of the foreign body, corneal abrasion, if present, is treated. Treatment includes antibacterial eyedrops or ointment and patching of the eye. A mydriatic is indicated if there is significant pain. Follow-up care in 24 hours is indicated if pain remains. Assessment of visual acuity should be completed and recorded before discharge.

OCULAR AVULSION

Avulsion of the eye from its socket may result from either blunt or penetrating trauma. The eye will be extruded from the orbit with obvious deformity and pain. However, even with rapid and expert care, the probability of preserving vision in the affected eye is slim.

The eye must be protected from drying by gently applying sterile dressings moistened with warm saline. An eye protector (cone, shield, paper cup) should be applied and secured gently to the head with gauze Kling or Kerlix. The nurse should patch the unaffected eye, and immobilize the head. Reassurance should be provided, but the nurse should not give false hopes about saving the eye. A prompt ophthalmologist referral should be obtained. The client should be prepared for surgery and kept NPO.

Musculoskeletal Emergencies

Musculoskeletal emergencies include fractures, amputations, joint dislocations, muscle strains, and ligament and tendon damage. These disorders are discussed in Chapter 46.

TRAUMATIC AMPUTATIONS

Traumatic amputations involve obvious total or partial severing of an extremity or digit. The severity of bleeding depends on the extent of trauma to surrounding tissues. A crush injury may not bleed profusely because of muscle spasms in the arterial walls. The artery constricts, and bleeding is decreased. Complete amputations usually do not bleed profusely because the vessels retract. However, a partially severed limb may require a tourniquet for control of bleeding.

Hypotension, shock, and tachycardia may be present if the client sustained significant blood loss. The nurse should be sure to maintain and support the ABCs; initiate intravenous and fluid resuscitation; control hemorrhage by direct pressure with use of a clean, sterile dressing if possible; draw blood for laboratory studies (CBC, T & C); and prepare the client for surgery.

The amputated part should accompany the client to the hospital because replantation with microsurgery is sometimes possible. The nurse must wrap the amputated part in saline-soaked gauze and place it in a plastic bag or container; place the container on ice; not place the amputated part directly in ice; and not use dry ice or freeze or totally submerge the tissue. In addition, the part should not be cleaned, disinfected, debrided, or perfused before transportation.

Soft Tissue Emergencies

Damage to the skin and soft tissues is a common emergency. The types of soft tissue injury are contusions, abrasions, puncture wounds, lacerations, and avulsions.

The nurse must always assess and maintain the ABCs; assess the wound for location, size, depth, and degree of contamination; assess for associated injuries, amount of tissue loss, and viability of wound edges and of amputated tissue; determine the history and mechanism of injury; include information about where the injury occurred, length of time since the injury, and allergies; obtain immunization history and the need for a tetanus booster; assess the range of motion and sensation distal to the wound; and ascertain how the injury may affect the client's activities of daily living.

Management

Bleeding should be stopped by direct pressure or application of a pressure dressing. The area around the wound should be cleaned and irrigated well with normal saline. Anesthesia may be needed to clean the wound properly.

The area around the wound should be shaved if necessary. The eyebrows should not be shaved because they are used as landmarks in situations in which extensive repair is needed. The nurse should scrub with a soft brush and normal saline; use forceps to remove imbedded foreign material; excise the wound if necessary; copiously irrigate the wound with normal saline; and leave the wound area open, if it is small. For larger areas, or areas in which friction may occur (waistline), the nurse dresses with gauze layers and covers with outer wrap.

The wound may be closed either noninvasively or with sutures. After closure, a thin layer of Neosporin,

TABLE 57–5 Summary of Tetanus Prophylaxis in Routine Wound Management

HISTORY OF TETANUS IMMUNIZATION (DOSES)	CLEAN, MINOR WOUNDS		ALL OTHER WOUNDS	
	Td	TIG	Td	TIG
Uncertain	Yes	No	Yes	Yes
0–1	Yes	No	Yes	Yes
2	Yes	No	Yes	No
3 or more	No	No	No	No

Td, tetanus and diphtheria toxoid; TIG, tetanus immune globulin.
Recommendations of the Centers for Disease Control. (1986). *Morbidity and Mortality Weekly Report*, Vol. 35.

CLIENT EDUCATION GUIDE

Wound Care

Client teaching should include the following points:

- Tissue swelling continues 8 to 12 hours after the injury. Therefore, keep the pressure dressing on, elevate the injured area, and apply cool packs.
- Keep the dressing clean and dry.
- Protect the dressing while carrying out activities of daily living (e.g., wear rubber gloves, place a plastic bag over the dressing while showering or bathing).
- Take all prescribed medications (e.g., antibiotics, analgesics) as directed.
- Report any signs of infection: swelling, increasing pain, redness, drainage, fever.
- Keep the scheduled appointment for suture removal.

Vaseline, or silver sulfadiazine (Silvadene) should be applied to prevent crusting. (The nurse must be certain to determine whether the client has any allergies to these medications.) An appropriate dressing should be applied. Air-permeable transparent dressings (i.e., Op-Site, Tegaderm) or a layered dressing may be used. A pressure dressing with tubular gauze should be used on fingers and toes and the digit protected with an aluminum splint.

Because of potential exposure to anaerobic organisms, tetanus prophylaxis is given. For wound management, the need for active immunization depends on the client's immunization history and condition of the wound. The recommendations for tetanus prophylaxis are outlined in Table 57–5.

Tetanus and diphtheria toxoid (Td) is the preferred preparation for active tetanus immunization in adults. If passive immunization is needed, human tetanus immune globulin (TIG) is given. The recommended dose of TIG for wounds with average severity is 250 units intramuscularly. When TIG and Td are given concurrently, separate syringes and separate sites should be used.[9]

Wound Closure

Noninvasive wound closure may be accomplished with the use of adhesive strips, often reinforced with nylon thread. Adhesive strips are used alone to approximate edges in small, superficial wounds not subject to a great amount of tension.

Wounds that require suturing include those with gaping wound edges; with visible subcutaneous or deeper structures; and located over joints, where joint movement opens the wound edges. Sutures remove dead space, stop hemorrhage, and give physical strength to a discontinuous surface.

After wound closure, the area should be cleaned and a layered dressing applied. The first layer should promote drainage but not adhere to the wound (Owen's silk, fine mesh gauze). The second layer promotes absorption (gauze sponges). The third layer minimizes dead space and provides slight pressure. A woven roller gauze (Kling or Kerlix) may be held in place by either adhesive tape or elastic net. The nurse should avoid placing adhesive tape over the wound area; occlusive tape may foster moisture accumulation and maceration of wound edges. A petroleum-based ointment is often applied directly to wound edges for minimizing crusting and promoting a thinner scar. A transparent dressing may be used in wounds not expected to swell or have large amounts of drainage.

If sutured wound edges are perfectly opposed and not disturbed or manipulated, adhesion of the edges occurs in about 6 hours, and infection cannot enter. Dry skin is more resistant to infection than is moist skin, and friction increases the potential for infection. The dressing should be left in place until time for suture removal. Dressings should be removed only if there is excessive bleeding, drainage, unexplained fever, or other indications of infection. (See Client Education Guide: Wound Care.)

HEAT EMERGENCIES

Exposure to increased environmental temperature may lead to heat emergencies (Box 57–3). As the temperature increases, the sweat glands attempt to cool the body through diaphoresis (sweating). As the temperature continues to increase, the body compensates with profuse sweating. Unless fluids and salts are replaced, hypotension, dehydration, sodium depletion, and electrolyte imbalances may occur from excess fluid loss through perspiration.

Clients who are very young, elderly, or receiving diuretics or anticholinergic and phototaxic drug regimens are at greater risk for heat emergencies. The nurse should be sure to assess the client's history for cardiac, pulmonary, or renal diseases and drug regimens. At discharge, these clients need to be taught about side effects of drug regimens and ways to avoid or reduce exposure to extremes in temperature.

BOX 57-3

Types of Heat Emergencies

Heat Cramps. Heat cramps are muscle spasms of arms, legs, and occasionally abdomen related to sodium depletion from excessive perspiration. The nurse must remove the client from the hot environment and administer oral fluids containing salt.

Heat Exhaustion. Heat exhaustion results from heat-induced hypotension caused by excessive fluid loss through sweating. Symptoms include headache, dizziness, faintness, anorexia, and nausea; skin may be cool and clammy. Vital signs will vary depending on the degree of volume depletion. The nurse must remove the client from the heat and administer oral or intravenous fluids as needed.

Heat Stroke. Heat stroke is an emergency and requires immediate treatment for survival. There are two forms of heat stroke: classic and exertional. Classic heat stroke is seen most commonly in the poor, the elderly, the chronically ill, clients with heart disease, the obese, and alcoholics. Hot, humid weather lasting 3 days or more increases the risk of heat stroke in these clients. The stress of the heat increases the demand on the heart. In addition, certain medications decrease the ability to sweat, including antihistamines, beta blockers, anticholinergics, and phenothiazines. Other medications, such as amphetamines and neuroleptics, increase heat production.

Exertional heat stroke is more common in laborers, farmers, military recruits, athletes (especially football players and long distance runners), and clients who work in boiler rooms or foundries. Symptoms of this form of heat stroke are similar to those of classic heat stroke except these clients sweat. They tend to experience lactic acidosis and have more severe bleeding problems.

Burns. Burn injury is discussed in Chapter 49.

Management

The nurse rapidly reduces body temperature (immerse or sponge with cool water). A hypothermia blanket may be used. The physician may order an intravenous catheter, a cardiac monitor, frequent measurement of vital signs, and chlorpromazine or diazepam to reduce shivering. Supplemental oxygen and a urinary catheter may also be ordered.

COLD EMERGENCIES

Hypothermia

Hypothermia is defined as a lowered core body temperature, usually below 34.4° C (94° F). It may occur in divers, clients exposed to cold weather, and near-drowning victims. Some clients appear dead yet have a feeble pulse. Pupils may be fixed and dilated. Symptoms depend on the client's core temperature:

- 34.4° C (94° F): amnesia or sluggishness
- 32.2° C (90° F): cardiac dysrhythmias, especially premature ventricular contractions
- 30° C (86° F): loss of muscle coordination, possible unconsciousness
- 25° C (77° F): cardiac arrest

Endotracheal intubation and cardiopulmonary resuscitation may be indicated. The nurse should insert an esophageal thermometer or rectal thermometer probe; insert an intravenous catheter and a central venous pressure catheter if hypothermia is severe; draw blood for laboratory studies (CBC, electrolytes, BUN, sugar, creatinine, coagulation screen, amylase, and ABGs); monitor the cardiac rhythm and obtain a 12-lead ECG; and insert a urinary catheter and monitor output every 30 minutes.

Core rewarming is performed by use of heated oxygen and gastric, urinary bladder, and peritoneal lavage with heated fluids.

CRITICAL TO REMEMBER

One must not apply heat to a profoundly hypothermic client. It causes vasodilation and further cardiovascular collapse.

Peripheral rewarming is usually delayed until the client's core temperature has been raised. Resuscitation is not usually successful until adequate core rewarming has been achieved and efforts should not be abandoned until rewarming is accomplished.

Frostbite

Frostbite is damage to tissues and blood vessels as a result of prolonged exposure to cold. Fingers, toes, nose, and ears are often affected. There may be initial numbness, paresthesia, and pallor of the affected part. Often, severe pain, swelling, erythema, and blistering (similar to a second-degree, partial-thickness burn) occurs once the client is in a warm environment. Necrosis and gangrene may develop in severe cases.

The tissues must be handled gently. The affected part must be rewarmed with use of tepid water (about 105° F).

CRITICAL TO REMEMBER

Massage should never be performed on frostbitten tissue; this may result in further tissue damage.

Bulky dressings should be applied to permit drainage and provide protection. A bed cradle may be needed.

SNAKE BITES

Four poisonous snakes are found in the United States. Three of these are pit vipers (rattlesnakes, copperheads, and water moccasins), and the other is a coral snake. Not all persons who are bitten are envenomated. Snake bites in the spring may be more severe because the venom is more concentrated at that time of year.

Local reactions are an intense burning pain immediately after the bite. There is swelling and copious bleeding. Blisters and blebs develop within 1 hour and become large and hemorrhagic. Significant swelling occurs. Generalized reactions may be present. The nurse assesses for muscle twitching and fasciculation, especially around the mouth. There may be a metallic taste, nausea, vomiting, and gastrointestinal tract bleeding. There may be diaphoresis, tachycardia, and hypotension as the client develops shock. The nurse must perform a neurologic assessment for syncope and coma and carefully monitor respirations; they may become shallow and progress to respiratory arrest as the envenomation spreads.

Management

The nurse must maintain and support the ABCs; act calmly and reassure the client; position the client at rest, immobilize the involved part, and place it at heart level; and apply a constricting band above the site to minimize lymphatic and superficial venous return (it should not be tighter than a watchband). The physician may order one to two large-bore intravenous catheters and Ringer's lactate. Blood must be drawn for laboratory studies (CBC, T & C, coagulation screen, electrolytes, BUN, sugar, erythrocyte sedimentation rate). If whole blood is needed, fresh rather than stored blood should be used. A urinalysis should be performed.

The nurse washes the skin. Incision and suction of wounds are accomplished next. (Note: incision should be done within 20 minutes after the bite; beyond that time, it is probably ineffective.) Initial wound care should be limited to cleansing and dressing with large absorbent, bulky dressings.

The nurse must administer antivenin by intravenous drip within 1 hour. Dosages range from 3 to 40 vials, depending on the degree of envenomation and the client's age and size. One must be sure to perform skin (or eye) allergy testing before administration; measure the girth of the extremity proximal to the bite every 15 to 30 minutes as a guide for additional antivenin; administer tetanus prophylaxis; provide pain relief; observe the client for respiratory depression after narcotic administration; and teach the client to wear high leather boots and thick trousers when walking through known areas for snakes. Heavy gloves should be worn by persons climbing in rocky areas.

ANIMAL BITES

Animal bites may result in puncture wounds, lacerations, and avulsions, especially if the client pulled away from the animal while its teeth were clenched. There is a potential for infection from bacteria normally residing in the animal's mouth (i.e., *Pasteurella multocida*). The nurse must be sure to assess the possibility of rabies from the biting animal. Rabies is an infectious virus that affects the central nervous system, especially the brain. The incidence of rabies in domesticated animals is very low in the United States, but the disease is fatal.

The nurse must obtain the history of the bite, including the type of animal, owner of the animal, description of the incident (provoked or unprovoked), location of the animal, and the animal's immunization history and state of health; assess the type of wound and amount of tissue damage; and be sure to include a neurovascular and musculoskeletal assessment.

The nurse must also carefully clean, irrigate, and debride the wound; assess for possible associated fractures, especially of the hand or head; apply a bulky, fluffy, and absorbent dressing; place fingers in the position of function; and administer tetanus prophylaxis and antibiotics as prescribed. Rabies prophylaxis is used if the animal cannot be found and kept for observation, in areas where rabies is endemic, or if there is a high index of suspicion for rabies. The incident must be reported to public health officials, animal control services, or police. The nurse must be sure to provide psychosocial support for the client and significant others.

HUMAN BITES

Human bites may be self-induced (tongue laceration), result from dental abrasions (usually superficial at the metacarpophalangeal joint and incurred during a fist fight if the client's knuckle hit the opponent's tooth), or be penetrating bites causing puncture wounds and tissue loss. Human bites can cause severe necrotizing infections and require vigorous intervention.

The history of the bite should be determined and the neurovascular and musculoskeletal function carefully assessed. Increased pain over the site may indicate a fracture. Fractures and tendon lacerations, especially of the hand, are common. Obtain x-ray studies if indicated.

The nurse must carefully clean and vigorously irrigate the wound and open and debride puncture wounds. Wounds are usually not sutured unless they are large or located on the face. Loosely placed sutures or adhesive strips may be used. Broad-spectrum antibiotics and tetanus prophylaxis are usually administered.

Poisoning and Overdose

Accidental or intentional poisonings (overdoses) requiring emergency care occur frequently. Telephone inquiries are often received by emergency department staff regarding poisonings. It is important that nurses responsible for emergency care be knowledgeable about the management and complications of poisoning and overdoses. Various resources are available (Poison Control Centers, Poison Index, and toxicology tests). An emergency nurse needs a working knowledge of agents commonly used or abused, especially currently popular street drugs.

The nurse must obtain an accurate history, including the following questions:

- Was the substance inhaled, injected, ingested, sniffed, or confined to skin surfaces?
- How long ago was the event, and what was the amount?
- In what kind of environment was the client found?
- Were there any associated incidents (fire, trauma, near-drowning)?
- Is there a history of prescribed medications, allergies, or medical problems?
- What is the state of physical and mental health?

The nurse must keep in mind that, despite careful fact finding and detailed questioning, a history of the nature and amount of the toxic substance and the time since ingestion may be grossly inaccurate. Clients with toxic substance ingestion may exaggerate or minimize the conditions of an overdose to achieve other goals. The history is considered in planning the care. However, reliance on physical examination is also important.

TABLE 57–6 Assessment Findings Associated with Various Toxins

PHYSICAL SIGNS OR SYMPTOMS	TOXINS TO BE CONSIDERED
Vomiting, nausea, diarrhea	Heavy metals (lead, arsenic); alcohols (ethanol, methanol, ethylene glycol); salicylates; digitalis; morphine and its analogs
Coma	Barbiturates; chloral hydrate; paraldehyde; bromide; ethchlorvynol; carbon monoxide; salicylates; atropine; scopolamine; ethanol
Delirium, agitation	Atropine; scopolamine; alcohol; amphetamines; barbiturates; physostigmine
Convulsions	Phenothiazines; strychnine; propoxyphene; amphetamines; alcohols (ethanol, methanol, ethylene glycol); salicylates; carbon monoxide; cholinesterase inhibitors; hydrocarbons
Dilated pupils	Amphetamines; glutethimide; alcohols; belladonna group; meperidine; cocaine; ephedrine; sympathomimetics; parasympatholytics; cyanide; botulin toxin
Constricted pupils	Morphine; propoxyphene; barbiturates; chloral hydrate
Partial or total blindness	Methanol
Pink skin	Carbon monoxide; cyanide; atropine (skin flushed and dry); phenothiazine
Kussmaul's respiration	Salicylates; methanol; ethanol; ethylene glycol
Dry mouth	Belladonna group; botulin toxin; antihistamines; morphine; phenothiazines; tricyclic antidepressants
Hematemesis	Mercuric chloride; salicylates; phosphorus; fluoride
Diaphoresis	Alcohol; insulin; fluoride; physostigmine salicylate
Extrapyramidal tremor	Phenothiazines

Modified from Cohen, A. S., et al. (1977). *Medical emergencies: Diagnostic and management procedures from Boston City Hospital.* Boston: Little, Brown.

Management

The acronym SIRES is an aid in remembering the essential care in cases of poisoning:

- S Stabilize the client.
- I Identify the toxic substance.
- R Reverse its effect.
- E Eliminate the substance from the body.
- S Support the client and significant others (physically and psychosocially).

The nurse must maintain the ABCs. Assessment findings associated with various toxins and antidotes are included in Table 57–6. The nurse must be sure to stabilize the ABCs; perform a rapid physical examination; start intravenous catheters and obtain appropriate laboratory studies, including toxicology screen; initiate a cardiac monitor and obtain an ECG; and insert a urinary catheter.

An appropriate means of reversing or eliminating the toxic substance must be selected. The safest and most effective method of inducing emesis is through administering syrup of ipecac.

Syrup of ipecac is safe and effective when used in properly selected clients (Box 57–4). The dose is 15 to 30 mL (1–10 years, 15 ml; over 10 years, 30 ml), administered orally, preceded or followed by several hundred milliliters of water or other solution (juice). Emesis usually occurs within 15 to 20 minutes. However, a second dose can be given 20 minutes after the first dose. More than two doses should not be given.

BOX 57–4

Cautions in the Use of Ipecac

The nurse must note the following:

- Use only syrup of ipecac, not ipecac fluid extract.
- Always ensure an intact gag reflex before giving ipecac. Do not assume a physician has done this.
- Ipecac may be ineffective in inducing emesis after ingestion of substances with antiemetic properties.
- Ipecac in large doses may be cardiotoxic. Lavage may be necessary if emesis does not occur.
- Frequently reassess the client. The client may become obtunded when the emesis occurs, and aspiration may result.
- Ipecac is most effective when adequate amounts of oral fluids are administered.

CRITICAL TO REMEMBER

It is important that enough oral fluid be given to prevent retching and possible esophageal tears.

Stomach contents should be saved for possible toxicologic analysis and the presence or absence of pill particles should be noted.

Gastric lavage may be indicated. However, it is believed to be less effective than emesis in removing ingested substances from the stomach. Thus, it is reserved for use in clients with central nervous system depression, those with diminished or absent gag reflex, and those unable to cooperate with emetic therapy. The nurse should remember that gastric lavage is not a deterrent to future overdose attempts and should not be used as a punitive measure.

Absorptives are also used. Activated charcoal powder, usually mixed with water, can be administered.

Antidotes and antagonists may be used in selected cases for management or diagnosis of the toxic substance (Table 57–7). One must remember that, although an antidote may produce significant results initially, the half-life of the toxic substance may be longer than the antidote. Clients receiving antidotes or antagonists must be observed for several hours before being discharged.

Other measures, depending on the client's condition, may include diuresis, fluid loading, cooling or warming, anticonvulsive therapy, antidysrhythmic therapy, hemodialysis, hemoperfusion, or exchange transfusions. Nursing care involves assessing the client and the responses, carrying out therapies, and providing supportive care. One must remember that an accidental or intentional poisoning may be reported to a poison control facility or additional agency.

For the client who intentionally overdoses, empathy and understanding are necessary. The nurse should remember the suicidal attempt may be repeated while the client is receiving care for the overdose and should be sure to implement suicide precautions.

A psychiatric evaluation is indicated for all clients who intentionally overdose or whose intentions seem unclear. The evaluation should occur before discharge, and plans for follow-up care should be well established. The nurse should investigate and use available support systems. Someone should stay with the client for the next several days. A telephone number for the crisis team or clinic and written instructions for follow-up care should be provided.

TABLE 57–7 Antidotes Commonly Used in Managing Poisoned or Overdosed Clients

SUBSTANCE	ANTIDOTE
Cholinesterase inhibitors (e.g., organophosphate insecticides, nerve gases, carbamates)	Atropine
Iron	Deferoxamine
Insulin	Dextrose 50%
Mercury, arsenic, lead, heavy metals	Dimercaprol, disodium edetate, penicillamine
Methanol, ethylene glycol	Ethanol
Lead	EDTA (ethylenediaminetetraacetic acid)
Acetaminophen	*N*-Acetylcysteine (Mucomyst)
Narcotics and narcotic derivatives, opiates	Naloxone (Narcan)
Cyanide	Amyl nitrite, sodium nitrite, sodium thiosulfate
Carbon monoxide	Oxygen
Cholinesterase inhibitors	2-PAM (Protopam)
Atropine, scopolamine, tricyclic antidepressants	Physostigmine (Antilirium)
Anticoagulants, (e.g., warfarin [Coumadin])	Vitamin K

EDTA = edetic acid.

Death and Dying in Emergency Care Settings

Death in the emergency department presents different problems to significant others and health-care givers than death from a prolonged illness (Box 57–5). There is often little time to interact with the dying client or to provide grief and loss counseling. Significant others may be overwhelmed by the suddenness of the event and feel there is not enough time to resolve their "unfinished business" with the dying person.

Medical Examiner's or Coroner's Jurisdiction

In the United States, deaths associated with the following are reported to the medical examiner's office:

- Suspected suicides or homicides
- Deaths in which the deceased has not been attended by a physician within 24 hours before death
- Deaths with suspicious circumstances
- Deaths caused by accidents
- Deaths after surgery
- Deaths associated with firearms or other weapons
- Deaths occurring as a result of crime
- Stillbirths
- Deaths resulting from drugs
- Deaths possibly associated with hazards to public safety (infectious diseases that may cause epidemics)

When notified of death, the medical examiner may accept or decline jurisdiction for determining the manner and cause of death. If jurisdiction is accepted, the medical examiner may conduct an autopsy or other investigation or grant the hospital caring for the deceased permission to perform an autopsy. Permission from significant others for postmortem examination in these circumstances is not required.

BOX 57-5

Considerations Related to Death and Dying in the Emergency Department

The nurse must note the following:

- Because there may not be much time before death actually takes place, make sure the dying client and significant others have ample opportunity to be together. If possible, delay procedures that will disrupt communication between the dying patient and significant others, such as endotracheal intubation.
- Allowing the presence of significant others during resuscitation is not necessarily disruptive, as traditionally thought, and can help survivors move through grief work in a less traumatic way. It can lessen their doubts about the loved one's receiving the best care and can involve them in decisions regarding termination of protracted and futile resuscitation measures.
- Religious support can be extremely important for the client and significant others, and nurses should have a clear understanding of how to access that support.
- The client's condition should be communicated to significant others in periodic updates containing clearly stated factual information.
- Viewing the body, particularly in instances of sudden death or trauma, is encouraged. This process can facilitate the grieving process.
- Because preservation of legal evidence is often important in sudden death, significant others are advised beforehand of the various tubes and devices present.
- The client's wishes concerning organ donation must be determined. Required Request Laws (federal and state) facilitate this procedure because all hospitalized clients are asked about organ donation.
- A follow-up telephone call or visit may be beneficial in answering the questions or concerns of the significant others.
- Referral to a support group that assists survivors is often helpful. The health-care facility or community social service agency can provide a list of the support groups in each area.

When the medical examiner plans to conduct the autopsy, it is important that all evidence be preserved. Therefore, all tubes, instruments, and devices are left in place, especially intravenous catheters. The deceased is not washed, nails are not cleaned, and any body fluids on the deceased at the time of death are left on, including clothing. Clothing that has been removed is carefully placed in a paper bag so that decomposition does not obscure any evidence. When removing clothing, the nurse should not cut through bullet holes, stab wound tears, or other tears. The clothing should not be washed. All valuables and clothing must be inventoried with the medical examiner's staff. Only they may release these items to significant others. Refer to specimen collection and chain of custody earlier in this chapter. A copy of the medical record is given to the medical examiner's staff. The record must be detailed, with special attention given to injuries and marks noted on arrival of the deceased and a description of and location of tubes, surgical incisions, venipunctures, and other therapeutic interventions.

STUDY QUESTIONS

1. Which of the following assessment findings indicate an immediate need for care in an emergency setting?
   A. A gradual loss of vision
   B. Persistent, chronic pain
   C. Chemical burns to the skin
   D. Mild chest pain in clients younger than 30 years

2. A client has a sucking chest wound. A dressing is applied. The client begins to manifest severe dyspnea, tachypnea, and crepitus. The nurse should suspect
   A. Laryngeal spasm
   B. Tension pneumothorax
   C. Fractured ribs
   D. Mediastinal shift

3. Management of clients who sustain minor head trauma includes teaching the family or significant others to
   A. Wake the client every 2 hours for at least 24 hours
   B. Give the client a soft, bland diet for the first 8 hours
   C. Give the client an anti-inflammatory drug or acetaminophen if the client has a headache
   D. Have the client consult a physician if the client has continued vomiting

4. A client has just been taught first aid for snake bites. Which of the following statements indicates he understands the appropriate management of an individual who has been bitten by a poisonous snake?
   A. "I'll immobilize the part that has been bitten and place it above heart level."
   B. "I'll apply a constricting band above the site, making sure it is very tight to stop the flow of venom to other areas of the body."
   C. "I'll put warm compresses on the wound."
   D. "I'll place the person at rest and apply a loosely constrictive band above the site."

5. To implement an effective plan of care for a client who has ingested a poisonous substance, the nurse will
   A. Use ipecac fluid extract
   B. Check pupillary response
   C. Administer no more than 500 mL of fluid along with the extract of ipecac
   D. Monitor the adequacy of the client's gag reflex

CRITICAL THINKING EXERCISES

SCENARIO A

You are making rounds on the 11 to 7 shift and find a 75-year-old client in acute distress. He was admitted with pneumonia. He has a history of chronic obstructive pulmonary disease (COPD) brought on by a 50-year history of cigarette smoking. When admitted, his vital signs were as follows: pulse, 106; blood pressure, 146/88; respiration, 24. You now find him in a very anxious state. He says that every time he tries to take a deep breath his pain gets worse. He says that he had a "coughing fit" that lasted a long time just before you entered his room. You notice he is diaphoretic and tachypneic and is becoming more and more restless. You determine his blood pressure is 86/62, his respirations are 28, and his pulse is 130 and weak. Whereas on admission he had equal breath sounds bilaterally, he now has no breath sounds on his right side.

1. What do clinical findings indicate?
2. What other observations would you make?
3. What is the difference between his situation and that of a client who has been a victim of trauma and has sustained chest trauma?
4. What will your immediate interventions be for this client?
5. What would you teach this client during the intervention stage and before he is discharged?

SCENARIO B

A young female client is admitted to the emergency room with a contusion to the left abdomen. She has no other injuries, is conscious, has stable vital signs, and has an otherwise unremarkable history. Her chief complaint is pain in her left shoulder. She is admitted to an observation unit for 24 hours. Later in the afternoon she tells you the pain in her shoulder is getting worse and that her abdomen now hurts. You assess her and find her abdomen to be soft and her left upper quadrant to be normal to percussion but tender when palpated. Her vital signs are as follows: pulse, 122 and thready; blood pressure, 88/46; and respiration, 20 and labored. You palpate her abdomen and find rebound tenderness in the left upper quadrant along with generalized abdominal tenderness. You report your findings to the physician.

1. What would you suspect from the client's signs and symptoms and the nature of her accident?
2. Why is this client's injury a common one? (Answer should be based on conclusions in question 1.)
3. What will you do to support the medical-surgical treatment of this client's condition?

BIBLIOGRAPHY

1. American College of Surgeons Committee on Trauma (1990). *Advanced trauma life support course manual.* Chicago: Author.
2. American Heart Association. (1994). *Textbook of advanced cardiac life support.* Dallas: Author.
3. American Hospital Association. (1990). Emergency transfer (patient dumping): Provisions of budget bill. *Washington Watch, 11,* 9–10.
4. Beachly, M., & Farrar, J. (1993). Abdominal trauma: Putting the pieces together. *American Journal of Nursing, 93(11),* 26–35.
5. Bobb, J. (1994). Trauma in the elderly. In V. Cardona et al. (Eds.), *Trauma nursing: From resuscitation through rehabilitation* (2nd ed.). Philadelphia: W. B. Saunders.
6. Bullock, B. (1988). Metabolic and immunologic response to trauma. In E. Howell et al. (Eds.), *Comprehensive trauma nursing: Theory and practice.* Chicago: Scott, Foresman.
7. Cardona, V., & Von Rueden, K. (1994). Nursing practice through the trauma cycles. In V. Cardona et al. (Eds.), *Trauma nursing: From resuscitation through rehabilitation* (2nd ed.). Philadelphia: W. B. Saunders.
8. Emergency Nurses Association. (1993). *Emergency nursing core curriculum* (4th ed.). Philadelphia: W. B. Saunders.
9. Emergency Nurses Association. (1994). *Standards of emergency nursing practice* (3rd ed.). St. Louis: Mosby-Year Book.
10. Fadale, J. (1990). Overcrowding, comfort, consideration, convenience. *Journal of Emergency Nursing, 16(3),* 132–133.
11. Faylor, J., & Royer, C. (1991). Intraosseous infusion for emergency intravascular access. *Trauma Talk Newsletter* (fall). Omaha: Saint Joseph Hospital at Creighton University Medical Center.
12. Fraser, S., & Atkins, J. (1990). Survivors' recollection of helpful and unhelpful nursing activities surrounding sudden death of a loved one. *Journal of Emergency Nursing, 16(1),* 13–16.
13. Greenberg, L. (1994). Emergency! Fast action for splenic rupture. *American Journal of Nursing, 94(2),* 51.
14. Halpern, J. (1989). Mechanisms and patterns of trauma. *Journal of Emergency Nursing, 15(5),* 380–388.
15. Hammond, S. C. (1990). Chest injuries in the trauma patient. *Nursing Clinics of North America, 25(1),* 35–44.
16. Harchelroad, S. (1990). *Comparing the role of the emergency nurse involved in trauma resuscitations* (unpublished thesis). Pittsburgh: University of Pittsburgh.
17. Harrahill, M., & Bartkus, E. (1990). Preparing the trauma patient for transfer. *Journal of Emergency Nursing, 16(1),* 25–28.
18. Howell, E., et al. (1988). *Comprehensive trauma nursing: Theory and practice.* Chicago: Scott, Foresman.

19. Hoyt, D., et al. (1988). Video recording trauma resuscitations: An effective teaching technique. *The Journal of Trauma, 28(4),* 435–440.

20. Ilano, A., & Raffin, T. (1990). Management of carbon monoxide poisoning. *Chest, 97(1),* 165–169.

21. Judkins, D., & Iserson, K. (1991). Rapid admixture blood warming. *Journal of Emergency Nursing, 17(3),* 146–151.

22. Kinkle, S. (1993). Violence in the ER: How to stop it before it starts. *American Journal of Nursing, 93(7),* 22–24.

23. Laskowski-Jones, L. (1993). Acute spinal cord injury: How to minimize the damage. *American Journal of Nursing, 93(12),* 22–33.

24. Lenehan, G. P. (1989). ED gridlock and blaming the victim. *Journal of Emergency Nursing, 15(3),* 211–213.

25. LoCicero, J., & Mattox, K. (1989). Epidemiology of chest trauma. *Surgical Clinics of North America, 69(1),* 15–19.

26. McCaffery, M., & Beebe, A. (1989). *Pain: Clinical manual for nursing practice.* St. Louis: C. V. Mosby.

27. McQuillan, K. (1994). Initial management of traumatic shock. In V. Cardona et al. (Eds.), *Trauma nursing: From resuscitation through rehabilitation* (2nd ed.). Philadelphia: W. B. Saunders.

28. Mitchell, P. (1994). Central nervous system I: Closed head injuries. In V. Cardona et al. (Eds.), *Trauma nursing: From resuscitation through rehabilitation* (2nd ed.). Philadelphia: W. B. Saunders.

29. Morris, J. A., et al. (1991). Trauma patients return to productivity. *The Journal of Trauma, 31(6),* 827–833.

30. National Safety Council. (1991). *Accident facts.* Chicago: Author.

31. Orlowski, J., et al. (1989). The hemodynamic and cardiovascular effects of near drowning in hypotonic, isotonic or hypertonic solutions. *Annals of Emergency Medicine, 18(10),* 1044–1049.

32. Potter, D. (Ed.). (1989). *Emergencies.* Springhouse, PA: Springhouse Corporation.

33. Ramler, C. (1990). Triage. In S. Kitt & J. Kaiser (Eds.), *Emergency nursing: A physiologic and clinical perspective.* Philadelphia: W. B. Saunders.

34. Repasky, T. (1994). Emergency! Tension pneumothorax. *American Journal of Nursing, 94(9),* 47.

35. Shingleton, B. (1991). Eye injuries. *The New England Journal of Medicine, 325(6),* 408–413.

36. Smith, L., & Glowac, B. (1989). New frontiers in the management of the multiply injured patient. *Critical Care Nursing Clinics of North America, 1(1),* 1–9.

37. Thom, S., & Keim, L. (1989). Carbon monoxide poisoning: A review of epidemiology, pathophysiology, clinical findings and treatment options including hyperbaric oxygen therapy. *Clinical Toxicology, 27(3),* 141–156.

38. Turnes, C. (1992). Geriatric trauma: A case study. *Geriatric Nursing, 13(4),* 210–213.

39. West, J. G., et al. (1988). Trauma systems: Current status —Future challenges. *Journal of the American Medical Association, 259(24),* 3597–3600.

Appendix A
Answers to Study Questions and Critical Thinking Exercises

Chapter 1, Acute and Chronic Illness

Study Questions

1. *Answer:* A
   Rationale: A physical assessment should include an assessment of the client's ability to function. The other choices are elements of a psychosocial assessment.
   Level: Knowledge
   Refer to Learning Outcome #1

2. *Answer:* B
   Rationale: A functional orientation to health means that the client seeks medical care only when he or she feels unwell or when symptoms interfere with the ability to carry out activities of daily living.
   Level: Application
   Refer to Learning Outcome #2

3. *Answer:* A
   Rationale: The first stage of adjustment to chronic illness or disability is disbelief or denial. The other choices are characteristics of developing awareness (B); integration (C); or maladaption (D).
   Level: Comprehension
   Refer to Learning Outcome #3

4. *Answer:* C
   Rationale: Although the overall data may indicate that all of the nursing diagnoses are appropriate, only Self-Care Deficit is specific to the data provided in the stem of the question.
   Level: Analysis
   Refer to Learning Outcome #4

5. *Answer:* C
   Rationale: This response is an adaptive response to a chronic condition. It indicates that the client is adjusting to the limitations of his condition and is incorporating new behaviors into his life-style in order to return to an optimal level of functioning. All the other responses are maladaptive.
   Level: Analysis
   Refer to Learning Outcome #6

Critical Thinking Exercises

Scenario A

1. The client is probably in the phase of developing awareness. She could demonstrate: withdrawal, preoccupation with self, crying, depression, expressions of anger toward others, feelings of guilt, anger, being different, and being alone.

   She is grieving over another loss. She feels a loss of control—a control she had previously attained with her old regimen.

2. There are many developmental tasks of young adulthood. Accepting self and stabilizing self-concept and body image are probably a major task related to the client's current attempt to manage the exacerbation of her illness. Change is viewed suspiciously by many Spanish-speaking cultures. Suffering is seen as one's destiny. It is difficult to control that destiny. However, the client may not "fit" into this cultural picture. It is therefore imperative for the nurse to assess this client without preconceived values.

3. The nurse should allow the client ample time to discuss her fears and concerns. The nurse must also utilize his or her knowledge of chronic illness in order to assist the client to integrate the additional regimen into her life-style. Listening and well planned counseling and teaching sessions are of utmost importance.

Scenario B

1. Personal values will be very influential in the response of any nurse to this client. What you feel about aging, chronic illness, the value of life, and the quality of life are only some of the issues that may influence your response.

2. After examining both your own value systems and the client's, you should assess how the client has adapted to previous crises and what types of coping mechanisms he has used.

Chapter 2, Health-Care Delivery

Study Questions

1. *Answer:* A
   Rationale: Prevention of illness requires that the individual accept responsibility for his or her own care. Ultimately, a healthier population will place less demand on health-care services.
   Level: Knowledge
   Refer to Learning Outcome #2

2. *Answer:* D
   Rationale: To improve care and decrease costs, the health-care delivery system focuses on achievement of client outcomes as clients pass through the system.
   Level: Comprehension
   Refer to Learning Outcome #3

3. *Answer:* C
   Rationale: While health-care reform is being debated, market-driven changes are responsible for many cost-cutting measures currently in effect.
   Level: Application
   Refer to Learning Outcome #2

Critical Thinking Exercises

1. The hospital will coordinate planning and implementation of health care from admission through treatment in the health-care setting to follow-up care in the home. Education of the client and significant others in self-care and methods of preventing illness is paramount. Personal responsibility for accepting and maintaining a healthy life-style will become an expectation.

2. The cost of care (length of stay, readmission rates, the incidence of complications, etc.) is monitored and evaluated on an ongoing basis. More care will be provided in the home, thus necessitating increased client responsibility for self-care. With the implementation of case management and clinical pathways, hospitals and other health-care institutions can more readily discover changes in the systems

that have an impact on cost and recovery and can quickly take action to contain and/or reduce the cost of care.

3. Health-care delivery systems place more emphasis on client rights, such as providing more information so that informed choices can be made, striving to provide a restraint-free environment, teaching about advance directives, ensuring client confidentiality in view of the electronic explosion of information access, and ensuring competency of health-care workers. The consumer is viewed as a person who is using a service, is capable of making informed choices, and, with education, will accept responsibility for positive health-care outcomes.

Chapter 3, Fluid and Electrolyte Balance

Study Questions

1. *Answer:* C
Rationale: Decreased blood flow from decreased circulatory volume would cause decreased glomerular filtration and increased fluid retention, along with decreasing urinary output. (A) is not an abnormal pulse range for the elderly. (B) is a poor indicator, especially in the elderly. (D) is normal in many elderly clients. Skin turgor can be a reliable indicator only if it is assessed carefully. (The tongue should be used as a focal point.)
Level: Comprehension
Refer to Learning Outcome #1

2. *Answer:* C
Rationale: Hand vein engorgement may indicate edema. Cyanosis (A) is a remote possibility; however, it is not a major sign of ECFVE. Instant hot cereals and vegetable juice are high in sodium and thus are contraindicated (B). Dizziness and lightheadedness are associated with ECFVD (D).
Level: Application
Refer to Learning Outcomes #2 and #6

3. *Answer:* D
Rationale: Potassium is irritating to the tissue. It must be well diluted in intravenous fluid, but it may still cause burning and tingling at the insertion site. (A) lists foods that are low in potassium. Although safety is a factor, bed rest is not necessary (B). **POTASSIUM IS NEVER ADMINISTERED IN AN INTRAMUSCULAR INJECTION!** (C)
Level: Application
Refer to Learning Outcome #3

4. *Answer:* A
Rationale: These laboratory values are associated with hypocalcemia. (B) is related to ECFVE. (C) and (D) are collaborative diagnoses, besides being inappropriate considering the data.
Level: Analysis
Refer to Learning Outcome #4

5. *Answer:* A
Rationale: Insulin helps promote potassium uptake by the cells. If the client does not have enough insulin, he or she could develop hyperkalemia. Therefore, every diabetic, especially those who take insulin, should be aware of foods high in potassium.
Level: Application
Refer to Learning Outcome #5

Critical Thinking Exercises

Scenario A

1. Extracellular fluid volume shift to the third space is a possible complication because of the client's age and his impending major abdominal procedure. Signs and symptoms of shock should be included in the tool (see Chap.56).

2. Consult each of the tables included in the chapter to determine the major clinical manifestations of each of the listed complications. Notice that all the major body systems are included. When you design your tool, make it inclusive of all the major signs and symptoms. Also include a section that allows the nurses to check lab results.

3. Directions given to the staff should include
   A. Baseline assessment
   B. Review of the client's concurrent illnesses and medications
   C. Review of the client's emotional status before surgery
   D. Geriatric physiology (Refer to geriatric nursing journals.)

   Although most nurses are able to recognize postoperative complications, many nurses may not have updated knowledge of aging physiology.

Scenario B

It is important for the nurse not to make assumptions. For some clients, culture may play a minor role, while for others it may be very significant. The nurse should consult articles and texts that clearly define cultural preferences. Also, before proceeding with the teaching process, the nurse should ascertain how the client views his dietary preferences.

Chapter 4, Acid-Base Imbalances

Study Questions

1. *Answer:* B
Rationale: The findings presented indicate respiratory alkalosis.
(A) indicates respiratory acidosis. (C) indicates metabolic acidosis. (D) indicates metabolic alkalosis.
Level: Analysis
Refer to Learning Outcome #1

2. *Answer:* B
Rationale: Excessive consumption of carbohydrates may cause respiratory acidosis.
(A) is the treatment for respiratory alkalosis. (C) could cause respiratory acidosis. (D) could cause respiratory alkalosis.
Level: Application
Refer to Learning Outcomes #2, #3, and #6

3. *Answer:* D
Rationale: Safety needs take priority, especially considering the client's age and laboratory data. (A), (B), and (C) are not related to the data.
Level: Analysis
Refer to Learning Outcome #4

4. *Answer:* C
Rationale: Dysrhythmia is the only sign associated with metabolic alkalosis.
(A), (B), and (D) are associated with metabolic acidosis.
Level: Comprehension
Refer to Learning Outcome #5

Critical Thinking Exercises

Scenario A

Age causes changes in all systems of the body. The major buffering systems (blood, lungs, and kidneys) decrease in their ability to maintain acid-base balance. Because the client had ingested large amounts of aspirin, she is at risk for respiratory alkalosis as well as gastric bleeding and altered clotting times.

A nurse should explain the major side effects of aspirin ingestion and provide instructions on proper body mechanics. While the nurse is teaching this client, he or she should also review the client's life-style practices, including diet and medication usage. Signs and symptoms that might appear as a result of respiratory alkalosis are tachypnea, dizziness, syncope, weakness, paresthesia, and tetany.

The nurse should perform a basic physical assessment, with emphasis on assessment of the client's neurologic function. This assessment would include more than assessing level of consciousness. It should include questions that would determine the client's ability to solve problems and make simple judgments. The nurse must also have baseline assessment data to judge whether the client's neurologic status is deteriorating as a result of respiratory alkalosis or aspirin intoxication.

Scenario B

1. Respiratory acidosis–uncompensated
2. Normal
3. Metabolic acidosis–uncompensated

Chapter 5, Perioperative Nursing

Study Questions

1. *Answer:* C
   Rationale: Obese clients are more susceptible to postoperative and pulmonary complications because of decreased lung capacity and weak pulmonary muscle tone. (A), (B), and (D) may occur but are not specific to obese individuals.
   Level: Knowledge
   Refer to Learning Outcome #1
2. *Answer:* C
   Rationale: Deep breathing exercises prior to coughing help produce a more effective cough. The client should breathe through pursed lips (A). The exercises should be performed at least a dozen times each hour (B). The incentive spirometer is an excellent adjunct to coughing and deep breathing exercises, but it does not replace coughing and deep breathing (D).
   Level: Comprehension
   Refer to Learning Outcome #2
3. *Answer:* C
   Rationale: Spinal anesthesia may cause hypotension postoperatively. (A) is true of other types of anesthesia. Spinal anesthesia numbs the feet first (B). Spinal anesthesia does have side effects (D).
   Level: Application
   Refer to Learning Outcomes #3 and #6
4. *Answer:* D
   Rationale: An elderly client's color may appear pale to slightly cyanotic. Therefore, the nurse must assess other parameters to determine shock. Also, one sign or symptom should not be the determinant of shock.
   Level: Analysis
   Refer to Learning Outcome #5
5. *Answer:* B
   Rationale: This is the safest position to ensure patency of an airway. All other choices are incorrect and unsafe.
   Level: Comprehension
   Refer to Learning Outcome #4

Critical Thinking Exercises

Scenario A

Developing an effective teaching plan requires careful assessment of the learners. Developing a useful plan of care for postoperative complications requires not only listing the complications but presenting them in order of severity and incidence. The nurse must not include rare or infrequently seen complications. The experienced nurse must also emphasize the importance of anticipating emergencies and carry out mock drills that will keep the new graduates confident when assessing and intervening in client care.

Scenario B

Because of the large dressing, the nature of the surgery, and the doses of narcotics, the client is at greatest risk for respiratory complications. He may also have abdominal distention. These complications could lead to atelectasis, pneumonia, and bronchitis. The nurse should assess blood values and blood gases as well as the quality of the client's respirations, his color, and his alertness and ability to follow commands. Further assessment should include the dressing and the client's ability to move and participate in deep breathing and coughing exercises and the level of his pain. Nursing interventions will depend on the outcome of the assessment. Some of the interventions might include: repositioning, ambulation, encouragement, and teaching.

Remember that the client's pain is his pain. The nurse should not place value judgments on the client's pain. It is the nurse's responsibility to assess for pain, know how the pain medication works and its side effects, and provide the medication with as little delay as possible. The physician should be informed as soon as possible if the medication is not effective or is causing side effects or toxic effects.

Chapter 6, Basic Concepts of Neoplastic Disorders

Study Questions

1. *Answer:* C
   Rationale: Asbestos is the only physical agent listed; the others are chemical agents.
   Level: Knowledge
   Refer to Learning Outcome #1
2. *Answer:* C
   Rationale: Anxiety and depression are the most common psychosocial reactions among clients with cancer. Support groups can be used early in the course of treatment. Medical insurance may not cover the entire cost of treatment. Physical changes often occur before the diagnosis of cancer is confirmed.
   Level: Comprehension
   Refer to Learning Outcome #2
3. *Answer:* B
   Rationale: Malignant cells can grow in the presence of necrosis as well as inflammation. The other choices describe characteristics of normal cells.
   Level: Application
   Refer to Learning Outcome #3
4. *Answer:* A
   Rationale: Metastases occur with malignant tumors, not with benign tumors.
   Level: Application
   Refer to Learning Outcome #4
5. *Answer:* C
   Rationale: Although this test was first developed to detect early cancer of the cervix, it is also used to detect respiratory, digestive, and renal cancers.
   Level: Knowledge
   Refer to Learning Outcome #5
6. *Answer:* B
   Rationale: Pain can occur when a tumor obstructs a body organ or causes increased pressure to body tissues. The other responses do not address the concern of the client.
   Level: Application
   Refer to Learning Outcome #6
7. *Answer:* C
   Rationale: Radioisotopes are given in very small doses that will not cause harm to the body's tissues. The remaining statements are false.
   Level: Application
   Refer to Learning Outcome #7

Critical Thinking Exercises

Scenario A

1. Both are terms used to describe a tumor or growth in the body. Neoplasm, which means growth of new tissue, is another term used when discussing cancer. A malignant neoplasm usually grows rapidly and invades surrounding tissue, whereas a benign tumor grows slowly by enlarging and expanding but not invading surrounding tissue.
2. Explain the terms associated with neoplastic disorders. Allow the client time to decide which term he prefers and encourage him to use the term consistently. If the client is able, he may

want to teach his significant others about the terms used and why he has chosen to use a certain term. Other concerns for this client are the reaction of friends and family to the diagnosis of cancer and the client's expressed fear of cancer.

3. A nursing history that details life-style information such as smoking and substance abuse practices, stress, type and length of employment, dietary habits, and health practices such as recommended physical examinations with screening tests for cancer should be conducted. Encourage the client to elaborate on certain elements of his life-style and their effects on his health; the client may express anger and guilt as well as resignation.

4. Most people are aware of and understand that chemical or physical agents are carcinogenic. Although viruses as carcinogens are under study today, most researchers believe that cancer results from multiple agents working together. The history of viral infection should be documented in the client's nursing history and brought to the attention of the physician if it is new information.

Scenario B

1. A variety of tests are performed so that the extent of the cancer can be determined. Some tests look at the structure of the body (e.g., whether organs are being infiltrated or crowded out), whereas some determine the function of the particular organ being studied (e.g., whether the results are within expected limits). It is important to determine the primary site of the cancer, and, if the cancer has progressed, the presence of metastasis. The prognosis and course of treatment are determined from the results of the diagnostic studies.

2. The nurse should explain which scheduled tests may cause pain or discomfort. The nurse should further teach the client how intense the expected pain might be and inform her that medication may be ordered (before or during the test). The client should also be taught how to use relaxation and imagery as methods to help control the response to pain. Psychological stress caused by anticipation can be alleviated by encouraging the client to talk about feelings and how she handles any pain experience.

3. During a biopsy, a sample of body tissue is excised and studied under a microscope. A pathologist is able to determine whether the cells seen under the microscope are normal or not. A biopsy can be performed under local or general anesthesia; it may also be done during surgery when a tissue sample known as a frozen section is excised. When performed during surgery, a biopsy can verify the presence of cancer cells in the tissue sample.

Chapter 7, Treatment Modalities for Neoplastic Disorders

Study Questions

1. *Answer:* A
   Rationale: An assessment for coping strategies must be done before any plans for intervention are developed.
   Level: Comprehension
   Refer to Learning Outcome #1

2. *Answer:* A
   Rationale: The client presents a realistic view with plans for coping with the progress of the cancer.
   Level: Application
   Refer to Learning Outcome #2

3. *Answer:* C
   Rationale: This statement reflects current thinking. (B) and (D) are not correct; (A) does not respond to the client's concern.
   Level: Application
   Refer to Learning Outcome #3

4. *Answer:* A
   Rationale: As a primary treatment modality, radiation therapy is the only treatment used and it provides local cure of the cancer.
   Level: Knowledge
   Refer to Learning Outcome #3

5. *Answer:* C
   Rationale: Because the assessment reflects the infusion of a chemotherapeutic agent, nausea, and two episodes of vomiting, the nurse should wear a pair of clean gloves in anticipation of contact with body secretions.
   Level: Application
   Refer to Learning Outcome #3

6. *Answer:* B
   Rationale: Because the client is receiving radiation from an unsealed source, the potential for contamination from body excretions is present.
   Level: Application
   Refer to Learning Outcome #4

7. *Answer:* D
   Rationale: Diminished white blood cell and platelet production are myelosuppressive effects that cause infection and hemorrhage (as a result of chemotherapy), which can be lethal.
   Level: Knowledge
   Refer to Learning Outcome #5

Critical Thinking Exercises

Scenario A

1. A great area of exposure for the myelosuppressed client occurs when the person interacts with large numbers of people. Children in a classroom setting would expose the client to high risk for infection, and the teacher may be forced by the presence of this side effect to avoid being in the classroom for periods of time. The following psychosocial aspects should be considered when assessing and caring for the client with this side effect: temporary or permanent loss of employment, the financial impact of such a loss, anger that myelosuppression is interfering with her life-style, change in self-image, changes in mood leading to depression because of the losses, and worry or obsession that infection or bleeding can be lethal.

2. The client would need to report to the physician even the slightest sore throat, fever, cough, and so on that might indicate that an infectious process is occurring. Most people in our society treat themselves without seeking a physician's advice; it may be a financial hardship to seek medical assistance frequently. In addition, the client may become overly protective of her body in view of the possibility of bleeding as a side effect.

3. The client should be taught the information on side effects of chemotherapy at the beginning of the course of treatment. Written materials should be used to reinforce the teaching. Telephone numbers of contact people in the medical and psychosocial support community should be given to the client. The client may deny that side effects as described might happen to her and pay scant attention to the teaching. The client may need to be retaught the information on side effects when they become more apparent with progression of treatment. Until the client is accepting of the disease and treatment, she may need to have ongoing teaching and learning to protect her from injury.

Scenario B

1. Men and women experience a change in self-image with hair loss. Clients of either sex may react with a sense of helplessness and loss of control. They are helpless to resist the loss of hair and have no control over how much will be lost or when it will grow back. Either sex may choose to shave the head. While bald, or until the hair regrows, men may wear baseball caps indoors and outdoors, whereas women

may wear wigs or scarves. Clients may become reclusive until hair growth resumes.

2. Complete hair loss is often associated with having cancer or a lesser known disease that has the same effect. A person may be stereotyped as having cancer and when in public may be treated with pity or covert glances and may even be ignored. A woman who is bald and wearing a scarf may be mistakenly identified as a cancer client. People in society may be uncomfortable in communicating with a person who has cancer because, even though the cure rates for cancer are improving with early detection and new treatments, cancer as a diagnosis may be perceived as a death sentence.

3. People with cancer are simply people who are as normal as anyone else but are experiencing side effects associated with cancer treatment. They need to be treated with the same courtesy, respect, caring, and compassion shown any other individual.

Chapter 8, Assessment of the Immune System

Study Questions

1. *Answer:* D
   Rationale: Bone marrow is the only organ of those listed that is directly related to immune function.
   Level: Comprehension
   Refer to Learning Outcome #1

2. *Answer:* C
   Rationale: Immunoglobin G is a major antibody that is readily available to provide primary and secondary immune responses signaled by the body. Immunoglobin A is found in tears, mucus, and breast milk.
   Level: Knowledge
   Refer to Learning Outcome #1

3. *Answer:* A
   Rationale: All of the clients are at risk. The client most at risk, however, is the infant with an adenosine deaminase deficiency because he or she has little if any immunocompetence and is highly susceptible to any pathogen.
   Level: Application
   Refer to Learning Outcome #1

4. *Answer:* B
   Rationale: Adequate nutrition is vital to promote optimum immune function. All other options put the client at risk for immunocompromise.
   Level: Analysis
   Refer to Learning Outcomes #2 and #3

5. *Answer:* C
   Rationale: A complete blood count with differential gives an indication of white blood cell production and distribution. The other tests do not directly demonstrate immune system function.
   Level: Application
   Refer to Learning Outcome #4

Critical Thinking Exercises

Scenario A

1. Hematologic malignancies, aplastic anemia, malignantly transferred cells, eosinophilia, and viral infections that target the immune system (e.g., human immunodeficiency virus) suppress the immune system.

2. Cytotoxic therapies, anti-inflammatory drugs, glucocorticoids, immunosuppressive drugs (e.g., cyclosporin), medications with bone marrow suppression as a side effect (e.g., antibiotics such as cephalosporins and penicillin and antipsychotics such as phenothiazines) suppress the immune system.

3. Alterations in the immune system are diagnosed using a complete blood count with differential, enzyme-linked immunosorbent assay, Western blot, CD4 cell count, history and physical, T-cell levels, immunoglobulin levels, monoclonal antibody levels, and food and skin allergy testing.

4. Infection and antigenic stimulus activate an immune response.

Scenario B

1. Asthma, infection, dexamethasone, acetaminophen, aminophylline, erythromycin, a clear liquid diet, and an intravenous line put the client at risk for immune system compromise.

2. The immunoglobulins, especially IgE, are specifically involved in reactive airway disease.

3. The infection must be of sufficient strength or concentration to overwhelm the immune system, or the immune system must be compromised so that an infection can take over the host.

4. Selecting a balanced diet, balancing exercise and rest, maintaining skin integrity, and removing infectious sources will enhance immune systems.

Chapter 9, Nursing Care of Clients with Altered Immune Systems

Study Questions

1. *Answer:* A
   Rationale: Clients who are HIV positive historically are asymptomatic throughout the seroconversion phase or experience mononucleosis-like symptoms such as fever, malaise, lymphadenopathy, rash, and, at times, aseptic meningitis. All other options address symptoms that are not indicative of the HIV disease.
   Level: Application
   Refer to Learning Outcome #1

2. *Answer:* C
   Rationale: The mode of transmission for HIV is through body fluids. Some body fluids are more concentrated than others, and contact with these fluids puts the person at higher risk. No other mode has been proven to transmit the disease.
   Level: Comprehension
   Refer to Learning Outcome #4

3. *Answer:* D
   Rationale: Tachycardia and hypotension are the only symptoms listed that are classic symptoms of a blood transfusion reaction.
   Level: Comprehension
   Refer to Learning Outcome #5

4. *Answer:* B
   Rationale: The client most able to donate organs is one who was healthy up to the point of death and received prompt medical attention. Systemic disease decreases the number and type of organs a potential donor may donate.
   Level: Analysis
   Refer to Learning Outcome #5

5. *Answer:* C
   Rationale: The work at a computer center would decrease the number and type of exposures to clients who are more likely to transmit disease.
   Level: Analysis
   Refer to Learning Outcome #3

6. *Answer:* C
   Rationale: All answers relate to the client who is HIV positive. HIV wasting relates to significant weight loss, which results in further compromise of the client's immune system. The best answer is the one concerning nutrition because this is what needs to be addressed to remedy the problem.
   Level: Analysis
   Refer to Learning Outcome #2

Critical Thinking Exercises

Scenario A

1. A differential diagnosis of *Pneumocystis carinii* pneumonia is made by examination of bronchial secretions or lung tissue. The client needs to know that this can be accomplished by bronchoscopy, transbronchial lung biopsy, or sputum induction.
2. Treatment for PCP includes a 3-week course of trimethoprim-sulfamethoxazole (Bactrim or Septra), parenteral pentamidine, or dapsone-trimethoprim. There is a high incidence of rash or fever reaction with trimethoprim-sulfamethoxazole.
3. Clients who are treated prophylactically for PCP include those who are HIV positive with fewer than 200 T4 lymphocytes.
4. The treatment for systemic candidiasis includes antifungals: ketoconazole and fluconazole.

Scenario B

1. This client is in group 1, laboratory category 2 (See Box 9–1), clinical category B (See Box 9–1).
2. No, this client does not have AIDS.
3. The nurse should prevent further infection, promote balanced nutrition, promote a balance of rest and activity based on the client's condition, administer medications as ordered and observe for side effects, and teach the client about behaviors that would further compromise his or her status and how to prevent them.
4. The client should take body substance precautions if in contact with the secretions from others, wash hands, avoid further at-risk behaviors as other diseases could be introduced, eat a balanced diet, balance rest and exercise, and report bodily changes as soon as possible for prompt diagnosis and treatment.

Chapter 10, Nursing Care of Clients with Infectious Diseases

Study Questions

1. *Answer:* C
   Rationale: Meningitis is a disease transmitted by air droplet. The isolation is respiratory, and gloves and gowns are not necessary. A private room is necessary.
   Level: Knowledge
   Refer to Learning Outcome #4
2. *Answer:* A
   Rationale: The skin is the first line of bodily defense. That is one of many reasons that hand washing is so important.
   Level: Application
   Refer to Learning Outcome #2
3. *Answer:* B
   Rationale: The latent period is defined as the period in which the pathogen is replicating, before it can be shed from the host. An asymptomatic host and a symptomatic host can both have colonization and may spread disease. At the end of incubation, the host is infectious and can shed the pathogen.
   Level: Analysis
   Refer to Learning Outcome #3
4. *Answer:* D
   Rationale: Smallpox requires strict isolation because of its virulence. Masks, gowns, gloves, and a private room are required for this type of isolation, as is hand washing. The other diseases do not require as stringent an isolation precaution.
   Level: Analysis
   Refer to Learning Outcome #1
5. *Answer:* A
   Rationale: Determining what specific type of infectious process the client has will guide the clinician to the most effective treatment. History and physical, possible sources of infection, and client behaviors will give clues but will not identify specific organisms or possible resistance to treatment.
   Level: Analysis
   Refer to Learning Outcome #5
6. *Answer:* C
   Rationale: Clients need to complete their therapeutic regimen, which includes educational participation for success in treatment. Asymptomatic clients, those who either improve or deteriorate in their hand-washing techniques, and those who can identify how to prevent further reinfection will not be successful if they have not accurately completed their primary therapeutic regimen.
   Level: Analysis
   Refer to Learning Outcome #6

Critical Thinking Exercises

Scenario A

1. Enteric precautions would be most appropriate.
2. Gloves are indicated for touching infectious materials. Hands must be washed after touching the client or potentially contaminated articles and before caring for another client. Articles contaminated with infectious material should be discarded or bagged and labeled before being sent for decontamination or reprocessing. A private room is indicated if the client's hygiene is poor.
3. Yes. At the moment, the reason for the diarrhea has not been determined. If there is an infectious process, to leave infectious gastrointestinal contents in the body longer than necessary would worsen the client's condition.
4. A private room is indicated if the client's hygiene is poor. In general, clients infected with the same organism may share a room. At this time, the client has not been diagnosed as having an infection.

Chapter 11, Nursing Care of Clients with Connective Tissue Disorders

Study Questions

1. *Answer:* B
   Rationale: Corticosteroids are used to decrease the inflammation that results in joint pain. The other answers are side effects of the medication that might further compromise the client.
   Level: Application
   Refer to Learning Outcome #2
2. *Answer:* C
   Rationale: Systemic lupus erythematosus (SLE) is most commonly found in black women between the ages of 15 and 40 years. Drug-induced SLE is associated with the use of drugs such as procainamide (Pronestyl), hydralazine (Apresoline), phenytoin (Dilantin), and phenobarbital. The client in (C) has the most risk factors.
   Level: Analysis
   Refer to Learning Outcome #1
3. *Answer:* D
   Rationale: Control of stress is the only option that would prevent an exacerbation of SLE. Exposure to sunlight, pregnancy, and anticonvulsant medications all could precipitate an attack.
   Level: Application
   Refer to Learning Outcome #3
4. *Answer:* A
   Rationale: The most common cause of death in SLE clients is renal failure from kidney involvement. Multiple systems are involved in the progression of SLE. Cardiac and nervous system involvement are the second and third causes of death in SLE clients.
   Level: Application
   Refer to Learning Outcome #4
5. *Answer:* A
   Rationale: Antibiotics are given prophylactically in surgery to prevent infection postoperatively. The other drugs may be given for symptoms or

are not given routinely for prophylaxis.
Level: Application
Refer to Learning Outcome #5

6. *Answer:* B
Rationale: For a client with rheumatoid arthritis who has joint pain, relief of pain is the primary goal. The other options may improve as well but if the pain does not subside, the treatment has not been effective.
Level: Application
Refer to Learning Outcome #6

Critical Thinking Exercises

Scenario A

1. C. *Rationale:* Aspirin or another nonsteroidal anti-inflammatory drug is the drug of choice for rheumatoid arthritis in the initial stages. Range-of-motion exercises should not be continuous. Massaging the involved joints furthers the inflammation. Surgery is not the treatment of choice in an acute exacerbation.

2. C. *Rationale:* Clients who have rheumatoid arthritis need to plan for rest when scheduling their daily activities. Rest prevents overexertion of involved joints. Heavy lifting and repetitive motion of affected joints will worsen symptoms. Planning should be done to keep necessary items within reach to minimize strain on the affected joint.

3. B. *Rationale:* Gastrointestinal irritation is a common side effect among clients being treated with nonsteroidal anti-inflammatory drugs. Therefore, it is suggested that these medications be taken with food. This is also why they are sometimes given with histamine receptor antagonists.

4. C. *Rationale:* Clients with postoperative hip joint replacement are to be kept aligned in a neutral position with no rotation of their hips, with less than 90 degrees of hip flexion and with legs *abducted.* Neurovascular assessments should be performed routinely on the affected side for the postoperative client with hip joint replacement.

Scenario B

1. B. *Rationale:* A male client who is not identified as the first client's husband or significant other would be inappropriate as a roommate. The client taking diuretics would need close access to the bathroom, as would the first client. This could create conflict unless a commode was available and one client chose to use it. The client on dialysis would not need quick access to the bathroom and does not have any infectious process at this time. The diabetic legally blind amputee would need extra time to access the bathroom and would not tolerate changes in the physical environment as well as another client.

2. A. *Rationale:* Both clients have under lying diseases that suggest compromise of their immune system. Any client with an infectious disease such as pneumonia would not be appropriate for either of these clients as a roommate.

3. Yes. *Rationale:* Both clients have diseases that compromise their immune system because of their disease process and treatment (corticosteroid and histamine blocker). At this time, there is no mention of an active infectious process in either client.

4. The client with systemic lupus erythematosus is most at risk.
Rationale: This client has major organ dysfunction because of the disease and is on a more potent immunosuppressant.

Chapter 12, Assessment of Clients with Neurologic Disorders

Study Questions

1. *Answer:* D
Rationale: Problem-solving ability and reasoning ability are functions of the prefrontal cortex of the frontal lobe.
Level: Knowledge
Refer to Learning Outcome #1

2. *Answer:* C
Rationale: To check pupillary reflex or pupil response, the nurse should approach the pupil with the light from the temporal side while the client looks straight ahead.
Level: Comprehension
Refer to Learning Outcomes #1 and #4

3. *Answer:* A
Rationale: The level of consciousness is best documented by stating a description of the client's behavior in response to stimulation. Terms such as stupor and obtundation should be avoided as they are often interpreted differently.
Level: Comprehension
Refer to Learning Outcomes #2 and #4

4. *Answer:* C
Rationale: During a lumbar puncture, the client is positioned lying on the side, with the back close to the edge of the bed. The knees are drawn up to the abdomen and the head is positioned with the chin to the chest. This position separates the vertebrae to allow for the needle to be inserted more easily.
Level: Comprehension
Refer to Learning Outcome #3

5. *Answer:* B
Rationale: Prior to an electroencephalogram (EEG), the client should avoid all stimulants such as coffee, tea, cola, cigarettes, and alcohol for 24 to 48 hours. The other options are not appropriate preparations for an EEG.
Refer to Learning Outcome #3

Critical Thinking Exercises

Scenario A

1. The parietal lobes contain a primary tactile reception area and tactile association areas. Concept formation and abstraction are carried out by the parietal association areas. The left parietal areas deal with written language or reading, right-left orientation, and mathematics. Damage to the parietal area could impair any of these functions.

2. The temporal lobe contains an auditory receptive area and an auditory association area. Spoken language memories are stored in the left temporal auditory association areas. Damage to these areas may leave the client unable to understand the spoken language.

3. The left cortex is better able to carry out sequential analysis involving an orderly, logical, systematic assessment of the parts. The left cortex deals with language, mathematics, abstraction, and reasoning. The right cortex is best at using the entire sensory experience at one time. The right cortex deals well with visual-spatial information and activities such as dancing, gymnastics, and art appreciation.

Scenario B

1. Magnetic resonance imaging (MRI) uses a powerful magnetic field and computers to produce an image. It does not use radiation like x-rays. Before the MRI, you will be asked to remove all metal objects including your watch, hair pins, and other jewelry. Because of the strong magnetic field, these objects may be pulled into the magnet and become harmful projectiles. You will lie on your back on the padded table and will move into the MRI machine. You will be asked to lie still during the examination, which may take up to an hour. During the examination, you will hear banging noises while the images are being

taken. After the MRI, you may resume your normal activities.

2. *Advantages:* No exposure to radiation, cost-effective, able to detect disorders that cause loss of myelin, able to detect disorders of blood flow, able to visualize the optic chiasm, posterior fossa, brain stem, and spinal cord
Disadvantages: Expensive, not available in all areas, requires the client to lie still, not able to be used on clients with pacemakers, ear or eye implants, cardiac valve replacements, or metal fragments in the body.

3. Client preparation for an MRI includes teaching about the purpose of the test, what the client should expect to experience, and what sensations to report. Sensations that the client should report include the feeling of claustrophobia or "that the walls are closing in" due to the small interior size of the scanner. Clients should be aware that sedation can often be given to combat this feeling. Additionally, client preparation should include a careful screening of the client for metal implants, pacemakers, and foreign objects such as metal fragments in the eyes of sheet metal workers, or shrapnel or retained bullet fragments. The powerful magnet can interfere with the functioning and position of these objects. Intravenous fluid pumps, some ventilators, or any equipment that contains metal or a computer chip for functioning have to be removed prior to the client's entering the magnetic field. Clients with pulse oximeters should be carefully assessed to ensure that the cord from the sensor is not wrapped around body parts, as it may cause a burn.

Chapter 13, Nursing Care of Clients with Loss of Protective Function

Study Questions

1. *Answer:* B
Rationale: Placing the comatose client lying flat on the back may lead to airway obstruction. The client's tongue may fall into the posterior pharynx, occluding the airway. Additionally, secretions may pool in the pharynx and be aspirated.
Level: Knowledge
Refer to Learning Outcome #2

2. *Answer:* A
Rationale: Checking residual volume prior to tube feedings helps to prevent gastrointestinal distension, which can lead to increased intracranial pressure.
Level: Comprehension
Refer to Learning Outcome #2

3. *Answer:* C
Rationale: Short, simple explanations are best for the confused client. These explanations may have to be repeated frequently. Long, complex explanations will be neither remembered nor understood by the confused client.
Level: Comprehension
Refer to Learning Outcome #3

4. *Answer:* B
Rationale: Elevation of the head 30 to 45 degrees prevents venous obstruction by allowing the blood to drain from the brain. The nurse should avoid turning the client's head sharply to either side and keep the head in alignment with the rest of the body.
Level: Analysis
Refer to Learning Outcome #5

5. *Answer:* C
Rationale: A decrease in the level of consciousness is evidenced in that the client is now only responding to painful stimuli. A decrease in the level of consciousness is often the first sign that the client's condition is deteriorating.
Level: Comprehension
Refer to Learning Outcome #5

Critical Thinking Exercises

Scenario A

1. In collecting data for the nursing history, the nurse should include information about the onset of the confusion, past medical illnesses, work and occupational history, and past injuries. If the client is not able to answer each question, the nurse may need to rely on the family or significant others to provide the information. Information about how well the client was able to handle the activities of daily living, financial transactions, and home safety will help determine whether it is safe for the client to return home or move in with a family member, or whether she will need placement in a nursing home at the time of discharge.

2. The confused client will benefit from a consistent routine and environment. If at all possible, the nursing staff members caring for the client should be consistent as well. The client should be reoriented as often as necessary. Clocks and calendars in the room will also help with reorientation. If possible, familiar objects from the client's home may be used to help the client recognize the room as his or her own. Unfamiliar noise should be reduced because it adds to confusion.
The nurse should also recognize that the client may become more disoriented at night, in unfamiliar surroundings, and in situations in which restraints are used.

Scenario B

1. Although suctioning may elevate intracranial pressure (ICP), it is necessary to maintain a patent airway. Clients should be adequately oxygenated before the passage of a suction catheter. The passage of the suction catheter should be as brief as possible and should not exceed 15 seconds. The nurse may also obtain a physician's order for lidocaine administered via the endotracheal tube. Endotracheal lidocaine decreases the cough reflex, thereby decreasing the rise in ICP during suctioning.

2. Advantages of ICP monitoring include the following: increases in ICP can be recognized and treated prior to the onset of clinical signs and symptoms; some monitoring systems allow for fluid drainage and can be used as a treatment for ICP increases; ICP monitoring can be used to evaluate the effectiveness of other treatments; the effect of nursing interventions on ICP can be monitored; and monitoring can provide assessment information for clients who require paralyzing drugs, barbiturate coma, or induced hypothermia.

3. D_5W would not be an acceptable fluid for the client. Currently the tendency is to use slightly hypertonic solutions, as these fluids tend to remain in the vascular space and therefore contribute less to cerebral edema. D_5W tends to move rapidly into the brain to cause edema.

Chapter 14, Nursing Care of Clients with Cerebral Disorders

Study Questions

1. *Answer:* B
Rationale: Risk factors associated with stroke include increasing age (usually above age 40), cardiac disease, diabetes, atherosclerosis, hypertension, hypercholesterolemia, obesity, and family history. Although smoking is a risk factor, cessation of smoking lowers the risk. The incidence of stroke is also higher in the black than in the white population.
Level: Application
Refer to Learning Outcome #2

2. *Answer:* C
Rationale: Both benign and malignant tumors are potentially fatal. The out-

come depends on the tumor location, size, and type. Brain tumors progressively increase intracranial pressure, which causes brain stem herniation and death.
Level: Application
Refer to Learning Outcomes #2 and #6

3. *Answer:* C
Rationale: Clear instruction must be given if the client is sent home after a head injury. Any client who has sustained a head injury should be observed for 24 hours. The client should be taken to the hospital immediately if any of the following things occur: increased drowsiness or confusion, inability to be awakened, vomiting, convulsions, bleeding or drainage from the nose or ears, weakness in the arms or legs, loss of feeling in the extremities, blurring of vision, slurred speech, enlargement or shrinkage of one pupil.
Level: Application
Refer to Learning Outcome #4

4. *Answer:* C
Rationale: Intravenous Ativan depresses respiratory function, and emergency ventilation equipment should be readily available.
Level: Comprehension
Refer to Learning Outcome #3

5. *Answer:* C
Rationale: Clinical manifestations of meningitis include headache, prostration, chills, fever, nausea, vomiting, stiff neck, and generalized seizures. Clients appear acutely ill and confused. Temperature is moderately elevated and the pulse and respiratory rate are increased. Blood pressure is usually normal.
Level: Knowledge
Refer to Learning Outcome #1

Critical Thinking Exercises

Scenario A

1. Clients experiencing a subarachnoid hemorrhage (SAH) may have mild premonitory indications such as mild headache, confusion, fainting, or vertigo. The onset is usually sudden, with the client experiencing a sudden, severe headache, typically in the occipital area and often accompanied by vomiting. The client may lose consciousness immediately, may become confused and lethargic and gradually comatose within hours, or may remain conscious and coherent. Generalized seizures may occur. There are signs of meningeal irritation due to blood in the subarachnoid space. Focal neurologic deficits include cranial nerve involvement and motor weakness.

2. Fusiform and saccular aneurysms are the two most common types of cerebral aneurysm. Both are caused by congenital weakness in artery walls. Saccular (berry) aneurysms usually have a neck or narrowed portion attached to the vessel. Most develop around the anterior portion of the circle of Willis. Fusiform aneurysms most often occur on the larger basilar and carotid arteries.

3. The client with SAH should be kept in a quiet environment with the head of the bed elevated 15 to 30 degrees. The client should be advised to avoid straining, so necessary items should be placed within reach. Valsalva's maneuvers should be avoided, so stool softeners and increased liquids and mild laxatives should be administered. The nurse administers prescribed medications such as analgesics for comfort and sedatives to promote rest.

Scenario B

1. These seizures are also called psychomotor seizures. They frequently begin with an aura, or recognizable sensation, that helps localize the focus. The most characteristic parts of a psychomotor seizure are the automatisms during the seizure, purposeless, repetitive activities such as lip-smacking, chewing, and so on while the client is in a dreamlike state. Inappropriate or asocial behavior may automatically occur during the seizure. Temporal lobe seizures usually last 2 to 3 minutes but may last up to 15 minutes. The client is usually unaware of any activity during the seizure and may be confused or drowsy postictally.

2. Criteria for resection include (1) failure of the medical approach and (2) localization and identification of a focus of abnormal discharge that is easily accessible surgically and is located in dispensable cortex. Thorough assessment is necessary prior to cortical resection, including several electroencephalograms to locate the epileptogenic site, neuropsychological testing, computed tomographic scan, and cerebral angiogram with Wada's procedure to determine cerebral dominance and speech center location.

Chapter 15, Nursing Care of Clients with Degenerative Neurologic Disorders

Study Questions

1. *Answer:* B
Rationale: Memory deficit occurs in all stages of dementia of the Alzheimer's type. Because long-term memory is retained longer than short-term memory in this type of disorder, the nurse should allow the client to reminisce. The nurse should be aware of the client's past so that experiences can be shared meaningfully.
Level: Comprehension
Refer to Learning Outcome #3

2. *Answer:* B
Rationale: The random distribution of multiple sclerosis (MS) plaques and demyelination leads to a variety of clinical manifestations, including weakness in the extremities, double vision, and urinary retention. Sudden bursts of energy are not typical of MS; the usual manifestation is fatigue.
Level: Comprehension
Refer to Learning Outcome #1

3. *Answer:* A
Rationale: The face of someone with advanced Parkinson's disease appears stiff, masklike, and without expression. Saliva may flow involuntarily from the mouth because of the lack of spontaneous swallowing.
Level: Knowledge
Refer to Learning Outcome #1

4. *Answer:* A
Rationale: In myasthenia gravis, weakness is usually greatest after exercise and at the end of the day. Activities should be carefully planned to include rest periods so that energy is conserved and the muscles have a chance to regain their strength.
Level: Application
Refer to Learning Outcome #2

5. *Answer:* B
Rationale: The characteristic feature of Guillain-Barré syndrome is ascending weakness, usually beginning in the lower extremities and spreading, sometimes rapidly, to the trunk, upper extremities, and even the face.
Level: Knowledge
Refer to Learning Outcome #1

Critical Thinking Exercises

Scenario A

1. Any environment can be unsafe for the client with dementia of the Alzheimer's type. In the home, electrical devices, toxic substances, loose rugs, inadequate lighting, and unlocked doors and windows can be sources of injury. Dangerous objects should be kept out of reach, and potentially dangerous activities like cooking should be supervised. It is recommended that alarms be installed or some method implemented to ensure that the client cannot leave the premises without being noticed. Additionally, some

form of identification, such as a bracelet, can be worn by the client in case she becomes lost.

2. Having clear, bright signs indicating where the bathroom is and leaving the light on at night may help the client to find the bathroom. Additionally, restricting fluid intake after the evening meal and frequently taking the client to the bathroom before bedtime may decrease the need for nighttime urination.

3. Angry and hostile behavior may be exhibited by an increase in motor activity, rattling doorknobs, frowning, raising voice volume and pitch, and so on. Interventions include decreasing environmental stimuli, approaching the client calmly and with assurance, taking care not to place more demands on the client, and distraction. If removed from the situation and provided a calm, nonthreatening environment, the client may forget why he or she was upset. Nurses and family members can often elicit listening behavior by reaching out and touching, holding a hand, or in some way maintaining physical contact.

Scenario B

1. Multiple sclerosis (MS) has two major courses: exacerbating remitting and chronic progressive. In exacerbating remitting MS, the client has episodes of neurologic dysfunction from which he or she recovers. In some cases, the recovery from each exacerbation is not complete, causing a stepwise decline with each exacerbation. In chronic progressive MS, the client experiences a steady decline in neurologic function that can occur over several years. Life expectancy is about 85% of that of the general population, with the usual cause of death being bacterial infection of the lungs, bladder, or pressure ulcers.

2. Fatigue in clients with MS usually worsens as the day progresses. Additionally, fatigue can be precipitated by warm temperatures such as hot weather or hot showers, so these should be avoided. Air conditioning and cool baths may decrease fatigue. Activities should be planned for the client's peak energy level, usually in the morning. Rest periods should be planned throughout the day to alleviate fatigue.

3. The nurse should assess the client's problem-solving strategies to identify coping behavior strengths and defense mechanisms such as denial, avoidance, or intellectualization, which the client may use to mask depression. The client's social support system should be evaluated because this contributes to his or her sense of well-being. Grieving the loss of function in MS can lead to a reactive depression and require provision of support group therapy for the client and significant others.

Chapter 16, Nursing Care of Clients with Spinal Cord and Peripheral and Cranial Nerve Disorders

Study Questions

1. *Answer:* B
   Rationale: Severe headache, nausea, nasal congestion, bradycardia, and hypertension are clinical manifestations of autonomic dysreflexia. It is often precipitated by a noxious stimulus such as a distended bladder.
   Level: Application
   Refer to Learning Outcome #2

2. *Answer:* C
   Rationale: Incomplete spinal cord lesions cause varying degrees of motor and sensory loss below the level of the lesion. Central cord syndrome, anterior cord syndrome, and Brown-Séquard syndrome are all types of incomplete spinal cord lesions.
   Level: Comprehension
   Refer to Learning Outcome #1

3. *Answer:* D
   Rationale: Heavy physical labor, strenuous exercise, and weak abdominal and back muscles all increase the risk of herniated disc. Use of proper body mechanics is the foundation of primary prevention of back injuries.
   Level: Knowledge
   Refer to Learning Outcome #4

4. *Answer:* B
   Rationale: Although there will be incisional pain, often the pain in an extremity that is associated with a herniated disc will be significantly decreased after surgery. In addition, many surgeons inject long-acting local anesthetics into the disc space during surgery. Often the pain recurs on the second postoperative day because of the increase in swelling and the fact that the local anesthetic is wearing off.
   Level: Comprehension
   Refer to Learning Outcome #5

5. *Answer:* B
   Rationale: Trigeminal neuralgia is characterized by intermittent episodes of intense pain with sudden onset. This pain is not relieved by analgesics.
   Level: Knowledge
   Refer to Learning Outcome #3

Critical Thinking Exercises

Scenario A

1. The nurse should gather information about the hemodynamic status of the client, including stability and adequacy of circulation. Information about the respiratory status of the client should include adequacy, use of accessory muscles, diaphragmatic breathing, nostril flaring, shortness of breath, and oxygen saturation. Assessment of spinal cord function should include the level at which the function is diminished or absent and the level at which sensation is diminished or absent. Assessment of urinary and bowel status is also done at this time.

2. Priority nursing diagnoses for this client include the following: Ventilatory Insufficiency or Atelectasis, Risk for; Aspiration, Risk for R/T ineffective airway clearance; Injury, Risk for R/T uncompensated sensory deficit; and Physical Mobility, Impaired R/T paralysis.

3. Nursing care for the client in a halo brace includes ensuring that the wrench that comes with the jacket is always taped to the jacket front to allow for quick removal in case of emergency. The nurse should also ensure that the nursing staff, ancillary personnel, and family members or significant others never grasp the rods to help in turning the client because this may displace the alignment of the client's neck. If the client has mobility, the nurse should assist the client with any activity. The halo jacket changes the client's center of gravity and makes it easier to fall. Additionally, the nurse should assist the client in assessing the condition of the skin under the brace, looking for areas of redness, abrasions, or signs of pressure sores.

Scenario B

1. Because the client is often admitted the day of the surgery, the amount of time nurses have for preoperative teaching is significantly decreased. The nurse should include the family or significant others in the teaching. The client should be taught that frequent turning follows surgery and that correct turning protects the back. The logrolling method of turning is explained. Coughing and deep breathing are explained with a return demonstration by the client. Additionally, the client is taught to roll to the side and to push the torso from the bed with the arms to rise from the bed.

2. Activity after lumbar laminectomy depends on the physician's orders. However, the usual activity progression allows the client to begin logrolling 1 hour after surgery. After microdiscectomy, the client may have the head of the bed elevated to whatever position is comfortable. However, if dural tear was repaired, the surgeon may order the client to remain flat to minimize the risk of cerebrospinal fluid leak. Clients with laminectomies are typically out of bed by the first or second postoperative day.

3. Discharge planning should include instructions on ability to walk, lift, drive, and return to work. Most clients can resume activity 6 weeks after surgery. The client should ask the surgeon when it will be safe to perform activities that could damage the back (climbing stairs, lifting weights greater than 5 lbs, prolonged travel, sexual activity, sports, exercises, driving a car). See Client Education Guide: Back Care.

Chapter 17, Assessment and Nursing Care of Clients with Eye Disorders

Study Questions

1. *Answer:* B
Rationale: It is critical to remember that normal intraocular pressure is maintained as long as the balance between aqueous production and aqueous outflow is maintained.
Level: Knowledge
Refer to Learning Outcome #1

2. *Answer:* A
Rationale: The use of eye drops on a daily basis might indicate that the client has glaucoma. Glaucoma is an ocular disorder that requires daily medication.
Level: Assessment
Refer to Learning Outcome #3

3. *Answer:* C
Rationale: The slit-lamp examination is the only one of those listed that permits direct visualization of the foreign body. It is often used in conjunction with fluorescein dye to highlight irregularities.
Level: Application
Refer to Learning Outcome #4

4. *Answer:* C
Rationale: The increased intraocular pressure would result in a person with angle-closure glaucoma seeing rainbow halos around lights.
Level: Assessment
Refer to Learning Outcome #5

5. *Answer:* A
Rationale: Because a mature cataract significantly reduces vision, the client should not drive a car.
Level: Application
Refer to Learning Outcome #7

6. *Answer:* B
Rationale: Trauma is a predisposing factor in the development of retinal detachment. A yearly examination does not prevent retinal detachment; pain, dizziness, and nausea are not clinical manifestations of retinal detachment; and increasing age does not predispose a person to the development of a retinal detachment.
Level: Application
Refer to Learning Outcome #6

7. *Answer:* A
Rationale: The usual treatment for the client with glaucoma is instillation of miotic eye drops. Lens implantation is performed for the client with a cataract; eye shields are worn after surgery; and vision, once lost, cannot be restored.
Level: Application
Refer to Learning Outcome #9

8. *Answer:* A
Rationale: Clinical manifestations of a cataract include blurred vision, monocular diplopia, photophobia, and glare.
Level: Knowledge
Refer to Learning Outcome #6

9. *Answer:* B
Rationale: Sleeping on the operative side increases pressure. There are restrictions on lifting (A); acetaminophen is recommended, as aspirin increases bleeding tendencies (C); and antibiotic or corticosteroid eye drops, or both, may be ordered postoperatively (D).
Level: Application
Refer to Learning Outcome #9

10. *Answer:* C
Rationale: Acetazolamide decreases the secretion of aqueous humor. The other medications do not exhibit this action.
Level: Comprehension
Refer to Learning Outcome #8

11. *Answer:* D
Rationale: The most important expectation is that the client or a significant other must have the manual dexterity needed to instill eye drops.
Level: Application
Refer to Learning Outcome #7

Critical Thinking Exercises

Scenario A

1. Untreated glaucoma may result in irreversible blindness.

2. Tonometry should be performed to ascertain the intraocular pressure. A Snellen eye chart should be used to determine whether visual changes have occurred. The nurse should assess the client's financial ability to purchase the prescription medications, the ability and dexterity to instill his own eye drops or whether a significant other must be relied upon, lack of understanding about the need for daily medication and consequences of noncompliance, and feelings about having the disease and accepting the change in life-style that daily medication may entail. The presence of signs and symptoms of glaucoma should also be assessed.

3. The client should be retaught about the action of the medication and how it is needed to prevent intraocular pressure. Simple drawings might be explained to the client and given for him to take home. He may need to be retaught how to instill the eye drops and asked for a redemonstration. The nurse should reteach the client about the signs and symptoms of glaucoma and to whom to report if they occur. A follow up appointment should be scheduled with the ophthalmologist. The client should be informed that the nurse will telephone his home to ascertain progress, answer any questions, and offer general support. The client should also be given information on how to reach the nurse at the clinic in case questions or problems arise.

Scenario B

1. The client should be given printed discharge instructions that indicate any limits on activity (no straining) and lifting (not more than 5 pounds). Special instructions for sleeping are also necessary (no sleeping on the affected side). A schedule of times for medication instillation should be given to the client, and the client is taught to self-medicate with eye drops. Also the clinical manifestations of infection (redness, swelling, drainage, blurred vision, and pain) and increased intraocular pressure (unrelieved pain, nausea, and decreased vision) should be taught and written on the discharge instruction sheet. A follow-up appointment is scheduled and the time is written on the discharge instruction sheet.

2. The client is instructed to cleanse the eye with warm tap water using a clean wash cloth. The application of warm compresses and an eye shield is discussed, as is the avoidance of heavy lifting and vigorous activity. Ways to create a safe home environment are also discussed. A follow-up appointment is scheduled, and the time is written on the discharge instruction sheet.
3. The elderly client may be unable to instill the eye drops as required. If no family member or significant other is available, a social service referral should be initiated so that home health-care nurses can ensure that the eye drops are given as scheduled. The nurse may be able to enlist the help of others in instilling the medication. If the elderly client needs assistance (e.g., dressing, eating, toileting, shopping) to function at home, a home health aide may be hired. The social service professionals will assess the client for financial ability and make the necessary referrals for financial assistance according to need and assistance with medication administration and activities of daily living in the home.

Chapter 18, Assessment and Nursing Care of Clients with Ear Disorders

Study Questions

1. *Answer:* A
   Rationale: The labyrinth is located in the inner ear; the suffix "itis" indicates the presence of infection.
   Level: Application
   Refer to Learning Outcomes #1 and #6
2. *Answer:* A
   Rationale: Pain, tinnitus, and loss of balance are classic symptoms of ear disorder. Headache and impaired visual acuity are not associated with ear disorders.
   Level: Comprehension
   Refer to Learning Outcomes #3 and #5
3. *Answer:* A
   Rationale: The Romberg test, which requires that a client stand while balance is tested, is used to assess the inner ear for balance.
   Level: Application
   Refer to Learning Outcome #4
4. *Answer:* C
   Rationale: An otoscope will help visualize perforations of the tympanic membrane. The normal color of the membrane is a pearly gray (A); the oval window is in the inner ear and cannot be visualized (B); and pressure within the eustachian tube cannot be visualized (D).
   Level: Application
   Refer to Learning Outcome #5
5. *Answer:* C
   Rationale: Since water would cause the insect to swell, it would not be used (B). Mineral oil is the fluid of choice. The use of alcohol is inappropriate (A); an insect in the ear canal usually causes pain, so allowing time for it to leave is not appropriate (D).
   Level: Application
   Refer to Learning Outcome #9
6. *Answer:* A
   Rationale: Ototoxic drugs damage the vestibulocochlear nerve (eighth cranial nerve).
   Level: Comprehension
   Refer to Learning Outcomes #8 and #9
7. *Answer:* C
   Rationale: The presence of water in the ear canal could interfere with healing by providing a medium for the growth of pathogens, thus the client must keep the ear dry for the required amount of time.
   Level: Application
   Refer to Learning Outcome #9

Critical Thinking Exercises

Scenario A

1. The nurse should gather more information on the history of ear infections. When did the infections start? How often did they occur? If medical treatment was sought, what medications and procedures were ordered and followed by the client? Was pain, drainage, loss of balance, or dizziness associated with the infections? What symptoms are of concern to the client right now? The nurse should also perform a general inspection of the ear and ear canal to check for the presence of excessive cerumen and abnormalities. He or she uses the fingers to palpate the external ear to determine if pain is present. The nurse could also perform the Weber and Rinne tests. The nurse should review the client's chart for other clues that may assist in care for the recurring infections.
2. The nurse should elicit concerns about the hearing loss from the client. She should also explain the term "presbycusis," how it occurs, and explain that there is no medical or surgical treatment to correct it. The client should be informed about the possibility of improving hearing ability (in some cases) with a hearing aid.
3. Recurrent ear infections can result in hearing loss. The client is at high risk for losing her hearing because of the history of recurrent infections as well as her advancing age.
4. If she has taken any ototoxic medications in the past, she may have experienced damage of the eighth cranial nerve. Her chart should be reviewed to discern if ototoxic medications have been administered in the past. If these have been used, the client's history should be examined for dizziness, nausea, vomiting with motion, vertigo, ear pain, nystagmus, and so on.
5. The nurse should first ask the client to review the dosage schedule for the eardrops and ask the client to demonstrate how she is instilling the drops. If the client needs a review of her medication schedule (for the eardrops), it should be completed at this time. If she needs to relearn how to instill the drops, she should be retaught and asked for a redemonstration at this time. If she cannot instill her own eardrops, arrangements will need to be made for a family member or friend to assist. The client also needs to be instructed in the importance of finishing all medications in a prescription even though she is feeling better. The nurse can explain, in simple terms, about the life cycle of the cell and why it is important to finish taking the medication so that all microorganisms are destroyed.

Scenario B

1. The nurse should elicit a history of the dizziness. How often does it occur? When did it start? Is this the first time the dizziness has interfered with the client's work? The nurse should further explore the client's description of feeling like he is at the center of a spinning plate. Vital signs should be measured and recorded as a baseline. The nurse should also assess for increased intracranial pressure because the client struck his head on an object while falling. Both ears should be checked for drainage.
2. The client should be informed about safety risks in the home, on the job, and in the environment. His illness (vertigo) should be reported to his employer. The diagnostic tests (audiometry, vestibular tests, imaging evaluation, and laboratory tests) should be explained to the client.
3. The client might react with disbelief that he could be afflicted with a prob-

lem at a young age and possibly without any previous history of illness. The client might use denial and not admit he has a problem (he is healthy, strong, and rarely ill). He might also rationalize about the situation and the problem. Because he may deny the possibility of vertigo, he may delay or cancel the necessary tests; not inform his employer of the problem; and not take heed of his personal environment by taking safety precautions until a diagnosis is confirmed.

Chapter 19, Assessment of Clients with Respiratory Disorders

Study Questions

1. *Answer:* D
   Rationale: The larynx connects the upper and lower airways. It contains the vocal cords and the epiglottis. When these are removed, the client is unable to vocalize or to close the epiglottis during coughing. Because the upper airways are bypassed, the inspired air is not filtered or humidified.
   Level: Comprehension
   Refer to Learning Outcome #2

2. *Answer:* C
   Rationale: Chemoreceptors on the brain side of the blood-brain barrier are sensitive to the hydrogen ion content of brain extracellular fluid as well as to CO_2 levels.
   Level: Application
   Refer to Learning Outcome #1

3. *Answer:* B
   Rationale: To obtain a specimen by the direct method, the client first brushes the teeth to reduce contamination, then he or she coughs into a sputum specimen container. The client should be encouraged to cough and not spit so as to obtain sputum. Sputum specimens should be collected before antimicrobial therapy is begun, but sputum is usually more plentiful and concentrated in the morning.
   Level: Comprehension
   Refer to Learning Outcome #3

4. *Answer:* C
   Rationale: Fine crackles are described as discontinuous, high-pitched, short, crackling, popping sounds heard during inspiration.
   Level: Knowledge
   Refer to Learning Outcome #5

5. *Answer:* C
   Rationale: A pulmonary embolus creates a dead space unit because there is ventilation without perfusion.
   Level: Analysis
   Refer to Learning Outcome #4

Critical Thinking Exercises

Scenario A

1. The bronchoscope is inserted via an endotracheal tube inserted in either the nose or the throat. It passes down through the larynx, into the trachea, and investigates all of the bronchi and lobes of the lung.

2. A bronchoscopy is an invasive procedure and requires informed consent. The nurse needs to evaluate the client's knowledge of the procedure, reasons for performing it, and potential complications. The client is maintained NPO (nothing by mouth) for at least 6 hours prior to the test.

3. Prior to the exam, the client is sedated to reduce the cough reflex, and a topical anesthetic is used on the oropharynx. The client is maintained NPO until he or she is alert and the cough and gag reflexes have returned.

4. After the bronchoscopy, the client is monitored for signs of respiratory distress including dyspnea, changes in respiratory rate, use of accessory muscles, and changes in or absent lung sounds. Expectorated secretions are inspected for evidence of any hemoptysis.

Scenario B

1. A thoracentesis is an invasive procedure and requires informed consent. The nurse needs to evaluate the client's knowledge of the procedure, reasons for performing it, and potential complications. The client is also instructed about the importance of holding still during the procedure.

2. The client is placed in the upright position with her arms on an overbed table. An alternate position is in the recumbent position with her arms under her head.

3. The entire left side of the chest will be exposed. The doctor will insert the thoracentesis needle in the midclavicular line between the second and third intercostal spaces. Remember: air rises!

4. After the procedure, the client is usually turned onto the unaffected side for about 1 hour to facilitate lung expansion. Vital signs should be assessed frequently according to agency policy. The respiratory rate and character and lung sounds should be assessed carefully. Tachypnea, dyspnea, cyanosis, retractions, or diminished breath sounds should be reported to the physician.

Chapter 20, Common Respiratory Interventions

Study Questions

1. *Answer:* D
   Rationale: Pursed lip breathing during exhalation prevents early airway collapse. Postural drainage uses gravity to drain specific lung segments of retained secretions and can be performed under the supervision of either a nurse or the respiratory therapist. Auscultating the lungs before and after the procedure allows the nurse or respiratory therapist to monitor the effectiveness of the treatment, and coughing after each position assists the client in mobilizing the secretions.
   Level: Application
   Refer to Learning Outcome #2

2. *Answer:* B
   Rationale: Indications of oxygen toxicity may include mild tracheobronchitis that begins as a substernal soreness, nasal congestion, pain or inspiration, and increased coughing. As the condition worsens, the cough becomes more severe, substernal soreness increases, and dyspnea develops.
   Level: Application
   Refer to Learning Outcome #1

3. *Answer:* A
   Rationale: Effective tracheal suctioning is a gentle yet swift procedure in which timing is very important. Tracheal suctioning removes oxygen and therefore lowers the PaO_2, which may trigger cardiac dysrhythmias.
   Level: Knowledge
   Refer to Learning Outcome #4

4. *Answer:* D
   Rationale: Bronchodilators cause tachycardia, palpitations, tremors, insomnia, nervousness, anxiety, gastrointestinal upset, esophageal reflux, and diarrhea.
   Level: Application
   Refer to Learning Outcome #3

5. *Answer:* B
   Rationale: Expected benefits of diaphragmatic breathing include an increased tidal volume, a decreased respiratory rate, an increased exercise tolerance, and an increase in alveolar ventilation.
   Level: Application
   Refer to Learning Outcome #3

Critical Thinking Exercises

Scenario A

1. All family members need to be taught about the oxygen therapy regardless of culture. However, Hispanic males are traditionally the head of the

household and therefore the decision-makers. The women of the house are usually responsible for work like cleaning and cooking. Care of the oxygen unit will probably be delegated to the client's wife so the nurse should make sure that the wife can give return demonstrations on all aspects of its maintenance.

2. The following information needs to be taught about the care of the concentrator unit:
   a. Wash hands with a bacteriostatic soap prior to changing the humidification chamber on the machine.
   b. Use distilled water and change the chamber every 24 hours. Wash the chamber in warm soapy water, rinse well, and allow to dry.
   c. Change the air filter weekly.
   d. Check the oxygen tubing for condensation, and change periodically.
3. All respiratory clients need to be taught the following infection control measures:
   a. Proper handwashing technique with a bacteriostatic soap.
   b. Activity, coughing, and deep breathing to mobilize secretion.
   c. Restrict contact with crowds and/or people with respiratory or other infections.
   d. Adequate rest, nutrition, and hydration are important to maintain resistance to infection.
   e. Wear warm, dry, protective clothing while outside in damp or cold weather.
   f. Avoid smoke-filled environments and quit smoking.
   g. The pneumonia vaccine (Pneumovax) is a one-time vaccine but influenza shots should be received annually.
   h. Monitor sputum production for changes in color, consistency, or odor.

Scenario B

1. The two main indications for mechanical ventilation include inadequate ventilation and hypoxemia. Because the client's injuries included multiple fractured ribs, he began with splinting of his respirations, which decreased his ventilation and resulted in hypoxemia. Inadequate ventilation leads to a decreasing pH and a stable or increasing $PaCO_2$.
2. Parameters for weaning include:

Inspiratory force	> -20 mm Hg
Tidal volume	10–15 mL/kg
Vital capacity	$>$10–15 mL/kg
Expiratory force	$> +60$ cm H_2O
Resting minute volume	$>$10 L/min
$PaCO_2$	within normal limits
PaO_2	minimally 70–80 mm Hg

3. For successful weaning by the rapid technique, the nurse needs to:
   a. Start after the client has had a good night's sleep.
   b. Place the client in the semi-Fowler's position.
   c. Reduce the respiratory rate to one half the original rate.
   d. Obtain ABGs in 30 minutes.
   e. If ABGs are at or near the client's baseline, place the client on a T-piece with "blowby" oxygen at the same FIO_2.
   f. Obtain ABGs in 30 minutes.
   g. If the ABGs are again at or near baseline and the respiratory rate is below 25 to 30 breaths per minute, extubate and place the client on supplemental O_2.

Chapter 21, Nursing Care of Clients with Upper Airway Disorders

Study Questions

1. *Answer:* B
   Rationale: Hoarseness that lasts longer than 2 weeks should be evaluated.
   Level: Knowledge
   Refer to Learning Outcome #1
2. *Answer:* D
   Rationale: The greatest problem for the client after laryngectomy is loss of voice. Because the trachea and pharynx are permanently separated by surgery, there is no risk of aspiration.
   Level: Analysis
   Refer to Learning Outcome #2
3. *Answer:* B
   Rationale: The client should be positioned in semi-Fowler's to high-Fowler's position to decrease edema of the airway, facilitate breathing, and improve comfort.
   Level: Application
   Refer to Learning Outcomes #4 and #6
4. *Answer:* D
   Rationale: Some blood-tinged sputum is expected in the tracheal secretions for the first 48 hours, but frank bleeding from the tracheostomy site or tube is a sign of hemorrhage and must be reported immediately.
   Level: Application
   Refer to Learning Outcome #3
5. *Answer:* D
   Rationale: A visit from a member of community support groups, like the Lost Chord Club or the International Association of Laryngectomees, may offer needed reassurance.
   Level: Application
   Refer to Learning Outcome #5
6. *Answer:* B
   Rationale: Trauma involving the head and neck can cause a complete or partial airway obstruction related to edema or bleeding or both.
   Level: Knowledge
   Refer to Learning Outcome #1
7. *Answer:* C
   Rationale: Few outward signs may be present. Observe for increased dyspnea, intercostal muscle retraction, stridor, inability to speak, and change in respiratory patterns.
   Level: Application
   Refer to Learning Outcome #5
8. *Answer:* C
   Rationale: The initial treatment for epistaxis is application of pressure by pinching the anterior portion of the nose for a minimum of 5 to 10 minutes. In addition, the application of ice compresses to produce vasoconstriction may also decrease bleeding.
   Level: Application
   Refer to Learning Outcome #3

Scenario A

1. Risk factors related to laryngeal cancer include tobacco and alcohol use. Considerable data indicate that the etiologic agent of laryngeal cancer is cigarette smoking. The risk is increased in the client who smokes and drinks alcohol. Other risk factors are voice abuse, chronic laryngitis, industrial exposure, and heredity.
2. The warning signs of head and neck cancer include change in voice quality; a lump anywhere in the neck or body; persistent cough, sore throat, or earache; hemoptysis; sores within the throat that do not heal; and difficulty swallowing or breathing.
3. Preoperative teaching should include the following:
   - Identifying a means of communication between the client and his caregivers because the client will have no voice after surgery; even if the client refuses the surgery, he needs to know that the voice quality will worsen as the tumor spreads
   - Making sure that the client knows he will require a permanent tracheal stoma
   - Teaching the client deep-breathing and coughing techniques to help him clear mucus from the tracheostomy tube postoperatively
   - Teaching the client all of the usual postoperative techniques: turning

every 2 hours, performing leg exercises to prevent deep vein thrombosis, and getting out of bed without putting strain on his neck incision

4. Immediately after surgery, a nasogastric tube will be used to remove gastric secretions until bowel activity resumes. Some clients will then be tube fed with commercial supplements. When the client exhibits signs of swallowing his own secretions and the edema has subsided, the oral feeding can begin. The diet usually begins with soft or semisoft foods and progresses as healing occurs.

Scenario B

1. Initial treatment of epistaxis includes the following:
    - Applying continuous pressure to the soft anterior nose against the internal septum for approximately 5 to 10 minutes
    - Keeping the client sitting upright but with her head tilted forward so that she does not swallow or aspirate the blood
    - Instructing the client to breathe through her mouth and not to talk
    - Applying ice compresses to the nose to promote vasoconstriction
2. If the initial steps do not stop bleeding, nasal packing may be inserted. With anterior bleeding, anterior nasal packing may be all that is needed. An antibacterial ointment such as bacitracin or Neosporin is applied to the gauze and then gently, but firmly, inserted into the anterior nasal cavities to apply pressure to the bleeding vessels. Nasal packing should remain in place for a minimum of 48 to 72 hours. If the location of the bleeding vessel can be identified, cauterization can be performed using silver nitrate, and then nasal packing can be inserted.
3. Insertion of posterior packing is very uncomfortable and requires a mild analgesic to reduce anxiety and discomfort. The client is admitted to the hospital and monitored closely for hypoxia. General comfort measures include humidification, the use of a drip pad to collect bloody drainage and mucus, and lubrication of the nares with a water-soluble ointment to alleviate some of the discomfort. The client must be monitored closely for signs of bleeding. The nurse should inspect the oral cavity for blood and placement of the posterior packing. The posterior packing should not be visible; if it is, the physician should be notified for readjustment. The packing should remain in place for 5 days, and prophylactic antibiotics are used to prevent toxic shock syndrome and sinusitis.

Chapter 22, Nursing Care of Clients with Lower Airway Disorders

Study Questions

1. *Answer:* C
   Rationale: The key to increasing the survival rate of clients with lung cancer is early detection. However, a tumor must be at least 1 cm in diameter before it is detectable on chest film. Unfortunately, invasion and metastasis have usually already occurred. Radiation may be used in clients with locally advanced disease who are poor surgical risks. It may also be used in combination with surgery or chemotherapy to improve treatment outcomes. Surgical intervention is the treatment of choice in early stage non–small cell lung cancer. Cure is possible if the disease is still localized to the thoracic cavity and no distant metastases are present.
   Level: Knowledge
   Refer to Learning Outcome #4
2. *Answer:* B
   Rationale: The signs and symptoms of impending respiratory problems associated with hypoxemia and hypercapnia (e.g., increased confusion or drowsiness, and increasing dyspnea) should be reviewed with the client and significant others prior to discharge. They need to be taught that prompt intervention is necessary.
   Level: Analysis
   Refer to Learning Outcome #1
3. *Answer:* C
   Rationale: This procedure involves removal of the entire lung. Because the mediastinum is no longer held in place on both sides by lung tissue, extreme turning may cause mediastinal shift and compression of the remaining lung.
   Level: Application
   Refer to Learning Outcome #5
4. *Answer:* D
   Rationale: Clients with pneumonia are at risk for a fluid volume deficit related to insensible fluid losses because of increased respiratory rate and fever. The nurse must monitor the client's fluid volume status carefully. Interventions aimed at keeping the secretions thinned and easier to mobilize should also help with the fluid volume.
   Level: Analysis
   Refer to Learning Outcome #1
5. *Answer:* C
   Rationale: Culture of *Mycobacterium tuberculosis* from sputum or other body secretions or tissue is the only method of confirming the diagnosis. Chest x-rays are used for detecting old lesions or new ones once they are large enough to be seen. The Mantoux test is also used in the diagnosis.
   Level: Knowledge
   Refer to Learning Outcome #2
6. *Answer:* B
   Rationale: Elderly clients frequently have other chronic medical conditions that complicate the course of the disease.
   Level: Synthesis
   Refer to Learning Outcome #2
7. *Answer:* C
   Rationale: The risk of cancer is increased when the smoker is also exposed to other carcinogenic agents, such as radioactive isotopes. Air pollution has also been implicated in increasing the risk of lung cancer. The primary cause of chronic airflow limitations is also cigarette smoking. Chewing tobacco has been implicated in the development of maxillofacial cancers.
   Level: Knowledge
   Refer to Learning Outcome #2 and #3
8. *Answer:* B
   Rationale: All other choices cite incorrect parameters.
   Level: Application
   Refer to Learning Outcome #4

Critical Thinking Exercises

Scenario A

1. The earliest clinical sign of adult respiratory distress syndrome (ARDS) is usually an increased respiratory rate. Breathing becomes increasingly labored; the client may exhibit air hunger, retractions, and cyanosis. Chest auscultation may or may not reveal the presence of adventitious sounds. At the client's age, dysrhythmias and hypotension are also to be expected.
2. The nurse assesses the elderly client for changes in cognition (confusion and lethargy), anorexia, tachypnea, and deterioration of any pre-existing disorders.
3. The nasal cannula is considered a low-flow delivery system and is used at flow rates from 1 to 6 L/minute. At those rates it delivers between 24 and 44 per cent oxygen.
4. The key to successful management of ARDS is early detection and initiation

of treatment. When blood gas analysis reveals increasing hypoxemia (PaO < 70 mm Hg when $FIO_2 > 0.4$) and the respiratory rate is greater than 35 breaths per minute, endotracheal intubation is considered a necessary intervention.

5. Endotracheal intubation, mechanical ventilation, and positive end expiratory pressure are usually required to maintain adequate blood oxygen levels. Positive end expiratory pressure is used to keep the small airways open, increase functional residual capacity and decrease shunting.

Scenario B

1. *Streptococcus pneumoniae* is the most common cause of community-acquired pneumonia. It often follows influenza and is frequently seen in clients with chronic diseases, immunosuppression, and alcohol abuse.

2. The clinical manifestations of bacterial pneumonia include sudden onset with a single shaking chill, high fever, stabbing, pleuritic chest pain, malaise, weakness, occasional vomiting, tachypnea, dyspnea, and elevated white blood cell count; single or multiple lobar consolidation on the chest film; and cough productive of rusty brown or blood-streaked sputum that turns yellow and mucoid.

3. The primary antibiotic is either penicillin G intravenously or penicillin V orally. Alternatively, cephalosporins or erythromycin may be used. Peak blood levels of antibiotic can be achieved about 30 to 60 minutes after ingestion. The client should begin to feel a response in 1 to 2 days. The client should be instructed to complete the full course of the antibiotic. She needs to be taught to report to the physician if there is no improvement in her symptoms or if they are still present after the full course of antibiotic therapy. More and more strains of bacteria are becoming resistant to penicillin.

Chapter 23, Assessment of Clients with Cardiovascular Disorders

Study Questions

1. *Answer:* D
   Rationale: All of the questions are important to determine the probable cause of the pain and to prioritize the nursing care of the client.
   Level: Assessment
   Refer to Learning Outcome #2

2. *Answer:* A
   Rationale: S_1 occurs with or just before the carotid pulse. This is the beginning of systole. Palpation of the carotid pulse is helpful in identifying the S_1 heart sound, particularly in rapid heart rates.
   Level: Assessment
   Refer to Learning Outcome #3

3. *Answer:* D
   Rationale: Depolarization of the ventricles is represented by the ST segment on the electrocardiogram.
   Level: Knowledge
   Refer to Learning Outcome #1

4. *Answer:* C
   Rationale: Myocardial ischemia is aggravated by exercise and alleviated by rest. Infarction pain is not relieved by rest. Pain associated with pericarditis and musculoskeletal deformity is not generally aggravated by exercise and alleviated by rest.
   Level: Assessment
   Refer to Learning Outcome #2

5. *Answer:* B
   Rationale: These are classic signs of impaired circulation and the physician should be notified. Infection of the site would be associated with increased pain and redness at the insertion site. Although the decreased circulation may be caused by spasm, the nurse cannot determine that at the bedside. The condition could also be associated with hematoma formation or other causes.
   Level: Assessment
   Refer to Learning Outcome #5

Critical Thinking Exercises

Scenario A

1. Diabetic clients, along with the elderly, do not always complain of chest pain with myocardial ischemia or infarction. In up to 25 per cent of clients, the chief complaint is shortness of breath. In addition, the nurse is aware that diabetes is a risk factor for coronary ischemia resulting from the development of atherosclerosis.

2. Because of the serious complications of myocardial ischemia and infarction (sudden death, dysrythmias), the client with a history of coronary artery disease is always treated according to myocardial infarction protocols until otherwise is proven by laboratory studies, tests, and medical examination.

Scenario B

It is true that family history is a nonmodifiable risk factor for cardiovascular disease, but that does not mean that an individual will acquire the disease. It only means that, statistically, an individual is at risk. On the other hand, we do know that life-style and health habits do have a major effect on the development of coronary artery disease. We also know that the risk increases greatly when cigarette smoking is combined with other risk factors. In this case, because a person cannot change family history, he or she should attempt to offset the risk by eliminating habits that can lead to a greater risk for coronary artery disease and early death.

Chapter 24, Nursing Care of Clients with Disorders of Cardiac Function

Study Questions

1. *Answer:* C
   Rationale: Diabetes mellitus is not a modifiable risk factor for coronary artery disease (CAD) because diabetes mellitus is not curable. Clients with diabetes mellitus have an increased incidence of CAD; however, clients can choose to modify smoking habits, dietary intake, and life-style.
   Level: Knowledge
   Refer to Learning Outcome #2

2. *Answer:* B
   Rationale: The client is displaying symptoms of fluid volume overload and congestive heart failure. Planning rest periods after meals is appropriate because digestion is work for the heart and increases cardiac oxygen demand. The other interventions all increase the workload of the heart.
   Level: Intervention
   Refer to Learning Outcome #4

3. *Answer:* B
   Rationale: Storing nitroglycerine in the original container prevents a decrease in the potency of the drug. The medication should never be kept close to the body (A) and is always dissolved under the tongue (D). The physician is notified if the client takes three tablets, 5 minutes apart, without relief (C).
   Level: Planning
   Refer to Learning Outcome #5

4. *Answer:* C
   Rationale: Myocardial infarction pain is unrelieved by rest or nitroglycerine. Ischemia is relieved by both; the other symptoms are common to both.
   Level: Application
   Refer to Learning Outcome #6

5. *Answer:* B
   Rationale: The ventricular pacemaker does not coordinate the natural atrial

and ventricular contraction. These clients lose "atrial kick" and can develop signs of decreased cardiac output. The atrioventricular physiologic pacemaker closely mimics the natural conduction and contraction of the atrium followed by the ventricle.
Level: Application
Refer to Learning Outcome #5

6. *Answer:* C
Rationale: In ventricular hypertrophy, the walls of the heart thicken and the weight of the heart increases. A hypertrophied heart does far greater work than a normal-sized heart.
Level: Comprehension
Refer to Learning Outcome #1

7. *Answer:* B
Rationale: Diuretics enhance renal excretion of sodium and water so that circulating blood volume is reduced, preload is diminished, and systemic and pulmonary congestion is lessened.
Level: Comprehension
Refer to Learning Outcome #5

8. *Answer:* A
Rationale: Dysrhythmias are disorders of the heart rate and rhythm and are caused by disturbances in the conduction system. The conduction system includes the pacemaker of the heart, the transmission of impulses through the heart, and the pathway of conduction.
Level: Knowledge
Refer to Learning Outcome #3

Critical Thinking Exercises

Scenario A

The client should not be restricted from driving based only on the incident of syncope since the cause was related to heart block. The properly functioning pacemaker should prevent further episodes of fainting. The client needs complete instructions in how to assess the functioning of the pacemaker to include taking a pulse, follow-up visits to the physician, and possibly use of the phone electrocardiographic system.

Activity is restricted during the first 6 weeks to active range of motion on the operative side and not lifting over 10 pounds. Once cleared by the physician, the client should be able to resume all activity except contact sports and holding a rifle butt against the pacer shoulder. Remaining active is an important part of the elderly client's quality of life.

Scenario B

Black males have the highest incidence of coronary artery disease (CAD) in the United States. Diabetic clients are at high risk, as are those suffering from hypertension and those who smoke. The history of shortness of breath with palpitations during exercises is suspicious of ischemia. The elderly and the diabetic client does not always present with chest pain.

During this visit the nurse should do a complete assessment including heart and lung sounds and should alert the physician to the new symptoms. The nurse should explain to the client any tests that the physician orders. Since the client has multiple nonmodifiable risk factors for CAD, the nurse needs to discuss with the client what life-style changes he can make to decrease the risk. Together they should set goals to stop smoking (refer to smoke stoppers) and decrease fat in the diet. The client must help set the priority of these activities. It is very difficult and often unsuccessful to attempt to change all habits at the same time.

Chapter 25, Nursing Care of Clients with Cardiac Structure Disorders

Study Questions

1. *Answer:* B
Rationale: Elderly clients are at risk because of degenerative changes of the valves that allow bacteria from the urinary tract to be trapped and multiply. Intravenous drug users bolus the blood stream with materials that can infect a previously healthy valve. Coronary artery bypass graft clients are not at increased risk.
Level: Knowledge
Refer to Learning Outcome #2

2. *Answer:* B
Rationale: The client is at risk for reinfection and additional heart damage. Signs and symptoms of infection or decreased cardiac function must be reported immediately. Tachycardia could be a sign of heart failure or the increased metabolic rate related to infection.
Level: Evaluation
Refer to Learning Outcome #6

3. *Answer:* B
Rationale: Atrial hypertrophy occurs with mitral insufficiency. The clients have symptoms of left and right ventricular failure. Increased afterload is associated with aortic stenosis.
Level: Knowledge
Refer to Learning Outcome #1

4. *Answer:* D
Rationale: Pansystolic murmur is assessed in the client with mitral insufficiency.
Level: Assessment
Refer to Learning Outcome #1

5. *Answer:* A
Rationale: Assessment data show fluid volume deficit. The client requires volume replacement. Inotropic medications may increase tachycardia and cardiac oxygen needs. There is not evidence of pain. Pain is generally associated with elevated blood pressure (BP) and anxiety. Intravenous nitropresside would decrease BP further and would not improve the urine output.
Level: Application
Refer to Learning Outcome #5

6. *Answer:* C
Rationale: The client displays signs of fluid volume overload. A high Fowler's position facilitates lung expansion. Input and output measurement is a valuable tool for monitoring renal function and fluid status. Lasix and digoxin are given in congestive heart failure (CHF). The client with CHF has activity intolerance because of decreased oxygenation. Bedrest is prescribed in the acute stages.
Level: Application
Refer to Learning Outcome #5

Critical Thinking Exercises

Scenario A

Previously healthy elderly clients are good candidates for valve replacement. These clients tend to have a longer hospital stay but benefit from early ambulation and a progressive exercise program. Age is not a contraindication for valve replacement.

Scenario B

Transplantation is the only option for survival for many clients with end-stage disease. Availability of organs remains a major block for many clients. Often it is the nurse who works closely with the family of critically ill clients. The nurse is the member of the health-care team who has the best opportunity to develop rapport with families of dying clients. Although this is a sensitive subject, nurses do have the ethical responsibility to make available donor information in a sensitive and appropriate manner, or to alert designated members of the health-care team of possible donors.

Chapter 26, Nursing Care of Clients with Peripheral Vascular Disorders

Study Questions

1. *Answer:* A
Rationale: Weight reduction is the

most important nonpharmacologic intervention for blood pressure reduction. Decreasing the fat content to less than 30 per cent of total calories has been shown to be the most effective way to decrease weight and to maintain lower weight. Although exercise is beneficial and may enhance the weight reduction and sense of well-being, it is not the initial intervention. The client does not require a no-salt diet. This is a difficult diet to maintain.
Level: Planning
Refer to Learning Outcome #5

2. *Answer:* D
Rationale: All are important aspects of the assessment of the client.
Level: Application
Refer to Learning Outcome #1

3. *Answer:* B
Rationale: Statements 1 and 2 address the problem directly. Although involvement of the significant other may be helpful, this should be done with the knowledge and permission of the client. The client does not display lack of understanding.
Level: Application
Refer to Learning Outcome #6

4. *Answer:* A
Rationale: The client displays signs and symptoms of occluded graft and requires medical intervention. Answers B and C delay definitive therapy and risk viability of the limb. Warming the leg is contraindicated because it may decrease oxygen supply to the muscle and increase flow to the skin. It also delays medical intervention.
Level: Application
Refer to Learning Outcome #5

5. *Answer:* B
Rationale: Phantom pain is common, hard to control, and may last weeks to years.
Level: Knowledge
Refer to Learning Outcome #2

Critical Thinking Exercises

Scenario A

The nurse needs to gather more information about why the client demonstrates poor compliance. The possible reasons are multiple and may include the following:

- Knowledge deficit
- Access to and availability of place of distribution of medication
- Intolerable side effects to medication

Appropriate intervention cannot be initiated until further information is available to the nurse. Intervention must be prioritized on the basis of client needs and client perception of the problem. Multiple pharmacologic and nonpharmacologic interventions are available. The goal is to develop a holistic plan that controls the blood pressure with few side effects and is available to the client.

Scenario B

The nurse needs to assess the client for postoperative complications of hemorrhage, occluded graft, or occluded extremity artery. The nurse should assess the pulse with Doppler ultrasonography. In addition, the nurse needs to complete a total neurovascular assessment including, but not limited to, temperature, capillary refill, edema, proprioception, sensation, and mobility. The client should be assessed for hypovolemia and hypothermia. If the nurse suspects hypovolemia or an occluded graft or extremity, the physician should be notified.

Chapter 27, Basic Concepts of Hematology

Study Questions

1. *Answer:* B
Rationale: Vitamin B_{12} is involved with red cell maturation and nervous system function; folic acid is responsible for red cell formation and maturation but does not play a role in nervous system function.
Level: Knowledge
Refer to Learning Outcome #1

2. *Answer:* B
Rationale: The AB blood type has antigens A and B present in the blood. Major antibodies are found in the serum; the individual cannot safely receive all types of blood; and the AB blood type is the least common of the blood types.
Level: Comprehension
Refer to Learning Outcome #2

3. *Answer:* A
Rationale: Fruits and vegetables are major sources of folic acid; thus, a decreased (or no) intake puts the client at risk for folic acid deficiency. Animal products are the source for vitamin B_{12}. Lack of folic acid is not involved in coagulation or an increase in the risk for infection.
Level: Application
Refer to Learning Outcome #3

4. *Answer:* C
Rationale: Because this is an invasive procedure with possible complications, the client is required to sign a consent for the procedure. The procedure is done with local anesthesia; a biopsy may be taken during aspiration; and bone marrow aspiration does not scrape the bone, it removes a specimen of bone marrow.
Level: Application
Refer to Learning Outcome #4

Critical Thinking Exercise

1. Any surgeries involving tumor removal, cardiac valve replacement, splenectomy, or resection of the gastrointestinal system should alert the nurse to bleeding problems or problems with absorption of vitamin B_{12}.
2. The client who does not eat a well-balanced diet is at risk for various anemias; thus, a complete diet history may alert the nurse to the possibility of an anemia caused by a dietary deficiency.
3. The client's problems may be caused by previous exposure to environmental toxins. A thorough work history should be explored with the client.
4. Disorders associated with the hematologic system affect all organs and tissues throughout the body.
5. General symptoms include fatigue, apathy, lethargy, malaise, weakness, heat intolerance, chills, fever, night sweats, and delayed wound healing. Some of these same symptoms may occur in relation to the aging process; the client may not realize a disease process is present, so the nurse should be alert for problems of this nature.

Chapter 28, Nursing Care of Clients with Hematologic Disorders

Study Questions

1. *Answer:* C
Rationale: Dysphagia (difficulty in swallowing) occurs in severe iron deficiency anemia. Stomatitis, an inflamed, smooth tongue, and small (microcytic) red blood cells are other hallmarks of severe anemia.
Level: Application
Refer to Learning Outcome #1

2. *Answer:* A
Rationale: The body needs vitamin B_{12} for gastrointestinal and neurologic functions. The person with pernicious anemia cannot absorb vitamin B_{12} because there is a lack of the intrinsic factor. To maintain body function, B_{12} must be supplied from outside sources on a regular basis. It is not present in red blood cells, does not respond to a special diet, and is not caused by environmental exposure to toxins.
Level: Application
Refer to Learning Outcome #2

3. *Answer:* D
   Rationale: Any exposure to low oxygen tensions eventually results in deformed red blood cells. Strenuous exercise elicits this response. Drinking fluid, driving a car, and eating fatty foods do not expose the body to low oxygen tension.
   Level: Application
   Refer to Learning Outcome #2

4. *Answer:* C
   Rationale: The client and her partner should be tested for sickle cell anemia; the couple would be counseled as to the expectations of children being born without sickle cell or with sickle cell anemia or trait. Pregnancy for women with sickle cell anemia carries a very high risk, a red blood cell count is not necessary every 6 months, and anticoagulant therapy has proven unsuccessful as a treatment for sickle cell anemia.
   Level: Application
   Refer to Learning Outcome #3

5. *Answer:* C
   Rationale: Since the immune system is malfunctioning, the client will be at risk for infection. The client is placed in reverse isolation; body temperature is assessed every 4 hours; and raw fruits and vegetables are excluded from the diet because of potential exposure to bacteria.
   Level: Application
   Refer to Learning Outcome #4

6. *Answer:* D
   Rationale: The client is experiencing a transfusion reaction and the primary nursing intervention is to stop the transfusion and keep an intravenous line open. The saline infusion rate would not be increased; double-checks should be carried out before the transfusion is begun; and vital signs should be taken after the transfusion is stopped.
   Level: Application
   Refer to Learning Outcome #5

7. *Answer:* B
   Rationale: The clotting ability of the blood is impaired, so the nurse should expect prolonged bleeding from the site. Pressure on the skin might cause an ecchymotic area; ecchymotic areas may be present as part of the disease process; and vitamin K would not be a stat order for this condition.
   Level: Application
   Refer to Learning Outcome #5

8. *Answer:* D
   Rationale: An application of ice or manual pressure will help promote hemostasis over a bleeding site. The teeth can be brushed regularly with a soft toothbrush; NSAIDs should be avoided because they prolong bleeding time; and the Valsalva maneuver should be avoided because of the increase in pressure it causes (related to capillary fragility).
   Level: Application
   Refer to Learning Outcome #6

Critical Thinking Exercises

Scenario A

1. The elderly may have financial constraints and may cut corners on the food budget. Other factors that impact on dietary intake are inability to drive and shop for groceries, inability to prepare nutritious, appealing meals, and inability to properly chew foods. The number of taste buds is reduced, so food might no longer taste the same. An elderly person may also be on a special diet that limits intake or is not as appealing as the person's life-long diet.

2. Some of the factors discussed in the first answer could be caused by the client's fatigue and shortness of breath, which result from the iron deficiency. Less oxygen is available so the client may reserve strength by doing only the necessary activities of daily living. Keep in mind that as one ages, the body's functions also decrease, for example, respiratory reserves decrease with age.

3. If the couple was eating the same type of diet, he would be at high risk for iron deficiency anemia. The fatigue seen in persons with iron deficiency anemia is also manifested in chronic myelogenous leukemia (CML). If, as a result of the wife's diagnosis, they both ate iron-rich foods, his risk would be reduced unless blood loss occurred.

4. Before teaching, the nurse should assess for risk factors that might have an impact on how the client is able to comply with treatment. A social worker may need to arrange for help with shopping, meal preparation, and other activities of daily living unless family members or friends are available to assist. The nurse should discuss the side effects of iron supplements (for example constipation, tarry stools, and upset stomach) and the importance of taking the supplement for at least 6 months on a daily basis. Remember to explain the function of the red blood cell in carrying oxygen and how the life cycle of the red blood cell (120 days) necessitates taking a supplement for at least 6 months. Teach to take the supplement with meals and how to prevent constipation (diet, fluids, and exercise such as walking).

5. CML is a disease of the white blood cells, in particular, increased numbers of both mature and slightly immature lymphocytes, while iron deficiency anemia affects the red blood cells. The symptoms of CML are characteristic of anemia, thrombocytopenia, and leukopenia.

6. The client should be assessed for present compliance with taking medications for the CML. The nurse should discuss the risk for bleeding and the need to prevent exposure to infection. The nurse should complete any reteaching required by the spouse at this time (refer to the Client Education Guide: The Immunosuppressed Client).

Scenario B

1. Due to low oxygen tension, the client becomes hypoxic, and due to the increased concentration of sickled cell, the blood is more viscous. A vicious circle ensues wherein the sickled cells clump together in the smaller blood vessels and occlude the microcirculation, causing hypoxia. The lack of oxygen causes more cells to sickle, and the cycle begins again.

2. The brain and kidneys demand a constant supply of oxygen so are at risk for infarction and necrosis when the supply of oxygen decreases. The bone marrow and spleen, because they have normally sluggish circulation, are also vulnerable to infarction and necrosis.

3. Both siblings and their partners should receive counseling to ascertain if children will be affected by the disease. The sister should also receive information regarding the risks of childbearing. They may also need psychological counseling to help them accept the decision they make.

4. The test is effective for mass screening, but it does not differentiate between sickle cell disease and the trait.

5. Since the individual with sickle cell trait generally has few or no symptoms, the brother in the example is more likely to develop sickle cell crisis.

6. Events that lower the oxygen tension of the blood (flying at high altitudes, for example) and changes in body function that cause dehydration lead to sickle cell crisis.

Chapter 29, Assessment of Clients with Urinary Disorders

Study Questions

1. *Answer:* C
   Rationale: The statement is correct in its anatomic description. The female urethra is 3.5 to 4.0 cm long (A); the urethra is the outlet from the bladder to the meatus (B); and peristaltic action in the ureters moves urine down and into the bladder (D).
   Level: Knowledge
   Refer to Learning Outcome #1

2. *Answer:* D
   Rationale: The most common result of trauma to the abdomen and pelvic area is hematuria because of injury to the urinary tract.
   Level: Comprehension
   Refer to Learning Outcome #2

3. *Answer:* A
   Rationale: Premedication with a steroid allows the test to proceed. Restriction of iodine-rich foods is already practiced by the client (B); withholding medications is not an appropriate choice (C); and the contrast medium for this test is given intravenously (D).
   Level: Application
   Refer to Learning Outcome #4

4. *Answer:* C
   Rationale: Typical ureteral pain is exhibited as back pain and may be colicky; it is often referred to the genitals.
   Level: Application
   Refer to Learning Outcome #3

5. *Answer:* A
   Rationale: Bleeding in the upper urinary tract may be a smokey gray or dark red color. Lower urinary tract bleeding appears as red urine (B), urobilinogen or bilirubin results in a dark yellow or green urine (C), absence of either would not affect urine color (D).
   Level: Comprehension
   Refer to Learning Outcome #3

6. *Answer:* D
   Rationale: To provide effective and appropriate treatment, the organism must be eradicated with an antibiotic to which it is susceptible.
   Level: Application
   Refer to Learning Outcome #4

Critical Thinking Exercises

Scenario A

1. The older male is more likely to report problems with dribbling and starting the stream.
2. Normal findings in a routine urinalysis do not change over a person's lifetime.
3. Results of diagnostic testing done during hospitalization would provide valuable baseline data for assessment of the current problem. Illnesses such as diabetes mellitus and hypertension can ultimately affect renal function and need to be considered in planning medical treatment for the client.

Scenario B

Answers:

1. N	4. A	7. UTI
2. A, ARF	5. A, B, TE	8. UTI, B, BS
3. A, UTI	6. N	9. A, B

Chapter 30, Nursing Care of Clients with Disorders of the Ureters, Bladder, and Urethra

Study Questions

1. *Answer:* B
   Rationale: Nitrofurantoin is known to cause changes in the color of urine. It is not photosensitive. Fluid intake should be encouraged to ensure high urine output. The medication is ordered for a period of 10 to 14 days.
   Level: Application
   Refer to Learning Outcome #5
2. *Answer:* B
   Rationale: Learning Kegel exercises begins with an understanding of which muscles are used. This is accomplished by stopping the urine several times when voiding.
   Level: Application
   Refer to Learning Outcome #4
3. *Answer:* A
   Rationale: The inability to void is one of the cardinal symptoms of cystitis. Painless hematuria is associated with neoplasms of the bladder, bladder retention is usually not associated with cystitis, and pain referred to the shoulder is associated with bladder trauma.
   Level: Comprehension
   Refer to Learning Outcome #1
4. *Answer:* A
   Rationale: Smoking is a major risk factor associated with development of bladder neoplasms. None of the other choices have been linked to the development of bladder neoplasm.
   Level: Knowledge
   Refer to Learning Outcome #2
5. *Answer:* B
   Rationale: The client with any urinary diversion needs to make special adaptations when traveling. The client with recurrent cystitis may need to adopt an acid-ash diet. Credé's maneuver and stimulation of the micturition reflex are not appropriate for the client with a urinary diversion.
   Level: Application
   Refer to Learning Outcome #6

Critical Thinking Exercises

Scenario A

1. When sexual activity is resumed, there is a high risk for impotence in the male. He may be able to attain an erection but will be unable to ejaculate. The female can expect decreased libido as a result of the removal of the uterus. The change in the anterior wall of the vagina may also impact on sexual enjoyment. The client and partner may need to be taught about different forms of sexual expression that may be acceptable to both partners. A sex therapist can be consulted if problems persist for a period of time after recovery from the surgery.
2. Although the pouch may retain as much as 800 mL of urine, emptying needs to be done around the clock. The technique used for urethral self-catheterization is used for urinary catheterization through a stoma into an artificially created pouch that stores urine. The nurse must teach basic principles about washing hands, avoiding infections, caring for equipment, intake of fluids, and complying with medications when ordered. The client is taught to observe for color, clarity, odor, and amount of the urine as well as condition of the stoma and external appliance.
3. The client can wear any clothing that is loose-fitting in the area of the stoma. Before the surgery, the client and entorostomal therapist discuss life-style and type of dress the client is used to. On the basis of this information, the stoma is created in an area that allows comfortable attachment of an appliance that will not show through the client's style of dress. The client may need to experiment somewhat to discover which of his or her

clothing is suitable to wear during and after the recovery phase.

Scenario B

1. Any client who has a urinary tract infection (UTI) at least once remains susceptible to recurrent UTIs. She may have experienced a first episode when catheterized after surgery or delivery of a child. Some female clients can trace recurrent UTIs to childhood; the infections may have started because of poor hygienic habits as a child.
2. The client most likely wiped back to front after voiding and emptying the bowels at the same time. *Escherichia coli* is common flora in the intestine but causes infection when it enters the sterile environment of the bladder. If the client or significant other is able, installing a stabilizing bar in the bathroom near the toilet may help. The client can steady herself while wiping with one hand and grabbing onto the bar with the other after voiding. The nurse must teach or reteach proper hygienic care after voiding; a person who has not learned proper perineal cleansing may need teaching and reinforcement to reduce the incidence of recurrence. Until the client is able to stand without assistance, a significant other may need to be taught about the proper methods of cleansing after toileting.
3. Clients who experience recurrent UTIs can certainly recognize the symptoms associated with infection. The client could be given a prescription to use in the event the symptoms appear. The client would need to be taught to make an appointment to have a culture completed to ensure that the urine has resumed the normal sterility.
4. When large amounts of fluid are ingested, the body will produce a correspondingly large amount to excrete. When small amounts are ingested, smaller amounts will be excreted. The elderly client needs to understand the importance of adequate fluid intake in keeping the kidneys flushed. The elderly person may limit the intake of fluid if there are problems associated with voiding (e.g., accessibility of toilet facilities, ability to toilet oneself) and should be taught the positive benefits of adequate fluid intake.

Chapter 31, Nursing Care of Clients with Renal Disorders

Study Questions

1. *Answer:* D
   Rationale: Antibiotics can be nephrotoxic and cause acute renal failure.
   Level: Comprehension
   Refer to Learning Outcome #1
2. *Answer:* B
   Rationale: Fluid control is a priority because the kidney is no longer able to perform this function effectively.
   Level: Comprehension
   Refer to Learning Outcome #6
3. *Answer:* B
   Rationale: Only hypertension is an extrarenal result.
   Level: Comprehension
   Refer to Learning Outcome #1
4. *Answer:* A
   Rationale: In most cases, kidneys retain sodium; infrequently, sodium wasting can occur.
   Level: Knowledge
   Refer to Learning Outcome #2
5. *Answer:* C
   Rationale: Large amounts of drainage are expected for days and weeks.
   Refer to Learning Outcome #5
6. *Answer:* A
   Rationale: Cola contains a high oxalate concentration and should be avoided when oxalate stones are produced by the body.
   Level: Knowledge
   Refer to Learning Outcome #5

Critical Thinking Exercises

Scenario A

Answers:

1. Restriction, to slow progression of renal failure, to prevent catabolism.
2. Decrease, to prevent retention of fluid by the kidney.
3. Restriction, to prevent osteodystrophy.
4. Restriction, to prevent hyperkalemia.
5. Restriction, to avoid increased levels.
6. Restriction, to prevent osteodystrophy.
7. Restriction, to prevent fluid overload.

Scenario B

Answer:

Glomeruli filter blood
↓
Complexes become trapped in glomeruli
↓
Inflammation/infection occurs
↓
Decreased glomerular function/selective permeability results
↓
Signs and symptoms

Chapter 32, Assessment of Clients with Gastrointestinal Disorders

Study Questions

1. *Answer:* C
   Rationale: In the elderly, the secretion of hydrochloric acid, digestive enzymes, and bile decrease. Bacterial growth in the gut can increase.
   Level: Comprehension
   Refer to Learning Outcome #1
2. *Answer:* D
   Rationale: The esophagus is located posterior to the trachea and larynx. Answers A and B refer to the location of the stomach and the fundus of the stomach, respectively. The duodenum of the small intestine begins at the pyloric valve and extends to the jejunum.
   Level: Knowledge
   Refer to Learning Outcome #1
3. *Answer:* D
   Rationale: The end products of digestion are absorbed in the small intestine. In the mouth, chewing begins digestion. The esophagus serves as a passage for food from mouth to stomach. The stomach liquefies the bolus of food into chyme and controls its passage into the duodenum.
   Level: Knowledge
   Refer to Learning Outcome #1
4. *Answer:* A
   Rationale: Although (B), (C), and (D) are true regarding the elderly, a decrease in hydrochloric acid secretion causes a decrease in the absorption of iron.
   Level: Comprehension
   Refer to Learning Outcome #4
5. *Answer:* B
   Rationale: The client with an upper gastrointestinal endoscopy receives a local anesthetic on the posterior pharynx, which suppresses the gag reflex. Until this reflex returns (2–4 hours), the client can have nothing by mouth (NPO). The client will have local anesthesia and medication for sedation. The client remains NPO after midnight before the test. Bleeding and fever may indicate the complication of perforation.
   Level: Application
   Refer to Learning Outcome #5

Critical Thinking Exercises

Scenario A

1. The components of the health history that contribute to identifying the diagnosis include demographic data such

as age, gender, and religion, as well as personal and family history, diet history, specific questions about the chief complaint, medical history, and psychosocial history and life-style.

2. Pertinent subjective data include information about the client's complaint of epigastric pain. These include onset, duration, quality and characteristics, severity, location, precipitating factors, relieving factors, and any associated symptoms.

3. The nurse should explain to the client why the test is used and what problems it can detect. The nurse must instruct the client about pretest preparation, the procedure itself, and follow-up care.

Scenario B

1. Data include condition of the mouth, teeth, gums, dentures, and chewing and swallowing. A diet history, including food and fluid intake, is essential. The nurse must assess the client's exercise habits. Does the client chronically use laxatives?

2. Changes such as loose teeth and decreased output of salivary glands can occur in the mouth. In the large intestine, peristalsis decreases and nerve impulses are dulled. There is decreased muscle tone in the abdominal wall.

3. Dietary changes to assist the client in managing constipation include instituting a high-residue diet by adding 2 g bran to the daily intake; decreasing the use of soft, processed foods that are low in fiber; and increasing fluid intake to six to eight glasses per day, if not contraindicated.

Chapter 33, Nursing Care of Clients with Ingestive Disorders

Study Questions

1. *Answer:* B
Rationale: The nature of the surgery mandates that respiratory care is a priority; thus, respiratory assessment is very important.
Level: Application
Refer to Learning Outcome #1

2. *Answer:* D
Rationale: Liquid or pureed foods may decrease the discomfort of eating. Hot liquids, citrus juices, and alcohol will increase the discomfort of drinking and should be avoided until the lesions heal.
Level: Comprehension
Refer to Learning Outcome #5

3. *Answer:* B
Rationale: Pain medication will be ordered postoperatively and should be administered before meals to facilitate eating. Temporary tracheostomies may be performed intraoperatively in cases of extensive resections. They remain in place until the edema subsides and then are removed. Oral hygiene should be performed every 4 hours with one-half strength hydrogen peroxide and saline. With extensive resections, care must be taken to protect the suture line from trauma. The client will be out of bed on the first postoperative day to prevent the complications of immobility.
Level: Comprehension
Refer to Learning Outcome #3

4. *Answer:* C
Rationale: Antacids interfere with absorption of H_2 receptor antagonists such as ranitidine. Taking the medications at the same time or 30 minutes apart would not allow adequate time for absorption. Taking the medications on alternate days would not contribute to the therapeutic plan.
Level: Application
Refer to Learning Outcome #3

5. *Answer:* A
Rationale: Nicotine increases the occurrence of reflux. Answers (B), (C), and (D) would not affect the lower esophageal sphincter.
Level: Application
Refer to Learning Outcome #5

Critical Thinking Exercises

Scenario A

1. The client should avoid heavy lifting, climbing stairs, and straining. She should avoid lying flat in bed by elevating the head of the bed on blocks.

2. She should be taught the mechanism of action for each medication. In addition, the nurse should review dosage and frequency. Antacids are taken 1 hour before meals and 2 hours after meals. Ranitidine may be taken with meals and at bedtime. They should not be taken simultaneously because antacids will decrease absorption of ranitidine.

3. The client should restrict foods and fluid close to bedtime. She should eat several small meals throughout the day rather than three large meals and avoid foods that might cause symptoms of reflux to recur, such as coffee, spicy foods, alcohol, and citrus juices. The client should follow a nutritionally sound diet with a reduction in calories, which will aid in weight loss.

Scenario B

1. Etiologic factors include increased incidence in males, blacks, Chinese, and Japanese; nutritional deficiencies in fruits and vegetables; contaminants in the soil and food; heavy smoking; habitual alcohol intake; and other esophageal problems.

2. Modifications include discontinuing use of alcohol and tobacco and improving oral hygiene and nutritional intake. Seeking care and treatment of other esophageal diseases will reduce the risk of esophageal cancer.

3. An early symptom of the disease is dysphagia, or difficulty swallowing. Initially, this is mild but slowly progresses until signs of esophageal obstruction are noticed.

Chapter 34, Nursing Care of Clients with Gastric Disorders

Study Questions

1. *Answer:* B
Rationale: Peptic ulcer disease may cause gastrointestinal bleeding, often manifested by melena and hematemesis. Increases in gastric acid secretion cause epigastric pain.
Level: Application
Refer to Learning Outcome #1

2. *Answer:* D
Rationale: The client must remain upright after a bolus tube feeding to prevent reflux and aspiration of the feeding, which could lead to ineffective gas exchange. It is important to check tube patency and placement before initiating the feeding.
Level: Application
Refer to Learning Outcome #5

3. *Answer:* A
Rationale: The client with acute gastritis should avoid spicy foods, caffeine, and large, heavy meals. A simple diet is usually well tolerated in acute gastritis until the client slowly returns to a normal diet.
Level: Comprehension
Refer to Learning Outcome #4

4. *Answer:* C
Rationale: H_2-receptor antagonists and anticholinergics cause a reduction in acid secretions. Mucosal barrier protectors form complexes with proteins at the base of a peptic ulcer that prevent digestive action of acid and pepsin.
Level: Knowledge
Refer to Learning Outcome #4

5. *Answer:* D
Rationale: When perforation occurs, clients experience sharp, severe pain

in the midepigastrium. When peritonitis develops, pain spreads over the entire abdomen.
Level: Comprehension
Refer to Learning Outcome #2

Critical Thinking Exercises

Scenario A

1. The nurse must assess for a history of smoking; use of steroids, aspirin, caffeine, and alcohol; and stress.
2. Antacids neutralize gastric acid and increase gastric pH. They should be taken 1 to 2 hours after meals. Some side effects may include constipation, diarrhea, anorexia, and electrolyte imbalances.
3. The client with a duodenal ulcer should be advised to avoid spicy foods, alcohol, milk, and caffeine. Other foods that cause discomfort should be avoided.
4. The following complications can occur with duodenal ulcer: hemorrhage, which usually manifests as melena; perforation, which causes severe epigastric pain; and obstruction, manifested by pain at night and vomiting.

Scenario B

1. The nurse should teach the daughter to flush the tube with water after each feeding.
2. She should observe for cramping, nausea, diarrhea, and tube displacement. Tube displacement could lead to aspiration of feedings.
3. The daughter should check for tube placement by aspirating gastric contents or by listening over the stomach while injecting air from a syringe.

Chapter 35, Nursing Care of Clients with Intestinal Disorders

Study Questions

1. *Answer:* A
   Rationale: Appendicitis may occur in any age group but reaches a peak between the ages of 20 and 30 years. It is uncommon in children younger than 2 years and in older adults.
   Level: Comprehension
   Refer to Learning Outcome #2
2. *Answer:* C
   Rationale: Abdominal pain and rebound tenderness in the presence of fever are indicative of peritonitis. Nausea, vomiting, and diarrhea may be associated with the condition resulting in peritonitis or may occur during the treatment for peritonitis.
   Level: Knowledge
   Refer to Learning Outcome #1
3. *Answer:* B
   Rationale: The mucosa of the small intestine becomes thickened and has an erythematous, cobblestone-like appearance. Clients with Crohn's disease often have bloody diarrhea leading to perianal ulceration. The malabsorption associated with Crohn's often leads to malnutrition.
   Level: Knowledge
   Refer to Learning Outcome #2
4. *Answer:* C
   Rationale: By maintaining a high-fiber diet, clients at risk for diverticular disease avoid constipation. Low-residue diets and decreased fluid intake contribute to constipation. Daily laxative use may lead to laxative abuse and fluid and electrolyte imbalances.
   Level: Application
   Refer to Learning Outcome #4
5. *Answer:* D
   Rationale: A reducible hernia sac can be replaced into the abdominal cavity by manipulation whereas an incarcerated hernia cannot. An incarcerated hernia becomes a surgical emergency if it becomes strangulated.
   Level: Knowledge
   Refer to Learning Outcome #2

Critical Thinking Exercises

Scenario A

1. Factors influencing nutritional status include a reduced absorptive surface in the intestines; impaired absorption of fat, fat-soluble vitamins, vitamin B_{12}, and minerals; and some medications.
2. Because metabolic requirements increase and food moves more rapidly through the gastrointestinal tract, clients should maintain a high-calorie, high-protein diet. Vitamin and mineral deficiencies should be corrected with dietary intake.
3. Foods that are chemically or mechanically irritating such as cola, chocolate, nuts, popcorn, citrus juices, and alcohol should be avoided. Foods should be bland and easily digested to promote absorption.

Scenario B

1. These clients should avoid those foods that cause gas, such as nuts, cabbage, corn, and legumes. Drinking carbonated beverages may also cause flatus.
2. Interventions include cleansing the skin around the stoma and changing the pouch every 4 to 5 days. When leakage occurs, the pouch should be changed.
3. A healthy stoma is red and slightly raised, and the surrounding skin is clean without redness or irritation.

Chapter 36, Assessment of Clients with Hepatic, Biliary, and Exocrine Pancreatic Disorders

Study Questions

1. *Answer:* C
   Rationale: Although carbohydrate and fat metabolism are important, human survival depends on the liver's role in protein metabolism.
   Level: Knowledge
   Refer to Learning Outcome #1
2. *Answer:* A
   Rationale: Abnormal function and location of the diseased organ affects the client's breathing.
   Level: Comprehension
   Refer to Learning Outcome #2
3. *Answer:* D
   Rationale: The enzymes that digest fats, proteins, and carbohydrates are secreted by the pancreas; any process that interferes with enzyme secretion has an impact on the client's response to disease.
   Level: Application
   Refer to Learning Outcome #3
4. *Answer:* B
   Rationale: The presence of fat in the duodenum is the signal for the release of bile from the gallbladder.
   Level: Application
   Refer to Learning Outcome #3
5. *Answer:* B
   Rationale: Since the liver is highly vascular, hemorrhage is a risk factor to consider following a percutaneous liver biopsy.
   Level: Application
   Refer to Learning Outcome #4

Critical Thinking Exercises

Scenario A

1. General assessments should be completed according to the agency's protocol. In addition, the main focus of assessment should be on the gastrointestinal, neurologic, genitourinary, integumentary, and cardiovascular functioning.
2. Family history should be explored for members who have had cancer, jaundice, hepatitis, alcoholism, obesity, or gallbladder problems.
3. The nurse should inspect the abdomen for distention and tight, glisten-

ing skin. The presence of bulging flanks and prominent abdominal veins should also be noted.

4. The client should be taught that failure of the dye to pass through the bile ducts indicates the presence of a duct obstruction.

Scenario B

1. A closed biopsy is more simple than an open biopsy. A needle is inserted into the liver and a sample of tissue is removed and sent to the laboratory so that cells can be studied for abnormalities. The client should be taught the importance of remaining still during the procedure because movement may cause the surgeon to accidentally puncture an organ. The client should be informed of monitoring and rationales for postprocedural care (such as vital sign measurements, activity, and the possibility of pain).

2. The greatest risks arise from hemorrhage and/or puncture of adjacent organs or body structures. Hemorrhage may occur during the first 24 hours, thus it is important to gain the client's confidence in the need for bed rest for 24 hours after completion of the procedure. The client should be informed by the physician of the risks. The nurse should observe for any bleeding and change in baseline vital signs.

Chapter 37, Nursing Care of Clients with Hepatic Disorders

Study Questions

1. *Answer:* B
   Rationale: Hepatic jaundice is caused by a defect in the uptake, conjugation, or transport of bilirubin within the liver, causing clay-colored stools and tea-colored urine. A strong odor to the breath is associated with cirrhosis.
   Level: Comprehension
   Refer to Learning Outcome #1

2. *Answer:* A
   Rationale: Hepatitis A is transmitted via the oral-fecal route and contaminated shellfish. Hepatitis B virus is transmitted through sexual contact; hepatitis C virus is transmitted through blood and body fluid contact; delta hepatitis virus is transmitted as a result of coinfection with hepatitis B.
   Level: Knowledge
   Refer to Learning Outcome #2

3. *Answer:* D
   Rationale: Because the client has cardiac cirrhosis and is on restricted fluid, fluids high in sodium should be restricted. (A), (B), and (C) are all fluids that are high in sodium.
   Level: Analysis
   Refer to Learning Outcome #3

4. *Answer:* D
   Rationale: Because the hepatitis is of unknown cause, all of these questions should help to pinpoint specific causes.
   Level: Application
   Refer to Learning Outcome #4

5. *Answer:* C
   Rationale: Infections can be a serious complication after a liver transplant. The client should be able to state why *all* of his medications are important (A). A high-protein diet is not necessary (B). The client should resume exercise slowly and carefully (D).
   Level: Analysis
   Refer to Learning Outcome #6

Critical Thinking Exercises

Scenario A

1. The nurse should encourage a diet high in protein (75–100 g), carbohydrate (300–400 g), and moderate fat (60–100 g).

2. The husband should be instructed to prepare small, frequent meals and plan for a protein-rich breakfast because breakfast is usually the best tolerated meal. He should be encouraged to give his wife choices and to use preprepared meals with caution because of high fat and sodium content.

3. The husband should be taught that while his wife is recovering, she needs a well-balanced diet so that her liver may recover. His wife will probably lose weight from a lack of appetite and sudden weight loss could increase the stress in her biliary system.

4. A diabetic diet is restricted in fats and carbohydrates as well as proteins. Collaboration with a dietitian is necessary, but nursing measures that emphasize prevention of nausea and emotional support are critical to ensure the ingestion of a diet.

Scenario B

1. Vasopressin is used to treat massive gastrointestinal bleeding. It is classified as a pituitary hormone. Propranolol (Inderal), the other agent that is used to decrease gastric bleeding, is classified as a beta-blocker. Vasopressin causes constriction and spasms of the coronary arteries, which require nitroglycerin to prevent these side effects.

2. For the client taking propranolol, the nurse should assess pulse strength, quality and rate of pulse, blood pressure, and electrocardiogram. Bradycardia is a serious side effect of propranolol. For the client taking vasopressin, the nurse should assess pulse, blood pressure, and the electrocardiogram. Cardiac arrest is a life-threatening side effect for the client taking vasopressin. Both of these medications require more extensive monitoring that would also include the client's alertness and orientation, intake and output, and weight. **Neither drug should be withdrawn suddenly.**

3. Because anxiety increases the stress response, it is imperative that the client be as calm as possible. Adding medication to decrease anxiety places added stress on the liver. Nursing procedures should be organized so that constant interruptions are avoided. Simple directions and constant, appropriate reassurance should be given.

Chapter 38, Nursing Care of Clients with Biliary and Exocrine Pancreatic Disorders

Study Questions

1. *Answer:* B
   Rationale: The suffix "-ostomy" indicates an opening; thus, choledochostomy is an opening or exploration of the common bile duct.
   Level: Knowledge
   Refer to Learning Outcome #1

2. *Answer:* D
   Rationale: The client with acute cholecystitis is usually hospitalized, and initially antibiotics effective against organisms found in the bile are administered.
   Level: Application
   Refer to Learning Outcome #2

3. *Answer:* A
   Rationale: All other choices contain some form of fat.
   Level: Comprehension
   Refer to Learning Outcome #3

4. *Answer:* D
   Rationale: A low-fat dietary intake is encouraged following a cholecystectomy. Neither bleeding tendencies nor abdominal cramping occur as a result of a cholecystectomy. A T-tube is inserted to help drain bile postoperatively.
   Level: Application
   Refer to Learning Outcome #4

5. *Answer:* A
   Rationale: Although the serum amylase study is most widely used, a serum lipase study is the most accurate indica-

tor of pancreatitis. A creatinine clearance study and complete blood count are not ordered to rule out pancreatitis.
Level: Knowledge
Refer to Learning Outcome #2

6. *Answer:* A
Rationale: (A) is the only true statement. The presence of nasogastric suction does not relieve thirst; the client would not be kept NPO strictly for purposes of enzyme replacement; and permitting any ice chips and other food or fluid will increase the client's pain.
Level: Application
Refer to Learning Outcome #6

7. *Answer:* B
Rationale: Diabetes is a complication of pancreatitis, thus the client and significant others must be taught the signs and symptoms and blood glucose monitoring of diabetes.
Level: Analysis
Refer to Learning Outcome #5

8. *Answer:* B
Rationale: The ingestion of alcohol will precipitate a recurrence of pancreatitis. The client should resume a normal diet once he or she is no longer on NPO status. Infection of another body organ may or may not cause illness associated with the pancreas.
Level: Analysis
Refer to Learning Outcome #8

Critical Thinking Exercises

Scenario A

1. The nurse should elicit support from the family by teaching about the need for healthy living by planning for and eating low-fat meals and increasing exercise so that a healthy weight is maintained. The nurse should teach the client to get the family more involved in the planning, shopping, and preparation of food; teach about the benefits for everyone from exercise like walking or swimming; and teach about psychologic support and how a healthy life-style will benefit each member of the family.

2. The nurse should interview the client for information about the family's dietary and food shopping habits. The dietitian should be consulted to explain alternatives to use in planning the family meals and keeping within a budget. The nurse can use the hospital menus as a means of demonstrating how to choose low-fat items for the family. The food advertisement section of the newspaper can be used to help show how planning will help the family save money as well as calories.

3. The client and family should be taught about care of the wound site and dressing changes, if indicated. The dressing change can be demonstrated to the husband and older children to include them in the provision of care. The level of activity should be discussed according to the surgeon's instructions for the client. The control of pain should also be discussed. The client needs teaching about signs and symptoms of infection and to whom problems with the wound, continued pain, possible infection, and eating should be reported. The information about dietary teaching should be reinforced with the client and family members.

Scenario B

1. The client can expect recurrent bouts of pancreatitis, the possibility of surgery for removal of the pancreas, the replacement of pancreatic enzymes, damage to surrounding body organs, and development of diabetes.

2. The family should be included in the teaching about the disease. The nurse should assess family members for their reaction to the illness and its implications and explain the need for psychological support. The client needs frequent positive reinforcement, to be able to attend Alcoholics Anonymous for peer support, support during times of regression, and encouragement to replace the drinking behavior with a positive satisfying behavior (such as playing with the grandchildren, chewing gum, taking up a new hobby, etc.)

3. The client should be taught about the destruction of the pancreatic tissue by the enzymes that it secretes. Pancreatic enzyme replacement results in increased digestion of fats, carbohydrates, and proteins in the digestive tract. Generally, a high-calorie, high-protein, and low-fat diet should be followed. The dose of the enzyme replacement may be adjusted for fat content in the diet.

4. Reteaching about the pathophysiology of the disease needs to occur. The nurse should explain how the pancreatic tissue destroys itself and will not regenerate. Use a drawing to make the explanation more vivid; many individuals are aware that the pancreas has some relationship to diabetes. The teaching about the occurrence of diabetes should be reinforced.

5. The client should be taught about pain control and the need to report comfort levels to the physician. When pain cannot be controlled, surgery may be indicated. Teaching about enzyme replacement should occur (see #3 above). The client and family should be taught about glucose monitoring and how to observe for the signs and symptoms of diabetes. The client and family will need further teaching about care if diabetes is diagnosed.

Chapter 39, Assessment of Clients with Metabolic Disorders

Study Questions

1. *Answer:* D
Rationale: Cortisol causes sodium retention and potassium excretion. Excessive glucocorticoid secretion results in hypervolemia and hypertension due to sodium and water retention.
Level: Comprehension
Refer to Learning Outcome #2

2. *Answer:* A
Rationale: The hormones that regulate carbohydrate metabolism include insulin, glucagon, adrenocorticotropic hormone (ACTH), corticosteroids, epinephrine, and thyroid hormone. The mineralocorticoids, primarily aldosterone, regulate electrolyte balance by promoting sodium retention and potassium excretion.
Level: Knowledge
Refer to Learning Outcome #2

3. *Answer:* B
Rationale: Exophthalmos (bulging eyes) is an important characteristic of hyperthyroidism. It is a manifestation of Graves' disease (hyperthyroidism) and is due to the accumulation of fluid in the fat pads and muscles that lie behind the eyeballs.
Level: Comprehension
Refer to Learning Outcome #1

4. *Answer:* C
Rationale: Drugs and foods that are high in iodine may interfere with the test by lowering uptake (see Fischbach, F. [1992]. *A Manual of Laboratory & Diagnostic Tests* [4th ed.; p. 616]. Philadelphia: J.B. Lippincott).
Level: Evaluation
Refer to Learning Outcome #3

5. *Answer:* A
Rationale: Insufficient antidiuretic hormone (ADH) from the pituitary gland can cause dehydration. When ADH is absent, large amounts of diluted urine are produced.
Level: Knowledge
Refer to Learning Outcome #4

Critical Thinking Exercises

Scenario A

1. This direct test of the function of the thyroid gland measures ability of the gland to concentrate and retain iodine. When radioactive iodine is administered, it is rapidly absorbed into the bloodstream. This procedure measures the rate of accumulation, incorporation, and release of iodine by the thyroid. The rate of absorption of the radioactive iodine (which is determined by an increase in radioactivity of the thyroid gland) is a measure of the ability of the thyroid gland to concentrate iodide from the plasma. The radioactive isotopes of iodine usually used are either ^{131}I or ^{123}I.
2. This procedure is indicated in the evaluation of hypothyroidism, hyperthyroidism, thyroiditis, goiter, pituitary failure, and post-treatment evaluation.
3. The patient who is a candidate for this test may have a "lumpy" or swollen neck or complain of pain in the neck, be jittery and ultrasensitive to heat, or may be sluggish and ultrasensitive to cold.
4. Factors that may interfere with the results of this test are:
   a. chemicals, drugs, and foods that interfere with the test by lowering uptake:
      1) iodized foods and iodine-containing drugs such as Lugol's solution, expectorants, saturated solutions of potassium iodide, and vitamin preparations that contain minerals
      2) radiographic contrast media such as Diodrast, Hypaque, Renografin, Lipiodal, Ethiodol, Pantopaque, Telepaque
      3) antithyroid drugs such as propylthiouracil and related compounds
      4) thyroid medications such as cytomel, desiccated thyroid, thyroxine, synthroid
      5) miscellaneous drugs: thiocyanate, nitrates, orinase, corticosteroids, para-aminosalicylic acid, isoniazid, Pentothal, adrenocorticotropic hormone, antihistamines

   b. the compounds and conditions that interfere by enhancing uptake: thyroid-stimulating hormone, pregnancy, cirrhosis, barbiturates, lithium carbonate, phenothiazines, iodine-deficient diets, renal failure. (According to Fischbach, F. [1992]. A Manual of Laboratory & Diagnostic Tests [4th ed.; pp. 616, 617]. Philadelphia: J.B. Lippincott).

Scenario B

1. Cortisol is the major glucocorticoid in humans.
2. a. Cortisol raises the blood glucose level by converting amino acids, lactate, and pyruvate to glucose in the liver.
   b. Tissue catabolism increases, and tissue wasting is the result. Amino acids are transported into the extracellular fluid and to the liver, where they are converted to glucose.
   c. Sodium retention and potassium excretion increase. Excessive glucocorticoid secretion results in hypervolemia and hypertension due to sodium and water retention.
   d. Cortisol suppresses the inflammatory response to tissue injury and the protective immune response to invasion by infectious agents.
   e. Cortisol is needed for the body to maintain balance in times of stress. Insufficient cortisol decreases resistance to stress. Such individuals can die in shock following relatively minor trauma unless they quickly receive an injection of glucocorticoid.
3. All clients should be monitored for signs and symptoms of hyperglycemia and glycosuria, to identify those at risk for steroid-induced diabetes and exacerbation of diabetes mellitus symptoms. Persistant hyperglycemia should be reported, since supplemental or increased doses of hypoglycemic drugs may be needed to restore normal carbohydrate metabolism during glucocorticoid therapy in diabetic clients.
4. Clients should be monitored for antianabolic effects and instructed to report muscle weakness. It is important to instruct clients to report slow wound healing and to make them aware that routine skeletal x-rays should be taken during prolonged therapy to assess for osteoporosis. The nurse should inform postmenopausal women (and others at risk for skeletal wasting) of their risk status during the course of glucocorticoid therapy. Advise clients to report symptomatic back or chest pain and to sleep on a firm mattress. Instruct clients to eat a high-protein diet and to take calcium and vitamin D supplements to antagonize the bone wasting effects of cortisol.
5. Glucocorticoid therapy with any agent that is given more than a few times for systemic effects poses the risk of adrenal suppression when drug treatment is stopped. For this reason, it is necessary to discontinue steroid therapy gradually, with slow daily dosage reductions. If systemic therapy is to be stopped, it may be necessary to taper the dose over several weeks or months before stopping administration altogether.

Chapter 40, Nursing Care of Clients with Endocrine Disorders of the Pancreas

Study Questions

1. *Answer:* A
   Rationale: In mild hypoglycemia, as the blood glucose level falls, the sympathetic nervous system is stimulated. The surge of adrenalin causes symptoms such as sweating, tremor, tachycardia, palpitation, nervousness, and hunger.
   Level: Knowledge
   Refer to Learning Outcome #1
2. *Answer:* C
   Rationale: Once diabetes develops, eating too much sugar can cause the glucose level to rise. However, the reason that diabetes develops initially is that there is a decrease in the amount of insulin in the body or a decrease in the ability of insulin to control the blood glucose level. These problems are *not* caused by eating too much sugar.
   Level: Knowledge
   Refer to Learning Outcome #2
3. *Answer:* B
   Rationale: The onset of intermediate-acting insulin is 3 to 4 hours; peak is 8 to 16 hours; and duration is 20 to 24 hours. It is important for the client to have eaten some food around the time of the onset and peak of the action of these insulins. The fruit sugar in juice contains enough simple carbohydrates to sufficiently raise the blood glucose level.
   Level: Comprehension
   Refer to Learning Outcome #5
4. *Answer:* D
   Rationale: The American Diabetes Association Exchange Diet lists each exchange with an overall heading of the grams of carbohydrates, protein, and fat and the number of calories. For example, List 1 Milk Exchanges: one exchange of milk contains 12 grams of carbohydrate, 8 grams of protein, a trace of fat, and 80 calories.
   Level: Knowledge
   Refer to Learning Outcome #4
5. *Answer:* C
   Rationale: Carbohydrate replacement: a fruit exchange is equal to approxi-

mately 15 g of carbohydrate, e.g., $\frac{1}{2}$ banana, 15 grapes, $\frac{1}{3}$ cup pineapple, etc.
Level: Application
Refer to Learning Outcome #4

6. *Answer:* D
Rationale: Three diabetic complications contribute to the increased risk of foot infections: neuropathy, peripheral vascular disease, and immunocompromise. The typical sequence of events in the development of a diabetic foot ulcer begins with a soft-tissue injury of the foot. Clients should be taught to wear well-fitting, closed-toe shoes.
Level: Application
Refer to Learning Outcome #6

Critical Thinking Exercises

Scenario A

1. Short-acting and intermediate-acting insulins are used together because their onset, peak, and duration of action differ. Short-acting insulins begin to act in 30 minutes to 1 hour, peak in 2 to 4 hours, and have a duration of 6 to 8 hours. Intermediate-acting insulins begin to act in 1 to 2 hours, peak in 6 to 12 hours, and have a duration of 18 to 26 hours. The split-dose regimen is used to mimic the normal pancreas. Semilente and Lente may be mixed. When regular insulin is mixed with Lente or Ultralente, the zinc in the intermediate and long acting insulin can cause prolonged actions of the regular insulin.
2. The bottle of insulin being used should be stored at room temperature, not to exceed 80 degrees. Extra bottles should be kept refrigerated, but not frozen. Insulin may be kept at room temperature for 1 month. If it is not used within 1 month, it should be refrigerated. Clients should be instructed never to leave their insulin in a car or in the baggage compartment of an airplane because of possible temperature alterations.
Insulin injections are administered into subcutaneous tissue.
a. Properly mix the two insulins into one syringe
b. Cleanse the injection site with alcohol
c. Stabilize the skin: compress or bunch
d. Insert the needle at a 90-degree angle and inject the insulin
e. Withdraw the needle and press over the site for several seconds
f. Dispose of needle and syringe into an appropriate container
3. Snacks are placed in relation to the peak time of the insulins being given. For example, if a client is receiving an intermediate-acting insulin at 8:00 AM and the peak action is in 6 to 8 hours, it would be appropriate to advise the client to have the snack somewhere in the late afternoon (3:00 to 4:00 PM). Snacks usually are best when they contain both protein and carbohydrate to slow down their absorption and lower the glycemic response. Appropriate snacks may include, but are not limited to, half a turkey sandwich, cheese and crackers, or graham crackers and milk. Because this client is a business executive who commutes, he would want to carry nonperishable snacks that do not need to be refrigerated, such as prepackaged cheese and crackers.

Scenario B

1. The nurse should tell the client never to omit her insulin. Infection is a stressor that causes a release of epinephrine, which causes glycogen to be converted to glucose which will raise her blood sugar.
2. The nurse should tell the client to take liquids every hour. Tell her to keep a record of all food and fluid taken and retained and to report this information to the physician. The client should be advised to take liquids or semi-liquids such as broth, gingerale, eggnog, or sherbet. If she is still unable to eat after replacing 4 to 5 meals with liquids or semi-liquids, she should call her physician.
3. The nurse should advise the client to go to bed and keep warm. Because she lives alone, she should call a family member or a friend to come over and stay with her. She should also test her blood glucose and urine ketones every 3 to 4 hours.

Chapter 41, Nursing Care of Clients with Thyroid or Parathyroid Disorders

Study Questions

1. *Answer:* D
Rationale: Thyrocalcitonin is the noniodinated hormone. T_3 and T_4 depend on the presence of both iodine and the amino acid tyrosine for their synthesis.
Level: Knowledge
Refer to Learning Outcome #2
2. *Answer:* A
Rationale: Constipation and fecal impaction due to slow peristaltic action and lack of normal physical activity constitute serious problems. The other three symptoms are characteristic of hyperthyroidism and reflect the increased metabolic rate caused by excess secretion of thyroid hormone.
Level: Comprehension
Refer to Learning Outcome #2
3. *Answer:* B
Rationale: Hyperthyroidism is predominantly a disorder of women, especially young women between the ages of 20 and 40 years of age.
Level: Knowledge
Refer to Learning Outcome #3
4. *Answer:* C
Rationale: The presence of Trousseau's sign (i.e. carpal spasms of the fingers and hand after application of a blood pressure cuff to the arm) may be indicative of hypoparathyroidism and may be a signal of an impending attack of tetany. The symptoms are caused by low serum calcium levels and elevation of serum phosphate levels secondary to deficient parathormone secretion.
Level: Comprehension
Refer to Learning Outcome #4
5. *Answer:* C
Rationale: Synthroid is a thyroid hormone supplied exogenously for the treatment of hypothyroidism.
Level: Knowledge
Refer to Learning Outcome #6
6. *Answer:* B
Rationale: Aspirin should not be given to clients in thyroid crisis, as it has a synergistic effect with thyronine. Aspirin displaces T_3 and T_4 from the thyroxine binding globulin, leading to an increased amount of free thyroid hormones in the blood stream.
Level: Application
Refer to Learning Outcome #6

Critical Thinking Exercises

Scenario A

1. Major side effects of Synthroid include but are not limited to the following:
   - CNS: anxiety, insomnia, tremors, irritability
   - CV: tachycardia, palpitations, angina, arrhythmias
   - GI: nausea, diarrhea
   - GYN: menstrual irregularities
   - DERM: sweating, heat intolerance
   - MISC: weight loss
2. Therapeutic response is evaluated on the absence of depression, increased weight loss, diuresis, vital signs within normal limits, absence of constipation, increased appetite, warm, moist skin, decreased lethargy, and increased sense of well-being.

3. General information that the nurse should give to the client and significant others includes but is not limited to:
   - inform the physician immediately of any palpitations or chest pain
   - report to the physician excitability or irritability, diarrhea, heat intolerance, or a weight loss of more than 2 pounds per week, which may mean that the dose of medication is too high
   - do not switch brands of thyroid replacement hormone or go from a generic brand to a name brand and vice versa without first consulting the physician
   - read labels of over-the-counter medications and check with nurse or physician before taking them
   - avoid iodine-containing foods such as iodized salt, turnips, and seafood
   - do not stop taking the medication without first consulting with the physician
   - take pulse before medication, at least initially; notify the physician if heart rate is greater than 100 beats per minute.

Scenario B

1. Preoperative preparation for the client undergoing a subtotal thyroidectomy may include:
   a. The use of antithyroid medications. The thioamides (propylthiouracil/Propacil and methimazole/Tapazole) may be used to block the production of thyroid hormone by blocking the utilization of iodine. These medications may be used in conjunction with the iodines (Lugol's solution and potassium iodide) which interfere with proteolysis of thyroglobulin and thus block the release of thyroid hormones. Iodines also cause the thyroid gland to involute and become less vascular, which diminishes the chance of hemorrhage. Thyroid hormones (e.g. Synthroid, Proloid) may be given with antithyroid medications in an attempt to put the thyroid gland at rest by providing an exogenous source of thyroid hormones. The goal is to have the gland in a euthyroid state.
   b. The client should eat a well-balanced, high-calorie diet. The calories should total between 4000 and 5000 per day. The client may need six full meals a day plus snacks to obtain adequate calories. Foods that increase peristalsis and may lead to diarrhea, such as bulky, fibrous, or highly seasoned foods, should be discouraged. Supplemental vitamins and minerals may be needed. The goal is to have the client at optimal weight before surgery.
   c. The client needs to be adequately rested before surgery. Nursing interventions to accomplish this goal are as many and varied as the clients themselves. Suggestions to aid the client to rest or relax include: promoting continuation of usual practices related to rest and sleep unless contraindicated, decrease the environmental stimuli, administer frequent backrubs, approach the client calmly and unhurredly, encourage quiet diversions (e.g., soft music), encourage frequent short walks during the day, encourage maintenance of usual bedtime rituals, administer sedatives as needed, eliminate caffeine (e.g., coffee, tea, cola, chocolate) from the diet; assigning a consistent staff member may be beneficial.

2. Possible postoperative complications that the nurse should be aware of are:
   a. respiratory obstruction: due to edema or bleeding at the operative site. The client should be placed in semi-Fowler's position and an endotracheal or tracheostomy tube, oxygen, and suctioning should be available at the bedside.
   b. hemorrhage: the nurse should check for bleeding especially behind the neck, as the blood will drain downward. The dressing may be dry, so be sure to gently place your hand behind the client's neck to check for blood there. Vital signs also need to be closely monitored. Characteristic signs of hemorrhage include a drop in blood pressure and an elevation in pulse. Remember that restlessness is an early sign of hemorrhage.
   c. vocal cord paralysis: the laryngeal nerve lies behind the thyroid next to the trachea and may become damaged during surgery. Check the client's voice and report any hoarseness to the physician.
   d. hypoparathyroidism (tetany): due to inadvertent removal of the parathyroid glands during surgery. Be aware of symptoms of tetany due to decreasing calcium levels. Intravenous calcium gluconate should be available.
   e. permanent hypothyroidism: if the remaining portion of thyroid gland does not hypertrophy and the client is left deficient in thyroid hormone. The client will have to be on life-long thyroid replacement therapy.

3. Many clients are discharged after a short hospital stay.
   a. Sutures are usually removed on the third to fourth hospital day and the client is instructed to inspect the area for any signs of redness, tenderness or drainage. Should any of these signs appear, the client should call his or her physician. Once the incision line has healed, lanolin may help to lessen the scar and keep the area soft.
   b. The client should be instructed that the rest, relaxation, and well-balanced diet begun preoperatively need to be continued into the postoperative period.
   c. Before the client leaves the hospital, written instructions will be given as to follow-up visits to the physician or clinic. The client should be encouraged to keep the appointments.
   d. It is expected that the client will be able to resume all presurgical activities once the suture line has healed and he or she has recovered from the surgery.

Chapter 42, Nursing Care of Clients with Adrenal, Pituitary, and Gonadal Disorders

Study Questions

1. *Answer:* C
   Rationale: Aldosterone is a mineralocorticoid secreted by the adrenal cortex. It functions in the regulation of sodium, chloride, and potassium. If too much aldosterone is secreted, sodium will be retained and potassium excreted.
   Level: Knowledge
   Refer to Learning Outcome #1
2. *Answer:* B
   Rationale: Clients with Addison's disease have decreased amounts of aldosterone, leading to sodium excretion and potassium retention. All of the answers with the exception of (B) relate to this sodium-potassium imbalance.
   Level: Comprehension
   Refer to Learning Outcome #1
3. *Answer:* D
   Rationale: One of the major risk factors for increased levels of cortisol is the administration of exogenous steroids. Whenever steroids are administered, a degree of excess is present. It is wise to place the client on the lowest amount of steroids possible to control the problem.

Level: Comprehension
Refer to Learning Outcome #2

4. *Answer:* A
Rationale: Aldosterone is the most powerful mineralocorticoid. Its primary role is to conserve sodium. It also promotes potassium excretion. Diagnosis of primary hyperaldosteronism is based on low serum potassium, alkalosis, and elevated urinary or plasma aldosterone with low plasma renin levels.
Level: Comprehension
Refer to Learning Outcome #3

5. *Answer:* A
Rationale: Diabetes insipidus is a deficiency of antidiuretic hormone resulting in a physiologic imbalance of water. Assessment of the client should center on monitoring intake and output. The client should be questioned about excessive thirst or urination, and his or her fluid and electrolyte balance must be monitored closely.
Level: Application
Refer to Learning Outcome #5

Critical Thinking Exercises

Scenario A

The nurse should instruct the client to do the following:

1. Wear a Medic Alert tag or bracelet or carry an identification card stating the medication and dosage that he is on. The physician's name, address, and telephone number plus instructions for emergency treatment should be available. In case of an accident or injury, additional steroids may need to be given.
2. Carry an emergency kit that contains a prepared syringe of hydrocortisone and an alcohol swab. The nurse should ensure that another family member or significant other is able to administer the medication if necessary.
3. Advise any other health-care providers (i.e., dentist, physician, nurse practitioner, pharmacist) that a steroid is being taken on a long-term basis.
4. Maintain regular medical check-ups so that the physician can monitor the effects of the medication and detect any adverse reactions. Periodic blood tests may have to be done.
5. Take no other medications (prescribed or over-the-counter) without first consulting with the physician who prescribed the steroid. Other medications may increase or decrease the expected therapeutic effects of the steroids.
6. Check with his physician about appropriate exercises. Osteoporosis is a side effect of long-term steroid therapy. Bones under stress tend to give up less calcium.
7. Take the steroid after a meal or with milk or food, not on an empty stomach. Gastrointestinal disorders are a possible side effect of long-term steroid therapy.
8. Learn about diabetes mellitus, which can complicate the picture. (Chapter 40).
9. Recognize stress and any situations that may precipitate stress. If the client is unable to avoid stressful situations, he needs to discuss with his physician the increased amount of medication to be taken at these times. Open and honest communication between the client and physician is necessary.
10. Never decrease the dosage or stop taking this medication because this could precipitate an addisonian crisis, vasomotor collapse, and death.
11. Maintain good grooming and pride in one's appearance, which are helpful if cushingoid features develop. Counseling may be necessary to help the client cope.

Scenario B

The nurse should explain the following:

1. Hyperaldosteronism is excessive production of aldosterone by the adrenal gland. Aldosterone is the most powerful mineralocorticoid, which causes sodium to be conserved by the body and potassium to be excreted. Because the aldosterone levels are high, the client retains sodium and loses potassium through the urine. The client may experience episodes of tetany, weakness, paralysis, hypertension, cardiac irregularity, polyuria, and polydipsia.
2. Possible foods to eat and those to be avoided on a low-sodium, high-potassium diet. Foods high in sodium that should be avoided are
   - Those in which salt is used as a preservative (e.g., luncheon meat, pickles, olives, bacon, ham, hot dogs, sausage, salted or smoked fish [anchovies, caviar, herring, sardines], sauerkraut)
   - Those that are highly salted (e.g., crackers, pretzels, potato chips, corn chips, salted nuts, salted popcorn)
   - Spices and condiments (e.g., bouillon cubes, ketchup, celery salt, garlic salt, onion salt, monosodium glutamate, meat tenderizers, soy sauce)
   - Cheese, peanut butter
   - Canned vegetables or canned vegetable juices that are not salt-free
   - Vegetables with high sodium content (e.g., artichokes, beets, carrots, celery, dandelion greens, kale, spinach)
   - Regular breads, rolls, crackers
   - Dry cereals
   - Shellfish
   - Salted butter and margarine
   - Commercial salad dressings or candies

   Meat, milk, and eggs should be consumed in small portions because these are foods with higher natural sodium content. Do not cook with or add salt to the food at the table. Food sources of potassium include fruits, vegetables, legumes, nuts, whole grains, meat, and salt substitutes. The client should be advised to consult with a registered dietitian.
3. Know the signs and symptoms of fluid retention and how this may be monitored. Tell the client to weigh himself daily on the same scale at the same time and in the same amount of clothing. Weight is one of the best indicators of fluid gain or loss. Advise the client to keep a record of his intake and output. They should be equal for a 24-hour period. Tell the client to observe for puffiness around the eyes when arising in the morning or swelling of the feet, ankles or hands at the end of the day. The client may complain that shoes or rings are too tight. Advise the client to have his blood pressure taken periodically. An increase in blood pressure may signal increased water retention.
4. Know signs and symptoms of hypokalemia, including episodes of muscular weakness or paralysis, tetany, or postural hypotension. The client may also complain of tingling around the mouth or of increased urination. These symptoms should be reported to the physician.
5. Know that spironolactone (Aldactone) is warranted. Tell the client that spironolactone causes him to lose sodium but that this diuretic conserves potassium (potassium sparing). This diuretic specifically antagonizes the effects of aldosterone and is the drug of choice for hyperaldosteronism. Some of the major side effects of spironolactone are nausea, vomiting, diarrhea, anorexia, and hyperkalemia.

Chapter 43, Assessment of Clients with Musculoskeletal Disorders

Study Questions

1. *Answer:* A
   Rationale: This choice indicates that limited movement often accompanies soft-tissue injury. All other choices are not correct or are not specific to acute soft-tissue injury.
   Level: Comprehension
   Refer to Learning Outcome #1

2. *Answer:* A
   Rationale: Asymmetry is a common finding in normal people. All other choices are incorrect.
   Level: Knowledge
   Refer to Learning Outcome #3

3. *Answer:* A
   Rationale: Because of decreased muscle strength and the rigidity of cartilage, older adults' chest walls do not elongate and expand maximally. The vertebral column decreases because of bone loss (B). Muscle strength is diminished in all muscles (C). Nodules are pathologic, not a result of aging (D).
   Level: Comprehension
   Refer to Learning Outcome #2

4. *Answer:* C
   Rationale: A compression bandage and rest of the affected joint for from 8 to 24 hours is the usual procedure.
   Level: Knowledge
   Refer to Learning Outcome #4

5. *Answer:* D
   Rationale: Because of the client's history, which places her at risk for osteoporosis, anticonvulsants could increase her risk because they may cause osteomalacia.
   Level: Analysis
   Refer to Learning Outcome #1

Critical Thinking Exercises

Scenario A

Begin by modifying the environment. The temperature should be comfortably warm, the lighting should be adequate so that the client can see without glare, and all extraneous noises should be excluded. The physical examination should be modified by asking the client about his chief complaint and directing his conversation to include a typical day's activity. Remember that consonants are difficult to discern for older adults. Older adults tire easily and may be confused by long, complex questions. The nurse should focus questions on vital information and keep the questions simple. Questions should include inquiries concerning his daily habits and ingestion of over-the-counter medications.

Just as questions would be kept simple, so also should the physical examination. You should face the client, so as to see his expression. This will make it easier to give directions to the client. Consolidation of parts of the examination will help the client to expend less energy. (Do not have the client stand and walk several times. Think carefully before giving directions.) The nurse should always keep the chief complaint in mind and use subjective information to direct the physical examination, remembering that subjective data provide more than 95 per cent of the data needed to formulate diagnoses.

Scenario B

Exercise should be consistent and gradual. Sporadic exercise may cause injury to muscles and joints, resulting in spasms and strain. Warm-ups and cool-downs are very important because older muscles and joints have less elasticity. Warming up before exercise prepares muscles and joints for further stress of aerobic exercise. Cool-downs help to redirect blood back to the heart and rid the body of lactic acid. Drinking plenty of water before and during exercise increases the water content of muscles and joints. Carbohydrates before exercise provides needed calories for energy. A banana is especially helpful because it not only increases the blood sugar but provides added potassium for muscles.

Chapter 44, Common Musculoskeletal Interventions

Study Questions

1. *Answer:* D
   Rationale: A baseline neurovascular assessment is essential before the insertion of the pin. The nurse needs to know what was "normal" before insertion of the pin and application of the traction.
   Level: Knowledge
   Refer to Learning Outcome #1

2. *Answer:* C
   Rationale: After remaining relatively flat for several days and having been on an antihypertensive medication, orthostatic hypotension is a probable complication. Sitting for several minutes before ambulating will help to offset the hypotensive response and create a safer environment for ambulating.
   Level: Analysis
   Refer to Learning Outcome #3

3. *Answer:* D
   Rationale: Musty odor is a prominent sign of infection.
   Level: Comprehension
   Refer to Learning Outcome #2

4. *Answer:* C
   Rationale: Supporting the entire arm and keeping the fingers higher than the elbow will help to reduce edema. This is the first action the nurse should take, considering there are no other signs or symptoms present. If the edema does not reduce in approximately 30 minutes, a physician should be notified.
   Level: Application
   Refer to Learning Outcome #5

5. *Answer:* C
   Rationale: The walker is lifted and placed ahead of the client and the client walks up to the walker.
   Level: Comprehension
   Refer to Learning Outcome #6

6. *Answer:* C
   Rationale: Because the shoulder supports the weight of the casted arm, the shoulder may become "frozen" unless the client regularly exercises the shoulder.
   Level: Comprehension
   Refer to Learning Outcome #4

Critical Thinking Exercises

Scenario A

1. Because the client is active and is clearly unwilling to take the time to learn all of the details of her care, the nurse might try to solicit the help of her children, her husband, or significant others. The nurse would teach her along with at least one member of her family. The nurse would tell her to

   - Keep the cast dry and wrap it in plastic when bathing
   - Use no talcum powder or sharp objects in or around the cast
   - Use a damp cloth and a small amount of cleansing powder to clean the outside of the cast

   The nurse would emphasize that the client should notify her physician immediately if she experiences edema or pain or detects any unusual odors.

2. Pain on passive movement and edema are signs of compartmental syndrome. This complication, although not exceedingly common, is a possibility that could cause permanent nerve and muscle damage. Because muscle compartments are bound by dense fascial sheaths, extreme pressure can result in

massive neurovascular damage and muscle necrosis. Pressure sources can be either internal (edema or bleeding) or external (casts, dressings, or crushing weights). Individuals who have sustained fractures or extensive soft tissue injury are vulnerable. The injury is usually in the lower leg or arm because distal portions of the extremities contain more compartments than proximal portions.

Scenario B

Keeping any client as independent as possible is usually an important consideration. However, in this case, the client will have only one functional limb and will have to keep her position in bed with relatively few position changes. Skin care will become vital, especially because of the client's age. The nurse should help the client to bathe. A total bath will be unnecessary unless excessive soiling or perspiration is present. Creams that are absorbed by the skin should be applied. The bed should be kept dry and free of crumbs and wrinkles. The client should be handled gently to reduce any shearing force when her position is changed. Geriatric clients are especially vulnerable to complications of immobility. Although the answer to this question seems simple, many nurses overlook the need for very specific skin care for older adults. New research stresses the importance of such care.

Chapter 45, Nursing Care of Clients with Musculoskeletal Disorders

Study Questions

1. *Answer:* C
   Rationale: Cheese, yogurt, and acidophilus milk are processed in such a way that they are tolerated even if a person is lactose intolerant.
   Level: Knowledge
   Refer to Learning Outcome #4

2. *Answer:* D
   Rationale: From the client history, the only risk factor aside from her sex is her diet rich in protein.
   Level: Comprehension
   Refer to Learning Outcome #2

3. *Answer:* A
   Rationale: Kyphosis, back pain, bone loss in the jaw, and loss of bone in the vertebrae and bones of the pelvis, leg, and arm are manifestations of osteoporosis.
   Level: Knowledge
   Refer to Learning Outcome #1

4. *Answer:* D
   Rationale: A sedentary client should begin a program of exercise that is easy to accomplish with relatively little risk. It should be weightbearing and consistent. (A) and (B) are not weightbearing. (C) is impractical for this client and is dangerous.
   Level: Application
   Refer to Learning Outcome #3

5. *Answer:* B
   Rationale: Restlessness may be a sign of diminished oxygen that can be caused by hemorrhage or emboli as well as acid-base imbalances. (A) is a dangerous practice. The physician should **always** be consulted if additional analgesia is necessary. (C) and (D) are inappropriate and dangerous.
   Level: Analysis
   Refer to Learning Outcome #5

6. *Answer:* B
   Rationale: This practice helps to relieve pressure on the foot. (A), (C), and (D) are all unsafe practices.
   Level: Application
   Refer to Learning Outcome #6

Critical Thinking Exercises

Scenario A

1. The nurse should assess the client's learning style, review her medical therapies, and determine her major concerns and goals. She should be taught how exercise and diet are very important in decreasing bone loss. Diet should emphasize calcium-rich, low-fat, easily digestible foods. The client should be taught that any vegetables growing above the ground contain higher amounts of calcium. She must be reminded that overconsumption of alcohol, cigarettes, and coffee will increase bone loss. Exercise should be in moderation, consistent, and weightbearing. The nurse should ask the client what she likes to do. Walking is excellent. Remember to caution her about approved footwear. No matter what information is provided, it should be tailored to the client. Make certain that the client makes major decisions. The nurse must not tell her what she must do. Finally, the nurse should consider any stressors that may contribute to decreased health and further bone loss.

2. Designing a teaching plan for the daughters should, once again, consider their life-styles, learning styles, and goals. Teenagers rarely believe they are vulnerable. The teaching plan should include diet, exercise, and stress reduction; making the teaching plan fun will help to instill good health practices. Many computer programs are available on diet and exercise. Books, audiotapes, and videos are also available. However, the nurse should not recommend any of these aids unless he or she has previously reviewed them. Excellent assessment, teaching, and follow-up could make a difference in the prevention and treatment of osteoporosis.

Scenario B

First, because the client is lactose intolerant, the nurse should recommend cheese, yogurt, and acidophilus milk. The nurse should encourage her to include sources of vitamin D and recommend that she spend some time in the sunshine each day. Vitamin D and ultraviolet light are necessary for the absorption and utilization of calcium. Dietary selections should be low in fat, sugar, and spices because of the client's hiatal hernia. Also, selection should include foods that she likes and can afford. Acidophilus milk and calcium-enriched orange juice may be too expensive. To construct a well-balanced diet that considers her health and economic needs, the nurse must do his or her "homework."

Chapter 46, Nursing Care of Clients with Musculoskeletal Trauma or Overuse

Study Questions

1. *Answer:* A
   Rationale: Anesthesia or paralysis distal to the fracture (in the absence of known neurologic injury) is a sign of arterial damage. (B) and (D) would be correct if they referred to the distal rather than the proximal end of the fracture. (C) should read "poorly filled vein."
   Level: Knowledge
   Refer to Learning Outcome #1

2. *Answer:* C
   Rationale: These are classic signs of fat embolism syndrome caused by fat liberation from the fracturing of a long bone.
   Level: Analysis
   Refer to Learning Outcome #5

3. *Answer:* A
   Rationale: Extreme flexion should be avoided. All other choices are inappropriate.
   Level: Application
   Refer to Learning Outcomes #2 and #3

4. *Answer:* A
   Rationale: (A) is the preferred position for an anterior approach. (B) is appro-

priate for a posterior approach. (C) and (D) are totally inappropriate.
Level: Knowledge
Refer to Learning Outcome #4

5. *Answer:* A
Rationale: Deep vein thrombosis is a major complication that can occur after a surgical repair of an intertrochanteric femoral repair. All other choices are not possible with the remote possibility of a fat embolus.
Level: Comprehension
Refer to Learning Outcome #6

Critical Thinking Exercises

Scenario A

1. This type of injury is considered an emergency because the retinocular vessels that supply blood to the femoral head may cut off the blood supply to bone cells in the area. Also, the sciatic nerve can become contused or disrupted, causing permanent, partial or complete sensory or motor loss in the dislocated leg. Another problem would be the possible fracture of the acetabulum.
2. The nurse would expect to see pain, deformity, and asymmetry of the hip joint; restricted mobility or the inability to move; reduced sensation; and absent or diminished pulses. If the client's hip were dislocated posteriorly, the client will hold his hip in a flexed and internally rotated position. If the client's hip were dislocated anteriorly, he would keep the hip extended and externally rotated.
3. The nurse should immediately assess the color, temperature, and position of the leg. Dorsalis pedis and posterior tibial pulses should be palpated. The nurse should also check capillary refill and sensation. The client should be asked to try dorsiflexion and plantar flexion of his affected foot. The nurse should compare the findings of the affected leg with the "normal" leg.

Scenario B

1. Age is not the major deciding factor. Older adults have a slower response to stress. Physiologic reserves decrease consistently from the age of 30 years. This is especially true of the client's cardiac, pulmonary, and renal reserves. She would be more susceptible to cardiogenic shock and deep vein thrombosis.
2. First, the nurse should not assume anything. One must use knowledge of aging physiology and remember that advanced age does not mean a client will not or cannot recover.

Chapter 47, Assessment of Clients with Integumentary Disorders

Study Questions

1. *Answer:* A
Rationale: According to the definition, eccrine glands are the sweat-producing glands of the body. Apocrine glands' function is not known; sebaceous glands release sebum; there are no epocrine glands in the body.
Level: Knowledge
Refer to Learning Outcome #1
2. *Answer:* A
Rationale: Poison ivy is a result of allergic contact dermatitis. Walking through the woods would not result in poison ivy unless there was direct contact; the environment is not a causative factor, although it may be a contributing factor to poison ivy. The last question does not respond to the client's request for knowledge.
Level: Application
Refer to Learning Outcome #2
3. *Answer:* A
Rationale: The skin of the entire body can be assessed during the bed bath. Asking the client about skin condition results in subjective data only. One does not use percussion to assess the skin. Reviewing the chart and assessing under a good light are incomplete methods of assessment.
Level: Comprehension
Refer to Learning Outcome #3
4. *Answer:* B
Rationale: The removal of skin tissue causes bleeding; certain medications such as aspirin, ibuprofen, or anticoagulants may affect bleeding tendencies if the client is taking them at the time of the biopsy.
Level: Application
Refer to Learning Outcome #4

Critical Thinking Exercises

Scenario A

1. The client should be taught that the skin is the body's first line of defense against infection and that it should be smooth, without breaks in integrity.
2. Physical examination methods used are inspection, palpation, and olfaction.
3. The client should be prepared for a scraping of the lesion. He should be taught that it will be done without anesthesia and that some fine bleeding and discomfort may occur following the scraping.
4. The nurse needs to assess for use of medications such as aspirin and anticoagulants. If a history of cardiac valve replacement is discovered, antibiotics will be ordered before a biopsy is scheduled. When the biopsy is performed, dressings and ointment are applied as ordered. The client should be informed that a follow-up appointment is needed, at which the results of the diagnostic studies will be discussed.

Scenario B

1. The nurse could explain how the skin is made up of layers and show the client several thin layers of clear plastic (or similar material). The nurse could further explain that the skin protects the body from germs that cause infection and, in order to do this, must not have any scratches or sores. The clear plastic could be used to demonstrate how water and solids do not penetrate to the other side. The use of simple terms and analogies would assist the client in understanding a portion of the skin's structure and function.
2. The nurse could ask the client to wash her face and hands while observing the sequence in which the body parts are washed and how the client washes, rinses, and dries her skin. This action would provide a baseline for teaching.

Chapter 48, Nursing Care of Clients with Integumentary Disorders

Study Questions

1. *Answer:* B
Rationale: The skin of a person with atopic dermatitis is reddened from scratching.
Level: Comprehension
Refer to Learning Outcome #1
2. *Answer:* D
Rationale: Changes associated with sunburn are dermatopathologic and are cumulative over the lifespan.
Level: Knowledge
Refer to Learning Outcome #2
3. *Answer:* C
Rationale: The client is communicating that he understands the implications of complying with the recommended treatment.
Level: Application
Refer to Learning Outcome #3
4. *Answer:* B
Rationale: Anyone who has pruritus is at increased risk for infection. Self-examination of the skin is a screening measure. Although distraction and antianxiety agents may help decrease

scratching, the higher risk is the possible infection from damage to the protective function of the skin.
Level: Application
Refer to Learning Outcome #4

5. *Answer:* D
Rationale: The nurse needs to show acceptance of the client by attending to needs and communicating in an open manner.
Level: Application
Refer to Learning Outcome #5

6. *Answer:* D
Rationale: An important part of teaching includes information on assessing the skin and promptly reporting any changes noted.
Level: Application
Refer to Learning Outcome #6

Critical Thinking Exercises

Scenario A

1. The client needs to be informed about the basics of sunbathing. The information in the Client Education Guide: Simple Guidelines for Protection Against the Damaging Rays of the Sun should be adapted to the client. Important information for this client includes the appropriate time of day to sunbathe, the length of time for exposure to the sun, the use of sunscreen (even on overcast days), and the cancer risks associated with frequent and prolonged exposure to the sun. She should also be given printed information on how to protect herself from sunburn as well as how to care for the sunburn she currently has.

2. For many young people, a sunburn has connotations of the beach, vacations, good health, and beauty. A suntan is something to be admired, and a tanned person may be given status by how dark he or she is tanned. Most people in society admire those who are suntanned.
Although a person may be taught the implications of repeated exposure to the sun's rays, cultural and societal beliefs may block learning. Teaching needs to include reference to cultural and societal beliefs and how one undertakes decision-making for the actions that may result in consequences in the distant future.

3. Certain medications, such as birth control pills, may cause photosensitivity as a side effect. Photosensitivity is an abnormally heightened sensitivity to sunlight; the skin may react to sunlight more than usual when medications are being taken that produce this side effect. A medication history should be taken on all clients, who should then be instructed about this particular side effect. The client should use sunscreen, avoid prolonged exposure, and wear protective clothing.

4. The client needs to know that tanning booths can cause sunburn and premature aging. Tanning booths also increase the risk for skin cancer. It would help the client to know that each unprotected exposure to sunlight causes damage that accumulates over a lifetime.

Scenario B

1. The client's beliefs were not correct and show that he needs more instruction on the normal aging process. He incorrectly based his belief on the fact that a parent experienced the same changes.

2. People need more information on the normal changes one can expect with aging. Aging does not mean illness; it means changes in the way the body functions. Education can occur through public channels such as advertising, journal reports, and television specials as well as private channels such as church and social group sponsorship of health education for seniors.

3. If this client were a farmer, he would be at high risk for development of skin cancer. This client may have spent time playing tennis in the sun and experienced lengthy and frequent exposure to the sun's rays. One could also conclude that lack of information is also a risk factor: if he had knowledge of normal aging and how to inspect the skin and report changes, the disease may have been treated much earlier.

4. The diagnosis was determined on the basis of clinical manifestations such as induration, erythema, and erosion and results of either a shave or excisional biopsy.

5. The excision will be wide enough to remove the affected tissue as well as a small margin of unaffected tissue. If the area is too large for the edges to be sewn together, a skin graft of flaps will be used. The area may be large enough to cause disfigurement.

6. Self-image may be affected by the disfigurement caused by the surgery, especially if it occurs in a visible area, such as the face, neck, or ears. The client may need the help of significant others and a support group to learn how to accept his altered image. His reaction to future health needs depends on the type of health-care teaching he received during the course of treatment for the melanoma. He should have been taught the warning signs of cancer and instructed to report to the physician any changes in body function whether related to the skin problem or not. Life expectancy is based on the level of invasion of the lesion. If diagnosed in stages I and II, the life expectancy is 90 per cent survival; diagnosis in stage V is 30 per cent survival.

Chapter 49, Nursing Care of Clients with Burn Injury

Study Questions

1. *Answer:* A
Rationale: The age and employment of the person are risk factors for a thermal burn; the others are at risk for none (B), chemical (C), and electrical (D) burn injuries.
Level: Knowledge
Refer to Learning Outcome #1

2. *Answer:* C
Rationale: The fluid shift from intravascular to tissue causes edema during the first 12 to 24 hours (emergency phase) after the burn. Dyspnea is associated with inhalation injury, scarring occurs in the rehabilitation phase, while diaphoresis occurs 48 to 72 hours (acute phase) after burn.
Level: Comprehension
Refer to Learning Outcome #2

3. *Answer:* C
Rationale: The affected areas are composed of anterior thorax (18%), the head (9%), and the left upper extremity (9%), for a total of 36%.
Level: Knowledge
Refer to Learning Outcome #3

4. *Answer:* C
Rationale: General health at the time of the injury would reveal information relating to both severity and plan of care.
Level: Comprehension
Refer to Learning Outcome #4

5. *Answer:* A
Rationale: Cadaver skin is known as an allograft.
Level: Knowledge
Refer to Learning Outcome #5

6. *Answer:* A
Rationale: Explanations can reduce anxiety; anxiety can increase pain. Oxygen administration may help the person with an inhalation injury, but does not reduce pain. Topical anesthetic agents are not used to reduce pain resulting from burns. Intramus-

cular meperidine is not an appropriate choice because edema occurs 12 hours after a burn, so nonabsorption is an issue.
Level: Application
Refer to Learning Outcome #5

Critical Thinking Exercises

Scenario A

1. Some reasons that elderly persons are at increased risk for burn injuries include frailty (inability to remove oneself from danger), decreased hand-eye coordination (over-reaching for something), decreased muscle strength (picking up items that are unexpectedly heavy), decreased sensation (unawareness of temperature of items), decreased visual and auditory acuity (unable to see danger or hear warnings of danger), and cloudy judgment (misjudging things like personal strength, distance, time, etc.).

2. The kitchen and bathroom are areas where a burn injury can occur. On the stove, handles of cookware should be turned inward, and two hands protected by oven mitts should be used to move heated cookware from stove to table or countertop. Food should be permitted to cool slightly to avoid oral injuries. The water heater thermostat should be adjusted at about 130 degrees or lower to prevent scald burns in the sink or tub. A sufficient number of smoke detectors should be installed and batteries should be checked on an easy to remember schedule such as the first day of the month when pension checks are deposited. Care should be taken if wood is used as a source for heating in cold weather. Sparks and ashes are always a danger. Cigarette smoking should be discouraged especially when the client is drowsy or ill.

3. The elderly person might not know immediately (due to altered pain perception) that a scald injury has occurred. The elderly person should be taught to inspect the skin at least daily for changes such as redness, blistering, and swelling that could indicate injury.

4. Home remedies can include everything from sprinkling pepper or spreading butter on the burn to breaking the blister of a serious burn. Most home remedies provide an environment conducive to the growth of bacteria. Elderly people need to be taught to seek medical assistance because of their lowered immune response as well as the presence of diseases (such as diabetes) that could impede healing.

Scenario B

1. The head (9%), the arms (18%), the anterior thorax (18%) equal a total body surface area (TBSA) of 45%.

2. The greatest concerns are fluid status; intravenous lines are established as a priority for fluid resuscitation. Care of the wounds begins by using sterile technique to clean and dress the wounds. Since the fire caused burns of the face, another concern is for the client's breathing status; oxygen would be started and an endotracheal or tracheostomy set-up may be prepared and used if indicated.

3. Pain management would begin in the Trauma Center and be continued during the healing process. The intravenous route is the route of choice.

4. A nasogastric tube is inserted to prevent emesis and aspiration. An indwelling urinary catheter is inserted to measure hourly urine output. Vital signs are measured to monitor for cardiac, respiratory, and thermoregulatory functioning. Baseline diagnostic studies are ordered to monitor for status as well as for changes as the healing process occurs. A prophylactic tetanus injection would also be administered.

Chapter 50, Nursing Care of Clients Undergoing Plastic Surgery

Study Questions

1. *Answer:* B
   Rationale: Assessment of the client's perception of body image is important because it may indicate how the client will respond to the changes resulting from the surgery as well as provide the health-care team with information about the psychosocial needs of the client. The physical deformity is known to be present; baseline vital signs are part of the preoperative routine; and discharge teaching should begin on admission to the unit.
   Level: Application
   Refer to Learning Outcome #1

2. *Answer:* C
   Rationale: Incisions parallel to the skin lines will camouflage scars, whereas incisions perpendicular to the skin lines will result in more obvious scars.
   Level: Knowledge
   Refer to Learning Outcome #2

3. *Answer:* B
   Rationale: The occurrence of infection may necessitate the removal of the implant.
   Level: Knowledge
   Refer to Learning Outcome #3

4. *Answer:* C
   Rationale: A patent airway is the most important assessment to make after any surgery. Facial surgery often involves the bones of the nose. The blood pressure is measured routinely after surgery (A). Blurred vision (B) and dryness of the eyes (D) may be experienced after facial surgery but are not life threatening.
   Level: Application
   Refer to Learning Outcome #4

5. *Answer:* C
   Rationale: Continued assessment for psychosocial needs is important for the client who is at risk for body image disturbance. The nurse should encourage the client to walk in the halls. The nurse should initiate discussion of disfigurement and not wait for the client or significant others to do so. The client needs to know that the nurse is available to discuss problems with perceptions about body image.
   Level: Application
   Refer to Learning Outcome #5

6. *Answer:* C
   Rationale: Warmth prevents vasoconstriction. Exposure to cold and tobacco use cause vasoconstriction. Sensory-motor nerve function may be damaged during the surgery, and its return is an indicator of successful replantation.
   Level: Application
   Refer to Learning Outcome #6

Critical Thinking Exercises

Scenario A

1. The nurse needs to be supportive of the client's decision to ask for the implant to be placed at the time of surgery. The nurse should make time to discuss with the client feelings about the surgery, how she perceives the change in her body image, and how she feels about her husband's perceptions about her body. The nurse could also refer the client to a community support group so that she can talk with others who have experienced the same kind of surgery and who could help her with her own acceptance of the change. Such a group may also include the spouse so that he can learn about changes in body image and how to respond to perceptions and feelings regarding the changes.

2. The nurse needs to approach the husband by asking him directly about his feelings about the surgery. He may be fearful about the changes and anxious about how his wife will respond to the surgery. The nurse needs to discover what "disfigurement" means to the husband. To him, the disfigurement might signify a form of mutilation or might be a visible reminder of the cause (a lesion), or he might fear a change in the couple's sex life. He needs more information, with drawings and photographs of a successful implant. He needs to resolve his feelings so his spouse will receive the support she needs for healing of her body and emotions.

3. The husband needs to be instructed about the natural asymmetry of the body, not only of the female breast but other areas of the body, such as the eyes and so on.

Scenario B

1. The client must realize the significance of general anesthesia as compared to simple suturing of minor lacerations. She may strongly suspect that there might be permanent damage to the skin of her face and arms. She might also hope that the plastic surgeon was able to effect a repair that minimized the amount of damage done. She might feel helpless because this surgery was a necessity and she had no control in the matter. Feelings about not appearing in public may surface.

   The nurse can help by accepting the client as she is and using a calm, positive approach to care. The nurse should allow the client to see herself in a mirror and should explain how healing occurs and how the surgeon made the repair to minimize scarring. The nurse should discuss feelings and expectations with the client, family members, and significant other.

2. Healing of inflicted trauma and surgical trauma should progress according to the client's level of wellness. A well-balanced diet will contribute to healing. Conditions such as diabetes mellitus and bleeding tendencies may impede the healing process. The ability to follow instructions regarding care at home may also affect healing.

3. The way society generally responds to disfigurement might influence how the family and visitors accept and respond to a person's disfigurement. They may view the client as helpless and may react with distaste on the initial visit. The nurse would plan to spend time with the family and visitors who are noticeably distressed by the client's appearance. The family and visitors may need to be taught how to approach the disfigurement and how to deal with it in public.

Chapter 51, Assessment of Clients with Reproductive Disorders

Study Questions

1. *Answer:* C
   Rationale: It will be important to first establish rapport before expecting the client to be willing to share what may seem private, embarrassing, or sensitive information or exposure.
   Level: Application
   Refer to Learning Outcome #1

2. *Answer:* C
   Rationale: Although family history of obesity may affect a client's nutritional status, family history alone will not affect reproductive functioning. All the other factors would.
   Level: Knowledge
   Refer to Learning Outcome #2

3. *Answer:* C
   Rationale: Attention to chief complaint demonstrates to the client that the nurse is interested in meeting the client's most pressing needs, thus making her cooperation more likely, with more detailed assessment to follow. History taking should precede physical examination, and the nurse should inquire about allergies early in the assessment.
   Level: Comprehension
   Refer to Learning Outcome #2

4. *Answer:* A
   Rationale: Abnormal findings are most likely to be recognized with thorough knowledge of one's own anatomy. The use of scare tactics (D) or other incentives (C) will be less effective than encouragement of self-knowledge. When the nurse gives the impression that she or he has all the knowledge (B), the client may be less likely to respond.
   Level: Application
   Refer to Learning Outcome #3

5. *Answer:* B
   Rationale: Maintaining an open posture and attitude is most effective for relaxation. The client has not indicated a concern for more privacy (A) or explanation (D), as she apparently understands what to expect because of previous experience. Bearing down will increase her tension (C); opening her hands and eyes are effective relaxation techniques.
   Level: Analysis
   Refer to Learning Outcome #3

Critical Thinking Exercises

Scenario A

1. Whether she has a family history or not, each woman who presents to a health-care facility should be encouraged in breast self-examination (BSE). In this case, the nurse should invite the woman to show how she actually performs BSE to determine adequacy as well as to encourage her in the likelihood of her being able to find any deviation from normal as long as she is faithful in monthly checks. She should also be advised about mammography.

2. While exploring the quality, location, intensity, and other factors in relation to her complaint of pain, the nurse must be careful to listen actively and with sensitivity to include all relevant data. She might be questioned about bowel and bladder status, with changes being of particular import. Once a comfortable rapport is established, the client should be encouraged to discuss sexual activity and satisfaction. There may be some concerns about having children, which could only be discussed if a trusting relationship has been established. Exercise, adequacy of rest and relaxation, and well-balanced meals all play a role in the promotion of normal immune function and thus become important areas of assessment.

3. Practice is key in the development of good assessment technique. By practicing history taking, by developing a normal routine that follows a pattern, and by active listening and thoughtful observation, a thorough and efficient assessment will result in accuracy of nursing diagnoses and appropriateness of interventions.

Scenario B

1. Is it necessary to ask the husband to leave? The client should be invited to make decisions about who will be in the room and how she can be made most comfortable. In the Vietnamese culture, the husband is usually expected to remain at the wife's side in a situation such as this one. Whether he speaks English or not is irrelevant, as long as the nurse can communicate effectively with the client. She can then interpret for him what you are saying and doing. Including the hus-

band will make the wife more comfortable.

2. Careful attention to modesty should be a priority, as with any client of any culture, but especially in this situation.

Chapter 52, Nursing Care of Men with Reproductive and Urinary Disorders

Study Questions

1. *Answer:* C
Rationale: Frequency of urination, an objective finding, will increase in men with prostatic enlargement. The subjective evaluations of dysuria (A) and odor (D) may provide important information but are not considered objective data. (B) is a judgmental question that would be unlikely to elicit much useful information and may interfere with further communication.
Level: Analysis
Refer to Learning Outcome #1

2. *Answer:* C
Rationale: There has been considerable evidence of the deleterious effects of environmental and occupational exposure and the resultant infertility in men. Avoidance of alcohol and tobacco have been shown to improve sperm count and motility (A). Heat will destroy sperm, not improve motility, so tight clothing should be avoided (B & D).
Level: Application
Refer to Learning Outcome #3

3. *Answer:* B
Rationale: Benign prostatic hyperplasia (BPH) is one of the most common disorders affecting men. It is more common in white men than in black men and is estimated that, by 50 years of age, 50% of men have some degree of BPH. Prostate cancer is the most common cancer among men, but the incidence is significantly lower than that of BPH.
Level: Knowledge
Refer to Learning Outcome #2

4. *Answer:* C
Rationale: Early detection of prostate cancer is essential and wise because cancer of the prostate is the most common cancer in men. Testicular cancer is more prevalent in younger men (ages 15–40 years) and thus testicular self-examination is an important part of any man's preventive health plan (A). Until the sperm in the ampulla of vas either die or are ejaculated, the postvasectomy client could still be fertile (B). Although sexual dysfunction is not always a result of prostatectomy, the client needs to be prepared for that possibility (D).
Level: Analysis
Refer to Learning Outcome #2

5. *Answer:* D
Rationale: Assessment every 3 hours is not often enough to monitor vital signs in a postoperative client, particularly when the potential for bleeding and fluid and electrolyte disturbance is as great as it is with surgery for BPH, such as transurethral resection. This type of surgery is particularly painful, and adequate analgesia is needed immediately after surgery. If bladder distension, an urgent postoperative complication, occurs, catheterization may be required. Because many of these clients are older men, it is especially important to differentiate acute dementia anxiety from the critical condition associated with this surgery, which results in fluid and electrolyte disturbance.
Level: Application
Refer to Learning Outcome #5

6. *Answer:* A
Rationale: Unless the most recent hourly output is determined, the first voiding after removal of an indwelling catheter cannot be as effective as planned. If the bladder is allowed to overdistend or does not contain enough urine, the initial act of voiding may be unsuccessful, leading to further need for catheterization. If the nurse can estimate when the bladder will contain 350 mL of urine, the client is provided the optimal chance for success in initial voiding. Adequate oral fluid intake should have been a part of routine care all along, especially when the client has an indwelling catheter (B). The catheter can be removed whether the client is ambulatory or not (C). Checking laboratory values is also a part of routine care and not specifically related to the removal of an indwelling catheter (D). Naturally, the catheter would not be removed without checking for physician's orders.
Level: Analysis
Refer to Learning Outcome #5

Critical Thinking Exercises

Scenario A

1. A sensitive, professional approach that allows the client opportunity to express concerns as the nurse provides privacy and invites the client to include his wife, should he desire, will help to establish the rapport necessary to conduct a thorough assessment.

2. Because the disease is more prevalent with advancing age, regular checkups with digital rectal examination of the prostate will help to detect discrete, hard nodules or asymmetry of the lobes. Laboratory studies will show elevated acid phosphatase, alkaline phosphatase, and prostatic-specific antigen in the presence of prostatic cancer. Finally, microscopic examination of tissue bits produced during transurethral resection of the prostate for BPH will reveal the presence of cancer cells.

3. The medication finasteride (Proscar) is being used to reduce glandular hyperplasia and is often combined with terazosin (Hytrin) to block or antagonize alpha-adrenergic receptors, thus relaxing the bladder outlet and reducing symptoms of obstruction of the proximal urethra. The dosage may be gradually increased to minimize the effects on systemic blood pressure. The client and his wife also need to be taught the catheterization technique because urinary retention can become an emergency.

4. Both the client and his wife need to be encouraged that expression of sexuality and affection can take many forms. The interference of circulation that generally accompanies the progression of BPH often results in impotence. The man should be allowed to express his concerns, and the nurse should be alert for signs of altered self-esteem.

Scenario B

1. A thorough assessment of the client's perception of his dysfunction, including cultural and social factors, drug use and abuse, expectations of self, and daily activities would help identify the problem.

2. Depending on the results of the assessment, the client could be encouraged to consult with an endocrinologist and a urologist, avoid alcohol and other substances that interfere with sexual function, or whatever appropriate intervention would be determined. Counseling may be helpful if the problem is psychological or related to social or cultural conflict. The client should be commended for seeking help.

Chapter 53, Nursing Care of Women with Gynecologic Disorders

Study Questions

1. *Answer:* B
Rationale: Historically, women have been discouraged from taking respon-

sibility for gynecologic health screening, either because it was considered to be all in their heads or related to role dysfunction, so the client who becomes informed and accountable for her own well-being should be encouraged and commended. It is not always without some discomfort (A) that screening is accomplished, and the time involved in a thorough examination may be greater than when the focus is on symptoms (D). Beginning a nurse-client relationship with instructions to undress (C) is unlikely to be effective.
Level: Analysis
Refer to Learning Outcome #1

2. *Answer:* D
Rationale: Although research has only recently been focused on treatment of menstrual disorders, more data are now available, so that effective treatment is likely. Medical management of symptoms may well reduce anxiety, further alleviating symptoms. It is no longer appropriate to suggest that the symptoms are psychosomatic (A) or the result of myths and evil spells (B) or even related to sexual function (C).
Level: Analysis
Refer to Learning Outcome #2

3. *Answer:* B
Rationale: The nurse may believe that the client should use hormone replacement therapy (A & C), but it is the informed client who should be making the decision, once the physician, certified nurse-midwife, or nurse discusses with the client the considerable research data now available (D).
Level: Analysis
Refer to Learning Outcome #3

4. *Answer:* A
Rationale: One of the most common presenting complaints is inability to conceive after several months of unprotected sex. As months go by without pregnancy, the pain of menstruation associated with endometriosis (B) often is intensified with increasing anxiety. Endometriosis has nothing to do with life-style (C), nor is it an emotional disorder (D).
Level: Comprehension
Refer to Learning Outcome #4

5. *Answer:* D
Rationale: The radical nature of this surgery will require adjustments in sexual function, but it is not helpful to suggest that the client must redefine her personhood (B) nor should she or the nurse be expected to accept death as inevitable (A); otherwise, the surgery would be pointless. There is no radiation involved (C), but there will be urinary or bowel diversion, or both.
Level: Analysis
Refer to Learning Outcome #5

6. *Answer:* D
Rationale: The client will have concerns about body function with such disfiguring surgery, but if she can look at the wound and share her concerns, she is achieving an appropriate goal of care related to body image. Crying is not inappropriate or unhealthy (C) and preparing a meal has to do with role function, not body image (B). There should not be a disturbance in body temperature related to this procedure (A).
Level: Analysis
Refer to Learning Outcome #6

Critical Thinking Exercises

Scenario A

1. In assisting the physician, the nurse is expected to provide support and encouragement to the client at the same time. As a client advocate, the nurse might offer to complete the examination by assessing the external genitalia to make both the physician and client more comfortable.

2. The physician needs to be aware of the importance of vulvar examination. If he is not doing it, it is appropriate for the nurse, privately and tactfully, to emphasize to the physician the importance of regular, thorough vulvar exams by offering current research findings or your own understanding, or both.

3. Here is an opportunity to introduce the client to the concept of regular self-examination of the vulva. The client can be taught to use a mirror to check for vulvar lesions or changes at the same time that she is performing monthly breast self-examinations. By explaining the very high cure rate for vulvar cancer that is detected early, the nurse can provide the client with a valuable means of disease prevention.

Scenario B

1. Before you make any judgments about the client's reluctance to have surgery, it is essential that a thorough psychosocial assessment be carried out. Until the nurse identifies cultural, social, or emotional factors, the nurse cannot meet the client's needs. Many women believe their personhood, not just their sexuality, would be affected by the removal of the female organs of reproduction. Nurses have an obligation to protect that which is important to the client. The nurse should help the client get a second opinion.

2. You may believe that the client is finished with her uterus, would feel great without it, and could use hormone replacement therapy if the ovarian function is affected, which it may not be. You may even feel that she is being foolish to want to go through surgery that may only reduce the tumors temporarily. As long as you are confident that she has been given as much accurate information as she desires, it is not the nurse's responsibility to change her mind. Nurses must allow women to be responsible for their own bodies and, in fact, equip them to be so.

3. It is important to help the client recognize the physical and mental effects these laboratory findings will have on her. If she can appreciate how fatigue and decreased energy levels can affect her, she may feel differently about the suggested surgery. If not, the nurse should help her find someone who will remove the fibroids without removing her uterus. Consider the term "hysterical." Can you appreciate why the removal of the uterus (hysterectomy) may be a problem for a woman today?

Chapter 54, Nursing Care of Clients with Sexually Transmitted Diseases

Study Questions

1. *Answer:* C
Rationale: Since the client is seeking treatment before symptoms become severe, she should be encouraged in the fact that she may be able to avoid serious, irreversible consequences. She will also need to be tested for gonorrhea since the two infections so often occur simultaneously. False reassurance (A) is never appropriate and "telling her" (D) will be as unlikely to be productive as avoidance (B) of a critical part of her assessment would be irresponsible.
Level: Analysis
Refer to Learning Outcome #1

2. *Answer:* B
Rationale: Although genital herpes is usually transmitted by direct sexual contact, transmission is possible by fomites such as towels used by an infected individual. There is a cure for syphilis (A) in the early stages, so it is imperative that the individual seek treatment for a "sore." Genital herpes cannot be cured (C) and genital warts cannot be cured by "home remedies"

(D). It is especially important for the client to be seen by a professional, as women with genital warts are at increased risk for genital malignancy.
Level: Application
Refer to Learning Outcome #2

3. *Answer:* B
Rationale: Because the challenge of treatment for gonorrhea is related to the increasingly resistant strains of organisms, it is especially important for the client to understand the need to complete all courses of antibiotic therapy. It may be important to teach proper use of condoms (A), but the priority at this point is to eradicate all infecting organisms. It is probably pointless to insist on abstinence (C), although many clients will take responsibility for abstaining from sexual activity until treatment has been shown to be effective, especially if the client is treated with respect. You are going to come across as judgmental and moralizing and may even cause a client to decide to refuse health care if you start in on the economic costs of STDs (D).
Level: Comprehension
Refer to Learning Outcome #3

4. *Answer:* A
Rationale: Honest, direct answers to questions relay to the client an attitude of trust and respect. You cannot accomplish compliance by insisting on changes in life-style (B). (C) and (D) are wrong because treatment will not protect the client from reinfection.
Level: Comprehension
Refer to Learning Outcome #4

5. *Answer:* A
Rationale: Since there is evidence that HSV-II predisposes to carcinoma of the cervix, the woman who makes an appointment for annual Pap smear and pelvic examination has demonstrated understanding and has taken responsibility for her health. Genital herpes cannot be cured (B) and there are several things that can be done for palliative treatment of the symptoms (C). Although sexual contact is certainly the most common mode of transmission, poor hand washing and exposure by fomites is also possible (D).
Level: Analysis
Refer to Learning Outcome #5

Critical Thinking Exercises

Scenario A

1. The assessment data for this client are no different than for any client presenting to an STD clinic or physician's office. Psychosocial findings, physical findings, and laboratory data are needed. All this can be accomplished by establishing an effective nurse-client rapport. The nurse needs to know what protection the client uses during sexual activity and inquire about medications she currently takes, including birth control pills and vitamins.

2. Obviously, this client will need current, accurate information about prevention of STDs. It is interesting to note, however, that she is at lower risk for STDs than most women. Prostitutes usually are more careful about hygiene and protection against STDs and pregnancy than the individual who participates in "casual sex" without either information or preparation.

3. As previously indicated, this is not usually the client who is in greatest need for health teaching and disease prevention. She is more likely to take responsibility for regular preventive health screening and to be proactive in relation to protecting herself. She is also more likely to appreciate the erroneous term "safe sex" and take extra precautions.

Scenario B

1. Gonorrhea is treated aggressively with antibiotics, usually one dose of Rocephin IM, followed by 7 days of oral tetracycline or doxycycline hyclate to treat the commonly occurring chlamydial coinfection. As the gonorrhea organisms become more resistant, antibiotic therapy may have to be changed.

2. The client needs to know to take the medication 1 to 2 hours after meals and to avoid iron, dairy products, and antacids. He also needs to identify all sexual partners within 30 days of diagnosis in order to provide examination and treatment. He should be encouraged to avoid all sexual activity until cured, and thereafter to use condoms for prevention of reinfection. Finally, he needs to be made aware of the seriousness of the infection and the concern about resistant strains in order to enhance compliance.

3. A professional, caring, and nonjudgmental approach is most likely to promote effective, therapeutic communication that will allow the client to ask questions, listen actively, and desire to follow instructions and return for follow-up. Only if the client chooses to take responsibility for his own health and chooses to accept your help can you consider that you can have any influence on his preventing reinfection.

Chapter 55, Nursing Care of Clients with Breast Disorders

Study Questions

1. *Answer:* A
Rationale: Nipple discharge is a common complaint, ranking only behind lumps and pain. The presence of a mass is the most significant other finding in relation to serious breast disease.
Level: Comprehension
Refer to Learning Outcome #1

2. *Answer:* C
Rationale: There is still controversy over the relationship of caffeine intake and breast disease, but many women do find that cutting down helps. There would be increased risk of breast cancer for a client whose mother has had it (A), and the client who has had chemotherapy should be especially careful to use sunscreen or avoid sun exposure (B). All women should practice monthly breast self-examination no matter what other screening is done (D).
Level: Analysis
Refer to Learning Outcome #2

3. *Answer:* B
Rationale: The client should be encouraged to take an active role in determining the course of treatment for any health problem, particularly one that has such a large impact on body image and self-esteem. You cannot tell someone to trust a physician; the physician—or nurse for that matter—will need to earn the client's trust (A). Using such scare tactics (C) will only serve to increase anxiety and decrease rapport and judgment. Breast cancer may or may not be curable in an individual situation. (D) includes false reassurance and giving advice, both of which are inappropriate.
Level: Analysis
Refer to Learning Outcome #3

4. *Answer:* B
Rationale: Because there is likelihood of lymphedema, the client should take precautions to avoid burns or other injuries. She should be encouraged to resume normal activities as much as possible, however, as well as enjoy friends and hope for a positive future.
Level: Analysis
Refer to Learning Outcome #4

5. *Answer:* D
Rationale: Although each is appropriate, none will be effective until the nurse has worked through his or her own feelings about breast cancer, life, death, and such issues.
Level: Analysis
Refer to Learning Outcome #5

Critical Thinking Exercises

Scenario A

1. The nurse should be empathetic and yet help the client recognize the value of mammography as part of responsible health screening. If the nurse is female and older than 40 years, she should be able to discuss the discomfort of mammography from her own experience. Perhaps if the client were given more information about how the x-rays are taken and why compression is necessary, she might be more willing to tolerate the discomfort.
2. Besides the need for regular mammography and physical examinations with Papanicolaou smear, the client should be assessed for understanding of the need for and method of breast self-examination. The nurse must never miss an opportunity to help a client become more knowledgeable about his or her own body and the means of attaining a higher level of preventive health care.
3. The nurse serves as role model, teacher, and advocate.

Scenario B

1. It is important for the nurse to identify his or her own feelings before attempting to become involved with this client and her family and significant others. Once those feelings, attitudes, and biases are identified, the nurse is in a position to help the client and her family work through the challenge of solving such an emotional and personal issue. Ultimately, the client should be allowed to decide what her treatment will or will not be. Ideally, the nurse would guide the family members to the point of acceptance of the client's decision and involvement in her care, whatever that will be.
2. The American Cancer Society, the National Cancer Institute, and local cancer support groups are but a few of the many resources available for information and support. Once a thorough assessment is made, the nurse can determine the specific resources needed in such areas as spiritual, financial, or informational. Obviously, the more accurate the assessment, the more appropriate the resource is likely to be.
3. The nurse must maintain careful documentation of all interviews as well as interventions to minimize legal risk. Unfortunately, in stressful and emotional situations, the client, family member, or significant others may misinterpret or misunderstand parts of a conversation. It is in everyone's best interest to record as much of these interactions as possible because even the nurse cannot be expected to remember details.

Chapter 56, Shock

Study Questions

1. *Answer:* B
   Rationale: One of the earliest signs of cardiogenic shock is a falling blood pressure with a rising pulse rate. All of the other choices are not indicative of cardiogenic shock, based on the data provided.
   Level: Analysis
   Refer to Learning Outcome #1
2. *Answer:* B
   Rationale: Diminished cardiac output will affect urinary output, dropping it to less than 20 mL/hour. All other choices are indicative of normal or hypervolemic states.
   Level: Comprehension
   Refer to Learning Outcome #2
3. *Answer:* A
   Rationale: In septic shock, every intervention is directed at restoring adequate oxygenation throughout the body. Hyperthermia, hypermetabolism, and circulatory abnormalities impair the cells' ability to consume oxygen. All other choices, while important, are secondary to restoring adequate oxygenation.
   Level: Knowledge
   Refer to Learning Outcome #3
4. *Answer:* C
   Rationale: Once again, a client in septic shock has an immediate need to restore oxygenation throughout his body. (A) would be contraindicated because pain medication could increase the severity of the shock. Restlessness in traumatic situations can easily be mistaken for pain.
   Level: Analysis
   Refer to Learning Outcome #3
5. *Answer:* D
   Rationale: With improved tissue perfusion, kidney output should be within normal limits. All other choices indicate that pathology is still present.
   Level: Comprehension
   Refer to Learning Outcome #4

Critical Thinking Exercises

Scenario A

1. The client is immunosupressed as a result of corticosteroid therapy and has a severe infection caused by a gram-negative bacteria. Also, vital organs necessary for regulation of fluid and electrolytes, blood pressure, and so on are severely compromised.
2. The client is a good candidate for septic shock. A molecule called lipid A, contained within the bacterial endotoxin, initiates the inflammatory process.
3. The client's temperature is not elevated to the level one would expect for a severe kidney infection. This is a direct result of the corticosteroid therapy. If the nurse did not realize the connection between the immune system and fever in the presence of corticosteroids, he or she might overlook the significance of temperature as being an early sign of impending septic shock.
   The client's respirations—hyperventilation—are also an early sign of shock caused by direct stimulation of hypothalamus by the endotoxin.
   Blood pressure—hypotension—is caused by generalized vasodilatation from the body's immune response to the bacterial endotoxin. The client's blood pressure may not drop as low as that of other clients because of the corticosteroid therapy.
   Pulse increases to compensate for massive vasodilatation.
4. The lungs are extremely susceptible to injury during septic shock. Therefore, the nurse should monitor lung sounds and blood gases. Lactate (serum) levels, if above 2 mmol/L would indicate anaerobic metabolism, a grave prognosis. Because antibiotics are not effective for the first 48 hours, the client's symptoms may worsen. Once antibiotics begin destroying bacterial cell membranes, the endotoxins may rise 50-fold. The nurse will have to assess vital signs, intake and output and numerous lab values for indications of organ malfunction. Fluid therapy will correct the balance between the delivery and consumption, besides correcting hypovolemia and hypotension. When intravascular volume is resolved, venous return to the heart increases, increasing cardiac output. Increased cardiac output will increase tissue perfusion and oxygen delivery. Aside from dependent and interdependent intervention, the nurse must also carry out independent functions that further support the client. These include positioning to optimize pulmonary function and providing complete nursing care in order to conserve the client's energy.

Scenario B

The 80-year-old is at greatest risk because his vital neuroendocrine, immune, and cardiovascular-renal systems are slower to respond and much less efficient. He is not only at risk for hypervolemic shock, but septic and cardiogenic shock as well.

Chapter 57, Nursing Care of Clients During Medical-Surgical Emergencies

Study Questions

1. *Answer:* C
Rationale: Chemical burns will worsen if left untreated. (A) would be a priority if the vision loss were sudden. (B) would be a priority if the pain were severe. (D) would be a priority if it were moderate to severe and in a client older than 35 years.
Level: Comprehension
Refer to Learning Outcome #1

2. *Answer:* B
Rationale: An open pneumothorax can easily become a tension pneumothorax. Considering the client's symptoms and history, the other choices are not viable.
Level: Analysis
Refer to Learning Outcome #4

3. *Answer:* D
Rationale: Persistent vomiting is an indication of increased intracranial pressure. (A) would be correct if the choice read "for the first 8 hours." (B) would be correct if the choice was to administer fluids only for the first 8 hours. Acetaminophen is usually the drug of choice for headache because it produces the fewest side effects and will not mask signs and symptoms that may indicate a deterioration of the client's condition (C).
Level: Application
Refer to Learning Outcome #3

4. *Answer:* D
Rationale: (D) is the correct emergency treatment for an individual who has just been bitten by a poisonous snake because it delays the circulation of the venom in the individual's general circulation. (A) and (C) would increase the circulation of the venom. (B) could cause permanent tissue and nerve damage.
Level: Comprehension
Refer to Learning Outcomes #2 and #6

5. *Answer:* D
Rationale: Syrup of ipecac will cause vomiting, making aspiration a possibility. Therefore, the client's gag reflex should always be checked before the syrup is administered. One should administer syrup of ipecac, not the extract (A). Pupillary response may be important for some poisons, but in general, the nurse should be more concerned with monitoring the client's cardiovascular status because ipecac can be cardiotoxic (B). It is important to administer as much fluid as possible with syrup of ipecac to assist with the removal of the poisonous substance (C).
Level: Comprehension
Refer to Learning Outcome #5

Critical Thinking Exercises

Scenario A

1. Considering the client's history and the current status of your assessment, the client has probably sustained a tension pneumothorax.

2. You would observe his respiratory efforts in general (i.e., how he breathes and the expansion and contraction of his chest). Asymmetry of the chest may be noted because of the air trapped on the affected side. You would also note whether he has any jugular vein engorgement. This would indicate increased pressure on his heart and great vessels, causing a backup in the venous system. You would also monitor for tracheal deviation, which would indicate pressure against the mediastinum that would shift the trachea out of midline.

3. The client's problem has resulted from hyperinflation or air trapping in a portion of his right lung, which causes a rupture to occur. In the case of an individual who has sustained trauma to the chest wall, the traumatic pneumothorax may be caused by a broken rib, penetrating trauma, a closed pleural biopsy, a puncture during the insertion of a central venous pressure catheter, or a barotrauma in mechanically ventilated patients.

4. You would quickly carry out the physician's stat orders. The orders would probably include placing the client on oxygen and, if time permits, obtaining a chest x-ray. You would also constantly monitor the client and have resuscitation equipment available. The physician will insert a chest tube. The client will need a local anesthetic and an antibacterial cleanser for the skin. After the chest tube is inserted, it will be connected to underwater seal drainage. The tube will be sutured in place, a sterile dressing applied, and tubes taped in place if institutional protocol so requires. An x-ray will be taken to confirm the position of the tube.

5. Even though the client may be very anxious, it is the nurse's responsibility to remain calm and give simple explanations of the procedure. You would try to help him remain still during the insertion of the chest tube, and instruct him to take several deep breaths to help him reinflate his collapsed lung and push air out the pleural space. Remember that, because of his age and weakened state, the client may need instruction and support when trying to take these deep breaths. On discharge, the nurse would teach the client to return to his physician immediately if any of the signs and symptoms of tension pneumothorax occur again. He is particularly vulnerable because of his history of smoking, his chronic obstructive pulmonary disease, and his age.

Scenario B

1. The clinical findings indicate peritonitis and, along with the intense left shoulder pain, (Kehr's sign), it is highly likely that the client has a ruptured spleen.

2. The spleen is the organ most likely to be injured in trauma of the abdomen. A rib fracture can cause splenic rupture. Because the spleen can encapsulate bleeding, there will be a delay in overt signs and symptoms of splenic rupture.

3. Surgery will be the immediate treatment. The nurse will carry out the physician's orders, which will probably include: oxygen by nonrebreather mask, blood transfusions, administration of lactated Ringer's solution (250 mL at first, followed by another 250 mL until the blood pressure rises to above 100). The physician may also order the client to be placed in a modified Trendelenburg position or lying flat to direct the blood back to the heart. A nasogastric tube and a urinary catheter may also be inserted. The nurse's independent role will require her or him to monitor for signs and symptoms of fluid overload when administering the lactated Ringer's solution. The nurse will also be expected to notify the operating room and contact the x-ray department. The most important intervention, along with carrying out emergency measures, is to make certain that the client is given simple, direct explanations and constant support. The family and significant others should also be given information and support.

Appendix B
Reference Laboratory Values

Reference Values in Hematology

Acid hemolysis test (Ham)	No hemolysis	
Alkaline phosphatase, leukocyte	Total score 14–100	
Cell counts		
Erythrocytes		
Males	4.8–5.5 million/mm³	
Females	4.0–5.0 million/mm³	
Children (varies with age)	4.5–5.1 million/mm³	
Leukocytes		
Total	5000–10,000 mm³	
Differential	*Percentage*	Absolute
Myelocytes	0	0/mm³
Band neutrophils	3–5	150–400/mm³
Segmented neutrophils	60–70	3000–5800/mm³
Lymphocytes	20–40	1500–3000/mm³
Monocytes	2–6	300–500/mm³
Eosinophils	1–4	50–250/mm³
Basophils	0–1	15–50/mm³
Platelets	150,000–400,000/mm³	
Reticulocytes	25,000–75,000/mm³	
	0.5–1.5% of erythrocytes	
Coagulation tests		
Bleeding time (template)	2.75–8.0 min	
Coagulation time (glass tubes)	5–15 min	
Factor VIII and other coagulation factors	50–150% of normal	
Fibrin split products (Thrombo-Welco test)	< 10 μg/mL	
Fibrinogen	200–400 mg/dL	
Partial thromboplastin time (PTT)	30–45 sec	
Prothrombin time (PT)	10–12.5 sec	

Coombs' test	
Direct	Negative
Indirect	Negative
Corpuscular values of erythrocytes	
Mean corpuscular hemoglobin (MCH)	26–34 pg
Mean corpuscular volume (MCV)	80–96 μm³
Mean corpuscular hemoglobin concentration (MCHC)	32–36%
Erythrocyte sedimentation rate (ESR)	
Wintrobe method: Males	0–9 mm/hr
Females	0–15 mm/hr
Westergren method: Males	0–15 mm/hr
Females	0–20 mm/hr
Haptoglobin	26–185 mg/dL
Hematocrit	
Males	40–54 mL/dL
Females	37–47 mL/dL
Newborns	49–54 mL/dL
Children (varies with age)	35–49 mL/dL
Hemoglobin	
Males	14.0–18.0 gm/dL
Females	12.0–16.0 gm/dL
Newborns	16.5–19.5 gm/dL
Children (varies with age)	11.2–16.5 gm/dL
Hemoglobin, fetal	< 1.0% of total
Hemoglobin A_{1C}	3–5% of total
Hemoglobin A_2	1.5–3.0% of total
Hemoglobin, plasma	0–5.0 mg/dL
Methemoglobin	30–130 mg/dL

Reference Values for Blood, Plasma, and Serum*

Acetoacetate plus acetone, serum	
Qualitative	Negative
Quantitative	0.3–2.0 mg/dL
Acid phosphatase (thymolphthalein monophosphate substrate), serum	0.11–0.60 mU/mL
Adrenocorticotropin (ACTH), plasma	
6 AM	10–80 pg/mL
6 PM	< 50 pg/mL
Alanine aminotransferase (ALT, SGPT), serum	5–35 U/L
Albumin, serum	3.5–5.5 gm/dL

Reference Values for Blood, Plasma, and Serum* *(continued)*

Albumin/globulin (A/G) ratio	1.5:1–2.5:1
Aldolase, serum	1.3–8.2 U/dL
Aldosterone, plasma	
Supine	3–10 ng/dL
Standing	
Males	6–22 ng/dL
Females	5–30 ng/dL
Alkaline phosphatase (ALP), serum	20–90 mU/mL
Alpha-fetoprotein (AFP)	< 10 ng/mL
Ammonia nitrogen, plasma	15–49 μg/dL
Amylase, serum	60–160 Somogyi U/dL
Anion gap	8–16 mEq/L
Ascorbic acid, blood	0.4–1.5 mg/dL
Aspartate aminotransferase (AST, SGOT), serum	10–50 mU/mL
Base excess, blood	0 ± 2 mEq/L
Bicarbonate	
Venous plasma	
Arterial blood	18–23 mEq/L
Bile acids, serum	0.3–3.0 mg/dL
Bilirubin, serum	
Conjugated	0.1–0.3 mg/dL
Unconjugated	0.2–0.8 mg/dL
Total	0.1–1.0 mg/dL
Ca-125	< 35 U
Calcitonin	< 100 pg/mL
Calcium, serum	9.0–11.0 mg/dL
Calcium, ionized, serum	4.25–5.25 mg/dL
Carbon dioxide, total, serum or plasma	24–30 mEq/L
Carbon dioxide tension (P_{CO_2}), blood	35–45 mmHg
Carcinoembryonic antigen	
Nonsmokers	0–2.5 ng/mL
Smokers	< 3.0 ng/mL
β-Carotene, serum	40–200 μg/dL
Ceruloplasmin, serum	23–44 mg/dL
Chloride, serum or plasma	96–106 mEq/L
Cholesterol, serum or EDTA plasma	
Desirable range	< 200 mg/dL
LDL cholesterol	60–180 mg/dL
HDL cholesterol	30–80 mg/dL
Copper	
Males	70–140 μg/dL
Females	85–155 μg/dL
Cortisol, plasma	
8 AM	6–23 μg/dL
4 PM	3–15 μg/dL
10 PM	< 50% of 8 AM value
Creatine, serum	0.7–1.4 mg/dL
Creatine kinase (CK, CPK), serum	
Males	55–170 U/L
Females	30–135 U/L
Creatine kinase MB isozyme, serum	0.0–4.7 ng/mL
Creatinine, serum	0.6–1.2 mg/dL
D-Xylase	Blood levels peak (25–40 mg/dL) 2 hours after ingestion; 80–95% excreted in 5 hours
Estrogen receptors	Positive > 10 fmol/mg
Ferritin, serum	20–200 ng/mL
Fibrinogen, plasma	200–400 mg/dL
Folate, serum	1.8–9.0 ng/mL
Erythrocytes	150–450 ng/mL
Follicle-stimulating hormone (FSH), plasma	
Males	4–25 mU/mL
Females	4–30 mU/mL
Postmenopausal	40–250 mU/mL
γ-Glutamyltransferase, serum	
Males	5–38 U/L
Females	5–29 U/L
Gastrin, serum	< 200 pg/mL
Glucose (fasting), plasma or serum	60–100 mg/dL
Growth hormone (hGH), plasma	3 μg/mL
Haptoglobin, serum	26–185 mg/dL
Hepatitis antigens and antibodies	Negative for antigens; positive or negative for antibodies, depending on history
Human chorionic gonadotropin (HCG)	0–5 IU/L
Immunoglobulins, serum	
IgG	500–1900 mg/dL
IgA	60–333 mg/dL
IgM	45–145 mg/dL
IgD	0.5–3.0 mg/dL
IgE	500 ng/mL
Insulin (fasting), plasma	5–25 μU/mL
Iron, serum	50–150 μg/dL
Iron binding capacity, serum	
Total	250–350 μg/dL
Saturation	20–55%
Lactate	
Venous blood	4.5–19.8 mg/dL
Arterial blood	4.5–14.4 mg/dL
Lactate dehydrogenase (LD, LDH), serum	60–150 IU/L
Lipase, serum	0–110 U/L
Lipids, total, serum	450–850 mg/dL
Luteinizing (LH), serum	
Males	6–18 IU/L
Females	
Premenopausal	5–22 IU/L
Mid-cycle	3 times baseline
Postmenopausal	> 30 IU/L
Lysozyme	2.8–15.8 μg/mL
Magnesium, serum	1.8–3.0 mg/dL
Metalbumin	Absent
Osmolality	286–295 mOsm/kg water
Oxygen, blood	
Capacity (varies with hemoglobin)	16–24 vol%
Content, arterial	15–23 vol %
Saturation, arterial	94–100%
Oxygen tension (P_{O_2}), blood	75–100 mmHg
P_{50}	26–27 mmHg
Parathyroid hormone	430–1860 ng/dL
pH, arterial blood	7.35–7.45
Phenylalanine, serum	< 3 mg/dL
Phosphate, inorganic, serum	3.0–4.5 mg/dL
Potassium, serum or plasma	3.5–5.0 mEq/L
Prolactin	
Males	1–20 ng/mL
Females	1–25 ng/mL
Protein, serum	
Total	6.0–8.0 gm/dL

Reference Values for Blood, Plasma, and Serum* *(continued)*

Albumin	3.5–5.5 gm/dL
α_1-globulin	0.2–0.4 gm/dL
α_2-globulin	0.5–0.9 gm/dL
β-globulin	0.6–1.1 gm/dL
γ-globulin	0.7–1.7 gm/dL
Pyruvate, blood	0.3–0.9 mg/dL
Serotonin	50–200 ng/dL
Serum 5′-nucleotidase	0.3–3.2 Bodansky units
Serum gamma-glutamyl transpeptidase (GGTP)	<65 IU/L
Sodium, serum or plasma	135–145 mEq/L
Testosterone, plasma	
Males	275–875 ng/dL
Females	23–75 ng/dL
Pregnant	38–190 ng/dL
Thyroid-stimulating hormone (TSH), serum	1–10 μU/mL
Thyroxine, free (FT), serum	0.8–2.4 ng/dL
Thyroxine (T_4), serum	4.5–11.5 μg/dL
Triglycerides, serum	40–150 mg/dL
Triiodothyronine (T_3), serum	70–220 ng/dL
Triiodothyronine uptake, resin (T_3RU)	25–38% uptake
Urate, serum	
Males	2.5–8.0 mg/dL
Females	1.5–7.0 mg/dL
Urea, serum or plasma	24–49 mg/dL
Urea nitrogen, serum or plasma	10–20 mg/dL
Uric acid	
Males	2.5–8.0 mg/dL
Females	1.4–7.0 mg/dL
Viscosity, serum	1.4–1.8 times water
Vitamin A, serum	20–80 μg/dL
Vitamin B_{12}, serum	180–900 pg/mL

* For some procedures, the reference values may vary depending on the method used.

Reference Values for Urine*

Acetone and acetoacetate, qualitative	Negative
Albumin	
Qualitative	Negative
Quantitative	10–100 mg/24 hr
Aldosterone	3–20 μg/24 hr
δ-Aminolevulinic acid	1.3–7.0 mg/24 hr
Amylase	3–35 IU/hr
Amylase/creatinine clearance ratio	1–4%
Bilirubin, qualitative	Negative
Calcium (usual diet)	<250 mg/24 hr
Catecholamines	
Epinephrine	<10 μg/24 hr
Norepinephrine	<100 μg/24 hr
Total free catecholamines	4–126 μg/24 hr
Total metanephrines	0.1–1.6 mg/24 hr
Chloride (varies with intake)	110–250 mEq/24 hr
Copper	0–50 μg/24 hr
Cortisol, free	10–100 μg/24 hr
Creatinine	15–25 mg/kg body weight/24 hr
Creatinine clearance (corrected to 1.73 m^2 body surface area)	
Males	110–150 mL/min
Females	105–132 mL/min
Dehydroepiandrosterone	
Males	0.2–2.0 mg/24 hr
Females	0.2–1.8 mg/24 hr
Estrogens, total	
Males	4–25 μg/24 hr
Females	5–100 μg/24 hr
Glucose	
Random specimen	Negative
24-hour specimen	<0.5 g/24 hr
Hemoglobin and myoglobin, qualitative	Negative
17-Hydroxycorticosteroids	
Males	3–9 mg/24 hr
Females	2–8 mg/24 hr
5-Hydroxyindoleacetic acid	
Qualitative	Negative
Quantitative	<9 mg/24 hr
17-Ketosteroids	
Males	6–18 mg/24 hr
Females	4–13 mg/24 hr
Magnesium	6.0–8.5 mEq/24 hr
Metanephrines (see Catecholamines)	
Osmolality	275–295 mOsm/L
pH	4.5–8.0
Phenylpyruvic acid, qualitative	Negative
Phosphate	0.9–1.3 grams/24 hr
Porphobilinogen	
Qualitative	Negative
Quantitative	<2.0 mg/24 hr
Porphyrins	
Coproporphyrin	50–250 μg/24 hr
Uroporphyrin	10–30 μg/24 hr
Potassium	25–100 mEq/24 hr
Pregnanediol	
Males	0.4–1.4 mg/24 hr
Females	
Proliferative phase	0.5–1.5 mg/24 hr
Luteal phase	2.0–7.0 mg/24 hr
Postmenopausal	0.2–1.0 mg/24 hr
Pregnanetriol	<2.5 mg/24 hr
Protein	
Qualitative	Negative
Quantitative	10–150 mg/24 hr
Sodium	130–260 mEq/24 hr
Specific gravity	1.002–1.035
Urate	200–500 mg/24 hr
Urobilinogen	0–4 mg/24 hr
Vanillylmandelic acid (VMA, 4-hydroxy-3-methoxymandelic acid)	1–8 mg/24 hr

* For some procedures, the reference values may vary depending on the method used.

Reference Values for Cerebrospinal Fluid

Cells	< 5/mm³; all mononuclear	IgG index $\left(\frac{\text{CSF/serum IgG ratio}}{\text{CSF/serum albumin ratio}}\right)$	0.3–0.6
Electrophoresis	Predominantly albumin		
Glucose	50–75 mg/dL (20 mg/dL less than serum)	Oligoclonal banding on electrophoresis	Absent
IgG			
Children under 14	< 8% of total protein	Pressure	70–180 mm water
Adults	< 14% of total protein	Protein, total	15–45 mg/dL

Appendix C
Sample Clinical Pathways

Pathway	Source
Total Knee Replacement	Carolinas Medical Center
Total Hip Replacement	New England Baptist Hospital
Ischemic Cerebrovascular Accident (CVA)	North Carolina Baptist Hospitals
Transient Ischemic Attack (TIA)	University of Iowa Hospitals and Clinics
Spinal Cord Injury—Paraplegic Patient	University of Virginia Health Sciences Center
Ventilator Patient—Respiratory Failure	University of Iowa Hospitals and Clinics
Cardiac Surgery	North Carolina Baptist Hospitals
Coronary Artery Bypass Graft (CABG)	Carolinas Medical Center
Acute Leukemia	North Carolina Baptist Hospitals
Kidney Transplantation	North Carolina Baptist Hospitals
Gastrointestinal Hemorrhage With Complications	North Carolina Baptist Hospitals

CAROLINAS MEDICAL CENTER
TOTAL KNEE REPLACEMENT
CLINICAL PATH

Addressograph

Expected LOS: 5 Days **DRG 209 ICD.9 81.54; 81.55**

	Date: OR Day	Date: Postop Day 1	Date: Postop Day 2
Outcomes	Performs incentive spirometry (IS). Breath sounds clear. Dressing dry/intact. Equal pulses in lower extremities. Drain (if present) patent. Skin dry/intact . Pt. verbalizes knowledge of surgical procedure and post-op care. Pain controlled w/PCA.	Vital signs stable. Temp max < 101.5. Surgical site without s/s of infection. Dressing dry/intact. Equal pulses in lower extremities. Skin dry/intact. Pain controlled with PCA. Up in chair as tolerated.	Vital signs stable. Incision dry/well approx., w/o redness or inflammation. Dressing dry/intact. Equal pulses in lower ext. Skin dry/intact. Pain controlled with po meds. Weight-bearing on affected leg.
Teaching	Discuss plan of care with patient and family. Instruct/Reinforce incentive spirometry/ TCDB. Continuous Passive Motion (CPM).	Discuss plan of care with patient and family. Instruct/reinforce incentive spirometry/ TCDB. Reinforce CPM purpose and active ROM.	Discuss plan of care with patient and family. Instruct/reinforce incentive spirometry/ TCDB. Reinforce CPM purpose and active ROM.
Consults	MSW/DCP. PT. OT.		
Assess/Tx/Tests	TCDB Q2H. Circulation checks Q2H. Antiembolism. exercise Q1H. Incentive spirometry Q1H. I&O IV. Foley catheter. Skin care Q8H. Trapeze. CPM TED Hose **Physical Therapy:** Post flow sheet and antiembolism exercise sheet. Instruct in anti-embolism exercises. Issue ankle roll. Instruct in use of CPM and adjust settings.	Hgb/Hct. Prothrombin time. Circulation checks Q4H. Antiembolism exercise. IS. I&O. IV. D/C Drain. D/C Foley. CPM. Change dressing **Physical Therapy:** Document knee ROM and ambulation on flow sheet. Assist w/anti-embolism exercises. Review CPM use and adjust settings. Instruct in weight bearing status. OOB to hip chair w/assist & using walker.	Hgb/Hct. Prothrombin time. Circulation checks Q4H. Antiembolism exercise. IS. I&O. D/C IV. CPM. Change Op dsg **Physical Therapy:** Document knee ROM and ambulation on flow sheet. Assist w/anti-embolism exercises. Increase CPM settings as tolerated. Ambulate up to 50ft. Instruct and perform SLRs, TKEs and standing exercises BID. May go to PT gym.
Meds	Antibiotics. Warfarin (dosage per physician order). PCA Meds as at home.	Antibiotics Warfarin (as ordered by physician). PCA. Meds as at home.	Pain meds po. D/C PCA. Warfarin (as ordered by physician). Meds as at home.
Diet	Clear liquids.	Advance as tolerated.	Diet as tolerated.
Activity	Antiembolism exercises.	Antiembolism exercises. Weight bearing as tolerated. Ambulate with walker. Active ROM.	Antiembolism exercise routine. Weight bearing as tolerated. Ambulate with walker. Active ROM.
Spirit/Psy/Soc	Anxiety related to hospitalization and condition. Encourage pt. to verbalize feelings.	Pt. verbalizes feelings related to hospitalization and participates in plan of care. Encourage pt. to verbalize feelings.	Pt. verbalizes feelings related to hospitalization and participates in plan of care. Encourage pt. to verbalize feelings.
Discharge	Assessment of conditions at home.	Assessment of conditions at home.	Assessment of conditions at home. MSW dischg planning consult completed.
Signatures	7-3 3-11 11-7 7A-7P 7P-7A	7-3 3-11 11-7 7A-7P 7P-7A	7-3 3-11 11-7 7A-7P 7P-7A

This clinical path is a suggested guideline of care. The physician may change this plan at any time depending on the patient's individual needs.

c:\knee.wk4 Revised 10/10/95

Clinical pathway: Total knee replacement. (Courtesy of Carolinas Medical Center, Charlotte, NC.)

CAROLINAS MEDICAL CENTER
TOTAL KNEE REPLACEMENT
CLINICAL PATH

Expected LOS: 5 Days | DRG 209 ICD.9 81.54; 81.55 | Procedure 81.54

	Date: Postop Day 3	Date: Postop Day 4	Date: Postop Day 5
Outcomes	Vital signs stable. Dressing dry/intact. Pain controlled with po medications. Equal pulses in lower ext. Pt. verbalizes activity restrictions. Skin dry/intact. Weight-bearing on affected leg. Ambulates with walker.	Vital signs stable. Dressing dry/intact. Pain controlled with po medications. Equal pulses in lower extremities. Weight-bearing on affected leg. Skin dry/intact. Pt. acknowledges foods to avoid while on anti-coagulants. Ambulates with walker. Demonstrates home exercises.	Incision dry/well approximated, w/o redness or inflammation. Staples out/ Steri-strips Pain controlled Equal pulses in lower extremeties. Ambulates indep. w/assistive devices. **Pt. verbalizes knowledge of:** Exercises, diet, follow-up appointments, meds, anti-coagulation protocol. Follow-up physical therapy.
Teaching	Discuss plan of care with patient and family. Reinforce CPM purpose and active ROM.	Discuss plan of care with patient and family. Reinforce CPM purpose and active ROM. Review: Warfarin, exercises, signs of infection.	Anticoagulation protocol. Instruct on: Dose, dosage times, side effects, food/drug interactions, other meds. Follow-up appointments and other prescriptions written.
Consults			Escort service. Pt. needs: (wheelchair w/elevated leg, cart, assistance.
Assess/Tx/Tests	Hgb/Hct. Prothrombin time. Circulation checks Q4H. Antiembolism exercise. IS. I&O. CPM. Change dressing PRN. **Physical Therapy:** Document knee ROM and ambulation on flow sheet. Assist w/anti-embolism exercises. Increase CPM settings as tolerated. Ambulate 50 ft. Instruct and perform SLRs, TKEs and standing exercises BID. May go to PT gym.	Prothrombin time. Circulation checks Q4H. Antiembolism exercise. IS. I&O. CPM. Change dressing PRN. **Physical Therapy:** Document knee ROM and ambulation on flow sheet. Assist w/anti-embolism exercises. Increase CPM settings as tolerated. Ambulate 100 ft. Instruct and perform SLRs, TKEs and standing exercises BID. May go to PT gym. Meet with family and instruct in home exercise program.	Prothrombin time. Circulation checks Q4H. Antiembolism exercise. IS. I&O. CPM. Change dressing PRN. **Physical Therapy:** Knee flexion to 90 degrees. Document knee ROM and ambul. on flow sheet. Assist w/anti-embolism exercises. Increase CPM settings as tolerated. If independent with ambulation and >150ft. decrease ambulation to 1x day. Instruct and perform SLRs, TKEs and standing exercises BID. Instruct in stair climbing. Meet with family and instruct in home exercise program.
Meds	Pain meds po. Warfarin (as ordered by physician). Laxative of choice, PRN. Meds as at home	Pain meds po. Warfarin (as ordered by physician). Laxative of choice, PRN. Meds as at home.	Pain meds po. Warfarin (as ordered by physician). Laxative of choice, PRN. Meds as at home.
Diet	Diet as tolerated.	Diet as tolerated.	Diet as tolerated.
Activity	Antiembolism exercise routine. Weight bearing as tolerated. Ambulate with walker. Active ROM.	Antiembolism exercise routine. Weight bearing as tolerated. Ambulate with walker. Active ROM.	Antiembolism exercise routine. Weight bearing as tolerated. Ambulate once at least with PT.
Spirit/Psy/Soc	Pt. verbalizes feelings related to hospitalization and participates in plan of care. Encourage pt. to verbalize feelings.	Pt. verbalizes feelings related to hospitalization and participates in plan of care. Encourage pt. to verbalize feelings.	Pt. verbalizes feelings related to hospitalization and participates in plan of care. Encourage pt. to verbalize feelings.
Discharge	Assessment of conditions at home.	Assessment of conditions at home.	Pt. has return office appt. 3 weeks post day of surgery. Pt. has appropriate ADL equipment per OT. Discharged after morning physical therapy.
Signatures	7-3 3-11 11-7 7A-7P 7P-7A	7-3 3-11 11-7 7A-7P 7P-7A	7-3 3-11 11-7 7A-7P 7P-7A

This clinical path is a suggested guideline of care. The physician may change this plan at any time depending on the patient's individual needs.

c:\knee.wk4 Revised 10/10/95

KEY: M= MET U= NOT MET(ORDERED BY MD) N/A = NOT ORDERED **REPEAT OF DAY:** RECORD SECOND DATE, CIRCLE ALL INDICATORS

Patient Problems	Outcomes DOS (DATE: TIME:)	Outcomes Day 1 (DATE: TIME:)	Outcomes Day 2 (DATE: TIME:)
1. Risk injury 2	Absence bleeding	Absence bleeding	Absence bleeding
anticoagulation therapy	Pt within protocol	Pt within protocol	Pt within protocol
2. Tissue perfusion risk for alt.: Cardio Pulmonary	BP/P ± 20 baseline	BP/P ± 20 baseline	BP/P ± 20 baseline
	O2 Sat ≥ 90% O2 ______L.	O2 Sat ≥ 90% O2 ______L.	O2 Sat ≥ 90% O2 ______L.
	BS at baseline HCT ≥30	BS at baseline HCT ≥30	BS at baseline HCT ≥30
3. Potential alteration neurovascular status	N/V status at baseline	N/V status at baseline	N/V status at baseline
4. Risk for infection R/T surgery	Temp ≤ 101.5 ∅ sign of infection	Temp ≤ 101.5 ∅ sign of infection	Temp ≤ 101.5 ∅ sign of infection
5. Potential alteration nutrition	Tolerates NPO/clear liquids	Tolerates NPO/ clear liquids	Tolerates normal diet
6. Potential alteration	DTV @______	Bowel sounds ⊕	Bowel sounds ⊕
elimination	Or Foley→ dd; u/o q s.	Foley→ dd; u/o q s.	± Foley - DTV ______ u/o q s.
7. Alteration comfort	Verbalizes acceptable level comfort	Verbalizes acceptable level comfort	Verbalizes acceptable level comfort
8. Knowledge deficit R/T surgery, illness, +/or treatments	Verbalizes/demonstrates I/S BS Analgesia Tests/treatments	Verbalizes/demonstrates I/S BS Analgesia Tests/treatments	Verbalizes/demonstrates I/S Analgesia Tests/treatments
9. Impaired physical mobility	Demonst. safe bed mobility & understanding of B/S	Demonst. safe bed mobility & understanding of B/S	Demonstr. safe bed mobility Understanding of B/S
		Demonstrates bed & sling exercises	Demonstrates bed, sling and chair exercises
		Dangles at bedside	Demonstrates bed↔chair with assist
		Stands at bedside with walker	Demonstrates amb. in room with walker and assist
10. Impaired home maintenance	Verbalizes understanding discharge plan	Verbalizes understanding discharge plan	Verbalizes understanding discharge plan
Unmet Outcomes Continued			
Clinical Pathway	**DOS**	**Day 1**	**Day 2**
TESTS/RESULTS	IN P.A.C.U.	CBC	CBC
	AP/PELVIS	PT, PTT	PT
	K, CBC	± TRANSFUSION	± TRANSFUSION

Clinical pathway: Total hip replacement. (Courtesy of New England Baptist Hospital, Boston, MA.)

TREATMENTS	VS PER MD ORDERED	VS PER UNIT PROTOCOL	VS PER UNIT PROTOCOL
	INCENTIVE SPIROMETRY	INCENTIVE SPIROMETRY	INCENTIVE SPIROMETRY
	BREATH SOUNDS	BREATH SOUNDS	BREATH SOUNDS
	VENODYNE STOCKING/TEDS	VENODYNE STOCKING/TEDS	VENODYNE STOCKING/TEDS
	NV CKS Q 4°	NV CKS Q 4°	NV CKS Q 4°
	SKIN ASSESS Q SHIFT	SKIN ASSESS Q SHIFT	SKIN ASSESS Q SHIFT
	SOFT CARE	SOFT CARE	SOFT CARE
	HEMOVAC DRAIN	HEMOVAC DRAIN D/C'D	
	DRESSING ASSESS	ASSESS DRESSING	OPEN WOUND TO AIR
ACTIVITY	B.R. BALANCE SUSPENSION	B/S @ NOC	
	PT CONSULT	REINFORCE EXERCISE PROGRAM	REINFORCE EXERCISE PROGRAM
	OT CONSULT	DANGLE	AMBULATE WITH WALKER
	BED MOBILITY/TOTAL JOINT PRECAUTIONS		
REHAB		BED MOBIITY / TOTAL JOINT PRECAUTIONS	BED MOBIITY / TOTAL JOINT PRECAUTIONS
		BS @ NOC	BS @ D/C
		DANGLE @ BEDSIDE	B↔CHAIR OR COMMODE
		STAND WITH WALKER	AMB IN ROOM WITH WALKER
		SLING EXERCISES	CHAIR EXERCISES
		BED EXERCISES	
MEDICATIONS	IV ________@ ______cc/hr	IV ________@ ______cc/hr	IV ________@ ______cc/hr
	ANALGESICS:	ANALGESICS:	
	PCA/EPIDURAL / IM/ IT	PCA/EPIDURAL / IM/ IT/po	ASSESS READINESS CHANGE PO MEDS
	COUMADIN DOSE ________	COUMADIN DOSE ________	COUMADIN DOSE ________
	ROUTINE MEDS	ROUTINE MEDS	ROUTINE MEDS
NUTRITION/ ELIMINATION	NPO / CLEARS (Note if modified diet necessary, eg, ada) ____	CLEARS, FULL-SOFT, HOUSE OR MOD. DIET	FULL, SOFT- HOUSE OR, MODI. DIET
			IF NO BM MOM @ HS
	I & O	I & O	I & O
LEARNING /PSYCHO SOCIAL	REVIEW I/S, C & DB	REVIEW I/S, C & DB	
	REVIEW PCA	REVIEW PCA	
	REVIEW POSITIONING HIP PRECAUTIONS	REVIEW POSITIONING HIP PRECAUTIONS	REVIEW PO PAIN MEDS
		REVIEW PROGRESS IN RELATION TO D/C PLANNING	REVIEW PROGRESS IN RELATION TO D/C PLANNING
DISCHARGE PLANNING		PATIENT ASSESSMENT	D/C PLANNING ONGOING
		INITIATE REFERRALS TO APPRO. FACILITIES	INITIATE REFERRAL FORMS
	PROGRESS	**PROGRESS**	**PROGRESS**
	UNABLE TO PROGRESS	**UNABLE TO PROGRESS**	**UNABLE TO PROGRESS**

KEY: M= MET U= NOT MET(ORDERED BY MD) **N/A** = NOT ORDERED **REPEAT OF DAY:** RECORD SECOND DATE, CIRCLE ALL INDICATORS

	DATE: TIME:					DATE: TIME:					DATE: TIME:				
Patient Problems	**Outcomes Day 3**					**Outcomes Day 4**					**Outcomes Day 5**				
1. Risk injury 2 anticoagulation therapy	Absence bleeding					Absence bleeding					Verbalizes signs & symptoms of bleeding				
	Pt within protocol					Pt within protocol					Pt within protocol				
2. Tissue perfusion risk for alt.: Cardio Pulmonary	BP/P ± 20 baseline					BP/P ± 20 baseline					BP/P ± 20 baseline				
	O2 Sat ≥ 90% O2 ______ L.					O2 Sat ≥ 90% O2 ______ L.					O2 Sat ≥ 90% O2 ______ L.				
	BS at baseline HCT ≥30					BS at baseline HCT ≥30					BS at baseline HCT ≥30				
3. Potential alteration neurovascular status	N/V status at baseline					N/V status at baseline					N/V status at baseline				
4. Risk for infection R/T surgery	afebrile ∅ signs of infection					afebrile ∅ signs of infection					afebrile ∅ signs of infection				
5. Potential alteration nutrition	Tolerates normal diet					Tolerates normal diet					Tolerates normal diet				
6. Potential alteration elimination	Return to normal elimination pattern					Return to normal elimination pattern					Return to normal elimination pattern				
7. Alteration comfort	Verbalizes acceptable level comfort oral pain meds					Verbalizes acceptable level comfort oral pain meds					Verbalizes acceptable level comfort oral pain meds				
8. Knowledge deficit R/T, surgery, illness, +/or treatments	Verbalizes/demonstrates: IS Analgesia Tests/Treatment					Verbalizes understanding joint precautions					Verbalizes understanding joint precautions				
9. Impaired physical mobility	Demonstrates exercise program with supervision					Demonstrates exercise program with supervision					Demonstrates exercise program with supervision				
	Amb. with walker increasing distance					Amb. with walker increasing distance					Amb. with walker increasing distance				
	Review d/c instructions for Jordan transfers										Review d/c instructions				
10. Impaired home maintenance	Accepts D/C plan					Accepts D/C plan					Accepts D/C plan				
Unmet Outcomes Continued															

Clinical Pathway	Day 3	Day 4	Day 5
TESTS/RESUTLS	CBC	D/C FILM (IF D/C OUTSIDE REHAB)	
	PT	PT, PTT	PT
	± TRANSFUSION		
TREATMENTS	VS PER UNIT PROTOCOL	VS PER UNIT PROTOCOL	VS PER UNIT PROTOCOL
	INCENTIVE SPIROMETRY	INCENTIVE SPIROMETRY	INCENTIVE SPIROMETRY
	BREATH SOUNDS	BREATH SOUNDS	BREATH SOUNDS
	VENODYNE STOCKING/TEDS	VENODYNE STOCKING/TEDS	VENODYNE STOCKING/TEDS
	NV CKS Q SHIFT	NV CKS Q SHIFT	NV CKS Q SHIFT
	SKIN ASSESS Q SHIFT	SKIN ASSESS Q SHIFT	SKIN ASSESS Q SHIFT
	SOFT CARE	SOFT CARE	SOFT CARE
	INSPECT WOUND	INSPECT WOUND	INSPECT WOUND
		± CENTRAL OR INTERNAL JUGULAR LINE	
ACTIVITY	REINFORCE EXERCISES PROGRAM	REINFORCE EXERCISES PROGRAM	REINFORCE EXERCISES PROGRAM
	AMBULATE WITH WALKER	AMBULATE WITH WALKER	AMBULATE WITH CRUTCHES
REHAB	AMBULATE WITH WALKER	AMBULATE WITH WALKER	AMBULATE WITH WALKER
	REINFORCE EXERCISE PROGRAM	REINFORCE EXERCISE PROGRAM	REINFORCE EXERCISE PROGRAM
	OT EVALUATION		
	BRP		
MEDICATIONS	PO PAIN MEDS	PO PAIN MEDS	PO PAIN MEDS
	COUMADIN DOSE ________	COUMADIN DOSE ________	COUMADIN DOSE ________
	ROUTINE MEDS	ROUTINE MEDS	ROUTINE MEDS
NUTRITION/ ELIMINATION	HOUSE OR MODI. DIET	HOUSE OR MODI. DIET	HOUSE OR MODI. DIET
	IF PT. REMAINS CLEAR LIQUIDS GI CONSULT		
	IF NO BM DUCOLAX		
LEARNING / PSYCHO SOCIAL	REVIEW PROGRESS IN RELATION TO D/C PLANNING	REVIEW PROGRESS IN RELATION TO D/C PLANNING	REVIEW D/C INSTRUCTIONS
	REVIEW JOINT PRECAUTIONS	REVIEW JOINT PRECAUTIONS	REVIEW JOINT PRECAUTIONS
	REVIEW D/C INSTRUCTION (JORDAN Pt.)		
DISCHARGE PLANNING	ONGOING D/C PLANNING		
	TRANSFER TO JORDAN	TRANSFER TO JORDAN	TRANSFER TO JORDAN
	TRANSFER TO OUTSIDE FACILITY	TRANSFER TO OUTSIDE FACILITY	TRANSFER TO OUTSIDE FACILITY
	PROGRESS	**PROGRESS**	**PROGRESS**
	UNABLE TO PROGRESS	**UNABLE TO PROGRESS**	**UNABLE TO PROGRESS**

THE NORTH CAROLINA BAPTIST HOSPITALS, INC
ISCHEMIC CVA CLINICAL PATHWAY
DRG #14

Admission Date and Time____________________
Date/time of transfer to 11NT__________________
Date transferred to Rehab____________________
Discharged to:__________________________
Discharge Date/Time______________________

Baseline Barthel Score:	Admission Barthel Score:	Discharge Barthel Score:
1.____	1.____	1.____
2.____	2.____	2.____
3.____	3.____	3.____
4.____	4.____	4.____
5.____	5.____	5.____
6.____	6.____	6.____
7.____	7.____	7.____
8.____	8.____	8.____
9.____	9.____	9.____
10.___	10.___	10.___
Total ___	Total ___	Total ___

	Day 1	Day 2	Day 3	Day 4	Day 5	Day 6
Diagnostic Tests/Labs	•SMAC, CBC or CDP •FLP, Hgb A_1C if indicated (Day 1 or Day 2) •PT/PTT •Unenhanced CT (ED) Per diagnostic algorithm: •TTE •Carotid ultrasound/TCD •EKG,CXR •R/o MI Protocol if indicated •Cardiac monitor if indicated x 24° •Nursing functional assessment	•Evaluate need for labs •Per diagnostic algorithm •MR with contrast if indicated •LP/EEG if indicated •TEE if indicated •Angiogram or MR-A if indicated •Stroke in young pt w/u if indicated •PTT 6 hrs after heparin initiation and any dosage change •Cardiac monitor only if necessary •MBS per ST rec.	---------> •u/a after d/c foley ----------> ----------> •PT qd if on coumadin	----------> •Plt ct q3d while on heparin •Repeat CT or MRI with justification PTT qd once PTT therapeutic ----------> ---------->	----------> ----------> ----------> ---------->	----------> ----------> ----------> •Nursing functional assessment ---------->
Activity	•Bedrest with HOB ↑ 30°; OOB if tolerated •Turn q2h while in bed	•OOB to chair bid ---------->	----------> ---------->	•Begin progressive ambulation as tolerated ---------->	----------> ---------->	----------> ---------->
Diet	•Diet per nursing dysphagia screen results	•Enteral fdgs if NPO x 24 hrs	---------->	---------->	---------->	•Enteral fdgs +/-po per ST
Consults	•Speech swallowing/communication screen •PT/OT per nursing screen results •Recreation Therapy	•Nutrition (if require enteral fdgs)		•Rehab consult if appropriate •Nutrition (teaching)		•Transfer to Rehab if accepted •GI consult for PEG placement if indicated

Effective: March, 1995
Revised: September, 1995
* Not a part of the permanent record.

Clinical pathway: Ischemic cerebrovascular accident (CVA). (Copyright 1995, North Carolina Baptist Hospitals, Winston-Salem, NC. Used by permission.)

	Day 1	Day 2	Day 3	Day 4	Day 5	Day 6
Treatments/ Procedures	•NG for meds if needed	---------->	---------->	---------->	---------->	---------->
	•Neuro checks as ordered	---------->	---------->	---------->	---------->	---------->
	•RT/Suction PRN	---------->	---------->	---------->	---------->	---------->
	•O_2/pulse oximetry q 8 h prn	---------->	D/C 0_2 when sats > 93%	---------->	---------->	---------->
	•Pneumatic compression hose if indicated	---------->	---------->	---------->	---------->	---------->
	•IVF or saline lock/I&O	---------->	•Convert to saline lock with diet toleration, completion of IV meds	D/C IV if not on heparin		
	•Bladder management protocol/foley if needed	---------->	•-->(D/C foley; ✓ PVR's)	---------->	---------->	---------->
	•Skin care as applicable	---------->	---------->	---------->	---------->	---------->
	•Bowel management protocol	---------->	---------->	---------->	---------->	---------->
			•Splint care per OT	---------->	---------->	---------->
			•OHF & T prn	---------->	---------->	---------->
	•ROM bid as per PT criteria	---------->	---------->	---------->	---------->	---------->
	•Hemetest stools while on IV Heparin and/or Coumadin	---------->	---------->	---------->	---------->	---------->
	•Bedside glucose monitoring AC&HS if indicated	---------->	---------->	---------->	---------->	---------->
Medications	•IV Heparin as indicated	---------->	---------->	---------->	D/C Heparin	
	•SQ Heparin as indicated	---------->	---------->	---------->	---------->	---------->
	•ASA+/or Ticlid as indicated	---------->	---------->	---------->	---------->	---------->
	•Antihypertensives as indicated	---------->	---------->	---------->	---------->	---------->
	with parameters	•Start coumadin	---------->	---------->	---------->	---------->
Discharge Planning	•Social Work Services Consult •Psychosocial screening assessment	•Team formulation of disposition plan	•Full Psychosocial assessment of high-risk patients •Referring physician contact	•Contact Rehab Centers/SNF/other facilities as per team plan •Complete FL-2	•Arrange for home needs: equipment, services, etc.	•Discharge •Send discharge progress note and diagnostic test results to primary physician and neurologist
Teaching	•Stroke	---------->	---------->	---------->	---------->Reinforce	Stroke education instrument - intervene as needed
	•Diagnostic testing	---------->	---------->			
	•Dysphagia	•Mobility				
	•Skin Care	•Safety	•Bowel/Bladder Elimination	---------->	---------->	----->Reinforce
	*See standardized patient education packet for daily written materials/ videos/classes, according to deficits	•Meds, including coumadin	---------->	----------> •Dietary •Risk factors/prevention •Rehab	----------> ----------> ----------> •Local resources/ support group	----->Reinforce ----->Reinforce ----->Reinforce

path14.stk/cc4/mc

A-20

MULTIDISCIPLINARY CAREMAP

TRANSIENT ISCHEMIC ATTACK

Map ID No. 26
Page 1

• File most recent sheet of this number ON BOTTOM

DATE
HOSP. NO.
NAME
BIRTH DATE
ADDRESS
SOCIAL SECURITY NUMBER

IF NOT IMPRINTED, PLEASE PRINT DATE, HOSP. NO., NAME AND LOCATION

Unit(s) 2 Carver West and Acute Care Stroke Monitoring Unit ______
Case Manager(s) ______

Physician(s) ______

Date/Time/Name Reviewed by MD/RN - Initial Review ______

Date/Time/Name RN Who Reviewed with Patient ______

Secondary Diagnoses ______

UIHC Expected LOS ______
Date/Time of Surgery ______
Discharge Date ______

Definition TIA: No deficits on admission but has experienced neurological symptoms lasting less than 24 hrs in the previous 2 weeks

☐ Discontinue Map (date) ______
☐ Transfer to Other Map (date) ______
☐ Return to This Map (date) ______

Other Map Name ______

MULTIDISCIPLINARY PLAN OF CARE (Critical path is on reverse side)

	INTERMEDIATE GOALS		OUTCOMES
	Admission Day	**Day 2**	**Day 3**
Date			
	Check the Met or Unmet box for each goal and outcome. Complete each day by 2300.		
PatientProblem	Met Unmet	Met Unmet	Met Unmet
Knowledge Deficit	Pt/family verbalize understanding of disease process ☐ ☐	Pt/family verbalize warning signs and symptoms of TIA's ☐ ☐	Pt/family verbalize own risk factors and ways to reduce or eliminate risk factors Pt.family verbalize understanding of need to seek medical attention if symptoms/warning signs reoccur Pt/family verbalize understanding of: • Names of discharge medication(s) • Doses of discharge medication(s) • Uses of discharge medication(s) • Schedule of discharge medication(s) • Side effects of discharge medication(s) ☐ ☐

2/95 Version 1

A-20 | B CLIN. NOTES | C LABORATORY | D X-RAY EXAM | E CONSULTATION | F SPEC. EXAM | G THERAPY | H PATHOLOGY | I DIAGNOSIS

Clinical pathway: Transient ischemic attack (TIA). (Copyright 1995, University of Iowa Hospitals and Clinics, Iowa City, IA. Used by permission.)

A-20

MULTIDISCIPLINARY CAREMAP
TRANSIENT ISCHEMIC ATTACK

Map ID No. 26
Page 2

PATIENT NAME ______________________

HOSP. NO. ______________________

CRITICAL PATH (Care plan is on reverse side)

	Admission Day	Day 2	Day 3
Date			
	Put initials in columns when ordered, sent, or completed. Ordered / Sent / Completed	Ordered / Sent / Completed	Ordered / Sent / Completed
Consults	Social service - if psychosocial needs identified	Dietary if patient on coumadin	
Tests	Doppler Echo CT scan EKG Chest x-ray ABG as indicated Stool hemocult per physician pt/PTT International Normalized Ratio (INR) ESR CBC General screen & cholesterol Lipid profile if <70 y.o. UA	Lipid panel if not drawn day 1	
Treatments/ Interventions	Vital signs q4h x 24h Neuro checks q4h x 24h O_2 spot check - if less than 95% obtain ABG Cardiac monitor x 24h Saline lock IV fluids as ordered O_2 as needed	Vital signs and neuro checks q 8h DC cardiac monitor if in NSR	DC saline lock
Medications	Anticoagulant/antiplatelet medications as ordered	d/c prescriptions written and sent to pharmacy	
Diet	Pre-admit diet unless NPO for lipid profile	Pre-admit diet	
Activity	UAL with assist as needed	UAL if neuro status stable	
Teaching	Unit orientation Diagnostic tests TIA teaching Distribute Physical Therapy activity survey	TIA risk factors Risk factor control/elimination TIA warning signs Brain Attack bookmarker Stroke: Reducing Your Risk Know the Warning Signs of Stroke Little Known Signs of a Stroke Tape: Reducing Your Stroke Risk Dietary pamphlets	Discharge medications Diet Physical Therapy survey returned
Discharge Planning	Social Service arrange for return to facility (if necessary)	If from a facility, begin medical discharge summary RX written and sent to pharmacy if needed Nursing discharge referral started	Dietary teaching arranged if appropriate d/c instruction sheet, form B19 completed, reviewed and signed or nursing discharge referral completed and report called to receiving facility Medical discharge summary sent with patient to facility if applicable Medication/RX given to patient by pharmacy

INITIALS/ SIGNATURE/ POSITION ______/______ ______/______ ______/______

1/95 Version

University of Virginia Medical Center - Patient Care Services
Clinical pathway: Spinal Cord Injury - Paraplegic Patient
Attending: **L.O.S. 6-7**
Medical Diagnosis: **ICD9 code:**

Patient's/Significant Other's learning needs are identified and documented on P.E.P.

	Date: E.R.	Init	Date: Within first 24°	Init	Date: Pre-Stabilization	Init	Date: D.O.S./ Decision	Init	Date: POD 1	Init	Date: POD 2	Init	Date POD 3-4	Init	Date: POD 5-6-7	Init
Interdisciplinary Communication (Consults)	• Consults: SCI Coord. ER - SW Orthopaedics or Neurosurgery Trauma Nurse Coordinator • Trauma Medicine to clear • Chaplain follows as indicated		• Consult: PM&R PT, OT Inform: SW SCI team Nutrition RT • Plan for fixation • Consults: Medical specialty as indicated Psych support Consider Acute Pain service consult		Consider P&O consult Nutrition Consult Service (if b.s. negative)											
Assessments	Resp. status (Poss. pulmonary consult) (NSG,RT) Pain (NSG) Alignment (NSG) NLI/ASIA (MD) VS per order set Trauma Protocol (MD) Home Meds (MD) PMH (MD)		→ Pt/family conference Urology consult - Uro Trauma Decub assm't (consult ostomy as indicated) → → O_2 sats per methylprednisolone Protocol I&O q1° Bowel sounds q4° Vital Capacity (RT) Pt Database (NSG)		→ Psych. assm't (Psych support) Anesthesia → → PT/OT assmt I&O q shift Presence of autonomic dysreflexia Spiritual assmt (Chaplain)		→ Evoked potentials (intra-operative) NLI/ASIA VS per post-op protocol → Pre-op check list →		→ Pt/fam resource assmt. (SW) → VS w/O_2 sat q shift → If b.s. neg.12° post-op eval. for hyperal nutrition support → Presence of spasticity/need for med consult PMR		Need for W/C (PT,NSG) → → → →		Renal Ultrasound NLI/ASIA daily → → →		→ → → →	
Diagnostics (LAB, RADIOL)	Trauma Labs Plain films of spine, chest pelvis/other as indicated MRI or CT spine		Chem 20		CBC Chem 13				Clear with 90° xrays							

Clinical pathway: Spinal cord injury—paraplegic patient. (Courtesy of University of Virginia Health Sciences Center, Charlottesville, VA.)

Medications	Acute Pain mgt & protocol (1.2) SCI meds Methylprednisolone in transit per order set or in OR w/in 8° of injury Consider Vasopressors (to keep Systolic ↑90 & HR ↑40)	→ → SCI bowel protocol (1.77) Heparin 5000 u q 8° sub q DVT prophy & protocol (1.21)	→ → → → →	→ → → Heparin 5000 u q 8° sub q →	→ → → → →	→ → → → →	→ → → → →	→ → → → →
Dressings Tubes/Drains	NG to intermittent suction (1.29) Foley & protocol (1.29) IV & protocol (1.40)	NG tube until + b.s. SCI Bladder protocol (1.93) →	→ →	Dsg ck w/ v.s. → → Chest tube care if anterior approach w/ protocol (1.17)	→ → → →	→ → → →	Dsg. change prn (NSG) Initiate I&O caths q4° D/C Foley & protocol if output <3000 cc & start I&O cath protocol →	Dsg. change prn (NSG) → →
Interventions Treatments	Alignment (NSG) Vent Protocol PRN (RT) (#1.87) Respiratory Protocol	SCI Resp. protocol (1.59) Incentive spirometry q1° SCD stockings protocol (1.63) Space boots External pneumatic compression sleeves both legs	Mold brace if indicated → Incentive spirometry w/ vs → Psych interventions as indicated (Psych support)	→ → → →	Brace fitting as indicated → Assistive cough tech-niques w/ spirometry (OT, PT,NSG) → →	→ → → →	→ → → Sitting OOB x 30" w/ press. relief prog. to activ. protocol →	→ → → →
Activity	Protocol: • Immobilized Pt. (1.36) • Alteration Skin Integrity (1.91) Logroll q 2° (NSG) Consider Rotorest Bed (MD,NSG)	→	PROM, strengthening w/ unstable spine precautions (PT,NSG) →	Bedrest Logroll q 2° (post-op)	When cleared by xray: • PROM • SLR • HOB ↑ per order (MD, NSG) • Strengthening w/ resistence (PT)	Sitting schedule w/ pressure relief per protocol for 30" (PT, OT, NSG) → Lower body bathing (OT) → Initiate functional activi-ties as tol. (PT,OT,NSG)	Sitting OOB w/ 30" ↑ 1X q d pressure relief c 30" per activity protocol → Progress func. activity (PT, OT,NSG) → →	Sitting OOB BID x 1°(PT, OT, NSG) → → → →
Nutrition	NPO IV Fluids 2 IV lines (1 16 gauge)	Order diet if b.s. present; if negative, nutrition support services	NPO for OR after midnight	IV fluids as indicated post-op	Diet as tolerated if b.s.+; if b.s. negative hyperal	Maintain balanced I&O (Intake <2400 cc output <500 cc q 4 h)	→	→

Discharge Preparation	Pt/Fam Support Conference (SW, NSG) Rehab options explored	Psychosocial Assessment (SW) Home support assmt (OT,PT) Team Conference D/C planning Coping skills & Self-Regulation Training (Psych support)	→ →	Eligibility Referrals (SW) → →	Specific Rehab options identified & Rehab tour offered Contact Rehab facility (SW) → → Family Conference	Final Discharge Coordination (SW, NSG, OT, PT, PMR MD) → Urology follow up for Urodynamics →	→ → →
Educational Activities	SCI PEP (3.92) Fam educ/ support group (WED) (SW, RN, Chaplain)	→ Relaxation exercises Self-Regulation Training →	→ →	→ Once cleared, Feeding, Grooming, Bathing (upper) training Daily activity schedule (RN) Pt demonstrates knowledge of hypo-tension & autonomic dysreflexia	→ Bathing (lower) training → →	→ → → →	→ → → →

PROCESS & DISCHARGE OUTCOMES

Concern	Desired Outcome	Date Met/Initials
Pain Mgt	Pain level managed to allow full participation in prescribed activity schedule	
DVT	Free of s/s DVT	
Infection	Free of s/s infection	
Alt. elimination	BM every other day	
	Safe & effective Bowel/Bladder Programs	
	Able to do I&O cath w/ minimal assistance	
	I&O cath schedule (urine vol. < 500 cc.)	
Alt nutrition	Calorie intake supports full activity	
Skin integrity	Intact skin w/ sitting schedule	
Orthostatic Hypotension	B/P will allow full prescribed activity	

HOME EQUIPMENT/DISCHARGE NEEDS (date, initial)

	ASSESSED	NEEDED	PROVIDED
Splints as appropriate			
Shell/external spine brace			

Pulmonary Function	Clears airway independently	
	Inspir. volumes >1200 cc-10 cc/Kgm Body Wt	
	O_2 Sats > 95% by oximetry	
Neurological Status	Pt. will initiate appropriate intervention for dysreflexia symptoms	
	Pt. will maintain or improve neurological status documented by ASIA standards	
Body image/ sexuality	Pt. will express feelings of change	
ADL's	ADL needs will be at expected level with adaptive devices & assistance as needed	
Anxiety	Pt. will learn & use appropriate coping techniques	
Psycho social adjustment	Communicated needs met - emotional & spiritual needs will be addressed	
Mobility	Sitting OOB 1°BID	
	Mobility & activity to expected level with supportive devices	
	Full passive ROM w/in limits of stabiliza tion	
Education	Pt. and family will demonstrate an understanding NLI.	
	Family will be taught ROM	
Social Service	Pt will be screened for resource eligibility	

Altered/Additional Outcomes

Altered Pathway Course (note in Progress Notes)

Note	Date; Sign

*This form is a documentation and decision support tool only.

A-20

MULTIDISCIPLINARY CAREMAP
VENTILATOR PATIENT
RESPIRATORY FAILURE

Map ID 22
Page 2

PATIENT NAME ______________________

HOSP. NO. ______________________

	Acute Respiratory Dysfunction Phase I/Stabilization -0-90 min.	Pre-Weaning Phase II/Treatment-90 min. - 1 week
Date		
	Please put initials in met or unmet box. If unmet, describe reason on variance tracking form. Met Unmet	Met Unmet
Outcomes	Patient ventilated HR <___>___ SBP <___>___ dbp <___>___ ABG's pH-7.33-7.48 pO2 > 60	Albumin > 2.5 gm, Magnesium >1.5, PO4 >2.5, Hgb ≥ 11 Burns weaning assessment protocol (BWAP) score = ____ ;VS w/in baseline Elec. stable Rested -____- hrs of sleep FiO2 ≤ 50%, PaO2 ≥ 60, PEEP ≤ 5, pH 7.33-7.48 Fluid balance: I-O ≤ 200 wt w/in baseline V_E < 12l/min Wean parameters: rr < 30, vc > 1l, NIF <-25, TV 8-10ml/kg, PIP ≤ 35 If ready to wean but doesn't meet criteria think about failure to wean caremap
Consults	Anesthesia (if appropriate) Chaplain	Social Services Physical Therapy w/in 24 hrs
Tests	ABG (*ASAP, & q 30 min x 3,) 5 min after intubation CxR w/in 30 min EKG Gen. Screen, CBC with diff, pt/PTT, Magnesium, Blood cultures if febrile, Cardiac Enzymes: q 8 hrs x 3 with cp, Cardiac Disease with pulmonary edema, or EKG changes UA, C&S of urine if indicated Sputum GS, C&S if indicated	ABG - 30 min after q ordered V_E change, ≥ 10% FiO2 change, SaO2 ≤ 91 or ≥ 3% change CxR q/day & q acute episode Sputum if color/texture/volume change Blood cultures q 24 hrs if T > 38.5°C, CBC with diff & e2 q day, Calcium, Magnesium, PO4 q 5 days, glucose/accu check if steroids/CVN Gent peak and trough with 4th dose, if Cr ↑, check with pharmacist about dosing
Treatments/ Interventions	Assessments: VS q 15 min Resp. assess q 15 min SaO2 monitor Glascow coma scale Fluid balance assess Intubation with ≥#8.0, suction Vent settings initial: Modes: Pressure control or Volume control TV 8 ml/kg of ideal body weight, Peak inspiratory pressure (PIP) ≤ 35: 5 PEEP, FiO2 start at 100% wean down/ ABG's, rr 10-20, cuff <20mmHg Start IV: (Central vs PIV) Consider: foley, art. line, PAP catheter, NG Implement nursing protocols: (Sux, line care, drsg & site cares, personal cares)	Pull up caremap for specific diagnosis Assessments: Resp. assess - see protocol sheet, con't SaO2 monitor, hemodynamics, infection, GI, pain, sleep, anxiety Vent settings: Con't to adjust using same parameters as in Phase I, pH >7.2 & < 7.45 Institute BWAP > 72 hrs on vent DVT prophylaxis (SCD vs Heparin) NG/Nasal intestinal tube, Assess functional status/PT w/in 24 hrs of intubation Implement nursing protocols (CPT q ____, suction with bs/crackles, supportive positioning, personal cares, line & drsg cares) I&O Daily wt
Medication	IV rate: D5.2 NaCl at 1 L/8 hrs Sedation for intubation: Midazolam 2-10 mg **and** If indicated: Succinylocholine .6 mg/kg (40-60 mg) PRN **or** Pancuronium 0.1 mg/kg IV PRN **or** Vecuronium .08-.1mg/kg IV PRN Bronchodilators if indicated: Metered dosed inhalers **or** Nebs - Albuterol 2.5 mg-5 mg if indicated Antibiotics, if indicated: Erythromycin 500 mg-1gm q 6 hrs **and** either Ceftriaxone 1 gm q 24 hrs **or** Piperacillin 3 gm q 6 hrs with Gentamicin	IV: Adjust to volume status Bronchodilators: Con't as indicated Steroids if indicated ATB: Con't & adjust/culture results Analgesics: per order and nrsg pain protocol Gastric protection: histamine blockers or Sucralfate 1 gm qid, NG/fdging tube QID Anti-anxiety prn - agitation/fighting vent Midazolam, Lorazepam, Morphine, Haloperidol DVT prophylaxis-Heparin 5,000 U subq q 12 hrs vs SCD
Diet	NPO except meds	Nutritional support: Tube feedings vs. CVN/Peripheral venous nutrition (Electrolytes q day: Na <70 mEq, K+ 40-50 mEq, Cl 110-130 mEq) If tube feeding, initiate @ 25 cc/hr for 4-6 hrs then increase 50 cc/hr to maximum per order. If pt is CO_2 retainer, initiate pulmonary formula.
Activity	Bedrest, Restraints prn	Active/passive ROM - initiate w/in 48 hrs Position/turn q 2 hrs, Kinetic therapy as indicated - Up as tolerated
Teaching	Orient to unit (pt & family) Family update/education MICU booklet, boards in unit & waiting room	Continue to teach pt/family to Unit, Cares, & Equipment
Discharge Planning	Advanced directives	Patient/family psychosocial resources and support systems Identify d/c resources

7/95 Version 1

Clinical pathway: Ventilator patient—respiratory failure. (Copyright 1995, University of Iowa Hospitals and Clinics, Iowa City, IA. Used by permission.)

A-20

MULTIDISCIPLINARY CAREMAP/ TRACKING RECORD

VENTILATOR PATIENT
RESPIRATORY FAILURE

Map ID No. 22
Page 3

DATE
HOSP. NO.
NAME
BIRTH DATE
ADDRESS
SS#

• **File most recent sheet of this number ON BOTTOM**

IF NOT IMPRINTED, PLEASE PRINT DATE, HOSP. NO., NAME AND LOCATION

	Acute Respiratory Dysfunction Phase IIIA/Weaning: 0 - 72 hrs	Phase IV/Extubation - 24 hrs
Date		
	Please put initials in met or unmet box. If unmet, describe reason on variance tracking form. Met / Unmet	Met / Unmet
Outcomes	Patient able to clear/protect airway - FVC >15ml/kg Lungs ausc clear Gag & swallow reflex intact ABG's baseline: pH 7.35-7.45, PO2 ≥ 60, FiO2 ≤ 50%, V_E 6-12 l/min nl elec. HR ____ SBP ____ dbp ____ rr < 30 Pt lucid	Breathe on own CDB & able to clear own secretions Lung sounds ausc clear
Consults	PT	
Tests	ABG: q AM before weaning trials & prn CxR q day, OET > 5 days with T> 38.5°C, consider sinus films EKG: if ectopy, P>120, or cp Blood cultures q 24 hrs if T >38.5°C; CBC, e2, Glu q day; calcium, magnesium, PO4 q 5 days Sputum - color/texture/volume change	ABG - ≤30 min after extubate & prn SaO2 ≤90 or > 3% change or rr >30 CxR: - 8 or + 24 hours with extubation (within 8 hrs before or 24 hrs after extubation) Sputum ifcolor/texture/volume change Labs: Blood culture q 24 hrs if T > 38.5°C, CBC & e2 qod, Calcium, Magnesium, PO4 q 5 days
Treatments/ Interventions	Assessments: Routine q 2 hr Resp. assess-, SaO2 monitor, hemodynamics, infection, GI, pain, sleep, anxiety FiO2 ≤ 50%, 5 PEEP PS trials- as. tol. between 0600-2000. Initial PS- match PIP, titrate to keep SpVT ≥ 5-7 ml/kg, rr<30, VE <12l/min, rest on pressure control or Assist control minimum 2 hr between trials & 2000-0600 NG/Nasointestinal, I&O, daily wt Implement nursing protocols: (Sux, line care, drsg & site cares, Personal cares)	Assessments: Resp. assess- q15 min x 4 after extubation then q 2 hr, SaO2 monitor, hemodynamics, infection, GI, pain, sleep, anxiety Con't SaO2, Extubate after suctioning Face mask ≤ 50% FiO2, Incentive spirometery ≥ TID, CDB hourly while awake Implement nursing protocols (assess need for CPTq ____, suction with breath sounds/crackles, supportive positioning HOB up, personal cares, line & drsg cares) NG/Nasointestinal, I&O, daily wt
Medication	IV rate ____________ Bronchodialators As indicated: Metered dose inhalers ____________ Nebs- Albuterol 2.5 mg-5 mg adventitous breath sounds Antibiotics: Same Anti-anxiety agitation/fighting vent - Midazolam, Lorazepam, Morphine, &/or Haldol Gastric Prophylaxis Same Steroids: Same	IV: ____________ Bronchodialators As indicated: Metered dose Inhalers ____________ Nebs- Albuterol 2.5 mg-5 mg adventitous breath sounds
Diet	Nutritional support con't	Begin ice chips to sips of water Cl. liq. 6 hrs after extubation Advance as tolerated
Activity	ROM encourage participation in ADL Incorporate individualized schedule Position to enhance breathing	ROM encourage participation in ADL Position to enhance breathing Resume functional status
Teaching	Weaning process Relaxation & Imagery techniques Pt/family support	Continue to teach pt/family about resp care Reinforce relaxation techniques
Discharge Planning	Patient/family psychosocial resources and support systems	Pt. satisfaction survey Transfer

INITIALS/
SIGNATURES

____/ ____________ ____/ ____________ ____/ ____________
____/ ____________ ____/ ____________ ____/ ____________
____/ ____________ ____/ ____________ ____/ ____________

CareMap® is adapted from The Center for Case Management, South Natick, MA and is used by permission.

7/95 Version 1

A-20 B CLIN. NOTES C LABORATORY D X-RAY EXAM E CONSULTATION F SPEC. EXAM G THERAPY H PATHOLOGY I DIAGNOSIS

The North Carolina Baptist Hospitals, Incorporated
Division of Nursing
Patient Progress Record

Adult Cardiac Surgery

<table>
<tr><td colspan="2">DAY OF SURGERY</td></tr>
<tr><td>Date/Time Admission to ICU:
Admission Note:

Legal Signature:
Please place a check (√) beside any of the conditions listed below which the patient has and that might impact postoperative progress:
[ ] IDDM
[ ] NIDDM
[ ] COPD
[ ] Renal insufficiency
[ ] MI in past 2 weeks
[ ] Pneumonia in past 2 weeks
[ ] Low ejection fraction [%]
[ ] Emergency operation
[ ] Previous dysrhythmia ________
[ ] Other:________</td><td>Problem #1: Airway/Respiratory
Date/Time of Extubation:___
Patient extubated within 4-8 hours of admission?
[ ] Met goal
[ ] Did not meet goal, patient was:
[ ] Hypercarbic
[ ] Hypoxic
[ ] Too sleepy
[ ] Bleeding >100cc/hr
[ ] Hemodynamically unstable
[ ] Other: (describe)

Action taken if goal not met:
[ ] See Patient Care Record
[ ] See MAR/IAR
[ ] See Integrated Progress Notes (IPN)
Date/Initial when completed:<hr>Problem #2: Mobility
Patient OOB within 4-8 hours of extubation?
[ ] Met goal
[ ] Did not meet goal, patient had:
[ ] Femoral A-line
[ ] IABP
[ ] Hemodynamic instability
[ ] Other:________

Action taken if goal not met:
[ ] See Patient Care Record
[ ] See MAR/IAR
[ ] See IPN
Comments:
Date/Initial when completed:</td></tr>
<tr><td>Signature/Initials:</td><td>Signature/Initials:</td></tr>
</table>

Clinical pathway: Cardiac surgery. (Copyright 1995, North Carolina Baptist Hospitals, Winston-Salem, NC.)

Date of Surgery:____________

Type of Surgery:____________

Surgeon:____________

	TRANSFER NOTE
Problem #3: Pain Patient communicating relief of pain? [ ] Met goal [ ] Did not meet goal Action taken if goal not met: [ ] See PCR [ ] See MAR/IAR [ ] See IPN Date/Initial when completed:	Date/Time of Transfer:__________ Patient transferred POD #1: [ ] Met goal [ ] Did not meet goal, patient was: [ ] Not extubated [ ] Extubated late AM [ ] Hemodynamically unstable [ ] Other: (describe) Comments: Date/Initial when completed:
Problem #4: Impaired Skin Integrity Patient dressing clean, dry and intact? [ ] Met goal [ ] Did not meet goal Action taken if goal not met: [ ] See PCR [ ] See MAR/IAR [ ] See IPN Date/Initial when completed: Problem #5: Knowledge Deficit Patient/family taught per Patient/Family Education Documentation Form (PFEDF) [ ] Met goal [ ] Did not meet goal Action taken if goal not met: [ ] See PFEDF [ ] IPN Comments: Date/Initial when completed:	If patient not transferred by POD 2, revert to documentation of progress in the Integrated Progress Notes (IPN). Transfer/Transfer Acceptance Notes:
Signature/Initials:	Signature/Initials:

PROBLEM AND GOAL	POD 1 Date/Time:__________	POD 2 Date/Time:__________
Problem #1: Ineffective Airway Clearance Post Cardiac Surgery Goal: Patient meets goal of performing breathing exercises every 2 hours while awake Problem resolved: Bilateral lung fields clear or at baseline per auscultation, or activity tolerance at or near baseline. Date/Time/Initials:________	[ ] Meets goal [ ] Does not meet goal, patient is: [ ] Too nauseous [ ] Too SOB [ ] Noncompliant [ ] Other: (describe)_________ __________________ Action taken if goal not met: [ ] See Patient Care Record (PCR) [ ] See MAR/IAR [ ] See IPN	[ ] Meets goal [ ] Does not meet goal, patient is: [ ] Too nauseous [ ] Too SOB [ ] Noncompliant [ ] Other: (describe)_________ __________________ Action taken if goal not met: [ ] See PCR [ ] See MAR/IAR [ ] See IPN
Problem #2: Impaired Mobility Post Cardiac Surgery Goal: Patient meets daily mobility goals Problem resolved: Patient walking in hall at/near baseline level of functioning Date/Time/Initials:________	Patient meets goal of OOB, up in room 3 times today? [ ] Meets goal [ ] Does not meet goal, patient is: [ ] Connected to femoral A-line [ ] On IABP [ ] Hemodynamically unstable [ ] Noncompliant [ ] Other: (describe)_________ __________________ Action taken if goal not met: [ ] See PCR [ ] See MAR/IAR [ ] See IPN	Patient meets goal of ambulation 1/4-1/2 hall QID today? [ ] Meets goal [ ] Does not meet goal, patient is: [ ] Having respiratory problems [ ] Having rate/rhythm problems [ ] Hemodynamically unstable [ ] Noncompliant [ ] Other: (describe)_________ __________________ Action taken if goal not met: [ ] See PCR [ ] See MAR/IAR [ ] See IPN
Problem #3: Pain post Cardiac Surgery Goal: Patient communicating relief from pain? Problem resolved: Patient denies pain for 24 hours or more Date/Time/Initials:________	[ ] Meets goal [ ] Does not meet goal Action taken if goal not met: [ ] See PCR [ ] See MAR/IAR [ ] See IPN	[ ] Meets goal [ ] Does not meet goal Action taken if goal not met: [ ] See PCR [ ] See MAR/IAR [ ] See IPN
Problem #4: Impaired Skin Integrity Goal: Patient's surgical incisions meet the following goals: dry, intact, not edematous nor reddened. Describe incisions at time of discharge in discharge note.	[ ] Meets goal [ ] Does not meet goal Action taken if goal not met: [ ] See PCR [ ] See MAR/IAR [ ] See IPN	[ ] Meets goal [ ] Does not meet goal Action taken if goal not met: [ ] See PCR [ ] See MAR/IAR [ ] See IPN
Problem #5: Knowledge Deficit Post Cardiac Surgery Goal: Patient/Family taught per PFEDF? Problem Resolved: See PFEDF Date/Time/Initials:________	[ ] Meets goal [ ] Does not meet goal Action taken if goal not met: [ ] See PCR [ ] See MAR/IAR [ ] See IPN	[ ] Meets goal [ ] Does not meet goal Action taken if goal not met: [ ] See PCR [ ] See MAR/IAR [ ] See IPN
Problem #6: Slowed Gastrointestinal Motility Post Cardiac Surgery Goal: Bowel Movement by POD #2 Problem Resolved: Patient had bowel movement Date/Time/Initials:________		Bowel Movement by POD #2? [ ] Meets goal [ ] Does not meet goal Action taken if goal not met: [ ] See Patient Care Record [ ] See MAR/IAR [ ] See IPN
Problem #7: Goal: Problem Resolved: Date/Time/Initials:________	Response: Action:	Response: Action:
Problem #8: Goal: Problem Resolved: Date/Time/Initials:________	Response: Action:	Response: Action:
Signature/Initials:	Signature/Initials:	Signature/Initials:

POD 3 Date/Time:_________	POD 4 Date/Time:_________	POD 5 Date/Time:_________
[ ] Meets goal [ ] Does not meet goal, patient is: [ ] Too nauseous [ ] Too SOB [ ] Noncompliant [ ] Other: (describe)_________ _________ Action taken if goal not met: [ ] See PCR [ ] See MAR/IAR [ ] See IPN	[ ] Meets goal [ ] Does not meet goal, patient is: [ ] Too nauseous [ ] Too SOB [ ] Noncompliant [ ] Other: (describe)_________ _________ Action taken if goal not met: [ ] See PCR [ ] See MAR/IAR [ ] See IPN	Patient discharged by POD #5? [ ] Meets goal [ ] Does not meet goal, patient has: [ ] Rate, rhythm problems (describe) [ ] Respiratory problems [ ] Renal insufficiency [ ] Home care problems [ ] Been to weak to meet activity goals [ ] Other: (describe)_________ _________ Action taken if goals not met: [ ] See PCR [ ] See MAR/IAR [ ] See IPN
Patient meets goal of ambulation ½ - 1 hall QID? [ ] Meets goal [ ] Does not meet goal, patient is: [ ] Having respiratory problems [ ] Having rate/rhythm problems [ ] Hemodynamically unstable [ ] Noncompliant [ ] Other: (describe)_________ _________ Action taken if goal not met: [ ] See PCR [ ] See MAR/IAR [ ] See IPN	Patient meets goal of ambulation ½ - 1 hall QID? [ ] Meets goal [ ] Does not meet goal, patient is: [ ] Having respiratory problems [ ] Having rate/rhythm problems [ ] Hemodynamically unstable [ ] Noncompliant [ ] Other: (describe)_________ _________ Action taken if goal not met: [ ] See PCR [ ] See MAR/IAR [ ] See IPN	Discharge Note: (If patient discharged on or before POD #5. If patient not discharged by POD #5, revert to documentation of progress in the IPN.)
[ ] Meets goal [ ] Does not meet goal Action taken if goal not met: [ ] See PCR [ ] See MAR/IAR [ ] See IPN	[ ] Meets goal [ ] Does not meet goal Action taken if goal not met: [ ] See PCR [ ] See MAR/IAR [ ] See IPN	
[ ] Meets goal [ ] Does not meet goal Action taken if goal not met: [ ] See PCR [ ] See MAR/IAR [ ] See IPN	[ ] Meets goal [ ] Does not meet goal Action taken if goal not met: [ ] See PCR [ ] See MAR/IAR [ ] See IPN	
[ ] Meets goal [ ] Does not meet goal Action taken if goal not met: [ ] See PCR [ ] See MAR/IAR [ ] See IPN		
Bowel Movement by POD #3? [ ] Meets goal [ ] Does not meet goal Action taken if goal not met: [ ] See PCR [ ] See MAR/IAR [ ] See IPN		
Response: Action:	Response: Action:	
Response: Action:	Response: Action:	
Signature/Initials:	Signature/Initials:	Signature/Initials:

Carolinas Heart Institute
Carolinas Medical Center
Cardiac Surgery Clinical Path
(CABG)

Addressograph

Expected LOS: 5 Days DRG 106 & 107

	Pre-Hospitalization	Date: Day of Surgery	Date: Post-op Day 1	Date: Post-op Day 2
Outcomes	Pt. voices understanding of: CV Surgery. Plan of care. Post-op care. Pt. verbalizes/demonstrates: Leg Exercises. Use of Incentive Spirometry (IS). TCDB.	Within 12H of arrival to CVRU: Pt. hemodynamics WNL. Extubated. Normal breathing patterns. Pt. acknowledges pain controlled with IV meds. Turns and performs ROM exercises.	Pt. alert and oriented. Breath sounds clear. PERRLA SBP > or = 100. UOP > or = 30cc/H. Resp Rate <or=24/MIN Pt. performs IS effectively. Turns and performs ROM.	Pt. verbalizes: Pain control with oral analgesics. Incision w/o redness/inflammation. Performs: IS; TCDB; leg exercises. Breath sounds clear. VS WNL. Uses O2 3-5L/min. Sits in chair 30 min. BID. Pt. tolerates HDPD/ADA.
Teaching	Enable discussion of surgery and post-op care. Provide patient education booklet. Teach patient: Leg Exercises. IS. TCDB.	Review Pt. plan of care with family. Explain availability/usage of pain meds. Explain turning, ROM. Ventilator care. Extubation process.	Review Pt. plan of care with patient/family. Review: availability/usage of pain meds; IS; TCDB; ROM exercises.	Review Pt. plan of care with patient/family. Review availability/usage of pain meds. Reinforce: IS; TCDB; ROM exercises. Instruct pt./family to view "Pt TV Channel": Cardiac Risk Factors . Heart Disease & Diet . Cardiac Rehab . Teach pt. activity expectations.
Consults	Anesthesia Clinic Evaluation.	Respiratory Care. Pastoral Care consult if needed.	Pt. & Family Services if needed. Pastoral Care consult if needed.	Pt. & Family Services if needed. RD. Pastoral Care consult if needed. Physical Therapy consult if needed.
Assess/Treatments/Tests	Per anesthesiologist. Pre-op weight.	**Pre-op weight.** Labs: Hgb, K, Mg, ABG/admission and ABG prior to extubation. CXR, EKG monitor. Chest tube to suction; NG tube to suction. (D/C NG when extubated.) Check Foley Q1H. I&O Q1H. Check IV site Q1H. VS Q15 MIN. Cardiac output w/in 1H of admission. Pacer on demand. Check Q8H. Autotransfusion (D/C after 12H). Monitor SwanGanz/art line. Monitor surgical site. Extubate per Anesthesia then O2 @ 3-5L/min. Apply aerosol mask.	Weight post-op QAM. EKG monitor. Chest tube to suction. Check Foley Q1H. I&O Q1H. Check IV site Q1H. VS Q15MIN. Pacer on demand. Check Q8H. Monitor SwanGanz/art line. O2 @3-5L/MIN. Anti-embolitic stockings.	Weight post-op QAM. D/C Chest Tubes. CXR post chest tube removal. D/C foley when chest tube removed. UPON TRANSFER TO 6T: D/C pressure lines. Telemetry. Remove pacer box. Ground pacer wires to chest. VS Q4H. I&O QSHIFT. Remove wound dressing. Begin weaning O2. Anti-embolitic stockings.
Meds	Per MD instructions.	Cefazolin 1gm IV Q8H x3. Vancomycin 500 mg IV Q8H x3, if allergic to PCN. Famotidine 20 mg IV Q12H. NTG Drip proph., D/C w/ extubation. D5W 1/4 NS w/ 30meQ KCL @ 50cc/H. IV pain med.	Famotidine 20mg PO BID. IV to KVO w/ adequate po intake. IV/po pain med. D/C KCL if K >4.7 & UOP 5cc/kg/H. ASA / Beta Blockers per MD order.	Oral Analgesics prn. Resume home meds per MD order. IV Flush intermittent device. D/C Famotidine when transferred to 6T.
Diet	NPO after MN day before surgery.	NPO while intubated. Full liquids after extubation.	Progress as tolerated to Heart Disease Preventive Diet (HPDA) or HPDA/ADA. 2000 cc fluid restriction.	HDPD or HDPD/ADA.
Activity	As tolerated.	Bedrest. Tilt side to side prn. (to facilitate chest tube drainage).	ROM in bed. Turn Q2H. Bedrest. Head of bed elevated.	Sit in chair BID. BRP w/ assist. Pillow under legs when in chair.
Spirit/Psy/Soc	Provide emotional support. Encourage patient and family to share feelings/expectations.	Assess spiritual needs. Provide emotional support. Encourage patient and family to share feelings/expectations.	Provide emotional support. Encourage patient and family to share feelings/expectations.	Reassess spiritual needs. Provide emotional support. Encourage patient and family to share feelings/expectations.
Discharge	Introduce Booklet and plan of care. Assess caregiver availability.	Assess caregiver availability.	Assess discharge needs. Begin discharge instructions w/ family.	Reassess discharge needs. Reinforce discharge instructions w/ pt and family.
Signatures	7-3 3-11 11-7 7A-7P 7P-7A	7-3 3-11 11-7 7A-7P 7P-7A	7-3 3-11 11-7 7A-7P 7P-7A	7-3 3-11 11-7 7A-7P 7P-7A

This clinical path is a suggested guideline of care. The physician may change this plan at any time depending on the patient's individual needs.

cabg.wk4 Revised:. 10/09/95

Clinical pathway: Coronary artery bypass graft (CABG). (Courtesy of Carolinas Medical Center, Charlotte, NC.)

Carolinas Heart Institute
Carolinas Medical Center
Cardiac Surgery Clinical Path
(CABG)

Addressograph

Expected LOS: 5 Days DRG 106 & 107 CABG

	Date: Post-op Day 3	Date: Post-op Day 4	Date: Post-op Day 5
Outcomes	Pt. verbalizes s/s infection. Incision w/o redness/inflam. Performs: IS; TCDB; leg exercises. Pt. tolerates : ambulating 50-100' BID. out of bed for meals TID.	Incision w/o redness/inflammation. Performs: IS; TCDB; leg exercises. NSR. AP rate <100. Postop weight <or= pre-op weight. Pt. tolerates ambulating w/o assistance 100-150' x4. Pt./family attend CMC Diet class. Pt verbalizes risk factors/diet.	Incision w/o redness/inflammation. Pt. ambulates 200' x4. NSR w/ occas. PVC/PAC. Pt verbalizes : absence of pain. knowledge of medications. understanding of discharge instructions.
Teaching	Review Pt. plan of care with patient/family. Review availability/usage of pain meds. Reinforce: IS; TCDB; ROM exercises. Instruct pt./family to view "Pt TV Channel": Cardiac Risk Factors . Heart Disease & Diet . Cardiac Rehab . Teach pt. activity expectations. Teach pt. s/s infection.	Review Pt. plan of care with patient/family. Review availability/usage of pain meds. Reinforce: IS; TCDB; ROM exercises. Ensure pt. attends CMC Diet Class. Instruct pt./family to view "Pt TV Channel" Cardiac Risk Factors . Heart Disease & Diet. Cardiac Rehab. Reinforce pt. activity expectations.	Review Pt. plan of care with patient/family. Reinforce: IS; TCDB; ROM exercises. Instruct pt./family to view "Pt TV Channel" Cardiac Risk Factors. Heart Disease & Diet. Cardiac Rehab. Review pt. activity expectations. Discharge instructions.
Consults	Pt. & Family Services if needed. RD . Pastoral Care consult if needed. Physical Therapy consult if needed. Cardiac Rehab assessment.	Pt. & Family Services if needed. RD. Pastoral Care consult if needed. Physical Therapy consult if needed.	Patient and Family Services if needed. RD.
Assess/Treatments/Tests	Weight post-op QAM. Telemetry. VS QSHIFT. IS Q4H. I&O QSHIFT. Anti-embolitic stockings. Wean/D/C O2 per pulse oximetry.	Weight post-op QAM. Per MD Order: Telemetry. D/C Pacer wires. CBC. Lytes. CXR. VS QSHIFT. I&O QSHIFT. Anti-embolitic stockings.	Weight post-op QAM. Telemetry. VS QSHIFT. I&O QSHIFT. Anti-embolitic stockings.
Meds	Oral Analgesics prn. Resume home meds per MD order. IV Flush intermittent device.	Oral Analgesics prn. Resume home meds per MD order. IV Flush intermittent device.	Oral Analgesics prn. Resume home meds per MD order. D/C IV intermittent device.
Diet	HDPD or HDPD/ADA.	HDPD or HDPD/ADA.	HDPD or HDPD/ADA.
Activity	Ambulate 50-100' BID. In chair, out of bed for meals TID.	Ambulate 100-150' x 4. In chair, out of bed for meals TID. Performs self AM care.	Ambulate 200' x 4.
Spirit/Psy/Soc	Provide emotional support. Encourage patient and family to share feelings and expectations.	Provide emotional support. Encourage patient and family to share feelings and expectations.	Provide emotional support. Encourage patient and family to share feelings and expectations.
Discharge	Reassess discharge needs. Reinforce discharge instr. w/ pt and family.	Reassess discharge needs. Reinforce discharge instr. w/ pt and family.	Ensure patient understanding of: meds, diet, risk factors, incision care, activity level, and food/drug interactions. Return appointment and Rx. S/S to notify MD. Review discharge instr. sheet.
Signatures	7-3 3-11 11-7 7A-7P 7P-7A	7-3 3-11 11-7 7A-7P 7P-7A	7-3 3-11 11-7 7A-7P 7P-7A

This clinical path is a suggested guideline of care. The physician may change this plan at any time depending on the patient's individual needs.

cabg.wk4 Revised:. 10/09/95

NORTH CAROLINA BAPTIST HOSPITALS, INC.
CLINICAL PATHWAY
ACUTE LEUKEMIA DRG 473

Date and time of admission____________________
Date and time of discharge____________________
Clinical Path Initiated____________________
Expected LOS________ **Actual LOS**________
Reviewed with Parents/Patient/Family__________
Case Manager____________________

	Day 1	Day 2-8	Day 9-21	Day 22-33
Diagnostic Tests	CBC/D, Plts, SMAC, Mg+ PT, PTT, Dimer, Fibrinogen HSV, CMV, HLA typing Serum Lysozyme Urine Lysozyme, UA, & C&S EKG, MUGA, CXR PA & LAT BC/fungal cultures (if fever)	CBC/D, Plts, SMAC, Mg++	------------------------> d/c diff Day 10-18	------------------------>
Activity	Ad lib	Ad lib Ambulate in hall	------------------------> ------------------------>	------------------------> ------------------------>
Diet	Oncology Select			
Consults	Dentistry, Surgery Dietary, Social Service Recreational Therapy Pharmacy			Home care referrals, Home phyisican
Treatments/ Procedures	BM Biopsy Weights every MWF Sitz Baths	Transfuse RBC's, Plts Weights every MWF Oncology Standards in effect Catheter placed Chemotherapy 7+3	BM Biopsy ------------------------> Catheter Care	------------------------> Catheter Care
Medications	Allopurinol Acyclovir Fluconazole Broad spectrum antibiotics	------------------------> ------------------------> ------------------------> ------------------------> ------------------------>	------------------------> ------------------------> Ampho-B	

Clinical pathway: Acute leukemia. (Copyright 1993, North Carolina Baptist Hospitals, Winston-Salem, NC. Used by permission.)

	Day 1	Day 2-8	Day 9-21	Day 22-23
Medications				
Teaching	- Your Health Care Team - CVC - Understanding Chemotherapy - AML - Nutrition and You - Blood Counts - Neutropenia Precautions	Reinforce Patient Education Material	------------------------------>	------------------------------>
Discharge Planning				Review CVC Procecure Nutritional Support Pharmacy - Review Meds
Acuity				

mrb\Drg473.frm/SA#2

NORTH CAROLINA BAPTIST HOSPITALS, INC.
CLINICAL PATHWAY
KIDNEY TRANSPLANTATION (DRG 302)

Date of admission ____________
Date of discharge ____________
Clinical Path Initiated ____________
Expected LOS ______ Actual LOS ________
LOS ICU _____ LOS 5 West _____
Reviewed with Parents/Patient/Family ________

	Date:						
	Day of Surgery	Day 1	Day 2	Day 3	Day 4	Day 5	Day 6-14
Diagnostic Tests	FB, creat., CBC with diff. CXR Renal ultrasound Y ____ N ____	CBC with diff., SMAC, Mg.	------------------->	------------------->	----------------->	----------------->	----------------> CYA Level ----------> (begin am 24° after CYA started)
Activity	Bedrest	OOB to chair --->	------------------->	Begin Amb. ------->	----------------->	Walk in hall ---->	---------------->
Diet	NPO with ice	cl. liq. --------->	Advance to prudent ------------>	------------------->	----------------->	----------------->	---------------->
Consults	Nephrology		Recreation Therapy Dietician (Prudent)				
Treatments/ Procedures	Incentive Spirometry ------>	Daily wt. --------> ------------------> D/C NG	-------------------> ------------------->	-------------------> ------------------->	-----------------> -----------------> D/C foley	-----------------> ----------------->	---------------->
Medications	D5 1/2 NS at 75 cc/hr - ----------> Urine replacement with .45 NaCl --------------> Dopamine gtt __Y __N	------------------> ------------------> ------------------>	-------------------> -------------------> ------------------->	Heplock IV --------> D/C Central line ->	----------------->	----------------->	------> D/C Heplock

jhb/kidneytx/shdsk2

Clinical pathway: Kidney transplantation. (Copyright 1995, North Carolina Baptist Hospitals, Winston-Salem, NC. Used by permission.)

	Date:						
	Day of Surgery	Day 1	Day 2	Day 3	Day 4	Day 5	Day 6-14
Medications	OKT_3 [Pre/Post Med (OKT_3) X 1st 3 doses] Rocephin Imuran Solumedrol BP meds 40% FS	----------------------> ----------------------> change to PO ----------------------> Acyclovir Carafate ----------------------> Ketoconazole D/C O_2	----------------------> ----------------------> ----------------------> ----------------------> ----------------------> ----------------------> ----------------------> ---------------------->	----------------------> ----------------------> ----------------------> ----------------------> ----------------------> ----------------------> ----------------------> ---------------------->	------------------> ------------------> change to prednisone ------------------> ------------------> ------------------> ------------------>	------------------> ------------------> ------------------> ------------------> ------------------> ------------------> ------------------>	----------------> CYA -------------> (when Cr. <4) POD: ______ ----------------> ----------------> ----------------> ----------------> ----------------> ---------------->
Discharge Planning		Social Services (To Floor)	Evaluate home situation Arrange for discharge meds				Discharge
Teaching	Pulmonary Toilet	----------------------> D/C teaching: infection, rejection, activity, etc. -----------------> Pt. ed. materials given on admission to 5 West	---------------------->	---------------------->	------------------>	------------------>	---------------->

Comments:

jhb/kidneytx/shdsk2

THE NORTH CAROLINA BAPTIST HOSPITALS, INCORPORATED
Clinical Pathway
GI Hemorrhage with complication
DRG 174

Medical Record # ____________
Admission Date ____________
Discharge Date ____________
Actual LOS ____________
LOS in ICU ____________

Principal Diagnosis ____________
Principal Procedure ____________

Path Category	ED - Day of Admission	Day # 1	Day # 2
Assessment/Diagnostic Tests	CBC, diff then Hct q6° PT, PTT SMAC Type & screen	Hct (q6° - 12° if actively bleeding)	Hct
Activity	Bedrest if actively bleeding	As tolerated (unless still bleeding)	-------------->
Diet	NPO exc. meds	Resume diet	-------------->
Consults	GI consult or admit to service Surgical consult if necessary		
Treatments/Procedures	Upper GI endoscopy IV fluids - transfuse as needed NG to LWS - if indicated I & O	Lower GI endoscopy if necessary Saline lock - if bleeding ceases D/C NG - if bleeding ceases -------------->	Discharge if no active bleeding by endoscopy Follow up diagnostics in WFUP
Patient Teaching/ Discharge Planning	Medications	Instructions re diagnosis, prevention, care at home, reportable symptoms	
Medications	Empiric H_2 blockers until endoscopy Continue patient's usual meds unless contraindicated	Zantac as continuous drip only if endoscopy confirms PUD. Change Zantac to po ASAP. -------------->	-------------->

CLINPATH.174/PP#1/MC

Clinical pathway: Gastrointestinal hemorrhage with complications. (Copyright 1995, North Carolina Baptist Hospitals, Winston-Salem, NC. Used by permission.)

Index

Note: Page numbers in *italics* indicate illustrations; those followed by t indicate tables; those followed by b indicate boxed material.

B

C

F

M

O

P

Q

R

S

T

U

V

American Nurses Association Standards of Clinical Nursing Practice

Standards of Care

Standard I. Assessment

The Nurse Collects Client Health Data.

Standard II. Diagnosis

The Nurse Analyzes the Assessment Data in Determining Diagnoses.

Standard III. Outcome Identification

The Nurse Identifies Expected Outcomes Individualized to the Client.

Standard IV. Planning

The Nurse Develops a Plan of Care That Prescribes Interventions to Attain Expected Outcomes.

Standard V. Implementation

The Nurse Implements the Interventions Identified in the Plan of Care.

Standard VI. Evaluation

The Nurse Evaluates the Client's Progress Toward Attainment of Outcomes.

Standards of Professional Performance

Standard I. Quality of Care

The Nurse Systematically Evaluates the Quality and Effectiveness of Nursing Practice.

Standard II. Performance Appraisal

The Nurse Evaluates His or Her Own Nursing Practice in Relation to Professional Practice Standards and Relevant Statutes and Regulations.

Standard III. Education

The Nurse Acquires and Maintains Current Knowledge in Nursing Practice.

Standard IV. Collegiality

The Nurse Contributes to the Professional Development of Peers, Colleagues, and Others.

Standard V. Ethics

The Nurse's Decisions and Actions on Behalf of Clients Are Determined in an Ethical Manner.

Standard VI. Collaboration

The Nurse Collaborates with the Client, Significant Others, and Health Care Providers in Providing Client Care.

Standard VII. Research

The Nurse Uses Research Findings in Practice.

Standard VIII. Resource Utilization

The Nurse Considers Factors Related to Safety, Effectiveness, and Cost in Planning and Delivering Client Care.